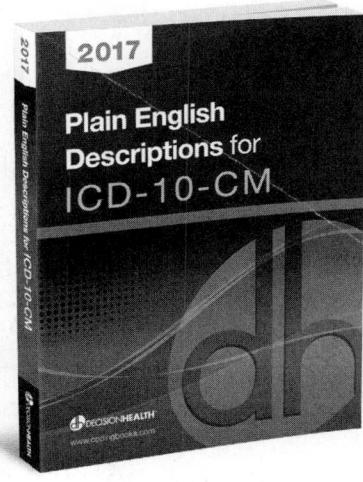

2017

International Classification of Diseases
10th Revision Clinical Modification

ICD-10-CM Expert for Physicians

ICD-1Ø-CM Expert for Physicians, 2Ø17

International Classification of Diseases, 1Øth Revision, Clinical Modification

Published by DecisionHealth
9737 Washingtonian Blvd., Ste. 5Ø2
Gaithersburg, MD 2Ø878-7364
www.codingbooks.com

Please call 8ØØ.334.5724 for questions or technical support

Printed in the United States of America

ISBN: 978-1-58383-857-Ø

Item Number: MPB-MICD1Ø-17

Disclaimer

Acknowledgements

Tonya Nevin, *Vice President, Medical Practice Group*
Renee Dudash, *Senior Director of Operations*
Brian Edlinski, *Production Manager*
Lori Becks, *RHIA, Clinical Technical Editor*
Michelle Suitor, *Clinical Technical Editor*
Ruby Woodward, *CPC, CPMA, COSC, CSFAC, Clinical Technical Editor*
Juli Folk, *Books Manager*
Bethany Angleberger, *Desktop Publisher*
Bradley H. Clark, *Artist/Medical Illustrator*

Table of Contents

Introduction to ICD-1Ø-CM

The International Classification of Diseases (ICD) is designed to promote international comparability in the collection, processing, classification, and presentation of mortality statistics. This includes providing a format for reporting causes of death on the death certificate. The reported conditions are translated into medical codes through use of the classification structure and the selection and modification rules contained in the applicable revision of the ICD, published by the World Health Organization (WHO). These coding rules improve the usefulness of mortality statistics by giving preference to certain categories, consolidating conditions, and systematically selecting a single cause of death from a reported sequence of conditions.

ICD-1Ø is used to code and classify mortality data from death certificates, having replaced ICD-9 for this purpose as of January 1, 1999.The ICD-1Ø is copyrighted by the World Health Organization (WHO), which owns and publishes the classification. WHO has authorized the development of an adaptation of ICD-1Ø for use in the United States for U.S. government purposes.

ICD-1Ø to ICD-9 Comparison

The ICD has been revised periodically to incorporate changes in the medical field. The Tenth Revision (ICD-1Ø) differs from the Ninth Revision (ICD-9) in its organization and structure, code composition, and level of detail, although the overall content is similar:

- ICD-1Ø has alphanumeric categories rather than strictly numeric categories
- Some chapters in ICD-1Ø have been rearranged, some titles have been changed, and conditions have been regrouped, forming 21 chapters
- ICD-1Ø has almost twice as many categories as ICD-9
- Minor changes have been made in the coding rules for mortality

Development of ICD-1Ø-CM

The National Center for Health Statistics (NCHS) is the Federal agency responsible for use of the *International Statistical Classification of Diseases and Related Health Problems*, 10th revision (ICD-1Ø) in the United States. The NCHS has developed a clinical modification of the classification for morbidity purposes (ICD-1Ø-CM). As agreed, all modifications to the ICD-1Ø (ICD-1Ø-CM) must conform to WHO conventions for the ICD. ICD-1Ø-CM was developed following a thorough evaluation by a Technical Advisory Panel and extensive additional consultation with physicians, clinical coders, and others to assure clinical accuracy and utility.

The entire draft of the Tabular List of ICD-1Ø-CM, and the preliminary crosswalk between ICD-9-CM and ICD-1Ø-CM were made available on the NCHS website for public comment. The public comment period ran from December 1997 through February 1998. The American Hospital Association (AHA) and the American Health Information Management Association (AHIMA) conducted a field test for ICD-1Ø-CM in the summer of 2003, with a subsequent report. All comments and suggestions from the open comment period and the field test were reviewed, and additional modifications to ICD-1Ø-CM were made based on these comments and suggestions. Additionally, new concepts have been added to ICD-1Ø-CM based on the established update process for ICD-9-CM (the ICD-9-CM Coordination and Maintenance Committee) and the World Health Organization's ICD-10 (the Update and Revision Committee).

On August 22, 2008, Health and Human Services (HHS) published a proposed rule to adopt ICD-10-CM (and ICD-10-PCS) to replace ICD-9-CM in HIPAA transactions. The proposed rule is available at the *Federal Register*:
http://edocket.access.gpo.gov/2008/pdf/E8-19298.pdf

The comment period for this proposed rule closed October 21, 2008. On January 16, 2009, the final rule on adoption of ICD-10-CM and ICD-10-PCS was published, specifying an anticipated implementation date of October 1, 2013. On August 24, 2012, the HHS announced a final rule delaying the implementation date for one year. The new implementation date was October 1, 2015.

The ICD-10-CM Coordination and Maintenance Committee

Annual modifications are made through the ICD-10-CM Coordination and Maintenance Committee. The Committee is made up of representatives from two Federal Government agencies, the National Center for Health Statistics (NCHS) and the Centers for Medicare and Medicaid Services (CMS). The Committee holds meetings twice a year which are open to the public. Modification proposals submitted to the Committee for consideration are presented at the meetings for public discussion. Approved modification proposals are incorporated into the official government version and become effective for use October 1 of the following year.

General Equivalence Mappings – ICD-9-CM to ICD-10-CM

The General Equivalence Mappings provide the conversion of ICD-9-CM diagnosis codes to ICD-10-CM diagnosis codes. The Mappings were developed as a tool to assist with the transition of *International Classification of Diseases, 9th Edition, Clinical Modification* (ICD-9-CM) codes to *International Classification of Diseases, 10th Edition* (ICD-10-CM).

ICD-10-CM Code Set Improvements

The clinical modification of ICD-10 represents a significant improvement over ICD-9-CM. Some of the specific organizational improvements that provide greater specificity in code assignment include:

- The addition of information relevant to ambulatory and managed care encounters
- Expanded injury codes, grouped by anatomical site rather than injury category
- The creation of combination diagnosis/symptom or manifestation codes to reduce the number of codes needed to fully describe a condition as well as combination codes for poisonings and external causes
- The addition of 6th and 7th characters with the seventh digit extensions representing visit encounter or sequelae for injuries and external causes
- Added laterality
- Full code titles for all codes with the incorporation of common 4th and 5th digit subclassifications (no more referring back to common fourth and fifth digits to understand the full code)
- V and E codes are no longer supplemental classifications
- Postoperative complications have been grouped within a procedure-specific body system chapter

How to Use the ICD-10-CM

Structure of ICD-10-CM

The new structure will allow further expansion than was possible with ICD-9-CM as more positions in more chapters are left open and available for future modifications.

ICD-10-CM has an index and tabular list similar to ICD-9-CM; however, the alphabetic index is more in-depth. ICD-10-CM also uses an indented format for both the index and tabular list. The Tabular List is similar to the ICD-9-CM version of the Tabular List, containing categories, subcategories, codes and descriptors, arranged numerically within the 21 separate chapters. The coding guidelines outlining coding conventions for ICD-10-CM are in the index, which consists of two parts: the index to diseases and injury and the index to external causes of injury. The former 'V' and 'E' code classifications that were previously considered supplemental to ICD-9-CM are incorporated into the Tabular List in the ICD-10-CM code set as individual chapters. The Neoplasm Table and the Table of Drugs and Chemicals are located in the Alphabetic Index to Diseases and Injury. Additionally, the Index to External Causes has been included.

Alphabetic Index of Diseases and Injuries

The Alphabetic List contains terms in the ICD-10-CM code set and the corresponding code. This List is divided into two parts: 'Index to Diseases and Injuries' and 'Index to External Causes of Injuries'. Within the Index there is a Neoplasm Table and a Table of Drugs and Chemicals.

Alphabetic Index Instructional Notations
Abbreviations

NEC   Not elsewhere classifiable – represents 'other specified.' When a specific code is not available for a condition, the Index directs the user to the 'other specified' code in the Tabular List.

Punctuation

( )   Parentheses – used in the Alphabetic Index to enclose supplementary words that may be present or absent in the statement of a disease/condition without affecting the code number to which is is assigned. The terms within the parentheses are referred to as nonessential modifiers.

Fainting (fit) R55

Manifestation codes

Conditions/diseases that are considered manifestation codes have a specific entry structure. Both conditions/diseases are listed together with the etiology code sequenced first, followed by the manifestation code second.

Trichinellosis, trichiniasis, trichinelliasis, trichinosis B75

with muscle disorder B75 [M63.80]

Morphology Codes

Some neoplasms contained in the Alphabetic Index include the morphology code or the histologic type. These codes are derived from the second edition of the International Classification of Diseases for Oncology (ICD-O). The correct morphology code can be found under the main term and subterm for the type of neoplasm, adenocarcinoma, sarcoma, etc.

Melanoma (malignant) (M8720/3) C43.9

Default Code

A code that is listed next to a main term in the Index is referred to as a default code. The default code represents the condition/disease that is most commonly associated with the main term, or the unspecified code for that condition. If a condition is documented in the medical record without any additional information (e.g., acute or chronic), the default code should be assigned.

Appendicitis (pneumococcal) (retrocecal) K37

Tabular List of Diseases and Injuries

The Tabular List consists of categories, subcategories, and valid codes. Valid ICD-10-CM codes contain letters (alpha) and numbers (numeric) and may be 3-7 characters long. The following describes the content of the specific digits:

- First Character – alpha. The only letter not used is the letter 'U', which is reserved for newly discovered diseases of unknown etiology.
- Second Character – numeric
- Third Character – numeric or alpha (not case sensitive)
- Fourth through Seventh Characters – numeric or alpha (not case sensitive). *Note: For some ICD-10-CM codes, an 'X' is used as a 4th-6th digit character place holder.*

The Letter 'x' as a Place Holder

If the code indicates there is a required 7th character and there are less than six (6) characters in the code, a place holder of 'X' should be assigned for all missing characters, in order to keep the 7th character of a code always in position 7. These placeholders have been included in the Tabular List to enable users to code more accurately. The ❼ icon noted in front of a code indicates the code has a 7th character, such as an encounter, sequela, tophus, fetus, etc.

Example:

W11.XXXA Fall on and from ladder, initial encounter

The ICD-10-CM system also utilizes the 'X' as a place holder with certain codes to allow for future expansion. An example of this is found in the poisoning, adverse effect, and underdosing codes, categories T36-T50. Where a placeholder exists, the 'X' must be used in order for the code to be considered valid.

Punctuation

[ ]   Brackets – used in the Tabular List to enclose synonyms, alternative wording, or explanatory phrases.

E87.5   Hyperkalemia

Potassium [K] excess
Potassium [K] overload

( )   Parentheses – used in the Tabular List to enclose supplementary words that may be present or absent in the statement of a disease/condition without affecting the code number to which it is assigned. The terms within the parentheses are referred to as nonessential modifiers.

G89.3   Neoplasm related pain (acute) (chronic)

:   Colons – used in the Tabular List after an incomplete term, which needs one or more of the modifiers following the colon to make it assignable to a given category.

Abbreviations

NEC Not elsewhere classifiable. This abbreviation represents 'other specified'. When a specific code is not available for a condition, the Tabular List includes an NEC entry under a code to identify it as an 'other specified' code.

NOS Not otherwise specified. This is equivalent to an unspecified code.

Includes

The word Includes appears immediately under certain categories to add further definition, or give examples of the content of the category.

Example: K27   Peptic ulcer, site unspecified

Includes   gastroduodenal ulcer NOS
peptic ulcer NOS

Inclusion Terms

A list of terms is included under some codes. These terms are the conditions for which that code number is to be used. The terms may be synonyms of the code title, or in the case of 'other specified' codes, the terms are a list of the various specified conditions assigned to that code. The inclusion terms are not necessarily exhaustive.

Excludes

The ICD-10-CM has two types of excludes notes. Each note has a different definition for use but they are both similar in the fact that they indicate those particular codes that are either mutually exclusive or independent of each other.

Excludes1

An *Excludes1* note is a pure excludes, which means both codes should not be used together under any circumstance. The excluded code should never be used at the same time as the code above the *Excludes1* note. An *Excludes1* type note is for used when two conditions cannot occur together, such as a congenital form versus an acquired form of the same condition.

Example: K14.0   Glossitis

Excludes1 atrophic glossitis (K14.4)

Excludes2

An *Excludes2* note represents "not included here". An *Excludes2* note indicates that the excluded condition is not inherently part of the referenced condition from which it is being excluded, but a patient may have both conditions at the same time. When an *Excludes2* note appears under a code, it is acceptable to use both the code and the excluded code together, as long as the patient has both conditions/diseases and both are clearly documented.

Example: N32   Other disorder of bladder

Excludes2 calculus of bladder (N21.0)
cystocele (N81.1-)
hernia or prolapse of bladder, female (N81.1-)

Code First/Use Additional Code

Code First/Use Additional Code notes (etiology/manifestation paired codes) mean that certain conditions have both an underlying etiology and multiple body system manifestations due to the underlying etiology. For such conditions, the ICD-10-CM has a coding convention that requires the underlying condition be sequenced first, followed by the manifestation. Wherever such a combination exists there is a "Use additional code" note at the etiology code, and a "Code first" note at the manifestation code. These instructional notes indicate the proper sequencing order of the codes – etiology followed by manifestation.

Example: F05   Delirium due to known physiological condition
Code first underlying physiological condition

G30   Alzheimer's Disease
Use additional code to identify
delirium, if applicable (F05)
dementia with behavioral disturbance (F02.81)
dementia without behavioral disturbance (F02.80)

In most cases, the manifestation codes will state "in diseases classified elsewhere" somewhere in the code title. Codes with this title are a component of the etiology/manifestation convention. The code title indicates that it is a manifestation code. "In diseases classified elsewhere" codes are never permitted to be used as first listed or principle diagnosis codes. They must be used in conjunction with an underlying condition code and they must be listed following the underlying condition.

Code Also

A *Code Also* note instructs that two codes may be required to fully describe a condition, but the sequencing of the two codes is discretionary, depending on the severity of the conditions and the reason for the encounter.

Example: E71.42   Carnitine deficiency due to inborn errors of metabolism
Code also associated inborn error or metabolism

And

If the word 'and' appears in a code description, it is inferred as and/or.

Example: G06.1   Intraspinal abscess and granuloma

ICD-1Ø-CM Official Guidelines/Reporting

Editor's Note: The FY2017 ICD-10-CM Coding Guidelines (effective Oct. 1, 2016) were not available as this coding manual went to press. When the new Guidelines are released, they will be posted on the DecisionHealth website at *https://www.codingbooks.com/errata-technical-corrections* as well as on the CMS website at *https://www.cms.gov/Medicare/Coding/ICD10/2017-ICD-10-CM-and-GEMs.html*.

The Centers for Medicare and Medicaid Services (CMS) and the National Center for Health Statistics (NCHS), two departments within the U.S. Federal Government's Department of Health and Human Services (DHHS) provide the following guidelines for coding and reporting using the *International Classification of Diseases, 10th Revision, Clinical Modification* (ICD-10-CM). These guidelines should be used as a companion document to the official version of the ICD-10-CM as published on the NCHS website. The ICD-10-CM is a morbidity classification published by the United States for classifying diagnoses and reason for visits in all health care settings. The ICD-10-CM is based on the ICD-10, the statistical classification of disease published by the World Health Organization (WHO).

These guidelines have been approved by the four organizations that make up the Cooperating Parties for the ICD-10-CM: the American Hospital Association (AHA), the American Health Information Management Association (AHIMA), CMS, and NCHS.

These guidelines are a set of rules that have been developed to accompany and complement the official conventions and instructions provided within the ICD-10-CM itself. The instructions and conventions of the classification take precedence over guidelines. These guidelines are based on the coding and sequencing instructions in the Tabular List and Alphabetic Index of ICD-10-CM, but provide additional instruction. Adherence to these guidelines when assigning ICD-10-CM diagnosis codes is required under the Health Insurance Portability and Accountability Act (HIPAA). The diagnosis codes (Tabular List and Alphabetic Index) have been adopted under HIPAA for all healthcare settings. A joint effort between the healthcare provider and the coder is essential to achieve complete and accurate documentation, code assignment, and reporting of diagnoses and procedures. These guidelines have been developed to assist both the healthcare provider and the coder in identifying those diagnoses that are to be reported. The importance of consistent, complete documentation in the medical record cannot be overemphasized. Without such documentation accurate coding cannot be achieved. The entire record should be reviewed to determine the specific reason for the encounter and the conditions treated.

The term encounter is used for all settings, including hospital admissions. In the context of these guidelines, the term provider is used throughout the guidelines to mean physician or any qualified health care practitioner who is legally accountable for establishing the patient's diagnosis. Only this set of guidelines, approved by the Cooperating Parties, is official.

The guidelines are organized into sections. Section I includes the structure and conventions of the classification and general guidelines that apply to the entire classification, and chapter-specific guidelines that correspond to the chapters as they are arranged in the classification. Section II includes guidelines for selection of principal diagnosis for non-outpatient settings. Section III includes guidelines for reporting additional diagnoses in non-outpatient settings. Section IV is for outpatient coding and reporting. It is necessary to review all sections

of the guidelines to fully understand all of the rules and instructions needed to code properly.

Section I. ICD-10-CM Official Guidelines for Coding and Reporting

The conventions, general guidelines and chapter-specific guidelines are applicable to all health care settings unless otherwise indicated. The conventions and instructions of the classification take precedence over guidelines.

A. Conventions for the ICD-10-CM

The conventions for the ICD-10-CM are the general rules for use of the classification independent of the guidelines. These conventions are incorporated within the Alphabetic Index and Tabular List of the ICD-10-CM as instructional notes.

1. The Alphabetic Index and Tabular List

The ICD-10-CM is divided into the Alphabetic Index, an alphabetical list of terms and their corresponding code, and the Tabular List, a structured list of codes divided into chapters based on body system or condition. The Alphabetic Index consists of the following parts: the Index of Diseases and Injury, the Index of External Causes of Injury, the Table of Neoplasms and the Table of Drugs and Chemicals.

See Section I.C2. General guidelines

See Section I.C.19. Adverse effects, poisoning, underdosing and toxic effects

2. Format and Structure:

The ICD-10-CM Tabular List contains categories, subcategories and codes. Characters for categories, subcategories and codes may be either a letter or a number. All categories are 3 characters. A three-character category that has no further subdivision is equivalent to a code. Subcategories are either 4 or 5 characters. Codes may be 3, 4, 5, 6 or 7 characters. That is, each level of subdivision after a category is a subcategory. The final level of subdivision is a code. Codes that have applicable 7th characters are still referred to as codes, not subcategories. A code that has an applicable 7th character is considered invalid without the 7th character.

The ICD-10-CM uses an indented format for ease in reference.

3. Use of codes for reporting purposes

For reporting purposes only codes are permissible, not categories or subcategories, and any applicable 7th character is required.

4. Placeholder character

The ICD-10-CM utilizes a placeholder character "X". The "X" is used as a placeholder at certain codes to allow for future expansion. An example of this is at the poisoning, adverse effect and underdosing codes, categories T36-T50.

Where a placeholder exists, the X must be used in order for the code to be considered a valid code.

5. 7th Characters

Certain ICD-10-CM categories have applicable 7th characters. The applicable 7th character is required for all codes within the category, or as the notes in the Tabular List instruct. The 7th character must always be the 7th character in the data field. If a code that requires a 7th character is not 6 characters, a placeholder X must be used to fill in the empty characters.

6. Abbreviations

a. Alphabetic Index abbreviations

NEC "Not elsewhere classifiable"

This abbreviation in the Alphabetic Index represents "other specified". When a specific code is not available for a condition, the Alphabetic Index directs the coder to the "other specified" code in the Tabular List.

NOS "Not otherwise specified"
This abbreviation is the equivalent of unspecified.

b. Tabular List abbreviations

NEC "Not elsewhere classifiable"

This abbreviation in the Tabular List represents "other specified". When a specific code is not available for a condition the Tabular List includes an NEC entry under a code to identify the code as the "other specified" code.

NOS "Not otherwise specified"
This abbreviation is the equivalent of unspecified.

7. Punctuation

[ ] Brackets are used in the Tabular List to enclose synonyms, alternative wording or explanatory phrases. Brackets are used in the Alphabetic Index to identify manifestation codes.

( ) Parentheses are used in both the Alphabetic Index and Tabular List to enclose supplementary words that may be present or absent in the statement of a disease or procedure without affecting the code number to which it is assigned. The terms within the parentheses are referred to as nonessential modifiers. The nonessential modifiers in the Alphabetic Index to Diseases apply to subterms following a main term except when a nonessential modifier and a subentry are mutually exclusive, the subentry takes precedence. For example, in the ICD-10-CM Alphabetic Index under the main term Enteritis, "acute" is a nonessential modifier and "chronic" is a subentry. In this case, the nonessential modifier "acute" does not apply to the subentry "chronic".

: Colons are used in the Tabular List after an incomplete term which needs one or more of the modifiers following the colon to make it assignable to a given category.

8. Use of "and"

See Section I.A.14. Use of the term "And"

9. Other and Unspecified codes

a. "Other" codes

Codes titled "other" or "other specified" are for use when the information in the medical record provides detail for which a specific code does not exist. Alphabetic Index entries with NEC in the line designate "other" codes in the Tabular List. These Alphabetic Index entries represent specific disease entities for which no specific code exists so the term is included within an "other" code.

b. "Unspecified" codes

Codes titled "unspecified" are for use when the information in the medical record is insufficient to assign a more specific code. For those categories for which an unspecified code is not provided, the "other specified" code may represent both other and unspecified.

See Section I.B.18 Use of Signs/Symptom/Unspecified Codes

10. Includes Notes

This note appears immediately under a three character code title to further define, or give examples of, the content of the category.

11. Inclusion terms

List of terms is included under some codes. These terms are the conditions for which that code is to be used. The terms may be synonyms of the code title, or, in the case of "other specified" codes, the terms are a list of the various conditions assigned to that code. The inclusion terms are not necessarily exhaustive. Additional terms found only in the Alphabetic Index may also be assigned to a code.

12. Excludes Notes

The ICD-10-CM has two types of excludes notes. Each type of note has a different definition for use but they are all similar in that they indicate that codes excluded from each other are independent of each other.

a. Excludes1

A type 1 Excludes note is a pure excludes note. It means "NOT CODED HERE!" An Excludes1 note indicates that the code excluded should never be used at the same time as the code above the Excludes1 note. An Excludes1 is used when two conditions cannot occur together, such as a congenital form versus an acquired form of the same condition.

b. Excludes2

A type 2 excludes note represents "Not included here". An excludes2 note indicates that the condition excluded is not part of the condition represented by the code, but a patient may have both conditions at the same time. When an Excludes2 note appears under a code, it is acceptable to use both the code and the excluded code together, when appropriate.

13. Etiology/manifestation convention ("code first", "use additional code" and "in diseases classified elsewhere" notes)

Certain conditions have both an underlying etiology and multiple body system manifestations due to the underlying etiology. For such conditions, the ICD-10-CM has a coding convention that requires the underlying condition be sequenced first followed by the manifestation. Wherever such a combination exists, there is a "use additional code" note at the etiology code, and a "code first" note at the manifestation code. These instructional notes indicate the proper sequencing order of the codes, etiology followed by manifestation.

In most cases the manifestation codes will have in the code title, "in diseases classified elsewhere." Codes with this title are a component of the etiology/ manifestation convention. The code title indicates that it is a manifestation code. "In diseases classified elsewhere" codes are never permitted to be used as first-listed or principal diagnosis codes. They must be used in conjunction with an underlying condition code and they must be listed following the underlying condition. See category F02, Dementia in other diseases classified elsewhere, for an example of this convention.

There are manifestation codes that do not have "in diseases classified elsewhere" in the title. For such codes, there is a "use additional code" note at the etiology code and a "code first" note at the manifestation code and the rules for sequencing apply.

In addition to the notes in the Tabular List, these conditions also have a specific Alphabetic Index entry structure. In the Alphabetic Index both conditions are listed together with the etiology code first followed by the manifestation codes in brackets. The code in brackets is always to be sequenced second.

An example of the etiology/manifestation convention is dementia in Parkinson's disease. In the Alphabetic Index, code G20 is listed first, followed by code F02.80 or F02.81 in brackets. Code G20 represents the underlying etiology, Parkinson's disease, and must be sequenced first, whereas codes F02.80 and F02.81 represent the manifestation of dementia in diseases classified elsewhere, with or without behavioral disturbance.

"Code first" and "Use additional code" notes are also used as sequencing rules in the classification for certain codes that are not part of an etiology/ manifestation combination.

See Section I.B.7. Multiple coding for a single condition.

14. "And"

The word "and" should be interpreted to mean either "and" or "or" when it appears in a title. For example, cases of "tuberculosis of bones", "tuberculosis of joints" and "tuberculosis of bones and joints" are classified to subcategory A18.0, Tuberculosis of bones and joints.

15. "With"

The word "with" should be interpreted to mean "associated with" or "due to" when it appears in a code title, the Alphabetic Index, or an instructional note in the Tabular List.

The word "with" in the Alphabetic Index is sequenced immediately following the main term, not in alphabetical order.

16. "See" and "See Also"

The "see" instruction following a main term in the Alphabetic Index indicates that another term should be referenced. It is necessary to go to the main term referenced with the "see" note to locate the correct code.

A "see also" instruction following a main term in the Alphabetic Index instructs that there is another main term that may also be referenced that may provide additional Alphabetic Index entries that may be useful. It is not necessary to follow the "see also" note when the original main term provides the necessary code.

17. "Code also note"

A "code also" note instructs that two codes may be required to fully describe a condition, but this note does not provide sequencing direction.

18. Default codes

A code listed next to a main term in the ICD-10-CM Alphabetic Index is referred to as a default code. The default code represents that condition that is most commonly associated with the main term, or is the unspecified code for the condition. If a condition is documented in a medical record (for example, appendicitis) without any additional information, such as acute or chronic, the default code should be assigned.

B. General Coding Guidelines

1. Locating a code in the ICD-10-CM

To select a code in the classification that corresponds to a diagnosis or reason for visit documented in a medical record, first locate the term in the Alphabetic Index, and then verify the code in the Tabular List. Read and be guided by instructional notations that appear in both the Alphabetic Index and the Tabular List.

It is essential to use both the Alphabetic Index and Tabular List when locating and assigning a code. The Alphabetic Index does not always provide the full code. Selection of the full code, including laterality and any applicable 7th character can only be done in the Tabular List. A dash (-) at the end of an Alphabetic Index entry indicates that additional characters are required. Even if a dash is not included at the Alphabetic Index entry, it is necessary to refer to the Tabular List to verify that no 7th character is required.

2. Level of Detail in Coding

Diagnosis codes are to be used and reported at their highest number of characters available.

ICD-10-CM diagnosis codes are composed of codes with 3, 4, 5, 6 or 7 characters. Codes with three characters are included in ICD-10-CM as the heading of a category of codes that may be further subdivided by the use of fourth and/or fifth characters and/or sixth characters, which provide greater detail.

A three-character code is to be used only if it is not further subdivided. A code is invalid if it has not been coded to the full number of characters required for that code, including the 7th character, if applicable.

3. Code or codes from A00.0 through T88.9, Z00-Z99.8

The appropriate code or codes from A00.0 through T88.9, Z00-Z99.8 must be used to identify diagnoses, symptoms, conditions, problems, complaints or other reason(s) for the encounter/visit.

4. Signs and symptoms

Codes that describe symptoms and signs, as opposed to diagnoses, are acceptable for reporting purposes when a related definitive diagnosis has not been established (confirmed) by the provider. Chapter 18 of ICD-10-CM, Symptoms, Signs, and Abnormal Clinical and Laboratory Findings, Not Elsewhere Classified (codes R00.0 - R99) contains many, but not all codes for symptoms.

See Section I.B.18 Use of Signs/Symptom/Unspecified Codes

5. Conditions that are an integral part of a disease process

Signs and symptoms that are associated routinely with a disease process should not be assigned as additional codes, unless otherwise instructed by the classification.

6. Conditions that are not an integral part of a disease process

Additional signs and symptoms that may not be associated routinely with a disease process should be coded when present.

7. Multiple coding for a single condition

In addition to the etiology/manifestation convention that requires two codes to fully describe a single condition that affects multiple body systems, there are other single conditions that also require more than one code. "Use additional code" notes are found in the Tabular List at codes that are not part of an etiology/manifestation pair where a secondary code is useful to fully describe a condition. The sequencing rule is the same as the etiology/manifestation pair, "use additional code" indicates that a secondary code should be added.

For example, for bacterial infections that are not included in chapter 1, a secondary code from category B95, Streptococcus, Staphylococcus, and Enterococcus, as the cause of diseases classified elsewhere, or B96, Other bacterial agents as the cause of diseases classified elsewhere, may be required to identify the bacterial organism causing the infection. A "use additional code" note will normally be found at the infectious disease code, indicating a need for the organism code to be added as a secondary code.

"Code first" notes are also under certain codes that are not specifically manifestation codes but may be due to an underlying cause. When there is a "code first" note and an underlying condition is present, the underlying condition should be sequenced first.

"Code, if applicable, any causal condition first", notes indicate that this code may be assigned as a principal diagnosis when the causal condition is unknown or not applicable. If a causal condition is known, then the code for that condition should be sequenced as the principal or first-listed diagnosis.

Multiple codes may be needed for sequela, complication codes and obstetric codes to more fully describe a condition. See the specific guidelines for these conditions for further instruction.

8. Acute and Chronic Conditions

If the same condition is described as both acute (subacute) and chronic, and separate subentries exist in the Alphabetic Index at the same indentation level, code both and sequence the acute (subacute) code first.

9. Combination Code

A combination code is a single code used to classify:

> Two diagnoses, or
> A diagnosis with an associated secondary process (manifestation)
> A diagnosis with an associated complication

Combination codes are identified by referring to subterm entries in the Alphabetic Index and by reading the inclusion and exclusion notes in the Tabular List.

Assign only the combination code when that code fully identifies the diagnostic conditions involved or when the Alphabetic Index so directs. Multiple coding should not be used when the classification provides a combination code that clearly identifies all of the elements documented in the diagnosis. When the combination code lacks necessary specificity in describing the manifestation or complication, an additional code should be used as a secondary code.

10. Sequela (Late Effects)

A sequela is the residual effect (condition produced) after the acute phase of an illness or injury has terminated. There is no time limit on when a sequela code can be used. The residual may be apparent early, such as in cerebral infarction, or it may occur months or years later, such as that due to a previous injury. Examples of sequela include: scar formation resulting from a burn, deviated septum due to a nasal fracture, and infertility due to tubal occlusion from old tuberculosis. Coding of sequela generally requires two codes sequenced in the following order: the condition or nature of the sequela is sequenced first. The sequela code is sequenced second.

An exception to the above guidelines are those instances where the code for the sequela is followed by a manifestation code identified in the Tabular List and title, or the sequela code has been expanded (at the fourth, fifth or sixth character levels) to include the manifestation(s). The code for the acute phase of an illness or injury that led to the sequela is never used with a code for the late effect.

See Section I.C.9. Sequelae of cerebrovascular disease

See Section I.C.15. Sequelae of complication of pregnancy, childbirth and the puerperium

See Section I.C.19. Application of 7th characters for Chapter 19

11. Impending or Threatened Condition

Code any condition described at the time of discharge as "impending" or "threatened" as follows:

- If it did occur, code as confirmed diagnosis.
- If it did not occur, reference the Alphabetic Index to determine if the condition has a subentry term for "impending" or "threatened" and also reference main term entries for "Impending" and for "Threatened."
- If the subterms are listed, assign the given code.
- If the subterms are not listed, code the existing underlying condition(s) and not the condition described as impending or threatened.

12. Reporting Same Diagnosis Code More than Once

Each unique ICD-10-CM diagnosis code may be reported only once for an encounter. This applies to bilateral conditions when there are no distinct codes identifying laterality or two different conditions classified to the same ICD-10-CM diagnosis code.

13. Laterality

Some ICD-10-CM codes indicate laterality, specifying whether the condition occurs on the left, right or is bilateral. If no bilateral code is provided and the condition is bilateral, assign separate codes for both the left and right side. If the side is not identified in the medical record, assign the code for the unspecified side.

14. Documentation for BMI and Pressure Ulcer Stages

For the Body Mass Index (BMI), depth of non-pressure chronic ulcers and pressure ulcer stage codes, code assignment may be based on medical record documentation from clinicians who are not the patient's provider (i.e., physician or other qualified healthcare practitioner legally accountable for establishing the patient's diagnosis), since this information is typically documented by other clinicians involved in the care of the patient (e.g., a dietitian often documents the BMI and nurses often documents the pressure ulcer stages). However, the associated diagnosis (such as overweight, obesity, or pressure ulcer) must be documented by the patient's provider. If there is conflicting medical record documentation, either from the same clinician or different clinicians, the patient's attending provider should be queried for clarification.

The BMI codes should only be reported as secondary diagnoses. As with all other secondary diagnosis codes, the BMI codes should only be assigned when they meet the definition of a reportable additional diagnosis (see Section III, Reporting Additional Diagnoses).

15. Syndromes

Follow the Alphabetic Index guidance when coding syndromes. In the absence of Alphabetic Index guidance, assign codes for the documented manifestations of the syndrome. Additional codes for manifestations that are not an integral part of the disease process may also be assigned when the condition does not have a unique code.

16. Documentation of Complications of Care

Codes assignment is based on the provider's documentation of the relationship between the condition and the care or procedure. The guideline extends to any complications of care, regardless of the chapter the code is located in. It is important to note that not all conditions that occur during or following medical care or surgery are classified as complications. There must be a cause-and-effect relationship between the care provided and the condition, and an indication in the documentation that it is a complication. Query the provider for clarification, if the complication is not clearly documented.

17. Borderline Diagnosis

If the provider documents a "borderline" diagnosis at the time of discharge, the diagnosis is coded as confirmed, unless the classification provides a specific entry (e.g., borderline diabetes). If a borderline condition has a specific index entry in ICD-10-CM, it should be coded as such. Since borderline conditions are not uncertain diagnoses, no distinction is made between the care setting (inpatient versus outpatient). Whenever the documentation is unclear regarding a borderline condition, coders are encouraged to query for clarification.

18. Use of Sign/Symptom/ Unspecified Codes

Sign/symptom and "unspecified" codes have acceptable, even necessary, uses. While specific diagnosis codes should be reported when they are supported by the available medical record documentation and clinical knowledge of the patient's health condition, there are instances when signs/symptoms or unspecified codes are the best choices for accurately reflecting the healthcare encounter. Each healthcare encounter should be coded to the level of certainty known for that encounter.

If a definitive diagnosis has not been established by the end of the encounter, it is appropriate to report codes for sign(s) and/or symptom(s) in lieu of a definitive diagnosis. When sufficient clinical information isn't known or available about a particular health condition to assign a more specific code, it is acceptable to report the appropriate "unspecified" code (e.g., a diagnosis of pneumonia has been determined, but not the specific type). Unspecified codes should be reported when they are the codes that most accurately reflect what is known about the patient's condition at the time of that particular encounter. It would be inappropriate to select a specific code that is not supported by the medical record documentation or conduct medically unnecessary diagnostic testing in order to determine a more specific code.

C. Chapter-Specific Coding Guidelines

In addition to general coding guidelines, there are guidelines for specific diagnoses and/or conditions in the classification. Unless otherwise indicated, these guidelines apply to all health care settings. Please refer to Section II for guidelines on the selection of principal diagnosis.

Chapter 1: Certain Infectious and Parasitic Diseases (A00-B99)

a. Human Immunodeficiency Virus (HIV) Infections

1) Code only confirmed cases

Code only confirmed cases of HIV infection/illness. This is an exception to the hospital inpatient guideline Section II, H.

In this context, "confirmation" does not require documentation of positive serology or culture for HIV; the provider's diagnostic statement that the patient is HIV positive, or has an HIV-related illness is sufficient.

2) Selection and sequencing of HIV codes

(a) Patient admitted for HIV-related condition

If a patient is admitted for an HIV-related condition, the principal diagnosis should be B20, *Human immunodeficiency virus [HIV] disease* followed by additional diagnosis codes for all reported HIV-related conditions.

(b) Patient with HIV disease admitted for unrelated condition

If a patient with HIV disease is admitted for an unrelated condition (such as a traumatic injury), the code for the unrelated condition (e.g., the nature of injury code) should be the principal diagnosis. Other diagnoses would be B20 followed by additional diagnosis codes for all reported HIV-related conditions.

(c) Whether the patient is newly diagnosed

Whether the patient is newly diagnosed or has had previous admissions/encounters for HIV conditions is irrelevant to the sequencing decision.

(d) Asymptomatic human immunodeficiency virus

Z21, *Asymptomatic human immunodeficiency virus [HIV] infection status*, is to be applied when the patient without any documentation of symptoms is listed as being "HIV positive," "known HIV," "HIV test positive," or similar terminology. Do not use this code if the term "AIDS" is used or if the patient is treated for any HIV-related illness or is described as having any condition(s) resulting from his/her HIV positive status; use B20 in these cases.

(e) Patients with inconclusive HIV serology

Patients with inconclusive HIV serology, but no definitive diagnosis or manifestations of the illness, may be assigned code R75, *Inconclusive laboratory evidence of human immunodeficiency virus [HIV]*.

(f) Previously diagnosed HIV-related illness

Patients with any known prior diagnosis of an HIV-related illness should be coded to B20. Once a patient has developed an HIV-related illness, the patient should always be assigned code B20 on every subsequent admission/ encounter. Patients previously diagnosed with any HIV illness (B20) should never be assigned to R75 or Z21, *Asymptomatic human immunodeficiency virus [HIV] infection status*.

(g) HIV Infection in Pregnancy, Childbirth and the Puerperium

During pregnancy, childbirth or the puerperium, a patient admitted (or presenting for a health care encounter) because of an HIV-related illness should receive a principal diagnosis code of O98.7-, Human immunodeficiency [HIV] disease complicating pregnancy, childbirth and the puerperium, followed by B20 and the code(s) for the HIV-related illness(es). Codes from Chapter 15 always take sequencing priority.

Patients with asymptomatic HIV infection status admitted (or presenting for a health care encounter) during pregnancy, childbirth, or the puerperium should receive codes of O98.7- and Z21.

(h) Encounters for testing for HIV

If a patient is being seen to determine his/her HIV status, use code Z11.4, *Encounter for screening for human immunodeficiency virus [HIV]*. Use additional codes for any associated high risk behavior.

If a patient with signs or symptoms is being seen for HIV testing, code the signs and symptoms. An additional counseling code Z71.7, *Human immunodeficiency virus [HIV] counseling*, may be used if counseling is provided during the encounter for the test.

When a patient returns to be informed of his/her HIV test results and the test result is negative, use code Z71.7, *Human immunodeficiency virus [HIV] counseling*.

If the results are positive, see previous guidelines and assign codes as appropriate.

b. Infectious agents as the cause of diseases classified to other chapters

Certain infections are classified in chapters other than Chapter 1 and no organism is identified as part of the infection code. In these instances, it is necessary to use an additional code from Chapter 1 to identify the organism. A code from category B95, *Streptococcus, Staphylococcus, and Enterococcus* as the cause of diseases classified to other chapters, B96, *Other bacterial agents as the cause of diseases classified to other chapters,* or B97, *Viral agents as the cause of diseases classified to other chapters,* is to be used as an additional code to identify the organism. An instructional note will be found at the infection code advising that an additional organism code is required.

c. Infections resistant to antibiotics

Many bacterial infections are resistant to current antibiotics. It is necessary to identify all infections documented as antibiotic resistant. Assign a code from category Z16, *Resistance to antimicrobial drugs,* following the infection code only if the infection codes does not identify drug resistance.

d. Sepsis, Severe Sepsis, and Septic Shock

1) Coding of Sepsis and Severe Sepsis

(a) Sepsis

For a diagnosis of sepsis, assign the appropriate code for the underlying systemic infection. If the type of infection or causal organism is not further specified, assign code A41.9, *Sepsis, unspecified organism.*

A code from subcategory R65.2, *Severe sepsis*, should not be assigned unless severe sepsis or an associated acute organ dysfunction is documented.

(i) Negative or inconclusive blood cultures and sepsis

Negative or inconclusive blood cultures do not preclude a diagnosis of sepsis in patients with clinical evidence of the condition, however, the provider should be queried.

(ii) Urosepsis

The term urosepsis is a nonspecific term. It is not to be considered synonymous with sepsis. It has no default code in the Alphabetic Index. Should a provider use this term, he/she must be queried for clarification.

(iii) Sepsis with organ dysfunction

If a patient has sepsis and associated acute organ dysfunction or multiple organ dysfunction (MOD), follow the instructions for coding severe sepsis.

(iv) Acute organ dysfunction that is not clearly associated with the sepsis

If a patient has sepsis and an acute organ dysfunction, but the medical record documentation indicates that the acute organ dysfunction is related to a medical condition other than the sepsis, do not assign a code from subcategory R65.2, Severe sepsis. An acute organ dysfunction must be associated with the sepsis in order to assign the severe sepsis code. If the documentation is not clear as to whether an acute organ dysfunction is related to the sepsis or another medical condition, query the provider.

(b) Severe sepsis

The coding of severe sepsis requires a minimum of 2 codes: first a code for the underlying systemic infection, followed by a code from subcategory R65.2, *Severe sepsis.*

If the causal organism is not documented, assign code A41.9, *Sepsis, unspecified organism*, for the infection. Additional code(s) for the associated acute organ dysfunction are also required.

Due to the complex nature of severe sepsis, some cases may require querying the provider prior to assignment of the codes.

2) Septic shock

Septic shock generally refers to circulatory failure associated with severe sepsis, and therefore, it represents a type of acute organ dysfunction.

For cases of septic shock, the code for the systemic infection should be sequenced first, followed by code R65.21, *Severe sepsis with septic shock* or code T81.12, *Postprocedural septic shock.* Any additional codes for the other acute organ dysfunctions should also be assigned. As noted in the sequencing instructions in the Tabular List, the code for septic shock cannot be assigned as a principal diagnosis.

3) Sequencing of severe sepsis

If severe sepsis is present on admission, and meets the definition of principal diagnosis, the underlying systemic infection should be assigned as principal diagnosis followed by the appropriate code from subcategory R65.2 as required by the sequencing rules in the Tabular List. A code from subcategory R65.2 can never be assigned as a principal diagnosis.

When severe sepsis develops during an encounter (it was not present on admission) the underlying systemic infection and the appropriate code from subcategory R65.2 should be assigned as secondary diagnoses.

Severe sepsis may be present on admission but the diagnosis may not be confirmed until sometime after admission. If the documentation is not clear whether severe sepsis was present on admission, the provider should be queried.

4) Sepsis and severe sepsis with a localized infection

If the reason for admission is both sepsis or severe sepsis and a localized infection, such as pneumonia or cellulitis, a code(s) for the underlying systemic infection should be assigned first and the code for the localized infection should be assigned as a secondary diagnosis. If the patient has severe sepsis, a code from subcategory R65.2 should also be assigned as a secondary diagnosis. If the patient is admitted with a localized infection, such as pneumonia, and sepsis/severe sepsis doesn't develop until after admission, the localized infection should be assigned first, followed by the appropriate sepsis/severe sepsis codes.

5) Sepsis due to a postprocedural infection

(a) Documentation of causal relationship

As with all postprocedural complications, code assignment is based on the provider's documentation of the relationship between the infection and the procedure.

(b) Sepsis due to a postprocedural infection

For such cases, the postprocedural infection code, such as, T80.2, *Infections following infusion, transfusion, and therapeutic injection*, T81.4, *Infection following a procedure*, T88.0, *Infection following immunization*, or O86.0, *Infection of obstetric surgical wound*, should be coded first, followed by the code for the specific infection. If the patient has severe sepsis the appropriate code from subcategory R65.2 should also be assigned with the additional code(s) for any acute organ dysfunction.

(c) Postprocedural infection and postprocedural septic shock

In cases where a postprocedural infection has occurred and has resulted in severe sepsis the code for the precipitating complication such as code T81.4, *Infection following a procedure*, or O86.0, *Infection of obstetrical surgical wound* should be coded first followed by code R65.20, Severe sepsis without septic shock. A code for the systemic infection should also be assigned.

If a postprocedural infection has resulted in postprocedural septic shock, the code for the precipitating complication such as code T81.4, *Infection following a procedure*, or O86.0, *Infection of obstetrical surgical wound* should be coded first followed by code T81.12-, *Postprocedural septic shock*. A code for the systemic infection should also be assigned.

6) Sepsis and severe sepsis associated with a noninfectious process (condition)

In some cases a noninfectious process (condition), such as trauma, may lead to an infection which can result in sepsis or severe sepsis. If sepsis or severe sepsis is documented as associated with a noninfectious condition, such as a burn or serious injury, and this condition meets the definition for principal diagnosis, the code for the noninfectious condition should be sequenced first, followed by the code for the resulting infection. If severe sepsis, is present a code from subcategory R65.2 should also be assigned with any associated organ dysfunction(s) codes. It is not necessary to assign a code from subcategory R65.1, *Systemic inflammatory response syndrome (SIRS) of non-infectious origin*, for these cases.

If the infection meets the definition of principal diagnosis it should be sequenced before the non-infectious condition. When both the associated non-infectious condition and the infection meet the definition of principal diagnosis either may be assigned as principal diagnosis.

Only one code from category R65, *Symptoms and signs specifically associated with systemic inflammation and infection*, should be assigned. Therefore, when a non-infectious condition leads to an infection resulting in severe sepsis, assign the appropriate code from subcategory R65.2, *Severe sepsis*. Do not additionally assign a code from subcategory R65.1, *Systemic inflammatory response syndrome (SIRS) of non-infectious origin*.

See Section I.C.18. SIRS due to non-infectious process

7) Sepsis and septic shock complicating abortion, pregnancy, childbirth, and the puerperium

See Section I.C.15. Sepsis and septic shock complicating abortion, pregnancy, childbirth and the puerperium

8) Newborn sepsis

See Section I.C.16. f. Bacterial sepsis of Newborn

e. Methicillin Resistant *Staphylococcus aureus* (MRSA) Conditions

1) Selection and sequencing of MRSA codes

(a) Combination codes for MRSA infection

When a patient is diagnosed with an infection that is due to methicillin resistant Staphylococcus aureus (MRSA), and that infection has a combination code that includes the causal organism (e.g., sepsis, pneumonia) assign the appropriate combination code for the condition (e.g., code

A41.02, *Sepsis due to Methicillin resistant Staphylococcus aureus* or code J15.212, *Pneumonia due to Methicillin resistant Staphylococcus aureus*). Do not assign code B95.62, Methicillin resistant Staphylococcus aureus infection as the cause of diseases classified elsewhere, as an additional code because the combination code includes the type of infection and the MRSA organism. Do not assign a code from subcategory Z16.11, Resistance to penicillins, as an additional diagnosis.

See Section C.1. for instructions on coding and sequencing of sepsis and severe sepsis.

(b) Other codes for MRSA infection

When there is documentation of a current infection (e.g., wound infection, stitch abscess, urinary tract infection) due to MRSA, and that infection does not have a combination code that includes the causal organism, assign the appropriate code to identify the condition along with code B95.62, *Methicillin resistant Staphylococcus aureus infection* as the cause of diseases classified elsewhere for the MRSA infection. Do not assign a code from subcategory Z16.11, *Resistance to penicillins.*

(c) Methicillin susceptible Staphylococcus aureus (MSSA) and MRSA colonization

The condition or state of being colonized or carrying MSSA or MRSA is called colonization or carriage, while an individual person is described as being colonized or being a carrier. Colonization means that MSSA or MSRA is present on or in the body without necessarily causing illness. A positive MRSA colonization test might be documented by the provider as "MRSA screen positive" or "MRSA nasal swab positive".

Assign code Z22.322, *Carrier or suspected carrier of Methicillin resistant Staphylococcus aureus*, for patients documented as having MRSA colonization. Assign code Z22.321, *Carrier or suspected carrier of Methicillin susceptible Staphylococcus aureus*, for patient documented as having MSSA colonization. Colonization is not necessarily indicative of a disease process or as the cause of a specific condition the patient may have unless documented as such by the provider

(d) MRSA colonization and infection

If a patient is documented as having both MRSA colonization and infection during a hospital admission, code Z22.322, *Carrier or suspected carrier of Methicillin resistant Staphylococcus aureus*, and a code for the MRSA infection may both be assigned.

Chapter 2: Neoplasms (C00-D49)
General Guidelines

Chapter 2 of the ICD-10-CM contains the codes for most benign and all malignant neoplasms. Certain benign neoplasms, such as prostatic adenomas, may be found in the specific body system chapters. To properly code a neoplasm it is necessary to determine from the record if the neoplasm is benign, in-situ, malignant, or of uncertain histologic behavior. If malignant, any secondary (metastatic) sites should also be determined.

Primary malignant neoplasms overlapping site boundaries

A primary malignant neoplasm that overlaps two or more contiguous (next to each other) sites should be classified to the subcategory/code .8 ('overlapping lesion'), unless the combination is specifically indexed elsewhere. For multiple neoplasms of the same site that are not contiguous such as tumors in different quadrants of the same breast, codes for each site should be assigned.

Malignant neoplasm of ectopic tissue

Malignant neoplasms of ectopic tissue are to be coded to the site of origin mentioned, e.g., ectopic pancreatic malignant neoplasms involving the stomach are coded to pancreas, unspecified (C25.9).

The neoplasm table in the Alphabetic Index should be referenced first. However, if the histological term is documented, that term should be referenced first, rather than going immediately to the Neoplasm Table, in order to determine which column in the Neoplasm Table is appropriate. For example, if the documentation indicates "adenoma," refer to the term in the Alphabetic Index to review the entries under this term and the instructional note to "see also neoplasm, by site, benign." The table provides the proper code based on the type of neoplasm and the site. It is important to select the proper column in the table that corresponds to the type of neoplasm. The Tabular List should then be referenced to verify that the correct code has been selected from the table and that a more specific site code does not exist.

See Section I.C.21. Factors influencing health status and contact with health services, Status, for information regarding Z15.0, codes for genetic susceptibility to cancer.

a. Treatment directed at the malignancy

If the treatment is directed at the malignancy, designate the malignancy as the principal diagnosis.

The only exception to this guideline is if a patient admission/encounter is solely for the administration of chemotherapy, immunotherapy or radiation therapy, assign the appropriate Z51.-- code as the first-listed or principal diagnosis, and the diagnosis or problem for which the service is being performed as a secondary diagnosis.

b. Treatment of secondary site

When a patient is admitted because of a primary neoplasm with metastasis and treatment is directed toward the secondary site only, the secondary neoplasm is designated as the principal diagnosis even though the primary malignancy is still present.

c. Coding and sequencing of complications

Coding and sequencing of complications associated with the malignancies or with the therapy thereof are subject to the following guidelines:

1) Anemia associated with malignancy

When admission/encounter is for management of an anemia associated with the malignancy, and the treatment is only for anemia, the appropriate code for the malignancy is sequenced as the principal or first-listed diagnosis followed by the appropriate code for the anemia (such as code D63.0, *Anemia* in neoplastic disease).

2) Anemia associated with chemotherapy, immunotherapy and radiation therapy

When the admission/encounter is for management of an anemia associated with an adverse effect of the administration of chemotherapy or immunotherapy and the only treatment is for the anemia, the anemia code is sequenced first followed by the appropriate codes for the neoplasm and the adverse effect (T45.1X5, *Adverse effect of antineoplastic and immunosuppressive drugs*).

When the admission/encounter is for management of an anemia associated with an adverse effect of radiotherapy, the anemia code should be sequenced first, followed by the appropriate neoplasm code and code Y84.2, *Radiological procedure and radiotherapy* as the cause of abnormal reaction of the patient, or of later complication, without mention of misadventure at the time of the procedure.

3) Management of dehydration due to the malignancy

When the admission/encounter is for management of dehydration due to the malignancy and only the dehydration is being treated (intravenous rehydration), the dehydration is sequenced first, followed by the code(s) for the malignancy.

4) Treatment of a complication resulting from a surgical procedure

When the admission/encounter is for treatment of a complication resulting from a surgical procedure, designate the complication as the principal or first-listed diagnosis if treatment is directed at resolving the complication.

d. Primary malignancy previously excised

When a primary malignancy has been previously excised or eradicated from its site and there is no further treatment directed to that site and there is no evidence of any existing primary malignancy, a code from category Z85, *Personal history of malignant neoplasm*, should be used to indicate the former site of the malignancy. Any mention of extension, invasion, or metastasis to another site is coded as a secondary malignant neoplasm to that site. The secondary site may be the principal or first-listed with the Z85 code used as a secondary code.

e. Admissions/Encounters involving chemotherapy, immunotherapy and radiation therapy

1) Episode of care involves surgical removal of neoplasm

When an episode of care involves the surgical removal of a neoplasm, primary or secondary site, followed by adjunct chemotherapy or radiation treatment during the same episode of care, the code for the neoplasm should be assigned as principal or first-listed diagnosis.

2) Patient admission/encounter solely for administration of chemotherapy, immunotherapy and radiation therapy

If a patient admission/encounter is solely for the administration of chemotherapy, immunotherapy or radiation therapy assign code Z51.0, *Encounter for antineoplastic radiation therapy*, or Z51.11, *Encounter for antineoplastic chemotherapy*, or Z51.12, *Encounter for antineoplastic immunotherapy as the first-listed or principal diagnosis*. If a patient receives more than one of these therapies during the same admission more than one of these codes may be assigned, in any sequence.

The malignancy for which the therapy is being administered should be assigned as a secondary diagnosis.

3) Patient admitted for radiation therapy, chemotherapy or immunotherapy and develops complications

When a patient is admitted for the purpose of radiotherapy, immunotherapy or chemotherapy and develops complications such as uncontrolled nausea and vomiting or dehydration, the principal or first-listed diagnosis is Z51.0, *Encounter for antineoplastic radiation therapy*, or Z51.11, *Encounter for antineoplastic chemotherapy*, or Z51.12, *Encounter for antineoplastic immunotherapy* followed by any codes for the complications.

f. Admission/encounter to determine extent of malignancy

When the reason for admission/encounter is to determine the extent of the malignancy, or for a procedure such as paracentesis or thoracentesis, the primary malignancy or appropriate metastatic site is designated as the principal or first-listed diagnosis, even though chemotherapy or radiotherapy is administered.

g. Symptoms, signs, and abnormal findings listed in Chapter 18 associated with neoplasms

Symptoms, signs, and ill-defined conditions listed in Chapter 18 characteristic of, or associated with, an existing primary or secondary site malignancy cannot be used to replace the malignancy as principal or first-listed diagnosis, regardless of the number of admissions or encounters for treatment and care of the neoplasm.

See Section I.C.21. Factors influencing health status and contact with health services, Encounter for prophylactic organ removal.

h. Admission/encounter for pain control/management

See Section I.C.6. for information on coding admission/encounter for pain control/management.

i. Malignancy in two or more noncontiguous sites

A patient may have more than one malignant tumor in the same organ. These tumors may represent different primaries or metastatic disease, depending on the site. Should the documentation be unclear, the provider should be queried as to the status of each tumor so that the correct codes can be assigned.

j. Disseminated malignant neoplasm, unspecified

Code C80.0, *Disseminated malignant neoplasm*, unspecified, is for use only in those cases where the patient has advanced metastatic disease and no known primary or secondary sites are specified. It should not be used in place of assigning codes for the primary site and all known secondary sites.

k. Malignant neoplasm without specification of site

Code C80.1, *Malignant (primary) neoplasm*, unspecified, equates to Cancer, unspecified. This code should only be used when no determination can be made as to the primary site of a malignancy. This code should rarely be used in the inpatient setting.

l. Sequencing of neoplasm codes

1) Encounter for treatment of primary malignancy

If the reason for the encounter is for treatment of a primary malignancy, assign the malignancy as the principal/first-listed diagnosis. The primary site is to be sequenced first, followed by any metastatic sites.

2) Encounter for treatment of secondary malignancy

When an encounter is for a primary malignancy with metastasis and treatment is directed toward the metastatic (secondary) site(s) only, the metastatic site(s) is designated as the principal/first-listed diagnosis. The primary malignancy is coded as an additional code.

3) Malignant neoplasm in a pregnant patient

When a pregnant woman has a malignant neoplasm, a code from subcategory O9A.1-, *Malignant neoplasm complicating pregnancy, childbirth, and the puerperium*, should be sequenced first, followed by the appropriate code from Chapter 2 to indicate the type of neoplasm.

4) Encounter for complication associated with a neoplasm

When an encounter is for management of a complication associated with a neoplasm, such as dehydration, and the treatment is only for the complication, the complication is coded first, followed by the appropriate code(s) for the neoplasm.

The exception to this guideline is anemia. When the admission/encounter is for management of an anemia associated with the malignancy, and the treatment is only for anemia, the appropriate code for the malignancy is sequenced as the principal or first-listed diagnosis followed by code D63.0, *Anemia* in neoplastic disease.

5) Complication from surgical procedure for treatment of a neoplasm

When an encounter is for treatment of a complication resulting from a surgical procedure performed for the treatment of the neoplasm, designate the complication as the principal/first-listed diagnosis. See guideline regarding the coding of a current malignancy versus personal history to determine if the code for the neoplasm should also be assigned.

6) Pathologic fracture due to a neoplasm

When an encounter is for a pathological fracture due to a neoplasm and the focus of treatment is the fracture, a code from subcategory M84.5, *Pathological fracture in neoplastic disease*, should be sequenced first, followed by the code for the neoplasm.

If the focus of treatment is the neoplasm with an associated pathological fracture, the neoplasm code should be sequenced first, followed by a code from M84.5 for the pathological fracture.

m. Current malignancy versus personal history of malignancy

When a primary malignancy has been excised but further treatment, such as an additional surgery for the malignancy, radiation therapy or chemotherapy is directed to that site, the primary malignancy code should be used until treatment is completed.

When a primary malignancy has been previously excised or eradicated from its site, there is no further treatment (of the malignancy) directed to that site, and there is no evidence of any existing primary malignancy, a code from category Z85, *Personal history of malignant neoplasm*, should be used to indicate the former site of the malignancy.

See Section I.C.21. Factors influencing health status and contact with health services, History (of)

n. Leukemia, Multiple Myeloma, and Malignant Plasma Cell Neoplasms in remission versus personal history

The categories for leukemia, and category C90, *Multiple myeloma and malignant plasma cell neoplasms*, have codes indicating whether or not the leukemia has achieved remission. There are also codes Z85.6, Personal history of leukemia, and Z85.79, *Personal history of other malignant neoplasms of lymphoid, hematopoietic and related tissues*. If the documentation is unclear, as to whether the leukemia has achieved remission, the provider should be queried.

See Section I.C.21. Factors influencing health status and contact with health services, History (of)

o. Aftercare following surgery for neoplasm

See Section I.C.21. Factors influencing health status and contact with health services, Aftercare

p. Follow-up care for completed treatment of a malignancy

See Section I.C.21. Factors influencing health status and contact with health services, Follow-up

q. Prophylactic organ removal for prevention of malignancy

See Section I.C. 21, Factors influencing health status and contact with health services, Prophylactic organ removal

r. Malignant neoplasm associated with transplanted organ

A malignant neoplasm of a transplanted organ should be coded as a transplant complication. Assign first the appropriate code from category T86.-, *Complications of transplanted organs and tissue*, followed by code C80.2, *Malignant neoplasm associated with transplanted organ*. Use an additional code for the specific malignancy.

Chapter 3: Disease of the blood and blood-forming organs and certain disorders involving the immune mechanism (D50-D89)

Reserved for future guideline expansion

Chapter 4: Endocrine, Nutritional, and Metabolic Diseases (E00-E89)

a. Diabetes mellitus

The diabetes mellitus codes are combination codes that include the type of diabetes mellitus, the body system affected, and the complications affecting that body system. As many codes within a particular category as are necessary to describe all of the complications of the disease may be used. They should be sequenced based on the reason for a particular encounter. Assign as many codes from categories E08 – E13 as needed to identify all of the associated conditions that the patient has.

1) Type of diabetes

The age of a patient is not the sole determining factor, though most type 1 diabetics develop the condition before reaching puberty. For this reason type 1 diabetes mellitus is also referred to as juvenile diabetes.

2) Type of diabetes mellitus not documented

If the type of diabetes mellitus is not documented in the medical record the default is E11.-, *Type 2 diabetes mellitus*.

3) Diabetes mellitus and the use of insulin

If the documentation in a medical record does not indicate the type of diabetes but does indicate that the patient uses insulin, code E11, *Type 2 diabetes mellitus*, should be assigned. Code Z79.4, Long-term (current) use of insulin, should also be assigned to indicate that the patient uses insulin. Code Z79.4 should not be assigned if insulin is given temporarily to bring a type 2 patient's blood sugar under control during an encounter.

4) Diabetes mellitus in pregnancy and gestational diabetes

See Section I.C.15. Diabetes mellitus in pregnancy.

See Section I.C.15. Gestational (pregnancy induced) diabetes

5) Complications due to insulin pump malfunction

(a) Underdose of insulin due to insulin pump failure

An underdose of insulin due to an insulin pump failure should be assigned to a code from subcategory T85.6, *Mechanical complication of other specified internal and external prosthetic devices, implants and grafts*, that specifies the type of pump malfunction, as the principal or first-listed code, followed by code T38.3x6-, *Underdosing of insulin and oral hypoglycemic [antidiabetic] drugs*. Additional codes for the type of diabetes mellitus and any associated complications due to the underdosing should also be assigned.

(b) Overdose of insulin due to insulin pump failure

The principal or first-listed code for an encounter due to an insulin pump malfunction resulting in an overdose of insulin, should also be T85.6-, *Mechanical complication of other*

specified internal and external prosthetic devices, implants and grafts, followed by code T38.3x1-, *Poisoning by insulin and oral hypoglycemic [antidiabetic] drugs, accidental (unintentional)*.

6) Secondary diabetes mellitus

Codes under categories E08, *Diabetes mellitus due to underlying condition*, and E09, *Drug or chemical induced diabetes mellitus*, and E13, *other specified diabetes mellitus*, identify complications/manifestations associated with secondary diabetes mellitus. Secondary diabetes is always caused by another condition or event (e.g., cystic fibrosis, malignant neoplasm of pancreas, pancreatectomy, adverse effect of drug, or poisoning).

(a) Secondary diabetes mellitus and the use of insulin

For patients who routinely use insulin, code Z79.4, *Long-term (current) use of insulin*, should also be assigned. Code Z79.4 should not be assigned if insulin is given temporarily to bring a patient's blood sugar under control during an encounter.

(b) Assigning and sequencing secondary diabetes codes and its causes

The sequencing of the secondary diabetes codes in relationship to codes for the cause of the diabetes is based on the Tabular List instructions for categories E08, E09 and E13.

(i) Secondary diabetes mellitus due to pancreatectomy

For postpancreatectomy diabetes mellitus (lack of insulin due to the surgical removal of all or part of the pancreas), assign code E89.1, *Postprocedural hypoinsulinemia*. Assign a code from category E13 and a code from subcategory Z90.41-, *Acquired absence of pancreas*, as additional codes.

(ii) Secondary diabetes due to drugs

Secondary diabetes may be caused by an adverse effect of correctly administered medications, poisoning or sequela of poisoning.

See Section I.C.19.e for coding of adverse effects and poisoning, and Section I.C.20 for external cause code reporting.

Chapter 5: Mental, Behavioral and Neurodevelopmental disorders (F01 – F99)

a. Pain disorders related to psychological factors

Assign code F45.41, for pain that is exclusively related to psychological disorders. As indicated by the Excludes 1 note under category G89, a code from category G89 should not be assigned with code F45.41

Code F45.42, *Pain disorders with related psychological factors*, should be used with a code from category G89, *Pain, not elsewhere classified*, if there is documentation of a psychological component for a patient with acute or chronic pain.

See Section I.C.6. Pain

b. Mental and behavioral disorders due to psychoactive substance use

1) In Remission

Selection of codes for "in remission" for categories F10-F19, Mental and behavioral disorders due to psychoactive substance use (categories F10-F19 with -.21) requires the provider's clinical judgment. The appropriate codes for "in remission" are assigned only on the basis of provider documentation (as defined in the *Official Guidelines for Coding and Reporting*).

2) Psychoactive Substance Use, Abuse And Dependence

When the provider documentation refers to use, abuse and dependence of the same substance (e.g. alcohol, opioid, cannabis, etc.), only one code should be assigned to identify the pattern of use based on the following hierarchy:

- If both use and abuse are documented, assign only the code for abuse

- If both abuse and dependence are documented, assign only the code for dependence

- If use, abuse and dependence are all documented, assign only the code for dependence

- If both use and dependence are documented, assign only the code for dependence.

3) Psychoactive Substance Use

As with all other diagnoses, the codes for psychoactive substance use (F10.9-, F11.9-, F12.9-, F13.9-, F14.9-, F15.9-, F16.9-) should only be assigned based on provider documentation and when they meet the definition of a reportable diagnosis (see *Section III, Reporting Additional Diagnoses*). The codes are to be used only when the psychoactive substance use is associated with a mental or behavioral disorder, and such a relationship is documented by the provider.

Chapter 6: Diseases of Nervous System and Sense Organs (G00-G99)

a. Dominant/nondominant side

Codes from category G81, *Hemiplegia and hemiparesis*, and subcategories, G83.1, *Monoplegia of lower limb*, G83.2, *Monoplegia of upper limb*, and G83.3, *Monoplegia, unspecified*, identify whether the dominant or nondominant side is affected. Should the affected side be documented, but not specified as dominant or nondominant, and the classification system does not indicate a default, code selection is as follows:

- For ambidextrous patients, the default should be dominant.

- If the left side is affected, the default is non-dominant.

- If the right side is affected, the default is dominant.

b. Pain - Category G89

1) General coding information

Codes in category G89, *Pain, not elsewhere classified*, may be used in conjunction with codes from other categories and chapters to provide more detail about acute or chronic pain and neoplasm-related pain, unless otherwise indicated below.

If the pain is not specified as acute or chronic, post-thoracotomy, postprocedural, or neoplasm-related, do not assign codes from category G89.

A code from category G89 should not be assigned if the underlying (definitive) diagnosis is known, unless the reason for the encounter is pain control/ management and not management of the underlying condition.

When an admission or encounter is for a procedure aimed at treating the underlying condition (e.g., spinal fusion, kyphoplasty), a code for the underlying condition (e.g., vertebral fracture, spinal stenosis) should be assigned as the principal diagnosis. No code from category G89 should be assigned.

(a) Category G89 Codes as Principal or First-Listed Diagnosis

Category G89 codes are acceptable as principal diagnosis or the first-listed code:

- When pain control or pain management is the reason for the admission/encounter (e.g., a patient with displaced intervertebral disc, nerve impingement and severe back pain presents for injection of steroid into the spinal canal). The underlying cause of the pain should be reported as an additional diagnosis, if known.

- When a patient is admitted for the insertion of a neurostimulator for pain control, assign the appropriate pain code as the principal or first-listed diagnosis. When an admission or encounter is for a procedure aimed at treating the underlying condition and a neurostimulator is inserted for pain control during the same admission/encounter, a code for the underlying condition should be assigned as the principal diagnosis and the appropriate pain code should be assigned as a secondary diagnosis.

(b) Use of Category G89 Codes in Conjunction with Site Specific Pain Codes

(i) Assigning Category G89 and Site-Specific Pain Codes

Codes from category G89 may be used in conjunction with codes that identify the site of pain (including codes from chapter 18) if the category G89 code provides additional information. For example, if the code describes the site of the pain, but does not fully describe whether the pain is acute or chronic, then both codes should be assigned.

(ii) Sequencing of Category G89 Codes with Site-Specific Pain Codes

The sequencing of category G89 codes with site-specific pain codes (including chapter 18 codes), is dependent on the circumstances of the encounter/admission as follows:

- If the encounter is for pain control or pain management, assign the code from category G89 followed by the code identifying the specific site of pain (e.g., encounter for pain management for acute neck pain from trauma is assigned code G89.11, Acute pain due to trauma, followed by code M54.2, Cervicalgia, to identify the site of pain).

- If the encounter is for any other reason except pain control or pain management, and a related definitive diagnosis has not been established (confirmed) by the provider, assign the code for the specific site of pain first, followed by the appropriate code from category G89.

2) Pain due to devices, implants and grafts

See Section I.C.19. Pain due to medical devices

3) Postoperative Pain

The provider's documentation should be used to guide the coding of postoperative pain, as well as *Section III. Reporting Additional Diagnoses and Section IV. Diagnostic Coding and Reporting in the Outpatient Setting*.

The default for post-thoracotomy and other postoperative pain not specified as acute or chronic is the code for the acute form.

Routine or expected postoperative pain immediately after surgery should not be coded.

(a) Postoperative pain not associated with specific postoperative complication

Postoperative pain not associated with a specific postoperative complication is assigned to the appropriate postoperative pain code in category G89.

(b) Postoperative pain associated with specific postoperative complication

Postoperative pain associated with a specific postoperative complication (such as painful wire sutures) is assigned to the appropriate code(s) found in Chapter 19, Injury, Poisoning, and Certain Other Consequences of External Causes. If appropriate, use additional code(s) from category G89 to identify acute or chronic pain (G89.18 or G89.28).

4) Chronic pain

Chronic pain is classified to subcategory G89.2. There is no time frame defining when pain becomes chronic pain. The provider's documentation should be used to guide use of these codes.

5) Neoplasm Related Pain

Code G89.3 is assigned to pain documented as being related, associated or due to cancer, primary or secondary malignancy, or tumor. This code is assigned regardless of whether the pain is acute or chronic.

This code may be assigned as the principal or first-listed code when the stated reason for the admission/encounter is documented as pain control/pain management. The underlying neoplasm should be reported as an additional diagnosis.

When the reason for the admission/encounter is management of the neoplasm and the pain associated with the neoplasm is also documented, code G89.3 may be assigned as an additional diagnosis. It is not necessary to assign an additional code for the site of the pain.

See Section I.C.2 for instructions on the sequencing of neoplasms for all other stated reasons for the admission/encounter (except for pain control/pain management).

6) Chronic pain syndrome

Central pain syndrome (G89.0) and chronic pain syndrome (G89.4) are different than the term "chronic pain," and therefore codes should only be used when the provider has specifically documented this condition.

See Section I.C.5. Pain disorders related to psychological factors

Chapter 7: Diseases of Eye and Adnexa (H00-H59)
a. Glaucoma
1) Assigning Glaucoma Codes

Assign as many codes from category H40, Glaucoma, as needed to identify the type of glaucoma, the affected eye, and the glaucoma stage.

2) Bilateral glaucoma with same type and stage

When a patient has bilateral glaucoma and both eyes are documented as being the same type and stage, and there is a code for bilateral glaucoma, report only the code for the type of glaucoma, bilateral, with the seventh character for the stage.

When a patient has bilateral glaucoma and both eyes are documented as being the same type and stage, and the classification does not provide a code for bilateral glaucoma (i.e. subcategories H40.10, H40.11 and H40.20) report only

one code for the type of glaucoma with the appropriate seventh character for the stage.

3) Bilateral glaucoma stage with different types or stages

When a patient has bilateral glaucoma and each eye is documented as having a different type or stage, and the classification distinguishes laterality, assign the appropriate code for each eye rather than the code for bilateral glaucoma.

When a patient has bilateral glaucoma and each eye is documented as having a different type, and the classification does not distinguish laterality (i.e. subcategories H40.10, H40.11 and H40.20), assign one code for each type of glaucoma with the appropriate seventh character for the stage.

When a patient has bilateral glaucoma and each eye is documented as having the same type, but different stage, and the classification does not distinguish laterality (i.e. subcategories H40.10, H40.11 and H40.20), assign a code for the type of glaucoma for each eye with the seventh character for the specific glaucoma stage documented for each eye.

4) Patient admitted with glaucoma and stage evolves during the admission

If a patient is admitted with glaucoma and the stage progresses during the admission, assign the code for highest stage documented.

5) Indeterminate stage glaucoma

Assignment of the seventh character "4" for "indeterminate stage" should be based on the clinical documentation. The seventh character "4" is used for glaucomas whose stage cannot be clinically determined. This seventh character should not be confused with the seventh character "0", unspecified, which should be assigned when there is no documentation regarding the stage of the glaucoma.

Chapter 8: Diseases of Ear and Mastoid Process (H60-H95)
Reserved for future guideline expansion

Chapter 9: Diseases of Circulatory System (I00-I99)
a. Hypertension
1) Hypertension with Heart Disease

Heart conditions classified to I50.- or I51.4-I51.9, are assigned to, a code from category I11, *Hypertensive heart disease*, when a causal relationship is stated (due to hypertension) or implied (hypertensive). Use an additional code from category I50, Heart failure, to identify the type of heart failure in those patients with heart failure.

The same heart conditions (I50.-, I51.4-I51.9) with hypertension, but without a stated causal relationship, are coded separately. Sequence according to the circumstances of the admission/encounter.

2) Hypertensive Chronic Kidney Disease

Assign codes from category I12, *Hypertensive chronic kidney disease*, when both hypertension and a condition classifiable to category N18, Chronic kidney disease (CKD), are present. Unlike hypertension with heart disease, ICD-10-CM presumes a cause-and-effect relationship and classifies chronic kidney disease with hypertension as hypertensive chronic kidney disease.

The appropriate code from category N18 should be used as a secondary code with a code from category I12 to identify the stage of chronic kidney disease.

See Section I.C.14. Chronic kidney disease.

If a patient has hypertensive chronic kidney disease and acute renal failure, an additional code for the acute renal failure is required.

3) Hypertensive Heart and Chronic Kidney Disease

Assign codes from combination category I13, *Hypertensive heart and chronic kidney disease*, when both hypertensive kidney disease and hypertensive heart disease are stated in the diagnosis. Assume a relationship between the hypertension and the chronic kidney disease, whether or not the condition is so designated. If heart failure is present, assign an additional code from category I50 to identify the type of heart failure.

The appropriate code from category N18, *Chronic kidney disease*, should be used as a secondary code with a code from category I13 to identify the stage of chronic kidney disease.

See Section I.C.14. Chronic kidney disease.

The codes in category I13, *Hypertensive heart and chronic kidney disease*, are combination codes that include hypertension, heart disease and chronic kidney disease. The Includes note at I13 specifies that the conditions included at I11 and I12 are included together in I13. If a patient has hypertension, heart disease and chronic kidney disease then a code from I13 should be used, not individual codes for hypertension, heart disease and chronic kidney disease, or codes from I11 or I12.

For patients with both acute renal failure and chronic kidney disease an additional code for acute renal failure is required.

4) Hypertensive Cerebrovascular Disease

For hypertensive cerebrovascular disease, first assign the appropriate code from categories I60-I69, followed by the appropriate hypertension code.

5) Hypertensive Retinopathy

Subcategory H35.0, *Background retinopathy and retinal vascular changes*, should be used with a code from category I10 – I15, Hypertensive disease to include the systemic hypertension. The sequencing is based on the reason for the encounter.

6) Hypertension, Secondary

Secondary hypertension is due to an underlying condition. Two codes are required: one to identify the underlying etiology and one from category I15 to identify the hypertension. Sequencing of codes is determined by the reason for admission/encounter.

7) Hypertension, Transient

Assign code R03.0, *Elevated blood pressure reading without diagnosis of hypertension*, unless patient has an established diagnosis of hypertension. Assign code O13.-, *Gestational [pregnancy-induced] hypertension without significant proteinuria*, or O14.-, *Pre-eclampsia*, for transient hypertension of pregnancy.

8) Hypertension, Controlled

This diagnostic statement usually refers to an existing state of hypertension under control by therapy. Assign the appropriate code from categories I10-I15, *Hypertensive diseases*.

9) Hypertension, Uncontrolled

Uncontrolled hypertension may refer to untreated hypertension or hypertension not responding to current therapeutic regimen.

In either case, assign the appropriate code from categories I10-I15, Hypertensive diseases.

b. Atherosclerotic Coronary Artery Disease and Angina

ICD-10-CM has combination codes for atherosclerotic heart disease with angina pectoris. The subcategories for these codes are I25.11, *Atherosclerotic heart disease of native coronary artery with angina pectoris* and I25.7, *Atherosclerosis of coronary artery bypass graft(s) and coronary artery of transplanted heart with angina pectoris*.

When using one of these combination codes it is not necessary to use an additional code for angina pectoris. A causal relationship can be assumed in a patient with both atherosclerosis and angina pectoris, unless the documentation indicates the angina is due to something other than the atherosclerosis.

If a patient with coronary artery disease is admitted due to an acute myocardial infarction (AMI), the AMI should be sequenced before the coronary artery disease.

See Section I.C.9. Acute myocardial infarction (AMI)

c. Intraoperative and Postprocedural Cerebrovascular Accident

Medical record documentation should clearly specify the cause-and-effect relationship between the medical intervention and the cerebrovascular accident in order to assign a code for intraoperative or postprocedural cerebrovascular accident.

Proper code assignment depends on whether it was an infarction or hemorrhage and whether it occurred intraoperatively or postoperatively. If it was a cerebral hemorrhage, code assignment depends on the type of procedure performed.

d. Sequelae of Cerebrovascular Disease

1) Category I69, Sequelae of Cerebrovascular disease

Category I69 is used to indicate conditions classifiable to categories I60-I67 as the causes of sequela (neurologic deficits), themselves classified elsewhere. These "late effects" include neurologic deficits that persist after initial onset of conditions classifiable to categories I60-I67. The neurologic deficits caused by cerebrovascular disease may be present from the onset or may arise at any time after the onset of the condition classifiable to categories I60-I67.

Codes from category I69, *Sequelae of cerebrovascular disease*, that specify hemiplegia, hemiparesis and monoplegia identify whether the dominant or nondominant side is affected. Should the affected side be documented, but not specified as dominant or nondominant, and the classification system does not indicate a default, code selection is as follows:

- For ambidextrous patients, the default should be dominant.
- If the left side is affected, the default is non-dominant.
- If the right side is affected, the default is dominant.

2) Codes from category I69 with codes from I60-I67

Codes from category I69 may be assigned on a health care record with codes from I60-I67, if the patient has a current cerebrovascular disease and deficits from an old cerebrovascular disease.

3) Codes from category I69 and Personal history of transient ischemic attack (TIA) and cerebral infarction (Z86.73)

Codes from category I69 should not be assigned if the patient does not have neurologic deficits.

See Section I.C.21. 4. History (of) for use of personal history codes.

e. Acute myocardial infarction (AMI)

1) ST elevation myocardial infarction (STEMI) and non ST elevation myocardial infarction (NSTEMI)

The ICD-10-CM codes for acute myocardial infarction (AMI) identify the site, such as anterolateral wall or true posterior wall. Subcategories I21.0-I21.2 and code I21.4 are used for ST elevation myocardial infarction (STEMI). Code I21.4, *Non-ST elevation (NSTEMI) myocardial infarction*, is used for non ST elevation myocardial infarction (NSTEMI) and nontransmural MIs.

If NSTEMI evolves to STEMI, assign the STEMI code. If STEMI converts to NSTEMI due to thrombolytic therapy, it is still coded as STEMI.

For encounters occurring while the myocardial infarction is equal to, or less than, four weeks old, including transfers to another acute setting or a postacute setting, and the patient requires continued care for the myocardial infarction, codes from category I21 may continue to be reported. For encounters after the 4 week time frame and the patient is still receiving care related to the myocardial infarction, the appropriate aftercare code should be assigned, rather than a code from category I21. For old or healed myocardial infarctions not requiring further care, code I25.2, *Old myocardial infarction*, may be assigned.

2) Acute myocardial infarction, unspecified

Code I21.3, ST elevation (STEMI) myocardial infarction of unspecified site, is the default for the unspecified term acute myocardial infarction. If only STEMI or transmural MI without the site is documented, query the provider as to the site, or assign code I21.3.

3) AMI documented as nontransmural or subendocardial but site provided

If an AMI is documented as nontransmural or subendocardial, but the site is provided, it is still coded as a subendocardial AMI.

See Section I.C.21.3 for information on coding status post administration of tPA in a different facility within the last 24 hours.

4) Subsequent acute myocardial infarction

A code from category I22, *Subsequent ST elevation (STEMI) and non ST elevation (NSTEMI) myocardial infarction*, is to be used when a patient who has suffered an AMI has a new AMI within the 4 week time frame of the initial AMI. A code from category I22 must be used in conjunction with a code from category I21. The sequencing of the I22 and I21 codes depends on the circumstances of the encounter.

Chapter 10: Diseases of the Respiratory System (J00-J99)

a. Chronic Obstructive Pulmonary Disease [COPD] and Asthma

1) Acute exacerbation of chronic obstructive bronchitis and asthma

The codes in categories J44 and J45 distinguish between uncomplicated cases and those in acute exacerbation. An acute exacerbation is a worsening or a decompensation of a chronic condition. An acute exacerbation is not equivalent to an infection superimposed on a chronic condition, though an exacerbation may be triggered by an infection.

b. Acute Respiratory Failure

1) Acute respiratory failure as principal diagnosis

A code from subcategory J96.0, *Acute respiratory failure*, or subcategory J96.2, *Acute and chronic respiratory failure*, may be assigned as a principal diagnosis when it is the condition established after study to be chiefly responsible for occasioning the admission to the hospital, and the selection is supported by the Alphabetic Index and Tabular List. However, chapter-specific coding guidelines (such as obstetrics, poisoning, HIV, newborn) that provide sequencing direction take precedence.

2) Acute respiratory failure as secondary diagnosis

Respiratory failure may be listed as a secondary diagnosis if it occurs after admission, or if it is present on admission, but does not meet the definition of principal diagnosis.

3) Sequencing of acute respiratory failure and another acute condition

When a patient is admitted with respiratory failure and another acute condition, (e.g., myocardial infarction, cerebrovascular accident, aspiration pneumonia), the principal diagnosis will not be the same in every situation. This applies whether the other acute condition is a respiratory or nonrespiratory condition. Selection of the principal diagnosis will be dependent on the circumstances of admission. If both the respiratory failure and the other acute condition are equally responsible for occasioning the admission to the hospital, and there are no chapter-specific sequencing rules, the guideline regarding two or more diagnoses that equally meet the definition for principal diagnosis *(Section II, C.)* may be applied in these situations.

If the documentation is not clear as to whether acute respiratory failure and another condition are equally responsible for occasioning the admission, query the provider for clarification.

c. Influenza due to certain identified influenza influenza viruses

Code only confirmed cases of influenza due to certain identified influenza viruses (category J09), and due to other identified influenza virus (category J10). This is an exception to the hospital inpatient guideline Section II, H. (Uncertain Diagnosis).

In this context, "confirmation" does not require documentation of positive laboratory testing specific for avian or other novel influenza A or other identified influenza virus. However, coding should be based on the provider's diagnostic statement that the patient has avian influenza, or other novel influenza A for category J09, or has another particular identified strain of influenza, such as H1N1 or H3N2, but not identified as novel or variant, for category J10..

If the provider records "suspected" or "possible" or "probable" avian influenza," or novel influenza, or other identified influenza, then the appropriate influenza code from category J11, Influenza due to unidentified influenza virus, should be assigned. A code from category J09, Influenza due to certain identified influenza viruses, should not be assigned nor should a code from category J10, Influenza due to other identified influenza virus.

d. Ventilator associated Pneumonia

1) Documentation of Ventilator associated Pneumonia

As with all procedural or postprocedural complications, code assignment is based on the provider's documentation of the relationship between the condition and the procedure.

Code J95.851, *Ventilator associated pneumonia*, should be assigned only when the provider has documented ventilator associated pneumonia (VAP). An additional code to identify the organism (e.g., Pseudomonas aeruginosa, code B96.5) should also be assigned. Do not assign an additional code from categories J12-J18 to identify the type of pneumonia.

Code J95.851 should not be assigned for cases where the patient has pneumonia and is on a mechanical ventilator and the provider has not specifically stated that the pneumonia is ventilator-associated pneumonia. If the documentation is unclear as to whether the patient has a pneumonia that is a complication attributable to the mechanical ventilator, query the provider.

2) Ventilator associated Pneumonia Develops after Admission

A patient may be admitted with one type of pneumonia (e.g., code J13, *Pneumonia due to Streptococcus pneumonia*) and subsequently develop VAP. In this instance, the principal diagnosis would be the appropriate code from categories J12-J18 for the pneumonia diagnosed at the time of admission. Code J95.851, Ventilator associated pneumonia, would be assigned as an additional diagnosis when the provider has also documented the presence of ventilator associated pneumonia.

Chapter 11: Diseases of the Digestive System (K00-K95)

Reserved for future guideline expansion

Chapter 12: Diseases of the Skin and Subcutaneous Tissue (L00-L99)

a. Pressure ulcer stage codes

1) Pressure ulcer stages

Codes from category L89, *Pressure ulcer*, are combination codes that identify the site of the pressure ulcer as well as the stage of the ulcer.

The ICD-10-CM classifies pressure ulcer stages based on severity, which is designated by stages 1-4, unspecified stage and unstageable.

Assign as many codes from category L89 as needed to identify all the pressure ulcers the patient has, if applicable.

2) Unstageable pressure ulcers

Assignment of the code for unstageable pressure ulcer (L89.--0) should be based on the clinical documentation. These codes are used for pressure ulcers whose stage cannot be clinically determined (e.g., the ulcer is covered by eschar or has been treated with a skin or muscle graft) and pressure ulcers that are documented as deep tissue injury but not documented as due to trauma. This code should not be confused with the codes for unspecified stage (L89.--9). When there is no documentation regarding the stage of the pressure ulcer, assign the appropriate code for unspecified stage (L89.--9).

3) Documented pressure ulcer stage

Assignment of the pressure ulcer stage code should be guided by clinical documentation of the stage or documentation of the terms found in the Alphabetic Index. For clinical terms describing the stage that are not found in the Alphabetic Index, and there is no documentation of the stage, the provider should be queried.

4) Patients admitted with pressure ulcers documented as healed

No code is assigned if the documentation states that the pressure ulcer is completely healed.

5) Patients admitted with pressure ulcers documented as healing

Pressure ulcers described as healing should be assigned the appropriate pressure ulcer stage code based on the documentation in the medical record. If the documentation does not provide information about the stage of the healing pressure ulcer, assign the appropriate code for unspecified stage.

If the documentation is unclear as to whether the patient has a current (new) pressure ulcer or if the patient is being treated for a healing pressure ulcer, query the provider.

6) Patient admitted with pressure ulcer evolving into another stage during the admission

If a patient is admitted with a pressure ulcer at one stage and it progresses to a higher stage, assign the code for the highest stage reported for that site.

Chapter 13: Diseases of the Musculoskeletal System and Connective Tissue (M00-M99)

a. Site and laterality

Most of the codes within Chapter 13 have site and laterality designations. The site represents the bone, joint or the muscle involved. For some conditions where more than one bone, joint or muscle is usually involved, such as osteoarthritis, there is a "multiple sites" code available. For categories where no multiple site code is provided and more than one bone, joint or muscle is involved, multiple codes should be used to indicate the different sites involved.

1) Bone versus joint

For certain conditions, the bone may be affected at the upper or lower end, (e.g., avascular necrosis of bone, M87, Osteoporosis, M80, M81). Though the portion of the bone affected may be at the joint, the site designation will be the bone, not the joint.

b. Acute traumatic versus chronic or recurrent musculoskeletal conditions

Many musculoskeletal conditions are a result of previous injury or trauma to a site, or are recurrent conditions. Bone, joint or muscle conditions that are the result of a healed injury are usually found in chapter 13. Recurrent bone, joint or muscle conditions are also usually found in chapter 13. Any current, acute injury should be coded to the appropriate injury code from chapter 19. Chronic or recurrent conditions should generally be coded with a code from chapter 13. If it is difficult to determine from the documentation in the record which code is best to describe a condition, query the provider.

c. Coding of Pathologic Fractures

7th character A is for use as long as the patient is receiving active treatment for the fracture. Examples of active treatment are: surgical treatment, emergency department encounter, evaluation and continuing treatment by the same or a different physician. While the patient may be seen by a new or different provider over the course of treatment for a pathological fracture, assignment of the 7th character is based on whether the patient is undergoing active treatment and not whether the provider is seeing the patient for the first time.

7th character, D is to be used for encounters after the patient has completed active treatment. The other 7th characters, listed under each subcategory in the Tabular List, are to be used for subsequent encounters for treatment of problems associated with the healing, such as malunions, nonunions, and sequelae.

Care for complications of surgical treatment for fracture repairs during the healing or recovery phase should be coded with the appropriate complication codes.

See Section I.C.19. Coding of traumatic fractures.

d. Osteoporosis

Osteoporosis is a systemic condition, meaning that all bones of the musculoskeletal system are affected. Therefore, site is not a component of the codes under category M81, *Osteoporosis without current pathological fracture*. The site codes under category M80, *Osteoporosis with current pathological fracture*, identify the site of the fracture, not the osteoporosis.

1) Osteoporosis without pathological fracture

Category M81, *Osteoporosis without current pathological fracture*, is for use for patients with osteoporosis who do not currently have a pathologic fracture due to the osteoporosis, even if they have had a fracture in the past. For patients with a history of osteoporosis fractures, status code Z87.310, *Personal history of (healed) osteoporosis fracture*, should follow the code from M81.

2) Osteoporosis with current pathological fracture

Category M80, *Osteoporosis with current pathological fracture*, is for patients who have a current pathologic fracture at the time of an encounter. The codes under M80 identify the site of the fracture. A code from category M80, not a traumatic fracture code, should be used for any patient with known osteoporosis who suffers a fracture, even if the patient had a minor fall or trauma, if that fall or trauma would not usually break a normal, healthy bone.

Chapter 14: Diseases of Genitourinary System (N00-N99)

a. Chronic kidney disease

1) Stages of chronic kidney disease (CKD)

The ICD-10-CM classifies CKD based on severity. The severity of CKD is designated by stages 1-5. Stage 2, code N18.2, equates to mild CKD; stage 3, code N18.3, equates to moderate CKD; and stage 4, code N18.4, equates to severe CKD. Code N18.6, *End stage renal disease (ESRD)*, is assigned when the provider has documented end-stage-renal disease (ESRD).

If both a stage of CKD and ESRD are documented, assign code N18.6 only.

2) Chronic kidney disease and kidney transplant status

Patients who have undergone kidney transplant may still have some form of chronic kidney disease (CKD) because the kidney transplant may not fully restore kidney function. Therefore, the presence of CKD alone does not constitute a transplant complication. Assign the appropriate N18 code for the patient's stage of CKD and code Z94.0, *Kidney transplant status*. If a transplant complication such as failure or rejection or other transplant complication is documented, see section I.C.19.g for information on coding complications of a kidney transplant. If the documentation is unclear as to whether the patient has a complication of the transplant, query the provider.

3) Chronic kidney disease with other conditions

Patients with CKD may also suffer from other serious conditions, most commonly diabetes mellitus and hypertension. The sequencing of the CKD code in relationship to codes for other contributing conditions is based on the conventions in the Tabular List.

See Section I.C.9. Hypertensive chronic kidney disease.

See Section I.C.19. Chronic kidney disease and kidney transplant complications.

Chapter 15: Pregnancy, Childbirth, and the Puerperium (O00-O9A)

a. General Rules for Obstetric Cases

1) Codes from chapter 15 and sequencing priority

Obstetric cases require codes from chapter 15, codes in the range O00-O9A, *Pregnancy, Childbirth, and the Puerperium*. Chapter 15 codes have sequencing priority over codes from other chapters. Additional codes from other chapters may be used in conjunction with chapter 15 codes to further specify conditions. Should the provider document that the pregnancy is incidental to the encounter, then code Z33.1, *Pregnant state, incidental*, should be used in place of any chapter 15 codes. It is the provider's responsibility to state that the condition being treated is not affecting the pregnancy.

2) Chapter 15 codes used only on the maternal record

Chapter 15 codes are to be used only on the maternal record, never on the record of the newborn.

3) Final character for trimester

The majority of codes in Chapter 15 have a final character indicating the trimester of pregnancy. The timeframes for the trimesters are indicated at the beginning of the chapter. If trimester is not a component of a code it is because the condition always occurs in a specific trimester, or the concept of trimester of pregnancy is not applicable. Certain codes have characters for only certain trimesters because the condition does not occur in all trimesters, but it may occur in more than just one.

Assignment of the final character for trimester should be based on the provider's documentation of the trimester (or number of weeks) for the current admission/encounter. This applies to the assignment of trimester for pre-existing conditions as well as those that develop during or are due to the pregnancy. The provider's documentation of the number of weeks may be used to assign the appropriate code identifying the trimester.

Whenever delivery occurs during the current admission, and there is an "in childbirth" option for the obstetric complication being coded, the "in childbirth" code should be assigned.

4) Selection of trimester for inpatient admissions that encompass more than one trimesters

In instances when a patient is admitted to a hospital for complications of pregnancy during one trimester and remains in the hospital into a subsequent trimester, the trimester character for the antepartum complication code should be assigned on the basis of the trimester when the complication developed, not the trimester of the discharge. If the condition developed prior to the current admission/encounter or represents a pre-existing condition, the trimester character for the trimester at the time of the admission/encounter should be assigned.

5) Unspecified trimester

Each category that includes codes for trimester has a code for "unspecified trimester." The "unspecified trimester" code should rarely be used, such as when the documentation in the record is insufficient to determine the trimester and it is not possible to obtain clarification.

6) 7th character for Fetus Identification

Where applicable, a 7th character is to be assigned for certain categories (O31, O32, O33.3 - O33.6, O35, O36, O40, O41, O60.1, O60.2, O64, and O69) to identify the fetus for which the complication code applies.

Assign 7th character "0":

- For single gestations
- When the documentation in the record is insufficient to determine the fetus affected and it is not possible to obtain clarification.
- When it is not possible to clinically determine which fetus is affected.

b. Selection of OB Principal or First-listed Diagnosis

1) Routine outpatient prenatal visits

For routine outpatient prenatal visits when no complications are present, a code from category Z34, *Encounter for supervision of normal pregnancy*, should be used as the first-listed diagnosis. These codes should not be used in conjunction with chapter 15 codes.

2) Prenatal outpatient visits for high-risk patients

For routine prenatal outpatient visits for patients with high-risk pregnancies, a code from category O09, *Supervision of high-risk pregnancy*, should be used as the first-listed diagnosis. Secondary chapter 15 codes may be used in conjunction with these codes if appropriate.

3) Episodes when no delivery occurs

In episodes when no delivery occurs, the principal diagnosis should correspond to the principal complication of the pregnancy which necessitated the encounter. Should more than one complication exist, all of which are treated or monitored, any of the complications codes may be sequenced first.

4) When a delivery occurs

When a delivery occurs, the principal diagnosis should correspond to the main circumstances or complication of the delivery. In cases of cesarean delivery, the selection of the principal diagnosis should be the condition established after study that was responsible for the patient's admission. If the patient was admitted with a condition that resulted in the performance of a cesarean procedure, that condition should be selected as the principal diagnosis. If the reason for the admission/encounter was unrelated to the condition resulting in the cesarean delivery, the condition related to the reason for the admission/encounter should be selected as the principal diagnosis.

5) Outcome of delivery

A code from category Z37, *Outcome of delivery*, should be included on every maternal record when a delivery has occurred. These codes are not to be used on subsequent records or on the newborn record.

c. Pre-existing conditions versus conditions due to the pregnancy

Certain categories in Chapter 15 distinguish between conditions of the mother that existed prior to pregnancy (pre-existing) and those that are a direct result of pregnancy. When assigning codes from Chapter 15, it is important to assess if a condition was pre-existing prior to pregnancy or developed during or due to the pregnancy in order to assign the correct code.

Categories that do not distinguish between pre-existing and pregnancy-related conditions may be used for either. It is acceptable to use codes specifically for the puerperium with codes complicating pregnancy and childbirth if a condition arises postpartum during the delivery encounter.

d. Pre-existing hypertension in pregnancy

Category O10, *Pre-existing hypertension complicating pregnancy, childbirth and the puerperium*, includes codes for hypertensive heart and hypertensive chronic kidney disease. When assigning one of the O10 codes that includes hypertensive heart disease or hypertensive chronic kidney disease, it is necessary to add a secondary code from the appropriate hypertension category to specify the type of heart failure or chronic kidney disease.

See Section I.C.9. Hypertension.

e. Fetal Conditions Affecting the Management of the Mother

1) Codes from categories O35 and O36

Codes from categories O35, *Maternal care for known or suspected fetal abnormality and damage*, and O36, *Maternal care for other fetal problems*, are assigned only when the fetal condition is actually responsible for modifying the management of the mother, i.e., by requiring diagnostic studies, additional observation, special care, or termination of pregnancy. The fact that the fetal condition exists does not justify assigning a code from this series to the mother's record.

2) In utero surgery

In cases when surgery is performed on the fetus, a diagnosis code from category O35, *Maternal care for known or suspected fetal abnormality and damage*, should be assigned identifying the fetal condition. Assign the appropriate procedure code for the procedure performed.

No code from Chapter 16, the perinatal codes, should be used on the mother's record to identify fetal conditions. Surgery performed in utero on a fetus is still to be coded as an obstetric encounter.

f. HIV Infection in Pregnancy, Childbirth and the Puerperium

During pregnancy, childbirth or the puerperium, a patient admitted because of an HIV-related illness should receive a principal diagnosis from subcategory O98.7-, *Human immunodeficiency [HIV] disease complicating pregnancy, childbirth and the puerperium*, followed by the code(s) for the HIV-related illness(es).

Patients with asymptomatic HIV infection status admitted during pregnancy, childbirth, or the puerperium should receive codes of O98.7- and Z21, *Asymptomatic human immunodeficiency virus [HIV] infection status*.

g. Diabetes mellitus in pregnancy

Diabetes mellitus is a significant complicating factor in pregnancy. Pregnant women who are diabetic should be assigned a code from category O24, *Diabetes mellitus in pregnancy, childbirth, and the puerperium*, first, followed by the appropriate diabetes code(s) (E08-E13) from Chapter 4.

h. Long-term use of insulin

Code Z79.4, *Long-term (current) use of insulin*, should also be assigned if the diabetes mellitus is being treated with insulin.

i. Gestational (pregnancy induced) diabetes

Gestational (pregnancy induced) diabetes can occur during the second and third trimester of pregnancy in women who were not diabetic prior to pregnancy. Gestational diabetes can cause complications in the pregnancy similar to those of pre-existing diabetes mellitus. It also puts the woman at greater risk of developing diabetes after the pregnancy. Codes for gestational diabetes are in subcategory O24.4, *Gestational diabetes mellitus*. No other code from category O24, *Diabetes mellitus in pregnancy, childbirth, and the puerperium*, should be used with a code from O24.4

The codes under subcategory O24.4 include diet controlled and insulin controlled. If a patient with gestational diabetes is treated with both diet and insulin, only the code for insulin-controlled is required.

Code Z79.4, *Long-term (current) use of insulin*, should not be assigned with codes from subcategory O24.4.

An abnormal glucose tolerance in pregnancy is assigned a code from subcategory O99.81, *Abnormal glucose complicating pregnancy, childbirth, and the puerperium*.

j. Sepsis and septic shock complicating abortion, pregnancy, childbirth and the puerperium

When assigning a chapter 15 code for sepsis complicating abortion, pregnancy, childbirth, and the puerperium, a code for the specific type of infection should be assigned as an additional diagnosis. If severe sepsis is present, a code from subcategory R65.2, *Severe sepsis*, and code(s) for associated organ dysfunction(s) should also be assigned as additional diagnoses.

k. Puerperal sepsis

Code O85, *Puerperal sepsis*, should be assigned with a secondary code to identify the causal organism (e.g., for a bacterial infection, assign a code from category B95-B96, *Bacterial infections in conditions classified elsewhere*). A code from category A40, *Streptococcal sepsis*, or A41, *Other sepsis*, should not be used for puerperal sepsis. If applicable, use additional codes to identify severe sepsis (R65.2-) and any associated acute organ dysfunction.

l. Alcohol and tobacco use during pregnancy, childbirth and the puerperium

1) Alcohol use during pregnancy, childbirth and the puerperium

Codes under subcategory O99.31, *Alcohol use complicating pregnancy, childbirth, and the puerperium*, should be assigned for any pregnancy case when a mother uses alcohol during the pregnancy or postpartum. A secondary code from category F10, Alcohol related disorders, should also be assigned to identify manifestations of the alcohol use.

2) Tobacco use during pregnancy, childbirth and the puerperium

Codes under subcategory O99.33, *Smoking (tobacco) complicating pregnancy, childbirth, and the puerperium*, should be assigned for any pregnancy case when a mother uses any type of tobacco product during the pregnancy or postpartum. A secondary code from category F17, *Nicotine dependence*, or code Z72.0, *Tobacco use*, should also be assigned to identify the type of nicotine dependence.

m. Poisoning, toxic effects, adverse effects and underdosing in a pregnant patient

A code from subcategory O9A.2, *Injury, poisoning and certain other consequences of external causes complicating pregnancy*, childbirth, and the puerperium, should be sequenced first, followed by the appropriate injury, poisoning, toxic effect, adverse effect or underdosing code, and then the additional code(s) that specifies the condition caused by the poisoning, toxic effect, adverse effect or underdosing.

See Section I.C.19. Adverse effects, poisoning, underdosing and toxic effects.

n. Normal Delivery, Code O80

1) Encounter for full term uncomplicated delivery

Code O80 should be assigned when a woman is admitted for a full-term normal delivery and delivers a single, healthy infant without any complications antepartum, during the delivery, or postpartum during the delivery episode. Code O80 is always a principal diagnosis. It is not to be used if any other code from chapter 15 is needed to describe a current complication of the antenatal, delivery, or perinatal period. Additional codes from other chapters may be used with code O80 if they are not related to or are in any way complicating the pregnancy.

2) Uncomplicated delivery with resolved antepartum complication

Code O80 may be used if the patient had a complication at some point during the pregnancy, but the complication is not present at the time of the admission for delivery.

3) Outcome of delivery for O80

Z37.0, *Single live birth*, is the only outcome of delivery code appropriate for use with O80.

o. The Peripartum and Postpartum Periods

1) Peripartum and Postpartum periods

The postpartum period begins immediately after delivery and continues for six weeks following delivery. The peripartum period is defined as the last month of pregnancy to five months postpartum.

2) Peripartum and postpartum complication

A postpartum complication is any complication occurring within the six-week period.

3) Pregnancy-related complications after 6 week period

Chapter 15 codes may also be used to describe pregnancy-related complications after the peripartum or postpartum period if the provider documents that a condition is pregnancy related.

4) Admission for routine postpartum care following delivery outside hospital

When the mother delivers outside the hospital prior to admission and is admitted for routine postpartum care and no complications are noted, code Z39.0, *Encounter for care and examination of mother immediately after delivery*, should be assigned as the principal diagnosis.

5) Pregnancy associated cardiomyopathy

Pregnancy associated cardiomyopathy, code O90.3, is unique in that it may be diagnosed in the third trimester of pregnancy but may continue to progress months after delivery. For this reason, it is referred to as peripartum cardiomyopathy. Code O90.3 is only for use when the cardiomyopathy develops as a result of pregnancy in a woman who did not have pre-existing heart disease.

p. Code O94, Sequelae of complication of pregnancy, childbirth, and the puerperium

1) Code O94

Code O94, *Sequelae of complication of pregnancy, childbirth, and the puerperium*, is for use in those cases when an initial complication of a pregnancy develops a sequelae requiring care or treatment at a future date.

2) After the initial postpartum period

This code may be used at any time after the initial postpartum period.

3) Sequencing of Code O94

This code, like all sequela codes, is to be sequenced following the code describing the sequelae of the complication.

q. Termination of Pregnancy and Spontaneous abortions

1) Abortion with Liveborn Fetus

When an attempted termination of pregnancy results in a liveborn fetus, assign code Z33.2, *Encounter for elective termination of pregnancy* and a code from category Z37, Outcome of Delivery.

2) Retained Products of Conception following an abortion

Subsequent encounters for retained products of conception following a spontaneous abortion or elective termination of pregnancy are assigned the appropriate code from category O03, *Spontaneous abortion*, or codes O07.4, *Failed attempted termination of pregnancy without complication* and Z33.2, *Encounter for elective termination of pregnancy*. This advice is appropriate even when the patient was discharged previously with a discharge diagnosis of complete abortion.

3) Complications leading to abortion

Codes from Chapter 15 may be used as additional codes to identify any documented complications of the pregnancy in conjunction with codes in categories in O07 and O08.

r. Abuse in a pregnant patient

For suspected or confirmed cases of abuse of a pregnant patient, a code(s) from subcategories O9A.3, *Physical abuse complicating pregnancy, childbirth, and the puerperium*, O9A.4, *Sexual abuse complicating pregnancy, childbirth, and the puerperium*, and O9A.5, *Psychological abuse complicating pregnancy, childbirth, and the puerperium*, should be sequenced first, followed by the appropriate codes (if applicable) to identify any associated current injury due to physical abuse, sexual abuse, and the perpetrator of abuse.

See Section I.C.19.f. Adult and child abuse, neglect and other maltreatment.

Chapter 16: Certain Conditions Originating in the Perinatal Period (P00-P96)

For coding and reporting purposes the perinatal period is defined as before birth through the 28th day following birth. The following guidelines are provided for reporting purposes

a. General Perinatal Rules

1) Use of Chapter 16 Codes

Codes in this chapter are never for use on the maternal record. Codes from Chapter 15, the obstetric chapter, are never permitted on the newborn record. Chapter 16 codes may be used throughout the life of the patient if the condition is still present.

2) Principal Diagnosis for Birth Record

When coding the birth episode in a newborn record, assign a code from category Z38, *Liveborn infants according to place of birth and type of delivery*, as the principal diagnosis. A code from category Z38 is assigned only once, to a newborn at the time of birth. If a newborn is transferred to another institution, a code from category Z38 should not be used at the receiving hospital.

A code from category Z38 is used only on the newborn record, not on the mother's record.

3) Use of Codes from other Chapters with Codes from Chapter 16

Codes from other chapters may be used with codes from chapter 16 if the codes from the other chapters provide more specific detail. Codes for signs and symptoms may be assigned when a definitive diagnosis has not been established. If the reason for the encounter is a perinatal condition, the code from chapter 16 should be sequenced first.

4) Use of Chapter 16 Codes after the Perinatal Period

Should a condition originate in the perinatal period, and continue throughout the life of the patient, the perinatal code should continue to be used regardless of the patient's age.

5) Birth process or community acquired conditions

If a newborn has a condition that may be either due to the birth process or community acquired and the documentation does not indicate which it is, the default is due to the birth process and the code from Chapter 16 should be used. If the condition is community-acquired, a code from Chapter 16 should not be assigned.

6) Code all clinically significant conditions

All clinically significant conditions noted on routine newborn examination should be coded. A condition is clinically significant if it requires:

- clinical evaluation; or
- therapeutic treatment; or
- diagnostic procedures; or
- extended length of hospital stay; or
- increased nursing care and/or monitoring; or
- has implications for future health care needs

Note: The perinatal guidelines listed above are the same as the general coding guidelines for "additional diagnoses", except for the final point regarding implications for future health care needs. Codes should be assigned for conditions that have been specified by the provider as having implications for future health care needs.

b. Observation and Evaluation of Newborns for Suspected Conditions not Found

Reserved for future expansion

c. Coding Additional Perinatal Diagnoses

1) Assigning codes for conditions that require treatment

Assign codes for conditions that require treatment or further investigation, prolong the length of stay, or require resource utilization.

2) Codes for conditions specified as having implications for future health care needs

Assign codes for conditions that have been specified by the provider as having implications for future health care needs.

Note: This guideline should not be used for adult patients.

d. Prematurity and Fetal Growth Retardation

Providers utilize different criteria in determining prematurity. A code for prematurity should not be assigned unless it is documented. Assignment of codes in categories P05, *Disorders of newborn related to slow fetal growth and fetal malnutrition*, and P07, *Disorders of newborn related to short gestation and low birth weight, not elsewhere classified*, should be based on the recorded birth weight and estimated gestational age. Codes from category P05 should not be assigned with codes from category P07.

When both birth weight and gestational age are available, two codes from category P07 should be assigned, with the code for birth weight sequenced before the code for gestational age.

e. Low birth weight and immaturity status

Codes from category P07, *Disorders of newborn related to short gestation and low birth weight*, not elsewhere classified, are for use for a child or adult who was premature or had a low birth weight as a newborn and this is affecting the patient's current health status.

See Section I.C.21. Factors influencing health status and contact with health services, Status.

f. Bacterial Sepsis of Newborn

Category P36, *Bacterial sepsis of newborn*, includes congenital sepsis. If a perinate is documented as having sepsis without documentation of congenital or community acquired, the default is congenital and a code from category P36 should be assigned. If the P36 code includes the causal organism, an additional code from category B95, *Streptococcus, Staphylococcus, and Enterococcus as the cause of diseases classified elsewhere*, or B96, *Other bacterial agents as the cause of diseases classified elsewhere*, should not be assigned. If the P36 code does not include the causal organism, assign an additional code from category B96. If applicable, use additional codes to identify severe sepsis (R65.2-) and any associated acute organ dysfunction.

g. Stillbirth

Code P95, *Stillbirth*, is only for use in institutions that maintain separate records for stillbirths. No other code should be used with P95. Code P95 should not be used on the mother's record.

Chapter 17: Congenital malformations, deformations, and chromosomal abnormalities (Q00-Q99)

Assign an appropriate code(s) from categories Q00-Q99, Congenital malformations, deformations, and chromosomal abnormalities when a malformation/deformation or chromosomal abnormality is documented. A malformation/deformation/or chromosomal abnormality may be the principal/first-listed diagnosis on a record or a secondary diagnosis.

When a malformation/deformation/or chromosomal abnormality does not have a unique code assignment, assign additional code(s) for any manifestations that may be present.

When the code assignment specifically identifies the malformation/deformation/or chromosomal abnormality, manifestations that are an inherent component of the anomaly should not be coded separately. Additional codes should be assigned for manifestations that are not an inherent component.

Codes from Chapter 17 may be used throughout the life of the patient. If a congenital malformation or deformity has been corrected, a personal history code should be used to identify the history of the malformation or deformity. Although present at birth, malformation/deformation/or chromosomal abnormality may not be identified until later in life. Whenever the condition is diagnosed by the physician, it is appropriate to assign a code from codes Q00-Q99.

For the birth admission, the appropriate code from category Z38, *Liveborn infants, according to place of birth and type of delivery*, should be sequenced as the principal diagnosis, followed by any congenital anomaly codes, Q00-Q99.

Chapter 18: Symptoms, signs, and abnormal clinical and laboratory findings, not elsewhere classified (R00-R99)

Chapter 18 includes symptoms, signs, abnormal results of clinical or other investigative procedures, and ill-defined conditions regarding which no diagnosis classifiable elsewhere is recorded. Signs and symptoms that point to a specific diagnosis have been assigned to a category in other chapters of the classification.

a. Use of symptom codes

Codes that describe symptoms and signs are acceptable for reporting purposes when a related definitive diagnosis has not been established (confirmed) by the provider.

b. Use of a symptom code with a definitive diagnosis code

Codes for signs and symptoms may be reported in addition to a related definitive diagnosis when the sign or symptom is not routinely associated with that diagnosis, such as the various signs and symptoms associated with complex syndromes. The definitive diagnosis code should be sequenced before the symptom code.

Signs or symptoms that are associated routinely with a disease process should not be assigned as additional codes, unless otherwise instructed by the classification.

c. Combination codes that include symptoms

ICD-10-CM contains a number of combination codes that identify both the definitive diagnosis and common symptoms of that diagnosis. When using one of these combination codes, an additional code should not be assigned for the symptom.

d. Repeated falls

Code R29.6, *Repeated falls*, is for use for encounters when a patient has recently fallen and the reason for the fall is being investigated.

Code Z91.81, *History of falling*, is for use when a patient has fallen in the past and is at risk for future falls. When appropriate, both codes R29.6 and Z91.81 may be assigned together.

e. Coma scale

The coma scale codes (R40.2-) can be used in conjunction with traumatic brain injury codes, acute cerebrovascular disease or sequelae of cerebrovascular disease codes. These codes are primarily for use by trauma registries, but they may be used in any setting where this information is collected. The coma scale codes should be sequenced after the diagnosis code(s).

These codes, one from each subcategory, are needed to complete the scale. The 7th character indicates when the scale was recorded. The 7th character should match for all three codes.

At a minimum, report the initial score documented on presentation at your facility. This may be a score from the emergency medicine technician (EMT) or in the emergency department. If desired, a facility may choose to capture multiple Glasgow coma scale scores.

Assign code R40.24, Glasgow coma scale, total score, when only the total score is documented in the medical record and not the individual score(s).

f. Functional quadriplegia

Functional quadriplegia (code R53.2) is the lack of ability to use one's limbs or to ambulate due to extreme debility. It is not associated with neurologic deficit or injury, and code R53.2 should not be used for cases of neurologic quadriplegia. It should only be assigned if functional quadriplegia is specifically documented in the medical record.

g. SIRS due to Non-Infectious Process

The systemic inflammatory response syndrome (SIRS) can develop as a result of certain non-infectious disease processes, such as trauma, malignant neoplasm, or pancreatitis. When SIRS is documented with a noninfectious condition, and no subsequent infection is documented, the code for the underlying condition, such as an injury, should be assigned, followed by code R65.10, *Systemic inflammatory response syndrome (SIRS) of non-infectious origin without acute organ dysfunction*, or code R65.11, *Systemic inflammatory response syndrome (SIRS) of non-infectious origin with acute organ dysfunction*. If an associated acute organ dysfunction is documented, the appropriate code(s) for the specific type of organ dysfunction(s) should be assigned in addition to code R65.11. If acute organ dysfunction is documented, but it cannot be determined if the acute organ dysfunction is associated with SIRS or due to another condition (e.g., directly due to the trauma), the provider should be queried.

h. Death NOS

Code R99, *Ill-defined and unknown cause of mortality*, is only for use in the very limited circumstance when a patient who has already died is brought into an emergency department or other healthcare facility and is pronounced dead upon arrival. It does not represent the discharge disposition of death.

Chapter 19: Injury, poisoning, and certain other consequences of external causes (S00-T88)

a. Application of 7th Characters in Chapter 19

Most categories in chapter 19 have a 7th character requirement for each applicable code. Most categories in this chapter have three 7th character values (with the exception of fractures): A, initial encounter, D, subsequent encounter and S, sequela. Categories for traumatic fractures have additional 7th character values. While the patient may be seen by a new or different provider over the course of treatment for an injury, assignment of the 7th character is based on whether the patient is undergoing active treatment and not whether the provider is seeing the patient for the first time.

For complication codes, active treatment refers to treatment for the condition described by the code, even though it may be related to an earlier precipitating problem. For example, code T84.50XA, Infection and inflammatory reaction due to unspecified internal joint prosthesis, initial encounter, is used when active treatment is provided for the infection, even though the condition relates to the prosthetic device, implant or graft that was placed at a previous encounter.

7th character "A", initial encounter is used while the patient is receiving active treatment for the condition. Examples of active treatment are: surgical treatment, emergency department encounter, and evaluation and continuing treatment by the same or a different physician.

7th character "D" subsequent encounter is used for encounters after the patient has received active treatment of the condition and is receiving routine care for the condition during the healing or recovery phase. Examples of subsequent care are: cast change or removal, an x-ray to check healing status of fracture, removal of external or internal fixation device, medication adjustment, other aftercare and follow up visits following treatment of the injury or condition.

The aftercare Z codes should not be used for aftercare for conditions such as injuries or poisonings, where 7th characters are provided to identify subsequent care. For example, for aftercare of an injury, assign the acute injury code with the 7th character "D" (subsequent encounter).

7th character "S", sequela, is for use for complications or conditions that arise as a direct result of a condition, such as scar formation after a burn. The scars are sequelae of the burn. When using 7th character "S", it is necessary to use both the injury code that precipitated the sequela and the code for the sequela itself. The "S" is added only to the injury code, not the sequela code. The 7th character "S" identifies the injury responsible for the sequela. The specific type of sequela (e.g. scar) is sequenced first, followed by the injury code.

b. Coding of Injuries

When coding injuries, assign separate codes for each injury unless a combination code is provided, in which case the combination code is assigned. Code T07, *Unspecified multiple injuries* should not be assigned in the inpatient setting unless information for a more specific code is not available. Traumatic injury codes (S00-T14.9) are not to be used for normal, healing surgical wounds or to identify complications of surgical wounds.

The code for the most serious injury, as determined by the provider and the focus of treatment, is sequenced first.

1) Superficial injuries

Superficial injuries such as abrasions or contusions are not coded when associated with more severe injuries of the same site.

2) Primary injury with damage to nerves/blood vessels

When a primary injury results in minor damage to peripheral nerves or blood vessels, the primary injury is sequenced first with additional code(s) for injuries to nerves and spinal cord (such as category S04), and/or injury to blood vessels (such as category S15). When the primary injury is to the blood vessels or nerves, that injury should be sequenced first.

c. Coding of Traumatic Fractures

The principles of multiple coding of injuries should be followed in coding fractures. Fractures of specified sites are coded individually by site in accordance with both the provisions within categories S02, S12, S22, S32, S42, S49, S52, S59, S62, S72, S79, S82, S89, S92 and the level of detail furnished by medical record content.

A fracture not indicated as open or closed should be coded to closed. A fracture not indicated whether displaced or not displaced should be coded to displaced.

More specific guidelines are as follows:

1) Initial vs. Subsequent Encounter for Fractures

Traumatic fractures are coded using the appropriate 7th character for initial encounter (A, B, C) while the patient is receiving active treatment for the fracture. Examples of active treatment are: surgical treatment, emergency department encounter, and evaluation and continuing (ongoing) treatment by the same or different physician. The appropriate 7th character for initial encounter should also be assigned for a patient who delayed seeking treatment for the fracture or nonunion.

Fractures are coded using the appropriate 7th character for subsequent care for encounters after the patient has completed active treatment of the fracture and is receiving routine care for the fracture during the healing or recovery phase. Examples of fracture aftercare are: cast change or removal, an x-ray to check healing status of fracture, removal of external or internal fixation device, medication adjustment, and follow-up visits following fracture treatment.

Care for complications of surgical treatment for fracture repairs during the healing or recovery phase should be coded with the appropriate complication codes.

Care of complications of fractures, such as malunion and nonunion, should be reported with the appropriate 7th character for subsequent care with nonunion (K, M, N,) or subsequent care with malunion (P, Q, R).

Malunion/nonunion: The appropriate 7th character for initial encounter should also be assigned for a patient who delayed seeking treatment for the fracture or nonunion.

A code from category M80, not a traumatic fracture code, should be used for any patient with known osteoporosis who suffers a fracture, even if the patient had a minor fall or trauma, if that fall or trauma would not usually break a normal, healthy bone.

See Section I.C.13. Osteoporosis.

The aftercare Z codes should not be used for aftercare for traumatic fractures. For aftercare of a traumatic fracture, assign the acute fracture code with the appropriate 7th character.

2) Multiple fractures sequencing

Multiple fractures are sequenced in accordance with the severity of the fracture.

d. Coding of Burns and Corrosions

The ICD-10-CM makes a distinction between burns and corrosions. The burn codes are for thermal burns, except sunburns, that come from a heat source, such as a fire or hot appliance. The burn codes are also for burns resulting from electricity and radiation. Corrosions are burns due to chemicals. The guidelines are the same for burns and corrosions.

Current burns (T20-T25) are classified by depth, extent and by agent (X code). Burns are classified by depth as first degree (erythema), second degree (blistering), and third degree (full-thickness involvement). Burns of the eye and internal organs (T26-T28) are classified by site, but not by degree.

1) Sequencing of burn and related condition codes

Sequence first the code that reflects the highest degree of burn when more than one burn is present.

a. When the reason for the admission or encounter is for treatment of external multiple burns, sequence first the code that reflects the burn of the highest degree.

b. When a patient has both internal and external burns, the circumstances of admission govern the selection of the principal diagnosis or first-listed diagnosis.

c. When a patient is admitted for burn injuries and other related conditions such as smoke inhalation and/or respiratory failure, the circumstances of admission govern the selection of the principal or first-listed diagnosis.

2) Burns of the same local site

Classify burns of the same local site (three-character category level, T20-T28) but of different degrees to the subcategory identifying the highest degree recorded in the diagnosis.

3) Non-healing burns

Non-healing burns are coded as acute burns.

Necrosis of burned skin should be coded as a non-healed burn.

4) Infected Burn

For any documented infected burn site, use an additional code for the infection.

5) Assign separate codes for each burn site

When coding burns, assign separate codes for each burn site. Category T30, *Burn and corrosion, body region unspecified* is extremely vague and should rarely be used.

6) Burns and Corrosions Classified According to Extent of Body Surface Involved

Assign codes from category T31, *Burns classified according to extent of body surface involved*, or T32, *Corrosions classified according to extent of body surface involved*, when the site of the burn is not specified or when there is a need for additional data. It is advisable to use category T31 as additional coding when needed to provide data for evaluating burn mortality, such as that needed by burn units. It is also advisable to use category T31 as an additional code for reporting purposes when there is mention of a third-degree burn involving 20 percent or more of the body surface.

Categories T31 and T32 are based on the classic "rule of nines" in estimating body surface involved: head and neck are assigned nine percent, each arm nine percent, each leg 18 percent, the anterior trunk 18 percent, posterior trunk 18 percent, and genitalia one percent. Providers may change these percentage assignments where necessary to accommodate infants and children who have proportionately larger heads than adults, and patients who have large buttocks, thighs, or abdomen that involve burns.

7) Encounters for treatment of sequela of burns

Encounters for the treatment of the late effects of burns or corrosions (i.e., scars or joint contractures) should be coded with a burn or corrosion code with the 7th character "S" for sequela.

8) Sequelae with a late effect code and current burn

When appropriate, both a code for a current burn or corrosion with 7th character "A" or "D" and a burn or corrosion code with 7th character "S" may be assigned on the same record (when both a current burn and sequelae of an old burn exist). Burns and corrosions do not heal at the same rate and a current healing wound may still exist with sequela of a healed burn or corrosion.

9) Use of an external cause code with burns and corrosions

An external cause code should be used with burns and corrosions to identify the source and intent of the burn, as well as the place where it occurred.

e. Adverse Effects, Poisoning , Underdosing and Toxic Effects

Codes in categories T36-T65 are combination codes that include the substance that was taken as well as the intent. No additional external cause code is required for poisonings, toxic effects, adverse effects and underdosing codes.

1) Do not code directly from the Table of Drugs

Do not code directly from the Table of Drugs and Chemicals. Always refer back to the Tabular List.

2) Use as many codes as necessary to describe

Use as many codes as necessary to describe completely all drugs, medicinal or biological substances.

3) If the same code would describe the causative agent

If the same code would describe the causative agent for more than one adverse reaction, poisoning, toxic effect or underdosing, assign the code only once.

4) If two or more drugs, medicinal or biological substances

If two or more drugs, medicinal or biological substances are reported, code each individually unless a combination code is listed in the Table of Drugs and Chemicals.

5) The occurrence of drug toxicity is classified in ICD-10-CM as follows:

(a) Adverse Effect

When coding an adverse effect of a drug that has been correctly prescribed and properly administered, assign the appropriate code for the nature of the adverse effect followed by the appropriate code for the adverse effect of the drug (T36-T50). The code for the drug should have a 5th or 6th character "5" (for example T36.0X5-) Examples of the nature of an adverse effect are tachycardia, delirium, gastrointestinal hemorrhaging, vomiting, hypokalemia, hepatitis, renal failure, or respiratory failure.

(b) Poisoning

When coding a poisoning or reaction to the improper use of a medication (e.g., overdose, wrong substance given or taken in error, wrong route of administration), first assign the appropriate code from categories T36-T50. The poisoning codes have an associated intent as their 5th or 6th character (accidental, intentional self-harm, assault and undetermined). Use additional code(s) for all manifestations of poisonings.

If there is also a diagnosis of abuse or dependence of the substance, the abuse or dependence is assigned as an additional code.

Examples of poisoning include:

(i) Error was made in drug prescription

Errors made in drug prescription or in the administration of the drug by provider, nurse, patient, or other person.

(ii) Overdose of a drug intentionally taken

If an overdose of a drug was intentionally taken or administered and resulted in drug toxicity, it would be coded as a poisoning.

(iii) Nonprescribed drug taken with correctly prescribed and properly administered drug

If a nonprescribed drug or medicinal agent was taken in combination with a correctly prescribed and properly administered drug, any drug toxicity or other reaction resulting from the interaction of the two drugs would be classified as a poisoning.

(iv) Interaction of drug(s) and alcohol

When a reaction results from the interaction of a drug(s) and alcohol, this would be classified as poisoning.

See Section I.C.4. if poisoning is the result of insulin pump malfunctions.

(c) Underdosing

Underdosing refers to taking less of a medication than is prescribed by a provider or a manufacturer's instruction.

For underdosing, assign the code from categories T36-T50 (fifth or sixth character "6").

Codes for underdosing should never be assigned as principal or first-listed codes. If a patient has a relapse or exacerbation of the medical condition for which the drug is prescribed because of the reduction in dose, then the medical condition itself should be coded.

Noncompliance (Z91.12-, Z91.13-) or complication of care (Y63.61, Y63.8-Y63.9) codes are to be used with an underdosing code to indicate intent, if known.

(d) Toxic Effects

When a harmful substance is ingested or comes in contact with a person, this is classified as a toxic effect. The toxic effect codes are in categories T51-T65.

Toxic effect codes have an associated intent: accidental, intentional self-harm, assault and undetermined.

f. Adult and child abuse, neglect and other maltreatment

Sequence first the appropriate code from categories T74.- (Adult and child abuse, neglect and other maltreatment, confirmed) or T76.- (Adult and child abuse, neglect and other maltreatment, suspected) for abuse, neglect and other maltreatment, followed by any accompanying mental health or injury code(s).

If the documentation in the medical record states abuse or neglect it is coded as confirmed (T74.-).
It is coded as suspected if it is documented as suspected (T76.-).

For cases of confirmed abuse or neglect an external cause code from the assault section (X92-Y08) should be added to identify the cause of any physical injuries. A perpetrator code (Y07) should be added when the perpetrator of the abuse is known. For suspected cases of abuse or neglect, do not report external cause or perpetrator code.

If a suspected case of abuse, neglect or mistreatment is ruled out during an encounter code Z04.71, Encounter for examination and observation following alleged physical adult abuse, ruled out, or code Z04.72, Encounter for examination and observation following alleged child physical abuse, ruled out, should be used, not a code from T76.

If a suspected case of alleged rape or sexual abuse is ruled out during an encounter code Z04.41, Encounter for examination and observation following alleged physical adult abuse, ruled out, or code Z04.42, Encounter for examination and observation following alleged rape or sexual abuse, ruled out, should be used, not a code from T76.

See Section I.C.15.r Abuse in a pregnant patient.

g. Complications of care

1) General guidelines for complications of care

(a) Documentation of complications of care

See Section I.B.16. for information on documentation of complications of care.

2) Pain due to medical devices

Pain associated with devices, implants or grafts left in a surgical site (for example painful hip prosthesis) is assigned to the appropriate code(s) found in Chapter 19, Injury, poisoning, and certain other consequences of external causes. Specific codes for pain due to medical devices are found in the T code section of the ICD-10-CM. Use additional code(s) from category G89 to identify acute or chronic pain due to presence of the device, implant or graft (G89.18 or G89.28).

3) Transplant complications

(a) Transplant complications other than kidney

Codes under category T86, Complications of transplanted organs and tissues, are for use for both complications and rejection of transplanted organs. A transplant complication code is only assigned if the complication affects the function of the transplanted organ. Two codes are required to fully describe a transplant complication: the appropriate code from category T86 and a secondary code that identifies the complication.

Pre-existing conditions or conditions that develop after the transplant are not coded as complications unless they affect the function of the transplanted organs.

See I.C.21.c.3 for transplant organ removal status

See I.C.2.r for malignant neoplasm associated with transplanted organ.

(b) Kidney transplant complications

Patients who have undergone kidney transplant may still have some form of chronic kidney disease (CKD) because the kidney transplant may not fully restore kidney function. Code T86.1- should be assigned for documented complications of a kidney transplant, such as transplant failure or rejection or other transplant complication. Code T86.1- should not be assigned for post kidney transplant patients who have chronic kidney (CKD) unless a transplant complication such as transplant failure or rejection is documented. If the documentation is unclear as to whether the patient has a complication of the transplant, query the provider.

Conditions that affect the function of the transplanted kidney, other than CKD, should be assigned a code from subcategory T86.1, *Complications of transplanted organ, Kidney*, and a secondary code that identifies the complication.

For patients with CKD following a kidney transplant, but who do not have a complication such as failure or rejection, *see Section I.C.14. Chronic kidney disease and kidney transplant status.*

4) Complication codes that include the external cause

As with certain other T codes, some of the complications of care codes have the external cause included in the code. The code includes the nature of the complication as well as the type of procedure that caused the complication. No external cause code indicating the type of procedure is necessary for these codes.

5) Complications of care codes within the body system chapters

Intraoperative and postprocedural complication codes are found within the body system chapters with codes specific to the organs and structures of that body system. These codes should be sequenced first, followed by a code(s) for the specific complication, if applicable.

Chapter 20: External Causes of Morbidity (V01-Y99)

The external causes of morbidity codes should never be sequenced as the first-listed or principal diagnosis.

External cause codes are intended to provide data for injury research and evaluation of injury prevention strategies. These codes capture how the injury or health condition happened (cause), the intent (unintentional or accidental; or intentional, such as suicide or assault), the place where the event occurred the activity of the patient at the time of the event, and the person's status (e.g., civilian, military).

There is no national requirement for mandatory ICD-10-CM external cause code reporting. Unless a provider is subject to a state-based external cause code reporting mandate or these codes are required by a particular payer, reporting of ICD-10-CM codes in Chapter 20, External Causes of Morbidity, is not required. In the absence of a mandatory reporting requirement, providers are encouraged to voluntarily report external cause codes, as they provide valuable data for injury research and evaluation of injury prevention strategies.

a. General External Cause Coding Guidelines

1) Used with any code in the range of A00.0-T88.9, Z00-Z99

An external cause code may be used with any code in the range of A00.0-T88.9, Z00-Z99, classification that is a health condition due to an external cause. Though they are most applicable to injuries, they are also valid for use with such things as infections or diseases due to an external source, and other health conditions, such as a heart attack that occurs during strenuous physical activity.

2) External cause code used for length of treatment

Assign the external cause code, with the appropriate 7th character (initial encounter, subsequent encounter or sequela) for each encounter for which the injury or condition is being treated.

Most categories in this chapter have three 7th character values: A, initial encounter, D, subsequent encounter and S, sequela. While the patient may be seen by a new or different provider over the course of treatment for an injury or condition, assignment of the 7th character for external cause should match the 7th character of the code assigned for the associated injury or condition for the encounter.

3) Use the full range of external cause codes

Use the full range of external cause codes to completely describe the cause, the intent, the place of occurrence, and if applicable, the activity of the patient at the time of the event, and the patient's status, for all injuries, and other health conditions due to an external cause.

4) Assign as many external cause codes as necessary

Assign as many external cause codes as necessary to fully explain each cause. If only one external code can be recorded, assign the code most related to the principal diagnosis.

5) The selection of the appropriate external cause code

The selection of the appropriate external cause code is guided by the Alphabetic Index of External Causes and by Inclusion and Exclusion notes in the Tabular List.

6) External cause code can never be a principal diagnosis

An external cause code can never be a principal (first-listed) diagnosis.

7) Combination external cause codes

Certain of the external cause codes are combination codes that identify sequential events that result in an injury, such as a fall which results in striking against an object. The injury may be due to either event or both. The combination external cause code used should correspond to the sequence of events regardless of which caused the most serious injury.

8) No external cause code needed in certain circumstances

No external cause code from Chapter 20 is needed if the external cause and intent are included in a code from another chapter (e.g. T36.0x1- Poisoning by penicillins, accidental (unintentional)).

b. Place of Occurrence Guideline

Codes from category Y92, *Place of occurrence of the external cause*, are secondary codes for use after other external cause codes to identify the location of the patient at the time of injury or other condition.

Generally, a place of occurrence code is assigned only once, at the initial encounter for treatment. However, in the rare instance that a new injury occurs during hospitalization, an additional place of occurrence code may be assigned. No 7th characters are used for Y92.

Do not use place of occurrence code Y92.9 if the place is not stated or is not applicable.

c. Activity Code

Assign a code from category Y93, Activity code, to describe the activity of the patient at the time the injury or other health condition occurred.

An activity code is used only once, at the initial encounter for treatment. Only one code from Y93 should be recorded on a medical record. An activity code should be used in conjunction with a place of occurrence code, Y92.

The activity codes are not applicable to poisonings, adverse effects, misadventures or sequela.

Do not assign Y93.9, *Unspecified activity*, if the activity is not stated.

A code from category Y93 is appropriate for use with external cause and intent codes if identifying the activity provides additional information about the event.

d. Place of Occurrence, Activity, and Status Codes Used with other External Cause Code

When applicable, place of occurrence, activity, and external cause status codes are sequenced after the main external cause code(s). Regardless of the number of external cause codes assigned, there should be only one place of occurrence code, one activity code, and one external cause status code assigned to an encounter.

e. If the Reporting Format Limits the Number of External Cause Codes

If the reporting format limits the number of external cause codes that can be used in reporting clinical data, report the code for the cause/intent most related to the principal diagnosis. If the format permits capture of additional external cause codes, the cause/intent, including medical misadventures, of the additional events should be reported rather than the codes for place, activity, or external status.

f. Multiple External Cause Coding Guidelines

More than one external cause code is required to fully describe the external cause of an illness or injury. The assignment of external cause codes should be sequenced in the following priority:

If two or more events cause separate injuries, an external cause code should be assigned for each cause. The first-listed external cause code will be selected in the following order:

External codes for child and adult abuse take priority over all other external cause codes.

See Section I.C.19., Child and Adult abuse guidelines.

External cause codes for terrorism events take priority over all other external cause codes except child and adult abuse.

External cause codes for cataclysmic events take priority over all other external cause codes except child and adult abuse and terrorism.

External cause codes for transport accidents take priority over all other external cause codes except cataclysmic events, child and adult abuse and terrorism.

Activity and external cause status codes are assigned following all causal (intent) external cause codes.

The first-listed external cause code should correspond to the cause of the most serious diagnosis due to an assault, accident, or self-harm, following the order of hierarchy listed above.

g. Child and Adult Abuse Guideline

Adult and child abuse, neglect and maltreatment are classified as assault. Any of the assault codes may be used to indicate the external cause of any injury resulting from the confirmed abuse.

For confirmed cases of abuse, neglect and maltreatment, when the perpetrator is known, a code from Y07, Perpetrator of maltreatment and neglect, should accompany any other assault codes.

See Section I.C.19. Adult and child abuse, neglect and other maltreatment

h. Unknown or Undetermined Intent Guideline

If the intent (accident, self-harm, assault) of the cause of an injury or other condition is unknown or unspecified, code the intent as accidental intent. All transport accident categories assume accidental intent.

1) Use of undetermined intent

External cause codes for events of undetermined intent are only for use if the documentation in the record specifies that the intent cannot be determined.

i. Sequelae (Late Effects)of External Cause Guidelines

1) Sequelae external cause codes

Sequela are reported using the external cause code with the 7th character "S" for sequela. These codes should be used with any report of a late effect or sequela resulting from a previous injury.

2) Sequela external cause code with a related current injury

A sequela external cause code should never be used with a related current nature of injury code.

3) Use of sequela external cause codes for subsequent visits

Use a late effect external cause code for subsequent visits when a late effect of the initial injury is being treated. Do not use a late effect external cause code for subsequent visits for follow-up care (e.g., to assess healing, to receive rehabilitative therapy) of the injury when no late effect of the injury has been documented.

j. Terrorism Guidelines

1) Cause of injury identified by the Federal Government (FBI) as terrorism

When the cause of an injury is identified by the Federal Government (FBI) as terrorism, the first-listed external cause code should be a code from category Y38, *Terrorism*. The definition of terrorism employed by the FBI is found at the inclusion note at the beginning of category Y38. Use additional code for place of occurrence (Y92.-). More than one Y38 code may be assigned if the injury is the result of more than one mechanism of terrorism.

2) Cause of an injury is suspected to be the result of terrorism

When the cause of an injury is suspected to be the result of terrorism a code from category Y38 should not be assigned. Suspected cases should be classified as assault.

3) Code Y38.9, *Terrorism, secondary effects*

Assign code Y38.9, *Terrorism, secondary effects*, for conditions occurring subsequent to the terrorist event. This code should not be assigned for conditions that are due to the initial terrorist act.

It is acceptable to assign code Y38.9 with another code from Y38 if there is an injury due to the initial terrorist event and an injury that is a subsequent result of the terrorist event.

k. External cause status

A code from category Y99, *External cause status*, should be assigned whenever any other external cause code is assigned for an encounter, including an Activity code, except for the events noted below. Assign a code from category Y99, *External cause status*, to indicate the work status of the person at the time the event occurred. The status code indicates whether the event occurred during military activity, whether a non-military person was at work, whether an individual including a student or volunteer was involved in a non-work activity at the time of the causal event.

A code from Y99, *External cause status*, should be assigned, when applicable, with other external cause codes, such as transport accidents and falls. The external cause status codes are not applicable to poisonings, adverse effects, misadventures or late effects.

Do not assign a code from category Y99 if no other external cause codes (cause, activity) are applicable for the encounter.

An external cause status code is used only once, at the initial encounter for treatment. Only one code from Y99 should be recorded on a medical record.

Do not assign code Y99.9, *Unspecified external cause status*, if the status is not stated.

Chapter 21: Factors influencing health status and contact with health services (Z00-Z99)

Note: The chapter specific guidelines provide additional information about the use of Z codes for specified encounters.

a. Use of Z codes in any healthcare setting

Z codes are for use in any healthcare setting. Z codes may be used as either a first-listed (principal diagnosis code in the inpatient setting) or secondary code, depending on the circumstances of the encounter. Certain Z codes may only be used as first-listed or principal diagnosis.

b. Z Codes indicate a reason for an encounter

Z codes are not procedure codes. A corresponding procedure code must accompany a Z code to describe any procedure performed.

c. Categories of Z Codes

1) Contact/Exposure

Category Z20 indicates contact with, and suspected exposure to, communicable diseases. These codes are for patients who do not show any sign or symptom of a disease **but** are suspected to have been exposed to it by close personal contact with an infected individual or are in an area where a disease is epidemic.

Category Z77, Other contact with and (suspected) exposures hazardous to health, indicates contact with and suspected exposures hazardous to health.

Contact/exposure codes may be used as a first-listed code to explain an encounter for testing, or, more commonly, as a secondary code to identify a potential risk.

2) Inoculations and vaccinations

Code Z23 is for encounters for inoculations and vaccinations. It indicates that a patient is being seen to receive a prophylactic inoculation against a disease. Procedure codes are required to identify the actual administration of the injection and the type(s) of immunizations given. Code Z23 may be used as a secondary code if the inoculation is given as a routine part of preventive health care, such as a well-baby visit.

3) Status

Status codes indicate that a patient is either a carrier of a disease or has the sequelae or residual of a past disease or condition. This includes such things as the presence of prosthetic or mechanical devices resulting from past treatment. A status code is informative, because the status may affect the course of treatment and its outcome. A status code is distinct from a history code. The history code indicates that the patient no longer has the condition.

A status code should not be used with a diagnosis code from one of the body system chapters, if the diagnosis code includes the information provided by the status code. For example, code Z94.1, *Heart transplant status*, should not be used with a code from subcategory T86.2, *Complications of heart transplant*. The status code does not provide additional information. The complication code indicates that the patient is a heart transplant patient.

For encounters for weaning from a mechanical ventilator, assign a code from subcategory J96.1, *Chronic respiratory failure*, followed by code Z99.11, *Dependence on respirator [ventilator] status*.

The status Z codes/categories are:

Z14 *Genetic carrier*

Genetic carrier status indicates that a person carries a gene, associated with a particular disease, which may be passed to offspring who may develop that disease. The person does not have the disease and is not at risk of developing the disease.

Z15 *Genetic susceptibility to disease*

Genetic susceptibility indicates that a person has a gene that increases the risk of that person developing the disease.

Codes from category Z15 should not be used as principal or first-listed codes. If the patient has the condition to which he/she is susceptible, and that condition is the reason for the encounter, the code for the current condition should be sequenced first. If the patient is being seen for follow-up after completed treatment for this condition, and the condition no longer exists, a follow-up code should be sequenced first, followed by the appropriate personal history and genetic susceptibility codes. If the purpose of the encounter is genetic counseling associated with procreative management, code Z31.5, *Encounter for genetic counseling*, should be assigned as the first-listed code, followed by a code from category Z15. Additional codes should be assigned for any applicable family or personal history.

Z16   *Resistance to antimicrobial drugs*
This code indicates that a patient has a condition that is resistant to antimicrobial drug treatment. Sequence the infection code first.

Z17   *Estrogen receptor status*

Z18   *Retained foreign body fragments*

Z21   *Asymptomatic HIV infection status*
This code indicates that a patient has tested positive for HIV but has manifested no signs or symptoms of the disease.

Z22   *Carrier of infectious disease*
Carrier status indicates that a person harbors the specific organisms of a disease without manifest symptoms and is capable of transmitting the infection.

Z28.3   *Underimmunization status*

Z33.1   *Pregnant state, incidental*
This code is a secondary code only for use when the pregnancy is in no way complicating the reason for visit. Otherwise, a code from the obstetric chapter is required.

Z66   *Do not resuscitate*
This code may be used when it is documented by the provider that a patient is on do not resuscitate status at any time during the stay.

Z67   *Blood type*

Z68   *Body mass index (BMI)*

Z74.01   *Bed confinement status*

Z76.82   *Awaiting organ transplant status*

Z78   *Other specified health status*
Code Z78.1, Physical restraint status, may be used when it is documented by the provider that a patient has been put in restraints during the current encounter. Please note that this code should not be reported when it is documented by the provider that a patient is temporarily restrained during a procedure.

Z79   *Long-term (current) drug therapy*
Codes from this category indicate a patient's continuous use of a prescribed drug (including such things as aspirin therapy) for the long-term treatment of a condition or for prophylactic use. It is not for use for patients who have addictions to drugs. This subcategory is not for use of medications for detoxification or maintenance programs to prevent withdrawal symptoms in patients with drug dependence (e.g., methadone maintenance for opiate dependence). Assign the appropriate code for the drug dependence instead.

Assign a code from Z79 if the patient is receiving a medication for an extended period as a prophylactic measure (such as for the prevention of deep vein thrombosis) or as treatment of a chronic condition (such as arthritis) or a disease requiring a lengthy course of treatment (such as cancer). Do not assign a code from category Z79 for medication being administered for a brief period of time to treat an acute illness or injury (such as a course of antibiotics to treat acute bronchitis).

Z88   *Allergy status to drugs, medicaments and biological substances*
Except: Z88.9, Allergy status to unspecified drugs, medicaments and biological substances status

Z89   *Acquired absence of limb*

Z90   *Acquired absence of organs, not elsewhere classified*

Z91.0-   *Allergy status, other than to drugs and biological substances*

Z92.82   *Status post administration of tPA (rtPA) in a different facility within the last 24 hours prior to admission to a current facility*

Assign code Z92.82, *Status post administration of tPA (rtPA) in a different facility within the last 24 hours prior to admission to current facility*, as a secondary diagnosis when a patient is received by transfer into a facility and documentation indicates they were administered tissue plasminogen activator (tPA) within the last 24 hours prior to admission to the current facility.

This guideline applies even if the patient is still receiving the tPA at the time they are received into the current facility.

The appropriate code for the condition for which the tPA was administered (such as cerebrovascular disease or myocardial infarction) should be assigned first.

Code Z92.82 is only applicable to the receiving facility record and not to the transferring facility record.

Z93   *Artificial opening status*

Z94   *Transplanted organ and tissue status*

Z95   *Presence of cardiac and vascular implants and grafts*

Z96   *Presence of other functional implants*

Z97   *Presence of other devices*

Z98   *Other postprocedural states*
Assign code Z98.85, *Transplanted organ removal status*, to indicate that a transplanted organ has been previously removed. This code should not be assigned for the encounter in which the transplanted organ is removed. The complication necessitating removal of the transplant organ should be assigned for that encounter.

See Section I.C19. for information on the coding of organ transplant complications.

Z99   *Dependence on enabling machines and devices, not elsewhere classified*
Note: Categories Z89-Z90 and Z93-Z99 are for use only if there are no complications or malfunctions of the organ or tissue replaced, the amputation site or the equipment on which the patient is dependent.

4) History (of)

There are two types of history Z codes, personal and family. Personal history codes explain a patient's past medical condition that no longer exists and is not receiving any treatment, but that has the potential for recurrence, and therefore may require continued monitoring.

Family history codes are for use when a patient has a family member(s) who has had a particular disease that causes the patient to be at higher risk of also contracting the disease.

Personal history codes may be used in conjunction with follow-up codes and family history codes may be used in conjunction with screening codes to explain the need for a test or procedure. History codes are also acceptable on any medical record regardless of the reason for visit. A history of an illness, even if no longer present, is important information that may alter the type of treatment ordered.

The history Z code categories are:

Z80 Family history of primary malignant neoplasm

Z81 *Family history of mental and behavioral disorders*

Z82 *Family history of certain disabilities and chronic diseases (leading to disablement)*

Z83 *Family history of other specific disorders*

Z84 *Family history of other conditions*

Z85 *Personal history of malignant neoplasm*

Z86 *Personal history of certain other diseases*

Z87 *Personal history of other diseases and conditions*

Z91.4- *Personal history of psychological trauma, not elsewhere classified*

Z91.5 *Personal history of self-harm*

Z91.8- *Other specified personal risk factors, not elsewhere classified*

Exception: Z91.83, Wandering in diseases classified elsewhere

Z92 *Personal history of medical treatment*

Except: Z92.0, Personal history of contraception

Except: Z92.82, Status post administration of tPA (rtPA) in a different facility within the last 24 hours prior to admission to a current facility

5) Screening

Screening is the testing for disease or disease precursors in seemingly well individuals so that early detection and treatment can be provided for those who test positive for the disease (e.g., screening mammogram).

The testing of a person to rule out or confirm a suspected diagnosis because the patient has some sign or symptom is a diagnostic examination, not a screening. In these cases, the sign or symptom is used to explain the reason for the test.

A screening code may be a first-listed code if the reason for the visit is specifically the screening exam. It may also be used as an additional code if the screening is done during an office visit for other health problems. A screening code is not necessary if the screening is inherent to a routine examination, such as a pap smear done during a routine pelvic examination.

Should a condition be discovered during the screening then the code for the condition may be assigned as an additional diagnosis.

The Z code indicates that a screening exam is planned. A procedure code is required to confirm that the screening was performed.

The screening Z codes/categories:

Z11 *Encounter for screening for infectious and parasitic diseases*

Z12 *Encounter for screening for malignant neoplasms*

Z13 *Encounter for screening for other diseases and disorders*

Except: Z13.9, Encounter for screening, unspecified

Z36 *Encounter for antenatal screening for mother*

6) Observation

There are two observation Z code categories. They are for use in very limited circumstances when a person is being observed for a suspected condition that is ruled out. The observation codes are not for use if an injury or illness or any signs or symptoms related to the suspected condition are present. In such cases the diagnosis/symptom code is used with the corresponding external cause code.

The observation codes are to be used as principal diagnosis only. Additional codes may be used in addition to the observation code but only if they are unrelated to the suspected condition being observed.

Codes from subcategory Z03.7, **Encounter for suspected maternal and fetal conditions ruled out,** may either be used as a first-listed or as an additional code assignment depending on the case. They are for use in very limited circumstances on a maternal record when an encounter is for a suspected maternal or fetal condition that is ruled out during that encounter (for example, a maternal or fetal condition may be suspected due to an abnormal test result). These codes should not be used when the condition is confirmed. In those cases, the confirmed condition should be coded. In addition, these codes are not for use if an illness or any signs or symptoms related to the suspected condition or problem are present. In such cases the diagnosis/symptom code is used.

Additional codes may be used in addition to the code from subcategory Z03.7, but only if they are unrelated to the suspected condition being evaluated.

Codes from subcategory Z03.7 may not be used for encounters for antenatal screening of mother.

See Section I.C.21.c.5, Screening.

For encounters for suspected fetal condition that are inconclusive following testing and evaluation, assign the appropriate code from category O35, O36, O40 or O41.

The observation Z code categories:

Z03 *Encounter for medical observation for suspected diseases and conditions ruled out*

Z04 *Encounter for examination and observation for other reasons*
Except: Z04.9, Encounter for examination and observation for unspecified reason

7) Aftercare

Aftercare visit codes cover situations when the initial treatment of a disease has been performed and the patient requires continued care during the healing or recovery phase, or for the long-term consequences of the disease. The aftercare Z code should not be used if treatment is directed at a current, acute disease. The diagnosis code is to be used in these cases. Exceptions to this rule are codes Z51.0, *Encounter for antineoplastic radiation therapy*, and codes from subcategory Z51.1, *Encounter for antineoplastic chemotherapy and immunotherapy*. These codes are to be first-listed, followed by the diagnosis code when a patient's encounter is solely to receive radiation therapy, chemotherapy, or immunotherapy for the treatment of a neoplasm. If the reason for the encounter is more than one type of antineoplastic therapy, code Z51.0 and a code from subcategory Z51.1 may be assigned together, in which case one of these codes would be reported as a secondary diagnosis.

The aftercare Z codes should also not be used for aftercare for injuries. For aftercare of an injury, assign the acute injury code with the appropriate 7th character (for subsequent encounter).

The aftercare codes are generally first-listed to explain the specific reason for the encounter. An aftercare code may be used as an additional code when some type of aftercare is provided in addition to the reason for admission and no diagnosis code is applicable. An example of this would be the closure of a colostomy during an encounter for treatment of another condition.

Aftercare codes should be used in conjunction with other aftercare codes or diagnosis codes to provide better detail on the specifics of an aftercare encounter visit, unless otherwise directed by the classification. Should a patient receive multiple types of antineoplastic therapy during the same encounter, code Z51.0, *Encounter for antineoplastic radiation therapy*, and codes from subcategory Z51.1, *Encounter for antineoplastic chemotherapy and immunotherapy*, may be used together on a record. The sequencing of multiple aftercare codes depends on the circumstances of the encounter.

Certain aftercare Z code categories need a secondary diagnosis code to describe the resolving condition or sequelae. For others, the condition is included in the code title.

Additional Z code aftercare category terms include fitting and adjustment, and attention to artificial openings.

Status Z codes may be used with aftercare Z codes to indicate the nature of the aftercare. For example code Z95.1, *Presence of aortocoronary bypass graft*, may be used with code Z48.812, *Encounter for surgical aftercare following surgery on the circulatory system*, to indicate the surgery for which the aftercare is being performed. A status code should not be used when the aftercare code indicates the type of status, such as using Z43.0, *Encounter for attention to tracheostomy*, with Z93.0, *Tracheostomy status*.

The aftercare Z category/codes:

Z42   *Encounter for plastic and reconstructive surgery following medical procedure or healed injury*

Z43   *Encounter for attention to artificial openings*

Z44   *Encounter for fitting and adjustment of external prosthetic device*

Z45   *Encounter for adjustment and management of implanted device*

Z46   *Encounter for fitting and adjustment of other devices*

Z47   *Orthopedic aftercare*

Z48   *Encounter for other postprocedural aftercare*

Z49   *Encounter for care involving renal dialysis*

Z51   *Encounter for other aftercare*

8) Follow-up

The follow-up codes are used to explain continuing surveillance following completed treatment of a disease, condition, or injury. They imply that the condition has been fully treated and no longer exists. They should not be confused with aftercare codes, or injury codes with a 7th character for subsequent encounter, that explain ongoing care of a healing condition or its sequelae. Follow-up codes may be used in conjunction with history codes to provide the full picture of the healed condition and its treatment. The follow-up code is sequenced first, followed by the history code.

A follow-up code may be used to explain multiple visits. Should a condition be found to have recurred on the follow-up visit, then the diagnosis code for the condition should be assigned in place of the follow-up code.

The follow-up Z code categories:

Z08   *Encounter for follow-up examination after completed treatment for malignant neoplasm*

Z09   *Encounter for follow-up examination after completed treatment for conditions other than malignant neoplasm*

Z39   *Encounter for maternal postpartum care and examination*

9) Donor

Codes in category Z52, *Donors of organs and tissues*, are used for living individuals who are donating blood or other body tissue. These codes are only for individuals donating for others, not for self-donations. They are not used to identify cadaveric donations.

10) Counseling

Counseling Z codes are used when a patient or family member receives assistance in the aftermath of an illness or injury, or when support is required in coping with family or social problems. They are not used in conjunction with a diagnosis code when the counseling component of care is considered integral to standard treatment.

The counseling Z codes/categories:

Z30.0-   *Encounter for general counseling and advice on contraception*

Z31.5   *Encounter for genetic counseling*

Z31.6-   *Encounter for general counseling and advice on procreation*

Z32.2   *Encounter for childbirth instruction*

Z32.3   *Encounter for childcare instruction*

Z69   *Encounter for mental health services for victim and perpetrator of abuse*

Z70   *Counseling related to sexual attitude, behavior and orientation*

Z71   *Persons encountering health services for other counseling and medical advice, not elsewhere classified*

Z76.81   *Expectant mother prebirth pediatrician visit*

11) Encounters for Obstetrical and Reproductive Services

See Section I.C.15. Pregnancy, Childbirth, and the Puerperium, for further instruction on the use of these codes.

Z codes for pregnancy are for use in those circumstances when none of the problems or complications included in the codes from the Obstetrics chapter exist (a routine prenatal visit or postpartum care). Codes in category Z34, *Encounter for supervision of normal pregnancy*, are always first-listed and are not to be used with any other code from the OB chapter.

Codes in category Z3A, Weeks of gestation, may be assigned to provide additional information about the pregnancy. The date of the admission should be used to determine weeks of gestation for inpatient admissions that encompass more than one gestational week.

The outcome of delivery, category Z37, should be included on all maternal delivery records. It is always a secondary code. Codes in category Z37 should not be used on the newborn record.

Z codes for family planning (contraceptive) or procreative management and counseling should be included on an obstetric record either during the pregnancy or the postpartum stage, if applicable.

Z codes/categories for obstetrical and reproductive services:

Z30   *Encounter for contraceptive management*

Z31   *Encounter for procreative management*

Z32.2   *Encounter for childbirth instruction*

Z32.3   *Encounter for childcare instruction*

Z33   *Pregnant state*

Z34   *Encounter for supervision of normal pregnancy*

Z36   *Encounter for antenatal screening of mother*

Z3A   *Weeks of gestation*

Z37   *Outcome of delivery*

Z39   *Encounter for maternal postpartum care and examination*

Z76.81 *Expectant mother prebirth pediatrician visit*

12) Newborns and Infants

See Section I.C.16. Newborn (Perinatal) Guidelines, for further instruction on the use of these codes.

Newborn Z codes/categories:

Z76.1   *Encounter for health supervision and care of foundling*

Z00.1- *Encounter for routine child health examination*

Z38   *Liveborn infants according to place of birth and type of delivery*

13) Routine and administrative examinations

The Z codes allow for the description of encounters for routine examinations, such as, a general check-up, or, examinations for administrative purposes, such as, a pre-employment physical. The codes are not to be used if the examination is for diagnosis of a suspected condition or for treatment purposes. In such cases the diagnosis code is used. During a routine exam, should a diagnosis or condition be discovered, it should be coded as an additional code. Pre-existing and chronic conditions and history codes may also be included as additional codes as long as the examination is for administrative purposes and not focused on any particular condition.

Some of the codes for routine health examinations distinguish between "with" and "without" abnormal findings. Code assignment depends on the information that is known at the time the encounter is being coded. For example, if no abnormal findings were found during the examination, but the encounter is being coded before test results are back, it is acceptable to assign the code for "without abnormal findings." When assigning a code for "with abnormal findings," additional code(s) should be assigned to identify the specific abnormal finding(s).

Pre-operative examination and pre-procedural laboratory examination Z codes are for use only in those situations when a patient is being cleared for a procedure or surgery and no treatment is given.

The Z codes/categories for routine and administrative examinations:

Z00   *Encounter for general examination without complaint, suspected or reported diagnosis*

Z01   *Encounter for other special examination without complaint, suspected or reported diagnosis*

Z02   *Encounter for administrative examination* Except: Z02.9, Encounter for administrative examinations, unspecified

Z32.0- *Encounter for pregnancy test*

14) Miscellaneous Z codes

The miscellaneous Z codes capture a number of other health care encounters that do not fall into one of the other categories. Certain of these codes identify the reason for the encounter; others are for use as additional codes that provide useful information on circumstances that may affect a patient's care and treatment.

Prophylactic Organ Removal

For encounters specifically for prophylactic removal of an organ (such as prophylactic removal of breasts due to a genetic susceptibility to cancer or a family history of cancer), the principal or first-listed code should be a code from category Z40, *Encounter for prophylactic surgery*, followed by the appropriate codes to identify the associated risk factor (such as genetic susceptibility or family history).

If the patient has a malignancy of one site and is having prophylactic removal at another site to prevent either a new primary malignancy or metastatic disease, a code for the malignancy should also be assigned in addition to a code from subcategory Z40.0, Encounter for prophylactic surgery for risk factors related to malignant neoplasms. A Z40.0 code should not be assigned if the patient is having organ removal for treatment of a malignancy, such as the removal of the testes for the treatment of prostate cancer.

Miscellaneous Z codes/categories:

Z28   *Immunization not carried out* Except: Z28.3, Underimmunization status

Z40   *Encounter for prophylactic surgery*

Z41   *Encounter for procedures for purposes other than remedying health state* Except: Z41.9, Encounter for procedure for purposes other than remedying health state, unspecified

Z53   *Persons encountering health services for specific procedures and treatment, not carried out*

Z55	Problems related to education and literacy
Z56	Problems related to employment and unemployment
Z57	Occupational exposure to risk factors
Z58	Problems related to physical environment
Z59	Problems related to housing and economic circumstances
Z60	Problems related to social environment
Z62	Problems related to upbringing
Z63	Other problems related to primary support group, including family circumstances
Z64	Problems related to certain psychosocial circumstances
Z65	Problems related to other psychosocial circumstances
Z72	Problems related to lifestyle
Z73	Problems related to life management difficulty
Z74	Problems related to care provider dependency Except: Z74.01, Bed confinement status
Z75	Problems related to medical facilities and other health care
Z76.0	Encounter for issue of repeat prescription
Z76.3	Healthy person accompanying sick person
Z76.4	Other boarder to healthcare facility
Z76.5	Malingerer [conscious simulation]
Z91.1-	Patient's noncompliance with medical treatment and regimen
Z91.83	Wandering in diseases classified elsewhere
Z91.89	Other specified personal risk factors, not elsewhere classified

15) Nonspecific Z codes

Certain Z codes are so non-specific, or potentially redundant with other codes in the classification, that there can be little justification for their use in the inpatient setting. Their use in the outpatient setting should be limited to those instances when there is no further documentation to permit more precise coding. Otherwise, any sign or symptom or any other reason for visit that is captured in another code should be used.

Nonspecific Z codes/categories:

Z02.9	Encounter for administrative examinations, unspecified
Z04.9	Encounter for examination and observation for unspecified reason
Z13.9	Encounter for screening, unspecified
Z41.9	Encounter for procedure for purposes other than remedying health state, unspecified
Z52.9	Donor of unspecified organ or tissue
Z86.59	Personal history of other mental and behavioral disorders
Z88.9	Allergy status to unspecified drugs, medicaments and biological substances status
Z92.0	Personal history of contraception

16) Z Codes That May Only be Principal/First-Listed Diagnosis

The following Z codes/categories may only be reported as the principal/first-listed diagnosis, except when there are multiple encounters on the same day and the medical records for the encounters are combined:

Z00	Encounter for general examination without complaint, suspected or reported diagnosis
Z01	Encounter for other special examination without complaint, suspected or reported diagnosis
Z02	Encounter for administrative examination
Z03	Encounter for medical observation for suspected diseases and conditions ruled out
Z04	Encounter for examination and observation for other reasons
Z33.2	Encounter for elective termination of pregnancy
Z31.81	Encounter for male factor infertility in female patient
Z31.82	Encounter for Rh incompatibility status
Z31.83	Encounter for assisted reproductive fertility procedure cycle
Z31.84	Encounter for fertility preservation procedure
Z34	Encounter for supervision of normal pregnancy
Z39	Encounter for maternal postpartum care and examination
Z38	Liveborn infants according to place of birth and type of delivery
Z42	Encounter for plastic and reconstructive surgery following medical procedure or healed injury
Z51.0	Encounter for antineoplastic radiation therapy
Z51.1-	Encounter for antineoplastic chemotherapy and immunotherapy
Z52	Donors of organs and tissues Except: Z52.9, Donor of unspecified organ or tissue
Z76.1	Encounter for health supervision and care of foundling
Z76.2	Encounter for health supervision and care of other healthy infant and child
Z99.12	Encounter for respirator [ventilator] dependence during power failure

Section II. Selection of Principal Diagnosis

The circumstances of inpatient admission always govern the selection of principal diagnosis. The principal diagnosis is defined in the Uniform Hospital Discharge Data Set (UHDDS) as "that condition established after study to be chiefly responsible for occasioning the admission of the patient to the hospital for care."

The UHDDS definitions are used by hospitals to report inpatient data elements in a standardized manner. These data elements and their definitions can be found in the July 31, 1985, *Federal Register* (Vol. 50, No, 147), pp. 31038-40.

Since that time the application of the UHDDS definitions has been expanded to include all non-outpatient settings (acute care, short term, long term care and psychiatric hospitals; home health agencies; rehab facilities; nursing homes, etc).

In determining principal diagnosis the coding conventions in the ICD-10-CM, the Tabular List and Alphabetic Index take precedence over these official coding guidelines. (*See Section I.A., Conventions for the ICD-10-CM*)

The importance of consistent, complete documentation in the medical record cannot be overemphasized. Without such documentation the application of all coding guidelines is a difficult, if not impossible, task.

A. Codes for symptoms, signs, and ill-defined conditions

Codes for symptoms, signs, and ill-defined conditions from Chapter 18 are not to be used as principal diagnosis when a related definitive diagnosis has been established.

B. Two or more interrelated conditions, each potentially meeting the definition for principal diagnosis.

When there are two or more interrelated conditions (such as diseases in the same ICD-10-CM chapter or manifestations characteristically associated with a certain disease) potentially meeting the definition of principal diagnosis, either condition may be sequenced first, unless the circumstances of the admission, the therapy provided, the Tabular List, or the Alphabetic Index indicate otherwise.

C. Two or more diagnoses that equally meet the definition for principal diagnosis

In the unusual instance when two or more diagnoses equally meet the criteria for principal diagnosis as determined by the circumstances of admission, diagnostic workup and/or therapy provided, and the Alphabetic Index, Tabular List, or another coding guidelines does not provide sequencing direction, any one of the diagnoses may be sequenced first.

D. Two or more comparative or contrasting conditions.

In those rare instances when two or more contrasting or comparative diagnoses are documented as "either/or" (or similar terminology), they are coded as if the diagnoses were confirmed and the diagnoses are sequenced according to the circumstances of the admission. If no further determination can be made as to which diagnosis should be principal, either diagnosis may be sequenced first.

E. A symptom(s) followed by contrasting/comparative diagnoses

GUIDELINE HAS BEEN DELETED EFFECTIVE OCTOBER 1, 2014

F. Original treatment plan not carried out

Sequence as the principal diagnosis the condition, which after study occasioned the admission to the hospital, even though treatment may not have been carried out due to unforeseen circumstances.

G. Complications of surgery and other medical care

When the admission is for treatment of a complication resulting from surgery or other medical care, the complication code is sequenced as the principal diagnosis. If the complication is classified to the T80-T88 series and the code lacks the necessary specificity in describing the complication, an additional code for the specific complication should be assigned.

H. Uncertain Diagnosis

If the diagnosis documented at the time of discharge is qualified as "probable", "suspected", "likely", "questionable", "possible", or "still to be ruled out", or other similar terms indicating uncertainty, code the condition as if it existed or was established. The bases for these guidelines are the diagnostic workup, arrangements for further workup or observation, and initial therapeutic approach that correspond most closely with the established diagnosis.

Note: This guideline is applicable only to inpatient admissions to short-term, acute, long-term care and psychiatric hospitals.

I. Admission from Observation Unit

1. Admission Following Medical Observation

   When a patient is admitted to an observation unit for a medical condition, which either worsens or does not improve, and is subsequently admitted as an inpatient of the same hospital for this same medical condition, the principal diagnosis would be the medical condition which led to the hospital admission.

2. Admission Following Post-Operative Observation

   When a patient is admitted to an observation unit to monitor a condition (or complication) that develops following outpatient surgery, and then is subsequently admitted as an inpatient of the same hospital, hospitals should apply the Uniform Hospital Discharge Data Set (UHDDS) definition of principal diagnosis as "that condition established after study to be chiefly responsible for occasioning the admission of the patient to the hospital for care."

J. Admission from Outpatient Surgery

When a patient receives surgery in the hospital's outpatient surgery department and is subsequently admitted for continuing inpatient care at the same hospital, the following guidelines should be followed in selecting the principal diagnosis for the inpatient admission:

If the reason for the inpatient admission is a complication, assign the complication as the principal diagnosis.

If no complication, or other condition, is documented as the reason for the inpatient admission, assign the reason for the outpatient surgery as the principal diagnosis.

If the reason for the inpatient admission is another condition unrelated to the surgery, assign the unrelated condition as the principal diagnosis.

K. Admissions/Encounters for Rehabilitation

When the purpose for the admission/encounter is rehabilitation, sequence first the code for the condition for which the service is being performed. For example, for an admission/encounter for rehabilitation for right-sided dominant hemiplegia following a cerebrovascular infarction, report code I69.351, *Hemiplegia and hemiparesis following cerebral infarction affecting right dominant side*, as the first-listed or principal diagnosis.

If the condition for which the rehabilitation service is no longer present, report the appropriate aftercare code as the first-listed or principal diagnosis. For example, if a patient with severe degenerative osteoarthritis of the hip, underwent hip replacement and the current encounter/admission is for rehabilitation, report code Z47.1, *Aftercare following joint replacement surgery*, as the first-listed or principal diagnosis.

See Section I.C.21.c.7, Factors influencing health states and contact with health services, Aftercare.

Section III. Reporting Additional Diagnoses

GENERAL RULES FOR OTHER (ADDITIONAL) DIAGNOSES

For reporting purposes the definition for "other diagnoses" is interpreted as additional conditions that affect patient care in terms of requiring:

- clinical evaluation; or
- therapeutic treatment; or
- diagnostic procedures; or
- extended length of hospital stay; or
- increased nursing care and/or monitoring.

The UHDDS item #11-b defines Other Diagnoses as "all conditions that coexist at the time of admission, that develop subsequently, or that affect the treatment received and/or the length of stay. Diagnoses that relate to an earlier episode which have no bearing on the current hospital stay are to be excluded." UHDDS definitions apply to inpatients in acute care, short-term, long term care and psychiatric hospital setting. The UHDDS definitions are used by acute care short-term hospitals to report inpatient data elements in a standardized manner. These data elements and their definitions can be found in the July 31, 1985, *Federal Register* (Vol. 50, No, 147), pp. 31038-40.

Since that time the application of the UHDDS definitions has been expanded to include all non-outpatient settings (acute care, short term, long term care and psychiatric hospitals; home health agencies; rehab facilities; nursing homes, etc).

The following guidelines are to be applied in designating "other diagnoses" when neither the Alphabetic Index nor the Tabular List in ICD-10-CM provide direction. The listing of the diagnoses in the patient record is the responsibility of the attending provider.

A. Previous conditions

If the provider has included a diagnosis in the final diagnostic statement, such as the discharge summary or the face sheet, it should ordinarily be coded. Some providers include in the diagnostic statement resolved conditions or diagnoses and status-post procedures from previous admission that have no bearing on the current stay. Such conditions are not to be reported and are coded only if required by hospital policy.

However, history codes (categories Z80-Z87) may be used as secondary codes if the historical condition or family history has an impact on current care or influences treatment.

B. Abnormal findings

Abnormal findings (laboratory, x-ray, pathologic, and other diagnostic results) are not coded and reported unless the provider indicates their clinical significance. If the findings are outside the normal range and the attending provider has ordered other tests to evaluate the condition or prescribed treatment, it is appropriate to ask the provider whether the abnormal finding should be added.

Please note: This differs from the coding practices in the outpatient setting for coding encounters for diagnostic tests that have been interpreted by a provider.

C. Uncertain Diagnosis

If the diagnosis documented at the time of discharge is qualified as "probable", "suspected", "likely", "questionable", "possible", or "still to be ruled out" or other similar terms indicating uncertainty, code the condition as if it existed or was established. The bases for these guidelines are the diagnostic workup, arrangements for further workup or observation, and initial therapeutic approach that correspond most closely with the established diagnosis.

Note: This guideline is applicable only to inpatient admissions to short-term, acute, long-term care and psychiatric hospitals.

Section IV. Diagnostic Coding and Reporting Guidelines for Outpatient Services

These coding guidelines for outpatient diagnoses have been approved for use by hospitals/ providers in coding and reporting hospital-based outpatient services and provider-based office visits.

Information about the use of certain abbreviations, punctuation, symbols, and other conventions used in the ICD-10-CM Tabular List (code numbers and titles), can be found in Section IA of these guidelines, under "Conventions Used in the Tabular List." Section I.B. contains general guidelines that apply to the entire classification. Section I.C. contains chapter-specific guidelines that correspond to the chapters as they are arranged in the classification. Information about the correct sequence to use in finding a code is also described in Section I.

The terms encounter and visit are often used interchangeably in describing outpatient service contacts and, therefore, appear together in these guidelines without distinguishing one from the other.

Though the conventions and general guidelines apply to all settings, coding guidelines for outpatient and provider reporting of diagnoses will vary in a number of instances from those for inpatient diagnoses, recognizing that:

The Uniform Hospital Discharge Data Set (UHDDS) definition of principal diagnosis applies only to inpatients in acute, short-term, long-term care and psychiatric hospitals.

Coding guidelines for inconclusive diagnoses (probable, suspected, rule out, etc.) were developed for inpatient reporting and do not apply to outpatients.

A. Selection of first-listed condition

In the outpatient setting, the term first-listed diagnosis is used in lieu of principal diagnosis.

In determining the first-listed diagnosis the coding conventions of ICD-10-CM, as well as the general and disease specific guidelines take precedence over the outpatient guidelines.

Diagnoses often are not established at the time of the initial encounter/ visit. It may take two or more visits before the diagnosis is confirmed.

The most critical rule involves beginning the search for the correct code assignment through the Alphabetic Index. Never begin searching initially in the Tabular List as this will lead to coding errors.

1. Outpatient Surgery

When a patient presents for outpatient surgery (same day surgery), code the reason for the surgery as the first-listed diagnosis (reason for the encounter), even if the surgery is not performed due to a contraindication.

2. Observation Stay

When a patient is admitted for observation for a medical condition, assign a code for the medical condition as the first-listed diagnosis.

When a patient presents for outpatient surgery and develops complications requiring admission to observation, code the reason for the surgery as the first reported diagnosis (reason for the encounter), followed by codes for the complications as secondary diagnoses.

B. Codes from A00.0 through T88.9, Z00-Z99

The appropriate code(s) from A00.0 through T88.9, Z00-Z99 must be used to identify diagnoses, symptoms, conditions, problems, complaints, or other reason(s) for the encounter/visit.

C. Accurate reporting of ICD-10-CM diagnosis codes

For accurate reporting of ICD-10-CM diagnosis codes, the documentation should describe the patient's condition, using terminology which includes specific diagnoses as well as symptoms, problems, or reasons for the encounter. There are ICD-10-CM codes to describe all of these.

D. Codes that describe symptoms and signs

Codes that describe symptoms and signs, as opposed to diagnoses, are acceptable for reporting purposes when a diagnosis has not been established (confirmed) by the provider. Chapter 18 of ICD-10-CM, Symptoms, Signs, and Abnormal Clinical and Laboratory Findings Not Elsewhere Classified (codes R00-R99) contain many, but not all codes for symptoms.

E. Encounters for circumstances other than a disease or injury

ICD-10-CM provides codes to deal with encounters for circumstances other than a disease or injury. The Factors Influencing Health Status and Contact with Health Services codes (Z00-Z99) are provided to deal with occasions when circumstances other than a disease or injury are recorded as diagnosis or problems.

See Section I.C.21. Factors influencing health status and contact with health services.

F. Level of Detail in Coding

1. ICD-10-CM codes with 3, 4, 5, 6 or 7 characters

ICD-10-CM is composed of codes with 3, 4, 5, 6 or 7 characters. Codes with three characters are included in ICD-10-CM as the heading of a category of codes that may be further subdivided by the use of fourth, fifth, sixth or seventh characters to provide greater specificity.

2. Use of full number of characters required for a code

A three-character code is to be used only if it is not further subdivided. A code is invalid if it has not been coded to the full number of characters required for that code, including the 7th character, if applicable.

G. ICD-10-CM code for the diagnosis, condition, problem, or other reason for encounter/visit

List first the ICD-10-CM code for the diagnosis, condition, problem, or other reason for encounter/visit shown in the medical record to be chiefly responsible for the services provided. List additional codes that describe any coexisting conditions. In some cases the first-listed diagnosis may be a symptom when a diagnosis has not been established (confirmed) by the physician.

H. Uncertain diagnosis

Do not code diagnoses documented as "probable", "suspected," "questionable," "rule out," or "working diagnosis" or other similar terms indicating uncertainty. Rather, code the condition(s) to the highest degree of certainty for that encounter/visit, such as symptoms, signs, abnormal test results, or other reason for the visit.

Please note: This differs from the coding practices used by short-term, acute care, long-term care and psychiatric hospitals. ICD-10-CM Official

I. Chronic diseases

Chronic diseases treated on an ongoing basis may be coded and reported as many times as the patient receives treatment and care for the condition(s)

J. Code all documented conditions that coexist

Code all documented conditions that coexist at the time of the encounter/visit, and require or affect patient care treatment or management. Do not code conditions that were previously treated and no longer exist. However, history codes (categories Z80-Z87) may be used as secondary codes if the historical condition or family history has an impact on current care or influences treatment.

K. Patients receiving diagnostic services only

For patients receiving diagnostic services only during an encounter/visit, sequence first the diagnosis, condition, problem, or other reason for encounter/visit shown in the medical record to be chiefly responsible for the outpatient services provided during the encounter/visit. Codes for other diagnoses (e.g., chronic conditions) may be sequenced as additional diagnoses.

For encounters for routine laboratory/radiology testing in the absence of any signs, symptoms, or associated diagnosis, assign Z01.89, Encounter for other specified special examinations. If routine testing is performed during the same encounter as a test to evaluate a sign, symptom, or diagnosis, it is appropriate to assign both the Z code and the code describing the reason for the non-routine test.

For outpatient encounters for diagnostic tests that have been interpreted by a physician, and the final report is available at the time of coding, code any confirmed or definitive diagnosis(es) documented in the interpretation. Do not code related signs and symptoms as additional diagnoses.

Please note: This differs from the coding practice in the hospital inpatient setting regarding abnormal findings on test results.

L. Patients receiving therapeutic services only

For patients receiving therapeutic services only during an encounter/visit, sequence first the diagnosis, condition, problem, or other reason for encounter/visit shown in the medical record to be chiefly responsible for the outpatient services provided during the encounter/visit. Codes for other diagnoses (e.g., chronic conditions) may be sequenced as additional diagnoses.

The only exception to this rule is that when the primary reason for the admission/encounter is chemotherapy or radiation therapy, the appropriate Z code for the service is listed first, and the diagnosis or problem for which the service is being performed listed second.

M. Patients receiving preoperative evaluations only

For patients receiving preoperative evaluations only, sequence first a code from subcategory Z01.81, *Encounter for pre-procedural examinations*, to describe the pre-op consultations. Assign a code for the condition to describe the reason for the surgery as an additional diagnosis. Code also any findings related to the pre-op evaluation.

N. Ambulatory surgery

For ambulatory surgery, code the diagnosis for which the surgery was performed. If the postoperative diagnosis is known to be different from the preoperative diagnosis at the time the diagnosis is confirmed, select the postoperative diagnosis for coding, since it is the most definitive.

O. Routine outpatient prenatal visits

See Section I.C.15. Routine outpatient prenatal visits.

P. Encounters for general medical examinations with abnormal findings

The subcategories for encounters for general medical examinations, Z00.0-, provide codes for with and without abnormal findings. Should a general medical examination result in an abnormal finding, the code for general medical examination with abnormal finding should be assigned as the first-listed diagnosis. A secondary code for the abnormal finding should also be coded.

Q. Encounters for routine health screenings

See Section I.C.21. Factors influencing health status and contact with health services, Screening

A

Aarskog's syndrome Q87.1
Abandonment — *see* Maltreatment
Abasia (-astasia) (hysterical) F44.4
Abderhalden-Kaufmann-Lignac syndrome
(cystinosis) E72.04
Abdomen, abdominal — *see also* condition
acute R10.0
angina K55.1
muscle deficiency syndrome Q79.4
Abdominalgia — *see* Pain, abdominal
Abduction contracture, hip or other joint — *see*
Contraction, joint
Aberrant (congenital) — *see also* Malposition,
congenital
adrenal gland Q89.1
artery (peripheral) Q27.8
basilar NEC Q28.1
cerebral Q28.3
coronary Q24.5
digestive system Q27.8
eye Q15.8
lower limb Q27.8
precerebral Q28.1
pulmonary Q25.79
renal Q27.2
retina Q14.1
specified site NEC Q27.8
subclavian Q27.8
upper limb Q27.8
vertebral Q28.1
breast Q83.8
endocrine gland NEC Q89.2
hepatic duct Q44.5
pancreas Q45.3
parathyroid gland Q89.2
pituitary gland Q89.2
sebaceous glands, mucous membrane, mouth,
congenital Q38.6
spleen Q89.09
subclavian artery Q27.8
thymus (gland) Q89.2
thyroid gland Q89.2
vein (peripheral) NEC Q27.8
cerebral Q28.3
digestive system Q27.8
lower limb Q27.8
precerebral Q28.1
specified site NEC Q27.8
upper limb Q27.8
Aberration
distantial — *see* Disturbance, visual
mental F99
Abetalipoproteinemia E78.6
Abiotrophy R68.89
Ablatio, ablation
retinae — *see* Detachment, retina
Ablepharia, ablepharon Q10.3
Abnormal, abnormality, abnormalities — *see
also* Anomaly
acid-base balance (mixed) E87.4
albumin R77.0
alphafetoprotein R77.2
alveolar ridge K08.9
anatomical relationship Q89.9
apertures, congenital, diaphragm Q79.1
auditory perception H93.29-
diplacusis — *see* Diplacusis
hyperacusis — *see* Hyperacusis
recruitment — *see* Recruitment, auditory
threshold shift — *see* Shift, auditory threshold
autosomes Q99.9
fragile site Q95.5
basal metabolic rate R94.8
biosynthesis, testicular androgen E29.1
bleeding time R79.1
blood-gas level R79.81
blood level (of)
cobalt R79.0
copper R79.0
iron R79.0
lithium R78.89
magnesium R79.0
mineral NEC R79.0
zinc R79.0
blood pressure
elevated R03.0
low reading (nonspecific) R03.1
blood sugar R73.09
bowel sounds R19.15
absent R19.11
hyperactive R19.12

Abnormal, abnormality, abnormalities - *continued*
brain scan R94.02
breathing R06.9
caloric test R94.138
cerebrospinal fluid R83.9
cytology R83.6
drug level R83.2
enzyme level R83.0
hormones R83.1
immunology R83.4
microbiology R83.5
nonmedicinal level R83.3
specified type NEC R83.8
chemistry, blood R79.9
C-reactive protein R79.82
drugs — *see* Findings, abnormal, in blood
gas level R79.81
minerals R79.0
pancytopenia D61.818
PTT R79.1
specified NEC R79.89
toxins — *see* Findings, abnormal, in blood
chest sounds (friction) (rales) R09.89
chromosome, chromosomal Q99.9
with more than three X chromosomes,
female Q97.1
analysis result R89.8
bronchial washings R84.8
cerebrospinal fluid R83.8
cervix uteri NEC R87.89
nasal secretions R84.8
nipple discharge R89.8
peritoneal fluid R85.89
pleural fluid R84.8
prostatic secretions R86.8
saliva R85.89
seminal fluid R86.8
sputum R84.8
synovial fluid R89.8
throat scrapings R84.8
vagina R87.89
vulva R87.89
wound secretions R89.8
dicentric replacement Q93.2
ring replacement Q93.2
sex Q99.8
female phenotype Q97.9
specified NEC Q97.8
male phenotype Q98.9
specified NEC Q98.8
structural male Q98.6
specified NEC Q99.8
clinical findings NEC R68.89
coagulation D68.9
newborn, transient P61.6
profile R79.1
time R79.1
communication — *see* Fistula
conjunctiva, vascular H11.41-
coronary artery Q24.5
cortisol-binding globulin E27.8
course, eustachian tube Q17.8
creatinine clearance R94.4
cytology
anus R85.619
atypical squamous cells cannot exclude high
grade squamous intraepithelial lesion (ASC-
H) R85.611
atypical squamous cells of undetermined
significance (ASC-US) R85.610
cytologic evidence of malignancy R85.614
high grade squamous intraepithelial lesion
(HGSIL) R85.613
human papillomavirus (HPV) DNA test
high risk positive R85.81
low risk postive R85.82
inadequate smear R85.615
low grade squamous intraepithelial lesion
(LGSIL) R85.612
satisfactory anal smear but lacking transformation
zone R85.616
specified NEC R85.618
unsatisfactory smear R85.615
female genital organs — *see* Abnormal,
Papanicolaou (smear)
dark adaptation curve H53.61
dentofacial NEC — *see* Anomaly, dentofacial
development, developmental Q89.9
central nervous system Q07.9
diagnostic imaging
abdomen, abdominal region NEC R93.5
biliary tract R93.2
bladder R93.41

Abnormal, abnormality, abnormalities - *continued*
diagnostic imaging - *continued*
breast R92.8
central nervous system NEC R90.89
cerebrovascular NEC R90.89
coronary circulation R93.1
digestive tract NEC R93.3
gastrointestinal (tract) R93.3
genitourinary organs R93.8
head R93.0
heart R93.1
intrathoracic organ NEC R93.8
kidney R93.42-
limbs R93.6
liver R93.2
lung (field) R91.8
musculoskeletal system NEC R93.7
renal pelvis R93.41
retroperitoneum R93.5
site specified NEC R93.8
skin and subcutaneous tissue R93.8
skull R93.0
urinary organs specified NEC R93.49
ureter R93.41
direction, teeth, fully erupted M26.30
ear ossicles, acquired NEC H74.39-
ankylosis — *see* Ankylosis, ear ossicles
discontinuity — *see* Discontinuity, ossicles, ear
partial loss — *see* Loss, ossicles, ear (partial)
Ebstein Q22.5
echocardiogram R93.1
echoencephalogram R90.81
echogram — *see* Abnormal, diagnostic imaging
electrocardiogram [ECG] [EKG] R94.31
electroencephalogram [EEG] R94.01
electrolyte — *see* Imbalance, electrolyte
electromyogram [EMG] R94.131
electro-oculogram [EOG] R94.110
electrophysiological intracardiac studies R94.39
electroretinogram [ERG] R94.111
erythrocytes
congenital, with perinatal jaundice D58.9
feces (color) (contents) (mucus) R19.5
finding — *see* Findings, abnormal, without
diagnosis
fluid
amniotic — *see* Abnormal, specimen, specified
cerebrospinal — *see* Abnormal, cerebrospinal fluid
peritoneal — *see* Abnormal, specimen, digestive
organs
pleural — *see* Abnormal, specimen, respiratory
organs
synovial — *see* Abnormal, specimen, specified
thorax (bronchial washings) (pleural fluid) — *see*
Abnormal, specimen, respiratory organs
vaginal — *see* Abnormal, specimen, female genital
organs
form
teeth K00.2
uterus — *see* Anomaly, uterus
function studies
auditory R94.120
bladder R94.8
brain R94.09
cardiovascular R94.30
ear R94.128
endocrine NEC R94.7
eye NEC R94.118
kidney R94.4
liver R94.5
nervous system
central NEC R94.09
peripheral NEC R94.138
pancreas R94.8
placenta R94.8
pulmonary R94.2
special senses NEC R94.128
spleen R94.8
thyroid R94.6
vestibular R94.121
gait — *see* Gait
hysterical F44.4
gastrin secretion E16.4
globulin R77.1
cortisol-binding E27.8
thyroid-binding E07.89
glomerular, minor — *see also* N00-N07 with fourth
character .0 N05.0
glucagon secretion E16.3
glucose tolerance (test) (non-fasting) R73.09
gravitational (G) forces or states (effect of) T75.81
hair (color) (shaft) L67.9
specified NEC L67.8

Abnormal, abnormality, abnormalities - *continued*
  hard tissue formation in pulp (dental) K04.3
  head movement R25.0
  heart
    rate R00.9
      specified NEC R00.8
    shadow R93.1
    sounds NEC R01.2
  hemoglobin (disease) — *see also* Disease,
    hemoglobin D58.2
    trait — *see* Trait, hemoglobin, abnormal
  histology NEC R89.7
  immunological findings R89.4
    in serum R76.9
      specified NEC R76.8
  increase in appetite R63.2
  involuntary movement — *see* Abnormal, movement,
    involuntary
  jaw closure M26.51
  karyotype R89.8
  kidney function test R94.4
  knee jerk R29.2
  leukocyte (cell) (differential) NEC D72.9
  liver
  loss of
    height R29.890
    weight R63.4
  mammogram NEC R92.8
    calcification (calculus) R92.1
    microcalcification R92.0
  Mantoux test R76.11
  movement (disorder) — *see also* Disorder,
    movement
    head R25.0
    involuntary R25.9
      fasciculation R25.3
      of head R25.0
      spasm R25.2
      specified type NEC R25.8
      tremor R25.1
  myoglobin (Aberdeen) (Annapolis) R89.7
  neonatal screening P09
  oculomotor study R94.113
  palmar creases Q82.8
  Papanicolaou (smear)
    anus R85.619
      atypical squamous cells cannot exclude high
        grade squamous intraepithelial lesion (ASC-
        H) R85.611
      atypical squamous cells of undetermined
        significance (ASC-US) R85.610
      cytologic evidence of malignancy R85.614
      high grade squamous intraepithelial lesion
        (HGSIL) R85.613
      human papillomavirus (HPV) DNA test
        high risk positive R85.81
        low risk postive R85.82
      inadequate smear R85.615
      low grade squamous intraepithelial lesion
        (LGSIL) R85.612
      satisfactory anal smear but lacking transformation
        zone R85.616
      specified NEC R85.618
      unsatisfactory smear R85.615
    bronchial washings R84.6
    cerebrospinal fluid R83.6
    cervix R87.619
      atypical squamous cells cannot exclude high
        grade squamous intraepithelial lesion (ASC-
        H) R87.611
      atypical squamous cells of undetermined
        significance (ASC-US) R87.610
      cytologic evidence of malignancy R87.614
      high grade squamous intraepithelial lesion
        (HGSIL) R87.613
      inadequate smear R87.615
      low grade squamous intraepithelial lesion
        (LGSIL) R87.612
      non-atypical endometrial cells R87.618
      satisfactory cervical smear but lacking
        transformation zone R87.616
      specified NEC R87.618
      thin preparaton R87.619
      unsatisfactory smear R87.615
    nasal secretions R84.6
    nipple discharge R89.6
    peritoneal fluid R85.69
    pleural fluid R84.6
    prostatic secretions R86.6
    saliva R85.69
    seminal fluid R86.6
    sites NEC R89.6
    sputum R84.6

Abnormal, abnormality, abnormalities - *continued*
  Papanicolaou (smear) - *continued*
    synovial fluid R89.6
    throat scrapings R84.6
    vagina R87.629
      atypical squamous cells cannot exclude high
        grade squamous intraepithelial lesion (ASC-
        H) R87.621
      atypical squamous cells of undetermined
        significance (ASC-US) R87.620
      cytologic evidence of malignancy R87.624
      high grade squamous intraepithelial lesion
        (HGSIL) R87.623
      inadequate smear R87.625
      low grade squamous intraepithelial lesion
        (LGSIL) R87.622
      specified NEC R87.628
      thin preparation R87.629
      unsatisfactory smear R87.625
    vulva R87.69
    wound secretions R89.6
  partial thromboplastin time (PTT) R79.1
  pelvis (bony) — *see* Deformity, pelvis
  percussion, chest (tympany) R09.89
  periods (grossly) — *see* Menstruation
  phonocardiogram R94.39
  plantar reflex R29.2
  plasma
    protein R77.9
      specified NEC R77.8
    viscosity R70.1
  pleural (folds) Q34.0
  posture R29.3
  product of conception O02.9
    specified type NEC O02.89
  prothrombin time (PT) R79.1
  pulmonary
    artery, congenital Q25.79
    function, newborn P28.89
    test results R94.2
  pulsations in neck R00.2
  pupillary H21.56-
    function (reaction) (reflex) — *see* Anomaly, pupil,
      function
  radiological examination — *see* Abnormal,
    diagnostic imaging
  red blood cell (s) (morphology) (volume) R71.8
  reflex — *see* Reflex
  renal function test R94.4
  response to nerve stimulation R94.130
  retinal correspondence H53.31
  retinal function study R94.111
  rhythm, heart — *see also* Arrhythmia
  saliva — *see* Abnormal, specimen, digestive organs
  scan
    kidney R94.4
    liver R93.2
    thyroid R94.6
  secretion
    gastrin E16.4
    glucagon E16.3
  semen, seminal fluid — *see* Abnormal, specimen,
    male genital organs
  serum level (of)
    acid phosphatase R74.8
    alkaline phosphatase R74.8
    amylase R74.8
    enzymes R74.9
      specified NEC R74.8
    lipase R74.8
    triacylglycerol lipase R74.8
  shape
    gravid uterus — *see* Anomaly, uterus
  sinus venosus Q21.1
  size, tooth, teeth K00.2
  spacing, tooth, teeth, fully erupted M26.30
  specimen
    digestive organs (peritoneal fluid) (saliva) R85.9
      cytology R85.69
      drug level R85.2
      enzyme level R85.0
      histology R85.7
      hormones R85.1
      immunology R85.4
      microbiology R85.5
      nonmedicinal level R85.3
      specified type NEC R85.89
    female genital organs (secretions) (smears) R87.9
      cytology R87.69
        cervix R87.619
          human papillomavirus (HPV) DNA test
            high risk positive R87.810
            low risk positive R87.820

Abnormal, abnormality, abnormalities - *continued*
  specimen - *continued*
    female genital organs (secretions) (smears) -
      continued
      cytology - *continued*
        cervix - *continued*
          inadequate (unsatisfactory) smear R87.615
          non-atypical endometrial cells R87.618
          specified NEC R87.618
        vagina R87.629
          human papillomavirus (HPV) DNA test
            high risk positive R87.811
            low risk positive R87.821
          inadequate (unsatisfactory) smear R87.625
        vulva R87.69
      drug level R87.2
      enzyme level R87.0
      histological R87.7
      hormones R87.1
      immunology R87.4
      microbiology R87.5
      nonmedicinal level R87.3
      specified type NEC R87.89
    male genital organs (prostatic secretions)
      (semen) R86.9
      cytology R86.6
      drug level R86.2
      enzyme level R86.0
      histological R86.7
      hormones R86.1
      immunology R86.4
      microbiology R86.5
      nonmedicinal level R86.3
      specified type NEC R86.8
    nipple discharge — *see* Abnormal, specimen,
      specified
    respiratory organs (bronchial washings) (nasal
      secretions) (pleural fluid) (sputum) R84.9
      cytology R84.6
      drug level R84.2
      enzyme level R84.0
      histology R84.7
      hormones R84.1
      immunology R84.4
      microbiology R84.5
      nonmedicinal level R84.3
      specified type NEC R84.8
    specified organ, system and tissue NOS R89.9
      cytology R89.6
      drug level R89.2
      enzyme level R89.0
      histology R89.7
      hormones R89.1
      immunology R89.4
      microbiology R89.5
      nonmedicinal level R89.3
      specified type NEC R89.8
    synovial fluid — *see* Abnormal, specimen,
      specified
    thorax (bronchial washings) (pleural fluids) — *see*
      Abnormal, specimen, respiratory organs
    vagina (secretion) (smear) R87.629
    vulva (secretion) (smear) R87.69
    wound secretion — *see* Abnormal, specimen,
      specified
  spermatozoa — *see* Abnormal, specimen, male
    genital organs
  sputum (amount) (color) (odor) R09.3
  stool (color) (contents) (mucus) R19.5
    bloody K92.1
    guaiac positive R19.5
  synchondrosis Q78.8
  thermography — *see also* Abnormal, diagnostic
    imaging R93.8
  thyroid-binding globulin E07.89
  tooth, teeth (form) (size) K00.2
  toxicology (findings) R78.9
  transport protein E88.09
  tumor marker NEC R97.8
  ultrasound results — *see* Abnormal, diagnostic
    imaging
  umbilical cord complicating delivery O69.9
  urination NEC R39.198
  urine (constituents) R82.90
    bile R82.2
    cytological examination R82.8
    drugs R82.5
    fat R82.0
    glucose R81
    heavy metals R82.6
    hemoglobin R82.3
    histological examination R82.8
    ketones R82.4

Abnormal, abnormality, abnormalities - *continued*
  urine (constituents) - *continued*
    microbiological examination (culture) R82.79
    myoglobin R82.1
    positive culture R82.79
    protein — *see* Proteinuria
    specified substance NEC R82.99
      chromoabnormality NEC R82.91
    substances nonmedical R82.6
  uterine hemorrhage — *see* Hemorrhage, uterus
  vectorcardiogram R94.39
  visually evoked potential (VEP) R94.112
  white blood cells D72.9
    specified NEC D72.89
  X-ray examination — *see* Abnormal, diagnostic imaging
Abnormity (any organ or part) — *see* Anomaly
Abocclusion M26.29
  hemolytic disease (newborn) P55.1
  incompatibility reaction ABO — *see* Complication(s), transfusion, incompatibility reaction, ABO
Abolition, language R48.8
Aborter, habitual or recurrent — *see* Loss (of), pregnancy, recurrent
Abortion (complete) (spontaneous) O03.9
  with
    retained products of conception — *see* Abortion, incomplete
  attempted (elective) (failed) O07.4
    complicated by O07.30
      afibrinogenemia O07.1
      cardiac arrest O07.36
      chemical damage of pelvic organ (s) O07.34
      circulatory collapse O07.31
      cystitis O07.38
      defibrination syndrome O07.1
      electrolyte imbalance O07.33
      embolism (air) (amniotic fluid) (blood clot) (fat) (pulmonary) (septic) (soap) O07.2
      endometritis O07.0
      genital tract and pelvic infection O07.0
      hemolysis O07.1
      hemorrhage (delayed) (excessive) O07.1
      infection
        genital tract or pelvic O07.0
        urinary tract tract O07.38
      intravascular coagulation O07.1
      laceration of pelvic organ (s) O07.34
      metabolic disorder O07.33
      oliguria O07.32
      oophoritis O07.0
      parametritis O07.0
      pelvic peritonitis O07.0
      perforation of pelvic organ (s) O07.34
      renal failure or shutdown O07.32
      salpingitis or salpingo-oophoritis O07.0
      sepsis O07.37
      shock O07.31
      specified condition NEC O07.39
      tubular necrosis (renal) O07.32
      uremia O07.32
      urinary tract infection O07.38
      venous complication NEC O07.35
        embolism (air) (amniotic fluid) (blood clot) (fat) (pulmonary) (septic) (soap) O07.2
  complicated (by) (following) O03.80
    afibrinogenemia O03.6
    cardiac arrest O03.86
    chemical damage of pelvic organ (s) O03.84
    circulatory collapse O03.81
    cystitis O03.88
    defibrination syndrome O03.6
    electrolyte imbalance O03.83
    embolism (air) (amniotic fluid) (blood clot) (fat) (pulmonary) (septic) (soap) O03.7
    endometritis O03.5
    genital tract and pelvic infection O03.5
    hemolysis O03.6
    hemorrhage (delayed) (excessive) O03.6
    infection
      genital tract or pelvic O03.5
      urinary tract O03.88
    intravascular coagulation O03.6
    laceration of pelvic organ (s) O03.84
    metabolic disorder O03.83
    oliguria O03.82
    oophoritis O03.5
    parametritis O03.5
    pelvic peritonitis O03.5
    perforation of pelvic organ (s) O03.84
    renal failure or shutdown O03.82
    salpingitis or salpingo-oophoritis O03.5

Abortion (complete) (spontaneous) - *continued*
  complicated (by) (following) - *continued*
    sepsis O03.87
    shock O03.81
    specified condition NEC O03.89
    tubular necrosis (renal) O03.82
    uremia O03.82
    urinary tract infection O03.88
    venous complication NEC O03.85
      embolism (air) (amniotic fluid) (blood clot) (fat) (pulmonary) (septic) (soap) O03.7
  failed — *see* Abortion, attempted
  habitual or recurrent N96
    with current abortion — *see* categories O03-O06
    without current pregnancy N96
    care in current pregnancy O26.2-
  incomplete (spontaneous) O03.4
    complicated (by) (following) O03.30
      afibrinogenemia O03.1
      cardiac arrest O03.36
      chemical damage of pelvic organ (s) O03.34
      circulatory collapse O03.31
      cystitis O03.38
      defibrination syndrome O03.1
      electrolyte imbalance O03.33
      embolism (air) (amniotic fluid) (blood clot) (fat) (pulmonary) (septic) (soap) O03.2
      endometritis O03.0
      genital tract and pelvic infection O03.0
      hemolysis O03.1
      hemorrhage (delayed) (excessive) O03.1
      infection
        genital tract or pelvic O03.0
        urinary tract O03.38
      intravascular coagulation O03.1
      laceration of pelvic organ (s) O03.34
      metabolic disorder O03.33
      oliguria O03.32
      oophoritis O03.0
      parametritis O03.0
      pelvic peritonitis O03.0
      perforation of pelvic organ (s) O03.34
      renal failure or shutdown O03.32
      salpingitis or salpingo-oophoritis O03.0
      sepsis O03.37
      shock O03.31
      specified condition NEC O03.39
      tubular necrosis (renal) O03.32
      uremia O03.32
      urinary infection O03.38
      venous complication NEC O03.35
        embolism (air) (amniotic fluid) (blood clot) (fat) (pulmonary) (septic) (soap) O03.2
  induced (encounter for) Z33.2
    complicated by O04.80
      afibrinogenemia O04.6
      cardiac arrest O04.86
      chemical damage of pelvic organ (s) O04.84
      circulatory collapse O04.81
      cystitis O04.88
      defibrination syndrome O04.6
      electrolyte imbalance O04.83
      embolism (air) (amniotic fluid) (blood clot) (fat) (pulmonary) (septic) (soap) O04.7
      endometritis O04.5
      genital tract and pelvic infection O04.5
      hemolysis O04.6
      hemorrhage (delayed) (excessive) O04.6
      infection
        genital tract or pelvic O04.5
        urinary tract O04.88
      intravascular coagulation O04.6
      laceration of pelvic organ (s) O04.84
      metabolic disorder O04.83
      oliguria O04.82
      oophoritis O04.5
      parametritis O04.5
      pelvic peritonitis O04.5
      perforation of pelvic organ (s) O04.84
      renal failure or shutdown O04.82
      salpingitis or salpingo-oophoritis O04.5
      sepsis O04.87
      shock O04.81
      specified condition NEC O04.89
      tubular necrosis (renal) O04.82
      uremia O04.82
      urinary tract infection O04.88
      venous complication NEC O04.85
        embolism (air) (amniotic fluid) (blood clot) (fat) (pulmonary) (septic) (soap) O04.7
  missed O02.1
  spontaneous — *see* Abortion (complete) (spontaneous)

Abortion (complete) (spontaneous) - *continued*
  spontaneous - *continued*
    threatened O20.0
  threatened (spontaneous) O20.0
  tubal O00.10
    with intrauterine pregnancy O00.11
Abortus fever A23.1
Aboulomania F60.7
Abrami's disease D59.8
Abramov-Fiedler myocarditis (acute isolated myocarditis) I40.1
Abrasion T14.8
  abdomen, abdominal (wall) S30.811
  alveolar process S00.512
  ankle S90.51-
  antecubital space — *see* Abrasion, elbow
  anus S30.817
  arm (upper) S40.81-
    auditory canal — *see* Abrasion, ear
  auricle — *see* Abrasion, ear
  axilla — *see* Abrasion, arm
  back, lower S30.810
  breast S20.11-
  brow S00.81
  buttock S30.810
  calf — *see* Abrasion, leg
  canthus — *see* Abrasion, eyelid
  cheek S00.81
    internal S00.512
  chest wall — *see* Abrasion, thorax
  chin S00.81
  clitoris S30.814
  cornea S05.0-
  costal region — *see* Abrasion, thorax
  dental K03.1
  digit (s)
    foot — *see* Abrasion, toe
    hand — *see* Abrasion, finger
  ear S00.41-
  elbow S50.31-
  epididymis S30.813
  epigastric region S30.811
  epiglottis S10.11
  esophagus (thoracic) S27.818
    cervical S10.11
  eyebrow — *see* Abrasion, eyelid
  eyelid S00.21-
  face S00.81
  finger (s) S60.41-
    index S60.41-
    little S60.41-
    middle S60.41-
    ring S60.41-
  flank S30.811
  foot (except toe (s) alone) S90.81-
    toe — *see* Abrasion, toe
  forearm S50.81-
    elbow only — *see* Abrasion, elbow
  forehead S00.81
  genital organs, external
    female S30.816
    male S30.815
  groin S30.811
  gum S00.512
  hand S60.51-
  head S00.91
    ear — *see* Abrasion, ear
    eyelid — *see* Abrasion, eyelid
    lip S00.511
    nose S00.31
    oral cavity S00.512
    scalp S00.01
    specified site NEC S00.81
  heel — *see* Abrasion, foot
  hip S70.21-
  inguinal region S30.811
  interscapular region S20.419
  jaw S00.81
  knee S80.21-
  labium (majus) (minus) S30.814
  larynx S10.11
  leg (lower) S80.81-
    knee — *see* Abrasion, knee
    upper — *see* Abrasion, thigh
  lip S00.511
  lower back S30.810
  lumbar region S30.810
  malar region S00.81
  mammary — *see* Abrasion, breast
  mastoid region S00.81
  mouth S00.512
  nail
    finger — *see* Abrasion, finger

Abrasion - *continued*
nail - *continued*
  toe — *see* Abrasion, toe
nape S10.81
nasal S00.31
neck S10.91
  specified site NEC S10.81
  throat S10.11
nose S00.31
occipital region S00.01
oral cavity S00.512
orbital region — *see* Abrasion, eyelid
palate S00.512
palm — *see* Abrasion, hand
parietal region S00.01
pelvis S30.810
penis S30.812
perineum
  female S30.814
  male S30.810
periocular area — *see* Abrasion, eyelid
phalanges
  finger — *see* Abrasion, finger
  toe — *see* Abrasion, toe
pharynx S10.11
pinna — *see* Abrasion, ear
popliteal space — *see* Abrasion, knee
prepuce S30.812
pubic region S30.810
pudendum
  female S30.816
  male S30.815
sacral region S30.810
scalp S00.01
scapular region — *see* Abrasion, shoulder
scrotum S30.813
shin — *see* Abrasion, leg
shoulder S40.21-
skin NEC T14.8
sternal region S20.319
submaxillary region S00.81
submental region S00.81
subungual
  finger (s) — *see* Abrasion, finger
  toe (s) — *see* Abrasion, toe
supraclavicular fossa S10.81
supraorbital S00.81
temple S00.81
temporal region S00.81
testis S30.813
thigh S70.31-
thorax, thoracic (wall) S20.91
  back S20.41-
  front S20.31-
throat S10.11
thumb S60.31-
toe (s) (lesser) S90.416
  great S90.41-
tongue S00.512
tooth, teeth (dentifrice) (habitual) (hard tissues) (occupational) (ritual) (traditional) K03.1
trachea S10.11
tunica vaginalis S30.813
tympanum, tympanic membrane — *see* Abrasion, ear
uvula S00.512
vagina S30.814
vocal cords S10.11
vulva S30.814
wrist S60.81-
Abrism — *see* Poisoning, food, noxious, plant
Abruptio placentae O45.9-
with
  afibrinogenemia O45.01-
  coagulation defect O45.00-
    specified NEC O45.09-
  disseminated intravascular coagulation O45.02-
  hypofibrinogenemia O45.01-
  specified NEC O45.8-
Abruption, placenta — *see* Abruptio placentae
Abscess (connective tissue) (embolic) (fistulous) (infective) (metastatic) (multiple) (pernicious) (pyogenic) (septic) L02.91
with
  diverticular disease (intestine) K57.80
    with bleeding K57.81
    large intestine K57.20
      with
        bleeding K57.21
        small intestine K57.40
          with bleeding K57.41
    small intestine K57.00
      with

Abscess (connective tissue) (embolic) (fistulous) (infective) (metastatic) (multiple) (pernicious) (pyogenic) (septic) - *continued*
with - *continued*
  diverticular disease (intestine) - *continued*
    small intestine - *continued*
      with - *continued*
        bleeding K57.01
        large intestine K57.40
          with bleeding K57.41
  lymphangitis - code by site under Abscess
abdomen, abdominal
  cavity K65.1
  wall L02.211
abdominopelvic K65.1
accessory sinus — *see* Sinusitis
adrenal (capsule) (gland) E27.8
alveolar K04.7
  with sinus K04.6
ambic A06.4
  brain (and liver or lung abscess) A06.6
  genitourinary tract A06.82
  liver (without mention of brain or lung abscess) A06.4
  lung (and liver) (without mention of brain abscess) A06.5
  specified site NEC A06.89
  spleen A06.89
anerobic A48.0
ankle — *see* Abscess, lower limb
anorectal K61.2
antecubital space — *see* Abscess, upper limb
antrum (chronic) (Highmore) — *see* Sinusitis, maxillary
anus K61.0
apical (tooth) K04.7
  with sinus (alveolar) K04.6
appendix K35.3
areola (acute) (chronic) (nonpuerperal) N61.1
  puerperal, postpartum or gestational — *see* Infection, nipple
arm (any part) — *see* Abscess, upper limb
artery (wall) I77.89
atheromatous I77.2
auricle, ear — *see* Abscess, ear, external
axilla (region) L02.41-
  lymph gland or node L04.2
back (any part, except buttock) L02.212
Bartholin's gland N75.1
  with
    abortion — *see* Abortion, by type complicated by, sepsis
    ectopic or molar pregnancy O08.0
  following ectopic or molar pregnancy O08.0
Bezold's — *see* Mastoiditis, acute
bilharziasis B65.1
bladder (wall) — *see* Cystitis, specified type NEC
bone (subperiosteal) — *see also* Osteomyelitis, specified type NEC
  accessory sinus (chronic) — *see* Sinusitis
  chronic or old — *see* Osteomyelitis, chronic
  jaw (lower) (upper) M27.2
  mastoid — *see* Mastoiditis, acute, subperiosteal
  petrous — *see* Petrositis
  spinal (tuberculous) A18.01
    nontuberculous — *see* Osteomyelitis, vertebra
bowel K63.0
brain (any part) (cystic) (otogenic) G06.0
  ambic (with abscess of any other site) A06.6
  gonococcal A54.82
  pheomycotic (chromomycotic) B43.1
  tuberculous A17.81
breast (acute) (chronic) (nonpuerperal) N61.1
  newborn P39.0
  puerperal, postpartum, gestational — *see* Mastitis, obstetric, purulent
broad ligament N73.2
  acute N73.0
  chronic N73.1
Brodie's (localized) (chronic) M86.8X-
bronchi J98.09
buccal cavity K12.2
bulbourethral gland N34.0
bursa M71.00
  ankle M71.07-
  elbow M71.02-
  foot M71.07-
  hand M71.04-
  hip M71.05-
  knee M71.06-
  multiple sites M71.09
  pharyngeal J39.1
  shoulder M71.01-

Abscess (connective tissue) (embolic) (fistulous) (infective) (metastatic) (multiple) (pernicious) (pyogenic) (septic) - *continued*
bursa - *continued*
  specified site NEC M71.08
  wrist M71.03-
buttock L02.31
canthus — *see* Blepharoconjunctivitis
cartilage — *see* Disorder, cartilage, specified type NEC
cecum K35.3
cerebellum, cerebellar G06.0
  sequelae G09
cerebral (embolic) G06.0
  sequelae G09
cervical (meaning neck) L02.11
  lymph gland or node L04.0
cervix (stump) (uteri) — *see* Cervicitis
cheek (external) L02.01
  inner K12.2
chest J86.9
  with fistula J86.0
  wall L02.213
chin L02.01
choroid — *see* Inflammation, chorioretinal
circumtonsillar J36
cold (lung) (tuberculous) — *see also* Tuberculosis, abscess, lung
  articular — *see* Tuberculosis, joint
colon (wall) K63.0
colostomy K94.02
conjunctiva — *see* Conjunctivitis, acute
cornea H16.31-
corpus
  cavernosum N48.21
  luteum — *see* Oophoritis
Cowper's gland N34.0
cranium G06.0
cul-de-sac (Douglas') (posterior) — *see* Peritonitis, pelvic, female
cutaneous — *see* Abscess, by site
dental K04.7
  with sinus (alveolar) K04.6
dentoalveolar K04.7
  with sinus K04.6
diaphragm, diaphragmatic K65.1
Douglas' cul-de-sac or pouch — *see* Peritonitis, pelvic, female
Dubois A50.59
ear (middle) — *see also* Otitis, media, suppurative
  acute — *see* Otitis, media, suppurative, acute
  external H60.0-
entamebic — *see* Abscess, amebic
enterostomy K94.12
epidural G06.2
  brain G06.0
  spinal cord G06.1
epiglottis J38.7
epiploon, epiploic K65.1
erysipelatous — *see* Erysipelas
esophagus K20.8
ethmoid (bone) (chronic) (sinus) J32.2
external auditory canal — *see* Abscess, ear, external
extradural G06.2
  brain G06.0
    sequelae G09
  spinal cord G06.1
extraperitoneal K68.19
eye — *see* Endophthalmitis, purulent
eyelid H00.03-
face (any part, except ear, eye and nose) L02.01
fallopian tube — *see* Salpingitis
fascia M72.8
fauces J39.1
fecal K63.0
femoral (region) — *see* Abscess, lower limb
filaria, filarial — *see* Infestation, filarial
finger (any) — *see also* Abscess, hand
  nail — *see* Cellulitis, finger
foot L02.61-
forehead L02.01
frontal sinus (chronic) J32.1
gallbladder K81.0
genital organ or tract
  female (external) N76.4
  male N49.9
    multiple sites N49.8
    specified NEC N49.8
gestational mammary O91.11-
gestational subareolar O91.11-
gingival — *see* Peridontitis, aggressive, localized

Abscess (connective tissue) (embolic) (fistulous) (infective) (metastatic) (multiple) (pernicious) (pyogenic) (septic) - *continued*
 gland, glandular (lymph) (acute) — *see* Lymphadenitis, acute
 gluteal (region) L02.31
 gonorrheal — *see* Gonococcus
 groin L02.214
 gum — *see* Peridontitis, aggressive, localized
 hand L02.51-
 head NEC L02.811
  face (any part, except ear, eye and nose) L02.01
 heart — *see* Carditis
 heel — *see* Abscess, foot
 helminthic — *see* Infestation, helminth
 hepatic (cholangitic) (hematogenic) (lymphogenic) (pylephlebitic) K75.0
  amebic A06.4
 hip (region) — *see* Abscess, lower limb
 ileocecal K35.3
 ileostomy (bud) K94.12
 iliac (region) L02.214
  fossa K35.3
 infraclavicular (fossa) — *see* Abscess, upper limb
 inguinal (region) L02.214
  lymph gland or node L04.1
 intestine, intestinal NEC K63.0
  rectal K61.1
 intra-abdominal — *see also* Abscess, peritoneum K65.1
  postprocedural T81.43
  retroperitoneal K68.11
 intracranial G06.0
 intramammary — *see* Abscess, breast
 intra-muscular, postprocedural T81.42
 intraorbital — *see* Abscess, orbit
 intraperitoneal K65.1
 intrasphincteric (anus) K61.4
 intraspinal G06.1
 intratonsillar J36
 ischiorectal (fossa) K61.3
 jaw (bone) (lower) (upper) M27.2
 joint — *see* Arthritis, pyogenic or pyemic
  spine (tuberculous) A18.01
   nontuberculous — *see* Spondylopathy, infective
 kidney N15.1
  with calculus N20.0
   with hydronephrosis N13.6
  puerperal (postpartum) O86.21
 knee — *see also* Abscess, lower limb
  joint M00.9
 labium (majus) (minus) N76.4
 lacrimal
  caruncle — *see* Inflammation, lacrimal, passages, acute
  gland — *see* Dacryoadenitis
  passages (duct) (sac) — *see* Inflammation, lacrimal, passages, acute
 lacunar N34.0
 larynx J38.7
 lateral (alveolar) K04.7
  with sinus K04.6
 leg (any part) — *see* Abscess, lower limb
 lens H27.8
 lingual K14.0
  tonsil J36
 lip K13.0
 Littre's gland N34.0
 liver (cholangitic) (hematogenic) (lymphogenic) (pylephlebitic) (pyogenic) K75.0
  amebic (due to Entamoeba histolytica) (dysenteric) (tropical) A06.4
   with
    brain abscess (and liver or lung abscess) A06.6
    lung abscess A06.5
 loin (region) L02.211
 lower limb L02.41-
 lumbar (tuberculous) A18.01
  nontuberculous L02.212
 lung (miliary) (putrid) J85.2
  with pneumonia J85.1
   due to specified organism (see Pneumonia, in (due to))
  amebic (with liver abscess) A06.5
   with
    brain abscess A06.6
    pneumonia A06.5
 lymph, lymphatic, gland or node (acute) — *see also* Lymphadenitis, acute
  mesentery I88.0
 malar M27.2
 mammary gland — *see* Abscess, breast
 marginal, anus K61.0

Abscess (connective tissue) (embolic) (fistulous) (infective) (metastatic) (multiple) (pernicious) (pyogenic) (septic) - *continued*
 mastoid — *see* Mastoiditis, acute
 maxilla, maxillary M27.2
  molar (tooth) K04.7
   with sinus K04.6
  premolar K04.7
  sinus (chronic) J32.0
 mediastinum J85.3
 meibomian gland — *see* Hordeolum
 meninges G06.2
 mesentery, mesenteric K65.1
 mesosalpinx — *see* Salpingitis
 mons pubis L02.215
 mouth (floor) K12.2
 muscle — *see* Myositis, infective
 myocardium I40.0
 nabothian (follicle) — *see* Cervicitis
 nasal J32.9
 nasopharyngeal J39.1
 navel L02.216
  newborn P38.9
   with mild hemorrhage P38.1
   without hemorrhage P38.9
 neck (region) L02.11
  lymph gland or node L04.0
 nephritic — *see* Abscess, kidney
 nipple N61.1
  associated with
   lactation — *see* Pregnancy, complicated by
   pregnancy — *see* Pregnancy, complicated by
 nose (external) (fossa) (septum) J34.0
  sinus (chronic) — *see* Sinusitis
 omentum K65.1
 operative wound T81.40
 orbit, orbital — *see* Cellulitis, orbit
 otogenic G06.0
 ovary, ovarian (corpus luteum) — *see* Oophoritis
 oviduct — *see* Oophoritis
 palate (soft) K12.2
  hard M27.2
 palmar (space) — *see* Abscess, hand
 pancreas (duct) — *see* Pancreatitis, acute
 parafrenal N48.21
 parametric, parametrium N73.2
  acute N73.0
  chronic N73.1
 paranephric N15.1
 parapancreatic — *see* Pancreatitis, acute
 parapharyngeal J39.0
 pararectal K61.1
 parasinus — *see* Sinusitis
 parauterine — *see also* Disease, pelvis, inflammatory N73.2
 paravaginal — *see* Vaginitis
 parietal region (scalp) L02.811
 parodontal — *see* Peridontitis, aggressive, localized
 parotid (duct) (gland) K11.3
  region K12.2
 pectoral (region) L02.213
 pelvis, pelvic
  female — *see* Disease, pelvis, inflammatory
  male, peritoneal K65.1
 penis N48.21
  gonococcal (accessory gland) (periurethral) A54.1
 perianal K61.0
 periapical K04.7
  with sinus (alveolar) K04.6
 periappendicular K35.3
 pericardial I30.1
 pericecal K35.3
 pericemental — *see* Peridontitis, aggressive, localized
 pericholecystic — *see* Cholecystitis, acute
 pericoronal — *see* Peridontitis, aggressive, localized
 peridental — *see* Peridontitis, aggressive, localized
 perimetric — *see also* Disease, pelvis, inflammatory N73.2
 perinephric, perinephritic — *see* Abscess, kidney
 perineum, perineal (superficial) L02.215
  urethra N34.0
 periodontal (parietal) — *see* Peridontitis, aggressive, localized
  apical K04.7
 periosteum, periosteal — *see also* Osteomyelitis, specified type NEC
  with osteomyelitis — *see also* Osteomyelitis, specified type NEC
   acute — *see* Osteomyelitis, acute
   chronic — *see* Osteomyelitis, chronic
 peripharyngeal J39.0
 peripleuritic J86.9

Abscess (connective tissue) (embolic) (fistulous) (infective) (metastatic) (multiple) (pernicious) (pyogenic) (septic) - *continued*
 peripleuritic - *continued*
  with fistula J86.0
 periprostatic N41.2
 perirectal K61.1
 perirenal (tissue) — *see* Abscess, kidney
 perisinuous (nose) — *see* Sinusitis
 peritoneum, peritoneal (perforated) (ruptured) K65.1
  with appendicitis K35.3
  pelvic
   female — *see* Peritonitis, pelvic, female
   male K65.1
  postoperative T81.43
  puerperal, postpartum, childbirth O85
  tuberculous A18.31
 peritonsillar J36
 perityphlic K35.3
 periureteral N28.89
 periurethral N34.0
  gonococcal (accessory gland) (periurethral) A54.1
 periuterine — *see also* Disease, pelvis, inflammatory N73.2
 perivesical — *see* Cystitis, specified type NEC
 petrous bone — *see* Petrositis
 phagedenic NOS L02.91
  chancroid A57
 pharynx, pharyngeal (lateral) J39.1
 pilonidal L05.01
 pituitary (gland) E23.6
 pleura J86.9
  with fistula J86.0
 popliteal — *see* Abscess, lower limb
 postcecal K35.3
 postlaryngeal J38.7
 postnasal J34.0
 postoperative (any site) T81.40
  retroperitoneal K68.11
 postpharyngeal J39.0
 posttonsillar J36
 post-typhoid A01.09
 pouch of Douglas — *see* Peritonitis, pelvic, female
 premammary — *see* Abscess, breast
 prepatellar — *see* Abscess, lower limb
 prostate N41.2
  gonococcal (acute) (chronic) A54.22
 psoas muscle K68.12
 puerperal - code by site under Puerperal, abscess
 pulmonary — *see* Abscess, lung
 pulp, pulpal (dental) K04.01
  irreversible K04.02
  reversible K04.01
 rectovaginal septum K63.0
 rectovesical — *see* Cystitis, specified type NEC
 rectum K61.1
 renal — *see* Abscess, kidney
 retina — *see* Inflammation, chorioretinal
 retrobulbar — *see* Abscess, orbit
 retrocecal K65.1
 retrolaryngeal J38.7
 retromammary — *see* Abscess, breast
 retroperitoneal NEC K68.19
  postprocedural K68.11
 retropharyngeal J39.0
 retrouterine — *see* Peritonitis, pelvic, female
 retrovesical — *see* Cystitis, specified type NEC
 root, tooth K04.7
  with sinus (alveolar) K04.6
 round ligament — *see also* Disease, pelvis, inflammatory N73.2
 rupture (spontaneous) NOS L02.91
 sacrum (tuberculous) A18.01
  nontuberculous M46.28
 salivary (duct) (gland) K11.3
 scalp (any part) L02.811
 scapular — *see* Osteomyelitis, specified type NEC
 sclera — *see* Scleritis
 scrofulous (tuberculous) A18.2
 scrotum N49.2
 seminal vesicle N49.0
 septal, dental K04.7
  with sinus (alveolar) K04.6
 serous — *see* Periostitis
 shoulder (region) — *see* Abscess, upper limb
 sigmoid K63.0
 sinus (accessory) (chronic) (nasal) — *see also* Sinusitis
  intracranial venous (any) G06.0
 Skene's duct or gland N34.0
 skin — *see* Abscess, by site
 specified site NEC L02.818
 spermatic cord N49.1

Abscess (connective tissue) (embolic) (fistulous) (infective) (metastatic) (multiple) (pernicious) (pyogenic) (septic) - *continued*
- sphenoidal (sinus) (chronic) J32.3
- spinal cord (any part) (staphylococcal) G06.1
  - tuberculous A17.81
- spine (column) (tuberculous) A18.01
  - epidural G06.1
  - nontuberculous — *see* Osteomyelitis, vertebra
- spleen D73.3
  - amebic A06.89
- stitch T81.48
- subarachnoid G06.2
  - brain G06.0
  - spinal cord G06.1
- subareolar — *see* Abscess, breast
- subcecal K35.3
- subcutaneous — *see also* Abscess, by site
  - pheomycotic (chromomycotic) B43.2
  - postprocedural T81.41
- subdiaphragmatic K65.1
- subdural G06.2
  - brain G06.0
    - sequelae G09
  - spinal cord G06.1
- subgaleal L02.811
- subhepatic K65.1
- sublingual K12.2
  - gland K11.3
- submammary — *see* Abscess, breast
- submandibular (region) (space) (triangle) K12.2
  - gland K11.3
- submaxillary (region) L02.01
  - gland K11.3
- submental L02.01
  - gland K11.3
- subperiosteal — *see* Osteomyelitis, specified type NEC
- subphrenic K65.1
  - postoperative T81.43
- suburethral N34.0
- sudoriparous L75.8
- supraclavicular (fossa) — *see* Abscess, upper limb
- suprapelvic, acute N73.0
- suprarenal (capsule) (gland) E27.8
- sweat gland L74.8
- tear duct — *see* Inflammation, lacrimal, passages, acute
- temple L02.01
- temporal region L02.01
- temporosphenoidal G06.0
- tendon (sheath) M65.00
  - ankle M65.07-
  - foot M65.07-
  - forearm M65.03-
  - hand M65.04-
  - lower leg M65.06-
  - pelvic region M65.05-
  - shoulder region M65.01-
  - specified site NEC M65.08
  - thigh M65.05-
  - upper arm M65.02-
- testis N45.4
- thigh — *see* Abscess, lower limb
- thorax J86.9
  - with fistula J86.0
- throat J39.1
- thumb — *see also* Abscess, hand
  - nail — *see* Cellulitis, finger
- thymus (gland) E32.1
- thyroid (gland) E06.0
- toe (any) — *see also* Abscess, foot
  - nail — *see* Cellulitis, toe
- tongue (staphylococcal) K14.0
- tonsil (s) (lingual) J36
- tonsillopharyngeal J36
- tooth, teeth (root) K04.7
  - with sinus (alveolar) K04.6
  - supporting structures NEC — *see* Peridontitis, aggressive, localized
- trachea J39.8
- trunk L02.219
  - abdominal wall L02.211
  - back L02.212
  - chest wall L02.213
  - groin L02.214
  - perineum L02.215
  - umbilicus L02.216
- tubal — *see* Salpingitis
- tuberculous — *see* Tuberculosis, abscess
- tubo-ovarian — *see* Salpingo-oophoritis
- tunica vaginalis N49.1
- umbilicus L02.216

Abscess (connective tissue) (embolic) (fistulous) (infective) (metastatic) (multiple) (pernicious) (pyogenic) (septic) - *continued*
- upper
  - limb L02.41-
    - respiratory J39.8
- urethral (gland) N34.0
- urinary N34.0
- uterus, uterine (wall) — *see also* Endometritis
  - ligament — *see also* Disease, pelvis, inflammatory N73.2
  - neck — *see* Cervicitis
- uvula K12.2
- vagina (wall) — *see* Vaginitis
- vaginorectal — *see* Vaginitis
- vas deferens N49.1
- vermiform appendix K35.3
- vertebra (column) (tuberculous) A18.01
  - nontuberculous — *see* Osteomyelitis, vertebra
- vesical — *see* Cystitis, specified type NEC
- vesico-uterine pouch — *see* Peritonitis, pelvic, female
- vitreous (humor) — *see* Endophthalmitis, purulent
- vocal cord J38.3
- von Bezold's — *see* Mastoiditis, acute
- vulva N76.4
- vulvovaginal gland N75.1
- web space — *see* Abscess, hand
- wound T81.40
- wrist — *see* Abscess, upper limb

Absence (of) (organ or part) (complete or partial)
- adrenal (gland) (congenital) Q89.1
  - acquired E89.6
- albumin in blood E88.09
- alimentary tract (congenital) Q45.8
  - upper Q40.8
- alveolar process (acquired) — *see* Anomaly, alveolar
- ankle (acquired) Z89.44-
- anus (congenital) Q42.3
  - with fistula Q42.2
- aorta (congenital) Q25.41
- appendix, congenital Q42.8
- arm (acquired) Z89.20-
  - above elbow Z89.22-
    - congenital (with hand present) — *see* Agenesis, arm, with hand present
    - and hand — *see* Agenesis, forearm, and hand
  - below elbow Z89.21-
    - congenital (with hand present) — *see* Agenesis, arm, with hand present
    - and hand — *see* Agenesis, forearm, and hand
  - congenital — *see* Defect, reduction, upper limb
  - shoulder (following explantation of shoulder joint prosthesis) (joint) (with or without presence of antibiotic-impregnated cement spacer) Z89.23-
    - congenital (with hand present) — *see* Agenesis, arm, with hand present
- artery (congenital) (peripheral) Q27.8
  - brain Q28.3
  - coronary Q24.5
  - pulmonary Q25.79
  - specified NEC Q27.8
  - umbilical Q27.0
- atrial septum (congenital) Q21.1
- auditory canal (congenital) (external) Q16.1
- auricle (ear) , congenital Q16.0
- bile, biliary duct, congenital Q44.5
- bladder (acquired) Z90.6
  - congenital Q64.5
- bowel sounds R19.11
- brain Q00.0
  - part of Q04.3
- breast (s) (and nipple (s)) (acquired) Z90.1-
  - congenital Q83.8
- broad ligament Q50.6
- bronchus (congenital) Q32.4
- canaliculus lacrimalis, congenital Q10.4
- cerebellum (vermis) Q04.3
- cervix (acquired) (with uterus) Z90.710
  - with remaining uterus Z90.712
  - congenital Q51.5
- chin, congenital Q18.8
- cilia (congenital) Q10.3
  - acquired — *see* Madarosis
- clitoris (congenital) Q52.6
- coccyx, congenital Q76.49
- cold sense R20.8
- congenital
  - lumen — *see* Atresia
  - organ or site NEC — *see* Agenesis
  - septum — *see* Imperfect, closure
- corpus callosum Q04.0
- cricoid cartilage, congenital Q31.8

Absence (of) (organ or part) (complete or partial) - *continued*
- diaphragm (with hernia) , congenital Q79.1
- digestive organ (s) or tract, congenital Q45.8
  - acquired NEC Z90.49
  - upper Q40.8
- ductus arteriosus Q28.8
- duodenum (acquired) Z90.49
  - congenital Q41.0
- ear, congenital Q16.9
  - acquired H93.8-
  - auricle Q16.0
  - external Q16.0
  - inner Q16.5
  - lobe, lobule Q17.8
  - middle, except ossicles Q16.4
    - ossicles Q16.3
  - ossicles Q16.3
- ejaculatory duct (congenital) Q55.4
- endocrine gland (congenital) NEC Q89.2
  - acquired E89.89
- epididymis (congenital) Q55.4
  - acquired Z90.79
- epiglottis, congenital Q31.8
- esophagus (congenital) Q39.8
  - acquired (partial) Z90.49
- eustachian tube (congenital) Q16.2
- extremity (acquired) Z89.9
  - congenital Q73.0
  - knee (following explantation of knee joint prosthesis) (joint) (with or without presence of antibiotic-impregnated cement spacer) Z89.52-
  - lower (above knee) Z89.619
    - below knee Z89.51-
  - upper — *see* Absence, arm
- eye (acquired) Z90.01
  - congenital Q11.1
  - muscle (congenital) Q10.3
- eyeball (acquired) Z90.01
- eyelid (fold) (congenital) Q10.3
  - acquired Z90.01
- face, specified part NEC Q18.8
- fallopian tube (s) (acquired) Z90.79
  - congenital Q50.6
- family member (causing problem in home) NEC — *see also* Disruption, family Z63.32
- femur, congenital — *see* Defect, reduction, lower limb, longitudinal, femur
- fibrinogen (congenital) D68.2
  - acquired D65
- finger (s) (acquired) Z89.02-
  - congenital — *see* Agenesis, hand
- foot (acquired) Z89.43-
  - congenital — *see* Agenesis, foot
- forearm (acquired) — *see* Absence, arm, below elbow
- gallbladder (acquired) Z90.49
  - congenital Q44.0
- gamma globulin in blood D80.1
  - hereditary D80.0
- genital organs
  - acquired (female) (male) Z90.79
  - female, congenital Q52.8
    - external Q52.71
    - internal NEC Q52.8
  - male, congenital Q55.8
- genitourinary organs, congenital NEC
  - female Q52.8
  - male Q55.8
- globe (acquired) Z90.01
  - congenital Q11.1
- glottis, congenital Q31.8
- hand and wrist (acquired) Z89.11-
  - congenital — *see* Agenesis, hand
- head, part (acquired) NEC Z90.09
- heat sense R20.8
- hip (following explantation of hip joint prosthesis) (joint) (with or without presence of antibiotic-impregnated cement spacer) Z89.62-
- hymen (congenital) Q52.4
- ileum (acquired) Z90.49
  - congenital Q41.2
- immunoglobulin, isolated NEC D80.3
  - IgA D80.2
  - IgG D80.3
  - IgM D80.4
- incus (acquired) — *see* Loss, ossicles, ear
  - congenital Q16.3
- inner ear, congenital Q16.5
- intestine (acquired) (small) Z90.49
  - congenital Q41.9
    - specified NEC Q41.8
  - large Z90.49

Absence (of) (organ or part) (complete or partial) - *continued*
  intestine (acquired) (small) - *continued*
    large - *continued*
      congenital Q42.9
        specified NEC Q42.8
  iris, congenital Q13.1
  jejunum (acquired) Z90.49
    congenital Q41.1
  joint
    acquired
      hip (following explantation of hip joint prosthesis) (with or without presence of antibiotic-impregnated cement spacer) Z89.62-
      knee (following explantation of knee joint prosthesis) (with or without presence of antibiotic-impregnated cement spacer) Z89.52-
      shoulder (following explantation of shoulder joint prosthesis) (with or without presence of antibiotic-impregnated cement spacer) Z89.23-
    congenital NEC Q74.8
  kidney (s) (acquired) Z90.5
    congenital Q60.2
      bilateral Q60.1
      unilateral Q60.0
  knee (following explantation of knee joint prosthesis) (joint) (with or without presence of antibiotic-impregnated cement spacer) Z89.52-
  labyrinth, membranous Q16.5
  larynx (congenital) Q31.8
    acquired Z90.02
  leg (acquired) (above knee) Z89.61-
    below knee (acquired) Z89.51-
    congenital — *see* Defect, reduction, lower limb
  lens (acquired) — *see also* Aphakia
    congenital Q12.3
    post cataract extraction Z98.4-
  limb (acquired) — *see* Absence, extremity
  lip Q38.6
  liver (congenital) Q44.7
  lung (fissure) (lobe) (bilateral) (unilateral) (congenital) Q33.3
    acquired (any part) Z90.2
  menstruation — *see* Amenorrhea
  muscle (congenital) (pectoral) Q79.8
    ocular Q10.3
  neck, part Q18.8
  neutrophil — *see* Agranulocytosis
  nipple (s) (with breast (s)) (acquired) Z90.1-
    congenital Q83.2
  nose (congenital) Q30.1
    acquired Z90.09
  organ
    of Corti, congenital Q16.5
    or site, congenital NEC Q89.8
      acquired NEC Z90.89
  osseous meatus (ear) Q16.4
  ovary (acquired)
    bilateral Z90.722
    congenital
      bilateral Q50.02
      unilateral Q50.01
    unilateral Z90.721
  oviduct (acquired)
    bilateral Z90.722
    congenital Q50.6
    unilateral Z90.721
  pancreas (congenital) Q45.0
    acquired Z90.410
      complete Z90.410
      partial Z90.411
      total Z90.410
  parathyroid gland (acquired) E89.2
    congenital Q89.2
  patella, congenital Q74.1
  penis (congenital) Q55.5
    acquired Z90.79
  pericardium (congenital) Q24.8
  pituitary gland (congenital) Q89.2
    acquired E89.3
  prostate (acquired) Z90.79
    congenital Q55.4
  pulmonary valve Q22.0
  punctum lacrimale (congenital) Q10.4
  radius, congenital — *see* Defect, reduction, upper limb, longitudinal, radius
  rectum (congenital) Q42.1
    with fistula Q42.0
    acquired Z90.49
  respiratory organ NOS Q34.9
  rib (acquired) Z90.89
    congenital Q76.6
  sacrum, congenital Q76.49

Absence (of) (organ or part) (complete or partial) - *continued*
  salivary gland (s) , congenital Q38.4
  scrotum, congenital Q55.29
  seminal vesicles (congenital) Q55.4
    acquired Z90.79
  septum
    atrial (congenital) Q21.1
    between aorta and pulmonary artery Q21.4
    ventricular (congenital) Q20.4
  sex chromosome
    female phenotype Q97.8
    male phenotype Q98.8
  skull bone (congenital) Q75.8
    with
      anencephaly Q00.0
      encephalocele — *see* Encephalocele
      hydrocephalus Q03.9
        with spina bifida — *see* Spina bifida, by site, with hydrocephalus
      microcephaly Q02
  spermatic cord, congenital Q55.4
  spine, congenital Q76.49
  spleen (congenital) Q89.01
    acquired Z90.81
  sternum, congenital Q76.7
  stomach (acquired) (partial) Z90.3
    congenital Q40.2
  superior vena cava, congenital Q26.8
  teeth, tooth (congenital) K00.0
    acquired (complete) K08.109
      class I K08.101
      class II K08.102
      class III K08.103
      class IV K08.104
      due to
        caries K08.139
          class I K08.131
          class II K08.132
          class III K08.133
          class IV K08.134
        periodontal disease K08.129
          class I K08.121
          class II K08.122
          class III K08.123
          class IV K08.124
        specified NEC K08.199
          class I K08.191
          class II K08.192
          class III K08.193
          class IV K08.194
        trauma K08.119
          class I K08.111
          class II K08.112
          class III K08.113
          class IV K08.114
      partial K08.409
        class I K08.401
        class II K08.402
        class III K08.403
        class IV K08.404
        due to
          caries K08.439
            class I K08.431
            class II K08.432
            class III K08.433
            class IV K08.434
          periodontal disease K08.429
            class I K08.421
            class II K08.422
            class III K08.423
            class IV K08.424
          specified NEC K08.499
            class I K08.491
            class II K08.492
            class III K08.493
            class IV K08.494
          trauma K08.419
            class I K08.411
            class II K08.412
            class III K08.413
            class IV K08.414
  tendon (congenital) Q79.8
  testis (congenital) Q55.0
    acquired Z90.79
  thumb (acquired) Z89.01-
    congenital — *see* Agenesis, hand
  thymus gland Q89.2
  thyroid (gland) (acquired) E89.0
    cartilage, congenital Q31.8
    congenital E03.1
  toe (s) (acquired) Z89.42-
    with foot — *see* Absence, foot and ankle

Absence (of) (organ or part) (complete or partial) - *continued*
  toe (s) (acquired) - *continued*
    congenital — *see* Agenesis, foot
    great Z89.41-
  tongue, congenital Q38.3
  trachea (cartilage) , congenital Q32.1
  transverse aortic arch, congenital Q25.49
  tricuspid valve Q22.4
  umbilical artery, congenital Q27.0
  upper arm and forearm with hand present, congenital — *see* Agenesis, arm, with hand present
  ureter (congenital) Q62.4
    acquired Z90.6
  urethra, congenital Q64.5
  uterus (acquired) Z90.710
    with cervix Z90.710
    with remaining cervical stump Z90.711
    congenital Q51.0
  uvula, congenital Q38.5
  vagina, congenital Q52.0
  vas deferens (congenital) Q55.4
    acquired Z90.79
  vein (peripheral) congenital NEC Q27.8
    cerebral Q28.3
    digestive system Q27.8
    great Q26.8
    lower limb Q27.8
    portal Q26.5
    precerebral Q28.1
    specified site NEC Q27.8
    upper limb Q27.8
  vena cava (inferior) (superior) , congenital Q26.8
  ventricular septum Q20.4
  vertebra, congenital Q76.49
  vulva, congenital Q52.71
  wrist (acquired) Z89.12-
Absorbent system disease I87.8
Absorption
  carbohydrate, disturbance K90.49
  chemical — *see* Table of Drugs and Chemicals
    through placenta (newborn) P04.9
      environmental substance P04.6
      nutritional substance P04.5
      obstetric anesthetic or analgesic drug P04.0
  drug NEC — *see* Table of Drugs and Chemicals
    addictive
      through placenta (newborn) P04.49
        cocaine P04.41
    medicinal
      through placenta (newborn) P04.1
      through placenta (newborn) P04.1
        obstetric anesthetic or analgesic drug P04.0
  fat, disturbance K90.49
    pancreatic K90.3
  noxious substance — *see* Table of Drugs and Chemicals
  protein, disturbance K90.49
  starch, disturbance K90.49
  toxic substance — *see* Table of Drugs and Chemicals
  uremic — *see* Uremia
Abstinence symptoms, syndrome
  alcohol F10.239
    with delirium F10.231
  cocaine F14.23
  neonatal P96.1
  nicotine — *see* Dependence, drug, nicotine, with, withdrawal
  opioid F11.93
    with dependence F11.23
  psychoactive NEC F19.939
    with
      delirium F19.931
      dependence F19.239
        with
          delirium F19.231
          perceptual disturbance F19.232
          uncomplicated F19.230
      perceptual disturbance F19.932
    uncomplicated F19.930
  sedative F13.939
    with
      delirium F13.931
      dependence F13.239
        with
          delirium F13.231
          perceptual disturbance F13.232
          uncomplicated F13.230
      perceptual disturbance F13.932
    uncomplicated F13.930
  stimulant NEC F15.93
    with dependence F15.23

Abulia R68.89
Abulomania F60.7
Abuse
  adult — *see* Maltreatment, adult
  as reason for
    couple seeking advice (including offender) Z63.0
  alcohol (non-dependent) F10.10
    with
      anxiety disorder F10.180
      intoxication F10.129
        with delirium F10.121
        uncomplicated F10.120
      mood disorder F10.14
      other specified disorder F10.188
      psychosis F10.159
        delusions F10.150
        hallucinations F10.151
      sexual dysfunction F10.181
      sleep disorder F10.182
      unspecified disorder F10.19
    counseling and surveillance Z71.41
  amphetamine (or related substance) — *see* Abuse, drug, stimulant NEC
  analgesics (non-prescribed) (over the counter) F55.8
  antacids F55.0
  antidepressants — *see* Abuse, drug, psychoactive NEC
  anxiolytic — *see* Abuse, drug, sedative
  barbiturates — *see* Abuse, drug, sedative
  caffeine — *see* Abuse, drug, stimulant NEC
  cannabis, cannabinoids — *see* Abuse, drug, cannabis
  child — *see* Maltreatment, child
  cocaine — *see* Abuse, drug, cocaine
  drug NEC (non-dependent) F19.10
    with sleep disorder F19.182
    amphetamine type — *see* Abuse, drug, stimulant NEC
    analgesics (non-prescribed) (over the counter) F55.8
    antacids F55.0
    antidepressants — *see* Abuse, drug, psychoactive NEC
    anxiolytics — *see* Abuse, drug, sedative
    barbiturates — *see* Abuse, drug, sedative
    caffeine — *see* Abuse, drug, stimulant NEC
    cannabis F12.10
      with
        anxiety disorder F12.180
        intoxication F12.129
          with
            delirium F12.121
            perceptual disturbance F12.122
          uncomplicated F12.120
        other specified disorder F12.188
        psychosis F12.159
          delusions F12.150
          hallucinations F12.151
        unspecified disorder F12.19
    cocaine F14.10
      with
        anxiety disorder F14.180
        intoxication F14.129
          with
            delirium F14.121
            perceptual disturbance F14.122
          uncomplicated F14.120
        mood disorder F14.14
        other specified disorder F14.188
        psychosis F14.159
          delusions F14.150
          hallucinations F14.151
        sexual dysfunction F14.181
        sleep disorder F14.182
        unspecified disorder F14.19
    counseling and surveillance Z71.51
    hallucinogen F16.10
      with
        anxiety disorder F16.180
        flashbacks F16.183
        intoxication F16.129
          with
            delirium F16.121
            perceptual disturbance F16.122
          uncomplicated F16.120
        mood disorder F16.14
        other specified disorder F16.188
        perception disorder, persisting F16.183
        psychosis F16.159
          delusions F16.150
          hallucinations F16.151
        unspecified disorder F16.19
    hashish — *see* Abuse, drug, cannabis
    herbal or folk remedies F55.1

Abuse - *continued*
  drug NEC (non-dependent) - *continued*
    hormones F55.3
    hypnotics — *see* Abuse, drug, sedative
    inhalant F18.10
      with
        anxiety disorder F18.180
        dementia, persisting F18.17
        intoxication F18.129
          with delirium F18.121
          uncomplicated F18.120
        mood disorder F18.14
        other specified disorder F18.188
        psychosis F18.159
          delusions F18.150
          hallucinations F18.151
        unspecified disorder F18.19
    laxatives F55.2
    LSD — *see* Abuse, drug, hallucinogen
    marihuana — *see* Abuse, drug, cannabis
    morphine type (opioids) — *see* Abuse, drug, opioid
    opioid F11.10
      with
        intoxication F11.129
          with
            delirium F11.121
            perceptual disturbance F11.122
          uncomplicated F11.120
        mood disorder F11.14
        other specified disorder F11.188
        psychosis F11.159
          delusions F11.150
          hallucinations F11.151
        sexual dysfunction F11.181
        sleep disorder F11.182
        unspecified disorder F11.19
    PCP (phencyclidine) (or related substance) — *see* Abuse, drug, hallucinogen
    psychoactive NEC F19.10
      with
        amnestic disorder F19.16
        anxiety disorder F19.180
        dementia F19.17
        intoxication F19.129
          with
            delirium F19.121
            perceptual disturbance F19.122
          uncomplicated F19.120
        mood disorder F19.14
        other specified disorder F19.188
        psychosis F19.159
          delusions F19.150
          hallucinations F19.151
        sexual dysfunction F19.181
        sleep disorder F19.182
        unspecified disorder F19.19
    sedative, hypnotic or anxiolytic F13.10
      with
        anxiety disorder F13.180
        intoxication F13.129
          with delirium F13.121
          uncomplicated F13.120
        mood disorder F13.14
        other specified disorder F13.188
        psychosis F13.159
          delusions F13.150
          hallucinations F13.151
        sexual dysfunction F13.181
        sleep disorder F13.182
        unspecified disorder F13.19
    solvent — *see* Abuse, drug, inhalant
    steroids F55.3
    stimulant NEC F15.10
      with
        anxiety disorder F15.180
        intoxication F15.129
          with
            delirium F15.121
            perceptual disturbance F15.122
          uncomplicated F15.120
        mood disorder F15.14
        other specified disorder F15.188
        psychosis F15.159
          delusions F15.150
          hallucinations F15.151
        sexual dysfunction F15.181
        sleep disorder F15.182
        unspecified disorder F15.19
    tranquilizers — *see* Abuse, drug, sedative
    vitamins F55.4
  hallucinogens — *see* Abuse, drug, hallucinogen
  hashish — *see* Abuse, drug, cannabis
  herbal or folk remedies F55.1

Abuse - *continued*
  hormones F55.3
  hypnotic — *see* Abuse, drug, sedative
  inhalant — *see* Abuse, drug, inhalant
  laxatives F55.2
  LSD — *see* Abuse, drug, hallucinogen
  marihuana — *see* Abuse, drug, cannabis
  morphine type (opioids) — *see* Abuse, drug, opioid
  non-psychoactive substance NEC F55.8
    antacids F55.0
    folk remedies F55.1
    herbal remedies F55.1
    hormones F55.3
    laxatives F55.2
    steroids F55.3
    vitamins F55.4
  opioids — *see* Abuse, drug, opioid
  PCP (phencyclidine) (or related substance) — *see* Abuse, drug, hallucinogen
  physical (adult) (child) — *see* Maltreatment
  psychoactive substance — *see* Abuse, drug, psychoactive NEC
  psychological (adult) (child) — *see* Maltreatment
  sedative — *see* Abuse, drug, sedative
  sexual — *see* Maltreatment
  solvent — *see* Abuse, drug, inhalant
  steroids F55.3
  vitamins F55.4
Acalculia R48.8
  developmental F81.2
Acanthamebiasis (with) B60.10
  conjunctiva B60.12
  keratoconjunctivitis B60.13
  meningoencephalitis B60.11
  other specified B60.19
Acanthocephaliasis B83.8
Acanthocheilonemiasis B74.4
Acanthocytosis E78.6
Acantholysis L11.9
Acanthosis (acquired) (nigricans) L83
  benign Q82.8
  congenital Q82.8
  seborrheic L82.1
    inflamed L82.0
  tongue K14.3
Acapnia E87.3
Acarbia E87.2
Acardia, acardius Q89.8
Acardiacus amorphus Q89.8
Acardiotrophia I51.4
Acariasis B88.0
  scabies B86
Acarodermatitis (urticarioides) B88.0
Acarophobia F40.218
Acatalasemia, acatalasia E80.3
Acathisia (drug induced) G25.71
Accelerated atrioventricular conduction I45.6
Accentuation of personality traits (type A) Z73.1
Accessory (congenital)
  adrenal gland Q89.1
  anus Q43.4
  appendix Q43.4
  atrioventricular conduction I45.6
  auditory ossicles Q16.3
  auricle (ear) Q17.0
  biliary duct or passage Q44.5
  bladder Q64.79
  blood vessels NEC Q27.9
    coronary Q24.5
  bone NEC Q79.8
  breast tissue, axilla Q83.1
  carpal bones Q74.0
  cecum Q43.4
  chromosome (s) NEC (nonsex) Q92.9
    with complex rearrangements NEC Q92.5
      seen only at prometaphase Q92.8
    partial Q92.9
    sex
      female phenotype Q97.8
      13 — *see* Trisomy, 13
      18 — *see* Trisomy, 18
      21 — *see* Trisomy, 21
  coronary artery Q24.5
  cusp (s) , heart valve NEC Q24.8
    pulmonary Q22.3
  cystic duct Q44.5
  digit (s) Q69.9
  ear (auricle) (lobe) Q17.0
  endocrine gland NEC Q89.2
  eye muscle Q10.3
  eyelid Q10.3
  face bone (s) Q75.8
  fallopian tube (fimbria) (ostium) Q50.6

Accessory (congenital) - *continued*
finger (s) Q69.0
foreskin N47.8
frontonasal process Q75.8
gallbladder Q44.1
genital organ (s)
female Q52.8
external Q52.79
internal NEC Q52.8
male Q55.8
genitourinary organs NEC Q89.8
female Q52.8
male Q55.8
hallux Q69.2
heart Q24.8
valve NEC Q24.8
pulmonary Q22.3
hepatic ducts Q44.5
hymen Q52.4
intestine (large) (small) Q43.4
kidney Q63.0
lacrimal canal Q10.6
leaflet, heart valve NEC Q24.8
ligament, broad Q50.6
liver Q44.7
duct Q44.5
lobule (ear) Q17.0
lung (lobe) Q33.1
muscle Q79.8
navicular of carpus Q74.0
nervous system, part NEC Q07.8
nipple Q83.3
nose Q30.8
organ or site not listed — *see* Anomaly, by site
ovary Q50.31
oviduct Q50.6
pancreas Q45.3
parathyroid gland Q89.2
parotid gland (and duct) Q38.4
pituitary gland Q89.2
preauricular appendage Q17.0
prepuce N47.8
renal arteries (multiple) Q27.2
rib Q76.6
cervical Q76.5
roots (teeth) K00.2
salivary gland Q38.4
sesamoid bones Q74.8
foot Q74.2
hand Q74.0
skin tags Q82.8
spleen Q89.09
sternum Q76.7
submaxillary gland Q38.4
tarsal bones Q74.2
teeth, tooth K00.1
tendon Q79.8
thumb Q69.1
thymus gland Q89.2
thyroid gland Q89.2
toes Q69.2
tongue Q38.3
tooth, teeth K00.1
tragus Q17.0
ureter Q62.5
urethra Q64.79
urinary organ or tract NEC Q64.8
uterus Q51.2
vagina Q52.10
valve, heart NEC Q24.8
pulmonary Q22.3
vertebra Q76.49
vocal cords Q31.8
vulva Q52.79
Accident
birth — *see* Birth, injury
cardiac — *see* Infarct, myocardium
cerebral I63.9
cerebrovascular (embolic) (ischemic)
(thrombotic) I63.9
aborted I63.9
hemorrhagic — *see* Hemorrhage, intracranial, intracerebral
old (without sequelae) Z86.73
with sequelae (of) — *see* Sequelae, infarction, cerebral
coronary — *see* Infarct, myocardium
craniovascular I63.9
vascular, brain I63.9
Accidental — *see* condition
Accommodation (disorder) — *see also* condition
hysterical paralysis of F44.89
insufficiency of H52.4

Accommodation (disorder) - *continued*
paresis — *see* Paresis, of accommodation
spasm — *see* Spasm, of accommodation
Accouchement — *see* Delivery
Accreta placenta O43.21-
Accretio cordis (nonrheumatic) I31.0
Accretions, tooth, teeth K03.6
Acculturation difficulty Z60.3
Accumulation secretion, prostate N42.89
Acephalia, acephalism, acephalus, acephaly Q00.0
Acephalobrachia monster Q89.8
Acephalochirus monster Q89.8
Acephalogaster Q89.8
Acephalostomus monster Q89.8
Acephalothorax Q89.8
Acerophobia F40.298
Acetonemia R79.89
in Type 1 diabetes E10.10
with coma E10.11
Acetonuria R82.4
Achalasia (cardia) (esophagus) K22.0
congenital Q39.5
pylorus Q40.0
sphincteral NEC K59.8
Ache (s) — *see* Pain
Acheilia Q38.6
Achillobursitis — *see* Tendinitis, Achilles
Achillodynia — *see* Tendinitis, Achilles
Achlorhydria, achlorhydric (neurogenic) K31.83
anemia D50.8
diarrhea K31.83
psychogenic F45.8
secondary to vagotomy K91.1
Achluophobia F40.228
Acholia K82.8
Acholuric jaundice (familial) (splenomegalic) —
see also Spherocytosis
acquired D59.8
Achondrogenesis Q77.0
Achondroplasia (osteosclerosis congenita) Q77.4
Achroma, cutis L80
Achromat (ism), **achromatopsia** (acquired)
(congenital) H53.51
Achromia parasitica B36.0
Achromia, congenital — *see* Albinism
Achylia gastrica K31.89
psychogenic F45.8
Acid
burn — *see* Corrosion
deficiency
amide nicotinic E52
ascorbic E54
folic E53.8
nicotinic E52
pantothenic E53.8
intoxication E87.2
peptic disease K30
phosphatase deficiency E83.39
stomach K30
psychogenic F45.8
Acidemia E87.2
argininosuccinic E72.22
isovaleric E71.110
metabolic (newborn) P19.9
first noted before onset of labor P19.0
first noted during labor P19.1
noted at birth P19.2
methylmalonic E71.120
pipecolic E72.3
propionic E71.121
Acidity, gastric (high) K30
psychogenic F45.8
Acidocytopenia — *see* Agranulocytosis
Acidocytosis D72.1
Acidopenia — *see* Agranulocytosis
Acidosis (lactic) (respiratory) E87.2
in Type 1 diabetes E10.10
with coma E10.11
kidney, tubular N25.89
lactic E87.2
metabolic NEC E87.2
with respiratory acidosis E87.4
late, of newborn P74.0
mixed metabolic and respiratory, newborn P84
newborn P84
renal (hyperchloremic) (tubular) N25.89
respiratory E87.2
complicated by
metabolic
acidosis E87.4
alkalosis E87.4
Aciduria
argininosuccinic E72.22

Aciduria - *continued*
glutaric (type I) E72.3
type II E71.313
type III E71.5-
orotic (congenital) (hereditary) (pyrimidine deficiency) E79.8
anemia D53.0
Acladiosis (skin) B36.0
Aclasis, diaphyseal Q78.6
Acleistocardia Q21.1
Aclusion — *see* Anomaly, dentofacial, malocclusion
Acne L70.9
artificialis L70.8
atrophica L70.2
cachecticorum (Hebra) L70.8
conglobata L70.1
cystic L70.0
decalvans L66.2
excoriée (des jeunes filles) L70.5
frontalis L70.2
indurata L70.0
infantile L70.4
keloid L73.0
lupoid L70.2
necrotic, necrotica (miliaris) L70.2
neonatal L70.4
nodular L70.0
occupational L70.8
picker's L70.5
pustular L70.0
rodens L70.2
rosacea L71.9
specified NEC L70.8
tropica L70.3
varioliformis L70.2
vulgaris L70.0
Acnitis (primary) A18.4
Acosta's disease T70.29
Acoustic — *see* condition
Acousticophobia F40.298
Acquired — *see also* condition
immunodeficiency syndrome (AIDS) B20
Acrania Q00.0
Acroangiodermatitis I78.9
Acroasphyxia, chronic I73.89
Acrobystitis N47.7
Acrocephalopolysyndactyly Q87.0
Acrocephalosyndactyly Q87.0
Acrocephaly Q75.0
Acrochondrohyperplasia — *see* Syndrome, Marfan's
Acrocyanosis I73.8
newborn P28.2
meaning transient blue hands and feet - omit code
Acrodermatitis L30.8
atrophicans (chronica) L90.4
continua (Hallopeau) L40.2
enteropathica (hereditary) E83.2
Hallopeau's L40.2
infantile papular L44.4
perstans L40.2
pustulosa continua L40.2
recalcitrant pustular L40.2
Acrodynia — *see* Poisoning, mercury
Acromegaly, acromegalia E22.0
Acromelalgia I73.81
Acromicria, acromikria Q79.8
Acronyx L60.0
Acropachy, thyroid — *see* Thyrotoxicosis
Acroparesthesia (simple) (vasomotor) I73.89
Acropathy, thyroid — *see* Thyrotoxicosis
Acrophobia F40.241
Acroposthitis N47.7
Acroscleriasis, acroscleroderma, acrosclerosis — *see* Sclerosis, systemic
Acrosphacelus I96
Acrospiroma, eccrine — *see* Neoplasm, skin, benign
Acrostealgia — *see* Osteochondropathy
Acrotrophodynia — *see* Immersion
ACTH ectopic syndrome E24.3
Actinic — *see* condition
Actinobacillosis, actinobacillus A28.8
mallei A24.0
muris A25.1
Actinomyces israelii (infection) — *see* Actinomycosis
Actinomycetoma (foot) B47.1
Actinomycosis, actinomycotic A42.9
with pneumonia A42.0
abdominal A42.1
cervicofacial A42.2
cutaneous A42.89
gastrointestinal A42.1
pulmonary A42.0

Actinomycosis, actinomycotic - *continued*
sepsis A42.7
specified site NEC A42.89
Actinoneuritis G62.82
Action, heart
disorder I49.9
irregular I49.9
psychogenic F45.8
Activated protein C resistance D68.51
Activation
mast cell (disorder) (syndrome) D89.40
idiopathic D89.42
monoclonal D89.41
secondary D89.43
specified type NEC D89.49
Active — *see* condition
Acute — *see also* condition
abdomen R10.0
gallbladder — *see* Cholecystitis, acute
Acyanotic heart disease (congenital) Q24.9
Acystia Q64.5
Adair-Dighton syndrome
(brittle bones and blue sclera, deafness) Q78.0
Adamantinoblastoma — *see* Ameloblastoma
Adamantinoma — *see also* Cyst, calcifying
odontogenic
long bones C40.90
lower limb C40.2-
upper limb C40.0-
malignant C41.1
jaw (bone) (lower) C41.1
upper C41.0
tibial C40.2-
Adamantoblastoma — *see* Ameloblastoma
Adams-Stokes (-Morgagni) **disease or syndrome** I45.9
Adaption reaction — *see* Disorder, adjustment
Addiction — *see also* Dependence F19.20
alcohol, alcoholic (ethyl) (methyl) (wood) (without remission) F10.20
with remission F10.21
drug — *see* Dependence, drug
ethyl alcohol (without remission) F10.20
with remission F10.21
heroin — *see* Dependence, drug, opioid
methyl alcohol (without remission) F10.20
with remission F10.21
methylated spirit (without remission) F10.20
with remission F10.21
morphine (-like substances) — *see* Dependence, drug, opioid
nicotine — *see* Dependence, drug, nicotine
opium and opioids — *see* Dependence, drug, opioid
tobacco — *see* Dependence, drug, nicotine
Addison-Biermer anemia (pernicious) D51.0
Addisonian crisis E27.2
Addison's
anemia (pernicious) D51.0
disease (bronze) or syndrome E27.1
tuberculous A18.7
keloid L94.0
Addison-Schilder complex E71.528
Additional — *see also* Accessory
chromosome (s) Q99.8
sex — *see* Abnormal, chromosome, sex
21 — *see* Trisomy, 21
Adduction contracture, hip or other joint — *see* Contraction, joint
Adenitis — *see also* Lymphadenitis
acute, unspecified site L04.9
axillary I88.9
acute L04.2
chronic or subacute I88.1
Bartholin's gland N75.8
bulbourethral gland — *see* Urethritis
cervical I88.9
acute L04.0
chronic or subacute I88.1
chancroid (Hemophilus ducreyi) A57
chronic, unspecified site I88.1
Cowper's gland — *see* Urethritis
due to Pasteurella multocida (p. septica) A28.0
epidemic, acute B27.09
gangrenous L04.9
gonorrheal NEC A54.89
groin I88.9
acute L04.1
chronic or subacute I88.1
infectious (acute) (epidemic) B27.09
inguinal I88.9
acute L04.1
chronic or subacute I88.1
lymph gland or node, except mesenteric I88.9

Adenitis - *continued*
lymph gland or node, except mesenteric - *continued*
acute — *see* Lymphadenitis, acute
chronic or subacute I88.1
mesenteric (acute) (chronic) (nonspecific) (subacute) I88.0
parotid gland (suppurative) — *see* Sialoadenitis
salivary gland (any) (suppurative) — *see* Sialoadenitis
scrofulous (tuberculous) A18.2
Skene's duct or gland — *see* Urethritis
strumous, tuberculous A18.2
subacute, unspecified site I88.1
sublingual gland (suppurative) — *see* Sialoadenitis
submandibular gland (suppurative) — *see* Sialoadenitis
submaxillary gland (suppurative) — *see* Sialoadenitis
tuberculous — *see* Tuberculosis, lymph gland
urethral gland — *see* Urethritis
Wharton's duct (suppurative) — *see* Sialoadenitis
Adenoacanthoma — *see* Neoplasm, malignant, by site
Adenoameloblastoma — *see* Cyst, calcifying odontogenic
Adenocarcinoid (tumor) — *see* Neoplasm, malignant, by site
Adenocarcinoma — *see also* Neoplasm, malignant, by site
acidophil
specified site — *see* Neoplasm, malignant, by site
unspecified site C75.1
adrenal cortical C74.0-
alveolar — *see* Neoplasm, lung, malignant
apocrine
breast — *see* Neoplasm, breast, malignant
in situ
breast D05.8-
specified site NEC — *see* Neoplasm, skin, in situ
unspecified site D04.9
specified site NEC — *see* Neoplasm, skin, malignant
unspecified site C44.99
basal cell
specified site — *see* Neoplasm, skin, malignant
unspecified site C08.9
basophil
specified site — *see* Neoplasm, malignant, by site
unspecified site C75.1
bile duct type C22.1
liver C22.1
specified site NEC — *see* Neoplasm, malignant, by site
unspecified site C22.1
bronchiolar — *see* Neoplasm, lung, malignant
bronchioloalveolar — *see* Neoplasm, lung, malignant
ceruminous C44.29-
cervix, in situ — *see also* Carcinoma, cervix uteri, in situ D06.9
chromophobe
specified site — *see* Neoplasm, malignant, by site
unspecified site C75.1
diffuse type
specified site — *see* Neoplasm, malignant, by site
unspecified site C16.9
duct
infiltrating
with Paget's disease — *see* Neoplasm, breast, malignant
specified site — *see* Neoplasm, malignant, by site
unspecified site (female) C50.91-
male C50.92-
specified site — *see* Neoplasm, malignant, by site
unspecified site
female C56.9
male C61
eosinophil
specified site — *see* Neoplasm, malignant, by site
unspecified site C75.1
follicular
with papillary C73
moderately differentiated C73
specified site — *see* Neoplasm, malignant, by site
trabecular C73
unspecified site C73
well differentiated C73
Hurthle cell C73
in
adenomatous
polyposis coli C18.9
infiltrating duct

Adenocarcinoma - *continued*
infiltrating duct - *continued*
with Paget's disease — *see* Neoplasm, breast, malignant
specified site — *see* Neoplasm, by site, malignant
unspecified site (female) C50.91-
male C50.92-
inflammatory
specified site — *see* Neoplasm, by site, malignant
unspecified site (female) C50.91-
male C50.92-
intestinal type
specified site — *see* Neoplasm, by site, malignant
unspecified site C16.9
intracystic papillary
intraductal
breast D05.1-
noninfiltrating
breast D05.1-
papillary
with invasion
specified site — *see* Neoplasm, by site, malignant
unspecified site (female) C50.91-
male C50.92-
breast D05.1-
specified site NEC — *see* Neoplasm, in situ, by site
unspecified site D05.1-
specified site NEC — *see* Neoplasm, in situ, by site
unspecified site D05.1-
papillary
with invasion
specified site — *see* Neoplasm, malignant, by site
unspecified site (female) C50.91-
male C50.92-
breast D05.1-
specified site — *see* Neoplasm, in situ, by site
unspecified site D05.1-
specified site NEC — *see* Neoplasm, in situ, by site
unspecified site D05.1-
islet cell
with exocrine, mixed
specified site — *see* Neoplasm, malignant, by site
unspecified site C25.9
pancreas C25.4
specified site NEC — *see* Neoplasm, malignant, by site
unspecified site C25.4
lobular
in situ
breast D05.0-
specified site NEC — *see* Neoplasm, in situ, by site
unspecified site D05.0-
specified site — *see* Neoplasm, malignant, by site
unspecified site (female) C50.91-
male C50.92-
mucoid — *see also* Neoplasm, malignant, by site
cell
specified site — *see* Neoplasm, malignant, by site
unspecified site C75.1
nonencapsulated sclerosing C73
papillary
with follicular C73
follicular variant C73
intraductal (noninfiltrating)
with invasion
specified site — *see* Neoplasm, malignant, by site
unspecified site (female) C50.91-
male C50.92-
breast D05.1-
specified site NEC — *see* Neoplasm, in situ, by site
unspecified site D05.1-
serous
specified site — *see* Neoplasm, malignant, by site
unspecified site C56.9
papillocystic
specified site — *see* Neoplasm, malignant, by site
unspecified site C56.9
pseudomucinous
specified site — *see* Neoplasm, malignant, by site
unspecified site C56.9
renal cell C64-
sebaceous — *see* Neoplasm, skin, malignant
serous — *see also* Neoplasm, malignant, by site
papillary
specified site — *see* Neoplasm, malignant, by site

Adenocarcinoma - *continued*
  serous - *continued*
    papillary - *continued*
      unspecified site C56.9
    sweat gland — *see* Neoplasm, skin, malignant
    water-clear cell C75.0
Adenocarcinoma-in-situ — *see also* Neoplasm, in situ, by site
  breast D05.9-
Adenofibroma
  clear cell — *see* Neoplasm, benign, by site
  endometrioid D27.9
    borderline malignancy D39.10
    malignant C56-
  mucinous
    specified site — *see* Neoplasm, benign, by site
    unspecified site D27.9
  papillary
    specified site — *see* Neoplasm, benign, by site
    unspecified site D27.9
  prostate — *see* Enlargement, enlarged, prostate
  serous
    specified site — *see* Neoplasm, benign, by site
    unspecified site D27.9
  specified site — *see* Neoplasm, benign, by site
  unspecified site D27.9
Adenofibrosis
  breast — *see* Fibroadenosis, breast
  endometrioid N80.0
Adenoiditis (chronic) J35.02
  with tonsillitis J35.03
  acute J03.90
    recurrent J03.91
    specified organism NEC J03.80
      recurrent J03.81
    staphylococcal J03.80
      recurrent J03.81
    streptococcal J03.00
      recurrent J03.01
Adenoids — *see* condition
Adenolipoma — *see* Neoplasm, benign, by site
Adenolipomatosis, Launois-Bensaude E88.89
Adenolymphoma
  specified site — *see* Neoplasm, benign, by site
  unspecified site D11.9
Adenoma — *see also* Neoplasm, benign, by site
  acidophil
    specified site — *see* Neoplasm, benign, by site
    unspecified site D35.2
  acidophil-basophil, mixed
    specified site — *see* Neoplasm, benign, by site
    unspecified site D35.2
  adrenal (cortical) D35.00
    clear cell D35.00
    compact cell D35.00
    glomerulosa cell D35.00
    heavily pigmented variant D35.00
    mixed cell D35.00
  alpha-cell
    pancreas D13.7
    specified site NEC — *see* Neoplasm, benign, by site
    unspecified site D13.7
  alveolar D14.30
  apocrine
    breast D24-
    specified site NEC — *see* Neoplasm, skin, benign, by site
    unspecified site D23.9
  basal cell D11.9
  basophil
    specified site — *see* Neoplasm, benign, by site
    unspecified site D35.2
  basophil-acidophil, mixed
    specified site — *see* Neoplasm, benign, by site
    unspecified site D35.2
  beta-cell
    pancreas D13.7
    specified site NEC — *see* Neoplasm, benign, by site
    unspecified site D13.7
  bile duct D13.4
    common D13.5
    extrahepatic D13.5
    intrahepatic D13.4
    specified site NEC — *see* Neoplasm, benign, by site
    unspecified site D13.4
  black D35.00
  bronchial D38.1
    cylindroid type — *see* Neoplasm, lung, malignant
  ceruminous D23.2-
  chief cell D35.1

Adenoma - *continued*
  chromophobe
    specified site — *see* Neoplasm, benign, by site
    unspecified site D35.2
  colloid
    specified site — *see* Neoplasm, benign, by site
    unspecified site D34
  duct
  eccrine, papillary — *see* Neoplasm, skin, benign
  endocrine, multiple
    single specified site — *see* Neoplasm, uncertain behavior, by site
    two or more specified sites D44-
    unspecified site D44.9
  endometrioid — *see also* Neoplasm, benign
    borderline malignancy — *see* Neoplasm, uncertain behavior, by site
  eosinophil
    specified site — *see* Neoplasm, benign, by site
    unspecified site D35.2
  fetal
    specified site — *see* Neoplasm, benign, by site
    unspecified site D34
  follicular
    specified site — *see* Neoplasm, benign, by site
    unspecified site D34
  hepatocellular D13.4
  Hurthle cell D34
  islet cell
    pancreas D13.7
    specified site NEC — *see* Neoplasm, benign, by site
    unspecified site D13.7
  liver cell D13.4
  macrofollicular
    specified site — *see* Neoplasm, benign, by site
    unspecified site D34
  malignant, malignum — *see* Neoplasm, malignant, by site
  microcystic
    pancreas D13.6
    specified site NEC — *see* Neoplasm, benign, by site
    unspecified site D13.6
  microfollicular
    specified site — *see* Neoplasm, benign, by site
    unspecified site D34
  mucoid cell
    specified site — *see* Neoplasm, benign, by site
    unspecified site D35.2
  multiple endocrine
    single specified site — *see* Neoplasm, uncertain behavior, by site
    two or more specified sites D44-
    unspecified site D44.9
  nipple D24-
  papillary — *see also* Neoplasm, benign, by site
    eccrine — *see* Neoplasm, skin, benign, by site
  Pick's tubular
    specified site — *see* Neoplasm, benign, by site
    unspecified site
      female D27.9
      male D29.20
  pleomorphic
    carcinoma in — *see* Neoplasm, salivary gland, malignant
    specified site — *see* Neoplasm, malignant, by site
    unspecified site C08.9
  polypoid — *see also* Neoplasm, benign
    adenocarcinoma in — *see* Neoplasm, malignant, by site
    adenocarcinoma in situ — *see* Neoplasm, in situ, by site
  prostate — *see* Neoplasm, benign, prostate
  rete cell D29.20
  sebaceous — *see* Neoplasm, skin, benign
  Sertoli cell
    specified site — *see* Neoplasm, benign, by site
    unspecified site
      female D27.9
      male D29.20
  skin appendage — *see* Neoplasm, skin, benign
  sudoriferous gland — *see* Neoplasm, skin, benign
  sweat gland — *see* Neoplasm, skin, benign
  testicular
    specified site — *see* Neoplasm, benign, by site
    unspecified site
      female D27.9
      male D29.20
  tubular — *see also* Neoplasm, benign, by site
    adenocarcinoma in — *see* Neoplasm, malignant, by site

Adenoma - *continued*
  tubular - *continued*
    adenocarcinoma in situ — *see* Neoplasm, in situ, by site
    Pick's
      specified site — *see* Neoplasm, benign, by site
      unspecified site
        female D27.9
        male D29.20
  tubulovillous — *see also* Neoplasm, benign, by site
    adenocarcinoma in — *see* Neoplasm, malignant, by site
    adenocarcinoma in situ — *see* Neoplasm, in situ, by site
  villous — *see* Neoplasm, uncertain behavior, by site
    adenocarcinoma in — *see* Neoplasm, malignant, by site
    adenocarcinoma in situ — *see* Neoplasm, in situ, by site
  water-clear cell D35.1
Adenomatosis
  endocrine (multiple) E31.20
    single specified site — *see* Neoplasm, uncertain behavior, by site
  erosive of nipple D24-
  pluriendocrine — *see* Adenomatosis, endocrine
  pulmonary D38.1
    malignant — *see* Neoplasm, lung, malignant
  specified site — *see* Neoplasm, benign, by site
  unspecified site D12.6
Adenomatous
  goiter (nontoxic) E04.9
    with hyperthyroidism — *see* Hyperthyroidism, with, goiter, nodular
    toxic — *see* Hyperthyroidism, with, goiter, nodular
Adenomyoma — *see also* Neoplasm, benign, by site
  prostate — *see* Enlarged, prostate
Adenomyometritis N80.0
Adenomyosis N80.0
Adenopathy (lymph gland) R59.9
  generalized R59.1
  inguinal R59.0
  localized R59.0
  mediastinal R59.0
  mesentery R59.0
  syphilitic (secondary) A51.49
  tracheobronchial R59.0
    tuberculous A15.4
      primary (progressive) A15.7
  tuberculous — *see also* Tuberculosis, lymph gland
    tracheobronchial A15.4
      primary (progressive) A15.7
Adenosalpingitis — *see* Salpingitis
Adenosarcoma — *see* Neoplasm, malignant, by site
Adenosclerosis I88.8
Adenosis (sclerosing) **breast** — *see* Fibroadenosis, breast
Adenovirus, as cause of disease classified elsewhere B97.0
Adentia (complete) (partial) — *see* Absence, teeth
Adherent — *see also* Adhesions
  labia (minora) N90.89
  pericardium (nonrheumatic) I31.0
    rheumatic I09.2
  placenta (with hemorrhage) O72.0
    without hemorrhage O73.0
  prepuce, newborn N47.0
  scar (skin) L90.5
  tendon in scar L90.5
Adhesions, adhesive (postinfective) K66.0
  with intestinal obstruction K56.5
  abdominal (wall) — *see* Adhesions, peritoneum
  appendix K38.8
  bile duct (common) (hepatic) K83.8
  bladder (sphincter) N32.89
  bowel — *see* Adhesions, peritoneum
  cardiac I31.0
    rheumatic I09.2
  cecum — *see* Adhesions, peritoneum
  cervicovaginal N88.1
    congenital Q52.8
    postpartal O90.89
    old N88.1
  cervix N88.1
  ciliary body NEC — *see* Adhesions, iris
  clitoris N90.89
  colon — *see* Adhesions, peritoneum
  common duct K83.8
  congenital — *see also* Anomaly, by site
    fingers — *see* Syndactylism, complex, fingers
    omental, anomalous Q43.3
    peritoneal Q43.3
    tongue (to gum or roof of mouth) Q38.3

Adhesions, adhesive (postinfective) - *continued*
  conjunctiva (acquired) H11.21-
    congenital Q15.8
  cystic duct K82.8
  diaphragm — *see* Adhesions, peritoneum
  due to foreign body — *see* Foreign body
  duodenum — *see* Adhesions, peritoneum
  ear
    middle H74.1-
  epididymis N50.89
  epidural — *see* Adhesions, meninges
  epiglottis J38.7
  eyelid H02.59
  female pelvis N73.6
  gallbladder K82.8
  globe H44.89
  heart I31.0
    rheumatic I09.2
  ileocecal (coil) — *see* Adhesions, peritoneum
  ileum — *see* Adhesions, peritoneum
  intestine — *see also* Adhesions, peritoneum
    with obstruction K56.5
  intra-abdominal — *see* Adhesions, peritoneum
  iris H21.50-
    anterior H21.51-
    goniosynechiae H21.52-
    posterior H21.54-
    to corneal graft T85.898
  joint — *see* Ankylosis
    knee M23.8X
    temporomandibular M26.61-
  labium (majus) (minus) , congenital Q52.5
  liver — *see* Adhesions, peritoneum
  lung J98.4
  mediastinum J98.59
  meninges (cerebral) (spinal) G96.12
    congenital Q07.8
    tuberculous (cerebral) (spinal) A17.0
  mesenteric — *see* Adhesions, peritoneum
  nasal (septum) (to turbinates) J34.89
  ocular muscle — *see* Strabismus, mechanical
  omentum — *see* Adhesions, peritoneum
  ovary N73.6
    congenital (to cecum, kidney or omentum) Q50.39
  paraovarian N73.6
  pelvic (peritoneal)
    female N73.6
      postprocedural N99.4
    male — *see* Adhesions, peritoneum
    postpartal (old) N73.6
    tuberculous A18.17
  penis to scrotum (congenital) Q55.8
  periappendiceal — *see also* Adhesions, peritoneum
  pericardium (nonrheumatic) I31.0
    focal I31.8
    rheumatic I09.2
    tuberculous A18.84
  pericholecystic K82.8
  perigastric — *see* Adhesions, peritoneum
  periovarian N73.6
  periprostatic N42.89
  perirectal — *see* Adhesions, peritoneum
  perirenal N28.89
  peritoneum, peritoneal (postinfective)
    (postprocedural) K66.0
    with obstruction (intestinal) K56.5
    congenital Q43.3
    pelvic, female N73.6
      postprocedural N99.4
    postpartal, pelvic N73.6
    to uterus N73.6
  peritubal N73.6
  periureteral N28.89
  periuterine N73.6
  perivesical N32.89
  perivesicular (seminal vesicle) N50.89
  pleura, pleuritic J94.8
    tuberculous NEC A15.6
  pleuropericardial J94.8
  postoperative (gastrointestinal tract) K66.0
    with obstruction K91.3
    due to foreign body accidentally left in
      wound — *see* Foreign body, accidentally left
      during a procedure
    pelvic peritoneal N99.4
    urethra — *see* Stricture, urethra, postprocedural
    vagina N99.2
  postpartal, old (vulva or perineum) N90.89
  preputial, prepuce N47.5
  pulmonary J98.4
  pylorus — *see* Adhesions, peritoneum
  sciatic nerve — *see* Lesion, nerve, sciatic
  seminal vesicle N50.89

Adhesions, adhesive (postinfective) - *continued*
  shoulder (joint) — *see* Capsulitis, adhesive
  sigmoid flexure — *see* Adhesions, peritoneum
  spermatic cord (acquired) N50.89
    congenital Q55.4
  spinal canal G96.12
  stomach — *see* Adhesions, peritoneum
  subscapular — *see* Capsulitis, adhesive
  temporomandibular M26.61-
  tendinitis — *see also* Tenosynovitis, specified type
    NEC
    shoulder — *see* Capsulitis, adhesive
  testis N44.8
  tongue, congenital (to gum or roof of mouth) Q38.3
    acquired K14.8
  trachea J39.8
  tubo-ovarian N73.6
  tunica vaginalis N44.8
  uterus N73.6
    internal N85.6
    to abdominal wall N73.6
  vagina (chronic) N89.5
    postoperative N99.2
  vitreomacular H43.82-
  vitreous H43.89
  vulva N90.89
Adiaspiromycosis B48.8
Adie (-Holmes) **pupil or syndrome** — *see* Anomaly,
  pupil, function, tonic pupil
Adiponecrosis neonatorum P83.8
Adiposis — *see also* Obesity
  cerebralis E23.6
  dolorosa E88.2
Adiposity — *see also* Obesity
  heart — *see* Degeneration, myocardial
  localized E65
Adiposogenital dystrophy E23.6
Adjustment
  disorder — *see* Disorder, adjustment
  implanted device — *see* Encounter (for), adjustment
    (of)
  prosthesis, external — *see* Fitting
  reaction — *see* Disorder, adjustment
Administration of tPA (rtPA)
  **in a different facility within the last 24 hours
  prior to admission to current facility** Z92.82
Admission (for) — *see also* Encounter (for)
  adjustment (of)
    artificial
      arm Z44.00-
        complete Z44.01-
        partial Z44.02-
      eye Z44.2
      leg Z44.10-
        complete Z44.11-
        partial Z44.12-
    brain neuropacemaker Z46.2
      implanted Z45.42
    breast
      implant Z45.81
      prosthesis (external) Z44.3
    colostomy belt Z46.89
    contact lenses Z46.0
    cystostomy device Z46.6
    dental prosthesis Z46.3
    device NEC
      abdominal Z46.89
      implanted Z45.89
        cardiac Z45.09
          defibrillator (with synchronous cardiac
            pacemaker) Z45.02
          pacemaker (cardiac resynchronization therapy
            (CRT-P)) Z45.018
          pulse generator Z45.010
          resynchronization therapy defibrillator (CRT-
            D) Z45.02
        hearing device Z45.328
          bone conduction Z45.320
          cochlear Z45.321
        infusion pump Z45.1
        nervous system Z45.49
          CSF drainage Z45.41
          hearing device — *see* Admission, adjustment,
            device, implanted, hearing device
          neuropacemaker Z45.42
          visual substitution Z45.31
        specified NEC Z45.89
        vascular access Z45.2
        visual substitution Z45.31
      nervous system Z46.2
        implanted — *see* Admission, adjustment,
          device, implanted, nervous system
      orthodontic Z46.4

Admission (for) - *continued*
  adjustment (of) - *continued*
    device NEC - *continued*
      prosthetic Z44.9
        arm — *see* Admission, adjustment, artificial,
          arm
        breast Z44.3
        dental Z46.3
        eye Z44.2
        leg — *see* Admission, adjustment, artificial, leg
        specified type NEC Z44.8
      substitution
        auditory Z46.2
          implanted — *see* Admission, adjustment,
            device, implanted, hearing device
        nervous system Z46.2
          implanted — *see* Admission, adjustment,
            device, implanted, nervous system
        visual Z46.2
          implanted Z45.31
      urinary Z46.6
    hearing aid Z46.1
      implanted — *see* Admission, adjustment, device,
        implanted, hearing device
    ileostomy device Z46.89
    intestinal appliance or device NEC Z46.89
    neuropacemaker (brain) (peripheral nerve) (spinal
      cord) Z46.2
      implanted Z45.42
    orthodontic device Z46.4
    orthopedic (brace) (cast) (device) (shoes) Z46.89
    pacemaker (cardiac resynchronization therapy
      (CRT-P))
      cardiac Z45.018
        pulse generator Z45.010
      nervous system Z46.2
        implanted Z45.42
    portacath (port-a-cath) Z45.2
    prosthesis Z44.9
      arm — *see* Admission, adjustment, artificial, arm
      breast Z44.3
      dental Z46.3
      eye Z44.2
      leg — *see* Admission, adjustment, artificial, leg
      specified NEC Z44.8
    spectacles Z46.0
  aftercare — *see also* Aftercare Z51.89
    postpartum
      immediately after delivery Z39.0
      routine follow-up Z39.2
    radiation therapy (antineoplastic) Z51.0
  attention to artificial opening (of) Z43.9
    artificial vagina Z43.7
    colostomy Z43.3
    cystostomy Z43.5
    enterostomy Z43.4
    gastrostomy Z43.1
    ileostomy Z43.2
    jejunostomy Z43.4
    nephrostomy Z43.6
    specified site NEC Z43.8
      intestinal tract Z43.4
      urinary tract Z43.6
    tracheostomy Z43.0
    ureterostomy Z43.6
    urethrostomy Z43.6
  breast augmentation or reduction Z41.1
  breast reconstruction following mastectomy Z42.1
  change of
    dressing (nonsurgical) Z48.00
    neuropacemaker device (brain) (peripheral nerve)
      (spinal cord) Z46.2
      implanted Z45.42
    surgical dressing Z48.01
  circumcision, ritual or routine (in absence of
    diagnosis) Z41.2
  clinical research investigation (control) (normal
    comparison) (participant) Z00.6
  contraceptive management Z30.9
  cosmetic surgery NEC Z41.1
  counseling — *see also* Counseling
    dietary Z71.3
    gestational carrier Z31.7
    HIV Z71.7
    human immunodeficiency virus Z71.7
    nonattending third party Z71.0
    procreative management NEC Z31.69
  delivery, full-term, uncomplicated O80
    cesarean, without indication O82
  desensitization to allergens Z51.6
  dietary surveillance and counseling Z71.3
  ear piercing Z41.3

Admission (for) - *continued*
  examination at health care facility (adult) — *see*
    also Examination Z00.00
    with abnormal findings Z00.01
    clinical research investigation (control) (normal
     comparison) (participant) Z00.6
    dental Z01.20
     with abnormal findings Z01.21
    donor (potential) Z00.5
    ear Z01.10
     with abnormal findings NEC Z01.118
    eye Z01.00
     with abnormal findings Z01.01
    general, specified reason NEC Z00.8
    hearing Z01.10
     with abnormal findings NEC Z01.118
    postpartum checkup Z39.2
    psychiatric (general) Z00.8
     requested by authority Z04.6
    vision Z01.00
     with abnormal findings Z01.01
  fitting (of)
    artificial
     arm — *see* Admission, adjustment, artificial, arm
     eye Z44.2
     leg — *see* Admission, adjustment, artificial, leg
    brain neuropacemaker Z46.2
     implanted Z45.42
    breast prosthesis (external) Z44.3
    colostomy belt Z46.89
    contact lenses Z46.0
    cystostomy device Z46.6
    dental prosthesis Z46.3
    dentures Z46.3
    device NEC
     abdominal Z46.89
     nervous system Z46.2
      implanted — *see* Admission, adjustment,
       device, implanted, nervous system
     orthodontic Z46.4
     prosthetic Z44.9
      breast Z44.3
      dental Z46.3
      eye Z44.2
     substitution
      auditory Z46.2
       implanted — *see* Admission, adjustment,
        device, implanted, hearing device
      nervous system Z46.2
       implanted — *see* Admission, adjustment,
        device, implanted, nervous system
      visual Z46.2
       implanted Z45.31
    hearing aid Z46.1
    ileostomy device Z46.89
    intestinal appliance or device NEC Z46.89
    neuropacemaker (brain) (peripheral nerve) (spinal
     cord) Z46.2
     implanted Z45.42
    orthodontic device Z46.4
    orthopedic device (brace) (cast) (shoes) Z46.89
    prosthesis Z44.9
     arm — *see* Admission, adjustment, artificial, arm
     breast Z44.3
     dental Z46.3
     eye Z44.2
     leg — *see* Admission, adjustment, artificial, leg
     specified type NEC Z44.8
    spectacles Z46.0
  follow-up examination Z09
  intrauterine device management Z30.431
    initial prescription Z30.014
  mental health evaluation Z00.8
    requested by authority Z04.6
  observation — *see* Observation
  Papanicolaou smear, cervix Z12.4
    for suspected malignant neoplasm Z12.4
  plastic and reconstructive surgery following medical
    procedure or healed injury NEC Z42.8
  plastic surgery, cosmetic NEC Z41.1
  postpartum observation
    immediately after delivery Z39.0
    routine follow-up Z39.2
  poststerilization (for restoration) Z31.0
    aftercare Z31.42
  procreative management Z31.9
  prophylactic (measure) — *see also* Encounter,
    prophylactic measures
    organ removal Z40.00
     breast Z40.01
     ovary Z40.02
     specified organ NEC Z40.09
     testes Z40.09

Admission (for) - *continued*
  prophylactic (measure) - *continued*
    vaccination Z23
  psychiatric examination (general) Z00.8
    requested by authority Z04.6
  radiation therapy (antineoplastic) Z51.0
  reconstructive surgery following medical procedure
    or healed injury NEC Z42.8
  removal of
    cystostomy catheter Z43.5
    drains Z48.03
    dressing (nonsurgical) Z48.00
    implantable subdermal contraceptive Z30.46
    intrauterine contraceptive device Z30.432
    neuropacemaker (brain) (peripheral nerve) (spinal
     cord) Z46.2
     implanted Z45.42
    staples Z48.02
    surgical dressing Z48.01
    sutures Z48.02
    ureteral stent Z46.6
  respirator [ventilator] use during power
    failure Z99.12
  restoration of organ continuity
    (poststerilization) Z31.0
    aftercare Z31.42
  sensitivity test — *see also* Test, skin
    allergy NEC Z01.82
    Mantoux Z11.1
  tuboplasty following previous sterilization Z31.0
    aftercare Z31.42
  vasoplasty following previous sterilization Z31.0
    aftercare Z31.42
  vision examination Z01.00
    with abnormal findings Z01.01
  waiting period for admission to other facility Z75.1
Adnexitis (suppurative) — *see* Salpingo-oophoritis
Adolescent X-linked
  adrenoleukodystrophy E71.521
Adrenal (gland) — *see* condition
Adrenalism, tuberculous A18.7
Adrenalitis, adrenitis E27.8
  autoimmune E27.1
  meningococcal, hemorrhagic A39.1
Adrenarche, premature E27.0
Adrenocortical syndrome — *see* Cushing's,
  syndrome
Adrenogenital syndrome E25.9
  acquired E25.8
  congenital E25.0
  salt loss E25.0
Adrenogenitalism, congenital E25.0
Adrenoleukodystrophy E71.529
  neonatal E71.511
  X-linked E71.529
    Addison only phenotype E71.528
    Addison-Schilder E71.528
    adolescent E71.521
    adrenomyeloneuropathy E71.522
    childhood cerebral E71.520
    other specified E71.528
Adrenomyeloneuropathy E71.522
Adventitious bursa — *see* Bursopathy, specified type
  NEC
Adverse effect — *see* Table of Drugs and Chemicals,
  categories T36-T50, with 6th character 5
Advice — *see* Counseling
Adynamia (episodica) (hereditary) (periodic) G72.3
Aeration lung imperfect, newborn — *see*
  Atelectasis
Aerobullosis T70.3
Aerocele — *see* Embolism, air
Aerodermectasia
  subcutaneous (traumatic) T79.7
Aerodontalgia T70.29
Aeroembolism T70.3
Aerogenes capsulatus infection A48.0
Aero-otitis media T70.0
Aerophagy, aerophagia (psychogenic) F45.8
Aerophobia F40.228
Aerosinusitis T70.1
Aerotitis T70.0
Affection — *see* Disease
Afibrinogenemia — *see also* Defect,
  coagulation D68.8
  acquired D65
  congenital D68.2
  following ectopic or molar pregnancy O08.1
  in abortion — *see* Abortion, by type, complicated
    by, afibrinogenemia
  puerperal O72.3
African
  sleeping sickness B56.9

African - *continued*
  tick fever A68.1
  trypanosomiasis B56.9
    gambian B56.0
    rhodesian B56.1
Aftercare — *see also* Care Z51.89
  following surgery (for) (on)
    amputation Z47.81
    attention to
     drains Z48.03
     dressings (nonsurgical) Z48.00
      surgical Z48.01
     sutures Z48.02
    circulatory system Z48.812
    delayed (planned) wound closure Z48.1
    digestive system Z48.815
    explanation of joint prosthesis (staged procedure)
     hip Z47.32
     knee Z47.33
     shoulder Z47.31
    genitourinary system Z48.816
    joint replacement Z47.1
    neoplasm Z48.3
    nervous system Z48.811
    oral cavity Z48.814
    organ transplant
     bone marrow Z48.290
     heart Z48.21
     heart-lung Z48.280
     kidney Z48.22
     liver Z48.23
     lung Z48.24
     multiple organs NEC Z48.288
     specified NEC Z48.298
    orthopedic NEC Z47.89
    planned wound closure Z48.1
    removal of internal fixation device Z47.2
    respiratory system Z48.813
    scoliosis Z47.82
    sense organs Z48.810
    skin and subcutaneous tissue Z48.817
    specified body system
     circulatory Z48.812
     digestive Z48.815
     genitourinary Z48.816
     nervous Z48.811
     oral cavity Z48.814
     respiratory Z48.813
     sense organs Z48.810
     skin and subcutaneous tissue Z48.817
     teeth Z48.814
    specified NEC Z48.89
    spinal Z48.89
    teeth Z48.814
  fracture - code to fracture with seventh character D
  involving
    removal of
     drains Z48.03
     dressings (nonsurgical) Z48.00
     staples Z48.02
     surgical dressings Z48.01
     sutures Z48.02
  neuropacemaker (brain) (peripheral nerve) (spinal
    cord) Z46.2
    implanted Z45.42
  orthopedic NEC Z47.89
  postprocedural — *see* Aftercare, following surgery
After-cataract — *see* Cataract, secondary
Agalactia (primary) O92.3
  elective, secondary or therapeutic O92.5
Agammaglobulinemia (acquired (secondary))
  (nonfamilial) (nonfamilial) D80.1
  with
    immunoglobulin-bearing B-lymphocytes D80.1
    lymphopenia D81.9
  autosomal recessive (Swiss type) D80.0
  Bruton's X-linked D80.0
  common variable (CVAgamma) D80.1
  congenital sex-linked D80.0
  hereditary D80.0
  lymphopenic D81.9
  Swiss type (autosomal recessive) D80.0
  X-linked (with growth hormone deficiency)
    (Bruton) D80.0
Aganglionosis (bowel) (colon) Q43.1
Age (old) — *see* Senility
Agenesis
  adrenal (gland) Q89.1
  alimentary tract (complete) (partial) NEC Q45.8
    upper Q40.8
  anus, anal (canal) Q42.3
    with fistula Q42.2
  aorta Q25.41

Agenesis - *continued*
appendix Q42.8
arm (complete) Q71.0-
  with hand present Q71.1-
artery (peripheral) Q27.9
  brain Q28.3
  coronary Q24.5
  pulmonary Q25.79
  specified NEC Q27.8
  umbilical Q27.0
auditory (canal) (external) Q16.1
auricle (ear) Q16.0
bile duct or passage Q44.5
bladder Q64.5
bone Q79.9
brain Q00.0
  part of Q04.3
breast (with nipple present) Q83.8
  with absent nipple Q83.0
bronchus Q32.4
canaliculus lacrimalis Q10.4
carpus — *see* Agenesis, hand
cartilage Q79.9
cecum Q42.8
cerebellum Q04.3
cervix Q51.5
chin Q18.8
cilia Q10.3
circulatory system, part NOS Q28.9
clavicle Q74.0
clitoris Q52.6
coccyx Q76.49
colon Q42.9
  specified NEC Q42.8
corpus callosum Q04.0
cricoid cartilage Q31.8
diaphragm (with hernia) Q79.1
digestive organ (s) or tract (complete) (partial)
  NEC Q45.8
  upper Q40.8
ductus arteriosus Q28.8
duodenum Q41.0
ear Q16.9
  auricle Q16.0
  lobe Q17.8
ejaculatory duct Q55.4
endocrine (gland) NEC Q89.2
epiglottis Q31.8
esophagus Q39.8
eustachian tube Q16.2
eye Q11.1
  adnexa Q15.8
eyelid (fold) Q10.3
face
  bones NEC Q75.8
  specified part NEC Q18.8
fallopian tube Q50.6
femur — *see* Defect, reduction, lower limb,
  longitudinal, femur
fibula — *see* Defect, reduction, lower limb,
  longitudinal, fibula
finger (complete) (partial) — *see* Agenesis, hand
foot (and toes) (complete) (partial) Q72.3-
forearm (with hand present) — *see* Agenesis, arm,
  with hand present
  and hand Q71.2-
gallbladder Q44.0
gastric Q40.2
genitalia, genital (organ (s))
  female Q52.8
    external Q52.71
    internal NEC Q52.8
  male Q55.8
glottis Q31.8
hair Q84.0
hand (and fingers) (complete) (partial) Q71.3-
heart Q24.8
  valve NEC Q24.8
    pulmonary Q22.0
hepatic Q44.7
humerus — *see* Defect, reduction, upper limb
hymen Q52.4
ileum Q41.2
incus Q16.3
intestine (small) Q41.9
  large Q42.9
    specified NEC Q42.8
iris (dilator fibers) Q13.1
jaw M26.09
jejunum Q41.1
kidney (s) (partial) Q60.2
  bilateral Q60.1
  unilateral Q60.0

Agenesis - *continued*
labium (majus) (minus) Q52.71
labyrinth, membranous Q16.5
lacrimal apparatus Q10.4
larynx Q31.8
leg (complete) Q72.0-
  with foot present Q72.1-
  lower leg (with foot present) — *see* Agenesis, leg,
    with foot present
    and foot Q72.2-
lens Q12.3
limb (complete) Q73.0
  lower — *see* Agenesis, leg
  upper — *see* Agenesis, arm
lip Q38.0
liver Q44.7
lung (fissure) (lobe) (bilateral) (unilateral) Q33.3
mandible, maxilla M26.09
metacarpus — *see* Agenesis, hand
metatarsus — *see* Agenesis, foot
muscle Q79.8
  eyelid Q10.3
  ocular Q15.8
musculoskeletal system NEC Q79.8
nail (s) Q84.3
neck, part Q18.8
nerve Q07.8
nervous system, part NEC Q07.8
nipple Q83.2
nose Q30.1
nuclear Q07.8
organ
  of Corti Q16.5
  or site not listed — *see* Anomaly, by site
osseous meatus (ear) Q16.1
ovary
  bilateral Q50.02
  unilateral Q50.01
oviduct Q50.6
pancreas Q45.0
parathyroid (gland) Q89.2
parotid gland (s) Q38.4
patella Q74.1
pelvic girdle (complete) (partial) Q74.2
penis Q55.5
pericardium Q24.8
pituitary (gland) Q89.2
prostate Q55.4
punctum lacrimale Q10.4
radioulnar — *see* Defect, reduction, upper limb
radius — *see* Defect, reduction, upper limb,
  longitudinal, radius
rectum Q42.1
  with fistula Q42.0
renal Q60.2
  bilateral Q60.1
  unilateral Q60.0
respiratory organ NEC Q34.8
rib Q76.6
roof of orbit Q75.8
round ligament Q52.8
sacrum Q76.49
salivary gland Q38.4
scapula Q74.0
scrotum Q55.29
seminal vesicles Q55.4
septum
  atrial Q21.1
  between aorta and pulmonary artery Q21.4
  ventricular Q20.4
shoulder girdle (complete) (partial) Q74.0
skull (bone) Q75.8
  with
    anencephaly Q00.0
    encephalocele — *see* Encephalocele
    hydrocephalus Q03.9
      with spina bifida — *see* Spina bifida, by site,
        with hydrocephalus
    microcephaly Q02
spermatic cord Q55.4
spinal cord Q06.0
spine Q76.49
spleen Q89.01
sternum Q76.7
stomach Q40.2
submaxillary gland (s) (congenital) Q38.4
tarsus — *see* Agenesis, foot
tendon Q79.8
testicle Q55.0
thymus (gland) Q89.2
thyroid (gland) E03.1
  cartilage Q31.8

Agenesis - *continued*
tibia — *see* Defect, reduction, lower limb,
  longitudinal, tibia
tibiofibular — *see* Defect, reduction, lower limb,
  specified type NEC
toe (and foot) (complete) (partial) — *see* Agenesis,
  foot
tongue Q38.3
trachea (cartilage) Q32.1
ulna — *see* Defect, reduction, upper limb,
  longitudinal, ulna
upper limb — *see* Agenesis, arm
ureter Q62.4
urethra Q64.5
urinary tract NEC Q64.8
uterus Q51.0
uvula Q38.5
vagina Q52.0
vas deferens Q55.4
vein (s) (peripheral) Q27.9
  brain Q28.3
  great NEC Q26.8
  portal Q26.5
vena cava (inferior) (superior) Q26.8
vermis of cerebellum Q04.3
vertebra Q76.49
vulva Q52.71
Ageusia R43.2
Agitated — *see* condition
Agitation R45.1
Aglossia (congenital) Q38.3
Aglossia-adactylia syndrome Q87.0
Aglycogenosis E74.00
Agnosia (body image) (other senses) (tactile) R48.1
developmental F88
verbal R48.1
  auditory R48.1
    developmental F80.2
  developmental F80.2
visual (object) R48.3
Agoraphobia F40.00
with panic disorder F40.01
without panic disorder F40.02
Agrammatism R48.8
Agranulocytopenia — *see* Agranulocytosis
Agranulocytosis (chronic) (cyclical) (genetic)
  (infantile) (periodic) (pernicious) — *see*
  also Neutropenia D70.9
congenital D70.0
cytoreductive cancer chemotherapy sequela D70.1
drug-induced D70.2
  due to cytoreductive cancer chemotherapy D70.1
due to infection D70.3
secondary D70.4
  drug-induced D70.2
    due to cytoreductive cancer chemotherapy D70.1
Agraphia (absolute) R48.8
with alexia R48.0
developmental F81.81
Ague (dumb) — *see* Malaria
Agyria Q04.3
Ahumada-del Castillo syndrome E23.0
Aichomophobia F40.298
AIDS (related complex) B20
Ailment heart — *see* Disease, heart
Ailurophobia F40.218
AIN — *see* Neoplasia, intraepithelial, anal
Ainhum (disease) L94.6
AIPHI
  (acute idiopathic pulmonary hemorrhage in infants
  (over 28 days old)) R04.81
Air
anterior mediastinum J98.2
compressed, disease T70.3
conditioner lung or pneumonitis J67.7
embolism (artery) (cerebral) (any site) T79.0
  with ectopic or molar pregnancy O08.2
  due to implanted device NEC — *see*
    Complications, by site and type, specified NEC
  following
    abortion — *see* Abortion by type, complicated by,
      embolism
    ectopic or molar pregnancy O08.2
    infusion, therapeutic injection or
      transfusion T80.0
  in pregnancy, childbirth or puerperium — *see*
    Embolism, obstetric
  traumatic T79.0
hunger, psychogenic F45.8
rarefied, effects of — *see* Effect, adverse, high
  altitude
sickness T75.3
Airplane sickness T75.3

Akathisia (drug-induced) (treatment-induced) G25.71
  neuroleptic induced (acute) G25.71
Akinesia R29.898
Akinetic mutism R41.89
Akureyri's disease G93.3
Alactasia, congenital E73.0
Alagille's syndrome Q44.7
Alastrim B03
Albers-Schönberg syndrome Q78.2
Albert's syndrome — *see* Tendinitis, Achilles
Albinism, albino E70.30
  with hematologic abnormality E70.339
    Chédiak-Higashi syndrome E70.330
    Hermansky-Pudlak syndrome E70.331
    other specified E70.338
  I E70.320
  II E70.321
  ocular E70.319
    autosomal recessive E70.311
    other specified E70.318
    X-linked E70.310
  oculocutaneous E70.329
    other specified E70.328
    tyrosinase (ty) negative E70.320
    tyrosinase (ty) positive E70.321
  other specified E70.39
Albinismus E70.30
Albright (-McCune) (-Sternberg) **syndrome** Q78.1
Albuminous — *see* condition
Albuminuria, albuminuric (acute) (chronic)
  (subacute) — *see also* Proteinuria R80.9
  complicating pregnancy — *see* Proteinuria,
    gestational
    with
      gestational hypertension — *see* Pre-eclampsia
      pre-existing hypertension — *see* Hypertension,
        complicating pregnancy, pre-existing, with, pre-
        eclampsia
  gestational — *see* Proteinuria, gestational
    with
      gestational hypertension — *see* Pre-eclampsia
      pre-existing hypertension — *see* Hypertension,
        complicating pregnancy, pre-existing, with, pre-
        eclampsia
  orthostatic R80.2
  postural R80.2
  pre-eclamptic — *see* Pre-eclampsia
  scarlatinal A38.8
Albuminurophobia F40.298
Alcaptonuria E70.29
Alcohol, alcoholic, alcohol-induced
  addiction (without remission) F10.20
    with remission F10.21
  amnestic disorder, persisting F10.96
    with dependence F10.26
  anxiety disorder F10.980
  bipolar and related disorder F10.94
  depressive disorder F10.94
  major neurocognitive disorder, amnestic-
    confabulatory type F10.96
  major neurocognitive disorder, nonamnestic-
    confabulatory type F10.97
  mild neurocognitive disorder F10.988
  psychotic disorder F10.959
  sexual dysfunction F10.981
  sleep disorder F10.982
  brain syndrome, chronic F10.97
    with dependence F10.27
  cardiopathy I42.6
  counseling and surveillance Z71.41
    family member Z71.42
  delirium (acute) (tremens) (withdrawal) F10.231
    with intoxication F10.921
      in
        abuse F10.121
        dependence F10.221
  dementia F10.97
    with dependence F10.27
  deterioration F10.97
    with dependence F10.27
  hallucinosis (acute) F10.951
    in
      abuse F10.151
      dependence F10.251
  insanity F10.959
  intoxication (acute) (without dependence) F10.129
    with
      delirium F10.121
      dependence F10.229
        with delirium F10.221
        uncomplicated F10.220
      uncomplicated F10.120
  jealousy F10.988

Alcohol, alcoholic, alcohol-induced - *continued*
  Korsakoff's, Korsakov's, Korsakow's F10.26
  liver K70.9
    acute — *see* Disease, liver, alcoholic, hepatitis
  mania (acute) (chronic) F10.959
  paranoia, paranoid (type) psychosis F10.950
  pellagra E52
  poisoning, accidental (acute) NEC — *see* Table of
    Drugs and Chemicals, alcohol, poisoning
  psychosis — *see* Psychosis, alcoholic
  withdrawal (without convulsions) F10.239
    with delirium F10.231
Alcoholism (chronic) (without remission) F10.20
  with
    psychosis — *see* Psychosis, alcoholic
    remission F10.21
    Korsakov's F10.96
    with dependence F10.26
Alder (-Reilly) **anomaly or syndrome**
  (leukocyte granulation) D72.0
Aldosteronism E26.9
  familial (type I) E26.02
  glucocorticoid-remediable E26.02
  primary (due to (bilateral) adrenal
    hyperplasia) E26.09
  primary NEC E26.09
  secondary E26.1
  specified NEC E26.89
Aldosteronoma D44.10
Aldrich (-Wiskott) **syndrome**
  (eczema-thrombocytopenia) D82.0
Alektorophobia F40.218
Aleppo boil B55.1
Aleukemic — *see* condition
Aleukia
  congenital D70.0
  hemorrhagica D61.9
    congenital D61.09
  splenica D73.1
Alexia R48.0
  developmental F81.0
  secondary to organic lesion R48.0
Algoneurodystrophy M89.00
  ankle M89.07-
  foot M89.07-
  forearm M89.03-
  hand M89.04-
  lower leg M89.06-
  multiple sites M89.0-
  shoulder M89.01-
  specified site NEC M89.08
  thigh M89.05-
  upper arm M89.02-
Algophobia F40.298
Alienation, mental — *see* Psychosis
Alkalemia E87.3
Alkalosis E87.3
  metabolic E87.3
    with respiratory acidosis E87.4
  respiratory E87.3
Alkaptonuria E70.29
Allen-Masters syndrome N83.8
Allergy, allergic (reaction) (to) T78.40
  air-borne substance NEC (rhinitis) J30.89
  alveolitis (extrinsic) J67.9
    due to
      Aspergillus clavatus J67.4
      Cryptostroma corticale J67.6
      organisms (fungal, thermophilic actinomycete)
        growing in ventilation (air conditioning)
        systems J67.7
    specified type NEC J67.8
  anaphylactic reaction or shock T78.2
  angioneurotic edema T78.3
  animal (dander) (epidermal) (hair) (rhinitis) J30.81
  bee sting (anaphylactic shock) — *see* Toxicity,
    venom, arthropod, bee
  biological — *see* Allergy, drug
  colitis — *see also* Colitis, allergic K52.29
  dander (animal) (rhinitis) J30.81
  dandruff (rhinitis) J30.81
  dental restorative material (existing) K08.55
  dermatitis — *see* Dermatitis, contact, allergic
  diathesis — *see* History, allergy
  drug, medicament & biological (any) (external)
    (internal) T78.40
    correct substance properly administered — *see*
      Table of Drugs and Chemicals, by drug, adverse
      effect
    wrong substance given or taken NEC (by
      accident) — *see* Table of Drugs and Chemicals,
      by drug, poisoning
  due to pollen J30.1

Allergy, allergic (reaction) (to) - *continued*
  dust (house) (stock) (rhinitis) J30.89
    with asthma — *see* Asthma, allergic extrinsic
  eczema — *see* Dermatitis, contact, allergic
  epidermal (animal) (rhinitis) J30.81
  feathers (rhinitis) J30.89
  food (any) (ingested) NEC T78.1
    anaphylactic shock — *see* Shock, anaphylactic,
      due to food
    dermatitis — *see* Dermatitis, due to, food
    dietary counseling and surveillance Z71.3
    in contact with skin L23.6
    rhinitis J30.5
    status (without reaction) Z91.018
      eggs Z91.012
      milk products Z91.011
      peanuts Z91.010
      seafood Z91.013
      specified NEC Z91.018
  gastrointestinal — *see also* specific type of allergic
    reaction
    meaning colitis — *see also* Colitis, allergic K52.29
    meaning gastroenteritis — *see also* Gastroenteritis,
      allergic K52.29
    meaning other adverse food reaction not elsewhere
      classified T78.1
  grain J30.1
  grass (hay fever) (pollen) J30.1
    asthma — *see* Asthma, allergic extrinsic
  hair (animal) (rhinitis) J30.81
  history (of) — *see* History, allergy
  horse serum — *see* Allergy, serum
  inhalant (rhinitis) J30.89
    pollen J30.1
  kapok (rhinitis) J30.89
  medicine — *see* Allergy, drug
  milk protein — *see also* Allergy, food Z91.011
    anaphylactic reaction T78.07
    dermatitis L27.2
    enterocolitis syndrome K52.21
    enteropathy K52.22
    gastroenteritis K52.29
    gastroesophageal reflux — *see also* Reaction,
      adverse, food K21.9
      with esophagitis K21.0
    proctocolitis K52.82
  nasal, seasonal due to pollen J30.1
  pneumonia J82
  pollen (any) (hay fever) J30.1
    asthma — *see* Asthma, allergic extrinsic
  primrose J30.1
  primula J30.1
  proctocolitis K52.82
  purpura D69.0
  ragweed (hay fever) (pollen) J30.1
    asthma — *see* Asthma, allergic extrinsic
  rose (pollen) J30.1
  seasonal NEC J30.2
  Senecio jacobae (pollen) J30.1
  serum — *see also* Reaction, serum T80.69
    anaphylactic shock T80.59
  shock (anaphylactic) T78.2
    due to
      administration of blood and blood
        products T80.51
      adverse effect of correct medicinal substance
        properly administered T88.6
      immunization T80.52
      serum NEC T80.59
      vaccination T80.52
    specific NEC T78.49
  tree (any) (hay fever) (pollen) J30.1
    asthma — *see* Asthma, allergic extrinsic
  upper respiratory J30.9
  urticaria L50.0
  vaccine — *see* Allergy, serum
  wheat — *see* Allergy, food
Allescheriasis B48.2
Alligator skin disease Q80.9
Allocheiria, allochiria R20.8
Almeida's disease — *see* Paracoccidioidomycosis
Alopecia (hereditaria) (seborrheica) L65.9
  androgenic L64.9
    drug-induced L64.0
    specified NEC L64.8
  areata L63.9
    ophiasis L63.2
    specified NEC L63.8
    totalis L63.0
    universalis L63.1
  cicatricial L66.9
    specified NEC L66.8
  circumscripta L63.9

Alopecia (hereditaria) (seborrheica) - *continued*
  congenital, congenitalis Q84.0
  due to cytotoxic drugs NEC L65.8
  mucinosa L65.2
  postinfective NEC L65.8
  postpartum L65.0
  premature L64.8
  specific (syphilitic) A51.32
  specified NEC L65.8
  syphilitic (secondary) A51.32
  totalis (capitis) L63.0
  universalis (entire body) L63.1
  X-ray L58.1
Alpers' disease G31.81
Alpine sickness T70.29
Alport syndrome Q87.81
ALTE (apparent life threatening event)
  in newborn and infant R68.13
Alteration (of) , **Altered**
  awareness
    transient R40.4
    unintended under general anesthesia, during
      procedureT88.53
  mental status R41.82
  pattern of family relationships affecting
    child Z62.898
  sensation
    following
      cerebrovascular disease I69.998
        cerebral infarction I69.398
        intracerebral hemorrhage I69.198
        nontraumatic intracranial hemorrhage
          NEC I69.298
        specified disease NEC I69.898
        subarachnoid hemorrhage I69.098
Alternating — *see* condition
Altitude, high (effects) — *see* Effect, adverse, high
  altitude
Aluminosis (of lung) J63.0
Alveolitis
  allergic (extrinsic) — *see* Pneumonitis,
    hypersensitivity
  due to
    Aspergillus clavatus J67.4
    Cryptostroma corticale J67.6
  fibrosing (cryptogenic) (idiopathic) J84.112
  jaw M27.3
  sicca dolorosa M27.3
Alveolus, alveolar — *see* condition
Alymphocytosis D72.810
  thymic (with immunodeficiency) D82.1
Alymphoplasia, thymic D82.1
Alzheimer's disease or sclerosis — *see* Disease,
  Alzheimer's
Amastia (with nipple present) Q83.8
  with absent nipple Q83.0
Amathophobia F40.228
Amaurosis (acquired) (congenital) — *see*
  also Blindness
  fugax G45.3
  hysterical F44.6
  Leber's congenital H35.50
  uremic — *see* Uremia
Amaurotic idiocy (infantile) (juvenile) (late) E75.4
Amaxophobia F40.248
Ambiguous genitalia Q56.4
Amblyopia (congenital) (ex anopsia) (partial)
  (suppression) H53.00-
  anisometropic — *see* Amblyopia, refractive
  deprivation H53.01-
  hysterical F44.6
  nocturnal — *see also* Blindness, night
    vitamin A deficiency E50.5
  refractive H53.02-
  strabismic H53.03-
  suspect H53.04-
  tobacco H53.8
  toxic NEC H53.8
  uremic — *see* Uremia
Ameba, amebic (histolytica) — *see also* Amebiasis
  abscess (liver) A06.4
Amebiasis A06.9
  with abscess — *see* Abscess, amebic
  acute A06.0
  chronic (intestine) A06.1
    with abscess — *see* Abscess, amebic
  cutaneous A06.7
  cutis A06.7
  cystitis A06.81
  genitourinary tract NEC A06.82
  hepatic — *see* Abscess, liver, amebic
  intestine A06.0
  nondysenteric colitis A06.2

Amebiasis - *continued*
  skin A06.7
  specified site NEC A06.89
Ameboma (of intestine) A06.3
Amelia Q73.0
  lower limb — *see* Agenesis, leg
  upper limb — *see* Agenesis, arm
Ameloblastoma — *see also* Cyst, calcifying
  odontogenic
  long bones C40.9-
    lower limb C40.2-
    upper limb C40.0-
  malignant C41.1
    jaw (bone) (lower) C41.1
      upper C41.0
  tibial C40.2-
Amelogenesis imperfecta K00.5
  nonhereditaria (segmentalis) K00.4
Amenorrhea N91.2
  hyperhormonal E28.8
  primary N91.0
  secondary N91.1
Amentia — *see* Disability, intellectual
  Meynert's (nonalcoholic) F04
American
  leishmaniasis B55.2
  mountain tick fever A93.2
Ametropia — *see* Disorder, refraction
AMH (asymptomatic microscopic hematuria) R31.21
Amianthosis J61
Amimia R48.8
Amino-acid disorder E72.9
  anemia D53.0
Aminoacidopathy E72.9
Aminoaciduria E72.9
Amnes (t) **ic syndrome** (post-traumatic) F04
  induced by
    alcohol F10.96
      with dependence F10.26
    psychoactive NEC F19.96
      with
        abuse F19.16
        dependence F19.26
    sedative F13.96
      with dependence F13.26
Amnesia R41.3
  anterograde R41.1
  auditory R48.8
  dissociative F44.0
    with dissociative fugue F44.1
  hysterical F44.0
  postictal in epilepsy — *see* Epilepsy
  psychogenic F44.0
  retrograde R41.2
  transient global G45.4
Amnion, amniotic — *see* condition
Amnionitis — *see* Pregnancy, complicated by
Amok F68.8
Amoral traits F60.89
Amphetamine (or other stimulant) **-induced**
  anxiety disorder F15.980
  bipolar and related disorder F15.94
  delirium F15.921
  depressive disorder F15.94
  obsessive-compulsive and related disorder F15.988
  psychotic disorder F15.959
  sexual dysfunction F15.981
  sleep disorder F15.982
  stimulant withdrawal F15.23
Ampulla
  lower esophagus K22.8
  phrenic K22.8
Amputation — *see also* Absence, by site, acquired
  neuroma (postoperative) (traumatic) — *see*
    Complications, amputation stump, neuroma
  stump (surgical)
    abnormal, painful, or with complication
      (late) — *see* Complications, amputation stump
    healed or old NOS Z89.9
  traumatic (complete) (partial)
    arm (upper) (complete) S48.91-
      at
        elbow S58.01-
          partial S58.02-
        shoulder joint (complete) S48.01-
          partial S48.02-
      between
        elbow and wrist (complete) S58.11-
          partial S58.12-
        shoulder and elbow (complete) S48.11-
          partial S48.12-
      partial S48.92-
    breast (complete) S28.21-

Amputation - *continued*
  traumatic (complete) (partial) - *continued*
    breast (complete) - *continued*
      partial S28.22-
    clitoris (complete) S38.211
      partial S38.212
    ear (complete) S08.11-
      partial S08.12-
    finger (complete) (metacarpophalangeal) S68.11-
      index S68.11-
      little S68.11-
      middle S68.11-
      partial S68.12-
        index S68.12-
        little S68.12-
        middle S68.12-
        ring S68.12-
      ring S68.11-
      thumb — *see* Amputation, traumatic, thumb
      transphalangeal (complete) S68.61-
        index S68.61-
        little S68.61-
        middle S68.61-
        partial S68.62-
          index S68.62-
          little S68.62-
          middle S68.62-
          ring S68.62-
        ring S68.61-
    foot (complete) S98.91-
      at ankle level S98.01-
        partial S98.02-
      midfoot S98.31-
        partial S98.32-
      partial S98.92-
    forearm (complete) S58.91-
      at elbow level (complete) S58.01-
        partial S58.02-
      between elbow and wrist (complete) S58.11-
        partial S58.12-
      partial S58.92-
    genital organ (s) (external)
      female (complete) S38.211
        partial S38.212
      male
        penis (complete) S38.221
          partial S38.222
        scrotum (complete) S38.231
          partial S38.232
        testes (complete) S38.231
          partial S38.232
    hand (complete) (wrist level) S68.41-
      finger (s) alone — *see* Amputation, traumatic,
        finger
      partial S68.42-
      thumb alone — *see* Amputation, traumatic,
        thumb
      transmetacarpal (complete) S68.71-
        partial S68.72-
    head
      ear — *see* Amputation, traumatic, ear
      nose (partial) S08.812
        complete S08.811
        part S08.89
        scalp S08.0
    hip (and thigh) (complete) S78.91-
      at hip joint (complete) S78.01-
        partial S78.02-
      between hip and knee (complete) S78.11-
        partial S78.12-
      partial S78.92-
    labium (majus) (minus) (complete) S38.21-
      partial S38.21-
    leg (lower) S88.91-
      at knee level S88.01-
        partial S88.02-
      between knee and ankle S88.11-
        partial S88.12-
      partial S88.92-
    nose (partial) S08.812
      complete S08.811
    penis (complete) S38.221
      partial S38.222
    scrotum (complete) S38.231
      partial S38.232
    shoulder — *see* Amputation, traumatic, arm
      at shoulder joint — *see* Amputation, traumatic,
        arm, at shoulder joint
    testes (complete) S38.231
      partial S38.232
    thigh — *see* Amputation, traumatic, hip
    thorax, part of S28.1
      breast — *see* Amputation, traumatic, breast

Amputation - *continued*
  traumatic (complete) (partial) - *continued*
    thumb (complete) (metacarpophalangeal) S68.01-
      partial S68.02-
      transphalangeal (complete) S68.51-
        partial S68.52-
    toe (lesser) S98.13-
      great S98.11-
        partial S98.12-
      more than one S98.21-
        partial S98.22-
        partial S98.14-
    vulva (complete) S38.211
      partial S38.212
Amputee (bilateral) (old) Z89.9
Amsterdam dwarfism Q87.1
Amusia R48.8
  developmental F80.89
Amyelencephalus, amyelencephaly Q00.0
Amyelia Q06.0
Amygdalitis — *see* Tonsillitis
Amygdalolith J35.8
Amyloid heart (disease) E85.4 *[I43]*
Amyloidosis (generalized) (primary) E85.9
  with lung involvement E85.4 *[J99]*
  familial E85.2
  genetic E85.2
  heart E85.4 *[I43]*
  hemodialysis-associated E85.3
  liver E85.4 *[K77]*
  localized E85.4
  neuropathic heredofamilial E85.1
  non-neuropathic heredofamilial E85.0
  organ limited E85.4
  Portuguese E85.1
  pulmonary E85.4 *[J99]*
  secondary systemic E85.3
  skin (lichen) (macular) E85.4 *[L99]*
  specified NEC E85.8
  subglottic E85.4 *[J99]*
Amylopectinosis (brancher enzyme
    deficiency) E74.03
Amylophagia — *see* Pica
Amyoplasia congenita Q79.8
Amyotonia M62.89
  congenita G70.2
Amyotrophia, amyotrophy, amyotrophic G71.8
  congenita Q79.8
  diabetic — *see* Diabetes, amyotrophy
  lateral sclerosis G12.21
  neuralgic G54.5
  spinal progressive G12.21
Anacidity, gastric K31.83
  psychogenic F45.8
Anaerosis of newborn P28.89
Analbuminemia E88.09
Analgesia — *see* Anesthesia
Analphalipoproteinemia E78.6
Anaphylactic
  purpura D69.0
  shock or reaction — *see* Shock, anaphylactic
Anaphylactoid shock or reaction — *see* Shock,
    anaphylactic
Anaphylactoid syndrome of pregnancy O88.01-
Anaphylaxis — *see* Shock, anaphylactic
Anaplasia cervix — *see also* Dysplasia, cervix N87.9
Anaplasmosis, human A77.49
Anarthria R47.1
Anasarca R60.1
  cardiac — *see* Failure, heart, congestive
  lung J18.2
  newborn P83.2
  nutritional E43
  pulmonary J18.2
  renal N04.9
Anastomosis
  aneurysmal — *see* Aneurysm
  arteriovenous ruptured brain I60.8
  intestinal K63.89
    complicated NEC K91.89
      involving urinary tract N99.89
  retinal and choroidal vessels (congenital) Q14.8
Anatomical narrow angle H40.03-
Ancylostoma, ancylostomiasis (braziliense)
    (caninum) (ceylanicum) (duodenale) B76.0
  Necator americanus B76.1
Andersen's disease (glycogen storage) E74.09
Anderson-Fabry disease E75.21
Andes disease T70.29
Andrews' disease (bacterid) L08.89
Androblastoma
  benign
    specified site — *see* Neoplasm, benign, by site

Androblastoma - *continued*
  benign - *continued*
    unspecified site
      female D27.9
      male D29.20
  malignant
    specified site — *see* Neoplasm, malignant, by site
    unspecified site
      female C56.9
      male C62.90
  specified site — *see* Neoplasm, uncertain behavior,
    by site
  tubular
    with lipid storage
      specified site — *see* Neoplasm, benign, by site
      unspecified site
        female D27.9
        male D29.20
    specified site — *see* Neoplasm, benign, by site
    unspecified site
      female D27.9
      male D29.20
  unspecified site
    female D39.10
    male D40.10
Androgen insensitivity syndrome — *see*
    also Syndrome, androgen insensitivity E34.50
Androgen resistance syndrome — *see*
    also Syndrome, androgen insensitivity E34.50
Android pelvis Q74.2
  with disproportion (fetopelvic) O33.3
    causing obstructed labor O65.3
Androphobia F40.290
Anectasis, pulmonary (newborn) — *see* Atelectasis
Anemia (essential) (general) (hemoglobin deficiency)
    (infantile) (primary) (profound) D64.9
  with (due to) (in)
    disorder of
      anaerobic glycolysis D55.2
      pentose phosphate pathway D55.1
    koilonychia D50.9
  achlorhydric D50.8
  achrestic D53.1
  Addison (-Biermer) (pernicious) D51.0
  agranulocytic — *see* Agranulocytosis
  amino-acid-deficiency D53.0
  aplastic D61.9
    congenital D61.09
    drug-induced D61.1
    due to
      drugs D61.1
      external agents NEC D61.2
      infection D61.2
      radiation D61.2
    idiopathic D61.3
    red cell (pure) D60.9
      chronic D60.0
      congenital D61.01
      specified type NEC D60.8
      transient D60.1
    specified type NEC D61.89
    toxic D61.2
  aregenerative
    congenital D61.09
  asiderotic D50.9
  atypical (primary) D64.9
  Baghdad spring D55.0
  Balantidium coli A07.0
  Biermer's (pernicious) D51.0
  blood loss (chronic) D50.0
    acute D62
  bothriocephalus B70.0 *[D63.8]*
  brickmaker's B76.9 *[D63.8]*
  cerebral I67.89
  childhood D58.9
  chlorotic D50.8
  chronic
    blood loss D50.0
    hemolytic D58.9
      idiopathic D59.9
    simple D53.9
  chronica congenita aregenerativa D61.09
  combined system disease NEC D51.0 *[G32.0]*
    due to dietary vitamin B12
      deficiency D51.3 *[G32.0]*
  complicating pregnancy, childbirth or
    puerperium — *see* Pregnancy, complicated by
    (management affected by), anemia
  congenital P61.4
    aplastic D61.09
    due to isoimmunization NOS P55.9
    dyserythropoietic, dyshematopoietic D64.4
    following fetal blood loss P61.3

Anemia (essential) (general) (hemoglobin deficiency)
    (infantile) (primary) (profound) - *continued*
  congenital - *continued*
    Heinz body D58.2
    hereditary hemolytic NOS D58.9
    pernicious D51.0
    spherocytic D58.0
  Cooley's (erythroblastic) D56.1
  cytogenic D51.0
  deficiency D53.9
    2, 3 diphosphoglycurate mutase D55.2
    2, 3 PG D55.2
    6 phosphogluconate dehydrogenase D55.1
    6-PGD D55.1
    amino-acid D53.0
    combined B12 and folate D53.1
    enzyme D55.9
      drug-induced (hemolytic) D59.2
      glucose-6-phosphate dehydrogenase
        (G6PD) D55.0
      glycolytic D55.2
      nucleotide metabolism D55.3
      related to hexose monophosphate (HMP) shunt
        pathway NEC D55.1
      specified type NEC D55.8
    erythrocytic glutathione D55.1
    folate D52.9
      dietary D52.0
      drug-induced D52.1
    folic acid D52.9
      dietary D52.0
      drug-induced D52.1
    G SH D55.1
    GGS-R D55.1
    glucose-6-phosphate dehydrogenase D55.0
    glutathione reductase D55.1
    glyceraldehyde phosphate dehydrogenase D55.2
    G6PD D55.0
    hexokinase D55.2
    iron D50.9
      secondary to blood loss (chronic) D50.0
    nutritional D53.9
      with
        poor iron absorption D50.8
        specified deficiency NEC D53.8
    phosphofructo-aldolase D55.2
    phosphoglycerate kinase D55.2
    PK D55.2
    protein D53.0
    pyruvate kinase D55.2
    transcobalamin II D51.2
    triose-phosphate isomerase D55.2
    vitamin B12 NOS D51.9
      dietary D51.3
      due to
        intrinsic factor deficiency D51.0
        selective vitamin B12 malabsorption with
          proteinuria D51.1
      pernicious D51.0
      specified type NEC D51.8
  Diamond-Blackfan (congenital hypoplastic) D61.01
  dibothriocephalus B70.0 *[D63.8]*
  dimorphic D53.1
  diphasic D53.1
  Diphyllobothrium
    (Dibothriocephalus) B70.0 *[D63.8]*
  due to (in) (with)
    antineoplastic chemotherapy D64.81
    blood loss (chronic) D50.0
      acute D62
    chemotherapy, antineoplastic D64.81
    chronic disease classified elsewhere NEC D63.8
    chronic kidney disease D63.1
    deficiency
      amino-acid D53.0
      copper D53.8
      folate (folic acid) D52.9
        dietary D52.0
        drug-induced D52.1
      molybdenum D53.8
      protein D53.0
      zinc D53.8
    dietary vitamin B12 deficiency D51.3
    disorder of
      glutathione metabolism D55.1
      nucleotide metabolism D55.3
    drug — *see* Anemia, by type — *see also* Table of
      Drugs and Chemicals
    end stage renal disease D63.1
    enzyme disorder D55.9
    fetal blood loss P61.3
    fish tapeworm (D.latum) infestation B70.0 *[D63.8]*
  hemorrhage (chronic) D50.0

Anemia (essential) (general) (hemoglobin deficiency) (infantile) (primary) (profound) - *continued*
due to (in) (with) - *continued*
hemorrhage (chronic) - *continued*
acute D62
impaired absorption D50.9
loss of blood (chronic) D50.0
acute D62
myxedema E03.9 *[D63.8]*
Necator americanus B76.1 *[D63.8]*
prematurity P61.2
selective vitamin B12 malabsorption with
proteinuria D51.1
transcobalamin II deficiency D51.2
Dyke-Young type (secondary) (symptomatic) D59.1
dyserythropoietic (congenital) D64.4
dyshematopoietic (congenital) D64.4
Egyptian B76.9 *[D63.8]*
elliptocytosis — *see* Elliptocytosis
enzyme-deficiency, drug-induced D59.2
epidemic — *see*
also Ancylostomiasis B76.9 *[D63.8]*
erythroblastic
familial D56.1
newborn — *see also* Disease, hemolytic P55.9
of childhood D56.1
erythrocytic glutathione deficiency D55.1
erythropoietin-resistant anemia (EPO resistant
anemia) D63.1
Faber's (achlorhydric anemia) D50.9
factitious (self-induced blood letting) D50.0
familial erythroblastic D56.1
Fanconi's (congenital pancytopenia) D61.09
favism D55.0
fish tapeworm (D. latum) infestation B70.0 *[D63.8]*
folate (folic acid) deficiency D52.9
glucose-6-phosphate dehydrogenase (G6PD)
deficiency D55.0
glutathione-reductase deficiency D55.1
goat's milk D52.0
granulocytic — *see* Agranulocytosis
Heinz body, congenital D58.2
hemolytic D58.9
acquired D59.9
with hemoglobinuria NEC D59.6
autoimmune NEC D59.1
infectious D59.4
specified type NEC D59.8
toxic D59.4
acute D59.9
due to enzyme deficiency specified type
NEC D55.8
Lederer's D59.1
autoimmune D59.1
drug-induced D59.0
chronic D58.9
idiopathic D59.9
cold type (secondary) (symptomatic) D59.1
congenital (spherocytic) — *see* Spherocytosis
due to
cardiac conditions D59.4
drugs (nonautoimmune) D59.2
autoimmune D59.0
enzyme disorder D55.9
drug-induced D59.2
presence of shunt or other internal prosthetic
device D59.4
familial D58.9
hereditary D58.9
due to enzyme disorder D55.9
specified type NEC D55.8
specified type NEC D58.8
idiopathic (chronic) D59.9
mechanical D59.4
microangiopathic D59.4
nonautoimmune D59.4
drug-induced D59.2
nonspherocytic
congenital or hereditary NEC D55.8
glucose-6-phosphate dehydrogenase
deficiency D55.0
pyruvate kinase deficiency D55.2
type
I D55.1
II D55.2
type
I D55.1
II D55.2
secondary D59.4
autoimmune D59.1
specified (hereditary) type NEC D58.8
Stransky-Regala type — *see*
also Hemoglobinopathy D58.8

Anemia (essential) (general) (hemoglobin deficiency) (infantile) (primary) (profound) - *continued*
hemolytic - *continued*
symptomatic D59.4
autoimmune D59.1
toxic D59.4
warm type (secondary) (symptomatic) D59.1
hemorrhagic (chronic) D50.0
acute D62
Herrick's D57.1
hexokinase deficiency D55.2
hookworm B76.9 *[D63.8]*
hypochromic (idiopathic) (microcytic)
(normoblastic) D50.9
due to blood loss (chronic) D50.0
acute D62
familial sex-linked D64.0
pyridoxine-responsive D64.3
sideroblastic, sex-linked D64.0
hypoplasia, red blood cells D61.9
congenital or familial D61.01
hypoplastic (idiopathic) D61.9
congenital or familial (of childhood) D61.01
hypoproliferative (refractive) D61.9
idiopathic D64.9
aplastic D61.3
hemolytic, chronic D59.9
in (due to) (with)
chronic kidney disease D63.1
end stage renal disease D63.1
failure, kidney (renal) D63.1
neoplastic disease — *see also* Neoplasm D63.0
intertropical — *see also* Ancylostomiasis D63.8
iron deficiency D50.9
secondary to blood loss (chronic) D50.0
acute D62
specified type NEC D50.8
Joseph-Diamond-Blackfan (congenital
hypoplastic) D61.01
Lederer's (hemolytic) D59.1
leukoerythroblastic D61.82
macrocytic D53.9
nutritional D52.0
tropical D52.8
malarial — *see also* Malaria B54 *[D63.8]*
malignant (progressive) D51.0
malnutrition D53.9
marsh — *see also* Malaria B54 *[D63.8]*
Mediterranean (with other
hemoglobinopathy) D56.9
megaloblastic D53.1
combined B12 and folate deficiency D53.1
hereditary D51.1
nutritional D52.0
orotic aciduria D53.0
refractory D53.1
specified type NEC D53.1
megalocytic D53.1
microcytic (hypochromic) D50.9
due to blood loss (chronic) D50.0
acute D62
familial D56.8
microdrepanocytosis D57.40
microelliptopoikilocytic (Rietti-Greppi-
Micheli) D56.9
miner's B76.9 *[D63.8]*
myelodysplastic D46.9
myelofibrosis D75.81
myelogenous D64.89
myelopathic D64.89
myelophthisic D61.82
myeloproliferative D47.Z9
newborn P61.4
due to
ABO (antibodies, isoimmunization,
maternal/fetal incompatibility) P55.1
Rh (antibodies, isoimmunization, maternal/fetal
incompatibility) P55.0
following fetal blood loss P61.3
posthemorrhagic (fetal) P61.3
nonspherocytic hemolytic — *see* Anemia,
hemolytic, nonspherocytic
normocytic (infectional) D64.9
due to blood loss (chronic) D50.0
acute D62
myelophthisic D61.82
nutritional (deficiency) D53.9
with
poor iron absorption D50.8
specified deficiency NEC D53.8
megaloblastic D52.0
of prematurity P61.2
orotaciduric (congenital) (hereditary) D53.0

Anemia (essential) (general) (hemoglobin deficiency) (infantile) (primary) (profound) - *continued*
osteosclerotic D64.89
ovalocytosis (hereditary) — *see* Elliptocytosis
paludal — *see also* Malaria B54 *[D63.8]*
pernicious (congenital) (malignant)
(progressive) D51.0
pleochromic D64.89
of sprue D52.8
posthemorrhagic (chronic) D50.0
acute D62
newborn P61.3
postoperative (postprocedural)
due to (acute) blood loss D62
chronic blood loss D50.0
specified NEC D64.9
postpartum O90.81
pressure D64.89
progressive D64.9
malignant D51.0
pernicious D51.0
protein-deficiency D53.0
pseudoleukemica infantum D64.89
pure red cell D60.9
congenital D61.01
pyridoxine-responsive D64.3
pyruvate kinase deficiency D55.2
refractory D46.4
with
excess of blasts D46.20
1 (RAEB 1) D46.21
2 (RAEB 2) D46.22
in transformation (RAEB T) — *see* Leukemia,
acute myeloblastic
hemochromatosis D46.1
sideroblasts (ring) (RARS) D46.1
megaloblastic D53.1
sideroblastic D46.1
sideropenic D50.9
without ring sideroblasts, so stated D46.0
without sideroblasts without excess of blasts D46.0
Rietti-Greppi-Micheli D56.9
scorbutic D53.2
secondary to
blood loss (chronic) D50.0
acute D62
hemorrhage (chronic) D50.0
acute D62
semiplastic D61.89
sickle-cell — *see* Disease, sickle-cell
sideroblastic D64.3
hereditary D64.0
hypochromic, sex-linked D64.0
pyridoxine-responsive NEC D64.3
refractory D46.1
secondary (due to)
disease D64.1
drugs and toxins D64.2
specified type NEC D64.3
sideropenic (refractory) D50.9
due to blood loss (chronic) D50.0
acute D62
simple chronic D53.9
specified type NEC D64.89
spherocytic (hereditary) — *see* Spherocytosis
splenic D64.89
splenomegalic D64.89
stomatocytosis D58.8
syphilitic (acquired) (late) A52.79 *[D63.8]*
target cell D64.89
thalassemia D56.9
thrombocytopenic — *see* Thrombocytopenia
toxic D61.2
tropical B76.9 *[D63.8]*
macrocytic D52.8
tuberculous A18.89 *[D63.8]*
vegan D51.3
vitamin
B6-responsive D64.3
B12 deficiency (dietary) pernicious D51.0
von Jaksch's D64.89
Witts' (achlorhydric anemia) D50.8
Anemophobia F40.228
Anencephalus, anencephaly Q00.0
Anergasia — *see* Psychosis, organic
Anesthesia, anesthetic R20.0
complication or reaction NEC — *see*
also Complications, anesthesia T88.59
due to
correct substance properly administered — *see*
Table of Drugs and Chemicals, by drug, adverse
effect

Anesthesia, anesthetic - *continued*
complication or reaction NEC - *continued*
due to - *continued*
overdose or wrong substance given — *see* Table of Drugs and Chemicals, by drug, poisoning
unintended awareness under general anesthesia during procedure T88.53
personal history of Z92.84
cornea H18.81-
dissociative F44.6
functional (hysterical) F44.6
hyperesthetic, thalamic G89.0
hysterical F44.6
local skin lesion R20.0
sexual (psychogenic) F52.1
shock (due to) T88.2
skin R20.0
testicular N50.9
Anetoderma (maculosum) (of) L90.8
Jadassohn-Pellizzari L90.2
Schweniger-Buzzi L90.1
Aneurin deficiency E51.9
Aneurysm (anastomotic) (artery) (cirsoid) (diffuse) (false) (fusiform) (multiple) (saccular) I72.9
abdominal (aorta) I71.4
ruptured I71.3
syphilitic A52.01
aorta, aortic (nonsyphilitic) I71.9
abdominal I71.4
ruptured I71.3
arch I71.2
ruptured I71.1
arteriosclerotic I71.9
ruptured I71.8
ascending I71.2
ruptured I71.1
congenital Q25.43
descending I71.9
abdominal I71.4
ruptured I71.3
ruptured I71.8
thoracic I71.2
ruptured I71.1
root Q25.43
ruptured I71.8
sinus, congenital Q25.43
syphilitic A52.01
thoracic I71.2
ruptured I71.1
thoracoabdominal I71.6
ruptured I71.5
thorax, thoracic (arch) I71.2
ruptured I71.1
transverse I71.2
ruptured I71.1
valve (heart) — *see also* Endocarditis, aortic I35.8
arteriosclerotic I72.9
cerebral I67.1
ruptured — *see* Hemorrhage, intracranial, subarachnoid
arteriovenous (congenital) — *see also* Malformation, arteriovenous
acquired I77.0
brain I67.1
coronary I25.41
pulmonary I28.0
brain Q28.2
ruptured I60.8
peripheral — *see* Malformation, arteriovenous, peripheral
precerebral vessels Q28.0
specified site NEC — *see also* Malformation, arteriovenous
acquired I77.0
basal — *see* Aneurysm, brain
basilar (trunk) I72.5
berry (congenital) (nonruptured) I67.1
ruptured I60.7
brain I67.1
arteriosclerotic I67.1
ruptured — *see* Hemorrhage, intracranial, subarachnoid
arteriovenous (congenital) (nonruptured) Q28.2
acquired I67.1
ruptured I60.8
ruptured I60.8
berry (congenital) (nonruptured) I67.1
ruptured — *see also* Hemorrhage, intracranial, subarachnoid I60.7
congenital Q28.3
ruptured I60.7
meninges I67.1
ruptured I60.8

Aneurysm (anastomotic) (artery) (cirsoid) (diffuse) (false) (fusiform) (multiple) (saccular) - *continued*
brain - *continued*
miliary (congenital) (nonruptured) I67.1
ruptured — *see also* Hemorrhage, intracranial, subarachnoid I60.7
mycotic I33.0
ruptured — *see* Hemorrhage, intracranial, subarachnoid
syphilitic (hemorrhage) A52.05
cardiac (false) — *see also* Aneurysm, heart I25.3
carotid artery (common) (external) I72.0
internal (intracranial) I67.1
extracranial portion I72.0
ruptured into brain I60.0-
syphilitic A52.09
intracranial A52.05
cavernous sinus I67.1
arteriovenous (congenital) (nonruptured) Q28.3
ruptured I60.8
celiac I72.8
central nervous system, syphilitic A52.05
cerebral — *see* Aneurysm, brain
chest — *see* Aneurysm, thorax
circle of Willis I67.1
congenital Q28.3
ruptured I60.6
ruptured I60.6
common iliac artery I72.3
congenital (peripheral) Q27.8
aorta (root) (sinus) Q25.43
brain Q28.3
ruptured I60.7
coronary Q24.5
digestive system Q27.8
lower limb Q27.8
pulmonary Q25.79
retina Q14.1
specified site NEC Q27.8
upper limb Q27.8
conjunctiva — *see* Abnormality, conjunctiva, vascular
conus arteriosus — *see* Aneurysm, heart
coronary (arteriosclerotic) (artery) I25.41
arteriovenous, congenital Q24.5
congenital Q24.5
ruptured — *see* Infarct, myocardium
syphilitic A52.06
vein I25.89
cylindroid (aorta) I71.9
ruptured I71.8
syphilitic A52.01
ductus arteriosus Q25.0
endocardial, infective (any valve) I33.0
femoral (artery) (ruptured) I72.4
gastroduodenal I72.8
gastroepiploic I72.8
heart (wall) (chronic or with a stated duration of over 4 weeks) I25.3
valve — *see* Endocarditis
hepatic I72.8
iliac (common) (artery) (ruptured) I72.3
infective I72.9
endocardial (any valve) I33.0
innominate (nonsyphilitic) I72.8
syphilitic A52.09
interauricular septum — *see* Aneurysm, heart
interventricular septum — *see* Aneurysm, heart
intrathoracic (nonsyphilitic) I71.2
ruptured I71.1
syphilitic A52.01
lower limb I72.4
lung (pulmonary artery) I28.1
mediastinal (nonsyphilitic) I72.8
syphilitic A52.09
miliary (congenital) I67.1
ruptured — *see* Hemorrhage, intracerebral, subarachnoid, intracranial
mitral (heart) (valve) I34.8
mural — *see* Aneurysm, heart
mycotic I72.9
endocardial (any valve) I33.0
ruptured, brain — *see* Hemorrhage, intracerebral, subarachnoid
myocardium — *see* Aneurysm, heart
neck I72.0
pancreaticoduodenal I72.8
patent ductus arteriosus Q25.0
peripheral NEC I72.8
congenital Q27.8
digestive system Q27.8
lower limb Q27.8
specified site NEC Q27.8

Aneurysm (anastomotic) (artery) (cirsoid) (diffuse) (false) (fusiform) (multiple) (saccular) - *continued*
peripheral NEC - *continued*
congenital - *continued*
upper limb Q27.8
popliteal (artery) (ruptured) I72.4
precerebral
congenital (nonruptured) Q28.1
specified site, NEC I72.5
pulmonary I28.1
arteriovenous Q25.72
acquired I28.0
syphilitic A52.09
valve (heart) — *see* Endocarditis, pulmonary
racemose (peripheral) I72.9
congenital — *see* Aneurysm, congenital
radial I72.1
Rasmussen NEC A15.0
renal (artery) I72.2
retina — *see also* Disorder, retina, microaneurysms
congenital Q14.1
diabetic — *see* Diabetes, microaneurysms, retinal
sinus of Valsalva Q25.49
specified NEC I72.8
spinal (cord) I72.8
syphilitic (hemorrhage) A52.09
splenic I72.8
subclavian (artery) (ruptured) I72.8
syphilitic A52.09
superior mesenteric I72.8
syphilitic (aorta) A52.01
central nervous system A52.05
congenital (late) A50.54 *[I79.0]*
spine, spinal A52.09
thoracoabdominal (aorta) I71.6
ruptured I71.5
syphilitic A52.01
thorax, thoracic (aorta) (arch) (nonsyphilitic) I71.2
ruptured I71.1
syphilitic A52.01
traumatic (complication) (early) , specified site — *see* Injury, blood vessel
tricuspid (heart) (valve) I07.8
ulnar I72.1
upper limb (ruptured) I72.1
valve, valvular — *see* Endocarditis
venous — *see also* Varix I86.8
congenital Q27.8
digestive system Q27.8
lower limb Q27.8
specified site NEC Q27.8
upper limb Q27.8
ventricle — *see* Aneurysm, heart
vertebral artery I72.6
visceral NEC I72.8
Angelman syndrome Q93.5
Anger R45.4
Angiectasis, angiectopia I99.8
Angiitis I77.6
allergic granulomatous M30.1
hypersensitivity M31.0
necrotizing M31.9
specified NEC M31.8
nervous system, granulomatous I67.7
Angina (attack) (cardiac) (chest) (heart) (pectoris) (syndrome) (vasomotor) I20.9
with
atherosclerotic heart disease — *see* Arteriosclerosis, coronary (artery), documented spasm I20.1
abdominal K55.1
accelerated — *see* Angina, unstable
agranulocytic — *see* Agranulocytosis
angiospastic — *see* Angina, with documented spasm
aphthous B08.5
crescendo — *see* Angina, unstable
croupous J05.0
cruris I73.9
de novo effort — *see* Angina, unstable
diphtheritic, membranous A36.0
equivalent I20.8
exudative, chronic J37.0
following acute myocardial infarction I23.7
gangrenous diphtheritic A36.0
intestinal K55.1
Ludovici K12.2
Ludwig's K12.2
malignant diphtheritic A36.0
membranous J05.0
diphtheritic A36.0
Vincent's A69.1
mesenteric K55.1
monocytic — *see* Mononucleosis, infectious

Angina (attack) (cardiac) (chest) (heart) (pectoris) (syndrome) (vasomotor) - *continued*
  of effort — *see* Angina, specified NEC
  phlegmonous J36
    diphtheritic A36.0
  post-infarctional I23.7
  pre-infarctional — *see* Angina, unstable
  Prinzmetal — *see* Angina, with documented spasm
  progressive — *see* Angina, unstable
  pseudomembranous A69.1
  pultaceous, diphtheritic A36.0
  spasm-induced — *see* Angina, with documented spasm
  specified NEC I20.8
  stable I20.8
  stenocardia — *see* Angina, specified NEC
  stridulous, diphtheritic A36.2
  tonsil J36
  trachealis J05.0
  unstable I20.0
  variant — *see* Angina, with documented spasm
  Vincent's A69.1
  worsening effort — *see* Angina, unstable
Angioblastoma — *see* Neoplasm, connective tissue, uncertain behavior
Angiocholecystitis — *see* Cholecystitis, acute
Angiocholitis — *see also* Cholecystitis, acute K83.0
Angiodysgenesis spinalis G95.19
Angiodysplasia (cecum) (colon) K55.20
  with bleeding K55.21
  duodenum (and stomach) K31.819
    with bleeding K31.811
  stomach (and duodenum) K31.819
    with bleeding K31.811
Angioedema (allergic) (any site) (with urticaria) T78.3
  hereditary D84.1
Angioendothelioma — *see* Neoplasm, uncertain behavior, by site
  benign D18.00
    intra-abdominal D18.03
    intracranial D18.02
    skin D18.01
    specified site NEC D18.09
  bone — *see* Neoplasm, bone, malignant
  Ewing's — *see* Neoplasm, bone, malignant
Angioendotheliomatosis C85.8-
Angiofibroma — *see also* Neoplasm, benign, by site
  juvenile
    specified site — *see* Neoplasm, benign, by site
    unspecified site D10.6
Angiohemophilia (A) (B) D68.0
Angioid streaks (choroid) (macula) (retina) H35.33
Angiokeratoma — *see* Neoplasm, skin, benign
  corporis diffusum E75.21
Angioleiomyoma — *see* Neoplasm, connective tissue, benign
Angiolipoma — *see also* Lipoma
  infiltrating — *see* Lipoma
Angioma — *see also* Hemangioma, by site
  capillary I78.1
  hemorrhagicum hereditaria I78.0
  intra-abdominal D18.03
  intracranial D18.02
  malignant — *see* Neoplasm, connective tissue, malignant
  plexiform D18.00
    intra-abdominal D18.03
    intracranial D18.02
    skin D18.01
    specified site NEC D18.09
  senile I78.1
  serpiginosum L81.7
  skin D18.01
  specified site NEC D18.09
  spider I78.1
  stellate I78.1
  venous Q28.3
Angiomatosis Q82.8
  bacillary A79.89
  encephalotrigeminal Q85.8
  hemorrhagic familial I78.0
  hereditary familial I78.0
  liver K76.4
Angiomyolipoma — *see* Lipoma
Angiomyoliposarcoma — *see* Neoplasm, connective tissue, malignant
Angiomyoma — *see* Neoplasm, connective tissue, benign
Angiomyosarcoma — *see* Neoplasm, connective tissue, malignant
Angiomyxoma — *see* Neoplasm, connective tissue, uncertain behavior

Angioneurosis F45.8
Angioneurotic edema (allergic) (any site) (with urticaria) T78.3
  hereditary D84.1
Angiopathia, angiopathy I99.9
  cerebral I67.9
    amyloid E85.4 *[I68.0]*
  diabetic (peripheral) — *see* Diabetes, angiopathy
  peripheral I73.9
    diabetic — *see* Diabetes, angiopathy
    specified type NEC I73.89
  retinae syphilitica A52.05
  retinalis (juvenilis)
    diabetic — *see* Diabetes, retinopathy
    proliferative — *see* Retinopathy, proliferative
Angiosarcoma — *see also* Neoplasm, connective tissue, malignant
  liver C22.3
Angiosclerosis — *see* Arteriosclerosis
Angiospasm (peripheral) (traumatic) (vessel) I73.9
  brachial plexus G54.0
  cerebral G45.9
  cervical plexus G54.2
  nerve
    arm — *see* Mononeuropathy, upper limb
      axillary G54.0
      median — *see* Lesion, nerve, median
      ulnar — *see* Lesion, nerve, ulnar
    axillary G54.0
    leg — *see* Mononeuropathy, lower limb
    median — *see* Lesion, nerve, median
    plantar — *see* Lesion, nerve, plantar
    ulnar — *see* Lesion, nerve, ulnar
Angiospastic disease or edema I73.9
Angiostrongyliasis
  due to
    Parastrongylus
      cantonensis B83.2
      costaricensis B81.3
  intestinal B81.3
Anguillulosis — *see* Strongyloidiasis
Angulation
  cecum — *see* Obstruction, intestine
  coccyx (acquired) (*see also* subcategory) M43.8
    congenital NEC Q76.49
  femur (acquired) — *see also* Deformity, limb, specified type NEC, thigh
    congenital Q74.2
  intestine (large) (small) — *see* Obstruction, intestine
  sacrum (acquired) (*see also* subcategory) M43.8
    congenital NEC Q76.49
  sigmoid (flexure) — *see* Obstruction, intestine
  spine — *see* Dorsopathy, deforming, specified NEC
  tibia (acquired) — *see also* Deformity, limb, specified type NEC, lower leg
    congenital Q74.2
  ureter N13.5
    with infection N13.6
  wrist (acquired) — *see also* Deformity, limb, specified type NEC, forearm
    congenital Q74.0
Angulus infectiosus (lips) K13.0
Anhedonia R45.84
  sexual F52.0
Anhidrosis L74.4
Anhydration E86.0
Anhydremia E86.0
Anidrosis L74.4
Aniridia (congenital) Q13.1
Anisakiasis (infection) (infestation) B81.0
Anisakis larvae infestation B81.0
Aniseikonia H52.32
Anisocoria (pupil) H57.02
  congenital Q13.2
Anisocytosis R71.8
Anisometropia (congenital) H52.31
Ankle — *see* condition
Ankyloblepharon (eyelid) (acquired) — *see also* Blepharophimosis
  filiforme (adnatum) (congenital) Q10.3
  total Q10.3
Ankyloglossia Q38.1
Ankylosis (fibrous) (osseous) (joint) M24.60
  ankle M24.67-
  arthrodesis status Z98.1
  cricoarytenoid (cartilage) (joint) (larynx) J38.7
  dental K03.5
  ear ossicles H74.31-
  elbow M24.62-
  foot M24.67-
  hand M24.64-
  hip M24.65-

Ankylosis (fibrous) (osseous) (joint) - *continued*
  incostapedial joint (infectional) — *see* Ankylosis, ear ossicles
  jaw (temporomandibular) M26.61-
  knee M24.66-
  lumbosacral (joint) M43.27
  postoperative (status) Z98.1
  produced by surgical fusion, status Z98.1
  sacro-iliac (joint) M43.28
  shoulder M24.61-
  spine (joint) — *see also* Fusion, spine
    spondylitic — *see* Spondylitis, ankylosing
  surgical Z98.1
  temporomandibular M26.61-
  tooth, teeth (hard tissues) K03.5
  wrist M24.63-
Ankylostoma — *see* Ancylostoma
Ankylostomiasis — *see* Ancylostomiasis
Ankylurethria — *see* Stricture, urethra
Annular — *see also* condition
  detachment, cervix N88.8
  organ or site, congenital NEC — *see* Distortion
  pancreas (congenital) Q45.1
Anodontia (complete) (partial) (vera) K00.0
  acquired K08.10
Anomaly, anomalous (congenital) (unspecified type) Q89.9
  abdominal wall NEC Q79.59
  acoustic nerve Q07.8
  adrenal (gland) Q89.1
  Alder (-Reilly) (leukocyte granulation) D72.0
  alimentary tract Q45.9
    upper Q40.9
  alveolar M26.70
    hyperplasia M26.79
      mandibular M26.72
      maxillary M26.71
    hypoplasia M26.79
      mandibular M26.74
      maxillary M26.73
    ridge (process) M26.79
    specified NEC M26.79
  ankle (joint) Q74.2
  anus Q43.9
  aorta (arch) NEC Q25.40
    coarctation (preductal) (postductal) Q25.1
  aortic cusp or valve Q23.9
  appendix Q43.8
  apple peel syndrome Q41.1
  aqueduct of Sylvius Q03.0
    with spina bifida — *see* Spina bifida, with hydrocephalus
  arm Q74.0
  arteriovenous NEC
    coronary Q24.5
    gastrointestinal Q27.33
      acquired — *see* Angiodysplasia
  artery (peripheral) Q27.9
    basilar NEC Q28.1
    cerebral Q28.3
    coronary Q24.5
    digestive system Q27.8
    eye Q15.8
    great Q25.9
      specified NEC Q25.8
    lower limb Q27.8
    peripheral Q27.9
      specified NEC Q27.8
    pulmonary NEC Q25.79
    renal Q27.2
    retina Q14.1
    specified site NEC Q27.8
    subclavian Q27.8
      origin Q25.48
    umbilical Q27.0
    upper limb Q27.8
    vertebral NEC Q28.1
  aryteno-epiglottic folds Q31.8
  atrial
    bands or folds Q20.8
    septa Q21.1
  atrioventricular
    excitation I45.6
    septum Q21.0
  auditory canal Q17.8
  auricle
    ear Q17.8
      causing impairment of hearing Q16.9
    heart Q20.8
  Axenfeld's Q15.0
  back Q89.9
  band
    atrial Q20.8

Anomaly, anomalous (congenital) (unspecified type)
- *continued*
  - band - *continued*
    - heart Q24.8
    - ventricular Q24.8
  - Bartholin's duct Q38.4
  - biliary duct or passage Q44.5
  - bladder Q64.70
    - absence Q64.5
    - diverticulum Q64.6
    - exstrophy Q64.10
      - cloacal Q64.12
      - extroversion Q64.19
      - specified type NEC Q64.19
      - supravesical fissure Q64.11
    - neck obstruction Q64.31
    - specified type NEC Q64.79
  - bone Q79.9
    - arm Q74.0
    - face Q75.9
    - leg Q74.2
    - pelvic girdle Q74.2
    - shoulder girdle Q74.0
    - skull Q75.9
      - with
        - anencephaly Q00.0
        - encephalocele — *see* Encephalocele
        - hydrocephalus Q03.9
          - with spina bifida — *see* Spina bifida, by site, with hydrocephalus
        - microcephaly Q02
  - brain (multiple) Q04.9
    - vessel Q28.3
  - breast Q83.9
  - broad ligament Q50.6
  - bronchus Q32.4
  - bulbus cordis Q21.9
  - bursa Q79.9
  - canal of Nuck Q52.4
  - canthus Q10.3
  - capillary Q27.9
  - cardiac Q24.9
    - chambers Q20.9
      - specified NEC Q20.8
    - septal closure Q21.9
      - specified NEC Q21.8
    - valve NEC Q24.8
      - pulmonary Q22.3
  - cardiovascular system Q28.8
  - carpus Q74.0
  - caruncle, lacrimal Q10.6
  - cascade stomach Q40.2
  - cauda equina Q06.3
  - cecum Q43.9
  - cerebral Q04.9
    - vessels Q28.3
  - cervix Q51.9
  - Chédiak-Higashi (-Steinbrinck) (congenital gigantism of peroxidase granules) E70.330
  - cheek Q18.9
  - chest wall Q67.8
    - bones Q76.9
  - chin Q18.9
  - chordae tendineae Q24.8
  - choroid Q14.3
    - plexus Q07.8
  - chromosomes, chromosomal Q99.9
    - D (1) — *see* condition, chromosome 13
    - E (3) — *see* condition, chromosome 18
    - G — *see* condition, chromosome 21
    - sex
      - female phenotype Q97.8
      - gonadal dysgenesis (pure) Q99.1
      - Klinefelter's Q98.4
      - male phenotype Q98.9
      - Turner's Q96.9
    - specified NEC Q99.8
  - cilia Q10.3
  - circulatory system Q28.9
  - clavicle Q74.0
  - clitoris Q52.6
  - coccyx Q76.49
  - colon Q43.9
  - common duct Q44.5
  - communication
    - coronary artery Q24.5
    - left ventricle with right atrium Q21.0
  - concha (ear) Q17.3
  - connection
    - portal vein Q26.5
    - pulmonary venous Q26.4
      - partial Q26.3
      - total Q26.2

Anomaly, anomalous (congenital) (unspecified type)
- *continued*
  - connection - *continued*
    - renal artery with kidney Q27.2
  - cornea (shape) Q13.4
  - coronary artery or vein Q24.5
  - cranium — *see* Anomaly, skull
  - cricoid cartilage Q31.8
  - cystic duct Q44.5
  - dental
    - alveolar — *see* Anomaly, alveolar
    - arch relationship M26.20
      - specified NEC M26.29
  - dentofacial M26.9
    - alveolar — *see* Anomaly, alveolar
    - dental arch relationship M26.20
      - specified NEC M26.29
    - functional M26.50
      - specified NEC M26.59
    - jaw-cranial base relationship M26.10
      - asymmetry M26.12
        - maxillary M26.11
      - specified type NEC M26.19
    - jaw size M26.00
      - macrogenia M26.05
      - mandibular
        - hyperplasia M26.03
        - hypoplasia M26.04
      - maxillary
        - hyperplasia M26.01
        - hypoplasia M26.02
      - microgenia M26.06
      - specified type NEC M26.09
    - malocclusion M26.4
      - dental arch relationship NEC M26.29
      - jaw-cranial base relationship — *see* Anomaly, dentofacial, jaw-cranial base relationship
      - jaw size — *see* Anomaly, dentofacial, jaw size
      - specified type NEC M26.89
    - temporomandibular joint M26.60-
      - adhesions M26.61-
      - ankylosis M26.61-
      - arthralgia M26.62-
      - articular disc M26.63-
      - specified type NEC M26.69
    - tooth position, fully erupted M26.30
      - specified NEC M26.39
  - dermatoglyphic Q82.8
  - diaphragm (apertures) NEC Q79.1
  - digestive organ (s) or tract Q45.9
    - lower Q43.9
    - upper Q40.9
  - distance, interarch (excessive) (inadequate) M26.25
  - distribution, coronary artery Q24.5
  - ductus
    - arteriosus Q25.0
    - botalli Q25.0
  - duodenum Q43.9
  - dura (brain) Q04.9
    - spinal cord Q06.9
  - ear (external) Q17.9
    - causing impairment of hearing Q16.9
    - inner Q16.5
    - middle (causing impairment of hearing) Q16.4
    - ossicles Q16.3
  - Ebstein's (heart) (tricuspid valve) Q22.5
  - ectodermal Q82.9
  - Eisenmenger's (ventricular septal defect) Q21.8
  - ejaculatory duct Q55.4
  - elbow Q74.0
  - endocrine gland NEC Q89.2
  - epididymis Q55.4
  - epiglottis Q31.8
  - esophagus Q39.9
  - eustachian tube Q17.8
  - eye Q15.9
    - anterior segment Q13.9
      - specified NEC Q13.89
    - posterior segment Q14.9
      - specified NEC Q14.8
    - ptosis (eyelid) Q10.0
    - specified NEC Q15.8
  - eyebrow Q18.8
  - eyelid Q10.3
    - ptosis Q10.0
  - face Q18.9
    - bone (s) Q75.9
  - fallopian tube Q50.6
  - fascia Q79.9
  - femur NEC Q74.2
  - fibula NEC Q74.2
  - finger Q74.0
  - fixation, intestine Q43.3

Anomaly, anomalous (congenital) (unspecified type)
- *continued*
  - flexion (joint) NOS Q74.9
    - hip or thigh Q65.89
  - foot NEC Q74.2
    - varus (congenital) Q66.3
  - foramen
    - Botalli Q21.1
    - ovale Q21.1
  - forearm Q74.0
  - forehead Q75.8
  - form, teeth K00.2
  - fovea centralis Q14.1
  - frontal bone — *see* Anomaly, skull
  - gallbladder (position) (shape) (size) Q44.1
  - Gartner's duct Q52.4
  - gastrointestinal tract Q45.9
  - genitalia, genital organ (s) or system
    - female Q52.9
      - external Q52.70
      - internal NOS Q52.9
    - male Q55.9
      - hydrocele P83.5
      - specified NEC Q55.8
  - genitourinary NEC
    - female Q52.9
    - male Q55.9
  - Gerbode Q21.0
  - glottis Q31.8
  - granulation or granulocyte, genetic (constitutional) (leukocyte) D72.0
  - gum Q38.6
  - gyri Q07.9
  - hair Q84.2
  - hand Q74.0
  - hard tissue formation in pulp K04.3
  - head — *see* Anomaly, skull
  - heart Q24.9
    - auricle Q20.8
    - bands or folds Q24.8
    - fibroelastosis cordis I42.4
    - obstructive NEC Q22.6
    - patent ductus arteriosus (Botalli) Q25.0
    - septum Q21.9
      - auricular Q21.1
      - interatrial Q21.1
      - interventricular Q21.0
        - with pulmonary stenosis or atresia, dextraposition of aorta and hypertrophy of right ventricle Q21.3
      - specified NEC Q21.8
      - ventricular Q21.0
        - with pulmonary stenosis or atresia, dextraposition of aorta and hypertrophy of right ventricle Q21.3
    - tetralogy of Fallot Q21.3
    - valve NEC Q24.8
      - aortic
        - bicuspid valve Q23.1
        - insufficiency Q23.1
        - stenosis Q23.0
          - subaortic Q24.4
      - mitral
        - insufficiency Q23.3
        - stenosis Q23.2
      - pulmonary Q22.3
        - atresia Q22.0
        - insufficiency Q22.2
        - stenosis Q22.1
          - infundibular Q24.3
          - subvalvular Q24.3
      - tricuspid
        - atresia Q22.4
        - stenosis Q22.4
    - ventricle Q20.8
  - heel NEC Q74.2
  - Hegglin's D72.0
  - hemianencephaly Q00.0
  - hemicephaly Q00.0
  - hemicrania Q00.0
  - hepatic duct Q44.5
  - hip NEC Q74.2
  - hourglass stomach Q40.2
  - humerus Q74.0
  - hydatid of Morgagni
    - female Q50.5
    - male (epididymal) Q55.4
    - testicular Q55.29
  - hymen Q52.4
  - hypersegmentation of neutrophils, hereditary D72.0
  - hypophyseal Q89.2
  - ileocecal (coil) (valve) Q43.9
  - ileum Q43.9

Anomaly, anomalous (congenital) (unspecified type)
- *continued*
  ilium NEC Q74.2
  integument Q84.9
    specified NEC Q84.8
  interarch distance (excessive) (inadequate) M26.25
  intervertebral cartilage or disc Q76.49
  intestine (large) (small) Q43.9
    with anomalous adhesions, fixation or malrotation Q43.3
  iris Q13.2
  ischium NEC Q74.2
  jaw — *see* Anomaly, dentofacial
    alveolar — *see* Anomaly, alveolar
  jaw-cranial base relationship — *see* Anomaly, dentofacial, jaw-cranial base relationship
  jejunum Q43.8
  joint Q74.9
    specified NEC Q74.8
  Jordan's D72.0
  kidney (s) (calyx) (pelvis) Q63.9
    artery Q27.2
    specified NEC Q63.8
  Klippel-Feil (brevicollis) Q76.1
  knee Q74.1
  labium (majus) (minus) Q52.70
  labyrinth, membranous Q16.5
  lacrimal apparatus or duct Q10.6
  larynx, laryngeal (muscle) Q31.9
    web (bed) Q31.0
  lens Q12.9
  leukocytes, genetic D72.0
    granulation (constitutional) D72.0
  lid (fold) Q10.3
  ligament Q79.9
    broad Q50.6
    round Q52.8
  limb Q74.9
    lower NEC Q74.2
      reduction deformity — *see* Defect, reduction, lower limb
    upper Q74.0
  lip Q38.0
  liver Q44.7
    duct Q44.5
  lower limb NEC Q74.2
  lumbosacral (joint) (region) Q76.49
    kyphosis — *see* Kyphosis, congenital
    lordosis — *see* Lordosis, congenital
  lung (fissure) (lobe) Q33.9
  mandible — *see* Anomaly, dentofacial
  maxilla — *see* Anomaly, dentofacial
  May (-Hegglin) D72.0
  meatus urinarius NEC Q64.79
  meningeal bands or folds Q07.9
    constriction of Q07.8
    spinal Q06.9
  meninges Q07.9
    cerebral Q04.8
    spinal Q06.9
  meningocele Q05.9
  mesentery Q45.9
  metacarpus Q74.0
  metatarsus NEC Q74.2
  middle ear Q16.4
    ossicles Q16.3
  mitral (leaflets) (valve) Q23.9
    insufficiency Q23.3
    specified NEC Q23.8
    stenosis Q23.2
  mouth Q38.6
  Müllerian — *see also* Anomaly, by site
    uterus NEC Q51.818
  multiple NEC Q89.7
  muscle Q79.9
    eyelid Q10.3
  musculoskeletal system, except limbs Q79.9
  myocardium Q24.8
  nail Q84.6
  narrowness, eyelid Q10.3
  nasal sinus (wall) Q30.8
  neck (any part) Q18.9
  nerve Q07.9
    acoustic Q07.8
    optic Q07.8
  nervous system (central) Q07.9
  nipple Q83.9
  nose, nasal (bones) (cartilage) (septum) (sinus) Q30.9
    specified NEC Q30.8
  ocular muscle Q15.8
  omphalomesenteric duct Q43.0
  opening, pulmonary veins Q26.4

Anomaly, anomalous (congenital) (unspecified type)
- *continued*
  optic
    disc Q14.2
    nerve Q07.8
  opticociliary vessels Q13.2
  orbit (eye) Q10.7
  organ Q89.9
    of Corti Q16.5
  origin
    artery
      innominate Q25.8
      pulmonary Q25.79
      renal Q27.2
      subclavian Q25.48
  osseous meatus (ear) Q16.1
  ovary Q50.39
  oviduct Q50.6
  palate (hard) (soft) NEC Q38.5
  pancreas or pancreatic duct Q45.3
  papillary muscles Q24.8
  parathyroid gland Q89.2
  paraurethral ducts Q64.79
  parotid (gland) Q38.4
  patella Q74.1
  Pelger-Huët (hereditary hyposegmentation) D72.0
  pelvic girdle NEC Q74.2
  pelvis (bony) NEC Q74.2
    rachitic E64.3
  penis (glans) Q55.69
  pericardium Q24.8
  peripheral vascular system Q27.9
  Peter's Q13.4
  pharynx Q38.8
  pigmentation L81.9
    congenital Q82.8
  pituitary (gland) Q89.2
  pleural (folds) Q34.0
  portal vein Q26.5
    connection Q26.5
  position, tooth, teeth, fully erupted M26.30
    specified NEC M26.39
  precerebral vessel Q28.1
  prepuce Q55.69
  prostate Q55.4
  pulmonary Q33.9
    artery NEC Q25.79
    valve Q22.3
      atresia Q22.0
      insufficiency Q22.2
      specified type NEC Q22.3
      stenosis Q22.1
        infundibular Q24.3
        subvalvular Q24.3
    venous connection Q26.4
      partial Q26.3
      total Q26.2
  pupil Q13.2
    function H57.00
      anisocoria H57.02
      Argyll Robertson pupil H57.01
      miosis H57.03
      mydriasis H57.04
      specified type NEC H57.09
      tonic pupil H57.05-
  pylorus Q40.3
  radius Q74.0
  rectum Q43.9
  reduction (extremity) (limb)
    femur (longitudinal) — *see* Defect, reduction, lower limb, longitudinal, femur
    fibula (longitudinal) — *see* Defect, reduction, lower limb, longitudinal, fibula
    lower limb — *see* Defect, reduction, lower limb
    radius (longitudinal) — *see* Defect, reduction, upper limb, longitudinal, radius
    tibia (longitudinal) — *see* Defect, reduction, lower limb, longitudinal, tibia
    ulna (longitudinal) — *see* Defect, reduction, upper limb, longitudinal, ulna
    upper limb — *see* Defect, reduction, upper limb
  refraction — *see* Disorder, refraction
  renal Q63.9
    artery Q27.2
    pelvis Q63.9
    specified NEC Q63.8
  respiratory system Q34.9
    specified NEC Q34.8
  retina Q14.1
  rib Q76.6
    cervical Q76.5
  Rieger's Q13.81
  rotation — *see* Malrotation

Anomaly, anomalous (congenital) (unspecified type)
- *continued*
  rotation - *continued*
    hip or thigh Q65.89
    round ligament Q52.8
  sacroiliac (joint) NEC Q74.2
  sacrum NEC Q76.49
    kyphosis — *see* Kyphosis, congenital
    lordosis — *see* Lordosis, congenital
  saddle nose, syphilitic A50.57
  salivary duct or gland Q38.4
  scapula Q74.0
  scrotum — *see* Malformation, testis and scrotum
  sebaceous gland Q82.9
  seminal vesicles Q55.4
  sense organs NEC Q07.8
  sex chromosomes NEC — *see also* Anomaly, chromosomes
    female phenotype Q97.8
    male phenotype Q98.9
  shoulder (girdle) (joint) Q74.0
  sigmoid (flexure) Q43.9
  simian crease Q82.8
  sinus of Valsalva Q25.49
  skeleton generalized Q78.9
  skin (appendage) Q82.9
  skull Q75.9
    with
      anencephaly Q00.0
      encephalocele — *see* Encephalocele
      hydrocephalus Q03.9
        with spina bifida — *see* Spina bifida, by site, with hydrocephalus
      microcephaly Q02
  specified organ or site NEC Q89.8
  spermatic cord Q55.4
  spine, spinal NEC Q76.49
    column NEC Q76.49
      kyphosis — *see* Kyphosis, congenital
      lordosis — *see* Lordosis, congenital
    cord Q06.9
    nerve root Q07.8
  spleen Q89.09
    agenesis Q89.01
  stenonian duct Q38.4
  sternum NEC Q76.7
  stomach Q40.3
  submaxillary gland Q38.4
  tarsus NEC Q74.2
  tendon Q79.9
  testis — *see* Malformation, testis and scrotum
  thigh NEC Q74.2
  thorax (wall) Q67.8
    bony Q76.9
  throat Q38.8
  thumb Q74.0
  thymus gland Q89.2
  thyroid (gland) Q89.2
    cartilage Q31.8
  tibia NEC Q74.2
    saber A50.56
  toe Q74.2
  tongue Q38.3
  tooth, teeth K00.9
    eruption K00.6
    position, fully erupted M26.30
    spacing, fully erupted M26.30
  trachea (cartilage) Q32.1
  tragus Q17.9
  tricuspid (leaflet) (valve) Q22.9
    atresia or stenosis Q22.4
    Ebstein's Q22.5
  Uhl's (hypoplasia of myocardium, right ventricle) Q24.8
  ulna Q74.0
  umbilical artery Q27.0
  union
    cricoid cartilage and thyroid cartilage Q31.8
    thyroid cartilage and hyoid bone Q31.8
    trachea with larynx Q31.8
  upper limb Q74.0
  urachus Q64.4
  ureter Q62.8
    obstructive NEC Q62.39
      cecoureterocele Q62.32
      orthotopic ureterocele Q62.31
  urethra Q64.70
    absence Q64.5
    double Q64.74
    fistula to rectum Q64.73
    obstructive Q64.39
      stricture Q64.32
    prolapse Q64.71

Anomaly, anomalous (congenital) (unspecified type) - *continued*
  urethra - *continued*
    specified type NEC Q64.79
  urinary tract Q64.9
  uterus Q51.9
    with only one functioning horn Q51.4
  uvula Q38.5
  vagina Q52.4
  valleculae Q31.8
  valve (heart) NEC Q24.8
    coronary sinus Q24.5
    inferior vena cava Q24.8
    pulmonary Q22.3
    sinus coronario Q24.5
    venae cavae inferioris Q24.8
  vas deferens Q55.4
  vascular Q27.9
    brain Q28.3
    ring Q25.45
  vein (s) (peripheral) Q27.9
    brain Q28.3
    cerebral Q28.3
    coronary Q24.5
    developmental Q28.3
    great Q26.9
      specified NEC Q26.8
  vena cava (inferior) (superior) Q26.9
  venous — *see* Anomaly, vein(s)
  venous return Q26.8
  ventricular
    bands or folds Q24.8
    septa Q21.0
  vertebra Q76.49
    kyphosis — *see* Kyphosis, congenital
    lordosis — *see* Lordosis, congenital
  vesicourethral orifice Q64.79
  vessel (s) Q27.9
    optic papilla Q14.2
    precerebral Q28.1
  vitelline duct Q43.0
  vitreous body or humor Q14.0
  vulva Q52.70
  wrist (joint) Q74.0
Anomia R48.8
Anonychia (congenital) Q84.3
  acquired L60.8
Anophthalmos, anophthalmus (congenital) (globe) Q11.1
  acquired Z90.01
Anopia, anopsia H53.46-
  quadrant H53.46-
Anorchia, anorchism, anorchidism Q55.0
Anorexia R63.0
  hysterical F44.89
  nervosa F50.00
    atypical F50.9
    binge-eating type F50.2
      with purging F50.02
    restricting type F50.01
Anorgasmy, psychogenic (female) F52.31
  male F52.32
Anosmia R43.0
  hysterical F44.6
  postinfectional J39.8
Anosognosia R41.89
Anosteoplasia Q78.9
Anovulatory cycle N97.0
Anoxemia R09.02
  newborn P84
Anoxia (pathological) R09.02
  altitude T70.29
  cerebral G93.1
    complicating
      anesthesia (general) (local) or other sedation T88.59
        in labor and delivery O74.3
        in pregnancy O29.21-
        postpartum, puerperal O89.2
      delivery (cesarean) (instrumental) O75.4
    during a procedure G97.81
    newborn P84
    resulting from a procedure G97.82
  due to
    drowning T75.1
    high altitude T70.29
  heart — *see* Insufficiency, coronary
  intrauterine P84
  myocardial — *see* Insufficiency, coronary
  newborn P84
  spinal cord G95.11
  systemic (by suffocation) (low content in atmosphere) — *see* Asphyxia, traumatic

Anteflexion — *see* Anteversion
Antenatal
  care (normal pregnancy) Z34.90
  screening (encounter for) of mother Z36
Antepartum — *see* condition
Anterior — *see* condition
Antero-occlusion M26.220
Anteversion
  cervix — *see* Anteversion, uterus
  femur (neck) , congenital Q65.89
  uterus, uterine (cervix) (postinfectional) (postpartal, old) N85.4
    congenital Q51.818
    in pregnancy or childbirth — *see* Pregnancy, complicated by
Anthophobia F40.228
Anthracosilicosis J60
Anthracosis (lung) (occupational) J60
  lingua K14.3
Anthrax A22.9
  with pneumonia A22.1
  cerebral A22.8
  colitis A22.2
  cutaneous A22.0
  gastrointestinal A22.2
  inhalation A22.1
  intestinal A22.2
  meningitis A22.8
  pulmonary A22.1
  respiratory A22.1
  sepsis A22.7
  specified manifestation NEC A22.8
Anthropoid pelvis Q74.2
  with disproportion (fetopelvic) O33.0
Anthropophobia F40.10
  generalized F40.11
Antibodies, maternal (blood group) — *see* Isoimmunization, affecting management of pregnancy
  anti-D — *see* Isoimmunization, affecting management of pregnancy, Rh
  newborn P55.0
Antibody
  anticardiolipin R76.0
    with
      hemorrhagic disorder D68.312
      hypercoagulable state D68.61
  antiphosphatidylglycerol R76.0
    with
      hemorrhagic disorder D68.312
      hypercoagulable state D68.61
  antiphosphatidylinositol R76.0
    with
      hemorrhagic disorder D68.312
      hypercoagulable state D68.61
  antiphosphatidylserine R76.0
    with
      hemorrhagic disorder D68.312
      hypercoagulable state D68.61
  antiphospholipid R76.0
    with
      hemorrhagic disorder D68.312
      hypercoagulable state D68.61
Anticardiolipin syndrome D68.61
Anticoagulant, circulating (intrinsic) — *see also* - Disorder, hemorrhagic D68.318
  drug-induced (extrinsic) — *see also* - Disorder, hemorrhagic D68.32
  iatrogenic D68.32
Antidiuretic hormone syndrome E22.2
Antimonial cholera — *see* Poisoning, antimony
Antiphospholipid
  antibody
    with hemorrhagic disorder D68.312
  syndrome D68.61
Antisocial personality F60.2
Antithrombinemia — *see* Circulating anticoagulants
Antithromboplastinemia D68.318
Antithromboplastinogenemia D68.318
Antitoxin complication or reaction — *see* Complications, vaccination
Antlophobia F40.228
Antritis J32.0
  maxilla J32.0
    acute J01.00
      recurrent J01.01
  stomach K29.60
    with bleeding K29.61
Antrum, antral — *see* condition
Anuria R34
  calculous (impacted) (recurrent) — *see also* Calculus, urinary N20.9
  following

Anuria - *continued*
  following - *continued*
    abortion — *see* Abortion by type complicated by, renal failure
    ectopic or molar pregnancy O08.4
  newborn P96.0
  postprocedural N99.0
  postrenal N13.8
  traumatic (following crushing) T79.5
Anus, anal — *see* condition
Anusitis K62.89
Anxiety F41.9
  depression F41.8
  episodic paroxysmal F41.0
  generalized F41.1
  hysteria F41.8
  neurosis F41.1
  panic type F41.0
  reaction F41.1
  separation, abnormal (of childhood) F93.0
  specified NEC F41.8
  state F41.1
Aorta, aortic — *see* condition
Aortectasia — *see* Ectasia, aorta
  with aneurysm — *see* Aneurysm, aorta
Aortitis (nonsyphilitic) (calcific) I77.6
  arteriosclerotic I70.0
  Doehle-Heller A52.02
  luetic A52.02
  rheumatic — *see* Endocarditis, acute, rheumatic
  specific (syphilitic) A52.02
  syphilitic A52.02
    congenital A50.54 [*I79.1*]
Apathetic thyroid storm — *see* Thyrotoxicosis
Apathy R45.3
Apeirophobia F40.228
Apepsia K30
  psychogenic F45.8
Aperistalsis, esophagus K22.0
Apertognathia M26.29
Apert's syndrome Q87.0
Aphagia R13.0
  psychogenic F50.9
Aphakia (acquired) (postoperative) H27.0-
  congenital Q12.3
Aphasia (amnestic) (global) (nominal) (semantic) (syntactic) R47.01
  acquired, with epilepsy (Landau-Kleffner syndrome) — *see* Epilepsy, specified NEC
  auditory (developmental) F80.2
  developmental (receptive type) F80.2
    expressive type F80.1
    Wernicke's F80.2
  following
    cerebrovascular disease I69.920
      cerebral infarction I69.320
      intracerebral hemorrhage I69.120
      nontraumatic intracranial hemorrhage NEC I69.220
      specified disease NEC I69.820
      subarachnoid hemorrhage I69.020
  primary progressive G31.01 [*F02.80*]
    with behavioral disturbance G31.01 [*F02.81*]
  progressive isolated G31.01 [*F02.80*]
    with behavioral disturbance G31.01 [*F02.81*]
  sensory F80.2
  syphilis, tertiary A52.19
  Wernicke's (developmental) F80.2
Aphonia (organic) R49.1
  hysterical F44.4
  psychogenic F44.4
Aphthae, aphthous — *see also* condition
  Bednar's K12.0
  cachectic K14.0
  epizootic B08.8
  fever B08.8
  oral (recurrent) K12.0
  stomatitis (major) (minor) K12.0
  thrush B37.0
  ulcer (oral) (recurrent) K12.0
    genital organ (s) NEC
      female N76.6
      male N50.89
    larynx J38.7
Apical — *see* condition
Apiphobia F40.218
Aplasia — *see also* Agenesis
  abdominal muscle syndrome Q79.4
  alveolar process (acquired) — *see* Anomaly, alveolar
    congenital Q38.6
  aorta (congenital) Q25.41
  axialis extracorticalis (congenita) E75.29
  bone marrow (myeloid) D61.9

Aplasia - *continued*
bone marrow (myeloid) - *continued*
  congenital D61.01
brain Q00.0
  part of Q04.3
bronchus Q32.4
cementum K00.4
cerebellum Q04.3
cervix (congenital) Q51.5
congenital pure red cell D61.01
corpus callosum Q04.0
cutis congenita Q84.8
erythrocyte congenital D61.01
extracortical axial E75.29
eye Q11.1
fovea centralis (congenital) Q14.1
gallbladder, congenital Q44.0
iris Q13.1
labyrinth, membranous Q16.5
limb (congenital) Q73.8
  lower — *see* Defect, reduction, lower limb
  upper — *see* Agenesis, arm
lung, congenital (bilateral) (unilateral) Q33.3
pancreas Q45.0
parathyroid-thymic D82.1
Pelizaeus-Merzbacher E75.29
penis Q55.5
prostate Q55.4
red cell (with thymoma) D60.9
  acquired D60.9
    due to drugs D60.9
  adult D60.9
  chronic D60.0
  congenital D61.01
  constitutional D61.01
  due to drugs D60.9
  hereditary D61.01
  of infants D61.01
  primary D61.01
  pure D61.01
    due to drugs D60.9
  specified type NEC D60.8
  transient D60.1
round ligament Q52.8
skin Q84.8
spermatic cord Q55.4
spleen Q89.01
testicle Q55.0
thymic, with immunodeficiency D82.1
thyroid (congenital) (with myxedema) E03.1
uterus Q51.0
ventral horn cell Q06.1
Apnea, apneic (of) (spells) R06.81
newborn NEC P28.4
  obstructive P28.4
  sleep (central) (obstructive) (primary) P28.3
prematurity P28.4
sleep G47.30
  central (primary) G47.31
    in conditions classified elsewhere G47.37
  obstructive (adult) (pediatric) G47.33
  primary central G47.31
  specified NEC G47.39
Apneumatosis, newborn P28.0
Apocrine metaplasia (breast) — *see* Dysplasia,
  mammary, specified type NEC
Apophysitis (bone) — *see also* Osteochondropathy
  calcaneus M92.8
  juvenile M92.9
Apoplectiform convulsions (cerebral
  ischemia) I67.82
Apoplexia, apoplexy, apoplectic
  adrenal A39.1
  heart (auricle) (ventricle) — *see* Infarct,
    myocardium
  heat T67.0
  hemorrhagic (stroke) — *see* Hemorrhage,
    intracranial
  meninges, hemorrhagic — *see* Hemorrhage,
    intracranial, subarachnoid
  uremic N18.9 [I68.8]
Appearance
  bizarre R46.1
  specified NEC R46.89
  very low level of personal hygiene R46.0
Appendage
  epididymal (organ of Morgagni) Q55.4
  intestine (epiploic) Q43.8
  preauricular Q17.0
  testicular (organ of Morgagni) Q55.29
Appendicitis (pneumococcal) (retrocecal) K37
  with
    perforation or rupture K35.2

Appendicitis (pneumococcal) (retrocecal) - *continued*
with - *continued*
    peritoneal abscess K35.3
    peritonitis NEC K35.3
      generalized (with perforation or rupture) K35.2
      localized (with perforation or rupture) K35.3
  acute (catarrhal) (fulminating) (gangrenous)
    (obstructive) (retrocecal) (suppurative) K35.80
    with
      peritoneal abscess K35.3
      peritonitis NEC K35.3
        generalized (with perforation or rupture) K35.2
        localized (with perforation or rupture) K35.3
      specified NEC K35.89
  amebic A06.89
  chronic (recurrent) K36
  exacerbation — *see* Appendicitis, acute
  gangrenous — *see* Appendicitis, acute
  healed (obliterative) K36
  interval K36
  neurogenic K36
  obstructive K36
  recurrent K36
  relapsing K36
  subacute (adhesive) K36
  subsiding K36
  suppurative — *see* Appendicitis, acute
  tuberculous A18.32
Appendicopathia oxyurica B80
Appendix, appendicular — *see also* condition
  epididymis Q55.4
  Morgagni
    female Q50.5
    male (epididymal) Q55.4
      testicular Q55.29
  testis Q55.29
Appetite
  depraved — *see* Pica
  excessive R63.2
  lack or loss — *see also* Anorexia R63.0
    nonorganic origin F50.89
    psychogenic F50.89
  perverted (hysterical) — *see* Pica
Apple peel syndrome Q41.1
Apprehension state F41.1
Apprehensiveness, abnormal F41.9
Approximal wear K03.0
Apraxia (classic) (ideational) (ideokinetic)
  (ideomotor) (motor) (verbal) R48.2
  following
    cerebrovascular disease I69.990
      cerebral infarction I69.390
      intracerebral hemorrhage I69.190
      nontraumatic intracranial hemorrhage
        NEC I69.290
      specified disease NEC I69.890
      subarachnoid hemorrhage I69.090
  oculomotor, congenital H51.8
Aptyalism K11.7
Apudoma — *see* Neoplasm, uncertain behavior, by
  site
Aqueous misdirection H40.83-
Arabicum elephantiasis — *see* Infestation, filarial
Arachnitis — *see* Meningitis
Arachnodactyly — *see* Syndrome, Marfan's
Arachnoiditis (acute) (adhesive) (basal) (brain)
  (cerebrospinal) — *see* Meningitis
Arachnophobia F40.210
Arboencephalitis, Australian A83.4
Arborization block (heart) I45.5
ARC (AIDS-related complex) B20
Arches — *see* condition
Arcuate uterus Q51.810
Arcuatus uterus Q51.810
Arcus (cornea) senilis — *see* Degeneration, cornea,
  senile
Arc-welder's lung J63.4
Areflexia R29.2
Areola — *see* condition
Argentaffinoma — *see also* Neoplasm, uncertain
  behavior, by site
  malignant — *see* Neoplasm, malignant, by site
  syndrome E34.0
Argininemia E72.21
Arginosuccinic aciduria E72.22
Argyll Robertson phenomenon, pupil or syndrome
  (syphilitic) A52.19
  atypical H57.09
  nonsyphilitic H57.09
Argyria, argyriasis
  conjunctival H11.13-
  from drug or medicament — *see* Table of Drugs and
    Chemicals, by substance

Argyrosis, conjunctival H11.13-
Arhinencephaly Q04.1
Ariboflavinosis E53.0
Arm — *see* condition
Arnold-Chiari disease, obstruction or syndrome
  (type II) Q07.00
  with
    hydrocephalus Q07.02
      with spina bifida Q07.03
    spina bifida Q07.01
      with hydrocephalus Q07.03
  type III — *see* Encephalocele
  type IV Q04.8
Aromatic amino-acid metabolism disorder E70.9
  specified NEC E70.8
Arousals, confusional G47.51
Arrest, arrested
  cardiac I46.9
    complicating
      abortion — *see* Abortion, by type, complicated
        by, cardiac arrest
      anesthesia (general) (local) or other
        sedation — *see* Table of Drugs and Chemicals,
          by drug,
        in labor and delivery O74.2
        in pregnancy O29.11-
          postpartum, puerperal O89.1
      delivery (cesarean) (instrumental) O75.4
    due to
      cardiac condition I46.2
      specified condition NEC I46.8
    intraoperative I97.71-
    newborn P29.81
    postprocedural I97.12-
      obstetric procedure O75.4
  cardiorespiratory — *see* Arrest, cardiac
  circulatory — *see* Arrest, cardiac
  deep transverse O64.0
  development or growth
    bone — *see* Disorder, bone, development or growth
    child R62.50
    tracheal rings Q32.1
  epiphyseal
    complete
      femur M89.15-
      humerus M89.12-
      tibia M89.16-
      ulna M89.13-
    forearm M89.13-
      specified NEC M89.13-
      ulna — *see* Arrest, epiphyseal, by type, ulna
    lower leg M89.16-
      specified NEC M89.168
      tibia — *see* Arrest, epiphyseal, by type, tibia
    partial
      femur M89.15-
      humerus M89.12-
      tibia M89.16-
      ulna M89.13-
    specified NEC M89.18
  granulopoiesis — *see* Agranulocytosis
  growth plate — *see* Arrest, epiphyseal
  heart — *see* Arrest, cardiac
  legal, anxiety concerning Z65.3
  physeal — *see* Arrest, epiphyseal
  respiratory R09.2
    newborn P28.81
  sinus I45.5
  spermatogenesis (complete) — *see* Azoospermia
    incomplete — *see* Oligospermia
  transverse (deep) O64.0
Arrhenoblastoma
  benign
    specified site — *see* Neoplasm, benign, by site
    unspecified site
      female D27.9
      male D29.20
  malignant
    specified site — *see* Neoplasm, malignant, by site
    unspecified site
      female C56.9
      male C62.90
  specified site — *see* Neoplasm, uncertain behavior,
    by site
  unspecified site
    female D39.10
    male D40.10
Arrhythmia (auricle) (cardiac) (juvenile) (nodal)
  (reflex) (sinus) (supraventricular) (transitory)
  (ventricle) I49.9
  block I45.9
  extrasystolic I49.49
  newborn

Arrhythmia (auricle) (cardiac) (juvenile) (nodal) (reflex) (sinus) (supraventricular) (transitory) (ventricle) - *continued*
  newborn - *continued*
    bradycardia P29.12
      occurring before birth P03.819
        before onset of labor P03.810
        during labor P03.811
    tachycardia P29.11
  psychogenic F45.8
  specified NEC I49.8
  vagal R55
  ventricular re-entry I47.0
Arrillaga-Ayerza syndrome
  (pulmonary sclerosis with pulmonary hypertension) I27.0
Arsenical pigmentation L81.8
  from drug or medicament — *see* Table of Drugs and Chemicals
Arsenism — *see* Poisoning, arsenic
Arterial — *see* condition
Arteriofibrosis — *see* Arteriosclerosis
Arteriolar sclerosis — *see* Arteriosclerosis
Arteriolith — *see* Arteriosclerosis
Arteriolitis I77.6
  necrotizing, kidney I77.5
  renal — *see* Hypertension, kidney
Arteriolosclerosis — *see* Arteriosclerosis
Arterionephrosclerosis — *see* Hypertension, kidney
Arteriopathy I77.9
Arteriosclerosis, arteriosclerotic (diffuse) (obliterans) (of) (senile) (with calcification) I70.90
  aorta I70.0
  arteries of extremities — *see* Arteriosclerosis, extremities
  brain I67.2
  bypass graft
    coronary — *see* Arteriosclerosis, coronary, bypass graft
    extremities — *see* Arteriosclerosis, extremities, bypass graft
  cardiac — *see* Disease, heart, ischemic, atherosclerotic
  cardiopathy — *see* Disease, heart, ischemic, atherosclerotic
  cardiorenal — *see* Hypertension, cardiorenal
  cardiovascular — *see* Disease, heart, ischemic, atherosclerotic
  carotid — *see also* Occlusion, artery, carotid I65.2-
  central nervous system I67.2
  cerebral I67.2
  cerebrovascular I67.2
  coronary (artery) I25.10
    due to
      calcified coronary lesion (severely) I25.84
      lipid rich plaque I25.83
    bypass graft I25.810
      with
        angina pectoris I25.709
          with documented spasm I25.701
          specified type NEC I25.708
          unstable I25.700
        ischemic chest pain I25.709
      autologous artery I25.810
        with
          angina pectoris I25.729
            with documented spasm I25.721
            specified type I25.728
            unstable I25.720
          ischemic chest pain I25.729
        autologous vein I25.810
          with
            angina pectoris I25.719
              with documented spasm I25.711
              specified type I25.718
              unstable I25.710
            ischemic chest pain I25.719
          nonautologous biological I25.810
            with
              angina pectoris I25.739
                with documented spasm I25.731
                specified type I25.738
                unstable I25.730
              ischemic chest pain I25.739
            specified type NEC I25.810
              with
                angina pectoris I25.799
                  with documented spasm I25.791
                  specified type I25.798
                  unstable I25.790
                ischemic chest pain I25.799
    native vessel
      with

Arteriosclerosis, arteriosclerotic (diffuse) (obliterans) (of) (senile) (with calcification) - *continued*
  coronary (artery) - *continued*
    native vessel - *continued*
      with - *continued*
        angina pectoris I25.119
          with documented spasm I25.111
          specified type NEC I25.118
          unstable I25.110
        ischemic chest pain I25.119
    transplanted heart I25.811
      bypass graft I25.812
        with
          angina pectoris I25.769
            with documented spasm I25.761
            specified type I25.768
            unstable I25.760
          ischemic chest pain I25.769
      native coronary artery I25.811
        with
          angina pectoris I25.759
            with documented spasm I25.751
            specified type I25.758
            unstable I25.750
          ischemic chest pain I25.759
  extremities (native arteries) I70.209
    bypass graft I70.309
      autologous vein graft I70.409
        leg I70.409
          with
            gangrene (and intermittent claudication, rest pain and ulcer) I70.469
            intermittent claudication I70.419
            rest pain (and intermittent claudication) I70.429
          bilateral I70.403
            with
              gangrene (and intermittent claudication, rest pain and ulcer) I70.463
              intermittent claudication I70.413
              rest pain (and intermittent claudication) I70.423
              specified type NEC I70.493
          left I70.402
            with
              gangrene (and intermittent claudication, rest pain and ulcer) I70.462
              intermittent claudication I70.412
              rest pain (and intermittent claudication) I70.422
              ulceration (and intermittent claudication and rest pain) I70.449
                ankle I70.443
                calf I70.442
                foot site NEC I70.445
                heel I70.444
                lower leg NEC I70.448
                midfoot I70.444
                thigh I70.441
              specified type NEC I70.492
          right I70.401
            with
              gangrene (and intermittent claudication, rest pain and ulcer) I70.461
              intermittent claudication I70.411
              rest pain (and intermittent claudication) I70.421
              ulceration (and intermittent claudication and rest pain) I70.439
                ankle I70.433
                calf I70.432
                foot site NEC I70.435
                heel I70.434
                lower leg NEC I70.438
                midfoot I70.434
                thigh I70.431
              specified type NEC I70.491
          specified type NEC I70.499
        specified NEC I70.408
          with
            gangrene (and intermittent claudication, rest pain and ulcer) I70.468
            intermittent claudication I70.418
            rest pain (and intermittent claudication) I70.428
            ulceration (and intermittent claudication and rest pain) I70.45
            specified type NEC I70.498
        leg I70.309
          with
            gangrene (and intermittent claudication, rest pain and ulcer) I70.369

Arteriosclerosis, arteriosclerotic (diffuse) (obliterans) (of) (senile) (with calcification) - *continued*
  extremities (native arteries) - *continued*
    bypass graft - *continued*
      leg - *continued*
        with - *continued*
          intermittent claudication I70.319
          rest pain (and intermittent claudication) I70.329
        bilateral I70.303
          with
            gangrene (and intermittent claudication, rest pain and ulcer) I70.363
            intermittent claudication I70.313
            rest pain (and intermittent claudication) I70.323
            specified type NEC I70.393
        left I70.302
          with
            gangrene (and intermittent claudication, rest pain and ulcer) I70.362
            intermittent claudication I70.312
            rest pain (and intermittent claudication) I70.322
            ulceration (and intermittent claudication and rest pain) I70.349
              ankle I70.343
              calf I70.342
              foot site NEC I70.345
              heel I70.344
              lower leg NEC I70.348
              midfoot I70.344
              thigh I70.341
            specified type NEC I70.392
        right I70.301
          with
            gangrene (and intermittent claudication, rest pain and ulcer) I70.361
            intermittent claudication I70.311
            rest pain (and intermittent claudication) I70.321
            ulceration (and intermittent claudication and rest pain) I70.339
              ankle I70.333
              calf I70.332
              foot site NEC I70.335
              heel I70.334
              lower leg NEC I70.338
              midfoot I70.334
              thigh I70.331
            specified type NEC I70.391
        specified type NEC I70.399
      nonautologous biological graft I70.509
        leg I70.509
          with
            gangrene (and intermittent claudication, rest pain and ulcer) I70.569
            intermittent claudication I70.519
            rest pain (and intermittent claudication) I70.529
          bilateral I70.503
            with
              gangrene (and intermittent claudication, rest pain and ulcer) I70.563
              intermittent claudication I70.513
              rest pain (and intermittent claudication) I70.523
              specified type NEC I70.593
          left I70.502
            with
              gangrene (and intermittent claudication, rest pain and ulcer) I70.562
              intermittent claudication I70.512
              rest pain (and intermittent claudication) I70.522
              ulceration (and intermittent claudication and rest pain) I70.549
                ankle I70.543
                calf I70.542
                foot site NEC I70.545
                heel I70.544
                lower leg NEC I70.548
                midfoot I70.544
                thigh I70.541
              specified type NEC I70.592
          right I70.501
            with
              gangrene (and intermittent claudication, rest pain and ulcer) I70.561
              intermittent claudication I70.511
              rest pain (and intermittent claudication) I70.521

Arteriosclerosis, arteriosclerotic (diffuse) (obliterans) (of) (senile) (with calcification) - continued
  extremities (native arteries) - continued
    bypass graft - continued
      nonautologous biological graft - continued
        leg - continued
          right - continued
            with - continued
              ulceration (and intermittent claudication and rest pain) I70.539
                ankle I70.533
                calf I70.532
                foot site NEC I70.535
                heel I70.534
                lower leg NEC I70.538
                midfoot I70.534
                thigh I70.531
            specified type NEC I70.591
          specified type NEC I70.599
      specified NEC I70.508
        with
          gangrene (and intermittent claudication, rest pain and ulcer) I70.568
          intermittent claudication I70.518
          rest pain (and intermittent claudication) I70.528
          ulceration (and intermittent claudication and rest pain) I70.55
        specified type NEC I70.598
      nonbiological graft I70.609
        leg I70.609
          with
            gangrene (and intermittent claudication, rest pain and ulcer) I70.669
            intermittent claudication I70.619
            rest pain (and intermittent claudication) I70.629
          bilateral I70.603
            with
              gangrene (and intermittent claudication, rest pain and ulcer) I70.663
              intermittent claudication I70.613
              rest pain (and intermittent claudication) I70.623
            specified type NEC I70.693
          left I70.602
            with
              gangrene (and intermittent claudication, rest pain and ulcer) I70.662
              intermittent claudication I70.612
              rest pain (and intermittent claudication) I70.622
              ulceration (and intermittent claudication and rest pain) I70.649
                ankle I70.643
                calf I70.642
                foot site NEC I70.645
                heel I70.644
                lower leg NEC I70.648
                midfoot I70.644
                thigh I70.641
            specified type NEC I70.692
          right I70.601
            with
              gangrene (and intermittent claudication, rest pain and ulcer) I70.661
              intermittent claudication I70.611
              rest pain (and intermittent claudication) I70.621
              ulceration (and intermittent claudication and rest pain) I70.639
                ankle I70.633
                calf I70.632
                foot site NEC I70.635
                heel I70.634
                lower leg NEC I70.638
                midfoot I70.634
                thigh I70.631
            specified type NEC I70.691
          specified type NEC I70.699
        specified NEC I70.608
          with
            gangrene (and intermittent claudication, rest pain and ulcer) I70.668
            intermittent claudication I70.618
            rest pain (and intermittent claudication) I70.628
            ulceration (and intermittent claudication and rest pain) I70.65
          specified type NEC I70.698
      specified graft NEC I70.709
        leg I70.709

Arteriosclerosis, arteriosclerotic (diffuse) (obliterans) (of) (senile) (with calcification) - continued
  extremities (native arteries) - continued
    bypass graft - continued
      specified graft NEC - continued
        leg - continued
          with
            gangrene (and intermittent claudication, rest pain and ulcer) I70.769
            intermittent claudication I70.719
            rest pain (and intermittent claudication) I70.729
          bilateral I70.703
            with
              gangrene (and intermittent claudication, rest pain and ulcer) I70.763
              intermittent claudication I70.713
              rest pain (and intermittent claudication) I70.723
            specified type NEC I70.793
          left I70.702
            with
              gangrene (and intermittent claudication, rest pain and ulcer) I70.762
              intermittent claudication I70.712
              rest pain (and intermittent claudication) I70.722
              ulceration (and intermittent claudication and rest pain) I70.749
                ankle I70.743
                calf I70.742
                foot site NEC I70.745
                heel I70.744
                lower leg NEC I70.748
                midfoot I70.744
                thigh I70.741
            specified type NEC I70.792
          right I70.701
            with
              gangrene (and intermittent claudication, rest pain and ulcer) I70.761
              intermittent claudication I70.711
              rest pain (and intermittent claudication) I70.721
              ulceration (and intermittent claudication and rest pain) I70.739
                ankle I70.733
                calf I70.732
                foot site NEC I70.735
                heel I70.734
                lower leg NEC I70.738
                midfoot I70.734
                thigh I70.731
            specified type NEC I70.791
          specified type NEC I70.799
        specified NEC I70.708
          with
            gangrene (and intermittent claudication, rest pain and ulcer) I70.768
            intermittent claudication I70.718
            rest pain (and intermittent claudication) I70.728
            ulceration (and intermittent claudication and rest pain) I70.75
          specified type NEC I70.798
        specified NEC I70.308
          with
            gangrene (and intermittent claudication, rest pain and ulcer) I70.368
            intermittent claudication I70.318
            rest pain (and intermittent claudication) I70.328
            ulceration (and intermittent claudication and rest pain) I70.35
          specified type NEC I70.398
      leg I70.209
        with
          gangrene (and intermittent claudication, rest pain and ulcer) I70.269
          intermittent claudication I70.219
          rest pain (and intermittent claudication) I70.229
        bilateral I70.203
          with
            gangrene (and intermittent claudication, rest pain and ulcer) I70.263
            intermittent claudication I70.213
            rest pain (and intermittent claudication) I70.223
          specified type NEC I70.293
        left I70.202
          with

Arteriosclerosis, arteriosclerotic (diffuse) (obliterans) (of) (senile) (with calcification) - continued
  extremities (native arteries) - continued
    leg - continued
      left - continued
        with - continued
          gangrene (and intermittent claudication, rest pain and ulcer) I70.262
          intermittent claudication I70.212
          rest pain (and intermittent claudication) I70.222
          ulceration (and intermittent claudication and rest pain) I70.249
            ankle I70.243
            calf I70.242
            foot site NEC I70.245
            heel I70.244
            lower leg NEC I70.248
            midfoot I70.244
            thigh I70.241
        specified type NEC I70.292
      right I70.201
        with
          gangrene (and intermittent claudication, rest pain and ulcer) I70.261
          intermittent claudication I70.211
          rest pain (and intermittent claudication) I70.221
          ulceration (and intermittent claudication and rest pain) I70.239
            ankle I70.233
            calf I70.232
            foot site NEC I70.235
            heel I70.234
            lower leg NEC I70.238
            midfoot I70.234
            thigh I70.231
        specified type NEC I70.291
      specified type NEC I70.299
    specified site NEC I70.208
      with
        gangrene (and intermittent claudication, rest pain and ulcer) I70.268
        intermittent claudication I70.218
        rest pain (and intermittent claudication) I70.228
        ulceration (and intermittent claudication and rest pain) I70.25
      specified type NEC I70.298
  generalized I70.91
  heart (disease) — see Arteriosclerosis, coronary (artery),
  kidney — see Hypertension, kidney
  medial — see Arteriosclerosis, extremities
  mesenteric (artery) K55.1
  Mönckeberg's — see Arteriosclerosis, extremities
  myocarditis I51.4
  peripheral (of extremities) — see Arteriosclerosis, extremities
  pulmonary (idiopathic) I27.0
  renal (arterioles) — see also Hypertension, kidney
    artery I70.1
  retina (vascular) I70.8 [H35.0-]
  specified artery NEC I70.8
  spinal (cord) G95.19
  vertebral (artery) I67.2
Arteriospasm I73.9
Arteriovenous — see condition
Arteritis I77.6
  allergic M31.0
  aorta (nonsyphilitic) I77.6
    syphilitic A52.02
  aortic arch M31.4
  brachiocephalic M31.4
  brain I67.7
    syphilitic A52.04
  cerebral I67.7
    in
      diseases classified elsewhere I68.2
      systemic lupus erythematosus M32.19
    listerial A32.89
    syphilitic A52.04
    tuberculous A18.89
  coronary (artery) I25.89
    rheumatic I01.8
      chronic I09.89
    syphilitic A52.06
  cranial (left) (right) , giant cell M31.6
  deformans — see Arteriosclerosis
  giant cell NEC M31.6
    with polymyalgia rheumatica M31.5
  necrosing or necrotizing M31.9
    specified NEC M31.8

Arteritis - *continued*
nodosa M30.0
obliterans — *see* Arteriosclerosis
pulmonary I28.8
rheumatic — *see* Fever, rheumatic
senile — *see* Arteriosclerosis
suppurative I77.2
syphilitic (general) A52.09
brain A52.04
coronary A52.06
spinal A52.09
temporal, giant cell M31.6
young female aortic arch syndrome M31.4
Artery, arterial — *see also* condition
abscess I77.89
single umbilical Q27.0
Arthralgia (allergic) — *see also* Pain, joint
in caisson disease T70.3
temporomandibular M26.62-
Arthritis, arthritic (acute) (chronic) (nonpyogenic)
(subacute) M19.90
allergic — *see* Arthritis, specified form NEC
ankylosing (crippling) (spine) — *see*
also Spondylitis, ankylosing
sites other than spine — *see* Arthritis, specified
form NEC
atrophic — *see* Osteoarthritis
spine — *see* Spondylitis, ankylosing
back — *see* Spondylopathy, inflammatory
blennorrhagic (gonococcal) A54.42
Charcot's — *see* Arthropathy, neuropathic
diabetic — *see* Diabetes, arthropathy, neuropathic
syringomyelic G95.0
chylous (filarial) (*see also* category M01) B74.9
climacteric (any site) NEC — *see* Arthritis, specified
form NEC
crystal (-induced) — *see* Arthritis, in, crystals
deformans — *see* Osteoarthritis
degenerative — *see* Osteoarthritis
due to or associated with
acromegaly E22.0
brucellosis — *see* Brucellosis
caisson disease T70.3
diabetes — *see* Diabetes, arthropathy
dracontiasis (*see also* category M01) B72
enteritis NEC
regional — *see* Enteritis, regional
erysipelas (*see also* category M01) A46
erythema
epidemic A25.1
nodosum L52
filariasis NOS B74.9
glanders A24.0
helminthiasis (*see also* category M01) B83.9
hemophilia D66 [M36.2]
Henoch- (Schönlein) purpura D69.0 [M36.4]
human parvovirus (*see also* category M01) B97.6
infectious disease NEC — *see* category M01
leprosy (see also category M01) — *see*
also Leprosy A30.9
Lyme disease A69.23
mycobacteria (*see also* category M01) A31.8
parasitic disease NEC (*see also* category M01) B89
paratyphoid fever (see also category M01) —
see also Fever, paratyphoid A01.4
rat bite fever (*see also* category M01) A25.1
regional enteritis — *see* Enteritis, regional
respiratory disorder NOS J98.9
serum sickness — *see also* Reaction, serum T80.69
syringomyelia G95.0
typhoid fever A01.04
epidemic erythema A25.1
febrile — *see* Fever, rheumatic
gonococcal A54.42
gouty (acute) — *see* Gout
in (due to)
acromegaly (*see also* subcategory M14.8-) E22.0
amyloidosis (*see also* subcategory M14.8-) E85.4
bacterial disease (*see also* subcategory M01) A49.9
Behçet's syndrome M35.2
caisson disease (*see also*
subcategory M14.8-) T70.3
coliform bacilli (Escherichia coli) — *see* Arthritis,
in, pyogenic organism NEC
crystals M11.9
dicalcium phosphate — *see* Arthritis, in, crystals,
specified type NEC
hydroxyapatite M11.0-
pyrophosphate — *see* Arthritis, in, crystals,
specified type NEC
specified type NEC M11.80
ankle M11.87-
elbow M11.82-

Arthritis, arthritic (acute) (chronic) (nonpyogenic)
(subacute) - *continued*
in (due to) - *continued*
crystals - *continued*
specified type NEC - *continued*
foot joint M11.87-
hand joint M11.84-
hip M11.85-
knee M11.86-
multiple sites M11.8-
shoulder M11.81-
vertebrae M11.88
wrist M11.83-
dermatoarthritis, lipoid E78.81
dracontiasis (dracunculiasis)
(*see also* category M01) B72
endocrine disorder NEC
(*see also* subcategory M14.8-) E34.9
enteritis, infectious NEC (*see also* category
M01) A09
specified organism NEC (*see also* category
M01) A08.8
erythema
multiforme (*see also* subcategory M14.8-) L51.9
nodosum (*see also* subcategory M14.8-) L52
gout — *see* Gout
helminthiasis NEC (*see also* category M01) B83.9
hemochromatosis (*see also*
subcategory M14.8-) E83.118
hemoglobinopathy NEC D58.2 [M36.3]
hemophilia NEC D66 [M36.2]
Hemophilus influenzae M00.8- [B96.3]
Henoch (-Schönlein) purpura D69.0 [M36.4]
hyperparathyroidism NEC
(*see also* subcategory M14.8-) E21.3
hypersensitivity reaction NEC T78.49 [M36.4]
hypogammaglobulinemia
(*see also* subcategory M14.8-) D80.1
hypothyroidism NEC
(*see also* subcategory M14.8-) E03.9
infection — *see* Arthritis, pyogenic or pyemic
spine — *see* Spondylopathy, infective
infectious disease NEC — *see* category M01
leprosy (*see also* category M01) A30.9
leukemia NEC C95.9- [M36.1]
lipoid dermatoarthritis E78.81
Lyme disease A69.23
Mediterranean fever, familial
(*see also* subcategory M14.8-) M04.1
Meningococcus A39.83
metabolic disorder NEC
(*see also* subcategory M14.8-) E88.9
multiple myelomatosis C90.0- [M36.1]
mumps B26.85
mycosis NEC (*see also* category M01) B49
myelomatosis (multiple) C90.0- [M36.1]
neurological disorder NEC G98.0
ochronosis (*see also* subcategory M14.8-) E70.29
O'nyong-nyong (*see also* category M01) A92.1
parasitic disease NEC (*see also* category M01) B89
paratyphoid fever (*see also* category M01) A01.4
Pseudomonas — *see* Arthritis, pyogenic, bacterial
NEC
psoriasis L40.50
pyogenic organism NEC — *see* Arthritis,
pyogenic, bacterial NEC
Reiter's disease — *see* Reiter's disease
respiratory disorder NEC
(*see also* subcategory M14.8-) J98.9
reticulosis, malignant
(*see also* subcategory M14.8-) C86.0
rubella B06.82
Salmonella (arizonae) (cholerae-suis) (enteritidis)
(typhimurium) A02.23
sarcoidosis D86.86
specified bacteria NEC — *see* Arthritis, pyogenic,
bacterial NEC
sporotrichosis B42.82
syringomyelia G95.0
thalassemia NEC D56.9 [M36.3]
tuberculosis — *see* Tuberculosis, arthritis
typhoid fever A01.04
urethritis, Reiter's — *see* Reiter's disease
viral disease NEC (*see also* category M01) B34.9
infectious or infective — *see also* Arthritis, pyogenic
or pyemic
spine — *see* Spondylopathy, infective
juvenile M08.90
with systemic onset — *see* Still's disease
ankle M08.97-
elbow M08.92-
foot joint M08.97-
hand joint M08.94-

Arthritis, arthritic (acute) (chronic) (nonpyogenic)
(subacute) - *continued*
juvenile - *continued*
hip M08.95-
knee M08.96-
multiple site M08.99
pauciarticular M08.40
ankle M08.47-
elbow M08.42-
foot joint M08.47-
hand joint M08.44-
hip M08.45-
knee M08.46-
shoulder M08.41-
vertebrae M08.48
wrist M08.43-
psoriatic L40.54
rheumatoid — *see* Arthritis, rheumatoid, juvenile
shoulder M08.91-
vertebra M08.98
specified type NEC M08.80
ankle M08.87-
elbow M08.82-
foot joint M08.87-
hand joint M08.84-
hip M08.85-
knee M08.86-
multiple site M08.89
shoulder M08.81-
specified joint NEC M08.88
vertebrae M08.88
wrist M08.83-
wrist M08.93-
meaning osteoarthritis — *see* Osteoarthritis
meningococcal A39.83
menopausal (any site) NEC — *see* Arthritis,
specified form NEC
mutilans (psoriatic) L40.52
mycotic NEC (*see also* category M01) B49
neuropathic (Charcot) — *see* Arthropathy,
neuropathic
diabetic — *see* Diabetes, arthropathy, neuropathic
nonsyphilitic NEC G98.0
syringomyelic G95.0
ochronotic (*see also* subcategory M14.8-) E70.29
palindromic (any site) — *see* Rheumatism,
palindromic
pneumococcal M00.10
ankle M00.17-
elbow M00.12-
foot joint — *see* Arthritis, pneumococcal, ankle
hand joint M00.14-
hip M00.15-
knee M00.16-
multiple site M00.19
shoulder M00.11-
vertebra M00.18
wrist M00.13-
postdysenteric — *see* Arthropathy, postdysenteric
postmeningococcal A39.84
postrheumatic, chronic — *see* Arthropathy,
postrheumatic, chronic
primary progressive — *see also* Arthritis, specified
form NEC
spine — *see* Spondylitis, ankylosing
psoriatic L40.50
purulent (any site except spine) — *see* Arthritis,
pyogenic or pyemic
spine — *see* Spondylopathy, infective
pyogenic or pyemic (any site except spine) M00.9
bacterial NEC M00.80
ankle M00.87-
elbow M00.82-
foot joint — *see* Arthritis, pyogenic, bacterial
NEC, ankle
hand joint M00.84-
hip M00.85-
knee M00.86-
multiple site M00.89
shoulder M00.81-
vertebra M00.88
wrist M00.83-
pneumococcal — *see* Arthritis, pneumococcal
spine — *see* Spondylopathy, infective
staphylococcal — *see* Arthritis, staphylococcal
streptococcal — *see* Arthritis, streptococcal NEC
pneumococcal — *see* Arthritis, pneumococcal
reactive — *see* Reiter's disease
rheumatic — *see also* Arthritis, rheumatoid
acute or subacute — *see* Fever, rheumatic
rheumatoid M06.9
with
carditis — *see* Rheumatoid, carditis

Arthritis, arthritic (acute) (chronic) (nonpyogenic) (subacute) - *continued*
- rheumatoid - *continued*
  - with - *continued*
    - endocarditis — *see* Rheumatoid, carditis
    - heart involvement NEC — *see* Rheumatoid, carditis
    - lung involvement — *see* Rheumatoid, lung
    - myocarditis — *see* Rheumatoid, carditis
    - myopathy — *see* Rheumatoid, myopathy
    - pericarditis — *see* Rheumatoid, carditis
    - polyneuropathy — *see* Rheumatoid, polyneuropathy
    - rheumatoid factor — *see* Arthritis, rheumatoid, seropositive
    - splenoadenomegaly and leukopenia — *see* Felty's syndrome
    - vasculitis — *see* Rheumatoid, vasculitis
    - visceral involvement NEC — *see* Rheumatoid, arthritis, with involvement of organs NEC
  - juvenile (with or without rheumatoid factor) M08.00
    - ankle M08.07-
    - elbow M08.02-
    - foot joint M08.07-
    - hand joint M08.04-
    - hip M08.05-
    - knee M08.06-
    - multiple site M08.09
    - shoulder M08.01-
    - vertebra M08.08
    - wrist M08.03-
  - seronegative M06.00
    - ankle M06.07-
    - elbow M06.02-
    - foot joint M06.07-
    - hand joint M06.04-
    - hip M06.05-
    - knee M06.06-
    - multiple site M06.09
    - shoulder M06.01-
    - vertebra M06.08
    - wrist M06.03-
  - seropositive M05.9
    - specified NEC M05.80
      - ankle M05.87-
      - elbow M05.82-
      - foot joint M05.87-
      - hand joint M05.84-
      - hip M05.85-
      - knee M05.86-
      - multiple sites M05.89
      - shoulder M05.81-
      - vertebra — *see* Spondylitis, ankylosing
      - wrist M05.83-
    - without organ involvement M05.70
      - ankle M05.77-
      - elbow M05.72-
      - foot joint M05.77-
      - hand joint M05.74-
      - hip M05.75-
      - knee M05.76-
      - multiple sites M05.79
      - shoulder M05.71-
      - vertebra — *see* Spondylitis, ankylosing
      - wrist M05.73-
  - specified type NEC M06.80
    - ankle M06.87-
    - elbow M06.82-
    - foot joint M06.87-
    - hand joint M06.84-
    - hip M06.85-
    - knee M06.86-
    - multiple site M06.89
    - shoulder M06.81-
    - vertebra M06.88
    - wrist M06.83-
  - spine — *see* Spondylitis, ankylosing
  - rubella B06.82
  - scorbutic (*see also* subcategory M14.8-) E54
  - senile or senescent — *see* Osteoarthritis
  - septic (any site except spine) — *see* Arthritis, pyogenic or pyemic
  - spine — *see* Spondylopathy, infective
  - serum (nontherapeutic) (therapeutic) — *see* Arthropathy, postimmunization
  - specified form NEC M13.80
    - ankle M13.87-
    - elbow M13.82-
    - foot joint M13.87-
    - hand joint M13.84-
    - hip M13.85-
    - knee M13.86-

Arthritis, arthritic (acute) (chronic) (nonpyogenic) (subacute) - *continued*
- specified form NEC - *continued*
  - multiple site M13.89
  - shoulder M13.81-
  - specified joint NEC M13.88
  - wrist M13.83-
- spine — *see also* Spondylopathy, inflammatory
  - infectious or infective NEC — *see* Spondylopathy, infective
  - Marie-Strümpell — *see* Spondylitis, ankylosing
  - pyogenic — *see* Spondylopathy, infective
  - rheumatoid — *see* Spondylitis, ankylosing
  - traumatic (old) — *see* Spondylopathy, traumatic
  - tuberculous A18.01
- staphylococcal M00.00
  - ankle M00.07-
  - elbow M00.02-
  - foot joint — *see* Arthritis, staphylococcal, ankle
  - hand joint M00.04-
  - hip M00.05-
  - knee M00.06-
  - multiple site M00.09
  - shoulder M00.01-
  - vertebra M00.08
  - wrist M00.03-
- streptococcal NEC M00.20
  - ankle M00.27-
  - elbow M00.22-
  - foot joint — *see* Arthritis, streptococcal, ankle
  - hand joint M00.24-
  - hip M00.25-
  - knee M00.26-
  - multiple site M00.29
  - shoulder M00.21-
  - vertebra M00.28
  - wrist M00.23-
- suppurative — *see* Arthritis, pyogenic or pyemic
- syphilitic (late) A52.16
  - congenital A50.55 [M12.80]
- syphilitica deformans (Charcot) A52.16
- temporomandibular M26.69
- toxic of menopause (any site) — *see* Arthritis, specified form NEC
- transient — *see* Arthropathy, specified form NEC
- traumatic (chronic) — *see* Arthropathy, traumatic
- tuberculous A18.02
  - spine A18.01
- uratic — *see* Gout
- urethritica (Reiter's) — *see* Reiter's disease
- vertebral — *see* Spondylopathy, inflammatory
- villous (any site) — *see* Arthropathy, specified form NEC

Arthrocele — *see* Effusion, joint
Arthrodesis status Z98.1
Arthrodynia — *see also* Pain, joint
Arthrodysplasia Q74.9
Arthrofibrosis, joint — *see* Ankylosis
Arthrogryposis (congenital) Q68.8
- multiplex congenita Q74.3
Arthrokatadysis M24.7
Arthropathy — *see also* Arthritis M12.9
- Charcot's — *see* Arthropathy, neuropathic
  - diabetic — *see* Diabetes, arthropathy, neuropathic
  - syringomyelic G95.0
- cricoarytenoid J38.7
- crystal (-induced) — *see* Arthritis, in, crystals
- diabetic NEC — *see* Diabetes, arthropathy
- distal interphalangeal, psoriatic L40.51
- enteropathic M07.60
  - ankle M07.67-
  - elbow M07.62-
  - foot joint M07.67-
  - hand joint M07.64-
  - hip M07.65-
  - knee M07.66-
  - multiple site M07.69
  - shoulder M07.61-
  - vertebra M07.68
  - wrist M07.63-
- following intestinal bypass M02.00
  - ankle M02.07-
  - elbow M02.02-
  - foot joint M02.07-
  - hand joint M02.04-
  - hip M02.05-
  - knee M02.06-
  - multiple site M02.09
  - shoulder M02.01-
  - vertebra M02.08
  - wrist M02.03-
- gouty — *see also* Gout
  - in (due to)

Arthropathy - *continued*
- gouty - *continued*
  - in (due to) - *continued*
    - Lesch-Nyhan syndrome E79.1 [M14.8-]
    - sickle-cell disorders D57- [M14.8-]
- hemophilic NEC D66 [M36.2]
  - in (due to)
    - hyperparathyroidism NEC E21.3 [M14.8-]
    - metabolic disease NOS E88.9 [M14.8-]
- in (due to)
  - acromegaly E22.0 [M14.8-]
  - amyloidosis E85.4 [M14.8-]
  - blood disorder NOS D75.9 [M36.3]
  - diabetes — *see* Diabetes, arthropathy
  - endocrine disease NOS E34.9 [M14.8-]
  - erythema
    - multiforme L51.9 [M14.8-]
    - nodosum L52 [M14.8-]
  - hemochromatosis E83.118 [M14.8-]
  - hemoglobinopathy NEC D58.2 [M36.3]
  - hemophilia NEC D66 [M36.2]
  - Henoch-Schönlein purpura D69.0 [M36.4]
  - hyperthyroidism E05.90 [M14.8-]
  - hypothyroidism E03.9 [M14.8-]
  - infective endocarditis I33.0 [M12.80]
  - leukemia NEC C95.9- [M36.1]
  - malignant histiocytosis C96.A [M36.1]
  - metabolic disease NOS E88.9 [M14.8-]
  - multiple myeloma C90.0- [M36.1]
  - neoplastic disease NOS (see also Neoplasm) D49.9 [M36.1]
  - nutritional deficiency (*see also* subcategory M14.8-) E63.9
  - psoriasis NOS L40.50
  - sarcoidosis D86.86
  - syphilis (late) A52.77
    - congenital A50.55 [M12.80]
  - thyrotoxicosis (*see also* subcategory M14.8-) E05.90
  - ulcerative colitis K51.90 [M07.60]
  - viral hepatitis (postinfectious) NEC B19.9 [M12.80]
  - Whipple's disease (*see also* subcategory M14.8-) K90.81
- Jaccoud — *see* Arthropathy, postrheumatic, chronic
- juvenile — *see* Arthritis, juvenile
  - psoriatic L40.54
- mutilans (psoriatic) L40.52
- neuropathic (Charcot) M14.60
  - ankle M14.67-
  - diabetic — *see* Diabetes, arthropathy, neuropathic
  - elbow M14.62-
  - foot joint M14.67-
  - hand joint M14.64-
  - hip M14.65-
  - knee M14.66-
  - multiple site M14.69
  - nonsyphilitic NEC G98.0
  - shoulder M14.61-
  - syringomyelic G95.0
  - vertebra M14.68
  - wrist M14.63-
- osteopulmonary — *see* Osteoarthropathy, hypertrophic, specified NEC
- postdysenteric M02.10
  - ankle M02.17-
  - elbow M02.12-
  - foot joint M02.17-
  - hand joint M02.14-
  - hip M02.15-
  - knee M02.16-
  - multiple site M02.19
  - shoulder M02.11-
  - vertebra M02.18
  - wrist M02.13-
- postimmunization M02.20
  - ankle M02.27-
  - elbow M02.22-
  - foot joint M02.27-
  - hand joint M02.24-
  - hip M02.25-
  - knee M02.26-
  - multiple site M02.29
  - shoulder M02.21-
  - vertebra M02.28
  - wrist M02.23-
- postinfectious NEC B99 [M12.80]
  - in (due to)
    - enteritis due to Yersinia enterocolitica A04.6 [M12.80]
    - syphilis A52.77
    - viral hepatitis NEC B19.9 [M12.80]
- postrheumatic, chronic (Jaccoud) M12.00

Arthropathy - *continued*
  postrheumatic, chronic (Jaccoud) - *continued*
    ankle M12.07-
    elbow M12.02-
    foot joint M12.07-
    hand joint M12.04-
    hip M12.05-
    knee M12.06-
    multiple site M12.09
    shoulder M12.01-
    specified joint NEC M12.08
    vertebrae M12.08
    wrist M12.03-
  psoriatic NEC L40.59
    interphalangeal, distal L40.51
  reactive M02.9
    in (due to)
      infective endocarditis I33.0 *[M02.9]*
    specified type NEC M02.80
      ankle M02.87-
      elbow M02.82-
      foot joint M02.87-
      hand joint M02.84-
      hip M02.85-
      knee M02.86-
      multiple site M02.89
      shoulder M02.81-
      vertebra M02.88
      wrist M02.83-
  specified form NEC M12.80
    ankle M12.87-
    elbow M12.82-
    foot joint M12.87-
    hand joint M12.84-
    hip M12.85-
    knee M12.86-
    multiple site M12.89
    shoulder M12.81-
    specified joint NEC M12.88
    vertebrae M12.88
    wrist M12.83-
  syringomyelic G95.0
  tabes dorsalis A52.16
  tabetic A52.16
  transient — *see* Arthropathy, specified form NEC
  traumatic M12.50
    ankle M12.57-
    elbow M12.52-
    foot joint M12.57-
    hand joint M12.54-
    hip M12.55-
    knee M12.56-
    multiple site M12.59
    shoulder M12.51-
    specified joint NEC M12.58
    vertebrae M12.58
    wrist M12.53-
Arthropyosis — *see* Arthritis, pyogenic or pyemic
Arthrosis (deformans) (degenerative)
  (localized) — *see also* Osteoarthritis M19.90
  spine — *see* Spondylosis
Arthus' phenomenon or reaction T78.41
  due to
    drug — *see* Table of Drugs and Chemicals, by drug
Articular — *see* condition
Articulation, reverse (teeth) M26.24
Artificial
  insemination complication — *see* Complications, artificial, fertilization
  opening status (functioning) (without complication) Z93.9
    anus (colostomy) Z93.3
    colostomy Z93.3
    cystostomy Z93.50
      appendico-vesicostomy Z93.52
      cutaneous Z93.51
      specified NEC Z93.59
    enterostomy Z93.4
    gastrostomy Z93.1
    ileostomy Z93.2
    intestinal tract NEC Z93.4
    jejunostomy Z93.4
    nephrostomy Z93.6
    specified site NEC Z93.8
    tracheostomy Z93.0
    ureterostomy Z93.6
    urethrostomy Z93.6
    urinary tract NEC Z93.6
    vagina Z93.8
  vagina status Z93.8
Arytenoid — *see* condition
Asbestosis (occupational) J61

Ascariasis B77.9
  with
    complications NEC B77.89
    intestinal complications B77.0
    pneumonia, pneumonitis B77.81
Ascaridosis, ascaridiasis — *see* Ascariasis
Ascaris (infection) (infestation) (lumbricoides) — *see* Ascariasis
Ascending — *see* condition
ASC-H
  (atypical squamous cells cannot exclude high grade squamous intraepithelial lesion on cytologic smear)
  anus R85.611
  cervix R87.611
  vagina R87.621
Aschoff's bodies — *see* Myocarditis, rheumatic
Ascites (abdominal) R18.8
  cardiac I50.9
  chylous (nonfilarial) I89.8
    filarial — *see* Infestation, filarial
    due to
      cirrhosis, alcoholic K70.31
      hepatitis
        alcoholic K70.11
        chronic active K71.51
      S. japonicum B65.2
  heart I50.9
  malignant R18.0
  pseudochylous R18.8
  syphilitic A52.74
  tuberculous A18.31
ASC-US
  (atypical squamous cells of undetermined significance on cytologic smear)
  anus R85.610
  cervix R87.610
  vagina R87.620
Aseptic — *see* condition
Asherman's syndrome N85.6
Asialia K11.7
Asiatic cholera — *see* Cholera
Asimultagnosia (simultanagnosia) R48.3
Askin's tumor — *see* Neoplasm, connective tissue, malignant
Asocial personality F60.2
Asomatognosia R41.4
Aspartylglucosaminuria E77.1
Asperger's disease or syndrome F84.5
Aspergilloma — *see* Aspergillosis
Aspergillosis (with pneumonia) B44.9
  bronchopulmonary, allergic B44.81
  disseminated B44.7
  generalized B44.7
  pulmonary NEC B44.1
    allergic B44.81
    invasive B44.0
  specified NEC B44.89
  tonsillar B44.2
Aspergillus (flavus) (fumigatus) (infection) (terreus) — *see* Aspergillosis
Aspermatogenesis — *see* Azoospermia
Aspermia (testis) — *see* Azoospermia
Asphyxia, asphyxiation (by) R09.01
  antenatal P84
  birth P84
  bunny bag — *see* Asphyxia, due to, mechanical threat to breathing, trapped in bed clothes
  crushing S28.0
  drowning T75.1
  gas, fumes, or vapor — *see* Table of Drugs and Chemicals
  inhalation — *see* Inhalation
  intrauterine P84
  local I73.00
    with gangrene I73.01
  mucus — *see also* Foreign body, respiratory tract, causing asphyxia
  newborn P84
  pathological R09.01
  postnatal P84
    mechanical — *see* Asphyxia, due to, mechanical threat to breathing
  prenatal P84
  reticularis R23.1
  strangulation — *see* Asphyxia, due to, mechanical threat to breathing
  submersion T75.1
  traumatic T71.9
    due to
      crushed chest S28.0
      foreign body (in) — *see* Foreign body, respiratory tract, causing asphyxia
      low oxygen content of ambient air T71.20

Asphyxia, asphyxiation (by) - *continued*
  traumatic - *continued*
    due to - *continued*
      low oxygen content of ambient air - *continued*
        due to
          being trapped in
            low oxygen environment T71.29
              in car trunk T71.221
                circumstances undetermined T71.224
                done with intent to harm by
                  another person T71.223
                  self T71.222
              in refrigerator T71.231
                circumstances undetermined T71.234
                done with intent to harm by
                  another person T71.233
                  self T71.232
          cave-in T71.21
      mechanical threat to breathing
        (accidental) T71.191
        circumstances undetermined T71.194
        done with intent to harm by
          another person T71.193
          self T71.192
        hanging T71.161
          circumstances undetermined T71.164
          done with intent to harm by
            another person T71.163
            self T71.162
        plastic bag T71.121
          circumstances undetermined T71.124
          done with intent to harm by
            another person T71.123
            self T71.122
        smothering
          in furniture T71.151
            circumstances undetermined T71.154
            done with intent to harm by
              another person T71.153
              self T71.152
          under
            another person's body T71.141
              circumstances undetermined T71.144
              done with intent to harm T71.143
            pillow T71.111
              circumstances undetermined T71.114
              done with intent to harm by
                another person T71.113
                self T71.112
        trapped in bed clothes T71.131
          circumstances undetermined T71.134
          done with intent to harm by
            another person T71.133
            self T71.132
  vomiting, vomitus — *see* Foreign body, respiratory tract, causing asphyxia
Aspiration
  amniotic (clear) fluid (newborn) P24.10
    with
      pneumonia (pneumonitis) P24.11
      respiratory symptoms P24.11
  blood
    newborn (without respiratory symptoms) P24.20
      with
        pneumonia (pneumonitis) P24.21
        respiratory symptoms P24.21
    specified age NEC — *see* Foreign body, respiratory tract
  bronchitis J69.0
  food or foreign body (with asphyxiation) — *see* Asphyxia, food
  liquor (amnii) (newborn) P24.10
    with
      pneumonia (pneumonitis) P24.11
      respiratory symptoms P24.11
  meconium (newborn) (without respiratory symptoms) P24.00
    with
      pneumonitis (pneumonitis) P24.01
      respiratory symptoms P24.01
  milk (newborn) (without respiratory symptoms) P24.30
    with
      pneumonia (pneumonitis) P24.31
      respiratory symptoms P24.31
    specified age NEC — *see* Foreign body, respiratory tract
  mucus — *see also* Foreign body, by site, causing asphyxia
    newborn P24.10
      with
        pneumonia (pneumonitis) P24.11
        respiratory symptoms P24.11

Aspiration - *continued*
neonatal P24.9
specific NEC (without respiratory symptoms) P24.80
with
pneumonia (pneumonitis) P24.81
respiratory symptoms P24.81
newborn P24.9
specific NEC (without respiratory symptoms) P24.80
with
pneumonia (pneumonitis) P24.81
respiratory symptoms P24.81
pneumonia J69.0
pneumonitis J69.0
syndrome of newborn — *see* Aspiration, by substance, with pneumonia
vernix caseosa (newborn) P24.80
with
pneumonia (pneumonitis) P24.81
respiratory symptoms P24.81
vomitus — *see also* Foreign body, respiratory tract
newborn (without respiratory symptoms) P24.30
with
pneumonia (pneumonitis) P24.31
respiratory symptoms P24.31
Asplenia (congenital) Q89.01
postsurgical Z90.81
Assam fever B55.0
Assault, sexual — *see* Maltreatment
Assmann's focus NEC A15.0
Astasia (-abasia) (hysterical) F44.4
Asteatosis cutis L85.3
Astereognosia, astereognosis R48.1
Asterixis R27.8
in liver disease K71.3
Asteroid hyalitis — *see* Deposit, crystalline
Asthenia, asthenic R53.1
cardiac — *see also* Failure, heart I50.9
psychogenic F45.8
cardiovascular — *see also* Failure, heart I50.9
psychogenic F45.8
heart — *see also* Failure, heart I50.9
psychogenic F45.8
hysterical F44.4
myocardial — *see also* Failure, heart I50.9
psychogenic F45.8
nervous F48.8
neurocirculatory F45.8
neurotic F48.8
psychogenic F48.8
psychoneurotic F48.8
psychophysiologic F48.8
reaction (psychophysiologic) F48.8
senile R54
Asthenopia — *see also* Discomfort, visual
hysterical F44.6
psychogenic F44.6
Asthenospermia — *see* Abnormal, specimen, male genital organs
Asthma, asthmatic (bronchial) (catarrh) (spasmodic) J45.909
with
chronic obstructive bronchitis J44.9
with
acute lower respiratory infection J44.0
exacerbation (acute) J44.1
chronic obstructive pulmonary disease J44.9
with
acute lower respiratory infection J44.0
exacerbation (acute) J44.1
exacerbation (acute) J45.901
hay fever — *see* Asthma, allergic extrinsic
rhinitis, allergic — *see* Asthma, allergic extrinsic
status asthmaticus J45.902
allergic extrinsic J45.909
with
exacerbation (acute) J45.901
status asthmaticus J45.902
atopic — *see* Asthma, allergic extrinsic
cardiac — *see* Failure, ventricular, left
cardiobronchial I50.1
childhood J45.909
with
exacerbation (acute) J45.901
status asthmaticus J45.902
chronic obstructive J44.9
with
acute lower respiratory infection J44.0
exacerbation (acute) J44.1
collier's J60
cough variant J45.991
detergent J69.8

Asthma, asthmatic (bronchial) (catarrh) (spasmodic) - *continued*
due to
detergent J69.8
inhalation of fumes J68.3
eosinophilic J82
extrinsic, allergic — *see* Asthma, allergic extrinsic
grinder's J62.8
hay — *see* Asthma, allergic extrinsic
heart I50.1
idiosyncratic — *see* Asthma, nonallergic
intermittent (mild) J45.20
with
exacerbation (acute) J45.21
status asthmaticus J45.22
intrinsic, nonallergic — *see* Asthma, nonallergic
Kopp's E32.8
late-onset J45.909
with
exacerbation (acute) J45.901
status asthmaticus J45.902
mild intermittent J45.20
with
exacerbation (acute) J45.21
status asthmaticus J45.22
mild persistent J45.30
with
exacerbation (acute) J45.31
status asthmaticus J45.32
Millar's (laryngismus stridulus) J38.5
miner's J60
mixed J45.909
with
exacerbation (acute) J45.901
status asthmaticus J45.902
moderate persistent J45.40
with
exacerbation (acute) J45.41
status asthmaticus J45.42
nervous — *see* Asthma, nonallergic
nonallergic (intrinsic) J45.909
with
exacerbation (acute) J45.901
status asthmaticus J45.902
persistent
mild J45.30
with
exacerbation (acute) J45.31
status asthmaticus J45.32
moderate J45.40
with
exacerbation (acute) J45.41
status asthmaticus J45.42
severe J45.50
with
exacerbation (acute) J45.51
status asthmaticus J45.52
platinum J45.998
pneumoconiotic NEC J64
potter's J62.8
predominantly allergic J45.909
psychogenic F54
pulmonary eosinophilic J82
red cedar J67.8
Rostan's I50.1
sandblaster's J62.8
sequoiosis J67.8
severe persistent J45.50
with
exacerbation (acute) J45.51
status asthmaticus J45.52
specified NEC J45.998
stonemason's J62.8
thymic E32.8
tuberculous — *see* Tuberculosis, pulmonary
Wichmann's (laryngismus stridulus) J38.5
wood J67.8
Astigmatism (compound) (congenital) H52.20-
irregular H52.21-
regular H52.22-
Astraphobia F40.220
Astroblastoma
specified site — *see* Neoplasm, malignant, by site
unspecified site C71.9
Astrocytoma (cystic)
anaplastic
specified site — *see* Neoplasm, malignant, by site
unspecified site C71.9
fibrillary
specified site — *see* Neoplasm, malignant, by site
unspecified site C71.9
fibrous
specified site — *see* Neoplasm, malignant, by site

Astrocytoma (cystic) - *continued*
fibrous - *continued*
unspecified site C71.9
gemistocytic
specified site — *see* Neoplasm, malignant, by site
unspecified site C71.9
juvenile
specified site — *see* Neoplasm, malignant, by site
unspecified site C71.9
pilocytic
specified site — *see* Neoplasm, malignant, by site
unspecified site C71.9
piloid
specified site — *see* Neoplasm, malignant, by site
unspecified site C71.9
protoplasmic
specified site — *see* Neoplasm, malignant, by site
unspecified site C71.9
specified site NEC — *see* Neoplasm, malignant, by site
subependymal D43.2
giant cell
specified site — *see* Neoplasm, uncertain behavior, by site
unspecified site D43.2
specified site — *see* Neoplasm, uncertain behavior, by site
unspecified site D43.2
unspecified site C71.9
Astroglioma
specified site — *see* Neoplasm, malignant, by site
unspecified site C71.9
Asymbolia R48.8
Asymmetry — *see also* Distortion
between native and reconstructed breast N65.1
face Q67.0
jaw (lower) — *see* Anomaly, dentofacial, jaw-cranial base relationship, asymmetry
Asynergia, asynergy R27.8
ventricular I51.89
Asystole (heart) — *see* Arrest, cardiac
At risk
for falling Z91.81
Ataxia, ataxy, ataxic R27.0
acute R27.8
brain (hereditary) G11.9
cerebellar (hereditary) G11.9
with defective DNA repair G11.3
alcoholic G31.2
early-onset G11.1
in
alcoholism G31.2
myxedema E03.9 *[G13.2]*
neoplastic disease — *see also* Neoplasm D49.9 *[G32.81]*
specified disease NEC G32.81
late-onset (Marie's) G11.2
cerebral (hereditary) G11.9
congenital nonprogressive G11.0
family, familial — *see* Ataxia, hereditary
following
cerebrovascular disease I69.993
cerebral infarction I69.393
intracerebral hemorrhage I69.193
nontraumatic intracranial hemorrhage NEC I69.293
specified disease NEC I69.893
subarachnoid hemorrhage I69.093
Friedreich's (heredofamilial) (cerebellar) (spinal) G11.1
gait R26.0
hysterical F44.4
general R27.8
gluten M35.9 *[G32.81]*
with celiac disease K90.0 *[G32.81]*
hereditary G11.9
with neuropathy G60.2
cerebellar — *see* Ataxia, cerebellar
spastic G11.4
specified NEC G11.8
spinal (Friedreich's) G11.1
heredofamilial — *see* Ataxia, hereditary
Hunt's G11.1
hysterical F44.4
locomotor (progressive) (syphilitic) (partial) (spastic) A52.11
diabetic — *see* Diabetes, ataxia
Marie's (cerebellar) (heredofamilial) (late-onset) G11.2
nonorganic origin F44.4
nonprogressive, congenital G11.0
psychogenic F44.4
Roussy-Lévy G60.0

Ataxia, ataxy, ataxic - *continued*
  Sanger-Brown's (hereditary) G11.2
  spastic hereditary G11.4
  spinal
    hereditary (Friedreich's) G11.1
    progressive (syphilitic) A52.11
  spinocerebellar, X-linked recessive G11.1
  telangiectasia (Louis-Bar) G11.3
Ataxia-telangiectasia (Louis-Bar) G11.3
Atelectasis (massive) (partial) (pressure)
    (pulmonary) J98.11
  newborn P28.10
    due to resorption P28.11
    partial P28.19
    primary P28.0
    secondary P28.19
  primary (newborn) P28.0
  tuberculous — *see* Tuberculosis, pulmonary
Atelocardia Q24.9
Atelomyelia Q06.1
Atheroembolism
  of
    extremities
      lower I75.02-
      upper I75.01-
    kidney I75.81
    specified NEC I75.89
Atheroma, atheromatous — *see*
    also Arteriosclerosis I70.90
  aorta, aortic I70.0
    valve — *see also* Endocarditis, aortic I35.8
  aorto-iliac I70.0
  artery — *see* Arteriosclerosis
  basilar (artery) I67.2
  carotid (artery) (common) (internal) I67.2
  cerebral (arteries) I67.2
  coronary (artery) I25.10
    with angina pectoris — *see* Arteriosclerosis,
      coronary (artery),
    degeneration — *see* Arteriosclerosis
  heart, cardiac — *see* Disease, heart, ischemic,
      atherosclerotic
  mitral (valve) I34.8
  myocardium, myocardial — *see* Disease, heart,
      ischemic, atherosclerotic
  pulmonary valve (heart) — *see also* Endocarditis,
      pulmonary I37.8
  tricuspid (heart) (valve) I36.8
  valve, valvular — *see* Endocarditis
  vertebral (artery) I67.2
Atheromatosis — *see* Arteriosclerosis
Atherosclerosis — *see also* Arteriosclerosis
  coronary
    artery I25.10
      with angina pectoris — *see* Arteriosclerosis,
        coronary (artery),
      due to
        calcified coronary lesion (severely) I25.84
        lipid rich plaque I25.83
    transplanted heart I25.811
      bypass graft I25.812
        with angina pectoris — *see* Arteriosclerosis,
          coronary (artery),
      native coronary artery I25.811
        with angina pectoris — *see* Arteriosclerosis,
          coronary (artery),
Athetosis (acquired) R25.8
  bilateral (congenital) G80.3
  congenital (bilateral) (double) G80.3
  double (congenital) G80.3
  unilateral R25.8
Athlete's
  foot B35.3
  heart I51.7
Athrepsia E41
Athyrea (acquired) — *see also* Hypothyroidism
  congenital E03.1
Atonia, atony, atonic
  bladder (sphincter) (neurogenic) N31.2
  capillary I78.8
  cecum K59.8
    psychogenic F45.8
  colon — *see* Atony, intestine
  congenital P94.2
  esophagus K22.8
  intestine K59.8
    psychogenic F45.8
  stomach K31.89
    neurotic or psychogenic F45.8
  uterus (during labor) O62.2
    with hemorrhage (postpartum) O72.1
    postpartum (with hemorrhage) O72.1
      without hemorrhage O75.89

Atopy — *see* History, allergy
Atransferrinemia, congenital E88.09
Atresia, atretic
  alimentary organ or tract NEC Q45.8
    upper Q40.8
  ani, anus, anal (canal) Q42.3
    with fistula Q42.2
  aorta (ring) Q25.29
  aortic (orifice) (valve) Q23.0
    arch Q25.21
    congenital with hypoplasia of ascending aorta and
      defective development of left ventricle (with
      mitral stenosis) Q23.4
    in hypoplastic left heart syndrome Q23.4
  aqueduct of Sylvius Q03.0
    with spina bifida — *see* Spina bifida, with
      hydrocephalus
  artery NEC Q27.8
    cerebral Q28.3
    coronary Q24.5
    digestive system Q27.8
    eye Q15.8
    lower limb Q27.8
    pulmonary Q25.5
    specified site NEC Q27.8
    umbilical Q27.0
    upper limb Q27.8
  auditory canal (external) Q16.1
  bile duct (common) (congenital) (hepatic) Q44.2
    acquired — *see* Obstruction, bile duct
  bladder (neck) Q64.39
    obstruction Q64.31
  bronchus Q32.4
  cecum Q42.8
  cervix (acquired) N88.2
    congenital Q51.828
    in pregnancy or childbirth — *see* Anomaly, cervix,
      in pregnancy or childbirth
    causing obstructed labor O65.5
  choana Q30.0
  colon Q42.9
    specified NEC Q42.8
  common duct Q44.2
  cricoid cartilage Q31.8
  cystic duct Q44.2
    acquired K82.8
      with obstruction K82.0
  digestive organs NEC Q45.8
  duodenum Q41.0
  ear canal Q16.1
  ejaculatory duct Q55.4
  epiglottis Q31.8
  esophagus Q39.0
    with tracheoesophageal fistula Q39.1
  eustachian tube Q17.8
  fallopian tube (congenital) Q50.6
    acquired N97.1
  follicular cyst N83.0-
  foramen of
    Luschka Q03.1
      with spina bifida — *see* Spina bifida, with
        hydrocephalus
    Magendie Q03.1
      with spina bifida — *see* Spina bifida, with
        hydrocephalus
  gallbladder Q44.1
  genital organ
    external
      female Q52.79
      male Q55.8
    internal
      female Q52.8
      male Q55.8
  glottis Q31.8
  gullet Q39.0
    with tracheoesophageal fistula Q39.1
  heart valve NEC Q24.8
    pulmonary Q22.0
    tricuspid Q22.4
  hymen Q52.3
    acquired (postinfective) N89.6
  ileum Q41.2
  intestine (small) Q41.9
    large Q42.9
      specified NEC Q42.8
  iris, filtration angle Q15.0
  jejunum Q41.1
  lacrimal apparatus Q10.4
  larynx Q31.8
  meatus urinarius Q64.33
  mitral valve Q23.2
    in hypoplastic left heart syndrome Q23.4
  nares (anterior) (posterior) Q30.0

Atresia, atretic - *continued*
  nasopharynx Q34.8
  nose, nostril Q30.0
    acquired J34.89
  organ or site NEC Q89.8
  osseous meatus (ear) Q16.1
  oviduct (congenital) Q50.6
    acquired N97.1
  parotid duct Q38.4
    acquired K11.8
  pulmonary (artery) Q25.5
    valve Q22.0
  pulmonic Q22.0
  pupil Q13.2
  rectum Q42.1
    with fistula Q42.0
  salivary duct Q38.4
    acquired K11.8
  sublingual duct Q38.4
    acquired K11.8
  submandibular duct Q38.4
    acquired K11.8
  submaxillary duct Q38.4
    acquired K11.8
  thyroid cartilage Q31.8
  trachea Q32.1
  tricuspid valve Q22.4
  ureter Q62.10
    pelvic junction Q62.11
    vesical orifice Q62.12
  ureteropelvic junction Q62.11
  ureterovesical orifice Q62.12
  urethra (valvular) Q64.39
    stricture Q64.32
  urinary tract NEC Q64.8
  uterus Q51.818
    acquired N85.8
  vagina (congenital) Q52.4
    acquired (postinfectional) (senile) N89.5
  vas deferens Q55.3
  vascular NEC Q27.8
    cerebral Q28.3
    digestive system Q27.8
    lower limb Q27.8
    specified site NEC Q27.8
    upper limb Q27.8
  vein NEC Q27.8
    digestive system Q27.8
    great Q26.8
    lower limb Q27.8
    portal Q26.5
    pulmonary Q26.3
    specified site NEC Q27.8
    upper limb Q27.8
  vena cava (inferior) (superior) Q26.8
  vesicourethral orifice Q64.31
  vulva Q52.79
    acquired N90.5
Atrichia, atrichosis — *see* Alopecia
Atrophia — *see also* Atrophy
  cutis senilis L90.8
    due to radiation L57.8
  gyrata of choroid and retina H31.23
  senilis R54
    dermatological L90.8
      due to radiation (nonionizing) (solar) L57.8
  unguium L60.3
    congenita Q84.6
Atrophie blanche (en plaque) (de Milian) L95.0
Atrophoderma, atrophodermia (of) L90.9
  diffusum (idiopathic) L90.4
  maculatum L90.8
    et striatum L90.8
      due to syphilis A52.79
    syphilitic A51.39
  neuriticum L90.8
  Pasini and Pierini L90.3
  pigmentosum Q82.1
  reticulatum symmetricum faciei L66.4
  senile L90.8
    due to radiation (nonionizing) (solar) L57.8
  vermiculata (cheeks) L66.4
Atrophy, atrophic (of)
  adrenal (capsule) (gland) E27.49
    primary (autoimmune) E27.1
  alveolar process or ridge (edentulous) K08.20
  anal sphincter (disuse) N81.84
  appendix K38.8
  arteriosclerotic — *see* Arteriosclerosis
  bile duct (common) (hepatic) K83.8
  bladder N32.89
    neurogenic N31.8
  blanche (en plaque) (of Milian) L95.0

Atrophy, atrophic (of) - *continued*
  bone (senile) NEC — *see also* Disorder, bone,
    specified type NEC
    due to
      tabes dorsalis (neurogenic) A52.11
  brain (cortex) (progressive) G31.9
    frontotemporal circumscribed G31.01 *[F02.80]*
      with behavioral disturbance G31.01 *[F02.81]*
    senile NEC G31.1
  breast N64.2
    obstetric — *see* Disorder, breast, specified type
      NEC
  buccal cavity K13.79
  cardiac — *see* Degeneration, myocardial
  cartilage (infectional) (joint) — *see* Disorder,
    cartilage, specified NEC
  cerebellar — *see* Atrophy, brain
  cerebral — *see* Atrophy, brain
  cervix (mucosa) (senile) (uteri) N88.8
    menopausal N95.8
  Charcot-Marie-Tooth G60.0
  choroid (central) (macular) (myopic) (retina) H31.10
    -
    diffuse secondary H31.12-
    gyrate H31.23
    senile H31.11-
  ciliary body — *see* Atrophy, iris
  conjunctiva (senile) H11.89
  corpus cavernosum N48.89
  cortical — *see* Atrophy, brain
  cystic duct K82.8
  Déjérine-Thomas G23.8
  disuse NEC — *see* Atrophy, muscle
  Duchenne-Aran G12.21
  ear H93.8-
  edentulous alveolar ridge K08.20
  endometrium (senile) N85.8
    cervix N88.8
  enteric K63.89
  epididymis N50.89
  eyeball — *see* Disorder, globe, degenerated
    condition, atrophy
  eyelid (senile) — *see* Disorder, eyelid, degenerative
  facial (skin) L90.9
  fallopian tube (senile) N83.32-
    with ovary N83.33-
  fascioscapulohumeral (Landouzy- Déjérine) G71.0
  fatty, thymus (gland) E32.8
  gallbladder K82.8
  gastric K29.40
    with bleeding K29.41
  gastrointestinal K63.89
  glandular I89.8
  globe H44.52-
  gum — *see also* Recession, gingival K06.0
  hair L67.8
  heart (brown) — *see* Degeneration, myocardial
  hemifacial Q67.4
    Romberg G51.8
  infantile E41
    paralysis, acute — *see* Poliomyelitis, paralytic
  intestine K63.89
  iris (essential) (progressive) H21.26-
    specified NEC H21.29
  kidney (senile) (terminal) — *see also* Sclerosis,
    renal N26.1
    congenital or infantile Q60.5
      bilateral Q60.4
      unilateral Q60.3
    hydronephrotic — *see* Hydronephrosis
  lacrimal gland (primary) H04.14-
    secondary H04.15-
  Landouzy-Déjérine G71.0
  laryngitis, infective J37.0
  larynx J38.7
  Leber's optic (hereditary) H47.22
  lip K13.0
  liver (yellow) K72.90
    with coma K72.91
    acute, subacute K72.00
      with coma K72.01
    chronic K72.10
      with coma K72.11
  lung (senile) J98.4
  macular (dermatological) L90.8
    syphilitic, skin A51.39
    striated A52.79
  mandible (edentulous) K08.20
    minimal K08.21
    moderate K08.22
    severe K08.23
  maxilla K08.20
    minimal K08.24

Atrophy, atrophic (of) - *continued*
  maxilla - *continued*
    moderate K08.25
    severe K08.26
  muscle, muscular (diffuse) (general) (idiopathic)
    (primary) M62.50
    ankle M62.57-
    Duchenne-Aran G12.21
    foot M62.57-
    forearm M62.53-
    hand M62.54-
    infantile spinal G12.0
    lower leg M62.56-
    multiple sites M62.59
    myelopathic — *see* Atrophy, muscle, spinal
    myotonic G71.11
    neuritic G58.9
    neuropathic (peroneal) (progressive) G60.0
    pelvic (disuse) N81.84
    peroneal G60.0
    progressive (bulbar) G12.21
      adult G12.1
      infantile (spinal) G12.0
      spinal G12.9
        adult G12.1
        infantile G12.0
    pseudohypertrophic G71.0
    shoulder region M62.51-
    specified site NEC M62.58
    spinal G12.9
      adult form G12.1
      Aran-Duchenne G12.21
      childhood form, type II G12.1
      distal G12.1
      hereditary NEC G12.1
      infantile, type I (Werdnig-Hoffmann) G12.0
      juvenile form, type III (Kugelberg-
        Welander) G12.1
      progressive G12.21
      scapuloperoneal form G12.1
      specified NEC G12.8
    syphilitic A52.78
    thigh M62.55-
    upper arm M62.52-
  myocardium — *see* Degeneration, myocardial
  myometrium (senile) N85.8
    cervix N88.8
  myopathic NEC — *see* Atrophy, muscle
  myotonia G71.11
  nail L60.3
  nasopharynx J31.1
  nerve — *see also* Disorder, nerve
    abducens — *see* Strabismus, paralytic, sixth nerve
    accessory G52.8
    acoustic or auditory — *see* subcategory H93.3
    cranial G52.9
      eighth (auditory) — *see* subcategory H93.3
      eleventh (accessory) G52.8
      fifth (trigeminal) G50.8
      first (olfactory) G52.0
      fourth (trochlear) — *see* Strabismus, paralytic,
        fourth nerve
      second (optic) H47.20
      sixth (abducens) — *see* Strabismus, paralytic,
        sixth nerve
      tenth (pneumogastric) (vagus) G52.2
      third (oculomotor) — *see* Strabismus, paralytic,
        third nerve
      twelfth (hypoglossal) G52.3
    hypoglossal G52.3
    oculomotor — *see* Strabismus, paralytic, third
      nerve
    olfactory G52.0
    optic (papillomacular bundle)
      syphilitic (late) A52.15
        congenital A50.44
    pneumogastric G52.2
    trigeminal G50.8
    trochlear — *see* Strabismus, paralytic, fourth nerve
    vagus (pneumogastric) G52.2
  neurogenic, bone, tabetic A52.11
  nutritional E41
  old age R54
  olivopontocerebellar G23.8
  optic (nerve) H47.20
    glaucomatous H47.23-
    hereditary H47.22
    primary H47.21-
    specified type NEC H47.29-
    syphilitic (late) A52.15
      congenital A50.44
  orbit H05.31-
  ovary (senile) N83.31-

Atrophy, atrophic (of) - *continued*
  ovary (senile) - *continued*
    with fallopian tube N83.33-
    oviduct (senile) — *see* Atrophy, fallopian tube
  palsy, diffuse (progressive) G12.22
  pancreas (duct) (senile) K86.89
  parotid gland K11.0
  pelvic muscle N81.84
  penis N48.89
  pharynx J39.2
  pluriglandular E31.8
    autoimmune E31.0
  polyarthritis M15.9
  prostate N42.89
  pseudohypertrophic (muscle) G71.0
  renal — *see also* Sclerosis, renal N26.1
  retina, retinal (postinfectional) H35.89
  rhinitis J31.0
  salivary gland K11.0
  scar L90.5
  sclerosis, lobar (of brain) G31.09 *[F02.80]*
    with behavioral disturbance G31.09 *[F02.81]*
  scrotum N50.89
  seminal vesicle N50.89
  senile R54
    due to radiation (nonionizing) (solar) L57.8
  skin (patches) (spots) L90.9
    degenerative (senile) L90.8
    due to radiation (nonionizing) (solar) L57.8
    senile L90.8
  spermatic cord N50.89
  spinal (acute) (cord) G95.89
    muscular — *see* Atrophy, muscle, spinal
    paralysis G12.20
      acute — *see* Poliomyelitis, paralytic
      meaning progressive muscular atrophy G12.21
  spine (column) — *see* Spondylopathy, specified
    NEC
  spleen (senile) D73.0
  stomach K29.40
    with bleeding K29.41
  striate (skin) L90.6
    syphilitic A52.79
  subcutaneous L90.9
  sublingual gland K11.0
  submandibular gland K11.0
  submaxillary gland K11.0
  Sudeck's — *see* Algoneurodystrophy
  suprarenal (capsule) (gland) E27.49
    primary E27.1
  systemic affecting central nervous system
    in
      myxedema E03.9 *[G13.2]*
      neoplastic disease — *see*
        also Neoplasm D49.9 *[G13.1]*
      specified disease NEC G13.8
  tarso-orbital fascia, congenital Q10.3
  testis N50.0
  thenar, partial — *see* Syndrome, carpal tunnel
  thymus (fatty) E32.8
  thyroid (gland) (acquired) E03.4
    with cretinism E03.1
    congenital (with myxedema) E03.1
  tongue (senile) K14.8
    papillae K14.4
  trachea J39.8
  tunica vaginalis N50.89
  turbinate J34.89
  tympanic membrane (nonflaccid) H73.82-
    flaccid H73.81-
  upper respiratory tract J39.8
  uterus, uterine (senile) N85.8
    cervix N88.8
    due to radiation (intended effect) N85.8
      adverse effect or misadventure N99.89
  vagina (senile) N95.2
  vas deferens N50.89
  vascular I99.8
  vertebra (senile) — *see* Spondylopathy, specified
    NEC
  vulva (senile) N90.5
  Werdnig-Hoffmann G12.0
  yellow — *see* Failure, hepatic
Attack, attacks
  with alteration of consciousness (with
    automatisms) — *see* Epilepsy, localization-related,
    symptomatic, with complex partial seizures
  Adams-Stokes I45.9
  akinetic — *see* Epilepsy, generalized, specified NEC
  angina — *see* Angina
  atonic — *see* Epilepsy, generalized, specified NEC
  benign shuddering G25.83
  cataleptic — *see* Catalepsy

Attack, attacks - *continued*
  coronary — *see* Infarct, myocardium
  cyanotic, newborn P28.2
  drop NEC R55
  epileptic — *see* Epilepsy
  heart — *see* infarct, myocardium
  hysterical F44.9
  jacksonian — *see* Epilepsy, localization-related,
    symptomatic, with simple partial seizures
  myocardium, myocardial — *see* Infarct,
    myocardium
  myoclonic — *see* Epilepsy, generalized, specified
    NEC
  panic F41.0
  psychomotor — *see* Epilepsy, localization-related,
    symptomatic, with complex partial seizures
  salaam — *see* Epilepsy, spasms
  schizophreniform, brief F23
  shuddering, benign G25.83
  Stokes-Adams I45.9
  syncope R55
  transient ischemic (TIA) G45.9
    specified NEC G45.8
  unconsciousness R55
    hysterical F44.89
  vasomotor R55
  vasovagal (paroxysmal) (idiopathic) R55
  without alteration of consciousness — *see* Epilepsy,
    localization-related, symptomatic, with simple
    partial seizures
Attention (to)
  artificial
    opening (of) Z43.9
      digestive tract NEC Z43.4
        colon Z43.3
        ilium Z43.2
        stomach Z43.1
      specified NEC Z43.8
      trachea Z43.0
      urinary tract NEC Z43.6
        cystostomy Z43.5
        nephrostomy Z43.6
        ureterostomy Z43.6
        urethrostomy Z43.6
      vagina Z43.7
  colostomy Z43.3
  cystostomy Z43.5
  deficit disorder or syndrome F98.8
    with hyperactivity — *see* Disorder, attention-deficit
      hyperactivity
  gastrostomy Z43.1
  ileostomy Z43.2
  jejunostomy Z43.4
  nephrostomy Z43.6
  surgical dressings Z48.01
  sutures Z48.02
  tracheostomy Z43.0
  ureterostomy Z43.6
  urethrostomy Z43.6
Attrition
  gum — *see also* Recession, gingival K06.0
  tooth, teeth (excessive) (hard tissues) K03.0
Atypical, atypism — *see also* condition
  cells (on cytolgocial smear) (endocervical)
    (endometrial) (glandular)
    cervix R87.619
      vagina R87.629
  cervical N87.9
  endometrium N85.9
    hyperplasia N85.00
  parenting situation Z62.9
Auditory — *see* condition
Aujeszky's disease B33.8
Aurantiasis, cutis E67.1
Auricle, auricular — *see also* condition
  cervical Q18.2
Auriculotemporal syndrome G50.8
Austin Flint murmur (aortic insufficiency) I35.1
Australian
  Q fever A78
  X disease A83.4
Autism, autistic (childhood) (infantile) F84.0
  atypical F84.9
  spectrum disorder F84.0
Autodigestion R68.89
Autoerythrocyte sensitization (syndrome) D69.2
Autographism L50.3
Autoimmune
  disease (systemic) M35.9
  inhibitors to clotting factors D68.311
  lymphoproliferative syndrome [ALPS] D89.82
  thyroiditis E06.3
Autointoxication R68.89

Automatism G93.89
  with temporal sclerosis G93.81
  epileptic — *see* Epilepsy, localization-related,
    symptomatic, with complex partial seizures
  paroxysmal, idiopathic — *see* Epilepsy, localization-
    related, symptomatic, with complex partial seizures
Autonomic, autonomous
  bladder (neurogenic) N31.2
  hysteria seizure F44.5
Autosensitivity, erythrocyte D69.2
Autosensitization, cutaneous L30.2
Autosome — *see* condition by chromosome involved
Autotopagnosia R48.1
Autotoxemia R68.89
Autumn — *see* condition
Avellis' syndrome G46.8
Aversion
  oral R63.3
    newborn P92.-
    nonorganic origin F98.2
  sexual F52.1
Aviator's
  disease or sickness — *see* Effect, adverse, high
    altitude
  ear T70.0
Avitaminosis (multiple) — *see also* Deficiency,
  vitamin E56.9
  B E53.9
    with
      beriberi E51.11
      pellagra E52
    B2 E53.0
    B6 E53.1
    B12 E53.8
    D E55.9
      with rickets E55.0
    G E53.0
    K E56.1
    nicotinic acid E52
AVNRT
  (atrioventricular nodal re-entrant tachycardia) I47.1
AVRT (atrioventricular nodal re-entrant
  tachycardia) I47.1
Avulsion (traumatic)
  blood vessel — *see* Injury, blood vessel
  bone — *see* Fracture, by site
  cartilage — *see also* Dislocation, by site
    symphyseal (inner) , complicating delivery O71.6
  external site other than limb — *see* Wound, open, by
    site
  eye S05.7-
  head (intracranial)
    external site NEC S08.89
    scalp S08.0
  internal organ or site — *see* Injury, by site
  joint — *see also* Dislocation, by site
    capsule — *see* Sprain, by site
  kidney S37.06-
  ligament — *see* Sprain, by site
  limb — *see also* Amputation, traumatic, by site
    skin and subcutaneous tissue — *see* Wound, open,
      by site
  muscle — *see* Injury, muscle
  nerve (root) — *see* Injury, nerve
  scalp S08.0
  skin and subcutaneous tissue — *see* Wound, open,
    by site
  spleen S36.032
  symphyseal cartilage (inner) , complicating
    delivery O71.6
  tendon — *see* Injury, muscle
  tooth S03.2
Awareness of heart beat R00.2
Axenfeld's
  anomaly or syndrome Q15.0
  degeneration (calcareous) Q13.4
Axilla, axillary — *see also* condition
  breast Q83.1
Axonotmesis — *see* Injury, nerve
Ayerza's disease or syndrome
  (pulmonary artery sclerosis with pulmonary
  hypertension) I27.0
Azoospermia (organic) N46.01
  due to
    drug therapy N46.021
    efferent duct obstruction N46.023
    infection N46.022
    radiation N46.024
    specified cause NEC N46.029
    systemic disease N46.025
Azotemia R79.89
  meaning uremia N19
Aztec ear Q17.3

Azygos
  continuation inferior vena cava Q26.8
  lobe (lung) Q33.1

B

Baastrup's disease — *see* Kissing spine
Babesiosis B60.0
Babington's disease
  (familial hemorrhagic telangiectasia) I78.0
Babinski's syndrome A52.79
Baby
  crying constantly R68.11
  floppy (syndrome) P94.2
Bacillary — *see* condition
Bacilluria R82.71
Bacillus — *see also* Infection, bacillus
  abortus infection A23.1
  anthracis infection A22.9
  coli infection — *see also* Escherichia coli B96.20
  Flexner's A03.1
  mallei infection A24.0
  Shiga's A03.0
  suipestifer infection — *see* Infection, salmonella
Back — *see* condition
Backache (postural) M54.9
  sacroiliac M53.3
  specified NEC M54.89
Backflow — *see* Reflux
Backward reading (dyslexia) F81.0
Bacteremia R78.81
  with sepsis — *see* Sepsis
Bactericholia — *see* Cholecystitis, acute
Bacterid, bacteride (pustular) L40.3
Bacterium, bacteria, bacterial
  agent NEC, as cause of disease classified
    elsewhere B96.89
  in blood — *see* Bacteremia
  in urine — *see* Bacteriuria
Bacteriuria, bacteruria R82.71
  asymptomatic R82.71
Bacteroides
  fragilis, as cause of disease classified
    elsewhere B96.6
Bad
  heart — *see* Disease, heart
  trip
    due to drug abuse — *see* Abuse, drug, hallucinogen
    due to drug dependence — *see* Dependence, drug,
      hallucinogen
Baelz's disease (cheilitis glandularis
  apostematosa) K13.0
Baerensprung's disease (eczema marginatum) B35.6
Bagasse disease or pneumonitis J67.1
Bagassosis J67.1
Baker's cyst — *see* Cyst, Baker's
Bakwin-Krida syndrome (metaphyseal
  dysplasia) Q78.5
Balancing side interference M26.56
Balanitis (circinata) (erosiva) (gangrenosa)
  (phagedenic) (vulgaris) N48.1
  amebic A06.82
  candidal B37.42
  due to Haemophilus ducreyi A57
  gonococcal (acute) (chronic) A54.09
  xerotica obliterans N48.0
Balanoposthitis N47.6
  gonococcal (acute) (chronic) A54.09
  ulcerative (specific) A63.8
Balanorrhagia — *see* Balanitis
Balantidiasis, balantidiosis A07.0
Bald tongue K14.4
Baldness — *see also* Alopecia
  male-pattern — *see* Alopecia, androgenic
Balkan grippe A78
Balloon disease — *see* Effect, adverse, high altitude
Balo's disease (concentric sclerosis) G37.5
Bamberger-Marie disease — *see* Osteoarthropathy,
  hypertrophic, specified type NEC
Bancroft's filariasis B74.0
Band (s)
  adhesive — *see* Adhesions, peritoneum
  anomalous or congenital — *see also* Anomaly, by
    site
    heart (atrial) (ventricular) Q24.8
    intestine Q43.3
    omentum Q43.3
  cervix N88.1
  constricting, congenital Q79.8
  gallbladder (congenital) Q44.1
  intestinal (adhesive) — *see* Adhesions, peritoneum
  obstructive
    intestine K56.5
    peritoneum K56.5

Band (s) - *continued*
  periappendiceal, congenital Q43.3
  peritoneal (adhesive) — *see* Adhesions, peritoneum
  uterus N73.6
    internal N85.6
  vagina N89.5
Bandemia D72.825
Bandl's ring (contraction) **, complicating delivery** O62.4
Bangkok hemorrhagic fever A91
Bang's disease (brucella abortus) A23.1
Bankruptcy, anxiety concerning Z59.8
Bannister's disease T78.3
  hereditary D84.1
Banti's disease or syndrome (with cirrhosis) (with portal hypertension) K76.6
Bar, median, prostate — *see* Enlargement, enlarged, prostate
Barcoo disease or rot — *see* Ulcer, skin
Barlow's disease E54
Barodontalgia T70.29
Baron Münchausen syndrome — *see* Disorder, factitious
Barosinusitis T70.1
Barotitis T70.0
Barotrauma T70.29
  odontalgia T70.29
  otitic T70.0
  sinus T70.1
Barraquer (-Simons) **disease or syndrome** (progressive lipodystrophy) E88.1
Barré-Guillain disease or syndrome G61.0
Barrel chest M95.4
Barré-Liéou syndrome (posterior cervical sympathetic) M53.0
Barrett's
  disease — *see* Barrett's, esophagus
  esophagus K22.70
    with dysplasia K22.719
      high grade K22.711
      low grade K22.710
    without dysplasia K22.70
  syndrome — *see* Barrett's, esophagus
  ulcer K22.10
    with bleeding K22.11
    without bleeding K22.10
Bársony (-Polgár) (-Teschendorf) **syndrome** (corkscrew esophagus) K22.4
Barth syndrome E78.71
Bartholinitis (suppurating) N75.8
  gonococcal (acute) (chronic) (with abscess) A54.1
Bartonellosis A44.9
  cutaneous A44.1
  mucocutaneous A44.1
  specified NEC A44.8
  systemic A44.0
Barton's fracture S52.56-
Bartter's syndrome E26.81
Basal — *see* condition
Basan's (hidrotic) **ectodermal dysplasia** Q82.4
Baseball finger — *see* Dislocation, finger
Basedow's disease (exophthalmic goiter) — *see* Hyperthyroidism, with, goiter
Basic — *see* condition
Basilar — *see* condition
Bason's (hidrotic) **ectodermal dysplasia** Q82.4
Basopenia — *see* Agranulocytosis
Basophilia D72.824
Basophilism (cortico-adrenal) (Cushing's) (pituitary) E24.0
Bassen-Kornzweig disease or syndrome E78.6
Bat ear Q17.5
Bateman's
  disease B08.1
  purpura (senile) D69.2
Bathing cramp T75.1
Bathophobia F40.248
Batten (-Mayou) **disease** E75.4
  retina E75.4 [*H36*]
Batten-Steinert syndrome G71.11
Battered — *see* Maltreatment
Battey Mycobacterium infection A31.0
Battle exhaustion F43.0
Battledore placenta O43.19-
Baumgarten-Cruveilhier cirrhosis, disease or syndrome K74.69
Bauxite fibrosis (of lung) J63.1
Bayle's disease (general paresis) A52.17
Bazin's disease (primary) (tuberculous) A18.4
Beach ear — *see* Swimmer's, ear
Beaded hair (congenital) Q84.1
Béal conjunctivitis or syndrome B30.2
Beard's disease (neurasthenia) F48.8

Beat (s)
  atrial, premature I49.1
  ectopic I49.49
  elbow — *see* Bursitis, elbow
  escaped, heart I49.49
  hand — *see* Bursitis, hand
  knee — *see* Bursitis, knee
  premature I49.40
    atrial I49.1
    auricular I49.1
    supraventricular I49.1
Beau's
  disease or syndrome — *see* Degeneration, myocardial
  lines (transverse furrows on fingernails) L60.4
Bechterev's syndrome — *see* Spondylitis, ankylosing
Becker's
  cardiomyopathy I42.8
  disease
    idiopathic mural endomyocardial disease I42.3
    myotonia congenita, recessive form G71.12
  dystrophy G71.0
  pigmented hairy nevus D22.5
Beck's syndrome (anterior spinal artery occlusion) I65.8
Beckwith-Wiedemann syndrome Q87.3
Bed confinement status Z74.01
Bed sore — *see* Ulcer, pressure, by site
Bedbug bite (s) — *see* Bite(s), by site, superficial, insect
Bedclothes, asphyxiation or suffocation by — *see* Asphyxia, traumatic, due to, mechanical, trapped
Bednar's
  aphthae K12.0
  tumor — *see* Neoplasm, malignant, by site
Bedridden Z74.01
Bedsore — *see* Ulcer, pressure, by site
Bedwetting — *see* Enuresis
Bee sting (with allergic or anaphylactic shock) — *see* Toxicity, venom, arthropod, bee
Beer drinker's heart (disease) I42.6
Begbie's disease (exophthalmic goiter) — *see* Hyperthyroidism, with, goiter
Behavior
  antisocial
    adult Z72.811
    child or adolescent Z72.810
  disorder, disturbance — *see* Disorder, conduct
  disruptive — *see* Disorder, conduct
  drug seeking Z76.5
  inexplicable R46.2
  marked evasiveness R46.5
  obsessive-compulsive R46.81
  overactivity R46.3
  poor responsiveness R46.4
  self-damaging (life-style) Z72.89
  sleep-incompatible Z72.821
  slowness R46.4
  specified NEC R46.89
  strange (and inexplicable) R46.2
  suspiciousness R46.5
  type A pattern Z73.1
  undue concern or preoccupation with stressful events R46.6
  verbosity and circumstantial detail obscuring reason for contact R46.7
Behçet's disease or syndrome M35.2
Behr's disease — *see* Degeneration, macula
Beigel's disease or morbus (white piedra) B36.2
Bejel A65
Bekhterev's syndrome — *see* Spondylitis, ankylosing
Belching — *see* Eructation
Bell's
  mania F30.8
  palsy, paralysis G51.0
    infant or newborn P11.3
  spasm G51.3
Bence Jones albuminuria or proteinuria NEC R80.3
Bends T70.3
Benedikt's paralysis or syndrome G46.3
Benign — *see also* condition
  prostatic hyperplasia — *see* Hyperplasia, prostate
Bennett's fracture (displaced) S62.21-
Benson's disease — *see* Deposit, crystalline
Bent
  back (hysterical) F44.4
  nose M95.0
    congenital Q67.4
Bereavement (uncomplicated) Z63.4
Bergeron's disease (hysterical chorea) F44.4
Berger's disease — *see* Nephropathy, IgA

Beriberi (dry) E51.11
  heart (disease) E51.12
  polyneuropathy E51.11
  wet E51.12
    involving circulatory system E51.11
Berlin's disease or edema (traumatic) S05.8X-
Berlock (berloque) **dermatitis** L56.2
Bernard-Horner syndrome G90.2
Bernard-Soulier disease or thrombopathia D69.1
Bernhardt (-Roth) **disease** — *see* Mononeuropathy, lower limb, meralgia paresthetica
Bernheim's syndrome — *see* Failure, heart, congestive
Bertielliasis B71.8
Berylliosis (lung) J63.2
Besnier-Boeck (-Schaumann) **disease** — *see* Sarcoidosis
Besnier's
  lupus pernio D86.3
  prurigo L20.0
Bestiality F65.89
Best's disease H35.50
Betalipoproteinemia, broad or floating E78.2
Beta-mercaptolactate-cysteine disulfiduria E72.09
Betting and gambling Z72.6
  pathological (compulsive) F63.0
Bezoar T18.9
  intestine T18.3
  stomach T18.2
Bezold's abscess — *see* Mastoiditis, acute
Bianchi's syndrome R48.8
Bicornate or bicornis uterus Q51.3
  in pregnancy or childbirth O34.0-
    causing obstructed labor O65.5
Bicuspid aortic valve Q23.1
Biedl-Bardet syndrome Q87.89
Bielschowsky (-Jansky) **disease** E75.4
Biermer's (pernicious) **anemia or disease** D51.0
Biett's disease L93.0
Bifid (congenital)
  apex, heart Q24.8
  clitoris Q52.6
  kidney Q63.8
  nose Q30.2
  patella Q74.1
  scrotum Q55.29
  toe NEC Q74.2
  tongue Q38.3
  ureter Q62.8
  uterus Q51.3
  uvula Q35.7
Biforis uterus (suprasimplex) Q51.3
Bifurcation (congenital)
  gallbladder Q44.1
  kidney pelvis Q63.8
  renal pelvis Q63.8
  rib Q76.6
  tongue, congenital Q38.3
  trachea Q32.1
  ureter Q62.8
  urethra Q64.74
  vertebra Q76.49
Big spleen syndrome D73.1
Bigeminal pulse R00.8
Bilateral — *see* condition
Bile
  duct — *see* condition
  pigments in urine R82.2
Bilharziasis — *see also* Schistosomiasis
  chyluria B65.0
  cutaneous B65.3
  galacturia B65.0
  hematochyluria B65.0
  intestinal B65.1
  lipemia B65.9
  lipuria B65.0
  oriental B65.2
  piarhemia B65.9
  pulmonary NOS B65.9 [*J99*]
    pneumonia B65.9 [*J17*]
  tropical hematuria B65.0
  vesical B65.0
Biliary — *see* condition
Bilirubin metabolism disorder E80.7
  specified NEC E80.6
Bilirubinemia, familial nonhemolytic E80.4
Bilirubinuria R82.2
Biliuria R82.2
Bilocular stomach K31.2
Binswanger's disease I67.3
Biparta, bipartite
  carpal scaphoid Q74.0
  patella Q74.1

Biparta, bipartite - *continued*
  vagina Q52.10
Bird
  face Q75.8
  fancier's disease or lung J67.2
Birth
  complications in mother — *see* Delivery,
    complicated
  compression during NOS P15.9
  defect — *see* Anomaly
  immature (less than 37 completed weeks) — *see*
    Preterm, newborn
    extremely (less than 28 completed weeks) — *see*
      Immaturity, extreme
  inattention, at or after — *see* Maltreatment, child,
    neglect
  injury NOS P15.9
    basal ganglia P11.1
    brachial plexus NEC P14.3
    brain (compression) (pressure) P11.2
    central nervous system NOS P11.9
    cerebellum P11.1
    cerebral hemorrhage P10.1
    external genitalia P15.5
    eye P15.3
    face P15.4
    fracture
      bone P13.9
        specified NEC P13.8
      clavicle P13.4
      femur P13.2
      humerus P13.3
      long bone, except femur P13.3
      radius and ulna P13.3
      skull P13.0
      spine P11.5
      tibia and fibula P13.3
    intracranial P11.2
      laceration or hemorrhage P10.9
        specified NEC P10.8
    intraventricular hemorrhage P10.2
    laceration
      brain P10.1
      by scalpel P15.8
      peripheral nerve P14.9
    liver P15.0
    meninges
      brain P11.1
      spinal cord P11.5
    nerve
      brachial plexus P14.3
      cranial NEC (except facial) P11.4
      facial P11.3
      peripheral P14.9
      phrenic (paralysis) P14.2
    paralysis
      facial nerve P11.3
      spinal P11.5
    penis P15.5
    rupture
      spinal cord P11.5
    scalp P12.9
    scalpel wound P15.8
    scrotum P15.5
    skull NEC P13.1
      fracture P13.0
    specified type NEC P15.8
    spinal cord P11.5
    spine P11.5
    spleen P15.1
    sternomastoid (hematoma) P15.2
    subarachnoid hemorrhage P10.3
    subcutaneous fat necrosis P15.6
    subdural hemorrhage P10.0
    tentorial tear P10.4
    testes P15.5
    vulva P15.5
  lack of care, at or after — *see* Maltreatment, child,
    neglect
  neglect, at or after — *see* Maltreatment, child,
    neglect
  palsy or paralysis, newborn, NOS (birth
    injury) P14.9
  premature (infant) — *see* Preterm, newborn
  shock, newborn P96.89
  trauma — *see* Birth, injury
  weight
    low (2499 grams or less) — *see* Low, birthweight
      extremely (999 grams or less) — *see* Low,
        birthweight, extreme
    4000 grams to 4499 grams P08.1
    4500 grams or more P08.0
Birthmark Q82.5

Birt-Hogg-Dube syndrome Q87.89
Bisalbuminemia E88.09
Biskra's button B55.1
Bite (s) (animal) (human)
  abdomen, abdominal
    wall S31.159
      with penetration into peritoneal cavity S31.659
      epigastric region S31.152
        with penetration into peritoneal cavity S31.652
      left
        lower quadrant S31.154
          with penetration into peritoneal cavity S31.654
        upper quadrant S31.151
          with penetration into peritoneal cavity S31.651
      periumbilic region S31.155
        with penetration into peritoneal cavity S31.655
      right
        lower quadrant S31.153
          with penetration into peritoneal cavity S31.653
        upper quadrant S31.150
          with penetration into peritoneal cavity S31.650
      superficial NEC S30.871
        insect S30.861
  alveolar (process) — *see* Bite, oral cavity
  amphibian (venomous) — *see* Venom, bite,
    amphibian
  animal — *see also* Bite, by site
    venomous — *see* Venom
  ankle S91.05-
    superficial NEC S90.57-
      insect S90.56-
  antecubital space — *see* Bite, elbow
  anus S31.835
    superficial NEC S30.877
      insect S30.867
  arm (upper) S41.15-
    lower — *see* Bite, forearm
    superficial NEC S40.87-
      insect S40.86-
  arthropod NEC — *see* Venom, bite, arthropod
  auditory canal (external) (meatus) — *see* Bite, ear
  auricle, ear — *see* Bite, ear
  axilla — *see* Bite, arm
  back — *see also* Bite, thorax, back
    lower S31.050
      with penetration into retroperitoneal
        space S31.051
    superficial NEC S30.870
      insect S30.860
  bedbug — *see* Bite(s), by site, superficial, insect
  breast S21.05-
    superficial NEC S20.17-
      insect S20.16-
  brow — *see* Bite, head, specified site NEC
  buttock S31.805
    left S31.825
    right S31.815
    superficial NEC S30.870
      insect S30.860
  calf — *see* Bite, leg
  canaliculus lacrimalis — *see* Bite, eyelid
  canthus, eye — *see* Bite, eyelid
  centipede — *see* Toxicity, venom, arthropod,
    centipede
  cheek (external) S01.45-
    superficial NEC S00.87
      insect S00.86
    internal — *see* Bite, oral cavity
  chest wall — *see* Bite, thorax
  chigger B88.0
  chin — *see* Bite, head, specified site NEC
  clitoris — *see* Bite, vulva
  costal region — *see* Bite, thorax
  digit (s)
    hand — *see* Bite, finger
    toe — *see* Bite, toe
  ear (canal) (external) S01.35-
    superficial NEC S00.47-
      insect S00.46-
  elbow S51.05-
    superficial NEC S50.37-
      insect S50.36-
  epididymis — *see* Bite, testis
  epigastric region — *see* Bite, abdomen
  epiglottis — *see* Bite, neck, specified site NEC
  esophagus, cervical S11.25
    superficial NEC S10.17
      insect S10.16
  eyebrow — *see* Bite, eyelid
  eyelid S01.15-
    superficial NEC S00.27-
      insect S00.26-
  face NEC — *see* Bite, head, specified site NEC

Bite (s) (animal) (human) - *continued*
  finger (s) S61.259
    with
      damage to nail S61.359
    index S61.258
      with
        damage to nail S61.358
    left S61.251
      with
        damage to nail S61.351
    right S61.250
      with
        damage to nail S61.350
    superficial NEC S60.478
      insect S60.46-
    little S61.25-
      with
        damage to nail S61.35-
      superficial NEC S60.47-
        insect S60.46-
    middle S61.25-
      with
        damage to nail S61.35-
      superficial NEC S60.47-
        insect S60.46-
    ring S61.25-
      with
        damage to nail S61.35-
      superficial NEC S60.47-
        insect S60.46-
    superficial NEC S60.479
      insect S60.469
    thumb — *see* Bite, thumb
  flank — *see* Bite, abdomen, wall
  flea — *see* Bite, by site, superficial, insect
  foot (except toe (s) alone) S91.35-
    superficial NEC S90.87-
      insect S90.86-
    toe — *see* Bite, toe
  forearm S51.85-
    elbow only — *see* Bite, elbow
    superficial NEC S50.87-
      insect S50.86-
  forehead — *see* Bite, head, specified site NEC
  genital organs, external
    female S31.552
      superficial NEC S30.876
        insect S30.866
      vagina and vulva — *see* Bite, vulva
    male S31.551
      penis — *see* Bite, penis
      scrotum — *see* Bite, scrotum
      superficial NEC S30.875
        insect S30.865
      testes — *see* Bite, testis
  groin — *see* Bite, abdomen, wall
  gum — *see* Bite, oral cavity
  hand S61.45-
    finger — *see* Bite, finger
    superficial NEC S60.57-
      insect S60.56-
    thumb — *see* Bite, thumb
  head S01.95
    cheek — *see* Bite, cheek
    ear — *see* Bite, ear
    eyelid — *see* Bite, eyelid
    lip — *see* Bite, lip
    nose — *see* Bite, nose
    oral cavity — *see* Bite, oral cavity
    scalp — *see* Bite, scalp
    specified site NEC S01.85
      superficial NEC S00.87
        insect S00.86
    superficial NEC S00.97
      insect S00.96
    temporomandibular area — *see* Bite, cheek
  heel — *see* Bite, foot
  hip S71.05-
    superficial NEC S70.27-
      insect S70.26-
  hymen S31.45
  hypochondrium — *see* Bite, abdomen, wall
  hypogastric region — *see* Bite, abdomen, wall
  inguinal region — *see* Bite, abdomen, wall
  insect — *see* Bite, by site, superficial, insect
  instep — *see* Bite, foot
  interscapular region — *see* Bite, thorax, back
  jaw — *see* Bite, head, specified site NEC
  knee S81.05-
    superficial NEC S80.27-
      insect S80.26-
  labium (majus) (minus) — *see* Bite, vulva
  lacrimal duct — *see* Bite, eyelid

Bite (s) (animal) (human) - *continued*
- larynx S11.015
  - superficial NEC S10.17
    - insect S10.16
- leg (lower) S81.85-
  - ankle — *see* Bite, ankle
  - foot — *see* Bite, foot
  - knee — *see* Bite, knee
  - superficial NEC S80.87-
    - insect S80.86-
  - toe — *see* Bite, toe
  - upper — *see* Bite, thigh
- lip S01.551
  - superficial NEC S00.571
    - insect S00.561
- lizard (venomous) — *see* Venom, bite, reptile
- loin — *see* Bite, abdomen, wall
- lower back — *see* Bite, back, lower
- lumbar region — *see* Bite, back, lower
- malar region — *see* Bite, head, specified site NEC
- mammary — *see* Bite, breast
- marine animals (venomous) — *see* Toxicity, venom, marine animal
- mastoid region — *see* Bite, head, specified site NEC
- mouth — *see* Bite, oral cavity
- nail
  - finger — *see* Bite, finger
  - toe — *see* Bite, toe
- nape — *see* Bite, neck, specified site NEC
- nasal (septum) (sinus) — *see* Bite, nose
- nasopharynx — *see* Bite, head, specified site NEC
- neck S11.95
  - involving
    - cervical esophagus — *see* Bite, esophagus, cervical
    - larynx — *see* Bite, larynx
    - pharynx — *see* Bite, pharynx
    - thyroid gland S11.15
    - trachea — *see* Bite, trachea
  - specified site NEC S11.85
    - superficial NEC S10.87
      - insect S10.86
  - superficial NEC S10.97
    - insect S10.96
  - throat S11.85
    - superficial NEC S10.17
      - insect S10.16
- nose (septum) (sinus) S01.25
  - superficial NEC S00.37
    - insect S00.36
- occipital region — *see* Bite, scalp
- oral cavity S01.552
  - superficial NEC S00.572
    - insect S00.562
- orbital region — *see* Bite, eyelid
- palate — *see* Bite, oral cavity
- palm — *see* Bite, hand
- parietal region — *see* Bite, scalp
- pelvis S31.050
  - with penetration into retroperitoneal space S31.051
  - superficial NEC S30.870
    - insect S30.860
- penis S31.25
  - superficial NEC S30.872
    - insect S30.862
- perineum
  - female — *see* Bite, vulva
  - male — *see* Bite, pelvis
- periocular area (with or without lacrimal passages) — *see* Bite, eyelid
- phalanges
  - finger — *see* Bite, finger
  - toe — *see* Bite, toe
- pharynx S11.25
  - superficial NEC S10.17
    - insect S10.16
- pinna — *see* Bite, ear
- poisonous — *see* Venom
- popliteal space — *see* Bite, knee
- prepuce — *see* Bite, penis
- pubic region — *see* Bite, abdomen, wall
- rectovaginal septum — *see* Bite, vulva
- red bug B88.0
- reptile NEC — *see also* Venom, bite, reptile
  - nonvenomous — *see* Bite, by site
  - snake — *see* Venom, bite, snake
- sacral region — *see* Bite, back, lower
- sacroiliac region — *see* Bite, back, lower
- salivary gland — *see* Bite, oral cavity
- scalp S01.05
  - superficial NEC S00.07
    - insect S00.06
- scapular region — *see* Bite, shoulder

Bite (s) (animal) (human) - *continued*
- scrotum S31.35
  - superficial NEC S30.873
    - insect S30.863
- sea-snake (venomous) — *see* Toxicity, venom, snake, sea snake
- shin — *see* Bite, leg
- shoulder S41.05-
  - superficial NEC S40.27-
    - insect S40.26-
- snake — *see also* Venom, bite, snake
  - nonvenomous — *see* Bite, by site
- spermatic cord — *see* Bite, testis
- spider (venomous) — *see* Toxicity, venom, spider
  - nonvenomous — *see* Bite, by site, superficial, insect
- sternal region — *see* Bite, thorax, front
- submaxillary region — *see* Bite, head, specified site NEC
- submental region — *see* Bite, head, specified site NEC
- subungual
  - finger (s) — *see* Bite, finger
  - toe — *see* Bite, toe
- superficial — *see* Bite, by site, superficial
- supraclavicular fossa S11.85
- supraorbital — *see* Bite, head, specified site NEC
- temple, temporal region — *see* Bite, head, specified site NEC
- temporomandibular area — *see* Bite, cheek
- testis S31.35
  - superficial NEC S30.873
    - insect S30.863
- thigh S71.15-
  - superficial NEC S70.37-
    - insect S70.36-
- thorax, thoracic (wall) S21.95
  - back S21.25-
    - with penetration into thoracic cavity S21.45-
  - breast — *see* Bite, breast
  - front S21.15-
    - with penetration into thoracic cavity S21.35-
  - superficial NEC S20.97
    - back S20.47-
    - front S20.37-
    - insect S20.96
      - back S20.46-
      - front S20.36-
- throat — *see* Bite, neck, throat
- thumb S61.05-
  - with
    - damage to nail S61.15-
  - superficial NEC S60.37-
    - insect S60.36-
- thyroid S11.15
  - superficial NEC S10.87
    - insect S10.86
- toe (s) S91.15-
  - with
    - damage to nail S91.25-
  - great S91.15-
    - with
      - damage to nail S91.25-
  - lesser S91.15-
    - with
      - damage to nail S91.25-
  - superficial NEC S90.47-
    - great S90.47-
    - insect S90.46-
      - great S90.46-
- tongue S01.552
- trachea S11.025
  - superficial NEC S10.17
    - insect S10.16
- tunica vaginalis — *see* Bite, testis
- tympanum, tympanic membrane — *see* Bite, ear
- umbilical region S31.155
- uvula — *see* Bite, oral cavity
- vagina — *see* Bite, vulva
- venomous — *see* Venom
- vocal cords S11.035
  - superficial NEC S10.17
    - insect S10.16
- vulva S31.45
  - superficial NEC S30.874
    - insect S30.864
- wrist S61.55-
  - superficial NEC S60.87-
    - insect S60.86-

Biting, cheek or lip K13.1
Biventricular failure (heart) I50.9
Björck (-Thorson) **syndrome** (malignant carcinoid) E34.0

Black
- death A20.9
- eye S00.1-
- hairy tongue K14.3
- heel (foot) S90.3-
- lung (disease) J60
- palm (hand) S60.22-
Blackfan-Diamond anemia or syndrome (congenital hypoplastic anemia) D61.01
Blackhead L70.0
Blackout R55
Bladder — *see* condition
Blast (air) (hydraulic) (immersion) (underwater)
- blindness S05.8X-
- injury
  - abdomen or thorax — *see* Injury, by site
  - ear (acoustic nerve trauma) — *see* Injury, nerve, acoustic, specified type NEC
- syndrome NEC T70.8
Blastoma — *see* Neoplasm, malignant, by site
- pulmonary — *see* Neoplasm, lung, malignant
Blastomycosis, blastomycotic B40.9
- Brazilian — *see* Paracoccidioidomycosis
- cutaneous B40.3
- disseminated B40.7
- European — *see* Cryptococcosis
- generalized B40.7
- keloidal B48.0
- North American B40.9
- primary pulmonary B40.0
- pulmonary B40.2
  - acute B40.0
  - chronic B40.1
- skin B40.3
- South American — *see* Paracoccidioidomycosis
- specified NEC B40.89
Bleb (s) R23.8
- emphysematous (lung) (solitary) J43.9
- endophthalmitis H59.43
- filtering (vitreous) , after glaucoma surgery Z98.83
- inflamed (infected) , postprocedural H59.40
  - stage 1 H59.41
  - stage 2 H59.42
  - stage 3 H59.43
- lung (ruptured) J43.9
  - congenital — *see* Atelectasis
  - newborn P25.8
- subpleural (emphysematous) J43.9
Blebitis, postprocedural H59.40
- stage 1 H59.41
- stage 2 H59.42
- stage 3 H59.43
Bleeder (familial) (hereditary) — *see* Hemophilia
Bleeding — *see also* Hemorrhage
- anal K62.5
- anovulatory N97.0
- atonic, following delivery O72.1
- capillary I78.8
  - puerperal O72.2
- contact (postcoital) N93.0
- due to uterine subinvolution N85.3
- ear — *see* Otorrhagia
- excessive, associated with menopausal onset N92.4
- familial — *see* Defect, coagulation
- following intercourse N93.0
- gastrointestinal K92.2
- hemorrhoids — *see* Hemorrhoids
- intermenstrual (regular) N92.3
  - irregular N92.1
- intraoperative — *see* Complication, intraoperative, hemorrhage
- irregular N92.6
- menopausal N92.4
- newborn, intraventricular — *see* Newborn, affected by, hemorrhage, intraventricular
- nipple N64.59
- nose R04.0
- ovulation N92.3
- postclimacteric N95.0
- postcoital N93.0
- postmenopausal N95.0
- postoperative — *see* Complication, postprocedural, hemorrhage
- preclimacteric N92.4
- pre-pubertal vaginal N93.1
- puberty (excessive, with onset of menstrual periods) N92.2
- rectum, rectal K62.5
  - newborn P54.2
- tendencies — *see* Defect, coagulation
- throat R04.1
- tooth socket (post-extraction) K91.840
- umbilical stump P51.9

Bleeding - *continued*
uterus, uterine NEC N93.9
climacteric N92.4
dysfunctional of functional N93.8
menopausal N92.4
preclimacteric or premenopausal N92.4
unrelated to menstrual cycle N93.9
vagina, vaginal (abnormal) N93.9
dysfunctional or functional N93.8
newborn P54.6
pre-pubertal N93.1
vicarious N94.89
Blennorrhagia, blennorrhagic — *see* Gonorrhea
Blennorrhea (acute) (chronic) — *see also* Gonorrhea
inclusion (neonatal) (newborn) P39.1
lower genitourinary tract (gonococcal) A54.00
neonatorum (gonococcal ophthalmia) A54.31
Blepharelosis — *see* Entropion
Blepharitis (angularis) (ciliaris) (eyelid) (marginal) (nonulcerative) H01.009
herpes zoster B02.39
left H01.006
lower H01.005
upper H01.004
right H01.003
lower H01.002
upper H01.001
squamous H01.029
left H01.026
lower H01.025
upper H01.024
right H01.023
lower H01.022
upper H01.021
ulcerative H01.019
left H01.016
lower H01.015
upper H01.014
right H01.013
lower H01.012
upper H01.011
Blepharochalasis H02.30
congenital Q10.0
left H02.36
lower H02.35
upper H02.34
right H02.33
lower H02.32
upper H02.31
Blepharoclonus H02.59
Blepharoconjunctivitis H10.50-
angular H10.52-
contact H10.53-
ligneous H10.51-
Blepharophimosis (eyelid) H02.529
congenital Q10.3
left H02.526
lower H02.525
upper H02.524
right H02.523
lower H02.522
upper H02.521
Blepharoptosis H02.40-
congenital Q10.0
mechanical H02.41-
myogenic H02.42-
neurogenic H02.43-
paralytic H02.43-
Blepharopyorrhea, gonococcal A54.39
Blepharospasm G24.5
drug induced G24.01
Blighted ovum O02.0
Blind — *see also* Blindness
bronchus (congenital) Q32.4
loop syndrome K90.2
congenital Q43.8
sac, fallopian tube (congenital) Q50.6
spot, enlarged — *see* Defect, visual field, localized, scotoma, blind spot area
tract or tube, congenital NEC — *see* Atresia, by site
Blindness (acquired) (congenital) (both eyes) H54.0
blast S05.8X-
color — *see* Deficiency, color vision
concussion S05.8X-
cortical H47.619
left brain H47.612
right brain H47.611
day H53.11
due to injury (current episode) S05.9-
sequelae -- code to injury with seventh character S
eclipse (total) — *see* Retinopathy, solar
emotional (hysterical) F44.6
face H53.16

Blindness (acquired) (congenital) (both eyes) - *continued*
hysterical F44.6
legal (both eyes) (USA definition) H54.8
mind R48.8
night H53.60
abnormal dark adaptation curve H53.61
acquired H53.62
congenital H53.63
specified type NEC H53.69
vitamin A deficiency E50.5
one eye (other eye normal) H54.40
left (normal vision on right) H54.42
low vision on right H54.12
low vision, other eye H54.10
right (normal vision on left) H54.41
low vision on left H54.11
psychic R48.8
river B73.01
snow — *see* Photokeratitis
sun, solar — *see* Retinopathy, solar
transient — *see* Disturbance, vision, subjective, loss, transient
traumatic (current episode) S05.9-
word (developmental) F81.0
acquired R48.0
secondary to organic lesion R48.0
Blister (nonthermal)
abdominal wall S30.821
alveolar process S00.522
ankle S90.52-
antecubital space — *see* Blister, elbow
anus S30.827
arm (upper) S40.82-
auditory canal — *see* Blister, ear
auricle — *see* Blister, ear
axilla — *see* Blister, arm
back, lower S30.820
beetle dermatitis L24.89
breast S20.12-
brow S00.82
calf — *see* Blister, leg
canthus — *see* Blister, eyelid
cheek S00.82
internal S00.522
chest wall — *see* Blister, thorax
chin S00.82
costal region — *see* Blister, thorax
digit (s)
foot — *see* Blister, toe
hand — *see* Blister, finger
due to burn — *see* Burn, by site, second degree
ear S00.42-
elbow S50.32-
epiglottis S10.12
esophagus, cervical S10.12
eyebrow — *see* Blister, eyelid
eyelid S00.22-
face S00.82
fever B00.1
finger (s) S60.429
index S60.42-
little S60.42-
middle S60.42-
ring S60.42-
foot (except toe (s) alone) S90.82-
toe — *see* Blister, toe
forearm S50.82-
elbow only — *see* Blister, elbow
forehead S00.82
fracture - omit code
genital organ
female S30.826
male S30.825
gum S00.522
hand S60.52-
head S00.92
ear — *see* Blister, ear
eyelid — *see* Blister, eyelid
lip S00.521
nose S00.32
oral cavity S00.522
scalp S00.02
specified site NEC S00.82
heel — *see* Blister, foot
hip S70.22-
interscapular region S20.429
jaw S00.82
knee S80.22-
larynx S10.12
leg (lower) S80.82-
knee — *see* Blister, knee
upper — *see* Blister, thigh

Blister (nonthermal) - *continued*
lip S00.521
malar region S00.82
mammary — *see* Blister, breast
mastoid region S00.82
mouth S00.522
multiple, skin, nontraumatic R23.8
nail
finger — *see* Blister, finger
toe — *see* Blister, toe
nasal S00.32
neck S10.92
specified site NEC S10.82
throat S10.12
nose S00.32
occipital region S00.02
oral cavity S00.522
orbital region — *see* Blister, eyelid
palate S00.522
palm — *see* Blister, hand
parietal region S00.02
pelvis S30.820
penis S30.822
periocular area — *see* Blister, eyelid
phalanges
finger — *see* Blister, finger
toe — *see* Blister, toe
pharynx S10.12
pinna — *see* Blister, ear
popliteal space — *see* Blister, knee
scalp S00.02
scapular region — *see* Blister, shoulder
scrotum S30.823
shin — *see* Blister, leg
shoulder S40.22-
sternal region S20.329
submaxillary region S00.82
submental region S00.82
subungual
finger (s) — *see* Blister, finger
toe (s) — *see* Blister, toe
supraclavicular fossa S10.82
supraorbital S00.82
temple S00.82
temporal region S00.82
testis S30.823
thermal — *see* Burn, second degree, by site
thigh S70.32-
thorax, thoracic (wall) S20.92
back S20.42-
front S20.32-
throat S10.12
thumb S60.32-
toe (s) S90.42-
great S90.42-
tongue S00.522
trachea S10.12
tympanum, tympanic membrane — *see* Blister, ear
upper arm — *see* Blister, arm (upper)
uvula S00.522
vagina S30.824
vocal cords S10.12
vulva S30.824
wrist S60.82-
Bloating R14.0
Bloch-Sulzberger disease or syndrome Q82.3
Block, blocked
alveolocapillary J84.10
arborization (heart) I45.5
arrhythmic I45.9
atrioventricular (incomplete) (partial) I44.30
with atrioventricular dissociation I44.2
complete I44.2
congenital Q24.6
congenital Q24.6
first degree I44.0
second degree (types I and II) I44.1
specified NEC I44.39
third degree I44.2
types I and II I44.1
auriculoventricular — *see* Block, atrioventricular
bifascicular (cardiac) I45.2
bundle-branch (complete) (false) (incomplete) I45.4
bilateral I45.2
left I44.7
with right bundle branch block I45.2
hemiblock I44.60
anterior I44.4
posterior I44.5
incomplete I44.7
with right bundle branch block I45.2
right I45.10
with

Block, blocked - *continued*
bundle-branch (complete) (false) (incomplete) -
continued
right - *continued*
with - *continued*
left bundle branch block I45.2
left fascicular block I45.2
specified NEC I45.19
Wilson's type I45.19
cardiac I45.9
conduction I45.9
complete I44.2
fascicular (left) I44.60
anterior I44.4
posterior I44.5
right I45.0
specified NEC I44.69
foramen Magendie (acquired) G91.1
congenital Q03.1
with spina bifida — *see* Spina bifida, by site, with
hydrocephalus
heart I45.9
bundle branch I45.4
bilateral I45.2
complete (atrioventricular) I44.2
congenital Q24.6
first degree (atrioventricular) I44.0
second degree (atrioventricular) I44.1
specified type NEC I45.5
third degree (atrioventricular) I44.2
hepatic vein I82.0
intraventricular (nonspecific) I45.4
bundle branch
bilateral I45.2
kidney N28.9
postcystoscopic or postprocedural N99.0
Mobitz (types I and II) I44.1
myocardial — *see* Block, heart
nodal I45.5
organ or site, congenital NEC — *see* Atresia, by site
portal (vein) I81
second degree (types I and II) I44.1
sinoatrial I45.5
sinoauricular I45.5
third degree I44.2
trifascicular I45.3
tubal N97.1
vein NOS I82.90
Wenckebach (types I and II) I44.1
Blockage — *see* Obstruction
Blocq's disease F44.4
Blood
constituents, abnormal R78.9
disease D75.9
donor — *see* Donor, blood
dyscrasia D75.9
with
abortion — *see* Abortion, by type, complicated
by, hemorrhage
ectopic pregnancy O08.1
molar pregnancy O08.1
following ectopic or molar pregnancy O08.1
newborn P61.9
puerperal, postpartum O72.3
flukes NEC — *see* Schistosomiasis
in
feces K92.1
occult R19.5
urine — *see* Hematuria
mole O02.0
occult in feces R19.5
pressure
decreased, due to shock following injury T79.4
examination only Z01.30
fluctuating I99.8
high — *see* Hypertension
borderline R03.0
incidental reading, without diagnosis of
hypertension R03.0
low — *see also* Hypotension
incidental reading, without diagnosis of
hypotension R03.1
spitting — *see* Hemoptysis
staining cornea — *see* Pigmentation, cornea, stromal
transfusion
reaction or complication — *see* Complications,
transfusion
type
A (Rh positive) Z67.10
Rh negative Z67.11
AB (Rh positive) Z67.30
Rh negative Z67.31
B (Rh positive) Z67.20

Blood - *continued*
type - *continued*
B (Rh positive) - *continued*
Rh negative Z67.21
O (Rh positive) Z67.40
Rh negative Z67.41
Rh (positive) Z67.90
negative Z67.91
vessel rupture — *see* Hemorrhage
vomiting — *see* Hematemesis
Blood-forming organs, disease D75.9
Bloodgood's disease — *see* Mastopathy, cystic
Bloom (-Machacek) (-Torre) **syndrome** Q82.8
Blount's disease or osteochondrosis — *see*
Osteochondrosis, juvenile, tibia
Blue
baby Q24.9
diaper syndrome E72.09
dome cyst (breast) — *see* Cyst, breast
dot cataract Q12.0
nevus D22.9
sclera Q13.5
with fragility of bone and deafness Q78.0
toe syndrome I75.02-
Blueness — *see* Cyanosis
Blues, postpartal O90.6
baby O90.6
Blurring, visual H53.8
Blushing (abnormal) (excessive) R23.2
BMI — *see* Body, mass index
Boarder, hospital NEC Z76.4
accompanying sick person Z76.3
healthy infant or child Z76.2
foundling Z76.1
Bockhart's impetigo L01.02
Bodechtel-Guttman disease
(subacute sclerosing panencephalitis) A81.1
Boder-Sedgwick syndrome (ataxia
-telangiectasia) G11.3
Body, bodies
Aschoff's — *see* Myocarditis, rheumatic
asteroid, vitreous — *see* Deposit, crystalline
cytoid (retina) — *see* Occlusion, artery, retina
drusen (degenerative) (macula) (retinal) — *see*
also Degeneration, macula, drusen
optic disc — *see* Drusen, optic disc
foreign — *see* Foreign body
loose
joint, except knee — *see* Loose, body, joint
knee M23.4-
sheath, tendon — *see* Disorder, tendon, specified
type NEC
mass index (BMI)
adult
19 or less Z68.1
20.0-20.9 Z68.20
21.0-21.9 Z68.21
22.0-22.9 Z68.22
23.0-23.9 Z68.23
24.0-24.9 Z68.24
25.0-25.9 Z68.25
26.0-26.9 Z68.26
27.0-27.9 Z68.27
28.0-28.9 Z68.28
29.0-29.9 Z68.29
30.0-30.9 Z68.30
31.0-31.9 Z68.31
32.0-32.9 Z68.32
33.0-33.9 Z68.33
34.0-34.9 Z68.34
35.0-35.9 Z68.35
36.0-36.9 Z68.36
37.0-37.9 Z68.37
38.0-38.9 Z68.38
39.0-39.9 Z68.39
40.0-44.9 Z68.41
45.0-49.9 Z68.42
50.0-59.9 Z68.43
60.0-69.9 Z68.44
70 and over Z68.45
pediatric
5th percentile to less than 85th percentile for
age Z68.52
85th percentile to less than 95th percentile for
age Z68.53
greater than or equal to ninety-fifth percentile for
age Z68.54
less than fifth percentile for age Z68.51
Mooser's A75.2
rice — *see also* Loose, body, joint
knee M23.4-
rocking F98.4

Boeck's
disease or sarcoid — *see* Sarcoidosis
lupoid (miliary) D86.3
Boerhaave's syndrome
(spontaneous esophageal rupture) K22.3
Boggy
cervix N88.8
uterus N85.8
Boil — *see also* Furuncle, by site
Aleppo B55.1
Baghdad B55.1
Delhi B55.1
lacrimal
gland — *see* Dacryoadenitis
passages (duct) (sac) — *see* Inflammation,
lacrimal, passages, acute
Natal B55.1
orbit, orbital — *see* Abscess, orbit
tropical B55.1
Bold hives — *see* Urticaria
Bombé, iris — *see* Membrane, pupillary
Bone — *see* condition
Bonnevie-Ullrich syndrome — *see also* Turner's
syndrome Q87.1
Bonnier's syndrome — *see* subcategory H81.8
Bonvale dam fever T73.3
Bony block of joint — *see* Ankylosis
BOOP
(bronchiolitis obliterans organized
pneumonia) J84.89
Borderline
diabetes mellitus R73.03
hypertension R03.0
osteopenia M85.8-
pelvis, with obstruction during labor O65.1
personality F60.3
Borna disease A83.9
Bornholm disease B33.0
Boston exanthem A88.0
Botalli, ductus (patent) (persistent) Q25.0
Bothriocephalus latus infestation B70.0
Botulism (foodborne intoxication) A05.1
infant A48.51
non-foodborne A48.52
wound A48.52
Bouba — *see* Yaws
Bouchard's nodes (with arthropathy) M15.2
Bouffée délirante F23
Bouillaud's disease or syndrome
(rheumatic heart disease) I01.9
Bourneville's disease Q85.1
Boutonniere deformity (finger) — *see* Deformity,
finger, boutonniere
Bouveret (-Hoffmann) **syndrome**
(paroxysmal tachycardia) I47.9
Bovine heart — *see* Hypertrophy, cardiac
Bowel — *see* condition
Bowen's
dermatosis (precancerous) — *see* Neoplasm, skin, in
situ
disease — *see* Neoplasm, skin, in situ
epithelioma — *see* Neoplasm, skin, in situ
type
epidermoid carcinoma-in-situ — *see* Neoplasm,
skin, in situ
intraepidermal squamous cell carcinoma — *see*
Neoplasm, skin, in situ
Bowing
femur — *see also* Deformity, limb, specified type
NEC, thigh
congenital Q68.3
fibula — *see also* Deformity, limb, specified type
NEC, lower leg
congenital Q68.4
forearm — *see* Deformity, limb, specified type NEC,
forearm
leg (s) , long bones, congenital Q68.5
radius — *see* Deformity, limb, specified type NEC,
forearm
tibia — *see also* Deformity, limb, specified type
NEC, lower leg
congenital Q68.4
Bowleg (s) (acquired) M21.16-
congenital Q68.5
rachitic E64.3
Boyd's dysentery A03.2
Brachial — *see* condition
Brachycardia R00.1
Brachycephaly Q75.0
Bradley's disease A08.19
Bradyarrhythmia, cardiac I49.8
Bradycardia (sinoatrial) (sinus) (vagal) R00.1
neonatal P29.12

Bradycardia (sinoatrial) (sinus) (vagal) - *continued*
  reflex G90.09
  tachycardia syndrome I49.5
Bradykinesia R25.8
Bradypnea R06.89
Bradytachycardia I49.5
Brailsford's disease or osteochondrosis — *see*
  Osteochondrosis, juvenile, radius
Brain — *see also* condition
  death G93.82
  syndrome — *see* Syndrome, brain
Branched-chain amino-acid disorder E71.2
Branchial — *see* condition
  cartilage, congenital Q18.2
Branchiogenic remnant (in neck) Q18.0
Brandt's syndrome (acrodermatitis
  enteropathica) E83.2
Brash (water) R12
Bravais-jacksonian epilepsy — *see* Epilepsy,
  localization-related, symptomatic, with simple
  partial seizures
Braxton Hicks contractions — *see* False, labor
Brazilian leishmaniasis B55.2
BRBPR K62.5
Break, retina (without detachment) H33.30-
  with retinal detachment — *see* Detachment, retina
  horseshoe tear H33.31-
  multiple H33.33-
  round hole H33.32-
Breakdown
  device, graft or implant — *see also* Complications,
    by site and type, mechanical T85.618
    arterial graft NEC — *see* Complication,
      cardiovascular device, mechanical, vascular
    breast (implant) T85.41
    catheter NEC T85.618
      cystostomy T83.010
      Hopkins T83.018
      ileostomy T83.018
      dialysis (renal) T82.41
        intraperitoneal T85.611
      infusion NEC T82.514
        cranial T85.610
        epidural T85.610
        intrathecal T85.610
        spinal T85.610
        subarachnoid T85.610
        subdural T85.610
      nephrostomy T83.012
      urethral indwelling T83.011
      urinary NEC T83.018
      urostomy T83.018
    electronic (electrode) (pulse generator) (stimulator)
      bone T84.310
      cardiac T82.119
        electrode T82.110
        pulse generator T82.111
        specified type NEC T82.118
      nervous system — *see* Complication, prosthetic
        device, mechanical, electronic nervous system
        stimulator
      urinary — *see* Complication, genitourinary,
        device, urinary, mechanical
    fixation, internal (orthopedic) NEC — *see*
      Complication, fixation device, mechanical
    gastrointestinal — *see* Complications, prosthetic
      device, mechanical, gastrointestinal device
    genital NEC T83.418
      intrauterine contraceptive device T83.31
      penile prosthesis (cylinder) (implanted) (pump)
        (resevoir) T83.410
      testicular prosthesis T83.411
    heart NEC — *see* Complication, cardiovascular
      device, mechanical
    intrathecal infusion pump T85.615
    joint prosthesis — *see* Complications..., joint
      prosthesis,internal, mechanical, by site
    nervous system, specified device NEC T85.615
    ocular NEC — *see* Complications, prosthetic
      device, mechanical, ocular device
    orthopedic NEC — *see* Complication, orthopedic,
      device, mechanical
    specified NEC T85.618
    subcutaneous device pocket
      nervous system prosthetic device, implant, or
        graft T85.890
      other internal prosthetic device, implant, or
        graft T85.898
    sutures, permanent T85.612
      used in bone repair — *see* Complications,
        fixation device, internal (orthopedic),
        mechanical
    urinary NEC T83.118

Breakdown - *continued*
  device, graft or implant - *continued*
    urinary NEC - *continued*
      graft T83.21
      sphincter, implanted T83.111
      stent (ileal conduit) (nephroureteral) T83.113
        ureteral indwelling T83.112
      vascular NEC — *see* Complication, cardiovascular
        device, mechanical
      ventricular intracranial shunt T85.01
    nervous F48.8
    perineum O90.1
    respirator J95.850
      specified NEC J95.859
    ventilator J95.850
      specified NEC J95.859
Breast — *see also* condition
  buds E30.1
    in newborn P96.89
  dense R92.2
  nodule N63
Breath
  foul R19.6
  holder, child R06.89
  holding spell R06.89
  shortness R06.02
Breathing
  labored — *see* Hyperventilation
  mouth R06.5
    causing malocclusion M26.5
  periodic R06.3
    high altitude G47.32
Breathlessness R06.81
Breda's disease — *see* Yaws
Breech presentation (mother) O32.1
  causing obstructed labor O64.1
  footling O32.8
    causing obstructed labor O64.8
  incomplete O32.8
    causing obstructed labor O64.8
Breisky's disease N90.4
Brennemann's syndrome I88.0
Brenner
  tumor (benign) D27.9
    borderline malignancy D39.1-
    malignant C56
    proliferating D39.1-
Bretonneau's disease or angina A36.0
Breus' mole O02.0
Brevicollis Q76.49
Brickmakers' anemia B76.9 [D63.8]
Bridge, myocardial Q24.5
Bright red blood per rectum (BRBPR) K62.5
Bright's disease — *see also* Nephritis
  arteriosclerotic — *see* Hypertension, kidney
Brill (-Zinsser) **disease** (recrudescent typhus) A75.1
  flea-borne A75.2
  louse-borne A75.1
Brill-Symmers' disease C82.90
Brion-Kayser disease — *see* Fever, parathyroid
Briquet's disorder or syndrome F45.0
Brissaud's
  infantilism or dwarfism E23.0
  motor-verbal tic F95.2
Brittle
  bones disease Q78.0
  nails L60.3
    congenital Q84.6
Broad — *see also* condition
  beta disease E78.2
  ligament laceration syndrome N83.8
Broad- or floating-betalipoproteinemia E78.2
Brock's syndrome
  (atelectasis due to enlarged lymph nodes) J98.19
Brocq-Duhring disease (dermatitis
  herpetiformis) L13.0
Brodie's abscess or disease M86.8X-
Broken
  arches — *see also* Deformity, limb, flat foot
  arm (meaning upper limb) — *see* Fracture, arm
  back — *see* Fracture, vertebra
  bone — *see* Fracture
  implant or internal device — *see* Complications, by
    site and type, mechanical
  leg (meaning lower limb) — *see* Fracture, leg
  nose S02.2
  tooth, teeth — *see* Fracture, tooth
Bromhidrosis, bromidrosis L75.0
Bromidism, bromism G92
  due to
    correct substance properly administered — *see*
      Table of Drugs and Chemicals, by drug, adverse
      effect

Bromidism, bromism - *continued*
  due to - *continued*
    overdose or wrong substance given or taken — *see*
      Table of Drugs and Chemicals, by drug,
      poisoning
  chronic (dependence) F13.20
Bromidrosiphobia F40.298
Bronchi, bronchial — *see* condition
Bronchiectasis (cylindrical) (diffuse) (fusiform)
  (localized) (saccular) J47.9
  with
    acute
      bronchitis J47.0
      lower respiratory infection J47.0
    exacerbation (acute) J47.1
  congenital Q33.4
  tuberculous NEC — *see* Tuberculosis, pulmonary
Bronchiolectasis — *see* Bronchiectasis
Bronchiolitis (acute) (infective) (subacute) J21.9
  with
    bronchospasm or obstruction J21.9
    influenza, flu or grippe — *see* Influenza, with,
      respiratory manifestations NEC
  chemical (chronic) J68.4
    acute J68.0
  chronic (fibrosing) (obliterative) J44.9
  due to
    external agent — *see* Bronchitis, acute, due to
    human metapneumovirus J21.1
    respiratory syncytial virus J21.0
    specified organism NEC J21.8
  fibrosa obliterans J44.9
  influenzal — *see* Influenza, with, respiratory
    manifestations NEC
  obliterans J42
    with organizing pneumonia (BOOP) J84.89
  obliterative (chronic) (subacute) J44.9
    due to fumes or vapors J68.4
    due to chemicals, gases, fumes or vapors
      (inhalation) J68.4
  respiratory, interstitial lung disease J84.115
Bronchitis (diffuse) (fibrinous) (hypostatic)
  (infective) (membranous) J40
  with
    influenza, flu or grippe — *see* Influenza, with,
      respiratory manifestations NEC
    obstruction (airway) (lung) J44.9
    tracheitis (15 years of age and above) J40
      acute or subacute J20.9
      chronic J42
      under 15 years of age J20.9
  acute or subacute (with bronchospasm or
    obstruction) J20.9
    with
      bronchiectasis J47.0
      chronic obstructive pulmonary disease J44.0
    chemical (due to gases, fumes or vapors) J68.0
    due to
      fumes or vapors J68.0
      Haemophilus influenzae J20.1
      Mycoplasma pneumoniae J20.0
      radiation J70.0
      specified organism NEC J20.8
      Streptococcus J20.2
      virus
        coxsackie J20.3
        echovirus J20.7
        parainfluenzae J20.4
        respiratory syncytial J20.5
        rhinovirus J20.6
      viral NEC J20.8
  allergic (acute) J45.909
    with
      exacerbation (acute) J45.901
      status asthmaticus J45.902
  arachidic T17.528
  aspiration (due to fumes or vapors) J68.0
  asthmatic J45.9
    chronic J44.9
      with
        acute lower respiratory infection J44.0
        exacerbation (acute) J44.1
  capillary — *see* Pneumonia, broncho
  caseous (tuberculous) A15.5
  Castellani's A69.8
  catarrhal (15 years of age and above) J40
    acute — *see* Bronchitis, acute
    chronic J41.0
    under 15 years of age J20.9
  chemical (acute) (subacute) J68.0
    chronic J68.4
    due to fumes or vapors J68.0
    chronic J68.4

Bronchitis (diffuse) (fibrinous) (hypostatic) (infective) (membranous) - *continued*
  chronic J42
    with
      airways obstruction J44.9
      tracheitis (chronic) J42
    asthmatic (obstructive) J44.9
    catarrhal J41.0
    chemical (due to fumes or vapors) J68.4
    due to
      chemicals, gases, fumes or vapors (inhalation) J68.4
      radiation J70.1
      tobacco smoking J41.0
    emphysematous J44.9
    mucopurulent J41.1
    non-obstructive J41.0
    obliterans J44.9
    obstructive J44.9
    purulent J41.1
    simple J41.0
  croupous — *see* Bronchitis, acute
  due to gases, fumes or vapors (chemical) J68.0
  emphysematous (obstructive) J44.9
  exudative — *see* Bronchitis, acute
  fetid J41.1
  grippal — *see* Influenza, with, respiratory manifestations NEC
  in those under l5 years age — *see* Bronchitis, acute
    chronic — *see* Bronchitis, chronic
  influenzal — *see* Influenza, with, respiratory manifestations NEC
  mixed simple and mucopurulent J41.8
  moulder's J62.8
  mucopurulent (chronic) (recurrent) J41.1
    acute or subacute J20.9
    simple (mixed) J41.8
  obliterans (chronic) J44.9
  obstructive (chronic) (diffuse) J44.9
  pituitous J41.1
  pneumococcal, acute or subacute J20.2
  pseudomembranous, acute or subacute — *see* Bronchitis, acute
  purulent (chronic) (recurrent) J41.1
    acute or subacute — *see* Bronchitis, acute
  putrid J41.1
  senile (chronic) J42
  simple and mucopurulent (mixed) J41.8
  smokers' J41.0
  spirochetal NEC A69.8
  subacute — *see* Bronchitis, acute
  suppurative (chronic) J41.1
    acute or subacute — *see* Bronchitis, acute
  tuberculous A15.5
  under l5 years of age — *see* Bronchitis, acute
    chronic — *see* Bronchitis, chronic
  viral NEC, acute or subacute — *see also* Bronchitis, acute J20.8
Bronchoalveolitis J18.0
Bronchoaspergillosis B44.1
Bronchocele meaning goiter E04.0
Broncholithiasis J98.09
  tuberculous NEC A15.5
Bronchomalacia J98.09
  congenital Q32.2
Bronchomycosis NOS B49 *[J99]*
  candidal B37.1
Bronchopleuropneumonia — *see* Pneumonia, broncho
Bronchopneumonia — *see* Pneumonia, broncho
Bronchopneumonitis — *see* Pneumonia, broncho
Bronchopulmonary — *see* condition
Bronchopulmonitis — *see* Pneumonia, broncho
Bronchorrhagia (see Hemoptysis)
Bronchorrhea J98.09
  acute J20.9
  chronic (infective) (purulent) J42
Bronchospasm (acute) J98.01
  with
    bronchiolitis, acute J21.9
    bronchitis, acute (conditions in J20) — *see* Bronchitis, acute
  due to external agent — *see* condition, respiratory, acute, due to
    exercise induced J45.990
Bronchospirochetosis A69.8
  Castellani A69.8
Bronchostenosis J98.09
Bronchus — *see* condition
Brontophobia F40.220
Bronze baby syndrome P83.8
Brooke's tumor — *see* Neoplasm, skin, benign
Brown enamel of teeth (hereditary) K00.5

Brown's sheath syndrome H50.61-
Brown-Séquard disease, paralysis or syndrome G83.81
Bruce sepsis A23.0
Brucellosis (infection) A23.9
  abortus A23.1
  canis A23.3
  dermatitis A23.9
  melitensis A23.0
  mixed A23.8
  sepsis A23.9
    melitensis A23.0
    specified NEC A23.8
  suis A23.2
Bruck-de Lange disease Q87.1
Bruck's disease — *see* Deformity, limb
Brugsch's syndrome Q82.8
Bruise (skin surface intact) — *see also* Contusion
  with
    open wound — *see* Wound, open
  internal organ — *see* Injury, by site
  newborn P54.5
  scalp, due to birth injury, newborn P12.3
  umbilical cord O69.5
Bruit (arterial) R09.89
  cardiac R01.1
Brush burn — *see* Abrasion, by site
Bruton's X-linked agammaglobulinemia D80.0
Bruxism
  psychogenic F45.8
  sleep related G47.63
Bubbly lung syndrome P27.0
Bubo I88.8
  blennorrhagic (gonococcal) A54.89
  chancroidal A57
  climatic A55
  due to Haemophilus ducreyi A57
  gonococcal A54.89
  indolent (nonspecific) I88.8
  inguinal (nonspecific) I88.8
    chancroidal A57
    climatic A55
    due to H. ducreyi A57
    infective I88.8
  scrofulous (tuberculous) A18.2
  soft chancre A57
  suppurating — *see* Lymphadenitis, acute
  syphilitic (primary) A51.0
    congenital A50.07
  tropical A55
  virulent (chancroidal) A57
Bubonic plague A20.0
Bubonocele — *see* Hernia, inguinal
Buccal — *see* condition
Buchanan's disease or osteochondrosis M91.0
Buchem's syndrome (hyperostosis corticalis) M85.2
Bucket-handle fracture or tear (semilunar cartilage) — *see* Tear, meniscus
Budd-Chiari syndrome (hepatic vein thrombosis) I82.0
Budgerigar fancier's disease or lung J67.2
Buds
  breast E30.1
    in newborn P96.89
Buerger's disease (thromboangiitis obliterans) I73.1
Bulbar — *see* condition
Bulbus cordis (left ventricle) (persistent) Q21.8
Bulimia (nervosa) F50.2
  atypical F50.9
  normal weight F50.9
Bulky
  stools R19.5
  uterus N85.2
Bulla (e) R23.8
  lung (emphysematous) (solitary) J43.9
    newborn P25.8
Bullet wound — *see also* Wound, open
  fracture - code as Fracture, by site
  internal organ — *see* Injury, by site
Bundle
  branch block (complete) (false) (incomplete) — *see* Block, bundle-branch
  of His — *see* condition
Bunion M21.61-
  tailor's M21.62-
Bunionette M21.62-
Buphthalmia, buphthalmos (congenital) Q15.0
Burdwan fever B55.0
Bürger-Grütz disease or syndrome E78.3
Buried
  penis (congenital) Q55.64
    acquired N48.83
  roots K08.3

Burke's syndrome K86.89
Burkitt
  cell leukemia C91.0-
  lymphoma (malignant) C83.7-
    small noncleaved, diffuse C83.7-
    spleen C83.77
    undifferentiated C83.7-
  tumor C83.7-
  type
    acute lymphoblastic leukemia C91.0-
    undifferentiated C83.7-
Burn (electricity) (flame) (hot gas, liquid or hot object) (radiation) (steam) (thermal) T30.0
  abdomen, abdominal (muscle) (wall) T21.02
    first degree T21.12
    second degree T21.22
    third degree T21.32
  above elbow T22.039
    first degree T22.139
    left T22.032
      first degree T22.132
      second degree T22.232
      third degree T22.332
    right T22.031
      first degree T22.131
      second degree T22.231
      third degree T22.331
    second degree T22.239
    third degree T22.339
  acid (caustic) (external) (internal) — *see* Corrosion, by site
  alimentary tract NEC T28.2
    esophagus T28.1
    mouth T28.0
    pharynx T28.0
  alkaline (caustic) (external) (internal) — *see* Corrosion, by site
  ankle T25.019
    first degree T25.119
    left T25.012
      first degree T25.112
      second degree T25.212
      third degree T25.312
    multiple with foot — *see* Burn, lower, limb, multiple, ankle and foot
    right T25.011
      first degree T25.111
      second degree T25.211
      third degree T25.311
    second degree T25.219
    third degree T25.319
  anus — *see* Burn, buttock
  arm (lower) (upper) — *see* Burn, upper, limb
  axilla T22.049
    first degree T22.149
    left T22.042
      first degree T22.142
      second degree T22.242
      third degree T22.342
    right T22.041
      first degree T22.141
      second degree T22.241
      third degree T22.341
    second degree T22.249
    third degree T22.349
  back (lower) T21.04
    first degree T21.14
    second degree T21.24
    third degree T21.34
    upper T21.03
      first degree T21.13
      second degree T21.23
      third degree T21.33
  blisters - code as Burn, second degree, by site
  breast (s) — *see* Burn, chest wall
  buttock (s) T21.05
    first degree T21.15
    second degree T21.25
    third degree T21.35
  calf T24.039
    first degree T24.139
    left T24.032
      first degree T24.132
      second degree T24.232
      third degree T24.332
    right T24.031
      first degree T24.131
      second degree T24.231
      third degree T24.331
    second degree T24.239
    third degree T24.339
  canthus (eye) — *see* Burn, eyelid

Burn (electricity) (flame)
(hot gas, liquid or hot object) (radiation) (steam)
(thermal) - *continued*
caustic acid or alkaline — *see* Corrosion, by site
cervix T28.3
cheek T20.06
  first degree T20.16
  second degree T20.26
  third degree T20.36
chemical (acids) (alkalines) (caustics) (external)
  (internal) — *see* Corrosion, by site
chest wall T21.01
  first degree T21.11
  second degree T21.21
  third degree T21.31
chin T20.03
  first degree T20.13
  second degree T20.23
  third degree T20.33
colon T28.2
conjunctiva (and cornea) — *see* Burn, cornea
cornea (and conjunctiva) T26.1-
  chemical — *see* Corrosion, cornea
corrosion (external) (internal) — *see* Corrosion, by
  site
deep necrosis of underlying tissue - code as Burn,
  third degree, by site
dorsum of hand T23.069
  first degree T23.169
  left T23.062
    first degree T23.162
    second degree T23.262
    third degree T23.362
  right T23.061
    first degree T23.161
    second degree T23.261
    third degree T23.361
  second degree T23.269
  third degree T23.369
due to ingested chemical agent — *see* Corrosion, by
  site
ear (auricle) (external) (canal) T20.01
  first degree T20.11
  second degree T20.21
  third degree T20.31
elbow T22.029
  first degree T22.129
  left T22.022
    first degree T22.122
    second degree T22.222
    third degree T22.322
  right T22.021
    first degree T22.121
    second degree T22.221
    third degree T22.321
  second degree T22.229
  third degree T22.329
epidermal loss - code as Burn, second degree, by site
erythema, erythematous - code as Burn, first degree,
  by site
esophagus T28.1
extent (percentage of body surface)
  less than 10 percent T31.0
  10-19 percent T31.10
    with 0-9 percent third degree burns T31.10
    with 10-19 percent third degree burns T31.11
  20-29 percent T31.20
    with 0-9 percent third degree burns T31.20
    with 10-19 percent third degree burns T31.21
    with 20-29 percent third degree burns T31.22
  30-39 percent T31.30
    with 0-9 percent third degree burns T31.30
    with 10-19 percent third degree burns T31.31
    with 20-29 percent third degree burns T31.32
    with 30-39 percent third degree burns T31.33
  40-49 percent T31.40
    with 0-9 percent third degree burns T31.40
    with 10-19 percent third degree burns T31.41
    with 20-29 percent third degree burns T31.42
    with 30-39 percent third degree burns T31.43
    with 40-49 percent third degree burns T31.44
  50-59 percent T31.50
    with 0-9 percent third degree burns T31.50
    with 10-19 percent third degree burns T31.51
    with 20-29 percent third degree burns T31.52
    with 30-39 percent third degree burns T31.53
    with 40-49 percent third degree burns T31.54
    with 50-59 percent third degree burns T31.55
  60-69 percent T31.60
    with 0-9 percent third degree burns T31.60
    with 10-19 percent third degree burns T31.61
    with 20-29 percent third degree burns T31.62
    with 30-39 percent third degree burns T31.63

Burn (electricity) (flame) (hot gas, liquid or hot
object) (radiation) (steam) (thermal) - *continued*
  extent (percentage of body surface) - *continued*
  60-69 percent - *continued*
    with 40-49 percent third degree burns T31.64
    with 50-59 percent third degree burns T31.65
    with 60-69 percent third degree burns T31.66
  70-79 percent T31.70
    with 0-9 percent third degree burns T31.70
    with 10-19 percent third degree burns T31.71
    with 20-29 percent third degree burns T31.72
    with 30-39 percent third degree burns T31.73
    with 40-49 percent third degree burns T31.74
    with 50-59 percent third degree burns T31.75
    with 60-69 percent third degree burns T31.76
    with 70-79 percent third degree burns T31.77
  80-89 percent T31.80
    with 0-9 percent third degree burns T31.80
    with 10-19 percent third degree burns T31.81
    with 20-29 percent third degree burns T31.82
    with 30-39 percent third degree burns T31.83
    with 40-49 percent third degree burns T31.84
    with 50-59 percent third degree burns T31.85
    with 60-69 percent third degree burns T31.86
    with 70-79 percent third degree burns T31.87
    with 80-89 percent third degree burns T31.88
  90 percent or more T31.90
    with 0-9 percent third degree burns T31.90
    with 10-19 percent third degree burns T31.91
    with 20-29 percent third degree burns T31.92
    with 30-39 percent third degree burns T31.93
    with 40-49 percent third degree burns T31.94
    with 50-59 percent third degree burns T31.95
    with 60-69 percent third degree burns T31.96
    with 70-79 percent third degree burns T31.97
    with 80-89 percent third degree burns T31.98
    with 90 percent or more third degree
    burns T31.99
extremity — *see* Burn, limb
eye (s) and adnexa T26.4-
  with resulting rupture and destruction of
    eyeball T26.2-
  conjunctival sac — *see* Burn, cornea
  cornea — *see* Burn, cornea
  lid — *see* Burn, eyelid
  periocular area — *see* Burn, eyelid
  specified site NEC T26.3-
eyeball — *see* Burn, eye
eyelid (s) T26.0-
  chemical — *see* Corrosion, eyelid
face — *see* Burn, head
finger T23.029
  first degree T23.129
  left T23.022
    first degree T23.122
    second degree T23.222
    third degree T23.322
  multiple sites (without thumb) T23.039
    with thumb T23.049
      first degree T23.149
      left T23.042
        first degree T23.142
        second degree T23.242
        third degree T23.342
      right T23.041
        first degree T23.141
        second degree T23.241
        third degree T23.341
      second degree T23.249
      third degree T23.349
    first degree T23.139
    left T23.032
      first degree T23.132
      second degree T23.232
      third degree T23.332
    right T23.031
      first degree T23.131
      second degree T23.231
      third degree T23.331
    second degree T23.239
    third degree T23.339
  right T23.021
    first degree T23.121
    second degree T23.221
    third degree T23.321
  second degree T23.229
  third degree T23.329
flank — *see* Burn, abdominal wall
foot T25.029
  first degree T25.129
  left T25.022
    first degree T25.122
    second degree T25.222

Burn (electricity) (flame) (hot gas, liquid or hot
object) (radiation) (steam) (thermal) - *continued*
  foot - *continued*
  left - *continued*
    third degree T25.322
    multiple with ankle — *see* Burn, lower, limb,
    multiple, ankle and foot
  right T25.021
    first degree T25.121
    second degree T25.221
    third degree T25.321
  second degree T25.229
  third degree T25.329
forearm T22.019
  first degree T22.119
  left T22.012
    first degree T22.112
    second degree T22.212
    third degree T22.312
  right T22.011
    first degree T22.111
    second degree T22.211
    third degree T22.311
  second degree T22.219
  third degree T22.319
forehead T20.06
  first degree T20.16
  second degree T20.26
  third degree T20.36
fourth degree - code as Burn, third degree, by site
friction — *see* Burn, by site
from swallowing caustic or corrosive substance
  NEC — *see* Corrosion, by site
full thickness skin loss - code as Burn, third degree,
  by site
gastrointestinal tract NEC T28.2
  from swallowing caustic or corrosive
    substance T28.7
genital organs
  external
    female T21.07
      first degree T21.17
      second degree T21.27
      third degree T21.37
    male T21.06
      first degree T21.16
      second degree T21.26
      third degree T21.36
  internal T28.3
    from caustic or corrosive substance T28.8
groin — *see* Burn, abdominal wall
hand (s) T23.009
  back — *see* Burn, dorsum of hand
  finger — *see* Burn, finger
  first degree T23.109
  left T23.002
    first degree T23.102
    second degree T23.202
    third degree T23.302
  multiple sites with wrist T23.099
    first degree T23.199
    left T23.092
      first degree T23.192
      second degree T23.292
      third degree T23.392
    right T23.091
      first degree T23.191
      second degree T23.291
      third degree T23.391
    second degree T23.299
    third degree T23.399
  palm — *see* Burn, palm
  right T23.001
    first degree T23.101
    second degree T23.201
    third degree T23.301
  second degree T23.209
  third degree T23.309
  thumb — *see* Burn, thumb
head (and face) (and neck) T20.00
  cheek — *see* Burn, cheek
  chin — *see* Burn, chin
  ear — *see* Burn, ear
  eye (s) only — *see* Burn, eye
  first degree T20.10
  forehead — *see* Burn, forehead
  lip — *see* Burn, lip
  multiple sites T20.09
    first degree T20.19
    second degree T20.29
    third degree T20.39
  neck — *see* Burn, neck
  nose — *see* Burn, nose

Burn (electricity) (flame) (hot gas, liquid or hot object) (radiation) (steam) (thermal) - *continued*
head (and face) (and neck) - *continued*
scalp — *see* Burn, scalp
second degree T20.20
third degree T20.30
hip (s) — *see* Burn, thigh
inhalation — *see* Burn, respiratory tract
caustic or corrosive substance (fumes) — *see* Corrosion, respiratory tract
internal organ (s) T28.40
alimentary tract T28.2
esophagus T28.1
eardrum T28.41
esophagus T28.1
from caustic or corrosive substance (swallowing) NEC — *see* Corrosion, by site
genitourinary T28.3
mouth T28.0
pharynx T28.0
respiratory tract — *see* Burn, respiratory tract
specified organ NEC T28.49
interscapular region — *see* Burn, back, upper
intestine (large) (small) T28.2
knee T24.029
first degree T24.129
left T24.022
first degree T24.122
second degree T24.222
third degree T24.322
right T24.021
first degree T24.121
second degree T24.221
third degree T24.321
second degree T24.229
third degree T24.329
labium (majus) (minus) — *see* Burn, genital organs, external, female
lacrimal apparatus, duct, gland or sac — *see* Burn, eye, specified site NEC
larynx T27.0
with lung T27.1
leg (s) (lower) (upper) — *see* Burn, lower, limb
lightning — *see* Burn, by site
limb (s)
lower (except ankle or foot alone) — *see* Burn, lower, limb
upper — *see* Burn, upper limb
lip (s) T20.02
first degree T20.12
second degree T20.22
third degree T20.32
lower
back — *see* Burn, back
limb T24.009
ankle — *see* Burn, ankle
calf — *see* Burn, calf
first degree T24.109
foot — *see* Burn, foot
hip — *see* Burn, thigh
knee — *see* Burn, knee
left T24.002
first degree T24.102
second degree T24.202
third degree T24.302
multiple sites, except ankle and foot T24.099
ankle and foot T25.099
first degree T25.199
left T25.092
first degree T25.192
second degree T25.292
third degree T25.392
right T25.091
first degree T25.191
second degree T25.291
third degree T25.391
second degree T25.299
third degree T25.399
first degree T24.199
left T24.092
first degree T24.192
second degree T24.292
third degree T24.392
right T24.091
first degree T24.191
second degree T24.291
third degree T24.391
second degree T24.299
third degree T24.399
right T24.001
first degree T24.101
second degree T24.201
third degree T24.301

Burn (electricity) (flame) (hot gas, liquid or hot object) (radiation) (steam) (thermal) - *continued*
lower - *continued*
limb - *continued*
second degree T24.209
thigh — *see* Burn, thigh
third degree T24.309
toe — *see* Burn, toe
lung (with larynx and trachea) T27.1
mouth T28.0
neck T20.07
first degree T20.17
second degree T20.27
third degree T20.37
nose (septum) T20.04
first degree T20.14
second degree T20.24
third degree T20.34
ocular adnexa — *see* Burn, eye
orbit region — *see* Burn, eyelid
palm T23.059
first degree T23.159
left T23.052
first degree T23.152
second degree T23.252
third degree T23.352
right T23.051
first degree T23.151
second degree T23.251
third degree T23.351
second degree T23.259
third degree T23.359
partial thickness - code as Burn, unspecified degree, by site
pelvis — *see* Burn, trunk
penis — *see* Burn, genital organs, external, male
perineum
female — *see* Burn, genital organs, external, female
male — *see* Burn, genital organs, external, male
periocular area — *see* Burn, eyelid
pharynx T28.0
rectum T28.2
respiratory tract T27.3
larynx — *see* Burn, larynx
specified part NEC T27.2
trachea — *see* Burn, trachea
sac, lacrimal — *see* Burn, eye, specified site NEC
scalp T20.05
first degree T20.15
second degree T20.25
third degree T20.35
scapular region T22.069
first degree T22.169
left T22.062
first degree T22.162
second degree T22.262
third degree T22.362
right T22.061
first degree T22.161
second degree T22.261
third degree T22.361
second degree T22.269
third degree T22.369
sclera — *see* Burn, eye, specified site NEC
scrotum — *see* Burn, genital organs, external, male
shoulder T22.059
first degree T22.159
left T22.052
first degree T22.152
second degree T22.252
third degree T22.352
right T22.051
first degree T22.151
second degree T22.251
third degree T22.351
second degree T22.259
third degree T22.359
stomach T28.2
temple — *see* Burn, head
testis — *see* Burn, genital organs, external, male
thigh T24.019
first degree T24.119
left T24.012
first degree T24.112
second degree T24.212
third degree T24.312
right T24.011
first degree T24.111
second degree T24.211
third degree T24.311
second degree T24.219
third degree T24.319

Burn (electricity) (flame) (hot gas, liquid or hot object) (radiation) (steam) (thermal) - *continued*
thorax (external) — *see* Burn, trunk
throat (meaning pharynx) T28.0
thumb (s) T23.019
first degree T23.119
left T23.012
first degree T23.112
second degree T23.212
third degree T23.312
multiple sites with fingers T23.049
first degree T23.149
left T23.042
first degree T23.142
second degree T23.242
third degree T23.342
right T23.041
first degree T23.141
second degree T23.241
third degree T23.341
second degree T23.249
third degree T23.349
right T23.011
first degree T23.111
second degree T23.211
third degree T23.311
second degree T23.219
third degree T23.319
toe T25.039
first degree T25.139
left T25.032
first degree T25.132
second degree T25.232
third degree T25.332
right T25.031
first degree T25.131
second degree T25.231
third degree T25.331
second degree T25.239
third degree T25.339
tongue T28.0
tonsil (s) T28.0
trachea T27.0
with lung T27.1
trunk T21.00
abdominal wall — *see* Burn, abdominal wall
anus — *see* Burn, buttock
axilla — *see* Burn, upper limb
back — *see* Burn, back
breast — *see* Burn, chest wall
buttock — *see* Burn, buttock
chest wall — *see* Burn, chest wall
first degree T21.10
flank — *see* Burn, abdominal wall
genital
female — *see* Burn, genital organs, external, female
male — *see* Burn, genital organs, external, male
groin — *see* Burn, abdominal wall
interscapular region — *see* Burn, back, upper
labia — *see* Burn, genital organs, external, female
lower back — *see* Burn, back
penis — *see* Burn, genital organs, external, male
perineum
female — *see* Burn, genital organs, external, female
male — *see* Burn, genital organs, external, male
scapula region — *see* Burn, scapular region
scrotum — *see* Burn, genital organs, external, male
second degree T21.20
specified site NEC T21.09
first degree T21.19
second degree T21.29
third degree T21.39
testes — *see* Burn, genital organs, external, male
third degree T21.30
upper back — *see* Burn, back, upper
vulva — *see* Burn, genital organs, external, female
unspecified site with extent of body surface involved specified
less than 10 per cent T31.0
10-19 per cent (0-9 percent third degree) T31.10
with 10-19 percent third degree T31.11
20-29 per cent (0-9 percent third degree) T31.20
with
10-19 percent third degree T31.21
20-29 percent third degree T31.22
30-39 per cent (0-9 percent third degree) T31.30
with
10-19 percent third degree T31.31
20-29 percent third degree T31.32
30-39 percent third degree T31.33
40-49 per cent (0-9 percent third degree) T31.40

Burn (electricity) (flame) (hot gas, liquid or hot object) (radiation) (steam) (thermal) - *continued*
unspecified site with extent of body surface involved specified - *continued*
40-49 per cent (0-9 percent third degree) - *continued*
with
10-19 percent third degree T31.41
20-29 percent third degree T31.42
30-39 percent third degree T31.43
40-49 percent third degree T31.44
50-59 per cent (0-9 percent third degree) T31.50
with
10-19 percent third degree T31.51
20-29 percent third degree T31.52
30-39 percent third degree T31.53
40-49 percent third degree T31.54
50-59 percent third degree T31.55
60-69 per cent (0-9 percent third degree) T31.60
with
10-19 percent third degree T31.61
20-29 percent third degree T31.62
30-39 percent third degree T31.63
40-49 percent third degree T31.64
50-59 percent third degree T31.65
60-69 percent third degree T31.66
70-79 per cent (0-9 percent third degree) T31.70
with
10-19 percent third degree T31.71
20-29 percent third degree T31.72
30-39 percent third degree T31.73
40-49 percent third degree T31.74
50-59 percent third degree T31.75
60-69 percent third degree T31.76
70-79 percent third degree T31.77
80-89 per cent (0-9 percent third degree) T31.80
with
10-19 percent third degree T31.81
20-29 percent third degree T31.82
30-39 percent third degree T31.83
40-49 percent third degree T31.84
50-59 percent third degree T31.85
60-69 percent third degree T31.86
70-79 percent third degree T31.87
80-89 percent third degree T31.88
90 per cent or more (0-9 percent third degree) T31.90
with
10-19 percent third degree T31.91
20-29 percent third degree T31.92
30-39 percent third degree T31.93
40-49 percent third degree T31.94
50-59 percent third degree T31.95
60-69 percent third degree T31.96
70-79 percent third degree T31.97
80-89 percent third degree T31.98
90-99 percent third degree T31.99
upper limb T22.00
above elbow — *see* Burn, above elbow
axilla — *see* Burn, axilla
elbow — *see* Burn, elbow
first degree T22.10
forearm — *see* Burn, forearm
hand — *see* Burn, hand
interscapular region — *see* Burn, back, upper
multiple sites T22.099
first degree T22.199
left T22.092
first degree T22.192
second degree T22.292
third degree T22.392
right T22.091
first degree T22.191
second degree T22.291
third degree T22.391
second degree T22.299
third degree T22.399
scapular region — *see* Burn, scapular region
second degree T22.20
shoulder — *see* Burn, shoulder
third degree T22.30
wrist — *see* Burn, wrist
uterus T28.3
vagina T28.3
vulva — *see* Burn, genital organs, external, female
wrist T23.079
first degree T23.179
left T23.072
first degree T23.172
second degree T23.272
third degree T23.372
multiple sites with hand T23.099
first degree T23.199

Burn (electricity) (flame) (hot gas, liquid or hot object) (radiation) (steam) (thermal) - *continued*
wrist - *continued*
multiple sites with hand - *continued*
left T23.092
first degree T23.192
second degree T23.292
third degree T23.392
right T23.091
first degree T23.191
second degree T23.291
third degree T23.391
second degree T23.299
third degree T23.399
right T23.071
first degree T23.171
second degree T23.271
third degree T23.371
second degree T23.279
third degree T23.379
Burnett's syndrome E83.52
Burning
feet syndrome E53.9
sensation R20.8
tongue K14.6
Burn-out (state) Z73.0
Burns' disease or osteochondrosis — *see* Osteochondrosis, juvenile, ulna
Bursa — *see* condition
Bursitis M71.9
Achilles — *see* Tendinitis, Achilles
adhesive — *see* Bursitis, specified NEC
ankle — *see* Enthesopathy, lower limb, ankle, specified type NEC
calcaneal — *see* Enthesopathy, foot, specified type NEC
collateral ligament, tibial — *see* Bursitis, tibial collateral
due to use, overuse, pressure — *see also* Disorder, soft tissue, due to use, specified type NEC
specified NEC — *see* Disorder, soft tissue, due to use, specified NEC
Duplay's M75.0
elbow NEC M70.3-
olecranon M70.2-
finger — *see* Disorder, soft tissue, due to use, specified type NEC, hand
foot — *see* Enthesopathy, foot, specified type NEC
gonococcal A54.49
gouty — *see* Gout
hand M70.1-
hip NEC M70.7-
trochanteric M70.6-
infective NEC M71.10
abscess — *see* Abscess, bursa
ankle M71.17-
elbow M71.12-
foot M71.17-
hand M71.14-
hip M71.15-
knee M71.16-
multiple sites M71.19
shoulder M71.11-
specified site NEC M71.18
wrist M71.13-
ischial — *see* Bursitis, hip
knee NEC M70.5-
prepatellar M70.4-
occupational NEC — *see also* Disorder, soft tissue, due to, use
olecranon — *see* Bursitis, elbow, olecranon
pharyngeal J39.1
popliteal — *see* Bursitis, knee
prepatellar M70.4-
radiohumeral M77.8
rheumatoid M06.20
ankle M06.27-
elbow M06.22-
foot joint M06.27-
hand joint M06.24-
hip M06.25-
knee M06.26-
multiple site M06.29
shoulder M06.21-
vertebra M06.28
wrist M06.23-
scapulohumeral — *see* Bursitis, shoulder
semimembranous muscle (knee) — *see* Bursitis, knee
shoulder M75.5-
adhesive — *see* Capsulitis, adhesive
specified NEC M71.50
ankle M71.57-

Bursitis - *continued*
specified NEC - *continued*
due to use, overuse or pressure — *see* Disorder, soft tissue, due to, use
elbow M71.52-
foot M71.57-
hand M71.54-
hip M71.55-
knee M71.56-
shoulder — *see* Bursitis, shoulder
specified site NEC M71.58
tibial collateral M76.4-
wrist M71.53-
subacromial — *see* Bursitis, shoulder
subcoracoid — *see* Bursitis, shoulder
subdeltoid — *see* Bursitis, shoulder
syphilitic A52.78
Thornwaldt, Tornwaldt J39.2
tibial collateral M76.4-
toe — *see* Enthesopathy, foot, specified type NEC
trochanteric (area) — *see* Bursitis, hip, trochanteric
wrist — *see* Bursitis, hand
Bursopathy M71.9
specified type NEC M71.80
ankle M71.87-
elbow M71.82-
foot M71.87-
hand M71.84-
hip M71.85-
knee M71.86-
multiple sites M71.89
shoulder M71.81-
specified site NEC M71.88
wrist M71.83-
Burst stitches or sutures (complication of surgery) T81.31
external operation wound T81.31
internal operation wound T81.32
Buruli ulcer A31.1
Bury's disease L95.1
Buschke's
disease B45.3
scleredema — *see* Sclerosis, systemic
Busse-Buschke disease B45.3
Buttock — *see* condition
Button
Biskra B55.1
Delhi B55.1
oriental B55.1
Buttonhole deformity (finger) — *see* Deformity, finger, boutonniere
Bwamba fever A92.8
Byssinosis J66.0
Bywaters' syndrome T79.5

C

Cachexia R64
cancerous R64
cardiac — *see* Disease, heart
dehydration E86.0
due to malnutrition R64
exophthalmic — *see* Hyperthyroidism
heart — *see* Disease, heart
hypophyseal E23.0
hypopituitary E23.0
lead — *see* Poisoning, lead
malignant R64
marsh — *see* Malaria
nervous F48.8
old age R54
paludal — *see* Malaria
pituitary E23.0
renal N28.9
saturnine — *see* Poisoning, lead
senile R54
Simmonds' E23.0
splenica D73.0
strumipriva E03.4
tuberculous NEC — *see* Tuberculosis
Café, au lait spots L81.3
Caffeine-induced
anxiety disorder F15.980
sleep disorder F15.982
Caffey's syndrome Q78.8
Caisson disease T70.3
Cake kidney Q63.1
Caked breast (puerperal, postpartum) O92.79
Calabar swelling B74.3
Calcaneal spur — *see* Spur, bone, calcaneal
Calcaneo-apophysitis M92.8
Calcareous — *see* condition
Calcicosis J62.8

Calciferol (vitamin D) deficiency E55.9
  with rickets E55.0
Calcification
  adrenal (capsule) (gland) E27.49
    tuberculous E35 [B90.8]
  aorta I70.0
  artery (annular) — see Arteriosclerosis
  auricle (ear) — see Disorder, pinna, specified type
    NEC
  basal ganglia G23.8
  bladder N32.89
    due to Schistosoma hematobium B65.0
  brain (cortex) — see Calcification, cerebral
  bronchus J98.09
  bursa M71.40
    ankle M71.47-
    elbow M71.42-
    foot M71.47-
    hand M71.44-
    hip M71.45-
    knee M71.46-
    multiple sites M71.49
    shoulder M75.3-
    specified site NEC M71.48
    wrist M71.43-
  cardiac — see Degeneration, myocardial
  cerebral (cortex) G93.89
    artery I67.2
  cervix (uteri) N88.8
  choroid plexus G93.89
  conjunctiva — see Concretion, conjunctiva
  corpora cavernosa (penis) N48.89
  cortex (brain) — see Calcification, cerebral
  dental pulp (nodular) K04.2
  dentinal papilla K00.4
  fallopian tube N83.8
  falx cerebri G96.19
  gallbladder K82.8
  general E83.59
  heart — see also Degeneration, myocardial
    valve — see Endocarditis
  idiopathic infantile arterial (IIAC) Q28.8
  intervertebral cartilage or disc (postinfective) — see
    Disorder, disc, specified NEC
  intracranial — see Calcification, cerebral
  joint — see Disorder, joint, specified type NEC
  kidney N28.89
    tuberculous N29 [B90.1]
  larynx (senile) J38.7
  lens — see Cataract, specified NEC
  lung (active) (postinfectional) J98.4
    tuberculous B90.9
  lymph gland or node (postinfectional) I89.8
    tuberculous — see also Tuberculosis, lymph
      gland B90.8
  mammographic R92.1
  massive (paraplegic) — see Myositis, ossificans, in,
    quadriplegia
  medial — see Arteriosclerosis, extremities
  meninges (cerebral) (spinal) G96.19
  metastatic E83.59
  Mönckeberg's — see Arteriosclerosis, extremities
  muscle M61.9
    due to burns — see Myositis, ossificans, in, burns
    paralytic — see Myositis, ossificans, in,
      quadriplegia
    specified type NEC M61.40
      ankle M61.47-
      foot M61.47-
      forearm M61.43-
      hand M61.44-
      lower leg M61.46-
      multiple sites M61.49
      pelvic region M61.45-
      shoulder region M61.41-
      specified site NEC M61.48
      thigh M61.45-
      upper arm M61.42-
  myocardium, myocardial — see Degeneration,
    myocardial
  ovary N83.8
  pancreas K86.89
  penis N48.89
  periarticular — see Disorder, joint, specified type
    NEC
  pericardium — see also Pericarditis I31.1
  pineal gland E34.8
  pleura J94.8
    postinfectional J94.8
    tuberculous NEC B90.9
  pulpal (dental) (nodular) K04.2
  sclera H15.89
  spleen D73.89

Calcification - continued
  subcutaneous L94.2
  suprarenal (capsule) (gland) E27.49
  tendon (sheath) — see also Tenosynovitis, specified
    type NEC
    with bursitis, synovitis or tenosynovitis — see
      Tendinitis, calcific
  trachea J39.8
  ureter N28.89
  uterus N85.8
  vitreous — see Deposit, crystalline
Calcified — see Calcification
Calcinosis (interstitial) (tumoral) (universalis) E83.59
  with Raynaud's phenomenon, esophageal
    dysfunction, sclerodactyly, telangiectasia (CREST
    syndrome) M34.1
  circumscripta (skin) L94.2
  cutis L94.2
Calciphylaxis — see also Calcification, by
  site E83.59
Calcium
  deposits — see Calcification, by site
  metabolism disorder E83.50
  salts or soaps in vitreous — see Deposit, crystalline
Calciuria R82.99
Calculi — see Calculus
Calculosis, intrahepatic — see Calculus, bile duct
Calculus, calculi, calculous
  ampulla of Vater — see Calculus, bile duct
  anuria (impacted) (recurrent) — see also Calculus,
    urinary N20.9
  appendix K38.1
  bile duct (common) (hepatic) K80.50
    with
      calculus of gallbladder — see Calculus,
        gallbladder and bile duct
      cholangitis K80.30
        with
          cholecystitis — see Calculus, bile duct, with
            cholecystitis
          obstruction K80.31
        acute K80.32
          with
            chronic cholangitis K80.36
              with obstruction K80.37
            obstruction K80.33
        chronic K80.34
          with
            acute cholangitis K80.36
              with obstruction K80.37
            obstruction K80.35
      cholecystitis (with cholangitis) K80.40
        with obstruction K80.41
        acute K80.42
          with
            chronic cholecystitis K80.46
              with obstruction K80.47
            obstruction K80.43
        chronic K80.44
          with
            acute cholecystitis K80.46
              with obstruction K80.47
            obstruction K80.45
      obstruction K80.51
    biliary — see also Calculus, gallbladder
      specified NEC K80.80
        with obstruction K80.81
    bilirubin, multiple — see Calculus, gallbladder
    bladder (encysted) (impacted) (urinary)
      (diverticulum) N21.0
    bronchus J98.09
    calyx (kidney) (renal) — see Calculus, kidney
    cholesterol (pure) (solitary) — see Calculus,
      gallbladder
    common duct (bile) — see Calculus, bile duct
    conjunctiva — see Concretion, conjunctiva
    cystic N21.0
      duct — see Calculus, gallbladder
    dental (subgingival) (supragingival) K03.6
    diverticulum
      bladder N21.0
      kidney N20.0
    epididymis N50.89
    gallbladder K80.20
      with
        bile duct calculus — see Calculus, gallbladder
          and bile duct
        cholecystitis K80.10
          with obstruction K80.11
          acute K80.00
            with
              chronic cholecystitis K80.12
                with obstruction K80.13

Calculus, calculi, calculous - continued
  gallbladder - continued
    with - continued
      cholecystitis - continued
        acute - continued
          with - continued
            obstruction K80.01
        chronic K80.10
          with
            acute cholecystitis K80.12
              with obstruction K80.13
            obstruction K80.11
        specified NEC K80.18
          with obstruction K80.19
      obstruction K80.21
  gallbladder and bile duct K80.70
    with
      cholecystitis K80.60
        with obstruction K80.61
        acute K80.62
          with
            chronic cholecystitis K80.66
              with obstruction K80.67
            obstruction K80.63
        chronic K80.64
          with
            acute cholecystitis K80.66
              with obstruction K80.67
            obstruction K80.65
      obstruction K80.71
  hepatic (duct) — see Calculus, bile duct
  hepatobiliary K80.80
    with obstruction K80.81
  ileal conduit N21.8
  intestinal (impaction) (obstruction) K56.49
  kidney (impacted) (multiple) (pelvis) (recurrent)
    (staghorn) N20.0
    with calculus, ureter N20.2
    congenital Q63.8
  lacrimal passages — see Dacryolith
  liver (impacted) — see Calculus, bile duct
  lung J98.4
  mammographic R92.1
  nephritic (impacted) (recurrent) — see Calculus,
    kidney
  nose J34.89
  pancreas (duct) K86.89
  parotid duct or gland K11.5
  pelvis, encysted — see Calculus, kidney
  prostate N42.0
  pulmonary J98.4
  pyelitis (impacted) (recurrent) N20.0
    with hydronephrosis N13.2
  pyelonephritis (impacted) (recurrent) — see
    category N20
    with hydronephrosis N13.2
  renal (impacted) (recurrent) — see Calculus, kidney
  salivary (duct) (gland) K11.5
  seminal vesicle N50.89
  staghorn — see Calculus, kidney
  Stensen's duct K11.5
  stomach K31.89
  sublingual duct or gland K11.5
    congenital Q38.4
  submandibular duct, gland or region K11.5
  submaxillary duct, gland or region K11.5
  suburethral N21.8
  tonsil J35.8
  tooth, teeth (subgingival) (supragingival) K03.6
  tunica vaginalis N50.89
  ureter (impacted) (recurrent) N20.1
    with calculus, kidney N20.2
      with hydronephrosis N13.2
        with infection N13.6
  urethra (impacted) N21.1
  urinary (duct) (impacted) (passage) (tract) N20.9
    with hydronephrosis N13.2
      with infection N13.6
    in (due to)
    lower N21.9
      specified NEC N21.8
  vagina N89.8
  vesical (impacted) N21.0
  Wharton's duct K11.5
  xanthine E79.8 [N22]
Calicectasis N28.89
Caliectasis N28.89
California
  disease B38.9
  encephalitis A83.5
Caligo cornea — see Opacity, cornea, central
Callositas, callosity (infected) L84

Callus (infected) L84
 bone — *see* Osteophyte
 excessive, following fracture - code as Sequelae of
 fracture
CALME
 (childhood asymmetric labium majus
 enlargement) N90.61
Calorie deficiency or malnutrition — *see
 also* Malnutrition E46
Calvé-Perthes disease — *see* Legg-Calvé-Perthes
 disease
Calvé's disease — *see* Osteochondrosis, juvenile,
 spine
Calvities — *see* Alopecia, androgenic
Cameroon fever — *see* Malaria
Camptocormia (hysterical) F44.4
Camurati-Engelmann syndrome Q78.3
Canal — *see also* condition
 atrioventricular common Q21.2
Canaliculitis (lacrimal) (acute) (subacute) H04.33-
 Actinomyces A42.89
 chronic H04.42-
Canavan's disease E75.29
Canceled procedure (surgical) Z53.9
 because of
 contraindication Z53.09
 smoking Z53.01
 left against medical advice (AMA) Z53.21
 patient's decision Z53.20
 for reasons of belief or group pressure Z53.1
 specified reason NEC Z53.29
 specified reason NEC Z53.8
Cancer — *see also* Neoplasm, by site, malignant
 bile duct type liver C22.1
 blood — *see* Leukemia
 breast — *see also* Neoplasm, breast,
 malignant C50.91-
 hepatocellular C22.0
 lung — *see also* Neoplasm, lung, malignant C34.90-
 ovarian — *see also* Neoplasm ovary,
 malignant C56.9-
 unspecified site (primary) C80.1
Cancerous — *see* Neoplasm, malignant, by site
Cancer (o) phobia F45.29
Cancrum oris A69.0
Candidiasis, candidal B37.9
 balanitis B37.42
 bronchitis B37.1
 cheilitis B37.83
 congenital P37.5
 cystitis B37.41
 disseminated B37.7
 endocarditis B37.6
 enteritis B37.82
 esophagitis B37.81
 intertrigo B37.2
 lung B37.1
 meningitis B37.5
 mouth B37.0
 nails B37.2
 neonatal P37.5
 onychia B37.2
 oral B37.0
 osteomyelitis B37.89
 otitis externa B37.84
 paronychia B37.2
 perionyxis B37.2
 pneumonia B37.1
 proctitis B37.82
 pulmonary B37.1
 pyelonephritis B37.49
 sepsis B37.7
 skin B37.2
 specified site NEC B37.89
 stomatitis B37.0
 systemic B37.7
 urethritis B37.41
 urogenital site NEC B37.49
 vagina B37.3
 vulva B37.3
 vulvovaginitis B37.3
Candidid L30.2
Candidosis — *see* Candidiasis
Candiru infection or infestation B88.8
Canities (premature) L67.1
 congenital Q84.2
Canker (mouth) (sore) K12.0
 rash A38.9
Cannabinosis J66.2
Cannabis induced
 anxiety disorder F12.980
 psychotic disorder F12.959
 sleep disorder F12.988

Canton fever A75.9
Cantrell's syndrome Q87.89
Capillariasis (intestinal) B81.1
 hepatic B83.8
Capillary — *see* condition
Caplan's syndrome — *see* Rheumatoid, lung
Capsule — *see* condition
Capsulitis (joint) — *see also* Enthesopathy
 adhesive (shoulder) M75.0-
 hepatic K65.8
 labyrinthine — *see* Otosclerosis, specified NEC
 thyroid E06.9
Caput
 crepitus Q75.8
 medusae I86.8
 succedaneum P12.81
Car sickness T75.3
Carapata (disease) A68.0
Carate — *see* Pinta
Carbon lung J60
Carbuncle L02.93
 abdominal wall L02.231
 anus K61.0
 auditory canal, external — *see* Abscess, ear, external
 auricle ear — *see* Abscess, ear, external
 axilla L02.43-
 back (any part) L02.232
 breast N61.1
 buttock L02.33
 cheek (external) L02.03
 chest wall L02.233
 chin L02.03
 corpus cavernosum N48.21
 ear (any part) (external) (middle) — *see* Abscess,
 ear, external
 external auditory canal — *see* Abscess, ear, external
 eyelid — *see* Abscess, eyelid
 face NEC L02.03
 femoral (region) — *see* Carbuncle, lower limb
 finger — *see* Carbuncle, hand
 flank L02.231
 foot L02.63-
 forehead L02.03
 genital — *see* Abscess, genital
 gluteal (region) L02.33
 groin L02.234
 hand L02.53-
 head NEC L02.831
 heel — *see* Carbuncle, foot
 hip — *see* Carbuncle, lower limb
 kidney — *see* Abscess, kidney
 knee — *see* Carbuncle, lower limb
 labium (majus) (minus) N76.4
 lacrimal
 gland — *see* Dacryoadenitis
 passages (duct) (sac) — *see* Inflammation,
 lacrimal, passages, acute
 leg — *see* Carbuncle, lower limb
 lower limb L02.43-
 malignant A22.0
 navel L02.236
 neck L02.13
 nose (external) (septum) J34.0
 orbit, orbital — *see* Abscess, orbit
 palmar (space) — *see* Carbuncle, hand
 partes posteriores L02.33
 pectoral region L02.233
 penis N48.21
 perineum L02.235
 pinna — *see* Abscess, ear, external
 popliteal — *see* Carbuncle, lower limb
 scalp L02.831
 seminal vesicle N49.0
 shoulder — *see* Carbuncle, upper limb
 specified site NEC L02.838
 temple (region) L02.03
 thumb — *see* Carbuncle, hand
 toe — *see* Carbuncle, foot
 trunk L02.239
 abdominal wall L02.231
 back L02.232
 chest wall L02.233
 groin L02.234
 perineum L02.235
 umbilicus L02.236
 umbilicus L02.236
 upper limb L02.43-
 urethra N34.0
 vulva N76.4
Carbunculus — *see* Carbuncle
Carcinoid (tumor) — *see* Tumor, carcinoid
Carcinoidosis E34.0

Carcinoma (malignant) — *see also* Neoplasm, by
 site, malignant
 acidophil
 specified site — *see* Neoplasm, malignant, by site
 unspecified site C75.1
 acidophil-basophil, mixed
 specified site — *see* Neoplasm, malignant, by site
 unspecified site C75.1
 adnexal (skin) — *see* Neoplasm, skin, malignant
 adrenal cortical C74.0-
 alveolar — *see* Neoplasm, lung, malignant
 cell — *see* Neoplasm, lung, malignant
 ameloblastic C41.1
 upper jaw (bone) C41.0
 apocrine
 breast — *see* Neoplasm, breast, malignant
 specified site NEC — *see* Neoplasm, skin,
 malignant
 unspecified site C44.99
 basal cell (pigmented) (see also Neoplasm, skin,
 malignant) C44.91
 fibro-epithelial — *see* Neoplasm, skin, malignant
 morphea — *see* Neoplasm, skin, malignant
 multicentric — *see* Neoplasm, skin, malignant
 basaloid
 basal-squamous cell, mixed — *see* Neoplasm, skin,
 malignant
 basophil
 specified site — *see* Neoplasm, malignant, by site
 unspecified site C75.1
 basophil-acidophil, mixed
 specified site — *see* Neoplasm, malignant, by site
 unspecified site C75.1
 basosquamous — *see* Neoplasm, skin, malignant
 bile duct
 with hepatocellular, mixed C22.0
 liver C22.1
 specified site NEC — *see* Neoplasm, malignant, by
 site
 unspecified site C22.1
 branchial or branchiogenic C10.4
 bronchial or bronchogenic — *see* Neoplasm, lung,
 malignant
 bronchiolar — *see* Neoplasm, lung, malignant
 bronchioloalveolar — *see* Neoplasm, lung,
 malignant
 C cell
 specified site — *see* Neoplasm, malignant, by site
 unspecified site C73
 ceruminous C44.29-
 cervix uteri
 in situ D06.9
 endocervix D06.0
 exocervix D06.1
 specified site NEC D06.7
 chorionic
 specified site — *see* Neoplasm, malignant, by site
 unspecified site
 female C58
 male C62.90
 chromophobe
 specified site — *see* Neoplasm, malignant, by site
 unspecified site C75.1
 cloacogenic
 specified site — *see* Neoplasm, malignant, by site
 unspecified site C21.2
 diffuse type
 specified site — *see* Neoplasm, malignant, by site
 unspecified site C16.9
 duct (cell)
 with Paget's disease — *see* Neoplasm, breast,
 malignant
 infiltrating
 with lobular carcinoma (in situ)
 specified site — *see* Neoplasm, malignant, by
 site
 unspecified site (female) C50.91-
 male C50.92-
 specified site — *see* Neoplasm, malignant, by site
 unspecified site (female) C50.91-
 male C50.92-
 ductal
 with lobular
 specified site — *see* Neoplasm, malignant, by site
 unspecified site (female) C50.91-
 male C50.92-
 ductular, infiltrating
 specified site — *see* Neoplasm, malignant, by site
 unspecified site (female) C50.91-
 male C50.92-
 embryonal
 liver C22.7
 endometrioid

Carcinoma (malignant) - *continued*
  endometrioid - *continued*
    specified site — *see* Neoplasm, malignant, by site
    unspecified site
      female C56.9
      male C61
  eosinophil
    specified site — *see* Neoplasm, malignant, by site
    unspecified site C75.1
  epidermoid — *see also* Neoplasm, skin malignant
    in situ, Bowen's type — *see* Neoplasm, skin, in situ
  fibroepithelial, basal cell — *see* Neoplasm, skin, malignant
  follicular
    with papillary (mixed) C73
    moderately differentiated C73
    pure follicle C73
    specified site — *see* Neoplasm, malignant, by site
    trabecular C73
    unspecified site C73
    well differentiated C73
  generalized, with unspecified primary site C80.0
  glycogen-rich — *see* Neoplasm, breast, malignant
  granulosa cell C56-
  hepatic cell C22.0
  hepatocellular C22.0
    with bile duct, mixed C22.0
    fibrolamellar C22.0
  hepatocholangiolitic C22.0
  Hurthle cell C73
  in
    adenomatous
      polyposis coli C18.9
    pleomorphic adenoma — *see* Neoplasm, salivary glands, malignant
    situ — *see* Carcinoma-in-situ
  infiltrating
    duct
      with lobular
        specified site — *see* Neoplasm, malignant, by site
        unspecified site (female) C50.91-
          male C50.92-
      with Paget's disease — *see* Neoplasm, breast, malignant
      specified site — *see* Neoplasm, malignant
      unspecified site (female) C50.91-
        male C50.92-
    ductular
      specified site — *see* Neoplasm, malignant
      unspecified site (female) C50.91-
        male C50.92-
    lobular
      specified site — *see* Neoplasm, malignant
      unspecified site (female) C50.91-
        male C50.92-
  inflammatory
    specified site — *see* Neoplasm, malignant
    unspecified site (female) C50.91-
      male C50.92-
  intestinal type
    specified site — *see* Neoplasm, malignant, by site
    unspecified site C16.9
  intracystic
    noninfiltrating — *see* Neoplasm, in situ, by site
  intraductal (noninfiltrating)
    with Paget's disease — *see* Neoplasm, breast, malignant
    breast D05.1-
    papillary
      with invasion
        specified site — *see* Neoplasm, malignant, by site
        unspecified site (female) C50.91-
          male C50.92-
      breast D05.1-
      specified site NEC — *see* Neoplasm, in situ, by site
      unspecified site (female) D05.1-
    specified site NEC — *see* Neoplasm, in situ, by site
    unspecified site (female) D05.1-
  intraepidermal — *see* Neoplasm, in situ
    squamous cell, Bowen's type — *see* Neoplasm, skin, in situ
  intraepithelial — *see* Neoplasm, in situ, by site
    squamous cell — *see* Neoplasm, in situ, by site
  intraosseous C41.1
    upper jaw (bone) C41.0
  islet cell
    with exocrine, mixed
      specified site — *see* Neoplasm, malignant, by site
      unspecified site C25.9

Carcinoma (malignant) - *continued*
  islet cell - *continued*
    pancreas C25.4
    specified site NEC — *see* Neoplasm, malignant, by site
    unspecified site C25.4
  juvenile, breast — *see* Neoplasm, breast, malignant
  large cell
    small cell
      specified site — *see* Neoplasm, malignant, by site
      unspecified site C34.90
  Leydig cell (testis)
    specified site — *see* Neoplasm, malignant, by site
    unspecified site
      female C56.9
      male C62.90
  lipid-rich (female) C50.91-
    male C50.92-
  liver cell C22.0
  liver NEC C22.7
  lobular (infiltrating)
    with intraductal
      specified site — *see* Neoplasm, malignant, by site
      unspecified site (female) C50.91-
        male C50.92-
    noninfiltrating
      breast D05.0-
      specified site NEC — *see* Neoplasm, in situ, by site
      unspecified site D05.0-
    specified site — *see* Neoplasm, malignant, by site
    unspecified site (female) C50.91-
      male C50.92-
  medullary
    with
      amyloid stroma
        specified site — *see* Neoplasm, malignant, by site
        unspecified site C73
      lymphoid stroma
        specified site — *see* Neoplasm, malignant, by site
        unspecified site (female) C50.91-
          male C50.92-
  Merkel cell C4A.9
    anal margin C4A.51
    anal skin C4A.51
    canthus C4A.1-
    ear and external auricular canal C4A.2-
    external auricular canal C4A.2-
    eyelid, including canthus C4A.1-
    face C4A.30
      specified NEC C4A.39
    hip C4A.7-
    lip C4A.0
    lower limb, including hip C4A.7-
    neck C4A.4
    nodal presentation C7B.1
    nose C4A.31
    overlapping sites C4A.8
    perianal skin C4A.51
    scalp C4A.4
    secondary C7B.1
    shoulder C4A.6-
    skin of breast C4A.52
    trunk NEC C4A.59
    upper limb, including shoulder C4A.6-
    visceral metastatic C7B.1
  metastatic — *see* Neoplasm, secondary, by site
  metatypical — *see* Neoplasm, skin, malignant
  morphea, basal cell — *see* Neoplasm, skin, malignant
  mucoid
    cell
      specified site — *see* Neoplasm, malignant, by site
      unspecified site C75.1
  neuroendocrine — *see also* Tumor, neuroendocrine
    high grade, any site C7A.1
    poorly differentiated, any site C7A.1
  nonencapsulated sclerosing C73
  noninfiltrating
    intracystic — *see* Neoplasm, in situ, by site
    intraductal
      breast D05.1-
      papillary
        breast D05.1-
        specified site NEC — *see* Neoplasm, in situ, by site
        unspecified site D05.1-
      specified site — *see* Neoplasm, in situ, by site
      unspecified site D05.1-
    lobular
      breast D05.0-

Carcinoma (malignant) - *continued*
  noninfiltrating - *continued*
    lobular - *continued*
      specified site NEC — *see* Neoplasm, in situ, by site
      unspecified site (female) D05.0-
  oat cell
    specified site — *see* Neoplasm, malignant, by site
    unspecified site C34.90
  odontogenic C41.1
    upper jaw (bone) C41.0
  papillary
    with follicular (mixed) C73
    follicular variant C73
    intraductal (noninfiltrating)
      with invasion
        specified site — *see* Neoplasm, malignant, by site
        unspecified site (female) C50.91-
          male C50.92-
      breast D05.1-
      specified site NEC — *see* Neoplasm, in situ, by site
      unspecified site D05.1-
    serous
      specified site — *see* Neoplasm, malignant, by site
      surface
        specified site — *see* Neoplasm, malignant, by site
        unspecified site C56.9
      unspecified site C56.9
  papillocystic
    specified site — *see* Neoplasm, malignant, by site
    unspecified site C56.9
  parafollicular cell
    specified site — *see* Neoplasm, malignant, by site
    unspecified site C73
  pilomatrix — *see* Neoplasm, skin, malignant
  pseudomucinous
    specified site — *see* Neoplasm, malignant, by site
    unspecified site C56.9
  renal cell C64-
  Schmincke — *see* Neoplasm, nasopharynx, malignant
  Schneiderian
    specified site — *see* Neoplasm, malignant, by site
    unspecified site C30.0
  sebaceous — *see* Neoplasm, skin, malignant
  secondary — *see also* Neoplasm, secondary, by site
    Merkel cell C7B.1
  secretory, breast — *see* Neoplasm, breast, malignant
  serous
    papillary
      specified site — *see* Neoplasm, malignant, by site
      unspecified site C56.9
    surface, papillary
      specified site — *see* Neoplasm, malignant, by site
      unspecified site C56.9
  Sertoli cell
    specified site — *see* Neoplasm, malignant, by site
    unspecified site C62.90
      female C56.9
      male C62.90
  skin appendage — *see* Neoplasm, skin, malignant
  small cell
    fusiform cell
      specified site — *see* Neoplasm, malignant, by site
      unspecified site C34.90
    intermediate cell
      specified site — *see* Neoplasm, malignant, by site
      unspecified site C34.90
    large cell
      specified site — *see* Neoplasm, malignant, by site
      unspecified site C34.90
  solid
    with amyloid stroma
      specified site — *see* Neoplasm, malignant, by site
      unspecified site C73
    microinvasive
      specified site — *see* Neoplasm, malignant, by site
      unspecified site C53.9
  sweat gland — *see* Neoplasm, skin, malignant
  theca cell C56.-
  thymic C37
  unspecified site (primary) C80.1
  water-clear cell C75.0
Carcinoma-in-situ — *see also* Neoplasm, in situ, by site
  breast NOS D05.9-
    specified type NEC D05.8-
  epidermoid — *see also* Neoplasm, in situ, by site
    with questionable stromal invasion
      cervix D06.9

Carcinoma-in-situ - *continued*
  epidermoid - *continued*
    with questionable stromal invasion - *continued*
      specified site NEC — *see* Neoplasm, in situ, by site
      unspecified site D06.9
    Bowen's type — *see* Neoplasm, skin, in situ
    intraductal
      breast D05.1-
      specified site NEC — *see* Neoplasm, in situ, by site
      unspecified site D05.1-
    lobular
      with
        infiltrating duct
          breast (female) C50.91-
            male C50.92-
          specified site NEC — *see* Neoplasm, malignant
          unspecified site (female) C50.91-
            male C50.92-
        intraductal
          breast D05.8-
          specified site NEC — *see* Neoplasm, in situ, by site
          unspecified site (female) D05.8-
      breast D05.0-
      specified site NEC — *see* Neoplasm, in situ, by site
      unspecified site D05.0-
    squamous cell — *see also* Neoplasm, in situ, by site
      with questionable stromal invasion
        cervix D06.9
      specified site NEC — *see* Neoplasm, in situ, by site
      unspecified site D06.9
Carcinomaphobia F45.29
Carcinomatosis C80.0
  peritonei C78.6
  unspecified site (primary) (secondary) C80.0
Carcinosarcoma — *see* Neoplasm, malignant, by site
  embryonal — *see* Neoplasm, malignant, by site
Cardia, cardial — *see* condition
Cardiac — *see also* condition
  death, sudden — *see* Arrest, cardiac
  pacemaker
    in situ Z95.0
    management or adjustment Z45.018
  tamponade I31.4
Cardialgia — *see* Pain, precordial
Cardiectasis — *see* Hypertrophy, cardiac
Cardiochalasia K21.9
Cardiomalacia I51.5
Cardiomegalia glycogenica diffusa E74.02 *[I43]*
Cardiomegaly — *see also* Hypertrophy, cardiac
  congenital Q24.8
  glycogen E74.02 *[I43]*
  idiopathic I51.7
Cardiomyoliposis I51.5
Cardiomyopathy (familial) (idiopathic) I42.9
  alcoholic I42.6
  amyloid E85.4 *[I43]*
  arteriosclerotic — *see* Disease, heart, ischemic, atherosclerotic
  beriberi E51.12
  cobalt-beer I42.6
  congenital I42.4
  congestive I42.0
  constrictive NOS I42.5
  dilated I42.0
  due to
    alcohol I42.6
    beriberi E51.12
    cardiac glycogenosis E74.02 *[I43]*
    drugs I42.7
    external agents NEC I42.7
    Friedreich's ataxia G11.1
    myotonia atrophica G71.11 *[I43]*
    progressive muscular dystrophy G71.0
  glycogen storage E74.02 *[I43]*
  hypertensive — *see* Hypertension, heart
  hypertrophic (nonobstructive) I42.2
    obstructive I42.1
      congenital Q24.8
  in
    Chagas' disease (chronic) B57.2
      acute B57.0
    sarcoidosis D86.85
  ischemic I25.5
  metabolic E88.9 *[I43]*
    thyrotoxic E05.90 *[I43]*
      with thyroid storm E05.91 *[I43]*
  newborn I42.8
    congenital I42.4

Cardiomyopathy (familial) (idiopathic) - *continued*
  nutritional E63.9 *[I43]*
    beriberi E51.12
  obscure of Africa I42.8
  peripartum O90.3
  postpartum O90.3
  restrictive NEC I42.5
  rheumatic I09.0
  secondary I42.9
  stress induced I51.81
  takotsubo I51.81
  thyrotoxic E05.90 *[I43]*
    with thyroid storm E05.91 *[I43]*
  toxic NEC I42.7
  tuberculous A18.84
  viral B33.24
Cardionephritis — *see* Hypertension, cardiorenal
Cardionephropathy — *see* Hypertension, cardiorenal
Cardionephrosis — *see* Hypertension, cardiorenal
Cardiopathia nigra I27.0
Cardiopathy — *see also* Disease, heart I51.9
  idiopathic I42.9
  mucopolysaccharidosis E76.3 *[I52]*
Cardiopericarditis — *see* Pericarditis
Cardiophobia F45.29
Cardiorenal — *see* condition
Cardiorrhexis — *see* Infarct, myocardium
Cardiosclerosis — *see* Disease, heart, ischemic, atherosclerotic
Cardiosis — *see* Disease, heart
Cardiospasm (esophagus) (reflex) (stomach) K22.0
  congenital Q39.5
    with megaesophagus Q39.5
Cardiostenosis — *see* Disease, heart
Cardiosymphysis I31.0
Cardiovascular — *see* condition
Carditis (acute) (bacterial) (chronic) (subacute) I51.89
  meningococcal A39.50
  rheumatic — *see* Disease, heart, rheumatic
  rheumatoid — *see* Rheumatoid, carditis
  viral B33.20
Care (of) (for) (following)
  child (routine) Z76.2
  family member (handicapped) (sick)
    creating problem for family Z63.6
    provided away from home for holiday relief Z75.5
    unavailable, due to
      absence (person rendering care) (sufferer) Z74.2
      inability (any reason) of person rendering care Z74.2
  foundling Z76.1
  holiday relief Z75.5
  improper — *see* Maltreatment
  lack of (at or after birth) (infant) — *see* Maltreatment, child, neglect
  lactating mother Z39.1
  palliative Z51.5
  postpartum
    immediately after delivery Z39.0
    routine follow-up Z39.2
  respite Z75.5
  unavailable, due to
    absence of person rendering care Z74.2
    inability (any reason) of person rendering care Z74.2
  well-baby Z76.2
Caries
  bone NEC A18.03
  dental (dentino enamel junction) (early childhood) (of dentine) (pre-eruptive) (recurrent) (to the pulp) K02.9
    arrested (coronal) (root) K02.3
    chewing surface
      limited to enamel K02.51
      penetrating into dentin K02.52
      penetrating into pulp K02.53
    coronal surface
      chewing surface
        limited to enamel K02.51
        penetrating into dentin K02.52
        penetrating into pulp K02.53
      pit and fissure surface
        limited to enamel K02.51
        penetrating into dentin K02.52
        penetrating into pulp K02.53
      smooth surface
        limited to enamel K02.61
        penetrating into dentin K02.62
        penetrating into pulp K02.63
    pit and fissure surface
      limited to enamel K02.51

Caries - *continued*
  dental (dentino enamel junction) (early childhood) (of dentine) (pre-eruptive) (recurrent) (to the pulp) - *continued*
    pit and fissure surface - *continued*
      penetrating into dentin K02.52
      penetrating into pulp K02.53
      primary, cervical origin K02.52
      root K02.7
    smooth surface
      limited to enamel K02.61
      penetrating into dentin K02.62
      penetrating into pulp K02.63
  external meatus — *see* Disorder, ear, external, specified type NEC
  hip (tuberculous) A18.02
  initial (tooth)
    chewing surface K02.51
    pit and fissure surface K02.51
    smooth surface K02.61
  knee (tuberculous) A18.02
  labyrinth — *see* subcategory H83.8
  limb NEC (tuberculous) A18.03
  mastoid process (chronic) — *see* Mastoiditis, chronic
    tuberculous A18.03
  middle ear — *see* subcategory H74.8
  nose (tuberculous) A18.03
  orbit (tuberculous) A18.03
  ossicles, ear — *see* Abnormal, ear ossicles
  petrous bone — *see* Petrositis
  root (dental) (tooth) K02.7
  sacrum (tuberculous) A18.01
  spine, spinal (column) (tuberculous) A18.01
  syphilitic A52.77
    congenital (early) A50.02 *[M90.80]*
  tooth, teeth — *see* Caries, dental
  tuberculous A18.03
  vertebra (column) (tuberculous) A18.01
Carious teeth — *see* Caries, dental
Carneous mole O02.0
Carnitine insufficiency E71.40
Carotid body or sinus syndrome G90.01
Carotidynia G90.01
Carotinemia (dietary) E67.1
Carotinosis (cutis) (skin) E67.1
Carpal tunnel syndrome — *see* Syndrome, carpal tunnel
Carpenter's syndrome Q87.0
Carpopedal spasm — *see* Tetany
Carr-Barr-Plunkett syndrome Q97.1
Carrier (suspected) of
  amebiasis Z22.1
  bacterial disease NEC Z22.39
    diphtheria Z22.2
    intestinal infectious NEC Z22.1
      typhoid Z22.0
    meningococcal Z22.31
    sexually transmitted Z22.4
    specified NEC Z22.39
    staphylococcal (Methicillin susceptible) Z22.321
      Methicillin resistant Z22.322
    streptococcal Z22.338
      group B Z22.330
        complicating pregnancy or delivery O99.82-
    typhoid Z22.0
  cholera Z22.1
  diphtheria Z22.2
  gastrointestinal pathogens NEC Z22.1
  genetic Z14.8
    cystic fibrosis Z14.1
    hemophilia A (asymptomatic) Z14.01
      symptomatic Z14.02
  gestational, pregnant Z33.1
  gonorrhea Z22.4
  HAA (hepatitis Australian-antigen) B18.8
  HB (c) (s) -AG B18.1
  hepatitis (viral) B18.9
    Australia-antigen (HAA) B18.8
    B surface antigen (HBsAg) B18.1
      with acute delta- (super) infection B17.0
    C B18.2
    specified NEC B18.8
  human T-cell lymphotropic virus type-1 (HTLV-1) infection Z22.6
  infectious organism Z22.9
    specified NEC Z22.8
  meningococci Z22.31
  Salmonella typhosa Z22.0
  serum hepatitis — *see* Carrier, hepatitis
  staphylococci (Methicillin susceptible) Z22.321
    Methicillin resistant Z22.322
  streptococci Z22.338

Carrier (suspected) **of** - *continued*
 streptococci - *continued*
  group B Z22.330
   complicating pregnancy or delivery O99.82-
 syphilis Z22.4
 typhoid Z22.0
 venereal disease NEC Z22.4
Carrion's disease A44.0
Carter's relapsing fever (Asiatic) A68.1
Cartilage — *see* condition
Caruncle (inflamed)
 conjunctiva (acute) — *see* Conjunctivitis, acute
 labium (majus) (minus) N90.89
 lacrimal — *see* Inflammation, lacrimal, passages
 myrtiform N89.8
 urethral (benign) N36.2
Cascade stomach K31.2
Caseation lymphatic gland (tuberculous) A18.2
Cassidy (-Scholte) **syndrome** (malignant
  carcinoid) E34.0
Castellani's disease A69.8
Castration, traumatic, male S38.231
Casts in urine R82.99
Cat
 cry syndrome Q93.4
 ear Q17.3
 eye syndrome Q92.8
Catabolism, senile R54
Catalepsy (hysterical) F44.2
 schizophrenic F20.2
Cataplexy (idiopathic) — *see* - Narcolepsy
Cataract (cortical) (immature) (incipient) H26.9
 with
  neovascularization — *see* Cataract, complicated
 age-related — *see* Cataract, senile
 anterior
  and posterior axial embryonal Q12.0
  pyramidal Q12.0
 associated with
  galactosemia E74.21 *[H28]*
  myotonic disorders G71.19 *[H28]*
 blue Q12.0
 central Q12.0
 cerulean Q12.0
 complicated H26.20
  with
   neovascularization H26.21-
   ocular disorder H26.22-
  glaucomatous flecks H26.23-
 congenital Q12.0
 coraliform Q12.0
 coronary Q12.0
 crystalline Q12.0
 diabetic — *see* Diabetes, cataract
 drug-induced H26.3-
 due to
  ocular disorder — *see* Cataract, complicated
  radiation H26.8
 electric H26.8
 extraction status Z98.4-
 glass-blower's H26.8
 heat ray H26.8
 heterochromic — *see* Cataract, complicated
 hypermature — *see* Cataract, senile, morgagnian
  type
 in (due to)
  chronic iridocyclitis — *see* Cataract, complicated
  diabetes — *see* Diabetes, cataract
  endocrine disease E34.9 *[H28]*
  eye disease — *see* Cataract, complicated
  hypoparathyroidism E20.9 *[H28]*
  malnutrition-dehydration E46 *[H28]*
  metabolic disease E88.9 *[H28]*
  myotonic disorders G71.19 *[H28]*
  nutritional disease E63.9 *[H28]*
 infantile — *see* Cataract, presenile
 irradiational — *see* Cataract, specified NEC
 juvenile — *see* Cataract, presenile
 malnutrition-dehydration E46 *[H28]*
 morgagnian — *see* Cataract, senile, morgagnian type
 myotonic G71.19 *[H28]*
 myxedema E03.9 *[H28]*
 nuclear
  embryonal Q12.0
  sclerosis — *see* Cataract, senile, nuclear
 presenile H26.00-
  combined forms H26.06-
  cortical H26.01-
  lamellar — *see* Cataract, presenile, cortical
  nuclear H26.03-
  specified NEC H26.09
  subcapsular polar (anterior) H26.04-
   posterior H26.05-

Cataract (cortical) (immature) (incipient) - *continued*
 presenile - *continued*
  zonular — *see* Cataract, presenile, cortical
 secondary H26.40
  Soemmering's ring H26.41-
  specified NEC H26.49-
  to eye disease — *see* Cataract, complicated
 senile H25.9
  brunescens — *see* Cataract, senile, nuclear
  combined forms H25.81-
  coronary — *see* Cataract, senile, incipient
  cortical H25.01-
   hypermature — *see* Cataract, senile, morgagnian
    type
  incipient (mature) (total) H25.09-
   cortical — *see* Cataract, senile, cortical
   subcapsular — *see* Cataract, senile, subcapsular
  morgagnian type (hypermature) H25.2-
  nuclear (sclerosis) H25.1-
  polar subcapsular (anterior) (posterior) — *see*
   Cataract, senile, incipient
  punctate — *see* Cataract, senile, incipient
  specified NEC H25.89
  subcapsular polar (anterior) H25.03-
   posterior H25.04-
 snowflake — *see* Diabetes, cataract
 specified NEC H26.8
 toxic — *see* Cataract, drug-induced
 traumatic H26.10-
  localized H26.11-
  partially resolved H26.12-
  total H26.13-
 zonular (perinuclear) Q12.0
Cataracta — *see also* Cataract
 brunescens — *see* Cataract, senile, nuclear
 centralis pulverulenta Q12.0
 cerulea Q12.0
 complicata — *see* Cataract, complicated
 congenita Q12.0
 coralliformis Q12.0
 coronaria Q12.0
 diabetic — *see* Diabetes, cataract
 membranacea
  accreta — *see* Cataract, secondary
  congenita Q12.0
 nigra — *see* Cataract, senile, nuclear
 sunflower — *see* Cataract, complicated
Catarrh, catarrhal (acute) (febrile) (infectious)
 (inflammation) — *see also* condition J00
 bronchial — *see* Bronchitis
 chest — *see* Bronchitis
 chronic J31.0
 due to congenital syphilis A50.03
 enteric — *see* Enteritis
 eustachian H68.009
 fauces — *see* Pharyngitis
 gastrointestinal — *see* Enteritis
 gingivitis K05.00
  nonplaque induced K05.01
  plaque induced K05.00
 hay — *see* Fever, hay
 intestinal — *see* Enteritis
 larynx, chronic J37.0
 liver B15.9
  with hepatic coma B15.0
 lung — *see* Bronchitis
 middle ear, chronic — *see* Otitis, media,
  nonsuppurative, chronic, serous
 mouth K12.1
 nasal (chronic) — *see* Rhinitis
 nasobronchial J31.1
 nasopharyngeal (chronic) J31.1
  acute J00
 pulmonary — *see* Bronchitis
 spring (eye) (vernal) — *see* Conjunctivitis, acute,
  atopic
 summer (hay) — *see* Fever, hay
 throat J31.2
 tubotympanal — *see also* Otitis, media,
  nonsuppurative
  chronic — *see* Otitis, media, nonsuppurative,
   chronic, serous
Catatonia (schizophrenic) F20.2
Catatonic
 disorder due to known physiologic condition F06.1
 schizophrenia F20.2
 stupor R40.1
Cat-scratch — *see also* Abrasion
 disease or fever A28.1
Cauda equina — *see* condition
Cauliflower ear M95.1-
Causalgia (upper limb) G56.4-
 lower limb G57.7-

Cause
 external, general effects T75.89
Caustic burn — *see* Corrosion, by site
Cavare's disease (familial periodic paralysis) G72.3
Cave-in, injury
 crushing (severe) — *see* Crush
 suffocation — *see* Asphyxia, traumatic, due to low
  oxygen, due to cave-in
Cavernitis (penis) N48.29
Cavernositis N48.29
Cavernous — *see* condition
Cavitation of lung — *see also* Tuberculosis,
 pulmonary
 nontuberculous J98.4
Cavities, dental — *see* Caries, dental
Cavity
 lung — *see* Cavitation of lung
 optic papilla Q14.2
 pulmonary — *see* Cavitation of lung
Cavovarus foot, congenital Q66.1
Cavus foot (congenital) Q66.7
 acquired — *see* Deformity, limb, foot, specified
  NEC
Cazenave's disease L10.2
Cecitis K52.9
 with perforation, peritonitis, or rupture K65.8
Cecum — *see* condition
Celiac
 artery compression syndrome I77.4
 disease (with steatorrhea) K90.0
 infantilism K90.0
Cell (s) **, cellular** — *see also* condition
 in urine R82.99
Cellulitis (diffuse) (phlegmonous) (septic)
 (suppurative) L03.90
 abdominal wall L03.311
 anaerobic A48.0
 ankle — *see* Cellulitis, lower limb
 anus K61.0
 arm — *see* Cellulitis, upper limb
 auricle (ear) — *see* Cellulitis, ear
 axilla L03.11-
 back (any part) L03.312
 breast (acute) (nonpuerperal) (subacute) N61.0
  nipple N61.0
 broad ligament
  acute N73.0
 buttock L03.317
 cervical (meaning neck) L03.221
 cervix (uteri) — *see* Cervicitis
 cheek (external) L03.211
  internal K12.2
 chest wall L03.313
 chronic L03.90
 clostridial A48.0
 corpus cavernosum N48.22
 digit
  finger — *see* Cellulitis, finger
  toe — *see* Cellulitis, toe
 Douglas' cul-de-sac or pouch
  acute N73.0
 drainage site (following operation) T81.48
 ear (external) H60.1-
 eosinophilic (granulomatous) L98.3
 erysipelatous — *see* Erysipelas
 external auditory canal — *see* Cellulitis, ear
 eyelid — *see* Abscess, eyelid
 face NEC L03.211
 finger (intrathecal) (periosteal) (subcutaneous)
  (subcuticular) L03.01-
 foot — *see* Cellulitis, lower limb
 gangrenous — *see* Gangrene
 genital organ NEC
  female (external) N76.4
  male N49.9
   multiple sites N49.8
   specified NEC N49.8
 gluteal (region) L03.317
 gonococcal A54.89
 groin L03.314
 hand — *see* Cellulitis, upper limb
 head NEC L03.811
  face (any part, except ear, eye and nose) L03.211
 heel — *see* Cellulitis, lower limb
 hip — *see* Cellulitis, lower limb
 jaw (region) L03.211
 knee — *see* Cellulitis, lower limb
 labium (majus) (minus) — *see* Vulvitis
 lacrimal passages — *see* Inflammation, lacrimal,
  passages
 larynx J38.7
 leg — *see* Cellulitis, lower limb
 lip K13.0

Cellulitis (diffuse) (phlegmonous) (septic) (suppurative) - *continued*
 lower limb L03.11-
  toe — *see* Cellulitis, toe
 mouth (floor) K12.2
 multiple sites, so stated L03.90
 nasopharynx J39.1
 navel L03.316
  newborn P38.9
   with mild hemorrhage P38.1
   without hemorrhage P38.9
 neck (region) L03.221
 nipple (acute) (nonpuerperal) (subacute) N61.0
 nose (septum) (external) J34.0
 orbit, orbital H05.01-
 palate (soft) K12.2
 pectoral (region) L03.313
 pelvis, pelvic (chronic)
  female — *see also* Disease, pelvis, inflammatory N73.2
   acute N73.0
  following ectopic or molar pregnancy O08.0
  male K65.0
 penis N48.22
 perineal, perineum L03.315
 periorbital L03.213
 perirectal K61.1
 peritonsillar J36
 periurethral N34.0
 periuterine — *see also* Disease, pelvis, inflammatory N73.2
  acute N73.0
 pharynx J39.1
 preseptal L03.213
 rectum K61.1
 retroperitoneal K68.9
 round ligament
  acute N73.0
 scalp (any part) L03.811
 scrotum N49.2
 seminal vesicle N49.0
 shoulder — *see* Cellulitis, upper limb
 specified site NEC L03.818
 submandibular (region) (space) (triangle) K12.2
  gland K11.3
 submaxillary (region) K12.2
  gland K11.3
 thigh — *see* Cellulitis, lower limb
 thumb (intrathecal) (periosteal) (subcutaneous) (subcuticular) — *see* Cellulitis, finger
 toe (intrathecal) (periosteal) (subcutaneous) (subcuticular) L03.03-
 tonsil J36
 trunk L03.319
  abdominal wall L03.311
  back (any part) L03.312
  buttock L03.317
  chest wall L03.313
  groin L03.314
  perineal, perineum L03.315
  umbilicus L03.316
 tuberculous (primary) A18.4
 umbilicus L03.316
 upper limb L03.11-
  axilla — *see* Cellulitis, axilla
  finger — *see* Cellulitis, finger
  thumb — *see* Cellulitis, finger
 vaccinal T88.0
 vocal cord J38.3
 vulva — *see* Vulvitis
 wrist — *see* Cellulitis, upper limb
Cementoblastoma, benign — *see* Cyst, calcifying odontogenic
Cementoma — *see* Cyst, calcifying odontogenic
Cementoperiostitis — *see* Periodontitis
Cementosis K03.4
Central auditory processing disorder H93.25
Central pain syndrome G89.0
Cephalematocele, cephal (o) **hematocele**
 newborn P52.8
  birth injury P10.8
  traumatic — *see* Hematoma, brain
Cephalematoma, cephalhematoma (calcified)
 newborn (birth injury) P12.0
 traumatic — *see* Hematoma, brain
Cephalgia, cephalalgia — *see also* Headache
 histamine G44.009
  intractable G44.001
  not intractable G44.009
 trigeminal autonomic (TAC) NEC G44.099
  intractable G44.091
  not intractable G44.099
Cephalic — *see* condition

Cephalitis — *see* Encephalitis
Cephalocele — *see* Encephalocele
Cephalomenia N94.89
Cephalopelvic — *see* condition
Cerclage (with cervical incompetence) **in pregnancy** — *see* Incompetence, cervix, in pregnancy
Cerebellitis — *see* Encephalitis
Cerebellum, cerebellar — *see* condition
Cerebral — *see* condition
Cerebritis — *see* Encephalitis
Cerebro-hepato-renal syndrome Q87.89
Cerebromalacia — *see* Softening, brain
 sequelae of cerebrovascular disease I69.398
Cerebroside lipidosis E75.22
Cerebrospasticity (congenital) G80.1
Cerebrospinal — *see* condition
Cerebrum — *see* condition
Ceroid-lipofuscinosis, neuronal E75.4
Cerumen (accumulation) (impacted) H61.2-
Cervical — *see also* condition
 auricle Q18.2
 dysplasia in pregnancy — *see* Abnormal, cervix, in pregnancy or childbirth
 erosion in pregnancy — *see* Abnormal, cervix, in pregnancy or childbirth
 fibrosis in pregnancy — *see* Abnormal, cervix, in pregnancy or childbirth
 fusion syndrome Q76.1
 rib Q76.5
 shortening (complicating pregnancy) O26.87-
Cervicalgia M54.2
Cervicitis (acute) (chronic) (nonvenereal) (senile (atrophic)) (subacute) (subacute) (with ulceration) N72
 with
  abortion — *see* Abortion, by type complicated by genital tract and pelvic infection
  ectopic pregnancy O08.0
  molar pregnancy O08.0
 chlamydial A56.09
 gonococcal A54.03
 herpesviral A60.03
 puerperal (postpartum) O86.11
 syphilitic A52.76
 trichomonal A59.09
 tuberculous A18.16
Cervicocolpitis (emphysematosa) (see also Cervicitis) N72
Cervix — *see* condition
Cesarean delivery, previous, affecting management of pregnancy O34.219
 classical (vertical) scar O34.212
 low transverse scar O34.211
Céstan (-Chenais) **paralysis or syndrome** G46.3
Céstan-Raymond syndrome I65.8
Cestode infestation B71.9
 specified type NEC B71.8
Cestodiasis B71.9
Chabert's disease A22.9
Chacaleh E53.8
Chafing L30.4
Chagas' (-Mazza) **disease** (chronic) B57.2
 with
  cardiovascular involvement NEC B57.2
  digestive system involvement B57.30
   megacolon B57.32
   megaesophagus B57.31
   other specified B57.39
  megacolon B57.32
  megaesophagus B57.31
  myocarditis B57.2
  nervous system involvement B57.40
   meningitis B57.41
   meningoencephalitis B57.42
   other specified B57.49
  specified organ involvement NEC B57.5
 acute (with) B57.1
  cardiovascular NEC B57.0
  myocarditis B57.0
Chagres fever B50.9
Chairridden Z74.09
Chalasia (cardiac sphincter) K21.9
Chalazion H00.19
 left H00.16
  lower H00.15
  upper H00.14
 right H00.13
  lower H00.12
  upper H00.11
Chalcosis — *see also* Disorder, globe, degenerative, chalcosis
 cornea — *see* Deposit, cornea

Chalcosis - *continued*
 crystalline lens — *see* Cataract, complicated
 retina H35.89
Chalicosis (pulmonum) J62.8
Chancre (any genital site) (hard) (hunterian) (mixed) (primary) (seronegative) (seropositive) (syphilitic) A51.0
 congenital A50.07
 conjunctiva NEC A51.2
 Ducrey's A57
 extragenital A51.2
 eyelid A51.2
 lip A51.2
 nipple A51.2
 Nisbet's A57
 of
  carate A67.0
  pinta A67.0
  yaws A66.0
 palate, soft A51.2
 phagedenic A57
 simple A57
 soft A57
  bubo A57
  palate A51.2
 urethra A51.0
 yaws A66.0
Chancroid (anus) (genital) (penis) (perineum) (rectum) (urethra) (vulva) A57
Chandler's disease (osteochondritis dissecans, hip) — *see* Osteochondritis, dissecans, hip
Change (s) (in) (of) — *see also* Removal
 arteriosclerotic — *see* Arteriosclerosis
 bone — *see also* Disorder, bone
  diabetic — *see* Diabetes, bone change
 bowel habit R19.4
 cardiorenal (vascular) — *see* Hypertension, cardiorenal
 cardiovascular — *see* Disease, cardiovascular
 circulatory I99.9
 cognitive (mild) (organic) R41.89
 color, tooth, teeth
  during formation K00.8
  posteruptive K03.7
 contraceptive device Z30.433
 corneal membrane H18.30
  Bowman's membrane fold or rupture H18.31-
  Descemet's membrane
   fold H18.32-
   rupture H18.33-
 coronary — *see* Disease, heart, ischemic
 degenerative, spine or vertebra — *see* Spondylosis
 dental pulp, regressive K04.2
 dressing (nonsurgical) Z48.00
  surgical Z48.01
 heart — *see* Disease, heart
 hip joint — *see* Derangement, joint, hip
 hyperplastic larynx J38.7
 hypertrophic
  nasal sinus J34.89
  turbinate, nasal J34.3
  upper respiratory tract J39.8
 indwelling catheter Z46.6
 inflammatory — *see also* Inflammation
  sacroiliac M46.1
 job, anxiety concerning Z56.1
 joint — *see* Derangement, joint
 life — *see* Menopause
 mental status R41.82
 minimal (glomerular) — *see also* N00-N07 with fourth character .0 N05.0
 myocardium, myocardial — *see* Degeneration, myocardial
 of life — *see* Menopause
 pacemaker Z45.018
  pulse generator Z45.010
 personality (enduring) F68.8
  due to (secondary to)
   general medical condition F07.0
  secondary (nonspecific) F60.89
 regressive, dental pulp K04.2
 renal — *see* Disease, renal
 retina H35.9
  myopic H44.2-
 sacroiliac joint M53.3
 senile — *see also* condition R54
 sensory R20.8
 skin R23.9
  acute, due to ultraviolet radiation L56.9
   specified NEC L56.8
  chronic, due to nonionizing radiation L57.9
   specified NEC L57.8
  cyanosis R23.0

Change (s) (in) (of) - *continued*
  skin - *continued*
    flushing R23.2
    pallor R23.1
    petechiae R23.3
    specified change NEC R23.8
    swelling — *see* Mass, localized
    texture R23.4
  trophic
    arm — *see* Mononeuropathy, upper limb
    leg — *see* Mononeuropathy, lower limb
  vascular I99.9
  vasomotor I73.9
  voice R49.9
    psychogenic F44.4
    specified NEC R49.8
Changing sleep-work schedule, affecting sleep G47.26
Changuinola fever A93.1
Chapping skin T69.8
Charcot-Marie-Tooth disease, paralysis or syndrome G60.0
Charcot's
  arthropathy — *see* Arthropathy, neuropathic
  cirrhosis K74.3
  disease (tabetic arthropathy) A52.16
  joint (disease) (tabetic) A52.16
    diabetic — *see* Diabetes, with, arthropathy
    syringomyelic G95.0
  syndrome (intermittent claudication) I73.9
CHARGE association Q89.8
Charley-horse (quadriceps) M62.831
  traumatic (quadriceps) S76.11-
Charlouis' disease — *see* Yaws
Cheadle's disease E54
Checking (of)
  cardiac pacemaker (battery) (electrode (s)) Z45.018
    pulse generator Z45.010
  implantable subdermal contraceptive Z30.46
  intrauterine contraceptive device Z30.431
Check-up — *see* Examination
Chédiak-Higashi (-Steinbrinck) **syndrome** (congenital gigantism of peroxidase granules) E70.330
Cheek — *see* condition
Cheese itch B88.0
Cheese-washer's lung J67.8
Cheese-worker's lung J67.8
Cheilitis (acute) (angular) (catarrhal) (chronic) (exfoliative) (gangrenous) (glandular) (infectional) (suppurative) (ulcerative) (vesicular) K13.0
  actinic (due to sun) L56.8
    other than from sun L59.8
  candidal B37.83
Cheilodynia K13.0
Cheiloschisis — *see* Cleft, lip
Cheilosis (angular) K13.0
  with pellagra E52
  due to
    vitamin B2 (riboflavin) deficiency E53.0
Cheiromegaly M79.89
Cheiropompholyx L30.1
Cheloid — *see* Keloid
Chemical burn — *see* Corrosion, by site
Chemodectoma — *see* Paraganglioma, nonchromaffin
Chemosis, conjunctiva — *see* Edema, conjunctiva
Chemotherapy (session) (for)
  cancer Z51.11
  neoplasm Z51.11
Cherubism M27.8
Chest — *see* condition
Cheyne-Stokes breathing (respiration) R06.3
Chiari's
  disease or syndrome (hepatic vein thrombosis) I82.0
  malformation
    type I G93.5
    type II — *see* Spina bifida
    net Q24.8
Chicago disease B40.9
Chickenpox — *see* Varicella
Chiclero ulcer or sore B55.1
Chigger (infestation) B88.0
Chignon (disease) B36.8
  newborn (from vacuum extraction) (birth injury) P12.1
Chilaiditi's syndrome (subphrenic displacement, colon) Q43.3
Chilblain (s) (lupus) T69.1
Child
  custody dispute Z65.3
Childbirth — *see* Delivery

Childhood
  cerebral X-linked adrenoleukodystrophy E71.520
  period of rapid growth Z00.2
Chill (s) R68.83
  with fever R50.9
  congestive in malarial regions B54
  without fever R68.83
Chilomastigiasis A07.8
Chimera 46,XX/46,XY Q99.0
Chin — *see* condition
Chinese dysentery A03.9
Chionophobia F40.228
Chitral fever A93.1
Chlamydia, chlamydial A74.9
  cervicitis A56.09
  conjunctivitis A74.0
  cystitis A56.01
  endometritis A56.11
  epididymitis A56.19
  female
    pelvic inflammatory disease A56.11
    pelviperitonitis A56.11
  orchitis A56.19
  peritonitis A74.81
  pharyngitis A56.4
  proctitis A56.3
  psittaci (infection) A70
  salpingitis A56.11
  sexually-transmitted infection NEC A56.8
  specified NEC A74.89
  urethritis A56.01
  vulvovaginitis A56.02
Chlamydiosis — *see* Chlamydia
Chloasma (skin) (idiopathic) (symptomatic) L81.1
  eyelid H02.719
    hyperthyroid E05.90 *[H02.719]*
      with thyroid storm E05.91 *[H02.719]*
    left H02.716
      lower H02.715
      upper H02.714
    right H02.713
      lower H02.712
      upper H02.711
Chloroma C92.3-
Chlorosis D50.9
  Egyptian B76.9 *[D63.8]*
  miner's B76.9 *[D63.8]*
Chlorotic anemia D50.8
Chocolate cyst (ovary) N80.1
Choked
  disc or disk — *see* Papilledema
  on food, phlegm, or vomitus NOS — *see* Foreign body, by site
  while vomiting NOS — *see* Foreign body, by site
Chokes (resulting from bends) T70.3
Choking sensation R09.89
Cholangiectasis K83.8
Cholangiocarcinoma
  with hepatocellular carcinoma, combined C22.0
  liver C22.1
  specified site NEC — *see* Neoplasm, malignant, by site
  unspecified site C22.1
Cholangiohepatitis K83.8
  due to fluke infestation B66.1
Cholangiohepatoma C22.0
Cholangiolitis (acute) (chronic) (extrahepatic) (gangrenous) (intrahepatic) K83.0
  paratyphoidal — *see* Fever, paratyphoid
  typhoidal A01.09
Cholangioma D13.4
  malignant — *see* Cholangiocarcinoma
Cholangitis (ascending) (primary) (recurrent) (sclerosing) (secondary) (stenosing) (suppurative) K83.0
  with calculus, bile duct — *see* Calculus, bile duct, with cholangitis
  chronic nonsuppurative destructive K74.3
Cholecystectasia K82.8
Cholecystitis K81.9
  with
    calculus, stones in
      bile duct (common) (hepatic) — *see* Calculus, bile duct, with cholecystitis
      cystic duct — *see* Calculus, gallbladder, with cholecystitis
      gallbladder — *see* Calculus, gallbladder, with cholecystitis
      choledocholithiasis — *see* Calculus, bile duct, with cholecystitis
      cholelithiasis — *see* Calculus, gallbladder, with cholecystitis

Cholecystitis - *continued*
  acute (emphysematous) (gangrenous) (suppurative) K81.0
    with
      calculus, stones in
        cystic duct — *see* Calculus, gallbladder, with cholecystitis, acute
        gallbladder — *see* Calculus, gallbladder, with cholecystitis, acute
      choledocholithiasis — *see* Calculus, bile duct, with cholecystitis, acute
      cholelithiasis — *see* Calculus, gallbladder, with cholecystitis, acute
    chronic cholecystitis K81.2
      with gallbladder calculus K80.12
        with obstruction K80.13
  chronic K81.1
    with acute cholecystitis K81.2
      with gallbladder calculus K80.12
        with obstruction K80.13
  emphysematous (acute) — *see* Cholecystitis, acute
  gangrenous — *see* Cholecystitis, acute
  paratyphoidal, current A01.4
  suppurative — *see* Cholecystitis, acute
  typhoidal A01.09
Cholecystolithiasis — *see* Calculus, gallbladder
Choledochitis (suppurative) K83.0
Choledocholith — *see* Calculus, bile duct
Choledocholithiasis (common duct) (hepatic duct) — *see* Calculus, bile duct
  cystic — *see* Calculus, gallbladder
  typhoidal A01.09
Cholelithiasis (cystic duct) (gallbladder) (impacted) (multiple) — *see* Calculus, gallbladder
  bile duct (common) (hepatic) — *see* Calculus, bile duct
  hepatic duct — *see* Calculus, bile duct
  specified NEC K80.80
    with obstruction K80.81
Cholemia — *see also* Jaundice
  familial (simple) (congenital) E80.4
  Gilbert's E80.4
Choleperitoneum, choleperitonitis K65.3
Cholera (Asiatic) (epidemic) (malignant) A00.9
  antimonial — *see* Poisoning, antimony
  classical A00.0
  due to Vibrio cholerae 01 A00.9
    biovar cholerae A00.0
    biovar eltor A00.1
    el tor A00.1
  el tor A00.1
Cholerine — *see* Cholera
Cholestasis NEC K83.1
  with hepatocyte injury K71.0
  due to total parenteral nutrition (TPN) K76.89
  pure K71.0
Cholesteatoma (ear) (middle) (with reaction) H71.9-
  attic H71.0-
  external ear (canal) H60.4-
  mastoid H71.2-
  postmastoidectomy cavity (recurrent) — *see* Complications, postmastoidectomy, recurrent cholesteatoma
  recurrent (postmastoidectomy) — *see* Complications, postmastoidectomy, recurrent cholesteatoma
  tympanum H71.1-
Cholesteatosis, diffuse H71.3-
Cholesteremia E78.00
Cholesterin in vitreous — *see* Deposit, crystalline
Cholesterol
  deposit
    retina H35.89
    vitreous — *see* Deposit, crystalline
  elevated (high) E78.00
    with elevated (high) triglycerides E78.2
    screening for Z13.220
  imbibition of gallbladder K82.4
Cholesterolemia (essential) (pure) E78.00
  familial E78.01
  hereditary E78.01
Cholesterolosis, cholesterosis (gallbladder) K82.4
  cerebrotendinous E75.5
Cholocolic fistula K82.3
Choluria R82.2
Chondritis M94.8X9
  auricular H61.03-
  costal (Tietze's) M94.0
  external ear H61.03-
  patella, posttraumatic — *see* Chondromalacia, patella
  pinna H61.03-
  purulent M94.8X-

Chondritis - *continued*
  tuberculous NEC A18.02
    intervertebral A18.01
Chondroblastoma — *see also* Neoplasm, bone, benign
  malignant — *see* Neoplasm, bone, malignant
Chondrocalcinosis M11.20
  ankle M11.27-
  elbow M11.22-
  familial M11.10
    ankle M11.17-
    elbow M11.12-
    foot joint M11.17-
    hand joint M11.14-
    hip M11.15-
    knee M11.16-
    multiple site M11.19
    shoulder M11.11-
    vertebrae M11.18
    wrist M11.13-
  foot joint M11.27-
  hand joint M11.24-
  hip M11.25-
  knee M11.26-
  multiple site M11.29
  shoulder M11.21-
  vertebrae M11.28
  specified type NEC M11.20
    ankle M11.27-
    elbow M11.22-
    foot joint M11.27-
    hand joint M11.24-
    hip M11.25-
    knee M11.26-
    multiple site M11.29
    shoulder M11.21-
    vertebrae M11.28
    wrist M11.23-
  wrist M11.23-
Chondrodermatitis nodularis helicis or anthelicis — *see* Perichondritis, ear
Chondrodysplasia Q78.9
  with hemangioma Q78.4
  calcificans congenita Q77.3
  fetalis Q77.4
  metaphyseal (Jansen's) (McKusick's) (Schmid's) Q78.8
  punctata Q77.3
Chondrodystrophy, chondrodystrophia (familial) (fetalis) (hypoplastic) Q78.9
  calcificans congenita Q77.3
  myotonic (congenital) G71.13
  punctata Q77.3
Chondroectodermal dysplasia Q77.6
Chondrogenesis imperfecta Q77.4
Chondrolysis M94.35-
Chondroma — *see also* Neoplasm, cartilage, benign
  juxtacortical — *see* Neoplasm, bone, benign
  periosteal — *see* Neoplasm, bone, benign
Chondromalacia (systemic) M94.20
  acromioclavicular joint M94.21-
  ankle M94.27-
  elbow M94.22-
  foot joint M94.27-
  glenohumeral joint M94.21-
  hand joint M94.24-
  hip M94.25-
  knee M94.26-
    patella M22.4-
  multiple sites M94.29
  patella M22.4-
  rib M94.28
  sacroiliac joint M94.259
  shoulder M94.21-
  sternoclavicular joint M94.21-
  vertebral joint M94.28
  wrist M94.23-
Chondromatosis — *see also* Neoplasm, cartilage, uncertain behavior
  internal Q78.4
Chondromyxosarcoma — *see* Neoplasm, cartilage, malignant
Chondro-osteodysplasia (Morquio-Brailsford type) E76.219
Chondro-osteodystrophy E76.29
Chondro-osteoma — *see* Neoplasm, bone, benign
Chondropathia tuberosa M94.0
Chondrosarcoma — *see* Neoplasm, cartilage, malignant
  juxtacortical — *see* Neoplasm, bone, malignant
  mesenchymal — *see* Neoplasm, connective tissue, malignant
  myxoid — *see* Neoplasm, cartilage, malignant

Chordee (nonvenereal) N48.89
  congenital Q54.4
  gonococcal A54.09
Chorditis (fibrinous) (nodosa) (tuberosa) J38.2
Chordoma — *see* Neoplasm, vertebral (column), malignant
Chorea (chronic) (gravis) (posthemiplegic) (senile) (spasmodic) G25.5
  with
    heart involvement I02.0
      active or acute (conditions in I01-) I02.0
      rheumatic I02.9
        with valvular disorder I02.0
    rheumatic heart disease (chronic) (inactive) (quiescent) - code to rheumatic heart condition involved
  drug-induced G25.4
  habit F95.8
  hereditary G10
  Huntington's G10
  hysterical F44.4
  minor I02.9
    with heart involvement I02.0
  progressive G25.5
    hereditary G10
  rheumatic (chronic) I02.9
    with heart involvement I02.0
  Sydenham's I02.9
    with heart involvement — *see* Chorea, with rheumatic heart disease
    nonrheumatic G25.5
Choreoathetosis (paroxysmal) G25.5
Chorioadenoma (destruens) D39.2
Chorioamnionitis O41.12-
Chorioangioma D26.7
Choriocarcinoma — *see* Neoplasm, malignant, by site
  combined with
    embryonal carcinoma — *see* Neoplasm, malignant, by site
    other germ cell elements — *see* Neoplasm, malignant, by site
    teratoma — *see* Neoplasm, malignant, by site
  specified site — *see* Neoplasm, malignant, by site
  unspecified site
    female C58
    male C62.90
Chorioencephalitis (acute) (lymphocytic) (serous) A87.2
Chorioepithelioma — *see* Choriocarcinoma
Choriomeningitis (acute) (lymphocytic) (serous) A87.2
Chorionepithelioma — *see* Choriocarcinoma
Chorioretinitis — *see also* Inflammation, chorioretinal
  disseminated — *see also* Inflammation, chorioretinal, disseminated
    in neurosyphilis A52.19
  Egyptian B76.9 *[D63.8]*
  focal — *see also* Inflammation, chorioretinal, focal
  histoplasmic B39.9 *[H32]*
  in (due to)
    histoplasmosis B39.9 *[H32]*
    syphilis (secondary) A51.43
      late A52.71
    toxoplasmosis (acquired) B58.01
      congenital (active) P37.1 *[H32]*
    tuberculosis A18.53
  juxtapapillary, juxtapapillaris — *see* Inflammation, chorioretinal, focal, juxtapapillary
  leprous A30.9 *[H32]*
  miner's B76.9 *[D63.8]*
  progressive myopia (degeneration) H44.2-
  syphilitic (secondary) A51.43
    congenital (early) A50.01 *[H32]*
      late A50.32
    late A52.71
  tuberculous A18.53
Chorioretinopathy, central serous H35.71-
Choroid — *see* condition
Choroideremia H31.21
Choroiditis — *see* Chorioretinitis
Choroidopathy — *see* Disorder, choroid
Choroidoretinitis — *see* Chorioretinitis
Choroidoretinopathy, central serous — *see* Chorioretinopathy, central serous
Christian-Weber disease M35.6
Christmas disease D67
Chromaffinoma — *see also* Neoplasm, benign, by site
  malignant — *see* Neoplasm, malignant, by site
Chromatopsia — *see* Deficiency, color vision
Chromhidrosis, chromidrosis L75.1

Chromoblastomycosis — *see* Chromomycosis
Chromoconversion R82.91
Chromomycosis B43.9
  brain abscess B43.1
  cerebral B43.1
  cutaneous B43.0
  skin B43.0
  specified NEC B43.8
  subcutaneous abscess or cyst B43.2
Chromophytosis B36.0
Chromosome — *see* condition by chromosome involved
  D (1) — *see* condition, chromosome 13
  E (3) — *see* condition, chromosome 18
  G — *see* condition, chromosome 21
Chromotrichomycosis B36.8
Chronic — *see* condition
  fracture — *see* Fracture, pathological
Churg-Strauss syndrome M30.1
Chyle cyst, mesentery I89.8
Chylocele (nonfilarial) I89.8
  filarial — *see also* Infestation, filarial B74.9 *[N51]*
  tunica vaginalis N50.89
    filarial — *see also* Infestation, filarial B74.9 *[N51]*
Chylomicronemia (fasting) (with hyperprebetalipoproteinemia) E78.3
Chylopericardium I31.3
  acute I30.9
Chylothorax (nonfilarial) I89.8
  filarial — *see also* Infestation, filarial B74.9 *[J91.8]*
Chylous — *see* condition
Chyluria (nonfilarial) R82.0
  due to
    bilharziasis B65.0
    Brugia (malayi) B74.1
      timori B74.2
    schistosomiasis (bilharziasis) B65.0
    Wuchereria (bancrofti) B74.0
  filarial — *see* Infestation, filarial
Cicatricial (deformity) — *see* Cicatrix
Cicatrix (adherent) (contracted) (painful) (vicious) — *see also* Scar L90.5
  adenoid (and tonsil) J35.8
  alveolar process M26.79
  anus K62.89
  auricle — *see* Disorder, pinna, specified type NEC
  bile duct (common) (hepatic) K83.8
  bladder N32.89
  bone — *see* Disorder, bone, specified type NEC
  brain G93.89
  cervix (postoperative) (postpartal) N88.1
  common duct K83.8
  cornea H17.9
    tuberculous A18.59
  duodenum (bulb) , obstructive K31.5
  esophagus K22.2
  eyelid — *see* Disorder, eyelid function
  hypopharynx J39.2
  lacrimal passages — *see* Obstruction, lacrimal
  larynx J38.7
  lung J98.4
  middle ear — *see* subcategory H74.8
  mouth K13.79
  muscle M62.89
    with contracture — *see* Contraction, muscle NEC
  nasopharynx J39.2
  palate (soft) K13.79
  penis N48.89
  pharynx J39.2
  prostate N42.89
  rectum K62.89
  retina — *see* Scar, chorioretinal
  semilunar cartilage — *see* Derangement, meniscus
  seminal vesicle N50.89
  skin L90.5
    infected L08.89
    postinfective L90.5
    tuberculous B90.8
  specified site NEC L90.5
  throat J39.2
  tongue K14.8
  tonsil (and adenoid) J35.8
  trachea J39.8
  tuberculous NEC B90.9
  urethra N36.8
  uterus N85.8
    postoperative N99.2
  vagina N89.8
    postoperative N99.2
  vocal cord J38.3
  wrist, constricting (annular) L90.5
CIDP
  (chronic inflammatory demyelinating polyneuropathy) G61.81

CIN — *see* Neoplasia, intraepithelial, cervix
CINCA
(chronic infantile neurological, cutaneous and articular syndrome) M04.2
Cinchonism — *see* Deafness, ototoxic
correct substance properly administered — *see* Table of Drugs and Chemicals, by drug, adverse effect
overdose or wrong substance given or taken — *see* Table of Drugs and Chemicals, by drug, poisoning
Circle of Willis — *see* condition
Circular — *see* condition
Circulating anticoagulants — *see also* - Disorder, hemorrhagic D68.318
due to drugs — *see also* - Disorder, hemorrhagic D68.32
following childbirth O72.3
Circulation
collateral, any site I99.8
defective (lower extremity) I99.8
congenital Q28.9
embryonic Q28.9
failure (peripheral) R57.9
newborn P29.89
fetal, persistent P29.3
heart, incomplete Q28.9
Circulatory system — *see* condition
Circulus senilis (cornea) — *see* Degeneration, cornea, senile
Circumcision (in absence of medical indication) (ritual) (routine) Z41.2
Circumscribed — *see* condition
Circumvallate placenta O43.11-
Cirrhosis, cirrhotic (hepatic) (liver) K74.60
alcoholic K70.30
with ascites K70.31
atrophic — *see* Cirrhosis, liver
Baumgarten-Cruveilhier K74.69
biliary (cholangiolitic) (cholangitic) (hypertrophic) (obstructive) (pericholangiolitic) K74.5
due to
Clonorchiasis B66.1
flukes B66.3
primary K74.3
secondary K74.4
cardiac (of liver) K76.1
Charcot's K74.3
cholangiolitic, cholangitic, cholostatic (primary) K74.3
congestive K76.1
Cruveilhier-Baumgarten K74.69
cryptogenic (liver) K74.69
due to
hepatolenticular degeneration E83.01
Wilson's disease E83.01
xanthomatosis E78.2
fatty K76.0
alcoholic K70.0
Hanot's (hypertrophic) K74.3
hepatic — *see* Cirrhosis, liver
hypertrophic K74.3
Indian childhood K74.69
kidney — *see* Sclerosis, renal
Laennec's K70.30
with ascites K70.31
alcoholic K70.30
with ascites K70.31
nonalcoholic K74.69
liver K74.60
alcoholic K70.30
with ascites K70.31
fatty K70.0
congenital P78.81
syphilitic A52.74
lung (chronic) J84.10
macronodular K74.69
alcoholic K70.30
with ascites K70.31
micronodular K74.69
alcoholic K70.30
with ascites K70.31
mixed type K74.69
monolobular K74.3
nephritis — *see* Sclerosis, renal
nutritional K74.69
alcoholic K70.30
with ascites K70.31
obstructive — *see* Cirrhosis, biliary
ovarian N83.8
pancreas (duct) K86.89
pigmentary E83.110
portal K74.69
alcoholic K70.30
with ascites K70.31

Cirrhosis, cirrhotic (hepatic) (liver) - *continued*
postnecrotic K74.69
alcoholic K70.30
with ascites K70.31
pulmonary J84.10
renal — *see* Sclerosis, renal
spleen D73.2
stasis K76.1
Todd's K74.3
unilobar K74.3
xanthomatous (biliary) K74.5
due to xanthomatosis (familial) (metabolic) (primary) E78.2
Cistern, subarachnoid R93.0
Citrullinemia E72.23
Citrullinuria E72.23
Civatte's disease or poikiloderma L57.3
Clam digger's itch B65.3
Clammy skin R23.1
Clap — *see* Gonorrhea
Clarke-Hadfield syndrome (pancreatic infantilism) K86.89
Clark's paralysis G80.9
Clastothrix L67.8
Claude Bernard-Horner syndrome G90.2
traumatic — *see* Injury, nerve, cervical sympathetic
Claude's disease or syndrome G46.3
Claudicatio venosa intermittens I87.8
Claudication (intermittent) I73.9
cerebral (artery) G45.9
spinal cord (arteriosclerotic) G95.19
syphilitic A52.09
venous (axillary) I87.8
Claustrophobia F40.240
Clavus (infected) L84
Clawfoot (congenital) Q66.89
acquired — *see* Deformity, limb, clawfoot
Clawhand (acquired) — *see also* Deformity, limb, clawhand
congenital Q68.1
Clawtoe (congenital) Q66.89
acquired — *see* Deformity, toe, specified NEC
Clay eating — *see* Pica
Cleansing of artificial opening — *see* Attention to, artificial, opening
Cleft (congenital) — *see also* Imperfect, closure
alveolar process M26.79
branchial (cyst) (persistent) Q18.2
cricoid cartilage, posterior Q31.8
foot Q72.7
hand Q71.6
lip (unilateral) Q36.9
with cleft palate Q37.9
hard Q37.1
with soft Q37.5
soft Q37.3
with hard Q37.5
bilateral Q36.0
with cleft palate Q37.8
hard Q37.1
with soft Q37.4
soft Q37.2
with hard Q37.4
median Q36.1
nose Q30.2
palate Q35.9
with cleft lip (unilateral) Q37.9
bilateral Q37.8
hard Q35.1
with
cleft lip (unilateral) Q37.1
bilateral Q37.0
soft Q35.5
with cleft lip (unilateral) Q37.5
bilateral Q37.4
medial Q35.5
soft Q35.3
with
cleft lip (unilateral) Q37.3
bilateral Q37.2
hard Q35.5
with cleft lip (unilateral) Q37.5
bilateral Q37.4
penis Q55.69
scrotum Q55.29
thyroid cartilage Q31.8
uvula Q35.7
Cleidocranial dysostosis Q74.0
Cleptomania F63.2
Clicking hip (newborn) R29.4
Climacteric (female) — *see also* Menopause
arthritis (any site) NEC — *see* Arthritis, specified form NEC

Climacteric (female) - *continued*
depression (single episode) F32.89
recurrent episode F33.8
melancholia (single episode) F32.89
recurrent episode F33.8
male (symptoms) (syndrome) NEC N50.89
paranoid state F22
polyarthritis NEC — *see* Arthritis, specified form NEC
symptoms (female) N95.1
Clinical research investigation (clinical trial) (control subject) (normal comparison) (participant) Z00.6
Clitoris — *see* condition
Cloaca (persistent) Q43.7
Clonorchiasis, clonorchis infection (liver) B66.1
Clonus R25.8
Closed bite M26.29
Clostridium (C.)
perfringens, as cause of disease classified elsewhere B96.7
Closure
congenital, nose Q30.0
cranial sutures, premature Q75.0
defective or imperfect NEC — *see* Imperfect, closure
fistula, delayed — *see* Fistula
foramen ovale, imperfect Q21.1
hymen N89.6
interauricular septum, defective Q21.1
interventricular septum, defective Q21.0
lacrimal duct — *see also* Stenosis, lacrimal, duct
congenital Q10.5
nose (congenital) Q30.0
acquired M95.0
of artificial opening — *see* Attention to, artificial, opening
primary angle, without glaucoma damage H40.06-
vagina N89.5
valve — *see* Endocarditis
vulva N90.5
Clot (blood) — *see also* Embolism
artery (obstruction) (occlusion) — *see* Embolism
bladder N32.89
brain (intradural or extradural) — *see* Occlusion, artery, cerebral
circulation I74.9
heart — *see also* Infarct, myocardium
not resulting in infarction I51.3
vein — *see* Thrombosis
Clouded state R40.1
epileptic — *see* Epilepsy, specified NEC
paroxysmal — *see* Epilepsy, specified NEC
Cloudy antrum, antra J32.0
Clouston's (hidrotic) ectodermal dysplasia Q82.4
Clubbed nail pachydermoperiostosis M89.40 *[L62]*
Clubbing of finger (s) (nails) R68.3
Clubfinger R68.3
congenital Q68.1
Clubfoot (congenital) Q66.89
acquired — *see* Deformity, limb, clubfoot
equinovarus Q66.0
paralytic — *see* Deformity, limb, clubfoot
Clubhand (congenital) (radial) Q71.4-
acquired — *see* Deformity, limb, clubhand
Clubnail R68.3
congenital Q84.6
Clump, kidney Q63.1
Clumsiness, clumsy child syndrome F82
Cluttering F80.81
Clutton's joints A50.51 *[M12.80]*
Coagulation, intravascular (diffuse) (disseminated) — *see also* Defibrination syndrome
complicating abortion — *see* Abortion, by type, complicated by, intravascular coagulation
following ectopic or molar pregnancy O08.1
Coagulopathy — *see also* Defect, coagulation
consumption D65
intravascular D65
newborn P60
Coalition
calcaneo-scaphoid Q66.89
tarsal Q66.89
Coalminer's
elbow — *see* Bursitis, elbow, olecranon
lung or pneumoconiosis J60
Coalworker's lung or pneumoconiosis J60
Coarctation
aorta (preductal) (postductal) Q25.1
pulmonary artery Q25.71
Coated tongue K14.3
Coats' disease (exudative retinopathy) — *see* Retinopathy, exudative

Cocaine-induced
anxiety disorder F14.980
bipolar and related disorder F14.94
depressive disorder F14.94
obsessive-compulsive and related disorder F14.988
psychotic disorder F14.959
sleep disorder F14.982
sexual dysfunction F14.981
Cocainism — *see* Disorder, cocaine use
Coccidioidomycosis B38.9
cutaneous B38.3
disseminated B38.7
generalized B38.7
meninges B38.4
prostate B38.81
pulmonary B38.2
acute B38.0
chronic B38.1
skin B38.3
specified NEC B38.89
Coccidioidosis — *see* Coccidioidomycosis
Coccidiosis (intestinal) A07.3
Coccydynia, coccygodynia M53.3
Coccyx — *see* condition
Cochin-China diarrhea K90.1
Cockayne's syndrome Q87.1
Cocked up toe — *see* Deformity, toe, specified NEC
Cock's peculiar tumor L72.3
Codman's tumor — *see* Neoplasm, bone, benign
Coenurosis B71.8
Coffee-worker's lung J67.8
Cogan's syndrome H16.32-
oculomotor apraxia H51.8
Coitus, painful (female) N94.10
male N53.12
psychogenic F52.6
Cold J00
with influenza, flu, or grippe — *see* Influenza, with, respiratory manifestations NEC
agglutinin disease or hemoglobinuria (chronic) D59.1
bronchial — *see* Bronchitis
chest — *see* Bronchitis
common (head) J00
effects of T69.9
specified effect NEC T69.8
excessive, effects of T69.9
specified effect NEC T69.8
exhaustion from T69.8
exposure to T69.9
specified effect NEC T69.8
head J00
injury syndrome (newborn) P80.0
on lung — *see* Bronchitis
rose J30.1
sensitivity, auto-immune D59.1
virus J00
Coldsore B00.1
Colibacillosis A49.8
as the cause of other disease — *see also* Escherichia coli B96.20
generalized A41.50
Colic (bilious) (infantile) (intestinal) (recurrent) (spasmodic) R10.83
abdomen R10.83
psychogenic F45.8
appendix, appendicular K38.8
bile duct — *see* Calculus, bile duct
biliary — *see* Calculus, bile duct
common duct — *see* Calculus, bile duct
cystic duct — *see* Calculus, gallbladder
Devonshire NEC — *see* Poisoning, lead
gallbladder — *see* Calculus, gallbladder
gallstone — *see* Calculus, gallbladder
gallbladder or cystic duct — *see* Calculus, gallbladder
hepatic (duct) — *see* Calculus, bile duct
hysterical F45.8
kidney N23
lead NEC — *see* Poisoning, lead
mucous K58.9
with diarrhea K58.0
psychogenic F54
nephritic N23
painter's NEC — *see* Poisoning, lead
pancreas K86.89
psychogenic F45.8
renal N23
saturnine NEC — *see* Poisoning, lead
ureter N23
urethral N36.8
due to calculus N21.1
uterus NEC N94.89

Colic (bilious) (infantile) (intestinal) (recurrent) (spasmodic) - *continued*
uterus NEC - *continued*
menstrual — *see* Dysmenorrhea
worm NOS B83.9
Colicystitis — *see* Cystitis
Colitis (acute) (catarrhal) (chronic) (noninfective) (hemorrhagic) — *see also* Enteritis K52.9
allergic K52.29
with
food protein-induced enterocolitis syndrome K52.21
proctocolitis K52.82
amebic (acute) — *see also* Amebiasis A06.0
nondysenteric A06.2
anthrax A22.2
bacillary — *see* Infection, Shigella
balantidial A07.0
Clostridium difficile A04.7
coccidial A07.3
collagenous K52.831
cystica superficialis K52.89
dietary counseling and surveillance (for) Z71.3
dietetic — *see also* Colitis, allergic K52.29
drug-induced K52.1
due to radiation K52.0
eosinophilic K52.82
food hypersensitivity — *see also* Colitis, allergic K52.29
giardial A07.1
granulomatous — *see* Enteritis, regional, large intestine
indeterminate, so stated K52.3
infectious — *see* Enteritis, infectious
ischemic K55.9
acute (subacute) — *see also* Ischemia, intestine, acute K55.039
chronic K55.1
due to mesenteric artery insufficiency K55.1
fulminant (acute) — *see also* Ischemia, intestine, acute K55.039
left sided K51.50
with
abscess K51.514
complication K51.519
specified NEC K51.518
fistula K51.513
obstruction K51.512
rectal bleeding K51.511
lymphocytic K52.832
membranous
psychogenic F54
microscopic K52.839
specified NEC K52.838
mucous — *see* Syndrome, irritable, bowel
psychogenic F54
noninfective K52.9
specified NEC K52.89
polyposa — *see* Polyp, colon, inflammatory
protozoal A07.9
pseudomembranous A04.7
pseudomucinous — *see* Syndrome, irritable, bowel
regional — *see* Enteritis, regional, large intestine
segmental — *see* Enteritis, regional, large intestine
septic — *see* Enteritis, infectious
spastic K58.9
with diarrhea K58.0
psychogenic F54
staphylococcal A04.8
foodborne A05.0
subacute ischemic — *see also* Ischemia, intestine, acute K55.039
thromboulcerative — *see also* Ischemia, intestine, acute K55.039
toxic NEC K52.1
due to Clostridium difficile A04.7
transmural — *see* Enteritis, regional, large intestine
trichomonal A07.8
tuberculous (ulcerative) A18.32
ulcerative (chronic) K51.90
with
complication K51.919
abscess K51.914
fistula K51.913
obstruction K51.912
rectal bleeding K51.911
specified complication NEC K51.918
enterocolitis — *see* Enterocolitis, ulcerative
ileocolitis — *see* Ileocolitis, ulcerative
mucosal proctocolitis — *see* Proctocolitis, mucosal
proctitis — *see* Proctitis, ulcerative
pseudopolyposis — *see* Polyp, colon, inflammatory

Colitis (acute) (catarrhal) (chronic) (noninfective) (hemorrhagic) - *continued*
ulcerative (chronic) - *continued*
psychogenic F54
rectosigmoiditis — *see* Rectosigmoiditis, ulcerative
specified type NEC K51.80
with
complication K51.819
abscess K51.814
fistula K51.813
obstruction K51.812
rectal bleeding K51.811
specified complication NEC K51.818
Collagenosis, collagen disease (nonvascular) (vascular) M35.9
cardiovascular I42.8
reactive perforating L87.1
specified NEC M35.8
Collapse R55
adrenal E27.2
cardiorespiratory R57.0
cardiovascular R57.0
newborn P29.89
circulatory (peripheral) R57.9
during or after labor and delivery O75.1
following ectopic or molar pregnancy O08.3
newborn P29.89
during or
after labor and delivery O75.1
resulting from a procedure, not elsewhere classified T81.10
external ear canal — *see* Stenosis, external ear canal
general R55
heart — *see* Disease, heart
heat T67.1
hysterical F44.89
labyrinth, membranous (congenital) Q16.5
lung (massive) — *see also* Atelectasis J98.19
pressure due to anesthesia (general) (local) or other sedation T88.2
during labor and delivery O74.1
in pregnancy O29.02-
postpartum, puerperal O89.09
myocardial — *see* Disease, heart
nervous F48.8
neurocirculatory F45.8
nose M95.0
postoperative T81.10
pulmonary — *see also* Atelectasis J98.19
newborn — *see* Atelectasis
trachea J39.8
tracheobronchial J98.09
valvular — *see* Endocarditis
vascular (peripheral) R57.9
during or after labor and delivery O75.1
following ectopic or molar pregnancy O08.3
newborn P29.89
vertebra M48.50-
cervical region M48.52-
cervicothoracic region M48.53-
in (due to)
metastasis — *see* Collapse, vertebra, in, specified disease NEC
osteoporosis — *see also* Osteoporosis M80.88
cervical region M80.88
cervicothoracic region M80.88
lumbar region M80.88
lumbosacral region M80.88
multiple sites M80.88
occipito-atlanto-axial region M80.88
sacrococcygeal region M80.88
thoracic region M80.88
thoracolumbar region M80.88
specified disease NEC M48.50-
cervical region M48.52-
cervicothoracic region M48.53-
lumbar region M48.56-
lumbosacral region M48.57-
occipito-atlanto-axial region M48.51-
sacrococcygeal region M48.58-
thoracic region M48.54-
thoracolumbar region M48.55-
lumbar region M48.56-
lumbosacral region M48.57-
occipito-atlanto-axial region M48.51-
sacrococcygeal region M48.58-
thoracic region M48.54-
thoracolumbar region M48.55-
Collateral — *see also* condition
circulation (venous) I87.8
dilation, veins I87.8
Colles' fracture S52.53-

Collet (-Sicard) **syndrome** G52.7
Collier's asthma or lung J60
Collodion baby Q80.2
Colloid nodule (of thyroid) (cystic) E04.1
Coloboma (iris) Q13.0
  eyelid Q10.3
  fundus Q14.8
  lens Q12.2
  optic disc (congenital) Q14.2
    acquired H47.31-
Coloenteritis — *see* Enteritis
Colon — *see* condition
Colonization
  MRSA (Methicillin resistant Staphylococcus
    aureus) Z22.322
  MSSA (Methicillin susceptible Staphylococcus
    aureus) Z22.321
  status — *see* Carrier (suspected) of
Coloptosis K63.4
Color blindness — *see* Deficiency, color vision
Colostomy
  attention to Z43.3
  fitting or adjustment Z46.89
  malfunctioning K94.03
  status Z93.3
Colpitis (acute) — *see* Vaginitis
Colpocele N81.5
Colpocystitis — *see* Vaginitis
Colpospasm N94.2
Column, spinal, vertebral — *see* condition
Coma R40.20
  with
    motor response (none) R40.231
      abnormal R40.233
      extension R40.232
      flexion withdrawal R40.234
      localizes pain R40.235
      obeys commands R40.236
    opening of eyes (never) R40.211
      in response to
        pain R40.212
        sound R40.213
      spontaneous R40.214
    verbal response (none) R40.221
      confused conversation R40.224
      inappropriate words R40.223
      incomprehensible words R40.222
      oriented R40.225
  eclamptic — *see* Eclampsia
  epileptic — *see* Epilepsy
  Glasgow, scale score — *see* Glasgow coma scale
  hepatic — *see* Failure, hepatic, by type, with coma
  hyperglycemic (diabetic) — *see* Diabetes, by type,
    with hyperosmolarity, with coma
  hyperosmolar (diabetic) — *see* Diabetes, by type,
    with hyperosmolarity, with coma
  hypoglycemic (diabetic) — *see* Diabetes, by type,
    with hypoglycemia, with coma
    nondiabetic E15
  in diabetes — *see* Diabetes, coma
  insulin-induced — *see* Coma, hypoglycemic
  myxedematous E03.5
  newborn P91.5
  persistent vegetative state R40.3
  specified NEC, without documented Glasgow coma
    scale score, or with partial Glasgow coma scale
    score reported R40.244
Comatose — *see* Coma
Combat fatigue F43.0
Combined — *see* condition
Comedo, comedones (giant) L70.0
Comedocarcinoma — *see also* Neoplasm, breast,
  malignant
  noninfiltrating
    breast D05.8-
    specified site — *see* Neoplasm, in situ, by site
    unspecified site D05.8-
Comedomastitis — *see* Ectasia, mammary duct
Comminuted fracture - code as Fracture, closed
Common
  arterial trunk Q20.0
  atrioventricular canal Q21.2
  atrium Q21.1
  cold (head) J00
  truncus (arteriosus) Q20.0
  variable immunodeficiency — *see*
    Immunodeficiency, common variable
  ventricle Q20.4
Commotio, commotion (current)
  brain — *see* Injury, intracranial, concussion
  cerebri — *see* Injury, intracranial, concussion
  retinae S05.8X-
  spinal cord — *see* Injury, spinal cord, by region

Commotio, commotion (current) - *continued*
  spinalis — *see* Injury, spinal cord, by region
Communication
  between
    base of aorta and pulmonary artery Q21.4
    left ventricle and right atrium Q20.5
    pericardial sac and pleural sac Q34.8
    pulmonary artery and pulmonary vein,
      congenital Q25.72
  congenital between uterus and digestive or urinary
    tract Q51.7
Compartment syndrome (deep) (posterior)
  (traumatic) T79.A0
  abdomen T79.A3
  lower extremity (hip, buttock, thigh, leg, foot,
    toes) T79.A2
  nontraumatic
    abdomen M79.A3
    lower extremity (hip, buttock, thigh, leg, foot,
      toes) M79.A2-
    specified site NEC M79.A9
    upper extremity (shoulder, arm, forearm, wrist,
      hand, fingers) M79.A1-
  specified site NEC T79.A9
  upper extremity (shoulder, arm, forearm, wrist, hand,
    fingers) T79.A1
Compensation
  failure — *see* Disease, heart
  neurosis, psychoneurosis — *see* Disorder, factitious
Complaint — *see also* Disease
  bowel, functional K59.9
    psychogenic F45.8
  intestine, functional K59.9
    psychogenic F45.8
  kidney — *see* Disease, renal
  miners' J60
Complete — *see* condition
Complex
  Addison-Schilder E71.528
  cardiorenal — *see* Hypertension, cardiorenal
  Costen's M26.69
  disseminated mycobacterium avium- intracellulare
    (DMAC) A31.2
  Eisenmenger's (ventricular septal defect) I27.89
  hypersexual F52.8
  jumped process, spine — *see* Dislocation, vertebra
  primary, tuberculous A15.7
  Schilder-Addison E71.528
  subluxation (vertebral) M99.19
    abdomen M99.19
    acromioclavicular M99.17
    cervical region M99.11
    cervicothoracic M99.11
    costochondral M99.18
    costovertebral M99.18
    head region M99.10
    hip M99.15
    lower extremity M99.16
    lumbar region M99.13
    lumbosacral M99.13
    occipitocervical M99.10
    pelvic region M99.15
    pubic M99.15
    rib cage M99.18
    sacral region M99.14
    sacrococcygeal M99.14
    sacroiliac M99.14
    specified NEC M99.19
    sternochondral M99.18
    sternoclavicular M99.17
    thoracic region M99.12
    thoracolumbar M99.12
    upper extremity M99.17
  Taussig-Bing (transposition, aorta and overriding
    pulmonary artery) Q20.1
Complication (s) (from) (of)
  accidental puncture or laceration during a procedure
    (of) — *see* Complications, intraoperative
    (intraprocedural), puncture or laceration
  amputation stump (surgical) (late) NEC T87.9
    dehiscence T87.81
    infection or inflammation T87.40
      lower limb T87.4-
      upper limb T87.4-
    necrosis T87.50
      lower limb T87.5-
      upper limb T87.5-
    neuroma T87.30
      lower limb T87.3-
      upper limb T87.3-
    specified type NEC T87.89
  anastomosis (and bypass) — *see also* Complications,
    prosthetic device or implant

Complication (s) (from) (of) - *continued*
  anastomosis (and bypass) - *continued*
    intestinal (internal) NEC K91.89
      involving urinary tract N99.89
    urinary tract (involving intestinal tract) N99.89
    vascular — *see* Complications, cardiovascular
      device or implant
  anesthesia, anesthetic — *see also* Anesthesia,
    complication T88.59
    brain, postpartum, puerperal O89.2
    cardiac
      in
        labor and delivery O74.2
        pregnancy O29.19-
      postpartum, puerperal O89.1
    central nervous system
      in
        labor and delivery O74.3
        pregnancy O29.29-
      postpartum, puerperal O89.2
    difficult or failed intubation T88.4
      in pregnancy O29.6-
    failed sedation (conscious) (moderate) during
      procedure T88.52
    general, unintended awareness during
      procedure T88.53
    hyperthermia, malignant T88.3
    hypothermia T88.51
    intubation failure T88.4
    malignant hyperthermia T88.3
    pulmonary
      in
        labor and delivery O74.1
        pregnancy NEC O29.09-
      postpartum, puerperal O89.09
    shock T88.2
    spinal and epidural
      in
        labor and delivery NEC O74.6
          headache O74.5
        pregnancy NEC O29.5X-
      postpartum, puerperal NEC O89.5
        headache O89.4
    unintended awareness under general anesthesia
      during procedure T88.53
  anti-reflux device — *see* Complications, esophageal
    anti-reflux device
  aortic (bifurcation) graft — *see* Complications, graft,
    vascular
  aortocoronary (bypass) graft — *see* Complications,
    coronary artery (bypass) graft
  aortofemoral (bypass) graft — *see* Complications,
    extremity artery (bypass) graft
  arteriovenous
    fistula, surgically created T82.9
      embolism T82.818
      fibrosis T82.828
      hemorrhage T82.838
      infection or inflammation T82.7
      mechanical
        breakdown T82.510
        displacement T82.520
        leakage T82.530
        malposition T82.520
        obstruction T82.590
        perforation T82.590
        protrusion T82.590
      pain T82.848
      specified type NEC T82.898
      stenosis T82.858
      thrombosis T82.868
    shunt, surgically created T82.9
      embolism T82.818
      fibrosis T82.828
      hemorrhage T82.838
      infection or inflammation T82.7
      mechanical
        breakdown T82.511
        displacement T82.521
        leakage T82.531
        malposition T82.521
        obstruction T82.591
        perforation T82.591
        protrusion T82.591
      pain T82.848
      specified type NEC T82.898
      stenosis T82.858
      thrombosis T82.868
  arthroplasty — *see* Complications, joint prosthesis
  artificial
    fertilization or insemination N98.9
      attempted introduction (of)
        embryo in embryo transfer N98.3

Complication (s) (from) (of) - *continued*
  artificial - *continued*
    fertilization or insemination - *continued*
      attempted introduction (of) - *continued*
        ovum following in vitro fertilization N98.2
      hyperstimulation of ovaries N98.1
      infection N98.0
      specified NEC N98.8
    heart T82.9
      embolism T82.817
      fibrosis T82.827
      hemorrhage T82.837
      infection or inflammation T82.7
      mechanical
        breakdown T82.512
        displacement T82.522
        leakage T82.532
        malposition T82.522
        obstruction T82.592
        perforation T82.592
        protrusion T82.592
      pain T82.847
      specified type NEC T82.897
      stenosis T82.857
      thrombosis T82.867
    opening
      cecostomy — *see* Complications, colostomy
      colostomy — *see* Complications, colostomy
      cystostomy — *see* Complications, cystostomy
      enterostomy — *see* Complications, enterostomy
      gastrostomy — *see* Complications, gastrostomy
      ileostomy — *see* Complications, enterostomy
      jejunostomy — *see* Complications, enterostomy
      nephrostomy — *see* Complications, stoma, urinary tract
      tracheostomy — *see* Complications, tracheostomy
      ureterostomy — *see* Complications, stoma, urinary tract
      urethrostomy — *see* Complications, stoma, urinary tract
  balloon implant or device
    gastrointestinal T85.9
      embolism T85.818
      fibrosis T85.828
      hemorrhage T85.838
      infection and inflammation T85.79
      pain T85.848
      specified type NEC T85.898
      stenosis T85.858
      thrombosis T85.868
    vascular (counterpulsation) T82.9
      embolism T82.818
      fibrosis T82.828
      hemorrhage T82.838
      infection or inflammation T82.7
      mechanical
        breakdown T82.513
        displacement T82.523
        leakage T82.533
        malposition T82.523
        obstruction T82.593
        perforation T82.593
        protrusion T82.593
      pain T82.848
      specified type NEC T82.898
      stenosis T82.858
      thrombosis T82.868
  bariatric procedure
    gastric band procedure K95.09
      infection K95.01
    specified procedure NEC K95.89
      infection K95.81
  bile duct implant (prosthetic) T85.9
    embolism T85.818
    fibrosis T85.828
    hemorrhage T85.838
    infection and inflammation T85.79
    mechanical
      breakdown T85.510
      displacement T85.520
      malfunction T85.510
      malposition T85.520
      obstruction T85.590
      perforation T85.590
      protrusion T85.590
      specified NEC T85.590
    pain T85.848
    specified type NEC T85.898
    stenosis T85.858
    thrombosis T85.868
  bladder device (auxiliary) — *see* Complications, genitourinary, device or implant, urinary system

Complication (s) (from) (of) - *continued*
  bleeding (postoperative) — *see* Complication, postoperative, hemorrhage
    intraoperative — *see* Complication, intraoperative, hemorrhage
  blood vessel graft — *see* Complications, graft, vascular
  bone
    device NEC T84.9
      embolism T84.81
      fibrosis T84.82
      hemorrhage T84.83
      infection or inflammation T84.7
      mechanical
        breakdown T84.318
        displacement T84.328
        malposition T84.328
        obstruction T84.398
        perforation T84.398
        protrusion T84.398
      pain T84.84
      specified type NEC T84.89
      stenosis T84.85
      thrombosis T84.86
    graft — *see* Complications, graft, bone
    growth stimulator (electrode) — *see* Complications, electronic stimulator device, bone
    marrow transplant — *see* Complications, transplant, bone, marrow
  brain neurostimulator (electrode) — *see* Complications, electronic stimulator device, brain
  breast implant (prosthetic) T85.9
    capsular contracture T85.44
    embolism T85.818
    fibrosis T85.828
    hemorrhage T85.838
    infection and inflammation T85.79
    mechanical
      breakdown T85.41
      displacement T85.42
      leakage T85.43
      malposition T85.42
      obstruction T85.49
      perforation T85.49
      protrusion T85.49
      specified NEC T85.49
    pain T85.848
    specified type NEC T85.898
    stenosis T85.858
    thrombosis T85.868
  bypass — *see also* Complications, prosthetic device or implant
    aortocoronary — *see* Complications, coronary artery (bypass) graft
    arterial — *see also* Complications, graft, vascular
      extremity — *see* Complications, extremity artery (bypass) graft
  cardiac — *see also* Disease, heart
    device, implant or graft T82.9
      embolism T82.817
      fibrosis T82.827
      hemorrhage T82.837
      infection or inflammation T82.7
        valve prosthesis T82.6
      mechanical
        breakdown T82.519
          specified device NEC T82.518
        displacement T82.529
          specified device NEC T82.528
        leakage T82.539
          specified device NEC T82.538
        malposition T82.529
          specified device NEC T82.528
        obstruction T82.599
          specified device NEC T82.598
        perforation T82.599
          specified device NEC T82.598
        protrusion T82.599
          specified device NEC T82.598
      pain T82.847
      specified type NEC T82.897
      stenosis T82.857
      thrombosis T82.867
  cardiovascular device, graft or implant T82.9
    aortic graft — *see* Complications, graft, vascular
    arteriovenous
      fistula, artificial — *see* Complication, arteriovenous, fistula, surgically created
      shunt — *see* Complication, arteriovenous, shunt, surgically created
    artificial heart — *see* Complication, artificial, heart
    balloon (counterpulsation) device — *see* Complication, balloon implant, vascular

Complication (s) (from) (of) - *continued*
  cardiovascular device, graft or implant - *continued*
    carotid artery graft — *see* Complications, graft, vascular
    coronary bypass graft — *see* Complication, coronary artery (bypass) graft
    dialysis catheter (vascular) — *see* Complication, catheter, dialysis
    electronic T82.9
      electrode T82.9
        embolism T82.817
        fibrosis T82.827
        hemorrhage T82.837
        infection T82.7
        mechanical
          breakdown T82.110
          displacement T82.120
          leakage T82.190
          obstruction T82.190
          perforation T82.190
          protrusion T82.190
          specified type NEC T82.190
        pain T82.847
        specified NEC T82.897
        stenosis T82.857
        thrombosis T82.867
      embolism T82.817
      fibrosis T82.827
      hemorrhage T82.837
      infection T82.7
      mechanical
        breakdown T82.119
        displacement T82.129
        leakage T82.199
        obstruction T82.199
        perforation T82.199
        protrusion T82.199
        specified type NEC T82.199
      pain T82.847
      pulse generator T82.9
        embolism T82.817
        fibrosis T82.827
        hemorrhage T82.837
        infection T82.7
        mechanical
          breakdown T82.111
          displacement T82.121
          leakage T82.191
          obstruction T82.191
          perforation T82.191
          protrusion T82.191
          specified type NEC T82.191
        pain T82.847
        specified NEC T82.897
        stenosis T82.857
        thrombosis T82.867
      specified condition NEC T82.897
      specified device NEC T82.9
        embolism T82.817
        fibrosis T82.827
        hemorrhage T82.837
        infection T82.7
        mechanical
          breakdown T82.118
          displacement T82.128
          leakage T82.198
          obstruction T82.198
          perforation T82.198
          protrusion T82.198
          specified type NEC T82.198
        pain T82.847
        specified NEC T82.897
        stenosis T82.857
        thrombosis T82.867
      stenosis T82.857
      thrombosis T82.867
    extremity artery graft — *see* Complication, extremity artery (bypass) graft
    femoral artery graft — *see* Complication, extremity artery (bypass) graft
    heart-lung transplant — *see* Complication, transplant, heart, with lung
    heart
      transplant — *see* Complication, transplant, heart
      valve — *see* Complication, prosthetic device, heart valve
        graft — *see* Complication, heart, valve, graft
    infection or inflammation T82.7
    umbrella device — *see* Complication, umbrella device, vascular
    vascular graft (or anastomosis) — *see* Complication, graft, vascular

Complication (s) (from) (of) - *continued*
 carotid artery (bypass) graft — *see* Complications,
  graft, vascular
 catheter (device) NEC — *see also* Complications,
  prosthetic device or implant
  cranial infusion
   infection and inflammation T85.735
   mechanical
    breakdown T85.610
    displacement T85.620
    leakage T85.630
    malfunction T85.690
    malposition T85.620
    obstruction T85.690
    perforation T85.690
    protrusion T85.690
    specified NEC T85.690
  cystostomy T83.9
   embolism T83.81
   fibrosis T83.82
   hemorrhage T83.83
   infection and inflammation T83.510
   mechanical
    breakdown T83.010
    displacement T83.020
    leakage T83.030
    malposition T83.020
    obstruction T83.090
    perforation T83.090
    protrusion T83.090
    specified NEC T83.090
   pain T83.84
   specified type NEC T83.89
   stenosis T83.85
   thrombosis T83.86
  dialysis (vascular) T82.9
   embolism T82.818
   fibrosis T82.828
   hemorrhage T82.838
   infection and inflammation T82.7
   intraperitoneal — *see* Complications, catheter,
    intraperitoneal
   mechanical
    breakdown T82.41
    displacement T82.42
    leakage T82.43
    malposition T82.42
    obstruction T82.49
    perforation T82.49
    protrusion T82.49
   pain T82.848
   specified type NEC T82.898
   stenosis T82.858
   thrombosis T82.868
  epidural infusion T85.9
   embolism T85.810
   fibrosis T85.820
   hemorrhage T85.830
   infection and inflammation T85.735
   mechanical
    breakdown T85.610
    displacement T85.620
    leakage T85.630
    malfunction T85.610
    malposition T85.620
    obstruction T85.690
    perforation T85.690
    protrusion T85.690
    specified NEC T85.690
   pain T85.840
   specified type NEC T85.890
   stenosis T85.850
   thrombosis T85.860
  intraperitoneal dialysis T85.9
   embolism T85.818
   fibrosis T85.828
   hemorrhage T85.838
   infection and inflammation T85.71
   mechanical
    breakdown T85.611
    displacement T85.621
    leakage T85.631
    malfunction T85.611
    malposition T85.621
    obstruction T85.691
    perforation T85.691
    protrusion T85.691
    specified NEC T85.691
   pain T85.848
   specified type NEC T85.898
   stenosis T85.858
   thrombosis T85.868
  intrathecal infusion

Complication (s) (from) (of) - *continued*
 catheter (device) NEC
  intrathecal infusion - *continued*
   infection and inflammation T85.735
   mechanical
    breakdown T85.610
    displacement T85.620
    leakage T85.630
    malfunction T85.690
    malposition T85.620
    obstruction T85.690
    perforation T85.690
    protrusion T85.690
    specified NEC T85.690
  intravenous infusion T82.9
   embolism T82.818
   fibrosis T82.828
   hemorrhage T82.838
   infection or inflammation T82.7
   mechanical
    breakdown T82.514
    displacement T82.524
    leakage T82.534
    malposition T82.524
    obstruction T82.594
    perforation T82.594
    protrusion T82.594
   pain T82.848
   specified type NEC T82.898
   stenosis T82.858
   thrombosis T82.868
  spinal infusion
   infection and inflammation T85.735
   mechanical
    breakdown T85.610
    displacement T85.620
    leakage T85.630
    malfunction T85.690
    malposition T85.620
    obstruction T85.690
    perforation T85.690
    protrusion T85.690
    specified NEC T85.690
  subarachnoid infusion
   infection and inflammation T85.735
   mechanical
    breakdown T85.610
    displacement T85.620
    leakage T85.630
    malfunction T85.690
    malposition T85.620
    obstruction T85.690
    perforation T85.690
    protrusion T85.690
    specified NEC T85.690
  subdural infusion T85.9
   embolism T85.810
   fibrosis T85.820
   hemorrhage T85.830
   infection and inflammation T85.735
   mechanical
    breakdown T85.610
    displacement T85.620
    leakage T85.630
    malfunction T85.610
    malposition T85.620
    obstruction T85.690
    perforation T85.690
    protrusion T85.690
    specified NEC T85.690
   pain T85.840
   specified type NEC T85.890
   stenosis T85.850
   thrombosis T85.860
  urethral T83.9
   displacement T83.028
   embolism T83.81
   fibrosis T83.82
   hemorrhage T83.83
   indwelling
    breakdown T83.011
    displacement T83.021
    infection and inflammation T83.511
    leakage T83.031
    specified complication NEC T83.091
   infection and inflammation T83.511
   leakage T83.038
   malposition T83.028
   mechanical
    breakdown T83.011
   obstruction (mechanical) T83.091
   pain T83.84
   perforation T83.091

Complication (s) (from) (of) - *continued*
 catheter (device) NEC - *continued*
  urethral - *continued*
   protrusion T83.091
   specified type NEC T83.091
   stenosis T83.85
   thrombosis T83.86
  urinary NEC
   breakdown T83.018
   displacement T83.028
   infection and inflammation T83.518
   leakage T83.038
   specified complication NEC T83.098
 cecostomy (stoma) — *see* Complications, colostomy
 cesarean delivery wound NEC O90.89
  disruption O90.0
  hematoma O90.2
  infection (following delivery) O86.0
 chemotherapy (antineoplastic) NEC T88.7
 chin implant (prosthetic) — *see* Complication,
  prosthetic device or implant, specified NEC
 circulatory system I99.8
  intraoperative I97.88
  postprocedural I97.89
   following cardiac surgery I97.19-
    postcardiotomy syndrome I97.0
   hypertension I97.3
   lymphedema after mastectomy I97.2
   postcardiotomy syndrome I97.0
   specified NEC I97.89
 colostomy (stoma) K94.00
  hemorrhage K94.01
  infection K94.02
  malfunction K94.03
  mechanical K94.03
  specified complication NEC K94.09
 contraceptive device, intrauterine — *see*
  Complications, intrauterine, contraceptive device
 cord (umbilical) — *see* Complications, umbilical
  cord
 corneal graft — *see* Complications, graft, cornea
 coronary artery (bypass) graft T82.9
  atherosclerosis — *see* Arteriosclerosis, coronary
   (artery)
  embolism T82.818
  fibrosis T82.828
  hemorrhage T82.838
  infection and inflammation T82.7
  mechanical
   breakdown T82.211
   displacement T82.212
   leakage T82.213
   malposition T82.212
   obstruction T82.218
   perforation T82.218
   protrusion T82.218
   specified NEC T82.218
  pain T82.848
  specified type NEC T82.898
  stenosis T82.858
  thrombosis T82.868
 counterpulsation device (balloon) , intra-
  aortic — *see* Complications, balloon implant,
  vascular
 cystostomy (stoma) N99.518
  catheter — *see* Complications, catheter,
   cystostomy
  hemorrhage N99.510
  infection N99.511
  malfunction N99.512
  specified type NEC N99.518
 delivery — *see also* Complications, obstetric O75.9
  procedure (instrumental) (manual) (surgical) O75.4
  specified NEC O75.89
 dialysis (peritoneal) (renal) — *see*
  also Complications, infusion
  catheter (vascular) — *see* Complication, catheter,
   dialysis
  peritoneal, intraperitoneal — *see* Complications,
   catheter, intraperitoneal
 dorsal column (spinal) neurostimulator — *see*
  Complications, electronic stimulator device, spinal
  cord
 drug NEC T88.7
 ear procedure — *see also* Disorder, ear
  intraoperative H95.88
   hematoma — *see* Complications, intraoperative,
    hemorrhage (hematoma) (of), ear
   hemorrhage — *see* Complications, intraoperative,
    hemorrhage (hematoma) (of), ear
   laceration — *see* Complications, intraoperative,
    puncture or laceration..., ear
   specified NEC H95.88

Complication (s) (from) (of) - *continued*
ear procedure - *continued*
postoperative H95.89
external ear canal stenosis H95.81-
hematoma — *see* Complications, postprocedural, hematoma (of), ear
hemorrhage — *see* Complications, postprocedural, hemorrhage (of), ear
postmastoidectomy — *see* Complications, postmastoidectomy
seroma — *see* Complications, postprocedural, seroma (of), mastoid process
specified NEC H95.89
ectopic pregnancy O08.9
damage to pelvic organs O08.6
embolism O08.2
genital infection O08.0
hemorrhage (delayed) (excessive) O08.1
metabolic disorder O08.5
renal failure O08.4
shock O08.3
specified type NEC O08.0
venous complication NEC O08.7
electronic stimulator device
bladder (urinary) — *see* Complications, electronic stimulator device, urinary
bone T84.9
breakdown T84.310
displacement T84.320
embolism T84.81
fibrosis T84.82
hemorrhage T84.83
infection or inflammation T84.7
malfunction T84.310
malposition T84.320
mechanical NEC T84.390
obstruction T84.390
pain T84.84
perforation T84.390
protrusion T84.390
specified type NEC T84.89
stenosis T84.85
thrombosis T84.86
brain T85.9
embolism T85.810
fibrosis T85.820
hemorrhage T85.830
infection and inflammation T85.731
mechanical
breakdown T85.110
displacement T85.120
leakage T85.190
malposition T85.120
obstruction T85.190
perforation T85.190
protrusion T85.190
specified NEC T85.190
pain T85.840
specified type NEC T85.890
stenosis T85.850
thrombosis T85.860
cardiac (defibrillator) (pacemaker) — *see* Complications, cardiovascular device or implant, electronic
generator (brain) (gastric) (peripheral) (sacral) (spinal)
breakdown T85.113
displacement T85.123
leakage T85.193
malposition T85.123
obstruction T85.193
perforation T85.193
protrusion T85.193
specified type NEC T85.193
muscle T84.9
breakdown T84.418
displacement T84.428
embolism T84.81
fibrosis T84.82
hemorrhage T84.83
infection or inflammation T84.7
mechanical NEC T84.498
pain T84.84
specified type NEC T84.89
stenosis T84.85
thrombosis T84.86
nervous system T85.9
brain — *see* Complications, electronic stimulator device, brain
cranial nerve — *see* Complications, electronic stimulator device, peripheral nerve
embolism T85.810
fibrosis T85.820

Complication (s) (from) (of) - *continued*
electronic stimulator device - *continued*
nervous system - *continued*
gastric nerve — *see* Complications, electronic stimulator device, peripheral nerve
hemorrhage T85.830
infection and inflammation T85.738
mechanical
breakdown T85.118
displacement T85.128
leakage T85.199
malposition T85.128
obstruction T85.199
perforation T85.199
protrusion T85.199
specified NEC T85.199
pain T85.840
peripheral nerve — *see* Complications, electronic stimulator device, peripheral nerve
sacral nerve — *see* Complications, electronic stimulator device, peripheral nerve
specified type NEC T85.890
spinal cord — *see* Complications, electronic stimulator device, spinal cord
stenosis T85.850
thrombosis T85.860
vagal nerve — *see* Complications, electronic stimulator device, peripheral nerve
peripheral nerve T85.9
embolism T85.810
fibrosis T85.820
hemorrhage T85.830
infection and inflammation T85.732
mechanical
breakdown T85.111
displacement T85.121
leakage T85.191
malposition T85.121
obstruction T85.191
perforation T85.191
protrusion T85.191
specified NEC T85.191
pain T85.840
specified type NEC T85.890
stenosis T85.850
thrombosis T85.860
spinal cord T85.9
embolism T85.810
fibrosis T85.820
hemorrhage T85.830
infection and inflammation T85.733
mechanical
breakdown T85.112
displacement T85.122
leakage T85.192
malposition T85.122
obstruction T85.192
perforation T85.192
protrusion T85.192
specified NEC T85.192
pain T85.840
specified type NEC T85.890
stenosis T85.850
thrombosis T85.860
urinary T83.9
embolism T83.81
fibrosis T83.82
hemorrhage T83.83
infection and inflammation T83.598
mechanical
breakdown T83.110
displacement T83.120
malposition T83.120
perforation T83.190
protrusion T83.190
specified NEC T83.190
pain T83.84
specified type NEC T83.89
stenosis T83.85
thrombosis T83.86
electroshock therapy T88.9
specified NEC T88.8
endocrine E34.9
postprocedural
adrenal hypofunction E89.6
hypoinsulinemia E89.1
hypoparathyroidism E89.2
hypopituitarism E89.3
hypothyroidism E89.0
ovarian failure E89.40
asymptomatic E89.40
symptomatic E89.41
specified NEC E89.89

Complication (s) (from) (of) - *continued*
endocrine - *continued*
postprocedural - *continued*
testicular hypofunction E89.5
endodontic treatment NEC M27.59
enterostomy (stoma) K94.10
hemorrhage K94.11
infection K94.12
malfunction K94.13
mechanical K94.13
specified complication NEC K94.19
episiotomy, disruption O90.1
esophageal anti-reflux device T85.9
embolism T85.818
fibrosis T85.828
hemorrhage T85.838
infection and inflammation T85.79
mechanical
breakdown T85.511
displacement T85.521
malfunction T85.511
malposition T85.521
obstruction T85.591
perforation T85.591
protrusion T85.591
specified NEC T85.591
pain T85.848
specified type NEC T85.898
stenosis T85.858
thrombosis T85.868
esophagostomy K94.30
hemorrhage K94.31
infection K94.32
malfunction K94.33
mechanical K94.33
specified complication NEC K94.39
extracorporeal circulation T80.90
extremity artery (bypass) graft T82.9
arteriosclerosis — *see* Arteriosclerosis, extremities, bypass graft
embolism T82.818
fibrosis T82.828
hemorrhage T82.838
infection and inflammation T82.7
mechanical
breakdown T82.318
femoral artery T82.312
displacement T82.328
femoral artery T82.322
leakage T82.338
femoral artery T82.332
malposition T82.328
femoral artery T82.322
obstruction T82.398
femoral artery T82.392
perforation T82.398
femoral artery T82.392
protrusion T82.398
femoral artery T82.392
pain T82.848
specified type NEC T82.898
stenosis T82.858
thrombosis T82.868
eye H57.9
corneal graft — *see* Complications, graft, cornea
implant (prosthetic) T85.9
embolism T85.818
fibrosis T85.828
hemorrhage T85.838
infection and inflammation T85.79
mechanical
breakdown T85.318
displacement T85.328
leakage T85.398
malposition T85.328
obstruction T85.398
perforation T85.398
protrusion T85.398
specified NEC T85.398
pain T85.848
specified type NEC T85.898
stenosis T85.858
thrombosis T85.868
intraocular lens — *see* Complications, intraocular lens
orbital prosthesis — *see* Complications, orbital prosthesis
female genital N94.9
device, implant or graft NEC — *see* Complications, genitourinary, device or implant, genital tract
femoral artery (bypass) graft — *see* Complication, extremity artery (bypass) graft

Complication (s) (from) (of) - *continued*
  fixation device, internal (orthopedic) T84.9
    infection and inflammation T84.60
      arm T84.61-
        humerus T84.61-
        radius T84.61-
        ulna T84.61-
      leg T84.629
        femur T84.62-
        fibula T84.62-
        tibia T84.62-
      specified site NEC T84.69
      spine T84.63
    mechanical
      breakdown
        limb T84.119
          carpal T84.210
          femur T84.11-
          fibula T84.11-
          humerus T84.11-
          metacarpal T84.210
          metatarsal T84.213
          phalanx
            foot T84.213
            hand T84.210
          radius T84.11-
          tarsal T84.213
          tibia T84.11-
          ulna T84.11-
        specified bone NEC T84.218
        spine T84.216
      displacement
        limb T84.129
          carpal T84.220
          femur T84.12-
          fibula T84.12-
          humerus T84.12-
          metacarpal T84.220
          metatarsal T84.223
          phalanx
            foot T84.223
            hand T84.220
          radius T84.12-
          tarsal T84.223
          tibia T84.12-
          ulna T84.12-
        specified bone NEC T84.228
        spine T84.226
      malposition — *see* Complications, fixation
        device, internal, mechanical, displacement
      obstruction — *see* Complications, fixation device,
        internal, mechanical, specified type NEC
      perforation — *see* Complications, fixation device,
        internal, mechanical, specified type NEC
      protrusion — *see* Complications, fixation device,
        internal, mechanical, specified type NEC
      specified type NEC
        limb T84.199
          carpal T84.290
          femur T84.19-
          fibula T84.19-
          humerus T84.19-
          metacarpal T84.290
          metatarsal T84.293
          phalanx
            foot T84.293
            hand T84.290
          radius T84.19-
          tarsal T84.293
          tibia T84.19-
          ulna T84.19-
        specified bone NEC T84.298
        vertebra T84.296
    specified type NEC T84.89
      embolism T84.81
      fibrosis T84.82
      hemorrhage T84.83
      pain T84.84
      specified complication NEC T84.89
      stenosis T84.85
      thrombosis T84.86
  following
    acute myocardial infarction NEC I23.8
      aneurysm (false) (of cardiac wall) (of heart wall)
        (ruptured) I23.3
      angina I23.7
      atrial
        septal defect I23.1
        thrombosis I23.6
      cardiac wall rupture I23.3
      chordae tendinae rupture I23.4
      defect
        septal

Complication (s) (from) (of) - *continued*
  following - *continued*
    acute myocardial infarction NEC - *continued*
      defect - *continued*
        septal - *continued*
          atrial (heart) I23.1
          ventricular (heart) I23.2
      hemopericardium I23.0
      papillary muscle rupture I23.5
      rupture
        cardiac wall I23.3
          with hemopericardium I23.0
        chordae tendineae I23.4
        papillary muscle I23.5
      specified NEC I23.8
      thrombosis
        atrium I23.6
        auricular appendage I23.6
        ventricle (heart) I23.6
      ventricular
        septal defect I23.2
        thrombosis I23.6
    ectopic or molar pregnancy O08.9
      cardiac arrest O08.81
      sepsis O08.82
      specified type NEC O08.89
      urinary tract infection O08.83
    termination of pregnancy — *see* Abortion
  gastrointestinal K92.9
    bile duct prosthesis — *see* Complications, bile duct
      implant
    esophageal anti-reflux device — *see*
      Complications, esophageal anti-reflux device
    postoperative
      colostomy — *see* Complications, colostomy
      dumping syndrome K91.1
      enterostomy — *see* Complications, enterostomy
      gastrostomy — *see* Complications, gastrostomy
      malabsorption NEC K91.2
      obstruction K91.3
      postcholecystectomy syndrome K91.5
      specified NEC K91.89
      vomiting after GI surgery K91.0
    prosthetic device or implant
      bile duct prosthesis — *see* Complications, bile
        duct implant
      esophageal anti-reflux device — *see*
        Complications, esophageal anti-reflux device
      specified type NEC
        embolism T85.818
        fibrosis T85.828
        hemorrhage T85.838
        mechanical
          breakdown T85.518
          displacement T85.528
          malfunction T85.518
          malposition T85.528
          obstruction T85.598
          perforation T85.598
          protrusion T85.598
          specified NEC T85.598
        pain T85.848
        specified complication NEC T85.898
        stenosis T85.858
        thrombosis T85.868
    gastrostomy (stoma) K94.20
      hemorrhage K94.21
      infection K94.22
      malfunction K94.23
      mechanical K94.23
      specified complication NEC K94.29
  genitourinary
    device or implant T83.9
      genital tract T83.9
        infection or inflammation T83.69
        intrauterine contraceptive device — *see*
          Complications, intrauterine, contraceptive
          device
        mechanical — *see* Complications, by device,
          mechanical
        mesh — *see* Complications, mesh
        penile prosthesis — *see* Complications,
          prosthetic device, penile
        specified type NEC T83.89
          embolism T83.81
          fibrosis T83.82
          hemorrhage T83.83
          pain T83.84
          specified complication NEC T83.89
          stenosis T83.85
          thrombosis T83.86
        vaginal mesh — *see* Complications, mesh
      urinary system T83.9

Complication (s) (from) (of) - *continued*
  genitourinary - *continued*
    device or implant - *continued*
      urinary system - *continued*
        cystostomy catheter — *see* Complication,
          catheter, cystostomy
        electronic stimulator — *see* Complications,
          electronic stimulator device, urinary
        indwelling urethral catheter — *see*
          Complications, catheter, urethral, indwelling
        infection or inflammation T83.598
          indwelling urethral catheter T83.511
        kidney transplant — *see* Complication,
          transplant, kidney
        organ graft — *see* Complication, graft, urinary
          organ
        specified type NEC T83.89
          embolism T83.81
          fibrosis T83.82
          hemorrhage T83.83
          mechanical T83.198
            breakdown T83.118
            displacement T83.128
            malfunction T83.118
            malposition T83.128
            obstruction T83.198
            perforation T83.198
            protrusion T83.198
            specified NEC T83.198
          sphincter, implanted T83.191
          stent (ileal conduit) (nephroureteral) T83.193
            ureteral indwelling T83.192
          pain T83.84
          specified complication NEC T83.89
          stenosis T83.85
          thrombosis T83.86
        sphincter implant — *see* Complications,
          implant, urinary sphincter
    postprocedural
      pelvic peritoneal adhesions N99.4
      renal failure N99.0
      specified NEC N99.89
      stoma — *see* Complications, stoma, urinary tract
      urethral stricture — *see* Stricture, urethra,
        postprocedural
      vaginal
        adhesions N99.2
        vault prolapse N99.3
  graft (bypass) (patch) — *see also* Complications,
    prosthetic device or implant
    aorta — *see* Complications, graft, vascular
    arterial — *see* Complication, graft, vascular
    bone T86.839
      failure T86.831
      infection T86.832
      mechanical T84.318
        breakdown T84.318
        displacement T84.328
        protrusion T84.398
        specified type NEC T84.398
      rejection T86.830
      specified type NEC T86.838
    carotid artery — *see* Complications, graft, vascular
    cornea T86.849
      failure T86.841
      infection T86.842
      mechanical T85.398
        breakdown T85.318
        displacement T85.328
        protrusion T85.398
        specified type NEC T85.398
      rejection T86.840
      retroprosthetic membrane T85.398
      specified type NEC T86.848
    femoral artery (bypass) — *see* Complication,
      extremity artery (bypass) graft
    genital organ or tract — *see* Complications,
      genitourinary, device or implant, genital tract
    muscle T84.9
      breakdown T84.410
      displacement T84.420
      embolism T84.81
      fibrosis T84.82
      hemorrhage T84.83
      infection and inflammation T84.7
      mechanical NEC T84.490
      pain T84.84
      specified type NEC T84.89
      stenosis T84.85
      thrombosis T84.86
    nerve — *see* Complication, prosthetic device or
      implant, specified NEC

Complication (s) (from) (of) - *continued*
  graft (bypass) (patch) - *continued*
    skin — *see* Complications, prosthetic device or
      implant, skin graft
    tendon T84.9
      breakdown T84.410
      displacement T84.420
      embolism T84.81
      fibrosis T84.82
      hemorrhage T84.83
      infection and inflammation T84.7
      mechanical NEC T84.490
      pain T84.84
      specified type NEC T84.89
      stenosis T84.85
      thrombosis T84.86
    urinary organ T83.9
      embolism T83.81
      fibrosis T83.82
      hemorrhage T83.83
      infection and inflammation T83.598
        indwelling urethral catheter T83.511
      mechanical
        breakdown T83.21
        displacement T83.22
        erosion T83.24
        exposure T83.25
        leakage T83.23
        malposition T83.22
        obstruction T83.29
        perforation T83.29
        protrusion T83.29
        specified NEC T83.29
      pain T83.84
      specified type NEC T83.89
      stenosis T83.85
      thrombosis T83.86
    vascular T82.9
      embolism T82.818
      femoral artery — *see* Complication, extremity
        artery (bypass) graft
      fibrosis T82.828
      hemorrhage T82.838
      mechanical
        breakdown T82.319
          aorta (bifurcation) T82.310
          carotid artery T82.311
          specified vessel NEC T82.318
        displacement T82.329
          aorta (bifurcation) T82.320
          carotid artery T82.321
          specified vessel NEC T82.328
        leakage T82.339
          aorta (bifurcation) T82.330
          carotid artery T82.331
          specified vessel NEC T82.338
        malposition T82.329
          aorta (bifurcation) T82.320
          carotid artery T82.321
          specified vessel NEC T82.328
        obstruction T82.399
          aorta (bifurcation) T82.390
          carotid artery T82.391
          specified vessel NEC T82.398
        perforation T82.399
          aorta (bifurcation) T82.390
          carotid artery T82.391
          specified vessel NEC T82.398
        protrusion T82.399
          aorta (bifurcation) T82.390
          carotid artery T82.391
          specified vessel NEC T82.398
      pain T82.848
      specified complication NEC T82.898
      stenosis T82.858
      thrombosis T82.868
  heart I51.9
    assist device
      infection and inflammation T82.7
    following acute myocardial infarction — *see*
      Complications, following, acute myocardial
      infarction
    postoperative — *see* Complications, circulatory
      system
    transplant — *see* Complication, transplant, heart
      and lung (s) — *see* Complications, transplant,
      heart, with lung
    valve
      graft (biological) T82.9
        embolism T82.817
        fibrosis T82.827
        hemorrhage T82.837
        infection and inflammation T82.7

Complication (s) (from) (of) - *continued*
  heart - *continued*
    valve - *continued*
      graft (biological) - *continued*
        mechanical T82.228
          breakdown T82.221
          displacement T82.222
          leakage T82.223
          malposition T82.222
          obstruction T82.228
          perforation T82.228
          protrusion T82.228
        pain T82.847
        specified type NEC T82.897
        stenosis T82.857
        thrombosis T82.867
      prosthesis T82.9
        embolism T82.817
        fibrosis T82.827
        hemorrhage T82.837
        infection or inflammation T82.6
        mechanical T82.09
          breakdown T82.01
          displacement T82.02
          leakage T82.03
          malposition T82.02
          obstruction T82.09
          perforation T82.09
          protrusion T82.09
        pain T82.847
        specified type NEC T82.897
          mechanical T82.09
        stenosis T82.857
        thrombosis T82.867
  hematoma
    intraoperative — *see* Complication, intraoperative,
      hemorrhage
    postprocedural — *see* Complication,
      postprocedural, hematoma
  hemodialysis — *see* Complications, dialysis
  hemorrhage
    intraoperative — *see* Complication, intraoperative,
      hemorrhage
    postprocedural — *see* Complication,
      postprocedural, hemorrhage
  ileostomy (stoma) — *see* Complications,
    enterostomy
  immunization (procedure) — *see* Complications,
    vaccination
  implant — *see also* Complications, by site and type
    urinary sphincter T83.9
      embolism T83.81
      fibrosis T83.82
      hemorrhage T83.83
      infection and inflammation T83.591
      mechanical
        breakdown T83.111
        displacement T83.121
        leakage T83.191
        malposition T83.121
        obstruction T83.191
        perforation T83.191
        protrusion T83.191
        specified NEC T83.191
      pain T83.84
      specified type NEC T83.89
      stenosis T83.85
      thrombosis T83.86
  infusion (procedure) T80.90
    air embolism T80.0
    blood — *see* Complications, transfusion
    catheter — *see* Complications, catheter
    infection T80.29
    pump — *see* Complications, cardiovascular, device
      or implant
    sepsis T80.29
    serum reaction — *see also* Reaction, serum T80.69
      anaphylactic shock — *see also* Shock,
        anaphylactic T80.59
    specified type NEC T80.89
  inhalation therapy NEC T81.81
  injection (procedure) T80.90
    drug reaction — *see* Reaction, drug
    infection T80.29
    sepsis T80.29
    serum (prophylactic) (therapeutic) — *see*
      Complications, vaccination
    specified type NEC T80.89
    vaccine (any) — *see* Complications, vaccination
  inoculation (any) — *see* Complications, vaccination
  insulin pump
    infection and inflammation T85.72
    mechanical

Complication (s) (from) (of) - *continued*
  insulin pump - *continued*
    mechanical - *continued*
      breakdown T85.614
      displacement T85.624
      leakage T85.633
      malposition T85.624
      obstruction T85.694
      perforation T85.694
      protrusion T85.694
      specified NEC T85.694
  intestinal pouch NEC K91.858
  intraocular lens (prosthetic) T85.9
    embolism T85.818
    fibrosis T85.828
    hemorrhage T85.838
    infection and inflammation T85.79
    mechanical
      breakdown T85.21
      displacement T85.22
      malposition T85.22
      obstruction T85.29
      perforation T85.29
      protrusion T85.29
      specified NEC T85.29
    pain T85.848
    specified type NEC T85.898
    stenosis T85.858
    thrombosis T85.868
  intraoperative (intraprocedural)
    cardiac arrest
      during cardiac surgery I97.710
      during other surgery I97.711
    cardiac functional disturbance NEC
      during cardiac surgery I97.790
      during other surgery I97.791
    hemorrhage (hematoma) (of)
      circulatory system organ or structure
        during cardiac bypass I97.411
        during cardiac catheterization I97.410
        during other circulatory system
          procedure I97.418
        during other procedure I97.42
      digestive system organ
        during procedure on digestive system K91.61
        during procedure on other organ K91.62
      ear
        during procedure on ear and mastoid
          process H95.21
        during procedure on other organ H95.22
      endocrine system organ or structure
        during procedure on endocrine system organ or
          structure E36.01
        during procedure on other organ E36.02
      eye and adnexa
        during ophthalmic procedure H59.11-
        during other procedure H59.12-
      genitourinary organ or structure
        during procedure on genitourinary organ or
          structure N99.61
        during procedure on other organ N99.62
      mastoid process
        during procedure on ear and mastoid
          process H95.21
        during procedure on other organ H95.22
      musculoskeletal structure
        during musculoskeletal surgery M96.810
        during non-orthopedic surgery M96.811
        during orthopedic surgery M96.810
      nervous system
        during a nervous system procedure G97.31
        during other procedure G97.32
      respiratory system
        during other procedure J95.62
        during procedure on respiratory system organ or
          structure J95.61
      skin and subcutaneous tissue
        during a dermatologic procedure L76.01
        during a procedure on other organ L76.02
      spleen
        during a procedure on other organ D78.02
        during a procedure on the spleen D78.01
    puncture or laceration (accidental) (unintentional)
      (of)
      brain
        during a nervous system procedure G97.48
        during other procedure G97.49
      circulatory system organ or structure
        during circulatory system procedure I97.51
        during other procedure I97.52
      digestive system
        during procedure on digestive system K91.71
        during procedure on other organ K91.72

Complication (s) (from) (of) - *continued*
  intraoperative (intraprocedural) - *continued*
    puncture or laceration (accidental) (unintentional) (of) - *continued*
      ear
        during procedure on ear and mastoid process H95.31
        during procedure on other organ H95.32
      endocrine system organ or structure
        during procedure on endocrine system organ or structure E36.11
        during procedure on other organ E36.12
      eye and adnexa
        during ophthalmic procedure H59.21-
        during other procedure H59.22-
      genitourinary organ or structure
        during procedure on genitourinary organ or structure N99.71
        during procedure on other organ N99.72
      mastoid process
        during procedure on ear and mastoid process H95.31
        during procedure on other organ H95.32
      musculoskeletal structure
        during musculoskeletal surgery M96.820
        during non-orthopedic surgery M96.821
        during orthopedic surgery M96.820
      nervous system
        during a nervous system procedure G97.48
        during other procedure G97.49
      respiratory system
        during other procedure J95.72
        during procedure on respiratory system organ or structure J95.71
      skin and subcutaneous tissue
        during a dermatologic procedure L76.11
        during a procedure on other organ L76.12
      spleen
        during a procedure on other organ D78.12
        during a procedure on the spleen D78.11
    specified NEC
      circulatory system I97.88
      digestive system K91.81
      ear H95.88
      endocrine system E36.8
      eye and adnexa H59.88
      genitourinary system N99.81
      mastoid process H95.88
      musculoskeletal structure M96.89
      nervous system G97.81
      respiratory system J95.88
      skin and subcutaneous tissue L76.81
      spleen D78.81
  intraperitoneal catheter (dialysis) (infusion) — *see* Complications, catheter, intraperitoneal
  intrathecal infusion pump
    infection and inflammation T85.738
    mechanical
      breakdown T85.615
      displacement T85.625
      leakage T85.635
      malfunction T85.695
      malposition T85.625
      obstruction T85.695
      perforation T85.695
      protrusion T85.695
      specified NEC T85.695
  intrauterine
    contraceptive device
      embolism T83.81
      fibrosis T83.82
      hemorrhage T83.83
      infection and inflammation T83.69
      mechanical
        breakdown T83.31
        displacement T83.32
        malposition T83.32
        obstruction T83.39
        perforation T83.39
        protrusion T83.39
        specified NEC T83.39
      pain T83.84
      specified type NEC T83.89
      stenosis T83.85
      thrombosis T83.86
    procedure (fetal) , to newborn P96.5
  jejunostomy (stoma) — *see* Complications, enterostomy
  joint prosthesis, internal T84.9
    breakage (fracture) T84.01-
    dislocation T84.02-
    fracture T84.01-
    infection or inflammation T84.50

Complication (s) (from) (of) - *continued*
  joint prosthesis, internal - *continued*
    infection or inflammation - *continued*
      hip T84.5-
      knee T84.5-
      specified joint NEC T84.59
    instability T84.02-
    malposition — *see* Complications, joint prosthesis, mechanical, displacement
    mechanical
      breakage, broken T84.01-
      dislocation T84.02-
      fracture T84.01-
      instability T84.02-
      leakage — *see* Complications, joint prosthesis, mechanical, specified NEC
      loosening T84.039
        hip T84.03-
        knee T84.03-
        specified joint NEC T84.038
      obstruction — *see* Complications, joint prosthesis, mechanical, specified NEC
      perforation — *see* Complications, joint prosthesis, mechanical, specified NEC
      osteolysis T84.059
        hip T84.05-
        knee T84.05-
        other specified joint T84.058
      protrusion — *see* Complications, joint prosthesis, mechanical, specified NEC
      specified complication NEC T84.099
        hip T84.09-
        knee T84.09-
        other specified joint T84.098
      subluxation T84.02-
      wear of articular bearing surface T84.069
        hip T84.06-
        knee T84.06-
        other specified joint T84.068
    specified joint NEC T84.89
      embolism T84.81
      fibrosis T84.82
      hemorrhage T84.83
      pain T84.84
      specified complication NEC T84.89
      stenosis T84.85
      thrombosis T84.86
    subluxation T84.02-
  kidney transplant — *see* Complications, transplant, kidney
  labor O75.9
    specified NEC O75.89
  liver transplant (immune or nonimmune) — *see* Complications, transplant, liver
  lumbar puncture G97.1
    cerebrospinal fluid leak G97.0
    headache or reaction G97.1
  lung transplant — *see* Complications, transplant, lung
    and heart — *see* Complications, transplant, lung, with heart
  male genital N50.9
    device, implant or graft — *see* Complications, genitourinary, device or implant, genital tract
    postprocedural or postoperative — *see* Complications, genitourinary, postprocedural
    specified NEC N99.89
  mastoid (process) procedure
    intraoperative H95.88
      hematoma — *see* Complications, intraoperative, hemorrhage (hematoma) (of), mastoid process
      hemorrhage — *see* Complications, intraoperative, hemorrhage (hematoma) (of), mastoid process
      laceration — *see* Complications, intraoperative, puncture or laceration..., mastoid process
      specified NEC H95.88
    postmastoidectomy — *see* Complications, postmastoidectomy
    postoperative H95.89
      external ear canal stenosis H95.81-
      hematoma — *see* Complications..., postprocedural, hematoma (of), mastoid process
      hemorrhage — *see* Complications..., postprocedural, hemorrhage (of), mastoid process
      postmastoidectomy — *see* Complications, postmastoidectomy
      seroma — *see* Complications, postprocedural, seroma (of), mastoid process
      specified NEC H95.89
  mastoidectomy cavity — *see* Complications, postmastoidectomy

Complication (s) (from) (of) - *continued*
  mechanical — *see* Complications, by site and type, mechanical
  medical procedures — *see also* Complication(s), intraoperative T88.9
  metabolic E88.9
    postoperative E89.89
    specified NEC E89.89
  molar pregnancy NOS O08.9
    damage to pelvic organs O08.6
    embolism O08.2
    genital infection O08.0
    hemorrhage (delayed) (excessive) O08.1
    metabolic disorder O08.5
    renal failure O08.4
    shock O08.3
    specified type NEC O08.0
    venous complication NEC O08.7
  musculoskeletal system — *see also* Complication, intraoperative (intraprocedural), by site
    device, implant or graft NEC — *see* Complications, orthopedic, device or implant
    internal fixation (nail) (plate) (rod) — *see* Complications, fixation device, internal
    joint prosthesis — *see* Complications, joint prosthesis
    postoperative (postprocedural) M96.89
      with osteoporosis — *see* Osteoporosis
      fracture following insertion of device — *see* Fracture, following insertion of orthopedic implant, joint prosthesis or bone plate
      joint instability after prosthesis removal M96.89
      lordosis M96.4
      postlaminectomy syndrome NEC M96.1
        kyphosis M96.3
      pseudarthrosis M96.0
      specified complication NEC M96.89
    post radiation M96.89
      kyphosis M96.2
      scoliosis M96.5
      specified complication NEC M96.89
  nephrostomy (stoma) — *see* Complications, stoma, urinary tract, external NEC
  nervous system G98.8
    central G96.9
    device, implant or graft — *see also* Complication, prosthetic device or implant, specified NEC
      electronic stimulator (electrode (s)) — *see* Complications, electronic stimulator device
      specified NEC
        infection and inflammation T85.738
        mechanical T85.695
          breakdown T85.615
          displacement T85.625
          leakage T85.635
          malfunction T85.695
          malposition T85.625
          obstruction T85.695
          perforation T85.695
          protrusion T85.695
          specified NEC T85.695
      ventricular shunt — *see* Complications, ventricular shunt
    electronic stimulator (electrode (s)) — *see* Complications, electronic stimulator device
    postprocedural G97.82
      intracranial hypotension G97.2
      specified NEC G97.82
      spinal fluid leak G97.0
  newborn, due to intrauterine (fetal) procedure P96.5
  nonabsorbable (permanent) sutures — *see* Complication, sutures, permanent
  obstetric O75.9
    procedure (instrumental) (manual) (surgical)
      specified NEC O75.4
    specified NEC O75.89
    surgical wound NEC O90.89
      hematoma O90.2
      infection O86.0
  ocular lens implant — *see* Complications, intraocular lens
  ophthalmologic
    postprocedural bleb — *see* Blebitis
  orbital prosthesis T85.9
    embolism T85.818
    fibrosis T85.828
    hemorrhage T85.838
    infection and inflammation T85.79
    mechanical
      breakdown T85.31-
      displacement T85.32-
      malposition T85.32-
      obstruction T85.39-

Complication (s) (from) (of) - *continued*
orbital prosthesis - *continued*
mechanical - *continued*
perforation T85.39-
protrusion T85.39-
specified NEC T85.39-
pain T85.848
specified type NEC T85.898
stenosis T85.858
thrombosis T85.868
organ or tissue transplant (partial) (total) — *see* Complications, transplant
orthopedic — *see also* Disorder, soft tissue
device or implant T84.9
bone
device or implant — *see* Complication, bone, device NEC
graft — *see* Complication, graft, bone
breakdown T84.418
displacement T84.428
electronic bone stimulator — *see* Complications, electronic stimulator device, bone
embolism T84.81
fibrosis T84.82
fixation device — *see* Complication, fixation device, internal
hemorrhage T84.83
infection or inflammation T84.7
joint prosthesis — *see* Complication, joint prosthesis, internal
malfunction T84.418
malposition T84.428
mechanical NEC T84.498
muscle graft — *see* Complications, graft, muscle
obstruction T84.498
pain T84.84
perforation T84.498
protrusion T84.498
specified complication NEC T84.89
stenosis T84.85
tendon graft — *see* Complications, graft, tendon
thrombosis T84.86
fracture (following insertion of device) — *see* Fracture, following insertion of orthopedic implant, joint prosthesis or bone plate
postprocedural M96.89
fracture — *see* Fracture, following insertion of orthopedic implant, joint prosthesis or bone plate
postlaminectomy syndrome NEC M96.1
kyphosis M96.3
lordosis M96.4
postradiation
kyphosis M96.2
scoliosis M96.5
pseudarthrosis post-fusion M96.0
specified type NEC M96.89
pacemaker (cardiac) — *see* Complications, cardiovascular device or implant, electronic
pancreas transplant — *see* Complications, transplant, pancreas
penile prosthesis (implant) — *see* Complications, prosthetic device, penile
perfusion NEC T80.90
perineal repair (obstetrical) NEC O90.89
disruption O90.1
hematoma O90.2
infection (following delivery) O86.0
phototherapy T88.9
specified NEC T88.8
postmastoidectomy NEC H95.19-
cyst, mucosal H95.13-
granulation H95.12-
inflammation, chronic H95.11-
recurrent cholesteatoma H95.0-
postoperative — *see* Complications, postprocedural
circulatory — *see* Complications, circulatory system
ear — *see* Complications, ear
endocrine — *see* Complications, endocrine
eye — *see* Complications, eye
lumbar puncture G97.1
cerebrospinal fluid leak G97.0
nervous system (central) (peripheral) — *see* Complications, nervous system
respiratory system — *see* Complications, respiratory system
postprocedural — *see also* Complications, surgical procedure
cardiac arrest
following cardiac surgery I97.120
following other surgery I97.121
cardiac functional disturbance NEC

Complication (s) (from) (of) - *continued*
postprocedural - *continued*
cardiac functional disturbance NEC - *continued*
following cardiac surgery I97.190
following other surgery I97.191
cardiac insufficiency
following cardiac surgery I97.110
following other surgery I97.111
chorioretinal scars following retinal surgery H59.81-
following cataract surgery
cataract (lens) fragments H59.02-
cystoid macular edema H59.03-
specified NEC H59.09-
vitreous (touch) syndrome H59.01-
heart failure
following cardiac surgery I97.130
following other surgery I97.131
hematoma (of)
circulatory system organ or structure
following cardiac bypass I97.631
following cardiac catheterization I97.630
following other circulatory system procedure I97.638
following other procedure I97.621
digestive system
following procedure on digestive system K91.870
following procedure on other organ K91.871
ear
following other procedure H95.52
following procedure on ear and mastoid process H95.51
endocrine system
following endocrine system procedure E89.820
following other procedure E89.821
eye and adnexa
following ophthalmic procedure H59.33-
following other procedure H59.34-
genitourinary organ or structure
following procedure on genitourinary organ or structure N99.840
following procedure on other organ N99.841
mastoid process
following other procedure H95.52
following procedure on ear and mastoid process H95.51
musculoskeletal structure
following musculoskeletal surgery M96.840
following non-orthopedic surgery M96.841
following orthopedic surgery M96.840
nervous system
following nervous system procedure G97.61
following other procedure G97.62
respiratory system
following other procedure J95.861
following procedure on respiratory system organ or structure J95.860
skin and subcutaneous tissue
following dermatologic procedure L76.31
following procedure on other organ L76.32
spleen
following procedure on other organ D78.32
following procedure on the spleen D78.31
hemorrhage (of)
circulatory system organ or structure
following cardiac bypass I97.611
following cardiac catheterization I97.610
following other circulatory system procedure I97.618
following other procedure I97.620
digestive system
following procedure on digestive system K91.840
following procedure on other organ K91.841
ear
following other procedure H95.42
following procedure on ear and mastoid process H95.41
endocrine system
following endocrine system procedure E89.810
following other procedure E89.811
eye and adnexa
following ophthalmic procedure H59.31-
following other procedure H59.32-
genitourinary organ or structure
following procedure on genitourinary organ or structure N99.820
following procedure on other organ N99.821
mastoid process
following other procedure H95.42
following procedure on ear and mastoid process H95.41

Complication (s) (from) (of) - *continued*
postprocedural - *continued*
hemorrhage (of) - *continued*
musculoskeletal structure
following musculoskeletal surgery M96.830
following non-orthopedic surgery M96.831
following orthopedic surgery M96.830
nervous system
following nervous system procedure G97.51
following other procedure G97.52
respiratory system
following other procedure J95.831
following procedure on respiratory system organ or structure J95.830
skin and subcutaneous tissue
following dermatologic procedure L76.21
following a procedure on other organ L76.22
spleen
following procedure on other organ D78.22
following procedure on the spleen D78.21
seroma (of)
circulatory system organ or structure
following cardiac bypass I97.641
following cardiac catheterization I97.640
following other circulatory system procedure I97.648
following other procedure I97.622
digestive system
following procedure on digestive system K91.872
following procedure on other organ K91.873
ear
following other procedure H95.54
following procedure on ear and mastoid process H95.53
endocrine system
following endocrine system procedure E89.822
following other procedure E89.823
eye and adnexa
following ophthalmic procedure H59.35-
following other procedure H59.36-
genitourinary organ or structure
following procedure on genitourinary organ or structure N99.842
following procedure on other organ N99.843
mastoid process
following other procedure H95.54
following procedure on ear and mastoid process H95.53
musculoskeletal structure
following musculoskeletal surgery M96.842
following non-orthopedic surgery M96.843
following orthopedic surgery M96.842
nervous system
following nervous system procedure G97.63
following other procedure G97.64
respiratory system
following other procedure J95.863
following procedure on respiratory system organ or structure J95.862
skin and subcutaneous tissue
following dermatologic procedure L76.33
following procedure on other organ L76.34
spleen
following procedure on other organ D78.34
following procedure on the spleen D78.33
specified NEC
circulatory system I97.89
digestive K91.89
ear H95.89
endocrine E89.89
eye and adnexa H59.89
genitourinary N99.89
mastoid process H95.89
metabolic E89.89
musculoskeletal structure M96.89
nervous system G97.82
respiratory system J95.89
skin and subcutaneous tissue L76.82
spleen D78.89
pregnancy NEC — *see* Pregnancy, complicated by
prosthetic device or implant T85.9
bile duct — *see* Complications, bile duct implant
breast — *see* Complications, breast implant
bulking agent
ureteral
erosion T83.714
exposure T83.724
urethral
erosion T83.713
exposure T83.723
cardiac and vascular NEC — *see* Complications, cardiovascular device or implant

Complication (s) (from) (of) - *continued*
  prosthetic device or implant - *continued*
    corneal transplant — *see* Complications, graft, cornea
    electronic nervous system stimulator — *see* Complications, electronic stimulator device
    epidural infusion catheter — *see* Complications, catheter, epidural
    esophageal anti-reflux device — *see* Complications, esophageal anti-reflux device
    genital organ or tract — *see* Complications, genitourinary, device or implant, genital tract
      specified NEC T83.79
    heart valve — *see* Complications, heart, valve, prosthesis
    infection or inflammation T85.79
      intestine transplant T86.892
      liver transplant T86.43
      lung transplant T86.812
      pancreas transplant T86.892
      skin graft T86.822
    intraocular lens — *see* Complications, intraocular lens
    intraperitoneal (dialysis) catheter — *see* Complications, catheter, intraperitoneal
    joint — *see* Complications, joint prosthesis, internal
    mechanical NEC T85.698
      dialysis catheter (vascular) — *see also* Complication, catheter, dialysis, mechanical
        peritoneal — *see* Complication, catheter, intraperitoneal, mechanical
      gastrointestinal device T85.598
      ocular device T85.398
      subdural (infusion) catheter T85.690
      suture, permanent T85.692
        that for bone repair — *see* Complications, fixation device, internal (orthopedic), mechanical
      ventricular shunt
        breakdown T85.01
        displacement T85.02
        leakage T85.03
        malposition T85.02
        obstruction T85.09
        perforation T85.09
        protrusion T85.09
        specified NEC T85.09
    mesh
      erosion (to surrounding organ or tissue) T83.717
        urethral (into pelvic floor muscles) T83.712
        vaginal (into pelvic floor muscles) T83.711
      exposure (into surrounding organ or tissue) T83.727
        urethral (through urethral wall) T83.722
        vaginal (into vagina) (through vaginal wall) T83.721
    orbital — *see* Complications, orbital prosthesis
    penile T83.9
      embolism T83.81
      fibrosis T83.82
      hemorrhage T83.83
      infection and inflammation T83.61
      mechanical
        breakdown T83.410
        displacement T83.420
        leakage T83.490
        malposition T83.420
        obstruction T83.490
        perforation T83.490
        protrusion T83.490
        specified NEC T83.490
      pain T83.84
      specified type NEC T83.89
      stenosis T83.85
      thrombosis T83.86
    prosthetic materials NEC
      erosion (to surrounding organ or tissue) T83.718
      exposure (into surrounding organ or tissue) T83.728
    skin graft T86.829
      artificial skin or decellularized allodermis
        embolism T85.818
        fibrosis T85.828
        hemorrhage T85.838
        infection and inflammation T85.79
        mechanical
          breakdown T85.613
          displacement T85.623
          malfunction T85.613
          malposition T85.623
          obstruction T85.693

Complication (s) (from) (of) - *continued*
  prosthetic device or implant - *continued*
    skin graft - *continued*
      artificial skin or decellularized allodermis - *continued*
        mechanical - *continued*
          perforation T85.693
          protrusion T85.693
          specified NEC T85.693
        pain T85.848
        specified type NEC T85.898
        stenosis T85.858
        thrombosis T85.868
      failure T86.821
      infection T86.822
      rejection T86.820
      specified NEC T86.828
    sling
      urethral (female) (male)
        erosion T83.712
        exposure T83.722
      specified NEC T85.9
        embolism T85.818
        fibrosis T85.828
        hemorrhage T85.838
        infection and inflammation T85.79
        mechanical
          breakdown T85.618
          displacement T85.628
          leakage T85.638
          malfunction T85.618
          malposition T85.628
          obstruction T85.698
          perforation T85.698
          protrusion T85.698
          specified NEC T85.698
        pain T85.848
        specified type NEC T85.898
        stenosis T85.858
        thrombosis T85.868
    subdural infusion catheter — *see* Complications, catheter, subdural
    sutures — *see* Complications, sutures
    urinary organ or tract NEC — *see* Complications, genitourinary, device or implant, urinary system
    vascular — *see* Complications, cardiovascular device or implant
    ventricular shunt — *see* Complications, ventricular shunt (device)
  puerperium — *see* Puerperal
  puncture, spinal G97.1
    cerebrospinal fluid leak G97.0
    headache or reaction G97.1
  pyelogram N99.89
  radiation
    kyphosis M96.2
    scoliosis M96.5
  reattached
    extremity (infection) (rejection)
      lower T87.1X-
      upper T87.0X-
    specified body part NEC T87.2
  reconstructed breast
    asymmetry between native and reconstructed breast N65.1
    deformity N65.0
    disproportion between native and reconstructed breast N65.1
    excess tissue N65.0
    misshappen N65.0
  reimplant NEC — *see also* Complications, prosthetic device or implant
    limb (infection) (rejection) — *see* Complications, reattached, extremity
    organ (partial) (total) — *see* Complications, transplant
    prosthetic device NEC — *see* Complications, prosthetic device
  renal N28.9
    allograft — *see* Complications, transplant, kidney
    dialysis — *see* Complications, dialysis
  respirator
    mechanical J95.850
      specified NEC J95.859
  respiratory system J98.9
    device, implant or graft — *see* Complication, prosthetic device or implant, specified NEC
    lung transplant — *see* Complications, prosthetic device or implant, lung transplant
    postoperative J95.89
      air leak J95.812
      Mendelson's syndrome (chemical pneumonitis) J95.4

Complication (s) (from) (of) - *continued*
  respiratory system - *continued*
    postoperative - *continued*
      pneumothorax J95.811
      pulmonary insufficiency (acute) (after nonthoracic surgery) J95.2
        chronic J95.3
        following thoracic surgery J95.1
      respiratory failure (acute) J95.821
        acute and chronic J95.822
        specified NEC J95.89
      subglottic stenosis J95.5
      tracheostomy complication — *see* Complications, tracheostomy
    therapy T81.89
  sedation during labor and delivery O74.9
    cardiac O74.2
    central nervous system O74.3
    pulmonary NEC O74.1
  shunt — *see also* Complications, prosthetic device or implant
    arteriovenous — *see* Complications, arteriovenous, shunt
    ventricular (communicating) — *see* Complications, ventricular shunt
  skin
    graft T86.829
      failure T86.821
      infection T86.822
      rejection T86.820
      specified type NEC T86.828
  spinal
    anesthesia — *see* Complications, anesthesia, spinal
    catheter (epidural) (subdural) — *see* Complications, catheter
    puncture or tap G97.1
      cerebrospinal fluid leak G97.0
      headache or reaction G97.1
  stent
    bile duct — *see* Complications, bile duct prosthesis
    ureteral indwelling
      breakdown T83.112
      displacement T83.122
      leakage T83.192
      malposition T83.122
      obstruction T83.192
      perforation T83.192
      protrusion T83.192
      specified NEC T83.192
    urinary NEC (ileal conduit) (nephroureteral) T83.193
      embolism T83.81
      fibrosis T83.82
      hemorrhage T83.83
      infection and inflammation T83.593
      mechanical
        breakdown T83.113
        displacement T83.123
        leakage T83.193
        malposition T83.123
        obstruction T83.193
        perforation T83.193
        protrusion T83.193
        specified NEC T83.193
      pain T83.84
      specified type NEC T83.89
      stenosis T83.85
      thrombosis T83.86
    vascular
      end stent stenosis — *see* Restenosis, stent
      in stent stenosis — *see* Restenosis, stent
  stoma
    digestive tract
      colostomy — *see* Complications, colostomy
      enterostomy — *see* Complications, enterostomy
      esophagostomy — *see* Complications, esophagostomy
      gastrostomy — *see* Complications, gastrostomy
    urinary tract N99.528
      continent N99.538
        hemorrhage N99.530
        herniation N99.533
        infection N99.531
        malfunction N99.532
        specified type NEC N99.538
        stenosis N99.534
      cystostomy — *see* Complications, cystostomy
      external NOS N99.528
        hemorrhage N99.520
        herniation N99.523
      incontinent N99.528
        hemorrhage N99.520
        herniation N99.523

Complication (s) (from) (of) - *continued*
  stoma - *continued*
    urinary tract - *continued*
      incontinent - *continued*
        infection N99.521
        malfunction N99.522
        specified type NEC N99.528
        stenosis N99.524
      infection N99.521
      malfunction N99.522
      specified type NEC N99.528
      stenosis N99.524
  stomach banding — *see* Complication(s), bariatric procedure
  stomach stapling — *see* Complication(s), bariatric procedure
  surgical material, nonabsorbable — *see* Complication, suture, permanent
  surgical procedure (on) T81.9
    amputation stump (late) — *see* Complications, amputation stump
    cardiac — *see* Complications, circulatory system
    cholesteatoma, recurrent — *see* Complications, postmastoidectomy, recurrent cholesteatoma
    circulatory (early) — *see* Complications, circulatory system
    digestive system — *see* Complications, gastrointestinal
    dumping syndrome (postgastrectomy) K91.1
    ear — *see* Complications, ear
    elephantiasis or lymphedema I97.89
      postmastectomy I97.2
    emphysema (surgical) T81.82
    endocrine — *see* Complications, endocrine
    eye — *see* Complications, eye
    fistula (persistent postoperative) T81.83
    foreign body inadvertently left in wound (sponge) (suture) (swab) — *see* Foreign body, accidentally left during a procedure
    gastrointestinal — *see* Complications, gastrointestinal
    genitourinary NEC N99.89
    hematoma
      intraoperative — *see* Complication, intraoperative, hemorrhage
      postprocedural — *see* Complication, postprocedural, hematoma
    hemorrhage
      intraoperative — *see* Complication, intraoperative, hemorrhage
      postprocedural — *see* Complication, postprocedural, hemorrhage
    hepatic failure K91.82
    hyperglycemia (postpancreatectomy) E89.1
    hypoinsulinemia (postpancreatectomy) E89.1
    hypoparathyroidism (postparathyroidectomy) E89.2
    hypopituitarism (posthypophysectomy) E89.3
    hypothyroidism (post-thyroidectomy) E89.0
    intestinal obstruction K91.3
    intracranial hypotension following ventricular shunting (ventriculostomy) G97.2
    lymphedema I97.89
      postmastectomy I97.2
    malabsorption (postsurgical) NEC K91.2
      osteoporosis — *see* Osteoporosis, postsurgical malabsorption
    mastoidectomy cavity NEC — *see* Complications, postmastoidectomy
    metabolic E89.89
      specified NEC E89.89
    musculoskeletal — *see* Complications, musculoskeletal system
    nervous system (central) (peripheral) — *see* Complications, nervous system
    ovarian failure E89.40
      asymptomatic E89.40
      symptomatic E89.41
    peripheral vascular — *see* Complications, surgical procedure, vascular
    postcardiotomy syndrome I97.0
    postcholecystectomy syndrome K91.5
    postcommissurotomy syndrome I97.0
    postgastrectomy dumping syndrome K91.1
    postlaminectomy syndrome NEC M96.1
      kyphosis M96.3
    postmastectomy lymphedema syndrome I97.2
    postmastoidectomy cholesteatoma — *see* Complications, postmastoidectomy, recurrent cholesteatoma
    postvagotomy syndrome K91.1
    postvalvulotomy syndrome I97.0
    pulmonary insufficiency (acute) J95.2

Complication (s) (from) (of) - *continued*
  surgical procedure (on) - *continued*
    pulmonary insufficiency (acute) - *continued*
      chronic J95.3
      following thoracic surgery J95.1
    reattached body part — *see* Complications, reattached
    respiratory — *see* Complications, respiratory system
    shock (hypovolemic) T81.19
    spleen (postoperative) D78.89
      intraoperative D78.81
    stitch abscess T81.48
    subglottic stenosis (postsurgical) J95.5
    testicular hypofunction E89.5
    transplant — *see* Complications, organ or tissue transplant
    urinary NEC N99.89
    vaginal vault prolapse (posthysterectomy) N99.3
    vascular (peripheral)
      artery T81.719
        mesenteric T81.710
        renal T81.711
        specified NEC T81.718
      vein T81.72
    wound infection T81.40
  suture, permanent (wire) NEC T85.9
    with repair of bone — *see* Complications, fixation device, internal
    embolism T85.818
    fibrosis T85.828
    hemorrhage T85.838
    infection and inflammation T85.79
    mechanical
      breakdown T85.612
      displacement T85.622
      malfunction T85.612
      malposition T85.622
      obstruction T85.692
      perforation T85.692
      protrusion T85.692
      specified NEC T85.692
    pain T85.848
    specified type NEC T85.898
    stenosis T85.858
    thrombosis T85.868
  tracheostomy J95.00
    granuloma J95.09
    hemorrhage J95.01
    infection J95.02
    malfunction J95.03
    mechanical J95.03
    obstruction J95.03
    specified type NEC J95.09
    tracheo-esophageal fistula J95.04
  transfusion (blood) (lymphocytes) (plasma) T80.92
    air embolism T80.0
    circulatory overload E87.71
    febrile nonhemolytic transfusion reaction R50.84
    hemolysis T80.89
    hemochromatosis E83.111
    hemolytic reaction (antigen unspecified) T80.919
    incompatibility reaction (antigen unspecified) T80.919
      ABO T80.30
        delayed serologic (DSTR) T80.39
        hemolytic transfusion reaction (HTR) (unspecified time after transfusion) T80.319
          acute (AHTR) (less than 24 hours after transfusion) T80.310
          delayed (DHTR) (24 hours or more after transfusion) T80.311
        specified NEC T80.39
      acute (antigen unspecified) T80.910
      delayed (antigen unspecified) T80.911
      delayed serologic (DSTR) T80.89
      Non-ABO (minor antigens (Duffy) (Kell) (Kidd) (Lewis) (M) (N) (P) (S)) T80.A0
        delayed serologic (DSTR) T80.A9
        hemolytic transfusion reaction (HTR) (unspecified time after transfusion) T80.A19
          acute (AHTR) (less than 24 hours after transfusion) T80.A10
          delayed (DHTR) (24 hours or more after transfusion) T80.A11
        specified NEC T80.A9
      Rh (antigens (C) (c) (D) (E) (e)) (factor) T80.40
        delayed serologic (DSTR) T80.49
        hemolytic transfusion reaction (HTR) (unspecified time after transfusion) T80.419
          acute (AHTR) (less than 24 hours after transfusion) T80.410

Complication (s) (from) (of) - *continued*
  transfusion (blood) (lymphocytes) (plasma) - *continued*
    incompatibility reaction (antigen unspecified) - *continued*
      Rh (antigens (C) (c) (D) (E) (e)) (factor) - *continued*
        hemolytic transfusion reaction (HTR) (unspecified time after transfusion) - *continued*
          delayed (DHTR) (24 hours or more after transfusion) T80.411
        specified NEC T80.49
    infection T80.29
      acute T80.22
    reaction NEC T80.89
    sepsis T80.29
    shock T80.89
  transplant T86.90
    bone T86.839
      failure T86.831
      infection T86.832
      rejection T86.830
      specified type NEC T86.838
    bone marrow T86.00
      failure T86.02
      infection T86.03
      rejection T86.01
      specified type NEC T86.09
    cornea T86.849
      failure T86.841
      infection T86.842
      rejection T86.840
      specified type NEC T86.848
    failure T86.92
    heart T86.20
      with lung T86.30
      cardiac allograft vasculopathy T86.290
        failure T86.32
        infection T86.33
        rejection T86.31
        specified type NEC T86.39
      failure T86.22
      infection T86.23
      rejection T86.21
      specified type NEC T86.298
    infection T86.93
    intestine T86.859
      failure T86.851
      infection T86.852
      rejection T86.850
      specified type NEC T86.858
    kidney T86.10
      failure T86.12
      infection T86.13
      rejection T86.11
      specified type NEC T86.19
    liver T86.40
      failure T86.42
      infection T86.43
      rejection T86.41
      specified type NEC T86.49
    lung T86.819
      with heart T86.30
        failure T86.32
        infection T86.33
        rejection T86.31
        specified type NEC T86.39
      failure T86.811
      infection T86.812
      rejection T86.810
      specified type NEC T86.818
    malignant neoplasm C80.2
    pancreas T86.899
      failure T86.891
      infection T86.892
      rejection T86.890
      specified type NEC T86.898
    peripheral blood stem cells T86.5
    post-transplant lymphoproliferative disorder (PTLD) D47.Z1
    rejection T86.91
    skin T86.829
      failure T86.821
      infection T86.822
      rejection T86.820
      specified type NEC T86.828
    specified
      tissue T86.899
        failure T86.891
        infection T86.892
        rejection T86.890
        specified type NEC T86.898
      type NEC T86.99

Complication (s) (from) (of) - *continued*
transplant - *continued*
stem cell (from peripheral blood) (from umbilical cord) T86.5
umbilical cord stem cells T86.5
trauma (early) T79.9
specified NEC T79.8
ultrasound therapy NEC T88.9
umbilical cord NEC
complicating delivery O69.9
specified NEC O69.89
umbrella device, vascular T82.9
embolism T82.818
fibrosis T82.828
hemorrhage T82.838
infection or inflammation T82.7
mechanical
breakdown T82.515
displacement T82.525
leakage T82.535
malposition T82.525
obstruction T82.595
perforation T82.595
protrusion T82.595
pain T82.848
specified type NEC T82.898
stenosis T82.858
thrombosis T82.868
urethral catheter — *see* Complications, catheter, urethral, indwelling
vaccination T88.1
anaphylaxis NEC T80.52
arthropathy — *see* Arthropathy, postimmunization
cellulitis T88.0
encephalitis or encephalomyelitis G04.02
infection (general) (local) NEC T88.0
meningitis G03.8
myelitis G04.02
protein sickness T80.62
rash T88.1
reaction (allergic) T88.1
serum T80.62
sepsis T88.0
serum intoxication, sickness, rash, or other serum reaction NEC T80.62
anaphylactic shock T80.52
shock (allergic) (anaphylactic) T80.52
vaccinia (generalized) (localized) T88.1
vas deferens device or implant — *see* Complications, genitourinary, device or implant, genital tract
vascular I99.9
device or implant T82.9
embolism T82.818
fibrosis T82.828
hemorrhage T82.838
infection or inflammation T82.7
mechanical
breakdown T82.519
specified device NEC T82.518
displacement T82.529
specified device NEC T82.528
leakage T82.539
specified device NEC T82.538
malposition T82.529
specified device NEC T82.528
obstruction T82.599
specified device NEC T82.598
perforation T82.599
specified device NEC T82.598
protrusion T82.599
specified device NEC T82.598
pain T82.848
specified type NEC T82.898
stenosis T82.858
thrombosis T82.868
dialysis catheter — *see* Complication, catheter, dialysis
following infusion, therapeutic injection or transfusion T80.1
graft T82.9
embolism T82.818
fibrosis T82.828
hemorrhage T82.838
mechanical
breakdown T82.319
aorta (bifurcation) T82.310
carotid artery T82.311
specified vessel NEC T82.318
displacement T82.329
aorta (bifurcation) T82.320
carotid artery T82.321
specified vessel NEC T82.328

Complication (s) (from) (of) - *continued*
vascular - *continued*
graft - *continued*
mechanical - *continued*
leakage T82.339
aorta (bifurcation) T82.330
carotid artery T82.331
specified vessel NEC T82.338
malposition T82.329
aorta (bifurcation) T82.320
carotid artery T82.321
specified vessel NEC T82.328
obstruction T82.399
aorta (bifurcation) T82.390
carotid artery T82.391
specified vessel NEC T82.398
perforation T82.399
aorta (bifurcation) T82.390
carotid artery T82.391
specified vessel NEC T82.398
protrusion T82.399
aorta (bifurcation) T82.390
carotid artery T82.391
specified vessel NEC T82.398
pain T82.848
specified complication NEC T82.898
stenosis T82.858
thrombosis T82.868
postoperative — *see* Complications, postoperative, circulatory
vena cava device (filter) (sieve) (umbrella) — *see* Complications, umbrella device, vascular
ventilation therapy NEC T81.81
ventilator
mechanical J95.850
specified NEC J95.859
ventricular (communicating) shunt (device) T85.9
embolism T85.810
fibrosis T85.820
hemorrhage T85.830
infection and inflammation T85.730
mechanical
breakdown T85.01
displacement T85.02
leakage T85.03
malposition T85.02
obstruction T85.09
perforation T85.09
protrusion T85.09
specified NEC T85.09
pain T85.840
specified type NEC T85.890
stenosis T85.850
thrombosis T85.860
wire suture, permanent (implanted) — *see* Complications, suture, permanent
Compressed air disease T70.3
Compression
with injury - code by Nature of injury
artery I77.1
celiac, syndrome I77.4
brachial plexus G54.0
brain (stem) G93.5
due to
contusion (diffuse) — *see* Injury, intracranial, diffuse
focal — *see* Injury, intracranial, focal
injury NEC — *see* Injury, intracranial, diffuse
traumatic — *see* Injury, intracranial, diffuse
bronchus J98.09
cauda equina G83.4
celiac (artery) (axis) I77.4
cerebral — *see* Compression, brain
cervical plexus G54.2
cord
spinal — *see* Compression, spinal
umbilical — *see* Compression, umbilical cord
cranial nerve G52.9
eighth — *see* subcategory H93.3
eleventh G52.8
fifth G50.8
first G52.0
fourth — *see* Strabismus, paralytic, fourth nerve
ninth G52.1
second — *see* Disorder, nerve, optic
seventh G52.8
sixth — *see* Strabismus, paralytic, sixth nerve
tenth G52.2
third — *see* Strabismus, paralytic, third nerve
twelfth G52.3
diver's squeeze T70.3
during birth (newborn) P15.9
esophagus K22.2

Compression - *continued*
eustachian tube — *see* Obstruction, eustachian tube, cartilaginous
facies Q67.1
fracture
nontraumatic NOS — *see* Collapse, vertebra
pathological — *see* Fracture, pathological
traumatic — *see* Fracture, traumatic
heart — *see* Disease, heart
intestine — *see* Obstruction, intestine
laryngeal nerve, recurrent G52.2
with paralysis of vocal cords and larynx J38.00
bilateral J38.02
unilateral J38.01
lumbosacral plexus G54.1
lung J98.4
lymphatic vessel I89.0
medulla — *see* Compression, brain
nerve — *see also* Disorder, nerve G58.9
arm NEC — *see* Mononeuropathy, upper limb
axillary G54.0
cranial — *see* Compression, cranial nerve
leg NEC — *see* Mononeuropathy, lower limb
median (in carpal tunnel) — *see* Syndrome, carpal tunnel
optic — *see* Disorder, nerve, optic
plantar — *see* Lesion, nerve, plantar
posterior tibial (in tarsal tunnel) — *see* Syndrome, tarsal tunnel
root or plexus NOS (in) G54.9
intervertebral disc disorder NEC — *see* Disorder, disc, with, radiculopathy
with myelopathy — *see* Disorder, disc, with, myelopathy
neoplastic disease — *see also* Neoplasm D49.9 *[G55]*
spondylosis — *see* Spondylosis, with radiculopathy
sciatic (acute) — *see* Lesion, nerve, sciatic
sympathetic G90.8
traumatic — *see* Injury, nerve
ulnar — *see* Lesion, nerve, ulnar
upper extremity NEC — *see* Mononeuropathy, upper limb
spinal (cord) G95.20
by displacement of intervertebral disc NEC — *see also* Disorder, disc, with, myelopathy
nerve root NOS G54.9
due to displacement of intervertebral disc NEC — *see* Disorder, disc, with, radiculopathy
with myelopathy — *see* Disorder, disc, with, myelopathy
specified NEC G95.29
spondylogenic (cervical) (lumbar, lumbosacral) (thoracic) — *see* Spondylosis, with myelopathy NEC
anterior — *see* Syndrome, anterior, spinal artery, compression
traumatic — *see* Injury, spinal cord, by region
subcostal nerve (syndrome) — *see* Mononeuropathy, upper limb, specified NEC
sympathetic nerve NEC G90.8
syndrome T79.5
trachea J39.8
ulnar nerve (by scar tissue) — *see* Lesion, nerve, ulnar
umbilical cord
complicating delivery O69.2
cord around neck O69.1
prolapse O69.0
specified NEC O69.2
ureter N13.5
vein I87.1
vena cava (inferior) (superior) I87.1
Compulsion, compulsive
gambling F63.0
neurosis F42.8
personality F60.5
states F42.8
swearing F42.8
in Gilles de la Tourette's syndrome F95.2
tics and spasms F95.9
Concato's disease (pericardial polyserositis) A19.9
nontubercular I31.1
pleural — *see* Pleurisy, with effusion
Concavity chest wall M95.4
Concealed penis Q55.69
Concern (normal) **about sick person in family** Z63.6
Concrescence (teeth) K00.2
Concretio cordis I31.1
rheumatic I09.2
Concretion — *see also* Calculus
appendicular K38.1

Concretion - *continued*
canaliculus — *see* Dacryolith
clitoris N90.89
conjunctiva H11.12-
eyelid — *see* Disorder, eyelid, specified type NEC
lacrimal passages — *see* Dacryolith
prepuce (male) N47.8
salivary gland (any) K11.5
seminal vesicle N50.89
tonsil J35.8
Concussion (brain) (cerebral) (current) S06.0X9
with
loss of consciousness of 30 minutes or less S06.0X1
loss of consciousness of unspecified durationS06.0X9
blast (air) (hydraulic) (immersion) (underwater)
abdomen or thorax — *see* Injury, blast, by site
ear with acoustic nerve injury — *see* Injury, nerve, acoustic, specified type NEC
cauda equina S34.3
conus medullaris S34.02
ocular S05.8X-
spinal (cord)
cervical S14.0
lumbar S34.01
sacral S34.02
thoracic S24.0
syndrome F07.81
without loss of consciousness S06.0X0
Condition — *see* Disease
Conditions arising in the perinatal period — *see* Newborn, affected by
Conduct disorder — *see* Disorder, conduct
Condyloma A63.0
acuminatum A63.0
gonorrheal A54.09
latum A51.31
syphilitic A51.31
congenital A50.07
venereal, syphilitic A51.31
Conflagration — *see also* Burn
asphyxia (by inhalation of gases, fumes or vapors) — *see also* Table of Drugs and Chemicals T59.9-
Conflict (with) — *see also* Discord
family Z73.9
marital Z63.0
involving divorce or estrangement Z63.5
parent-child Z62.820
parent-adopted child Z62.821
parent-biological child Z62.820
parent-foster child Z62.822
social role NEC Z73.5
Confluent — *see* condition
Confusion, confused R41.0
epileptic F05
mental state (psychogenic) F44.89
psychogenic F44.89
reactive (from emotional stress, psychological trauma) F44.89
Confusional arousals G47.51
Congelation T69.9
Congenital — *see also* condition
aortic septum Q25.49
intrinsic factor deficiency D51.0
malformation — *see* Anomaly
Congestion, congestive
bladder N32.89
bowel K63.89
brain G93.89
breast N64.59
bronchial J98.09
catarrhal J31.0
chest R09.89
chill, malarial — *see* Malaria
circulatory NEC I99.8
duodenum K31.89
eye — *see* Hyperemia, conjunctiva
facial, due to birth injury P15.4
general R68.89
glottis J37.0
heart — *see* Failure, heart, congestive
hepatic K76.1
hypostatic (lung) — *see* Edema, lung
intestine K63.89
kidney N28.89
labyrinth — *see* subcategory H83.8
larynx J37.0
liver K76.1
lung R09.89
active or acute — *see* Pneumonia
malaria, malarial — *see* Malaria

Congestion, congestive - *continued*
nasal R09.81
nose R09.81
orbit, orbital — *see also* Exophthalmos
inflammatory (chronic) — *see* Inflammation, orbit
ovary N83.8
pancreas K86.89
pelvic, female N94.89
pleural J94.8
prostate (active) N42.1
pulmonary — *see* Congestion, lung
renal N28.89
retina H35.81
seminal vesicle N50.1
spinal cord G95.19
spleen (chronic) D73.2
stomach K31.89
trachea — *see* Tracheitis
urethra N36.8
uterus N85.8
with subinvolution N85.3
venous (passive) I87.8
viscera R68.89
Congestive — *see* Congestion
Conical
cervix (hypertrophic elongation) N88.4
cornea — *see* Keratoconus
teeth K00.2
Conjoined twins Q89.4
Conjugal maladjustment Z63.0
involving divorce or estrangement Z63.5
Conjunctiva — *see* condition
Conjunctivitis (staphylococcal) (streptococcal) **NOS** H10.9
Acanthamoeba B60.12
acute H10.3-
atopic H10.1-
mucopurulent H10.02-
follicular H10.01-
chemical — *see also* Corrosion, cornea H10.21-
pseudomembranous H10.22-
serous except viral H10.23-
viral — *see* Conjunctivitis, viral
toxic H10.21-
adenoviral (acute) (follicular) B30.1
allergic (acute) — *see* Conjunctivitis, acute, atopic
chronic H10.45
vernal H10.44
anaphylactic — *see* Conjunctivitis, acute, atopic
Apollo B30.3
atopic (acute) — *see* Conjunctivitis, acute, atopic
Béal's B30.2
blennorrhagic (gonococcal) (neonatorum) A54.31
chemical (acute) — *see also* Corrosion, cornea H10.21-
chlamydial A74.0
due to trachoma A71.1
neonatal P39.1
chronic (nodosa) (petrificans) (phlyctenular) H10.40-
allergic H10.45
vernal H10.44
follicular H10.43-
giant papillary H10.41-
simple H10.42-
vernal H10.44
coxsackievirus 24 B30.3
diphtheritic A36.86
due to
dust — *see* Conjunctivitis, acute, atopic
filariasis B74.9
mucocutaneous leishmaniasis B55.2
enterovirus type 70 (hemorrhagic) B30.3
epidemic (viral) B30.9
hemorrhagic B30.3
gonococcal (neonatorum) A54.31
granular (trachomatous) A71.1
sequelae (late effect) B94.0
hemorrhagic (acute) (epidemic) B30.3
herpes zoster B02.31
in (due to)
Acanthamoeba B60.12
adenovirus (acute) (follicular) B30.1
Chlamydia A74.0
coxsackievirus 24 B30.3
diphtheria A36.86
enterovirus type 70 (hemorrhagic) B30.3
filariasis B74.9
gonococci A54.31
herpes (simplex) virus B00.53
zoster B02.31
infectious disease NEC B99
meningococci A39.89

Conjunctivitis (staphylococcal) (streptococcal) **NOS** - *continued*
in (due to) - *continued*
mucocutaneous leishmaniasis B55.2
rosacea L71.9
syphilis (late) A52.71
zoster B02.31
inclusion A74.0
infantile P39.1
gonococcal A54.31
Koch-Weeks' — *see* Conjunctivitis, acute, mucopurulent
light — *see* Conjunctivitis, acute, atopic
ligneous — *see* Blepharoconjunctivitis, ligneous
meningococcal A39.89
mucopurulent — *see* Conjunctivitis, acute, mucopurulent
neonatal P39.1
gonococcal A54.31
Newcastle B30.8
of Béal B30.2
parasitic
filariasis B74.9
mucocutaneous leishmaniasis B55.2
Parinaud's H10.89
petrificans H10.89
rosacea L71.9
specified NEC H10.89
swimming-pool B30.1
trachomatous A71.1
acute A71.0
sequelae (late effect) B94.0
traumatic NEC H10.89
tuberculous A18.59
tularemic A21.1
tularensis A21.1
viral B30.9
due to
adenovirus B30.1
enterovirus B30.3
specified NEC B30.8
Conjunctivochalasis H11.82-
Connective tissue — *see* condition
Conn's syndrome E26.01
Conradi (-Hunermann) **disease** Q77.3
Consanguinity Z84.3
counseling Z71.89
Conscious simulation (of illness) Z76.5
Consecutive — *see* condition
Consolidation lung (base) — *see* Pneumonia, lobar
Constipation (atonic) (neurogenic) (simple) (spastic) K59.00
chronic K59.09
idiopathic K59.04
drug-induced K59.03
functional K59.04
outlet dysfunction K59.02
psychogenic F45.8
slow transit K59.01
specified NEC K59.09
Constitutional — *see also* condition
substandard F60.7
Constitutionally substandard F60.7
Constriction — *see also* Stricture
auditory canal — *see* Stenosis, external ear canal
bronchial J98.09
duodenum K31.5
esophagus K22.2
external
abdomen, abdominal (wall) S30.841
alveolar process S00.542
ankle S90.54-
antecubital space — *see* Constriction, external, forearm
arm (upper) S40.84-
auricle — *see* Constriction, external, ear
axilla — *see* Constriction, external, arm
back, lower S30.840
breast S20.14-
brow S00.84
buttock S30.840
calf — *see* Constriction, external, leg
canthus — *see* Constriction, external, eyelid
cheek S00.84
internal S00.542
chest wall — *see* Constriction, external, thorax
chin S00.84
clitoris S30.844
costal region — *see* Constriction, external, thorax
digit (s)
foot — *see* Constriction, external, toe
hand — *see* Constriction, external, finger
ear S00.44-

Constriction - *continued*
external - *continued*
elbow S50.34-
epididymis S30.843
epigastric region S30.841
esophagus, cervical S10.14
eyebrow — *see* Constriction, external, eyelid
eyelid S00.24-
face S00.84
finger (s) S60.44-
index S60.44-
little S60.44-
middle S60.44-
ring S60.44-
flank S30.841
foot (except toe (s) alone) S90.84-
toe — *see* Constriction, external, toe
forearm S50.84-
elbow only — *see* Constriction, external, elbow
forehead S00.84
genital organs, external
female S30.846
male S30.845
groin S30.841
gum S00.542
hand S60.54-
head S00.94
ear — *see* Constriction, external, ear
eyelid — *see* Constriction, external, eyelid
lip S00.541
nose S00.34
oral cavity S00.542
scalp S00.04
specified site NEC S00.84
heel — *see* Constriction, external, foot
hip S70.24-
inguinal region S30.841
interscapular region S20.449
jaw S00.84
knee S80.24-
labium (majus) (minus) S30.844
larynx S10.14
leg (lower) S80.84-
knee — *see* Constriction, external, knee
upper — *see* Constriction, external, thigh
lip S00.541
lower back S30.840
lumbar region S30.840
malar region S00.84
mammary — *see* Constriction, external, breast
mastoid region S00.84
mouth S00.542
nail
finger — *see* Constriction, external, finger
toe — *see* Constriction, external, toe
nasal S00.34
neck S10.94
specified site NEC S10.84
throat S10.14
nose S00.34
occipital region S00.04
oral cavity S00.542
orbital region — *see* Constriction, external, eyelid
palate S00.542
palm — *see* Constriction, external, hand
parietal region S00.04
pelvis S30.840
penis S30.842
perineum
female S30.844
male S30.840
periocular area — *see* Constriction, external, eyelid
phalanges
finger — *see* Constriction, external, finger
toe — *see* Constriction, external, toe
pharynx S10.14
pinna — *see* Constriction, external, ear
popliteal space — *see* Constriction, external, knee
prepuce S30.842
pubic region S30.840
pudendum
female S30.846
male S30.845
sacral region S30.840
scalp S00.04
scapular region — *see* Constriction, external, shoulder
scrotum S30.843
shin — *see* Constriction, external, leg
shoulder S40.24-
sternal region S20.349
submaxillary region S00.84
submental region S00.84

Constriction - *continued*
external - *continued*
subungual
finger (s) — *see* Constriction, external, finger
toe (s) — *see* Constriction, external, toe
supraclavicular fossa S10.84
supraorbital S00.84
temple S00.84
temporal region S00.84
testis S30.843
thigh S70.34-
thorax, thoracic (wall) S20.94
back S20.44-
front S20.34-
throat S10.14
thumb S60.34-
toe (s) (lesser) S90.44-
great S90.44-
tongue S00.542
trachea S10.14
tunica vaginalis S30.843
uvula S00.542
vagina S30.844
vulva S30.844
wrist S60.84-
gallbladder — *see* Obstruction, gallbladder
intestine — *see* Obstruction, intestine
larynx J38.6
congenital Q31.8
specified NEC Q31.8
subglottic Q31.1
organ or site, congenital NEC — *see* Atresia, by site
prepuce (acquired) (congenital) N47.1
pylorus (adult hypertrophic) K31.1
congenital or infantile Q40.0
newborn Q40.0
ring dystocia (uterus) O62.4
spastic — *see also* Spasm
ureter N13.5
ureter N13.5
with infection N13.6
urethra — *see* Stricture, urethra
visual field (peripheral) (functional) — *see* Defect, visual field
Constrictive — *see* condition
Consultation
medical — *see* Counseling, medical
religious Z71.81
specified reason NEC Z71.89
spiritual Z71.81
without complaint or sickness Z71.9
feared complaint unfounded Z71.1
specified reason NEC Z71.89
Consumption — *see* Tuberculosis
Contact (with) — *see also* Exposure (to)
acariasis Z20.7
AIDS virus Z20.6
air pollution Z77.110
algae and algae toxins Z77.121
algae bloom Z77.121
anthrax Z20.810
aromatic amines Z77.020
aromatic (hazardous) compounds NEC Z77.028
aromatic dyes NOS Z77.028
arsenic Z77.010
asbestos Z77.090
bacterial disease NEC Z20.818
benzene Z77.021
blue-green algae bloom Z77.121
body fluids (potentially hazardous) Z77.21
brown tide Z77.121
chemicals (chiefly nonmedicinal) (hazardous) NEC Z77.098
cholera Z20.09
chromium compounds Z77.018
communicable disease Z20.9
bacterial NEC Z20.818
specified NEC Z20.89
viral NEC Z20.828
cyanobacteria bloom Z77.121
dyes Z77.098
Escherichia coli (E. coli) Z20.01
fiberglass — *see* Table of Drugs and Chemicals, fiberglass
German measles Z20.4
gonorrhea Z20.2
hazardous metals NEC Z77.018
hazardous substances NEC Z77.29
hazards in the physical environment NEC Z77.128
hazards to health NEC Z77.9
HIV Z20.6
HTLV-III/LAV Z20.6
human immunodeficiency virus (HIV) Z20.6

Contact (with) - *continued*
infection Z20.9
specified NEC Z20.89
infestation (parasitic) NEC Z20.7
intestinal infectious disease NEC Z20.09
Escherichia coli (E. coli) Z20.01
lead Z77.011
meningococcus Z20.811
mold (toxic) Z77.120
nickel dust Z77.018
noise Z77.122
parasitic disease Z20.7
pediculosis Z20.7
pfiesteria piscicida Z77.121
poliomyelitis Z20.89
pollution
air Z77.110
environmental NEC Z77.118
soil Z77.112
water Z77.111
polycyclic aromatic hydrocarbons Z77.028
rabies Z20.3
radiation, naturally occurring NEC Z77.123
radon Z77.123
red tide (Florida) Z77.121
rubella Z20.4
sexually-transmitted disease Z20.2
smallpox (laboratory) Z20.89
syphilis Z20.2
tuberculosis Z20.1
uranium Z77.012
varicella Z20.820
venereal disease Z20.2
viral disease NEC Z20.828
viral hepatitis Z20.5
water pollution Z77.111
Contamination, food — *see* Intoxication, foodborne
Contraception, contraceptive
advice Z30.09
counseling Z30.09
device (intrauterine) (in situ) Z97.5
causing menorrhagia T83.83
checking Z30.431
complications — *see* Complications, intrauterine, contraceptive device
in place Z97.5
initial prescription Z30.014
reinsertion Z30.433
removal Z30.432
replacement Z30.433
emergency (postcoital) Z30.012
initial prescription Z30.019
barrier Z30.018
diaphragm Z30.018
injectable Z30.013
intrauterine device Z30.014
pills Z30.011
postcoital (emergency) Z30.012
specified type NEC Z30.018
subdermal implantable Z30.017
transdermal patch hormonal Z30.016
vaginal ring hormonal Z30.015
maintenance Z30.40
barrier Z30.49
diaphragm Z30.49
examination Z30.8
injectable Z30.42
intrauterine device Z30.431
pills Z30.41
specified type NEC Z30.49
subdermal implantable Z30.46
transdermal patch hormonal Z30.45
vaginal ring hormonal Z30.44
management Z30.9
specified NEC Z30.8
postcoital (emergency) Z30.012
prescription Z30.019
repeat Z30.40
sterilization Z30.2
surveillance (drug) — *see* Contraception, maintenance
Contraction (s) , contracture, contracted
Achilles tendon — *see also* Short, tendon, Achilles
congenital Q66.89
amputation stump (surgical) (flexion) (late) (next proximal joint) T87.89
anus K59.8
bile duct (common) (hepatic) K83.8
bladder N32.89
neck or sphincter N32.0
bowel, cecum, colon or intestine, any part — *see* Obstruction, intestine
Braxton Hicks — *see* False, labor

Contraction (s) , contracture, contracted - *continued*
- breast implant, capsular T85.44
- bronchial J98.09
- burn (old) — *see* Cicatrix
- cervix — *see* Stricture, cervix
- cicatricial — *see* Cicatrix
- conjunctiva, trachomatous, active A71.1
  - sequelae (late effect) B94.0
- Dupuytren's M72.0
- eyelid — *see* Disorder, eyelid function
- fascia (lata) (postural) M72.8
  - Dupuytren's M72.0
  - palmar M72.0
  - plantar M72.2
- finger NEC — *see also* Deformity, finger
  - congenital Q68.1
  - joint — *see* Contraction, joint, hand
- flaccid — *see* Contraction, paralytic
- gallbladder K82.0
- heart valve — *see* Endocarditis
- hip — *see* Contraction, joint, hip
- hourglass
  - bladder N32.89
    - congenital Q64.79
  - gallbladder K82.0
    - congenital Q44.1
  - stomach K31.89
    - congenital Q40.2
    - psychogenic F45.8
  - uterus (complicating delivery) O62.4
- hysterical F44.4
- internal os — *see* Stricture, cervix
- joint (abduction) (acquired) (adduction) (flexion) (rotation) M24.50
  - ankle M24.57-
  - congenital NEC Q68.8
    - hip Q65.89
  - elbow M24.52-
  - foot joint M24.57-
  - hand joint M24.54-
  - hip M24.55-
    - congenital Q65.89
  - hysterical F44.4
  - knee M24.56-
  - shoulder M24.51-
  - wrist M24.53-
- kidney (granular) (secondary) N26.9
  - congenital Q63.8
  - hydronephritic — *see* Hydronephrosis
  - Page N26.2
  - pyelonephritic — *see* Pyelitis, chronic
  - tuberculous A18.11
- ligament — *see also* Disorder, ligament
  - congenital Q79.8
- muscle (postinfective) (postural) NEC M62.40
  - with contracture of joint — *see* Contraction, joint
  - ankle M62.47-
  - congenital Q79.8
    - sternocleidomastoid Q68.0
  - extraocular — *see* Strabismus
  - eye (extrinsic) — *see* Strabismus
  - foot M62.47-
  - forearm M62.43-
  - hand M62.44-
  - hysterical F44.4
  - ischemic (Volkmann's) T79.6
  - lower leg M62.46-
  - multiple sites M62.49
  - pelvic region M62.45-
  - posttraumatic — *see* Strabismus, paralytic
  - psychogenic F45.8
    - conversion reaction F44.4
  - shoulder region M62.41-
  - specified site NEC M62.48
  - thigh M62.45-
  - upper arm M62.42-
- neck — *see* Torticollis
- ocular muscle — *see* Strabismus
- organ or site, congenital NEC — *see* Atresia, by site
- outlet (pelvis) — *see* Contraction, pelvis
- palmar fascia M72.0
- paralytic
  - joint — *see* Contraction, joint
  - muscle — *see also* Contraction, muscle NEC
    - ocular — *see* Strabismus, paralytic
- pelvis (acquired) (general) M95.5
  - with disproportion (fetopelvic) O33.1
    - causing obstructed labor O65.1
    - inlet O33.2
    - mid-cavity O33.3
    - outlet O33.3
- plantar fascia M72.2

Contraction (s) , contracture, contracted - *continued*
- premature
  - atrium I49.1
  - auriculoventricular I49.49
  - heart I49.49
  - junctional I49.2
  - supraventricular I49.1
  - ventricular I49.3
- prostate N42.89
- pylorus NEC — *see also* Pylorospasm
  - psychogenic F45.8
- rectum, rectal (sphincter) K59.8
- ring (Bandl's) (complicating delivery) O62.4
- scar — *see* Cicatrix
- spine — *see* Dorsopathy, deforming
- sternocleidomastoid (muscle) , congenital Q68.0
- stomach K31.89
  - hourglass K31.89
    - congenital Q40.2
    - psychogenic F45.8
  - psychogenic F45.8
- tendon (sheath) M62.40
  - with contracture of joint — *see* Contraction, joint
    - Achilles — *see* Short, tendon, Achilles
  - ankle M62.47-
    - Achilles — *see* Short, tendon, Achilles
  - foot M62.47-
  - forearm M62.43-
  - hand M62.44-
  - lower leg M62.46-
  - multiple sites M62.49
  - neck M62.48
  - pelvic region M62.45-
  - shoulder region M62.41-
  - specified site NEC M62.48
  - thigh M62.45-
  - thorax M62.48
  - trunk M62.48
  - upper arm M62.42-
- toe — *see* Deformity, toe, specified NEC
- ureterovesical orifice (postinfectional) N13.5
  - with infection N13.6
- urethra — *see also* Stricture, urethra
  - orifice N32.0
- uterus N85.8
  - abnormal NEC O62.9
  - clonic (complicating delivery) O62.4
  - dyscoordinate (complicating delivery) O62.4
  - hourglass (complicating delivery) O62.4
  - hypertonic O62.4
  - hypotonic NEC O62.2
  - inadequate
    - primary O62.0
    - secondary O62.1
  - incoordinate (complicating delivery) O62.4
  - poor O62.2
  - tetanic (complicating delivery) O62.4
- vagina (outlet) N89.5
- vesical N32.89
  - neck or urethral orifice N32.0
- visual field — *see* Defect, visual field, generalized
- Volkmann's (ischemic) T79.6

Contusion (skin surface intact) T14.8
- abdomen, abdominal (muscle) (wall) S30.1
- adnexa, eye NEC S05.8X-
- adrenal gland S37.812
- alveolar process S00.532
- ankle S90.0-
- antecubital space — *see* Contusion, forearm
- anus S30.3
- arm (upper) S40.02-
  - lower (with elbow) — *see* Contusion, forearm
- auditory canal — *see* Contusion, ear
- auricle — *see* Contusion, ear
- axilla — *see* Contusion, arm, upper
- back — *see also* Contusion, thorax, back
  - lower S30.0
- bile duct S36.13
- bladder S37.22
- bone NEC T14.8
- brain (diffuse) — *see* Injury, intracranial, diffuse
  - focal — *see* Injury, intracranial, focal
- brainstem S06.38-
- breast S20.0-
- broad ligament S37.892
- brow S00.83
- buttock S30.0
- canthus, eye S00.1-
- cauda equina S34.3
- cerebellar, traumatic S06.37-
- cerebral S06.33-
  - left side S06.32-

Contusion (skin surface intact) - *continued*
- cerebral - *continued*
  - right side S06.31-
- cheek S00.83
  - internal S00.532
- chest (wall) — *see* Contusion, thorax
- chin S00.83
- clitoris S30.23
- colon — *see* Injury, intestine, large, contusion
- common bile duct S36.13
- conjunctiva S05.1-
  - with foreign body (in conjunctival sac) — *see* Foreign body, conjunctival sac
- conus medullaris (spine) S34.139
- cornea — *see* Contusion, eyeball
  - with foreign body — *see* Foreign body, cornea
- corpus cavernosum S30.21
- cortex (brain) (cerebral) — *see* Injury, intracranial, diffuse
  - focal — *see* Injury, intracranial, focal
- costal region — *see* Contusion, thorax
- cystic duct S36.13
- diaphragm S27.802
- duodenum S36.420
- ear S00.43-
- elbow S50.0-
  - with forearm — *see* Contusion, forearm
- epididymis S30.22
- epigastric region S30.1
- epiglottis S10.0
- esophagus (thoracic) S27.812
  - cervical S10.0
- eyeball S05.1-
- eyebrow S00.1-
- eyelid (and periocular area) S00.1-
- face NEC S00.83
- fallopian tube S37.529
  - bilateral S37.522
  - unilateral S37.521
- femoral triangle S30.1
- finger (s) S60.00
  - with damage to nail (matrix) S60.10
  - index S60.02-
    - with damage to nail S60.12-
  - little S60.05-
    - with damage to nail S60.15-
  - middle S60.03-
    - with damage to nail S60.13-
  - ring S60.04-
    - with damage to nail S60.14-
  - thumb — *see* Contusion, thumb
- flank S30.1
- foot (except toe (s) alone) S90.3-
  - toe — *see* Contusion, toe
- forearm S50.1-
  - elbow only — *see* Contusion, elbow
- forehead S00.83
- gallbladder S36.122
- genital organs, external
  - female S30.202
  - male S30.201
- globe (eye) — *see* Contusion, eyeball
- groin S30.1
- gum S00.532
- hand S60.22-
  - finger (s) — *see* Contusion, finger
  - wrist — *see* Contusion, wrist
- head S00.93
  - ear — *see* Contusion, ear
  - eyelid — *see* Contusion, eyelid
  - lip S00.531
  - nose S00.33
  - oral cavity S00.532
  - scalp S00.03
  - specified part NEC S00.83
- heart — *see also* Injury, heart S26.91
- heel — *see* Contusion, foot
- hepatic duct S36.13
- hip S70.0-
- ileum S36.428
- iliac region S30.1
- inguinal region S30.1
- interscapular region S20.229
- intra-abdominal organ S36.92
  - colon — *see* Injury, intestine, large, contusion
  - liver S36.112
  - pancreas — *see* Contusion, pancreas
  - rectum S36.62
  - small intestine — *see* Injury, intestine, small, contusion
  - specified organ NEC S36.892
  - spleen — *see* Contusion, spleen
  - stomach S36.32

Contusion (skin surface intact) - *continued*
  iris (eye) — *see* Contusion, eyeball
  jaw S00.83
  jejunum S36.428
  kidney S37.01-
    major (greater than 2 cm) S37.02-
    minor (less than 2 cm) S37.01-
  knee S80.0-
  labium (majus) (minus) S30.23
  lacrimal apparatus, gland or sac S05.8X-
  larynx S10.0
  leg (lower) S80.1-
    knee — *see* Contusion, knee
  lens — *see* Contusion, eyeball
  lip S00.531
  liver S36.112
  lower back S30.0
  lumbar region S30.0
  lung S27.329
    bilateral S27.322
    unilateral S27.321
  malar region S00.83
  mastoid region S00.83
  membrane, brain — *see* Injury, intracranial, diffuse
    focal — *see* Injury, intracranial, focal
  mesentery S36.892
  mesosalpinx S37.892
  mouth S00.532
  muscle — *see* Contusion, by site
  nail
    finger — *see* Contusion, finger, with damage to nail
    toe — *see* Contusion, toe, with damage to nail
  nasal S00.33
  neck S10.93
    specified site NEC S10.83
    throat S10.0
  nerve — *see* Injury, nerve
  newborn P54.5
  nose S00.33
  occipital
    lobe (brain) — *see* Injury, intracranial, diffuse
    focal — *see* Injury, intracranial, focal
    region (scalp) S00.03
  orbit (region) (tissues) S05.1-
  ovary S37.429
    bilateral S37.422
    unilateral S37.421
  palate S00.532
  pancreas S36.229
    body S36.221
    head S36.220
    tail S36.222
  parietal
    lobe (brain) — *see* Injury, intracranial, diffuse
    focal — *see* Injury, intracranial, focal
    region (scalp) S00.03
  pelvic organ S37.92
    adrenal gland S37.812
    bladder S37.22
    fallopian tube — *see* Contusion, fallopian tube
    kidney — *see* Contusion, kidney
    ovary — *see* Contusion, ovary
    prostate S37.822
    specified organ NEC S37.892
    ureter S37.12
    urethra S37.32
    uterus S37.62
  pelvis S30.0
  penis S30.21
  perineum
    female S30.23
    male S30.0
  periocular area S00.1-
  peritoneum S36.81
  periurethral tissue — *see* Contusion, urethra
  pharynx S10.0
  pinna — *see* Contusion, ear
  popliteal space — *see* Contusion, knee
  prepuce S30.21
  prostate S37.822
  pubic region S30.1
  pudendum
    female S30.202
    male S30.201
  quadriceps femoris — *see* Contusion, thigh
  rectum S36.62
  retroperitoneum S36.892
  round ligament S37.892
  sacral region S30.0
  scalp S00.03
    due to birth injury P12.3
  scapular region — *see* Contusion, shoulder

Contusion (skin surface intact) - *continued*
  sclera — *see* Contusion, eyeball
  scrotum S30.22
  seminal vesicle S37.892
  shoulder S40.01-
  skin NEC T14.8
  small intestine — *see* Injury, intestine, small, contusion
  spermatic cord S30.22
  spinal cord — *see* Injury, spinal cord, by region
    cauda equina S34.3
    conus medullaris S34.139
  spleen S36.029
    major S36.021
    minor S36.020
  sternal region S20.219
  stomach S36.32
  subconjunctival S05.1-
  subcutaneous NEC T14.8
  submaxillary region S00.83
  submental region S00.83
  subperiosteal NEC T14.8
  subungual
    finger — *see* Contusion, finger, with damage to nail
    toe — *see* Contusion, toe, with damage to nail
  supraclavicular fossa S10.83
  supraorbital S00.83
  suprarenal gland S37.812
  temple (region) S00.83
  temporal
    lobe (brain) — *see* Injury, intracranial, diffuse
    focal — *see* Injury, intracranial, focal
    region S00.83
  testis S30.22
  thigh S70.1-
  thorax (wall) S20.20
    back S20.22-
    front S20.21-
  throat S10.0
  thumb S60.01-
    with damage to nail S60.11-
  toe (s) (lesser) S90.12-
    with damage to nail S90.22-
    great S90.11-
      with damage to nail S90.21-
      specified type NEC S90.221
  tongue S00.532
  trachea (cervical) S10.0
    thoracic S27.52
  tunica vaginalis S30.22
  tympanum, tympanic membrane — *see* Contusion, ear
  ureter S37.12
  urethra S37.32
  urinary organ NEC S37.892
  uterus S37.62
  uvula S00.532
  vagina S30.23
  vas deferens S37.892
  vesical S37.22
  vocal cord (s) S10.0
  vulva S30.23
  wrist S60.21-
Conus (congenital) (any type) Q14.8
  cornea — *see* Keratoconus
  medullaris syndrome G95.81
Conversion hysteria, neurosis or reaction F44.9
Converter, tuberculosis (test reaction) R76.11
Conviction (legal) **, anxiety concerning** Z65.0
  with imprisonment Z65.1
Convulsions (idiopathic) — *see also* Seizure(s) R56.9
  apoplectiform (cerebral ischemia) I67.82
  dissociative F44.5
  epileptic — *see* Epilepsy
  epileptiform, epileptoid — *see* Seizure, epileptiform
  ether (anesthetic) — *see* Table of Drugs and Chemicals, by drug
  febrile R56.00
    with status epilepticus G40.901
    complex R56.01
      with status epilepticus G40.901
    simple R56.00
  hysterical F44.5
  infantile P90
    epilepsy — *see* Epilepsy
  jacksonian — *see* Epilepsy, localization-related, symptomatic, with simple partial seizures
  myoclonic G25.3
  newborn P90
  obstetrical (nephritic) (uremic) — *see* Eclampsia
  paretic A52.17
  post traumatic R56.1

Convulsions (idiopathic) - *continued*
  psychomotor — *see* Epilepsy, localization-related, symptomatic, with complex partial seizures
  recurrent R56.9
  reflex R25.8
  scarlatinal A38.8
  tetanus, tetanic — *see* Tetanus
  thymic E32.8
Convulsive — *see also* Convulsions
Cooley's anemia D56.1
Coolie itch B76.9
Cooper's
  disease — *see* Mastopathy, cystic
  hernia — *see* Hernia, abdomen, specified site NEC
Copra itch B88.0
Coprophagy F50.89
Coprophobia F40.298
Coproporphyria, hereditary E80.29
Cor
  biloculare Q20.8
  bovis, bovinum — *see* Hypertrophy, cardiac
  pulmonale (chronic) I27.81
    acute I26.09
  triatriatum, triatrium Q24.2
  triloculare Q20.8
    biatrium Q20.4
    biventriculare Q21.1
Corbus' disease (gangrenous balanitis) N48.1
Cord — *see also* condition
  around neck (tightly) (with compression) complicating delivery O69.1
  bladder G95.89
  tabetic A52.19
Cordis ectopia Q24.8
Corditis (spermatic) N49.1
Corectopia Q13.2
Cori's disease (glycogen storage) E74.03
Corkhandler's disease or lung J67.3
Corkscrew esophagus K22.4
Corkworker's disease or lung J67.3
Corn (infected) L84
Cornea — *see also* condition
  donor Z52.5
  plana Q13.4
Cornelia de Lange syndrome Q87.1
Cornu cutaneum L85.8
Cornual gestation or pregnancy O00.80
  with intrauterine pregnancy O00.81
Coronary (artery) — *see* condition
Coronavirus, as cause of disease classified elsewhere B97.29
  SARS-associated B97.21
Corpora — *see also* condition
  amylacea, prostate N42.89
  cavernosa — *see* condition
Corpulence — *see* Obesity
Corpus — *see* condition
Corrected transposition Q20.5
Corrosion (injury) (acid) (caustic) (chemical) (lime) (external) (internal) T30.4
  abdomen, abdominal (muscle) (wall) T21.42
    first degree T21.52
    second degree T21.62
    third degree T21.72
  above elbow T22.439
    first degree T22.539
    left T22.432
      first degree T22.532
      second degree T22.632
      third degree T22.732
    right T22.431
      first degree T22.531
      second degree T22.631
      third degree T22.731
    second degree T22.639
    third degree T22.739
  alimentary tract NEC T28.7
  ankle T25.419
    first degree T25.519
    left T25.412
      first degree T25.512
      second degree T25.612
      third degree T25.712
    multiple with foot — *see* Corrosion, lower, limb, multiple, ankle and foot
    right T25.411
      first degree T25.511
      second degree T25.611
      third degree T25.711
    second degree T25.619
    third degree T25.719
  anus — *see* Corrosion, buttock

Corrosion (injury) (acid) (caustic) (chemical) (lime) (external) (internal) - *continued*
  arm (s) (meaning upper limb (s)) — *see* Corrosion, upper limb
  axilla T22.449
    first degree T22.549
    left T22.442
      first degree T22.542
      second degree T22.642
      third degree T22.742
    right T22.441
      first degree T22.541
      second degree T22.641
      third degree T22.741
    second degree T22.649
    third degree T22.749
  back (lower) T21.44
    first degree T21.54
    second degree T21.64
    third degree T21.74
    upper T21.43
      first degree T21.53
      second degree T21.63
      third degree T21.73
  blisters - code as Corrosion, second degree, by site
  breast (s) — *see* Corrosion, chest wall
  buttock (s) T21.45
    first degree T21.55
    second degree T21.65
    third degree T21.75
  calf T24.439
    first degree T24.539
    left T24.432
      first degree T24.532
      second degree T24.632
      third degree T24.732
    right T24.431
      first degree T24.531
      second degree T24.631
      third degree T24.731
    second degree T24.639
    third degree T24.739
  canthus (eye) — *see* Corrosion, eyelid
  cervix T28.8
  cheek T20.46
    first degree T20.56
    second degree T20.66
    third degree T20.76
  chest wall T21.41
    first degree T21.51
    second degree T21.61
    third degree T21.71
  chin T20.43
    first degree T20.53
    second degree T20.63
    third degree T20.73
  colon T28.7
  conjunctiva (and cornea) — *see* Corrosion, cornea
  cornea (and conjunctiva) T26.6-
  deep necrosis of underlying tissue - code as Corrosion, third degree, by site
  dorsum of hand T23.469
    first degree T23.569
    left T23.462
      first degree T23.562
      second degree T23.662
      third degree T23.762
    right T23.461
      first degree T23.561
      second degree T23.661
      third degree T23.761
    second degree T23.669
    third degree T23.769
  ear (auricle) (external) (canal) T20.41
    drum T28.91
    first degree T20.51
    second degree T20.61
    third degree T20.71
  elbow T22.429
    first degree T22.529
    left T22.422
      first degree T22.522
      second degree T22.622
      third degree T22.722
    right T22.421
      first degree T22.521
      second degree T22.621
      third degree T22.721
    second degree T22.629
    third degree T22.729
  entire body — *see* Corrosion, multiple body regions
  epidermal loss - code as Corrosion, second degree, by site

Corrosion (injury) (acid) (caustic) (chemical) (lime) (external) (internal) - *continued*
  epiglottis T27.4
  erythema, erythematous - code as Corrosion, first degree, by site
  esophagus T28.6
  extent (percentage of body surface)
    less than 10 per cent T32.0
    10-19 per cent (0-9 percent third degree) T32.10
      with 10-19 percent third degree T32.11
    20-29 per cent (0-9 percent third degree) T32.20
      with
        10-19 percent third degree T32.21
        20-29 percent third degree T32.22
    30-39 per cent (0-9 percent third degree) T32.30
      with
        10-19 percent third degree T32.31
        20-29 percent third degree T32.32
        30-39 percent third degree T32.33
    40-49 per cent (0-9 percent third degree) T32.40
      with
        10-19 percent third degree T32.41
        20-29 percent third degree T32.42
        30-39 percent third degree T32.43
        40-49 percent third degree T32.44
    50-59 per cent (0-9 percent third degree) T32.50
      with
        10-19 percent third degree T32.51
        20-29 percent third degree T32.52
        30-39 percent third degree T32.53
        40-49 percent third degree T32.54
        50-59 percent third degree T32.55
    60-69 per cent (0-9 percent third degree) T32.60
      with
        10-19 percent third degree T32.61
        20-29 percent third degree T32.62
        30-39 percent third degree T32.63
        40-49 percent third degree T32.64
        50-59 percent third degree T32.65
        60-69 percent third degree T32.66
    70-79 per cent (0-9 percent third degree) T32.70
      with
        10-19 percent third degree T32.71
        20-29 percent third degree T32.72
        30-39 percent third degree T32.73
        40-49 percent third degree T32.74
        50-59 percent third degree T32.75
        60-69 percent third degree T32.76
        70-79 percent third degree T32.77
    80-89 per cent (0-9 percent third degree) T32.80
      with
        10-19 percent third degree T32.81
        20-29 percent third degree T32.82
        30-39 percent third degree T32.83
        40-49 percent third degree T32.84
        50-59 percent third degree T32.85
        60-69 percent third degree T32.86
        70-79 percent third degree T32.87
        80-89 percent third degree T32.88
    90 per cent or more (0-9 percent third degree) T32.90
      with
        10-19 percent third degree T32.91
        20-29 percent third degree T32.92
        30-39 percent third degree T32.93
        40-49 percent third degree T32.94
        50-59 percent third degree T32.95
        60-69 percent third degree T32.96
        70-79 percent third degree T32.97
        80-89 percent third degree T32.98
        90-99 percent third degree T32.99
  extremity — *see* Corrosion, limb
  eye (s) and adnexa T26.9-
    with resulting rupture and destruction of eyeball T26.7-
    conjunctival sac — *see* Corrosion, cornea
    cornea — *see* Corrosion, cornea
    lid — *see* Corrosion, eyelid
    periocular area — *see* Corrosion eyelid
    specified site NEC T26.8-
  eyeball — *see* Corrosion, eye
  eyelid (s) T26.5-
  face — *see* Corrosion, head
  finger T23.429
    first degree T23.529
    left T23.422
      first degree T23.522
      second degree T23.622
      third degree T23.722
    multiple sites (without thumb) T23.439
      with thumb T23.449
        first degree T23.549
        left T23.442

Corrosion (injury) (acid) (caustic) (chemical) (lime) (external) (internal) - *continued*
  finger - *continued*
    multiple sites (without thumb) - *continued*
      with thumb - *continued*
        left - *continued*
          first degree T23.542
          second degree T23.642
          third degree T23.742
        right T23.441
          first degree T23.541
          second degree T23.641
          third degree T23.741
        second degree T23.649
        third degree T23.749
      first degree T23.539
      left T23.432
        first degree T23.532
        second degree T23.632
        third degree T23.732
      right T23.431
        first degree T23.531
        second degree T23.631
        third degree T23.731
      second degree T23.639
      third degree T23.739
    right T23.421
      first degree T23.521
      second degree T23.621
      third degree T23.721
    second degree T23.629
    third degree T23.729
  flank — *see* Corrosion, abdomen
  foot T25.429
    first degree T25.529
    left T25.422
      first degree T25.522
      second degree T25.622
      third degree T25.722
    multiple with ankle — *see* Corrosion, lower, limb, multiple, ankle and foot
    right T25.421
      first degree T25.521
      second degree T25.621
      third degree T25.721
    second degree T25.629
    third degree T25.729
  forearm T22.419
    first degree T22.519
    left T22.412
      first degree T22.512
      second degree T22.612
      third degree T22.712
    right T22.411
      first degree T22.511
      second degree T22.611
      third degree T22.711
    second degree T22.619
    third degree T22.719
  forehead T20.46
    first degree T20.56
    second degree T20.66
    third degree T20.76
  fourth degree - code as Corrosion, third degree, by site
  full thickness skin loss - code as Corrosion, third degree, by site
  gastrointestinal tract NEC T28.7
  genital organs
    external
      female T21.47
        first degree T21.57
        second degree T21.67
        third degree T21.77
      male T21.46
        first degree T21.56
        second degree T21.66
        third degree T21.76
    internal T28.8
  groin — *see* Corrosion, abdominal wall
  hand (s) T23.409
    back — *see* Corrosion, dorsum of hand
    finger — *see* Corrosion, finger
    first degree T23.509
    left T23.402
      first degree T23.502
      second degree T23.602
      third degree T23.702
    multiple sites with wrist T23.499
      first degree T23.599
      left T23.492
        first degree T23.592
        second degree T23.692

Corrosion (injury) (acid) (caustic) (chemical) (lime) (external) (internal) - *continued*
  hand (s) - *continued*
    multiple sites with wrist - *continued*
      left - *continued*
        third degree T23.792
      right T23.491
        first degree T23.591
        second degree T23.691
        third degree T23.791
      second degree T23.699
      third degree T23.799
    palm — *see* Corrosion, palm
    right T23.401
      first degree T23.501
      second degree T23.601
      third degree T23.701
    second degree T23.609
    third degree T23.709
    thumb — *see* Corrosion, thumb
  head (and face) (and neck) T20.40
    cheek — *see* Corrosion, cheek
    chin — *see* Corrosion, chin
    ear — *see* Corrosion, ear
    eye (s) only — *see* Corrosion, eye
    first degree T20.50
    forehead — *see* Corrosion, forehead
    lip — *see* Corrosion, lip
    multiple sites T20.49
      first degree T20.59
      second degree T20.69
      third degree T20.79
    neck — *see* Corrosion, neck
    nose — *see* Corrosion, nose
    scalp — *see* Corrosion, scalp
    second degree T20.60
    third degree T20.70
  hip (s) — *see* Corrosion, lower, limb
  inhalation — *see* Corrosion, respiratory tract
  internal organ (s) — *see also* Corrosion, by
    site T28.90
    alimentary tract T28.7
      esophagus T28.6
    esophagus T28.6
    genitourinary T28.8
    mouth T28.5
    pharynx T28.5
    specified organ NEC T28.99
  interscapular region — *see* Corrosion, back, upper
  intestine (large) (small) T28.7
  knee T24.429
    first degree T24.529
    left T24.422
      first degree T24.522
      second degree T24.622
      third degree T24.722
    right T24.421
      first degree T24.521
      second degree T24.621
      third degree T24.721
    second degree T24.629
    third degree T24.729
  labium (majus) (minus) — *see* Corrosion, genital organs, external, female
  lacrimal apparatus, duct, gland or sac — *see* Corrosion, eye, specified site NEC
  larynx T27.4
    with lung T27.5
  leg (s) (meaning lower limb (s)) — *see* Corrosion, lower limb
  limb (s)
    lower — *see* Corrosion, lower, limb
    upper — *see* Corrosion, upper limb
  lip (s) T20.42
    first degree T20.52
    second degree T20.62
    third degree T20.72
  lower
    back — *see* Corrosion, back
    limb T24.409
      ankle — *see* Corrosion, ankle
      calf — *see* Corrosion, calf
      first degree T24.509
      foot — *see* Corrosion, foot
      knee — *see* Corrosion, knee
      left T24.402
        first degree T24.502
        second degree T24.602
        third degree T24.702
      multiple sites, except ankle and foot T24.499
        ankle and foot T25.499
          first degree T25.599
          left T25.492

Corrosion (injury) (acid) (caustic) (chemical) (lime) (external) (internal) - *continued*
  lower - *continued*
    limb - *continued*
      multiple sites, except ankle and foot - *continued*
        ankle and foot - *continued*
          left - *continued*
            first degree T25.592
            second degree T25.692
            third degree T25.792
          right T25.491
            first degree T25.591
            second degree T25.691
            third degree T25.791
          second degree T25.699
          third degree T25.799
        first degree T24.599
        left T24.492
          first degree T24.592
          second degree T24.692
          third degree T24.792
        right T24.491
          first degree T24.591
          second degree T24.691
          third degree T24.791
        second degree T24.699
        third degree T24.799
      right T24.401
        first degree T24.501
        second degree T24.601
        third degree T24.701
      second degree T24.609
      hip — *see* Corrosion, thigh
      thigh — *see* Corrosion, thigh
      third degree T24.709
  lung (with larynx and trachea) T27.5
  mouth T28.5
  neck T20.47
    first degree T20.57
    second degree T20.67
    third degree T20.77
  nose (septum) T20.44
    first degree T20.54
    second degree T20.64
    third degree T20.74
  ocular adnexa — *see* Corrosion, eye
  orbit region — *see* Corrosion, eyelid
  palm T23.459
    first degree T23.559
    left T23.452
      first degree T23.552
      second degree T23.652
      third degree T23.752
    right T23.451
      first degree T23.551
      second degree T23.651
      third degree T23.751
    second degree T23.659
    third degree T23.759
  partial thickness - code as Corrosion, unspecified degree, by site
  pelvis — *see* Corrosion, trunk
  penis — *see* Corrosion, genital organs, external, male
  perineum
    female — *see* Corrosion, genital organs, external, female
    male — *see* Corrosion, genital organs, external, male
  periocular area — *see* Corrosion, eyelid
  pharynx T28.5
  rectum T28.7
  respiratory tract T27.7
    larynx — *see* Corrosion, larynx
    specified part NEC T27.6
    trachea — *see* Corrosion, larynx
  sac, lacrimal — *see* Corrosion, eye, specified site NEC
  scalp T20.45
    first degree T20.55
    second degree T20.65
    third degree T20.75
  scapular region T22.469
    first degree T22.569
    left T22.462
      first degree T22.562
      second degree T22.662
      third degree T22.762
    right T22.461
      first degree T22.561
      second degree T22.661
      third degree T22.761
    second degree T22.669

Corrosion (injury) (acid) (caustic) (chemical) (lime) (external) (internal) - *continued*
  scapular region - *continued*
    third degree T22.769
  sclera — *see* Corrosion, eye, specified site NEC
  scrotum — *see* Corrosion, genital organs, external, male
  shoulder T22.459
    first degree T22.559
    left T22.452
      first degree T22.552
      second degree T22.652
      third degree T22.752
    right T22.451
      first degree T22.551
      second degree T22.651
      third degree T22.751
    second degree T22.659
    third degree T22.759
  stomach T28.7
  temple — *see* Corrosion, head
  testis — *see* Corrosion, genital organs, external, male
  thigh T24.419
    first degree T24.519
    left T24.412
      first degree T24.512
      second degree T24.612
      third degree T24.712
    right T24.411
      first degree T24.511
      second degree T24.611
      third degree T24.711
    second degree T24.619
    third degree T24.719
  thorax (external) — *see* Corrosion, trunk
  throat (meaning pharynx) T28.5
  thumb (s) T23.419
    first degree T23.519
    left T23.412
      first degree T23.512
      second degree T23.612
      third degree T23.712
    multiple sites with fingers T23.449
      first degree T23.549
      left T23.442
        first degree T23.542
        second degree T23.642
        third degree T23.742
      right T23.441
        first degree T23.541
        second degree T23.641
        third degree T23.741
      second degree T23.649
      third degree T23.749
    right T23.411
      first degree T23.511
      second degree T23.611
      third degree T23.711
    second degree T23.619
    third degree T23.719
  toe T25.439
    first degree T25.539
    left T25.432
      first degree T25.532
      second degree T25.632
      third degree T25.732
    right T25.431
      first degree T25.531
      second degree T25.631
      third degree T25.731
    second degree T25.639
    third degree T25.739
  tongue T28.5
  tonsil (s) T28.5
  total body — *see* Corrosion, multiple body regions
  trachea T27.4
    with lung T27.5
  trunk T21.40
    abdominal wall — *see* Corrosion, abdominal wall
    anus — *see* Corrosion, buttock
    axilla — *see* Corrosion, upper limb
    back — *see* Corrosion, back
    breast — *see* Corrosion, chest wall
    buttock — *see* Corrosion, buttock
    chest wall — *see* Corrosion, chest wall
    first degree T21.50
    flank — *see* Corrosion, abdominal wall
    genital
      female — *see* Corrosion, genital organs, external, female
      male — *see* Corrosion, genital organs, external, male

Corrosion (injury) (acid) (caustic) (chemical) (lime) (external) (internal) - *continued*
  trunk - *continued*
    groin — *see* Corrosion, abdominal wall
    interscapular region — *see* Corrosion, back, upper
    labia — *see* Corrosion, genital organs, external, female
    lower back — *see* Corrosion, back
    penis — *see* Corrosion, genital organs, external, male
    perineum
      female — *see* Corrosion, genital organs, external, female
      male — *see* Corrosion, genital organs, external, male
    scapular region — *see* Corrosion, upper limb
    scrotum — *see* Corrosion, genital organs, external, male
    second degree T21.60
    shoulder — *see* Corrosion, upper limb
    specified site NEC T21.49
      first degree T21.59
      second degree T21.69
      third degree T21.79
    testes — *see* Corrosion, genital organs, external, male
    third degree T21.70
    upper back — *see* Corrosion, back, upper
    vagina T28.8
    vulva — *see* Corrosion, genital organs, external, female
  unspecified site with extent of body surface involved specified
    less than 10 per cent T32.0
    10-19 per cent (0-9 percent third degree) T32.10
      with 10-19 percent third degree T32.11
    20-29 per cent (0-9 percent third degree) T32.20
      with
        10-19 percent third degree T32.21
        20-29 percent third degree T32.22
    30-39 per cent (0-9 percent third degree) T32.30
      with
        10-19 percent third degree T32.31
        20-29 percent third degree T32.32
        30-39 percent third degree T32.33
    40-49 per cent (0-9 percent third degree) T32.40
      with
        10-19 percent third degree T32.41
        20-29 percent third degree T32.42
        30-39 percent third degree T32.43
        40-49 percent third degree T32.44
    50-59 per cent (0-9 percent third degree) T32.50
      with
        10-19 percent third degree T32.51
        20-29 percent third degree T32.52
        30-39 percent third degree T32.53
        40-49 percent third degree T32.54
        50-59 percent third degree T32.55
    60-69 per cent (0-9 percent third degree) T32.60
      with
        10-19 percent third degree T32.61
        20-29 percent third degree T32.62
        30-39 percent third degree T32.63
        40-49 percent third degree T32.64
        50-59 percent third degree T32.65
        60-69 percent third degree T32.66
    70-79 per cent (0-9 percent third degree) T32.70
      with
        10-19 percent third degree T32.71
        20-29 percent third degree T32.72
        30-39 percent third degree T32.73
        40-49 percent third degree T32.74
        50-59 percent third degree T32.75
        60-69 percent third degree T32.76
        70-79 percent third degree T32.77
    80-89 per cent (0-9 percent third degree) T32.80
      with
        10-19 percent third degree T32.81
        20-29 percent third degree T32.82
        30-39 percent third degree T32.83
        40-49 percent third degree T32.84
        50-59 percent third degree T32.85
        60-69 percent third degree T32.86
        70-79 percent third degree T32.87
        80-89 percent third degree T32.88
    90 per cent or more (0-9 percent third degree) T32.90
      with
        10-19 percent third degree T32.91
        20-29 percent third degree T32.92
        30-39 percent third degree T32.93
        40-49 percent third degree T32.94
        50-59 percent third degree T32.95

Corrosion (injury) (acid) (caustic) (chemical) (lime) (external) (internal) - *continued*
  unspecified site with extent of body surface involved specified - *continued*
    90 per cent or more (0-9 percent third degree) - *continued*
      with - *continued*
        60-69 percent third degree T32.96
        70-79 percent third degree T32.97
        80-89 percent third degree T32.98
        90-99 percent third degree T32.99
  upper limb (axilla) (scapular region) T22.40
    above elbow — *see* Corrosion, above elbow
    axilla — *see* Corrosion, axilla
    elbow — *see* Corrosion, elbow
    first degree T22.50
    forearm — *see* Corrosion, forearm
    hand — *see* Corrosion, hand
    interscapular region — *see* Corrosion, back, upper
    multiple sites T22.499
      first degree T22.599
      left T22.492
        first degree T22.592
        second degree T22.692
        third degree T22.792
      right T22.491
        first degree T22.591
        second degree T22.691
        third degree T22.791
      second degree T22.699
      third degree T22.799
    scapular region — *see* Corrosion, scapular region
    second degree T22.60
    shoulder — *see* Corrosion, shoulder
    third degree T22.70
    wrist — *see* Corrosion, hand
  uterus T28.8
  vagina T28.8
  vulva — *see* Corrosion, genital organs, external, female
  wrist T23.479
    first degree T23.579
    left T23.472
      first degree T23.572
      second degree T23.672
      third degree T23.772
    multiple sites with hand T23.499
      first degree T23.599
      left T23.492
        first degree T23.592
        second degree T23.692
        third degree T23.792
      right T23.491
        first degree T23.591
        second degree T23.691
        third degree T23.791
      second degree T23.699
      third degree T23.799
    right T23.471
      first degree T23.571
      second degree T23.671
      third degree T23.771
    second degree T23.679
    third degree T23.779
Corrosive burn — *see* Corrosion
Corsican fever — *see* Malaria
Cortical — *see* condition
Cortico-adrenal — *see* condition
Coryza (acute) J00
  with grippe or influenza — *see* Influenza, with, respiratory manifestations NEC
  syphilitic
    congenital (chronic) A50.05
Costen's syndrome or complex M26.69
Costiveness — *see* Constipation
Costochondritis M94.0
Cot death R99
Cotard's syndrome F22
Cotia virus B08.8
Cotton wool spots (retinal) H35.81
Cotungo's disease — *see* Sciatica
Cough (affected) (chronic) (epidemic) (nervous) R05
  with hemorrhage — *see* Hemoptysis
  bronchial R05
    with grippe or influenza — *see* Influenza, with, respiratory manifestations NEC
  functional F45.8
  hysterical F45.8
  laryngeal, spasmodic R05
  psychogenic F45.8
  smokers' J41.0
  tea taster's B49

Counseling (for) Z71.9
  abuse NEC
    perpetrator Z69.82
    victim Z69.81
  alcohol abuser Z71.41
    family Z71.42
  child abuse
    nonparental
      perpetrator Z69.021
      victim Z69.020
    parental
      perpetrator Z69.011
      victim Z69.010
  consanguinity Z71.89
  contraceptive Z30.09
  dietary Z71.3
  drug abuser Z71.51
    family member Z71.52
  family Z71.89
  fertility preservation (prior to cancer therapy) (prior to removal of gonads) Z31.62
  for non-attending third party Z71.0
    related to sexual behavior or orientation Z70.2
  genetic NEC Z31.5
  gestational carrier Z31.7
  health (advice) (education) (instruction) — *see* Counseling, medical
  human immunodeficiency virus (HIV) Z71.7
  impotence Z70.1
  insulin pump use Z46.81
  medical (for) Z71.9
    boarding school resident Z59.3
    consanguinity Z71.89
    feared complaint and no disease found Z71.1
    human immunodeficiency virus (HIV) Z71.7
    institutional resident Z59.3
    on behalf of another Z71.0
      related to sexual behavior or orientation Z70.2
    person living alone Z60.2
    specified reason NEC Z71.89
  natural family planning
    procreative Z31.61
    to avoid pregnancy Z30.02
  perpetrator (of)
    abuse NEC Z69.82
    child abuse
      non-parental Z69.021
      parental Z69.011
    rape NEC Z69.82
    spousal abuse Z69.12
  procreative NEC Z31.69
    fertility preservation (prior to cancer therapy) (prior to removal of gonads) Z31.62
    using natural family planning Z31.61
  promiscuity Z70.1
  rape victim Z69.81
  religious Z71.81
  sex, sexual (related to) Z70.9
    attitude (s) Z70.0
    behavior or orientation Z70.1
    combined concerns Z70.3
    non-responsiveness Z70.1
    on behalf of third party Z70.2
    specified reason NEC Z70.8
  specified reason NEC Z71.89
  spiritual Z71.81
  spousal abuse (perpetrator) Z69.12
    victim Z69.11
  substance abuse Z71.89
    alcohol Z71.41
    drug Z71.51
    tobacco Z71.6
  tobacco use Z71.6
  use (of)
    insulin pump Z46.81
  victim (of)
    abuse Z69.81
    child abuse
      by parent Z69.010
      non-parental Z69.020
    rape NEC Z69.81
Coupled rhythm R00.8
Couvelaire syndrome or uterus
  (complicating delivery) O45.8X-
Cowperitis — *see* Urethritis
Cowper's gland — *see* condition
Cowpox B08.010
  due to vaccination T88.1
Coxa
  magna M91.4-
  plana M91.2-
  valga (acquired) — *see also* Deformity, limb, specified type NEC, thigh

Coxa - *continued*
valga (acquired) - *continued*
congenital Q65.81
sequelae (late effect) of rickets E64.3
vara (acquired) — *see also* Deformity, limb,
specified type NEC, thigh
congenital Q65.82
sequelae (late effect) of rickets E64.3
Coxalgia, coxalgic (nontuberculous) — *see also* Pain,
joint, hip
tuberculous A18.02
Coxitis — *see* Monoarthritis, hip
Coxsackie (virus) (infection) B34.1
as cause of disease classified elsewhere B97.11
carditis B33.20
central nervous system NEC A88.8
endocarditis B33.21
enteritis A08.39
meningitis (aseptic) A87.0
myocarditis B33.22
pericarditis B33.23
pharyngitis B08.5
pleurodynia B33.0
specific disease NEC B33.8
Crabs, meaning pubic lice B85.3
Crack baby P04.41
Cracked nipple N64.0
associated with
lactation O92.13
pregnancy O92.11-
puerperium O92.12
Cracked tooth K03.81
Cradle cap L21.0
Craft neurosis F48.8
Cramp (s) R25.2
abdominal — *see* Pain, abdominal
bathing T75.1
colic R10.83
psychogenic F45.8
due to immersion T75.1
fireman T67.2
heat T67.2
immersion T75.1
intestinal — *see* Pain, abdominal
psychogenic F45.8
leg, sleep related G47.62
limb (lower) (upper) NEC R25.2
sleep related G47.62
linotypist's F48.8
organic G25.89
muscle (limb) (general) R25.2
due to immersion T75.1
psychogenic F45.8
occupational (hand) F48.8
organic G25.89
salt-depletion E87.1
sleep related, leg G47.62
stoker's T67.2
swimmer's T75.1
telegrapher's F48.8
organic G25.89
typist's F48.8
organic G25.89
uterus N94.89
menstrual — *see* Dysmenorrhea
writer's F48.8
organic G25.89
Cranial — *see* condition
Craniocleidodysostosis Q74.0
Craniofenestria (skull) Q75.8
Craniolacunia (skull) Q75.8
Craniopagus Q89.4
Craniopathy, metabolic M85.2
Craniopharyngeal — *see* condition
Craniopharyngioma D44.4
Craniorachischisis (totalis) Q00.1
Cranioschisis Q75.8
Craniostenosis Q75.0
Craniosynostosis Q75.0
Craniotabes (cause unknown) M83.8
neonatal P96.3
rachitic E64.3
syphilitic A50.56
Cranium — *see* condition
Craw-craw — *see* Onchocerciasis
Creaking joint — *see* Derangement, joint, specified
type NEC
Creeping
eruption B76.9
palsy or paralysis G12.22
Crenated tongue K14.8
Creotoxism A05.9

Crepitus
caput Q75.8
joint — *see* Derangement, joint, specified type NEC
Crescent or conus choroid, congenital Q14.3
CREST syndrome M34.1
Cretin, cretinism (congenital) (endemic)
(nongoitrous) (sporadic) E00.9
pelvis
with disproportion (fetopelvic) O33.0
causing obstructed labor O65.0
type
hypothyroid E00.1
mixed E00.2
myxedematous E00.1
neurological E00.0
Creutzfeldt-Jakob disease or syndrome
(with dementia) A81.00
familial A81.09
iatrogenic A81.09
specified NEC A81.09
sporadic A81.09
variant (vCJD) A81.01
Crib death R99
Cribriform hymen Q52.3
Cri-du-chat syndrome Q93.4
Crigler-Najjar disease or syndrome E80.5
Crime, victim of Z65.4
Crimean hemorrhagic fever A98.0
Criminalism F60.2
Crisis
abdomen R10.0
acute reaction F43.0
addisonian E27.2
adrenal (cortical) E27.2
celiac K90.0
Dietl's N13.8
emotional — *see also* Disorder, adjustment
acute reaction to stress F43.0
specific to childhood and adolescence F93.8
glaucomatocyclitic — *see* Glaucoma, secondary,
inflammation
heart — *see* Failure, heart
nitritoid I95.2
correct substance properly administered — *see*
Table of Drugs and Chemicals, by drug, adverse
effect
overdose or wrong substance given or taken — *see*
Table of Drugs and Chemicals, by drug,
poisoning
oculogyric H51.8
psychogenic F45.8
Pel's (tabetic) A52.11
psychosexual identity F64.2
renal N28.0
sickle-cell D57.00
with
acute chest syndrome D57.01
splenic sequestration D57.02
state (acute reaction) F43.0
tabetic A52.11
thyroid — *see* Thyrotoxicosis with thyroid storm
thyrotoxic — *see* Thyrotoxicosis with thyroid storm
Crocq's disease (acrocyanosis) I73.89
Crohn's disease — *see* Enteritis, regional
Crooked septum, nasal J34.2
Cross syndrome E70.328
Crossbite (anterior) (posterior) M26.24
Cross-eye — *see* Strabismus, convergent concomitant
Croup, croupous (catarrhal) (infectious)
(inflammatory) (nondiphtheritic) J05.0
bronchial J20.9
diphtheritic A36.2
false J38.5
spasmodic J38.5
diphtheritic A36.2
stridulous J38.5
diphtheritic A36.2
Crouzon's disease Q75.1
Crowding, tooth, teeth, fully erupted M26.31
CRST syndrome M34.1
Cruchet's disease A85.8
Cruelty in children — *see also* Disorder, conduct
Crural ulcer — *see* Ulcer, lower limb
Crush, crushed, crushing T14.8
abdomen S38.1
ankle S97.0-
arm (upper) (and shoulder) S47.-
axilla — *see* Crush, arm
back, lower S38.1
buttock S38.1
cheek S07.0
chest S28.0
cranium S07.1

Crush, crushed, crushing - *continued*
ear S07.0
elbow S57.0-
extremity
lower
ankle — *see* Crush, ankle
below knee — *see* Crush, leg
foot — *see* Crush, foot
hip — *see* Crush, hip
knee — *see* Crush, knee
thigh — *see* Crush, thigh
toe — *see* Crush, toe
upper
below elbow S67.9-
elbow — *see* Crush, elbow
finger — *see* Crush, finger
forearm — *see* Crush, forearm
hand — *see* Crush, hand
thumb — *see* Crush, thumb
upper arm — *see* Crush, arm
wrist — *see* Crush, wrist
face S07.0
finger (s) S67.1-
with hand (and wrist) — *see* Crush, hand, specified
site NEC
index S67.19-
little S67.19-
middle S67.19-
ring S67.19-
thumb — *see* Crush, thumb
foot S97.8-
toe — *see* Crush, toe
forearm S57.8-
genitalia, external
female S38.002
vagina S38.03
vulva S38.03
male S38.001
penis S38.01
scrotum S38.02
testis S38.02
hand (except fingers alone) S67.2-
with wrist S67.4-
head S07.9
specified NEC S07.8
heel — *see* Crush, foot
hip S77.0-
with thigh S77.2-
internal organ (abdomen, chest, or pelvis)
NEC T14.8
knee S87.0-
labium (majus) (minus) S38.03
larynx S17.0
leg (lower) S87.8-
knee — *see* Crush, knee
lip S07.0
lower
back S38.1
leg — *see* Crush, leg
neck S17.9
nerve — *see* Injury, nerve
nose S07.0
pelvis S38.1
penis S38.01
scalp S07.8
scapular region — *see* Crush, arm
scrotum S38.02
severe, unspecified site T14.8
shoulder (and upper arm) — *see* Crush, arm
skull S07.1
syndrome (complication of trauma) T79.5
testis S38.02
thigh S77.1-
with hip S77.2-
throat S17.8
thumb S67.0-
with hand (and wrist) — *see* Crush, hand, specified
site NEC
toe (s) S97.10-
great S97.11-
lesser S97.12-
trachea S17.0
vagina S38.03
vulva S38.03
wrist S67.3-
with hand S67.4-
Crusta lactea L21.0
Crusts R23.4
Crutch paralysis — *see* Injury, brachial plexus
**Cruveilhier-Baumgarten cirrhosis, disease or
syndrome** K74.69
Cruveilhier's atrophy or disease G12.8

Crying (constant) (continuous) (excessive)
  child, adolescent, or adult R45.83
  infant (baby) (newborn) R68.11
Cryofibrinogenemia D89.2
Cryoglobulinemia (essential) (idiopathic) (mixed)
    (primary) (purpura) (secondary) (vasculitis) D89.1
  with lung involvement D89.1 *[J99]*
Cryptitis (anal) (rectal) K62.89
Cryptococcosis, cryptococcus (infection)
    (neoformans) B45.9
  bone B45.3
  cerebral B45.1
  cutaneous B45.2
  disseminated B45.7
  generalized B45.7
  meningitis B45.1
  meningocerebralis B45.1
  osseous B45.3
  pulmonary B45.0
  skin B45.2
  specified NEC B45.8
Cryptopapillitis (anus) K62.89
Cryptophthalmos Q11.2
  syndrome Q87.0
Cryptorchid, cryptorchism, cryptorchidism Q53.9
  bilateral Q53.20
    abdominal Q53.21
    perineal Q53.22
  unilateral Q53.10
    abdominal Q53.11
    perineal Q53.12
Cryptosporidiosis A07.2
  hepatobiliary B88.8
  respiratory B88.8
Cryptostromosis J67.6
Crystalluria R82.99
Cubitus
  congenital Q68.8
  valgus (acquired) M21.0-
    congenital Q68.8
    sequelae (late effect) of rickets E64.3
  varus (acquired) M21.1-
    congenital Q68.8
    sequelae (late effect) of rickets E64.3
Cultural deprivation or shock Z60.3
Curling esophagus K22.4
Curling's ulcer — *see* Ulcer, peptic, acute
Curschmann (-Batten) (-Steinert)
  disease or syndrome G71.11
Curse, Ondine's — *see* Apnea, sleep
Curvature
  organ or site, congenital NEC — *see* Distortion
  penis (lateral) Q55.61
  Pott's (spinal) A18.01
  radius, idiopathic, progressive (congenital) Q74.0
  spine (acquired) (angular) (idiopathic) (incorrect)
      (postural) — *see* Dorsopathy, deforming
    congenital Q67.5
    due to or associated with
      Charcot-Marie-Tooth disease
        (*see also* subcategory M49.8) G60.0
      osteitis
        deformans M88.88
        fibrosa cystica (*see also* subcategory
          M49.8) E21.0
      tuberculosis (Pott's curvature) A18.01
    sequelae (late effect) of rickets E64.3
    tuberculous A18.01
Cushingoid due to steroid therapy E24.2
  correct substance properly administered — *see* Table
    of Drugs and Chemicals, by drug, adverse effect
  overdose or wrong substance given or taken — *see*
    Table of Drugs and Chemicals, by drug, poisoning
Cushing's
  syndrome or disease E24.9
    drug-induced E24.2
    iatrogenic E24.2
    pituitary-dependent E24.0
    specified NEC E24.8
  ulcer — *see* Ulcer, peptic, acute
Cusp, Carabelli - omit code
Cut (external) — *see also* Laceration
  muscle — *see* Injury, muscle
Cutaneous — *see also* condition
  hemorrhage R23.3
  larva migrans B76.9
Cutis — *see also* condition
  hyperelastica Q82.8
    acquired L57.4
  laxa (hyperelastica) — *see* Dermatolysis
  marmorata R23.8
  osteosis L94.2
  pendula — *see* Dermatolysis

Cutis - *continued*
  rhomboidalis nuchae L57.2
  verticis gyrata Q82.8
    acquired L91.8
Cyanosis R23.0
  due to
    patent foramen botalli Q21.1
    persistent foramen ovale Q21.1
  enterogenous D74.8
  paroxysmal digital — *see* Raynaud's disease
    with gangrene I73.01
  retina, retinal H35.89
Cyanotic heart disease I24.9
  congenital Q24.9
Cycle
  anovulatory N97.0
  menstrual, irregular N92.6
Cyclencephaly Q04.9
Cyclical vomiting — *see also* Vomiting,
  cyclical G43.A0
  psychogenic F50.89
Cyclitis — *see also* Iridocyclitis H20.9
  chronic — *see* Iridocyclitis, chronic
  Fuchs' heterochromic H20.81-
  granulomatous — *see* Iridocyclitis, chronic
  lens-induced — *see* Iridocyclitis, lens-induced
  posterior H30.2-
Cycloid personality F34.0
Cyclophoria H50.54
Cyclopia, cyclops Q87.0
Cyclopism Q87.0 ˙
Cyclosporidiasis A07.4
Cyclothymia F34.0
Cyclothymic personality F34.0
Cyclotropia H50.41-
Cylindroma — *see also* Neoplasm, malignant, by site
  eccrine dermal — *see* Neoplasm, skin, benign
  skin — *see* Neoplasm, skin, benign
Cylindruria R82.99
Cynanche
  diphtheritic A36.2
  tonsillaris J36
Cynophobia F40.218
Cynorexia R63.2
Cyphosis — *see* Kyphosis
Cyprus fever — *see* Brucellosis
Cyst (colloid) (mucous) (simple) (retention)
  adenoid (infected) J35.8
  adrenal gland E27.8
    congenital Q89.1
  air, lung J98.4
  allantoic Q64.4
  alveolar process (jaw bone) M27.40
  amnion, amniotic O41.8X-
  aneurysmal M27.49
  anterior
    chamber (eye) — *see* Cyst, iris
    nasopalatine K09.1
  antrum J34.1
  anus K62.89
  apical (tooth) (periodontal) K04.8
  appendix K38.8
  arachnoid, brain (acquired) G93.0
    congenital Q04.6
  arytenoid J38.7
  Baker's M71.2-
    ruptured M66.0
    tuberculous A18.02
  Bartholin's gland N75.0
  bile duct (common) (hepatic) K83.5
  bladder (multiple) (trigone) N32.89
  blue dome (breast) — *see* Cyst, breast
  bone (local) NEC M85.60
    aneurysmal M85.50
      ankle M85.57-
      foot M85.57-
      forearm M85.53-
      hand M85.54-
      jaw M27.49
      lower leg M85.56-
      multiple site M85.59
      neck M85.58
      rib M85.58
      shoulder M85.51-
      skull M85.58
      specified site NEC M85.58
      thigh M85.55-
      toe M85.57-
      upper arm M85.52-
      vertebra M85.58
    solitary M85.40
      ankle M85.47-
      fibula M85.46-

Cyst (colloid) (mucous) (simple) (retention) -
    continued
  bone (local) NEC - *continued*
    solitary - *continued*
      foot M85.47-
      hand M85.44-
      humerus M85.42-
      jaw M27.49
      neck M85.48
      pelvis M85.45-
      radius M85.43-
      rib M85.48
      shoulder M85.41-
      skull M85.48
      specified site NEC M85.48
      tibia M85.46-
      toe M85.47-
      ulna M85.43-
      vertebra M85.48
    specified type NEC M85.60
      ankle M85.67-
      foot M85.67-
      forearm M85.63-
      hand M85.64-
      jaw M27.40
        developmental (nonodontogenic) K09.1
          odontogenic K09.0
        latent M27.0
      lower leg M85.66-
      multiple site M85.69
      neck M85.68
      rib M85.68
      shoulder M85.61-
      skull M85.68
      specified site NEC M85.68
      thigh M85.65-
      toe M85.67-
      upper arm M85.62-
      vertebra M85.68
  brain (acquired) G93.0
    congenital Q04.6
    hydatid B67.99 *[G94]*
    third ventricle (colloid) , congenital Q04.6
  branchial (cleft) Q18.0
  branchiogenic Q18.0
  breast (benign) (blue dome) (pedunculated)
      (solitary) N60.0-
    involution — *see* Dysplasia, mammary, specified
      type NEC
    sebaceous — *see* Dysplasia, mammary, specified
      type NEC
  broad ligament (benign) N83.8
  bronchogenic (mediastinal) (sequestration) J98.4
    congenital Q33.0
  buccal K09.8
  bulbourethral gland N36.8
  bursa, bursal NEC M71.30
    with rupture — *see* Rupture, synovium
    ankle M71.37-
    elbow M71.32-
    foot M71.37-
    hand M71.34-
    hip M71.35-
    multiple sites M71.39
    pharyngeal J39.2
    popliteal space — *see* Cyst, Baker's
    shoulder M71.31-
    specified site NEC M71.38
    wrist M71.33-
  calcifying odontogenic D16.5
    upper jaw (bone) (maxilla) D16.4
  canal of Nuck (female) N94.89
    congenital Q52.4
  canthus — *see* Cyst, conjunctiva
  carcinomatous — *see* Neoplasm, malignant, by site
  cauda equina G95.89
  cavum septi pellucidi — *see* Cyst, brain
  celomic (pericardium) Q24.8
  cerebellopontine (angle) — *see* Cyst, brain
  cerebellum — *see* Cyst, brain
  cerebral — *see* Cyst, brain
  cervical lateral Q18.0
  cervix NEC N88.8
    embryonic Q51.6
    nabothian N88.8
  chiasmal optic NEC — *see* Disorder, optic, chiasm
  chocolate (ovary) N80.1
  choledochus, congenital Q44.4
  chorion O41.8X-
  choroid plexus G93.0
  ciliary body — *see* Cyst, iris
  clitoris N90.7
  colon K63.89

Cyst (colloid) (mucous) (simple) (retention) - *continued*
 common (bile) duct K83.5
 congenital NEC Q89.8
  adrenal gland Q89.1
  epiglottis Q31.8
  esophagus Q39.8
  fallopian tube Q50.4
  kidney Q61.00
   more than one (multiple) Q61.02
    specified as polycystic Q61.3
     adult type Q61.2
     infantile type NEC Q61.19
      collecting duct dilation Q61.11
   solitary Q61.01
  larynx Q31.8
  liver Q44.6
  lung Q33.0
  mediastinum Q34.1
  ovary Q50.1
  oviduct Q50.4
  periurethral (tissue) Q64.79
  prepuce Q55.69
  salivary gland (any) Q38.4
  sublingual Q38.6
  submaxillary gland Q38.6
  thymus (gland) Q89.2
  tongue Q38.3
  ureterovesical orifice Q62.8
  vulva Q52.79
 conjunctiva H11.44-
 cornea H18.89-
 corpora quadrigemina G93.0
 corpus
  albicans N83.29-
  luteum (hemorrhagic) (ruptured) N83.1-
 Cowper's gland (benign) (infected) N36.8
 cranial meninges G93.0
 craniobuccal pouch E23.6
 craniopharyngeal pouch E23.6
 cystic duct K82.8
 Cysticercus — *see* Cysticercosis
 Dandy-Walker Q03.1
  with spina bifida — *see* Spina bifida
 dental (root) K04.8
  developmental K09.0
  eruption K09.0
  primordial K09.0
 dentigerous (mandible) (maxilla) K09.0
 dermoid — *see* Neoplasm, benign, by site
  with malignant transformation C56.-
  implantation
   external area or site (skin) NEC L72.0
   iris — *see* Cyst, iris, implantation
   vagina N89.8
   vulva N90.7
  mouth K09.8
  oral soft tissue K09.8
  sacrococcygeal — *see* Cyst, pilonidal
 developmental K09.1
  odontogenic K09.0
  oral region (nonodontogenic) K09.1
  ovary, ovarian Q50.1
 dura (cerebral) G93.0
  spinal G96.19
 ear (external) Q18.1
 echinococcal — *see* Echinococcus
 embryonic
  cervix uteri Q51.6
  fallopian tube Q50.4
  vagina Q51.6
 endometrium, endometrial (uterus) N85.8
  ectopic — *see* Endometriosis
 enterogenous Q43.8
 epidermal, epidermoid (inclusion) (see also Cyst, skin) L72.0
  mouth K09.8
  oral soft tissue K09.8
 epididymis N50.3
 epiglottis J38.7
 epiphysis cerebri E34.8
 epithelial (inclusion) L72.0
 epoophoron Q50.5
 eruption K09.0
 esophagus K22.8
 ethmoid sinus J34.1
 external female genital organs NEC N90.7
 eye NEC H57.8
  congenital Q15.8
 eyelid (sebaceous) H02.829
  infected — *see* Hordeolum
  left H02.826
   lower H02.825

Cyst (colloid) (mucous) (simple) (retention) - *continued*
 eyelid (sebaceous) - *continued*
  left - *continued*
   upper H02.824
  right H02.823
   lower H02.822
   upper H02.821
 fallopian tube N83.8
  congenital Q50.4
 fimbrial (twisted) Q50.4
 fissural (oral region) K09.1
 follicle (graafian) (hemorrhagic) N83.0-
  nabothian N88.8
 follicular (atretic) (hemorrhagic) (ovarian) N83.0-
  dentigerous K09.0
  odontogenic K09.0
  skin L72.9
   specified NEC L72.8
 frontal sinus J34.1
 gallbladder K82.8
 ganglion — *see* Ganglion
 Gartner's duct Q52.4
 gingiva K09.0
 gland of Moll — *see* Cyst, eyelid
 globulomaxillary K09.1
 graafian follicle (hemorrhagic) N83.0-
 granulosal lutein (hemorrhagic) N83.1-
 hemangiomatous D18.00
  intra-abdominal D18.03
  intracranial D18.02
  skin D18.01
  specified site NEC D18.09
 hemorrhagic M27.49
 hydatid — *see also* Echinococcus B67.90
  brain B67.99 *[G94]*
  liver — *see* Cyst, liver, hydatid B67.8
  lung NEC B67.99 *[J99]*
  Morgagni
   female Q50.5
   male (epididymal) Q55.4
    testicular Q55.29
  specified site NEC B67.99
 hymen N89.8
  embryonic Q52.4
 hypopharynx J39.2
 hypophysis, hypophyseal (duct) (recurrent) E23.6
  cerebri E23.6
 implantation (dermoid)
  external area or site (skin) NEC L72.0
  iris — *see* Cyst, iris, implantation
  vagina N89.8
  vulva N90.7
 incisive canal K09.1
 inclusion (epidermal) (epithelial) (epidermoid) (squamous) L72.0
  not of skin - code under Cyst, by site
 intestine (large) (small) K63.89
 intracranial — *see* Cyst, brain
 intraligamentous — *see also* Disorder, ligament
  knee — *see* Derangement, knee
 intrasellar E23.6
 iris H21.309
  exudative H21.31-
  idiopathic H21.30-
  implantation H21.32-
  parasitic H21.33-
  pars plana (primary) H21.34-
   exudative H21.35-
 jaw (bone) M27.40
  aneurysmal M27.49
  hemorrhagic M27.49
  traumatic M27.49
  developmental (odontogenic) K09.0
  fissural K09.1
 joint NEC — *see* Disorder, joint, specified type NEC
 kidney (acquired) N28.1
  calyceal — *see* Hydronephrosis
  congenital Q61.00
   more than one (multiple) Q61.02
    specified as polycystic Q61.3
     adult type (autosomal dominant) Q61.2
     infantile type (autosomal recessive) NEC Q61.19
      collecting duct dilation Q61.11
  pyelogenic — *see* Hydronephrosis
  simple N28.1
  solitary (single) Q61.01
   acquired N28.1
 labium (majus) (minus) N90.7
  sebaceous N90.7
 lacrimal — *see also* Disorder, lacrimal system, specified NEC

Cyst (colloid) (mucous) (simple) (retention) - *continued*
 lacrimal - *continued*
  gland H04.13-
  passages or sac — *see* Disorder, lacrimal system, specified NEC
 larynx J38.7
 lateral periodontal K09.0
 lens H27.8
  congenital Q12.8
 lip (gland) K13.0
 liver (idiopathic) (simple) K76.89
  congenital Q44.6
  hydatid B67.8
   granulosus B67.0
   multilocularis B67.5
 lung J98.4
  congenital Q33.0
  giant bullous J43.9
 lutein N83.1-
 lymphangiomatous D18.1
 lymphoepithelial, oral soft tissue K09.8
 macula — *see* Degeneration, macula, hole
 malignant — *see* Neoplasm, malignant, by site
 mammary gland — *see* Cyst, breast
 mandible M27.40
  dentigerous K09.0
  radicular K04.8
 maxilla M27.40
  dentigerous K09.0
  radicular K04.8
 medial, face and neck Q18.8
 median
  anterior maxillary K09.1
  palatal K09.1
 mediastinum, congenital Q34.1
 meibomian (gland) — *see* Chalazion
  infected — *see* Hordeolum
 membrane, brain G93.0
 meninges (cerebral) G93.0
  spinal G96.19
 meniscus, knee — *see* Derangement, knee, meniscus, cystic
 mesentery, mesenteric K66.8
  chyle I89.8
 mesonephric duct
  female Q50.5
  male Q55.4
 milk N64.89
 Morgagni (hydatid)
  female Q50.5
  male (epididymal) Q55.4
   testicular Q55.29
 mouth K09.8
 Müllerian duct Q50.4
  appendix testis Q55.29
  cervix Q51.6
  fallopian tube Q50.4
  female Q50.4
  male Q55.29
  prostatic utricle Q55.4
  vagina (embryonal) Q52.4
 multilocular (ovary) D39.10
  benign — *see* Neoplasm, benign, by site
 myometrium N85.8
 nabothian (follicle) (ruptured) N88.8
 nasoalveolar K09.1
 nasolabial K09.1
 nasopalatine (anterior) (duct) K09.1
 nasopharynx J39.2
 neoplastic — *see* Neoplasm, uncertain behavior, by site
  benign — *see* Neoplasm, benign, by site
 nervous system NEC G96.8
 neuroenteric (congenital) Q06.8
 nipple — *see* Cyst, breast
 nose (turbinates) J34.1
  sinus J34.1
 odontogenic, developmental K09.0
 omentum (lesser) K66.8
  congenital Q45.8
 ora serrata — *see* Cyst, retina, ora serrata
 oral
  region K09.9
   developmental (nonodontogenic) K09.1
   specified NEC K09.8
  soft tissue K09.9
   specified NEC K09.8
 orbit H05.81-
 ovary, ovarian (twisted) N83.20-
  adherent N83.20-
  chocolate N80.1
  corpus

Cyst (colloid) (mucous) (simple) (retention) - *continued*
  ovary, ovarian (twisted) - *continued*
    corpus - *continued*
      albicans N83.29-
        luteum (hemorrhagic) N83.1-
      dermoid D27.9
      developmental Q50.1
      due to failure of involution NEC N83.20-
      endometrial N80.1
      follicular (graafian) (hemorrhagic) N83.0-
      hemorrhagic N83.20-
      in pregnancy or childbirth O34.8-
        with obstructed labor O65.5
      multilocular D39.10
      pseudomucinous D27.9
      retention N83.29-
      serous N83.20-
      specified NEC N83.29-
      theca lutein (hemorrhagic) N83.1-
      tuberculous A18.18
  oviduct N83.8
  palate (median) (fissural) K09.1
  palatine papilla (jaw) K09.1
  pancreas, pancreatic (hemorrhagic) (true) K86.2
    congenital Q45.2
    false K86.3
  paralabral
    hip M24.85-
    shoulder S43.43-
  paramesonephric duct Q50.4
    female Q50.4
    male Q55.29
  paranephric N28.1
  paraphysis, cerebri, congenital Q04.6
  parasitic B89
  parathyroid (gland) E21.4
  paratubal N83.8
  paraurethral duct N36.8
  paroophoron Q50.5
  parotid gland K11.6
  parovarian Q50.5
  pelvis, female N94.89
    in pregnancy or childbirth O34.8-
      causing obstructed labor O65.5
  penis (sebaceous) N48.89
  periapical K04.8
  pericardial (congenital) Q24.8
    acquired (secondary) I31.8
  pericoronal K09.0
  periodontal K04.8
    lateral K09.0
  peripelvic (lymphatic) N28.1
  peritoneum K66.8
    chylous I89.8
  periventricular, acquired, newborn P91.1
  pharynx (wall) J39.2
  pilar L72.11
  pilonidal (infected) (rectum) L05.91
    with abscess L05.01
    malignant C44.59-
  pituitary (duct) (gland) E23.6
  placenta O43.19-
  pleura J94.8
  popliteal — *see* Cyst, Baker's
  porencephalic Q04.6
    acquired G93.0
  postanal (infected) — *see* Cyst, pilonidal
  postmastoidectomy cavity (mucosal) — *see*
    Complications, postmastoidectomy, cyst
  preauricular Q18.1
  prepuce N47.4
    congenital Q55.69
  primordial (jaw) K09.0
  prostate N42.83
  pseudomucinous (ovary) D27.9
  pupillary, miotic H21.27-
  radicular (residual) K04.8
  radiculodental K04.8
  ranular K11.8
  Rathke's pouch E23.6
  rectum (epithelium) (mucous) K62.89
  renal — *see* Cyst, kidney
  residual (radicular) K04.8
  retention (ovary) N83.29-
    salivary gland K11.6
  retina H33.19-
    ora serrata H33.11-
    parasitic H33.12-
  retroperitoneal K68.9
  sacrococcygeal (dermoid) — *see* Cyst, pilonidal
  salivary gland or duct (mucous extravasation or
    retention) K11.6

Cyst (colloid) (mucous) (simple) (retention) - *continued*
  Sampson's N80.1
  sclera H15.89
  scrotum L72.9
    sebaceous L72.3
  sebaceous (duct) (gland) L72.3
    breast — *see* Dysplasia, mammary, specified type
      NEC
    eyelid — *see* Cyst, eyelid
    genital organ NEC
      female N94.89
      male N50.89
    scrotum L72.3
  semilunar cartilage (knee) (multiple) — *see*
    Derangement, knee, meniscus, cystic
  seminal vesicle N50.89
  serous (ovary) N83.20-
  sinus (accessory) (nasal) J34.1
  Skene's gland N36.8
  skin L72.9
    breast — *see* Dysplasia, mammary, specified type
      NEC
    epidermal, epidermoid L72.0
    epithelial L72.0
    eyelid — *see* Cyst, eyelid
    genital organ NEC
      female N90.7
      male N50.89
    inclusion L72.0
    scrotum L72.9
    sebaceous L72.3
    sweat gland or duct L74.8
  solitary
    bone — *see* Cyst, bone, solitary
    jaw M27.40
    kidney N28.1
  spermatic cord N50.89
  sphenoid sinus J34.1
  spinal meninges G96.19
  spleen NEC D73.4
    congenital Q89.09
    hydatid — *see also* Echinococcus B67.99 [D77]
  Stafne's M27.0
  subarachnoid intrasellar R93.0
  subcutaneous, pheomycotic (chromomycotic) B43.2
  subdural (cerebral) G93.0
    spinal cord G96.19
  sublingual gland K11.6
  submandibular gland K11.6
  submaxillary gland K11.6
  suburethral N36.8
  suprarenal gland E27.8
  suprasellar — *see* Cyst, brain
  sweat gland or duct L74.8
  synovial — *see also* Cyst, bursa
    ruptured — *see* Rupture, synovium
  tarsal — *see* Chalazion
  tendon (sheath) — *see* Disorder, tendon, specified
    type NEC
  testis N44.2
    tunica albuginea N44.1
  theca lutein (ovary) N83.1-
  Thornwaldt's J39.2
  thymus (gland) E32.8
  thyroglossal duct (infected) (persistent) Q89.2
  thyrolingual duct (infected) (persistent) Q89.2
  thyroid (gland) E04.1
  tongue K14.8
  tonsil J35.8
  tooth — *see* Cyst, dental
  Tornwaldt's J39.2
  trichilemmal (proliferating) L72.12
  trichodermal L72.12
  tubal (fallopian) N83.8
    inflammatory — *see* Salpingitis, chronic
  tubo-ovarian N83.8
    inflammatory N70.13
  tunica
    albuginea testis N44.1
    vaginalis N50.89
  turbinate (nose) J34.1
  Tyson's gland N48.89
  urachus, congenital Q64.4
  ureter N28.89
  ureterovesical orifice N28.89
  urethra, urethral (gland) N36.8
  uterine ligament N83.8
  uterus (body) (corpus) (recurrent) N85.8
    embryonic Q51.818
    cervix Q51.6
  vagina, vaginal (implantation) (inclusion) (squamous
    cell) (wall) N89.8

Cyst (colloid) (mucous) (simple) (retention) - *continued*
  vagina, vaginal (implantation) (inclusion) (squamous
    cell) (wall) - *continued*
    embryonic Q52.4
  vallecula, vallecular (epiglottis) J38.7
  vesical (orifice) N32.89
  vitreous body H43.89
  vulva (implantation) (inclusion) N90.7
    congenital Q52.79
    sebaceous gland N90.7
  vulvovaginal gland N90.7
  wolffian
    female Q50.5
    male Q55.4
Cystadenocarcinoma — *see* Neoplasm, malignant,
  by site
  bile duct C22.1
  endometrioid — *see* Neoplasm, malignant, by site
    specified site — *see* Neoplasm, malignant, by site
    unspecified site
      female C56.9
      male C61
  mucinous
    papillary
      specified site — *see* Neoplasm, malignant, by site
      unspecified site C56.9
    specified site — *see* Neoplasm, malignant, by site
    unspecified site C56.9
  papillary
    mucinous
      specified site — *see* Neoplasm, malignant, by site
      unspecified site C56.9
    pseudomucinous
      specified site — *see* Neoplasm, malignant, by site
      unspecified site C56.9
    serous
      specified site — *see* Neoplasm, malignant, by site
      unspecified site C56.9
    specified site — *see* Neoplasm, malignant, by site
    unspecified site C56.9
  pseudomucinous
    papillary
      specified site — *see* Neoplasm, malignant, by site
      unspecified site C56.9
    specified site — *see* Neoplasm, malignant, by site
    unspecified site C56.9
  serous
    papillary
      specified site — *see* Neoplasm, malignant, by site
      unspecified site C56.9
    specified site — *see* Neoplasm, malignant, by site
    unspecified site C56.9
Cystadenofibroma
  clear cell — *see* Neoplasm, benign, by site
  endometrioid D27.9
    borderline malignancy D39.1-
    malignant C56.-
  mucinous
    specified site — *see* Neoplasm, benign, by site
    unspecified site D27.9
  serous
    specified site — *see* Neoplasm, benign, by site
    unspecified site D27.9
  specified site — *see* Neoplasm, benign, by site
  unspecified site D27.9
Cystadenoma — *see also* Neoplasm, benign, by site
  bile duct D13.4
  endometrioid — *see* Neoplasm, benign, by site
    borderline malignancy — *see* Neoplasm, uncertain
      behavior, by site
    malignant — *see* Neoplasm, malignant, by site
  mucinous
    borderline malignancy
      ovary C56.-
      specified site NEC — *see* Neoplasm, uncertain
        behavior, by site
      unspecified site C56.9
    papillary
      borderline malignancy
        ovary C56.-
        specified site NEC — *see* Neoplasm, uncertain
          behavior, by site
        unspecified site C56.9
      specified site — *see* Neoplasm, benign, by site
      unspecified site D27.9
    specified site — *see* Neoplasm, benign, by site
    unspecified site D27.9
  papillary
    borderline malignancy
      ovary C56.-
      specified site NEC — *see* Neoplasm, uncertain
        behavior, by site

Cystadenoma - *continued*
  papillary - *continued*
    borderline malignancy - *continued*
      unspecified site C56.9
    lymphomatosum
      specified site — *see* Neoplasm, benign, by site
      unspecified site D11.9
    mucinous
      borderline malignancy
        ovary C56.-
        specified site NEC — *see* Neoplasm, uncertain behavior, by site
        unspecified site C56.9
      specified site — *see* Neoplasm, benign, by site
      unspecified site D27.9
    pseudomucinous
      borderline malignancy
        ovary C56.-
        specified site NEC — *see* Neoplasm, uncertain behavior, by site
        unspecified site C56.9
      specified site — *see* Neoplasm, benign, by site
      unspecified site D27.9
    serous
      borderline malignancy
        ovary C56.-
        specified site NEC — *see* Neoplasm, uncertain behavior, by site
        unspecified site C56.9
      specified site — *see* Neoplasm, benign, by site
      unspecified site D27.9
    specified site — *see* Neoplasm, benign, by site
    unspecified site D27.9
  pseudomucinous
    borderline malignancy
      ovary C56.-
      specified site NEC — *see* Neoplasm, uncertain behavior, by site
      unspecified site C56.9
    papillary
      borderline malignancy
        ovary C56.-
        specified site NEC — *see* Neoplasm, uncertain behavior, by site
        unspecified site C56.9
      specified site — *see* Neoplasm, benign, by site
      unspecified site D27.9
    specified site — *see* Neoplasm, benign, by site
    unspecified site D27.9
  serous
    borderline malignancy
      ovary C56.-
      specified site NEC — *see* Neoplasm, uncertain behavior, by site
      unspecified site C56.9
    papillary
      borderline malignancy
        ovary C56.-
        specified site NEC — *see* Neoplasm, uncertain behavior, by site
        unspecified site C56.9
      specified site — *see* Neoplasm, benign, by site
      unspecified site D27.9
    specified site — *see* Neoplasm, benign, by site
    unspecified site D27.9
Cystathionine synthase deficiency E72.11
Cystathioninemia E72.19
Cystathioninuria E72.19
Cystic — *see also* condition
  breast (chronic) — *see* Mastopathy, cystic
  corpora lutea (hemorrhagic) N83.1-
  duct — *see* condition
  eyeball (congenital) Q11.0
  fibrosis — *see* Fibrosis, cystic
  kidney (congenital) Q61.9
    adult type Q61.2
    infantile type NEC Q61.19
      collecting duct dilatation Q61.11
    medullary Q61.5
  liver, congenital Q44.6
  lung disease J98.4
    congenital Q33.0
  mastitis, chronic — *see* Mastopathy, cystic
  medullary, kidney Q61.5
  meniscus — *see* Derangement, knee, meniscus, cystic
  ovary N83.20-
Cysticercosis, cysticerciasis B69.9
  with
    epileptiform fits B69.0
    myositis B69.81
  brain B69.0
  central nervous system B69.0

Cysticercosis, cysticerciasis - *continued*
  cerebral B69.0
  ocular B69.1
  specified NEC B69.89
Cysticercus cellulose infestation — *see* Cysticercosis
Cystinosis (malignant) E72.04
Cystinuria E72.01
Cystitis (exudative) (hemorrhagic) (septic) (suppurative) N30.90
  with
    fibrosis — *see* Cystitis, chronic, interstitial
    hematuria N30.91
    leukoplakia — *see* Cystitis, chronic, interstitial
    malakoplakia — *see* Cystitis, chronic, interstitial
    metaplasia — *see* Cystitis, chronic, interstitial
    prostatitis N41.3
  acute N30.00
    with hematuria N30.01
    of trigone N30.30
      with hematuria N30.31
  allergic — *see* Cystitis, specified type NEC
  amebic A06.81
  bilharzial B65.9 [N33]
  blennorrhagic (gonococcal) A54.01
  bullous — *see* Cystitis, specified type NEC
  calculous N21.0
  chlamydial A56.01
  chronic N30.20
    with hematuria N30.21
    interstitial N30.10
      with hematuria N30.11
    of trigone N30.30
      with hematuria N30.31
    specified NEC N30.20
      with hematuria N30.21
  cystic (a) — *see* Cystitis, specified type NEC
  diphtheritic A36.85
  echinococcal
    granulosus B67.39
    multilocularis B67.69
  emphysematous — *see* Cystitis, specified type NEC
  encysted — *see* Cystitis, specified type NEC
  eosinophilic — *see* Cystitis, specified type NEC
  follicular — *see* Cystitis, of trigone
  gangrenous — *see* Cystitis, specified type NEC
  glandularis — *see* Cystitis, specified type NEC
  gonococcal A54.01
  incrusted — *see* Cystitis, specified type NEC
  interstitial (chronic) — *see* Cystitis, chronic, interstitial
  irradiation N30.40
    with hematuria N30.41
  irritation — *see* Cystitis, specified type NEC
  malignant — *see* Cystitis, specified type NEC
  of trigone N30.30
    with hematuria N30.31
  panmural — *see* Cystitis, chronic, interstitial
  polyposa — *see* Cystitis, specified type NEC
  prostatic N41.3
  puerperal (postpartum) O86.22
  radiation — *see* Cystitis, irradiation
  specified type NEC N30.80
    with hematuria N30.81
  subacute — *see* Cystitis, chronic
  submucous — *see* Cystitis, chronic, interstitial
  syphilitic (late) A52.76
  trichomonal A59.03
  tuberculous A18.12
  ulcerative — *see* Cystitis, chronic, interstitial
Cystocele (-urethrocele)
  female N81.10
    with prolapse of uterus — *see* Prolapse, uterus
    lateral N81.12
    midline N81.11
    paravaginal N81.12
  in pregnancy or childbirth O34.8-
    causing obstructed labor O65.5
  male N32.89
Cystolithiasis N21.0
Cystoma — *see also* Neoplasm, benign, by site
  endometrial, ovary N80.1
  mucinous
    specified site — *see* Neoplasm, benign, by site
    unspecified site D27.9
  serous
    specified site — *see* Neoplasm, benign, by site
    unspecified site D27.9
  simple (ovary) N83.29-
Cystoplegia N31.2
Cystoptosis N32.89
Cystopyelitis — *see* Pyelonephritis
Cystorrhagia N32.89

Cystosarcoma phyllodes D48.6-
  benign D24-
  malignant — *see* Neoplasm, breast, malignant
Cystostomy
  attention to Z43.5
  complication — *see* Complications, cystostomy
  status Z93.50
    appendico-vesicostomy Z93.52
    cutaneous Z93.51
    specified NEC Z93.59
Cystourethritis — *see* Urethritis
Cystourethrocele — *see also* Cystocele
  female N81.10
    with uterine prolapse — *see* Prolapse, uterus
    lateral N81.12
    midline N81.11
    paravaginal N81.12
  male N32.89
Cytomegalic inclusion disease
  congenital P35.1
Cytomegalovirus infection B25.9
Cytomycosis (reticuloendothelial) B39.4
Cytopenia D75.9
  refractory
    with multilineage dysplasia D46.A
    and ring sideroblasts (RCMD RS) D46.B
Czerny's disease (periodic hydrarthrosis of the knee) — *see* Effusion, joint, knee

D

Da Costa's syndrome F45.8
Daae (-Finsen) **disease** (epidemic pleurodynia) B33.0
Dabney's grip B33.0
Dacryoadenitis, dacryadenitis H04.00-
  acute H04.01-
  chronic H04.02-
Dacryocystitis H04.30-
  acute H04.32-
  chronic H04.41-
  neonatal P39.1
  phlegmonous H04.31-
  syphilitic A52.71
    congenital (early) A50.01
  trachomatous, active A71.1
    sequelae (late effect) B94.0
Dacryocystoblenorrhea — *see* Inflammation, lacrimal, passages, chronic
Dacryocystocele — *see* Disorder, lacrimal system, changes
Dacryolith, dacryolithiasis H04.51-
Dacryoma — *see* Disorder, lacrimal system, changes
Dacryopericystitis — *see* Dacryocystitis
Dacryops H04.11-
Dacryostenosis — *see also* Stenosis, lacrimal
  congenital Q10.5
Dactylitis
  bone — *see* Osteomyelitis
  sickle-cell D57.00
    Hb C D57.219
    Hb SS D57.00
    specified NEC D57.819
  skin L08.9
  syphilitic A52.77
  tuberculous A18.03
Dactylolysis spontanea (ainhum) L94.6
Dactylosymphysis Q70.9
  fingers — *see* Syndactylism, complex, fingers
  toes — *see* Syndactylism, complex, toes
Damage
  arteriosclerotic — *see* Arteriosclerosis
  brain (nontraumatic) G93.9
    anoxic, hypoxic G93.1
      resulting from a procedure G97.82
    child NEC G80.9
    due to birth injury P11.2
  cardiorenal (vascular) — *see* Hypertension, cardiorenal
  cerebral NEC — *see* Damage, brain
  coccyx, complicating delivery O71.6
  coronary — *see* Disease, heart, ischemic
  eye, birth injury P15.3
  liver (nontraumatic) K76.9
    alcoholic K70.9
    due to drugs — *see* Disease, liver, toxic
    toxic — *see* Disease, liver, toxic
  medication T88.7
  pelvic
    joint or ligament, during delivery O71.6
    organ NEC
      during delivery O71.5
      following ectopic or molar pregnancy O08.6
  renal — *see* Disease, renal

Damage - *continued*
  subendocardium, subendocardial — *see* Degeneration, myocardial
  vascular I99.9
Dana-Putnam syndrome (subacute combined sclerosis with pernicious anemia) — *see* Degeneration, combined
Danbolt (-Cross) syndrome (acrodermatitis enteropathica) E83.2
Dandruff L21.0
Dandy-Walker syndrome Q03.1
  with spina bifida — *see* Spina bifida
Danlos' syndrome Q79.6
Darier (-White) disease (congenital) Q82.8
  meaning erythema annulare centrifugum L53.1
Darier-Roussy sarcoid D86.3
Darling's disease or histoplasmosis B39.4
Darwin's tubercle Q17.8
Dawson's (inclusion body) **encephalitis** A81.1
De Beurmann (-Gougerot) **disease** B42.1
De la Tourette's syndrome F95.2
De Lange's syndrome Q87.1
De Morgan's spots (senile angiomas) I78.1
De Quervain's
  disease (tendon sheath) M65.4
  syndrome E34.51
  thyroiditis (subacute granulomatous thyroiditis) E06.1
De Toni-Fanconi (-Debré) syndrome E72.09
  with cystinosis E72.04
Dead
  fetus, retained (mother) O36.4
    early pregnancy O02.1
  labyrinth — *see* subcategory H83.2
  ovum, retained O02.0
Deaf nonspeaking NEC H91.3
Deafmutism (acquired) (congenital) **NEC** H91.3
  hysterical F44.6
  syphilitic, congenital (*see also* subcategory H94.8) A50.09
Deafness (acquired) (complete) (hereditary) (partial) H91.9-
  with blue sclera and fragility of bone Q78.0
  auditory fatigue — *see* Deafness, specified type NEC
  aviation T70.0
  nerve injury — *see* Injury, nerve, acoustic, specified type NEC
  boilermaker's — *see* subcategory H83.3
  central — *see* Deafness, sensorineural
  conductive H90.2
    and sensorineural
      mixed H90.8
        bilateral H90.6
      bilateral H90.0
      unilateral H90.1-
        with restricted hearing on the contralateral side H90.A-
    congenital H90.5
      with blue sclera and fragility of bone Q78.0
  due to toxic agents — *see* Deafness, ototoxic
  emotional (hysterical) F44.6
  functional (hysterical) F44.6
  high frequency H91.9-
  hysterical F44.6
  low frequency H91.9-
  mental R48.8
  mixed conductive and sensorineural H90.8
    bilateral H90.6
    unilateral H90.7-
  nerve — *see* Deafness, sensorineural
  neural — *see* Deafness, sensorineural
  noise-induced (*see also* subcategory) H83.3
    nerve injury — *see* Injury, nerve, acoustic, specified type NEC
  nonspeaking H91.3
  ototoxic — *see* subcategory H91.0
  perceptive — *see* Deafness, sensorineural
  psychogenic (hysterical) F44.6
  sensorineural H90.5
    and conductive
      mixed H90.8
        bilateral H90.6
      bilateral H90.3
      unilateral H90.4-
        with restricted hearing on the contralateral side H90.A-
  sensory — *see* Deafness, sensorineural
  specified type NEC — *see* subcategory H91.8
  sudden (idiopathic) H91.2-
  syphilitic A52.15
  transient ischemic H93.01-

Deafness (acquired) (complete) (hereditary) (partial) - *continued*
  traumatic — *see* Injury, nerve, acoustic, specified type NEC
  word (developmental) H93.25
Death (cause unknown) (of) (unexplained) (unspecified cause) R99
  brain G93.82
  cardiac (sudden) (with successful resuscitation) - code to underlying disease
    family history of Z82.41
    personal history of Z86.74
  family member (assumed) Z63.4
Debility (chronic) (general) (nervous) R53.81
  congenital or neonatal NOS P96.9
  nervous R53.81
  old age R54
  senile R54
Débove's disease (splenomegaly) R16.1
Decalcification
  bone — *see* Osteoporosis
  teeth K03.89
Decapsulation, kidney N28.89
Decay
  dental — *see* Caries, dental
  senile R54
  tooth, teeth — *see* Caries, dental
Deciduitis (acute)
  following ectopic or molar pregnancy O08.0
Decline (general) — *see* Debility
  cognitive, age-associated R41.81
Decompensation
  cardiac (acute) (chronic) — *see* Disease, heart
  cardiovascular — *see* Disease, cardiovascular
  heart — *see* Disease, heart
  hepatic — *see* Failure, hepatic
  myocardial (acute) (chronic) — *see* Disease, heart
  respiratory J98.8
Decompression sickness T70.3
Decrease (d)
  absolute neutrophile count — *see* Neutropenia
  blood
    platelets — *see* Thrombocytopenia
    pressure R03.1
      due to shock following
        injury T79.4
        operation T81.19
  estrogen E28.39
    postablative E89.40
      asymptomatic E89.40
      symptomatic E89.41
  fragility of erythrocytes D58.8
  function
    lipase (pancreatic) K90.3
    ovary in hypopituitarism E23.0
    parenchyma of pancreas K86.89
    pituitary (gland) (anterior) (lobe) E23.0
      posterior (lobe) E23.0
  functional activity R68.89
  glucose R73.09
  hematocrit R71.0
  hemoglobin R71.0
  leukocytes D72.819
    specified NEC D72.818
  libido R68.82
  lymphocytes D72.810
  platelets D69.6
  respiration, due to shock following injury T79.4
  sexual desire R68.82
  tear secretion NEC — *see* Syndrome, dry eye
  tolerance
    fat K90.49
    glucose R73.09
    pancreatic K90.3
    salt and water E87.8
  vision NEC H54.7
  white blood cell count D72.819
    specified NEC D72.818
Decubitus (ulcer) — *see* Ulcer, pressure, by site
  cervix N86
Deepening acetabulum — *see* Derangement, joint, specified type NEC, hip
Defect, defective Q89.9
  3-beta-hydroxysteroid dehydrogenase E25.0
  11-hydroxylase E25.0
  21-hydroxylase E25.0
  abdominal wall, congenital Q79.59
  antibody immunodeficiency D80.9
  aorticopulmonary septum Q21.4
  atrial septal (ostium secundum type) Q21.1
    following acute myocardial infarction (current complication) I23.1
    ostium primum type Q21.2

Defect, defective - *continued*
  atrioventricular
    canal Q21.2
    septum Q21.2
  auricular septal Q21.1
  bilirubin excretion NEC E80.6
  biosynthesis, androgen (testicular) E29.1
  bulbar septum Q21.0
  catalase E80.3
  cell membrane receptor complex (CR3) D71
  circulation I99.9
    congenital Q28.9
    newborn Q28.9
  coagulation (factor) — *see also* Deficiency, factor D68.9
    with
      ectopic pregnancy O08.1
      molar pregnancy O08.1
    acquired D68.4
    antepartum with hemorrhage — *see* Hemorrhage, antepartum, with coagulation defect
    due to
      liver disease D68.4
      vitamin K deficiency D68.4
    hereditary NEC D68.2
    intrapartum O67.0
    newborn, transient P61.6
    postpartum O72.3
    specified type NEC D68.8
  complement system D84.1
  conduction (heart) I45.9
    bone — *see* Deafness, conductive
  congenital, organ or site not listed — *see* Anomaly, by site
  coronary sinus Q21.1
  cushion, endocardial Q21.2
  degradation, glycoprotein E77.1
  dental bridge, crown, fillings — *see* Defect, dental restoration
  dental restoration K08.50
    specified NEC K08.59
  dentin (hereditary) K00.5
  Descemet's membrane, congenital Q13.89
  developmental — *see also* Anomaly
    cauda equina Q06.3
  diaphragm
    with elevation, eventration or hernia — *see* Hernia, diaphragm
    congenital Q79.1
      with hernia Q79.0
      gross (with hernia) Q79.0
  ectodermal, congenital Q82.9
  Eisenmenger's Q21.8
  enzyme
    catalase E80.3
    peroxidase E80.3
  esophagus, congenital Q39.9
  extensor retinaculum M62.89
  fibrin polymerization D68.2
  filling
    bladder R93.41
    kidney R93.42-
    renal pelvis R93.41
    stomach R93.3
    ureter R93.41
    urinary organs, specified NEC R93.49
  Gerbode Q21.0
  glycoprotein degradation E77.1
  Hageman (factor) D68.2
  hearing — *see* Deafness
  high grade F70
  interatrial septal Q21.1
  interauricular septal Q21.1
  interventricular septal Q21.0
    with dextroposition of aorta, pulmonary stenosis and hypertrophy of right ventricle Q21.3
    in tetralogy of Fallot Q21.3
  learning (specific) — *see* Disorder, learning
  lymphocyte function antigen-1 (LFA-1) D84.0
  lysosomal enzyme, post-translational modification E77.0
  major osseous M89.70
    ankle M89.77-
    carpus M89.74-
    clavicle M89.71-
    femur M89.75-
    fibula M89.76-
    fingers M89.74-
    foot M89.77-
    forearm M89.73-
    hand M89.74-
    humerus M89.72-
    lower leg M89.76-

Defect, defective - *continued*
major osseous - *continued*
  metacarpus M89.74-
  metatarsus M89.77-
  multiple sites M89.79
  pelvic region M89.75-
  pelvis M89.75-
  radius M89.73-
  scapula M89.71-
  shoulder region M89.71-
  specified NEC M89.78
  tarsus M89.77-
  thigh M89.75-
  tibia M89.76-
  toes M89.77-
  ulna M89.73-
mental — *see* Disability, intellectual
modification, lysosomal enzymes, post-
  translational E77.0
obstructive, congenital
  renal pelvis Q62.39
  ureter Q62.39
    atresia — *see* Atresia, ureter
    cecoureterocele Q62.32
    megaureter Q62.2
    orthotopic ureterocele Q62.31
osseous, major M89.70
  ankle M89.77-
  carpus M89.74-
  clavicle M89.71-
  femur M89.75-
  fibula M89.76-
  fingers M89.74-
  foot M89.77-
  forearm M89.73-
  hand M89.74-
  humerus M89.72-
  lower leg M89.76-
  metacarpus M89.74-
  metatarsus M89.77-
  multiple sites M89.9
  pelvic region M89.75-
  pelvis M89.75-
  radius M89.73-
  scapula M89.71-
  shoulder region M89.71-
  specified NEC M89.78
  tarsus M89.77-
  thigh M89.75-
  tibia M89.76-
  toes M89.77-
  ulna M89.73-
osteochondral NEC — *see also* Deformity M95.8
ostium
  primum Q21.2
  secundum Q21.1
peroxidase E80.3
placental blood supply — *see* Insufficiency,
  placental
platelets, qualitative D69.1
  constitutional D68.0
postural NEC, spine — *see* Dorsopathy, deforming
reduction
  limb Q73.8
    lower Q72.9-
      absence — *see* Agenesis, leg
        foot — *see* Agenesis, foot
      longitudinal
        femur Q72.4-
        fibula Q72.6-
        tibia Q72.5-
      specified type NEC Q72.89-
      split foot Q72.7-
    specified type NEC Q73.8
    upper Q71.9-
      absence — *see* Agenesis, arm
        forearm — *see* Agenesis, forearm
        hand — *see* Agenesis, hand
      lobster-claw hand Q71.6-
      longitudinal
        radius Q71.4-
        ulna Q71.5-
      specified type NEC Q71.89-
renal pelvis Q63.8
  obstructive Q62.39
respiratory system, congenital Q34.9
restoration, dental K08.50
  specified NEC K08.59
retinal nerve bundle fibers H35.89
septal (heart) NOS Q21.9
  acquired (atrial) (auricular) (ventricular) (old) I51.0
  atrial Q21.1

Defect, defective - *continued*
septal (heart) NOS - *continued*
  atrial - *continued*
    concurrent with acute myocardial
      infarction — *see* Infarct, myocardium
    following acute myocardial infarction (current
      complication) I23.1
    ventricular — *see also* Defect, ventricular
      septal Q21.0
  sinus venosus Q21.1
  speech R47.9
    developmental F80.9
    specified NEC R47.89
  Taussig-Bing (aortic transposition and overriding
    pulmonary artery) Q20.1
  teeth, wedge K03.1
  vascular (local) I99.9
    congenital Q27.9
  ventricular septal Q21.0
    concurrent with acute myocardial infarction — *see*
      Infarct, myocardium
    following acute myocardial infarction (current
      complication) I23.2
    in tetralogy of Fallot Q21.3
  vision NEC H54.7
  visual field H53.40
    bilateral
      heteronymous H53.47
      homonymous H53.46-
    generalized contraction H53.48-
    localized
      arcuate H53.43-
      scotoma (central area) H53.41-
        blind spot area H53.42-
      sector H53.43-
      specified type NEC H53.45-
  voice R49.9
    specified NEC R49.8
  wedge, tooth, teeth (abrasion) K03.1
Deferentitis N49.1
  gonorrheal (acute) (chronic) A54.23
Defibrination (syndrome) D65
  antepartum — *see* Hemorrhage, antepartum, with
    coagulation defect, disseminated intravascular
    coagulation
  following ectopic or molar pregnancy O08.1
  intrapartum O67.0
  newborn P60
  postpartum O72.3
Deficiency, deficient
  3-beta hydroxysteroid dehydrogenase E25.0
  5-alpha reductase (with male
    pseudohermaphroditism) E29.1
  11-hydroxylase E25.0
  21-hydroxylase E25.0
  abdominal muscle syndrome Q79.4
  accelerator globulin (Ac G) (blood) D68.2
  AC globulin (congenital) (hereditary) D68.2
    acquired D68.4
  acid phosphatase E83.39
  activating factor (blood) D68.2
  adenosine deaminase (ADA) D81.3
  aldolase (hereditary) E74.19
  alpha-1-antitrypsin E88.01
  amino-acids E72.9
  anemia — *see* Anemia
  aneurin E51.9
  antibody with
    hyperimmunoglobulinemia D80.6
    near-normal immunoglobins D80.6
  antidiuretic hormone E23.2
  anti-hemophilic
    factor (A) D66
      B D67
      C D68.1
    globulin (AHG) NEC D66
  antithrombin (antithrombin III) D68.59
  ascorbic acid E54
  attention (disorder) (syndrome) F98.8
    with hyperactivity — *see* Disorder, attention-deficit
      hyperactivity
  autoprothrombin
    I D68.2
    II D67
    C D68.2
  beta-glucuronidase E76.29
  biotin E53.8
  biotin-dependent carboxylase D81.819
  biotinidase D81.810
  brancher enzyme (amylopectinosis) E74.03
  calciferol E55.9
    with
      adult osteomalacia M83.8

Deficiency, deficient - *continued*
calciferol - *continued*
  with - *continued*
    rickets — *see* Rickets
calcium (dietary) E58
calorie, severe E43
  with marasmus E41
    and kwashiorkor E42
cardiac — *see* Insufficiency, myocardial
carnitine E71.40
  due to
    hemodialysis E71.43
    inborn errors of metabolism E71.42
    Valproic acid therapy E71.43
  iatrogenic E71.43
  muscle palmityltransferase E71.314
  primary E71.41
  secondary E71.448
carotene E50.9
central nervous system G96.8
ceruloplasmin (Wilson) E83.01
choline E53.8
Christmas factor D67
chromium E61.4
clotting (blood) — *see also* Deficiency, coagulation
  factor D68.9
clotting factor NEC (hereditary) — *see
  also* Deficiency, factor D68.2
coagulation NOS D68.9
  with
    ectopic pregnancy O08.1
    molar pregnancy O08.1
  acquired (any) D68.4
  antepartum hemorrhage — *see* Hemorrhage,
    antepartum, with coagulation defect
  clotting factor NEC — *see also* Deficiency,
    factor D68.2
  due to
    hyperprothrombinemia D68.4
    liver disease D68.4
    vitamin K deficiency D68.4
  newborn, transient P61.6
  postpartum O72.3
  specified NEC D68.8
cognitive F09
color vision H53.50
  achromatopsia H53.51
  acquired H53.52
  deuteranomaly H53.53
  protanomaly H53.54
  specified type NEC H53.59
  tritanomaly H53.55
combined glucocorticoid and
  mineralocorticoid E27.49
contact factor D68.2
copper (nutritional) E61.0
corticoadrenal E27.40
  primary E27.1
craniofacial axis Q75.0
cyanocobalamin E53.8
C1 esterase inhibitor (C1-INH) D84.1
debrancher enzyme (limit dextrinosis) E74.03
dehydrogenase
  long chain/very long chain acyl CoA E71.310
  medium chain acyl CoA E71.311
  short chain acyl CoA E71.312
diet E63.9
dihydropyrimidine dehydrogenase (DPD) E88.89
disaccharidase E73.9
edema — *see* Malnutrition, severe
endocrine E34.9
energy-supply — *see* Malnutrition
enzymes, circulating NEC E88.09
ergosterol E55.9
  with
    adult osteomalacia M83.8
    rickets — *see* Rickets
essential fatty acid (EFA) E63.0
factor — *see also* Deficiency, coagulation
  Hageman D68.2
  I (congenital) (hereditary) D68.2
  II (congenital) (hereditary) D68.2
  IX (congenital) (functional) (hereditary) (with
    functional defect) D67
  multiple (congenital) D68.8
    acquired D68.4
  V (congenital) (hereditary) D68.2
  VII (congenital) (hereditary) D68.2
  VIII (congenital) (functional) (hereditary) (with
    functional defect) D66
    with vascular defect D68.0
  X (congenital) (hereditary) D68.2
  XI (congenital) (hereditary) D68.1

Deficiency, deficient - *continued*
factor - *continued*
XII (congenital) (hereditary) D68.2
XIII (congenital) (hereditary) D68.2
femoral, proximal focal (congenital) — *see* Defect, reduction, lower limb, longitudinal, femur
fibrin-stabilizing factor (congenital) (hereditary) D68.2
acquired D68.4
fibrinase D68.2
fibrinogen (congenital) (hereditary) D68.2
acquired D65
folate E53.8
folic acid E53.8
foreskin N47.3
fructokinase E74.11
fructose 1,6-diphosphatase E74.19
fructose-1-phosphate aldolase E74.19
galactokinase E74.29
galactose-1-phosphate uridyl transferase E74.29
gammaglobulin in blood D80.1
hereditary D80.0
glass factor D68.2
glucocorticoid E27.49
mineralocorticoid E27.49
glucose-6-phosphatase E74.01
glucose-6-phosphate dehydrogenase anemia D55.0
glucuronyl transferase E80.5
glycogen synthetase E74.09
gonadotropin (isolated) E23.0
growth hormone (idiopathic) (isolated) E23.0
Hageman factor D68.2
hemoglobin D64.9
hepatophosphorylase E74.09
homogentisate 1,2-dioxygenase E70.29
hormone
anterior pituitary (partial) NEC E23.0
growth E23.0
growth (isolated) E23.0
pituitary E23.0
testicular E29.1
hypoxanthine- (guanine) -phosphoribosyltransferase (HG- PRT) (total H-PRT) E79.1
immunity D84.9
cell-mediated D84.8
with thrombocytopenia and eczema D82.0
combined D81.9
humoral D80.9
IgA (secretory) D80.2
IgG D80.3
IgM D80.4
immuno — *see* Immunodeficiency
immunoglobulin, selective
A (IgA) D80.2
G (IgG) (subclasses) D80.3
M (IgM) D80.4
inositol (B complex) E53.8
intrinsic
factor (congenital) D51.0
sphincter N36.42
with urethral hypermobility N36.43
iodine E61.8
congenital syndrome — *see* Syndrome, iodine-deficiency, congenital
iron E61.1
anemia D50.9
kalium E87.6
kappa-light chain D80.8
labile factor (congenital) (hereditary) D68.2
acquired D68.4
lacrimal fluid (acquired) — *see also* Syndrome, dry eye
congenital Q10.6
lactase
congenital E73.0
secondary E73.1
Laki-Lorand factor D68.2
lecithin cholesterol acyltransferase E78.6
lipocaic K86.89
lipoprotein (familial) (high density) E78.6
liver phosphorylase E74.09
lysosomal alpha-1, 4 glucosidase E74.02
magnesium E61.2
major histocompatibility complex
class I D81.6
class II D81.7
manganese E61.3
menadione (vitamin K) E56.1
newborn P53
mental (familial) (hereditary) — *see* Disability, intellectual
methylenetetrahydrofolate reductase (MTHFR) E72.12

Deficiency, deficient - *continued*
mevalonate kinase M04.1
mineral NEC E61.8
mineralocorticoid E27.49
with glucocorticoid E27.49
molybdenum (nutritional) E61.5
moral F60.2
multiple nutrient elements E61.7
muscle
carnitine (palmityltransferase) E71.314
phosphofructokinase E74.09
myoadenylate deaminase E79.2
myocardial — *see* Insufficiency, myocardial
myophosphorylase E74.04
NADH diaphorase or reductase (congenital) D74.0
NADH-methemoglobin reductase (congenital) D74.0
natrium E87.1
niacin (amide) (-tryptophan) E52
nicotinamide E52
nicotinic acid E52
number of teeth — *see* Anodontia
nutrient element E61.9
multiple E61.7
specified NEC E61.8
nutrition, nutritional E63.9
sequelae — *see* Sequelae, nutritional deficiency
specified NEC E63.8
of interleukin 1 receptor antagonist [DIRA] M04.8
ornithine transcarbamylase E72.4
ovarian E28.39
oxygen — *see* Anoxia
pantothenic acid E53.8
parathyroid (gland) E20.9
perineum (female) N81.89
phenylalanine hydroxylase E70.1
phosphoenolpyruvate carboxykinase E74.4
phosphofructokinase E74.19
phosphomannomutuse E74.8
phosphomannose isomerase E74.8
phosphomannosyl mutase E74.8
phosphorylase kinase, liver E74.09
pituitary hormone (isolated) E23.0
plasma thromboplastin
antecedent (PTA) D68.1
component (PTC) D67
platelet NEC D69.1
constitutional D68.0
polyglandular E31.8
autoimmune E31.0
potassium (K) E87.6
prepuce N47.3
proaccelerin (congenital) (hereditary) D68.2
acquired D68.4
proconvertin factor (congenital) (hereditary) D68.2
acquired D68.4
protein — *see also* Malnutrition E46
anemia D53.0
C D68.59
S D68.59
prothrombin (congenital) (hereditary) D68.2
acquired D68.4
Prower factor D68.2
pseudocholinesterase E88.09
PTA (plasma thromboplastin antecedent) D68.1
PTC (plasma thromboplastin component) D67
purine nucleoside phosphorylase (PNP) D81.5
pyracin (alpha) (beta) E53.1
pyridoxal E53.1
pyridoxamine E53.1
pyridoxine (derivatives) E53.1
pyruvate
carboxylase E74.4
dehydrogenase E74.4
riboflavin (vitamin B2) E53.0
salt E87.1
secretion
ovary E28.39
salivary gland (any) K11.7
urine R34
selenium (dietary) E59
serum antitrypsin, familial E88.01
short stature homeobox gene (SHOX)
with
dyschondrosteosis Q78.8
short stature (idiopathic) E34.3
Turner's syndrome Q96.9
sodium (Na) E87.1
SPCA (factor VII) D68.2
sphincter, intrinsic N36.42
with urethral hypermobility N36.43
stable factor (congenital) (hereditary) D68.2
acquired D68.4

Deficiency, deficient - *continued*
Stuart-Prower (factor X) D68.2
sucrase E74.39
sulfatase E75.29
sulfite oxidase E72.19
thiamin, thiaminic (chloride) E51.9
beriberi (dry) E51.11
wet E51.12
thrombokinase D68.2
newborn P53
thyroid (gland) — *see* Hypothyroidism
tocopherol E56.0
tooth bud K00.0
transcobalamine II (anemia) D51.2
vanadium E61.6
vascular I99.9
vasopressin E23.2
vertical ridge K06.8
viosterol — *see* Deficiency, calciferol
vitamin (multiple) NOS E56.9
A E50.9
with
Bitot's spot (corneal) E50.1
follicular keratosis E50.8
keratomalacia E50.4
manifestations NEC E50.8
night blindness E50.5
scar of cornea, xerophthalmic E50.6
xeroderma E50.8
xerophthalmia E50.7
xerosis
conjunctival E50.0
and Bitot's spot E50.1
cornea E50.2
and ulceration E50.3
sequelae E64.1
B (complex) NOS E53.9
with
beriberi (dry) E51.11
wet E51.12
pellagra E52
B1 NOS E51.9
beriberi (dry) E51.11
with circulatory system manifestations E51.11
wet E51.12
B12 E53.8
B2 (riboflavin) E53.0
B6 E53.1
C E54
sequelae E64.2
D E55.9
with
adult osteomalacia M83.8
rickets — *see* Rickets
25-hydroxylase E83.32
E E56.0
folic acid E53.8
G E53.0
group B E53.9
specified NEC E53.8
H (biotin) E53.8
K E56.1
of newborn P53
nicotinic E52
P E56.8
PP (pellagra-preventing) E52
specified NEC E56.8
thiamin E51.9
beriberi — *see* Beriberi
zinc, dietary E60
Deficit — *see also* Deficiency
attention and concentration R41.840
following
cerebral infarction I69.310
cerebrovascular disease I69.910
specified disease NEC I69.810
nontraumatic
intracerebral hemorrhage I69.110
specified intracranial hemorrhage NEC I69.210
subarachnoid hemorrhage I69.010
disorder — *see* Attention, deficit
cognitive
communication R41.841
emotional
following
cerebral infarction I69.315
cerebrovascular disease I69.915
specified disease NEC I69.815
nontraumatic
intracerebral hemorrhage I69.115
specified intracranial hemorrhage NEC I69.215
subarachnoid hemorrhage I69.015

Deficit - *continued*
cognitive - *continued*
  following
    cerebral infarction I69.319
    cerebrovascular disease I69.919
      specified disease NEC I69.819
    nontraumatic
      intracerebral hemorrhage I69.119
      specified intracranial hemorrhage NEC I69.219
      subarachnoid hemorrhage I69.019
  social
    following
      cerebral infarction I69.315
      cerebrovascular disease I69.915
        specified disease NEC I69.815
      nontraumatic
        intracerebral hemorrhage I69.115
        specified intracranial hemorrhage NEC I69.215
        subarachnoid hemorrhage I69.015
  cognitive NEC R41.89
    following
      cerebral infarction I69.318
      cerebrovascular disease I69.918
        specified disease NEC I69.818
      nontraumatic
        intracerebral hemorrhage I69.118
        specified intracranial hemorrhage NEC I69.218
        subarachnoid hemorrhage I69.018
  concentration R41.840
  executive function R41.844
    following
      cerebral infarction I69.314
      cerebrovascular disease I69.914
        specified disease NEC I69.814
      nontraumatic
        intracerebral hemorrhage I69.114
        specified intracranial hemorrhage NEC I69.214
        subarachnoid hemorrhage I69.014
  frontal lobe R41.844
    following
      cerebral infarction I69.314
      cerebrovascular disease I69.914
        specified disease NEC I69.814
      nontraumatic
        intracerebral hemorrhage I69.114
        specified intracranial hemorrhage NEC I69.214
        subarachnoid hemorrhage I69.014
  memory
    following
      cerebral infarction I69.311
      cerebrovascular disease I69.911
        specified disease NEC I69.811
      nontraumatic
        intracerebral hemorrhage I69.111
        specified intracranial hemorrhage NEC I69.211
        subarachnoid hemorrhage I69.011
  neurologic NEC R29.818
    ischemic
      reversible (RIND) I63.9
      prolonged (PRIND) I63.9
  oxygen R09.02
  prolonged reversible ischemic neurologic (PRIND) I63.9
  psychomotor R41.843
    following
      cerebral infarction I69.313
      cerebrovascular disease I69.913
        specified disease NEC I69.813
      nontraumatic
        intracerebral hemorrhage I69.113
        specified intracranial hemorrhage NEC I69.213
        subarachnoid hemorrhage I69.013
  visuospatial R41.842
    following
      cerebral infarction I69.312
      cerebrovascular disease I69.912
        specified disease NEC I69.812
      nontraumatic
        intracerebral hemorrhage I69.112
        specified intracranial hemorrhage NEC I69.212
        subarachnoid hemorrhage I69.012

Deflection
radius — *see* Deformity, limb, specified type NEC, forearm
septum (acquired) (nasal) (nose) J34.2
spine — *see* Curvature, spine
turbinate (nose) J34.2

Defluvium
capillorum — *see* Alopecia
ciliorum — *see* Madarosis
unguium L60.8

Deformity Q89.9
abdomen, congenital Q89.9
abdominal wall
  acquired M95.8
  congenital Q79.59
acquired (unspecified site) M95.9
adrenal gland Q89.1
alimentary tract, congenital Q45.9
  upper Q40.9
ankle (joint) (acquired) — *see also* Deformity, limb, lower leg
  abduction — *see* Contraction, joint, ankle
  congenital Q68.8
  contraction — *see* Contraction, joint, ankle
  specified type NEC — *see* Deformity, limb, foot, specified NEC
anus (acquired) K62.89
  congenital Q43.9
aorta (arch) (congenital) Q25.40
  acquired I77.89
aortic
  arch, acquired I77.89
  cusp or valve (congenital) Q23.8
    acquired — *see also* Endocarditis, aortic I35.8
arm (acquired) (upper) — *see also* Deformity, limb, upper arm
  congenital Q68.8
  forearm — *see* Deformity, limb, forearm
artery (congenital) (peripheral) NOS Q27.9
  acquired I77.89
  coronary (acquired) I25.9
    congenital Q24.5
  umbilical Q27.0
atrial septal Q21.1
auditory canal (external) (congenital) — *see also* Malformation, ear, external
  acquired — *see* Disorder, ear, external, specified type NEC
auricle
  ear (congenital) — *see also* Malformation, ear, external
    acquired — *see* Disorder, pinna, deformity
back — *see* Dorsopathy, deforming
bile duct (common) (congenital) (hepatic) Q44.5
  acquired K83.8
biliary duct or passage (congenital) Q44.5
  acquired K83.8
bladder (neck) (trigone) (sphincter) (acquired) N32.89
  congenital Q64.79
bone (acquired) NOS M95.9
  congenital Q79.9
  turbinate M95.0
brain (congenital) Q04.9
  acquired G93.89
  reduction Q04.3
breast (acquired) N64.89
  congenital Q83.9
  reconstructed N65.0
bronchus (congenital) Q32.4
  acquired NEC J98.09
bursa, congenital Q79.9
canaliculi (lacrimalis) (acquired) — *see also* Disorder, lacrimal system, changes
  congenital Q10.6
canthus, acquired — *see* Disorder, eyelid, specified type NEC
capillary (acquired) I78.8
cardiovascular system, congenital Q28.9
caruncle, lacrimal (acquired) — *see also* Disorder, lacrimal system, changes
  congenital Q10.6
cascade, stomach K31.2
cecum (congenital) Q43.9
  acquired K63.89
cerebral, acquired G93.89
  congenital Q04.9
cervix (uterus) (acquired) NEC N88.8
  congenital Q51.9
cheek (acquired) M95.2
  congenital Q18.9
chest (acquired) (wall) M95.4
  congenital Q67.8
  sequelae (late effect) of rickets E64.3
chin (acquired) M95.2
  congenital Q18.9
choroid (congenital) Q14.3
  acquired H31.8
  plexus Q07.8
    acquired G96.19
cicatricial — *see* Cicatrix
cilia, acquired — *see* Disorder, eyelid, specified type NEC

Deformity - *continued*
clavicle (acquired) M95.8
  congenital Q68.8
clitoris (congenital) Q52.6
  acquired N90.89
clubfoot — *see* Clubfoot
coccyx (acquired) — *see* subcategory M43.8
colon (congenital) Q43.9
  acquired K63.89
concha (ear) , congenital — *see also* Malformation, ear, external
  acquired — *see* Disorder, pinna, deformity
cornea (acquired) H18.70
  congenital Q13.4
  descemetocele — *see* Descemetocele
  ectasia — *see* Ectasia, cornea
  specified NEC H18.79-
  staphyloma — *see* Staphyloma, cornea
coronary artery (acquired) I25.9
  congenital Q24.5
cranium (acquired) — *see* Deformity, skull
cricoid cartilage (congenital) Q31.8
  acquired J38.7
cystic duct (congenital) Q44.5
  acquired K82.8
Dandy-Walker Q03.1
  with spina bifida — *see* Spina bifida
diaphragm (congenital) Q79.1
  acquired J98.6
digestive organ NOS Q45.9
ductus arteriosus Q25.0
duodenal bulb K31.89
duodenum (congenital) Q43.9
  acquired K31.89
dura — *see* Deformity, meninges
ear (acquired) — *see also* Disorder, pinna, deformity
  congenital (external) Q17.9
    internal Q16.5
    middle Q16.4
      ossicles Q16.3
    ossicles Q16.3
ectodermal (congenital) NEC Q84.9
ejaculatory duct (congenital) Q55.4
  acquired N50.89
elbow (joint) (acquired) — *see also* Deformity, limb, upper arm
  congenital Q68.8
  contraction — *see* Contraction, joint, elbow
endocrine gland NEC Q89.2
epididymis (congenital) Q55.4
  acquired N50.89
epiglottis (congenital) Q31.8
  acquired J38.7
esophagus (congenital) Q39.9
  acquired K22.8
eustachian tube (congenital) NEC Q17.8
eye, congenital Q15.9
eyebrow (congenital) Q18.8
eyelid (acquired) — *see also* Disorder, eyelid, specified type NEC
  congenital Q10.3
face (acquired) M95.2
  congenital Q18.9
fallopian tube, acquired N83.8
femur (acquired) — *see* Deformity, limb, specified type NEC, thigh
fetal
  with fetopelvic disproportion O33.7
  causing obstructed labor O66.3
finger (acquired) M20.00-
  boutonniere M20.02-
  congenital Q68.1
  flexion contracture — *see* Contraction, joint, hand
  mallet finger M20.01-
  specified NEC M20.09-
  swan-neck M20.03-
flexion (joint) (acquired) — *see also* Deformity, limb, flexion M21.20
  congenital NOS Q74.9
    hip Q65.89
foot (acquired) — *see also* Deformity, limb, lower leg
  cavovarus (congenital) Q66.1
  congenital NOS Q66.9
    specified type NEC Q66.89
  specified type NEC — *see* Deformity, limb, foot, specified NEC
  valgus (congenital) Q66.6
    acquired — *see* Deformity, valgus, ankle
  varus (congenital) NEC Q66.3
    acquired — *see* Deformity, varus, ankle
forearm (acquired) — *see also* Deformity, limb, forearm

Deformity - *continued*
  forearm (acquired) - *continued*
    congenital Q68.8
  forehead (acquired) M95.2
    congenital Q75.8
  frontal bone (acquired) M95.2
    congenital Q75.8
  gallbladder (congenital) Q44.1
    acquired K82.8
  gastrointestinal tract (congenital) NOS Q45.9
    acquired K63.89
  genitalia, genital organ (s) or system NEC
    female (congenital) Q52.9
      acquired N94.89
      external Q52.70
    male (congenital) Q55.9
      acquired N50.89
  globe (eye) (congenital) Q15.8
    acquired H44.89
  gum, acquired NEC K06.8
  hand (acquired) — *see* Deformity, limb, hand
    congenital Q68.1
  head (acquired) M95.2
    congenital Q75.8
  heart (congenital) Q24.9
    septum Q21.9
      auricular Q21.1
      ventricular Q21.0
    valve (congenital) NEC Q24.8
      acquired — *see* Endocarditis
  heel (acquired) — *see* Deformity, foot
  hepatic duct (congenital) Q44.5
    acquired K83.8
  hip (joint) (acquired) — *see also* Deformity, limb, thigh
    congenital Q65.9
    due to (previous) juvenile osteochondrosis — *see* Coxa, plana
    flexion — *see* Contraction, joint, hip
  hourglass — *see* Contraction, hourglass
  humerus (acquired) M21.82-
    congenital Q74.0
  hypophyseal (congenital) Q89.2
  ileocecal (coil) (valve) (acquired) K63.89
    congenital Q43.9
  ileum (congenital) Q43.9
    acquired K63.89
  ilium (acquired) M95.5
    congenital Q74.2
  integument (congenital) Q84.9
  intervertebral cartilage or disc (acquired) — *see* Disorder, disc, specified NEC
  intestine (large) (small) (congenital) NOS Q43.9
    acquired K63.89
  intrinsic minus or plus (hand) — *see* Deformity, limb, specified type NEC, forearm
  iris (acquired) H21.89
    congenital Q13.2
  ischium (acquired) M95.5
    congenital Q74.2
  jaw (acquired) (congenital) M26.9
  joint (acquired) NEC M21.90
    congenital Q68.8
    elbow M21.92-
    hand M21.94-
    hip M21.95-
    knee M21.96-
    shoulder M21.92-
    wrist M21.93-
  kidney (s) (calyx) (pelvis) (congenital) Q63.9
    acquired N28.89
    artery (congenital) Q27.2
      acquired I77.89
  Klippel-Feil (brevicollis) Q76.1
  knee (acquired) NEC — *see also* Deformity, limb, lower leg
    congenital Q68.2
  labium (majus) (minus) (congenital) Q52.79
    acquired N90.89
  lacrimal passages or duct (congenital) NEC Q10.6
    acquired — *see* Disorder, lacrimal system, changes
  larynx (muscle) (congenital) Q31.8
    acquired J38.7
    web (glottic) Q31.0
  leg (upper) (acquired) NEC — *see also* Deformity, limb, thigh
    congenital Q68.8
    lower leg — *see* Deformity, limb, lower leg
  lens (acquired) H27.8
    congenital Q12.9
  lid (fold) (acquired) — *see also* Disorder, eyelid, specified type NEC
    congenital Q10.3

Deformity - *continued*
  ligament (acquired) — *see* Disorder, ligament
    congenital Q79.9
  limb (acquired) M21.90
    clawfoot M21.53-
    clawhand M21.51-
    clubfoot M21.54-
    clubhand M21.52-
    congenital, except reduction deformity Q74.9
    flat foot M21.4-
    flexion M21.20
      ankle M21.27-
      elbow M21.22-
      finger M21.24-
      hip M21.25-
      knee M21.26-
      shoulder M21.21-
      toe M21.27-
      wrist M21.23-
    foot
      claw — *see* Deformity, limb, clawfoot
      club — *see* Deformity, limb, clubfoot
      drop M21.37-
      flat — *see* Deformity, limb, flat foot
      specified NEC M21.6X-
    forearm M21.93-
    hand M21.94-
    lower leg M21.96-
    specified type NEC M21.80
      forearm M21.83-
      lower leg M21.86-
      thigh M21.85-
      upper arm M21.82-
    thigh M21.95-
    unequal length M21.70
      short site is
        femur M21.75-
        fibula M21.76-
        humerus M21.72-
        radius M21.73-
        tibia M21.76-
        ulna M21.73-
    upper arm M21.92-
    valgus — *see* Deformity, valgus
    varus — *see* Deformity, varus
    wrist drop M21.33-
  lip (acquired) NEC K13.0
    congenital Q38.0
  liver (congenital) Q44.7
    acquired K76.89
  lumbosacral (congenital) (joint) (region) Q76.49
    acquired — *see* subcategory M43.8
    kyphosis — *see* Kyphosis, congenital
    lordosis — *see* Lordosis, congenital
  lung (congenital) Q33.9
    acquired J98.4
  lymphatic system, congenital Q89.9
  Madelung's (radius) Q74.0
  mandible (acquired) (congenital) M26.9
  maxilla (acquired) (congenital) M26.9
  meninges or membrane (congenital) Q07.9
    cerebral Q04.8
      acquired G96.19
    spinal cord (congenital) G96.19
      acquired G96.19
  metacarpus (acquired) — *see* Deformity, limb, forearm
    congenital Q74.0
  metatarsus (acquired) — *see* Deformity, foot
    congenital Q66.9
  middle ear (congenital) Q16.4
    ossicles Q16.3
  mitral (leaflets) (valve) I05.8
    parachute Q23.2
    stenosis, congenital Q23.2
  mouth (acquired) K13.79
    congenital Q38.6
  multiple, congenital NEC Q89.7
  muscle (acquired) M62.89
    congenital Q79.9
    sternocleidomastoid Q68.0
  musculoskeletal system (acquired) M95.9
    congenital Q79.9
    specified NEC M95.8
  nail (acquired) L60.8
    congenital Q84.6
  nasal — *see* Deformity, nose
  neck (acquired) M95.3
    congenital Q18.9
    sternocleidomastoid Q68.0
  nervous system (congenital) Q07.9
  nipple (congenital) Q83.9
    acquired N64.89

Deformity - *continued*
  nose (acquired) (cartilage) M95.0
    bone (turbinate) M95.0
    congenital Q30.9
      bent or squashed Q67.4
    saddle M95.0
      syphilitic A50.57
    septum (acquired) J34.2
      congenital Q30.8
    sinus (wall) (congenital) Q30.8
      acquired M95.0
    syphilitic (congenital) A50.57
      late A52.73
  ocular muscle (congenital) Q10.3
    acquired — *see* Strabismus, mechanical
  opticociliary vessels (congenital) Q13.2
  orbit (eye) (acquired) H05.30
    atrophy — *see* Atrophy, orbit
    congenital Q10.7
    due to
      bone disease NEC H05.32-
      trauma or surgery H05.33-
    enlargement — *see* Enlargement, orbit
    exostosis — *see* Exostosis, orbit
  organ of Corti (congenital) Q16.5
  ovary (congenital) Q50.39
    acquired N83.8
  oviduct, acquired N83.8
  palate (congenital) Q38.5
    acquired M27.8
    cleft (congenital) — *see* Cleft, palate
  pancreas (congenital) Q45.3
    acquired K86.89
  parathyroid (gland) Q89.2
  parotid (gland) (congenital) Q38.4
    acquired K11.8
  patella (acquired) — *see* Disorder, patella, specified NEC
  pelvis, pelvic (acquired) (bony) M95.5
    with disproportion (fetopelvic) O33.0
      causing obstructed labor O65.0
    congenital Q74.2
    rachitic sequelae (late effect) E64.3
  penis (glans) (congenital) Q55.69
    acquired N48.89
  pericardium (congenital) Q24.8
    acquired — *see* Pericarditis
  pharynx (congenital) Q38.8
    acquired J39.2
  pinna, acquired — *see also* Disorder, pinna, deformity
    congenital Q17.9
  pituitary (congenital) Q89.2
  posture — *see* Dorsopathy, deforming
  prepuce (congenital) Q55.69
    acquired N47.8
  prostate (congenital) Q55.4
    acquired N42.89
  pupil (congenital) Q13.2
    acquired — *see* Abnormality, pupillary
  pylorus (congenital) Q40.3
    acquired K31.89
  rachitic (acquired) , old or healed E64.3
  radius (acquired) — *see also* Deformity, limb, forearm
    congenital Q68.8
  rectum (congenital) Q43.9
    acquired K62.89
  reduction (extremity) (limb) , congenital — *see also* condition and site Q73.8
    brain Q04.3
    lower — *see* Defect, reduction, lower limb
    upper — *see* Defect, reduction, upper limb
  renal — *see* Deformity, kidney
  respiratory system (congenital) Q34.9
  rib (acquired) M95.4
    congenital Q76.6
    cervical Q76.5
  rotation (joint) (acquired) — *see* Deformity, limb, specified site NEC
    congenital Q74.9
    hip — *see* Deformity, limb, specified type NEC, thigh
      congenital Q65.89
  sacroiliac joint (congenital) Q74.2
    acquired — *see* subcategory M43.8
  sacrum (acquired) — *see* subcategory M43.8
  saddle
    back — *see* Lordosis
    nose M95.0
      syphilitic A50.57
  salivary gland or duct (congenital) Q38.4
    acquired K11.8

Deformity - *continued*
scapula (acquired) M95.8
  congenital Q68.8
scrotum (congenital) — *see also* Malformation, testis and scrotum
  acquired N50.89
seminal vesicles (congenital) Q55.4
  acquired N50.89
septum, nasal (acquired) J34.2
shoulder (joint) (acquired) — *see* Deformity, limb, upper arm
  congenital Q74.0
  contraction — *see* Contraction, joint, shoulder
sigmoid (flexure) (congenital) Q43.9
  acquired K63.89
skin (congenital) Q82.9
skull (acquired) M95.2
  congenital Q75.8
    with
      anencephaly Q00.0
      encephalocele — *see* Encephalocele
      hydrocephalus Q03.9
        with spina bifida — *see* Spina bifida, by site, with hydrocephalus
      microcephaly Q02
soft parts, organs or tissues (of pelvis)
  in pregnancy or childbirth NEC O34.8-
    causing obstructed labor O65.5
spermatic cord (congenital) Q55.4
  acquired N50.89
  torsion — *see* Torsion, spermatic cord
spinal — *see* Dorsopathy, deforming
  column (acquired) — *see* Dorsopathy, deforming
    congenital Q67.5
  cord (congenital) Q06.9
    acquired G95.89
  nerve root (congenital) Q07.9
spine (acquired) — *see also* Dorsopathy, deforming
  congenital Q67.5
  rachitic E64.3
  specified NEC — *see* Dorsopathy, deforming, specified NEC
spleen
  acquired D73.89
  congenital Q89.09
Sprengel's (congenital) Q74.0
sternocleidomastoid (muscle) , congenital Q68.0
sternum (acquired) M95.4
  congenital NEC Q76.7
stomach (congenital) Q40.3
  acquired K31.89
submandibular gland (congenital) Q38.4
submaxillary gland (congenital) Q38.4
  acquired K11.8
talipes — *see* Talipes
testis (congenital) — *see also* Malformation, testis and scrotum
  acquired N44.8
  torsion — *see* Torsion, testis
thigh (acquired) — *see also* Deformity, limb, thigh
  congenital NEC Q68.8
thorax (acquired) (wall) M95.4
  congenital Q67.8
  sequelae of rickets E64.3
thumb (acquired) — *see also* Deformity, finger
  congenital NEC Q68.1
thymus (tissue) (congenital) Q89.2
thyroid (gland) (congenital) Q89.2
  cartilage Q31.8
    acquired J38.7
tibia (acquired) — *see also* Deformity, limb, specified type NEC, lower leg
  congenital NEC Q68.8
  saber (syphilitic) A50.56
toe (acquired) M20.6-
  congenital Q66.9
  hallux rigidus M20.2-
  hallux valgus M20.1-
  hallux varus M20.3-
  hammer toe M20.4-
  specified NEC M20.5X-
tongue (congenital) Q38.3
  acquired K14.8
tooth, teeth K00.2
trachea (rings) (congenital) Q32.1
  acquired J39.8
transverse aortic arch (congenital) Q25.49
tricuspid (leaflets) (valve) I07.8
  atresia or stenosis Q22.4
  Ebstein's Q22.5
trunk (acquired) M95.8
  congenital Q89.9
ulna (acquired) — *see also* Deformity, limb, forearm

Deformity - *continued*
ulna (acquired) - *continued*
  congenital NEC Q68.8
urachus, congenital Q64.4
ureter (opening) (congenital) Q62.8
  acquired N28.89
urethra (congenital) Q64.79
  acquired N36.8
urinary tract (congenital) Q64.9
  urachus Q64.4
uterus (congenital) Q51.9
  acquired N85.8
uvula (congenital) Q38.5
vagina (acquired) N89.8
  congenital Q52.4
valgus NEC M21.00
  ankle M21.07-
  elbow M21.02-
  hip M21.05-
  knee M21.06-
valve, valvular (congenital) (heart) Q24.8
  acquired — *see* Endocarditis
varus NEC M21.10
  ankle M21.17-
  elbow M21.12-
  hip M21.15
  knee M21.16-
  tibia — *see* Osteochondrosis, juvenile, tibia
vas deferens (congenital) Q55.4
  acquired N50.89
vein (congenital) Q27.9
  great Q26.9
vertebra — *see* Dorsopathy, deforming
vertical talus (congenital) Q66.80
  left foot Q66.82
  right foot Q66.81
vesicourethral orifice (acquired) N32.89
  congenital NEC Q64.79
vessels of optic papilla (congenital) Q14.2
visual field (contraction) — *see* Defect, visual field
vitreous body, acquired H43.89
vulva (congenital) Q52.79
  acquired N90.89
wrist (joint) (acquired) — *see also* Deformity, limb, forearm
  congenital Q68.8
  contraction — *see* Contraction, joint, wrist

Degeneration, degenerative
adrenal (capsule) (fatty) (gland) (hyaline) (infectional) E27.8
amyloid — *see also* Amyloidosis E85.9
anterior cornua, spinal cord G12.29
anterior labral S43.49-
aorta, aortic I70.0
  fatty I77.89
aortic valve (heart) — *see* Endocarditis, aortic
arteriovascular — *see* Arteriosclerosis
artery, arterial (atheromatous) (calcareous) — *see also* Arteriosclerosis
  cerebral, amyloid E85.4 *[I68.0]*
  medial — *see* Arteriosclerosis, extremities
articular cartilage NEC — *see* Derangement, joint, articular cartilage, by site
atheromatous — *see* Arteriosclerosis
basal nuclei or ganglia G23.9
  specified NEC G23.8
bone NEC — *see* Disorder, bone, specified type NEC
brachial plexus G54.0
brain (cortical) (progressive) G31.9
  alcoholic G31.2
  arteriosclerotic I67.2
  childhood G31.9
    specified NEC G31.89
  cystic G31.89
    congenital Q04.6
  in
    alcoholism G31.2
    beriberi E51.2
    cerebrovascular disease I67.9
    congenital hydrocephalus Q03.9
      with spina bifida — *see also* Spina bifida
    Fabry-Anderson disease E75.21
    Gaucher's disease E75.22
    Hunter's syndrome E76.1
    lipidosis
      cerebral E75.4
      generalized E75.6
    mucopolysaccharidosis — *see* Mucopolysaccharidosis
    myxedema E03.9 *[G32.89]*
    neoplastic disease — *see also* Neoplasm D49.6 *[G32.89]*

Degeneration, degenerative - *continued*
brain (cortical) (progressive) - *continued*
  in - *continued*
    Niemann-Pick disease E75.249 *[G32.89]*
    sphingolipidosis E75.3 *[G32.89]*
    vitamin B12 deficiency E53.8 *[G32.89]*
  senile NEC G31.1
breast N64.89
Bruch's membrane — *see* Degeneration, choroid
capillaries (fatty) I78.8
  amyloid E85.8 *[I79.8]*
cardiac — *see also* Degeneration, myocardial
  valve, valvular — *see* Endocarditis
cardiorenal — *see* Hypertension, cardiorenal
cardiovascular — *see also* Disease, cardiovascular
  renal — *see* Hypertension, cardiorenal
cerebellar NOS G31.9
  alcoholic G31.2
  primary (hereditary) (sporadic) G11.9
cerebral — *see* Degeneration, brain
cerebrovascular I67.9
  due to hypertension I67.4
cervical plexus G54.2
cervix N88.8
  due to radiation (intended effect) N88.8
    adverse effect or misadventure N99.89
chamber angle H21.21-
changes, spine or vertebra — *see* Spondylosis
chorioretinal — *see also* Degeneration, choroid
  hereditary H31.20
choroid (colloid) (drusen) H31.10-
  atrophy — *see* Atrophy, choroidal
  hereditary — *see* Dystrophy, choroidal, hereditary
ciliary body H21.22-
cochlear — *see* subcategory H83.8
combined (spinal cord) (subacute) E53.8 *[G32.0]*
  with anemia (pernicious) D51.0 *[G32.0]*
    due to dietary vitamin B12 deficiency D51.3 *[G32.0]*
  in (due to)
    vitamin B12 deficiency E53.8 *[G32.0]*
      anemia D51.9 *[G32.0]*
conjunctiva H11.10
  concretions — *see* Concretion, conjunctiva
  deposits — *see* Deposit, conjunctiva
  pigmentations — *see* Pigmentation, conjunctiva
  pinguecula — *see* Pinguecula
  xerosis — *see* Xerosis, conjunctiva
cornea H18.40
  calcerous H18.43
    band keratopathy H18.42-
  familial, hereditary — *see* Dystrophy, cornea
  hyaline (of old scars) H18.49
  keratomalacia — *see* Keratomalacia
  nodular H18.45-
  peripheral H18.46-
  senile H18.41-
  specified type NEC H18.49
cortical (cerebellar) (parenchymatous) G31.89
  alcoholic G31.2
  diffuse, due to arteriopathy I67.2
corticobasal G31.85
cutis L98.8
  amyloid E85.4 *[L99]*
dental pulp K04.2
disc disease — *see* Degeneration, intervertebral disc NEC
dorsolateral (spinal cord) — *see* Degeneration, combined
extrapyramidal G25.9
eye, macular — *see also* Degeneration, macula
  congenital or hereditary — *see* Dystrophy, retina
facet joints — *see* Spondylosis
fatty
  liver NEC K76.0
    alcoholic K70.0
grey matter (brain) (Alpers') G31.81
heart — *see also* Degeneration, myocardial
  amyloid E85.4 *[I43]*
  atheromatous — *see* Disease, heart, ischemic, atherosclerotic
  ischemic — *see* Disease, heart, ischemic
hepatolenticular (Wilson's) E83.01
hepatorenal K76.7
hyaline (diffuse) (generalized)
  localized — *see* Degeneration, by site
infrapatellar fat pad M79.4
intervertebral disc NOS
  with
    myelopathy — *see* Disorder, disc, with, myelopathy
    radiculitis or radiculopathy — *see* Disorder, disc, with, radiculopathy

Degeneration, degenerative - *continued*
  intervertebral disc NOS - *continued*
    cervical, cervicothoracic — *see* Disorder, disc, cervical, degeneration
      with
        myelopathy — *see* Disorder, disc, cervical, with myelopathy
        neuritis, radiculitis or radiculopathy — *see* Disorder, disc, cervical, with neuritis
    lumbar region M51.36
      with
        myelopathy M51.06
        neuritis, radiculitis, radiculopathy or sciatica M51.16
    lumbosacral region M51.37
      with
        neuritis, radiculitis, radiculopathy or sciatica M51.17
    sacrococcygeal region M53.3
    thoracic region M51.34
      with
        myelopathy M51.04
        neuritis, radiculitis, radiculopathy M51.14
    thoracolumbar region M51.35
      with
        myelopathy M51.05
        neuritis, radiculitis, radiculopathy M51.15
  intestine, amyloid E85.4
  iris (pigmentary) H21.23-
  ischemic — *see* Ischemia
  joint disease — *see* Osteoarthritis
  kidney N28.89
    amyloid E85.4 [N29]
    cystic, congenital Q61.9
    fatty N28.89
    polycystic Q61.3
      adult type (autosomal dominant) Q61.2
      infantile type (autosomal recessive) NEC Q61.19
        collecting duct dilatation Q61.11
  Kuhnt-Junius — *see also* Degeneration, macula H35.32-
  lens — *see* Cataract
  lenticular (familial) (progressive) (Wilson's) (with cirrhosis of liver) E83.01
  liver (diffuse) NEC K76.89
    amyloid E85.4 [K77]
    cystic K76.89
      congenital Q44.6
    fatty NEC K76.0
      alcoholic K70.0
    hypertrophic K76.89
    parenchymatous, acute or subacute K72.00
      with coma K72.01
    pigmentary K76.89
    toxic (acute) K71.9
  lung J98.4
  lymph gland I89.8
    hyaline I89.8
  macula, macular (acquired) (age-related) (senile) H35.30
    angioid streaks H35.33
    atrophic age-related H35.31-
    congenital or hereditary — *see* Dystrophy, retina
    cystoid H35.35-
    drusen H35.36-
    dry age-related H35.31-
    exudative H35.32-
    hole H35.34-
    nonexudative H35.31-
    puckering H35.37-
    toxic H35.38-
    wet age-related H35.32-
  membranous labyrinth, congenital (causing impairment of hearing) Q16.5
  meniscus — *see* Derangement, meniscus
  mitral — *see* Insufficiency, mitral
  Mönckeberg's — *see* Arteriosclerosis, extremities
  motor centers, senile G31.1
  multi-system G90.3
  mural — *see* Degeneration, myocardial
  muscle (fatty) (fibrous) (hyaline) (progressive) M62.89
    heart — *see* Degeneration, myocardial
  myelin, central nervous system G37.9
  myocardial, myocardium (fatty) (hyaline) (senile) I51.5
    with rheumatic fever (conditions in I00) I09.0
      active, acute or subacute I01.2
        with chorea I02.0
      inactive or quiescent (with chorea) I09.0
    hypertensive — *see* Hypertension, heart
    rheumatic — *see* Degeneration, myocardial, with rheumatic fever

Degeneration, degenerative - *continued*
  myocardial, myocardium (fatty) (hyaline) (senile) - *continued*
    syphilitic A52.06
  nasal sinus (mucosa) J32.9
    frontal J32.1
    maxillary J32.0
  nerve — *see* Disorder, nerve
  nervous system G31.9
    alcoholic G31.2
    amyloid E85.4 [G99.8]
    autonomic G90.9
    fatty G31.89
    specified NEC G31.89
  nipple N64.89
  olivopontocerebellar (hereditary) (familial) G23.8
  osseous labyrinth — *see* subcategory H83.8
  ovary N83.8
    cystic N83.20-
    microcystic N83.20-
  pallidal pigmentary (progressive) G23.0
  pancreas K86.89
    tuberculous A18.83
  penis N48.89
  pigmentary (diffuse) (general)
    localized — *see* Degeneration, by site
    pallidal (progressive) G23.0
  pineal gland E34.8
  pituitary (gland) E23.6
  popliteal fat pad M79.4
  posterolateral (spinal cord) — *see* Degeneration, combined
  pulmonary valve (heart) I37.8
  pulp (tooth) K04.2
  pupillary margin H21.24-
  renal — *see* Degeneration, kidney
  retina H35.9
    hereditary (cerebroretinal) (congenital) (juvenile) (macula) (peripheral) (pigmentary) — *see* Dystrophy, retina
    Kuhnt-Junius — *see also* Degeneration, macula H35.32-
    macula (cystic) (exudative) (hole) (nonexudative) (pseudohole) (senile) (toxic) — *see* Degeneration, macula
    peripheral H35.40
      lattice H35.41-
      microcystoid H35.42-
      paving stone H35.43-
      secondary
        pigmentary H35.45-
        vitreoretinal H35.46-
      senile reticular H35.44-
    pigmentary (primary) — *see also* Dystrophy, retina
      secondary — *see* Degeneration, retina, peripheral, secondary
    posterior pole — *see* Degeneration, macula
  saccule, congenital (causing impairment of hearing) Q16.5
  senile R54
    brain G31.1
    cardiac, heart or myocardium — *see* Degeneration, myocardial
    motor centers G31.1
    vascular — *see* Arteriosclerosis
  sinus (cystic) — *see also* Sinusitis
    polypoid J33.1
  skin L98.8
    amyloid E85.4 [L99]
    colloid L98.8
  spinal (cord) G31.89
    amyloid E85.4 [G32.89]
    combined (subacute) — *see* Degeneration, combined
    dorsolateral — *see* Degeneration, combined
    familial NEC G31.89
    fatty G31.89
    funicular — *see* Degeneration, combined
    posterolateral — *see* Degeneration, combined
    subacute combined — *see* Degeneration, combined
    tuberculous A17.81
  spleen D73.0
    amyloid E85.4 [D77]
  stomach K31.89
  striatonigral G23.2
  suprarenal (capsule) (gland) E27.8
  synovial membrane (pulpy) — *see* Disorder, synovium, specified type NEC
  tapetoretinal — *see* Dystrophy, retina
  thymus (gland) E32.8
    fatty E32.8
  thyroid (gland) E07.89
  tricuspid (heart) (valve) I07.9

Degeneration, degenerative - *continued*
  tuberculous NEC — *see* Tuberculosis
  turbinate J34.89
  uterus (cystic) N85.8
  vascular (senile) — *see* Arteriosclerosis
    hypertensive — *see* Hypertension
  vitreoretinal, secondary — *see* Degeneration, retina, peripheral, secondary, vitreoretinal
  vitreous (body) H43.81-
  Wallerian — *see* Disorder, nerve
  Wilson's hepatolenticular E83.01
Deglutition
  paralysis R13.0
    hysterical F44.4
  pneumonia J69.0
Degos' disease I77.89
Dehiscence (of)
  amputation stump T87.81
  cesarean wound O90.0
  closure of
    cornea T81.31
    craniotomy T81.32
    fascia (muscular) (superficial) T81.32
    internal organ or tissue T81.32
    laceration (external) (internal) T81.33
    ligament T81.32
    mucosa T81.31
    muscle or muscle flap T81.32
    ribs or rib cage T81.32
    skin and subcutaneous tissue (full-thickness) (superficial) T81.31
    skull T81.32
    sternum (sternotomy) T81.32
    tendon T81.32
    traumatic laceration (external) (internal) T81.33
  episiotomy O90.1
  operation wound NEC T81.31
    external operation wound (superficial) T81.31
    internal operation wound (deep) T81.32
  perineal wound (postpartum) O90.1
  traumatic injury wound repair T81.33
  wound T81.30
    traumatic repair T81.33
Dehydration E86.0
  newborn P74.1
Déjérine-Roussy syndrome G89.0
Déjérine-Sottas disease or neuropathy (hypertrophic) G60.0
Déjérine-Thomas atrophy G23.8
Delay, delayed
  any plane in pelvis
    complicating delivery O66.9
  birth or delivery NOS O63.9
  closure, ductus arteriosus (Botalli) P29.3
  coagulation — *see* Defect, coagulation
  conduction (cardiac) (ventricular) I45.9
  delivery, second twin, triplet, etc O63.2
  development R62.50
    global F88
    intellectual (specific) F81.9
    language F80.9
      due to hearing loss F80.4
    learning F81.9
    pervasive F84.9
    physiological R62.50
      specified stage NEC R62.0
    reading F81.0
    sexual E30.0
    speech F80.9
      due to hearing loss F80.4
    spelling F81.81
  ejaculation F52.32
  gastric emptying K30
  menarche E30.0
  menstruation (cause unknown) N91.0
  milestone R62.0
  passage of meconium (newborn) P76.0
  primary respiration P28.9
  puberty (constitutional) E30.0
  separation of umbilical cord P96.82
  sexual maturation, female E30.0
  sleep phase syndrome G47.21
  union, fracture — *see* Fracture, by site
  vaccination Z28.9
Deletion (s)
  autosome Q93.9
    identified by fluorescence in situ hybridization (FISH) Q93.89
    identified by in situ hybridization (ISH) Q93.89
  chromosome
    with complex rearrangements NEC Q93.7
    part of NEC Q93.5
    seen only at prometaphase Q93.89

Deletion (s) - *continued*
chromosome - *continued*
short arm
4 Q93.3
5p Q93.4
22q11.2 Q93.81
specified NEC Q93.89
long arm chromosome 18 or 21 Q93.89
with complex rearrangements NEC Q93.7
microdeletions NEC Q93.88
Delhi boil or button B55.1
Delinquency (juvenile) (neurotic) F91.8
group Z72.810
Delinquent immunization status Z28.3
Delirium, delirious (acute or subacute)
(not alcohol-or drug-induced) (with dementia) R41.0
alcoholic (acute) (tremens) (withdrawal) F10.921
with intoxication F10.921
in
abuse F10.121
dependence F10.221
due to (secondary to)
alcohol
intoxication F10.921
in
abuse F10.121
dependence F10.221
withdrawal F10.231
amphetamine intoxication F15.921
in
abuse F15.121
dependence F15.221
anxiolytic
intoxication F13.921
in
abuse F13.121
dependence F13.221
withdrawal F13.231
cannabis intoxication (acute) F12.921
in
abuse F12.121
dependence F12.221
cocaine intoxication (acute) F14.921
in
abuse F14.121
dependence F14.221
general medical condition F05
hallucinogen intoxication F16.921
in
abuse F16.121
dependence F16.221
hypnotic
intoxication F13.921
in
abuse F13.121
dependence F13.221
withdrawal F13.231
inhalant intoxication (acute) F18.921
in
abuse F18.121
dependence F18.221
multiple etiologies F05
opioid intoxication (acute) F11.921
in
abuse F11.121
dependence F11.221
other (or unknown) substance F19.921
phencyclidine intoxication (acute) F16.921
in
abuse F16.121
dependence F16.221
psychoactive substance NEC intoxication
(acute) F19.921
in
abuse F19.121
dependence F19.221
sedative
intoxication F13.921
in
abuse F13.121
dependence F13.221
withdrawal F13.231
unknown etiology F05
exhaustion F43.0
hysterical F44.89
postprocedural (postoperative) F05
puerperal F05
thyroid — *see* Thyrotoxicosis with thyroid storm
traumatic — *see* Injury, intracranial
tremens (alcohol-induced) F10.231
sedative-induced F13.231
Delivery (childbirth) (labor)
arrested active phase O62.1

Delivery (childbirth) (labor) - *continued*
cesarean (for)
abnormal
pelvis (bony) (deformity) (major) NEC with
disproportion (fetopelvic) O33.0
with obstructed labor O65.0
presentation or position O32.9
abruptio placentae — *see also* Abruptio
placentae O45.9-
acromion presentation O32.2
atony, uterus O62.2
breech presentation O32.1
incomplete O32.8
brow presentation O32.3
cephalopelvic disproportion O33.9
cerclage O34.3-
chin presentation O32.3
cicatrix of cervix O34.4-
contracted pelvis (general)
inlet O33.2
outlet O33.3
cord presentation or prolapse O69.0
cystocele O34.8-
deformity (acquired) (congenital)
pelvic organs or tissues NEC O34.8-
pelvis (bony) NEC O33.0
disproportion NOS O33.9
eclampsia — *see* Eclampsia
face presentation O32.3
failed
forceps O66.5
induction of labor O61.9
instrumental O61.1
mechanical O61.1
medical O61.0
specified NEC O61.8
surgical O61.1
trial of labor NOS O66.40
following previous cesarean delivery O66.41
vacuum extraction O66.5
ventouse O66.5
fetal-maternal hemorrhage O43.01-
hemorrhage (intrapartum) O67.9
with coagulation defect O67.0
specified cause NEC O67.8
high head at term O32.4
hydrocephalic fetus O33.6
incarceration of uterus O34.51-
incoordinate uterine action O62.4
increased size, fetus O33.5
inertia, uterus O62.2
primary O62.0
secondary O62.1
lateroversion, uterus O34.59-
mal lie O32.9
malposition
fetus O32.9
pelvic organs or tissues NEC O34.8-
uterus NEC O34.59-
malpresentation NOS O32.9
oblique presentation O32.2
occurring after 37 completed weeks of gestation
but before 39 completed weeks gestation due to
(spontaneous) onset of labor O75.82
oversize fetus O33.5
pelvic tumor NEC O34.8-
placenta previa O44.0-
complete O44.0-
with hemorrhage O44.1-
placental insufficiency O36.51-
planned, occurring after 37 completed weeks of
gestation but before 39 completed weeks
gestation due to (spontaneous) onset of
labor O75.82
polyp, cervix O34.4-
causing obstructed labor O65.5
poor dilatation, cervix O62.0
pre-eclampsia O14.94
mild O14.04
moderate O14.04
severe O14.14
with hemolysis, elevated liver enzymes and low
platelet count (HELLP) O14.24
previous
cesarean delivery O34.219
classical (vertical) scar O34.212
low transverse scar O34.211
surgery (to)
cervix O34.4-
gynecological NEC O34.8-
rectum O34.7-
uterus O34.29
vagina O34.6-

Delivery (childbirth) (labor) - *continued*
cesarean (for) - *continued*
prolapse
arm or hand O32.2
uterus O34.52-
prolonged labor NOS O63.9
rectocele O34.8-
retroversion
uterus O34.53-
rigid
cervix O34.4-
pelvic floor O34.8-
perineum O34.7-
vagina O34.6-
vulva O34.7-
sacculation, pregnant uterus O34.59-
scar (s)
cervix O34.4-
cesarean delivery O34.219
classical (vertical) O34.212
low transverse O34.211
transmural uterine O34.29
uterus O34.29
Shirodkar suture in situ O34.3-
shoulder presentation O32.2
stenosis or stricture, cervix O34.4-
streptococcus group B (GBS) carrier state O99.824
transmural uterine scar O34.29
transverse presentation or lie O32.2
tumor, pelvic organs or tissues NEC O34.8-
cervix O34.4-
umbilical cord presentation or prolapse O69.0
without indication O82
completely normal case O80
complicated O75.9
by
abnormal, abnormality (of)
forces of labor O62.9
specified type NEC O62.8
glucose O99.814
uterine contractions NOS O62.9
abruptio placentae — *see also* Abruptio
placentae O45.9-
abuse
physical O9A.32
psychological O9A.52
sexual O9A.42
adherent placenta O72.0
without hemorrhage O73.0
alcohol use O99.314
anemia (pre-existing) O99.02
anesthetic death O74.8
annular detachment of cervix O71.3
atony, uterus O62.2
attempted vacuum extraction and forceps O66.5
Bandl's ring O62.4
bariatric surgery status O99.844
biliary tract disorder O26.62
bleeding — *see* Delivery, complicated by,
hemorrhage
blood disorder NEC O99.12
cervical dystocia (hypotonic) O62.2
primary O62.0
secondary O62.1
circulatory system disorder O99.42
compression of cord (umbilical) NEC O69.2
condition NEC O99.89
contraction, contracted ring O62.4
cord (umbilical)
around neck
with compression O69.1
without compression O69.81
bruising O69.5
complication O69.9
specified NEC O69.89
compression NEC O69.2
entanglement O69.2
without compression O69.82
hematoma O69.5
presentation O69.0
prolapse O69.0
short O69.3
thrombosis (vessels) O69.5
vascular lesion O69.5
Couvelaire uterus O45.8X-
damage to (injury to) NEC
perineum O71.82
periurethral tissue O71.82
vulva O71.82
delay following rupture of membranes
(spontaneous) — *see* Pregnancy, complicated
by, premature rupture of membranes
depressed fetal heart tones O76

Delivery (childbirth) (labor) - *continued*
  complicated - *continued*
    by - *continued*
      diabetes O24.92
        gestational O24.429
          diet controlled O24.420
          insulin controlled O24.424
          oral drug controlled (antidiabetic)
            (hypoglycemic) O24.425
        pre-existing O24.32
          specified NEC O24.82
          type 1 O24.02
          type 2 O24.12
      diastasis recti (abdominis) O71.89
      dilatation
        bladder O66.8
        cervix incomplete, poor or slow O62.0
      disease NEC O99.89
      disruptio uteri — *see* Delivery, complicated by,
        rupture, uterus
      drug use O99.324
      dysfunction, uterus NOS O62.9
        hypertonic O62.4
        hypotonic O62.2
          primary O62.0
          secondary O62.1
        incoordinate O62.4
      eclampsia O15.1
      embolism (pulmonary) — *see* Embolism,
        obstetric
      endocrine, nutritional or metabolic disease
        NEC O99.284
      failed
        attempted vaginal birth after previous cesarean
          delivery O66.41
        induction of labor O61.9
          instrumental O61.1
          mechanical O61.1
          medical O61.0
          specified NEC O61.8
          surgical O61.1
        trial of labor O66.40
      female genital mutilation O65.5
      fetal
        abnormal acid-base balance O68
        acidemia O68
        acidosis O68
        alkalosis O68
        death, early O02.1
        deformity O66.3
        heart rate or rhythm (abnormal) (non-
          reassuring) O76
        hypoxia O77.8
        stress O77.9
          due to drug administration O77.1
          electrocardiographic evidence of O77.8
          specified NEC O77.8
          ultrasound evidence of O77.8
      fever during labor O75.2
      gastric banding status O99.844
      gastric bypass status O99.844
      gastrointestinal disease NEC O99.62
      gestational
        diabetes O24.429
          diet controlled O24.420
          insulin (and diet) controlled O24.424
          oral drug controlled (antidiabetic)
            (hypoglycemic) O24.425
        edema O12.04
          with proteinuria O12.24
        proteinuria O12.14
      gonorrhea O98.22
      hematoma O71.7
        ischial spine O71.7
        pelvic O71.7
        vagina O71.7
        vulva or perineum O71.7
      hemorrhage (uterine) O67.9
        associated with
          afibrinogenemia O67.0
          coagulation defect O67.0
          hyperfibrinolysis O67.0
          hypofibrinogenemia O67.0
        due to
          low implantation of placenta O44.5-
          low lying placenta O44.5-
          placenta previa O44.1-
            marginal O44.3-
            partial O44.3-
          premature separation of placenta (normally
            implanted) — *see also* Abruptio
            placentae O45.9-
          retained placenta O72.0

Delivery (childbirth) (labor) - *continued*
  complicated - *continued*
    by - *continued*
      hemorrhage (uterine) - *continued*
        due to - *continued*
          uterine leiomyoma O67.8
          placenta NEC O67.8
        postpartum NEC (atonic) (immediate) O72.1
          with retained or trapped placenta O72.0
          delayed O72.2
          secondary O72.2
          third stage O72.0
      hourglass contraction, uterus O62.4
      hypertension, hypertensive (pre-existing) — *see*
        Hypertension, complicated by, childbirth (labor)
      hypotension O26.5-
      incomplete dilatation (cervix) O62.0
      incoordinate uterine contractions O62.4
      inertia, uterus O62.2
        during latent phase of labor O62.0
        primary O62.0
        secondary O62.1
      infection (maternal) O98.92
        carrier state NEC O99.834
        gonorrhea O98.22
        human immunodeficiency virus (HIV) O98.72
        sexually transmitted NEC O98.32
        specified NEC O98.82
        syphilis O98.12
        tuberculosis O98.02
        viral hepatitis O98.42
        viral NEC O98.52
      injury (to mother) — *see also* Delivery,
        complicated, by, damage to O71.9
        nonobstetric O9A.22
        caused by abuse — *see* Delivery, complicated
          by, abuse
      intrauterine fetal death, early O02.1
      inversion, uterus O71.2
      laceration (perineal) O70.9
        anus (sphincter) O70.4
          with third degree laceration — *see
            also* Delivery, complicated, by, laceration,
            perineum, third degree O70.20
            with mucosa O70.3
          without third degree laceration O70.4
        bladder (urinary) O71.5
        bowel O71.5
        cervix (uteri) O71.3
        fourchette O70.0
        hymen O70.0
        labia O70.0
        pelvic
          floor O70.1
          organ NEC O71.5
        perineum, perineal O70.9
          first degree O70.0
          fourth degree O70.3
          muscles O70.1
          second degree O70.1
          skin O70.0
          slight O70.0
          third degree O70.20
            with
              both external anal sphincter (EAS) and
                internal anal sphincter (IAS) torn
                (IIIc) O70.23
              less than 50% of external anal sphincter
                (EAS) thickness torn (IIIa) O70.21
              more than 50% external anal sphincter
                (EAS) thickness torn (IIIb) O70.22
            IIIa O70.21
            IIIb O70.22
            IIIc O70.23
        peritoneum (pelvic) O71.5
        rectovaginal (septum) (without perineal
          laceration) O71.4
          with perineum — *see also* Delivery,
            complicated, by, laceration, perineum, third
            degree O70.20
          with anal or rectal mucosa O70.3
        specified NEC O71.89
        sphincter ani — *see* Delivery, complicated, by,
          laceration, anus (sphincter)
        urethra O71.5
        uterus O71.81
          before labor O71.81
        vagina, vaginal (deep) (high) (without perineal
          laceration) O71.4
          with perineum O70.0
            muscles, with perineum O70.1
        vulva O70.0
      liver disorder O26.62

Delivery (childbirth) (labor) - *continued*
  complicated - *continued*
    by - *continued*
      malignancy O9A.12
      malnutrition O25.2
      malposition, malpresentation
        placenta O44.0-
          with hemorrhage O44.1-
        uterus or cervix O65.5
        without obstruction — *see also* Delivery,
          complicated by, obstruction O32.9
          breech O32.1
          compound O32.6
          face (brow) (chin) O32.3
          footling O32.8
          high head O32.4
          oblique O32.2
          specified NEC O32.8
          transverse O32.2
          unstable lie O32.0
      meconium in amniotic fluid O77.0
      mental disorder NEC O99.344
      metrorrhexis — *see* Delivery, complicated by,
        rupture, uterus
      nervous system disorder O99.354
      obesity (pre-existing) O99.214
      obesity surgery status O99.844
      obstetric trauma O71.9
        specified NEC O71.89
      obstructed labor
        due to
          breech (complete) (frank) presentation O64.1
            incomplete O64.8
          brow presentation O64.3
          buttock presentation O64.1
          chin presentation O64.2
          compound presentation O64.5
          contracted pelvis O65.1
          deep transverse arrest O64.0
          deformed pelvis O65.0
          dystocia (fetal) O66.9
            due to
              conjoined twins O66.3
              fetal
                abnormality NEC O66.3
                ascites O66.3
                hydrops O66.3
                meningomyelocele O66.3
                sacral teratoma O66.3
                tumor O66.3
                hydrocephalic fetus O66.3
            shoulder O66.0
          face presentation O64.2
          fetopelvic disproportion O65.4
          footling presentation O64.8
          impacted shoulders O66.0
          incomplete rotation of fetal head O64.0
          large fetus O66.2
          locked twins O66.1
          malposition O64.9
            specified NEC O64.8
          malpresentation O64.9
            specified NEC O64.8
          multiple fetuses NEC O66.6
          pelvic
            abnormality (maternal) O65.9
              organ O65.5
              specified NEC O65.8
            contraction
              inlet O65.2
              mid-cavity O65.3
              outlet O65.3
          persistent (position)
            occipitoiliac O64.0
            occipitoposterior O64.0
            occipitosacral O64.0
            occipitotransverse O64.0
          prolapsed arm O64.4
          shoulder presentation O64.4
          specified NEC O66.8
      pathological retraction ring, uterus O62.4
      penetration, pregnant uterus by instrument O71.1
      perforation — *see* Delivery, complicated by,
        laceration
      placenta, placental
        ablatio — *see also* Abruptio placentae O45.9-
        abnormality O43.9-
          specified NEC O43.89-
        abruptio — *see also* Abruptio placentae O45.9-
        accreta O43.21-
        adherent (with hemorrhage) O72.0
          without hemorrhage O73.0

Delivery (childbirth) (labor) - *continued*
complicated - *continued*
  by - *continued*
    placenta, placental - *continued*
      detachment (premature) — *see also* Abruptio
        placentae O45.9-
      disorder O43.9-
        specified NEC O43.89-
      hemorrhage NEC O67.8
      increta O43.22-
      low (implantation) (lying) O44.4-
        with hemorrhage O44.5-
      malformation O43.10-
      malposition O44.0-
        without hemorrhage O44.1-
      percreta O43.23-
      previa (central) (complete) (lateral)
        (total) O44.0-
        with hemorrhage O44.1-
        marginal O44.2-
          with hemorrhage O44.3-
        partial O44.2-
          with hemorrhage O44.3-
      retained (with hemorrhage) O72.0
        without hemorrhage O73.0
      separation (premature) O45.9-
        specified NEC O45.8X-
      vicious insertion O44.1-
    precipitate labor O62.3
    premature rupture, membranes — *see*
      also Pregnancy, complicated by, premature
      rupture of membranes O42.90
    prolapse
      arm or hand O32.2
      cord (umbilical) O69.0
      foot or leg O32.8
      uterus O34.52-
    prolonged labor O63.9
      first stage O63.0
      second stage O63.1
    protozoal disease (maternal) O98.62
    respiratory disease NEC O99.52
    retained membranes or portions of
      placenta O72.2
      without hemorrhage O73.1
    retarded birth O63.9
    retention of secundines (with hemorrhage) O72.0
      without hemorrhage O73.0
      partial O72.2
        without hemorrhage O73.1
    rupture
      bladder (urinary) O71.5
      cervix O71.3
      pelvic organ NEC O71.5
      urethra O71.5
      uterus (during or after labor) O71.1
        before labor O71.0-
    separation, pubic bone (symphysis pubis) O71.6
    shock O75.1
    shoulder presentation O64.4
    skin disorder NEC O99.72
    spasm, cervix O62.4
    stenosis or stricture, cervix O65.5
    streptococcus group B (GBS) carrier
      state O99.824
    subluxation of symphysis (pubis) O26.72
    syphilis (maternal) O98.12
    tear — *see* Delivery, complicated by, laceration
    tetanic uterus O62.4
    trauma (obstetrical) — *see also* Delivery,
      complicated, by, damage to O71.9
      non-obstetric O9A.22
      periurethral O71.82
      specified NEC O71.89
    tuberculosis (maternal) O98.02
    tumor, pelvic organs or tissues NEC O65.5
    umbilical cord around neck
      with compression O69.1
      without compression O69.81
    uterine inertia O62.2
      during latent phase of labor O62.0
      primary O62.0
      secondary O62.1
    vasa previa O69.4
    velamentous insertion of cord O43.12-
  specified complication NEC O75.89
delayed NOS O63.9
  following rupture of membranes
    artificial O75.5
  second twin, triplet, etc. O63.2
forceps, low following failed vacuum
  extraction O66.5
missed (at or near term) O36.4

Delivery (childbirth) (labor) - *continued*
normal O80
obstructed — *see* Delivery, complicated by,
  obstruction
precipitate O62.3
preterm — *see also* Pregnancy, complicated by,
  preterm labor O60.10
spontaneous O80
term pregnancy NOS O80
uncomplicated O80
vaginal, following previous cesarean
  delivery O34.219
  classical (vertical) scar O34.212
  low transverse scar O34.211
Delusions (paranoid) — *see* Disorder, delusional
Dementia (degenerative (primary)) (old age)
(old age) (persisting) F03.90
  with
    aggressive behavior F03.91
    behavioral disturbance F03.91
    combative behavior F03.91
    Lewy bodies G31.83 *[F02.80]*
      with behavioral disturbance G31.83 *[F02.81]*
    Parkinsonism G31.83 *[F02.80]*
      with behavioral disturbance G31.83 *[F02.81]*
    Parkinson's disease G20 *[F02.80]*
      with behavioral disturbance G20 *[F02.81]*
    violent behavior F03.91
  alcoholic F10.97
    with dependence F10.27
  Alzheimer's type — *see* Disease, Alzheimer's
  arteriosclerotic — *see* Dementia, vascular
  atypical, Alzheimer's type — *see* Disease,
    Alzheimer's, specified NEC
  congenital — *see* Disability, intellectual
  frontal (lobe) G31.09 *[F02.80]*
    with behavioral disturbance G31.09 *[F02.81]*
  frontotemporal G31.09 *[F02.80]*
    with behavioral disturbance G31.09 *[F02.81]*
    specified NEC G31.09 *[F02.80]*
      with behavioral disturbance G31.09 *[F02.81]*
  in (due to)
    alcohol F10.97
      with dependence F10.27
    Alzheimer's disease — *see* Disease, Alzheimer's
    arteriosclerotic brain disease — *see* Dementia,
      vascular
    cerebral lipidoses E75.- *[F02.80]*
      with behavioral disturbance E75.- *[F02.81]*
    Creutzfeldt-Jakob disease — *see also* Creutzfeldt-
      Jakob disease or syndrome (with
      dementia) A81.00
    epilepsy G40.- *[F02.80]*
      with behavioral disturbance G40.- *[F02.81]*
    hepatolenticular degeneration E83.01 *[F02.80]*
      with behavioral disturbance E83.01 *[F02.81]*
    human immunodeficiency virus (HIV)
      disease B20 *[F02.80]*
      with behavioral disturbance B20 *[F02.81]*
    Huntington's disease or chorea G10
    hypercalcemia E83.52 *[F02.80]*
      with behavioral disturbance E83.52 *[F02.81]*
    hypothyroidism, acquired E03.9 *[F02.80]*
      with behavioral disturbance E03.9 *[F02.81]*
      due to iodine deficiency E01.8 *[F02.80]*
        with behavioral disturbance E01.8 *[F02.81]*
    inhalants F18.97
      with dependence F18.27
    multiple
      etiologies F03
      sclerosis G35 *[F02.80]*
        with behavioral disturbance G35 *[F02.81]*
    neurosyphilis A52.17 *[F02.80]*
      with behavioral disturbance A52.17 *[F02.81]*
      juvenile A50.49 *[F02.80]*
        with behavioral disturbance A50.49 *[F02.81]*
    niacin deficiency E52 *[F02.80]*
      with behavioral disturbance E52 *[F02.81]*
    paralysis agitans G20 *[F02.80]*
      with behavioral disturbance G20 *[F02.81]*
    Parkinson's disease G20 *[F02.80]*
    pellagra E52 *[F02.80]*
      with behavioral disturbance E52 *[F02.81]*
    Pick's G31.01 *[F02.80]*
      with behavioral disturbance G31.01 *[F02.81]*
    polyarteritis nodosa M30.0 *[F02.80]*
      with behavioral disturbance M30.0 *[F02.81]*
    psychoactive drug F19.97
      with dependence F19.27
      inhalants F18.97
        with dependence F18.27
      sedatives, hypnotics or anxiolytics F13.97
        with dependence F13.27

Dementia (degenerative (primary)) (old age)
(old age) (persisting) - *continued*
  in (due to) - *continued*
    sedatives, hypnotics or anxiolytics F13.97
      with dependence F13.27
    systemic lupus erythematosus M32.- *[F02.80]*
      with behavioral disturbance M32.- *[F02.81]*
    trypanosomiasis
      African B56.9 *[F02.80]*
        with behavioral disturbance B56.9 *[F02.81]*
    unknown etiology F03
    vitamin B12 deficiency E53.8 *[F02.80]*
      with behavioral disturbance E53.8 *[F02.81]*
    volatile solvents F18.97
      with dependence F18.27
      with behavioral disturbance G31.83 *[F02.81]*
  infantile, infantilis F84.3
  Lewy body G31.83 *[F02.80]*
    with behavioral disturbance G31.83 *[F02.81]*
  multi-infarct — *see* Dementia, vascular
  paralytica, paralytic (syphilitic) A52.17 *[F02.80]*
    with behavioral disturbance A52.17 *[F02.81]*
    juvenilis A50.45
  paretic A52.17
  praecox — *see* Schizophrenia
  presenile F03
    Alzheimer's type — *see* Disease, Alzheimer's,
      early onset
  primary degenerative F03
  progressive, syphilitic A52.17
  senile F03
    with acute confusional state F05
    Alzheimer's type — *see* Disease, Alzheimer's, late
      onset
    depressed or paranoid type F03
  vascular (acute onset) (mixed) (multi-infarct)
    (subcortical) F01.50
    with behavioral disturbance F01.51
Demineralization, bone — *see* Osteoporosis
Demodex folliculorum (infestation) B88.0
Demophobia F40.248
Demoralization R45.3
Demyelination, demyelinization
  central nervous system G37.9
    specified NEC G37.8
  corpus callosum (central) G37.1
  disseminated, acute G36.9
    specified NEC G36.8
  global G35
  in optic neuritis G36.0
Dengue (classical) (fever) A90
  hemorrhagic A91
  sandfly A93.1
Dennie-Marfan syphilitic syndrome A50.45
Dens evaginatus, in dente or invaginatus K00.2
Dense breasts R92.2
Density
  increased, bone (disseminated) (generalized)
    (spotted) — *see* Disorder, bone, density and
    structure, specified type NEC
  lung (nodular) J98.4
Dental — *see also* condition
  examination Z01.20
    with abnormal findings Z01.21
  restoration
    aesthetically inadequate or displeasing K08.56
    defective K08.50
      specified NEC K08.59
    failure of marginal integrity K08.51
    failure of periodontal anatomical integrity K08.54
Dentia praecox K00.6
Denticles (pulp) K04.2
Dentigerous cyst K09.0
Dentin
  irregular (in pulp) K04.3
  opalescent K00.5
  secondary (in pulp) K04.3
  sensitive K03.89
Dentinogenesis imperfecta K00.5
Dentinoma — *see* Cyst, calcifying odontogenic
Dentition (syndrome) K00.7
  delayed K00.6
  difficult K00.7
  precocious K00.6
  premature K00.6
  retarded K00.6
Dependence (on) (syndrome) F19.20
  with remission F19.21
  alcohol (ethyl) (methyl) (without remission) F10.20
    with
      amnestic disorder, persisting F10.26
      anxiety disorder F10.280
      dementia, persisting F10.27

Dependence (on) (syndrome) - *continued*
alcohol (ethyl) (methyl) (without remission) - *continued*
with - *continued*
intoxication F10.229
with delirium F10.221
uncomplicated F10.220
mood disorder F10.24
psychotic disorder F10.259
with
delusions F10.250
hallucinations F10.251
remission F10.21
sexual dysfunction F10.281
sleep disorder F10.282
specified disorder NEC F10.288
withdrawal F10.239
with
delirium F10.231
perceptual disturbance F10.232
uncomplicated F10.230
counseling and surveillance Z71.41
amobarbital — *see* Dependence, drug, sedative
amphetamine (s) (type) — *see* Dependence, drug, stimulant NEC
amytal (sodium) — *see* Dependence, drug, sedative
analgesic NEC F55.8
anesthetic (agent) (gas) (general) (local) NEC — *see* Dependence, drug, psychoactive NEC
anxiolytic NEC — *see* Dependence, drug, sedative
barbital (s) — *see* Dependence, drug, sedative
barbiturate (s) (compounds) (drugs classifiable to T42) — *see* Dependence, drug, sedative
benzedrine — *see* Dependence, drug, stimulant NEC
bhang — *see* Dependence, drug, cannabis
bromide (s) NEC — *see* Dependence, drug, sedative
caffeine — *see* Dependence, drug, stimulant NEC
cannabis (sativa) (indica) (resin) (derivatives) (type) — *see* Dependence, drug, cannabis
chloral (betaine) (hydrate) — *see* Dependence, drug, sedative
chlordiazepoxide — *see* Dependence, drug, sedative
coca (leaf) (derivatives) — *see* Dependence, drug, cocaine
cocaine — *see* Dependence, drug, cocaine
codeine — *see* Dependence, drug, opioid
combinations of drugs F19.20
dagga — *see* Dependence, drug, cannabis
demerol — *see* Dependence, drug, opioid
dexamphetamine — *see* Dependence, drug, stimulant NEC
dexedrine — *see* Dependence, drug, stimulant NEC
dextromethorphan — *see* Dependence, drug, opioid
dextromoramide — *see* Dependence, drug, opioid
dextro-nor-pseudo-ephedrine — *see* Dependence, drug, stimulant NEC
dextrorphan — *see* Dependence, drug, opioid
diazepam — *see* Dependence, drug, sedative
dilaudid — *see* Dependence, drug, opioid
D-lysergic acid diethylamide — *see* Dependence, drug, hallucinogen
drug NEC F19.20
with sleep disorder F19.282
cannabis F12.20
with
anxiety disorder F12.280
intoxication F12.229
with
delirium F12.221
perceptual disturbance F12.222
uncomplicated F12.220
other specified disorder F12.288
psychosis F12.259
delusions F12.250
hallucinations F12.251
unspecified disorder F12.29
in remission F12.21
cocaine F14.20
with
anxiety disorder F14.280
intoxication F14.229
with
delirium F14.221
perceptual disturbance F14.222
uncomplicated F14.220
mood disorder F14.24
other specified disorder F14.288
psychosis F14.259
delusions F14.250
hallucinations F14.251
sexual dysfunction F14.281
sleep disorder F14.282
unspecified disorder F14.29

Dependence (on) (syndrome) - *continued*
drug NEC - *continued*
cocaine - *continued*
with - *continued*
withdrawal F14.23
in remission F14.21
withdrawal symptoms in newborn P96.1
counseling and surveillance Z71.51
hallucinogen F16.20
with
anxiety disorder F16.280
flashbacks F16.283
intoxication F16.229
with delirium F16.221
uncomplicated F16.220
mood disorder F16.24
other specified disorder F16.288
perception disorder, persisting F16.283
psychosis F16.259
delusions F16.250
hallucinations F16.251
unspecified disorder F16.29
in remission F16.21
inhalant F18.20
with
anxiety disorder F18.280
dementia, persisting F18.27
intoxication F18.229
with delirium F18.221
uncomplicated F18.220
mood disorder F18.24
other specified disorder F18.288
psychosis F18.259
delusions F18.250
hallucinations F18.251
unspecified disorder F18.29
in remission F18.21
nicotine F17.200
with disorder F17.209
remission F17.201
specified disorder NEC F17.208
withdrawal F17.203
chewing tobacco F17.220
with disorder F17.229
remission F17.221
specified disorder NEC F17.228
withdrawal F17.223
cigarettes F17.210
with disorder F17.219
remission F17.211
specified disorder NEC F17.218
withdrawal F17.213
specified product NEC F17.290
with disorder F17.299
remission F17.291
specified disorder NEC F17.298
withdrawal F17.293
opioid F11.20
with
intoxication F11.229
with
delirium F11.221
perceptual disturbance F11.222
uncomplicated F11.220
mood disorder F11.24
other specified disorder F11.288
psychosis F11.259
delusions F11.250
hallucinations F11.251
sexual dysfunction F11.281
sleep disorder F11.282
unspecified disorder F11.29
withdrawal F11.23
in remission F11.21
psychoactive NEC F19.20
with
amnestic disorder F19.26
anxiety disorder F19.280
dementia F19.27
intoxication F19.229
with
delirium F19.221
perceptual disturbance F19.222
uncomplicated F19.220
mood disorder F19.24
other specified disorder F19.288
psychosis F19.259
delusions F19.250
hallucinations F19.251
sexual dysfunction F19.281
sleep disorder F19.282
unspecified disorder F19.29

Dependence (on) (syndrome) - *continued*
drug NEC - *continued*
psychoactive NEC - *continued*
with - *continued*
withdrawal F19.239
with
delirium F19.231
perceptual disturbance F19.232
uncomplicated F19.230
sedative, hypnotic or anxiolytic F13.20
with
amnestic disorder F13.26
anxiety disorder F13.280
dementia, persisting F13.27
intoxication F13.229
with delirium F13.221
uncomplicated F13.220
mood disorder F13.24
other specified disorder F13.288
psychosis F13.259
delusions F13.250
hallucinations F13.251
sexual dysfunction F13.281
sleep disorder F13.282
unspecified disorder F13.29
withdrawal F13.239
with
delirium F13.231
perceptual disturbance F13.232
uncomplicated F13.230
in remission F13.21
stimulant NEC F15.20
with
anxiety disorder F15.280
intoxication F15.229
with
delirium F15.221
perceptual disturbance F15.222
uncomplicated F15.220
mood disorder F15.24
other specified disorder F15.288
psychosis F15.259
delusions F15.250
hallucinations F15.251
sexual dysfunction F15.281
sleep disorder F15.282
unspecified disorder F15.29
withdrawal F15.23
in remission F15.21
ethyl
alcohol (without remission) F10.20
with remission F10.21
bromide — *see* Dependence, drug, sedative
carbamate F19.20
chloride F19.20
morphine — *see* Dependence, drug, opioid
ganja — *see* Dependence, drug, cannabis
glue (airplane) (sniffing) — *see* Dependence, drug, inhalant
glutethimide — *see* Dependence, drug, sedative
hallucinogenics — *see* Dependence, drug, hallucinogen
hashish — *see* Dependence, drug, cannabis
hemp — *see* Dependence, drug, cannabis
heroin (salt) (any) — *see* Dependence, drug, opioid
hypnotic NEC — *see* Dependence, drug, sedative
Indian hemp — *see* Dependence, drug, cannabis
inhalants — *see* Dependence, drug, inhalant
khat — *see* Dependence, drug, stimulant NEC
laudanum — *see* Dependence, drug, opioid
LSD (-25) (derivatives) — *see* Dependence, drug, hallucinogen
luminal — *see* Dependence, drug, sedative
lysergic acid — *see* Dependence, drug, hallucinogen
maconha — *see* Dependence, drug, cannabis
marihuana — *see* Dependence, drug, cannabis
meprobamate — *see* Dependence, drug, sedative
mescaline — *see* Dependence, drug, hallucinogen
methadone — *see* Dependence, drug, opioid
methamphetamine (s) — *see* Dependence, drug, stimulant NEC
methaqualone — *see* Dependence, drug, sedative
methyl
alcohol (without remission) F10.20
with remission F10.21
bromide — *see* Dependence, drug, sedative
morphine — *see* Dependence, drug, opioid
phenidate — *see* Dependence, drug, stimulant NEC
sulfonal — *see* Dependence, drug, sedative
morphine (sulfate) (sulfite) (type) — *see* Dependence, drug, opioid

Dependence (on) (syndrome) - *continued*
 narcotic (drug) NEC — *see* Dependence, drug, opioid
 nembutal — *see* Dependence, drug, sedative
 neraval — *see* Dependence, drug, sedative
 neravan — *see* Dependence, drug, sedative
 neurobarb — *see* Dependence, drug, sedative
 nicotine — *see* Dependence, drug, nicotine
 nitrous oxide F19.20
 nonbarbiturate sedatives and tranquilizers with
  similar effect — *see* Dependence, drug, sedative
 on
  artificial heart (fully implantable)
   (mechanical) Z95.812
  aspirator Z99.0
  care provider (because of) Z74.9
   impaired mobility Z74.09
   need for
    assistance with personal care Z74.1
    continuous supervision Z74.3
   no other household member able to render
    care Z74.2
   specified reason NEC Z74.8
  machine Z99.89
   enabling NEC Z99.89
   specified type NEC Z99.89
  renal dialysis (hemodialysis) (peritoneal) Z99.2
  respirator Z99.11
  ventilator Z99.11
  wheelchair Z99.3
 opiate — *see* Dependence, drug, opioid
 opioids — *see* Dependence, drug, opioid
 opium (alkaloids) (derivatives) (tincture) — *see*
  Dependence, drug, opioid
 oxygen (long-term) (supplemental) Z99.81
 paraldehyde — *see* Dependence, drug, sedative
 paregoric — *see* Dependence, drug, opioid
 PCP (phencyclidine) (or related substance) — *see*
  Dependence, drug, hallucinogen
 pentobarbital — *see* Dependence, drug, sedative
 pentobarbitone (sodium) — *see* Dependence, drug,
  sedative
 pentothal — *see* Dependence, drug, sedative
 peyote — *see* Dependence, drug, hallucinogen
 phencyclidine (PCP) (or related substance) — *see*
  Dependence, drug, hallucinogen
 phenmetrazine — *see* Dependence, drug, stimulant
  NEC
 phenobarbital — *see* Dependence, drug, sedative
 polysubstance F19.20
 psilocibin, psilocin, psilocyn, psilocyline — *see*
  Dependence, drug, hallucinogen
 psychostimulant NEC — *see* Dependence, drug,
  stimulant NEC
 secobarbital — *see* Dependence, drug, sedative
 seconal — *see* Dependence, drug, sedative
 sedative NEC — *see* Dependence, drug, sedative
 specified drug NEC — *see* Dependence, drug
 stimulant NEC — *see* Dependence, drug, stimulant
  NEC
 substance NEC — *see* Dependence, drug
 supplemental oxygen Z99.81
 tobacco — *see* Dependence, drug, nicotine
  counseling and surveillance Z71.6
 tranquilizer NEC — *see* Dependence, drug, sedative
 vitamin B6 E53.1
 volatile solvents — *see* Dependence, drug, inhalant
Dependency
 care-provider Z74.9
 passive F60.7
 reactions (persistent) F60.7
Depersonalization (in neurotic state) (neurotic)
 (syndrome) F48.1
Depletion
 extracellular fluid E86.9
 plasma E86.1
 potassium E87.6
  nephropathy N25.89
 salt or sodium E87.1
  causing heat exhaustion or prostration T67.4
  nephropathy N28.9
 volume NOS E86.9
Deployment (current) (military) **status** Z56.82
 in theater or in support of military war, peacekeeping
  and humanitarian operations Z56.82
 personal history of Z91.82
  military war, peacekeeping and humanitarian
   deployment (current or past conflict) Z91.82
  returned from Z91.82
Depolarization, premature I49.40
 atrial I49.1
 junctional I49.2
 specified NEC I49.49

Depolarization, premature - *continued*
 ventricular I49.3
Deposit
 bone in Boeck's sarcoid D86.89
 calcareous, calcium — *see* Calcification
 cholesterol
  retina H35.89
  vitreous (body) (humor) — *see* Deposit, crystalline
 conjunctiva H11.11-
 cornea H18.00-
  argentous H18.02-
  due to metabolic disorder H18.03-
  Kayser-Fleischer ring H18.04-
  pigmentation — *see* Pigmentation, cornea
 crystalline, vitreous (body) (humor) H43.2-
 hemosiderin in old scars of cornea — *see*
  Pigmentation, cornea, stromal
 metallic in lens — *see* Cataract, specified NEC
 skin R23.8
 tooth, teeth (betel) (black) (green) (materia alba)
  (orange) (tobacco) K03.6
 urate, kidney — *see* Calculus, kidney
Depraved appetite — *see* Pica
Depressed
 HDL cholesterol E78.6
Depression (acute) (mental) F32.9
 agitated (single episode) F32.2
 anaclitic — *see* Disorder, adjustment
 anxiety F41.8
  persistent F34.1
 arches — *see also* Deformity, limb, flat foot
 atypical (single episode) F32.89
  recurrent episode F33.8
 basal metabolic rate R94.8
 bone marrow D75.89
 central nervous system R09.2
 cerebral R29.818
  newborn P91.4
 cerebrovascular I67.9
 chest wall M95.4
 climacteric (single episode) F32.89
  recurrent episode F33.8
 endogenous (without psychotic symptoms) F33.2
  with psychotic symptoms F33.3
 functional activity R68.89
 hysterical F44.89
 involutional (single episode) F32.89
  recurrent episode F33.8
 major F32.9
  with psychotic symptoms F32.3
  recurrent — *see* Disorder, depressive, recurrent
 manic-depressive — *see* Disorder, depressive,
  recurrent
 masked (single episode) F32.89
 medullary G93.89
 menopausal (single episode) F32.89
  recurrent episode F33.8
 metatarsus — *see* Depression, arches
 monopolar F33.9
 nervous F34.1
 neurotic F34.1
 nose M95.0
 postnatal F53
 postpartum F53
 post-psychotic of schizophrenia F32.89
 post-schizophrenic F32.89
 psychogenic (reactive) (single episode) F32.9
 psychoneurotic F34.1
 psychotic (single episode) F32.3
  recurrent F33.3
 reactive (psychogenic) (single episode) F32.9
  psychotic (single episode) F32.3
 recurrent — *see* Disorder, depressive, recurrent
 respiratory center G93.89
 seasonal — *see* Disorder, depressive, recurrent
 senile F03
 severe, single episode F32.2
 situational F43.21
 skull Q67.4
 specified NEC (single episode) F32.89
 sternum M95.4
 visual field — *see* Defect, visual field
 vital (recurrent) (without psychotic
  symptoms) F33.2
  with psychotic symptoms F33.3
  single episode F32.2
Deprivation
 cultural Z60.3
 effects NOS T73.9
  specified NEC T73.8
 emotional NEC Z65.8
  affecting infant or child — *see* Maltreatment, child,
   psychological

Deprivation - *continued*
 food T73.0
 protein — *see* Malnutrition
 sleep Z72.820
 social Z60.4
  affecting infant or child — *see* Maltreatment, child,
   psychological
 specified NEC T73.8
 vitamins — *see* Deficiency, vitamin
 water T73.1
Derangement
 ankle (internal) — *see* Derangement, joint, ankle
 cartilage (articular) NEC — *see* Derangement, joint,
  articular cartilage, by site
  recurrent — *see* Dislocation, recurrent
 cruciate ligament, anterior, current injury — *see*
  Sprain, knee, cruciate, anterior
 elbow (internal) — *see* Derangement, joint, elbow
 hip (joint) (internal) (old) — *see* Derangement, joint,
  hip
 joint (internal) M24.9
  ankylosis — *see* Ankylosis
  articular cartilage M24.10
   ankle M24.17-
   elbow M24.12-
   foot M24.17-
   hand M24.14-
   hip M24.15-
   knee NEC M23.9-
   loose body — *see* Loose, body
   shoulder M24.11-
   wrist M24.13-
  contracture — *see* Contraction, joint
  current injury — *see also* Dislocation
   knee, meniscus or cartilage — *see* Tear, meniscus
  dislocation
   pathological — *see* Dislocation, pathological
   recurrent — *see* Dislocation, recurrent
  knee — *see* Derangement, knee
  ligament — *see* Disorder, ligament
  loose body — *see* Loose, body
  recurrent — *see* Dislocation, recurrent
  specified type NEC M24.80
   ankle M24.87-
   elbow M24.82-
   foot joint M24.87-
   hand joint M24.84-
   hip M24.85-
   shoulder M24.81-
   wrist M24.83-
  temporomandibular M26.69
 knee (recurrent) M23.9-
  ligament disruption, spontaneous M23.60-
   anterior cruciate M23.61-
   capsular M23.67-
   instability, chronic M23.5-
   lateral collateral M23.64-
   medial collateral M23.63-
   posterior cruciate M23.62-
  loose body M23.4-
  meniscus M23.30-
   cystic M23.00-
    lateral M23.002
     anterior horn M23.04-
     posterior horn M23.05-
     specified NEC M23.06-
    medial M23.005
     anterior horn M23.01-
     posterior horn M23.02-
     specified NEC M23.03-
   degenerate — *see* Derangement, knee, meniscus,
    specified NEC
   detached — *see* Derangement, knee, meniscus,
    specified NEC
   due to old tear or injury M23.20-
    lateral M23.20-
     anterior horn M23.24-
     posterior horn M23.25-
     specified NEC M23.26-
    medial M23.20-
     anterior horn M23.21-
     posterior horn M23.22-
     specified NEC M23.23-
   retained — *see* Derangement, knee, meniscus,
    specified NEC
   specified NEC M23.30-
    lateral M23.30-
     anterior horn M23.34-
     posterior horn M23.35-
     specified NEC M23.36-
    medial M23.30-
     anterior horn M23.31-
     posterior horn M23.32-

Derangement - *continued*
  knee (recurrent) - *continued*
    meniscus - *continued*
      specified NEC - *continued*
        medial - *continued*
          specified NEC M23.33-
        old M23.8X-
      specified NEC — *see* subcategory M23.8
    low back NEC — *see* Dorsopathy, specified NEC
    meniscus — *see* Derangement, knee, meniscus
    mental — *see* Psychosis
    patella, specified NEC — *see* Disorder, patella, derangement NEC
    semilunar cartilage (knee) — *see* Derangement, knee, meniscus, specified NEC
    shoulder (internal) — *see* Derangement, joint, shoulder
Dercum's disease E88.2
Derealization (neurotic) F48.1
Dermal — *see* condition
Dermaphytid — *see* Dermatophytosis
Dermatitis (eczematous) L30.9
  ab igne L59.0
  acarine B88.0
  actinic (due to sun) L57.8
    other than from sun L59.8
  allergic — *see* Dermatitis, contact, allergic
  ambustionis, due to burn or scald — *see* Burn
  amebic A06.7
  ammonia L22
  arsenical (ingested) L27.8
  artefacta L98.1
    psychogenic F54
  atopic L20.9
    psychogenic F54
    specified NEC L20.89
  autoimmune progesterone L30.8
  berlock, berloque L56.2
  blastomycotic B40.3
  blister beetle L24.89
  bullous, bullosa L13.9
    mucosynechial, atrophic L12.1
    seasonal L30.8
    specified NEC L13.8
  calorica L59.0
    due to burn or scald — *see* Burn
  caterpillar L24.89
  cercarial B65.3
  combustionis L59.0
    due to burn or scald — *see* Burn
  congelationis T69.1
  contact (occupational) L25.9
    allergic L23.9
      due to
        adhesives L23.1
        cement L23.5
        chemical products NEC L23.5
        chromium L23.0
        cosmetics L23.2
        dander (cat) (dog) L23.81
        drugs in contact with skin L23.3
        dyes L23.4
        food in contact with skin L23.6
        hair (cat) (dog) L23.81
        insecticide L23.5
        metals L23.0
        nickel L23.0
        plants, non-food L23.7
        plastic L23.5
        rubber L23.5
        specified agent NEC L23.89
    due to
      cement L25.3
      chemical products NEC L25.3
      cosmetics L25.0
      dander (cat) (dog) L23.81
      drugs in contact with skin L25.1
      dyes L25.2
      food in contact with skin L25.4
      hair (cat) (dog) L23.81
      plants, non-food L25.5
      specified agent NEC L25.8
    irritant L24.9
      due to
        cement L24.5
        chemical products NEC L24.5
        cosmetics L24.3
        detergents L24.0
        drugs in contact with skin L24.4
        food in contact with skin L24.6
        oils and greases L24.1
        plants, non-food L24.7
        solvents L24.2

Dermatitis (eczematous) - *continued*
  contact (occupational) - *continued*
    irritant - *continued*
      due to - *continued*
        specified agent NEC L24.89
  contusiformis L52
  diabetic — *see* E08-E13 with .620
  diaper L22
  diphtheritica A36.3
  dry skin L85.3
  due to
    acetone (contact) (irritant) L24.2
    acids (contact) (irritant) L24.5
    adhesive (s) (allergic) (contact) (plaster) L23.1
      irritant L24.5
    alcohol (irritant) (skin contact) (substances in category T51) L24.2
      taken internally L27.8
    alkalis (contact) (irritant) L24.5
    arsenic (ingested) L27.8
    carbon disulfide (contact) (irritant) L24.2
    caustics (contact) (irritant) L24.5
    cement (contact) L25.3
    cereal (ingested) L27.2
    chemical (s) NEC L25.3
      taken internally L27.8
    chlorocompounds L24.2
    chromium (contact) (irritant) L24.81
    coffee (ingested) L27.2
    cold weather L30.8
    cosmetics (contact) L25.0
      allergic L23.2
      irritant L24.3
    cyclohexanes L24.2
    dander (cat) (dog) L23.81
    Demodex species B88.0
    Dermanyssus gallinae B88.0
    detergents (contact) (irritant) L24.0
    dichromate L24.81
    drugs and medicaments (generalized) (internal use) L27.0
      external — *see* Dermatitis, due to, drugs, in contact with skin
      in contact with skin L25.1
        allergic L23.3
        irritant L24.4
      localized skin eruption L27.1
      specified substance — *see* Table of Drugs and Chemicals
    dyes (contact) L25.2
      allergic L23.4
      irritant L24.89
    epidermophytosis — *see* Dermatophytosis
    esters L24.2
    external irritant NEC L24.9
    fish (ingested) L27.2
    flour (ingested) L27.2
    food (ingested) L27.2
      in contact with skin L25.4
    fruit (ingested) L27.2
    furs (allergic) (contact) L23.81
    glues — *see* Dermatitis, due to, adhesives
    glycols L24.2
    greases NEC (contact) (irritant) L24.1
    hair (cat) (dog) L23.81
    hot
      objects and materials — *see* Burn
      weather or places L59.0
    hydrocarbons L24.2
    infrared rays L59.8
    ingestion, ingested substance L27.9
      chemical NEC L27.8
      drugs and medicaments — *see* Dermatitis, due to, drugs
      food L27.2
      specified NEC L27.8
    insecticide in contact with skin L24.5
    internal agent L27.9
      drugs and medicaments (generalized) — *see* Dermatitis, due to, drugs
      food L27.2
    irradiation — *see* Dermatitis, due to, radioactive substance
    ketones L24.2
    lacquer tree (allergic) (contact) L23.7
    light (sun) NEC L57.8
      acute L56.8
      other L59.8
    Liponyssoides sanguineus B88.0
    low temperature L30.8
    meat (ingested) L27.2
    metals, metal salts (contact) (irritant) L24.81
    milk (ingested) L27.2

Dermatitis (eczematous) - *continued*
  due to - *continued*
    nickel (contact) (irritant) L24.81
    nylon (contact) (irritant) L24.5
    oils NEC (contact) (irritant) L24.1
    paint solvent (contact) (irritant) L24.2
    petroleum products (contact) (irritant) (substances in T52.0) L24.2
    plants NEC (contact) L25.5
      allergic L23.7
      irritant L24.7
    plasters (adhesive) (any) (allergic) (contact) L23.1
      irritant L24.5
    plastic (contact) L25.3
    preservatives (contact) — *see* Dermatitis, due to, chemical, in contact with skin
    primrose (allergic) (contact) L23.7
    primula (allergic) (contact) L23.7
    radiation L59.8
      nonionizing (chronic exposure) L57.8
      sun NEC L57.8
        acute L56.8
    radioactive substance L58.9
      acute L58.0
      chronic L58.1
    radium L58.9
      acute L58.0
      chronic L58.1
    ragweed (allergic) (contact) L23.7
    Rhus (allergic) (contact) (diversiloba) (radicans) (toxicodendron) (venenata) (verniciflua) L23.7
    rubber (contact) L24.5
    Senecio jacobaea (allergic) (contact) L23.7
    solvents (contact) (irritant) (substances in categories T52) L24.2
    specified agent NEC (contact) L25.8
      allergic L23.89
      irritant L24.89
    sunshine NEC L57.8
      acute L56.8
    tetrachlorethylene (contact) (irritant) L24.2
    toluene (contact) (irritant) L24.2
    turpentine (contact) L24.2
    ultraviolet rays (sun NEC) (chronic exposure) L57.8
      acute L56.8
    vaccine or vaccination L27.0
      specified substance — *see* Table of Drugs and Chemicals
    varicose veins — *see* Varix, leg, with, inflammation
    X-rays L58.9
      acute L58.0
      chronic L58.1
  dyshydrotic L30.1
  dysmenorrheica N94.6
  escharotica — *see* Burn
  exfoliative, exfoliativa (generalized) L26
    neonatorum L00
  eyelid — *see also* Dermatosis, eyelid
    allergic H01.119
      left H01.116
        lower H01.115
        upper H01.114
      right H01.113
        lower H01.112
        upper H01.111
    contact — *see* Dermatitis, eyelid, allergic
    due to
      Demodex species B88.0
      herpes (zoster) B02.39
        simplex B00.59
    eczematous H01.139
      left H01.136
        lower H01.135
        upper H01.134
      right H01.133
        lower H01.132
        upper H01.131
  facta, factitia, factitial L98.1
    psychogenic F54
  flexural NEC L20.82
  friction L30.4
  fungus B36.9
    specified type NEC B36.8
  gangrenosa, gangrenous infantum L08.0
  harvest mite B88.0
  heat L59.0
  herpesviral, vesicular (ear) (lip) B00.1
  herpetiformis (bullous) (erythematous) (pustular) (vesicular) L13.0
    juvenile L12.2
    senile L12.0

Dermatitis (eczematous) - *continued*
hiemalis L30.8
hypostatic, hypostatica — *see* Varix, leg, with, inflammation
infectious eczematoid L30.3
infective L30.3
irritant — *see* Dermatitis, contact, irritant
Jacquet's (diaper dermatitis) L22
Leptus B88.0
lichenified NEC L28.0
medicamentosa (generalized) (internal use) — *see* Dermatitis, due to drugs
mite B88.0
multiformis L13.0
juvenile L12.2
napkin L22
neurotica L13.0
nummular L30.0
papillaris capillitii L73.0
pellagrous E52
perioral L71.0
photocontact L56.2
polymorpha dolorosa L13.0
pruriginosa L13.0
pruritic NEC L30.8
psychogenic F54
purulent L08.0
pustular
contagious B08.02
subcorneal L13.1
pyococcal L08.0
pyogenica L08.0
repens L40.2
Ritter's (exfoliativa) L00
Schamberg's L81.7
schistosome B65.3
seasonal bullous L30.8
seborrheic L21.9
infantile L21.1
specified NEC L21.8
sensitization NOS L23.9
septic L08.0
solare L57.8
specified NEC L30.8
stasis I87.2
with
varicose ulcer — *see* Varix, leg, with ulcer, with inflammation
varicose veins — *see* Varix, leg, with, inflammation
due to postthrombotic syndrome — *see* Syndrome, postthrombotic
suppurative L08.0
traumatic NEC L30.4
trophoneurotica L13.0
ultraviolet (sun) (chronic exposure) L57.8
acute L56.8
varicose — *see* Varix, leg, with, inflammation
vegetans L10.1
verrucosa B43.0
vesicular, herpesviral B00.1
Dermatoarthritis, lipoid E78.81
Dermatochalasis, eyelid H02.839
left H02.836
lower H02.835
upper H02.834
right H02.833
lower H02.832
upper H02.831
Dermatofibroma (lenticulare) — *see* Neoplasm, skin, benign
protuberans — *see* Neoplasm, skin, uncertain behavior
Dermatofibrosarcoma (pigmented) (protuberans) — *see* Neoplasm, skin, malignant
Dermatographia L50.3
Dermatolysis (exfoliativa) (congenital) Q82.8
acquired L57.4
eyelids — *see* Blepharochalasis
palpebrarum — *see* Blepharochalasis
senile L57.4
Dermatomegaly NEC Q82.8
Dermatomucosomyositis M33.10
with
myopathy M33.12
respiratory involvement M33.11
specified organ involvement NEC M33.19
Dermatomycosis B36.9
furfuracea B36.0
specified type NEC B36.8

Dermatomyositis (acute) (chronic) — *see also* Dermatopolymyositis
in (due to) neoplastic disease — *see also* Neoplasm D49.9 *[M36.0]*
Dermatoneuritis of children — *see* Poisoning, mercury
Dermatophilosis A48.8
Dermatophytid L30.2
Dermatophytide — *see* Dermatophytosis
Dermatophytosis (epidermophyton) (infection) (Microsporum) (tinea) (Trichophyton) B35.9
beard B35.0
body B35.4
capitis B35.0
corporis B35.4
deep-seated B35.8
disseminated B35.8
foot B35.3
granulomatous B35.8
groin B35.6
hand B35.2
nail B35.1
perianal (area) B35.6
scalp B35.0
specified NEC B35.8
Dermatopolymyositis M33.90
with
myopathy M33.92
respiratory involvement M33.91
specified organ involvement NEC M33.99
in neoplastic disease — *see also* Neoplasm D49.9 *[M36.0]*
juvenile M33.00
with
myopathy M33.02
respiratory involvement M33.01
specified organ involvement NEC M33.09
specified NEC M33.10
myopathy M33.12
respiratory involvement M33.11
specified organ involvement NEC M33.19
Dermatopolyneuritis — *see* Poisoning, mercury
Dermatorrhexis Q79.6
acquired L57.4
Dermatosclerosis — *see also* Scleroderma
localized L94.0
Dermatosis L98.9
Andrews' L08.89
Bowen's — *see* Neoplasm, skin, in situ
bullous L13.9
specified NEC L13.8
exfoliativa L26
eyelid (noninfectious)
dermatitis — *see* Dermatitis, eyelid
discoid lupus erythematosus — *see* Lupus, erythematosus, eyelid
xeroderma — *see* Xeroderma, acquired, eyelid
factitial L98.1
febrile neutrophilic L98.2
gonococcal A54.89
herpetiformis L13.0
juvenile L12.2
linear IgA L13.8
menstrual NEC L98.8
neutrophilic, febrile L98.2
occupational — *see* Dermatitis, contact
papulosa nigra L82.1
pigmentary L81.9
progressive L81.7
Schamberg's L81.7
psychogenic F54
purpuric, pigmented L81.7
pustular, subcorneal L13.1
transient acantholytic L11.1
Dermographia, dermographism L50.3
Dermoid (cyst) — *see also* Neoplasm, benign, by site
with malignant transformation C56-
due to radiation (nonionizing) L57.8
Dermopathy
infiltrative with thyrotoxicosis — *see* Thyrotoxicosis
nephrogenic fibrosing L90.8
Dermophytosis — *see* Dermatophytosis
Descemetocele H18.73-
Descemet's membrane — *see* condition
Descending — *see* condition
Descensus uteri — *see* Prolapse, uterus
Desert
rheumatism B38.0
sore — *see* Ulcer, skin
Desertion (newborn) — *see* Maltreatment
Desmoid (extra-abdominal) (tumor) — *see* Neoplasm, connective tissue, uncertain behavior
abdominal D48.1

Despondency F32.9
Desquamation, skin R23.4
Destruction, destructive — *see also* Damage
articular facet — *see also* Derangement, joint, specified type NEC
knee M23.8X-
vertebra — *see* Spondylosis
bone — *see also* Disorder, bone, specified type NEC
syphilitic A52.77
joint — *see also* Derangement, joint, specified type NEC
sacroiliac M53.3
rectal sphincter K62.89
septum (nasal) J34.89
tuberculous NEC — *see* Tuberculosis
tympanum, tympanic membrane (nontraumatic) — *see* Disorder, tympanic membrane, specified NEC
vertebral disc — *see* Degeneration, intervertebral disc
Destructiveness — *see also* Disorder, conduct
adjustment reaction — *see* Disorder, adjustment
Desultory labor O62.2
Detachment
cartilage — *see* Sprain
cervix, annular N88.8
complicating delivery O71.3
choroid (old) (postinfectional) (simple) (spontaneous) H31.40-
hemorrhagic H31.41-
serous H31.42-
ligament — *see* Sprain
meniscus (knee) — *see also* Derangement, knee, meniscus, specified NEC
current injury — *see* Tear, meniscus
due to old tear or injury — *see* Derangement, knee, meniscus, due to old tear
retina (without retinal break) (serous) H33.2-
with retinal:
break H33.00-
giant H33.03-
multiple H33.02-
single H33.01-
dialysis H33.04-
pigment epithelium — *see* Degeneration, retina, separation of layers, pigment epithelium detachment
rhegmatogenous — *see* Detachment, retina, with retinal, break
specified NEC H33.8
total H33.05-
traction H33.4-
vitreous (body) H43.81
Detergent asthma J69.8
Deterioration
epileptic F06.8
general physical R53.81
heart, cardiac — *see* Degeneration, myocardial
mental — *see* Psychosis
myocardial, myocardium — *see* Degeneration, myocardial
senile (simple) R54
Deuteranomaly (anomalous trichromat) H53.53
Deuteranopia (complete) (incomplete) H53.53
Development
abnormal, bone Q79.9
arrested R62.50
bone — *see* Arrest, development or growth, bone
child R62.50
due to malnutrition E45
defective, congenital — *see also* Anomaly, by site
cauda equina Q06.3
left ventricle Q24.8
in hypoplastic left heart syndrome Q23.4
valve Q24.8
pulmonary Q22.3
delayed — *see also* Delay, development R62.50
arithmetical skills F81.2
language (skills) (expressive) F80.1
learning skill F81.9
mixed skills F88
motor coordination F82
reading F81.0
specified learning skill NEC F81.89
speech F80.9
spelling F81.81
written expression F81.81
imperfect, congenital — *see also* Anomaly, by site
heart Q24.9
lungs Q33.6
incomplete
bronchial tree Q32.4
organ or site not listed — *see* Hypoplasia, by site

Development - *continued*
  incomplete - *continued*
    respiratory system Q34.9
    sexual, precocious NEC E30.1
    tardy, mental — *see also* Disability, intellectual F79
Developmental — *see* condition
  testing, infant or child — *see* Examination, child
Devergie's disease (pityriasis rubra pilaris) L44.0
Deviation (in)
  conjugate palsy (eye) (spastic) H51.0
  esophagus (acquired) K22.8
  eye, skew H51.8
  midline (jaw) (teeth) (dental arch) M26.29
    specified site NEC — *see* Malposition
  nasal septum J34.2
    congenital Q67.4
  opening and closing of the mandible M26.53
  organ or site, congenital NEC — *see* Malposition, congenital
  septum (nasal) (acquired) J34.2
    congenital Q67.4
  sexual F65.9
    bestiality F65.89
    erotomania F52.8
    exhibitionism F65.2
    fetishism, fetishistic F65.0
     transvestism F65.1
    frotteurism F65.81
    masochism F65.51
    multiple F65.89
    necrophilia F65.89
    nymphomania F52.8
    pederosis F65.4
    pedophilia F65.4
    sadism, sadomasochism F65.52
    satyriasis F52.8
    specified type NEC F65.89
    transvestism F64.1
    voyeurism F65.3
  teeth, midline M26.29
  trachea J39.8
  ureter, congenital Q62.61
Device
  cerebral ventricle (communicating) in situ Z98.2
  contraceptive — *see* Contraceptive, device
  drainage, cerebrospinal fluid, in situ Z98.2
Devic's disease G36.0
Devil's
  grip B33.0
  pinches (purpura simplex) D69.2
Devitalized tooth K04.99
Devonshire colic — *see* Poisoning, lead
Dextraposition, aorta Q20.3
  in tetralogy of Fallot Q21.3
Dextrinosis, limit (debrancher enzyme deficiency) E74.03
Dextrocardia (true) Q24.0
  with
    complete transposition of viscera Q89.3
    situs inversus Q89.3
Dextrotransposition, aorta Q20.3
d-glycericacidemia E72.59
Dhat syndrome F48.8
Dhobi itch B35.6
Di George's syndrome D82.1
Di Guglielmo's disease C94.0-
Diabetes, diabetic (mellitus) (sugar) E11.9
  with
    amyotrophy E11.44
    arthropathy NEC E11.618
    autonomic (poly) neuropathy E11.43
    cataract E11.36
    Charcot's joints E11.610
    chronic kidney disease E11.22
    circulatory complication NEC E11.59
    complication E11.8
     specified NEC E11.69
    dermatitis E11.620
    foot ulcer E11.621
    gangrene E11.52
    gastroparalysis E11.43
    gastroparesis E11.43
    glomerulonephrosis, intracapillary E11.21
    glomerulosclerosis, intercapillary E11.21
    hyperglycemia E11.65
    hyperosmolarity E11.00
     with coma E11.01
    hypoglycemia E11.649
     with coma E11.641
    kidney complications NEC E11.29
    Kimmelstiel-Wilson disease E11.21
    loss of protective sensation (LOPS) — *see* Diabetes, by type, with neuropathy

Diabetes, diabetic (mellitus) (sugar) - *continued*
  with - *continued*
    mononeuropathy E11.41
    myasthenia E11.44
    necrobiosis lipoidica E11.620
    nephropathy E11.21
    neuralgia E11.42
    neurologic complication NEC E11.49
    neuropathic arthropathy E11.610
    neuropathy E11.40
    ophthalmic complication NEC E11.39
    oral complication NEC E11.638
    osteomyelitis E11.69
    periodontal disease E11.630
    peripheral angiopathy E11.51
     with gangrene E11.52
    polyneuropathy E11.42
    renal complication NEC E11.29
    renal tubular degeneration E11.29
    retinopathy E11.319
     with macular edema E11.311
      resolved following treatment E11.37
     nonproliferative E11.329
      with macular edema E11.321
      mild E11.329
       with macular edema E11.321
      moderate E11.339
       with macular edema E11.331
      severe E11.349
       with macular edema E11.341
     proliferative E11.359
      with
       combined traction retinal detachment and rhegmatogenous retinal detachment E11.354
       macular edema E11.351
       stable proliferative diabetic retinopathy E11.355
       traction retinal detachment involving the macula E11.352
       traction retinal detachment not involving the macula E11.353
    skin complication NEC E11.628
    skin ulcer NEC E11.622
  brittle — *see* Diabetes, type 1
  bronzed E83.110
  complicating pregnancy — *see* Pregnancy, complicated by, diabetes
  dietary counseling and surveillance Z71.3
  due to
    autoimmune process — *see* Diabetes, type 1
    immune mediated pancreatic islet beta-cell destruction — *see* Diabetes, type 1
  due to drug or chemical E09.9
    with
     amyotrophy E09.44
     arthropathy NEC E09.618
     autonomic (poly) neuropathy E09.43
     cataract E09.36
     Charcot's joints E09.610
     chronic kidney disease E09.22
     circulatory complication NEC E09.59
     complication E09.8
      specified NEC E09.69
     dermatitis E09.620
     foot ulcer E09.621
     gangrene E09.52
     gastroparalysis E09.43
     gastroparesis E09.43
     glomerulonephrosis, intracapillary E09.21
     glomerulosclerosis, intercapillary E09.21
     hyperglycemia E09.65
     hyperosmolarity E09.00
      with coma E09.01
     hypoglycemia E09.649
      with coma E09.641
     ketoacidosis E09.10
      with coma E09.11
     kidney complications NEC E09.29
     Kimmelstiel-Wilson disease E09.21
     mononeuropathy E09.41
     myasthenia E09.44
     necrobiosis lipoidica E09.620
     nephropathy E09.21
     neuralgia E09.42
     neurologic complication NEC E09.49
     neuropathic arthropathy E09.610
     neuropathy E09.40
     ophthalmic complication NEC E09.39
     oral complication NEC E09.638
     periodontal disease E09.630
     peripheral angiopathy E09.51
      with gangrene E09.52
     polyneuropathy E09.42

Diabetes, diabetic (mellitus) (sugar) - *continued*
  due to drug or chemical - *continued*
    with - *continued*
     renal complication NEC E09.29
     renal tubular degeneration E09.29
     retinopathy E09.319
      with macular edema E09.311
      resolved following treatment E09.37
      nonproliferative E09.329
       with macular edema E09.321
       mild E09.329
        with macular edema E09.321
       moderate E09.339
        with macular edema E09.331
       severe E09.349
        with macular edema E09.341
      proliferative E09.359
       with
        combined traction retinal detachment and rhegmatogenous retinal detachment E09.354
        macular edema E09.351
        stable proliferative diabetic retinopathy E09.355
        traction retinal detachment involving the macula E09.352
        traction retinal detachment not involving the macula E09.353
     skin complication NEC E09.628
     skin ulcer NEC E09.622
  due to underlying condition E08.9
    with
     amyotrophy E08.44
     arthropathy NEC E08.618
     autonomic (poly) neuropathy E08.43
     cataract E08.36
     Charcot's joints E08.610
     chronic kidney disease E08.22
     circulatory complication NEC E08.59
     complication E08.8
      specified NEC E08.69
     dermatitis E08.620
     foot ulcer E08.621
     gangrene E08.52
     gastroparalysis E08.43
     gastroparesis E08.43
     glomerulonephrosis, intracapillary E08.21
     glomerulosclerosis, intercapillary E08.21
     hyperglycemia E08.65
     hyperosmolarity E08.00
      with coma E08.01
     hypoglycemia E08.649
      with coma E08.641
     ketoacidosis E08.10
      with coma E08.11
     kidney complications NEC E08.29
     Kimmelstiel-WIlson disease E08.21
     mononeuropathy E08.41
     myasthenia E08.44
     necrobiosis lipoidica E08.620
     nephropathy E08.21
     neuralgia E08.42
     neurologic complication NEC E08.49
     neuropathic arthropathy E08.610
     neuropathy E08.40
     ophthalmic complication NEC E08.39
     oral complication NEC E08.638
     periodontal disease E08.630
     peripheral angiopathy E08.51
      with gangrene E08.52
     polyneuropathy E08.42
     renal complication NEC E08.29
     renal tubular degeneration E08.29
     retinopathy E08.319
      with macular edema E08.311
      resolved following treatment E08.37
      nonproliferative E08.329
       with macular edema E08.321
       mild E08.329
        with macular edema E08.321
       moderate E08.339
        with macular edema E08.331
       severe E08.349
        with macular edema E08.341
      proliferative E08.359
       with
        combined traction retinal detachment and rhegmatogenous retinal detachment E08.354
        macular edema E08.351
        stable proliferative diabetic retinopathy E08.355

Diabetes, diabetic (mellitus) (sugar) - *continued*
  due to underlying condition - *continued*
    with - *continued*
      retinopathy - *continued*
        proliferative - *continued*
          with - *continued*
            traction retinal detachment involving the macula E08.352
            traction retinal detachment not involving the macula E08.353
      skin complication NEC E08.628
      skin ulcer NEC E08.622
  gestational (in pregnancy) O24.419
    affecting newborn P70.0
    diet controlled O24.410
    in childbirth O24.429
      diet controlled O24.420
      insulin (and diet) controlled O24.424
      oral drug controlled (antidiabetic) (hypoglycemic) O24.425
    insulin (and diet) controlled O24.414
    oral drug controlled (antidiabetic) (hypoglycemic) O24.415
    puerperal O24.439
      diet controlled O24.430
      insulin (and diet) controlled O24.434
      oral drug controlled (antidiabetic) (hypoglycemic) O24.435
  hepatogenous E13.9
  idiopathic — *see* Diabetes, type 1
  inadequately controlled - code to Diabetes, by type, with hyperglycemia
  insipidus E23.2
    nephrogenic N25.1
    pituitary E23.2
    vasopressin resistant N25.1
  insulin dependent - code to type of diabetes
  juvenile-onset — *see* Diabetes, type 1
  ketosis-prone — *see* Diabetes, type 1
  latent R73.03
  neonatal (transient) P70.2
  non-insulin dependent - code to type of diabetes
  out of control - code to Diabetes, by type, with hyperglycemia
  phosphate E83.39
  poorly controlled - code to Diabetes, by type, with hyperglycemia
  postpancreatectomy — *see* Diabetes, specified type NEC
  postprocedural — *see* Diabetes, specified type NEC
  secondary diabetes mellitus NEC — *see* Diabetes, specified type NEC
  specified type NEC E13.9
    with
      amyotrophy E13.44
      arthropathy NEC E13.618
      autonomic (poly) neuropathy E13.43
      cataract E13.36
      Charcot's joints E13.610
      chronic kidney disease E13.22
      circulatory complication NEC E13.59
      complication E13.8
        specified NEC E13.69
      dermatitis E13.620
      foot ulcer E13.621
      gangrene E13.52
      gastroparalysis E13.43
      gastroparesis E13.43
      glomerulonephrosis, intracapillary E13.21
      glomerulosclerosis, intercapillary E13.21
      hyperglycemia E13.65
      hyperosmolarity E13.00
        with coma E13.01
      hypoglycemia E13.649
        with coma E13.641
      ketoacidosis E13.10
        with coma E13.11
      kidney complications NEC E13.29
      Kimmelstiel-Wilson disease E13.21
      mononeuropathy E13.41
      myasthenia E13.44
      necrobiosis lipoidica E13.620
      nephropathy E13.21
      neuralgia E13.42
      neurologic complication NEC E13.49
      neuropathic arthropathy E13.610
      neuropathy E13.40
      ophthalmic complication NEC E13.39
      oral complication NEC E13.638
      periodontal disease E13.630
      peripheral angiopathy E13.51
        with gangrene E13.52
      polyneuropathy E13.42

Diabetes, diabetic (mellitus) (sugar) - *continued*
  specified type NEC - *continued*
    with - *continued*
      renal complication NEC E13.29
      renal tubular degeneration E13.29
      retinopathy E13.319
        with macular edema E13.311
        resolved following treatment E13.37
        nonproliferative E13.329
          with macular edema E13.321
          mild E13.329
            with macular edema E13.321
          moderate E13.339
            with macular edema E13.331
          severe E13.349
            with macular edema E13.341
        proliferative E13.359
          with
            combined traction retinal detachment and rhegmatogenous retinal detachment E13.354
            macular edema E13.351
            stable proliferative diabetic retinopathy E13.355
            traction retinal detachment involving the macula E13.352
            traction retinal detachment not involving the macula E13.353
      skin complication NEC E13.628
      skin ulcer NEC E13.622
  steroid-induced — *see* Diabetes, due to, drug or chemical
  type 1 E10.9
    with
      amyotrophy E10.44
      arthropathy NEC E10.618
      autonomic (poly) neuropathy E10.43
      cataract E10.36
      Charcot's joints E10.610
      chronic kidney disease E10.22
      circulatory complication NEC E10.59
      complication E10.8
        specified NEC E10.69
      dermatitis E10.620
      foot ulcer E10.621
      gangrene E10.52
      gastroparalysis E10.43
      gastroparesis E10.43
      glomerulonephrosis, intracapillary E10.21
      glomerulosclerosis, intercapillary E10.21
      hyperglycemia E10.65
      hypoglycemia E10.649
        with coma E10.641
      ketoacidosis E10.10
        with coma E10.11
      kidney complications NEC E10.29
      Kimmelstiel-Wilson disease E10.21
      mononeuropathy E10.41
      myasthenia E10.44
      necrobiosis lipoidica E10.620
      nephropathy E10.21
      neuralgia E10.42
      neurologic complication NEC E10.49
      neuropathic arthropathy E10.610
      neuropathy E10.40
      ophthalmic complication NEC E10.39
      oral complication NEC E10.638
      periodontal disease E10.630
      peripheral angiopathy E10.51
        with gangrene E10.52
      polyneuropathy E10.42
      renal complication NEC E10.29
      renal tubular degeneration E10.29
      retinopathy E10.319
        with macular edema E10.311
        resolved following treatment E10.37
        nonproliferative E10.329
          with macular edema E10.321
          mild E10.329
            with macular edema E10.321
          moderate E10.339
            with macular edema E10.331
          severe E10.349
            with macular edema E10.341
        proliferative E10.359
          with
            combined traction retinal detachment and rhegmatogenous retinal detachment E10.354
            macular edema E10.351
            stable proliferative diabetic retinopathy E10.355

Diabetes, diabetic (mellitus) (sugar) - *continued*
  type 1 - *continued*
    with - *continued*
      retinopathy - *continued*
        proliferative - *continued*
          with - *continued*
            traction retinal detachment involving the macula E10.352
            traction retinal detachment not involving the macula E10.353
      skin complication NEC E10.628
      skin ulcer NEC E10.622
  type 2 E11.9
    with
      amyotrophy E11.44
      arthropathy NEC E11.618
      autonomic (poly) neuropathy E11.43
      cataract E11.36
      Charcot's joints E11.610
      chronic kidney disease E11.22
      circulatory complication NEC E11.59
      complication E11.8
        specified NEC E11.69
      dermatitis E11.620
      foot ulcer E11.621
      gangrene E11.52
      gastroparalysis E11.43
      gastroparesis E11.43
      glomerulonephrosis, intracapillary E11.21
      glomerulosclerosis, intercapillary E11.21
      hyperglycemia E11.65
      hyperosmolarity E11.00
        with coma E11.01
      hypoglycemia E11.649
        with coma E11.641
      kidney complications NEC E11.29
      Kimmelstiel-Wilson disease E11.21
      mononeuropathy E11.41
      myasthenia E11.44
      necrobiosis lipoidica E11.620
      nephropathy E11.21
      neuralgia E11.42
      neurologic complication NEC E11.49
      neuropathic arthropathy E11.610
      neuropathy E11.40
      ophthalmic complication NEC E11.39
      oral complication NEC E11.638
      periodontal disease E11.630
      peripheral angiopathy E11.51
        with gangrene E11.52
      polyneuropathy E11.42
      renal complication NEC E11.29
      renal tubular degeneration E11.29
      retinopathy E11.319
        with macular edema E11.311
        resolved following treatment E11.37
        nonproliferative E11.329
          with macular edema E11.321
          mild E11.329
            with macular edema E11.321
          moderate E11.339
            with macular edema E11.331
          severe E11.349
            with macular edema E11.341
        proliferative E11.359
          with
            combined traction retinal detachment and rhegmatogenous retinal detachment E11.354
            macular edema E11.351
            stable proliferative diabetic retinopathy E11.355
            traction retinal detachment involving the macula E11.352
            traction retinal detachment not involving the macula E11.353
      skin complication NEC E11.628
      skin ulcer NEC E11.622
  uncontrolled
    meaning
      hyperglycemia — *see* Diabetes, by type, with, hyperglycemia
      hypoglycemia — *see* Diabetes, by type, with, hypoglycemia
Diacyclothrombopathia D69.1
Diagnosis deferred R69
Dialysis (intermittent) (treatment)
  noncompliance (with) Z91.15
  renal (hemodialysis) (peritoneal) , status Z99.2
  retina, retinal — *see* Detachment, retina, with retinal, dialysis
Diamond-Blackfan anemia (congenital hypoplastic) D61.01

Diamond-Gardener syndrome
  (autoerythrocyte sensitization) D69.2
Diaper rash L22
Diaphoresis (excessive) R61
Diaphragm — *see* condition
Diaphragmalgia R07.1
Diaphragmatitis, diaphragmitis J98.6
Diaphysial aclasis Q78.6
Diaphysitis — *see* Osteomyelitis, specified type NEC
Diarrhea, diarrheal (disease) (infantile)
  (inflammatory) R19.7
  achlorhydric K31.83
  allergic K52.29
    due to
      colitis — *see* Colitis, allergic
      enteritis — *see* Enteritis, allergic
  amebic — *see also* Amebiasis A06.0
    with abscess — *see* Abscess, amebic
    acute A06.0
    chronic A06.1
    nondysenteric A06.2
  bacillary — *see* Dysentery, bacillary
  balantidial A07.0
  cachectic NEC K52.89
  Chilomastix A07.8
  choleriformis A00.1
  chronic (noninfectious) K52.9
  coccidial A07.3
  Cochin-China K90.1
    strongyloidiasis B78.0
  dietetic — *see also* Diarrhea, allergic K52.29
  drug-induced K52.1
  due to
    bacteria A04.9
      specified NEC A04.8
    Campylobacter A04.5
    Capillaria philippinensis B81.1
    Clostridium difficile A04.7
    Clostridium perfringens (C) (F) A04.8
    Cryptosporidium A07.2
    drugs K52.1
    Escherichia coli A04.4
      enteroaggregative A04.4
      enterohemorrhagic A04.3
      enteroinvasive A04.2
      enteropathogenic A04.0
      enterotoxigenic A04.1
      specified NEC A04.4
    food hypersensitivity — *see also* Diarrhea,
      allergic K52.29
    Necator americanus B76.1
    S. japonicum B65.2
    specified organism NEC A08.8
      bacterial A04.8
      viral A08.39
    Staphylococcus A04.8
    Trichuris trichiuria B79
    virus — *see* Enteritis, viral
    Yersinia enterocolitica A04.6
  dysenteric A09
  endemic A09
  epidemic A09
  flagellate A07.9
  Flexner's (ulcerative) A03.1
  functional K59.1
    following gastrointestinal surgery K91.89
    psychogenic F45.8
  Giardia lamblia A07.1
  giardial A07.1
  hill K90.1
  infectious A09
  malarial — *see* Malaria
  mite B88.0
  mycotic NEC B49
  neonatal (noninfectious) P78.3
  nervous F45.8
  neurogenic K59.1
  noninfectious K52.9
  postgastrectomy K91.1
  postvagotomy K91.1
  protozoal A07.9
    specified NEC A07.8
  psychogenic F45.8
  specified
    bacterium NEC A04.8
    virus NEC A08.39
  strongyloidiasis B78.0
  toxic K52.1
  trichomonal A07.8
  tropical K90.1
  tuberculous A18.32
  viral — *see* Enteritis, viral

Diastasis
  cranial bones M84.88
    congenital NEC Q75.8
  joint (traumatic) — *see* Dislocation
  muscle M62.00
    ankle M62.07-
    congenital Q79.8
    foot M62.07-
    forearm M62.03-
    hand M62.04-
    lower leg M62.06-
    pelvic region M62.05-
    shoulder region M62.01-
    specified site NEC M62.08
    thigh M62.05-
    upper arm M62.02-
  recti (abdomen)
    complicating delivery O71.89
    congenital Q79.59
Diastema, tooth, teeth, fully erupted M26.32
Diastematomyelia Q06.2
Diataxia, cerebral G80.4
Diathesis
  allergic — *see* History, allergy
  bleeding (familial) D69.9
  cystine (familial) E72.00
  gouty — *see* Gout
  hemorrhagic (familial) D69.9
    newborn NEC P53
  spasmophilic R29.0
Diaz's disease or osteochondrosis (juvenile)
  (talus) — *see* Osteochondrosis, juvenile, tarsus
Dibothriocephalus, dibothriocephaliasis (latus)
  (infection) (infestation) B70.0
  larval B70.1
Dicephalus, dicephaly Q89.4
Dichotomy, teeth K00.2
Dichromat, dichromatopsia (congenital) — *see*
  Deficiency, color vision
Dichuchwa A65
Dicroceliasis B66.2
Didelphia, didelphys — *see* Double uterus
Didymytis N45.1
  with orchitis N45.3
Dietary
  inadequacy or deficiency E63.9
  surveillance and counseling Z71.3
Dietl's crisis N13.8
Dieulafoy lesion (hemorrhagic)
  duodenum K31.82
  esophagus K22.8
  intestine (colon) K63.81
  stomach K31.82
Difficult, difficulty (in)
  acculturation Z60.3
  feeding R63.3
    newborn P92.9
      breast P92.5
      specified NEC P92.8
    nonorganic (infant or child) F98.29
  intubation, in anesthesia T88.4
  mechanical, gastroduodenal stoma K91.89
    causing obstruction K91.3
  micturition
    need to immediately re-void R39.191
    position dependent R39.192
    specified NEC R39.198
  reading (developmental) F81.0
    secondary to emotional disorders F93.9
  spelling (specific) F81.81
    with reading disorder F81.89
    due to inadequate teaching Z55.8
  swallowing — *see* Dysphagia
  walking R26.2
  work
    conditions NEC Z56.5
    schedule Z56.3
Diffuse — *see* condition
DiGeorge's syndrome (thymic hypoplasia) D82.1
Digestive — *see* condition
Dihydropyrimidine dehydrogenase disease
  (DPD) E88.89
Diktyoma — *see* Neoplasm, malignant, by site
Dilaceration, tooth K00.4
Dilatation
  anus K59.8
    venule — *see* Hemorrhoids
  aorta (focal) (general) — *see* Ectasia, aorta
    with aneuysm — *see* Aneurysm, aorta
    congenital Q25.44
  artery — *see* Aneurysm
  bladder (sphincter) N32.89
    congenital Q64.79

Dilatation - *continued*
  blood vessel I99.8
  bronchial J47.9
    with
      exacerbation (acute) J47.1
      lower respiratory infection J47.0
  calyx (due to obstruction) — *see* Hydronephrosis
  capillaries I78.8
  cardiac (acute) (chronic) — *see also* Hypertrophy,
    cardiac
    congenital Q24.8
      valve NEC Q24.8
        pulmonary Q22.3
    valve — *see* Endocarditis
  cavum septi pellucidi Q06.8
  cervix (uteri) — *see also* Incompetency, cervix
    incomplete, poor, slow complicating
      delivery O62.0
  colon K59.39
    congenital Q43.1
    psychogenic F45.8
    toxic K59.31
  common duct (acquired) K83.8
    congenital Q44.5
  cystic duct (acquired) K82.8
    congenital Q44.5
  duct, mammary — *see* Ectasia, mammary duct
  duodenum K59.8
  esophagus K22.8
    congenital Q39.5
    due to achalasia K22.0
  eustachian tube, congenital Q17.8
  gallbladder K82.8
  gastric — *see* Dilatation, stomach
  heart (acute) (chronic) — *see also* Hypertrophy,
    cardiac
    congenital Q24.8
    valve — *see* Endocarditis
  ileum K59.8
    psychogenic F45.8
  jejunum K59.8
    psychogenic F45.8
  kidney (calyx) (collecting structures) (cystic)
    (parenchyma) (pelvis) (idiopathic) N28.89
  lacrimal passages or duct — *see* Disorder, lacrimal
    system, changes
  lymphatic vessel I89.0
  mammary duct — *see* Ectasia, mammary duct
  Meckel's diverticulum (congenital) Q43.0
    malignant — *see* Table of Neoplasms, small
      intestine, malignant
  myocardium (acute) (chronic) — *see* Hypertrophy,
    cardiac
  organ or site, congenital NEC — *see* Distortion
  pancreatic duct K86.89
  pericardium — *see* Pericarditis
  pharynx J39.2
  prostate N42.89
  pulmonary
    artery (idiopathic) I28.8
    valve, congenital Q22.3
  pupil H57.04
  rectum K59.39
  saccule, congenital Q16.5
  salivary gland (duct) K11.8
  sphincter ani K62.89
  stomach K31.89
    acute K31.0
    psychogenic F45.8
  submaxillary duct K11.8
  trachea, congenital Q32.1
  ureter (idiopathic) N28.82
    congenital Q62.2
    due to obstruction N13.4
  urethra (acquired) N36.8
  vasomotor I73.9
  vein I86.8
  ventricular, ventricle (acute) (chronic) — *see*
    also Hypertrophy, cardiac
    cerebral, congenital Q04.8
  venule NEC I86.8
  vesical orifice N32.89
Dilated, dilation — *see* Dilatation
Diminished, diminution
  hearing (acuity) — *see* Deafness
  sense or sensation (cold) (heat) (tactile)
    (vibratory) R20.8
  vision NEC H54.7
  vital capacity R94.2
Diminuta taenia B71.0
Dimitri-Sturge-Weber disease Q85.8
Dimple
  congenital sacral Q82.6

Dimple - *continued*
  parasacral Q82.6
  pilonidal or postanal — *see* Cyst, pilonidal
Dioctophyme renalis (infection) (infestation) B83.8
Dipetalonemiasis B74.4
Diphallus Q55.69
Diphtheria, diphtheritic (gangrenous)
    (hemorrhagic) A36.9
  carrier (suspected) Z22.2
  cutaneous A36.3
  faucial A36.0
  infection of wound A36.3
  laryngeal A36.2
  myocarditis A36.81
  nasal, anterior A36.89
  nasopharyngeal A36.1
  neurological complication A36.89
  pharyngeal A36.0
  specified site NEC A36.89
  tonsillar A36.0
Diphyllobothriasis (intestine) B70.0
  larval B70.1
Diplacusis H93.22-
Diplegia (upper limbs) G83.0
  congenital (cerebral) G80.8
  facial G51.0
  lower limbs G82.20
  spastic G80.1
Diplococcus, diplococcal — *see* condition
Diplopia H53.2
Dipsomania F10.20
  with
    psychosis — *see* Psychosis, alcoholic
    remission F10.21
Dipylidiasis B71.1
DIRA
    (deficiency of interleukin 1 receptor
    antagonist) M04.8
Direction, teeth, abnormal, fully erupted M26.30
Dirofilariasis B74.8
Dirt-eating child F98.3
Disability, disabilities
  heart — *see* Disease, heart
  intellectual F79
    with
      autistic features F84.9
    mild (I.Q.50-69) F70
    moderate (I.Q.35-49) F71
    profound (I.Q. under 20) F73
    severe (I.Q.20-34) F72
    specified level NEC F78
  knowledge acquisition F81.9
  learning F81.9
  limiting activities Z73.6
  spelling, specific F81.81
Disappearance of family member Z63.4
Disarticulation — *see* Amputation
  meaning traumatic amputation — *see* Amputation,
    traumatic
Discharge (from)
  abnormal finding in — *see* Abnormal, specimen
  breast (female) (male) N64.52
  diencephalic autonomic idiopathic — *see* Epilepsy,
    specified NEC
  ear — *see also* Otorrhea
    blood — *see* Otorrhagia
  excessive urine R35.8
  nipple N64.52
  penile R36.9
  postnasal R09.82
  prison, anxiety concerning Z65.2
  urethral R36.9
    without blood R36.0
    hematospermia R36.1
  vaginal N89.8
Discitis, diskitis M46.40
  cervical region M46.42
  cervicothoracic region M46.43
  lumbar region M46.46
  lumbosacral region M46.47
  multiple sites M46.49
  occipito-atlanto-axial region M46.41
  pyogenic — *see* Infection, intervertebral disc,
    pyogenic
  sacrococcygeal region M46.48
  thoracic region M46.44
  thoracolumbar region M46.45
Discoid
  meniscus (congenital) Q68.6
  semilunar cartilage (congenital) —
    Derangement, knee, meniscus, specified NEC
Discoloration
  nails L60.8

Discoloration - *continued*
  teeth (posteruptive) K03.7
    during formation K00.8
Discomfort
  chest R07.89
  visual H53.14-
Discontinuity, ossicles, ear H74.2-
Discord (with)
  boss Z56.4
  classmates Z55.4
  counselor Z64.4
  employer Z56.4
  family Z63.8
  fellow employees Z56.4
  in-laws Z63.1
  landlord Z59.2
  lodgers Z59.2
  neighbors Z59.2
  probation officer Z64.4
  social worker Z64.4
  teachers Z55.4
  workmates Z56.4
Discordant connection
  atrioventricular (congenital) Q20.5
  ventriculoarterial Q20.3
Discrepancy
  centric occlusion maximum intercuspation M26.55
  leg length (acquired) — *see* Deformity, limb,
    unequal length
    congenital — *see* Defect, reduction, lower limb
  uterine size date O26.84-
Discrimination
  ethnic Z60.5
  political Z60.5
  racial Z60.5
  religious Z60.5
  sex Z60.5
Disease, diseased — *see also* Syndrome
  absorbent system I87.8
  acid-peptic K30
  Acosta's T70.29
  Adams-Stokes (-Morgagni) (syncope with heart
    block) I45.9
  Addison's anemia (pernicious) D51.0
  adenoids (and tonsils) J35.9
  adrenal (capsule) (cortex) (gland) (medullary) E27.9
    hyperfunction E27.0
    specified NEC E27.8
  ainhum L94.6
  airway
    obstructive, chronic J44.9
      due to
        cotton dust J66.0
        specific organic dusts NEC J66.8
    reactive — *see* Asthma
  akamushi (scrub typhus) A75.3
  Albers-Schönberg (marble bones) Q78.2
  Albert's — *see* Tendinitis, Achilles
  alimentary canal K63.9
  alligator-skin Q80.9
    acquired L85.0
  alpha heavy chain C88.3
  alpine T70.29
  altitude T70.20
  alveolar ridge
    edentulous K06.9
      specified NEC K06.8
  alveoli, teeth K08.9
  Alzheimer's G30.9 *[F02.80]*
    with behavioral disturbance G30.9 *[F02.81]*
    early onset G30.0 *[F02.80]*
      with behavioral disturbance G30.0 *[F02.81]*
    late onset G30.1 *[F02.80]*
      with behavioral disturbance G30.1 *[F02.81]*
    specified NEC G30.8 *[F02.80]*
      with behavioral disturbance G30.8 *[F02.81]*
  amyloid — *see* Amyloidosis
  Andersen's (glycogenosis IV) E74.09
  Andes T70.29
  Andrews' (bacterid) L08.89
  angiospastic I73.9
    cerebral G45.9
    vein I87.8
  anterior
    chamber H21.9
    horn cell G12.29
  antiglomerular basement membrane (anti- GBM)
    antibody M31.0
    tubulo-interstitial nephritis N12
  antral — *see* Sinusitis, maxillary
  anus K62.9
    specified NEC K62.89
  aorta (nonsyphilitic) I77.9

Disease, diseased - *continued*
  aorta (nonsyphilitic) - *continued*
    syphilitic NEC A52.02
  aortic (heart) (valve) I35.9
    rheumatic I06.9
  Apollo B30.3
  aponeuroses — *see* Enthesopathy
  appendix K38.9
    specified NEC K38.8
  aqueous (chamber) H21.9
  Arnold-Chiari — *see* Arnold-Chiari disease
  arterial I77.9
    occlusive — *see* Occlusion, by site
    due to stricture or stenosis I77.1
  arteriocardiorenal — *see* Hypertension, cardiorenal
  arteriolar (generalized) (obliterative) I77.9
  arteriorenal — *see* Hypertension, kidney
  arteriosclerotic — *see also* Arteriosclerosis
    cardiovascular — *see* Disease, heart, ischemic,
      atherosclerotic
    coronary (artery) — *see* Disease, heart, ischemic,
      atherosclerotic
    heart — *see* Disease, heart, ischemic,
      atherosclerotic
  artery I77.9
    cerebral I67.9
    coronary I25.10
      with angina pectoris — *see* Arteriosclerosis,
        coronary (artery)
  arthropod-borne NOS (viral) A94
    specified type NEC A93.8
  atticoantral, chronic H66.20
    left H66.22
      with right H66.23
    right H66.21
      with left H66.23
  auditory canal — *see* Disorder, ear, external
  auricle, ear NEC — *see* Disorder, pinna
  Australian X A83.4
  autoimmune (systemic) NOS M35.9
    hemolytic (cold type) (warm type) D59.1
      drug-induced D59.0
    thyroid E06.3
  aviator's — *see* Effect, adverse, high altitude
  Ayerza's (pulmonary artery sclerosis with pulmonary
    hypertension) I27.0
  Babington's (familial hemorrhagic
    telangiectasia) I78.0
  bacterial A49.9
    specified NEC A48.8
    zoonotic A28.9
      specified type NEC A28.8
  Baelz's (cheilitis glandularis apostematosa) K13.0
  bagasse J67.1
  balloon — *see* Effect, adverse, high altitude
  Bang's (brucella abortus) A23.1
  Bannister's T78.3
  barometer makers' — *see* Poisoning, mercury
  Barraquer (-Simons') (progressive
    lipodystrophy) E88.1
  Barrett's — *see* Barrett's, esophagus
  Bartholin's gland N75.9
  basal ganglia G25.9
    degenerative G23.9
      specified NEC G23.8
    specified NEC G25.89
  Basedow's (exophthalmic goiter) — *see*
    Hyperthyroidism, with, goiter (diffuse)
  Bateman's B08.1
  Batten-Steinert G71.11
  Battey A31.0
  Beard's (neurasthenia) F48.8
  Becker
    idiopathic mural endomyocardial I42.3
    myotonia congenita G71.12
  Begbie's (exophthalmic goiter) — *see*
    Hyperthyroidism, with, goiter (diffuse)
  behavioral, organic F07.9
  Beigel's (white piedra) B36.2
  Benson's — *see* Deposit, crystalline
  Bernard-Soulier (thrombopathy) D69.1
  Bernhardt (-Roth) — *see* Mononeuropathy, lower
    limb, meralgia paresthetica
  Biermer's (pernicious anemia) D51.0
  bile duct (common) (hepatic) K83.9
    with calculus, stones — *see* Calculus, bile duct
    specified NEC K83.8
  biliary (tract) K83.9
    specified NEC K83.8
  Billroth's — *see* Spina bifida
  bird fancier's J67.2
  black lung J60
  bladder N32.9

Disease, diseased - *continued*
  bladder - *continued*
    in (due to)
      schistosomiasis (bilharziasis) B65.0 *[N33]*
    specified NEC N32.89
  bleeder's D66
  blood D75.9
    forming organs D75.9
    vessel I99.9
  Bloodgood's — *see* Mastopathy, cystic
  Bodechtel-Guttmann (subacute sclerosing
    panencephalitis) A81.1
  bone — *see also* Disorder, bone
    aluminum M83.4
    fibrocystic NEC
      jaw M27.49
  bone-marrow D75.9
  Borna A83.9
  Bornholm (epidemic pleurodynia) B33.0
  Bouchard's (myopathic dilatation of the
    stomach) K31.0
  Bouillaud's (rheumatic heart disease) I01.9
  Bourneville (-Brissaud) (tuberous sclerosis) Q85.1
  Bouveret (-Hoffmann) (paroxysmal
    tachycardia) I47.9
  bowel K63.9
    functional K59.9
      psychogenic F45.8
  brain G93.9
    arterial, artery I67.9
    arteriosclerotic I67.2
    congenital Q04.9
    degenerative — *see* Degeneration, brain
    inflammatory — *see* Encephalitis
    organic G93.9
      arteriosclerotic I67.2
    parasitic NEC B71.9 *[G94]*
    senile NEC G31.1
    specified NEC G93.89
  breast — *see also* Disorder, breast N64.9
    cystic (chronic) — *see* Mastopathy, cystic
    fibrocystic — *see* Mastopathy, cystic
    Paget's
      female, unspecified side C50.91-
      male, unspecified side C50.92-
    specified NEC N64.89
  Breda's — *see* Yaws
  Bretonneau's (diphtheritic malignant angina) A36.0
  Bright's — *see* Nephritis
    arteriosclerotic — *see* Hypertension, kidney
  Brill's (recrudescent typhus) A75.1
  Brill-Zinsser (recrudescent typhus) A75.1
  Brion-Kayser — *see* Fever, paratyphoid
  broad
    beta E78.2
    ligament (noninflammatory) N83.9
      inflammatory — *see* Disease, pelvis,
        inflammatory
    specified NEC N83.8
  Brocq-Duhring (dermatitis herpetiformis) L13.0
  Brocq's
    meaning
      dermatitis herpetiformis L13.0
      prurigo L28.2
  bronchopulmonary J98.4
  bronchus NEC J98.09
  bronze Addison's E27.1
    tuberculous A18.7
  budgerigar fancier's J67.2
  bullous L13.9
    chronic of childhood L12.2
    specified NEC L13.8
  Buerger's (thromboangiitis obliterans) I73.1
  Bürger-Grütz (essential familial hyperlipemia) E78.3
  bursa — *see* Bursopathy
  caisson T70.3
  California — *see* Coccidioidomycosis
  capillaries I78.9
    specified NEC I78.8
  Carapata A68.0
  cardiac — *see* Disease, heart
  cardiopulmonary, chronic I27.9
  cardiorenal (hepatic) (hypertensive)
    (vascular) — *see* Hypertension, cardiorenal
  cardiovascular (atherosclerotic) I25.10
    with angina pectoris — *see* Arteriosclerosis,
      coronary (artery)
    congenital Q28.9
    newborn P29.9
      specified NEC P29.89
    hypertensive — *see* Hypertension, heart
    renal (hypertensive) — *see* Hypertension,
      cardiorenal

Disease, diseased - *continued*
  cardiovascular (atherosclerotic) - *continued*
    syphilitic (asymptomatic) A52.00
  cartilage — *see* Disorder, cartilage
  Castellani's A69.8
  Castleman (unicentric) (multicentric) D47.Z2
    HHV-8-associated — *see also* Herpesvirus,
      human, 8 D47.Z2
  cat-scratch A28.1
  Cavare's (familial periodic paralysis) G72.3
  cecum K63.9
  celiac (adult) (infantile) (with steatorrhea) K90.0
  cellular tissue L98.9
  central core G71.2
  cerebellar, cerebellum — *see* Disease, brain
  cerebral — *see also* Disease, brain
    degenerative — *see* Degeneration, brain
  cerebrospinal G96.9
  cerebrovascular I67.9
    acute I67.89
      embolic I63.4-
      thrombotic I63.3-
    arteriosclerotic I67.2
    specified NEC I67.89
  cervix (uteri) (noninflammatory) N88.9
    inflammatory — *see* Cervicitis
    specified NEC N88.8
  Chabert's A22.9
  Chandler's (osteochondritis dissecans, hip) — *see*
    Osteochondritis, dissecans, hip
  Charlouis — *see* Yaws
  Chédiak-Steinbrinck (-Higashi) (congenital
    gigantism of peroxidase granules) E70.330
  chest J98.9
  Chiari's (hepatic vein thrombosis) I82.0
  Chicago B40.9
  Chignon B36.8
  chigo, chigoe B88.1
  childhood granulomatous D71
  Chinese liver fluke B66.1
  chlamydial A74.9
    specified NEC A74.89
  cholecystic K82.9
  choroid H31.9
    specified NEC H31.8
  Christmas D67
  chronic bullous of childhood L12.2
  chylomicron retention E78.3
  ciliary body H21.9
    specified NEC H21.89
  circulatory (system) NEC I99.8
    newborn P29.9
    syphilitic A52.00
      congenital A50.54
  coagulation factor deficiency (congenital) — *see*
    Defect, coagulation
  coccidioidal — *see* Coccidioidomycosis
  cold
    agglutinin or hemoglobinuria D59.1
      paroxysmal D59.6
    hemagglutinin (chronic) D59.1
  collagen NOS (nonvascular) (vascular) M35.9
    specified NEC M35.8
  colon K63.9
    functional K59.9
      congenital Q43.2
    ischemic — *see also* Ischemia, intestine,
      acute K55.039
  colonic inflammatory bowel, unclassified
    (IBDU) K52.3
  combined system — *see* Degeneration, combined
  compressed air T70.3
  Concato's (pericardial polyserositis) A19.9
    nontubercular I31.1
    pleural — *see* Pleurisy, with effusion
  conjunctiva H11.9
    chlamydial A74.0
    specified NEC H11.89
    viral B30.9
      specified NEC B30.8
  connective tissue, systemic (diffuse) M35.9
    in (due to)
      hypogammaglobulinemia D80.1 *[M36.8]*
      ochronosis E70.29 *[M36.8]*
    specified NEC M35.8
  Conor and Bruch's (boutonneuse fever) A77.1
  Cooper's — *see* Mastopathy, cystic
  Cori's (glycogenosis III) E74.03
  corkhandler's or corkworker's J67.3
  cornea H18.9
    specified NEC H18.89-
  coronary (artery) — *see* Disease, heart, ischemic,
    atherosclerotic

Disease, diseased - *continued*
  coronary (artery) - *continued*
    congenital Q24.5
    ostial, syphilitic (aortic) (mitral)
      (pulmonary) A52.03
  corpus cavernosum N48.9
    specified NEC N48.89
  Cotugno's — *see* Sciatica
  coxsackie (virus) NEC B34.1
  cranial nerve NOS G52.9
  Creutzfeldt-Jakob — *see* Creutzfeldt-Jakob disease
    or syndrome
  Crocq's (acrocyanosis) I73.89
  Crohn's — *see* Enteritis, regional
  Curschmann G71.11
  cystic
    breast (chronic) — *see* Mastopathy, cystic
    kidney, congenital Q61.9
    liver, congenital Q44.6
    lung J98.4
      congenital Q33.0
  cytomegalic inclusion (generalized) B25.9
    with pneumonia B25.0
    congenital P35.1
  cytomegaloviral B25.9
    specified NEC B25.8
  Czerny's (periodic hydrarthrosis of the knee) — *see*
    Effusion, joint, knee
  Daae (-Finsen) (epidemic pleurodynia) B33.0
  Darling's — *see* Histoplasmosis capsulati
  deer fly — *see* Tularemia
  Degos' I77.89
  demyelinating, demyelinizating (nervous
    system) G37.9
    multiple sclerosis G35
    specified NEC G37.8
  dense deposit — *see also* N00-N07 with fourth
    character .6 N05.6
  deposition, hydroxyapatite — *see* Disease,
    hydroxyapatite deposition
  de Quervain's (tendon sheath) M65.4
    thyroid (subacute granulomatous thyroiditis) E06.1
  Devergie's (pityriasis rubra pilaris) L44.0
  Devic's G36.0
  diaphorase deficiency D74.0
  diaphragm J98.6
  diarrheal, infectious NEC A09
  digestive system K92.9
    specified NEC K92.89
  disc, degenerative — *see* Degeneration,
    intervertebral disc
  discogenic — *see also* Displacement, intervertebral
    disc NEC
    with myelopathy — *see* Disorder, disc, with,
      myelopathy
  diverticular — *see* Diverticula
  Dubois (thymus) A50.59 *[E35]*
  Duchenne-Griesinger G71.0
  Duchenne's
    muscular dystrophy G71.0
    pseudohypertrophy, muscles G71.0
  ductless glands E34.9
  Duhring's (dermatitis herpetiformis) L13.0
  duodenum K31.9
    specified NEC K31.89
  Dupré's (meningism) R29.1
  Dupuytren's (muscle contracture) M72.0
  Durand-Nicholas-Favre (climatic bubo) A55
  Duroziez's (congenital mitral stenosis) Q23.2
  ear — *see* Disorder, ear
  Eberth's — *see* Fever, typhoid
  Ebola (virus) A98.4
  Ebstein's heart Q22.5
  Echinococcus — *see* Echinococcus
  echovirus NEC B34.1
  Eddowes' (brittle bones and blue sclera) Q78.0
  edentulous (alveolar) ridge K06.9
    specified NEC K06.8
  Edsall's T67.2
  Eichstedt's (pityriasis versicolor) B36.0
  Ellis-van Creveld (chondroectodermal
    dysplasia) Q77.6
  end stage renal (ESRD) N18.6
    due to hypertension I12.0
  endocrine glands or system NEC E34.9
  endomyocardial (eosinophilic) I42.3
  English (rickets) E55.0
  enteroviral, enterovirus NEC B34.1
    central nervous system NEC A88.8
  epidemic B99.9
    specified NEC B99.8
  epididymis N50.9

Disease, diseased - *continued*
Erb (-Landouzy) G71.0
Erdheim-Chester (ECD) E88.89
esophagus K22.9
  functional K22.4
  psychogenic F45.8
  specified NEC K22.8
Eulenburg's (congenital paramyotonia) G71.19
eustachian tube — *see* Disorder, eustachian tube
external
  auditory canal — *see* Disorder, ear, external
  ear — *see* Disorder, ear, external
extrapyramidal G25.9
  specified NEC G25.89
eye H57.9
  anterior chamber H21.9
  inflammatory NEC H57.8
  muscle (external) — *see* Strabismus
  specified NEC H57.8
  syphilitic — *see* Oculopathy, syphilitic
eyeball H44.9
  specified NEC H44.89
eyelid — *see* Disorder, eyelid
  specified NEC — *see* Disorder, eyelid, specified
   type NEC
eyeworm of Africa B74.3
facial nerve (seventh) G51.9
  newborn (birth injury) P11.3
Fahr (of brain) G23.8
Fahr Volhard (of kidney) I12.-
fallopian tube (noninflammatory) N83.9
  inflammatory — *see* Salpingo-oophoritis
  specified NEC N83.8
familial periodic paralysis G72.3
Fanconi's (congenital pancytopenia) D61.09
fascia NEC — *see also* Disorder, muscle
  inflammatory — *see* Myositis
  specified NEC M62.89
Fauchard's (periodontitis) — *see* Periodontitis
Favre-Durand-Nicolas (climatic bubo) A55
Fede's K14.0
Feer's — *see* Poisoning, mercury
female pelvic inflammatory — *see also* Disease,
  pelvis, inflammatory N73.9
  syphilitic (secondary) A51.42
  tuberculous A18.17
Fernels' (aortic aneurysm) I71.9
fibrocaseous of lung — *see* Tuberculosis, pulmonary
fibrocystic — *see* Fibrocystic disease
Fiedler's (leptospiral jaundice) A27.0
fifth B08.3
file-cutter's — *see* Poisoning, lead
fish-skin Q80.9
  acquired L85.0
Flajani (-Basedow) (exophthalmic goiter) — *see*
  Hyperthyroidism, with, goiter (diffuse)
flax-dresser's J66.1
fluke — *see* Infestation, fluke
foot and mouth B08.8
foot process N04.9
Forbes' (glycogenosis III) E74.03
Fordyce-Fox (apocrine miliaria) L75.2
Fordyce's (ectopic sebaceous glands) (mouth) Q38.6
Forestier's (rhizomelic pseudopolyarthritis) M35.3
  meaning ankylosing hyperostosis — *see*
   Hyperostosis, ankylosing
Fothergill's
  neuralgia — *see* Neuralgia, trigeminal
  scarlatina anginosa A38.9
Fournier (gangrene) N49.3
  female N76.89
fourth B08.8
Fox (-Fordyce) (apocrine miliaria) L75.2
Francis' — *see* Tularemia
Franklin C88.2
Frei's (climatic bubo) A55
Friedreich's
  combined systemic or ataxia G11.1
  myoclonia G25.3
frontal sinus — *see* Sinusitis, frontal
fungus NEC B49
Gaisböck's (polycythemia hypertonica) D75.1
gallbladder K82.9
  calculus — *see* Calculus, gallbladder
  cholecystitis — *see* Cholecystitis
  cholesterolosis K82.4
  fistula — *see* Fistula, gallbladder
  hydrops K82.1
  obstruction — *see* Obstruction, gallbladder
  perforation K82.2
  specified NEC K82.8
gamma heavy chain C88.2
Gamna's (siderotic splenomegaly) D73.2

Disease, diseased - *continued*
Gamstorp's (adynamia episodica hereditaria) G72.3
Gandy-Nanta (siderotic splenomegaly) D73.2
ganister J62.8
gastric — *see* Disease, stomach
gastroesophageal reflux (GERD) K21.9
  with esophagitis K21.0
gastrointestinal (tract) K92.9
  amyloid E85.4
  functional K59.9
   psychogenic F45.8
  specified NEC K92.89
Gee (-Herter) (-Heubner) (-Thaysen) (nontropical
  sprue) K90.0
genital organs
  female N94.9
  male N50.9
Gerhardt's (erythromelalgia) I73.81
Gibert's (pityriasis rosea) L42
Gierke's (glycogenosis I) E74.01
Gilles de la Tourette's (motor-verbal tic) F95.2
gingiva K06.9
  plaque induced K05.00
  specified NEC K06.8
gland (lymph) I89.9
Glanzmann's (hereditary hemorrhagic
  thrombasthenia) D69.1
glass-blower's (cataract) — *see* Cataract, specified
  NEC
  salivary gland hypertrophy K11.1
Glisson's — *see* Rickets
globe H44.9
  specified NEC H44.89
glomerular — *see also* Glomerulonephritis
  with edema — *see* Nephrosis
  acute — *see* Nephritis, acute
  chronic — *see* Nephritis, chronic
  minimal change N05.0
  rapidly progressive N01.9
glycogen storage E74.00
  Andersen's E74.09
  Cori's E74.03
  Forbes' E74.03
  generalized E74.00
  glucose-6-phosphatase deficiency E74.01
  heart E74.02 *[I43]*
  hepatorenal E74.09
  Hers' E74.09
  liver and kidney E74.09
  McArdle's E74.04
  muscle phosphofructokinase E74.09
  myocardium E74.02 *[I43]*
  Pompe's E74.02
  Tauri's E74.09
  type 0 E74.09
  type I E74.01
  type II E74.02
  type III E74.03
  type IV E74.09
  type V E74.04
  type VI-XI E74.09
  Von Gierke's E74.01
Goldstein's (familial hemorrhagic
  telangiectasia) I78.0
gonococcal NOS A54.9
graft-versus-host (GVH) D89.813
  acute D89.810
  acute on chronic D89.812
  chronic D89.811
grainhandler's J67.8
granulomatous (childhood) (chronic) D71
Graves' (exophthalmic goiter) — *see*
  Hyperthyroidism, with, goiter (diffuse)
Griesinger's — *see* Ancylostomiasis
Grisel's M43.6
Gruby's (tinea tonsurans) B35.0
Guillain-Barré G61.0
Guinon's (motor-verbal tic) F95.2
gum K06.9
gynecological N94.9
H (Hartnup's) E72.02
Haff — *see* Poisoning, mercury
Hageman (congenital factor XII deficiency) D68.2
hair (color) (shaft) L67.9
  follicles L73.9
   specified NEC L73.8
Hamman's (spontaneous mediastinal
  emphysema) J98.2
hand, foot and mouth B08.4
Hansen's — *see* Leprosy
Hantavirus, with pulmonary manifestations B33.4
  with renal manifestations A98.5
Harada's H30.81-

Disease, diseased - *continued*
Hartnup (pellagra-cerebellar ataxia-renal
  aminoaciduria) E72.02
Hart's (pellagra-cerebellar ataxia-renal
  aminoaciduria) E72.02
Hashimoto's (struma lymphomatosa) E06.3
Hb — *see* Disease, hemoglobin
heart (organic) I51.9
  with
   pulmonary edema (acute) — *see also* Failure,
    ventricular, left I50.1
   rheumatic fever (conditions in I00)
    active I01.9
     with chorea I02.0
     specified NEC I01.8
    inactive or quiescent (with chorea) I09.9
     specified NEC I09.89
  amyloid E85.4 *[I43]*
  aortic (valve) I35.9
  arteriosclerotic or sclerotic (senile) — *see* Disease,
   heart, ischemic, atherosclerotic
  artery, arterial — *see* Disease, heart, ischemic,
   atherosclerotic
  beer drinkers' I42.6
  beriberi (wet) E51.12
  black I27.0
  congenital Q24.9
   cyanotic Q24.9
   specified NEC Q24.8
  coronary — *see* Disease, heart, ischemic
  cryptogenic I51.9
  fibroid — *see* Myocarditis
  functional I51.89
   psychogenic F45.8
  glycogen storage E74.02 *[I43]*
  gonococcal A54.83
  hypertensive — *see* Hypertension, heart
  hyperthyroid — *see*
   also Hyperthyroidism E05.90 *[I43]*
   with thyroid storm E05.91 *[I43]*
  ischemic (chronic or with a stated duration of over
   4 weeks) I25.9
   atherosclerotic (of) I25.10
    with angina pectoris — *see* Arteriosclerosis,
     coronary (artery)
    coronary artery bypass graft — *see*
     Arteriosclerosis, coronary (artery),
     cardiomyopathy I25.5
   diagnosed on ECG or other special investigation,
    but currently presenting no symptoms I25.6
   silent I25.6
   specified form NEC I25.89
  kyphoscoliotic I27.1
  meningococcal A39.50
   endocarditis A39.51
   myocarditis A39.52
   pericarditis A39.53
  mitral I05.9
   specified NEC I05.8
  muscular — *see* Degeneration, myocardial
  psychogenic (functional) F45.8
  pulmonary (chronic) I27.9
   in schistosomiasis B65.9 *[I52]*
   specified NEC I27.89
  rheumatic (chronic) (inactive) (old) (quiescent)
   (with chorea) I09.9
   active or acute I01.9
    with chorea (acute) (rheumatic)
     (Sydenham's) I02.0
   specified NEC I09.89
  senile — *see* Myocarditis
  syphilitic A52.06
   aortic A52.03
    aneurysm A52.01
   congenital A50.54 *[I52]*
  thyrotoxic — *see also* Thyrotoxicosis E05.90 *[I43]*
   with thyroid storm E05.91 *[I43]*
  valve, valvular (obstructive) (regurgitant) —
   see also Endocarditis
   congenital NEC Q24.8
   pulmonary Q22.3
  vascular — *see* Disease, cardiovascular
heavy chain NEC C88.2
  alpha C88.3
  gamma C88.2
  mu C88.2
Hebra's
  pityriasis
   maculata et circinata L42
   rubra pilaris L44.0
  prurigo L28.2
hematopoietic organs D75.9
hemoglobin or Hb

Disease, diseased - *continued*
  hemoglobin or Hb - *continued*
    abnormal (mixed) NEC D58.2
      with thalassemia D56.9
    AS genotype D57.3
    Bart's D56.0
    C (Hb-C) D58.2
      with other abnormal hemoglobin NEC D58.2
      elliptocytosis D58.1
      Hb-S D57.2-
        sickle-cell D57.2-
      thalassemia D56.8
    Constant Spring D58.2
    D (Hb-D) D58.2
    E (Hb-E) D58.2
    E-beta thalassemia D56.5
    elliptocytosis D58.1
    H (Hb-H) (thalassemia) D56.0
      with other abnormal hemoglobin NEC D56.9
      Constant Spring D56.0
    I thalassemia D56.9
    M D74.0
    S or SS D57.1
    SC D57.2-
    SD D57.8-
    SE D57.8-
    spherocytosis D58.0
    unstable, hemolytic D58.2
  hemolytic (newborn) P55.9
    autoimmune (cold type) (warm type) D59.1
    drug-induced D59.0
    due to or with
      incompatibility
        ABO (blood group) P55.1
        blood (group) (Duffy) (K (ell)) (Kidd) (Lewis) (M) (S) NEC P55.8
        Rh (blood group) (factor) P55.0
        Rh negative mother P55.0
      specified type NEC P55.8
    unstable hemoglobin D58.2
  hemorrhagic D69.9
    newborn P53
  Henoch (-Schönlein) (purpura nervosa) D69.0
  hepatic — *see* Disease, liver
  hepatobiliary K83.9
    toxic K71.9
  hepatolenticular E83.01
  heredodegenerative NEC
    spinal cord G95.89
  herpesviral, disseminated B00.7
  Hers' (glycogenosis VI) E74.09
  Herter (-Gee) (-Heubner) (nontropical sprue) K90.0
  Heubner-Herter (nontropical sprue) K90.0
  high fetal gene or hemoglobin thalassemia D56.9
  Hildenbrand's — *see* Typhus
  hip (joint) M25.9
    congenital Q65.89
    suppurative M00.9
    tuberculous A18.02
  His (-Werner) (trench fever) A79.0
  Hodgson's I71.2
    ruptured I71.1
  Holla — *see* Spherocytosis
  hookworm B76.9
    specified NEC B76.8
  host-versus-graft D89.813
    acute D89.810
    acute on chronic D89.812
    chronic D89.811
  human immunodeficiency virus (HIV) B20
  Huntington's G10
  Hutchinson's (cheiropompholyx) — *see* Hutchinson's disease
  hyaline (diffuse) (generalized)
    membrane (lung) (newborn) P22.0
      adult J80
  hydatid — *see* Echinococcus
  hydroxyapatite deposition M11.00
    ankle M11.07-
    elbow M11.02-
    foot joint M11.07-
    hand joint M11.04-
    hip M11.05-
    knee M11.06-
    multiple site M11.09
    shoulder M11.01-
    vertebra M11.08
    wrist M11.03-
  hyperkinetic — *see* Hyperkinesia
  hypertensive — *see* Hypertension
  hypophysis E23.7
  Iceland G93.3
  I-cell E77.0

Disease, diseased - *continued*
  immune D89.9
  immunoproliferative (malignant) C88.9
    small intestinal C88.3
    specified NEC C88.8
  inclusion B25.9
    salivary gland B25.9
  infectious, infective B99.9
    congenital P37.9
      specified NEC P37.8
      viral P35.9
        specified type NEC P35.8
    specified NEC B99.8
  inflammatory
    penis N48.29
      abscess N48.21
      cellulitis N48.22
    prepuce N47.7
      balanoposthitis N47.6
    tubo-ovarian — *see* Salpingo-oophoritis
  intervertebral disc — *see also* Disorder, disc
    with myelopathy — *see* Disorder, disc, with, myelopathy
    cervical, cervicothoracic — *see* Disorder, disc, cervical
      with
        myelopathy — *see* Disorder, disc, cervical, with myelopathy
        neuritis, radiculitis or radiculopathy — *see* Disorder, disc, cervical, with neuritis
        specified NEC — *see* Disorder, disc, cervical, specified type NEC
    lumbar (with)
      myelopathy M51.06
      neuritis, radiculitis, radiculopathy or sciatica M51.16
      specified NEC M51.86
    lumbosacral (with)
      neuritis, radiculitis, radiculopathy or sciatica M51.17
      specified NEC M51.87
    specified NEC — *see* Disorder, disc, specified NEC
    thoracic (with)
      myelopathy M51.04
      neuritis, radiculitis or radiculopathy M51.14
      specified NEC M51.84
    thoracolumbar (with)
      myelopathy M51.05
      neuritis, radiculitis or radiculopathy M51.15
      specified NEC M51.85
  intestine K63.9
    functional K59.9
      psychogenic F45.8
      specified NEC K59.8
    organic K63.9
    protozoal A07.9
    specified NEC K63.89
  iris H21.9
    specified NEC H21.89
  iron metabolism or storage E83.10
  island (scrub typhus) A75.3
  itai-itai — *see* Poisoning, cadmium
  Jakob-Creutzfeldt — *see* Creutzfeldt-Jakob disease or syndrome
  jaw M27.9
    fibrocystic M27.49
    specified NEC M27.8
  jigger B88.1
  joint — *see also* Disorder, joint
    Charcot's — *see* Arthropathy, neuropathic (Charcot)
    degenerative — *see* Osteoarthritis
      multiple M15.9
      spine — *see* Spondylosis
    hypertrophic — *see* Osteoarthritis
    sacroiliac M53.3
    specified NEC — *see* Disorder, joint, specified type NEC
    spine NEC — *see* Dorsopathy
    suppurative — *see* Arthritis, pyogenic or pyemic
  Jourdain's (acute gingivitis) K05.00
    nonplaque induced K05.01
    plaque induced K05.00
  Kaschin-Beck (endemic polyarthritis) M12.10
    ankle M12.17-
    elbow M12.12-
    foot joint M12.17-
    hand joint M12.14-
    hip M12.15-
    knee M12.16-
    multiple site M12.19
    shoulder M12.11-

Disease, diseased - *continued*
  Kaschin-Beck (endemic polyarthritis) - *continued*
    vertebra M12.18
    wrist M12.13-
  Katayama B65.2
  Kedani (scrub typhus) A75.3
  Keshan E59
  kidney (functional) (pelvis) N28.9
    chronic N18.9
      hypertensive — *see* Hypertension, kidney
      stage 1 N18.1
      stage 2 (mild) N18.2
      stage 3 (moderate) N18.3
      stage 4 (severe) N18.4
      stage 5 N18.5
    complicating pregnancy — *see* Pregnancy, complicated by, renal disease
    cystic (congenital) Q61.9
    diabetic — *see* E08-E13 with .22
    fibrocystic (congenital) Q61.8
    hypertensive — *see* Hypertension, kidney
    in (due to)
      schistosomiasis (bilharziasis) B65.9 *[N29]*
    multicystic Q61.4
    polycystic Q61.3
      adult type Q61.2
      childhood type NEC Q61.19
        collecting duct dilatation Q61.11
  Kimmelstiel (-Wilson) (intercapillary polycystic (congenital) glomerulosclerosis) — *see* E08-E13 with .21
  Kimura D21.9
    specified site (see Neoplasm, connective tissue benign)
  Kinnier Wilson's (hepatolenticular degeneration) E83.01
  kissing — *see* Mononucleosis, infectious
  Klebs' — *see also* Glomerulonephritis N05.-
  Klippel-Feil (brevicollis) Q76.1
  Köhler-Pellegrini-Stieda (calcification, knee joint) — *see* Bursitis, tibial collateral
  Kok Q89.8
  König's (osteochondritis dissecans) — *see* Osteochondritis, dissecans
  Korsakoff's (nonalcoholic) F04
    alcoholic F10.96
      with dependence F10.26
  Kostmann's (infantile genetic agranulocytosis) D70.0
  kuru A81.81
  Kyasanur Forest A98.2
  labyrinth, ear — *see* Disorder, ear, inner
  lacrimal system — *see* Disorder, lacrimal system
  Lafora's — *see* Epilepsy, generalized, idiopathic
  Lancereaux-Mathieu (leptospiral jaundice) A27.0
  Landry's G61.0
  Larrey-Weil (leptospiral jaundice) A27.0
  larynx J38.7
  legionnaires' A48.1
    nonpneumonic A48.2
  Lenegre's I44.2
  lens H27.9
    specified NEC H27.8
  Lev's (acquired complete heart block) I44.2
  Lewy body (dementia) G31.83 *[F02.80]*
    with behavioral disturbance G31.83 *[F02.81]*
  Lichtheim's (subacute combined sclerosis with pernicious anemia) D51.0
  Lightwood's (renal tubular acidosis) N25.89
  Lignac's (cystinosis) E72.04
  lip K13.0
  lipid-storage E75.6
    specified NEC E75.5
  Lipschütz's N76.6
  liver (chronic) (organic) K76.9
    alcoholic (chronic) K70.9
      acute — *see* Disease, liver, alcoholic, hepatitis
      cirrhosis K70.30
        with ascites K70.31
      failure K70.40
        with coma K70.41
      fatty liver K70.0
      fibrosis K70.2
      hepatitis K70.10
        with ascites K70.11
      sclerosis K70.2
    cystic, congenital Q44.6
    drug-induced (idiosyncratic) (toxic) (predictable) (unpredictable) — *see* Disease, liver, toxic
    end stage K72.90
      due to hepatitis — *see* Hepatitis
    fatty, nonalcoholic (NAFLD) K76.0
      alcoholic K70.0

Disease, diseased - *continued*
  liver (chronic) (organic) - *continued*
    fibrocystic (congenital) Q44.6
    fluke
      Chinese B66.1
      oriental B66.1
      sheep B66.3
    glycogen storage E74.09 [K77]
    in (due to)
      schistosomiasis (bilharziasis) B65.9 [K77]
    inflammatory K75.9
      alcoholic K70.1
      specified NEC K75.89
    polycystic (congenital) Q44.6
    toxic K71.9
      with
        cholestasis K71.0
        cirrhosis (liver) K71.7
        fibrosis (liver) K71.7
        focal nodular hyperplasia K71.8
        hepatic granuloma K71.8
        hepatic necrosis K71.10
          with coma K71.11
        hepatitis NEC K71.6
          acute K71.2
          chronic
            active K71.50
              with ascites K71.51
            lobular K71.4
            persistent K71.3
          lupoid K71.50
            with ascites K71.51
        peliosis hepatis K71.8
        veno-occlusive disease (VOD) of liver K71.8
    veno-occlusive K76.5
  Lobo's (keloid blastomycosis) B48.0
  Lobstein's (brittle bones and blue sclera) Q78.0
  Ludwig's (submaxillary cellulitis) K12.2
  lumbosacral region M53.87
  lung J98.4
    black J60
    congenital Q33.9
    cystic J98.4
      congenital Q33.0
    fibroid (chronic) — *see* Fibrosis, lung
    fluke B66.4
      oriental B66.4
    in
      amyloidosis E85.4 [J99]
      sarcoidosis D86.0
      Sjögren's syndrome M35.02
      systemic
        lupus erythematosus M32.13
        sclerosis M34.81
    interstitial J84.9
      of childhood, specified NEC J84.848
      respiratory bronchiolitis J84.115
      specified NEC J84.89
    obstructive (chronic) J44.9
      with
        acute
          bronchitis J44.0
          exacerbation NEC J44.1
          lower respiratory infection J44.0
        alveolitis, allergic J67.9
        asthma J44.9
        bronchiectasis J47.9
          with
            exacerbation (acute) J47.1
            lower respiratory infection J47.0
        bronchitis J44.9
          with
            exacerbation (acute) J44.1
            lower respiratory infection J44.0
        emphysema J44.9
        hypersensitivity pneumonitis J67.9
      decompensated J44.1
        with
          exacerbation (acute) J44.1
    polycystic J98.4
      congenital Q33.0
    rheumatoid (diffuse) (interstitial) — *see* Rheumatoid, lung
  Lutembacher's (atrial septal defect with mitral stenosis) Q21.1
  Lyme A69.20
  lymphatic (gland) (system) (channel) (vessel) I89.9
  lymphoproliferative D47.9
    specified NEC D47.Z9
    T-gamma D47.Z9
    X-linked D82.3
  Magitot's M27.2
  malarial — *see* Malaria

Disease, diseased - *continued*
  malignant — *see also* Neoplasm, malignant, by site
  Manson's B65.1
  maple bark J67.6
  maple-syrup-urine E71.0
  Marburg (virus) A98.3
  Marion's (bladder neck obstruction) N32.0
  Marsh's (exophthalmic goiter) — *see* Hyperthyroidism, with, goiter (diffuse)
  mastoid (process) — *see* Disorder, ear, middle
  Mathieu's (leptospiral jaundice) A27.0
  Maxcy's A75.2
  McArdle (-Schmid-Pearson) (glycogenosis V) E74.04
  mediastinum J98.59
  medullary center (idiopathic) (respiratory) G93.89
  Meige's (chronic hereditary edema) Q82.0
  meningococcal — *see* Infection, meningococcal
  mental F99
    organic F09
  mesenchymal M35.9
  mesenteric embolic — *see also* Ischemia, intestine, acute K55.039
  metabolic, metabolism E88.9
    bilirubin E80.7
  metal-polisher's J62.8
  metastatic — *see also* Neoplasm, secondary, by site C79.9
  microvascular - code to condition
  microvillus
    atrophy Q43.8
    inclusion (MVD) Q43.8
  middle ear — *see* Disorder, ear, middle
  Mikulicz' (dryness of mouth, absent or decreased lacrimation) K11.8
  Milroy's (chronic hereditary edema) Q82.0
  Minamata — *see* Poisoning, mercury
  minicore G71.2
  Minor's G95.19
  Minot's (hemorrhagic disease, newborn) P53
  Minot-von Willebrand-Jürgens (angiohemophilia) D68.0
  Mitchell's (erythromelalgia) I73.81
  mitral (valve) I05.9
    nonrheumatic I34.9
  mixed connective tissue M35.1
  moldy hay J67.0
  Monge's T70.29
  Morgagni-Adams-Stokes (syncope with heart block) I45.9
  Morgagni's (syndrome) (hyperostosis frontalis interna) M85.2
  Morton's (with metatarsalgia) — *see* Lesion, nerve, plantar
  Morvan's G60.8
  motor neuron (bulbar) (familial) (mixed type) (spinal) G12.20
    amyotrophic lateral sclerosis G12.21
    progressive bulbar palsy G12.22
    specified NEC G12.29
  moyamoya I67.5
  mu heavy chain disease C88.2
  multicore G71.2
  muscle — *see also* Disorder, muscle
    inflammatory — *see* Myositis
    ocular (external) — *see* Strabismus
  musculoskeletal system, soft tissue — *see also* Disorder, soft tissue
    specified NEC — *see* Disorder, soft tissue, specified type NEC
  mushroom workers' J67.5
  mycotic B49
  myelodysplastic, not classified C94.6
  myeloproliferative, not classified C94.6
    chronic D47.1
  myocardium, myocardial — *see also* Degeneration, myocardial I51.5
    primary (idiopathic) I42.9
  myoneural G70.9
  Naegeli's D69.1
  nails L60.9
    specified NEC L60.8
  Nairobi (sheep virus) A93.8
  nasal J34.9
  nemaline body G71.2
  nerve — *see* Disorder, nerve
  nervous system G98.8
    autonomic G90.9
    central G96.9
      specified NEC G96.8
    congenital Q07.9
    parasympathetic G90.9
    specified NEC G98.8

Disease, diseased - *continued*
  nervous system - *continued*
    sympathetic G90.9
    vegetative G90.9
  neuromuscular system G70.9
  Newcastle B30.8
  Nicolas (-Durand) -Favre (climatic bubo) A55
  nipple N64.9
    Paget's C50.01-
      female C50.01-
      male C50.02-
  Nishimoto (-Takeuchi) I67.5
  nonarthropod-borne NOS (viral) B34.9
    enterovirus NEC B34.1
  nonautoimmune hemolytic D59.4
    drug-induced D59.2
  Nonne-Milroy-Meige (chronic hereditary edema) Q82.0
  nose J34.9
  nucleus pulposus — *see* Disorder, disc
  nutritional E63.9
  oast-house-urine E72.19
  ocular
    herpesviral B00.50
    zoster B02.30
  obliterative vascular I77.1
  Ohara's — *see* Tularemia
  Opitz's (congestive splenomegaly) D73.2
  Oppenheim-Urbach (necrobiosis lipoidica diabeticorum) — *see* E08-E13 with .620
  optic nerve NEC — *see* Disorder, nerve, optic
  orbit — *see* Disorder, orbit
  Oriental liver fluke B66.1
  Oriental lung fluke B66.4
  Ormond's N13.5
  Oropouche virus A93.0
  Osler-Rendu (familial hemorrhagic telangiectasia) I78.0
  osteofibrocystic E21.0
  Otto's M24.7
  outer ear — *see* Disorder, ear, external
  ovary (noninflammatory) N83.9
    cystic N83.20-
    inflammatory — *see* Salpingo-oophoritis
    polycystic E28.2
    specified NEC N83.8
  Owren's (congenital) — *see* Defect, coagulation
  pancreas K86.9
    cystic K86.2
    fibrocystic E84.9
    specified NEC K86.89
  panvalvular I08.9
    specified NEC I08.8
  parametrium (noninflammatory) N83.9
  parasitic B89
    cerebral NEC B71.9 [G94]
    intestinal NOS B82.9
    mouth B37.0
    skin NOS B88.9
    specified type — *see* Infestation
    tongue B37.0
  parathyroid (gland) E21.5
    specified NEC E21.4
  Parkinson's G20
  parodontal K05.6
  Parrot's (syphilitic osteochondritis) A50.02
  Parry's (exophthalmic goiter) — *see* Hyperthyroidism, with, goiter (diffuse)
  Parson's (exophthalmic goiter) — *see* Hyperthyroidism, with, goiter (diffuse)
  Paxton's (white piedra) B36.2
  pearl-worker's — *see* Osteomyelitis, specified type NEC
  Pellegrini-Stieda (calcification, knee joint) — *see* Bursitis, tibial collateral
  pelvis, pelvic
    female NOS N94.9
      specified NEC N94.89
    gonococcal (acute) (chronic) A54.24
    inflammatory (female) N73.9
      acute N73.0
      chlamydial A56.11
      chronic N73.1
      specified NEC N73.8
      syphilitic (secondary) A51.42
        late A52.76
      tuberculous A18.17
    organ, female N94.9
    peritoneum, female NEC N94.89
  penis N48.9
    inflammatory N48.29
      abscess N48.21
      cellulitis N48.22

Disease, diseased - *continued*
  penis - *continued*
    specified NEC N48.89
  periapical tissues NOS K04.90
  periodontal K05.6
    specified NEC K05.5
  periosteum — *see* Disorder, bone, specified type NEC
  peripheral
    arterial I73.9
    autonomic nervous system G90.9
    nerves — *see* Polyneuropathy
    vascular NOS I73.9
  peritoneum K66.9
    pelvic, female NEC N94.89
    specified NEC K66.8
  persistent mucosal (middle ear) H66.20
    left H66.22
      with right H66.23
    right H66.21
      with left H66.23
  Petit's — *see* Hernia, abdomen, specified site NEC
  pharynx J39.2
    specified NEC J39.2
  Phocas' — *see* Mastopathy, cystic
  photochromogenic (acid-fast bacilli) (pulmonary) A31.0
    nonpulmonary A31.9
  Pick's G31.01 *[F02.80]*
    with behavioral disturbance G31.01 *[F02.81]*
    brain G31.01 *[F02.80]*
      with behavioral disturbance G31.01 *[F02.81]*
    of pericardium (pericardial pseudocirrhosis of liver) I31.1
  pigeon fancier's J67.2
  pineal gland E34.8
  pink — *see* Poisoning, mercury
  Pinkus' (lichen nitidus) L44.1
  pinworm B80
  Piry virus A93.8
  pituitary (gland) E23.7
  pituitary-snuff-taker's J67.8
  pleura (cavity) J94.9
    specified NEC J94.8
  pneumatic drill (hammer) T75.21
  Pollitzer's (hidradenitis suppurativa) L73.2
  polycystic
    kidney or renal Q61.3
      adult type Q61.2
      childhood type NEC Q61.19
        collecting duct dilatation Q61.11
    liver or hepatic Q44.6
    lung or pulmonary J98.4
      congenital Q33.0
    ovary, ovaries E28.2
    spleen Q89.09
  polyethylene T84.05-
  Pompe's (glycogenosis II) E74.02
  Posadas-Wernicke B38.9
  Potain's (pulmonary edema) — *see* Edema, lung
  prepuce N47.8
    inflammatory N47.7
      balanoposthitis N47.6
  Pringle's (tuberous sclerosis) Q85.1
  prion, central nervous system A81.9
    specified NEC A81.89
  prostate N42.9
    specified NEC N42.89
  protozoal B64
    acanthamebiasis — *see* Acanthamebiasis
    African trypanosomiasis — *see* African trypanosomiasis
    babesiosis B60.0
    Chagas disease — *see* Chagas disease
    intestine, intestinal A07.9
    leishmaniasis — *see* Leishmaniasis
    malaria — *see* Malaria
    naegleriasis B60.2
    pneumocystosis B59
    specified organism NEC B60.8
    toxoplasmosis — *see* Toxoplasmosis
  pseudo-Hurler's E77.0
  psychiatric F99
  psychotic — *see* Psychosis
  Puente's (simple glandular cheilitis) K13.0
  puerperal — *see also* Puerperal O90.89
  pulmonary — *see also* Disease, lung
    artery I28.9
    chronic obstructive J44.9
      with
        acute bronchitis J44.0
        exacerbation (acute) J44.1
        lower respiratory infection (acute) J44.0

Disease, diseased - *continued*
  pulmonary - *continued*
    chronic obstructive - *continued*
      decompensated J44.1
        with
          exacerbation (acute) J44.1
    heart I27.9
      specified NEC I27.89
    hypertensive (vascular) I27.0
    valve I37.9
      rheumatic I09.89
    pulp (dental) NOS K04.90
    pulseless M31.4
  Putnam's (subacute combined sclerosis with pernicious anemia) D51.0
  Pyle (-Cohn) (metaphyseal dysplasia) Q78.5
  ragpicker's or ragsorter's A22.1
  Raynaud's — *see* Raynaud's disease
  reactive airway — *see* Asthma
  Reclus' (cystic) — *see* Mastopathy, cystic
  rectum K62.9
    specified NEC K62.89
  Refsum's (heredopathia atactica polyneuritiformis) G60.1
  renal (functional) (pelvis) — *see also* Disease, kidney N28.9
    with
      edema — *see* Nephrosis
      glomerular lesion — *see* Glomerulonephritis
        with edema — *see* Nephrosis
      interstitial nephritis N12
    acute N28.9
    chronic — *see also* Disease, kidney, chronic N18.9
    cystic, congenital Q61.9
    diabetic — *see* E08-E13 with .22
    end-stage (failure) N18.6
      due to hypertension I12.0
    fibrocystic (congenital) Q61.8
    hypertensive — *see* Hypertension, kidney
    lupus M32.14
    phosphate-losing (tubular) N25.0
    polycystic (congenital) Q61.3
      adult type Q61.2
      childhood type NEC Q61.19
        collecting duct dilatation Q61.11
    rapidly progressive N01.9
    subacute N01.9
  Rendu-Osler-Weber (familial hemorrhagic telangiectasia) I78.0
  renovascular (arteriosclerotic) — *see* Hypertension, kidney
  respiratory (tract) J98.9
    acute or subacute NOS J06.9
      due to
        chemicals, gases, fumes or vapors (inhalation) J68.3
        external agent J70.9
          specified NEC J70.8
        radiation J70.0
        smoke inhalation J70.5
      noninfectious J39.8
    chronic NOS J98.9
      due to
        chemicals, gases, fumes or vapors J68.4
        external agent J70.9
          specified NEC J70.8
        radiation J70.1
      newborn P27.9
        specified NEC P27.8
    due to
      chemicals, gases, fumes or vapors J68.9
        acute or subacute NEC J68.3
        chronic J68.4
      external agent J70.9
        specified NEC J70.8
    newborn P28.9
      specified type NEC P28.89
    upper J39.9
      acute or subacute J06.9
      noninfectious NEC J39.8
      specified NEC J39.8
      streptococcal J06.9
  retina, retinal H35.9
    Batten's or Batten-Mayou E75.4 *[H36]*
    specified NEC H35.89
  rheumatoid — *see* Arthritis, rheumatoid
  rickettsial NOS A79.9
    specified type NEC A79.89
  Riga (-Fede) (cachectic aphthae) K14.0
  Riggs' (compound periodontitis) — *see* Periodontitis
  Ritter's L00
  Rivalta's (cervicofacial actinomycosis) A42.2
  Robles' (onchocerciasis) B73.01

Disease, diseased - *continued*
  Roger's (congenital interventricular septal defect) Q21.0
  Rosenthal's (factor XI deficiency) D68.1
  Rossbach's (hyperchlorhydria) K30
  Ross River B33.1
  Rotes Quérol — *see* Hyperostosis, ankylosing
  Roth (-Bernhardt) — *see* Mononeuropathy, lower limb, meralgia paresthetica
  Runeberg's (progressive pernicious anemia) D51.0
  sacroiliac NEC M53.3
  salivary gland or duct K11.9
    inclusion B25.9
    specified NEC K11.8
    virus B25.9
  sandworm B76.9
  Schimmelbusch's — *see* Mastopathy, cystic
  Schmorl's — *see* Schmorl's disease or nodes
  Schönlein (-Henoch) (purpura rheumatica) D69.0
  Schottmüller's — *see* Fever, paratyphoid
  Schultz's (agranulocytosis) — *see* Agranulocytosis
  Schwalbe-Ziehen-Oppenheim G24.1
  Schwartz-Jampel G71.13
  sclera H15.9
    specified NEC H15.89
  scrofulous (tuberculous) A18.2
  scrotum N50.9
  sebaceous glands L73.9
  semilunar cartilage, cystic — *see also* Derangement, knee, meniscus, cystic
  seminal vesicle N50.9
  serum NEC — *see* Reaction, serum T80.69
  sexually transmitted A64
    anogenital
      herpesviral infection — *see* Herpes, anogenital
      warts A63.0
    chancroid A57
    chlamydial infection — *see* Chlamydia
    gonorrhea — *see* Gonorrhea
    granuloma inguinale A58
    specified organism NEC A63.8
    syphilis — *see* Syphilis
    trichomoniasis — *see* Trichomoniasis
  Sézary C84.1-
  shimamushi (scrub typhus) A75.3
  shipyard B30.0
  sickle-cell D57.1
    with crisis (vasoocclusive pain) D57.00
      with
        acute chest syndrome D57.01
        splenic sequestration D57.02
    elliptocytosis D57.8-
    Hb-C D57.20
      with crisis (vasoocclusive pain) D57.219
        with
          acute chest syndrome D57.211
          splenic sequestration D57.212
      without crisis D57.20
    Hb-SD D57.80
      with crisis D57.819
        with
          acute chest syndrome D57.811
          splenic sequestration D57.812
    Hb-SE D57.80
      with crisis D57.819
        with
          acute chest syndrome D57.811
          splenic sequestration D57.812
    specified NEC D57.80
      with crisis D57.819
        with
          acute chest syndrome D57.811
          splenic sequestration D57.812
    spherocytosis D57.80
      with crisis D57.819
        with
          acute chest syndrome D57.811
          splenic sequestration D57.812
    thalassemia D57.40
      with crisis (vasoocclusive pain) D57.419
        with
          acute chest syndrome D57.411
          splenic sequestration D57.412
      without crisis D57.40
  silo-filler's J68.8
    bronchitis J68.0
    pneumonitis J68.0
    pulmonary edema J68.1
  simian B B00.4
  Simons' (progressive lipodystrophy) E88.1
  sin nombre virus B33.4
  sinus — *see* Sinusitis
  Sirkari's B55.0

Disease, diseased - *continued*
sixth B08.20
  due to human herpesvirus 6 B08.21
  due to human herpesvirus 7 B08.22
skin L98.9
  due to metabolic disorder NEC E88.9 *[L99]*
  specified NEC L98.8
slim (HIV) B20
small vessel I73.9
Sneddon-Wilkinson (subcorneal pustular
  dermatosis) L13.1
South African creeping B88.0
spinal (cord) G95.9
  congenital Q06.9
  specified NEC G95.89
spine — *see also* Spondylopathy
  joint — *see* Dorsopathy
  tuberculous A18.01
spinocerebellar (hereditary) G11.9
  specified NEC G11.8
spleen D73.9
  amyloid E85.4 *[D77]*
  organic D73.9
  polycystic Q89.09
  postinfectional D73.89
sponge-diver's — *see* Toxicity, venom, marine
  animal, sea anemone
Startle Q89.8
Steinert's G71.11
Sticker's (erythema infectiosum) B08.3
Stieda's (calcification, knee joint) — *see* Bursitis,
  tibial collateral
Stokes' (exophthalmic goiter) — *see*
  Hyperthyroidism, with, goiter (diffuse)
Stokes-Adams (syncope with heart block) I45.9
stomach K31.9
  functional, psychogenic F45.8
  specified NEC K31.89
stonemason's J62.8
storage
  glycogen — *see* Disease, glycogen storage
  mucopolysaccharide — *see*
    Mucopolysaccharidosis
striatopallidal system NEC G25.89
Stuart-Prower (congenital factor X
  deficiency) D68.2
Stuart's (congenital factor X deficiency) D68.2
subcutaneous tissue — *see* Disease, skin
supporting structures of teeth K08.9
  specified NEC K08.89
suprarenal (capsule) (gland) E27.9
  hyperfunction E27.0
  specified NEC E27.8
sweat glands L74.9
  specified NEC L74.8
Sweeley-Klionsky E75.21
Swift (-Feer) — *see* Poisoning, mercury
swimming-pool granuloma A31.1
Sylvest's (epidemic pleurodynia) B33.0
sympathetic nervous system G90.9
synovium — *see* Disorder, synovium
syphilitic — *see* Syphilis
systemic tissue mast cell C96.2
tanapox (virus) B08.71
Tangier E78.6
Tarral-Besnier (pityriasis rubra pilaris) L44.0
Tauri's E74.09
tear duct — *see* Disorder, lacrimal system
tendon, tendinous — *see also* Disorder, tendon
  nodular — *see* Trigger finger
terminal vessel I73.9
testis N50.9
thalassemia Hb-S — *see* Disease, sickle-cell,
  thalassemia
Thaysen-Gee (nontropical sprue) K90.0
Thomsen G71.12
throat J39.2
  septic J02.0
thromboembolic — *see* Embolism
thymus (gland) E32.9
  specified NEC E32.8
thyroid (gland) E07.9
  heart — *see also* Hyperthyroidism E05.90 *[I43]*
    with thyroid storm E05.91 *[I43]*
  specified NEC E07.89
Tietze's M94.0
tongue K14.9
  specified NEC K14.8
tonsils, tonsillar (and adenoids) J35.9
tooth, teeth K08.9
  hard tissues K03.9
    specified NEC K03.89
  pulp NEC K04.99

Disease, diseased - *continued*
tooth, teeth - *continued*
  specified NEC K08.89
Tourette's F95.2
trachea NEC J39.8
tricuspid I07.9
  nonrheumatic I36.9
triglyceride-storage E75.5
trophoblastic — *see* Mole, hydatidiform
tsutsugamushi A75.3
tube (fallopian) (noninflammatory) N83.9
  inflammatory — *see* Salpingitis
  specified NEC N83.8
tuberculous NEC — *see* Tuberculosis
tubo-ovarian (noninflammatory) N83.9
  inflammatory — *see* Salpingo-oophoritis
  specified NEC N83.8
tubotympanic, chronic — *see* Otitis, media,
  suppurative, chronic, tubotympanic
tubulo-interstitial N15.9
  specified NEC N15.8
tympanum — *see* Disorder, tympanic membrane
Uhl's Q24.8
Underwood's (sclerema neonatorum) P83.0
Unverricht (-Lundborg) — *see* Epilepsy,
  generalized, idiopathic
Urbach-Oppenheim (necrobiosis lipoidica
  diabeticorum) — *see* E08-E13 with .620
ureter N28.9
  in (due to)
    schistosomiasis (bilharziasis) B65.0 *[N29]*
urethra N36.9
  specified NEC N36.8
urinary (tract) N39.9
  bladder N32.9
    specified NEC N32.89
  specified NEC N39.8
uterus (noninflammatory) N85.9
  infective — *see* Endometritis
  inflammatory — *see* Endometritis
  specified NEC N85.8
uveal tract (anterior) H21.9
  posterior H31.9
vagabond's B85.1
vagina, vaginal (noninflammatory) N89.9
  inflammatory NEC N76.89
  specified NEC N89.8
valve, valvular I38
  multiple I08.9
    specified NEC I08.8
van Creveld-von Gierke (glycogenosis I) E74.01
vas deferens N50.9
vascular I99.9
  arteriosclerotic — *see* Arteriosclerosis
  ciliary body NEC — *see* Disorder, iris, vascular
  hypertensive — *see* Hypertension
  iris NEC — *see* Disorder, iris, vascular
  obliterative I77.1
    peripheral I73.9
  occlusive I99.8
  peripheral (occlusive) I73.9
    in diabetes mellitus — *see* E08-E13 with .51
  vasomotor I73.9
  vasospastic I73.9
vein I87.9
venereal — *see also* Disease, sexually
  transmitted A64
  chlamydial NEC A56.8
    anus A56.3
    genitourinary NOS A56.2
    pharynx A56.4
    rectum A56.3
  fifth A55
  sixth A55
  specified nature or type NEC A63.8
vertebra, vertebral — *see also* Spondylopathy
  disc — *see* Disorder, disc
vibration — *see* Vibration, adverse effects
viral, virus — *see also* Disease, by type of
  virus B34.9
  arbovirus NOS A94
  arthropod-borne NOS A94
  congenital P35.9
    specified NEC P35.8
  Hanta (with renal manifestations) (Dobrava)
    (Puumala) (Seoul) A98.5
      with pulmonary manifestations (Andes) (Bayou)
        (Bermejo) (Black Creek Canal) (Choclo)
        (Juquitiba) (Laguna negra) (Lechiguanas) (New
        York) (Oran) (Sin nombre) B33.4
  Hantaan (Korean hemorrhagic fever) A98.5
  human immunodeficiency (HIV) B20
  Kunjin A83.4

Disease, diseased - *continued*
viral, virus - *continued*
  nonarthropod-borne NOS B34.9
  Powassan A84.8
  Rocio (encephalitis) A83.6
  Sin nombre (Hantavirus) (cardio) -pulmonary
    syndrome) B33.4
  Tahyna B33.8
  vesicular stomatitis A93.8
vitreous H43.9
  specified NEC H43.89
vocal cord J38.3
Volkmann's, acquired T79.6
von Eulenburg's (congenital paramyotonia) G71.19
von Gierke's (glycogenosis I) E74.01
von Graefe's — *see* Strabismus, paralytic,
  ophthalmoplegia, progressive
von Willebrand (-Jürgens) (angiohemophilia) D68.0
Vrolik's (osteogenesis imperfecta) Q78.0
vulva (noninflammatory) N90.9
  inflammatory NEC N76.89
  specified NEC N90.89
Wallgren's (obstruction of splenic vein with
  collateral circulation) I87.8
Wassilieff's (leptospiral jaundice) A27.0
wasting NEC R64
  due to malnutrition E41
Waterhouse-Friderichsen A39.1
Wegner's (syphilitic osteochondritis) A50.02
Weil's (leptospiral jaundice of lung) A27.0
Weir Mitchell's (erythromelalgia) I73.81
Werdnig-Hoffmann G12.0
Wermer's E31.21
Werner-His (trench fever) A79.0
Werner-Schultz (neutropenic splenomegaly) D73.81
Wernicke-Posadas B38.9
whipworm B79
white blood cells D72.9
  specified NEC D72.89
white matter R90.82
white-spot, meaning lichen sclerosus et
  atrophicus L90.0
  penis N48.0
  vulva N90.4
Wilkie's K55.1
Wilkinson-Sneddon (subcorneal pustular
  dermatosis) L13.1
Willis' — *see* Diabetes
Wilson's (hepatolenticular degeneration) E83.01
woolsorter's A22.1
yaba monkey tumor B08.72
yaba pox (virus) B08.72
Zika virus A92.5
zoonotic, bacterial A28.9
  specified type NEC A28.8
Disfigurement (due to scar) L90.5
Disgerminoma — *see* Dysgerminoma
DISH (diffuse idiopathic skeletal hyperostosis) — *see*
  Hyperostosis, ankylosing
Disinsertion, retina — *see* Detachment, retina
Dislocatable hip, congenital Q65.6
Dislocation (articular)
with fracture — *see* Fracture
acromioclavicular (joint) S43.10-
  with displacement
    100%-200% S43.12-
    more than 200% S43.13-
  inferior S43.14-
  posterior S43.15-
ankle S93.0-
astragalus — *see* Dislocation, ankle
atlantoaxial S13.121
atlantooccipital S13.111
atloidooccipital S13.111
breast bone S23.29
capsule, joint - code by site under Dislocation
carpal (bone) — *see* Dislocation, wrist
carpometacarpal (joint) NEC S63.05-
  thumb S63.04-
cartilage (joint) - code by site under Dislocation
cervical spine (vertebra) — *see* Dislocation,
  vertebra, cervical
chronic — *see* Dislocation, recurrent
clavicle — *see* Dislocation, acromioclavicular joint
coccyx S33.2
congenital NEC Q68.8
coracoid — *see* Dislocation, shoulder
costal cartilage S23.29
costochondral S23.29
cricoarytenoid articulation S13.29
cricothyroid articulation S13.29
dorsal vertebra — *see* Dislocation, vertebra, thoracic
ear ossicle — *see* Discontinuity, ossicles, ear

Dislocation (articular) - *continued*
elbow S53.10-
  congenital Q68.8
  pathological — *see* Dislocation, pathological NEC, elbow
  radial head alone — *see* Dislocation, radial head
  recurrent — *see* Dislocation, recurrent, elbow
  traumatic S53.10-
    anterior S53.11-
    lateral S53.14-
    medial S53.13-
    posterior S53.12-
    specified type NEC S53.19-
eye, nontraumatic — *see* Luxation, globe
eyeball, nontraumatic — *see* Luxation, globe
femur
  distal end — *see* Dislocation, knee
  proximal end — *see* Dislocation, hip
fibula
  distal end — *see* Dislocation, ankle
  proximal end — *see* Dislocation, knee
finger S63.25-
  index S63.25-
  interphalangeal S63.27-
    distal S63.29-
      index S63.29-
      little S63.29-
      middle S63.29-
      ring S63.29-
    index S63.27-
    little S63.27-
    middle S63.27-
    proximal S63.28-
      index S63.28-
      little S63.28-
      middle S63.28-
      ring S63.28-
    ring S63.27-
  little S63.25-
  metacarpophalangeal S63.26-
    index S63.26-
    little S63.26-
    middle S63.26-
    ring S63.26-
  middle S63.25-
  recurrent — *see* Dislocation, recurrent, finger
  ring S63.25-
  thumb — *see* Dislocation, thumb
foot S93.30-
  recurrent — *see* Dislocation, recurrent, foot
  specified site NEC S93.33-
  tarsal joint S93.31-
  tarsometatarsal joint S93.32-
  toe — *see* Dislocation, toe
fracture — *see* Fracture
glenohumeral (joint) — *see* Dislocation, shoulder
glenoid — *see* Dislocation, shoulder
habitual — *see* Dislocation, recurrent
hip S73.00-
  anterior S73.03-
    obturator S73.02-
  central S73.04-
  congenital (total) Q65.2
    bilateral Q65.1
    partial Q65.5
      bilateral Q65.4
      unilateral Q65.3-
    unilateral Q65.0-
  developmental M24.85-
  pathological — *see* Dislocation, pathological NEC, hip
  posterior S73.01-
  recurrent — *see* Dislocation, recurrent, hip
humerus, proximal end — *see* Dislocation, shoulder
incomplete — *see* Subluxation, by site
incus — *see* Discontinuity, ossicles, ear
infracoracoid — *see* Dislocation, shoulder
innominate (pubic junction) (sacral junction) S33.39
  acetabulum — *see* Dislocation, hip
interphalangeal (joint (s))
  finger S63.279
    distal S63.29-
      index S63.29-
      little S63.29-
      middle S63.29-
      ring S63.29-
    index S63.27-
    little S63.27-
    middle S63.27-
    proximal S63.28-
      index S63.28-
      little S63.28-
      middle S63.28-

Dislocation (articular) - *continued*
interphalangeal (joint (s)) - *continued*
  finger - *continued*
    proximal - *continued*
      ring S63.28-
    ring S63.27-
  foot or toe — *see* Dislocation, toe
  thumb S63.12-
    distal S63.14-
    proximal joint S63.13-
jaw (cartilage) (meniscus) S03.0-
joint prosthesis — *see* Complications, joint prosthesis, mechanical, displacement, by site
knee S83.106
  cap — *see* Dislocation, patella
  congenital Q68.2
  old M23.8X-
  patella — *see* Dislocation, patella
  pathological — *see* Dislocation, pathological NEC, knee
  proximal tibia
    anteriorly S83.11-
    laterally S83.14-
    medially S83.13-
    posteriorly S83.12-
  recurrent — *see also* Derangement, knee, specified NEC
  specified type NEC S83.19-
lacrimal gland H04.16-
lens (complete) H27.10
  anterior H27.12-
  congenital Q12.1
  ocular implant — *see* Complications, intraocular lens
  partial H27.11-
  posterior H27.13-
  traumatic S05.8X-
ligament - code by site under Dislocation
lumbar (vertebra) — *see* Dislocation, vertebra, lumbar
lumbosacral (vertebra) — *see also* Dislocation, vertebra, lumbar
  congenital Q76.49
mandible S03.0-
meniscus (knee) — *see* Tear, meniscus
  other sites - code by site under Dislocation
metacarpal (bone)
  distal end — *see* Dislocation, finger
  proximal end S63.06-
metacarpophalangeal (joint)
  finger S63.26-
    index S63.26-
    little S63.26-
    middle S63.26-
    ring S63.26-
  thumb S63.11-
metatarsal (bone) — *see* Dislocation, foot
metatarsophalangeal (joint (s)) — *see* Dislocation, toe
midcarpal (joint) S63.03-
midtarsal (joint) — *see* Dislocation, foot
neck S13.20
  specified site NEC S13.29
  vertebra — *see* Dislocation, vertebra, cervical
nose (septal cartilage) S03.1
occipitoatloid S13.111
old — *see* Derangement, joint, specified type NEC
ossicles, ear — *see* Discontinuity, ossicles, ear
partial — *see* Subluxation, by site
patella S83.006
  congenital Q74.1
  lateral S83.01-
  recurrent (nontraumatic) M22.0-
    incomplete M22.1-
  specified type NEC S83.09-
pathological NEC M24.30
  ankle M24.37-
  elbow M24.32-
  foot joint M24.37-
  hand joint M24.34-
  hip M24.35-
  knee M24.36-
  lumbosacral joint — *see* subcategory M53.2
  pelvic region — *see* Dislocation, pathological, hip
  sacroiliac — *see* subcategory M53.2
  shoulder M24.31-
  wrist M24.33-
pelvis NEC S33.30
  specified NEC S33.39
phalanx
  finger or hand — *see* Dislocation, finger
  foot or toe — *see* Dislocation, toe

Dislocation (articular) - *continued*
prosthesis, internal — *see* Complications, prosthetic device, by site, mechanical
radial head S53.006
  anterior S53.01-
  posterior S53.02-
  specified type NEC S53.09-
radiocarpal (joint) S63.02-
radiohumeral (joint) — *see* Dislocation, radial head
radioulnar (joint)
  distal S63.01-
  proximal — *see* Dislocation, elbow
radius
  distal end — *see* Dislocation, wrist
  proximal end — *see* Dislocation, radial head
recurrent M24.40
  ankle M24.47-
  elbow M24.42-
  finger M24.44-
  foot joint M24.47-
  hand joint M24.44-
  hip M24.45-
  knee M24.46-
    patella — *see* Dislocation, patella, recurrent
  patella — *see* Dislocation, patella, recurrent
  sacroiliac — *see* subcategory M53.2
  shoulder M24.41-
  toe M24.47-
  vertebra (*see also* subcategory) M43.5
    atlantoaxial M43.4
      with myelopathy M43.3
  wrist M24.43-
rib (cartilage) S23.29
sacrococcygeal S33.2
sacroiliac (joint) (ligament) S33.2
  congenital Q74.2
  recurrent — *see* subcategory M53.2
sacrum S33.2
scaphoid (bone) (hand) (wrist) — *see* Dislocation, wrist
  foot — *see* Dislocation, foot
scapula — *see* Dislocation, shoulder, girdle, scapula
semilunar cartilage, knee — *see* Tear, meniscus
septal cartilage (nose) S03.1
septum (nasal) (old) J34.2
sesamoid bone - code by site under Dislocation
shoulder (blade) (ligament) (joint)
  (traumatic) S43.006
  acromioclavicular — *see* Dislocation, acromioclavicular
  chronic — *see* Dislocation, recurrent, shoulder
  congenital Q68.8
  girdle S43.30-
    scapula S43.31-
    specified site NEC S43.39-
  humerus S43.00-
    anterior S43.01-
    inferior S43.03-
    posterior S43.02-
  pathological — *see* Dislocation, pathological NEC, shoulder
  recurrent — *see* Dislocation, recurrent, shoulder
  specified type NEC S43.08-
spine
  cervical — *see* Dislocation, vertebra, cervical
  congenital Q76.49
  due to birth trauma P11.5
  lumbar — *see* Dislocation, vertebra, lumbar
  thoracic — *see* Dislocation, vertebra, thoracic
  spontaneous — *see* Dislocation, pathological
sternoclavicular (joint) S43.206
  anterior S43.21-
  posterior S43.22-
sternum S23.29
subglenoid — *see* Dislocation, shoulder
symphysis pubis S33.4
talus — *see* Dislocation, ankle
tarsal (bone (s)) (joint (s)) — *see* Dislocation, foot
tarsometatarsal (joint (s)) — *see* Dislocation, foot
temporomandibular (joint) S03.0-
thigh, proximal end — *see* Dislocation, hip
thorax S23.20
  specified site NEC S23.29
  vertebra — *see* Dislocation, vertebra
thumb S63.10-
  interphalangeal joint — *see* Dislocation, interphalangeal (joint), thumb
  metacarpophalangeal joint — *see* Dislocation, metacarpophalangeal (joint), thumb
thyroid cartilage S13.29
tibia
  distal end — *see* Dislocation, ankle
  proximal end — *see* Dislocation, knee

Dislocation (articular) - *continued*
 tibiofibular (joint)
  distal — *see* Dislocation, ankle
  superior — *see* Dislocation, knee
 toe (s) S93.106
  great S93.10-
   interphalangeal joint S93.11-
   metatarsophalangeal joint S93.12-
  interphalangeal joint S93.119
  lesser S93.106
   interphalangeal joint S93.11-
   metatarsophalangeal joint S93.12-
  metatarsophalangeal joint S93.12-
 tooth S03.2
 trachea S23.29
 ulna
  distal end S63.07-
  proximal end — *see* Dislocation, elbow
 ulnohumeral (joint) — *see* Dislocation, elbow
 vertebra (articular process) (body) (traumatic)
  cervical S13.101
   atlantoaxial joint S13.121
   atlantooccipital joint S13.111
   atloidooccipital joint S13.111
   joint between
    C0 and C1 S13.111
    C1 and C2 S13.121
    C2 and C3 S13.131
    C3 and C4 S13.141
    C4 and C5 S13.151
    C5and C6 S13.161
    C6and C7 S13.171
    C7and T1 S13.181
   occipitoatloid joint S13.111
  congenital Q76.49
  lumbar S33.101
   joint between
    L1and L2 S33.111
    L2and L3 S33.121
    L3 and L4 S33.131
    L4and L5 S33.141
  nontraumatic — *see* Displacement, intervertebral disc
  partial — *see* Subluxation, by site
  recurrent NEC — *see* subcategory M43.5
  thoracic S23.101
   joint between
    T1 and T2 S23.111
    T2 and T3 S23.121
    T3 and T4 S23.123
    T4 and T5 S23.131
    T5 and T6 S23.133
    T6 and T7 S23.141
    T7 and T8 S23.143
    T8 and T9 S23.151
    T9 and T10 S23.153
    T10 and T11 S23.161
    T11 and T12 S23.163
    T12 and L1 S23.171
 wrist (carpal bone) S63.006
  carpometacarpal joint — *see* Dislocation, carpometacarpal (joint)
  distal radioulnar joint — *see* Dislocation, radioulnar (joint), distal
  metacarpal bone, proximal — *see* Dislocation, metacarpal (bone), proximal end
  midcarpal — *see* Dislocation, midcarpal (joint)
  radiocarpal joint — *see* Dislocation, radiocarpal (joint)
  recurrent — *see* Dislocation, recurrent, wrist
  specified site NEC S63.09-
  ulna — *see* Dislocation, ulna, distal end
 xiphoid cartilage S23.29
Disorder (of) — *see also* Disease
 acantholytic L11.9
  specified NEC L11.8
 acute
  psychotic — *see* Psychosis, acute
  stress F43.0
 adjustment (grief) F43.20
  with
   anxiety F43.22
    with depressed mood F43.23
   conduct disturbance F43.24
    with emotional disturbance F43.25
   depressed mood F43.21
    with anxiety F43.23
   other specified symptom F43.29
 adrenal (capsule) (gland) (medullary) E27.9
  specified NEC E27.8
 adrenogenital E25.9
  drug-induced E25.8
  iatrogenic E25.8

Disorder (of) - *continued*
 adrenogenital - *continued*
  idiopathic E25.8
 adult personality (and behavior) F69
  specified NEC F68.8
 affective (mood) — *see* Disorder, mood
 aggressive, unsocialized F91.1
 alcohol-related F10.99
  with
   amnestic disorder, persisting F10.96
   anxiety disorder F10.980
   dementia, persisting F10.97
   intoxication F10.929
    with delirium F10.921
    uncomplicated F10.920
   mood disorder F10.94
   other specified F10.988
   psychotic disorder F10.959
    with
     delusions F10.950
     hallucinations F10.951
   sexual dysfunction F10.981
   sleep disorder F10.982
 alcohol use
  mild F10.10
   with
    alcohol-induced
     anxiety disorder F10.180
     bipolar and related disorder F10.14
     depressive disorder F10.14
     psychotic disorder F10.159
     sexual dysfunction F10.181
     sleep disorder F10.182
    alcohol intoxication F10.129
     delirium F10.121
  moderate or severe F10.20
   with
    alcohol-induced
     anxiety disorder F10.280
     bipolar and related disorder F10.24
     depressive disorder F10.24
     major neurocognitive disorder, amnestic-confabulatory type F10.26
     major neurocognitive disorder, nonamnestic-confabulatory type F10.27
     mild neurocognitive disorder F10.288
     psychotic disorder F10.259
     sexual dysfunction F10.281
     sleep disorder F10.282
    alcohol intoxication F10.229
     delirium F10.221
 allergic — *see* Allergy
 alveolar NEC J84.09
 amino-acid
  cystathioninuria E72.19
  cystinosis E72.04
  cystinuria E72.01
  glycinuria E72.09
  homocystinuria E72.11
  metabolism — *see* Disturbance, metabolism, amino-acid
   specified NEC E72.8
  neonatal, transitory P74.8
  renal transport NEC E72.09
  transport NEC E72.09
 amnesic, amnestic
  alcohol-induced F10.96
   with dependence F10.26
  due to (secondary to) general medical condition F04
  psychoactive NEC-induced F19.96
   with
    abuse F19.16
    dependence F19.26
  sedative, hypnotic or anxiolytic-induced F13.96
   with dependence F13.26
 amphetamine-type substance use
  mild F15.10
  moderate F15.20
  severe F15.20
 amphetamine (or other stimulant) use
  mild
   with
    amphetamine (or other stimulant) -induced
     anxiety disorder F15.180
     bipolar and related disorder F15.14
     depressive disorder F15.14
     obsessive-compulsive and related disorder F15.188
     psychotic disorder F15.159
     sexual dysfunction F15.181
    amphetamine, cocaine, or other stimulant intoxication

Disorder (of) - *continued*
 amphetamine (or other stimulant) use - *continued*
  mild - *continued*
   with - *continued*
    amphetamine, cocaine, or other stimulant intoxication - *continued*
     with perceptual disturbances F15.122
     without perceptual disturbances F15.129
    intoxication delirium F15.121
  moderate or severe
   with
    amphetamine (or other stimulant) -induced
     anxiety disorder F15.280
     obsessive-compulsive and related disorder F15.288
     sexual dysfunction F15.281
     bipolar and related disorder F15.24
     depressive disorder F15.24
     psychotic disorder F15.259
    amphetamine, cocaine, or other stimulant intoxication
     with perceptual disturbances F15.222
     without perceptual disturbances F15.229
    intoxication delirium F15.221
 anaerobic glycolysis with anemia D55.2
 anxiety F41.9
  due to (secondary to)
   alcohol F10.980
   amphetamine F15.980
    in
     abuse F15.180
     dependence F15.280
   anxiolytic F13.980
    in
     abuse F13.180
     dependence F13.280
   caffeine F15.980
    in
     abuse F15.180
     dependence F15.280
   cannabis F12.980
    in
     abuse F12.180
     dependence F12.280
   cocaine F14.980
    in
     abuse F14.180
     dependence F14.180
   general medical condition F06.4
   hallucinogen F16.980
    in
     abuse F16.180
     dependence F16.280
   hypnotic F13.980
    in
     abuse F13.180
     dependence F13.280
   inhalant F18.980
    in
     abuse F18.180
     dependence F18.280
   phencyclidine F16.980
    in
     abuse F16.180
     dependence F16.280
   psychoactive substance NEC F19.980
    in
     abuse F19.180
     dependence F19.280
   sedative F13.980
    in
     abuse F13.180
     dependence F13.280
   volatile solvents F18.980
    in
     abuse F18.180
     dependence F18.280
  generalized F41.1
  illness F45.21
  mixed
   with depression (mild) F41.8
   specified NEC F41.3
  organic F06.4
  phobic F40.9
   of childhood F40.8
  specified NEC F41.8
 aortic valve — *see* Endocarditis, aortic
 aromatic amino-acid metabolism E70.9
  specified NEC E70.8
 arteriole NEC I77.89
 artery NEC I77.89
 articulation — *see* Disorder, joint
 attachment (childhood)

Disorder (of) - *continued*
  attachment (childhood) - *continued*
    disinhibited F94.2
    reactive F94.1
  attention-deficit hyperactivity (adolescent) (adult)
    (child) F90.9
    combined type F90.2
    hyperactive type F90.1
    inattentive type F90.0
    specified type NEC F90.8
  attention-deficit without hyperactivity (adolescent)
    (adult) (child) F98.8
  auditory processing (central) H93.25
  autistic F84.0
  autism spectrum F84.0
  autonomic nervous system G90.9
    specified NEC G90.8
  avoidant
    child or adolescent F40.10
    restrictive food intake F50.89
  balance
    acid-base E87.8
      mixed E87.4
    electrolyte E87.8
    fluid NEC E87.8
  behavioral (disruptive) — *see* Disorder, conduct
  beta-amino-acid metabolism E72.8
  bile acid and cholesterol metabolism E78.70
    Barth syndrome E78.71
    other specified E78.79
    Smith-Lemli-Opitz syndrome E78.72
  bilirubin excretion E80.6
  binge eating F50.81
  binocular
    movement H51.9
      convergence
        excess H51.12
        insufficiency H51.11
      internuclear ophthalmoplegia — *see*
        Ophthalmoplegia, internuclear
      palsy of conjugate gaze H51.0
      specified type NEC H51.8
    vision NEC — *see* Disorder, vision, binocular
  bipolar (I) F31.9
    current episode
      depressed F31.9
        with psychotic features F31.5
        without psychotic features F31.30
          mild F31.31
          moderate F31.32
          severe (without psychotic features) F31.4
            with psychotic features F31.5
      hypomanic F31.0
      manic F31.9
        with psychotic features F31.2
        without psychotic features F31.10
          mild F31.11
          moderate F31.12
          severe (without psychotic features) F31.13
            with psychotic features F31.2
      mixed F31.60
        mild F31.61
        moderate F31.62
        severe (without psychotic features) F31.63
          with psychotic features F31.64
      severe depression (without psychotic
        features) F31.4
        with psychotic features F31.5
    in remission (currently) F31.70
      in full remission
        most recent episode
          depressed F31.76
          hypomanic F31.72
          manic F31.74
          mixed F31.78
      in partial remission
        most recent episode
          depressed F31.75
          hypomanic F31.71
          manic F31.73
          mixed F31.77
    specified NEC F31.89
    II F31.81
    organic F06.30
    single manic episode F30.9
      mild F30.11
      moderate F30.12
      severe (without psychotic symptoms) F30.13
        with psychotic symptoms F30.2
  bladder N32.9
    functional NEC N31.9
    in schistosomiasis B65.0 *[N33]*
    specified NEC N32.89

Disorder (of) - *continued*
  bleeding D68.9
  blood D75.9
    in congenital early syphilis A50.09 *[D77]*
  body dysmorphic F45.22
  bone M89.9
    continuity M84.9
      specified type NEC M84.80
        ankle M84.87-
        fibula M84.86-
        foot M84.87-
        hand M84.84-
        humerus M84.82-
        neck M84.88
        pelvis M84.859
        radius M84.83-
        rib M84.88
        shoulder M84.81-
        skull M84.88
        thigh M84.85-
        tibia M84.86-
        ulna M84.83-
        vertebra M84.88
    density and structure M85.9
      cyst — *see also* Cyst, bone, specified type NEC
        aneurysmal — *see* Cyst, bone, aneurysmal
        solitary — *see* Cyst, bone, solitary
      diffuse idiopathic skeletal hyperostosis — *see*
        Hyperostosis, ankylosing
      fibrous dysplasia (monostotic) — *see* Dysplasia,
        fibrous, bone
      fluorosis — *see* Fluorosis, skeletal
      hyperostosis of skull M85.2
      osteitis condensans — *see* Osteitis, condensans
      specified type NEC M85.8-
        ankle M85.87-
        foot M85.87-
        forearm M85.83-
        hand M85.84-
        lower leg M85.86-
        multiple sites M85.89
        neck M85.88
        rib M85.88
        shoulder M85.81-
        skull M85.88
        thigh M85.85-
        upper arm M85.82-
        vertebra M85.88
    development and growth NEC M89.20
      carpus M89.24-
      clavicle M89.21-
      femur M89.25-
      fibula M89.26-
      finger M89.24-
      humerus M89.22-
      ilium M89.259
      ischium M89.259
      metacarpus M89.24-
      metatarsus M89.27-
      multiple sites M89.29
      neck M89.28
      radius M89.23-
      rib M89.28
      scapula M89.21-
      skull M89.28
      tarsus M89.27-
      tibia M89.26-
      toe M89.27-
      ulna M89.23-
      vertebra M89.28
    specified type NEC M89.8X-
  brachial plexus G54.0
  branched-chain amino-acid metabolism E71.2
    specified NEC E71.19
  breast N64.9
    agalactia — *see* Agalactia
    associated with
      lactation O92.70
        specified NEC O92.79
      pregnancy O92.20
        specified NEC O92.29
      puerperium O92.20
        specified NEC O92.29
    cracked nipple — *see* Cracked nipple
    galactorrhea — *see* Galactorrhea
    hypogalactia O92.4
    lactation disorder NEC O92.79
    mastitis — *see* Mastitis
    nipple infection — *see* Infection, nipple
    retracted nipple — *see* Retraction, nipple
    specified type NEC N64.89
  Briquet's F45.0
  bullous, in diseases classified elsewhere L14

Disorder (of) - *continued*
  caffeine use
    mild
      with
        caffeine-induced
          anxiety disorder F15.180
          sleep disorder F15.182
    moderate or severe
      with
        caffeine-induced
          anxiety disorder F15.280
          sleep disorder F15.282
  cannabis use
    mild F12.10
      with
        cannabis-induced
          anxiety disorder F12.180
          psychotic disorder F12.159
          sleep disorder F12.188
        cannabis intoxication delirium F12.121
          with perceptual disturbances F12.122
          without perceptual disturbances F12.129
    moderate or severe F12.20
      with
        cannabis-induced
          anxiety disorder F12.280
          psychotic disorder F12.259
          sleep disorder F12.288
        cannabis intoxication
          with perceptual disturbances F12.222
          without perceptual disturbances F12.229
        delirium F12.221
  carbohydrate
    absorption, intestinal NEC E74.39
    metabolism (congenital) E74.9
      specified NEC E74.8
  cardiac, functional I51.89
  carnitine metabolism E71.40
  cartilage M94.9
    articular NEC — *see* Derangement, joint, articular
      cartilage
    chondrocalcinosis — *see* Chondrocalcinosis
    specified type NEC M94.8X-
      articular — *see* Derangement, joint, articular
        cartilage
      multiple sites M94.8X0
  catatonia (due to known physiological condition)
    (with another mental disorder) F06.1
  catatonic
    due to (secondary to) known physiological
      condition F06.1
    organic F06.1
  central auditory processing H93.25
  cervical
    region NEC M53.82
    root (nerve) NEC G54.2
  character NOS F60.9
  childhood disintegrative NEC F84.3
  cholesterol and bile acid metabolism E78.70
    Barth syndrome E78.71
    other specified E78.79
    Smith-Lemli-Opitz syndrome E78.72
  choroid H31.9
    atrophy — *see* Atrophy, choroid
    degeneration — *see* Degeneration, choroid
    detachment — *see* Detachment, choroid
    dystrophy — *see* Dystrophy, choroid
    hemorrhage — *see* Hemorrhage, choroid
    rupture — *see* Rupture, choroid
    scar — *see* Scar, chorioretinal
    solar retinopathy — *see* Retinopathy, solar
    specified type NEC H31.8
  ciliary body — *see* Disorder, iris
    degeneration — *see* Degeneration, ciliary body
  coagulation (factor) — *see also* Defect,
    coagulation D68.9
    newborn, transient P61.6
  cocaine use
    mild F14.10
      with
        amphetamine, cocaine, or other stimulant
          intoxication
          with perceptual disturbances F14.122
          without perceptual disturbances F14.129
        cocaine-induced
          anxiety disorder F14.180
          bipolar and related disorder F14.14
          depressive disorder F14.14
          obsessive-compulsive and related
           disorder F14.188
          psychotic disorder F14.159
          sexual dysfunction F14.181
          sleep disorder F14.182

Disorder (of) - *continued*
cocaine use - *continued*
  mild - *continued*
    with - *continued*
      cocaine intoxication delirium F14.121
  moderate or severe F14.20
    with
      amphetamine, cocaine, or other stimulant
        intoxication
        with perceptual disturbances F14.222
        without perceptual disturbances F14.229
      cocaine-induced
        anxiety disorder F14.280
        bipolar and related disorder F14.24
        depressive disorder F14.24
        obsessive-compulsive and related
          disorder F14.288
        psychotic disorder F14.259
        sexual dysfunction F14.281
        sleep disorder F14.282
      cocaine intoxication delirium F14.221
  coccyx NEC M53.3
cognitive F09
  due to (secondary to) general medical
    condition F09
  persisting R41.89
    due to
      alcohol F10.97
        with dependence F10.27
      anxiolytics F13.97
        with dependence F13.27
      hypnotics F13.97
        with dependence F13.27
      sedatives F13.97
        with dependence F13.27
      specified substance NEC F19.97
        with
          abuse F19.17
          dependence F19.27
communication F80.9
  social pragmatic F80.82
conduct (childhood) F91.9
  adjustment reaction — *see* Disorder, adjustment
  adolescent onset type F91.2
  childhood onset type F91.1
  compulsive F63.9
  confined to family context F91.0
  depressive F91.8
  group type F91.2
  hyperkinetic — *see* Disorder, attention-deficit
    hyperactivity
  oppositional defiance F91.3
  socialized F91.2
  solitary aggressive type F91.1
  specified NEC F91.8
  unsocialized (aggressive) F91.1
conduction, heart I45.9
congenital glycosylation (CDG) E74.8
conjunctiva H11.9
  infection — *see* Conjunctivitis
connective tissue, localized L94.9
  specified NEC L94.8
conversion (functional neurological symptom
  disorder)
  with
    abnormal movement F44.4
    anesthesia or sensory loss F44.6
    attacks or seizures F44.5
    mixed symptoms F44.7
    special sensory symptoms F44.6
    speech symptoms F44.4
    swallowing symptoms F44.4
    weakness or paralysis F44.4
convulsive (secondary) — *see* Convulsions
cornea H18.9
  deformity — *see* Deformity, cornea
  degeneration — *see* Degeneration, cornea
  deposits — *see* Deposit, cornea
  due to contact lens H18.82-
    specified as edema — *see* Edema, cornea
  edema — *see* Edema, cornea
  keratitis — *see* Keratitis
  keratoconjunctivitis — *see* Keratoconjunctivitis
  membrane change — *see* Change, corneal
    membrane
  neovascularization — *see* Neovascularization,
    cornea
  scar — *see* Opacity, cornea
  specified type NEC H18.89-
  ulcer — *see* Ulcer, cornea
corpus cavernosum N48.9
cranial nerve — *see* Disorder, nerve, cranial
cyclothymic F34.0

Disorder (of) - *continued*
defiant oppositional F91.3
delusional (persistent) (systematized) F22
  induced F24
depersonalization F48.1
depressive F32.9
  major F32.9
    with psychotic symptoms F32.3
    in remission (full) F32.5
      partial F32.4
    recurrent F33.9
    single episode F32.9
      mild F32.0
      moderate F32.1
      severe (without psychotic symptoms) F32.2
        with psychotic symptoms F32.3
  organic F06.31
  persistent F34.1
  recurrent F33.9
    current episode
      mild F33.0
      moderate F33.1
      severe (without psychotic symptoms) F33.2
        with psychotic symptoms F33.3
    in remission F33.40
      full F33.42
      partial F33.41
    specified NEC F33.8
  single episode — *see* Episode, depressive
  specified NEC F32.89
developmental F89
  arithmetical skills F81.2
  coordination (motor) F82
  expressive writing F81.81
  language F80.9
    expressive F80.1
    mixed receptive and expressive F80.2
    receptive type F80.2
    specified NEC F80.89
  learning F81.9
    arithmetical F81.2
    reading F81.0
  mixed F88
  motor coordination or function F82
  pervasive F84.9
    specified NEC F84.8
  phonological F80.0
  reading F81.0
  scholastic skills — *see also* Disorder, learning
    mixed F81.89
  specified NEC F88
  speech F80.9
    articulation F80.0
    specified NEC F80.89
  written expression F81.81
diaphragm J98.6
digestive (system) K92.9
  newborn P78.9
    specified NEC P78.89
  postprocedural — *see* Complication,
    gastrointestinal
  psychogenic F45.8
disc (intervertebral) M51.9
  with
    myelopathy
      cervical region M50.00
      cervicothoracic region M50.03
      high cervical region M50.01
      lumbar region M51.06
      mid-cervical region M50.020
      sacrococcygeal region M53.3
      thoracic region M51.04
      thoracolumbar region M51.05
    radiculopathy
      cervical region M50.10
      cervicothoracic region M50.13
      high cervical region M50.11
      lumbar region M51.16
      lumbosacral region M51.17
      mid-cervical region M50.120
      sacrococcygeal region M53.3
      thoracic region M51.14
      thoracolumbar region M51.15
  cervical M50.90
    with
      myelopathy M50.00
        C2-C3 M50.01
        C3-C4 M50.01
        C4-C5 M50.021
        C5-C6 M50.022
        C6-C7 M50.023
        C7-T1 M50.03
        cervicothoracic region M50.03

Disorder (of) - *continued*
disc (intervertebral) - *continued*
  cervical - *continued*
    with - *continued*
      myelopathy - *continued*
        high cervical region M50.01
        mid-cervical region M50.020
      neuritis, radiculitis or radiculopathy M50.10
        C2-C3 M50.11
        C3-C4 M50.11
        C4-C5 M50.121
        C5-C6 M50.122
        C6-C7 M50.123
        C7-T1 M50.13
        cervicothoracic region M50.13
        high cervical region M50.11
        mid-cervical region M50.120
      C2-C3 M50.91
      C3-C4 M50.91
      C4-C5 M50.921
      C5-C6 M50.922
      C6-C7 M50.923
      C7-T1 M50.93
      cervicothoracic region M50.93
      degeneration M50.30
        C2-C3 M50.31
        C3-C4 M50.31
        C4-C5 M50.321
        C5-C6 M50.322
        C6-C7 M50.323
        C7-T1 M50.33
        cervicothoracic region M50.33
        high cervical region M50.31
        mid-cervical region M50.320
      displacement M50.20
        C2-C3 M50.21
        C3-C4 M50.21
        C4-C5 M50.221
        C5-C6 M50.222
        C6-C7 M50.223
        C7-T1 M50.23
        cervicothoracic region M50.23
        high cervical region M50.21
        mid-cervical region M50.220
      high cervical region M50.91
      mid-cervical region M50.920
      specified type NEC M50.80
        C2-C3 M50.81
        C3-C4 M50.81
        C4-C5 M50.821
        C5-C6 M50.822
        C6-C7 M50.823
        C7-T1 M50.83
        cervicothoracic region M50.83
        high cervical region M50.81
        mid-cervical region M50.820
  specified NEC
    lumbar region M51.86
    lumbosacral region M51.87
    sacrococcygeal region M53.3
    thoracic region M51.84
    thoracolumbar region M51.85
disinhibited attachment (childhood) F94.2
disintegrative, childhood NEC F84.3
disruptive F91.9
  mood dysregulation F34.81
  specified NEC F91.8
disruptive behavior F91.9
dissocial personality F60.2
dissociative F44.9
  affecting
    motor function F44.4
      and sensation F44.7
    sensation F44.6
      and motor function F44.7
  brief reactive F43.0
  due to (secondary to) general medical
    condition F06.8
  mixed F44.7
  organic F06.8
  other specified NEC F44.89
double heterozygous sickling — *see* Disease, sickle-
  cell
dream anxiety F51.5
drug induced hemorrhagic D68.32
drug related F19.99
  abuse — *see* Abuse, drug
  dependence — *see* Dependence, drug
dysmorphic body F45.22
dysthymic F34.1
ear H93.9-
  bleeding — *see* Otorrhagia
  deafness — *see* Deafness

Disorder (of) - *continued*
ear - *continued*
  degenerative H93.09-
  discharge — *see* Otorrhea
  external H61.9-
    auditory canal stenosis — *see* Stenosis, external ear canal
    exostosis — *see* Exostosis, external ear canal
    impacted cerumen — *see* Impaction, cerumen
    otitis — *see* Otitis, externa
    perichondritis — *see* Perichondritis, ear
    pinna — *see* Disorder, pinna
    specified type NEC H61.89-
    in diseases classified elsewhere H62.8X-
  inner H83.9-
    vestibular dysfunction — *see* Disorder, vestibular function
  middle H74.9-
    adhesive H74.1-
    ossicle — *see* Abnormal, ear ossicles
    polyp — *see* Polyp, ear (middle)
    specified NEC, in diseases classified elsewhere H75.8-
  postprocedural — *see* Complications, ear, procedure
  specified NEC, in diseases classified elsewhere H94.8-
eating (adult) (psychogenic) F50.9
  anorexia — *see* Anorexia
  binge F50.81
  bulimia F50.2
  child F98.29
    pica F98.3
    rumination disorder F98.21
  pica F50.89
    childhood F98.3
electrolyte (balance) NEC E87.8
  with
    abortion — *see* Abortion by type complicated by specified condition NEC
    ectopic pregnancy O08.5
    molar pregnancy O08.5
  acidosis (metabolic) (respiratory) E87.2
  alkalosis (metabolic) (respiratory) E87.3
elimination, transepidermal L87.9
  specified NEC L87.8
emotional (persistent) F34.9
  of childhood F93.9
    specified NEC F93.8
endocrine E34.9
  postprocedural E89.89
  specified NEC E89.89
erectile (male) (organic) — *see also* Dysfunction, sexual, male, erectile N52.9
  nonorganic F52.21
erythematous — *see* Erythema
esophagus K22.9
  functional K22.4
  psychogenic F45.8
eustachian tube H69.9-
  infection — *see* Salpingitis, eustachian
  obstruction — *see* Obstruction, eustachian tube
  patulous — *see* Patulous, eustachian tube
  specified NEC H69.8-
extrapyramidal G25.9
  in diseases classified elsewhere — *see* category G26
  specified type NEC G25.89
eye H57.9
  postprocedural — *see* Complication, postprocedural, eye
eyelid H02.9
  cyst — *see* Cyst, eyelid
  degenerative H02.70
    chloasma — *see* Chloasma, eyelid
    madarosis — *see* Madarosis
    specified type NEC H02.79
    vitiligo — *see* Vitiligo, eyelid
    xanthelasma — *see* Xanthelasma
  dermatochalasis — *see* Dermatochalasis
  edema — *see* Edema, eyelid
  elephantiasis — *see* Elephantiasis, eyelid
  foreign body, retained — *see* Foreign body, retained, eyelid
  function H02.59
    abnormal innervation syndrome — *see* Syndrome, abnormal innervation
    blepharochalasis — *see* Blepharochalasis
    blepharoclonus — *see* Blepharoclonus
    blepharophimosis — *see* Blepharophimosis
    blepharoptosis — *see* Blepharoptosis
    lagophthalmos — *see* Lagophthalmos
    lid retraction — *see* Retraction, lid

Disorder (of) - *continued*
eyelid - *continued*
  hypertrichosis — *see* Hypertrichosis, eyelid
  specified type NEC H02.89
  vascular H02.879
    left H02.876
      lower H02.875
      upper H02.874
    right H02.873
      lower H02.872
      upper H02.871
factitious F68.10
  with predominantly
    psychological symptoms F68.11
      with physical symptoms F68.13
    physical symptoms F68.12
      with psychological symptoms F68.13
factor, coagulation — *see* Defect, coagulation
fatty acid
  metabolism E71.30
    specified NEC E71.39
  oxidation
    LCAD E71.310
    MCAD E71.311
    SCAD E71.312
    specified deficiency NEC E71.318
feeding (infant or child) — *see also* Disorder, eating R63.3
feigned (with obvious motivation) Z76.5
  without obvious motivation — *see* Disorder, factitious
female
  hypoactive sexual desire F52.0
  orgasmic F52.31
  sexual arousal F52.22
fibroblastic M72.9
  specified NEC M72.8
fluency
  adult onset F98.5
  childhood onset F80.81
  following
    cerebral infarction I69.323
    cerebrovascular disease I69.923
      specified disease NEC I69.823
    intracerebral hemorrhage I69.123
    nontraumatic intracranial hemorrhage NEC I69.223
    subarachnoid hemorrhage I69.023
  in conditions classified elsewhere R47.82
fluid balance E87.8
follicular (skin) L73.9
  specified NEC L73.8
fructose metabolism E74.10
  essential fructosuria E74.11
  fructokinase deficiency E74.11
  fructose-1, 6-diphosphatase deficiency E74.19
  hereditary fructose intolerance E74.12
  other specified E74.19
functional polymorphonuclear neutrophils D71
gallbladder, biliary tract and pancreas in diseases classified elsewhere K87
gamma-glutamyl cycle E72.8
gastric (functional) K31.9
  motility K30
  psychogenic F45.8
  secretion K30
gastrointestinal (functional) NOS K92.9
  newborn P78.9
  psychogenic F45.8
gender-identity or -role F64.9
  childhood F64.2
  effect on relationship F66
  of adolescence or adulthood F64.0
    nontranssexual F64.8
  specified NEC F64.8
  uncertainty F66
genito-pelvic pain penetration F52.6
genitourinary system
  female N94.9
  male N50.9
  psychogenic F45.8
globe H44.9
  degenerated condition H44.50
    absolute glaucoma H44.51-
    atrophy H44.52-
    leucocoria H44.53-
  degenerative H44.30
    chalcosis H44.31-
    myopia H44.2-
    siderosis H44.32-
    specified type NEC H44.39-
  endophthalmitis — *see* Endophthalmitis

Disorder (of) - *continued*
globe - *continued*
  foreign body, retained — *see* Foreign body, intraocular, old, retained
  hemophthalmos — *see* Hemophthalmos
  hypotony H44.40
    due to
      ocular fistula H44.42-
      specified disorder NEC H44.43-
    flat anterior chamber H44.41-
    primary H44.44-
  luxation — *see* Luxation, globe
  specified type NEC H44.89
glomerular (in) N05.9
  amyloidosis E85.4 *[N08]*
  cryoglobulinemia D89.1 *[N08]*
  disseminated intravascular coagulation D65 *[N08]*
  Fabry's disease E75.21 *[N08]*
  familial lecithin cholesterol acyltransferase deficiency E78.6 *[N08]*
  Goodpasture's syndrome M31.0
  hemolytic-uremic syndrome D59.3
  Henoch (-Schönlein) purpura D69.0 *[N08]*
  malariae malaria B52.0
  microscopic polyangiitis M31.7 *[N08]*
  multiple myeloma C90.0- *[N08]*
  mumps B26.83
  schistosomiasis B65.9 *[N08]*
  sepsis NEC A41.- *[N08]*
    streptococcal A40.- *[N08]*
  sickle-cell disorders D57.- *[N08]*
  strongyloidiasis B78.9 *[N08]*
  subacute bacterial endocarditis I33.0 *[N08]*
  syphilis A52.75
  systemic lupus erythematosus M32.14
  thrombotic thrombocytopenic purpura M31.1 *[N08]*
  Waldenström macroglobulinemia C88.0 *[N08]*
  Wegener's granulomatosis M31.31
gluconeogenesis E74.4
glucosaminoglycan metabolism — *see* Disorder, metabolism, glucosaminoglycan
glycine metabolism E72.50
  d-glycericacidemia E72.59
  hyperhydroxyprolinemia E72.59
  hyperoxaluria E72.53
  hyperprolinemia E72.59
  non-ketotic hyperglycinemia E72.51
  oxalosis E72.53
  oxaluria E72.53
  sarcosinemia E72.59
  trimethylaminuria E72.52
glycoprotein metabolism E77.9
  specified NEC E77.8
habit (and impulse) F63.9
  involving sexual behavior NEC F65.9
  specified NEC F63.89
hallucinogen use
  mild F16.10
    with
      hallucinogen-induced
        anxiety disorder F16.180
        bipolar and related disorder F16.14
        depressive disorder F16.14
        psychotic disorder F16.159
      hallucinogen intoxication delirium F16.121
      other hallucinogen intoxication F16.129
  moderate or severe F16.20
    with
      hallucinogen-induced
        anxiety disorder F16.280
        bipolar and related disorder F16.24
        depressive disorder F16.24
        psychotic disorder F16.259
      hallucinogen intoxication delirium F16.221
      other hallucinogen intoxication F16.229
heart action I49.9
hematological D75.9
  newborn (transient) P61.9
    specified NEC P61.8
hematopoietic organs D75.9
hemorrhagic NEC D69.9
  drug-induced D68.32
  due to
    extrinsic circulating anticoagulants D68.32
      increase in
        anti-IIa D68.32
        anti-Xa D68.32
    intrinsic
      circulating anticoagulants D68.318
        increase in
          antithrombin D68.318
          anti-VIIIa D68.318

Disorder (of) - *continued*
hemorrhagic NEC - *continued*
  due to - *continued*
    intrinsic - *continued*
      increase in - *continued*
        anti-IXa D68.318
        anti-XIa D68.318
    following childbirth O72.3
  hemostasis — *see* Defect, coagulation
histidine metabolism E70.40
  histidinemia E70.41
  other specified E70.49
hoarding F42.3
hyperkinetic — *see* Disorder, attention-deficit
  hyperactivity
hyperleucine-isoleucinemia E71.19
hypervalinemia E71.19
hypoactive sexual desire F52.0
hypochondriacal F45.20
  body dysmorphic F45.22
  neurosis F45.21
  other specified F45.29
identity
  dissociative F44.81
  of childhood F93.8
  illness anxiety F45.21
immune mechanism (immunity) D89.9
  specified type NEC D89.89
impaired renal tubular function N25.9
  specified NEC N25.89
impulse (control) F63.9
inflammatory
  pelvic, in diseases classified elsewhere — *see*
    category N74
  penis N48.29
    abscess N48.21
    cellulitis N48.22
inhalant use
  mild F18.10
    with
      inhalant-induced
        anxiety disorder F18.180
        depressive disorder F18.14
        major neurocognitive disorder F18.17
        mild neurocognitive disorder F18.188
        psychotic disorder F18.159
      inhalant intoxication F18.129
      inhalant intoxication delirium F18.121
  moderate or severe F18.20
    with
      inhalant-induced
        anxiety disorder F18.280
        depressive disorder F18.24
        major neurocognitive disorder F18.27
        mild neurocognitive disorder F18.288
        psychotic disorder F18.259
      inhalant intoxication F18.229
      inhalant intoxication delirium F18.221
integument, newborn P83.9
  specified NEC P83.8
intermittent explosive F63.81
internal secretion pancreas — *see* Increased,
  secretion, pancreas, endocrine
intestine, intestinal
  carbohydrate absorption NEC E74.39
    postoperative K91.2
  functional NEC K59.9
    postoperative K91.89
  psychogenic F45.8
  vascular K55.9
    chronic K55.1
    specified NEC K55.8
intraoperative (intraprocedural) — *see*
  Complications, intraoperative
involuntary emotional expression (IEED) F48.2
iris H21.9
  adhesions — *see* Adhesions, iris
  atrophy — *see* Atrophy, iris
  chamber angle recession — *see* Recession,
    chamber angle
  cyst — *see* Cyst, iris
  degeneration — *see* Degeneration, iris
  in diseases classified elsewhere H22
  iridodialysis — *see* Iridodialysis
  iridoschisis — *see* Iridoschisis
  miotic pupillary cyst — *see* Cyst, pupillary
  pupillary
    abnormality — *see* Abnormality, pupillary
    membrane — *see* Membrane, pupillary
  specified type NEC H21.89
  vascular NEC H21.1X-
iron metabolism E83.10
  specified NEC E83.19

Disorder (of) - *continued*
isovaleric acidemia E71.110
jaw, developmental M27.0
  temporomandibular — *see also* Anomaly,
    dentofacial, temporomandibular joint M26.60-
joint M25.9
  derangement — *see* Derangement, joint
  effusion — *see* Effusion, joint
  fistula — *see* Fistula, joint
  hemarthrosis — *see* Hemarthrosis
  instability — *see* Instability, joint
  osteophyte — *see* Osteophyte
  pain — *see* Pain, joint
  psychogenic F45.8
  specified type NEC M25.80
    ankle M25.87-
    elbow M25.82-
    foot joint M25.87-
    hand joint M25.84-
    hip M25.85-
    knee M25.86-
    shoulder M25.81-
    wrist M25.83-
  stiffness — *see* Stiffness, joint
ketone metabolism E71.32
kidney N28.9
  functional (tubular) N25.9
  in
    schistosomiasis B65.9 *[N29]*
  tubular function N25.9
    specified NEC N25.89
lacrimal system H04.9
  changes H04.69
  fistula — *see* Fistula, lacrimal
  gland H04.19
    atrophy — *see* Atrophy, lacrimal gland
    cyst — *see* Cyst, lacrimal, gland
    dacryops — *see* Dacryops
    dislocation — *see* Dislocation, lacrimal gland
    dry eye syndrome — *see* Syndrome, dry eye
    infection — *see* Dacryoadenitis
  granuloma — *see* Granuloma, lacrimal
  inflammation — *see* Inflammation, lacrimal
  obstruction — *see* Obstruction, lacrimal
  specified NEC H04.89
lactation NEC O92.79
language (developmental) F80.9
  expressive F80.1
  mixed receptive and expressive F80.2
  receptive F80.2
late luteal phase dysphoric N94.89
learning (specific) F81.9
  acalculia R48.8
  alexia R48.0
  mathematics F81.2
  reading F81.0
  specified NEC F81.89
  spelling F81.81
  written expression F81.81
lens H27.9
  aphakia — *see* Aphakia
  cataract — *see* Cataract
  dislocation — *see* Dislocation, lens
  specified type NEC H27.8
ligament M24.20
  ankle M24.27-
  attachment, spine — *see* Enthesopathy, spinal
  elbow M24.22-
  foot joint M24.27-
  hand joint M24.24-
  hip M24.25-
  knee — *see* Derangement, knee, specified NEC
  shoulder M24.21-
  vertebra M24.28
  wrist M24.23-
ligamentous attachments — *see also* Enthesopathy
  spine — *see* Enthesopathy, spinal
lipid
  metabolism, congenital E78.9
  storage E75.6
    specified NEC E75.5
lipoprotein
  deficiency (familial) E78.6
  metabolism E78.9
    specified NEC E78.89
liver K76.9
  malarial B54 *[K77]*
low back — *see also* Dorsopathy, specified NEC
lumbosacral
  plexus G54.1
  root (nerve) NEC G54.4
lung, interstitial, drug-induced J70.4
  acute J70.2

Disorder (of) - *continued*
lung, interstitial, drug-induced - *continued*
  chronic J70.3
lymphoproliferative, post-transplant (PTLD) D47.Z1
lysine and hydroxylysine metabolism E72.3
major neurocognitive — *see* Dementia, in (due to)
male
  erectile (organic) — *see also* Dysfunction, sexual,
    male, erectile N52.9
    nonorganic F52.21
  hypoactive sexual desire F52.0
  orgasmic F52.32
manic F30.9
  organic F06.33
mast cell activation — *see* Activation, mast cell
mastoid — *see also* Disorder, ear, middle
  postprocedural — *see* Complications, ear,
    procedure
meniscus — *see* Derangement, knee, meniscus
menopausal N95.9
  specified NEC N95.8
menstrual N92.6
  psychogenic F45.8
  specified NEC N92.5
mental (or behavioral) (nonpsychotic) F99
  due to (secondary to)
    amphetamine
      due to drug abuse — *see* Abuse, drug, stimulant
      due to drug dependence — *see* Dependence,
        drug, stimulant
    brain disease, damage and dysfunction F09
    caffeine use
      due to drug abuse — *see* Abuse, drug, stimulant
      due to drug dependence — *see* Dependence,
        drug, stimulant
    cannabis use
      due to drug abuse — *see* Abuse, drug, cannabis
      due to drug dependence — *see* Dependence,
        drug, cannabis
    general medical condition F09
    sedative or hypnotic use
      due to drug abuse — *see* Abuse, drug, sedative
      due to drug dependence — *see* Dependence,
        drug, sedative
    tobacco (nicotine) use — *see* Dependence, drug,
      nicotine
  following organic brain damage F07.9
    frontal lobe syndrome F07.0
    personality change F07.0
    postconcussional syndrome F07.81
    specified NEC F07.89
  infancy, childhood or adolescence F98.9
  neurotic — *see* Neurosis
  organic or symptomatic F09
  presenile, psychotic F03
  problem NEC
  psychoneurotic — *see* Neurosis
  psychotic — *see* Psychosis
  puerperal F53
  senile, psychotic NEC F03
metabolic, amino acid, transitory, newborn P74.8
metabolism NOS E88.9
  amino-acid E72.9
    aromatic E70.9
      albinism — *see* Albinism
      histidine E70.40
        histidinemia E70.41
        other specified E70.49
      hyperphenylalaninemia E70.1
        classical phenylketonuria E70.0
      other specified E70.8
      tryptophan E70.5
      tyrosine E70.20
        hypertyrosinemia E70.21
        other specified E70.29
    branched chain E71.2
      3-methylglutaconic aciduria E71.111
      hyperleucine-isoleucinemia E71.19
      hypervalinemia E71.19
      isovaleric acidemia E71.110
      maple syrup urine disease E71.0
      methylmalonic acidemia E71.120
      organic aciduria NEC E71.118
      other specified E71.19
      propionate NEC E71.128
      propronic acidemia E71.121
    glycine E72.50
      d-glycericacidemia E72.59
      hyperhydroxyprolinemia E72.59
      hyperoxaluria E72.53
      hyperprolinemia E72.59
      non-ketotic hyperglycinemia E72.51
      other specified E72.59

Disorder (of) - *continued*
  metabolism NOS - *continued*
    amino-acid - *continued*
      glycine - *continued*
        sarcosinemia E72.59
        trimethylaminuria E72.52
      hydroxylysine E72.3
      lysine E72.3
      ornithine E72.4
      other specified E72.8
        beta-amino acid E72.8
        gamma-glutamyl cycle E72.8
        straight-chain E72.8
        sulfur-bearing E72.10
          homocystinuria E72.11
          methylenetetrahydrofolate reductase
            deficiency E72.12
          other specified E72.19
    bile acid and cholesterol metabolism E78.70
    bilirubin E80.7
      specified NEC E80.6
    calcium E83.50
      hypercalcemia E83.52
      hypocalcemia E83.51
      other specified E83.59
    carbohydrate E74.9
      specified NEC E74.8
    cholesterol and bile acid metabolism E78.70
    congenital E88.9
    copper E83.00
      Wilson's disease E83.01
      specified type NEC E83.09
    cystinuria E72.01
    fructose E74.10
    galactose E74.20
    glucosaminoglycan E76.9
      mucopolysaccharidosis — *see*
        Mucopolysaccharidosis
      specified NEC E76.8
    glutamine E72.8
    glycine E72.50
    glycogen storage (hepatorenal) E74.09
    glycoprotein E77.9
      specified NEC E77.8
    glycosaminoglycan E76.9
      specified NEC E76.8
    in labor and delivery O75.89
    iron E83.10
    isoleucine E71.19
    leucine E71.19
    lipoid E78.9
    lipoprotein E78.9
      specified NEC E78.89
    magnesium E83.40
      hypermagnesemia E83.41
      hypomagnesemia E83.42
      other specified E83.49
    mineral E83.9
      specified NEC E83.89
    mitochondrial E88.40
      MELAS syndrome E88.41
      MERRF syndrome (myoclonic epilepsy
        associated with ragged-red fibers) E88.42
      other specified E88.49
    ornithine E72.4
    phosphatases E83.30
    phosphorus E83.30
      acid phosphatase deficiency E83.39
      hypophosphatasia E83.39
      hypophosphatemia E83.39
        familial E83.31
      other specified E83.39
      pseudovitamin D deficiency E83.32
    plasma protein NEC E88.09
    porphyrin — *see* Porphyria
    postprocedural E89.89
      specified NEC E89.89
    purine E79.9
      specified NEC E79.8
    pyrimidine E79.9
      specified NEC E79.8
    pyruvate E74.4
    serine E72.8
    sodium E87.8
      specified NEC E88.89
    threonine E72.8
    valine E71.19
    zinc E83.2
  methylmalonic acidemia E71.120
  micturition NEC — *see also* Difficulty,
    micturition R39.198
    feeling of incomplete emptying R39.14
    hesitancy R39.11

Disorder (of) - *continued*
  micturition NEC - *continued*
    poor stream R39.12
    psychogenic F45.8
    split stream R39.13
    straining R39.16
    urgency R39.15
  mild neurocognitive G31.84
  mitochondrial metabolism E88.40
  mitral (valve) — *see* Endocarditis, mitral
  mixed
    anxiety and depressive F41.8
    of scholastic skills (developmental) F81.89
    receptive expressive language F80.2
  mood F39
    bipolar — *see* Disorder, bipolar
    depressive — *see* Disorder, depressive
    due to (secondary to)
      alcohol F10.94
      amphetamine F15.94
        in
          abuse F15.14
          dependence F15.24
      anxiolytic F13.94
        in
          abuse F13.14
          dependence F13.24
      cocaine F14.94
        in
          abuse F14.14
          dependence F14.24
      general medical condition F06.30
      hallucinogen F16.94
        in
          abuse F16.14
          dependence F16.24
      hypnotic F13.94
        in
          abuse F13.14
          dependence F13.24
      inhalant F18.94
        in
          abuse F18.14
          dependence F18.24
      opioid F11.94
        in
          abuse F11.14
          dependence F11.24
      phencyclidine (PCP) F16.94
        in
          abuse F16.14
          dependence F16.24
      physiological condition F06.30
        with
          depressive features F06.31
          major depressive-like episode F06.32
          manic features F06.33
          mixed features F06.34
      psychoactive substance NEC F19.94
        in
          abuse F19.14
          dependence F19.24
      sedative F13.94
        in
          abuse F13.14
          dependence F13.24
      volatile solvents F18.94
        in
          abuse F18.14
          dependence F18.24
    manic episode F30.9
      with psychotic symptoms F30.2
      in remission (full) F30.4
        partial F30.3
      specified type NEC F30.8
      without psychotic symptoms F30.10
        mild F30.11
        moderate F30.12
        severe F30.13
    organic F06.30
      right hemisphere F07.89
    persistent F34.9
      cyclothymia F34.0
      dysthymia F34.1
      specified type NEC F34.89
    recurrent F39
    right hemisphere organic F07.89
  movement G25.9
    drug-induced G25.70
      akathisia G25.71
      specified NEC G25.79
    hysterical F44.4

Disorder (of) - *continued*
  movement - *continued*
    in diseases classified elsewhere — *see* category
      G26
    periodic limb G47.61
      sleep related G47.61
    specified NEC G25.89
    sleep related NEC G47.69
    stereotyped F98.4
    treatment-induced G25.9
  multiple personality F44.81
  muscle M62.9
    attachment, spine — *see* Enthesopathy, spinal
    in trichinellosis — *see* Trichinellosis, with muscle
      disorder
    psychogenic F45.8
    specified type NEC M62.89
    tone, newborn P94.9
      specified NEC P94.8
  muscular
    attachments — *see also* Enthesopathy
      spine — *see* Enthesopathy, spinal
    urethra N36.44
  musculoskeletal system, soft tissue — *see* Disorder,
    soft tissue
    postprocedural M96.89
    psychogenic F45.8
  myoneural G70.9
    due to lead G70.1
    specified NEC G70.89
    toxic G70.1
  myotonic NEC G71.19
  nail, in diseases classified elsewhere L62
  neck region NEC — *see* Dorsopathy, specified NEC
  neonatal onset multisystemic inflammatory
    (NOMID) M04.2
  nerve G58.9
    abducent NEC — *see* Strabismus, paralytic, sixth
      nerve
    accessory G52.8
    acoustic — *see* subcategory H93.3
    auditory — *see* subcategory H93.3
    auriculotemporal G50.8
    axillary G54.0
    cerebral — *see* Disorder, nerve, cranial
    cranial G52.9
      eighth — *see* subcategory H93.3
      eleventh G52.8
      fifth G50.9
      first G52.0
      fourth NEC — *see* Strabismus, paralytic, fourth
        nerve
      multiple G52.7
      ninth G52.1
      second NEC — *see* Disorder, nerve, optic
      seventh NEC G51.8
      sixth NEC — *see* Strabismus, paralytic, sixth
        nerve
      specified NEC G52.8
      tenth G52.2
      third NEC — *see* Strabismus, paralytic, third
        nerve
      twelfth G52.3
    entrapment — *see* Neuropathy, entrapment
    facial G51.9
      specified NEC G51.8
    femoral — *see* Lesion, nerve, femoral
    glossopharyngeal NEC G52.1
    hypoglossal G52.3
    intercostal G58.0
    lateral
      cutaneous of thigh — *see* Mononeuropathy, lower
        limb, meralgia paresthetica
      popliteal — *see* Lesion, nerve, popliteal
    lower limb — *see* Mononeuropathy, lower limb
    medial popliteal — *see* Lesion, nerve, popliteal,
      medial
    median NEC — *see* Lesion, nerve, median
    multiple G58.7
    oculomotor NEC — *see* Strabismus, paralytic,
      third nerve
    olfactory G52.0
    optic NEC H47.09-
      hemorrhage into sheath — *see* Hemorrhage, optic
        nerve
      ischemic H47.01-
    peroneal — *see* Lesion, nerve, popliteal
    phrenic G58.8
    plantar — *see* Lesion, nerve, plantar
    pneumogastric G52.2
    posterior tibial — *see* Syndrome, tarsal tunnel
    radial — *see* Lesion, nerve, radial
    recurrent laryngeal G52.2

Disorder (of) - *continued*
 nerve - *continued*
  root G54.9
   cervical G54.2
   lumbosacral G54.1
   specified NEC G54.8
   thoracic G54.3
  sciatic NEC — *see* Lesion, nerve, sciatic
  specified NEC G58.8
   lower limb — *see* Mononeuropathy, lower limb,
    specified NEC
   upper limb — *see* Mononeuropathy, upper limb,
    specified NEC
  sympathetic G90.9
  tibial –- *see* Lesion, nerve, popliteal, medial
  trigeminal G50.9
   specified NEC G50.8
  trochlear NEC — *see* Strabismus, paralytic, fourth
    nerve — *see* Lesion, nerve, ulnar
  ulnar — *see* Lesion, nerve, ulnar
  upper limb — *see* Mononeuropathy, upper limb
  vagus G52.2
 nervous system G98.8
  autonomic (peripheral) G90.9
   specified NEC G90.8
  central G96.9
   specified NEC G96.8
  parasympathetic G90.9
   specified NEC G98.8
  sympathetic G90.9
  vegetative G90.9
 neurocognitive
  major
   with
    aggressive behavior F01.51
    combative behavior F01.51
    violent behavior F01.51
   due to vascular disease, with behavioral
     disturbance F01.51
   in (due to) (other diseases classified
     elsewhere) — *see also* Dementia, in (due
     to) F02.80
    with
     aggressive behavior F02.81
     combative behavior F02.81
     violent behavior F02.81
    without behavioral disturbance F01.50
  mild G31.84
 neurodevelopmental F89
  specified NEC F88
 neurohypophysis NEC E23.3
 neurological NEC R29.818
 neuromuscular G70.9
  hereditary NEC G71.9
  specified NEC G70.89
  toxic G70.1
 neurotic F48.9
  specified NEC F48.8
 neutrophil, polymorphonuclear D71
 nicotine use — *see* Dependence, drug, nicotine
 nightmare F51.5
 nose J34.9
  specified NEC J34.89
 obsessive-compulsive F42.9
 odontogenesis NOS K00.9
 opioid use
  with
   opioid-induced psychotic disorder F11.959
    with
     delusions F11.950
     hallucinations F11.951
  due to drug abuse — *see* Abuse, drug, opioid
  due to drug dependence — *see* Dependence, drug,
    opioid
  mild F11.10
   with
    opioid-induced
     anxiety disorder F11.188
     depressive disorder F11.14
     sexual dysfunction F11.181
    opioid intoxication
     with perceptual disturbances F11.122
     delirium F11.121
     without perceptual disturbances F11.129
   moderate or severe F11.20
    with
     opioid-induced
      anxiety disorder F11.288
      anxiety disorder F11.988
      depressive disorder F11.24
      depressive disorder F11.94
      sexual dysfunction F11.281
      sexual dysfunction F11.981

Disorder (of) - *continued*
 opioid use - *continued*
  moderate or severe - *continued*
   with - *continued*
    opioid intoxication
     with perceptual disturbances F11.222
     delirium F11.221
     without perceptual disturbances F11.229
 oppositional defiant F91.3
 optic
  chiasm H47.49
   due to
    inflammatory disorder H47.41
    neoplasm H47.42
    vascular disorder H47.43
  disc H47.39-
   coloboma — *see* Coloboma, optic disc
   drusen — *see* Drusen, optic disc
   pseudopapilledema — *see* Pseudopapilledema
  radiations — *see* Disorder, visual, pathway
  tracts — *see* Disorder, visual, pathway
 orbit H05.9
  cyst — *see* Cyst, orbit
  deformity — *see* Deformity, orbit
  edema — *see* Edema, orbit
  enophthalmos — *see* Enophthalmos
  exophthalmos — *see* Exophthalmos
  hemorrhage — *see* Hemorrhage, orbit
  inflammation — *see* Inflammation, orbit
  myopathy — *see* Myopathy, extraocular muscles
  retained foreign body — *see* Foreign body, orbit,
    old
  specified type NEC H05.89
 organic
  anxiety F06.4
  catatonic F06.1
  delusional F06.2
  dissociative F06.8
  emotionally labile (asthenic) F06.8
  mood (affective) F06.30
  schizophrenia-like F06.2
 orgasmic (female) F52.31
  male F52.32
 ornithine metabolism E72.4
 overanxious F41.1
  of childhood F93.8
 pain
  with related psychological factors F45.42
  exclusively related to psychological factors F45.41
  genito-pelvic penetration disorder F52.6
 pancreatic internal secretion E16.9
  specified NEC E16.8
 panic F41.0
  with agoraphobia F40.01
 papulosquamous L44.9
  in diseases classified elsewhere L45
  specified NEC L44.8
 paranoid F22
  induced F24
  shared F24
 parathyroid (gland) E21.5
  specified NEC E21.4
 parietoalveolar NEC J84.09
 paroxysmal, mixed R56.9
 patella M22.9-
  chondromalacia — *see* Chondromalacia, patella
  derangement NEC M22.3X-
  recurrent
   dislocation — *see* Dislocation, patella, recurrent
   subluxation — *see* Dislocation, patella, recurrent,
     incomplete
  specified NEC M22.8X-
 patellofemoral M22.2X-
 pentose phosphate pathway with anemia D55.1
 perception, due to hallucinogens F16.983
  in
   abuse F16.183
   dependence F16.283
 peripheral nervous system NEC G64
 peroxisomal E71.50
  biogenesis
   neonatal adrenoleukodystrophy E71.511
   specified disorder NEC E71.518
   Zellweger syndrome E71.510
  rhizomelic chondrodysplasia punctata E71.540
  specified form NEC E71.548
   group 1 E71.518
   group 2 E71.53
   group 3 E71.542
  X-linked adrenoleukodystrophy E71.529
   adolescent E71.521
   adrenomyeloneuropathy E71.522
   childhood E71.520

Disorder (of) - *continued*
 peroxisomal - *continued*
  X-linked adrenoleukodystrophy - *continued*
   specified form NEC E71.528
  Zellweger-like syndrome E71.541
 persistent
  (somatoform) pain F45.41
  affective (mood) F34.9
 personality — *see also* Personality F60.9
  affective F34.0
  aggressive F60.3
  amoral F60.2
  anankastic F60.5
  antisocial F60.2
  anxious F60.6
  asocial F60.2
  asthenic F60.7
  avoidant F60.6
  borderline F60.3
  change (secondary) due to general medical
    condition F07.0
  compulsive F60.5
  cyclothymic F34.0
  dependent (passive) F60.7
  depressive F34.1
  dissocial F60.2
  emotional instability F60.3
  expansive paranoid F60.0
  explosive F60.3
  following organic brain damage F07.9
  histrionic F60.4
  hyperthymic F34.0
  hypothymic F34.1
  hysterical F60.4
  immature F60.89
  inadequate F60.7
  labile F60.3
  mixed (nonspecific) F60.89
  moral deficiency F60.2
  narcissistic F60.81
  negativistic F60.89
  obsessional F60.5
  obsessive (-compulsive) F60.5
  organic F07.9
  overconscientious F60.5
  paranoid F60.0
  passive (-dependent) F60.7
  passive-aggressive F60.89
  pathological NEC F60.9
  pseudosocial F60.2
  psychopathic F60.2
  schizoid F60.1
  schizotypal F21
  self-defeating F60.7
  specified NEC F60.89
  type A F60.5
  unstable (emotional) F60.3
 pervasive, developmental F84.9
 phencyclidine use
  mild F16.10
   with
    phencyclidine-induced
     anxiety disorder F16.180
     bipolar and related disorder F16.14
     depressive disorder F16.14
     psychotic disorder F16.159
    phencyclidine intoxication F16.129
    phencyclidine intoxication delirium F16.121
  moderate or severe F16.20
   with
    phencyclidine-induced
     anxiety disorder F16.280
     bipolar and related disorder F16.24
     depressive disorder F16.24
     psychotic disorder F16.259
    phencyclidine intoxication F16.229
    phencyclidine intoxication delirium F16.221
 phobic anxiety, childhood F40.8
 phosphate-losing tubular N25.0
 pigmentation L81.9
  choroid, congenital Q14.3
  diminished melanin formation L81.6
  iron L81.8
  specified NEC L81.8
 pinna (noninfective) H61.10-
  deformity, acquired H61.11-
  hematoma H61.12-
  perichondritis — *see* Perichondritis, ear
  specified type NEC H61.19-
 pituitary gland E23.7
  iatrogenic (postprocedural) E89.3
  specified NEC E23.6
 platelets D69.1

Disorder (of) - *continued*
plexus G54.9
  specified NEC G54.8
polymorphonuclear neutrophils D71
porphyrin metabolism — *see* Porphyria
postconcussional F07.81
posthallucinogen perception F16.983
  in
    abuse F16.183
    dependence F16.283
postmenopausal N95.9
  specified NEC N95.8
postprocedural (postoperative) — *see*
  Complications, postprocedural
post-transplant lymphoproliferative D47.Z1
post-traumatic stress (PTSD) F43.10
  acute F43.11
  chronic F43.12
premenstrual dysphoric (PMDD) F32.81
prepuce N47.8
propionic acidemia E71.121
prostate N42.9
  specified NEC N42.89
psychogenic NOS — *see also* condition F45.9
  anxiety F41.8
  appetite F50.9
  asthenic F48.8
  cardiovascular (system) F45.8
  compulsive F42.8
  cutaneous F54
  depressive F32.9
  digestive (system) F45.8
  dysmenorrheic F45.8
  dyspneic F45.8
  endocrine (system) F54
  eye NEC F45.8
  feeding — *see* Disorder, eating
  functional NEC F45.8
  gastric F45.8
  gastrointestinal (system) F45.8
  genitourinary (system) F45.8
  heart (function) (rhythm) F45.8
  hyperventilatory F45.8
  hypochondriacal — *see* Disorder, hypochondriacal
  intestinal F45.8
  joint F45.8
  learning F81.9
  limb F45.8
  lymphatic (system) F45.8
  menstrual F45.8
  micturition F45.8
  monoplegic NEC F44.4
  motor F44.4
  muscle F45.8
  musculoskeletal F45.8
  neurocirculatory F45.8
  obsessive F42.8
  occupational F48.8
  organ or part of body NEC F45.8
  paralytic NEC F44.4
  phobic F40.9
  physical NEC F45.8
  rectal F45.8
  respiratory (system) F45.8
  rheumatic F45.8
  sexual (function) F52.9
  skin (allergic) (eczematous) F54
  sleep F51.9
  specified part of body NEC F45.8
  stomach F45.8
psychological F99
  associated with
    disease classified elsewhere F54
    sexual
      development F66
      relationship F66
      uncertainty about gender identity F64.9
psychomotor NEC F44.4
  hysterical F44.4
psychoneurotic — *see also* Neurosis
  mixed NEC F48.8
psychophysiologic — *see* Disorder, somatoform
psychosexual F65.9
  development F66
  identity of childhood F64.2
psychosomatic NOS — *see* Disorder, somatoform
  multiple F45.0
  undifferentiated F45.1
psychotic — *see* Psychosis
  transient (acute) F23
puberty E30.9
  specified NEC E30.8
pulmonary (valve) — *see* Endocarditis, pulmonary

Disorder (of) - *continued*
purine metabolism E79.9
pyrimidine metabolism E79.9
pyruvate metabolism E74.4
reactive attachment (childhood) F94.1
reading R48.0
  developmental (specific) F81.0
receptive language F80.2
receptor, hormonal, peripheral — *see
also* Syndrome, androgen insensitivity E34.50
recurrent brief depressive F33.8
reflex R29.2
refraction H52.7
  aniseikonia H52.32
  anisometropia H52.31
  astigmatism — *see* Astigmatism
  hypermetropia — *see* Hypermetropia
  myopia — *see* Myopia
  presbyopia H52.4
  specified NEC H52.6
relationship F68.8
  due to sexual orientation F66
REM sleep behavior G47.52
renal function, impaired (tubular) N25.9
resonance R49.9
  specified NEC R49.8
respiratory function, impaired — *see also* Failure,
respiration
  postprocedural — *see* Complication, postoperative,
  respiratory system
  psychogenic F45.8
retina H35.9
  angioid streaks H35.33
  changes in vascular appearance H35.01-
  degeneration — *see* Degeneration, retina
  dystrophy (hereditary) — *see* Dystrophy, retina
  edema H35.81
  hemorrhage — *see* Hemorrhage, retina
  ischemia H35.82
  macular degeneration — *see* Degeneration, macula
  microaneurysms H35.04-
  microvascular abnormality NEC H35.09
  neovascularization — *see* Neovascularization,
  retina
  retinopathy — *see* Retinopathy
  separation of layers H35.70
    central serous chorioretinopathy H35.71-
    pigment epithelium detachment (serous) H35.72-
    hemorrhagic H35.73-
  specified type NEC H35.89
  telangiectasis — *see* Telangiectasis, retina
  vasculitis — *see* Vasculitis, retina
retroperitoneal K68.9
right hemisphere organic affective F07.89
rumination (infant or child) F98.21
sacrum, sacrococcygeal NEC M53.3
schizoaffective F25.9
  bipolar type F25.0
  depressive type F25.1
  manic type F25.0
  mixed type F25.0
  specified NEC F25.8
schizoid of childhood F84.5
schizophreniform F20.81
  brief F23
schizotypal (personality) F21
secretion, thyrocalcitonin E07.0
sedative, hypnotic, or anxiolytic use
  mild F13.10
    with
      sedative, hypnotic, or anxiolytic-induced
        anxiety disorder F13.180
        bipolar and related disorder F13.14
        depressive disorder F13.14
        psychotic disorder F13.159
        sexual dysfunction F13.181
      sedative, hypnotic, or anxiolytic
        intoxication F13.129
      sedative, hypnotic, or anxiolytic intoxication
        delirium F13.121
  moderate or severe F13.20
    with
      sedative, hypnotic, or anxiolytic-induced
        anxiety disorder F13.280
        bipolar and related disorder F13.24
        depressive disorder F13.24
        major neurocognitive disorder F13.27
        mild neurocognitive disorder F13.288
        psychotic disorder F13.259
        sexual dysfunction F13.281
      sedative, hypnotic, or anxiolytic
        intoxication F13.229

Disorder (of) - *continued*
sedative, hypnotic, or anxiolytic use - *continued*
  moderate or severe - *continued*
    with - *continued*
      sedative, hypnotic, or anxiolytic intoxication
        delirium F13.221
seizure — *see also* Epilepsy G40.909
  intractable G40.919
    with status epilepticus G40.911
semantic pragmatic F80.89
  with autism F84.0
sense of smell R43.1
  psychogenic F45.8
separation anxiety, of childhood F93.0
sexual
  arousal, female F52.22
  aversion F52.1
  function, psychogenic F52.9
  maturation F66
  nonorganic F52.9
  preference — *see also* Deviation, sexual F65.9
    fetishistic transvestism F65.1
  relationship F66
shyness, of childhood and adolescence F40.10
sibling rivalry F93.8
sickle-cell (sickling) (homozygous) — *see* Disease,
  sickle-cell
  heterozygous D57.3
  specified type NEC D57.8-
  trait D57.3
sinus (nasal) J34.9
  specified NEC J34.89
skin L98.9
  atrophic L90.9
    specified NEC L90.8
  granulomatous L92.9
    specified NEC L92.8
  hypertrophic L91.9
    specified NEC L91.8
  infiltrative NEC L98.6
  newborn P83.9
    specified NEC P83.8
  picking F42.4
  psychogenic (allergic) (eczematous) F54
sleep G47.9
  breathing-related — *see* Apnea, sleep
  circadian rhythm G47.20
    advance sleep phase type G47.22
    delayed sleep phase type G47.21
    due to
      alcohol
        abuse F10.182
        dependence F10.282
        use F10.982
      amphetamines
        abuse F15.182
        dependence F15.282
        use F15.982
      caffeine
        abuse F15.182
        dependence F15.282
        use F15.982
      cocaine
        abuse F14.182
        dependence F14.282
        use F14.982
      drug NEC
        abuse F19.182
        dependence F19.282
        use F19.982
      opioid
        abuse F11.182
        dependence F11.282
        use F11.982
      psychoactive substance NEC
        abuse F19.182
        dependence F19.282
        use F19.982
      sedative, hypnotic, or anxiolytic
        abuse F13.182
        dependence F13.282
        use F13.982
      stimulant NEC
        abuse F15.182
        dependence F15.282
        use F15.982
    free running type G47.24
    in conditions classified elsewhere G47.27
    irregular sleep wake type G47.23
    jet lag type G47.25
    shift work type G47.26
    specified NEC G47.29
  due to

Disorder (of) - *continued*
 sleep - *continued*
  due to - *continued*
   alcohol
    abuse F10.182
    dependence F10.282
    use F10.982
   amphetamine
    abuse F15.182
    dependence F15.282
    use F15.982
   anxiolytic
    abuse F13.182
    dependence F13.282
    use F13.982
   caffeine
    abuse F15.182
    dependence F15.282
    use F15.982
   cocaine
    abuse F14.182
    dependence F14.282
    use F14.982
   drug NEC
    abuse F19.182
    dependence F19.282
    use F19.982
   hypnotic
    abuse F13.182
    dependence F13.282
    use F13.982
   opioid
    abuse F11.182
    dependence F11.282
    use F11.982
   psychoactive substance NEC
    abuse F19.182
    dependence F19.282
    use F19.982
   sedative
    abuse F13.182
    dependence F13.282
    use F13.982
   stimulant NEC
    abuse F15.182
    dependence F15.282
    use F15.982
  emotional F51.9
  excessive somnolence — *see* Hypersomnia
  hypersomnia type — *see* Hypersomnia
  initiating or maintaining — *see* Insomnia
  nightmares F51.5
  nonorganic F51.9
   specified NEC F51.8
  parasomnia type G47.50
   specified NEC G47.8
  terrors F51.4
  walking F51.3
 sleep-wake pattern or schedule — *see* Disorder, sleep, circadian rhythm
 social
  anxiety of childhood F40.10
  functioning in childhood F94.9
   specified NEC F94.8
  pragmatic F80.82
 soft tissue M79.9
  ankle M79.9
  due to use, overuse and pressure M70.90
   ankle M70.97-
   bursitis — *see* Bursitis
   foot M70.97-
   forearm M70.93-
   hand M70.94-
   lower leg M70.96-
   multiple sites M70.99
   pelvic region M70.95-
   shoulder region M70.91-
   specified site NEC M70.98
   specified type NEC M70.80
    ankle M70.87-
    foot M70.87-
    forearm M70.83-
    hand M70.84-
    lower leg M70.86-
    multiple sites M70.89
    pelvic region M70.85-
    shoulder region M70.81-
    specified site NEC M70.88
    thigh M70.85-
    upper arm M70.82-
   thigh M70.95-
   upper arm M70.92-
  foot M79.9

Disorder (of) - *continued*
 soft tissue - *continued*
  forearm M79.9
  hand M79.9
  lower leg M79.9
  multiple sites M79.9
  occupational — *see* Disorder, soft tissue, due to use, overuse and pressure
  pelvic region M79.9
  shoulder region M79.9
  specified type NEC M79.89
  thigh M79.9
  upper arm M79.9
 somatic symptom F45.1
 somatization F45.0
 somatoform F45.9
  pain (persistent) F45.41
  somatization (multiple) (long-lasting) F45.0
  specified NEC F45.8
  undifferentiated F45.1
 somnolence, excessive — *see* Hypersomnia
 specific
  arithmetical F81.2
  developmental, of motor F82
  reading F81.0
  speech and language F80.9
  spelling F81.81
  written expression F81.81
 speech R47.9
  articulation (functional) (specific) F80.0
  developmental F80.9
  specified NEC R47.89
 speech-sound F80.0
 spelling (specific) F81.81
 spine — *see also* Dorsopathy
  ligamentous or muscular attachments, peripheral — *see* Enthesopathy, spinal
  specified NEC — *see* Dorsopathy, specified NEC
 stereotyped, habit or movement F98.4
 stimulant use (other) (unspecified)
  mild F15.10
  moderate or severe F15.20
 stomach (functional) — *see* Disorder, gastric
 stress F43.9
  acute F43.0
  post-traumatic F43.10
   acute F43.11
   chronic F43.12
 substance use (other) (unknown)
  mild F19.10
   with substance-induced
    anxiety disorder F19.180
    bipolar and related disorder F19.14
    depressive disorder F19.14
    major neurocognitive disorder F19.17
    mild neurocognitive disorder F19.188
    obsessive-compulsive and related disorder F19.188
    sexual dysfunction F19.181
    substance intoxication F19.129
    substance intoxication delirium F19.121
  moderate or severe F19.20
   with substance-induced
    anxiety disorder F19.280
    bipolar and related disorder F19.24
    depressive disorder F19.24
    major neurocognitive disorder F19.27
    mild neurocognitive disorder F19.288
    obsessive-compulsive and related disorder F19.288
    sexual dysfunction F19.281
    substance intoxication F19.229
    substance intoxication delirium F19.221
 sulfur-bearing amino-acid metabolism E72.10
 sweat gland (eccrine) L74.9
  apocrine L75.9
   specified NEC L75.8
  specified NEC L74.8
 synovium M67.90
  acromioclavicular M67.91-
  ankle M67.97-
  elbow M67.92-
  foot M67.97-
  forearm M67.93-
  hand M67.94-
  hip M67.95-
  knee M67.96-
  multiple sites M67.99
  rupture — *see* Rupture, synovium
  shoulder M67.91-
  specified type NEC M67.80
   acromioclavicular M67.81-
   ankle M67.87-

Disorder (of) - *continued*
 synovium - *continued*
  specified type NEC - *continued*
   elbow M67.82-
   foot M67.87-
   hand M67.84-
   hip M67.85-
   knee M67.86-
   multiple sites M67.89
   wrist M67.83-
  synovitis — *see* Synovitis
  upper arm M67.92-
  wrist M67.93-
 temperature regulation, newborn P81.9
  specified NEC P81.8
 temporomandibular joint M26.60-
 tendon M67.90
  acromioclavicular M67.91-
  ankle M67.97-
  contracture — *see* Contracture, tendon
  elbow M67.92-
  foot M67.97-
  forearm M67.93-
  hand M67.94-
  hip M67.95-
  knee M67.96-
  multiple sites M67.99
  rupture — *see* Rupture, tendon
  shoulder M67.91-
  specified type NEC M67.80
   acromioclavicular M67.81-
   ankle M67.87-
   elbow M67.82-
   foot M67.87-
   hand M67.84-
   hip M67.85-
   knee M67.86-
   multiple sites M67.89
   trunk M67.88
   wrist M67.83-
  synovitis — *see* Synovitis
  tendinitis — *see* Tendinitis
  tenosynovitis — *see* Tenosynovitis
  trunk M67.98
  upper arm M67.92-
  wrist M67.93-
 thoracic root (nerve) NEC G54.3
 thyrocalcitonin hypersecretion E07.0
 thyroid (gland) E07.9
  function NEC, neonatal, transitory P72.2
  iodine-deficiency related E01.8
  specified NEC E07.89
 tic — *see* Tic
 tobacco use
  mild Z72.0
  moderate F17.200
  severe F17.200
 tooth K08.9
  development K00.9
   specified NEC K00.8
  eruption K00.6
 Tourette's F95.2
 trance and possession F44.89
 trauma and stressor-related F43.9
  other specified F43.8
 tricuspid (valve) — *see* Endocarditis, tricuspid
 tryptophan metabolism E70.5
 tubular, phosphate-losing N25.0
 tubulo-interstitial (in)
  brucellosis A23.9 *[N16]*
  cystinosis E72.04
  diphtheria A36.84
  glycogen storage disease E74.00 *[N16]*
  leukemia NEC C95.9- *[N16]*
  lymphoma NEC C85.9- *[N16]*
  mixed cryoglobulinemia D89.1 *[N16]*
  multiple myeloma C90.0- *[N16]*
  Salmonella infection A02.25
  sarcoidosis D86.84
  sepsis A41.9 *[N16]*
   streptococcal A40.9 *[N16]*
  systemic lupus erythematosus M32.15
  toxoplasmosis B58.83
  transplant rejection T86.91 *[N16]*
  Wilson's disease E83.01 *[N16]*
 tubulo-renal function, impaired N25.9
  specified NEC N25.89
 tympanic membrane H73.9-
  atrophy — *see* Atrophy, tympanic membrane
  infection — *see* Myringitis
  perforation — *see* Perforation, tympanum
  specified NEC H73.89-
 unsocialized aggressive F91.1

Disorder (of) - *continued*
  urea cycle metabolism E72.20
    arginimemia E72.21
    arginosuccinic aciduria E72.22
    citrullinemia E72.23
    ornithine transcarbamylase deficiency E72.4
    other specified E72.29
  ureter (in) N28.9
    schistosomiasis B65.0 *[N29]*
    tuberculosis A18.11
  urethra N36.9
    specified NEC N36.8
  urinary system N39.9
    specified NEC N39.8
  valve, heart
    aortic — *see* Endocarditis, aortic
    mitral — *see* Endocarditis, mitral
    pulmonary — *see* Endocarditis, pulmonary
    rheumatic
      aortic — *see* Endocarditis, aortic, rheumatic
      mitral — *see* Endocarditis, mitral
      pulmonary — *see* Endocarditis, pulmonary, rheumatic
      tricuspid — *see* Endocarditis, tricuspid
    tricuspid — *see* Endocarditis, tricuspid
  vestibular function H81.9-
    specified NEC — *see* subcategory H81.8
    in diseases classified elsewhere H82.-
    vertigo — *see* Vertigo
  vision, binocular H53.30
    abnormal retinal correspondence H53.31
    diplopia H53.2
    fusion with defective stereopsis H53.32
    simultaneous perception H53.33
    suppression H53.34
  visual
    cortex
      blindness H47.619
        left brain H47.612
        right brain H47.611
      due to
        inflammatory disorder H47.629
          left brain H47.622
          right brain H47.621
        neoplasm H47.639
          left brain H47.632
          right brain H47.631
        vascular disorder H47.649
          left brain H47.642
          right brain H47.641
    pathway H47.9
      due to
        inflammatory disorder H47.51-
        neoplasm H47.52-
        vascular disorder H47.53-
    optic chiasm — *see* Disorder, optic, chiasm
  vitreous body H43.9
    crystalline deposits — *see* Deposit, crystalline
    degeneration — *see* Degeneration, vitreous
    hemorrhage — *see* Hemorrhage, vitreous
    opacities — *see* Opacity, vitreous
    prolapse — *see* Prolapse, vitreous
    specified type NEC H43.89
  voice R49.9
    specified type NEC R49.8
  volatile solvent use
    due to drug abuse — *see* Abuse, drug, inhalant
    due to drug dependence — *see* Dependence, drug, inhalant
  white blood cells D72.9
    specified NEC D72.89
  withdrawing, child or adolescent F40.10
Disorientation R41.0
Displacement, displaced
  acquired traumatic of bone, cartilage, joint, tendon NEC — *see* Dislocation
  adrenal gland (congenital) Q89.1
  appendix, retrocecal (congenital) Q43.8
  auricle (congenital) Q17.4
  bladder (acquired) N32.89
    congenital Q64.19
  brachial plexus (congenital) Q07.8
  brain stem, caudal (congenital) Q04.8
  canaliculus (lacrimalis) , congenital Q10.6
  cardia through esophageal hiatus (congenital) Q40.1
  cerebellum, caudal (congenital) Q04.8
  cervix — *see* Malposition, uterus
  colon (congenital) Q43.3
  device, implant or graft — *see also* Complications, by site and type, mechanical T85.628
    arterial graft NEC — *see* Complication, cardiovascular device, mechanical, vascular
    breast (implant) T85.42

Displacement, displaced - *continued*
  device, implant or graft - *continued*
    catheter NEC T85.628
      dialysis (renal) T82.42
        intraperitoneal T85.621
      infusion NEC T82.524
        spinal (epidural) (subdural) T85.620
      urinary
        cystostomy T83.020
        Hopkins T83.028
        ileostomy T83.028
        indwelling T83.021
        nephrostomy T83.022
        specified NEC T83.028
        urostomy T83.028
    electronic (electrode) (pulse generator) (stimulator) — *see* Complication, electronic stimulator
    fixation, internal (orthopedic) NEC — *see* Complication, fixation device, mechanical
    gastrointestinal — *see* Complications, prosthetic device, mechanical, gastrointestinal device
    genital NEC T83.428
      intrauterine contraceptive device (string) T83.32
      penile prosthesis (cylinder) (implanted) (pump) (resevoir) T83.420
      testicular prosthesis T83.421
    heart NEC — *see* Complication, cardiovascular device, mechanical
    joint prosthesis — *see* Complications, joint prosthesis, mechanical
    ocular — *see* Complications, prosthetic device, mechanical, ocular device
    orthopedic NEC — *see* Complication, orthopedic, device or graft, mechanical
    specified NEC T85.628
    urinary NEC T83.128
      graft T83.22
      sphincter, implanted T83.121
      stent (ileal conduit) (nephroureteral) T83.123
        ureteral indwelling T83.122
    vascular NEC — *see* Complication, cardiovascular device, mechanical
    ventricular intracranial shunt T85.02
  electronic stimulator
    bone T84.320
    cardiac — *see* Complications, cardiac device, electronic
    nervous system — *see* Complication, prosthetic device, mechanical, electronic nervous system stimulator
    urinary — *see* Complications, electronic stimulator, urinary
  esophageal mucosa into cardia of stomach, congenital Q39.8
  esophagus (acquired) K22.8
    congenital Q39.8
  eyeball (acquired) (lateral) (old) — *see* Displacement, globe
    congenital Q15.8
    current — *see* Avulsion, eye
  fallopian tube (acquired) N83.4-
    congenital Q50.6
    opening (congenital) Q50.6
  gallbladder (congenital) Q44.1
  gastric mucosa (congenital) Q40.2
  globe (acquired) (old) (lateral) H05.21-
    current — *see* Avulsion, eye
  heart (congenital) Q24.8
    acquired I51.89
  hymen (upward) (congenital) Q52.4
  intervertebral disc NEC
    with myelopathy — *see* Disorder, disc, with, myelopathy
    cervical, cervicothoracic (with) M50.20
      myelopathy — *see* Disorder, disc, cervical, with myelopathy
      neuritis, radiculitis or radiculopathy — *see* Disorder, disc, cervical, with neuritis
    due to trauma — *see* Dislocation, vertebra
    lumbar region M51.26
      with
        myelopathy M51.06
        neuritis, radiculitis, radiculopathy or sciatica M51.16
    lumbosacral region M51.27
      with
        neuritis, radiculitis, radiculopathy or sciatica M51.17
    sacrococcygeal region M53.3
    thoracic region M51.24
      with
        myelopathy M51.04

Displacement, displaced - *continued*
  intervertebral disc NEC - *continued*
    thoracic region - *continued*
      with - *continued*
        neuritis, radiculitis, radiculopathy M51.14
    thoracolumbar region M51.25
      with
        myelopathy M51.05
        neuritis, radiculitis, radiculopathy M51.15
  intrauterine device (string) T83.32
  kidney (acquired) N28.83
    congenital Q63.2
  lachrymal, lacrimal apparatus or duct (congenital) Q10.6
  lens, congenital Q12.1
  macula (congenital) Q14.1
  Meckel's diverticulum Q43.0
    malignant — *see* Table of Neoplasms, small intestine, malignant
  nail (congenital) Q84.6
    acquired L60.8
  opening of Wharton's duct in mouth Q38.4
  organ or site, congenital NEC — *see* Malposition, congenital
  ovary (acquired) N83.4-
    congenital Q50.39
    free in peritoneal cavity (congenital) Q50.39
    into hernial sac N83.4-
  oviduct (acquired) N83.4-
    congenital Q50.6
  parathyroid (gland) E21.4
  parotid gland (congenital) Q38.4
  punctum lacrimale (congenital) Q10.6
  sacro-iliac (joint) (congenital) Q74.2
    current injury S33.2
    old — *see* subcategory M53.2
  salivary gland (any) (congenital) Q38.4
  spleen (congenital) Q89.09
  stomach, congenital Q40.2
  sublingual duct Q38.4
  tongue (downward) (congenital) Q38.3
  tooth, teeth, fully erupted M26.30
    horizontal M26.33
    vertical M26.34
  trachea (congenital) Q32.1
  ureter or ureteric opening or orifice (congenital) Q62.62
  uterine opening of oviducts or fallopian tubes Q50.6
  uterus, uterine — *see* Malposition, uterus
  ventricular septum Q21.0
    with rudimentary ventricle Q20.4
Disproportion
  between native and reconstructed breast N65.1
  fiber-type G71.2
Disruptio uteri — *see* Rupture, uterus
Disruption (of)
  ciliary body NEC H21.89
  closure of
    cornea T81.31
    craniotomy T81.32
    fascia (muscular) (superficial) T81.32
    internal organ or tissue T81.32
    laceration (external) (internal) T81.33
    ligament T81.32
    mucosa T81.31
    muscle or muscle flap T81.32
    ribs or rib cage T81.32
    skin and subcutaneous tissue (full-thickness) (superficial) T81.31
    skull T81.32
    sternum (sternotomy) T81.32
    tendon T81.32
    traumatic laceration (external) (internal) T81.33
  family Z63.8
    due to
      absence of family member due to military deployment Z63.31
      absence of family member NEC Z63.32
      alcoholism and drug addiction in family Z63.72
      bereavement Z63.4
      death (assumed) or disappearance of family member Z63.4
      divorce or separation Z63.5
      drug addiction in family Z63.72
      return of family member from military deployment (current or past conflict) Z63.71
      stressful life events NEC Z63.79
  iris NEC H21.89
  ligament (s) — *see also* Sprain
  knee
    current injury — *see* Dislocation, knee
    old (chronic) — *see* Derangement, knee, ligament, instability, chronic

Disruption (of) - *continued*
ligament (s) - *continued*
knee - *continued*
spontaneous NEC — *see* Derangement, knee, disruption ligament
ossicular chain — *see* Discontinuity, ossicles, ear
pelvic ring (stable) S32.810
unstable S32.811
wound T81.30
episiotomy O90.1
operation T81.31
cesarean O90.0
external operation wound (superficial) T81.31
internal operation wound (deep) T81.32
perineal (obstetric) O90.1
traumatic injury repair T81.33
traumatic injury wound repair T81.33
Dissatisfaction with
employment Z56.9
school environment Z55.4
Dissecting — *see* condition
Dissection
aorta I71.00
abdominal I71.02
thoracic I71.01
thoracoabdominal I71.03
artery I77.70
basilar (trunk) I77.75
carotid I77.71
cerebral (nonruptured) I67.0
ruptured — *see* Hemorrhage, intracranial, subarachnoid
coronary I25.42
extremity
lower I77.77
upper I77.76
iliac I77.72
precerebral
congenital (nonruptured) Q28.1
specified site NEC I77.75
renal I77.73
specified NEC I77.79
vertebral I77.74
traumatic — *see* Wound, open, by site
vascular I99.8
wound — *see* Wound, open
Disseminated — *see* condition
Dissociation
auriculoventricular or atrioventricular (AV) (any degree) (isorhythmic) I45.89
with heart block I44.2
interference I45.89
Dissociative reaction, state F44.9
Dissolution, vertebra — *see* Osteoporosis
Distension, distention
abdomen R14.0
bladder N32.89
cecum K63.89
colon K63.89
gallbladder K82.8
intestine K63.89
kidney N28.89
liver K76.89
seminal vesicle N50.89
stomach K31.89
acute K31.0
psychogenic F45.8
ureter — *see* Dilatation, ureter
uterus N85.8
Distoma hepaticum infestation B66.3
Distomiasis B66.9
bile passages B66.3
hemic B65.9
hepatic B66.3
due to Clonorchis sinensis B66.1
intestinal B66.5
liver B66.3
due to Clonorchis sinensis B66.1
lung B66.4
pulmonary B66.4
Distomolar (fourth molar) K00.1
Disto-occlusion (Division I) (Division II) M26.212
Distortion (s) (congenital)
adrenal (gland) Q89.1
arm NEC Q68.8
bile duct or passage Q44.5
bladder Q64.79
brain Q04.9
cervix (uteri) Q51.9
chest (wall) Q67.8
bones Q76.8
clavicle Q74.0
clitoris Q52.6

Distortion (s) (congenital) - *continued*
coccyx Q76.49
common duct Q44.5
coronary Q24.5
cystic duct Q44.5
ear (auricle) (external) Q17.3
inner Q16.5
middle Q16.4
ossicles Q16.3
endocrine NEC Q89.2
eustachian tube Q17.8
eye (adnexa) Q15.8
face bone (s) NEC Q75.8
fallopian tube Q50.6
femur NEC Q68.8
fibula NEC Q68.8
finger (s) Q68.1
foot Q66.9
genitalia, genital organ (s)
female Q52.8
external Q52.79
internal NEC Q52.8
gyri Q04.8
hand bone (s) Q68.1
heart (auricle) (ventricle) Q24.8
valve (cusp) Q24.8
hepatic duct Q44.5
humerus NEC Q68.8
hymen Q52.4
intrafamilial communications Z63.8
jaw NEC M26.89
labium (majus) (minus) Q52.79
leg NEC Q68.8
lens Q12.8
liver Q44.7
lumbar spine Q76.49
with disproportion O33.8
causing obstructed labor O65.0
lumbosacral (joint) (region) Q76.49
kyphosis — *see* Kyphosis, congenital
lordosis — *see* Lordosis, congenital
nerve Q07.8
nose Q30.8
organ
of Corti Q16.5
or site not listed — *see* Anomaly, by site
ossicles, ear Q16.3
oviduct Q50.6
pancreas Q45.3
parathyroid (gland) Q89.2
pituitary (gland) Q89.2
radius NEC Q68.8
sacroiliac joint Q74.2
sacrum Q76.49
scapula Q74.0
shoulder girdle Q74.0
skull bone (s) NEC Q75.8
with
anencephalus Q00.0
encephalocele — *see* Encephalocele
hydrocephalus Q03.9
with spina bifida — *see* Spina bifida, with hydrocephalus
microcephaly Q02
spinal cord Q06.8
spine Q76.49
kyphosis — *see* Kyphosis, congenital
lordosis — *see* Lordosis, congenital
spleen Q89.09
sternum NEC Q76.7
thorax (wall) Q67.8
bony Q76.8
thymus (gland) Q89.2
thyroid (gland) Q89.2
tibia NEC Q68.8
toe (s) Q66.9
tongue Q38.3
trachea (cartilage) Q32.1
ulna NEC Q68.8
ureter Q62.8
urethra Q64.79
causing obstruction Q64.39
uterus Q51.9
vagina Q52.4
vertebra Q76.49
kyphosis — *see* Kyphosis, congenital
lordosis — *see* Lordosis, congenital
visual — *see also* Disturbance, vision
shape and size H53.15
vulva Q52.79
wrist (bones) (joint) Q68.8
Distress
abdomen — *see* Pain, abdominal

Distress - *continued*
acute respiratory R06.00
syndrome (adult) (child) J80
epigastric R10.13
fetal P84
complicating pregnancy — *see* Stress, fetal
gastrointestinal (functional) K30
psychogenic F45.8
intestinal (functional) NOS K59.9
psychogenic F45.8
maternal, during labor and delivery O75.0
respiratory (adult) (child) R06.00
newborn P22.9
specified NEC P22.8
orthopnea R06.01
psychogenic F45.8
shortness of breath R06.02
specified type NEC R06.09
Distribution vessel, atypical Q27.9
coronary artery Q24.5
precerebral Q28.1
Districhiasis L68.8
Disturbance (s) — *see also* Disease
absorption K90.9
calcium E58
carbohydrate K90.49
fat K90.49
pancreatic K90.3
protein K90.49
starch K90.49
vitamin — *see* Deficiency, vitamin
acid-base equilibrium E87.8
mixed E87.4
activity and attention (with hyperkinesis) — *see* Disorder, attention-deficit hyperactivity
amino acid transport E72.00
assimilation, food K90.9
auditory nerve, except deafness — *see* subcategory H93.3
behavior — *see* Disorder, conduct
blood clotting (mechanism) — *see also* Defect, coagulation D68.9
cerebral
nerve — *see* Disorder, nerve, cranial
status, newborn P91.9
specified NEC P91.8
circulatory I99.9
conduct — *see also* Disorder, conduct F91.9
adjustment reaction — *see* Disorder, adjustment
compulsive F63.9
disruptive F91.9
hyperkinetic — *see* Disorder, attention-deficit hyperactivity
socialized F91.2
specified NEC F91.8
unsocialized F91.1
coordination R27.8
cranial nerve — *see* Disorder, nerve, cranial
deep sensibility — *see* Disturbance, sensation
digestive K30
psychogenic F45.8
electrolyte — *see also* Imbalance, electrolyte
newborn, transitory P74.4
hyperammonemia P74.6
potassium balance P74.3
sodium balance P74.2
specified type NEC P74.4
emotions specific to childhood and adolescence F93.9
with
anxiety and fearfulness NEC F93.8
elective mutism F94.0
oppositional disorder F91.3
sensitivity (withdrawal) F40.10
shyness F40.10
social withdrawal F40.10
involving relationship problems F93.8
mixed F93.8
specified NEC F93.8
endocrine (gland) E34.9
neonatal, transitory P72.9
specified NEC P72.8
equilibrium R42
fructose metabolism E74.10
gait — *see* Gait
hysterical F44.4
psychogenic F44.4
gastrointestinal (functional) K30
psychogenic F45.8
habit, child F98.9
hearing, except deafness and tinnitus — *see* Abnormal, auditory perception
heart, functional (conditions in I44-I50)

Disturbance (s) - *continued*
  heart, functional (conditions in I44-I50) - *continued*
    due to presence of (cardiac) prosthesis I97.19-
      postoperative I97.89
        cardiac surgery I97.19-
  hormones E34.9
  innervation uterus (parasympathetic) (sympathetic) N85.8
  keratinization NEC
    gingiva K05.10
      nonplaque induced K05.11
      plaque induced K05.10
    lip K13.0
    oral (mucosa) (soft tissue) K13.29
    tongue K13.29
  learning (specific) — *see* Disorder, learning
  memory — *see* Amnesia
    mild, following organic brain damage F06.8
  mental F99
    associated with diseases classified elsewhere F54
  metabolism E88.9
    with
      abortion — *see* Abortion, by type with other specified complication
      ectopic pregnancy O08.5
      molar pregnancy O08.5
    amino-acid E72.9
      aromatic E70.9
      branched-chain E71.2
      straight-chain E72.8
      sulfur-bearing E72.10
    ammonia E72.20
    arginine E72.21
    arginosuccinic acid E72.22
    carbohydrate E74.9
    cholesterol E78.9
    citrulline E72.23
    cystathionine E72.19
    general E88.9
    glutamine E72.8
    histidine E70.40
    homocystine E72.19
    hydroxylysine E72.3
    in labor or delivery O75.89
    iron E83.10
    lipoid E78.9
    lysine E72.3
    methionine E72.19
    neonatal, transitory P74.9
      calcium and magnesium P71.9
        specified type NEC P71.8
      carbohydrate metabolism P70.9
        specified type NEC P70.8
      specified NEC P74.8
    ornithine E72.4
    phosphate E83.39
    sodium NEC E87.8
    threonine E72.8
    tryptophan E70.5
    tyrosine E70.20
    urea cycle E72.20
  motor R29.2
  nervous, functional R45.0
  neuromuscular mechanism (eye) , due to syphilis A52.15
  nutritional E63.9
    nail L60.3
  ocular motion H51.9
    psychogenic F45.8
  oculogyric H51.8
    psychogenic F45.8
  oculomotor H51.9
    psychogenic F45.8
  olfactory nerve R43.1
  optic nerve NEC — *see* Disorder, nerve, optic
  oral epithelium, including tongue NEC K13.29
  perceptual due to
    alcohol withdrawal F10.232
    amphetamine intoxication F15.922
      in
        abuse F15.122
        dependence F15.222
    anxiolytic withdrawal F13.232
    cannabis intoxication (acute) F12.922
      in
        abuse F12.122
        dependence F12.222
    cocaine intoxication (acute) F14.922
      in
        abuse F14.122
        dependence F14.222
    hypnotic withdrawal F13.232
    opioid intoxication (acute) F11.922

Disturbance (s) - *continued*
  perceptual due to - *continued*
    opioid intoxication (acute) - *continued*
      in
        abuse F11.122
        dependence F11.222
    phencyclidine intoxication (acute) F16.122
    sedative withdrawal F13.232
  personality (pattern) (trait) — *see also* Disorder, personality F60.9
    following organic brain damage F07.9
  polyglandular E31.9
    specified NEC E31.8
  potassium balance, newborn P74.3
  psychogenic F45.9
  psychomotor F44.4
  psychophysical visual H53.16
  pupillary — *see* Anomaly, pupil, function
  reflex R29.2
  rhythm, heart I49.9
  salivary secretion K11.7
  sensation (cold) (heat) (localization) (tactile discrimination) (texture) (vibratory) NEC R20.9
    hysterical F44.6
    skin R20.9
      anesthesia R20.0
      hyperesthesia R20.3
      hypoesthesia R20.1
      paresthesia R20.2
      specified type NEC R20.8
    smell R43.9
      and taste (mixed) R43.8
      anosmia R43.0
      parosmia R43.1
      specified NEC R43.8
    taste R43.9
      and smell (mixed) R43.8
      parageusia R43.2
      specified NEC R43.8
  sensory — *see* Disturbance, sensation
  situational (transient) — *see also* Disorder, adjustment
    acute F43.0
  sleep G47.9
    nonorganic origin F51.9
  smell — *see* Disturbance, sensation, smell
  sociopathic F60.2
  sodium balance, newborn P74.2
  speech R47.9
    developmental F80.9
    specified NEC R47.89
  stomach (functional) K31.9
  sympathetic (nerve) G90.9
  taste — *see* Disturbance, sensation, taste
  temperature
    regulation, newborn P81.9
      specified NEC P81.8
    sense R20.8
      hysterical F44.6
  tooth
    eruption K00.6
    formation K00.4
    structure, hereditary NEC K00.5
  touch — *see* Disturbance, sensation
  vascular I99.9
    arteriosclerotic — *see* Arteriosclerosis
  vasomotor I73.9
  vasospastic I73.9
  vision, visual H53.9
    following
      cerebral infarction I69.398
      cerebrovascular disease I69.998
        specified NEC I69.898
      intracerebral hemorrhage I69.198
      nontraumatic intracranial hemorrhage NEC I69.298
      specified disease NEC I69.898
      subarachnoid hemorrhage I69.098
    psychophysical H53.16
    specified NEC H53.8
    subjective H53.10
      day blindness H53.11
      discomfort H53.14-
      distortions of shape and size H53.15
      loss
        sudden H53.13-
        transient H53.12-
      specified type NEC H53.19
  voice R49.9
    psychogenic F44.4
    specified NEC R49.8
Diuresis R35.8
Diver's palsy, paralysis or squeeze T70.3

Diverticulitis (acute) K57.92
  bladder — *see* Cystitis
  ileum — *see* Diverticulitis, intestine, small
  intestine K57.92
    with
      abscess, perforation or peritonitis K57.80
        with bleeding K57.81
      bleeding K57.93
    congenital Q43.8
    large K57.32
      with
        abscess, perforation or peritonitis K57.20
          with bleeding K57.21
        bleeding K57.33
        small intestine K57.52
          with
            abscess, perforation or peritonitis K57.40
              with bleeding K57.41
            bleeding K57.53
    small K57.12
      with
        abscess, perforation or peritonitis K57.00
          with bleeding K57.01
        bleeding K57.13
        large intestine K57.52
          with
            abscess, perforation or peritonitis K57.40
              with bleeding K57.41
            bleeding K57.53
Diverticulosis K57.90
  with bleeding K57.91
  large intestine K57.30
    with
      bleeding K57.31
      small intestine K57.50
        with bleeding K57.51
  small intestine K57.10
    with
      bleeding K57.11
      large intestine K57.50
        with bleeding K57.51
Diverticulum, diverticula (multiple) K57.90
  appendix (noninflammatory) K38.2
  bladder (sphincter) N32.3
    congenital Q64.6
  bronchus (congenital) Q32.4
    acquired J98.09
  calyx, calyceal (kidney) N28.89
  cardia (stomach) K31.4
  cecum — *see* Diverticulosis, intestine, large
    congenital Q43.8
  colon — *see* Diverticulosis, intestine, large
    congenital Q43.8
  duodenum — *see* Diverticulosis, intestine, small
    congenital Q43.8
  epiphrenic (esophagus) K22.5
  esophagus (congenital) Q39.6
    acquired (epiphrenic) (pulsion) (traction) K22.5
  eustachian tube — *see* Disorder, eustachian tube, specified NEC
  fallopian tube N83.8
  gastric K31.4
  heart (congenital) Q24.8
  ileum — *see* Diverticulosis, intestine, small
  jejunum — *see* Diverticulosis, intestine, small
  kidney (pelvis) (calyces) N28.89
    with calculus — *see* Calculus, kidney
  Meckel's (displaced) (hypertrophic) Q43.0
    malignant — *see* Table of Neoplasms, small intestine, malignant
  midthoracic K22.5
  organ or site, congenital NEC — *see* Distortion
  pericardium (congenital) (cyst) Q24.8
    acquired I31.8
  pharyngoesophageal (congenital) Q39.6
    acquired K22.5
  pharynx (congenital) Q38.7
  rectosigmoid — *see* Diverticulosis, intestine, large
    congenital Q43.8
  rectum — *see* Diverticulosis, intestine, large
  Rokitansky's K22.5
  seminal vesicle N50.89
  sigmoid — *see* Diverticulosis, intestine, large
    congenital Q43.8
  stomach (acquired) K31.4
    congenital Q40.2
  trachea (acquired) J39.8
  ureter (acquired) N28.89
    congenital Q62.8
  ureterovesical orifice N28.89
  urethra (acquired) N36.1
    congenital Q64.79
  ventricle, left (congenital) Q24.8

Diverticulum, diverticula (multiple) - *continued*
vesical N32.3
congenital Q64.6
Zenker's (esophagus) K22.5
Division
cervix uteri (acquired) N88.8
glans penis Q55.69
labia minora (congenital) Q52.79
ligament (partial or complete) (current) — *see also* Sprain
with open wound — *see* Wound, open
muscle (partial or complete) (current) — *see also* Injury, muscle
with open wound — *see* Wound, open
nerve (traumatic) — *see* Injury, nerve
spinal cord — *see* Injury, spinal cord, by region
vein I87.8
Divorce, causing family disruption Z63.5
Dix-Hallpike neurolabyrinthitis — *see* Neuronitis, vestibular
Dizziness R42
hysterical F44.89
psychogenic F45.8
DMAC
(disseminated mycobacterium avium-intracellulare complex) A31.2
DNR (do not resuscitate) Z66
Doan-Wiseman syndrome
(primary splenic neutropenia) — *see* Agranulocytosis
Doehle-Heller aortitis A52.02
Dog bite — *see* Bite
Dohle body panmyelopathic syndrome D72.0
Dolichocephaly Q67.2
Dolichocolon Q43.8
Dolichostenomelia — *see* Syndrome, Marfan's
Donohue's syndrome E34.8
Donor (organ or tissue) Z52.9
blood (whole) Z52.000
autologous Z52.010
specified component (lymphocytes) (platelets) NEC Z52.008
autologous Z52.018
specified donor NEC Z52.098
specified donor NEC Z52.090
stem cells Z52.001
autologous Z52.011
specified donor NEC Z52.091
bone Z52.20
autologous Z52.21
marrow Z52.3
specified type NEC Z52.29
cornea Z52.5
egg (Oocyte) Z52.819
age 35 and over Z52.812
anonymous recipient Z52.812
designated recipient Z52.813
under age 35 Z52.810
anonymous recipient Z52.810
designated recipient Z52.811
kidney Z52.4
liver Z52.6
lung Z52.89
lymphocyte — *see* Donor, blood, specified components NEC
Oocyte — *see* Donor, egg
platelets Z52.008
potential, examination of Z00.5
semen Z52.89
skin Z52.10
autologous Z52.11
specified type NEC Z52.19
specified organ or tissue NEC Z52.89
sperm Z52.89
Donovanosis A58
Dorsalgia M54.9
psychogenic F45.41
specified NEC M54.89
Dorsopathy M53.9
deforming M43.9
specified NEC — *see* subcategory M43.8
specified NEC M53.80
cervical region M53.82
cervicothoracic region M53.83
lumbar region M53.86
lumbosacral region M53.87
occipito-atlanto-axial region M53.81
sacrococcygeal region M53.88
thoracic region M53.84
thoracolumbar region M53.85
Double
albumin E88.09
aortic arch Q25.45

Double - *continued*
auditory canal Q17.8
auricle (heart) Q20.8
bladder Q64.79
cervix Q51.820
with doubling of uterus (and vagina) Q51.10
with obstruction Q51.11
inlet ventricle Q20.4
kidney with double pelvis (renal) Q63.0
meatus urinarius Q64.75
monster Q89.4
outlet
left ventricle Q20.2
right ventricle Q20.1
pelvis (renal) with double ureter Q62.5
tongue Q38.3
ureter (one or both sides) Q62.5
with double pelvis (renal) Q62.5
urethra Q64.74
urinary meatus Q64.75
uterus Q51.2
with
doubling of cervix (and vagina) Q51.10
with obstruction Q51.11
in pregnancy or childbirth O34.59-
causing obstructed labor O65.5
vagina Q52.10
with doubling of uterus (and cervix) Q51.10
with obstruction Q51.11
vision H53.2
vulva Q52.79
Douglas' pouch, cul-de-sac — *see* condition
Down syndrome Q90.9
meiotic nondisjunction Q90.0
mitotic nondisjunction Q90.1
mosaicism Q90.1
translocation Q90.2
DPD (dihydropyrimidine dehydrogenase deficiency) E88.89
Dracontiasis B72
Dracunculiasis, dracunculosis B72
Dream state, hysterical F44.89
Drepanocytic anemia — *see* Disease, sickle-cell
Dresbach's syndrome (elliptocytosis) D58.1
Dreschlera (hawaiiensis) (infection) B43.8
Dressler's syndrome I24.1
Drift, ulnar — *see* Deformity, limb, specified type NEC, forearm
Drinking (alcohol)
excessive, to excess NEC (without dependence) F10.10
habitual (continual) (without remission) F10.20
with remission F10.21
Drip, postnasal (chronic) R09.82
due to
allergic rhinitis — *see* Rhinitis, allergic
common cold J00
gastroesophageal reflux — *see* Reflux, gastroesophageal
nasopharyngitis — *see* Nasopharyngitis
other know condition - code to condition
sinusitis — *see* Sinusitis
Droop
facial R29.810
cerebrovascular disease I69.992
cerebral infarction I69.392
intracerebral hemorrhage I69.192
nontraumatic intracranial hemorrhage NEC I69.292
specified disease NEC I69.892
subarachnoid hemorrhage I69.092
Drop (in)
attack NEC R55
finger — *see* Deformity, finger
foot — *see* Deformity, limb, foot, drop
hematocrit (precipitous) R71.0
hemoglobin R71.0
toe — *see* Deformity, toe, specified NEC
wrist — *see* Deformity, limb, wrist drop
Dropped heart beats I45.9
Dropsy, dropsical — *see also* Hydrops
abdomen R18.8
brain — *see* Hydrocephalus
cardiac, heart — *see* Failure, heart, congestive
gangrenous — *see* Gangrene
heart — *see* Failure, heart, congestive
kidney — *see* Nephrosis
lung — *see* Edema, lung
newborn due to isoimmunization P56.0
pericardium — *see* Pericarditis
Drowned, drowning (near) T75.1
Drowsiness R40.0

Drug
abuse counseling and surveillance Z71.51
addiction — *see* Dependence
dependence — *see* Dependence
habit — *see* Dependence
harmful use — *see* Abuse, drug
induced fever R50.2
overdose — *see* Table of Drugs and Chemicals, by drug, poisoning
poisoning — *see* Table of Drugs and Chemicals, by drug, poisoning
resistant organism infection — *see also* Resistant, organism, to, drug Z16.30
therapy
long term (current) (prophylactic) — *see* Therapy, drug long-term (current) (prophylactic)
short term - omit code
wrong substance given or taken in error — *see* Table of Drugs and Chemicals, by drug, poisoning
Drunkenness (without dependence) F10.129
acute in alcoholism F10.229
chronic (without remission) F10.20
with remission F10.21
pathological (without dependence) F10.129
with dependence F10.229
sleep F51.9
Drusen
macula (degenerative) (retina) — *see* Degeneration, macula, drusen
optic disc H47.32-
Dry, dryness — *see also* condition
larynx J38.7
mouth R68.2
due to dehydration E86.0
nose J34.89
socket (teeth) M27.3
throat J39.2
DSAP L56.5
Duane's syndrome H50.81-
Dubin-Johnson disease or syndrome E80.6
Dubois' disease (thymus gland) A50.59 *[E35]*
Dubowitz' syndrome Q87.1
Duchenne-Aran muscular atrophy G12.21
Duchenne-Griesinger disease G71.0
Duchenne's
disease or syndrome
motor neuron disease G12.22
muscular dystrophy G71.0
locomotor ataxia (syphilitic) A52.11
paralysis
birth injury P14.0
due to or associated with
motor neuron disease G12.22
muscular dystrophy G71.0
Ducrey's chancre A57
Duct, ductus — *see* condition
Duhring's disease (dermatitis herpetiformis) L13.0
Dullness, cardiac (decreased) (increased) R01.2
Dumb ague — *see* Malaria
Dumbness — *see* Aphasia
Dumdum fever B55.0
Dumping syndrome (postgastrectomy) K91.1
Duodenitis (nonspecific) (peptic) K29.80
with bleeding K29.81
Duodenocholangitis — *see* Cholangitis
Duodenum, duodenal — *see* condition
Duplay's bursitis or periarthritis — *see* Tendinitis, calcific, shoulder
Duplication, duplex — *see also* Accessory
alimentary tract Q45.8
anus Q43.4
appendix (and cecum) Q43.4
biliary duct (any) Q44.5
bladder Q64.79
cecum (and appendix) Q43.4
cervix Q51.820
chromosome NEC
with complex rearrangements NEC Q92.5
seen only at prometaphase Q92.8
cystic duct Q44.5
digestive organs Q45.8
esophagus Q39.8
frontonasal process Q75.8
intestine (large) (small) Q43.4
kidney Q63.0
liver Q44.7
pancreas Q45.3
penis Q55.69
respiratory organs NEC Q34.8
salivary duct Q38.4
spinal cord (incomplete) Q06.2
stomach Q40.2
Dupré's disease (meningism) R29.1

Dupuytren's contraction or disease M72.0
Durand-Nicolas-Favre disease A55
Durotomy (inadvertent) (incidental) G97.41
Duroziez's disease (congenital mitral stenosis) Q23.2
Dutton's relapsing fever (West African) A68.1
Dwarfism E34.3
  achondroplastic Q77.4
  congenital E34.3
  constitutional E34.3
  hypochondroplastic Q77.4
  hypophyseal E23.0
  infantile E34.3
  Laron-type E34.3
  Lorain (-Levi) type E23.0
  metatropic Q77.8
  nephrotic-glycosuric (with hypophosphatemic
    rickets) E72.09
  nutritional E45
  pancreatic K86.89
  pituitary E23.0
  renal N25.0
  thanatophoric Q77.1
Dyke-Young anemia (secondary)
  (symptomatic) D59.1
Dysacusis — see Abnormal, auditory perception
Dysadrenocortism E27.9
  hyperfunction E27.0
Dysarthria R47.1
  following
    cerebral infarction I69.322
    cerebrovascular disease I69.922
      specified disease NEC I69.822
    intracerebral hemorrhage I69.122
    nontraumatic intracranial hemorrhage
      NEC I69.222
    subarachnoid hemorrhage I69.022
Dysautonomia (familial) G90.1
Dysbarism T70.3
Dysbasia R26.2
  angiosclerotica intermittens I73.9
  hysterical F44.4
  lordotica (progressiva) G24.1
  nonorganic origin F44.4
  psychogenic F44.4
Dysbetalipoproteinemia (familial) E78.2
Dyscalculia R48.8
  developmental F81.2
Dyschezia K59.00
Dyschondroplasia (with hemangiomata) Q78.4
Dyschromia (skin) L81.9
Dyscollagenosis M35.9
Dyscranio-pygo-phalangy Q87.0
Dyscrasia
  blood (with) D75.9
    antepartum hemorrhage — see Hemorrhage,
      antepartum, with coagulation defect
    newborn P61.9
      specified type NEC P61.8
    intrapartum hemorrhage O67.0
    puerperal, postpartum O72.3
  polyglandular, pluriglandular E31.9
Dysendocrinism E34.9
Dysentery, dysenteric (catarrhal) (diarrhea)
  (epidemic) (hemorrhagic) (infectious) (sporadic)
  (tropical) A09
  abscess, liver A06.4
  amebic — see also Amebiasis A06.0
    with abscess — see Abscess, amebic
    acute A06.0
    chronic A06.1
  arthritis (see also category M01) A09
    bacillary (see also category M01) A03.9
  bacillary A03.9
    arthritis (see also category M01) A03.9
    Boyd A03.2
    Flexner A03.1
    Schmitz (-Stutzer) A03.0
    Shiga (-Kruse) A03.0
    Shigella A03.9
      boydii A03.2
      dysenteriae A03.0
      flexneri A03.1
      group A A03.0
      group B A03.1
      group C A03.2
      group D A03.3
      sonnei A03.3
      specified type NEC A03.8
    Sonne A03.3
    specified type NEC A03.8
  balantidial A07.0
    Balantidium coli A07.0
  Boyd's A03.2

Dysentery, dysenteric (catarrhal) (diarrhea)
  (epidemic) (hemorrhagic) (infectious) (sporadic)
  (tropical) - continued
  candidal B37.82
  Chilomastix A07.8
  Chinese A03.9
  coccidial A07.3
  Dientamoeba (fragilis) A07.8
  Embadomonas A07.8
  Entamoeba, entambic — see Dysentery, amebic
  Flexner-Boyd A03.2
  Flexner's A03.1
  Giardia lamblia A07.1
  Hiss-Russell A03.1
  Lamblia A07.1
  leishmanial B55.0
  malarial — see Malaria
  metazoal B82.0
  monilial B37.82
  protozoal A07.9
  Salmonella A02.0
  schistosomal B65.1
  Schmitz (-Stutzer) A03.0
  Shiga (-Kruse) A03.0
  Shigella NOS — see Dysentery, bacillary
  Sonne A03.3
  strongyloidiasis B78.0
  trichomonal A07.8
  viral — see also Enteritis, viral A08.4
Dysequilibrium R42
Dysesthesia R20.8
  hysterical F44.6
Dysfibrinogenemia (congenital) D68.2
Dysfunction
  adrenal E27.9
    hyperfunction E27.0
  autonomic
    due to alcohol G31.2
    somatoform F45.8
  bladder N31.9
    neurogenic NOS — see Dysfunction, bladder,
      neuromuscular
    neuromuscular NOS N31.9
      atonic (motor) (sensory) N31.2
      autonomous N31.2
      flaccid N31.2
      nonreflex N31.2
      reflex N31.1
      specified NEC N31.8
      uninhibited N31.0
  bleeding, uterus N93.8
  cerebral G93.89
  colon K59.9
    psychogenic F45.8
  colostomy K94.03
  cystic duct K82.8
  cystostomy (stoma) — see Complications,
    cystostomy
  ejaculation N53.19
    anejaculatory orgasm N53.13
    painful N53.12
    premature F52.4
    retarded N53.11
  endocrine NOS E34.9
  endometrium N85.8
  enterostomy K94.13
  erectile — see Dysfunction, sexual, male, erectile
  gallbladder K82.8
  gastrostomy (stoma) K94.23
  gland, glandular NOS E34.9
  heart I51.89
  hemoglobin D75.89
  hepatic K76.89
  hypophysis E23.7
  hypothalamic NEC E23.3
  ileostomy (stoma) K94.13
  jejunostomy (stoma) K94.13
  kidney — see Disease, renal
  labyrinthine — see subcategory H83.2
  left ventricular, following sudden emotional
    stress I51.81
  liver K76.89
  male — see Dysfunction, sexual, male
  orgasmic (female) F52.31
    male F52.32
  ovary E28.9
    specified NEC E28.8
  papillary muscle I51.89
  parathyroid E21.4
  physiological NEC R68.89
    psychogenic F59
  pineal gland E34.8
  pituitary (gland) E23.3

Dysfunction - continued
  platelets D69.1
  polyglandular E31.9
    specified NEC E31.8
  psychophysiologic F59
  psychosexual F52.9
    with
      dyspareunia F52.6
      premature ejaculation F52.4
      vaginismus F52.5
  pylorus K31.9
  rectum K59.9
    psychogenic F45.8
  reflex (sympathetic) — see Syndrome, pain,
    complex regional I
  segmental — see Dysfunction, somatic
  senile R54
  sexual (due to) R37
    alcohol F10.981
    amphetamine F15.981
      in
        abuse F15.181
        dependence F15.281
    anxiolytic F13.981
      in
        abuse F13.181
        dependence F13.281
    cocaine F14.981
      in
        abuse F14.181
        dependence F14.281
    excessive sexual drive F52.8
    failure of genital response (male) F52.21
      female F52.22
    female N94.9
      aversion F52.1
      dyspareunia N94.10
        psychogenic F52.6
      frigidity F52.22
      nymphomania F52.8
      orgasmic F52.31
      psychogenic F52.9
        aversion F52.1
        dyspareunia F52.6
        frigidity F52.22
        nymphomania F52.8
        orgasmic F52.31
        vaginismus F52.5
      vaginismus N94.2
        psychogenic F52.5
    hypnotic F13.981
      in
        abuse F13.181
        dependence F13.281
    inhibited orgasm (female) F52.31
      male F52.32
    lack
      of sexual enjoyment F52.1
      or loss of sexual desire F52.0
    male N53.9
      anejaculatory orgasm N53.13
      ejaculatory N53.19
        painful N53.12
        premature F52.4
        retarded N53.11
      erectile N52.9
        drug induced N52.2
        due to
          disease classified elsewhere N52.1
          drug N52.2
          postoperative (postprocedural) N52.39
            following
              cryotherapy N52.37
              interstitial seed therapy N52.36
              prostate ablative therapy N52.37
              prostatectomy N52.34
                radical N52.31
              radiation therapy N52.35
              radical cystectomy N52.32
              ultrasound ablative therapy N52.37
              urethral surgery N52.33
        psychogenic F52.21
        specified cause NEC N52.8
        vasculogenic
          arterial insufficiency N52.01
            with corporo-venous occlusive N52.03
          corporo-venous occlusive N52.02
            with arterial insufficiency N52.03
      impotence — see Dysfunction, sexual, male,
        erectile
      psychogenic F52.9
        aversion F52.1
        erectile F52.21

Dysfunction - *continued*
  sexual (due to) - *continued*
    male - *continued*
      psychogenic - *continued*
        orgasmic F52.32
        premature ejaculation F52.4
        satyriasis F52.8
        specified type NEC F52.8
      specified type NEC N53.8
    nonorganic F52.9
      specified NEC F52.8
    opioid F11.981
      in
        abuse F11.181
        dependence F11.281
    orgasmic dysfunction (female) F52.31
      male F52.32
    premature ejaculation F52.4
    psychoactive substances NEC F19.981
      in
        abuse F19.181
        dependence F19.281
    psychogenic F52.9
    sedative F13.981
      in
        abuse F13.181
        dependence F13.281
    sexual aversion F52.1
    vaginismus (nonorganic) (psychogenic) F52.5
  sinoatrial node I49.5
  somatic M99.09
    abdomen M99.09
    acromioclavicular M99.07
    cervical region M99.01
    cervicothoracic M99.01
    costochondral M99.08
    costovertebral M99.08
    head region M99.00
    hip M99.05
    lower extremity M99.06
    lumbar region M99.03
    lumbosacral M99.03
    occipitocervical M99.00
    pelvic region M99.05
    pubic M99.05
    rib cage M99.08
    sacral region M99.04
    sacrococcygeal M99.04
    sacroiliac M99.04
    specified NEC M99.09
    sternochondral M99.08
    sternoclavicular M99.07
    thoracic region M99.02
    thoracolumbar M99.02
    upper extremity M99.07
  somatoform autonomic F45.8
  stomach K31.89
    psychogenic F45.8
  suprarenal E27.9
    hyperfunction E27.0
  symbolic R48.9
    specified type NEC R48.8
  temporomandibular (joint) M26.69
    joint-pain syndrome M26.62-
  testicular (endocrine) E29.9
    specified NEC E29.8
  thymus E32.9
  thyroid E07.9
  ureterostomy (stoma) — *see* Complications, stoma, urinary tract
  urethrostomy (stoma) — *see* Complications, stoma, urinary tract
  uterus, complicating delivery O62.9
    hypertonic O62.4
    hypotonic O62.2
      primary O62.0
      secondary O62.1
  ventricular I51.9
    with congestive heart failure I50.9- - left, reversible, following sudden emotional stress I51.81
Dysgenesis
  gonadal (due to chromosomal anomaly) Q96.9
    pure Q99.1
  renal Q60.5
    bilateral Q60.4
    unilateral Q60.3
  reticular D72.0
  tidal platelet D69.3
Dysgerminoma
  specified site — *see* Neoplasm, malignant, by site
  unspecified site
    female C56.9

Dysgerminoma - *continued*
  unspecified site - *continued*
    male C62.90
Dysgeusia R43.2
Dysgraphia R27.8
Dyshidrosis, dysidrosis L30.1
Dyskaryotic cervical smear R87.619
Dyskeratosis L85.8
  cervix — *see* Dysplasia, cervix
  congenital Q82.8
  uterus NEC N85.8
Dyskinesia G24.9
  biliary (cystic duct or gallbladder) K82.8
  drug induced
    orofacial G24.01
  esophagus K22.4
  hysterical F44.4
  intestinal K59.8
  nonorganic origin F44.4
  orofacial (idiopathic) G24.4
    drug induced G24.01
  psychogenic F44.4
  subacute, drug induced G24.01
  tardive G24.01
    neuroleptic induced G24.01
  trachea J39.8
  tracheobronchial J98.09
Dyslalia (developmental) F80.0
Dyslexia R48.0
  developmental F81.0
Dyslipidemia E78.5
  depressed HDL cholesterol E78.6
  elevated fasting triglycerides E78.1
Dysmaturity — *see also* Light for dates
  pulmonary (newborn) (Wilson-Mikity) P27.0
Dysmenorrhea (essential) (exfoliative) N94.6
  congestive (syndrome) N94.6
  primary N94.4
  psychogenic F45.8
  secondary N94.5
Dysmetabolic syndrome X E88.81
Dysmetria R27.8
Dysmorphism (due to)
  alcohol Q86.0
  exogenous cause NEC Q86.8
  hydantoin Q86.1
  warfarin Q86.2
Dysmorphophobia (nondelusional) F45.22
  delusional F22
Dysnomia R47.01
Dysorexia R63.0
  psychogenic F50.89
Dysostosis
  cleidocranial, cleidocranialis Q74.0
  craniofacial Q75.1
  Fairbank's (idiopathic familial generalized osteophytosis) Q78.9
  mandibulofacial (incomplete) Q75.4
  multiplex E76.01
  oculomandibular Q75.5
Dyspareunia (female) N94.10
  deep N94.12
  male N53.12
  nonorganic F52.6
  psychogenic F52.6
  secondary N94.19
  specified NEC N94.19
  superficial (introital) N94.11
Dyspepsia R10.13
  atonic K30
  functional (allergic) (congenital) (gastrointestinal) (occupational) (reflex) K30
  intestinal K59.8
  nervous F45.8
  neurotic F45.8
  psychogenic F45.8
Dysphagia R13.10
  cervical R13.19
  following
    cerebral infarction I69.391
    cerebrovascular disease I69.991
      specified NEC I69.891
    intracerebral hemorrhage I69.191
    nontraumatic intracranial hemorrhage NEC I69.291
    specified disease NEC I69.891
    subarachnoid hemorrhage I69.091
  functional (hysterical) F45.8
  hysterical F45.8
  nervous (hysterical) F45.8
  neurogenic R13.19
  oral phase R13.11
  oropharyngeal phase R13.12

Dysphagia - *continued*
  pharyneal phase R13.13
  pharyngoesophageal phase R13.14
  psychogenic F45.8
  sideropenic D50.1
  spastica K22.4
  specified NEC R13.19
Dysphagocytosis, congenital D71
Dysphasia R47.02
  developmental
    expressive type F80.1
    receptive type F80.2
  following
    cerebrovascular disease I69.921
      cerebral infarction I69.321
      intracerebral hemorrhage I69.121
      nontraumatic intracranial hemorrhage NEC I69.221
      specified disease NEC I69.821
      subarachnoid hemorrhage I69.021
Dysphonia R49.0
  functional F44.4
  hysterical F44.4
  psychogenic F44.4
  spastica J38.3
Dysphoria
  gender
    in
      adolescence and adulthood F64.0
      children F64.2
  postpartal O90.6
Dyspituitarism E23.3
Dysplasia — *see also* Anomaly
  acetabular, congenital Q65.89
  alveolar capillary, with vein misalignment J84.843
  anus (histologically confirmed) (mild) (moderate) K62.82
    severe D01.3
  arrhythmogenic right ventricular I42.8
  arterial, fibromuscular I77.3
  asphyxiating thoracic (congenital) Q77.2
  brain Q07.9
  bronchopulmonary, perinatal P27.1
  cervix (uteri) N87.9
    mild N87.0
    moderate N87.1
    severe D06.9
  chondroectodermal Q77.6
  colon D12.6
  craniometaphyseal Q78.8
  dentinal K00.5
  diaphyseal, progressive Q78.3
  dystrophic Q77.5
  ectodermal (anhidrotic) (congenital) (hereditary) Q82.4
  hydrotic Q82.8
  epithelial, uterine cervix — *see* Dysplasia, cervix
  eye (congenital) Q11.2
  fibrous
    bone NEC (monostotic) M85.00
      ankle M85.07-
      foot M85.07-
      forearm M85.03-
      hand M85.04-
      lower leg M85.06-
      multiple site M85.09
      neck M85.08
      rib M85.08
      shoulder M85.01-
      skull M85.08
      specified site NEC M85.08
      thigh M85.05-
      toe M85.07-
      upper arm M85.02-
      vertebra M85.08
  diaphyseal, progressive Q78.3
  jaw M27.8
  polyostotic Q78.1
  florid osseous — *see also* Cyst, calcifying odontogenic
  high grade, focal D12.6
  hip, congenital Q65.89
  joint, congenital Q74.8
  kidney Q61.4
    multicystic Q61.4
  leg Q74.2
  lung, congenital (not associated with short gestation) Q33.6
  mammary (gland) (benign) N60.9-
    cyst (solitary) — *see* Cyst, breast
    cystic — *see* Mastopathy, cystic
    duct ectasia — *see* Ectasia, mammary duct
    fibroadenosis — *see* Fibroadenosis, breast

Dysplasia - *continued*
  mammary (gland) (benign) - *continued*
    fibrosclerosis — *see* Fibrosclerosis, breast
    specified type NEC N60.8-
  metaphyseal Q78.5
  muscle Q79.8
  oculodentodigital Q87.0
  periapical (cemental) (cemento-osseous) — *see*
    Cyst, calcifying odontogenic
  periosteum — *see* Disorder, bone, specified type
    NEC
  polyostotic fibrous Q78.1
  prostate — *see also* Neoplasia, intraepithelial,
    prostate N42.30
    severe D07.5
    specified NEC N42.39
  renal Q61.4
    multicystic Q61.4
  retinal, congenital Q14.1
  right ventricular, arrhythmogenic I42.8
  septo-optic Q04.4
  skin L98.8
  spinal cord Q06.1
  spondyloepiphyseal Q77.7
  thymic, with immunodeficiency D82.1
  vagina N89.3
    mild N89.0
    moderate N89.1
    severe NEC D07.2
  vulva N90.3
    mild N90.0
    moderate N90.1
    severe NEC D07.1
Dyspnea (nocturnal) (paroxysmal) R06.00
  asthmatic (bronchial) J45.909
    with
      exacerbation (acute) J45.901
      bronchitis J45.909
        with
          exacerbation (acute) J45.901
          status asthmaticus J45.902
          chronic J44.9
      status asthmaticus J45.902
    cardiac — *see* Failure, ventricular, left
  cardiac — *see* Failure, ventricular, left
  functional F45.8
  hyperventilation R06.4
  hysterical F45.8
  newborn P28.89
  orthopnea R06.01
  psychogenic F45.8
  shortness of breath R06.02
  specified type NEC R06.09
Dyspraxia R27.8
  developmental (syndrome) F82
Dysproteinemia E88.09
Dysreflexia, autonomic G90.4
Dysrhythmia
  cardiac I49.9
    newborn
      bradycardia P29.12
        occurring before birth P03.819
          before onset of labor P03.810
          during labor P03.811
      tachycardia P29.11
    postoperative I97.89
  cerebral or cortical — *see* Epilepsy
Dyssomnia — *see* Disorder, sleep
Dyssynergia
  biliary K83.3
  bladder sphincter N36.44
  cerebellaris myoclonica (Hunt's ataxia) G11.1
Dysthymia F34.1
Dysthyroidism E07.9
Dystocia O66.9
  affecting newborn P03.1
  cervical (hypotonic) O62.2
    affecting newborn P03.6
    primary O62.0
    secondary O62.1
  contraction ring O62.4
  fetal O66.9
    abnormality NEC O66.3
    conjoined twins O66.3
    oversize O66.2
  maternal O66.9
  positional O64.9
  shoulder (girdle) O66.0
    causing obstructed labor O66.0
  uterine NEC O62.4
Dystonia G24.9
  deformans progressiva G24.1
  drug induced NEC G24.09

Dystonia - *continued*
  drug induced NEC - *continued*
    acute G24.02
    specified NEC G24.09
  familial G24.1
  idiopathic G24.1
    familial G24.1
    nonfamilial G24.2
    orofacial G24.4
  lenticularis G24.8
  musculorum deformans G24.1
  neuroleptic induced (acute) G24.02
  orofacial (idiopathic) G24.4
  oromandibular G24.4
    due to drug G24.01
  specified NEC G24.8
  torsion (familial) (idiopathic) G24.1
    acquired G24.8
    genetic G24.1
  symptomatic (nonfamilial) G24.2
Dystonic movements R25.8
Dystrophy, dystrophia
  adiposogenital E23.6
  Becker's type G71.0
  cervical sympathetic G90.2
  choroid (hereditary) H31.20
    central areolar H31.22
    choroideremia H31.21
    gyrate atrophy H31.23
    specified type NEC H31.29
  cornea (hereditary) H18.50
    endothelial H18.51
    epithelial H18.52
    granular H18.53
    lattice H18.54
    macular H18.55
    specified type NEC H18.59
  Duchenne's type G71.0
  due to malnutrition E45
  Erb's G71.0
  Fuchs' H18.51
  Gower's muscular G71.0
  hair L67.8
  infantile neuroaxonal G31.89
  Landouzy-Déjérine G71.0
  Leyden-Möbius G71.0
  muscular G71.0
    benign (Becker type) G71.0
    congenital (hereditary) (progressive) (with specific
      morphological abnormalities of the muscle
      fiber) G71.0
      myotonic G71.11
    distal G71.0
    Duchenne type G71.0
    Emery-Dreifuss G71.0
    Erb type G71.0
    facioscapulohumeral G71.0
    Gower's G71.0
    hereditary (progressive) G71.0
    Landouzy-Déjérine type G71.0
    limb-girdle G71.0
    myotonic G71.11
    progressive (hereditary) G71.0
      Charcot-Marie (-Tooth) type G60.0
    pseudohypertrophic (infantile) G71.0
    severe (Duchenne type) G71.0
  myocardium, myocardial — *see* Degeneration,
    myocardial
  myotonic, myotonica G71.11
  nail L60.3
    congenital Q84.6
  nutritional E45
  ocular G71.0
  oculocerebrorenal E72.03
  oculopharyngeal G71.0
  ovarian N83.8
  polyglandular E31.8
  reflex (neuromuscular) (sympathetic) — *see*
    Syndrome, pain, complex regional I
  retinal (hereditary) H35.50
    in
      lipid storage disorders E75.6 *[H36]*
      systemic lipidoses E75.6 *[H36]*
    involving
      pigment epithelium H35.54
      sensory area H35.53
    pigmentary H35.52
    vitreoretinal H35.51
  Salzmann's nodular — *see* Degeneration, cornea,
    nodular
  scapuloperoneal G71.0
  skin NEC L98.8

Dystrophy, dystrophia - *continued*
  sympathetic (reflex) — *see* Syndrome, pain,
    complex regional I
    cervical G90.2
  tapetoretinal H35.54
  thoracic, asphyxiating Q77.2
  unguium L60.3
    congenital Q84.6
  vitreoretinal H35.51
  vulva N90.4
  yellow (liver) — *see* Failure, hepatic
Dysuria R30.0
  psychogenic F45.8

E

Eales' disease H35.06-
Ear — *see also* condition
  piercing Z41.3
  tropical NEC B36.9 *[H62.40]*
    in
      aspergillosis B44.89
      candidiasis B37.84
      moniliasis B37.84
  wax (impacted) H61.20
    left H61.22
      with right H61.23
    right H61.21
      with left H61.23
Earache — *see* subcategory H92.0
Early satiety R68.81
Eaton-Lambert syndrome — *see* Syndrome,
  Lambert-Eaton
Eberth's disease (typhoid fever) A01.00
Ebola virus disease A98.4
Ebstein's anomaly or syndrome (heart) Q22.5
Eccentro-osteochondrodysplasia E76.29
Ecchondroma — *see* Neoplasm, bone, benign
Ecchondrosis D48.0
Ecchymosis R58
  conjunctiva — *see* Hemorrhage, conjunctiva
  eye (traumatic) — *see* Contusion, eyeball
  eyelid (traumatic) — *see* Contusion, eyelid
  newborn P54.5
  spontaneous R23.3
  traumatic — *see* Contusion
Echinococciasis — *see* Echinococcus
Echinococcosis — *see* Echinococcus
Echinococcus (infection) B67.90
  granulosus B67.4
    bone B67.2
    liver B67.0
    lung B67.1
    multiple sites B67.32
    specified site NEC B67.39
    thyroid B67.31
  liver NOS B67.8
    granulosus B67.0
    multilocularis B67.5
  lung NEC B67.99
    granulosus B67.1
    multilocularis B67.69
  multilocularis B67.7
    liver B67.5
    multiple sites B67.61
    specified site NEC B67.69
  specified site NEC B67.99
    granulosus B67.39
    multilocularis B67.69
  thyroid NEC B67.99
    granulosus B67.31
    multilocularis B67.69 *[E35]*
Echinorhynchiasis B83.8
Echinostomiasis B66.8
Echolalia R48.8
**Echovirus, as cause of disease classified
  elsewhere** B97.12
Eclampsia, eclamptic (coma) (convulsions)
  (delirium) (with hypertension) **NEC** O15.9
  complicating
    labor and delivery O15.1
    postpartum O15.2
    pregnancy O15.0-
    puerperium O15.2
Economic circumstances affecting care Z59.9
Economo's disease A85.8
Ectasia, ectasis
  annuloaortic I35.8
  aorta I77.819
    with aneurysm — *see* Aneurysm, aorta
    abdominal I77.811
    thoracic I77.810
    thoracoabdominal I77.812
  breast — *see* Ectasia, mammary duct

Ectasia, ectasis - *continued*
capillary I78.8
cornea H18.71-
gastric antral vascular (GAVE) K31.819
with hemorrhage K31.811
without hemorrhage K31.819
mammary duct N60.4-
salivary gland (duct) K11.8
sclera — *see* Sclerectasia
Ecthyma L08.0
contagiosum B08.02
gangrenosum L08.0
infectiosum B08.02
Ectocardia Q24.8
Ectodermal dysplasia (anhidrotic) Q82.4
Ectodermosis erosiva pluriorificialis L51.1
Ectopic, ectopia (congenital)
abdominal viscera Q45.8
due to defect in anterior abdominal wall Q79.59
ACTH syndrome E24.3
adrenal gland Q89.1
anus Q43.5
atrial beats I49.1
beats I49.49
atrial I49.1
ventricular I49.3
bladder Q64.10
bone and cartilage in lung Q33.5
brain Q04.8
breast tissue Q83.8
cardiac Q24.8
cerebral Q04.8
cordis Q24.8
endometrium — *see* Endometriosis
gastric mucosa Q40.2
gestation — *see* Pregnancy, by site
heart Q24.8
hormone secretion NEC E34.2
kidney (crossed) (pelvis) Q63.2
lens, lentis Q12.1
mole — *see* Pregnancy, by site
organ or site NEC — *see* Malposition, congenital
pancreas Q45.3
pregnancy — *see* Pregnancy, ectopic
pupil — *see* Abnormality, pupillary
renal Q63.2
sebaceous glands of mouth Q38.6
spleen Q89.09
testis Q53.00
bilateral Q53.02
unilateral Q53.01
thyroid Q89.2
tissue in lung Q33.5
ureter Q62.63
ventricular beats I49.3
vesicae Q64.10
Ectromelia Q73.8
lower limb — *see* Defect, reduction, limb, lower, specified type NEC
upper limb — *see* Defect, reduction, limb, upper, specified type NEC
Ectropion H02.109
cervix N86
with cervicitis N72
congenital Q10.1
eyelid (paralytic) H02.109
cicatricial H02.119
left H02.116
lower H02.115
upper H02.114
right H02.113
lower H02.112
upper H02.111
congenital Q10.1
left H02.106
lower H02.105
upper H02.104
mechanical H02.129
left H02.126
lower H02.125
upper H02.124
right H02.123
lower H02.122
upper H02.121
right H02.103
lower H02.102
upper H02.101
senile H02.139
left H02.136
lower H02.135
upper H02.134
right H02.133
lower H02.132

Ectropion - *continued*
eyelid (paralytic) - *continued*
senile - *continued*
right - *continued*
upper H02.131
spastic H02.149
left H02.146
lower H02.145
upper H02.144
right H02.143
lower H02.142
upper H02.141
iris H21.89
lip (acquired) K13.0
congenital Q38.0
urethra N36.8
uvea H21.89
Eczema (acute) (chronic) (erythematous) (fissum) (rubrum) (squamous) — *see also* Dermatitis L30.9
contact — *see* Dermatitis, contact
dyshydrotic L30.1
external ear — *see* Otitis, externa, acute, eczematoid
flexural L20.82
herpeticum B00.0
hypertrophicum L28.0
hypostatic — *see* Varix, leg, with, inflammation
impetiginous L01.1
infantile (due to any substance) L20.83
intertriginous L21.1
seborrheic L21.1
intertriginous NEC L30.4
infantile L21.1
intrinsic (allergic) L20.84
lichenified NEC L28.0
marginatum (hebrae) B35.6
pustular L30.3
stasis I87.2
with varicose veins — *see* Varix, leg, with, inflammation
vaccination, vaccinatum T88.1
varicose — *see* Varix, leg, with, inflammation
Eczematid L30.2
Eddowes (-Spurway) **syndrome** Q78.0
Edema, edematous (infectious) (pitting) (toxic) R60.9
with nephritis — *see* Nephrosis
allergic T78.3
amputation stump (surgical) (sequelae (late effect)) T87.89
angioneurotic (allergic) (any site) (with urticaria) T78.3
hereditary D84.1
angiospastic I73.9
Berlin's (traumatic) S05.8X-
brain (cytotoxic) (vasogenic) G93.6
due to birth injury P11.0
newborn (anoxia or hypoxia) P52.4
birth injury P11.0
traumatic — *see* Injury, intracranial, cerebral edema
cardiac — *see* Failure, heart, congestive
cardiovascular — *see* Failure, heart, congestive
cerebral — *see* Edema, brain
cerebrospinal — *see* Edema, brain
cervix (uteri) (acute) N88.8
puerperal, postpartum O90.89
chronic hereditary Q82.0
circumscribed, acute T78.3
hereditary D84.1
conjunctiva H11.42-
cornea H18.2-
idiopathic H18.22-
secondary H18.23-
due to contact lens H18.21-
due to
lymphatic obstruction I89.0
salt retention E87.0
epiglottis — *see* Edema, glottis
essential, acute T78.3
hereditary D84.1
extremities, lower — *see* Edema, legs
eyelid NEC H02.849
left H02.846
lower H02.845
upper H02.844
right H02.843
lower H02.842
upper H02.841
familial, hereditary Q82.0
famine — *see* Malnutrition, severe
generalized R60.1
glottis, glottic, glottidis (obstructive) (passive) J38.4
allergic T78.3

Edema, edematous (infectious) (pitting) (toxic) - *continued*
glottis, glottic, glottidis (obstructive) (passive) - *continued*
allergic - *continued*
hereditary D84.1
heart — *see* Failure, heart, congestive
heat T67.7
hereditary Q82.0
inanition — *see* Malnutrition, severe
intracranial G93.6
iris H21.89
joint — *see* Effusion, joint
larynx — *see* Edema, glottis
legs R60.0
due to venous obstruction I87.1
hereditary Q82.0
localized R60.0
due to venous obstruction I87.1
lower limbs — *see* Edema, legs
lung J81.1
with heart condition or failure — *see* Failure, ventricular, left
acute J81.0
chemical (acute) J68.1
chronic J68.1
chronic J81.1
due to
chemicals, gases, fumes or vapors (inhalation) J68.1
external agent J70.9
specified NEC J70.8
radiation J70.1
due to
chemicals, fumes or vapors (inhalation) J68.1
external agent J70.9
specified NEC J70.8
high altitude T70.29
near drowning T75.1
radiation J70.0
meaning failure, left ventricle I50.1
lymphatic I89.0
due to mastectomy I97.2
macula H35.81
cystoid, following cataract surgery — *see* Complications, postprocedural, following cataract surgery
diabetic — *see* Diabetes, by type, with, retinopathy, with macular edema
malignant — *see* Gangrene, gas
Milroy's Q82.0
nasopharynx J39.2
newborn P83.30
hydrops fetalis — *see* Hydrops, fetalis
specified NEC P83.39
nutritional — *see also* Malnutrition, severe
with dyspigmentation, skin and hair E40
optic disc or nerve — *see* Papilledema
orbit H05.22-
pancreas K86.89
papilla, optic — *see* Papilledema
penis N48.89
periodic T78.3
hereditary D84.1
pharynx J39.2
pulmonary — *see* Edema, lung
Quincke's T78.3
hereditary D84.1
renal — *see* Nephrosis
retina H35.81
diabetic — *see* Diabetes, by type, with, retinopathy, with macular edema
salt E87.0
scrotum N50.89
seminal vesicle N50.89
spermatic cord N50.89
spinal (cord) (vascular) (nontraumatic) G95.19
starvation — *see* Malnutrition, severe
stasis — *see* Hypertension, venous, (chronic)
subglottic — *see* Edema, glottis
supraglottic — *see* Edema, glottis
testis N44.8
tunica vaginalis N50.89
vas deferens N50.89
vulva (acute) N90.89
Edentulism — *see* Absence, teeth, acquired
Edsall's disease T67.2
Educational handicap Z55.9
specified NEC Z55.8
Edward's syndrome — *see* Trisomy, 18
Effect (s) (of) (from) — *see* Effect, adverse NEC
Effect, adverse
abnormal gravitational (G) forces or states T75.81

Effect, adverse - *continued*
  abuse — *see* Maltreatment
  air pressure T70.9
    specified NEC T70.8
  altitude (high) — *see* Effect, adverse, high altitude
  anesthesia — *see also* Anesthesia T88.59
    in labor and delivery O74.9
    local, toxic
      in labor and delivery O74.4
      in pregnancy NEC O29.3-
      postpartum, puerperal O89.3
    postpartum, puerperal O89.9
    specified NEC T88.59
      in labor and delivery O74.8
      postpartum, puerperal O89.8
    spinal and epidural T88.59
      headache T88.59
        in labor and delivery O74.5
        postpartum, puerperal O89.4
      specified NEC
        in labor and delivery O74.6
        postpartum, puerperal O89.5
  antitoxin — *see* Complications, vaccination
  atmospheric pressure T70.9
    due to explosion T70.8
    high T70.3
    low — *see* Effect, adverse, high altitude
    specified effect NEC T70.8
  biological, correct substance properly
    administered — *see* Effect, adverse, drug
  blood (derivatives) (serum) (transfusion) —
    see Complications, transfusion
  chemical substance — *see* Table of Drugs and
    Chemicals
  cold (temperature) (weather) T69.9
    chilblains T69.1
    frostbite — *see* Frostbite
    specified effect NEC T69.8
  drugs and medicaments T88.7
    specified drug — *see* Table of Drugs and
      Chemicals, by drug, adverse effect
    specified effect - code to condition
  electric current, electricity (shock) T75.4
    burn — *see* Burn
  exertion (excessive) T73.3
  exposure — *see* Exposure
  external cause NEC T75.89
  foodstuffs T78.1
    allergic reaction — *see* Allergy, food
      causing anaphylaxis — *see* Shock, anaphylactic,
        due to food
    noxious — *see* Poisoning, food, noxious
  gases, fumes, or vapors T59.9-
    specified agent — *see* Table of Drugs and
      Chemicals
  glue (airplane) sniffing
    due to drug abuse — *see* Abuse, drug, inhalant
    due to drug dependence — *see* Dependence, drug,
      inhalant
  heat — *see* Heat
  high altitude NEC T70.29
    anoxia T70.29
    on
      ears T70.0
      sinuses T70.1
    polycythemia D75.1
  high pressure fluids T70.4
  hot weather — *see* Heat
  hunger T73.0
  immersion, foot — *see* Immersion
  immunization — *see* Complications, vaccination
  immunological agents — *see* Complications,
    vaccination
  infrared (radiation) (rays) NOS T66
    dermatitis or eczema L59.8
  infusion — *see* Complications, infusion
  lack of care of infants — *see* Maltreatment, child
  lightning — *see* Lightning
  medical care T88.9
    specified NEC T88.8
  medicinal substance, correct, properly
    administered — *see* Effect, adverse, drug
  motion T75.3
  noise, on inner ear — *see* subcategory H83.3
  overheated places — *see* Heat
  psychosocial, of work environment Z56.5
  radiation (diagnostic) (infrared) (natural source)
    (therapeutic) (ultraviolet) (X-ray) NOS T66
    dermatitis or eczema — *see* Dermatitis, due to,
      radiation
    fibrosis of lung J70.1
    pneumonitis J70.0
    pulmonary manifestations

Effect, adverse - *continued*
  radiation (diagnostic) (infrared) (natural source)
  (therapeutic) (ultraviolet) (X-ray) NOS - *continued*
    pulmonary manifestations - *continued*
      acute J70.0
      chronic J70.1
    skin L59.9
  radioactive substance NOS
    dermatitis or eczema — *see* Radiodermatitis
  reduced temperature T69.9
    immersion foot or hand — *see* Immersion
    specified effect NEC T69.8
  serum NEC — *see also* Reaction, serum T80.69
  specified NEC T78.8
    external cause NEC T75.89
  strangulation — *see* Asphyxia, traumatic
  submersion T75.1
  thirst T73.1
  toxic — *see* Toxicity
  transfusion — *see* Complications, transfusion
  ultraviolet (radiation) (rays) NOS T66
    burn — *see* Burn
    dermatitis or eczema — *see* Dermatitis, due to,
      ultraviolet rays
      acute L56.8
  vaccine (any) — *see* Complications, vaccination
  vibration — *see* Vibration, adverse effects
  water pressure NEC T70.9
    specified NEC T70.8
  weightlessness T75.82
  whole blood — *see* Complications, transfusion
  work environment Z56.5
Effects, late — *see* Sequelae
Effluvium
  anagen L65.1
  telogen L65.0
Effort syndrome (psychogenic) F45.8
Effusion
  amniotic fluid — *see* Pregnancy, complicated by,
    prematue rupture of membranes
  brain (serous) G93.6
  bronchial — *see* Bronchitis
  cerebral G93.6
  cerebrospinal — *see also* Meningitis
    vessel G93.6
  chest — *see* Effusion, pleura
  chylous, chyliform (pleura) J94.0
  intracranial G93.6
  joint M25.40
    ankle M25.47-
    elbow M25.42-
    foot joint M25.47-
    hand joint M25.44-
    hip M25.45-
    knee M25.46-
    shoulder M25.41-
    specified joint NEC M25.48
    wrist M25.43-
  malignant pleural J91.0
  meninges — *see* Meningitis
  pericardium, pericardial (noninflammatory) I31.3
    acute — *see* Pericarditis, acute
  peritoneal (chronic) R18.8
  pleura, pleurisy, pleuritic, pleuropericardial J90
    chylous, chyliform J94.0
    due to systemic lupus erythematosis M32.13
    influenzal — *see* Influenza, with, respiratory
      manifestations NEC
    malignant J91.0
    newborn P28.89
    tuberculous NEC A15.6
      primary (progressive) A15.7
  spinal — *see* Meningitis
  thorax, thoracic — *see* Effusion, pleura
Egg shell nails L60.3
  congenital Q84.6
Egyptian splenomegaly B65.1
Ehlers-Danlos syndrome Q79.6
Ehrlichiosis A77.40
  due to
    E. chafeensis A77.41
    E. sennetsu A79.81
    specified organism NEC A77.49
Eichstedt's disease B36.0
Eisenmenger's
  complex or syndrome I27.89
  defect Q21.8
Ejaculation
  delayed F52.32
  painful N53.12
  premature F52.4
  retarded N53.11
  retrograde N53.14

Ejaculation - *continued*
  semen, painful N53.12
    psychogenic F52.6
Ekbom's syndrome (restless legs) G25.81
Ekman's syndrome (brittle bones and blue
  sclera) Q78.0
Elastic skin Q82.8
  acquired L57.4
Elastofibroma — *see* Neoplasm, connective tissue,
  benign
Elastoma (juvenile) Q82.8
  Miescher's L87.2
Elastomyofibrosis I42.4
Elastosis
  actinic, solar L57.8
  atrophicans (senile) L57.4
  perforans serpiginosa L87.2
  senilis L57.4
Elbow — *see* condition
Electric current, electricity, effects (concussion)
  (fatal) (nonfatal) (shock) T75.4
  burn — *see* Burn
Electric feet syndrome E53.8
Electrocution T75.4
  from electroshock gun (taser) T75.4
Electrolyte imbalance E87.8
  with
    abortion — *see* Abortion by type, complicated by,
      electrolyte imbalance
    ectopic pregnancy O08.5
    molar pregnancy O08.5
Elephantiasis (nonfilarial) I89.0
  arabicum — *see* Infestation, filarial
  bancroftian B74.0
  congenital (any site) (hereditary) Q82.0
  due to
    Brugia (malayi) B74.1
      timori B74.2
    mastectomy I97.2
    Wuchereria (bancrofti) B74.0
  eyelid H02.859
    left H02.856
      lower H02.855
      upper H02.854
    right H02.853
      lower H02.852
      upper H02.851
  filarial, filariensis — *see* Infestation, filarial
  glandular I89.0
  graecorum A30.9
  lymphangiectatic I89.0
  lymphatic vessel I89.0
    due to mastectomy I97.2
  scrotum (nonfilarial) I89.0
  streptococcal I89.0
  surgical I97.89
    postmastectomy I97.2
  telangiectodes I89.0
  vulva (nonfilarial) N90.89
Elevated, elevation
  antibody titer R76.0
  basal metabolic rate R94.8
  blood pressure — *see also* Hypertension
    reading (incidental) (isolated) (nonspecific) , no
      diagnosis of hypertension R03.0
  blood sugar R73.9
  body temperature (of unknown origin) R50.9
  C-reactive protein (CRP) R79.82
  cancer antigen 125 [CA 125] R97.1
  carcinoembryonic antigen [CEA] R97.0
  cholesterol E78.00
    with high triglycerides E78.2
  conjugate, eye H51.0
  diaphragm, congenital Q79.1
  erythrocyte sedimentation rate R70.0
  fasting glucose R73.01
  fasting triglycerides E78.1
  finding on laboratory examination — *see* Findings,
    abnormal, inconclusive, without diagnosis, by type
    of exam
  GFR (glomerular filtration rate) — *see* Findings,
    abnormal, inconclusive, without diagnosis, by type
    of exam
  glucose tolerance (oral) R73.02
  immunoglobulin level R76.8
  indoleacetic acid R82.5
  lactic acid dehydrogenase (LDH) level R74.0
  leukocytes D72.829
  lipoprotein a level E78.8
  liver function
    study R94.5
    test R79.89
      alkaline phosphatase R74.8

Elevated, elevation - *continued*
liver function - *continued*
test - *continued*
aminotransferase R74.0
bilirubin R17
hepatic enzyme R74.8
lactate dehydrogenase R74.0
lymphocytes D72.820
prostate specific antigen [PSA] R97.20
Rh titer — *see* Complication(s), transfusion,
incompatibility reaction, Rh (factor)
scapula, congenital Q74.0
sedimentation rate R70.0
SGOT R74.0
SGPT R74.0
transaminase level R74.0
triglycerides E78.1
with high cholesterol E78.2
tumor associated antigens [TAA] NEC R97.8
tumor specific antigens [TSA] NEC R97.8
urine level of
catecholamine R82.5
indoleacetic acid R82.5
17-ketosteroids R82.5
steroids R82.5
vanillylmandelic acid (VMA) R82.5
venous pressure I87.8
white blood cell count D72.829
specified NEC D72.828
Elliptocytosis (congenital) (hereditary) D58.1
Hb C (disease) D58.1
hemoglobin disease D58.1
sickle-cell (disease) D57.8-
trait D57.3
Ellison-Zollinger syndrome E16.4
Ellis-van Creveld syndrome
(chondroectodermal dysplasia) Q77.6
Elongated, elongation (congenital) — *see
also* Distortion
bone Q79.9
cervix (uteri) Q51.828
acquired N88.4
hypertrophic N88.4
colon Q43.8
common bile duct Q44.5
cystic duct Q44.5
frenulum, penis Q55.69
labia minora (acquired) N90.69
ligamentum patellae Q74.1
petiolus (epiglottidis) Q31.8
tooth, teeth K00.2
uvula Q38.6
Eltor cholera A00.1
Emaciation (due to malnutrition) E41
Embadomoniasis A07.8
Embedded tooth, teeth K01.0
root only K08.3
Embolic — *see* condition
Embolism (multiple) (paradoxical) I74.9
air (any site) (traumatic) T79.0
following
abortion — *see* Abortion by type complicated by
embolism
ectopic pregnancy O08.2
infusion, therapeutic injection or
transfusion T80.0
molar pregnancy O08.2
procedure NEC
artery T81.719
mesenteric T81.710
renal T81.711
specified NEC T81.718
vein T81.72
in pregnancy, childbirth or puerperium — *see*
Embolism, obstetric
amniotic fluid (pulmonary) — *see also* Embolism,
obstetric
following
abortion — *see* Abortion by type complicated by
embolism
ectopic pregnancy O08.2
molar pregnancy O08.2
aorta, aortic I74.10
abdominal I74.09
saddle I74.01
bifurcation I74.09
saddle I74.01
thoracic I74.11
artery I74.9
auditory, internal I65.8
basilar — *see* Occlusion, artery, basilar
carotid (common) (internal) — *see* Occlusion,
artery, carotid

Embolism (multiple) (paradoxical) - *continued*
artery - *continued*
cerebellar (anterior inferior) (posterior inferior)
(superior) I66.3
cerebral — *see* Occlusion, artery, cerebral
choroidal (anterior) I66.8
communicating posterior I66.8
coronary — *see also* Infarct, myocardium
not resulting in infarction I24.0
extremity I74.4
lower I74.3
upper I74.2
hypophyseal I66.8
iliac I74.5
limb I74.4
lower I74.3
upper I74.2
mesenteric (with gangrene) — *see also* Ischemia,
intestine, acute K55.059
ophthalmic — *see* Occlusion, artery, retina
peripheral I74.4
pontine I66.8
precerebral — *see* Occlusion, artery, precerebral
pulmonary — *see* Embolism, pulmonary
renal N28.0
retinal — *see* Occlusion, artery, retina
septic I76
specified NEC I74.8
vertebral — *see* Occlusion, artery, vertebral
basilar (artery) I65.1
blood clot
following
abortion — *see* Abortion by type complicated by
embolism
ectopic or molar pregnancy O08.2
in pregnancy, childbirth or puerperium — *see*
Embolism, obstetric
brain — *see also* Occlusion, artery, cerebral
following
abortion — *see* Abortion by type complicated by
embolism
ectopic or molar pregnancy O08.2
puerperal, postpartum, childbirth — *see* Embolism,
obstetric
capillary I78.8
cardiac — *see also* Infarct, myocardium
not resulting in infarction I51.3
carotid (artery) (common) (internal) — *see*
Occlusion, artery, carotid
cavernous sinus (venous) — *see* Embolism,
intracranial venous sinus
cerebral — *see* Occlusion, artery, cerebral
cholesterol — *see* Atheroembolism
coronary (artery or vein) (systemic) — *see*
Occlusion, coronary
due to device, implant or graft — *see
also* Complications, by site and type, specified
NEC
arterial graft NEC T82.818
breast (implant) T85.818
catheter NEC T85.818
dialysis (renal) T82.818
intraperitoneal T85.818
infusion NEC T82.818
spinal (epidural) (subdural) T85.810
urinary (indwelling) T83.81
electronic (electrode) (pulse generator) (stimulator)
bone T84.81
cardiac T82.817
nervous system (brain) (peripheral nerve)
(spinal) T85.810
urinary T83.81
fixation, internal (orthopedic) NEC T84.81
gastrointestinal (bile duct) (esophagus) T85.818
genital NEC T83.81
heart (graft) (valve) T82.817
joint prosthesis T84.81
ocular (corneal graft) (orbital implant) T85.818
orthopedic (bone graft) NEC T86.838
specified NEC T85.818
urinary (graft) NEC T83.81
vascular NEC T82.818
ventricular intracranial shunt T85.810
extremities
lower — *see* Embolism, vein, lower extremity
arterial I74.3
upper I74.2
eye H34.9
fat (cerebral) (pulmonary) (systemic) T79.1
following
abortion — *see* Abortion by type complicated by
embolism
ectopic or molar pregnancy O08.2

Embolism (multiple) (paradoxical) - *continued*
fat (cerebral) (pulmonary) (systemic) - *continued*
complicating delivery — *see* Embolism, obstetric
following
abortion — *see* Abortion by type complicated by
embolism
ectopic or molar pregnancy O08.2
infusion, therapeutic injection or transfusion
air T80.0
heart (fatty) — *see also* Infarct, myocardium
not resulting in infarction I51.3
hepatic (vein) I82.0
in pregnancy, childbirth or puerperium — *see*
Embolism, obstetric
intestine (artery) (vein) (with gangrene) — *see
also* Ischemia, intestine, acute K55.039
intracranial — *see also* Occlusion, artery, cerebral
venous sinus (any) G08
nonpyogenic I67.6
intraspinal venous sinuses or veins G08
nonpyogenic G95.19
kidney (artery) N28.0
lateral sinus (venous) — *see* Embolism, intracranial,
venous sinus
leg — *see* Embolism, vein, lower extremity
arterial I74.3
longitudinal sinus (venous) — *see* Embolism,
intracranial, venous sinus
lung (massive) — *see* Embolism, pulmonary
meninges I66.8
mesenteric (artery) (vein) (with gangrene) —
see also Ischemia, intestine, acute K55.059
obstetric (in) (pulmonary)
childbirth O88.22
air O88.02
amniotic fluid O88.12
blood clot O88.22
fat O88.82
pyemic O88.32
septic O88.32
specified type NEC O88.82
pregnancy O88.21-
air O88.01-
amniotic fluid O88.11-
blood clot O88.21-
fat O88.81-
pyemic O88.31-
septic O88.31-
specified type NEC O88.81-
puerperal O88.23
air O88.03
amniotic fluid O88.13
blood clot O88.23
fat O88.83
pyemic O88.33
septic O88.33
specified type NEC O88.83
ophthalmic — *see* Occlusion, artery, retina
penis N48.81
peripheral artery NOS I74.4
pituitary E23.6
popliteal (artery) I74.3
portal (vein) I81
postoperative, postprocedural
artery T81.719
mesenteric T81.710
renal T81.711
specified NEC T81.718
vein T81.72
precerebral artery — *see* Occlusion, artery,
precerebral
puerperal — *see* Embolism, obstetric
pulmonary (acute) (artery) (vein) I26.99
with acute cor pulmonale I26.09
chronic I27.82
following
abortion — *see* Abortion by type complicated by
embolism
ectopic or molar pregnancy O08.2
healed or old Z86.711
in pregnancy, childbirth or puerperium — *see*
Embolism, obstetric
personal history of Z86.711
saddle I26.92
with acute cor pulmonale I26.02
septic I26.90
with acute cor pulmonale I26.01
pyemic (multiple) I76
following
abortion — *see* Abortion by type complicated by
embolism
ectopic or molar pregnancy O08.2
Hemophilus influenzae A41.3

Embolism (multiple) (paradoxical) - *continued*
pyemic (multiple) - *continued*
  pneumococcal A40.3
    with pneumonia J13
  puerperal, postpartum, childbirth (any
    organism) — *see* Embolism, obstetric
  specified organism NEC A41.89
  staphylococcal A41.2
  streptococcal A40.9
renal (artery) N28.0
  vein I82.3
retina, retinal — *see* Occlusion, artery, retina
saddle
  abdominal aorta I74.01
  pulmonary artery I26.92
    with acute cor pulmonale I26.02
septic (arterial) I76
  complicating abortion — *see* Abortion, by type,
    complicated by, embolism
sinus — *see* Embolism, intracranial, venous sinus
soap complicating abortion — *see* Abortion, by type,
  complicated by, embolism
spinal cord G95.19
  pyogenic origin G06.1
spleen, splenic (artery) I74.8
upper extremity I74.2
vein (acute) I82.90
  antecubital I82.61-
    chronic I82.71-
  axillary I82.A1-
    chronic I82.A2-
  basilic I82.61-
    chronic I82.71-
  brachial I82.62-
    chronic I82.72-
  brachiocephalic (innominate) I82.290
    chronic I82.291
  cephalic I82.61-
    chronic I82.71-
  chronic I82.91
  deep (DVT) I82.40-
    calf I82.4Z-
      chronic I82.5Z-
    lower leg I82.4Z-
      chronic I82.5Z-
    thigh I82.4Y-
      chronic I82.5Y-
    upper leg I82.4Y
      chronic I82.5y--
  femoral I82.41-
    chronic I82.51-
  iliac (iliofemoral) I82.42-
    chronic I82.52-
  innominate I82.290
    chronic I82.291
  internal jugular I82.C1-
    chronic I82.C2-
  lower extremity
    deep I82.40-
      chronic I82.50-
      specified NEC I82.49-
        chronic NEC I82.59-
    distal
      deep I82.4Z-
    proximal
      deep I82.4Y-
        chronic I82.5Y-
    superficial I82.81-
  popliteal I82.43-
    chronic I82.53-
  radial I82.62-
    chronic I82.72-
  renal I82.3
  saphenous (greater) (lesser) I82.81-
  specified NEC I82.890
    chronic NEC I82.891
  subclavian I82.B1-
    chronic I82.B2-
  thoracic NEC I82.290
    chronic I82.291
  tibial I82.44-
    chronic I82.54-
  ulnar I82.62-
    chronic I82.72-
  upper extremity I82.60-
    chronic I82.70-
    deep I82.62-
      chronic I82.72-
    superficial I82.61-
      chronic I82.71-
vena cava
  inferior (acute) I82.220
    chronic I82.221

Embolism (multiple) (paradoxical) - *continued*
vena cava - *continued*
  superior (acute) I82.210
    chronic I82.211
  venous sinus G08
  vessels of brain — *see* Occlusion, artery, cerebral
Embolus — *see* Embolism
Embryoma — *see also* Neoplasm, uncertain
behavior, by site
benign — *see* Neoplasm, benign, by site
kidney C64.-
liver C22.0
malignant — *see also* Neoplasm, malignant, by site
  kidney C64.-
  liver C22.0
  testis C62.9-
    descended (scrotal) C62.1-
    undescended C62.0-
testis C62.9-
  descended (scrotal) C62.1-
  undescended C62.0-
Embryonic
circulation Q28.9
heart Q28.9
vas deferens Q55.4
Embryopathia NOS Q89.9
Embryotoxon Q13.4
Emesis — *see* Vomiting
Emotional lability R45.86
Emotionality, pathological F60.3
Emotogenic disease — *see* Disorder, psychogenic
Emphysema (atrophic) (bullous) (chronic)
  (interlobular) (lung) (obstructive) (pulmonary)
  (senile) (vesicular) J43.9
cellular tissue (traumatic) T79.7
  surgical T81.82
centrilobular J43.2
compensatory J98.3
congenital (interstitial) P25.0
conjunctiva H11.89
connective tissue (traumatic) T79.7
  surgical T81.82
due to chemicals, gases, fumes or vapors J68.4
eyelid (s) — *see* Disorder, eyelid, specified type
  NEC
  surgical T81.82
  traumatic T79.7
interstitial J98.2
  congenital P25.0
  perinatal period P25.0
laminated tissue T79.7
  surgical T81.82
mediastinal J98.2
  newborn P25.2
orbit, orbital — *see* Disorder, orbit, specified type
  NEC
panacinar J43.1
panlobular J43.1
specified NEC J43.8
subcutaneous (traumatic) T79.7
  nontraumatic J98.2
  postprocedural T81.82
  surgical T81.82
surgical T81.82
thymus (gland) (congenital) E32.8
traumatic (subcutaneous) T79.7
unilateral J43.0
Empty nest syndrome Z60.0
Empyema (acute) (chest) (double) (pleura)
  (supradiaphragmatic) (thorax) J86.9
with fistula J86.0
accessory sinus (chronic) — *see* Sinusitis
antrum (chronic) — *see* Sinusitis, maxillary
brain (any part) — *see* Abscess, brain
ethmoidal (chronic) (sinus) — *see* Sinusitis,
  ethmoidal
extradural — *see* Abscess, extradural
frontal (chronic) (sinus) — *see* Sinusitis, frontal
gallbladder K81.0
mastoid (process) (acute) — *see* Mastoiditis, acute
maxilla, maxillary M27.2
  sinus (chronic) — *see* Sinusitis, maxillary
nasal sinus (chronic) — *see* Sinusitis
sinus (accessory) (chronic) (nasal) — *see* Sinusitis
sphenoidal (sinus) (chronic) — *see* Sinusitis,
  sphenoidal
subarachnoid — *see* Abscess, extradural
subdural — *see* Abscess, subdural
tuberculous A15.6
ureter — *see* Ureteritis
ventricular — *see* Abscess, brain
En coup de sabre lesion L94.1
Enamel pearls K00.2

Enameloma K00.2
Enanthema, viral B09
Encephalitis (chronic) (hemorrhagic) (idiopathic)
  (nonepidemic) (spurious) (subacute) G04.90
acute — *see also* Encephalitis, viral A86
  disseminated G04.00
    infectious G04.01
    noninfectious G04.81
    postimmunization (postvaccination) G04.02
    postinfectious G04.01
  inclusion body A85.8
  necrotizing hemorrhagic G04.30
    postimmunization G04.32
    postinfectious G04.31
    specified NEC G04.39
arboviral, arbovirus NEC A85.2
arthropod-borne NEC (viral) A85.2
Australian A83.4
California (virus) A83.5
Central European (tick-borne) A84.1
Czechoslovakian A84.1
Dawson's (inclusion body) A81.1
diffuse sclerosing A81.1
disseminated, acute G04.00
due to
  cat scratch disease A28.1
  human immunodeficiency virus (HIV)
    disease B20 *[G05.3]*
  malaria — *see* Malaria
  rickettsiosis — *see* Rickettsiosis
  smallpox inoculation G04.02
  typhus — *see* Typhus
Eastern equine A83.2
endemic (viral) A86
epidemic NEC (viral) A86
equine (acute) (infectious) (viral) A83.9
  Eastern A83.2
  Venezuelan A92.2
  Western A83.1
Far Eastern (tick-borne) A84.0
following vaccination or other immunization
  procedure G04.02
herpes zoster B02.0
herpesviral B00.4
  due to herpesvirus 6 B10.01
  due to herpesvirus 7 B10.09
  specified NEC B10.09
Ilheus (virus) A83.8
inclusion body A81.1
in (due to)
  actinomycosis A42.82
  adenovirus A85.1
  African trypanosomiasis B56.9 *[G05.3]*
  Chagas' disease (chronic) B57.42
  cytomegalovirus B25.8
  enterovirus A85.0
  herpes (simplex) virus B00.4
    due to herpesvirus 6 B10.01
    due to herpesvirus 7 B10.09
    specified NEC B10.09
  infectious disease NEC B99 *[G05.3]*
  influenza — *see* Influenza, with, encephalopathy
  listeriosis A32.12
  measles B05.0
  mumps B26.2
  naegleriasis B60.2
  parasitic disease NEC B89 *[G05.3]*
  poliovirus A80.9 *[G05.3]*
  rubella B06.01
  syphilis
    congenital A50.42
    late A52.14
  systemic lupus erythematosus M32.19
  toxoplasmosis (acquired) B58.2
    congenital P37.1
  tuberculosis A17.82
  zoster B02.0
infectious (acute) (virus) NEC A86
Japanese (B type) A83.0
La Crosse A83.5
lead — *see* Poisoning, lead
lethargica (acute) (infectious) A85.8
louping ill A84.8
lupus erythematosus, systemic M32.19
lymphatica A87.2
Mengo A85.8
meningococcal A39.81
Murray Valley A83.4
otitic NEC H66.40 *[G05.3]*
parasitic NOS B71.9
periaxial G37.0
periaxialis (concentrica) (diffuse) G37.5
postchickenpox B01.11

Encephalitis (chronic) (hemorrhagic) (idiopathic) (nonepidemic) (spurious) (subacute) - *continued*
  postexanthematous NEC B09
  postimmunization G04.02
  postinfectious NEC G04.01
  postmeasles B05.0
  postvaccinal G04.02
  postvaricella B01.11
  postviral NEC A86
  Powassan A84.8
  Rasmussen G04.81
  Rio Bravo A85.8
  Russian
    autumnal A83.0
    spring-summer (taiga) A84.0
  saturnine — *see* Poisoning, lead
  specified NEC G04.81
  St. Louis A83.3
  subacute sclerosing A81.1
  summer A83.0
  suppurative G04.81
  tick-borne A84.9
  Torula, torular (cryptococcal) B45.1
  toxic NEC G92
  trichinosis B75 *[G05.3]*
  type
    B A83.0
    C A83.3
  van Bogaert's A81.1
  Venezuelan equine A92.2
  Vienna A85.8
  viral, virus A86
    arthropod-borne NEC A85.2
      mosquito-borne A83.9
        Australian X disease A83.4
        California virus A83.5
        Eastern equine A83.2
        Japanese (B type) A83.0
        Murray Valley A83.4
        specified NEC A83.8
        St. Louis A83.3
        type B A83.0
        type C A83.3
        Western equine A83.1
      tick-borne A84.9
        biundulant A84.1
        central European A84.1
        Czechoslovakian A84.1
        diphasic meningoencephalitis A84.1
        Far Eastern A84.0
        Russian spring-summer (taiga) A84.0
        specified NEC A84.8
      specified type NEC A85.8
  Western equine A83.1
Encephalocele Q01.9
  frontal Q01.0
  nasofrontal Q01.1
  occipital Q01.2
  specified NEC Q01.8
Encephalocystocele — *see* Encephalocele
Encephaloduroarteriomyosynangiosis (EDAMS) I67.5
Encephalomalacia (brain) (cerebellar) (cerebral) — *see* Softening, brain
Encephalomeningitis — *see* Meningoencephalitis
Encephalomeningocele — *see* Encephalocele
Encephalomeningomyelitis — *see* Meningoencephalitis
Encephalomyelitis — *see also* Encephalitis G04.90
  acute disseminated G04.00
    infectious G04.01
    noninfectious G04.81
    postimmunization G04.02
    postinfectious G04.01
  acute necrotizing hemorrhagic G04.30
    postimmunization G04.32
    postinfectious G04.31
    specified NEC G04.39
  benign myalgic G93.3
  equine A83.9
    Eastern A83.2
    Venezuelan A92.2
    Western A83.1
  in diseases classified elsewhere G05.3
  myalgic, benign G93.3
  postchickenpox B01.11
  postinfectious NEC G04.01
  postmeasles B05.0
  postvaccinal G04.02
  postvaricella B01.11
  rubella B06.01
  specified NEC G04.81
  Venezuelan equine A92.2

Encephalomyelocele — *see* Encephalocele
Encephalomyelomeningitis — *see* Meningoencephalitis
Encephalomyelopathy G96.9
Encephalomyeloradiculitis (acute) G61.0
Encephalomyeloradiculoneuritis (acute) (Guillain-Barré) G61.0
Encephalomyeloradiculopathy G96.9
Encephalopathia hyperbilirubinemica, newborn P57.9
  due to isoimmunization (conditions in P55) P57.0
Encephalopathy (acute) G93.40
  acute necrotizing hemorrhagic G04.30
    postimmunization G04.32
    postinfectious G04.31
    specified NEC G04.39
  alcoholic G31.2
  anoxic — *see* Damage, brain, anoxic
  arteriosclerotic I67.2
  centrolobar progressive (Schilder) G37.0
  congenital Q07.9
  degenerative, in specified disease NEC G32.89
  demyelinating callosal G37.1
  due to
    drugs - — *see also* Table of Drugs and Chemicals G92
  hepatic — *see* Failure, hepatic
  hyperbilirubinemic, newborn P57.9
    due to isoimmunization (conditions in P55) P57.0
  hypertensive I67.4
  hypoglycemic E16.2
  hypoxic — *see* Damage, brain, anoxic
  hypoxic ischemic P91.60
    mild P91.61
    moderate P91.62
    severe P91.63
  in (due to) (with)
    birth injury P11.1
    hyperinsulinism E16.1 *[G94]*
    influenza — *see* Influenza, with, encephalopathy
    lack of vitamin — *see also* Deficiency, vitamin E56.9 *[G32.89]*
    neoplastic disease (see also Neoplasm) D49.9 *[G13.1]*
    serum — *see also* Reaction, serum T80.69
    syphilis A52.17
    trauma (postconcussional) F07.81
      current injury — *see* Injury, intracranial
    vaccination G04.02
  lead — *see* Poisoning, lead
  metabolic G93.41
    drug induced G92
    toxic G92
  myoclonic, early, symptomatic — *see* Epilepsy, generalized, specified NEC
  necrotizing, subacute (Leigh) G31.82
  pellagrous E52 *[G32.89]*
  portosystemic — *see* Failure, hepatic
  postcontusional F07.81
    current injury — *see* Injury, intracranial, diffuse
  posthypoglycemic (coma) E16.1 *[G94]*
  postradiation G93.89
  saturnine — *see* Poisoning, lead
  septic G93.41
  specified NEC G93.49
  spongioform, subacute (viral) A81.09
  toxic G92
    metabolic G92
  traumatic (postconcussional) F07.81
    current injury — *see* Injury, intracranial
  vitamin B deficiency NEC E53.9 *[G32.89]*
    vitamin B1 E51.2
  Wernicke's E51.2
Encephalorrhagia — *see* Hemorrhage, intracranial, intracerebral
Encephalosis, posttraumatic F07.81
Enchondroma — *see also* Neoplasm, bone, benign
Enchondromatosis (cartilaginous) (multiple) Q78.4
Encopresis R15.9
  functional F98.1
  nonorganic origin F98.1
  psychogenic F98.1
Encounter (with health service) (for) Z76.89
  adjustment and management (of)
    breast implant Z45.81
    implanted device NEC Z45.89
    myringotomy device (stent) (tube) Z45.82
  administrative purpose only Z02.9
    examination for
      adoption Z02.82
      armed forces Z02.3
      disability determination Z02.71
      driving license Z02.4

Encounter (with health service) (for) - *continued*
  administrative purpose only - *continued*
    examination for - *continued*
      employment Z02.1
      insurance Z02.6
      medical certificate NEC Z02.79
      paternity testing Z02.81
      residential institution admission Z02.2
      school admission Z02.0
      sports Z02.5
      specified reason NEC Z02.89
  aftercare — *see* Aftercare
  antenatal screening Z36
  assisted reproductive fertility procedure cycle Z31.83
  blood typing Z01.83
    Rh typing Z01.83
  breast augmentation or reduction Z41.1
  breast implant exchange (different material) (different size) Z45.81
  breast reconstruction following mastectomy Z42.1
  check-up — *see* Examination
  chemotherapy for neoplasm Z51.11
  colonoscopy, screening Z12.11
  counseling — *see* Counseling
  delivery, full-term, uncomplicated O80
    cesarean, without indication O82
  desensitization to allergens Z51.6
  ear piercing Z41.3
  examination — *see* Examination
  expectant parent (s) (adoptive) pre-birth pediatrician visit Z76.81
  fertility preservation procedure (prior to cancer therapy) (prior to removal of gonads) Z31.84
  fitting (of) — *see* Fitting (and adjustment) (of)
  genetic
    counseling Z31.5
    testing — *see* Test, genetic
  hearing conservation and treatment Z01.12
  immunotherapy for neoplasm Z51.12
  in vitro fertilization cycle Z31.83
  instruction (in)
    childbirth Z32.2
    child care (postpartal) (prenatal) Z32.3
    natural family planning
      procreative Z31.61
      to avoid pregnancy Z30.02
  insulin pump titration Z46.81
  joint prosthesis insertion following prior explantation of joint prosthesis (staged procedure)
    hip Z47.32
    knee Z47.33
    shoulder Z47.31
  laboratory (as part of a general medical examination) Z00.00
    with abnormal findings Z00.01
  mental health services (for)
    abuse NEC
      perpetrator Z69.82
      victim Z69.81
    child abuse
      nonparental
        perpetrator Z69.021
        victim Z69.020
      parental
        perpetrator Z69.011
        victim Z69.010
    spousal or partner abuse
      perpetrator Z69.12
      victim Z69.11
  observation (for) (ruled out)
    exposure to (suspected)
      anthrax Z03.810
      biological agent NEC Z03.818
  pediatrician visit, by expectant parent (s) (adoptive) Z76.81
  plastic and reconstructive surgery following medical procedure or healed injury NEC Z42.8
  pregnancy
    supervision of — *see* Pregnancy, supervision of
    test Z32.00
      result negative Z32.02
      result positive Z32.01
  procreative management and counseling for gestational carrier Z31.7
  prophylactic measures Z29.9
    antivenin Z29.12
    fluoride administration Z29.3
    immunotherapy for respiratory syncytial virus (RSV) Z29.11
    rabies immune globin Z29.14
    Rho (D) immune globulin Z29.13
    specified NEC Z29.8

Encounter (with health service) (for) - *continued*
  radiation therapy (antineoplastic) Z51.0
  radiological (as part of a general medical
    examination) Z00.00
    with abnormal findings Z00.01
  reconstructive surgery following medical procedure
    or healed injury NEC Z42.8
  removal (of) — *see also* Removal
    artificial
      arm Z44.00-
        complete Z44.01-
        partial Z44.02-
      eye Z44.2-
      leg Z44.10-
        complete Z44.11-
        partial Z44.12-
    breast implant Z45.81
      tissue expander (without synchronous insertion of
        permanent implant) Z45.81
    device Z46.9
      specified NEC Z46.89
    external
      fixation device - code to fracture with seventh
        character D
      prosthesis, prosthetic device Z44.9
        breast Z44.3-
        specified NEC Z44.8
    implanted device NEC Z45.89
    insulin pump Z46.81
    internal fixation device Z47.2
    myringotomy device (stent) (tube) Z45.82
    nervous system device NEC Z46.2
      brain neuropacemaker Z46.2
      visual substitution device Z46.2
        implanted Z45.31
    non-vascular catheter Z46.82
    orthodontic device Z46.4
    stent
      ureteral Z46.6
    urinary device Z46.6
  repeat cervical smear to confirm findings of recent
    normal smear following initial abnormal
    smear Z01.42
  respirator [ventilator] use during power
    failure Z99.12
  Rh typing Z01.83
  screening — *see* Screening
  specified NEC Z76.89
  sterilization Z30.2
  suspected condition, ruled out
    amniotic cavity and membrane Z03.71
    cervical shortening Z03.75
    fetal anomaly Z03.73
    fetal growth Z03.74
    maternal and fetal conditions NEC Z03.79
    oligohydramnios Z03.71
    placental problem Z03.72
    polyhydramnios Z03.71
  suspected exposure (to) , ruled out
    anthrax Z03.810
    biological agents NEC Z03.818
  termination of pregnancy, elective Z33.2
  testing — *see* Test
  therapeutic drug level monitoring Z51.81
  titration, insulin pump Z46.81
  to determine fetal viability of pregnancy O36.80
  training
    insulin pump Z46.81
  X-ray of chest (as part of a general medical
    examination) Z00.00
    with abnormal findings Z00.01
Encystment — *see* Cyst
Endarteritis (bacterial, subacute) (infective) I77.6
  brain I67.7
  cerebral or cerebrospinal I67.7
  deformans — *see* Arteriosclerosis
  embolic — *see* Embolism
  obliterans — *see also* Arteriosclerosis
    pulmonary I28.8
  pulmonary I28.8
  retina — *see* Vasculitis, retina
  senile — *see* Arteriosclerosis
  syphilitic A52.09
    brain or cerebral A52.04
    congenital A50.54 *[179.8]*
  tuberculous A18.89
Endemic — *see* condition
Endocarditis (chronic) (marantic) (nonbacterial)
  (thrombotic) (valvular) I38
  with rheumatic fever (conditions in I00)
    active — *see* Endocarditis, acute, rheumatic
    inactive or quiescent (with chorea) I09.1
  acute or subacute I33.9

Endocarditis (chronic) (marantic) (nonbacterial)
(thrombotic) (valvular) - *continued*
  acute or subacute - *continued*
    infective I33.0
    rheumatic (aortic) (mitral) (pulmonary)
      (tricuspid) I01.1
      with chorea (acute) (rheumatic)
        (Sydenham's) I02.0
  aortic (heart) (nonrheumatic) (valve) I35.8
    with
      mitral disease I08.0
        with tricuspid (valve) disease I08.3
        active or acute I01.1
          with chorea (acute) (rheumatic)
            (Sydenham's) I02.0
      rheumatic fever (conditions in I00)
        active — *see* Endocarditis, acute, rheumatic
        inactive or quiescent (with chorea) I06.9
      tricuspid (valve) disease I08.2
        with mitral (valve) disease I08.3
    acute or subacute I33.9
    arteriosclerotic I35.8
    rheumatic I06.9
      with mitral disease I08.0
        with tricuspid (valve) disease I08.3
        active or acute I01.1
          with chorea (acute) (rheumatic)
            (Sydenham's) I02.0
      active or acute I01.1
        with chorea (acute) (rheumatic)
          (Sydenham's) I02.0
      specified NEC I06.8
    specified cause NEC I35.8
    syphilitic A52.03
  arteriosclerotic I38
  atypical verrucous (Libman-Sacks) M32.11
  bacterial (acute) (any valve) (subacute) I33.0
  candidal B37.6
  congenital Q24.8
  constrictive I33.0
  Coxiella burnetii A78 *[139]*
  Coxsackie B33.21
  due to
    prosthetic cardiac valve T82.6
    Q fever A78 *[139]*
    Serratia marcescens I33.0
    typhoid (fever) A01.02
  gonococcal A54.83
  infectious or infective (acute) (any valve)
    (subacute) I33.0
  lenta (acute) (any valve) (subacute) I33.0
  Libman-Sacks M32.11
  listerial A32.82
  Löffler's I42.3
  malignant (acute) (any valve) (subacute) I33.0
  meningococcal A39.51
  mitral (chronic) (double) (fibroid) (heart) (inactive)
    (valve) (with chorea) I05.9
    with
      aortic (valve) disease I08.0
        with tricuspid (valve) disease I08.3
        active or acute I01.1
          with chorea (acute) (rheumatic)
            (Sydenham's) I02.0
      rheumatic fever (conditions in I00)
        active — *see* Endocarditis, acute, rheumatic
        inactive or quiescent (with chorea) I05.9
      tricuspid (valve) disease I08.1
        with aortic (valve) disease I08.3
    active or acute I01.1
      with chorea (acute) (rheumatic)
        (Sydenham's) I02.0
    bacterial I33.0
    arteriosclerotic I34.8
    nonrheumatic I34.8
      acute or subacute I33.9
    specified NEC I05.8
  monilial B37.6
  multiple valves I08.9
    specified disorders I08.8
  mycotic (acute) (any valve) (subacute) I33.0
  pneumococcal (acute) (any valve) (subacute) I33.0
  pulmonary (chronic) (heart) (valve) I37.8
    with rheumatic fever (conditions in I00)
      active — *see* Endocarditis, acute, rheumatic
      inactive or quiescent (with chorea) I09.89
        with aortic, mitral or tricuspid disease I08.8
    acute or subacute I33.9
    rheumatic I01.1
      with chorea (acute) (rheumatic)
        (Sydenham's) I02.0
    arteriosclerotic I37.8
    congenital Q22.2

Endocarditis (chronic) (marantic) (nonbacterial)
(thrombotic) (valvular) - *continued*
  pulmonary (chronic) (heart) (valve) - *continued*
    rheumatic (chronic) (inactive) (with chorea) I09.89
      active or acute I01.1
        with chorea (acute) (rheumatic)
          (Sydenham's) I02.0
      syphilitic A52.03
  purulent (acute) (any valve) (subacute) I33.0
  Q fever A78 *[139]*
  rheumatic (chronic) (inactive) (with chorea) I09.1
    active or acute (aortic) (mitral) (pulmonary)
      (tricuspid) I01.1
      with chorea (acute) (rheumatic)
        (Sydenham's) I02.0
  rheumatoid — *see* Rheumatoid, carditis
  septic (acute) (any valve) (subacute) I33.0
  streptococcal (acute) (any valve) (subacute) I33.0
  subacute — *see* Endocarditis, acute
  suppurative (acute) (any valve) (subacute) I33.0
  syphilitic A52.03
  toxic I33.9
  tricuspid (chronic) (heart) (inactive) (rheumatic)
    (valve) (with chorea) I07.9
    with
      aortic (valve) disease I08.2
        mitral (valve) disease I08.3
      mitral (valve) disease I08.1
        aortic disease I08.3
      rheumatic fever (conditions in I00)
        active — *see* Endocarditis, acute, rheumatic
        inactive or quiescent (with chorea) I07.8
    active or acute I01.1
      with chorea (acute) (rheumatic)
        (Sydenham's) I02.0
    arteriosclerotic I36.8
    nonrheumatic I36.8
      acute or subacute I33.9
    specified cause, except rheumatic I36.8
  tuberculous — *see* Tuberculosis, endocarditis
  typhoid A01.02
  ulcerative (acute) (any valve) (subacute) I33.0
  vegetative (acute) (any valve) (subacute) I33.0
  verrucous (atypical) (nonbacterial)
    (nonrheumatic) M32.11
Endocardium, endocardial — *see also* condition
  cushion defect Q21.2
Endocervicitis — *see also* Cervicitis
  due to intrauterine (contraceptive) device T83.69
  hyperplastic N72
Endocrine — *see* condition
Endocrinopathy, pluriglandular E31.9
Endodontic
  overfill M27.52
  underfill M27.53
Endodontitis K04.01
  irreversible K04.02
  reversible K04.01
Endomastoiditis — *see* Mastoiditis
Endometrioma N80.9
Endometriosis N80.9
  appendix N80.5
  bladder N80.8
  bowel N80.5
  broad ligament N80.3
  cervix N80.0
  colon N80.5
  cul-de-sac (Douglas') N80.3
  exocervix N80.0
  fallopian tube N80.2
  female genital organ NEC N80.8
  gallbladder N80.8
  in scar of skin N80.6
  internal N80.0
  intestine N80.5
  lung N80.8
  myometrium N80.0
  ovary N80.1
  parametrium N80.3
  pelvic peritoneum N80.3
  peritoneal (pelvic) N80.3
  rectovaginal septum N80.4
  rectum N80.5
  round ligament N80.3
  skin (scar) N80.6
  specified site NEC N80.8
  stromal D39.0
  umbilicus N80.8
  uterus (internal) N80.0
  vagina N80.4
  vulva N80.8

Endometritis (decidual) (nonspecific) (purulent) (senile) (atrophic) (suppurative) N71.9
  with ectopic pregnancy O08.0
  acute N71.0
  blenorrhagic (gonococcal) (acute) (chronic) A54.24
  cervix, cervical (with erosion or ectropion) — *see also* Cervicitis
    hyperplastic N72
  chlamydial A56.11
  chronic N71.1
  following
    abortion — *see* Abortion by type complicated by genital infection
    ectopic or molar pregnancy O08.0
  gonococcal, gonorrheal (acute) (chronic) A54.24
  hyperplastic — *see also* Hyperplasia, endometrial N85.00-
    cervix N72
  puerperal, postpartum, childbirth O86.12
  subacute N71.0
  tuberculous A18.17
Endometrium — *see* condition
Endomyocardiopathy, South African I42.3
Endomyocarditis — *see* Endocarditis
Endomyofibrosis I42.3
Endomyometritis — *see* Endometritis
Endopericarditis — *see* Endocarditis
Endoperineuritis — *see* Disorder, nerve
Endophlebitis — *see* Phlebitis
Endophthalmia — *see* Endophthalmitis, purulent
Endophthalmitis (acute) (infective) (metastatic) (subacute) H44.009
  bleb associated H59.4 — *see also* Bleb, inflamed (infected), postprocedural
  gonorrheal A54.39
  in (due to)
    cysticercosis B69.1
    onchocerciasis B73.01
    toxocariasis B83.0
  panuveitis — *see* Panuveitis
  parasitic H44.12-
  purulent H44.00-
    panophthalmitis — *see* Panophthalmitis
    vitreous abscess H44.02-
  specified NEC H44.19
  sympathetic — *see* Uveitis, sympathetic
Endosalpingioma D28.2
Endosalpingiosis N94.89
Endosteitis — *see* Osteomyelitis
Endothelioma, bone — *see* Neoplasm, bone, malignant
Endotheliosis (hemorrhagic infectional) D69.8
Endotoxemia - code to condition
Endotrachelitis — *see* Cervicitis
Engelmann (-Camurati) **syndrome** Q78.3
English disease — *see* Rickets
Engman's disease L30.3
Engorgement
  breast N64.59
    newborn P83.4
    puerperal, postpartum O92.79
  lung (passive) — *see* Edema, lung
  pulmonary (passive) — *see* Edema, lung
  stomach K31.89
  venous, retina — *see* Occlusion, retina, vein, engorgement
Enlargement, enlarged — *see also* Hypertrophy
  adenoids J35.2
    with tonsils J35.3
  alveolar ridge K08.89
    congenital — *see* Anomaly, alveolar
  apertures of diaphragm (congenital) Q79.1
  gingival K06.1
  heart, cardiac — *see* Hypertrophy, cardiac
  labium majus, childhood asymmetric (CALME) N90.61
  lacrimal gland, chronic H04.03-
  liver — *see* Hypertrophy, liver
  lymph gland or node R59.9
    generalized R59.1
    localized R59.0
  orbit H05.34-
  organ or site, congenital NEC — *see* Anomaly, by site
  parathyroid (gland) E21.0
  pituitary fossa R93.0
  prostate N40.0
    with lower urinary tract symptoms (LUTS) N40.1
    without lower urinary tract symtpoms (LUTS) N40.0
  sella turcica R93.0
  spleen — *see* Splenomegaly
  thymus (gland) (congenital) E32.0

Enlargement, enlarged - *continued*
  thyroid (gland) — *see* Goiter
  tongue K14.8
  tonsils J35.1
    with adenoids J35.3
  uterus N85.2
Enophthalmos H05.40-
  due to
    orbital tissue atrophy H05.41-
    trauma or surgery H05.42-
Enostosis M27.8
Entamebic, entamebiasis — *see* Amebiasis
Entanglement
  umbilical cord (s) O69.2
    with compression O69.2
      without compression O69.82
    around neck (with compression) O69.1
      without compression O69.81
    of twins in monoamniotic sac O69.2
Enteralgia — *see* Pain, abdominal
Enteric — *see* condition
Enteritis (acute) (diarrheal) (hemorrhagic) (noninfective) K52.9
  adenovirus A08.2
  aertrycke infection A02.0
  allergic K52.29
    with
      eosinophilic gastritis or gastroenteritis K52.81
      food protein-induced enterocolitis syndrome K52.21
      food protein-induced enteropathy K52.22
  amebic (acute) A06.0
    with abscess — *see* Abscess, amebic
    chronic A06.1
      with abscess — *see* Abscess, amebic
      nondysenteric A06.2
    nondysenteric A06.2
  astrovirus A08.32
  bacillary NOS A03.9
  bacterial A04.9
    specified NEC A04.8
  calicivirus A08.31
  candidal B37.82
  Chilomastix A07.8
  choleriformis A00.1
  chronic (noninfectious) K52.9
    ulcerative — *see* Colitis, ulcerative
  cicatrizing (chronic) — *see* Enteritis, regional, small intestine
  Clostridium
    botulinum (food poisoning) A05.1
    difficile A04.7
  coccidial A07.3
  coxsackie virus A08.39
  dietetic — *see also* Enteritis, allergic K52.29
  drug-induced K52.1
  due to
    astrovirus A08.32
    calicivirus A08.31
    coxsackie virus A08.39
    drugs K52.1
    echovirus A08.39
    enterovirus NEC A08.39
    food hypersensitivity — *see also* Enteritis, allergic K52.29
    infectious organism (bacterial) (viral) — *see* Enteritis, infectious
    torovirus A08.39
    Yersinia enterocolitica A04.6
  echovirus A08.39
  eltor A00.1
  enterovirus NEC A08.39
  eosinophilic K52.81
  epidemic (infectious) A09
  fulminant — *see also* Ischemia, intestine, acute K55.019
  gangrenous — *see* Enteritis, infectious
  giardial A07.1
  infectious NOS A09
    due to
      adenovirus A08.2
      Aerobacter aerogenes A04.8
      Arizona (bacillus) A02.0
      bacteria NOS A04.9
        specified NEC A04.8
      Campylobacter A04.5
      Clostridium difficile A04.7
      Clostridium perfringens A04.8
      Enterobacter aerogenes A04.8
      enterovirus A08.39
      Escherichia coli A04.4
        enteroaggregative A04.4
        enterohemorrhagic A04.3

Enteritis (acute) (diarrheal) (hemorrhagic) (noninfective) - *continued*
  infectious NOS - *continued*
    due to - *continued*
      Escherichia coli - *continued*
        enteroinvasive A04.2
        enteropathogenic A04.0
        enterotoxigenic A04.1
        specified NEC A04.4
      specified
        bacteria NEC A04.8
        virus NEC A08.39
      Staphylococcus A04.8
      virus NEC A08.4
        specified type NEC A08.39
      Yersinia enterocolitica A04.6
    specified organism NEC A08.8
  influenzal — *see* Influenza, with, digestive manifestations
  ischemic K55.9
    acute — *see also* Ischemia, intestine, acute K55.019
    chronic K55.1
  microsporidial A07.8
  mucomembranous, myxomembranous — *see* Syndrome, irritable bowel
  mucous — *see* Syndrome, irritable bowel
  necroticans A05.2
  necrotizing of newborn — *see* Enterocolitis, necrotizing, in newborn
  neurogenic — *see* Syndrome, irritable bowel
  newborn necrotizing — *see* Enterocolitis, necrotizing, in newborn
  noninfectious K52.9
  norovirus A08.11
  parasitic NEC B82.9
  paratyphoid (fever) — *see* Fever, paratyphoid
  protozoal A07.9
    specified NEC A07.8
  radiation K52.0
  regional (of) K50.90
    with
      complication K50.919
        abscess K50.914
        fistula K50.913
        intestinal obstruction K50.912
        rectal bleeding K50.911
        specified complication NEC K50.918
    colon — *see* Enteritis, regional, large intestine
    duodenum — *see* Enteritis, regional, small intestine
    ileum — *see* Enteritis, regional, small intestine
    jejunum — *see* Enteritis, regional, small intestine
    large bowel — *see* Enteritis, regional, large intestine
    large intestine (colon) (rectum) K50.10
      with
        complication K50.119
          abscess K50.114
          fistula K50.113
          intestinal obstruction K50.112
          rectal bleeding K50.111
          small intestine (duodenum) (ileum) (jejunum) involvement K50.80
            with
              complication K50.819
                abscess K50.814
                fistula K50.813
                intestinal obstruction K50.812
                rectal bleeding K50.811
                specified complication NEC K50.818
          specified complication NEC K50.118
    rectum — *see* Enteritis, regional, large intestine
    small intestine (duodenum) (ileum) (jejunum) K50.00
      with
        complication K50.019
          abscess K50.014
          fistula K50.013
          intestinal obstruction K50.012
          large intestine (colon) (rectum) involvement K50.80
            with
              complication K50.819
                abscess K50.814
                fistula K50.813
                intestinal obstruction K50.812
                rectal bleeding K50.811
                specified complication NEC K50.818
          rectal bleeding K50.011
          specified complication NEC K50.018
  rotaviral A08.0

Enteritis (acute) (diarrheal) (hemorrhagic) (noninfective) - *continued*
  Salmonella, salmonellosis (arizonae) (cholerae-suis) (enteritidis) (typhimurium) A02.0
  segmental — *see* Enteritis, regional
  septic A09
  Shigella — *see* Infection, Shigella
  small round structured NEC A08.19
  spasmodic, spastic — *see* Syndrome, irritable bowel
  staphylococcal A04.8
    due to food A05.0
  torovirus A08.39
  toxic NEC K52.1
    due to Clostridium difficile A04.7
  trichomonal A07.8
  tuberculous A18.32
  typhosa A01.00
  ulcerative (chronic) — *see* Colitis, ulcerative
  viral A08.4
    adenovirus A08.2
    enterovirus A08.39
    Rotavirus A08.0
    small round structured NEC A08.19
    specified NEC A08.39
    virus specified NEC A08.39
Enterobiasis B80
Enterobius vermicularis (infection) (infestation) B80
Enterocele — *see also* Hernia, abdomen
  pelvic, pelvis (acquired) (congenital) N81.5
  vagina, vaginal (acquired) (congenital) NEC N81.5
Enterocolitis — *see also* Enteritis K52.9
  due to Clostridium difficile A04.7
  fulminant ischemic — *see also* Ischemia, intestine, acute K55.059
  granulomatous — *see* Enteritis, regional
  hemorrhagic (acute) — *see also* Ischemia, intestine, acute K55.059
    chronic K55.1
  infectious NEC A09
  ischemic K55.9
  necrotizing K55.30
    with
      perforation K55.33
      pneumatosis K55.32
        and perforation K55.33
    due to Clostridium difficile A04.7
    in non-newborn K55.30
      stage 1 (without pneumatosis, without perforation) K55.31
      stage 2 (with pneumatosis, without perforation) K55.32
      stage 3 (with pneumatosis, with perforation) K55.33
    in newborn P77.9
      stage 1 (without pneumatosis, without perforation) P77.1
      stage 2 (with pneumatosis, without perforation) P77.2
      stage 3 (with pneumatosis, with perforation) P77.3
    without pneumatosis or perforation K55.31
  noninfectious K52.9
  newborn — *see* Enterocolitis, necrotizing, in newborn
  pseudomembranous (newborn) A04.7
  radiation K52.0
    newborn — *see* Enterocolitis, necrotizing, in newborn
  ulcerative (chronic) — *see* Pancolitis, ulcerative (chronic)
Enterogastritis — *see* Enteritis
Enteropathy K63.9
  food protein-induced enterocolitis K52.22
  gluten-sensitive K90.0
    non-celiac K90.41
  hemorrhagic, terminal — *see also* Ischemia, intestine, acute K55.059
  protein-losing K90.49
Enteroperitonitis — *see* Peritonitis
Enteroptosis K63.4
Enterorrhagia K92.2
Enterospasm — *see also* Syndrome, irritable, bowel
  psychogenic F45.8
Enterostenosis –– *see also* Obstruction, intestine K56.69
Enterostomy
  complication — *see* Complication, enterostomy
  status Z93.4
Enterovirus, as cause of disease classified elsewhere B97.10
  coxsackievirus B97.11
  echovirus B97.12

Enterovirus, as cause of disease classified elsewhere - *continued*
  other specified B97.19
Enthesopathy (peripheral) M77.9
  Achilles tendinitis — *see* Tendinitis, Achilles
  ankle and tarsus M77.9
    specified type NEC — *see* Enthesopathy, foot, specified type NEC
  anterior tibial syndrome M76.81-
  calcaneal spur — *see* Spur, bone, calcaneal
  elbow region M77.8
    lateral epicondylitis — *see* Epicondylitis, lateral
    medial epicondylitis — *see* Epicondylitis, medial
  foot NEC M77.9
    metatarsalgia — *see* Metatarsalgia
    specified type NEC M77.5-
  forearm M77.9
  gluteal tendinitis — *see* Tendinitis, gluteal
  hand M77.9
  hip — *see* Enthesopathy, lower limb, specified type NEC
  iliac crest spur — *see* Spur, bone, iliac crest
  iliotibial band syndrome — *see* Syndrome, iliotibial band
  knee — *see* Enthesopathy, lower limb, lower leg, specified type NEC
  lateral epicondylitis — *see* Epicondylitis, lateral
  lower limb (excluding foot) M76.9
    Achilles tendinitis — *see* Tendinitis, Achilles
    anterior tibial syndrome M76.81-
    gluteal tendinitis — *see* Tendinitis, gluteal
    iliac crest spur — *see* Spur, bone, iliac crest
    iliotibial band syndrome — *see* Syndrome, iliotibial band
    patellar tendinitis — *see* Tendinitis, patellar
    pelvic region — *see* Enthesopathy, lower limb, specified type NEC
    peroneal tendinitis — *see* Tendinitis, peroneal
    posterior tibial syndrome M76.82-
    psoas tendinitis — *see* Tendinitis, psoas
    shoulder M77.9
    specified type NEC M76.89-
    tibial collateral bursitis — *see* Bursitis, tibial collateral
  medial epicondylitis — *see* Epicondylitis, medial
  metatarsalgia — *see* Metatarsalgia
  multiple sites M77.9
  patellar tendinitis — *see* Tendinitis, patellar
  pelvis M77.9
  periarthritis of wrist — *see* Periarthritis, wrist
  peroneal tendinitis — *see* Tendinitis, peroneal
  posterior tibial syndrome M76.82-
  psoas tendinitis — *see* Tendinitis, psoas
  shoulder region — *see* Lesion, shoulder
  specified site NEC M77.9
  specified type NEC M77.8
  spinal M46.00
    cervical region M46.02
    cervicothoracic region M46.03
    lumbar region M46.06
    lumbosacral region M46.07
    multiple sites M46.09
    occipito-atlanto-axial region M46.01
    sacrococcygeal region M46.08
    thoracic region M46.04
    thoracolumbar region M46.05
  tibial collateral bursitis — *see* Bursitis, tibial collateral
  upper arm M77.9
  wrist and carpus NEC M77.8
    calcaneal spur — *see* Spur, bone, calcaneal
    periarthritis of wrist — *see* Periarthritis, wrist
Entomophobia F40.218
Entomophthoromycosis B46.8
Entrance, air into vein — *see* Embolism, air
Entrapment, nerve — *see* Neuropathy, entrapment
Entropion (eyelid) (paralytic) H02.009
  cicatricial H02.019
    left H02.016
      lower H02.015
      upper H02.014
    right H02.013
      lower H02.012
      upper H02.011
  congenital Q10.2
  left H02.006
    lower H02.005
    upper H02.004
  mechanical H02.029
    left H02.026
      lower H02.025
      upper H02.024
    right H02.023

Entropion (eyelid) (paralytic) - *continued*
  mechanical - *continued*
    right - *continued*
      lower H02.022
      upper H02.021
  right H02.003
    lower H02.002
    upper H02.001
  senile H02.039
    left H02.036
      lower H02.035
      upper H02.034
    right H02.033
      lower H02.032
      upper H02.031
  spastic H02.049
    left H02.046
      lower H02.045
      upper H02.044
    right H02.043
      lower H02.042
      upper H02.041
Enucleated eye (traumatic, current) S05.7-
Enuresis R32
  functional F98.0
  habit disturbance F98.0
  nocturnal N39.44
    psychogenic F98.0
  nonorganic origin F98.0
  psychogenic F98.0
Eosinopenia — *see* Agranulocytosis
Eosinophilia (allergic) (hereditary) (idiopathic) (secondary) D72.1
  with
    angiolymphoid hyperplasia (ALHE) D18.01
  infiltrative J82
  Löffler's J82
  peritoneal — *see* Peritonitis, eosinophilic
  pulmonary NEC J82
  tropical (pulmonary) J82
Eosinophilia-myalgia syndrome M35.8
Ependymitis (acute) (cerebral) (chronic) (granular) — *see* Encephalomyelitis
Ependymoblastoma
  specified site — *see* Neoplasm, malignant, by site
  unspecified site C71.9
Ependymoma (epithelial) (malignant)
  anaplastic
    specified site — *see* Neoplasm, malignant, by site
    unspecified site C71.9
  benign
    specified site — *see* Neoplasm, benign, by site
    unspecified site D33.2
  myxopapillary D43.2
    specified site — *see* Neoplasm, uncertain behavior, by site
    unspecified site D43.2
  papillary D43.2
    specified site — *see* Neoplasm, uncertain behavior, by site
    unspecified site D43.2
  specified site — *see* Neoplasm, malignant, by site
  unspecified site C71.9
Ependymopathy G93.89
Ephelis, ephelides L81.2
Epiblepharon (congenital) Q10.3
Epicanthus, epicanthic fold (eyelid) (congenital) Q10.3
Epicondylitis (elbow)
  lateral M77.1-
  medial M77.0-
Epicystitis — *see* Cystitis
Epidemic — *see* condition
Epidermidalization, cervix — *see* Dysplasia, cervix
Epidermis, epidermal — *see* condition
Epidermodysplasia verruciformis B07.8
Epidermolysis
  bullosa (congenital) Q81.9
    acquired L12.30
      drug-induced L12.31
      specified cause NEC L12.35
    dystrophica Q81.2
    letalis Q81.1
    simplex Q81.0
    specified NEC Q81.8
  necroticans combustiformis L51.2
    due to drug — *see* Table of Drugs and Chemicals, by drug
Epidermophytid — *see* Dermatophytosis
Epidermophytosis (infected) — *see* Dermatophytosis
Epididymis — *see* condition

Epididymitis (acute) (nonvenereal) (recurrent) (residual) N45.1
  with orchitis N45.3
  blennorrhagic (gonococcal) A54.23
  caseous (tuberculous) A18.15
  chlamydial A56.19
  filarial — see also Infestation, filarial B74.9 [N51]
  gonococcal A54.23
  syphilitic A52.76
  tuberculous A18.15
Epididymo-orchitis — see also Epididymitis N45.3
Epidural — see condition
Epigastrium, epigastric — see condition
Epigastrocele — see Hernia, ventral
Epiglottis — see condition
Epiglottitis, epiglottiditis (acute) J05.10
  with obstruction J05.11
  chronic J37.0
Epignathus Q89.4
Epilepsia partialis continua — see also Kozhevnikof's epilepsy G40.1-
Epilepsy, epileptic, epilepsia (attack) (cerebral) (convulsion) (fit) (seizure) G40.909
  Note: the following terms are to be considered equivalent to intractable: pharmacoresistant (pharmacologically resistant) , treatment resistant, refractory (medically) and poorly controlled
  with
    complex partial seizures — see Epilepsy, localization-related, symptomatic, with complex partial seizures
    grand mal seizures on awakening — see Epilepsy, generalized, specified NEC
    myoclonic absences — see Epilepsy, generalized, specified NEC
    myoclonic-astatic seizures — see Epilepsy, generalized, specified NEC
    simple partial seizures — see Epilepsy, localization-related, symptomatic, with simple partial seizures
  akinetic — see Epilepsy, generalized, specified NEC
  benign childhood with centrotemporal EEG spikes — see Epilepsy, localization-related, idiopathic
  benign myoclonic in infancy G40.80-
  Bravais-jacksonian — see Epilepsy, localization-related, symptomatic, with simple partial seizures
  childhood
    with occipital EEG paroxysms — see Epilepsy, localization-related, idiopathic
    absence G40.A09
      intractable G40.A19
        with status epilepticus G40.A11
        without status epilepticus G40.A19
      not intractable G40.A09
        with status epilepticus G40.A01
        without status epilepticus G40.A09
  climacteric — see Epilepsy, specified NEC
  cysticercosis B69.0
  deterioration (mental) F06.8
  due to syphilis A52.19
  focal — see Epilepsy, localization-related, symptomatic, with simple partial seizures
  generalized
    idiopathic G40.309
      intractable G40.319
        with status epilepticus G40.311
        without status epilepticus G40.319
      not intractable G40.309
        with status epilepticus G40.301
        without status epilepticus G40.309
    specified NEC G40.409
      intractable G40.419
        with status epilepticus G40.411
        without status epilepticus G40.419
      not intractable G40.409
        with status epilepticus G40.401
        without status epilepticus G40.409
  impulsive petit mal — see Epilepsy, juvenile myoclonic
  intractable G40.919
    with status epilepticus G40.911
    without status epilepticus G40.919
  juvenile absence G40.A09
    intractable G40.A19
      with status epilepticus G40.A11
      without status epilepticus G40.A19
    not intractable G40.A09
      with status epilepticus G40.A01
      without status epilepticus G40.A09
  juvenile myoclonic G40.B09
    intractable G40.B19
      with status epilepticus G40.B11

Epilepsy, epileptic, epilepsia (attack) (cerebral) (convulsion) (fit) (seizure) - continued
  juvenile myoclonic - continued
    intractable - continued
      without status epilepticus G40.B19
    not intractable G40.B09
      with status epilepticus G40.B01
      without status epilepticus G40.B09
  localization-related (focal) (partial)
    idiopathic G40.009
      with seizures of localized onset G40.009
      intractable G40.019
        with status epilepticus G40.011
        without status epilepticus G40.019
      not intractable G40.009
        with status epilepticus G40.001
        without status epilepticus G40.009
    symptomatic
      with complex partial seizures G40.209
      intractable G40.219
        with status epilepticus G40.211
        without status epilepticus G40.219
      not intractable G40.209
        with status epilepticus G40.201
        without status epilepticus G40.209
      with simple partial seizures G40.109
      intractable G40.119
        with status epilepticus G40.111
        without status epilepticus G40.119
      not intractable G40.109
        with status epilepticus G40.101
        without status epilepticus G40.109
  myoclonus, myoclonic — see Epilepsy, generalized, specified NEC
    progressive — see Epilepsy, generalized, idiopathic
  not intractable G40.909
    with status epilepticus G40.901
    without status epilepticus G40.909
  on awakening — see Epilepsy, generalized, specified NEC
  parasitic NOS B71.9 [G94]
  partialis continua — see also Kozhevnikof's epilepsy G40.1-
  peripheral — see Epilepsy, specified NEC
  procursiva — see Epilepsy, localization-related, symptomatic, with simple partial seizures
  progressive (familial) myoclonic — see Epilepsy, generalized, idiopathic
  reflex — see Epilepsy, specified NEC
  related to
    alcohol G40.509
      not intractable G40.509
        with status epilepticus G40.501
        without status epliepticus G40.509
    drugs G40.509
      not intractable G40.509
        with status epilepticus G40.501
        without status epliepticus G40.509
    external causes G40.509
      not intractable G40.509
        with status epilepticus G40.501
        without status epliepticus G40.509
    hormonal changes G40.509
      not intractable G40.509
        with status epilepticus G40.501
        without status epliepticus G40.509
    sleep deprivation G40.509
      not intractable G40.509
        with status epilepticus G40.501
        without status epliepticus G40.509
    stress G40.509
      not intractable G40.509
        with status epilepticus G40.501
        without status epilepticus G40.509
  somatomotor — see Epilepsy, localization-related, symptomatic, with simple partial seizures
  somatosensory — see Epilepsy, localization-related, symptomatic, with simple partial seizures
  spasms G40.822
    intractable G40.824
      with status epilepticus G40.823
      without status epilepticus G40.824
    not intractable G40.822
      with status epilepticus G40.821
      without status epilepticus G40.822
  specified NEC G40.802
    intractable G40.804
      with status epilepticus G40.803
      without status epilepticus G40.804
    not intractable G40.802
      with status epilepticus G40.801
      without status epilepticus G40.802
  syndromes

Epilepsy, epileptic, epilepsia (attack) (cerebral) (convulsion) (fit) (seizure) - continued
  syndromes - continued
    generalized
      idiopathic G40.309
        intractable G40.319
          with status epilepticus G40.311
          without status epilepticus G40.319
        not intractable G40.309
          with status epilepticus G40.301
          without status epilepticus G40.309
      specified NEC G40.409
        intractable G40.419
          with status epilepticus G40.411
          without status epilepticus G40.419
        not intractable G40.409
          with status epilepticus G40.401
          without status epilepticus G40.409
    localization-related (focal) (partial)
      idiopathic G40.009
        with seizures of localized onset G40.009
        intractable G40.019
          with status epilepticus G40.011
          without status epilepticus G40.019
        not intractable G40.009
          with status epilepticus G40.001
          without status epilepticus G40.009
      symptomatic
        with complex partial seizures G40.209
        intractable G40.219
          with status epilepticus G40.211
          without status epilepticus G40.219
        not intractable G40.209
          with status epilepticus G40.201
          without status epilepticus G40.209
        with simple partial seizures G40.109
        intractable G40.119
          with status epilepticus G40.111
          without status epilepticus G40.119
        not intractable G40.109
          with status epilepticus G40.101
          without status epilepticus G40.109
    specified NEC G40.802
      intractable G40.804
        with status epilepticus G40.803
        without status epilepticus G40.804
      not intractable G40.802
        with status epilepticus G40.801
        without status epilepticus G40.802
  tonic (-clonic) — see Epilepsy, generalized, specified NEC
  twilight F05
  uncinate (gyrus) — see Epilepsy, localization-related, symptomatic, with complex partial seizures
  Unverricht (-Lundborg) (familial myoclonic) — see Epilepsy, generalized, idiopathic
  visceral — see Epilepsy, specified NEC
  visual — see Epilepsy, specified NEC
Epiloia Q85.1
Epimenorrhea N92.0
Epipharyngitis — see Nasopharyngitis
Epiphora H04.20-
  due to
    excess lacrimation H04.21-
    insufficient drainage H04.22-
Epiphyseal arrest — see Arrest, epiphyseal
Epiphyseolysis, epiphysiolysis — see Osteochondropathy
Epiphysitis — see also Osteochondropathy
  juvenile M92.9
  syphilitic (congenital) A50.02
Epiplocele — see Hernia, abdomen
Epiploitis — see Peritonitis
Epiplosarcomphalocele — see Hernia, umbilicus
Episcleritis (suppurative) H15.10-
  in (due to)
    syphilis A52.71
    tuberculosis A18.51
  nodular H15.12-
  periodica fugax H15.11-
    angioneurotic — see Edema, angioneurotic
  syphilitic (late) A52.71
  tuberculous A18.51
Episode
  affective, mixed F39
  depersonalization (in neurotic state) F48.1
  depressive F32.9
    major F32.9
    mild F32.0
    moderate F32.1
    severe (without psychotic symptoms) F32.2
      with psychotic symptoms F32.3
    recurrent F33.9

Episode - *continued*
  depressive - *continued*
    recurrent - *continued*
      brief F33.8
      specified NEC F32.89
  hypomanic F30.8
  manic F30.9
    with
      psychotic symptoms F30.2
      remission (full) F30.4
        partial F30.3
    other specified F30.8
    recurrent F31.89
    without psychotic symptoms F30.10
      mild F30.11
      moderate F30.12
      severe (without psychotic symptoms) F30.13
        with psychotic symptoms F30.2
  psychotic F23
    organic F06.8
  schizophrenic (acute) NEC, brief F23
Epispadias (female) (male) Q64.0
Episplenitis D73.89
Epistaxis (multiple) R04.0
  hereditary I78.0
  vicarious menstruation N94.89
Epithelioma (malignant) — *see also* Neoplasm,
  malignant, by site
  adenoides cysticum — *see* Neoplasm, skin, benign
  basal cell — *see* Neoplasm, skin, malignant
  benign — *see* Neoplasm, benign, by site
  Bowen's — *see* Neoplasm, skin, in situ
  calcifying, of Malherbe — *see* Neoplasm, skin,
    benign
  external site — *see* Neoplasm, skin, malignant
  intraepidermal, Jadassohn — *see* Neoplasm, skin,
    benign
  squamous cell — *see* Neoplasm, malignant, by site
Epitheliomatosis pigmented Q82.1
Epitheliopathy, multifocal placoid pigment H30.14-
Epithelium, epithelial — *see* condition
Epituberculosis (with atelectasis) (allergic) A15.7
Eponychia Q84.6
Epstein's
  nephrosis or syndrome — *see* Nephrosis
  pearl K09.8
Epulis (gingiva) (fibrous) (giant cell) K06.8
Equinia A24.0
Equinovarus (congenital) (talipes) Q66.0
  acquired — *see* Deformity, limb, clubfoot
Equivalent
  convulsive (abdominal) — *see* Epilepsy, specified
    NEC
  epileptic (psychic) — *see* Epilepsy, localization-
    related, symptomatic, with complex partial seizures
Erb (-Duchenne) **paralysis** (birth injury)
  (newborn) P14.0
Erb-Goldflam disease or syndrome G70.00
  with exacerbation (acute) G70.01
  in crisis G70.01
Erb's
  disease G71.0
  palsy, paralysis (brachial) (birth) (newborn) P14.0
  spinal (spastic) syphilitic A52.17
  pseudohypertrophic muscular dystrophy G71.0
Erdheim's syndrome (acromegalic
  macrospondylitis) E22.0
Erection, painful (persistent) — *see* Priapism
Ergosterol deficiency (vitamin D) E55.9
  with
    adult osteomalacia M83.8
    rickets — *see* Rickets
Ergotism — *see also* Poisoning, food, noxious, plant
  from ergot used as drug (migraine therapy) — *see*
    Table of Drugs and Chemicals
Erosio interdigitalis blastomycetica B37.2
Erosion
  artery I77.2
    without rupture I77.89
  bone — *see* Disorder, bone, density and structure,
    specified NEC
  bronchus J98.09
  cartilage (joint) — *see* Disorder, cartilage, specified
    type NEC
  cervix (uteri) (acquired) (chronic) (congenital) N86
    with cervicitis N72
  cornea (nontraumatic) — *see* Ulcer, cornea
    recurrent H18.83-
    traumatic — *see* Abrasion, cornea
  dental (idiopathic) (occupational) (due to diet, drugs
    or vomiting) K03.2
  duodenum, postpyloric — *see* Ulcer, duodenum
  esophagus K22.10

Erosion - *continued*
  esophagus - *continued*
    with bleeding K22.11
  gastric — *see* Ulcer, stomach
  gastrojejunal — *see* Ulcer, gastrojejunal
  implanted mesh — *see* Complications, mesh
  intestine K63.3
  lymphatic vessel I89.8
  pylorus, pyloric (ulcer) — *see* Ulcer, stomach
  spine, aneurysmal A52.09
  stomach — *see* Ulcer, stomach
  subcutaneous device pocket
    nervous system prosthetic device, implant, or
      graft T85.890
    other internal prosthetic device, implant, or
      graft T85.898
  teeth (idiopathic) (occupational) (due to diet, drugs
    or vomiting) K03.2
  urethra N36.8
  uterus N85.8
Erotomania F52.8
Error
  metabolism, inborn -- se Disorder, metabolism
  refractive — *see* Disorder, refraction
Eructation R14.2
  nervous or psychogenic F45.8
Eruption
  creeping B76.9
  drug (generalized) (taken internally) L27.0
    fixed L27.1
    in contact with skin — *see* Dermatitis, due to drugs
    localized L27.1
  Hutchinson, summer L56.4
  Kaposi's varicelliform B00.0
  napkin L22
  polymorphous light (sun) L56.4
  recalcitrant pustular L13.8
  ringed R23.8
  skin (nonspecific) R21
    creeping (meaning hookworm) B76.9
    due to inoculation/vaccination (generalized) —
      see also Dermatitis, due to, vaccine L27.0
      localized L27.1
    erysipeloid A26.0
    feigned L98.1
    Kaposi's varicelliform B00.0
    lichenoid L28.0
    meaning dermatitis — *see* Dermatitis
    toxic NEC L53.0
  tooth, teeth, abnormal (incomplete) (late)
    (premature) (sequence) K00.6
  vesicular R23.8
Erysipelas (gangrenous) (infantile) (newborn)
  (phlegmonous) (suppurative) A46
  external ear A46 *[H62.40]*
  puerperal, postpartum O86.89
Erysipeloid A26.9
  cutaneous (Rosenbach's) A26.0
  disseminated A26.8
  sepsis A26.7
  specified NEC A26.8
Erythema, erythematous (infectional)
  (inflammation) L53.9
  ab igne L59.0
  annulare (centrifugum) (rheumaticum) L53.1
  arthriticum epidemicum A25.1
  brucellum — *see* Brucellosis
  chronic figurate NEC L53.3
  chronicum migrans (Borrelia burgdorferi) A69.20
  diaper L22
  due to
    chemical NEC L53.0
      in contact with skin L24.5
    drug (internal use) — *see* Dermatitis, due to, drugs
  elevatum diutinum L95.1
  endemic E52
  epidemic, arthritic A25.1
  figuratum perstans L53.3
  gluteal L22
  heat - code by site under Burn, first degree
  ichthyosiforme congenitum bullous Q80.3
  in diseases classified elsewhere L54
  induratum (nontuberculous) L52
    tuberculous A18.4
  infectiosum B08.3
  intertrigo L30.4
  iris L51.9
  marginatum L53.2
    in (due to) acute rheumatic fever I00
  medicamentosum — *see* Dermatitis, due to, drugs
  migrans A26.0
    chronicum A69.20
    tongue K14.1

Erythema, erythematous (infectional)
(inflammation) - *continued*
  multiforme (major) (minor) L51.9
    bullous, bullosum L51.1
    conjunctiva L51.1
    nonbullous L51.0
    pemphigoides L12.0
    specified NEC L51.8
  napkin L22
  neonatorum P83.8
    toxic P83.1
  nodosum L52
    tuberculous A18.4
  palmar L53.8
  pernio T69.1
  rash, newborn P83.8
  scarlatiniform (recurrent) (exfoliative) L53.8
  solare L55.0
  specified NEC L53.8
  toxic, toxicum NEC L53.0
    newborn P83.1
  tuberculous (primary) A18.4
Erythematous, erythematosus — *see* condition
Erythermalgia (primary) I73.81
Erythralgia I73.81
Erythrasma L08.1
Erythredema (polyneuropathy) — *see* Poisoning,
  mercury
Erythremia (acute) C94.0-
  chronic D45
  secondary D75.1
Erythroblastopenia — *see also* Aplasia, red
  cell D60.9
  congenital D61.01
Erythroblastophthisis D61.09
Erythroblastosis (fetalis) (newborn) P55.9
  due to
    ABO (antibodies) (incompatibility)
      (isoimmunization) P55.1
    Rh (antibodies) (incompatibility)
      (isoimmunization) P55.0
Erythrocyanosis (crurum) I73.89
Erythrocythemia — *see* Erythremia
Erythrocytosis (megalosplenic) (secondary) D75.1
  familial D75.0
  oval, hereditary — *see* Elliptocytosis
  secondary D75.1
  stress D75.1
Erythroderma (secondary) — *see*
  also Erythema L53.9
  bullous ichthyosiform, congenital Q80.3
  desquamativum L21.1
  ichthyosiform, congenital (bullous) Q80.3
  neonatorum P83.8
  psoriaticum L40.8
Erythrodysesthesia, palmar plantar (PPE) L27.1
Erythrogenesis imperfecta D61.09
Erythroleukemia C94.0-
Erythromelalgia I73.81
Erythrophagocytosis D75.89
Erythrophobia F40.298
Erythroplakia, oral epithelium, and tongue K13.29
Erythroplasia (Queyrat) D07.4
  specified site — *see* Neoplasm, skin, in situ
  unspecified site D07.4
Escherichia coli (E. coli)
  , as cause of disease classified elsewhere B96.20
  non-O157 Shiga toxin-producing (with known O
    group) B96.22
  non-Shiga toxin-producing B96.29
  O157 with confirmation of Shiga toxin when H
    antigen is unknown, or is not H7 B96.21
  O157:H- (nonmotile) with confirmation of Shiga
    toxin B96.21
  O157:H7 with or without confirmation of Shiga
    toxin-production B96.21
  Shiga toxin-producing (with unspecified O group)
    (STEC) B96.23
  O157 B96.21
  O157:H7 with or without confirmation of Shiga
    toxin-production B96.21
    specified NEC B96.22
  specified NEC B96.29
Esophagismus K22.4
Esophagitis (acute) (alkaline) (chemical) (chronic)
  (infectional) (necrotic) (peptic)
  (postoperative) K20.9
  candidal B37.81
  due to gastrointestinal reflux disease K21.0
  eosinophilic K20.0
  reflux K21.0
  specified NEC K20.8
  tuberculous A18.83

Esophagitis (acute) (alkaline) (chemical) (chronic) (infectional) (necrotic) (peptic) (postoperative) - *continued*
  ulcerative K22.10
    with bleeding K22.11
Esophagocele K22.5
Esophagomalacia K22.8
Esophagospasm K22.4
Esophagostenosis K22.2
Esophagostomiasis B81.8
Esophagotracheal — *see* condition
Esophagus — *see* condition
Esophoria H50.51
  convergence, excess H51.12
  divergence, insufficiency H51.8
Esotropia — *see* Strabismus, convergent concomitant
Espundia B55.2
Essential — *see* condition
Esthesioneuroblastoma C30.0
Esthesioneurocytoma C30.0
Esthesioneuroepithelioma C30.0
Esthiomene A55
Estivo-autumnal malaria (fever) B50.9
Estrangement (marital) Z63.5
  parent-child NEC Z62.890
Estriasis — *see* Myiasis
Ethanolism — *see* Alcoholism
Etherism — *see* Dependence, drug, inhalant
Ethmoid, ethmoidal — *see* condition
Ethmoiditis (chronic) (nonpurulent) (purulent)
  see also Sinusitis, ethmoidal
  influenzal — *see* Influenza, with, respiratory manifestations NEC
  Woakes' J33.1
Ethylism — *see* Alcoholism
Eulenburg's disease (congenital paramyotonia) G71.19
Eumycetoma B47.0
Eunuchoidism E29.1
  hypogonadotropic E23.0
European blastomycosis — *see* Cryptococcosis
Eustachian — *see* condition
Evaluation (for) (of)
  development state
    adolescent Z00.3
    period of
      delayed growth in childhood Z00.70
        with abnormal findings Z00.71
      rapid growth in childhood Z00.2
    puberty Z00.3
  growth and developmental state (period of rapid growth) Z00.2
    delayed growth Z00.70
      with abnormal findings Z00.71
  mental health (status) Z00.8
    requested by authority Z04.6
  period of
    delayed growth in childhood Z00.70
      with abnormal findings Z00.71
    rapid growth in childhood Z00.2
  suspected condition — *see* Observation
Evans syndrome D69.41
Event, apparent life threatening in newborn and infant (ALTE) R68.13
Eventration — *see also* Hernia, ventral
  colon into chest — *see* Hernia, diaphragm
  diaphragm (congenital) Q79.1
Eversion
  bladder N32.89
  cervix (uteri) N86
    with cervicitis N72
  foot NEC — *see also* Deformity, valgus, ankle
    congenital Q66.6
  punctum lacrimale (postinfectional) (senile) H04.52-
  ureter (meatus) N28.89
  urethra (meatus) N36.8
  uterus N81.4
Evidence
  cytologic
    of malignancy on anal smear R85.614
    of malignancy on cervical smear R87.614
    of malignancy on vaginal smear R87.624
Evisceration
  birth injury P15.8
  traumatic NEC
    eye — *see* Enucleated eye
Evulsion — *see* Avulsion
Ewing's sarcoma or tumor - — *see* Neoplasm, bone, malignant
Examination (for) (following) (general) (of) (routine) Z00.00
  with abnormal findings Z00.01
  abuse, physical (alleged) , ruled out

Examination (for) (following) (general) (of) (routine) - *continued*
  abuse, physical (alleged) , ruled out - *continued*
    adult Z04.71
    child Z04.72
  adolescent (development state) Z00.3
  alleged rape or sexual assault (victim) , ruled out
    adult Z04.41
    child Z04.42
  allergy Z01.82
  annual (adult) (periodic) (physical) Z00.00
    with abnormal findings Z00.01
    gynecological Z01.419
      with abnormal findings Z01.411
  antibody response Z01.84
  blood — *see* Examination, laboratory
  blood pressure Z01.30
    with abnormal findings Z01.31
  cancer staging — *see* Neoplasm, malignant, by site
  cervical Papanicolaou smear Z12.4
    as part of routine gynecological examination Z01.419
      with abnormal findings Z01.411
  child (over 28 days old) Z00.129
    with abnormal findings Z00.121
    under 28 days old — *see* Newborn, examination
  clinical research control or normal comparison (control) (participant) Z00.6
  contraceptive (drug) maintenance (routine) Z30.8
    device (intrauterine) Z30.431
  dental Z01.20
    with abnormal findings Z01.21
  developmental — *see* Examination, child
  donor (potential) Z00.5
  ear Z01.10
    with abnormal findings NEC Z01.118
  eye Z01.00
    with abnormal findings Z01.01
  following
    accident NEC Z04.3
      transport Z04.1
      work Z04.2
    assault, alleged, ruled out
      adult Z04.71
      child Z04.72
    motor vehicle accident Z04.1
    treatment (for) Z09
      combined NEC Z09
        fracture Z09
        malignant neoplasm Z08
      malignant neoplasm Z08
      mental disorder Z09
      specified condition NEC Z09
  follow-up (routine) (following) Z09
    chemotherapy NEC Z09
      malignant neoplasm Z08
    fracture Z09
    malignant neoplasm Z08
    postpartum Z39.2
    psychotherapy Z09
    radiotherapy NEC Z09
      malignant neoplasm Z08
    surgery NEC Z09
      malignant neoplasm Z08
  gynecological Z01.419
    with abnormal findings Z01.411
    for contraceptive maintenance Z30.8
  health — *see* Examination, medical
  hearing Z01.10
    with abnormal findings NEC Z01.118
    following failed hearing screening Z01.110
  immunity status testing Z01.84
  laboratory (as part of a general medical examination) Z00.00
    with abnormal findings Z00.01
    preprocedural Z01.812
  lactating mother Z39.1
  medical (adult) (for) (of) Z00.00
    with abnormal findings Z00.01
    administrative purpose only Z02.9
      specified NEC Z02.89
    admission to
      armed forces Z02.3
      old age home Z02.2
      prison Z02.89
      residential institution Z02.2
      school Z02.0
        following illness or medical treatment Z02.0
      summer camp Z02.89
    adoption Z02.82
    blood alcohol or drug level Z02.83
    camp (summer) Z02.89

Examination (for) (following) (general) (of) (routine) - *continued*
  medical (adult) (for) (of) - *continued*
    clinical research, normal subject (control) (participant) Z00.6
    control subject in clinical research (normal comparison) (participant) Z00.6
    donor (potential) Z00.5
    driving license Z02.4
    general (adult) Z00.00
      with abnormal findings Z00.01
    immigration Z02.89
    insurance purposes Z02.6
    marriage Z02.89
    medicolegal reasons NEC Z04.8
    naturalization Z02.89
    participation in sport Z02.5
    paternity testing Z02.81
    population survey Z00.8
    pre-employment Z02.1
    pre-operative — *see* Examination, pre-procedural
    pre-procedural
      cardiovascular Z01.810
      respiratory Z01.811
      specified NEC Z01.818
    preschool children
      for admission to school Z02.0
    prisoners
      for entrance into prison Z02.89
    recruitment for armed forces Z02.3
    specified NEC Z00.8
    sport competition Z02.5
  medicolegal reason NEC Z04.8
  newborn — *see* Newborn, examination
  pelvic (annual) (periodic) Z01.419
    with abnormal findings Z01.411
  period of rapid growth in childhood Z00.2
  periodic (adult) (annual) (routine) Z00.00
    with abnormal findings Z00.01
  physical (adult) — *see also* Examination, medical Z00.00
    sports Z02.5
  postpartum
    immediately after delivery Z39.0
    routine follow-up Z39.2
  prenatal (normal pregnancy) — *see also* Pregnancy, normal Z34.9-
  pre-chemotherapy (antineoplastic) Z01.818
  pre-procedural (pre-operative)
    cardiovascular Z01.810
    laboratory Z01.812
    respiratory Z01.811
    specified NEC Z01.818
  prior to chemotherapy (antineoplastic) Z01.818
  psychiatric NEC Z00.8
    follow-up not needing further care Z09
    requested by authority Z04.6
  radiological (as part of a general medical examination) Z00.00
    with abnormal findings Z00.01
  repeat cervical smear to confirm findings of recent normal smear following initial abnormal smear Z01.42
  skin (hypersensitivity) Z01.82
  special — *see also* Examination, by type Z01.89
    specified type NEC Z01.89
  specified type or reason NEC Z04.8
  teeth Z01.20
    with abnormal findings Z01.21
  urine — *see* Examination, laboratory
  vision Z01.00
    with abnormal findings Z01.01
Exanthem, exanthema — *see also* Rash
  with enteroviral vesicular stomatitis B08.4
  Boston A88.0
  epidemic with meningitis A88.0 *[G02]*
  subitum B08.20
    due to human herpesvirus 6 B08.21
    due to human herpesvirus 7 B08.22
  viral, virus B09
    specified type NEC B08.8
Excess, excessive, excessively
  alcohol level in blood R78.0
  androgen (ovarian) E28.1
  attrition, tooth, teeth K03.0
  carotene, carotin (dietary) E67.1
  cold, effects of T69.9
    specified effect NEC T69.8
  convergence H51.12
  crying
    in child, adolescent, or adult R45.83
    in infant R68.11
  development, breast N62

Excess, excessive, excessively - *continued*
divergence H51.8
drinking (alcohol) NEC (without
dependence) F10.10
habitual (continual) (without remission) F10.20
eating R63.2
estrogen E28.0
fat — *see also* Obesity
in heart — *see* Degeneration, myocardial
localized E65
foreskin N47.8
gas R14.0
glucagon E16.3
heat — *see* Heat
intermaxillary vertical dimension of fully erupted
teeth M26.37
interocclusal distance of fully erupted teeth M26.37
kalium E87.5
large
colon K59.39
congenital Q43.8
infant P08.0
organ or site, congenital NEC — *see* Anomaly, by
site
long
organ or site, congenital NEC — *see* Anomaly, by
site
menstruation (with regular cycle) N92.0
with irregular cycle N92.1
napping Z72.821
natrium E87.0
number of teeth K00.1
nutrient (dietary) NEC R63.2
potassium (K) E87.5
salivation K11.7
secretion — *see also* Hypersecretion
milk O92.6
sputum R09.3
sweat R61
sexual drive F52.8
short
organ or site, congenital NEC — *see* Anomaly, by
site
umbilical cord in labor or delivery O69.3
skin L98.7
and subcutaneous tissue L98.7
eyelid (acquired) — *see* Blepharochalasis
congenital Q10.3
sodium (Na) E87.0
spacing of fully erupted teeth M26.32
sputum R09.3
sweating R61
thirst R63.1
due to deprivation of water T73.1
tuberosity of jaw M26.07
vitamin
A (dietary) E67.0
administered as drug (prolonged intake) — *see*
Table of Drugs and Chemicals, vitamins,
adverse effect
overdose or wrong substance given or
taken — *see* Table of Drugs and Chemicals,
vitamins, poisoning
D (dietary) E67.3
administered as drug (prolonged intake) — *see*
Table of Drugs and Chemicals, vitamins,
adverse effect
overdose or wrong substance given or
taken — *see* Table of Drugs and Chemicals,
vitamins, poisoning
weight
gain R63.5
loss R63.4
Excitability, abnormal, under minor stress
(personality disorder) F60.3
Excitation
anomalous atrioventricular I45.6
psychogenic F30.8
reactive (from emotional stress, psychological
trauma) F30.8
Excitement
hypomanic F30.8
manic F30.9
mental, reactive (from emotional stress,
psychological trauma) F30.8
state, reactive (from emotional stress, psychological
trauma) F30.8
Excoriation (traumatic) — *see also* Abrasion
neurotic L98.1
skin picking disorder F42.4
Exfoliation
due to erythematous conditions according to extent
of body surface involved L49.0

Exfoliation - *continued*
due to erythematous conditions according to extent
of body surface involved - *continued*
10-19 percent of body surface L49.1
20-29 percent of body surface L49.2
30-39 percent of body surface L49.3
40-49 percent of body surface L49.4
50-59 percent of body surface L49.5
60-69 percent of body surface L49.6
70-79 percent of body surface L49.7
80-89 percent of body surface L49.8
90-99 percent of body surface L49.9
less than 10 percent of body surface L49.0
teeth, due to systemic causes K08.0
Exfoliative — *see* condition
Exhaustion, exhaustive (physical NEC) R53.83
battle F43.0
cardiac — *see* Failure, heart
delirium F43.0
due to
cold T69.8
excessive exertion T73.3
exposure T73.2
neurasthenia F48.8
heart — *see* Failure, heart
heat — *see also* Heat, exhaustion T67.5
due to
salt depletion T67.4
water depletion T67.3
maternal, complicating delivery O75.81
mental F48.8
myocardium, myocardial — *see* Failure, heart
nervous F48.8
old age R54
psychogenic F48.8
psychosis F43.0
senile R54
vital NEC Z73.0
Exhibitionism F65.2
Exocervicitis — *see* Cervicitis
Exomphalos Q79.2
meaning hernia — *see* Hernia, umbilicus
Exophoria H50.52
convergence, insufficiency H51.11
divergence, excess H51.8
Exophthalmos H05.2-
congenital Q15.8
constant NEC H05.24-
displacement, globe — *see* Displacement, globe
due to thyrotoxicosis (hyperthyroidism) — *see*
Hyperthyroidism, with, goiter (diffuse)
dysthyroid — *see* Hyperthyroidism, with, goiter
(diffuse)
goiter — *see* Hyperthyroidism, with, goiter (diffuse)
intermittent NEC H05.25-
malignant — *see* Hyperthyroidism, with, goiter
(diffuse)
orbital
edema — *see* Edema, orbit
hemorrhage — *see* Hemorrhage, orbit
pulsating NEC H05.26-
thyrotoxic, thyrotropic — *see* Hyperthyroidism,
with, goiter (diffuse)
Exostosis — *see also* Disorder, bone
cartilaginous — *see* Neoplasm, bone, benign
congenital (multiple) Q78.6
external ear canal H61.81-
gonococcal A54.49
jaw (bone) M27.8
multiple, congenital Q78.6
orbit H05.35-
osteocartilaginous — *see* Neoplasm, bone, benign
syphilitic A52.77
Exotropia — *see* Strabismus, divergent concomitant
Explanation of
investigation finding Z71.2
medication Z71.89
Exposure (to) — *see also* Contact, with T75.89
acariasis Z20.7
AIDS virus Z20.6
air pollution Z77.110
algae and algae toxins Z77.121
algae bloom Z77.121
anthrax Z20.810
aromatic amines Z77.020
aromatic (hazardous) compounds NEC Z77.028
aromatic dyes NOS Z77.028
arsenic Z77.010
asbestos Z77.090
bacterial disease NEC Z20.818
benzene Z77.021
blue-green algae bloom Z77.121
body fluids (potentially hazardous) Z77.21

Exposure (to) - *continued*
brown tide Z77.121
chemicals (chiefly nonmedicinal) (hazardous)
NEC Z77.098
cholera Z20.09
chromium compounds Z77.018
cold, effects of T69.9
specified effect NEC T69.8
communicable disease Z20.9
bacterial NEC Z20.818
specified NEC Z20.89
viral NEC Z20.828
cyanobacteria bloom Z77.121
disaster Z65.5
discrimination Z60.5
dyes Z77.098
effects of T73.9
environmental tobacco smoke (acute)
(chronic) Z77.22
Escherichia coli (E. coli) Z20.01
exhaustion due to T73.2
fiberglass — *see* Table of Drugs and Chemicals,
fiberglass
German measles Z20.4
gonorrhea Z20.2
hazardous metals NEC Z77.018
hazardous substances NEC Z77.29
hazards in the physical environment NEC Z77.128
hazards to health NEC Z77.9
human immunodeficiency virus (HIV) Z20.6
human T-lymphotropic virus type-1 (HTLV-
1) Z20.89
implanted
mesh — *see* Complications, mesh
prosthetic materials NEC — *see* Complications,
prosthetic materials NEC
infestation (parasitic) NEC Z20.7
intestinal infectious disease NEC Z20.09
Escherichia coli (E. coli) Z20.01
lead Z77.011
meningococcus Z20.811
mold (toxic) Z77.120
nickel dust Z77.018
noise Z77.122
occupational
air contaminants NEC Z57.39
dust Z57.2
environmental tobacco smoke Z57.31
extreme temperature Z57.6
noise Z57.0
radiation Z57.1
risk factors Z57.9
specified NEC Z57.8
toxic agents (gases) (liquids) (solids) (vapors) in
agriculture Z57.4
toxic agents (gases) (liquids) (solids) (vapors) in
industry NEC Z57.5
vibration Z57.7
parasitic disease NEC Z20.7
pediculosis Z20.7
persecution Z60.5
pfiesteria piscicida Z77.121
poliomyelitis Z20.89
polycyclic aromatic hydrocarbons Z77.028
pollution
air Z77.110
environmental NEC Z77.118
soil Z77.112
water Z77.111
prenatal (drugs) (toxic chemicals) — *see* Newborn,
affected by, noxious substances transmitted via
placenta or breast milk
rabies Z20.3
radiation, naturally occurring NEC Z77.123
radon Z77.123
red tide (Florida) Z77.121
rubella Z20.4
second hand tobacco smoke (acute) (chronic) Z77.22
in the perinatal period P96.81
sexually-transmitted disease Z20.2
smallpox (laboratory) Z20.89
syphilis Z20.2
terrorism Z65.4
torture Z65.4
tuberculosis Z20.1
uranium Z77.012
varicella Z20.820
venereal disease Z20.2
viral disease NEC Z20.828
war Z65.5
water pollution Z77.111
Exsanguination — *see* Hemorrhage

Exstrophy
  abdominal contents Q45.8
  bladder Q64.10
    cloacal Q64.12
    specified type NEC Q64.19
    supravesical fissure Q64.11
Extensive — *see* condition
Extra — *see also* Accessory
  marker chromosomes (normal individual) Q92.61
    in abnormal individual Q92.62
  rib Q76.6
    cervical Q76.5
Extrasystoles (supraventricular) I49.49
  atrial I49.1
  auricular I49.1
  junctional I49.2
  ventricular I49.3
Extrauterine gestation or pregnancy - — *see*
  Pregnancy, by site
Extravasation
  blood R58
  chyle into mesentery I89.8
  pelvicalyceal N13.8
  pyelosinus N13.8
  urine (from ureter) R39.0
  vesicant agent
    antineoplastic chemotherapy T80.810
    other agent NEC T80.818
Extremity — *see* condition, limb
Extrophy — *see* Exstrophy
Extroversion
  bladder Q64.19
  uterus N81.4
    complicating delivery O71.2
    postpartal (old) N81.4
Extruded tooth (teeth) M26.34
Extrusion
  breast implant (prosthetic) T85.42
  eye implant (globe) (ball) T85.328
  intervertebral disc — *see* Displacement,
    intervertebral disc
  ocular lens implant (prosthetic) — *see*
    Complications, intraocular lens
  vitreous — *see* Prolapse, vitreous
Exudate
  pleural — *see* Effusion, pleura
  retina H35.89
Exudative — *see* condition
Eye, eyeball, eyelid — *see* condition
Eyestrain — *see* Disturbance, vision, subjective
Eyeworm disease of Africa B74.3

F

Faber's syndrome (achlorhydric anemia) D50.9
Fabry (-Anderson) **disease** E75.21
Faciocephalalgia, autonomic — *see*
  also Neuropathy, peripheral, autonomic G90.09
Factor (s)
  psychic, associated with diseases classified
    elsewhere F54
  psychological
    affecting physical conditions F54
    or behavioral
      affecting general medical condition F54
      associated with disorders or diseases classified
      elsewhere F54
Fahr disease (of brain) G23.8
Fahr Volhard disease (of kidney) I12.-
Failure, failed
  abortion — *see* Abortion, attempted
  aortic (valve) I35.8
    rheumatic I06.8
  attempted abortion — *see* Abortion, attempted
  biventricular I50.9
  bone marrow — *see* Anemia, aplastic
  cardiac — *see* Failure, heart
  cardiorenal (chronic) I50.9
    hypertensive I13.2
  cardiorespiratory — *see also* Failure, heart R09.2
  cardiovascular (chronic) — *see* Failure, heart
  cerebrovascular I67.9
  cervical dilatation in labor O62.0
  circulation, circulatory (peripheral) R57.9
    newborn P29.89
  compensation — *see* Disease, heart
  compliance with medical treatment or
    regimen — *see* Noncompliance
  congestive — *see* Failure, heart, congestive
  dental implant (endosseous) M27.69
    due to
      failure of dental prosthesis M27.63
      lack of attached gingiva M27.62
      occlusal trauma (poor prosthetic design) M27.62

Failure, failed - *continued*
  dental implant (endosseous) - *continued*
    due to - *continued*
      parafunctional habits M27.62
      periodontal infection (peri-implantitis) M27.62
      poor oral hygiene M27.62
      osseointegration M27.61
      due to
        complications of systemic disease M27.61
        poor bone quality M27.61
      iatrogenic M27.61
    post-osseointegration
      biological M27.62
      due to complications of systemic disease M27.62
      iatrogenic M27.62
      mechanical M27.63
    pre-integration M27.61
    pre-osseointegration M27.61
    specified NEC M27.69
  descent of head (at term) of pregnancy
    (mother) O32.4
  endosseous dental implant — *see* Failure, dental
    implant
  engagement of head (term of pregnancy)
    (mother) O32.4
  erection (penile) — *see also* Dysfunction, sexual,
    male, erectile N52.9
    nonorganic F52.21
  examination (s) , anxiety concerning Z55.2
  expansion terminal respiratory units (newborn)
    (primary) P28.0
  forceps NOS (with subsequent cesarean
    delivery) O66.5
  gain weight (child over 28 days old) R62.51
    adult R62.7
    newborn P92.6
  genital response (male) F52.21
    female F52.22
  heart (acute) (senile) (sudden) I50.9
    with
      acute pulmonary edema — *see* Failure,
        ventricular, left
      decompensation — *see* Failure, heart, congestive
      dilatation — *see* Disease, heart
    arteriosclerotic I70.90
    biventricular I50.9
    combined left-right sided I50.9
    compensated I50.9
    complicating
      anesthesia (general) (local) or other sedation
        in labor and delivery O74.2
        in pregnancy O29.12-
        postpartum, puerperal O89.1
      delivery (cesarean) (instrumental) O75.4
    congestive (compensated) (decompensated) I50.9
      with rheumatic fever (conditions in I00)
        active I01.8
        inactive or quiescent (with chorea) I09.81
      newborn P29.0
      rheumatic (chronic) (inactive) (with
        chorea) I09.81
        active or acute I01.8
          with chorea I02.0
    decompensated I50.9
    degenerative — *see* Degeneration, myocardial
    diastolic (congestive) I50.30
      acute (congestive) I50.31
        and (on) chronic (congestive) I50.33
      chronic (congestive) I50.32
        and (on) acute (congestive) I50.33
      combined with systolic (congestive) I50.40
        acute (congestive) I50.41
          and (on) chronic (congestive) I50.43
        chronic (congestive) I50.42
          and (on) acute (congestive) I50.43
    due to presence of cardiac prosthesis I97.13-
    following cardiac surgery I97.13-
    high output NOS I50.9
    hypertensive — *see* Hypertension, heart
    left (ventricular) — *see* Failure, ventricular, left
    low output (syndrome) NOS I50.9
    newborn P29.0
    organic — *see* Disease, heart
    peripartum O90.3
    postprocedural I97.13-
    rheumatic (chronic) (inactive) I09.9
    right (ventricular) (secondary to left heart
      failure) — *see* Failure, heart, congestive
    systolic (congestive) I50.20
      acute (congestive) I50.21
        and (on) chronic (congestive) I50.23
      chronic (congestive) I50.22
        and (on) acute (congestive) I50.23

Failure, failed - *continued*
  heart (acute) (senile) (sudden) - *continued*
    systolic (congestive) - *continued*
      combined with diastolic (congestive) I50.40
        acute (congestive) I50.41
          and (on) chronic (congestive) I50.43
        chronic (congestive) I50.42
          and (on) acute (congestive) I50.43
    thyrotoxic — *see also* Thyrotoxicosis E05.90 *[I43]*
      with thyroid storm E05.91 *[I43]*
    valvular — *see* Endocarditis
  hepatic K72.90
    with coma K72.91
    acute or subacute K72.00
      with coma K72.01
      due to drugs K71.10
        with coma K71.11
    alcoholic (acute) (chronic) (subacute) K70.40
      with coma K70.41
    chronic K72.10
      with coma K72.11
      due to drugs (acute) (subacute) (chronic) K71.10
        with coma K71.11
    due to drugs (acute) (subacute) (chronic) K71.10
      with coma K71.11
    postprocedural K91.82
  hepatorenal K76.7
  induction (of labor) O61.9
    abortion — *see* Abortion, attempted
    by
      oxytocic drugs O61.0
      prostaglandins O61.0
    instrumental O61.1
    mechanical O61.1
    medical O61.0
    specified NEC O61.8
    surgical O61.1
  intubation during anesthesia T88.4
    in pregnancy O29.6-
    labor and delivery O74.7
    postpartum, puerperal O89.6
  involution, thymus (gland) E32.0
  kidney — *see also* Disease, kidney, chronic N19
    acute — *see also* Failure, renal, acute N17.9-
    diabetic — *see* E08-E13 with .22
  lactation (complete) O92.3
    partial O92.4
  Leydig's cell, adult E29.1
  liver — *see* Failure, hepatic
  menstruation at puberty N91.0
  mitral I05.8
  myocardial, myocardium — *see also* Failure,
    heart I50.9
    chronic — *see also* Failure, heart, congestive I50.9
    congestive — *see also* Failure, heart,
      congestive I50.9
  orgasm (female) (psychogenic) F52.31
    male F52.32
  ovarian (primary) E28.39
    iatrogenic E89.40
      asymptomatic E89.40
      symptomatic E89.41
    postprocedural (postablative) (postirradiation)
      (postsurgical) E89.40
      asymptomatic E89.40
      symptomatic E89.41
  ovulation causing infertility N97.0
  polyglandular, autoimmune E31.0
  prosthetic joint implant — *see* Complications, joint
    prosthesis, mechanical, breakdown, by site
  renal N19
    with
      tubular necrosis (acute) N17.0
    acute N17.9
      with
        cortical necrosis N17.1
        medullary necrosis N17.2
        tubular necrosis N17.0
      specified NEC N17.8
    chronic N18.9
      hypertensive — *see* Hypertension, kidney
    congenital P96.0
    end stage (chronic) N18.6
      due to hypertension I12.0
    following
      abortion — *see* Abortion by type complicated by
        specified condition NEC
      crushing T79.5
      ectopic or molar pregnancy O08.4
      labor and delivery (acute) O90.4
    hypertensive — *see* Hypertension, kidney
    postprocedural N99.0
  respiration, respiratory J96.90

Failure, failed - *continued*
  respiration, respiratory - *continued*
    with
      hypercapnia J96.92
      hypoxia J96.91
    acute J96.00
      with
        hypercapnia J96.02
        hypoxia J96.01
      center G93.89
    acute and (on) chronic J96.20
      with
        hypercapnia J96.22
        hypoxia J96.21
    chronic J96.10
      with
        hypercapnia J96.12
        hypoxia J96.11
    newborn P28.5
    postprocedural (acute) J95.821
      acute and chronic J95.822
  rotation
    cecum Q43.3
    colon Q43.3
    intestine Q43.3
    kidney Q63.2
  sedation (conscious) (moderate) during
    procedure T88.52
    history of Z92.83
  segmentation — *see also* Fusion
    fingers — *see* Syndactylism, complex, fingers
    vertebra Q76.49
      with scoliosis Q76.3
  seminiferous tubule, adult E29.1
  senile (general) R54
  sexual arousal (male) F52.21
    female F52.22
  testicular endocrine function E29.1
  to thrive (child over 28 days old) R62.51
    adult R62.7
    newborn P92.6
  transplant T86.92
    bone T86.831
      marrow T86.02
    cornea T86.841
    heart T86.22
      with lung (s) T86.32
    intestine T86.851
    kidney T86.12
    liver T86.42
    lung (s) T86.811
      with heart T86.32
    pancreas T86.891
    skin (allograft) (autograft) T86.821
    specified organ or tissue NEC T86.891
    stem cell (peripheral blood) (umbilical cord) T86.5
  trial of labor (with subsequent cesarean
    delivery) O66.40
    following previous cesarean delivery O66.41
  tubal ligation N99.89
  urinary — *see* Disease, kidney, chronic
  vacuum extraction NOS (with subsequent cesarean
    delivery) O66.5
  vasectomy N99.89
  ventouse NOS (with subsequent cesarean
    delivery) O66.5
  ventricular — *see also* Failure, heart I50.9
    left I50.1
      with rheumatic fever (conditions in I00)
        active I01.8
          with chorea I02.0
        inactive or quiescent (with chorea) I09.81
      rheumatic (chronic) (inactive) (with
        chorea) I09.81
        active or acute I01.8
          with chorea I02.0
    right — *see also* Failure, heart, congestive I50.9
  vital centers, newborn P91.8
Fainting (fit) R55
Fallen arches — *see* Deformity, limb, flat foot
Falling, falls (repeated) R29.6
  any organ or part — *see* Prolapse
Fallopian
  insufflation Z31.41
  tube — *see* condition
Fallot's
  pentalogy Q21.8
  tetrad or tetralogy Q21.3
  triad or trilogy Q22.3
False — *see also* condition
  croup J38.5
  joint — *see* Nonunion, fracture
  labor (pains) O47.9

False - *continued*
  labor (pains) - *continued*
    at or after 37 completed weeks of gestation O47.1
    before 37 completed weeks of gestation O47.0-
  passage, urethra (prostatic) N36.5
  pregnancy F45.8
Family, familial — *see also* condition
  disruption Z63.8
    involving divorce or separation Z63.5
  Li-Fraumeni (syndrome) Z15.01
  planning advice Z30.09
  problem Z63.9
    specified NEC Z63.8
  retinoblastoma C69.2-
Famine (effects of) T73.0
  edema — *see* Malnutrition, severe
Fanconi (-de Toni) (-Debré) **syndrome** E72.09
  with cystinosis E72.04
Fanconi's anemia (congenital pancytopenia) D61.09
Farber's disease or syndrome E75.29
Farcy A24.0
Farmer's
  lung J67.0
  skin L57.8
Farsightedness — *see* Hypermetropia
Fascia — *see* condition
Fasciculation R25.3
Fasciitis M72.9
  diffuse (eosinophilic) M35.4
  infective M72.8
    necrotizing M72.6
  necrotizing M72.6
  nodular M72.4
  perirenal (with ureteral obstruction) N13.5
    with infection N13.6
  plantar M72.2
  specified NEC M72.8
  traumatic (old) M72.8
    current - code by site under Sprain
Fascioliasis B66.3
Fasciolopsis, fasciolopsiasis (intestinal) B66.5
Fascioscapulohumeral myopathy G71.0
Fast pulse R00.0
Fat
  embolism — *see* Embolism, fat
  excessive — *see also* Obesity
    in heart — *see* Degeneration, myocardial
  in stool R19.5
  localized (pad) E65
    heart — *see* Degeneration, myocardial
    knee M79.4
    retropatellar M79.4
  necrosis
    breast N64.1
    mesentery K65.4
    omentum K65.4
  pad E65
    knee M79.4
Fatigue R53.83
  auditory deafness — *see* Deafness
  chronic R53.82
  combat F43.0
  general R53.83
    psychogenic F48.8
  heat (transient) T67.6
  muscle M62.89
  myocardium — *see* Failure, heart
  neoplasm-related R53.0
  nervous, neurosis F48.8
  operational F48.8
  psychogenic (general) F48.8
  senile R54
  voice R49.8
Fatness — *see* Obesity
Fatty — *see also* condition
  apron E65
  degeneration — *see* Degeneration, fatty
  heart (enlarged) — *see* Degeneration, myocardial
  liver NEC K76.0
    alcoholic K70.0
    nonalcoholic K76.0
  necrosis — *see* Degeneration, fatty
Fauces — *see* condition
Fauchard's disease (periodontitis) — *see*
  Periodontitis
Faucitis J02.9
Favism (anemia) D55.0
Favus — *see* Dermatophytosis
Fazio-Londe disease or syndrome G12.1
Fear complex or reaction F40.9
Fear of — *see* Phobia
Feared complaint unfounded Z71.1

Febris, febrile — *see also* Fever
  flava — *see also* Fever, yellow A95.9
  melitensis A23.0
  pestis — *see* Plague
  recurrens — *see* Fever, relapsing
  rubra A38.9
Fecal
  incontinence R15.9
  smearing R15.1
  soiling R15.1
  urgency R15.2
Fecalith (impaction) K56.41
  appendix K38.1
  congenital P76.8
Fede's disease K14.0
**Feeble rapid pulse due to shock following
  injury** T79.4
Feeble-minded F70
Feeding
  difficulties R63.3
  problem R63.3
    newborn P92.9
      specified NEC P92.8
  nonorganic (adult) — *see* Disorder, eating
Feeling (of)
  foreign body in throat R09.89
Feer's disease — *see* Poisoning, mercury
Feet — *see* condition
Feigned illness Z76.5
Feil-Klippel syndrome (brevicollis) Q76.1
Feinmesser's (hidrotic) **ectodermal dysplasia** Q82.4
Felinophobia F40.218
Felon — *see also* Cellulitis, digit
  with lymphangitis — *see* Lymphangitis, acute, digit
Felty's syndrome M05.00
  ankle M05.07-
  elbow M05.02-
  foot joint M05.07-
  hand joint M05.04-
  hip M05.05-
  knee M05.06-
  multiple site M05.09
  shoulder M05.01-
  vertebra — *see* Spondylitis, ankylosing
  wrist M05.03-
Female genital cutting status — *see* Female genital
  mutilation status (FGM)
Female genital mutilation status (FGM) N90.810
  specified NEC N90.818
  type I (clitorectomy status) N90.811
  type II (clitorectomy with excision of labia minora
    status) N90.812
  type III (infibulation status) N90.813
  type IV N90.818
Femur, femoral — *see* condition
Fenestration, fenestrated — *see also* Imperfect,
  closure
  aortico-pulmonary Q21.4
  cusps, heart valve NEC Q24.8
    pulmonary Q22.3
  pulmonic cusps Q22.3
Fernell's disease (aortic aneurysm) I71.9
Fertile eunuch syndrome E23.0
Fetid
  breath R19.6
  sweat L75.0
Fetishism F65.0
  transvestic F65.1
Fetus, fetal — *see also* condition
  alcohol syndrome (dysmorphic) Q86.0
  compressus O31.0-
  hydantoin syndrome Q86.1
  lung tissue P28.0
  papyraceous O31.0-
Fever (inanition) (of unknown origin) (persistent)
  (with chills) (with rigor) R50.9
  abortus A23.1
  Aden (dengue) A90
  African tick-borne A68.1
  American
    mountain (tick) A93.2
    spotted A77.0
  aphthous B08.8
  arbovirus, arboviral A94
    hemorrhagic A94
    specified NEC A93.8
  Argentinian hemorrhagic A96.0
  Assam B55.0
  Australian Q A78
  Bangkok hemorrhagic A91
  Barmah forest A92.8
  Bartonella A44.0
  bilious, hemoglobinuric B50.8

Fever (inanition) (of unknown origin) (persistent)
(with chills) (with rigor) - *continued*
  blackwater B50.8
  blister B00.1
  Bolivian hemorrhagic A96.1
  Bonvale dam T73.3
  boutonneuse A77.1
  brain — *see* Encephalitis
  Brazilian purpuric A48.4
  breakbone A90
  Bullis A77.0
  Bunyamwera A92.8
  Burdwan B55.0
  Bwamba A92.8
  Cameroon — *see* Malaria
  Canton A75.9
  catarrhal (acute) J00
    chronic J31.0
  cat-scratch A28.1
  Central Asian hemorrhagic A98.0
  cerebral — *see* Encephalitis
  cerebrospinal meningococcal A39.0
  Chagres B50.9
  Chandipura A92.8
  Changuinola A93.1
  Charcot's (biliary) (hepatic) (intermittent) - — *see*
    Calculus, bile duct
  Chikungunya (viral) (hemorrhagic) A92.0
  Chitral A93.1
  Colombo — *see* Fever, paratyphoid
  Colorado tick (virus) A93.2
  congestive (remittent) — *see* Malaria
  Congo virus A98.0
  continued malarial B50.9
  Corsican — *see* Malaria
  Crimean-Congo hemorrhagic A98.0
  Cyprus — *see* Brucellosis
  dandy A90
  deer fly — *see* Tularemia
  dengue (virus) A90
    hemorrhagic A91
    sandfly A93.1
  desert B38.0
  drug induced R50.2
  due to
    conditions classified elsewhere R50.81
    heat T67.0
  enteric A01.00
  enteroviral exanthematous (Boston exanthem) A88.0
  ephemeral (of unknown origin) R50.9
  epidemic hemorrhagic A98.5
  erysipelatous — *see* Erysipelas
  estivo-autumnal (malarial) B50.9
  famine A75.0
  five day A79.0
  following delivery O86.4
  Fort Bragg A27.89
  gastroenteric A01.00
  gastromalarial — *see* Malaria
  Gibraltar — *see* Brucellosis
  glandular — *see* Mononucleosis, infectious
  Guama (viral) A92.8
  Haverhill A25.1
  hay (allergic) J30.1
    with asthma (bronchial) J45.909
      with
        exacerbation (acute) J45.901
        status asthmaticus J45.902
      due to
        allergen other than pollen J30.89
        pollen, any plant or tree J30.1
  heat (effects) T67.0
  hematuric, bilious B50.8
  hemoglobinuric (malarial) (bilious) B50.8
  hemorrhagic (arthropod-borne) NOS A94
    with renal syndrome A98.5
    arenaviral A96.9
      specified NEC A96.8
    Argentinian A96.0
    Bangkok A91
    Bolivian A96.1
    Central Asian A98.0
    Chikungunya A92.0
    Crimean-Congo A98.0
    dengue (virus) A91
    epidemic A98.5
    Junin (virus) A96.0
    Korean A98.5
    Kyasanur forest A98.2
    Machupo (virus) A96.1
    mite-borne A93.8
    mosquito-borne A92.8
    Omsk A98.1

Fever (inanition) (of unknown origin) (persistent)
(with chills) (with rigor) - *continued*
  hemorrhagic (arthropod-borne) NOS - *continued*
    Philippine A91
    Russian A98.5
    Singapore A91
    Southeast Asia A91
    Thailand A91
    tick-borne NEC A93.8
    viral A99
      specified NEC A98.8
  hepatic — *see* Cholecystitis
  herpetic — *see* Herpes
  icterohemorrhagic A27.0
  Indiana A93.8
  infective B99.9
    specified NEC B99.8
  intermittent (bilious) — *see also* Malaria
    of unknown origin R50.9
    pernicious B50.9
  iodide R50.2
  Japanese river A75.3
  jungle — *see also* Malaria
    yellow A95.0
  Junin (virus) hemorrhagic A96.0
  Katayama B65.2
  kedani A75.3
  Kenya (tick) A77.1
  Kew Garden A79.1
  Korean hemorrhagic A98.5
  Lassa A96.2
  Lone Star A77.0
  Machupo (virus) hemorrhagic A96.1
  malaria, malarial — *see* Malaria
  Malta A23.9
  Marseilles A77.1
  marsh — *see* Malaria
  Mayaro (viral) A92.8
  Mediterranean — *see also* Brucellosis A23.9
    familial M04.1
    tick A77.1
  meningeal — *see* Meningitis
  Meuse A79.0
  Mexican A75.2
  mianeh A68.1
  miasmatic — *see* Malaria
  mosquito-borne (viral) A92.9
    hemorrhagic A92.8
  mountain — *see also* Brucellosis
    meaning Rocky Mountain spotted fever A77.0
    tick (American) (Colorado) (viral) A93.2
  Mucambo (viral) A92.8
  mud A27.9
  Neapolitan — *see* Brucellosis
  neutropenic D70.9
  newborn P81.9
    environmental P81.0
  Nine-Mile A78
  non-exanthematous tick A93.2
  North Asian tick-borne A77.2
  Omsk hemorrhagic A98.1
  O'nyong-nyong (viral) A92.1
  Oropouche (viral) A93.0
  Oroya A44.0
  paludal — *see* Malaria
  Panama (malarial) B50.9
  Pappataci A93.1
  paratyphoid A01.4
    A A01.1
    B A01.2
    C A01.3
  parrot A70
  periodic (Mediterranean) M04.1
  persistent (of unknown origin) R50.9
  petechial A39.0
  pharyngoconjunctival B30.2
  Philippine hemorrhagic A91
  phlebotomus A93.1
  Piry (virus) A93.8
  Pixuna (viral) A92.8
  Plasmodium ovale B53.0
  polioviral (nonparalytic) A80.4
  Pontiac A48.2
  postimmunization R50.83
  postoperative R50.82
    due to infection T81.40
  posttransfusion R50.84
  postvaccination R50.83
  presenting with conditions classified
    elsewhere R50.81
  pretibial A27.89
  puerperal O86.4
  Q A78

Fever (inanition) (of unknown origin) (persistent)
(with chills) (with rigor) - *continued*
  quadrilateral A78
  quartan (malaria) B52.9
  Queensland (coastal) (tick) A77.3
  quintan A79.0
  rabbit — *see* Tularemia
  rat-bite A25.9
    due to
      Spirillum A25.0
      Streptobacillus moniliformis A25.1
  recurrent — *see* Fever, relapsing
  relapsing (Borrelia) A68.9
    Carter's (Asiatic) A68.1
    Dutton's (West African) A68.1
    Koch's A68.9
    louse-borne A68.0
    Novy's
      louse-borne A68.0
      tick-borne A68.1
    Obermeyer's (European) A68.0
    tick-borne A68.1
  remittent (bilious) (congestive) (gastric) — *see*
    Malaria
  rheumatic (active) (acute) (chronic) (subacute) I00
    with central nervous system involvement I02.9
    active with heart involvement — *see* category I01
    inactive or quiescent with
      cardiac hypertrophy I09.89
      carditis I09.9
      endocarditis I09.1
        aortic (valve) I06.9
          with mitral (valve) disease I08.0
        mitral (valve) I05.9
          with aortic (valve) disease I08.0
        pulmonary (valve) I09.89
        tricuspid (valve) I07.8
      heart disease NEC I09.89
      heart failure (congestive) (conditions in
        I50.9) I09.81
      left ventricular failure (conditions in I50.1) I09.81
      myocarditis, myocardial degeneration (conditions
        in I51.4) I09.0
      pancarditis I09.9
      pericarditis I09.2
  Rift Valley (viral) A92.4
  Rocky Mountain spotted A77.0
  rose J30.1
  Ross River B33.1
  Russian hemorrhagic A98.5
  San Joaquin (Valley) B38.0
  sandfly A93.1
  Sao Paulo A77.0
  scarlet A38.9
  seven day (leptospirosis) (autumnal)
    (Japanese) A27.89
    dengue A90
  shin-bone A79.0
  Singapore hemorrhagic A91
  solar A90
  Songo A98.5
  sore B00.1
  South African tick-bite A68.1
  Southeast Asia hemorrhagic A91
  spinal — *see* Meningitis
  spirillary A25.0
  splenic — *see* Anthrax
  spotted A77.9
    American A77.0
    Brazilian A77.0
    cerebrospinal meningitis A39.0
    Colombian A77.0
    due to Rickettsia
      australis A77.3
      conorii A77.1
      rickettsii A77.0
      sibirica A77.2
      specified type NEC A77.8
    Ehrlichiosis A77.40
      due to
        E. chafeensis A77.41
        specified organism NEC A77.49
    Rocky Mountain A77.0
  steroid R50.2
  streptobacillary A25.1
  subtertian B50.9
  Sumatran mite A75.3
  sun A90
  swamp A27.9
  swine A02.8
  sylvatic, yellow A95.0
  Tahyna B33.8
  tertian — *see* Malaria, tertian

Fever (inanition) (of unknown origin) (persistent) (with chills) (with rigor) - *continued*
  Thailand hemorrhagic A91
  thermic T67.0
  three-day A93.1
  tick
    American mountain A93.2
    Colorado A93.2
    Kemerovo A93.8
    Mediterranean A77.1
    mountain A93.2
    nonexanthematous A93.2
    Quaranfil A93.8
  tick-bite NEC A93.8
  tick-borne (hemorrhagic) NEC A93.8
  trench A79.0
  tsutsugamushi A75.3
  typhogastric A01.00
  typhoid (abortive) (hemorrhagic) (intermittent) (malignant) A01.00
    complicated by
      arthritis A01.04
      heart involvement A01.02
      meningitis A01.01
      osteomyelitis A01.05
      pneumonia A01.03
      specified NEC A01.09
  typhomalarial — *see* Malaria
  typhus — *see* Typhus (fever)
  undulant — *see* Brucellosis
  unknown origin R50.9
  uveoparotid D86.89
  valley B38.0
  Venezuelan equine A92.2
  vesicular stomatitis A93.8
  viral hemorrhagic — *see* Fever, hemorrhagic, by type of virus
  Volhynian A79.0
  Wesselsbron (viral) A92.8
  West
    African B50.8
    Nile (viral) A92.30
      with
        complications NEC A92.39
        cranial nerve disorders A92.32
        encephalitis A92.31
        encephalomyelitis A92.31
        neurologic manifestation NEC A92.32
        optic neuritis A92.32
        polyradiculitis A92.32
  Whitmore's — *see* Melioidosis
  Wolhynian A79.0
  worm B83.9
  yellow A95.9
    jungle A95.0
    sylvatic A95.0
    urban A95.1
  Zika virus A92.5

Fibrillation
  atrial or auricular (established) I48.91
    chronic I48.2
    paroxysmal I48.0
    permanent I48.2
    persistent I48.1
  cardiac I49.8
  heart I49.8
  muscular M62.89
  ventricular I49.01

Fibrin
  ball or bodies, pleural (sac) J94.1
  chamber, anterior (eye) (gelatinous exudate) — *see* Iridocyclitis, acute

Fibrinogenolysis — *see* Fibrinolysis
Fibrinogenopenia D68.8
  acquired D65
  congenital D68.2
Fibrinolysis (hemorrhagic) (acquired) D65
  antepartum hemorrhage — *see* Hemorrhage, antepartum, with coagulation defect
  following
    abortion — *see* Abortion by type complicated by hemorrhage
    ectopic or molar pregnancy O08.1
  intrapartum O67.0
  newborn, transient P60
  postpartum O72.3
Fibrinopenia (hereditary) D68.2
  acquired D68.4
Fibrinopurulent — *see* condition
Fibrinous — *see* condition
Fibroadenoma
  cellular intracanalicular D24-
  giant D24-

Fibroadenoma - *continued*
  intracanalicular
    cellular D24-
    giant D24-
    specified site — *see* Neoplasm, benign, by site
    unspecified site D24-
  juvenile D24-
  pericanalicular
    specified site — *see* Neoplasm, benign, by site
    unspecified site D24-
  phyllodes D24-
  prostate D29.1
  specified site NEC — *see* Neoplasm, benign, by site
  unspecified site D24-
Fibroadenosis, breast (chronic) (cystic) (diffuse) (periodic) (segmental) N60.2-
Fibroangioma — *see also* Neoplasm, benign, by site
  juvenile
    specified site — *see* Neoplasm, benign, by site
    unspecified site D10.6
Fibrochondrosarcoma — *see* Neoplasm, cartilage, malignant
Fibrocystic
  disease — *see also* Fibrosis, cystic
    breast — *see* Mastopathy, cystic
    jaw M27.49
    kidney (congenital) Q61.8
    liver Q44.6
    pancreas E84.9
  kidney (congenital) Q61.8
Fibrodysplasia ossificans progressiva - *see* Myositis, ossificans, progressiva
Fibroelastosis (cordis) (endocardial) (endomyocardial) I42.4
Fibroid (tumor) — *see also* Neoplasm, connective tissue, benign
  disease, lung (chronic) — *see* Fibrosis, lung
  heart (disease) — *see* Myocarditis
  in pregnancy or childbirth O34.1-
    causing obstructed labor O65.5
  induration, lung (chronic) — *see* Fibrosis, lung
  lung — *see* Fibrosis, lung
  pneumonia (chronic) — *see* Fibrosis, lung
  uterus D25.9
Fibrolipoma — *see* Lipoma
Fibroliposarcoma — *see* Neoplasm, connective tissue, malignant
Fibroma — *see also* Neoplasm, connective tissue, benign
  ameloblastic — *see* Cyst, calcifying odontogenic
  bone (nonossifying) — *see* Disorder, bone, specified type NEC
    ossifying — *see* Neoplasm, bone, benign
  cementifying — *see* Neoplasm, bone, benign
  chondromyxoid — *see* Neoplasm, bone, benign
  desmoplastic — *see* Neoplasm, connective tissue, uncertain behavior
  durum — *see* Neoplasm, connective tissue, benign
  fascial — *see* Neoplasm, connective tissue, benign
  invasive — *see* Neoplasm, connective tissue, uncertain behavior
  molle — *see* Lipoma
  myxoid — *see* Neoplasm, connective tissue, benign
  nasopharynx, nasopharyngeal (juvenile) D10.6
  nonosteogenic (nonossifying) — *see* Dysplasia, fibrous
  odontogenic (central) — *see* Cyst, calcifying odontogenic
  ossifying — *see* Neoplasm, bone, benign
  periosteal — *see* Neoplasm, bone, benign
  soft — *see* Lipoma
Fibromatosis M72.9
  abdominal — *see* Neoplasm, connective tissue, uncertain behavior
  aggressive — *see* Neoplasm, connective tissue, uncertain behavior
  congenital generalized — *see* Neoplasm, connective tissue, uncertain behavior
  Dupuytren's M72.0
  gingival K06.1
  palmar (fascial) M72.0
  plantar (fascial) M72.2
  pseudosarcomatous (proliferative) (subcutaneous) M72.4
  retroperitoneal D48.3
  specified NEC M72.8
Fibromyalgia M79.7
Fibromyoma — *see also* Neoplasm, connective tissue, benign
  uterus (corpus) — *see also* Leiomyoma, uterus
    in pregnancy or childbirth — *see* Fibroid, in pregnancy or childbirth
      causing obstructed labor O65.5

Fibromyositis M79.7
Fibromyxolipoma D17.9
Fibromyxoma — *see* Neoplasm, connective tissue, benign
Fibromyxosarcoma — *see* Neoplasm, connective tissue, malignant
Fibro-odontoma, ameloblastic — *see* Cyst, calcifying odontogenic
Fibro-osteoma — *see* Neoplasm, bone, benign
Fibroplasia, retrolental H35.17-
Fibropurulent — *see* condition
Fibrosarcoma — *see also* Neoplasm, connective tissue, malignant
  ameloblastic C41.1
    upper jaw (bone) C41.0
  congenital — *see* Neoplasm, connective tissue, malignant
  fascial — *see* Neoplasm, connective tissue, malignant
  infantile — *see* Neoplasm, connective tissue, malignant
  odontogenic C41.1
    upper jaw (bone) C41.0
  periosteal — *see* Neoplasm, bone, malignant
Fibrosclerosis
  breast N60.3-
  multifocal M35.5
  penis (corpora cavernosa) N48.6
Fibrosis, fibrotic
  adrenal (gland) E27.8
  amnion O41.8X-
  anal papillae K62.89
  arteriocapillary — *see* Arteriosclerosis
  bladder N32.89
    interstitial — *see* Cystitis, chronic, interstitial
    localized submucosal — *see* Cystitis, chronic, interstitial
    panmural — *see* Cystitis, chronic, interstitial
  breast — *see* Fibrosclerosis, breast
  capillary — *see also* Arteriosclerosis I70.90
    lung (chronic) — *see* Fibrosis, lung
  cardiac — *see* Myocarditis
  cervix N88.8
  chorion O41.8X-
  corpus cavernosum (sclerosing) N48.6
  cystic (of pancreas) E84.9
    with
      distal intestinal obstruction syndrome E84.19
      fecal impaction E84.19
      intestinal manifestations NEC E84.19
      pulmonary manifestations E84.0
      specified manifestations NEC E84.8
  due to device, implant or graft — *see also* Complications, by site and type, specified NEC T85.828
    arterial graft NEC T82.828
    breast (implant) T85.828
    catheter NEC T85.828
      dialysis (renal) T82.828
        intraperitoneal T85.828
      infusion NEC T82.828
        spinal (epidural) (subdural) T85.820
      urinary (indwelling) T83.82
    electronic (electrode) (pulse generator) (stimulator)
      bone T84.82
      cardiac T82.827
      nervous system (brain) (peripheral nerve) (spinal) T85.820
      urinary T83.82
    fixation, internal (orthopedic) NEC T84.82
    gastrointestinal (bile duct) (esophagus) T85.828
    genital NEC T83.82
    heart NEC T82.827
    joint prosthesis T84.82
    ocular (corneal graft) (orbital implant) NEC T85.828
    orthopedic NEC T84.82
    specified NEC T85.828
    urinary NEC T83.82
    vascular NEC T82.828
    ventricular intracranial shunt T85.820
  ejaculatory duct N50.89
  endocardium — *see* Endocarditis
  endomyocardial (tropical) I42.3
  epididymis N50.89
  eye muscle — *see* Strabismus, mechanical
  heart — *see* Myocarditis
  hepatic — *see* Fibrosis, liver
  hepatolienal (portal hypertension) K76.6
  hepatosplenic (portal hypertension) K76.6
  infrapatellar fat pad M79.4
  intrascrotal N50.89
  kidney N26.9

Fibrosis, fibrotic - *continued*
- liver K74.0
  - with sclerosis K74.2
  - alcoholic K70.2
- lung (atrophic) (chronic) (confluent) (massive) (perialveolar) (peribronchial) J84.10
  - with
    - anthracosilicosis J60
    - anthracosis J60
    - asbestosis J61
    - bagassosis J67.1
    - bauxite J63.1
    - berylliosis J63.2
    - byssinosis J66.0
    - calcicosis J62.8
    - chalicosis J62.8
    - dust reticulation J64
    - farmer's lung J67.0
    - ganister disease J62.8
    - graphite J63.3
    - pneumoconiosis NOS J64
    - siderosis J63.4
    - silicosis J62.8
  - capillary J84.10
  - congenital P27.8
  - diffuse (idiopathic) J84.10
    - chemicals, gases, fumes or vapors (inhalation) J68.4
    - interstitial J84.10
      - acute J84.114
    - talc J62.0
  - following radiation J70.1
  - idiopathic J84.112
  - postinflammatory J84.10
  - silicotic J62.8
  - tuberculous — *see* Tuberculosis, pulmonary
- lymphatic gland I89.8
- median bar — *see* Hyperplasia, prostate
- mediastinum (idiopathic) J98.59
- meninges G96.19
- myocardium, myocardial — *see* Myocarditis
- ovary N83.8
- oviduct N83.8
- pancreas K86.89
- penis NEC N48.6
- pericardium I31.0
- perineum, in pregnancy or childbirth O34.7-
  - causing obstructed labor O65.5
- pleura J94.1
- popliteal fat pad M79.4
- prostate (chronic) — *see* Hyperplasia, prostate
- pulmonary — *see also* Fibrosis, lung J84.10
  - congenital P27.8
  - idiopathic J84.112
- rectal sphincter K62.89
- retroperitoneal, idiopathic (with ureteral obstruction) N13.5
  - with infection N13.6
- sclerosing mesenteric (idiopathic) K65.4
- scrotum N50.89
- seminal vesicle N50.89
- senile R54
- skin L90.5
- spermatic cord N50.89
- spleen D73.89
  - in schistosomiasis (bilharziasis) B65.9 *[D77]*
- subepidermal nodular — *see* Neoplasm, skin, benign
- submucous (oral) (tongue) K13.5
- testis N44.8
  - chronic, due to syphilis A52.76
- thymus (gland) E32.8
- tongue, submucous K13.5
- tunica vaginalis N50.89
- uterus (non-neoplastic) N85.8
- vagina N89.8
- valve, heart — *see* Endocarditis
- vas deferens N50.89
- vein I87.8

Fibrositis (periarticular) M79.7
- nodular, chronic (Jaccoud's) (rheumatoid) — *see* Arthropathy, postrheumatic, chronic

Fibrothorax J94.1

Fibrotic — *see* Fibrosis

Fibrous — *see* condition

Fibroxanthoma — *see also* Neoplasm, connective tissue, benign
- atypical — *see* Neoplasm, connective tissue, uncertain behavior
- malignant — *see* Neoplasm, connective tissue, malignant

Fibroxanthosarcoma — *see* Neoplasm, connective tissue, malignant

Fiedler's
- disease (icterohemorrhagic leptospirosis) A27.0
- myocarditis (acute) I40.1

Fifth disease B08.3
- venereal A55

Filaria, filarial, filariasis — *see* Infestation, filarial

Filatov's disease — *see* Mononucleosis, infectious

File-cutter's disease — *see* Poisoning, lead

Filling defect
- biliary tract R93.2
- bladder R93.41
- duodenum R93.3
- gallbladder R93.2
- gastrointestinal tract R93.3
- intestine R93.3
- kidney R93.42-
- stomach R93.3
- ureter R93.41
- urinary organs, specified NEC R93.49

Fimbrial cyst Q50.4

Financial problem affecting care NOS Z59.9
- bankruptcy Z59.8
- foreclosure on loan Z59.8

Findings, abnormal, inconclusive, without diagnosis — *see also* Abnormal
- 17-ketosteroids, elevated R82.5
- acetonuria R82.4
- alcohol in blood R78.0
- anisocytosis R71.8
- antenatal screening of mother O28.9
  - biochemical O28.1
  - chromosomal O28.5
  - cytological O28.2
  - genetic O28.5
  - hematological O28.0
  - radiological O28.4
  - specified NEC O28.8
  - ultrasonic O28.3
- antibody titer, elevated R76.0
- anticardiolipin antibody R76.0
- antiphosphatidylglycerol antibody R76.0
- antiphosphatidylinositol antibody R76.0
- antiphosphatidylserine antibody R76.0
- antiphospholipid antibody R76.0
- bacteriuria R82.71
- bicarbonate E87.8
- bile in urine R82.2
- blood sugar R73.09
  - high R73.9
  - low (transient) E16.2
- body fluid or substance, specified NEC R88.8
- casts, urine R82.99
- catecholamines R82.5
- cells, urine R82.99
- chloride E87.8
- cholesterol E78.9
  - high E78.00
    - with high triglycerides E78.2
- chyluria R82.0
- cloudy
  - dialysis effluent R88.0
  - urine R82.90
- creatinine clearance R94.4
- crystals, urine R82.99
- culture
  - blood R78.81
  - positive — *see* Positive, culture
- echocardiogram R93.1
- electrolyte level, urinary R82.99
- function study NEC R94.8
  - bladder R94.8
  - endocrine NEC R94.7
    - thyroid R94.6
  - kidney R94.4
  - liver R94.5
  - pancreas R94.8
  - placenta R94.8
  - pulmonary R94.2
  - spleen R94.8
- gallbladder, nonvisualization R93.2
- glucose (tolerance test) (non-fasting) R73.09
- glycosuria R81
- heart
  - shadow R93.1
  - sounds R01.2
- hematinuria R82.3
- hematocrit drop (precipitous) R71.0
- hemoglobinuria R82.3
- human papillomavirus (HPV) DNA test positive
  - cervix
    - high risk R87.810
    - low risk R87.820
  - vagina

Findings, abnormal, inconclusive, without diagnosis - *continued*
- human papillomavirus (HPV) DNA test positive - *continued*
  - vagina - *continued*
    - high risk R87.811
    - low risk R87.821
- in blood (of substance not normally found in blood) R78.9
  - addictive drug NEC R78.4
  - alcohol (excessive level) R78.0
  - cocaine R78.2
  - hallucinogen R78.3
  - heavy metals (abnormal level) R78.79
  - lead R78.71
  - lithium (abnormal level) R78.89
  - opiate drug R78.1
  - psychotropic drug R78.5
  - specified substance NEC R78.89
  - steroid agent R78.6
- indoleacetic acid, elevated R82.5
- ketonuria R82.4
- lactic acid dehydrogenase (LDH) R74.0
- liver function test R79.89
- mammogram NEC R92.8
  - calcification (calculus) R92.1
  - inconclusive result (due to dense breasts) R92.2
  - microcalcification R92.0
- mediastinal shift R93.8
- melanin, urine R82.99
- myoglobinuria R82.1
- neonatal screening P09
- nonvisualization of gallbladder R93.2
- odor of urine NOS R82.90
- Papanicolaou cervix R87.619
  - non-atypical endometrial cells R87.618
- pneumoencephalogram R93.0
- poikilocytosis R71.8
- potassium (deficiency) E87.6
  - excess E87.5
- PPD R76.11
- radiologic (X-ray) R93.8
  - abdomen R93.5
  - biliary tract R93.2
  - breast R92.8
  - gastrointestinal tract R93.3
  - genitourinary organs R93.8
  - head R93.0
  - inconclusive due to excess body fat of patient R93.9
  - intrathoracic organs NEC R93.1
  - placenta R93.8
  - retroperitoneum R93.5
  - skin R93.8
  - skull R93.0
  - subcutaneous tissue R93.8
- red blood cell (count) (morphology) (sickling) (volume) R71.8
- scan NEC R94.8
  - bladder R94.8
  - bone R94.8
  - kidney R94.4
  - liver R93.2
  - lung R94.2
  - pancreas R94.8
  - placental R94.8
  - spleen R94.8
  - thyroid R94.6
- sedimentation rate, elevated R70.0
- SGOT R74.0
- SGPT R74.0
- sodium (deficiency) E87.1
  - excess E87.0
- specified body fluid NEC R88.8
- stress test R94.39
- thyroid (function) (metabolic rate) (scan) (uptake) R94.6
- transaminase (level) R74.0
- triglycerides E78.9
  - high E78.1
    - with high cholesterol E78.2
- tuberculin skin test (without active tuberculosis) R76.11
- urine R82.90
  - acetone R82.4
  - bacteria R82.71
  - bile R82.2
  - casts or cells R82.99
  - chyle R82.0
  - culture positive R82.79
  - glucose R81
  - hemoglobin R82.3
  - ketone R82.4

Findings, abnormal, inconclusive, without diagnosis - *continued*
  urine - *continued*
    sugar R81
    vanillylmandelic acid (VMA) , elevated R82.5
    vectorcardiogram (VCG) R94.39
    ventriculogram R93.0
    white blood cell (count) (differential) (morphology) D72.9
    xerography R92.8
Finger — *see* condition
Fire, Saint Anthony's — *see* Erysipelas
Fire-setting
  pathological (compulsive) F63.1
Fish hook stomach K31.89
Fishmeal-worker's lung J67.8
Fissure, fissured
  anus, anal K60.2
    acute K60.0
    chronic K60.1
    congenital Q43.8
  ear, lobule, congenital Q17.8
  epiglottis (congenital) Q31.8
  larynx J38.7
    congenital Q31.8
  lip K13.0
    congenital — *see* Cleft, lip
  nipple N64.0
    associated with
      lactation O92.13
      pregnancy O92.11-
      puerperium O92.12
  nose Q30.2
  palate (congenital) — *see* Cleft, palate
  skin R23.4
  spine (congenital) — *see also* Spina bifida
    with hydrocephalus — *see* Spina bifida, by site, with hydrocephalus
  tongue (acquired) K14.5
    congenital Q38.3
Fistula (cutaneous) L98.8
  abdomen (wall) K63.2
    bladder N32.2
    intestine NEC K63.2
    ureter N28.89
    uterus N82.5
  abdominorectal K63.2
  abdominosigmoidal K63.2
  abdominothoracic J86.0
  abdominouterine N82.5
    congenital Q51.7
  abdominovesical N32.2
  accessory sinuses — *see* Sinusitis
  actinomycotic — *see* Actinomycosis
  alveolar antrum — *see* Sinusitis, maxillary
  alveolar process K04.6
  anorectal K60.5
  antrobuccal — *see* Sinusitis, maxillary
  antrum — *see* Sinusitis, maxillary
  anus, anal (recurrent) (infectional) K60.3
    congenital Q43.6
      with absence, atresia and stenosis Q42.2
    tuberculous A18.32
  aorta-duodenal I77.2
  appendix, appendicular K38.3
  arteriovenous (acquired) (nonruptured) I77.0
    brain I67.1
      congenital Q28.2
        ruptured I60.8
      ruptured I60.8
    cerebral — *see* Fistula, arteriovenous, brain
    congenital (peripheral) — *see also* Malformation, arteriovenous
      brain Q28.2
        ruptured I60.8
      coronary Q24.5
      pulmonary Q25.72
    coronary I25.41
      congenital Q24.5
    pulmonary I28.0
      congenital Q25.72
    surgically created (for dialysis) Z99.2
      complication — *see* Complication, arteriovenous, fistula, surgically created
    traumatic — *see* Injury, blood vessel
  artery I77.2
  aural (mastoid) — *see* Mastoiditis, chronic
  auricle — *see also* Disorder, pinna, specified type NEC
    congenital Q18.1
  Bartholin's gland N82.8
  bile duct (common) (hepatic) K83.3
    with calculus, stones — *see* Calculus, bile duct

Fistula (cutaneous) - *continued*
  biliary (tract) — *see* Fistula, bile duct
  bladder (sphincter) NEC — *see also* Fistula, vesico- N32.2
    into seminal vesicle N32.2
  bone — *see also* Disorder, bone, specified type NEC
    with osteomyelitis, chronic — *see* Osteomyelitis, chronic, with draining sinus
  brain G93.89
    arteriovenous (acquired) I67.1
      congenital Q28.2
  branchial (cleft) Q18.0
  branchiogenous Q18.0
  breast N61.0
    puerperal, postpartum or gestational, due to mastitis (purulent) — *see* Mastitis, obstetric, purulent
  bronchial J86.0
  bronchocutaneous, bronchomediastinal, bronchopleural, bronchopleuromediastinal (infective) J86.0
    tuberculous NEC A15.5
  bronchoesophageal J86.0
    congenital Q39.2
      with atresia of esophagus Q39.1
  bronchovisceral J86.0
  buccal cavity (infective) K12.2
  cecosigmoidal K63.2
  cecum K63.2
  cerebrospinal (fluid) G96.0
  cervical, lateral Q18.1
  cervicoaural Q18.1
  cervicosigmoidal N82.4
  cervicovesical N82.1
  cervix N82.8
  chest (wall) J86.0
  cholecystenteric — *see* Fistula, gallbladder
  cholecystocolic — *see* Fistula, gallbladder
  cholecystocolonic — *see* Fistula, gallbladder
  cholecystoduodenal — *see* Fistula, gallbladder
  cholecystogastric — *see* Fistula, gallbladder
  cholecystointestinal — *see* Fistula, gallbladder
  choledochoduodenal — *see* Fistula, bile duct
  cholocolic K82.3
  coccyx — *see* Sinus, pilonidal
  colon K63.2
  colostomy K94.09
  common duct — *see* Fistula, bile duct
  congenital, site not listed — *see* Anomaly, by site
  coronary, arteriovenous I25.41
    congenital Q24.5
  costal region J86.0
  cul-de-sac, Douglas' N82.8
  cystic duct — *see also* Fistula, gallbladder
    congenital Q44.5
  dental K04.6
  diaphragm J86.0
  duodenum K31.6
  ear (external) (canal) — *see* Disorder, ear, external, specified type NEC
  enterocolic K63.2
  enterocutaneous K63.2
  enterouterine N82.4
    congenital Q51.7
  enterovaginal N82.4
    congenital Q52.2
    large intestine N82.3
    small intestine N82.2
  enterovesical N32.1
  epididymis N50.89
    tuberculous A18.15
  esophagobronchial J86.0
    congenital Q39.2
      with atresia of esophagus Q39.1
  esophagocutaneous K22.8
  esophagopleural-cutaneous J86.0
  esophagotracheal J86.0
    congenital Q39.2
      with atresia of esophagus Q39.1
  esophagus K22.8
    congenital Q39.2
      with atresia of esophagus Q39.1
  ethmoid — *see* Sinusitis, ethmoidal
  eyeball (cornea) (sclera) — *see* Disorder, globe, hypotony
  eyelid H01.8
  fallopian tube, external N82.5
  fecal K63.2
    congenital Q43.6
  from periapical abscess K04.6
  frontal sinus — *see* Sinusitis, frontal
  gallbladder K82.3

Fistula (cutaneous) - *continued*
  gallbladder - *continued*
    with calculus, cholelithiasis, stones — *see* Calculus, gallbladder
  gastric K31.6
  gastrocolic K31.6
    congenital Q40.2
    tuberculous A18.32
  gastroenterocolic K31.6
  gastroesophageal K31.6
  gastrojejunal K31.6
  gastrojejunocolic K31.6
  genital tract (female) N82.9
    specified NEC N82.8
    to intestine NEC N82.4
    to skin N82.5
  hepatic artery-portal vein, congenital Q26.6
  hepatopleural J86.0
  hepatopulmonary J86.0
  ileorectal or ileosigmoidal K63.2
  ileovaginal N82.2
  ileovesical N32.1
  ileum K63.2
  in ano K60.3
    tuberculous A18.32
  inner ear (labyrinth) — *see* subcategory H83.1
  intestine NEC K63.2
  intestinocolonic (abdominal) K63.2
  intestinoureteral N28.89
  intestinouterine N82.4
  intestinovaginal N82.4
    large intestine N82.3
    small intestine N82.2
  intestinovesical N32.1
  ischiorectal (fossa) K61.3
  jejunum K63.2
  joint M25.10
    ankle M25.17-
    elbow M25.12-
    foot joint M25.17-
    hand joint M25.14-
    hip M25.15-
    knee M25.16-
    shoulder M25.11-
    specified joint NEC M25.18
    tuberculous — *see* Tuberculosis, joint
    vertebrae M25.18
    wrist M25.13-
  kidney N28.89
  labium (majus) (minus) N82.8
  labyrinth — *see* subcategory H83.1
  lacrimal (gland) (sac) H04.61-
  lacrimonasal duct — *see* Fistula, lacrimal
  laryngotracheal, congenital Q34.8
  larynx J38.7
  lip K13.0
    congenital Q38.0
  lumbar, tuberculous A18.01
  lung J86.0
  lymphatic I89.8
  mammary (gland) N61.0
  mastoid (process) (region) — *see* Mastoiditis, chronic
  maxillary J32.0
  medial, face and neck Q18.8
  mediastinal J86.0
  mediastinobronchial J86.0
  mediastinocutaneous J86.0
  middle ear — *see* subcategory H74.8
  mouth K12.2
  nasal J34.89
    sinus — *see* Sinusitis
  nasopharynx J39.2
  nipple N64.0
  nose J34.89
  oral (cutaneous) K12.2
    maxillary J32.0
    nasal (with cleft palate) — *see* Cleft, palate
  orbit, orbital — *see* Disorder, orbit, specified type NEC
  oroantral J32.0
  oviduct, external N82.5
  palate (hard) M27.8
  pancreatic K86.89
  pancreaticoduodenal K86.89
  parotid (gland) K11.4
    region K12.2
  penis N48.89
  perianal K60.3
  pericardium (pleura) (sac) — *see* Pericarditis
  pericecal K63.2
  perineorectal K60.4
  perineosigmoidal K63.2

Fistula (cutaneous) - *continued*
perineum, perineal (with urethral involvement)
  NEC N36.0
    tuberculous A18.13
  ureter N28.89
perirectal K60.4
  tuberculous A18.32
peritoneum K65.9
pharyngoesophageal J39.2
pharynx J39.2
  branchial cleft (congenital) Q18.0
pilonidal (infected) (rectum) — *see* Sinus, pilonidal
pleura, pleural, pleurocutaneous,
  pleuroperitoneal J86.0
    tuberculous NEC A15.6
pleuropericardial I31.8
portal vein-hepatic artery, congenital Q26.6
postauricular H70.81-
postoperative, persistent T81.83
  specified site — *see* Fistula, by site
preauricular (congenital) Q18.1
prostate N42.89
pulmonary J86.0
  arteriovenous I28.0
    congenital Q25.72
  tuberculous — *see* Tuberculosis, pulmonary
pulmonoperitoneal J86.0
rectolabial N82.4
rectosigmoid (intercommunicating) K63.2
rectoureteral N28.89
rectourethral N36.0
  congenital Q64.73
rectouterine N82.4
  congenital Q51.7
rectovaginal N82.3
  congenital Q52.2
  tuberculous A18.18
rectovesical N32.1
  congenital Q64.79
rectovesicovaginal N82.3
rectovulval N82.4
  congenital Q52.79
rectum (to skin) K60.4
  congenital Q43.6
    with absence, atresia and stenosis Q42.0
  tuberculous A18.32
renal N28.89
retroauricular — *see* Fistula, postauricular
salivary duct or gland (any) K11.4
  congenital Q38.4
scrotum (urinary) N50.89
  tuberculous A18.15
semicircular canals — *see* subcategory H83.1
sigmoid K63.2
  to bladder N32.1
sinus — *see* Sinusitis
skin L98.8
  to genital tract (female) N82.5
splenocolic D73.89
stercoral K63.2
stomach K31.6
sublingual gland K11.4
submandibular gland K11.4
submaxillary (gland) K11.4
  region K12.2
thoracic J86.0
  duct I89.8
thoracoabdominal J86.0
thoracogastric J86.0
thoracointestinal J86.0
thorax J86.0
thyroglossal duct Q89.2
thyroid E07.89
trachea, congenital (external) (internal) Q32.1
tracheoesophageal J86.0
  congenital Q39.2
    with atresia of esophagus Q39.1
  following tracheostomy J95.04
traumatic arteriovenous — *see* Injury, blood vessel,
  by site
tuberculous - code by site under Tuberculosis
typhoid A01.09
umbilicourinary Q64.8
urachus, congenital Q64.4
ureter (persistent) N28.89
ureteroabdominal N28.89
ureterorectal N28.89
ureterosigmoido-abdominal N28.89
ureterovaginal N82.1
ureterovesical N32.2
urethra N36.0
  congenital Q64.79
  tuberculous A18.13

Fistula (cutaneous) - *continued*
urethroperineal N36.0
urethroperineovesical N32.2
urethrorectal N36.0
  congenital Q64.73
urethroscrotal N50.89
urethrovaginal N82.1
urethrovesical N32.2
urinary (tract) (persistent) (recurrent) N36.0
uteroabdominal N82.5
  congenital Q51.7
uteroenteric, uterointestinal N82.4
  congenital Q51.7
uterorectal N82.4
  congenital Q51.7
uteroureteric N82.1
uterourethral Q51.7
uterovaginal N82.8
uterovesical N82.1
  congenital Q51.7
uterus N82.8
vagina (postpartal) (wall) N82.8
vaginocutaneous (postpartal) N82.5
vaginointestinal NEC N82.4
  large intestine N82.3
  small intestine N82.2
vaginoperineal N82.5
vasocutaneous, congenital Q55.7
vesical NEC N32.2
vesicoabdominal N32.2
vesicocervicovaginal N82.1
vesicocolic N32.1
vesicocutaneous N32.2
vesicoenteric N32.1
vesicointestinal N32.1
vesicometrorectal N82.4
vesicoperineal N32.2
vesicorectal N32.1
  congenital Q64.79
vesicosigmoidal N32.1
vesicosigmoidovaginal N82.3
vesicoureteral N32.2
vesicoureterovaginal N82.1
vesicourethral N32.2
vesicourethrorectal N32.1
vesicouterine N82.1
  congenital Q51.7
vesicovaginal N82.0
vulvorectal N82.4
  congenital Q52.79

Fit R56.9
epileptic — *see* Epilepsy
fainting R55
hysterical F44.5
newborn P90

Fitting (and adjustment) (of)
artificial
  arm — *see* Admission, adjustment, artificial, arm
  breast Z44.3
  eye Z44.2
  leg — *see* Admission, adjustment, artificial, leg
automatic implantable cardiac defibrillator (with
  synchronous cardiac pacemaker) Z45.02
brain neuropacemaker Z46.2
  implanted Z45.42
cardiac defibrillator — *see* Fitting (and adjustment)
  (of), automatic implantable cardiac defibrillator
catheter, non-vascular Z46.82
colostomy belt Z46.89
contact lenses Z46.0
CRT-D (resynchronization therapy
  defibrillator) Z45.02
CRT-P (cardiac resynchronization therapy
  pacemaker) Z45.018
  pulse generator Z45.010
cystostomy device Z46.6
defibrillator, cardiac — *see* Fitting (and adjustment)
  (of), automatic implantable cardiac defibrillator
dentures Z46.3
device NOS Z46.9
  abdominal Z46.89
    gastrointestinal NEC Z46.59
  implanted NEC Z45.89
  nervous system Z46.2
    implanted — *see* Admission, adjustment, device,
    implanted, nervous system
  orthodontic Z46.4
  orthoptic Z46.0
  orthotic Z46.89
  prosthetic (external) Z44.9
    breast Z44.3
    dental Z46.3
    eye Z44.2

Fitting (and adjustment) (of) - *continued*
device NOS - *continued*
  prosthetic (external) - *continued*
    specified NEC Z44.8
  specified NEC Z46.89
  substitution
    auditory Z46.2
      implanted — *see* Admission, adjustment,
      device, implanted, hearing device
    nervous system Z46.2
      implanted — *see* Admission, adjustment,
      device, implanted, nervous system
    visual Z46.2
      implanted Z45.31
  urinary Z46.2
gastric lap band Z46.51
gastrointestinal appliance NEC Z46.59
glasses (reading) Z46.0
hearing aid Z46.1
ileostomy device Z46.89
insulin pump Z46.81
intestinal appliance NEC Z46.89
myringotomy device (stent) (tube) Z45.82
neuropacemaker Z46.2
  implanted Z45.42
non-vascular catheter Z46.82
orthodontic device Z46.4
orthopedic device (brace) (cast) (corset)
  (shoes) Z46.89
pacemaker (cardiac) (cardiac resynchronization
  therapy (CRT-P)) Z45.018
  nervous system (brain) (peripheral nerve) (spinal
    cord) Z46.2
    implanted Z45.42
  pulse generator Z45.010
portacath (port-a-cath) Z45.2
prosthesis (external) Z44.9
  arm — *see* Admission, adjustment, artificial, arm
  breast Z44.3
  dental Z46.3
  eye Z44.2
  leg — *see* Admission, adjustment, artificial, leg
  specified NEC Z44.8
spectacles Z46.0
wheelchair Z46.89

Fitzhugh-Curtis syndrome
due to
  Chlamydia trachomatis A74.81
  Neisseria gonorrhorea (gonococcal
    peritonitis) A54.85

Fitz's syndrome (acute hemorrhagic
pancreatitis) — *see also* Pancreatitis, acute K85.80

Fixation
joint — *see* Ankylosis
larynx J38.7
stapes — *see* Ankylosis, ear ossicles
  deafness — *see* Deafness, conductive
uterus (acquired) — *see* Malposition, uterus
vocal cord J38.3

Flabby ridge K06.8

Flaccid — *see also* condition
palate, congenital Q38.5

Flail
chest S22.5
  newborn (birth injury) P13.8
joint (paralytic) M25.20
  ankle M25.27-
  elbow M25.22-
  foot joint M25.27-
  hand joint M25.24-
  hip M25.25-
  knee M25.26-
  shoulder M25.21-
  specified joint NEC M25.28
  wrist M25.23-

Flajani's disease — *see* Hyperthyroidism, with,
goiter (diffuse)

Flap, liver K71.3

Flashbacks (residual to hallucinogen use) F16.283

Flat
chamber (eye) — *see* Disorder, globe, hypotony, flat
  anterior chamber
chest, congenital Q67.8
foot (acquired) (fixed type) (painful)
  (postural) — *see also* Deformity, limb, flat foot
  congenital (rigid) (spastic (everted)) Q66.5-
  rachitic sequelae (late effect) E64.3
organ or site, congenital NEC — *see* Anomaly, by
  site
pelvis M95.5
  with disproportion (fetopelvic) O33.0
    causing obstructed labor O65.0
  congenital Q74.2

Flatau-Schilder disease G37.0
Flatback syndrome M40.30
  lumbar region M40.36
  lumbosacral region M40.37
  thoracolumbar region M40.35
Flattening
  head, femur M89.8X5
  hip — *see* Coxa, plana
  lip (congenital) Q18.8
  nose (congenital) Q67.4
    acquired M95.0
Flatulence R14.3
  psychogenic F45.8
Flatus R14.3
  vaginalis N89.8
Flax-dresser's disease J66.1
Flea bite — *see* Injury, bite, by site, superficial, insect
Flecks, glaucomatous (subcapsular) — *see* Cataract, complicated
Fleischer (-Kayser) **ring** (cornea) H18.04-
Fleshy mole O02.0
Flexibilitas cerea — *see* Catalepsy
Flexion
  amputation stump (surgical) T87.89
  cervix — *see* Malposition, uterus
  contracture, joint — *see* Contraction, joint
  deformity, joint — *see also* Deformity, limb, flexion M21.20
    hip, congenital Q65.89
  uterus — *see also* Malposition, uterus
    lateral — *see* Lateroversion, uterus
Flexner-Boyd dysentery A03.2
Flexner's dysentery A03.1
Flexure — *see* Flexion
Flint murmur (aortic insufficiency) I35.1
Floater, vitreous — *see* Opacity, vitreous
Floating
  cartilage (joint) — *see also* Loose, body, joint
    knee — *see* Derangement, knee, loose body
  gallbladder, congenital Q44.1
  kidney N28.89
    congenital Q63.8
  spleen D73.89
Flooding N92.0
Floor — *see* condition
Floppy
  baby syndrome (nonspecific) P94.2
  iris syndrome (intraoperative) (IFIS) H21.81
  nonrheumatic mitral valve syndrome I34.1
Flu — *see also* Influenza
  avian — *see also* Influenza, due to, identified novel influenza A virus J09.X2
  bird — *see also* Influenza, due to, identified novel influenza A virus J09.X2
  intestinal NEC A08.4
  swine (viruses that normally cause infections in pigs) — *see also* Influenza, due to, identified novel influenza A virus J09.X2
Fluctuating blood pressure I99.8
Fluid
  abdomen R18.8
  chest J94.8
  heart — *see* Failure, heart, congestive
  joint — *see* Effusion, joint
  loss (acute) E86.9
  lung — *see* Edema, lung
  overload E87.70
    specified NEC E87.79
  peritoneal cavity R18.8
  pleural cavity J94.8
  retention R60.9
Flukes NEC — *see also* Infestation, fluke
  blood NEC — *see* Schistosomiasis
  liver B66.3
Fluor (vaginalis) N89.8
  trichomonal or due to Trichomonas (vaginalis) A59.00
Fluorosis
  dental K00.3
  skeletal M85.10
    ankle M85.17-
    foot M85.17-
    forearm M85.13-
    hand M85.14-
    lower leg M85.16-
    multiple site M85.19
    neck M85.18
    rib M85.18
    shoulder M85.11-
    skull M85.18
    specified site NEC M85.18
    thigh M85.15-
    toe M85.17-

Fluorosis - *continued*
  skeletal - *continued*
    upper arm M85.12-
    vertebra M85.18
Flush syndrome E34.0
Flushing R23.2
  menopausal N95.1
Flutter
  atrial or auricular I48.92
    atypical I48.4
    type I I48.3
    type II I48.4
    typical I48.3
  heart I49.8
    atrial or auricular I48.92
      atypical I48.4
      type I I48.3
      type II I48.4
      typical I48.3
    ventricular I49.02
  ventricular I49.02
FNHTR (febrile nonhemolytic transfusion reaction) R50.84
Fochier's abscess - code by site under Abscess
Focus, Assmann's — *see* Tuberculosis, pulmonary
Fogo selvagem L10.3
Foix-Alajouanine syndrome G95.19
Fold, folds (anomalous) — *see also* Anomaly, by site
  Descemet's membrane — *see* Change, corneal membrane, Descemet's, fold
  epicanthic Q10.3
  heart Q24.8
Folie à deux F24
Follicle
  cervix (nabothian) (ruptured) N88.8
  graafian, ruptured, with hemorrhage N83.0-
  nabothian N88.8
Follicular — *see* condition
Folliculitis (superficial) L73.9
  abscedens et suffodiens L66.3
  cyst N83.0-
  decalvans L66.2
  deep — *see* Furuncle, by site
  gonococcal (acute) (chronic) A54.01
  keloid, keloidalis L73.0
  pustular L01.02
  ulerythematosa reticulata L66.4
Folliculome lipidique
  specified site — *see* Neoplasm, benign, by site
  unspecified site
    female D27.9
    male D29.20
Følling's disease E70.0
Follow-up — *see* Examination, follow-up
Fong's syndrome (hereditary osteo-onychodysplasia) Q87.2
Food
  allergy L27.2
  asphyxia (from aspiration or inhalation) — *see* Foreign body, by site
  choked on — *see* Foreign body, by site
  deprivation T73.0
    specified kind of food NEC E63.8
  intoxication — *see* Poisoning, food
  lack of T73.0
  poisoning — *see* Poisoning, food
  rejection NEC — *see* Disorder, eating
  strangulation or suffocation — *see* Foreign body, by site
  toxemia — *see* Poisoning, food
Foot — *see* condition
Foramen ovale (nonclosure) (patent) (persistent) Q21.1
Forbes' glycogen storage disease E74.03
Fordyce-Fox disease L75.2
Fordyce's disease (mouth) Q38.6
Forearm — *see* condition
Foreign body
  with
    laceration — *see* Laceration, by site, with foreign body
    puncture wound — *see* Puncture, by site, with foreign body
  accidentally left following a procedure T81.509
    aspiration T81.506
      resulting in
        adhesions T81.516
        obstruction T81.526
        perforation T81.536
        specified complication NEC T81.596
    cardiac catheterization T81.505
      resulting in
        acute reaction T81.60

Foreign body - *continued*
  accidentally left following a procedure - *continued*
    cardiac catheterization - *continued*
      resulting in - *continued*
        acute reaction - *continued*
          aseptic peritonitis T81.61
          specified NEC T81.69
        adhesions T81.515
        obstruction T81.525
        perforation T81.535
        specified complication NEC T81.595
    causing
      acute reaction T81.60
        aseptic peritonitis T81.61
        specified complication NEC T81.69
      adhesions T81.519
      aseptic peritonitis T81.61
      obstruction T81.529
      perforation T81.539
      specified complication NEC T81.599
    endoscopy T81.504
      resulting in
        adhesions T81.514
        obstruction T81.524
        perforation T81.534
        specified complication NEC T81.594
    immunization T81.503
      resulting in
        adhesions T81.513
        obstruction T81.523
        perforation T81.533
        specified complication NEC T81.593
    infusion T81.501
      resulting in
        adhesions T81.511
        obstruction T81.521
        perforation T81.531
        specified complication NEC T81.591
    injection T81.503
      resulting in
        adhesions T81.513
        obstruction T81.523
        perforation T81.533
        specified complication NEC T81.593
    kidney dialysis T81.502
      resulting in
        adhesions T81.512
        obstruction T81.522
        perforation T81.532
        specified complication NEC T81.592
    packing removal T81.507
      resulting in
        acute reaction T81.60
          aseptic peritonitis T81.61
          specified NEC T81.69
        adhesions T81.517
        obstruction T81.527
        perforation T81.537
        specified complication NEC T81.597
    puncture T81.506
      resulting in
        adhesions T81.516
        obstruction T81.526
        perforation T81.536
        specified complication NEC T81.596
    specified procedure NEC T81.508
      resulting in
        acute reaction T81.60
          aseptic peritonitis T81.61
          specified NEC T81.69
        adhesions T81.518
        obstruction T81.528
        perforation T81.538
        specified complication NEC T81.598
    surgical operation T81.500
      resulting in
        acute reaction T81.60
          aseptic peritonitis T81.61
          specified NEC T81.69
        adhesions T81.510
        obstruction T81.520
        perforation T81.530
        specified complication NEC T81.590
    transfusion T81.501
      resulting in
        adhesions T81.511
        obstruction T81.521
        perforation T81.531
        specified complication NEC T81.591
  alimentary tract T18.9
  anus T18.5
  colon T18.4
  esophagus — *see* Foreign body, esophagus

Foreign body - *continued*
alimentary tract - *continued*
  mouth T18.0
  multiple sites T18.8
  rectosigmoid (junction) T18.5
  rectum T18.5
  small intestine T18.3
  specified site NEC T18.8
  stomach T18.2
anterior chamber (eye) S05.5-
auditory canal — *see* Foreign body, entering through orifice, ear
bronchus T17.508
  causing
    asphyxiation T17.500
      food (bone) (seed) T17.520
      gastric contents (vomitus) T17.510
      specified type NEC T17.590
    injury NEC T17.508
      food (bone) (seed) T17.528
      gastric contents (vomitus) T17.518
      specified type NEC T17.598
canthus — *see* Foreign body, conjunctival sac
ciliary body (eye) S05.5-
conjunctival sac T15.1-
cornea T15.0-
entering through orifice
  accessory sinus T17.0
  alimentary canal T18.9
    multiple parts T18.8
    specified part NEC T18.8
  alveolar process T18.0
  antrum (Highmore's) T17.0
  anus T18.5
  appendix T18.4
  auditory canal — *see* Foreign body, entering through orifice, ear
  auricle — *see* Foreign body, entering through orifice, ear
  bladder T19.1
  bronchioles — *see* Foreign body, respiratory tract, specified site NEC
  bronchus (main) — *see* Foreign body, bronchus
  buccal cavity T18.0
  canthus (inner) — *see* Foreign body, conjunctival sac
  cecum T18.4
  cervix (canal) (uteri) T19.3
  colon T18.4
  conjunctival sac — *see* Foreign body, conjunctival sac
  cornea — *see* Foreign body, cornea
  digestive organ or tract NOS T18.9
    multiple parts T18.8
    specified part NEC T18.8
  duodenum T18.3
  ear (external) T16.-
  esophagus — *see* Foreign body, esophagus
  eye (external) NOS T15.9-
    conjunctival sac — *see* Foreign body, conjunctival sac
    cornea — *see* Foreign body, cornea
    specified part NEC T15.8-
  eyeball — *see also* Foreign body, entering through orifice, eye, specified part NEC
    with penetrating wound — *see* Puncture, eyeball
  eyelid — *see also* Foreign body, conjunctival sac
    with
      laceration — *see* Laceration, eyelid, with foreign body
      puncture — *see* Puncture, eyelid, with foreign body
      superficial injury — *see* Foreign body, superficial, eyelid
  gastrointestinal tract T18.9
    multiple parts T18.8
    specified part NEC T18.8
  genitourinary tract T19.9
    multiple parts T19.8
    specified part NEC T19.8
  globe — *see* Foreign body, entering through orifice, eyeball
  gum T18.0
  Highmore's antrum T17.0
  hypopharynx — *see* Foreign body, pharynx
  ileum T18.3
  intestine (small) T18.3
    large T18.4
  lacrimal apparatus (punctum) — *see* Foreign body, entering through orifice, eye, specified part NEC
  large intestine T18.4
  larynx — *see* Foreign body, larynx

Foreign body - *continued*
entering through orifice - *continued*
  lung — *see* Foreign body, respiratory tract, specified site NEC
  maxillary sinus T17.0
  mouth T18.0
  nasal sinus T17.0
  nasopharynx — *see* Foreign body, pharynx
  nose (passage) T17.1
  nostril T17.1
  oral cavity T18.0
  palate T18.0
  penis T19.4
  pharynx — *see* Foreign body, pharynx
  piriform sinus — *see* Foreign body, pharynx
  rectosigmoid (junction) T18.5
  rectum T18.5
  respiratory tract — *see* Foreign body, respiratory tract
  sinus (accessory) (frontal) (maxillary) (nasal) T17.0
    piriform — *see* Foreign body, pharynx
  small intestine T18.3
  stomach T18.2
  suffocation by — *see* Foreign body, by site
  tear ducts or glands — *see* Foreign body, entering through orifice, eye, specified part NEC
  throat — *see* Foreign body, pharynx
  tongue T18.0
  tonsil, tonsillar (fossa) — *see* Foreign body, pharynx
  trachea — *see* Foreign body, trachea
  ureter T19.8
  urethra T19.0
  uterus (any part) T19.3
  vagina T19.2
  vulva T19.2
esophagus T18.108
  causing
    injury NEC T18.108
      food (bone) (seed) T18.128
      gastric contents (vomitus) T18.118
      specified type NEC T18.198
    tracheal compression T18.100
      food (bone) (seed) T18.120
      gastric contents (vomitus) T18.110
      specified type NEC T18.190
felling of, in throat R09.89
fragment — *see* Retained, foreign body fragments (type of)
genitourinary tract T19.9
  bladder T19.1
  multiple parts T19.8
  penis T19.4
  specified site NEC T19.8
  urethra T19.0
  uterus T19.3
    IUD Z97.5
  vagina T19.2
    contraceptive device Z97.5
  vulva T19.2
granuloma (old) (soft tissue) — *see also* Granuloma, foreign body
  skin L92.3
in
  laceration — *see* Laceration, by site, with foreign body
  puncture wound — *see* Puncture, by site, with foreign body
  soft tissue (residual) M79.5
inadvertently left in operation wound — *see* Foreign body, accidentally left during a procedure
ingestion, ingested NOS T18.9
inhalation or inspiration — *see* Foreign body, by site
internal organ, not entering through a natural orifice - code as specific injury with foreign body
intraocular S05.5-
  old, retained (nonmagnetic) H44.70-
    anterior chamber H44.71-
    ciliary body H44.72-
    iris H44.72-
    lens H44.73-
    magnetic H44.60-
      anterior chamber H44.61-
      ciliary body H44.62-
      iris H44.62-
      lens H44.63-
      posterior wall H44.64-
      specified site NEC H44.69-
      vitreous body H44.65-
    posterior wall H44.74-
    specified site NEC H44.79-
    vitreous body H44.75-

Foreign body - *continued*
iris — *see* Foreign body, intraocular
lacrimal punctum — *see* Foreign body, entering through orifice, eye, specified part NEC
larynx T17.308
  causing
    asphyxiation T17.300
      food (bone) (seed) T17.320
      gastric contents (vomitus) T17.310
      specified type NEC T17.390
    injury NEC T17.308
      food (bone) (seed) T17.328
      gastric contents (vomitus) T17.318
      specified type NEC T17.398
lens — *see* Foreign body, intraocular
ocular muscle S05.4-
  old, retained — *see* Foreign body, orbit, old
old or residual
  soft tissue (residual) M79.5
operation wound, left accidentally — *see* Foreign body, accidentally left during a procedure
orbit S05.4-
  old, retained H05.5-
pharynx T17.208
  causing
    asphyxiation T17.200
      food (bone) (seed) T17.220
      gastric contents (vomitus) T17.210
      specified type NEC T17.290
    injury NEC T17.208
      food (bone) (seed) T17.228
      gastric contents (vomitus) T17.218
      specified type NEC T17.298
respiratory tract T17.908
  bronchioles — *see* Foreign body, respiratory tract, specified site NEC
  bronchus — *see* Foreign body, bronchus
  causing
    asphyxiation T17.900
      food (bone) (seed) T17.920
      gastric contents (vomitus) T17.910
      specified type NEC T17.990
    injury NEC T17.908
      food (bone) (seed) T17.928
      gastric contents (vomitus) T17.918
      specified type NEC T17.998
  larynx — *see* Foreign body, larynx
  lung — *see* Foreign body, respiratory tract, specified site NEC
  multiple parts — *see* Foreign body, respiratory tract, specified site NEC
  nasal sinus T17.0
  nasopharynx — *see* Foreign body, pharynx
  nose T17.1
  nostril T17.1
  pharynx — *see* Foreign body, pharynx
  specified site NEC T17.808
    causing
      asphyxiation T17.800
        food (bone) (seed) T17.820
        gastric contents (vomitus) T17.810
        specified type NEC T17.890
      injury NEC T17.808
        food (bone) (seed) T17.828
        gastric contents (vomitus) T17.818
        specified type NEC T17.898
  throat — *see* Foreign body, pharynx
  trachea — *see* Foreign body, trachea
retained (old) (nonmagnetic) (in)
  anterior chamber (eye) — *see* Foreign body, intraocular, old, retained, anterior chamber
    magnetic — *see* Foreign body, intraocular, old, retained, magnetic, anterior chamber
  ciliary body — *see* Foreign body, intraocular, old, retained, ciliary body
    magnetic — *see* Foreign body, intraocular, old, retained, magnetic, ciliary body
  eyelid H02.819
    left H02.816
      lower H02.815
      upper H02.814
    right H02.813
      lower H02.812
      upper H02.811
  fragments — *see* Retained, foreign body fragments (type of)
  globe — *see* Foreign body, intraocular, old, retained
    magnetic — *see* Foreign body, intraocular, old, retained, magnetic
  intraocular — *see* Foreign body, intraocular, old, retained

Foreign body - *continued*
  retained (old) (nonmagnetic) (in) - *continued*
    intraocular - *continued*
      magnetic — *see* Foreign body, intraocular, old, retained, magnetic
      iris — *see* Foreign body, intraocular, old, retained, iris
        magnetic — *see* Foreign body, intraocular, old, retained, magnetic, iris
      lens — *see* Foreign body, intraocular, old, retained, lens
        magnetic — *see* Foreign body, intraocular, old, retained, magnetic, lens
      muscle — *see* Foreign body, retained, soft tissue
      orbit — *see* Foreign body, orbit, old
      posterior wall of globe — *see* Foreign body, intraocular, old, retained, posterior wall
        magnetic — *see* Foreign body, intraocular, old, retained, magnetic, posterior wall
      retrobulbar — *see* Foreign body, orbit, old, retrobulbar
      soft tissue M79.5
      vitreous — *see* Foreign body, intraocular, old, retained, vitreous body
        magnetic — *see* Foreign body, intraocular, old, retained, magnetic, vitreous body
    retina S05.5-
  superficial, without open wound
    abdomen, abdominal (wall) S30.851
    alveolar process S00.552
    ankle S90.55-
    antecubital space — *see* Foreign body, superficial, forearm
    anus S30.857
    arm (upper) S40.85-
    auditory canal — *see* Foreign body, superficial, ear
    auricle — *see* Foreign body, superficial, ear
    axilla — *see* Foreign body, superficial, arm
    back, lower S30.850
    breast S20.15-
    brow S00.85
    buttock S30.850
    calf — *see* Foreign body, superficial, leg
    canthus — *see* Foreign body, superficial, eyelid
    cheek S00.85
      internal S00.552
    chest wall — *see* Foreign body, superficial, thorax
    chin S00.85
    clitoris S30.854
    costal region — *see* Foreign body, superficial, thorax
    digit (s)
      hand — *see* Foreign body, superficial, finger
      foot — *see* Foreign body, superficial, toe
    ear S00.45-
    elbow S50.35-
    epididymis S30.853
    epigastric region S30.851
    epiglottis S10.15
    esophagus, cervical S10.15
    eyebrow — *see* Foreign body, superficial, eyelid
    eyelid S00.25-
    face S00.85
    finger (s) S60.459
      index S60.45-
      little S60.45-
      middle S60.45-
      ring S60.45-
    flank S30.851
    foot (except toe (s) alone) S90.85-
      toe — *see* Foreign body, superficial, toe
    forearm S50.85-
      elbow only — *see* Foreign body, superficial, elbow
    forehead S00.85
    genital organs, external
      female S30.856
      male S30.855
    groin S30.851
    gum S00.552
    hand S60.55-
    head S00.95
      ear — *see* Foreign body, superficial, ear
      eyelid — *see* Foreign body, superficial, eyelid
      lip S00.551
      nose S00.35
      oral cavity S00.552
      scalp S00.05
      specified site NEC S00.85
    heel — *see* Foreign body, superficial, foot
    hip S70.25-
    inguinal region S30.851
    interscapular region S20.459

Foreign body - *continued*
  superficial, without open wound - *continued*
    jaw S00.85
    knee S80.25-
    labium (majus) (minus) S30.854
    larynx S10.15
    leg (lower) S80.85-
      knee — *see* Foreign body, superficial, knee
      upper — *see* Foreign body, superficial, thigh
    lip S00.551
    lower back S30.850
    lumbar region S30.850
    malar region S00.85
    mammary — *see* Foreign body, superficial, breast
    mastoid region S00.85
    mouth S00.552
    nail
      finger — *see* Foreign body, superficial, finger
      toe — *see* Foreign body, superficial, toe
    nape S10.85
    nasal S00.35
    neck S10.95
      specified site NEC S10.85
      throat S10.15
    nose S00.35
    occipital region S00.05
    oral cavity S00.552
    orbital region — *see* Foreign body, superficial, eyelid
    palate S00.552
    palm — *see* Foreign body, superficial, hand
    parietal region S00.05
    pelvis S30.850
    penis S30.852
    perineum
      female S30.854
      male S30.850
    periocular area — *see* Foreign body, superficial, eyelid
    phalanges
      finger — *see* Foreign body, superficial, finger
      toe — *see* Foreign body, superficial, toe
    pharynx S10.15
    pinna — *see* Foreign body, superficial, ear
    popliteal space — *see* Foreign body, superficial, knee
    prepuce S30.852
    pubic region S30.850
    pudendum
      female S30.856
      male S30.855
    sacral region S30.850
    scalp S00.05
    scapular region — *see* Foreign body, superficial, shoulder
    scrotum S30.853
    shin — *see* Foreign body, superficial, leg
    shoulder S40.25-
    sternal region S20.359
    submaxillary region S00.85
    submental region S00.85
    subungual
      finger (s) — *see* Foreign body, superficial, finger
      toe (s) — *see* Foreign body, superficial, toe
    supraclavicular fossa S10.85
    supraorbital S00.85
    temple S00.85
    temporal region S00.85
    testis S30.853
    thigh S70.35-
    thorax, thoracic (wall) S20.95
      back S20.45-
      front S20.35-
    throat S10.15
    thumb S60.35-
    toe (s) (lesser) S90.456
      great S90.45-
    tongue S00.552
    trachea S10.15
    tunica vaginalis S30.853
    tympanum, tympanic membrane — *see* Foreign body, superficial, ear
    uvula S00.552
    vagina S30.854
    vocal cords S10.15
    vulva S30.854
    wrist S60.85-
  swallowed T18.9
  trachea T17.408
    causing
      asphyxiation T17.400
        food (bone) (seed) T17.420
        gastric contents (vomitus) T17.410

Foreign body - *continued*
  trachea - *continued*
    causing - *continued*
      asphyxiation - *continued*
        specified type NEC T17.490
      injury NEC T17.408
        food (bone) (seed) T17.428
        gastric contents (vomitus) T17.418
        specified type NEC T17.498
    type of fragment — *see* Retained, foreign body fragments (type of)
    vitreous (humor) S05.5-
Forestier's disease (rhizomelic pseudopolyarthritis) M35.3
  meaning ankylosing hyperostosis — *see* Hyperostosis, ankylosing
Formation
  hyalin in cornea — *see* Degeneration, cornea
  sequestrum in bone (due to infection) — *see* Osteomyelitis, chronic
  valve
    colon, congenital Q43.8
    ureter (congenital) Q62.39
Formication R20.2
Fort Bragg fever A27.89
Fossa — *see also* condition
  pyriform — *see* condition
Foster-Kennedy syndrome H47.14-
Fothergill's
  disease (trigeminal neuralgia) — *see also* Neuralgia, trigeminal
  scarlatina anginosa A38.9
Foul breath R19.6
Foundling Z76.1
Fournier disease or gangrene N49.3
  female N76.89
Fourth
  cranial nerve — *see* condition
  molar K00.1
Foville's (peduncular) **disease or syndrome** G46.3
Fox (-Fordyce) **disease** (apocrine miliaria) L75.2
Fracture, burst — *see* Fracture, traumatic, by site
Fracture, chronic — *see* Fracture, pathological
Fracture, insufficiency — *see* Fracture, pathologic, by site
Fracture, nontraumatic, NEC
  atypical
    femur M84.750-
      complete
        oblique M84.759
          left side M84.758
          right side M84.757
        transverse M84.756
          left side M84.755
          right side M84.754
      incomplete M84.753
        left side M84.752
        right side M84.751
Fracture, pathological (pathologic) — *see also* Fracture, traumatic M84.40
  ankle M84.47-
  carpus M84.44-
  clavicle M84.41-
  compression (not due to trauma) — *see also* Collapse, vertebra M48.50-
  dental implant M27.63
  dental restorative material K08.539
    with loss of material K08.531
    without loss of material K08.530
  due to
    neoplastic disease NEC — *see also* Neoplasm M84.50
      ankle M84.57-
      carpus M84.54-
      clavicle M84.51-
      femur M84.55-
      fibula M84.56-
      finger M84.54-
      hip M84.559
      humerus M84.52-
      ilium M84.550
      ischium M84.550
      metacarpus M84.54-
      metatarsus M84.57-
      neck M84.58
      pelvis M84.550
      radius M84.53-
      rib M84.58
      scapula M84.51-
      skull M84.58
      specified site NEC M84.58
      tarsus M84.57-
      tibia M84.56-

Fracture, pathological (pathologic) - *continued*
due to - *continued*
neoplastic disease NEC - *continued*
toe M84.57-
ulna M84.53-
vertebra M84.58
osteoporosis M80.00
disuse — *see* Osteoporosis, specified type NEC, with pathological fracture
drug-induced — *see* Osteoporosis, drug induced, with pathological fracture
idiopathic — *see* Osteoporosis, specified type NEC, with pathological fracture
postmenopausal — *see* Osteoporosis, postmenopausal, with pathological fracture
postoophorectomy — *see* Osteoporosis, postoophorectomy, with pathological fracture
postsurgical malabsorption — *see* Osteoporosis, specified type NEC, with pathological fracture
specified cause NEC — *see* Osteoporosis, specified type NEC, with pathological fracture
specified disease NEC M84.60
ankle M84.67-
carpus M84.64-
clavicle M84.61-
femur M84.65-
fibula M84.66-
finger M84.64-
hip M84.65-
humerus M84.62-
ilium M84.650
ischium M84.650
metacarpus M84.64-
metatarsus M84.67-
neck M84.68
radius M84.63-
rib M84.68
scapula M84.61-
skull M84.68
tarsus M84.67-
tibia M84.66-
toe M84.67-
ulna M84.63-
vertebra M84.68
femur M84.45-
fibula M84.46-
finger M84.44-
hip M84.459
humerus M84.42-
ilium M84.454
ischium M84.454
joint prosthesis — *see* Complications, joint prosthesis, mechanical, breakdown, by site
periprosthetic — *see* Fracture, pathological, periprosthetic
metacarpus M84.44-
metatarsus M84.47-
neck M84.48
pelvis M84.454
periprosthetic M97.9
ankle M97.2-
elbow M97.4-
finger M97.8
hip M97.0-
knee M97.1-
other specified joint M97.8
shoulder M97.3-
spinal joint M97.8
toe joint M97.8
wrist joint M97.8
radius M84.43-
restorative material (dental) K08.539
with loss of material K08.531
without loss of material K08.530
rib M84.48
scapula M84.41-
skull M84.48
tarsus M84.47-
tibia M84.46-
toe M84.47-
ulna M84.43-
vertebra M84.48

Fracture, traumatic (abduction) (adduction) (separation) — *see also* Fracture, pathological T14.8
acetabulum S32.40-
column
anterior (displaced) (iliopubic) S32.43-
nondisplaced S32.436
posterior (displaced) (ilioischial) S32.443
nondisplaced S32.44-
dome (displaced) S32.48-
nondisplaced S32.48
specified NEC S32.49-

Fracture, traumatic (abduction) (adduction) (separation) - *continued*
acetabulum - *continued*
transverse (displaced) S32.45-
with associated posterior wall fracture (displaced) S32.46-
nondisplaced S32.46-
nondisplaced S32.45-
wall
anterior (displaced) S32.41-
nondisplaced S32.41-
medial (displaced) S32.47-
nondisplaced S32.47-
posterior (displaced) S32.42-
with associated transverse fracture (displaced) S32.46-
nondisplaced S32.46-
nondisplaced S32.42-
acromion — *see* Fracture, scapula, acromial process
ankle S82.899
bimalleolar (displaced) S82.84-
nondisplaced S82.84-
lateral malleolus only (displaced) S82.6-
nondisplaced S82.6-
medial malleolus (displaced) S82.5-
associated with Maisonneuve's fracture — *see* Fracture, Maisonneuve's
nondisplaced S82.5-
talus — *see* Fracture, tarsal, talus
trimalleolar (displaced) S82.85-
nondisplaced S82.85-
arm (upper) — *see also* Fracture, humerus, shaft
humerus — *see* Fracture, humerus
radius — *see* Fracture, radius
ulna — *see* Fracture, ulna
astragalus — *see* Fracture, tarsal, talus
atlas — *see* Fracture, neck, cervical vertebra, first
axis — *see* Fracture, neck, cervical vertebra, second
back — *see* Fracture, vertebra
Barton's — *see* Barton's fracture
base of skull — *see* Fracture, skull, base
basicervical (basal) (femoral) S72.0
Bennett's — *see* Bennett's fracture
bimalleolar — *see* Fracture, ankle, bimalleolar
blow-out S02.3-
bone NEC T14.8
birth injury P13.9
following insertion of orthopedic implant, joint prosthesis or bone plate — *see* Fracture, following insertion of orthopedic implant, joint prosthesis or bone plate
in (due to) neoplastic disease NEC — *see* Fracture, pathological, due to, neoplastic disease
pathological (cause unknown) — *see* Fracture, pathological
breast bone — *see* Fracture, sternum
bucket handle (semilunar cartilage) — *see* Tear, meniscus
burst — *see* Fracture, traumatic, by site
calcaneus — *see* Fracture, tarsal, calcaneus
carpal bone (s) S62.10-
capitate (displaced) S62.13-
nondisplaced S62.13-
cuneiform — *see* Fracture, carpal bone, triquetrum
hamate (body) (displaced) S62.143
hook process (displaced) S62.15-
nondisplaced S62.15-
nondisplaced S62.14-
larger multangular — *see* Fracture, carpal bones, trapezium
lunate (displaced) S62.12-
nondisplaced S62.12-
navicular S62.00-
distal pole (displaced) S62.01-
nondisplaced S62.01-
middle third (displaced) S62.02-
nondisplaced S62.02-
proximal third (displaced) S62.03-
nondisplaced S62.03-
volar tuberosity — *see* Fracture, carpal bones, navicular, distal pole
os magnum — *see* Fracture, carpal bones, capitate
pisiform (displaced) S62.16-
nondisplaced S62.16-
semilunar — *see* Fracture, carpal bones, lunate
smaller multangular — *see* Fracture, carpal bones, trapezoid
trapezium (displaced) S62.17-
nondisplaced S62.17-
trapezoid (displaced) S62.18-
nondisplaced S62.18-
triquetrum (displaced) S62.11-
nondisplaced S62.11-

Fracture, traumatic (abduction) (adduction) (separation) - *continued*
carpal bone (s) - *continued*
unciform — *see* Fracture, carpal bones, hamate
cervical — *see* Fracture, vertebra, cervical
clavicle S42.00-
acromial end (displaced) S42.03-
nondisplaced S42.03-
birth injury P13.4
lateral end — *see* Fracture, clavicle, acromial end
shaft (displaced) S42.02-
nondisplaced S42.02-
sternal end (anterior) (displaced) S42.01-
nondisplaced S42.01-
posterior S42.01-
coccyx S32.2
collapsed — *see* Collapse, vertebra
collar bone — *see* Fracture, clavicle
Colles' — *see* Colles' fracture
coronoid process — *see* Fracture, ulna, upper end, coronoid process
corpus cavernosum penis S39.840
costochondral cartilage S23.41
costochondral, costosternal junction — *see* Fracture, rib
cranium — *see* Fracture, skull
cricoid cartilage S12.8
cuboid (ankle) — *see* Fracture, tarsal, cuboid
cuneiform
foot — *see* Fracture, tarsal, cuneiform
wrist — *see* Fracture, carpal, triquetrum
delayed union — *see* Delay, union, fracture
dental restorative material K08.539
with loss of material K08.531
without loss of material K08.530
due to
birth injury — *see* Birth, injury, fracture
osteoporosis — *see* Osteoporosis, with fracture
Dupuytren's — *see* Fracture, ankle, lateral malleolus
elbow S42.40-
ethmoid (bone) (sinus) — *see* Fracture, skull, base
face bone S02.92
fatigue — *see also* Fracture, stress
vertebra M48.40
cervical region M48.42
cervicothoracic region M48.43
lumbar region M48.46
lumbosacral region M48.47
occipito-atlanto-axial region M48.41
sacrococcygeal region M48.48
thoracic region M48.44
thoracolumbar region M48.45
femur, femoral S72.9-
basicervical (basal) S72.0
birth injury P13.2
capital epiphyseal S79.01-
condyles, epicondyles — *see* Fracture, femur, lower end
distal end — *see* Fracture, femur, lower end
epiphysis
head — *see* Fracture, femur, upper end, epiphysis
lower — *see* Fracture, femur, lower end, epiphysis
upper — *see* Fracture, femur, upper end, epiphysis
following insertion of implant, prosthesis or plate M96.66-
head — *see* Fracture, femur, upper end, head
intertrochanteric — *see* Fracture, femur, trochanteric
intratrochanteric — *see* Fracture, femur, trochanteric
lower end S72.40-
condyle (displaced) S72.41-
lateral (displaced) S72.42-
nondisplaced S72.42-
medial (displaced) S72.43-
nondisplaced S72.43-
nondisplaced S72.41-
epiphysis (displaced) S72.44-
nondisplaced S72.44-
physeal S79.10-
Salter-Harris
Type I S79.11-
Type II S79.12-
Type III S79.13-
Type IV S79.14-
specified NEC S79.19-
specified NEC S72.49-
supracondylar (displaced) S72.45-
with intracondylar extension (displaced) S72.46-
nondisplaced S72.46-

Fracture, traumatic (abduction) (adduction) (separation) - *continued*
  femur, femoral - *continued*
    lower end - *continued*
      supracondylar (displaced) - *continued*
        nondisplaced S72.45-
        torus S72.47-
      neck — *see* Fracture, femur, upper end, neck
      pertrochanteric — *see* Fracture, femur, trochanteric
    shaft (lower third) (middle third) (upper third) S72.30-
      comminuted (displaced) S72.35-
        nondisplaced S72.35-
      oblique (displaced) S72.33-
        nondisplaced S72.33-
      segmental (displaced) S72.36-
        nondisplaced S72.36-
      specified NEC S72.39-
      spiral (displaced) S72.34-
        nondisplaced S72.34-
      transverse (displaced) S72.32-
        nondisplaced S72.32-
    specified site NEC — *see* subcategory S72.8
    subcapital (displaced) S72.01-
    subtrochanteric (region) (section) (displaced) S72.2-
      nondisplaced S72.2-
    transcervical — *see* Fracture, femur, upper end, neck
    transtrochanteric — *see* Fracture, femur, trochanteric
    trochanteric S72.10-
      apophyseal (displaced) S72.13-
        nondisplaced S72.13-
      greater trochanter (displaced) S72.11-
        nondisplaced S72.11-
      intertrochanteric (displaced) S72.14-
        nondisplaced S72.14-
      lesser trochanter (displaced) S72.12-
        nondisplaced S72.12-
    upper end S72.00-
      apophyseal (displaced) S72.13-
        nondisplaced S72.13-
      cervicotrochanteric — *see* Fracture, femur, upper end, neck, base
      epiphysis (displaced) S72.02-
        nondisplaced S72.02-
      head S72.05-
        articular (displaced) S72.06-
          nondisplaced S72.06-
        specified NEC S72.09-
      intertrochanteric (displaced) S72.14-
        nondisplaced S72.14-
      intracapsular S72.01-
      midcervical (displaced) S72.03-
        nondisplaced S72.03-
      neck S72.00-
        base (displaced) S72.04-
          nondisplaced S72.04-
        specified NEC S72.09-
      pertrochanteric — *see* Fracture, femur, upper end, trochanteric
      physeal S79.00-
        Salter-Harris type I S79.01-
        specified NEC S79.09-
      subcapital (displaced) S72.01-
      subtrochanteric (displaced) S72.2-
        nondisplaced S72.2-
      transcervical — *see* Fracture, femur, upper end, midcervical
      trochanteric S72.10-
        greater (displaced) S72.11-
          nondisplaced S72.11-
        lesser (displaced) S72.12-
          nondisplaced S72.12-
  fibula (shaft) (styloid) S82.40-
    comminuted (displaced) S82.45-
      nondisplaced S82.45-
    following insertion of implant, prosthesis or plate M96.67-
    involving ankle or malleolus — *see* Fracture, fibula, lateral malleolus
    lateral malleolus (displaced) S82.6-
      nondisplaced S82.6-
    lower end
      physeal S89.30-
        Salter-Harris
          Type I S89.31-
          Type II S89.32-
        specified NEC S89.39-
      specified NEC S82.83-
      torus S82.82-
    oblique (displaced) S82.43-

Fracture, traumatic (abduction) (adduction) (separation) - *continued*
  fibula (shaft) (styloid) - *continued*
    oblique (displaced) - *continued*
      nondisplaced S82.43-
    segmental (displaced) S82.46-
      nondisplaced S82.46-
    specified NEC S82.49-
    spiral (displaced) S82.44-
      nondisplaced S82.44-
    transverse (displaced) S82.42-
      nondisplaced S82.42-
    upper end
      physeal S89.20-
        Salter-Harris
          Type I S89.21-
          Type II S89.22-
        specified NEC S89.29-
      specified NEC S82.83-
      torus S82.81-
  finger (except thumb) S62.60-
    distal phalanx (displaced) S62.63-
      nondisplaced S62.66-
    index S62.60-
      distal phalanx (displaced) S62.63-
        nondisplaced S62.66-
      medial phalanx (displaced) S62.62-
        nondisplaced S62.65-
      proximal phalanx (displaced) S62.61-
        nondisplaced S62.64-
    little S62.60-
      distal phalanx (displaced) S62.63-
        nondisplaced S62.66-
      medial phalanx (displaced) S62.62-
        nondisplaced S62.65-
      proximal phalanx (displaced) S62.61-
        nondisplaced S62.64-
    medial phalanx (displaced) S62.62-
      nondisplaced S62.65-
    middle S62.60-
      distal phalanx (displaced) S62.63-
        nondisplaced S62.66-
      medial phalanx (displaced) S62.62-
        nondisplaced S62.65-
      proximal phalanx (displaced) S62.61-
        nondisplaced S62.64-
    proximal phalanx (displaced) S62.61-
      nondisplaced S62.64-
    ring S62.60-
      distal phalanx (displaced) S62.63-
        nondisplaced S62.66-
      medial phalanx (displaced) S62.62-
        nondisplaced S62.65-
      proximal phalanx (displaced) S62.61-
        nondisplaced S62.64-
    thumb — *see* Fracture, thumb
  following insertion (intraoperative) (postoperative) of orthopedic implant, joint prosthesis or bone plate M96.69
    femur M96.66-
    fibula M96.67-
    humerus M96.62-
    pelvis M96.65
    radius M96.63-
    specified bone NEC M96.69
    tibia M96.67-
    ulna M96.63-
  foot S92.90-
    astragalus — *see* Fracture, tarsal, talus
    calcaneus — *see* Fracture, tarsal, calcaneus
    cuboid — *see* Fracture, tarsal, cuboid
    cuneiform — *see* Fracture, tarsal, cuneiform
    metatarsal — *see* Fracture, metatarsal
    navicular — *see* Fracture, tarsal, navicular
    sesamoid S92.81-
    specified NEC S92.81-
    talus — *see* Fracture, tarsal, talus
    tarsal — *see* Fracture, tarsal
    toe — *see* Fracture, toe
  forearm S52.9-
    radius — *see* Fracture, radius
    ulna — *see* Fracture, ulna
  fossa (anterior) (middle) (posterior) S02.19
  frontal (bone) (skull) S02.0
    sinus S02.19
  glenoid (cavity) (scapula) — *see* Fracture, scapula, glenoid cavity
  greenstick — *see* Fracture, by site
  hallux — *see* Fracture, toe, great
  hand S62.9-
    carpal — *see* Fracture, carpal bone
    finger (except thumb) — *see* Fracture, finger
    metacarpal — *see* Fracture, metacarpal

Fracture, traumatic (abduction) (adduction) (separation) - *continued*
  hand - *continued*
    navicular (scaphoid) (hand) — *see* Fracture, carpal bone, navicular
    thumb — *see* Fracture, thumb
  healed or old
    with complications - code by Nature of the complication
  heel bone — *see* Fracture, tarsal, calcaneus
  Hill-Sachs S42.29-
  hip — *see* Fracture, femur, neck
  humerus S42.30-
    anatomical neck — *see* Fracture, humerus, upper end
    articular process — *see* Fracture, humerus, lower end
    capitellum — *see* Fracture, humerus, lower end, condyle, lateral
    distal end — *see* Fracture, humerus, lower end
    epiphysis
      lower — *see* Fracture, humerus, lower end, physeal
      upper — *see* Fracture, humerus, upper end, physeal
    external condyle — *see* Fracture, humerus, lower end, condyle, lateral
    following insertion of implant, prosthesis or plate M96.62-
    great tuberosity — *see* Fracture, humerus, upper end, greater tuberosity
    intercondylar — *see* Fracture, humerus, lower end
    internal epicondyle — *see* Fracture, humerus, lower end, epicondyle, medial
    lesser tuberosity — *see* Fracture, humerus, upper end, lesser tuberosity
    lower end S42.40-
      condyle
        lateral (displaced) S42.45-
          nondisplaced S42.45-
        medial (displaced) S42.46-
          nondisplaced S42.46-
      epicondyle
        lateral (displaced) S42.43-
          nondisplaced S42.43-
        medial (displaced) S42.44-
          incarcerated S42.44-
          nondisplaced S42.44-
      physeal S49.10-
        Salter-Harris
          Type I S49.11-
          Type II S49.12-
          Type III S49.13-
          Type IV S49.14-
        specified NEC S49.19-
      specified NEC (displaced) S42.49-
        nondisplaced S42.49-
      supracondylar (simple) (displaced) S42.41-
        with intercondylar fracture — *see* Fracture, humerus, lower end
        comminuted (displaced) S42.42-
          nondisplaced S42.42-
          nondisplaced S42.41-
        torus S42.48-
      transcondylar (displaced) S42.47-
        nondisplaced S42.47-
    proximal end — *see* Fracture, humerus, upper end
    shaft S42.30-
      comminuted (displaced) S42.35-
        nondisplaced S42.35-
      greenstick S42.31-
      oblique (displaced) S42.33-
        nondisplaced S42.33-
      segmental (displaced) S42.36-
        nondisplaced S42.36-
      specified NEC S42.39-
      spiral (displaced) S42.34-
        nondisplaced S42.34-
      transverse (displaced) S42.32-
        nondisplaced S42.32-
    supracondylar — *see* Fracture, humerus, lower end
    surgical neck — *see* Fracture, humerus, upper end, surgical neck
    trochlea — *see* Fracture, humerus, lower end, condyle, medial
    tuberosity — *see* Fracture, humerus, upper end
    upper end S42.20-
      anatomical neck — *see* Fracture, humerus, upper end, specified NEC
      articular head — *see* Fracture, humerus, upper end, specified NEC
      epiphysis — *see* Fracture, humerus, upper end, physeal

Fracture, traumatic (abduction) (adduction) (separation) - *continued*
  humerus - *continued*
    upper end - *continued*
      greater tuberosity (displaced) S42.25-
        nondisplaced S42.25-
      lesser tuberosity (displaced) S42.26-
        nondisplaced S42.26-
      physeal S49.00-
        Salter-Harris
          Type I S49.01-
          Type II S49.02-
          Type III S49.03-
          Type IV S49.04-
          specified NEC S49.09-
      specified NEC (displaced) S42.29-
        nondisplaced S42.29-
      surgical neck (displaced) S42.21-
        four-part S42.24-
        nondisplaced S42.21-
        three-part S42.23-
        two-part (displaced) S42.22-
          nondisplaced S42.22-
      torus S42.27-
      transepiphyseal — *see* Fracture, humerus, upper end, physeal
  hyoid bone S12.8
  ilium S32.30-
    with disruption of pelvic ring — *see* Disruption, pelvic ring
    avulsion (displaced) S32.31-
      nondisplaced S32.31-
    specified NEC S32.39-
  impaction, impacted - code as Fracture, by site
  innominate bone — *see* Fracture, ilium
  instep — *see* Fracture, foot
  ischium S32.60-
    with disruption of pelvic ring — *see* Disruption, pelvic ring
    avulsion (displaced) S32.61-
      nondisplaced S32.61-
    specified NEC S32.69-
  jaw (bone) (lower) — *see* Fracture, mandible
    upper — *see* Fracture, maxilla
  joint prosthesis — *see* Complications, joint prosthesis, mechanical, breakdown, by site
    periprosthetic — *see* Fracture, traumatic, periprosthetic
  knee cap — *see* Fracture, patella
  larynx S12.8
  late effects — *see* Sequelae, fracture
  leg (lower) S82.9-
    ankle — *see* Fracture, ankle
    femur — *see* Fracture, femur
    fibula — *see* Fracture, fibula
    malleolus — *see* Fracture, ankle
    patella — *see* Fracture, patella
    specified site NEC S82.89-
    tibia — *see* Fracture, tibia
  lumbar spine — *see* Fracture, vertebra, lumbar
  lumbosacral spine S32.9
  Maisonneuve's (displaced) S82.86-
    nondisplaced S82.86-
  malar bone — *see also* Fracture, maxilla S02.400
    left side S02.40B
    right side S02.40A
  malleolus — *see* Fracture, ankle
  malunion — *see* Fracture, by site
  mandible (lower jaw (bone)) S02.609
    alveolus S02.67-
    angle (of jaw) S02.65-
    body, unspecified S02.600
      left side S02.602
      right side S02.601
    condylar process S02.61-
    coronoid process S02.63-
    ramus, unspecified S02.64-
    specified site NEC S02.69
    subcondylar process S02.62-
    symphysis S02.66
  manubrium (sterni) S22.21
    dissociation from sternum S22.23
  march — *see* Fracture, traumatic, stress, by site
  maxilla, maxillary (bone) (sinus) (superior) (upper jaw) S02.401
    alveolus S02.42
    inferior — *see* Fracture, mandible
    LeFort I S02.411
    LeFort II S02.412
    LeFort III S02.413
    left side S02.40D
    right side S02.40C
  metacarpal S62.309

Fracture, traumatic (abduction) (adduction) (separation) - *continued*
  metacarpal - *continued*
    base (displaced) S62.319
      nondisplaced S62.349
    fifth S62.30-
      base (displaced) S62.31-
        nondisplaced S62.34-
      neck (displaced) S62.33-
        nondisplaced S62.36-
      shaft (displaced) S62.32-
        nondisplaced S62.35-
      specified NEC S62.398
    first S62.20-
      base NEC (displaced) S62.23-
        nondisplaced S62.23-
      Bennett's — *see* Bennett's fracture
      neck (displaced) S62.25-
        nondisplaced S62.25-
      shaft (displaced) S62.24-
        nondisplaced S62.24-
      specified NEC S62.29-
    fourth S62.30-
      base (displaced) S62.31-
        nondisplaced S62.34-
      neck (displaced) S62.33-
        nondisplaced S62.36-
      shaft (displaced) S62.32-
        nondisplaced S62.35-
      specified NEC S62.39-
    neck (displaced) S62.33-
      nondisplaced S62.36-
    Rolando's — *see* Rolando's fracture
    second S62.30-
      base (displaced) S62.31-
        nondisplaced S62.34-
      neck (displaced) S62.33-
        nondisplaced S62.36-
      shaft (displaced) S62.32-
        nondisplaced S62.35-
      specified NEC S62.39-
    shaft (displaced) S62.32-
      nondisplaced S62.35-
    third S62.30-
      base (displaced) S62.31-
        nondisplaced S62.34-
      neck (displaced) S62.33-
        nondisplaced S62.36-
      shaft (displaced) S62.32-
        nondisplaced S62.35-
      specified NEC S62.39-
    specified NEC S62.399
  metastatic — *see* Fracture, pathological, due to, neoplastic disease — *see also* Neoplasm
  metatarsal bone S92.30-
    fifth (displaced) S92.35-
      nondisplaced S92.35-
    first (displaced) S92.31-
      nondisplaced S92.31-
    fourth (displaced) S92.34-
      nondisplaced S92.34-
    physeal S99.10-
      Salter-Harris
        Type I S99.11-
        Type II S99.12-
        Type III S99.13-
        Type IV S99.14-
        specified NEC S99.19-
    second (displaced) S92.32-
      nondisplaced S92.32-
    third (displaced) S92.33-
      nondisplaced S92.33-
  Monteggia's — *see* Monteggia's fracture
  multiple
    hand (and wrist) NEC — *see* Fracture, by site
    ribs — *see* Fracture, rib, multiple
  nasal (bone (s)) S02.2
  navicular (scaphoid) (foot) — *see also* Fracture, tarsal, navicular
    hand — *see* Fracture, carpal, navicular
  neck S12.9
    cervical vertebra S12.9
      fifth (displaced) S12.400
        nondisplaced S12.401
        specified type NEC (displaced) S12.490
          nondisplaced S12.491
      first (displaced) S12.000
        burst (stable) S12.01
          unstable S12.02
        lateral mass (displaced) S12.040
          nondisplaced S12.041
        nondisplaced S12.001
        posterior arch (displaced) S12.030

Fracture, traumatic (abduction) (adduction) (separation) - *continued*
  neck - *continued*
    cervical vertebra - *continued*
      first (displaced) - *continued*
        posterior arch (displaced) - *continued*
          nondisplaced S12.031
        specified type NEC (displaced) S12.090
          nondisplaced S12.091
      fourth (displaced) S12.300
        nondisplaced S12.301
        specified type NEC (displaced) S12.390
          nondisplaced S12.391
      second (displaced) S12.100
        nondisplaced S12.101
        dens (anterior) (displaced) (type II) S12.110
          nondisplaced S12.112
          posterior S12.111
          specified type NEC (displaced) S12.120
            nondisplaced S12.121
        specified type NEC (displaced) S12.190
          nondisplaced S12.191
      seventh (displaced) S12.600
        nondisplaced S12.601
        specified type NEC (displaced) S12.690
          nondisplaced S12.691
      sixth (displaced) S12.500
        nondisplaced S12.501
        specified type NEC (displaced) S12.590
          nondisplaced S12.591
      third (displaced) S12.200
        nondisplaced S12.201
        specified type NEC (displaced) S12.290
          nondisplaced S12.291
    hyoid bone S12.8
    larynx S12.8
    specified site NEC S12.8
    thyroid cartilage S12.8
    trachea S12.8
  neoplastic NEC — *see* Fracture, pathological, due to, neoplastic disease
  neural arch — *see* Fracture, vertebra
  newborn — *see* Birth, injury, fracture
  nontraumatic — *see* Fracture, pathological
  nonunion — *see* Nonunion, fracture
  nose, nasal (bone) (septum) S02.2
  occiput — *see* Fracture, skull, base, occiput
  odontoid process — *see* Fracture, neck, cervical vertebra, second
  olecranon (process) (ulna) — *see* Fracture, ulna, upper end, olecranon process
  orbit, orbital (bone) (region) S02.8-
    floor (blow-out) S02.3-
    roof S02.19
  os
    calcis — *see* Fracture, tarsal, calcaneus
    magnum — *see* Fracture, carpal, capitate
    pubis — *see* Fracture, pubis
  palate S02.8-
  parietal bone (skull) S02.0
  patella S82.00-
    comminuted (displaced) S82.04-
      nondisplaced S82.04-
    longitudinal (displaced) S82.02-
      nondisplaced S82.02-
    osteochondral (displaced) S82.01-
      nondisplaced S82.01-
    specified NEC S82.09-
    transverse (displaced) S82.03-
      nondisplaced S82.03-
  pedicle (of vertebral arch) — *see* Fracture, vertebra
  pelvis, pelvic (bone) S32.9
    acetabulum — *see* Fracture, acetabulum
    circle — *see* Disruption, pelvic ring
    following insertion of implant, prosthesis or plate M96.65
    ilium — *see* Fracture, ilium
    ischium — *see* Fracture, ischium
    multiple
      with disruption of pelvic ring (circle) — *see* Disruption, pelvic ring
      without disruption of pelvic ring (circle) S32.82
    pubis — *see* Fracture, pubis
    specified site NEC S32.89
    sacrum — *see* Fracture, sacrum
  periprosthetic, around internal prosthetic joint M97.9
    ankle M97.2-
    elbow M97.4-
    finger M97.8
    hip M97.0-
    knee M97.1--
    shoulder M97.3-
    specified joint NEC M97.8

Fracture, traumatic (abduction) (adduction) (separation) - *continued*
- periprosthetic, around internal prosthetic joint - *continued*
  - spine M97.8
  - toe M97.8
  - wrist M97.8
- phalanx
  - foot — *see* Fracture, toe
  - hand — *see* Fracture, finger
- pisiform — *see* Fracture, carpal, pisiform
- pond — *see* Fracture, skull
- prosthetic device, internal — *see* Complications, prosthetic device, by site, mechanical
- pubis S32.50-
  - with disruption of pelvic ring — *see* Disruption, pelvic ring
  - specified site NEC S32.59-
  - superior rim S32.51-
- radius S52.9-
  - distal end — *see* Fracture, radius, lower end
  - following insertion of implant, prosthesis or plate M96.63-
  - head — *see* Fracture, radius, upper end, head
  - lower end S52.50-
    - Barton's — *see* Barton's fracture
    - Colles' — *see* Colles' fracture
    - extraarticular NEC S52.55-
    - intraarticular NEC S52.57-
    - physeal S59.20-
      - Salter-Harris
        - Type I S59.21-
        - Type II S59.22-
        - Type III S59.23-
        - Type IV S59.24-
      - specified NEC S59.29-
    - Smith's — *see* Smith's fracture
    - specified NEC S52.59-
    - styloid process (displaced) S52.51-
      - nondisplaced S52.51-
    - torus S52.52-
  - neck — *see* Fracture, radius, upper end
  - proximal end — *see* Fracture, radius, upper end
  - shaft S52.30-
    - bent bone S52.38-
    - comminuted (displaced) S52.35-
      - nondisplaced S52.35-
    - Galeazzi's — *see* Galeazzi's fracture
    - greenstick S52.31-
    - oblique (displaced) S52.33-
      - nondisplaced S52.33-
    - segmental (displaced) S52.36-
      - nondisplaced S52.36-
    - specified NEC S52.39-
    - spiral (displaced) S52.34-
      - nondisplaced S52.34-
    - transverse (displaced) S52.32-
      - nondisplaced S52.32-
  - upper end S52.10-
    - head (displaced) S52.12-
      - nondisplaced S52.12-
    - neck (displaced) S52.13-
      - nondisplaced S52.13-
    - specified NEC S52.18-
    - physeal S59.10-
      - Salter-Harris
        - Type I S59.11-
        - Type II S59.12-
        - Type III S59.13-
        - Type IV S59.14-
      - specified NEC S59.19-
    - torus S52.11-
- ramus
  - inferior or superior, pubis — *see* Fracture, pubis
  - mandible — *see* Fracture, mandible
- restorative material (dental) K08.539
  - with loss of material K08.531
  - without loss of material K08.530
- rib S22.3-
  - with flail chest — *see* Flail, chest
  - multiple S22.4-
    - with flail chest — *see* Flail, chest
- root, tooth — *see* Fracture, tooth
- sacrum S32.10
  - specified NEC S32.19
  - Type
    - 1 S32.14
    - 2 S32.15
    - 3 S32.16
    - 4 S32.17
  - Zone
    - I S32.119
      - displaced (minimally) S32.111

Fracture, traumatic (abduction) (adduction) (separation) - *continued*
- sacrum - *continued*
  - Zone - *continued*
    - I - *continued*
      - displaced (minimally) - *continued*
        - severely S32.112
      - nondisplaced S32.110
    - II S32.129
      - displaced (minimally) S32.121
        - severely S32.122
      - nondisplaced S32.120
    - III S32.139
      - displaced (minimally) S32.131
        - severely S32.132
      - nondisplaced S32.130
- scaphoid (hand) — *see also* Fracture, carpal, navicular
  - foot — *see* Fracture, tarsal, navicular
- scapula S42.10-
  - acromial process (displaced) S42.12-
    - nondisplaced S42.12-
  - body (displaced) S42.11-
    - nondisplaced S42.11-
  - coracoid process (displaced) S42.13-
    - nondisplaced S42.13-
  - glenoid cavity (displaced) S42.14-
    - nondisplaced S42.14-
  - neck (displaced) S42.15-
    - nondisplaced S42.15-
  - specified NEC S42.19-
- semilunar bone, wrist — *see* Fracture, carpal, lunate
- sequelae — *see* Sequelae, fracture
- sesamoid bone
  - foot S92.81-
  - hand — *see* Fracture, carpal
  - other — *see* Fracture, traumatic, by site
- shepherd's — *see* Fracture, tarsal, talus
- shoulder (girdle) S42.9-
  - blade — *see* Fracture, scapula
- sinus (ethmoid) (frontal) S02.19
- skull S02.91
  - base S02.10-
    - occiput S02.119
      - condyle S02.113
        - type I S02.110
          - left side S02.11B
          - right side S02.11A
        - type II S02.111
          - left side S02.11D
          - right side S02.11C
        - type III S02.112
          - left side S02.11F
          - right side S02.11E
        - specified NEC S02.118
          - left side S02.11H
          - right side S02.11G
      - specified NEC S02.19
    - birth injury P13.0
    - frontal bone S02.0
    - parietal bone S02.0
    - specified site NEC S02.8-
    - temporal bone S02.19
    - vault S02.0
- Smith's — *see* Smith's fracture
- sphenoid (bone) (sinus) S02.19
- spine — *see* Fracture, vertebra
- spinous process — *see* Fracture, vertebra
- spontaneous (cause unknown) — *see* Fracture, pathological
- stave (of thumb) — *see* Fracture, metacarpal, first
- sternum S22.20
  - with flail chest — *see* Flail, chest
  - body S22.22
  - manubrium S22.21
  - xiphoid (process) S22.24
- stress M84.30
  - ankle M84.37-
  - carpus M84.34-
  - clavicle M84.31-
  - femoral neck M84.359
  - femur M84.35-
  - fibula M84.36-
  - finger M84.34-
  - hip M84.359
  - humerus M84.32-
  - ilium M84.350
  - ischium M84.350
  - metacarpus M84.34-
  - metatarsus M84.37-
  - neck — *see* Fracture, fatigue, vertebra
  - pelvis M84.350
  - radius M84.33-

Fracture, traumatic (abduction) (adduction) (separation) - *continued*
- stress - *continued*
  - rib M84.38
  - scapula M84.31-
  - skull M84.38
  - tarsus M84.37-
  - tibia M84.36-
  - toe M84.37-
  - ulna M84.33-
  - vertebra — *see* Fracture, fatigue, vertebra
- supracondylar, elbow — *see* Fracture, humerus, lower end, supracondylar
- symphysis pubis — *see* Fracture, pubis
- talus (ankle bone) — *see* Fracture, tarsal, talus
- tarsal bone (s) S92.20-
  - astragalus — *see* Fracture, tarsal, talus
  - calcaneus S92.00-
    - anterior process (displaced) S92.02-
      - nondisplaced S92.02-
    - body (displaced) S92.01-
      - nondisplaced S92.01-
    - extraarticular NEC (displaced) S92.05-
      - nondisplaced S92.05-
    - intraarticular (displaced) S92.06-
      - nondisplaced S92.06-
    - physeal S99.00-
      - Salter-Harris
        - Type I S99.01-
        - Type II S99.02-
        - Type III S99.03-
        - Type IV S99.04-
      - specified NEC S99.09-
    - tuberosity (displaced) S92.04-
      - avulsion (displaced) S92.03-
        - nondisplaced S92.03-
      - nondisplaced S92.04-
  - cuboid (displaced) S92.21-
    - nondisplaced S92.21-
  - cuneiform
    - intermediate (displaced) S92.23-
      - nondisplaced S92.23-
    - lateral (displaced) S92.22-
      - nondisplaced S92.22-
    - medial (displaced) S92.24-
      - nondisplaced S92.24-
  - navicular (displaced) S92.25-
    - nondisplaced S92.25-
  - scaphoid — *see* Fracture, tarsal, navicular
  - talus S92.10-
    - avulsion (displaced) S92.15-
      - nondisplaced S92.15-
    - body (displaced) S92.12-
      - nondisplaced S92.12-
    - dome (displaced) S92.14-
      - nondisplaced S92.14-
    - head (displaced) S92.12-
      - nondisplaced S92.12-
    - lateral process (displaced) S92.14-
      - nondisplaced S92.14-
    - neck (displaced) S92.11-
      - nondisplaced S92.11-
    - posterior process (displaced) S92.13-
      - nondisplaced S92.13-
    - specified NEC S92.19-
- temporal bone (styloid) S02.19
- thorax (bony) S22.9
  - with flail chest — *see* Flail, chest
  - rib S22.3-
    - multiple S22.4-
      - with flail chest — *see* Flail, chest
  - sternum S22.20
    - body S22.22
    - manubrium S22.21
    - xiphoid process S22.24
  - vertebra (displaced) S22.009
    - burst (stable) S22.001
      - unstable S22.002
    - eighth S22.069
      - burst (stable) S22.061
        - unstable S22.062
      - specified type NEC S22.068
      - wedge compression S22.060
    - eleventh S22.089
      - burst (stable) S22.081
        - unstable S22.082
      - specified type NEC S22.088
      - wedge compression S22.080
    - fifth S22.059
      - burst (stable) S22.051
        - unstable S22.052
      - specified type NEC S22.058
      - wedge compression S22.050

Fracture, traumatic (abduction) (adduction) (separation) - *continued*
  thorax (bony) - *continued*
    vertebra (displaced) - *continued*
      first S22.019
        burst (stable) S22.011
          unstable S22.012
        specified type NEC S22.018
        wedge compression S22.010
      fourth S22.049
        burst (stable) S22.041
          unstable S22.042
        specified type NEC S22.048
        wedge compression S22.040
      ninth S22.079
        burst (stable) S22.071
          unstable S22.072
        specified type NEC S22.078
        wedge compression S22.070
      nondisplaced S22.001
      second S22.029
        burst (stable) S22.021
          unstable S22.022
        specified type NEC S22.028
        wedge compression S22.020
      seventh S22.069
        burst (stable) S22.061
          unstable S22.062
        specified type NEC S22.068
        wedge compression S22.060
      sixth S22.059
        burst (stable) S22.051
          unstable S22.052
        specified type NEC S22.058
        wedge compression S22.050
      specified type NEC S22.008
      tenth S22.079
        burst (stable) S22.071
          unstable S22.072
        specified type NEC S22.078
        wedge compression S22.070
      third S22.039
        burst (stable) S22.031
          unstable S22.032
        specified type NEC S22.038
        wedge compression S22.030
      twelfth S22.089
        burst (stable) S22.081
          unstable S22.082
        specified type NEC S22.088
        wedge compression S22.080
      wedge compression S22.000
  thumb S62.50-
    distal phalanx (displaced) S62.52-
      nondisplaced S62.52-
    proximal phalanx (displaced) S62.51-
      nondisplaced S62.51-
  thyroid cartilage S12.8
  tibia (shaft) S82.20-
    comminuted (displaced) S82.25-
      nondisplaced S82.25-
    condyles — *see* Fracture, tibia, upper end
    distal end — *see* Fracture, tibia, lower end
    epiphysis
      lower — *see* Fracture, tibia, lower end
      upper — *see* Fracture, tibia, upper end
    following insertion of implant, prosthesis or plate M96.67-
    head (involving knee joint) — *see* Fracture, tibia, upper end
    intercondyloid eminence — *see* Fracture, tibia, upper end
    involving ankle or malleolus — *see* Fracture, ankle, medial malleolus
    lower end S82.30-
      physeal S89.10-
        Salter-Harris
          Type I S89.11-
          Type II S89.12-
          Type III S89.13-
          Type IV S89.14-
          specified NEC S89.19-
      pilon (displaced) S82.87-
        nondisplaced S82.87-
      specified NEC S82.39-
      torus S82.31-
    malleolus — *see* Fracture, ankle, medial malleolus
    oblique (displaced) S82.23-
      nondisplaced S82.23-
    pilon — *see* Fracture, tibia, lower end, pilon
    proximal end — *see* Fracture, tibia, upper end
    segmental (displaced) S82.26-
      nondisplaced S82.26-

Fracture, traumatic (abduction) (adduction) (separation) - *continued*
  tibia (shaft) - *continued*
    specified NEC S82.29-
    spine — *see* Fracture, upper end, spine
    spiral (displaced) S82.24-
      nondisplaced S82.24-
    transverse (displaced) S82.22-
      nondisplaced S82.22-
    tuberosity — *see* Fracture, tibia, upper end, tuberosity
    upper end S82.10-
      bicondylar (displaced) S82.14-
        nondisplaced S82.14-
      lateral condyle (displaced) S82.12-
        nondisplaced S82.12-
      medial condyle (displaced) S82.13-
        nondisplaced S82.13-
      physeal S89.00-
        Salter-Harris
          Type I S89.01-
          Type II S89.02-
          Type III S89.03-
          Type IV S89.04-
          specified NEC S89.09-
      plateau — *see* Fracture, tibia, upper end, bicondylar
      spine (displaced) S82.11-
        nondisplaced S82.11-
      torus S82.16-
      specified NEC S82.19-
      tuberosity (displaced) S82.15-
        nondisplaced S82.15-
  toe S92.91-
    great (displaced) S92.40-
      distal phalanx (displaced) S92.42-
        nondisplaced S92.42-
      nondisplaced S92.40-
      proximal phalanx (displaced) S92.41-
        nondisplaced S92.41-
      specified NEC S92.49-
    lesser (displaced) S92.50-
      distal phalanx (displaced) S92.53-
        nondisplaced S92.53-
      medial phalanx (displaced) S92.52-
        nondisplaced S92.52-
      nondisplaced S92.50-
      proximal phalanx (displaced) S92.51-
        nondisplaced S92.51-
      specified NEC S92.59-
    physeal
      phalanx S99.20-
        Salter-Harris
          Type I S99.21-
          Type II S99.22-
          Type III S99.23-
          Type IV S99.24-
          specified NEC S99.29-
  tooth (root) S02.5
  trachea (cartilage) S12.8
  transverse process — *see* Fracture, vertebra
  trapezium or trapezoid bone — *see* Fracture, carpal
  trimalleolar — *see* Fracture, ankle, trimalleolar
  triquetrum (cuneiform of carpus) — *see* Fracture, carpal, triquetrum
  trochanter — *see* Fracture, femur, trochanteric
  tuberosity (external) — *see* Fracture, traumatic, by site
  ulna (shaft) S52.20-
    bent bone S52.28-
    coronoid process — *see* Fracture, ulna, upper end, coronoid process
    distal end — *see* Fracture, ulna, lower end
    following insertion of implant, prosthesis or plate M96.63-
    head S52.00-
    lower end S52.60-
      physeal S59.00-
        Salter-Harris
          Type I S59.01-
          Type II S59.02-
          Type III S59.03-
          Type IV S59.04-
          specified NEC S59.09-
      specified NEC S52.69-
      styloid process (displaced) S52.61-
        nondisplaced S52.61-
      torus S52.62-
    proximal end — *see* Fracture, ulna, upper end
    shaft S52.20-
      comminuted (displaced) S52.25-
        nondisplaced S52.25-
      greenstick S52.21-

Fracture, traumatic (abduction) (adduction) (separation) - *continued*
  ulna (shaft) - *continued*
    shaft - *continued*
      Monteggia's — *see* Monteggia's fracture
      oblique (displaced) S52.23-
        nondisplaced S52.23-
      segmental (displaced) S52.26-
        nondisplaced S52.26-
      specified NEC S52.29-
      spiral (displaced) S52.24-
        nondisplaced S52.24-
      transverse (displaced) S52.22-
        nondisplaced S52.22-
    upper end S52.00-
      coronoid process (displaced) S52.04-
        nondisplaced S52.04-
      olecranon process (displaced) S52.02-
        with intraarticular extension S52.03-
        nondisplaced S52.02-
          with intraarticular extension S52.03-
      specified NEC S52.09-
      torus S52.01-
  unciform — *see* Fracture, carpal, hamate
  vault of skull S02.0
  vertebra, vertebral (arch) (body) (column) (neural arch) (pedicle) (spinous process) (transverse process)
    atlas — *see* Fracture, neck, cervical vertebra, first
    axis — *see* Fracture, neck, cervical vertebra, second
    cervical (teardrop) S12.9
      axis — *see* Fracture, neck, cervical vertebra, second
      first (atlas) — *see* Fracture, neck, cervical vertebra, first
      second (axis) — *see* Fracture, neck, cervical vertebra, second
    chronic M84.48
    coccyx S32.2
    dorsal — *see* Fracture, thorax, vertebra
    lumbar S32.009
      burst (stable) S32.001
        unstable S32.002
      fifth S32.059
        burst (stable) S32.051
          unstable S32.052
        specified type NEC S32.058
        wedge compression S32.050
      first S32.019
        burst (stable) S32.011
          unstable S32.012
        specified type NEC S32.018
        wedge compression S32.010
      fourth S32.049
        burst (stable) S32.041
          unstable S32.042
        specified type NEC S32.048
        wedge compression S32.040
      second S32.029
        burst (stable) S32.021
          unstable S32.022
        specified type NEC S32.028
        wedge compression S32.020
      specified type NEC S32.008
      third S32.039
        burst (stable) S32.031
          unstable S32.032
        specified type NEC S32.038
        wedge compression S32.030
      wedge compression S32.000
    metastatic — *see* Collapse, vertebra, in, specified disease NEC — *see also* Neoplasm
    newborn (birth injury) P11.5
    sacrum S32.10
      specified NEC S32.19
      Type
        1 S32.14
        2 S32.15
        3 S32.16
        4 S32.17
      Zone
        I S32.119
          displaced (minimally) S32.111
            severely S32.112
          nondisplaced S32.110
        II S32.129
          displaced (minimally) S32.121
            severely S32.122
          nondisplaced S32.120
        III S32.139
          displaced (minimally) S32.131
            severely S32.132

Fracture, traumatic (abduction) (adduction) (separation) - *continued*
vertebra, vertebral (arch) (body) (column) (neural arch) (pedicle) (spinous process) (transverse process) - *continued*
  sacrum - *continued*
    Zone - *continued*
      III - *continued*
        nondisplaced S32.130
  thoracic — *see* Fracture, thorax, vertebra
  vertex S02.0
  vomer (bone) S02.2
  wrist S62.10-
    carpal — *see* Fracture, carpal bone
    navicular (scaphoid) (hand) — *see* Fracture, carpal, navicular
  xiphisternum, xiphoid (process) S22.24
  zygoma S02.402
    left side S02.40F
    right side S02.40E
Fragile, fragility
  autosomal site Q95.5
  bone, congenital (with blue sclera) Q78.0
  capillary (hereditary) D69.8
  hair L67.8
  nails L60.3
  non-sex chromosome site Q95.5
  X chromosome Q99.2
Fragilitas
  crinium L67.8
  ossium (with blue sclerae) (hereditary) Q78.0
  unguium L60.3
    congenital Q84.6
Fragments, cataract (lens)
  , following cataract surgery H59.02-
  retained foreign body — *see* Retained, foreign body fragments (type of)
Frailty (frail) R54
  mental R41.81
Frambesia, frambesial (tropica) — *see also* Yaws
  initial lesion or ulcer A66.0
  primary A66.0
Frambeside
  gummatous A66.4
  of early yaws A66.2
Frambesioma A66.1
Franceschetti-Klein (-Wildervanck)
  disease or syndrome Q75.4
Francis' disease — *see* Tularemia
Franklin disease C88.2
Frank's essential thrombocytopenia D69.3
Fraser's syndrome Q87.0
Freckle (s) L81.2
  malignant melanoma in — *see* Melanoma
  melanotic (Hutchinson's) — *see* Melanoma, in situ
  retinal D49.81
Frederickson's hyperlipoproteinemia, type
  I and V E78.3
  IIA E78.00
  IIB and III E78.2
  IV E78.1
Freeman Sheldon syndrome Q87.0
Freezing — *see also* Effect, adverse, cold T69.9
Freiberg's disease
  (infraction of metatarsal head or osteochondrosis) — *see* Osteochondrosis, juvenile, metatarsus
Frei's disease A55
Fremitus, friction, cardiac R01.2
Frenum, frenulum
  external os Q51.828
  tongue (shortening) (congenital) Q38.1
Frequency micturition (nocturnal) R35.0
  psychogenic F45.8
Frey's syndrome
  auriculotemporal G50.8
  hyperhidrosis L74.52
Friction
  burn — *see* Burn, by site
  fremitus, cardiac R01.2
  precordial R01.2
  sounds, chest R09.89
Friderichsen-Waterhouse syndrome or disease A39.1
Friedländer's B (bacillus) **NEC** — *see also* condition A49.8
Friedreich's
  ataxia G11.1
  combined systemic disease G11.1
  facial hemihypertrophy Q67.4
  sclerosis (cerebellum) (spinal cord) G11.1
Frigidity F52.22
Fröhlich's syndrome E23.6

Frontal — *see also* condition
  lobe syndrome F07.0
Frostbite (superficial) T33.90
  with
    partial thickness skin loss — *see* Frostbite (superficial), by site
    tissue necrosis T34.90
  abdominal wall T33.3
    with tissue necrosis T34.3
  ankle T33.81-
    with tissue necrosis T34.81-
  arm T33.4-
    with tissue necrosis T34.4-
    finger (s) — *see* Frostbite, finger
    hand — *see* Frostbite, hand
    wrist — *see* Frostbite, wrist
  ear T33.01-
    with tissue necrosis T34.01-
  face T33.09
    with tissue necrosis T34.09
  finger T33.53-
    with tissue necrosis T34.53-
  foot T33.82-
    with tissue necrosis T34.82-
  hand T33.52-
    with tissue necrosis T34.52-
  head T33.09
    with tissue necrosis T34.09
    ear — *see* Frostbite, ear
    nose — *see* Frostbite, nose
  hip (and thigh) T33.6-
    with tissue necrosis T34.6-
  knee T33.7-
    with tissue necrosis T34.7-
  leg T33.9-
    with tissue necrosis T34.9-
    ankle — *see* Frostbite, ankle
    foot — *see* Frostbite, foot
    knee — *see* Frostbite, knee
    lower T33.7-
      with tissue necrosis T34.7-
    thigh — *see* Frostbite, hip
    toe — *see* Frostbite, toe
  limb
    lower T33.99
      with tissue necrosis T34.99
    upper — *see* Frostbite, arm
  neck T33.1
    with tissue necrosis T34.1
  nose T33.02
    with tissue necrosis T34.02
  pelvis T33.3
    with tissue necrosis T34.3
  specified site NEC T33.99
    with tissue necrosis T34.99
  thigh — *see* Frostbite, hip
  thorax T33.2
    with tissue necrosis T34.2
  toes T33.83-
    with tissue necrosis T34.83-
  trunk T33.99
    with tissue necrosis T34.99
  wrist T33.51-
    with tissue necrosis T34.51-
Frotteurism F65.81
Frozen — *see also* Effect, adverse, cold T69.9
  pelvis (female) N94.89
    male K66.8
  shoulder — *see* Capsulitis, adhesive
Fructokinase deficiency E74.11
Fructose 1,6 diphosphatase deficiency E74.19
Fructosemia (benign) (essential) E74.12
Fructosuria (benign) (essential) E74.11
Fuchs'
  black spot (myopic) H44.2-
  dystrophy (corneal endothelium) H18.51
  heterochromic cyclitis — *see* Cyclitis, Fuchs' heterochromic
Fucosidosis E77.1
Fugue R68.89
  dissociative F44.1
  hysterical (dissociative) F44.1
  postictal in epilepsy — *see* Epilepsy
  reaction to exceptional stress (transient) F43.0
Fulminant, fulminating — *see* condition
Functional — *see also* condition
  bleeding (uterus) N93.8
Functioning, intellectual, borderline R41.83
Fundus — *see* condition
Fungemia NOS B49
Fungus, fungous
  cerebral G93.89
  disease NOS B49

Fungus, fungous - *continued*
  infection — *see* Infection, fungus
Funiculitis (acute) (chronic) (endemic) N49.1
  gonococcal (acute) (chronic) A54.23
  tuberculous A18.15
Funnel
  breast (acquired) M95.4
    congenital Q67.6
    sequelae (late effect) of rickets E64.3
  chest (acquired) M95.4
    congenital Q67.6
    sequelae (late effect) of rickets E64.3
  pelvis (acquired) M95.5
    with disproportion (fetopelvic) O33.3
      causing obstructed labor O65.3
    congenital Q74.2
FUO (fever of unknown origin) R50.9
Furfur L21.0
  microsporon B36.0
Furrier's lung J67.8
Furrowed K14.5
  nail (s) (transverse) L60.4
    congenital Q84.6
  tongue K14.5
    congenital Q38.3
Furuncle L02.92
  abdominal wall L02.221
  ankle — *see* Furuncle, lower limb
  anus K61.0
  antecubital space — *see* Furuncle, upper limb
  arm — *see* Furuncle, upper limb
  auditory canal, external — *see* Abscess, ear, external
  auricle (ear) — *see* Abscess, ear, external
  axilla (region) L02.42-
  back (any part) L02.222
  breast N61.1
  buttock L02.32
  cheek (external) L02.02
  chest wall L02.223
  chin L02.02
  corpus cavernosum N48.21
  ear, external — *see* Abscess, ear, external
  external auditory canal — *see* Abscess, ear, external
  eyelid — *see* Abscess, eyelid
  face L02.02
  femoral (region) — *see* Furuncle, lower limb
  finger — *see* Furuncle, hand
  flank L02.221
  foot L02.62-
  forehead L02.02
  gluteal (region) L02.32
  groin L02.224
  hand L02.52-
  head L02.821
    face L02.02
  hip — *see* Furuncle, lower limb
  kidney — *see* Abscess, kidney
  knee — *see* Furuncle, lower limb
  labium (majus) (minus) N76.4
  lacrimal
    gland — *see* Dacryoadenitis
    passages (duct) (sac) — *see* Inflammation, lacrimal, passages, acute
  leg (any part) — *see* Furuncle, lower limb
  lower limb L02.42-
  malignant A22.0
  mouth K12.2
  navel L02.226
  neck L02.12
  nose J34.0
  orbit, orbital — *see* Abscess, orbit
  palmar (space) — *see* Furuncle, hand
  partes posteriores L02.32
  pectoral region L02.223
  penis N48.21
  perineum L02.225
  pinna — *see* Abscess, ear, external
  popliteal — *see* Furuncle, lower limb
  prepatellar — *see* Furuncle, lower limb
  scalp L02.821
  seminal vesicle N49.0
  shoulder — *see* Furuncle, upper limb
  specified site NEC L02.828
  submandibular K12.2
  temple (region) L02.02
  thumb — *see* Furuncle, hand
  toe — *see* Furuncle, foot
  trunk L02.229
    abdominal wall L02.221
    back L02.222
    chest wall L02.223
    groin L02.224
    perineum L02.225

Furuncle - *continued*
trunk - *continued*
umbilicus L02.226
umbilicus L02.226
upper limb L02.42-
vulva N76.4
Furunculosis — *see* Furuncle
Fused — *see* Fusion, fused
Fusion, fused (congenital)
astragaloscaphoid Q74.2
atria Q21.1
auditory canal Q16.1
auricles, heart Q21.1
binocular with defective stereopsis H53.32
bone Q79.8
cervical spine M43.22
choanal Q30.0
commissure, mitral valve Q23.2
cusps, heart valve NEC Q24.8
mitral Q23.2
pulmonary Q22.1
tricuspid Q22.4
ear ossicles Q16.3
fingers Q70.0-
hymen Q52.3
joint (acquired) — *see also* Ankylosis
congenital Q74.8
kidneys (incomplete) Q63.1
labium (majus) (minus) Q52.5
larynx and trachea Q34.8
limb, congenital Q74.8
lower Q74.2
upper Q74.0
lobes, lung Q33.8
lumbosacral (acquired) M43.27
arthrodesis status Z98.1
congenital Q76.49
postprocedural status Z98.1
nares, nose, nasal, nostril (s) Q30.0
organ or site not listed — *see* Anomaly, by site
ossicles Q79.9
auditory Q16.3
pulmonic cusps Q22.1
ribs Q76.6
sacroiliac (joint) (acquired) M43.28
arthrodesis status Z98.1
congenital Q74.2
postprocedural status Z98.1
spine (acquired) NEC M43.20
arthrodesis status Z98.1
cervical region M43.22
cervicothoracic region M43.23
congenital Q76.49
lumbar M43.26
lumbosacral region M43.27
occipito-atlanto-axial region M43.21
postoperative status Z98.1
sacrococcygeal region M43.28
thoracic region M43.24
thoracolumbar region M43.25
sublingual duct with submaxillary duct at opening in
mouth Q38.4
testes Q55.1
toes Q70.2-
tooth, teeth K00.2
trachea and esophagus Q39.8
twins Q89.4
vagina Q52.4
ventricles, heart Q21.0
vertebra (arch) — *see* Fusion, spine
vulva Q52.5
Fusospirillosis (mouth) (tongue) (tonsil) A69.1
Fussy baby R68.12

G

Gain in weight (abnormal) (excessive) — *see
also* Weight, gain
Gaisböck's disease (polycythemia
hypertonica) D75.1
Gait abnormality R26.9
ataxic R26.0
falling R29.6
hysterical (ataxic) (staggering) F44.4
paralytic R26.1
spastic R26.1
specified type NEC R26.89
staggering R26.0
unsteadiness R26.81
walking difficulty NEC R26.2
Galactocele (breast) N64.89
puerperal, postpartum O92.79
Galactokinase deficiency E74.29

Galactophoritis N61.0
gestational, puerperal, postpartum O91.2-
Galactorrhea O92.6
not associated with childbirth N64.3
Galactosemia (classic) (congenital) E74.21
Galactosuria E74.29
Galacturia R82.0
schistosomiasis (bilharziasis) B65.0
Galeazzi's fracture S52.37-
Galen's vein — *see* condition
Gall duct — *see* condition
Gallbladder — *see also* condition
acute K81.0
Gallop rhythm R00.8
Gallstone (colic) (cystic duct) (gallbladder)
(impacted) (multiple) — *see also* Calculus,
gallbladder
with
cholecystitis — *see* Calculus, gallbladder, with
cholecystitis
bile duct (common) (hepatic) — *see* Calculus, bile
duct
causing intestinal obstruction K56.3
specified NEC K80.80
with obstruction K80.81
Gambling Z72.6
pathological (compulsive) F63.0
Gammopathy
(of undetermined significance [MGUS]) D47.2
associated with lymphoplasmacytic dyscrasia D47.2
monoclonal D47.2
polyclonal D89.0
Gamna's disease (siderotic splenomegaly) D73.1
Gamophobia F40.298
Gampsodactylia (congenital) Q66.7
Gamstorp's disease (adynamia episodica
hereditaria) G72.3
Gandy-Nanta disease (siderotic
splenomegaly) D73.1
Gang
membership offenses Z72.810
Gangliocytoma D36.10
Ganglioglioma — *see* Neoplasm, uncertain behavior,
by site
Ganglion (compound) (diffuse) (joint)
(tendon (sheath)) M67.40
ankle M67.47-
foot M67.47-
forearm M67.43-
hand M67.44-
lower leg M67.46-
multiple sites M67.49
of yaws (early) (late) A66.6
pelvic region M67.45-
periosteal — *see* Periostitis
shoulder region M67.41-
specified site NEC M67.48
thigh region M67.45-
tuberculous A18.09
upper arm M67.42-
wrist M67.43-
Ganglioneuroblastoma — *see* Neoplasm, nerve,
malignant
Ganglioneuroma D36.10
malignant — *see* Neoplasm, nerve, malignant
Ganglioneuromatosis D36.10
Ganglionitis
fifth nerve — *see* Neuralgia, trigeminal
gasserian (postherpetic) (postzoster) B02.21
geniculate G51.1
newborn (birth injury) P11.3
postherpetic, postzoster B02.21
herpes zoster B02.21
postherpetic geniculate B02.21
Gangliosidosis E75.10
GM1 E75.19
GM2 E75.00
other specified E75.09
Sandhoff disease E75.01
Tay-Sachs disease E75.02
GM3 E75.19
mucolipidosis IV E75.11
Gangosa A66.5
Gangrene, gangrenous (connective tissue)
(dropsical) (dry) (moist) (skin) (ulcer) — *see
also* Necrosis I96
with diabetes (mellitus) — *see* Diabetes, gangrene
abdomen (wall) I96
alveolar M27.3
appendix K35.80
with
perforation or rupture K35.2

Gangrene, gangrenous (connective tissue)
(dropsical) (dry) (moist) (skin) (ulcer) - *continued*
appendix - *continued*
with - *continued*
peritoneal abscess K35.3
peritonitis NEC K35.3
generalized (with perforation or rupture) K35.2
localized (with perforation or rupture) K35.3
arteriosclerotic (general) (senile) — *see*
Arteriosclerosis, extremities, with, gangrene
auricle I96
Bacillus welchii A48.0
bladder (infectious) — *see* Cystitis, specified type
NEC
bowel, cecum, or colon — *see* Gangrene, intestine
Clostridium perfringens or welchii A48.0
cornea H18.89-
corpora cavernosa N48.29
noninfective N48.89
cutaneous, spreading I96
decubital — *see* Ulcer, pressure, by site
diabetic (any site) — *see* Diabetes, gangrene
epidemic — *see* Poisoning, food, noxious, plant
epididymis (infectional) N45.1
erysipelas — *see* Erysipelas
emphysematous — *see* Gangrene, gas
extremity (lower) (upper) I96
Fournier N49.3
female N76.89
fusospirochetal A69.0
gallbladder — *see* Cholecystitis, acute
gas (bacillus) A48.0
following
abortion — *see* Abortion by type complicated by
infection
ectopic or molar pregnancy O08.0
glossitis K14.0
hernia — *see* Hernia, by site, with gangrene
intestine, intestinal (hemorrhagic) (massive) —
see also Infarct, intestine K55.069
with
mesenteric embolism — *see also* Infarct,
intestine K55.069
obstruction — *see* Obstruction, intestine
laryngitis J04.0
limb (lower) (upper) I96
lung J85.0
spirochetal A69.8
lymphangitis I89.1
Meleney's (synergistic) — *see* Ulcer, skin
mesentery — *see also* Infarct, intestine K55.069
with
embolism — *see also* Infarct, intestine K55.069
intestinal obstruction — *see* Obstruction,
intestine
mouth A69.0
ovary — *see* Oophoritis
pancreas — *see* Pancreatitis, acute
penis N48.29
noninfective N48.89
perineum I96
pharynx — *see also* Pharyngitis
Vincent's A69.1
presenile I73.1
progressive synergistic — *see* Ulcer, skin
pulmonary J85.0
pulpal (dental) K04.1
quinsy J36
Raynaud's (symmetric gangrene) I73.01
retropharyngeal J39.2
scrotum N49.3
noninfective N50.89
senile (atherosclerotic) — *see* Arteriosclerosis,
extremities, with, gangrene
spermatic cord N49.1
noninfective N50.89
spine I96
spirochetal NEC A69.8
spreading cutaneous I96
stomatitis A69.0
symmetrical I73.01
testis (infectional) N45.2
noninfective N44.8
throat — *see also* Pharyngitis
diphtheritic A36.0
Vincent's A69.1
thyroid (gland) E07.89
tooth (pulp) K04.1
tuberculous NEC — *see* Tuberculosis
tunica vaginalis N49.1
noninfective N50.89
umbilicus I96
uterus — *see* Endometritis

Gangrene, gangrenous (connective tissue)
(dropsical) (dry) (moist) (skin) (ulcer) - *continued*
  uvulitis K12.2
  vas deferens N49.1
    noninfective N50.89
  vulva N76.89
Ganister disease J62.8
Ganser's syndrome (hysterical) F44.89
Gardner-Diamond syndrome
  (autoerythrocyte sensitization) D69.2
Gargoylism E76.01
Garré's disease, osteitis (sclerosing) ,
  osteomyelitis — *see* Osteomyelitis, specified type
  NEC
Garrod's pad, knuckle M72.1
Gartner's duct
  cyst Q52.4
  persistent Q50.6
Gas R14.3
  asphyxiation, inhalation, poisoning, suffocation
    NEC — *see* Table of Drugs and Chemicals
  excessive R14.0
  gangrene A48.0
  following
    abortion — *see* Abortion by type complicated by
      infection
    ectopic or molar pregnancy O08.0
  on stomach R14.0
  pains R14.1
Gastralgia — *see also* Pain, abdominal
Gastrectasis K31.0
  psychogenic F45.8
Gastric — *see* condition
Gastrinoma
  malignant
    pancreas C25.4
    specified site NEC — *see* Neoplasm, malignant, by
      site
    unspecified site C25.4
  specified site — *see* Neoplasm, uncertain behavior
  unspecified site D37.9
Gastritis (simple) K29.70
  with bleeding K29.71
  acute (erosive) K29.00
    with bleeding K29.01
  alcoholic K29.20
    with bleeding K29.21
  allergic K29.60
    with bleeding K29.61
  atrophic (chronic) K29.40
    with bleeding K29.41
  chronic (antral) (fundal) K29.50
    with bleeding K29.51
    atrophic K29.40
      with bleeding K29.41
    superficial K29.30
      with bleeding K29.31
  dietary counseling and surveillance Z71.3
  due to diet deficiency E63.9
  eosinophilic K52.81
  giant hypertrophic K29.60
    with bleeding K29.61
  granulomatous K29.60
    with bleeding K29.61
  hypertrophic (mucosa) K29.60
    with bleeding K29.61
  nervous F54
  spastic K29.60
    with bleeding K29.61
  specified NEC K29.60
    with bleeding K29.61
  superficial chronic K29.30
    with bleeding K29.31
  tuberculous A18.83
  viral NEC A08.4
Gastrocarcinoma — *see* Neoplasm, malignant,
  stomach
Gastrocolic — *see* condition
Gastrodisciasis, gastrodiscoidiasis B66.8
Gastroduodenitis K29.90
  with bleeding K29.91
  virus, viral A08.4
    specified type NEC A08.39
Gastrodynia — *see* Pain, abdominal
Gastroenteritis (acute) (chronic)
  (noninfectious) — *see also* Enteritis K52.9
  allergic K52.29
  with
    eosinophilic gastritis or gastroenteritis K52.81
    food protein-induced enterocolitis
      syndrome K52.21
    food protein-induced enteropathy K52.22
  dietetic — *see also* Gastroenteritis, allergic K52.29

Gastroenteritis (acute) (chronic) (noninfectious) -
continued
  drug-induced K52.1
  due to
    Cryptosporidium A07.2
    drugs K52.1
    food poisoning — *see* Intoxication, foodborne
    radiation K52.0
  eosinophilic K52.81
  epidemic (infectious) A09
  food hypersensitivity — *see also* Gastroenteritis,
    allergic K52.29
  infectious — *see* Enteritis, infectious
  influenzal — *see* Influenza, with gastroenteritis
  noninfectious K52.9
    specified NEC K52.89
  rotaviral A08.0
  Salmonella A02.0
  toxic K52.1
  viral NEC A08.4
    acute infectious A08.39
      type Norwalk A08.11
    infantile (acute) A08.39
    Norwalk agent A08.11
    rotaviral A08.0
    severe of infants A08.39
    specified type NEC A08.39
Gastroenteropathy — *see also* Gastroenteritis K52.9
  acute, due to Norwalk agent A08.11
  acute, due to Norovirus A08.11
  infectious A09
Gastroenteroptosis K63.4
Gastroesophageal laceration- hemorrhage
  syndrome K22.6
Gastrointestinal — *see* condition
Gastrojejunal — *see* condition
Gastrojejunitis — *see also* Enteritis K52.9
Gastrojejunocolic — *see* condition
Gastroliths K31.89
Gastromalacia K31.89
Gastroparalysis K31.84
  diabetic — *see* Diabetes, gastroparalysis
Gastroparesis K31.84
  diabetic — *see* Diabetes, by type, with gastroparesis
Gastropathy K31.9
  congestive portal K31.89
  erythematous K29.70
  exudative K90.89
  portal hypertensive K31.89
Gastroptosis K31.89
Gastrorrhagia K92.2
  psychogenic F45.8
Gastroschisis (congenital) Q79.3
Gastrospasm (neurogenic) (reflex) K31.89
  neurotic F45.8
  psychogenic F45.8
Gastrostaxis — *see* Gastritis, with bleeding
Gastrostenosis K31.89
Gastrostomy
  attention to Z43.1
  status Z93.1
Gastrosuccorrhea (continuous) (intermittent) K31.89
  neurotic F45.8
  psychogenic F45.8
Gatophobia F40.218
Gaucher's disease or splenomegaly (adult)
  (infantile) E75.22
Gee (-Herter) (-Thaysen) **disease** (nontropical
  sprue) K90.0
Gélineau's syndrome G47.419
  with cataplexy G47.411
Gemination, tooth, teeth K00.2
Gemistocytoma
  specified site — *see* Neoplasm, malignant, by site
  unspecified site C71.9
General, generalized — *see* condition
Genetic
  carrier (status)
    cystic fibrosis Z14.1
    hemophilia A (asymptomatic) Z14.01
      symptomatic Z14.02
    specified NEC Z14.8
  susceptibility to disease NEC Z15.89
    malignant neoplasm Z15.09
      breast Z15.01
      endometrium Z15.04
      ovary Z15.02
      prostate Z15.03
      specified NEC Z15.09
    multiple endocrine neoplasia Z15.81
Genital — *see* condition
Genito-anorectal syndrome A55
Genitourinary system — *see* condition

Genu
  congenital Q74.1
  extrorsum (acquired) — *see also* Deformity, varus,
    knee
    congenital Q74.1
    sequelae (late effect) of rickets E64.3
  introrsum (acquired) — *see also* Deformity, valgus,
    knee
    congenital Q74.1
    sequelae (late effect) of rickets E64.3
  rachitic (old) E64.3
  recurvatum (acquired) — *see also* Deformity, limb,
    specified type NEC, lower leg
    congenital Q68.2
    sequelae (late effect) of rickets E64.3
  valgum (acquired) (knock-knee) M21.06-
    congenital Q74.1
    sequelae (late effect) of rickets E64.3
  varum (acquired) (bowleg) M21.16-
    congenital Q74.1
    sequelae (late effect) of rickets E64.3
Geographic tongue K14.1
Geophagia — *see* Pica
Geotrichosis B48.3
  stomatitis B48.3
Gephyrophobia F40.242
Gerbode defect Q21.0
GERD (gastroesophageal reflux disease) K21.9
Gerhardt's
  disease (erythromelalgia) I73.81
  syndrome (vocal cord paralysis) J38.00
    bilateral J38.02
    unilateral J38.01
German measles — *see also* Rubella
  exposure to Z20.4
Germinoblastoma (diffuse) C85.9-
  follicular C82.9-
Germinoma — *see* Neoplasm, malignant, by site
Gerontoxon — *see* Degeneration, cornea, senile
Gerstmann's syndrome R48.8
  developmental F81.2
Gerstmann-Sträussler-Scheinker syndrome
  (GSS) A81.82
Gestation (period) — *see also* Pregnancy
  ectopic — *see* Pregnancy, by site
  multiple O30.9-
    greater than quadruplets — *see* Pregnancy,
      multiple (gestation), specified NEC
    specified NEC — *see* Pregnancy, multiple
      (gestation), specified NEC
Gestational
  mammary abscess O91.11-
  purulent mastitis O91.11-
  subareolar abscess O91.11-
Ghon tubercle, primary infection A15.7
Ghost
  teeth K00.4
  vessels (cornea) H16.41-
Ghoul hand A66.3
Gianotti-Crosti disease L44.4
Giant
  cell
    epulis K06.8
    peripheral granuloma K06.8
  esophagus, congenital Q39.5
  kidney, congenital Q63.3
  urticaria T78.3
    hereditary D84.1
Giardiasis A07.1
Gibert's disease or pityriasis L42
Giddiness R42
  hysterical F44.89
  psychogenic F45.8
Gierke's disease (glycogenosis I) E74.01
Gigantism (cerebral) (hypophyseal) (pituitary) E22.0
  constitutional E34.4
Gilbert's disease or syndrome E80.4
Gilchrist's disease B40.9
Gilford-Hutchinson disease E34.8
Gilles de la Tourette's disease or syndrome
  (motor-verbal tic) F95.2
Gingivitis K05.10
  acute (catarrhal) K05.00
    necrotizing A69.1
    nonplaque induced K05.01
    plaque induced K05.00
  chronic (desquamative) (hyperplastic) (simple
    marginal) (pregnancy associated)
    (ulcerative) K05.10
    nonplaque induced K05.11
    plaque induced K05.10
  expulsiva — *see* Periodontitis
  necrotizing ulcerative (acute) A69.1

Gingivitis - *continued*
pellagrous E52
acute necrotizing A69.1
Vincent's A69.1
Gingivoglossitis K14.0
Gingivopericementitis — *see* Periodontitis
Gingivosis — *see* Gingivitis, chronic
Gingivostomatitis K05.10
herpesviral B00.2
necrotizing ulcerative (acute) A69.1
Gland, glandular — *see* condition
Glanders A24.0
Glanzmann (-Naegeli) **disease or thrombasthenia** D69.1
Glasgow coma scale
total score
3-8 R40.243
9-12 R40.242
13-15 R40.241
Glass-blower's disease (cataract) — *see* Cataract, specified NEC
Glaucoma H40.9
with
increased episcleral venous pressure H40.81-
pseudoexfoliation of lens — *see* Glaucoma, open angle, primary, capsular
absolute H44.51-
angle-closure (primary) H40.20-
acute (attack) (crisis) H40.21-
chronic H40.22-
intermittent H40.23-
residual stage H40.24-
borderline H40.00-
capsular (with pseudoexfoliation of lens) — *see* Glaucoma, open angle, primary, capsular
childhood Q15.0
closed angle — *see* Glaucoma, angle-closure
congenital Q15.0
corticosteroid-induced — *see* Glaucoma, secondary, drugs
hypersecretion H40.82-
in (due to)
amyloidosis E85.4 *[H42]*
aniridia Q13.1 *[H42]*
concussion of globe — *see* Glaucoma, secondary, trauma
dislocation of lens — *see* Glaucoma, secondary
disorder of lens NEC — *see* Glaucoma, secondary
drugs — *see* Glaucoma, secondary, drugs
endocrine disease NOS E34.9 *[H42]*
eye
inflammation — *see* Glaucoma, secondary, inflammation
trauma — *see* Glaucoma, secondary, trauma
hypermature cataract — *see* Glaucoma, secondary
iridocyclitis — *see* Glaucoma, secondary, inflammation
lens disorder — *see* Glaucoma, secondary,
Lowe's syndrome E72.03 *[H42]*
metabolic disease NOS E88.9 *[H42]*
ocular disorders NEC — *see* Glaucoma, secondary
onchocerciasis B73.02
pupillary block — *see* Glaucoma, secondary
retinal vein occlusion — *see* Glaucoma, secondary
Rieger's anomaly Q13.81 *[H42]*
rubeosis of iris — *see* Glaucoma, secondary
tumor of globe — *see* Glaucoma, secondary
infantile Q15.0
low tension — *see* Glaucoma, open angle, primary, low-tension
malignant H40.83-
narrow angle — *see* Glaucoma, angle-closure
newborn Q15.0
noncongestive (chronic) — *see* Glaucoma, open angle
nonobstructive — *see* Glaucoma, open angle
obstructive — *see also* Glaucoma, angle-closure
due to lens changes — *see* Glaucoma, secondary
open angle H40.10-
primary H40.11-
capsular (with pseudoexfoliation of lens) H40.14-
low-tension H40.12-
pigmentary H40.13-
residual stage H40.15-
phacolytic — *see* Glaucoma, secondary
pigmentary — *see* Glaucoma, open angle, primary, pigmentary
postinfectious — *see* Glaucoma, secondary, inflammation
secondary (to) H40.5-
drugs H40.6-
inflammation H40.4-
trauma H40.3-

Glaucoma - *continued*
simple (chronic) H40.11-
simplex H40.11-
specified type NEC H40.89
suspect H40.00-
syphilitic A52.71
traumatic — *see also* Glaucoma, secondary, trauma
newborn (birth injury) P15.3
tuberculous A18.59
Glaucomatous flecks (subcapsular) — *see* Cataract, complicated
Glazed tongue K14.4
Gleet (gonococcal) A54.01
Glénard's disease K63.4
Glioblastoma (multiforme)
with sarcomatous component
specified site — *see* Neoplasm, malignant, by site
unspecified site C71.9
giant cell
specified site — *see* Neoplasm, malignant, by site
unspecified site C71.9
specified site — *see* Neoplasm, malignant, by site
unspecified site C71.9
Glioma (malignant)
astrocytic
specified site — *see* Neoplasm, malignant, by site
unspecified site C71.9
mixed
specified site — *see* Neoplasm, malignant, by site
unspecified site C71.9
nose Q30.8
specified site NEC — *see* Neoplasm, malignant, by site
subependymal D43.2
specified site — *see* Neoplasm, uncertain behavior, by site
unspecified site D43.2
unspecified site C71.9
Gliomatosis cerebri C71.0
Glioneuroma — *see* Neoplasm, uncertain behavior, by site
Gliosarcoma
specified site — *see* Neoplasm, malignant, by site
unspecified site C71.9
Gliosis (cerebral) G93.89
spinal G95.89
Glisson's disease — *see* Rickets
Globinuria R82.3
Globus (hystericus) F45.8
Glomangioma D18.00
intra-abdominal D18.03
intracranial D18.02
skin D18.01
specified site NEC D18.09
Glomangiomyoma D18.00
intra-abdominal D18.03
intracranial D18.02
skin D18.01
specified site NEC D18.09
Glomangiosarcoma — *see* Neoplasm, connective tissue, malignant
Glomerular
disease in syphilis A52.75
nephritis — *see* Glomerulonephritis
Glomerulitis — *see* Glomerulonephritis
Glomerulonephritis — *see also* Nephritis N05.9
with
edema — *see* Nephrosis
minimal change N05.0
minor glomerular abnormality N05.0
acute N00.9
chronic N03.9
crescentic (diffuse) NEC — *see also* N00-N07 with fourth character .7 N05.7
dense deposit — *see also* N00-N07 with fourth character .6 N05.6
diffuse
crescentic — *see also* N00-N07 with fourth character .7 N05.7
endocapillary proliferative — *see also* N00-N07 with fourth character .4 N05.4
membranous — *see also* N00-N07 with fourth character .2 N05.2
mesangial proliferative — *see also* N00-N07 with fourth character .3 N05.3
mesangiocapillary — *see also* N00-N07 with fourth character .5 N05.5
sclerosing N05.8
endocapillary proliferative (diffuse) NEC — *see also* N00-N07 with fourth character .4 N05.4
extracapillary NEC — *see also* N00-N07 with fourth character .7 N05.7

Glomerulonephritis - *continued*
focal (and segmental) — *see also* N00-N07 with fourth character .1 N05.1
hypocomplementemic — *see* Glomerulonephritis, membranoproliferative
IgA — *see* Nephropathy, IgA
immune complex (circulating) NEC N05.8
in (due to)
amyloidosis E85.4 *[N08]*
bilharziasis B65.9 *[N08]*
cryoglobulinemia D89.1 *[N08]*
defibrination syndrome D65 *[N08]*
diabetes mellitus — *see* Diabetes, glomerulosclerosis
disseminated intravascular coagulation D65 *[N08]*
Fabry (-Anderson) disease E75.21 *[N08]*
Goodpasture's syndrome M31.0
hemolytic-uremic syndrome D59.3
Henoch (-Schönlein) purpura D69.0 *[N08]*
lecithin cholesterol acyltransferase deficiency E78.6 *[N08]*
microscopic polyangiitis M31.7 *[N08]*
multiple myeloma C90.0- *[N08]*
Plasmodium malariae B52.0
schistosomiasis B65.9 *[N08]*
sepsis A41.9 *[N08]*
streptococcal A40- *[N08]*
sickle-cell disorders D57.- *[N08]*
strongyloidiasis B78.9 *[N08]*
subacute bacterial endocarditis I33.0 *[N08]*
syphilis (late) congenital A50.59 *[N08]*
systemic lupus erythematosus M32.14
thrombotic thrombocytopenic purpura M31.1 *[N08]*
typhoid fever A01.09
Waldenström macroglobulinemia C88.0 *[N08]*
Wegener's granulomatosis M31.31
latent or quiescent N03.9
lobular, lobulonodular — *see* Glomerulonephritis, membranoproliferative
membranoproliferative (diffuse) (type 1 or 3) — *see also* N00-N07 with fourth character .5 N05.5
dense deposit (type 2) NEC — *see also* N00-N07 with fourth character .6 N05.6
membranous (diffuse) NEC — *see also* N00-N07 with fourth character .2 N05.2
mesangial
IgA/IgG — *see* Nephropathy, IgA
proliferative (diffuse) NEC — *see also* N00-N07 with fourth character .3 N05.3
mesangiocapillary (diffuse) NEC — *see also* N00-N07 with fourth character .5 N05.5
necrotic, necrotizing NEC — *see also* N00-N07 with fourth character .8 N05.8
nodular — *see* Glomerulonephritis, membranoproliferative
poststreptococcal NEC N05.9
acute N00.9
chronic N03.9
rapidly progressive N01.9
proliferative NEC — *see also* N00-N07 with fourth character .8 N05.8
diffuse (lupus) M32.14
rapidly progressive N01.9
sclerosing, diffuse N05.8
specified pathology NEC — *see also* N00-N07 with fourth character .8 N05.8
subacute N01.9
Glomerulopathy — *see* Glomerulonephritis
Glomerulosclerosis — *see also* Sclerosis, renal
intercapillary (nodular) (with diabetes) — *see* Diabetes, glomerulosclerosis
intracapillary — *see* Diabetes, glomerulosclerosis
Glossagra K14.6
Glossalgia K14.6
Glossitis (chronic superficial) (gangrenous) (Moeller's) K14.0
areata exfoliativa K14.1
atrophic K14.4
benign migratory K14.1
cortical superficial, sclerotic K14.0
Hunter's D51.0
interstitial, sclerous K14.0
median rhomboid K14.2
pellagrous E52
superficial, chronic K14.0
Glossocele K14.8
Glossodynia K14.6
exfoliativa K14.4
Glossoncus K14.8
Glossopathy K14.9
Glossophytia K14.3
Glossoplegia K14.8

Glossoptosis K14.8
Glossopyrosis K14.6
Glossotrichia K14.3
Glossy skin L90.8
Glottis — *see* condition
Glottitis — *see also* Laryngitis J04.0
Glucagonoma
  pancreas
    benign D13.7
    malignant C25.4
    uncertain behavior D37.8
  specified site NEC
    benign — *see* Neoplasm, benign, by site
    malignant — *see* Neoplasm, malignant, by site
    uncertain behavior — *see* Neoplasm, uncertain
      behavior, by site
  unspecified site
    benign D13.7
    malignant C25.4
    uncertain behavior D37.8
Glucoglycinuria E72.51
Glucose-galactose malabsorption E74.39
Glue
  ear — *see* Otitis, media, nonsuppurative, chronic,
    mucoid
  sniffing (airplane) — *see* Abuse, drug, inhalant
    dependence — *see* Dependence, drug, inhalant
Glutaric aciduria E72.3
Glycinemia E72.51
Glycinuria (renal) (with ketosis) E72.09
Glycogen
  infiltration — *see* Disease, glycogen storage
  storage disease — *see* Disease, glycogen storage
Glycogenosis (diffuse) (generalized) — *see*
  also Disease, glycogen storage
  cardiac E74.02 *[143]*
  diabetic, secondary — *see* Diabetes, glycogenosis,
    secondary
  pulmonary interstitial J84.842
Glycopenia E16.2
Glycosuria R81
  renal E74.8
Gnathostoma spinigerum (infection) (infestation)
, gnathostomiasis (wandering swelling) B83.1
Goiter (plunging) (substernal) E04.9
  with
    hyperthyroidism (recurrent) — *see*
      Hyperthyroidism, with, goiter
    thyrotoxicosis — *see* Hyperthyroidism, with, goiter
  adenomatous — *see* Goiter, nodular
  cancerous C73
  congenital (nontoxic) E03.0
    diffuse E03.0
    parenchymatous E03.0
    transitory, with normal functioning P72.0
  cystic E04.2
    due to iodine-deficiency E01.1
  due to
    enzyme defect in synthesis of thyroid
      hormone E07.1
    iodine-deficiency (endemic) E01.2
  dyshormonogenetic (familial) E07.1
  endemic (iodine-deficiency) E01.2
    diffuse E01.0
    multinodular E01.1
  exophthalmic — *see* Hyperthyroidism, with, goiter
  iodine-deficiency (endemic) E01.2
    diffuse E01.0
    multinodular E01.1
    nodular E01.1
  lingual Q89.2
  lymphadenoid E06.3
  malignant C73
  multinodular (cystic) (nontoxic) E04.2
    toxic or with hyperthyroidism E05.20
      with thyroid storm E05.21
  neonatal NEC P72.0
  nodular (nontoxic) (due to) E04.9
    with
      hyperthyroidism E05.20
        with thyroid storm E05.21
      thyrotoxicosis E05.20
        with thyroid storm E05.21
    endemic E01.1
    iodine-deficiency E01.1
    sporadic E04.9
    toxic E05.20
      with thyroid storm E05.21
  nontoxic E04.9
    diffuse (colloid) E04.0
    multinodular E04.2
    simple E04.0
    specified NEC E04.8

Goiter (plunging) (substernal) - *continued*
  nontoxic - *continued*
    uninodular E04.1
    simple E04.0
  toxic — *see* Hyperthyroidism, with, goiter
  uninodular (nontoxic) E04.1
    toxic or with hyperthyroidism E05.10
      with thyroid storm E05.11
Goiter-deafness syndrome E07.1
Goldberg syndrome Q89.8
Goldberg-Maxwell syndrome E34.51
Goldblatt's hypertension or kidney I70.1
Goldenhar (-Gorlin) **syndrome** Q87.0
Goldflam-Erb disease or syndrome G70.00
  with exacerbation (acute) G70.01
  in crisis G70.01
Goldscheider's disease Q81.8
Goldstein's disease
  (familial hemorrhagic telangiectasia) I78.0
Golfer's elbow — *see* Epicondylitis, medial
Gonadoblastoma
  specified site — *see* Neoplasm, uncertain behavior,
    by site
  unspecified site
    female D39.10
    male D40.10
Gonecystitis — *see* Vesiculitis
Gongylonemiasis B83.8
Goniosynechiae — *see* Adhesions, iris,
  goniosynechiae
Gonococcemia A54.86
Gonococcus, gonococcal (disease) (infection) —
  see also condition A54.9
  anus A54.6
  bursa, bursitis A54.49
  conjunctiva, conjunctivitis (neonatorum) A54.31
  endocardium A54.83
  eye A54.30
    conjunctivitis A54.31
    iridocyclitis A54.32
    keratitis A54.33
    newborn A54.31
    other specified A54.39
  fallopian tubes (acute) (chronic) A54.24
  genitourinary (organ) (system) (tract) (acute)
    lower A54.00
      with abscess (accessory gland)
        (periurethral) A54.1
    upper — *see also* condition A54.29
  heart A54.83
  iridocyclitis A54.32
  joint A54.42
  lymphatic (gland) (node) A54.89
  meninges, meningitis A54.81
  musculoskeletal A54.40
    arthritis A54.42
    osteomyelitis A54.43
    other specified A54.49
    spondylopathy A54.41
  pelviperitonitis A54.24
  pelvis (acute) (chronic) A54.24
  pharynx A54.5
  proctitis A54.6
  pyosalpinx (acute) (chronic) A54.24
  rectum A54.6
  skin A54.89
  specified site NEC A54.89
  tendon sheath A54.49
  throat A54.5
  urethra (acute) (chronic) A54.01
    with abscess (accessory gland) (periurethral) A54.1
  vulva (acute) (chronic) A54.02
Gonocytoma
  specified site — *see* Neoplasm, uncertain behavior,
    by site
  unspecified site
    female D39.10
    male D40.10
Gonorrhea (acute) (chronic) A54.9
  Bartholin's gland (acute) (chronic) (purulent) A54.02
    with abscess (accessory gland) (periurethral) A54.1
  bladder A54.01
  cervix A54.03
  conjunctiva, conjunctivitis (neonatorum) A54.31
  contact Z20.2
  Cowper's gland (with abscess) A54.1
  exposure to Z20.2
  fallopian tube (acute) (chronic) A54.24
  kidney (acute) (chronic) A54.21
  lower genitourinary tract A54.00
    with abscess (accessory gland) (periurethral) A54.1
  ovary (acute) (chronic) A54.24
  pelvis (acute) (chronic) A54.24

Gonorrhea (acute) (chronic) - *continued*
  pelvis (acute) (chronic) - *continued*
    female pelvic inflammatory disease A54.24
  penis A54.09
  prostate (acute) (chronic) A54.22
  seminal vesicle (acute) (chronic) A54.23
  specified site not listed — *see*
    also Gonococcus A54.89
  spermatic cord (acute) (chronic) A54.23
  urethra A54.01
    with abscess (accessory gland) (periurethral) A54.1
  vagina A54.02
  vas deferens (acute) (chronic) A54.23
  vulva A54.02
Goodall's disease A08.19
Goodpasture's syndrome M31.0
Gopalan's syndrome (burning feet) E53.0
Gorlin-Chaudry-Moss syndrome Q87.0
Gottron's papules L94.4
Gougerot-Blum syndrome
  (pigmented purpuric lichenoid dermatitis) L81.7
Gougerot-Carteaud disease or syndrome
  (confluent reticulate papillomatosis) L83
Gougerot's syndrome (trisymptomatic) L81.7
Gouley's syndrome (constrictive pericarditis) I31.1
Goundou A66.6
Gout, chronic — *see also* Gout, gouty M1A.9
  drug-induced M1A.20
    ankle M1A.27-
    elbow M1A.22-
    foot joint M1A.27-
    hand joint M1A.24-
    hip M1A.25-
    knee M1A.26-
    multiple site M1A.29-
    shoulder M1A.21-
    vertebrae M1A.28
    wrist M1A.23-
  idiopathic M1A.00
    ankle M1A.07-
    elbow M1A.02-
    foot joint M1A.07-
    hand joint M1A.04-
    hip M1A.05-
    knee M1A.06-
    multiple site M1A.09-
    shoulder M1A.01-
    vertebrae M1A.08
    wrist M1A.03-
  in (due to) renal impairment M1A.30
    ankle M1A.37-
    elbow M1A.32-
    foot joint M1A.37-
    hand joint M1A.34-
    hip M1A.35-
    knee M1A.36-
    multiple site M1A.39-
    shoulder M1A.31-
    vertebrae M1A.38
    wrist M1A.33-
  lead-induced M1A.10
    ankle M1A.17-
    elbow M1A.12-
    foot joint M1A.17-
    hand joint M1A.14-
    hip M1A.15-
    knee M1A.16-
    multiple site M1A.19-
    shoulder M1A.11-
    vertebrae M1A.18
    wrist M1A.13-
  primary — *see* Gout, chronic, idiopathic
  saturnine — *see* Gout, chronic, lead-induced
  secondary NEC M1A.40
    ankle M1A.47-
    elbow M1A.42-
    foot joint M1A.47-
    hand joint M1A.44-
    hip M1A.45-
    knee M1A.46-
    multiple site M1A.49-
    shoulder M1A.41-
    vertebrae M1A.48
    wrist M1A.43-
  syphilitic (*see also* subcategory M14.8-) A52.77
  tophi M1A.9
Gout, gouty (acute) (attack) (flare) — *see also* Gout,
  chronic M10.9
  drug-induced M10.20
    ankle M10.27-
    elbow M10.22-
    foot joint M10.27-
    hand joint M10.24-

Gout, gouty (acute) (attack) (flare) - *continued*
  drug-induced - *continued*
    hip M10.25-
    knee M10.26-
    multiple site M10.29
    shoulder M10.21-
    vertebrae M10.28
    wrist M10.23-
  idiopathic M10.00
    ankle M10.07-
    elbow M10.02-
    foot joint M10.07-
    hand joint M10.04-
    hip M10.05-
    knee M10.06-
    multiple site M10.09
    shoulder M10.01-
    vertebrae M10.08
    wrist M10.03-
  in (due to) renal impairment M10.30
    ankle M10.37-
    elbow M10.32-
    foot joint M10.37-
    hand joint M10.34-
    hip M10.35-
    knee M10.36-
    multiple site M10.39
    shoulder M10.31-
    vertebrae M10.38
    wrist M10.33-
  lead-induced M10.10
    ankle M10.17-
    elbow M10.12-
    foot joint M10.17-
    hand joint M10.14-
    hip M10.15-
    knee M10.16-
    multiple site M10.19
    shoulder M10.11-
    vertebrae M10.18
    wrist M10.13-
  primary — *see* Gout, idiopathic
  saturnine — *see* Gout, lead-induced
  secondary NEC M10.40
    ankle M10.47-
    elbow M10.42-
    foot joint M10.47-
    hand joint M10.44-
    hip M10.45-
    knee M10.46-
    multiple site M10.49
    shoulder M10.41-
    vertebrae M10.48
    wrist M10.43-
  syphilitic (*see also* subcategory M14.8-) A52.77
  tophi — *see* Gout, chronic
Gower's
  muscular dystrophy G71.0
  syndrome (vasovagal attack) R55
Gradenigo's syndrome — *see* Otitis, media, suppurative, acute
Graefe's disease — *see* Strabismus, paralytic, ophthalmoplegia, progressive
Graft-versus-host disease D89.813
  acute D89.810
  acute on chronic D89.812
  chronic D89.811
Grain mite (itch) B88.0
Grainhandler's disease or lung J67.8
Grand mal — *see* Epilepsy, generalized, specified NEC
Grand multipara status only (not pregnant) Z64.1
  pregnant — *see* Pregnancy, complicated by, grand multiparity
Granite worker's lung J62.8
Granular — *see also* condition
  inflammation, pharynx J31.2
  kidney (contracting) — *see* Sclerosis, renal
  liver K74.69
Granulation tissue (abnormal) (excessive) L92.9
  postmastoidectomy cavity — *see* Complications, postmastoidectomy, granulation
Granulocytopenia (primary) (malignant) — *see* Agranulocytosis
Granuloma L92.9
  abdomen K66.8
    from residual foreign body L92.3
    pyogenicum L98.0
  actinic L57.5
  annulare (perforating) L92.0
  apical K04.5
  aural — *see* Otitis, externa, specified NEC
  beryllium (skin) L92.3

Granuloma - *continued*
  bone
    eosinophilic C96.6
    from residual foreign body — *see* Osteomyelitis, specified type NEC
    lung C96.6
  brain (any site) G06.0
    schistosomiasis B65.9 [G07]
  canaliculus lacrimalis — *see* Granuloma, lacrimal
  candidal (cutaneous) B37.2
  cerebral (any site) G06.0
  coccidioidal (primary) (progressive) B38.7
    lung B38.1
    meninges B38.4
  colon K63.89
  conjunctiva H11.22-
  dental K04.5
  ear, middle — *see* Cholesteatoma
  eosinophilic C96.6
    bone C96.6
    lung C96.6
    oral mucosa K13.4
    skin L92.2
  eyelid H01.8
  facial (e) L92.2
  foreign body (in soft tissue) NEC M60.20
    ankle M60.27-
    foot M60.27-
    forearm M60.23-
    hand M60.24-
    in operation wound — *see* Foreign body, accidentally left during a procedure
    lower leg M60.26-
    pelvic region M60.25-
    shoulder region M60.21-
    skin L92.3
    specified site NEC M60.28
    subcutaneous tissue L92.3
    thigh M60.25-
    upper arm M60.22-
  gangraenescens M31.2
  genito-inguinale A58
  giant cell (central) (reparative) (jaw) M27.1
    gingiva (peripheral) K06.8
  gland (lymph) I88.8
  hepatic NEC K75.3
    in (due to)
      berylliosis J63.2 [K77]
      sarcoidosis D86.89
  Hodgkin C81.9
  ileum K63.89
  infectious B99.9
    specified NEC B99.8
  inguinale (Donovan) (venereal) A58
  intestine NEC K63.89
  intracranial (any site) G06.0
  intraspinal (any part) G06.1
  iridocyclitis — *see* Iridocyclitis, chronic
  jaw (bone) (central) M27.1
    reparative giant cell M27.1
  kidney — *see also* Infection, kidney N15.8
  lacrimal H04.81-
  larynx J38.7
  lethal midline (faciale (e)) M31.2
  liver NEC — *see* Granuloma, hepatic
  lung (infectious) — *see also* Fibrosis, lung
    coccidioidal B38.1
    eosinophilic C96.6
  Majocchi's B35.8
  malignant (facial (e)) M31.2
  mandible (central) M27.1
  midline (lethal) M31.2
  monilial (cutaneous) B37.2
  nasal sinus — *see* Sinusitis
  operation wound T81.89
    foreign body — *see* Foreign body, accidentally left during a procedure
    stitch T81.89
    talc — *see* Foreign body, accidentally left during a procedure
  oral mucosa K13.4
  orbit, orbital H05.11-
  paracoccidioidal B41.8
  penis, venereal A58
  periapical K04.5
  peritoneum K66.8
    due to ova of helminths NOS — *see also* Helminthiasis B83.9 [K67]
  postmastoidectomy cavity — *see* Complications, postmastoidectomy, recurrent cholesteatoma
  prostate N42.89
  pudendi (ulcerating) A58
  pulp, internal (tooth) K03.3

Granuloma - *continued*
  pyogenic, pyogenicum (of) (skin) L98.0
    gingiva K06.8
    maxillary alveolar ridge K04.5
    oral mucosa K13.4
  rectum K62.89
  reticulohistiocytic D76.3
  rubrum nasi L74.8
  Schistosoma — *see* Schistosomiasis
  septic (skin) L98.0
  silica (skin) L92.3
  sinus (accessory) (infective) (nasal) — *see* Sinusitis
  skin L92.9
    from residual foreign body L92.3
    pyogenicum L98.0
  spine
    syphilitic (epidural) A52.19
    tuberculous A18.01
  stitch (postoperative) T81.89
  suppurative (skin) L98.0
  swimming pool A31.1
  talc — *see also* Granuloma, foreign body
    in operation wound — *see* Foreign body, accidentally left during a procedure
  telangiectaticum (skin) L98.0
  tracheostomy J95.09
  trichophyticum B35.8
  tropicum A66.4
  umbilicus L92.9
  urethra N36.8
  uveitis — *see* Iridocyclitis, chronic
  vagina A58
  venereum A58
  vocal cord J38.3
Granulomatosis L92.9
  lymphoid C83.8-
  miliary (listerial) A32.89
  necrotizing, respiratory M31.30
  progressive septic D71
  specified NEC L92.8
  Wegener's M31.30
    with renal involvement M31.31
Granulomatous tissue (abnormal) (excessive) L92.9
Granulosis rubra nasi L74.8
Graphite fibrosis (of lung) J63.3
Graphospasm F48.8
  organic G25.89
Grating scapula M89.8X1
Gravel (urinary) — *see* Calculus, urinary
Graves' disease — *see* Hyperthyroidism, with, goiter
Gravis — *see* condition
Grawitz tumor C64.-
Gray syndrome (newborn) P93.0
Grayness, hair (premature) L67.1
  congenital Q84.2
Green sickness D50.8
Greenfield's disease
  meaning
    concentric sclerosis (encephalitis periaxialis concentrica) G37.5
    metachromatic leukodystrophy E75.25
Greenstick fracture - code as Fracture, by site
Grey syndrome (newborn) P93.0
Grief F43.21
  prolonged F43.29
  reaction — *see also* Disorder, adjustment F43.20
Griesinger's disease B76.9
Grinder's lung or pneumoconiosis J62.8
Grinding, teeth
  psychogenic F45.8
  sleep related G47.63
Grip
  Dabney's B33.0
  devil's B33.0
Grippe, grippal — *see also* Influenza
  Balkan A78
  summer, of Italy A93.1
Grisel's disease M43.6
Groin — *see* condition
Grooved tongue K14.5
Ground itch B76.9
Grover's disease or syndrome L11.1
Growing pains, children R29.898
Growth (fungoid) (neoplastic) (new) — *see also* Neoplasm
  adenoid (vegetative) J35.8
  benign — *see* Neoplasm, benign, by site
  malignant — *see* Neoplasm, malignant, by site
  rapid, childhood Z00.2
  secondary — *see* Neoplasm, secondary, by site
Gruby's disease B35.0
Gubler-Millard paralysis or syndrome G46.3
Guerin-Stern syndrome Q74.3

Guidance, insufficient anterior (occlusal) M26.54
Guillain-Barré disease or syndrome G61.0
  sequelae G65.0
Guinea worms (infection) (infestation) B72
Guinon's disease (motor-verbal tic) F95.2
Gull's disease E03.4
Gum — *see* condition
Gumboil K04.7
  with sinus K04.6
Gumma (syphilitic) A52.79
  artery A52.09
    cerebral A52.04
  bone A52.77
    of yaws (late) A66.6
  brain A52.19
  cauda equina A52.19
  central nervous system A52.3
  ciliary body A52.71
  congenital A50.59
  eyelid A52.71
  heart A52.06
  intracranial A52.19
  iris A52.71
  kidney A52.75
  larynx A52.73
  leptomeninges A52.19
  liver A52.74
  meninges A52.19
  myocardium A52.06
  nasopharynx A52.73
  neurosyphilitic A52.3
  nose A52.73
  orbit A52.71
  palate (soft) A52.79
  penis A52.76
  pericardium A52.06
  pharynx A52.73
  pituitary A52.79
  scrofulous (tuberculous) A18.4
  skin A52.79
  specified site NEC A52.79
  spinal cord A52.19
  tongue A52.79
  tonsil A52.73
  trachea A52.73
  tuberculous A18.4
  ulcerative due to yaws A66.4
  ureter A52.75
  yaws A66.4
    bone A66.6
Gunn's syndrome Q07.8
Gunshot wound — *see also* Wound, open
  fracture - code as Fracture, by site
  internal organs — *see* Injury, by site
Gynandrism Q56.0
Gynandroblastoma
  specified site — *see* Neoplasm, uncertain behavior, by site
  unspecified site
    female D39.10
    male D40.10
Gynecological examination (periodic) (routine) Z01.419
  with abnormal findings Z01.411
Gynecomastia N62
Gynephobia F40.291
Gyrate scalp Q82.8

H

H (Hartnup's) **disease** E72.02
Haas' disease or osteochondrosis (juvenile) (head of humerus) — *see* Osteochondrosis, juvenile, humerus
Habit, habituation
  bad sleep Z72.821
  chorea F95.8
  disturbance, child F98.9
  drug — *see* Dependence, drug
  irregular sleep Z72.821
  laxative F55.2
  spasm — *see* Tic
  tic — *see* Tic
Haemophilus (H.)
  influenzae, as cause of disease classified elsewhere B96.3
Haff disease — *see* Poisoning, mercury
Hageman's factor defect, deficiency or disease D68.2
Haglund's disease or osteochondrosis (juvenile) (os tibiale externum) — *see* Osteochondrosis, juvenile, tarsus
Hailey-Hailey disease Q82.8

Hair — *see also* condition
  plucking F63.3
    in stereotyped movement disorder F98.4
  tourniquet syndrome — *see also* Constriction, external, by site
    finger S60.44-
    penis S30.842
    thumb S60.34-
    toe S90.44-
Hairball in stomach T18.2
Hair-pulling, pathological (compulsive) F63.3
Hairy black tongue K14.3
Half vertebra Q76.49
Halitosis R19.6
Hallerman-Streiff syndrome Q87.0
Hallervorden-Spatz disease G23.0
Hallopeau's acrodermatitis or disease L40.2
Hallucination R44.3
  auditory R44.0
  gustatory R44.2
  olfactory R44.2
  specified NEC R44.2
  tactile R44.2
  visual R44.1
Hallucinosis (chronic) F28
  alcoholic (acute) F10.951
    in
      abuse F10.151
      dependence F10.251
  drug-induced F19.951
    cannabis F12.951
    cocaine F14.951
    hallucinogen F16.151
    in
      abuse F19.151
        cannabis F12.151
        cocaine F14.151
        hallucinogen F16.151
        inhalant F18.151
        opioid F11.151
        sedative, anxiolytic or hypnotic F13.151
        stimulant NEC F15.151
      dependence F19.251
        cannabis F12.251
        cocaine F14.251
        hallucinogen F16.251
        inhalant F18.251
        opioid F11.251
        sedative, anxiolytic or hypnotic F13.251
        stimulant NEC F15.251
    inhalant F18.951
    opioid F11.951
    sedative, anxiolytic or hypnotic F13.951
    stimulant NEC F15.951
  organic F06.0
Hallux
  deformity (acquired) NEC M20.5X-
  limitus M20.5X-
  malleus (acquired) NEC M20.3-
  rigidus (acquired) M20.2-
    congenital Q74.2
    sequelae (late effect) of rickets E64.3
  valgus (acquired) M20.1-
    congenital Q66.6
  varus (acquired) M20.3-
    congenital Q66.3
Halo, visual H53.19
Hamartoma, hamartoblastoma Q85.9
  epithelial (gingival) , odontogenic, central or peripheral — *see* Cyst, calcifying odontogenic
Hamartosis Q85.9
Hamman-Rich syndrome J84.114
Hammer toe (acquired) **NEC** — *see also* Deformity, toe, hammer toe
  congenital Q66.89
  sequelae (late effect) of rickets E64.3
Hand — *see* condition
Hand-foot syndrome L27.1
Handicap, handicapped
  educational Z55.9
  specified NEC Z55.8
Hand-Schüller-Christian disease or syndrome C96.5
Hanging (asphyxia) (strangulation) (suffocation) — *see* Asphyxia, traumatic, due to mechanical threat
Hangnail — *see also* Cellulitis, digit
  with lymphangitis — *see* Lymphangitis, acute, digit
Hangover (alcohol) F10.129
Hanhart's syndrome Q87.0
Hanot-Chauffard (-Troisier) **syndrome** E83.19
Hanot's cirrhosis or disease K74.3
Hansen's disease — *see* Leprosy

Hantaan virus disease (Korean hemorrhagic fever) A98.5
Hantavirus disease (with renal manifestations) (Dobrava) (Puumala) (Seoul) A98.5
  with pulmonary manifestations (Andes) (Bayou) (Bermejo) (Black Creek Canal) (Choclo) (Juquitiba) (Laguna negra) (Lechiguanas) (New York) (Oran) (Sin nombre) B33.4
Happy puppet syndrome Q93.5
Harada's disease or syndrome H30.81-
Hardening
  artery — *see* Arteriosclerosis
  brain G93.89
Harelip (complete) (incomplete) — *see* Cleft, lip
Harlequin (newborn) Q80.4
Harley's disease D59.6
Harmful use (of)
  alcohol F10.10
  anxiolytics — *see* Abuse, drug, sedative
  cannabinoids — *see* Abuse, drug, cannabis
  cocaine — *see* Abuse, drug, cocaine
  drug — *see* Abuse, drug
  hallucinogens — *see* Abuse, drug, hallucinogen
  hypnotics — *see* Abuse, drug, sedative
  opioids — *see* Abuse, drug, opioid
  PCP (phencyclidine) — *see* Abuse, drug, hallucinogen
  sedatives — *see* Abuse, drug, sedative
  stimulants NEC — *see* Abuse, drug, stimulant
Harris' lines — *see* Arrest, epiphyseal
Hartnup's disease E72.02
Harvester's lung J67.0
Harvesting ovum for in vitro fertilization Z31.83
Hashimoto's disease or thyroiditis E06.3
Hashitoxicosis (transient) E06.3
Hassal-Henle bodies or warts (cornea) H18.49
Haut mal — *see* Epilepsy, generalized, specified NEC
Haverhill fever A25.1
Hay fever — *see also* Fever, hay J30.1
Hayem-Widal syndrome D59.8
Haygarth's nodes M15.8
Haymaker's lung J67.0
Hb (abnormal)
  Bart's disease D56.0
  disease — *see* Disease, hemoglobin
  trait — *see* Trait
Head — *see* condition
Headache R51
  allergic NEC G44.89
  associated with sexual activity G44.82
  chronic daily R51
  cluster G44.009
    chronic G44.029
      intractable G44.021
      not intractable G44.029
    episodic G44.019
      intractable G44.011
      not intractable G44.019
    intractable G44.001
    not intractable G44.009
  cough (primary) G44.83
  daily chronic R51
  drug-induced NEC G44.40
    intractable G44.41
    not intractable G44.40
  exertional (primary) G44.84
  histamine G44.009
    intractable G44.001
    not intractable G44.009
  hypnic G44.81
  lumbar puncture G97.1
  medication overuse G44.40
    intractable G44.41
    not intractable G44.40
  menstrual — *see* Migraine, menstrual
  migraine (type) — *see also* Migraine G43.909
  nasal septum R51
  neuralgiform, short lasting unilateral, with conjunctival injection and tearing (SUNCT) G44.059
    intractable G44.051
    not intractable G44.059
  new daily persistent (NDPH) G44.52
  orgasmic G44.82
  periodic syndromes in adults and children G43.C0
    with refractory migraine G43.C1
      intractable G43.C1
      not intractable G43.C0
    without refractory migraine G43.C0
  postspinal puncture G97.1
  post-traumatic G44.309
    acute G44.319

Headache - *continued*
  post-traumatic - *continued*
    acute - *continued*
      intractable G44.311
      not intractable G44.319
    chronic G44.329
      intractable G44.321
      not intractable G44.329
    intractable G44.301
    not intractable G44.309
  pre-menstrual — *see* Migraine, menstrual
  preorgasmic G44.82
  primary
    cough G44.83
    exertional G44.84
    stabbing G44.85
    thunderclap G44.53
  rebound G44.40
    intractable G44.41
    not intractable G44.40
  short lasting unilateral neuralgiform, with
    conjunctival injection and tearing
    (SUNCT) G44.059
    intractable G44.051
    not intractable G44.059
  specified syndrome NEC G44.89
  spinal and epidural anesthesia - induced T88.59
    in labor and delivery O74.5
    in pregnancy O29.4-
    postpartum, puerperal O89.4
  spinal fluid loss (from puncture) G97.1
  stabbing (primary) G44.85
  tension (-type) G44.209
    chronic G44.229
      intractable G44.221
      not intractable G44.229
    episodic G44.219
      intractable G44.211
      not intractable G44.219
    intractable G44.201
    not intractable G44.209
  thunderclap (primary) G44.53
  vascular NEC G44.1
Healthy
  infant
    accompanying sick mother Z76.3
    receiving care Z76.2
  person accompanying sick person Z76.3
Hearing examination Z01.10
  with abnormal findings NEC Z01.118
  following failed hearing screening Z01.110
  for hearing conservation and treatment Z01.12
Heart — *see* condition
Heart beat
  abnormality R00.9
    specified NEC R00.8
  awareness R00.2
  rapid R00.0
  slow R00.1
Heartburn R12
  psychogenic F45.8
Heat (effects) T67.9
  apoplexy T67.0
  burn — *see also* Burn L55.9
  collapse T67.1
  cramps T67.2
  dermatitis or eczema L59.0
  edema T67.7
  erythema - code by site under Burn, first degree
  excessive T67.9
    specified effect NEC T67.8
  exhaustion T67.5
    anhydrotic T67.3
    due to
      salt (and water) depletion T67.4
      water depletion T67.3
        with salt depletion T67.4
  fatigue (transient) T67.6
  fever T67.0
  hyperpyrexia T67.0
  prickly L74.0
  prostration — *see* Heat, exhaustion
  pyrexia T67.0
  rash L74.0
  specified effect NEC T67.8
  stroke T67.0
  sunburn — *see* Sunburn
  syncope T67.1
Heavy-for-dates NEC (infant) (4000g to 4499g) P08.1
  exceptionally (4500g or more) P08.0
Hebephrenia, hebephrenic (schizophrenia) F20.1

Heberden's disease or nodes (with arthropathy) M15.1
Hebra's
  pityriasis L26
  prurigo L28.2
Heel — *see* condition
Heerfordt's disease D86.89
Hegglin's anomaly or syndrome D72.0
Heilmeyer-Schoner disease D45
Heine-Medin disease A80.9
Heinz body anemia, congenital D58.2
Heliophobia F40.228
Heller's disease or syndrome F84.3
HELLP syndrome
  (hemolysis, elevated liver enzymes and low platelet count) O14.2-
  complicating
    childbirth O14.24
    puerperium O14.25
Helminthiasis — *see also* Infestation, helminth
  Ancylostoma B76.0
  intestinal B82.0
    mixed types (types classifiable to more than one of the titles B65.0-B81.3 and B81.8) B81.4
    specified type NEC B81.8
  mixed types (intestinal) (types classifiable to more than one of the titles B65.0-B81.3 and B81.8) B81.4
  Necator (americanus) B76.1
  specified type NEC B83.8
Heloma L84
Hemangioblastoma — *see* Neoplasm, connective tissue, uncertain behavior
  malignant — *see* Neoplasm, connective tissue, malignant
Hemangioendothelioma — *see also* Neoplasm, uncertain behavior, by site
  benign D18.00
    intra-abdominal D18.03
    intracranial D18.02
    skin D18.01
    specified site NEC D18.09
  bone (diffuse) — *see* Neoplasm, bone, malignant
  epithelioid — *see also* Neoplasm, uncertain behavior, by site
    malignant — *see* Neoplasm, malignant, by site
  malignant — *see* Neoplasm, connective tissue, malignant
Hemangiofibroma — *see* Neoplasm, benign, by site
Hemangiolipoma — *see* Lipoma
Hemangioma D18.00
  arteriovenous D18.00
    intra-abdominal D18.03
    intracranial D18.02
    skin D18.01
    specified site NEC D18.09
  capillary D18.00
    intra-abdominal D18.03
    intracranial D18.02
    skin D18.01
    specified site NEC D18.09
  cavernous D18.00
    intra-abdominal D18.03
    intracranial D18.02
    skin D18.01
    specified site NEC D18.09
  epithelioid D18.00
    intra-abdominal D18.03
    intracranial D18.02
    skin D18.01
    specified site NEC D18.09
  histiocytoid D18.00
    intra-abdominal D18.03
    intracranial D18.02
    skin D18.01
    specified site NEC D18.09
  infantile D18.00
    intra-abdominal D18.03
    intracranial D18.02
    skin D18.01
    specified site NEC D18.09
  intra-abdominal D18.03
  intracranial D18.02
  intramuscular D18.00
    intra-abdominal D18.03
    intracranial D18.02
    skin D18.01
    specified site NEC D18.09
  intrathoracic structures D18.09
  juvenile D18.00
  malignant — *see* Neoplasm,connective tissue, malignant
  plexiform D18.00

Hemangioma - *continued*
  plexiform - *continued*
    intra-abdominal D18.03
    intracranial D18.02
    skin D18.01
    specified site NEC D18.09
  racemose D18.00
    intra-abdominal D18.03
    intracranial D18.02
    skin D18.01
    specified site NEC D18.09
  sclerosing — *see* Neoplasm,skin, benign
  simplex D18.00
    intra-abdominal D18.03
    intracranial D18.02
    skin D18.01
    specified site NEC D18.09
  skin D18.01
  specified site NEC D18.09
  venous D18.00
    intra-abdominal D18.03
    intracranial D18.02
    skin D18.01
    specified site NEC D18.09
  verrucous keratotic D18.00
    intra-abdominal D18.03
    intracranial D18.02
    skin D18.01
    specified site NEC D18.09
Hemangiomatosis (systemic) I78.8
  involving single site — *see* Hemangioma
Hemangiopericytoma — *see also* Neoplasm, connective tissue, uncertain behavior
  benign — *see* Neoplasm, connective tissue, benign
  malignant — *see* Neoplasm, connective tissue, malignant
Hemangiosarcoma — *see* Neoplasm, connective tissue, malignant
Hemarthrosis (nontraumatic) M25.00
  ankle M25.07-
  elbow M25.02-
  foot joint M25.07-
  hand joint M25.04-
  hip M25.05-
  in hemophilic arthropathy — *see* Arthropathy, hemophilic
  knee M25.06-
  shoulder M25.01-
  specified joint NEC M25.08
  traumatic — *see* Sprain, by site
  vertebrae M25.08
  wrist M25.03-
Hematemesis K92.0
  with ulcer - code by site under Ulcer, with hemorrhage K27.4
  newborn, neonatal P54.0
    due to swallowed maternal blood P78.2
Hematidrosis L74.8
Hematinuria — *see also* Hemoglobinuria
  malarial B50.8
Hematobilia K83.8
Hematocele
  female NEC N94.89
    with ectopic pregnancy O00.90
      with intrauterine pregnancy O00.91
    ovary N83.8
  male N50.1
Hematochezia — *see also* Melena K92.1
Hematochyluria — *see also* Infestation, filarial
  schistosomiasis (bilharziasis) B65.0
Hematocolpos (with hematometra or hematosalpinx) N89.7
Hematocornea — *see* Pigmentation, cornea, stromal
Hematogenous — *see* condition
Hematoma (traumatic) (skin surface intact) — *see also* Contusion
  with
    injury of internal organs — *see* Injury, by site
    open wound — *see* Wound, open
  amputation stump (surgical) (late) T87.89
  aorta, dissecting I71.00
    abdominal I71.02
    thoracic I71.01
    thoracoabdominal I71.03
  aortic intramural — *see* Dissection, aorta
  arterial (complicating trauma) — *see* Injury, blood vessel, by site
  auricle — *see* Contusion, ear
    nontraumatic — *see* Disorder, pinna, hematoma
  birth injury NEC P15.8
  brain (traumatic)
    with

Hematoma (traumatic) (skin surface intact) - *continued*
  brain (traumatic) - *continued*
    with - *continued*
      cerebral laceration or contusion (diffuse) — *see* Injury, intracranial, diffuse
        focal — *see* Injury, intracranial, focal
    cerebellar, traumatic S06.37-
    newborn NEC P52.4
      birth injury P10.1
    intracerebral, traumatic — *see* Injury, intracranial, intracerebral hemorrhage
    nontraumatic — *see* Hemorrhage, intracranial
    subarachnoid, arachnoid, traumatic — *see* Injury, intracranial, subarachnoid hemorrhage
    subdural, traumatic — *see* Injury, intracranial, subdural hemorrhage
  breast (nontraumatic) N64.89
  broad ligament (nontraumatic) N83.7
    traumatic S37.892
  cerebellar, traumatic S06.37-
  cerebral — *see* Hematoma, brain
  cerebrum S06.36-
    left S06.35-
    right S06.34-
  cesarean delivery wound O90.2
  complicating delivery (perineal) (pelvic) (vagina) (vulva) O71.7
  corpus cavernosum (nontraumatic) N48.89
  epididymis (nontraumatic) N50.1
  epidural (traumatic) — *see* Injury, intracranial, epidural hemorrhage
    spinal — *see* Injury, spinal cord, by region
  episiotomy O90.2
  face, birth injury P15.4
  genital organ NEC (nontraumatic)
    female (nonobstetric) N94.89
      traumatic S30.202
    male N50.1
      traumatic S30.201
  internal organs — *see* Injury, by site
  intracerebral, traumatic — *see* Injury, intracranial, intracerebral hemorrhage
  intraoperative — *see* Complications, intraoperative, hemorrhage
  labia (nontraumatic) (nonobstetric) N90.89
  liver (subcapsular) (nontraumatic) K76.89
    birth injury P15.0
  mediastinum — *see* Injury, intrathoracic
  mesosalpinx (nontraumatic) N83.7
    traumatic S37.898
  muscle - code by site under Contusion
  nontraumatic
    muscle M79.81
    soft tissue M79.81
  obstetrical surgical wound O90.2
  orbit, orbital (nontraumatic) — *see also* Hemorrhage, orbit
    traumatic — *see* Contusion, orbit
  pelvis (female) (nontraumatic) (nonobstetric) N94.89
    obstetric O71.7
    traumatic — *see* Injury, by site
  penis (nontraumatic) N48.89
    birth injury P15.5
  perianal (nontraumatic) K64.5
  perineal S30.23
    complicating delivery O71.7
  perirenal — *see* Injury, kidney
  pinna — *see* Contusion, ear
    nontraumatic — *see* Disorder, pinna, hematoma
  placenta O43.89-
  postoperative (postprocedural) — *see* Complication, postprocedural, hematoma
  retroperitoneal (nontraumatic) K66.1
    traumatic S36.892
  scrotum, superficial S30.22
    birth injury P15.5
  seminal vesicle (nontraumatic) N50.1
    traumatic S37.892
  spermatic cord (traumatic) S37.892
    nontraumatic N50.1
  spinal (cord) (meninges) — *see also* Injury, spinal cord, by region
    newborn (birth injury) P11.5
  spleen D73.5
    intraoperative — *see* Complications, intraoperative, hemorrhage, spleen
    postprocedural (postoperative) — *see* Complications, postprocedural, hemorrhage, spleen
  sternocleidomastoid, birth injury P15.2
  sternomastoid, birth injury P15.2

Hematoma (traumatic) (skin surface intact) - *continued*
  subarachnoid (traumatic) — *see* Injury, intracranial, subarachnoid hemorrhage
    newborn (nontraumatic) P52.5
      due to birth injury P10.3
    nontraumatic — *see* Hemorrhage, intracranial, subarachnoid
  subdural (traumatic) — *see* Injury, intracranial, subdural hemorrhage
    newborn (localized) P52.8
      birth injury P10.0
    nontraumatic — *see* Hemorrhage, intracranial, subdural
    superficial, newborn P54.5
  testis (nontraumatic) N50.1
    birth injury P15.5
  tunica vaginalis (nontraumatic) N50.1
  umbilical cord, complicating delivery O69.5
  uterine ligament (broad) (nontraumatic) N83.7
    traumatic S37.892
  vagina (ruptured) (nontraumatic) N89.8
    complicating delivery O71.7
  vas deferens (nontraumatic) N50.1
    traumatic S37.892
  vitreous — *see* Hemorrhage, vitreous
  vulva (nontraumatic) (nonobstetric) N90.89
    complicating delivery O71.7
    newborn (birth injury) P15.5
Hematometra N85.7
  with hematocolpos N89.7
Hematomyelia (central) G95.19
  newborn (birth injury) P11.5
  traumatic T14.8
Hematomyelitis G04.90
Hematoperitoneum — *see* Hemoperitoneum
Hematophobia F40.230
Hematopneumothorax (see Hemothorax)
Hematopoiesis, cyclic D70.4
Hematoporphyria — *see* Porphyria
Hematorachis, hematorrhachis G95.19
  newborn (birth injury) P11.5
Hematosalpinx N83.6
  with
    hematocolpos N89.7
    hematometra N85.7
      with hematocolpos N89.7
  infectional — *see* Salpingitis
Hematospermia R36.1
Hematothorax (see Hemothorax)
Hematuria R31.9
  due to sulphonamide, sulfonamide — *see* Table of Drugs and Chemicals, by drug
  benign (familial) (of childhood) — *see also* Hematuria, idiopathic
    essential microscopic R31.1
  endemic — *see also* Schistosomiasis B65.0
  gross R31.0
  idiopathic N02.9
    with glomerular lesion
      crescentic (diffuse) glomerulonephritis N02.7
      dense deposit disease N02.6
      endocapillary proliferative glomerulonephritis N02.4
      focal and segmental hyalinosis or sclerosis N02.1
      membranoproliferative (diffuse) N02.5
      membranous (diffuse) N02.2
      mesangial proliferative (diffuse) N02.3
      mesangiocapillary (diffuse) N02.5
      minor abnormality N02.0
      proliferative NEC N02.8
      specified pathology NEC N02.8
  intermittent — *see* Hematuria, idiopathic
  malarial B50.8
  microscopic NEC (with symptoms) R31.29
    asymptomatic R31.21
    benign essential R31.1
  paroxysmal — *see also* Hematuria, idiopathic
    nocturnal D59.5
  persistent — *see* Hematuria, idiopathic
  recurrent — *see* Hematuria, idiopathic
  tropical — *see also* Schistosomiasis B65.0
  tuberculous A18.13
Hemeralopia (day blindness) H53.11
  vitamin A deficiency E50.5
Hemi-akinesia R41.4
Hemianalgesia R20.0
Hemianencephaly Q00.0
Hemianesthesia R20.0
Hemianopia, hemianopsia (heteronymous) H53.47
  homonymous H53.46-
  syphilitic A52.71
Hemiathetosis R25.8

Hemiatrophy R68.89
  cerebellar G31.9
  face, facial, progressive (Romberg) G51.8
  tongue K14.8
Hemiballism (us) G25.5
Hemicardia Q24.8
Hemicephalus, hemicephaly Q00.0
Hemichorea G25.5
Hemicolitis, left — *see* Colitis, left sided
Hemicrania
  congenital malformation Q00.0
  continua G44.51
  meaning migraine — *see also* Migraine G43.909
  paroxysmal G44.039
    chronic G44.049
      intractable G44.041
      not intractable G44.049
    episodic G44.039
      intractable G44.031
      not intractable G44.039
    intractable G44.031
    not intractable G44.039
Hemidystrophy — *see* Hemiatrophy
Hemiectromelia Q73.8
Hemihypalgesia R20.8
Hemihypesthesia R20.1
Hemi-inattention R41.4
Hemimelia Q73.8
  lower limb — *see* Defect, reduction, lower limb, specified type NEC
  upper limb — *see* Defect, reduction, upper limb, specified type NEC
Hemiparalysis — *see* Hemiplegia
Hemiparesis — *see* Hemiplegia
Hemiparesthesia R20.2
Hemiparkinsonism G20
Hemiplegia G81.9-
  alternans facialis G83.89
  ascending NEC G81.90
    spinal G95.89
  congenital (cerebral) G80.8
    spastic G80.2
  embolic (current episode) I63.4-
  flaccid G81.0-
  following
    cerebrovascular disease I69.959
      cerebral infarction I69.35-
      intracerebral hemorrhage I69.15-
      nontraumatic intracranial hemorrhage NEC I69.25-
      specified disease NEC I69.85-
      stroke NOS I69.35-
      subarachnoid hemorrhage I69.05-
  hysterical F44.4
  newborn NEC P91.8
    birth injury P11.9
  spastic G81.1-
    congenital G80.2
  thrombotic (current episode) I63.3-
Hemisection, spinal cord — *see* Injury, spinal cord, by region
Hemispasm (facial) R25.2
Hemisporosis B48.8
Hemitremor R25.1
Hemivertebra Q76.49
  failure of segmentation with scoliosis Q76.3
  fusion with scoliosis Q76.3
Hemochromatosis E83.119
  with refractory anemia D46.1
  due to repeated red blood cell transfusion E83.111
  hereditary (primary) E83.110
  primary E83.110
  specified NEC E83.118
Hemoglobin — *see also* condition
  abnormal (disease) — *see* Disease, hemoglobin
  AS genotype D57.3
  Constant Spring D58.2
  E-beta thalassemia D56.5
  fetal, hereditary persistence (HPFH) D56.4
  H Constant Spring D56.0
  low NOS D64.9
  S (Hb S), heterozygous D57.3
Hemoglobinemia D59.9
  due to blood transfusion T80.89
  paroxysmal D59.6
    nocturnal D59.5
Hemoglobinopathy (mixed) D58.2
  with thalassemia D56.8
  sickle-cell D57.1
    with thalassemia D57.40
      with crisis (vasoocclusive pain) D57.419
      with
        acute chest syndrome D57.411

Hemoglobinopathy (mixed) - *continued*
  sickle-cell - *continued*
    with thalassemia - *continued*
      with crisis (vasoocclusive pain) - *continued*
        with - *continued*
          splenic sequestration D57.412
        without crisis D57.40
Hemoglobinuria R82.3
  with anemia, hemolytic, acquired (chronic) NEC D59.6
  cold (agglutinin) (paroxysmal) (with Raynaud's syndrome) D59.6
  due to exertion or hemolysis NEC D59.6
  intermittent D59.6
  malarial B50.8
  march D59.6
  nocturnal (paroxysmal) D59.5
  paroxysmal (cold) D59.6
    nocturnal D59.5
Hemolymphangioma D18.1
Hemolysis
  intravascular
    with
      abortion — *see* Abortion, by type, complicated by, hemorrhage
      ectopic or molar pregnancy O08.1
      hemorrhage
        antepartum — *see* Hemorrhage, antepartum, with coagulation defect
        intrapartum — *see also* Hemorrhage, complicating, delivery O67.0
      postpartum O72.3
  neonatal (excessive) P58.9
    specified NEC P58.8
Hemolytic — *see* condition
Hemopericardium I31.2
  following acute myocardial infarction (current complication) I23.0
  newborn P54.8
  traumatic — *see* Injury, heart, with hemopericardium
Hemoperitoneum K66.1
  infectional K65.9
  traumatic S36.899
    with open wound — *see* Wound, open, with penetration into peritoneal cavity
Hemophilia (classical) (familial) (hereditary) D66
  A D66
  B D67
  C D68.1
  acquired D68.311
  autoimmune D68.311
  calcipriva — *see also* Defect, coagulation D68.4
  nonfamilial — *see also* Defect, coagulation D68.4
  secondary D68.311
  vascular D68.0
Hemophthalmos H44.81-
Hemopneumothorax — *see also* Hemothorax
  traumatic S27.2
Hemoptysis R04.2
  newborn P26.9
  tuberculous — *see* Tuberculosis, pulmonary
Hemorrhage, hemorrhagic (concealed) R58
  abdomen R58
  accidental antepartum — *see* Hemorrhage, antepartum
  acute idiopathic pulmonary, in infants R04.81
  adenoid J35.8
  adrenal (capsule) (gland) E27.49
    medulla E27.8
    newborn P54.4
  after delivery — *see* Hemorrhage, postpartum
  alveolar
    lung, newborn P26.8
    process K08.89
  alveolus K08.89
  amputation stump (surgical) T87.89
  anemia (chronic) D50.0
    acute D62
  antepartum (with) O46.90
    with coagulation defect O46.00-
      afibrinogenemia O46.01-
      disseminated intravascular coagulation O46.02-
      hypofibrinogenemia O46.01-
      specified defect NEC O46.09-
    before 20 weeks gestation O20.9
      specified type NEC O20.8
      threatened abortion O20.0
    due to
      abruptio placenta — *see also* Abruptio placentae O45.9-
      leiomyoma, uterus — *see* Hemorrhage, antepartum, specified cause NEC

Hemorrhage, hemorrhagic (concealed) - *continued*
  antepartum (with) - *continued*
    due to - *continued*
      placenta previa O44.1-
      specified cause NEC — *see* subcategory O46.8X-
  anus (sphincter) K62.5
  apoplexy (stroke) — *see* Hemorrhage, intracranial, intracerebral
  arachnoid — *see* Hemorrhage, intracranial, subarachnoid
  artery R58
    brain — *see* Hemorrhage, intracranial, intracerebral
  basilar (ganglion) I61.0
  bladder N32.89
  bowel K92.2
    newborn P54.3
  brain (miliary) (nontraumatic) — *see* Hemorrhage, intracranial, intracerebral
    due to
      birth injury P10.1
      syphilis A52.05
    epidural or extradural (traumatic) — *see* Injury, intracranial, epidural hemorrhage
      newborn P52.4
        birth injury P10.1
    subarachnoid — *see* Hemorrhage, intracranial, subarachnoid
    subdural — *see* Hemorrhage, intracranial, subdural
  brainstem (nontraumatic) I61.3
    traumatic S06.38-
  breast N64.59
  bronchial tube — *see* Hemorrhage, lung
  bronchopulmonary — *see* Hemorrhage, lung
  bronchus — *see* Hemorrhage, lung
  bulbar I61.5
  capillary I78.8
    primary D69.8
  cecum K92.2
  cerebellar, cerebellum (nontraumatic) I61.4
    newborn P52.6
    traumatic S06.37-
  cerebral, cerebrum — *see also* Hemorrhage, intracranial, intracerebral
    newborn (anoxic) P52.4
      birth injury P10.1
    lobe I61.1
  cerebromeningeal I61.8
  cerebrospinal — *see* Hemorrhage, intracranial, intracerebral
  cervix (uteri) (stump) NEC N88.8
  chamber, anterior (eye) — *see* Hyphema
  childbirth — *see* Hemorrhage, complicating, delivery
  choroid H31.30-
    expulsive H31.31-
  ciliary body — *see* Hyphema
  cochlea — *see* subcategory H83.8
  colon K92.2
  complicating
    abortion — *see* Abortion, by type, complicated by, hemorrhage
    delivery O67.9
      associated with coagulation defect (afibrinogenemia) (DIC) (hyperfibrinolysis) O67.0
      specified cause NEC O67.8
    surgical procedure — *see* Hemorrhage, intraoperative
  conjunctiva H11.3-
    newborn P54.8
  cord, newborn (stump) P51.9
  corpus luteum (ruptured) cyst N83.1-
  cortical (brain) I61.1
  cranial — *see* Hemorrhage, intracranial
  cutaneous R23.3
    due to autosensitivity, erythrocyte D69.2
    newborn P54.5
  delayed
    following ectopic or molar pregnancy O08.1
    postpartum O72.2
  diathesis (familial) D69.9
  disease D69.9
    newborn P53
    specified type NEC D69.8
  due to or associated with
    afibrinogenemia or other coagulation defect (conditions in categories D65-D69)
      antepartum — *see* Hemorrhage, antepartum, with coagulation defect
      intrapartum O67.0
    dental implant M27.61

Hemorrhage, hemorrhagic (concealed) - *continued*
  due to or associated with - *continued*
    device, implant or graft — *see also* Complications, by site and type, specified NEC T85.838
      arterial graft NEC T82.838
      breast T85.838
      catheter NEC T85.838
        dialysis (renal) T82.838
          intraperitoneal T85.838
        infusion NEC T82.838
          spinal (epidural) (subdural) T85.830
        urinary (indwelling) T83.83
      electronic (electrode) (pulse generator) (stimulator)
        bone T84.83
        cardiac T82.837
        nervous system (brain) (peripheral nerve) (spinal) T85.830
        urinary T83.83
      fixation, internal (orthopedic) NEC T84.83
      gastrointestinal (bile duct) (esophagus) T85.838
      genital NEC T83.83
      heart NEC T82.837
      joint prosthesis T84.83
      ocular (corneal graft) (orbital implant) NEC T85.838
      orthopedic NEC T84.83
        bone graft T86.838
      specified NEC T85.838
      urinary NEC T83.83
      vascular NEC T82.838
      ventricular intracranial shunt T85.830
  duodenum, duodenal K92.2
    ulcer — *see* Ulcer, duodenum, with hemorrhage
  dura mater — *see* Hemorrhage, intracranial, subdural
  endotracheal — *see* Hemorrhage, lung
  epicranial subaponeurotic (massive) , birth injury P12.2
  epidural (traumatic) — *see also* Injury, intracranial, epidural hemorrhage
    nontraumatic I62.1
  esophagus K22.8
    varix I85.01
      secondary I85.11
  excessive, following ectopic gestation (subsequent episode) O08.1
  extradural (traumatic) — *see* Injury, intracranial, epidural hemorrhage
    birth injury P10.8
    newborn (anoxic) (nontraumatic) P52.8
    nontraumatic I62.1
  eye NEC H57.8
    fundus — *see* Hemorrhage, retina
    lid — *see* Disorder, eyelid, specified type NEC
  fallopian tube N83.6
  fibrinogenolysis — *see* Fibrinolysis
  fibrinolytic (acquired) — *see* Fibrinolysis
  from
    ear (nontraumatic) — *see* Otorrhagia
    tracheostomy stoma J95.01
  fundus, eye — *see* Hemorrhage, retina
  funis — *see* Hemorrhage, umbilicus, cord
  gastric — *see* Hemorrhage, stomach
  gastroenteric K92.2
    newborn P54.3
  gastrointestinal (tract) K92.2
    newborn P54.3
  genital organ, male N50.1
  genitourinary (tract) NOS R31.9
  gingiva K06.8
  globe (eye) — *see* Hemophthalmos
  graafian follicle cyst (ruptured) N83.0-
  gum K06.8
  heart I51.89
  hypopharyngeal (throat) R04.1
  intermenstrual (regular) N92.3
    irregular N92.1
  internal (organs) NEC R58
    capsule I61.0
    ear — *see* subcategory H83.8
    newborn P54.8
  intestine K92.2
    newborn P54.3
  intra-abdominal R58
  intra-alveolar (lung) , newborn P26.8
  intracerebral (nontraumatic) — *see* Hemorrhage, intracranial, intracerebral
  intracranial (nontraumatic) I62.9
    birth injury P10.9
    epidural, nontraumatic I62.1
    extradural, nontraumatic I62.1
    newborn P52.9

Hemorrhage, hemorrhagic (concealed) - *continued*
  intracranial (nontraumatic) - *continued*
    newborn - *continued*
      specified NEC P52.8
    intracerebral (nontraumatic) (in) I61.9
      brain stem I61.3
      cerebellum I61.4
      newborn P52.4
        birth injury P10.1
      hemisphere I61.2
        cortical (superficial) I61.1
        subcortical (deep) I61.0
      intraoperative
        during a nervous system procedure G97.31
        during other procedure G97.32
      intraventricular I61.5
      multiple localized I61.6
      postprocedural
        following a nervous system procedure G97.51
        following other procedure G97.52
      specified NEC I61.8
      superficial I61.1
      traumatic (diffuse) — *see* Injury, intracranial, diffuse
        focal — *see* Injury, intracranial, focal
    subarachnoid (nontraumatic) (from) I60.9
      newborn P52.5
        birth injury P10.3
      intracranial (cerebral) artery I60.7
        anterior communicating I60.2
        basilar I60.4
        carotid siphon and bifurcation I60.0-
        communicating I60.7
          anterior I60.2
          posterior I60.3-
        middle cerebral I60.1-
        posterior communicating I60.3-
        specified artery NEC I60.6
        vertebral I60.5-
      specified NEC I60.8
      traumatic S06.6X-
    subdural (nontraumatic) I62.00
      acute I62.01
      birth injury P10.0
      chronic I62.03
      newborn (anoxic) (hypoxic) P52.8
        birth injury P10.0
      spinal G95.19
      subacute I62.02
      traumatic — *see* Injury, intracranial, subdural hemorrhage
    traumatic — *see* Injury, intracranial, focal brain injury
  intramedullary NEC G95.19
  intraocular — *see* Hemophthalmos
  intraoperative, intraprocedural — *see* Complication, hemorrhage (hematoma), intraoperative (intraprocedural), by site
  intrapartum — *see* Hemorrhage, complicating, delivery
  intrapelvic
    female N94.89
    male K66.1
  intraperitoneal K66.1
  intrapontine I61.3
  intraprocedural — *see* Complication, hemorrhage (hematoma), intraoperative (intraprocedural), by site
  intrauterine N85.7
    complicating delivery — *see also* Hemorrhage, complicating, delivery O67.9
    postpartum — *see* Hemorrhage, postpartum
  intraventricular I61.5
    newborn (nontraumatic) — *see also* Newborn, affected by, hemorrhage P52.3
      due to birth injury P10.2
      grade
        1 P52.0
        2 P52.1
        3 P52.21
        4 P52.22
  intravesical N32.89
  iris (postinfectional) (postinflammatory) (toxic) — *see* Hyphema
  joint (nontraumatic) — *see* Hemarthrosis
  kidney N28.89
  knee (joint) (nontraumatic) — *see* Hemarthrosis, knee
  labyrinth — *see* subcategory H83.8
  lenticular striate artery I61.0
  ligature, vessel — *see* Hemorrhage, postoperative
  liver K76.89
  lung R04.89

Hemorrhage, hemorrhagic (concealed) - *continued*
  lung - *continued*
    newborn P26.9
      massive P26.1
      specified NEC P26.8
    tuberculous — *see* Tuberculosis, pulmonary
  massive umbilical, newborn P51.0
  mediastinum — *see* Hemorrhage, lung
  medulla I61.3
  membrane (brain) I60.8
    spinal cord — *see* Hemorrhage, spinal cord
  meninges, meningeal (brain) (middle) I60.8
    spinal cord — *see* Hemorrhage, spinal cord
  mesentery K66.1
  metritis — *see* Endometritis
  mouth K13.79
  mucous membrane NEC R58
    newborn P54.8
  muscle M62.89
  nail (subungual) L60.8
  nasal turbinate R04.0
    newborn P54.8
  navel, newborn P51.9
  newborn P54.9
    specified NEC P54.8
  nipple N64.59
  nose R04.0
    newborn P54.8
  omentum K66.1
  optic nerve (sheath) H47.02-
  orbit, orbital H05.23-
  ovary NEC N83.8
  oviduct N83.6
  pancreas K86.89
  parathyroid (gland) (spontaneous) E21.4
  parturition — *see* Hemorrhage, complicating, delivery
  penis N48.89
  pericardium, pericarditis I31.2
  peritoneum, peritoneal K66.1
  peritonsillar tissue J35.8
    due to infection J36
  petechial R23.3
    due to autosensitivity, erythrocyte D69.2
  pituitary (gland) E23.6
  pleura — *see* Hemorrhage, lung
  polioencephalitis, superior E51.2
  polymyositis — *see* Polymyositis
  pons, pontine I61.3
  posterior fossa (nontraumatic) I61.8
    newborn P52.6
  postmenopausal N95.0
  postnasal R04.0
  postoperative — *see* Complications, postprocedural, hemorrhage, by site
  postpartum NEC (following delivery of placenta) O72.1
    delayed or secondary O72.2
    retained placenta O72.0
    third stage O72.0
  pregnancy — *see* Hemorrhage, antepartum
  preretinal — *see* Hemorrhage, retina
  prostate N42.1
  puerperal — *see* Hemorrhage, postpartum
    delayed or secondary O72.2
  pulmonary R04.89
    newborn P26.9
      massive P26.1
      specified NEC P26.8
    tuberculous — *see* Tuberculosis, pulmonary
  purpura (primary) D69.3
  rectum (sphincter) K62.5
    newborn P54.2
  recurring, following initial hemorrhage at time of injury T79.2
  renal N28.89
  respiratory passage or tract R04.9
    specified NEC R04.89
  retina, retinal (vessels) H35.6-
    diabetic — *see* Diabetes, retinal, hemorrhage
  retroperitoneal R58
  scalp R58
  scrotum N50.1
  secondary (nontraumatic) R58
    following initial hemorrhage at time of injury T79.2
  seminal vesicle N50.1
  skin R23.3
    newborn P54.5
  slipped umbilical ligature P51.8
  spermatic cord N50.1
  spinal (cord) G95.19
    newborn (birth injury) P11.5

Hemorrhage, hemorrhagic (concealed) - *continued*
  spleen D73.5
    intraoperative — *see* Complications, intraoperative, hemorrhage, spleen
    postprocedural — *see* Complications, postprocedural, hemorrhage, spleen
  stomach K92.2
    newborn P54.3
    ulcer — *see* Ulcer, stomach, with hemorrhage
  subarachnoid (nontraumatic) — *see* Hemorrhage, intracranial, subarachnoid
  subconjunctival — *see also* Hemorrhage, conjunctiva
    birth injury P15.3
  subcortical (brain) I61.0
  subcutaneous R23.3
  subdiaphragmatic R58
  subdural (acute) (nontraumatic) — *see* Hemorrhage, intracranial, subdural
  subependymal
    newborn P52.0
      with intraventricular extension P52.1
        and intracerebral extension P52.22
  subgaleal P12.2
  subhyaloid — *see* Hemorrhage, retina
  subperiosteal — *see* Disorder, bone, specified type NEC
  subretinal — *see* Hemorrhage, retina
  subtentorial — *see* Hemorrhage, intracranial, subdural
  subungual L60.8
  suprarenal (capsule) (gland) E27.49
    newborn P54.4
  tentorium (traumatic) NEC — *see* Hemorrhage, brain
    newborn (birth injury) P10.4
  testis N50.1
  third stage (postpartum) O72.0
  thorax — *see* Hemorrhage, lung
  throat R04.1
  thymus (gland) E32.8
  thyroid (cyst) (gland) E07.89
  tongue K14.8
  tonsil J35.8
  trachea — *see* Hemorrhage, lung
  tracheobronchial R04.89
    newborn P26.0
  traumatic - code to specific injury
    cerebellar — *see* Hemorrhage, brain
    intracranial — *see* Hemorrhage, brain
    recurring or secondary (following initial hemorrhage at time of injury) T79.2
  tuberculous NEC — *see also* Tuberculosis, pulmonary A15.0
  tunica vaginalis N50.1
  ulcer - code by site under Ulcer, with hemorrhage K27.4
  umbilicus, umbilical
    cord
      after birth, newborn P51.9
      complicating delivery O69.5
    newborn P51.9
      massive P51.0
      slipped ligature P51.8
    stump P51.9
  urethra (idiopathic) N36.8
  uterus, uterine (abnormal) N93.9
    climacteric N92.4
    complicating delivery — *see* Hemorrhage, complicating, delivery
    dysfunctional or functional N93.8
    intermenstrual (regular) N92.3
      irregular N92.1
    postmenopausal N95.0
    postpartum — *see* Hemorrhage, postpartum
    preclimacteric or premenopausal N92.4
    prepubertal N93.8
    pubertal N92.2
  vagina (abnormal) N93.9
    newborn P54.6
  vas deferens N50.1
  vasa previa O69.4
  ventricular I61.5
  vesical N32.89
  viscera NEC R58
    newborn P54.8
  vitreous (humor) (intraocular) H43.1-
  vulva N90.89

Hemorrhoids (bleeding) (without mention of degree) K64.9
  1st degree (grade/stage I) (without prolapse outside of anal canal) K64.0

Hemorrhoids (bleeding) (without mention of degree)
- continued
 2nd degree (grade/stage II) (that prolapse with
  straining but retract spontaneously) K64.1
 3rd degree (grade/stage III) (that prolapse with
  straining and require manual replacement back
  inside anal canal) K64.2
 4th degree (grade/stage IV) (with prolapsed tissue
  that cannot be manually replaced) K64.3
 complicating
  pregnancy O22.4
  puerperium O87.2
 external K64.4
  with
   thrombosis K64.5
 internal (without mention of degree) K64.8
 prolapsed K64.8
 skin tags
  anus K64.4
  residual K64.4
 specified NEC K64.8
 strangulated — see also Hemorrhoids, by
  degree K64.8
 thrombosed — see also Hemorrhoids, by
  degree K64.5
 ulcerated — see also Hemorrhoids, by degree K64.8
Hemosalpinx N83.6
 with
  hematocolpos N89.7
  hematometra N85.7
   with hematocolpos N89.7
Hemosiderosis (dietary) E83.19
 pulmonary, idiopathic E83.1- [J84.03]
 transfusion T80.89
Hemothorax (bacterial) (nontuberculous) J94.2
 newborn P54.8
 traumatic S27.1
  with pneumothorax S27.2
 tuberculous NEC A15.6
Henoch (-Schönlein) **disease or syndrome**
 (purpura) D69.0
Henpue, henpuye A66.6
Hepar lobatum (syphilitic) A52.74
Hepatalgia K76.89
Hepatitis K75.9
 acute B17.9
  with coma K72.01
  with hepatic failure — see Failure, hepatic
  alcoholic — see Hepatitis, alcoholic
  infectious B17.9
  non-viral K72.0
  viral B17.9
 alcoholic (acute) (chronic) K70.10
  with ascites K70.11
 amebic — see Abscess, liver, amebic
 anicteric, (viral) — see Hepatitis, viral
 antigen-associated (HAA) — see Hepatitis, B
 Australia-antigen (positive) — see Hepatitis, B
 autoimmune K75.4
 B B19.10
  with hepatic coma B19.11
  acute B16.9
   with
    delta-agent (coinfection) (without hepatic
     coma) B16.1
     with hepatic coma B16.0
    hepatic coma (without delta-agent
     coinfection) B16.2
  chronic B18.1
   with delta-agent B18.0
 bacterial NEC K75.89
 C (viral) B19.20
  with hepatic coma B19.21
  acute B17.10
   with hepatic coma B17.11
  chronic B18.2
 catarrhal (acute) B15.9
  with hepatic coma B15.0
 cholangiolitic K75.89
 cholestatic K75.89
 chronic K73.9
  active NEC K73.2
  lobular NEC K73.1
  persistent NEC K73.0
  specified NEC K73.8
 cytomegaloviral B25.1
 due to ethanol (acute) (chronic) — see Hepatitis,
  alcoholic
 epidemic B15.9
  with hepatic coma B15.0
 fulminant NEC (viral) — see Hepatitis, viral
 neonatal giant cell P59.29
 granulomatous NEC K75.3

Hepatitis - continued
 herpesviral B00.81
 history of
  B Z86.19
  C Z86.19
 homologous serum — see Hepatitis, viral, type B
 in (due to)
  mumps B26.81
  toxoplasmosis (acquired) B58.1
   congenital (active) P37.1 [K77]
 infectious, infective B15.9
  acute (subacute) B17.9
  chronic B18.9
 inoculation — see Hepatitis, viral, type B
 interstitial (chronic) K74.69
 lupoid NEC K75.4
 malignant NEC (with hepatic failure) K72.90
  with coma K72.91
 neonatal (idiopathic) (toxic) P59.29
 newborn P59.29
 postimmunization — see Hepatitis, viral, type B
 post-transfusion — see Hepatitis, viral, type B
 reactive, nonspecific K75.2
 serum — see Hepatitis, viral, type B
 specified type NEC
  with hepatic failure — see Failure, hepatic
 syphilitic (late) A52.74
  congenital (early) A50.08 [K77]
   late A50.59 [K77]
  secondary A51.45
 toxic — see also Disease, liver, toxic K71.6
 tuberculous A18.83
 viral, virus B19.9
  with hepatic coma B19.0
  acute B17.9
  chronic B18.9
   specified NEC B18.8
  type
   B B18.1
    with delta-agent B18.0
   C B18.2
  congenital P35.3
  coxsackie B33.8 [K77]
  cytomegalic inclusion B25.1
  in remission, any type - code to Hepatitis, chronic,
   by type
  non-A, non-B B17.8
  specified type NEC (with or without coma) B17.8
  type
   A B15.9
    with hepatic coma B15.0
   B B19.10
    with hepatic coma B19.11
    acute B16.9
     with
      delta-agent (coinfection) (without hepatic
       coma) B16.1
       with hepatic coma B16.0
      hepatic coma (without delta-agent
       coinfection) B16.2
    chronic B18.1
     with delta-agent B18.0
   C B19.20
    with hepatic coma B19.21
    acute B17.10
     with hepatic coma B17.11
    chronic B18.2
   E B17.2
   non-A, non-B B17.8
Hepatization lung (acute) — see Pneumonia, lobar
Hepatoblastoma C22.2
Hepatocarcinoma C22.0
Hepatocholangiocarcinoma C22.0
Hepatocholangioma, benign D13.4
Hepatocholangitis K75.89
Hepatolenticular degeneration E83.01
Hepatoma (malignant) C22.0
 benign D13.4
 embryonal C22.0
Hepatomegaly — see also Hypertrophy, liver
 with splenomegaly R16.2
 congenital Q44.7
 in mononucleosis
  gammaherpesviral B27.09
  infectious specified NEC B27.89
Hepatoptosis K76.89
**Hepatorenal syndrome following labor and
delivery** O90.4
Hepatosis K76.89
Hepatosplenomegaly R16.2
 hyperlipemic (Bürger-Grütz type) E78.3 [K77]
Hereditary — see condition

Heredodegeneration, macular — see Dystrophy,
retina
Heredopathia atactica polyneuritiformis G60.1
Heredosyphilis — see Syphilis, congenital
Herlitz' syndrome Q81.1
Hermansky-Pudlak syndrome E70.331
Hermaphrodite, hermaphroditism (true) Q56.0
 46,XX with streak gonads Q99.1
 46,XX/46,XY Q99.0
 46,XY with streak gonads Q99.1
 chimera 46,XX/46,XY Q99.0
Hernia, hernial (acquired) (recurrent) K46.9
 with
  gangrene — see Hernia, by site, with, gangrene
  incarceration — see Hernia, by site, with,
   obstruction
  irreducible — see Hernia, by site, with, obstruction
  obstruction — see Hernia, by site, with,
   obstruction
  strangulation — see Hernia, by site, with,
   obstruction
 abdomen, abdominal K46.9
  with
   gangrene (and obstruction) K46.1
   obstruction K46.0
  femoral — see Hernia, femoral
  incisional — see Hernia, incisional
  inguinal — see Hernia, inguinal
  specified site NEC K45.8
   with
    gangrene (and obstruction) K45.1
    obstruction K45.0
  umbilical — see Hernia, umbilical
  wall — see Hernia, ventral
 appendix — see Hernia, abdomen
 bladder (mucosa) (sphincter)
  congenital (female) (male) Q79.51
  female — see Cystocele
  male N32.89
 brain, congenital — see Encephalocele
 cartilage, vertebra — see Displacement,
  intervertebral disc
 cerebral, congenital — see also Encephalocele
  endaural Q01.8
 ciliary body (traumatic) S05.2-
 colon — see Hernia, abdomen
 Cooper's — see Hernia, abdomen, specified site
  NEC
 crural — see Hernia, femoral
 diaphragm, diaphragmatic K44.9
  with
   gangrene (and obstruction) K44.1
   obstruction K44.0
  congenital Q79.0
 direct (inguinal) — see Hernia, inguinal
 diverticulum, intestine — see Hernia, abdomen
 double (inguinal) — see Hernia, inguinal, bilateral
 due to adhesions (with obstruction) K56.5
 epigastric — see also Hernia, ventral K43.9
 esophageal hiatus — see Hernia, hiatal
 external (inguinal) — see Hernia, inguinal
 fallopian tube N83.4-
 fascia M62.89
 femoral K41.90
  with
   gangrene (and obstruction) K41.40
    not specified as recurrent K41.40
    recurrent K41.41
   obstruction K41.30
    not specified as recurrent K41.30
    recurrent K41.31
  bilateral K41.20
   with
    gangrene (and obstruction) K41.10
     not specified as recurrent K41.10
     recurrent K41.11
    obstruction K41.00
     not specified as recurrent K41.00
     recurrent K41.01
   not specified as recurrent K41.20
   recurrent K41.21
  unilateral K41.90
   with
    gangrene (and obstruction) K41.40
     not specified as recurrent K41.40
     recurrent K41.41
    obstruction K41.30
     not specified as recurrent K41.30
     recurrent K41.31
   not specified as recurrent K41.90
   recurrent K41.91
  not specified as recurrent K41.90
  recurrent K41.91

Hernia, hernial (acquired) (recurrent) - *continued*
foramen magnum G93.5
congenital Q01.8
funicular (umbilical) — *see also* Hernia, umbilicus
spermatic (cord) — *see* Hernia, inguinal
gastrointestinal tract — *see* Hernia, abdomen
Hesselbach's — *see* Hernia, femoral, specified site
NEC
hiatal (esophageal) (sliding) K44.9
with
gangrene (and obstruction) K44.1
obstruction K44.0
congenital Q40.1
hypogastric — *see* Hernia, ventral
incarcerated — *see also* Hernia, by site, with
obstruction
with gangrene — *see* Hernia, by site, with
gangrene
incisional K43.2
with
gangrene (and obstruction) K43.1
obstruction K43.0
indirect (inguinal) — *see* Hernia, inguinal
inguinal (direct) (external) (funicular) (indirect)
(internal) (oblique) (scrotal) (sliding) K40.90
with
gangrene (and obstruction) K40.40
not specified as recurrent K40.40
recurrent K40.41
obstruction K40.30
not specified as recurrent K40.30
recurrent K40.31
not specified as recurrent K40.90
recurrent K40.91
bilateral K40.20
with
gangrene (and obstruction) K40.10
not specified as recurrent K40.10
recurrent K40.11
obstruction K40.00
not specified as recurrent K40.00
recurrent K40.01
not specified as recurrent K40.20
recurrent K40.21
unilateral K40.90
with
gangrene (and obstruction) K40.40
not specified as recurrent K40.40
recurrent K40.41
obstruction K40.30
not specified as recurrent K40.30
recurrent K40.31
not specified as recurrent K40.90
recurrent K40.91
internal — *see also* Hernia, abdomen
inguinal — *see* Hernia, inguinal
interstitial — *see* Hernia, abdomen
intervertebral cartilage or disc — *see* Displacement,
intervertebral disc
intestine, intestinal — *see* Hernia, by site
intra-abdominal — *see* Hernia, abdomen
iris (traumatic) S05.2-
irreducible — *see also* Hernia, by site, with
obstruction
with gangrene — *see* Hernia, by site, with
gangrene
ischiatic — *see* Hernia, abdomen, specified site NEC
ischiorectal — *see* Hernia, abdomen, specified site
NEC
lens (traumatic) S05.2-
linea (alba) (semilunaris) — *see* Hernia, ventral
Littre's — *see* Hernia, abdomen
lumbar — *see* Hernia, abdomen, specified site NEC
lung (subcutaneous) J98.4
mediastinum J98.59
mesenteric (internal) — *see* Hernia, abdomen
midline — *see* Hernia, ventral
muscle (sheath) M62.89
nucleus pulposus — *see* Displacement,
intervertebral disc
oblique (inguinal) — *see* Hernia, inguinal
obstructive — *see also* Hernia, by site, with
obstruction
with gangrene — *see* Hernia, by site, with
gangrene
obturator — *see* Hernia, abdomen, specified site
NEC
omental — *see* Hernia, abdomen
ovary N83.4-
oviduct N83.4-
paraesophageal — *see also* Hernia, diaphragm
congenital Q40.1
parastomal K43.5

Hernia, hernial (acquired) (recurrent) - *continued*
parastomal - *continued*
with
gangrene (and obstruction) K43.4
obstruction K43.3
paraumbilical — *see* Hernia, umbilicus
perineal — *see* Hernia, abdomen, specified site NEC
Petit's — *see* Hernia, abdomen, specified site NEC
postoperative — *see* Hernia, incisional
pregnant uterus — *see* Abnormal, uterus in
pregnancy or childbirth
prevesical N32.89
properitoneal — *see* Hernia, abdomen, specified site
NEC
pudendal — *see* Hernia, abdomen, specified site
NEC
rectovaginal N81.6
retroperitoneal — *see* Hernia, abdomen, specified
site NEC
Richter's — *see* Hernia, abdomen, with obstruction
Rieux's, Riex's — *see* Hernia, abdomen, specified
site NEC
sac condition (adhesion) (dropsy) (inflammation)
(laceration) (suppuration) - code by site under
Hernia
sciatic — *see* Hernia, abdomen, specified site NEC
scrotum, scrotal — *see* Hernia, inguinal
sliding (inguinal) — *see also* Hernia, inguinal
hiatus — *see* Hernia, hiatal
spigelian — *see* Hernia, ventral
spinal — *see* Spina bifida
strangulated — *see also* Hernia, by site, with
obstruction
with gangrene — *see* Hernia, by site, with
gangrene
subxiphoid — *see* Hernia, ventral
supra-umbilicus — *see* Hernia, ventral
tendon — *see* Disorder, tendon, specified type NEC
Treitz's (fossa) — *see* Hernia, abdomen, specified
site NEC
tunica vaginalis Q55.29
umbilicus, umbilical K42.9
with
gangrene (and obstruction) K42.1
obstruction K42.0
ureter N28.89
urethra, congenital Q64.79
urinary meatus, congenital Q64.79
uterus N81.4
pregnant — *see* Abnormal, uterus in pregnancy or
childbirth
vaginal (anterior) (wall) — *see* Cystocele
Velpeau's — *see* Hernia, femoral
ventral K43.9
with
gangrene (and obstruction) K43.7
obstruction K43.6
recurrent — *see* Hernia, incisional
incisional K43.2
with
gangrene (and obstruction) K43.1
obstruction K43.0
specified NEC K43.9
with
gangrene (and obstruction) K43.7
obstruction K43.6
vesical
congenital (female) (male) Q79.51
female — *see* Cystocele
male N32.89
vitreous (into wound) S05.2-
into anterior chamber — *see* Prolapse, vitreous
Herniation — *see also* Hernia
brain (stem) G93.5
cerebral G93.5
mediastinum J98.59
nucleus pulposus — *see* Displacement,
intervertebral disc
Herpangina B08.5
Herpes, herpesvirus, herpetic B00.9
anogenital A60.9
perianal skin A60.1
rectum A60.1
urogenital tract A60.00
cervix A60.03
male genital organ NEC A60.02
penis A60.01
specified site NEC A60.09
vagina A60.04
vulva A60.04
blepharitis (zoster) B02.39
simplex B00.59
circinatus B35.4

Herpes, herpesvirus, herpetic - *continued*
circinatus - *continued*
bullosus L12.0
conjunctivitis (simplex) B00.53
zoster B02.31
cornea B02.33
encephalitis B00.4
due to herpesvirus 6 B10.01
due to herpesvirus 7 B10.09
specified NEC B10.09
eye (zoster) B02.30
simplex B00.50
eyelid (zoster) B02.39
simplex B00.59
facialis B00.1
febrilis B00.1
geniculate ganglionitis B02.21
genital, genitalis A60.00
female A60.09
male A60.02
gestational, gestationis O26.4-
gingivostomatitis B00.2
human B00.9
1 — *see* Herpes, simplex
2 — *see* Herpes, simplex
3 — *see* Varicella
4 — *see* Mononucleosis, Epstein-Barr (virus)
5 — *see* Disease, cytomegalic inclusion
(generalized)
6
encephalitis B10.01
specified NEC B10.81
7
encephalitis B10.09
specified NEC B10.82
8 B10.89
infection NEC B10.89
Kaposi's sarcoma associated B10.89
iridocyclitis (simplex) B00.51
zoster B02.32
iris (vesicular erythema multiforme) L51.9
iritis (simplex) B00.51
Kaposi's sarcoma associated B10.89
keratitis (simplex) (dendritic) (disciform)
(interstitial) B00.52
zoster (interstitial) B02.33
keratoconjunctivitis (simplex) B00.52
zoster B02.33
labialis B00.1
lip B00.1
meningitis (simplex) B00.3
zoster B02.1
ophthalmicus (zoster) NEC B02.30
simplex B00.50
penis A60.01
perianal skin A60.1
pharyngitis, pharyngotonsillitis B00.2
rectum A60.1
scrotum A60.02
sepsis B00.7
simplex B00.9
complicated NEC B00.89
congenital P35.2
conjunctivitis B00.53
external ear B00.1
eyelid B00.59
hepatitis B00.81
keratitis (interstitial) B00.52
myleitis B00.82
specified complication NEC B00.89
visceral B00.89
stomatitis B00.2
tonsurans B35.0
visceral B00.89
vulva A60.04
whitlow B00.89
zoster — *see also* condition B02.9
auricularis B02.21
complicated NEC B02.8
conjunctivitis B02.31
disseminated B02.7
encephalitis B02.0
eye (lid) B02.39
geniculate ganglionitis B02.21
keratitis (interstitial) B02.33
meningitis B02.1
myelitis B02.24
neuritis, neuralgia B02.29
ophthalmicus NEC B02.30
oticus B02.21
polyneuropathy B02.23
specified complication NEC B02.8
trigeminal neuralgia B02.22

Herpesvirus (human) — *see* Herpes
Herpetophobia F40.218
Herrick's anemia — *see* Disease, sickle-cell
Hers' disease E74.09
Herter-Gee syndrome K90.0
Herxheimer's reaction R68.89
Hesitancy
  of micturition R39.11
  urinary R39.11
Hesselbach's hernia — *see* Hernia, femoral,
  specified site NEC
Heterochromia (congenital) Q13.2
  cataract — *see* Cataract, complicated
  cyclitis (Fuchs) — *see* Cyclitis, Fuchs'
    heterochromic
  hair L67.1
  iritis — *see* Cyclitis, Fuchs' heterochromic
  retained metallic foreign body (nonmagnetic) — *see*
    Foreign body, intraocular, old, retained
    magnetic — *see* Foreign body, intraocular, old,
      retained, magnetic
  uveitis — *see* Cyclitis, Fuchs' heterochromic
Heterophoria — *see* Strabismus, heterophoria
Heterophyes, heterophyiasis (small intestine) B66.8
Heterotopia, heterotopic — *see also* Malposition,
  congenital
  cerebralis Q04.8
Heterotropia — *see* Strabismus
Heubner-Herter disease K90.0
Hexadactylism Q69.9
HGSIL (cytology finding)
  (high grade squamous intraepithelial lesion on
  cytologic smear) (Pap smear finding)
  anus R85.613
  cervix R87.613
    biopsy (histology) finding — *see* Neoplasia,
      intraepithelial, cervix, grade II or grade III
  vagina R87.623
    biopsy (histology) finding — *see* Neoplasia,
      intraepithelial, vagina, grade II or grade III
Hibernoma — *see* Lipoma
Hiccup, hiccough R06.6
  epidemic B33.0
  psychogenic F45.8
Hidden penis (congenital) Q55.64
  acquired N48.83
Hidradenitis (axillaris) (suppurative) L73.2
Hidradenoma (nodular) — *see also* Neoplasm, skin,
  benign
  clear cell — *see* Neoplasm, skin, benign
  papillary — *see* Neoplasm, skin, benign
Hidrocystoma — *see* Neoplasm, skin, benign
High
  altitude effects T70.20
    anoxia T70.29
    on
      ears T70.0
      sinuses T70.1
    polycythemia D75.1
  arch
    foot Q66.7
    palate, congenital Q38.5
  arterial tension — *see* Hypertension
  basal metabolic rate R94.8
  blood pressure — *see also* Hypertension
    borderline R03.0
    reading (incidental) (isolated) (nonspecific) ,
      without diagnosis of hypertension R03.0
  cholesterol E78.00
    with high triglycerides E78.2
  diaphragm (congenital) Q79.1
  expressed emotional level within family Z63.8
  head at term O32.4
  palate, congenital Q38.5
  risk
    infant NEC Z76.2
    sexual behavior (heterosexual) Z72.51
      bisexual Z72.53
      homosexual Z72.52
  temperature (of unknown origin) R50.9
  thoracic rib Q76.6
  triglycerides E78.1
    with high cholesterol E78.2
Hildenbrand's disease A75.0
Hilum — *see* condition
Hip — *see* condition
Hippel's disease Q85.8
Hippophobia F40.218
Hippus H57.09
Hirschsprung's disease or megacolon Q43.1
Hirsutism, hirsuties L68.0
Hirudiniasis
  external B88.3

Hirudiniasis - *continued*
  internal B83.4
Hiss-Russell dysentery A03.1
Histidinemia, histidinuria E70.41
Histiocytoma — *see also* Neoplasm, skin, benign
  fibrous — *see also* Neoplasm, skin, benign
    atypical — *see* Neoplasm, connective tissue,
      uncertain behavior
    malignant — *see* Neoplasm, connective tissue,
      malignant
Histiocytosis D76.3
  acute differentiated progressive C96.0
  Langerhans' cell NEC C96.6
    multifocal X
      multisystemic (disseminated) C96.0
      unisystemic C96.5
    pulmonary, adult (adult PLCH) J84.82
    unifocal (X) C96.6
  lipid, lipoid D76.3
    essential E75.29
  malignant C96.A
  mononuclear phagocytes NEC D76.1
    Langerhans' cells C96.6
  non-Langerhans cell D76.3
  polyostotic sclerosing D76.3
  sinus, with massive lymphadenopathy D76.3
  syndrome NEC D76.3
  X NEC C96.6
    acute (progressive) C96.0
    chronic C96.6
    multifocal C96.5
    multisystemic C96.0
    unifocal C96.6
Histoplasmosis B39.9
  with pneumonia NEC B39.2
  African B39.5
  American — *see* Histoplasmosis, capsulati
  capsulati B39.4
    disseminated B39.3
    generalized B39.3
    pulmonary B39.2
      acute B39.0
      chronic B39.1
  Darling's B39.4
  duboisii B39.5
  lung NEC B39.2
History
  family (of) — *see also* History, personal (of)
    alcohol abuse Z81.1
    allergy NEC Z84.89
    anemia Z83.2
    arthritis Z82.61
    asthma Z82.5
    blindness Z82.1
    cardiac death (sudden) Z82.41
    carrier of genetic disease Z84.81
    chromosomal anomaly Z82.79
    chronic
      disabling disease NEC Z82.8
      lower respiratory disease Z82.5
    colonic polyps Z83.71
    congenital malformations and deformations Z82.79
      polycystic kidney Z82.71
    consanguinity Z84.3
    deafness Z82.2
    diabetes mellitus Z83.3
    disability NEC Z82.8
    disease or disorder (of)
      allergic NEC Z84.89
      behavioral NEC Z81.8
      blood and blood-forming organs Z83.2
      cardiovascular NEC Z82.49
      chronic disabling NEC Z82.8
      digestive Z83.79
      ear NEC Z83.52
      endocrine NEC Z83.49
      eye NEC Z83.518
        glaucoma Z83.511
      familial hypercholesterolemia Z83.42
      genitourinary NEC Z84.2
      glaucoma Z83.511
      hematological Z83.2
      immune mechanism Z83.2
      infectious NEC Z83.1
      ischemic heart Z82.49
      kidney Z84.1
      mental NEC Z81.8
      metabolic Z83.49
      musculoskeletal NEC Z82.69
      neurological NEC Z82.0
      nutritional Z83.49
      parasitic NEC Z83.1
      psychiatric NEC Z81.8

History - *continued*
  family (of) - *continued*
    disease or disorder (of) - *continued*
      respiratory NEC Z83.6
      skin and subcutaneous tissue NEC Z84.0
      specified NEC Z84.89
    drug abuse NEC Z81.3
    epilepsy Z82.0
    familial hypercholesterolemia Z83.42
    genetic disease carrier Z84.81
    glaucoma Z83.511
    hearing loss Z82.2
    human immunodeficiency virus (HIV)
      infection Z83.0
    Huntington's chorea Z82.0
    intellectual disability Z81.0
    leukemia Z80.6
    malignant neoplasm (of) NOS Z80.9
      bladder Z80.52
      breast Z80.3
      bronchus Z80.1
      digestive organ Z80.0
      gastrointestinal tract Z80.0
      genital organ Z80.49
        ovary Z80.41
        prostate Z80.42
        specified organ NEC Z80.49
        testis Z80.43
      hematopoietic NEC Z80.7
      intrathoracic organ NEC Z80.2
      kidney Z80.51
      lung Z80.1
      lymphatic NEC Z80.7
      ovary Z80.41
      prostate Z80.42
      respiratory organ NEC Z80.2
      specified site NEC Z80.8
      testis Z80.43
      trachea Z80.1
      urinary organ or tract Z80.59
        bladder Z80.52
        kidney Z80.51
    mental
      disorder NEC Z81.8
    multiple endocrine neoplasia (MEN)
      syndrome Z83.41
    osteoporosis Z82.62
    polycystic kidney Z82.71
    polyps (colon) Z83.71
    psychiatric disorder Z81.8
    psychoactive substance abuse NEC Z81.3
    respiratory condition NEC Z83.6
      asthma and other lower respiratory
        conditions Z82.5
    self-harmful behavior Z81.8
    SIDS (sudden infant death syndrome) Z84.82
    skin condition Z84.0
    specified condition NEC Z84.89
    stroke (cerebrovascular) Z82.3
    substance abuse NEC Z81.4
      alcohol Z81.1
      drug NEC Z81.3
      psychoactive NEC Z81.3
      tobacco Z81.2
    sudden
      cardiac death Z82.41
      infant death syndrome (SIDS) Z84.82
    tobacco abuse Z81.2
    violence, violent behavior Z81.8
    visual loss Z82.1
  personal (of) — *see also* History, family (of)
    abuse
      childhood Z62.819
        physical Z62.810
        psychological Z62.811
        sexual Z62.810
      adult Z91.419
        physical and sexual Z91.410
        psychological Z91.411
    alcohol dependence F10.21
    allergy (to) Z88.9
      analgesic agent NEC Z88.6
      anesthetic Z88.4
      antibiotic agent NEC Z88.1
      anti-infective agent NEC Z88.3
      contrast media Z91.041
      drugs, medicaments and biological
        substances Z88.9
        specified NEC Z88.8
      food Z91.018
        additives Z91.02
        eggs Z91.012
        milk products Z91.011

History - *continued*
  personal (of) - *continued*
    allergy (to) - *continued*
      food - *continued*
        peanuts Z91.010
        seafood Z91.013
        specified food NEC Z91.018
      insect Z91.038
        bee Z91.030
      latex Z91.040
      medicinal agents Z88.9
        specified NEC Z88.8
      narcotic agent NEC Z88.5
      nonmedicinal agents Z91.048
      penicillin Z88.0
      serum Z88.7
      specified NEC Z91.09
      sulfonamides Z88.2
      vaccine Z88.7
    anaphylactic shock Z87.892
    anaphylaxis Z87.892
    behavioral disorders Z86.59
    benign carcinoid tumor Z86.012
    benign neoplasm Z86.018
      carcinoid Z86.012
      brain Z86.011
      colonic polyps Z86.010
    brain injury (traumatic) Z87.820
    breast implant removal Z98.86
    calculi, renal Z87.442
    cancer — *see* History, personal (of), malignant
      neoplasm (of)
    cardiac arrest (death) , successfully
      resuscitated Z86.74
    cerebral infarction without residual deficit Z86.73
    cervical dysplasia Z87.410
    chemotherapy for neoplastic condition Z92.21
    childhood abuse — *see* History, personal (of),
      abuse
    cleft lip (corrected) Z87.730
    cleft palate (corrected) Z87.730
    collapsed vertebra (healed) Z87.311
      due to osteoporosis Z87.310
    combat and operational stress reaction Z86.51
    congenital malformation (corrected) Z87.798
      circulatory system (corrected) Z87.74
      digestive system (corrected) NEC Z87.738
      ear (corrected) Z87.720
      eye (corrected) Z87.721
      face and neck (corrected) Z87.790
      genitourinary system (corrected) NEC Z87.718
      heart (corrected) Z87.74
      integument (corrected) Z87.76
      limb (s) (corrected) Z87.76
      musculoskeletal system (corrected) Z87.76
      neck (corrected) Z87.790
      nervous system (corrected) NEC Z87.728
      respiratory system (corrected) Z87.75
      sense organs (corrected) NEC Z87.728
      specified NEC Z87.798
    contraception Z92.0
    deployment (military) Z91.82
    diabetic foot ulcer Z86.31
    disease or disorder (of) Z87.898
      blood and blood-forming organs Z86.2
      circulatory system Z86.79
        specified condition NEC Z86.79
      connective tissue NEC Z87.39
      digestive system Z87.19
        colonic polyp Z86.010
        peptic ulcer disease Z87.11
        specified condition NEC Z87.19
      ear Z86.69
      endocrine Z86.39
        diabetic foot ulcer Z86.31
        gestational diabetes Z86.32
        specified type NEC Z86.39
      eye Z86.69
      genital (track) system NEC
        female Z87.42
        male Z87.438
      hematological Z86.2
      Hodgkin Z85.71
      immune mechanism Z86.2
      infectious Z86.19
        malaria Z86.13
        Methicillin resistant Staphylococcus aureus
          (MRSA) Z86.14
        poliomyelitis Z86.12
        specified NEC Z86.19
        tuberculosis Z86.11
      mental NEC Z86.59
      metabolic Z86.39

History - *continued*
  personal (of) - *continued*
    disease or disorder (of) - *continued*
      metabolic - *continued*
        diabetic foot ulcer Z86.31
        gestational diabetes Z86.32
        specified type NEC Z86.39
      musculoskeletal NEC Z87.39
      nervous system Z86.69
      nutritional Z86.39
      parasitic Z86.19
      respiratory system NEC Z87.09
      sense organs Z86.69
      skin Z87.2
      specified site or type NEC Z87.898
      subcutaneous tissue Z87.2
      trophoblastic Z87.59
      urinary system NEC Z87.448
    drug dependence — *see* Dependence, drug, by
      type, in remission
    drug therapy
      antineoplastic chemotherapy Z92.21
      estrogen Z92.23
      immunosupression Z92.25
      inhaled steroids Z92.240
      monoclonal drug Z92.22
      specified NEC Z92.29
      steroid Z92.241
      systemic steroids Z92.241
    dysplasia
      cervical (mild) (moderate) Z87.410
        severe (grade III) Z86.001
      prostatic Z87.430
      vaginal (mild) (moderate) Z87.411
        severe (grade III) Z86.008
      vulvar (mild) (moderate) Z87.412
        severe (grade III) Z86.008
    embolism (venous) Z86.718
      pulmonary Z86.711
    encephalitis Z86.61
    estrogen therapy Z92.23
    extracorporeal membrane oxygenation
      (ECMO) Z92.81
    failed moderate sedation Z92.83
    failed conscious sedation Z92.83
    fall, falling Z91.81
    fracture (healed)
      fatigue Z87.312
      fragility Z87.310
      osteoporosis Z87.310
      pathological NEC Z87.311
      stress Z87.312
      traumatic Z87.81
    gestational diabetes Z86.32
    hepatitis
      B Z86.19
      C Z86.19
    Hodgkin disease Z85.71
    hyperthermia, malignant Z88.4
    hypospadias (corrected) Z87.710
    hysterectomy Z90.710
    immunosupression therapy Z92.25
    in situ neoplasm
      breast Z86.000
      cervix uteri Z86.001
      specified NEC Z86.008
    infection NEC Z86.19
      central nervous system Z86.61
      Methicillin resistant Staphylococcus aureus
        (MRSA) Z86.14
      urinary (recurrent) (tract) Z87.440
    injury NEC Z87.828
    in utero procedure during pregnancy Z98.870
    in utero procedure while a fetus Z98.871
    irradiation Z92.3
    kidney stones Z87.442
    leukemia Z85.6
    lymphoma (non-Hodgkin) Z85.72
    malignant melanoma (skin) Z85.820
    malignant neoplasm (of) Z85.9
      accessory sinuses Z85.22
      anus NEC Z85.048
        carcinoid Z85.040
      bladder Z85.51
      bone Z85.830
      brain Z85.841
      breast Z85.3
      bronchus NEC Z85.118
        carcinoid Z85.110
      carcinoid — *see* History, personal (of), malignant
        neoplasm, by site, carcinioid
      cervix Z85.41
      colon NEC Z85.038

History - *continued*
  personal (of) - *continued*
    malignant neoplasm (of) - *continued*
      colon NEC - *continued*
        carcinoid Z85.030
      digestive organ Z85.00
        specified NEC Z85.09
      endocrine gland NEC Z85.858
      epididymis Z85.48
      esophagus Z85.01
      eye Z85.840
      gastrointestinal tract — *see* History, malignant
        neoplasm, digestive organ
      genital organ
        female Z85.40
          specified NEC Z85.44
        male Z85.45
          specified NEC Z85.49
      hematopoietic NEC Z85.79
      intrathoracic organ Z85.20
      kidney NEC Z85.528
        carcinoid Z85.520
      large intestine NEC Z85.038
        carcinoid Z85.030
      larynx Z85.21
      liver Z85.05
      lung NEC Z85.118
        carcinoid Z85.110
      mediastinum Z85.29
      Merkel cell Z85.821
      middle ear Z85.22
      nasal cavities Z85.22
      nervous system NEC Z85.848
      oral cavity Z85.819
        specified site NEC Z85.818
      ovary Z85.43
      pancreas Z85.07
      pharynx Z85.819
        specified site NEC Z85.818
      pelvis Z85.53
      pleura Z85.29
      prostate Z85.46
      rectosigmoid junction NEC Z85.048
        carcinoid Z85.040
      rectum NEC Z85.048
        carcinoid Z85.040
      respiratory organ Z85.20
      sinuses, accessory Z85.22
      skin NEC Z85.828
        melanoma Z85.820
        Merkel cell Z85.821
      small intestine NEC Z85.068
        carcinoid Z85.060
      soft tissue Z85.831
      specified site NEC Z85.89
      stomach NEC Z85.028
        carcinoid Z85.020
      testis Z85.47
      thymus NEC Z85.238
        carcinoid Z85.230
      thyroid Z85.850
      tongue Z85.810
      trachea Z85.12
      ureter Z85.54
      urinary organ or tract Z85.50
        specified NEC Z85.59
      uterus Z85.42
    maltreatment Z91.89
    medical treatment NEC Z92.89
    melanoma (malignant) (skin) Z85.820
    meningitis Z86.61
    mental disorder Z86.59
    Merkel cell carcinoma (skin) Z85.821
    Methicillin resistant Staphylococcus aureus
      (MRSA) Z86.14
    military deployment Z91.82
    military war, peacekeeping and humanitarian
      deployment (current or past conflict) Z91.82
    myocardial infarction (old) I25.2
    neglect (in)
      adult Z91.412
      childhood Z62.812
    neoplasm
      benign Z86.018
        brain Z86.011
        colon polyp Z86.010
      in situ
        breast Z86.000
        cervix uteri Z86.001
        specified NEC Z86.008
      malignant — *see* History of, malignant neoplasm
      uncertain behavior Z86.03
    nephrotic syndrome Z87.441

History - *continued*
  personal (of) - *continued*
    nicotine dependence Z87.891
    noncompliance with medical treatment or regimen — *see* Noncompliance
    nutritional deficiency Z86.39
    obstetric complications Z87.59
      childbirth Z87.59
      pregnancy Z87.59
      pre-term labor Z87.51
      puerperium Z87.59
    osteoporosis fractures Z87.31
    parasuicide (attempt) Z91.5
    physical trauma NEC Z87.828
      self-harm or suicide attempt Z91.5
    poisoning NEC Z91.89
      self-harm or suicide attempt Z91.5
    poor personal hygiene Z91.89
    pneumonia (recurrent) Z87.01
    preterm labor Z87.51
    prolonged reversible ischemic neurologic deficit (PRIND) Z86.73
    procedure during pregnancy Z98.870
    procedure while a fetus Z98.871
    prostatic dysplasia Z87.430
    psychological
      abuse
        adult Z91.411
        child Z62.811
      trauma, specified NEC Z91.49
    radiation therapy Z92.3
    removal
      implant
        breast Z98.86
    renal calculi Z87.442
    respiratory condition NEC Z87.09
    retained foreign body fully removed Z87.821
    risk factors NEC Z91.89
    self-harm Z91.5
    self-poisoning attempt Z91.5
    sex reassignment Z87.890
    sleep-wake cycle problem Z72.821
    specified NEC Z87.898
    steroid therapy (systemic) Z92.241
      inhaled Z92.240
    stroke without residual deficits Z86.73
    substance abuse NEC F10-F19 with fifth character 1
    sudden cardiac arrest Z86.74
    sudden cardiac death successfully resuscitated Z86.74
    suicide attempt Z91.5
    surgery NEC Z98.890
      with uterine scar Z98.891
      sex reassignment Z87.890
      transplant — *see* Transplant
    thrombophlebitis Z86.72
    thrombosis (venous) Z86.718
      pulmonary Z86.711
    tobacco dependence Z87.891
    transient ischemic attack (TIA) without residual deficits Z86.73
    trauma (physical) NEC Z87.828
      psychological NEC Z91.49
      self-harm Z91.5
    traumatic brain injury Z87.820
    unhealthy sleep-wake cycle Z72.821
    unintended awareness under general anesthesia Z92.84
    urinary calculi Z87.442
    urinary (recurrent) (tract) infection (s) Z87.440
    uterine scar from previous surgery Z98.891
    vaginal dysplasia Z87.411
    venous thrombosis or embolism Z86.718
      pulmonary Z86.711
    vulvar dysplasia Z87.412
His-Werner disease A79.0
HIV — *see also* Human, immunodeficiency virus B20
  laboratory evidence (nonconclusive) R75
  positive, seropositive Z21
  nonconclusive test (in infants) R75
Hives (bold) — *see* Urticaria
Hoarseness R49.0
Hobo Z59.0
Hodgkin disease — *see* Lymphoma, Hodgkin
Hodgson's disease I71.2
  ruptured I71.1
Hoffa-Kastert disease E88.89
Hoffa's disease E88.89
Hoffmann-Bouveret syndrome I47.9
Hoffmann's syndrome E03.9 *[G73.7]*

Hole (round)
  macula H35.34-
  retina (without detachment) — *see* Break, retina, round hole
    with detachment — *see* Detachment, retina, with retinal, break
Holiday relief care Z75.5
Hollenhorst's plaque — *see* Occlusion, artery, retina
Hollow foot (congenital) Q66.7
  acquired — *see* Deformity, limb, foot, specified NEC
Holoprosencephaly Q04.2
Holt-Oram syndrome Q87.2
Homelessness Z59.0
Homesickness — *see* Disorder, adjustment
Homocystinemia, homocystinuria E72.11
Homogentisate 1,2-dioxygenase deficiency E70.29
Homologous serum hepatitis (prophylactic) (therapeutic) — *see* Hepatitis, viral, type B
Honeycomb lung J98.4
  congenital Q33.0
Hooded
  clitoris Q52.6
  penis Q55.69
Hookworm (anemia) (disease) (infection) (infestation) B76.9
  specified NEC B76.8
Hordeolum (eyelid) (externum) (recurrent) H00.019
  internum H00.029
    left H00.026
      lower H00.025
      upper H00.024
    right H00.023
      lower H00.022
      upper H00.021
    left H00.016
      lower H00.015
      upper H00.014
    right H00.013
      lower H00.012
      upper H00.011
Horn
  cutaneous L85.8
  nail L60.2
    congenital Q84.6
Horner (-Claude Bernard) **syndrome** G90.2
  traumatic — *see* Injury, nerve, cervical sympathetic
Horseshoe kidney (congenital) Q63.1
Horton's headache or neuralgia G44.099
  intractable G44.091
  not intractable G44.099
Hospital hopper syndrome — *see* Disorder, factitious
Hospitalism in children — *see* Disorder, adjustment
Hostility R45.5
  towards child Z62.3
Hot flashes
  menopausal N95.1
Hourglass (contracture) — *see also* Contraction, hourglass
  stomach K31.89
    congenital Q40.2
    stricture K31.2
Household, housing circumstance affecting care Z59.9
  specified NEC Z59.8
Housemaid's knee — *see* Bursitis, prepatellar
Hudson (-Stähli) **line** (cornea) — *see* Pigmentation, cornea, anterior
Human
  bite (open wound) — *see also* Bite
    intact skin surface — *see* Bite, superficial
  herpesvirus — *see* Herpes
  immunodeficiency virus (HIV) disease (infection) B20
    asymptomatic status Z21
    contact Z20.6
    counseling Z71.7
    dementia B20 *[F02.80]*
      with behavioral disturbance B20 *[F02.81]*
    exposure to Z20.6
    laboratory evidence R75
    type-2 (HIV 2) as cause of disease classified elsewhere B97.35
  papillomavirus (HPV)
    DNA test positive
      high risk
        cervix R87.810
        vagina R87.811
      low risk
        cervix R87.820
        vagina R87.821
    screening for Z11.51

Human - *continued*
  T-cell lymphotropic virus
    type-1 (HTLV-I) infection B33.3
      as cause of disease classified elsewhere B97.33
      carrier Z22.6
    type-2 (HTLV-II) as cause of disease classified elsewhere B97.34
Humidifier lung or pneumonitis J67.7
Humiliation (experience) **in childhood** Z62.898
Humpback (acquired) — *see* Kyphosis
Hunchback (acquired) — *see* Kyphosis
Hunger T73.0
  air, psychogenic F45.8
Hungry bone syndrome E83.81
Hunner's ulcer — *see* Cystitis, chronic, interstitial
Hunter's
  glossitis D51.0
  syndrome E76.1
Huntington's disease or chorea G10
  with dementia G10 *[F02.80]*
    with behavioral disturbance G10 *[F02.81]*
Hunt's
  disease or syndrome (herpetic geniculate ganglionitis) B02.21
  dyssynergia cerebellaris myoclonica G11.1
  neuralgia B02.21
Hurler (-Scheie) **disease or syndrome** E76.02
Hurst's disease G36.1
Hurthle cell
  adenocarcinoma C73
  adenoma D34
  carcinoma C73
  tumor D34
Hutchinson-Boeck disease or syndrome — *see* Sarcoidosis
Hutchinson-Gilford disease or syndrome E34.8
Hutchinson's
  disease, meaning
    angioma serpiginosum L81.7
    pompholyx (cheiropompholyx) L30.1
    prurigo estivalis L56.4
    summer eruption or summer prurigo L56.4
  melanotic freckle — *see* Melanoma, in situ
    malignant melanoma in — *see* Melanoma
  teeth or incisors (congenital syphilis) A50.52
  triad (congenital syphilis) A50.53
Hyalin plaque, sclera, senile H15.89
Hyaline membrane (disease) (lung) (pulmonary) (newborn) P22.0
Hyalinosis
  cutis (et mucosae) E78.89
  focal and segmental (glomerular) — *see also* N00-N07 with fourth character .1 N05.1
Hyalitis, hyalosis, asteroid — *see also* Deposit, crystalline
  syphilitic (late) A52.71
Hydatid
  cyst or tumor — *see* Echinococcus
  mole — *see* Hydatidiform mole
  Morgagni
    female Q50.5
    male (epididymal) Q55.4
    testicular Q55.29
Hydatidiform mole (benign) (complicating pregnancy) (delivered) (undelivered) O01.9
  classical O01.0
  complete O01.0
  incomplete O01.1
  invasive D39.2
  malignant D39.2
  partial O01.1
Hydatidosis — *see* Echinococcus
Hydradenitis (axillaris) (suppurative) L73.2
Hydradenoma — *see* Hidradenoma
Hydramnios O40.-
Hydrancephaly, hydranencephaly Q04.3
  with spina bifida — *see* Spina bifida, with hydrocephalus
Hydrargyrism NEC — *see* Poisoning, mercury
Hydrarthrosis — *see also* Effusion, joint
  gonococcal A54.42
  intermittent M12.40
    ankle M12.47-
    elbow M12.42-
    foot joint M12.47-
    hand joint M12.44-
    hip M12.45-
    knee M12.46-
    multiple site M12.49
    shoulder M12.41-
    specified joint NEC M12.48
    wrist M12.43-

Hydrarthrosis - *continued*
of yaws (early) (late) (*see also*
subcategory M14.8-) A66.6
syphilitic (late) A52.77
congenital A50.55 *[M12.80]*
Hydremia D64.89
Hydrencephalocele (congenital) — *see*
Encephalocele
Hydrencephalomeningocele (congenital) — *see*
Encephalocele
Hydroa R23.8
aestivale L56.4
vacciniforme L56.4
Hydroadenitis (axillaris) (suppurative) L73.2
Hydrocalycosis — *see* Hydronephrosis
Hydrocele (spermatic cord) (testis) (tunica
vaginalis) N43.3
canal of Nuck N94.89
communicating N43.2
congenital P83.5
congenital P83.5
encysted N43.0
female NEC N94.89
infected N43.1
newborn P83.5
round ligament N94.89
specified NEC N43.2
spinalis — *see* Spina bifida
vulva N90.89
Hydrocephalus (acquired) (external) (internal)
(malignant) (recurrent) G91.9
aqueduct Sylvius stricture Q03.0
causing disproportion O33.6
with obstructed labor O66.3
communicating G91.0
congenital (external) (internal) Q03.9
with spina bifida Q05.4
cervical Q05.0
dorsal Q05.1
lumbar Q05.2
lumbosacral Q05.2
sacral Q05.3
thoracic Q05.1
thoracolumbar Q05.1
specified NEC Q03.8
due to toxoplasmosis (congenital) P37.1
foramen Magendie block (acquired) G91.1
congenital — *see also* Hydrocephalus,
congenital Q03.1
in (due to)
infectious disease NEC B89 *[G91.4]*
neoplastic disease NEC (see also Neoplasm) G91.4
parasitic disease B89 *[G91.4]*
newborn Q03.9
with spina bifida — *see* Spina bifida, with
hydrocephalus
noncommunicating G91.1
normal pressure G91.2
secondary G91.0
obstructive G91.1
otitic G93.2
post-traumatic NEC G91.3
secondary G91.4
post-traumatic G91.3
specified NEC G91.8
syphilitic, congenital A50.49
Hydrocolpos (congenital) N89.8
Hydrocystoma — *see* Neoplasm, skin, benign
Hydroencephalocele (congenital) — *see*
Encephalocele
Hydroencephalomeningocele (congenital) — *see*
Encephalocele
Hydrohematopneumothorax — *see* Hemothorax
Hydromeningitis — *see* Meningitis
Hydromeningocele (spinal) — *see also* Spina bifida
cranial — *see* Encephalocele
Hydrometra N85.8
Hydrometrocolpos N89.8
Hydromicrocephaly Q02
Hydromphalos (since birth) Q45.8
Hydromyelia Q06.4
Hydromyelocele — *see* Spina bifida
Hydronephrosis (atrophic) (early) (functionless)
(intermittent) (primary) (secondary) **NEC** N13.30
with
infection N13.6
obstruction (by) (of)
renal calculus N13.2
with infection N13.6
ureteral NEC N13.1
with infection N13.6
calculus N13.2
with infection N13.6

Hydronephrosis (atrophic) (early) (functionless)
(intermittent) (primary) (secondary) **NEC** - *continued*
with - *continued*
obstruction (by) (of) - *continued*
ureteropelvic junction (congenital) Q62.0
acquired N13.0
with infection N13.6
ureteral stricture NEC N13.1
with infection N13.6
congenital Q62.0
due to acquired occlusion of ureteropelvic
junction N13.0
specified type NEC N13.39
tuberculous A18.11
Hydropericarditis — *see* Pericarditis
Hydropericardium — *see* Pericarditis
Hydroperitoneum R18.8
Hydrophobia — *see* Rabies
Hydrophthalmos Q15.0
Hydropneumohemothorax — *see* Hemothorax
Hydropneumopericarditis — *see* Pericarditis
Hydropneumopericardium — *see* Pericarditis
Hydropneumothorax J94.8
traumatic — *see* Injury, intrathoracic, lung
tuberculous NEC A15.6
Hydrops R60.9
abdominis R18.8
articulorum intermittens — *see* Hydrarthrosis,
intermittent
cardiac — *see* Failure, heart, congestive
causing obstructed labor (mother) O66.3
endolymphatic H81.0-
fetal — *see* Pregnancy, complicated by, hydrops,
fetalis
fetalis P83.2
due to
ABO isoimmunization P56.0
alpha thalassemia D56.0
hemolytic disease P56.90
specified NEC P56.99
isoimmunization (ABO) (Rh) P56.0
other specified nonhemolytic disease NEC P83.2
Rh incompatibility P56.0
during pregnancy — *see* Pregnancy, complicated
by, hydrops, fetalis
gallbladder K82.1
joint — *see* Effusion, joint
labyrinth H81.0-
newborn (idiopathic) P83.2
due to
ABO isoimmunization P56.0
alpha thalassemia D56.0
hemolytic disease P56.90
specified NEC P56.99
isoimmunization (ABO) (Rh) P56.0
Rh incompatibility P56.0
nutritional — *see* Malnutrition, severe
pericardium — *see* Pericarditis
pleura — *see* Hydrothorax
spermatic cord — *see* Hydrocele
Hydropyonephrosis N13.6
Hydrorachis Q06.4
Hydrorrhea (nasal) J34.89
pregnancy — *see* Rupture, membranes, premature
Hydrosadenitis (axillaris) (suppurative) L73.2
Hydrosalpinx (fallopian tube) (follicularis) N70.11
Hydrothorax (double) (pleura) J94.8
chylous (nonfilarial) I89.8
filarial — *see also* Infestation,
filarial B74.9 *[J91.8]*
traumatic — *see* Injury, intrathoracic
tuberculous NEC (non primary) A15.6
Hydroureter — *see also* Hydronephrosis N13.4
with infection N13.6
congenital Q62.39
Hydroureteronephrosis — *see* Hydronephrosis
Hydrourethra N36.8
Hydroxykynureninuria E70.8
Hydroxylysinemia E72.3
Hydroxyprolinemia E72.59
Hygiene, sleep
abuse Z72.821
inadequate Z72.821
poor Z72.821
Hygroma (congenital) (cystic) D18.1
praepatellare, prepatellar — *see* Bursitis, prepatellar
Hymen — *see* condition
Hymenolepis, hymenolepiasis (diminuta) (infection)
(infestation) (nana) B71.0
Hypalgesia R20.8
Hyperacidity (gastric) K31.89
psychogenic F45.8

Hyperactive, hyperactivity F90.9
basal cell, uterine cervix — *see* Dysplasia, cervix
bowel sounds R19.12
cervix epithelial (basal) — *see* Dysplasia, cervix
child F90.9
attention deficit — *see* Disorder, attention-deficit
hyperactivity
detrusor muscle N32.81
gastrointestinal K31.89
psychogenic F45.8
nasal mucous membrane J34.3
stomach K31.89
thyroid (gland) — *see* Hyperthyroidism
Hyperacusis H93.23-
Hyperadrenalism E27.5
Hyperadrenocorticism E24.9
congenital E25.0
iatrogenic E24.2
correct substance properly administered — *see*
Table of Drugs and Chemicals, by drug, adverse
effect
overdose or wrong substance given or taken — *see*
Table of Drugs and Chemicals, by drug,
poisoning
not associated with Cushing's syndrome E27.0
pituitary-dependent E24.0
Hyperaldosteronism E26.9
familial (type I) E26.02
glucocorticoid-remediable E26.02
primary (due to (bilateral) adrenal
hyperplasia) E26.09
primary NEC E26.09
secondary E26.1
specified NEC E26.89
Hyperalgesia R20.8
Hyperalimentation R63.2
carotene, carotin E67.1
specified NEC E67.8
vitamin
A E67.0
D E67.3
Hyperaminoaciduria
arginine E72.21
cystine E72.01
lysine E72.3
ornithine E72.4
Hyperammonemia (congenital) E72.20
Hyperazotemia — *see* Uremia
Hyperbetalipoproteinemia (familial) E78.00
with prebetalipoproteinemia E78.2
Hyperbilirubinemia
constitutional E80.6
familial conjugated E80.6
neonatal (transient) — *see* Jaundice, newborn
Hypercalcemia, hypocalciuric, familial E83.52
Hypercalciuria, idiopathic E83.52
Hypercapnia R06.89
newborn P84
Hypercarotenemia, hypercarotinemia
(dietary) E67.1
Hypercementosis K03.4
Hyperchloremia E87.8
Hyperchlorhydria K31.89
neurotic F45.8
psychogenic F45.8
Hypercholesterinemia — *see* Hypercholesterolemia
Hypercholesterolemia (essential) (primary)
(pure) E78.00
with hyperglyceridemia, endogenous E78.2
dietary counseling and surveillance Z71.3
familial E78.01
hereditary E78.01
Hyperchylia gastrica, psychogenic F45.8
Hyperchylomicronemia (familial) (primary) E78.3
with hyperbetalipoproteinemia E78.3
Hypercoagulable (state) D68.59
activated protein C resistance D68.51
antithrombin (III) deficiency D68.59
factor V Leiden mutation D68.51
primary NEC D68.59
protein C deficiency D68.59
protein S deficiency D68.59
prothrombin gene mutation D68.52
secondary D68.69
specified NEC D68.69
Hypercoagulation (state) D68.59
Hypercorticalism, pituitary-dependent E24.0
Hypercorticosolism — *see* Cushing's, syndrome
Hypercorticosteronism E24.2
correct substance properly administered — *see* Table
of Drugs and Chemicals, by drug, adverse effect
overdose or wrong substance given or taken — *see*
Table of Drugs and Chemicals, by drug, poisoning

Hypercortisonism E24.2
correct substance properly administered — *see* Table of Drugs and Chemicals, by drug, adverse effect
overdose or wrong substance given or taken — *see* Table of Drugs and Chemicals, by drug, poisoning
Hyperekplexia Q89.8
Hyperelectrolytemia E87.8
Hyperemesis R11.10
with nausea R11.2
gravidarum (mild) O21.0
with
carbohydrate depletion O21.1
dehydration O21.1
electrolyte imbalance O21.1
metabolic disturbance O21.1
severe (with metabolic disturbance) O21.1
projectile R11.12
psychogenic F45.8
Hyperemia (acute) (passive) R68.89
anal mucosa K62.89
bladder N32.89
cerebral I67.89
conjunctiva H11.43-
ear internal, acute — *see* subcategory H83.0
enteric K59.8
eye — *see* Hyperemia, conjunctiva
eyelid (active) (passive) — *see* Disorder, eyelid, specified type NEC
intestine K59.8
iris — *see* Disorder, iris, vascular
kidney N28.89
labyrinth — *see* subcategory H83.0
liver (active) K76.89
lung (passive) — *see* Edema, lung
pulmonary (passive) — *see* Edema, lung
renal N28.89
retina H35.89
stomach K31.89
Hyperesthesia (body surface) R20.3
larynx (reflex) J38.7
hysterical F44.89
pharynx (reflex) J39.2
hysterical F44.89
Hyperestrogenism (drug-induced) (iatrogenic) E28.0
Hyperexplexia Q89.8
Hyperfibrinolysis — *see* Fibrinolysis
Hyperfructosemia E74.19
Hyperfunction
adrenal cortex, not associated with Cushing's syndrome E27.0
medulla E27.5
adrenomedullary E27.5
virilism E25.9
congenital E25.0
ovarian E28.8
pancreas K86.89
parathyroid (gland) E21.3
pituitary (gland) (anterior) E22.9
specified NEC E22.8
polyglandular E31.1
testicular E29.0
Hypergammaglobulinemia D89.2
polyclonal D89.0
Waldenström D89.0
Hypergastrinemia E16.4
Hyperglobulinemia R77.1
Hyperglycemia, hyperglycemic (transient) R73.9
coma — *see* Diabetes, by type, with coma
postpancreatectomy E89.1
Hyperglyceridemia (endogenous) (essential) (familial) (hereditary) (pure) E78.1
mixed E78.3
Hyperglycinemia (non-ketotic) E72.51
Hypergonadism
ovarian E28.8
testicular (primary) (infantile) E29.0
Hyperheparinemia D68.32
Hyperhidrosis, hyperidrosis R61
focal
primary L74.519
axilla L74.510
face L74.511
palms L74.512
soles L74.513
secondary L74.52
generalized R61
localized
primary L74.519
axilla L74.510
face L74.511
palms L74.512
soles L74.513
secondary L74.52

Hyperhidrosis, hyperidrosis - *continued*
psychogenic F45.8
secondary R61
focal L74.52
Hyperhistidinemia E70.41
Hyperhomocysteinemia E72.11
Hyperhydroxyprolinemia E72.59
Hyperinsulinism (functional) E16.1
with
coma (hypoglycemic) E15
encephalopathy E16.1 *[G94]*
ectopic E16.1
therapeutic misadventure (from administration of insulin) — *see* subcategory T38.3
Hyperkalemia E87.5
Hyperkeratosis — *see also* Keratosis L85.9
cervix N88.0
due to yaws (early) (late) (palmar or plantar) A66.3
follicularis Q82.8
penetrans (in cutem) L87.0
palmoplantaris climacterica L85.1
pinta A67.1
senile (with pruritus) L57.0
universalis congenita Q80.8
vocal cord J38.3
vulva N90.4
Hyperkinesia, hyperkinetic (disease) (reaction) (syndrome) (childhood) (adolescence) — *see also* Disorder, attention-deficit hyperactivity
heart I51.89
Hyperleucine-isoleucinemia E71.19
Hyperlipemia, hyperlipidemia E78.5
combined E78.2
familial E78.4
group
A E78.00
B E78.1
C E78.2
D E78.3
mixed E78.2
specified NEC E78.4
Hyperlipidosis E75.6
hereditary NEC E75.5
Hyperlipoproteinemia E78.5
Fredrickson's type
I E78.3
IIa E78.00
IIb E78.2
III E78.2
IV E78.1
V E78.3
low-density-lipoprotein-type (LDL) E78.00
very-low-density-lipoprotein-type (VLDL) E78.1
Hyperlucent lung, unilateral J43.0
Hyperlysinemia E72.3
Hypermagnesemia E83.41
neonatal P71.8
Hypermenorrhea N92.0
Hypermethioninemia E72.19
Hypermetropia (congenital) H52.0-
Hypermobility, hypermotility
cecum — *see* Syndrome, irritable bowel
coccyx — *see* subcategory M53.2
colon — *see* Syndrome, irritable bowel
psychogenic F45.8
ileum K58.9
intestine — *see also* Syndrome, irritable bowel K58.9
psychogenic F45.8
meniscus (knee) — *see* Derangement, knee, meniscus
scapula — *see* Instability, joint, shoulder
stomach K31.89
psychogenic F45.8
syndrome M35.7
urethra N36.41
with intrinsic sphincter deficiency N36.43
Hypernasality R49.21
Hypernatremia E87.0
Hypernephroma C64.-
Hyperopia — *see* Hypermetropia
Hyperorexia nervosa F50.2
Hyperornithinemia E72.4
Hyperosmia R43.1
Hyperosmolality E87.0
Hyperostosis (monomelic) — *see also* Disorder, bone, density and structure, specified NEC
ankylosing (spine) M48.10
cervical region M48.12
cervicothoracic region M48.13
lumbar region M48.16
lumbosacral region M48.17
multiple sites M48.19

Hyperostosis (monomelic) - *continued*
ankylosing (spine) - *continued*
occipito-atlanto-axial region M48.11
sacrococcygeal region M48.18
thoracic region M48.14
thoracolumbar region M48.15
cortical (skull) M85.2
infantile M89.8X-
frontal, internal of skull M85.2
interna frontalis M85.2
skeletal, diffuse idiopathic — *see* Hyperostosis, ankylosing
skull M85.2
congenital Q75.8
vertebral, ankylosing — *see* Hyperostosis, ankylosing
Hyperovarism E28.8
Hyperoxaluria (primary) E72.53
Hyperparathyroidism E21.3
primary E21.0
secondary (renal) N25.81
non-renal E21.1
specified NEC E21.2
tertiary E21.2
Hyperpathia R20.8
Hyperperistalsis R19.2
psychogenic F45.8
Hyperpermeability, capillary I78.8
Hyperphagia R63.2
Hyperphenylalaninemia NEC E70.1
Hyperphoria (alternating) H50.53
Hyperphosphatemia E83.39
Hyperpiesis, hyperpiesia — *see* Hypertension
Hyperpigmentation — *see also* Pigmentation
melanin NEC L81.4
postinflammatory L81.0
Hyperpinealism E34.8
Hyperpituitarism E22.9
Hyperplasia, hyperplastic
adenoids J35.2
adrenal (capsule) (cortex) (gland) E27.8
with
sexual precocity (male) E25.9
congenital E25.0
virilism, adrenal E25.9
congenital E25.0
virilization (female) E25.9
congenital E25.0
congenital E25.0
salt-losing E25.0
adrenomedullary E27.5
angiolymphoid, eosinophilia (ALHE) D18.01
appendix (lymphoid) K38.0
artery, fibromuscular I77.3
bone — *see also* Hypertrophy, bone
marrow D75.89
breast — *see also* Hypertrophy, breast
ductal (atypical) N60.9-
C-cell, thyroid E07.0
cementation (tooth) (teeth) K03.4
cervical gland R59.0
cervix (uteri) (basal cell) (endometrium) (polypoid) — *see also* Dysplasia, cervix
congenital Q51.828
clitoris, congenital Q52.6
denture K06.2
endocervicitis N72
endometrium, endometrial (adenomatous) (benign) (cystic) (glandular) (glandular-cystic) (polypoid) N85.00
with atypia N85.02
cervix — *see* Dysplasia, cervix
complex (without atypia) N85.01
simple (without atypia) N85.01
epithelial L85.9
focal, oral, including tongue K13.29
nipple N62
skin L85.9
tongue K13.29
vaginal wall N89.3
erythroid D75.89
fibromuscular of artery (carotid) (renal) I77.3
genital
female NEC N94.89
male N50.89
gingiva K06.1
glandularis cystica uteri (interstitialis) — *see also* Hyperplasia, endometrial N85.00-
gum K06.1
hymen, congenital Q52.4
irritative, edentulous (alveolar) K06.2
jaw M26.09
alveolar M26.79

Hyperplasia, hyperplastic - *continued*
jaw - *continued*
lower M26.03
alveolar M26.72
upper M26.01
alveolar M26.71
kidney (congenital) Q63.3
labia N90.69
epithelial N90.3
liver (congenital) Q44.7
nodular, focal K76.89
lymph gland or node R59.9
mandible, mandibular M26.03
alveolar M26.72
unilateral condylar M27.8
maxilla, maxillary M26.01
alveolar M26.71
myometrium, myometrial N85.2
neuroendocrine cell, of infancy J84.841
nose
lymphoid J34.89
polypoid J33.9
oral mucosa (irritative) K13.6
organ or site, congenital NEC — *see* Anomaly, by site
ovary N83.8
palate, papillary (irritative) K13.6
pancreatic islet cells E16.9
alpha E16.8
with excess
gastrin E16.4
glucagon E16.3
beta E16.1
parathyroid (gland) E21.0
pharynx (lymphoid) J39.2
prostate (adenofibromatous) (nodular) N40.0
with lower urinary tract symptoms (LUTS) N40.1
without lower urinary tract symtpoms (LUTS) N40.0
renal artery I77.89
reticulo-endothelial (cell) D75.89
salivary gland (any) K11.1
Schimmelbusch's — *see* Mastopathy, cystic
suprarenal capsule (gland) E27.8
thymus (gland) (persistent) E32.0
thyroid (gland) — *see* Goiter
tonsils (faucial) (infective) (lingual) (lymphoid) J35.1
with adenoids J35.3
unilateral condylar M27.8
uterus, uterine N85.2
endometrium (glandular) — *see also* Hyperplasia, endometrial N85.00-
vulva N90.69
epithelial N90.3
Hyperpnea — *see* Hyperventilation
Hyperpotassemia E87.5
Hyperprebetalipoproteinemia (familial) E78.1
Hyperprolactinemia E22.1
Hyperprolinemia (type I) (type II) E72.59
Hyperproteinemia E88.09
Hyperprothrombinemia, causing coagulation factor deficiency D68.4
Hyperpyrexia R50.9
heat (effects) T67.0
malignant, due to anesthetic T88.3
rheumatic — *see* Fever, rheumatic
unknown origin R50.9
Hyper-reflexia R29.2
Hypersalivation K11.7
Hypersecretion
ACTH (not associated with Cushing's syndrome) E27.0
pituitary E24.0
adrenaline E27.5
adrenomedullary E27.5
androgen (testicular) E29.0
ovarian (drug-induced) (iatrogenic) E28.1
calcitonin E07.0
catecholamine E27.5
corticoadrenal E24.9
cortisol E24.9
epinephrine E27.5
estrogen E28.0
gastric K31.89
psychogenic F45.8
gastrin E16.4
glucagon E16.3
hormone (s)
ACTH (not associated with Cushing's syndrome) E27.0
pituitary E24.0
antidiuretic E22.2

Hypersecretion - *continued*
hormone (s) - *continued*
growth E22.0
intestinal NEC E34.1
ovarian androgen E28.1
pituitary E22.9
testicular E29.0
thyroid stimulating E05.80
with thyroid storm E05.81
insulin — *see* Hyperinsulinism
lacrimal glands — *see* Epiphora
medulloadrenal E27.5
milk O92.6
ovarian androgens E28.1
salivary gland (any) K11.7
thyrocalcitonin E07.0
upper respiratory J39.8
Hypersegmentation, leukocytic, hereditary D72.0
Hypersensitive, hypersensitiveness, hypersensitivity — *see also* Allergy
carotid sinus G90.01
colon — *see* Irritable, colon
drug T88.7
gastrointestinal K52.29
immediate K52.29
psychogenic F45.8
labyrinth — *see* subcategory H83.2
pain R20.8
pneumonitis — *see* Pneumonitis, allergic
reaction T78.40
upper respiratory tract NEC J39.3
Hypersomnia (organic) G47.10
due to
alcohol
abuse F10.182
dependence F10.282
use F10.982
amphetamines
abuse F15.182
dependence F15.282
use F15.982
caffeine
abuse F15.182
dependence F15.282
use F15.982
cocaine
abuse F14.182
dependence F14.282
use F14.982
drug NEC
abuse F19.182
dependence F19.282
use F19.982
medical condition G47.14
mental disorder F51.13
opioid
abuse F11.182
dependence F11.282
use F11.982
psychoactive substance NEC
abuse F19.182
dependence F19.282
use F19.982
sedative, hypnotic, or anxiolytic
abuse F13.182
dependence F13.282
use F13.982
stimulant NEC
abuse F15.182
dependence F15.282
use F15.982
idiopathic G47.11
with long sleep time G47.11
without long sleep time G47.12
menstrual related G47.13
nonorganic origin F51.11
specified NEC F51.19
not due to a substance or known physiological condition F51.11
specified NEC F51.19
primary F51.11
recurrent G47.13
specified NEC G47.19
Hypersplenia, hypersplenism D73.1
Hyperstimulation, ovaries (associated with induced ovulation) N98.1
Hypersusceptibility — *see* Allergy
Hypertelorism (ocular) (orbital) Q75.2
Hypertension, hypertensive (accelerated) (benign) (essential) (idiopathic) (malignant) (systemic) I10
with
heart involvement (conditions in I51.4- I51.9 due to hypertension) — *see* Hypertension, heart

Hypertension, hypertensive (accelerated) (benign) (essential) (idiopathic) (malignant) (systemic) - *continued*
with - *continued*
kidney involvement — *see* Hypertension, kidney
benign, intracranial G93.2
borderline R03.0
cardiorenal (disease) I13.10
with heart failure I13.0
with stage 1 through stage 4 chronic kidney disease I13.0
with stage 5 or end stage renal disease I13.2
without heart failure I13.10
with stage 1 through stage 4 chronic kidney disease I13.10
with stage 5 or end stage renal disease I13.11
cardiovascular
disease (arteriosclerotic) (sclerotic) — *see* Hypertension, heart
renal (disease) — *see* Hypertension, cardiorenal
chronic venous — *see* Hypertension, venous (chronic)
complicating
childbirth (labor) O16.4
pre-existing O10.92
with
heart disease O10.12
with renal disease O10.32
pre-eclampsia O11.4
renal disease O10.22
with heart disease O10.32
essential O10.02
secondary O10.42
pregnancy O16.-
with edema — *see also* Pre-eclampsia O14.9-
gestational (pregnancy induced) (without proteinuria) O13.-
with proteinuria O14.9-
mild pre-eclampsia O14.0-
moderate pre-eclampsia O14.0-
severe pre-eclampsia O14.1-
with hemolysis, elevated liver enzymes and low platelet count (HELLP) O14.2-
pre-existing O10.91-
with
heart disease O10.11-
with renal disease O10.31-
pre-eclampsia — *see* category O11
renal disease O10.21-
with heart disease O10.31-
essential O10.01-
secondary O10.41-
transient O13.-
puerperium, pre-existing O16.5
pre-existing
with
heart disease O10.13
with renal disease O10.33
pre-eclampsia O11.5
renal disease O10.23
with heart disease O10.33
essential O10.03
pregnancy-induced O13.9
secondary O10.43
crisis I16.9
due to
endocrine disorders I15.2
pheochromocytoma I15.2
renal disorders NEC I15.1
arterial I15.0
renovascular disorders I15.0
specified disease NEC I15.8
emergency I16.2
encephalopathy I67.4
gestational (without significant proteinuria) (pregnancy-induced) (transient) O13.-
with significant proteinuria — *see* Pre-eclampsia
complicating
delivery O13.4
puerperium O13.5
Goldblatt's I70.1
heart (disease) (conditions in I51.4-I51.9 due to hypertension) I11.9
with
heart failure (congestive) I11.0
kidney disease (chronic) — *see* Hypertension, cardiorenal
intracranial (benign) G93.2
kidney I12.9
with
heart disease — *see* Hypertension, cardiorenal
stage 5 chronic kidney disease (CKD) or end stage renal disease (ESRD) I12.0

Hypertension, hypertensive (accelerated) (benign)
(essential) (idiopathic) (malignant) (systemic) -
continued
  kidney - *continued*
    with - *continued*
      stage 1 through stage 4 chronic kidney
        disease I12.9
  lesser circulation I27.0
  maternal O16.-
  newborn P29.2
    pulmonary (persistent) P29.3
  ocular H40.05-
  pancreatic duct - code to underlying condition
    with chronic pancreatitis K86.1
  portal (due to chronic liver disease)
    (idiopathic) K76.6
    gastropathy K31.89
    in (due to) schistosomiasis
      (bilharziasis) B65.9 [K77]
  postoperative I97.3
  psychogenic F45.8
  pulmonary (artery) (secondary) NEC I27.2
    with
      cor pulmonale (chronic) I27.2
        acute I26.09
      right heart ventricular strain/failure I27.2
        acute I26.09
    of newborn (persistent) P29.3
    primary (idiopathic) I27.0
  renal — *see* Hypertension, kidney
  renovascular I15.0
  secondary NEC I15.9
    due to
      endocrine disorders I15.2
      pheochromocytoma I15.2
      renal disorders NEC I15.1
        arterial I15.0
      renovascular disorders I15.0
    specified NEC I15.8
  transient, of pregnancy O13.-
  urgency I16.0
  venous (chronic)
    due to
      deep vein thrombosis — *see* Syndrome,
        postthrombotic
    idiopathic I87.309
      with
        inflammation I87.32-
          with ulcer I87.33-
        specified complication NEC I87.39-
        ulcer I87.31-
          with inflammation I87.33-
      asymptomatic I87.30-
Hypertensive urgency — *see* Hypertension
Hyperthecosis ovary E28.8
Hyperthermia (of unknown origin) — *see*
also Hyperpyrexia
  malignant, due to anesthesia T88.3
  newborn P81.9
    environmental P81.0
Hyperthyroid (recurrent) — *see* Hyperthyroidism
Hyperthyroidism (latent) (pre-adult)
(recurrent) E05.90
  with
    goiter (diffuse) E05.00
      with thyroid storm E05.01
      nodular (multinodular) E05.20
        with thyroid storm E05.21
        uninodular E05.10
          with thyroid storm E05.11
    storm E05.91
  due to ectopic thyroid tissue E05.30
    with thyroid storm E05.31
  neonatal, transitory P72.1
  specified NEC E05.80
    with thyroid storm E05.81
Hypertony, hypertonia, hypertonicity
  bladder N31.8
  congenital P94.1
  stomach K31.89
    psychogenic F45.8
  uterus, uterine (contractions) (complicating
    delivery) O62.4
Hypertrichosis L68.9
  congenital Q84.2
  eyelid H02.869
    left H02.866
      lower H02.865
      upper H02.864
    right H02.863
      lower H02.862
      upper H02.861
  lanuginosa Q84.2

Hypertrichosis - *continued*
  lanuginosa - *continued*
    acquired L68.1
    localized L68.2
    specified NEC L68.8
Hypertriglyceridemia, essential E78.1
Hypertrophy, hypertrophic
  adenofibromatous, prostate — *see* Enlargement,
    enlarged, prostate
  adenoids (infective) J35.2
    with tonsils J35.3
  adrenal cortex E27.8
  alveolar process or ridge — *see* Anomaly, alveolar
  anal papillae K62.89
  artery I77.89
    congenital NEC Q27.8
      digestive system Q27.8
      lower limb Q27.8
      specified site NEC Q27.8
      upper limb Q27.8
  auricular — *see* Hypertrophy, cardiac
  Bartholin's gland N75.8
  bile duct (common) (hepatic) K83.8
  bladder (sphincter) (trigone) N32.89
  bone M89.30
    carpus M89.34-
    clavicle M89.31-
    femur M89.35-
    fibula M89.36-
    finger M89.34-
    humerus M89.32-
    ilium M89.359
    ischium M89.359
    metacarpus M89.34-
    metatarsus M89.37-
    multiple sites M89.39
    neck M89.38
    radius M89.33-
    rib M89.38
    scapula M89.31-
    skull M89.38
    tarsus M89.37-
    tibia M89.36-
    toe M89.37-
    ulna M89.33-
    vertebra M89.38
  brain G93.89
  breast N62
    cystic — *see* Mastopathy, cystic
    newborn P83.4
    pubertal, massive N62
    puerperal, postpartum — *see* Disorder, breast,
      specified type NEC
    senile (parenchymatous) N62
  cardiac (chronic) (idiopathic) I51.7
    with rheumatic fever (conditions in I00)
      active I01.8
      inactive or quiescent (with chorea) I09.89
    congenital NEC Q24.8
    fatty — *see* Degeneration, myocardial
    hypertensive — *see* Hypertension, heart
    rheumatic (with chorea) I09.89
      active or acute I01.8
        with chorea I02.0
    valve — *see* Endocarditis
  cartilage — *see* Disorder, cartilage, specified type
    NEC
  cecum — *see* Megacolon
  cervix (uteri) N88.8
    congenital Q51.828
    elongation N88.4
  clitoris (cirrhotic) N90.89
    congenital Q52.6
  colon — *see also* Megacolon
    congenital Q43.2
  conjunctiva, lymphoid H11.89
  corpora cavernosa N48.89
  cystic duct K82.8
  duodenum K31.89
  endometrium (glandular) — *see also* Hyperplasia,
    endometrial N85.00-
    cervix N88.8
  epididymis N50.89
  esophageal hiatus (congenital) Q79.1
    with hernia — *see* Hernia, hiatal
  eyelid — *see* Disorder, eyelid, specified type NEC
  fat pad E65
    knee (infrapatellar) (popliteal) (prepatellar)
      (retropatellar) M79.4
  foot (congenital) Q74.2
  frenulum, frenum (tongue) K14.8
    lip K13.0
  gallbladder K82.8

Hypertrophy, hypertrophic - *continued*
  gastric mucosa K29.60
    with bleeding K29.61
  gland, glandular R59.9
    generalized R59.1
    localized R59.0
  gum (mucous membrane) K06.1
  heart (idiopathic) — *see also* Hypertrophy, cardiac
    valve — *see also* Endocarditis I38
  hemifacial Q67.4
  hepatic — *see* Hypertrophy, liver
  hiatus (esophageal) Q79.1
  hilus gland R59.0
  hymen, congenital Q52.4
  ileum K63.89
  intestine NEC K63.89
  jejunum K63.89
  kidney (compensatory) N28.81
    congenital Q63.3
  labium (majus) (minus) N90.60
  ligament — *see* Disorder, ligament
  lingual tonsil (infective) J35.1
    with adenoids J35.3
  lip K13.0
    congenital Q18.6
  liver R16.0
    acute K76.89
    congenital Q44.7
    cirrhotic — *see* Cirrhosis, liver
    fatty — *see* Fatty, liver
  lymph, lymphatic gland R59.9
    generalized R59.1
    localized R59.0
    tuberculous — *see* Tuberculosis, lymph gland
  mammary gland — *see* Hypertrophy, breast
  Meckel's diverticulum (congenital) Q43.0
    malignant — *see* Table of Neoplasms, small
      intestine, malignant
  median bar — *see* Hyperplasia, prostate
  meibomian gland — *see* Chalazion
  meniscus, knee, congenital Q74.1
  metatarsal head — *see* Hypertrophy, bone,
    metatarsus
  metatarsus — *see* Hypertrophy, bone, metatarsus
  mucous membrane
    alveolar ridge K06.2
    gum K06.1
    nose (turbinate) J34.3
  muscle M62.89
  muscular coat, artery I77.89
  myocardium — *see also* Hypertrophy, cardiac
    idiopathic I42.2
  myometrium N85.2
  nail L60.2
    congenital Q84.5
  nasal J34.89
    alae J34.89
    bone J34.89
    cartilage J34.89
    mucous membrane (septum) J34.3
    sinus J34.89
    turbinate J34.3
  nasopharynx, lymphoid (infectional) (tissue)
    (wall) J35.2
  nipple N62
  organ or site, congenital NEC — *see* Anomaly, by
    site
  ovary N83.8
  palate (hard) M27.8
    soft K13.79
  pancreas, congenital Q45.3
  parathyroid (gland) E21.0
  parotid gland K11.1
  penis N48.89
  pharyngeal tonsil J35.2
  pharynx J39.2
    lymphoid (infectional) (tissue) (wall) J35.2
  pituitary (anterior) (fossa) (gland) E23.6
  prepuce (congenital) N47.8
    female N90.89
  prostate — *see* Enlargement, enlarged, prostate
    congenital Q55.4
  pseudomuscular G71.0
  pylorus (adult) (muscle) (sphincter) K31.1
    congenital or infantile Q40.0
  rectal, rectum (sphincter) K62.89
  rhinitis (turbinate) J31.0
  salivary gland (any) K11.1
    congenital Q38.4
  scaphoid (tarsal) — *see* Hypertrophy, bone, tarsus
  scar L91.0
  scrotum N50.89
  seminal vesicle N50.89

Hypertrophy, hypertrophic - *continued*
  sigmoid — *see* Megacolon
  skin L91.9
    specified NEC L91.8
  spermatic cord N50.89
  spleen — *see* Splenomegaly
  spondylitis — *see* Spondylosis
  stomach K31.89
  sublingual gland K11.1
  submandibular gland K11.1
  suprarenal cortex (gland) E27.8
  synovial NEC M67.20
    acromioclavicular M67.21-
    ankle M67.27-
    elbow M67.22-
    foot M67.27-
    hand M67.24-
    hip M67.25-
    knee M67.26-
    multiple sites M67.29
    specified site NEC M67.28
    wrist M67.23-
  tendon — *see* Disorder, tendon, specified type NEC
  testis N44.8
    congenital Q55.29
  thymic, thymus (gland) (congenital) E32.0
  thyroid (gland) — *see* Goiter
  toe (congenital) Q74.2
    acquired — *see also* Deformity, toe, specified NEC
  tongue K14.8
    congenital Q38.2
    papillae (foliate) K14.3
  tonsils (faucial) (infective) (lingual) (lymphoid) J35.1
    with adenoids J35.3
  tunica vaginalis N50.89
  ureter N28.89
  urethra N36.8
  uterus N85.2
    neck (with elongation) N88.4
    puerperal O90.89
  uvula K13.79
  vagina N89.8
  vas deferens N50.89
  vein I87.8
  ventricle, ventricular (heart) — *see also* Hypertrophy, cardiac
    congenital Q24.8
    in tetralogy of Fallot Q21.3
  verumontanum N36.8
  vocal cord J38.3
  vulva N90.60
    stasis (nonfilarial) N90.69
Hypertropia H50.2-
Hypertyrosinemia E70.21
Hyperuricemia (asymptomatic) E79.0
Hypervalinemia E71.19
Hyperventilation (tetany) R06.4
  hysterical F45.8
  psychogenic F45.8
  syndrome F45.8
Hypervitaminosis (dietary) **NEC** E67.8
  A E67.0
    administered as drug (prolonged intake) — *see* Table of Drugs and Chemicals, vitamins, adverse effect
    overdose or wrong substance given or taken — *see* Table of Drugs and Chemicals, vitamins, poisoning
  B6 E67.2
  D E67.3
    administered as drug (prolonged intake) — *see* Table of Drugs and Chemicals, vitamins, adverse effect
    overdose or wrong substance given or taken — *see* Table of Drugs and Chemicals, vitamins, poisoning
  K E67.8
    administered as drug (prolonged intake) — *see* Table of Drugs and Chemicals, vitamins, adverse effect
    overdose or wrong substance given or taken — *see* Table of Drugs and Chemicals, vitamins, poisoning
Hypervolemia E87.70
  specified NEC E87.79
Hypesthesia R20.1
  cornea — *see* Anesthesia, cornea
Hyphema H21.0-
  traumatic S05.1-
Hypoacidity, gastric K31.89
  psychogenic F45.8

Hypoadrenalism, hypoadrenia E27.40
  primary E27.1
  tuberculous A18.7
Hypoadrenocorticism E27.40
  pituitary E23.0
  primary E27.1
Hypoalbuminemia E88.09
Hypoaldosteronism E27.40
Hypoalphalipoproteinemia E78.6
Hypobarism T70.29
Hypobaropathy T70.29
Hypobetalipoproteinemia (familial) E78.6
Hypocalcemia E83.51
  dietary E58
  neonatal P71.1
    due to cow's milk P71.0
  phosphate-loading (newborn) P71.1
Hypochloremia E87.8
Hypochlorhydria K31.89
  neurotic F45.8
  psychogenic F45.8
Hypochondria, hypochondriac, hypochondriasis (reaction) F45.21
  sleep F51.03
Hypochondrogenesis Q77.0
Hypochondroplasia Q77.4
Hypochromasia, blood cells D50.8
Hypodontia — *see* Anodontia
Hypoeosinophilia D72.89
Hypoesthesia R20.1
Hypofibrinogenemia D68.8
  acquired D65
  congenital (hereditary) D68.2
Hypofunction
  adrenocortical E27.40
    drug-induced E27.3
    postprocedural E89.6
    primary E27.1
  adrenomedullary, postprocedural E89.6
  cerebral R29.818
  corticoadrenal NEC E27.40
  intestinal K59.8
  labyrinth — *see* subcategory H83.2
  ovary E28.39
  pituitary (gland) (anterior) E23.0
  testicular E29.1
    postprocedural (postsurgical) (postirradiation) (iatrogenic) E89.5
Hypogalactia O92.4
Hypogammaglobulinemia — *see also* Agammaglobulinemia D80.1
  hereditary D80.0
  nonfamilial D80.1
  transient, of infancy D80.7
Hypogenitalism (congenital) — *see* Hypogonadism
Hypoglossia Q38.3
Hypoglycemia (spontaneous) E16.2
  coma E15
    diabetic — *see* Diabetes, coma
  diabetic — *see* Diabetes, hypoglycemia
  dietary counseling and surveillance Z71.3
  drug-induced E16.0
    with coma (nondiabetic) E15
  due to insulin E16.0
    with coma (nondiabetic) E15
    therapeutic misadventure — *see* subcategory T38.3
  functional, nonhyperinsulinemic E16.1
  iatrogenic E16.0
    with coma (nondiabetic) E15
  in infant of diabetic mother P70.1
    gestational diabetes P70.0
  infantile E16.1
  leucine-induced E71.19
  neonatal (transitory) P70.4
    iatrogenic P70.3
  reactive (not drug-induced) E16.1
  transitory neonatal P70.4
Hypogonadism
  female E28.39
  hypogonadotropic E23.0
  male E29.1
  ovarian (primary) E28.39
  pituitary E23.0
  testicular (primary) E29.1
Hypohidrosis, hypoidrosis L74.4
Hypoinsulinemia, postprocedural E89.1
Hypokalemia E87.6
Hypoleukocytosis — *see* Agranulocytosis
Hypolipoproteinemia (alpha) (beta) E78.6
Hypomagnesemia E83.42
  neonatal P71.2
Hypomania, hypomanic reaction F30.8
Hypomenorrhea — *see* Oligomenorrhea

Hypometabolism R63.8
Hypomotility
  gastrointestinal (tract) K31.89
    psychogenic F45.8
  intestine K59.8
    psychogenic F45.8
  stomach K31.89
    psychogenic F45.8
Hyponasality R49.22
Hyponatremia E87.1
Hypo-osmolality E87.1
Hypo-ovarianism, hypo-ovarism E28.39
Hypoparathyroidism E20.9
  familial E20.8
  idiopathic E20.0
  neonatal, transitory P71.4
  postprocedural E89.2
  specified NEC E20.8
Hypoperfusion (in)
  newborn P96.89
Hypopharyngitis — *see* Laryngopharyngitis
Hypophoria H50.53
Hypophosphatemia, hypophosphatasia (acquired) (congenital) (renal) E83.39
  familial E83.31
Hypophyseal, hypophysis — *see also* condition
  dwarfism E23.0
  gigantism E22.0
Hypopiesis — *see* Hypotension
Hypopinealism E34.8
Hypopituitarism (juvenile) E23.0
  drug-induced E23.1
  due to
    hypophysectomy E89.3
    radiotherapy E89.3
  iatrogenic NEC E23.1
  postirradiation E89.3
  postpartum O99.285
  postprocedural E89.3
Hypoplasia, hypoplastic
  adrenal (gland) , congenital Q89.1
  alimentary tract, congenital Q45.8
    upper Q40.8
  anus, anal (canal) Q42.3
    with fistula Q42.2
  aorta, aortic Q25.42
    ascending, in hypoplastic left heart syndrome Q23.4
    valve Q23.1
      in hypoplastic left heart syndrome Q23.4
  areola, congenital Q83.8
  arm (congenital) — *see* Defect, reduction, upper limb
  artery (peripheral) Q27.8
    brain (congenital) Q28.3
    coronary Q24.5
    digestive system Q27.8
    lower limb Q27.8
    pulmonary Q25.79
      functional, unilateral J43.0
    retinal (congenital) Q14.1
    specified site NEC Q27.8
    umbilical Q27.0
    upper limb Q27.8
  auditory canal Q17.8
    causing impairment of hearing Q16.9
  biliary duct or passage Q44.5
  bone NOS Q79.9
    face Q75.8
    marrow D61.9
      megakaryocytic D69.49
    skull — *see* Hypoplasia, skull
  brain Q02
    gyri Q04.3
    part of Q04.3
  breast (areola) N64.82
  bronchus Q32.4
  cardiac Q24.8
  carpus — *see* Defect, reduction, upper limb, specified type NEC
  cartilage hair Q78.8
  cecum Q42.8
  cementum K00.4
  cephalic Q02
  cerebellum Q04.3
  cervix (uteri) , congenital Q51.821
  clavicle (congenital) Q74.0
  coccyx Q76.49
  colon Q42.9
    specified NEC Q42.8
  corpus callosum Q04.0
  cricoid cartilage Q31.2
  digestive organ (s) or tract NEC Q45.8

Hypoplasia, hypoplastic - *continued*
digestive organ (s) or tract NEC - *continued*
  upper (congenital) Q40.8
ear (auricle) (lobe) Q17.2
  middle Q16.4
enamel of teeth (neonatal) (postnatal)
  (prenatal) K00.4
endocrine (gland) NEC Q89.2
endometrium N85.8
epididymis (congenital) Q55.4
epiglottis Q31.2
erythroid, congenital D61.01
esophagus (congenital) Q39.8
eustachian tube Q17.8
eye Q11.2
eyelid (congenital) Q10.3
face Q18.8
  bone (s) Q75.8
femur (congenital) — *see* Defect, reduction, lower
  limb, specified type NEC
fibula (congenital) — *see* Defect, reduction, lower
  limb, specified type NEC
finger (congenital) — *see* Defect, reduction, upper
  limb, specified type NEC
focal dermal Q82.8
foot — *see* Defect, reduction, lower limb, specified
  type NEC
gallbladder Q44.0
genitalia, genital organ (s)
  female, congenital Q52.8
    external Q52.79
    internal NEC Q52.8
  in adiposogenital dystrophy E23.6
glottis Q31.2
hair Q84.2
hand (congenital) — *see* Defect, reduction, upper
  limb, specified type NEC
heart Q24.8
humerus (congenital) — *see* Defect, reduction,
  upper limb, specified type NEC
intestine (small) Q41.9
  large Q42.9
    specified NEC Q42.8
jaw M26.09
  alveolar M26.79
  lower M26.04
    alveolar M26.74
  upper M26.02
    alveolar M26.73
kidney (s) Q60.5
  bilateral Q60.4
  unilateral Q60.3
labium (majus) (minus) , congenital Q52.79
larynx Q31.2
left heart syndrome Q23.4
leg (congenital) — *see* Defect, reduction, lower limb
limb Q73.8
  lower (congenital) — *see* Defect, reduction, lower
    limb
  upper (congenital) — *see* Defect, reduction, upper
    limb
liver Q44.7
lung (lobe) (not associated with short
  gestation) Q33.6
  associated with immaturity, low birth weight,
    prematurity, or short gestation P28.0
mammary (areola) , congenital Q83.8
mandible, mandibular M26.04
  alveolar M26.74
  unilateral condylar M27.8
maxillary M26.02
  alveolar M26.73
medullary D61.9
megakaryocytic D69.49
metacarpus — *see* Defect, reduction, upper limb,
  specified type NEC
metatarsus — *see* Defect, reduction, lower limb,
  specified type NEC
muscle Q79.8
nail (s) Q84.6
nose, nasal Q30.1
optic nerve H47.03-
osseous meatus (ear) Q17.8
ovary, congenital Q50.39
pancreas Q45.0
parathyroid (gland) Q89.2
parotid gland Q38.4
patella Q74.1
pelvis, pelvic girdle Q74.2
penis (congenital) Q55.62
peripheral vascular system Q27.8
  digestive system Q27.8
  lower limb Q27.8

Hypoplasia, hypoplastic - *continued*
peripheral vascular system - *continued*
  specified site NEC Q27.8
  upper limb Q27.8
pituitary (gland) (congenital) Q89.2
pulmonary (not associated with short
  gestation) Q33.6
  artery, functional J43.0
  associated with short gestation P28.0
radioulnar — *see* Defect, reduction, upper limb,
  specified type NEC
radius — *see* Defect, reduction, upper limb
rectum Q42.1
  with fistula Q42.0
respiratory system NEC Q34.8
rib Q76.6
right heart syndrome Q22.6
sacrum Q76.49
scapula Q74.0
scrotum Q55.1
shoulder girdle Q74.0
skin Q82.8
skull (bone) Q75.8
  with
    anencephaly Q00.0
    encephalocele — *see* Encephalocele
    hydrocephalus Q03.9
      with spina bifida — *see* Spina bifida, by site,
      with hydrocephalus
    microcephaly Q02
spinal (cord) (ventral horn cell) Q06.1
spine Q76.49
sternum Q76.7
tarsus — *see* Defect, reduction, lower limb, specified
  type NEC
testis Q55.1
thymic, with immunodeficiency D82.1
thymus (gland) Q89.2
  with immunodeficiency D82.1
thyroid (gland) E03.1
  cartilage Q31.2
tibiofibular (congenital) — *see* Defect, reduction,
  lower limb, specified type NEC
toe — *see* Defect, reduction, lower limb, specified
  type NEC
tongue Q38.3
Turner's K00.4
ulna (congenital) — *see* Defect, reduction, upper
  limb
umbilical artery Q27.0
unilateral condylar M27.8
ureter Q62.8
uterus, congenital Q51.811
vagina Q52.4
vascular NEC peripheral Q27.8
  brain Q28.3
  digestive system Q27.8
  lower limb Q27.8
  specified site NEC Q27.8
  upper limb Q27.8
vein (s) (peripheral) Q27.8
  brain Q28.3
  digestive system Q27.8
  great Q26.8
  lower limb Q27.8
  specified site NEC Q27.8
  upper limb Q27.8
vena cava (inferior) (superior) Q26.8
vertebra Q76.49
vulva, congenital Q52.79
zonule (ciliary) Q12.8
Hypopotassemia E87.6
Hypoproconvertinemia, congenital
  (hereditary) D68.2
Hypoproteinemia E77.8
Hypoprothrombinemia (congenital) (hereditary)
  (idiopathic) D68.2
  acquired D68.4
  newborn, transient P61.6
Hypoptyalism K11.7
Hypopyon (eye) (anterior chamber) — *see*
  Iridocyclitis, acute, hypopyon
Hypopyrexia R68.0
Hyporeflexia R29.2
Hyposecretion
  ACTH E23.0
  antidiuretic hormone E23.2
  ovary E28.39
  salivary gland (any) K11.7
  vasopressin E23.2
Hyposegmentation, leukocytic, hereditary D72.0
Hyposiderinemia D50.9

Hypospadias Q54.9
balanic Q54.0
coronal Q54.0
glandular Q54.0
penile Q54.1
penoscrotal Q54.2
perineal Q54.3
specified NEC Q54.8
Hypospermatogenesis — *see* Oligospermia
Hyposplenism D73.0
Hypostasis pulmonary, passive — *see* Edema, lung
Hypostatic — *see* condition
Hyposthenuria N28.89
Hypotension (arterial) (constitutional) I95.9
chronic I95.89
due to (of) hemodialysis I95.3
drug-induced I95.2
iatrogenic I95.89
idiopathic (permanent) I95.0
intracranial, following ventricular shunting
  (ventriculostomy) G97.2
intra-dialytic I95.3
maternal, syndrome (following labor and
  delivery) O26.5-
neurogenic, orthostatic G90.3
orthostatic (chronic) I95.1
  due to drugs I95.2
  neurogenic G90.3
postoperative I95.81
postural I95.1
specified NEC I95.89
Hypothermia (accidental) T68
due to anesthesia, anesthetic T88.51
low environmental temperature T68
neonatal P80.9
  environmental (mild) NEC P80.8
  mild P80.8
  severe (chronic) (cold injury syndrome) P80.0
  specified NEC P80.8
not associated with low environmental
  temperature R68.0
Hypothyroidism (acquired) E03.9
congenital (without goiter) E03.1
  with goiter (diffuse) E03.0
due to
  exogenous substance NEC E03.2
  iodine-deficiency, acquired E01.8
    subclinical E02
  irradiation therapy E89.0
  medicament NEC E03.2
  P-aminosalicylic acid (PAS) E03.2
  phenylbutazone E03.2
  resorcinol E03.2
  sulfonamide E03.2
  surgery E89.0
  thiourea group drugs E03.2
iatrogenic NEC E03.2
iodine-deficiency (acquired) E01.8
  congenital — *see* Syndrome, iodine- deficiency,
    congenital
  subclinical E02
neonatal, transitory P72.2
postinfectious E03.3
postirradiation E89.0
postprocedural E89.0
postsurgical E89.0
specified NEC E03.8
subclinical, iodine-deficiency related E02
Hypotonia, hypotonicity, hypotony
bladder N31.2
congenital (benign) P94.2
eye — *see* Disorder, globe, hypotony
Hypotrichosis — *see* Alopecia
Hypotropia H50.2-
Hypoventilation R06.89
congenital central alveolar G47.35
sleep related
  idiopathic nonobstructive alveolar G47.34
  in conditions classified elsewhere G47.36
Hypovitaminosis — *see* Deficiency, vitamin
Hypovolemia E86.1
surgical shock T81.19
traumatic (shock) T79.4
Hypoxemia R09.02
newborn P84
sleep related, in conditions classified
  elsewhere G47.36
Hypoxia — *see also* Anoxia R09.02
cerebral, during a procedure NEC G97.81
  postprocedural NEC G97.82
intrauterine P84
myocardial — *see* Insufficiency, coronary
newborn P84

Hypoxia - *continued*
    sleep-related G47.34
Hypsarhythmia — *see* Epilepsy, generalized,
        specified NEC
Hysteralgia, pregnant uterus O26.89-
Hysteria, hysterical (conversion) (dissociative
        state) F44.9
    anxiety F41.8
    convulsions F44.5
    psychosis, acute F44.9
Hysteroepilepsy F44.5

I

I.Q.
    under 20 F73
    20-34 F72
    35-49 F71
    50-69 F70
IBDU
    (colonic inflammatory bowel disease
        unclassified) K52.3
Ichthyoparasitism due to Vandellia cirrhosa B88.8
Ichthyosis (congenital) Q80.9
    acquired L85.0
    fetalis Q80.4
    hystrix Q80.8
    lamellar Q80.2
    lingual K13.29
    palmaris and plantaris Q82.8
    simplex Q80.0
    vera Q80.8
    vulgaris Q80.0
    X-linked Q80.1
Ichthyotoxism — *see* Poisoning, fish
    bacterial — *see* Intoxication, foodborne
Icteroanemia, hemolytic (acquired) D59.9
    congenital — *see* Spherocytosis
Icterus — *see also* Jaundice
    conjunctiva R17
    newborn P59.9
    gravis, newborn P55.0
    hematogenous (acquired) D59.9
    hemolytic (acquired) D59.9
        congenital — *see* Spherocytosis
    hemorrhagic (acute) (leptospiral) (spirochetal) A27.0
        newborn P53
    infectious B15.9
        with hepatic coma B15.0
        leptospiral A27.0
        spirochetal A27.0
    neonatorum — *see* Jaundice, newborn
    spirochetal A27.0
Ictus solaris, solis T67.0
Id reaction (due to bacteria) L30.2
Ideation
    homicidal R45.850
    suicidal R45.851
Identity disorder (child) F64.9
    gender role F64.2
    psychosexual F64.2
Idioglossia F80.0
Idiopathic — *see* condition
Idiot, idiocy (congenital) F73
    amaurotic (Bielschowsky (-Jansky)) (family)
        (infantile (late)) (juvenile (late)) (Vogt-
        Spielmeyer) E75.4
    microcephalic Q02
IgE asthma J45.909
IIAC (idiopathic infantile arterial calcification) Q28.8
Ileitis (chronic) (noninfectious) — *see*
    also Enteritis K52.9
    backwash — *see* Pancolitis, ulcerative (chronic)
    infectious A09
    regional (ulcerative) — *see* Enteritis, regional, small
        intestine
    segmental — *see* Enteritis, regional
    terminal (ulcerative) — *see* Enteritis, regional, small
        intestine
Ileocolitis — *see also* Enteritis K52.9
    regional — *see* Enteritis, regional
    infectious A09
Ileostomy
    attention to Z43.2
    malfunctioning K94.13
    status Z93.2
        with complication — *see* Complications,
            enterostomy
Ileotyphus — *see* Typhoid
Ileum — *see* condition
Ileus (bowel) (colon) (inhibitory) (intestine) K56.7
    adynamic K56.0
    due to gallstone (in intestine) K56.3
    duodenal (chronic) K31.5

Ileus (bowel) (colon) (inhibitory) (intestine) -
continued
    gallstone K56.3
    mechanical NEC K56.69
    meconium P76.0
        in cystic fibrosis E84.11
        meaning meconium plug (without cystic
            fibrosis) P76.0
    myxedema K59.8
    neurogenic K56.0
        Hirschsprung's disease or megacolon Q43.1
    newborn
        due to meconium P76.0
            in cystic fibrosis E84.11
            meaning meconium plug (without cystic
                fibrosis) P76.0
        transitory P76.1
    obstructive K56.69
    paralytic K56.0
Iliac — *see* condition
Iliotibial band syndrome M76.3-
Illiteracy Z55.0
Illness — *see also* Disease R69
    manic-depressive — *see* Disorder, bipolar
Imbalance R26.89
    autonomic G90.8
    constituents of food intake E63.1
    electrolyte E87.8
        with
            abortion — *see* Abortion by type, complicated by,
                electrolyte imbalance
            molar pregnancy O08.5
        due to hyperemesis gravidarum O21.1
        following ectopic or molar pregnancy O08.5
        neonatal, transitory NEC P74.4
            potassium P74.3
            sodium P74.2
    endocrine E34.9
    eye muscle NOS H50.9
    hormone E34.9
    hysterical F44.4
    labyrinth — *see* subcategory H83.2
    posture R29.3
    protein-energy — *see* Malnutrition
    sympathetic G90.8
Imbecile, imbecility (I.Q.35-49) F71
Imbedding, intrauterine device T83.39
Imbibition, cholesterol (gallbladder) K82.4
Imbrication, teeth,, fully erupted M26.30
Imerslund (-Gräsbeck) **syndrome** D51.1
Immature — *see also* Immaturity
    birth (less than 37 completed weeks) — *see* Preterm,
        newborn
    extremely (less than 28 completed weeks) — *see*
        Immaturity, extreme
    personality F60.89
Immaturity (less than 37 completed weeks) —
    see also Preterm, newborn
    extreme of newborn (less than 28 completed weeks
        of gestation) (less than 196 completed days of
        gestation) (unspecified weeks of gestation) P07.20
        gestational age
            23 completed weeks (23 weeks, 0 days through
                23 weeks, 6 days) P07.22
            24 completed weeks (24 weeks, 0 days through
                24 weeks, 6 days) P07.23
            25 completed weeks (25 weeks, 0 days through
                25 weeks, 6 days) P07.24
            26 completed weeks (26 weeks, 0 days through
                26 weeks, 6 days) P07.25
            27 completed weeks (27 weeks, 0 days through
                27 weeks, 6 days) P07.26
            less than 23 completed weeks P07.21
    fetus or infant light-for-dates — *see* Light-for-dates
    lung, newborn P28.0
    organ or site NEC — *see* Hypoplasia
    pulmonary, newborn P28.0
    reaction F60.89
    sexual (female) (male) , after puberty E30.0
Immersion T75.1
    hand T69.01-
    foot T69.02-
Immobile, immobility
    complete, due to severe physical disability or
        frailty R53.2
    intestine K59.8
    syndrome (paraplegic) M62.3
Immune reconstitution (inflammatory)
    syndrome [IRIS] D89.3
Immunization — *see also* Vaccination
    ABO — *see* Incompatibility, ABO
        in newborn P55.1
    complication — *see* Complications, vaccination

Immunization - *continued*
    encounter for Z23
    not done (not carried out) Z28.9
        because (of)
            acute illness of patient Z28.01
            allergy to vaccine (or component) Z28.04
            caregiver refusal Z28.82
            chronic illness of patient Z28.02
            contraindication NEC Z28.09
            group pressure Z28.1
            guardian refusal Z28.82
            immune compromised state of patient Z28.03
            parent refusal Z28.82
            patient's belief Z28.1
            patient had disease being vaccinated
                against Z28.81
            patient refusal Z28.21
            religious beliefs of patient Z28.1
            specified reason NEC Z28.89
                of patient Z28.29
            unspecified patient reason Z28.20
    Rh factor
        affecting management of pregnancy NEC O36.09-
            anti-D antibody O36.01-
        from transfusion — *see* Complication(s),
            transfusion, incompatibility reaction, Rh (factor)
Immunocytoma C83.0-
Immunodeficiency D84.9
    with
        adenosine-deaminase deficiency D81.3
        antibody defects D80.9
            specified type NEC D80.8
        hyperimmunoglobulinemia D80.6
        increased immunoglobulin M (IgM) D80.5
        major defect D82.9
            specified type NEC D82.8
        partial albinism D82.8
        short-limbed stature D82.2
        thrombocytopenia and eczema D82.0
    antibody with
        hyperimmunoglobulinemia D80.6
        near-normal immunoglobulins D80.6
    autosomal recessive, Swiss type D80.0
    combined D81.9
        biotin-dependent carboxylase D81.819
            biotinidase D81.810
            holocarboxylase synthetase D81.818
            specified type NEC D81.818
        severe (SCID) D81.9
            with
                low or normal B-cell numbers D81.2
                low T- and B-cell numbers D81.1
                reticular dysgenesis D81.0
        specified type NEC D81.89
    common variable D83.9
        with
            abnormalities of B-cell numbers and
                function D83.0
            autoantibodies to B- or T-cells D83.2
            immunoregulatory T-cell disorders D83.1
        specified type NEC D83.8
    following hereditary defective response to Epstein-
        Barr virus (EBV) D82.3
    selective, immunoglobulin
        A (IgA) D80.2
        G (IgG) (subclasses) D80.3
        M (IgM) D80.4
    severe combined (SCID) D81.9
    specified type NEC D84.8
    X-linked, with increased IgM D80.5
Immunotherapy (encounter for)
    antineoplastic Z51.12
Impaction, impacted
    bowel, colon, rectum — *see also* Impaction,
        fecal K56.49
        by gallstone K56.3
    calculus — *see* Calculus
    cerumen (ear) (external) H61.2-
    cuspid — *see* Impaction, tooth
    dental (same or adjacent tooth) K01.1
    fecal, feces K56.41
    fracture — *see* Fracture, by site
    gallbladder — *see* Calculus, gallbladder
    gallstone (s) — *see* Calculus, gallbladder
        bile duct (common) (hepatic) — *see* Calculus, bile
            duct
        cystic duct — *see* Calculus, gallbladder
        in intestine, with obstruction (any part) K56.3
    intestine (calculous) NEC — *see also* Impaction,
        fecal K56.49
        gallstone, with ileus K56.3
    intrauterine device (IUD) T83.39
    molar — *see* Impaction, tooth

Impaction, impacted - *continued*
shoulder, causing obstructed labor O66.0
tooth, teeth K01.1
turbinate J34.89
Impaired, impairment (function)
auditory discrimination — *see* Abnormal, auditory perception
cognitive, mild, so stated G31.84
dual sensory Z73.82
fasting glucose R73.01
glucose tolerance (oral) R73.02
hearing — *see* Deafness
heart — *see* Disease, heart
kidney N28.9
disorder resulting from N25.9
specified NEC N25.89
liver K72.90
with coma K72.91
mastication K08.89
mild cognitive, so stated G31.84
mobility
ear ossicles — *see* Ankylosis, ear ossicles
requiring care provider Z74.09
myocardium, myocardial — *see* Insufficiency, myocardial
rectal sphincter R19.8
renal (acute) (chronic) N28.9
disorder resulting from N25.9
specified NEC N25.89
vision NEC H54.7
both eyes H54.3
Impediment, speech R47.9
psychogenic (childhood) F98.8
slurring R47.81
specified NEC R47.89
Impending
coronary syndrome I20.0
delirium tremens F10.239
myocardial infarction I20.0
Imperception auditory (acquired) — *see also* Deafness
congenital H93.25
Imperfect
aeration, lung (newborn) NEC — *see* Atelectasis
closure (congenital)
alimentary tract NEC Q45.8
lower Q43.8
upper Q40.8
atrioventricular ostium Q21.2
atrium (secundum) Q21.1
branchial cleft or sinus Q18.0
choroid Q14.3
cricoid cartilage Q31.8
cusps, heart valve NEC Q24.8
pulmonary Q22.3
ductus
arteriosus Q25.0
Botalli Q25.0
ear drum (causing impairment of hearing) Q16.4
esophagus with communication to bronchus or trachea Q39.1
eyelid Q10.3
foramen
botalli Q21.1
ovale Q21.1
genitalia, genital organ (s) or system
female Q52.8
external Q52.79
internal NEC Q52.8
male Q55.8
glottis Q31.8
interatrial ostium or septum Q21.1
interauricular ostium or septum Q21.1
interventricular ostium or septum Q21.0
larynx Q31.8
lip — *see* Cleft, lip
nasal septum Q30.3
nose Q30.2
omphalomesenteric duct Q43.0
optic nerve entry Q14.2
organ or site not listed — *see* Anomaly, by site
ostium
interatrial Q21.1
interauricular Q21.1
interventricular Q21.0
palate — *see* Cleft, palate
preauricular sinus Q18.1
retina Q14.1
roof of orbit Q75.8
sclera Q13.5
septum
aorticopulmonary Q21.4
atrial (secundum) Q21.1

Imperfect - *continued*
closure (congenital) - *continued*
septum - *continued*
between aorta and pulmonary artery Q21.4
heart Q21.9
interatrial (secundum) Q21.1
interauricular (secundum) Q21.1
interventricular Q21.0
in tetralogy of Fallot Q21.3
nasal Q30.3
ventricular Q21.0
with pulmonary stenosis or atresia, dextraposition of aorta, and hypertrophy of right ventricle Q21.3
in tetralogy of Fallot Q21.3
skull Q75.0
with
anencephaly Q00.0
encephalocele — *see* Encephalocele
hydrocephalus Q03.9
with spina bifida — *see* Spina bifida, by site, with hydrocephalus
microcephaly Q02
spine (with meningocele) — *see* Spina bifida
trachea Q32.1
tympanic membrane (causing impairment of hearing) Q16.4
uterus Q51.818
vitelline duct Q43.0
erection — *see* Dysfunction, sexual, male, erectile
fusion — *see* Imperfect, closure
inflation, lung (newborn) — *see* Atelectasis
posture R29.3
rotation, intestine Q43.3
septum, ventricular Q21.0
Imperfectly descended testis — *see* Cryptorchid
Imperforate (congenital) — *see also* Atresia
anus Q42.3
with fistula Q42.2
cervix (uteri) Q51.828
esophagus Q39.0
with tracheoesophageal fistula Q39.1
hymen Q52.3
jejunum Q41.1
pharynx Q38.8
rectum Q42.1
with fistula Q42.0
urethra Q64.39
vagina Q52.4
Impervious (congenital) — *see also* Atresia
anus Q42.3
with fistula Q42.2
bile duct Q44.2
esophagus Q39.0
with tracheoesophageal fistula Q39.1
intestine (small) Q41.9
large Q42.9
specified NEC Q42.8
rectum Q42.1
with fistula Q42.0
ureter — *see* Atresia, ureter
urethra Q64.39
Impetiginization of dermatoses L01.1
Impetigo (any organism) (any site) (circinate) (contagiosa) (simplex) (vulgaris) L01.00
Bockhart's L01.02
bullous, bullosa L01.03
external ear L01.00 *[H62.40]*
follicularis L01.02
furfuracea L30.5
herpetiformis L40.1
nonobstetrical L40.1
neonatorum L01.03
nonbullous L01.01
specified type NEC L01.09
ulcerative L01.09
Impingement (on teeth)
soft tissue
anterior M26.81
posterior M26.82
Implant, endometrial N80.9
Implantation
anomalous — *see* Anomaly, by site
ureter Q62.63
cyst
external area or site (skin) NEC L72.0
iris — *see* Cyst, iris, implantation
vagina N89.8
vulva N90.7
dermoid (cyst) — *see* Implantation, cyst
Impotence (sexual) N52.9
counseling Z70.1

Impotence (sexual) - *continued*
organic origin — *see also* Dysfunction, sexual, male, erectile N52.9
psychogenic F52.21
Impression, basilar Q75.8
Imprisonment, anxiety concerning Z65.1
Improper care (child) (newborn) — *see* Maltreatment
Improperly tied umbilical cord (causing hemorrhage) P51.8
Impulsiveness (impulsive) R45.87
Inability to swallow — *see* Aphagia
Inaccessible, inaccessibility
health care NEC Z75.3
due to
waiting period Z75.2
for admission to facility elsewhere Z75.1
other helping agencies Z75.4
Inactive — *see* condition
Inadequate, inadequacy
aesthetics of dental restoration K08.56
biologic, constitutional, functional, or social F60.7
development
child R62.50
genitalia
after puberty NEC E30.0
congenital
female Q52.8
external Q52.79
internal Q52.8
male Q55.8
lungs Q33.6
associated with short gestation P28.0
organ or site not listed — *see* Anomaly, by site
diet (causing nutritional deficiency) E63.9
eating habits Z72.4
environment, household Z59.1
family support Z63.8
food (supply) NEC Z59.4
hunger effects T73.0
functional F60.7
household care, due to
family member
handicapped or ill Z74.2
on vacation Z75.5
temporarily away from home Z74.2
technical defects in home Z59.1
temporary absence from home of person rendering care Z74.2
housing (heating) (space) Z59.1
income (financial) Z59.6
intrafamilial communication Z63.8
material resources Z59.9
mental — *see* Disability, intellectual
parental supervision or control of child Z62.0
personality F60.7
pulmonary
function R06.89
newborn P28.5
ventilation, newborn P28.5
sample of cytologic smear
anus R85.615
cervix R87.615
vagina R87.625
social F60.7
insurance Z59.7
skills NEC Z73.4
supervision of child by parent Z62.0
teaching affecting education Z55.8
welfare support Z59.7
Inanition R64
with edema — *see* Malnutrition, severe
due to
deprivation of food T73.0
malnutrition — *see* Malnutrition
fever R50.9
Inappropriate
change in quantitative human chorionic gonadotropin (hCG) in early pregnancy O02.81
diet or eating habits Z72.4
level of quantitative human chorionic gonadotropin (hCG) for gestational age in early pregnancy O02.81
secretion
antidiuretic hormone (ADH) (excessive) E22.2
deficiency E23.2
pituitary (posterior) E22.2
Inattention at or after birth — *see* Neglect
Incarceration, incarcerated
enterocele K46.0
gangrenous K46.1
epiplocele K46.0
gangrenous K46.1

Incarceration, incarcerated - *continued*
exomphalos K42.0
gangrenous K42.1
hernia — *see also* Hernia, by site, with obstruction
with gangrene — *see* Hernia, by site, with
gangrene
iris, in wound — *see* Injury, eye, laceration, with
prolapse
lens, in wound — *see* Injury, eye, laceration, with
prolapse
omphalocele K42.0
prison, anxiety concerning Z65.1
rupture — *see* Hernia, by site
sarcoepiplocele K46.0
gangrenous K46.1
sarcoepiplomphalocele K42.0
with gangrene K42.1
uterus N85.8
gravid O34.51-
causing obstructed labor O65.5
Incised wound
external — *see* Laceration
internal organs — *see* Injury, by site
Incision, incisional
hernia K43.2
with
gangrene (and obstruction) K43.1
obstruction K43.0
surgical, complication — *see* Complications,
surgical procedure
traumatic
external — *see* Laceration
internal organs — *see* Injury, by site
Inclusion
azurophilic leukocytic D72.0
blennorrhea (neonatal) (newborn) P39.1
gallbladder in liver (congenital) Q44.1
Incompatibility
ABO
affecting management of pregnancy O36.11-
anti-A sensitization O36.11-
anti-B sensitization O36.19-
specified NEC O36.19-
infusion or transfusion reaction — *see*
Complication(s), transfusion, incompatibility
reaction, ABO
newborn P55.1
blood (group) (Duffy) (K (ell)) (Kidd) (Lewis) (M)
(S) NEC
affecting management of pregnancy O36.11-
anti-A sensitization O36.11-
anti-B sensitization O36.19-
infusion or transfusion reaction T80.89
newborn P55.8
divorce or estrangement Z63.5
Rh (blood group) (factor) Z31.82
affecting management of pregnancy NEC O36.09-
anti-D antibody O36.01-
infusion or transfusion reaction — *see*
Complication(s), transfusion, incompatibility
reaction, Rh (factor)
newborn P55.0
rhesus — *see* Incompatibility, Rh
Incompetency, incompetent, incompetence
annular
aortic (valve) — *see* Insufficiency, aortic
mitral (valve) I34.0
pulmonary valve (heart) I37.1
aortic (valve) — *see* Insufficiency, aortic
cardiac valve — *see* Endocarditis
cervix, cervical (os) N88.3
in pregnancy O34.3-
chronotropic I45.89
with
autonomic dysfunction G90.8
ischemic heart disease I25.89
left ventricular dysfunction I51.89
sinus node dysfunction I49.8
esophagogastric (junction) (sphincter) K22.0
mitral (valve) — *see* Insufficiency, mitral
pelvic fundus N81.89
pubocervical tissue N81.82
pulmonary valve (heart) I37.1
congenital Q22.3
rectovaginal tissue N81.83
tricuspid (annular) (valve) — *see* Insufficiency,
tricuspid
valvular — *see* Endocarditis
congenital Q24.8
vein, venous (saphenous) (varicose) — *see* Varix, leg
Incomplete — *see also* condition
bladder, emptying R33.9
defecation R15.0

Incomplete - *continued*
expansion lungs (newborn) NEC — *see* Atelectasis
rotation, intestine Q43.3
Inconclusive
diagnostic imaging due to excess body fat of
patient R93.9
findings on diagnostic imaging of breast NEC R92.8
mammogram (due to dense breasts) R92.2
Incontinence R32
anal sphincter R15.9
coital N39.491
feces R15.9
nonorganic origin F98.1
insensible (urinary) N39.42
overflow N39.490
postural (urinary) N39.492
psychogenic F45.8
rectal R15.9
reflex N39.498
stress (female) (male) N39.3
and urge N39.46
urethral sphincter R32
urge N39.41
and stress (female) (male) N39.46
urine (urinary) R32
continuous N39.45
due to cognitive impairment, or severe physical
disability or immobility R39.81
functional R39.81
insensible N39.42
mixed (stress and urge) N39.46
nocturnal N39.44
nonorganic origin F98.0
overflow N39.490
post dribbling N39.43
postural N39.492
reflex N39.498
specified NEC N39.498
stress (female) (male) N39.3
and urge N39.46
total N39.498
unaware N39.42
urge N39.41
and stress (female) (male) N39.46
Incontinentia pigmenti Q82.3
Incoordinate, incoordination
esophageal-pharyngeal (newborn) — *see* Dysphagia
muscular R27.8
uterus (action) (contractions) (complicating
delivery) O62.4
Increase, increased
abnormal, in development R63.8
androgens (ovarian) E28.1
anticoagulants (antithrombin) (anti-VIIIa) (anti-IXa)
(anti-Xa) (anti-XIa) — *see* Circulating
anticoagulants
cold sense R20.8
estrogen E28.0
function
adrenal
cortex — *see* Cushing's, syndrome
medulla E27.5
pituitary (gland) (anterior) (lobe) E22.9
posterior E22.2
heat sense R20.8
intracranial pressure (benign) G93.2
permeability, capillaries I78.8
pressure, intracranial G93.2
secretion
gastrin E16.4
glucagon E16.3
pancreas, endocrine E16.9
growth hormone-releasing hormone E16.8
pancreatic polypeptide E16.8
somatostatin E16.8
vasoactive-intestinal polypeptide E16.8
sphericity, lens Q12.4
splenic activity D73.1
venous pressure I87.8
portal K76.6
Increta placenta O43.22-
Incrustation, cornea, foreign body (lead)
(zinc) — *see* Foreign body, cornea
Incyclophoria H50.54
Incyclotropia — *see* Cyclotropia
Indeterminate sex Q56.4
India rubber skin Q82.8
Indigestion (acid) (bilious) (functional) K30
catarrhal K31.89
due to decomposed food NOS A05.9
nervous F45.8
psychogenic F45.8
Indirect — *see* condition

Induratio penis plastica N48.6
Induration, indurated
brain G93.89
breast (fibrous) N64.51
puerperal, postpartum O92.29
broad ligament N83.8
chancre
anus A51.1
congenital A50.07
extragenital NEC A51.2
corpora cavernosa (penis) (plastic) N48.6
liver (chronic) K76.89
lung (black) (chronic) (fibroid) — *see also* Fibrosis,
lung J84.10
essential brown J84.03
penile (plastic) N48.6
phlebitic — *see* Phlebitis
skin R23.4
Inebriety (without dependence) — *see* Alcohol,
intoxication
Inefficiency, kidney N28.9
Inelasticity, skin R23.4
Inequality, leg (length) (acquired) — *see*
also Deformity, limb, unequal length
congenital — *see* Defect, reduction, lower limb
lower leg — *see* Deformity, limb, unequal length
Inertia
bladder (neurogenic) N31.2
stomach R14.0
psychogenic F45.8
uterus, uterine during labor O62.2
during latent phase of labor O62.0
primary O62.0
secondary O62.1
vesical (neurogenic) N31.2
Infancy, infantile, infantilism — *see also* condition
celiac K90.0
genitalia, genitals (after puberty) E30.0
Herter's (nontropical sprue) K90.0
intestinal K90.0
Lorain E23.0
pancreatic K86.89
pelvis M95.5
with disproportion (fetopelvic) O33.1
causing obstructed labor O65.1
pituitary E23.0
renal N25.0
uterus — *see* Infantile, genitalia
Infant (s) — *see also* Infancy
excessive crying R68.11
irritable child R68.12
lack of care — *see* Neglect
liveborn (singleton) Z38.2
born in hospital Z38.00
by cesarean Z38.01
born outside hospital Z38.1
multiple NEC Z38.8
born in hospital Z38.68
by cesarean Z38.69
born outside hospital Z38.7
quadruplet Z38.8
born in hospital Z38.63
by cesarean Z38.64
born outside hospital Z38.7
quintuplet Z38.8
born in hospital Z38.65
by cesarean Z38.66
born outside hospital Z38.7
triplet Z38.8
born in hospital Z38.61
by cesarean Z38.62
born outside hospital Z38.7
twin Z38.5
born in hospital Z38.30
by cesarean Z38.31
born outside hospital Z38.4
of diabetic mother (syndrome of) P70.1
gestational diabetes P70.0
Infantile — *see also* condition
genitalia, genitals E30.0
os, uterine E30.0
penis E30.0
testis E29.1
uterus E30.0
Infantilism — *see* Infancy
Infarct, infarction
adrenal (capsule) (gland) E27.49
appendices epiploicae — *see also* Infarct,
intestine K55.069
bowel — *see also* Infarct, intestine K55.069
brain (stem) — *see* Infarct, cerebral
breast N64.89
brewer's (kidney) N28.0

Infarct, infarction - *continued*
- cardiac — *see* Infarct, myocardium
- cerebellar — *see* Infarct, cerebral
- cerebral — *see also* Occlusion, artery cerebral or precerebral, with infarction I63.9-
  - aborted I63.9
  - cortical I63.9
  - due to
    - cerebral venous thrombosis, nonpyogenic I63.6
    - embolism
      - cerebral arteries I63.4-
      - precerebral arteries I63.1-
    - occlusion NEC
      - cerebral arteries I63.5-
      - precerebral arteries I63.2-
    - stenosis NEC
      - cerebral arteries I63.5-
      - precerebral arteries I63.2-
    - thrombosis
      - cerebral artery I63.3-
      - precerebral artery I63.0-
  - intraoperative
    - during cardiac surgery I97.810
    - during other surgery I97.811
  - postprocedural
    - following cardiac surgery I97.820
    - following other surgery I97.821
  - specified NEC I63.8
- colon (acute) (agnogenic) (embolic) (hemorrhagic) (nonocclusive) (nonthrombotic) (occlusive) (segmental) (thrombotic) (with gangrene) — *see also* Infarct, intestine K55.049
- coronary artery — *see* Infarct, myocardium
- embolic — *see* Embolism
- fallopian tube N83.8
- gallbladder K82.8
- heart — *see* Infarct, myocardium
- hepatic K76.3
- hypophysis (anterior lobe) E23.6
- impending (myocardium) I20.0
- intestine (acute) (agnogenic) (embolic) (hemorrhagic) (nonocclusive) (nonthrombotic) (occlusive) (thrombotic) (with gangrene) K55.069
  - diffuse K55.062
  - focal K55.061
  - large K55.049
    - diffuse K55.042
    - focal K55.041
  - small K55.029
    - diffuse K55.022
    - focal K55.021
- kidney N28.0
- liver K76.3
- lung (embolic) (thrombotic) — *see* Embolism, pulmonary
- lymph node I89.8
- mesentery, mesenteric (embolic) (thrombotic) (with gangrene) — *see also* Infarct, intestine K55.069
- muscle (ischemic) M62.20
  - ankle M62.27-
  - foot M62.27-
  - forearm M62.23-
  - hand M62.24-
  - lower leg M62.26-
  - pelvic region M62.25-
  - shoulder region M62.21-
  - specified site NEC M62.28
  - thigh M62.25-
  - upper arm M62.22-
- myocardium, myocardial (acute) (with stated duration of 4 weeks or less) I21.3
  - diagnosed on ECG, but presenting no symptoms I25.2
  - healed or old I25.2
  - intraoperative
    - during cardiac surgery I97.790
    - during other surgery I97.791
  - non-Q wave I21.4
  - non-ST elevation (NSTEMI) I21.4
    - subsequent I22.2
  - nontransmural I21.4
  - past (diagnosed on ECG or other investigation, but currently presenting no symptoms) I25.2
  - postprocedural
    - following cardiac surgery I97.190
    - following other surgery I97.191
  - Q wave (see also, Infarct, myocardium, by site) I21.3
  - ST elevation (STEMI) I21.3
    - anterior (anteroapical) (anterolateral) (anteroseptal) (Q wave) (wall) I21.09
      - subsequent I22.0

Infarct, infarction - *continued*
- myocardium, myocardial (acute) (with stated duration of 4 weeks or less) - *continued*
  - ST elevation (STEMI) - *continued*
    - inferior (diaphragmatic) (inferolateral) (inferoposterior) (wall) NEC I21.19
      - subsequent I22.1
    - inferoposterior transmural (Q wave) I21.11
    - involving
      - coronary artery of anterior wall NEC I21.09
      - coronary artery of inferior wall NEC I21.19
      - diagonal coronary artery I21.02
      - left anterior descending coronary artery I21.02
      - left circumflex coronary artery I21.21
      - left main coronary artery I21.01
      - oblique marginal coronary artery I21.21
      - right coronary artery I21.11
    - lateral (apical-lateral) (basal-lateral) (high) I21.29
      - subsequent I22.8
    - posterior (posterobasal) (posterolateral) (posteroseptal) (true) I21.29
      - subsequent I22.8
    - septal I21.29
      - subsequent I22.8
    - specified NEC I21.29
      - subsequent I22.8
    - subsequent I22.9
  - subsequent (recurrent) (reinfarction) I22.9
    - anterior (anteroapical) (anterolateral) (anteroseptal) (wall) I22.0
    - diaphragmatic (wall) I22.1
    - inferior (diaphragmatic) (inferolateral) (inferoposterior) (wall) I22.1
    - lateral (apical-lateral) (basal-lateral) (high) I22.8
    - non-ST elevation (NSTEMI) I22.2
    - posterior (posterobasal) (posterolateral) (posteroseptal) (true) I22.8
    - septal I22.8
    - specified NEC I22.8
    - ST elevation I22.9
      - anterior (anteroapical) (anterolateral) (anteroseptal) (wall) I22.0
      - inferior (diaphragmatic) (inferolateral) (inferoposterior) (wall) I22.1
      - specified NEC I22.8
    - subendocardial I22.2
    - transmural I22.9
      - anterior (anteroapical) (anterolateral) (anteroseptal) (wall) I22.0
      - diaphragmatic (wall) I22.1
      - inferior (diaphragmatic) (inferolateral) (inferoposterior) (wall) I22.1
      - lateral (apical-lateral) (basal-lateral) (high) I22.8
      - posterior (posterobasal) (posterolateral) (posteroseptal) (true) I22.8
      - specified NEC I22.8
  - syphilitic A52.06
  - transmural I21.3
    - anterior (anteroapical) (anterolateral) (anteroseptal) (Q wave) (wall) NEC I21.09
    - inferior (diaphragmatic) (inferolateral) (inferoposterior) (Q wave) (wall) NEC I21.19
    - inferoposterior (Q wave) I21.11
    - lateral (apical-lateral) (basal-lateral) (high) NEC I21.29
    - posterior (posterobasal) (posterolateral) (posteroseptal) (true) NEC I21.29
    - septal NEC I21.29
    - specified NEC I21.29
  - nontransmural I21.4
- omentum — *see also* Infarct, intestine K55.069
- ovary N83.8
- pancreas K86.89
- papillary muscle — *see* Infarct, myocardium
- parathyroid gland E21.4
- pituitary (gland) E23.6
- placenta O43.81-
- prostate N42.89
- pulmonary (artery) (vein) (hemorrhagic) — *see* Embolism, pulmonary
- renal (embolic) (thrombotic) N28.0
- retina, retinal (artery) — *see* Occlusion, artery, retina
- spinal (cord) (acute) (embolic) (nonembolic) G95.11
- spleen D73.5
  - embolic or thrombotic I74.8
- subendocardial (acute) (nontransmural) I21.4
- suprarenal (capsule) (gland) E27.49
- testis N50.1
- thrombotic — *see also* Thrombosis
  - artery, arterial — *see* Embolism
- thyroid (gland) E07.89
- ventricle (heart) — *see* Infarct, myocardium

Infecting — *see* condition
Infection, infected, infective (opportunistic) B99.9
- with
  - drug resistant organism — *see* Resistance (to), drug — *see also* specific organism
  - lymphangitis — *see* Lymphangitis
  - organ dysfunction (acute) R65.20
    - with septic shock R65.21
- abscess (skin) - code by site under Abscess
- Absidia — *see* Mucormycosis
- Acanthamoeba — *see* Acanthamebiasis
- Acanthocheilonema (perstans) (streptocerca) B74.4
- accessory sinus (chronic) — *see* Sinusitis
- achorion — *see* Dermatophytosis
- Acremonium falciforme B47.0
- acromioclavicular M00.9
- Actinobacillus (actinomycetem-comitans) A28.8
  - mallei A24.0
  - muris A25.1
- Actinomadura B47.1
- Actinomyces (israelii) — *see also* Actinomycosis A42.9
- Actinomycetales — *see* Actinomycosis
- actinomycotic NOS — *see* Actinomycosis
- adenoid (and tonsil) J03.90
  - chronic J35.02
- adenovirus NEC
  - as cause of disease classified elsewhere B97.0
  - unspecified nature or site B34.0
- aerogenes capsulatus A48.0
- aertrycke — *see* Infection, salmonella
- alimentary canal NOS — *see* Enteritis, infectious
- Allescheria boydii B48.2
- Alternaria B48.8
- alveolus, alveolar (process) K04.7
- Ameba, amebic (histolytica) — *see* Amebiasis
- amniotic fluid, sac or cavity O41.10-
  - chorioamnionitis O41.12-
  - placentitis O41.14-
- amputation stump (surgical) — *see* Complication, amputation stump, infection
- Ancylostoma (duodenalis) B76.0
- Anisakiasis, Anisakis larvae B81.0
- anthrax — *see* Anthrax
- antrum (chronic) — *see* Sinusitis, maxillary
- anus, anal (papillae) (sphincter) K62.89
- arbovirus (arbor virus) A94
  - specified type NEC A93.8
- artificial insemination N98.0
- Ascaris lumbricoides — *see* Ascariasis
- Ascomycetes B47.0
- Aspergillus (flavus) (fumigatus) (terreus) — *see* Aspergillosis
- atypical
  - acid-fast (bacilli) — *see* Mycobacterium, atypical
  - mycobacteria — *see* Mycobacterium, atypical
  - virus A81.9
    - specified type NEC A81.89
- auditory meatus (external) — *see* Otitis, externa, infective
- auricle (ear) — *see* Otitis, externa, infective
- axillary gland (lymph) L04.2
- Bacillus A49.9
  - abortus A23.1
  - anthracis — *see* Anthrax
  - Ducrey's (any location) A57
  - Flexner's A03.1
  - Friedländer's NEC A49.8
  - gas (gangrene) A48.0
  - mallei A24.0
  - melitensis A23.0
  - paratyphoid, paratyphosus A01.4
    - A A01.1
    - B A01.2
    - C A01.3
  - Shiga (-Kruse) A03.0
  - suipestifer — *see* Infection, salmonella
  - swimming pool A31.1
  - typhosa A01.00
  - welchii — *see* Gangrene, gas
- bacterial NOS A49.9
  - as cause of disease classified elsewhere B96.89
    - Clostridium perfringens [C. perfringens] B96.7
    - Bacteroides fragilis [B. fragilis] B96.6
    - Enterobacter sakazakii B96.89
    - Enterococcus B95.2
    - Escherichia coli [E. coli] — *see also* Escherichia coli B96.20
    - Helicobacter pylori [H.pylori] B96.81
    - Hemophilus influenzae [H. influenzae] B96.3
    - Klebsiella pneumoniae [K. pneumoniae] B96.1
    - Mycoplasma pneumoniae [M. pneumoniae] B96.0

Infection, infected, infective (opportunistic) - *continued*
  bacterial NOS - *continued*
    as cause of disease classified elsewhere - *continued*
      Proteus (mirabilis) (morganii) B96.4
      Pseudomonas (aeruginosa) (mallei) (pseudomallei) B96.5
      Staphylococcus B95.8
        aureus (methicillin susceptible) (MSSA) B95.61
          methicillin resistant (MRSA) B95.62
        specified NEC B95.7
      Streptococcus B95.5
        group A B95.0
        group B B95.1
        pneumoniae B95.3
        specified NEC B95.4
      Vibrio vulnificus B96.82
    specified NEC A48.8
  Bacterium
    paratyphosum A01.4
      A A01.1
      B A01.2
      C A01.3
    typhosum A01.00
  Bacteroides NEC A49.8
    fragilis, as cause of disease classified elsewhere B96.6
  Balantidium coli A07.0
  Bartholin's gland N75.8
  Basidiobolus B46.8
  bile duct (common) (hepatic) — *see* Cholangitis
  bladder — *see* Cystitis
  Blastomyces, blastomycotic — *see also* Blastomycosis
    brasiliensis — *see* Paracoccidioidomycosis
    dermatitidis — *see* Blastomycosis
    European — *see* Cryptococcosis
    Loboi B48.0
    North American B40.9
    South American — *see* Paracoccidioidomycosis
  bleb, postprocedure — *see* Blebitis
  bone — *see* Osteomyelitis
  Bordetella — *see* Whooping cough
  Borrelia bergdorfi A69.20
  brain — *see also* Encephalitis G04.90
    membranes — *see* Meningitis
    septic G06.0
      meninges — *see* Meningitis, bacterial
  branchial cyst Q18.0
  breast — *see* Mastitis
  bronchus — *see* Bronchitis
  Brucella A23.9
    abortus A23.1
    canis A23.3
    melitensis A23.0
    mixed A23.8
    specified NEC A23.8
    suis A23.2
  Brugia (malayi) B74.1
    timori B74.2
  bursa — *see* Bursitis, infective
  buttocks (skin) L08.9
  Campylobacter, intestinal A04.5
    as cause of disease classified elsewhere B96.81
  Candida (albicans) (tropicalis) — *see* Candidiasis
  candiru B88.8
  Capillaria (intestinal) B81.1
    hepatica B83.8
    philippinensis B81.1
  cartilage — *see* Disorder, cartilage, specified type NEC
  catheter-related bloodstream (CRBSI) T80.211
  cat liver fluke B66.0
  cellulitis - code by site under Cellulitis
  central line-associated T80.219
    bloodstream (CLABSI) T80.211
    specified NEC T80.218
  Cephalosporium falciforme B47.0
  cerebrospinal — *see* Meningitis
  cervical gland (lymph) L04.0
  cervix — *see* Cervicitis
  cesarean delivery wound (puerperal) O86.0
  cestodes — *see* Infestation, cestodes
  chest J22
  Chilomastix (intestinal) A07.8
  Chlamydia, chlamydial A74.9
    anus A56.3
    genitourinary tract A56.2
      lower A56.00
        specified NEC A56.19
    lymphogranuloma A55
    pharynx A56.4
    psittaci A70

Infection, infected, infective (opportunistic) - *continued*
  Chlamydia, chlamydial - *continued*
    rectum A56.3
    sexually transmitted NEC A56.8
  cholera — *see* Cholera
  Cladosporium
    bantianum (brain abscess) B43.1
    carrionii B43.0
    castellanii B36.1
    trichoides (brain abscess) B43.1
    werneckii B36.1
  Clonorchis (sinensis) (liver) B66.1
  Clostridium NEC
    bifermentans A48.0
    botulinum (food poisoning) A05.1
      infant A48.51
      wound A48.52
    difficile
      as cause of disease classified elsewhere B96.89
      foodborne (disease) A04.7
      gas gangrene A48.0
      necrotizing enterocolitis A04.7
      sepsis A41.4
    gas-forming NEC A48.0
    histolyticum A48.0
    novyi, causing gas gangrene A48.0
    oedematiens A48.0
    perfringens
      as cause of disease classified elsewhere B96.7
      due to food A05.2
      foodborne (disease) A05.2
      gas gangrene A48.0
      sepsis A41.4
    septicum, causing gas gangrene A48.0
    sordellii, causing gas gangrene A48.0
    welchii
      as cause of disease classified elsewhere B96.7
      foodborne (disease) A05.2
      gas gangrene A48.0
      necrotizing enteritis A05.2
      sepsis A41.4
  Coccidioides (immitis) — *see* Coccidioidomycosis
  colon — *see* Enteritis, infectious
  colostomy K94.02
  common duct — *see* Cholangitis
  congenital P39.9
    Candida (albicans) P37.5
    cytomegalovirus P35.1
    hepatitis, viral P35.3
    herpes simplex P35.2
    infectious or parasitic disease P37.9
      specified NEC P37.8
    listeriosis (disseminated) P37.2
    malaria NEC P37.4
      falciparum P37.3
    Plasmodium falciparum P37.3
    poliomyelitis P35.8
    rubella P35.0
    skin P39.4
    toxoplasmosis (acute) (subacute) (chronic) P37.1
    tuberculosis P37.0
    urinary (tract) P39.3
    vaccinia P35.8
    virus P35.9
      specified type NEC P35.8
  Conidiobolus B46.8
  coronavirus NEC B34.2
    as cause of disease classified elsewhere B97.29
    severe acute respiratory syndrome (SARS associated) B97.21
  corpus luteum — *see* Salpingo-oophoritis
  Corynebacterium diphtheriae — *see* Diphtheria
  cotia virus B08.8
  Coxiella burnetii A78
  coxsackie — *see* Coxsackie
  Cryptococcus neoformans — *see* Cryptococcosis
  Cryptosporidium A07.2
  Cunninghamella — *see* Mucormycosis
  cyst — *see* Cyst
  cystic duct — *see also* Cholecystitis K81.9
  Cysticercus cellulosae — *see* Cysticercosis
  cytomegalovirus, cytomegaloviral B25.9
    congenital P35.1
    maternal, maternal care for (suspected) damage to fetus O35.3
    mononucleosis B27.10
      with
        complication NEC B27.19
        meningitis B27.12
        polyneuropathy B27.11
  delta-agent (acute) , in hepatitis B carrier B17.0
  dental (pulpal origin) K04.7

Infection, infected, infective (opportunistic) - *continued*
  Deuteromycetes B47.0
  Dicrocoelium dendriticum B66.2
  Dipetalonema (perstans) (streptocerca) B74.4
  diphtherial — *see* Diphtheria
  Diphyllobothrium (adult) (latum) (pacificum) B70.0
    larval B70.1
  Diplogonoporus (grandis) B71.8
  Dipylidium caninum B67.4
  Dirofilaria B74.8
  Dracunculus medinensis B72
  Drechslera (hawaiiensis) B43.8
  Ducrey Haemophilus (any location) A57
  due to or resulting from
    artificial insemination N98.0
    central venous catheter T80.219
      bloodstream T80.211
      exit or insertion site T80.212
      localized T80.212
      port or reservoir T80.212
      specified NEC T80.218
      tunnel T80.212
    device, implant or graft — *see also* Complications, by site and type, infection or inflammation T85.79
      arterial graft NEC T82.7
      breast (implant) T85.79
      catheter NEC T85.79
        dialysis (renal) T82.7
          intraperitoneal T85.71
        infusion NEC T82.7
          cranial T85.735
          intrathecal T85.735
          spinal (epidural) (subdural) T85.735
          subarachnoid T85.735
        urinary T83.518
          cystostomy T83.510
          Hopkins T83.518
          ileostomy T83.518
          nephrostomy T83.512
          specified NEC T83.518
          urethral indwelling T83.511
          urostomy T83.518
      electronic (electrode) (pulse generator) (stimulator)
        bone T84.7
        cardiac T82.7
        nervous system T85.738
          brain T85.731
          cranial nerve T85.732
          gastric nerve T85.732
          generator pocket T85.734
          neurostimulator generator T85.734
          peripheral nerve T85.732
          sacral nerve T85.732
          spinal cord T85.733
          vagal nerve T85.732
        urinary T83.590
      fixation, internal (orthopedic) NEC — *see* Complication, fixation device, infection
      gastrointestinal (bile duct) (esophagus) T85.79
        neurostimulator electrode (lead) T85.732
      genital NEC T83.69
      heart NEC T82.7
        valve (prosthesis) T82.6
          graft T82.7
      joint prosthesis — *see* Complication, joint prosthesis, infection
      ocular (corneal graft) (orbital implant) NEC T85.79
      orthopedic NEC T84.7
      penile (cylinder) (pump) (resevoir) T83.61
      specified NEC T85.79
      testicular T83.62
      urinary NEC T83.598
        ileal conduit stent T83.593
        implanted neurostimulation T83.590
        implanted sphincter T83.591
        indwelling ureteral stent T83.592
        nephroureteral stent T83.593
        specified stent NEC T83.593
      vascular NEC T82.7
      ventricular intracranial (communicating) shunt T85.730
    Hickman catheter T80.219
      bloodstream T80.211
      localized T80.212
      specified NEC T80.218
    immunization or vaccination T88.0
    infusion, injection or transfusion NEC T80.29
      acute T80.22
    injury NEC - code by site under Wound, open

Infection, infected, infective (opportunistic) - *continued*
  due to or resulting from - *continued*
    peripherally inserted central catheter (PICC) T80.219
      bloodstream T80.211
      localized T80.212
      specified NEC T80.218
    portacath (port-a-cath) T80.219
      bloodstream T80.211
      localized T80.212
      specified NEC T80.218
    pulmonary artery catheter — *see* Infection, due to or resulting from, central venous catheter
    surgery T81.40
    Swan Ganz catheter — *see* Infection, due to or resulting from, central venous catheter
    triple lumen catheter T80.219
      bloodstream T80.211
      localized T80.212
      specified NEC T80.218
    umbilical venous catheter T80.219
      bloodstream T80.211
      localized T80.212
      specified NEC T80.218
  during labor NEC O75.3
  ear (middle) — *see also* Otitis media
    external — *see* Otitis, externa, infective
    inner — *see* subcategory H83.0
  Eberthella typhosa A01.00
  Echinococcus — *see* Echinococcus
  echovirus
    as cause of disease classified elsewhere B97.12
    unspecified nature or site B34.1
  endocardium I33.0
  endocervix — *see* Cervicitis
  Entamoeba — *see* Amebiasis
  enteric — *see* Enteritis, infectious
  Enterobacter sakazakii B96.89
  Enterobius vermicularis B80
  enterostomy K94.12
  enterovirus B34.1
    as cause of disease classified elsewhere B97.10
      coxsackievirus B97.11
      echovirus B97.12
      specified NEC B97.19
  Entomophthora B46.8
  Epidermophyton — *see* Dermatophytosis
  epididymis — *see* Epididymitis
  episiotomy (puerperal) O86.0
  Erysipelothrix (insidiosa) (rhusiopathiae) — *see* Erysipeloid
  erythema infectiosum B08.3
  Escherichia (E.) coli NEC A49.8
    as cause of disease classified elsewhere — *see also* Escherichia coli B96.20
    congenital P39.8
      sepsis P36.4
    generalized A41.51
    intestinal — *see* Enteritis, infectious, due to, Escherichia coli
  ethmoidal (chronic) (sinus) — *see* Sinusitis, ethmoidal
  eustachian tube (ear) — *see* Salpingitis, eustachian
  external auditory canal (meatus) NEC — *see* Otitis, externa, infective
  eye (purulent) — *see* Endophthalmitis, purulent
  eyelid — *see* Inflammation, eyelid
  fallopian tube — *see* Salpingo-oophoritis
  Fasciola (gigantica) (hepatica) (indica) B66.3
  Fasciolopsis (buski) B66.5
  filarial — *see* Infestation, filarial
  finger (skin) L08.9
    nail L03.01-
      fungus B35.1
  fish tapeworm B70.0
    larval B70.1
  flagellate, intestinal A07.9
  fluke — *see* Infestation, fluke
  focal
    teeth (pulpal origin) K04.7
    tonsils J35.01
  Fonsecaea (compactum) (pedrosoi) B43.0
  food — *see* Intoxication, foodborne
  foot (skin) L08.9
    dermatophytic fungus B35.3
  Francisella tularensis — *see* Tularemia
  frontal (sinus) (chronic) — *see* Sinusitis, frontal
  fungus NOS B49
    beard B35.0
    dermatophytic — *see* Dermatophytosis
    foot B35.3
    groin B35.6

Infection, infected, infective (opportunistic) - *continued*
  fungus NOS - *continued*
    hand B35.2
    nail B35.1
    pathogenic to compromised host only B48.8
    perianal (area) B35.6
    scalp B35.0
    skin B36.9
      foot B35.3
      hand B35.2
      toenails B35.1
  Fusarium B48.8
  gallbladder — *see* Cholecystitis
  gas bacillus — *see* Gangrene, gas
  gastrointestinal — *see* Enteritis, infectious
  generalized NEC — *see* Sepsis
  generator pocket, implanted electronic neurostimulator T85.734
  genital organ or tract
    female — *see* Disease, pelvis, inflammatory
    male N49.9
      multiple sites N49.8
      specified NEC N49.8
  Ghon tubercle, primary A15.7
  Giardia lamblia A07.1
  gingiva (chronic) K05.10
    acute K05.00
      nonplaque induced K05.01
      plaque induced K05.00
    nonplaque induced K05.11
    plaque induced K05.10
  glanders A24.0
  glenosporopsis B48.0
  Gnathostoma (spinigerum) B83.1
  Gongylonema B83.8
  gonococcal — *see* Gonococcus
  gram-negative bacilli NOS A49.9
  guinea worm B72
  gum (chronic) K05.10
    acute K05.00
      nonplaque induced K05.01
      plaque induced K05.00
    nonplaque induced K05.11
    plaque induced K05.10
  Haemophilus — *see* Infection, Hemophilus
  heart — *see* Carditis
  Helicobacter pylori A04.8
    as cause of disease classified elsewhere B96.81
  helminths B83.9
    intestinal B82.0
      mixed (types classifiable to more than one of the titles B65.0-B81.3 and B81.8) B81.4
      specified type NEC B81.8
    specified type NEC B83.8
  Hemophilus
    aegyptius, systemic A48.4
    ducrey (any location) A57
    influenzae NEC A49.2
      as cause of disease classified elsewhere B96.3
    generalized A41.3
  herpes (simplex) — *see also* Herpes
    congenital P35.2
    disseminated B00.7
    zoster B02.9
  herpesvirus, herpesviral — *see* Herpes
  hip (joint) NEC M00.9
    due to internal joint prosthesis
      left T84.52
      right T84.51
    skin NEC L08.9
  Heterophyes (heterophyes) B66.8
  Histoplasma — *see* Histoplasmosis
    American B39.4
    capsulatum B39.4
  hookworm B76.9
  human
    papilloma virus A63.0
    T-cell lymphotropic virus type-1 (HTLV-1) B33.3
  hydrocele N43.0
  Hymenolepis B71.0
  hypopharynx — *see* Pharyngitis
  inguinal (lymph) glands L04.1
    due to soft chancre A57
  intervertebral disc, pyogenic M46.30
    cervical region M46.32
    cervicothoracic region M46.33
    lumbar region M46.36
    lumbosacral region M46.37
    multiple sites M46.39
    occipito-atlanto-axial region M46.31
    sacrococcygeal region M46.38
    thoracic region M46.34

Infection, infected, infective (opportunistic) - *continued*
  intervertebral disc, pyogenic - *continued*
    thoracolumbar region M46.35
  intestine, intestinal — *see* Enteritis, infectious
    specified NEC A08.8
  intra-amniotic affecting newborn NEC P39.2
  Isospora belli or hominis A07.3
  Japanese B encephalitis A83.0
  jaw (bone) (lower) (upper) M27.2
  joint NEC M00.9
    due to internal joint prosthesis T84.50
  kidney (cortex) (hematogenous) N15.9
    with calculus N20.0
      with hydronephrosis N13.6
    following ectopic gestation O08.83
    pelvis and ureter (cystic) N28.85
    puerperal (postpartum) O86.21
    specified NEC N15.8
  Klebsiella (K.) pneumoniae NEC A49.8
    as cause of disease classified elsewhere B96.1
  knee (joint) NEC M00.9
    joint M00.9
    due to internal joint prosthesis
      left T84.54
      right T84.53
    skin L08.9
  Koch's — *see* Tuberculosis
  labia (majora) (minora) (acute) — *see* Vulvitis
  lacrimal
    gland — *see* Dacryoadenitis
    passages (duct) (sac) — *see* Inflammation, lacrimal, passages
  lancet fluke B66.2
  larynx NEC J38.7
  leg (skin) NOS L08.9
  Legionella pneumophila A48.1
    nonpneumonic A48.2
  Leishmania — *see also* Leishmaniasis
    aethiopica B55.1
    braziliensis B55.2
    chagasi B55.0
    donovani B55.0
    infantum B55.0
    major B55.1
    mexicana B55.1
    tropica B55.1
  lentivirus, as cause of disease classified elsewhere B97.31
  Leptosphaeria senegalensis B47.0
  Leptospira interrogans A27.9
    autumnalis A27.89
    canicola A27.89
    hebdomadis A27.89
    icterohaemorrhagiae A27.0
    pomona A27.89
    specified type NEC A27.89
  leptospirochetal NEC — *see* Leptospirosis
  Listeria monocytogenes — *see also* Listeriosis
    congenital P37.2
  Loa loa B74.3
    with conjunctival infestation B74.3
    eyelid B74.3
  Loboa loboi B48.0
  local, skin (staphylococcal) (streptococcal) L08.9
    abscess - code by site under Abscess
    cellulitis - code by site under Cellulitis
    specified NEC L08.89
    ulcer — *see* Ulcer, skin
  Loefflerella mallei A24.0
  lung — *see also* Pneumonia J18.9
    atypical Mycobacterium A31.0
    spirochetal A69.8
    tuberculous — *see* Tuberculosis, pulmonary
    virus — *see* Pneumonia, viral
  lymph gland — *see also* Lymphadenitis, acute
    mesenteric I88.0
  lymphoid tissue, base of tongue or posterior pharynx, NEC (chronic) J35.03
  Madurella (grisea) (mycetomii) B47.0
  major
    following ectopic or molar pregnancy O08.0
    puerperal, postpartum, childbirth O85
  Malassezia furfur B36.0
  Malleomyces
    mallei A24.0
    pseudomallei (whitmori) — *see* Melioidosis
  mammary gland N61.0
  Mansonella (ozzardi) (perstans) (streptocerca) B74.4
  mastoid — *see* Mastoiditis
  maxilla, maxillary M27.2
    sinus (chronic) — *see* Sinusitis, maxillary
  mediastinum J98.51

Infection, infected, infective (opportunistic) - *continued*
  Medina (worm) B72
  meibomian cyst or gland — *see* Hordeolum
  meninges — *see* Meningitis, bacterial
  meningococcal — *see also* condition A39.9
    adrenals A39.1
    brain A39.81
    cerebrospinal A39.0
    conjunctiva A39.89
    endocardium A39.51
    heart A39.50
      endocardium A39.51
      myocardium A39.52
      pericardium A39.53
    joint A39.83
    meninges A39.0
    meningococcemia A39.4
      acute A39.2
      chronic A39.3
    myocardium A39.52
    pericardium A39.53
    retrobulbar neuritis A39.82
    specified site NEC A39.89
  mesenteric lymph nodes or glands NEC I88.0
  Metagonimus B66.8
  metatarsophalangeal M00.9
  methicillin
    resistant Staphylococcus aureus (MRSA) A49.02
    susceptible Staphylococcus aureus (MSSA) A49.01
  Microsporum, microsporic — *see* Dermatophytosis
  mixed flora (bacterial) NEC A49.8
  Monilia — *see* Candidiasis
  Monosporium apiospermum B48.2
  mouth, parasitic B37.0
  Mucor — *see* Mucormycosis
  muscle NEC — *see* Myositis, infective
  mycelium NOS B49
  mycetoma B47.9
    actinomycotic NEC B47.1
    mycotic NEC B47.0
  Mycobacterium, mycobacterial — *see* Mycobacterium
  Mycoplasma NEC A49.3
    pneumoniae, as cause of disease classified elsewhere B96.0
  mycotic NOS B49
    pathogenic to compromised host only B48.8
    skin NOS B36.9
  myocardium NEC I40.0
  nail (chronic)
    with lymphangitis — *see* Lymphangitis, acute, digit
    finger L03.01-
      fungus B35.1
    ingrowing L60.0
    toe L03.03-
      fungus B35.1
  nasal sinus (chronic) — *see* Sinusitis
  nasopharynx — *see* Nasopharyngitis
  navel L08.82
  Necator americanus B76.1
  Neisseria — *see* Gonococcus
  Neotestudina rosatii B47.0
  newborn P39.9
    intra-amniotic NEC P39.2
    skin P39.4
    specified type NEC P39.8
  nipple N61.0
    associated with
      lactation O91.03
      pregnancy O91.01-
      puerperium O91.02
  Nocardia — *see* Nocardiosis
  obstetrical surgical wound (puerperal) O86.0
  Oesophagostomum (apiostomum) B81.8
  Oestrus ovis — *see* Myiasis
  Oidium albicans B37.9
  Onchocerca (volvulus) — *see* Onchocerciasis
  oncovirus, as cause of disease classified elsewhere B97.32
  operation wound T81.40
  Opisthorchis (felineus) (viverrini) B66.0
  orbit, orbital — *see* Inflammation, orbit
  orthopoxvirus NEC B08.09
  ovary — *see* Salpingo-oophoritis
  Oxyuris vermicularis B80
  pancreas (acute) — *see* Pancreatitis, acute
    abscess — *see* Pancreatitis, acute
    specified NEC — *see also* Pancreatitis, acute K85.80
  papillomavirus, as cause of disease classified elsewhere B97.7

Infection, infected, infective (opportunistic) - *continued*
  papovavirus NEC B34.4
  Paracoccidioides brasiliensis — *see* Paracoccidioidomycosis
  Paragonimus (westermani) B66.4
  parainfluenza virus B34.8
  parameningococcus NOS A39.9
  parapoxvirus B08.60
    specified NEC B08.69
  parasitic B89
  Parastrongylus
    cantonensis B83.2
    costaricensis B81.3
  paratyphoid A01.4
    Type A A01.1
    Type B A01.2
    Type C A01.3
  paraurethral ducts N34.2
  parotid gland — *see* Sialoadenitis
  parvovirus NEC B34.3
    as cause of disease classified elsewhere B97.6
  Pasteurella NEC A28.0
    multocida A28.0
    pestis — *see* Plague
    pseudotuberculosis A28.0
    septica (cat bite) (dog bite) A28.0
    tularensis — *see* Tularemia
  pelvic, female — *see* Disease, pelvis, inflammatory
  Penicillium (marneffei) B48.4
  penis (glans) (retention) NEC N48.29
  periapical K04.5
  peridental, periodontal K05.20
    generalized — *see* Peridontitis, aggressive, generalized
    localized — *see* Peridontitis, aggressive, localized
  perinatal period P39.9
    specified type NEC P39.8
  perineal repair (puerperal) O86.0
  periorbital — *see* Inflammation, orbit
  perirectal K62.89
  perirenal — *see* Infection, kidney
  peritoneal — *see* Peritonitis
  periureteral N28.89
  Petriellidium boydii B48.2
  pharynx — *see also* Pharyngitis
    coxsackievirus B08.5
    posterior, lymphoid (chronic) J35.03
  Phialophora
    gougerotii (subcutaneous abscess or cyst) B43.2
    jeanselmei (subcutaneous abscess or cyst) B43.2
    verrucosa (skin) B43.0
  Piedraia hortae B36.3
  pinta A67.9
    intermediate A67.1
    late A67.2
    mixed A67.3
    primary A67.0
  pinworm B80
  pityrosporum furfur B36.0
  pleuro-pneumonia-like organism (PPLO) NEC A49.3
    as cause of disease classified elsewhere B96.0
  pneumococcus, pneumococcal NEC A49.1
    as cause of disease classified elsewhere B95.3
    generalized (purulent) A40.3
      with pneumonia J13
  Pneumocystis carinii (pneumonia) B59
  Pneumocystis jiroveci (pneumonia) B59
  port or reservoir T80.212
  postoperative T81.40
  postoperative wound T81.40
  postprocedural T81.40
    deep incisional surgical site T81.42
    organ and space surgical site T81.43
    sepsis T81.49
    specified surgical site NEC T81.48
    superficial incisional surgical site T81.41
  postvaccinal T88.0
  prepuce NEC N47.7
    with penile inflammation N47.6
  prion — *see* Disease, prion, central nervous system
  prostate (capsule) — *see* Prostatitis
  Proteus (mirabilis) (morganii) (vulgaris) NEC A49.8
    as cause of disease classified elsewhere B96.4
  protozoal NEC B64
    intestinal A07.9
      specified NEC A07.8
    specified NEC B60.8
  Pseudoallescheria boydii B48.2
  Pseudomonas NEC A49.8
    as cause of disease classified elsewhere B96.5
    mallei A24.0

Infection, infected, infective (opportunistic) - *continued*
  Pseudomonas NEC - *continued*
    pneumonia J15.1
    pseudomallei — *see* Melioidosis
  puerperal O86.4
    genitourinary tract NEC O86.89
    major or generalized O85
    minor O86.4
    specified NEC O86.89
  pulmonary — *see* Infection, lung
  purulent — *see* Abscess
  Pyrenochaeta romeroi B47.0
  Q fever A78
  rectum (sphincter) K62.89
  renal — *see also* Infection, kidney
    pelvis and ureter (cystic) N28.85
  reovirus, as cause of disease classified elsewhere B97.5
  respiratory (tract) NEC J98.8
    acute J22
    chronic J98.8
    influenzal (upper) (acute) — *see* Influenza, with, respiratory manifestations NEC
    lower (acute) J22
      chronic — *see* Bronchitis, chronic
    rhinovirus J00
    syncytial virus, as cause of disease classified elsewhere B97.4
    upper (acute) NOS J06.9
      chronic J39.8
      streptococcal J06.9
      viral NOS J06.9
  resulting from
    presence of internal prosthesis, implant, graft — *see* Complications, by site and type, infection
  retortamoniasis A07.8
  retroperitoneal NEC K68.9
  retrovirus B33.3
    as cause of disease classified elsewhere B97.30
    human
      immunodeficiency, type 2 (HIV 2) B97.35
      T-cell lymphotropic
        type I (HTLV-I) B97.33
        type II (HTLV-II) B97.34
    lentivirus B97.31
    oncovirus B97.32
    specified NEC B97.39
  Rhinosporidium (seeberi) B48.1
  rhinovirus
    as cause of disease classified elsewhere B97.89
    unspecified nature or site B34.8
  Rhizopus — *see* Mucormycosis
  rickettsial NOS A79.9
  roundworm (large) NEC B82.0
    Ascariasis — *see also* Ascariasis B77.9
  rubella — *see* Rubella
  Saccharomyces — *see* Candidiasis
  salivary duct or gland (any) — *see* Sialoadenitis
  Salmonella (aertrycke) (arizonae) (callinarum) (cholerae-suis) (enteritidis) (suipestifer) (typhimurium) A02.9
    with
      (gastro) enteritis A02.0
      sepsis A02.1
      specified manifestation NEC A02.8
    due to food (poisoning) A02.9
    hirschfeldii A01.3
    localized A02.20
      arthritis A02.23
      meningitis A02.21
      osteomyelitis A02.24
      pneumonia A02.22
      pyelonephritis A02.25
      specified NEC A02.29
    paratyphi A01.4
      A A01.1
      B A01.2
      C A01.3
    schottmuelleri A01.2
    typhi, typhosa — *see* Typhoid
  Sarcocystis A07.8
  scabies B86
  Schistosoma — *see* Infestation, Schistosoma
  scrotum (acute) NEC N49.2
  seminal vesicle — *see* Vesiculitis
  septic
    localized, skin — *see* Abscess
  sheep liver fluke B66.3
  Shigella A03.9
    boydii A03.2
    dysenteriae A03.0

Infection, infected, infective (opportunistic) - *continued*

Shigella - *continued*
flexneri A03.1
group
A A03.0
B A03.1
C A03.2
D A03.3
Schmitz (-Stutzer) A03.0
schmitzii A03.0
shigae A03.0
sonnei A03.3
specified NEC A03.8
shoulder (joint) NEC M00.9
due to internal joint prosthesis T84.59
skin NEC L08.9
sinus (accessory) (chronic) (nasal) — *see also* Sinusitis
pilonidal — *see* Sinus, pilonidal
skin NEC L08.89
Skene's duct or gland — *see* Urethritis
skin (local) (staphylococcal) (streptococcal) L08.9
abscess - code by site under Abscess
cellulitis - code by site under Cellulitis
due to fungus B36.9
specified type NEC B36.8
mycotic B36.9
specified type NEC B36.8
newborn P39.4
ulcer — *see* Ulcer, skin
slow virus A81.9
specified NEC A81.89
Sparganum (mansoni) (proliferum) (baxteri) B70.1
specific — *see also* Syphilis
to perinatal period — *see* Infection, congenital
specified NEC B99.8
spermatic cord NEC N49.1
sphenoidal (sinus) — *see* Sinusitis, sphenoidal
spinal cord NOS — *see also* Myelitis G04.91
abscess G06.1
meninges — *see* Meningitis
streptococcal G04.89
Spirillum A25.0
spirochetal NOS A69.9
lung A69.8
specified NEC A69.8
Spirometra larvae B70.1
spleen D73.89
Sporotrichum, Sporothrix (schenckii) — *see* Sporotrichosis
staphylococcal, unspecified site
aureus (methicillin susceptible) (MSSA) A49.01
methicillin resistant (MRSA) A49.02
as cause of disease classified elsewhere B95.8
aureus (methicillin susceptible) (MSSA) B95.61
methicillin resistant (MRSA) B95.62
specified NEC B95.7
food poisoning A05.0
generalized (purulent) A41.2
pneumonia — *see* Pneumonia, staphylococcal
Stellantchasmus falcatus B66.8
streptobacillus moniliformis A25.1
streptococcal NEC A49.1
as cause of disease classified elsewhere B95.5
B genitourinary complicating
childbirth O98.82
pregnancy O98.81-
puerperium O98.83
congenital
sepsis P36.10
group B P36.0
specified NEC P36.19
generalized (purulent) A40.9
Streptomyces B47.1
Strongyloides (stercoralis) — *see* Strongyloidiasis
stump (amputation) (surgical) — *see* Complication, amputation stump, infection
subcutaneous tissue, local L08.9
suipestifer — *see* Infection, salmonella
swimming pool bacillus A31.1
Taenia — *see* Infestation, Taenia
Taeniarhynchus saginatus B68.1
tapeworm — *see* Infestation, tapeworm
tendon (sheath) — *see* Tenosynovitis, infective NEC
Ternidens diminutus B81.8
testis — *see* Orchitis
threadworm B80
throat — *see* Pharyngitis
thyroglossal duct K14.8
toe (skin) L08.9
cellulitis L03.03-
fungus B35.1

Infection, infected, infective (opportunistic) - *continued*

toe (skin) - *continued*
nail L03.03-
fungus B35.1
tongue NEC K14.0
parasitic B37.0
tonsil (and adenoid) (faucial) (lingual) (pharyngeal) — *see* Tonsillitis
tooth, teeth K04.7
periapical K04.7
peridental, periodontal K05.20
generalized — *see* Peridontitis, aggressive, generalized
localized — *see* Peridontitis, aggressive, localized
pulp K04.01
irreversible K04.02
reversible K04.01
socket M27.3
TORCH — *see* Infection, congenital
without active infection P00.2
Torula histolytica — *see* Cryptococcosis
Toxocara (canis) (cati) (felis) B83.0
Toxoplasma gondii — *see* Toxoplasma
trachea, chronic J42
trematode NEC — *see* Infestation, fluke
trench fever A79.0
Treponema pallidum — *see* Syphilis
Trichinella (spiralis) B75
Trichomonas A59.9
cervix A59.09
intestine A07.8
prostate A59.02
specified site NEC A59.8
urethra A59.03
urogenitalis A59.00
vagina A59.01
vulva A59.01
Trichophyton, trichophytic — *see* Dermatophytosis
Trichosporon (beigelii) cutaneum B36.2
Trichostrongylus B81.2
Trichuris (trichiura) B79
Trombicula (irritans) B88.0
Trypanosoma
brucei
gambiense B56.0
rhodesiense B56.1
cruzi — *see* Chagas' disease
tubal — *see* Salpingo-oophoritis
tuberculous NEC — *see* Tuberculosis
tubo-ovarian — *see* Salpingo-oophoritis
tunnel T80.212
tunica vaginalis N49.1
tympanic membrane NEC — *see* Myringitis
typhoid (abortive) (ambulant) (bacillus) — *see* Typhoid
typhus A75.9
flea-borne A75.2
mite-borne A75.3
recrudescent A75.1
tick-borne A77.9
African A77.1
North Asian A77.2
umbilicus L08.82
ureter N28.86
urethra — *see* Urethritis
urinary (tract) N39.0
bladder — *see* Cystitis
complicating
pregnancy O23.4-
specified type NEC O23.3-
kidney — *see* Infection, kidney
newborn P39.3
puerperal (postpartum) O86.20
tuberculous A18.13
urethra — *see* Urethritis
uterus, uterine — *see* Endometritis
vaccination T88.0
vaccinia not from vaccination B08.011
vagina (acute) — *see* Vaginitis
varicella B01.9
varicose veins — *see* Varix
vas deferens NEC N49.1
vesical — *see* Cystitis
Vibrio
cholerae A00.0
El Tor A00.1
parahaemolyticus (food poisoning) A05.3
vulnificus
as cause of disease classified elsewhere B96.82
foodborne intoxication A05.5
Vincent's (gum) (mouth) (tonsil) A69.1
virus, viral NOS B34.9

Infection, infected, infective (opportunistic) - *continued*

virus, viral NOS - *continued*
adenovirus
as cause of disease classified elsewhere B97.0
unspecified nature or site B34.0
arbovirus, arbovirus arthropod-borne A94
as cause of disease classified elsewhere B97.89
adenovirus B97.0
coronavirus B97.29
SARS-associated B97.21
coxsackievirus B97.11
echovirus B97.12
enterovirus B97.10
coxsackievirus B97.11
echovirus B97.12
specified NEC B97.19
human
immunodeficiency, type 2 (HIV 2) B97.35
T-cell lymphotropic, type I (HTLV-I) B97.33
type II (HTLV-II) B97.34
metapneumovirus B97.81
papillomavirus B97.7
parvovirus B97.6
reovirus B97.5
respiratory syncytial B97.4
retrovirus B97.30
human
immunodeficiency, type 2 (HIV 2) B97.35
T-cell lymphotropic, type I (HTLV-I) B97.33
type II (HTLV-II) B97.34
lentivirus B97.31
oncovirus B97.32
specified NEC B97.39
specified NEC B97.89
central nervous system A89
atypical A81.9
specified NEC A81.89
enterovirus NEC A88.8
meningitis A87.0
slow virus A81.9
specified NEC A81.89
specified NEC A88.8
chest J98.8
cotia B08.8
coxsackie — *see also* Infection, coxsackie B34.1
as cause of disease classified elsewhere B97.11
ECHO
as cause of disease classified elsewhere B97.12
unspecified nature or site B34.1
encephalitis, tick-borne A84.9
enterovirus, as cause of disease classified elsewhere B97.10
coxsackievirus B97.11
echovirus B97.12
specified NEC B97.19
exanthem NOS B09
human papilloma as cause of disease classified elsewhere B97.7
human metapneumovirus as cause of disease classified elsewhere B97.81
intestine — *see* Enteritis, viral
respiratory syncytial
as cause of disease classified elsewhere B97.4
bronchopneumonia J12.1
common cold syndrome J00
nasopharyngitis (acute) J00
rhinovirus
as cause of disease classified elsewhere B97.89
unspecified nature or site B34.8
slow A81.9
specified NEC A81.89
specified type NEC B33.8
as cause of disease classified elsewhere B97.89
unspecified nature or site B34.8
unspecified nature or site B34.9
West Nile — *see* Virus, West Nile
vulva (acute) — *see* Vulvitis
West Nile — *see* Virus, West Nile
whipworm B79
worms B83.9
specified type NEC B83.8
Wuchereria (bancrofti) B74.0
malayi B74.1
yatapoxvirus B08.70
specified NEC B08.79
yeast — *see also* Candidiasis B37.9
yellow fever — *see* Fever, yellow
Yersinia
enterocolitica (intestinal) A04.6
pestis — *see* Plague

Infection, infected, infective (opportunistic) - *continued*
  Yersinia - *continued*
    pseudotuberculosis A28.2
  Zeis' gland — *see* Hordeolum
  Zika virus A92.5
  zoonotic bacterial NOS A28.9
  Zopfia senegalensis B47.0
Infective, infectious — *see* condition
Infertility
  female N97.9
    age-related N97.8
    associated with
      anovulation N97.0
      cervical (mucus) disease or anomaly N88.3
      congenital anomaly
        cervix N88.3
        fallopian tube N97.1
        uterus N97.2
        vagina N97.8
      dysmucorrhea N88.3
      fallopian tube disease or anomaly N97.1
      pituitary-hypothalamic origin E23.0
      specified origin NEC N97.8
      Stein-Leventhal syndrome E28.2
      uterine disease or anomaly N97.2
      vaginal disease or anomaly N97.8
    due to
      cervical anomaly N88.3
      fallopian tube anomaly N97.1
      ovarian failure E28.39
      Stein-Leventhal syndrome E28.2
      uterine anomaly N97.2
      vaginal anomaly N97.8
    nonimplantation N97.2
    origin
      cervical N88.3
      tubal (block) (occlusion) (stenosis) N97.1
      uterine N97.2
      vaginal N97.8
  male N46.9
    azoospermia N46.01
      extratesticular cause N46.029
        drug therapy N46.021
        efferent duct obstruction N46.023
        infection N46.022
        radiation N46.024
        specified cause NEC N46.029
        systemic disease N46.025
    oligospermia N46.11
      extratesticular cause N46.129
        drug therapy N46.121
        efferent duct obstruction N46.123
        infection N46.122
        radiation N46.124
        specified cause NEC N46.129
        systemic disease N46.125
    specified type NEC N46.8
Infestation B88.9
  Acanthocheilonema (perstans) (streptocerca) B74.4
  Acariasis B88.0
    demodex folliculorum B88.0
    sarcoptes scabiei B86
    trombiculae B88.0
  Agamofilaria streptocerca B74.4
  Ancylostoma, ankylostoma (braziliense) (caninum) (ceylanicum) (duodenale) B76.0
    americanum B76.1
    new world B76.1
  Anisakis larvae, anisakiasis B81.0
  arthropod NEC B88.2
  Ascaris lumbricoides — *see* Ascariasis
  Balantidium coli A07.0
  beef tapeworm B68.1
  Bothriocephalus (latus) B70.0
    larval B70.1
  broad tapeworm B70.0
    larval B70.1
  Brugia (malayi) B74.1
    timori B74.2
  candiru B88.8
  Capillaria
    hepatica B83.8
    philippinensis B81.1
  cat liver fluke B66.0
  cestodes B71.9
    diphyllobothrium — *see* Infestation, diphyllobothrium
    dipylidiasis B71.1
    hymenolepiasis B71.0
    specified type NEC B71.8
  chigger B88.0
  chigo, chigoe B88.1

Infestation - *continued*
  Clonorchis (sinensis) (liver) B66.1
  coccidial A07.3
  crab-lice B85.3
  Cysticercus cellulosae — *see* Cysticercosis
  Demodex (folliculorum) B88.0
  Dermanyssus gallinae B88.0
  Dermatobia (hominis) — *see* Myiasis
  Dibothriocephalus (latus) B70.0
    larval B70.1
  Dicrocoelium dendriticum B66.2
  Diphyllobothrium (adult) (latum) (intestinal) (pacificum) B70.0
    larval B70.1
  Diplogonoporus (grandis) B71.8
  Dipylidium caninum B67.4
  Distoma hepaticum B66.3
  dog tapeworm B67.4
  Dracunculus medinensis B72
  dragon worm B72
  dwarf tapeworm B71.0
  Echinococcus — *see* Echinococcus
  Echinostomum ilocanum B66.8
  Entamoeba (histolytica) — *see* Infection, Ameba
  Enterobius vermicularis B80
  eyelid
    in (due to)
      leishmaniasis B55.1
      loiasis B74.3
      onchocerciasis B73.09
      phthiriasis B85.3
      parasitic NOS B89
  eyeworm B74.3
  Fasciola (gigantica) (hepatica) (indica) B66.3
  Fasciolopsis (buski) (intestine) B66.5
  filarial B74.9
    bancroftian B74.0
    conjunctiva B74.9
    due to
      Acanthocheilonema (perstans) (streptocerca) B74.4
      Brugia (malayi) B74.1
        timori B74.2
      Dracunculus medinensis B72
      guinea worm B72
      loa loa B74.3
      Mansonella (ozzardi) (perstans) (streptocerca) B74.4
      Onchocerca volvulus B73.00
        eye B73.00
        eyelid B73.09
      Wuchereria (bancrofti) B74.0
    Malayan B74.1
    ozzardi B74.4
    specified type NEC B74.8
  fish tapeworm B70.0
    larval B70.1
  fluke B66.9
    blood NOS — *see* Schistosomiasis
    cat liver B66.0
    intestinal B66.5
    liver (sheep) B66.3
      cat B66.0
      Chinese B66.1
      due to clonorchiasis B66.1
      oriental B66.1
    lancet B66.2
    lung (oriental) B66.4
    sheep liver B66.3
    specified type NEC B66.8
  fly larvae — *see* Myiasis
  Gasterophilus (intestinalis) — *see* Myiasis
  Gastrodiscoides hominis B66.8
  Giardia lamblia A07.1
  Gnathostoma (spinigerum) B83.1
  Gongylonema B83.8
  guinea worm B72
  helminth B83.9
    angiostrongyliasis B83.2
      intestinal B81.3
    gnathostomiasis B83.1
    hirudiniasis, internal B83.4
    intestinal B82.0
      angiostrongyliasis B81.3
      anisakiasis B81.0
      ascariasis — *see* Ascariasis
      capillariasis B81.1
      cysticercosis — *see* Cysticercosis
      diphyllobothriasis — *see* Infestation, diphyllobothriasis
      dracunculiasis B72
      echinococcus — *see* Echinococcosis
      enterobiasis B80

Infestation - *continued*
  helminth - *continued*
    intestinal - *continued*
      filariasis - — *see* Infestation, filarial
      fluke — *see* Infestation, fluke
      hookworm — *see* Infestation, hookworm
      mixed (types classifiable to more than one of the titles B65.0-B81.3 and B81.8) B81.4
      onchocerciasis — *see* Onchocerciasis
      schistosomiasis — *see* Infestation, schistosoma
      specified
        cestode NEC — *see* Infestation, cestode type NEC B81.8
      strongyloidiasis — *see* Strongyloidiasis
      taenia — *see* Infestation, taenia
      trichinellosis B75
      trichostrongyliasis B81.2
      trichuriasis B79
      specified type NEC B83.8
      syngamiasis B83.3
      visceral larva migrans B83.0
  Heterophyes (heterophyes) B66.8
  hookworm B76.9
    ancylostomiasis B76.0
    necatoriasis B76.1
    specified type NEC B76.8
  Hymenolepis (diminuta) (nana) B71.0
  intestinal NEC B82.9
  leeches (aquatic) (land) — *see* Hirudiniasis
  Leishmania — *see* Leishmaniasis
  lice, louse — *see* Infestation, Pediculus
  Linguatula B88.8
  Liponyssoides sanguineus B88.0
  Loa loa B74.3
    conjunctival B74.3
    eyelid B74.3
  louse — *see* Infestation, Pediculus
  maggots — *see* Myiasis
  Mansonella (ozzardi) (perstans) (streptocerca) B74.4
  Medina (worm) B72
  Metagonimus (yokogawai) B66.8
  microfilaria streptocerca — *see* Onchocerciasis
    eye B73.00
    eyelid B73.09
  mites B88.9
    scabic B86
  Monilia (albicans) — *see* Candidiasis
  mouth B37.0
  Necator americanus B76.1
  nematode NEC (intestinal) B82.0
    Ancylostoma B76.0
    conjunctiva NEC B83.9
    Enterobius vermicularis B80
    Gnathostoma spinigerum B83.1
    physaloptera B80
    specified NEC B81.8
    trichostrongylus B81.2
    trichuris (trichuria) B79
  Oesophagostomum (apiostomum) B81.8
  Oestrus ovis — *see also* Myiasis B87.9
  Onchocerca (volvulus) — *see* Onchocerciasis
  Opisthorchis (felineus) (viverrini) B66.0
  orbit, parasitic NOS B89
  Oxyuris vermicularis B80
  Paragonimus (westermani) B66.4
  parasite, parasitic B89
    eyelid B89
    intestinal NOS B82.9
    mouth B37.0
    skin B88.9
    tongue B37.0
  Parastrongylus
    cantonensis B83.2
    costaricensis B81.3
  Pediculus B85.2
    body B85.1
    capitis (humanus) (any site) B85.0
    corporis (humanus) (any site) B85.1
    head B85.0
    mixed (classifiable to more than one of the titles B85.0-B85.3) B85.4
    pubis (any site) B85.3
  Pentastoma B88.8
  Phthirus (pubis) (any site) B85.3
    with any infestation classifiable to B85.0-B85.2 B85.4
  pinworm B80
  pork tapeworm (adult) B68.0
  protozoal NEC B64
    intestinal A07.9
      specified NEC A07.8
    specified NEC B60.8
  pubic, louse B85.3

Infestation - *continued*

rat tapeworm B71.0
red bug B88.0
roundworm (large) NEC B82.0
  Ascariasis — *see also* Ascariasis B77.9
sandflea B88.1
Sarcoptes scabiei B86
scabies B86
Schistosoma B65.9
  bovis B65.8
  cercariae B65.3
  haematobium B65.0
  intercalatum B65.8
  japonicum B65.2
  mansoni B65.1
  mattheei B65.8
  mekongi B65.8
  specified type NEC B65.8
  spindale B65.8
screw worms — *see* Myiasis
skin NOS B88.9
Sparganum (mansoni) (proliferum) (baxteri) B70.1
  larval B70.1
specified type NEC B88.8
Spirometra larvae B70.1
Stellantchasmus falcatus B66.8
Strongyloides stercoralis — *see* Strongyloidiasis
Taenia B68.9
  diminuta B71.0
  echinococcus — *see* Echinococcus
  mediocanellata B68.1
  nana B71.0
  saginata B68.1
  solium (intestinal form) B68.0
   larval form — *see* Cysticercosis
Taeniarhynchus saginatus B68.1
tapeworm B71.9
  beef B68.1
  broad B70.0
   larval B70.1
  dog B67.4
  dwarf B71.0
  fish B70.0
   larval B70.1
  pork B68.0
  rat B71.0
Ternidens diminutus B81.8
Tetranychus molestissimus B88.0
threadworm B80
tongue B37.0
Toxocara (canis) (cati) (felis) B83.0
trematode (s) NEC — *see* Infestation, fluke
Trichinella (spiralis) B75
Trichocephalus B79
Trichomonas — *see* Trichomoniasis
Trichostrongylus B81.2
Trichuris (trichiura) B79
Trombicula (irritans) B88.0
Tunga penetrans B88.1
Uncinaria americana B76.1
Vandellia cirrhosa B88.8
whipworm B79
worms B83.9
  intestinal B82.0
Wuchereria (bancrofti) B74.0

Infiltrate, infiltration

amyloid (generalized) (localized) — *see* Amyloidosis
calcareous NEC R89.7
  localized — *see* Degeneration, by site
calcium salt R89.7
cardiac
  fatty — *see* Degeneration, myocardial
  glycogenic E74.02 *[I43]*
corneal — *see* Edema, cornea
eyelid — *see* Inflammation, eyelid
glycogen, glycogenic — *see* Disease, glycogen storage
heart, cardiac
  fatty — *see* Degeneration, myocardial
  glycogenic E74.02 *[I43]*
inflammatory in vitreous H43.89
kidney N28.89
leukemic — *see* Leukemia
liver K76.89
  fatty — *see* Fatty, liver NEC
  glycogen — *see also* Disease, glycogen storage E74.03 *[K77]*
lung R91.8
  eosinophilic J82
lymphatic — *see also* Leukemia, lymphatic C91.9-
  gland I88.9
muscle, fatty M62.89

Infiltrate, infiltration - *continued*

myocardium, myocardial
  fatty — *see* Degeneration, myocardial
  glycogenic E74.02 *[I43]*
on chest x-ray R91.8
pulmonary R91.8
  with eosinophilia J82
skin (lymphocytic) L98.6
thymus (gland) (fatty) E32.8
urine R39.0
vesicant agent
  antineoplastic chemotherapy T80.810
  other agent NEC T80.818
vitreous body H43.89

Infirmity R68.89

senile R54

Inflammation, inflamed, inflammatory

(with exudation)
abducent (nerve) — *see* Strabismus, paralytic, sixth nerve
accessory sinus (chronic) — *see* Sinusitis
adrenal (gland) E27.8
alveoli, teeth M27.3
  scorbutic E54
anal canal, anus K62.89
antrum (chronic) — *see* Sinusitis, maxillary
appendix — *see* Appendicitis
arachnoid — *see* Meningitis
areola
  puerperal, postpartum or gestational — *see* Infection, nipple
areolar tissue NOS L08.9
artery — *see* Arteritis
auditory meatus (external) — *see* Otitis, externa
Bartholin's gland N75.8
bile duct (common) (hepatic) or passage — *see* Cholangitis
bladder — *see* Cystitis
bone — *see* Osteomyelitis
brain — *see also* Encephalitis
  membrane — *see* Meningitis
breast N61.0
  puerperal, postpartum, gestational — *see* Mastitis, obstetric
broad ligament — *see* Disease, pelvis, inflammatory
bronchi — *see* Bronchitis
catarrhal J00
cecum — *see* Appendicitis
cerebral — *see also* Encephalitis
  membrane — *see* Meningitis
cerebrospinal
  meningococcal A39.0
cervix (uteri) — *see* Cervicitis
chest J98.8
chorioretinal H30.9-
  cyclitis — *see* Cyclitis
  disseminated H30.10-
   generalized H30.13-
   peripheral H30.12-
   posterior pole H30.11-
  epitheliopathy — *see* Epitheliopathy
  focal H30.00-
   juxtapapillary H30.01-
   macular H30.04-
   paramacular — *see* Inflammation, chorioretinal, focal, macular
   peripheral H30.03-
   posterior pole H30.02-
  specified type NEC H30.89-
choroid — *see* Inflammation, chorioretinal
chronic, postmastoidectomy cavity — *see* Complications, postmastoidectomy, inflammation
colon — *see* Enteritis
connective tissue (diffuse) NEC — *see* Disorder, soft tissue, specified type NEC
cornea — *see* Keratitis
corpora cavernosa N48.29
cranial nerve — *see* Disorder, nerve, cranial
Douglas' cul-de-sac or pouch (chronic) N73.0
due to device, implant or graft — *see also* Complications, by site and type, infection or inflammation
  arterial graft T82.7
  breast (implant) T85.79
  catheter T85.79
   dialysis (renal) T82.7
    intraperitoneal T85.71
   infusion T82.7
    cranial T85.735
    intrathecal T85.735
    spinal (epidural) (subdural) T85.735
    subarachnoid T85.735
   urinary T83.518

Inflammation, inflamed, inflammatory

(with exudation) - *continued*
due to device, implant or graft - *continued*
  catheter - *continued*
   urinary - *continued*
    cystostomy T83.510
    Hopkins T83.518
    ileostomy T83.518
    nephrostomy T83.512
    specified NEC T83.518
    urethral indwelling T83.511
    urostomy T83.518
  electronic (electrode) (pulse generator) (stimulator)
   bone T84.7
   cardiac T82.7
   nervous system T85.738
    brain T85.731
    cranial nerve T85.732
    gastric nerve T85.732
    neurostimulator generator T85.734
    peripheral nerve T85.732
    sacral nerve T85.732
    spinal cord T85.733
    vagal nerve T85.732
   urinary T83.590
  fixation, internal (orthopedic) NEC — *see* Complication, fixation device, infection
  gastrointestinal (bile duct) (esophagus) T85.79
   neurostimulator electrode (lead) T85.732
  genital NEC T83.69
  heart NEC T82.7
   valve (prosthesis) T82.6
    graft T82.7
  joint prosthesis — *see* Complication, joint prosthesis, infection
  ocular (corneal graft) (orbital implant) NEC T85.79
  orthopedic NEC T84.7
  penile (cylinder) (pump) (resevoir) T83.61
  specified NEC T85.79
  testicular T83.62
  urinary NEC T83.598
   ileal conduit stent T83.593
   implanted neurostimulation T83.590
   implanted sphincter T83.591
   indwelling ureteral stent T83.592
   nephroureteral stent T83.593
   specified stent NEC T83.593
  vascular NEC T82.7
  ventricular intracranial (communicating) shunt T85.730
duodenum K29.80
  with bleeding K29.81
dura mater — *see* Meningitis
ear (middle) — *see also* Otitis, media
  external — *see* Otitis, externa
  inner — *see* subcategory H83.0
epididymis — *see* Epididymitis
esophagus K20.9
ethmoidal (sinus) (chronic) — *see* Sinusitis, ethmoidal
eustachian tube (catarrhal) — *see* Salpingitis, eustachian
eyelid H01.9
  abscess — *see* Abscess, eyelid
  blepharitis — *see* Blepharitis
  chalazion — *see* Chalazion
  dermatosis (noninfectious) — *see* Dermatosis, eyelid
  hordeolum — *see* Hordeolum
  specified NEC H01.8
fallopian tube — *see* Salpingo-oophoritis
fascia — *see* Myositis
follicular, pharynx J31.2
frontal (sinus) (chronic) — *see* Sinusitis, frontal
gallbladder — *see* Cholecystitis
gastric — *see* Gastritis
gastrointestinal — *see* Enteritis
genital organ (internal) (diffuse)
  female — *see* Disease, pelvis, inflammatory
  male N49.9
   multiple sites N49.8
   specified NEC N49.8
gland (lymph) — *see* Lymphadenitis
glottis — *see* Laryngitis
granular, pharynx J31.2
gum K05.10
  nonplaque induced K05.11
  plaque induced K05.10
heart — *see* Carditis
hepatic duct — *see* Cholangitis
ileoanal (internal) pouch K91.850
ileum — *see also* Enteritis

Inflammation, inflamed, inflammatory (with exudation) - *continued*
  ileum - *continued*
    regional or terminal — *see* Enteritis, regional
    intestine (any part) — *see* Enteritis
  intestinal pouch K91.850
  jaw (acute) (bone) (chronic) (lower) (suppurative) (upper) M27.2
  joint NEC — *see* Arthritis
    sacroiliac M46.1
  kidney — *see* Nephritis
  knee (joint) M13.169
    tuberculous A18.02
  labium (majus) (minus) — *see* Vulvitis
  lacrimal
    gland — *see* Dacryoadenitis
    passages (duct) (sac) — *see also* Dacryocystitis
      canaliculitis — *see* Canaliculitis, lacrimal
  larynx — *see* Laryngitis
  leg NOS L08.9
  lip K13.0
  liver (capsule) — *see also* Hepatitis
    chronic K73.9
    suppurative K75.0
  lung (acute) — *see also* Pneumonia
    chronic J98.4
  lymph gland or node — *see* Lymphadenitis
  lymphatic vessel — *see* Lymphangitis
  maxilla, maxillary M27.2
    sinus (chronic) — *see* Sinusitis, maxillary
  membranes of brain or spinal cord — *see* Meningitis
  meninges — *see* Meningitis
  mouth K12.1
  muscle — *see* Myositis
  myocardium — *see* Myocarditis
  nasal sinus (chronic) — *see* Sinusitis
  nasopharynx — *see* Nasopharyngitis
  navel L08.82
  nerve NEC — *see* Neuralgia
  nipple N61.0
    puerperal, postpartum or gestational — *see* Infection, nipple
  nose — *see* Rhinitis
  oculomotor (nerve) — *see* Strabismus, paralytic, third nerve
  optic nerve — *see* Neuritis, optic
  orbit (chronic) H05.10
    acute H05.00
      abscess — *see* Abscess, orbit
      cellulitis — *see* Cellulitis, orbit
      osteomyelitis — *see* Osteomyelitis, orbit
      periostitis — *see* Periostitis, orbital
      tenonitis — *see* Tenonitis, eye
      granuloma — *see* Granuloma, orbit
      myositis — *see* Myositis, orbital
  ovary — *see* Salpingo-oophoritis
  oviduct — *see* Salpingo-oophoritis
  pancreas (acute) — *see* Pancreatitis
  parametrium N73.0
  parotid region L08.9
  pelvis, female — *see* Disease, pelvis, inflammatory
  penis (corpora cavernosa) N48.29
  perianal K62.89
  pericardium — *see* Pericarditis
  perineum (female) (male) L08.9
  periuterine — *see* Disease, pelvis, inflammatory
  perivesical — *see* Cystitis
  petrous bone (acute) (chronic) — *see* Petrositis
  pharynx (acute) — *see* Pharyngitis
  pia mater — *see* Meningitis
  pleura — *see* Pleurisy
  polyp, colon — *see also* Polyp, colon, inflammatory K51.40
  prostate — *see also* Prostatitis
    specified type NEC N41.8
  rectosigmoid — *see* Rectosigmoiditis
  rectum — *see also* Proctitis K62.89
  respiratory, upper — *see also* Infection, respiratory, upper J06.9
    acute, due to radiation J70.0
    chronic, due to external agent — *see* condition, respiratory, chronic, due to
    due to
      chemicals, gases, fumes or vapors (inhalation) J68.2
      radiation J70.1
  retina — *see* Chorioretinitis
  retrocecal — *see* Appendicitis
  retroperitoneal — *see* Peritonitis
  salivary duct or gland (any) (suppurative) — *see* Sialoadenitis

Inflammation, inflamed, inflammatory (with exudation) - *continued*
  scorbutic, alveoli, teeth E54
  scrotum N49.2
  seminal vesicle — *see* Vesiculitis
  sigmoid — *see* Enteritis
  sinus — *see* Sinusitis
  Skene's duct or gland — *see* Urethritis
  skin L08.9
  spermatic cord N49.1
  sphenoidal (sinus) — *see* Sinusitis, sphenoidal
  spinal
    cord — *see* Encephalitis
    membrane — *see* Meningitis
    nerve — *see* Disorder, nerve
  spine — *see* Spondylopathy, inflammatory
  spleen (capsule) D73.89
  stomach — *see* Gastritis
  subcutaneous tissue L08.9
  suprarenal (gland) E27.8
  synovial — *see* Tenosynovitis
  tendon (sheath) NEC — *see* Tenosynovitis
  testis — *see* Orchitis
  throat (acute) — *see* Pharyngitis
  thymus (gland) E32.8
  thyroid (gland) — *see* Thyroiditis
  tongue K14.0
  tonsil — *see* Tonsillitis
  trachea — *see* Tracheitis
  trochlear (nerve) — *see* Strabismus, paralytic, fourth nerve
  tubal — *see* Salpingo-oophoritis
  tuberculous NEC — *see* Tuberculosis
  tubo-ovarian — *see* Salpingo-oophoritis
  tunica vaginalis N49.1
  tympanic membrane — *see* Tympanitis
  umbilicus, umbilical L08.82
  uterine ligament — *see* Disease, pelvis, inflammatory
  uterus (catarrhal) — *see* Endometritis
  uveal tract (anterior) NOS — *see also* Iridocyclitis
    posterior — *see* Chorioretinitis
  vagina — *see* Vaginitis
  vas deferens N49.1
  vein — *see also* Phlebitis
    intracranial or intraspinal (septic) G08
    thrombotic I80.9
      leg — *see* Phlebitis, leg
      lower extremity — *see* Phlebitis, leg
  vocal cord J38.3
  vulva — *see* Vulvitis
  Wharton's duct (suppurative) — *see* Sialoadenitis
Inflation, lung, imperfect (newborn) — *see* Atelectasis
Influenza (bronchial) (epidemic) (respiratory (upper)) (unidentified influenza virus)
  (unidentified influenza virus) J11.1
  with
    digestive manifestations J11.2
    encephalopathy J11.81
    enteritis J11.2
    gastroenteritis J11.2
    gastrointestinal manifestations J11.2
    laryngitis J11.1
    myocarditis J11.82
    otitis media J11.83
    pharyngitis J11.1
    pneumonia J11.00
      specified type J11.08
    respiratory manifestations NEC J11.1
    specified manifestation NEC J11.89
  A/H5N1 — *see also* Influenza, due to, identified novel influenza A virus J09.X2
  avian — *see also* Influenza, due to, identified novel influenza A virus J09.X2
  bird — *see also* Influenza, due to, identified novel influenza A virus J09.X2
  novel (2009) H1N1 influenza — *see also* Influenza, due to, identified influenza virus NEC J10.1
  novel influenza A/H1N1 — *see also* Influenza, due to, identified influenza virus NEC J10.1
  due to
    avian — *see also* Influenza, due to, identified novel influenza A virus J09.X2
    identified influenza virus NEC J10.1
      with
        digestive manifestations J10.2
        encephalopathy J10.81
        enteritis J10.2
        gastroenteritis J10.2
        gastrointestinal manifestations J10.2
        laryngitis J10.1
        myocarditis J10.82

Influenza (bronchial) (epidemic) (respiratory (upper)) (unidentified influenza virus) (unidentified influenza virus) - *continued*
  due to - *continued*
    identified influenza virus NEC - *continued*
      with - *continued*
        otitis media J10.83
        pharyngitis J10.1
        pneumonia (unspecified type) J10.00
          with same identified influenza virus J10.01
          specified type NEC J10.08
        respiratory manifestations NEC J10.1
        specified manifestation NEC J10.89
    identified novel influenza A virus J09.X2
      with
        digestive manifestations J09.X3
        encephalopathy J09.X9
        enteritis J09.X3
        gastroenteritis J09.X3
        gastrointestinal manifestations J09.X3
        laryngitis J09.X2
        myocarditis J09.X9
        otitis media J09.X9
        pharyngitis J09.X2
        pneumonia J09.X1
        respiratory manifestations NEC J09.X2
        specified manifestation NEC J09.X9
        upper respiratory symptoms J09.X2
    of other animal origin, not bird or swine — *see also* Influenza, due to, identified novel influenza A virus J09.X2
    swine (viruses that normally cause infections in pigs) — *see also* Influenza, due to, identified novel influenza A virus J09.X2
Influenzal — *see* Influenza
Influenza-like disease — *see* Influenza
Infraction, Freiberg's (metatarsal head) — *see* Osteochondrosis, juvenile, metatarsus
Infraeruption of tooth (teeth) M26.34
Infusion complication, misadventure, or reaction — *see* Complications, infusion
Ingestion
  chemical — *see* Table of Drugs and Chemicals, by substance, poisoning
  drug or medicament
    correct substance properly administered — *see* Table of Drugs and Chemicals, by drug, adverse effect
    overdose or wrong substance given or taken — *see* Table of Drugs and Chemicals, by drug, poisoning
  foreign body — *see* Foreign body, alimentary tract
  tularemia A21.3
Ingrowing
  hair (beard) L73.1
  nail (finger) (toe) L60.0
Inguinal — *see also* condition
  testicle Q53.9
    bilateral Q53.21
    unilateral Q53.11
Inhalant-induced
  anxiety disorder F18.980
  depressive disorder F18.94
  major neurocognitive disorder F18.97
  mild neurocognitive disorder F18.988
  psychotic disorder F18.959
Inhalation
  anthrax A22.1
  flame T27.3
  food or foreign body — *see* Foreign body, by site
  gases, fumes, or vapors NEC T59.9-
    specified agent — *see* Table of Drugs and Chemicals, by substance
  liquid or vomitus — *see* Asphyxia
  meconium (newborn) P24.00
    with
      pneumonia (pneumonitis) P24.01
      with respiratory symptoms P24.01
  mucus — *see* Asphyxia, mucus
  oil or gasoline (causing suffocation) — *see* Foreign body, by site
  smoke J70.5
    due to chemicals, gases, fumes and vapors J68.9
  steam — *see* Toxicity, vapors
  stomach contents or secretions — *see* Foreign body, by site
    due to anesthesia (general) (local) or other sedation T88.59
      in labor and delivery O74.0
      in pregnancy O29.01-
      postpartum, puerperal O89.01
Inhibition, orgasm
  female F52.31

Inhibition, orgasm - *continued*
  male F52.32
Inhibitor, systemic lupus erythematosus
  (presence of) D68.62
Iniencephalus, iniencephaly Q00.2
Injection, traumatic jet (air) (industrial) (water)
  (paint or dye) T70.4
Injury — *see also* specified injury type T14.90
  abdomen, abdominal S39.91
    blood vessel — *see* Injury, blood vessel, abdomen
    cavity — *see* Injury, intra-abdominal
    contusion S30.1
    internal — *see* Injury, intra-abdominal
    intra-abdominal organ — *see* Injury, intra-
      abdominal
    nerve — *see* Injury, nerve, abdomen
    open — *see* Wound, open, abdomen
    specified NEC S39.81
    superficial — *see* Injury, superficial, abdomen
  Achilles tendon S86.00-
    laceration S86.02-
    specified type NEC S86.09-
    strain S86.01-
  acoustic, resulting in deafness — *see* Injury, nerve,
    acoustic
  adrenal (gland) S37.819
    contusion S37.812
    laceration S37.813
    specified type NEC S37.818
  alveolar (process) S09.93
  ankle S99.91-
    contusion — *see* Contusion, ankle
    dislocation — *see* Dislocation, ankle
    fracture — *see* Fracture, ankle
    nerve — *see* Injury, nerve, ankle
    open — *see* Wound, open, ankle
    specified type NEC S99.81-
    sprain — *see* Sprain, ankle
    superficial — *see* Injury, superficial, ankle
  anterior chamber, eye — *see* Injury, eye, specified
    site NEC
  anus — *see* Injury, abdomen
  aorta (thoracic) S25.00
    abdominal S35.00
      laceration (minor) (superficial) S35.01
        major S35.02
      specified type NEC S35.09
    laceration (minor) (superficial) S25.01
      major S25.02
    specified type NEC S25.09
  arm (upper) S49.9-
    blood vessel — *see* Injury, blood vessel, arm
    contusion — *see* Contusion, arm, upper
    fracture — *see* Fracture, humerus
    lower — *see* Injury, forearm
    muscle — *see* Injury, muscle, shoulder
    nerve — *see* Injury, nerve, arm
    open — *see* Wound, open, arm
    specified type NEC S49.8-
    superficial — *see* Injury, superficial, arm
  artery (complicating trauma) — *see also* Injury,
    blood vessel, by site
    cerebral or meningeal — *see* Injury, intracranial
  auditory canal (external) (meatus) S09.91
  auricle, auris, ear S09.91
  axilla — *see* Injury, shoulder
  back — *see* Injury, back, lower
  bile duct S36.13
  birth — *see also* Birth, injury P15.9
  bladder (sphincter) S37.20
    at delivery O71.5
    contusion S37.22
    laceration S37.23
    obstetrical trauma O71.5
    specified type NEC S37.29
  blast (air) (hydraulic) (immersion) (underwater)
    NEC T14.8
    acoustic nerve trauma — *see* Injury, nerve, acoustic
    bladder — *see* Injury, bladder
    brain — *see* Concussion
    colon — *see* Injury, intestine, large, blast injury
    ear (primary) S09.31-
      secondary S09.39-
    generalized T70.8
    lung — *see* Injury, intrathoracic, lung, blast injury
    multiple body organs T70.8
    peritoneum S36.81
    rectum S36.61
    retroperitoneum S36.898
    small intestine S36.419
      duodenum S36.410
      specified site NEC S36.418
    specified

Injury - *continued*
  blast (air) (hydraulic) (immersion) (underwater)
  NEC - *continued*
    specified - *continued*
      intra-abdominal organ NEC S36.898
      pelvic organ NEC S37.899
  blood vessel NEC T14.8
    abdomen S35.9-
      aorta — *see* Injury, aorta, abdominal
      celiac artery — *see* Injury, blood vessel, celiac
        artery
      iliac vessel — *see* Injury, blood vessel, iliac
      laceration S35.91
      mesenteric vessel — *see* Injury, mesenteric
      portal vein — *see* Injury, blood vessel, portal vein
      renal vessel — *see* Injury, blood vessel, renal
      specified vessel NEC S35.8X-
      splenic vessel — *see* Injury, blood vessel, splenic
      vena cava — *see* Injury, vena cava, inferior
    ankle — *see* Injury, blood vessel, foot
    aorta (abdominal) (thoracic) — *see* Injury, aorta
    arm (upper) NEC S45.90-
      forearm — *see* Injury, blood vessel, forearm
      laceration S45.91-
      specified
        site NEC S45.80-
          laceration S45.81-
          specified type NEC S45.89-
        type NEC S45.99-
      superficial vein S45.30-
        laceration S45.31-
        specified type NEC S45.39-
    axillary
      artery S45.00-
        laceration S45.01-
        specified type NEC S45.09-
      vein S45.20-
        laceration S45.21-
        specified type NEC S45.29-
    azygos vein — *see* Injury, blood vessel, thoracic,
      specified site NEC
    brachial
      artery S45.10-
        laceration S45.11-
        specified type NEC S45.19-
      vein S45.20-
        laceration S45.219
        specified type NEC S45.29-
    carotid artery (common) (external) (internal,
      extracranial) S15.00-
      internal, intracranial S06.8-
      laceration (minor) (superficial) S15.01-
        major S15.02-
      specified type NEC S15.09-
    celiac artery S35.219
      branch S35.299
        laceration (minor) (superficial) S35.291
          major S35.292
        specified NEC S35.298
      laceration (minor) (superficial) S35.211
        major S35.212
      specified type NEC S35.218
    cerebral — *see* Injury, intracranial
    deep plantar — *see* Injury, blood vessel, plantar
      artery
    digital (hand) — *see* Injury, blood vessel, finger
    dorsal
      artery (foot) S95.00-
        laceration S95.01-
        specified type NEC S95.09-
      vein (foot) S95.20-
        laceration S95.21-
        specified type NEC S95.29-
    due to accidental laceration during
      procedure — *see* Laceration, accidental
      complicating surgery
    extremity — *see* Injury, blood vessel, limb
    femoral
      artery (common) (superficial) S75.00-
        laceration (minor) (superficial) S75.01-
          major S75.02-
        specified type NEC S75.09-
      vein (hip level) (thigh level) S75.10-
        laceration (minor) (superficial) S75.11-
          major S75.12-
        specified type NEC S75.19-
    finger S65.50-
      index S65.50-
        laceration S65.51-
        specified type NEC S65.59-
      laceration S65.51-
      little S65.50-
        laceration S65.51-

Injury - *continued*
  blood vessel NEC - *continued*
    finger - *continued*
      little - *continued*
        specified type NEC S65.59-
      middle S65.50-
        laceration S65.51-
        specified type NEC S65.59-
      specified type NEC S65.59-
      thumb — *see* Injury, blood vessel, thumb
    foot S95.90-
      dorsal
        artery — *see* Injury, blood vessel, dorsal, artery
        vein — *see* Injury, blood vessel, dorsal, vein
      laceration S95.91-
      plantar artery — *see* Injury, blood vessel, plantar
        artery
      specified
        site NEC S95.80-
          laceration S95.81-
          specified type NEC S95.89-
        specified type NEC S95.99-
    forearm S55.90-
      laceration S55.91-
      radial artery — *see* Injury, blood vessel, radial
        artery
      specified
        site NEC S55.80-
          laceration S55.81-
          specified type NEC S55.89-
        type NEC S55.99-
      ulnar artery — *see* Injury, blood vessel, ulnar
        artery
      vein S55.20-
        laceration S55.21-
        specified type NEC S55.29-
    gastric
      artery — *see* Injury, mesenteric, artery, branch
      vein — *see* Injury, blood vessel, abdomen
    gastroduodenal artery — *see* Injury, mesenteric,
      artery, branch
    greater saphenous vein (lower leg level) S85.30-
      hip (and thigh) level S75.20-
        laceration (minor) (superficial) S75.21-
          major S75.22-
        specified type NEC S75.29-
      laceration S85.31-
      specified type NEC S85.39-
    hand (level) S65.90-
      finger — *see* Injury, blood vessel, finger
      laceration S65.91-
      palmar arch — *see* Injury, blood vessel, palmar
        arch
      radial artery — *see* Injury, blood vessel, radial
        artery, hand
      specified
        site NEC S65.80-
          laceration S65.81-
          specified type NEC S65.89-
        type NEC S65.99-
      thumb — *see* Injury, blood vessel, thumb
      ulnar artery — *see* Injury, blood vessel, ulnar
        artery, hand
    head S09.0
      intracranial — *see* Injury, intracranial
      multiple S09.0
    hepatic
      artery — *see* Injury, mesenteric, artery
      vein — *see* Injury, vena cava, inferior
    hip S75.90-
      femoral artery — *see* Injury, blood vessel,
        femoral, artery
      femoral vein — *see* Injury, blood vessel, femoral,
        vein
      greater saphenous vein — *see* Injury, blood
        vessel, greater saphenous, hip level
      laceration S75.91-
      specified
        site NEC S75.80-
          laceration S75.81-
          specified type NEC S75.89-
        type NEC S75.99-
    hypogastric (artery) (vein) — *see* Injury, blood
      vessel, iliac
    iliac S35.5-
      artery S35.51-
      specified vessel NEC S35.5-
      uterine vessel — *see* Injury, blood vessel, uterine
      vein S35.51-
    innominate — *see* Injury, blood vessel, thoracic,
      innominate
    intercostal (artery) (vein) — *see* Injury, blood
      vessel, thoracic, intercostal

Injury - *continued*
blood vessel NEC - *continued*
jugular vein (external) S15.20-
internal S15.30-
laceration (minor) (superficial) S15.31-
major S15.32-
specified type NEC S15.39-
laceration (minor) (superficial) S15.21-
major S15.22-
specified type NEC S15.29-
leg (level) (lower) S85.90-
greater saphenous — *see* Injury, blood vessel,
greater saphenous
laceration S85.91-
lesser saphenous — *see* Injury, blood vessel,
lesser saphenous
peroneal artery — *see* Injury, blood vessel,
peroneal artery
popliteal
artery — *see* Injury, blood vessel, popliteal,
artery
vein — *see* Injury, blood vessel, popliteal, vein
specified
site NEC S85.80-
laceration S85.81-
specified type NEC S85.89-
type NEC S85.99-
thigh — *see* Injury, blood vessel, hip
tibial artery — *see* Injury, blood vessel, tibial
artery
lesser saphenous vein (lower leg level) S85.40-
laceration S85.41-
specified type NEC S85.49-
limb
lower — *see* Injury, blood vessel, leg
upper — *see* Injury, blood vessel, arm
lower back — *see* Injury, blood vessel, abdomen
specified NEC — *see* Injury, blood vessel,
abdomen, specified, site NEC
mammary (artery) (vein) — *see* Injury, blood
vessel, thoracic, specified site NEC
mesenteric (inferior) (superior)
artery — *see* Injury, mesenteric, artery
vein — *see* Injury, mesenteric, vein
neck S15.9
specified site NEC S15.8
ovarian (artery) (vein) — *see* subcategory S35.8
palmar arch (superficial) S65.20-
deep S65.30-
laceration S65.31-
specified type NEC S65.39-
laceration S65.21-
specified type NEC S65.29-
pelvis — *see* Injury, blood vessel, abdomen
specified NEC — *see* Injury, blood vessel,
abdomen, specified, site NEC
peroneal artery S85.20-
laceration S85.21-
specified type NEC S85.29-
plantar artery (deep) (foot) S95.10-
laceration S95.11-
specified type NEC S95.19-
popliteal
artery S85.00-
laceration S85.01-
specified type NEC S85.09-
vein S85.50-
laceration S85.51-
specified type NEC S85.59-
portal vein S35.319
laceration S35.311
specified type NEC S35.318
precerebral — *see* Injury, blood vessel, neck
pulmonary (artery) (vein) — *see* Injury, blood
vessel, thoracic, pulmonary
radial artery (forearm level) S55.10-
hand and wrist (level) S65.10-
laceration S65.11-
specified type NEC S65.19-
laceration S55.11-
specified type NEC S55.19-
renal
artery S35.40-
laceration S35.41-
specified NEC S35.49-
vein S35.40-
laceration S35.41-
specified NEC S35.49-
saphenous vein (greater) (lower leg level) — *see*
Injury, blood vessel, greater saphenous
hip and thigh level — *see* Injury, blood vessel,
greater saphenous, hip level

Injury - *continued*
blood vessel NEC - *continued*
saphenous vein (greater) (lower leg level) -
continued
lesser — *see* Injury, blood vessel, lesser
saphenous
shoulder
specified NEC — *see* Injury, blood vessel, arm,
specified site NEC
superficial vein — *see* Injury, blood vessel, arm,
superficial vein
specified NEC T14.8
splenic
artery — *see* Injury, blood vessel, celiac artery,
branch
vein S35.329
laceration S35.321
specified NEC S35.328
subclavian — *see* Injury, blood vessel, thoracic,
innominate
thigh — *see* Injury, blood vessel, hip
thoracic S25.90
aorta S25.00
laceration (minor) (superficial) S25.01
major S25.02
specified type NEC S25.09
azygos vein — *see* Injury, blood vessel, thoracic,
specified, site NEC
innominate
artery S25.10-
laceration (minor) (superficial) S25.11-
major S25.12-
specified type NEC S25.19-
vein S25.30-
laceration (minor) (superficial) S25.31-
major S25.32-
specified type NEC S25.39-
intercostal S25.50-
laceration S25.51-
specified type NEC S25.59-
laceration S25.91
mammary vessel — *see* Injury, blood vessel,
thoracic, specified, site NEC
pulmonary S25.40-
laceration (minor) (superficial) S25.41-
major S25.42-
specified type NEC S25.49-
specified
site NEC S25.80-
laceration S25.81-
specified type NEC S25.89-
type NEC S25.99
subclavian — *see* Injury, blood vessel, thoracic,
innominate
vena cava (superior) S25.20
laceration (minor) (superficial) S25.21
major S25.22
specified type NEC S25.29
thumb S65.40-
laceration S65.41-
specified type NEC S65.49-
tibial artery S85.10-
anterior S85.13-
laceration S85.14-
specified injury NEC S85.15-
laceration S85.11-
posterior S85.16-
laceration S85.17-
specified injury NEC S85.18-
specified injury NEC S85.12-
ulnar artery (forearm level) S55.00-
hand and wrist (level) S65.00-
laceration S65.01-
specified type NEC S65.09-
laceration S55.01-
specified type NEC S55.09-
upper arm (level) — *see* Injury, blood vessel, arm
superficial vein — *see* Injury, blood vessel, arm,
superficial vein
uterine S35.5-
artery S35.53-
vein S35.53-
vena cava — *see* Injury, vena cava
vertebral artery S15.10-
laceration (minor) (superficial) S15.11-
major S15.12-
specified type NEC S15.19-
wrist (level) — *see* Injury, blood vessel, hand
brachial plexus S14.3
newborn P14.3
brain (traumatic) S06.9-
diffuse (axonal) S06.2X-
focal S06.30-

Injury - *continued*
brainstem S06.38-
breast NOS S29.9
broad ligament — *see* Injury, pelvic organ, specified
site NEC
bronchus, bronchi — *see* Injury, intrathoracic,
bronchus
brow S09.90
buttock S39.92
canthus, eye S05.90
cardiac plexus — *see* Injury, nerve, thorax,
sympathetic
cauda equina S34.3
cavernous sinus — *see* Injury, intracranial
cecum — *see* Injury, colon
celiac ganglion or plexus — *see* Injury, nerve,
lumbosacral, sympathetic
cerebellum — *see* Injury, intracranial
cerebral — *see* Injury, intracranial
cervix (uteri) — *see* Injury, uterus
cheek (wall) S09.93
chest — *see* Injury, thorax
childbirth (newborn) — *see also* Birth, injury
maternal NEC O71.9
chin S09.93
choroid (eye) — *see* Injury, eye, specified site NEC
clitoris S39.94
coccyx — *see also* Injury, back, lower
complicating delivery O71.6
colon — *see* Injury, intestine, large
common bile duct — *see* Injury, liver
conjunctiva (superficial) — *see* Injury, eye,
conjunctiva
conus medullaris — *see* Injury, spinal, sacral
cord
spermatic (pelvic region) S37.898
scrotal region S39.848
spinal — *see* Injury, spinal cord, by region
cornea — *see* Injury, eye, specified site NEC
abrasion — *see* Injury, eye, cornea, abrasion
cortex (cerebral) — *see also* Injury, intracranial
visual — *see* Injury, nerve, optic
costal region NEC S29.9
costochondral NEC S29.9
cranial
cavity — *see* Injury, intracranial
nerve — *see* Injury, nerve, cranial
crushing — *see* Crush
cutaneous sensory nerve
cystic duct — *see* Injury, liver
deep tissue — *see* Contusion, by site
meaning pressure ulcer — *see* Ulcer, pressure,
unstageable, by site
delivery (newborn) P15.9
maternal NEC O71.9
Descemet's membrane — *see* Injury, eyeball,
penetrating
diaphragm — *see* Injury, intrathoracic, diaphragm
duodenum — *see* Injury, intestine, small, duodenum
ear (auricle) (external) (canal) S09.91
abrasion — *see* Abrasion, ear
bite — *see* Bite, ear
blister — *see* Blister, ear
bruise — *see* Contusion, ear
contusion — *see* Contusion, ear
external constriction — *see* Constriction, external,
ear
hematoma — *see* Hematoma, ear
inner — *see* Injury, ear, middle
laceration — *see* Laceration, ear
middle S09.30-
blast — *see* Injury, blast, ear
specified NEC S09.39-
puncture — *see* Puncture, ear
superficial — *see* Injury, superficial, ear
eighth cranial nerve (acoustic or auditory) — *see*
Injury, nerve, acoustic
elbow S59.90-
contusion — *see* Contusion, elbow
dislocation — *see* Dislocation, elbow
fracture — *see* Fracture, ulna, upper end
open — *see* Wound, open, elbow
specified NEC S59.80-
sprain — *see* Sprain, elbow
superficial — *see* Injury, superficial, elbow
eleventh cranial nerve (accessory) — *see* Injury,
nerve, accessory
epididymis S39.94
epigastric region S39.91
epiglottis NEC S19.89
esophageal plexus — *see* Injury, nerve, thorax,
sympathetic

Injury - *continued*
esophagus (thoracic part) — *see also* Injury,
  intrathoracic, esophagus
  cervical NEC S19.85
eustachian tube S09.30-
eye S05.9-
  avulsion S05.7-
  ball — *see* Injury, eyeball
  conjunctiva S05.0-
  cornea
    abrasion S05.0-
  laceration S05.3-
    with prolapse S05.2-
  lacrimal apparatus S05.8X-
  orbit penetration S05.4-
  specified site NEC S05.8X-
eyeball S05.8X-
  contusion S05.1-
  penetrating S05.6-
    with
      foreign body S05.5-
      prolapse or loss of intraocular tissue S05.2-
    without prolapse or loss of intraocular
      tissue S05.3-
  specified type NEC S05.8-
eyebrow S09.93
eyelid S09.93
  abrasion — *see* Abrasion, eyelid
  contusion — *see* Contusion, eyelid
  open — *see* Wound, open, eyelid
face S09.93
fallopian tube S37.509
  bilateral S37.502
    blast injury S37.512
    contusion S37.522
    laceration S37.532
    specified type NEC S37.592
  blast injury (primary) S37.519
    bilateral S37.512
    secondary — *see* Injury, fallopian tube, specified
      type NEC
    unilateral S37.511
  contusion S37.529
    bilateral S37.522
    unilateral S37.521
  laceration S37.539
    bilateral S37.532
    unilateral S37.531
  specified type NEC S37.599
    bilateral S37.592
    unilateral S37.591
  unilateral S37.501
    blast injury S37.511
    contusion S37.521
    laceration S37.531
    specified type NEC S37.591
fascia — *see* Injury, muscle
fifth cranial nerve (trigeminal) — *see* Injury, nerve,
  trigeminal
finger (nail) S69.9-
  blood vessel — *see* Injury, blood vessel, finger
  contusion — *see* Contusion, finger
  dislocation — *see* Dislocation, finger
  fracture — *see* Fracture, finger
  muscle — *see* Injury, muscle, finger
  nerve — *see* Injury, nerve, digital, finger
  open — *see* Wound, open, finger
  specified NEC S69.8-
  sprain — *see* Sprain, finger
  superficial — *see* Injury, superficial, finger
first cranial nerve (olfactory) — *see* Injury, nerve,
  olfactory
flank — *see* Injury, abdomen
foot S99.92-
  blood vessel — *see* Injury, blood vessel, foot
  contusion — *see* Contusion, foot
  dislocation — *see* Dislocation, foot
  fracture — *see* Fracture, foot
  muscle — *see* Injury, muscle, foot
  open — *see* Wound, open, foot
  specified type NEC S99.82-
  sprain — *see* Sprain, foot
  superficial — *see* Injury, superficial, foot
forceps NOS P15.9
forearm S59.91-
  blood vessel — *see* Injury, blood vessel, forearm
  contusion — *see* Contusion, forearm
  fracture — *see* Fracture, forearm
  muscle — *see* Injury, muscle, forearm
  nerve — *see* Injury, nerve, forearm
  open — *see* Wound, open, forearm
  specified NEC S59.81-
  superficial — *see* Injury, superficial, forearm

Injury - *continued*
forehead S09.90
fourth cranial nerve (trochlear) — *see* Injury, nerve,
  trochlear
gallbladder S36.129
  contusion S36.122
  laceration S36.123
  specified NEC S36.128
ganglion
  celiac, coeliac — *see* Injury, nerve, lumbosacral,
    sympathetic
  gasserian — *see* Injury, nerve, trigeminal
  stellate — *see* Injury, nerve, thorax, sympathetic
  thoracic sympathetic — *see* Injury, nerve, thorax,
    sympathetic
gasserian ganglion — *see* Injury, nerve, trigeminal
gastric artery — *see* Injury, blood vessel, celiac
  artery, branch
gastroduodenal artery — *see* Injury, blood vessel,
  celiac artery, branch
gastrointestinal tract — *see* Injury, intra-abdominal
  with open wound into abdominal cavity — *see*
    Wound, open, with penetration into peritoneal
    cavity
  colon — *see* Injury, intestine, large
  rectum — *see* Injury, intestine, large, rectum
    with open wound into abdominal cavity S36.61
  specified site NEC — *see* Injury, intra-abdominal,
    specified, site NEC
  stomach — *see* Injury, stomach
  small intestine — *see* Injury, intestine, small
genital organ (s)
  external S39.94
    specified NEC S39.848
  internal S37.90
    fallopian tube — *see* Injury, fallopian tube
    ovary — *see* Injury, ovary
    prostate — *see* Injury, prostate
    seminal vesicle — *see* Injury, pelvis, organ,
      specified site NEC
    uterus — *see* Injury, uterus
    vas deferens — *see* Injury, pelvis, organ,
      specified site NEC
  obstetrical trauma O71.9
gland
  lacrimal laceration — *see* Injury, eye, specified site
    NEC
  salivary S09.93
  thyroid NEC S19.84
globe (eye) S05.90
  specified NEC S05.8X-
groin — *see* Injury, abdomen
gum S09.90
hand S69.9-
  blood vessel — *see* Injury, blood vessel, hand
  contusion — *see* Contusion, hand
  fracture — *see* Fracture, hand
  muscle — *see* Injury, muscle, hand
  nerve — *see* Injury, nerve, hand
  open — *see* Wound, open, hand
  specified NEC S69.8-
  sprain — *see* Sprain, hand
  superficial — *see* Injury, superficial, hand
head S09.90
  with loss of consciousness S06.9-
  specified NEC S09.8
heart S26.90
  with hemopericardium S26.00
    contusion S26.01
    laceration (mild) S26.020
      moderate S26.021
      major S26.022
    specified type NEC S26.09
  contusion S26.91
  laceration S26.92
  specified type NEC S26.99
  without hemopericardium S26.10
    contusion S26.11
    laceration S26.12
    specified type NEC S26.19
heel — *see* Injury, foot
hepatic
  artery — *see* Injury, blood vessel, celiac artery,
    branch
  duct — *see* Injury, liver
  vein — *see* Injury, vena cava, inferior
hip S79.91-
  blood vessel — *see* Injury, blood vessel, hip
  contusion — *see* Contusion, hip
  dislocation — *see* Dislocation, hip
  fracture — *see* Fracture, femur, neck
  muscle — *see* Injury, muscle, hip
  nerve — *see* Injury, nerve, hip

Injury - *continued*
hip - *continued*
  open — *see* Wound, open, hip
  sprain — *see* Sprain, hip
  superficial — *see* Injury, superficial, hip
  specified NEC S79.81-
hymen S39.94
hypogastric
  blood vessel — *see* Injury, blood vessel, iliac
  plexus — *see* Injury, nerve, lumbosacral,
    sympathetic
ileum — *see* Injury, intestine, small
iliac region S39.91
instrumental (during surgery) — *see* Laceration,
  accidental complicating surgery
  birth injury — *see* Birth, injury
  nonsurgical — *see* Injury, by site
  obstetrical O71.9
    bladder O71.5
    cervix O71.3
    high vaginal O71.4
    perineal NOS O70.9
    urethra O71.5
    uterus O71.5
      with rupture or perforation O71.1
internal T14.8
  aorta — *see* Injury, aorta
  bladder (sphincter) — *see* Injury, bladder
    with
      ectopic or molar pregnancy O08.6
      following ectopic or molar pregnancy O08.6
      obstetrical trauma O71.5
  bronchi, bronchi — *see* Injury, intrathoracic,
    bronchus
  cecum — *see* Injury, intestine, large
  cervix (uteri) — *see also* Injury, uterus
    with ectopic or molar pregnancy O08.6
    following ectopic or molar pregnancy O08.6
    obstetrical trauma O71.3
  chest — *see* Injury, intrathoracic
  gastrointestinal tract — *see* Injury, intra-abdominal
  heart — *see* Injury, heart
  intestine NEC — *see* Injury, intestine
  intrauterine — *see* Injury, uterus
  mesentery — *see* Injury, intra-abdominal,
    specified, site NEC
  pelvis, pelvic (organ) S37.90
    following ectopic or molar pregnancy
      (subsequent episode) O08.6
    obstetrical trauma NEC O71.5
      rupture or perforation O71.1
    specified NEC S39.83
  rectum — *see* Injury, intestine, large, rectum
  stomach — *see* Injury, stomach
  ureter — *see* Injury, ureter
  urethra (sphincter) following ectopic or molar
    pregnancy O08.6
  uterus — *see* Injury, uterus
interscapular area — *see* Injury, thorax
intestine
  large S36.509
    ascending (right) S36.500
      blast injury (primary) S36.510
        secondary S36.590
      contusion S36.520
      laceration S36.530
      specified type NEC S36.590
    blast injury (primary) S36.519
      ascending (right) S36.510
      descending (left) S36.512
      rectum S36.61
      sigmoid S36.513
      specified site NEC S36.518
      transverse S36.511
    contusion S36.529
      ascending (right) S36.520
      descending (left) S36.522
      rectum S36.62
      sigmoid S36.523
      specified site NEC S36.528
      transverse S36.521
    descending (left) S36.502
      blast injury (primary) S36.512
        secondary S36.592
      contusion S36.522
      laceration S36.532
      specified type NEC S36.592
    laceration S36.539
      ascending (right) S36.530
      descending (left) S36.532
      rectum S36.63
      sigmoid S36.533
      specified site NEC S36.538

Injury - *continued*
  intestine - *continued*
    large - *continued*
      laceration - *continued*
        transverse S36.531
      rectum S36.60
        blast injury (primary) S36.61
          secondary S36.69
        contusion S36.62
        laceration S36.63
        specified type NEC S36.69
      sigmoid S36.503
        blast injury (primary) S36.513
          secondary S36.593
        contusion S36.523
        laceration S36.533
        specified type NEC S36.593
      specified
        site NEC S36.508
          blast injury (primary) S36.518
            secondary S36.598
          contusion S36.528
          laceration S36.538
          specified type NEC S36.598
        type NEC S36.599
          ascending (right) S36.590
          descending (left) S36.592
          rectum S36.69
          sigmoid S36.593
          specified site NEC S36.598
          transverse S36.591
      transverse S36.501
        blast injury (primary) S36.511
          secondary S36.591
        contusion S36.521
        laceration S36.531
        specified type NEC S36.591
    small S36.409
      blast injury (primary) S36.419
        duodenum S36.410
        secondary S36.499
          duodenum S36.490
          specified site NEC S36.498
        specified site NEC S36.418
      contusion S36.429
        duodenum S36.420
        specified site NEC S36.428
      duodenum S36.400
        blast injury (primary) S36.410
          secondary S36.490
        contusion S36.420
        laceration S36.430
        specified NEC S36.490
      laceration S36.439
        duodenum S36.430
        specified site NEC S36.438
      specified
        type NEC S36.499
          duodenum S36.490
          specified site NEC S36.498
        site NEC S36.408
  intra-abdominal S36.90
    adrenal gland — *see* Injury, adrenal gland
    bladder — *see* Injury, bladder
    colon — *see* Injury, intestine, large
    contusion S36.92
    fallopian tube — *see* Injury, fallopian tube
    gallbladder — *see* Injury, gallbladder
    intestine — *see* Injury, intestine
    laceration S36.93
    liver — *see* Injury, liver
    kidney — *see* Injury, kidney
    ovary — *see* Injury, ovary
    pancreas — *see* Injury, pancreas
    pelvic NOS S37.90
    peritoneum — *see* Injury, intra-abdominal,
      specified, site NEC
    prostate — *see* Injury, prostate
    rectum — *see* Injury, intestine, large, rectum
    retroperitoneum — *see* Injury, intra-abdominal,
      specified, site NEC
    seminal vesicle — *see* Injury, pelvis, organ,
      specified site NEC
    small intestine — *see* Injury, intestine, small
    specified
      site NEC S36.899
        contusion S36.892
        laceration S36.893
        specified type NEC S36.898
      type NEC S36.99
      pelvic S37.90
        specified
          site NEC S37.899

Injury - *continued*
  intra-abdominal - *continued*
    specified - *continued*
      pelvic - *continued*
        specified - *continued*
          site NEC - *continued*
            specified type NEC S37.898
          type NEC S37.99
    spleen — *see* Injury, spleen
    stomach — *see* Injury, stomach
    ureter — *see* Injury, ureter
    urethra — *see* Injury, urethra
    uterus — *see* Injury, uterus
    vas deferens — *see* Injury, pelvis, organ, specified
      site NEC
  intracranial (traumatic) S06.9-
    cerebellar hemorrhage, traumatic — *see* Injury,
      intracranial, focal
    cerebral edema, traumatic S06.1X-
      diffuse S06.1X-
      focal S06.1X-
    diffuse (axonal) S06.2X-
    epidural hemorrhage (traumatic) S06.4X-
    focal brain injury S06.30-
      contusion — *see* Contusion, cerebral
      laceration — *see* Laceration, cerebral
      intracerebral hemorrhage, traumatic S06.36-
        left side S06.35-
        right side S06.34-
    subarachnoid hemorrhage, traumatic S06.6X-
    subdural hemorrhage, traumatic S06.5X-
  intraocular — *see* Injury, eyeball, penetrating
  intrathoracic S27.9
    bronchus S27.409
      bilateral S27.402
      blast injury (primary) S27.419
        bilateral S27.412
        secondary — *see* Injury, intrathoracic, bronchus,
          specified type NEC
        unilateral S27.411
      contusion S27.429
        bilateral S27.422
        unilateral S27.421
      laceration S27.439
        bilateral S27.432
        unilateral S27.431
      specified type NEC S27.499
        bilateral S27.492
        unilateral S27.491
      unilateral S27.401
    diaphragm S27.809
      contusion S27.802
      laceration S27.803
      specified type NEC S27.808
    esophagus (thoracic) S27.819
      contusion S27.812
      laceration S27.813
      specified type NEC S27.818
    heart — *see* Injury, heart
    hemopneumothorax S27.2
    hemothorax S27.1
    lung S27.309
      aspiration J69.0
      bilateral S27.302
      blast injury (primary) S27.319
        bilateral S27.312
        secondary — *see* Injury, intrathoracic, lung,
          specified type NEC
        unilateral S27.311
      contusion S27.329
        bilateral S27.322
        unilateral S27.321
      laceration S27.339
        bilateral S27.332
        unilateral S27.331
      specified type NEC S27.399
        bilateral S27.392
        unilateral S27.391
      unilateral S27.301
    pleura S27.60
      laceration S27.63
      specified type NEC S27.69
    pneumothorax S27.0
    specified organ NEC S27.899
      contusion S27.892
      laceration S27.893
      specified type NEC S27.898
    thoracic duct — *see* Injury, intrathoracic, specified
      organ NEC
    thymus gland — *see* Injury, intrathoracic, specified
      organ NEC
    trachea, thoracic S27.50
      blast (primary) S27.51

Injury - *continued*
  intrathoracic - *continued*
    trachea, thoracic - *continued*
      contusion S27.52
      laceration S27.53
      specified type NEC S27.59
  iris — *see* Injury, eye, specified site NEC
    penetrating — *see* Injury, eyeball, penetrating
  jaw S09.93
  jejunum — *see* Injury, intestine, small
  joint NOS T14.8
    old or residual — *see* Disorder, joint, specified
      type NEC
  kidney S37.00-
    acute (nontraumatic) N17.9
    contusion — *see* Contusion, kidney
    laceration — *see* Laceration, kidney
    specified NEC S37.09-
  knee S89.9-
    contusion — *see* Contusion, knee
    dislocation — *see* Dislocation, knee
    meniscus (lateral) (medial) — *see* Sprain, knee,
      specified site NEC
      old injury or tear — *see* Derangement, knee,
        meniscus, due to old injury
    open — *see* Wound, open, knee
    specified NEC S89.8-
    sprain — *see* Sprain, knee
    superficial — *see* Injury, superficial, knee
  labium (majus) (minus) S39.94
  labyrinth, ear S09.30-
  lacrimal apparatus, duct, gland, or sac — *see* Injury,
    eye, specified site NEC
  larynx NEC S19.81
  leg (lower) S89.9-
    blood vessel — *see* Injury, blood vessel, leg
    contusion — *see* Contusion, leg
    fracture — *see* Fracture, leg
    muscle — *see* Injury, muscle, leg
    nerve — *see* Injury, nerve, leg
    open — *see* Wound, open, leg
    specified NEC S89.8-
    superficial — *see* Injury, superficial, leg
  lens, eye — *see* Injury, eye, specified site NEC
    penetrating — *see* Injury, eyeball, penetrating
  limb NEC T14.8
  lip S09.93
  liver S36.119
    contusion S36.112
    laceration S36.113
      major (stellate) S36.116
      minor S36.114
      moderate S36.115
    specified NEC S36.118
  lower back S39.92
    specified NEC S39.82
  lumbar, lumbosacral (region) S39.92
    plexus — *see* Injury, lumbosacral plexus
  lumbosacral plexus S34.4
  lung — *see also* Injury, intrathoracic, lung
    aspiration J69.0
    transfusion-related (TRALI) J95.84
  lymphatic thoracic duct — *see* Injury, intrathoracic,
    specified organ NEC
  malar region S09.93
  mastoid region S09.90
  maxilla S09.93
  mediastinum — *see* Injury, intrathoracic, specified
    organ NEC
  membrane, brain — *see* Injury, intracranial
  meningeal artery — *see* Injury, intracranial, subdural
    hemorrhage
  meninges (cerebral) — *see* Injury, intracranial
  mesenteric
    artery
      branch S35.299
        laceration (minor) (superficial) S35.291
          major S35.292
          specified NEC S35.298
      inferior S35.239
        laceration (minor) (superficial) S35.231
          major S35.232
          specified NEC S35.238
      superior S35.229
        laceration (minor) (superficial) S35.221
          major S35.222
          specified NEC S35.228
    plexus (inferior) (superior) — *see* Injury, nerve,
      lumbosacral, sympathetic
    vein
      inferior S35.349
        laceration S35.341
        specified NEC S35.348

Injury - *continued*
mesenteric - *continued*
  vein - *continued*
    superior S35.339
     laceration S35.331
     specified NEC S35.338
  mesentery — *see* Injury, intra-abdominal, specified
   site NEC
  mesosalpinx — *see* Injury, pelvic organ, specified
   site NEC
  middle ear S09.30-
  midthoracic region NOS S29.9
  mouth S09.93
  multiple NOS T07
  muscle (and fascia) (and tendon)
   abdomen S39.001
    laceration S39.021
    specified type NEC S39.091
    strain S39.011
   abductor
    thumb, forearm level — *see* Injury, muscle,
     thumb, abductor
   adductor
    thigh S76.20-
     laceration S76.22-
     specified type NEC S76.29-
     strain S76.21-
   ankle — *see* Injury, muscle, foot
   anterior muscle group, at leg level (lower) S86.20-
    laceration S86.22-
    specified type NEC S86.29-
    strain S86.21-
   arm (upper) — *see* Injury, muscle, shoulder
   biceps (parts NEC) S46.20-
    laceration S46.22-
    long head S46.10-
     laceration S46.12-
     strain S46.11-
     specified type NEC S46.19-
    specified type NEC S46.29-
    strain S46.21-
   extensor
    finger (s) (other than thumb) — *see* Injury,
     muscle, finger by site, extensor
    forearm level, specified NEC — *see* Injury,
     muscle, forearm, extensor
    thumb — *see* Injury, muscle, thumb, extensor
    toe (large) (ankle level) (foot level) — *see* Injury,
     muscle, toe, extensor
   finger
    extensor (forearm level) S56.40-
     hand level S66.309
      laceration S66.329
      specified type NEC S66.399
      strain S66.319
     laceration S56.429
     specified type NEC S56.499
     strain S56.419
    flexor (forearm level) S56.10-
     hand level S66.109
      laceration S66.129
      specified type NEC S66.199
      strain S66.119
     laceration S56.129
     specified type NEC S56.199
     strain S56.119
    intrinsic S66.509
     laceration S66.529
     specified type NEC S66.599
     strain S66.519
   index
    extensor (forearm level)
     hand level S66.308
      laceration S66.32-
      specified type NEC S66.39-
      strain S66.31-
     specified type NEC S56.492-
    flexor (forearm level)
     hand level S66.108
      laceration S66.12-
      specified type NEC S66.19-
      strain S66.11-
     specified type NEC S56.19-
     strain S56.11-
    intrinsic S66.50-
     laceration S66.52-
     specified type NEC S66.59-
     strain S66.51-
   little
    extensor (forearm level)
     hand level S66.30-
      laceration S66.32-
      specified type NEC S66.39-

Injury - *continued*
muscle (and fascia) (and tendon) - *continued*
  finger - *continued*
   little - *continued*
    extensor (forearm level) - *continued*
     hand level - *continued*
      strain S66.31-
     laceration S56.42-
     specified type NEC S56.49-
     strain S56.41-
    flexor (forearm level)
     hand level S66.10-
      laceration S66.12-
      specified type NEC S66.19-
      strain S66.11-
     laceration S56.12-
     specified type NEC S56.19-
     strain S56.11-
    intrinsic S66.50-
     laceration S66.52-
     specified type NEC S66.59-
     strain S66.51-
   middle
    extensor (forearm level)
     hand level S66.30-
      laceration S66.32-
      specified type NEC S66.39-
      strain S66.31-
     laceration S56.42-
     specified type NEC S56.49-
     strain S56.41-
    flexor (forearm level)
     hand level S66.10-
      laceration S66.12-
      specified type NEC S66.19-
      strain S66.11-
     laceration S56.12-
     specified type NEC S56.19-
     strain S56.11-
    intrinsic S66.50-
     laceration S66.52-
     specified type NEC S66.59-
     strain S66.51-
   ring
    extensor (forearm level)
     hand level S66.30-
      laceration S66.32-
      specified type NEC S66.39-
      strain S66.31-
     laceration S56.42-
     specified type NEC S56.49-
     strain S56.41-
    flexor (forearm level)
     hand level S66.10-
      laceration S66.12-
      specified type NEC S66.19-
      strain S66.11-
     laceration S56.12-
     specified type NEC S56.19-
     strain S56.11-
    intrinsic S66.50-
     laceration S66.52-
     specified type NEC S66.59-
     strain S66.51-
  flexor
   finger (s) (other than thumb) — *see* Injury,
    muscle, finger
   forearm level, specified NEC — *see* Injury,
    muscle, forearm, flexor
   thumb — *see* Injury, muscle, thumb, flexor
   toe (long) (ankle level) (foot level) — *see* Injury,
    muscle, toe, flexor
  foot S96.90-
   intrinsic S96.20-
    laceration S96.22-
    specified type NEC S96.29-
    strain S96.21-
   laceration S96.92-
   long extensor, toe — *see* Injury, muscle, toe,
    extensor
   long flexor, toe — *see* Injury, muscle, toe, flexor
   specified
    site NEC S96.80-
     laceration S96.82-
     specified type NEC S96.89-
     strain S96.81-
    type NEC S96.99-
   strain S96.91-
  forearm (level) S56.90-
   extensor S56.50-
    laceration S56.52-
    specified type NEC S56.59-
    strain S56.51-

Injury - *continued*
muscle (and fascia) (and tendon) - *continued*
  forearm (level) - *continued*
   flexor S56.20-
    laceration S56.22-
    specified type NEC S56.29-
    strain S56.21-
   laceration S56.92-
   specified type NEC S56.99-
    site NEC S56.80-
     laceration S56.82-
     strain S56.81-
    type NEC S56.89-
   strain S56.91-
  hand (level) S66.90-
   laceration S66.92-
   specified
    site NEC S66.80-
     laceration S66.82-
     specified type NEC S66.89-
     strain S66.81-
    type NEC S66.99-
   strain S66.91-
  head S09.10
   laceration S09.12
   specified type NEC S09.19
   strain S09.11
  hip NEC S76.00-
   laceration S76.02-
   specified type NEC S76.09-
   strain S76.01-
  intrinsic
   ankle and foot level — *see* Injury, muscle, foot,
    intrinsic
   finger (other than thumb) — *see* Injury, muscle,
    finger by site, intrinsic
   foot (level) — *see* Injury, muscle, foot, intrinsic
   thumb — *see* Injury, muscle, thumb, intrinsic
  leg (level) (lower) S86.90-
   Achilles tendon — *see* Injury, Achilles tendon
   anterior muscle group — *see* Injury, muscle,
    anterior muscle group
   laceration S86.92-
   peroneal muscle group — *see* Injury, muscle,
    peroneal muscle group
   posterior muscle group — *see* Injury, muscle,
    posterior muscle group, leg level
   specified
    site NEC S86.80-
     laceration S86.82-
     specified type NEC S86.89-
     strain S86.81-
    type NEC S86.99-
   strain S86.91-
  long
   extensor toe, at ankle and foot level — *see* Injury,
    muscle, toe, extensor
   flexor, toe, at ankle and foot level — *see* Injury,
    muscle, toe, flexor
   head, biceps — *see* Injury, muscle, biceps, long
    head
  lower back S39.002
   laceration S39.022
   specified type NEC S39.092
   strain S39.012
  neck (level) S16.9
   laceration S16.2
   specified type NEC S16.8
   strain S16.1
  pelvis S39.003
   laceration S39.023
   specified type NEC S39.093
   strain S39.013
  peroneal muscle group, at leg level (lower) S86.30-
   laceration S86.32-
   specified type NEC S86.39-
   strain S86.31-
  posterior muscle (group)
   leg level (lower) S86.10-
    laceration S86.12-
    specified type NEC S86.19-
    strain S86.11-
   thigh level S76.30-
    laceration S76.32-
    specified type NEC S76.39-
    strain S76.31-
  quadriceps (thigh) S76.10-
   laceration S76.12-
   specified type NEC S76.19-
   strain S76.11-
  shoulder S46.90-
   laceration S46.92-
   rotator cuff — *see* Injury, rotator cuff

Injury - *continued*
muscle (and fascia) (and tendon) - *continued*
  shoulder - *continued*
    specified site NEC S46.80-
      laceration S46.82-
      strain S46.81-
      specified type NEC S46.89-
    strain S46.91-
    specified type NEC S46.99-
  thigh NEC (level) S76.90-
    adductor — *see* Injury, muscle, adductor, thigh
    laceration S76.92-
    posterior muscle (group) — *see* Injury, muscle, posterior muscle, thigh level
    quadriceps — *see* Injury, muscle, quadriceps
    specified
      site NEC S76.80-
        laceration S76.82-
        specified type NEC S76.89-
        strain S76.81-
      type NEC S76.99-
    strain S76.91-
  thorax (level) S29.009
    back wall S29.002
    front wall S29.001
    laceration S29.029
      back wall S29.022
      front wall S29.021
    specified type NEC S29.099
      back wall S29.092
      front wall S29.091
    strain S29.019
      back wall S29.012
      front wall S29.011
  thumb
    abductor (forearm level) S56.30-
      laceration S56.32-
      specified type NEC S56.39-
      strain S56.31-
    extensor (forearm level) S56.30-
      hand level S66.20-
        laceration S66.22-
        specified type NEC S66.29-
        strain S66.21-
      laceration S56.32-
      specified type NEC S56.39-
      strain S56.31-
    flexor (forearm level) S56.00-
      hand level S66.00-
        laceration S66.02-
        specified type NEC S66.09-
        strain S66.01-
      laceration S56.02-
      specified type NEC S56.09-
      strain S56.01-
      wrist level — *see* Injury, muscle, thumb, flexor, hand level
    intrinsic S66.40-
      laceration S66.42-
      specified type NEC S66.49-
      strain S66.41-
  toe — *see also* Injury, muscle, foot
    extensor, long S96.10-
      laceration S96.12-
      specified type NEC S96.19-
      strain S96.11-
    flexor, long S96.00-
      laceration S96.02-
      specified type NEC S96.09-
      strain S96.01-
  triceps S46.30-
    laceration S46.32-
    specified type NEC S46.39-
    strain S46.31-
  wrist (and hand) level — *see* Injury, muscle, hand
musculocutaneous nerve — *see* Injury, nerve, musculocutaneous
myocardium — *see* Injury, heart
nape — *see* Injury, neck
nasal (septum) (sinus) S09.92
nasopharynx S09.92
neck S19.9
  specified NEC S19.80
  specified site NEC S19.89
nerve NEC T14.8
  abdomen S34.9
    peripheral S34.6
    specified site NEC S34.8
  abducens S04.4-
    contusion S04.4-
    laceration S04.4-
    specified type NEC S04.4-
  abducent — *see* Injury, nerve, abducens

Injury - *continued*
nerve NEC - *continued*
  accessory S04.7-
    contusion S04.7-
    laceration S04.7-
    specified type NEC S04.7-
  acoustic S04.6-
    contusion S04.6-
    laceration S04.6-
    specified type NEC S04.6-
  ankle S94.9-
    cutaneous sensory S94.3-
    specified site NEC — *see* subcategory S94.8
  anterior crural, femoral — *see* Injury, nerve, femoral
  arm (upper) S44.9-
    axillary — *see* Injury, nerve, axillary
    cutaneous — *see* Injury, nerve, cutaneous, arm
    median — *see* Injury, nerve, median, upper arm
    musculocutaneous — *see* Injury, nerve, musculocutaneous
    radial — *see* Injury, nerve, radial, upper arm
    specified site NEC — *see* subcategory S44.8
    ulnar — *see* Injury, nerve, ulnar, arm
  auditory — *see* Injury, nerve, acoustic
  axillary S44.3-
  brachial plexus — *see* Injury, brachial plexus
  cervical sympathetic S14.5
  cranial S04.9
    contusion S04.9
    eighth (acoustic or auditory) — *see* Injury, nerve, acoustic
    eleventh (accessory) — *see* Injury, nerve, accessory
    fifth (trigeminal) — *see* Injury, nerve, trigeminal
    first (olfactory) — *see* Injury, nerve, olfactory
    fourth (trochlear) — *see* Injury, nerve, trochlear
    laceration S04.9
    ninth (glossopharyngeal) — *see* Injury, nerve, glossopharyngeal
    second (optic) — *see* Injury, nerve, optic
    seventh (facial) — *see* Injury, nerve, facial
    sixth (abducent) — *see* Injury, nerve, abducens
    specified
      nerve NEC S04.89-
        contusion S04.89-
        laceration S04.89-
        specified type NEC S04.89-
      type NEC S04.9
    tenth (pneumogastric or vagus) — *see* Injury, nerve, vagus
    third (oculomotor) — *see* Injury, nerve, oculomotor
    twelfth (hypoglossal) — *see* Injury, nerve, hypoglossal
  cutaneous sensory
    ankle (level) S94.3-
    arm (upper) (level) S44.5-
    foot (level) — *see* Injury, nerve, cutaneous sensory, ankle
    forearm (level) S54.3-
    hip (level) S74.2-
    leg (lower level) S84.2-
    shoulder (level) — *see* Injury, nerve, cutaneous sensory, arm
    thigh (level) — *see* Injury, nerve, cutaneous sensory, hip
  deep peroneal — *see* Injury, nerve, peroneal, foot
  digital
    finger S64.4-
      index S64.49-
      little S64.49-
      middle S64.49-
      ring S64.49-
      thumb S64.3-
    toe — *see* Injury, nerve, ankle, specified site NEC
  eighth cranial (acoustic or auditory) — *see* Injury, nerve, acoustic
  eleventh cranial (accessory) — *see* Injury, nerve, accessory
  facial S04.5-
    contusion S04.5-
    laceration S04.5-
    newborn P11.3
    specified type NEC S04.5-
  femoral (hip level) (thigh level) S74.1-
  fifth cranial (trigeminal) — *see* Injury, nerve, trigeminal
  finger (digital) — *see* Injury, nerve, digital, finger
  first cranial (olfactory) — *see* Injury, nerve, olfactory
  foot S94.9-
    cutaneous sensory S94.3-

Injury - *continued*
nerve NEC - *continued*
  foot - *continued*
    deep peroneal S94.2-
    lateral plantar S94.0-
    medial plantar S94.1-
    specified site NEC — *see* subcategory S94.8
  forearm (level) S54.9-
    cutaneous sensory — *see* Injury, nerve, cutaneous sensory, forearm
    median — *see* Injury, nerve, median
    radial — *see* Injury, nerve, radial
    specified site NEC — *see* subcategory S54.8
    ulnar — *see* Injury, nerve, ulnar
  fourth cranial (trochlear) — *see* Injury, nerve, trochlear
  glossopharyngeal S04.89-
    specified type NEC S04.89-
  hand S64.9-
    median — *see* Injury, nerve, median, hand
    radial — *see* Injury, nerve, radial, hand
    specified NEC — *see* subcategory S64.8
    ulnar — *see* Injury, nerve, ulnar, hand
  hip (level) S74.9-
    cutaneous sensory — *see* Injury, nerve, cutaneous sensory, hip
    femoral — *see* Injury, nerve, femoral
    sciatic — *see* Injury, nerve, sciatic
    specified site NEC — *see* subcategory S74.8
  hypoglossal S04.89-
    specified type NEC S04.89-
  lateral plantar S94.0-
  leg (lower) S84.9-
    cutaneous sensory — *see* Injury, nerve, cutaneous sensory, leg
    peroneal — *see* Injury, nerve, peroneal
    specified site NEC — *see* subcategory S84.8
    tibial — *see* Injury, nerve, tibial
    upper — *see* Injury, nerve, thigh
  lower
    back — *see* Injury, nerve, abdomen, specified site NEC
      peripheral — *see* Injury, nerve, abdomen, peripheral
    limb — *see* Injury, nerve, leg
  lumbar spinal — *see* Injury, nerve, spinal, lumbar
  lumbar plexus — *see* Injury, nerve, lumbosacral, sympathetic
  lumbosacral
    plexus — *see* Injury, nerve, lumbosacral, sympathetic
    sympathetic S34.5
  medial plantar S94.1-
  median (forearm level) S54.1-
    hand (level) S64.1-
    upper arm (level) S44.1-
    wrist (level) — *see* Injury, nerve, median, hand
  musculocutaneous S44.4-
  musculospiral (upper arm level) — *see* Injury, nerve, radial, upper arm
  neck S14.9
    peripheral S14.4
    specified site NEC S14.8
    sympathetic S14.5
  ninth cranial (glossopharyngeal) — *see* Injury, nerve, glossopharyngeal
  oculomotor S04.1-
    contusion S04.1-
    laceration S04.1-
    specified type NEC S04.1-
  olfactory S04.81-
    specified type NEC S04.81-
  optic S04.01-
    contusion S04.01-
    laceration S04.01-
    specified type NEC S04.01-
  pelvic girdle — *see* Injury, nerve, hip
  pelvis — *see* Injury, nerve, abdomen, specified site NEC
    peripheral — *see* Injury, nerve, abdomen, peripheral
  peripheral NEC T14.8
    abdomen — *see* Injury, nerve, abdomen, peripheral
    lower back — *see* Injury, nerve, abdomen, peripheral
    neck — *see* Injury, nerve, neck, peripheral
    pelvis — *see* Injury, nerve, abdomen, peripheral
    specified NEC T14.8
  peroneal (lower leg level) S84.1-
    foot S94.2-
  plexus
    brachial — *see* Injury, brachial plexus

Injury - *continued*
nerve NEC - *continued*
plexus - *continued*
celiac, coeliac — *see* Injury, nerve, lumbosacral, sympathetic
mesenteric, inferior — *see* Injury, nerve, lumbosacral, sympathetic
sacral — *see* Injury, lumbosacral plexus
spinal
brachial — *see* Injury, brachial plexus
lumbosacral — *see* Injury, lumbosacral plexus
pneumogastric — *see* Injury, nerve, vagus
radial (forearm level) S54.2-
hand (level) S64.2-
upper arm (level) S44.2-
wrist (level) — *see* Injury, nerve, radial, hand
root — *see* Injury, nerve, spinal, root
sacral plexus — *see* Injury, lumbosacral plexus
sacral spinal — *see* Injury, nerve, spinal, sacral
sciatic (hip level) (thigh level) S74.0-
second cranial (optic) — *see* Injury, nerve, optic
seventh cranial (facial) — *see* Injury, nerve, facial
shoulder — *see* Injury, nerve, arm
sixth cranial (abducent) — *see* Injury, nerve, abducens
spinal
plexus — *see* Injury, nerve, plexus, spinal
root
cervical S14.2
dorsal S24.2
lumbar S34.21
sacral S34.22
thoracic — *see* Injury, nerve, spinal, root, dorsal
splanchnic — *see* Injury, nerve, lumbosacral, sympathetic
sympathetic NEC — *see* Injury, nerve, lumbosacral, sympathetic
cervical — *see* Injury, nerve, cervical sympathetic
tenth cranial (pneumogastric or vagus) — *see* Injury, nerve, vagus
thigh (level) — *see* Injury, nerve, hip
cutaneous sensory — *see* Injury, nerve, cutaneous sensory, hip
femoral — *see* Injury, nerve, femoral
sciatic — *see* Injury, nerve, sciatic
specified NEC — *see* Injury, nerve, hip
third cranial (oculomotor) — *see* Injury, nerve, oculomotor
thorax S24.9
peripheral S24.3
specified site NEC S24.8
sympathetic S24.4
thumb, digital — *see* Injury, nerve, digital, thumb
tibial (lower leg level) (posterior) S84.0-
toe — *see* Injury, nerve, ankle
trigeminal S04.3-
contusion S04.3-
laceration S04.3-
specified type NEC S04.3-
trochlear S04.2-
contusion S04.2-
laceration S04.2-
specified type NEC S04.2-
twelfth cranial (hypoglossal) — *see* Injury, nerve, hypoglossal
ulnar (forearm level) S54.0-
arm (upper) (level) S44.0-
hand (level) S64.0-
wrist (level) — *see* Injury, nerve, ulnar, hand
vagus S04.89-
specified type NEC S04.89-
wrist (level) — *see* Injury, nerve, hand
ninth cranial nerve (glossopharyngeal) — *see* Injury, nerve, glossopharyngeal
nose (septum) S09.92
obstetrical O71.9
specified NEC O71.89
occipital (region) (scalp) S09.90
lobe — *see* Injury, intracranial
optic chiasm S04.02
optic radiation S04.03-
optic tract and pathways S04.03-
orbit, orbital (region) — *see* Injury, eye
penetrating (with foreign body) — *see* Injury, eye, orbit, penetrating
specified NEC — *see* Injury, eye, specified site NEC
ovary, ovarian S37.409
bilateral S37.402
contusion S37.422
laceration S37.432
specified type NEC S37.492
blood vessel — *see* Injury, blood vessel, ovarian

Injury - *continued*
ovary, ovarian - *continued*
contusion S37.429
bilateral S37.422
unilateral S37.421
laceration S37.439
bilateral S37.432
unilateral S37.431
specified type NEC S37.499
bilateral S37.492
unilateral S37.491
unilateral S37.401
contusion S37.421
laceration S37.431
specified type NEC S37.491
palate (hard) (soft) S09.93
pancreas S36.209
body S36.201
contusion S36.221
laceration S36.231
major S36.261
minor S36.241
moderate S36.251
specified type NEC S36.291
contusion S36.229
head S36.200
contusion S36.220
laceration S36.230
major S36.260
minor S36.240
moderate S36.250
specified type NEC S36.290
laceration S36.239
major S36.269
minor S36.249
moderate S36.259
specified type NEC S36.299
tail S36.202
contusion S36.222
laceration S36.232
major S36.262
minor S36.242
moderate S36.252
specified type NEC S36.292
parietal (region) (scalp) S09.90
lobe — *see* Injury, intracranial
patellar ligament (tendon) S76.10-
laceration S76.12-
specified NEC S76.19-
strain S76.11-
pelvis, pelvic (floor) S39.93
complicating delivery O70.1
joint or ligament, complicating delivery O71.6
organ S37.90
with ectopic or molar pregnancy O08.6
complication of abortion — *see* Abortion
contusion S37.92
following ectopic or molar pregnancy O08.6
laceration S37.93
obstetrical trauma NEC O71.5
specified
site NEC S37.899
contusion S37.892
laceration S37.893
specified type NEC S37.898
type NEC S37.99
specified NEC S39.83
penis S39.94
perineum S39.94
peritoneum S36.81
laceration S36.893
periurethral tissue — *see* Injury, urethra
complicating delivery O71.82
phalanges
foot — *see* Injury, foot
hand — *see* Injury, hand
pharynx NEC S19.85
pleura — *see* Injury, intrathoracic, pleura
plexus
brachial — *see* Injury, brachial plexus
cardiac — *see* Injury, nerve, thorax, sympathetic
celiac, coeliac — *see* Injury, nerve, lumbosacral, sympathetic
esophageal — *see* Injury, nerve, thorax, sympathetic
hypogastric — *see* Injury, nerve, lumbosacral, sympathetic
lumbar, lumbosacral — *see* Injury, lumbosacral plexus
mesenteric — *see* Injury, nerve, lumbosacral, sympathetic
pulmonary — *see* Injury, nerve, thorax, sympathetic

Injury - *continued*
postcardiac surgery (syndrome) I97.0
prepuce S39.94
prostate S37.829
contusion S37.822
laceration S37.823
specified type NEC S37.828
pubic region S39.94
pudendum S39.94
pulmonary plexus — *see* Injury, nerve, thorax, sympathetic
rectovaginal septum NEC S39.83
rectum — *see* Injury, intestine, large, rectum
retina — *see* Injury, eye, specified site NEC
penetrating — *see* Injury, eyeball, penetrating
retroperitoneal — *see* Injury, intra-abdominal, specified site NEC
rotator cuff (muscle (s)) (tendon (s)) S46.00-
laceration S46.02-
specified type NEC S46.09-
strain S46.01-
round ligament — *see* Injury, pelvic organ, specified site NEC
sacral plexus — *see* Injury, lumbosacral plexus
salivary duct or gland S09.93
scalp S09.90
newborn (birth injury) P12.9
due to monitoring (electrode) (sampling incision) P12.4
specified NEC P12.89
caput succedaneum P12.81
scapular region — *see* Injury, shoulder
sclera — *see* Injury, eye, specified site NEC
penetrating — *see* Injury, eyeball, penetrating
scrotum S39.94
second cranial nerve (optic) — *see* Injury, nerve, optic
seminal vesicle — *see* Injury, pelvic organ, specified site NEC
seventh cranial nerve (facial) — *see* Injury, nerve, facial
shoulder S49.9-
blood vessel — *see* Injury, blood vessel, arm
contusion — *see* Contusion, shoulder
dislocation — *see* Dislocation, shoulder
fracture — *see* Fracture, shoulder
muscle — *see* Injury, muscle, shoulder
nerve — *see* Injury, nerve, shoulder
open — *see* Wound, open, shoulder
specified type NEC S49.8-
sprain — *see* Sprain, shoulder girdle
superficial — *see* Injury, superficial, shoulder
sinus
cavernous — *see* Injury, intracranial
nasal S09.92
sixth cranial nerve (abducent) — *see* Injury, nerve, abducens
skeleton, birth injury P13.9
specified part NEC P13.8
skin NEC T14.8
surface intact — *see* Injury, superficial
skull NEC S09.90
specified NEC T14.8
spermatic cord (pelvic region) S37.898
scrotal region S39.848
spinal (cord)
cervical (neck) S14.109
anterior cord syndrome S14.139
C1 level S14.131
C2 level S14.132
C3 level S14.133
C4 level S14.134
C5 level S14.135
C6 level S14.136
C7 level S14.137
C8 level S14.138
Brown-Séquard syndrome S14.149
C1 level S14.141
C2 level S14.142
C3 level S14.143
C4 level S14.144
C5 level S14.145
C6 level S14.146
C7 level S14.147
C8 level S14.148
C1 level S14.101
C2 level S14.102
C3 level S14.103
C4 level S14.104
C5 level S14.105
C6 level S14.106
C7 level S14.107
C8 level S14.108

Injury - *continued*
  spinal (cord) - *continued*
    cervical (neck) - *continued*
      central cord syndrome S14.129
        C1 level S14.121
        C2 level S14.122
        C3 level S14.123
        C4 level S14.124
        C5 level S14.125
        C6 level S14.126
        C7 level S14.127
        C8 level S14.128
      complete lesion S14.119
        C1 level S14.111
        C2 level S14.112
        C3 level S14.113
        C4 level S14.114
        C5 level S14.115
        C6 level S14.116
        C7 level S14.117
        C8 level S14.118
      concussion S14.0
      edema S14.0
      incomplete lesion specified NEC S14.159
        C1 level S14.151
        C2 level S14.152
        C3 level S14.153
        C4 level S14.154
        C5 level S14.155
        C6 level S14.156
        C7 level S14.157
        C8 level S14.158
      posterior cord syndrome S14.159
        C1 level S14.151
        C2 level S14.152
        C3 level S14.153
        C4 level S14.154
        C5 level S14.155
        C6 level S14.156
        C7 level S14.157
        C8 level S14.158
    dorsal — *see* Injury, spinal, thoracic
    lumbar S34.109
      complete lesion S34.119
        L1 level S34.111
        L2 level S34.112
        L3 level S34.113
        L4 level S34.114
        L5 level S34.115
      concussion S34.01
      edema S34.01
      incomplete lesion S34.129
        L1 level S34.121
        L2 level S34.122
        L3 level S34.123
        L4 level S34.124
        L5 level S34.125
        L1 level S34.101
        L2 level S34.102
        L3 level S34.103
        L4 level S34.104
        L5 level S34.105
    nerve root NEC
      cervical — *see* Injury, nerve, spinal, root, cervical
      dorsal — *see* Injury, nerve, spinal, root, dorsal
      lumbar S34.21
      sacral S34.22
      thoracic — *see* Injury, nerve, spinal, root, dorsal
    plexus
      brachial — *see* Injury, brachial plexus
      lumbosacral — *see* Injury, lumbosacral plexus
    sacral S34.139
      complete lesion S34.131
      incomplete lesion S34.132
    thoracic S24.109
      anterior cord syndrome S24.139
        T1 level S24.131
        T2-T6 level S24.132
        T7-T10 level S24.133
        T11-T12 level S24.134
      Brown-Séquard syndrome S24.149
        T1 level S24.141
        T2-T6 level S24.142
        T7-T10 level S24.143
        T11-T12 level S24.144
      complete lesion S24.119
        T1 level S24.111
        T2-T6 level S24.112
        T7-T10 level S24.113
        T11-T12 level S24.114
      concussion S24.0
      edema S24.0
      incomplete lesion specified NEC S24.159

Injury - *continued*
  spinal (cord) - *continued*
    thoracic - *continued*
      incomplete lesion specified NEC - *continued*
        T1 level S24.151
        T2-T6 level S24.152
        T7-T10 level S24.153
        T11-T12 level S24.154
      posterior cord syndrome S24.159
        T1 level S24.151
        T2-T6 level S24.152
        T7-T10 level S24.153
        T11-T12 level S24.154
        T1 level S24.101
        T2-T6 level S24.102
        T7-T10 level S24.103
        T11-T12 level S24.104
    splanchnic nerve — *see* Injury, nerve, lumbosacral, sympathetic
    spleen S36.00
      contusion S36.029
        major S36.021
        minor S36.020
      laceration S36.039
        major (massive) (stellate) S36.032
        moderate S36.031
        superficial (capsular) (minor) S36.030
      specified type NEC S36.09
    splenic artery — *see* Injury, blood vessel, celiac artery, branch
    stellate ganglion — *see* Injury, nerve, thorax, sympathetic
    sternal region S29.9
    stomach S36.30
      contusion S36.32
      laceration S36.33
      specified type NEC S36.39
    subconjunctival — *see* Injury, eye, conjunctiva
    subcutaneous NEC T14.8
    submaxillary region S09.93
    submental region S09.93
    subungual
      fingers — *see* Injury, hand
      toes — *see* Injury, foot
    superficial NEC T14.8
      abdomen, abdominal (wall) S30.92
        abrasion S30.811
        bite S30.871
          insect S30.861
        contusion S30.1
        external constriction S30.841
        foreign body S30.851
      abrasion — *see* Abrasion, by site
      adnexa, eye NEC — *see* Injury, eye, specified site NEC
      alveolar process — *see* Injury, superficial, oral cavity
      ankle S90.91-
        abrasion — *see* Abrasion, ankle
        blister — *see* Blister, ankle
        bite — *see* Bite, ankle
        contusion — *see* Contusion, ankle
        external constriction — *see* Constriction, external, ankle
        foreign body — *see* Foreign body, superficial, ankle
      anus S30.98
      arm (upper) S40.92-
        abrasion — *see* Abrasion, arm
        bite — *see* Bite, superficial, arm
        blister — *see* Blister, arm (upper)
        contusion — *see* Contusion, arm
        external constriction — *see* Constriction, external, arm
        foreign body — *see* Foreign body, superficial, arm
      auditory canal (external) (meatus) — *see* Injury, superficial, ear
      auricle — *see* Injury, superficial, ear
      axilla — *see* Injury, superficial, arm
      back — *see also* Injury, superficial, thorax, back
        lower S30.91
          abrasion S30.810
          contusion S30.0
          external constriction S30.840
          superficial
            bite NEC S30.870
              insect S30.860
            foreign body S30.850
      bite NEC — *see* Bite, superficial NEC, by site
      blister — *see* Blister, by site
      breast S20.10-
        abrasion — *see* Abrasion, breast

Injury - *continued*
  superficial NEC - *continued*
    breast - *continued*
      bite — *see* Bite, superficial, breast
      contusion — *see* Contusion, breast
      external constriction — *see* Constriction, external, breast
      foreign body — *see* Foreign body, superficial, breast
    brow — *see* Injury, superficial, head, specified NEC
    buttock S30.91
    calf — *see* Injury, superficial, leg
    canthus, eye — *see* Injury, superficial, periocular area
    cheek (external) — *see* Injury, superficial, head, specified NEC
      internal — *see* Injury, superficial, oral cavity
    chest wall — *see* Injury, superficial, thorax
    chin — *see* Injury, superficial, head NEC
    clitoris S30.95
    conjunctiva — *see* Injury, eye, conjunctiva
      with foreign body (in conjunctival sac) — *see* Foreign body, conjunctival sac
    contusion — *see* Contusion, by site
    costal region — *see* Injury, superficial, thorax
    digit (s)
      hand — *see* Injury, superficial, finger
    ear (auricle) (canal) (external) S00.40-
      abrasion — *see* Abrasion, ear
      bite — *see* Bite, superficial, ear
      contusion — *see* Contusion, ear
      external constriction — *see* Constriction, external, ear
      foreign body — *see* Foreign body, superficial, ear
    elbow S50.90-
      abrasion — *see* Abrasion, elbow
      bite — *see* Bite, superficial, elbow
      blister — *see* Blister, elbow
      contusion — *see* Contusion, elbow
      external constriction — *see* Constriction, external, elbow
      foreign body — *see* Foreign body, superficial, elbow
    epididymis S30.94
    epigastric region S30.92
    epiglottis — *see* Injury, superficial, throat
    esophagus
      cervical — *see* Injury, superficial, throat
    external constriction — *see* Constriction, external, by site
    extremity NEC T14.8
    eyeball NEC — *see* Injury, eye, specified site NEC
    eyebrow — *see* Injury, superficial, periocular area
    eyelid S00.20-
      abrasion — *see* Abrasion, eyelid
      bite — *see* Bite, superficial, eyelid
      contusion — *see* Contusion, eyelid
      external constriction — *see* Constriction, external, eyelid
      foreign body — *see* Foreign body, superficial, eyelid
    face NEC — *see* Injury, superficial, head, specified NEC
    finger (s) S60.949
      abrasion — *see* Abrasion, finger
      bite — *see* Bite, superficial, finger
      blister — *see* Blister, finger
      contusion — *see* Contusion, finger
      external constriction — *see* Constriction, external, finger
      foreign body — *see* Foreign body, superficial, finger
      insect bite — *see* Bite, by site, superficial, insect
      index S60.94-
      little S60.94-
      middle S60.94-
      ring S60.94-
    flank S30.92
    foot S90.92-
      abrasion — *see* Abrasion, foot
      bite — *see* Bite, foot
      blister — *see* Blister, foot
      contusion — *see* Contusion, foot
      external constriction — *see* Constriction, external, foot
      foreign body — *see* Foreign body, superficial, foot
    forearm S50.91-
      abrasion — *see* Abrasion, forearm
      bite — *see* Bite, forearm, superficial
      blister — *see* Blister, forearm
      contusion — *see* Contusion, forearm

Injury - *continued*
superficial NEC - *continued*
forearm - *continued*
elbow only — *see* Injury, superficial, elbow
external constriction — *see* Constriction, external, forearm
foreign body — *see* Foreign body, superficial, forearm
forehead — *see* Injury, superficial, head NEC
foreign body — *see* Foreign body, superficial
genital organs, external
female S30.97
male S30.96
globe (eye) — *see* Injury, eye, specified site NEC
groin S30.92
gum — *see* Injury, superficial, oral cavity
hand S60.92-
abrasion — *see* Abrasion, hand
bite — *see* Bite, superficial, hand
contusion — *see* Contusion, hand
external constriction — *see* Constriction, external, hand
foreign body — *see* Foreign body, superficial, hand
head S00.90
ear — *see* Injury, superficial, ear
eyelid — *see* Injury, superficial, eyelid
nose S00.30
oral cavity S00.502
scalp S00.00
specified site NEC S00.80
heel — *see* Injury, superficial, foot
hip S70.91-
abrasion — *see* Abrasion, hip
bite — *see* Bite, superficial, hip
blister — *see* Blister, hip
contusion — *see* Contusion, hip
external constriction — *see* Constriction, external, hip
foreign body — *see* Foreign body, superficial, hip
iliac region — *see* Injury, superficial, abdomen
inguinal region — *see* Injury, superficial, abdomen
insect bite — *see* Bite, by site, superficial, insect
interscapular region — *see* Injury, superficial, thorax, back
jaw — *see* Injury, superficial, head, specified NEC
knee S80.91-
abrasion — *see* Abrasion, knee
bite — *see* Bite, superficial, knee
blister — *see* Blister, knee
contusion — *see* Contusion, knee
external constriction — *see* Constriction, external, knee
foreign body — *see* Foreign body, superficial, knee
labium (majus) (minus) S30.95
lacrimal (apparatus) (gland) (sac) — *see* Injury, eye, specified site NEC
larynx — *see* Injury, superficial, throat
leg (lower) S80.92-
abrasion — *see* Abrasion, leg
bite — *see* Bite, superficial, leg
contusion — *see* Contusion, leg
external constriction — *see* Constriction, external, leg
foreign body — *see* Foreign body, superficial, leg
knee — *see* Injury, superficial, knee
limb NEC T14.8
lip S00.501
lower back S30.91
lumbar region S30.91
malar region — *see* Injury, superficial, head, specified NEC
mammary — *see* Injury, superficial, breast
mastoid region — *see* Injury, superficial, head, specified NEC
mouth — *see* Injury, superficial, oral cavity
muscle NEC T14.8
nail NEC T14.8
finger — *see* Injury, superficial, finger
toe — *see* Injury, superficial, toe
nasal (septum) — *see* Injury, superficial, nose
neck S10.90
specified site NEC S10.80
nose (septum) S00.30
occipital region — *see* Injury, superficial, scalp
oral cavity S00.502
orbital region — *see* Injury, superficial, periocular area
palate — *see* Injury, superficial, oral cavity
palm — *see* Injury, superficial, hand
parietal region — *see* Injury, superficial, scalp
pelvis S30.91

Injury - *continued*
superficial NEC - *continued*
pelvis - *continued*
girdle — *see* Injury, superficial, hip
penis S30.93
perineum
female S30.95
male S30.91
periocular area S00.20-
abrasion — *see* Abrasion, eyelid
bite — *see* Bite, superficial, eyelid
contusion — *see* Contusion, eyelid
external constriction — *see* Constriction, external, eyelid
foreign body — *see* Foreign body, superficial, eyelid
phalanges
finger — *see* Injury, superficial, finger
toe — *see* Injury, superficial, toe
pharynx — *see* Injury, superficial, throat
pinna — *see* Injury, superficial, ear
popliteal space — *see* Injury, superficial, knee
prepuce S30.93
pubic region S30.91
pudendum
female S30.97
male S30.96
sacral region S30.91
scalp S00.00
scapular region — *see* Injury, superficial, shoulder
sclera — *see* Injury, eye, specified site NEC
scrotum S30.94
shin — *see* Injury, superficial, leg
shoulder S40.91-
abrasion — *see* Abrasion, shoulder
bite — *see* Bite, superficial, shoulder
blister — *see* Blister, shoulder
contusion — *see* Contusion, shoulder
external constriction — *see* Constriction, external, shoulder
foreign body — *see* Foreign body, superficial, shoulder
skin NEC T14.8
sternal region — *see* Injury, superficial, thorax, front
subconjunctival — *see* Injury, eye, specified site NEC
subcutaneous NEC T14.8
submaxillary region — *see* Injury, superficial, head, specified NEC
submental region — *see* Injury, superficial, head, specified NEC
subungual
finger (s) — *see* Injury, superficial, finger
toe (s) — *see* Injury, superficial, toe
supraclavicular fossa — *see* Injury, superficial, neck
supraorbital — *see* Injury, superficial, head, specified NEC
temple — *see* Injury, superficial, head, specified NEC
temporal region — *see* Injury, superficial, head, specified NEC
testis S30.94
thigh S70.92-
abrasion — *see* Abrasion, thigh
bite — *see* Bite, superficial, thigh
blister — *see* Blister, thigh
contusion — *see* Contusion, thigh
external constriction — *see* Constriction, external, thigh
foreign body — *see* Foreign body, superficial, thigh
thorax, thoracic (wall) S20.90
abrasion — *see* Abrasion, thorax
back S20.40-
bite — *see* Bite, thorax, superficial
blister — *see* Blister, thorax
contusion — *see* Contusion, thorax
external constriction — *see* Constriction, external, thorax
foreign body — *see* Foreign body, superficial, thorax
front S20.30-
throat S10.10
abrasion S10.11
bite S10.17
insect S10.16
blister S10.12
contusion S10.0
external constriction S10.14
foreign body S10.15
thumb S60.93-

Injury - *continued*
superficial NEC - *continued*
thumb - *continued*
abrasion — *see* Abrasion, thumb
bite — *see* Bite, superficial, thumb
blister — *see* Blister, thumb
contusion — *see* Contusion, thumb
external constriction — *see* Constriction, external, thumb
foreign body — *see* Foreign body, superficial, thumb
insect bite — *see* Bite, by site, superficial, insect
specified type NEC S60.39-
toe (s) S90.93-
abrasion — *see* Abrasion, toe
bite — *see* Bite, toe
blister — *see* Blister, toe
contusion — *see* Contusion, toe
external constriction — *see* Constriction, external, toe
foreign body — *see* Foreign body, superficial, toe
great S90.93-
tongue — *see* Injury, superficial, oral cavity
tooth, teeth — *see* Injury, superficial, oral cavity
trachea S10.10
tunica vaginalis S30.94
tympanum, tympanic membrane — *see* Injury, superficial, ear
uvula — *see* Injury, superficial, oral cavity
vagina S30.95
vocal cords — *see* Injury, superficial, throat
vulva S30.95
wrist S60.91-
supraclavicular region — *see* Injury, neck
supraorbital S09.93
suprarenal gland (multiple) — *see* Injury, adrenal
surgical complication (external or internal site) — *see* Laceration, accidental complicating surgery
temple S09.90
temporal region S09.90
tendon — *see also* Injury, muscle, by site
abdomen — *see* Injury, muscle, abdomen
Achilles — *see* Injury, Achilles tendon
lower back — *see* Injury, muscle, lower back
pelvic organs — *see* Injury, muscle, pelvis
tenth cranial nerve (pneumogastric or vagus) — *see* Injury, nerve, vagus
testis S39.94
thigh S79.92-
blood vessel — *see* Injury, blood vessel, hip
contusion — *see* Contusion, thigh
fracture — *see* Fracture, femur
muscle — *see* Injury, muscle, thigh
nerve — *see* Injury, nerve, thigh
open — *see* Wound, open, thigh
specified NEC S79.82-
superficial — *see* Injury, superficial, thigh
third cranial nerve (oculomotor) — *see* Injury, nerve, oculomotor
thorax, thoracic S29.9
blood vessel — *see* Injury, blood vessel, thorax
cavity — *see* Injury, intrathoracic
dislocation — *see* Dislocation, thorax
external (wall) S29.9
contusion — *see* Contusion, thorax
nerve — *see* Injury, nerve, thorax
open — *see* Wound, open, thorax
specified NEC S29.8
sprain — *see* Sprain, thorax
superficial — *see* Injury, superficial, thorax
fracture — *see* Fracture, thorax
internal — *see* Injury, intrathoracic
intrathoracic organ — *see* Injury, intrathoracic
sympathetic ganglion — *see* Injury, nerve, thorax, sympathetic
throat — *see also* Injury, neck S19.9
thumb S69.9-
blood vessel — *see* Injury, blood vessel, thumb
contusion — *see* Contusion, thumb
dislocation — *see* Dislocation, thumb
fracture — *see* Fracture, thumb
muscle — *see* Injury, muscle, thumb
nerve — *see* Injury, nerve, digital, thumb
open — *see* Wound, open, thumb
specified NEC S69.8-
sprain — *see* Sprain, thumb
superficial — *see* Injury, superficial, thumb
thymus (gland) — *see* Injury, intrathoracic, specified organ NEC
thyroid (gland) NEC S19.84
toe S99.92-
contusion — *see* Contusion, toe

Injury - *continued*
toe - *continued*
dislocation — *see* Dislocation, toe
fracture — *see* Fracture, toe
muscle — *see* Injury, muscle, toe
open — *see* Wound, open, toe
specified type NEC S99.82-
sprain — *see* Sprain, toe
superficial — *see* Injury, superficial, toe
tongue S09.93
tonsil S09.93
tooth S09.93
trachea (cervical) NEC S19.82
thoracic — *see* Injury, intrathoracic, trachea, thoracic
transfusion-related acute lung (TRALI) J95.84
tunica vaginalis S39.94
twelfth cranial nerve (hypoglossal) — *see* Injury, nerve, hypoglossal
ureter S37.10
contusion S37.12
laceration S37.13
specified type NEC S37.19
urethra (sphincter) S37.30
at delivery O71.5
contusion S37.32
laceration S37.33
specified type NEC S37.39
urinary organ S37.90
contusion S37.92
laceration S37.93
specified
site NEC S37.899
contusion S37.892
laceration S37.893
specified type NEC S37.898
type NEC S37.99
uterus, uterine S37.60
with ectopic or molar pregnancy O08.6
blood vessel — *see* Injury, blood vessel, iliac
contusion S37.62
laceration S37.63
cervix at delivery O71.3
rupture associated with obstetrics — *see* Rupture, uterus
specified type NEC S37.69
uvula S09.93
vagina S39.93
abrasion S30.814
bite S31.45
insect S30.864
superficial NEC S30.874
contusion S30.23
crush S38.03
during delivery — *see* Laceration, vagina, during delivery
external constriction S30.844
insect bite S30.864
laceration S31.41
with foreign body S31.42
open wound S31.40
puncture S31.43
with foreign body S31.44
superficial S30.95
foreign body S30.854
vas deferens — *see* Injury, pelvic organ, specified site NEC
vascular NEC T14.8
vein — *see* Injury, blood vessel
vena cava (superior) S25.20
inferior S35.10
laceration (minor) (superficial) S35.11
major S35.12
specified type NEC S35.19
laceration (minor) (superficial) S25.21
major S25.22
specified type NEC S25.29
vesical (sphincter) — *see* Injury, bladder
visual cortex S04.04-
vitreous (humor) S05.90
specified NEC S05.8X-
vocal cord NEC S19.83
vulva S39.94
abrasion S30.814
bite S31.45
insect S30.864
superficial NEC S30.874
contusion S30.23
crush S38.03
during delivery — *see* Laceration, perineum, female, during delivery
external constriction S30.844
insect bite S30.864

Injury - *continued*
vulva - *continued*
laceration S31.41
with foreign body S31.42
open wound S31.40
puncture S31.43
with foreign body S31.44
superficial S30.95
foreign body S30.854
whiplash (cervical spine) S13.4
wrist S69.9-
blood vessel — *see* Injury, blood vessel, hand
contusion — *see* Contusion, wrist
dislocation — *see* Dislocation, wrist
fracture — *see* Fracture, wrist
muscle — *see* Injury, muscle, hand
nerve — *see* Injury, nerve, hand
open — *see* Wound, open, wrist
specified NEC S69.8-
sprain — *see* Sprain, wrist
superficial — *see* Injury, superficial, wrist
Inoculation — *see also* Vaccination
complication or reaction — *see* Complications, vaccination
Insanity, insane — *see also* Psychosis
adolescent — *see* Schizophrenia
confusional F28
acute or subacute F05
delusional F22
senile F03
Insect
bite — *see* Bite, by site, superficial, insect
venomous, poisoning NEC (by) — *see* Venom, arthropod
Insensitivity
adrenocorticotropin hormone (ACTH) E27.49
androgen E34.50
complete E34.51
partial E34.52
Insertion
cord (umbilical) lateral or velamentous O43.12-
intrauterine contraceptive device (encounter for) — *see* Intrauterine contraceptive device
Insolation (sunstroke) T67.0
Insomnia (organic) G47.00
adjustment F51.02
adjustment disorder F51.02
behavioral, of childhood Z73.819
combined type Z73.812
limit setting type Z73.811
sleep-onset association type Z73.810
childhood Z73.819
chronic F51.04
somatized tension F51.04
conditioned F51.04
due to
alcohol
abuse F10.182
dependence F10.282
use F10.982
amphetamines
abuse F15.182
dependence F15.282
use F15.982
anxiety disorder F51.05
caffeine
abuse F15.182
dependence F15.282
use F15.982
cocaine
abuse F14.182
dependence F14.282
use F14.982
depression F51.05
drug NEC
abuse F19.182
dependence F19.282
use F19.982
medical condition G47.01
mental disorder NEC F51.05
opioid
abuse F11.182
dependence F11.282
use F11.982
psychoactive substance NEC
abuse F19.182
dependence F19.282
use F19.982
sedative, hypnotic, or anxiolytic
abuse F13.182
dependence F13.282
use F13.982
stimulant NEC

Insomnia (organic) - *continued*
due to - *continued*
stimulant NEC - *continued*
abuse F15.182
dependence F15.282
use F15.982
fatal familial (FFI) A81.83
idiopathic F51.01
learned F51.3
nonorganic origin F51.01
not due to a substance or known physiological condition F51.01
specified NEC F51.09
paradoxical F51.03
primary F51.01
psychiatric F51.05
psychophysiologic F51.04
related to psychopathology F51.05
short-term F51.02
specified NEC G47.09
stress-related F51.02
transient F51.02
without objective findings F51.02
Inspiration
food or foreign body — *see* Foreign body, by site
mucus — *see* Asphyxia, mucus
Inspissated bile syndrome (newborn) P59.1
Instability
emotional (excessive) F60.3
joint (post-traumatic) M25.30
ankle M25.37-
due to old ligament injury — *see* Disorder, ligament
elbow M25.32-
flail — *see* Flail, joint
foot M25.37-
hand M25.34-
hip M25.35-
knee M25.36-
lumbosacral — *see* subcategory M53.2
prosthesis — *see* Complications, joint prosthesis, mechanical, displacement, by site
sacroiliac — *see* subcategory M53.2
secondary to
old ligament injury — *see* Disorder, ligament
removal of joint prosthesis M96.89
shoulder (region) M25.31-
spine — *see* subcategory M53.2
wrist M25.33-
knee (chronic) M23.5-
lumbosacral — *see* subcategory M53.2
nervous F48.8
personality (emotional) F60.3
spine — *see* Instability, joint, spine
vasomotor R55
Institutional syndrome (childhood) F94.2
Institutionalization, affecting child Z62.22
disinhibited attachment F94.2
Insufficiency, insufficient
accommodation, old age H52.4
adrenal (gland) E27.40
primary E27.1
adrenocortical E27.40
drug-induced E27.3
iatrogenic E27.3
primary E27.1
anatomic crown height K08.89
anterior (occlusal) guidance M26.54
anus K62.89
aortic (valve) I35.1
with
mitral (valve) disease I08.0
with tricuspid (valve) disease I08.3
stenosis I35.2
tricuspid (valve) disease I08.2
with mitral (valve) disease I08.3
congenital Q23.1
rheumatic I06.1
with
mitral (valve) disease I08.0
with tricuspid (valve) disease I08.3
stenosis I06.2
with mitral (valve) disease I08.0
with tricuspid (valve) disease I08.3
tricuspid (valve) disease I08.2
with mitral (valve) disease I08.3
specified cause NEC I35.1
syphilitic A52.03
arterial I77.1
basilar G45.0
carotid (hemispheric) G45.1
cerebral I67.81
coronary (acute or subacute) I24.8

Insufficiency, insufficient - *continued*
arterial - *continued*
mesenteric K55.1
peripheral I73.9
precerebral (multiple) (bilateral) G45.2
vertebral G45.0
arteriovenous I99.8
biliary K83.8
cardiac — *see also* Insufficiency, myocardial
due to presence of (cardiac) prosthesis I97.11-
postprocedural I97.11-
cardiorenal, hypertensive I13.2
cardiovascular — *see* Disease, cardiovascular
cerebrovascular (acute) I67.81
with transient focal neurological signs and
symptoms G45.8
circulatory NEC I99.8
newborn P29.89
clinical crown length K08.89
convergence H51.11
coronary (acute or subacute) I24.8
chronic or with a stated duration of over 4
weeks I25.89
corticoadrenal E27.40
primary E27.1
dietary E63.9
divergence H51.8
food T73.0
gastroesophageal K22.8
gonadal
ovary E28.39
testis E29.1
heart — *see also* Insufficiency, myocardial
newborn P29.0
valve — *see* Endocarditis
hepatic — *see* Failure, hepatic
idiopathic autonomic G90.09
interocclusal distance of fully erupted teeth
(ridge) M26.36
kidney N28.9
acute N28.9
chronic N18.9
lacrimal (secretion) H04.12-
passages — *see* Stenosis, lacrimal
liver — *see* Failure, hepatic
lung — *see* Insufficiency, pulmonary
mental (congenital) — *see* Disability, intellectual
mesenteric K55.1
mitral (valve) I34.0
with
aortic valve disease I08.0
with tricuspid (valve) disease I08.3
obstruction or stenosis I05.2
with aortic valve disease I08.0
tricuspid (valve) disease I08.1
with aortic (valve) disease I08.3
congenital Q23.3
rheumatic I05.1
with
aortic valve disease I08.0
with tricuspid (valve) disease I08.3
obstruction or stenosis I05.2
with aortic valve disease I08.0
with tricuspid (valve) disease I08.3
tricuspid (valve) disease I08.1
with aortic (valve) disease I08.3
active or acute I01.1
with chorea, rheumatic (Sydenham's) I02.0
specified cause, except rheumatic I34.0
muscle — *see also* Disease, muscle
heart — *see* Insufficiency, myocardial
ocular NEC H50.9
myocardial, myocardium (with
arteriosclerosis) I50.9
with
rheumatic fever (conditions in I00) I09.0
active, acute or subacute I01.2
with chorea I02.0
inactive or quiescent (with chorea) I09.0
congenital Q24.8
hypertensive — *see* Hypertension, heart
newborn P29.0
rheumatic I09.0
active, acute, or subacute I01.2
syphilitic A52.06
nourishment T73.0
pancreatic K86.89
exocrine K86.81
parathyroid (gland) E20.9
peripheral vascular (arterial) I73.9
pituitary E23.0
placental (mother) O36.51-
platelets D69.6

Insufficiency, insufficient - *continued*
prenatal care affecting management of
pregnancy O09.3-
progressive pluriglandular E31.0
pulmonary J98.4
acute, following surgery (nonthoracic) J95.2
thoracic J95.1
chronic, following surgery J95.3
following
shock J98.4
trauma J98.4
newborn P28.5
valve I37.1
with stenosis I37.2
congenital Q22.2
rheumatic I09.89
with aortic, mitral or tricuspid (valve)
disease I08.8
pyloric K31.89
renal (acute) N28.9
chronic N18.9
respiratory R06.89
newborn P28.5
rotation — *see* Malrotation
sleep syndrome F51.12
social insurance Z59.7
suprarenal E27.40
primary E27.1
tarso-orbital fascia, congenital Q10.3
testis E29.1
thyroid (gland) (acquired) E03.9
congenital E03.1
tricuspid (valve) (rheumatic) I07.1
with
aortic (valve) disease I08.2
with mitral (valve) disease I08.3
mitral (valve) disease I08.1
with aortic (valve) disease I08.3
obstruction or stenosis I07.2
with aortic (valve) disease I08.2
with mitral (valve) disease I08.3
congenital Q22.8
nonrheumatic I36.1
with stenosis I36.2
urethral sphincter R32
valve, valvular (heart) — *see* Endocarditis
congenital Q24.8
vascular I99.8
intestine K55.9
acute — *see also* Ischemia, intestine,
acute K55.059
mesenteric K55.1
peripheral I73.9
renal — *see* Hypertension, kidney
velopharyngeal
acquired K13.79
congenital Q38.8
venous (chronic) (peripheral) I87.2
ventricular — *see* Insufficiency, myocardial
welfare support Z59.7
Insufflation, fallopian Z31.41
Insular — *see* condition
Insulinoma
pancreas
benign D13.7
malignant C25.4
uncertain behavior D37.8
specified site
benign — *see* Neoplasm, by site, benign
malignant — *see* Neoplasm, by site, malignant
uncertain behavior — *see* Neoplasm, by site,
uncertain behavior
unspecified site
benign D13.7
malignant C25.4
uncertain behavior D37.8
Insuloma — *see* Insulinoma
Interference
balancing side M26.56
non-working side M26.56
Intermenstrual — *see* condition
Intermittent — *see* condition
Internal — *see* condition
Interrogation
cardiac defibrillator (automatic)
(implantable) Z45.02
cardiac pacemaker Z45.018
cardiac (event) (loop) recorder Z45.09
infusion pump (implanted) (intrathecal) Z45.1
neurostimulator Z46.2
Interruption
aortic arch Q25.21
bundle of His I44.30

Interruption - *continued*
phase-shift, sleep cycle — *see* Disorder, sleep,
circadian rhythm
sleep phase-shift, or 24 hour sleep-wake cycle — *see*
Disorder, sleep, circadian rhythm
Interstitial — *see* condition
Intertrigo L30.4
labialis K13.0
Intervertebral disc — *see* condition
Intestine, intestinal — *see* condition
Intolerance
carbohydrate K90.49
disaccharide, hereditary E73.0
fat NEC K90.49
pancreatic K90.3
food K90.49
dietary counseling and surveillance Z71.3
fructose E74.10
hereditary E74.12
glucose (-galactose) E74.39
gluten K90.41
lactose E73.9
specified NEC E73.8
lysine E72.3
milk NEC K90.49
lactose E73.9
protein K90.49
starch NEC K90.49
sucrose (-isomaltose) E74.31
Intoxicated NEC (without dependence) — *see*
Alcohol, intoxication
Intoxication
acid E87.2
alcoholic (acute) (without dependence) — *see*
Alcohol, intoxication
alimentary canal K52.1
amphetamine (without dependence) — *see* Abuse,
drug, stimulant, with intoxication
with dependence — *see* Dependence, drug,
stimulant, with intoxication
anxiolytic (acute) (without dependence) — *see*
Abuse, drug, sedative, with intoxication
with dependence — *see* Dependence, drug,
sedative, with intoxication
caffeine F15.929
with dependence — *see* Dependence, drug,
stimulant, with intoxication
cannabinoids (acute) (without dependence) — *see*
Use, cannabis, with intoxication
with
abuse — *see* Abuse, drug, cannabis, with
intoxication
dependence — *see* Dependence, drug, cannabis,
with intoxication
chemical — *see* Table of Drugs and Chemicals
via placenta or breast milk — *see* - Absorption,
chemical, through placenta
cocaine (acute) (without dependence) — *see* Abuse,
drug, cocaine, with intoxication
with dependence — *see* Dependence, drug,
cocaine, with intoxication
drug
acute (without dependence) — *see* Abuse, drug, by
type with intoxication
with dependence — *see* Dependence, drug, by
type with intoxication
addictive
via placenta or breast milk — *see* Absorption,
drug, addictive, through placenta
newborn P93.8
gray baby syndrome P93.0
overdose or wrong substance given or taken — *see*
Table of Drugs and Chemicals, by drug,
poisoning
enteric K52.1
foodborne A05.9
bacterial A05.9
classical (Clostridium botulinum) A05.1
due to
Bacillus cereus A05.4
bacterium A05.9
specified NEC A05.8
Clostridium
botulinum A05.1
perfringens A05.2
welchii A05.2
Salmonella A02.9
with
(gastro) enteritis A02.0
localized infection (s) A02.20
arthritis A02.23
meningitis A02.21
osteomyelitis A02.24

Intoxication - *continued*
  foodborne - *continued*
    due to - *continued*
      Salmonella - *continued*
        with - *continued*
          localized infection (s) - *continued*
            pneumonia A02.22
            pyelonephritis A02.25
            specified NEC A02.29
          sepsis A02.1
          specified manifestation NEC A02.8
        Staphylococcus A05.0
        Vibrio
          parahaemolyticus A05.3
          vulnificus A05.5
      enterotoxin, staphylococcal A05.0
    noxious — *see* Poisoning, food, noxious
  gastrointestinal K52.1
  hallucinogenic (without dependence) — *see* Abuse, drug, hallucinogen, with intoxication
    with dependence — *see* Dependence, drug, hallucinogen, with intoxication
  hypnotic (acute) (without dependence) — *see* Abuse, drug, sedative, with intoxication
    with dependence — *see* Dependence, drug, sedative, with intoxication
  inhalant (acute) (without dependence) — *see* Abuse, drug, inhalant, with intoxication
    with dependence — *see* Dependence, drug, inhalant, with intoxication
  meaning
    inebriation — *see* category F10
    poisoning — *see* Table of Drugs and Chemicals
  methyl alcohol (acute) (without dependence) — *see* Alcohol, intoxication
  opioid (acute) (without dependence) — *see* Abuse, drug, opioid, with intoxication
    with dependence — *see* Dependence, drug, opioid, with intoxication
  pathologic NEC (without dependence) — *see* Alcohol, intoxication
  phencyclidine (without dependence) — *see* Abuse, drug, hallucinogen, with intoxication
    with dependence - — *see* Dependence, drug, hallucinogen, with intoxication
  potassium (K) E87.5
  psychoactive substance NEC (without dependence) — *see* Abuse, drug, psychoactive NEC, with intoxication
    with dependence — *see* Dependence, drug, psychoactive NEC, with intoxication
  sedative (acute) (without dependence) — *see* Abuse, drug, sedative, with intoxication
    with dependence — *see* Dependence, drug, sedative, with intoxication
  serum — *see also* Reaction, serum T80.69
  uremic — *see* Uremia
  volatile solvents (acute) (without dependence) — *see* Abuse, drug, inhalant, with intoxication
    with dependence — *see* Dependence, drug, inhalant, with intoxication
  water E87.79
Intracranial — *see* condition
Intrahepatic gallbladder Q44.1
Intraligamentous — *see* condition
Intrathoracic — *see also* condition
  kidney Q63.2
Intrauterine contraceptive device
  checking Z30.431
  insertion Z30.430
    immediately following removal Z30.433
  in situ Z97.5
  management Z30.431
  reinsertion Z30.433
  removal Z30.432
  replacement Z30.433
  retention in pregnancy O26.3-
Intraventricular — *see* condition
Intrinsic deformity — *see* Deformity
Intubation, difficult or failed T88.4
Intumescence, lens (eye) (cataract) — *see* Cataract
Intussusception (bowel) (colon) (enteric) (ileocecal) (ileocolic) (intestine) (rectum) K56.1
  appendix K38.8
  congenital Q43.8
  ureter (with obstruction) N13.5
Invagination (bowel, colon, intestine or rectum) K56.1
Inversion
  albumin-globulin (A-G) ratio E88.09
  bladder N32.89
  cecum — *see* Intussusception
  cervix N88.8

Inversion - *continued*
  chromosome in normal individual Q95.1
  circadian rhythm — *see* Disorder, sleep, circadian rhythm
  nipple N64.59
    congenital Q83.8
    gestational — *see* Retraction, nipple
    puerperal, postpartum — *see* Retraction, nipple
  nyctohemeral rhythm — *see* Disorder, sleep, circadian rhythm
  optic papilla Q14.2
  organ or site, congenital NEC — *see* Anomaly, by site
  sleep rhythm — *see* Disorder, sleep, circadian rhythm
  testis (congenital) Q55.29
  uterus (chronic) (postinfectional) (postpartal, old) N85.5
    postpartum O71.2
  vagina (posthysterectomy) N99.3
  ventricular Q20.5
Investigation — *see also* Examination Z04.9
  clinical research subject (control) (normal comparison) (participant) Z00.6
Involuntary movement, abnormal R25.9
Involution, involutional — *see also* condition
  breast, cystic — *see* Dysplasia, mammary, specified type NEC
  depression (single episode) F32.89
    recurrent episode F33.9
  melancholia (single episode) F32.89
    recurrent episode F33.8
  ovary, senile — *see* Atrophy, ovary
  thymus failure E32.8
IRDS (type I) P22.0
  type II P22.1
Irideremia Q13.1
Iridis rubeosis — *see* Disorder, iris, vascular
Iridochoroiditis (panuveitis) — *see* Panuveitis
Iridocyclitis H20.9
  acute H20.0-
    hypopyon H20.05-
    primary H20.01-
    recurrent H20.02-
    secondary (noninfectious) H20.04-
      infectious H20.03-
  chronic H20.1-
  due to allergy — *see* Iridocyclitis, acute, secondary
  endogenous — *see* Iridocyclitis, acute, primary
  Fuchs' — *see* Cyclitis, Fuchs' heterochromic
  gonococcal A54.32
  granulomatous — *see* Iridocyclitis, chronic
  herpes, herpetic (simplex) B00.51
    zoster B02.32
  hypopyon — *see* Iridocyclitis, acute, hypopyon
  in (due to)
    ankylosing spondylitis M45.9
    gonococcal infection A54.32
    herpes (simplex) virus B00.51
      zoster B02.32
    infectious disease NOS B99
    parasitic disease NOS B89 *[H22]*
    sarcoidosis D86.83
    syphilis A51.43
    tuberculosis A18.54
    zoster B02.32
  lens-induced H20.2-
  nongranulomatous — *see* Iridocyclitis, acute
  recurrent — *see* Iridocyclitis, acute, recurrent
  rheumatic — *see* Iridocyclitis, chronic
  subacute — *see* Iridocyclitis, acute
  sympathetic — *see* Uveitis, sympathetic
  syphilitic (secondary) A51.43
  tuberculous (chronic) A18.54
  Vogt-Koyanagi H20.82-
Iridocyclochoroiditis (panuveitis) — *see* Panuveitis
Iridodialysis H21.53-
Iridodonesis H21.89
Iridoplegia (complete) (partial) (reflex) H57.09
Iridoschisis H21.25-
Iris — *see also* condition
  bombé — *see* Membrane, pupillary
Iritis — *see also* Iridocyclitis
  chronic — *see* Iridocyclitis, chronic
  diabetic — *see* E08-E13 with .39
  due to
    herpes simplex B00.51
    leprosy A30.9 *[H22]*
  gonococcal A54.32
  gouty — *see also* Gout, by type M10.9 *[H22]*
  granulomatous — *see* Iridocyclitis, chronic
  lens induced — *see* Iridocyclitis, lens-induced
  papulosa (syphilitic) A52.71

Iritis - *continued*
  rheumatic — *see* Iridocyclitis, chronic
  syphilitic (secondary) A51.43
    congenital (early) A50.01
    late A52.71
  tuberculous A18.54
Iron — *see* condition
Iron-miner's lung J63.4
Irradiated enamel (tooth, teeth) K03.89
Irradiation effects, adverse T66
Irreducible, irreducibility — *see* condition
Irregular, irregularity
  action, heart I49.9
  alveolar process K08.89
  bleeding N92.6
  breathing R06.89
  contour of cornea (acquired) — *see* Deformity, cornea
    congenital Q13.4
  contour, reconstructed breast N65.0
  dentin (in pulp) K04.3
  eye movements H55.89
    nystagmus — *see* Nystagmus
    saccadic H55.81
  labor O62.2
  menstruation (cause unknown) N92.6
  periods N92.6
  prostate N42.9
  pupil — *see* Abnormality, pupillary
  reconstructed breast N65.0
  respiratory R06.89
  septum (nasal) J34.2
  shape, organ or site, congenital NEC — *see* Distortion
  sleep-wake pattern (rhythm) G47.23
Irritable, irritability R45.4
  bladder N32.89
  bowel (syndrome) K58.9
    with
      constipation K58.1
      diarrhea K58.0
    mixed K58.2
    psychogenic F45.8
    specified NEC K58.8
  bronchial — *see* Bronchitis
  cerebral, in newborn P91.3
  colon — *see also* Irritable, bowel K58.9
    with diarrhea K58.0
    psychogenic F45.8
  duodenum K59.8
  heart (psychogenic) F45.8
  hip — *see* Derangement, joint, specified type NEC, hip
  ileum K59.8
  infant R68.12
  jejunum K59.8
  rectum K59.8
  stomach K31.89
    psychogenic F45.8
  sympathetic G90.8
  urethra N36.8
Irritation
  anus K62.89
  axillary nerve G54.0
  bladder N32.89
  brachial plexus G54.0
  bronchial — *see* Bronchitis
  cervical plexus G54.2
  cervix — *see* Cervicitis
  choroid, sympathetic — *see* Endophthalmitis
  cranial nerve — *see* Disorder, nerve, cranial
  gastric K31.89
    psychogenic F45.8
  globe, sympathetic — *see* Uveitis, sympathetic
  labyrinth — *see* subcategory H83.2
  lumbosacral plexus G54.1
  meninges (traumatic) — *see* Injury, intracranial
    nontraumatic — *see* Meningismus
  nerve — *see* Disorder, nerve
  nervous R45.0
  penis N48.89
  perineum NEC L29.3
  peripheral autonomic nervous system G90.8
  peritoneum — *see* Peritonitis
  pharynx J39.2
  plantar nerve — *see* Lesion, nerve, plantar
  spinal (cord) (traumatic) — *see also* Injury, spinal cord, by region
    nerve G58.9
      root NEC — *see* Radiculopathy
    nontraumatic — *see* Myelopathy
  stomach K31.89
    psychogenic F45.8

Irritation - *continued*
  sympathetic nerve NEC G90.8
  ulnar nerve — *see* Lesion, nerve, ulnar
  vagina N89.8
Ischemia, ischemic I99.8
  brain — *see* Ischemia, cerebral
  bowel (transient)
    acute — *see also* Ischemia, intestine,
      acute K55.059
    chronic K55.1
    due to mesenteric artery insufficiency K55.1
  cardiac (see Disease, heart, ischemic)
  cardiomyopathy I25.5
  cerebral (chronic) (generalized) I67.82
    arteriosclerotic I67.2
    intermittent G45.9
    newborn P91.0
    recurrent focal G45.8
    transient G45.9
  colon chronic (due to mesenteric artery
    insufficiency) K55.1
  coronary — *see* Disease, heart, ischemic
  demand (coronary) — *see also* Angina I24.8
  heart (chronic or with a stated duration of over 4
    weeks) I25.9
    acute or with a stated duration of 4 weeks or
      less I24.9
    subacute I24.9
  infarction, muscle — *see* Infarct, muscle
  intestine (large) (small) (transient) K55.9
    acute K55.059
      diffuse K55.052
      focal K55.051
      large K55.039
        diffuse K55.032
        focal K55.031
      small K55.019
        diffuse K55.012
        focal K55.011
    chronic K55.1
    due to mesenteric artery insufficiency K55.1
  kidney N28.0
  mesenteric, acute — *see also* Ischemia, intestine,
    acute K55.059
  muscle, traumatic T79.6
  myocardium, myocardial (chronic or with a stated
    duration of over 4 weeks) I25.9
    acute, without myocardial infarction I51.3
    silent (asymptomatic) I25.6
    transient of newborn P29.4
  renal N28.0
  retina, retinal — *see* Occlusion, artery, retina
  small bowel
    acute K55.019
      diffuse K55.012
      focal K55.011
    chronic K55.1
    due to mesenteric artery insufficiency K55.1
  spinal cord G95.11
  subendocardial — *see* Insufficiency, coronary
  supply (coronary) — *see also* Angina I25.9
    due to vasospasm I20.1
Ischial spine — *see* condition
Ischialgia — *see* Sciatica
Ischiopagus Q89.4
Ischium, ischial — *see* condition
Ischuria R34
Iselin's disease or osteochondrosis — *see*
  Osteochondrosis, juvenile, metatarsus
Islands of
  parotid tissue in
    lymph nodes Q38.6
    neck structures Q38.6
  submaxillary glands in
    fascia Q38.6
    lymph nodes Q38.6
    neck muscles Q38.6
Islet cell tumor, pancreas D13.7
Isoimmunization NEC — *see also* Incompatibility
  affecting management of pregnancy (ABO) (with
    hydrops fetalis) O36.11-
    anti-A sensitization O36.11-
    anti-B sensitization O36.19-
    anti-c sensitization O36.09-
    anti-C sensitization O36.09-
    anti-e sensitization O36.09-
    anti-E sensitization O36.09-
    Rh NEC O36.09-
      anti-D antibody O36.01-
    specified NEC O36.19-
  newborn P55.9
    with
      hydrops fetalis P56.0

Isoimmunization NEC - *continued*
  newborn - *continued*
    with - *continued*
      kernicterus P57.0
      ABO (blood groups) P55.1
      Rhesus (Rh) factor P55.0
      specified type NEC P55.8
Isolation, isolated
  dwelling Z59.8
  family Z63.79
  social Z60.4
Isoleucinosis E71.19
Isomerism atrial appendages
  (with asplenia or polysplenia) Q20.6
Isosporiasis, isosporosis A07.3
Isovaleric acidemia E71.110
Issue of
  medical certificate Z02.79
    for disability determination Z02.71
  repeat prescription (appliance) (glasses) (medicinal
    substance, medicament, medicine) Z76.0
    contraception — *see* Contraception
Itch, itching — *see also* Pruritus
  baker's L23.6
  barber's B35.0
  bricklayer's L24.5
  cheese B88.0
  clam digger's B65.3
  coolie B76.9
  copra B88.0
  dew B76.9
  dhobi B35.6
  filarial — *see* Infestation, filarial
  grain B88.0
  grocer's B88.0
  ground B76.9
  harvest B88.0
  jock B35.6
  Malabar B35.5
    beard B35.0
    foot B35.3
    scalp B35.0
  meaning scabies B86
  Norwegian B86
  perianal L29.0
  poultrymen's B88.0
  sarcoptic B86
  scabies B86
  scrub B88.0
  straw B88.0
  swimmer's B65.3
  water B76.9
  winter L29.8
Ivemark's syndrome
  (asplenia with congenital heart disease) Q89.01
Ivory bones Q78.2
Ixodiasis NEC B88.8

J

Jaccoud's syndrome — *see* Arthropathy,
  postrheumatic, chronic
Jackson's
  membrane Q43.3
  paralysis or syndrome G83.89
  veil Q43.3
Jacquet's dermatitis (diaper dermatitis) L22
Jadassohn-Pellizari's disease or anetoderma L90.2
Jadassohn's
  blue nevus — *see* Nevus
  intraepidermal epithelioma — *see* Neoplasm, skin,
    benign
Jaffe-Lichtenstein (-Uehlinger) **syndrome** — *see*
  Dysplasia, fibrous, bone NEC
Jakob-Creutzfeldt disease or syndrome — *see*
  Creutzfeldt-Jakob disease or syndrome
Jaksch-Luzet disease D64.89
Jamaican
  neuropathy G92
  paraplegic tropical ataxic-spastic syndrome G92
Janet's disease F48.8
Janiceps Q89.4
Jansky-Bielschowsky amaurotic idiocy E75.4
Japanese
  B-type encephalitis A83.0
  river fever A75.3
Jaundice (yellow) R17
  acholuric (familial) (splenomegalic) — *see*
    also Spherocytosis
    acquired D59.8
  breast-milk (inhibitor) P59.3
  catarrhal (acute) B15.9
    with hepatic coma B15.0
  cholestatic (benign) R17

Jaundice (yellow) - *continued*
  due to or associated with
    delayed conjugation P59.8
      associated with (due to) preterm delivery P59.0
    preterm delivery P59.0
  epidemic (catarrhal) B15.9
    with hepatic coma B15.0
    leptospiral A27.0
    spirochetal A27.0
  familial nonhemolytic (congenital) (Gilbert) E80.4
    Crigler-Najjar E80.5
  febrile (acute) B15.9
    with hepatic coma B15.0
    leptospiral A27.0
    spirochetal A27.0
  hematogenous D59.9
  hemolytic (acquired) D59.9
    congenital — *see* Spherocytosis
  hemorrhagic (acute) (leptospiral) (spirochetal) A27.0
  infectious (acute) (subacute) B15.9
    with hepatic coma B15.0
    leptospiral A27.0
    spirochetal A27.0
  leptospiral (hemorrhagic) A27.0
  malignant (without coma) K72.90
    with coma K72.91
  newborn P59.9
    due to or associated with
      ABO
        antibodies P55.1
        incompatibility, maternal/fetal P55.1
        isoimmunization P55.1
      absence or deficiency of enzyme system for
        bilirubin conjugation (congenital) P59.8
      bleeding P58.1
      breast milk inhibitors to conjugation P59.3
        associated with preterm delivery P59.0
      bruising P58.0
      Crigler-Najjar syndrome E80.5
      delayed conjugation P59.8
        associated with preterm delivery P59.0
      drugs or toxins
        given to newborn P58.42
        transmitted from mother P58.41
      excessive hemolysis P58.9
        due to
          bleeding P58.1
          bruising P58.0
          drugs or toxins
            given to newborn P58.42
            transmitted from mother P58.41
          infection P58.2
          polycythemia P58.3
          swallowed maternal blood P58.5
        specified type NEC P58.8
      galactosemia E74.21
      Gilbert syndrome E80.4
      hemolytic disease P55.9
        ABO isoimmunization P55.1
        Rh isoimmunization P55.0
        specified NEC P55.8
      hepatocellular damage P59.20
        specified NEC P59.29
      hereditary hemolytic anemia P58.8
      hypothyroidism, congenital E03.1
      incompatibility, maternal/fetal NOS P55.9
      infection P58.2
      inspissated bile syndrome P59.1
      isoimmunization NOS P55.9
      mucoviscidosis E84.9
      polycythemia P58.3
      preterm delivery P59.0
      Rh
        antibodies P55.0
        incompatibility, maternal/fetal P55.0
        isoimmunization P55.0
      specified cause NEC P59.8
      swallowed maternal blood P58.5
    spherocytosis (congenital) D58.0
  neonatal — *see* Jaundice, newborn
  nonhemolytic congenital familial (Gilbert) E80.4
  nuclear, newborn — *see also* Kernicterus of
    newborn P57.9
  obstructive — *see also* Obstruction, bile duct K83.1
  post-immunization — *see* Hepatitis, viral, type, B
  post-transfusion — *see* Hepatitis, viral, type, B
  regurgitation — *see also* Obstruction, bile
    duct K83.1
  serum (homologous) (prophylactic)
    (therapeutic) — *see* Hepatitis, viral, type, B
  spirochetal (hemorrhagic) A27.0
  symptomatic R17
    newborn P59.9

Jaw — see condition
Jaw-winking phenomenon or syndrome Q07.8
Jealousy
　alcoholic F10.988
　childhood F93.8
　sibling F93.8
Jejunitis — see Enteritis
Jejunostomy status Z93.4
Jejunum, jejunal — see condition
Jensen's disease — see Inflammation, chorioretinal, focal, juxtapapillary
Jerks, myoclonic G25.3
Jervell-Lange-Nielsen syndrome I45.81
Jeune's disease Q77.2
Jigger disease B88.1
Job's syndrome (chronic granulomatous disease) D71
Joint — see also condition
　mice — see Loose, body, joint
　　knee M23.4-
Jordan's anomaly or syndrome D72.0
Joseph-Diamond-Blackfan anemia (congenital hypoplastic) D61.01
Jungle yellow fever A95.0
Jüngling's disease — see Sarcoidosis
Juvenile — see condition

K

Kahler's disease C90.0-
Kakke E51.11
Kala-azar B55.0
Kallmann's syndrome E23.0
Kanner's syndrome (autism) — see Psychosis, childhood
Kaposi's
　dermatosis (xeroderma pigmentosum) Q82.1
　lichen ruber L44.0
　　acuminatus L44.0
　sarcoma
　　colon C46.4
　　connective tissue C46.1
　　gastrointestinal organ C46.4
　　lung C46.5-
　　lymph node (multiple) C46.3
　　palate (hard) (soft) C46.2
　　rectum C46.4
　　skin (multiple sites) C46.0
　　specified site NEC C46.7
　　stomach C46.4
　　unspecified site C46.9
　varicelliform eruption B00.0
　　vaccinia T88.1
Kartagener's syndrome or triad (sinusitis, bronchiectasis, situs inversus) Q89.3
Karyotype
　with abnormality except iso (Xq) Q96.2
　45,X Q96.0
　46,X
　　iso (Xq) Q96.1
　46,XX Q98.3
　　with streak gonads Q50.32
　　hermaphrodite (true) Q99.1
　　male Q98.3
　46,XY
　　with streak gonads Q56.1
　　female Q97.3
　　hermaphrodite (true) Q99.1
　47,XXX Q97.0
　47,XXY Q98.0
　47,XYY Q98.5
Kaschin-Beck disease — see Disease, Kaschin-Beck
Katayama's disease or fever B65.2
Kawasaki's syndrome M30.3
Kayser-Fleischer ring (cornea) (pseudosclerosis) H18.04-
Kaznelson's syndrome (congenital hypoplastic anemia) D61.01
Kearns-Sayre syndrome H49.81-
Kedani fever A75.3
Kelis L91.0
Kelly (-Patterson) syndrome (sideropenic dysphagia) D50.1
Keloid, cheloid L91.0
　acne L73.0
　Addison's L94.0
　cornea — see Opacity, cornea
　Hawkin's L91.0
　scar L91.0
Keloma L91.0
Kenya fever A77.1
Keratectasia — see also Ectasia, cornea
　congenital Q13.4

Keratinization of alveolar ridge mucosa
　excessive K13.23
　minimal K13.22
Keratinized residual ridge mucosa
　excessive K13.23
　minimal K13.22
Keratitis (nodular) (nonulcerative) (simple) (zonular) H16.9
　with ulceration (central) (marginal) (perforated) (ring) — see Ulcer, cornea
　actinic — see Photokeratitis
　arborescens (herpes simplex) B00.52
　areolar H16.11-
　bullosa H16.8
　deep H16.309
　　specified type NEC H16.399
　dendritic (a) (herpes simplex) B00.52
　disciform (is) (herpes simplex) B00.52
　　varicella B01.81
　filamentary H16.12-
　gonococcal (congenital or prenatal) A54.33
　herpes, herpetic (simplex) B00.52
　　zoster B02.33
　in (due to)
　　acanthamebiasis B60.13
　　adenovirus B30.0
　　exanthema — see also Exanthem B09
　　herpes (simplex) virus B00.52
　　measles B05.81
　　syphilis A50.31
　　tuberculosis A18.52
　　zoster B02.33
　interstitial (nonsyphilitic) H16.30-
　　diffuse H16.32-
　　herpes, herpetic (simplex) B00.52
　　　zoster B02.33
　　sclerosing H16.33-
　　specified type NEC H16.39-
　　syphilitic (congenital) (late) A50.31
　　tuberculous A18.52
　macular H16.11-
　nummular H16.11-
　oyster shuckers' H16.8
　parenchymatous — see Keratitis, interstitial
　petrificans H16.8
　postmeasles B05.81
　punctata
　　leprosa A30.9 [H16.14-]
　　syphilitic (profunda) A50.31
　punctate H16.14-
　purulent H16.8
　rosacea L71.8
　sclerosing H16.33-
　　specified type NEC H16.8
　stellate H16.11-
　striate H16.11-
　superficial H16.10-
　　with conjunctivitis — see Keratoconjunctivitis
　　due to light — see Photokeratitis
　suppurative H16.8
　syphilitic (congenital) (prenatal) A50.31
　trachomatous A71.1
　　sequelae B94.0
　tuberculous A18.52
　vesicular H16.8
　xerotic — see also Keratomalacia H16.8
　　vitamin A deficiency E50.4
Keratoacanthoma L85.8
Keratocele — see Descemetocele
Keratoconjunctivitis H16.20-
　Acanthamoeba B60.13
　adenoviral B30.0
　epidemic B30.0
　exposure H16.21-
　herpes, herpetic (simplex) B00.52
　　zoster B02.33
　in exanthema — see also Exanthem B09
　infectious B30.0
　lagophthalmic — see Keratoconjunctivitis, specified type NEC
　neurotrophic H16.23-
　phlyctenular H16.25-
　postmeasles B05.81
　shipyard B30.0
　sicca (Sjogren's) M35.0-
　　not Sjogren's H16.22-
　specified type NEC H16.29-
　tuberculous (phlyctenular) A18.52
　vernal H16.26-
Keratoconus H18.60-
　congenital Q13.4
　stable H18.61-
　unstable H18.62-

Keratocyst (dental) (odontogenic) — see Cyst, calcifying odontogenic
Keratoderma, keratodermia (congenital) (palmaris et plantaris) (symmetrical) Q82.8
　acquired L85.1
　　in diseases classified elsewhere L86
　climactericum L85.1
　gonococcal A54.89
　gonorrheal A54.89
　punctata L85.2
　Reiter's — see Reiter's disease
Keratodermatocele — see Descemetocele
Keratoglobus H18.79
　congenital Q15.8
　　with glaucoma Q15.0
Keratohemia — see Pigmentation, cornea, stromal
Keratoiritis — see also Iridocyclitis
　syphilitic A50.39
　tuberculous A18.54
Keratoma L57.0
　palmaris and plantaris hereditarium Q82.8
　senile L57.0
Keratomalacia H18.44-
　vitamin A deficiency E50.4
Keratomegaly Q13.4
Keratomycosis B49
　nigrans, nigricans (palmaris) B36.1
Keratopathy H18.9
　band H18.42-
　bullous H18.1-
　bullous (aphakic), following cataract surgery H59.01-
Keratoscleritis, tuberculous A18.52
Keratosis L57.0
　actinic L57.0
　arsenical L85.8
　congenital, specified NEC Q80.8
　female genital NEC N94.89
　follicularis Q82.8
　　acquired L11.0
　　congenita Q82.8
　　et parafollicularis in cutem penetrans L87.0
　　spinulosa (decalvans) Q82.8
　　vitamin A deficiency E50.8
　gonococcal A54.89
　male genital (external) N50.89
　nigricans L83
　obturans, external ear (canal) — see Cholesteatoma, external ear
　palmaris et plantaris (inherited) (symmetrical) Q82.8
　　acquired L85.1
　penile N48.89
　pharynx J39.2
　pilaris, acquired L85.8
　punctata (palmaris et plantaris) L85.2
　scrotal N50.89
　seborrheic L82.1
　　inflamed L82.0
　senile L57.0
　solar L57.0
　tonsillaris J35.8
　vagina N89.4
　vegetans Q82.8
　vitamin A deficiency E50.8
　vocal cord J38.3
Kerato-uveitis — see Iridocyclitis
Kerion (celsi) B35.0
Kernicterus of newborn
　(not due to isoimmunization) P57.9
　due to isoimmunization (conditions in P55.0-P55.9) P57.0
　specified type NEC P57.8
Kerunoparalysis T75.09
Keshan disease E59
Ketoacidosis E87.2
　diabetic — see Diabetes, by type, with ketoacidosis
Ketonuria R82.4
Ketosis NEC E88.89
　diabetic — see Diabetes, by type, with with ketoacidosis
Kew Garden fever A79.1
Kidney — see condition
Kienböck's disease — see also Osteochondrosis, juvenile, hand, carpal lunate
　adult M93.1
Kimmelstiel (-Wilson) disease — see Diabetes, Kimmelstiel (-Wilson) disease
Kimura disease D21.9
　specified site (see Neoplasm, connective tissue benign)
Kink, kinking
　artery I77.1
　hair (acquired) L67.8

Kink, kinking - *continued*
  ileum or intestine — *see* Obstruction, intestine
  Lane's — *see* Obstruction, intestine
  organ or site, congenital NEC — *see* Anomaly, by
    site
  ureter (pelvic junction) N13.5
    with
      hydronephrosis N13.1
        with infection N13.6
      pyelonephritis (chronic) N11.1
    congenital Q62.39
  vein (s) I87.8
    caval I87.1
    peripheral I87.1
Kinnier Wilson's disease
  (hepatolenticular degeneration) E83.01
Kissing spine M48.20
  cervical region M48.22
  cervicothoracic region M48.23
  lumbar region M48.26
  lumbosacral region M48.27
  occipito-atlanto-axial region M48.21
  thoracic region M48.24
  thoracolumbar region M48.25
Klatskin's tumor C24.0
Klauder's disease A26.8
Klebs' disease — *see also* Glomerulonephritis N05.-
Klebsiella (K.)
  pneumoniae, as cause of disease classified
  elsewhere B96.1
Klein (e) **-Levin syndrome** G47.13
Kleptomania F63.2
Klinefelter's syndrome Q98.4
  karyotype 47,XXY Q98.0
  male with more than two X chromosomes Q98.1
Klippel-Feil deficiency, disease, or syndrome
  (brevicollis) Q76.1
Klippel's disease I67.2
Klippel-Trenaunay (-Weber) **syndrome** Q87.2
Klumpke (-Déjerine) **palsy, paralysis** (birth)
  (newborn) P14.1
Knee — *see* condition
Knock knee (acquired) M21.06-
  congenital Q74.1
Knot (s)
  intestinal, syndrome (volvulus) K56.2
  surfer S89.8-
  umbilical cord (true) O69.2
Knotting (of)
  hair L67.8
  intestine K56.2
Knuckle pad (Garrod's) M72.1
Koch's
  infection — *see* Tuberculosis
  relapsing fever A68.9
Koch-Weeks' conjunctivitis — *see* Conjunctivitis,
  acute, mucopurulent
Köebner's syndrome Q81.8
Köenig's disease (osteochondritis dissecans) — *see*
  Osteochondritis, dissecans
Köhler-Pellegrini-Steida disease or syndrome
  (calcification, knee joint) — *see* Bursitis, tibial
  collateral
Köhler's disease
  patellar — *see* Osteochondrosis, juvenile, patella
  tarsal navicular — *see* Osteochondrosis, juvenile,
    tarsus
Koilonychia L60.3
  congenital Q84.6
Kojevnikov's, epilepsy — *see* Kozhevnikof's epilepsy
Koplik's spots B05.9
Kopp's asthma E32.8
Korsakoff's (Wernicke)
  disease, psychosis or syndrome (alcoholic) F10.96
    with dependence F10.26
  drug-induced
    due to drug abuse — *see* Abuse, drug, by type,
      with amnestic disorder
    due to drug dependence — *see* Dependence, drug,
      by type, with amnestic disorder
  nonalcoholic F04
Korsakov's disease, psychosis or syndrome — *see*
  Korsakoff's disease
Korsakow's disease, psychosis or syndrome — *see*
  Korsakoff's disease
Kostmann's disease or syndrome
  (infantile genetic agranulocytosis) — *see*
  Agranulocytosis
Kozhevnikof's epilepsy G40.109
  intractable G40.119
    with status epilepticus G40.111
    without status epilepticus G40.119
  not intractable G40.109

Kozhevnikof's epilepsy - *continued*
  not intractable - *continued*
    with status epilepticus G40.101
    without status epilepticus G40.109
Krabbe's
  disease E75.23
  syndrome, congenital muscle hypoplasia Q79.8
Kraepelin-Morel disease — *see* Schizophrenia
Kraft-Weber-Dimitri disease Q85.8
Kraurosis
  ani K62.89
  penis N48.0
  vagina N89.8
  vulva N90.4
Kreotoxism A05.9
Krukenberg's
  spindle — *see* Pigmentation, cornea, posterior
  tumor C79.6-
Kufs' disease E75.4
Kugelberg-Welander disease G12.1
Kuhnt-Junius degeneration — *see*
  also Degeneration, macula H35.32-
Kümmell's disease or spondylitis — *see*
  Spondylopathy, traumatic
Kupffer cell sarcoma C22.3
Kuru A81.81
Kussmaul's
  disease M30.0
  respiration E87.2
    in diabetic acidosis — *see* Diabetes, by type, with
      ketoacidosis
Kwashiorkor E40
  marasmic, marasmus type E42
Kyasanur Forest disease A98.2
Kyphoscoliosis, kyphoscoliotic (acquired) —
  see also Scoliosis M41.9
  congenital Q67.5
  heart (disease) I27.1
  sequelae of rickets E64.3
  tuberculous A18.01
Kyphosis, kyphotic (acquired) M40.209
  cervical region M40.202
  cervicothoracic region M40.203
  congenital Q76.419
    cervical region Q76.412
    cervicothoracic region Q76.413
    occipito-atlanto-axial region Q76.411
    thoracic region Q76.414
    thoracolumbar region Q76.415
  Morquio-Brailsford type (spinal)
    (*see also* subcategory M49.8) E76.219
  postlaminectomy M96.3
  postradiation therapy M96.2
  postural (adolescent) M40.00
    cervicothoracic region M40.03
    thoracic region M40.04
    thoracolumbar region M40.05
  secondary NEC M40.10
    cervical region M40.12
    cervicothoracic region M40.13
    thoracic region M40.14
    thoracolumbar region M40.15
  sequelae of rickets E64.3
  specified type NEC M40.299
    cervical region M40.292
    cervicothoracic region M40.293
    thoracic region M40.294
    thoracolumbar region M40.295
  syphilitic, congenital A50.56
  thoracic region M40.204
  thoracolumbar region M40.205
  tuberculous A18.01
Kyrle disease L87.0

L

Labia, labium — *see* condition
Labile
  blood pressure R09.89
  vasomotor system I73.9
Labioglossal paralysis G12.29
Labium leporinum — *see* Cleft, lip
Labor — *see* Delivery
Labored breathing — *see* Hyperventilation
Labyrinthitis (circumscribed) (destructive) (diffuse)
  (inner ear) (latent) (purulent) (suppurative)
  (*see also* subcategory H83.0
  syphilitic A52.79
Laceration
  with abortion — *see* Abortion, by type, complicated
    by laceration of pelvic organs
  abdomen, abdominal
    wall S31.119
      with

Laceration - *continued*
  abdomen, abdominal - *continued*
    wall - *continued*
      with - *continued*
        foreign body S31.129
        penetration into peritoneal cavity S31.619
          with foreign body S31.629
      epigastric region S31.112
        with
          foreign body S31.122
          penetration into peritoneal cavity S31.612
            with foreign body S31.622
      left
        lower quadrant S31.114
          with
            foreign body S31.124
            penetration into peritoneal cavity S31.614
              with foreign body S31.624
        upper quadrant S31.111
          with
            foreign body S31.121
            penetration into peritoneal cavity S31.611
              with foreign body S31.621
      periumbilic region S31.115
        with
          foreign body S31.125
          penetration into peritoneal cavity S31.615
            with foreign body S31.625
      right
        lower quadrant S31.113
          with
            foreign body S31.123
            penetration into peritoneal cavity S31.613
              with foreign body S31.623
        upper quadrant S31.110
          with
            foreign body S31.120
            penetration into peritoneal cavity S31.610
              with foreign body S31.620
  accidental, complicating surgery — *see*
    Complications, surgical, accidental puncture or
    laceration
  Achilles tendon S86.02-
  adrenal gland S37.813
  alveolar (process) — *see* Laceration, oral cavity
  ankle S91.01-
    with
      foreign body S91.02-
  antecubital space — *see* Laceration, elbow
  anus (sphincter) S31.831
    with
      ectopic or molar pregnancy O08.6
      foreign body S31.832
    complicating delivery — *see* Delivery,
      complicated, by, laceration, anus (sphincter)
    following ectopic or molar pregnancy O08.6
    nontraumatic, nonpuerperal — *see* Fissure, anus
  arm (upper) S41.11-
    with foreign body S41.12-
    lower — *see* Laceration, forearm
  auditory canal (external) (meatus) — *see* Laceration,
    ear
  auricle, ear — *see* Laceration, ear
  axilla — *see* Laceration, arm
  back — *see also* Laceration, thorax, back
    lower S31.010
      with
        foreign body S31.020
          with penetration into retroperitoneal
            space S31.021
        penetration into retroperitoneal space S31.011
  bile duct S36.13
  bladder S37.23
    with ectopic or molar pregnancy O08.6
    following ectopic or molar pregnancy O08.6
    obstetrical trauma O71.5
  blood vessel — *see* Injury, blood vessel
  bowel — *see also* Laceration, intestine
    with ectopic or molar pregnancy O08.6
    complicating abortion — *see* Abortion, by type,
      complicated by, specified condition NEC
    following ectopic or molar pregnancy O08.6
    obstetrical trauma O71.5
  brain (any part) (cortex) (diffuse) (membrane) —
    see also Injury, intracranial, diffuse
    during birth P10.8
      with hemorrhage P10.1
    focal — *see* Injury, intracranial, focal brain injury
  brainstem S06.38-
  breast S21.01-
    with foreign body S21.02-
  broad ligament S37.893
    with ectopic or molar pregnancy O08.6

Laceration - *continued*
broad ligament - *continued*
  following ectopic or molar pregnancy O08.6
  laceration syndrome N83.8
  obstetrical trauma O71.6
  syndrome (laceration) N83.8
buttock S31.801
  with foreign body S31.802
  left S31.821
    with foreign body S31.822
  right S31.811
    with foreign body S31.812
calf — *see* Laceration, leg
canaliculus lacrimalis — *see* Laceration, eyelid
canthus, eye — *see* Laceration, eyelid
capsule, joint — *see* Sprain
causing eversion of cervix uteri (old) N86
central (perineal) , complicating delivery O70.9
cerebellum, traumatic S06.37-
cerebral S06.33-
  left side S06.32-
  during birth P10.8
    with hemorrhage P10.1
  right side S06.31-
cervix (uteri)
  with ectopic or molar pregnancy O08.6
  following ectopic or molar pregnancy O08.6
  nonpuerperal, nontraumatic N88.1
  obstetrical trauma (current) O71.3
  old (postpartal) N88.1
  traumatic S37.63
cheek (external) S01.41-
  with foreign body S01.42-
  internal — *see* Laceration, oral cavity
chest wall — *see* Laceration, thorax
chin — *see* Laceration, head, specified site NEC
chordae tendinae NEC I51.1
  concurrent with acute myocardial infarction — *see* Infarct, myocardium
  following acute myocardial infarction (current complication) I23.4
clitoris — *see* Laceration, vulva
colon — *see* Laceration, intestine, large, colon
common bile duct S36.13
cortex (cerebral) — *see* Injury, intracranial, diffuse
costal region — *see* Laceration, thorax
cystic duct S36.13
diaphragm S27.803
digit (s)
  hand — *see* Laceration, finger
  foot — *see* Laceration, toe
duodenum S36.430
ear (canal) (external) S01.31-
  with foreign body S01.32-
  drum S09.2-
elbow S51.01-
  with
    foreign body S51.02-
epididymis — *see* Laceration, testis
epigastric region — *see* Laceration, abdomen, wall, epigastric region
esophagus K22.8
  traumatic
    cervical S11.21
      with foreign body S11.22
    thoracic S27.813
eye (ball) S05.3-
  with prolapse or loss of intraocular tissue S05.2-
  penetrating S05.6-
eyebrow — *see* Laceration, eyelid
eyelid S01.11-
  with foreign body S01.12-
face NEC — *see* Laceration, head, specified site NEC
fallopian tube S37.539
  bilateral S37.532
  unilateral S37.531
finger (s) S61.219
  with
    damage to nail S61.319
      with
        foreign body S61.329
    foreign body S61.229
  index S61.218
    with
      damage to nail S61.318
        with
          foreign body S61.328
      foreign body S61.228
    left S61.211
      with
        damage to nail S61.311
        with

Laceration - *continued*
finger (s) - *continued*
  index - *continued*
    left - *continued*
      with - *continued*
        damage to nail - *continued*
          with - *continued*
            foreign body S61.321
        foreign body S61.221
    right S61.210
      with
        damage to nail S61.310
        with
          foreign body S61.320
        foreign body S61.220
  little S61.218
    with
      damage to nail S61.318
        with
          foreign body S61.328
      foreign body S61.228
    left S61.217
      with
        damage to nail S61.317
        with
          foreign body S61.327
      foreign body S61.227
    right S61.216
      with
        damage to nail S61.316
        with
          foreign body S61.326
      foreign body S61.226
  middle S61.218
    with
      damage to nail S61.318
        with
          foreign body S61.328
      foreign body S61.228
    left S61.213
      with
        damage to nail S61.313
        with
          foreign body S61.323
      foreign body S61.223
    right S61.212
      with
        damage to nail S61.312
        with
          foreign body S61.322
      foreign body S61.222
  ring S61.218
    with
      damage to nail S61.318
        with
          foreign body S61.328
      foreign body S61.228
    left S61.215
      with
        damage to nail S61.315
        with
          foreign body S61.325
      foreign body S61.225
    right S61.214
      with
        damage to nail S61.314
        with
          foreign body S61.324
      foreign body S61.224
flank S31.119
  with foreign body S31.129
foot (except toe (s) alone) S91.319
  with foreign body S91.329
  left S91.312
    with foreign body S91.322
  right S91.311
    with foreign body S91.321
  toe — *see* Laceration, toe
forearm S51.819
  with
    foreign body S51.829
  elbow only — *see* Laceration, elbow
  left S51.812
    with
      foreign body S51.822
  right S51.811
    with
      foreign body S51.821
forehead S01.81
  with foreign body S01.82
fourchette O70.0
  with ectopic or molar pregnancy O08.6
  complicating delivery O70.0

Laceration - *continued*
fourchette - *continued*
  following ectopic or molar pregnancy O08.6
gallbladder S36.123
genital organs, external
  female S31.512
    with foreign body S31.522
    vagina — *see* Laceration, vagina
    vulva — *see* Laceration, vulva
  male S31.511
    with foreign body S31.521
    penis — *see* Laceration, penis
    scrotum — *see* Laceration, scrotum
    testis — *see* Laceration, testis
groin — *see* Laceration, abdomen, wall
gum — *see* Laceration, oral cavity
hand S61.419
  with
    foreign body S61.429
  finger — *see* Laceration, finger
  left S61.412
    with
      foreign body S61.422
  right S61.411
    with
      foreign body S61.421
  thumb — *see* Laceration, thumb
head S01.91
  with foreign body S01.92
  cheek — *see* Laceration, cheek
  ear — *see* Laceration, ear
  eyelid — *see* Laceration, eyelid
  lip — *see* Laceration, lip
  nose — *see* Laceration, nose
  oral cavity — *see* Laceration, oral cavity
  scalp S01.01
    with foreign body S01.02
  specified site NEC S01.81
    with foreign body S01.82
  temporomandibular area — *see* Laceration, cheek
heart — *see* Injury, heart, laceration
heel — *see* Laceration, foot
hepatic duct S36.13
hip S71.019
  with foreign body S71.029
  left S71.012
    with foreign body S71.022
  right S71.011
    with foreign body S71.021
hymen — *see* Laceration, vagina
hypochondrium — *see* Laceration, abdomen, wall
hypogastric region — *see* Laceration, abdomen, wall
ileum S36.438
inguinal region — *see* Laceration, abdomen, wall
instep — *see* Laceration, foot
internal organ — *see* Injury, by site
interscapular region — *see* Laceration, thorax, back
intestine
  large
    colon S36.539
      ascending S36.530
      descending S36.532
      sigmoid S36.533
      specified site NEC S36.538
    rectum S36.63
    transverse S36.531
  small S36.439
    duodenum S36.430
    specified site NEC S36.438
intra-abdominal organ S36.93
  intestine — *see* Laceration, intestine
  liver — *see* Laceration, liver
  pancreas — *see* Laceration, pancreas
  peritoneum S36.81
  specified site NEC S36.893
  spleen — *see* Laceration, spleen
  stomach — *see* Laceration, stomach
intracranial NEC — *see also* Injury, intracranial, diffuse
  birth injury P10.9
jaw — *see* Laceration, head, specified site NEC
jejunum S36.438
joint capsule — *see* Sprain, by site
kidney S37.03-
  major (greater than 3 cm) (massive) (stellate) S37.06-
  minor (less than 1 cm) S37.04-
  moderate (1 to 3 cm) S37.05-
    multiple S37.06-
knee S81.01-
  with foreign body S81.02-
labium (majus) (minus) — *see* Laceration, vulva
lacrimal duct — *see* Laceration, eyelid

Laceration - *continued*
large intestine — *see* Laceration, intestine, large
larynx S11.011
  with foreign body S11.012
leg (lower) S81.819
  with foreign body S81.829
  foot — *see* Laceration, foot
  knee — *see* Laceration, knee
  left S81.812
    with foreign body S81.822
  right S81.811
    with foreign body S81.821
  upper — *see* Laceration, thigh
ligament — *see* Sprain
lip S01.511
  with foreign body S01.521
liver S36.113
  major (stellate) S36.116
  minor S36.114
  moderate S36.115
loin — *see* Laceration, abdomen, wall
lower back — *see* Laceration, back, lower
lumbar region — *see* Laceration, back, lower
lung S27.339
  bilateral S27.332
  unilateral S27.331
malar region — *see* Laceration, head, specified site NEC
mammary — *see* Laceration, breast
mastoid region — *see* Laceration, head, specified site NEC
meninges — *see* Injury, intracranial, diffuse
meniscus — *see* Tear, meniscus
mesentery S36.893
mesosalpinx S37.893
mouth — *see* Laceration, oral cavity
muscle — *see* Injury, muscle, by site, laceration
nail
  finger — *see* Laceration, finger, with damage to nail
  toe — *see* Laceration, toe, with damage to nail
nasal (septum) (sinus) — *see* Laceration, nose
nasopharynx — *see* Laceration, head, specified site NEC
neck S11.91
  with foreign body S11.92
  involving
    cervical esophagus S11.21
      with foreign body S11.22
    larynx — *see* Laceration, larynx
    pharynx — *see* Laceration, pharynx
    thyroid gland — *see* Laceration, thyroid gland
    trachea — *see* Laceration, trachea
  specified site NEC S11.81
    with foreign body S11.82
nerve — *see* Injury, nerve
nose (septum) (sinus) S01.21
  with foreign body S01.22
ocular NOS S05.3-
  adnexa NOS S01.11-
oral cavity S01.512
  with foreign body S01.522
orbit (eye) — *see* Wound, open, ocular, orbit
ovary S37.439
  bilateral S37.432
  unilateral S37.431
palate — *see* Laceration, oral cavity
palm — *see* Laceration, hand
pancreas S36.239
  body S36.231
    major S36.261
    minor S36.241
    moderate S36.251
  head S36.230
    major S36.260
    minor S36.240
    moderate S36.250
  major S36.269
  minor S36.249
  moderate S36.259
  tail S36.232
    major S36.262
    minor S36.242
    moderate S36.252
pelvic S31.010
  with
    foreign body S31.020
      penetration into retroperitoneal cavity S31.021
    penetration into retroperitoneal cavity S31.011
  floor — *see also* Laceration, back, lower
    with ectopic or molar pregnancy O08.6
    complicating delivery O70.1
    following ectopic or molar pregnancy O08.6

Laceration - *continued*
pelvic - *continued*
  floor - *continued*
    old (postpartal) N81.89
  organ S37.93
    with ectopic or molar pregnancy O08.6
    adrenal gland S37.813
    bladder S37.23
    fallopian tube — *see* Laceration, fallopian tube
    following ectopic or molar pregnancy O08.6
    kidney — *see* Laceration, kidney
    obstetrical trauma O71.5
    ovary — *see* Laceration, ovary
    prostate S37.823
    specified site NEC S37.893
    ureter S37.13
    urethra S37.33
    uterus S37.63
penis S31.21
  with foreign body S31.22
perineum
  female S31.41
    with
      ectopic or molar pregnancy O08.6
      foreign body S31.42
    during delivery O70.9
      first degree O70.0
      fourth degree O70.3
      second degree O70.1
      third degree — *see also* Delivery, complicated, by, laceration, perineum, third degree O70.20
    old (postpartal) N81.89
    postpartal N81.89
    secondary (postpartal) O90.1
  male S31.119
    with foreign body S31.129
periocular area (with or without lacrimal passages) — *see* Laceration, eyelid
peritoneum S36.893
periumbilic region — *see* Laceration, abdomen, wall, periumbilic
periurethral tissue — *see* Laceration, urethra
phalanges
  finger — *see* Laceration, finger
  toe — *see* Laceration, toe
pharynx S11.21
  with foreign body S11.22
pinna — *see* Laceration, ear
popliteal space — *see* Laceration, knee
prepuce — *see* Laceration, penis
prostate S37.823
pubic region S31.119
  with foreign body S31.129
pudendum — *see* Laceration, genital organs, external
rectovaginal septum — *see* Laceration, vagina
rectum S36.63
retroperitoneum S36.893
round ligament S37.893
sacral region — *see* Laceration, back, lower
sacroiliac region — *see* Laceration, back, lower
salivary gland — *see* Laceration, oral cavity
scalp S01.01
  with foreign body S01.02
scapular region — *see* Laceration, shoulder
scrotum S31.31
  with foreign body S31.32
seminal vesicle S37.893
shin — *see* Laceration, leg
shoulder S41.019
  with foreign body S41.029
  left S41.012
    with foreign body S41.022
  right S41.011
    with foreign body S41.021
small intestine — *see* Laceration, intestine, small
spermatic cord — *see* Laceration, testis
spinal cord (meninges) — *see also* Injury, spinal cord, by region
  due to injury at birth P11.5
  newborn (birth injury) P11.5
spleen S36.039
  major (massive) (stellate) S36.032
  moderate S36.031
  superficial (minor) S36.030
sternal region — *see* Laceration, thorax, front
stomach S36.33
submaxillary region — *see* Laceration, head, specified site NEC
submental region — *see* Laceration, head, specified site NEC
subungual

Laceration - *continued*
subungual - *continued*
  finger (s) — *see* Laceration, finger, with damage to nail
  toe (s) — *see* Laceration, toe, with damage to nail
suprarenal gland — *see* Laceration, adrenal gland
temple, temporal region — *see* Laceration, head, specified site NEC
temporomandibular area — *see* Laceration, cheek
tendon — *see* Injury, muscle, by site, laceration
  Achilles S86.02-
tentorium cerebelli — *see* Injury, intracranial, diffuse
testis S31.31
  with foreign body S31.32
thigh S71.11-
  with foreign body S71.12-
thorax, thoracic (wall) S21.91
  with foreign body S21.92
  back S21.22-
    with penetration into thoracic cavity S21.42-
  front S21.12-
    with penetration into thoracic cavity S21.32-
  back S21.21-
    with
      foreign body S21.22-
      with penetration into thoracic cavity S21.42-
    penetration into thoracic cavity S21.41-
  breast — *see* Laceration, breast
  front S21.11-
    with
      foreign body S21.12-
      with penetration into thoracic cavity S21.32-
    penetration into thoracic cavity S21.31-
thumb S61.019
  with
    damage to nail S61.119
      with
        foreign body S61.129
    foreign body S61.029
  left S61.012
    with
      damage to nail S61.112
        with
          foreign body S61.122
      foreign body S61.022
  right S61.011
    with
      damage to nail S61.111
        with
          foreign body S61.121
      foreign body S61.021
thyroid gland S11.11
  with foreign body S11.12
toe (s) S91.119
  with
    damage to nail S91.219
      with
        foreign body S91.229
    foreign body S91.129
  great S91.113
    with
      damage to nail S91.213
        with
          foreign body S91.223
      foreign body S91.123
    left S91.112
      with
        damage to nail S91.212
          with
            foreign body S91.222
        foreign body S91.122
    right S91.111
      with
        damage to nail S91.211
          with
            foreign body S91.221
        foreign body S91.121
  lesser S91.116
    with
      damage to nail S91.216
        with
          foreign body S91.226
      foreign body S91.126
    left S91.115
      with
        damage to nail S91.215
          with
            foreign body S91.225
        foreign body S91.125
    right S91.114
      with
        damage to nail S91.214

Laceration - *continued*
  toe (s) - *continued*
    lesser - *continued*
      right - *continued*
        with - *continued*
          damage to nail - *continued*
            with
              foreign body S91.224
            foreign body S91.124
  tongue — *see* Laceration, oral cavity
  trachea S11.021
    with foreign body S11.022
  tunica vaginalis — *see* Laceration, testis
  tympanum, tympanic membrane — *see* Laceration, ear, drum
  umbilical region S31.115
    with foreign body S31.125
  ureter S37.13
  urethra S37.33
    with or following ectopic or molar pregnancy O08.6
    obstetrical trauma O71.5
  urinary organ NEC S37.893
  uterus S37.63
    with ectopic or molar pregnancy O08.6
    following ectopic or molar pregnancy O08.6
    nonpuerperal, nontraumatic N85.8
    obstetrical trauma NEC O71.81
    old (postpartal) N85.8
  uvula — *see* Laceration, oral cavity
  vagina S31.41
    with
      ectopic or molar pregnancy O08.6
      foreign body S31.42
    during delivery O71.4
      with perineal laceration — *see* Laceration, perineum, female, during delivery
    following ectopic or molar pregnancy O08.6
    nonpuerperal, nontraumatic N89.8
    old (postpartal) N89.8
  vas deferens S37.893
  vesical — *see* Laceration, bladder
  vocal cords S11.031
    with foreign body S11.032
  vulva S31.41
    with
      ectopic or molar pregnancy O08.6
      foreign body S31.42
    complicating delivery O70.0
    following ectopic or molar pregnancy O08.6
    nonpuerperal, nontraumatic N90.89
    old (postpartal) N90.89
  wrist S61.519
    with
      foreign body S61.529
    left S61.512
      with
        foreign body S61.522
    right S61.511
      with
        foreign body S61.521

Lack of
  achievement in school Z55.3
  adequate
    food Z59.4
    intermaxillary vertical dimension of fully erupted teeth M26.36
    sleep Z72.820
  appetite (see Anorexia) R63.0
  awareness R41.9
  care
    in home Z74.2
    of infant (at or after birth) T76.02
      confirmed T74.02
  cognitive functions R41.9
  coordination R27.9
    ataxia R27.0
    specified type NEC R27.8
  development (physiological) R62.50
    failure to thrive (child over 28 days old) R62.51
      adult R62.7
      newborn P92.6
    short stature R62.52
    specified type NEC R62.59
  energy R53.83
  financial resources Z59.6
  food T73.0
  growth R62.52
  heating Z59.1
  housing (permanent) (temporary) Z59.0
    adequate Z59.1
  learning experiences in childhood Z62.898
  leisure time (affecting life-style) Z73.2

Lack of - *continued*
  material resources Z59.9
  memory — *see also* Amnesia
    mild, following organic brain damage F06.8
  ovulation N97.0
  parental supervision or control of child Z62.0
  person able to render necessary care Z74.2
  physical exercise Z72.3
  play experience in childhood Z62.898
  posterior occlusal support M26.57
  relaxation (affecting life-style) Z73.2
  sexual
    desire F52.0
    enjoyment F52.1
  shelter Z59.0
  sleep (adequate) Z72.820
  supervision of child by parent Z62.0
  support, posterior occlusal M26.57
  water T73.1
Lacrimal — *see* condition
Lacrimation, abnormal — *see* Epiphora
Lacrimonasal duct — *see* condition
Lactation, lactating (breast) (puerperal, postpartum)
  associated
    cracked nipple O92.13
    retracted nipple O92.03
  defective O92.4
  disorder NEC O92.79
  excessive O92.6
  failed (complete) O92.3
    partial O92.4
  mastitis NEC — *see* Mastitis, obstetric
  mother (care and/or examination) Z39.1
  nonpuerperal N64.3
Lacticemia, excessive E87.2
Lacunar skull Q75.8
Laennec's cirrhosis K70.30
  with ascites K70.31
  nonalcoholic K74.69
Lafora's disease — *see* Epilepsy, generalized, idiopathic
Lag, lid (nervous) — *see* Retraction, lid
Lagophthalmos (eyelid) (nervous) H02.209
  cicatricial H02.219
    left H02.216
      lower H02.215
      upper H02.214
    right H02.213
      lower H02.212
      upper H02.211
  keratoconjunctivitis — *see* Keratoconjunctivitis
  left H02.206
    lower H02.205
    upper H02.204
  mechanical H02.229
    left H02.226
      lower H02.225
      upper H02.224
    right H02.223
      lower H02.222
      upper H02.221
  paralytic H02.239
    left H02.236
      lower H02.235
      upper H02.234
    right H02.233
      lower H02.232
      upper H02.231
  right H02.203
    lower H02.202
    upper H02.201
Laki-Lorand factor deficiency — *see* Defect, coagulation, specified type NEC
Lalling F80.0
Lambert-Eaton syndrome — *see* Syndrome, Lambert-Eaton
Lambliasis, lambliosis A07.1
Landau-Kleffner syndrome — *see* Epilepsy, specified NEC
Landouzy-Déjérine dystrophy or facioscapulohumeral atrophy G71.0
Landouzy's disease (icterohemorrhagic leptospirosis) A27.0
Landry-Guillain-Barré, syndrome or paralysis G61.0
Landry's disease or paralysis G61.0
Lane's
  band Q43.3
  kink — *see* Obstruction, intestine
  syndrome K90.2
Langdon Down syndrome — *see* Trisomy, 21
Lapsed immunization schedule status Z28.3

Large
  baby (regardless of gestational age) (4000g to 4499g) P08.1
  ear, congenital Q17.1
  physiological cup Q14.2
  stature R68.89
Large-for-dates NEC (infant) (4000g to 4499g) P08.1
  affecting management of pregnancy O36.6-
  exceptionally (4500g or more) P08.0
Larsen-Johansson disease orosteochondrosis — *see* Osteochondrosis, juvenile, patella
Larsen's syndrome
  (flattened facies and multiple congenital dislocations) Q74.8
Larva migrans
  cutaneous B76.9
    Ancylostoma B76.0
  visceral B83.0
Laryngeal — *see* condition
Laryngismus (stridulus) J38.5
  congenital P28.89
  diphtheritic A36.2
Laryngitis (acute) (edematous) (fibrinous) (infective) (infiltrative) (malignant) (membranous) (phlegmonous) (pneumococcal) (pseudomembranous) (septic) (subglottic) (suppurative) (ulcerative) J04.0
  with
    influenza, flu, or grippe — *see* Influenza, with, laryngitis
    tracheitis (acute) — *see* Laryngotracheitis
  atrophic J37.0
  catarrhal J37.0
  chronic J37.0
    with tracheitis (chronic) J37.1
  diphtheritic A36.2
  due to external agent — *see* Inflammation, respiratory, upper, due to
  Hemophilus influenzae J04.0
  H. influenzae J04.0
  hypertrophic J37.0
  influenzal — *see* Influenza, with, respiratory manifestations NEC
  obstructive J05.0
  sicca J37.0
  spasmodic J05.0
    acute J04.0
  streptococcal J04.0
  stridulous J05.0
  syphilitic (late) A52.73
    congenital A50.59 *[J99]*
    early A50.03 *[J99]*
  tuberculous A15.5
  Vincent's A69.1
Laryngocele (congenital) (ventricular) Q31.3
Laryngofissure J38.7
  congenital Q31.8
Laryngomalacia (congenital) Q31.5
Laryngopharyngitis (acute) J06.0
  chronic J37.0
  due to external agent — *see* Inflammation, respiratory, upper, due to
Laryngoplegia J38.00
  bilateral J38.02
  unilateral J38.01
Laryngoptosis J38.7
Laryngospasm J38.5
Laryngostenosis J38.6
Laryngotracheitis (acute) (Infectional) (infective) (viral) J04.2
  atrophic J37.1
  catarrhal J37.1
  chronic J37.1
  diphtheritic A36.2
  due to external agent — *see* Inflammation, respiratory, upper, due to
  Hemophilus influenzae J04.2
  hypertrophic J37.1
  influenzal — *see* Influenza, with, respiratory manifestations NEC
  pachydermic J38.7
  sicca J37.1
  spasmodic J38.5
    acute J05.0
  streptococcal J04.2
  stridulous J38.5
  syphilitic (late) A52.73
    congenital A50.59 *[J99]*
    early A50.03 *[J99]*
  tuberculous A15.5
  Vincent's A69.1
Laryngotracheobronchitis — *see* Bronchitis

Larynx, laryngeal — *see* condition
Lassa fever A96.2
Lassitude — *see* Weakness
Late
  talker R62.0
  walker R62.0
Late effect (s) — *see* Sequelae
Latent — *see* condition
Laterocession — *see* Lateroversion
Lateroflexion — *see* Lateroversion
Lateroversion
  cervix — *see* Lateroversion, uterus
  uterus, uterine (cervix) (postinfectional) (postpartal, old) N85.4
    congenital Q51.818
    in pregnancy or childbirth O34.59-
Lathyrism — *see* Poisoning, food, noxious, plant
Launois' syndrome (pituitary gigantism) E22.0
Launois-Bensaude adenolipomatosis E88.89
Laurence-Moon (-Bardet) **-Biedl syndrome** Q87.89
Lax, laxity — *see also* Relaxation
  ligament (ous) — *see also* Disorder, ligament
    familial M35.7
    knee — *see* Derangement, knee
  skin (acquired) L57.4
    congenital Q82.8
Laxative habit F55.2
Lazy leukocyte syndrome D70.8
Lead miner's lung J63.6
Leak, leakage
  air NEC J93.82
    postprocedural J95.812
  amniotic fluid — *see* Rupture, membranes, premature
  blood (microscopic) , fetal, into maternal circulation affecting management of pregnancy — *see* Pregnancy, complicated by
  cerebrospinal fluid G96.0
    from spinal (lumbar) puncture G97.0
  device, implant or graft — *see also* Complications, by site and type, mechanical
    arterial graft NEC — *see* Complication, cardiovascular device, mechanical, vascular
    breast (implant) T85.43
    catheter NEC T85.638
      urinary T83.038
        cystostomy T83.030
        Hopkins T83.038
        ileostomy T83.038
        indwelling T83.031
        nephrostomy T83.032
        specified NEC T83.038
        urostomy T83.038
    dialysis (renal) T82.43
      intraperitoneal T85.631
    infusion NEC T82.534
      spinal (epidural) (subdural) T85.630
    gastrointestinal — *see* Complications, prosthetic device, mechanical, gastrointestinal device
    genital NEC T83.498
      penile prosthesis (cylinder) (implanted) (pump) (resevoir) T83.490
      testicular prosthesis T83.491
    heart NEC — *see* Complication, cardiovascular device, mechanical
    joint prosthesis — *see* Complications, joint prosthesis, mechanical, specified NEC, by site
    ocular NEC — *see* Complications, prosthetic device, mechanical, ocular device
    orthopedic NEC — *see* Complication, orthopedic, device, mechanical
    persistent air J93.82
    specified NEC T85.638
    urinary NEC — *see also* Complication, genitourinary, device, urinary, mechanical
      graft T83.23
    vascular NEC — *see* Complication, cardiovascular device, mechanical
    ventricular intracranial shunt T85.03
  urine — *see* Incontinence
Leaky heart — *see* Endocarditis
Learning defect (specific) F81.9
Leather bottle stomach C16.9
Leber's
  congenital amaurosis H35.50
  optic atrophy (hereditary) H47.22
Lederer's anemia D59.1
Leeches (external) — *see* Hirudiniasis
Leg — *see* condition
Legg (-Calvé)
  -Perthes disease, syndrome or osteochondrosis M91.1-

Legionellosis A48.1
  nonpneumonic A48.2
Legionnaires'
  disease A48.1
    nonpneumonic A48.2
  pneumonia A48.1
Leigh's disease G31.82
Leiner's disease L21.1
Leiofibromyoma — *see* Leiomyoma
Leiomyoblastoma — *see* Neoplasm, connective tissue, benign
Leiomyofibroma — *see also* Neoplasm, connective tissue, benign
  uterus (cervix) (corpus) D25.9
Leiomyoma — *see also* Neoplasm, connective tissue, benign
  bizarre — *see* Neoplasm, connective tissue, benign
  cellular — *see* Neoplasm, connective tissue, benign
  epithelioid — *see* Neoplasm, connective tissue, benign
  uterus (cervix) (corpus) D25.9
    intramural D25.1
    submucous D25.0
    subserosal D25.2
  vascular — *see* Neoplasm, connective tissue, benign
Leiomyoma, leiomyomatosis (intravascular) — *see* Neoplasm, connective tissue, uncertain behavior
Leiomyosarcoma — *see also* Neoplasm, connective tissue, malignant
  epithelioid — *see* Neoplasm, connective tissue, malignant
  myxoid — *see* Neoplasm, connective tissue, malignant
Leishmaniasis B55.9
  American (mucocutaneous) B55.2
    cutaneous B55.1
  Asian Desert B55.1
  Brazilian B55.2
  cutaneous (any type) B55.1
  dermal — *see also* Leishmaniasis, cutaneous
    post-kala-azar B55.0
  eyelid B55.1
  infantile B55.0
  Mediterranean B55.0
  mucocutaneous (American) (New World) B55.2
  naso-oral B55.2
  nasopharyngeal B55.2
  old world B55.1
  tegumentaria diffusa B55.1
  visceral B55.0
Leishmanoid, dermal — *see also* Leishmaniasis, cutaneous
  post-kala-azar B55.0
Lenegre's disease I44.2
Lengthening, leg — *see* Deformity, limb, unequal length
Lennert's lymphoma — *see* Lymphoma, Lennert's
Lennox-Gastaut syndrome G40.812
  intractable G40.814
    with status epilepticus G40.813
    without status epilepticus G40.814
  not intractable G40.812
    with status epilepticus G40.811
    without status epilepticus G40.812
Lens — *see* condition
Lenticonus (anterior) (posterior) (congenital) Q12.8
Lenticular degeneration, progressive E83.01
Lentiglobus (posterior) (congenital) Q12.8
Lentigo (congenital) L81.4
  maligna — *see also* Melanoma, in situ
    melanoma — *see* Melanoma
Lentivirus, as cause of disease classified elsewhere B97.31
Leontiasis
  ossium M85.2
  syphilitic (late) A52.78
    congenital A50.59
Lepothrix A48.8
Lepra — *see* Leprosy
Leprechaunism E34.8
Leprosy A30.-
  with muscle disorder A30.9 *[M63.80]*
    ankle A30.9 *[M63.87-]*
    foot A30.9 *[M63.87-]*
    forearm A30.9 *[M63.83-]*
    hand A30.9 *[M63.84-]*
    lower leg A30.9 *[M63.86-]*
    multiple sites A30.9 *[M63.89]*
    pelvic region A30.9 *[M63.85-]*
    shoulder region A30.9 *[M63.81-]*
    specified site NEC A30.9 *[M63.88]*
    thigh A30.9 *[M63.85-]*
    upper arm A30.9 *[M63.82-]*

Leprosy - *continued*
  anesthetic A30.9
  BB A30.3
  BL A30.4
  borderline (infiltrated) (neuritic) A30.3
    lepromatous A30.4
    tuberculoid A30.2
  BT A30.2
  dimorphous (infiltrated) (neuritic) A30.3
  I A30.0
  indeterminate (macular) (neuritic) A30.0
  lepromatous (diffuse) (infiltrated) (macular) (neuritic) (nodular) A30.5
  LL A30.5
  macular (early) (neuritic) (simple) A30.9
  maculoanesthetic A30.9
  mixed A30.3
  neural A30.9
  nodular A30.5
  primary neuritic A30.3
  specified type NEC A30.8
  TT A30.1
  tuberculoid (major) (minor) A30.1
Leptocytosis, hereditary D56.9
Leptomeningitis (chronic) (circumscribed) (hemorrhagic) (nonsuppurative) — *see* Meningitis
Leptomeningopathy G96.19
Leptospiral — *see* condition
Leptospirochetal — *see* condition
Leptospirosis A27.9
  canicola A27.89
  due to Leptospira interrogans serovar icterohaemorrhagiae A27.0
  icterohemorrhagica A27.0
  pomona A27.89
  Weil's disease A27.0
Leptus dermatitis B88.0
Leriche's syndrome (aortic bifurcation occlusion) I74.09
Leri's pleonosteosis Q78.8
Leri-Weill syndrome Q77.8
Lermoyez' syndrome — *see* Vertigo, peripheral NEC
Lesch-Nyhan syndrome E79.1
Leser-Trélat disease L82.1
  inflamed L82.0
Lesion (s) (nontraumatic)
  abducens nerve — *see* Strabismus, paralytic, sixth nerve
  alveolar process K08.9
  angiocentric immunoproliferative D47.Z9
  anorectal K62.9
  aortic (valve) I35.9
  auditory nerve — *see* subcategory H93.3
  basal ganglion G25.9
  bile duct — *see* Disease, bile duct
  biomechanical M99.9
    specified type NEC M99.89
      abdomen M99.89
      acromioclavicular M99.87
      cervical region M99.81
      cervicothoracic M99.81
      costochondral M99.88
      costovertebral M99.88
      head region M99.80
      hip M99.85
      lower extremity M99.86
      lumbar region M99.83
      lumbosacral M99.83
      occipitocervical M99.80
      pelvic region M99.85
      pubic M99.85
      rib cage M99.88
      sacral region M99.84
      sacrococcygeal M99.84
      sacroiliac M99.84
      specified NEC M99.89
      sternochondral M99.88
      sternoclavicular M99.87
      thoracic region M99.82
      thoracolumbar M99.82
      upper extremity M99.87
  bladder N32.9
  bone — *see* Disorder, bone
  brachial plexus G54.0
  brain G93.9
    congenital Q04.9
    vascular I67.9
      degenerative I67.9
      hypertensive I67.4
  buccal cavity K13.79
  calcified — *see* Calcification
  canthus — *see* Disorder, eyelid
  carate — *see* Pinta, lesions

Lesion (s) (nontraumatic) - *continued*
cardia K31.9
cardiac — *see also* Disease, heart I51.9
  congenital Q24.9
  valvular — *see* Endocarditis
cauda equina G83.4
cecum K63.9
cerebral — *see* Lesion, brain
cerebrovascular I67.9
  degenerative I67.9
  hypertensive I67.4
cervical (nerve) root NEC G54.2
chiasmal — *see* Disorder, optic, chiasm
chorda tympani G51.8
coin, lung R91.1
colon K63.9
combined periodontic - endodontic K05.5
congenital — *see* Anomaly, by site
conjunctiva H11.9
conus medullaris — *see* Injury, conus medullaris
coronary artery — *see* Ischemia, heart
cranial nerve G52.9
  eighth — *see* Disorder, ear
  eleventh G52.9
  fifth G50.9
  first G52.0
  fourth — *see* Strabismus, paralytic, fourth nerve
  seventh G51.9
  sixth — *see* Strabismus, paralytic, sixth nerve
  tenth G52.2
  twelfth G52.3
cystic — *see* Cyst
degenerative — *see* Degeneration
duodenum K31.9
edentulous (alveolar) ridge, associated with trauma, due to traumatic occlusion K06.2
en coup de sabre L94.1
eyelid — *see* Disorder, eyelid
gasserian ganglion G50.8
gastric K31.9
gastroduodenal K31.9
gastrointestinal K63.9
gingiva, associated with trauma K06.2
glomerular
  focal and segmental — *see also* N00-N07 with fourth character .1 N05.1
  minimal change — *see also* N00-N07 with fourth character .0 N05.0
heart (organic) — *see* Disease, heart
hyperchromic, due to pinta (carate) A67.1
hyperkeratotic — *see* Hyperkeratosis
hypothalamic E23.7
ileocecal K63.9
ileum K63.9
iliohypogastric nerve G57.8-
inflammatory — *see* Inflammation
intestine K63.9
intracerebral — *see* Lesion, brain
intrachiasmal (optic) — *see* Disorder, optic, chiasm
intracranial, space-occupying R90.0
joint — *see* Disorder, joint
  sacroiliac (old) M53.3
keratotic — *see* Keratosis
kidney — *see* Disease, renal
laryngeal nerve (recurrent) G52.2
lip K13.0
liver K76.9
lumbosacral
  plexus G54.1
  root (nerve) NEC G54.4
lung (coin) R91.1
maxillary sinus J32.0
mitral I05.9
Morel-Lavallée — *see* Hematoma, by site
motor cortex NEC G93.89
mouth K13.79
nerve G58.9
  femoral G57.2-
  median G56.1-
    carpal tunnel syndrome — *see* Syndrome, carpal tunnel
  plantar G57.6-
  popliteal (lateral) G57.3-
    medial G57.4-
  radial G56.3-
  sciatic G57.0-
  spinal — *see* Injury, nerve, spinal
  ulnar G56.2-
nervous system, congenital Q07.9
nonallopathic — *see* Lesion, biomechanical
nose (internal) J34.89
obstructive — *see* Obstruction
obturator nerve G57.8-

Lesion (s) (nontraumatic) - *continued*
oral mucosa K13.70
organ or site NEC — *see* Disease, by site
osteolytic — *see* Osteolysis
peptic K27.9
periodontal, due to traumatic occlusion K05.5
pharynx J39.2
pigment, pigmented (skin) L81.9
pinta — *see* Pinta, lesions
polypoid — *see* Polyp
prechiasmal (optic) — *see* Disorder, optic, chiasm
primary — *see also* Syphilis, primary A51.0
  carate A67.0
  pinta A67.0
  yaws A66.0
pulmonary J98.4
  valve I37.9
pylorus K31.9
rectosigmoid K63.9
retina, retinal H35.9
sacroiliac (joint) (old) M53.3
salivary gland K11.9
  benign lymphoepithelial K11.8
saphenous nerve G57.8-
sciatic nerve G57.0-
secondary — *see* Syphilis, secondary
shoulder (region) M75.9-
  specified NEC M75.8-
sigmoid K63.9
sinus (accessory) (nasal) J34.89
skin L98.9
  suppurative L08.0
SLAP S43.43-
spinal cord G95.9
  congenital Q06.9
spleen D73.89
stomach K31.9
superior glenoid labrum S43.43-
syphilitic — *see* Syphilis
tertiary — *see* Syphilis, tertiary
thoracic root (nerve) NEC G54.3
tonsillar fossa J35.9
tooth, teeth K08.9
  white spot
    chewing surface K02.51
    pit and fissure surface K02.51
    smooth surface K02.61
traumatic — *see* specific type of injury by site
tricuspid (valve) I07.9
  nonrheumatic I36.9
trigeminal nerve G50.9
ulcerated or ulcerative — *see* Ulcer, skin
uterus N85.9
vagus nerve G52.2
valvular — *see* Endocarditis
vascular I99.9
  affecting central nervous system I67.9
  following trauma NEC T14.8
  umbilical cord, complicating delivery O69.5
warty — *see* Verruca
white spot (tooth)
  chewing surface K02.51
  pit and fissure surface K02.51
  smooth surface K02.61
Lethargic — *see* condition
Lethargy R53.83
Letterer-Siwe's disease C96.0
Leukemia, leukemic C95.9-
acute basophilic C94.8-
acute bilineal C95.0-
acute erythroid C94.0-
acute lymphoblastic C91.0-
acute megakaryoblastic C94.2-
acute megakaryocytic C94.2-
acute mixed lineage C95.0-
acute monoblastic (monoblastic/monocytic) C93.0-
acute monocytic (monoblastic/monocytic) C93.0-
acute myeloblastic (minimal differentiation) (with maturation) C92.0-
acute myeloid
  with
    11q23-abnormality C92.6-
    dysplasia of remaining hematopoesis and/or myelodysplastic disease in its history C92.A-
    multilineage dysplasia C92.A-
    variation of MLL-gene C92.6-
  M6 (a) (b) C94.0-
  M7 C94.2-
acute myelomonocytic C92.5-
acute promyelocytic C92.4-
adult T-cell (HTLV-1-associated) (acute variant) (chronic variant) (lymphomatoid variant) (smouldering variant) C91.5-

Leukemia, leukemic - *continued*
aggressive NK-cell C94.8-
AML (1/ETO) (M0) (M1) (M2) (without a FAB classification) C92.0-
AML M3 C92.4-
AML M4 (Eo with inv (16) or t (16;16)) C92.5-
AML M5 C93.0-
AML M5a C93.0-
AML M5b C93.0-
AML Me with t (15;17) and variants C92.4-
atypical chronic myeloid, BCR/ABL-negative C92.2-
biphenotypic acute C95.0-
blast cell C95.0-
Burkitt-type, mature B-cell C91.A-
chronic lymphocytic, of B-cell type C91.1-
chronic monocytic C93.1-
chronic myelogenous (Philadelphia chromosome (Ph1) positive) (t (9;22)) (q34;q11) (with crisis of blast cells) C92.1-
chronic myeloid, BCR/ABL-positive C92.1-
  atypical, BCR/ABL-negative C92.2-
chronic myelomonocytic C93.1-
chronic neutrophilic D47.1
CMML (-1) (-2) (with eosinophilia) C93.1-
granulocytic (*see also* Category C92) C92.9-
hairy cell C91.4-
juvenile myelomonocytic C93.3-
lymphoid C91.9-
  specified NEC C91.Z-
mast cell C94.3-
mature B-cell, Burkitt-type C91.A-
monocytic (subacute) C93.9-
  specified NEC C93.Z-
myelogenous (*see also* Category C92) C92.9-
myeloid C92.9-
  specified NEC C92.Z-
plasma cell C90.1-
plasmacytic C90.1-
prolymphocytic
  of B-cell type C91.3-
  of T-cell type C91.6-
specified NEC C94.8-
stem cell, of unclear lineage C95.0-
subacute lymphocytic C91.9-
T-cell large granular lymphocytic C91.Z-
unspecified cell type C95.9-
  acute C95.0-
  chronic C95.1-
Leukemoid reaction — *see also* Reaction, leukemoid D72.823-
Leukoaraiosis (hypertensive) I67.81
Leukoariosis — *see* Leukoaraiosis
Leukocoria — *see* Disorder, globe, degenerated condition, leucocoria
Leukocytopenia D72.819
Leukocytosis D72.829
  eosinophilic D72.1
Leukoderma, leukodermia NEC L81.5
  syphilitic A51.39
  late A52.79
Leukodystrophy E75.29
Leukoedema, oral epithelium K13.29
Leukoencephalitis G04.81
  acute (subacute) hemorrhagic G36.1
    postimmunization or postvaccinal G04.02
  postinfectious G04.01
  subacute sclerosing A81.1
  van Bogaert's (sclerosing) A81.1
Leukoencephalopathy — *see*
  also Encephalopathy G93.49
  Binswanger's I67.3
  heroin vapor G92
  metachromatic E75.25
  multifocal (progressive) A81.2
  postimmunization and postvaccinal G04.02
  progressive multifocal A81.2
  reversible, posterior G93.6
  van Bogaert's (sclerosing) A81.1
  vascular, progressive I67.3
Leukoerythroblastosis D75.9
Leukokeratosis — *see also* Leukoplakia
  mouth K13.21
  nicotina palati K13.24
  oral mucosa K13.21
  tongue K13.21
  vocal cord J38.3
Leukokraurosis vulva (e) N90.4
Leukoma (cornea) — *see also* Opacity, cornea
  adherent H17.0-
  interfering with central vision — *see* Opacity, cornea, central

Leukomalacia, cerebral, newborn P91.2
  periventricular P91.2
Leukomelanopathy, hereditary D72.0
Leukonychia (punctata) (striata) L60.8
  congenital Q84.4
Leukopathia unguium L60.8
  congenital Q84.4
Leukopenia D72.819
  basophilic D72.818
  chemotherapy (cancer) induced D70.1
  congenital D70.0
  cyclic D70.0
  drug induced NEC D70.2
    due to cytoreductive cancer chemotherapy D70.1
  eosinophilic D72.818
  familial D70.0
  infantile genetic D70.0
  malignant D70.9
  periodic D70.0
  transitory neonatal P61.5
Leukopenic — see condition
Leukoplakia
  anus K62.89
  bladder (postinfectional) N32.89
  buccal K13.21
  cervix (uteri) N88.0
  esophagus K22.8
  gingiva K13.21
  hairy (oral mucosa) (tongue) K13.3
  kidney (pelvis) N28.89
  larynx J38.7
  lip K13.21
  mouth K13.21
  oral epithelium, including tongue (mucosa) K13.21
  palate K13.21
  pelvis (kidney) N28.89
  penis (infectional) N48.0
  rectum K62.89
  syphilitic (late) A52.79
  tongue K13.21
  ureter (postinfectional) N28.89
  urethra (postinfectional) N36.8
  uterus N85.8
  vagina N89.4
  vocal cord J38.3
  vulva N90.4
Leukorrhea N89.8
  due to Trichomonas (vaginalis) A59.00
  trichomonal A59.00
Leukosarcoma C85.9-
Levocardia (isolated) Q24.1
  with situs inversus Q89.3
Levotransposition Q20.5
Lev's disease or syndrome
  (acquired complete heart block) I44.2
Levulosuria — see Fructosuria
Levurid L30.2
Lewy body (ies) (dementia) (disease) G31.83
Leyden-Moebius dystrophy G71.0
Leydig cell
  carcinoma
    specified site — see Neoplasm, malignant, by site
    unspecified site
      female C56.9
      male C62.9-
  tumor
    benign
      specified site — see Neoplasm, benign, by site
      unspecified site
        female D27.-
        male D29.2-
    malignant
      specified site — see Neoplasm, malignant, by site
      unspecified site
        female C56.-
        male C62.9-
    specified site — see Neoplasm, uncertain behavior, by site
    unspecified site
      female D39.1-
      male D40.1-
Leydig-Sertoli cell tumor
  specified site — see Neoplasm, benign, by site
  unspecified site
    female D27.-
    male D29.2-
LGSIL
  (Low grade squamous intraepithelial lesion on cytologic smear of)
  anus R85.612
  cervix R87.612
  vagina R87.622
Liar, pathologic F60.2

Libido
  decreased R68.82
Libman-Sacks disease M32.11
Lice (infestation) B85.2
  body (Pediculus corporis) B85.1
  crab B85.3
  head (Pediculus capitis) B85.0
  mixed (classifiable to more than one of the titles B85.0-B85.3) B85.4
  pubic (Phthirus pubis) B85.3
Lichen L28.0
  albus L90.0
    penis N48.0
    vulva N90.4
  amyloidosis E85.4 [L99]
  atrophicus L90.0
    penis N48.0
    vulva N90.4
  congenital Q82.8
  myxedematosus L98.5
  nitidus L44.1
  pilaris Q82.8
    acquired L85.8
  planopilaris L66.1
  planus (chronicus) L43.9
    annularis L43.8
    bullous L43.1
    follicular L66.1
    hypertrophic L43.0
    moniliformis L44.3
    of Wilson L43.9
    specified NEC L43.8
    subacute (active) L43.3
    tropicus L43.3
  ruber
    acuminatus L44.0
    moniliformis L44.3
    planus L43.9
  sclerosus (et atrophicus) L90.0
    penis N48.0
    vulva N90.4
  scrofulosus (primary) (tuberculous) A18.4
  simplex (chronicus) (circumscriptus) L28.0
  striatus L44.2
  urticatus L28.2
Lichenification L28.0
Lichenoides tuberculosis (primary) A18.4
Lichtheim's disease or syndrome — see Degeneration, combined
Lien migrans D73.89
Ligament — see condition
Light
  for gestational age — see Light for dates
  headedness R42
Light-for-dates (infant) P05.00
  with weight of
    499 grams or less P05.01
    500-749 grams P05.02
    750-999 grams P05.03
    1000-1249 grams P05.04
    1250-1499 grams P05.05
    1500-1749 grams P05.06
    1750-1999 grams P05.07
    2000-2499 grams P05.08
    2500 grams and over P05.09
  specified NEC P05.09
  and small-for-dates — see Small for dates
  affecting management of pregnancy O36.59-
Lightning (effects) (stroke) (struck by) T75.00
  burn — see Burn
  foot E53.8
  shock T75.01
  specified effect NEC T75.09
Lightwood-Albright syndrome N25.89
Lightwood's disease or syndrome
  (renal tubular acidosis) N25.89
Lignac (-de Toni) (-Fanconi) (-Debré) **disease or syndrome** E72.09
  with cystinosis E72.04
Ligneous thyroiditis E06.5
Likoff's syndrome I20.8
Limb — see condition
Limbic epilepsy personality syndrome F07.0
Limitation, limited
  activities due to disability Z73.6
  cardiac reserve — see Disease, heart
  eye muscle duction, traumatic — see Strabismus, mechanical
  mandibular range of motion M26.52
Lindau (-von Hippel) **disease** Q85.8
Line (s)
  Beau's L60.4
  Harris' — see Arrest, epiphyseal

Line (s) - continued
  Hudson's (cornea) — see Pigmentation, cornea, anterior
  Stähli's (cornea) — see Pigmentation, cornea, anterior
Linea corneae senilis — see Change, cornea, senile
Lingua
  geographica K14.1
  nigra (villosa) K14.3
  plicata K14.5
  tylosis K13.29
Lingual — see condition
Linguatulosis B88.8
Linitis (gastric) **plastica C16.9**
Lip — see condition
Lipedema — see Edema
Lipemia — see also Hyperlipidemia
  retina, retinalis E78.3
Lipidosis E75.6
  cerebral (infantile) (juvenile) (late) E75.4
  cerebroretinal E75.4
  cerebroside E75.22
  cholesterol (cerebral) E75.5
  glycolipid E75.21
  hepatosplenomegalic E78.3
  sphingomyelin — see Niemann-Pick disease or syndrome
  sulfatide E75.29
Lipoadenoma — see Neoplasm, benign, by site
Lipoblastoma — see Lipoma
Lipoblastomatosis — see Lipoma
Lipochondrodystrophy E76.01
Lipochrome histiocytosis (familial) D71
Lipodermatosclerosis — see Varix, leg, with, inflammation
  ulcerated — see Varix, leg, with, ulcer, with inflammation by site
Lipodystrophia progressiva E88.1
Lipodystrophy (progressive) E88.1
  insulin E88.1
  intestinal K90.81
  mesenteric K65.4
Lipofibroma — see Lipoma
Lipofuscinosis, neuronal (with ceroidosis) E75.4
Lipogranuloma, sclerosing L92.8
Lipogranulomatosis E78.89
Lipoid — see also condition
  histiocytosis D76.3
    essential E75.29
  nephrosis N04.9
  proteinosis of Urbach E78.89
Lipoidemia — see Hyperlipidemia
Lipoidosis — see Lipidosis
Lipoma D17.9
  fetal D17.9
  fat cell D17.9
  infiltrating D17.9
  intramuscular D17.9
  pleomorphic D17.9
  site classification
    arms (skin) (subcutaneous) D17.2-
    connective tissue D17.30
      intra-abdominal D17.5
      intrathoracic D17.4
      peritoneum D17.79
      retroperitoneum D17.79
      specified site NEC D17.39
      spermatic cord D17.6
    face (skin) (subcutaneous) D17.0
    genitourinary organ NEC D17.72
    head (skin) (subcutaneous) D17.0
    intra-abdominal D17.5
    intrathoracic D17.4
    kidney D17.71
    legs (skin) (subcutaneous) D17.2-
    neck (skin) (subcutaneous) D17.0
    peritoneum D17.79
    retroperitoneum D17.79
    skin D17.30
      specified site NEC D17.39
    specified site NEC D17.79
    spermatic cord D17.6
    subcutaneous D17.30
      specified site NEC D17.39
    trunk (skin) (subcutaneous) D17.1
    unspecified D17.9
  spindle cell D17.9
Lipomatosis E88.2
  dolorosa (Dercum) E88.2
  fetal — see Lipoma
  Launois-Bensaude E88.89
Lipomyoma — see Lipoma
Lipomyxoma — see Lipoma

Lipomyxosarcoma — *see* Neoplasm, connective tissue, malignant
Lipoprotein metabolism disorder E78.9
Lipoproteinemia E78.5
  broad-beta E78.2
  floating-beta E78.2
  hyper-pre-beta E78.1
Liposarcoma — *see also* Neoplasm, connective tissue, malignant
  dedifferentiated — *see* Neoplasm, connective tissue, malignant
  differentiated type — *see* Neoplasm, connective tissue, malignant
  embryonal — *see* Neoplasm, connective tissue, malignant
  mixed type — *see* Neoplasm, connective tissue, malignant
  myxoid — *see* Neoplasm, connective tissue, malignant
  pleomorphic — *see* Neoplasm, connective tissue, malignant
  round cell — *see* Neoplasm, connective tissue, malignant
  well differentiated type — *see* Neoplasm, connective tissue, malignant
Liposynovitis prepatellaris E88.89
Lipping, cervix N86
Lipschütz disease or ulcer N76.6
Lipuria R82.0
  schistosomiasis (bilharziasis) B65.0
Lisping F80.0
Lissauer's paralysis A52.17
Lissencephalia, lissencephaly Q04.3
Listeriosis, listerellosis A32.9
  congenital (disseminated) P37.2
  cutaneous A32.0
  neonatal, newborn (disseminated) P37.2
  oculoglandular A32.81
  specified NEC A32.89
Lithemia E79.0
Lithiasis — *see* Calculus
Lithosis J62.8
Lithuria R82.99
Litigation, anxiety concerning Z65.3
Little leaguer's elbow — *see* Epicondylitis, medial
Little's disease G80.9
Littre's
  gland — *see* condition
  hernia — *see* Hernia, abdomen
Littritis — *see* Urethritis
Livedo (annularis) (racemosa) (reticularis) R23.1
Liver — *see* condition
Living alone (problems with) Z60.2
  with handicapped person Z74.2
Lloyd's syndrome — *see* Adenomatosis, endocrine
Loa loa, loaiasis, loasis B74.3
Lobar — *see* condition
Lobomycosis B48.0
Lobo's disease B48.0
Lobotomy syndrome F07.0
Lobstein (-Ekman) **disease or syndrome** Q78.0
Lobster-claw hand Q71.6-
Lobulation (congenital) — *see also* Anomaly, by site
  kidney, Q63.1
  liver, abnormal Q44.7
  spleen Q89.09
Lobule, lobular — *see* condition
Local, localized — *see* condition
Locked twins causing obstructed labor O66.1
Locked-in state G83.5
Locking
  joint — *see* Derangement, joint, specified type NEC
  knee — *see* Derangement, knee
Lockjaw — *see* Tetanus
Löffler's
  endocarditis I42.3
  eosinophilia J82
  pneumonia J82
  syndrome (eosinophilic pneumonitis) J82
Loiasis (with conjunctival infestation) (eyelid) B74.3
Lone Star fever A77.0
Long
  labor O63.9
    first stage O63.0
    second stage O63.1
  QT syndrome I45.81
Longitudinal stripes or grooves, nails L60.8
  congenital Q84.6
Long-term (current) (prophylactic) **drug therapy** (use of)
  agents affecting estrogen receptors and estrogen levels NEC Z79.818
  anastrozole (Arimidex) Z79.811

Long-term (current) (prophylactic) **drug therapy** (use of) - *continued*
  antibiotics Z79.2
    short-term use - omit code
  anticoagulants Z79.01
  anti-inflammatory, non-steroidal (NSAID) Z79.1
  antiplatelet Z79.02
  antithrombotics Z79.02
  aromatase inhibitors Z79.811
  aspirin Z79.82
  birth control pill or patch Z79.3
  bisphosphonates Z79.83
  contraceptive, oral Z79.3
  drug, specified NEC Z79.899
  estrogen receptor downregulators Z79.818
  Evista Z79.810
  exemestane (Aromasin) Z79.811
  Fareston Z79.810
  fulvestrant (Faslodex) Z79.818
  gonadotropin-releasing hormone (GnRH) agonist Z79.818
  goserelin acetate (Zoladex) Z79.818
  hormone replacement (postmenopausal) Z79.890
  insulin Z79.4
  letrozole (Femara) Z79.811
  leuprolide acetate (leuprorelin) (Lupron) Z79.818
  megestrol acetate (Megace) Z79.818
  methadone for pain management Z79.891
  Nolvadex Z79.810
  non-steroidal anti-inflammatories (NSAID) Z79.1
  opiate analgesic Z79.891
  oral
    antidiabetic Z79.84
    contraceptive Z79.3
    hypoglycemic Z79.84
  raloxifene (Evista) Z79.810
  selective estrogen receptor modulators (SERMs) Z79.810
  steroids
    inhaled Z79.51
    systemic Z79.52
  tamoxifen (Nolvadex) Z79.810
  toremifene (Fareston) Z79.810
Loop
  intestine — *see* Volvulus
  vascular on papilla (optic) Q14.2
Loose — *see also* condition
  body
    joint M24.00
      ankle M24.07-
      elbow M24.02-
      hand M24.04-
      hip M24.05-
      knee M23.4-
      shoulder (region) M24.01-
      specified site NEC M24.08
      vertebra M24.08
      toe M24.07-
      wrist M24.03-
    knee M23.4-
    sheath, tendon — *see* Disorder, tendon, specified type NEC
  cartilage — *see* Loose, body, joint
  skin and subcutaneous tissue (following bariatric surgery weight loss) (following dietary weight loss) L98.7
  tooth, teeth K08.89
Loosening
  aseptic
    joint prosthesis — *see* Complications, joint prosthesis, mechanical, loosening, by site
  epiphysis — *see* Osteochondropathy
  mechanical
    joint prosthesis — *see* Complications, joint prosthesis, mechanical, loosening, by site
Looser-Milkman (-Debray) **syndrome** M83.8
Lop ear (deformity) Q17.3
Lorain (-Levi) **short stature syndrome** E23.0
Lordosis M40.50
  acquired — *see* Lordosis, specified type NEC
  congenital Q76.429
    lumbar region Q76.426
    lumbosacral region Q76.427
    sacral region Q76.428
    sacrococcygeal region Q76.428
    thoracolumbar region Q76.425
  lumbar region M40.56
  lumbosacral region M40.57
  postsurgical M96.4
  postural — *see* Lordosis, specified type NEC
  rachitic (late effect) (sequelae) E64.3
  sequelae of rickets E64.3
  specified type NEC M40.40

Lordosis - *continued*
  specified type NEC - *continued*
    lumbar region M40.46
    lumbosacral region M40.47
    thoracolumbar region M40.45
    thoracolumbar region M40.55
    tuberculous A18.01
Loss (of)
  appetite (see Anorexia) R63.0
    hysterical F50.89
    nonorganic origin F50.89
    psychogenic F50.89
  blood — *see* Hemorrhage
  bone — *see* Loss, substance of, bone
  control, sphincter, rectum R15.9
    nonorganic origin F98.1
  consciousness, transient R55
    traumatic — *see* Injury, intracranial
  elasticity, skin R23.4
  family (member) in childhood Z62.898
  fluid (acute) E86.9
  function of labyrinth — *see* subcategory H83.2
  hair, nonscarring — *see* Alopecia
  hearing — *see also* Deafness
    central NOS H90.5
    conductive H90.2
      bilateral H90.0
      unilateral
        with
          restricted hearing on the contralateral side H90.A1-
          unrestricted hearing on the contralateral side H90.1-
    mixed conductive and sensorineural hearing loss H90.8
      bilateral H90.6
      unilateral
        with
          restricted hearing on the contralateral side H90.A3-
          unrestricted hearing on the contralateral side H90.7-
    neural NOS H90.5
    perceptive NOS H90.5
    sensorineural NOS H90.5
      bilateral H90.3
      unilateral
        with
          restricted hearing on the contralateral side H90.A2-
          unrestricted hearing on the contralateral side H90.4-
    sensory NOS H90.5
  height R29.890
  limb or member, traumatic, current — *see* Amputation, traumatic
  love relationship in childhood Z62.898
  memory — *see also* Amnesia
    mild, following organic brain damage F06.8
  mind — *see* Psychosis
  occlusal vertical dimension of fully erupted teeth M26.37
  organ or part — *see* Absence, by site, acquired
  ossicles, ear (partial) H74.32-
  parent in childhood Z63.4
  pregnancy, recurrent N96
    care in current pregnancy O26.2-
    without current pregnancy N96
  recurrent pregnancy — *see* Loss, pregnancy, recurrent
  self-esteem, in childhood Z62.898
  sense of
    smell — *see* Disturbance, sensation, smell
    taste — *see* Disturbance, sensation, taste
    touch R20.8
  sensory R44.9
    dissociative F44.6
  sexual desire F52.0
  sight (acquired) (complete) (congenital) — *see* Blindness
  substance of
    bone — *see* Disorder, bone, density and structure, specified NEC
      horizontal alveolar K06.3
    cartilage — *see* Disorder, cartilage, specified type NEC
      auricle (ear) — *see* Disorder, pinna, specified type NEC
    vitreous (humor) H15.89
  tooth, teeth — *see* Absence, teeth, acquired
  vision, visual H54.7
    both eyes H54.3
    one eye H54.60

Loss (of) - *continued*
  vision, visual - *continued*
    one eye - *continued*
      left (normal vision on right) H54.62
      right (normal vision on left) H54.61
    specified as blindness — *see* Blindness
    subjective
      sudden H53.13-
      transient H53.12-
  vitreous — *see* Prolapse, vitreous
  voice — *see* Aphonia
  weight (abnormal) (cause unknown) R63.4
Louis-Bar syndrome (ataxia-telangiectasia) G11.3
Louping ill (encephalitis) A84.8
Louse, lousiness — *see* Lice
Low
  achiever, school Z55.3
  back syndrome M54.5
  basal metabolic rate R94.8
  birthweight (2499 grams or less) P07.10
    with weight of
      1000-1249 grams P07.14
      1250-1499 grams P07.15
      1500-1749 grams P07.16
      1750-1999 grams P07.17
      2000-2499 grams P07.18
    extreme (999 grams or less) P07.00
      with weight of
        499 grams or less P07.01
        500-749 grams P07.02
        750-999 grams P07.03
    for gestational age — *see* Light for dates
  blood pressure — *see also* Hypotension
    reading (incidental) (isolated) (nonspecific) R03.1
  cardiac reserve — *see* Disease, heart
  function — *see also* Hypofunction
    kidney N28.9
  hematocrit D64.9
  hemoglobin D64.9
  income Z59.6
  level of literacy Z55.0
  lying
    kidney N28.89
    organ or site, congenital — *see* Malposition, congenital
  output syndrome (cardiac) — *see* Failure, heart
  platelets (blood) — *see* Thrombocytopenia
  reserve, kidney N28.89
  salt syndrome E87.1
  self esteem R45.81
  set ears Q17.4
  vision H54.2
    one eye (other eye normal) H54.50
      left (normal vision on right) H54.52
      other eye blind — *see* Blindness
      right (normal vision on left) H54.51
Low-density-lipoprotein-type (LDL)
  hyperlipoproteinemia E78.00
Lowe's syndrome E72.03
Lown-Ganong-Levine syndrome I45.6
LSD reaction (acute) (without dependence) F16.90
  with dependence F16.20
L-shaped kidney Q63.8
Ludwig's angina or disease K12.2
Lues (venerea) **, luetic** — *see* Syphilis
Luetscher's syndrome (dehydration) E86.0
Lumbago, lumbalgia M54.5
  with sciatica M54.4-
    due to intervertebral disc disorder M51.17
  due to displacement, intervertebral disc M51.27
    with sciatica M51.17
Lumbar — *see* condition
Lumbarization, vertebra, congenital Q76.49
Lumbermen's itch B88.0
Lump — *see* Mass
Lunacy — *see* Psychosis
Lung — *see* condition
Lupoid (miliary) **of Boeck** D86.3
Lupus
  anticoagulant D68.62
    with
      hemorrhagic disorder D68.312
      hypercoagulable state D68.62
    finding without diagnosis R76.0
  discoid (local) L93.0
  erythematosus (discoid) (local) L93.0
    disseminated — *see* Lupus, erythematosus, systemic
    eyelid H01.129
      left H01.126
        lower H01.125
        upper H01.124
      right H01.123

Lupus - *continued*
  erythematosus (discoid) (local) - *continued*
    eyelid - *continued*
      right - *continued*
        lower H01.122
        upper H01.121
    profundus L93.2
    specified NEC L93.2
    subacute cutaneous L93.1
    systemic M32.9
      with organ or system involvement M32.10
        endocarditis M32.11
        lung M32.13
        pericarditis M32.12
        renal (glomerular) M32.14
          tubulo-interstitial M32.15
        specified organ or system NEC M32.19
      drug-induced M32.0
      inhibitor (presence of) D68.62
        with
          hemorrhagic disorder D68.312
          hypercoagulable state D68.62
        finding without diagnosis R76.0
      specified NEC M32.8
    exedens A18.4
    hydralazine M32.0
      correct substance properly administered — *see* Table of Drugs and Chemicals, by drug, adverse effect
      overdose or wrong substance given or taken — *see* Table of Drugs and Chemicals, by drug, poisoning
    nephritis (chronic) M32.14
    nontuberculous, not disseminated L93.0
    panniculitis L93.2
    pernio (Besnier) D86.3
    systemic — *see* Lupus, erythematosus, systemic
    tuberculous A18.4
      eyelid A18.4
    vulgaris A18.4
      eyelid A18.4
Luteinoma D27.-
Lutembacher's disease or syndrome
  (atrial septal defect with mitral stenosis) Q21.1
Luteoma D27.-
Lutz (-Splendore-de Almeida) **disease** — *see* Paracoccidioidomycosis
Luxation — *see also* Dislocation
  eyeball (nontraumatic) — *see* Luxation, globe
    birth injury P15.3
  globe, nontraumatic H44.82-
  lacrimal gland — *see* Dislocation, lacrimal gland
  lens (old) (partial) (spontaneous)
    congenital Q12.1
    syphilitic A50.39
Lycanthropy F22
Lyell's syndrome L51.2
  due to drug L51.2
    correct substance properly administered — *see* Table of Drugs and Chemicals, by drug, adverse effect
    overdose or wrong substance given or taken — *see* Table of Drugs and Chemicals, by drug, poisoning
Lyme disease A69.20
Lymph
  gland or node — *see* condition
  scrotum — *see* Infestation, filarial
Lymphadenitis I88.9
  with ectopic or molar pregnancy O08.0
  acute L04.9
    axilla L04.2
    face L04.0
    head L04.0
    hip L04.3
    limb
      lower L04.3
      upper L04.2
    neck L04.0
    shoulder L04.2
    specified site NEC L04.8
    trunk L04.1
  anthracosis (occupational) J60
  any site, except mesenteric I88.9
    chronic I88.1
    subacute I88.1
  breast
    gestational — *see* Mastitis, obstetric
    puerperal, postpartum (nonpurulent) O91.22
  chancroidal (congenital) A57
  chronic I88.1
    mesenteric I88.0
  due to

Lymphadenitis - *continued*
  due to - *continued*
    Brugia (malayi) B74.1
      timori B74.2
    chlamydial lymphogranuloma A55
    diphtheria (toxin) A36.89
    lymphogranuloma venereum A55
    Wuchereria bancrofti B74.0
  following ectopic or molar pregnancy O08.0
  gonorrheal A54.89
  infective — *see* Lymphadenitis, acute
  mesenteric (acute) (chronic) (nonspecific) (subacute) I88.0
    due to Salmonella typhi A01.09
    tuberculous A18.39
  mycobacterial A31.8
  purulent — *see* Lymphadenitis, acute
  pyogenic — *see* Lymphadenitis, acute
  regional, nonbacterial I88.8
  septic — *see* Lymphadenitis, acute
  subacute, unspecified site I88.1
  suppurative — *see* Lymphadenitis, acute
  syphilitic (early) (secondary) A51.49
    late A52.79
  tuberculous — *see* Tuberculosis, lymph gland
  venereal (chlamydial) A55
Lymphadenoid goiter E06.3
Lymphadenopathy (generalized) R59.1
  angioimmunoblastic, with dysproteinemia (AILD) C86.5
  due to toxoplasmosis (acquired) B58.89
    congenital (acute) (subacute) (chronic) P37.1
  localized R59.0
  syphilitic (early) (secondary) A51.49
Lymphadenosis R59.1
Lymphangiectasis I89.0
  conjunctiva H11.89
  postinfectional I89.0
  scrotum I89.0
Lymphangiectatic elephantiasis, nonfilarial I89.0
Lymphangioendothelioma D18.1
  malignant — *see* Neoplasm, connective tissue, malignant
Lymphangioleiomyomatosis J84.81
Lymphangioma D18.1
  capillary D18.1
  cavernous D18.1
  cystic D18.1
  malignant — *see* Neoplasm, connective tissue, malignant
Lymphangiomyoma D18.1
Lymphangiomyomatosis J84.81
Lymphangiosarcoma — *see* Neoplasm, connective tissue, malignant
Lymphangitis I89.1
  with
    abscess - code by site under Abscess
    cellulitis - code by site under Cellulitis
    ectopic or molar pregnancy O08.0
  acute L03.91
    abdominal wall L03.321
    ankle — *see* Lymphangitis, acute, lower limb
    arm — *see* Lymphangitis, acute, upper limb
    auricle (ear) — *see* Lymphangitis, acute, ear
    axilla L03.12-
    back (any part) L03.322
    buttock L03.327
    cervical (meaning neck) L03.222
    cheek (external) L03.212
    chest wall L03.323
    digit
      finger — *see* Lymphangitis, acute, finger
      toe — *see* Lymphangitis, acute, toe
    ear (external) H60.1-
    external auditory canal — *see* Lymphangitis, acute, ear
    eyelid — *see* Abscess, eyelid
    face NEC L03.212
    finger (intrathecal) (periosteal) (subcutaneous) (subcuticular) L03.02-
    foot — *see* Lymphangitis, acute, lower limb
    gluteal (region) L03.327
    groin L03.324
    hand — *see* Lymphangitis, acute, upper limb
    head NEC L03.891
      face (any part, except ear, eye and nose) L03.212
    heel — *see* Lymphangitis, acute, lower limb
    hip — *see* Lymphangitis, acute, lower limb
    jaw (region) L03.212
    knee — *see* Lymphangitis, acute, lower limb
    leg — *see* Lymphangitis, acute, lower limb
    lower limb L03.12-
      toe — *see* Lymphangitis, acute, toe

Lymphangitis - *continued*
  acute - *continued*
    navel L03.326
    neck (region) L03.222
    orbit, orbital — *see* Cellulitis, orbit
    pectoral (region) L03.323
    perineal, perineum L03.325
    scalp (any part) L03.891
    shoulder — *see* Lymphangitis, acute, upper limb
    specified site NEC L03.898
    thigh — *see* Lymphangitis, acute, lower limb
    thumb (intrathecal) (periosteal) (subcutaneous)
      (subcuticular) — *see* Lymphangitis, acute, finger
    toe (intrathecal) (periosteal) (subcutaneous)
      (subcuticular) L03.04-
    trunk L03.329
      abdominal wall L03.321
      back (any part) L03.322
      buttock L03.327
      chest wall L03.323
      groin L03.324
      perineal, perineum L03.325
      umbilicus L03.326
    umbilicus L03.326
    upper limb L03.12-
      axilla — *see* Lymphangitis, acute, axilla
      finger — *see* Lymphangitis, acute, finger
      thumb — *see* Lymphangitis, acute, finger
      wrist — *see* Lymphangitis, acute, upper limb
  breast
    gestational — *see* Mastitis, obstetric
  chancroidal A57
  chronic (any site) I89.1
  due to
    Brugia (malayi) B74.1
    timori B74.2
    Wuchereria bancrofti B74.0
  following ectopic or molar pregnancy O08.89
  penis
    acute N48.29
    gonococcal (acute) (chronic) A54.09
  puerperal, postpartum, childbirth O86.89
  strumous, tuberculous A18.2
  subacute (any site) I89.1
  tuberculous — *see* Tuberculosis, lymph gland
Lymphatic (vessel) — *see* condition
Lymphatism E32.8
Lymphectasia I89.0
Lymphedema (acquired) — *see also* Elephantiasis
  congenital Q82.0
  hereditary (chronic) (idiopathic) Q82.0
  postmastectomy I97.2
  praecox I89.0
  secondary I89.0
  surgical NEC I97.89
    postmastectomy (syndrome) I97.2
Lymphoblastic — *see* condition
Lymphoblastoma (diffuse) — *see* Lymphoma,
  lymphoblastic (diffuse)
  giant follicular — *see* Lymphoma, lymphoblastic
    (diffuse)
  macrofollicular — *see* Lymphoma, lymphoblastic
    (diffuse)
Lymphocele I89.8
Lymphocytic
  chorioencephalitis (acute) (serous) A87.2
  choriomeningitis (acute) (serous) A87.2
  meningoencephalitis A87.2
Lymphocytoma, benign cutis L98.8
Lymphocytopenia D72.810
Lymphocytosis (symptomatic) D72.820
  infectious (acute) B33.8
Lymphoepithelioma — *see* Neoplasm, malignant, by
  site
Lymphogranuloma (malignant) — *see*
  also Lymphoma, Hodgkin
  chlamydial A55
  inguinale A55
  venereum (any site) (chlamydial) (with stricture of
    rectum) A55
Lymphogranulomatosis (malignant) — *see*
  also Lymphoma, Hodgkin
  benign (Boeck's sarcoid) (Schaumann's) D86.1
Lymphohistiocytosis, hemophagocytic
  (familial) D76.1
Lymphoid — *see* condition
Lymphoma (of) (malignant) C85.90
  adult (HTLV-1-associated) (acute variant)
    (chronic variant) (lymphomatoid variant)
    (smouldering variant) C91.5-
  anaplastic large cell
    ALK-negative C84.7-
    ALK-positive C84.6-

Lymphoma (of) (malignant) - *continued*
  anaplastic large cell - *continued*
    CD30-positive C84.6-
      primary cutaneous C86.6
  angioimmunoblastic T-cell C86.5
  BALT C88.4
  B-cell C85.1-
  B-precursor C83.5-
  blastic NK-cell C86.4
  bronchial-associated lymphoid tissue [BALT-
    lymphoma] C88.4
  Burkitt (atypical) C83.7-
  Burkitt-like C83.7-
  centrocytic C83.1-
  cutaneous follicle center C82.6-
  cutaneous T-cell C84.A-
  diffuse follicle center C82.5-
  diffuse large cell C83.3-
    anaplastic C83.3-
    B-cell C83.3-
    CD30-positive C83.3-
    centroblastic C83.3-
    immunoblastic C83.3-
    plasmablastic C83.3-
    subtype not specified C83.3-
    T-cell rich C83.3-
  enteropathy-type (associated) (intestinal) T-
    cell C86.2
  extranodal NK/T-cell, nasal type C86.0
  extranodal marginal zone B-cell lymphoma of
    mucosa-associated lymphoid tissue [MALT-
    lymphoma] C88.4
  follicular C82.9-
    grade
      I C82.0-
      II C82.1-
      III C82.2-
      IIIa C82.3-
      IIIb C82.4-
    specified NEC C82.8-
  hepatosplenic T-cell (alpha-beta) (gamma-
    delta) C86.1
  histiocytic C85.9-
    true C96.A
  Hodgkin C81.9
    lymphocyte-rich (classical) C81.4-
    lymphocyte depleted (classical) C81.3-
    mixed cellularity (classical) C81.2-
    nodular sclerosis (classical) C81.1-
    specified NEC (classical) C81.7-
    lymphocyte-rich classical C81.4-
    lymphocyte depleted classical C81.3-
    mixed cellularity classical C81.2-
    nodular
      lymphocyte predominant C81.0-
      sclerosis (classical) C81.1-
  intravascular large B-cell C83.8-
  Lennert's C84.4-
  lymphoblastic B-cell C83.5-
  lymphoblastic (diffuse) C83.5-
  lymphoblastic T-cell C83.5-
  lymphoepithelioid C84.4-
  lymphoplasmacytic C83.0-
    with IgM-production C88.0
  MALT C88.4
  mantle cell C83.1-
  mature T-cell NEC C84.4-
  mature T/NK-cell C84.9-
    specified NEC C84.Z-
  mediastinal (thymic) large B-cell C85.2-
  Mediterranean C88.3
  mucosa-associated lymphoid tissue [MALT-
    lymphoma] C88.4
  NK/T cell C84.9-
  nodal marginal zone C83.0-
  non-follicular (diffuse) C83.9-
    specified NEC C83.8-
  non-Hodgkin — *see also* Lymphoma, by type C85.9
    -
    specified NEC C85.8-
  non-leukemic variant of B-CLL C83.0-
  peripheral T-cell, not classified C84.4-
  primary cutaneous
    anaplastic large cell C86.6
    CD30-positive large T-cell C86.6
  primary effusion B-cell C83.8-
  SALT C88.4
  skin-associated lymphoid tissue [SALT-
    lymphoma] C88.4
  small cell B-cell C83.0-
  splenic marginal zone C83.0-
  subcutaneous panniculitis-like T-cell C86.3
  T-precursor C83.5-

Lymphoma (of) (malignant) - *continued*
  true histiocytic C96.A
Lymphomatosis — *see* Lymphoma
Lymphopathia venereum, veneris A55
Lymphopenia D72.810
Lymphoplasmacytic leukemia — *see* Leukemia,
  chronic lymphocytic, B-cell type
Lymphoproliferation, X-linked disease D82.3
Lymphoreticulosis, benign (of inoculation) A28.1
Lymphorrhea I89.8
Lymphosarcoma (diffuse) — *see*
  also Lymphoma C85.9-
Lymphostasis I89.8
Lypemania — *see* Melancholia
Lysine and hydroxylysine metabolism
  disorder E72.3
Lyssa — *see* Rabies

M

Macacus ear Q17.3
Maceration, wet feet, tropical (syndrome) T69.02-
MacLeod's syndrome J43.0
Macrocephalia, macrocephaly Q75.3
Macrocheilia, macrochilia (congenital) Q18.6
Macrocolon — *see also* Megacolon Q43.1
Macrocornea Q15.8
  with glaucoma Q15.0
Macrocytic — *see* condition
Macrocytosis D75.89
Macrodactylia, macrodactylism (fingers)
  (thumbs) Q74.0
  toes Q74.2
Macrodontia K00.2
Macrogenia M26.05
Macrogenitosomia (adrenal) (male) (praecox) E25.9
  congenital E25.0
Macroglobulinemia (idiopathic) (primary) C88.0
  monoclonal (essential) D47.2
  Waldenström C88.0
Macroglossia (congenital) Q38.2
  acquired K14.8
Macrognathia, macrognathism (congenital)
  (mandibular) (maxillary) M26.09
Macrogyria (congenital) Q04.8
Macrohydrocephalus — *see* Hydrocephalus
Macromastia — *see* Hypertrophy, breast
Macrophthalmos Q11.3
  in congenital glaucoma Q15.0
Macropsia H53.15
Macrosigmoid K59.39
  congenital Q43.2
Macrospondylitis , acromegalic E22.0
Macrostomia (congenital) Q18.4
Macrotia (external ear) (congenital) Q17.1
Macula
  cornea, corneal — *see* Opacity, cornea
  degeneration (atrophic) (exudative) (senile) —
    see also Degeneration, macula
    hereditary — *see* Dystrophy, retina
Maculae ceruleae -- B85.1
Maculopathy, toxic — *see* Degeneration, macula,
  toxic
Madarosis (eyelid) H02.729
  left H02.726
    lower H02.725
    upper H02.724
  right H02.723
    lower H02.722
    upper H02.721
Madelung's
  deformity (radius) Q74.0
  disease
    radial deformity Q74.0
    symmetrical lipomas, neck E88.89
Madness — *see* Psychosis
Madura
  foot B47.9
    actinomycotic B47.1
    mycotic B47.0
Maduromycosis B47.0
Maffucci's syndrome Q78.4
Magnesium metabolism disorder — *see* Disorder,
  metabolism, magnesium
Main en griffe (acquired) — *see also* Deformity,
  limb, clawhand
  congenital Q74.0
Maintenance (encounter for)
  antineoplastic chemotherapy Z51.11
  antineoplastic radiation therapy Z51.0
  methadone F11.20
Majocchi's
  disease L81.7
  granuloma B35.8

Major — see condition
Mal de los pintos — see Pinta
Mal de mer T75.3
Malabar itch (any site) B35.5
Malabsorption K90.9
  calcium K90.89
  carbohydrate K90.49
  disaccharide E73.9
  fat K90.49
  galactose E74.20
  glucose (-galactose) E74.39
  intestinal K90.9
    specified NEC K90.89
  isomaltose E74.31
  lactose E73.9
  methionine E72.19
  monosaccharide E74.39
  postgastrectomy K91.2
  postsurgical K91.2
  protein K90.49
  starch K90.49
  sucrose E74.39
  syndrome K90.9
    postsurgical K91.2
Malacia, bone (adult) M83.9
  juvenile — see Rickets
Malacoplakia
  bladder N32.89
  pelvis (kidney) N28.89
  ureter N28.89
  urethra N36.8
Malacosteon, juvenile — see Rickets
Maladaptation — see Maladjustment
Maladie de Roger Q21.0
Maladjustment
  conjugal Z63.0
    involving divorce or estrangement Z63.5
  educational Z55.4
  family Z63.9
  marital Z63.0
    involving divorce or estrangement Z63.5
  occupational NEC Z56.89
  simple, adult — see Disorder, adjustment
  situational — see Disorder, adjustment
  social Z60.9
    due to
      acculturation difficulty Z60.3
      discrimination and persecution (perceived) Z60.5
      exclusion and isolation Z60.4
      life-cycle (phase of life) transition Z60.0
      rejection Z60.4
      specified reason NEC Z60.8
Malaise R53.81
Malakoplakia — see Malacoplakia
Malaria, malarial (fever) B54
  with
    blackwater fever B50.8
      hemoglobinuric (bilious) B50.8
    hemoglobinuria B50.8
  accidentally induced (therapeutically) - code by type
    under Malaria
  algid B50.9
  cerebral B50.0 [G94]
  clinically diagnosed (without parasitological
    confirmation) B54
  congenital NEC P37.4
    falciparum P37.3
  congestion, congestive B54
  continued (fever) B50.9
  estivo-autumnal B50.9
  falciparum B50.9
    with complications NEC B50.8
      cerebral B50.0 [G94]
    severe B50.8
  hemorrhagic B54
  malariae B52.9
    with
      complications NEC B52.8
      glomerular disorder B52.0
  malignant (tertian) — see Malaria, falciparum
  mixed infections - code to first listed type in B50-
    B53
  ovale B53.0
  parasitologically confirmed NEC B53.8
  pernicious, acute — see Malaria, falciparum
  Plasmodium (P.)
    falciparum NEC — see Malaria, falciparum
    malariae NEC B52.9
      with Plasmodium
        falciparum (and or vivax) — see Malaria,
          falciparum
        vivax — see also Malaria, vivax
          and falciparum — see Malaria, falciparum

Malaria, malarial (fever) - continued
  Plasmodium (P.) - continued
    ovale B53.0
      with Plasmodium malariae — see also Malaria,
        malariae
        and vivax — see also Malaria, vivax
          and falciparum — see Malaria, falciparum
    simian B53.1
      with Plasmodium malariae — see also Malaria,
        malariae
        and vivax — see also Malaria, vivax
          and falciparum — see Malaria, falciparum
    vivax NEC B51.9
      with Plasmodium falciparum — see Malaria,
        falciparum
  quartan — see Malaria, malariae
  quotidian — see Malaria, falciparum
  recurrent B54
  remittent B54
  specified type NEC (parasitologically
    confirmed) B53.8
  spleen B54
  subtertian (fever) — see Malaria, falciparum
  tertian (benign) — see also Malaria, vivax
    malignant B50.9
  tropical B50.9
  typhoid B54
  vivax B51.9
    with
      complications NEC B51.8
      ruptured spleen B51.0
Malassez's disease (cystic) N50.89
Malassimilation K90.9
Maldescent, testis Q53.9
  bilateral Q53.20
    abdominal Q53.21
    perineal Q53.22
  unilateral Q53.10
    abdominal Q53.11
    perineal Q53.12
Maldevelopment — see also Anomaly
  brain Q07.9
  colon Q43.9
  hip Q74.2
    congenital dislocation Q65.2
      bilateral Q65.1
      unilateral Q65.0-
  mastoid process Q75.8
  middle ear Q16.4
    except ossicles Q16.4
    ossicles Q16.3
  ossicles Q16.3
  spine Q76.49
  toe Q74.2
Male type pelvis Q74.2
  with disproportion (fetopelvic) O33.3
    causing obstructed labor O65.3
Malformation (congenital) — see also Anomaly
  adrenal gland Q89.1
  affecting multiple systems with skeletal changes
    NEC Q87.5
  alimentary tract Q45.9
    specified type NEC Q45.8
    upper Q40.9
      specified type NEC Q40.8
  aorta Q25.40
    absence Q25.41
    aneurysm, congenital Q25.43
    aplasia Q25.41
    atresia Q25.29
      aortic arch Q25.21
    coarctation (preductal) (postductal) Q25.1
    dilatation, congenital Q25.44
    hypoplasia Q25.42
    patent ductus arteriosus Q25.0
    specified type NEC Q25.49
    stenosis Q25.1
      supravalvular Q25.3
  aortic valve Q23.9
    specified NEC Q23.8
  arteriovenous, aneurysmatic (congenital) Q27.30
    brain Q28.2
    cerebral Q28.2
    peripheral Q27.30
      digestive system Q27.33
      lower limb Q27.32
      other specified site Q27.39
      renal vessel Q27.34
      upper limb Q27.31
    precerebral vessels (nonruptured) Q28.0
  auricle
    ear (congenital) Q17.3
      acquired H61.119

Malformation (congenital) - continued
  auricle - continued
    ear (congenital) - continued
      acquired - continued
        left H61.112
          with right H61.113
        right H61.111
          with left H61.113
  bile duct Q44.5
  bladder Q64.79
    aplasia Q64.5
    diverticulum Q64.6
    exstrophy — see Exstrophy, bladder
    neck obstruction Q64.31
  bone Q79.9
    face Q75.9
      specified type NEC Q75.8
    skull Q75.9
      specified type NEC Q75.8
  brain (multiple) Q04.9
    arteriovenous Q28.2
    specified type NEC Q04.8
  branchial cleft Q18.2
  breast Q83.9
    specified type NEC Q83.8
  broad ligament Q50.6
  bronchus Q32.4
  bursa Q79.9
  cardiac
    chambers Q20.9
      specified type NEC Q20.8
    septum Q21.9
      specified type NEC Q21.8
  cerebral Q04.9
    vessels Q28.3
  cervix uteri Q51.9
    specified type NEC Q51.828
  Chiari
    Type I G93.5
    Type II Q07.01
  choroid (congenital) Q14.3
    plexus Q07.8
  circulatory system Q28.9
  cochlea Q16.5
  cornea Q13.4
  coronary vessels Q24.5
  corpus callosum (congenital) Q04.0
  diaphragm Q79.1
  digestive system NEC, specified type NEC Q45.8
  dura Q07.9
    brain Q04.9
    spinal Q06.9
  ear Q17.9
    causing impairment of hearing Q16.9
    external Q17.9
      accessory auricle Q17.0
      causing impairment of hearing Q16.9
      absence of
        auditory canal Q16.1
        auricle Q16.0
      macrotia Q17.1
      microtia Q17.2
      misplacement Q17.4
      misshapen NEC Q17.3
      prominence Q17.5
      specified type NEC Q17.8
    inner Q16.5
    middle Q16.4
      absence of eustachian tube Q16.2
      ossicles (fusion) Q16.3
      ossicles Q16.3
      specified type NEC Q17.8
  epididymis Q55.4
  esophagus Q39.9
    specified type NEC Q39.8
  eye Q15.9
    lid Q10.3
    specified NEC Q15.8
  fallopian tube Q50.6
  genital organ — see Anomaly, genitalia
  great
    artery Q25.9
      aorta — see Malformation, aorta
      pulmonary artery — see Malformation,
        pulmonary, artery
      specified type NEC Q25.8
    vein Q26.9
      anomalous
        portal venous connection Q26.5
        pulmonary venous connection Q26.4
          partial Q26.3
          total Q26.2
      persistent left superior vena cava Q26.1

Malformation (congenital) - *continued*
  great - *continued*
    vein - *continued*
      portal vein-hepatic artery fistula Q26.6
      specified type NEC Q26.8
      vena cava stenosis, congenital Q26.0
  gum Q38.6
  hair Q84.2
  heart Q24.9
    specified type NEC Q24.8
  integument Q84.9
    specified type NEC Q84.8
  internal ear Q16.5
  intestine Q43.9
    specified type NEC Q43.8
  iris Q13.2
  joint Q74.9
    ankle Q74.2
    lumbosacral Q76.49
    sacroiliac Q74.2
    specified type NEC Q74.8
  kidney Q63.9
    accessory Q63.0
    giant Q63.3
    horseshoe Q63.1
    hydronephrosis Q62.0
    malposition Q63.2
    specified type NEC Q63.8
  lacrimal apparatus Q10.6
  lip Q38.0
  lingual Q38.3
  liver Q44.7
  lung Q33.9
  meninges or membrane (congenital) Q07.9
    cerebral Q04.8
    spinal (cord) Q06.9
  middle ear Q16.4
    ossicles Q16.3
  mitral valve Q23.9
    specified type NEC Q23.8
  Mondini's (congenital) (malformation,
    cochlea) Q16.5
  mouth (congenital) Q38.6
  multiple types NEC Q89.7
  musculoskeletal system Q79.9
  myocardium Q24.8
  nail Q84.6
  nervous system (central) Q07.9
  nose Q30.9
    specified type NEC Q30.8
  optic disc Q14.2
  orbit Q10.7
  ovary Q50.39
  palate Q38.5
  parathyroid gland Q89.2
  pelvic organs or tissues NEC
    in pregnancy or childbirth O34.8-
      causing obstructed labor O65.5
  penis Q55.69
    aplasia Q55.5
    curvature (lateral) Q55.61
    hypoplasia Q55.62
  pericardium Q24.8
  peripheral vascular system Q27.9
    specified type NEC Q27.8
  pharynx Q38.8
  precerebral vessels Q28.1
  prostate Q55.4
  pulmonary
    arteriovenous Q25.72
    artery Q25.9
      atresia Q25.5
      specified type NEC Q25.79
      stenosis Q25.6
    valve Q22.3
  renal artery Q27.2
  respiratory system Q34.9
  retina Q14.1
  scrotum — *see* Malformation, testis and scrotum
  seminal vesicles Q55.4
  sense organs NEC Q07.9
  skin Q82.9
  specified NEC Q89.8
  spinal
    cord Q06.9
    nerve root Q07.8
  spine Q76.49
    kyphosis — *see* Kyphosis, congenital
    lordosis — *see* Lordosis, congenital
  spleen Q89.09
  stomach Q40.3
    specified type NEC Q40.2
  teeth, tooth K00.9

Malformation (congenital) - *continued*
  tendon Q79.9
  testis and scrotum Q55.20
    aplasia Q55.0
    hypoplasia Q55.1
    polyorchism Q55.21
    retractile testis Q55.22
    scrotal transposition Q55.23
    specified NEC Q55.29
  throat Q38.8
  thorax, bony Q76.9
  thyroid gland Q89.2
  tongue (congenital) Q38.3
    hypertrophy Q38.2
    tie Q38.1
  trachea Q32.1
  tricuspid valve Q22.9
    specified type NEC Q22.8
  umbilical cord NEC (complicating delivery) O69.89
  umbilicus Q89.9
  ureter Q62.8
    agenesis Q62.4
    duplication Q62.5
    malposition — *see* Malposition, congenital, ureter
    obstructive defect — *see* Defect, obstructive, ureter
    vesico-uretero-renal reflux Q62.7
  urethra Q64.79
    aplasia Q64.5
    duplication Q64.74
    posterior valves Q64.2
    prolapse Q64.71
    stricture Q64.32
  urinary system Q64.9
  uterus Q51.9
    specified type NEC Q51.818
  vagina Q52.4
  vascular system, peripheral Q27.9
  vas deferens Q55.4
    atresia Q55.3
  venous — *see* Anomaly, vein(s)
  vulva Q52.70
Malfunction — *see also* Dysfunction
  cardiac electronic device T82.119
    electrode T82.110
    pulse generator T82.111
    specified type NEC T82.118
  catheter device NEC T85.618
    cystostomy T83.010
    dialysis (renal) (vascular) T82.41
      intraperitoneal T85.611
    infusion NEC T82.514
      cranial T85.610
      epidural T85.610
      intrathecal T85.610
      spinal T85.610
      subarachnoid T85.610
      subdural T85.610
    urinary — *see also* Breakdown, device,
      catheter T83.018
  colostomy K94.03
    valve K94.03
  cystostomy (stoma) N99.512
    catheter T83.010
  enteric stoma K94.13
  enterostomy K94.13
  esophagostomy K94.33
  gastroenteric K31.89
  gastrostomy K94.23
  ileostomy K94.13
    valve K94.13
  intrathecal infusion pump T85.615
  jejunostomy K94.13
  nervous system device, implant or graft, specified
    NEC T85.615
  pacemaker — *see* Malfunction, cardiac electronic
    device
  prosthetic device, internal — *see* Complications,
    prosthetic device, by site, mechanical
  tracheostomy J95.03
  urinary device NEC — *see* Complication,
    genitourinary, device, urinary, mechanical
  valve
    colostomy K94.03
    heart T82.09
    ileostomy K94.13
  vascular graft or shunt NEC — *see* Complication,
    cardiovascular device, mechanical, vascular
  ventricular (communicating shunt) T85.01
Malherbe's tumor — *see* Neoplasm, skin, benign
Malibu disease L98.8
Malignancy — *see also* Neoplasm, malignant, by site
  unspecified site (primary) C80.1
Malignant — *see* condition

Malingerer, malingering Z76.5
Mallet finger (acquired) — *see* Deformity, finger,
  mallet finger
  congenital Q74.0
  sequelae of rickets E64.3
Malleus A24.0
Mallory's bodies R89.7
Mallory-Weiss syndrome K22.6
Malnutrition E46
  degree
    first E44.1
    mild (protein) E44.1
    moderate (protein) E44.0
    second E44.0
    severe (protein-energy) E43
      intermediate form E42
        with
          kwashiorkor (and marasmus) E42
          marasmus E41
    third E43
  following gastrointestinal surgery K91.2
  intrauterine
    light-for-dates — *see* Light for dates
    small-for-dates — *see* Small for dates
  lack of care, or neglect (child) (infant) T76.02
    confirmed T74.02
  malignant E40
  protein E46
    calorie E46
      mild E44.1
      moderate E44.0
      severe E43
        intermediate form E42
          with
            kwashiorkor (and marasmus) E42
            marasmus E41
    energy E46
      mild E44.1
      moderate E44.0
      severe E43
        intermediate form E42
          with
            kwashiorkor (and marasmus) E42
            marasmus E41
  severe (protein-energy) E43
    with
      kwashiorkor (and marasmus) E42
      marasmus E41
Malocclusion (teeth) M26.4
  Angle's M26.219
    class I M26.211
    class II M26.212
    class III M26.213
  due to
    abnormal swallowing M26.59
    mouth breathing M26.59
    tongue, lip or finger habits M26.59
  temporomandibular (joint) M26.69
Malposition
  cervix — *see* Malposition, uterus
  congenital
    adrenal (gland) Q89.1
    alimentary tract Q45.8
      lower Q43.8
      upper Q40.8
    aorta Q25.49
    appendix Q43.8
    arterial trunk Q20.0
    artery (peripheral) Q27.8
      coronary Q24.5
      digestive system Q27.8
      lower limb Q27.8
      pulmonary Q25.79
      specified site NEC Q27.8
      upper limb Q27.8
    auditory canal Q17.8
      causing impairment of hearing Q16.9
    auricle (ear) Q17.4
      causing impairment of hearing Q16.9
      cervical Q18.2
    biliary duct or passage Q44.5
    bladder (mucosa) — *see* Exstrophy, bladder
    brachial plexus Q07.8
    brain tissue Q04.8
    breast Q83.8
    bronchus Q32.4
    cecum Q43.8
    clavicle Q74.0
    colon Q43.8
    digestive organ or tract NEC Q45.8
      lower Q43.8
      upper Q40.8
    ear (auricle) (external) Q17.4

Malposition - *continued*
congenital - *continued*
  ear (auricle) (external) - *continued*
    ossicles Q16.3
  endocrine (gland) NEC Q89.2
  epiglottis Q31.8
  eustachian tube Q17.8
  eye Q15.8
  facial features Q18.8
  fallopian tube Q50.6
  finger (s) Q68.1
    supernumerary Q69.0
  foot Q66.9
  gallbladder Q44.1
  gastrointestinal tract Q45.8
  genitalia, genital organ (s) or tract
    female Q52.8
      external Q52.79
      internal NEC Q52.8
    male Q55.8
  glottis Q31.8
  hand Q68.1
  heart Q24.8
    dextrocardia Q24.0
      with complete transposition of viscera Q89.3
  hepatic duct Q44.5
  hip (joint) Q65.89
  intestine (large) (small) Q43.8
    with anomalous adhesions, fixation or malrotation Q43.3
  joint NEC Q68.8
  kidney Q63.2
  larynx Q31.8
  limb Q68.8
    lower Q68.8
    upper Q68.8
  liver Q44.7
  lung (lobe) Q33.8
  nail (s) Q84.6
  nerve Q07.8
  nervous system NEC Q07.8
  nose, nasal (septum) Q30.8
  organ or site not listed — *see* Anomaly, by site
  ovary Q50.39
  pancreas Q45.3
  parathyroid (gland) Q89.2
  patella Q74.1
  peripheral vascular system Q27.8
  pituitary (gland) Q89.2
  respiratory organ or system NEC Q34.8
  rib (cage) Q76.6
    supernumerary in cervical region Q76.5
  scapula Q74.0
  shoulder Q74.0
  spinal cord Q06.8
  spleen Q89.09
  sternum NEC Q76.7
  stomach Q40.2
  symphysis pubis Q74.2
  thymus (gland) Q89.2
  thyroid (gland) (tissue) Q89.2
    cartilage Q31.8
  toe (s) Q66.9
    supernumerary Q69.2
  tongue Q38.3
  trachea Q32.1
  ureter Q62.60
    deviation Q62.61
    displacement Q62.62
    ectopia Q62.63
    specified type NEC Q62.69
  uterus Q51.818
  vein (s) (peripheral) Q27.8
    great Q26.8
  vena cava (inferior) (superior) Q26.8
device, implant or graft — *see also* Complications, by site and type, mechanical T85.628
  arterial graft NEC — *see* Complication, cardiovascular device, mechanical, vascular
  breast (implant) T85.42
  catheter NEC T85.628
    cystostomy T83.020
    dialysis (renal) T82.42
      intraperitoneal T85.621
    infusion NEC T82.524
      spinal (epidural) (subdural) T85.620
    urinary — *see also* Displacement, device, catheter, urinary T83.028
  electronic (electrode) (pulse generator) (stimulator)
    bone T84.320
    cardiac T82.129
      electrode T82.120
      pulse generator T82.121

Malposition - *continued*
device, implant or graft - *continued*
  electronic (electrode) (pulse generator) (stimulator) - *continued*
    cardiac - *continued*
      specified type NEC T82.128
    nervous system — *see* Complication, prosthetic device, mechanical, electronic nervous system stimulator
    urinary — *see* Complication, genitourinary, device, urinary, mechanical
  fixation, internal (orthopedic) NEC — *see* Complication, fixation device, mechanical
  gastrointestinal — *see* Complications, prosthetic device, mechanical, gastrointestinal device
  genital NEC T83.428
    intrauterine contraceptive device (string) T83.32
    penile prosthesis (cylinder) (implanted) (pump) (resevoir) T83.420
    testicular prosthesis T83.421
  heart NEC — *see* Complication, cardiovascular device, mechanical
  joint prosthesis — *see* Complication, joint prosthesis, mechanical
  ocular NEC — *see* Complications, prosthetic device, mechanical, ocular device
  orthopedic NEC — *see* Complication, orthopedic, device, mechanical
  specified NEC T85.628
  urinary NEC — *see also* Complication, genitourinary, device, urinary, mechanical
    graft T83.22
  vascular NEC — *see* Complication, cardiovascular device, mechanical
  ventricular intracranial shunt T85.02
fetus — *see* Pregnancy, complicated by (management affected by), presentation, fetal
gallbladder K82.8
gastrointestinal tract, congenital Q45.8
heart, congenital NEC Q24.8
joint prosthesis — *see* Complications, joint prosthesis, mechanical, displacement, by site
stomach K31.89
  congenital Q40.2
tooth, teeth, fully erupted M26.30
uterus (acute) (acquired) (adherent) (asymptomatic) (postinfectional) (postpartal, old) N85.4
  anteflexion or anteversion N85.4
    congenital Q51.818
  flexion N85.4
    lateral — *see* Lateroversion, uterus
  inversion N85.5
  lateral (flexion) (version) — *see* Lateroversion, uterus
    in pregnancy or childbirth — *see* subcategory O34.5
  retroflexion or retroversion — *see* Retroversion, uterus
Malposture R29.3
Malrotation
  cecum Q43.3
  colon Q43.3
  intestine Q43.3
  kidney Q63.2
Malta fever — *see* Brucellosis
Maltreatment
adult
  abandonment
    confirmed T74.01
    suspected T76.01
  confirmed T74.91
  history of Z91.419
  neglect
    confirmed T74.01
    suspected T76.01
  physical abuse
    confirmed T74.11
    suspected T76.11
  psychological abuse
    confirmed T74.31
    suspected T76.31
    history of Z91.411
  sexual abuse
    confirmed T74.21
    suspected T76.21
    suspected T76.91
child
  abandonment
    confirmed T74.02
    suspected T76.02
  confirmed T74.92
  history of — *see* History, personal (of), abuse
  neglect

Maltreatment - *continued*
child - *continued*
  neglect - *continued*
    confirmed T74.02
    history of — *see* History, personal (of), abuse
    suspected T76.02
  physical abuse
    confirmed T74.12
    history of — *see* History, personal (of), abuse
    suspected T76.12
  psychological abuse
    confirmed T74.32
    history of — *see* History, personal (of), abuse
    suspected T76.32
  sexual abuse
    confirmed T74.22
    history of — *see* History, personal (of), abuse
    suspected T76.22
  suspected T76.92
  personal history of Z91.89
Maltworker's lung J67.4
Malunion, fracture — *see* Fracture, by site
Mammillitis N61.0
  puerperal, postpartum O91.02
Mammitis — *see* Mastitis
Mammogram (examination) Z12.39
  routine Z12.31
Mammoplasia N62
Management (of)
  bone conduction hearing device (implanted) Z45.320
  cardiac pacemaker NEC Z45.018
  cerebrospinal fluid drainage device Z45.41
  cochlear device (implanted) Z45.321
  contraceptive Z30.9
    specified NEC Z30.8
  implanted device Z45.9
    specified NEC Z45.89
  infusion pump Z45.1
  procreative Z31.9
    male factor infertility in female Z31.81
    specified NEC Z31.89
  prosthesis (external) — *see also* Fitting Z44.9
    implanted Z45.9
      specified NEC Z45.89
  renal dialysis catheter Z49.01
  vascular access device Z45.2
Mangled — *see* specified injury by site
Mania (monopolar) — *see also* Disorder, mood, manic episode
  with psychotic symptoms F30.2
  without psychotic symptoms F30.10
    mild F30.11
    moderate F30.12
    severe F30.13
  Bell's F30.8
  chronic (recurrent) F31.89
  hysterical F44.89
  puerperal F30.8
  recurrent F31.89
Manic-depressive insanity, psychosis, or syndrome — *see* Disorder, bipolar
Mannosidosis E77.1
Mansonelliasis, mansonellosis B74.4
Manson's
  disease B65.1
  schistosomiasis B65.1
Manual — *see* condition
Maple-bark-stripper's lung (disease) J67.6
Maple-syrup-urine disease E71.0
Marable's syndrome (celiac artery compression) I77.4
Marasmus E41
  due to malnutrition E41
  intestinal E41
  nutritional E41
  senile R54
  tuberculous NEC — *see* Tuberculosis
Marble
  bones Q78.2
  skin R23.8
Marburg virus disease A98.3
March
  fracture — *see* Fracture, traumatic, stress, by site
  hemoglobinuria D59.6
Marchesani (-Weill) **syndrome** Q87.0
Marchiafava (-Bignami) **syndrome or disease** G37.1
Marchiafava-Micheli syndrome D59.5
Marcus Gunn's syndrome Q07.8
Marfan's syndrome — *see* Syndrome, Marfan's
Marie-Bamberger disease — *see* Osteoarthropathy, hypertrophic, specified NEC
Marie-Charcot-Tooth neuropathic muscular atrophy G60.0

Marie's
cerebellar ataxia (late-onset) G11.2
disease or syndrome (acromegaly) E22.0
Marie-Strümpell arthritis, disease or
spondylitis — *see* Spondylitis, ankylosing
Marion's disease (bladder neck obstruction) N32.0
Marital conflict Z63.0
Mark
port wine Q82.5
raspberry Q82.5
strawberry Q82.5
stretch L90.6
tattoo L81.8
Marker heterochromatin — *see* Extra, marker
chromosomes
Maroteaux-Lamy syndrome (mild) (severe) E76.29
Marrow (bone)
arrest D61.9
poor function D75.89
Marseilles fever A77.1
Marsh fever — *see* Malaria
Marshall's (hidrotic) **ectodermal dysplasia** Q82.4
Marsh's disease (exophthalmic goiter) E05.00
with storm E05.01
Masculinization (female) **with adrenal**
hyperplasia E25.9
congenital E25.0
Masculinovoblastoma D27.-
Masochism (sexual) F65.51
Mason's lung J62.8
Mass
abdominal R19.00
epigastric R19.06
generalized R19.07
left lower quadrant R19.04
left upper quadrant R19.02
periumbilic R19.05
right lower quadrant R19.03
right upper quadrant R19.01
specified site NEC R19.09
breast N63
chest R22.2
cystic — *see* Cyst
ear H93.8-
head R22.0
intra-abdominal (diffuse) (generalized) — *see* Mass,
abdominal
kidney N28.89
liver R16.0
localized (skin) R22.9
chest R22.2
head R22.0
limb
lower R22.4-
upper R22.3-
neck R22.1
trunk R22.2
lung R91.8
malignant — *see* Neoplasm, malignant, by site
neck R22.1
pelvic (diffuse) (generalized) — *see* Mass,
abdominal
specified organ NEC — *see* Disease, by site
splenic R16.1
substernal thyroid — *see* Goiter
superficial (localized) R22.9
umbilical (diffuse) (generalized) R19.09
Massive — *see* condition
Mast cell
disease, systemic tissue D47.0
leukemia C94.3-
sarcoma C96.2
tumor D47.0
malignant C96.2
Mastalgia N64.4
Masters-Allen syndrome N83.8
Mastitis (acute) (diffuse) (nonpuerperal)
(subacute) N61.0
with abscess N61.1
chronic (cystic) — *see* Mastopathy, cystic
cystic (Schimmelbusch's type) — *see* Mastopathy,
cystic
fibrocystic — *see* Mastopathy, cystic
infective N61.0
newborn P39.0
interstitial, gestational or puerperal — *see* Mastitis,
obstetric
neonatal (noninfective) P83.4
infective P39.0
obstetric (interstitial) (nonpurulent)
associated with
lactation O91.23
pregnancy O91.21-

Mastitis (acute) (diffuse) (nonpuerperal) (subacute) -
continued
obstetric (interstitial) (nonpurulent) - *continued*
associated with - *continued*
puerperium O91.22
purulent
associated with
lactation O91.13
pregnancy O91.11-
puerperium O91.12
periductal — *see* Ectasia, mammary duct
phlegmonous — *see* Mastopathy, cystic
plasma cell — *see* Ectasia, mammary duct
without abscess N61.0
Mastocytoma D47.0
malignant C96.2
Mastocytosis Q82.2
aggressive systemic C96.2
indolent systemic D47.0
malignant C96.2
systemic, associated with clonal hematopoetic non-
mast-cell disease (SM-AHNMD) D47.0
Mastodynia N64.4
Mastoid — *see* condition
Mastoidalgia — *see* subcategory H92.0
Mastoiditis (coalescent) (hemorrhagic)
(suppurative) H70.9-
acute, subacute H70.00-
complicated NEC H70.09-
subperiosteal H70.01-
chronic (necrotic) (recurrent) H70.1-
in (due to)
infectious disease NEC B99 [H75.0-]
parasitic disease NEC B89 [H75.0-]
tuberculosis A18.03
petrositis — *see* Petrositis
postauricular fistula — *see* Fistula, postauricular
specified NEC H70.89-
tuberculous A18.03
Mastopathy, mastopathia N64.9
chronica cystica — *see* Mastopathy, cystic
cystic (chronic) (diffuse) N60.1-
with epithelial proliferation N60.3-
diffuse cystic — *see* Mastopathy, cystic
estrogenic, oestrogenica N64.89
ovarian origin N64.89
Mastoplasia, mastoplastia N62
Masturbation (excessive) F98.8
Maternal care (for) — *see* Pregnancy (complicated
by) (management affected by)
Matheiu's disease (leptospiral jaundice) A27.0
Mauclaire's disease or osteochondrosis — *see*
Osteochondrosis, juvenile, hand, metacarpal
Maxcy's disease A75.2
Maxilla, maxillary — *see* condition
May (-Hegglin) **anomaly or syndrome** D72.0
McArdle (-Schmid) (-Pearson) **disease**
(glycogen storage) E74.04
McCune-Albright syndrome Q78.1
McQuarrie's syndrome
(idiopathic familial hypoglycemia) E16.2
Meadow's syndrome Q86.1
Measles (black) (hemorrhagic) (suppressed) B05.9
with
complications NEC B05.89
encephalitis B05.0
intestinal complications B05.4
keratitis (keratoconjunctivitis) B05.81
meningitis B05.1
otitis media B05.3
pneumonia B05.2
French — *see* Rubella
German — *see* Rubella
Liberty — *see* Rubella
Meatitis, urethral — *see* Urethritis
Meatus, meatal — *see* condition
Meat-wrappers' asthma J68.9
Meckel-Gruber syndrome Q61.9
Meckel's diverticulitis, diverticulum (displaced)
(hypertrophic) Q43.0
malignant — *see* Table of Neoplasms, small
intestine, malignant
Meconium
ileus, newborn P76.0
in cystic fibrosis E84.11
meaning meconium plug (without cystic
fibrosis) P76.0
obstruction, newborn P76.9
due to fecaliths P76.0
in mucoviscidosis E84.11
peritonitis P78.0
plug syndrome (newborn) NEC P76.0

Median — *see also* condition
arcuate ligament syndrome I77.4
bar (prostate) (vesical orifice) — *see* Hyperplasia,
prostate
rhomboid glossitis K14.2
Mediastinal shift R93.8
Mediastinitis (acute) (chronic) J98.51
syphilitic A52.73
tuberculous A15.8
Mediastinopericarditis — *see also* Pericarditis
acute I30.9
adhesive I31.0
chronic I31.8
rheumatic I09.2
Mediastinum, mediastinal — *see* condition
Medicine poisoning — *see* Table of Drugs and
Chemicals, by drug, poisoning
Mediterranean
fever — *see* Brucellosis
familial M04.1
tick A77.1
kala-azar B55.0
leishmaniasis B55.0
tick fever A77.1
Medulla — *see* condition
Medullary cystic kidney Q61.5
Medullated fibers
optic (nerve) Q14.8
retina Q14.1
Medulloblastoma
desmoplastic C71.6
specified site — *see* Neoplasm, malignant, by site
unspecified site C71.6
Medulloepithelioma — *see also* Neoplasm,
malignant, by site
teratoid — *see* Neoplasm, malignant, by site
Medullomyoblastoma
specified site — *see* Neoplasm, malignant, by site
unspecified site C71.6
Meekeren-Ehlers-Danlos syndrome Q79.6
Megacolon (acquired) (functional)
(not Hirschsprung's disease) (in) K59.39
Chagas' disease B57.32
congenital, congenitum (aganglionic) Q43.1
Hirschsprung's (disease) Q43.1
toxic NEC K59.31
due to Clostridium difficile A04.7
Megaesophagus (functional) K22.0
congenital Q39.5
in (due to) Chagas' disease B57.31
Megalencephaly Q04.5
Megalerythema (epidemic) B08.3
Megaloappendix Q43.8
Megalocephalus, megalocephaly NEC Q75.3
Megalocornea Q15.8
with glaucoma Q15.0
Megalocytic anemia D53.1
Megalodactylia (fingers) (thumbs)
(congenital) Q74.0
toes Q74.2
Megaloduodenum Q43.8
Megaloesophagus (functional) K22.0
congenital Q39.5
Megalogastria (acquired) K31.89
congenital Q40.2
Megalophthalmos Q11.3
Megalopsia H53.15
Megalosplenia — *see* Splenomegaly
Megaloureter N28.82
congenital Q62.2
Megarectum K62.89
Megasigmoid K59.39
congenital Q43.2
Megaureter N28.82
congenital Q62.2
Megavitamin-B6 syndrome E67.2
Megrim — *see* Migraine
Meibomian
cyst, infected — *see* Hordeolum
gland — *see* condition
sty, stye — *see* Hordeolum
Meibomitis — *see* Hordeolum
Meige-Milroy disease (chronic hereditary
edema) Q82.0
Meige's syndrome Q82.0
Melalgia, nutritional E53.8
Melancholia F32.9
climacteric (single episode) F32.89
recurrent episode F33.8
hypochondriac F45.29
intermittent (single episode) F32.89
recurrent episode F33.8
involutional (single episode) F32.89

Melancholia - *continued*
  involutional (single episode) - *continued*
    recurrent episode F33.8
  menopausal (single episode) F32.89
    recurrent episode F33.8
  puerperal F32.89
  reactive (emotional stress or trauma) F32.3
  recurrent F33.9
  senile F03
  stuporous (single episode) F32.89
    recurrent episode F33.8
Melanemia R79.89
Melanoameloblastoma — *see* Neoplasm, bone, benign
Melanoblastoma — *see* Melanoma
Melanocarcinoma — *see* Melanoma
Melanocytoma, eyeball D31.9-
Melanocytosis, neurocutaneous Q82.8
Melanoderma, melanodermia L81.4
Melanodontia, infantile K03.89
Melanodontoclasia K03.89
Melanoepithelioma — *see* Melanoma
Melanoma (malignant) C43.9
  acral lentiginous, malignant — *see* Melanoma, skin, by site
  amelanotic — *see* Melanoma, skin, by site
  balloon cell — *see* Melanoma, skin, by site
  benign — *see* Nevus
  desmoplastic, malignant — *see* Melanoma, skin, by site
  epithelioid cell — *see* Melanoma, skin, by site
    with spindle cell, mixed — *see* Melanoma, skin, by site
  in
    giant pigmented nevus — *see* Melanoma, skin, by site
    Hutchinson's melanotic freckle — *see* Melanoma, skin, by site
    junctional nevus — *see* Melanoma, skin, by site
    precancerous melanosis — *see* Melanoma, skin, by site
  in situ D03.9
    abdominal wall D03.59
    ala nasi D03.39
    ankle D03.7-
    anus, anal (margin) (skin) D03.51
    arm D03.6-
    auditory canal D03.2-
    auricle (ear) D03.2-
    auricular canal (external) D03.2-
    axilla, axillary fold D03.59
    back D03.59
    breast D03.52
    brow D03.39
    buttock D03.59
    canthus (eye) D03.1-
    cheek (external) D03.39
    chest wall D03.59
    chin D03.39
    choroid D03.8
    conjunctiva D03.8
    ear (external) D03.2-
    external meatus (ear) D03.2-
    eye D03.8
    eyebrow D03.39
    eyelid (lower) (upper) D03.1-
    face D03.30
      specified NEC D03.39
    female genital organ (external) NEC D03.8
    finger D03.6-
    flank D03.59
    foot D03.7-
    forearm D03.6-
    forehead D03.39
    foreskin D03.8
    gluteal region D03.59
    groin D03.59
    hand D03.6-
    heel D03.7-
    helix D03.2-
    hip D03.7-
    interscapular region D03.59
    iris D03.8
    jaw D03.39
    knee D03.7-
    labium (majus) (minus) D03.8
    lacrimal gland D03.8
    leg D03.7-
    lip (lower) (upper) D03.0
    lower limb NEC D03.7-
    male genital organ (external) NEC D03.8
    nail D03.9
      finger D03.6-

Melanoma (malignant) - *continued*
  in situ - *continued*
    nail - *continued*
      toe D03.7-
    neck D03.4
    nose (external) D03.39
    orbit D03.8
    penis D03.8
    perianal skin D03.51
    perineum D03.51
    pinna D03.2-
    popliteal fossa or space D03.7-
    prepuce D03.8
    pudendum D03.8
    retina D03.8
    retrobulbar D03.8
    scalp D03.4
    scrotum D03.8
    shoulder D03.6-
    specified site NEC D03.8
    submammary fold D03.52
    temple D03.39
    thigh D03.7-
    toe D03.7-
    trunk NEC D03.59
    umbilicus D03.59
    upper limb NEC D03.6-
    vulva D03.8
  juvenile — *see* Nevus
  malignant, of soft parts except skin — *see* Neoplasm, connective tissue, malignant
  metastatic
    breast C79.81
    genital organ C79.82
    specified site NEC C79.89
  neurotropic, malignant — *see* Melanoma, skin, by site
  nodular — *see* Melanoma, skin, by site
  regressing, malignant — *see* Melanoma, skin, by site
  skin C43.9
    abdominal wall C43.59
    ala nasi C43.31
    ankle C43.7-
    anus, anal (skin) C43.51
    arm C43.6-
    auditory canal (external) C43.2-
    auricle (ear) C43.2-
    auricular canal (external) C43.2-
    axilla, axillary fold C43.59
    back C43.59
    breast (female) (male) C43.52
    brow C43.39
    buttock C43.59
    canthus (eye) C43.1-
    cheek (external) C43.39
    chest wall C43.59
    chin C43.39
    ear (external) C43.2-
    elbow C43.6-
    external meatus (ear) C43.2-
    eyebrow C43.39
    eyelid (lower) (upper) C43.1-
    face C43.30
      specified NEC C43.39
    female genital organ (external) NEC C51.9
    finger C43.6-
    flank C43.59
    foot C43.7-
    forearm C43.6-
    forehead C43.39
    foreskin C60.0
    glabella C43.39
    gluteal region C43.59
    groin C43.59
    hand C43.6-
    heel C43.7-
    helix C43.2-
    hip C43.7-
    interscapular region C43.59
    jaw (external) C43.39
    knee C43.7-
    labium C51.9
      majus C51.0
      minus C51.1
    leg C43.7-
    lip (lower) (upper) C43.0
    lower limb NEC C43.7-
    male genital organ (external) NEC C63.9
    nail
      finger C43.6-
      toe C43.7-
    nasolabial groove C43.39
    nates C43.59

Melanoma (malignant) - *continued*
  skin - *continued*
    neck C43.4
    nose (external) C43.31
    overlapping site C43.8
    palpebra C43.1-
    penis C60.9
    perianal skin C43.51
    perineum C43.51
    pinna C43.2-
    popliteal fossa or space C43.7-
    prepuce C60.0
    pudendum C51.9
    scalp C43.4
    scrotum C63.2
    shoulder C43.6-
    skin NEC C43.9
    submammary fold C43.52
    temple C43.39
    thigh C43.7-
    toe C43.7-
    trunk NEC C43.59
    umbilicus C43.59
    upper limb NEC C43.6-
    vulva C51.9
      overlapping sites C51.8
  spindle cell
    with epithelioid, mixed — *see* Melanoma, skin, by site
    type A C69.4-
    type B C69.4-
  superficial spreading — *see* Melanoma, skin, by site
Melanosarcoma — *see also* Melanoma
  epithelioid cell — *see* Melanoma
Melanosis L81.4
  addisonian E27.1
    tuberculous A18.7
  adrenal E27.1
  colon K63.89
  conjunctiva — *see* Pigmentation, conjunctiva
    congenital Q13.89
  cornea (presenile) (senile) — *see also* Pigmentation, cornea
    congenital Q13.4
  eye NEC H57.8
    congenital Q15.8
  lenticularis progressiva Q82.1
  liver K76.89
  precancerous — *see also* Melanoma, in situ
    malignant melanoma in — *see* Melanoma
  Riehl's L81.4
  sclera H15.89
    congenital Q13.89
  suprarenal E27.1
  tar L81.4
  toxic L81.4
Melanuria R82.99
MELAS syndrome E88.41
Melasma L81.1
  adrenal (gland) E27.1
  suprarenal (gland) E27.1
Melena K92.1
  with ulcer - code by site under Ulcer, with hemorrhage K27.4
  due to swallowed maternal blood P78.2
  newborn, neonatal P54.1
    due to swallowed maternal blood P78.2
Meleney's
  gangrene (cutaneous) — *see* Ulcer, skin
  ulcer (chronic undermining) — *see* Ulcer, skin
Melioidosis A24.9
  acute A24.1
  chronic A24.2
  fulminating A24.1
  pneumonia A24.1
  pulmonary (chronic) A24.2
    acute A24.1
    subacute A24.2
  sepsis A24.1
  specified NEC A24.3
  subacute A24.2
Melitensis, febris A23.0
Melkersson (-Rosenthal) **syndrome** G51.2
Mellitus, diabetes — *see* Diabetes
Melorheostosis (bone) — *see* Disorder, bone, density and structure, specified NEC
Meloschisis Q18.4
Melotia Q17.4
Membrana
  capsularis lentis posterior Q13.89
  epipapillaris Q14.2
Membranacea placenta O43.19-
Membranaceous uterus N85.8

Membrane (s) , membranous — see also condition
- cyclitic — see Membrane, pupillary
- folds, congenital — see Web
- Jackson's Q43.3
- over face of newborn P28.9
- premature rupture — see Rupture, membranes, premature
- pupillary H21.4-
  - persistent Q13.89
- retained (with hemorrhage) (complicating delivery) O72.2
  - without hemorrhage O73.1
- secondary cataract — see Cataract, secondary
- unruptured (causing asphyxia) — see Asphyxia, newborn
- vitreous — see Opacity, vitreous, membranes and strands

Membranitis — see Chorioamnionitis

Memory disturbance, lack or loss — see also Amnesia
- mild, following organic brain damage F06.8

Menadione deficiency E56.1

Menarche
- delayed E30.0
- precocious E30.1

Mendacity, pathologic F60.2

Mendelson's syndrome (due to anesthesia) J95.4
- in labor and delivery O74.0
- in pregnancy O29.01-
  - obstetric O74.0
- postpartum, puerperal O89.01

Ménétrier's disease or syndrome K29.60
- with bleeding K29.61

Ménière's disease, syndrome or vertigo H81.0-

Meninges, meningeal — see condition

Meningioma — see also Neoplasm, meninges, benign
- angioblastic — see Neoplasm, meninges, benign
- angiomatous — see Neoplasm, meninges, benign
- endotheliomatous — see Neoplasm, meninges, benign
- fibroblastic — see Neoplasm, meninges, benign
- fibrous — see Neoplasm, meninges, benign
- hemangioblastic — see Neoplasm, meninges, benign
- hemangiopericytic — see Neoplasm, meninges, benign
- malignant — see Neoplasm, meninges, malignant
- meningiothelial — see Neoplasm, meninges, benign
- meningotheliomatous — see Neoplasm, meninges, benign
- mixed — see Neoplasm, meninges, benign
- multiple — see Neoplasm, meninges, uncertain behavior
- papillary — see Neoplasm, meninges, uncertain behavior
- psammomatous — see Neoplasm, meninges, benign
- syncytial — see Neoplasm, meninges, benign
- transitional — see Neoplasm, meninges, benign

Meningiomatosis (diffuse) — see Neoplasm, meninges, uncertain behavior

Meningism — see Meningismus

Meningismus (infectional) (pneumococcal) R29.1
- due to serum or vaccine R29.1
- influenzal — see Influenza, with, manifestations NEC

Meningitis (basal) (basic) (brain) (cerebral) (cervical) (congestive) (diffuse) (hemorrhagic) (infantile) (membranous) (metastatic) (nonspecific) (pontine) (progressive) (simple) (spinal) (subacute) (sympathetic) (toxic) G03.9
- abacterial G03.0
- actinomycotic A42.81
- adenoviral A87.1
- arbovirus A87.8
- aseptic (acute) G03.0
- bacterial G00.9
  - Escherichia coli (E. coli) G00.8
  - Friedländer (bacillus) G00.8
  - gram-negative G00.9
  - H. influenzae G00.0
  - Klebsiella G00.8
  - pneumococcal G00.1
  - specified organism NEC G00.8
  - staphylococcal G00.3
  - streptococcal (acute) G00.2
- benign recurrent (Mollaret) G03.2
- candidal B37.5
- caseous (tuberculous) A17.0
- cerebrospinal A39.0
- chronic NEC G03.1
- clear cerebrospinal fluid NEC G03.0
- coxsackievirus A87.0
- cryptococcal B45.1

Meningitis (basal) (basic) (brain) (cerebral) (cervical) (congestive) (diffuse) (hemorrhagic) (infantile) (membranous) (metastatic) (nonspecific) (pontine) (progressive) (simple) (spinal) (subacute) (sympathetic) (toxic) - continued
- diplococcal (gram positive) A39.0
- echovirus A87.0
- enteroviral A87.0
- eosinophilic B83.2
- epidemic NEC A39.0
- Escherichia coli (E. coli) G00.8
- fibrinopurulent G00.9
  - specified organism NEC G00.8
- Friedländer (bacillus) G00.8
- gonococcal A54.81
- gram-negative cocci G00.9
- gram-positive cocci G00.9
- Haemophilus (influenzae) G00.0
- H. influenzae G00.0
- in (due to)
  - adenovirus A87.1
  - African trypanosomiasis B56.9 [G02]
  - anthrax A22.8
  - bacterial disease NEC A48.8 [G01]
  - Chagas' disease (chronic) B57.41
  - chickenpox B01.0
  - coccidioidomycosis B38.4
  - Diplococcus pneumoniae G00.1
  - enterovirus A87.0
  - herpes (simplex) virus B00.3
    - zoster B02.1
  - infectious mononucleosis B27.92
  - leptospirosis A27.81
  - Listeria monocytogenes A32.11
  - Lyme disease A69.21
  - measles B05.1
  - mumps (virus) B26.1
  - neurosyphilis (late) A52.13
  - parasitic disease NEC B89 [G02]
  - poliovirus A80.9 [G02]
  - preventive immunization, inoculation or vaccination G03.8
  - rubella B06.02
  - Salmonella infection A02.21
  - specified cause NEC G03.8
  - Streptococcal pneumoniae G00.1
  - typhoid fever A01.01
  - varicella B01.0
  - viral disease NEC A87.8
  - whooping cough A37.90
  - zoster B02.1
- infectious G00.9
- influenzal (H. influenzae) G00.0
- Klebsiella G00.8
- leptospiral (aseptic) A27.81
- lymphocytic (acute) (benign) (serous) A87.2
- meningococcal A39.0
- Mima polymorpha G00.8
- Mollaret (benign recurrent) G03.2
- monilial B37.5
- mycotic NEC B49 [G02]
- Neisseria A39.0
- nonbacterial G03.0
- nonpyogenic NEC G03.0
- ossificans G96.19
- pneumococcal streptococcus pneumoniae G00.1
- poliovirus A80.9 [G02]
- postmeasles B05.1
- purulent G00.9
  - specified organism NEC G00.8
- pyogenic G00.9
  - specified organism NEC G00.8
- Salmonella (arizonae) (Cholerae-Suis) (enteritidis) (typhimurium) A02.21
- septic G00.9
  - specified organism NEC G00.8
- serosa circumscripta NEC G03.0
- serous NEC G93.2
- specified organism NEC G00.8
- sporotrichosis B42.81
- staphylococcal G00.3
- sterile G03.0
- Streptococcal (acute) G00.2
  - pneumoniae G00.1
- suppurative G00.9
  - specified organism NEC G00.8
- syphilitic (late) (tertiary) A52.13
  - acute A51.41
  - congenital A50.41
  - secondary A51.41
- Torula histolytica (cryptococcal) B45.1
- traumatic (complication of injury) T79.8
- tuberculous A17.0

Meningitis (basal) (basic) (brain) (cerebral) (cervical) (congestive) (diffuse) (hemorrhagic) (infantile) (membranous) (metastatic) (nonspecific) (pontine) (progressive) (simple) (spinal) (subacute) (sympathetic) (toxic) - continued
- typhoid A01.01
- viral NEC A87.9
- Yersinia pestis A20.3

Meningocele (spinal) — see also Spina bifida
- with hydrocephalus — see Spina bifida, by site, with hydrocephalus
- acquired (traumatic) G96.19
- cerebral — see Encephalocele

Meningocerebritis — see Meningoencephalitis

Meningococcemia A39.4
- acute A39.2
- chronic A39.3

Meningococcus, meningococcal — see also condition A39.9
- adrenalitis, hemorrhagic A39.1
- carrier (suspected) of Z22.31
- meningitis (cerebrospinal) A39.0

Meningoencephalitis — see also Encephalitis G04.90
- acute NEC — see also Encephalitis, viral A86
- bacterial NEC G04.2
- California A83.5
- diphasic A84.1
- eosinophilic B83.2
- epidemic A39.81
- herpesviral, herpetic B00.4
  - due to herpesvirus 6 B10.01
  - due to herpesvirus 7 B10.09
  - specified NEC B10.09
- in (due to)
  - blastomycosis NEC B40.81
  - diseases classified elsewhere G05.3
  - free-living ameba B60.2
  - Hemophilus influenzae (H .influenzae) G00.0
  - herpes B00.4
    - due to herpesvirus 6 B10.01
    - due to herpesvirus 7 B10.09
    - specified NEC B10.09
  - H. influenzae G00.0
  - Lyme disease A69.22
  - mercury — see subcategory T56.1
  - mumps B26.2
  - Naegleria (amebae) (organisms) (fowleri) B60.2
  - Parastrongylus cantonensis B83.2
  - toxoplasmosis (acquired) B58.2
    - congenital P37.1
- infectious (acute) (viral) A86
- influenzal (H. influenzae) G00.0
- Listeria monocytogenes A32.12
- lymphocytic (serous) A87.2
- mumps B26.2
- parasitic NEC B89 [G05.3]
- pneumococcal G04.2
- primary amebic B60.2
- specific (syphilitic) A52.14
- specified organism NEC G04.81
- staphylococcal G04.2
- streptococcal G04.2
- syphilitic A52.14
- toxic NEC G92
  - due to mercury — see subcategory T56.1
- tuberculous A17.82
- virus NEC A86

Meningoencephalocele — see also Encephalocele
- syphilitic A52.19
- congenital A50.49

Meningoencephalomyelitis — see also Meningoencephalitis
- acute NEC (viral) A86
  - disseminated G04.00
    - postimmunization or postvaccination G04.02
    - postinfectious G04.01
- due to
  - actinomycosis A42.82
  - Torula B45.1
  - Toxoplasma or toxoplasmosis (acquired) B58.2
    - congenital P37.1
- postimmunization or postvaccination G04.02

Meningoencephalomyelopathy G96.9

Meningoencephalopathy G96.9

Meningomyelitis — see also Meningoencephalitis
- bacterial NEC G04.2
- blastomycotic NEC B40.81
- cryptococcal B45.1
- in diseases classified elsewhere G05.4
- meningococcal A39.81
- syphilitic A52.14
- tuberculous A17.82

Meningomyelocele — *see also* Spina bifida
  syphilitic A52.19
Meningomyeloneuritis — *see* Meningoencephalitis
Meningoradiculitis — *see* Meningitis
Meningovascular — *see* condition
Menkes' disease or syndrome E83.09
  meaning maple-syrup-urine disease E71.0
Menometrorrhagia N92.1
Menopause, menopausal (asymptomatic)
  (state) Z78.0
  arthritis (any site) NEC — *see* Arthritis, specified
    form NEC
  bleeding N92.4
  depression (single episode) F32.89
    agitated (single episode) F32.2
      recurrent episode F33.9
    psychotic (single episode) F32.89
      recurrent episode F33.9
    recurrent episode F33.8
  melancholia (single episode) F32.89
    recurrent episode F33.8
  paranoid state F22
  premature E28.319
    asymptomatic E28.319
      postirradiation E89.40
      postsurgical E89.40
    symptomatic E28.310
      postirradiation E89.41
      postsurgical E89.41
  psychosis NEC F28
  symptomatic N95.1
  toxic polyarthritis NEC — *see* Arthritis, specified
    form NEC
Menorrhagia (primary) N92.0
  climacteric N92.4
    menopausal N92.4
  menopausal N92.4
  postclimacteric N95.0
  postmenopausal N95.0
  preclimacteric or premenopausal N92.4
  pubertal (menses retained) N92.2
Menostaxis N92.0
Menses, retention N94.89
Menstrual — *see* Menstruation
Menstruation
  absent — *see* Amenorrhea
  anovulatory N97.0
  cycle, irregular N92.6
  delayed N91.0
  disorder N93.9
    psychogenic F45.8
  during pregnancy O20.8
  excessive (with regular cycle) N92.0
    with irregular cycle N92.1
      at puberty N92.2
  frequent N92.0
  infrequent — *see* Oligomenorrhea
  irregular N92.6
    specified NEC N92.5
  latent N92.5
  membranous N92.5
  painful — *see also* Dysmenorrhea N94.6
    primary N94.4
    psychogenic F45.8
    secondary N94.5
  passage of clots N92.0
  precocious E30.1
  protracted N92.5
  rare — *see* Oligomenorrhea
  retained N94.89
  retrograde N92.5
  scanty — *see* Oligomenorrhea
  suppression N94.89
  vicarious (nasal) N94.89
Mental — *see also* condition
  deficiency — *see* Disability, intellectual
  deterioration — *see* Psychosis
  disorder — *see* Disorder, mental
  exhaustion F48.8
  insufficiency (congenital) — *see* Disability,
    intellectual
  observation without need for further medical
    care Z03.89
  retardation — *see* Disability, intellectual
  subnormality — *see* Disability, intellectuall
  upset — *see* Disorder, mental
Meralgia paresthetica G57.1-
Mercurial — *see* condition
Mercurialism — *see* subcategory T56.1
Merkel cell tumor — *see* Carcinoma, Merkel cell
Merocele — *see* Hernia, femoral
Meromelia
  lower limb — *see* Defect, reduction, lower limb

Meromelia - *continued*
  lower limb - *continued*
    intercalary
      femur — *see* Defect, reduction, lower limb,
        specified type NEC
      tibiofibular (complete) (incomplete) — *see*
        Defect, reduction, lower limb
    upper limb — *see* Defect, reduction, upper limb
      intercalary, humeral, radioulnar — *see* Agenesis,
        arm, with hand present
MERRF syndrome
  (myoclonic epilepsy associated with ragged-red
  fiber) E88.42
Merzbacher-Pelizaeus disease E75.29
Mesaortitis — *see* Aortitis
Mesarteritis — *see* Arteritis
Mesencephalitis — *see* Encephalitis
Mesenchymoma — *see also* Neoplasm, connective
  tissue, uncertain behavior
  benign — *see* Neoplasm, connective tissue, benign
  malignant — *see* Neoplasm, connective tissue,
    malignant
Mesenteritis
  retractile K65.4
  sclerosing K65.4
Mesentery, mesenteric — *see* condition
Mesiodens, mesiodentes K00.1
Mesio-occlusion M26.213
Mesocolon — *see* condition
Mesonephroma (malignant) — *see* Neoplasm,
  malignant, by site
  benign — *see* Neoplasm, benign, by site
Mesophlebitis — *see* Phlebitis
Mesostromal dysgenesia Q13.89
Mesothelioma (malignant) C45.9
  benign
    mesentery D19.1
    mesocolon D19.1
    omentum D19.1
    peritoneum D19.1
    pleura D19.0
    specified site NEC D19.7
    unspecified site D19.9
  biphasic C45.9
    benign
      mesentery D19.1
      mesocolon D19.1
      omentum D19.1
      peritoneum D19.1
      pleura D19.0
      specified site NEC D19.7
      unspecified site D19.9
  cystic D48.4
  epithelioid C45.9
    benign
      mesentery D19.1
      mesocolon D19.1
      omentum D19.1
      peritoneum D19.1
      pleura D19.0
      specified site NEC D19.7
      unspecified site D19.9
  fibrous C45.9
    benign
      mesentery D19.1
      mesocolon D19.1
      omentum D19.1
      peritoneum D19.1
      pleura D19.0
      specified site NEC D19.7
      unspecified site D19.9
  site classification
    liver C45.7
    lung C45.7
    mediastinum C45.7
    mesentery C45.1
    mesocolon C45.1
    omentum C45.1
    pericardium C45.2
    peritoneum C45.1
    pleura C45.0
      parietal C45.0
    retroperitoneum C45.7
    specified site NEC C45.7
    unspecified C45.9
Metabolic syndrome E88.81
Metagonimiasis B66.8
Metagonimus infestation (intestine) B66.8
Metal
  pigmentation L81.8
  polisher's disease J62.8
Metamorphopsia H53.15

Metaplasia
  apocrine (breast) — *see* Dysplasia, mammary,
    specified type NEC
  cervix (squamous) — *see* Dysplasia, cervix
  endometrium (squamous) (uterus) N85.8
  esophagus K22.7-
  kidney (pelvis) (squamous) N28.89
  myelogenous D73.1
  myeloid (agnogenic) (megakaryocytic) D73.1
  spleen D73.1
  squamous cell, bladder N32.89
Metastasis, metastatic
  abscess — *see* Abscess
  calcification E83.59
  cancer
    from specified site — *see* Neoplasm, malignant, by
      site
    to specified site — *see* Neoplasm, secondary, by
      site
  deposits (in) — *see* Neoplasm, secondary, by site
  disease — *see also* Neoplasm, secondary, by
    site C79.9
  spread (to) — *see* Neoplasm, secondary, by site
Metastrongyliasis B83.8
Metatarsalgia M77.4-
  anterior G57.6-
  Morton's G57.6-
Metatarsus, metatarsal — *see also* condition
  adductus, congenital Q66.22
  valgus (abductus) , congenital Q66.6
  varus (congenital) Q66.22
    primus Q66.21
Methadone use — *see* Use, opioid
Methemoglobinemia D74.9
  acquired (with sulfhemoglobinemia) D74.8
  congenital D74.0
  enzymatic (congenital) D74.0
  Hb M disease D74.0
  hereditary D74.0
  toxic D74.8
Methemoglobinuria — *see* Hemoglobinuria
Methioninemia E72.19
Methylmalonic acidemia E71.120
Metritis (catarrhal) (hemorrhagic) (septic)
  (suppurative) — *see also* Endometritis
  cervical — *see* Cervicitis
Metropathia hemorrhagica N93.8
Metroperitonitis — *see* Peritonitis, pelvic, female
Metrorrhagia N92.1
  climacteric N92.4
  menopausal N92.4
  postpartum NEC (atonic) (following delivery of
    placenta) O72.1
    delayed or secondary O72.2
  preclimacteric or premenopausal N92.4
  psychogenic F45.8
Metrorrhexis — *see* Rupture, uterus
Metrosalpingitis N70.91
Metrostaxis N93.8
Metrovaginitis — *see* Endometritis
Meyer-Schwickerath and Weyers syndrome Q87.0
Meynert's amentia (nonalcoholic) F04
  alcoholic F10.96
    with dependence F10.26
Mibelli's disease (porokeratosis) Q82.8
Mice, joint — *see* Loose, body, joint
  knee M23.4-
Micrencephalon, micrencephaly Q02
Microalbuminuria R80.9
Microaneurysm, retinal — *see also* Disorder, retina,
  microaneurysms
  diabetic — *see* E08-E13 with .31
Microangiopathy (peripheral) I73.9
  thrombotic M31.1
Microcalcifications, breast R92.0
Microcephalus, microcephalic, microcephaly Q02
  due to toxoplasmosis (congenital) P37.1
Microcheilia Q18.7
Microcolon (congenital) Q43.8
Microcornea (congenital) Q13.4
Microcytic — *see* condition
Microdeletions NEC Q93.88
Microdontia K00.2
Microdrepanocytosis D57.40
  with crisis (vasoocclusive pain) D57.419
    with
      acute chest syndrome D57.411
      splenic sequestration D57.412
Microembolism
  atherothrombotic — *see* Atheroembolism
  retinal — *see* Occlusion, artery, retina
Microencephalon Q02

Microfilaria streptocerca infestation — *see* Onchocerciasis
Microgastria (congenital) Q40.2
Microgenia M26.06
Microgenitalia, congenital
  female Q52.8
  male Q55.8
Microglioma — *see* Lymphoma, non-Hodgkin, specified NEC
Microglossia (congenital) Q38.3
Micrognathia, micrognathism (congenital) (mandibular) (maxillary) M26.09
Microgyria (congenital) Q04.3
Microinfarct of heart — *see* Insufficiency, coronary
Microlentia (congenital) Q12.8
Microlithiasis, alveolar, pulmonary J84.02
Micromastia N64.82
Micromyelia (congenital) Q06.8
Micropenis Q55.62
Microphakia (congenital) Q12.8
Microphthalmos, microphthalmia (congenital) Q11.2
  due to toxoplasmosis P37.1
Micropsia H53.15
Microscopic polyangiitis (polyarteritis) M31.7
Microsporidiosis B60.8
  intestinal A07.8
Microsporon furfur infestation B36.0
Microsporosis — *see also* Dermatophytosis
  nigra B36.1
Microstomia (congenital) Q18.5
Microtia (congenital) (external ear) Q17.2
Microtropia H50.40
Microvillus inclusion disease (MVD) (MVID) Q43.8
Micturition
  disorder NEC — *see also* Difficulty, micturition R39.198
    psychogenic F45.8
  frequency R35.0
    psychogenic F45.8
  hesitancy R39.11
  incomplete emptying R39.14
  nocturnal R35.1
  painful R30.9
    dysuria R30.0
    psychogenic F45.8
    tenesmus R30.1
  poor stream R39.12
  position dependent R39.192
  split stream R39.13
  straining R39.16
  urgency R39.15
Mid plane — *see* condition
Middle
  ear — *see* condition
  lobe (right) syndrome J98.19
Miescher's elastoma L87.2
Mietens' syndrome Q87.2
Migraine (idiopathic) G43.909
  with refractory migraine G43.919
    with status migrainosus G43.911
    without status migrainosus G43.919
  with aura (acute-onset) (prolonged) (typical) (without headache) G43.109
    with refractory migraine G43.119
      with status migrainosus G43.111
      without status migrainosus G43.119
    intractable G43.119
      with status migrainosus G43.111
      without status migrainosus G43.119
    not intractable G43.109
      with status migrainosus G43.101
      without status migrainosus G43.109
    persistent G43.509
      with cerebral infarction G43.609
        with refractory migraine G43.619
          with status migrainosus G43.611
          without status migrainosus G43.619
        intractable G43.619
          with status migrainosus G43.611
          without status migrainosus G43.619
        not intractable G43.609
          with status migrainosus G43.601
          without status migrainosus G43.609
        without refractory migraine G43.609
          with status migrainosus G43.601
          without status migrainosus G43.609
      without cerebral infarction G43.509
        with refractory migraine G43.519
          with status migrainosus G43.511

Migraine (idiopathic) - *continued*
  with aura (acute-onset) (prolonged) (typical) (without headache) - *continued*
    persistent - *continued*
      without cerebral infarction - *continued*
        intractable - *continued*
          without status migrainosus G43.519
        not intractable G43.509
          with status migrainosus G43.501
          without status migrainosus G43.509
        without refractory migraine G43.509
          with status migrainosus G43.501
          without status migrainosus G43.509
    without mention of refractory migraine G43.109
      with status migrainosus G43.101
      without status migrainosus G43.109
  abdominal G43.D0
    with refractory migraine G43.D1
    intractable G43.D1
    not intractable G43.D0
    without refractory migraine G43.D0
  basilar — *see* Migraine, with aura
  classical — *see* Migraine, with aura
  common — *see* Migraine, without aura
  complicated G43.109
  equivalents — *see* Migraine, with aura
  familiar — *see* Migraine, hemiplegic
  hemiplegic G43.409
    with refractory migraine G43.419
      with status migrainosus G43.411
      without status migrainosus G43.419
    intractable G43.419
      with status migrainosus G43.411
      without status migrainosus G43.419
    not intractable G43.409
      with status migrainosus G43.401
      without status migrainosus G43.409
    without refractory migraine G43.409
      with status migrainosus G43.401
      without status migrainosus G43.409
    intractable G43.919
      with status migrainosus G43.911
      without status migrainosus G43.919
  menstrual G43.829
    with refractory migraine G43.839
      with status migrainosus G43.831
      without status migrainosus G43.839
    intractable G43.839
      with status migrainosus G43.831
      without status migrainosus G43.839
    not intractable 4G43.829
      with status migrainosus G43.821
      without status migrainosus G43.829
    without refractory migraine G43.829
      with status migrainosus G43.821
      without status migrainosus G43.829
  menstrually related — *see* Migraine, menstrual
  not intractable G43.909
    with status migrainosus G43.901
    without status migrainosus G43.919
  ophthalmoplegic G43.B0
    with refractory migraine G43.B1
    intractable G43.B1
    not intractable G43.B0
    without refractory migraine G43.B0
  persistent aura (with, without) cerebral infarction — *see* Migraine, with aura, persistent
  preceded or accompanied by transient focal neurological phenomena — *see* Migraine, with aura
  pre-menstrual — *see* Migraine, menstrual
  pure menstrual — *see* Migraine, menstrual
  retinal — *see* Migraine, with aura
  specified NEC G43.809
    intractable G43.819
      with status migrainosus G43.811
      without status migrainosus G43.819
    not intractable G43.809
      with status migrainosus G43.801
      without status migrainosus G43.809
  sporadic — *see* Migraine, hemiplegic
  transformed — *see* Migraine, without aura, chronic
  triggered seizures — *see* Migraine, with aura
  without aura G43.009
    with refractory migraine G43.019
      with status migrainosus G43.011
      without status migrainosus G43.019
    chronic G43.709
      with refractory migraine G43.719
        with status migrainosus G43.711
        without status migrainosus G43.719
      intractable
        with status migrainosus G43.711

Migraine (idiopathic) - *continued*
  without aura - *continued*
    chronic - *continued*
      intractable - *continued*
        without status migrainosus G43.719
      not intractable
        with status migrainosus G43.701
        without status migrainosus G43.709
      without refractory migraine G43.709
        with status migrainosus G43.701
        without status migrainosus G43.709
    intractable
      with status migrainosus G43.011
      without status migrainosus G43.019
    not intractable
      with status migrainosus G43.001
      without status migrainosus G43.009
    without mention of refractory migraine G43.009
      with status migrainosus G43.001
      without status migrainosus G43.009
    without refractory migraine G43.909
      with status migrainosus G43.901
      without status migrainosus G43.919
Migrant, social Z59.0
Migration, anxiety concerning Z60.3
Migratory, migrating — *see also* condition
  person Z59.0
  testis Q55.29
Mikity-Wilson disease or syndrome P27.0
Mikulicz' disease or syndrome K11.8
Miliaria L74.3
  alba L74.1
  apocrine L75.2
  crystallina L74.1
  profunda L74.2
  rubra L74.0
  tropicalis L74.2
Miliary — *see* condition
Milium L72.0
  colloid L57.8
Milk
  crust L21.0
  excessive secretion O92.6
  poisoning — *see* Poisoning, food, noxious
  retention O92.79
  sickness — *see* Poisoning, food, noxious
  spots I31.0
Milk-alkali disease or syndrome E83.52
Milk-leg (deep vessels) (nonpuerperal) — *see* Embolism, vein, lower extremity
  complicating pregnancy O22.3-
  puerperal, postpartum, childbirth O87.1
Milkman's disease or syndrome M83.8
Milky urine — *see* Chyluria
Millard-Gubler (-Foville) **paralysis or syndrome** G46.3
Millar's asthma J38.5
Miller Fisher syndrome G61.0
Mills' disease — *see* Hemiplegia
Millstone maker's pneumoconiosis J62.8
Milroy's disease (chronic hereditary edema) Q82.0
Minamata disease T56.1
Miners' asthma or lung J60
Minkowski-Chauffard syndrome — *see* Spherocytosis
Minor — *see* condition
Minor's disease (hematomyelia) G95.19
Minot's disease (hemorrhagic disease) , newborn P53
Minot-von Willebrand-Jurgens disease or syndrome (angiohemophilia) D68.0
Minus (and plus) **hand** (intrinsic) — *see* Deformity, limb, specified type NEC, forearm
Miosis (pupil) H57.03
Mirizzi's syndrome (hepatic duct stenosis) K83.1
Mirror writing F81.0
Misadventure (of) (prophylactic) (therapeutic) — *see also* Complications T88.9
  administration of insulin (by accident) — *see* subcategory T38.3
  infusion — *see* Complications, infusion
  local applications (of fomentations, plasters, etc.) T88.9
    burn or scald — *see* Burn
    specified NEC T88.8
  medical care (early) (late) T88.9
    adverse effect of drugs or chemicals — *see* Table of Drugs and Chemicals
  medical care (early) (late)
    burn or scald — *see* Burn
    specified NEC T88.8
  specified NEC T88.8

Misadventure (of) (prophylactic) (therapeutic) - *continued*
surgical procedure (early) (late) — *see* Complications, surgical procedure
transfusion — *see* Complications, transfusion
vaccination or other immunological procedure — *see* Complications, vaccination
Miscarriage O03.9
Misdirection, aqueous H40.83-
Misperception, sleep state F51.02
Misplaced, misplacement
ear Q17.4
kidney (acquired) N28.89
congenital Q63.2
organ or site, congenital NEC — *see* Malposition, congenital
Missed
abortion O02.1
delivery O36.4
Missing — *see also* Absence
string of intrauterine contraceptive device T83.32
Misuse of drugs F19.99
Mitchell's disease (erythromelalgia) I73.81
Mite (s) (infestation) B88.9
diarrhea B88.0
grain (itch) B88.0
hair follicle (itch) B88.0
in sputum B88.0
Mitral — *see* condition
Mittelschmerz N94.0
Mixed — *see* condition
MMN (multifocal motor neuropathy) G61.82
MNGIE
(Mitochondrial Neurogastrointestinal Encephalopathy) **syndrome** E88.49
Mobile, mobility
cecum Q43.3
excessive — *see* Hypermobility
gallbladder, congenital Q44.1
kidney N28.89
organ or site, congenital NEC — *see* Malposition, congenital
Mobitz heart block (atrioventricular) I44.1
Moebius, Möbius
disease (ophthalmoplegic migraine) — *see* Migraine, ophthalmoplegic
syndrome Q87.0
congenital oculofacial paralysis (with other anomalies) Q87.0
ophthalmoplegic migraine — *see* Migraine, ophthalmoplegic
Moeller's glossitis K14.0
Mohr's syndrome (Types I and II) Q87.0
Mola destruens D39.2
Molar pregnancy O02.0
Molarization of premolars K00.2
Molding, head (during birth) - **omit code**
Mole (pigmented) — *see also* Nevus
blood O02.0
Breus' O02.0
cancerous — *see* Melanoma
carneous O02.0
destructive D39.2
fleshy O02.0
hydatid, hydatidiform (benign) (complicating pregnancy) (delivered) (undelivered) O01.9
classical O01.0
complete O01.0
incomplete O01.1
invasive D39.2
malignant D39.2
partial O01.1
intrauterine O02.0
invasive (hydatidiform) D39.2
malignant
meaning
malignant hydatidiform mole D39.2
melanoma — *see* Melanoma
nonhydatidiform O02.0
nonpigmented — *see* Nevus
pregnancy NEC O02.0
skin — *see* Nevus
tubal O00.10
with intrauterine pregnancy O00.11
vesicular — *see* Mole, hydatidiform
Molimen, molimina (menstrual) N94.3
Molluscum contagiosum (epitheliale) B08.1
Mönckeberg's arteriosclerosis, disease, or sclerosis — *see* Arteriosclerosis, extremities
Mondini's malformation (cochlea) Q16.5
Mondor's disease I80.8
Monge's disease T70.29
Monilethrix (congenital) Q84.1

Moniliasis — *see also* Candidiasis B37.9
neonatal P37.5
Monitoring (encounter for)
therapeutic drug level Z51.81
Monkey malaria B53.1
Monkeypox B04
Monoarthritis M13.10
ankle M13.17-
elbow M13.12-
foot joint M13.17-
hand joint M13.14-
hip M13.15-
knee M13.16-
shoulder M13.11-
wrist M13.13-
Monoblastic — *see* condition
Monochromat (ism) **, monochromatopsia** (acquired) (congenital) H53.51
Monocytic — *see* condition
Monocytopenia D72.818
Monocytosis (symptomatic) D72.821
Monomania — *see* Psychosis
Mononeuritis G58.9
cranial nerve — *see* Disorder, nerve, cranial
femoral nerve G57.2-
lateral
cutaneous nerve of thigh G57.1-
popliteal nerve G57.3-
lower limb G57.9-
specified nerve NEC G57.8-
medial popliteal nerve G57.4-
median nerve G56.1-
multiplex G58.7
plantar nerve G57.6-
posterior tibial nerve G57.5-
radial nerve G56.3-
sciatic nerve G57.0-
specified NEC G58.8
tibial nerve G57.4-
ulnar nerve G56.2-
upper limb G56.9-
specified nerve NEC G56.8-
vestibular — *see* subcategory H93.3
Mononeuropathy G58.9
carpal tunnel syndrome — *see* Syndrome, carpal tunnel
diabetic NEC — *see* E08-E13 with .41
femoral nerve — *see* Lesion, nerve, femoral
ilioinguinal nerve G57.8-
in diseases classified elsewhere — *see* category G59
intercostal G58.0
lower limb G57.9-
causalgia — *see* Causalgia, lower limb
femoral nerve — *see* Lesion, nerve, femoral
meralgia paresthetica G57.1-
plantar nerve — *see* Lesion, nerve, plantar
popliteal nerve — *see* Lesion, nerve, popliteal
sciatic nerve — *see* Lesion, nerve, sciatic
specified NEC G57.8-
tarsal tunnel syndrome — *see* Syndrome, tarsal tunnel
median nerve — *see* Lesion, nerve, median
multiplex G58.7
obturator nerve G57.8-
popliteal nerve — *see* Lesion, nerve, popliteal
radial nerve — *see* Lesion, nerve, radial
saphenous nerve G57.8-
specified NEC G58.8
tarsal tunnel syndrome — *see* Syndrome, tarsal tunnel
tuberculous A17.83
ulnar nerve — *see* Lesion, nerve, ulnar
upper limb G56.9-
carpal tunnel syndrome — *see* Syndrome, carpal tunnel
causalgia — *see* Causalgia
median nerve — *see* Lesion, nerve, median
radial nerve — *see* Lesion, nerve, radial
specified site NEC G56.8-
ulnar nerve — *see* Lesion, nerve, ulnar
Mononucleosis, infectious B27.90
with
complication NEC B27.99
meningitis B27.92
polyneuropathy B27.91
cytomegaloviral B27.10
with
complication NEC B27.19
meningitis B27.12
polyneuropathy B27.11
Epstein-Barr (virus) B27.00
with
complication NEC B27.09

Mononucleosis, infectious - *continued*
Epstein-Barr (virus) - *continued*
with - *continued*
meningitis B27.02
polyneuropathy B27.01
gammaherpesviral B27.00
with
complication NEC B27.09
meningitis B27.02
polyneuropathy B27.01
specified NEC B27.80
with
complication NEC B27.89
meningitis B27.82
polyneuropathy B27.81
Monoplegia G83.3-
congenital (cerebral) G80.8
spastic G80.1
embolic (current episode) I63.4-
following
cerebrovascular disease
cerebral infarction
lower limb I69.34-
upper limb I69.33-
intracerebral hemorrhage
lower limb I69.14-
upper limb I69.13-
lower limb I69.94-
nontraumatic intracranial hemorrhage NEC
lower limb I69.24-
upper limb I69.23-
specified disease NEC
lower limb I69.84-
upper limb I69.83-
stroke NOS
lower limb I69.34-
upper limb I69.33-
subarachnoid hemorrhage
lower limb I69.04-
upper limb I69.03-
upper limb I69.93-
hysterical (transient) F44.4
lower limb G83.1-
psychogenic (conversion reaction) F44.4
thrombotic (current episode) I63.3-
transient R29.818
upper limb G83.2-
Monorchism, monorchidism Q55.0
Monosomy — *see also* Deletion, chromosome Q93.9
specified NEC Q93.89
whole chromosome
meiotic nondisjunction Q93.0
mitotic nondisjunction Q93.1
mosaicism Q93.1
X Q96.9
Monster, monstrosity (single) Q89.7
acephalic Q00.0
twin Q89.4
Monteggia's fracture (-dislocation) S52.27-
Mooren's ulcer (cornea) — *see* Ulcer, cornea, Mooren's
Moore's syndrome — *see* Epilepsy, specified NEC
Mooser-Neill reaction A75.2
Mooser's bodies A75.2
Morbidity not stated or unknown R69
Morbilli — *see* Measles
Morbus — *see also* Disease
angelicus, anglorum E55.0
Beigel B36.2
caducus — *see* Epilepsy
celiacus K90.0
comitialis — *see* Epilepsy
cordis — *see also* Disease, heart I51.9
valvulorum — *see* Endocarditis
coxae senilis M16.9
tuberculous A18.02
hemorrhagicus neonatorum P53
maculosus neonatorum P54.5
Morel (-Stewart) (-Morgagni) **syndrome** M85.2
Morel-Kraepelin disease — *see* Schizophrenia
Morel-Moore syndrome M85.2
Morgagni's
cyst, organ, hydatid, or appendage
female Q50.5
male (epididymal) Q55.4
testicular Q55.29
syndrome M85.2
Morgagni-Stewart-Morel syndrome M85.2
Morgagni-Stokes-Adams syndrome I45.9
Morgagni-Turner (-Albright) **syndrome** Q96.9
Moria F07.0
Moron (I.Q.50-69) F70
Morphea L94.0

Morphinism (without remission) F11.20
  with remission F11.21
Morphinomania (without remission) F11.20
  with remission F11.21
Morquio (-Ullrich) (-Brailsford)
  disease or syndrome — *see* Mucopolysaccharidosis
Mortification (dry) (moist) — *see* Gangrene
Morton's metatarsalgia (neuralgia) (neuroma)
  (syndrome) G57.6-
Morvan's disease or syndrome G60.8
Mosaicism, mosaic (autosomal) (chromosomal)
  45,X/other cell lines NEC with abnormal sex
    chromosome Q96.4
  45,X/46,XX Q96.3
  sex chromosome
    female Q97.8
    lines with various numbers of X
      chromosomes Q97.2
    male Q98.7
  XY Q96.3
Moschowitz' disease M31.1
Mother yaw A66.0
Motion sickness (from travel, any vehicle)
  (from roundabouts or swings) T75.3
Mottled, mottling, teeth (enamel) (endemic)
  (nonendemic) K00.3
Mounier-Kuhn syndrome Q32.4
  with bronchiectasis J47.9
    exacerbation (acute) J47.1
    lower respiratory infection J47.0
  acquired J98.09
    with bronchiectasis J47.9
      with
        exacerbation (acute) J47.1
        lower respiratory infection J47.0
Mountain
  sickness T70.29
    with polycythemia , acquired (acute) D75.1
  tick fever A93.2
Mouse, joint — *see* Loose, body, joint
  knee M23.4-
Mouth — *see* condition
Movable
  coccyx — *see* subcategory M53.2
  kidney N28.89
    congenital Q63.8
  spleen D73.89
Movements, dystonic R25.8
Moyamoya disease I67.5
MRSA (Methicillin resistant Staphylococcus aureus)
  infection A49.02
    as the cause of diseases classified
      elsewhere B95.62
  sepsis A41.02
MSSA
  (Methicillin susceptible Staphylococcus aureus)
  infection A49.01
    as the cause of diseases classified
      elsewhere B95.61
  sepsis A41.01
Mucha-Habermann disease L41.0
Mucinosis (cutaneous) (focal) (papular)
  (reticular erythematous) (skin) L98.5
  oral K13.79
Mucocele
  appendix K38.8
  buccal cavity K13.79
  gallbladder K82.1
  lacrimal sac, chronic H04.43-
  nasal sinus J34.1
  nose J34.1
  salivary gland (any) K11.6
  sinus (accessory) (nasal) J34.1
  turbinate (bone) (middle) (nasal) J34.1
  uterus N85.8
Mucolipidosis
  I E77.1
  II, III E77.0
  IV E75.11
Mucopolysaccharidosis E76.3
  beta-gluduronidase deficiency E76.29
  cardiopathy E76.3 *[I52]*
  Hunter's syndrome E76.1
  Hurler's syndrome E76.01
  Hurler-Scheie syndrome E76.02
  Maroteaux-Lamy syndrome E76.29
  Morquio syndrome E76.219
    A E76.210
    B E76.211
    classic E76.210
  Sanfilippo syndrome E76.22
  Scheie's syndrome E76.03
  specified NEC E76.29

Mucopolysaccharidosis - *continued*
  type
    I
      Hurler's syndrome E76.01
      Hurler-Scheie syndrome E76.02
      Scheie's syndrome E76.03
    II E76.1
    III E76.22
    IV E76.219
    IVA E76.210
    IVB E76.211
    VI E76.29
    VII E76.29
Mucormycosis B46.5
  cutaneous B46.3
  disseminated B46.4
  gastrointestinal B46.2
  generalized B46.4
  pulmonary B46.0
  rhinocerebral B46.1
  skin B46.3
  subcutaneous B46.3
Mucositis (ulcerative) K12.30
  due to drugs NEC K12.32
  gastrointestinal K92.81
  mouth (oral) (oropharyngeal) K12.30
    due to antineoplastic therapy K12.31
    due to drugs NEC K12.32
    due to radiation K12.33
    specified NEC K12.39
    viral K12.39
  nasal J34.81
  oral cavity — *see* Mucositis, mouth
  oral soft tissues — *see* Mucositis, mouth
  vagina and vulva N76.81
Mucositis necroticans agranulocytica — *see*
  Agranulocytosis
Mucous — *see also* condition
  patches (syphilitic) A51.39
    congenital A50.07
Mucoviscidosis E84.9
  with meconium obstruction E84.11
Mucus
  asphyxia or suffocation — *see* Asphyxia, mucus
  in stool R19.5
  plug — *see* Asphyxia, mucus
Muguet B37.0
Mulberry molars (congenital syphilis) A50.52
Müllerian mixed tumor
  specified site — *see* Neoplasm, malignant, by site
  unspecified site C54.9
Multicystic kidney (development) Q61.4
Multiparity (grand) Z64.1
  affecting management of pregnancy, labor and
    delivery (supervision only) O09.4-
  requiring contraceptive management — *see*
    Contraception
Multipartita placenta O43.19-
Multiple, multiplex — *see also* condition
  digits (congenital) Q69.9
  endocrine neoplasia — *see* Neoplasia, endocrine,
    multiple (MEN)
  personality F44.81
Mumps B26.9
  arthritis B26.85
  complication NEC B26.89
  encephalitis B26.2
  hepatitis B26.81
  meningitis (aseptic) B26.1
  meningoencephalitis B26.2
  myocarditis B26.82
  oophoritis B26.89
  orchitis B26.0
  pancreatitis B26.3
  polyneuropathy B26.84
Mumu — *see also* Infestation, filarial B74.9 *[N51]*
Münchhausen's syndrome — *see* Disorder,
  factitious
Münchmeyer's syndrome — *see* Myositis,
  ossificans, progressiva
Mural — *see* condition
Murmur (cardiac) (heart) (organic) R01.1
  abdominal R19.15
  aortic (valve) — *see* Endocarditis, aortic
  benign R01.0
  diastolic — *see* Endocarditis
  Flint I35.1
  functional R01.0
  Graham Steell I37.1
  innocent R01.0
  mitral (valve) — *see* Insufficiency, mitral
  nonorganic R01.0
  presystolic, mitral — *see* Insufficiency, mitral

Murmur (cardiac) (heart) (organic) - *continued*
  pulmonic (valve) I37.8
  systolic R01.1
  tricuspid (valve) I07.9
  valvular — *see* Endocarditis
Murri's disease (intermittent hemoglobinuria) D59.6
Muscle, muscular — *see also* condition
  carnitine (palmityltransferase) deficiency E71.314
Musculoneuralgia — *see* Neuralgia
Mushrooming hip — *see* Derangement, joint,
  specified NEC, hip
Mushroom-workers' (pickers') **disease or lung** J67.5
Mutation (s)
  factor V Leiden D68.51
  surfactant, of lung J84.83
  prothrombin gene D68.52
Mutism — *see also* Aphasia
  deaf (acquired) (congenital) NEC H91.3
  elective (adjustment reaction) (childhood) F94.0
  hysterical F44.4
  selective (childhood) F94.0
MVD (microvillus inclusion disease) Q43.8
MVID (microvillus inclusion disease) Q43.8
Myalgia M79.1
  epidemic (cervical) B33.0
  traumatic NEC T14.8
Myasthenia G70.9
  congenital G70.2
  cordis — *see* Failure, heart
  developmental G70.2
  gravis G70.00
    with exacerbation (acute) G70.01
    in crisis G70.01
  neonatal, transient P94.0
  pseudoparalytica G70.00
    with exacerbation (acute) G70.01
    in crisis G70.01
  stomach, psychogenic F45.8
  syndrome
    in
      diabetes mellitus — *see* E08-E13 with .44
      neoplastic disease — *see*
        also Neoplasm D49.9 *[G73.3]*
      pernicious anemia D51.0 *[G73.3]*
      thyrotoxicosis E05.90 *[G73.3]*
        with thyroid storm E05.91 *[G73.3]*
Myasthenic M62.81
Mycelium infection B49
Mycetismus — *see* Poisoning, food, noxious,
  mushroom
Mycetoma B47.9
  actinomycotic B47.1
  bone (mycotic) B47.9 *[M90.80]*
  eumycotic B47.0
  foot B47.9
    actinomycotic B47.1
    mycotic B47.0
  madurae NEC B47.9
    mycotic B47.0
  maduromycotic B47.0
  mycotic B47.0
  nocardial B47.1
Mycobacteriosis — *see* Mycobacterium
Mycobacterium, mycobacterial (infection) A31.9
  anonymous A31.9
  atypical A31.9
    cutaneous A31.1
    pulmonary A31.0
      tuberculous — *see* Tuberculosis, pulmonary
    specified site NEC A31.8
  avium (intracellulare complex) A31.0
  balnei A31.1
  Battey A31.0
  chelonei A31.8
  cutaneous A31.1
  extrapulmonary systemic A31.8
  fortuitum A31.8
  intracellulare (Battey bacillus) A31.0
  kansasii (yellow bacillus) A31.0
  kakaferifu A31.8
  kasongo A31.8
  leprae — *see also* Leprosy A30.9
  luciflavum A31.1
  marinum (M. balnei) A31.1
  nonspecific — *see* Mycobacterium, atypical
  pulmonary (atypical) A31.0
    tuberculous — *see* Tuberculosis, pulmonary
  scrofulaceum A31.8
  simiae A31.8
  systemic, extrapulmonary A31.8
  szulgai A31.8
  terrae A31.8
  triviale A31.8

Mycobacterium, mycobacterial (infection) - *continued*
tuberculosis (human, bovine) - see Tuberculosis
ulcerans A31.1
xenopi A31.8
Mycoplasma (M.)
pneumoniae, as cause of disease classified elsewhere B96.0
Mycosis, mycotic B49
cutaneous NEC B36.9
ear B36.9
in
aspergillosis B44.89
candidiasis B37.84
moniliasis B37.84
fungoides (extranodal) (solid organ) C84.0-
mouth B37.0
nails B35.1
opportunistic B48.8
skin NEC B36.9
specified NEC B48.8
stomatitis B37.0
vagina, vaginitis (candidal) B37.3
Mydriasis (pupil) H57.04
Myelatelia Q06.1
Myelinolysis, pontine, central G37.2
Myelitis (acute) (ascending) (childhood) (chronic) (descending) (diffuse) (disseminated) (idiopathic) (pressure) (progressive) (spinal cord) (subacute) — see also Encephalitis G04.91
herpes simplex B00.82
herpes zoster B02.24
in diseases classified elsewhere G05.4
necrotizing, subacute G37.4
optic neuritis in G36.0
postchickenpox B01.12
postherpetic B02.24
postimmunization G04.02
postinfectious NEC G04.89
postvaccinal G04.02
specified NEC G04.89
syphilitic (transverse) A52.14
toxic G92
transverse (in demyelinating diseases of central nervous system) G37.3
tuberculous A17.82
varicella B01.12
Myeloblastic — see condition
Myeloblastoma
granular cell — see also Neoplasm, connective tissue
malignant — see Neoplasm, connective tissue, malignant
tongue D10.1
Myelocele — see Spina bifida
Myelocystocele — see Spina bifida
Myelocytic — see condition
Myelodysplasia D46.9
specified NEC D46.Z
spinal cord (congenital) Q06.1
Myelodysplastic syndrome D46.9
with
5q deletion D46.C
isolated del (5q) chromosomal abnormality D46.C
specified NEC D46.Z
Myeloencephalitis — see Encephalitis
Myelofibrosis D75.81
with myeloid metaplasia D47.4
acute C94.4-
idiopathic (chronic) D47.4
primary D47.1
secondary D75.81
in myeloproliferative disease D47.4
Myelogenous — see condition
Myeloid — see condition
Myelokathexis D70.9
Myeloleukodystrophy E75.29
Myelolipoma — see Lipoma
Myeloma (multiple) C90.0-
monostotic C90.3
plasma cell C90.0-
plasma cell C90.0-
solitary — see also Plasmacytoma, solitary C90.3-
Myelomalacia G95.89
Myelomatosis C90.0-
Myelomeningitis — see Meningoencephalitis
Myelomeningocele (spinal cord) — see Spina bifida
Myelo-osteo-musculodysplasia hereditaria Q79.8
Myelopathic
anemia D64.89
muscle atrophy — see Atrophy, muscle, spinal
pain syndrome G89.0

Myelopathy (spinal cord) G95.9
drug-induced G95.89
in (due to)
degeneration or displacement, intervertebral disc NEC — see Disorder, disc, with, myelopathy
infection — see Encephalitis
intervertebral disc disorder — see also Disorder, disc, with, myelopathy
mercury — see subcategory T56.1
neoplastic disease — see also Neoplasm D49.9 [G99.2]
pernicious anemia D51.0 [G99.2]
spondylosis — see Spondylosis, with myelopathy NEC
necrotic (subacute) (vascular) G95.19
radiation-induced G95.89
spondylogenic NEC — see Spondylosis, with myelopathy NEC
toxic G95.89
transverse, acute G37.3
vascular G95.19
vitamin B12 E53.8 [G32.0]
Myelophthisis D61.82
Myeloradiculitis G04.91
Myeloradiculodysplasia (spinal) Q06.1
Myelosarcoma C92.3-
Myelosclerosis D75.89
with myeloid metaplasia D47.4
disseminated, of nervous system G35
megakaryocytic D47.4
with myeloid metaplasia D47.4
Myelosis
acute C92.0-
aleukemic C92.9-
chronic D47.1
erythremic (acute) C94.0-
megakaryocytic C94.2-
nonleukemic D72.828
subacute C92.9-
Myiasis (cavernous) B87.9
aural B87.4
creeping B87.0
cutaneous B87.0
dermal B87.0
ear (external) (middle) B87.4
eye B87.2
genitourinary B87.81
intestinal B87.82
laryngeal B87.3
nasopharyngeal B87.3
ocular B87.2
orbit B87.2
skin B87.0
specified site NEC B87.89
traumatic B87.1
wound B87.1
Myoadenoma, prostate — see Hyperplasia, prostate
Myoblastoma
granular cell — see also Neoplasm, connective tissue, benign
malignant — see Neoplasm, connective tissue, malignant
tongue D10.1
Myocardial — see condition
Myocardiopathy (congestive) (constrictive) (familial) (hypertrophic nonobstructive) (idiopathic) (infiltrative) (obstructive) (primary) (restrictive) (sporadic) — see also Cardiomyopathy I42.9
alcoholic I42.6
cobalt-beer I42.6
glycogen storage E74.02 [I43]
hypertrophic obstructive I42.1
in (due to)
beriberi E51.12
cardiac glycogenosis E74.02 [I43]
Friedreich's ataxia G11.1 [I43]
myotonia atrophica G71.11 [I43]
progressive muscular dystrophy G71.0 [I43]
obscure (African) I42.8
secondary I42.9
thyrotoxic E05.90 [I43]
with storm E05.91 [I43]
toxic NEC I42.7
Myocarditis (with arteriosclerosis) (chronic) (fibroid) (interstitial) (old) (progressive) (senile) I51.4
with
rheumatic fever (conditions in I00) I09.0
active — see Myocarditis, acute, rheumatic
inactive or quiescent (with chorea) I09.0
active I40.9
rheumatic I01.2
with chorea (acute) (rheumatic) (Sydenham's) I02.0

Myocarditis (with arteriosclerosis) (chronic) (fibroid) (interstitial) (old) (progressive) (senile) - *continued*
acute or subacute (interstitial) I40.9
due to
streptococcus (beta-hemolytic) I01.2
idiopathic I40.1
rheumatic I01.2
with chorea (acute) (rheumatic) (Sydenham's) I02.0
specified NEC I40.8
aseptic of newborn B33.22
bacterial (acute) I40.0
Coxsackie (virus) B33.22
diphtheritic A36.81
eosinophilic I40.1
epidemic of newborn (Coxsackie) B33.22
Fiedler's (acute) (isolated) I40.1
giant cell (acute) (subacute) I40.1
gonococcal A54.83
granulomatous (idiopathic) (isolated) (nonspecific) I40.1
hypertensive — see Hypertension, heart
idiopathic (granulomatous) I40.1
in (due to)
diphtheria A36.81
epidemic louse-borne typhus A75.0 [I41]
Lyme disease A69.29
sarcoidosis D86.85
scarlet fever A38.1
toxoplasmosis (acquired) B58.81
typhoid A01.02
typhus NEC A75.9 [I41]
infective I40.0
influenzal — see Influenza, with, myocarditis
isolated (acute) I40.1
meningococcal A39.52
mumps B26.82
nonrheumatic, active I40.9
parenchymatous I40.9
pneumococcal I40.0
rheumatic (chronic) (inactive) (with chorea) I09.0
active or acute I01.2
with chorea (acute) (rheumatic) (Sydenham's) I02.0
rheumatoid — see Rheumatoid, carditis
septic I40.0
staphylococcal I40.0
suppurative I40.0
syphilitic (chronic) A52.06
toxic I40.8
rheumatic — see Myocarditis, acute, rheumatic
tuberculous A18.84
typhoid A01.02
valvular — see Endocarditis
virus, viral I40.0
of newborn (Coxsackie) B33.22
Myocardium, myocardial — see condition
Myocardosis — see Cardiomyopathy
Myoclonus, myoclonic, myoclonia (familial) (essential) (multifocal) (simplex) G25.3
drug-induced G25.3
epilepsy — see also Epilepsy, generalized, specified NEC G40.4-
familial (progressive) G25.3
epileptica G40.409
with status epilepticus G40.401
facial G51.3
familial progressive G25.3
Friedreich's G25.3
jerks G25.3
massive G25.3
palatal G25.3
pharyngeal G25.3
Myocytolysis I51.5
Myodiastasis — see Diastasis, muscle
Myoendocarditis — see Endocarditis
Myoepithelioma — see Neoplasm, benign, by site
Myofasciitis (acute) — see Myositis
Myofibroma — see also Neoplasm, connective tissue, benign
uterus (cervix) (corpus) — see Leiomyoma
Myofibromatosis D48.1
infantile Q89.8
Myofibrosis M62.89
heart — see Myocarditis
scapulohumeral — see Lesion, shoulder, specified NEC
Myofibrositis M79.7
scapulohumeral — see Lesion, shoulder, specified NEC
Myoglobulinuria, myoglobinuria (primary) R82.1
Myokymia, facial G51.4
Myolipoma — see Lipoma

Myoma — *see also* Neoplasm, connective tissue, benign
  malignant — *see* Neoplasm, connective tissue, malignant
  prostate D29.1
  uterus (cervix) (corpus) — *see* Leiomyoma
Myomalacia M62.89
Myometritis — *see* Endometritis
Myometrium — *see* condition
Myonecrosis, clostridial A48.0
Myopathy G72.9
  acute
    necrotizing G72.81
    quadriplegic G72.81
  alcoholic G72.1
  benign congenital G71.2
  central core G71.2
  centronuclear G71.2
  congenital (benign) G71.2
  critical illness G72.81
  distal G71.0
  drug-induced G72.0
  endocrine NEC E34.9 *[G73.7]*
  extraocular muscles H05.82-
  facioscapulohumeral G71.0
  hereditary G71.9
    specified NEC G71.8
  immune NEC G72.49
  in (due to)
    Addison's disease E27.1 *[G73.7]*
    alcohol G72.1
    amyloidosis E85.0 *[G73.7]*
    cretinism E00.9 *[G73.7]*
    Cushing's syndrome E24.9 *[G73.7]*
    drugs G72.0
    endocrine disease NEC E34.9 *[G73.7]*
    giant cell arteritis M31.6 *[G73.7]*
    glycogen storage disease E74.00 *[G73.7]*
    hyperadrenocorticism E24.9 *[G73.7]*
    hyperparathyroidism NEC E21.3 *[G73.7]*
    hypoparathyroidism E20.9 *[G73.7]*
    hypopituitarism E23.0 *[G73.7]*
    hypothyroidism E03.9 *[G73.7]*
    infectious disease NEC B99 *[G73.7]*
    lipid storage disease E75.6 *[G73.7]*
    metabolic disease NEC E88.9 *[G73.7]*
    myxedema E03.9 *[G73.7]*
    parasitic disease NEC B89 *[G73.7]*
    polyarteritis nodosa M30.0 *[G73.7]*
    rheumatoid arthritis — *see* Rheumatoid, myopathy
    sarcoidosis D86.87
    scleroderma M34.82
    sicca syndrome M35.03
    Sjögren's syndrome M35.03
    systemic lupus erythematosus M32.19
    thyrotoxicosis (hyperthyroidism) E05.90 *[G73.7]*
      with thyroid storm E05.91 *[G73.7]*
    toxic agent NEC G72.2
  inflammatory NEC G72.49
  intensive care (ICU) G72.81
  limb-girdle G71.0
  mitochondrial NEC G71.3
  myotonic, proximal (PROMM) G71.11
  myotubular G71.2
  nemaline G71.2
  ocular G71.0
  oculopharyngeal G71.0
  of critical illness G72.81
  primary G71.9
    specified NEC G71.8
  progressive NEC G72.89
  proximal myotonic (PROMM) G71.11
  rod G71.2
  scapulohumeral G71.0
  specified NEC G72.89
  toxic G72.2
Myopericarditis — *see also* Pericarditis
  chronic rheumatic I09.2
Myopia (axial) (congenital) H52.1-
  degenerative (malignant) H44.2-
  malignant H44.2-
  pernicious H44.2-
  progressive high (degenerative) H44.2-
Myosarcoma — *see* Neoplasm, connective tissue, malignant
Myosis (pupil) H57.03
  stromal (endolymphatic) D39.0
Myositis M60.9
  clostridial A48.0
  due to posture — *see* Myositis, specified type NEC
  epidemic B33.0
  fibrosa or fibrous (chronic) , Volkmann's T79.6

Myositis - *continued*
  foreign body granuloma — *see* Granuloma, foreign body
  in (due to)
    bilharziasis B65.9 *[M63.8-]*
    cysticercosis B69.81
    leprosy A30.9 *[M63.8-]*
    mycosis B49 *[M63.8-]*
    sarcoidosis D86.87
    schistosomiasis B65.9 *[M63.8-]*
    syphilis
      late A52.78
      secondary A51.49
    toxoplasmosis (acquired) B58.82
    trichinellosis B75 *[M63.8-]*
    tuberculosis A18.09
  inclusion body [IBM] G72.41
  infective M60.009
    arm M60.002
      left M60.001
      right M60.000
    leg M60.005
      left M60.004
      right M60.003
    lower limb M60.005
      ankle M60.07-
      foot M60.07-
      lower leg M60.06-
      thigh M60.05-
      toe M60.07-
    multiple sites M60.09
    specified site NEC M60.08
    upper limb M60.002
      finger M60.04-
      forearm M60.03-
      hand M60.04-
      shoulder region M60.01-
      upper arm M60.02-
  interstitial M60.10
    ankle M60.17-
    foot M60.17-
    forearm M60.13-
    hand M60.14-
    lower leg M60.16-
    multiple sites M60.19
    shoulder region M60.11-
    specified site NEC M60.18
    thigh M60.15-
    upper arm M60.12-
  mycotic B49 *[M63.8-]*
  orbital, chronic H05.12-
  ossificans or ossifying (circumscripta) — *see also* Ossification, muscle, specified NEC
    in (due to)
      burns M61.30
        ankle M61.37-
        foot M61.37-
        forearm M61.33-
        hand M61.34-
        lower leg M61.36-
        multiple sites M61.39
        pelvic region M61.35-
        shoulder region M61.31-
        specified site NEC M61.38
        thigh M61.35-
        upper arm M61.32-
    quadriplegia or paraplegia M61.20
      ankle M61.27-
      foot M61.27-
      forearm M61.23-
      hand M61.24-
      lower leg M61.26-
      multiple sites M61.29
      pelvic region M61.25-
      shoulder region M61.21-
      specified site NEC M61.28
      thigh M61.25-
      upper arm M61.22-
    progressiva M61.10
      ankle M61.17-
      finger M61.14-
      foot M61.17-
      forearm M61.13-
      hand M61.14-
      lower leg M61.16-
      multiple sites M61.19
      pelvic region M61.15-
      shoulder region M61.11-
      specified site NEC M61.18
      thigh M61.15-
      toe M61.17-
      upper arm M61.12-
    traumatica M61.00

Myositis - *continued*
  ossificans or ossifying (circumscripta) - *continued*
    traumatica - *continued*
      ankle M61.07-
      foot M61.07-
      forearm M61.03-
      hand M61.04-
      lower leg M61.06-
      multiple sites M61.09
      pelvic region M61.05-
      shoulder region M61.01-
      specified site NEC M61.08
      thigh M61.05-
      upper arm M61.02-
  purulent — *see* Myositis, infective
  specified type NEC M60.80
    ankle M60.87-
    foot M60.87-
    forearm M60.83-
    hand M60.84-
    lower leg M60.86-
    multiple sites M60.89
    pelvic region M60.85-
    shoulder region M60.81-
    specified site NEC M60.88
    thigh M60.85-
    upper arm M60.82-
  suppurative — *see* Myositis, infective
  traumatic (old) — *see* Myositis, specified type NEC
Myospasia impulsiva F95.2
Myotonia (acquisita) (intermittens) M62.89
  atrophica G71.11
  chondrodystrophic G71.13
  congenita (acetazolamide responsive) (dominant) (recessive) G71.12
  drug-induced G71.14
  dystrophica G71.11
  fluctuans G71.19
  levior G71.12
  permanens G71.19
  symptomatic G71.19
Myotonic pupil — *see* Anomaly, pupil, function, tonic pupil
Myriapodiasis B88.2
Myringitis H73.2-
  with otitis media — *see* Otitis, media
  acute H73.00-
    bullous H73.01-
    specified NEC H73.09-
  bullous — *see* Myringitis, acute, bullous
  chronic H73.1-
Mysophobia F40.228
Mytilotoxism — *see* Poisoning, fish
Myxadenitis labialis K13.0
Myxedema (adult) (idiocy) (infantile) (juvenile) — *see also* Hypothyroidism E03.9
  circumscribed E05.90
    with storm E05.91
  coma E03.5
  congenital E00.1
  cutis L98.5
  localized (pretibial) E05.90
    with storm E05.91
  papular L98.5
Myxochondrosarcoma — *see* Neoplasm, cartilage, malignant
Myxofibroma — *see* Neoplasm, connective tissue, benign
  odontogenic — *see* Cyst, calcifying odontogenic
Myxofibrosarcoma — *see* Neoplasm, connective tissue, malignant
Myxolipoma D17.9
Myxoliposarcoma — *see* Neoplasm, connective tissue, malignant
Myxoma — *see also* Neoplasm, connective tissue, benign
  nerve sheath — *see* Neoplasm, nerve, benign
  odontogenic — *see* Cyst, calcifying odontogenic
Myxosarcoma — *see* Neoplasm, connective tissue, malignant

N

Naegeli's
  disease Q82.8
  leukemia, monocytic C93.1-
Naegleriasis (with meningoencephalitis) B60.2
Naffziger's syndrome G54.0
Naga sore — *see* Ulcer, skin
Nägele's pelvis M95.5
  with disproportion (fetopelvic) O33.0
    causing obstructed labor O65.0
Nail — *see also* condition
  biting F98.8

Nail - *continued*
patella syndrome Q87.2
Nanism, nanosomia — *see* Dwarfism
Nanophyetiasis B66.8
Nanukayami A27.89
Napkin rash L22
Narcolepsy G47.419
with cataplexy G47.411
in conditions classified elsewhere G47.429
with cataplexy G47.421
Narcosis R06.89
Narcotism — *see* Dependence
NARP (Neuropathy, Ataxia and Retinitis pigmentosa)
syndrome E88.49
Narrow
anterior chamber angle H40.03-
gingival width (of periodontal soft tissue) K05.5
pelvis — *see* Contraction, pelvis
Narrowing — *see also* Stenosis
artery I77.1
auditory, internal I65.8
basilar — *see* Occlusion, artery, basilar
carotid — *see* Occlusion, artery, carotid
cerebellar — *see* Occlusion, artery, cerebellar
cerebral — *see* Occlusion artery, cerebral
choroidal — *see* Occlusion, artery, cerebral,
specified NEC
communicating posterior — *see* Occlusion, artery,
cerebral, specified NEC
coronary — *see also* Disease, heart, ischemic,
atherosclerotic
congenital Q24.5
syphilitic A50.54 *[152]*
due to syphilis NEC A52.06
hypophyseal — *see* Occlusion, artery, cerebral,
specified NEC
pontine — *see* Occlusion, artery, cerebral,
specified NEC
precerebral — *see* Occlusion, artery, precerebral
vertebral — *see* Occlusion, artery, vertebral
auditory canal (external) — *see* Stenosis, external
ear canal
eustachian tube — *see* Obstruction, eustachian tube
eyelid — *see* Disorder, eyelid function
larynx J38.6
mesenteric artery — *see also* Ischemia, intestine,
acute K55.059
palate M26.89
palpebral fissure — *see* Disorder, eyelid function
ureter N13.5
with infection N13.6
urethra — *see* Stricture, urethra
Narrowness, abnormal, eyelid Q10.3
Nasal — *see* condition
Nasolachrymal, nasolacrimal — *see* condition
Nasopharyngeal — *see also* condition
pituitary gland Q89.2
torticollis M43.6
Nasopharyngitis (acute) (infective) (streptococcal)
(subacute) J00
chronic (suppurative) (ulcerative) J31.1
Nasopharynx, nasopharyngeal — *see* condition
Natal tooth, teeth K00.6
Nausea (without vomiting) R11.0
with vomiting R11.2
gravidarum — *see* Hyperemesis, gravidarum
marina T75.3
navalis T75.3
Navel — *see* condition
Neapolitan fever — *see* Brucellosis
Near drowning T75.1
Nearsightedness — *see* Myopia
Near-syncope R55
Nebula, cornea — *see* Opacity, cornea
Necator americanus infestation B76.1
Necatoriasis B76.1
Neck — *see* condition
Necrobiosis R68.89
lipoidica NEC L92.1
with diabetes — *see* E08-E13 with .620
Necrolysis, toxic epidermal L51.2
due to drug
correct substance properly administered — *see*
Table of Drugs and Chemicals, by drug, adverse
effect
overdose or wrong substance given or taken — *see*
Table of Drugs and Chemicals, by drug,
poisoning
Necrophilia F65.89
Necrosis, necrotic (ischemic) — *see also* Gangrene
adrenal (capsule) (gland) E27.49
amputation stump (surgical) (late) T87.50
arm T87.5-

Necrosis, necrotic (ischemic) - *continued*
amputation stump (surgical) (late) - *continued*
leg T87.5-
antrum J32.0
aorta (hyaline) — *see also* Aneurysm, aorta
cystic medial — *see* Dissection, aorta
artery I77.5
bladder (aseptic) (sphincter) N32.89
bone — *see also* Osteonecrosis M87.9
aseptic or avascular — *see* Osteonecrosis
idiopathic M87.00
ethmoid J32.2
jaw M27.2
tuberculous — *see* Tuberculosis, bone
brain I67.89
breast (aseptic) (fat) (segmental) N64.1
bronchus J98.09
central nervous system NEC I67.89
cerebellar I67.89
cerebral I67.89
colon — *see also* Infarct, intestine K55.049
cornea H18.89-
cortical (acute) (renal) N17.1
cystic medial (aorta) — *see* Dissection, aorta
dental pulp K04.1
esophagus K22.8
ethmoid (bone) J32.2
eyelid — *see* Disorder, eyelid, degenerative
fat, fatty (generalized) — *see also* Disorder, soft
tissue, specified type NEC
abdominal wall K65.4
breast (aseptic) (segmental) N64.1
localized — *see* Degeneration, by site, fatty
mesentery K65.4
omentum K65.4
pancreas K86.89
peritoneum K65.4
skin (subcutaneous) , newborn P83.0
subcutaneous, due to birth injury P15.6
gallbladder — *see* Cholecystitis, acute
heart — *see* Infarct, myocardium
hip, aseptic or avascular — *see* Osteonecrosis, by
type, femur
intestine (acute) (hemorrhagic) (massive) — *see
also* Infarct, intestine K55.069
jaw M27.2
kidney (bilateral) N28.0
acute N17.9
cortical (acute) (bilateral) N17.1
with ectopic or molar pregnancy O08.4
medullary (bilateral) (in acute renal failure)
(papillary) N17.2
papillary (bilateral) (in acute renal failure) N17.2
tubular N17.0
with ectopic or molar pregnancy O08.4
complicating
abortion — *see* Abortion, by type, complicated
by, tubular necrosis
ectopic or molar pregnancy O08.4
pregnancy — *see* Pregnancy, complicated by,
diseases of, specified type or system NEC
following ectopic or molar pregnancy O08.4
traumatic T79.5
larynx J38.7
liver (with hepatic failure) (cell) — *see* Failure,
hepatic
hemorrhagic, central K76.2
lung J85.0
lymphatic gland — *see* Lymphadenitis, acute
mammary gland (fat) (segmental) N64.1
mastoid (chronic) — *see* Mastoiditis, chronic
medullary (acute) (renal) N17.2
mesentery — *see also* Infarct, intestine K55.069
fat K65.4
mitral valve — *see* Insufficiency, mitral
myocardium, myocardial — *see* Infarct,
myocardium
nose J34.0
omentum (with mesenteric infarction) — *see
also* Infarct, intestine K55.069
fat K65.4
orbit, orbital — *see* Osteomyelitis, orbit
ossicles, ear — *see* Abnormal, ear ossicles
ovary N70.92
pancreas (aseptic) (duct) (fat) K86.89
acute (infective) — *see* Pancreatitis, acute
infective — *see* Pancreatitis, acute
papillary (acute) (renal) N17.2
perineum N90.89
peritoneum (with mesenteric infarction) — *see
also* Infarct, intestine K55.069
fat K65.4
pharynx J02.9

Necrosis, necrotic (ischemic) - *continued*
pharynx - *continued*
in granulocytopenia — *see* Neutropenia
Vincent's A69.1
phosphorus — *see* subcategory T54.2
pituitary (gland) E23.0
postpartum O99.285
Sheehan O99.285
pressure — *see* Ulcer, pressure, by site
pulmonary J85.0
pulp (dental) K04.1
radiation — *see* Necrosis, by site
radium — *see* Necrosis, by site
renal — *see* Necrosis, kidney
sclera H15.89
scrotum N50.89
skin or subcutaneous tissue NEC I96
spine, spinal (column) — *see also* Osteonecrosis, by
type, vertebra
cord G95.19
spleen D73.5
stomach K31.89
stomatitis (ulcerative) A69.0
subcutaneous fat, newborn P83.8
subendocardial (acute) I21.4
chronic I25.89
suprarenal (capsule) (gland) E27.49
testis N50.89
thymus (gland) E32.8
tonsil J35.8
trachea J39.8
tuberculous NEC — *see* Tuberculosis
tubular (acute) (anoxic) (renal) (toxic) N17.0
postprocedural N99.0
vagina N89.8
vertebra — *see also* Osteonecrosis, by type, vertebra
tuberculous A18.01
vulva N90.89
X-ray — *see* Necrosis, by site
Necrospermia — *see* Infertility, male
Need (for)
care provider because (of)
assistance with personal care Z74.1
continuous supervision required Z74.3
impaired mobility Z74.09
no other household member able to render
care Z74.2
specified reason NEC Z74.8
immunization — *see* Vaccination
vaccination — *see* Vaccination
Neglect
adult
confirmed T74.01
history of Z91.412
suspected T76.01
child (childhood)
confirmed T74.02
history of Z62.812
suspected T76.02
emotional, in childhood Z62.898
hemispatial R41.4
left-sided R41.4
sensory R41.4
visuospatial R41.4
Neisserian infection NEC — *see* Gonococcus
Nelaton's syndrome G60.8
Nelson's syndrome E24.1
Nematodiasis (intestinal) B82.0
Ancylostoma B76.0
Neonatal — *see also* Newborn
acne L70.4
bradycardia P29.12
tachycardia P29.11
screening, abnormal findings on P09
tooth, teeth K00.6
Neonatorum — *see* condition
Neoplasia
endocrine, multiple (MEN) E31.20
type I E31.21
type IIA E31.22
type IIB E31.23
intraepithelial (histologically confirmed)
anal (AIN) (histologically confirmed) K62.82
grade I K62.82
grade II K62.82
severe D01.3
cervical glandular (histologically confirmed) D06.9
cervix (uteri) (CIN) (histologically
confirmed) N87.9
glandular D06.9
grade I N87.0
grade II N87.1

Neoplasia - *continued*
  intraepithelial (histologically confirmed) - *continued*
   cervix (uteri) (CIN) (histologically confirmed) -
    continued
    grade III (severe dysplasia) — *see*
     also Carcinoma, cervix uteri, in situ D06.9
   prostate (histologically confirmed) (PIN) N42.31
    grade I N42.31
    grade II N42.31
    grade III (severe dysplasia) D07.5
   vagina (histologically confirmed) (VAIN) N89.3
    grade I N89.0
    grade II N89.1
    grade III (severe dysplasia) D07.2
   vulva (histologically confirmed) (VIN) N90.3
    grade I N90.0
    grade II N90.1
    grade III (severe dysplasia) D07.1
Neoplasm, neoplastic — *see also* Table of
  Neoplasms
  lipomatous, benign — *see* Lipoma

Table of Neoplasms *(side tab)*

abdomen, abdominal — bone *(side tab)*

Notes:

The list below gives the code numbers for neoplasms by anatomical site. For each site there are six possible code numbers according to whether the neoplasm in question is malignant, benign, in situ, of uncertain behavior, or of unspecified nature. The description of the neoplasm will often indicate which of the six columns is appropriate; e.g., malignant melanoma of skin, benign fibroadenoma of breast, carcinoma in situ of cervix uteri. Where such descriptors are not present, the remainder of the Index should be consulted where guidance is given to the appropriate column for each morphological (histological) variety listed; e.g., Mesonephroma -- see Neoplasm, malignant; Embryoma -- see also Neoplasm, uncertain behavior; Disease, Bowen's -- see Neoplasm, skin, in situ. However, the guidance in the Index can be overridden if one of the descriptors mentioned above is present; e.g., malignant adenoma of colon to C18.9 and not to D12.6 as the adjective "malignant" overrides the Index entry "Adenoma - see also Neoplasm, benign."

Codes listed with a dash -, following the code have a required additional character for laterality. The tabular must be reviewed for the complete code.

Neoplasm, neoplastic	Malignant Primary	Malignant Secondary	Ca in situ	Benign	Uncertain Behavior	Unspecified Behavior
Neoplasm, neoplastic	C80.1	C79.9	D09.9	D36.9	D48.9	D49.9
abdomen, abdominal	C76.2	C79.8-	D09.8	D36.7	D48.7	D49.89
cavity	C76.2	C79.8-	D09.8	D36.7	D48.7	D49.89
organ	C76.2	C79.8-	D09.8	D36.7	D48.7	D49.89
viscera	C76.2	C79.8-	D09.8	D36.7	D48.7	D49.89
wall — see also Neoplasm, abdomen, wall, skin	C44.509	C79.2-	D04.5	D23.5	D48.5	D49.2
connective tissue	C49.4	C79.8-		D21.4	D48.1	D49.2
skin	C44.509					
basal cell carcinoma	C44.519	-	-	-	-	-
specified type NEC	C44.599	-	-	-	-	-
squamous cell carcinoma	C44.529	-	-	-	-	-
abdominopelvic	C76.8	C79.8-		D36.7	D48.7	D49.89
accessory sinus — see Neoplasm, sinus						
acoustic nerve	C72.4-	C79.49	-	D33.3	D43.3	D49.7
adenoid (pharynx) (tissue)	C11.1	C79.89	D00.08	D10.6	D37.05	D49.0
adipose tissue — see also Neoplasm, connective tissue	C49.4	C79.89	-	D21.9	D48.1	D49.2
adnexa (uterine)	C57.4	C79.89	D07.39	D28.7	D39.8	D49.59
adrenal	C74.9-	C79.7-	D09.3	D35.0-	D44.1-	D49.7
capsule	C74.9-	C79.7-	D09.3	D35.0-	D44.1-	D49.7
cortex	C74.0-	C79.7-	D09.3	D35.0-	D44.1-	D49.7
gland	C74.9-	C79.7-	D09.3	D35.0-	D44.1-	D49.7
medulla	C74.1-	C79.7-	D09.3	D35.0-	D44.1-	D49.7
ala nasi (external) — see also Neoplasm, skin, nose	C44.301	C79.2	D04.39	D23.39	D48.5	D49.2
alimentary canal or tract NEC	C26.9	C78.80	D01.9	D13.9	D37.9	D49.0
alveolar	C03.9	C79.89	D00.03	D10.39	D37.09	D49.0
mucosa	C03.9	C79.89	D00.03	D10.39	D37.09	D49.0
lower	C03.1	C79.89	D00.03	D10.39	D37.09	D49.0
upper	C03.0	C79.89	D00.03	D10.39	D37.09	D49.0
ridge or process	C41.1	C79.51	-	D16.5-	D48.0	D49.2
carcinoma	C03.9	C79.8-	-	-	-	-
lower	C03.1	C79.8-	-	-	-	-
upper	C03.0	C79.8-	-	-	-	-
lower	C41.1	C79.51	-	D16.5-	D48.0	D49.2
mucosa	C03.9	C79.89	D00.03	D10.39	D37.09	D49.0
lower	C03.1	C79.89	D00.03	D10.39	D37.09	D49.0
upper	C03.0	C79.89	D00.03	D10.39	D37.09	D49.0
upper	C41.0	C79.51	-	D16.4-	D48.0	D49.2
sulcus	C06.1	C79.89	D00.02	D10.39	D37.09	D49.0
alveolus	C03.9	C79.89	D00.03	D10.39	D37.09	D49.0
lower	C03.1	C79.89	D00.03	D10.39	D37.09	D49.0
upper	C03.0	C79.89	D00.03	D10.39	D37.09	D49.0
ampulla of Vater	C24.1	C78.89	D01.5	D13.5	D37.6	D49.0
ankle NEC	C76.5-	C79.89	D04.7-	D36.7	D48.7	D49.89
anorectum, anorectal (junction)	C21.8	C78.5	D01.3	D12.9	D37.8	D49.0
antecubital fossa or space	C76.4-	C79.89	D04.6-	D36.7	D48.7	D49.89
antrum (Highmore) (maxillary)	C31.0	C78.39	D02.3	D14.0	D38.5	D49.1
pyloric	C16.3	C78.89	D00.2	D13.1	D37.1	D49.0
tympanicum	C30.1	C78.39	D02.3	D14.0	D38.5	D49.1
anus, anal	C21.0	C78.5	D01.3	D12.9	D37.8	D49.0
canal	C21.1	C78.5	D01.3	D12.9	D37.8	D49.0
cloacogenic zone	C21.2	C78.5	D01.3	D12.9	D37.8	D49.0
margin — see also Neoplasm, anus, skin	C44.500	C79.2	D04.5	D23.5	D48.5	D49.2
overlapping lesion with rectosigmoid junction or rectum	C21.8	-	-	-	-	-
skin	C44.500	C79.2	D04.5	D23.5	D48.5	D49.2
basal cell carcinoma	C44.510	-	-	-	-	-
specified type NEC	C44.590	-	-	-	-	-
squamous cell carcinoma	C44.520	-	-	-	-	-
sphincter	C21.1	C78.5	D01.3	D12.9	D37.8	D49.0

Neoplasm, neoplastic	Malignant Primary	Malignant Secondary	Ca in situ	Benign	Uncertain Behavior	Unspecified Behavior
aorta (thoracic)	C49.3	C79.89	-	D21.3	D48.1	D49.2
abdominal	C49.4	C79.89	-	D21.4	D48.1	D49.2
aortic body	C75.5	C79.89	-	D35.6	D44.7	D49.7
aponeurosis	C49.9	C79.89	-	D21.9	D48.1	D49.2
palmar	C49.1-	C79.89	-	D21.1-	D48.1	D49.2
plantar	C49.2-	C79.89	-	D21.2-	D48.1	D49.2
appendix	C18.1	C78.5	D01.0	D12.1	D37.3	D49.0
arachnoid	C70.9	C79.49	-	D32.9	D42.9	D49.7
cerebral	C70.0	C79.32	-	D32.0	D42.0	D49.7
spinal	C70.1	C79.49	-	D32.1	D42.1	D49.7
areola	C50.0-	C79.81	D05.-	D24.-	D48.6-	D49.3
arm NEC	C76.4-	C79.89	D04.6-	D36.7	D48.7	D49.89
artery — see Neoplasm, connective tissue						
aryepiglottic fold	C13.1	C79.89	D00.08	D10.7	D37.05	D49.0
hypopharyngeal aspect	C13.1	C79.89	D00.08	D10.7	D37.05	D49.0
laryngeal aspect	C32.1	C78.39	D02.0	D14.1	D38.0	D49.1
marginal zone	C13.1	C79.89	D00.08	D10.7	D37.05	D49.0
arytenoid (cartilage)	C32.3	C78.39	D02.0	D14.1	D38.0	D49.1
fold — see Neoplasm, aryepiglottic						
associated with transplanted organ	C80.2	-	-	-	-	-
atlas	C41.2	C79.51	-	D16.6	D48.0	D49.2
atrium, cardiac	C38.0	C79.89	-	D15.1	D48.7	D49.89
auditory						
canal (external) (skin)	C44.20-	C79.2	D04.2-	D23.2-	D48.5	D49.2
internal	C30.1	C78.39	D02.3	D14.0	D38.5	D49.1
nerve	C72.4-	C79.49	-	D33.3	D43.3	D49.7
tube	C30.1	C78.39	D02.3	D14.0	D38.5	D49.1
opening	C11.2	C79.89	D00.08	D10.6	D37.05	D49.0
auricle, ear — see also Neoplasm, skin, ear	C44.20-	C79.2	D04.2-	D23.2-	D48.5	D49.2
auricular canal (external) — see also Neoplasm, skin, ear	C44.20-	C79.2	D04.2-	D23.2-	D48.5	D49.2
internal	C30.1	C78.39	D02.3	D14.0	D38.5	D49.2
autonomic nerve or nervous system NEC (see Neoplasm, nerve, peripheral)						
axilla, axillary	C76.1	C79.89	D09.8	D36.7	D48.7	D49.89
fold — see also Neoplasm, skin, trunk	C44.509	C79.2	D04.5	D23.5	D48.5	D49.2
back NEC	C76.8	C79.89	D04.5	D36.7	D48.7	D49.89
Bartholin's gland	C51.0	C79.82	D07.1	D28.0	D39.8	D49.59
basal ganglia	C71.0	C79.31	-	D33.0	D43.0	D49.6
basis pedunculi	C71.7	C79.31	-	D33.1	D43.1	D49.6
bile or biliary (tract)	C24.9	C78.89	D01.5	D13.5	D37.6	D49.0
canaliculi (biliferi) (intrahepatic)	C22.1	C78.7	D01.5	D13.4	D37.6	D49.0
canals, interlobular	C22.1	C78.89	D01.5	D13.4	D37.6	D49.0
duct or passage (common) (cystic) (extrahepatic)	C24.0	C78.89	D01.5	D13.5	D37.6	D49.0
interlobular	C22.1	C78.89	D01.5	D13.4	D37.6	D49.0
intrahepatic	C22.1	C78.7	D01.5	D13.4	D37.6	D49.0
and extrahepatic	C24.8	C78.89	D01.5	D13.5	D37.6	D49.0
bladder (urinary)	C67.9	C79.11	D09.0	D30.3	D41.4	D49.4
dome	C67.1	C79.11	D09.0	D30.3	D41.4	D49.4
neck	C67.5	C79.11	D09.0	D30.3	D41.4	D49.4
orifice	C67.9	C79.11	D09.0	D30.3	D41.4	D49.4
ureteric	C67.6	C79.11	D09.0	D30.3	D41.4	D49.4
urethral	C67.5	C79.11	D09.0	D30.3	D41.4	D49.4
overlapping lesion	C67.8	-	-	-	-	-
sphincter	C67.8	C79.11	D09.0	D30.3	D41.4	D49.4
trigone	C67.0	C79.11	D09.0	D30.3	D41.4	D49.4
urachus	C67.7	C79.11	D09.0	D30.3	D41.4	D49.4
wall	C67.9	C79.11	D09.0	D30.3	D41.4	D49.4
anterior	C67.3	C79.11	D09.0	D30.3	D41.4	D49.4
lateral	C67.2	C79.11	D09.0	D30.3	D41.4	D49.4
posterior	C67.4	C79.11	D09.0	D30.3	D41.4	D49.4
blood vessel — see Neoplasm, connective tissue						
bone (periosteum)	C41.9	C79.51	-	D16.9-	D48.0	D49.2
acetabulum	C41.4	C79.51	-	D16.8-	D48.0	D49.2
ankle	C40.3-	C79.51	-	D16.3-	-	-
arm NEC	C40.0-	C79.51	-	D16.0-	-	-
astragalus	C40.3-	C79.51	-	D16.3-	-	-
atlas	C41.2	C79.51	-	D16.6-	D48.0	D49.2
axis	C41.2	C79.51	-	D16.6-	D48.0	D49.2
back NEC	C41.2	C79.51	-	D16.6-	D48.0	D49.2
calcaneus	C40.3-	C79.51	-	D16.3-	-	-
calvarium	C41.0	C79.51	-	D16.4-	D48.0	D49.2
carpus (any)	C40.1-	C79.51	-	D16.1-	-	-

Neoplasm, neoplastic	Malignant Primary	Malignant Secondary	Ca in situ	Benign	Uncertain Behavior	Unspecified Behavior
bone - continued						
cartilage NEC	C41.9	C79.51	-	D16.9-	D48.0	D49.2
clavicle	C41.3	C79.51	-	D16.7-	D48.0	D49.2
clivus	C41.0	C79.51	-	D16.4-	D48.0	D49.2
coccygeal vertebra	C41.4	C79.51	-	D16.8-	D48.0	D49.2
coccyx	C41.4	C79.51	-	D16.8-	D48.0	D49.2
costal cartilage	C41.3	C79.51	-	D16.7-	D48.0	D49.2
costovertebral joint	C41.3	C79.51	-	D16.7-	D48.0	D49.2
cranial	C41.0	C79.51	-	D16.4-	D48.0	D49.2
cuboid	C40.3-	C79.51	-	D16.3-	-	-
cuneiform	C41.9	C79.51	-	D16.9-	D48.0	D49.2
elbow	C40.0-	C79.51	-	D16.0-	-	-
ethmoid (labyrinth)	C41.0	C79.51	-	D16.4-	D48.0	D49.2
face	C41.0	C79.51	-	D16.4-	D48.0	D49.2
femur (any part)	C40.2-	C79.51	-	D16.2-	-	-
fibula (any part)	C40.2-	C79.51	-	D16.2-	-	-
finger (any)	C40.1-	C79.51	-	D16.1-	-	-
foot	C40.3-	C79.51	-	D16.3-	-	-
forearm	C40.0-	C79.51	-	D16.0-	-	-
frontal	C41.0	C79.51	-	D16.4-	D48.0	D49.2
hand	C40.1-	C79.51	-	D16.1-	-	-
heel	C40.3-	C79.51	-	D16.3-	-	-
hip	C41.4	C79.51	-	D16.8-	D48.0	D49.2
humerus (any part)	C40.0-	C79.51	-	D16.0-	-	-
hyoid	C41.0	C79.51	-	D16.4-	D48.0	D49.2
ilium	C41.4	C79.51	-	D16.8-	D48.0	D49.2
innominate	C41.4	C79.51	-	D16.8-	D48.0	D49.2
intervertebral cartilage or disc	C41.2	C79.51	-	D16.6-	D48.0	D49.2
ischium	C41.4	C79.51	-	D16.8-	D48.0	D49.2
jaw (lower)	C41.1	C79.51	-	D16.5-	D48.0	D49.2
knee	C40.2-	C79.51	-	D16.2-	-	-
leg NEC	C40.2-	C79.51	-	D16.2-	-	-
limb NEC	C40.9-	C79.51	-	D16.9-	-	-
lower (long bones)	C40.2-	C79.51	-	D16.2-	-	-
short bones	C40.3-	C79.51	-	D16.3-	-	-
upper (long bones)	C40.0-	C79.51	-	D16.0-	-	-
short bones	C40.1-	C79.51	-	D16.1-	-	-
malar	C41.0	C79.51	-	D16.4-	D48.0	D49.2
mandible	C41.1	C79.51	-	D16.5-	D48.0	D49.2
marrow NEC (any bone)	C96.9	C79.52	-	-	D47.9	D49.89
mastoid	C41.0	C79.51	-	D16.4-	D48.0	D49.2
maxilla, maxillary (superior)	C41.0	C79.51	-	D16.4-	D48.0	D49.2
inferior	C41.1	C79.51	-	D16.5-	D48.0	D49.2
metacarpus (any)	C40.1-	C79.51	-	D16.1-	-	-
metatarsus (any)	C40.3-	C79.51	-	D16.3-	-	-
overlapping sites	C40.8-	-	-	-	-	-
navicular						
ankle	C40.3-	C79.51	-	-	-	-
hand	C40.1-	C79.51	-	-	-	-
nose, nasal	C41.0	C79.51	-	D16.4-	D48.0	D49.2
occipital	C41.0	C79.51	-	D16.4-	D48.0	D49.2
orbit	C41.0	C79.51	-	D16.4-	D48.0	D49.2
parietal	C41.0	C79.51	-	D16.4-	D48.0	D49.2
patella	C40.2-	C79.51	-	-	-	-
pelvic	C41.4	C79.51	-	D16.8	D48.0	D49.2
phalanges						
foot	C40.3-	C79.51	-	-	-	-
hand	C40.1-	C79.51	-	-	-	-
pubic	C41.4	C79.51	-	D16.8	D48.0	D49.2
radius (any part)	C40.0-	C79.51	-	D16.0-	-	-
rib	C41.3	C79.51	-	D16.7	D48.0	D49.2
sacral vertebra	C41.4	C79.51	-	D16.8	D48.0	D49.2
sacrum	C41.4	C79.51	-	D16.8	D48.0	D49.2
scaphoid						
of ankle	C40.3-	C79.51	-	-	-	-
of hand	C40.1-	C79.51	-	-	-	-
scapula (any part)	C40.0-	C79.51	-	D16.0-	-	-
sella turcica	C41.0	C79.51	-	D16.4-	D48.0	D49.2
shoulder	C40.0-	C79.51	-	D16.0-	-	-
skull	C41.0	C79.51	-	D16.4-	D48.0	D49.2
sphenoid	C41.0	C79.51	-	D16.4-	D48.0	D49.2
spine, spinal (column)	C41.2	C79.51	-	D16.6	D48.0	D49.2
coccyx	C41.4	C79.51	-	D16.8	D48.0	D49.2
sacrum	C41.4	C79.51	-	D16.8	D48.0	D49.2
sternum	C41.3	C79.51	-	D16.7	D48.0	D49.2
tarsus (any)	C40.3-	C79.51	-	-	-	-
temporal	C41.0	C79.51	-	D16.4-	D48.0	D49.2
thumb	C40.1-	C79.51	-	-	-	-
tibia (any part)	C40.2-	C79.51	-	-	-	-

Neoplasm, neoplastic	Malignant Primary	Malignant Secondary	Ca in situ	Benign	Uncertain Behavior	Unspecified Behavior
bone - continued						
toe (any)	C40.3-	C79.51	-	-	-	-
trapezium	C40.1-	C79.51	-	-	-	-
trapezoid	C40.1-	C79.51	-	-	-	-
turbinate	C41.0	C79.51	-	D16.4-	D48.0	D49.2
ulna (any part)	C40.0-	C79.51	-	D16.0-	-	-
unciform	C40.1-	C79.51	-	-	-	-
vertebra (column)	C41.2	C79.51	-	D16.6	D48.0	D49.2
coccyx	C41.4	C79.51	-	D16.8	D48.0	D49.2
sacrum	C41.4	C79.51	-	D16.8	D48.0	D49.2
vomer	C41.0	C79.51	-	D16.4-	D48.0	D49.2
wrist	C40.1-	C79.51	-	-	-	-
xiphoid process	C41.3	C79.51	-	D16.7	D48.0	D49.2
zygomatic	C41.0	C79.51	-	D16.4-	D48.0	D49.2
book-leaf (mouth)	C06.89	C79.89	D00.00	D10.39	D37.09	D49.0
bowel — see Neoplasm, intestine						
brachial plexus	C47.1-	C79.89	-	D36.12	D48.2	D49.2
brain NEC	C71.9	C79.31	-	D33.2	D43.2	D49.6
basal ganglia	C71.0	C79.31	-	D33.0	D43.0	D49.6
cerebellopontine angle	C71.6	C79.31	-	D33.1	D43.1	D49.6
cerebellum NOS	C71.6	C79.31	-	D33.1	D43.1	D49.6
cerebrum	C71.0	C79.31	-	D33.0	D43.0	D49.6
choroid plexus	C71.7	C79.31	-	D33.1	D43.1	D49.6
corpus callosum	C71.8	C79.31	-	D33.2	D43.2	D49.6
corpus striatum	C71.0	C79.31	-	D33.0	D43.0	D49.6
cortex (cerebral)	C71.0	C79.31	-	D33.0	D43.0	D49.6
frontal lobe	C71.1	C79.31	-	D33.0	D43.0	D49.6
globus pallidus	C71.0	C79.31	-	D33.0	D43.0	D49.6
hippocampus	C71.2	C79.31	-	D33.0	D43.0	D49.6
hypothalamus	C71.0	C79.31	-	D33.0	D43.0	D49.6
internal capsule	C71.0	C79.31	-	D33.0	D43.0	D49.6
medulla oblongata	C71.7	C79.31	-	D33.1	D43.1	D49.6
meninges	C70.0	C79.32	-	D32.0	D42.0	D49.7
midbrain	C71.7	C79.31	-	D33.1	D43.1	D49.6
occipital lobe	C71.4	C79.31	-	D33.0	D43.0	D49.6
overlapping lesion	C71.8	C79.31	-	-	-	-
parietal lobe	C71.3	C79.31	-	D33.0	D43.0	D49.6
peduncle	C71.7	C79.31	-	D33.1	D43.1	D49.6
pons	C71.7	C79.31	-	D33.1	D43.1	D49.6
stem	C71.7	C79.31	-	D33.1	D43.1	D49.6
tapetum	C71.8	C79.31	-	D33.2	D43.2	D49.6
temporal lobe	C71.2	C79.31	-	D33.0	D43.0	D49.6
thalamus	C71.0	C79.31	-	D33.0	D43.0	D49.6
uncus	C71.2	C79.31	-	D33.0	D43.0	D49.6
ventricle (floor)	C71.5	C79.31	-	D33.0	D43.0	D49.6
fourth	C71.7	C79.31	-	D33.1	D43.1	D49.6
branchial (cleft) (cyst) (vestiges)	C10.4	C79.89	D00.08	D10.5	D37.05	D49.0
breast (connective tissue) (glandular tissue) (soft parts)	C50.9-	C79.81	D05.-	D24.-	D48.6-	D49.3
areola	C50.0-	C79.81	D05.-	D24.-	D48.6-	D49.3
axillary tail	C50.6-	C79.81	D05.-	D24.-	D48.6-	D49.3
central portion	C50.1-	C79.81	D05.-	D24.-	D48.6-	D49.3
inner	C50.8-	C79.81	D05.-	D24.-	D48.6-	D49.3
lower	C50.8-	C79.81	D05.-	D24.-	D48.6-	D49.3
lower-inner quadrant	C50.3-	C79.81	D05.-	D24.-	D48.6-	D49.3
lower-outer quadrant	C50.5-	C79.81	D05.-	D24.-	D48.6-	D49.3
mastectomy site (skin) — see also Neoplasm, breast, skin	C44.501	C79.2	-	-	-	-
specified as breast tissue	C50.8-	C79.81	-	-	-	-
midline	C50.8-	C79.81	D05.-	D24.-	D48.6-	D49.3
nipple	C50.0-	C79.81	D05.-	D24.-	D48.6-	D49.3
outer	C50.8-	C79.81	D05.-	D24.-	D48.6-	D49.3
overlapping lesion	C50.8-	-	-	-	-	-
skin	C44.501	C79.2	D04.5	D23.5	D48.5	D49.2
basal cell carcinoma	C44.511	-	-	-	-	-
specified type NEC	C44.591	-	-	-	-	-
squamous cell carcinoma	C44.521	-	-	-	-	-
tail (axillary)	C50.6-	C79.81	D05.-	D24.-	D48.6-	D49.3
upper	C50.8-	C79.81	D05.-	D24.-	D48.6-	D49.3
upper-inner quadrant	C50.2-	C79.81	D05.-	D24.-	D48.6-	D49.3
upper-outer quadrant	C50.4-	C79.81	D05.-	D24.-	D48.6-	D49.3
broad ligament	C57.1	C79.82	D07.39	D28.2	D39.8	D49.59
bronchiogenic, bronchogenic (lung)	C34.9-	C78.0-	D02.2-	D14.3-	D38.1	D49.1
bronchiole	C34.9-	C78.0-	D02.2-	D14.3-	D38.1	D49.1
bronchus	C34.9-	C78.0-	D02.2-	D14.3-	D38.1	D49.1
carina	C34.0-	C78.0-	D02.2-	D14.3-	D38.1	D49.1
lower lobe of lung	C34.3-	C78.0-	D02.2-	D14.3-	D38.1	D49.1
main	C34.0-	C78.0-	D02.2-	D14.3-	D38.1	D49.1
middle lobe of lung	C34.2	C78.0-	D02.21	D14.31	D38.1	D49.1

Neoplasm, neoplastic	Malignant Primary	Malignant Secondary	Ca in situ	Benign	Uncertain Behavior	Unspecified Behavior
bronchus - *continued*						
overlapping lesion	C34.8-	-	-	-	-	-
upper lobe of lung	C34.1-	C78.0-	D02.2-	D14.3-	D38.1	D49.1
brow	C44.309	C79.2	D04.39	D23.39	D48.5	D49.2
basal cell carcinoma	C44.319	-	-	-	-	-
specified type NEC	C44.399	-	-	-	-	-
squamous cell carcinoma	C44.329	-	-	-	-	-
buccal (cavity)	C06.9	C79.89	D00.00	D10.39	D37.09	D49.0
commissure	C06.0	C79.89	D00.02	D10.39	D37.09	D49.0
groove (lower) (upper)	C06.1	C79.89	D00.02	D10.39	D37.09	D49.0
mucosa	C06.0	C79.89	D00.02	D10.39	D37.09	D49.0
sulcus (lower) (upper)	C06.1	C79.89	D00.02	D10.39	D37.09	D49.0
bulbourethral gland	C68.0	C79.19	D09.19	D30.4	D41.3	D49.59
bursa — *see* Neoplasm, connective tissue						
buttock NEC	C76.3	C79.89	D04.5	D36.7	D48.7	D49.89
calf	C76.5-	C79.89	D04.7-	D36.7	D48.7	D49.89
calvarium	C41.0	C79.51	-	D16.4-	D48.0	D49.2
calyx, renal	C65.-	C79.0-	D09.19	D30.1-	D41.1-	D49.51-
canal						
anal	C21.1	C78.5	D01.3	D12.9	D37.8	D49.0
auditory (external) — *see also* Neoplasm, skin, ear	C44.20-	C79.2	D04.2-	D23.2-	D48.5	D49.2
auricular (external) — *see also* Neoplasm, skin, ear	C44.20-	C79.2	D04.2-	D23.2-	D48.5	D49.2
canaliculi, biliary (biliferi) (intrahepatic)	C22.1	C78.7	D01.5	D13.4	D37.6	D49.0
canthus (eye) (inner) (outer)	C44.10-	C79.2	D04.1-	D23.1-	D48.5	D49.2
basal cell carcinoma	C44.11-	-	-	-	-	-
specified type NEC	C44.19-	-	-	-	-	-
squamous cell carcinoma	C44.12-	-	-	-	-	-
capillary — *see* Neoplasm, connective tissue						
caput coli	C18.0	C78.5	D01.0	D12.0	D37.4	D49.0
carcinoid — *see* Tumor, carcinoid						
cardia (gastric)	C16.0	C78.89	D00.2	D13.1	D37.1	D49.0
cardiac orifice (stomach)	C16.0	C78.89	D00.2	D13.1	D37.1	D49.0
cardio-esophageal junction	C16.0	C78.89	D00.2	D13.1	D37.1	D49.0
cardio-esophagus	C16.0	C78.89	D00.2	D13.1	D37.1	D49.0
carina (bronchus)	C34.0-	C78.0-	D02.2-	D14.3-	D38.1	D49.1
carotid (artery)	C49.0	C79.89	-	D21.0	D48.1	D49.2
body	C75.4	C79.89	-	D35.5	D44.6	D49.7
carpus (any bone)	C40.1-	C79.51	-	D16.1-		
cartilage (articular) (joint) NEC — *see also* Neoplasm, bone	C41.9	C79.51	-	D16.9-	D48.0	D49.2
arytenoid	C32.3	C78.39	D02.0	D14.1	D38.0	D49.1
auricular	C49.0	C79.89	-	D21.0	D48.1	D49.2
bronchi	C34.0-	C78.39	-	D14.3-	D38.1	D49.1
costal	C41.3	C79.51	-	D16.7	D48.0	D49.2
cricoid	C32.3	C78.39	D02.0	D14.1	D38.0	D49.1
cuneiform	C32.3	C78.39	D02.0	D14.1	D38.0	D49.1
ear (external)	C49.0	C79.89	-	D21.0	D48.1	D49.2
ensiform	C41.3	C79.51	-	D16.7	D48.0	D49.2
epiglottis	C32.1	C78.39	D02.0	D14.1	D38.0	D49.1
anterior surface	C10.1	C79.89	D00.08	D10.5	D37.05	D49.0
eyelid	C49.0	C79.89	-	D21.0	D48.1	D49.2
intervertebral	C41.2	C79.51	-	D16.6	D48.0	D49.2
larynx, laryngeal	C32.3	C78.39	D02.0	D14.1	D38.0	D49.1
nose, nasal	C30.0	C78.39	D02.3	D14.0	D38.5	D49.1
pinna	C49.0	C79.89	-	D21.0	D48.1	D49.2
rib	C41.3	C79.51	-	D16.7	D48.0	D49.2
semilunar (knee)	C40.2-	C79.51	-	D16.2-	D48.0	D49.2
thyroid	C32.3	C78.39	D02.0	D14.1	D38.0	D49.1
trachea	C33	C78.39	D02.1	D14.2	D38.1	D49.1
cauda equina	C72.1	C79.49	-	D33.4	D43.4	D49.7
cavity						
buccal	C06.9	C79.89	D00.00	D10.30	D37.09	D49.0
nasal	C30.0	C78.39	D02.3	D14.0	D38.5	D49.1
oral	C06.9	C79.89	D00.00	D10.30	D37.09	D49.0
peritoneal	C48.2	C78.6	-	D20.1	D48.4	D49.0
tympanic	C30.1	C78.39	D02.3	D14.0	D38.5	D49.1
cecum	C18.0	C78.5	D01.0	D12.0	D37.4	D49.0
central nervous system	C72.9	C79.40	-	-	-	-
cerebellopontine (angle)	C71.6	C79.31	-	D33.1	D43.1	D49.6
cerebellum, cerebellar	C71.6	C79.31	-	D33.1	D43.1	D49.6
cerebrum, cerebral (cortex) (hemisphere) (white matter)	C71.0	C79.31	-	D33.0	D43.0	D49.6
meninges	C70.0	C79.32	-	D32.0	D42.0	D49.7
peduncle	C71.7	C79.31	-	D33.1	D43.1	D49.6

Neoplasm, neoplastic	Malignant Primary	Malignant Secondary	Ca in situ	Benign	Uncertain Behavior	Unspecified Behavior
cerebrum, cerebral - *continued*						
ventricle	C71.5	C79.31	-	D33.0	D43.0	D49.6
fourth	C71.7	C79.31	-	D33.1	D43.1	D49.6
cervical region	C76.0	C79.89	D09.8	D36.7	D48.7	D49.89
cervix (cervical) (uteri) (uterus)	C53.9	C79.82	D06.9	D26.0	D39.0	D49.59
canal	C53.0	C79.82	D06.0	D26.0	D39.0	D49.59
endocervix (canal) (gland)	C53.0	C79.82	D06.0	D26.0	D39.0	D49.59
exocervix	C53.1	C79.82	D06.1	D26.0	D39.0	D49.59
external os	C53.1	C79.82	D06.1	D26.0	D39.0	D49.59
internal os	C53.0	C79.82	D06.0	D26.0	D39.0	D49.59
nabothian gland	C53.0	C79.82	D06.0	D26.0	D39.0	D49.59
overlapping lesion	C53.8					
squamocolumnar junction	C53.8	C79.82	D06.7	D26.0	D39.0	D49.59
stump	C53.8	C79.82	D06.7	D26.0	D39.0	D49.59
cheek	C76.0	C79.89	D09.8	D36.7	D48.7	D49.89
external	C44.309	C79.2	D04.39	D23.39	D48.5	D49.2
basal cell carcinoma	C44.319	-	-	-	-	-
specified type NEC	C44.399	-	-	-	-	-
squamous cell carcinoma	C44.329	-	-	-	-	-
inner aspect	C06.0	C79.89	D00.02	D10.39	D37.09	D49.0
internal	C06.0	C79.89	D00.02	D10.39	D37.09	D49.0
mucosa	C06.0	C79.89	D00.02	D10.39	D37.09	D49.0
chest (wall) NEC	C76.1	C79.89	D09.8	D36.7	D48.7	D49.89
chiasma opticum	C72.3-	C79.49	-	D33.3	D43.3	D49.7
chin	C44.309	C79.2	D04.39	D23.39	D48.5	D49.2
basal cell carcinoma	C44.319	-	-	-	-	-
specified type NEC	C44.399	-	-	-	-	-
squamous cell carcinoma	C44.329	-	-	-	-	-
choana	C11.3	C79.89	D00.08	D10.6	D37.05	D49.0
cholangiole	C22.1	C78.89	D01.5	D13.4	D37.6	D49.0
choledochal duct	C24.0	C78.89	D01.5	D13.5	D37.6	D49.0
choroid	C69.3-	C79.49	D09.2-	D31.3-	D48.7	D49.81
plexus	C71.5	C79.31	-	D33.0	D43.0	D49.6
ciliary body	C69.4-	C79.49	D09.2-	D31.4-	D48.7	D49.89
clavicle	C41.3	C79.51	-	D16.7	D48.0	D49.2
clitoris	C51.2	C79.82	D07.1	D28.0	D39.8	D49.59
clivus	C41.0	C79.51	-	D16.4-	D48.0	D49.2
cloacogenic zone	C21.2	C78.5	D01.3	D12.9	D37.8	D49.0
coccygeal						
body or glomus	C49.5	C79.89	-	D21.5	D48.1	D49.2
vertebra	C41.4	C79.51	-	D16.8	D48.0	D49.2
coccyx	C41.4	C79.51	-	D16.8	D48.0	D49.2
colon — *see also* Neoplasm, intestine, large	C18.9	C78.5	-	-	-	-
with rectum	C19	C78.5	D01.1	D12.7	D37.5	D49.0
column, spinal — *see* Neoplasm, spine						
columnella — *see also* Neoplasm, skin, face	C44.390	C79.2	D04.39	D23.39	D48.5	D49.2
commissure						
labial, lip	C00.6	C79.89	D00.01	D10.39	D37.01	D49.0
laryngeal	C32.0	C78.39	D02.0	D14.1	D38.0	D49.0
common (bile) duct	C24.0	C78.89	D01.5	D13.5	D37.6	D49.0
concha — *see also* Neoplasm, skin, ear	C44.20-	C79.2	D04.2-	D23.2-	D48.5	D49.2
nose	C30.0	C78.39	D02.3	D14.0	D38.5	D49.1
conjunctiva	C69.0-	C79.49	D09.2-	D31.0-	D48.7	D49.89
connective tissue NEC	C49.9	C79.89	-	D21.9	D48.1	D49.2
Note: For neoplasms of connective tissue (blood vessel, bursa, fascia, ligament, muscle, peripheral nerves, sympathetic and parasympathetic nerves and ganglia, synovia, tendon, etc.) or of morphological types that indicate connective tissue, code according to the list under "Neoplasm, connective tissue". For sites that do not appear in this list, code to neoplasm of that site; e.g., fibrosarcoma, pancreas (C25.9)						
Note: Morphological types that indicate connective tissue appear in their proper place in the alphabetic index with the instruction "see Neoplasm, connective tissue ...."						
abdomen	C49.4	C79.89	-	D21.4	D48.1	D49.2
abdominal wall	C49.4	C79.89	-	D21.4	D48.1	D49.2

Neoplasm, neoplastic	Malignant Primary	Malignant Secondary	Ca in situ	Benign	Uncertain Behavior	Unspecified Behavior
connective tissue NEC - *continued*						
ankle	C49.2-	C79.89	-	D21.2-	D48.1	D49.2
antecubital fossa or space	C49.1-	C79.89	-	D21.1-	D48.1	D49.2
arm	C49.1-	C79.89	-	D21.1-	D48.1	D49.2
auricle (ear)	C49.0	C79.89	-	D21.0	D48.1	D49.2
axilla	C49.3	C79.89	-	D21.3	D48.1	D49.2
back	C49.6	C79.89	-	D21.6	D48.1	D49.2
breast — *see* Neoplasm, breast						
buttock	C49.5	C79.89	-	D21.5	D48.1	D49.2
calf	C49.2-	C79.89	-	D21.2-	D48.1	D49.2
cervical region	C49.0	C79.89	-	D21.0	D48.1	D49.2
cheek	C49.0	C79.89	-	D21.0	D48.1	D49.2
chest (wall)	C49.3	C79.89	-	D21.3	D48.1	D49.2
chin	C49.0	C79.89	-	D21.0	D48.1	D49.2
diaphragm	C49.3	C79.89	-	D21.3	D48.1	D49.2
ear (external)	C49.0	C79.89	-	D21.0	D48.1	D49.2
elbow	C49.1-	C79.89	-	D21.1-	D48.1	D49.2
extrarectal	C49.5	C79.89	-	D21.5	D48.1	D49.2
extremity	C49.9	C79.89	-	D21.9	D48.1	D49.2
lower	C49.2-	C79.89	-	D21.2-	D48.1	D49.2
upper	C49.1-	C79.89	-	D21.1-	D48.1	D49.2
eyelid	C49.0	C79.89	-	D21.0	D48.1	D49.2
face	C49.0	C79.89	-	D21.0	D48.1	D49.2
finger	C49.1-	C79.89	-	D21.1-	D48.1	D49.2
flank	C49.6	C79.89	-	D21.6	D48.1	D49.2
foot	C49.2-	C79.89	-	D21.2-	D48.1	D49.2
forearm	C49.1-	C79.89	-	D21.1-	D48.1	D49.2
forehead	C49.0	C79.89	-	D21.0	D48.1	D49.2
gastric	C49.4	C79.89	-	D21.4	D48.1	D49.2
gastrointestinal	C49.4	C79.89	-	D21.4	D48.1	D49.2
gluteal region	C49.5	C79.89	-	D21.5	D48.1	D49.2
great vessels NEC	C49.3	C79.89	-	D21.3	D48.1	D49.2
groin	C49.5	C79.89	-	D21.5	D48.1	D49.2
hand	C49.1-	C79.89	-	D21.1-	D48.1	D49.2
head	C49.0	C79.89	-	D21.0	D48.1	D49.2
heel	C49.2-	C79.89	-	D21.2-	D48.1	D49.2
hip	C49.2-	C79.89	-	D21.2-	D48.1	D49.2
hypochondrium	C49.4	C79.89	-	D21.4	D48.1	D49.2
iliopsoas muscle	C49.5	C79.89	-	D21.5	D48.1	D49.2
infraclavicular region	C49.3	C79.89	-	D21.3	D48.1	D49.2
inguinal (canal) (region)	C49.5	C79.89	-	D21.5	D48.1	D49.2
intestinal	C49.4	C79.89	-	D21.4	D48.1	D49.2
intrathoracic	C49.3	C79.89	-	D21.3	D48.1	D49.2
ischiorectal fossa	C49.5	C79.89	-	D21.5	D48.1	D49.2
jaw	C03.9	C79.89	D00.03	D10.39	D48.1	D49.0
knee	C49.2-	C79.89	-	D21.2-	D48.1	D49.2
leg	C49.2-	C79.89	-	D21.2-	D48.1	D49.2
limb NEC	C49.9	C79.89	-	D21.9	D48.1	D49.2
lower	C49.2-	C79.89	-	D21.2-	D48.1	D49.2
upper	C49.1-	C79.89	-	D21.1-	D48.1	D49.2
nates	C49.5	C79.89	-	D21.5	D48.1	D49.2
neck	C49.0	C79.89	-	D21.0	D48.1	D49.2
orbit	C69.6-	C79.49	D09.2-	D31.6-	D48.1	D49.89
overlapping lesion	C49.8	-	-	-	-	-
pararectal	C49.5	C79.89	-	D21.5	D48.1	D49.2
para-urethral	C49.5	C79.89	-	D21.5	D48.1	D49.2
paravaginal	C49.5	C79.89	-	D21.5	D48.1	D49.2
pelvis (floor)	C49.5	C79.89	-	D21.5	D48.1	D49.2
pelvo-abdominal	C49.8	C79.89	-	D21.6	D48.1	D49.2
perineum	C49.5	C79.89	-	D21.5	D48.1	D49.2
perirectal (tissue)	C49.5	C79.89	-	D21.5	D48.1	D49.2
periurethral (tissue)	C49.5	C79.89	-	D21.5	D48.1	D49.2
popliteal fossa or space	C49.2-	C79.89	-	D21.2-	D48.1	D49.2
presacral	C49.5	C79.89	-	D21.5	D48.1	D49.2
psoas muscle	C49.4	C79.89	-	D21.4	D48.1	D49.2
pterygoid fossa	C49.0	C79.89	-	D21.0	D48.1	D49.2
rectovaginal septum or wall	C49.5	C79.89	-	D21.5	D48.1	D49.2
rectovesical	C49.5	C79.89	-	D21.5	D48.1	D49.2
retroperitoneum	C48.0	C78.6	-	D20.0	D48.3	D49.0
sacrococcygeal region	C49.5	C79.89	-	D21.5	D48.1	D49.2
scalp	C49.0	C79.89	-	D21.0	D48.1	D49.2
scapular region	C49.3	C79.89	-	D21.3	D48.1	D49.2
shoulder	C49.1-	C79.89	-	D21.1-	D48.1	D49.2
skin (dermis) NEC — *see also* Neoplasm, skin, by site	C44.90	C79.2	D04.9	D23.9	D48.5	D49.2
stomach	C49.4	C79.89	-	D21.4	D48.1	D49.2
submental	C49.0	C79.89	-	D21.0	D48.1	D49.2
supraclavicular region	C49.0	C79.89	-	D21.0	D48.1	D49.2
temple	C49.0	C79.89	-	D21.0	D48.1	D49.2

Neoplasm, neoplastic	Malignant Primary	Malignant Secondary	Ca in situ	Benign	Uncertain Behavior	Unspecified Behavior
connective tissue NEC - *continued*						
temporal region	C49.0	C79.89	-	D21.0	D48.1	D49.2
thigh	C49.2-	C79.89	-	D21.2-	D48.1	D49.2
thoracic (duct) (wall)	C49.3	C79.89	-	D21.3	D48.1	D49.2
thorax	C49.3	C79.89	-	D21.3	D48.1	D49.2
thumb	C49.1-	C79.89	-	D21.1-	D48.1	D49.2
toe	C49.2-	C79.89	-	D21.2-	D48.1	D49.2
trunk	C49.6	C79.89	-	D21.6	D48.1	D49.2
umbilicus	C49.4	C79.89	-	D21.4	D48.1	D49.2
vesicorectal	C49.5	C79.89	-	D21.5	D48.1	D49.2
wrist	C49.1-	C79.89	-	D21.1-	D48.1	D49.2
conus medullaris	C72.0	C79.49	-	D33.4	D43.4	D49.7
cord (true) (vocal)	C32.0	C78.39	D02.0	D14.1	D38.0	D49.1
false	C32.1	C78.39	D02.0	D14.1	D38.0	D49.1
spermatic	C63.1-	C79.82	D07.69	D29.8	D40.8	D49.59
spinal (cervical) (lumbar) (thoracic)	C72.0	C79.49	-	D33.4	D43.4	D49.7
cornea (limbus)	C69.1-	C79.49	D09.2-	D31.1-	D48.7	D49.89
corpus						
albicans	C56.-	C79.6-	D07.39	D27.-	D39.1-	D49.59
callosum, brain	C71.0	C79.31	-	D33.0	D43.2	D49.6
cavernosum	C60.2	C79.82	D07.4	D29.0	D40.8	D49.59
gastric	C16.2	C78.89	D00.2	D13.1	D37.1	D49.0
overlapping sites	C54.8	-	-	-	-	-
penis	C60.2	C79.82	D07.4	D29.0	D40.8	D49.59
striatum, cerebrum	C71.0	C79.31	-	D33.0	D43.0	D49.6
uteri	C54.9	C79.82	D07.0	D26.1	D39.0	D49.59
isthmus	C54.0	C79.82	D07.0	D26.1	D39.0	D49.59
cortex						
adrenal	C74.0-	C79.7-	D09.3	D35.0-	D44.1-	D49.7
cerebral	C71.0	C79.31	-	D33.0	D43.0	D49.6
costal cartilage	C41.3	C79.51	-	D16.7	D48.0	D49.2
costovertebral joint	C41.3	C79.51	-	D16.7	D48.0	D49.2
Cowper's gland	C68.0	C79.19	D09.19	D30.4	D41.3	D49.59
cranial (fossa, any)	C71.9	C79.31	-	D33.2	D43.2	D49.6
meninges	C70.0	C79.32	-	D32.0	D42.0	D49.7
nerve	C72.50	C79.49	-	D33.3	D43.3	D49.7
specified NEC	C72.59	C79.49	-	D33.3	D43.3	D49.7
craniobuccal pouch	C75.2	C79.89	D09.3	D35.2	D44.3	D49.7
craniopharyngeal (duct) (pouch)	C75.2	C79.89	D09.3	D35.3	D44.4	D49.7
cricoid	C13.0	C79.89	D00.08	D10.7	D37.05	D49.0
cartilage	C32.3	C78.39	D02.0	D14.1	D38.0	D49.1
cricopharynx	C13.0	C79.89	D00.08	D10.7	D37.05	D49.0
crypt of Morgagni	C21.8	C78.5	D01.3	D12.9	D37.8	D49.0
crystalline lens	C69.4-	C79.49	D09.2-	D31.4-	D48.7	D49.89
cul-de-sac (Douglas')	C48.1	C78.6	-	D20.1	D48.4	D49.0
cuneiform cartilage	C32.3	C78.39	D02.0	D14.1	D38.0	D49.1
cutaneous — *see* Neoplasm, skin						
cutis — *see* Neoplasm, skin						
cystic (bile) duct (common)	C24.0	C78.89	D01.5	D13.5	D37.6	D49.0
dermis — *see* Neoplasm, skin						
diaphragm	C49.3	C79.89	-	D21.3	D48.1	D49.2
digestive organs, system, tube, or tract NEC	C26.9	C78.89	D01.9	D13.9	D37.9	D49.0
disc, intervertebral	C41.2	C79.51	-	D16.6	D48.0	D49.2
disease, generalized	C80.0	-	-	-	-	-
disseminated	C80.0	-	-	-	-	-
Douglas' cul-de-sac or pouch	C48.1	C78.6	-	D20.1	D48.4	D49.0
duodenojejunal junction	C17.8	C78.4	D01.49	D13.39	D37.2	D49.0
duodenum	C17.0	C78.4	D01.49	D13.2	D37.2	D49.0
dura (cranial) (mater)	C70.9	C79.49	-	D32.9	D42.9	D49.7
cerebral	C70.0	C79.32	-	D32.0	D42.0	D49.7
spinal	C70.1	C79.49	-	D32.1	D42.1	D49.7
ear (external) — *see also* Neoplasm, skin, ear	C44.20-	C79.2	D04.2-	D23.2-	D48.5	D49.2
auricle or auris — *see also* Neoplasm, skin, ear	C44.20-	C79.2	D04.2-	D23.2-	D48.5	D49.2
canal, external — *see also* Neoplasm, skin, ear	C44.20-	C79.2	D04.2-	D23.2-	D48.5	D49.2
cartilage	C49.0	C79.89	-	D21.0	D48.1	D49.2
external meatus — *see also* Neoplasm, skin, ear	C44.20-	C79.2	D04.2-	D23.2-	D48.5	D49.2
inner	C30.1	C78.39	D02.3	D14.0	D38.5	D49.1
lobule — *see also* Neoplasm, skin, ear	C44.20-	C79.2	D04.2-	D23.2-	D48.5	D49.2
middle	C30.1	C78.39	D02.3	D14.0	D38.5	D49.1
overlapping lesion with accessory sinuses	C31.8	-	-	-	-	-
skin	C44.20-	C79.2	D04.2-	D23.2-	D48.5	D49.2

Neoplasm, neoplastic	Malignant Primary	Malignant Secondary	Ca in situ	Benign	Uncertain Behavior	Unspecified Behavior
ear - *continued*						
basal cell carcinoma	C44.21-	-	-	-	-	-
specified type NEC	C44.29-	-	-	-	-	-
squamous cell carcinoma	C44.22-	-	-	-	-	-
earlobe	C44.20-	C79.2	D04.2-	D23.2-	D48.5	D49.2
basal cell carcinoma	C44.21-	-	-	-	-	-
specified type NEC	C44.29-	-	-	-	-	-
squamous cell carcinoma	C44.22-	-	-	-	-	-
ejaculatory duct	C63.7	C79.82	D07.69	D29.8	D40.8	D49.59
elbow NEC	C76.4-	C79.89	D04.6-	D36.7	D48.7	D49.89
endocardium	C38.0	C79.89	-	D15.1	D48.7	D49.89
endocervix (canal) (gland)	C53.0	C79.82	D06.0	D26.0	D39.0	D49.59
endocrine gland NEC	C75.9	C79.89	D09.3	D35.9	D44.9	D49.7
pluriglandular	C75.8	C79.89	D09.3	D35.7	D44.9	D49.7
endometrium (gland) (stroma)	C54.1	C79.82	D07.0	D26.1	D39.0	D49.59
ensiform cartilage	C41.3	C79.51	-	D16.7	D48.0	D49.2
enteric — *see* Neoplasm, intestine						
ependyma (brain)	C71.5	C79.31	-	D33.0	D43.0	D49.6
fourth ventricle	C71.7	C79.31	-	D33.1	D43.1	D49.6
epicardium	C38.0	C79.89	-	D15.1	D48.7	D49.89
epididymis	C63.0-	C79.82	D07.69	D29.3-	D40.8	D49.59
epidural	C72.9	C79.49	-	D33.9	D43.9	D49.7
epiglottis	C32.1	C78.39	D02.0	D14.1	D38.0	D49.1
anterior aspect or surface	C10.1	C79.89	D00.08	D10.5	D37.05	D49.0
cartilage	C32.3	C78.39	D02.0	D14.1	D38.0	D49.1
free border (margin)	C10.1	C79.89	D00.08	D10.5	D37.05	D49.0
junctional region	C10.8	C79.89	D00.08	D10.5	D37.05	D49.0
posterior (laryngeal) surface	C32.1	C78.39	D02.0	D14.1	D38.0	D49.1
suprahyoid portion	C32.1	C78.39	D02.0	D14.1	D38.0	D49.1
esophagogastric junction	C16.0	C78.89	D00.2	D13.1	D37.1	D49.0
esophagus	C15.9	C78.89	D00.1	D13.0	D37.8	D49.0
abdominal	C15.5	C78.89	D00.1	D13.0	D37.8	D49.0
cervical	C15.3	C78.89	D00.1	D13.0	D37.8	D49.0
distal (third)	C15.5	C78.89	D00.1	D13.0	D37.8	D49.0
lower (third)	C15.5	C78.89	D00.1	D13.0	D37.8	D49.0
middle (third)	C15.4	C78.89	D00.1	D13.0	D37.8	D49.0
overlapping lesion	C15.8	-				
proximal (third)	C15.3	C78.89	D00.1	D13.0	D37.8	D49.0
thoracic	C15.4	C78.89	D00.1	D13.0	D37.8	D49.0
upper (third)	C15.3	C78.89	D00.1	D13.0	D37.8	D49.0
ethmoid (sinus)	C31.1	C78.39	D02.3	D14.0	D38.5	D49.1
bone or labyrinth	C41.0	C79.51	-	D16.4-	D48.0	D49.2
eustachian tube	C30.1	C78.39	D02.3	D14.0	D38.5	D49.1
exocervix	C53.1	C79.82	D06.1	D26.0	D39.0	D49.59
external						
meatus (ear) — *see also* Neoplasm, skin, ear	C44.20-	C79.2	D04.2-	D23.2-	D48.5	D49.2
os, cervix uteri	C53.1	C79.82	D06.1	D26.0	D39.0	D49.59
extradural	C72.9	C79.49	-	D33.9	D43.9	D49.7
extrahepatic (bile) duct	C24.0	C78.89	D01.5	D13.5	D37.6	D49.0
overlapping lesion with gallbladder	C24.8					
extraocular muscle	C69.6-	C79.49	D09.2-	D31.6-	D48.7	D49.89
extrarectal	C76.3	C79.89	D09.8	D36.7	D48.7	D49.89
extremity	C76.8	C79.89	D04.8	D36.7	D48.7	D49.89
lower	C76.5-	C79.89	D04.7-	D36.7	D48.7	D49.89
upper	C76.4-	C79.89	D04.6-	D36.7	D48.7	D49.89
eye NEC	C69.9-	C79.49	D09.2	D31.9	D48.7	D49.89
overlapping sites	C69.8	-	-	-	-	-
eyeball	C69.9-	C79.49	D09.2-	D31.9-	D48.7	D49.89
eyebrow	C44.309	C79.2	D04.39	D23.39	D48.5	D49.2
basal cell carcinoma	C44.319	-	-	-	-	-
specified type NEC	C44.399	-	-	-	-	-
squamous cell carcinoma	C44.329	-	-	-	-	-
eyelid (lower) (skin) (upper)	C44.10-	-	-	-	-	-
basal cell carcinoma	C44.11-	-	-	-	-	-
specified type NEC	C44.19-	-	-	-	-	-
squamous cell carcinoma	C44.12-	-	-	-	-	-
cartilage	C49.0	C79.89	-	D21.0	D48.1	D49.2
face NEC	C76.0	C79.89	D04.39	D36.7	D48.7	D49.89
fallopian tube (accessory)	C57.0-	C79.82	D07.39	D28.2	D39.8	D49.59
falx (cerebella) (cerebri)	C70.0	C79.32	-	D32.0	D42.0	D49.7
fascia — *see also* Neoplasm, connective tissue						
palmar	C49.1-	C79.89	-	D21.1-	D48.1	D49.2
plantar	C49.2-	C79.89	-	D21.2-	D48.1	D49.2
fatty tissue — *see* Neoplasm, connective tissue						
fauces, faucial NEC	C10.9	C79.89	D00.08	D10.5	D37.05	D49.0
pillars	C09.1	C79.89	D00.08	D10.5	D37.05	D49.0

Neoplasm, neoplastic	Malignant Primary	Malignant Secondary	Ca in situ	Benign	Uncertain Behavior	Unspecified Behavior
fauces, faucial NEC - *continued*						
tonsil	C09.9	C79.89	D00.08	D10.4	D37.05	D49.0
femur (any part)	C40.2-			D16.2-		
fetal membrane	C58	C79.82	D07.0	D26.7	D39.2	D49.59
fibrous tissue — *see* Neoplasm, connective tissue						
fibula (any part)	C40.2-	C79.51	-	D16.2-	-	-
filum terminale	C72.0	C79.49	-	D33.4	D43.4	D49.7
finger NEC	C76.4-	C79.89	D04.6-	D36.7	D48.7	D49.89
flank NEC	C76.8	C79.89	D04.5	D36.7	D48.7	D49.89
follicle, nabothian	C53.0	C79.82	D06.0	D26.0	D39.0	D49.59
foot NEC	C76.5-	C79.89	D04.7-	D36.7	D48.7	D49.89
forearm NEC	C76.4-	C79.89	D04.6-	D36.7	D48.7	D49.89
forehead (skin)	C44.309	C79.2	D04.39	D23.39	D48.5	D49.2
basal cell carcinoma	C44.319	-	-	-	-	-
specified type NEC	C44.399	-	-	-	-	-
squamous cell carcinoma	C44.329	-	-	-	-	-
foreskin	C60.0	C79.82	D07.4	D29.0	D40.8	D49.59
fornix						
pharyngeal	C11.3	C79.89	D00.08	D10.6	D37.05	D49.0
vagina	C52	C79.82	D07.2	D28.1	D39.8	D49.59
fossa (of)						
anterior (cranial)	C71.9	C79.31	-	D33.2	D43.2	D49.6
cranial	C71.9	C79.31	-	D33.2	D43.2	D49.6
ischiorectal	C76.3	C79.89	D09.8	D36.7	D48.7	D49.89
middle (cranial)	C71.9	C79.31	-	D33.2	D43.2	D49.6
piriform	C12	C79.89	D00.08	D10.7	D37.05	D49.0
pituitary	C75.1	C79.89	D09.3	D35.2	D44.3	D49.7
posterior (cranial)	C71.9	C79.31	-	D33.2	D43.2	D49.6
pterygoid	C49.0	C79.89	-	D21.0	D48.1	D49.2
pyriform	C12	C79.89	D00.08	D10.7	D37.05	D49.0
Rosenmuller	C11.2	C79.89	D00.08	D10.6	D37.05	D49.0
tonsillar	C09.0	C79.89	D00.08	D10.5	D37.05	D49.0
fourchette	C51.9	C79.82	D07.1	D28.0	D39.8	D49.59
frenulum						
labii — *see* Neoplasm, lip, internal						
linguae	C02.2	C79.89	D00.07	D10.1	D37.02	D49.0
frontal						
bone	C41.0	C79.51	-	D16.4-	D48.0	D49.2
lobe, brain	C71.1	C79.31	-	D33.0	D43.0	D49.6
pole	C71.1	C79.31	-	D33.0	D43.0	D49.6
sinus	C31.2	C78.39	D02.3	D14.0	D38.5	D49.1
fundus						
stomach	C16.1	C78.89	D00.2	D13.1	D37.1	D49.0
uterus	C54.3	C79.82	D07.0	D26.1	D39.0	D49.59
gall duct (extrahepatic)	C24.0	C78.89	D01.5	D13.5	D37.6	D49.0
intrahepatic	C22.1	C78.7	D01.5	D13.4	D37.6	D49.0
gallbladder	C23	C78.89	D01.5	D13.5	D37.6	D49.0
overlapping lesion with extrahepatic bile ducts	C24.8					
ganglia — *see also* Neoplasm, nerve, peripheral	C47.9	C79.89	-	D36.10	D48.2	D49.2
basal	C71.0	C79.31	-	D33.0	D43.0	D49.6
cranial nerve	C72.50	C79.49	-	D33.3	D43.3	D49.7
Gartner's duct	C52	C79.82	D07.2	D28.1	D39.8	D49.59
gastric — *see* Neoplasm, stomach						
gastrocolic	C26.9	C78.89	D01.9	D13.9	D37.9	D49.0
gastroesophageal junction	C16.0	C78.89	D00.2	D13.1	D37.1	D49.0
gastrointestinal (tract) NEC	C26.9	C78.89	D01.9	D13.9	D37.9	D49.0
generalized	C80.0	-	-	-	-	-
genital organ or tract						
female NEC	C57.9	C79.82	D07.30	D28.9	D39.9	D49.59
overlapping lesion	C57.8	-	-	-	-	-
specified site NEC	C57.7	C79.82	D07.39	D28.7	D39.8	D49.59
male NEC	C63.9	C79.82	D07.60	D29.9	D40.9	D49.59
overlapping lesion	C63.8					
specified site NEC	C63.7	C79.82	D07.69	D29.8	D40.8	D49.59
genitourinary tract						
female	C57.9	C79.82	D07.30	D28.9	D39.9	D49.59
male	C63.9	C79.82	D07.60	D29.9	D40.9	D49.59
gingiva (alveolar) (marginal)	C03.9	C79.89	D00.03	D10.39	D37.09	D49.0
lower	C03.1	C79.89	D00.03	D10.39	D37.09	D49.0
mandibular	C03.1	C79.89	D00.03	D10.39	D37.09	D49.0
maxillary	C03.0	C79.89	D00.03	D10.39	D37.09	D49.0
upper	C03.0	C79.89	D00.03	D10.39	D37.09	D49.0
gland, glandular (lymphatic) (system) — *see also* Neoplasm, lymph gland						
endocrine NEC	C75.9	C79.89	D09.3	D35.9	D44.9	D49.7

Neoplasm, neoplastic	Malignant Primary	Malignant Secondary	Ca in situ	Benign	Uncertain Behavior	Unspecified Behavior
gland, glandular - *continued*						
salivary — *see* Neoplasm, salivary gland						
glans penis	C60.1	C79.82	D07.4	D29.0	D40.8	D49.59
globus pallidus	C71.0	C79.31	-	D33.0	D43.0	D49.6
glomus						
coccygeal	C49.5	C79.89	-	D21.5	D48.1	D49.2
jugularis	C75.5	C79.89	-	D35.6	D44.7	D49.7
glosso-epiglottic fold (s)	C10.1	C79.89	D00.08	D10.5	D37.05	D49.0
glossopalatine fold	C09.1	C79.89	D00.08	D10.5	D37.05	D49.0
glossopharyngeal sulcus	C09.0	C79.89	D00.08	D10.5	D37.05	D49.0
glottis	C32.0	C78.39	D02.0	D14.1	D38.0	D49.1
gluteal region	C76.3	C79.89	D04.5	D36.7	D48.7	D49.89
great vessels NEC	C49.3	C79.89	-	D21.3	D48.1	D49.2
groin NEC	C76.3	C79.89	D04.5	D36.7	D48.7	D49.89
gum	C03.9	C79.89	D00.03	D10.39	D37.09	D49.0
lower	C03.1	C79.89	D00.03	D10.39	D37.09	D49.0
upper	C03.0	C79.89	D00.03	D10.39	D37.09	D49.0
hand NEC	C76.4-	C79.89	D04.6-	D36.7	D48.7	D49.89
head NEC	C76.0	C79.89	D04.4	D36.7	D48.7	D49.89
heart	C38.0	C79.89	-	D15.1	D48.7	D49.89
heel NEC	C76.5-	C79.89	D04.7-	D36.7	D48.7	D49.89
helix — *see also* Neoplasm, skin, ear	C44.20-	C79.2	D04.2-	D23.2-	D48.5	D49.2
hematopoietic, hemopoietic tissue NEC	C96.9	-	-	-	-	-
specified NEC	C96.Z	-	-	-	-	-
hemisphere, cerebral	C71.0	C79.31	-	D33.0	D43.0	D49.6
hemorrhoidal zone	C21.1	C78.5	D01.3	D12.9	D37.8	D49.0
hepatic — *see also* Index to disease, by histology	C22.9	C78.7	D01.5	D13.4	D37.6	D49.0
duct (bile)	C24.0	C78.89	D01.5	D13.5	D37.6	D49.0
flexure (colon)	C18.3	C78.5	D01.0	D12.3	D37.4	D49.0
primary	C22.8	C78.7	D01.5	D13.4	D37.6	D49.0
hepatobiliary	C24.9	C78.89	D01.5	D13.5	D37.6	D49.0
hepatoblastoma	C22.2	C78.7	D01.5	D13.4	D37.6	D49.0
hepatoma	C22.0	C78.7	D01.5	D13.4	D37.6	D49.0
hilus of lung	C34.0-	C78.0-	D02.2-	D14.3-	D38.1	D49.1
hip NEC	C76.5-	C79.89	D04.7-	D36.7	D48.7	D49.89
hippocampus, brain	C71.2	C79.31	-	D33.0	D43.0	D49.6
humerus (any part)	C40.0-	C79.51	-	D16.0-	-	-
hymen	C52	C79.82	D07.2	D28.1	D39.8	D49.59
hypopharynx, hypopharyngeal NEC	C13.9	C79.89	D00.08	D10.7	D37.05	D49.0
overlapping lesion	C13.8	-	-	-	-	-
postcricoid region	C13.0	C79.89	D00.08	D10.7	D37.05	D49.0
posterior wall	C13.2	C79.89	D00.08	D10.7	D37.05	D49.0
pyriform fossa (sinus)	C12	C79.89	D00.08	D10.7	D37.05	D49.0
hypophysis	C75.1	C79.89	D09.3	D35.2	D44.3	D49.7
hypothalamus	C71.0	C79.31	-	D33.0	D43.0	D49.6
ileocecum, ileocecal (coil) (junction) (valve)	C18.0	C78.5	D01.0	D12.0	D37.4	D49.0
ileum	C17.2	C78.4	D01.49	D13.39	D37.2	D49.0
ilium	C41.4	C79.51	-	D16.8	D48.0	D49.2
immunoproliferative NEC	C88.9	-	-	-	-	-
infraclavicular (region)	C76.1	C79.89	D04.5	D36.7	D48.7	D49.89
inguinal (region)	C76.3	C79.89	D04.5	D36.7	D48.7	D49.89
insula	C71.0	C79.31	-	D33.0	D43.0	D49.6
insular tissue (pancreas)	C25.4	C78.89	D01.7	D13.7	D37.8	D49.0
brain	C71.0	C79.31	-	D33.0	D43.0	D49.6
interarytenoid fold	C13.1	C79.89	D00.08	D10.7	D37.05	D49.0
hypopharyngeal aspect	C13.1	C79.89	D00.08	D10.7	D37.05	D49.0
laryngeal aspect	C32.1	C78.39	D02.0	D14.1	D38.0	D49.1
marginal zone	C13.1	C79.89	D00.08	D10.7	D37.05	D49.0
interdental papillae	C03.9	C79.89	D00.03	D10.39	D37.09	D49.0
lower	C03.1	C79.89	D00.03	D10.39	D37.09	D49.0
upper	C03.0	C79.89	D00.03	D10.39	D37.09	D49.0
internal						
capsule	C71.0	C79.31	-	D33.0	D43.0	D49.6
os (cervix)	C53.0	C79.82	D06.0	D26.0	D39.0	D49.59
intervertebral cartilage or disc	C41.2	C79.51	-	D16.6	D48.0	D49.2
intestine, intestinal	C26.0	C78.80	D01.40	D13.9	D37.8	D49.0
large	C18.9	C78.5	D01.0	D12.6	D37.4	D49.0
appendix	C18.1	C78.5	D01.0	D12.1	D37.3	D49.0
caput coli	C18.0	C78.5	D01.0	D12.0	D37.4	D49.0
cecum	C18.0	C78.5	D01.0	D12.0	D37.4	D49.0
colon	C18.9	C78.5	D01.0	D12.6	D37.4	D49.0
and rectum	C19	C78.5	D01.1	D12.7	D37.5	D49.0
ascending	C18.2	C78.5	D01.0	D12.2	D37.4	D49.0
caput	C18.0	C78.5	D01.0	D12.0	D37.4	D49.0

Neoplasm, neoplastic	Malignant Primary	Malignant Secondary	Ca in situ	Benign	Uncertain Behavior	Unspecified Behavior
intestine, intestinal - *continued*						
descending	C18.6	C78.5	D01.0	D12.4	D37.4	D49.0
distal	C18.6	C78.5	D01.0	D12.4	D37.4	D49.0
left	C18.6	C78.5	D01.0	D12.4	D37.4	D49.0
overlapping lesion	C18.8	-	-	-	-	-
pelvic	C18.7	C78.5	D01.0	D12.5	D37.4	D49.0
right	C18.2	C78.5	D01.0	D12.2	D37.4	D49.0
sigmoid (flexure)	C18.7	C78.5	D01.0	D12.5	D37.4	D49.0
transverse	C18.4	C78.5	D01.0	D12.3	D37.4	D49.0
hepatic flexure	C18.3	C78.5	D01.0	D12.3	D37.4	D49.0
ileocecal (coil) (valve)	C18.0	C78.5	D01.0	D12.0	D37.4	D49.0
overlapping lesion	C18.8	-	-	-	-	-
sigmoid flexure (lower) (upper)	C18.7	C78.5	D01.0	D12.5	D37.4	D49.0
splenic flexure	C18.5	C78.5	D01.0	D12.3	D37.4	D49.0
small	C17.9	C78.4	D01.40	D13.30	D37.2	D49.0
duodenum	C17.0	C78.4	D01.49	D13.2	D37.2	D49.0
ileum	C17.2	C78.4	D01.49	D13.39	D37.2	D49.0
jejunum	C17.1	C78.4	D01.49	D13.39	D37.2	D49.0
overlapping lesion	C17.8	-	-	-	-	-
tract NEC	C26.0	C78.89	D01.40	D13.9	D37.8	D49.0
intra-abdominal	C76.2	C79.89	D09.8	D36.7	D48.7	D49.89
intracranial NEC	C71.9	C79.31	-	D33.2	D43.2	D49.6
intrahepatic (bile) duct	C22.1	C78.7	D01.5	D13.4	D37.6	D49.0
intraocular	C69.9-	C79.49	D09.2-	D31.9-	D48.7	D49.89
intraorbital	C69.6-	C79.49	D09.2-	D31.6-	D48.7	D49.89
intrasellar	C75.1	C79.89	D09.3	D35.2	D44.3	D49.7
intrathoracic (cavity) (organs)	C76.1	C79.89	D09.8	D15.9	D48.7	D49.89
specified NEC	C76.1	C79.89	D09.8	D15.7	-	-
iris	C69.4-	C79.49	D09.2-	D31.4-	D48.7	D49.89
ischiorectal (fossa)	C76.3	C79.89	D09.8	D36.7	D48.7	D49.89
ischium	C41.4	C79.51	-	D16.8	D48.0	D49.2
island of Reil	C71.0	C79.31	-	D33.0	D43.0	D49.6
islands or islets of Langerhans	C25.4	C78.89	D01.7	D13.7	D37.8	D49.0
isthmus uteri	C54.0	C79.82	D07.0	D26.1	D39.0	D49.59
jaw	C76.0	C79.89	D09.8	D36.7	D48.7	D49.89
bone	C41.1	C79.51	-	D16.5-	D48.0	D49.2
lower	C41.1	C79.51	-	D16.5-	-	-
upper	C41.0	C79.51	-	D16.4-	-	-
carcinoma (any type) (lower) (upper)	C76.0	C79.89				
skin — *see also* Neoplasm, skin, face	C44.309	C79.2	D04.39	D23.39	D48.5	D49.2
soft tissues	C03.9	C79.89	D00.03	D10.39	D37.09	D49.0
lower	C03.1	C79.89	D00.03	D10.39	D37.09	D49.0
upper	C03.0	C79.89	D00.03	D10.39	D37.09	D49.0
jejunum	C17.1	C78.4	D01.49	D13.39	D37.2	D49.0
joint NEC — *see also* Neoplasm, bone	C41.9	C79.51	-	D16.9-	D48.0	D49.2
acromioclavicular	C40.0-	C79.51	-	D16.0-	-	-
bursa or synovial membrane — *see* Neoplasm, connective tissue						
costovertebral	C41.3	C79.51	-	D16.7	D48.0	D49.2
sternocostal	C41.3	C79.51	-	D16.7	D48.0	D49.2
temporomandibular	C41.1	C79.51	-	D16.5-	D48.0	D49.2
junction						
anorectal	C21.8	C78.5	D01.3	D12.9	D37.8	D49.0
cardioesophageal	C16.0	C78.89	D00.2	D13.1	D37.1	D49.0
esophagogastric	C16.0	C78.89	D00.2	D13.1	D37.1	D49.0
gastroesophageal	C16.0	C78.89	D00.2	D13.1	D37.1	D49.0
hard and soft palate	C05.9	C79.89	D00.00	D10.39	D37.09	D49.0
ileocecal	C18.0	C78.5	D01.0	D12.0	D37.4	D49.0
pelvirectal	C19	C78.5	D01.1	D12.7	D37.5	D49.0
pelviureteric	C65.-	C79.0-	D09.19	D30.1-	D41.1-	D49.59
rectosigmoid	C19	C78.5	D01.1	D12.7	D37.5	D49.0
squamocolumnar, of cervix	C53.8	C79.82	D06.7	D26.0	D39.0	D49.59
Kaposi's sarcoma — *see* Kaposi's, sarcoma						
kidney (parenchymal)	C64.-	C79.0-	D09.19	D30.0-	D41.0-	D49.51-
calyx	C65.-	C79.0-	D09.19	D30.1-	D41.1-	D49.51-
hilus	C65.-	C79.0-	D09.19	D30.1-	D41.1-	D49.51-
pelvis	C65.-	C79.0-	D09.19	D30.1-	D41.1-	D49.51-
knee NEC	C76.5-	C79.89	D04.7-	D36.7	D48.7	D49.89
labia (skin)	C51.9	C79.82	D07.1	D28.0	D39.8	D49.59
majora	C51.0	C79.82	D07.1	D28.0	D39.8	D49.59
minora	C51.1	C79.82	D07.1	D28.0	D39.8	D49.59
labial — *see also* Neoplasm, lip	C00.9	C79.89	D00.01	D10.0	D37.01	D49.0
sulcus (lower) (upper)	C06.1	C79.89	D00.02	D10.39	D37.09	D49.0
labium (skin)	C51.9	C79.82	D07.1	D28.0	D39.8	D49.59

Neoplasm, neoplastic	Malignant Primary	Malignant Secondary	Ca in situ	Benign	Uncertain Behavior	Unspecified Behavior
labium - *continued*						
majus	C51.0	C79.82	D07.1	D28.0	D39.8	D49.59
minus	C51.1	C79.82	D07.1	D28.0	D39.8	D49.59
lacrimal						
canaliculi	C69.5-	C79.49	D09.2-	D31.5-	D48.7	D49.89
duct (nasal)	C69.5-	C79.49	D09.2-	D31.5-	D48.7	D49.89
gland	C69.5-	C79.49	D09.2-	D31.5-	D48.7	D49.89
punctum	C69.5-	C79.49	D09.2-	D31.5-	D48.7	D49.89
sac	C69.5-	C79.49	D09.2-	D31.5-	D48.7	D49.89
Langerhans, islands or islets	C25.4	C78.89	D01.7	D13.7	D37.8	D49.0
laryngopharynx	C13.9	C79.89	D00.08	D10.7	D37.05	D49.0
larynx, laryngeal NEC	C32.9	C78.39	D02.0	D14.1	D38.0	D49.1
aryepiglottic fold	C32.1	C78.39	D02.0	D14.1	D38.0	D49.1
cartilage (arytenoid) (cricoid) (cuneiform) (thyroid)	C32.3	C78.39	D02.0	D14.1	D38.0	D49.1
commissure (anterior) (posterior)	C32.0	C78.39	D02.0	D14.1	D38.0	D49.1
extrinsic NEC	C32.1	C78.39	D02.0	D14.1	D38.0	D49.1
meaning hypopharynx	C13.9	C79.89	D00.08	D10.7	D37.05	D49.0
interarytenoid fold	C32.1	C78.39	D02.0	D14.1	D38.0	D49.1
intrinsic	C32.0	C78.39	D02.0	D14.1	D38.0	D49.1
overlapping lesion	C32.8					
ventricular band	C32.1	C78.39	D02.0	D14.1	D38.0	D49.1
leg NEC	C76.5-	C79.89	D04.7-	D36.7	D48.7	D49.89
lens, crystalline	C69.4-	C79.49	D09.2-	D31.4-	D48.7	D49.89
lid (lower) (upper)	C44.10-	C79.2	D04.1-	D23.1-	D48.5	D49.2
basal cell carcinoma	C44.11-	-	-	-	-	-
specified type NEC	C44.19-	-	-	-	-	-
squamous cell carcinoma	C44.12-	-	-	-	-	-
ligament — *see also* Neoplasm, connective tissue						
broad	C57.1	C79.82	D07.39	D28.2	D39.8	D49.59
Mackenrodt's	C57.7	C79.82	D07.39	D28.7	D39.8	D49.59
non-uterine — *see* Neoplasm, connective tissue						
round	C57.2	C79.82	-	D28.2	D39.8	D49.59
sacro-uterine	C57.3	C79.82	-	D28.2	D39.8	D49.59
uterine	C57.3	C79.82	-	D28.2	D39.8	D49.59
utero-ovarian	C57.7	C79.82	D07.39	D28.2	D39.8	D49.59
uterosacral	C57.3	C79.82	-	D28.2	D39.8	D49.59
limb	C76.8	C79.89	D04.8	D36.7	D48.7	D49.89
lower	C76.5-	C79.89	D04.7-	D36.7	D48.7	D49.89
upper	C76.4-	C79.89	D04.6-	D36.7	D48.7	D49.89
limbus of cornea	C69.1-	C79.49	D09.2-	D31.1-	D48.7	D49.89
lingual NEC — *see also* Neoplasm, tongue	C02.9	C79.89	D00.07	D10.1	D37.02	D49.0
lingula, lung	C34.1-	C78.0-	D02.2-	D14.3-	D38.1	D49.1
lip	C00.9	C79.89	D00.01	D10.0	D37.01	D49.0
buccal aspect — *see* Neoplasm, lip, internal						
commissure	C00.6	C79.89	D00.01	D10.0	D37.01	D49.0
external	C00.2	C79.89	D00.01	D10.0	D37.01	D49.0
lower	C00.1	C79.89	D00.01	D10.0	D37.01	D49.0
upper	C00.0	C79.89	D00.01	D10.0	D37.01	D49.0
frenulum — *see* Neoplasm, lip, internal						
inner aspect — *see* Neoplasm, lip, internal						
internal	C00.5	C79.89	D00.01	D10.0	D37.01	D49.0
lower	C00.4	C79.89	D00.01	D10.0	D37.01	D49.0
upper	C00.3	C79.89	D00.01	D10.0	D37.01	D49.0
lipstick area	C00.2	C79.89	D00.01	D10.0	D37.01	D49.0
lower	C00.1	C79.89	D00.01	D10.0	D37.01	D49.0
upper	C00.0	C79.89	D00.01	D10.0	D37.01	D49.0
lower	C00.1	C79.89	D00.01	D10.0	D37.01	D49.0
internal	C00.4	C79.89	D00.01	D10.0	D37.01	D49.0
mucosa — *see* Neoplasm, lip, internal						
oral aspect — *see* Neoplasm, lip, internal						
overlapping lesion	C00.8	-	-	-	-	-
with oral cavity or pharynx	C14.8	-	-	-	-	-
skin (commissure) (lower) (upper)	C44.00	C79.2	D04.0	D23.0	D48.5	D49.2
basal cell carcinoma	C44.01	-	-	-	-	-
specified type NEC	C44.09	-	-	-	-	-
squamous cell carcinoma	C44.02	-	-	-	-	-
upper	C00.0	C79.89	D00.01	D10.0	D37.01	D49.0
internal	C00.3	C79.89	D00.01	D10.0	D37.01	D49.0
vermilion border	C00.2	C79.89	D00.01	D10.0	D37.01	D49.0
lower	C00.1	C79.89	D00.01	D10.0	D37.01	D49.0

Neoplasm, neoplastic	Malignant Primary	Malignant Secondary	Ca in situ	Benign	Uncertain Behavior	Unspecified Behavior
lip - *continued*						
upper	C00.0	C79.89	D00.01	D10.0	D37.01	D49.0
lipomatous — *see* Lipoma, by site						
liver — *see also* Index to disease, by histology	C22.9	C78.7	D01.5	D13.4	D37.6	D49.0
primary	C22.8	C78.7	D01.5	D13.4	D37.6	D49.0
lumbosacral plexus	C47.5	C79.89	-	D36.16	D48.2	D49.2
lung	C34.9-	C78.0-	D02.2-	D14.3-	D38.1	D49.1
azygos lobe	C34.1-	C78.0-	D02.2-	D14.3-	D38.1	D49.1
carina	C34.0-	C78.0-	D02.2-	D14.3-	D38.1	D49.1
hilus	C34.0-	C78.0-	D02.2-	D14.3-	D38.1	D49.1
lingula	C34.1-	C78.0-	D02.2-	D14.3-	D38.1	D49.1
lobe NEC	C34.9-	C78.0-	D02.2-	D14.3-	D38.1	D49.1
lower lobe	C34.3-	C78.0-	D02.2-	D14.3-	D38.1	D49.1
main bronchus	C34.0-	C78.0-	D02.2-	D14.3-	D38.1	D49.1
mesothelioma — *see* Mesothelioma						
middle lobe	C34.2	C78.0-	D02.21	D14.31	D38.1	D49.1
overlapping lesion	C34.8-	-	-	-	-	-
upper lobe	C34.1-	C78.0-	D02.2-	D14.3-	D38.1	D49.1
lymph, lymphatic channel NEC	C49.9	C79.89	-	D21.9	D48.1	D49.2
gland (secondary)	-	C77.9	-	D36.0	D48.7	D49.89
abdominal	-	C77.2	-	D36.0	D48.7	D49.89
aortic	-	C77.2	-	D36.0	D48.7	D49.89
arm	-	C77.3	-	D36.0	D48.7	D49.89
auricular (anterior) (posterior)	-	C77.0	-	D36.0	D48.7	D49.89
axilla, axillary	-	C77.3	-	D36.0	D48.7	D49.89
brachial	-	C77.3	-	D36.0	D48.7	D49.89
bronchial	-	C77.1	-	D36.0	D48.7	D49.89
bronchopulmonary	-	C77.1	-	D36.0	D48.7	D49.89
celiac	-	C77.2	-	D36.0	D48.7	D49.89
cervical	-	C77.0	-	D36.0	D48.7	D49.89
cervicofacial	-	C77.0	-	D36.0	D48.7	D49.89
Cloquet	-	C77.4	-	D36.0	D48.7	D49.89
colic	-	C77.2	-	D36.0	D48.7	D49.89
common duct	-	C77.2	-	D36.0	D48.7	D49.89
cubital	-	C77.3	-	D36.0	D48.7	D49.89
diaphragmatic	-	C77.1	-	D36.0	D48.7	D49.89
epigastric, inferior	-	C77.1	-	D36.0	D48.7	D49.89
epitrochlear	-	C77.3	-	D36.0	D48.7	D49.89
esophageal	-	C77.1	-	D36.0	D48.7	D49.89
face	-	C77.0	-	D36.0	D48.7	D49.89
femoral	-	C77.4	-	D36.0	D48.7	D49.89
gastric	-	C77.2	-	D36.0	D48.7	D49.89
groin	-	C77.4	-	D36.0	D48.7	D49.89
head	-	C77.0	-	D36.0	D48.7	D49.89
hepatic	-	C77.2	-	D36.0	D48.7	D49.89
hilar (pulmonary)	-	C77.1	-	D36.0	D48.7	D49.89
splenic	-	C77.2	-	D36.0	D48.7	D49.89
hypogastric	-	C77.5	-	D36.0	D48.7	D49.89
ileocolic	-	C77.2	-	D36.0	D48.7	D49.89
iliac	-	C77.5	-	D36.0	D48.7	D49.89
infraclavicular	-	C77.3	-	D36.0	D48.7	D49.89
inguina, inguinal	-	C77.4	-	D36.0	D48.7	D49.89
innominate	-	C77.1	-	D36.0	D48.7	D49.89
intercostal	-	C77.1	-	D36.0	D48.7	D49.89
intestinal	-	C77.2	-	D36.0	D48.7	D49.89
intrabdominal	-	C77.2	-	D36.0	D48.7	D49.89
intrapelvic	-	C77.5	-	D36.0	D48.7	D49.89
intrathoracic	-	C77.1	-	D36.0	D48.7	D49.89
jugular	-	C77.0	-	D36.0	D48.7	D49.89
leg	-	C77.4	-	D36.0	D48.7	D49.89
limb						
lower	-	C77.4	-	D36.0	D48.7	D49.89
upper	-	C77.3	-	D36.0	D48.7	D49.89
lower limb	-	C77.4	-	D36.0	D48.7	D49.89
lumbar	-	C77.2	-	D36.0	D48.7	D49.89
mandibular	-	C77.0	-	D36.0	D48.7	D49.89
mediastinal	-	C77.1	-	D36.0	D48.7	D49.89
mesenteric (inferior) (superior)	-	C77.2	-	D36.0	D48.7	D49.89
midcolic	-	C77.2	-	D36.0	D48.7	D49.89
multiple sites in categories C77.0 - C77.5	-	C77.8	-	D36.0	D48.7	D49.89
neck	-	C77.0	-	D36.0	D48.7	D49.89
obturator	-	C77.5	-	D36.0	D48.7	D49.89
occipital	-	C77.0	-	D36.0	D48.7	D49.89
pancreatic	-	C77.2	-	D36.0	D48.7	D49.89
para-aortic	-	C77.2	-	D36.0	D48.7	D49.89
paracervical	-	C77.5	-	D36.0	D48.7	D49.89

Neoplasm, neoplastic	Malignant Primary	Malignant Secondary	Ca in situ	Benign	Uncertain Behavior	Unspecified Behavior
lymph, lymphatic channel NEC - *continued*						
parametrial	-	C77.5	-	D36.0	D48.7	D49.89
parasternal	-	C77.1	-	D36.0	D48.7	D49.89
parotid	-	C77.0	-	D36.0	D48.7	D49.89
pectoral	-	C77.3	-	D36.0	D48.7	D49.89
pelvic	-	C77.5	-	D36.0	D48.7	D49.89
peri-aortic	-	C77.2	-	D36.0	D48.7	D49.89
peripancreatic	-	C77.2	-	D36.0	D48.7	D49.89
popliteal	-	C77.4	-	D36.0	D48.7	D49.89
porta hepatis	-	C77.2	-	D36.0	D48.7	D49.89
portal	-	C77.2	-	D36.0	D48.7	D49.89
preauricular	-	C77.0	-	D36.0	D48.7	D49.89
prelaryngeal	-	C77.0	-	D36.0	D48.7	D49.89
presymphysial	-	C77.5	-	D36.0	D48.7	D49.89
pretracheal	-	C77.0	-	D36.0	D48.7	D49.89
primary (any site) NEC	C96.9	-		-	-	-
pulmonary (hiler)	-	C77.1	-	D36.0	D48.7	D49.89
pyloric	-	C77.2	-	D36.0	D48.7	D49.89
retroperitoneal	-	C77.2	-	D36.0	D48.7	D49.89
retropharyngeal	-	C77.0	-	D36.0	D48.7	D49.89
Rosenmuller's	-	C77.4	-	D36.0	D48.7	D49.89
sacral	-	C77.5	-	D36.0	D48.7	D49.89
scalene	-	C77.0	-	D36.0	D48.7	D49.89
site NEC	-	C77.9	-	D36.0	D48.7	D49.89
splenic (hilar)	-	C77.2	-	D36.0	D48.7	D49.89
subclavicular	-	C77.3	-	D36.0	D48.7	D49.89
subinguinal	-	C77.4	-	D36.0	D48.7	D49.89
sublingual	-	C77.0	-	D36.0	D48.7	D49.89
submandibular	-	C77.0	-	D36.0	D48.7	D49.89
submaxillary	-	C77.0	-	D36.0	D48.7	D49.89
submental	-	C77.0	-	D36.0	D48.7	D49.89
subscapular	-	C77.3	-	D36.0	D48.7	D49.89
supraclavicular	-	C77.0	-	D36.0	D48.7	D49.89
thoracic	-	C77.1	-	D36.0	D48.7	D49.89
tibial	-	C77.4	-	D36.0	D48.7	D49.89
tracheal	-	C77.1	-	D36.0	D48.7	D49.89
tracheobronchial	-	C77.1	-	D36.0	D48.7	D49.89
upper limb	-	C77.3	-	D36.0	D48.7	D49.89
Virchow's	-	C77.0	-	D36.0	D48.7	D49.89
node — *see also* Neoplasm, lymph gland						
primary NEC	C96.9	-		-	-	-
vessel — *see also* Neoplasm, connective tissue	C49.9	C79.89	-	D21.9	D48.1	D49.2
Mackenrodt's ligament	C57.7	C79.82	D07.39	D28.7	D39.8	D49.59
malar	C41.0	C79.51		D16.4-	D48.0	D49.2
region — *see Neoplasm, cheek*						
mammary gland — *see* Neoplasm, breast						
mandible	C41.1	C79.51	-	D16.5-	D48.0	D49.2
alveolar						
mucosa (carcinoma)	C03.1	C79.89	D00.03	D10.39	D37.09	D49.0
ridge or process	C41.1	C79.51	-	D16.5-	D48.0	D49.2
marrow (bone) NEC	C96.9	C79.52	-	-	D47.9	D49.89
mastectomy site (skin) — *see also* Neoplasm, breast, skin	C44.501	C79.2	-	-	-	-
specified as breast tissue	C50.8-	C79.81	-	-	-	-
mastoid (air cells) (antrum) (cavity)	C30.1	C78.39	D02.3	D14.0	D38.5	D49.1
bone or process	C41.0	C79.51	-	D16.4-	D48.0	D49.2
maxilla, maxillary (superior)	C41.0	C79.51	-	D16.4-	D48.0	D49.2
alveolar						
mucosa	C03.0	C79.89	D00.03	D10.39	D37.09	D49.0
ridge or process (carcinoma)	C41.0	C79.51	-	D16.4-	D48.0	D49.2
antrum	C31.0	C78.39	D02.3	D14.0	D38.5	D49.1
carcinoma	C03.0	C79.51	-	-	-	-
inferior — *see* Neoplasm, mandible						
sinus	C31.0	C78.39	D02.3	D14.0	D38.5	D49.1
meatus external (ear) — *see also* Neoplasm, skin, ear	C44.20-	C79.2	D04.2-	D23.2-	D48.5	D49.2
Meckel diverticulum, malignant	C17.3	C78.4	D01.49	D13.39	D37.2	D49.0
mediastinum, mediastinal	C38.3	C78.1	-	D15.2	D38.3	D49.89
anterior	C38.1	C78.1	-	D15.2	D38.3	D49.89
posterior	C38.2	C78.1	-	D15.2	D38.3	D49.89
medulla						
adrenal	C74.1-	C79.7-	D09.3	D35.0-	D44.1-	D49.7
oblongata	C71.7	C79.31		D33.1	D43.1	D49.6
meibomian gland	C44.10-	C79.2	D04.1-	D23.1-	D48.5	D49.2

Neoplasm, neoplastic	Malignant Primary	Malignant Secondary	Ca in situ	Benign	Uncertain Behavior	Unspecified Behavior
meibomian gland - *continued*						
basal cell carcinoma	C44.11-	-	-	-	-	-
specified type NEC	C44.19-	-	-	-	-	-
squamous cell carcinoma	C44.12-	-	-	-	-	-
melanoma — *see* Melanoma						
meninges	C70.9	C79.49	-	D32.9	D42.9	D49.7
brain	C70.0	C79.32	-	D32.0	D42.0	D49.7
cerebral	C70.0	C79.32	-	D32.0	D42.0	D49.7
crainial	C70.0	C79.32	-	D32.0	D42.0	D49.7
intracranial	C70.0	C79.32	-	D32.0	D42.0	D49.7
spinal (cord)	C70.1	C79.49	-	D32.1	D42.1	D49.7
meniscus, knee joint (lateral) (medial)	C40.2-	C79.51	-	D16.2-	D48.0	D49.2
Merkel cell — *see* Carcinoma, Merkel cell						
mesentery, mesenteric	C48.1	C78.6	-	D20.1	D48.4	D49.0
mesoappendix	C48.1	C78.6	-	D20.1	D48.4	D49.0
mesocolon	C48.1	C78.6	-	D20.1	D48.4	D49.0
mesopharynx — *see* Neoplasm, oropharynx						
mesosalpinx	C57.1	C79.82	D07.39	D28.2	D39.8	D49.59
mesothelial tissue — *see* Mesothelioma						
mesothelioma — *see* Mesothelioma						
mesovarium	C57.1	C79.82	D07.39	D28.2	D39.8	D49.59
metacarpus (any bone)	C40.1-	C79.51	-	D16.1-	-	-
metastatic NEC — *see also* Neoplasm, by site, secondary	-	C79.9	-	-	-	-
metatarsus (any bone)	C40.3-	C79.51	-	D16.3-	-	-
midbrain	C71.7	C79.31	-	D33.1	D43.1	D49.6
milk duct — *see Neoplasm, breast*						
mons						
pubis	C51.9	C79.82	D07.1	D28.0	D39.8	D49.59
veneris	C51.9	C79.82	D07.1	D28.0	D39.8	D49.59
motor tract	C72.9	C79.49	-	D33.9	D43.9	D49.7
brain	C71.9	C79.31	-	D33.2	D43.2	D49.6
cauda equina	C72.1	C79.49	-	D33.4	D43.4	D49.7
spinal	C72.0	C79.49	-	D33.4	D43.4	D49.7
mouth	C06.9	C79.89	D00.00	D10.30	D37.09	D49.0
book-leaf	C06.89	C79.89				
floor	C04.9	C79.89	D00.06	D10.2	D37.09	D49.0
anterior portion	C04.0	C79.89	D00.06	D10.2	D37.09	D49.0
lateral portion	C04.1	C79.89	D00.06	D10.2	D37.09	D49.0
overlapping lesion	C04.8	-				
overlapping NEC	C06.80	-	-	-	-	-
roof	C05.9	C79.89	D00.00	D10.39	D37.09	D49.0
specified part NEC	C06.89	C79.89	D00.00	D10.39	D37.09	D49.0
vestibule	C06.1	C79.89	D00.00	D10.39	D37.09	D49.0
mucosa						
alveolar (ridge or process)	C03.9	C79.89	D00.03	D10.39	D37.09	D49.0
lower	C03.1	C79.89	D00.03	D10.39	D37.09	D49.0
upper	C03.0	C79.89	D00.03	D10.39	D37.09	D49.0
buccal	C06.0	C79.89	D00.02	D10.39	D37.09	D49.0
cheek	C06.0	C79.89	D00.02	D10.39	D37.09	D49.0
lip — *see Neoplasm, lip, internal*						
nasal	C30.0	C78.39	D02.3	D14.0	D38.5	D49.1
oral	C06.0	C79.89	D00.02	D10.39	D37.09	D49.0
Mullerian duct						
female	C57.7	C79.82	D07.39	D28.7	D39.8	D49.59
male	C63.7	C79.82	D07.69	D29.8	D40.8	D49.59
muscle — *see also* Neoplasm, connective tissue						
extraocular	C69.6-	C79.49	D09.2-	D31.6-	D48.7	D49.89
myocardium	C38.0	C79.89	-	D15.1	D48.7	D49.89
myometrium	C54.2	C79.82	D07.0	D26.1	D39.0	D49.59
myopericardium	C38.0	C79.89	-	D15.1	D48.7	D49.89
nabothian gland (follicle)	C53.0	C79.82	D06.0	D26.0	D39.0	D49.59
nail — *see also* Neoplasm, skin, limb	C44.90	C79.2	D04.9	D23.9	D48.5	D49.2
finger — *see also* Neoplasm, skin, limb, upper	C44.60-	C79.2	D04.6-	D23.6-	D48.5	D49.2
toe — *see also* Neoplasm, skin, limb, lower	C44.70-	C79.2	D04.7-	D23.7-	D48.5	D49.2
nares, naris (anterior) (posterior)	C30.0	C78.39	D02.3	D14.0	D38.5	D49.1
nasal — *see Neoplasm, nose*						
nasolabial groove — *see also* Neoplasm, skin, face	C44.309	C79.2	D04.39	D23.39	D48.5	D49.2
nasolacrimal duct	C69.5-	C79.49	D09.2-	D31.5-	D48.7	D49.89
nasopharynx, nasopharyngeal	C11.9	C79.89	D00.08	D10.6	D37.05	D49.0

Neoplasm, neoplastic	Malignant Primary	Malignant Secondary	Ca in situ	Benign	Uncertain Behavior	Unspecified Behavior
nasopharynx, nasopharyngeal - *continued*						
floor	C11.3	C79.89	D00.08	D10.6	D37.05	D49.0
overlapping lesion	C11.8	-	-	-	-	-
roof	C11.0	C79.89	D00.08	D10.6	D37.05	D49.0
wall	C11.9	C79.89	D00.08	D10.6	D37.05	D49.0
anterior	C11.3	C79.89	D00.08	D10.6	D37.05	D49.0
lateral	C11.2	C79.89	D00.08	D10.6	D37.05	D49.0
posterior	C11.1	C79.89	D00.08	D10.6	D37.05	D49.0
superior	C11.0	C79.89	D00.08	D10.6	D37.05	D49.0
nates — *see also* Neoplasm, skin, trunk	C44.509	C79.2	D04.5	D23.5	D48.5	D49.2
neck NEC	C76.0	C79.89	D09.8	D36.7	D48.7	D49.89
skin	C44.40	-	-	-	-	-
basal cell carcinoma	C44.41	-	-	-	-	-
specified type NEC	C44.49	-	-	-	-	-
squamous cell carcinoma	C44.42	-	-	-	-	-
nerve (ganglion)	C47.9	C79.89	-	D36.10	D48.2	D49.2
abducens	C72.59	C79.49	-	D33.3	D43.3	D49.7
accessory (spinal)	C72.59	C79.49	-	D33.3	D43.3	D49.7
acoustic	C72.4-	C79.49	-	D33.3	D43.3	D49.7
auditory	C72.4-	C79.49	-	D33.3	D43.3	D49.7
autonomic NEC — *see also* Neoplasm, nerve, peripheral	C47.9	C79.89	-	D36.10	D48.2	D49.2
brachial	C47.1-	C79.89	-	D36.12	D48.2	D49.2
cranial	C72.50	C79.49	-	D33.3	D43.3	D49.7
specified NEC	C72.59	C79.49	-	D33.3	D43.3	D49.7
facial	C72.59	C79.49	-	D33.3	D43.3	D49.7
femoral	C47.2-	C79.89	-	D36.13	D48.2	D49.2
ganglion NEC — *see also* Neoplasm, nerve, peripheral	C47.9	C79.89	-	D36.10	D48.2	D49.2
glossopharyngeal	C72.59	C79.49	-	D33.3	D43.3	D49.7
hypoglossal	C72.59	C79.49	-	D33.3	D43.3	D49.7
intercostal	C47.3	C79.89	-	D36.14	D48.2	D49.2
lumbar	C47.6	C79.89	-	D36.17	D48.2	D49.2
median	C47.1-	C79.89	-	D36.12	D48.2	D49.2
obturator	C47.2-	C79.89	-	D36.13	D48.2	D49.2
oculomotor	C72.59	C79.49	-	D33.3	D43.3	D49.7
olfactory	C47.2-	C79.49	-	D33.3	D43.3	D49.7
optic	C72.3-	C79.49	-	D33.3	D43.3	D49.7
parasympathetic NEC	C47.9	C79.89	-	D36.10	D48.2	D49.2
peripheral NEC	C47.9	C79.89	-	D36.10	D48.2	D49.2
abdomen	C47.4	C79.89	-	D36.15	D48.2	D49.2
abdominal wall	C47.4	C79.89	-	D36.15	D48.2	D49.2
ankle	C47.2-	C79.89	-	D36.13	D48.2	D49.2
antecubital fossa or space	C47.1-	C79.89	-	D36.12	D48.2	D49.2
arm	C47.1-	C79.89	-	D36.12	D48.2	D49.2
auricle (ear)	C47.0	C79.89	-	D36.11	D48.2	D49.2
axilla	C47.3	C79.89	-	D36.12	D48.2	D49.2
back	C47.6	C79.89	-	D36.17	D48.2	D49.2
buttock	C47.5	C79.89	-	D36.16	D48.2	D49.2
calf	C47.2-	C79.89	-	D36.13	D48.2	D49.2
cervical region	C47.0	C79.89	-	D36.11	D48.2	D49.2
cheek	C47.0	C79.89	-	D36.11	D48.2	D49.2
chest (wall)	C47.3	C79.89	-	D36.14	D48.2	D49.2
chin	C47.0	C79.89	-	D36.11	D48.2	D49.2
ear (external)	C47.0	C79.89	-	D36.11	D48.2	D49.2
elbow	C47.1-	C79.89	-	D36.12	D48.2	D49.2
extrarectal	C47.5	C79.89	-	D36.16	D48.2	D49.2
extremity	C47.9	C79.89	-	D36.10	D48.2	D49.2
lower	C47.2-	C79.89	-	D36.13	D48.2	D49.2
upper	C47.1-	C79.89	-	D36.12	D48.2	D49.2
eyelid	C47.0	C79.89	-	D36.11	D48.2	D49.2
face	C47.0	C79.89	-	D36.11	D48.2	D49.2
finger	C47.1-	C79.89	-	D36.12	D48.2	D49.2
flank	C47.6	C79.89	-	D36.17	D48.2	D49.2
foot	C47.2-	C79.89	-	D36.13	D48.2	D49.2
forearm	C47.1-	C79.89	-	D36.12	D48.2	D49.2
forehead	C47.0	C79.89	-	D36.11	D48.2	D49.2
gluteal region	C47.5	C79.89	-	D36.16	D48.2	D49.2
groin	C47.5	C79.89	-	D36.16	D48.2	D49.2
hand	C47.1-	C79.89	-	D36.12	D48.2	D49.2
head	C47.0	C79.89	-	D36.11	D48.2	D49.2
heel	C47.2-	C79.89	-	D36.13	D48.2	D49.2
hip	C47.2-	C79.89	-	D36.13	D48.2	D49.2
infraclavicular region	C47.3	C79.89	-	D36.14	D48.2	D49.2
inguinal (canal) (region)	C47.5	C79.89	-	D36.16	D48.2	D49.2
intrathoracic	C47.3	C79.89	-	D36.14	D48.2	D49.2
ischiorectal fossa	C47.5	C79.89	-	D36.16	D48.2	D49.2

Neoplasm, neoplastic	Malignant Primary	Malignant Secondary	Ca in situ	Benign	Uncertain Behavior	Unspecified Behavior
nerve - *continued*						
knee	C47.2-	C79.89	-	D36.13	D48.2	D49.2
leg	C47.2-	C79.89	-	D36.13	D48.2	D49.2
limb NEC	C47.9	C79.89	-	D36.10	D48.2	D49.2
lower	C47.2-	C79.89	-	D36.13	D48.2	D49.2
upper	C47.1-	C79.89	-	D36.12	D48.2	D49.2
nates	C47.5	C79.89	-	D36.16	D48.2	D49.2
neck	C47.0	C79.89	-	D36.11	D48.2	D49.2
orbit	C69.6-	C79.49	-	D31.6-	D48.7	D49.2
pararectal	C47.5	C79.89	-	D36.16	D48.2	D49.2
paraurethral	C47.5	C79.89	-	D36.16	D48.2	D49.2
paravaginal	C47.5	C79.89	-	D36.16	D48.2	D49.2
pelvis (floor)	C47.5	C79.89	-	D36.16	D48.2	D49.2
pelvoabdominal	C47.8	C79.89	-	D36.17	D48.2	D49.2
perineum	C47.5	C79.89	-	D36.16	D48.2	D49.2
perirectal (tissue)	C47.5	C79.89	-	D36.16	D48.2	D49.2
periurethral (tissue)	C47.5	C79.89	-	D36.16	D48.2	D49.2
popliteal fossa or space	C47.2-	C79.89	-	D36.13	D48.2	D49.2
presacral	C47.5	C79.89	-	D36.16	D48.2	D49.2
pterygoid fossa	C47.0	C79.89	-	D36.11	D48.2	D49.2
rectovaginal septum or wall	C47.5	C79.89	-	D36.16	D48.2	D49.2
rectovesical	C47.5	C79.89	-	D36.16	D48.2	D49.2
sacrococcygeal region	C47.5	C79.89	-	D36.16	D48.2	D49.2
scalp	C47.0	C79.89	-	D36.11	D48.2	D49.2
scapular region	C47.3	C79.89	-	D36.14	D48.2	D49.2
shoulder	C47.1-	C79.89	-	D36.12	D48.2	D49.2
submental	C47.0	C79.89	-	D36.11	D48.2	D49.2
supraclavicular region	C47.0	C79.89	-	D36.11	D48.2	D49.2
temple	C47.0	C79.89	-	D36.11	D48.2	D49.2
temporal region	C47.0	C79.89	-	D36.11	D48.2	D49.2
thigh	C47.2-	C79.89	-	D36.13	D48.2	D49.2
thoracic (duct) (wall)	C47.3	C79.89	-	D36.14	D48.2	D49.2
thorax	C47.3	C79.89	-	D36.14	D48.2	D49.2
thumb	C47.1-	C79.89	-	D36.12	D48.2	D49.2
toe	C47.2-	C79.89	-	D36.13	D48.2	D49.2
trunk	C47.6	C79.89	-	D36.17	D48.2	D49.2
umbilicus	C47.4	C79.89	-	D36.15	D48.2	D49.2
vesicorectal	C47.5	C79.89	-	D36.16	D48.2	D49.2
wrist	C47.1-	C79.89	-	D36.12	D48.2	D49.2
radial	C47.1-	C79.89	-	D36.12	D48.2	D49.2
sacral	C47.5	C79.89	-	D36.16	D48.2	D49.2
sciatic	C47.2-	C79.89	-	D36.13	D48.2	D49.2
spinal NEC	C47.9	C79.89	-	D36.10	D48.2	D49.2
accessory	C72.59	C79.49	-	D33.3	D43.3	D49.7
sympathetic NEC — *see also* Neoplasm, nerve, peripheral	C47.9	C79.89	-	D36.10	D48.2	D49.2
trigeminal	C72.59	C79.49	-	D33.3	D43.3	D49.7
trochlear	C72.59	C79.49	-	D33.3	D43.3	D49.7
ulnar	C47.1-	C79.89	-	D36.12	D48.2	D49.2
vagus	C72.59	C79.49	-	D33.3	D43.3	D49.7
nervous system (central)	C72.9	C79.40	-	D33.9	D43.9	D49.7
autonomic — *see* Neoplasm, nerve, peripheral						
parasympathetic — *see* Neoplasm, nerve, peripheral						
specified site NEC	-	C79.49	-	D33.7	D43.8	-
sympathetic — *see* Neoplasm, nerve, peripheral						
nevus — *see* Nevus						
nipple	C50.0-	C79.81	D05.-	D24.-	-	-
nose, nasal	C76.0	C79.89	D09.8	D36.7	D48.7	D49.89
ala (external) (nasi) — *see also* Neoplasm, nose, skin	C44.301	C79.2	D04.39	D23.39	D48.5	D49.2
bone	C41.0	C79.51	-	D16.4-	D48.0	D49.2
cartilage	C30.0	C78.39	D02.3	D14.0	D38.5	D49.1
cavity	C30.0	C78.39	D02.3	D14.0	D38.5	D49.1
choana	C11.3	C79.89	D00.08	D10.6	D37.05	D49.0
external (skin) — *see also* Neoplasm, nose, skin	C44.301	C79.2	D04.39	D23.39	D48.5	D49.2
fossa	C30.0	C78.39	D02.3	D14.0	D38.5	D49.1
internal	C30.0	C78.39	D02.3	D14.0	D38.5	D49.1
mucosa	C30.0	C78.39	D02.3	D14.0	D38.5	D49.1
septum	C30.0	C78.39	D02.3	D14.0	D38.5	D49.1
posterior margin	C11.3	C79.89	D00.08	D10.6	D37.05	D49.0
sinus — *see* Neoplasm, sinus						
skin	C44.301	C79.2	D04.39	D23.39	D48.5	D49.2
basal cell carcinoma	C44.311	-	-	-	-	-
specified type NEC	C44.391	-	-	-	-	-
squamous cell carcinoma	C44.321	-	-	-	-	-

Neoplasm, neoplastic	Malignant Primary	Malignant Secondary	Ca in situ	Benign	Uncertain Behavior	Unspecified Behavior
nose, nasal - *continued*						
turbinate (mucosa)	C30.0	C78.39	D02.3	D14.0	D38.5	D49.1
bone	C41.0	C79.51	-	D16.4-	D48.0	D49.2
vestibule	C30.0	C78.39	D02.3	D14.0	D38.5	D49.1
nostril	C30.0	C78.39	D02.3	D14.0	D38.5	D49.1
nucleus pulposus	C41.2	C79.51	-	D16.6	D48.0	D49.2
occipital						
bone	C41.0	C79.51	-	D16.4-	D48.0	D49.2
lobe or pole, brain	C71.4	C79.31	-	D33.0	D43.0	D49.6
odontogenic — *see* Neoplasm, jaw bone						
olfactory nerve or bulb	C72.2-	C79.49	-	D33.3	D43.3	D49.7
olive (brain)	C71.7	C79.31	-	D33.1	D43.1	D49.6
omentum	C48.1	C78.6	-	D20.1	D48.4	D49.0
operculum (brain)	C71.0	C79.31	-	D33.0	D43.0	D49.6
optic nerve, chiasm, or tract	C72.3-	C79.49	-	D33.3	D43.3	D49.7
oral (cavity)	C06.9	C79.89	D00.00	D10.30	D37.09	D49.0
ill-defined	C14.8	C79.89	D00.00	D10.30	D37.09	D49.0
mucosa	C06.0	C79.89	D00.02	D10.39	D37.09	D49.0
orbit	C69.6-	C79.49	D09.2-	D31.6-	D48.7	D49.89
autonomic nerve	C69.6-	C79.49	-	D31.6-	D48.7	D49.2
bone	C41.0	C79.51	-	D16.4-	D48.0	D49.2
eye	C69.6-	C79.49	D09.2-	D31.6-	D48.7	D49.89
peripheral nerves	C69.6-	C79.49	-	D31.6-	D48.7	D49.2
soft parts	C69.6-	C79.49	D09.2-	D31.6-	D48.7	D49.89
organ of Zuckerkandl	C75.5	C79.89	-	D35.6	D44.7	D49.7
oropharynx	C10.9	C79.89	D00.08	D10.5	D37.05	D49.0
branchial cleft (vestige)	C10.4	C79.89	D00.08	D10.5	D37.05	D49.0
junctional region	C10.8	C79.89	D00.08	D10.5	D37.05	D49.0
lateral wall	C10.2	C79.89	D00.08	D10.5	D37.05	D49.0
overlapping lesion	C10.8	-	-	-	-	-
pillars or fauces	C09.1	C79.89	D00.08	D10.5	D37.05	D49.0
posterior wall	C10.3	C79.89	D00.08	D10.5	D37.05	D49.0
vallecula	C10.0	C79.89	D00.08	D10.5	D37.05	D49.0
os						
external	C53.1	C79.82	D06.1	D26.0	D39.0	D49.59
internal	C53.0	C79.82	D06.0	D26.0	D39.0	D49.59
ovary	C56.-	C79.6-	D07.39	D27.-	D39.1-	D49.59
oviduct	C57.0-	C79.82	D07.39	D28.2	D39.8	D49.59
palate	C05.9	C79.89	D00.00	D10.39	D37.09	D49.0
hard	C05.0	C79.89	D00.05	D10.39	D37.09	D49.0
junction of hard and soft palate	C05.9	C79.89	D00.00	D10.39	D37.09	D49.0
overlapping lesions	C05.8	-	-	-	-	-
soft	C05.1	C79.89	D00.04	D10.39	D37.09	D49.0
nasopharyngeal surface	C11.3	C79.89	D00.08	D10.6	D37.05	D49.0
posterior surface	C11.3	C79.89	D00.08	D10.6	D37.05	D49.0
superior surface	C11.3	C79.89	D00.08	D10.6	D37.05	D49.0
palatoglossal arch	C09.1	C79.89	D00.00	D10.5	D37.09	D49.0
palatopharyngeal arch	C09.1	C79.89	D00.00	D10.5	D37.09	D49.0
pallium	C71.0	C79.31	-	D33.0	D43.0	D49.6
palpebra	C44.10-	C79.2	D04.1-	D23.1-	D48.5	D49.2
basal cell carcinoma	C44.11-	-	-	-	-	-
specified type NEC	C44.19-	-	-	-	-	-
squamous cell carcinoma	C44.12-	-	-	-	-	-
pancreas	C25.9	C78.89	D01.7	D13.6	D37.8	D49.0
body	C25.1	C78.89	D01.7	D13.6	D37.8	D49.0
duct (of Santorini) (of Wirsung)	C25.3	C78.89	D01.7	D13.6	D37.8	D49.0
ectopic tissue	C25.7	C78.89	-	D13.6	D37.8	D49.0
head	C25.0	C78.89	D01.7	D13.6	D37.8	D49.0
islet cells	C25.4	C78.89	D01.7	D13.7	D37.8	D49.0
neck	C25.7	C78.89	D01.7	D13.6	D37.8	D49.0
overlapping lesion	C25.8	-	-	-	-	-
tail	C25.2	C78.89	D01.7	D13.6	D37.8	D49.0
para-aortic body	C75.5	C79.89	-	D35.6	D44.7	D49.7
paraganglion NEC	C75.5	C79.89	-	D35.6	D44.7	D49.7
parametrium	C57.3	C79.82	-	D28.2	D39.8	D49.59
paranephric	C48.0	C78.6	-	D20.0	D48.3	D49.0
pararectal	C76.3	C79.89	-	D36.7	D48.7	D49.89
parasagittal (region)	C76.0	C79.89	D09.8	D36.7	D48.7	D49.89
parasellar	C72.9	C79.49	-	D33.9	D43.8	D49.7
parathyroid (gland)	C75.0	C79.89	D09.3	D35.1	D44.2	D49.7
paraurethral	C76.3	C79.89	-	D36.7	D48.7	D49.89
gland	C68.1	C79.19	D09.19	D30.8	D41.8	D49.59
paravaginal	C76.3	C79.89	-	D36.7	D48.7	D49.89
parenchyma, kidney	C64.-	C79.0-	D09.19	D30.0-	D41.0-	D49.51-
parietal						
bone	C41.0	C79.51	-	D16.4-	D48.0	D49.2
lobe, brain	C71.3	C79.31	-	D33.0	D43.0	D49.6
paroophoron	C57.1	C79.82	D07.39	D28.2	D39.8	D49.59

Neoplasm, neoplastic	Malignant Primary	Malignant Secondary	Ca in situ	Benign	Uncertain Behavior	Unspecified Behavior
parotid (duct) (gland)	C07	C79.89	D00.00	D11.0	D37.030	D49.0
parovarium	C57.1	C79.82	D07.39	D28.2	D39.8	D49.59
patella	C40.20	C79.51	-			
peduncle, cerebral	C71.7	C79.31	-	D33.1	D43.1	D49.6
pelvirectal junction	C19	C78.5	D01.1	D12.7	D37.5	D49.0
pelvis, pelvic	C76.3	C79.89	D09.8	D36.7	D48.7	D49.89
bone	C41.4	C79.51	-	D16.8	D48.0	D49.2
floor	C76.3	C79.89	D09.8	D36.7	D48.7	D49.89
renal	C65.-	C79.0-	D09.19	D30.1-	D41.1-	D49.51-
viscera	C76.3	C79.89	D09.8	D36.7	D48.7	D49.89
wall	C76.3	C79.89	D09.8	D36.7	D48.7	D49.89
pelvo-abdominal	C76.8	C79.89	D09.8	D36.7	D48.7	D49.89
penis	C60.9	C79.82	D07.4	D29.0	D40.8	D49.59
body	C60.2	C79.82	D07.4	D29.0	D40.8	D49.59
corpus (cavernosum)	C60.2	C79.82	D07.4	D29.0	D40.8	D49.59
glans	C60.1	C79.82	D07.4	D29.0	D40.8	D49.59
overlapping sites	C60.8					
skin NEC	C60.9	C79.82	D07.4	D29.0	D40.8	D49.59
periadrenal (tissue)	C48.0	C78.6	-	D20.0	D48.3	D49.0
perianal (skin) — *see also* Neoplasm, anus, skin	C44.500	C79.2	D04.5	D23.5	D48.5	D49.2
pericardium	C38.0	C79.89	-	D15.1	D48.7	D49.89
perinephric	C48.0	C78.6	-	D20.0	D48.3	D49.0
perineum	C76.3	C79.89	D09.8	D36.7	D48.7	D49.89
periodontal tissue NEC	C03.9	C79.89	D00.03	D10.39	D37.09	D49.0
periosteum — *see* Neoplasm, bone						
peripancreatic	C48.0	C78.6	-	D20.0	D48.3	D49.0
peripheral nerve NEC	C47.9	C79.89	-	D36.10	D48.2	D49.2
perirectal (tissue)	C76.3	C79.89	-	D36.7	D48.7	D49.89
perirenal (tissue)	C48.0	C78.6	-	D20.0	D48.3	D49.0
peritoneum, peritoneal (cavity)	C48.2	C78.6	-	D20.1	D48.4	D49.0
benign mesothelial tissue — *see* Mesothelioma, benign						
overlapping lesion	C48.8	-	-	-	-	-
with digestive organs	C26.9					
parietal	C48.1	C78.6	-	D20.1	D48.4	D49.0
pelvic	C48.1	C78.6	-	D20.1	D48.4	D49.0
specified part NEC	C48.1	C78.6	-	D20.1	D48.4	D49.0
peritonsillar (tissue)	C76.0	C79.89	D09.8	D36.7	D48.7	D49.89
periurethral tissue	C76.3	C79.89	-	D36.7	D48.7	D49.89
phalanges						
foot	C40.3-	C79.51	-	D16.3-	-	-
hand	C40.1-	C79.51	-	D16.1-	-	-
pharynx, pharyngeal	C14.0	C79.89	D00.08	D10.9	D37.05	D49.0
bursa	C11.1	C79.89	D00.08	D10.6	D37.05	D49.0
fornix	C11.3	C79.89	D00.08	D10.6	D37.05	D49.0
recess	C11.2	C79.89	D00.08	D10.6	D37.05	D49.0
region	C14.0	C79.89	D00.08	D10.9	D37.05	D49.0
tonsil	C11.1	C79.89	D00.08	D10.6	D37.05	D49.0
wall (lateral) (posterior)	C14.0	C79.89	D00.08	D10.9	D37.05	D49.0
pia mater	C70.9	C79.40	-	D32.9	D42.9	D49.7
cerebral	C70.0	C79.32	-	D32.0	D42.0	D49.7
cranial	C70.0	C79.32	-	D32.0	D42.0	D49.7
spinal	C70.1	C79.49	-	D32.1	D42.1	D49.7
pillars of fauces	C09.1	C79.89	D00.08	D10.5	D37.05	D49.0
pineal (body) (gland)	C75.3	C79.89	D09.3	D35.4	D44.5	D49.7
pinna (ear) NEC — *see also* Neoplasm, skin, ear	C44.20-	C79.2	D04.2-	D23.2-	D48.5	D49.2
piriform fossa or sinus	C12	C79.89	D00.08	D10.7	D37.05	D49.0
pituitary (body) (fossa) (gland) (lobe)	C75.1	C79.89	D09.3	D35.2	D44.3	D49.7
placenta	C58	C79.82	D07.0	D26.7	D39.2	D49.59
pleura, pleural (cavity)	C38.4	C78.2	-	D19.0	D38.2	D49.1
overlapping lesion with heart or mediastinum	C38.8	-	-	-	-	-
parietal	C38.4	C78.2	-	D19.0	D38.2	D49.1
visceral	C38.4	C78.2	-	D19.0	D38.2	D49.1
plexus						
brachial	C47.1-	C79.89	-	D36.12	D48.2	D49.2
cervical	C47.0	C79.89	-	D36.11	D48.2	D49.2
choroid	C71.5	C79.31	-	D33.0	D43.0	D49.6
lumbosacral	C47.5	C79.89	-	D36.16	D48.2	D49.2
sacral	C47.5	C79.89	-	D36.16	D48.2	D49.2
pluriendocrine	C75.8	C79.89	D09.3	D35.7	D44.9	D49.7
pole						
frontal	C71.1	C79.31	-	D33.0	D43.0	D49.6
occipital	C71.4	C79.31	-	D33.0	D43.0	D49.6
pons (varolii)	C71.7	C79.31	-	D33.1	D43.1	D49.6
popliteal fossa or space	C76.5-	C79.89	D04.7-	D36.7	D48.7	D49.89

Neoplasm, neoplastic	Malignant Primary	Malignant Secondary	Ca in situ	Benign	Uncertain Behavior	Unspecified Behavior
postcricoid (region)	C13.0	C79.89	D00.08	D10.7	D37.05	D49.0
posterior fossa (cranial)	C71.9	C79.31	-	D33.2	D43.2	D49.6
postnasal space	C11.9	C79.89	D00.08	D10.6	D37.05	D49.0
prepuce	C60.0	C79.82	D07.4	D29.0	D40.8	D49.59
prepylorus	C16.4	C78.89	D00.2	D13.1	D37.1	D49.0
presacral (region)	C76.3	C79.89	-	D36.7	D48.7	D49.89
prostate (gland)	C61	C79.82	D07.5	D29.1	D40.8	D49.59
utricle	C68.0	C79.19	D09.19	D30.4	D41.3	D49.59
pterygoid fossa	C49.0	C79.89	-	D21.0	D48.1	D49.2
pubic bone	C41.4	C79.51	-	D16.8	D48.0	D49.2
pudenda, pudendum (female)	C51.9	C79.82	D07.1	D28.0	D39.8	D49.59
pulmonary — see also Neoplasm, lung	C34.9-	C78.0-	D02.2-	D14.3-	D38.1	D49.1
putamen	C71.0	C79.31	-	D33.0	D43.0	D49.6
pyloric						
antrum	C16.3	C78.89	D00.2	D13.1	D37.1	D49.0
canal	C16.4	C78.89	D00.2	D13.1	D37.1	D49.0
pylorus	C16.4	C78.89	D00.2	D13.1	D37.1	D49.0
pyramid (brain)	C71.7	C79.31	-	D33.1	D43.1	D49.6
pyriform fossa or sinus	C12	C79.89	D00.08	D10.7	D37.05	D49.0
radius (any part)	C40.0-	C79.51	-	D16.0-	-	-
Rathke's pouch	C75.1	C79.89	D09.3	D35.2	D44.3	D49.7
rectosigmoid (junction)	C19	C78.5	D01.1	D12.7	D37.5	D49.0
overlapping lesion with anus or rectum	C21.8	-	-	-	-	-
rectouterine pouch	C48.1	C78.6	-	D20.1	D48.4	D49.0
rectovaginal septum or wall	C76.3	C79.89	D09.8	D36.7	D48.7	D49.89
rectovesical septum	C76.3	C79.89	D09.8	D36.7	D48.7	D49.89
rectum (ampulla)	C20	C78.5	D01.2	D12.8	D37.5	D49.0
and colon	C19	C78.5	D01.1	D12.7	D37.5	D49.0
overlapping lesion with anus or rectosigmoid junction	C21.8	-	-	-	-	-
renal	C64.-	C79.0-	D09.19	D30.0-	D41.0-	D49.51-
calyx	C65.-	C79.0-	D09.19	D30.1-	D41.1-	D49.51-
hilus	C65.-	C79.0-	D09.19	D30.1-	D41.1-	D49.51-
parenchyma	C64.-	C79.0-	D09.19	D30.0-	D41.0-	D49.51-
pelvis	C65.-	C79.0-	D09.19	D30.1-	D41.1-	D49.51-
respiratory						
organs or system NEC	C39.9	C78.30	D02.4	D14.4	D38.6	D49.1
tract NEC	C39.9	C78.30	D02.4	D14.4	D38.5	D49.1
upper	C39.0	C78.30	D02.4	D14.4	D38.5	D49.1
retina	C69.2-	C79.49	D09.2-	D31.2-	D48.7	D49.81
retrobulbar	C69.6-	C79.49	-	D31.6-	D48.7	D49.89
retrocecal	C48.0	C78.6	-	D20.0	D48.3	D49.0
retromolar (area) (triangle) (trigone)	C06.2	C79.89	D00.00	D10.39	D37.09	D49.0
retro-orbital	C76.0	C79.89	D09.8	D36.7	D48.7	D49.89
retroperitoneal (space) (tissue)	C48.0	C78.6	-	D20.0	D48.3	D49.0
retroperitoneum	C48.0	C78.6	-	D20.0	D48.3	D49.0
retropharyngeal	C14.0	C79.89	D00.08	D10.9	D37.05	D49.0
retrovesical (septum)	C76.3	C79.89	D09.8	D36.7	D48.7	D49.89
rhinencephalon	C71.0	C79.31	-	D33.0	D43.0	D49.6
rib	C41.3	C79.51	-	D16.7	D48.0	D49.2
Rosenmuller's fossa	C11.2	C79.89	D00.08	D10.6	D37.05	D49.0
round ligament	C57.2	C79.82	-	D28.2	D39.8	D49.59
sacrococcyx, sacrococcygeal	C41.4	C79.51	-	D16.8	D48.0	D49.2
region	C76.3	C79.89	D09.8	D36.7	D48.7	D49.89
sacrouterine ligament	C57.3	C79.82	-	D28.2	D39.8	D49.59
sacrum, sacral (vertebra)	C41.4	C79.51	-	D16.8	D48.0	D49.2
salivary gland or duct (major)	C08.9	C79.89	D00.00	D11.9	D37.039	D49.0
minor NEC	C06.9	C79.89	D00.00	D10.39	D37.04	D49.0
overlapping lesion	C08.9	-	-	-	-	-
parotid	C07	C79.89	D00.00	D11.0	D37.030	D49.0
pluriglandular	C08.9	C79.89	D00.00	D11.9	D37.039	D49.0
sublingual	C08.1	C79.89	D00.00	D11.7	D37.031	D49.0
submandibular	C08.0	C79.89	D00.00	D11.7	D37.032	D49.0
submaxillary	C08.0	C79.89	D00.00	D11.7	D37.032	D49.0
salpinx (uterine)	C57.0-	C79.82	D07.39	D28.2	D39.8	D49.59
Santorini's duct	C25.3	C78.89	D01.7	D13.6	D37.8	D49.0
scalp	C44.40	C79.2	D04.4	D23.4	D48.5	D49.2
basal cell carcinoma	C44.41	-	-	-	-	-
specified type NEC	C44.49	-	-	-	-	-
squamous cell carcinoma	C44.42	-	-	-	-	-
scapula (any part)	C40.0-	C79.51	-	D16.0-	-	-
scapular region	C76.1	C79.89	D09.8	D36.7	D48.7	D49.89
scar NEC — see also Neoplasm, skin, by site	C44.90	C79.2	D04.9	D23.9	D48.5	D49.2
sciatic nerve	C47.2-	C79.89	-	D36.13	D48.2	D49.2
sclera	C69.4-	C79.49	D09.2-	D31.4-	D48.7	D49.89

Neoplasm, neoplastic	Malignant Primary	Malignant Secondary	Ca in situ	Benign	Uncertain Behavior	Unspecified Behavior
scrotum (skin)	C63.2	C79.82	D07.61	D29.4	D40.8	D49.59
sebaceous gland — see Neoplasm, skin						
sella turcica	C75.1	C79.89	D09.3	D35.2	D44.3	D49.7
bone	C41.0	C79.51	-	D16.4-	D48.0	D49.2
semilunar cartilage (knee)	C40.2-	C79.51	-	D16.2-	D48.0	D49.2
seminal vesicle	C63.7	C79.82	D07.69	D29.8	D40.8	D49.59
septum						
nasal	C30.0	C78.39	D02.3	D14.0	D38.5	D49.1
posterior margin	C11.3	C79.89	D00.08	D10.6	D37.05	D49.0
rectovaginal	C76.3	C79.89	D09.8	D36.7	D48.7	D49.89
rectovesical	C76.3	C79.89	D09.8	D36.7	D48.7	D49.89
urethrovaginal	C57.9	C79.82	D07.30	D28.9	D39.9	D49.59
vesicovaginal	C57.9	C79.82	D07.30	D28.9	D39.9	D49.59
shoulder NEC	C76.4-	C79.89	D04.6-	D36.7	D48.7	D49.89
sigmoid flexure (lower) (upper)	C18.7	C78.5	D01.0	D12.5	D37.4	D49.0
sinus (accessory)	C31.9	C78.39	D02.3	D14.0	D38.5	D49.1
bone (any)	C41.0	C79.51	-	D16.4-	D48.0	D49.2
ethmoidal	C31.1	C78.39	D02.3	D14.0	D38.5	D49.1
frontal	C31.2	C78.39	D02.3	D14.0	D38.5	D49.1
maxillary	C31.0	C78.39	D02.3	D14.0	D38.5	D49.1
nasal, paranasal NEC	C31.9	C78.39	D02.3	D14.0	D38.5	D49.1
overlapping lesion	C31.8	-	-	-	-	-
pyriform	C12	C79.89	D00.08	D10.7	D37.05	D49.0
sphenoid	C31.3	C78.39	D02.3	D14.0	D38.5	D49.1
skeleton, skeletal NEC	C41.9	C79.51	-	D16.9-	D48.0	D49.2
Skene's gland	C68.1	C79.19	D09.19	D30.8	D41.8	D49.59
skin NOS	C44.90	C79.2	D04.9	D23.9	D48.5	D49.2
abdominal wall	C44.509	C79.2	D04.5	D23.5	D48.5	D49.2
basal cell carcinoma	C44.519	-	-	-	-	-
specified type NEC	C44.599	-	-	-	-	-
squamous cell carcinoma	C44.529	-	-	-	-	-
ala nasi — see also Neoplasm, nose, skin	C44.301	C79.2	D04.39	D23.39	D48.5	D49.2
ankle — see also Neoplasm, skin, limb, lower	C44.70-	C79.2	D04.7-	D23.7-	D48.5	D49.2
antecubital space — see also Neoplasm, skin, limb, upper	C44.60-	C79.2	D04.6-	D23.6-	D48.5	D49.2
anus	C44.500	C79.2	D04.5	D23.5	D48.5	D49.2
basal cell carcinoma	C44.510	-	-	-	-	-
specified type NEC	C44.590	-	-	-	-	-
squamous cell carcinoma	C44.520	-	-	-	-	-
arm — see also Neoplasm, skin, limb, upper	C44.60-	C79.2	D04.6-	D23.6-	D48.5	D49.2
auditory canal (external) — see also Neoplasm, skin, ear	C44.20-	C79.2	D04.2-	D23.2-	D48.5	D49.2
auricle (ear) — see also Neoplasm, skin, ear	C44.20-	C79.2	D04.2-	D23.2-	D48.5	D49.2
auricular canal (external) — see also Neoplasm, skin, ear	C44.20-	C79.2	D04.2-	D23.2-	D48.5	D49.2
axilla, axillary fold — see also Neoplasm, skin, trunk	C44.509	C79.2	D04.5	D23.5	D48.5	D49.2
back — see also Neoplasm, skin, trunk	C44.509	C79.2	D04.5	D23.5	D48.5	D49.2
basal cell carcinoma	C44.91					
breast	C44.501	C79.2	D04.5	D23.5	D48.5	D49.2
basal cell carcinoma	C44.511	-	-	-	-	-
specified type NEC	C44.591	-	-	-	-	-
squamous cell carcinoma	C44.521	-	-	-	-	-
brow — see also Neoplasm, skin, face	C44.309	C79.2	D04.39	D23.39	D48.5	D49.2
buttock — see also Neoplasm, skin, trunk	C44.509	C79.2	D04.5	D23.5	D48.5	D49.2
calf — see also Neoplasm, skin, limb, lower	C44.70-	C79.2	D04.7-	D23.7-	D48.5	D49.2
canthus (eye) (inner) (outer)	C44.10-	C79.2	D04.1-	D23.1-	D48.5	D49.2
basal cell carcinoma	C44.11-	-	-	-	-	-
specified type NEC	C44.19-	-	-	-	-	-
squamous cell carcinoma	C44.12-	-	-	-	-	-
cervical region — see also Neoplasm, skin, neck	C44.40	C79.2	D04.4	D23.4	D48.5	D49.2
cheek (external) — see also Neoplasm, skin, face	C44.309	C79.2	D04.39	D23.39	D48.5	D49.2
chest (wall) — see also Neoplasm, skin, trunk	C44.509	C79.2	D04.5	D23.5	D48.5	D49.2
chin — see also Neoplasm, skin, face	C44.309	C79.2	D04.39	D23.39	D48.5	D49.2
clavicular area — see also Neoplasm, skin, trunk	C44.509	C79.2	D04.5	D23.5	D48.5	D49.2
clitoris	C51.2	C79.82	D07.1	D28.0	D39.8	D49.59

Neoplasm, neoplastic	Malignant Primary	Malignant Secondary	Ca in situ	Benign	Uncertain Behavior	Unspecified Behavior
skin NOS - *continued*						
columnella — *see also* Neoplasm, skin, face	C44.309	C79.2	D04.39	D23.39	D48.5	D49.2
concha — *see also* Neoplasm, skin, ear	C44.20-	C79.2	D04.2-	D23.2-	D48.5	D49.2
ear (external)	C44.20-	C79.2	D04.2-	D23.2-	D48.5	D49.2
basal cell carcinoma	C44.21-	-	-	-	-	-
specified type NEC	C44.29-	-	-	-	-	-
squamous cell carcinoma	C44.22-	-	-	-	-	-
elbow — *see also* Neoplasm, skin, limb, upper	C44.60-	C79.2	D04.6-	D23.6-	D48.5	D49.2
eyebrow — *see also* Neoplasm, skin, face	C44.309	C79.2	D04.39	D23.39	D48.5	D49.2
eyelid	C44.10-	C79.2	D04.1-	D23.1-	D48.5	D49.2
basal cell carcinoma	C44.11-	-	-	-	-	-
specified type NEC	C44.19-	-	-	-	-	-
squamous cell carcinoma	C44.12-	-	-	-	-	-
face NOS	C44.300	C79.2	D04.30	D23.30	D48.5	D49.2
basal cell carcinoma	C44.310	-	-	-	-	-
specified type NEC	C44.390	-	-	-	-	-
squamous cell carcinoma	C44.320	-	-	-	-	-
female genital organs (external)	C51.9	C79.82	D07.1	D28.0	D39.8	D49.59
clitoris	C51.2	C79.82	D07.1	D28.0	D39.8	D49.59
labium NEC	C51.9	C79.82	D07.1	D28.0	D39.8	D49.59
majus	C51.0	C79.82	D07.1	D28.0	D39.8	D49.59
minus	C51.1	C79.82	D07.1	D28.0	D39.8	D49.59
pudendum	C51.9	C79.82	D07.1	D28.0	D39.8	D49.59
vulva	C51.9	C79.82	D07.1	D28.0	D39.8	D49.59
finger — *see also* Neoplasm, skin, limb, upper	C44.60-	C79.2	D04.6-	D23.6-	D48.5	D49.2
flank — *see also* Neoplasm, skin, trunk	C44.509	C79.2	D04.5	D23.5	D48.5	D49.2
foot — *see also* Neoplasm, skin, limb, lower	C44.70-	C79.2	D04.7-	D23.7-	D48.5	D49.2
forearm — *see also* Neoplasm, skin, limb, upper	C44.60-	C79.2	D04.6-	D23.6-	D48.5	D49.2
forehead — *see also* Neoplasm, skin, face	C44.309	C79.2	D04.39	D23.39	D48.5	D49.2
glabella — *see also* Neoplasm, skin, face	C44.309	C79.2	D04.39	D23.39	D48.5	D49.2
gluteal region — *see also* Neoplasm, skin, trunk	C44.509	C79.2	D04.5	D23.5	D48.5	D49.2
groin — *see also* Neoplasm, skin, trunk	C44.509	C79.2	D04.5	D23.5	D48.5	D49.2
hand — *see also* Neoplasm, skin, limb, upper	C44.60-	C79.2	D04.6-	D23.6-	D48.5	D49.2
head NEC — *see also* Neoplasm, skin, scalp	C44.40	C79.2	D04.4	D23.4	D48.5	D49.2
heel — *see also* Neoplasm, skin, limb, lower	C44.70-	C79.2	D04.7-	D23.7-	D48.5	D49.2
helix — *see also* Neoplasm, skin, ear	C44.20-	C79.2	D04.2-	D23.2-	D48.5	D49.2
hip — *see also* Neoplasm, skin, limb, lower	C44.70-	C79.2	D04.7-	D23.7-	D48.5	D49.2
infraclavicular region — *see also* Neoplasm, skin, trunk	C44.509	C79.2	D04.5	D23.5	D48.5	D49.2
inguinal region — *see also* Neoplasm, skin, trunk	C44.509	C79.2	D04.5	D23.5	D48.5	D49.2
jaw — *see also* Neoplasm, skin, face	C44.309	C79.2	D04.39	D23.39	D48.5	D49.2
Kaposi's sarcoma — *see* Kaposi's, sarcoma, skin						
knee — *see also* Neoplasm, skin, limb, lower	C44.70-	C79.2	D04.7-	D23.7-	D48.5	D49.2
labia						
majora	C51.0	C79.82	D07.1	D28.0	D39.8	D49.59
minora	C51.1	C79.82	D07.1	D28.0	D39.8	D49.59
leg — *see also* Neoplasm, skin, limb, lower	C44.70-	C79.2	D04.7-	D23.7-	D48.5	D49.2
lid (lower) (upper)	C44.10-	C79.2	D04.1-	D23.1-	D48.5	D49.2
basal cell carcinoma	C44.11-	-	-	-	-	-
specified type NEC	C44.19-	-	-	-	-	-
squamous cell carcinoma	C44.12-	-	-	-	-	-
limb NEC	C44.90	C79.2	D04.9	D23.9	D48.5	D49.2
basal cell carcinoma	C44.91					
lower	C44.70-	C79.2	D04.7-	D23.7-	D48.5	D49.2
basal cell carcinoma	C44.71-	-	-	-	-	-
specified type NEC	C44.79-	-	-	-	-	-
squamous cell carcinoma	C44.72-	-	-	-	-	-
upper	C44.60-	C79.2	D04.6-	D23.6-	D48.5	D49.2

Neoplasm, neoplastic	Malignant Primary	Malignant Secondary	Ca in situ	Benign	Uncertain Behavior	Unspecified Behavior
skin NOS - *continued*						
basal cell carcinoma	C44.61-	-	-	-	-	-
specified type NEC	C44.69-	-	-	-	-	-
squamous cell carcinoma	C44.62-	-	-	-	-	-
lip (lower) (upper)	C44.00	C79.2	D04.0	D23.0	D48.5	D49.2
basal cell carcinoma	C44.01	-	-	-	-	-
specified type NEC	C44.09	-	-	-	-	-
squamous cell carcinoma	C44.02	-	-	-	-	-
male genital organs	C63.9	C79.82	D07.60	D29.9	D40.8	D49.59
penis	C60.9	C79.82	D07.4	D29.0	D40.8	D49.59
prepuce	C60.0	C79.82	D07.4	D29.0	D40.8	D49.59
scrotum	C63.2	C79.82	D07.61	D29.4	D40.8	D49.59
mastectomy site (skin) — *see also* Neoplasm, skin, breast	C44.501	C79.2				
specified as breast tissue	C50.8-	C79.81	-	-	-	-
meatus, acoustic (external) — *see also* Neoplasm, skin, ear	C44.20-	C79.2	D04.2-	D23.2-	D48.5	D49.2
melanotic — *see* Melanoma						
Merkel cell — *see* Carcinoma, Merkel cell						
nates — *see also* Neoplasm, skin, trunk	C44.509	C79.2	D04.5	D23.5	D48.5	D49.2
neck	C44.40	C79.2	D04.4	D23.4	D48.5	D49.2
basal cell carcinoma	C44.41	-	-	-	-	-
specified type NEC	C44.49	-	-	-	-	-
squamous cell carcinoma	C44.42	-	-	-	-	-
nevus — *see* Nevus, skin						
nose (external) — *see also* Neoplasm, nose, skin	C44.301	C79.2	D04.39	D23.39	D48.5	D49.2
overlapping lesion	C44.80	-	-	-	-	-
basal cell carcinoma	C44.81	-	-	-	-	-
specified type NEC	C44.89	-	-	-	-	-
squamous cell carcinoma	C44.82	-	-	-	-	-
palm — *see also* Neoplasm, skin, limb, upper	C44.60-	C79.2	D04.6-	D23.6-	D48.5	D49.2
palpebra	C44.10-	C79.2	D04.1-	D23.1-	D48.5	D49.2
basal cell carcinoma	C44.11-	-	-	-	-	-
specified type NEC	C44.19-	-	-	-	-	-
squamous cell carcinoma	C44.12-	-	-	-	-	-
penis NEC	C60.9	C79.82	D07.4	D29.0	D40.8	D49.59
perianal — *see also* Neoplasm, skin, anus	C44.500	C79.2	D04.5	D23.5	D48.5	D49.2
perineum — *see also* Neoplasm, skin, anus	C44.500	C79.2	D04.5	D23.5	D48.5	D49.2
pinna — *see also* Neoplasm, skin, ear	C44.20-	C79.2	D04.2-	D23.2-	D48.5	D49.2
plantar — *see also* Neoplasm, skin, limb, lower	C44.70-	C79.2	D04.7-	D23.7-	D48.5	D49.2
popliteal fossa or space — *see also* Neoplasm, skin, limb, lower	C44.70-	C79.2	D04.7-	D23.7-	D48.5	D49.2
prepuce	C60.0	C79.82	D07.4	D29.0	D40.8	D49.59
pubes — *see also* Neoplasm, skin, trunk	C44.509	C79.2	D04.5	D23.5	D48.5	D49.2
sacrococcygeal region — *see also* Neoplasm, skin, trunk	C44.509	C79.2	D04.5	D23.5	D48.5	D49.2
scalp	C44.40	C79.2	D04.4	D23.4	D48.5	D49.2
basal cell carcinoma	C44.41	-	-	-	-	-
specified type NEC	C44.49	-	-	-	-	-
squamous cell carcinoma	C44.42	-	-	-	-	-
scapular region — *see also* Neoplasm, skin, trunk	C44.509	C79.2	D04.5	D23.5	D48.5	D49.2
scrotum	C63.2	C79.82	D07.61	D29.4	D40.8	D49.59
shoulder — *see also* Neoplasm, skin, limb, upper	C44.60-	C79.2	D04.6-	D23.6-	D48.5	D49.2
sole (foot) — *see also* Neoplasm, skin, limb, lower	C44.70-	C79.2	D04.7-	D23.7-	D48.5	D49.2
specified sites NEC	C44.80	C79.2	D04.8	D23.9	D48.5	D49.2
basal cell carcinoma	C44.81	-	-	-	-	-
specified type NEC	C44.89	-	-	-	-	-
squamous cell carcinoma	C44.82	-	-	-	-	-
specified type NEC	C44.99	-	-	-	-	-
squamous cell carcinoma	C44.92	-	-	-	-	-
submammary fold — *see also* Neoplasm, skin, trunk	C44.509	C79.2	D04.5	D23.5	D48.5	D49.2
supraclavicular region — *see also* Neoplasm, skin, neck	C44.40	C79.2	D04.4	D23.4	D48.5	D49.2
temple — *see also* Neoplasm, skin, face	C44.309	C79.2	D04.39	D23.39	D48.5	D49.2

Neoplasm, neoplastic	Malignant Primary	Malignant Secondary	Ca in situ	Benign	Uncertain Behavior	Unspecified Behavior
skin NOS - *continued*						
thigh — *see also* Neoplasm, skin, limb, lower	C44.70-	C79.2	D04.7-	D23.7-	D48.5	D49.2
thoracic wall — *see also* Neoplasm, skin, trunk	C44.509	C79.2	D04.5	D23.5	D48.5	D49.2
thumb — *see also* Neoplasm, skin, limb, upper	C44.60-	C79.2	D04.6-	D23.6-	D48.5	D49.2
toe — *see also* Neoplasm, skin, limb, lower	C44.70-	C79.2	D04.7-	D23.7-	D48.5	D49.2
tragus — *see also* Neoplasm, skin, ear	C44.20-	C79.2	D04.2-	D23.2-	D48.5	D49.2
trunk	C44.509	C79.2	D04.5	D23.5	D48.5	D49.2
basal cell carcinoma	C44.519	-	-	-	-	-
specified type NEC	C44.599	-	-	-	-	-
squamous cell carcinoma	C44.529	-	-	-	-	-
umbilicus — *see also* Neoplasm, skin, trunk	C44.509	C79.2	D04.5	D23.5	D48.5	D49.2
vulva	C51.9	C79.82	D07.1	D28.0	D39.8	D49.59
overlapping lesion	C51.8	-	-	-	-	-
wrist — *see also* Neoplasm, skin, limb, upper	C44.60-	C79.2	D04.6-	D23.6-	D48.5	D49.2
skull	C41.0	C79.51	-	D16.4-	D48.0	D49.2
soft parts or tissues — *see* Neoplasm, connective tissue						
specified site NEC	C76.8	C79.89	D09.8	D36.7	D48.7	D49.89
spermatic cord	C63.1-	C79.82	D07.69	D29.8	D40.8	D49.59
sphenoid	C31.3	C78.39	D02.3	D14.0	D38.5	D49.1
bone	C41.0	C79.51	-	D16.4-	D48.0	D49.2
sinus	C31.3	C78.39	D02.3	D14.0	D38.5	D49.1
sphincter						
anal	C21.1	C78.5	D01.3	D12.9	D37.8	D49.0
of Oddi	C24.0	C78.89	D01.5	D13.5	D37.6	D49.0
spine, spinal (column)	C41.2	C79.51	-	D16.6	D48.0	D49.2
bulb	C71.7	C79.31	-	D33.1	D43.1	D49.6
coccyx	C41.4	C79.51	-	D16.8	D48.0	D49.2
cord (cervical) (lumbar) (sacral) (thoracic)	C72.0	C79.49	-	D33.4	D43.4	D49.7
dura mater	C70.1	C79.49	-	D32.1	D42.1	D49.7
lumbosacral	C41.2	C79.51	-	D16.6	D48.0	D49.2
marrow NEC	C96.9	C79.52	-	D47.9		D49.89
membrane	C70.1	C79.49	-	D32.1	D42.1	D49.7
meninges	C70.1	C79.49	-	D32.1	D42.1	D49.7
nerve (root)	C47.9	C79.89	-	D36.10	D48.2	D49.2
pia mater	C70.1	C79.49	-	D32.1	D42.1	D49.7
root	C47.9	C79.89	-	D36.10	D48.2	D49.2
sacrum	C41.4	C79.51	-	D16.8	D48.0	D49.2
spleen, splenic NEC	C26.1	C78.89	D01.7	D13.9	D37.8	D49.0
flexure (colon)	C18.5	C78.5	D01.0	D12.3	D37.4	D49.0
stem, brain	C71.7	C79.31	-	D33.1	D43.1	D49.6
Stensen's duct	C07	C79.89	D00.00	D11.0	D37.030	D49.0
sternum	C41.3	C79.51	-	D16.7	D48.0	D49.2
stomach	C16.9	C78.89	D00.2	D13.1	D37.1	D49.0
antrum (pyloric)	C16.3	C78.89	D00.2	D13.1	D37.1	D49.0
body	C16.2	C78.89	D00.2	D13.1	D37.1	D49.0
cardia	C16.0	C78.89	D00.2	D13.1	D37.1	D49.0
cardiac orifice	C16.0	C78.89	D00.2	D13.1	D37.1	D49.0
corpus	C16.2	C78.89	D00.2	D13.1	D37.1	D49.0
fundus	C16.1	C78.89	D00.2	D13.1	D37.1	D49.0
greater curvature NEC	C16.6	C78.89	D00.2	D13.1	D37.1	D49.0
lesser curvature NEC	C16.5	C78.89	D00.2	D13.1	D37.1	D49.0
overlapping lesion	C16.8	-	-	-	-	-
prepylorus	C16.4	C78.89	D00.2	D13.1	D37.1	D49.0
pylorus	C16.4	C78.89	D00.2	D13.1	D37.1	D49.0
wall NEC	C16.9	C78.89	D00.2	D13.1	D37.1	D49.0
anterior NEC	C16.8	C78.89	D00.2	D13.1	D37.1	D49.0
posterior NEC	C16.8	C78.89	D00.2	D13.1	D37.1	D49.0
stroma, endometrial	C54.1	C79.82	D07.0	D26.1	D39.0	D49.59
stump, cervical	C53.8	C79.82	D06.7	D26.0	D39.0	D49.59
subcutaneous (nodule) (tissue) NEC — *see* Neoplasm, connective tissue						
subdural	C70.9	C79.32	-	D32.9	D42.9	D49.7
subglottis, subglottic	C32.2	C78.39	D02.0	D14.1	D38.0	D49.1
sublingual	C04.9	C79.89	D00.06	D10.2	D37.09	D49.0
gland or duct	C08.1	C79.89	D00.00	D11.7	D37.031	D49.0
submandibular gland	C08.0	C79.89	D00.00	D11.7	D37.032	D49.0
submaxillary gland or duct	C08.0	C79.89	D00.00	D11.7	D37.032	D49.0
submental	C76.0	C79.89	D09.8	D36.7	D48.7	D49.89
subpleural	C34.9-	C78.0-	D02.2-	D14.3-	D38.1	D49.1

Neoplasm, neoplastic	Malignant Primary	Malignant Secondary	Ca in situ	Benign	Uncertain Behavior	Unspecified Behavior
substernal	C38.1	C78.1	-	D15.2	D38.3	D49.89
sudoriferous, sudoriparous gland, site unspecified	C44.90	C79.2	D04.9	D23.9	D48.5	D49.2
specified site — *see* Neoplasm, skin						
supraclavicular region	C76.0	C79.89	D09.8	D36.7	D48.7	D49.89
supraglottis	C32.1	C78.39	D02.0	D14.1	D38.0	D49.1
suprarenal	C74.9-	C79.7-	D09.3	D35.0-	D44.1-	D49.7
capsule	C74.9-	C79.7-	D09.3	D35.0-	D44.1-	D49.7
cortex	C74.0-	C79.7-	D09.3	D35.0-	D44.1-	D49.7
gland	C74.9-	C79.7-	D09.3	D35.0-	D44.1-	D49.7
medulla	C74.1-	C79.7-	D09.3	D35.0-	D44.1-	D49.7
suprasellar (region)	C71.9	C79.31	-	D33.2	D43.2	D49.6
supratentorial (brain) NEC	C71.0	C79.31	-	D33.0	D43.0	D49.6
sweat gland (apocrine) (eccrine), site unspecified	C44.90	C79.2	D04.9	D23.9	D48.5	D49.2
specified site — *see* Neoplasm, skin						
sympathetic nerve or nervous system NEC	C47.9	C79.89	-	D36.10	D48.2	D49.2
symphysis pubis	C41.4	C79.51	-	D16.8	D48.0	D49.2
synovial membrane — *see* Neoplasm, connective tissue						
tapetum, brain	C71.8	C79.31	-	D33.2	D43.2	D49.6
tarsus (any bone)	C40.3-	C79.51	-	D16.3-	-	-
temple (skin) — *see also* Neoplasm, skin, face	C44.309	C79.2	D04.39	D23.39	D48.5	D49.2
temporal						
bone	C41.0	C79.51	-	D16.4-	D48.0	D49.2
lobe or pole	C71.2	C79.31	-	D33.0	D43.0	D49.6
region	C76.0	C79.89	D09.8	D36.7	D48.7	D49.89
skin — *see also* Neoplasm, skin, face	C44.309	C79.2	D04.39	D23.39	D48.5	D49.2
tendon (sheath) — *see* Neoplasm, connective tissue						
tentorium (cerebelli)	C70.0	C79.32	-	D32.0	D42.0	D49.7
testis, testes	C62.9-	C79.82	D07.69	D29.2-	D40.1-	D49.59
descended	C62.1-	C79.82	D07.69	D29.2-	D40.1-	D49.59
ectopic	C62.0-	C79.82	D07.69	D29.2-	D40.1-	D49.59
retained	C62.0-	C79.82	D07.69	D29.2-	D40.1-	D49.59
scrotal	C62.1-	C79.82	D07.69	D29.2-	D40.1-	D49.59
undescended	C62.0-	C79.82	D07.69	D29.2-	D40.1-	D49.59
unspecified whether descended or undescended	C62.9-	C79.82	D07.69	D29.2-	D40.1-	D49.59
thalamus	C71.0	C79.31	-	D33.0	D43.0	D49.6
thigh NEC	C76.5-	C79.89	D04.7-	D36.7	D48.7	D49.89
thorax, thoracic (cavity) (organs NEC)	C76.1	C79.89	D09.8	D36.7	D48.7	D49.89
duct	C49.3	C79.89	-	D21.3	D48.1	D49.2
wall NEC	C76.1	C79.89	D09.8	D36.7	D48.7	D49.89
throat	C14.0	C79.89	D00.08	D10.9	D37.05	D49.0
thumb NEC	C76.4-	C79.89	D04.6-	D36.7	D48.7	D49.89
thymus (gland)	C37	C79.89	D09.3	D15.0	D38.4	D49.89
thyroglossal duct	C73	C79.89	D09.3	D34	D44.0	D49.7
thyroid (gland)	C73	C79.89	D09.3	D34	D44.0	D49.7
cartilage	C32.3	C78.39	D02.0	D14.1	D38.0	D49.1
tibia (any part)	C40.2-	C79.51	-	D16.2-	-	-
toe NEC	C76.5-	C79.89	D04.7-	D36.7	D48.7	D49.89
tongue	C02.9	C79.89	D00.07	D10.1	D37.02	D49.0
anterior (two-thirds) NEC	C02.3	C79.89	D00.07	D10.1	D37.02	D49.0
dorsal surface	C02.0	C79.89	D00.07	D10.1	D37.02	D49.0
ventral surface	C02.2	C79.89	D00.07	D10.1	D37.02	D49.0
base (dorsal surface)	C01	C79.89	D00.07	D10.1	D37.02	D49.0
border (lateral)	C02.1	C79.89	D00.07	D10.1	D37.02	D49.0
dorsal surface NEC	C02.0	C79.89	D00.07	D10.1	D37.02	D49.0
fixed part NEC	C01	C79.89	D00.07	D10.1	D37.02	D49.0
foreamen cecum	C02.0	C79.89	D00.07	D10.1	D37.02	D49.0
frenulum linguae	C02.2	C79.89	D00.07	D10.1	D37.02	D49.0
junctional zone	C02.8	C79.89	D00.07	D10.1	D37.02	D49.0
margin (lateral)	C02.1	C79.89	D00.07	D10.1	D37.02	D49.0
midline NEC	C02.0	C79.89	D00.07	D10.1	D37.02	D49.0
mobile part NEC	C02.3	C79.89	D00.07	D10.1	D37.02	D49.0
overlapping lesion	C02.8					
posterior (third)	C01	C79.89	D00.07	D10.1	D37.02	D49.0
root	C01	C79.89	D00.07	D10.1	D37.02	D49.0
surface (dorsal)	C02.0	C79.89	D00.07	D10.1	D37.02	D49.0
base	C01	C79.89	D00.07	D10.1	D37.02	D49.0
ventral	C02.2	C79.89	D00.07	D10.1	D37.02	D49.0
tip	C02.1	C79.89	D00.07	D10.1	D37.02	D49.0

Neoplasm, neoplastic	Malignant Primary	Malignant Secondary	Ca in situ	Benign	Uncertain Behavior	Unspecified Behavior
tongue - continued						
tonsil	C02.4	C79.89	D00.07	D10.1	D37.02	D49.0
tonsil	C09.9	C79.89	D00.08	D10.4	D37.05	D49.0
fauces, faucial	C09.9	C79.89	D00.08	D10.4	D37.05	D49.0
lingual	C02.4	C79.89	D00.07	D10.1	D37.02	D49.0
overlapping sites	C09.8					
palatine	C09.9	C79.89	D00.08	D10.4	D37.05	D49.0
pharyngeal	C11.1	C79.89	D00.08	D10.6	D37.05	D49.0
pillar (anterior) (posterior)	C09.1	C79.89	D00.08	D10.5	D37.05	D49.0
tonsillar fossa	C09.0	C79.89	D00.08	D10.5	D37.05	D49.0
tooth socket NEC	C03.9	C79.89	D00.03	D10.39	D37.09	D49.0
trachea (cartilage) (mucosa)	C33	C78.39	D02.1	D14.2	D38.1	D49.1
overlapping lesion with bronchus or lung	C34.8-	-	-	-	-	-
tracheobronchial	C34.8-	C78.39	D02.1	D14.2	D38.1	D49.1
overlapping lesion with lung	C34.8-	-	-	-	-	-
tragus — see also Neoplasm, skin, ear	C44.20-	C79.2	D04.2-	D23.2-	D48.5	D49.2
trunk NEC	C76.8	C79.89	D04.5	D36.7	D48.7	D49.89
tubo-ovarian	C57.8	C79.82	D07.39	D28.7	D39.8	D49.59
tunica vaginalis	C63.7	C79.82	D07.69	D29.8	D40.8	D49.59
turbinate (bone)	C41.0	C79.51	-	D16.4-	D48.0	D49.2
nasal	C30.0	C78.39	D02.3	D14.0	D38.5	D49.1
tympanic cavity	C30.1	C78.39	D02.3	D14.0	D38.5	D49.1
ulna (any part)	C40.0-	C79.51	-	D16.0-	-	-
umbilicus, umbilical — see also Neoplasm, skin, trunk	C44.509	C79.2	D04.5	D23.5	D48.5	D49.2
uncus, brain	C71.2	C79.31	-	D33.0	D43.0	D49.6
unknown site or unspecified	C80.1	C79.9	D09.9	D36.9	D48.9	D49.9
urachus	C67.7	C79.11	D09.0	D30.3	D41.4	D49.4
ureter, ureteral	C66.-	C79.19	D09.19	D30.2-	D41.2-	D49.59
orifice (bladder)	C67.6	C79.11	D09.0	D30.3	D41.4	D49.4
ureter-bladder (junction)	C67.6	C79.11	D09.0	D30.3	D41.4	D49.4
urethra, urethral (gland)	C68.0	C79.19	D09.19	D30.4	D41.3	D49.59
orifice, internal	C67.5	C79.11	D09.0	D30.3	D41.4	D49.4
urethrovaginal (septum)	C57.9	C79.82	D07.30	D28.9	D39.8	D49.59
urinary organ or system	C68.9	C79.10	D09.10	D30.9	D41.9	D49.59
bladder — see Neoplasm, bladder						
overlapping lesion	C68.8	-	-	-	-	-
specified sites NEC	C68.8	C79.19	D09.19	D30.8	D41.8	D49.59
utero-ovarian	C57.8	C79.82	D07.39	D28.7	D39.8	D49.59
ligament	C57.1	C79.82	D07.39	D28.2	D39.8	D49.59
uterosacral ligament	C57.3	C79.82	-	D28.2	D39.8	D49.59
uterus, uteri, uterine	C55	C79.82	D07.0	D26.9	D39.0	D49.59
adnexa NEC	C57.4	C79.82	D07.39	D28.7	D39.8	D49.59
body	C54.9	C79.82	D07.0	D26.1	D39.0	D49.59
cervix	C53.9	C79.82	D06.9	D26.0	D39.0	D49.59
cornu	C54.9	C79.82	D07.0	D26.1	D39.0	D49.59
corpus	C54.9	C79.82	D07.0	D26.1	D39.0	D49.59
endocervix (canal) (gland)	C53.0	C79.82	D06.0	D26.0	D39.0	D49.59
endometrium	C54.1	C79.82	D07.0	D26.1	D39.0	D49.59
exocervix	C53.1	C79.82	D06.1	D26.0	D39.0	D49.59
external os	C53.1	C79.82	D06.1	D26.0	D39.0	D49.59
fundus	C54.3	C79.82	D07.0	D26.1	D39.0	D49.59
internal os	C53.0	C79.82	D06.0	D26.0	D39.0	D49.59
isthmus	C54.0	C79.82	D07.0	D26.1	D39.0	D49.59
ligament	C57.3	C79.82	-	D28.2	D39.8	D49.59
broad	C57.1	C79.82	D07.39	D28.2	D39.8	D49.59
round	C57.2	C79.82	-	D28.2	D39.8	D49.59
lower segment	C54.0	C79.82	D07.0	D26.1	D39.0	D49.59
myometrium	C54.2	C79.82	D07.0	D26.1	D39.0	D49.59
overlapping sites	C54.8	-	-	-	-	-
squamocolumnar junction	C53.8	C79.82	D06.7	D26.0	D39.0	D49.59
tube	C57.0-	C79.82	D07.39	D28.2	D39.8	D49.59
utricle, prostatic	C68.0	C79.19	D09.19	D30.4	D41.3	D49.59
uveal tract	C69.4-	C79.49	D09.2-	D31.4-	D48.7	D49.89
uvula	C05.2	C79.89	D00.04	D10.39	D37.09	D49.0
vagina, vaginal (fornix) (vault) (wall)	C52	C79.82	D07.2	D28.1	D39.8	D49.59
vaginovesical	C57.9	C79.82	D07.30	D28.9	D39.9	D49.59
septum	C57.9	C79.82	D07.30	D28.9	D39.9	D49.59
vallecula (epiglottis)	C10.0	C79.89	D00.08	D10.5	D37.05	D49.0
vas deferens	C63.1-	C79.82	D07.69	D29.8	D40.8	D49.59
vascular — see Neoplasm, connective tissue						
Vater's ampulla	C24.1	C78.89	D01.5	D13.5	D37.6	D49.0
vein, venous — see Neoplasm, connective tissue						
vena cava (abdominal) (inferior)	C49.4	C79.89	-	D21.4	D48.1	D49.2
superior	C49.3	C79.89	-	D21.3	D48.1	D49.2

Neoplasm, neoplastic	Malignant Primary	Malignant Secondary	Ca in situ	Benign	Uncertain Behavior	Unspecified Behavior
ventricle (cerebral) (floor) (lateral) (third)	C71.5	C79.31	-	D33.0	D43.0	D49.6
cardiac (left) (right)	C38.0	C79.89	-	D15.1	D48.7	D49.89
fourth	C71.7	C79.31	-	D33.1	D43.1	D49.6
ventricular band of larynx	C32.1	C78.39	D02.0	D14.1	D38.0	D49.1
ventriculus — see Neoplasm, stomach						
vermillion border — see Neoplasm, lip						
vermis, cerebellum	C71.6	C79.31	-	D33.1	D43.1	D49.6
vertebra (column)	C41.2	C79.51	-	D16.6	D48.0	D49.2
coccyx	C41.4	C79.51	-	D16.8-	D48.0	D49.2
marrow NEC	C96.9	C79.52	-	-	D47.9	D49.89
sacrum	C41.4	C79.51	-	D16.8-	D48.0	D49.2
vesical — see Neoplasm, bladder						
vesicle, seminal	C63.7	C79.82	D07.69	D29.8	D40.8	D49.59
vesicocervical tissue	C57.9	C79.82	D07.30	D28.9	D39.9	D49.59
vesicorectal	C76.3	C79.82	D09.8	D36.7	D48.7	D49.89
vesicovaginal	C57.9	C79.82	D07.30	D28.9	D39.9	D49.59
septum	C57.9	C79.82	D07.30	D28.9	D39.8	D49.59
vessel (blood) — see Neoplasm, connective tissue						
vestibular gland, greater	C51.0	C79.82	D07.1	D28.0	D39.8	D49.59
vestibule						
mouth	C06.1	C79.89	D00.00	D10.39	D37.09	D49.0
nose	C30.0	C78.39	D02.3	D14.0	D38.5	D49.1
Virchow's gland	C77.0	C77.0	-	D36.0	D48.7	D49.89
viscera NEC	C76.8	C79.89	D09.8	D36.7	D48.7	D49.89
vocal cords (true)	C32.0	C78.39	D02.0	D14.1	D38.0	D49.1
false	C32.1	C78.39	D02.0	D14.1	D38.0	D49.1
vomer	C41.0	C79.51	-	D16.4-	D48.0	D49.2
vulva	C51.9	C79.82	D07.1	D28.0	D39.8	D49.59
vulvovaginal gland	C51.0	C79.82	D07.1	D28.0	D39.8	D49.59
Waldeyer's ring	C14.2	C79.89	D00.08	D10.9	D37.05	D49.0
Wharton's duct	C08.0	C79.89	D00.00	D11.7	D37.032	D49.0
white matter (central) (cerebral)	C71.0	C79.31	-	D33.0	D43.0	D49.6
windpipe	C33	C78.39	D02.1	D14.2	D38.1	D49.1
Wirsung's duct	C25.3	C78.89	D01.7	D13.6	D37.8	D49.0
wolffian (body) (duct)						
female	C57.7	C79.82	D07.39	D28.7	D39.8	D49.59
male	C63.7	C79.82	D07.69	D29.8	D40.8	D49.59
womb — see Neoplasm, uterus						
wrist NEC	C76.4-	C79.89	D04.6-	D36.7	D48.7	D49.89
xiphoid process	C41.3	C79.51	-	D16.7	D48.0	D49.2
Zuckerkandl organ	C75.5	C79.89	-	D35.6	D44.7	D49.7

Neovascularization
ciliary body — *see* Disorder, iris, vascular
cornea H16.40-
  deep H16.44-
  ghost vessels — *see* Ghost, vessels
  localized H16.43-
  pannus — *see* Pannus
iris — *see* Disorder, iris, vascular
retina H35.05-
Nephralgia N23
Nephritis, nephritic (albuminuric) (azotemic)
(congenital) (disseminated) (epithelial) (familial)
(focal) (granulomatous) (hemorrhagic) (infantile)
(nonsuppurative, excretory) (uremic) N05.9
with
  dense deposit disease N05.6
  diffuse
    crescentic glomerulonephritis N05.7
    endocapillary proliferative
      glomerulonephritis N05.4
    membranous glomerulonephritis N05.2
    mesangial proliferative glomerulonephritis N05.3
    mesangiocapillary glomerulonephritis N05.5
  edema — *see* Nephrosis
  focal and segmental glomerular lesions N05.1
  foot process disease N04.9
  glomerular lesion
    diffuse sclerosing N05.8
    hypocomplementemic — *see* Nephritis,
      membranoproliferative
    IgA — *see* Nephropathy, IgA
    lobular, lobulonodular — *see* Nephritis,
      membranoproliferative
    nodular — *see* Nephritis, membranoproliferative
  lesion of
    glomerulonephritis, proliferative N05.8
    renal necrosis N05.9
  minor glomerular abnormality N05.0
  specified morphological changes NEC N05.8
acute N00.9
with
  dense deposit disease N00.6
  diffuse
    crescentic glomerulonephritis N00.7
    endocapillary proliferative
      glomerulonephritis N00.4
    membranous glomerulonephritis N00.2
    mesangial proliferative
      glomerulonephritis N00.3
    mesangiocapillary glomerulonephritis N00.5
  focal and segmental glomerular lesions N00.1
  minor glomerular abnormality N00.0
  specified morphological changes NEC N00.8
amyloid E85.4 *[N08]*
antiglomerular basement membrane (anti-GBM)
  antibody NEC
  in Goodpasture's syndrome M31.0
antitubular basement membrane (tubulo-interstitial)
  NEC N12
  toxic — *see* Nephropathy, toxic
arteriolar — *see* Hypertension, kidney
arteriosclerotic — *see* Hypertension, kidney
ascending — *see* Nephritis, tubulo-interstitial
atrophic N03.9
Balkan (endemic) N15.0
calculous, calculus — *see* Calculus, kidney
cardiac — *see* Hypertension, kidney
cardiovascular — *see* Hypertension, kidney
chronic N03.9
with
  dense deposit disease N03.6
  diffuse
    crescentic glomerulonephritis N03.7
    endocapillary proliferative
      glomerulonephritis N03.4
    membranous glomerulonephritis N03.2
    mesangial proliferative
      glomerulonephritis N03.3
    mesangiocapillary glomerulonephritis N03.5
  focal and segmental glomerular lesions N03.1
  minor glomerular abnormality N03.0
  specified morphological changes NEC N03.8
  arteriosclerotic — *see* Hypertension, kidney
cirrhotic N26.9
complicating pregnancy O26.83-
croupous N00.9
degenerative — *see* Nephrosis
diffuse sclerosing N05.8
due to
  diabetes mellitus — *see* E08-E13 with .21
  subacute bacterial endocarditis I33.0
  systemic lupus erythematosus (chronic) M32.14
  typhoid fever A01.09

Nephritis, nephritic (albuminuric) (azotemic)
(congenital) (disseminated) (epithelial) (familial)
(focal) (granulomatous) (hemorrhagic) (infantile)
(nonsuppurative, excretory) (uremic) - *continued*
gonococcal (acute) (chronic) A54.21
hypocomplementemic — *see* Nephritis,
  membranoproliferative
IgA — *see* Nephropathy, IgA
immune complex (circulating) NEC N05.8
infective — *see* Nephritis, tubulo-interstitial
interstitial — *see* Nephritis, tubulo-interstitial
lead N14.3
membranoproliferative (diffuse) (type 1 or 3) —
  see also N00-N07 with fourth character .5 N05.5
  type 2 — *see also* N00-N07 with fourth character
    .6 N05.6
minimal change N05.0
necrotic, necrotizing NEC — *see also* N00-N07 with
  fourth character .8 N05.8
nephrotic — *see* Nephrosis
nodular — *see* Nephritis, membranoproliferative
polycystic Q61.3
  adult type Q61.2
  autosomal
    dominant Q61.2
    recessive NEC Q61.19
  childhood type NEC Q61.19
  infantile type NEC Q61.19
poststreptococcal N05.9
  acute N00.9
  chronic N03.9
  rapidly progressive N01.9
proliferative NEC — *see also* N00-N07 with fourth
  character .8 N05.8
purulent — *see* Nephritis, tubulo-interstitial
rapidly progressive N01.9
with
  dense deposit disease N01.6
  diffuse
    crescentic glomerulonephritis N01.7
    endocapillary proliferative
      glomerulonephritis N01.4
    membranous glomerulonephritis N01.2
    mesangial proliferative
      glomerulonephritis N01.3
    mesangiocapillary glomerulonephritis N01.5
  focal and segmental glomerular lesions N01.1
  minor glomerular abnormality N01.0
  specified morphological changes NEC N01.8
salt losing or wasting NEC N28.89
saturnine N14.3
sclerosing, diffuse N05.8
septic — *see* Nephritis, tubulo-interstitial
specified pathology NEC — *see also* N00-N07 with
  fourth character .8 N05.8
subacute N01.9
suppurative — *see* Nephritis, tubulo-interstitial
syphilitic (late) A52.75
  congenital A50.59 *[N08]*
  early (secondary) A51.44
toxic — *see* Nephropathy, toxic
tubal, tubular — *see* Nephritis, tubulo-interstitial
tuberculous A18.11
tubulo-interstitial (in) N12
  acute (infectious) N10
  chronic (infectious) N11.9
    nonobstructive N11.8
      reflux-associated N11.0
    obstructive N11.1
    specified NEC N11.8
  due to
    brucellosis A23.9 *[N16]*
    cryoglobulinemia D89.1 *[N16]*
    glycogen storage disease E74.00 *[N16]*
    Sjögren's syndrome M35.04
  vascular — *see* Hypertension, kidney
war N00.9
Nephroblastoma (epithelial) (mesenchymal) C64-
Nephrocalcinosis E83.59 *[N29]*
Nephrocystitis, pustular — *see* Nephritis, tubulo-
interstitial
Nephrolithiasis (congenital) (pelvis)
(recurrent) — *see also* Calculus, kidney
Nephroma C64-
mesoblastic D41.0-
Nephronephritis — *see* Nephrosis
Nephronophthisis Q61.5
Nephropathia epidemica A98.5
Nephropathy — *see also* Nephritis N28.9
with
  edema — *see* Nephrosis
  glomerular lesion — *see* Glomerulonephritis
amyloid, hereditary E85.0

Nephropathy - *continued*
analgesic N14.0
  with medullary necrosis, acute N17.2
Balkan (endemic) N15.0
chemical — *see* Nephropathy, toxic
diabetic — *see* E08-E13 with .21
drug-induced N14.2
  specified NEC N14.1
focal and segmental hyalinosis or sclerosis N02.1
heavy metal-induced N14.3
hereditary NEC N07.9
with
  dense deposit disease N07.6
  diffuse
    crescentic glomerulonephritis N07.7
    endocapillary proliferative
      glomerulonephritis N07.4
    membranous glomerulonephritis N07.2
    mesangial proliferative
      glomerulonephritis N07.3
    mesangiocapillary glomerulonephritis N07.5
  focal and segmental glomerular lesions N07.1
  minor glomerular abnormality N07.0
  specified morphological changes NEC N07.8
hypercalcemic N25.89
hypertensive — *see* Hypertension, kidney
hypokalemic (vacuolar) N25.89
IgA N02.8
  with glomerular lesion N02.9
    focal and segmental hyalinosis or sclerosis N02.1
    membranoproliferative (diffuse) N02.5
    membranous (diffuse) N02.2
    mesangial proliferative (diffuse) N02.3
    mesangiocapillary (diffuse) N02.5
    proliferative NEC N02.8
    specified pathology NEC N02.8
lead N14.3
membranoproliferative (diffuse) N02.5
membranous (diffuse) N02.2
mesangial (IgA/IgG) — *see* Nephropathy, IgA
  proliferative (diffuse) N02.3
mesangiocapillary (diffuse) N02.5
obstructive N13.8
phenacetin N17.2
phosphate-losing N25.0
potassium depletion N25.89
pregnancy-related O26.83-
proliferative NEC — *see also* N00-N07 with fourth
  character .8 N05.8
protein-losing N25.89
saturnine N14.3
sickle-cell D57.- *[N08]*
toxic NEC N14.4
  due to
    drugs N14.2
      analgesic N14.0
      specified NEC N14.1
    heavy metals N14.3
vasomotor N17.0
water-losing N25.89
Nephroptosis N28.83
Nephropyosis — *see* Abscess, kidney
Nephrorrhagia N28.89
Nephrosclerosis (arteriolar) (arteriosclerotic)
(chronic) (hyaline) — *see also* Hypertension, kidney
hyperplastic — *see* Hypertension, kidney
senile N26.9
Nephrosis, nephrotic (Epstein's) (syndrome)
(congenital) N04.9
with
  foot process disease N04.9
  glomerular lesion N04.1
  hypocomplementemic N04.5
acute N04.9
anoxic — *see* Nephrosis, tubular
chemical — *see* Nephrosis, tubular
cholemic K76.7
diabetic — *see* E08-E13 with .21
Finnish type (congenital) Q89.8
hemoglobin N10
hemoglobinuric — *see* Nephrosis, tubular
in
  amyloidosis E85.4 *[N08]*
  diabetes mellitus — *see* E08-E13 with .21
  epidemic hemorrhagic fever A98.5
  malaria (malariae) B52.0
ischemic — *see* Nephrosis, tubular
lipoid N04.9
lower nephron — *see* Nephrosis, tubular
malarial (malariae) B52.0
minimal change N04.0
myoglobin N10
necrotizing — *see* Nephrosis, tubular

Nephrosis, nephrotic (Epstein's) (syndrome)
(congenital) - *continued*
  osmotic (sucrose) N25.89
  radiation N04.9
  syphilitic (late) A52.75
  toxic — *see* Nephrosis, tubular
  tubular (acute) N17.0
    postprocedural N99.0
    radiation N04.9
Nephrosonephritis, hemorrhagic (endemic) A98.5
Nephrostomy
  attention to Z43.6
  status Z93.6
Nerve — *see also* condition
  injury — *see* Injury, nerve, by body site
Nerves R45.0
Nervous — *see also* condition R45.0
  heart F45.8
  stomach F45.8
  tension R45.0
Nervousness R45.0
Nesidioblastoma
  pancreas D13.7
  specified site NEC — *see* Neoplasm, benign, by site
  unspecified site D13.7
Nettleship's syndrome Q82.2
Neumann's disease or syndrome L10.1
Neuralgia, neuralgic (acute) M79.2
  accessory (nerve) G52.8
  acoustic (nerve) — *see* subcategory H93.3
  auditory (nerve) — *see* subcategory H93.3
  ciliary G44.009
    intractable G44.001
    not intractable G44.009
  cranial
    nerve — *see also* Disorder, nerve, cranial
      fifth or trigeminal — *see* Neuralgia, trigeminal
    postherpetic, postzoster B02.29
  ear — *see* subcategory H92.0
  facialis vera G51.1
  Fothergill's — *see* Neuralgia, trigeminal
  glossopharyngeal (nerve) G52.1
  Horton's G44.099
    intractable G44.091
    not intractable G44.099
  Hunt's B02.21
  hypoglossal (nerve) G52.3
  infraorbital — *see* Neuralgia, trigeminal
  malarial — *see* Malaria
  migrainous G44.009
    intractable G44.001
    not intractable G44.009
  Morton's G57.6-
  nerve, cranial — *see* Disorder, nerve, cranial
  nose G52.0
  occipital M54.81
  olfactory G52.0
  penis N48.9
  perineum R10.2
  postherpetic NEC B02.29
    trigeminal B02.22
  pubic region R10.2
  scrotum R10.2
  Sluder's G44.89
  specified nerve NEC G58.8
  spermatic cord R10.2
  sphenopalatine (ganglion) G90.09
  trifacial — *see* Neuralgia, trigeminal
  trigeminal G50.0
    postherpetic, postzoster B02.22
  vagus (nerve) G52.2
  writer's F48.8
    organic G25.89
Neurapraxia — *see* Injury, nerve
Neurasthenia F48.8
  cardiac F45.8
  gastric F45.8
  heart F45.8
Neurilemmoma — *see also* Neoplasm, nerve, benign
  acoustic (nerve) D33.3
  malignant — *see also* Neoplasm, nerve, malignant
    acoustic (nerve) C72.4-
Neurilemmosarcoma — *see* Neoplasm, nerve, malignant
Neurinoma — *see* Neoplasm, nerve, benign
Neurinomatosis — *see* Neoplasm, nerve, uncertain behavior
Neuritis (rheumatoid) M79.2
  abducens (nerve) — *see* Strabismus, paralytic, sixth nerve
  accessory (nerve) G52.8
  acoustic (nerve) (*see also* subcategory) H93.3
    in (due to)

Neuritis (rheumatoid) - *continued*
  acoustic (nerve) - *continued*
    in (due to) - *continued*
      infectious disease NEC B99 [H94.0-]
      parasitic disease NEC B89 [H94.0-]
    syphilitic A52.15
  alcoholic G62.1
    with psychosis — *see* Psychosis, alcoholic
  amyloid, any site E85.4 [G63]
  auditory (nerve) — *see* subcategory H93.3
  brachial — *see* Radiculopathy
    due to displacement, intervertebral disc — *see* Disorder, disc, cervical, with neuritis
  cranial nerve
    due to Lyme disease A69.22
    eighth or acoustic or auditory — *see* subcategory H93.3
    eleventh or accessory G52.8
    fifth or trigeminal G51.0
    first or olfactory G52.0
    fourth or trochlear — *see* Strabismus, paralytic, fourth nerve
    second or optic — *see* Neuritis, optic
    seventh or facial G51.8
      newborn (birth injury) P11.3
    sixth or abducent — *see* Strabismus, paralytic, sixth nerve
    tenth or vagus G52.2
    third or oculomotor — *see* Strabismus, paralytic, third nerve
    twelfth or hypoglossal G52.3
  Déjérine-Sottas G60.0
  diabetic (mononeuropathy) — *see* E08-E13 with .41
    polyneuropathy — *see* E08-E13 with .42
  due to
    beriberi E51.11
    displacement, prolapse or rupture, intervertebral disc — *see* Disorder, disc, with, radiculopathy
    herniation, nucleus pulposus M51.9 [G55]
  endemic E51.11
  facial G51.8
    newborn (birth injury) P11.3
  general — *see* Polyneuropathy
  geniculate ganglion G51.1
    due to herpes (zoster) B02.21
  gouty — *see also* Gout, by type M10.9 [G63]
  hypoglossal (nerve) G52.3
  ilioinguinal (nerve) G57.9-
  infectious (multiple) NEC G61.0
  interstitial hypertrophic progressive G60.0
  lumbar M54.16
  lumbosacral M54.17
  multiple — *see also* Polyneuropathy
    endemic E51.11
    infective, acute G61.0
  multiplex endemica E51.11
  nerve root — *see* Radiculopathy
  oculomotor (nerve) — *see* Strabismus, paralytic, third nerve
  olfactory nerve G52.0
  optic (nerve) (hereditary) (sympathetic) H46.9
    with demyelination G36.0
    in myelitis G36.0
    nutritional H46.2
    papillitis — *see* Papillitis, optic
    retrobulbar H46.1-
    specified type NEC H46.8
    toxic H46.3
  peripheral (nerve) G62.9
    multiple — *see* Polyneuropathy
    single — *see* Mononeuritis
  pneumogastric (nerve) G52.2
  postherpetic, postzoster B02.29
  progressive hypertrophic interstitial G60.0
  retrobulbar — *see also* Neuritis, optic, retrobulbar
    in (due to)
      late syphilis A52.15
      meningococcal infection A39.82
    meningococcal A39.82
    syphilitic A52.15
  sciatic (nerve) — *see also* Sciatica
    due to displacement of intervertebral disc — *see* Disorder, disc, with, radiculopathy
  serum — *see also* Reaction, serum T80.69
  shoulder-girdle G54.5
  specified nerve NEC G58.8
  spinal (nerve) root — *see* Radiculopathy
  syphilitic A52.15
  thenar (median) G56.1-
  thoracic M54.14
  toxic NEC G62.2
  trochlear (nerve) — *see* Strabismus, paralytic, fourth nerve

Neuritis (rheumatoid) - *continued*
  vagus (nerve) G52.2
Neuroastrocytoma — *see* Neoplasm, uncertain behavior, by site
Neuroavitaminosis E56.9 [G99.8]
Neuroblastoma
  olfactory C30.0
  specified site — *see* Neoplasm, malignant, by site
  unspecified site C74.90
Neurochorioretinitis — *see* Chorioretinitis
Neurocirculatory asthenia F45.8
Neurocysticercosis B69.0
Neurocytoma — *see* Neoplasm, benign, by site
Neurodermatitis (circumscribed) (circumscripta) (local) L28.0
  atopic L20.81
  diffuse (Brocq) L20.81
  disseminated L20.81
Neuroencephalomyelopathy, optic G36.0
Neuroepithelioma — *see also* Neoplasm, malignant, by site
  olfactory C30.0
Neurofibroma — *see also* Neoplasm, nerve, benign
  melanotic — *see* Neoplasm, nerve, benign
  multiple — *see* Neurofibromatosis
  plexiform — *see* Neoplasm, nerve, benign
Neurofibromatosis (multiple) (nonmalignant) Q85.00
  acoustic Q85.02
  malignant — *see* Neoplasm, nerve, malignant
  specified NEC Q85.09
  type 1 (von Recklinghausen) Q85.01
  type 2 Q85.02
Neurofibrosarcoma — *see* Neoplasm, nerve, malignant
Neurogenic — *see also* condition
  bladder — *see also* Dysfunction, bladder, neuromuscular N31.9
    cauda equina syndrome G83.4
  bowel NEC K59.2
  heart F45.8
Neuroglioma — *see* Neoplasm, uncertain behavior, by site
Neurolabyrinthitis (of Dix and Hallpike) — *see* Neuronitis, vestibular
Neurolathyrism — *see* Poisoning, food, noxious, plant
Neuroleprosy A30.9
Neuroma — *see also* Neoplasm, nerve, benign
  acoustic (nerve) D33.3
  amputation (stump) (traumatic) (surgical complication) (late) T87.3-
    arm T87.3-
    leg T87.3-
  digital (toe) G57.6-
  interdigital G58.8
    lower limb (toe) G57.8-
    upper limb G56.8-
  intermetatarsal G57.8-
  Morton's G57.6-
  nonneoplastic
    arm G56.9-
    leg G57.9-
    lower extremity G57.9-
    upper extremity G56.9-
  optic (nerve) D33.3
  plantar G57.6-
  plexiform — *see* Neoplasm, nerve, benign
  surgical (nonneoplastic)
    arm G56.9-
    leg G57.9-
    lower extremity G57.9-
    upper extremity G56.9-
Neuromyalgia — *see* Neuralgia
Neuromyasthenia (epidemic) (postinfectious) G93.3
Neuromyelitis G36.9
  ascending G61.0
  optica G36.0
Neuromyopathy G70.9
  paraneoplastic D49.9 [G13.0]
Neuromyotonia (Isaacs) G71.19
Neuronevus — *see* Nevus
Neuronitis G58.9
  ascending (acute) G57.2-
  vestibular H81.2-
Neuroparalytic — *see* condition
Neuropathy, neuropathic G62.9
  acute motor G62.81
  alcoholic G62.1
    with psychosis — *see* Psychosis, alcoholic
  arm G56.9-
  autonomic, peripheral — *see* Neuropathy, peripheral, autonomic
  axillary G56.9-

Neuropathy, neuropathic - *continued*
bladder N31.9
 atonic (motor) (sensory) N31.2
 autonomous N31.2
 flaccid N31.2
 nonreflex N31.2
 reflex N31.1
 uninhibited N31.0
brachial plexus G54.0
cervical plexus G54.2
chronic
 progressive segmentally demyelinating G62.89
 relapsing demyelinating G62.89
Déjérine-Sottas G60.0
diabetic — *see* E08-E13 with .40
 mononeuropathy — *see* E08-E13 with .41
 polyneuropathy — *see* E08-E13 with .42
entrapment G58.9
 iliohypogastric nerve G57.8-
 ilioinguinal nerve G57.8-
 lateral cutaneous nerve of thigh G57.1-
 median nerve G56.0-
 obturator nerve G57.8-
 peroneal nerve G57.3-
 posterior tibial nerve G57.5-
 saphenous nerve G57.8-
 ulnar nerve G56.2-
facial nerve G51.9
hereditary G60.9
 motor and sensory (types I-IV) G60.0
 sensory G60.8
 specified NEC G60.8
hypertrophic G60.0
 Charcot-Marie-Tooth G60.0
 Déjérine-Sottas G60.0
 interstitial progressive G60.0
 of infancy G60.0
 Refsum G60.1
idiopathic G60.9
 progressive G60.3
 specified NEC G60.8
in association with hereditary ataxia G60.2
intercostal G58.0
ischemic — *see* Disorder, nerve
Jamaica (ginger) G62.2
leg NEC G57.9-
lower extremity G57.9-
lumbar plexus G54.1
median nerve G56.1-
motor and sensory — *see also* Polyneuropathy
 hereditary (types I-IV) G60.0
multifocal motor (MMN) G61.82
multiple (acute) (chronic) — *see* Polyneuropathy
optic (nerve) — *see also* Neuritis, optic
 ischemic H47.01-
paraneoplastic (sensorial) (Denny
 Brown) D49.9 *[G13.0]*
peripheral (nerve) — *see also* Polyneuropathy G62.9
 autonomic G90.9
  idiopathic G90.09
  in (due to)
   amyloidosis E85.4 *[G99.0]*
   diabetes mellitus — *see* E08-E13 with .43
   endocrine disease NEC E34.9 *[G99.0]*
   gout M10.00 *[G99.0]*
   hyperthyroidism E05.90 *[G99.0]*
    with thyroid storm E05.91 *[G99.0]*
   metabolic disease NEC E88.9 *[G99.0]*
  idiopathic G60.9
   progressive G60.3
  in (due to)
   antitetanus serum G62.0
   arsenic G62.2
   drugs NEC G62.0
   lead G62.2
   organophosphate compounds G62.2
   toxic agent NEC G62.2
plantar nerves G57.6-
progressive
 hypertrophic interstitial G60.0
 inflammatory G62.81
radicular NEC — *see* Radiculopathy
sacral plexus G54.1
sciatic G57.0-
serum G61.1
toxic NEC G62.2
trigeminal sensory G50.8
ulnar nerve G56.2-
uremic N18.9 *[G63]*
vitamin B12 E53.8 *[G63]*
 with anemia (pernicious) D51.0 *[G63]*
  due to dietary deficiency D51.3 *[G63]*

Neurophthisis — *see also* Disorder, nerve
 peripheral, diabetic — *see* E08-E13 with .42
Neuroretinitis — *see* Chorioretinitis
Neuroretinopathy, hereditary optic H47.22
Neurosarcoma — *see* Neoplasm, nerve, malignant
Neurosclerosis — *see* Disorder, nerve
Neurosis, neurotic F48.9
 anankastic F42.8
 anxiety (state) F41.1
  panic type F41.0
 asthenic F48.8
 bladder F45.8
 cardiac (reflex) F45.8
 cardiovascular F45.8
 character F60.9
 colon F45.8
 compensation F68.1
 compulsive, compulsion F42.8
 conversion F44.9
 craft F48.8
 cutaneous F45.8
 depersonalization F48.1
 depressive (reaction) (type) F34.1
 environmental F48.8
 excoriation L98.1
 fatigue F48.8
 functional — *see* Disorder, somatoform
 gastric F45.8
 gastrointestinal F45.8
 heart F45.8
 hypochondriacal F45.21
 hysterical F44.9
 incoordination F45.8
  larynx F45.8
  vocal cord F45.8
 intestine F45.8
 larynx (sensory) F45.8
  hysterical F44.4
 mixed NEC F48.8
 musculoskeletal F45.8
 obsessional F42.8
 obsessive-compulsive F42.8
 occupational F48.8
 ocular NEC F45.8
 organ — *see* Disorder, somatoform
 pharynx F45.8
 phobic F40.9
 posttraumatic (situational) F43.10
  acute F43.11
  chronic F43.12
 psychasthenic (type) F48.8
 railroad F48.8
 rectum F45.8
 respiratory F45.8
 rumination F45.8
 sexual F65.9
 situational F48.8
 social F40.10
  generalized F40.11
 specified type NEC F48.8
 state F48.9
  with depersonalization episode F48.1
 stomach F45.8
 traumatic F43.10
  acute F43.11
  chronic F43.12
 vasomotor F45.8
 visceral F45.8
 war F48.8
Neurospongioblastosis diffusa Q85.1
Neurosyphilis (arrested) (early) (gumma) (late)
 (latent) (recurrent) (relapse) A52.3
 with ataxia (cerebellar) (locomotor) (spastic)
  (spinal) A52.19
 aneurysm (cerebral) A52.05
 arachnoid (adhesive) A52.13
 arteritis (any artery) (cerebral) A52.04
 asymptomatic A52.2
 congenital A50.40
 dura (mater) A52.13
 general paresis A52.17
 hemorrhagic A52.05
 juvenile (asymptomatic) (meningeal) A50.40
 leptomeninges (aseptic) A52.13
 meningeal, meninges (adhesive) A52.13
 meningitis A52.13
 meningovascular (diffuse) A52.13
 optic atrophy A52.15
 parenchymatous (degenerative) A52.19
 paresis, paretic A52.17
  juvenile A50.45
 remission in (sustained) A52.3
 serological (without symptoms) A52.2

Neurosyphilis (arrested) (early) (gumma) (late)
(latent) (recurrent) (relapse) - *continued*
 specified nature or site NEC A52.19
 tabes, tabetic (dorsalis) A52.11
  juvenile A50.45
 taboparesis A52.17
  juvenile A50.45
 thrombosis (cerebral) A52.05
 vascular (cerebral) NEC A52.05
Neurothekeoma — *see* Neoplasm, nerve, benign
Neurotic — *see* Neurosis
Neurotoxemia — *see* Toxemia
Neutroclusion M26.211
Neutropenia, neutropenic (chronic) (genetic)
 (idiopathic) (immune) (infantile) (malignant)
 (pernicious) (splenic) D70.9
 congenital (primary) D70.0
 cyclic D70.4
 cytoreductive cancer chemotherapy sequela D70.1
 drug-induced D70.2
  due to cytoreductive cancer chemotherapy D70.1
 due to infection D70.3
 fever D70.9
 neonatal, transitory (isoimmune) (maternal
  transfer) P61.5
 periodic D70.4
 secondary (cyclic) (periodic) (splenic) D70.4
  drug-induced D70.2
  due to cytoreductive cancer chemotherapy D70.1
 toxic D70.8
Neutrophilia, hereditary giant D72.0
Nevocarcinoma — *see* Melanoma
Nevus D22.9
 achromic — *see* Neoplasm, skin, benign
 amelanotic — *see* Neoplasm, skin, benign
 angiomatousD18.00
  intra-abdominal D18.03
  intracranial D18.02
  skin D18.01
  specified site NEC D18.09
 araneus I78.1
 balloon cell — *see* Neoplasm, skin, benign
 bathing trunk D48.5
 blue — *see* Neoplasm, skin, benign
  cellular — *see* Neoplasm, skin, benign
  giant — *see* Neoplasm, skin, benign
  Jadassohn's — *see* Neoplasm, skin, benign
  malignant — *see* Melanoma
 capillary D18.00
  intra-abdominal D18.03
  intracranial D18.02
  skin D18.01
  specified site NEC D18.09
 cavernous D18.00
  intra-abdominal D18.03
  intracranial D18.02
  skin D18.01
  specified site NEC D18.09
 cellular — *see* Neoplasm, skin, benign
  blue — *see* Neoplasm, skin, benign
 choroid D31.3-
 comedonicus Q82.5
 conjunctiva D31.0-
 dermal — *see* Neoplasm, skin, benign
  with epidermal nevus — *see* Neoplasm, skin,
   benign
 dysplastic — *see* Neoplasm, skin, benign
 eye D31.9-
 flammeus Q82.5
 hemangiomatous D18.00
  intra-abdominal D18.03
  intracranial D18.02
  skin D18.01
  specified site NEC D18.09
 iris D31.4-
 lacrimal gland D31.5-
 lymphatic D18.1
 magnocellular
  specified site — *see* Neoplasm, benign, by site
  unspecified site D31.40
 malignant — *see* Melanoma
 meaning hemangioma D18.00
  intra-abdominal D18.03
  intracranial D18.02
  skin D18.01
  specified site NEC D18.09
 mouth (mucosa) D10.30
  specified site NEC D10.39
  white sponge Q38.6
 multiplex Q85.1
 non-neoplastic I78.1
 oral mucosa D10.30
  specified site NEC D10.39

Nevus - *continued*
  oral mucosa - *continued*
    white sponge Q38.6
  orbit D31.6-
  pigmented
    giant — *see also* Neoplasm, skin, uncertain
      behavior D48.5
      malignant melanoma in — *see* Melanoma
  portwine Q82.5
  retina D31.2-
  retrobulbar D31.6-
  sanguineous Q82.5
  senile I78.1
  skin D22.9
    abdominal wall D22.5
    ala nasi D22.39
    ankle D22.7-
    anus, anal D22.5
    arm D22.6-
    auditory canal (external) D22.2-
    auricle (ear) D22.2-
    auricular canal (external) D22.2-
    axilla, axillary fold D22.5
    back D22.5
    breast D22.5
    brow D22.39
    buttock D22.5
    canthus (eye) D22.1-
    cheek (external) D22.39
    chest wall D22.5
    chin D22.39
    ear (external) D22.2-
    external meatus (ear) D22.2-
    eyebrow D22.39
    eyelid (lower) (upper) D22.1-
    face D22.30
      specified NEC D22.39
    female genital organ (external) NEC D28.0
    finger D22.6-
    flank D22.5
    foot D22.7-
    forearm D22.6-
    forehead D22.39
    foreskin D29.0
    genital organ (external) NEC
      female D28.0
      male D29.9
    gluteal region D22.5
    groin D22.5
    hand D22.6-
    heel D22.7-
    helix D22.2-
    hip D22.7-
    interscapular region D22.5
    jaw D22.39
    knee D22.7-
    labium (majus) (minus) D28.0
    leg D22.7-
    lip (lower) (upper) D22.0
    lower limb D22.7-
    male genital organ (external) D29.9
    nail D22.9
      finger D22.6-
      toe D22.7-
    nasolabial groove D22.39
    nates D22.5
    neck D22.4
    nose (external) D22.39
    palpebra D22.1-
    penis D29.0
    perianal skin D22.5
    perineum D22.5
    pinna D22.2-
    popliteal fossa or space D22.7-
    prepuce D29.0
    pudendum D28.0
    scalp D22.4
    scrotum D29.4
    shoulder D22.6-
    submammary fold D22.5
    temple D22.39
    thigh D22.7-
    toe D22.7-
    trunk NEC D22.5
    umbilicus D22.5
    upper limb D22.6-
    vulva D28.0
  specified site NEC — *see* Neoplasm, by site, benign
  spider I78.1
  stellar I78.1
  strawberry Q82.5
  Sutton's — *see* Neoplasm, skin, benign
  unius lateris Q82.5

Nevus - *continued*
  Unna's Q82.5
  vascular Q82.5
  verrucous Q82.5
Newborn (infant) (liveborn) (singleton) Z38.2
  acne L70.4
  abstinence syndrome P96.1
  affected by
    abnormalities of membranes P02.9
      specified NEC P02.8
    abruptio placenta P02.1
    amino-acid metabolic disorder, transitory P74.8
    amniocentesis (while in utero) P00.6
    amnionitis P02.7
    apparent life threatening event (ALTE) R68.13
    bleeding (into)
      cerebral cortex P52.22
      germinal matrix P52.0
      ventricles P52.1
    breech delivery P03.0
    cardiac arrest P29.81
    cardiomyopathy I42.8
      congenital I42.4
    cerebral ischemia P91.0
    Cesarean delivery P03.4
    chemotherapy agents P04.1
    chorioamnionitis P02.7
    cocaine (crack) P04.41
    complications of labor and delivery P03.9
      specified NEC P03.89
    compression of umbilical cord NEC P02.5
    contracted pelvis P03.1
    delivery P03.9
      Cesarean P03.4
      forceps P03.2
      vacuum extractor P03.3
    environmental chemicals P04.6
    entanglement (knot) in umbilical cord P02.5
    fetal (intrauterine)
      growth retardation P05.9
      malnutrition not light or small for gestational
        age P05.2
    forceps delivery P03.2
    heart rate abnormalities
      bradycardia P29.12
      intrauterine P03.819
        before onset of labor P03.810
        during labor P03.811
      tachycardia P29.11
    hemorrhage (antepartum) P02.1
      cerebellar (nontraumatic) P52.6
      intracerebral (nontraumatic) P52.4
      intracranial (nontraumatic) P52.9
        specified NEC P52.8
      intraventricular (nontraumatic) P52.3
        grade 1 P52.0
        grade 2 P52.1
        grade 3 P52.21
        grade 4 P52.22
      posterior fossa (nontraumatic) P52.6
      subarachnoid (nontraumatic) P52.5
      subependymal P52.0
        with intracerebral extension P52.22
        with intraventricular extension P52.1
          with enlargment of ventricles P52.21
        without intraventricular extension P52.0
    hypoxic ischemic encephalopathy [HIE] P91.60
      mild P91.61
      moderate P91.62
      severe P91.63
    induction of labor P03.89
    intestinal perforation P78.0
    intrauterine (fetal) blood loss P50.9
      due to (from)
        cut end of co-twin cord P50.5
        hemorrhage into
          co-twin P50.3
          maternal circulation P50.4
        placenta P50.2
        ruptured cord blood P50.1
        vasa previa P50.0
        specified NEC P50.8
    intrauterine (fetal) hemorrhage P50.9
    intrauterine (in utero) procedure P96.5
    malpresentation (malposition) NEC P03.1
    maternal (complication of) (use of)
      alcohol P04.3
      analgesia (maternal) P04.0
      anesthesia (maternal) P04.0
      blood loss P02.1
      circulatory disease P00.3
      condition P00.9
        specified NEC P00.89

Newborn (infant) (liveborn) (singleton) - *continued*
  affected by - *continued*
    maternal (complication of) (use of) - *continued*
      delivery P03.9
        Cesarean P03.4
        forceps P03.2
        vacuum extractor P03.3
      diabetes mellitus (pre-existing) P70.1
      disorder P00.9
        specified NEC P00.89
      drugs (addictive) (illegal) NEC P04.49
      ectopic pregnancy P01.4
      gestational diabetes P70.0
      hemorrhage P02.1
      hypertensive disorder P00.0
      incompetent cervix P01.0
      infectious disease P00.2
      injury P00.5
      labor and delivery P03.9
      malpresentation before labor P01.7
      maternal death P01.6
      medical procedure P00.7
      medication P04.1
      multiple pregnancy P01.5
      nutritional disorder P00.4
      oligohydramnios P01.2
      parasitic disease P00.2
      periodontal disease P00.81
      placenta previa P02.0
      polyhydramnios P01.3
      precipitate delivery P03.5
      pregnancy P01.9
        specified P01.8
      premature rupture of membranes P01.1
      renal disease P00.1
      respiratory disease P00.3
      surgical procedure P00.6
      urinary tract disease P00.1
      uterine contraction (abnormal) P03.6
    meconium peritonitis P78.0
    medication (legal) (maternal use)
      (prescribed) P04.1
    membrane abnormalities P02.9
      specified NEC P02.8
    membranitis P02.7
    methamphetamine (s) P04.49
    mixed metabolic and respiratory acidosis P84
    neonatal abstinence syndrome P96.1
    noxious substances transmitted via placenta or
      breast milk P04.9
      specified NEC P04.8
    nutritional supplements P04.5
    placenta previa P02.0
    placental
      abnormality (functional) (morphological) P02.20
        specified NEC P02.29
      dysfunction P02.29
      infarction P02.29
      insufficiency P02.29
      separation NEC P02.1
      transfusion syndromes P02.3
    placentitis P02.7
    precipitate delivery P03.5
    prolapsed cord P02.4
    respiratory arrest P28.81
    slow intrauterine growth P05.9
    tobacco P04.2
    twin to twin transplacental transfusion P02.3
    umbilical cord (tightly) around neck P02.5
    umbilical cord condition P02.60
      short cord P02.69
      specified NEC P02.69
    uterine contractions (abnormal) P03.6
    vasa previa P02.69
      from intrauterine blood loss P50.0
  apnea P28.4
    primary P28.3
    obstructive P28.4
    sleep (central) (obstructive) (primary) P28.3
  born in hospital Z38.00
    by cesarean Z38.01
  born outside hospital Z38.1
  breast buds P96.89
  breast engorgement P83.4
  check-up — *see* Newborn, examination
  convulsion P90
  dehydration P74.1
  examination
    8 to 28 days old Z00.111
    under 8 days old Z00.110
  fever P81.9
    environmentally-induced P81.0
  hyperbilirubinemia P59.9

Newborn (infant) (liveborn) (singleton) - *continued*
hyperbilirubinemia - *continued*
of prematurity P59.0
hypernatremia P74.2
hyponatremia P74.2
infection P39.9
candidal P37.5
specified NEC P39.8
urinary tract P39.3
jaundice P59.9
due to
breast milk inhibitor P59.3
hepatocellular damage P59.20
specified NEC P59.29
preterm delivery P59.0
of prematurity P59.0
specified NEC P59.8
late metabolic acidosis P74.0
mastitis P39.0
infective P39.0
noninfective P83.4
multiple born NEC Z38.8
born in hospital Z38.68
by cesarean Z38.69
born outside hospital Z38.7
omphalitis P38.9
with mild hemorrhage P38.1
without hemorrhage P38.9
post-term P08.21
prolonged gestation (over 42 completed weeks) P08.22
quadruplet Z38.8
born in hospital Z38.63
by cesarean Z38.64
born outside hospital Z38.7
quintuplet Z38.8
born in hospital Z38.65
by cesarean Z38.66
born outside hospital Z38.7
seizure P90
sepsis (congenital) P36.9
due to
anaerobes NEC P36.5
Escherichia coli P36.4
Staphylococcus P36.30
aureus P36.2
specified NEC P36.39
Streptococcus P36.10
group B P36.0
specified NEC P36.19
specified NEC P36.8
triplet Z38.8
born in hospital Z38.61
by cesarean Z38.62
born outside hospital Z38.7
twin Z38.5
born in hospital Z38.30
by cesarean Z38.31
born outside hospital Z38.4
vomiting P92.09
bilious P92.01
weight check Z00.111
Newcastle conjunctivitis or disease B30.8
Nezelof's syndrome (pure alymphocytosis) D81.4
Niacin (amide) **deficiency** E52
Nicolas (-Durand) **-Favre disease** A55
Nicotine — *see* Tobacco
Nicotinic acid deficiency E52
Niemann-Pick disease or syndrome E75.249
specified NEC E75.248
type
A E75.240
B E75.241
C E75.242
D E75.243
Night
blindness — *see* Blindness, night
sweats R61
terrors (child) F51.4
Nightmares (REM sleep type) F51.5
NIHSS (National Institutes of Health Stroke Scale) **score** R29.7-
Nipple — *see* condition
Nisbet's chancre A57
Nishimoto (-Takeuchi) **disease** I67.5
Nitritoid crisis or reaction — *see* Crisis, nitritoid
Nitrosohemoglobinemia D74.8
Njovera A65
Nocardiosis, nocardiasis A43.9
cutaneous A43.1
lung A43.0
pneumonia A43.0
pulmonary A43.0

Nocardiosis, nocardiasis - *continued*
specified site NEC A43.8
Nocturia R35.1
psychogenic F45.8
Nocturnal — *see* condition
Nodal rhythm I49.8
Node (s) — *see also* Nodule
Bouchard's (with arthropathy) M15.2
Haygarth's M15.8
Heberden's (with arthropathy) M15.1
larynx J38.7
lymph — *see* condition
milker's B08.03
Osler's I33.0
Schmorl's — *see* Schmorl's disease
singer's J38.2
teacher's J38.2
tuberculous — *see* Tuberculosis, lymph gland
vocal cord J38.2
Nodule (s) **, nodular**
actinomycotic — *see* Actinomycosis
breast NEC N63
colloid (cystic) , thyroid E04.1
cutaneous — *see* Swelling, localized
endometrial (stromal) D26.1
Haygarth's M15.8
inflammatory — *see* Inflammation
juxta-articular
syphilitic A52.77
yaws A66.7
larynx J38.7
lung, solitary (subsegmental branch of the bronchial tree) R91.1
multiple R91.8
milker's B08.03
prostate N40.2
with lower urinary tract symptoms (LUTS) N40.3
without lower urinary tract symtpoms (LUTS) N40.2
pulmonary, solitary (subsegmental branch of the bronchial tree) R91.1
retrocardiac R09.89
rheumatoid M06.30
ankle M06.37-
elbow M06.32-
foot joint M06.37-
hand joint M06.34-
hip M06.35-
knee M06.36-
multiple site M06.39
shoulder M06.31-
vertebra M06.38
wrist M06.33-
scrotum (inflammatory) N49.2
singer's J38.2
solitary, lung (subsegmental branch of the bronchial tree) R91.1
multiple R91.8
subcutaneous — *see* Swelling, localized
teacher's J38.2
thyroid (cold) (gland) (nontoxic) E04.1
with thyrotoxicosis E05.20
with thyroid storm E05.21
toxic or with hyperthyroidism E05.20
with thyroid storm E05.21
vocal cord J38.2
Noma (gangrenous) (hospital) (infective) A69.0
auricle I96
mouth A69.0
pudendi N76.89
vulvae N76.89
Nomad, nomadism Z59.0
NOMID
(neonatal onset multisystemic inflammatory disorder) M04.2
Nonautoimmune hemolytic anemia D59.4
drug-induced D59.2
Nonclosure — *see also* Imperfect, closure
ductus arteriosus (Botallo's) Q25.0
foramen
botalli Q21.1
ovale Q21.1
Noncompliance Z91.19
with
dietary regimen Z91.11
dialysis Z91.15
medical treatment Z91.19
medication regimen NEC Z91.14
underdosing — *see also* Table of Drugs and Chemicals, categories T36-T50, with final character 6 Z91.14
intentional NEC Z91.128
due to financial hardship of patient Z91.120

Noncompliance - *continued*
with - *continued*
medication regimen NEC - *continued*
underdosing - *continued*
unintentional NEC Z91.138
due to patient's age related debility Z91.130
renal dialysis Z91.15
Nondescent (congenital) — *see also* Malposition, congenital
cecum Q43.3
colon Q43.3
testicle Q53.9
bilateral Q53.20
abdominal Q53.21
perineal Q53.22
unilateral Q53.10
abdominal Q53.11
perineal Q53.12
Nondevelopment
brain Q02
part of Q04.3
heart Q24.8
organ or site, congenital NEC — *see* Hypoplasia
Nonengagement
head NEC O32.4
in labor, causing obstructed labor O64.8
Nonexanthematous tick fever A93.2
Nonexpansion, lung (newborn) P28.0
Nonfunctioning
cystic duct — *see also* Disease, gallbladder K82.8
gallbladder — *see also* Disease, gallbladder K82.8
kidney N28.9
labyrinth — *see* subcategory H83.2
Non-Hodgkin lymphoma NEC — *see* Lymphoma, non-Hodgkin
Nonimplantation, ovum N97.2
Noninsufflation, fallopian tube N97.1
Non-ketotic hyperglycinemia E72.51
Nonne-Milroy syndrome Q82.0
Nonovulation N97.0
Nonpatent fallopian tube N97.1
Nonpneumatization, lung NEC P28.0
Nonrotation — *see* Malrotation
Nonsecretion, urine — *see* Anuria
Nonunion
fracture — *see* Fracture, by site
joint, following fusion or arthrodesis M96.0
organ or site, congenital NEC — *see* Imperfect, closure
symphysis pubis, congenital Q74.2
Nonvisualization, gallbladder R93.2
Nonvital, nonvitalized tooth K04.99
Non-working side interference M26.56
Noonan's syndrome Q87.1
Normocytic anemia (infectional) **due to blood loss** (chronic) D50.0
acute D62
Norrie's disease (congenital) Q15.8
North American blastomycosis B40.9
Norwegian itch B86
Nose, nasal — *see* condition
Nosebleed R04.0
Nose-picking F98.8
Nosomania F45.21
Nosophobia F45.22
Nostalgia F43.20
Notch of iris Q13.2
Notching nose, congenital (tip) Q30.2
Nothnagel's
syndrome — *see* Strabismus, paralytic, third nerve
vasomotor acroparesthesia I73.89
Novy's relapsing fever A68.9
louse-borne A68.0
tick-borne A68.1
Noxious
foodstuffs, poisoning by — *see* Poisoning, food, noxious, plant
substances transmitted through placenta or breast milk P04.9
Nucleus pulposus — *see* condition
Numbness R20.0
Nuns' knee — *see* Bursitis, prepatellar
Nursemaid's elbow S53.03-
Nutcracker esophagus K22.4
Nutmeg liver K76.1
Nutrient element deficiency E61.9
specified NEC E61.8
Nutrition deficient or insufficient — *see also* Malnutrition E46
due to
insufficient food T73.0
lack of
care (child) T76.02

Nutrition deficient or insufficient - *continued*
  due to - *continued*
    lack of - *continued*
      care (child) - *continued*
        adult T76.01
      food T73.0
Nutritional stunting E45
Nyctalopia (night blindness) — *see* Blindness, night
Nycturia R35.1
  psychogenic F45.8
Nymphomania F52.8
Nystagmus H55.00
  benign paroxysmal — *see* Vertigo, benign
    paroxysmal
  central positional H81.4-
  congenital H55.01
  dissociated H55.04
  latent H55.02
  miners' H55.09
  positional
    benign paroxysmal H81.4-
    central H81.4-
  specified form NEC H55.09
  visual deprivation H55.03

O

Obermeyer's relapsing fever (European) A68.0
Obesity E66.9
  with alveolar hypoventilation E66.2
  adrenal E27.8
  complicating
    childbirth O99.214
    pregnancy O99.21-
    puerperium O99.215
  constitutional E66.8
  dietary counseling and surveillance Z71.3
  drug-induced E66.1
  due to
    drug E66.1
    excess calories E66.09
      morbid E66.01
      severe E66.01
  endocrine E66.8
  endogenous E66.8
  exogenous E66.09
  familial E66.8
  glandular E66.8
  hypothyroid — *see* Hypothyroidism
  hypoventilation syndrome (OHS) E66.2
  morbid E66.01
    with
      alveolar hypoventilation E66.2
      obesity hypoventilation syndrome (OHS) E66.2
    due to excess calories E66.01
  nutritional E66.09
  pituitary E23.6
  severe E66.01
  specified type NEC E66.8
Oblique — *see* condition
Obliteration
  appendix (lumen) K38.8
  artery I77.1
  bile duct (noncalculous) K83.1
  common duct (noncalculous) K83.1
  cystic duct — *see* Obstruction, gallbladder
  disease, arteriolar I77.1
  endometrium N85.8
  eye, anterior chamber — *see* Disorder, globe,
    hypotony
  fallopian tube N97.1
  lymphatic vessel I89.0
    due to mastectomy I97.2
  organ or site, congenital NEC — *see* Atresia, by site
  ureter N13.5
    with infection N13.6
  urethra — *see* Stricture, urethra
  vein I87.8
  vestibule (oral) K08.89
Observation (following) (for)
  (without need for further medical care) Z04.9
  accident NEC Z04.3
    at work Z04.2
    transport Z04.1
  adverse effect of drug Z03.6
  alleged rape or sexual assault (victim) , ruled out
    adult Z04.41
    child Z04.42
  criminal assault Z04.8
  development state
    adolescent Z00.3
    period of rapid growth in childhood Z00.2
    puberty Z00.3
  disease, specified NEC Z03.89

Observation (following) (for)
(without need for further medical care) - *continued*
  following work accident Z04.2
  growth and development state — *see* Observation,
    development state
  injuries (accidental) NEC — *see also* Observation,
    accident
  newborn (for)
    suspected condition, related to exposure from the
      mother or birth process — *see* - Newborn,
      affected by, maternal
    ruled out Z05.9
      cardiac Z05.0
      connective tissue Z05.73
      gastrointestinal Z05.5
      genetic Z05.41
      genitourinary Z05.6
      immunologic Z05.43
      infectious Z05.1
      metabolic Z05.42
      musculoskeletal Z05.72
      neurological Z05.2
      respiratory Z05.3
      skin and subcutaneous tissue Z05.71
      specified condition NEC Z05.8
  postpartum
    immediately after delivery Z39.0
    routine follow-up Z39.2
  pregnancy (normal) (without complication) Z34.9-
    high risk O09.9-
  suicide attempt, alleged NEC Z03.89
    self-poisoning Z03.6
  suspected, ruled out — *see also* Suspected condition,
    ruled out
    abuse, physical
      adult Z04.71
      child Z04.72
    accident at work Z04.2
    adult battering victim Z04.71
    child battering victim Z04.72
    condition NEC Z03.89
      newborn — *see also* Observation, newborn (for),
        suspected condition, ruled out Z05.9
    drug poisoning or adverse effect Z03.6
    exposure (to)
      anthrax Z03.810
      biological agent NEC Z03.818
    inflicted injury NEC Z04.8
    suicide attempt, alleged Z03.89
      self-poisoning Z03.6
    toxic effects from ingested substance (drug)
      (poison) Z03.6
  toxic effects from ingested substance (drug)
    (poison) Z03.6
Obsession, obsessional state F42.8
  mixed thoughts and acts F42.2
Obsessive-compulsive neurosis or reaction F42.8
Obstetric embolism, septic — *see* Embolism,
  obstetric, septic
Obstetrical trauma (complicating delivery) O71.9
  with or following ectopic or molar pregnancy O08.6
  specified type NEC O71.89
Obstipation — *see* Constipation
Obstruction, obstructed, obstructive
  airway J98.8
    with
      allergic alveolitis J67.9
      asthma J45.909
        with
          exacerbation (acute) J45.901
          status asthmaticus J45.902
      bronchiectasis J47.9
        with
          exacerbation (acute) J47.1
          lower respiratory infection J47.0
      bronchitis (chronic) J44.9
      emphysema J43.9
    chronic J44.9
      with
        allergic alveolitis — *see* Pneumonitis,
          hypersensitivity
        bronchiectasis J47.9
          with
            exacerbation (acute) J47.1
            lower respiratory infection J47.0
    due to
      foreign body — *see* Foreign body, by site,
        causing asphyxia
      inhalation of fumes or vapors J68.9
      laryngospasm J38.5
  ampulla of Vater K83.1
  aortic (heart) (valve) — *see* Stenosis, aortic
  aortoiliac I74.09

Obstruction, obstructed, obstructive - *continued*
  aqueduct of Sylvius G91.1
    congenital Q03.0
      with spina bifida — *see* Spina bifida, by site, with
        hydrocephalus
  Arnold-Chiari — *see* Arnold-Chiari disease
  artery — *see also* Embolism, artery I74.9
    stent — *see* Restenosis, stent
    basilar (complete) (partial) — *see* Occlusion,
      artery, basilar
    carotid (complete) (partial) — *see* Occlusion,
      artery, carotid
    cerebellar — *see* Occlusion, artery, cerebellar
    cerebral (anterior) (middle) (posterior) — *see*
      Occlusion, artery, cerebral
    precerebral — *see* Occlusion, artery, precerebral
      renal N28.0
    retinal NEC — *see* Occlusion, artery, retina
    vertebral (complete) (partial) — *see* Occlusion,
      artery, vertebral
  band (intestinal) K56.69
  bile duct or passage (common) (hepatic)
    (noncalculous) K83.1
    with calculus K80.51
    congenital (causing jaundice) Q44.3
  biliary (duct) (tract) K83.1
    gallbladder K82.0
  bladder-neck (acquired) N32.0
    congenital Q64.31
    due to hyperplasia (hypertrophy) of prostate — *see*
      Hyperplasia, prostate
  bowel — *see* Obstruction, intestine
  bronchus J98.09
  canal, ear — *see* Stenosis, external ear canal
  cardia K22.2
  caval veins (inferior) (superior) I87.1
  cecum — *see* Obstruction, intestine
  circulatory I99.8
  colon — *see* Obstruction, intestine
  common duct (noncalculous) K83.1
  coronary (artery) — *see* Occlusion, coronary
  cystic duct — *see also* Obstruction, gallbladder
    with calculus K80.21
  device, implant or graft — *see also* Complications,
    by site and type, mechanical T85.698
    arterial graft NEC — *see* Complication,
      cardiovascular device, mechanical, vascular
    catheter NEC T85.628
      cystostomy T83.090
      dialysis (renal) T82.49
        intraperitoneal T85.691
      Hopkins T83.098
      ileostomy T83.098
      infusion NEC T82.594
        spinal (epidural) (subdural) T85.690
      nephrostomy T83.092
      urethral indwelling T83.091
      urinary T83.098
      urostomy T83.098
    due to infection T85.79
    gastrointestinal — *see* Complications, prosthetic
      device, mechanical, gastrointestinal device
    genital NEC T83.498
      intrauterine contraceptive device T83.39
      penile prosthesis (cylinder) (implanted) (pump)
        (resevoir) T83.490
      testicular prosthesis T83.491
    heart NEC — *see* Complication, cardiovascular
      device, mechanical
    joint prosthesis — *see* Complications, joint
      prosthesis, mechanical, specified NEC, by site
    orthopedic NEC — *see* Complication, orthopedic,
      device, mechanical
    specified NEC T85.628
    urinary NEC — *see also* Complication,
      genitourinary, device, urinary, mechanical
      graft T83.29
    vascular NEC — *see* Complication, cardiovascular
      device, mechanical
    ventricular intracranial shunt T85.09
  due to foreign body accidentally left in operative
    wound T81.529
  duodenum K31.5
  ejaculatory duct N50.89
  esophagus K22.2
  eustachian tube (complete) (partial) H68.10-
    cartilagenous (extrinsic) H68.13-
      intrinsic H68.12-
    osseous H68.11-
  fallopian tube (bilateral) N97.1
  fecal K56.41
    with hernia — *see* Hernia, by site, with obstruction
  foramen of Monro (congenital) Q03.8

Obstruction, obstructed, obstructive - *continued*
foramen of Monro (congenital) - *continued*
  with spina bifida — *see* Spina bifida, by site, with hydrocephalus
foreign body — *see* Foreign body
gallbladder K82.0
  with calculus, stones K80.21
  congenital Q44.1
gastric outlet K31.1
gastrointestinal — *see* Obstruction, intestine
hepatic K76.89
  duct (noncalculous) K83.1
hepatobiliary K83.1
ileum — *see* Obstruction, intestine
iliofemoral (artery) I74.5
intestine K56.60
  with
    adhesions (intestinal) (peritoneal) K56.5
  adynamic K56.0
  by gallstone K56.3
  congenital (small) Q41.9
    large Q42.9
      specified part NEC Q42.8
  neurogenic K56.0
    Hirschsprung's disease or megacolon Q43.1
  newborn P76.9
    due to
      fecaliths P76.8
      inspissated milk P76.2
      meconium (plug) P76.0
        in mucoviscidosis E84.11
      specified NEC P76.8
  postoperative K91.3
  reflex K56.0
  specified NEC K56.69
  volvulus K56.2
intracardiac ball valve prosthesis T82.09
jejunum — *see* Obstruction, intestine
joint prosthesis — *see* Complications, joint prosthesis, mechanical, specified NEC, by site
kidney (calices) N28.89
labor — *see* Delivery
lacrimal (passages) (duct)
  by
    dacryolith — *see* Dacryolith
    stenosis — *see* Stenosis, lacrimal
  congenital Q10.5
  neonatal H04.53-
lacrimonasal duct — *see* Obstruction, lacrimal
lacteal, with steatorrhea K90.2
laryngitis — *see* Laryngitis
larynx NEC J38.6
  congenital Q31.8
lung J98.4
  disease, chronic J44.9
lymphatic I89.0
meconium (plug)
  newborn P76.0
    due to fecaliths P76.0
    in mucoviscidosis E84.11
mitral — *see* Stenosis, mitral
nasal J34.89
nasolacrimal duct — *see also* Obstruction, lacrimal
  congenital Q10.5
nasopharynx J39.2
nose J34.89
organ or site, congenital NEC — *see* Atresia, by site
pancreatic duct K86.89
parotid duct or gland K11.8
pelviureteral junction N13.5
  with hydronephrosis N13.0
  congenital Q62.39
pharynx J39.2
portal (circulation) (vein) I81
prostate — *see also* Hyperplasia, prostate
  valve (urinary) N32.0
pulmonary valve (heart) I37.0
pyelonephritis (chronic) N11.1
pylorus
  adult K31.1
  congenital or infantile Q40.0
rectosigmoid — *see* Obstruction, intestine
rectum K62.4
renal N28.89
  outflow N13.8
  pelvis, congenital Q62.39
respiratory J98.8
  chronic J44.9
retinal (vessels) H34.9
salivary duct (any) K11.8
  with calculus K11.5
sigmoid — *see* Obstruction, intestine
sinus (accessory) (nasal) J34.89

Obstruction, obstructed, obstructive - *continued*
Stensen's duct K11.8
stomach NEC K31.89
  acute K31.0
  congenital Q40.2
  due to pylorospasm K31.3
submandibular duct K11.8
submaxillary gland K11.8
  with calculus K11.5
thoracic duct I89.0
thrombotic — *see* Thrombosis
trachea J39.8
tracheostomy airway J95.03
tricuspid (valve) — *see* Stenosis, tricuspid
upper respiratory, congenital Q34.8
ureter (functional) (pelvic junction) NEC N13.5
  with
    hydronephrosis N13.1
      with infection N13.6
    pyelonephritis (chronic) N11.1
  congenital Q62.39
  due to calculus — *see* Calculus, ureter
urethra NEC N36.8
  congenital Q64.39
urinary (moderate) N13.9
  due to hyperplasia (hypertrophy) of prostate — *see* Hyperplasia, prostate
  organ or tract (lower) N13.9
  prostatic valve N32.0
  specified NEC N13.8
uropathy N13.9
uterus N85.8
vagina N89.5
valvular — *see* Endocarditis
vein, venous I87.1
  caval (inferior) (superior) I87.1
  thrombotic — *see* Thrombosis
vena cava (inferior) (superior) I87.1
vesical NEC N32.0
vesicourethral orifice N32.0
  congenital Q64.31
vessel NEC I99.8
  stent — *see* Restenosis, stent
Obturator — *see* condition
Occlusal wear, teeth K03.0
Occlusio pupillae — *see* Membrane, pupillary
Occlusion, occluded
anus K62.4
  congenital Q42.3
    with fistula Q42.2
aortoiliac (chronic) I74.09
aqueduct of Sylvius G91.1
  congenital Q03.0
    with spina bifida — *see* Spina bifida, by site, with hydrocephalus
artery — *see also* Embolism, artery I74.9
  auditory, internal I65.8
  basilar I65.1
    with
      infarction I63.22
        due to
          embolism I63.12
          thrombosis I63.02
  brain or cerebral I66.9
    with infarction (due to) I63.5-
      embolism I63.4-
      thrombosis I63.3-
  carotid I65.2-
    with
      infarction I63.23-
        due to
          embolism I63.13-
          thrombosis I63.03-
  cerebellar (anterior inferior) (posterior inferior) (superior) I66.3
    with infarction I63.54-
      due to
        embolism I63.44-
        thrombosis I63.34-
  cerebral I66.9
    with infarction I63.50
      due to
        embolism I63.40
          specified NEC I63.49
        thrombosis I63.30
          specified NEC I63.39
    anterior I66.1-
      with infarction I63.52-
        due to
          embolism I63.42-
          thrombosis I63.32-
    middle I66.0-
      with infarction I63.51-

Occlusion, occluded - *continued*
artery - *continued*
  cerebral - *continued*
    middle - *continued*
      with infarction - *continued*
        due to
          embolism I63.41-
          thrombosis I63.31-
    posterior I66.2-
      with infarction I63.53-
        due to
          embolism I63.43-
          thrombosis I63.33-
    specified NEC I66.8
      with infarction I63.59
        due to
          embolism I63.4-
          thrombosis I63.3-
  choroidal (anterior) — *see* Occlusion, artery, precerebral, specified NEC
  communicating posterior — *see* Occlusion, artery, cerebral, specified NEC
  complete
    coronary I25.82
    extremities I70.92
  coronary (acute) (thrombotic) (without myocardial infarction) I24.0
    with myocardial infarction — *see* Infarction, myocardium
    chronic total I25.82
    complete I25.82
    healed or old I25.2
    total (chronic) I25.82
  hypophyseal — *see* Occlusion, artery, precerebral, specified NEC
  iliac I74.5
  lower extremities due to stenosis or stricture I77.1
  mesenteric (embolic) (thrombotic) — *see also* Infarct, intestine K55.069
  perforating — *see* Occlusion, artery, cerebral, specified NEC
  peripheral I77.9
    thrombotic or embolic I74.4
  pontine — *see* Occlusion, artery, cerebral, specified NEC
  precerebral I65.9
    with infarction I63.20
      specified NEC I63.29
      due to
        embolism I63.10
          specified NEC I63.19
        thrombosis I63.00
          specified NEC I63.09
    basilar — *see* Occlusion, artery, basilar
    carotid — *see* Occlusion, artery, carotid
    puerperal O88.23
    specified NEC I65.8
      with infarction I63.29
        due to
          embolism I63.19
          thrombosis I63.00
    vertebral — *see* Occlusion, artery, vertebral
  renal N28.0
  retinal
    central H34.1-
    partial H34.21-
    branch H34.23-
    transient H34.0-
  spinal — *see* Occlusion, artery, precerebral, vertebral
  total (chronic)
    coronary I25.82
    extremities I70.92
  vertebral I65.0-
    with
      infarction I63.21-
        due to
          embolism I63.11-
          thrombosis I63.01-
basilar artery — *see* Occlusion, artery, basilar
bile duct (common) (hepatic) (noncalculous) K83.1
bowel — *see* Obstruction, intestine
carotid (artery) (common) (internal) — *see* Occlusion, artery, carotid
centric (of teeth) M26.59
  maximum intercuspation discrepancy M26.55
cerebellar (artery) — *see* Occlusion, artery, cerebellar
cerebral (artery) — *see* Occlusion, artery, cerebral
cerebrovascular — *see also* Occlusion, artery, cerebral
  with infarction I63.5-
cervical canal — *see* Stricture, cervix

Occlusion, occluded - *continued*
  cervix (uteri) — *see* Stricture, cervix
  choanal Q30.0
  choroidal (artery) — *see* Occlusion, artery,
    precerebral, specified NEC
  colon — *see* Obstruction, intestine
  communicating posterior artery — *see* Occlusion,
    artery, precerebral, specified NEC
  coronary (artery) (vein) (thrombotic) — *see*
    also Infarct, myocardium
    chronic total I25.82
    healed or old I25.2
    not resulting in infarction I24.0
    total (chronic) I25.82
  cystic duct — *see* Obstruction, gallbladder
  embolic — *see* Embolism
  fallopian tube N97.1
    congenital Q50.6
  gallbladder — *see also* Obstruction, gallbladder
    congenital (causing jaundice) Q44.1
  gingiva, traumatic K06.2
  hymen N89.6
    congenital Q52.3
  hypophyseal (artery) — *see* Occlusion, artery,
    precerebral, specified NEC
  iliac artery I74.5
  intestine — *see* Obstruction, intestine
  lacrimal passages — *see* Obstruction, lacrimal
  lung J98.4
  lymph or lymphatic channel I89.0
  mammary duct N64.89
  mesenteric artery (embolic) (thrombotic) — *see*
    also Infarct, intestine K55.069
  nose J34.89
    congenital Q30.0
  organ or site, congenital NEC — *see* Atresia, by site
  oviduct N97.1
    congenital Q50.6
  peripheral arteries
    due to stricture or stenosis I77.1
    upper extremity I74.2
  pontine (artery) — *see* Occlusion, artery,
    precerebral, specified NEC
  posterior lingual, of mandibular teeth M26.29
  precerebral artery — *see* Occlusion, artery,
    precerebral
  punctum lacrimale — *see* Obstruction, lacrimal
  pupil — *see* Membrane, pupillary
  pylorus, adult — *see also* Stricture, pylorus K31.1
  renal artery N28.0
  retina, retinal
    artery — *see* Occlusion, artery, retinal
    vein (central) H34.81-
      engorgement H34.82-
      tributary H34.83-
    vessels H34.9
  spinal artery — *see* Occlusion, artery, precerebral,
    vertebral
  teeth (mandibular) (posterior lingual) M26.29
  thoracic duct I89.0
  thrombotic — *see* Thrombosis, artery
  traumatic
    edentulous (alveolar) ridge K06.2
    gingiva K06.2
    periodontal K05.5
  tubal N97.1
  ureter (complete) (partial) N13.5
    congenital Q62.10
  ureteropelvic junction N13.5
    congenital Q62.11
  ureterovesical orifice N13.5
    congenital Q62.12
  urethra — *see* Stricture, urethra
  uterus N85.8
  vagina N89.5
  vascular NEC I99.8
  vein — *see* Thrombosis
    retinal — *see* Occlusion, retinal, vein
  vena cava (inferior) (superior) — *see* Embolism,
    vena cava
  ventricle (brain) NEC G91.1
  vertebral (artery) — *see* Occlusion, artery, vertebral
  vessel (blood) I99.8
  vulva N90.5
Occult
  blood in feces (stools) R19.5
Occupational
  problems NEC Z56.89
Ochlophobia — *see* Agoraphobia
Ochronosis (endogenous) E70.29
Ocular muscle — *see* condition
Oculogyric crisis or disturbance H51.8
  psychogenic F45.8

Oculomotor syndrome H51.9
Oculopathy
  syphilitic NEC A52.71
    congenital
      early A50.01
      late A50.30
    early (secondary) A51.43
    late A52.71
Oddi's sphincter spasm K83.4
Odontalgia K08.89
Odontoameloblastoma — *see* Cyst, calcifying
  odontogenic
Odontoclasia K03.89
Odontodysplasia, regional K00.4
Odontogenesis imperfecta K00.5
Odontoma (ameloblastic) (complex) (compound)
  (fibroameloblastic) — *see* Cyst, calcifying
  odontogenic
Odontomyelitis (closed) (open) K04.01
  irreversible K04.02
  reversible K04.01
Odontorrhagia K08.89
Odontosarcoma, ameloblastic C41.1
  upper jaw (bone) C41.0
Oestriasis — *see* Myiasis
Oguchi's disease H53.63
Ohara's disease — *see* Tularemia
OHS (obesity hypoventilation syndrome) E66.2
Oidiomycosis — *see* Candidiasis
Oidium albicans infection — *see* Candidiasis
Old age (without mention of debility) R54
  dementia F03
Old (previous) **myocardial infarction** I25.2
Olfactory — *see* condition
Oligemia — *see* Anemia
Oligoastrocytoma
  specified site — *see* Neoplasm, malignant, by site
  unspecified site C71.9
Oligocythemia D64.9
Oligodendroblastoma
  specified site — *see* Neoplasm, malignant
  unspecified site C71.9
Oligodendroglioma
  anaplastic type
    specified site — *see* Neoplasm, malignant, by site
    unspecified site C71.9
  specified site — *see* Neoplasm, malignant, by site
  unspecified site C71.9
Oligodontia — *see* Anodontia
Oligoencephalon Q02
Oligohidrosis L74.4
Oligohydramnios O41.0-
Oligohydrosis L74.4
Oligomenorrhea N91.5
  primary N91.3
  secondary N91.4
Oligophrenia — *see also* Disability, intellectual
  phenylpyruvic E70.0
Oligospermia N46.11
  due to
    drug therapy N46.121
    efferent duct obstruction N46.123
    infection N46.122
    radiation N46.124
    specified cause NEC N46.129
    systemic disease N46.125
Oligotrichia — *see* Alopecia
Oliguria R34
  with, complicating or following ectopic or molar
    pregnancy O08.4
  postprocedural N99.0
Ollier's disease Q78.4
Omenotocele — *see* Hernia, abdomen, specified site
  NEC
Omentitis — *see* Peritonitis
Omentum, omental — *see* condition
Omphalitis (congenital) (newborn) P38.9
  with mild hemorrhage P38.1
  without hemorrhage P38.9
  not of newborn L08.82
  tetanus A33
Omphalocele Q79.2
Omphalomesenteric duct, persistent Q43.0
Omphalorrhagia, newborn P51.9
Omsk hemorrhagic fever A98.1
Onanism (excessive) F98.8
Onchocerciasis, onchocercosis B73.1
  with
    eye disease B73.00
      endophthalmitis B73.01
      eyelid B73.09
      glaucoma B73.02
      specified NEC B73.09

Onchocerciasis, onchocercosis - *continued*
    eye NEC B73.00
    eyelid B73.09
Oncocytoma — *see* Neoplasm, benign, by site
Oncovirus, as cause of disease classified
  elsewhere B97.32
Ondine's curse — *see* Apnea, sleep
Oneirophrenia F23
Onychauxis L60.2
  congenital Q84.5
Onychia — *see also* Cellulitis, digit
  with lymphangitis — *see* Lymphangitis, acute, digit
  candidal B37.2
  dermatophytic B35.1
Onychitis — *see also* Cellulitis, digit
  with lymphangitis — *see* Lymphangitis, acute, digit
Onychocryptosis L60.0
Onychodystrophy L60.3
  congenital Q84.6
Onychogryphosis, onychogryposis L60.2
Onycholysis L60.1
Onychomadesis L60.8
Onychomalacia L60.3
Onychomycosis (finger) (toe) B35.1
Onycho-osteodysplasia Q87.2
Onychophagia F98.8
Onychophosis L60.8
Onychoptosis L60.8
Onychorrhexis L60.3
  congenital Q84.6
Onychoschizia L60.3
Onyxis (finger) (toe) L60.0
Onyxitis — *see also* Cellulitis, digit
  with lymphangitis — *see* Lymphangitis, acute, digit
Oophoritis (cystic) (infectional) (interstitial) N70.92
  with salpingitis N70.93
  acute N70.02
    with salpingitis N70.03
  chronic N70.12
    with salpingitis N70.13
  complicating abortion — *see* Abortion, by type,
    complicated by, oophoritis
Oophorocele N83.4-
Opacity, opacities
  cornea H17.-
    central H17.1-
    congenital Q13.3
    degenerative — *see* Degeneration, cornea
    hereditary — *see* Dystrophy, cornea
    inflammatory — *see* Keratitis
    minor H17.81-
    peripheral H17.82-
    sequelae of trachoma (healed) B94.0
    specified NEC H17.89
  enamel (teeth) (fluoride) (nonfluoride) K00.3
  lens — *see* Cataract
  snowball — *see* Deposit, crystalline
  vitreous (humor) NEC H43.39-
    congenital Q14.0
    membranes and strands H43.31-
Opalescent dentin (hereditary) K00.5
Open, opening
  abnormal, organ or site, congenital — *see* Imperfect,
    closure
  angle with
    borderline
      findings
        high risk H40.02-
        low risk H40.01-
      intraocular pressure H40.00-
    cupping of discs H40.01-
    glaucoma (primary) — *see* Glaucoma, open angle
  bite
    anterior M26.220
    posterior M26.221
  false — *see* Imperfect, closure
  margin on tooth restoration K08.51
  restoration margins of tooth K08.51
  wound — *see* Wound, open
Operational fatigue F48.8
Operative — *see* condition
Operculitis — *see* Periodontitis
Operculum — *see* Break, retina
Ophiasis L63.2
Ophthalmia — *see also* Conjunctivitis H10.9
  actinic rays — *see* Photokeratitis
  allergic (acute) — *see* Conjunctivitis, acute, atopic
  blennorrhagic (gonococcal) (neonatorum) A54.31
  diphtheritic A36.86
  Egyptian A71.1
  electrica — *see* Photokeratitis
  gonococcal (neonatorum) A54.31
  metastatic — *see* Endophthalmitis, purulent

Ophthalmia - *continued*
  migraine — *see* Migraine, ophthalmoplegic
  neonatorum, newborn P39.1
    gonococcal A54.31
  nodosa H16.24-
  purulent — *see* Conjunctivitis, acute, mucopurulent
  spring — *see* Conjunctivitis, acute, atopic
  sympathetic — *see* Uveitis, sympathetic
Ophthalmitis — *see* Ophthalmia
Ophthalmocele (congenital) Q15.8
Ophthalmoneuromyelitis G36.0
Ophthalmoplegia — *see also* Strabismus, paralytic
  anterior internuclear — *see* Ophthalmoplegia, internuclear
  ataxia-areflexia G61.0
  diabetic — *see* E08-E13 with .39
  exophthalmic E05.00
    with thyroid storm E05.01
  external H49.88-
    progressive H49.4-
      with pigmentary retinopathy — *see* Kearns-Sayre syndrome
    total H49.3-
  internal (complete) (total) H52.51-
  internuclear H51.2-
  migraine — *see* Migraine, ophthalmoplegic
  Parinaud's H49.88-
  progressive external — *see* Ophthalmoplegia, external, progressive
  supranuclear, progressive G23.1
  total (external) — *see* Ophthalmoplegia, external, total
Opioid (s)
  abuse — *see* Abuse, drug, opioids
  dependence — *see* Dependence, drug, opioids
  induced, without use disorder
    anxiety disorder F11.988
    delirium F11.921
    depressive disorder F11.94
    sexual dysfunction F11.981
    sleep disorder F11.982
Opisthognathism M26.09
Opisthorchiasis (felineus) (viverrini) B66.0
Opitz' disease D73.2
Opiumism — *see* Dependence, drug, opioid
Oppenheim's disease G70.2
Oppenheim-Urbach disease (necrobiosis lipoidica diabeticorum) — *see* E08-E13 with .620
Optic nerve — *see* condition
Orbit — *see* condition
Orchioblastoma C62.9-
Orchitis (gangrenous) (nonspecific) (septic) (suppurative) N45.2
  blennorrhagic (gonococcal) (acute) (chronic) A54.23
  chlamydial A56.19
  filarial — *see also* Infestation, filarial B74.9 [N51]
  gonococcal (acute) (chronic) A54.23
  mumps B26.0
  syphilitic A52.76
  tuberculous A18.15
Orf (virus disease) B08.02
Organic — *see also* condition
  brain syndrome F09
  heart — *see* Disease, heart
  mental disorder F09
  psychosis F09
Orgasm
  anejaculatory N53.13
Oriental
  bilharziasis B65.2
  schistosomiasis B65.2
Orifice — *see* condition
Origin of both great vessels from right ventricle Q20.1
Ormond's disease (with ureteral obstruction) N13.5
  with infection N13.6
Ornithine metabolism disorder E72.4
Ornithinemia (Type I) (Type II) E72.4
Ornithosis A70
Orotaciduria, oroticaciduria (congenital) (hereditary) (pyrimidine deficiency) E79.8
  anemia D53.0
Orthodontics
  adjustment Z46.4
  fitting Z46.4
Orthopnea R06.01
Orthopoxvirus B08.09
  specified NEC B08.09
Os, uterus — *see* condition
Osgood-Schlatter disease or osteochondrosis — *see* Osteochondrosis, juvenile, tibia
Osler (-Weber) **-Rendu disease** I78.0

Osler's nodes I33.0
Osmidrosis L75.0
Osseous — *see* condition
Ossification
  artery — *see* Arteriosclerosis
  auricle (ear) — *see* Disorder, pinna, specified type NEC
  bronchial J98.09
  cardiac — *see* Degeneration, myocardial
  cartilage (senile) — *see* Disorder, cartilage, specified type NEC
  coronary (artery) — *see* Disease, heart, ischemic, atherosclerotic
  diaphragm J98.6
  ear, middle — *see* Otosclerosis
  falx cerebri G96.19
  fontanel, premature Q75.0
  heart — *see also* Degeneration, myocardial
    valve — *see* Endocarditis
  larynx J38.7
  ligament — *see* Disorder, tendon, specified type NEC
    posterior longitudinal — *see* Spondylopathy, specified NEC
  meninges (cerebral) (spinal) G96.19
  multiple, eccentric centers — *see* Disorder, bone, development or growth
  muscle — *see also* Calcification, muscle
    due to burns — *see* Myositis, ossificans, in, burns
    paralytic — *see* Myositis, ossificans, in, quadriplegia
    progressive — *see* Myositis, ossificans, progressiva
    specified NEC M61.50
      ankle M61.57-
      foot M61.57-
      forearm M61.53-
      hand M61.54-
      lower leg M61.56-
      multiple sites M61.59
      pelvic region M61.55-
      shoulder region M61.51-
      specified site NEC M61.58
      thigh M61.55-
      upper arm M61.52-
    traumatic — *see* Myositis, ossificans, traumatica
  myocardium, myocardial — *see* Degeneration, myocardial
  penis N48.89
  periarticular — *see* Disorder, joint, specified type NEC
  pinna — *see* Disorder, pinna, specified type NEC
  rider's bone — *see* Ossification, muscle, specified NEC
  sclera H15.89
  subperiosteal, post-traumatic M89.8X-
  tendon — *see* Disorder, tendon, specified type NEC
  trachea J39.8
  tympanic membrane — *see* Disorder, tympanic membrane, specified NEC
  vitreous (humor) — *see* Deposit, crystalline
Osteitis — *see also* Osteomyelitis
  alveolar M27.3
  condensans M85.30
    ankle M85.37-
    foot M85.37-
    forearm M85.33-
    hand M85.34-
    lower leg M85.36-
    multiple site M85.39
    neck M85.38
    rib M85.38
    shoulder M85.31-
    skull M85.38
    specified site NEC M85.38
    thigh M85.35-
    toe M85.37-
    upper arm M85.32-
    vertebra M85.38
  deformans M88.9
    in (due to)
      malignant neoplasm of bone C41.9 [M90.60]
      neoplastic disease — *see also* Neoplasm D49.9 [M90.60]
        carpus D49.9 [M90.64-]
        clavicle D49.9 [M90.61-]
        femur D49.9 [M90.65-]
        fibula D49.9 [M90.66-]
        finger D49.9 [M90.64-]
        humerus D49.9 [M90.62-]
        ilium D49.9 [M90.65-]
        ischium D49.9 [M90.65-]
        metacarpus D49.9 [M90.64-]
        metatarsus D49.9 [M90.67-]

Osteitis - *continued*
  deformans - *continued*
    in (due to) - *continued*
      neoplastic disease - *continued*
        multiple sites D49.9 [M90.69]
        neck D49.9 [M90.68]
        radius D49.9 [M90.63-]
        rib D49.9 [M90.68]
        scapula D49.9 [M90.61-]
        skull D49.9 [M90.68]
        tarsus D49.9 [M90.67-]
        tibia D49.9 [M90.66-]
        toe D49.9 [M90.67-]
        ulna D49.9 [M90.63-]
        vertebra D49.9 [M90.68]
    skull M88.0
    specified NEC — *see* Paget's disease, bone, by site
    vertebra M88.1
  due to yaws A66.6
  fibrosa NEC — *see* Cyst, bone, by site
    circumscripta — *see* Dysplasia, fibrous, bone NEC
    cystica (generalisata) E21.0
    disseminata Q78.1
    osteoplastica E21.0
  fragilitans Q78.0
  Garr's (sclerosing) — *see* Osteomyelitis, specified type NEC
  jaw (acute) (chronic) (lower) (suppurative) (upper) M27.2
  parathyroid E21.0
  petrous bone (acute) (chronic) — *see* Petrositis
  sclerotic, nonsuppurative — *see* Osteomyelitis, specified type NEC
  tuberculosa A18.09
    cystica D86.89
    multiplex cystoides D86.89
Osteoarthritis M19.90
  ankle M19.07-
  elbow M19.02-
  foot joint M19.07-
  generalized M15.9
    erosive M15.4
    primary M15.0
    specified NEC M15.8
  hand joint M19.04-
    first carpometacarpal joint M18.9
  hip M16.1-
    bilateral M16.0
    due to hip dysplasia (unilateral) M16.3-
      bilateral M16.2
  interphalangeal
    distal (Heberden) M15.1
    proximal (Bouchard) M15.2
  knee M17.9
    bilateral M17.0
  shoulder M19.01-
  spine — *see* Spondylosis
  wrist M19.03-
  post-traumatic NEC M19.92
    ankle M19.17-
    elbow M19.12-
    foot joint M19.17-
    hand joint M19.14-
      first carpometacarpal joint M18.3-
        bilateral M18.2
    hip M16.5-
      bilateral M16.4
    knee M17.3-
      bilateral M17.2
    shoulder M19.11-
    wrist M19.13-
  primary M19.91
    ankle M19.07-
    elbow M19.02-
    foot joint M19.07-
    hand joint M19.04-
      first carpometacarpal joint M18.1-
        bilateral M18.0
    hip M16.1-
      bilateral M16.0
    knee M17.1-
      bilateral M17.0
    shoulder M19.01-
    spine — *see* Spondylosis
    wrist M19.03-
  secondary M19.93
    ankle M19.27-
    elbow M19.22-
    foot joint M19.27-
    hand joint M19.24-
      first carpometacarpal joint M18.5-
        bilateral M18.4
    hip M16.7

Osteoarthritis - *continued*
  secondary - *continued*
    hip - *continued*
      bilateral M16.6
      knee M17.5
        bilateral M17.4
      multiple M15.3
      shoulder M19.21-
      spine — *see* Spondylosis
      wrist M19.23-
Osteoarthropathy (hypertrophic) M19.90
  ankle — *see* Osteoarthritis, primary, ankle
  elbow — *see* Osteoarthritis, primary, elbow
  foot joint — *see* Osteoarthritis, primary, foot
  hand joint — *see* Osteoarthritis, primary, hand joint
  knee joint — *see* Osteoarthritis, primary, knee
  multiple site — *see* Osteoarthritis, primary, multiple joint
  pulmonary — *see also* Osteoarthropathy, specified type NEC
    hypertrophic — *see* Osteoarthropathy, hypertrophic, specified type NEC
    secondary hypertrophic — *see* Osteoarthropathy, specified type NEC
  shoulder — *see* Osteoarthritis, primary, shoulder
  specified joint NEC — *see* Osteoarthritis, primary, specified joint NEC
  specified type NEC M89.40
    carpus M89.44-
    clavicle M89.41-
    femur M89.45-
    fibula M89.46-
    finger M89.44-
    humerus M89.42-
    ilium M89.459
    ischium M89.459
    metacarpus M89.44-
    metatarsus M89.47-
    multiple sites M89.49
    neck M89.48
    radius M89.43-
    rib M89.48
    scapula M89.41-
    skull M89.48
    tarsus M89.47-
    tibia M89.46-
    toe M89.47-
    ulna M89.43-
    vertebra M89.48
  secondary — *see* Osteoarthropathy, specified type NEC
  spine — *see* Spondylosis
  wrist — *see* Osteoarthritis, primary, wrist
Osteoarthrosis (degenerative) (hypertrophic) (joint) — *see also* Osteoarthritis
  deformans alkaptonurica E70.29 *[M36.8]*
  erosive M15.4
  generalized M15.9
    primary M15.0
  polyarticular M15.9
  spine — *see* Spondylosis
Osteoblastoma — *see* Neoplasm, bone, benign
  aggressive — *see* Neoplasm, bone, uncertain behavior
Osteochondritis — *see also* Osteochondropathy, by site
  Brailsford's — *see* Osteochondrosis, juvenile, radius
  dissecans M93.20
    ankle M93.27-
    elbow M93.22-
    foot M93.27-
    hand M93.24-
    hip M93.25-
    knee M93.26-
    multiple sites M93.29
    shoulder joint M93.21-
    specified site NEC M93.28
    wrist M93.23-
  juvenile M92.9
  patellar — *see* Osteochondrosis, juvenile, patella
  syphilitic (congenital) (early) A50.02 *[M90.80]*
    ankle A50.02 *[M90.87-]*
    elbow A50.02 *[M90.82-]*
    foot A50.02 *[M90.87-]*
    forearm A50.02 *[M90.83-]*
    hand A50.02 *[M90.84-]*
    hip A50.02 *[M90.85-]*
    knee A50.02 *[M90.86-]*
    multiple sites A50.02 *[M90.89]*
    shoulder joint A50.02 *[M90.81-]*
    specified site NEC A50.02 *[M90.88]*
Osteochondroarthrosis deformans endemica — *see* Disease, Kaschin-Beck

Osteochondrodysplasia Q78.9
  with defects of growth of tubular bones and spine Q77.9
    specified NEC Q77.8
  specified NEC Q78.8
Osteochondrodystrophy E78.9
Osteochondrolysis — *see* Osteochondritis, dissecans
Osteochondroma — *see* Neoplasm, bone, benign
Osteochondromatosis D48.0
  syndrome Q78.4
Osteochondromyxosarcoma — *see* Neoplasm, bone, malignant
Osteochondropathy M93.90
  ankle M93.97-
  elbow M93.92-
  foot M93.97-
  hand M93.94-
  hip M93.95-
  Kienböck's disease of adults M93.1
  knee M93.96-
  multiple joints M93.99
  osteochondritis dissecans — *see* Osteochondritis, dissecans
  osteochondrosis — *see* Osteochondrosis
  shoulder region M93.91-
  slipped upper femoral epiphysis — *see* Slipped, epiphysis, upper femoral
  specified joint NEC M93.98
  specified type NEC M93.80
    ankle M93.87-
    elbow M93.82-
    foot M93.87-
    hand M93.84-
    hip M93.85-
    knee M93.86-
    multiple joints M93.89
    shoulder region M93.81-
    specified joint NEC M93.88
    wrist M93.83-
  syphilitic, congenital
    early A50.02 *[M90.80]*
    late A50.56 *[M90.80]*
  wrist M93.93-
Osteochondrosarcoma — *see* Neoplasm, bone, malignant
Osteochondrosis — *see also* Osteochondropathy, by site
  acetabulum (juvenile) M91.0
  adult — *see* Osteochondropathy, specified type NEC, by site
  astragalus (juvenile) — *see* Osteochondrosis, juvenile, tarsus
  Blount's — *see* Osteochondrosis, juvenile, tibia
  Buchanan's M91.0
  Burns' — *see* Osteochondrosis, juvenile, ulna
  calcaneus (juvenile) — *see* Osteochondrosis, juvenile, tarsus
  capitular epiphysis (femur) (juvenile) — *see* Legg-Calvé-Perthes disease
  carpal (juvenile) (lunate) (scaphoid) — *see* Osteochondrosis, juvenile, hand, carpal lunate adult M93.1
  coxae juvenilis — *see* Legg-Calvé-Perthes disease
  deformans juvenilis, coxae — *see* Legg-Calvé-Perthes disease
  Diaz's — *see* Osteochondrosis, juvenile, tarsus
  dissecans (knee) (shoulder) — *see* Osteochondritis, dissecans
  femoral capital epiphysis (juvenile) — *see* Legg-Calvé-Perthes disease
  femur (head), juvenile — *see* Legg-Calvé-Perthes disease
  fibula (juvenile) — *see* Osteochondrosis, juvenile, fibula
  foot NEC (juvenile) M92.8
  Freiberg's — *see* Osteochondrosis, juvenile, metatarsus
  Haas' (juvenile) — *see* Osteochondrosis, juvenile, humerus
  Haglund's — *see* Osteochondrosis, juvenile, tarsus
  hip (juvenile) — *see* Legg-Calvé-Perthes disease
  humerus (capitulum) (head) (juvenile) — *see* Osteochondrosis, juvenile, humerus
  ilium, iliac crest (juvenile) M91.0
  ischiopubic synchondrosis M91.0
  Iselin's — *see* Osteochondrosis, juvenile, metatarsus
  juvenile, juvenilis M92.9
    after congenital dislocation of hip reduction — *see* Osteochondrosis, juvenile, hip, specified NEC
    arm — *see* Osteochondrosis, juvenile, upper limb NEC
    capitular epiphysis (femur) — *see* Legg-Calvé-Perthes disease

Osteochondrosis - *continued*
  juvenile, juvenilis - *continued*
    clavicle, sternal epiphysis — *see* Osteochondrosis, juvenile, upper limb NEC
    coxae — *see* Legg-Calvé-Perthes disease
    deformans M92.9
    fibula M92.5-
    foot NEC M92.8
    hand M92.20-
      carpal lunate M92.21-
      metacarpal head M92.22-
      specified site NEC M92.29-
    head of femur — *see* Legg-Calvé-Perthes disease
    hip and pelvis M91.9-
      coxa plana — *see* Coxa, plana
      femoral head — *see* Legg-Calvé-Perthes disease
      pelvis M91.0
      pseudocoxalgia — *see* Pseudocoxalgia
      specified NEC M91.8-
    humerus M92.0-
    limb
      lower NEC M92.8
      upper NEC — *see* Osteochondrosis, juvenile, upper limb NEC
    medial cuneiform bone — *see* Osteochondrosis, juvenile, tarsus
    metatarsus M92.7-
    patella M92.4-
    radius M92.1-
    specified site NEC M92.8
    spine M42.00
      cervical region M42.02
      cervicothoracic region M42.03
      lumbar region M42.06
      lumbosacral region M42.07
      multiple sites M42.09
      occipito-atlanto-axial region M42.01
      sacrococcygeal region M42.08
      thoracic region M42.04
      thoracolumbar region M42.05
    tarsus M92.6-
    tibia M92.5-
    ulna M92.1-
    upper limb NEC M92.3-
    vertebra (body) (epiphyseal plates) (Calvé's) (Scheuermann's) — *see* Osteochondrosis, juvenile, spine
  Kienböck's — *see* Osteochondrosis, juvenile, hand, carpal lunate adult M93.1
  Köhler's
    patellar — *see* Osteochondrosis, juvenile, patella
    tarsal navicular — *see* Osteochondrosis, juvenile, tarsus
  Legg-Perthes (-Calvé) (-Waldenström) — *see* Legg-Calvé-Perthes disease
  limb
    lower NEC (juvenile) M92.8
    upper NEC (juvenile) — *see* Osteochondrosis, juvenile, upper limb NEC
  lunate bone (carpal) (juvenile) — *see also* Osteochondrosis, juvenile, hand, carpal lunate adult M93.1
  Mauclaire's — *see* Osteochondrosis, juvenile, hand, metacarpal
  metacarpal (head) (juvenile) — *see* Osteochondrosis, juvenile, hand, metacarpal
  metatarsus (fifth) (head) (juvenile) (second) — *see* Osteochondrosis, juvenile, metatarsus
  navicular (juvenile) — *see* Osteochondrosis, juvenile, tarsus
  os
    calcis (juvenile) — *see* Osteochondrosis, juvenile, tarsus
    tibiale externum (juvenile) — *see* Osteochondrosis, juvenile, tarsus
  Osgood-Schlatter — *see* Osteochondrosis, juvenile, tibia
  Panner's — *see* Osteochondrosis, juvenile, humerus
  patellar center (juvenile) (primary) (secondary) — *see* Osteochondrosis, juvenile, patella
  pelvis (juvenile) M91.0
  Pierson's M91.0
  radius (head) (juvenile) — *see* Osteochondrosis, juvenile, radius
  Scheuermann's — *see* Osteochondrosis, juvenile, spine
  Sever's — *see* Osteochondrosis, juvenile, tarsus
  Sinding-Larsen — *see* Osteochondrosis, juvenile, patella
  spine M42.9
    adult M42.10

Osteochondrosis - *continued*
 spine - *continued*
  adult - *continued*
   cervical region M42.12
   cervicothoracic region M42.13
   lumbar region M42.16
   lumbosacral region M42.17
   multiple sites M42.19
   occipito-atlanto-axial region M42.11
   sacrococcygeal region M42.18
   thoracic region M42.14
   thoracolumbar region M42.15
  juvenile — *see* Osteochondrosis, juvenile, spine
 symphysis pubis (juvenile) M91.0
 syphilitic (congenital) A50.02
 talus (juvenile) — *see* Osteochondrosis, juvenile, tarsus
 tarsus (navicular) (juvenile) — *see* Osteochondrosis, juvenile, tarsus
 tibia (proximal) (tubercle) (juvenile) — *see* Osteochondrosis, juvenile, tibia
 tuberculous — *see* Tuberculosis, bone
 ulna (lower) (juvenile) — *see* Osteochondrosis, juvenile, ulna
 van Neck's M91.0
 vertebral — *see* Osteochondrosis, spine
Osteoclastoma D48.0
 malignant — *see* Neoplasm, bone, malignant
Osteodynia — *see* Disorder, bone, specified type NEC
Osteodystrophy Q78.9
 azotemic N25.0
 congenital Q78.9
 parathyroid, secondary E21.1
 renal N25.0
Osteofibroma — *see* Neoplasm, bone, benign
Osteofibrosarcoma — *see* Neoplasm, bone, malignant
Osteogenesis imperfecta Q78.0
Osteogenic — *see* condition
Osteolysis M89.50
 carpus M89.54-
 clavicle M89.51-
 femur M89.55-
 fibula M89.56-
 finger M89.54-
 humerus M89.52-
 ilium M89.559
 ischium M89.559
 joint prosthesis (periprosthetic) — *see* Complications, joint prosthesis, mechanical, periprosthetic, osteolysis, by site
 metacarpus M89.54-
 metatarsus M89.57-
 multiple sites M89.59
 neck M89.58
 periprosthetic — *see* Complications, joint prosthesis, mechanical, periprosthetic, osteolysis, by site
 radius M89.53-
 rib M89.58
 scapula M89.51-
 skull M89.58
 tarsus M89.57-
 tibia M89.56-
 toe M89.57-
 ulna M89.53-
 vertebra M89.58
Osteoma — *see also* Neoplasm, bone, benign
 osteoid — *see also* Neoplasm, bone, benign
 giant — *see* Neoplasm, bone, benign
Osteomalacia M83.9
 adult M83.9
  drug-induced NEC M83.5
  due to
   malabsorption (postsurgical) M83.2
   malnutrition M83.3
  specified NEC M83.8
 aluminium-induced M83.4
 infantile — *see* Rickets
 juvenile — *see* Rickets
 oncogenic E83.89
 pelvis M83.8
 puerperal M83.0
 senile M83.1
 vitamin-D-resistant in adults E83.31 *[M90.8-]*
  carpus E83.31 *[M90.84-]*
  clavicle E83.31 *[M90.81-]*
  femur E83.31 *[M90.85-]*
  fibula E83.31 *[M90.86-]*
  finger E83.31 *[M90.84-]*
  humerus E83.31 *[M90.82-]*
  ilium E83.31 *[M90.859]*
  ischium E83.31 *[M90.859]*

Osteomalacia - *continued*
 vitamin-D-resistant in adults - *continued*
  metacarpus E83.31 *[M90.84-]*
  metatarsus E83.31 *[M90.87-]*
  multiple sites E83.31 *[M90.89]*
  neck E83.31 *[M90.88]*
  radius E83.31 *[M90.83-]*
  rib E83.31 *[M90.88]*
  scapula E83.31 *[M90.819]*
  skull E83.31 *[M90.88]*
  tarsus E83.31 *[M90.879]*
  tibia E83.31 *[M90.869]*
  toe E83.31 *[M90.879]*
  ulna E83.31 *[M90.839]*
  vertebra E83.31 *[M90.88]*
Osteomyelitis (general) (infective) (localized) (neonatal) (purulent) (septic) (staphylococcal) (streptococcal) (suppurative) (with periostitis) M86.9
 acute M86.10
  carpus M86.14-
  clavicle M86.11-
  femur M86.15-
  fibula M86.16-
  finger M86.14-
  hematogenous M86.00
   carpus M86.04-
   clavicle M86.01-
   femur M86.05-
   fibula M86.06-
   finger M86.04-
   humerus M86.02-
   ilium M86.059
   ischium M86.059
   mandible M27.2
   metacarpus M86.04-
   metatarsus M86.07-
   multiple sites M86.09
   neck M86.08
   orbit H05.02-
   petrous bone — *see* Petrositis
   radius M86.03-
   rib M86.08
   scapula M86.01-
   skull M86.08
   tarsus M86.07-
   tibia M86.06-
   toe M86.07-
   ulna M86.03-
   vertebra — *see* Osteomyelitis, vertebra
  humerus M86.12-
  ilium M86.159
  ischium M86.159
  mandible M27.2
  metacarpus M86.14-
  metatarsus M86.17-
  multiple sites M86.19
  neck M86.18
  orbit H05.02-
  petrous bone — *see* Petrositis
  radius M86.13-
  rib M86.18
  scapula M86.11-
  skull M86.18
  tarsus M86.17-
  tibia M86.16-
  toe M86.17-
  ulna M86.13-
  vertebra — *see* Osteomyelitis, vertebra
 chronic (or old) M86.60
  with draining sinus M86.40
   carpus M86.44-
   clavicle M86.41-
   femur M86.45-
   fibula M86.46-
   finger M86.44-
   humerus M86.42-
   ilium M86.459
   ischium M86.459
   mandible M27.2
   metacarpus M86.44-
   metatarsus M86.47-
   multiple sites M86.49
   neck M86.48
   orbit H05.02-
   petrous bone — *see* Petrositis
   radius M86.43-
   rib M86.48
   scapula M86.41-
   skull M86.48
   tarsus M86.47-
   tibia M86.46-
   toe M86.47-

Osteomyelitis (general) (infective) (localized) (neonatal) (purulent) (septic) (staphylococcal) (streptococcal) (suppurative) (with periostitis) - *continued*
 chronic (or old) - *continued*
  with draining sinus - *continued*
   ulna M86.43-
   vertebra — *see* Osteomyelitis, vertebra
  carpus M86.64-
  clavicle M86.61-
  femur M86.65-
  fibula M86.66-
  finger M86.64-
  hematogenous NEC M86.50
   carpus M86.54-
   clavicle M86.51-
   femur M86.55-
   fibula M86.56-
   finger M86.54-
   humerus M86.52-
   ilium M86.559
   ischium M86.559
   mandible M27.2
   metacarpus M86.54-
   metatarsus M86.57-
   multifocal M86.30
    carpus M86.34-
    clavicle M86.31-
    femur M86.35-
    fibula M86.36-
    finger M86.34-
    humerus M86.32-
    ilium M86.359
    ischium M86.359
    metacarpus M86.34-
    metatarsus M86.37-
    multiple sites M86.39
    neck M86.38
    radius M86.33-
    rib M86.38
    scapula M86.31-
    skull M86.38
    tarsus M86.37-
    tibia M86.36-
    toe M86.37-
    ulna M86.33-
    vertebra — *see* Osteomyelitis, vertebra
   multiple sites M86.59
   neck M86.58
   orbit H05.02-
   petrous bone — *see* Petrositis
   radius M86.53-
   rib M86.58
   scapula M86.51-
   skull M86.58
   tarsus M86.57-
   tibia M86.56-
   toe M86.57-
   ulna M86.53-
   vertebra — *see* Osteomyelitis, vertebra
  humerus M86.62-
  ilium M86.659
  ischium M86.659
  mandible M27.2
  metacarpus M86.64-
  metatarsus M86.67-
  multifocal — *see* Osteomyelitis, chronic, hematogenous, multifocal
  multiple sites M86.69
  neck M86.68
  orbit H05.02-
  petrous bone — *see* Petrositis
  radius M86.63-
  rib M86.68
  scapula M86.61-
  skull M86.68
  tarsus M86.67-
  tibia M86.66-
  toe M86.67-
  ulna M86.63-
  vertebra — *see* Osteomyelitis, vertebra
 echinococcal B67.2
 Garr's — *see* Osteomyelitis, specified type NEC
 in diabetes mellitus — *see* E08-E13 with .69
 jaw (acute) (chronic) (lower) (neonatal) (suppurative) (upper) M27.2
 nonsuppurating — *see* Osteomyelitis, specified type NEC
 orbit H05.02-
 petrous bone — *see* Petrositis
 Salmonella (arizonae) (cholerae-suis) (enteritidis) (typhimurium) A02.24

Osteomyelitis (general) (infective) (localized)
(neonatal) (purulent) (septic) (staphylococcal)
(streptococcal) (suppurative) (with periostitis) -
continued
  sclerosing, nonsuppurative — *see* Osteomyelitis,
    specified type NEC
  specified type NEC (*see also* subcategory) M86.8X-
    mandible M27.2
    orbit H05.02-
    petrous bone — *see* Petrositis
    vertebra — *see* Osteomyelitis, vertebra
  subacute M86.20
    carpus M86.24-
    clavicle M86.21-
    femur M86.25-
    fibula M86.26-
    finger M86.24-
    humerus M86.22-
    mandible M27.2
    metacarpus M86.24-
    metatarsus M86.27-
    multiple sites M86.29
    neck M86.28
    orbit H05.02-
    petrous bone — *see* Petrositis
    radius M86.23-
    rib M86.28
    scapula M86.21-
    skull M86.28
    tarsus M86.27-
    tibia M86.26-
    toe M86.27-
    ulna M86.23-
    vertebra — *see* Osteomyelitis, vertebra
  syphilitic A52.77
    congenital (early) A50.02 *[M90.80]*
  tuberculous — *see* Tuberculosis, bone
  typhoid A01.05
  vertebra M46.20
    cervical region M46.22
    cervicothoracic region M46.23
    lumbar region M46.26
    lumbosacral region M46.27
    occipito-atlanto-axial region M46.21
    sacrococcygeal region M46.28
    thoracic region M46.24
    thoracolumbar region M46.25
Osteomyelofibrosis D47.4
Osteomyelosclerosis D75.89
Osteonecrosis M87.9
  due to
    drugs — *see* Osteonecrosis, secondary, due to,
      drugs
    trauma — *see* Osteonecrosis, secondary, due to,
      trauma
  idiopathic aseptic M87.00
    ankle M87.07-
    carpus M87.03-
    clavicle M87.01-
    femur M87.05-
    fibula M87.06-
    finger M87.04-
    humerus M87.02-
    ilium M87.050
    ischium M87.050
    metacarpus M87.04-
    metatarsus M87.07-
    multiple sites M87.09
    neck M87.08
    pelvis M87.050
    radius M87.03-
    rib M87.08
    scapula M87.01-
    skull M87.08
    tarsus M87.07-
    tibia M87.06-
    toe M87.07-
    ulna M87.03-
    vertebra M87.08
  secondary NEC M87.30
    carpus M87.33-
    clavicle M87.31-
    due to
      drugs M87.10
        carpus M87.13-
        clavicle M87.11-
        femur M87.15-
        fibula M87.16-
        finger M87.14-
        humerus M87.12-
        ilium M87.159
        ischium M87.159
        jaw M87.180

Osteonecrosis - *continued*
  secondary NEC - *continued*
    due to - *continued*
      drugs - *continued*
        metacarpus M87.14-
        metatarsus M87.17-
        multiple sites M87.19
        neck M87.18
        radius M87.13-
        rib M87.18
        scapula M87.11-
        skull M87.18
        tarsus M87.17-
        tibia M87.16-
        toe M87.17-
        ulna M87.13-
        vertebra M87.18
      hemoglobinopathy NEC D58.2 *[M90.50]*
        carpus D58.2 *[M90.54-]*
        clavicle D58.2 *[M90.51-]*
        femur D58.2 *[M90.55-]*
        fibula D58.2 *[M90.56-]*
        finger D58.2 *[M90.54-]*
        humerus D58.2 *[M90.52-]*
        ilium D58.2 *[M90.55-]*
        ischium D58.2 *[M90.55-]*
        metacarpus D58.2 *[M90.54-]*
        metatarsus D58.2 *[M90.57-]*
        multiple sites D58.2 *[M90.58]*
        neck D58.2 *[M90.58]*
        radius D58.2 *[M90.53-]*
        rib D58.2 *[M90.58]*
        scapula D58.2 *[M90.51-]*
        skull D58.2 *[M90.58]*
        tarsus D58.2 *[M90.57-]*
        tibia D58.2 *[M90.56-]*
        toe D58.2 *[M90.57-]*
        ulna D58.2 *[M90.53-]*
        vertebra D58.2 *[M90.58]*
      trauma (previous) M87.20
        carpus M87.23-
        clavicle M87.21-
        femur M87.25-
        fibula M87.26-
        finger M87.24-
        humerus M87.22-
        ilium M87.25-
        ischium M87.25-
        metacarpus M87.24-
        metatarsus M87.27-
        multiple sites M87.29
        neck M87.28
        radius M87.23-
        rib M87.28
        scapula M87.21-
        skull M87.28
        tarsus M87.27-
        tibia M87.26-
        toe M87.27-
        ulna M87.23-
        vertebra M87.28
    femur M87.35-
    fibula M87.36-
    finger M87.34-
    humerus M87.32-
    ilium M87.350
    in
      caisson disease T70.3 *[M90.50]*
        carpus T70.3 *[M90.54-]*
        clavicle T70.3 *[M90.51-]*
        femur T70.3 *[M90.55-]*
        fibula T70.3 *[M90.56-]*
        finger T70.3 *[M90.54-]*
        humerus T70.3 *[M90.52-]*
        ilium T70.3 *[M90.55-]*
        ischium T70.3 *[M90.55-]*
        metacarpus T70.3 *[M90.54-]*
        metatarsus T70.3 *[M90.57-]*
        multiple sites T70.3 *[M90.59]*
        neck T70.3 *[M90.58]*
        radius T70.3 *[M90.53-]*
        rib T70.3 *[M90.58]*
        scapula T70.3 *[M90.51-]*
        skull T70.3 *[M90.58]*
        tarsus T70.3 *[M90.57-]*
        tibia T70.3 *[M90.56-]*
        toe T70.3 *[M90.57-]*
        ulna T70.3 *[M90.53-]*
        vertebra T70.3 *[M90.58]*
    ischium M87.350
    metacarpus M87.34-
    metatarsus M87.37-
    multiple site M87.39

Osteonecrosis - *continued*
  secondary NEC - *continued*
    neck M87.38
    radius M87.33-
    rib M87.38
    scapula M87.319
    skull M87.38
    tarsus M87.379
    tibia M87.366
    toe M87.379
    ulna M87.33-
    vertebra M87.38
  specified type NEC M87.80
    carpus M87.83-
    clavicle M87.81-
    femur M87.85-
    fibula M87.86-
    finger M87.84-
    humerus M87.82-
    ilium M87.85-
    ischium M87.85-
    metacarpus M87.84-
    metatarsus M87.87-
    multiple sites M87.89
    neck M87.88
    radius M87.83-
    rib M87.88
    scapula M87.81-
    skull M87.88
    tarsus M87.87-
    tibia M87.86-
    toe M87.87-
    ulna M87.83-
    vertebra M87.88
Osteo-onycho-arthro-dysplasia Q87.2
Osteo-onychodysplasia, hereditary Q87.2
Osteopathia condensans disseminata Q78.8
Osteopathy — *see also* Osteomyelitis, Osteonecrosis,
  Osteoporosis
  after poliomyelitis M89.60
    carpus M89.64-
    clavicle M89.61-
    femur M89.65-
    fibula M89.66-
    finger M89.64-
    humerus M89.62-
    ilium M89.659
    ischium M89.659
    metacarpus M89.64-
    metatarsus M89.67-
    multiple sites M89.69
    neck M89.68
    radius M89.63-
    rib M89.68
    scapula M89.61-
    skull M89.68
    tarsus M89.67-
    tibia M89.66-
    toe M89.67-
    ulna M89.63-
    vertebra M89.68
  in (due to)
    renal osteodystrophy N25.0
    specified diseases classified elsewhere — *see*
      subcategory M90.8
Osteopenia M85.8-
  borderline M85.8-
Osteoperiostitis — *see* Osteomyelitis, specified type
  NEC
Osteopetrosis (familial) Q78.2
Osteophyte M25.70
  ankle M25.77-
  elbow M25.72-
  foot joint M25.77-
  hand joint M25.74-
  hip M25.75-
  knee M25.76-
  shoulder M25.71-
  spine M25.78
  vertebrae M25.78
  wrist M25.73-
Osteopoikilosis Q78.8
Osteoporosis (female) (male) M81.0
  with current pathological fracture M80.00
  age-related M81.0
    with current pathologic fracture M80.00
      carpus M80.04-
      clavicle M80.01-
      fibula M80.06-
      finger M80.04-
      humerus M80.02-
      ilium M80.05-
      ischium M80.05-

Osteoporosis (female) (male) - *continued*
  age-related - *continued*
    with current pathologic fracture - *continued*
      metacarpus M80.04-
      metatarsus M80.07-
      pelvis M80.05-
      radius M80.03-
      scapula M80.01-
      tarsus M80.07-
      tibia M80.06-
      toe M80.07-
      ulna M80.03-
      vertebra M80.08
    disuse M81.8
      with current pathological fracture M80.80
        carpus M80.84-
        clavicle M80.81-
        fibula M80.86-
        finger M80.84-
        humerus M80.82-
        ilium M80.85-
        ischium M80.85-
        metacarpus M80.84-
        metatarsus M80.87-
        pelvis M80.85-
        radius M80.83-
        scapula M80.81-
        tarsus M80.87-
        tibia M80.86-
        toe M80.87-
        ulna M80.83-
        vertebra M80.88
    drug-induced — *see* Osteoporosis, specified type NEC
    idiopathic — *see* Osteoporosis, specified type NEC
    involutional — *see* Osteoporosis, age-related
    Lequesne M81.6
    localized M81.6
    postmenopausal M81.0
      with pathological fracture M80.00
        carpus M80.04-
        clavicle M80.01-
        fibula M80.06-
        finger M80.04-
        humerus M80.02-
        ilium M80.05-
        ischium M80.05-
        metacarpus M80.04-
        metatarsus M80.07-
        pelvis M80.05-
        radius M80.03-
        scapula M80.01-
        tarsus M80.07-
        tibia M80.06-
        toe M80.07-
        ulna M80.03-
        vertebra M80.08
    postoophorectomy — *see* Osteoporosis, specified type NEC
    postsurgical malabsorption — *see* Osteoporosis, specified type NEC
    post-traumatic — *see* Osteoporosis, specified type NEC
    senile — *see* Osteoporosis, age-related
    specified type NEC M81.8
      with pathological fracture M80.80
        carpus M80.84-
        clavicle M80.81-
        fibula M80.86-
        finger M80.84-
        humerus M80.82-
        ilium M80.85-
        ischium M80.85-
        metacarpus M80.84-
        metatarsus M80.87-
        pelvis M80.85-
        radius M80.83-
        scapula M80.81-
        tarsus M80.87-
        tibia M80.86-
        toe M80.87-
        ulna M80.83-
        vertebra M80.88
Osteopsathyrosis (idiopathica) Q78.0
Osteoradionecrosis, jaw (acute) (chronic) (lower) (suppurative) (upper) M27.2
Osteosarcoma (any form) — *see* Neoplasm, bone, malignant
Osteosclerosis Q78.2
  acquired M85.8-
  congenita Q77.4
  fragilitas (generalisata) Q78.2
  myelofibrosis D75.81

Osteosclerotic anemia D64.89
Osteosis
  cutis L94.2
  renal fibrocystic N25.0
Österreicher-Turner syndrome Q87.2
Ostium
  atrioventriculare commune Q21.2
  primum (arteriosum) (defect) (persistent) Q21.2
  secundum (arteriosum) (defect) (patent) (persistent) Q21.1
Ostrum-Furst syndrome Q75.8
Otalgia — *see* subcategory H92.0
Otitis (acute) H66.90
  with effusion — *see also* Otitis, media, nonsuppurative
    purulent — *see* Otitis, media, suppurative
  adhesive — *see* subcategory H74.1
  chronic — *see also* Otitis, media, chronic
    with effusion — *see also* Otitis, media, nonsuppurative, chronic
  externa H60.9-
    abscess — *see* Abscess, ear, external
    acute (noninfective) H60.50-
      actinic H60.51-
      chemical H60.52-
      contact H60.53-
      eczematoid H60.54-
      infective — *see* Otitis, externa, infective
      reactive H60.55-
      specified NEC H60.59-
    cellulitis — *see* Cellulitis, ear
    chronic H60.6-
    diffuse — *see* Otitis, externa, infective, diffuse
    hemorrhagic — *see* Otitis, externa, infective, hemorrhagic
    in (due to)
      aspergillosis B44.89
      candidiasis B37.84
      erysipelas A46 *[H62.40]*
      herpes (simplex) virus infection B00.1
        zoster B02.8
      impetigo L01.00 *[H62.40]*
      infectious disease NEC B99 *[H62.4-]*
      mycosis NEC B36.9 *[H62.40]*
      parasitic disease NEC B89 *[H62.40]*
      viral disease NEC B34.9 *[H62.40]*
      zoster B02.8
    infective NEC H60.39-
      abscess — *see* Abscess, ear, external
      cellulitis — *see* Cellulitis, ear
      diffuse H60.31-
      hemorrhagic H60.32-
      swimmer's ear — *see* Swimmer's, ear
    malignant H60.2-
    mycotic NEC B36.9 *[H62.40]*
      in
        aspergillosis B44.89
        candidiasis B37.84
        moniliasis B37.84
    necrotizing — *see* Otitis, externa, malignant
    Pseudomonas aeruginosa — *see* Otitis, externa, malignant
    reactive — *see* Otitis, externa, acute, reactive
    specified NEC — *see* subcategory H60.8
    tropical NEC B36.9 *[H62.40]*
      in
        aspergillosis B44.89
        candidiasis B37.84
        moniliasis B37.84
  insidiosa — *see* Otosclerosis
  interna — *see* subcategory H83.0
  media (hemorrhagic) (staphylococcal) (streptococcal) H66.9-
    with effusion (nonpurulent) — *see* Otitis, media, nonsuppurative
    acute, subacute H66.90
      allergic — *see* Otitis, media, nonsuppurative, acute, allergic
      exudative — *see* Otitis, media, suppurative, acute
      mucoid — *see* Otitis, media, nonsuppurative, acute
      necrotizing — *see also* Otitis, media, suppurative, acute
        in
          measles B05.3
          scarlet fever A38.0
      nonsuppurative NEC — *see* Otitis, media, nonsuppurative, acute
      purulent — *see* Otitis, media, suppurative, acute
      sanguinous — *see* Otitis, media, nonsuppurative, acute
      secretory — *see* Otitis, media, nonsuppurative, acute, serous

Otitis (acute) - *continued*
  media (hemorrhagic) (staphylococcal) (streptococcal) - *continued*
    acute, subacute - *continued*
      seromucinous — *see* Otitis, media, nonsuppurative, acute
      serous — *see* Otitis, media, nonsuppurative, acute, serous
      suppurative — *see* Otitis, media, suppurative, acute
    allergic — *see* Otitis, media, nonsuppurative
    catarrhal — *see* Otitis, media, nonsuppurative
    chronic H66.90
      with effusion (nonpurulent) — *see* Otitis, media, nonsuppurative, chronic
      allergic — *see* Otitis, media, nonsuppurative, chronic, allergic
      benign suppurative — *see* Otitis, media, suppurative, chronic, tubotympanic
      catarrhal — *see* Otitis, media, nonsuppurative, chronic, serous
      exudative — *see* Otitis, media, nonsuppurative, chronic
      mucinous — *see* Otitis, media, nonsuppurative, chronic, mucoid
      mucoid — *see* Otitis, media, nonsuppurative, chronic, mucoid
      nonsuppurative NEC — *see* Otitis, media, nonsuppurative, chronic
      purulent — *see* Otitis, media, suppurative, chronic
      secretory — *see* Otitis, media, nonsuppurative, chronic, mucoid
      seromucinous — *see* Otitis, media, nonsuppurative, chronic
      serous — *see* Otitis, media, nonsuppurative, chronic, serous
      suppurative — *see* Otitis, media, suppurative, chronic
      transudative — *see* Otitis, media, nonsuppurative, chronic, mucoid
    exudative — *see* Otitis, media, suppurative
    in (due to) (with)
      influenza — *see* Influenza, with, otitis media
      measles B05.3
      scarlet fever A38.0
      tuberculosis A18.6
      viral disease NEC B34.- *[H67.-]*
    mucoid — *see* Otitis, media, nonsuppurative
    nonsuppurative H65.9-
      acute or subacute NEC H65.19-
        allergic H65.11-
          recurrent H65.11-
        recurrent H65.19-
        secretory — *see* Otitis, media, nonsuppurative, serous
        serous H65.0-
          recurrent H65.0-
      chronic H65.49-
        allergic H65.41-
        mucoid H65.3-
        serous H65.2-
      postmeasles B05.3
      purulent — *see* Otitis, media, suppurative
      secretory — *see* Otitis, media, nonsuppurative
      seromucinous — *see* Otitis, media, nonsuppurative
      serous — *see* Otitis, media, nonsuppurative
    suppurative H66.4-
      acute H66.00-
        with rupture of ear drum H66.01-
        recurrent H66.00-
          with rupture of ear drum H66.01-
      chronic (*see also* subcategory) H66.3
        atticoantral H66.2-
        benign — *see* Otitis, media, suppurative, chronic, tubotympanic
        tubotympanic H66.1-
      transudative — *see* Otitis, media, nonsuppurative
      tuberculous A18.6
Otocephaly Q18.2
Otolith syndrome — *see* subcategory H81.8
Otomycosis (diffuse) **NEC** B36.9 *[H62.40]*
  in
    aspergillosis B44.89
    candidiasis B37.84
    moniliasis B37.84
Otoporosis — *see* Otosclerosis
Otorrhagia (nontraumatic) H92.2-
  traumatic - code by Type of injury
Otorrhea H92.1-
  cerebrospinal G96.0
Otosclerosis (general) H80.9-
  cochlear (endosteal) H80.2-

Otosclerosis (general) - *continued*
  involving
    otic capsule — *see* Otosclerosis, cochlear
    oval window
      nonobliterative H80.0-
      obliterative H80.1-
    round window — *see* Otosclerosis, cochlear
    nonobliterative — *see* Otosclerosis, involving, oval window, nonobliterative
    obliterative — *see* Otosclerosis, involving, oval window, obliterative
    specified NEC H80.8-
Otospongiosis — *see* Otosclerosis
Otto's disease or pelvis M24.7
Outcome of delivery Z37.9
  multiple births Z37.9
    all liveborn Z37.50
      quadruplets Z37.52
      quintuplets Z37.53
      sextuplets Z37.54
      specified number NEC Z37.59
      triplets Z37.51
    all stillborn Z37.7
    some liveborn Z37.60
      quadruplets Z37.62
      quintuplets Z37.63
      sextuplets Z37.64
      specified number NEC Z37.69
      triplets Z37.61
  single NEC Z37.9
    liveborn Z37.0
    stillborn Z37.1
  twins NEC Z37.9
    both liveborn Z37.2
    both stillborn Z37.4
    one liveborn, one stillborn Z37.3
Outlet — *see* condition
Ovalocytosis (congenital) (hereditary) — *see* Elliptocytosis
Ovarian — *see* Condition
Ovariocele N83.4-
Ovaritis (cystic) — *see* Oophoritis
Ovary, ovarian — *see also* condition
  resistant syndrome E28.39
  vein syndrome N13.8
Overactive — *see also* Hyperfunction
  adrenal cortex NEC E27.0
  bladder N32.81
  hypothalamus E23.3
  thyroid — *see* Hyperthyroidism
Overactivity R46.3
  child — *see* Disorder, attention-deficit hyperactivity
Overbite (deep) (excessive) (horizontal) (vertical) M26.29
Overbreathing — *see* Hyperventilation
Overconscientious personality F60.5
Overdevelopment — *see* Hypertrophy
Overdistension — *see* Distension
Overdose, overdosage (drug) — *see* Table of Drugs and Chemicals, by drug, poisoning
Overeating R63.2
  nonorganic origin F50.89
  psychogenic F50.89
Overexertion (effects) (exhaustion) T73.3
Overexposure (effects) T73.9
  exhaustion T73.2
Overfeeding — *see* Overeating
  newborn P92.4
Overfill, endodontic M27.52
Overgrowth, bone — *see* Hypertrophy, bone
Overhanging of dental restorative material (unrepairable) K08.52
Overheated (places) (effects) — *see* Heat
Overjet (excessive horizontal) M26.29
Overlaid, overlying (suffocation) — *see* Asphyxia, traumatic, due to mechanical threat
Overlap, excessive horizontal (teeth) M26.23
Overlapping toe (acquired) — *see also* Deformity, toe, specified NEC
  congenital (fifth toe) Q66.89
Overload
  circulatory, due to transfusion (blood) (blood components) (TACO) E87.71
  fluid E87.70
    due to transfusion (blood) (blood components) E87.71
    specified NEC E87.79
  iron, due to repeated red blood cell transfusions E83.111
  potassium (K) E87.5
  sodium (Na) E87.0
Overnutrition — *see* Hyperalimentation

Overproduction — *see also* Hypersecretion
  ACTH E27.0
  catecholamine E27.5
  growth hormone E22.0
Overprotection, child by parent Z62.1
Overriding
  aorta Q25.49
  finger (acquired) — *see* Deformity, finger
    congenital Q68.1
  toe (acquired) — *see also* Deformity, toe, specified NEC
    congenital Q66.89
Overstrained R53.83
  heart — *see* Hypertrophy, cardiac
Overuse, muscle NEC M70.8-
Overweight E66.3
Overworked R53.83
Oviduct — *see* condition
Ovotestis Q56.0
Ovulation (cycle)
  failure or lack of N97.0
  pain N94.0
Ovum — *see* condition
Owren's disease or syndrome (parahemophilia) D68.2
Ox heart — *see* Hypertrophy, cardiac
Oxalosis E72.53
Oxaluria E72.53
Oxycephaly, oxycephalic Q75.0
  syphilitic, congenital A50.02
Oxyuriasis B80
Oxyuris vermicularis (infestation) B80
Ozena J31.0

P

Pachyderma, pachydermia L85.9
  larynx (verrucosa) J38.7
Pachydermatocele (congenital) Q82.8
Pachydermoperiostosis — *see also* Osteoarthropathy, hypertrophic, specified type NEC
  clubbed nail M89.40 *[L62]*
Pachygyria Q04.3
Pachymeningitis (adhesive) (basal) (brain) (cervical) (chronic) (circumscribed) (external) (fibrous) (hemorrhagic) (hypertrophic) (internal) (purulent) (spinal) (suppurative) — *see* Meningitis
Pachyonychia (congenital) Q84.5
Pacinian tumor — *see* Neoplasm, skin, benign
Pad, knuckle or Garrod's M72.1
Paget's disease
  with infiltrating duct carcinoma — *see* Neoplasm, breast, malignant
  bone M88.9
    carpus M88.84-
    clavicle M88.81-
    femur M88.85-
    fibula M88.86-
    finger M88.84-
    humerus M88.82-
    ilium M88.85-
    in neoplastic disease — *see* Osteitis, deformans, in neoplastic disease
    ischium M88.85-
    metacarpus M88.84-
    metatarsus M88.87-
    multiple sites M88.89
    neck M88.88
    radius M88.83-
    rib M88.88
    scapula M88.81-
    skull M88.0
    tarsus M88.87-
    tibia M88.86-
    toe M88.87-
    ulna M88.83-
    vertebra M88.88
  breast (female) C50.01-
    male C50.02-
  extramammary — *see also* Neoplasm, skin, malignant
    anus C21.0
      margin C44.590
      skin C44.590
  intraductal carcinoma — *see* Neoplasm, breast, malignant
  malignant — *see* Neoplasm, skin, malignant
    breast (female) C50.01-
      male C50.02-
    unspecified site (female) C50.01-
      male C50.02-
  mammary — *see* Paget's disease, breast
  nipple — *see* Paget's disease, breast

Paget's disease - *continued*
  osteitis deformans — *see* Paget's disease, bone
Paget-Schroetter syndrome I82.890
Pain (s) — *see also* Painful R52
  abdominal R10.9
    colic R10.83
    generalized R10.84
      with acute abdomen R10.0
    lower R10.30
      left quadrant R10.32
      pelvic or perineal R10.2
      periumbilical R10.33
      right quadrant R10.31
    rebound — *see* Tenderness, abdominal, rebound
    severe with abdominal rigidity R10.0
    tenderness — *see* Tenderness, abdominal
    upper R10.10
      epigastric R10.13
      left quadrant R10.12
      right quadrant R10.11
  acute R52
    due to trauma G89.11
    neoplasm related G89.3
    postprocedural NEC G89.18
    post-thoracotomy G89.12
    specified by site - code to Pain, by site
  adnexa (uteri) R10.2
  anginoid — *see* Pain, precordial
  anus K62.89
  arm — *see* Pain, limb, upper
  axillary (axilla) M79.62-
  back (postural) M54.9
  bladder R39.89
    associated with micturition — *see* Micturition, painful
    chronic R39.82
  bone — *see* Disorder, bone, specified type NEC
  breast N64.4
  broad ligament R10.2
  cancer associated (acute) (chronic) G89.3
  cecum — *see* Pain, abdominal
  cervicobrachial M53.1
  chest (central) R07.9
    anterior wall R07.89
    atypical R07.89
    ischemic I20.9
    musculoskeletal R07.89
    non-cardiac R07.89
    on breathing R07.1
    pleurodynia R07.81
    precordial R07.2
    wall (anterior) R07.89
  chronic G89.29
    associated with significant psychosocial dysfunction G89.4
    due to trauma G89.21
    neoplasm related G89.3
    postoperative NEC G89.28
    postprocedural NEC G89.28
    post-thoracotomy G89.22
    specified NEC G89.29
  coccyx M53.3
  colon — *see* Pain, abdominal
  coronary — *see* Angina
  costochondral R07.1
  diaphragm R07.1
  due to cancer G89.3
  due to device, implant or graft — *see also* Complications, by site and type, specified NEC T85.848
    arterial graft NEC T82.848
    breast (implant) T85.848
    catheter NEC T85.848
      dialysis (renal) T82.848
        intraperitoneal T85.848
      infusion NEC T82.848
        spinal (epidural) (subdural) T85.840
      urinary (indwelling) T83.84
    electronic (electrode) (pulse generator) (stimulator)
      bone T84.84
      cardiac T82.847
      nervous system (brain) (peripheral nerve) (spinal) T85.840
      urinary T83.84
    fixation, internal (orthopedic) NEC T84.84
    gastrointestinal (bile duct) (esophagus) T85.848
    genital NEC T83.84
    heart NEC T82.847
    infusion NEC T85.848
    joint prosthesis T84.84
    ocular (corneal graft) (orbital implant) NEC T85.848
    orthopedic NEC T84.84

Pain (s) - *continued*
  due to device, implant or graft - *continued*
    specified NEC T85.848
      urinary NEC T83.84
      vascular NEC T82.848
      ventricular intracranial shunt T85.840
  due to malignancy (primary) (secondary) G89.3
  ear — *see* subcategory H92.0
  epigastric, epigastrium R10.13
  eye — *see* Pain, ocular
  face, facial R51
    atypical G50.1
  female genital organs NEC N94.89
  finger — *see* Pain, limb, upper
  flank — *see* Pain, abdominal
  foot — *see* Pain, limb, lower
  gallbladder K82.9
  gas (intestinal) R14.1
  gastric — *see* Pain, abdominal
  generalized NOS R52
  genital organ
    female N94.89
    male N50.89
  groin — *see* Pain, abdominal, lower
  hand — *see* Pain, limb, upper
  head — *see* Headache
  heart — *see* Pain, precordial
  infra-orbital — *see* Neuralgia, trigeminal
  intercostal R07.82
  intermenstrual N94.0
  jaw R68.84
  joint M25.50
    ankle M25.57-
    elbow M25.52-
    finger M25.54-
    foot M25.57-
    hand M25.54-
    hip M25.55-
    knee M25.56-
    shoulder M25.51-
    toe M25.57-
    wrist M25.53-
  kidney N23
  laryngeal R07.0
  leg — *see* Pain, limb, lower
  limb M79.609
    lower M79.60-
      foot M79.67-
      lower leg M79.66-
      thigh M79.65-
      toe M79.67-
    upper M79.60-
      axilla M79.62-
      finger M79.64-
      forearm M79.63-
      hand M79.64-
      upper arm M79.62-
  loin M54.5
  low back M54.5
  lumbar region M54.5
  mandibular R68.84
  mastoid — *see* subcategory H92.0
  maxilla R68.84
  menstrual — *see also* Dysmenorrhea N94.6
  metacarpophalangeal (joint) — *see* Pain, joint, hand
  metatarsophalangeal (joint) — *see* Pain, joint, foot
  mouth K13.79
  muscle — *see* Myalgia
  musculoskeletal — *see also* Pain, by site M79.1
  myofascial M79.1
  nasal J34.89
  nasopharynx J39.2
  neck NEC M54.2
  nerve NEC — *see* Neuralgia
  neuromuscular — *see* Neuralgia
  nose J34.89
  ocular H57.1-
  ophthalmic — *see* Pain, ocular
  orbital region — *see* Pain, ocular
  ovary N94.89
  over heart — *see* Pain, precordial
  ovulation N94.0
  pelvic (female) R10.2
  penis N48.89
  pericardial — *see* Pain, precordial
  perineal, perineum R10.2
  pharynx J39.2
  pleura, pleural, pleuritic R07.81
  postoperative NOS G89.18
  postprocedural NOS G89.18
  post-thoracotomy G89.12
  precordial (region) R07.2
  premenstrual N94.3

Pain (s) - *continued*
  psychogenic (persistent) (any site) F45.41
  radicular (spinal) — *see* Radiculopathy
  rectum K62.89
  respiration R07.1
  retrosternal R07.2
  rheumatoid, muscular — *see* Myalgia
  rib R07.81
  root (spinal) — *see* Radiculopathy
  round ligament (stretch) R10.2
  sacroiliac M53.3
  sciatic — *see* Sciatica
  scrotum N50.82
  seminal vesicle N50.89
  shoulder M25.51-
  spermatic cord N50.89
  spinal root — *see* Radiculopathy
  spine M54.9
    cervical M54.2
    low back M54.5
      with sciatica M54.4-
    thoracic M54.6
  stomach — *see* Pain, abdominal
  substernal R07.2
  temporomandibular (joint) M26.62-
  testis N50.81-
  thoracic spine M54.6
    with radicular and visceral pain M54.14
  throat R07.0
  tibia — *see* Pain, limb, lower
  toe — *see* Pain, limb, lower
  tongue K14.6
  tooth K08.89
  trigeminal — *see* Neuralgia, trigeminal
  tumor associated G89.3
  ureter N23
  urinary (organ) (system) N23
  uterus NEC N94.89
  vagina R10.2
  vertebrogenic (syndrome) M54.89
  vesical R39.89
    associated with micturition — *see* Micturition, painful
  vulva R10.2
Painful — *see also* Pain
  coitus
    female N94.10
    male N53.12
    psychogenic F52.6
  ejaculation (semen) N53.12
    psychogenic F52.6
  erection — *see* Priapism
  feet syndrome E53.8
  joint replacement (hip) (knee) T84.84
  menstruation — *see* Dysmenorrhea
    psychogenic F45.8
  micturition — *see* Micturition, painful
  respiration R07.1
  scar NEC L90.5
  wire sutures T81.89
Painter's colic — *see* subcategory T56.0
Palate — *see* condition
Palatoplegia K13.79
Palatoschisis — *see* Cleft, palate
Palilalia R48.8
Palliative care Z51.5
Pallor R23.1
  optic disc, temporal — *see* Atrophy, optic
Palmar — *see also* condition
  fascia — *see* condition
Palpable
  cecum K63.89
  kidney N28.89
  ovary N83.8
  prostate N42.9
  spleen — *see* Splenomegaly
Palpitations (heart) R00.2
  psychogenic F45.8
Palsy — *see also* Paralysis G83.9
  atrophic diffuse (progressive) G12.22
  Bell's — *see also* Palsy, facial
    newborn P11.3
  brachial plexus NEC G54.0
    newborn (birth injury) P14.3
  brain — *see* Palsy, cerebral
  bulbar (progressive) (chronic) G12.22
    of childhood (Fazio-Londe) G12.1
    pseudo NEC G12.29
    supranuclear (progressive) G23.1
  cerebral (congenital) G80.9
    ataxic G80.4
    athetoid G80.3
    choreathetoid G80.3

Palsy - *continued*
  cerebral (congenital) - *continued*
    diplegic G80.8
      spastic G80.1
    dyskinetic G80.3
      athetoid G80.3
      choreathetoid G80.3
      distonic G80.3
    dystonic G80.3
    hemiplegic G80.8
      spastic G80.2
    mixed G80.8
    monoplegic G80.8
      spastic G80.1
    paraplegic G80.8
      spastic G80.1
    quadriplegic G80.8
      spastic G80.0
    spastic G80.1
      diplegic G80.1
      hemiplegic G80.2
      monoplegic G80.1
      quadriplegic G80.0
      specified NEC G80.1
      tetrapelgic G80.0
    specified NEC G80.8
    syphilitic A52.12
      congenital A50.49
    tetraplegic G80.8
      spastic G80.0
  cranial nerve — *see also* Disorder, nerve, cranial
    multiple G52.7
      in
        infectious disease B99 *[G53]*
        neoplastic disease — *see also* Neoplasm D49.9 *[G53]*
        parasitic disease B89 *[G53]*
        sarcoidosis D86.82
  creeping G12.22
  diver's T70.3
  Erb's P14.0
  facial G51.0
    newborn (birth injury) P11.3
  glossopharyngeal G52.1
  Klumpke (-Déjérine) P14.1
  lead — *see* subcategory T56.0
  median nerve (tardy) G56.1-
  nerve G58.9
    specified NEC G58.8
  peroneal nerve (acute) (tardy) G57.3-
  progressive supranuclear G23.1
  pseudobulbar NEC G12.29
  radial nerve (acute) G56.3-
  seventh nerve — *see also* Palsy, facial
    newborn P11.3
  shaking — *see* Parkinsonism
  spastic (cerebral) (spinal) G80.1
  ulnar nerve (tardy) G56.2-
  wasting G12.29
Paludism — *see* Malaria
Panangiitis M30.0
Panaris, panaritium — *see also* Cellulitis, digit
  with lymphangitis — *see* Lymphangitis, acute, digit
Panarteritis nodosa M30.0
  brain or cerebral I67.7
Pancake heart R93.1
  with cor pulmonale (chronic) I27.81
Pancarditis (acute) (chronic) I51.89
  rheumatic I09.89
    active or acute I01.8
Pancoast's syndrome or tumor C34.1-
Pancolitis, ulcerative (chronic) K51.00
  with
    complication K51.019
      abscess K51.014
      fistula K51.013
      obstruction K51.012
      rectal bleeding K51.011
      specified complication NEC K51.018
Pancreas, pancreatic — *see* condition
Pancreatitis (annular) (apoplectic) (calcareous) (edematous) (hemorrhagic) (malignant) (recurrent) (subacute) (suppurative) K85.90
  with necrosis (uninfected) K85.91
    infected K85.92
  acute (without necrosis or infection) K85.90
    with necrosis (uninfected) K85.91
      infected K85.92
    alcohol induced (without necrosis or infection) K85.20
      with necrosis (uninfected) K85.21
        infected K85.22
    biliary (without necrosis or infection) K85.10

Pancreatitis (annular) (apoplectic) (calcareous) (edematous) (hemorrhagic) (malignant) (recurrent) (subacute) (suppurative) - *continued*
  acute (without necrosis or infection) - *continued*
    biliary (without necrosis or infection) - *continued*
      with necrosis (uninfected) K85.11
        infected K85.12
     drug induced (without necrosis or infection) K85.30
      with necrosis (uninfected) K85.31
        infected K85.32
     gallstone (without necrosis or infection) K85.10
      with necrosis (uninfected) K85.11
        infected K85.12
     idiopathic (without necrosis or infection) K85.00
      with necrosis (uninfected) K85.01
        infected K85.02
     specified NEC (without necrosis or infection) K85.80
      with necrosis (uninfected) K85.81
        infected K85.82
  chronic (infectious) K86.1
    alcohol-induced K86.0
    recurrent K86.1
    relapsing K86.1
  cystic (chronic) K86.1
  cytomegaloviral B25.2
  fibrous (chronic) K86.1
  gangrenous — *see* Pancreatitis, acute
  gallstone (without necrosis or infection) K85.10
    with necrosis (uninfected) K85.11
      infected K85.12
  interstitial (chronic) K86.1
    acute — *see also* Pancreatitis, acute K85.80
  mumps B26.3
  recurrent (chronic) K86.1
  relapsing, chronic K86.1
  syphilitic A52.74
Pancreatoblastoma — *see* Neoplasm, pancreas, malignant
Pancreolithiasis K86.89
Pancytolysis D75.89
Pancytopenia (acquired) D61.818
  with
    malformations D61.09
    myelodysplastic syndrome — *see* Syndrome, myelodysplastic
  antineoplastic chemotherapy induced D61.810
  congenital D61.09
  drug-induced NEC D61.811
Panencephalitis, subacute, sclerosing A81.1
Panhematopenia D61.9
  congenital D61.09
  constitutional D61.09
  splenic, primary D73.1
Panhemocytopenia D61.9
  congenital D61.09
  constitutional D61.09
Panhypogonadism E29.1
Panhypopituitarism E23.0
  prepubertal E23.0
Panic (attack) (state) F41.0
  reaction to exceptional stress (transient) F43.0
Panmyelopathy, familial, constitutional D61.09
Panmyelophthisis D61.82
  congenital D61.09
Panmyelosis (acute) (with myelofibrosis) C94.4-
Panner's disease — *see* Osteochondrosis, juvenile, humerus
Panneuritis endemica E51.11
Panniculitis (nodular) (nonsuppurative) M79.3
  back M54.00
    cervical region M54.02
    cervicothoracic region M54.03
    lumbar region M54.06
    lumbosacral region M54.07
    multiple sites M54.09
    occipito-atlanto-axial region M54.01
    sacrococcygeal region M54.08
    thoracic region M54.04
    thoracolumbar region M54.05
  lupus L93.2
  mesenteric K65.4
  neck M54.02
    cervicothoracic region M54.03
    occipito-atlanto-axial region M54.01
  relapsing M35.6
Panniculus adiposus (abdominal) E65
Pannus (allergic) (cornea) (degenerativus) (keratic) H16.42-
  abdominal (symptomatic) E65
  trachomatosus, trachomatous (active) A71.1
Panophthalmitis H44.01-

Pansinusitis (chronic) (hyperplastic) (nonpurulent) (purulent) J32.4
  acute J01.40
    recurrent J01.41
  tuberculous A15.8
Panuveitis (sympathetic) H44.11-
Panvalvular disease I08.9
  specified NEC I08.8
PAPA
  (pyogenic arthritis, pyoderma gangrenosum, and acne syndrome) M04.8
Papanicolaou smear, cervix Z12.4
  as part of routine gynecological examination Z01.419
    with abnormal findings Z01.411
  for suspected neoplasm Z12.4
  nonspecific abnormal finding R87.619
  routine Z01.419
    with abnormal findings Z01.411
Papilledema (choked disc) H47.10
  associated with
    decreased ocular pressure H47.12
    increased intracranial pressure H47.11
    retinal disorder H47.13
  Foster-Kennedy syndrome H47.14-
Papillitis H46.00
  anus K62.89
  chronic lingual K14.4
  necrotizing, kidney N17.2
  optic H46.0-
  rectum K62.89
  renal, necrotizing N17.2
  tongue K14.0
Papilloma — *see also* Neoplasm, benign, by site
  acuminatum (female) (male) (anogenital) A63.0
  basal cell L82.1
    inflamed L82.0
  benign pinta (primary) A67.0
  bladder (urinary) (transitional cell) D41.4
  choroid plexus (lateral ventricle) (third ventricle) D33.0
    anaplastic C71.5
    fourth ventricle D33.1
    malignant C71.5
  renal pelvis (transitional cell) D41.1-
    benign D30.1-
  Schneiderian
    specified site — *see* Neoplasm, benign, by site
    unspecified site D14.0
  serous surface
    borderline malignancy
      specified site — *see* Neoplasm, uncertain behavior, by site
      unspecified site D39.10
    specified site — *see* Neoplasm, benign, by site
    unspecified site D27.9
  transitional (cell)
    bladder (urinary) D41.4
    inverted type — *see* Neoplasm, uncertain behavior, by site
    renal pelvis D41.1-
    ureter D41.2-
  ureter (transitional cell) D41.2-
    benign D30.2-
  urothelial — *see* Neoplasm, uncertain behavior, by site
  villous — *see* Neoplasm, uncertain behavior, by site
    adenocarcinoma in — *see* Neoplasm, malignant, by site
    in situ — *see* Neoplasm, in situ
  yaws, plantar or palmar A66.1
Papillomata, multiple, of yaws A66.1
Papillomatosis — *see also* Neoplasm, benign, by site
  confluent and reticulated L83
  cystic, breast — *see* Mastopathy, cystic
  ductal, breast — *see* Mastopathy, cystic
  intraductal (diffuse) — *see* Neoplasm, benign, by site
  subareolar duct D24-
Papillomavirus, as cause of disease classified elsewhere B97.7
Papillon-Léage and Psaume syndrome Q87.0
Papule (s) R23.8
  carate (primary) A67.0
  fibrous, of nose D22.39
  Gottron's L94.4
  pinta (primary) A67.0
Papulosis
  lymphomatoid C86.6
  malignant I77.89
Papyraceous fetus O31.0-
Para-albuminemia E88.09
Paracephalus Q89.7

Parachute mitral valve Q23.2
Paracoccidioidomycosis B41.9
  disseminated B41.7
  generalized B41.7
  mucocutaneous-lymphangitic B41.8
  pulmonary B41.0
  specified NEC B41.8
  visceral B41.8
Paradentosis K05.4
Paraffinoma T88.8
Paraganglioma D44.7
  adrenal D35.0-
    malignant C74.1-
  aortic body D44.7
    malignant C75.5
  carotid body D44.6
    malignant C75.4
  chromaffin — *see also* Neoplasm, benign, by site
    malignant — *see* Neoplasm, malignant, by site
  extra-adrenal D44.7
    malignant C75.5
      specified site — *see* Neoplasm, malignant, by site
      unspecified site C75.5
    specified site — *see* Neoplasm, uncertain behavior, by site
    unspecified site D44.7
  gangliocytic D13.2
    specified site — *see* Neoplasm, benign, by site
    unspecified site D13.2
  glomus jugulare D44.7
    malignant C75.5
  jugular D44.7
  malignant C75.5
    specified site — *see* Neoplasm, malignant, by site
    unspecified site C75.5
  nonchromaffin D44.7
    malignant C75.5
      specified site — *see* Neoplasm, malignant, by site
      unspecified site C75.5
    specified site — *see* Neoplasm, uncertain behavior, by site
    unspecified site D44.7
  parasympathetic D44.7
    specified site — *see* Neoplasm, uncertain behavior, by site
    unspecified site D44.7
  specified site — *see* Neoplasm, uncertain behavior, by site
  sympathetic D44.7
    specified site — *see* Neoplasm, uncertain behavior, by site
    unspecified site D44.7
  unspecified site D44.7
Parageusia R43.2
  psychogenic F45.8
Paragonimiasis B66.4
Paragranuloma, Hodgkin — *see* Lymphoma, Hodgkin, classical, specified NEC
Parahemophilia — *see also* Defect, coagulation D68.2
Parakeratosis R23.4
  variegata L41.0
Paralysis, paralytic (complete) (incomplete) G83.9
  with
    syphilis A52.17
  abducens, abducent (nerve) — *see* Strabismus, paralytic, sixth nerve
  abductor, lower extremity G57.9-
  accessory nerve G52.8
  accommodation — *see also* Paresis, of accommodation
    hysterical F44.89
  acoustic nerve (except Deafness) — *see* subcategory H93.3
  agitans — *see also* Parkinsonism G20
    arteriosclerotic G21.4
  alternating (oculomotor) G83.89
  amyotrophic G12.21
  ankle G57.9-
  anus (sphincter) K62.89
  arm — *see* Monoplegia, upper limb
  ascending (spinal), acute G61.0
  association G12.29
  asthenic bulbar G70.00
    with exacerbation (acute) G70.01
    in crisis G70.01
  ataxic (hereditary) G11.9
    general (syphilitic) A52.17
  atrophic G58.9
    infantile, acute — *see* Poliomyelitis, paralytic
    progressive G12.22
    spinal (acute) — *see* Poliomyelitis, paralytic
  axillary G54.0

Paralysis, paralytic (complete) (incomplete) - *continued*
  Babinski-Nageotte's G83.89
  Bell's G51.0
    newborn P11.3
  Benedikt's G46.3
  birth injury P14.9
    spinal cord P11.5
  bladder (neurogenic) (sphincter) N31.2
  bowel, colon or intestine K56.0
  brachial plexus G54.0
    birth injury P14.3
    newborn (birth injury) P14.3
  brain G83.9
    diplegia G83.0
    triplegia G83.89
  bronchial J98.09
  Brown-Séquard G83.81
  bulbar (chronic) (progressive) G12.22
    infantile — *see* Poliomyelitis, paralytic
    poliomyelitic — *see* Poliomyelitis, paralytic
    pseudo G12.29
  bulbospinal G70.00
    with exacerbation (acute) G70.01
    in crisis G70.01
  cardiac — *see also* Failure, heart I50.9
  cerebrocerebellar, diplegic G80.1
  cervical
    plexus G54.2
    sympathetic G90.09
  Céstan-Chenais G46.3
  Charcot-Marie-Tooth type G60.0
  Clark's G80.9
  colon K56.0
  compressed air T70.3
  compression
    arm G56.9-
    leg G57.9-
    lower extremity G57.9-
    upper extremity G56.9-
  congenital (cerebral) — *see* Palsy, cerebral
  conjugate movement (gaze) (of eye) H51.0
    cortical (nuclear) (supranuclear) H51.0
  cordis — *see* Failure, heart
  cranial or cerebral nerve G52.9
  creeping G12.22
  crossed leg G83.89
  crutch — *see* Injury, brachial plexus
  deglutition R13.0
    hysterical F44.4
  dementia A52.17
  descending (spinal) NEC G12.29
  diaphragm (flaccid) J98.6
    due to accidental dissection of phrenic nerve
      during procedure — *see* Puncture, accidental
      complicating surgery
  digestive organs NEC K59.8
  diplegic — *see* Diplegia
  divergence (nuclear) H51.8
  diver's T70.3
  Duchenne's
    birth injury P14.0
    due to or associated with
      motor neuron disease G12.22
      muscular dystrophy G71.0
  due to intracranial or spinal birth injury — *see* Palsy, cerebral
  embolic (current episode) I63.4-
  Erb (-Duchenne) (birth) (newborn) P14.0
  Erb's syphilitic spastic spinal A52.17
  esophagus K22.8
  eye muscle (extrinsic) H49.9
    intrinsic — *see also* Paresis, of accommodation
  facial (nerve) G51.0
    birth injury P11.3
    congenital P11.3
    following operation NEC — *see* Puncture, accidental complicating surgery
    newborn (birth injury) P11.3
  familial (recurrent) (periodic) G72.3
    spastic G11.4
  fauces J39.2
  finger G56.9-
  gait R26.1
  gastric nerve (nondiabetic) G52.2
  gaze, conjugate H51.0
  general (progressive) (syphilitic) A52.17
    juvenile A50.45
  glottis J38.00
    bilateral J38.02
    unilateral J38.01
  gluteal G54.1
  Gubler (-Millard) G46.3

Paralysis, paralytic (complete) (incomplete) - *continued*
  hand — *see* Monoplegia, upper limb
  heart — *see* Arrest, cardiac
  hemiplegic — *see* Hemiplegia
  hyperkalemic periodic (familial) G72.3
  hypoglossal (nerve) G52.3
  hypokalemic periodic G72.3
  hysterical F44.4
  ileus K56.0
  infantile — *see also* Poliomyelitis, paralytic A80.30
    bulbar — *see* Poliomyelitis, paralytic
    cerebral — *see* Palsy, cerebral
    spastic — *see* Palsy, cerebral, spastic
  infective — *see* Poliomyelitis, paralytic
  inferior nuclear G83.9
  internuclear — *see* Ophthalmoplegia, internuclear
  intestine K56.0
  iris H57.09
    due to diphtheria (toxin) A36.89
  ischemic, Volkmann's (complicating trauma) T79.6
  Jackson's G83.89
  jake — *see* Poisoning, food, noxious, plant
  Jamaica ginger (jake) G62.2
  juvenile general A50.45
  Klumpke (-Déjérine) (birth) (newborn) P14.1
  labioglossal (laryngeal) (pharyngeal) G12.29
  Landry's G61.0
  laryngeal nerve (recurrent) (superior) (unilateral) J38.00
    bilateral J38.02
    unilateral J38.01
  larynx J38.00
    bilateral J38.02
    due to diphtheria (toxin) A36.2
    unilateral J38.01
  lateral G12.21
  lead — *see* subcategory T56.0
  left side — *see* Hemiplegia
  leg G83.1-
    both — *see* Paraplegia
    crossed G83.89
    hysterical F44.4
    psychogenic F44.4
    transient or transitory R29.818
      traumatic NEC — *see* Injury, nerve, leg
  levator palpebrae superioris — *see* Blepharoptosis, paralytic
  limb — *see* Monoplegia
  lip K13.0
  Lissauer's A52.17
  lower limb — *see* Monoplegia, lower limb
    both — *see* Paraplegia
  lung J98.4
  median nerve G56.1-
  medullary (tegmental) G83.89
  mesencephalic G83.89
    tegmental G83.89
  middle alternating G83.89
  Millard-Gubler-Foville G46.3
  monoplegic — *see* Monoplegia
  motor G83.9
  muscle, muscular NEC G72.89
    due to nerve lesion G58.9
    eye (extrinsic) H49.9
      intrinsic — *see* Paresis, of accommodation
      oblique — *see* Strabismus, paralytic, fourth nerve
    iris sphincter H21.9
    ischemic (Volkmann's) (complicating trauma) T79.6
    progressive G12.21
    pseudohypertrophic G71.0
  musculocutaneous nerve G56.9-
  musculospiral G56.9-
  nerve — *see also* Disorder, nerve
    abducent — *see* Strabismus, paralytic, sixth nerve
    accessory G52.8
    auditory (except Deafness) — *see* subcategory H93.3
    birth injury P14.9
    cranial or cerebral G52.9
    facial G51.0
      birth injury P11.3
      congenital P11.3
      newborn (birth injury) P11.3
    fourth or trochlear — *see* Strabismus, paralytic, fourth nerve
    newborn (birth injury) P14.9
    oculomotor — *see* Strabismus, paralytic, third nerve
    phrenic (birth injury) P14.2
    radial G56.3-
    seventh or facial G51.0

Paralysis, paralytic (complete) (incomplete) - *continued*
  nerve - *continued*
    seventh or facial - *continued*
      newborn (birth injury) P11.3
    sixth or abducent — *see* Strabismus, paralytic, sixth nerve
    syphilitic A52.15
    third or oculomotor — *see* Strabismus, paralytic, third nerve
    trigeminal G50.9
    trochlear — *see* Strabismus, paralytic, fourth nerve
    ulnar G56.2-
  normokalemic periodic G72.3
  ocular H49.9
    alternating G83.89
  oculofacial, congenital (Moebius) Q87.0
  oculomotor (external bilateral) (nerve) — *see* Strabismus, paralytic, third nerve
  palate (soft) K13.79
  paratrigeminal G50.9
  periodic (familial) (hyperkalemic) (hypokalemic) (myotonic) (normokalemic) (potassium sensitive) (secondary) G72.3
  peripheral autonomic nervous system — *see* Neuropathy, peripheral, autonomic
  peroneal (nerve) G57.3-
  pharynx J39.2
  phrenic nerve G56.8-
  plantar nerve (s) G57.6-
  pneumogastric nerve G52.2
  poliomyelitis (current) — *see* Poliomyelitis, paralytic
  popliteal nerve G57.3-
  postepileptic transitory G83.84
  progressive (atrophic) (bulbar) (spinal) G12.22
    general A52.17
    infantile acute — *see* Poliomyelitis, paralytic
    supranuclear G23.1
  pseudobulbar G12.29
  pseudohypertrophic (muscle) G71.0
  psychogenic F44.4
  quadriceps G57.9-
  quadriplegic — *see* Tetraplegia
  radial nerve G56.3-
  rectus muscle (eye) H49.9
  recurrent isolated sleep G47.53
  respiratory (muscle) (system) (tract) R06.81
    center NEC G93.89
    congenital P28.89
    newborn P28.89
  right side — *see* Hemiplegia
  saturnine — *see* subcategory T56.0
  sciatic nerve G57.0-
  senile G83.9
  shaking — *see* Parkinsonism
  shoulder G56.9-
  sleep, recurrent isolated G47.53
  spastic G83.9
    cerebral — *see* Palsy, cerebral, spastic
    congenital (cerebral) — *see* Palsy, cerebral, spastic
    familial G11.4
    hereditary G11.4
    quadriplegic G80.0
    syphilitic (spinal) A52.17
  sphincter, bladder — *see* Paralysis, bladder
  spinal (cord) G83.9
    accessory nerve G52.8
    acute — *see* Poliomyelitis, paralytic
    ascending acute G61.0
    atrophic (acute) — *see also* Poliomyelitis, paralytic
      spastic, syphilitic A52.17
    congenital NEC — *see* Palsy, cerebral
    infantile — *see* Poliomyelitis, paralytic
    hereditary G95.89
    progressive G12.21
    sequelae NEC G83.89
  sternomastoid G52.8
  stomach K31.84
    diabetic — *see* Diabetes, by type, with gastroparesis
    nerve G52.2
      diabetic — *see* Diabetes, by type, with gastroparesis
  stroke — *see* Infarct, brain
  subcapsularis G56.8-
  supranuclear (progressive) G23.1
  sympathetic G90.8
    cervical G90.09
    nervous system — *see* Neuropathy, peripheral, autonomic
  syndrome G83.9
    specified NEC G83.89

Paralysis, paralytic (complete) (incomplete) - *continued*
  syphilitic spastic spinal (Erb's) A52.17
  thigh G57.9-
  throat J39.2
    diphtheritic A36.0
    muscle J39.2
  thrombotic (current episode) I63.3-
  thumb G56.9-
  tick — *see* Toxicity, venom, arthropod, specified NEC
  Todd's (postepileptic transitory paralysis) G83.84
  toe G57.6-
  tongue K14.8
  transient R29.5
    arm or leg NEC R29.818
    traumatic NEC — *see* Injury, nerve
  trapezius G52.8
  traumatic, transient NEC — *see* Injury, nerve
  trembling — *see* Parkinsonism
  triceps brachii G56.9-
  trigeminal nerve G50.9
  trochlear (nerve) — *see* Strabismus, paralytic, fourth nerve
  ulnar nerve G56.2-
  upper limb — *see* Monoplegia, upper limb
  uremic N18.9 *[G99.8]*
  uveoparotitic D86.89
  uvula K13.79
    postdiphtheritic A36.0
  vagus nerve G52.2
  vasomotor NEC G90.8
  velum palati K13.79
  vesical — *see* Paralysis, bladder
  vestibular nerve (except Vertigo) — *see* subcategory H93.3
  vocal cords J38.00
    bilateral J38.02
    unilateral J38.01
  Volkmann's (complicating trauma) T79.6
  wasting G12.29
  Weber's G46.3
  wrist G56.9-
Paramedial urethrovesical orifice Q64.79
Paramenia N92.6
Parametritis — *see also* Disease, pelvis, inflammatory N73.2
  acute N73.0
  complicating abortion — *see* Abortion, by type, complicated by, parametritis
Parametrium, parametric — *see* condition
Paramnesia — *see* Amnesia
Paramolar K00.1
Paramyloidosis E85.8
Paramyoclonus multiplex G25.3
Paramyotonia (congenita) G71.19
Parangi — *see* Yaws
Paranoia (querulans) F22
  senile F03
Paranoid
  dementia (senile) F03
    praecox — *see* Schizophrenia
  personality F60.0
  psychosis (climacteric) (involutional) (menopausal) F22
    psychogenic (acute) F23
    senile F03
  reaction (acute) F23
    chronic F22
  schizophrenia F20.0
  state (climacteric) (involutional) (menopausal) (simple) F22
    senile F03
  tendencies F60.0
  traits F60.0
  trends F60.0
  type, psychopathic personality F60.0
Paraparesis — *see* Paraplegia
Paraphasia R47.02
Paraphilia F65.9
Paraphimosis (congenital) N47.2
  chancroidal A57
Paraphrenia, paraphrenic (late) F22
  schizophrenia F20.0
Paraplegia (lower) G82.20
  ataxic — *see* Degeneration, combined, spinal cord
  complete G82.21
  congenital (cerebral) G80.8
    spastic G80.1
  familial spastic G11.4
  functional (hysterical) F44.4
  hereditary, spastic G11.4
  hysterical F44.4

Paraplegia (lower) - *continued*
  incomplete G82.22
  Pott's A18.01
  psychogenic F44.4
  spastic
    Erb's spinal, syphilitic A52.17
    hereditary G11.4
    tropical G04.1
  syphilitic (spastic) A52.17
  tropical spastic G04.1
Parapoxvirus B08.60
  specified NEC B08.69
Paraproteinemia D89.2
  benign (familial) D89.2
  monoclonal D47.2
  secondary to malignant disease D47.2
Parapsoriasis L41.9
  en plaques L41.4
  guttata L41.1
  large plaque L41.4
  retiform, retiformis L41.5
  small plaque L41.3
  specified NEC L41.8
  varioliformis (acuta) L41.0
Parasitic — *see also* condition
  disease NEC B89
  stomatitis B37.0
  sycosis (beard) (scalp) B35.0
  twin Q89.4
Parasitism B89
  intestinal B82.9
  skin B88.9
  specified — *see* Infestation
Parasitophobia F40.218
Parasomnia G47.50
  due to
    alcohol
      abuse F10.182
      dependence F10.282
      use F10.982
    amphetamines
      abuse F15.182
      dependence F15.282
      use F15.982
    caffeine
      abuse F15.182
      dependence F15.282
      use F15.982
    cocaine
      abuse F14.182
      dependence F14.282
      use F14.982
    drug NEC
      abuse F19.182
      dependence F19.282
      use F19.982
    opioid
      abuse F11.182
      dependence F11.282
      use F11.982
    psychoactive substance NEC
      abuse F19.182
      dependence F19.282
      use F19.982
    sedative, hypnotic, or anxiolytic
      abuse F13.182
      dependence F13.282
      use F13.982
    stimulant NEC
      abuse F15.182
      dependence F15.282
      use F15.982
  in conditions classified elsewhere G47.54
  nonorganic origin F51.8
  organic G47.50
  specified NEC G47.59
Paraspadias Q54.9
Paraspasmus facialis G51.8
Parasuicide (attempt)
  history of (personal) Z91.5
    in family Z81.8
Parathyroid gland — *see* condition
Parathyroid tetany E20.9
Paratrachoma A74.0
Paratyphilitis — *see* Appendicitis
Paratyphoid (fever) — *see* Fever, paratyphoid
Paratyphus — *see* Fever, paratyphoid
Paraurethral duct Q64.79
  nonorganic origin F51.5
Paraurethritis — *see also* Urethritis
  gonococcal (acute) (chronic) (with abscess) A54.1
Paravaccinia NEC B08.04
Paravaginitis — *see* Vaginitis

Parencephalitis — *see also* Encephalitis
  sequelae G09
Parent-child conflict — *see* Conflict, parent-child
  estrangement NEC Z62.890
Paresis — *see also* Paralysis
  accommodation — *see* Paresis, of accommodation
  Bernhardt's G57.1-
  bladder (sphincter) — *see also* Paralysis, bladder
    tabetic A52.17
  bowel, colon or intestine K56.0
  extrinsic muscle, eye H49.9
  general (progressive) (syphilitic) A52.17
    juvenile A50.45
  heart — *see* Failure, heart
  insane (syphilitic) A52.17
  juvenile (general) A50.45
  of accommodation H52.52-
  peripheral progressive (idiopathic) G60.3
  pseudohypertrophic G71.0
  senile G83.9
  syphilitic (general) A52.17
    congenital A50.45
  vesical NEC N31.2
Paresthesia — *see also* Disturbance, sensation
  Bernhardt G57.1-
Paretic — *see* condition
Parinaud's
  conjunctivitis H10.89
  oculoglandular syndrome H10.89
  ophthalmoplegia H49.88-
Parkinsonism (idiopathic) (primary) G20
  with neurogenic orthostatic hypotension (symptomatic) G90.3
  arteriosclerotic G21.4
  dementia G31.83 *[F02.80]*
    with behavioral disturbance G31.83 *[F02.81]*
  due to
    drugs NEC G21.19
      neuroleptic G21.11
  neuroleptic induced G21.11
  postencephalitic G21.3
  secondary G21.9
    due to
      arteriosclerosis G21.4
      drugs NEC G21.19
        neuroleptic G21.11
      encephalitis G21.3
      external agents NEC G21.2
      syphilis A52.19
    specified NEC G21.8
  syphilitic A52.19
  treatment-induced NEC G21.19
  vascular G21.4
Parkinson's disease, syndrome or tremor — *see* Parkinsonism
Parodontitis — *see* Periodontitis
Parodontosis K05.4
Paronychia — *see also* Cellulitis, digit
  with lymphangitis — *see* Lymphangitis, acute, digit
  candidal (chronic) B37.2
  tuberculous (primary) A18.4
Parorexia (psychogenic) F50.89
Parosmia R43.1
  psychogenic F45.8
Parotid gland — *see* condition
Parotitis, parotiditis (allergic) (nonspecific toxic) (purulent) (septic) (suppurative) — *see also* Sialoadenitis
  epidemic — *see* Mumps
  infectious — *see* Mumps
  postoperative K91.89
  surgical K91.89
Parrot fever A70
Parrot's disease
  (early congenital syphilitic pseudoparalysis) A50.02
Parry-Romberg syndrome G51.8
Parry's disease or syndrome E05.00
  with thyroid storm E05.01
Pars planitis — *see* Cyclitis
Parsonage (-Aldren)-Turner syndrome G54.5
Parson's disease (exophthalmic goiter) E05.00
  with thyroid storm E05.01
Particolored infant Q82.8
Parturition — *see* Delivery
Parulis K04.7
  with sinus K04.6
Parvovirus, as cause of disease classified elsewhere B97.6
Pasini and Pierini's atrophoderma L90.3
Passage
  false, urethra N36.5
  meconium (newborn) during delivery P03.82

Passage - *continued*
  of sounds or bougies — *see* Attention to, artificial,
    opening
Passive — *see* condition
  smoking Z77.22
Pasteurella septica A28.0
Pasteurellosis — *see* Infection, Pasteurella
PAT (paroxysmal atrial tachycardia) I47.1
Patau's syndrome — *see* Trisomy, 13
Patches
  mucous (syphilitic) A51.39
    congenital A50.07
  smokers' (mouth) K13.24
Patellar — *see* condition
Patent — *see also* Imperfect, closure
  canal of Nuck Q52.4
  cervix N88.3
  ductus arteriosus or Botallo's Q25.0
  foramen
    botalli Q21.1
    ovale Q21.1
  interauricular septum Q21.1
  interventricular septum Q21.0
  omphalomesenteric duct Q43.0
  os (uteri) — *see* Patent, cervix
  ostium secundum Q21.1
  urachus Q64.4
  vitelline duct Q43.0
Paterson (-Brown) (-Kelly) **syndrome or web** D50.1
Pathologic, pathological — *see also* condition
  asphyxia R09.01
  fire-setting F63.1
  gambling F63.0
  ovum O02.0
  resorption, tooth K03.3
  stealing F63.2
Pathology (of) — *see* Disease
  periradicular, associated with previous endodontic
    treatment NEC M27.59
Pattern, sleep-wake, irregular G47.23
Patulous — *see also* Imperfect, closure (congenital)
  alimentary tract Q45.8
    lower Q43.8
    upper Q40.8
  eustachian tube H69.0-
Pause, sinoatrial I49.5
Paxton's disease B36.2
Pearl (s)
  enamel K00.2
  Epstein's K09.8
Pearl-worker's disease — *see* Osteomyelitis,
  specified type NEC
Pectenosis K62.4
Pectoral — *see* condition
Pectus
  carinatum (congenital) Q67.7
    acquired M95.4
    rachitic sequelae (late effect) E64.3
  excavatum (congenital) Q67.6
    acquired M95.4
    rachitic sequelae (late effect) E64.3
  recurvatum (congenital) Q67.6
Pedatrophia E41
Pederosis F65.4
Pediculosis (infestation) B85.2
  capitis (head-louse) (any site) B85.0
  corporis (body-louse) (any site) B85.1
  eyelid B85.0
  mixed (classifiable to more than one of the titles
    B85.0-B85.3) B85.4
  pubis (pubic louse) (any site) B85.3
  vestimenti B85.1
  vulvae B85.3
Pediculus (infestation) — *see* Pediculosis
Pedophilia F65.4
Peg-shaped teeth K00.2
Pelade — *see* Alopecia, areata
Pelger-Huët anomaly or syndrome D72.0
Peliosis (rheumatica) D69.0
  hepatis K76.4
    with toxic liver disease K71.8
Pelizaeus-Merzbacher disease E75.29
Pellagra (alcoholic) (with polyneuropathy) E52
**Pellagra-cerebellar-ataxia-renal aminoaciduria
  syndrome** E72.02
Pellegrini (-Stieda) **disease or syndrome** — *see*
  Bursitis, tibial collateral
Pellizzi's syndrome E34.8
Pel's crisis A52.11
Pelvic — *see also* condition
  examination (periodic) (routine) Z01.419
    with abnormal findings Z01.411
  kidney, congenital Q63.2

Pelviolithiasis — *see* Calculus, kidney
Pelviperitonitis — *see also* Peritonitis, pelvic
  gonococcal A54.24
  puerperal O85
Pelvis — *see* condition or type
Pemphigoid L12.9
  benign, mucous membrane L12.1
  bullous L12.0
  cicatricial L12.1
  juvenile L12.2
  ocular L12.1
  specified NEC L12.8
Pemphigus L10.9
  benign familial (chronic) Q82.8
  Brazilian L10.3
  circinatus L13.0
  conjunctiva L12.1
  drug-induced L10.5
  erythematosus L10.4
  foliaceus L10.2
  gangrenous — *see* Gangrene
  neonatorum L01.03
  ocular L12.1
  paraneoplastic L10.81
  specified NEC L10.89
  syphilitic (congenital) A50.06
  vegetans L10.1
  vulgaris L10.0
  wildfire L10.3
Pendred's syndrome E07.1
Pendulous
  abdomen, in pregnancy — *see* Pregnancy,
    complicated by, abnormal, pelvic organs or tissues
    NEC
  breast N64.89
Penetrating wound — *see also* Puncture
  with internal injury — *see* Injury, by site
  eyeball — *see* Puncture, eyeball
  orbit (with or without foreign body) — *see* Puncture,
    orbit
  uterus by instrument with or following ectopic or
    molar pregnancy O08.6
Penicillosis B48.4
Penis — *see* condition
Penitis N48.29
Pentalogy of Fallot Q21.8
Pentasomy X syndrome Q97.1
Pentosuria (essential) E74.8
Percreta placenta O43.23-
Peregrinating patient — *see* Disorder, factitious
Perforation, perforated (nontraumatic) (of)
  accidental during procedure (blood vessel) (nerve)
    (organ) — *see* Complication, accidental puncture
    or laceration
  antrum — *see* Sinusitis, maxillary
  appendix K35.2
    with localized peritonitis K35.3
  atrial septum, multiple Q21.1
  attic, ear — *see* Perforation, tympanum, attic
  bile duct (common) (hepatic) K83.2
    cystic K82.2
  bladder (urinary)
    with or following ectopic or molar
      pregnancy O08.6
    obstetrical trauma O71.5
    traumatic S37.29
      at delivery O71.5
  bowel K63.1
    with or following ectopic or molar
      pregnancy O08.6
    newborn P78.0
    obstetrical trauma O71.5
    traumatic — *see* Laceration, intestine
  broad ligament N83.8
    with or following ectopic or molar
      pregnancy O08.6
    obstetrical trauma O71.6
  by
    device, implant or graft — *see also* Complications,
      by site and type, mechanical T85.628
      arterial graft NEC — *see* Complication,
        cardiovascular device, mechanical, vascular
      breast (implant) T85.49
      catheter NEC T85.698
        cystostomy T83.090
        dialysis (renal) T82.49
          intraperitoneal T85.691
        infusion NEC T82.594
          spinal (epidural) (subdural) T85.690
        urinary — *see also* Complications, catheter,
          urinary T83.098
      electronic (electrode) (pulse generator)
        (stimulator)

Perforation, perforated (nontraumatic) (of) -
continued
  by - *continued*
    device, implant or graft - *continued*
      electronic (electrode) (pulse generator)
        (stimulator) - *continued*
        bone T84.390
        cardiac T82.199
          electrode T82.190
          pulse generator T82.191
          specified type NEC T82.198
        nervous system — *see* Complication, prosthetic
          device, mechanical, electronic nervous system
          stimulator
        urinary — *see* Complication, genitourinary,
          device, urinary, mechanical
      fixation, internal (orthopedic) NEC — *see*
        Complication, fixation device, mechanical
      gastrointestinal — *see* Complication, prosthetic
        device, mechanical, gastrointestinal device
      genital NEC T83.498
        intrauterine contraceptive device T83.39
        penile prosthesis T83.490
      heart NEC — *see* Complication, cardiovascular
        device, mechanical
      joint prosthesis — *see* Complications, joint
        prosthesis, mechanical, specified NEC, by site
      ocular NEC — *see* Complications, prosthetic
        device, mechanical, ocular device
      orthopedic NEC — *see* Complication, orthopedic,
        device, mechanical
      specified NEC T85.628
      urinary NEC — *see also* Complication,
        genitourinary, device, urinary, mechanical
        graft T83.29
      vascular NEC — *see* Complication,
        cardiovascular device, mechanical
      ventricular intracranial shunt T85.09
    foreign body left accidentally in operative
      wound T81.539
    instrument (any) during a procedure,
      accidental — *see* Puncture, accidental
      complicating surgery
  cecum K35.2
    with localized peritonitis K35.3
  cervix (uteri) N88.8
    with or following ectopic or molar
      pregnancy O08.6
    obstetrical trauma O71.3
  colon K63.1
    newborn P78.0
    obstetrical trauma O71.5
    traumatic — *see* Laceration, intestine, large
  common duct (bile) K83.2
  cornea (due to ulceration) — *see* Ulcer, cornea,
    perforated
  cystic duct K82.2
  diverticulum (intestine) K57.80
    with bleeding K57.81
    large intestine K57.20
      with
        bleeding K57.21
        small intestine K57.40
          with bleeding K57.41
    small intestine K57.00
      with
        bleeding K57.01
        large intestine K57.40
          with bleeding K57.41
  ear drum — *see* Perforation, tympanum
  esophagus K22.3
  ethmoidal sinus — *see* Sinusitis, ethmoidal
  frontal sinus — *see* Sinusitis, frontal
  gallbladder K82.2
  heart valve — *see* Endocarditis
  ileum K63.1
    newborn P78.0
    obstetrical trauma O71.5
    traumatic — *see* Laceration, intestine, small
  instrumental, surgical (accidental) (blood vessel)
    (nerve) (organ) — *see* Puncture, accidental
    complicating surgery
  intestine NEC K63.1
    with ectopic or molar pregnancy O08.6
    newborn P78.0
    obstetrical trauma O71.5
    traumatic — *see* Laceration, intestine
    ulcerative NEC K63.1
      newborn P78.0
  jejunum, jejunal K63.1
    obstetrical trauma O71.5
    traumatic — *see* Laceration, intestine, small
  ulcer — *see* Ulcer, gastrojejunal, with perforation

Perforation, perforated (nontraumatic) (of) - *continued*
  joint prosthesis — *see* Complications, joint
    prosthesis, mechanical, specified NEC, by site
  mastoid (antrum) (cell) — *see* Disorder, mastoid,
    specified NEC
  maxillary sinus — *see* Sinusitis, maxillary
  membrana tympani — *see* Perforation, tympanum
  nasal
    septum J34.89
      congenital Q30.3
      syphilitic A52.73
    sinus J34.89
      congenital Q30.8
      due to sinusitis — *see* Sinusitis
  palate — *see also* Cleft, palate Q35.9
    syphilitic A52.79
  palatine vault — *see also* Cleft, palate, hard Q35.1
    syphilitic A52.79
      congenital A50.59
  pars flaccida (ear drum) — *see* Perforation,
    tympanum, attic
  pelvic
    floor S31.030
      with
        ectopic or molar pregnancy O08.6
        penetration into retroperitoneal space S31.031
        retained foreign body S31.040
          with penetration into retroperitoneal
            space S31.041
      following ectopic or molar pregnancy O08.6
      obstetrical trauma O70.1
    organ S37.99
      adrenal gland S37.818
      bladder — *see* Perforation, bladder
      fallopian tube S37.599
        bilateral S37.592
        unilateral S37.591
      kidney S37.09-
        obstetrical trauma O71.5
      ovary S37.499
        bilateral S37.492
        unilateral S37.491
      prostate S37.828
      specified organ NEC S37.898
      ureter — *see* Perforation, ureter
      urethra — *see* Perforation, urethra
      uterus — *see* Perforation, uterus
  perineum — *see* Laceration, perineum
  pharynx J39.2
  rectum K63.1
    newborn P78.0
    obstetrical trauma O71.5
    traumatic S36.63
  root canal space due to endodontic
    treatment M27.51
  sigmoid K63.1
    newborn P78.0
    obstetrical trauma O71.5
    traumatic S36.533
  sinus (accessory) (chronic) (nasal) J34.89
  sphenoidal sinus — *see* Sinusitis, sphenoidal
  surgical (accidental) (by instrument) (blood vessel)
    (nerve) (organ) — *see* Puncture, accidental
    complicating surgery
  traumatic
    external — *see* Puncture
    eye — *see* Puncture, eyeball
    internal organ — *see* Injury, by site
  tympanum, tympanic (membrane) (persistent post-
    traumatic) (postinflammatory) H72.9-
    attic H72.1-
      multiple — *see* Perforation, tympanum, multiple
      total — *see* Perforation, tympanum, total
    central H72.0-
      multiple — *see* Perforation, tympanum, multiple
      total — *see* Perforation, tympanum, total
    marginal NEC — *see* subcategory H72.2
    multiple H72.81-
    pars flaccida — *see* Perforation, tympanum, attic
    total H72.82-
    traumatic, current episode S09.2-
  typhoid, gastrointestinal — *see* Typhoid
  ulcer — *see* Ulcer, by site, with perforation
  ureter N28.89
    traumatic S37.19
  urethra N36.8
    with ectopic or molar pregnancy O08.6
    following ectopic or molar pregnancy O08.6
    obstetrical trauma O71.5
    traumatic S37.39
      at delivery O71.5
  uterus

Perforation, perforated (nontraumatic) (of) - *continued*
  uterus - *continued*
    with ectopic or molar pregnancy O08.6
    by intrauterine contraceptive device T83.39
    following ectopic or molar pregnancy O08.6
    obstetrical trauma O71.1
    traumatic S37.69
      obstetric O71.1
  uvula K13.79
    syphilitic A52.79
  vagina
    obstetrical trauma O71.4
    other trauma — *see* Puncture, vagina
Periadenitis mucosa necrotica recurrens K12.0
Periappendicitis (acute) — *see* Appendicitis
Periarteritis nodosa (disseminated) (infectious)
  (necrotizing) M30.0
Periarthritis (joint) — *see also* Enthesopathy
  Duplay's M75.0-
  gonococcal A54.42
  humeroscapularis — *see* Capsulitis, adhesive
  scapulohumeral — *see* Capsulitis, adhesive
  shoulder — *see* Capsulitis, adhesive
  wrist M77.2-
Periarthrosis (angioneural) — *see* Enthesopathy
Pericapsulitis, adhesive (shoulder) — *see* Capsulitis,
  adhesive
Pericarditis (with decompensation) (with
  effusion) I31.9
  with rheumatic fever (conditions in I00)
    active — *see* Pericarditis, rheumatic
    inactive or quiescent I09.2
  acute (hemorrhagic) (nonrheumatic) (Sicca) I30.9
    with chorea (acute) (rheumatic)
      (Sydenham's) I02.0
  benign I30.8
  nonspecific I30.0
  rheumatic I01.0
    with chorea (acute) (Sydenham's) I02.0
  adhesive or adherent (chronic) (external)
    (internal) I31.0
    acute — *see* Pericarditis, acute
    rheumatic I09.2
  bacterial (acute) (subacute) (with serous or
    seropurulent effusion) I30.1
  calcareous I31.1
  cholesterol (chronic) I31.8
    acute I30.9
  chronic (nonrheumatic) I31.9
    rheumatic I09.2
  constrictive (chronic) I31.1
  coxsackie B33.23
  fibrinocaseous (tuberculous) A18.84
  fibrinopurulent I30.1
  fibrinous I30.8
  fibrous I31.0
  gonococcal A54.83
  idiopathic I30.0
  in systemic lupus erythematosus M32.12
  infective I30.1
  meningococcal A39.53
  neoplastic (chronic) I31.8
    acute I30.9
  obliterans, obliterating I31.0
  plastic I31.0
  pneumococcal I30.1
  postinfarction I24.1
  purulent I30.1
  rheumatic (active) (acute) (with effusion) (with
    pneumonia) I01.0
    with chorea (acute) (rheumatic)
      (Sydenham's) I02.0
    chronic or inactive (with chorea) I09.2
  rheumatoid — *see* Rheumatoid, carditis
  septic I30.1
  serofibrinous I30.8
  staphylococcal I30.1
  streptococcal I30.1
  suppurative I30.1
  syphilitic A52.06
  tuberculous A18.84
  uremic N18.9 *[I32]*
  viral I30.1
Pericardium, pericardial — *see* condition
Pericellulitis — *see* Cellulitis
Pericementitis (chronic) (suppurative) — *see
  also* Periodontitis
  acute K05.20
    generalized — *see* Periodontitis, aggressive,
      generalized
    localized — *see* Peridontitis, aggressive, localized

Perichondritis
  auricle — *see* Perichondritis, ear
  bronchus J98.09
  ear (external) H61.00-
    acute H61.01-
    chronic H61.02-
  external auditory canal — *see* Perichondritis, ear
  larynx J38.7
    syphilitic A52.73
    typhoid A01.09
  nose J34.89
  pinna — *see* Perichondritis, ear
  trachea J39.8
Periclasia K05.4
Pericoronitis — *see* Periodontitis
Pericystitis N30.90
  with hematuria N30.91
Peridiverticulitis (intestine) K57.92
  cecum — *see* Diverticulitis, intestine, large
  colon — *see* Diverticulitis, intestine, large
  duodenum — *see* Diverticulitis, intestine, small
  intestine — *see* Diverticulitis, intestine
  jejunum — *see* Diverticulitis, intestine, small
  rectosigmoid — *see* Diverticulitis, intestine, large
  rectum — *see* Diverticulitis, intestine, large
  sigmoid — *see* Diverticulitis, intestine, large
Periendocarditis — *see* Endocarditis
Periepididymitis N45.1
Perifolliculitis L01.02
  abscedens, caput, scalp L66.3
  capitis, abscedens (et suffodiens) L66.3
  superficial pustular L01.02
Perihepatitis K65.8
Perilabyrinthitis (acute) — *see* subcategory H83.0
Perimeningitis — *see* Meningitis
Perimetritis — *see* Endometritis
Perimetrosalpingitis — *see* Salpingo-oophoritis
Perineocele N81.81
Perinephric, perinephritic — *see* condition
Perinephritis — *see also* Infection, kidney
  purulent — *see* Abscess, kidney
Perineum, perineal — *see* condition
Perineuritis NEC — *see* Neuralgia
Periodic — *see* condition
Periodontitis (chronic) (complex) (compound) (local)
  (simplex) K05.30
  acute K05.20
    generalized K05.229
      moderate K05.222
      severe K05.223
      slight K05.221
    localized K05.219
      moderate K05.212
      severe K05.213
      slight K05.211
  apical K04.5
    acute (pulpal origin) K04.4
  generalized K05.329
    moderate K05.322
    severe K05.323
    slight K05.321
  localized K05.319
    moderate K05.312
    severe K05.313
    slight K05.311
Periodontoclasia K05.4
Periodontosis (juvenile) K05.4
Periods — *see also* Menstruation
  heavy N92.0
  irregular N92.6
  shortened intervals (irregular) N92.1
Perionychia — *see also* Cellulitis, digit
  with lymphangitis — *see* Lymphangitis, acute, digit
Perioophoritis — *see* Salpingo-oophoritis
Periorchitis N45.2
Periosteum, periosteal — *see* condition
Periostitis (albuminosa) (circumscribed) (diffuse)
  (infective) (monomelic) — *see also* Osteomyelitis
  alveolar M27.3
  alveolodental M27.3
  dental M27.3
  gonorrheal A54.43
  jaw (lower) (upper) M27.2
  orbit H05.03-
  syphilitic A52.77
    congenital (early) A50.02 *[M90.80]*
    secondary A51.46
  tuberculous — *see* Tuberculosis, bone
  yaws (hypertrophic) (early) (late) A66.6 *[M90.80]*
Periostosis (hyperplastic) — *see also* Disorder, bone,
  specified type NEC
  with osteomyelitis — *see* Osteomyelitis, specified
    type NEC

Peripartum
  cardiomyopathy O90.3
Periphlebitis — *see* Phlebitis
Periproctitis K62.89
Periprostatitis — *see* Prostatitis
Perirectal — *see* condition
Perirenal — *see* condition
Perisalpingitis — *see* Salpingo-oophoritis
Perisplenitis (infectional) D73.89
Peristalsis, visible or reversed R19.2
Peritendinitis — *see* Enthesopathy
Peritoneum, peritoneal — *see* condition
Peritonitis (adhesive) (bacterial) (fibrinous)
    (hemorrhagic) (idiopathic) (localized) (perforative)
    (primary) (with adhesions) (with effusion) K65.9
  with or following
    abscess K65.1
    appendicitis K35.3
      with perforation or rupture K35.2
      generalized K35.2
      localized K35.3
    diverticular disease (intestine) K57.80
      with bleeding K57.81
      large intestine K57.20
        with
          bleeding K57.21
          small intestine K57.40
            with bleeding K57.41
      small intestine K57.00
        with
          bleeding K57.01
          large intestine K57.40
            with bleeding K57.41
    ectopic or molar pregnancy O08.0
  acute (generalized) K65.0
  aseptic T81.61
  bile, biliary K65.3
  chemical T81.61
  chlamydial A74.81
  complicating abortion — *see* Abortion, by type,
    complicated by, pelvic peritonitis
  congenital P78.1
  chronic proliferative K65.8
  diaphragmatic K65.0
  diffuse K65.0
  diphtheritic A36.89
  disseminated K65.0
  due to
    bile K65.3
    foreign
      body or object accidentally left during a
        procedure (instrument) (sponge)
        (swab) T81.599
      substance accidentally left during a procedure
        (chemical) (powder) (talc) T81.61
    talc T81.61
    urine K65.8
  eosinophilic K65.8
    acute K65.0
  fibrocaseous (tuberculous) A18.31
  fibropurulent K65.0
  following ectopic or molar pregnancy O08.0
  general (ized) K65.0
  gonococcal A54.85
  meconium (newborn) P78.0
  neonatal P78.1
    meconium P78.0
  pancreatic K65.0
  paroxysmal, familial E85.0
    benign E85.0
  pelvic
    female N73.5
      acute N73.3
      chronic N73.4
        with adhesions N73.6
    male K65.0
  periodic, familial E85.0
  proliferative, chronic K65.8
  puerperal, postpartum, childbirth O85
  purulent K65.0
  septic K65.0
  specified NEC K65.8
  spontaneous bacterial K65.2
  subdiaphragmatic K65.0
  subphrenic K65.0
  suppurative K65.0
  syphilitic A52.74
    congenital (early) A50.08 *[K67]*
  talc T81.61
  tuberculous A18.31
  urine K65.8
Peritonsillar — *see* condition
Peritonsillitis J36

Perityphlitis K37
Periureteritis N28.89
Periurethral — *see* condition
Periurethritis (gangrenous) — *see* Urethritis
Periuterine — *see* condition
Perivaginitis — *see* Vaginitis
Perivasculitis, retinal H35.06-
Perivasitis (chronic) N49.1
Perivesiculitis (seminal) — *see* Vesiculitis
Perlèche NEC K13.0
  due to
    candidiasis B37.83
    moniliasis B37.83
    riboflavin deficiency E53.0
    vitamin B2 (riboflavin) deficiency E53.0
Pernicious — *see* condition
Pernio, perniosis T69.1
Perpetrator (of abuse) — *see* Index to External
    Causes of Injury, Perpetrator
Persecution
  delusion F22
  social Z60.5
Perseveration (tonic) R48.8
Persistence, persistent (congenital)
  anal membrane Q42.3
    with fistula Q42.2
  arteria stapedia Q16.3
  atrioventricular canal Q21.2
  branchial cleft Q18.0
  bulbus cordis in left ventricle Q21.8
  canal of Cloquet Q14.0
  capsule (opaque) Q12.8
  ciliaretinal artery or vein Q14.8
  cloaca Q43.7
  communication — *see* Fistula, congenital
  convolutions
    aortic arch Q25.46
    fallopian tube Q50.6
    oviduct Q50.6
    uterine tube Q50.6
  double aortic arch Q25.45
  ductus arteriosus (Botalli) Q25.0
  fetal
    circulation P29.3
    form of cervix (uteri) Q51.828
    hemoglobin, hereditary (HPFH) D56.4
  foramen
    Botalli Q21.1
    ovale Q21.1
  Gartner's duct Q52.4
  hemoglobin, fetal (hereditary) (HPFH) D56.4
  hyaloid
    artery (generally incomplete) Q14.0
    system Q14.8
  hymen, in pregnancy or childbirth — *see* Pregnancy,
    complicated by, abnormal, vulva
  lanugo Q84.2
  left
    posterior cardinal vein Q26.8
    root with right arch of aorta Q25.49
    superior vena cava Q26.1
  Meckel's diverticulum Q43.0
    malignant — *see* Table of Neoplasms, small
      intestine, malignant
  mucosal disease (middle ear) — *see* Otitis, media,
    suppurative, chronic, tubotympanic
  nail (s) , anomalous Q84.6
  omphalomesenteric duct Q43.0
  organ or site not listed — *see* Anomaly, by site
  ostium
    atrioventriculare commune Q21.2
    primum Q21.2
    secundum Q21.1
  ovarian rests in fallopian tube Q50.6
  pancreatic tissue in intestinal tract Q43.8
  primary (deciduous)
    teeth K00.6
    vitreous hyperplasia Q14.0
  pupillary membrane Q13.89
  right aortic arch Q25.47
  rhesus (Rh) titer — *see* Complication(s), transfusion,
    incompatibility reaction, Rh (factor)
  sinus
    urogenitalis
      female Q52.8
      male Q55.8
    venosus with imperfect incorporation in right
      auricle Q26.8
  thymus (gland) (hyperplasia) E32.0
  thyroglossal duct Q89.2
  thyrolingual duct Q89.2
  truncus arteriosus or communis Q20.0
  tunica vasculosa lentis Q12.2

Persistence, persistent (congenital) - *continued*
  umbilical sinus Q64.4
  urachus Q64.4
  vitelline duct Q43.0
Person (with)
  admitted for clinical research, as a control subject
    (normal comparison) (participant) Z00.6
  awaiting admission to adequate facility
    elsewhere Z75.1
  concern (normal) about sick person in family Z63.6
  consulting on behalf of another Z71.0
  feigning illness Z76.5
  living (in)
    alone Z60.2
    boarding school Z59.3
    residential institution Z59.3
    without
      adequate housing (heating) (space) Z59.1
      housing (permanent) (temporary) Z59.0
      person able to render necessary care Z74.2
      shelter Z59.0
  on waiting list Z75.1
  sick or handicapped in family Z63.6
Personality (disorder) F60.9
  accentuation of traits (type A pattern) Z73.1
  affective F34.0
  aggressive F60.3
  amoral F60.2
  anacastic, anankastic F60.5
  antisocial F60.2
  anxious F60.6
  asocial F60.2
  asthenic F60.7
  avoidant F60.6
  borderline F60.3
  change due to organic condition (enduring) F07.0
  compulsive F60.5
  cycloid F34.0
  cyclothymic F34.0
  dependent F60.7
  depressive F34.1
  dissocial F60.2
  dual F44.81
  eccentric F60.89
  emotionally unstable F60.3
  expansive paranoid F60.0
  explosive F60.3
  fanatic F60.0
  haltose type F60.89
  histrionic F60.4
  hyperthymic F34.0
  hypothymic F34.1
  hysterical F60.4
  immature F60.89
  inadequate F60.7
  labile (emotional) F60.3
  mixed (nonspecific) F60.89
  morally defective F60.2
  multiple F44.81
  narcissistic F60.81
  obsessional F60.5
  obsessive (-compulsive) F60.5
  organic F07.0
  overconscientious F60.5
  paranoid F60.0
  passive (-dependent) F60.7
  passive-aggressive F60.89
  pathologic F60.9
  pattern defect or disturbance F60.9
  pseudopsychopathic (organic) F07.0
  pseudoretarded (organic) F07.0
  psychoinfantile F60.4
  psychoneurotic NEC F60.89
  psychopathic F60.2
  querulant F60.0
  sadistic F60.89
  schizoid F60.1
  self-defeating F60.7
  sensitive paranoid F60.0
  sociopathic (amoral) (antisocial) (asocial)
    (dissocial) F60.2
  specified NEC F60.89
  type A Z73.1
  unstable (emotional) F60.3
Perthes' disease — *see* Legg-Calvé-Perthes disease
Pertussis — *see also* Whooping cough A37.90
Perversion, perverted
  appetite F50.89
    psychogenic F50.89
  function
    pituitary gland E23.2
      posterior lobe E22.2
  sense of smell and taste R43.8

Perversion, perverted - *continued*
  sense of smell and taste - *continued*
    psychogenic F45.8
  sexual — *see* Deviation, sexual
Pervious, congenital — *see also* Imperfect, closure
  ductus arteriosus Q25.0
Pes (congenital) — *see also* Talipes
  acquired — *see also* Deformity, limb, foot, specified NEC
    planus — *see* Deformity, limb, flat foot
  adductus Q66.89
  cavus Q66.7
  deformity NEC, acquired — *see* Deformity, limb, foot, specified NEC
  planus (acquired) (any degree) — *see also* Deformity, limb, flat foot
    rachitic sequelae (late effect) E64.3
  valgus Q66.6
Pest, pestis — *see* Plague
Petechia, petechiae R23.3
  newborn P54.5
Petechial typhus A75.9
Peter's anomaly Q13.4
Petit mal seizure — *see* Epilepsy, generalized, specified NEC
Petit's hernia — *see* Hernia, abdomen, specified site NEC
Petrellidosis B48.2
Petrositis H70.20-
  acute H70.21-
  chronic H70.22-
Peutz-Jeghers disease or syndrome Q85.8
Peyronie's disease N48.6
PFAPA
  (periodic fever, aphthous stomatitis, pharyngitis, and adenopathy syndrome) M04.8
Pfeiffer's disease — *see* Mononucleosis, infectious
Phagedena (dry) (moist) (sloughing) — *see also* Gangrene
  geometric L88
  penis N48.29
  tropical — *see* Ulcer, skin
  vulva N76.6
Phagedenic — *see* condition
Phakoma H35.89
Phakomatosis — *see also* specific eponymous syndromes Q85.9
  Bourneville's Q85.1
  specified NEC Q85.8
Phantom limb syndrome (without pain) G54.7
  with pain G54.6
Pharyngeal pouch syndrome D82.1
Pharyngitis (acute) (catarrhal) (gangrenous) (infective) (malignant) (membranous) (phlegmonous) (pseudomembranous) (simple) (subacute) (suppurative) (ulcerative) (viral) J02.9
  with influenza, flu, or grippe — *see* Influenza, with, pharyngitis
  aphthous B08.5
  atrophic J31.2
  chlamydial A56.4
  chronic (atrophic) (granular) (hypertrophic) J31.2
  coxsackievirus B08.5
  diphtheritic A36.0
  enteroviral vesicular B08.5
  follicular (chronic) J31.2
  fusospirochetal A69.1
  gonococcal A54.5
  granular (chronic) J31.2
  herpesviral B00.2
  hypertrophic J31.2
  infectional, chronic J31.2
  influenzal — *see* Influenza, with, respiratory manifestations NEC
  lymphonodular, acute (enteroviral) B08.8
  pneumococcal J02.8
  purulent J02.9
  putrid J02.9
  septic J02.0
  sicca J31.2
  specified organism NEC J02.8
  staphylococcal J02.8
  streptococcal J02.0
  syphilitic, congenital (early) A50.03
  tuberculous A15.8
  vesicular, enteroviral B08.5
  viral NEC J02.8
Pharyngoconjunctivitis, viral B30.2
Pharyngolaryngitis (acute) J06.0
  chronic J37.0
Pharyngoplegia J39.2
Pharyngotonsillitis, herpesviral B00.2
Pharyngotracheitis, chronic J42

Pharynx, pharyngeal — *see* condition
Phencyclidine-induced
  anxiety disorder F16.980
  bipolar and related disorder F16.94
  depressive disorder F16.94
  psychotic disorder F16.959
Phenomenon
  Arthus' — *see* Arthus' phenomenon
  jaw-winking Q07.8
  lupus erythematosus (LE) cell M32.9
  Raynaud's (secondary) I73.00
    with gangrene I73.01
  vasomotor R55
  vasospastic I73.9
  vasovagal R55
  Wenckebach's I44.1
Phenylketonuria E70.1
  classical E70.0
  maternal E70.1
Pheochromoblastoma
  specified site — *see* Neoplasm, malignant, by site
  unspecified site C74.10
Pheochromocytoma
  malignant
    specified site — *see* Neoplasm, malignant, by site
    unspecified site C74.10
  specified site — *see* Neoplasm, benign, by site
  unspecified site D35.00
Pheohyphomycosis — *see* Chromomycosis
Pheomycosis — *see* Chromomycosis
Phimosis (congenital) (due to infection) N47.1
  chancroidal A57
Phlebectasia — *see also* Varix
  congenital Q27.4
Phlebitis (infective) (pyemic) (septic) (suppurative) I80.9
  antepartum — *see* Thrombophlebitis, antepartum
  blue — *see* Phlebitis, leg, deep
  breast, superficial I80.8
  cavernous (venous) sinus — *see* Phlebitis, intracranial (venous) sinus
  cerebral (venous) sinus — *see* Phlebitis, intracranial (venous) sinus
  chest wall, superficial I80.8
  cranial (venous) sinus — *see* Phlebitis, intracranial (venous) sinus
  deep (vessels) — *see* Phlebitis, leg, deep
  due to implanted device — *see* Complications, by site and type, specified NEC
  during or resulting from a procedure T81.72
  femoral vein (superficial) I80.1-
  femoropopliteal vein I80.0-
  gestational — *see* Phlebopathy, gestational
  hepatic veins I80.8
  iliofemoral — *see* Phlebitis, femoral vein
  intracranial (venous) sinus (any) G08
    nonpyogenic I67.6
  intraspinal venous sinuses and veins G08
    nonpyogenic G95.19
  lateral (venous) sinus — *see* Phlebitis, intracranial (venous) sinus
  leg I80.3
    antepartum — *see* Thrombophlebitis, antepartum
    deep (vessels) NEC I80.20-
      iliac I80.21-
      popliteal vein I80.22-
      specified vessel NEC I80.29-
      tibial vein I80.23-
    femoral vein (superficial) I80.1-
    superficial (vessels) I80.0-
  longitudinal sinus — *see* Phlebitis, intracranial (venous) sinus
  lower limb — *see* Phlebitis, leg
  migrans, migrating (superficial) I82.1
  pelvic
    with ectopic or molar pregnancy O08.0
    following ectopic or molar pregnancy O08.0
    puerperal, postpartum O87.1
  popliteal vein — *see* Phlebitis, leg, deep, popliteal
  portal (vein) K75.1
  postoperative T81.72
  pregnancy — *see* Thrombophlebitis, antepartum
  puerperal, postpartum, childbirth O87.0
    deep O87.1
    pelvic O87.1
    superficial O87.0
  retina — *see* Vasculitis, retina
  saphenous (accessory) (great) (long) (small) — *see* Phlebitis, leg, superficial
  sinus (meninges) — *see* Phlebitis, intracranial (venous) sinus
  specified site NEC I80.8
  syphilitic A52.09

Phlebitis (infective) (pyemic) (septic) (suppurative) - *continued*
  tibial vein — *see* Phlebitis, leg, deep, tibial
  ulcerative I80.9
    leg — *see* Phlebitis, leg
  umbilicus I80.8
  uterus (septic) — *see* Endometritis
  varicose (leg) (lower limb) — *see* Varix, leg, with, inflammation
Phlebofibrosis I87.8
Phleboliths I87.8
Phlebopathy,
  gestational O22.9-
  puerperal O87.9
Phlebosclerosis I87.8
Phlebothrombosis — *see also* Thrombosis
  antepartum — *see* Thrombophlebitis, antepartum
  pregnancy — *see* Thrombophlebitis, antepartum
  puerperal — *see* Thrombophlebitis, puerperal
Phlebotomus fever A93.1
Phlegmasia
  alba dolens O87.1
    nonpuerperal — *see* Phlebitis, femoral vein
  cerulea dolens — *see* Phlebitis, leg, deep
Phlegmon — *see* Abscess
Phlegmonous — *see* condition
Phlyctenulosis (allergic) (keratoconjunctivitis) (nontuberculous) — *see also* Keratoconjunctivitis
  cornea — *see* Keratoconjunctivitis
  tuberculous A18.52
Phobia, phobic F40.9
  animal F40.218
    spiders F40.210
  examination F40.298
  reaction F40.9
  simple F40.298
  social F40.10
    generalized F40.11
  specific (isolated) F40.298
    animal F40.218
      spiders F40.210
    blood F40.230
    injection F40.231
    injury F40.233
    men F40.290
    natural environment F40.228
      thunderstorms F40.220
    situational F40.248
      bridges F40.242
      closed in spaces F40.240
      flying F40.243
      heights F40.241
    specified focus NEC F40.298
    transfusion F40.231
    women F40.291
  specified NEC F40.8
    medical care NEC F40.232
  state F40.9
Phocas' disease — *see* Mastopathy, cystic
Phocomelia Q73.1
  lower limb — *see* Agenesis, leg, with foot present
  upper limb — *see* Agenesis, arm, with hand present
Phoria H50.50
Phosphate-losing tubular disorder N25.0
Phosphatemia E83.39
Phosphaturia E83.39
Photodermatitis (sun) L56.8
  chronic L57.8
  due to drug L56.8
  light other than sun L59.8
Photokeratitis H16.13-
Photophobia H53.14-
Photophthalmia — *see* Photokeratitis
Photopsia H53.19
Photoretinitis — *see* Retinopathy, solar
Photosensitivity, photosensitization (sun)
  skin L56.8
  light other than sun L59.8
Phrenitis — *see* Encephalitis
Phrynoderma (vitamin A deficiency) E50.8
Phthiriasis (pubis) B85.3
  with any infestation classifiable to B85.0-B85.2 B85.4
Phthirus infestation — *see* Phthiriasis
Phthisis — *see also* Tuberculosis
  bulbi (infectional) — *see* Disorder, globe, degenerated condition, atrophy
  eyeball (due to infection) — *see* Disorder, globe, degenerated condition, atrophy
Phycomycosis — *see* Zygomycosis
Physalopteriasis B81.8
Physical restraint status Z78.1

Phytobezoar T18.9
  intestine T18.3
  stomach T18.2
Pian — *see* Yaws
Pianoma A66.1
Pica F50.89
  in adults F50.89
  infant or child F98.3
Picking, nose F98.8
Pick-Niemann disease — *see* Niemann-Pick disease
    or syndrome
Pick's
  cerebral atrophy G31.01 *[F02.80]*
    with behavioral disturbance G31.01 *[F02.81]*
  disease or syndrome (brain) G31.01 *[F02.80]*
    with behavioral disturbance G31.01 *[F02.81]*
      brain G31.01 *[F02.80]*
        with behavioral disturbance G31.01 *[F02.81]*
      pericardium (pericardial pseudocirrhosis of
          liver) I31.1
  syndrome
    brain G31.01 *[F02.80]*
      with behavioral disturbance G31.01 *[F02.81]*
    of heart (pericardial pseudocirrhosis of liver) I31.1
Pickwickian syndrome E66.2
Piebaldism E70.39
Piedra (beard) (scalp) B36.8
  black B36.3
  white B36.2
Pierre Robin deformity or syndrome Q87.0
Pierson's disease or osteochondrosis M91.0
Pig-bel A05.2
Pigeon
  breast or chest (acquired) M95.4
    congenital Q67.7
    rachitic sequelae (late effect) E64.3
  breeder's disease or lung J67.2
  fancier's disease or lung J67.2
  toe — *see* Deformity, toe, specified NEC
Pigmentation (abnormal) (anomaly) L81.9
  conjunctiva H11.13-
  cornea (anterior) H18.01-
    posterior H18.05-
    stromal H18.06-
  diminished melanin formation NEC L81.6
  iron L81.8
  lids, congenital Q82.8
  limbus corneae — *see* Pigmentation, cornea
  metals L81.8
  optic papilla, congenital Q14.2
  retina, congenital (grouped) (nevoid) Q14.1
  scrotum, congenital Q82.8
  tattoo L81.8
Piles — *see also* Hemorrhoids K64.9
Pili
  annulati or torti (congenital) Q84.1
  incarnati L73.1
Pill roller hand (intrinsic) — *see* Parkinsonism
Pilomatrixoma — *see* Neoplasm, skin, benign
  malignant — *see* Neoplasm, skin, malignant
Pilonidal — *see* condition
Pimple R23.8
PIN — *see* Neoplasia, intraepithelial, prostate
Pinched nerve — *see* Neuropathy, entrapment
Pindborg tumor — *see* Cyst, calcifying odontogenic
Pineal body or gland — *see* condition
Pinealoblastoma C75.3
Pinealoma D44.5
  malignant C75.3
Pineoblastoma C75.3
Pineocytoma D44.5
Pinguecula H11.15-
Pingueculitis H10.81-
Pinhole meatus — *see also* Stricture, urethra N35.9
Pink
  disease — *see* subcategory T56.1
  eye — *see* Conjunctivitis, acute, mucopurulent
Pinkus' disease (lichen nitidus) L44.1
Pinpoint
  meatus — *see* Stricture, urethra
  os (uteri) — *see* Stricture, cervix
Pins and needles R20.2
Pinta A67.9
  cardiovascular lesions A67.2
  chancre (primary) A67.0
  erythematous plaques A67.1
  hyperchromic lesions A67.1
  hyperkeratosis A67.1
  lesions A67.9
    cardiovascular A67.2
    hyperchromic A67.1
    intermediate A67.1
    late A67.2

Pinta - *continued*
  lesions - *continued*
    mixed A67.3
    primary A67.0
    skin (achromic) (cicatricial) (dyschromic) A67.2
      hyperchromic A67.1
      mixed (achromic and hyperchromic) A67.3
    papule (primary) A67.0
    skin lesions (achromic) (cicatricial)
        (dyschromic) A67.2
      hyperchromic A67.1
      mixed (achromic and hyperchromic) A67.3
    vitiligo A67.2
Pintids A67.1
Pinworm (disease) (infection) (infestation) B80
Piroplasmosis B60.0
Pistol wound — *see* Gunshot wound
Pitchers' elbow — *see* Derangement, joint, specified
    type NEC, elbow
Pithecoid pelvis Q74.2
  with disproportion (fetopelvic) O33.0
    causing obstructed labor O65.0
Pithiatism F48.8
Pitted — *see* Pitting
Pitting — *see also* Edema R60.9
  lip R60.0
  nail L60.8
  teeth K00.4
Pituitary gland — *see* condition
Pituitary-snuff-taker's disease J67.8
Pityriasis (capitis) L21.0
  alba L30.5
  circinata (et maculata) L42
  furfuracea L21.0
  Hebra's L26
  lichenoides L41.0
    chronica L41.1
    et varioliformis (acuta) L41.0
  maculata (et circinata) L30.5
  nigra B36.1
  pilaris, Hebra's L44.0
  rosea L42
  rotunda L44.8
  rubra (Hebra) pilaris L44.0
  simplex L30.5
  specified type NEC L30.5
  streptogenes L30.5
  versicolor (scrotal) B36.0
Placenta, placental — *see* Pregnancy, complicated by
    (care of) (management affected by), specified
    condition
Placentitis O41.14-
Plagiocephaly Q67.3
Plague A20.9
  abortive A20.8
  ambulatory A20.8
  asymptomatic A20.8
  bubonic A20.0
  cellulocutaneous A20.1
  cutaneobubonic A20.1
  lymphatic gland A20.0
  meningitis A20.3
  pharyngeal A20.8
  pneumonic (primary) (secondary) A20.2
  pulmonary, pulmonic A20.2
  septicemic A20.7
  tonsillar A20.8
    septicemic A20.7
Planning, family
  contraception Z30.9
  procreation Z31.69
Plaque (s)
  artery, arterial — *see* Arteriosclerosis
  calcareous — *see* Calcification
  coronary, lipid rich I25.83
  epicardial I31.8
  erythematous, of pinta A67.1
  Hollenhorst's — *see* Occlusion, artery, retina
  lipid rich, coronary I25.83
  pleural (without asbestos) J92.9
    with asbestos J92.0
  tongue K13.29
Plasmacytoma C90.3-
  extramedullary C90.2-
  medullary C90.0-
  solitary C90.3-
Plasmacytopenia D72.818
Plasmacytosis D72.822
Plaster ulcer — *see* Ulcer, pressure, by site
Plateau iris syndrome (post-iridectomy)
    (postprocedural) (without glaucoma) H21.82
  with glaucoma H40.22-
Platybasia Q75.8

Platyonychia (congenital) Q84.6
  acquired L60.8
Platypelloid pelvis M95.5
  with disproportion (fetopelvic) O33.0
    causing obstructed labor O65.0
  congenital Q74.2
Platyspondylisis Q76.49
Plaut (-Vincent) **disease** — *see also* Vincent's A69.1
Plethora R23.2
  newborn P61.1
Pleura, pleural — *see* condition
Pleuralgia R07.81
Pleurisy (acute) (adhesive) (chronic) (costal)
    (diaphragmatic) (double) (dry) (fibrinous) (fibrous)
    (interlobar) (latent) (plastic) (primary) (residual)
    (sicca) (sterile) (subacute) (unresolved) R09.1
  with
    adherent pleura J86.0
    effusion J90
      chylous, chyliform J94.0
      tuberculous (non primary) A15.6
        primary (progressive) A15.7
    tuberculosis — *see* Pleurisy, tuberculous (non
        primary)
  encysted — *see* Pleurisy, with effusion
  exudative — *see* Pleurisy, with effusion
  fibrinopurulent, fibropurulent — *see* Pyothorax
  hemorrhagic — *see* Hemothorax
  pneumococcal J90
  purulent — *see* Pyothorax
  septic — *see* Pyothorax
  serofibrinous — *see* Pleurisy, with effusion
  seropurulent — *see* Pyothorax
  serous — *see* Pleurisy, with effusion
  staphylococcal J86.9
  streptococcal J90
  suppurative — *see* Pyothorax
  traumatic (post) (current) — *see* Injury,
      intrathoracic, pleura
  tuberculous (with effusion) (non primary) A15.6
    primary (progressive) A15.7
Pleuritis sicca — *see* Pleurisy
Pleurobronchopneumonia — *see* Pneumonia,
    broncho-
Pleurodynia R07.81
  epidemic B33.0
  viral B33.0
Pleuropericarditis — *see also* Pericarditis
  acute I30.9
Pleuropneumonia (acute) (bilateral) (double)
    (septic) — *see also* Pneumonia J18.8
  chronic — *see* Fibrosis, lung
Pleuro-pneumonia-like-organism (PPLO)
    , as cause of disease classified elsewhere B96.0
Pleurorrhea — *see* Pleurisy, with effusion
Plexitis, brachial G54.0
Plica
  polonica B85.0
  syndrome, knee M67.5-
  tonsil J35.8
Plicated tongue K14.5
Plug
  bronchus NEC J98.09
  meconium (newborn) NEC syndrome P76.0
  mucus — *see* Asphyxia, mucus
Plumbism — *see* subcategory T56.0
Plummer's disease E05.20
  with thyroid storm E05.21
Plummer-Vinson syndrome D50.1
Pluricarential syndrome of infancy E40
Plus (and minus) **hand** (intrinsic) — *see* Deformity,
    limb, specified type NEC, forearm
Pneumathemia — *see* Air, embolism
Pneumatic hammer (drill) **syndrome** T75.21
Pneumatocele (lung) J98.4
  intracranial G93.89
  tension J44.9
Pneumatosis
  cystoides intestinalis K63.89
  intestinalis K63.89
  peritonei K66.8
Pneumaturia R39.89
Pneumoblastoma — *see* Neoplasm, lung, malignant
Pneumocephalus G93.89
Pneumococcemia A40.3
Pneumococcus, pneumococcal — *see* condition
Pneumoconiosis (due to) (inhalation of) J64
  with tuberculosis (any type in A15) J65
  aluminum J63.0
  asbestos J61
  bagasse, bagassosis J67.1
  bauxite J63.1
  beryllium J63.2

Pneumoconiosis (due to) (inhalation of) - *continued*
coal miners' (simple) J60
coalworkers' (simple) J60
collier's J60
cotton dust J66.0
diatomite (diatomaceous earth) J62.8
dust
  inorganic NEC J63.6
  lime J62.8
  marble J62.8
  organic NEC J66.8
fumes or vapors (from silo) J68.9
graphite J63.3
grinder's J62.8
kaolin J62.8
mica J62.8
millstone maker's J62.8
mineral fibers NEC J61
miner's J60
moldy hay J67.0
potter's J62.8
rheumatoid — *see* Rheumatoid, lung
sandblaster's J62.8
silica, silicate NEC J62.8
  with carbon J60
stonemason's J62.8
talc (dust) J62.0
Pneumocystis carinii pneumonia B59
Pneumocystis jiroveci (pneumonia) B59
Pneumocystosis (with pneumonia) B59
Pneumohemopericardium I31.2
Pneumohemothorax J94.2
traumatic S27.2
Pneumohydropericardium — *see* Pericarditis
Pneumohydrothorax — *see* Hydrothorax
Pneumomediastinum J98.2
congenital or perinatal P25.2
Pneumomycosis B49 *[J99]*
Pneumonia (acute) (double) (migratory) (purulent)
(septic) (unresolved) J18.9
with
  lung abscess J85.1
    due to specified organism — *see* Pneumonia, in
    (due to)
  influenza — *see* Influenza, with, pneumonia
adenoviral J12.0
adynamic J18.2
alba A50.04
allergic (eosinophilic) J82
alveolar — *see* Pneumonia, lobar
anaerobes J15.8
anthrax A22.1
apex, apical — *see* Pneumonia, lobar
Ascaris B77.81
aspiration J69.0
  due to
    aspiration of microorganisms
      bacterial J15.9
      viral J12.9
    food (regurgitated) J69.0
    gastric secretions J69.0
    milk (regurgitated) J69.0
    oils, essences J69.1
    solids, liquids NEC J69.8
    vomitus J69.0
  newborn P24.81
    amniotic fluid (clear) P24.11
    blood P24.21
    liquor (amnii) P24.11
    meconium P24.01
    milk P24.31
    mucus P24.11
    food (regurgitated) P24.31
    specified NEC P24.81
    stomach contents P24.31
  postprocedural J95.4
atypical NEC J18.9
bacillus J15.9
  specified NEC J15.8
bacterial J15.9
  specified NEC J15.8
Bacteroides (fragilis) (oralis)
  (melaninogenicus) J15.8
basal, basic, basilar — *see* Pneumonia, by type
bronchiolitis obliterans organized (BOOP) J84.89
broncho-, bronchial (confluent) (croupous) (diffuse)
  (disseminated) (hemorrhagic) (involving lobes)
  (lobar) (terminal) J18.0
  allergic (eosinophilic) J82
  aspiration — *see* Pneumonia, aspiration
  bacterial J15.9
    specified NEC J15.8
  chronic — *see* Fibrosis, lung

Pneumonia (acute) (double) (migratory) (purulent)
(septic) (unresolved) - *continued*
broncho-, bronchial (confluent) (croupous) (diffuse)
  (disseminated) (hemorrhagic) (involving lobes)
  (lobar) (terminal) - *continued*
  diplococcal J13
  Eaton's agent J15.7
  Escherichia coli (E. coli) J15.5
  Friedländer's bacillus J15.0
  Hemophilus influenzae J14
  hypostatic J18.2
  inhalation — *see also* Pneumonia, aspiration
    due to fumes or vapors (chemical) J68.0
    of oils or essences J69.1
  Klebsiella (pneumoniae) J15.0
  lipid, lipoid J69.1
    endogenous J84.89
  Mycoplasma (pneumoniae) J15.7
  pleuro-pneumonia-like-organisms (PPLO) J15.7
  pneumococcal J13
  Proteus J15.6
  Pseudomonas J15.1
  Serratia marcescens J15.6
  specified organism NEC J16.8
  staphylococcal — *see* Pneumonia, staphylococcal
  streptococcal NEC J15.4
    group B J15.3
    pneumoniae J13
  viral, virus — *see* Pneumonia, viral
Butyrivibrio (fibriosolvens) J15.8
Candida B37.1
caseous — *see* Tuberculosis, pulmonary
catarrhal — *see* Pneumonia, broncho
chlamydial J16.0
  congenital P23.1
cholesterol J84.89
cirrhotic (chronic) — *see* Fibrosis, lung
Clostridium (haemolyticum) (novyi) J15.8
confluent — *see* Pneumonia, broncho
congenital (infective) P23.9
  due to
    bacterium NEC P23.6
    Chlamydia P23.1
    Escherichia coli P23.4
    Haemophilus influenzae P23.6
    infective organism NEC P23.8
    Klebsiella pneumoniae P23.6
    Mycoplasma P23.6
    Pseudomonas P23.5
    Staphylococcus P23.2
    Streptococcus (except group B) P23.6
      group B P23.3
    viral agent P23.0
    specified NEC P23.8
croupous — *see* Pneumonia, lobar
cryptogenic organizing J84.116
cytomegalic inclusion B25.0
cytomegaloviral B25.0
deglutition — *see* Pneumonia, aspiration
desquamative interstitial J84.117
diffuse — *see* Pneumonia, broncho
diplococcal, diplococcus (broncho-) (lobar) J13
disseminated (focal) — *see* Pneumonia, broncho
Eaton's agent J15.7
embolic, embolism — *see* Embolism, pulmonary
Enterobacter J15.6
eosinophilic J82
Escherichia coli (E. coli) J15.5
Eubacterium J15.8
fibrinous — *see* Pneumonia, lobar
fibroid, fibrous (chronic) — *see* Fibrosis, lung
Friedländer's bacillus J15.0
Fusobacterium (nucleatum) J15.8
gangrenous J85.0
giant cell (measles) B05.2
gonococcal A54.84
gram-negative bacteria NEC J15.6
  anaerobic J15.8
Hemophilus influenzae (broncho) (lobar) J14
human metapneumovirus J12.3
hypostatic (broncho) (lobar) J18.2
in (due to)
  actinomycosis A42.0
  adenovirus J12.0
  anthrax A22.1
  ascariasis B77.81
  aspergillosis B44.9
  Bacillus anthracis A22.1
  Bacterium anitratum J15.6
  candidiasis B37.1
  chickenpox B01.2
  Chlamydia J16.0
    neonatal P23.1

Pneumonia (acute) (double) (migratory) (purulent)
(septic) (unresolved) - *continued*
in (due to) - *continued*
  coccidioidomycosis B38.2
    acute B38.0
    chronic B38.1
  cytomegalovirus disease B25.0
  Diplococcus (pneumoniae) J13
  Eaton's agent J15.7
  Enterobacter J15.6
  Escherichia coli (E. coli) J15.5
  Friedländer's bacillus J15.0
  fumes and vapors (chemical) (inhalation) J68.0
  gonorrhea A54.84
  Hemophilus influenzae (H. influenzae) J14
  Herellea J15.6
  histoplasmosis B39.2
    acute B39.0
    chronic B39.1
  human metapneumovirus J12.3
  Klebsiella (pneumoniae) J15.0
  measles B05.2
  Mycoplasma (pneumoniae) J15.7
  nocardiosis, nocardiasis A43.0
  ornithosis A70
  parainfluenza virus J12.2
  pleuro-pneumonia-like-organism (PPLO) J15.7
  pneumococcus J13
  pneumocystosis (Pneumocystis carinii)
    (Pneumocystis jiroveci) B59
  Proteus J15.6
  Pseudomonas NEC J15.1
    pseudomallei A24.1
  psittacosis A70
  Q fever A78
  respiratory syncytial virus J12.1
  rheumatic fever I00 *[J17]*
  rubella B06.81
  Salmonella (infection) A02.22
    typhi A01.03
  schistosomiasis B65.9 *[J17]*
  Serratia marcescens J15.6
  specified
    bacterium NEC J15.8
    organism NEC J16.8
    spirochetal NEC A69.8
  Staphylococcus J15.20
    aureus (methicillin susceptible) (MSSA) J15.211
      methicillin resistant (MRSA) J15.212
    specified NEC J15.29
  Streptococcus J15.4
    group B J15.3
    pneumoniae J13
    specified NEC J15.4
  toxoplasmosis B58.3
  tularemia A21.2
  typhoid (fever) A01.03
  varicella B01.2
  virus — *see* Pneumonia, viral
  whooping cough A37.91
    due to
      Bordetella parapertussis A37.11
      Bordetella pertussis A37.01
      specified NEC A37.81
  Yersinia pestis A20.2
inhalation of food or vomit — *see* Pneumonia,
  aspiration
interstitial J84.9
  chronic J84.111
  desquamative J84.117
  due to
    collagen vascular disease J84.17
    known underlying cause J84.17
  idiopathic NOS J84.111
  in disease classified elsewhere J84.17
  lymphocytic (due to collagen vascular disease) (in
    diseases classified elsewhere) J84.17
  lymphoid J84.2
  non-specific J84.89
    due to
      collagen vascular disease J84.17
      known underlying cause J84.17
    idiopathic J84.113
    in diseases classified elsewhere J84.17
  plasma cell B59
  pseudomonas J15.1
  usual J84.112
    due to collagen vascular disease J84.17
    idiopathic J84.112
    in diseases classified elsewhere J84.17
Klebsiella (pneumoniae) J15.0
lipid, lipoid (exogenous) J69.1
  endogenous J84.89

Pneumonia (acute) (double) (migratory) (purulent) (septic) (unresolved) - *continued*
- lobar (disseminated) (double) (interstitial) J18.1
  - bacterial J15.9
    - specified NEC J15.8
  - chronic — *see* Fibrosis, lung
  - Escherichia coli (E. coli) J15.5
  - Friedländer's bacillus J15.0
  - Hemophilus influenzae J14
  - hypostatic J18.2
  - Klebsiella (pneumoniae) J15.0
  - pneumococcal J13
  - Proteus J15.6
  - Pseudomonas J15.1
  - specified organism NEC J16.8
  - staphylococcal — *see* Pneumonia, staphylococcal
  - streptococcal NEC J15.4
  - Streptococcus pneumoniae J13
  - viral, virus — *see* Pneumonia, viral
- lobular — *see* Pneumonia, broncho
- Löffler's J82
- lymphoid interstitial J84.2
- massive — *see* Pneumonia, lobar
- meconium P24.01
- MRSA (Methicillin resistant Staphylococcus aureus) J15.212
- MSSA (methicillin susceptible Staphylococcus aureus) J15.211
- multilobar — *see* Pneumonia, by type
- Mycoplasma (pneumoniae) J15.7
- necrotic J85.0
- neonatal P23.9
  - aspiration — *see* Aspiration, by substance, with pneumonia
- nitrogen dioxide J68.0
- organizing J84.89
  - due to
    - collagen vascular disease J84.17
    - known underlying cause J84.17
  - in diseases classified elsewhere J84.17
- orthostatic J18.2
- parainfluenza virus J12.2
- parenchymatous — *see* Fibrosis, lung
- passive J18.2
- patchy — *see* Pneumonia, broncho
- Peptococcus J15.8
- Peptostreptococcus J15.8
- plasma cell (of infants) B59
- pleurolobar — *see* Pneumonia, lobar
- pleuro-pneumonia-like organism (PPLO) J15.7
- pneumococcal (broncho) (lobar) J13
- Pneumocystis (carinii) (jiroveci) B59
- postinfectional NEC B99 *[J17]*
- postmeasles B05.2
- Proteus J15.6
- Pseudomonas J15.1
- psittacosis A70
- radiation J70.0
- respiratory syncytial virus J12.1
- resulting from a procedure J95.89
- rheumatic I00 *[J17]*
- Salmonella (arizonae) (cholerae-suis) (enteritidis) (typhimurium) A02.22
  - typhi A01.03
  - typhoid fever A01.03
- SARS-associated coronavirus J12.81
- segmented, segmental — *see* Pneumonia, broncho-
- Serratia marcescens J15.6
- specified NEC J18.8
  - bacterium NEC J15.8
  - organism NEC J16.8
  - virus NEC J12.89
- spirochetal NEC A69.8
- staphylococcal (broncho) (lobar) J15.20
  - aureus (methicillin susceptible) (MSSA) J15.211
    - methicillin resistant (MRSA) J15.212
  - specified NEC J15.29
- static, stasis J18.2
- streptococcal NEC (broncho) (lobar) J15.4
  - group
    - A J15.4
    - B J15.3
  - specified NEC J15.4
- Streptococcus pneumoniae J13
- syphilitic, congenital (early) A50.04
- traumatic (complication) (early) (secondary) T79.8
- tuberculous (any) — *see* Tuberculosis, pulmonary
- tularemic A21.2
- varicella B01.2
- Veillonella J15.8
- ventilator associated J95.851
- viral, virus (broncho) (interstitial) (lobar) J12.9
  - adenoviral J12.0

Pneumonia (acute) (double) (migratory) (purulent) (septic) (unresolved) - *continued*
- viral, virus (broncho) (interstitial) (lobar) - *continued*
  - congenital P23.0
  - human metapneumovirus J12.3
  - parainfluenza J12.2
  - respiratory syncytial J12.1
  - SARS-associated coronavirus J12.81
  - specified NEC J12.89
- white (congenital) A50.04
Pneumonic — *see* condition
Pneumonitis (acute) (primary) — *see also* Pneumonia
- air-conditioner J67.7
- allergic (due to) J67.9
  - organic dust NEC J67.8
  - red cedar dust J67.8
  - sequoiosis J67.8
  - wood dust J67.8
- aspiration J69.0
  - due to
    - anesthesia J95.4
      - during
        - labor and delivery O74.0
        - pregnancy O29.01-
        - puerperium O89.01
    - fumes or gases J68.0
  - obstetric O74.0
- chemical (due to gases, fumes or vapors) (inhalation) J68.0
  - due to anesthesia J95.4
- cholesterol J84.89
- crack (cocaine) J68.0
- chronic — *see* Fibrosis, lung
- congenital rubella P35.0
- due to
  - beryllium J68.0
  - cadmium J68.0
  - crack (cocaine) J68.0
  - detergent J69.8
  - fluorocarbon-polymer J68.0
  - food, vomit (aspiration) J69.0
  - fumes or vapors J68.0
  - gases, fumes or vapors (inhalation) J68.0
  - inhalation
    - blood J69.8
    - essences J69.1
    - food (regurgitated) , milk, vomit J69.0
    - oils, essences J69.1
    - saliva J69.0
    - solids, liquids NEC J69.8
  - manganese J68.0
  - nitrogen dioxide J68.0
  - oils, essences J69.1
  - solids, liquids NEC J69.8
  - toxoplasmosis (acquired) B58.3
    - congenital P37.1
  - vanadium J68.0
  - ventilator J95.851
- eosinophilic J82
- hypersensitivity J67.9
  - air conditioner lung J67.7
  - bagassosis J67.1
  - bird fancier's lung J67.2
  - farmer's lung J67.0
  - maltworker's lung J67.4
  - maple bark-stripper's lung J67.6
  - mushroom worker's lung J67.5
  - specified organic dust NEC J67.8
  - suberosis J67.3
- interstitial (chronic) J84.89
  - acute J84.114
  - lymphoid J84.2
  - non-specific J84.89
    - idiopathic J84.113
- lymphoid, interstitial J84.2
- meconium P24.01
- postanesthetic J95.4
  - correct substance properly administered — *see* Table of Drugs and Chemicals, by drug, adverse effect
  - in labor and delivery O74.0
  - in pregnancy O29.01-
  - obstetric O74.0
  - overdose or wrong substance given or taken (by accident) — *see* Table of Drugs and Chemicals, by drug, poisoning
- postpartum, puerperal O89.01
- postoperative J95.4
  - obstetric O74.0
- radiation J70.0
- rubella, congenital P35.0
- ventilation (air-conditioning) J67.7

Pneumonitis (acute) (primary) - *continued*
- ventilator associated J95.851
- wood-dust J67.8
Pneumonoconiosis — *see* Pneumoconiosis
Pneumoparotid K11.8
Pneumopathy NEC J98.4
- alveolar J84.09
- due to organic dust NEC J66.8
- parietoalveolar J84.09
Pneumopericarditis — *see also* Pericarditis
- acute I30.9
Pneumopericardium — *see also* Pericarditis
- congenital P25.3
- newborn P25.3
- traumatic (post) — *see* Injury, heart
Pneumophagia (psychogenic) F45.8
Pneumopleurisy, pneumopleuritis — *see also* Pneumonia J18.8
Pneumopyopericardium I30.1
Pneumopyothorax — *see* Pyopneumothorax
- with fistula J86.0
Pneumorrhagia — *see also* Hemorrhage, lung
- tuberculous — *see* Tuberculosis, pulmonary
Pneumothorax NOS J93.9
- acute J93.83
- chronic J93.81
- congenital P25.1
- perinatal period P25.1
- postprocedural J95.811
- specified NEC J93.83
- spontaneous NOS J93.83
  - newborn P25.1
  - primary J93.11
  - secondary J93.12
  - tension J93.0
- tense valvular, infectional J93.0
- tension (spontaneous) J93.0
- traumatic S27.0
  - with hemothorax S27.2
- tuberculous — *see* Tuberculosis, pulmonary
Podagra — *see also* Gout M10.9
Podencephalus Q01.9
Poikilocytosis R71.8
Poikiloderma L81.6
- Civatte's L57.3
- congenital Q82.8
- vasculare atrophicans L94.5
Poikilodermatomyositis M33.10
- with
  - myopathy M33.12
  - respiratory involvement M33.11
  - specified organ involvement NEC M33.19
Pointed ear (congenital) Q17.3
Poison ivy, oak, sumac or other plant dermatitis (allergic) (contact) L23.7
Poisoning (acute) — *see also* Table of Drugs and Chemicals
- algae and toxins T65.82-
- Bacillus B (aertrycke) (cholerae (suis)) (paratyphosus) (suipestifer) A02.9
- botulinus A05.1
- bacterial toxins A05.9
- berries, noxious — *see* Poisoning, food, noxious, berries
- botulism A05.1
- ciguatera fish T61.0-
- Clostridium botulinum A05.1
- death-cap (Amanita phalloides) (Amanita verna) — *see* Poisoning, food, noxious, mushrooms
- drug — *see* Table of Drugs and Chemicals, by drug, poisoning
- epidemic, fish (noxious) — *see* Poisoning, seafood bacterial A05.9
- fava bean D55.0
- fish (noxious) T61.9-
  - bacterial — *see* Intoxication, foodborne, by agent
  - ciguatera fish — *see* Poisoning, ciguatera fish
  - scombroid fish — *see* Poisoning, scombroid fish
  - specified type NEC T61.77-
- food (acute) (diseased) (infected) (noxious) NEC T62.9-
  - bacterial — *see* Intoxication, foodborne, by agent
  - due to
    - Bacillus (aertrycke) (choleraesuis) (paratyphosus) (suipestifer) A02.9
      - botulinus A05.1
    - Clostridium (perfringens) (Welchii) A05.2
    - salmonella (aertrycke) (callinarum) (choleraesuis) (enteritidis) (paratyphi) (suipestifer) A02.9
      - with
        - gastroenteritis A02.0
        - sepsis A02.1

Poisoning (acute) - *continued*
  food (acute) (diseased) (infected) (noxious) NEC - *continued*
    due to - *continued*
      staphylococcus A05.0
      Vibrio
        parahaemolyticus A05.3
        vulnificus A05.5
    noxious or naturally toxic T62.9-
      berries — *see* subcategory T62.1-
      fish — *see* Poisoning, seafood
      mushrooms — *see* subcategory T62.0X-
      plants NEC — *see* subcategory T62.2X-
      seafood — *see* Poisoning, seafood
      specified NEC — *see* subcategory T62.8X-
    ichthyotoxism — *see* Poisoning, seafood
  kreotoxism, food A05.9
  latex T65.81-
  lead T56.0-
  mushroom — *see* Poisoning, food, noxious, mushroom
  mussels — *see also* Poisoning, shellfish
    bacterial — *see* Intoxication, foodborne, by agent
  nicotine (tobacco) T65.2-
  noxious foodstuffs — *see* Poisoning, food, noxious
  plants, noxious — *see* Poisoning, food, noxious, plants NEC
  ptomaine — *see* Poisoning, food
  radiation J70.0
  Salmonella (arizonae) (cholerae-suis) (enteritidis) (typhimurium) A02.9
  scombroid fish T61.1-
  seafood (noxious) T61.9-
    bacterial — *see* Intoxication, foodborne, by agent
    fish — *see* Poisoning, fish
    shellfish — *see* Poisoning, shellfish
    specified NEC — *see* subcategory T61.8X-
  shellfish (amnesic) (azaspiracid) (diarrheic) (neurotoxic) (noxious) (paralytic) T61.78-
    bacterial — *see* Intoxication, foodborne, by agent
    ciguatera mollusk — *see* Poisoning, ciguatera fish
  specified substance NEC T65.891
  Staphylococcus, food A05.0
  tobacco (nicotine) T65.2-
  water E87.79
Poker spine — *see* Spondylitis, ankylosing
Poland syndrome Q79.8
Polioencephalitis (acute) (bulbar) A80.9
  inferior G12.22
  influenzal — *see* Influenza, with, encephalopathy
  superior hemorrhagic (acute) (Wernicke's) E51.2
    Wernicke's E51.2
Polioencephalomyelitis (acute) (anterior) A80.9
  with beriberi E51.2
Polioencephalopathy, superior hemorrhagic E51.2
  with
    beriberi E51.11
    pellagra E52
Poliomeningoencephalitis — *see* Meningoencephalitis
Poliomyelitis (acute) (anterior) (epidemic) A80.9
  with paralysis (bulbar) — *see* Poliomyelitis, paralytic
  abortive A80.4
  ascending (progressive) — *see* Poliomyelitis, paralytic
  bulbar (paralytic) — *see* Poliomyelitis, paralytic
  congenital P35.8
  nonepidemic A80.9
  nonparalytic A80.4
  paralytic A80.30
    specified NEC A80.39
    vaccine-associated A80.0
    wild virus
      imported A80.1
      indigenous A80.2
  spinal, acute A80.9
Poliosis (eyebrow) (eyelashes) L67.1
  circumscripta, acquired L67.1
Pollakiuria R35.0
  psychogenic F45.8
Pollinosis J30.1
Pollitzer's disease L73.2
Polyadenitis — *see also* Lymphadenitis
  malignant A20.0
Polyalgia M79.89
Polyangiitis M30.0
  microscopic M31.7
  overlap syndrome M30.8
Polyarteritis
  microscopic M31.7
  nodosa M30.0
    with lung involvement M30.1

Polyarteritis - *continued*
  nodosa - *continued*
    juvenile M30.2
    related condition NEC M30.8
Polyarthralgia — *see* Pain, joint
Polyarthritis, polyarthropathy — *see also* Arthritis M13.0
  due to or associated with other specified conditions — *see* Arthritis
  epidemic (Australian) (with exanthema) B33.1
  infective — *see* Arthritis, pyogenic or pyemic
  inflammatory M06.4
  juvenile (chronic) (seronegative) M08.3
  migratory — *see* Fever, rheumatic
  rheumatic, acute — *see* Fever, rheumatic
Polyarthrosis M15.9
  post-traumatic M15.3
  primary M15.0
  specified NEC M15.8
Polycarential syndrome of infancy E40
Polychondritis (atrophic) (chronic) — *see also* Disorder, cartilage, specified type NEC
  relapsing M94.1
Polycoria Q13.2
Polycystic (disease)
  degeneration, kidney Q61.3
    autosomal dominant (adult type) Q61.2
    autosomal recessive (infantile type) NEC Q61.19
  kidney Q61.3
    autosomal
      dominant Q61.2
      recessive NEC Q61.19
    autosomal dominant (adult type) Q61.2
    autosomal recessive (childhood type) NEC Q61.19
    infantile type NEC Q61.19
  liver Q44.6
  lung J98.4
    congenital Q33.0
  ovary, ovaries E28.2
  spleen Q89.09
Polycythemia (secondary) D75.1
  acquired D75.1
  benign (familial) D75.0
  due to
    donor twin P61.1
    erythropoietin D75.1
    fall in plasma volume D75.1
    high altitude D75.1
    maternal-fetal transfusion P61.1
    stress D75.1
  emotional D75.1
  erythropoietin D75.1
  familial (benign) D75.0
  Gaisböck's (hypertonica) D75.1
  high altitude D75.1
  hypertonica D75.1
  hypoxemic D75.1
  neonatorum P61.1
  nephrogenous D75.1
  relative D75.1
  secondary D75.1
  spurious D75.1
  stress D75.1
  vera D45
Polycytosis cryptogenica D75.1
Polydactylism, polydactyly Q69.9
  toes Q69.2
Polydipsia R63.1
Polydystrophy, pseudo-Hurler E77.0
Polyembryoma — *see* Neoplasm, malignant, by site
Polyglandular
  deficiency E31.0
  dyscrasia E31.9
  dysfunction E31.9
  syndrome E31.8
Polyhydramnios O40.-
Polymastia Q83.1
Polymenorrhea N92.0
Polymyalgia M35.3
  arteritica, giant cell M31.5
  rheumatica M35.3
    with giant cell arteritis M31.5
Polymyositis (acute) (chronic) (hemorrhagic) M33.20
  with
    myopathy M33.22
    respiratory involvement M33.21
    skin involvement — *see* Dermatopolymyositis
    specified organ involvement NEC M33.29
  ossificans (generalisata) (progressiva) — *see* Myositis, ossificans, progressiva
Polyneuritis, polyneuritic — *see also* Polyneuropathy
  acute (post-) infective G61.0

Polyneuritis, polyneuritic - *continued*
  alcoholic G62.1
  cranialis G52.7
  demyelinating, chronic inflammatory (CIDP) G61.81
  diabetic — *see* Diabetes, polyneuropathy
  diphtheritic A36.83
  due to lack of vitamin NEC E56.9 *[G63]*
  endemic E51.11
  erythredema — *see* subcategory T56.1
  febrile, acute G61.0
  hereditary ataxic G60.1
  idiopathic, acute G61.0
  infective (acute) G61.0
  inflammatory, chronic demyelinating (CIDP) G61.81
  nutritional E63.9 *[G63]*
  postinfective (acute) G61.0
  specified NEC G62.89
Polyneuropathy (peripheral) G62.9
  alcoholic G62.1
  amyloid (Portuguese) E85.1 *[G63]*
  arsenical G62.2
  critical illness G62.81
  demyelinating, chronic inflammatory (CIDP) G61.81
  diabetic — *see* Diabetes, polyneuropathy
  drug-induced G62.0
  hereditary G60.9
    specified NEC G60.8
  idiopathic G60.9
    progressive G60.3
  in (due to)
    alcohol G62.1
      sequelae G65.2
    amyloidosis, familial (Portuguese) E85.1 *[G63]*
    antitetanus serum G61.1
    arsenic G62.2
      sequelae G65.2
    avitaminosis NEC E56.9 *[G63]*
    beriberi E51.11
    collagen vascular disease NEC M35.9 *[G63]*
    deficiency (of)
      B (-complex) vitamins E53.9 *[G63]*
      vitamin B6 E53.1 *[G63]*
    diabetes — *see* Diabetes, polyneuropathy
    diphtheria A36.83
    drug or medicament G62.0
      correct substance properly administered — *see* Table of Drugs and Chemicals, by drug, adverse effect
      overdose or wrong substance given or taken — *see* Table of Drugs and Chemicals, by drug, poisoning
    endocrine disease NEC E34.9 *[G63]*
    herpes zoster B02.23
    hypoglycemia E16.2 *[G63]*
    infectious
      disease NEC B99 *[G63]*
      mononucleosis B27.91
    lack of vitamin NEC E56.9 *[G63]*
    lead G62.2
      sequelae G65.2
    leprosy A30.9 *[G63]*
    Lyme disease A69.22
    metabolic disease NEC E88.9 *[G63]*
    microscopic polyangiitis M31.7 *[G63]*
    mumps B26.84
    neoplastic disease — *see also* Neoplasm D49.9 *[G63]*
    nutritional deficiency NEC E63.9 *[G63]*
    organophosphate compounds G62.2
      sequelae G65.2
    parasitic disease NEC B89 *[G63]*
    pellagra E52 *[G63]*
    polyarteritis nodosa M30.0
    porphyria E80.20 *[G63]*
    radiation G62.82
    rheumatoid arthritis — *see* Rheumatoid, polyneuropathy
    sarcoidosis D86.89
    serum G61.1
    syphilis (late) A52.15
      congenital A50.43
    systemic
      connective tissue disorder M35.9 *[G63]*
      lupus erythematosus M32.19
    toxic agent NEC G62.2
      sequelae G65.2
    triorthocresyl phosphate G62.2
      sequelae G65.2
    tuberculosis A17.89
    uremia N18.9 *[G63]*

Polyneuropathy (peripheral) - *continued*
  in (due to) - *continued*
    vitamin B12 deficiency E53.8 *[G63]*
      with anemia (pernicious) D51.0 *[G63]*
        due to dietary deficiency D51.3 *[G63]*
    zoster B02.23
  inflammatory G61.9
    chronic demyelinating (CIDP) G61.81
    sequelae G65.1
    specified NEC G61.89
  lead G62.2
    sequelae G65.2
  nutritional NEC E63.9 *[G63]*
  postherpetic (zoster) B02.23
  progressive G60.3
  radiation-induced G62.82
  sensory (hereditary) (idiopathic) G60.8
  specified NEC G62.89
  syphilitic (late) A52.15
    congenital A50.43
Polyopia H53.8
Polyorchism, polyorchidism Q55.21
Polyosteoarthritis — *see also* Osteoarthritis,
  generalized M15.9-
  post-traumatic M15.3
  specified NEC M15.8
Polyostotic fibrous dysplasia Q78.1
Polyotia Q17.0
Polyp, polypus
  accessory sinus J33.8
  adenocarcinoma in — *see* Neoplasm, malignant, by
    site
  adenocarcinoma in situ in — *see* Neoplasm, in situ,
    by site
  adenoid tissue J33.0
  adenomatous — *see also* Neoplasm, benign, by site
    adenocarcinoma in — *see* Neoplasm, malignant,
      by site
    adenocarcinoma in situ in — *see* Neoplasm, in situ,
      by site
    carcinoma in — *see* Neoplasm, malignant, by site
    carcinoma in situ in — *see* Neoplasm, in situ, by
      site
    multiple — *see* Neoplasm, benign
      adenocarcinoma in — *see* Neoplasm, malignant,
        by site
      adenocarcinoma in situ in — *see* Neoplasm, in
        situ, by site
  antrum J33.8
  anus, anal (canal) K62.0
  Bartholin's gland N84.3
  bladder D41.4
  carcinoma in — *see* Neoplasm, malignant, by site
  carcinoma in situ in — *see* Neoplasm, in situ, by site
  cecum D12.0
  cervix (uteri) N84.1
    in pregnancy or childbirth — *see* Pregnancy,
      complicated by, abnormal, cervix
    mucous N84.1
    nonneoplastic N84.1
  choanal J33.0
  cholesterol K82.4
  clitoris N84.3
  colon K63.5
    adenomatous D12.6
    ascending D12.2
    cecum D12.0
    descending D12.4
    inflammatory K51.40
      with
        abscess K51.414
        complication K51.419
          specified NEC K51.418
        fistula K51.413
        intestinal obstruction K51.412
        rectal bleeding K51.411
    sigmoid D12.5
    transverse D12.3
  corpus uteri N84.0
  dental K04.01
    irreversible K04.02
    reversible K04.01
  duodenum K31.7
  ear (middle) H74.4-
  endometrium N84.0
  ethmoidal (sinus) J33.8
  fallopian tube N84.8
  female genital tract N84.9
    specified NEC N84.8
  frontal (sinus) J33.8
  gallbladder K82.4
  gingiva, gum K06.8
  labia, labium (majus) (minus) N84.3

Polyp, polypus - *continued*
  larynx (mucous) J38.1
    adenomatous D14.1
  malignant — *see* Neoplasm, malignant, by site
  maxillary (sinus) J33.8
  middle ear — *see* Polyp, ear (middle)
  myometrium N84.0
  nares
    anterior J33.9
    posterior J33.0
  nasal (mucous) J33.9
    cavity J33.0
    septum J33.0
  nasopharyngeal J33.0
  nose (mucous) J33.9
  oviduct N84.8
  pharynx J39.2
  placenta O90.89
  prostate — *see* Enlargement, enlarged, prostate
  pudenda, pudendum N84.3
  pulpal (dental) K04.01
    irreversible K04.02
    reversible K04.01
  rectum (nonadenomatous) K62.1
    adenomatous — *see* Polyp, adenomatous
  septum (nasal) J33.0
  sinus (accessory) (ethmoidal) (frontal) (maxillary)
    (sphenoidal) J33.8
  sphenoidal (sinus) J33.8
  stomach K31.7
    adenomatous D13.1
  tube, fallopian N84.8
  turbinate, mucous membrane J33.8
  umbilical, newborn P83.6
  ureter N28.89
  urethra N36.2
  uterus (body) (corpus) (mucous) N84.0
    cervix N84.1
    in pregnancy or childbirth — *see* Pregnancy,
      complicated by, tumor, uterus
  vagina N84.2
  vocal cord (mucous) J38.1
  vulva N84.3
Polyphagia R63.2
Polyploidy Q92.7
Polypoid — *see* condition
Polyposis — *see also* Polyp
  coli (adenomatous) D12.6
    adenocarcinoma in C18.9
    adenocarcinoma in situ in — *see* Neoplasm, in situ,
      by site
    carcinoma in C18.9
  colon (adenomatous) D12.6
  familial D12.6
    adenocarcinoma in situ in — *see* Neoplasm, in situ,
      by site
  intestinal (adenomatous) D12.6
  malignant lymphomatous C83.1-
  multiple, adenomatous — *see also* Neoplasm,
    benign D36.9
Polyradiculitis — *see* Polyneuropathy
Polyradiculoneuropathy (acute) (postinfective)
  (segmentally demyelinating) G61.0
Polyserositis
  due to pericarditis I31.1
  pericardial I31.1
  periodic, familial E85.0
  tuberculous A19.9
    acute A19.1
    chronic A19.8
Polysplenia syndrome Q89.09
Polysyndactyly — *see also* Syndactylism,
  syndactyly Q70.4
Polytrichia L68.3
Polyunguia Q84.6
Polyuria R35.8
  nocturnal R35.1
  psychogenic F45.8
Pompe's disease (glycogen storage) E74.02
Pompholyx L30.1
Poncet's disease (tuberculous rheumatism) A18.09
Pond fracture — *see* Fracture, skull
Ponos B55.0
Pons, pontine — *see* condition
Poor
  aesthetic of existing restoration of tooth K08.56
  contractions, labor O62.2
  gingival margin to tooth restoration K08.51
  personal hygiene R46.0
  prenatal care, affecting management of
    pregnancy — *see* Pregnancy, complicated by,
    insufficient, prenatal care
  sucking reflex (newborn) R29.2

Poor - *continued*
  urinary stream R39.12
  vision NEC H54.7
Poradenitis, nostras inguinalis or venerea A55
Porencephaly (congenital) (developmental)
  (true) Q04.6
  acquired G93.0
  nondevelopmental G93.0
  traumatic (post) F07.89
Porocephaliasis B88.8
Porokeratosis Q82.8
Poroma, eccrine — *see* Neoplasm, skin, benign
Porphyria (South African) E80.20
  acquired E80.20
  acute intermittent (hepatic) (Swedish) E80.21
  cutanea tarda (hereditary) (symptomatic) E80.1
  due to drugs E80.20
    correct substance properly administered — *see*
      Table of Drugs and Chemicals, by drug, adverse
      effect
    overdose or wrong substance given or taken — *see*
      Table of Drugs and Chemicals, by drug,
      poisoning
  erythropoietic (congenital) (hereditary) E80.0
  hepatocutaneous type E80.1
  secondary E80.20
  toxic NEC E80.20
  variegata E80.20
Porphyrinuria — *see* Porphyria
Porphyruria — *see* Porphyria
Port wine nevus, mark, or stain Q82.5
Portal — *see* condition
Posadas-Wernicke disease B38.9
Positive
  culture (nonspecific)
    blood R78.81
    bronchial washings R84.5
    cerebrospinal fluid R83.5
    cervix uteri R87.5
    nasal secretions R84.5
    nipple discharge R89.5
    nose R84.5
      staphylococcus (Methicillin susceptible) Z22.321
        Methicillin resistant Z22.322
    peritoneal fluid R85.5
    pleural fluid R84.5
    prostatic secretions R86.5
    saliva R85.5
    seminal fluid R86.5
    sputum R84.5
    synovial fluid R89.5
    throat scrapings R84.5
    urine R82.79
    vagina R87.5
    vulva R87.5
    wound secretions R89.5
  PPD (skin test) R76.11
  serology for syphilis A53.0
    false R76.8
    with signs or symptoms - code as Syphilis, by site
      and stage
  skin test, tuberculin (without active
    tuberculosis) R76.11
  test, human immunodeficiency virus (HIV) R75
  VDRL A53.0
    with signs or symptoms - code by site and stage
      under Syphilis A53.9
  Wassermann reaction A53.0
Postcardiotomy syndrome I97.0
Postcaval ureter Q62.62
Postcholecystectomy syndrome K91.5
Postclimacteric bleeding N95.0
Postcommissurotomy syndrome I97.0
Postconcussion syndrome F07.81
Postcontusional syndrome F07.81
Postcricoid region — *see* condition
Post-dates (40-42 weeks) (pregnancy)
  (mother) O48.0
  more than 42 weeks gestation O48.1
Postencephalitic syndrome F07.89
Posterior — *see* condition
Posterolateral sclerosis (spinal cord) — *see*
  Degeneration, combined
Postexanthematous — *see* condition
Postfebrile — *see* condition
Postgastrectomy dumping syndrome K91.1
Posthemiplegic chorea — *see* Monoplegia
Posthemorrhagic anemia (chronic) D50.0
  acute D62
  newborn P61.3
Postherpetic neuralgia (zoster) B02.29
  trigeminal B02.22
Posthitis N47.7

Postimmunization complication or reaction — *see* Complications, vaccination
Postinfectious — *see* condition
Postlaminectomy syndrome NEC M96.1
Postleukotomy syndrome F07.0
Postmastectomy lymphedema (syndrome) I97.2
Postmaturity, postmature (over 42 weeks)
  maternal (over 42 weeks gestation) O48.1
  newborn P08.22
Postmeasles complication NEC — *see also* condition B05.89
Postmenopausal
  endometrium (atrophic) N95.8
    suppurative — *see also* Endometritis N71.9
  osteoporosis — *see* Osteoporosis, postmenopausal
Postnasal drip R09.82
  due to
    allergic rhinitis — *see* Rhinitis, allergic
    common cold J00
    gastroesophageal reflux — *see* Reflux, gastroesophageal
    nasopharyngitis — *see* Nasopharyngitis
    other know condition - code to condition
    sinusitis — *see* Sinusitis
Postnatal — *see* condition
Postoperative (postprocedural) — *see* Complication, postoperative
  pneumothorax, therapeutic Z98.3
  state NEC Z98.890
Postpancreatectomy hyperglycemia E89.1
Postpartum — *see* Puerperal
Postphlebitic syndrome — *see* Syndrome, postthrombotic
Postpolio (myelitic) **syndrome** G14
Postpoliomyelitic — *see also* condition
  osteopathy — *see* Osteopathy, after poliomyelitis
Postprocedural — *see also* Postoperative
  hypoinsulinemia E89.1
Postschizophrenic depression F32.89
Postsurgery status — *see also* Status (post)
  pneumothorax, therapeutic Z98.3
Post-term (40-42 weeks) (pregnancy) (mother) O48.0
  infant P08.21
  more than 42 weeks gestation (mother) O48.1
Post-traumatic brain syndrome, nonpsychotic F07.81
Post-typhoid abscess A01.09
Postures, hysterical F44.2
Postvaccinal reaction or complication — *see* Complications, vaccination
Postvalvulotomy syndrome I97.0
Potain's
  disease (pulmonary edema) — *see* Edema, lung
  syndrome (gastrectasis with dyspepsia) K31.0
Potter's
  asthma J62.8
  facies Q60.6
  lung J62.8
  syndrome (with renal agenesis) Q60.6
Pott's
  curvature (spinal) A18.01
  disease or paraplegia A18.01
  spinal curvature A18.01
  tumor, puffy — *see* Osteomyelitis, specified type NEC
Pouch
  bronchus Q32.4
  Douglas' — *see* condition
  esophagus, esophageal, congenital Q39.6
    acquired K22.5
  gastric K31.4
  Hartmann's K82.8
  pharynx, pharyngeal (congenital) Q38.7
Pouchitis K91.850
Poultrymen's itch B88.0
Poverty NEC Z59.6
  extreme Z59.5
Poxvirus NEC B08.8
Prader-Willi syndrome Q87.1
Preauricular appendage or tag Q17.0
Prebetalipoproteinemia (acquired) (essential) (familial) (hereditary) (primary) (secondary) E78.1
  with chylomicronemia E78.3
Precipitate labor or delivery O62.3
Preclimacteric bleeding (menorrhagia) N92.4
Precocious
  adrenarche E30.1
  menarche E30.1
  menstruation E30.1
  pubarche E30.1
  puberty E30.1
    central E22.8
  sexual development NEC E30.1

Precocious - *continued*
  thelarche E30.8
Precocity, sexual (constitutional) (cryptogenic) (female) (idiopathic) (male) E30.1
  with adrenal hyperplasia E25.9
    congenital E25.0
Precordial pain R07.2
Predeciduous teeth K00.2
Prediabetes, prediabetic R73.03
  complicating
    pregnancy — *see* Pregnancy, complicated by, diseases of, specified type or system NEC
    puerperium O99.89
Predislocation status of hip at birth Q65.6
Pre-eclampsia O14.9-
  with pre-existing hypertension — *see* Hypertension, complicating pregnancy, pre-existing, with, pre-eclampsia
  complicating
    childbirth O14.94
    puerperium O14.95
  mild O14.0-
    complicating
      childbirth O14.04
      puerperium O14.05
  moderate O14.0-
    complicating
      childbirth O14.04
      puerperium O14.05
  severe O14.1-
    with hemolysis, elevated liver enzymes and low platelet count (HELLP) O14.2-
      complicating
        childbirth O14.24
        puerperium O14.25
    complicating
      childbirth O14.14
      puerperium O14.15
Pre-eruptive color change, teeth, tooth K00.8
Pre-excitation atrioventricular conduction I45.6
Preglaucoma H40.00-
Pregnancy (single) (uterine) — *see also* Delivery and Puerperal
  Note: The Tabular must be reviewed for assignment of the appropriate character indicating the trimester of the pregnancy
  Note: The Tabular must be reviewed for assignment of appropriate seventh character for multiple gestation codes in Chapter 15
  abdominal (ectopic) O00.00
    with intrauterine pregnancy O00.01
    with viable fetus O36.7-
  ampullar O00.10
    with intrauterine pregnancy O00.11
  biochemical O02.81
  broad ligament O00.80
    with intrauterine pregnancy O00.81
  cervical O00.80
    with intrauterine pregnancy O00.81
  chemical O02.81
  complicated NOS O26.9-
  complicated by (care of) (management affected by)
    abnormal, abnormality
      cervix O34.4-
        causing obstructed labor O65.5
      cord (umbilical) O69.9
      findings on antenatal screening of mother O28.9
        biochemical O28.1
        cytological O28.2
        chromosomal O28.5
        genetic O28.5
        hematological O28.0
        radiological O28.4
        specified NEC O28.8
        ultrasonic O28.3
      glucose (tolerance) NEC O99.810
      pelvic organs O34.9-
        specified NEC O34.8-
          causing obstructed labor O65.5
      pelvis (bony) (major) NEC O33.0
      perineum O34.7-
      position
        placenta O44.0-
          with hemorrhage O44.1-
        uterus O34.59-
      uterus O34.59-
        causing obstructed labor O65.5
        congenital O34.0-
      vagina O34.6-
        causing obstructed labor O65.5
      vulva O34.7-
        causing obstructed labor O65.5
    abruptio placentae — *see* Abruptio placentae

Pregnancy (single) (uterine) - *continued*
  complicated by (care of) (management affected by) - *continued*
    abscess or cellulitis
      bladder O23.1-
      breast O91.11-
      genital organ or tract O23.9-
    abuse
      physical O9A.31-
      psychological O9A.51-
      sexual O9A.41-
    adverse effect anesthesia O29.9-
      aspiration pneumonitis O29.01-
      cardiac arrest O29.11-
      cardiac complication NEC O29.19-
      cardiac failure O29.12-
      central nervous system complication NEC O29.29-
      cerebral anoxia O29.21-
      failed or difficult intubation O29.6-
      inhalation of stomach contents or secretions NOS O29.01-
      local, toxic reaction O29.3X
      Mendelson's syndrome O29.01-
      pressure collapse of lung O29.02-
      pulmonary complications NEC O29.09-
      specified NEC O29.8X-
      spinal and epidural type NEC O29.5X
        induced headache O29.4-
    albuminuria — *see also* Proteinuria, gestational O12.1-
    alcohol use O99.31-
    amnionitis O41.12-
    anaphylactoid syndrome of pregnancy O88.01-
    anemia (conditions in D50-D64) (pre-existing) O99.01-
      complicating the puerperium O99.03
    antepartum hemorrhage O46.9-
      with coagulation defect — *see* Hemorrhage, antepartum, with coagulation defect
      specified NEC O46.8X-
    appendicitis O99.61-
    atrophy (yellow) (acute) liver (subacute) O26.61-
    bariatric surgery status O99.84-
    bicornis or bicornuate uterus O34.0-
    biliary tract problems O26.61-
    breech presentation O32.1
    cardiovascular diseases (conditions in I00-I09, I20-I52, I70-I99) O99.41-
    cerebrovascular disorders (conditions in I60-I69) O99.41-
    cervical shortening O26.87-
    cervicitis O23.51-
    chloasma (gravidarum) O26.89-
    cholestasis (intrahepatic) O26.61-
    cholecystitis O99.61-
    chorioamnionitis O41.12-
    circulatory system disorder (conditions in I00-I09, I20-I99, O99.41-)
    compound presentation O32.6
    conjoined twins O30.02-
    connective system disorders (conditions in M00-M99) O99.89
    contracted pelvis (general) O33.1
      inlet O33.2
      outlet O33.3
    convulsions (eclamptic) (uremic) — *see also* Eclampsia O15.9-
    cracked nipple O92.11-
    cystitis O23.1-
    cystocele O34.8-
    death of fetus (near term) O36.4
      early pregnancy O02.1
      of one fetus or more in multiple gestation O31.2-
    deciduitis O41.14-
    decreased fetal movement O36.81-
    dental problems O99.61-
    diabetes (mellitus) O24.91-
      gestational (pregnancy induced) — *see* - Diabetes, gestational
      pre-existing O24.31-
        specified NEC O24.81-
        type 1 O24.01-
        type 2 O24.11-
    digestive system disorders (conditions in K00-K93) O99.61-
    diseases of — *see* Pregnancy, complicated by, specified body system disease
      biliary tract O26.61-
      blood NEC (conditions in D65-D77) O99.11-
      liver O26.61-
      specified NEC O99.89

Pregnancy (single) (uterine) - *continued*
  complicated by (care of) (management affected by) - *continued*
    disorders of — *see* Pregnancy, complicated by, specified body system disorder
    amniotic fluid and membranes O41.9-
      specified NEC O41.8X-
    biliary tract O26.61-
    ear and mastoid process (conditions in H60-H95) O99.89
    eye and adnexa (conditions in H00-H59) O99.89
    liver O26.61-
    skin (conditions in L00-L99) O99.71-
    specified NEC O99.89
    displacement, uterus NEC O34.59-
      causing obstructed labor O65.5
    disproportion (due to) O33.9
      fetal (ascites) (hydrops) (meningomyelocele) (sacral teratoma) (tumor) deformities NEC O33.7
      generally contracted pelvis O33.1
      hydrocephalic fetus O33.6
      inlet contraction of pelvis O33.2
      mixed maternal and fetal origin O33.4
      specified NEC O33.8
    double uterus O34.0-
      causing obstructed labor O65.5
    drug use (conditions in F11-F19) O99.32-
    eclampsia, eclamptic (coma) (convulsions) (delirium) (nephritis) (uremia) — *see also* Eclampsia O15.-
    ectopic pregnancy — *see* Pregnancy, ectopic
    edema O12.0-
      with
        gestational hypertension, mild — *see also* Pre-eclampsia O14.0-
        proteinuria O12.2-
    effusion, amniotic fluid — *see* Pregnancy, complicated by, premature rupture of membranes
    elderly
      multigravida O09.52-
      primigravida O09.51-
    embolism — *see also* Embolism, obstetric, pregnancy O88.-
    endocrine diseases NEC O99.28-
    endometritis O86.12
    excessive weight gain O26.0-
    exhaustion O26.81-
      during labor and delivery O75.81
    face presentation O32.3
    failed induction of labor O61.9
      instrumental O61.1
      mechanical O61.1
      medical O61.0
      specified NEC O61.8
      surgical O61.1
    failed or difficult intubation for anesthesia O29.6-
    false labor (pains) O47.9
      at or after 37 completed weeks of pregnancy O47.1
      before 37 completed weeks of pregnancy O47.0-
    fatigue O26.81-
      during labor and delivery O75.81
    fatty metamorphosis of liver O26.61-
    female genital mutilation O34.8- *[N90.81-]*
    fetal (maternal care for)
      abnormality or damage O35.9
        acid-base balance O68
        specified type NEC O35.8
      acidemia O68
      acidosis O68
      alkalosis O68
      anemia and thrombocytopenia O36.82-
      anencephaly O35.0
      chromosomal abnormality (conditions in Q90-Q99) O35.1
      conjoined twins O30.02-
      damage from
        amniocentesis O35.7
        biopsy procedures O35.7
        drug addiction O35.5
        hematological investigation O35.7
        intrauterine contraceptive device O35.7
        maternal
          alcohol addiction O35.4
          cytomegalovirus infection O35.3
          disease NEC O35.8
          drug addiction O35.5
          listeriosis O35.8
          rubella O35.3
          toxoplasmosis O35.8
          viral infection O35.3
        medical procedure NEC O35.7

Pregnancy (single) (uterine) - *continued*
  complicated by (care of) (management affected by) - *continued*
    fetal (maternal care for) - *continued*
      damage from - *continued*
        radiation O35.6
      death (near term) O36.4
        early pregnancy O02.1
      decreased movement O36.81-
      disproportion due to deformity (fetal) O33.7
      excessive growth (large for dates) O36.6-
      growth retardation O36.59-
        light for dates O36.59-
        small for dates O36.59-
      heart rate irregularity (bradycardia) (decelerations) (tachycardia) O76
      hereditary disease O35.2
      hydrocephalus O35.0
      intrauterine death O36.4
      poor growth O36.59-
        light for dates O36.59-
        small for dates O36.59-
      problem O36.9-
        specified NEC O36.89-
      reduction (elective) O31.3-
      selective termination O31.3-
      spina bifida O35.0
      thrombocytopenia O36.82-
    fibroid (tumor) (uterus) O34.1-
    fissure of nipple O92.11-
    gallstones O99.61-
    gastric banding status O99.84-
    gastric bypass status O99.84-
    genital herpes (asymptomatic) (history of) (inactive) O98.51-
    genital tract infection O23.9-
    glomerular diseases (conditions in N00-N07) O26.83-
      with hypertension, pre-existing — *see* Hypertension, complicating, pregnancy, pre-existing, with, renal disease
    gonorrhea O98.21-
    grand multiparity O09.4
    habitual aborter — *see* Pregnancy, complicated by, recurrent pregnancy loss
    HELLP syndrome (hemolysis, elevated liver enzymes and low platelet count) O14.2-
    hemorrhage
      antepartum — *see* Hemorrhage, antepartum
      before 20 completed weeks gestation O20.9
        specified NEC O20.8
      due to premature separation, placenta — *see also* Abruptio placentae O45.9-
      early O20.9
        specified NEC O20.8
      threatened abortion O20.0
    hemorrhoids O22.4-
    hepatitis (viral) O98.41-
    herniation of uterus O34.59-
    high
      head at term O32.4
      risk — *see* Supervision (of) (for), high-risk
    history of in utero procedure during previous pregnancy O09.82-
    HIV O98.71-
    human immunodeficiency virus (HIV) disease O98.71-
    hydatidiform mole — *see also* Mole, hydatidiform O01.9-
    hydramnios O40.-
    hydrocephalic fetus (disproportion) O33.6
    hydrops
      amnii O40.-
      fetalis O36.2-
        associated with isoimmunization — *see also* Pregnancy, complicated by, isoimmunization O36.11-
    hydrorrhea O42.90
    hyperemesis (gravidarum) (mild) — *see also* Hyperemesis, gravidarum O21.0-
    hypertension — *see* Hypertension, complicating pregnancy
    hypertensive
      heart and renal disease, pre-existing — *see* Hypertension, complicating, pregnancy, pre-existing, with, heart disease, with renal disease
      heart disease, pre-existing — *see* Hypertension, complicating, pregnancy, pre-existing, with, heart disease
      renal disease, pre-existing — *see* Hypertension, complicating, pregnancy, pre-existing, with, renal disease
    hypotension O26.5-

Pregnancy (single) (uterine) - *continued*
  complicated by (care of) (management affected by) - *continued*
    immune disorders NEC (conditions in D80-D89) O99.11-
    incarceration, uterus O34.51-
    incompetent cervix O34.3-
    inconclusive fetal viability O36.80
    infection (s) O98.91-
      amniotic fluid or sac O41.10-
      bladder O23.1-
      carrier state NEC O99.830
        streptococcus B O99.820
      genital organ or tract O23.9-
        specified NEC O23.59-
      genitourinary tract O23.9-
      gonorrhea O98.21-
      hepatitis (viral) O98.41-
      HIV O98.71-
      human immunodeficiency virus (HIV) O98.71-
      kidney O23.0-
      nipple O91.01-
      parasitic disease O98.91-
        specified NEC O98.81-
      protozoal disease O98.61-
      sexually transmitted NEC O98.31-
      specified type NEC O98.81-
      syphilis O98.11-
      tuberculosis O98.01-
      urethra O23.2-
      urinary (tract) O23.4-
        specified NEC O23.3-
      viral disease O98.51-
    injury or poisoning (conditions in S00-T88) O9A.21-
      due to abuse
        physical O9A.31-
        psychological O9A.51-
        sexual O9A.41-
    insufficient
      prenatal care O09.3-
      weight gain O26.1-
    insulin resistance O26.89
    intrauterine fetal death (near term) O36.4
      early pregnancy O02.1
      multiple gestation (one fetus or more) O31.2-
    isoimmunization O36.11-
      anti-A sensitization O36.11-
      anti-B sensitization O36.19-
      Rh O36.09-
        anti-D antibody O36.01-
      specified NEC O36.19-
    laceration of uterus NEC O71.81
    malformation
      placenta, placental (vessel) O43.10-
        specified NEC O43.19-
      uterus (congenital) O34.0-
    malnutrition (conditions in E40-E46) O25.1-
    maternal hypotension syndrome O26.5-
    mental disorders (conditions in F01-F09, F20-F99) O99.34-
      alcohol use O99.31-
      drug use O99.32-
      smoking O99.33-
    mentum presentation O32.3
    metabolic disorders O99.28-
    missed
      abortion O02.1
      delivery O36.4
    multiple gestations O30.9-
      conjoined twins O30.02-
      specified number of multiples NEC — *see* Pregnancy, multiple (gestation), specified NEC
      quadruplet — *see* Pregnancy, quadruplet
      specified complication NEC O31.8X-
      triplet — *see* Pregnancy, triplet
      twin — *see* Pregnancy, twin
    musculoskeletal condition (conditions is M00-M99) O99.89
    necrosis, liver (conditions in K72) O26.61-
    neoplasm
      benign
        cervix O34.4-
        corpus uteri O34.1-
        uterus O34.1-
      malignant O9A.11-
    nephropathy NEC O26.83-
    nervous system condition (conditions in G00-G99) O99.35-
    nutritional diseases NEC O99.28-
    obesity (pre-existing) O99.21-
    obesity surgery status O99.84-
    oblique lie or presentation O32.2

Pregnancy (single) (uterine) - *continued*
complicated by (care of) (management affected by) - *continued*
older mother — *see* Pregnancy, complicated by, elderly
oligohydramnios O41.0-
with premature rupture of membranes — *see also* Pregnancy, complicated by, premature rupture of membranes O42.-
onset (spontaneous) of labor after 37 completed weeks of gestation but before 39 completed weeks gestation, with delivery by (planned) cesarean section O75.82
oophoritis O23.52-
overdose, drug — *see also* Table of Drugs and Chemicals, by drug, poisoning O9A.21-
oversize fetus O33.5
papyraceous fetus O31.0-
pelvic inflammatory disease O99.89
periodontal disease O99.61-
peripheral neuritis O26.82-
peritoneal (pelvic) adhesions O99.89
phlebitis O22.9-
phlebopathy O22.9-
phlebothrombosis (superficial) O22.2-
deep O22.3-
placenta accreta O43.21-
placenta increta O43.22-
placenta percreta O43.23-
placenta previa O44.0-
complete O44.0-
with hemorrhage O44.1-
marginal O44.2-
with hemorrhage O44.3-
partial O44.2-
with hemorrhage O44.3-
placental disorder O43.9-
specified NEC O43.89-
placental dysfunction O43.89-
placental infarction O43.81-
placental insufficiency O36.51-
placental transfusion syndromes
fetomaternal O43.01-
fetus to fetus O43.02-
maternofetal O43.01-
placentitis O41.14-
pneumonia O99.51-
poisoning — *see also* Table of Drugs and Chemicals O9A.21-
polyhydramnios O40-
polymorphic eruption of pregnancy O26.86
poor obstetric history NEC O09.29-
postmaturity (post-term) (40 to 42 weeks) O48.0
more than 42 completed weeks gestation (prolonged) O48.1
pre-eclampsia O14.9-
mild O14.0-
moderate O14.0-
severe O14.1-
with hemolysis, elevated liver enzymes and low platelet count (HELLP) O14.2-
premature labor — *see* Pregnancy, complicated by, preterm labor
premature rupture of membranes O42.90
full-term, unspecified as to length of time between rupture and onset of labor O42.92
with onset of labor
within 24 hours O42.00
at or after 37 weeks gestation, onset of labor within 24 hours of rupture O42.02
pre-term (before 37 completed weeks of gestation) O42.01-
after 24 hours O42.10
at or after 37 weeks gestation, onset of labor more than 24 hours following rupture O42.12
pre-term (before 37 completed weeks of gestation) O42.11-
at or after 37 weeks gestation, unspecified as to length of time between rupture and onset of labor O42.92
pre-term (before 37 completed weeks of gestation) O42.91-
premature separation of placenta — *see also* Abruptio placentae O45.9-
presentation, fetal - — *see* Delivery, complicated by, malposition
preterm delivery O60.10
preterm labor
with delivery O60.10
preterm O60.10
term O60.20
second trimester
with term delivery O60.22

Pregnancy (single) (uterine) - *continued*
complicated by (care of) (management affected by) - *continued*
preterm labor - *continued*
second trimester - *continued*
without delivery O60.02
with preterm delivery
second trimester O60.12
third trimester O60.13
third trimester
with term delivery O60.23
without delivery O60.03
with third trimester preterm delivery O60.14
without delivery O60.00
second trimester O60.02
third trimester O60.03
previous history of — *see* Pregnancy, supervision of, high-risk
prolapse, uterus O34.52-
proteinuria (gestational) — *see also* Proteinuria, gestational O12.1-
with edema O12.2-
pruritic urticarial papules and plaques of pregnancy (PUPPP) O26.86
pruritus (neurogenic) O26.89-
psychosis or psychoneurosis (puerperal) F53
ptyalism O26.89-
PUPPP (pruritic urticarial papules and plaques of pregnancy) O26.86
pyelitis O23.0-
recurrent pregnancy loss O26.2-
renal disease or failure NEC O26.83-
with secondary hypertension, pre-existing — *see* Hypertension, complicating, pregnancy, pre-existing, secondary
hypertensive, pre-existing — *see* Hypertension, complicating, pregnancy, pre-existing, with, renal disease
respiratory condition (conditions in J00-J99) O99.51-
retained, retention
dead ovum O02.0
intrauterine contraceptive device O26.3-
retroversion, uterus O34.53-
Rh immunization, incompatibility or sensitization NEC O36.09-
anti-D antibody O36.01-
rupture
amnion (premature) — *see also* Pregnancy, complicated by, premature rupture of membranes O42-
membranes (premature) — *see also* Pregnancy, complicated by, premature rupture of membranes O42-
uterus (during labor) O71.1
before onset of labor O71.0-
salivation (excessive) O26.89-
salpingitis O23.52-
salpingo-oophoritis O23.52-
sepsis (conditions in A40, A41) O98.81-
size date discrepancy (uterine) O26.84-
skin condition (conditions in L00-L99) O99.71-
smoking (tobacco) O99.33-
social problem O09.7-
specified condition NEC O26.89-
spotting O26.85-
streptococcus group B (GBS) carrier state O99.820
subluxation of symphysis (pubis) O26.71-
syphilis (conditions in A50-A53) O98.11-
threatened
abortion O20.0
labor O47.9
at or after 37 completed weeks of gestation O47.1
before 37 completed weeks of gestation O47.0-
thrombophlebitis (superficial) O22.2-
thrombosis O22.9-
cerebral venous O22.5-
cerebrovenous sinus O22.5-
deep O22.3-
tobacco use disorder (smoking) O99.33-
torsion of uterus O34.59-
toxemia O14.9-
transverse lie or presentation O32.2
tuberculosis (conditions in A15-A19) O98.01-
tumor (benign)
cervix O34.4-
malignant O9A.11-
uterus O34.1-
unstable lie O32.0
upper respiratory infection O99.51-
urethritis O23.2-
uterine size date discrepancy O26.84-

Pregnancy (single) (uterine) - *continued*
complicated by (care of) (management affected by) - *continued*
vaginitis or vulvitis O23.59-
varicose veins (lower extremities) O22.0-
genitals O22.1-
legs O22.0-
perineal O22.1-
vaginal or vulval O22.1-
venereal disease NEC (conditions in A63.8) O98.31-
venous disorders O22.9-
specified NEC O22.8X-
viral diseases (conditions in A80-B09, B25-B34) O98.51-
very young mother — *see* Pregnancy, complicated by, young mother
vomiting O21.9
due to diseases classified elsewhere O21.8
hyperemesis gravidarum (mild) — *see also* Hyperemesis, gravidarum O21.0-
late (occurring after 20 weeks of gestation) O21.2
young mother
multigravida O09.62-
primigravida O09.61-
concealed O09.3-
continuing following
elective fetal reduction of one or more fetus O31.3-
intrauterine death of one or more fetus O31.2-
spontaneous abortion of one or more fetus O31.1-
cornual O00.80
with intrauterine pregnancy O00.81
ectopic (ruptured) O00.90
with intrauterine pregnancy O00.91
abdominal O00.00
with
intrauterine pregnancy O00.01
viable fetus O36.7-
cervical O00.80
with intrauterine pregnancy O00.81
complicated (by) O08.9
afibrinogenemia O08.1
cardiac arrest O08.81
chemical damage of pelvic organ (s) O08.6
circulatory collapse O08.3
defibrination syndrome O08.1
electrolyte imbalance O08.5
embolism (amniotic fluid) (blood clot) (pulmonary) (septic) O08.2
endometritis O08.0
genital tract and pelvic infection O08.0
hemorrhage (delayed) (excessive) O08.1
infection
genital tract or pelvic O08.0
kidney 008.83
urinary tract O08.83
intravascular coagulation O08.1
laceration of pelvic organ (s) O08.6
metabolic disorder O08.5
oliguria O08.4
oophoritis O08.0
parametritis O08.0
pelvic peritonitis O08.0
perforation of pelvic organ (s) O08.6
renal failure or shutdown O08.4
salpingitis or salpingo-oophoritis O08.0
sepsis O08.82
shock O08.83
septic O08.82
specified condition NEC O08.89
tubular necrosis (renal) O08.4
uremia O08.4
urinary infection O08.83
venous complication NEC O08.7
embolism O08.2
cornual O00.80
with intrauterine pregnancy O00.81
intraligamentous O00.80
with intrauterine pregnancy O00.81
mural O00.80
with intrauterine pregnancy O00.81
ovarian O00.20
with intrauterine pregnancy O00.21
specified site NEC O00.80
with intrauterine pregnancy O00.81
tubal (ruptured) O00.10
with intrauterine pregnancy O00.11
examination (normal) Z34.9-
high-risk — *see* Pregnancy, supervision of, high-risk
first Z34.0-
specified Z34.8-
extrauterine — *see* Pregnancy, ectopic

Pregnancy (single) (uterine) - *continued*
fallopian O00.10
  with intrauterine pregnancy O00.11
false F45.8
gestational carrier Z33.3
hidden O09.3-
high-risk — *see* Pregnancy, supervision of, high-risk
incidental finding Z33.1
interstitial O00.80
  with intrauterine pregnancy O00.81
intraligamentous O00.80
  with intrauterine pregnancy O00.81
intramural O00.80
  with intrauterine pregnancy O00.81
intraperitoneal O00.00
  with intrauterine pregnancy O00.01
isthmian O00.10
  with intrauterine pregnancy O00.11
mesometric (mural) O00.80
  with intrauterine pregnancy O00.81
molar NEC O02.0
complicated (by) O08.9
  afibrinogenemia O08.1
  cardiac arrest O08.81
  chemical damage of pelvic organ (s) O08.6
  circulatory collapse O08.3
  defibrination syndrome O08.1
  electrolyte imbalance O08.5
  embolism (amniotic fluid) (blood clot)
    (pulmonary) (septic) O08.2
  endometritis O08.0
  genital tract and pelvic infection O08.0
  hemorrhage (delayed) (excessive) O08.1
  infection
    genital tract or pelvic O08.0
    kidney O08.83
    urinary tract O08.83
  intravascular coagulation O08.1
  laceration of pelvic organ (s) O08.6
  metabolic disorder O08.5
  oliguria O08.4
  oophoritis O08.0
  parametritis O08.0
  pelvic peritonitis O08.0
  perforation of pelvic organ (s) O08.6
  renal failure or shutdown O08.4
  salpingitis or salpingo-oophoritis O08.0
  sepsis O08.82
  shock O08.3
    septic O08.82
  specified condition NEC O08.89
  tubular necrosis (renal) O08.4
  uremia O08.4
  urinary infection O08.83
  venous complication NEC O08.7
    embolism O08.2
hydatidiform — *see also* Mole, hydatidiform O01.9-
multiple (gestation) O30.9-
  greater than quadruplets — *see* Pregnancy, multiple (gestation), specified NEC
  specified NEC O30.80-
    with
      two or more monoamniotic fetuses O30.82-
      two or more monochorionic fetuses O30.81-
      two or more monoamniotic fetuses O30.82-
      two or more monochorionic fetuses O30.81-
      unable to determine number of placenta and number of amniotic sacs O30.89-
      unspecified number of placenta and unspecified number of amniotic sacs O30.80-
mural O00.80
  with intrauterine pregnancy O00.81
normal (supervision of) Z34.9-
  high-risk — *see* Pregnancy, supervision of, high-risk
  first Z34.0-
  specified Z34.8-
ovarian O00.20
  with intrauterine pregnancy O00.21
postmature (40 to 42 weeks) O48.0
  more than 42 weeks gestation O48.1
post-term (40 to 42 weeks) O48.0
prenatal care only Z34.9-
  high-risk — *see* Pregnancy, supervision of, high-risk
  first Z34.0-
  specified Z34.8-
prolonged (more than 42 weeks gestation) O48.1
quadruplet O30.20-
  with
    two or more monoamniotic fetuses O30.22-
    two or more monochorionic fetuses O30.21-

Pregnancy (single) (uterine) - *continued*
quadruplet - *continued*
  two or more monoamniotic fetuses O30.22-
  two or more monochorionic fetuses O30.21-
  unable to determine number of placenta and number of amniotic sacs O30.29-
  unspecified number of placenta and unspecified number of amniotic sacs O30.20-
quintuplet — *see* Pregnancy, multiple (gestation), specified NEC
sextuplet — *see* Pregnancy, multiple (gestation), specified NEC
supervision of
  concealed pregnancy O09.3-
  elderly mother
    multigravida O09.52-
    primigravida O09.51-
  hidden pregnancy O09.3-
  high-risk O09.9-
    due to (history of)
      ectopic pregnancy O09.1-
      elderly — *see* Pregnancy, supervision, elderly mother
      grand multiparity O09.4
      infertility O09.0-
      insufficient prenatal care O09.3-
      in utero procedure during previous pregnancy O09.82-
      in vitro fertilization O09.81-
      molar pregnancy O09.A-
      multiple previous pregnancies O09.4-
      older mother — *see* Pregnancy, supervision of, elderly mother
      poor reproductive or obstetric history NEC O09.29-
      pre-term labor O09.21-
      previous
        neonatal death O09.29-
      social problems O09.7-
      specified NEC O09.89-
      very young mother — *see* Pregnancy, supervision, young mother
    resulting from in vitro fertilization O09.81-
  normal Z34.9-
    first Z34.0-
    specified NEC Z34.8-
  young mother
    multigravida O09.62-
    primigravida O09.61-
triplet O30.10-
  with
    two or more monoamniotic fetuses O30.12-
    two or more monochrorionic fetuses O30.11-
    two or more monoamniotic fetuses O30.12-
    two or more monochrorionic fetuses O30.11-
    unable to determine number of placenta and number of amniotic sacs O30.19-
    unspecified number of placenta and unspecified number of amniotic sacs O30.10-
tubal (with abortion) (with rupture) O00.10
  with intrauterine pregnancy O00.11
twin O30.00-
  conjoined O30.02-
  dichorionic/diamniotic (two placenta, two amniotic sacs) O30.04-
  monochorionic/diamniotic (one placenta, two amniotic sacs) O30.03-
  monochorionic/monoamniotic (one placenta, one amniotic sac) O30.01-
  unable to determine number of placenta and number of amniotic sacs O30.09-
  unspecified number of placenta and unspecified number of amniotic sacs O30.00-
unwanted Z64.0
weeks of gestation
  8 weeks Z3A.08
  9 weeks Z3A.09
  10 weeks Z3A.10
  11 weeks Z3A.11
  12 weeks Z3A.12
  13 weeks Z3A.13
  14 weeks Z3A.14
  15 weeks Z3A.15
  16 weeks Z3A.16
  17 weeks Z3A.17
  18 weeks Z3A.18
  19 weeks Z3A.19
  20 weeks Z3A.20
  21 weeks Z3A.21
  22 weeks Z3A.22
  23 weeks Z3A.23
  24 weeks Z3A.24
  25 weeks Z3A.25

Pregnancy (single) (uterine) - *continued*
weeks of gestation - *continued*
  26 weeks Z3A.26
  27 weeks Z3A.27
  28 weeks Z3A.28
  29 weeks Z3A.29
  30 weeks Z3A.30
  31 weeks Z3A.31
  32 weeks Z3A.32
  33 weeks Z3A.33
  34 weeks Z3A.34
  35 weeks Z3A.35
  36 weeks Z3A.36
  37 weeks Z3A.37
  38 weeks Z3A.38
  39 weeks Z3A.39
  40 weeks Z3A.40
  41 weeks Z3A.41
  42 weeks Z3A.42
  greater than 42 weeks Z3A.49
  less than 8 weeks Z3A.01
  not specified Z3A.00
Preiser's disease — *see* Osteonecrosis, secondary, due to, trauma, metacarpus
Pre-kwashiorkor — *see* Malnutrition, severe
Preleukemia (syndrome) D46.9
Preluxation, hip, congenital Q65.6
Premature — *see also* condition
adrenarche E27.0
aging E34.8
beats I49.40
  atrial I49.1
  auricular I49.1
  supraventricular I49.1
birth NEC — *see* Preterm, newborn
closure, foramen ovale Q21.8
contraction
  atrial I49.1
  atrioventricular I49.2
  auricular I49.1
  auriculoventricular I49.49
  heart (extrasystole) I49.49
  junctional I49.2
  ventricular I49.3
delivery — *see also* Pregnancy, complicated by, preterm labor O60.10
ejaculation F52.4
infant NEC — *see* Preterm, newborn
  light-for-dates — *see* Light for dates
labor — *see* Pregnancy, complicated by, preterm labor
lungs P28.0
menopause E28.319
  asymptomatic E28.319
  symptomatic E28.310
newborn
  extreme (less than 28 completed weeks) — *see* Immaturity, extreme
  less than 37 completed weeks — *see* Preterm, newborn
puberty E30.1
rupture membranes or amnion — *see* Pregnancy, complicated by, premature rupture of membranes
senility E34.8
thelarche E30.8
ventricular systole I49.3
Prematurity NEC (less than 37 completed weeks) — *see* Preterm, newborn
extreme (less than 28 completed weeks) — *see* Immaturity, extreme
Premenstrual
dysphoric disorder (PMDD) F32.81
tension (syndrome) N94.3
Premolarization, cuspids K00.2
Prenatal
care, normal pregnancy — *see* Pregnancy, normal
screening of mother Z36
teeth K00.6
Preparatory care for subsequent treatment NEC
for dialysis Z49.01
peritoneal Z49.02
Prepartum — *see* condition
Preponderance, left or right ventricular I51.7
Prepuce — *see* condition
PRES
(posterior reversible encephalopathy syndrome) I67.83
Presbycardia R54
Presbycusis, presbyacusia H91.1-
Presbyesophagus K22.8
Presbyophrenia F03
Presbyopia H52.4

Prescription of contraceptives (initial) Z30.019
　barrier Z30.018
　diaphragm Z30.018
　emergency (postcoital) Z30.012
　implantable subdermal Z30.017
　injectable Z30.013
　intrauterine contraceptive device Z30.014
　pills Z30.011
　postcoital (emergency) Z30.012
　repeat Z30.40
　　barrier Z30.49
　　diaphragm Z30.49
　　implantable subdermal Z30.46
　　injectable Z30.42
　　pills Z30.41
　　specified type NEC Z30.49
　　transdermal patch hormonal Z30.45
　　vaginal ring hormonal Z30.44
　specified type NEC Z30.018
　　transdermal patch hormonal Z30.016
　　vaginal ring hormonal Z30.015
Presence (of)
　ankle-joint implant (functional) (prosthesis) Z96.66-
　aortocoronary (bypass) graft Z95.1
　arterial-venous shunt (dialysis) Z99.2
　artificial
　　eye (globe) Z97.0
　　heart (fully implantable) (mechanical) Z95.812
　　　valve Z95.2
　　larynx Z96.3
　　lens (intraocular) Z96.1
　　limb (complete) (partial) Z97.1-
　　　arm Z97.1-
　　　　bilateral Z97.15
　　　leg Z97.1-
　　　　bilateral Z97.16
　audiological implant (functional) Z96.29
　bladder implant (functional) Z96.0
　bone
　　conduction hearing device Z96.29
　　implant (functional) NEC Z96.7
　　joint (prosthesis) — *see* Presence, joint implant
　cardiac
　　defibrillator (functional) (with synchronous cardiac pacemaker) Z95.810
　　implant or graft Z95.9
　　　specified type NEC Z95.818
　　pacemaker Z95.0
　　resynchronization therapy
　　　defibrillator Z95.810
　　　pacemaker Z95.0
　cerebrospinal fluid drainage device Z98.2
　cochlear implant (functional) Z96.21
　contact lens (es) Z97.3
　coronary artery graft or prosthesis Z95.5
　CRT-D (cardiac resynchronization therapy defibrillator) Z95.810
　CRT-P (cardiac resynchronization therapy pacemaker) Z95.0
　cardioverter-defibrillator (ICD) Z95.810
　CSF shunt Z98.2
　dental prosthesis device Z97.2
　dentures Z97.2
　device (external) NEC Z97.8
　　cardiac NEC Z95.818
　　heart assist Z95.811
　　implanted (functional) Z96.9
　　　specified NEC Z96.89
　　prosthetic Z97.8
　ear implant Z96.20
　　cochlear implant Z96.21
　　myringotomy tube Z96.22
　　specified type NEC Z96.29
　elbow-joint implant (functional) (prosthesis) Z96.62-
　endocrine implant (functional) NEC Z96.49
　eustachian tube stent or device (functional) Z96.29
　external hearing-aid or device Z97.4
　finger-joint implant (functional) (prosthetic) Z96.69-
　functional implant Z96.9
　　specified NEC Z96.89
　graft
　　cardiac NEC Z95.818
　　vascular NEC Z95.828
　hearing-aid or device (external) Z97.4
　　implant (bone) (cochlear) (functional) Z96.21
　heart assist device Z95.811
　heart valve implant (functional) Z95.2
　　prosthetic Z95.2
　　specified type NEC Z95.4
　　xenogenic Z95.3
　hip-joint implant (functional) (prosthesis) Z96.64-
　ICD (cardioverter-defibrillator) Z95.810

Presence (of) - *continued*
　implanted device (artificial) (functional) (prosthetic) Z96.9
　　automatic cardiac defibrillator (with synchronous cardiac pacemaker) Z95.810
　　cardiac pacemaker Z95.0
　　cochlear Z96.21
　　dental Z96.5
　　heart Z95.812
　　heart valve Z95.2
　　　prosthetic Z95.2
　　　specified NEC Z95.4
　　　xenogenic Z95.3
　　insulin pump Z96.41
　　intraocular lens Z96.1
　　joint Z96.60
　　　ankle Z96.66-
　　　elbow Z96.62-
　　　finger Z96.69-
　　　hip Z96.64-
　　　knee Z96.65-
　　　shoulder Z96.61-
　　　specified NEC Z96.698
　　　wrist Z96.63-
　　larynx Z96.3
　　myringotomy tube Z96.22
　　otological Z96.20
　　　cochlear Z96.21
　　　eustachian stent Z96.29
　　　myringotomy Z96.22
　　　specified NEC Z96.29
　　　stapes Z96.29
　　skin Z96.81
　　skull plate Z96.7
　　specified NEC Z96.89
　　urogenital Z96.0
　insulin pump (functional) Z96.41
　intestinal bypass or anastomosis Z98.0
　intraocular lens (functional) Z96.1
　intrauterine contraceptive device (IUD) Z97.5
　intravascular implant (functional) (prosthetic) NEC Z95.9
　　coronary artery Z95.5
　　defibrillator (with synchronous cardiac pacemaker) Z95.810
　　peripheral vessel (with angioplasty) Z95.820
　joint implant (prosthetic) (any) Z96.60
　　ankle — *see* Presence, ankle joint implant
　　elbow — *see* Presence, elbow joint implant
　　finger — *see* Presence, finger joint implant
　　hip — *see* Presence, hip joint implant
　　knee — *see* Presence, knee joint implant
　　shoulder — *see* Presence, shoulder joint implant
　　specified joint NEC Z96.698
　　wrist — *see* Presence, wrist joint implant
　knee-joint implant (functional) (prosthesis) Z96.65-
　laryngeal implant (functional) Z96.3
　mandibular implant (dental) Z96.5
　myringotomy tube (s) Z96.22
　orthopedic-joint implant (prosthetic) (any) — *see* Presence, joint implant
　otological implant (functional) Z96.29
　shoulder-joint implant (functional) (prosthesis) Z96.61-
　skull-plate implant Z96.7
　spectacles Z97.3
　stapes implant (functional) Z96.29
　systemic lupus erythematosus [SLE] inhibitor D68.62
　tendon implant (functional) (graft) Z96.7
　tooth root (s) implant Z96.5
　ureteral stent Z96.0
　urethral stent Z96.0
　urogenital implant (functional) Z96.0
　vascular implant or device Z95.9
　　access port device Z95.828
　　specified type NEC Z95.828
　wrist-joint implant (functional) (prosthesis) Z96.63-
Presenile — *see also* condition
　dementia F03
　premature aging E34.8
Presentation, fetal — *see* Delivery , complicated by, malposition
Prespondylolisthesis (congenital) Q76.2
Pressure
　area, skin — *see* Ulcer, pressure, by site
　brachial plexus G54.0
　brain G93.5
　　injury at birth NEC P11.1
　cerebral — *see* Pressure, brain
　chest R07.89
　cone, tentorial G93.5
　hyposystolic — *see also* Hypotension

Pressure - *continued*
　hyposystolic - *continued*
　　incidental reading, without diagnosis of hypotension R03.1
　increased
　　intracranial (benign) G93.2
　　　injury at birth P11.0
　　intraocular H40.05-
　lumbosacral plexus G54.1
　mediastinum J98.59
　necrosis (chronic) — *see* Ulcer, pressure, by site
　parental, inappropriate (excessive) Z62.6
　sore (chronic) — *see* Ulcer, pressure, by site
　spinal cord G95.20
　ulcer (chronic) — *see* Ulcer, pressure, by site
　venous, increased I87.8
Pre-syncope R55
Preterm
　delivery — *see also* Pregnancy, complicated by, preterm labor O60.10
　labor — *see* Pregnancy, complicated by, preterm labor
　newborn (infant) P07.30
　　gestational age
　　　28 completed weeks (28 weeks, 0 days through 28 weeks, 6 days) P07.31
　　　29 completed weeks (29 weeks, 0 days through 29 weeks, 6 days) P07.32
　　　30 completed weeks (30 weeks, 0 days through 30 weeks, 6 days) P07.33
　　　31 completed weeks (31 weeks, 0 days through 31 weeks, 6 days) P07.34
　　　32 completed weeks (32 weeks, 0 days through 32 weeks, 6 days) P07.35
　　　33 completed weeks (33 weeks, 0 days through 33 weeks, 6 days) P07.36
　　　34 completed weeks (34 weeks, 0 days through 34 weeks, 6 days) P07.37
　　　35 completed weeks (35 weeks, 0 days through 35 weeks, 6 days) P07.38
　　　36 completed weeks (36 weeks, 0 days through 36 weeks, 6 days) P07.39
Previa
　placenta (total) (without hemorrhage) O44.0-
　　with hemorrhage O44.1-
　　complete O44.0-
　　　with hemorrhage O44.1-
　　low — *see also* Delivery, complicated, by, placenta, low O44.4-
　　　with hemorrhage O44.5-
　　marginal O44.2-
　　　with hemorrhage O44.3-
　　partial O44.2-
　　　with hemorrhage O44.3-
　vasa O69.4
Priapism N48.30
　due to
　　disease classified elsewhere N48.32
　　drug N48.33
　　specified cause NEC N48.39
　　trauma N48.31
Prickling sensation (skin) R20.2
Prickly heat L74.0
Primary — *see* condition
Primigravida
　elderly, affecting management of pregnancy, labor and delivery (supervision only) — *see* Pregnancy, complicated by, elderly, primigravida
　older, affecting management of pregnancy, labor and delivery (supervision only) — *see* Pregnancy, complicated by, elderly, primigravida
　very young, affecting management of pregnancy, labor and delivery (supervision only) — *see* Pregnancy, complicated by, young mother, primigravida
Primipara
　elderly, affecting management of pregnancy, labor and delivery (supervision only) — *see* Pregnancy, complicated by, elderly, primigravida
　older, affecting management of pregnancy, labor and delivery (supervision only) — *see* Pregnancy, complicated by, elderly, primigravida
　very young, affecting management of pregnancy, labor and delivery (supervision only) — *see* Pregnancy, complicated by, young mother, primigravida
Primus varus (bilateral) Q66.2
PRIND
　(Prolonged reversible ischemic neurologic deficit) I63.9
Pringle's disease (tuberous sclerosis) Q85.1
Prinzmetal angina I20.1
Prizefighter ear — *see* Cauliflower ear

Problem (with) (related to)
- academic Z55.8
- acculturation Z60.3
- adjustment (to)
  - change of job Z56.1
  - life-cycle transition Z60.0
  - pension Z60.0
  - retirement Z60.0
- adopted child Z62.821
- alcoholism in family Z63.72
- atypical parenting situation Z62.9
- bankruptcy Z59.8
- behavioral (adult) F69
  - drug seeking Z76.5
- birth of sibling affecting child Z62.898
- care (of)
  - provider dependency Z74.9
    - specified NEC Z74.8
  - sick or handicapped person in family or household Z63.6
- child
  - abuse (affecting the child) — see Maltreatment, child
  - custody or support proceedings Z65.3
  - in welfare custody Z62.21
  - in care of non-parental family member Z62.21
  - in foster care Z62.21
  - living in orphanage or group home Z62.22
- child-rearing Z62.9
  - specified NEC Z62.898
- communication (developmental) F80.9
- conflict or discord (with)
  - boss Z56.4
  - classmates Z55.4
  - counselor Z64.4
  - employer Z56.4
  - family Z63.9
    - specified NEC Z63.8
  - probation officer Z64.4
  - social worker Z64.4
  - teachers Z55.4
  - workmates Z56.4
- conviction in legal proceedings Z65.0
  - with imprisonment Z65.1
- counselor Z64.4
- creditors Z59.8
- digestive K92.9
- drug addict in family Z63.72
- ear — see Disorder, ear
- economic Z59.9
  - affecting care Z59.9
  - specified NEC Z59.8
- education Z55.9
  - specified NEC Z55.8
- employment Z56.9
  - change of job Z56.1
  - discord Z56.4
  - environment Z56.5
  - sexual harassment Z56.81
  - specified NEC Z56.89
  - stress NEC Z56.6
  - stressful schedule Z56.3
  - threat of job loss Z56.2
  - unemployment Z56.0
- enuresis, child F98.0
- eye H57.9
- failed examinations (school) Z55.2
- falling Z91.81
- family — see also Disruption, family Z63.9-
  - specified NEC Z63.8
- feeding (elderly) (infant) R63.3
  - newborn P92.9
    - breast P92.5
    - overfeeding P92.4
    - slow P92.2
    - specified NEC P92.8
    - underfeeding P92.3
  - nonorganic F50.89
- finance Z59.9
  - specified NEC Z59.8
- foreclosure on loan Z59.8
- foster child Z62.822
- frightening experience (s) in childhood Z62.898
- genital NEC
  - female N94.9
  - male N50.9
- health care Z75.9
  - specified NEC Z75.8
- hearing — see Deafness
- homelessness Z59.0
- housing Z59.9
  - inadequate Z59.1
  - isolated Z59.8

Problem (with) (related to) - continued
- housing - continued
  - specified NEC Z59.8
- identity (of childhood) F93.8
- illegitimate pregnancy (unwanted) Z64.0
- illiteracy Z55.0
- impaired mobility Z74.09
- imprisonment or incarceration Z65.1
- inadequate teaching affecting education Z55.8
- inappropriate (excessive) parental pressure Z62.6
- influencing health status NEC Z78.9
- in-law Z63.1
- institutionalization, affecting child Z62.22
- intrafamilial communication Z63.8
- jealousy, child F93.8
- landlord Z59.2
- language (developmental) F80.9
- learning (developmental) F81.9
- legal Z65.3
  - conviction without imprisonment Z65.0
  - imprisonment Z65.1
  - release from prison Z65.2
- life-management Z73.9
  - specified NEC Z73.89
- life-style Z72.9
  - gambling Z72.6
  - high-risk sexual behavior (heterosexual) Z72.51
    - bisexual Z72.53
    - homosexual Z72.52
  - inappropriate eating habits Z72.4
  - self-damaging behavior NEC Z72.89
  - specified NEC Z72.89
  - tobacco use Z72.0
- literacy Z55.9
  - low level Z55.0
  - specified NEC Z55.8
- living alone Z60.2
- lodgers Z59.2
- loss of love relationship in childhood Z62.898
- marital Z63.0
  - involving
    - divorce Z63.5
    - estrangement Z63.5
    - gender identity F66
- mastication K08.89
- medical
  - care, within family Z63.6
  - facilities Z75.9
    - specified NEC Z75.8
- mental F48.9
- multiparity Z64.1
- negative life events in childhood Z62.9
  - altered pattern of family relationships Z62.898
  - frightening experience Z62.898
  - loss of
    - love relationship Z62.898
    - self-esteem Z62.898
  - physical abuse (alleged) — see Maltreatment, child
  - removal from home Z62.29
  - specified event NEC Z62.898
- neighbor Z59.2
- neurological NEC R29.818
- new step-parent affecting child Z62.898
- none (feared complaint unfounded) Z71.1
- occupational NEC Z56.89
- parent-child — see Conflict, parent-child
- personal hygiene Z91.89
- personality F69
- phase-of-life transition, adjustment Z60.0
- presence of sick or disabled person in family or household Z63.79
  - needing care Z63.6
- primary support group (family) Z63.9
  - specified NEC Z63.8
- probation officer Z64.4
- psychiatric F99
- psychosexual (development) F66
- psychosocial Z65.9
  - specified NEC Z65.8
- relationship Z63.9
  - childhood F93.8
- release from prison Z65.2
- removal from home affecting child Z62.29
- seeking and accepting known hazardous and harmful behavioral or psychological interventions Z65.8
  - chemical, nutritional or physical interventions Z65.8
- sexual function (nonorganic) F52.9
- sight H54.7
- sleep disorder, child F51.9
- smell — see Disturbance, sensation, smell
- social
  - environment Z60.9

Problem (with) (related to) - continued
- social - continued
  - environment - continued
    - specified NEC Z60.8
  - exclusion and rejection Z60.4
  - worker Z64.4
- speech R47.9
  - developmental F80.9
  - specified NEC R47.89
- swallowing — see Dysphagia
- taste — see Disturbance, sensation, taste
- tic, child F95.0
- underachievement in school Z55.3
- unemployment Z56.0
  - threatened Z56.2
- unwanted pregnancy Z64.0
- upbringing Z62.9
  - specified NEC Z62.898
- urinary N39.9
- voice production R47.89
- work schedule (stressful) Z56.3

Procedure (surgical)
- converted
  - arthroscopic to open Z53.33
  - laparoscopic to open Z53.31
  - specified procedure NEC to open Z53.39
  - thoracoscopic to open Z53.32
- for purpose other than remedying health state Z41.9
  - specified NEC Z41.8
- not done Z53.9
  - because of
    - administrative reasons Z53.8
    - contraindication Z53.09
      - smoking Z53.01
    - patient's decision Z53.20
      - for reasons of belief or group pressure Z53.1
      - left against medical advice (AMA) Z53.21
      - specified reason NEC Z53.29
    - specified reason NEC Z53.8

Procidentia (uteri) N81.3

Proctalgia K62.89
- fugax K59.4
- spasmodic K59.4

Proctitis K62.89
- amebic (acute) A06.0
- chlamydial A56.3
- gonococcal A54.6
- granulomatous — see Enteritis, regional, large intestine
- herpetic A60.1
- radiation K62.7
- tuberculous A18.32
- ulcerative (chronic) K51.20
  - with
    - complication K51.219
      - abscess K51.214
      - fistula K51.213
      - obstruction K51.212
      - rectal bleeding K51.211
      - specified NEC K51.218

Proctocele
- female (without uterine prolapse) N81.6
  - with uterine prolapse N81.2
    - complete N81.3
- male K62.3

Proctocolitis
- food-induced eosinophilic K52.82
- food protein-induced K52.82
- milk protein-induced K52.82
- mucosal — see Rectosigmoiditis, ulcerative

Proctoptosis K62.3

Proctorrhagia K62.5

Proctosigmoiditis K63.89
- ulcerative (chronic) — see Rectosigmoiditis, ulcerative

Proctospasm K59.4
- psychogenic F45.8

Profichet's disease — see Disorder, soft tissue, specified type NEC

Progeria E34.8

Prognathism (mandibular) (maxillary) M26.19

Progonoma (melanotic) — see Neoplasm, benign, by site

Progressive — see condition

Prolactinoma
- specified site — see Neoplasm, benign, by site
- unspecified site D35.2

Prolapse, prolapsed
- anus, anal (canal) (sphincter) K62.2
- arm or hand O32.2
  - causing obstructed labor O64.4
- bladder (mucosa) (sphincter) (acquired)
  - congenital Q79.4

Prolapse, prolapsed - *continued*
  bladder (mucosa) (sphincter) (acquired) - *continued*
    female — *see* Cystocele
    male N32.89
  breast implant (prosthetic) T85.49
  cecostomy K94.09
  cecum K63.4
  cervix, cervical (hypertrophied) N81.2
    anterior lip, obstructing labor O65.5
    congenital Q51.828
    postpartal, old N81.2
    stump N81.85
  ciliary body (traumatic) — *see* Laceration, eye(ball),
    with prolapse or loss of interocular tissue
  colon (pedunculated) K63.4
  colostomy K94.09
  disc (intervertebral) — *see* Displacement,
    intervertebral disc
  eye implant (orbital) T85.398
    lens (ocular) — *see* Complications, intraocular lens
  fallopian tube N83.4-
  gastric (mucosa) K31.89
  genital, female N81.9
    specified NEC N81.89
  globe, nontraumatic — *see* Luxation, globe
  ileostomy bud K94.19
  intervertebral disc — *see* Displacement,
    intervertebral disc
  intestine (small) K63.4
  iris (traumatic) — *see* Laceration, eye(ball), with
    prolapse or loss of interocular tissue
    nontraumatic H21.89
  kidney N28.83
    congenital Q63.2
  laryngeal muscles or ventricle J38.7
  liver K76.89
  meatus urinarius N36.8
  mitral (valve) I34.1
  ocular lens implant — *see* Complications,
    intraocular lens
  organ or site, congenital NEC — *see* Malposition,
    congenital
  ovary N83.4-
  pelvic floor, female N81.89
  perineum, female N81.89
  rectum (mucosa) (sphincter) K62.3
    due to trichuris trichuria B79
  spleen D73.89
  stomach K31.89
  umbilical cord
    complicating delivery O69.0
  urachus, congenital Q64.4
  ureter N28.89
    with obstruction N13.5
      with infection N13.6
  ureterovesical orifice N28.89
  urethra (acquired) (infected) (mucosa) N36.8
    congenital Q64.71
  urinary meatus N36.8
    congenital Q64.72
  uterovaginal N81.4
    complete N81.3
    incomplete N81.2
  uterus (with prolapse of vagina) N81.4
    complete N81.3
    congenital Q51.818
    first degree N81.2
    in pregnancy or childbirth — *see* Pregnancy,
      complicated by, abnormal, uterus
    incomplete N81.2
    postpartal (old) N81.4
    second degree N81.2
    third degree N81.3
  uveal (traumatic) — *see* Laceration, eye(ball), with
    prolapse or loss of interocular tissue
  vagina (anterior) (wall) — *see* Cystocele
    with prolapse of uterus N81.4
      complete N81.3
      incomplete N81.2
    posterior wall N81.6
    posthysterectomy N99.3
  vitreous (humor) H43.0-
    in wound — *see* Laceration, eye(ball), with
      prolapse or loss of interocular tissue
  womb — *see* Prolapse, uterus
Prolapsus, female N81.9
  specified NEC N81.89
Proliferation (s)
  prostate, atypical small acinar N42.32
  primary cutaneous CD30-positive large T-cell C86.6
Proliferative — *see* condition
Prolonged, prolongation (of)
  bleeding (time) (idiopathic) R79.1

Prolonged, prolongation (of) - *continued*
  coagulation (time) R79.1
  gestation (over 42 completed weeks)
    mother O48.1
    newborn P08.22
  interval I44.0
  labor O63.9
    first stage O63.0
    second stage O63.1
  partial thromboplastin time (PTT) R79.1
  pregnancy (more than 42 weeks gestation) O48.1
  prothrombin time R79.1
  QT interval I45.81
  uterine contractions in labor O62.4
Prominence, prominent
  auricle (congenital) (ear) Q17.5
  ischial spine or sacral promontory
    with disproportion (fetopelvic) O33.0
      causing obstructed labor O65.0
  nose (congenital) acquired M95.0
Promiscuity — *see* High, risk, sexual behavior
Pronation
  ankle — *see* Deformity, limb, foot, specified NEC
  foot — *see also* Deformity, limb, foot, specified
    NEC
    congenital Q74.2
Prophylactic
  administration of
    antibiotics, long-term Z79.2
      short-term use - omit code
    drug — *see also* Long-term (current) drug therapy
      (use of) Z79.899-
  medication Z79.899
  organ removal (for neoplasia management) Z40.00
    breast Z40.01
    ovary Z40.02
    specified site NEC Z40.09
  surgery Z40.9
    for risk factors related to malignant
      neoplasm — *see* Prophylactic, organ removal
    specified NEC Z40.8
  vaccination Z23
Propionic acidemia E71.121
Proptosis (ocular) — *see also* Exophthalmos
  thyroid — *see* Hyperthyroidism, with goiter
Prosecution, anxiety concerning Z65.3
Prosopagnosia R48.3
Prostadynia N42.81
Prostate, prostatic — *see* condition
Prostatism — *see* Hyperplasia, prostate
Prostatitis (congestive) (suppurative) (with
  cystitis) N41.9
  acute N41.0
  cavitary N41.8
  chronic N41.1
  diverticular N41.8
  due to Trichomonas (vaginalis) A59.02
  fibrous N41.1
  gonococcal (acute) (chronic) A54.22
  granulomatous N41.4
  hypertrophic N41.1
  subacute N41.1
  trichomonal A59.02
  tuberculous A18.14
Prostatocystitis N41.3
Prostatorrhea N42.89
Prostatosis N42.82
Prostration R53.83
  heat — *see also* Heat, exhaustion
    anhydrotic T67.3
    due to
      salt (and water) depletion T67.4
      water depletion T67.3
  nervous F48.8
  senile R54
Protanomaly (anomalous trichromat) H53.54
Protanopia (complete) (incomplete) H53.54
Protection (against) (from) — *see* Prophylactic
Protein
  deficiency NEC — *see* Malnutrition
  malnutrition — *see* Malnutrition
  sickness — *see also* Reaction, serum T80.69
Proteinemia R77.9
Proteinosis
  alveolar (pulmonary) J84.01
  lipid or lipoid (of Urbach) E78.89
Proteinuria R80.9
  Bence Jones R80.3
  complicating pregnancy — *see* Proteinuria,
    gestational
  gestational
    complicating
      childbirth O12.14

Proteinuria - *continued*
  gestational - *continued*
    complicating - *continued*
      pregnancy O12.1-
        with edema O12.2-
      puerperium O12.15
  idiopathic R80.0
  isolated R80.0
    with glomerular lesion N06.9
      dense deposit disease N06.6
      diffuse
        crescentic glomerulonephritis N06.7
        endocapillary proliferative
          glomerulonephritis N06.4
        mesangiocapillary glomerulonephritis N06.5
      focal and segmental hyalinosis or sclerosis N06.1
      membranous (diffuse) N06.2
      mesangial proliferative (diffuse) N06.3
      minimal change N06.0
      specified pathology NEC N06.8
  orthostatic R80.2
    with glomerular lesion — *see* Proteinuria, isolated,
      with glomerular lesion
  persistent R80.1
    with glomerular lesion — *see* Proteinuria, isolated,
      with glomerular lesion
  postural R80.2
    with glomerular lesion — *see* Proteinuria, isolated,
      with glomerular lesion
  pre-eclamptic — *see* Pre-eclampsia
  puerperal O12.15
  specified type NEC R80.8
Proteolysis, pathologic D65
Proteus (mirabilis) (morganii)
  , as cause of disease classified elsewhere B96.4
Prothrombin gene mutation D68.52
Protoporphyria, erythropoietic E80.0
Protozoal — *see also* condition
  disease B64
    specified NEC B60.8
Protrusion, protrusio
  acetabuli M24.7
  acetabulum (into pelvis) M24.7
  device, implant or graft — *see also* Complications,
    by site and type, mechanical T85.698
    arterial graft NEC — *see* Complication,
      cardiovascular device, mechanical, vascular
    breast (implant) T85.49
    catheter NEC T85.698
      cystostomy T83.090
      dialysis (renal) T82.49
        intraperitoneal T85.691
      infusion NEC T82.594
        spinal (epidural) (subdural) T85.690
      urinary — *see also* Complications, catheter,
        urinary T83.098
    electronic (electrode) (pulse generator) (stimulator)
      bone T84.390
      nervous system — *see* Complication, prosthetic
        device, mechanical, electronic nervous system
        stimulator
    fixation, internal (orthopedic) NEC — *see*
      Complication, fixation device, mechanical
    gastrointestinal — *see* Complications, prosthetic
      device, mechanical, gastrointestinal device
    genital NEC T83.498
      intrauterine contraceptive device T83.39
      penile prosthesis (cylinder) (implanted) (pump)
        (resevoir) T83.490
      testicular prosthesis T83.491
    heart NEC — *see* Complication, cardiovascular
      device, mechanical
    joint prosthesis — *see* Complications, joint
      prosthesis, mechanical, specified NEC, by site
    ocular NEC — *see* Complications, prosthetic
      device, mechanical, ocular device
    orthopedic NEC — *see* Complication, orthopedic,
      device, mechanical
    specified NEC T85.628
    urinary NEC — *see also* Complication,
      genitourinary, device, urinary, mechanical
      graft T83.29
    vascular NEC — *see* Complication, cardiovascular
      device, mechanical
    ventricular intracranial shunt T85.09
  intervertebral disc — *see* Displacement,
    intervertebral disc
  joint prosthesis — *see* Complications, joint
    prosthesis, mechanical, specified NEC, by site
  nucleus pulposus — *see* Displacement,
    intervertebral disc
Prune belly (syndrome) Q79.4

Prurigo (ferox) (gravis) (Hebrae) (Hebra's) (mitis) (simplex) L28.2
  Besnier's L20.0
  estivalis L56.4
  nodularis L28.1
  psychogenic F45.8
Pruritus, pruritic (essential) L29.9
  ani, anus L29.0
    psychogenic F45.8
  anogenital L29.3
    psychogenic F45.8
  due to onchocerca volvulus B73.1
  gravidarum — *see* Pregnancy, complicated by, specified pregnancy-related condition NEC
  hiemalis L29.8
  neurogenic (any site) F45.8
  perianal L29.0
  psychogenic (any site) F45.8
  scroti, scrotum L29.1
    psychogenic F45.8
  senile, senilis L29.8
  specified NEC L29.8
    psychogenic F45.8
  Trichomonas A59.9
  vulva, vulvae L29.2
    psychogenic F45.8
Pseudarthrosis, pseudoarthrosis (bone) — *see* Nonunion, fracture
  clavicle, congenital Q74.0
  joint, following fusion or arthrodesis M96.0
Pseudoaneurysm — *see* Aneurysm
Pseudoangina (pectoris) — *see* Angina
Pseudoangioma I81
Pseudoarteriosus Q28.8
Pseudoarthrosis — *see* Pseudarthrosis
Pseudobulbar affect (PBA) F48.2
Pseudochromhidrosis L67.8
Pseudocirrhosis, liver, pericardial I31.1
Pseudocowpox B08.03
Pseudocoxalgia M91.3-
Pseudocroup J38.5
Pseudo-Cushing's syndrome, alcohol -induced E24.4
Pseudocyesis F45.8
Pseudocyst
  lung J98.4
  pancreas K86.3
  retina — *see* Cyst, retina
Pseudoelephantiasis neuroarthritica Q82.0
Pseudoexfoliation, capsule (lens) — *see* Cataract, specified NEC
Pseudofolliculitis barbae L73.1
Pseudoglioma H44.89
Pseudohemophilia (Bernuth's) (hereditary) (type B) D68.0
  Type A D69.8
  vascular D69.8
Pseudohermaphroditism Q56.3
  adrenal E25.8
  female Q56.2
    with adrenocortical disorder E25.8
    without adrenocortical disorder Q56.2
    adrenal (congenital) E25.0
  male Q56.1
    with
      adrenocortical disorder E25.8
      androgen resistance E34.51
      cleft scrotum Q56.1
      feminizing testis E34.51
      5-alpha-reductase deficiency E29.1
    without gonadal disorder Q56.1
    adrenal E25.8
Pseudo-Hurler's polydystrophy E77.0
Pseudohydrocephalus G93.2
Pseudohypertrophic muscular dystrophy (Erb's) G71.0
Pseudohypertrophy, muscle G71.0
Pseudohypoparathyroidism E20.1
Pseudoinsomnia F51.03
Pseudoleukemia, infantile D64.89
Pseudomembranous — *see* condition
Pseudomeningocele (cerebral) (infective) (post-traumatic) G96.19
  postprocedural (spinal) G97.82
Pseudomenses (newborn) P54.6
Pseudomenstruation (newborn) P54.6
Pseudomonas
  aeruginosa, as cause of disease classified elsewhere B96.5
  mallei infection A24.0
    as cause of disease classified elsewhere B96.5
  pseudomallei, as cause of disease classified elsewhere B96.5

Pseudomyotonia G71.19
Pseudomyxoma peritonei C78.6
Pseudoneuritis, optic (nerve) (disc) (papilla), congenital Q14.2
Pseudo-obstruction intestine (acute) (chronic) (idiopathic) (intermittent secondary) (primary) K59.8
Pseudopapilledema H47.33-
  congenital Q14.2
Pseudoparalysis
  arm or leg R29.818
  atonic, congenital P94.2
Pseudopelade L66.0
Pseudophakia Z96.1
Pseudopolyarthritis, rhizomelic M35.3
Pseudopolycythemia D75.1
Pseudopseudohypoparathyroidism E20.1
Pseudopterygium H11.81-
Pseudoptosis (eyelid) — *see* Blepharochalasis
Pseudopuberty, precocious
  female heterosexual E25.8
  male isosexual E25.8
Pseudorickets (renal) N25.0
Pseudorubella B08.20
Pseudosclerema, newborn P83.8
Pseudosclerosis (brain)
  of Westphal (Strümpell) E83.01
  Jakob's — *see* Creutzfeldt-Jakob disease or syndrome
  spastic — *see* Creutzfeldt-Jakob disease or syndrome
Pseudotetanus — *see* Convulsions
Pseudotetany R29.0
  hysterical F44.5
Pseudotruncus arteriosus Q25.49
Pseudotuberculosis A28.2
  enterocolitis A04.8
  pasteurella (infection) A28.0
Pseudotumor
  cerebri G93.2
  orbital H05.11-
Pseudoxanthoma elasticum Q82.8
Psilosis (sprue) (tropical) K90.1
  nontropical K90.0
Psittacosis A70
Psoitis M60.88
Psoriasis L40.9
  arthropathic L40.50
    arthritis mutilans L40.52
    distal interphalangeal L40.51
    juvenile L40.54
    other specified L40.59
    spondylitis L40.53
  buccal K13.29
  flexural L40.8
  guttate L40.4
  mouth K13.29
  nummular L40.0
  plaque L40.0
  psychogenic F54
  pustular (generalized) L40.1
    palmaris et plantaris L40.3
  specified NEC L40.8
  vulgaris L40.0
Psychasthenia F48.8
Psychiatric disorder or problem F99
Psychogenic — *see also* condition
  factors associated with physical conditions F54
Psychological and behavioral factors affecting medical condition F59
Psychoneurosis, psychoneurotic — *see also* Neurosis
  anxiety (state) F41.1
  depersonalization F48.1
  hypochondriacal F45.21
  hysteria F44.9
  neurasthenic F48.8
  personality NEC F60.89
Psychopathy, psychopathic
  affectionless F94.2
  autistic F84.5
  constitution, post-traumatic F07.81
  personality — *see* Disorder, personality
  sexual — *see* Deviation, sexual
  state F60.2
Psychosexual identity disorder of childhood F64.2
Psychosis, psychotic F29
  acute (transient) F23
    hysterical F44.9
  affective — *see* Disorder, mood
  alcoholic F10.959
    with
      abuse F10.159

Psychosis, psychotic - *continued*
  alcoholic - *continued*
    with - *continued*
      anxiety disorder F10.980
        with
          abuse F10.180
          dependence F10.280
      delirium tremens F10.231
      delusions F10.950
        with
          abuse F10.150
          dependence F10.250
      dementia F10.97
        with dependence F10.27
      dependence F10.259
      hallucinosis F10.951
        with
          abuse F10.151
          dependence F10.251
      mood disorder F10.94
        with
          abuse F10.14
          dependence F10.24
      paranoia F10.950
        with
          abuse F10.150
          dependence F10.250
      persisting amnesia F10.96
        with dependence F10.26
    amnestic confabulatory F10.96
      with dependence F10.26
    delirium tremens F10.231
    Korsakoff's, Korsakov's, Korsakow's F10.26
    paranoid type F10.950
      with
        abuse F10.150
        dependence F10.250
  anergastic — *see* Psychosis, organic
  arteriosclerotic (simple type) (uncomplicated) F01.50
    with behavioral disturbance F01.51
  childhood F84.0
    atypical F84.8
  climacteric — *see* Psychosis, involutional
  confusional F29
    acute or subacute F05
    reactive F23
  cycloid F23
  depressive — *see* Disorder, depressive
  disintegrative (childhood) F84.3
  drug-induced — *see* F11-F19 with .x59
    paranoid and hallucinatory states — *see* F11-F19 with .x50 or .x51
  due to or associated with
    addiction, drug — *see* F11-F19 with .x59
    dependence
      alcohol F10.259
      drug — *see* F11-F19 with .x59
    epilepsy F06.8
    Huntington's chorea F06.8
    ischemia, cerebrovascular (generalized) F06.8
    multiple sclerosis F06.8
    physical disease F06.8
    presenile dementia F03
    senile dementia F03
    vascular disease (arteriosclerotic) (cerebral) F01.50
      with behavioral disturbance F01.51
  epileptic F06.8
  episode F23
    due to or associated with physical condition F06.8
  exhaustive F43.0
  hallucinatory, chronic F28
  hypomanic F30.8
  hysterical (acute) F44.9
  induced F24
  infantile F84.0
    atypical F84.8
  infective (acute) (subacute) F05
  involutional F28
    depressive — *see* Disorder, depressive
    melancholic — *see* Disorder, depressive
    paranoid (state) F22
  Korsakoff's, Korsakov's, Korsakow's (nonalcoholic) F04
    alcoholic F10.96
      in dependence F10.26
  induced by other psychoactive substance — *see* categories F11-F19 with .x5x
  mania, manic (single episode) F30.2
    recurrent type F31.89
  manic-depressive — *see* Disorder, bipolar
  menopausal — *see* Psychosis, involutional
  mixed schizophrenic and affective F25.8

Psychosis, psychotic - *continued*
  multi-infarct (cerebrovascular) F01.50
    with behavioral disturbance F01.51
  nonorganic F29
    specified NEC F28
  organic F09
    due to or associated with
      arteriosclerosis (cerebral) — *see* Psychosis,
        arteriosclerotic
      cerebrovascular disease, arteriosclerotic — *see*
        Psychosis, arteriosclerotic
      childbirth — *see* Psychosis, puerperal
      Creutzfeldt-Jakob disease or syndrome — *see*
        Creutzfeldt-Jakob disease or syndrome
      dependence, alcohol F10.259
      disease
        alcoholic liver F10.259
        brain, arteriosclerotic — *see* Psychosis,
          arteriosclerotic
        cerebrovascular F01.50
          with behavioral disturbance F01.51
        Creutzfeldt-Jakob — *see* Creutzfeldt-Jakob
          disease or syndrome
        endocrine or metabolic F06.8
          acute or subacute F05
        liver, alcoholic F10.259
      epilepsy transient (acute) F05
      infection
        brain (intracranial) F06.8
          acute or subacute F05
      intoxication
        alcoholic (acute) F10.259
        drug F19 with .x59 F11-
      ischemia, cerebrovascular (generalized) — *see*
        Psychosis, arteriosclerotic
      puerperium — *see* Psychosis, puerperal
      trauma, brain (birth) (from electric current)
        (surgical) F06.8
        acute or subacute F05
    infective F06.8
      acute or subacute F05
    post-traumatic F06.8
      acute or subacute F05
  paranoiac F22
  paranoid (climacteric) (involutional)
    (menopausal) F22
    psychogenic (acute) F23
    schizophrenic F20.0
    senile F03
  postpartum F53
  presbyophrenic (type) F03
  presenile F03
  psychogenic (paranoid) F23
    depressive F32.3
  puerperal F53
    specified type — *see* Psychosis, by type
  reactive (brief) (transient) (emotional stress)
    (psychological trauma) F23
    depressive F32.3
      recurrent F33.3
    excitative type F30.8
  schizoaffective F25.9
    depressive type F25.1
    manic type F25.0
  schizophrenia, schizophrenic — *see* Schizophrenia
  schizophrenia-like, in epilepsy F06.2
  schizophreniform F20.81
    affective type F25.9
    brief F23
    confusional type F23
    depressive type F25.1
    manic type F25.0
    mixed type F25.0
  senile NEC F03
    depressed or paranoid type F03
    simple deterioration F03
    specified type - code to condition
  shared F24
  situational (reactive) F23
  symbiotic (childhood) F84.3
  symptomatic F09
Psychosomatic — *see* Disorder, psychosomatic
Psychosyndrome, organic F07.9
Psychotic episode due to or associated with
physical condition F06.8
Pterygium (eye) H11.00-
  amyloid H11.01-
  central H11.02-
  colli Q18.3
  double H11.03-
  peripheral
    progressive H11.05-
    stationary H11.04-

Pterygium (eye) - *continued*
  recurrent H11.06-
Ptilosis (eyelid) — *see* Madarosis
Ptomaine (poisoning) — *see* Poisoning, food
Ptosis — *see also* Blepharoptosis
  adiposa (false) — *see* Blepharoptosis
  breast N64.81
  cecum K63.4
  colon K63.4
  congenital (eyelid) Q10.0
    specified site NEC — *see* Anomaly, by site
  eyelid — *see* Blepharoptosis
    congenital Q10.0
  gastric K31.89
  intestine K63.4
  kidney N28.83
  liver K76.89
  renal N28.83
  splanchnic K63.4
  spleen D73.89
  stomach K31.89
  viscera K63.4
PTP D69.51
Ptyalism (periodic) K11.7
  hysterical F45.8
  pregnancy — *see* Pregnancy, complicated by,
    specified pregnancy-related condition NEC
  psychogenic F45.8
Ptyalolithiasis K11.5
Pubarche, precocious E30.1
Pubertas praecox E30.1
Puberty (development state) Z00.3
  bleeding (excessive) N92.2
  delayed E30.0
  precocious (constitutional) (cryptogenic)
    (idiopathic) E30.1
    central E22.8
    due to
      ovarian hyperfunction E28.1
        estrogen E28.0
      testicular hyperfunction E29.0
  premature E30.1
    due to
      adrenal cortical hyperfunction E25.8
      pineal tumor E34.8
      pituitary (anterior) hyperfunction E22.8
Puckering, macula — *see* Degeneration, macula,
  puckering
Pudenda, pudendum — *see* condition
Puente's disease (simple glandular cheilitis) K13.0
Puerperal, puerperium
  (complicated by, complications)
  abnormal glucose (tolerance test) O99.815
  abscess
    areola O91.02
      associated with lactation O91.03
    Bartholin's gland O86.19
    breast O91.12
      associated with lactation O91.13
    cervix (uteri) O86.11
    genital organ NEC O86.19
    kidney O86.21
    mammary O91.12
      associated with lactation O91.13
    nipple O91.02
      associated with lactation O91.03
    peritoneum O85
    subareolar O91.12
      associated with lactation O91.13
    urinary tract — *see* Puerperal, infection, urinary
    uterus O86.12
    vagina (wall) O86.13
    vaginorectal O86.13
    vulvovaginal gland O86.13
  adnexitis O86.19
  afibrinogenemia, or other coagulation defect O72.3
  albuminuria (acute) (subacute) — *see* Proteinuria,
    gestational
  alcohol use O99.315
  anemia O90.81
    pre-existing (pre-pregnancy) O99.03
  anesthetic death O89.8
  apoplexy O99.43
  bariatric surgery status O99.845
  blood disorder NEC O99.13
  blood dyscrasia O72.3
  cardiomyopathy O90.3
  cerebrovascular disorder (conditions in I60-
    I69) O99.43
  cervicitis O86.11
  circulatory system disorder O99.43
  coagulopathy (any) O72.3
  complications O90.9

Puerperal, puerperium
  (complicated by, complications) - *continued*
  complications - *continued*
    specified NEC O90.89
  convulsions — *see* Eclampsia
  cystitis O86.22
  cystopyelitis O86.29
  delirium NEC F05
  diabetes O24.93
    gestational — *see* Puerperal, gestational diabetes
    pre-existing O24.33
      specified NEC O24.83
      type 1 O24.03
      type 2 O24.13
  digestive system disorder O99.63
  disease O90.9
    breast NEC O92.29
    cerebrovascular (acute) O99.43
    nonobstetric NEC O99.89
    tubo-ovarian O86.19
    Valsuani's O99.03
  disorder O90.9
    biliary tract O26.63
    lactation O92.70
    liver O26.63
    nonobstetric NEC O99.89
  disruption
    cesarean wound O90.0
    episiotomy wound O90.1
    perineal laceration wound O90.1
  drug use O99.325
  eclampsia (with pre-existing hypertension) O15.2
  embolism (pulmonary) (blood clot) — *see*
    Embolism, obstetric, puerperal
  endocrine, nutritional or metabolic disease
    NEC O99.285
  endophlebitis — *see* Puerperal, phlebitis
  endotrachelitis O86.11
  failure
    lactation (complete) O92.3
      partial O92.4
    renal, acute O90.4
  fever (of unknown origin) O86.4
    septic O85
  fissure, nipple O92.12
    associated with lactation O92.13
  fistula
    breast (due to mastitis) O91.12
      associated with lactation O91.13
    nipple O91.02
      associated with lactation O91.03
  galactophoritis O91.22
    associated with lactation O91.23
  galactorrhea O92.6
  gastric banding status O99.845
  gastric bypass status O99.845
  gastrointestinal disease NEC O99.63
  gestational
    diabetes O24.439
      diet controlled O24.430
      insulin (and diet) controlled O24.434
      oral drug controlled (antidiabetic)
        (hypoglycemic) O24.435
    edema O12.05
      with proteinuria O12.25
    proteinuria O12.15
  gonorrhea O98.23
  hematoma, subdural O99.43
  hemiplegia, cerebral O99.355
    due to cerebrovascular disorder O99.43
  hemorrhage O72.1
    brain O99.43
    bulbar O99.43
    cerebellar O99.43
    cerebral O99.43
    cortical O99.43
    delayed or secondary O72.2
    extradural O99.43
    internal capsule O99.43
    intracranial O99.43
    intrapontine O99.43
    meningeal O99.43
    pontine O99.43
    retained placenta O72.0
    subarachnoid O99.43
    subcortical O99.43
    subdural O99.43
    third stage O72.0
    uterine, delayed O72.2
    ventricular O99.43
  hemorrhoids O87.2
  hepatorenal syndrome O90.4

Puerperal, puerperium (complicated by, complications) - *continued*
  hypertension — *see* Hypertension, complicating, puerperium
  hypertrophy, breast O92.29
  induration breast (fibrous) O92.29
  infection O86.4
    cervix O86.11
    generalized O85
    genital tract NEC O86.19
      obstetric surgical wound O86.0
    kidney (bacillus coli) O86.21
    maternal O98.93
      carrier state NEC O99.835
      gonorrhea O98.23
      human immunodeficiency virus (HIV) O98.73
      protozoal O98.63
      sexually transmitted NEC O98.33
      specified NEC O98.83
      streptococcus group B (GBS) carrier state O99.825
      syphilis O98.13
      tuberculosis O98.03
      viral hepatitis O98.43
      viral NEC O98.53
    nipple O91.02
      associated with lactation O91.03
    peritoneum O85
    renal O86.21
    specified NEC O86.89
    urinary (asymptomatic) (tract) NEC O86.20
      bladder O86.22
      kidney O86.21
      specified site NEC O86.29
      urethra O86.22
      vagina O86.13
    vein — *see* Puerperal, phlebitis
  ischemia, cerebral O99.43
  lymphangitis O86.89
    breast O91.22
      associated with lactation O91.23
  malignancy O9A.13
  malnutrition O25.3
  mammillitis O91.02
    associated with lactation O91.03
  mammitis O91.22
    associated with lactation O91.23
  mania F30.8
  mastitis O91.22
    associated with lactation O91.23
    purulent O91.12
      associated with lactation O91.13
  melancholia — *see* Disorder, depressive
  mental disorder NEC O99.345
  metroperitonitis O85
  metrorrhagia — *see* Hemorrhage, postpartum
  metrosalpingitis O86.19
  metrovaginitis O86.13
  milk leg O87.1
  monoplegia, cerebral O99.43
  mood disturbance O90.6
  necrosis, liver (acute) (subacute) (conditions in subcategory K72.0) O26.63
    with renal failure O90.4
  nervous system disorder O99.355
  neuritis O90.89
  obesity (pre-existing prior to pregnancy) O99.215
  obesity surgery status O99.845
  occlusion, precerebral artery O99.43
  paralysis
    bladder (sphincter) O90.89
    cerebral O99.43
  paralytic stroke O99.43
  parametritis O85
  paravaginitis O86.13
  pelviperitonitis O85
  perimetritis O86.12
  perimetrosalpingitis O86.19
  perinephritis O86.21
  periphlebitis — *see* Puerperal phlebitis
  peritoneal infection O85
  peritonitis (pelvic) O85
  perivaginitis O86.13
  phlebitis O87.0
    deep O87.1
    pelvic O87.1
    superficial O87.0
  phlebothrombosis, deep O87.1
  phlegmasia alba dolens O87.1
  placental polyp O90.89
  pneumonia, embolic — *see* Embolism, obstetric, puerperal
  pre-eclampsia — *see* Pre-eclampsia

Puerperal, puerperium (complicated by, complications) - *continued*
  psychosis F53
  pyelitis O86.21
  pyelocystitis O86.29
  pyelonephritis O86.21
  pyelonephrosis O86.21
  pyemia O85
  pyocystitis O86.29
  pyohemia O85
  pyometra O86.12
  pyonephritis O86.21
  pyosalpingitis O86.19
  pyrexia (of unknown origin) O86.4
  renal
    disease NEC O90.89
    failure O90.4
  respiratory disease NEC O99.53
  retention
    decidua — *see* Retention, decidua
    placenta O72.0
    secundines — *see* Retention, secundines
  retrated nipple O92.02
  salpingo-ovaritis O86.19
  salpingoperitonitis O85
  secondary perineal tear O90.1
  sepsis (pelvic) O85
  sepsis O85
  septic thrombophlebitis O86.81
  skin disorder NEC O99.73
  specified condition NEC O99.89
  stroke O99.43
  subinvolution (uterus) O90.89
  subluxation of symphysis (pubis) O26.73
  suppuration — *see* Puerperal, abscess
  tetanus A34
  thelitis O91.02
    associated with lactation O91.03
  thrombocytopenia O72.3
  thrombophlebitis (superficial) O87.0
    deep O87.1
    pelvic O87.1
    septic O86.81
  thrombosis (venous) — *see* Thrombosis, puerperal
  thyroiditis O90.5
  toxemia (eclamptic) (pre-eclamptic) (with convulsions) O15.2
  trauma, non-obstetric O9A.23
    caused by abuse (physical) (suspected) O9A.33
      confirmed O9A.33
    psychological (suspected) O9A.53
      confirmed O9A.53
    sexual (suspected) O9A.43
      confirmed O9A.43
  uremia (due to renal failure) O90.4
  urethritis O86.22
  vaginitis O86.13
  varicose veins (legs) O87.4
    vulva or perineum O87.8
  venous O87.9
  vulvitis O86.19
  vulvovaginitis O86.13
  white leg O87.1
Puerperium — *see* Puerperal
Pulmolithiasis J98.4
Pulmonary — *see* condition
Pulpitis (acute) (anachoretic) (chronic) (hyperplastic) (putrescent) (suppurative) (ulcerative) K04.01
  irreversible K04.02
  reversible K04.01
Pulpless tooth K04.99
Pulse
  alternating R00.8
  bigeminal R00.8
  fast R00.0
  feeble, rapid due to shock following injury T79.4
  rapid R00.0
  weak R09.89
Pulsus alternans or trigeminus R00.8
Punch drunk F07.81
Punctum lacrimale occlusion — *see* Obstruction, lacrimal
Puncture
  abdomen, abdominal
    wall S31.139
      with
        foreign body S31.149
        penetration into peritoneal cavity S31.639
          with foreign body S31.649
      epigastric region S31.132
        with
          foreign body S31.142
          penetration into peritoneal cavity S31.632

Puncture - *continued*
  abdomen, abdominal - *continued*
    wall - *continued*
      epigastric region - *continued*
        with - *continued*
          penetration into peritoneal cavity - *continued*
            with foreign body S31.642
      left
        lower quadrant S31.134
          with
            foreign body S31.144
            penetration into peritoneal cavity S31.634
              with foreign body S31.644
        upper quadrant S31.131
          with
            foreign body S31.141
            penetration into peritoneal cavity S31.631
              with foreign body S31.641
      periumbilic region S31.135
        with
          foreign body S31.145
          penetration into peritoneal cavity S31.635
            with foreign body S31.645
      right
        lower quadrant S31.133
          with
            foreign body S31.143
            penetration into peritoneal cavity S31.633
              with foreign body S31.643
        upper quadrant S31.130
          with
            foreign body S31.140
            penetration into peritoneal cavity S31.630
              with foreign body S31.640
  accidental, complicating surgery — *see* Complication, accidental puncture or laceration
  alveolar (process) — *see* Puncture, oral cavity
  ankle S91.039
    with
      foreign body S91.049
    left S91.032
      with
        foreign body S91.042
    right S91.031
      with
        foreign body S91.041
  anus S31.833
    with foreign body S31.834
  arm (upper) S41.139
    with foreign body S41.149
    left S41.132
      with foreign body S41.142
    lower — *see* Puncture, forearm
    right S41.131
      with foreign body S41.141
  auditory canal (external) (meatus) — *see* Puncture, ear
  auricle, ear — *see* Puncture, ear
  axilla — *see* Puncture, arm
  back — *see also* Puncture, thorax, back
    lower S31.030
      with
        foreign body S31.040
          with penetration into retroperitoneal space S31.041
        penetration into retroperitoneal space S31.031
  bladder (traumatic) S37.29
    nontraumatic N32.89
  breast S21.039
    with foreign body S21.049
    left S21.032
      with foreign body S21.042
    right S21.031
      with foreign body S21.041
  buttock S31.803
    with foreign body S31.804
    left S31.823
      with foreign body S31.824
    right S31.813
      with foreign body S31.814
  by
    device, implant or graft — *see* Complications, by site and type, mechanical
    foreign body left accidentally in operative wound T81.539
    instrument (any) during a procedure, accidental — *see* Puncture, accidental complicating surgery
  calf — *see* Puncture, leg
  canaliculus lacrimalis — *see* Puncture, eyelid
  canthus, eye — *see* Puncture, eyelid
  cervical esophagus S11.23
    with foreign body S11.24

Puncture - *continued*
  cheek (external) S01.439
    with foreign body S01.449
    left S01.432
      with foreign body S01.442
    right S01.431
      with foreign body S01.441
    internal — *see* Puncture, oral cavity
  chest wall — *see* Puncture, thorax
  chin — *see* Puncture, head, specified site NEC
  clitoris — *see* Puncture, vulva
  costal region — *see* Puncture, thorax
  digit (s)
    hand — *see* Puncture, finger
    foot — *see* Puncture, toe
  ear (canal) (external) S01.339
    with foreign body S01.349
    left S01.332
      with foreign body S01.342
    right S01.331
      with foreign body S01.341
    drum S09.2-
  elbow S51.039
    with
      foreign body S51.049
    left S51.032
      with
        foreign body S51.042
    right S51.031
      with
        foreign body S51.041
  epididymis — *see* Puncture, testis
  epigastric region — *see* Puncture, abdomen, wall, epigastric
  epiglottis S11.83
    with foreign body S11.84
  esophagus
    cervical S11.23
      with foreign body S11.24
    thoracic S27.818
  eyeball S05.6-
    with foreign body S05.5-
  eyebrow — *see* Puncture, eyelid
  eyelid S01.13-
    with foreign body S01.14-
    left S01.132
      with foreign body S01.142
    right S01.131
      with foreign body S01.141
  face NEC — *see* Puncture, head, specified site NEC
  finger (s) S61.239
    with
      damage to nail S61.339
        with
          foreign body S61.349
      foreign body S61.249
    index S61.238
      with
        damage to nail S61.338
          with
            foreign body S61.348
        foreign body S61.248
      left S61.231
        with
          damage to nail S61.331
            with
              foreign body S61.341
          foreign body S61.241
      right S61.230
        with
          damage to nail S61.330
            with
              foreign body S61.340
          foreign body S61.240
    little S61.238
      with
        damage to nail S61.338
          with
            foreign body S61.348
        foreign body S61.248
      left S61.237
        with
          damage to nail S61.337
            with
              foreign body S61.347
          foreign body S61.247
      right S61.236
        with
          damage to nail S61.336
            with
              foreign body S61.346
          foreign body S61.246
    middle S61.238

Puncture - *continued*
  finger (s) - *continued*
    middle - *continued*
      with
        damage to nail S61.338
          with
            foreign body S61.348
        foreign body S61.248
      left S61.233
        with
          damage to nail S61.333
            with
              foreign body S61.343
          foreign body S61.243
      right S61.232
        with
          damage to nail S61.332
            with
              foreign body S61.342
          foreign body S61.242
    ring S61.238
      with
        damage to nail S61.338
          with
            foreign body S61.348
        foreign body S61.248
      left S61.235
        with
          damage to nail S61.335
            with
              foreign body S61.345
          foreign body S61.245
      right S61.234
        with
          damage to nail S61.334
            with
              foreign body S61.344
          foreign body S61.244
  flank S31.139
    with foreign body S31.149
  foot (except toe (s) alone) S91.339
    with foreign body S91.349
    left S91.332
      with foreign body S91.342
    right S91.331
      with foreign body S91.341
    toe — *see* Puncture, toe
  forearm S51.839
    with
      foreign body S51.849
    elbow only — *see* Puncture, elbow
    left S51.832
      with
        foreign body S51.842
    right S51.831
      with
        foreign body S51.841
  forehead — *see* Puncture, head, specified site NEC
  genital organs, external
    female S31.532
      with foreign body S31.542
      vagina — *see* Puncture, vagina
      vulva — *see* Puncture, vulva
    male S31.531
      with foreign body S31.541
      penis — *see* Puncture, penis
      scrotum — *see* Puncture, scrotum
      testis — *see* Puncture, testis
  groin — *see* Puncture, abdomen, wall
  gum — *see* Puncture, oral cavity
  hand S61.439
    with
      foreign body S61.449
    finger — *see* Puncture, finger
    left S61.432
      with
        foreign body S61.442
    right S61.431
      with
        foreign body S61.441
    thumb — *see* Puncture, thumb
  head S01.93
    with foreign body S01.94
    cheek — *see* Puncture, cheek
    ear — *see* Puncture, ear
    eyelid — *see* Puncture, eyelid
    lip — *see* Puncture, oral cavity
    nose — *see* Puncture, nose
    oral cavity — *see* Puncture, oral cavity
    scalp S01.03
      with foreign body S01.04
    specified site NEC S01.83
      with foreign body S01.84

Puncture - *continued*
  head - *continued*
    temporomandibular area — *see* Puncture, cheek
    heart S26.99
      with hemopericardium S26.09
      without hemopericardium S26.19
    heel — *see* Puncture, foot
    hip S71.039
      with foreign body S71.049
      left S71.032
        with foreign body S71.042
      right S71.031
        with foreign body S71.041
    hymen — *see* Puncture, vagina
    hypochondrium — *see* Puncture, abdomen, wall
    hypogastric region — *see* Puncture, abdomen, wall
    inguinal region — *see* Puncture, abdomen, wall
    instep — *see* Puncture, foot
    internal organs — *see* Injury, by site
    interscapular region — *see* Puncture, thorax, back
    intestine
      large
        colon S36.599
          ascending S36.590
          descending S36.592
          sigmoid S36.593
          specified site NEC S36.598
          transverse S36.591
        rectum S36.69
      small S36.499
        duodenum S36.490
        specified site NEC S36.498
    intra-abdominal organ S36.99
      gallbladder S36.128
      intestine — *see* Puncture, intestine
      liver S36.118
      pancreas — *see* Puncture, pancreas
      peritoneum S36.81
      specified site NEC S36.898
      spleen S36.09
      stomach S36.39
    jaw — *see* Puncture, head, specified site NEC
    knee S81.039
      with foreign body S81.049
      left S81.032
        with foreign body S81.042
      right S81.031
        with foreign body S81.041
    labium (majus) (minus) — *see* Puncture, vulva
    lacrimal duct — *see* Puncture, eyelid
    larynx S11.013
      with foreign body S11.014
    leg (lower) S81.839
      with foreign body S81.849
      foot — *see* Puncture, foot
      knee — *see* Puncture, knee
      left S81.832
        with foreign body S81.842
      right S81.831
        with foreign body S81.841
      upper — *see* Puncture, thigh
    lip S01.531
      with foreign body S01.541
    loin — *see* Puncture, abdomen, wall
    lower back — *see* Puncture, back, lower
    lumbar region — *see* Puncture, back, lower
    malar region — *see* Puncture, head, specified site NEC
    mammary — *see* Puncture, breast
    mastoid region — *see* Puncture, head, specified site NEC
    mouth — *see* Puncture, oral cavity
    nail
      finger — *see* Puncture, finger, with damage to nail
      toe — *see* Puncture, toe, with damage to nail
    nasal (septum) (sinus) — *see* Puncture, nose
    nasopharynx — *see* Puncture, head, specified site NEC
    neck S11.93
      with foreign body S11.94
      involving
        cervical esophagus — *see* Puncture, cervical esophagus
        larynx — *see* Puncture, larynx
        pharynx — *see* Puncture, pharynx
        thyroid gland — *see* Puncture, thyroid gland
        trachea — *see* Puncture, trachea
      specified site NEC S11.83
        with foreign body S11.84
    nose (septum) (sinus) S01.23
      with foreign body S01.24
    ocular — *see* Puncture, eyeball
    oral cavity S01.532

Puncture - *continued*
oral cavity - *continued*
 with foreign body S01.542
orbit S05.4-
palate — *see* Puncture, oral cavity
palm — *see* Puncture, hand
pancreas S36.299
 body S36.291
 head S36.290
 tail S36.292
pelvis — *see* Puncture, back, lower
penis S31.23
 with foreign body S31.24
perineum
 female S31.43
 with foreign body S31.44
 male S31.139
 with foreign body S31.149
periocular area (with or without lacrimal passages) — *see* Puncture, eyelid
phalanges
 finger — *see* Puncture, finger
 toe — *see* Puncture, toe
pharynx S11.23
 with foreign body S11.24
pinna — *see* Puncture, ear
popliteal space — *see* Puncture, knee
prepuce — *see* Puncture, penis
pubic region S31.139
 with foreign body S31.149
pudendum — *see* Puncture, genital organs, external
rectovaginal septum — *see* Puncture, vagina
sacral region — *see* Puncture, back, lower
sacroiliac region — *see* Puncture, back, lower
salivary gland — *see* Puncture, oral cavity
scalp S01.03
 with foreign body S01.04
scapular region — *see* Puncture, shoulder
scrotum S31.33
 with foreign body S31.34
shin — *see* Puncture, leg
shoulder S41.039
 with foreign body S41.049
 left S41.032
 with foreign body S41.042
 right S41.031
 with foreign body S41.041
spermatic cord — *see* Puncture, testis
sternal region — *see* Puncture, thorax, front
submaxillary region — *see* Puncture, head, specified site NEC
submental region — *see* Puncture, head, specified site NEC
subungual
 finger (s) — *see* Puncture, finger, with damage to nail
 toe — *see* Puncture, toe, with damage to nail
supraclavicular fossa — *see* Puncture, neck, specified site NEC
temple, temporal region — *see* Puncture, head, specified site NEC
temporomandibular area — *see* Puncture, cheek
testis S31.33
 with foreign body S31.34
thigh S71.139
 with foreign body S71.149
 left S71.132
 with foreign body S71.142
 right S71.131
 with foreign body S71.141
thorax, thoracic (wall) S21.93
 with foreign body S21.94
 back S21.23-
 with
 foreign body S21.24-
 with penetration S21.44
 penetration S21.43
 breast — *see* Puncture, breast
 front S21.13-
 with
 foreign body S21.14-
 with penetration S21.34
 penetration S21.33
throat — *see* Puncture, neck
thumb S61.039
 with
 damage to nail S61.139
 with
 foreign body S61.149
 foreign body S61.049
 left S61.032
 with
 damage to nail S61.132

Puncture - *continued*
thumb - *continued*
 left - *continued*
 with - *continued*
 damage to nail - *continued*
 with
 foreign body S61.142
 foreign body S61.042
 right S61.031
 with
 damage to nail S61.131
 with
 foreign body S61.141
 foreign body S61.041
thyroid gland S11.13
 with foreign body S11.14
toe (s) S91.139
 with
 damage to nail S91.239
 with
 foreign body S91.249
 foreign body S91.149
 great S91.133
 with
 damage to nail S91.233
 with
 foreign body S91.243
 foreign body S91.143
 left S91.132
 with
 damage to nail S91.232
 with
 foreign body S91.242
 foreign body S91.142
 right S91.131
 with
 damage to nail S91.231
 with
 foreign body S91.241
 foreign body S91.141
 lesser S91.136
 with
 damage to nail S91.236
 with
 foreign body S91.246
 foreign body S91.146
 left S91.135
 with
 damage to nail S91.235
 with
 foreign body S91.245
 foreign body S91.145
 right S91.134
 with
 damage to nail S91.234
 with
 foreign body S91.244
 foreign body S91.144
tongue — *see* Puncture, oral cavity
trachea S11.023
 with foreign body S11.024
tunica vaginalis — *see* Puncture, testis
tympanum, tympanic membrane S09.2-
umbilical region S31.135
 with foreign body S31.145
uvula — *see* Puncture, oral cavity
vagina S31.43
 with foreign body S31.44
vocal cords S11.033
 with foreign body S11.034
vulva S31.43
 with foreign body S31.44
wrist S61.539
 with
 foreign body S61.549
 left S61.532
 with
 foreign body S61.542
 right S61.531
 with
 foreign body S61.541
PUO (pyrexia of unknown origin) R50.9
Pupillary membrane (persistent) Q13.89
Pupillotonia — *see* Anomaly, pupil, function, tonic pupil
Purpura D69.2
abdominal D69.0
allergic D69.0
anaphylactoid D69.0
annularis telangiectodes L81.7
arthritic D69.0
autoerythrocyte sensitization D69.2
autoimmune D69.0

Purpura - *continued*
bacterial D69.2
Bateman's (senile) D69.2
capillary fragility (hereditary) (idiopathic) D69.8
cryoglobulinemic D89.1
Devil's pinches D69.2
fibrinolytic — *see* Fibrinolysis
fulminans, fulminous D65
gangrenous D65
hemorrhagic, hemorrhagica D69.3
 not due to thrombocytopenia D69.0
Henoch (-Schönlein) (allergic) D69.0
hypergammaglobulinemic (benign) (Waldenström) D89.0
idiopathic (thrombocytopenic) D69.3
 nonthrombocytopenic D69.0
immune thrombocytopenic D69.3
infectious D69.0
malignant D69.0
neonatorum P54.5
nervosa D69.0
newborn P54.5
nonthrombocytopenic D69.2
 hemorrhagic D69.0
 idiopathic D69.0
nonthrombopenic D69.2
peliosis rheumatica D69.0
posttransfusion (post-transfusion) (from (fresh) whole blood or blood products) D69.51
primary D69.49
red cell membrane sensitivity D69.2
rheumatica D69.0
Schönlein (-Henoch) (allergic) D69.0
scorbutic E54 *[D77]*
senile D69.2
simplex D69.2
symptomatica D69.0
telangiectasia annularis L81.7
thrombocytopenic D69.49
 congenital D69.42
 hemorrhagic D69.3
 hereditary D69.42
 idiopathic D69.3
 immune D69.3
 neonatal, transitory P61.0
 thrombotic M31.1
thrombohemolytic — *see* Fibrinolysis
thrombolytic — *see* Fibrinolysis
thrombopenic D69.49
thrombotic, thrombocytopenic M31.1
toxic D69.0
vascular D69.0
visceral symptoms D69.0
Purpuric spots R23.3
Purulent — *see* condition
Pus
in
 stool R19.5
 urine N39.0
tube (rupture) — *see* Salpingo-oophoritis
Pustular rash L08.0
Pustule (nonmalignant) L08.9
malignant A22.0
Pustulosis palmaris et plantaris L40.3
Putnam (-Dana) **disease or syndrome** — *see* Degeneration, combined
Putrescent pulp (dental) K04.1
Pyarthritis, pyarthrosis — *see* Arthritis, pyogenic or pyemic
tuberculous — *see* Tuberculosis, joint
Pyelectasis — *see* Hydronephrosis
Pyelitis (congenital) (uremic) — *see also* Pyelonephritis
with
 calculus — *see* category N20
 with hydronephrosis N13.2
 contracted kidney N11.9
acute N10
chronic N11.9
 with calculus — *see* category N20
 with hydronephrosis N13.2
cystica N28.84
puerperal (postpartum) O86.21
tuberculous A18.11
Pyelocystitis — *see* Pyelonephritis
Pyelonephritis — *see also* Nephritis, tubulo-interstitial
with
 calculus — *see* category N20
 with hydronephrosis N13.2
 contracted kidney N11.9
acute N10
calculous — *see* category N20

Pyelonephritis - *continued*
  calculous - *continued*
    with hydronephrosis N13.2
  chronic N11.9
    with calculus — *see* category N20
      with hydronephrosis N13.2
    associated with ureteral obstruction or
      stricture N11.1
    nonobstructive N11.8
      with reflux (vesicoureteral) N11.0
    obstructive N11.1
    specified NEC N11.8
  in (due to)
    brucellosis A23.9 [N16]
    cryoglobulinemia (mixed) D89.1 [N16]
    cystinosis E72.04
    diphtheria A36.84
    glycogen storage disease E74.09 [N16]
    leukemia NEC C95.9- [N16]
    lymphoma NEC C85.90 [N16]
    multiple myeloma C90.0- [N16]
    obstruction N11.1
    Salmonella infection A02.25
    sarcoidosis D86.84
    sepsis A41.9 [N16]
    Sjögren's disease M35.04
    toxoplasmosis B58.83
    transplant rejection T86.91 [N16]
    Wilson's disease E83.01 [N16]
  nonobstructive N12
    with reflux (vesicoureteral) N11.0
    chronic N11.8
  syphilitic A52.75
Pyelonephrosis (obstructive) N11.1
  chronic N11.9
Pyelophlebitis I80.8
Pyeloureteritis cystica N28.85
Pyemia, pyemic (fever) (infection) (purulent) —
  see also Sepsis
  joint — *see* Arthritis, pyogenic or pyemic
  liver K75.1
  pneumococcal A40.3
  portal K75.1
  postvaccinal T88.0
  puerperal, postpartum, childbirth O85
  specified organism NEC A41.89
  tuberculous — *see* Tuberculosis, miliary
Pygopagus Q89.4
Pyknoepilepsy (idiopathic) — *see* Pyknolepsy
Pyknolepsy G40.A09
  intractable G40.A19
    with status epilepticus G40.A11
    without status epilepticus G40.A19
  not intractable G40.A09
    with status epilepticus G40.A01
    without status epilepticus G40.A09
Pylephlebitis K75.1
Pyle's syndrome Q78.5
Pylethrombophlebitis K75.1
Pylethrombosis K75.1
Pyloritis K29.90
  with bleeding K29.91
Pylorospasm (reflex) **NEC** K31.3
  congenital or infantile Q40.0
  newborn Q40.0
  neurotic F45.8
  psychogenic F45.8
Pylorus, pyloric — *see* condition
Pyoarthrosis — *see* Arthritis, pyogenic or pyemic
Pyocele
  mastoid — *see* Mastoiditis, acute
  sinus (accessory) — *see* Sinusitis
  turbinate (bone) J32.9
  urethra — *see also* Urethritis N34.0
Pyocolpos — *see* Vaginitis
Pyocystitis N30.80
  with hematuria N30.81
Pyoderma, pyodermia L08.0
  gangrenosum L88
  newborn P39.4
  phagedenic L88
  vegetans L08.81
Pyodermatitis L08.0
  vegetans L08.81
Pyogenic — *see* condition
Pyohydronephrosis N13.6
Pyometra, pyometrium, pyometritis — *see*
  Endometritis
Pyomyositis (tropical) — *see* Myositis, infective
Pyonephritis N12
Pyonephrosis N13.6
  tuberculous A18.11
Pyo-oophoritis — *see* Salpingo-oophoritis

Pyo-ovarium — *see* Salpingo-oophoritis
Pyopericarditis, pyopericardium I30.1
Pyophlebitis — *see* Phlebitis
Pyopneumopericardium I30.1
Pyopneumothorax (infective) J86.9
  with fistula J86.0
  tuberculous NEC A15.6
Pyosalpinx, pyosalpingitis — *see also* Salpingo-
  oophoritis
Pyothorax J86.9
  with fistula J86.0
  tuberculous NEC A15.6
Pyoureter N28.89
  tuberculous A18.11
Pyramidopallidonigral syndrome G20
Pyrexia (of unknown origin) R50.9
  atmospheric T67.0
  during labor NEC O75.2
  heat T67.0
  newborn P81.9
    environmentally-induced P81.0
  persistent R50.9
  puerperal O86.4
Pyroglobulinemia NEC E88.09
Pyromania F63.1
Pyrosis R12
Pyuria (bacterial) N39.0

Q

Q fever A78
  with pneumonia A78
Quadricuspid aortic valve Q23.8
Quadrilateral fever A78
Quadriparesis — *see* Quadriplegia
  meaning muscle weakness M62.81
Quadriplegia G82.50
  complete
    C1-C4 level G82.51
    C5-C7 level G82.53
  congenital (cerebral) (spinal) G80.8
    spastic G80.0
  embolic (current episode) I63.4-
  functional R53.2
  incomplete
    C1-C4 level G82.52
    C5-C7 level G82.54
  thrombotic (current episode) I63.3-
  traumatic -- code to injury with seventh character S
    current episode — *see* Injury, spinal (cord),
      cervical
Quadruplet, pregnancy — *see* Pregnancy,
  quadruplet
Quarrelsomeness F60.3
Queensland fever A77.3
Quervain's disease M65.4
  thyroid E06.1
Queyrat's erythroplasia D07.4
  penis D07.4
  specified site — *see* Neoplasm, skin, in situ
  unspecified site D07.4
Quincke's disease or edema T78.3
  hereditary D84.1
Quinsy (gangrenous) J36
Quintan fever A79.0
Quintuplet, pregnancy — *see* Pregnancy, quintuplet

R

Rabbit fever — *see* Tularemia
Rabies A82.9
  contact Z20.3
  exposure to Z20.3
  inoculation reaction — *see* Complications,
    vaccination
  sylvatic A82.0
  urban A82.1
Rachischisis — *see* Spina bifida
Rachitic — *see also* condition
  deformities of spine (late effect) (sequelae) E64.3
  pelvis (late effect) (sequelae) E64.3
    with disproportion (fetopelvic) O33.0
      causing obstructed labor O65.0
Rachitis, rachitism (acute) (tarda) — *see*
  also Rickets
  renalis N25.0
  sequelae E64.3
Radial nerve — *see* condition
Radiation
  burn — *see* Burn
  effects NOS T66
  sickness NOS T66
  therapy, encounter for Z51.0
Radiculitis (pressure) (vertebrogenic) — *see*
  Radiculopathy

Radiculomyelitis — *see also* Encephalitis
  toxic, due to
    Clostridium tetani A35
    Corynebacterium diphtheriae A36.82
Radiculopathy M54.10
  cervical region M54.12
  cervicothoracic region M54.13
  due to
    disc disorder
      C3 M50.11
      C4 M50.11
      C5 M50.121
      C6 M50.122
      C7 M50.123
      C8 M50.13
    displacement of intervertebral disc — *see* Disorder,
      disc, with, radiculopathy
  leg M54.1-
  lumbar region M54.16
  lumbosacral region M54.17
  occipito-atlanto-axial region M54.11
  postherpetic B02.29
  sacrococcygeal region M54.18
  syphilitic A52.11
  thoracic region (with visceral pain) M54.14
  thoracolumbar region M54.15
Radiodermal burns (acute, chronic, or
  occupational) — *see* Burn
Radiodermatitis L58.9
  acute L58.0
  chronic L58.1
Radiotherapy session Z51.0
RAEB (refractory anemia with excess blasts) D46.2-
Rage, meaning rabies — *see* Rabies
Ragpicker's disease A22.1
Ragsorter's disease A22.1
Raillietiniasis B71.8
Railroad neurosis F48.8
Railway spine F48.8
Raised — *see also* Elevated
  antibody titer R76.0
Rake teeth, tooth M26.39
Rales R09.89
Ramifying renal pelvis Q63.8
Ramsay-Hunt disease or syndrome — *see*
  also Hunt's disease B02.21
  meaning dyssynergia cerebellaris myoclonica G11.1
Ranula K11.6
  congenital Q38.4
Rape
  adult
    confirmed T74.21
    suspected T76.21
  alleged, observation or examination, ruled out
    adult Z04.41
    child Z04.42
  child
    confirmed T74.22
    suspected T76.22
Rapid
  feeble pulse, due to shock, following injury T79.4
  heart (beat) R00.0
    psychogenic F45.8
  second stage (delivery) O62.3
  time-zone change syndrome — *see* Disorder, sleep,
    circadian rhythm, psychogenic
Rarefaction, bone — *see* Disorder, bone, density and
  structure, specified NEC
Rash (toxic) R21
  canker A38.9
  diaper L22
  drug (internal use) L27.0
    contact — *see also* Dermatitis, due to, drugs,
      external L25.1
  following immunization T88.1
  food — *see* Dermatitis, due to, food
  heat L74.0
  napkin (psoriasiform) L22
  nettle — *see* Urticaria
  pustular L08.0
  rose R21
    epidemic B06.9
  scarlet A38.9
  serum — *see also* Reaction, serum T80.69
  wandering tongue K14.1
Rasmussen aneurysm — *see* Tuberculosis,
  pulmonary
Rasmussen encephalitis G04.81
Rat-bite fever A25.9
  due to Streptobacillus moniliformis A25.1
  spirochetal (morsus muris) A25.0
Rathke's pouch tumor D44.3
Raymond (-Céstan) **syndrome** I65.8

Raynaud's disease, phenomenon or syndrome
(secondary) I73.00
with gangrene (symmetric) I73.01
RDS (newborn) (type I) P22.0
type II P22.1
Reaction — *see also* Disorder
adaptation — *see* Disorder, adjustment
adjustment (anxiety) (conduct disorder)
(depressiveness) (distress) — *see* Disorder,
adjustment
with
mutism, elective (child) (adolescent) F94.0
adverse
food (any) (ingested) NEC T78.1
anaphylactic — *see* Shock, anaphylactic, due to
food
affective — *see* Disorder, mood
allergic — *see* Allergy
anaphylactic — *see* Shock, anaphylactic
anaphylactoid — *see* Shock, anaphylactic
anesthesia — *see* Anesthesia, complication
antitoxin (prophylactic) (therapeutic) — *see*
Complications, vaccination
anxiety F41.1
Arthus — *see* Arthus' phenomenon
asthenic F48.8
combat and operational stress F43.0
compulsive F42.8
conversion F44.9
crisis, acute F43.0
deoxyribonuclease (DNA) (DNase)
hypersensitivity D69.2
depressive (single episode) F32.9
affective (single episode) F31.4
recurrent episode F33.9
neurotic F34.1
psychoneurotic F34.1
psychotic F32.3
recurrent — *see* Disorder, depressive, recurrent
dissociative F44.9
drug NEC T88.7
addictive — *see* Dependence, drug
transmitted via placenta or breast milk — *see*
Absorption, drug, addictive, through placenta
allergic — *see* Allergy, drug
lichenoid L43.2
newborn P93.8
gray baby syndrome P93.0
overdose or poisoning (by accident) — *see* Table
of Drugs and Chemicals, by drug, poisoning
photoallergic L56.1
phototoxic L56.0
withdrawal — *see* Dependence, by drug, with,
withdrawal
infant of dependent mother P96.1
newborn P96.1
wrong substance given or taken (by
accident) — *see* Table of Drugs and Chemicals,
by drug, poisoning
fear F40.9
child (abnormal) F93.8
febrile nonhemolytic transfusion (FNHTR) R50.84
fluid loss, cerebrospinal G97.1
foreign
body NEC — *see* Granuloma, foreign body
in operative wound (inadvertently left) — *see*
Foreign body, accidentally left during a
procedure
substance accidentally left during a procedure
(chemical) (powder) (talc) T81.60
aseptic peritonitis T81.61
body or object (instrument) (sponge)
(swab) — *see* Foreign body, accidentally left
during a procedure
specified reaction NEC T81.69
grief — *see* Disorder, adjustment
Herxheimer's R68.89
hyperkinetic — *see* Hyperkinesia
hypochondriacal F45.20
hypoglycemic, due to insulin E16.0
with coma (diabetic) — *see* Diabetes, coma
nondiabetic E15
therapeutic misadventure — *see* subcategory T38.3
hypomanic F30.8
hysterical F44.9
immunization — *see* Complications, vaccination
incompatibility
ABO blood group (infusion) (transfusion) — *see*
Complication(s), transfusion, incompatibility
reaction, ABO
delayed serologic T80.39
minor blood group (Duffy) (E) (K (ell)) (Kidd)
(Lewis) (M) (N) (P) (S) T80.89

Reaction - *continued*
incompatibility - *continued*
Rh (factor) (infusion) (transfusion) — *see*
Complication(s), transfusion, incompatibility
reaction, Rh (factor)
inflammatory — *see* Infection
infusion — *see* Complications, infusion
inoculation (immune serum) — *see* Complications,
vaccination
insulin T38.3-
involutional psychotic — *see* Disorder, depressive
leukemoid D72.823
basophilic D72.823
lymphocytic D72.823
monocytic D72.823
myelocytic D72.823
neutrophilic D72.823
LSD (acute)
due to drug abuse — *see* Abuse, drug, hallucinogen
due to drug dependence — *see* Dependence, drug,
hallucinogen
lumbar puncture G97.1
manic-depressive — *see* Disorder, bipolar
neurasthenic F48.8
neurogenic — *see* Neurosis
neurotic F48.9
neurotic-depressive F34.1
nitritoid — *see* Crisis, nitritoid
nonspecific
to
cell mediated immunity measurement of gamma
interferon antigen response without active
tuberculosis R76.12
QuantiFERON-TB test (QFT) without active
tuberculosis R76.12
tuberculin test — *see also* Reaction, tuberculin
skin test R76.11
obsessive-compulsive F42.8
organic, acute or subacute — *see* Delirium
paranoid (acute) F23
chronic F22
senile F03
passive dependency F60.7
phobic F40.9
post-traumatic stress, uncomplicated Z73.3
psychogenic F99
psychoneurotic — *see also* Neurosis
compulsive F42.8
depersonalization F48.1
depressive F34.1
hypochondriacal F45.20
neurasthenic F48.8
obsessive F42.8
psychophysiologic — *see* Disorder, somatoform
psychosomatic — *see* Disorder, somatoform
psychotic — *see* Psychosis
scarlet fever toxin — *see* Complications, vaccination
schizophrenic F23
acute (brief) (undifferentiated) F23
latent F21
undifferentiated (acute) (brief) F23
serological for syphilis — *see* Serology for syphilis
serum T80.69
anaphylactic (immediate) — *see also* Shock,
anaphylactic T80.59
specified reaction NEC
due to
administration of blood and blood
products T80.61
immunization T80.62
serum specified NEC T80.69
vaccination T80.62
situational — *see* Disorder, adjustment
somatization — *see* Disorder, somatoform
spinal puncture G97.1
stress (severe) F43.9
acute (agitation) ("daze") (disorientation)
(disturbance of consciousness) (flight reaction)
(fugue) F43.0
specified NEC F43.8
surgical procedure — *see* Complications, surgical
procedure
tetanus antitoxin — *see* Complications, vaccination
toxic, to local anesthesia T88.59
in labor and delivery O74.4
in pregnancy O29.3X-
postpartum, puerperal O89.3
toxin-antitoxin — *see* Complications, vaccination
transfusion (blood) (bone marrow) (lymphocytes)
(allergic) — *see* Complications, transfusion
tuberculin skin test, abnormal R76.11
vaccination (any) — *see* Complications, vaccination
withdrawing, child or adolescent F93.8

Reactive airway disease — *see* Asthma
Reactive depression — *see* Reaction, depressive
Rearrangement
chromosomal
balanced (in) Q95.9
abnormal individual (autosomal) Q95.2
non-sex (autosomal) chromosomes Q95.2
sex/non-sex chromosomes Q95.3
specified NEC Q95.8
Recalcitrant patient — *see* Noncompliance
Recanalization, thrombus — *see* Thrombosis
Recession, receding
chamber angle (eye) H21.55-
chin M26.09
gingival (generalized) (localized) (postinfective)
(postoperative) K06.00
Miller Class I K06.01
Miller Class II K06.02
Miller Class III K06.03
Miller Class IV K06.04
Recklinghausen disease Q85.01
bones E21.0
Reclus' disease (cystic) — *see* Mastopathy, cystic
Recrudescent typhus (fever) A75.1
Recruitment, auditory H93.21-
Rectalgia K62.89
Rectitis K62.89
Rectocele
female (without uterine prolapse) N81.6
with uterine prolapse N81.4
incomplete N81.2
in pregnancy — *see* Pregnancy, complicated by,
abnormal, pelvic organs or tissues NEC
male K62.3
Rectosigmoid junction — *see* condition
Rectosigmoiditis K63.89
ulcerative (chronic) K51.30
with
complication K51.319
abscess K51.314
fistula K51.313
obstruction K51.312
rectal bleeding K51.311
specified NEC K51.318
Rectourethral — *see* condition
Rectovaginal — *see* condition
Rectovesical — *see* condition
Rectum, rectal — *see* condition
Recurrent — *see* condition
pregnancy loss — *see* Loss (of), pregnancy,
recurrent
Red bugs B88.0
Red tide — *see also* Table of Drugs and
Chemicals T65.82-
Red-cedar lung or pneumonitis J67.8
Reduced
mobility Z74.09
ventilatory or vital capacity R94.2
Redundant, redundancy
anus (congenital) Q43.8
clitoris N90.89
colon (congenital) Q43.8
foreskin (congenital) N47.8
intestine (congenital) Q43.8
labia N90.69
organ or site, congenital NEC — *see* Accessory
panniculus (abdominal) E65
prepuce (congenital) N47.8
pylorus K31.89
rectum (congenital) Q43.8
scrotum N50.89
sigmoid (congenital) Q43.8
skin L98.7
and subcutaneous tissue L98.7
of face L57.4
eyelids — *see* Blepharochalasis
stomach K31.89
Reduplication — *see* Duplication
Reflex R29.2
hyperactive gag J39.2
pupillary, abnormal — *see* Anomaly, pupil, function
vasoconstriction I73.9
vasovagal R55
Reflux K21.9
acid K21.9
esophageal K21.9
with esophagitis K21.0
newborn P78.83
gastroesophageal K21.9
with esophagitis K21.0
mitral — *see* Insufficiency, mitral
ureteral — *see* Reflux, vesicoureteral
vesicoureteral (with scarring) N13.70

Reflux - *continued*
  vesicoureteral (with scarring) - *continued*
    with
      nephropathy N13.729
        with hydroureter N13.739
          bilateral N13.732
          unilateral N13.731
          bilateral N13.722
          unilateral N13.721
        without hydroureter N13.729
          bilateral N13.722
          unilateral N13.721
      pyelonephritis (chronic) N11.0
    congenital Q62.7
    without nephropathy N13.71
Reforming, artificial openings — *see* Attention to, artificial, opening
Refractive error — *see* Disorder, refraction
Refsum's disease or syndrome G60.1
Refusal of
  food, psychogenic F50.89
  treatment (because of) Z53.20
    left against medical advice (AMA) Z53.21
    patient's decision NEC Z53.29
    reasons of belief or group pressure Z53.1
Regional — *see* condition
Regurgitation R11.10
  aortic (valve) — *see* Insufficiency, aortic
  food — *see also* Vomiting
    with reswallowing — *see* Rumination
    newborn P92.1
  gastric contents — *see* Vomiting
  heart — *see* Endocarditis
  mitral (valve) — *see* Insufficiency, mitral
    congenital Q23.3
  myocardial — *see* Endocarditis
  pulmonary (valve) (heart) I37.1
    congenital Q22.2
    syphilitic A52.03
  tricuspid — *see* Insufficiency, tricuspid
  valve, valvular — *see* Endocarditis
    congenital Q24.8
  vesicoureteral — *see* Reflux, vesicoureteral
Reichmann's disease or syndrome K31.89
Reifenstein syndrome E34.52
Reinsertion
  implantable subdermal contraceptive Z30.46
  intrauterine contraceptive device Z30.433
Reiter's disease, syndrome, or urethritis M02.30
  ankle M02.37-
  elbow M02.32-
  foot joint M02.37-
  hand joint M02.34-
  hip M02.35-
  knee M02.36-
  multiple site M02.39
  shoulder M02.31-
  vertebra M02.38
  wrist M02.33-
Rejection
  food, psychogenic F50.89
  transplant T86.91
    bone T86.830
      marrow T86.01
    cornea T86.840
    heart T86.21
      with lung (s) T86.31
    intestine T86.850
    kidney T86.11
    liver T86.41
    lung (s) T86.810
      with heart T86.31
    organ (immune or nonimmune cause) T86.91
    pancreas T86.890
    skin (allograft) (autograft) T86.820
    specified NEC T86.890
    stem cell (peripheral blood) (umbilical cord) T86.5
Relapsing fever A68.9
  Carter's (Asiatic) A68.1
  Dutton's (West African) A68.1
  Koch's A68.9
  louse-borne (epidemic) A68.0
  Novy's (American) A68.1
  Obermeyers's (European) A68.0
  Spirillum A68.9
  tick-borne (endemic) A68.1
Relationship
  occlusal
    open anterior M26.220
    open posterior M26.221
Relaxation
  anus (sphincter) K62.89
    psychogenic F45.8

Relaxation - *continued*
  arch (foot) — *see also* Deformity, limb, flat foot
  back ligaments — *see* Instability, joint, spine
  bladder (sphincter) N31.2
  cardioesophageal K21.9
  cervix — *see* Incompetency, cervix
  diaphragm J98.6
  joint (capsule) (ligament) (paralytic) — *see* Flail, joint
    congenital NEC Q74.8
  lumbosacral (joint) — *see* subcategory M53.2
  pelvic floor N81.89
  perineum N81.89
  posture R29.3
  rectum (sphincter) K62.89
  sacroiliac (joint) — *see* subcategory M53.2
  scrotum N50.89
  urethra (sphincter) N36.44
  vesical N31.2
Release from prison, anxiety concerning Z65.2
Remains
  canal of Cloquet Q14.0
  capsule (opaque) Q14.8
Remittent fever (malarial) B54
Remnant
  canal of Cloquet Q14.0
  capsule (opaque) Q14.8
  cervix, cervical stump (acquired) (postpartive) N88.8
  cystic duct, postcholecystectomy K91.5
  fingernail L60.8
    congenital Q84.6
  meniscus, knee — *see* Derangement, knee, meniscus, specified NEC
  thyroglossal duct Q89.2
  tonsil J35.8
    infected (chronic) J35.01
  urachus Q64.4
Removal (from) (of)
  artificial
    arm Z44.00-
      complete Z44.01-
      partial Z44.02-
    eye Z44.2-
    leg Z44.10-
      complete Z44.11-
      partial Z44.12-
  breast implant Z45.81
  cardiac pulse generator (battery) (end-of-life) Z45.010
  catheter (urinary) (indwelling) Z46.6
    from artificial opening — *see* Attention to, artificial, opening
    non-vascular Z46.82
    vascular NEC Z45.2
  drains Z48.03
  device Z46.9
    contraceptive Z30.432
      implantable subdermal Z30.46
    implanted NEC Z45.89
    specified NEC Z46.89
  dressing (nonsurgical) Z48.00
    surgical Z48.01
  external
    fixation device - code to fracture with seventh character D
    prosthesis, prosthetic device Z44.9
      breast Z44.3-
      specified NEC Z44.8
  home in childhood (to foster home or institution) Z62.29
  ileostomy Z43.2
  insulin pump Z46.81
  myringotomy device (stent) (tube) Z45.82
  nervous system device NEC Z46.2
    brain neuropacemaker Z46.2
    visual substitution device Z46.2
      implanted Z45.31
  non-vascular catheter Z46.82
  orthodontic device Z46.4
  organ, prophylactic (for neoplasia management) — *see* Prophylactic, organ removal
  staples Z48.02
  stent
    ureteral Z46.6
  suture Z48.02
  urinary device Z46.6
  vascular access device or catheter Z45.2
Ren
  arcuatus Q63.1
  mobile, mobilis N28.89
    congenital Q63.8
  unguliformis Q63.1

Renal — *see* condition
Rendu-Osler-Weber disease or syndrome I78.0
Reninoma D41.0-
Renon-Delille syndrome E23.3
Reovirus, as cause of disease classified elsewhere B97.5
Repeated falls NEC R29.6
Replaced chromosome by dicentric ring Q93.2
Replacement by artificial or mechanical device or prosthesis of
  bladder Z96.0
  blood vessel NEC Z95.828
  bone NEC Z96.7
  cochlea Z96.21
  coronary artery Z95.5
  eustachian tube Z96.29
  eye globe Z97.0
  heart Z95.812
    valve Z95.2
      prosthetic Z95.2
      specified NEC Z95.4
      xenogenic Z95.3
  intestine Z96.89
  joint Z96.60
    hip — *see* Presence, hip joint implant
    knee — *see* Presence, knee joint implant
    specified site NEC Z96.698
  larynx Z96.3
  lens Z96.1
  limb (s) — *see* Presence, artificial, limb
  mandible NEC (for tooth root implant (s)) Z96.5
  organ NEC Z96.89
  peripheral vessel NEC Z95.828
  stapes Z96.29
  teeth Z97.2
  tendon Z96.7
  tissue NEC Z96.89
  tooth root (s) Z96.5
  vessel NEC Z95.828
    coronary (artery) Z95.5
Request for expert evidence Z04.8
Reserve, decreased or low
  cardiac — *see* Disease, heart
  kidney N28.89
Residual — *see also* condition
  ovary syndrome N99.83
  state, schizophrenic F20.5
  urine R39.198
Resistance, resistant (to)
  activated protein C D68.51
  complicating pregnancy O26.89
  insulin E88.81
  organism (s)
    to
      drug Z16.30
        aminoglycosides Z16.29
        amoxicillin Z16.11
        ampicillin Z16.11
        antibiotic (s) Z16.20
          multiple Z16.24
          specified NEC Z16.29
        antifungal Z16.32
        antimicrobial (single) Z16.30
          multiple Z16.35
          specified NEC Z16.39
        antimycobacterial (single) Z16.341
          multiple Z16.342
        antiparasitic Z16.31
        antiviral Z16.33
        beta lactam antibiotics Z16.10
          specified NEC Z16.19
        cephalosporins Z16.19
        extended beta lactamase (ESBL) Z16.12
        fluoroquinolones Z16.23
        macrolides Z16.29
        methicillin — *see* MRSA
        multiple drugs (MDRO)
          antibiotics Z16.24
          antimicrobial Z16.35
          antimycobacterials Z16.342
        penicillins Z16.11
        quinine (and related compounds) Z16.31
        quinolones Z16.23
        sulfonamides Z16.29
        tetracyclines Z16.29
        tuberculostatics (single) Z16.341
          multiple Z16.342
        vancomycin Z16.21
          related antibiotics Z16.22
  thyroid hormone E07.89
Resorption
  dental (roots) K03.3
    alveoli M26.79

Resorption - *continued*
teeth (external) (internal) (pathological) (roots) K03.3
Respiration
Cheyne-Stokes R06.3
decreased due to shock, following injury T79.4
disorder of, psychogenic F45.8
insufficient, or poor R06.89
newborn P28.5
painful R07.1
sighing, psychogenic F45.8
Respiratory — *see also* condition
distress syndrome (newborn) (type I) P22.0
type II P22.1
syncytial virus, as cause of disease classified elsewhere B97.4
Respite care Z75.5
Response (drug)
photoallergic L56.1
phototoxic L56.0
Restenosis
stent
vascular
end stent
adjacent to stent — *see* Arteriosclerosis
within the stent
coronary T82.855
peripheral T82.856
in stent
coronary vessel T82.855
peripheral vessel T82.856
Restless legs (syndrome) G25.81
Restlessness R45.1
Restoration (of)
dental
aesthetically inadequate or displeasing K08.56
defective K08.50
specified NEC K08.59
failure of marginal integrity K08.51
failure of periodontal anatomical intergrity K08.54
organ continuity from previous sterilization (tuboplasty) (vasoplasty) Z31.0
aftercare Z31.42
tooth (existing)
contours biologically incompatible with oral health K08.54
open margins K08.51
overhanging K08.52
poor aesthetic K08.56
poor gingival margins K08.51
unsatisfactory, of tooth K08.50
specified NEC K08.59
Restorative material (dental)
allergy to K08.55
fractured K08.539
with loss of material K08.531
without loss of material K08.530
unrepairable overhanging of K08.52
Restriction of housing space Z59.1
Rests, ovarian, in fallopian tube Q50.6
Restzustand (schizophrenic) F20.5
Retained — *see also* Retention
cholelithiasis following cholecystectomy K91.86
foreign body fragments (type of) Z18.9
acrylics Z18.2
animal quill (s) or spines Z18.31
cement Z18.83
concrete Z18.83
crystalline Z18.83
depleted isotope Z18.09
depleted uranium Z18.01
diethylhexylphthalates Z18.2
glass Z18.81
isocyanate Z18.2
magnetic metal Z18.11
metal Z18.10
nonmagnectic metal Z18.12
nontherapeutic radioactive Z18.09
organic NEC Z18.39
plastic Z18.2
quill (s) (animal) Z18.31
radioactive (nontherapeutic) NEC Z18.09
specified NEC Z18.89
spine (s) (animal) Z18.31
stone Z18.83
tooth (teeth) Z18.32
wood Z18.33
fragments (type of) Z18.9
acrylics Z18.2
animal quill (s) or spines Z18.31
cement Z18.83
concrete Z18.83
crystalline Z18.83

Retained - *continued*
fragments (type of) - *continued*
depleted isotope Z18.09
depleted uranium Z18.01
diethylhexylphthalates Z18.2
glass Z18.81
isocyanate Z18.2
magnetic metal Z18.11
metal Z18.10
nonmagnectic metal Z18.12
nontherapeutic radioactive Z18.09
organic NEC Z18.39
plastic Z18.2
quill (s) (animal) Z18.31
radioactive (nontherapeutic) NEC Z18.09
specified NEC Z18.89
spine (s) (animal) Z18.31
stone Z18.83
tooth (teeth) Z18.32
wood Z18.33
gallstones, following cholecystectomy K91.86
Retardation
development, developmental, specific — *see* Disorder, developmental
endochondral bone growth — *see* Disorder, bone, development or growth
growth R62.50
due to malnutrition E45
mental — *see* Disability, intellectual
motor function, specific F82
physical (child) R62.52
due to malnutrition E45
reading (specific) F81.0
spelling (specific) (without reading disorder) F81.81
Retching — *see* Vomiting
Retention — *see also* Retained
bladder — *see* Retention, urine
carbon dioxide E87.2
cholelithiasis following cholecystectomy K91.86
cyst — *see* Cyst
dead
fetus (at or near term) (mother) O36.4
early fetal death O02.1
ovum O02.0
decidua (fragments) (following delivery) (with hemorrhage) O72.2
without hemorrhage O73.1
deciduous tooth K00.6
dental root K08.3
fecal — *see* Constipation
fetus
dead O36.4
early O02.1
fluid R60.9
foreign body — *see also* Foreign body, retained
current trauma - code as Foreign body, by site or type
gallstones, following cholecystectomy K91.86
gastric K31.89
intrauterine contraceptive device, in pregnancy — *see* Pregnancy, complicated by, retention, intrauterine device
membranes (complicating delivery) (with hemorrhage) O72.2
with abortion — *see* Abortion, by type
without hemorrhage O73.1
meniscus — *see* Derangement, meniscus
menses N94.89
milk (puerperal, postpartum) O92.79
nitrogen, extrarenal R39.2
ovary syndrome N99.83
placenta (total) (with hemorrhage) O72.0
without hemorrhage O73.0
portions or fragments (with hemorrhage) O72.2
without hemorrhage O73.1
products of conception
early pregnancy (dead fetus) O02.1
following
delivery (with hemorrhage) O72.2
without hemorrhage O73.1
secundines (following delivery) (with hemorrhage) O72.0
without hemorrhage O73.0
complicating puerperium (delayed hemorrhage) O72.2
partial O72.2
without hemorrhage O73.1
smegma, clitoris N90.89
urine R33.9
due to hyperplasia (hypertrophy) of prostate — *see* Hyperplasia, prostate
drug-induced R33.0
organic R33.8

Retention - *continued*
urine - *continued*
organic - *continued*
drug-induced R33.0
psychogenic F45.8
specified NEC R33.8
water (in tissues) — *see* Edema
Reticular erythematous mucinosis L98.5
Reticulation, dust — *see* Pneumoconiosis
Reticulocytosis R70.1
Reticuloendotheliosis
acute infantile C96.0
leukemic C91.4-
nonlipid C96.0
Reticulohistiocytoma (giant-cell) D76.3
Reticuloid, actinic L57.1
Reticulosis (skin)
acute of infancy C96.0
hemophagocytic, familial D76.1
histiocytic medullary C96.A
lipomelanotic I89.8
malignant (midline) C86.0
polymorphic C86.0
Sézary — *see* Sézary disease
Retina, retinal — *see also* condition
dark area D49.81
Retinitis — *see also* Inflammation, chorioretinal
albuminurica N18.9 *[H32]*
diabetic — *see* Diabetes, retinitis
disciformis — *see* Degeneration, macula
focal — *see* Inflammation, chorioretinal, focal
gravidarum — *see* Pregnancy, complicated by, specified pregnancy-related condition NEC
juxtapapillaris — *see* Inflammation, chorioretinal, focal, juxtapapillaris
luetic — *see* Retinitis, syphilitic
pigmentosa H35.52
proliferans — *see* Disorder, globe, degenerative, specified type NEC
proliferating — *see* Disorder, globe, degenerative, specified type NEC
renal N18.9 *[H32]*
syphilitic (early) (secondary) A51.43
central, recurrent A52.71
congenital (early) A50.01 *[H32]*
late A52.71
tuberculous A18.53
Retinoblastoma C69.2-
differentiated C69.2-
undifferentiated C69.2-
Retinochoroiditis — *see also* Inflammation, chorioretinal
disseminated — *see* Inflammation, chorioretinal, disseminated
syphilitic A52.71
focal — *see* Inflammation, chorioretinal, focal, juxtapapillaris
juxtapapillaris — *see* Inflammation, chorioretinal, focal, juxtapapillary
Retinopathy (background) H35.00
arteriosclerotic I70.8 *[H35.0-]*
atherosclerotic I70.8 *[H35.0-]*
central serous — *see* Chorioretinopathy, central serous
Coats H35.02-
diabetic — *see* Diabetes, retinopathy
exudative H35.02-
hypertensive H35.03-
in (due to)
diabetes — *see* Diabetes, retinopathy
sickle-cell disorders D57.- *[H36]*
of prematurity H35.10-
stage 0 H35.11-
stage 1 H35.12-
stage 2 H35.13-
stage 3 H35.14-
stage 4 H35.15-
stage 5 H35.16-
pigmentary, congenital — *see* Dystrophy, retina
proliferative NEC H35.2-
diabetic — *see* Diabetes, retinopathy, proliferative
sickle-cell D57.- *[H36]*
solar H31.02-
Retinoschisis H33.10-
congenital Q14.1
specified type NEC H33.19-
Retortamoniasis A07.8
Retractile testis Q55.22
Retraction
cervix — *see* Retroversion, uterus
drum (membrane) — *see* Disorder, tympanic membrane, specified NEC
finger — *see* Deformity, finger
lid H02.539

Retraction - *continued*
lid - *continued*
left H02.536
lower H02.535
upper H02.534
right H02.533
lower H02.532
upper H02.531
lung J98.4
mediastinum J98.59
nipple N64.53
associated with
lactation O92.03
pregnancy O92.01-
puerperium O92.02
congenital Q83.8
palmar fascia M72.0
pleura — *see* Pleurisy
ring, uterus (Bandl's) (pathological) O62.4
sternum (congenital) Q76.7
acquired M95.4
uterus — *see* Retroversion, uterus
valve (heart) — *see* Endocarditis
Retrobulbar — *see* condition
Retrocecal — *see* condition
Retrocession — *see* Retroversion
Retrodisplacement — *see* Retroversion
Retroflection, retroflexion — *see* Retroversion
Retrognathia, retrognathism (mandibular) (maxillary) M26.19
Retrograde menstruation N92.5
Retroperineal — *see* condition
Retroperitoneal — *see* condition
Retroperitonitis K68.9
Retropharyngeal — *see* condition
Retroplacental — *see* condition
Retroposition — *see* Retroversion
Retroprosthetic membrane T85.398
Retrosternal thyroid (congenital) Q89.2
Retroversion, retroverted
cervix — *see* Retroversion, uterus
female NEC — *see* Retroversion, uterus
iris H21.89
testis (congenital) Q55.29
uterus (acquired) (acute) (any degree) (asymptomatic) (cervix) (postinfectional) (postpartal, old) N85.4
congenital Q51.818
in pregnancy O34.53-
Retrovirus, as cause of disease classified elsewhere B97.30
human
immunodeficiency, type 2 (HIV 2) B97.35
T-cell lymphotropic
type I (HTLV-I) B97.33
type II (HTLV-II) B97.34
lentivirus B97.31
oncovirus B97.32
specified NEC B97.39
Retrusion, premaxilla (developmental) M26.09
Rett's disease or syndrome F84.2
Reverse peristalsis R19.2
Reye's syndrome G93.7
Rh (factor)
hemolytic disease (newborn) P55.0
incompatibility, immunization or sensitization
affecting management of pregnancy NEC O36.09-
anti-D antibody O36.01-
newborn P55.0
transfusion reaction — *see* Complication(s), transfusion, incompatibility reaction, Rh (factor)
negative mother affecting newborn P55.0
titer elevated — *see* Complication(s), transfusion, incompatibility reaction, Rh (factor)
transfusion reaction — *see* Complication(s), transfusion, incompatibility reaction, Rh (factor)
Rhabdomyolysis (idiopathic) **NEC** M62.82
traumatic T79.6
Rhabdomyoma — *see also* Neoplasm, connective tissue, benign
adult — *see* Neoplasm, connective tissue, benign
fetal — *see* Neoplasm, connective tissue, benign
glycogenic — *see* Neoplasm, connective tissue, benign
Rhabdomyosarcoma (any type) — *see* Neoplasm, connective tissue, malignant
Rhabdosarcoma — *see* Rhabdomyosarcoma
Rhesus (factor) **incompatibility** — *see* Rh, incompatibility
Rheumatic (acute) (subacute) (chronic)
adherent pericardium I09.2
coronary arteritis I01.9
degeneration, myocardium I09.0

Rheumatic (acute) (subacute) (chronic) - *continued*
fever (acute) — *see* Fever, rheumatic
heart — *see* Disease, heart, rheumatic
myocardial degeneration — *see* Degeneration, myocardium
myocarditis (chronic) (inactive) (with chorea) I09.0
active or acute I01.2
with chorea (acute) (rheumatic) (Sydenham's) I02.0
pancarditis, acute I01.8
with chorea (acute) (rheumatic) Sydenham's) I02.0
pericarditis (active) (acute) (with effusion) (with pneumonia) I01.0
with chorea (acute) (rheumatic) (Sydenham's) I02.0
chronic or inactive I09.2
pneumonia I00 *[J17]*
torticollis M43.6
typhoid fever A01.09
Rheumatism (articular) (neuralgic) (nonarticular) M79.0
gout — *see* Arthritis, rheumatoid
intercostal, meaning Tietze's disease M94.0
palindromic (any site) M12.30
ankle M12.37-
elbow M12.32-
foot joint M12.37-
hand joint M12.34-
hip M12.35-
knee M12.36-
multiple site M12.39
shoulder M12.31-
specified joint NEC M12.38
vertebrae M12.38
wrist M12.33-
sciatic M54.4-
Rheumatoid — *see also* condition
arthritis — *see also* Arthritis, rheumatoid
with involvement of organs NEC M05.60
ankle M05.67-
elbow M05.62-
foot joint M05.67-
hand joint M05.64-
hip M05.65-
knee M05.66-
multiple site M05.69
shoulder M05.61-
vertebra — *see* Spondylitis, ankylosing
wrist M05.63-
seronegative — *see* Arthritis, rheumatoid, seronegative
seropositive — *see* Arthritis, rheumatoid, seropositive
carditis M05.30
ankle M05.37-
elbow M05.32-
foot joint M05.37-
hand joint M05.34-
hip M05.35-
knee M05.36-
multiple site M05.39
shoulder M05.31-
vertebra — *see* Spondylitis, ankylosing
wrist M05.33-
endocarditis — *see* Rheumatoid, carditis
lung (disease) M05.10
ankle M05.17-
elbow M05.12-
foot joint M05.17-
hand joint M05.14-
hip M05.15-
knee M05.16-
multiple site M05.19
shoulder M05.11-
vertebra — *see* Spondylitis, ankylosing
wrist M05.13-
myocarditis — *see* Rheumatoid, carditis
myopathy M05.40
ankle M05.47-
elbow M05.42-
foot joint M05.47-
hand joint M05.44-
hip M05.45-
knee M05.46-
multiple site M05.49
shoulder M05.41-
vertebra — *see* Spondylitis, ankylosing
wrist M05.43-
pericarditis — *see* Rheumatoid, carditis
polyarthritis — *see* Arthritis, rheumatoid
polyneuropathy M05.50
ankle M05.57-
elbow M05.52-

Rheumatoid - *continued*
polyneuropathy - *continued*
foot joint M05.57-
hand joint M05.54-
hip M05.55-
knee M05.56-
multiple site M05.59
shoulder M05.51-
vertebra — *see* Spondylitis, ankylosing
wrist M05.53-
vasculitis M05.20
ankle M05.27-
elbow M05.22-
foot joint M05.27-
hand joint M05.24-
hip M05.25-
knee M05.26-
multiple site M05.29
shoulder M05.21-
vertebra — *see* Spondylitis, ankylosing
wrist M05.23-
Rhinitis (atrophic) (catarrhal) (chronic) (croupous) (fibrinous) (granulomatous) (hyperplastic) (hypertrophic) (membranous) (obstructive) (purulent) (suppurative) (ulcerative) J31.0
with
sore throat — *see* Nasopharyngitis
acute J00
allergic J30.9
with asthma J45.909
with
exacerbation (acute) J45.901
status asthmaticus J45.902
due to
food J30.5
pollen J30.1
nonseasonal J30.89
perennial J30.89
seasonal NEC J30.2
specified NEC J30.89
infective J00
pneumococcal J00
syphilitic A52.73
congenital A50.05 *[J99]*
tuberculous A15.8
vasomotor J30.0
Rhinoantritis (chronic) — *see* Sinusitis, maxillary
Rhinodacryolith — *see* Dacryolith
Rhinolith (nasal sinus) J34.89
Rhinomegaly J34.89
Rhinopharyngitis (acute) (subacute) — *see also* Nasopharyngitis
chronic J31.1
destructive ulcerating A66.5
mutilans A66.5
Rhinophyma L71.1
Rhinorrhea J34.89
cerebrospinal (fluid) G96.0
paroxysmal — *see* Rhinitis, allergic
spasmodic — *see* Rhinitis, allergic
Rhinosalpingitis — *see* Salpingitis, eustachian
Rhinoscleroma A48.8
Rhinosporidiosis B48.1
Rhinovirus infection NEC B34.8
Rhizomelic chondrodysplasia punctata E71.540
Rhythm
atrioventricular nodal I49.8
disorder I49.9
coronary sinus I49.8
ectopic I49.8
nodal I49.8
escape I49.9
heart, abnormal I49.9
idioventricular I44.2
nodal I49.8
sleep, inversion G47.2-
nonorganic origin — *see* Disorder, sleep, circadian rhythm, psychogenic
Rhytidosis facialis L98.8
Rib — *see also* condition
cervical Q76.5
Riboflavin deficiency E53.0
Rice bodies — *see also* Loose, body, joint
knee M23.4-
Richter syndrome — *see* Leukemia, chronic lymphocytic, B-cell type
Richter's hernia — *see* Hernia, abdomen, with obstruction
Ricinism — *see* Poisoning, food, noxious, plant
Rickets (active) (acute) (adolescent) (chest wall) (congenital) (current) (infantile) (intestinal) E55.0
adult — *see* Osteomalacia
celiac K90.0

Rickets (active) (acute) (adolescent) (chest wall) (congenital) (current) (infantile) (intestinal) - *continued*
  hypophosphatemic with nephrotic-glycosuric dwarfism E72.09
  inactive E64.3
  kidney N25.0
  renal N25.0
  sequelae, any E64.3
  vitamin-D-resistant E83.31 *[M90.80]*
Rickettsial disease A79.9
  specified type NEC A79.89
Rickettsialpox (Rickettsia akari) A79.1
Rickettsiosis A79.9
  due to
    Ehrlichia sennetsu A79.81
    Rickettsia akari (rickettsialpox) A79.1
  specified type NEC A79.89
  tick-borne A77.9
  vesicular A79.1
Rider's bone — *see* Ossification, muscle, specified NEC
Ridge, alveolus — *see also* condition
  flabby K06.8
Ridged ear, congenital Q17.3
Riedel's
  lobe, liver Q44.7
  struma, thyroiditis or disease E06.5
Rieger's anomaly or syndrome Q13.81
Riehl's melanosis L81.4
Rietti-Greppi-Micheli anemia D56.9
Rieux's hernia — *see* Hernia, abdomen, specified site NEC
Riga (-Fede) **disease** K14.0
Riggs' disease — *see* Periodontitis
Right aortic arch Q25.47
Right middle lobe syndrome J98.11
Rigid, rigidity — *see also* condition
  abdominal R19.30
    with severe abdominal pain R10.0
    epigastric R19.36
    generalized R19.37
    left lower quadrant R19.34
    left upper quadrant R19.32
    periumbilic R19.35
    right lower quadrant R19.33
    right upper quadrant R19.31
  articular, multiple, congenital Q68.8
  cervix (uteri) in pregnancy — *see* Pregnancy, complicated by, abnormal, cervix
  hymen (acquired) (congenital) N89.6
  nuchal R29.1
  pelvic floor in pregnancy — *see* Pregnancy, complicated by, abnormal, pelvic organs or tissues NEC
  perineum or vulva in pregnancy — *see* Pregnancy, complicated by, abnormal, vulva
  spine — *see* Dorsopathy, specified NEC
  vagina in pregnancy — *see* Pregnancy, complicated by, abnormal, vagina
Rigors R68.89
  with fever R50.9
Riley-Day syndrome G90.1
RIND (reversible ischemic neurologic deficit) I63.9
Ring (s)
  aorta (vascular) Q25.45
  Bandl's O62.4
  contraction, complicating delivery O62.4
  esophageal, lower (muscular) K22.2
  Fleischer's (cornea) H18.04-
  hymenal, tight (acquired) (congenital) N89.6
  Kayser-Fleischer (cornea) H18.04-
  retraction, uterus, pathological O62.4
  Schatzki's (esophagus) (lower) K22.2
    congenital Q39.3
  Soemmerring's — *see* Cataract, secondary
  vascular (congenital) Q25.8
    aorta Q25.45
Ringed hair (congenital) Q84.1
Ringworm B35.9
  beard B35.0
  black dot B35.0
  body B35.4
  Burmese B35.5
  corporeal B35.4
  foot B35.3
  groin B35.6
  hand B35.2
  honeycomb B35.0
  nails B35.1
  perianal (area) B35.6
  scalp B35.0
  specified NEC B35.8

Ringworm - *continued*
  Tokelau B35.5
Rise, venous pressure I87.8
Rising, PSA following treatment for malignant neoplasm of prostate R97.21
Risk, suicidal
  meaning personal history of attempted suicide Z91.5
  meaning suicidal ideation — *see* Ideation, suicidal
Ritter's disease L00
Rivalry, sibling Z62.891
Rivalta's disease A42.2
River blindness B73.01
Robert's pelvis Q74.2
  with disproportion (fetopelvic) O33.0
    causing obstructed labor O65.0
Robin (-Pierre) **syndrome** Q87.0
Robinow-Silvermann-Smith syndrome Q87.1
Robinson's (hidrotic) **ectodermal dysplasia or syndrome** Q82.4
Robles' disease B73.01
Rocky Mountain (spotted) **fever** A77.0
Roetheln — *see* Rubella
Roger's disease Q21.0
Rokitansky-Aschoff sinuses (gallbladder) K82.8
Rolando's fracture (displaced) S62.22-
  nondisplaced S62.22-
Romano-Ward (prolonged QT interval) **syndrome** I45.81
Romberg's disease or syndrome G51.8
Roof, mouth — *see* condition
Rosacea L71.9
  acne L71.9
  keratitis L71.8
  specified NEC L71.8
Rosary, rachitic E55.0
Rose
  cold J30.1
  fever J30.1
  rash R21
    epidemic B06.9
Rosenbach's erysipeloid A26.0
Rosenthal's disease or syndrome D68.1
Roseola B09
  infantum B08.20
    due to human herpesvirus 6 B08.21
    due to human herpesvirus 7 B08.22
Ross River disease or fever B33.1
Rossbach's disease K31.89
  psychogenic F45.8
Rostan's asthma (cardiac) — *see* Failure, ventricular, left
Rotation
  anomalous, incomplete or insufficient, intestine Q43.3
  cecum (congenital) Q43.3
  colon (congenital) Q43.3
  spine, incomplete or insufficient — *see* Dorsopathy, deforming, specified NEC
  tooth, teeth, fully erupted M26.35
  vertebra, incomplete or insufficient — *see* Dorsopathy, deforming, specified NEC
Rotes Quérol disease or syndrome — *see* Hyperostosis, ankylosing
Roth (-Bernhardt) **disease or syndrome** — *see* Meralgia paraesthetica
Rothmund (-Thomson) **syndrome** Q82.8
Rotor's disease or syndrome E80.6
Round
  back (with wedging of vertebrae) — *see* Kyphosis
    sequelae (late effect) of rickets E64.3
  worms (large) (infestation) NEC B82.0
    Ascariasis — *see also* Ascariasis B77.9
Roussy-Lévy syndrome G60.0
Rubella (German measles) B06.9
  complication NEC B06.09
    neurological B06.00
  congenital P35.0
  contact Z20.4
  exposure to Z20.4
  maternal
    manifest rubella in infant P35.0
    care for (suspected) damage to fetus O35.3
    suspected damage to fetus affecting management of pregnancy O35.3
  specified complications NEC B06.89
Rubeola (meaning measles) — *see* Measles
  meaning rubella — *see* Rubella
Rubeosis, iris — *see* Disorder, iris, vascular
Rubinstein-Taybi syndrome Q87.2
Rudimentary (congenital) — *see also* Agenesis
  arm — *see* Defect, reduction, upper limb
  bone Q79.9
  cervix uteri Q51.828

Rudimentary (congenital) - *continued*
  eye Q11.2
  lobule of ear Q17.3
  patella Q74.1
  respiratory organs in thoracopagus Q89.4
  tracheal bronchus Q32.4
  uterus Q51.818
    in male Q56.1
  vagina Q52.0
Ruled out condition — *see* Observation, suspected
Rumination R11.10
  with nausea R11.2
  disorder of infancy F98.21
  neurotic F42.8
  newborn P92.1
  obsessional F42.8
  psychogenic F42.8
Runeberg's disease D51.0
Runny nose R09.89
Rupia (syphilitic) A51.39
  congenital A50.06
  tertiary A52.79
Rupture, ruptured
  abscess (spontaneous) - code by site under Abscess
  aneurysm — *see* Aneurysm
  anus (sphincter) — *see* Laceration, anus
  aorta, aortic I71.8
    abdominal I71.3
    arch I71.1
    ascending I71.1
    descending I71.8
      abdominal I71.3
      thoracic I71.1
    syphilitic A52.01
    thoracoabdominal I71.5
    thorax, thoracic I71.1
    transverse I71.1
    traumatic — *see* Injury, aorta, laceration, major
    valve or cusp — *see also* Endocarditis, aortic I35.8
  appendix (with peritonitis) K35.2
    with localized peritonitis K35.3
  arteriovenous fistula, brain I60.8
  artery I77.2
    brain — *see* Hemorrhage, intracranial, intracerebral
    coronary — *see* Infarct, myocardium
    heart — *see* Infarct, myocardium
    pulmonary I28.8
    traumatic (complication) — *see* Injury, blood vessel
  bile duct (common) (hepatic) K83.2
    cystic K82.2
  bladder (sphincter) (nontraumatic) (spontaneous) N32.89
    following ectopic or molar pregnancy O08.6
    obstetrical trauma O71.5
    traumatic S37.29
  blood vessel — *see also* Hemorrhage
    brain — *see* Hemorrhage, intracranial, intracerebral
    heart — *see* Infarct, myocardium
    traumatic (complication) — *see* Injury, blood vessel, laceration, major, by site
  bone — *see* Fracture
  bowel (nontraumatic) K63.1
  brain
    aneurysm (congenital) — *see also* Hemorrhage, intracranial, subarachnoid
      syphilitic A52.05
    hemorrhagic — *see* Hemorrhage, intracranial, intracerebral
  capillaries I78.8
  cardiac (auricle) (ventricle) (wall) I23.3
    with hemopericardium I23.0
    infectional I40.9
    traumatic — *see* Injury, heart
  cartilage (articular) (current) — *see also* Sprain
    knee S83.3-
    semilunar — *see* Tear, meniscus
  cecum (with peritonitis) K65.0
    with peritoneal abscess K35.3
    traumatic S36.598
  celiac artery, traumatic — *see* Injury, blood vessel, celiac artery, laceration, major
  cerebral aneurysm (congenital) (see Hemorrhage, intracranial, subarachnoid)
  cervix (uteri)
    with ectopic or molar pregnancy O08.6
    following ectopic or molar pregnancy O08.6
    obstetrical trauma O71.3
    traumatic S37.69
  chordae tendineae NEC I51.1

Rupture, ruptured - *continued*
chordae tendineae NEC - *continued*
concurrent with acute myocardial infarction — *see* Infarct, myocardium
following acute myocardial infarction (current complication) I23.4
choroid (direct) (indirect) (traumatic) H31.32-
circle of Willis I60.6
colon (nontraumatic) K63.1
traumatic — *see* Injury, intestine, large
cornea (traumatic) — *see* Injury, eye, laceration
coronary (artery) (thrombotic) — *see* Infarct, myocardium
corpus luteum (infected) (ovary) N83.1-
cyst — *see* Cyst
cystic duct K82.2
Descemet's membrane — *see* Change, corneal membrane, Descemet's, rupture
traumatic — *see* Injury, eye, laceration
diaphragm, traumatic — *see* Injury, intrathoracic, diaphragm
disc — *see* Rupture, intervertebral disc
diverticulum (intestine) K57.80
with bleeding K57.81
bladder N32.3
large intestine K57.20
with
bleeding K57.21
small intestine K57.40
with bleeding K57.41
small intestine K57.00
with
bleeding K57.01
large intestine K57.40
with bleeding K57.41
duodenal stump K31.89
ear drum (nontraumatic) — *see also* Perforation, tympanum
traumatic S09.2-
due to blast injury — *see* Injury, blast, ear
esophagus K22.3
eye (without prolapse or loss of intraocular tissue) — *see* Injury, eye, laceration
fallopian tube NEC (nonobstetric) (nontraumatic) N83.8
due to pregnancy O00.10
with intrauterine pregnancy O00.11
fontanel P13.1
gallbladder K82.2
traumatic S36.128
gastric — *see also* Rupture, stomach
vessel K92.2
globe (eye) (traumatic) — *see* Injury, eye, laceration
graafian follicle (hematoma) N83.0-
heart — *see* Rupture, cardiac
hymen (nontraumatic) (nonintentional) N89.8
internal organ, traumatic — *see* Injury, by site
intervertebral disc — *see* Displacement, intervertebral disc
traumatic — *see* Rupture, traumatic, intervertebral disc
intestine NEC (nontraumatic) K63.1
traumatic — *see* Injury, intestine
iris — *see also* Abnormality, pupillary
traumatic — *see* Injury, eye, laceration
joint capsule, traumatic — *see* Sprain
kidney (traumatic) S37.06-
birth injury P15.8
nontraumatic N28.89
lacrimal duct (traumatic) — *see* Injury, eye, specified site NEC
lens (cataract) (traumatic) — *see* Cataract, traumatic
ligament, traumatic — *see* Rupture, traumatic, ligament, by site
liver S36.116
birth injury P15.0
lymphatic vessel I89.8
marginal sinus (placental) (with hemorrhage) — *see* Hemorrhage, antepartum, specified cause NEC
membrana tympani (nontraumatic) — *see* Perforation, tympanum
membranes (spontaneous)
artificial
delayed delivery following O75.5
delayed delivery following — *see* Pregnancy, complicated by, premature rupture of membranes
meningeal artery I60.8
meniscus (knee) — *see also* Tear, meniscus
old — *see* Derangement, meniscus
site other than knee - code as Sprain
mesenteric artery, traumatic — *see* Injury, mesenteric, artery, laceration, major
mesentery (nontraumatic) K66.8

Rupture, ruptured - *continued*
mesentery (nontraumatic) - *continued*
traumatic — *see* Injury, intra-abdominal, specified, site NEC
mitral (valve) I34.8
muscle (traumatic) — *see also* Strain
diastasis — *see* Diastasis, muscle
nontraumatic M62.10
ankle M62.17-
foot M62.17-
forearm M62.13-
hand M62.14-
lower leg M62.16-
pelvic region M62.15-
shoulder region M62.11-
specified site NEC M62.18
thigh M62.15-
upper arm M62.12-
traumatic — *see* Strain, by site
musculotendinous junction NEC, nontraumatic — *see* Rupture, tendon, spontaneous
mycotic aneurysm causing cerebral hemorrhage — *see* Hemorrhage, intracranial, subarachnoid
myocardium, myocardial — *see* Rupture, cardiac
traumatic — *see* Injury, heart
nontraumatic, meaning hernia — *see* Hernia
obstructed — *see* Hernia, by site, obstructed
operation wound — *see* Disruption, wound, operation
ovary, ovarian N83.8
corpus luteum cyst N83.1-
follicle (graafian) N83.0-
oviduct (nonobstetric) (nontraumatic) N83.8
due to pregnancy O00.10
with intrauterine pregnancy O00.11
pancreas (nontraumatic) K86.89
traumatic S36.299
papillary muscle NEC I51.2
following acute myocardial infarction (current complication) I23.5
pelvic
floor, complicating delivery O70.1
organ NEC, obstetrical trauma O71.5
perineum (nonobstetric) (nontraumatic) N90.89
complicating delivery — *see* Delivery, complicated, by, laceration, anus (sphincter)
postoperative wound — *see* Disruption, wound, operation
prostate (traumatic) S37.828
pulmonary
artery I28.8
valve (heart) I37.8
vein I28.8
vessel I28.8
pus tube — *see* Salpingitis
pyosalpinx — *see* Salpingitis
rectum (nontraumatic) K63.1
traumatic S36.69
retina, retinal (traumatic) (without detachment) — *see also* Break, retina
with detachment — *see* Detachment, retina, with retinal, break
rotator cuff (nontraumatic) M75.10-
complete M75.12-
incomplete M75.11-
sclera — *see* Injury, eye, laceration
sigmoid (nontraumatic) K63.1
traumatic S36.593
spinal cord — *see also* Injury, spinal cord, by region
due to injury at birth P11.5
newborn (birth injury) P11.5
spleen (traumatic) S36.09
birth injury P15.1
congenital (birth injury) P15.1
due to P. vivax malaria B51.0
nontraumatic D73.5
spontaneous D73.5
splenic vein R58
traumatic — *see* Injury, blood vessel, splenic vein
stomach (nontraumatic) (spontaneous) K31.89
traumatic S36.39
supraspinatus (complete) (incomplete) (nontraumatic) — *see* Tear, rotator cuff
symphysis pubis
obstetric O71.6
traumatic S33.4
synovium (cyst) M66.10
ankle M66.17-
elbow M66.12-
finger M66.14-
foot M66.17-
forearm M66.13-

Rupture, ruptured - *continued*
synovium (cyst) - *continued*
hand M66.14-
pelvic region M66.15-
shoulder region M66.11-
specified site NEC M66.18
thigh M66.15-
toe M66.17-
upper arm M66.12-
wrist M66.13-
tendon (traumatic) — *see* Strain
nontraumatic (spontaneous) M66.9
ankle M66.87-
extensor M66.20
ankle M66.27-
foot M66.27-
forearm M66.23-
hand M66.24-
lower leg M66.26-
multiple sites M66.29
pelvic region M66.25-
shoulder region M66.21-
specified site NEC M66.28
thigh M66.25-
upper arm M66.22-
flexor M66.30
ankle M66.37-
foot M66.37-
forearm M66.33-
hand M66.34-
lower leg M66.36-
multiple sites M66.39
pelvic region M66.35-
shoulder region M66.31-
specified site NEC M66.38
thigh M66.35-
upper arm M66.32-
foot M66.87-
forearm M66.83-
hand M66.84-
lower leg M66.86-
multiple sites M66.89
pelvic region M66.85-
shoulder region M66.81-
specified
site NEC M66.88
tendon M66.80
thigh M66.85-
upper arm M66.82-
thoracic duct I89.8
tonsil J35.8
traumatic
aorta — *see* Injury, aorta, laceration, major
diaphragm — *see* Injury, intrathoracic, diaphragm
external site — *see* Wound, open, by site
eye — *see* Injury, eye, laceration
internal organ — *see* Injury, by site
intervertebral disc
cervical S13.0
lumbar S33.0
thoracic S23.0
kidney S37.06-
ligament — *see also* Sprain
ankle — *see* Sprain, ankle
carpus — *see* Rupture, traumatic, ligament, wrist
collateral (hand) — *see* Rupture, traumatic, ligament, finger, collateral
finger (metacarpophalangeal) (interphalangeal) S63.40-
collateral S63.41-
index S63.41-
little S63.41-
middle S63.41-
ring S63.41-
index S63.40-
little S63.40-
middle S63.40-
palmar S63.42-
index S63.42-
little S63.42-
middle S63.42-
ring S63.42-
ring S63.40-
specified site NEC S63.499
index S63.49-
little S63.49-
middle S63.49-
ring S63.49-
volar plate S63.43-
index S63.43-
little S63.43-
middle S63.43-
ring S63.43-

Rupture, ruptured - *continued*
traumatic - *continued*
  ligament - *continued*
    foot — *see* Sprain, foot
    radial collateral S53.2-
    radiocarpal — *see* Rupture, traumatic, ligament, wrist, radiocarpal
    ulnar collateral S53.3-
    ulnocarpal — *see* Rupture, traumatic, ligament, wrist, ulnocarpal
    wrist S63.30-
      collateral S63.31-
      radiocarpal S63.32-
      specified site NEC S63.39-
      ulnocarpal (palmar) S63.33-
  liver S36.116
  membrana tympani — *see* Rupture, ear drum, traumatic
  muscle or tendon — *see* Strain
  myocardium — *see* Injury, heart
  pancreas S36.299
  rectum S36.69
  sigmoid S36.593
  spleen S36.09
  stomach S36.39
  symphysis pubis S33.4
  tympanum, tympanic (membrane) — *see* Rupture, ear drum, traumatic
  ureter S37.19
  uterus S37.69
  vagina — *see* Injury, vagina
  vena cava — *see* Injury, vena cava, laceration, major
tricuspid (heart) (valve) I07.8
tube, tubal (nonobstetric) (nontraumatic) N83.8
  abscess — *see* Salpingitis
  due to pregnancy O00.10
    with intrauterine pregnancy O00.11
tympanum, tympanic (membrane) (nontraumatic) — *see also* Perforation, tympanic membrane H72.9-
  traumatic — *see* Rupture, ear drum, traumatic
umbilical cord, complicating delivery O69.89
ureter (traumatic) S37.19
  nontraumatic N28.89
urethra (nontraumatic) N36.8
  with ectopic or molar pregnancy O08.6
  following ectopic or molar pregnancy O08.6
  obstetrical trauma O71.5
  traumatic S37.39
uterosacral ligament (nonobstetric) (nontraumatic) N83.8
uterus (traumatic) S37.69
  before labor O71.0-
  during or after labor O71.1
  nonpuerperal, nontraumatic N85.8
  pregnant (during labor) O71.1
    before labor O71.0-
vagina — *see* Injury, vagina
valve, valvular (heart) — *see* Endocarditis
varicose vein — *see* Varix
varix — *see* Varix
vena cava R58
  traumatic — *see* Injury, vena cava, laceration, major
vesical (urinary) N32.89
vessel (blood) R58
  pulmonary I28.8
  traumatic — *see* Injury, blood vessel
viscus R19.8
vulva complicating delivery O70.0
Russell-Silver syndrome Q87.1
Russian spring-summer type encephalitis A84.0
Rust's disease (tuberculous cervical spondylitis) A18.01
Ruvalcaba-Myhre-Smith syndrome E71.440
Rytand-Lipsitch syndrome I44.2

S

Saber, sabre shin or tibia (syphilitic) A50.56 *[M90.8-]*
Sac lacrimal — *see* condition
Saccharomyces infection B37.9
Saccharopinuria E72.3
Saccular — *see* condition
Sacculation
aorta (nonsyphilitic) — *see* Aneurysm, aorta
bladder N32.3
intralaryngeal (congenital) (ventricular) Q31.3
larynx (congenital) (ventricular) Q31.3
organ or site, congenital — *see* Distortion
pregnant uterus — *see* Pregnancy, complicated by, abnormal, uterus

Sacculation - *continued*
ureter N28.89
urethra N36.1
vesical N32.3
Sachs' amaurotic familial idiocy or disease E75.02
Sachs-Tay disease E75.02
Sacks-Libman disease M32.11
Sacralgia M53.3
Sacralization Q76.49
Sacrodynia M53.3
Sacroiliac joint — *see* condition
Sacroiliitis NEC M46.1
Sacrum — *see* condition
Saddle
back — *see* Lordosis
embolus
  abdominal aorta I74.01
  pulmonary artery I26.92
    with acute cor pulmonale I26.02
injury - code to condition
nose M95.0
  due to syphilis A50.57
Sadism (sexual) F65.52
Sadness, postpartal O90.6
Sadomasochism F65.50
Saemisch's ulcer (cornea) — *see* Ulcer, cornea, central
Sagging
skin and subcutaneous tissue (following bariatric surgery weight loss) (following dietary weight loss) L98.7
Sahib disease B55.0
Sailors' skin L57.8
Saint
Anthony's fire — *see* Erysipelas
triad — *see* Hernia, diaphragm
Vitus' dance — *see* Chorea, Sydenham's
Salaam
attack (s) — *see* Epilepsy, spasms
tic R25.8
Salicylism
abuse F55.8
overdose or wrong substance given — *see* Table of Drugs and Chemicals, by drug, poisoning
Salivary duct or gland — *see* condition
Salivation, excessive K11.7
Salmonella — *see* Infection, Salmonella
Salmonellosis A02.0
Salpingitis (catarrhal) (fallopian tube) (nodular) (pseudofollicular) (purulent) (septic) N70.91
with oophoritis N70.93
acute N70.01
  with oophoritis N70.03
chlamydial A56.11
chronic N70.11
  with oophoritis N70.13
complicating abortion — *see* Abortion, by type, complicated by, salpingitis
ear — *see* Salpingitis, eustachian
eustachian (tube) H68.00-
  acute H68.01-
  chronic H68.02-
follicularis N70.11
  with oophoritis N70.13
gonococcal (acute) (chronic) A54.24
interstitial, chronic N70.11
  with oophoritis N70.13
isthmica nodosa N70.11
  with oophoritis N70.13
specific (gonococcal) (acute) (chronic) A54.24
tuberculous (acute) (chronic) A18.17
venereal (gonococcal) (acute) (chronic) A54.24
Salpingocele N83.4-
Salpingo-oophoritis (catarrhal) (purulent) (ruptured) (septic) (suppurative) N70.93
acute N70.03
  with ectopic or molar pregnancy O08.0
  following ectopic or molar pregnancy O08.0
  gonococcal A54.24
chronic N70.13
following ectopic or molar pregnancy O08.0
gonococcal (acute) (chronic) A54.24
puerperal O86.19
specific (gonococcal) (acute) (chronic) A54.24
subacute N70.03
tuberculous (acute) (chronic) A18.17
venereal (gonococcal) (acute) (chronic) A54.24
Salpingo-ovaritis — *see* Salpingo-oophoritis
Salpingoperitonitis — *see* Salpingo-oophoritis
Salzmann's nodular dystrophy — *see* Degeneration, cornea, nodular
Sampson's cyst or tumor N80.1
San Joaquin (Valley) **fever** B38.0

Sandblaster's asthma, lung or pneumoconiosis J62.8
Sander's disease (paranoia) F22
Sandfly fever A93.1
Sandhoff's disease E75.01
Sanfilippo (Type B) (Type C) (Type D) **syndrome** E76.22
Sanger-Brown ataxia G11.2
Sao Paulo fever or typhus A77.0
Saponification, mesenteric K65.8
Sarcocele (benign)
syphilitic A52.76
  congenital A50.59
Sarcocystosis A07.8
Sarcoepiplocele — *see* Hernia
Sarcoepiplomphalocele Q79.2
Sarcoid — *see also* Sarcoidosis
arthropathy D86.86
Boeck's D86.9
Darier-Roussy D86.3
iridocyclitis D86.83
meningitis D86.81
myocarditis D86.85
myositis D86.87
pyelonephritis D86.84
Spiegler-Fendt L08.89
Sarcoidosis D86.9
with
  cranial nerve palsies D86.82
  hepatic granuloma D86.89
  polyarthritis D86.86
  tubulo-interstitial nephropathy D86.84
combined sites NEC D86.89
lung D86.0
  and lymph nodes D86.2
lymph nodes D86.1
  and lung D86.2
meninges D86.81
skin D86.3
specified type NEC D86.89
Sarcoma (of) — *see also* Neoplasm, connective tissue, malignant
alveolar soft part — *see* Neoplasm, connective tissue, malignant
ameloblastic C41.1
  upper jaw (bone) C41.0
botryoid — *see* Neoplasm, connective tissue, malignant
botryoides — *see* Neoplasm, connective tissue, malignant
cerebellar C71.6
  circumscribed (arachnoidal) C71.6
circumscribed (arachnoidal) cerebellar C71.6
clear cell — *see also* Neoplasm, connective tissue, malignant
  kidney C64.-
dendritic cells (accessory cells) C96.4
embryonal — *see* Neoplasm, connective tissue, malignant
endometrial (stromal) C54.1
  isthmus C54.0
epithelioid (cell) — *see* Neoplasm, connective tissue, malignant
Ewing's — *see* Neoplasm, bone, malignant
follicular dendritic cell C96.4
germinoblastic (diffuse) — *see* Lymphoma, diffuse large cell
  follicular — *see* Lymphoma, follicular, specified NEC
giant cell (except of bone) — *see also* Neoplasm, connective tissue, malignant
  bone — *see* Neoplasm, bone, malignant
glomoid — *see* Neoplasm, connective tissue, malignant
granulocytic C92.3-
hemangioendothelial — *see* Neoplasm, connective tissue, malignant
hemorrhagic, multiple — *see* Sarcoma, Kaposi's
histiocytic C96.A
Hodgkin — *see* Lymphoma, Hodgkin
immunoblastic (diffuse) — *see* Lymphoma, diffuse large cell
interdigitating dendritic cell C96.4
Kaposi's
  colon C46.4
  connective tissue C46.1
  gastrointestinal organ C46.4
  lung C46.5-
  lymph node (s) C46.3
  palate (hard) (soft) C46.2
  rectum C46.4
  skin C46.0
  specified site NEC C46.7

Sarcoma (of) - *continued*
  Kaposi's - *continued*
    stomach C46.4
    unspecified site C46.9
  Kupffer cell C22.3
  Langerhans cell C96.4
  leptomeningeal — *see* Neoplasm, meninges, malignant
  liver NEC C22.4
  lymphangioendothelial — *see* Neoplasm, connective tissue, malignant
  lymphoblastic — *see* Lymphoma, lymphoblastic (diffuse)
  lymphocytic — *see* Lymphoma, small cell B-cell
  mast cell C96.2
  melanotic — *see* Melanoma
  meningeal — *see* Neoplasm, meninges, malignant
  meningothelial — *see* Neoplasm, meninges, malignant
  mesenchymal — *see also* Neoplasm, connective tissue, malignant
    mixed — *see* Neoplasm, connective tissue, malignant
  mesothelial — *see* Mesothelioma
  monstrocellular
    specified site — *see* Neoplasm, malignant, by site
    unspecified site C71.9
  myeloid C92.3-
  neurogenic — *see* Neoplasm, nerve, malignant
  odontogenic C41.1
    upper jaw (bone) C41.0
  osteoblastic — *see* Neoplasm, bone, malignant
  osteogenic — *see also* Neoplasm, bone, malignant
    juxtacortical — *see* Neoplasm, bone, malignant
    periosteal — *see* Neoplasm, bone, malignant
  periosteal — *see also* Neoplasm, bone, malignant
    osteogenic — *see* Neoplasm, bone, malignant
  pleomorphic cell — *see* Neoplasm, connective tissue, malignant
  reticulum cell (diffuse) — *see* Lymphoma, diffuse large cell
    nodular — *see* Lymphoma, follicular
    pleomorphic cell type — *see* Lymphoma, diffuse large cell
  rhabdoid — *see* Neoplasm, malignant, by site
  round cell — *see* Neoplasm, connective tissue, malignant
  small cell — *see* Neoplasm, connective tissue, malignant
  soft tissue — *see* Neoplasm, connective tissue, malignant
  spindle cell — *see* Neoplasm, connective tissue, malignant
  stromal (endometrial) C54.1
    isthmus C54.0
  synovial — *see also* Neoplasm, connective tissue, malignant
    biphasic — *see* Neoplasm, connective tissue, malignant
    epithelioid cell — *see* Neoplasm, connective tissue, malignant
    spindle cell — *see* Neoplasm, connective tissue, malignant
Sarcomatosis
  meningeal — *see* Neoplasm, meninges, malignant
  specified site NEC — *see* Neoplasm, connective tissue, malignant
  unspecified site C80.1
Sarcopenia (age-related) M62.84
Sarcosinemia E72.59
Sarcosporidiosis (intestinal) A07.8
Satiety, early R68.81
Saturnine — *see* condition
Saturnism
  overdose or wrong substance given or taken — *see* Table of Drugs and Chemicals, by drug, poisoning
Satyriasis F52.8
Sauriasis — *see* Ichthyosis
SBE (subacute bacterial endocarditis) I33.0
Scabies (any site) B86
Scabs R23.4
Scaglietti-Dagnini syndrome E22.0
Scald — *see* Burn
Scalenus anticus (anterior) **syndrome** G54.0
Scales R23.4
Scaling, skin R23.4
Scalp — *see* condition
Scapegoating affecting child Z62.3
Scaphocephaly Q75.0
Scapulalgia M89.8X1
Scapulohumeral myopathy G71.0
Scar, scarring — *see also* Cicatrix L90.5
  adherent L90.5

Scar, scarring - *continued*
  atrophic L90.5
  cervix
    in pregnancy or childbirth — *see* Pregnancy, complicated by, abnormal cervix
  cheloid L91.0
  chorioretinal H31.00-
    posterior pole macula H31.01-
    postsurgical H59.81-
    solar retinopathy H31.02-
    specified type NEC H31.09-
  choroid — *see* Scar, chorioretinal
  conjunctiva H11.24-
  cornea H17.9
    xerophthalmic — *see also* Opacity, cornea
      vitamin A deficiency E50.6
  duodenum, obstructive K31.5
  hypertrophic L91.0
  keloid L91.0
  labia N90.89
  lung (base) J98.4
  macula — *see* Scar, chorioretinal, posterior pole
  muscle M62.89
  myocardium, myocardial I25.2
  painful L90.5
  posterior pole (eye) — *see* Scar, chorioretinal, posterior pole
  retina — *see* Scar, chorioretinal
  trachea J39.8
  transmural uterine, in pregnancy O34.29
  uterus N85.8
    in pregnancy O34.29
  vagina N89.8
    postoperative N99.2
  vulva N90.89
Scarabiasis B88.2
Scarlatina (anginosa) (maligna) (ulcerosa) A38.9
  myocarditis (acute) A38.1
  old — *see* Myocarditis
  otitis media A38.0
Scarlet fever (albuminuria) (angina) A38.9
Schamberg's disease
  (progressive pigmentary dermatosis) L81.7
Schatzki's ring (acquired) (esophagus) (lower) K22.2
  congenital Q39.3
Schaufenster krankheit I20.8
Schaumann's
  benign lymphogranulomatosis D86.1
  disease or syndrome — *see* Sarcoidosis
Scheie's syndrome E76.03
Schenck's disease B42.1
Scheuermann's disease or osteochondrosis — *see* Osteochondrosis, juvenile, spine
Schilder (-Flatau) **disease** G37.0
Schilling-type monocytic leukemia C93.0-
Schimmelbusch's disease, cystic mastitis, or hyperplasia — *see* Mastopathy, cystic
Schistosoma infestation — *see* Infestation, Schistosoma
Schistosomiasis B65.9
  with muscle disorder B65.9 [M63.80]
    ankle B65.9 [M63.87-]
    foot B65.9 [M63.87-]
    forearm B65.9 [M63.83-]
    hand B65.9 [M63.84-]
    lower leg B65.9 [M63.86-]
    multiple sites B65.9 [M63.89]
    pelvic region B65.9 [M63.85-]
    shoulder region B65.9 [M63.81-]
    specified site NEC B65.9 [M63.88]
    thigh B65.9 [M63.85-]
    upper arm B65.9 [M63.82-]
  Asiatic B65.2
  bladder B65.0
  chestermani B65.8
  colon B65.1
  cutaneous B65.3
  due to
    S. haematobium B65.0
    S. japonicum B65.2
    S. mansoni B65.1
    S. mattheii B65.8
  Eastern B65.2
  genitourinary tract B65.0
  intestinal B65.1
  lung NEC B65.9 [J99]
    pneumonia B65.9 [J17]
  Manson's (intestinal) B65.1
  oriental B65.2
  pulmonary NEC B65.9 [J99]
    pneumonia B65.9
  Schistosoma
    haematobium B65.0

Schistosomiasis - *continued*
  Schistosoma - *continued*
    japonicum B65.2
    mansoni B65.1
  specified type NEC B65.8
  urinary B65.0
  vesical B65.0
Schizencephaly Q04.6
Schizoaffective psychosis F25.9
Schizodontia K00.2
Schizoid personality F60.1
Schizophrenia, schizophrenic F20.9
  acute (brief) (undifferentiated) F23
  atypical (form) F20.3
  borderline F21
  catalepsy F20.2
  catatonic (type) (excited) (withdrawn) F20.2
  cenesthopathic, cenesthesiopathic F20.89
  childhood type F84.5
  chronic undifferentiated F20.5
  cyclic F25.0
  disorganized (type) F20.1
  flexibilitas cerea F20.2
  hebephrenic (type) F20.1
  incipient F21
  latent F21
  negative type F20.5
  paranoid (type) F20.0
  paraphrenic F20.0
  post-psychotic depression F32.89
  prepsychotic F21
  prodromal F21
  pseudoneurotic F21
  pseudopsychopathic F21
  reaction F23
  residual (state) (type) F20.5
  restzustand F20.5
  schizoaffective (type) — *see* Psychosis, schizoaffective
  simple (type) F20.89
  simplex F20.89
  specified type NEC F20.89
  stupor F20.2
  syndrome of childhood F84.5
  undifferentiated (type) F20.3
    chronic F20.5
Schizothymia (persistent) F60.1
Schlatter-Osgood disease or osteochondrosis — *see* Osteochondrosis, juvenile, tibia
Schlatter's tibia — *see* Osteochondrosis, juvenile, tibia
Schmidt's syndrome (polyglandular, autoimmune) E31.0
Schmincke's carcinoma or tumor — *see* Neoplasm, nasopharynx, malignant
Schmitz (-Stutzer) **dysentery** A03.0
Schmorl's disease or nodes
  lumbar region M51.46
  lumbosacral region M51.47
  sacrococcygeal region M53.3
  thoracic region M51.44
  thoracolumbar region M51.45
Schneiderian
  papilloma — *see* Neoplasm, nasopharynx, benign
    specified site — *see* Neoplasm, benign, by site
    unspecified site D14.0
    specified site — *see* Neoplasm, malignant, by site
    unspecified site C30.0
Scholte's syndrome (malignant carcinoid) E34.0
Scholz (-Bielchowsky-Henneberg) **disease or syndrome** E75.25
Schönlein (-Henoch) **disease or purpura** (primary) (rheumatic) D69.0
Schottmuller's disease A01.4
Schroeder's syndrome (endocrine hypertensive) E27.0
Schüller-Christian disease or syndrome C96.5
Schultze's type acroparesthesia, simple I73.89
Schultz's disease or syndrome — *see* Agranulocytosis
Schwalbe-Ziehen-Oppenheim disease G24.1
Schwannoma — *see also* Neoplasm, nerve, benign
  malignant — *see also* Neoplasm, nerve, malignant
    with rhabdomyoblastic differentiation — *see* Neoplasm, nerve, malignant
  melanocytic — *see* Neoplasm, nerve, benign
  pigmented — *see* Neoplasm, nerve, benign
Schwannomatosis Q85.03
Schwartz (-Jampel) **syndrome** G71.13
Schwartz-Bartter syndrome E22.2
Schweniger-Buzzi anetoderma L90.1
Sciatic — *see* condition

Sciatica (infective)
  with lumbago M54.4-
    due to intervertebral disc disorder — *see* Disorder, disc, with, radiculopathy
  due to displacement of intervertebral disc (with lumbago) — *see* Disorder, disc, with, radiculopathy
  wallet M54.3-
Scimitar syndrome Q26.8
Sclera — *see* condition
Scleredema
  adultorum — *see* Sclerosis, systemic
  Buschke's — *see* Sclerosis, systemic
  newborn P83.0
Sclerema (adiposum) (edematosum) (neonatorum) (newborn) P83.0
  adultorum — *see* Sclerosis, systemic
Scleriasis — *see* Scleroderma
Scleritis H15.00-
  with corneal involvement H15.04-
  anterior H15.01-
  brawny H15.02-
  in (due to) zoster B02.34
  posterior H15.03-
  specified type NEC H15.09-
  syphilitic A52.71
  tuberculous (nodular) A18.51
Sclerochoroiditis H31.8
Scleroconjunctivitis — *see* Scleritis
Sclerocystic ovary syndrome E28.2
Sclerodactyly, sclerodactylia L94.3
Scleroderma, sclerodermia (acrosclerotic) (diffuse) (generalized) (progressive) (pulmonary) — *see also* Sclerosis, systemic M34.9-
  circumscribed L94.0
  linear L94.1
  localized L94.0
  newborn P83.8
  systemic M34.9
Sclerokeratitis H16.8
  tuberculous A18.52
Scleroma nasi A48.8
Scleromalacia (perforans) H15.05-
Scleromyxedema L98.5
Sclérose en plaques G35
Sclerosis, sclerotic
  adrenal (gland) E27.8
  Alzheimer's — *see* Disease, Alzheimer's
  amyotrophic (lateral) G12.21
  aorta, aortic I70.0
    valve — *see* Endocarditis, aortic
  artery, arterial, arteriolar, arteriovascular — *see* Arteriosclerosis
  ascending multiple G35
  brain (generalized) (lobular) G37.9
    artery, arterial I67.2
    diffuse G37.0
    disseminated G35
    insular G35
    Krabbe's E75.23
    miliary G35
    multiple G35
    presenile (Alzheimer's) — *see* Disease, Alzheimer's, early onset
    senile (arteriosclerotic) I67.2
    stem, multiple G35
    tuberous Q85.1
  bulbar, multiple G35
  bundle of His I44.39
  cardiac — *see* Disease, heart, ischemic, atherosclerotic
  cardiorenal — *see* Hypertension, cardiorenal
  cardiovascular — *see also* Disease, cardiovascular
    renal — *see* Hypertension, cardiorenal
  cerebellar — *see* Sclerosis, brain
  cerebral — *see* Sclerosis, brain
  cerebrospinal (disseminated) (multiple) G35
  cerebrovascular I67.2
  choroid — *see* Degeneration, choroid
  combined (spinal cord) — *see also* Degeneration, combined
    multiple G35
  concentric (Balo) G37.5
  cornea — *see* Opacity, cornea
  coronary (artery) I25.10
    with angina pectoris — *see* Arteriosclerosis, coronary (artery),
  corpus cavernosum
    female N90.89
    male N48.6
  diffuse (brain) (spinal cord) G37.0
  disseminated G35

Sclerosis, sclerotic - *continued*
  dorsal G35
  dorsolateral (spinal cord) — *see* Degeneration, combined
  endometrium N85.5
  extrapyramidal G25.9
  eye, nuclear (senile) — *see* Cataract, senile, nuclear
  focal and segmental (glomerular) — *see also* N00-N07 with fourth character .1 N05.1
  Friedreich's (spinal cord) G11.1
  funicular (spermatic cord) N50.89
  general (vascular) — *see* Arteriosclerosis
  gland (lymphatic) I89.8
  hepatic K74.1
    alcoholic K70.2
  hereditary
    cerebellar G11.9
    spinal (Friedreich's ataxia) G11.1
  hippocampal G93.81
  insular G35
  kidney — *see* Sclerosis, renal
  larynx J38.7
  lateral (amyotrophic) (descending) (primary) (spinal) G12.21
  lens, senile nuclear — *see* Cataract, senile, nuclear
  liver K74.1
    with fibrosis K74.2
      alcoholic K70.2
    alcoholic K70.2
    cardiac K76.1
  lung — *see* Fibrosis, lung
  mastoid — *see* Mastoiditis, chronic
  mesial temporal G93.81
  mitral I05.8
  Mönckeberg's (medial) — *see* Arteriosclerosis, extremities
  multiple (brain stem) (cerebral) (generalized) (spinal cord) G35
  myocardium, myocardial — *see* Disease, heart, ischemic, atherosclerotic
  nuclear (senile) , eye — *see* Cataract, senile, nuclear
  ovary N83.8
  pancreas K86.89
  penis N48.6
  peripheral arteries — *see* Arteriosclerosis, extremities
  plaques G35
  pluriglandular E31.8
  polyglandular E31.8
  posterolateral (spinal cord) — *see* Degeneration, combined
  presenile (Alzheimer's) — *see* Disease, Alzheimer's, early onset
  primary, lateral G12.29
  progressive, systemic M34.0
  pulmonary — *see* Fibrosis, lung
    artery I27.0
    valve (heart) — *see* Endocarditis, pulmonary
  renal N26.9
    with
      cystine storage disease E72.09
      hypertensive heart disease (conditions in I11) — *see* Hypertension, cardiorenal
      arteriolar (hyaline) (hyperplastic) — *see* Hypertension, kidney
  retina (senile) (vascular) H35.00
  senile (vascular) — *see* Arteriosclerosis
  spinal (cord) (progressive) G95.89
    ascending G61.0
    combined — *see also* Degeneration, combined
      multiple G35
      syphilitic A52.11
    disseminated G35
    dorsolateral — *see* Degeneration, combined
    hereditary (Friedreich's) (mixed form) G11.1
    lateral (amyotrophic) G12.21
    multiple G35
    posterior (syphilitic) A52.11
  stomach K31.89
  subendocardial, congenital I42.4
  systemic M34.9
    with
      lung involvement M34.81
      myopathy M34.82
      polyneuropathy M34.83
    drug-induced M34.2
    due to chemicals NEC M34.2
    progressive M34.0
    specified NEC M34.89
  temporal (mesial) G93.81
  tricuspid (heart) (valve) I07.8
  tuberous (brain) Q85.1

Sclerosis, sclerotic - *continued*
  tympanic membrane — *see* Disorder, tympanic membrane, specified NEC
  valve, valvular (heart) — *see* Endocarditis
  vascular — *see* Arteriosclerosis
  vein I87.8
Scoliosis (acquired) (postural) M41.9
  adolescent (idiopathic) — *see* Scoliosis, idiopathic, adolescent
  congenital Q67.5
    due to bony malformation Q76.3
    failure of segmentation (hemivertebra) Q76.3
    hemivertebra fusion Q76.3
    postural Q67.5
  idiopathic M41.20
    adolescent M41.129
      cervical region M41.122
      cervicothoracic region M41.123
      lumbar region M41.126
      lumbosacral region M41.127
      thoracic region M41.124
      thoracolumbar region M41.125
    cervical region M41.22
    cervicothoracic region M41.23
    infantile M41.00
      cervical region M41.02
      cervicothoracic region M41.03
      lumbar region M41.06
      lumbosacral region M41.07
      sacrococcygeal region M41.08
      thoracic region M41.04
      thoracolumbar region M41.05
    juvenile M41.119
      cervical region M41.112
      cervicothoracic region M41.113
      lumbar region M41.116
      lumbosacral region M41.117
      thoracic region M41.114
      thoracolumbar region M41.115
    lumbar region M41.26
    lumbosacral region M41.27
    thoracic region M41.24
    thoracolumbar region M41.25
  infantile — *see* Scoliosis, idiopathic, infantile
  neuromuscular M41.40
    cervical region M41.42
    cervicothoracic region M41.43
    lumbar region M41.46
    lumbosacral region M41.47
    occipito-atlanto-axial region M41.41
    thoracic region M41.44
    thoracolumbar region M41.45
  paralytic — *see* Scoliosis, neuromuscular
  postradiation therapy M96.5
  rachitic (late effect or sequelae) E64.3 *[M49.80]*
    cervical region E64.3 *[M49.82]*
    cervicothoracic region E64.3 *[M49.83]*
    lumbar region E64.3 *[M49.86]*
    lumbosacral region E64.3 *[M49.87]*
    multiple sites E64.3 *[M49.89]*
    occipito-atlanto-axial region E64.3 *[M49.81]*
    sacrococcygeal region E64.3 *[M49.88]*
    thoracic region E64.3 *[M49.84]*
    thoracolumbar region E64.3 *[M49.85]*
  sciatic M54.4-
  secondary (to) NEC M41.50
    cerebral palsy, Friedreich's ataxia, poliomyelitis, neuromuscular disorders — *see* Scoliosis, neuromuscular
    cervical region M41.52
    cervicothoracic region M41.53
    lumbar region M41.56
    lumbosacral region M41.57
    thoracic region M41.54
    thoracolumbar region M41.55
  specified form NEC M41.80
    cervical region M41.82
    cervicothoracic region M41.83
    lumbar region M41.86
    lumbosacral region M41.87
    thoracic region M41.84
    thoracolumbar region M41.85
  thoracogenic M41.30
    thoracic region M41.34
    thoracolumbar region M41.35
  tuberculous A18.01
Scoliotic pelvis
  with disproportion (fetopelvic) O33.0
    causing obstructed labor O65.0
Scorbutus, scorbutic — *see also* Scurvy
  anemia D53.2
Score, NIHSS
  (National Institutes of Health Stroke Scale) R29.7-

Scotoma (arcuate) (Bjerrum) (central) (ring) —
see also Defect, visual field, localized, scotoma
scintillating H53.19
Scratch — *see* Abrasion
Scratchy throat R09.89
Screening (for) Z13.9
alcoholism Z13.89
anemia Z13.0
anomaly, congenital Z13.89
antenatal, of mother Z36
arterial hypertension Z13.6
arthropod-borne viral disease NEC Z11.59
bacteriuria, asymptomatic Z13.89
behavioral disorder Z13.89
brain injury, traumatic Z13.850
bronchitis, chronic Z13.83
brucellosis Z11.2
cardiovascular disorder Z13.6
cataract Z13.5
chlamydial diseases Z11.8
cholera Z11.0
chromosomal abnormalities (nonprocreative)
NEC Z13.79
colonoscopy Z12.11
congenital
dislocation of hip Z13.89
eye disorder Z13.5
malformation or deformation Z13.89
contamination NEC Z13.88
cystic fibrosis Z13.228
dengue fever Z11.59
dental disorder Z13.84
depression Z13.89
developmental handicap Z13.42
in early childhood Z13.42
infant Z13.41
diabetes mellitus Z13.1
diphtheria Z11.2
disability, intellectual Z13.42
infant Z13.41
disease or disorder Z13.9
bacterial NEC Z11.2
intestinal infectious Z11.0
respiratory tuberculosis Z11.1
blood or blood-forming organ Z13.0
cardiovascular Z13.6
Chagas' Z11.6
chlamydial Z11.8
dental Z13.89
developmental Z13.42
in child Z13.42
infant Z13.41
digestive tract NEC Z13.818
lower GI Z13.811
upper GI Z13.810
ear Z13.5
endocrine Z13.29
eye Z13.5
genitourinary Z13.89
heart Z13.6
human immunodeficiency virus (HIV)
infection Z11.4
immunity Z13.0
infection
intestinal Z11.0
specified NEC Z11.6
infectious Z11.9
mental Z13.89
metabolic Z13.228
neurological Z13.89
nutritional Z13.21
metabolic Z13.228
lipoid disorders Z13.220
protozoal Z11.6
intestinal Z11.0
respiratory Z13.83
rheumatic Z13.828
rickettsial Z11.8
sexually-transmitted NEC Z11.3
human immunodeficiency virus (HIV) Z11.4
sickle-cell (trait) Z13.0
skin Z13.89
specified NEC Z13.89
spirochetal Z11.8
thyroid Z13.29
vascular Z13.6
venereal Z11.3
viral NEC Z11.59
human immunodeficiency virus (HIV) Z11.4
intestinal Z11.0
elevated titer Z13.89
emphysema Z13.83
encephalitis, viral (mosquito- or tick-borne) Z11.59

Screening (for) - *continued*
exposure to contaminants (toxic) Z13.88
fever
dengue Z11.59
hemorrhagic Z11.59
yellow Z11.59
filariasis Z11.6
galactosemia Z13.228
gastrointestinal condition Z13.818
genetic (nonprocreative) - for procreative
management — *see* Testing, genetic, for
procreative management
disease carrier status (nonprocreative) Z13.71
specified NEC (nonprocreative) Z13.79
genitourinary condition Z13.89
glaucoma Z13.5
gonorrhea Z11.3
gout Z13.89
helminthiasis (intestinal) Z11.6
hematopoietic malignancy Z12.89
hemoglobinopathies NEC Z13.0
hemorrhagic fever Z11.59
Hodgkin disease Z12.89
human immunodeficiency virus (HIV) Z11.4
human papillomavirus Z11.51
hypertension Z13.6
immunity disorders Z13.0
infection
mycotic Z11.8
parasitic Z11.8
ingestion of radioactive substance Z13.88
intellectual disability Z13.42
infant Z13.41
intestinal
helminthiasis Z11.6
infectious disease Z11.0
leishmaniasis Z11.6
leprosy Z11.2
leptospirosis Z11.8
leukemia Z12.89
lymphoma Z12.89
malaria Z11.6
malnutrition Z13.29
metabolic Z13.228
nutritional Z13.21
measles Z11.59
mental disorder Z13.89
metabolic errors, inborn Z13.228
multiphasic Z13.89
musculoskeletal disorder Z13.828
osteoporosis Z13.820
mycoses Z11.8
myocardial infarction (acute) Z13.6
neoplasm (malignant) (of) Z12.9
bladder Z12.6
blood Z12.89
breast Z12.39
routine mammogram Z12.31
cervix Z12.4
colon Z12.11
genitourinary organs NEC Z12.79
bladder Z12.6
cervix Z12.4
ovary Z12.73
prostate Z12.5
testis Z12.71
vagina Z12.72
hematopoietic system Z12.89
intestinal tract Z12.10
colon Z12.11
rectum Z12.12
small intestine Z12.13
lung Z12.2
lymph (glands) Z12.89
nervous system Z12.82
oral cavity Z12.81
prostate Z12.5
rectum Z12.12
respiratory organs Z12.2
skin Z12.83
small intestine Z12.13
specified site NEC Z12.89
stomach Z12.0
nephropathy Z13.89
nervous system disorders NEC Z13.858
neurological condition Z13.89
osteoporosis Z13.820
parasitic infestation Z11.9
specified NEC Z11.8
phenylketonuria Z13.228
plague Z11.2
poisoning (chemical) (heavy metal) Z13.88
poliomyelitis Z11.59

Screening (for) - *continued*
postnatal, chromosomal abnormalities Z13.89
prenatal, of mother Z36
protozoal disease Z11.6
intestinal Z11.0
pulmonary tuberculosis Z11.1
radiation exposure Z13.88
respiratory condition Z13.83
respiratory tuberculosis Z11.1
rheumatoid arthritis Z13.828
rubella Z11.59
schistosomiasis Z11.6
sexually-transmitted disease NEC Z11.3
human immunodeficiency virus (HIV) Z11.4
sickle-cell disease or trait Z13.0
skin condition Z13.89
sleeping sickness Z11.6
special Z13.9
specified NEC Z13.89
syphilis Z11.3
tetanus Z11.2
trachoma Z11.8
traumatic brain injury Z13.850
trypanosomiasis Z11.6
tuberculosis, respiratory Z11.1
venereal disease Z11.3
viral encephalitis (mosquito- or tick-borne) Z11.59
whooping cough Z11.2
worms, intestinal Z11.6
yaws Z11.8
yellow fever Z11.59
Scrofula, scrofulosis
(tuberculosis of cervical lymph glands) A18.2
Scrofulide (primary) (tuberculous) A18.4
Scrofuloderma, scrofulodermia (any site)
(primary) A18.4
Scrofulosus lichen (primary) (tuberculous) A18.4
Scrofulous — *see* condition
Scrotal tongue K14.5
Scrotum — *see* condition
Scurvy, scorbutic E54
anemia D53.2
gum E54
infantile E54
rickets E55.0 *[M90.80]*
Sealpox B08.62
Seasickness T75.3
Seatworm (infection) (infestation) B80
Sebaceous — *see also* condition
cyst — *see* Cyst, sebaceous
Seborrhea, seborrheic L21.9
capillitii R23.8
capitis L21.0
dermatitis L21.9
infantile L21.1
eczema L21.9
infantile L21.1
sicca L21.0
Seckel's syndrome Q87.1
Seclusion, pupil — *see* Membrane, pupillary
Second hand tobacco smoke exposure (acute)
(chronic) Z77.22
in the perinatal period P96.81
Secondary
dentin (in pulp) K04.3
neoplasm, secondaries — *see* Table of Neoplasms,
secondary
Secretion
antidiuretic hormone, inappropriate E22.2
catecholamine, by pheochromocytoma E27.5
hormone
antidiuretic, inappropriate (syndrome) E22.2
by
carcinoid tumor E34.0
pheochromocytoma E27.5
ectopic NEC E34.2
urinary
excessive R35.8
suppression R34
Section
nerve, traumatic — *see* Injury, nerve
Sedative, hypnotic, or anxiolytic-induced
anxiety disorder F13.980
bipolar and related disorder F13.94
delirium F13.921
depressive disorder F13.94
major neurocognitive disorder F13.97
mild neurocognitive disorder F13.988
psychotic disorder F13.959
sexual dysfunction F13.981
sleep disorder F13.982

Segmentation, incomplete (congenital) — *see also* Fusion
  bone NEC Q78.8
  lumbosacral (joint) (vertebra) Q76.49
Seitelberger's syndrome
  (infantile neuraxonal dystrophy) G31.89
Seizure (s) — *see also* Convulsions R56.9
  akinetic — *see* Epilepsy, generalized, specified NEC
  atonic — *see* Epilepsy, generalized, specified NEC
  autonomic (hysterical) F44.5
  convulsive — *see* Convulsions
  cortical (focal) (motor) — *see* Epilepsy, localization-related, symptomatic, with simple partial seizures
  disorder — *see also* Epilepsy G40.909
  due to stroke — *see* Sequelae (of), disease, cerebrovascular, by type, specified NEC
  epileptic — *see* Epilepsy
  febrile (simple) R56.00
    with status epilepticus G40.901
    complex (atypical) (complicated) R56.01
     with status epilepticus G40.901
  grand mal G40.409
    intractable G40.419
     with status epilepticus G40.411
     without status epilepticus G40.419
    not intractable G40.409
     with status epilepticus G40.401
     without status epilepticus G40.409
  heart — *see* Disease, heart
  hysterical F44.5
  intractable G40.919
    with status epilepticus G40.911
  Jacksonian (focal) (motor type) (sensory type) — *see* Epilepsy, localization-related, symptomatic, with simple partial seizures
  newborn P90
  nonspecific epileptic
    atonic — *see* Epilepsy, generalized, specified NEC
    clonic — *see* Epilepsy, generalized, specified NEC
    myoclonic — *see* Epilepsy, generalized, specified NEC
    tonic — *see* Epilepsy, generalized, specified NEC
    tonic-clonic — *see* Epilepsy, generalized, specified NEC
  partial, developing into secondarily generalized seizures
    complex — *see* Epilepsy, localization-related, symptomatic, with complex partial seizures
    simple — *see* Epilepsy, localization-related, symptomatic, with simple partial seizures
  petit mal G40.409
    intractable G40.419
     with status epilepticus G40.411
     without status epilepticus G40.419
    not intractable G40.409
     with status epilepticus G40.401
     without status epilepticus G40.409
  post traumatic R56.1
  recurrent G40.909
  specified NEC G40.89
  uncinate — *see* Epilepsy, localization-related, symptomatic, with complex partial seizures
Selenium deficiency, dietary E59
Self-damaging behavior (life-style) Z72.89
Self-harm (attempted)
  history (personal) Z91.5
    in family Z81.8
Self-mutilation (attempted)
  history (personal) Z91.5
    in family Z81.8
Self-poisoning
  history (personal) Z91.5
    in family Z81.8
  observation following (alleged) attempt Z03.6
Semicoma R40.1
Seminal vesiculitis N49.0
Seminoma C62.9-
  specified site — *see* Neoplasm, malignant, by site
Senear-Usher disease or syndrome L10.4
Senectus R54
Senescence (without mention of psychosis) R54
Senile, senility — *see also* condition R41.81
  with
    acute confusional state F05
    mental changes NOS F03
    psychosis NEC — *see* Psychosis, senile
  asthenia R54
  cervix (atrophic) N88.8
  debility R54
  endometrium (atrophic) N85.8
  fallopian tube (atrophic) — *see* Atrophy, fallopian tube
  heart (failure) R54

Senile, senility - *continued*
  ovary (atrophic) — *see* Atrophy, ovary
  premature E34.8
  vagina, vaginitis (atrophic) N95.2
  wart L82.1
Sensation
  burning (skin) R20.8
    tongue K14.6
  loss of R20.8
  prickling (skin) R20.2
  tingling (skin) R20.2
Sense loss
  smell — *see* Disturbance, sensation, smell
  taste — *see* Disturbance, sensation, taste
  touch R20.8
Sensibility disturbance (cortical) (deep) (vibratory) R20.9
Sensitive, sensitivity — *see also* Allergy
  carotid sinus G90.01
  child (excessive) F93.8
  cold, autoimmune D59.1
  dentin K03.89
  gluten (non-celiac) K90.41
  latex Z91.040
  methemoglobin D74.8
  tuberculin, without clinical or radiological symptoms R76.11
  visual
    glare H53.71
    impaired contrast H53.72
Sensitiver Beziehungswahn F22
Sensitization, auto-erythrocytic D69.2
Separation
  anxiety, abnormal (of childhood) F93.0
  apophysis, traumatic - code as Fracture, by site
  choroid — *see* Detachment, choroid
  epiphysis, epiphyseal
    nontraumatic — *see also* Osteochondropathy, specified type NEC
     upper femoral — *see* Slipped, epiphysis, upper femoral
    traumatic - code as Fracture, by site
  fracture — *see* Fracture
  infundibulum cardiac from right ventricle by a partition Q24.3
  joint (traumatic) (current) - code by site under Dislocation
  pubic bone, obstetrical trauma O71.6
  retina, retinal — *see* Detachment, retina
  symphysis pubis, obstetrical trauma O71.6
  tracheal ring, incomplete, congenital Q32.1
Sepsis (generalized) (unspecified organism) A41.9
  with
    organ dysfunction (acute) (multiple) R65.20
     with septic shock R65.21
  actinomycotic A42.7
  adrenal hemorrhage syndrome (meningococcal) A39.1
  anaerobic A41.4
  Bacillus anthracis A22.7
  Brucella — *see also* Brucellosis A23.9
  candidal B37.7
  cryptogenic A41.9
  due to device, implant or graft T85.79
    arterial graft NEC T82.7
    breast (implant) T85.79
    catheter NEC T85.79
     dialysis (renal) T82.7
      intraperitoneal T85.71
     infusion NEC T82.7
      spinal (cranial) (epidural) (intrathecal) (spinal) (subarachnoid) (subdural) T85.735
     urethral indwelling T83.511
     urinary T83.518
    ectopic or molar pregnancy O08.82
    electronic (electrode) (pulse generator) (stimulator)
     bone T84.7
     cardiac T82.7
     nervous system T85.738
      brain T85.731
      neurostimulator generator T85.734
      peripheral nerve T85.732
      spinal cord T85.733
     urinary T83.590
    fixation, internal (orthopedic) — *see* Complication, fixation device, infection
    gastrointestinal (bile duct) (esophagus) T85.79
     neurostimulator electrode (lead) T85.732
    genital T83.69
    heart NEC T82.7
     valve (prosthesis) T82.6
      graft T82.7

Sepsis (generalized) (unspecified organism) - *continued*
  due to device, implant or graft - *continued*
    joint prosthesis — *see* Complication, joint prosthesis, infection
    ocular (corneal graft) (orbital implant) T85.79
    orthopedic NEC T84.7
     fixation device, internal — *see* Complication, fixation device, infection
    specified NEC T85.79
    vascular T82.7
    ventricular intracranial (communicating) shunt T85.730
  during labor O75.3
  Enterococcus A41.81
  Erysipelothrix (rhusiopathiae) (erysipeloid) A26.7
  Escherichia coli (E. coli) A41.5
  extraintestinal yersiniosis A28.2
  following
    abortion (subsequent episode) O08.0
     current episode — *see* Abortion
    ectopic or molar pregnancy O08.82
    immunization T88.0
    infusion, therapeutic injection or transfusion NEC T80.29
  gangrenous A41.9
  gonococcal A54.86
  Gram-negative (organism) A41.5
    anaerobic A41.4
  Haemophilus influenzae A41.3
  herpesviral B00.7
  intra-abdominal K65.1
  intraocular — *see* Endophthalmitis, purulent
  Listeria monocytogenes A32.7
  localized - code to specific localized infection
    in operation wound T81.49
    skin — *see* Abscess
  malleus A24.0
  melioidosis A24.1
  meningeal — *see* Meningitis
  meningococcal A39.4
    acute A39.2
    chronic A39.3
  MSSA (Methicillin susceptible Staphylococcus aureus) A41.01
  newborn P36.9
    due to
     anaerobes NEC P36.5
     Escherichia coli P36.4
     Staphylococcus P36.30
      aureus P36.2
      specified NEC P36.39
     Streptococcus P36.10
      group B P36.0
      specified NEC P36.19
     specified NEC P36.8
  Pasteurella multocida A28.0
  pelvic, puerperal, postpartum, childbirth O85
  postprocedural T81.49
  pneumococcal A40.3
  puerperal, postpartum, childbirth (pelvic) O85
  Salmonella (arizonae) (cholerae-suis) (enteritidis) (typhimurium) A02.1
  severe R65.20
    with septic shock R65.21
  skin, localized — *see* Abscess
  Shigella — *see also* Dysentery, bacillary A03.9
  specified organism NEC A41.89
  Staphylococcus, staphylococcal A41.2
    aureus (methicillin susceptible) (MSSA) A41.01
     methicillin resistant (MRSA) A41.02
    coagulase-negative A41.1
    specified NEC A41.1
  Streptococcus, streptococcal A40.9
    agalactiae A40.1
    group
     A A40.0
     B A40.1
     D A41.81
    neonatal P36.10
     group B P36.0
     specified NEC P36.19
    pneumoniae A40.3
    pyogenes A40.0
    specified NEC A40.8
  tracheostomy stoma J95.02
  tularemic A21.7
  umbilical, umbilical cord (newborn) — *see* Sepsis, newborn
  Yersinia pestis A20.7
Septate — *see* Septum
Septic — *see* condition
  arm — *see* Cellulitis, upper limb

Septic - *continued*
  arm - *continued*
    with lymphangitis — *see* Lymphangitis, acute, upper limb
  embolus — *see* Embolism
  finger — *see* Cellulitis, digit
    with lymphangitis — *see* Lymphangitis, acute, digit
  foot — *see* Cellulitis, lower limb
    with lymphangitis — *see* Lymphangitis, acute, lower limb
  gallbladder (acute) K81.0
  hand — *see* Cellulitis, upper limb
    with lymphangitis — *see* Lymphangitis, acute, upper limb
  joint — *see* Arthritis, pyogenic or pyemic
  leg — *see* Cellulitis, lower limb
    with lymphangitis — *see* Lymphangitis, acute, lower limb
  nail — *see also* Cellulitis, digit
    with lymphangitis — *see* Lymphangitis, acute, digit
  sore — *see also* Abscess
    throat J02.0
    streptococcal J02.0
  spleen (acute) D73.89
  teeth, tooth (pulpal origin) K04.4
  throat — *see* Pharyngitis
  thrombus — *see* Thrombosis
  toe — *see* Cellulitis, digit
    with lymphangitis — *see* Lymphangitis, acute, digit
  tonsils, chronic J35.01
    with adenoiditis J35.03
  uterus — *see* Endometritis
Septicemia A41.9
  meaning sepsis — *see* Sepsis
Septum, septate (congenital) — *see also* Anomaly, by site
  anal Q42.3
    with fistula Q42.2
  aqueduct of Sylvius Q03.0
    with spina bifida — *see* Spina bifida, by site, with hydrocephalus
  uterus (complete) (partial) Q51.2
  vagina Q52.10
    in pregnancy — *see* Pregnancy, complicated by, abnormal vagina
    causing obstructed labor O65.5
    longitudinal Q52.129
      microperforate
        left side Q52.124
        right side Q52.123
      nonobstruction Q52.120
      obstructing Q52.129
        left side Q52.122
        right side Q52.121
    transverse Q52.11
Sequelae (of) — *see also* condition
  abscess, intracranial or intraspinal (conditions in G06) G09
  amputation -- code to injury with seventh character S
  burn and corrosion -- code to injury with seventh character S
  calcium deficiency E64.8
  cerebrovascular disease — *see* Sequelae, disease, cerebrovascular
  childbirth O94
  contusion -- code to injury with seventh character S
  corrosion — *see* Sequelae, burn and corrosion
  crushing injury -- code to injury with seventh character S
  disease
    cerebrovascular I69.90
      alteration of sensation I69.998
      aphasia I69.920
      apraxia I69.990
      ataxia I69.993
      cognitive deficits I69.91
      disturbance of vision I69.998
      dysarthria I69.922
      dysphagia I69.991
      dysphasia I69.921
      facial droop I69.992
      facial weakness I69.992
      fluency disorder I69.923
      hemiplegia I69.95-
      hemorrhage
        intracerebral — *see* Sequelae, hemorrhage, intracerebral
        intracranial, nontraumatic NEC — *see* Sequelae, hemorrhage, intracranial, nontraumatic

Sequelae (of) - *continued*
  disease - *continued*
    cerebrovascular - *continued*
      hemorrhage - *continued*
        subarachnoid — *see* Sequelae, hemorrhage, subarachnoid
      language deficit I69.928
      monoplegia
        lower limb I69.84-
        upper limb I69.93-
      paralytic syndrome I69.96-
      specified effect NEC I69.998
      specified type NEC I69.80
        alteration of sensation I69.898
        aphasia I69.820
        apraxia I69.890
        ataxia I69.893
        cognitive deficits I69.81
        disturbance of vision I69.898
        dysarthria I69.822
        dysphagia I69.891
        dysphasia I69.821
        facial droop I69.892
        facial weakness I69.892
        fluency disorder I69.823
        hemiplegia I69.85-
        language deficit I69.828
        monoplegia
          lower limb I69.84-
          upper limb I69.83-
        paralytic syndrome I69.86-
        specified effect NEC I69.898
      speech deficit I69.928
        speech deficit I69.828
      stroke NOS — *see* Sequelae, stroke NOS
  dislocation -- code to injury with seventh character S
  encephalitis or encephalomyelitis (conditions in G04) G09
    in infectious disease NEC B94.8
    viral B94.1
  external cause -- code to injury with seventh character S
  foreign body entering natural orifice -- code to injury with seventh character S
  fracture -- code to injury with seventh character S
  frostbite -- code to injury with seventh character S
  Hansen's disease B92
  hemorrhage
    intracerebral I69.10
      alteration of sensation I69.198
      aphasia I69.120
      apraxia I69.190
      ataxia I69.193
      cognitive deficits I69.11
      disturbance of vision I69.198
      dysarthria I69.122
      dysphagia I69.191
      dysphasia I69.121
      facial droop I69.192
      facial weakness I69.192
      fluency disorder I69.123
      hemiplegia I69.15-
      language deficit NEC I69.128
      monoplegia
        lower limb I69.14-
        upper limb I69.13-
      paralytic syndrome I69.16-
      specified effect NEC I69.198
      speech deficit NEC I69.128
    intracranial, nontraumatic NEC I69.20
      alteration of sensation I69.298
      aphasia I69.220
      apraxia I69.290
      ataxia I69.293
      cognitive deficits I69.21
      disturbance of vision I69.298
      dysarthria I69.222
      dysphagia I69.291
      dysphasia I69.221
      facial droop I69.292
      facial weakness I69.292
      fluency disorder I69.223
      hemiplegia I69.25-
      language deficit NEC I69.228
      monoplegia
        lower limb I69.24-
        upper limb I69.23-
      paralytic syndrome I69.26-
      specified effect NEC I69.298
      speech deficit NEC I69.228
    subarachnoid I69.00
      alteration of sensation I69.098
      aphasia I69.020

Sequelae (of) - *continued*
  hemorrhage - *continued*
    subarachnoid - *continued*
      apraxia I69.090
      ataxia I69.093
      cognitive deficits — *see* subcategory I69.01-
      disturbance of vision I69.098
      dysarthria I69.022
      dysphagia I69.091
      dysphasia I69.021
      facial droop I69.092
      facial weakness I69.092
      fluency disorder I69.023
      hemiplegia I69.05-
      language deficit NEC I69.028
      monoplegia
        lower limb I69.04-
        upper limb I69.03-
      paralytic syndrome I69.06-
      specified effect NEC I69.098
      speech deficit NEC I69.028
  hepatitis, viral B94.2
  hyperalimentation E68
  infarction
    cerebral I69.30
      alteration of sensation I69.398
      aphasia I69.320
      apraxia I69.390
      ataxia I69.393
      cognitive deficits I69.31
      disturbance of vision I69.398
      dysarthria I69.322
      dysphagia I69.391
      dysphasia I69.321
      facial droop I69.392
      facial weakness I69.392
      fluency disorder I69.323
      hemiplegia I69.35-
      language deficit NEC I69.328
      monoplegia
        lower limb I69.34-
        upper limb I69.33-
      paralytic syndrome I69.36-
      specified effect NEC I69.398
      speech deficit NEC I69.328
  infection, pyogenic, intracranial or intraspinal G09
  infectious disease B94.9
    specified NEC B94.8
  injury -- code to injury with seventh character S
  leprosy B92
  meningitis
    bacterial (conditions in G00) G09
    other or unspecified cause (conditions in G03) G09
  muscle (and tendon) injury -- code to injury with seventh character S
  myelitis — *see* Sequelae, encephalitis
  niacin deficiency E64.8
  nutritional deficiency E64.9
    specified NEC E64.8
  obstetrical condition O94
  parasitic disease B94.9
  phlebitis or thrombophlebitis of intracranial or intraspinal venous sinuses and veins (conditions in G08) G09
  poisoning -- code to poisoning with seventh character S
    nonmedicinal substance — *see* Sequelae, toxic effect, nonmedicinal substance
  poliomyelitis (acute) B91
  pregnancy O94
  protein-energy malnutrition E64.0
  puerperium O94
  rickets E64.3
  selenium deficiency E64.8
  sprain and strain -- code to injury with seventh character S
  stroke NOS I69.30
    alteration in sensation I69.398
    aphasia I69.320
    apraxia I69.390
    ataxia I69.393
    cognitive deficits I69.31
    disturbance of vision I69.398
    dysarthria I69.322
    dysphagia I69.391
    dysphasia I69.321
    facial droop I69.392
    facial weakness I69.392
    hemiplegia I69.35-
    language deficit NEC I69.328
    monoplegia
      lower limb I69.34-
      upper limb I69.33-

Sequelae (of) - *continued*
  stroke NOS - *continued*
    paralytic syndrome I69.36-
    specified effect NEC I69.398
    speech deficit NEC I69.328
  tendon and muscle injury -- code to injury with seventh character S
  thiamine deficiency E64.8
  trachoma B94.0
  tuberculosis B90.9
    bones and joints B90.2
    central nervous system B90.0
    genitourinary B90.1
    pulmonary (respiratory) B90.9
    specified organs NEC B90.8
  viral
    encephalitis B94.1
    hepatitis B94.2
  vitamin deficiency NEC E64.8
    A E64.1
    B E64.8
    C E64.2
  wound, open -- code to injury with seventh character S
Sequestration — *see also* Sequestrum
  disk — *see* Displacement, intervertebral disk
  lung, congenital Q33.2
Sequestrum
  bone — *see* Osteomyelitis, chronic
  dental M27.2
  jaw bone M27.2
  orbit — *see* Osteomyelitis, orbit
  sinus (accessory) (nasal) — *see* Sinusitis
Sequoiosis lung or pneumonitis J67.8
Serology for syphilis
  doubtful
    with signs or symptoms - code by site and stage under Syphilis
    follow-up of latent syphilis — *see* Syphilis, latent
  negative, with signs or symptoms - code by site and stage under Syphilis
  positive A53.0
    with signs or symptoms - code by site and stage under Syphilis
  reactivated A53.0
Seroma — *see also* Hematoma
  postprocedural — *see* Complication, postprocedural, seroma
  traumatic, secondary and recurrent T79.2
Seropurulent — *see* condition
Serositis, multiple K65.8
  pericardial I31.1
  peritoneal K65.8
Serous — *see* condition
Sertoli cell
  adenoma
    specified site — *see* Neoplasm, benign, by site
    unspecified site
      female D27.9
      male D29.20
  carcinoma
    specified site — *see* Neoplasm, malignant, by site
    unspecified site (male) C62.9-
      female C56.9
  tumor
    with lipid storage
      specified site — *see* Neoplasm, benign, by site
      unspecified site
        female D27.9
        male D29.20
    specified site — *see* Neoplasm, benign, by site
    unspecified site
      female D27.9
      male D29.20
Sertoli-Leydig cell tumor — *see* Neoplasm, benign, by site
  specified site — *see* Neoplasm, benign, by site
  unspecified site
    female D27.9
    male D29.20
Serum
  allergy, allergic reaction — *see also* Reaction, serum T80.69
    shock — *see also* Shock, anaphylactic T80.59
  arthritis — *see also* Reaction, serum T80.69
  complication or reaction NEC — *see also* Reaction, serum T80.69
  disease NEC — *see also* Reaction, serum T80.69
  hepatitis — *see also* Hepatitis, viral, type B
    carrier (suspected) of B18.1
  intoxication — *see also* Reaction, serum T80.69
  neuritis — *see also* Reaction, serum T80.69
  neuropathy G61.1

Serum - *continued*
  poisoning NEC — *see also* Reaction, serum T80.69
  rash NEC — *see also* Reaction, serum T80.69
  reaction NEC — *see also* Reaction, serum T80.69
  sickness NEC — *see also* Reaction, serum T80.69
  urticaria — *see also* Reaction, serum T80.69
Sesamoiditis M25.8-
Severe sepsis R65.20
  with septic shock R65.21
Sever's disease or osteochondrosis — *see* Osteochondrosis, juvenile, tarsus
Sex
  chromosome mosaics Q97.8
    lines with various numbers of X chromosomes Q97.2
  education Z70.8
  reassignment surgery status Z87.890
Sextuplet pregnancy — *see* Pregnancy, sextuplet
Sexual
  function, disorder of (psychogenic) F52.9
  immaturity (female) (male) E30.0
  impotence (psychogenic) organic origin NEC — *see* Dysfunction, sexual, male
  precocity (constitutional) (cryptogenic) (female) (idiopathic) (male) E30.1
Sexuality, pathologic — *see* Deviation, sexual
Sézary disease C84.1-
Shadow, lung R91.8
Shaking palsy or paralysis — *see* Parkinsonism
Shallowness, acetabulum — *see* Derangement, joint, specified type NEC, hip
Shaver's disease J63.1
Sheath (tendon) — *see* condition
Sheathing, retinal vessels H35.01-
Shedding
  nail L60.8
  premature, primary (deciduous) teeth K00.6
Sheehan's disease or syndrome E23.0
Shelf, rectal K62.89
Shell teeth K00.5
Shellshock (current) F43.0
  lasting state — *see* Disorder, post-traumatic stress
Shield kidney Q63.1
Shift
  auditory threshold (temporary) H93.24-
  mediastinal R93.8
Shifting sleep-work schedule (affecting sleep) G47.26
Shiga (-Kruse) **dysentery** A03.0
Shiga's bacillus A03.0
Shigella (dysentery) — *see* Dysentery, bacillary
Shigellosis A03.9
  Group A A03.0
  Group B A03.1
  Group C A03.2
  Group D A03.3
Shin splints S86.89
Shingles — *see* Herpes, zoster
Shipyard disease or eye B30.0
Shirodkar suture, in pregnancy — *see* Pregnancy, complicated by, incompetent cervix
Shock R57.9
  with ectopic or molar pregnancy O08.3
  adrenal (cortical) (Addisonian) E27.2
  adverse food reaction (anaphylactic) — *see* Shock, anaphylactic, due to food
  allergic — *see* Shock, anaphylactic
  anaphylactic T78.2
    chemical — *see* Table of Drugs and Chemicals
    due to drug or medicinal substance
      correct substance properly administered T88.6
      overdose or wrong substance given or taken (by accident) — *see* Table of Drugs and Chemicals, by drug, poisoning
    due to food (nonpoisonous) T78.00
      additives T78.06
      dairy products T78.07
      eggs T78.08
      fish T78.03
        shellfish T78.02
      fruit T78.04
      milk T78.07
      nuts T78.05
        multiple types T78.05
        peanuts T78.01
      peanuts T78.01
      seeds T78.05
      specified type NEC T78.09
      vegetable T78.04
    following sting (s) — *see* Venom
    immunization T80.52
    serum T80.59
      blood and blood products T80.51

Shock - *continued*
  anaphylactic - *continued*
    serum - *continued*
      immunization T80.52
      specified NEC T80.59
      vaccination T80.52
  anaphylactoid — *see* Shock, anaphylactic
  anesthetic
    correct substance properly administered T88.2
    overdose or wrong substance given or taken — *see* Table of Drugs and Chemicals, by drug, poisoning
    specified anesthetic — *see* Table of Drugs and Chemicals, by drug, poisoning
  cardiogenic R57.0
  chemical substance — *see* Table of Drugs and Chemicals
  complicating ectopic or molar pregnancy O08.3
  culture — *see* Disorder, adjustment
  drug
    due to correct substance properly administered T88.6
    overdose or wrong substance given or taken (by accident) — *see* Table of Drugs and Chemicals, by drug, poisoning
  during or after labor and delivery O75.1
  electric T75.4
    (taser) T75.4
  endotoxic R65.21
    postprocedural (resulting from a procedure, not elsewhere classified) T81.12
  following
    ectopic or molar pregnancy O08.3
    injury (immediate) (delayed) T79.4
    labor and delivery O75.1
  food (anaphylactic) — *see* Shock, anaphylactic, due to food
  from electroshock gun (taser) T75.4
  gram-negative R65.21
    postprocedural (resulting from a procedure, not elsewhere classified) T81.12
  hematologic R57.8
  hemorrhagic
    surgery (intraoperative) (postoperative) T81.19
    trauma T79.4
  hypovolemic R57.1
    surgical T81.19
    traumatic T79.4
  insulin E15
    therapeutic misadventure — *see* subcategory T38.3
  kidney N17.0
    traumatic (following crushing) T79.5
  liver K72.00
  lightning T75.01
  lung J80
  obstetric O75.1
    with ectopic or molar pregnancy O08.3
    following ectopic or molar pregnancy O08.3
  pleural (surgical) T81.19
    due to trauma T79.4
  postprocedural (postoperative) T81.10
    with ectopic or molar pregnancy O08.3
    cardiogenic T81.11
    endotoxic T81.12
    following ectopic or molar pregnancy O08.3
    gram-negative T81.12
    hypovolemic T81.19
    septic T81.12
    specified type NEC T81.19
  psychic F43.0
  septic (due to severe sepsis) R65.21
  specified NEC R57.8
  surgical T81.10
  taser gun (taser) T75.4
  therapeutic misadventure NEC T81.10
  thyroxin
    overdose or wrong substance given or taken — *see* Table of Drugs and Chemicals, by drug, poisoning
  toxic, syndrome A48.3
  transfusion — *see* Complications, transfusion
  traumatic (immediate) (delayed) T79.4
Shoemaker's chest M95.4
Short, shortening, shortness
  arm (acquired) — *see also* Deformity, limb, unequal length
    congenital Q71.81-
    forearm — *see* Deformity, limb, unequal length
  bowel syndrome K91.2
  breath R06.02
  cervical (complicating pregnancy) O26.87-
    non-gravid uterus N88.3
  common bile duct, congenital Q44.5

Short, shortening, shortness - *continued*
cord (umbilical) , complicating delivery O69.3
cystic duct, congenital Q44.5
esophagus (congenital) Q39.8
femur (acquired) — *see* Deformity, limb, unequal length, femur
congenital — *see* Defect, reduction, lower limb, longitudinal, femur
frenum, frenulum, linguae (congenital) Q38.1
hip (acquired) — *see also* Deformity, limb, unequal length
congenital Q65.89
leg (acquired) — *see also* Deformity, limb, unequal length
congenital Q72.81-
lower leg — *see also* Deformity, limb, unequal length
limbed stature, with immunodeficiency D82.2
lower limb (acquired) — *see also* Deformity, limb, unequal length
congenital Q72.81-
organ or site, congenital NEC — *see* Distortion
palate, congenital Q38.5
radius (acquired) — *see also* Deformity, limb, unequal length
congenital — *see* Defect, reduction, upper limb, longitudinal, radius
rib syndrome Q77.2
stature (child) (hereditary) (idiopathic) NEC R62.52
constitutional E34.3
due to endocrine disorder E34.3
Laron-type E34.3
tendon — *see also* Contraction, tendon
with contracture of joint — *see* Contraction, joint
Achilles (acquired) M67.0-
congenital Q66.89
congenital Q79.8
thigh (acquired) — *see also* Deformity, limb, unequal length, femur
congenital — *see* Defect, reduction, lower limb, longitudinal, femur
tibialis anterior (tendon) — *see* Contraction, tendon
umbilical cord
complicating delivery O69.3
upper limb, congenital — *see* Defect, reduction, upper limb, specified type NEC
urethra N36.8
uvula, congenital Q38.5
vagina (congenital) Q52.4
Shortsightedness — *see* Myopia
Shoshin (acute fulminating beriberi) E51.11
Shoulder — *see* condition
Shovel-shaped incisors K00.2
Shower, thromboembolic — *see* Embolism
Shunt
arterial-venous (dialysis) Z99.2
arteriovenous, pulmonary (acquired) I28.0
congenital Q25.72
cerebral ventricle (communicating) in situ Z98.2
surgical, prosthetic, with complications — *see* Complications, cardiovascular, device or implant
Shutdown, renal N28.9
Shy-Drager syndrome G90.3
Sialadenitis, sialadenosis (any gland) (chronic) (periodic) (suppurative) — *see* Sialoadenitis
Sialectasia K11.8
Sialidosis E77.1
Sialitis, silitis (any gland) (chronic) (suppurative) — *see* Sialoadenitis
Sialoadenitis (any gland) (periodic) (suppurative) K11.20
acute K11.21
recurrent K11.22
chronic K11.23
Sialoadenopathy K11.9
Sialoangitis — *see* Sialoadenitis
Sialodochitis (fibrinosa) — *see* Sialoadenitis
Sialodocholithiasis K11.5
Sialolithiasis K11.5
Sialometaplasia, necrotizing K11.8
Sialorrhea — *see also* Ptyalism
periodic — *see* Sialoadenitis
Sialosis K11.7
Siamese twin Q89.4
Sibling rivalry Z62.891
Sicard's syndrome G52.7
Sicca syndrome M35.00
with
keratoconjunctivitis M35.01
lung involvement M35.02
myopathy M35.03
renal tubulo-interstitial disorders M35.04
specified organ involvement NEC M35.09

Sick R69
or handicapped person in family Z63.79
needing care at home Z63.6
sinus (syndrome) I49.5
Sick-euthyroid syndrome E07.81
Sickle-cell
anemia — *see* Disease, sickle-cell
trait D57.3
Sicklemia — *see also* Disease, sickle-cell
trait D57.3
Sickness
air (travel) T75.3
airplane T75.3
alpine T70.29
altitude T70.20
Andes T70.29
aviator's T70.29
balloon T70.29
car T75.3
compressed air T70.3
decompression T70.3
green D50.8
milk — *see* Poisoning, food, noxious
motion T75.3
mountain T70.29
acute D75.1
protein — *see also* Reaction, serum T80.69
radiation T66
roundabout (motion) T75.3
sea T75.3
serum NEC — *see also* Reaction, serum T80.69
sleeping (African) B56.9
by Trypanosoma B56.9
brucei
gambiense B56.0
rhodesiense B56.1
East African B56.1
Gambian B56.0
Rhodesian B56.1
West African B56.0
swing (motion) T75.3
train (railway) (travel) T75.3
travel (any vehicle) T75.3
Sideropenia — *see* Anemia, iron deficiency
Siderosilicosis J62.8
Siderosis (lung) J63.4
eye (globe) — *see* Disorder, globe, degenerative, siderosis
Siemens' syndrome (ectodermal dysplasia) Q82.8
Sighing R06.89
psychogenic F45.8
Sigmoid — *see also* condition
flexure — *see* condition
kidney Q63.1
Sigmoiditis — *see also* Enteritis K52.9
infectious A09
noninfectious K52.9
Silfversköld's syndrome Q78.9
Silicosiderosis J62.8
Silicosis, silicotic (simple) (complicated) J62.8
with tuberculosis J65
Silicotuberculosis J65
Silo-fillers' disease J68.8
bronchitis J68.0
pneumonitis J68.0
pulmonary edema J68.1
Silver's syndrome Q87.1
Simian malaria B53.1
Simmonds' cachexia or disease E23.0
Simons' disease or syndrome (progressive lipodystrophy) E88.1
Simple, simplex — *see* condition
Simulation, conscious (of illness) Z76.5
Simultanagnosia (asimultagnosia) R48.3
Sin Nombre virus disease (Hantavirus) (cardio-pulmonary syndrome) B33.4
Sinding-Larsen disease or osteochondrosis — *see* Osteochondrosis, juvenile, patella
Singapore hemorrhagic fever A91
Singer's node or nodule J38.2
Single
atrium Q21.2
coronary artery Q24.5
umbilical artery Q27.0
ventricle Q20.4
Singultus R06.6
epidemicus B33.0
Sinus — *see also* Fistula
abdominal K63.89
arrest I45.5
arrhythmia I49.8
bradycardia R00.1
branchial cleft (internal) (external) Q18.0

Sinus - *continued*
coccygeal — *see* Sinus, pilonidal
dental K04.6
dermal (congenital) Q06.8
with abscess Q06.8
coccygeal, pilonidal — *see* Sinus, coccygeal
infected, skin NEC L08.89
marginal, ruptured or bleeding — *see* Hemorrhage, antepartum, specified cause NEC
medial, face and neck Q18.8
pause I45.5
pericranii Q01.9
pilonidal (infected) (rectum) L05.92
with abscess L05.02
preauricular Q18.1
rectovaginal N82.3
Rokitansky-Aschoff (gallbladder) K82.8
sacrococcygeal (dermoid) (infected) — *see* Sinus, pilonidal
tachycardia R00.0
paroxysmal I47.1
tarsi syndrome M25.57-
testis N50.89
tract (postinfective) — *see* Fistula
urachus Q64.4
Sinusitis (accessory) (chronic) (hyperplastic) (nasal) (nonpurulent) (purulent) J32.9
acute J01.90
ethmoidal J01.20
recurrent J01.21
frontal J01.10
recurrent J01.11
involving more than one sinus, other than pansinusitis J01.80
recurrent J01.81
maxillary J01.00
recurrent J01.01
pansinusitis J01.40
recurrent J01.41
recurrent J01.91
specified NEC J01.80
recurrent J01.81
sphenoidal J01.30
recurrent J01.31
allergic — *see* Rhinitis, allergic
due to high altitude T70.1
ethmoidal J32.2
acute J01.20
recurrent J01.21
frontal J32.1
acute J01.10
recurrent J01.11
influenzal — *see* Influenza, with, respiratory manifestations NEC
involving more than one sinus but not pansinusitis J32.8
acute J01.80
recurrent J01.81
maxillary J32.0
acute J01.00
recurrent J01.01
sphenoidal J32.3
acute J01.30
recurrent J01.31
tuberculous, any sinus A15.8
Sinusitis-bronchiectasis-situs inversus (syndrome) (triad) Q89.3
Sipple's syndrome E31.22
Sirenomelia (syndrome) Q87.2
Siriasis T67.0
Sirkari's disease B55.0
Siti A65
Situation, psychiatric F99
Situational
disturbance (transient) — *see* Disorder, adjustment
acute F43.0
maladjustment — *see* Disorder, adjustment
reaction — *see* Disorder, adjustment
acute F43.0
Situs inversus or transversus (abdominalis) (thoracis) Q89.3
Sixth disease B08.20
due to human herpesvirus 6 B08.21
due to human herpesvirus 7 B08.22
Sjögren-Larsson syndrome Q87.1
Sjögren's syndrome or disease — *see* Sicca syndrome
Skeletal — *see* condition
Skene's gland — *see* condition
Skenitis — *see* Urethritis
Skerljevo A65
Skevas-Zerfus disease — *see* Toxicity, venom, marine animal, sea anemone

Skin — *see also* condition
clammy R23.1
donor — *see* Donor, skin
hidebound M35.9
Slate-dressers' or slate-miners' lung J62.8
Sleep
apnea — *see* Apnea, sleep
deprivation Z72.820
disorder or disturbance G47.9
child F51.9
nonorganic origin F51.9
specified NEC G47.8
disturbance G47.9
nonorganic origin F51.9
drunkenness F51.9
rhythm inversion G47.2-
terrors F51.4
walking F51.3
hysterical F44.89
Sleep hygiene
abuse Z72.821
inadequate Z72.821
poor Z72.821
Sleeping sickness — *see* Sickness, sleeping
Sleeplessness — *see* Insomnia
menopausal N95.1
Sleep-wake schedule disorder G47.20
Slim disease (in HIV infection) B20
Slipped, slipping
epiphysis (traumatic) — *see*
also Osteochondropathy, specified type NEC
capital femoral (traumatic)
acute (on chronic) S79.01-
current traumatic - code as Fracture, by site
upper femoral (nontraumatic) M93.00-
acute M93.01-
on chronic M93.03-
chronic M93.02-
intervertebral disc — *see* Displacement,
intervertebral disc
ligature, umbilical P51.8
patella — *see* Disorder, patella, derangement NEC
rib M89.8X8
sacroiliac joint — *see* subcategory M53.2
tendon — *see* Disorder, tendon
ulnar nerve, nontraumatic — *see* Lesion, nerve,
ulnar
vertebra NEC — *see* Spondylolisthesis
Slocumb's syndrome E27.0
Sloughing (multiple) (phagedena) (skin) — *see*
also Gangrene
abscess — *see* Abscess
appendix K38.8
fascia — *see* Disorder, soft tissue, specified type
NEC
scrotum N50.89
tendon — *see* Disorder, tendon
transplanted organ — *see* Rejection, transplant
ulcer — *see* Ulcer, skin
Slow
feeding, newborn P92.2
flow syndrome, coronary I20.8
heart (beat) R00.1
Slowing, urinary stream R39.198
Sluder's neuralgia (syndrome) G44.89
Slurred, slurring speech R47.81
Small (ness)
for gestational age — *see* Small for dates
introitus, vagina N89.6
kidney (unknown cause) N27.9
bilateral N27.1
unilateral N27.0
ovary (congenital) Q50.39
pelvis
with disproportion (fetopelvic) O33.1
causing obstructed labor O65.1
uterus N85.8
white kidney N03.9
Small-and-light-for-dates — *see* Small for dates
Small-for-dates (infant) P05.10
with weight of
499 grams or less P05.11
500-749 grams P05.12
750-999 grams P05.13
1000-1249 grams P05.14
1250-1499 grams P05.15
1500-1749 grams P05.16
1750-1999 grams P05.17
2000-2499 grams P05.18
2500 grams and over P05.19
specified NEC P05.19
Smallpox B03
Smearing, fecal R15.1

Smith-Lemli-Opitz syndrome E78.72
Smith's fracture S52.54-
Smoker — *see* Dependence, drug, nicotine
Smoker's
bronchitis J41.0
cough J41.0
palate K13.24
throat J31.2
tongue K13.24
Smoking
passive Z77.22
Smothering spells R06.81
Snaggle teeth, tooth M26.39
Snapping
finger — *see* Trigger finger
hip — *see* Derangement, joint, specified type NEC,
hip
involving the iliotibial band M76.3-
knee — *see* Derangement, knee
involving the iliotibial band M76.3-
Sneddon-Wilkinson disease or syndrome
(sub-corneal pustular dermatosis) L13.1
Sneezing (intractable) R06.7
Sniffing
cocaine
abuse — *see* Abuse, drug, cocaine
dependence — *see* Dependence, drug, cocaine
gasoline
abuse — *see* Abuse, drug, inhalant
dependence — *see* Dependence, drug, inhalant
glue (airplane)
abuse — *see* Abuse, drug, inhalant
drug dependence — *see* Dependence, drug,
inhalant
Sniffles R06.5
newborn P28.89
Snoring R06.83
Snow blindness — *see* Photokeratitis
Snuffles (non-syphilitic) R06.5
newborn P28.89
syphilitic (infant) A50.05 *[J99]*
Social
exclusion Z60.4
due to discrimination or persecution
(perceived) Z60.5
migrant Z59.0
acculturation difficulty Z60.3
rejection Z60.4
due to discrimination or persecution Z60.5
role conflict NEC Z73.5
skills inadequacy NEC Z73.4
transplantation Z60.3
Sodoku A25.0
Soemmerring's ring — *see* Cataract, secondary
Soft — *see also* condition
nails L60.3
Softening
bone — *see* Osteomalacia
brain (necrotic) (progressive) G93.89
congenital Q04.8
embolic I63.4-
hemorrhagic — *see* Hemorrhage, intracranial,
intracerebral
occlusive I63.5-
thrombotic I63.3-
cartilage M94.2-
patella M22.4-
cerebellar — *see* Softening, brain
cerebral — *see* Softening, brain
cerebrospinal — *see* Softening, brain
myocardial, heart — *see* Degeneration, myocardial
spinal cord G95.89
stomach K31.89
Soldier's
heart F45.8
patches I31.0
Solitary
cyst, kidney N28.1
kidney, congenital Q60.0
Solvent abuse — *see* Abuse, drug, inhalant
dependence — *see* Dependence, drug, inhalant
Somatization reaction, somatic reaction — *see*
Disorder, somatoform
Somnambulism F51.3
hysterical F44.89
Somnolence R40.0
nonorganic origin F51.11
Sonne dysentery A03.3
Soor B37.0
Sore
bed — *see* Ulcer, pressure, by site
chiclero B55.1
Delhi B55.1

Sore - *continued*
desert — *see* Ulcer, skin
eye H57.1-
Lahore B55.1
mouth K13.79
canker K12.0
muscle M79.1
Naga — *see* Ulcer, skin
of skin — *see* Ulcer, skin
oriental B55.1
pressure — *see* Ulcer, pressure, by site
skin L98.9
soft A57
throat (acute) — *see also* Pharyngitis
with influenza, flu, or grippe — *see* Influenza,
with, respiratory manifestations NEC
chronic J31.2
coxsackie (virus) B08.5
diphtheritic A36.0
herpesviral B00.2
influenzal — *see* Influenza, with, respiratory
manifestations NEC
septic J02.0
streptococcal (ulcerative) J02.0
viral NEC J02.8
coxsackie B08.5
tropical — *see* Ulcer, skin
veldt — *see* Ulcer, skin
Soto's syndrome (cerebral gigantism) Q87.3
South African cardiomyopathy syndrome I42.8
Southeast Asian hemorrhagic fever A91
Spacing
abnormal, tooth, teeth, fully erupted M26.30
excessive, tooth, fully erupted M26.32
Spade-like hand (congenital) Q68.1
Spading nail L60.8
congenital Q84.6
Spanish collar N47.1
Sparganosis B70.1
Spasm (s) , spastic, spasticity — *see*
also condition R25.2
accommodation — *see* Spasm, of accommodation
ampulla of Vater K83.4
anus, ani (sphincter) (reflex) K59.4
psychogenic F45.8
artery I73.9
cerebral G45.9
Bell's G51.3
bladder (sphincter, external or internal) N32.89
psychogenic F45.8
bronchus, bronchiole J98.01
cardia K22.0
cardiac I20.1
carpopedal — *see* Tetany
cerebral (arteries) (vascular) G45.9
cervix, complicating delivery O62.4
ciliary body (of accommodation) — *see* Spasm, of
accommodation
colon — *see also* Irritable, bowel K58.9
with diarrhea K58.0
psychogenic F45.8
common duct K83.8
compulsive — *see* Tic
conjugate H51.8
coronary (artery) I20.1
diaphragm (reflex) R06.6
epidemic B33.0
psychogenic F45.8
duodenum K59.8
epidemic diaphragmatic (transient) B33.0
esophagus (diffuse) K22.4
psychogenic F45.8
facial G51.3
fallopian tube N83.8
gastrointestinal (tract) K31.89
psychogenic F45.8
glottis J38.5
hysterical F44.4
psychogenic F45.8
conversion reaction F44.4
reflex through recurrent laryngeal nerve J38.5
habit — *see* Tic
heart I20.1
hemifacial (clonic) G51.3
hourglass — *see* Contraction, hourglass
hysterical F44.4
infantile — *see* Epilepsy, spasms
inferior oblique, eye H51.8
intestinal — *see also* Syndrome, irritable
bowel K58.9
psychogenic F45.8
larynx, laryngeal J38.5
hysterical F44.4

Spondylolysis (acquired) - *continued*
  occipito-atlanto-axial region M43.01
  sacrococcygeal region M43.08
  thoracic region M43.04
  thoracolumbar region M43.05
Spondylopathy M48.9
  infective NEC M46.50
    cervical region M46.52
    cervicothoracic region M46.53
    lumbar region M46.56
    lumbosacral region M46.57
    multiple sites M46.59
    occipito-atlanto-axial region M46.51
    sacrococcygeal region M46.58
    thoracic region M46.54
    thoracolumbar region M46.55
  inflammatory M46.90
    cervical region M46.92
    cervicothoracic region M46.93
    lumbar region M46.96
    lumbosacral region M46.97
    multiple sites M46.99
    occipito-atlanto-axial region M46.91
    sacrococcygeal region M46.98
    specified type NEC M46.80
      cervical region M46.82
      cervicothoracic region M46.83
      lumbar region M46.86
      lumbosacral region M46.87
      multiple sites M46.89
      occipito-atlanto-axial region M46.81
      sacrococcygeal region M46.88
      thoracic region M46.84
      thoracolumbar region M46.85
    thoracic region M46.94
    thoracolumbar region M46.95
  neuropathic, in
    syringomyelia and syringobulbia G95.0
    tabes dorsalis A52.11
  specified NEC — *see* subcategory M48.8
  traumatic M48.30
    cervical region M48.32
    cervicothoracic region M48.33
    lumbar region M48.36
    lumbosacral region M48.37
    occipito-atlanto-axial region M48.31
    sacrococcygeal region M48.38
    thoracic region M48.34
    thoracolumbar region M48.35
Spondylosis M47.9
  with
    disproportion (fetopelvic) O33.0
      causing obstructed labor O65.0
    myelopathy NEC M47.10
      cervical region M47.12
      cervicothoracic region M47.13
      lumbar region M47.16
      occipito-atlanto-axial region M47.11
      thoracic region M47.14
      thoracolumbar region M47.15
    radiculopathy M47.20
      cervical region M47.22
      cervicothoracic region M47.23
      lumbar region M47.26
      lumbosacral region M47.27
      occipito-atlanto-axial region M47.21
      sacrococcygeal region M47.28
      thoracic region M47.24
      thoracolumbar region M47.25
  specified NEC M47.899
    cervical region M47.892
    cervicothoracic region M47.893
    lumbar region M47.896
    lumbosacral region M47.897
    occipito-atlanto-axial region M47.891
    sacrococcygeal region M47.898
    thoracic region M47.894
    thoracolumbar region M47.895
  traumatic — *see* Spondylopathy, traumatic
  without myelopathy or radiculopathy M47.819
    cervical region M47.812
    cervicothoracic region M47.813
    lumbar region M47.816
    lumbosacral region M47.817
    occipito-atlanto-axial region M47.811
    sacrococcygeal region M47.818
    thoracic region M47.814
    thoracolumbar region M47.815
Sponge
  inadvertently left in operation wound — *see* Foreign body, accidentally left during a procedure
  kidney (medullary) Q61.5

Sponge-diver's disease — *see* Toxicity, venom, marine animal, sea anemone
Spongioblastoma (any type) — *see* Neoplasm, malignant, by site
  specified site — *see* Neoplasm, malignant, by site
  unspecified site C71.9
Spongioneuroblastoma — *see* Neoplasm, malignant, by site
Spontaneous — *see also* condition
  fracture (cause unknown) — *see* Fracture, pathological
Spoon nail L60.3
  congenital Q84.6
Sporadic — *see* condition
Sporothrix schenckii infection — *see* Sporotrichosis
Sporotrichosis B42.9
  arthritis B42.82
  disseminated B42.7
  generalized B42.7
  lymphocutaneous (fixed) (progressive) B42.1
  pulmonary B42.0
  specified NEC B42.89
Spots, spotting (in) (of)
  Bitot's — *see also* Pigmentation, conjunctiva
    in the young child E50.1
      vitamin A deficiency E50.1
  café, au lait L81.3
  Cayenne pepper I78.1
  cotton wool, retina — *see* Occlusion, artery, retina
  de Morgan's (senile angiomas) I78.1
  Fuchs' black (myopic) H44.2-
  intermenstrual (regular) N92.0
    irregular N92.1
  Koplik's B05.9
  liver L81.4
  pregnancy O26.85-
  purpuric R23.3
  ruby I78.1
Spotted fever — *see* Fever, spotted N92.3
Sprain (joint) (ligament)
  acromioclavicular joint or ligament S43.5-
  ankle S93.40-
    calcaneofibular ligament S93.41-
    deltoid ligament S93.42-
    internal collateral ligament — *see* Sprain, ankle, specified ligament NEC
    specified ligament NEC S93.49-
    talofibular ligament — *see* Sprain, ankle, specified ligament NEC
    tibiofibular ligament S93.43-
  anterior longitudinal, cervical S13.4
  atlas, atlanto-axial, atlanto-occipital S13.4
  breast bone — *see* Sprain, sternum
  calcaneofibular — *see* Sprain, ankle
  carpal — *see* Sprain, wrist
  carpometacarpal — *see* Sprain, hand, specified site NEC
  cartilage
    costal S23.41
    semilunar (knee) — *see* Sprain, knee, specified site NEC
      with current tear — *see* Tear, meniscus
    thyroid region S13.5
    xiphoid — *see* Sprain, sternum
  cervical, cervicodorsal, cervicothoracic S13.4
  chondrosternal S23.421
  coracoclavicular S43.8-
  coracohumeral S43.41-
  coronary, knee — *see* Sprain, knee, specified site NEC
  costal cartilage S23.41
  cricoarytenoid articulation or ligament S13.5
  cricothyroid articulation S13.5
  cruciate, knee — *see* Sprain, knee, cruciate
  deltoid, ankle — *see* Sprain, ankle
  dorsal (spine) S23.3
  elbow S53.40-
    radial collateral ligament S53.43-
    radiohumeral S53.41-
    rupture
      radial collateral ligament — *see* Rupture, traumatic, ligament, radial collateral
      ulnar collateral ligament — *see* Rupture, traumatic, ligament, ulnar collateral
    specified type NEC S53.49-
    ulnar collateral ligament S53.44-
    ulnohumeral S53.42-
  femur, head — *see* Sprain, hip
  fibular collateral, knee — *see* Sprain, knee, collateral
  fibulocalcaneal — *see* Sprain, ankle
  finger (s) S63.61-
    index S63.61-
    interphalangeal (joint) S63.63-

Sprain (joint) (ligament) - *continued*
  finger (s) - *continued*
    interphalangeal (joint) - *continued*
      index S63.63-
      little S63.63-
      middle S63.63-
      ring S63.63-
    little S63.61-
    middle S63.61-
    ring S63.61-
    metacarpophalangeal (joint) S63.65-
    specified site NEC S63.69-
      index S63.69-
      little S63.69-
      middle S63.69-
      ring S63.69-
  foot S93.60-
    specified ligament NEC S93.69-
    tarsal ligament S93.61-
    tarsometatarsal ligament S93.62-
    toe — *see* Sprain, toe
  hand S63.9-
    finger — *see* Sprain, finger
    specified site NEC — *see* subcategory S63.8
    thumb — *see* Sprain, thumb
  head S03.9
  hip S73.10-
    iliofemoral ligament S73.11-
    ischiocapsular (ligament) S73.12-
    specified NEC S73.19-
  iliofemoral — *see* Sprain, hip
  innominate
    acetabulum — *see* Sprain, hip
    sacral junction S33.6
  internal
    collateral, ankle — *see* Sprain, ankle
    semilunar cartilage — *see* Sprain, knee, specified site NEC
  interphalangeal
    finger — *see* Sprain, finger, interphalangeal (joint)
    toe — *see* Sprain, toe, interphalangeal joint
  ischiocapsular — *see* Sprain, hip
  ischiofemoral — *see* Sprain, hip
  jaw (articular disc) (cartilage) (meniscus) S03.4-
    old M26.69
  knee S83.9-
    collateral ligament S83.40-
      lateral (fibular) S83.42-
      medial (tibial) S83.41-
    cruciate ligament S83.50-
      anterior S83.51-
      posterior S83.52-
    lateral (fibular) collateral ligament S83.42-
    medial (tibial) collateral ligament S83.41-
    patellar ligament S76.11-
    specified site NEC S83.8X-
    superior tibiofibular joint (ligament) S83.6-
  lateral collateral, knee — *see* Sprain, knee, collateral
  lumbar (spine) S33.5
  lumbosacral S33.9
  mandible (articular disc) S03.4-
    old M26.69
  medial collateral, knee — *see* Sprain, knee, collateral
  meniscus
    jaw S03.4-
      old M26.69
    knee — *see* Sprain, knee, specified site NEC
      with current tear — *see* Tear, meniscus
      old — *see* Derangement, knee, meniscus, due to old tear
    mandible S03.4-
      old M26.69
  metacarpal (distal) (proximal) — *see* Sprain, hand, specified site NEC
  metacarpophalangeal — *see* Sprain, finger, metacarpophalangeal (joint)
  metatarsophalangeal — *see* Sprain, toe, metatarsophalangeal joint
  midcarpal — *see* Sprain, hand, specified site NEC
  midtarsal — *see* Sprain, foot, specified site NEC
  neck S13.9
    anterior longitudinal cervical ligament S13.4
    atlanto-axial joint S13.4
    atlanto-occipital joint S13.4
    cervical spine S13.4
    cricoarytenoid ligament S13.5
    cricothyroid ligament S13.5
    specified site NEC S13.8
    thyroid region (cartilage) S13.5
  nose S03.8
  orbicular, hip — *see* Sprain, hip
  patella — *see* Sprain, knee, specified site NEC

Sprain (joint) (ligament) - *continued*
　patellar ligament S76.11-
　pelvis NEC S33.8
　phalanx
　　finger — *see* Sprain, finger
　　toe — *see* Sprain, toe
　pubofemoral — *see* Sprain, hip
　radiocarpal — *see* Sprain, wrist
　radiohumeral — *see* Sprain, elbow
　radius, collateral — *see* Rupture, traumatic,
　　ligament, radial collateral
　rib (cage) S23.41
　rotator cuff (capsule) S43.42-
　sacroiliac (region)
　　chronic or old — *see* subcategory M53.2
　　joint S33.6
　scaphoid (hand) — *see* Sprain, hand, specified site
　　NEC
　scapula (r) — *see* Sprain, shoulder girdle, specified
　　site NEC
　semilunar cartilage (knee) — *see* Sprain, knee,
　　specified site NEC
　　with current tear — *see* Tear, meniscus
　　old — *see* Derangement, knee, meniscus, due to
　　　old tear
　shoulder joint S43.40-
　　acromioclavicular joint (ligament) — *see* Sprain,
　　　acromioclavicular joint
　　blade — *see* Sprain, shoulder, girdle, specified site
　　　NEC
　　coracoclavicular joint (ligament) — *see* Sprain,
　　　coracoclavicular joint
　　coracohumeral ligament — *see* Sprain,
　　　coracohumeral joint
　　girdle S43.9-
　　　specified site NEC S43.8-
　　rotator cuff — *see* Sprain, rotator cuff
　　specified site NEC S43.49-
　　sternoclavicular joint (ligament) — *see* Sprain,
　　　sternoclavicular joint
　spine
　　cervical S13.4
　　lumbar S33.5
　　thoracic S23.3
　sternoclavicular joint S43.6-
　sternum S23.429
　　chondrosternal joint S23.421
　　specified site NEC S23.428
　　sternoclavicular (joint) (ligament) S23.420
　symphysis
　　jaw S03.4-
　　　old M26.69
　　mandibular S03.4-
　　　old M26.69
　talofibular — *see* Sprain, ankle
　tarsal — *see* Sprain, foot, specified site NEC
　tarsometatarsal — *see* Sprain, foot, specified site
　　NEC
　temporomandibular S03.4-
　　old M26.69
　thorax S23.9
　　ribs S23.41
　　specified site NEC S23.8
　　spine S23.3
　　sternum — *see* Sprain, sternum
　thumb S63.60-
　　interphalangeal (joint) S63.62-
　　metacarpophalangeal (joint) S63.64-
　　specified site NEC S63.68-
　thyroid cartilage or region S13.5
　tibia (proximal end) — *see* Sprain, knee, specified
　　site NEC
　tibial collateral, knee — *see* Sprain, knee, collateral
　tibiofibular
　　distal — *see* Sprain, ankle
　　superior — *see* Sprain, knee, specified site NEC
　toe (s) S93.50-
　　great S93.50-
　　interphalangeal joint S93.51-
　　　great S93.51-
　　　lesser S93.51-
　　lesser S93.50-
　　metatarsophalangeal joint S93.52-
　　　great S93.52-
　　　lesser S93.52-
　ulna, collateral — *see* Rupture, traumatic, ligament,
　　ulnar collateral
　ulnohumeral — *see* Sprain, elbow
　wrist S63.50-
　　carpal S63.51-
　　radiocarpal S63.52-
　　specified site NEC S63.59-
　xiphoid cartilage — *see* Sprain, sternum

Sprengel's deformity (congenital) Q74.0
Sprue (tropical) K90.1
　celiac K90.0
　idiopathic K90.49
　meaning thrush B37.0
　nontropical K90.0
Spur, bone — *see also* Enthesopathy
　calcaneal M77.3-
　iliac crest M76.2-
　nose (septum) J34.89
Spurway's syndrome Q78.0
Sputum
　abnormal (amount) (color) (odor) (purulent) R09.3
　blood-stained R04.2
　excessive (cause unknown) R09.3
Squamous — *see also* condition
　epithelium in
　　cervical canal (congenital) Q51.828
　　uterine mucosa (congenital) Q51.818
Squashed nose M95.0
　congenital Q67.4
Squeeze, diver's T70.3
Squint — *see also* Strabismus
　accommodative — *see* Strabismus, convergent
　　concomitant
St. Hubert's disease A82.9
Stab — *see also* Laceration
　internal organs — *see* Injury, by site
Stafne's cyst or cavity M27.0
Staggering gait R26.0
　hysterical F44.4
Staghorn calculus — *see* Calculus, kidney
Stähli's line (cornea) (pigment) — *see* Pigmentation,
　cornea, anterior
Stain, staining
　meconium (newborn) P96.83
　port wine Q82.5
　tooth, teeth (hard tissues) (extrinsic) K03.6
　　due to
　　　accretions K03.6
　　　deposits (betel) (black) (green) (materia alba)
　　　　(orange) (soft) (tobacco) K03.6
　　　metals (copper) (silver) K03.7
　　　nicotine K03.6
　　　pulpal bleeding K03.7
　　　tobacco K03.6
　　intrinsic K00.8
Stammering — *see also* Disorder, fluency F80.81
Standstill
　auricular I45.5
　cardiac — *see* Arrest, cardiac
　sinoatrial I45.5
　ventricular — *see* Arrest, cardiac
Stannosis J63.5
Stanton's disease — *see* Melioidosis
Staphylitis (acute) (catarrhal) (chronic) (gangrenous)
　(membranous) (suppurative) (ulcerative) K12.2
Staphylococcal scalded skin syndrome L00
Staphylococcemia A41.2
Staphylococcus, staphylococcal — *see
　also* condition
　as cause of disease classified elsewhere B95.8
　　aureus (methicillin susceptible) (MSSA) B95.61
　　　methicillin resistant (MRSA) B95.62
　specified NEC, as cause of disease classified
　　elsewhere B95.7
Staphyloma (sclera)
　cornea H18.72-
　equatorial H15.81-
　localized (anterior) H15.82-
　posticum H15.83-
　ring H15.85-
Stargardt's disease — *see* Dystrophy, retina
Starvation (inanition) (due to lack of food) T73.0
　edema — *see* Malnutrition, severe
Stasis
　bile (noncalculous) K83.1
　bronchus J98.09
　　with infection — *see* Bronchitis
　cardiac — *see* Failure, heart, congestive
　cecum K59.8
　colon K59.8
　dermatitis I87.2
　　with
　　　varicose ulcer — *see* Varix, leg, with ulcer, with
　　　　inflammation
　　　varicose veins — *see* Varix, leg, with,
　　　　inflammation
　　due to postthrombotic syndrome — *see* Syndrome,
　　　postthrombotic
　duodenal K31.5
　eczema — *see* Varix, leg, with, inflammation

Stasis - *continued*
　edema — *see* Hypertension, venous (chronic),
　　idiopathic
　foot T69.0-
　ileocecal coil K59.8
　ileum K59.8
　intestinal K59.8
　jejunum K59.8
　kidney N19
　liver (cirrhotic) K76.1
　lymphatic I89.8
　pneumonia J18.2
　pulmonary — *see* Edema, lung
　rectal K59.8
　renal N19
　　tubular N17.0
　ulcer — *see* Varix, leg, with, ulcer
　　without varicose veins I87.2
　urine — *see* Retention, urine
　venous I87.8
State (of)
　affective and paranoid, mixed, organic
　　psychotic F06.8
　agitated R45.1
　　acute reaction to stress F43.0
　anxiety (neurotic) F41.1
　apprehension F41.1
　burn-out Z73.0
　climacteric, female Z78.0
　　symptomatic N95.1
　compulsive F42.8
　　mixed with obsessional thoughts F42.2
　confusional (psychogenic) F44.89
　　acute — *see also* Delirium
　　　with
　　　　arteriosclerotic dementia F01.50
　　　　　with behavioral disturbance F01.51
　　　　senility or dementia F05
　　　alcoholic F10.231
　　　epileptic F05
　　　reactive (from emotional stress, psychological
　　　　trauma) F44.89
　　　subacute — *see* Delirium
　　convulsive — *see* Convulsions
　　crisis F43.0
　depressive F32.9
　　neurotic F34.1
　dissociative F44.9
　emotional shock (stress) R45.7
　hypercoagulation — *see* Hypercoagulable
　locked-in G83.5
　menopausal Z78.0
　　symptomatic N95.1
　neurotic F48.9
　　with depersonalization F48.1
　obsessional F42.8
　oneiroid (schizophrenia-like) F23
　organic
　　hallucinatory (nonalcoholic) F06.0
　　paranoid (-hallucinatory) F06.2
　panic F41.0
　paranoid F22
　　climacteric F22
　　involutional F22
　　menopausal F22
　　organic F06.2
　　senile F03
　　simple F22
　persistent vegetative R40.3
　phobic F40.9
　postleukotomy F07.0
　pregnant
　　gestational carrier Z33.3
　　incidental Z33.1
　psychogenic, twilight F44.89
　psychopathic (constitutional) F60.2
　psychotic, organic — *see also* Psychosis, organic
　　mixed paranoid and affective F06.8
　　senile or presenile F03
　　transient NEC F06.8
　　　with
　　　　hallucinations F06.0
　　　　depression F06.31
　residual schizophrenic F20.5
　restlessness R45.1
　stress (emotional) R45.7
　tension (mental) F48.9
　　specified NEC F48.8
　transient organic psychotic NEC F06.8
　　depressive type F06.31
　　hallucinatory type F06.0
　twilight
　　epileptic F05

State (of) - *continued*
twilight - *continued*
psychogenic F44.89
vegetative, persistent R40.3
vital exhaustion Z73.0
withdrawal, — *see* Withdrawal, state
Status (post) — *see also* Presence (of)
absence, epileptic — *see* Epilepsy, by type, with
status epilepticus
administration of tPA (rtPA) in a different facility
within the last 24 hours prior to admission to
current facility Z92.82
adrenalectomy (unilateral) (bilateral) E89.6
anastomosis Z98.0
angioplasty (peripheral) Z98.62
with implant Z95.820
coronary artery Z98.61
with implant Z95.5
anginosus I20.9
aortocoronary bypass Z95.1
arthrodesis Z98.1
artificial opening (of) Z93.9
gastrointestinal tract Z93.4
specified NEC Z93.8
urinary tract Z93.6
vagina Z93.8
asthmaticus — *see* Asthma, by type, with status
asthmaticus
awaiting organ transplant Z76.82
bariatric surgery Z98.84
bed confinement Z74.01
bleb, filtering (vitreous) , after glaucoma
surgery Z98.83
breast implant Z98.82
removal Z98.86
cataract extraction Z98.4-
cholecystectomy Z90.49
clitorectomy N90.811
with excision of labia minora N90.812
colectomy (complete) (partial) Z90.49
colonization — *see* Carrier (suspected) of
colostomy Z93.3
convulsivus idiopathicus — *see* Epilepsy, by type,
with status epilepticus
coronary artery angioplasty — *see* Status,
angioplasty, coronary artery
cystectomy (urinary bladder) Z90.6
cystostomy Z93.50
appendico-vesicostomy Z93.52
cutaneous Z93.51
specified NEC Z93.59
delinquent immunization Z28.3
dental Z98.818
crown Z98.811
fillings Z98.811
restoration Z98.811
sealant Z98.810
specified NEC Z98.818
deployment (current) (military) Z56.82
dialysis (hemodialysis) (peritoneal) Z99.2
do not resuscitate (DNR) Z66
donor — *see* Donor
embedded fragments — *see* Retained, foreign body
fragments (type of)
embedded splinter — *see* Retained, foreign body
fragments (type of)
enterostomy Z93.4
epileptic, epilepticus — *see also* Epilepsy, by type,
with status epilepticus G40.901
estrogen receptor
negative Z17.1
positive Z17.0
female genital cutting — *see* Female genital
mutilation status
female genital mutilation — *see* Female genital
mutilation status
filtering (vitreous) bleb after glaucoma
surgery Z98.83
gastrectomy (complete) (partial) Z90.3
gastric banding Z98.84
gastric bypass for obesity Z98.84
gastrostomy Z93.1
human immunodeficiency virus (HIV) infection,
asymptomatic Z21
hysterectomy (complete) (total) Z90.710
partial (with remaining cervial stump) Z90.711
ileostomy Z93.2
implant
breast Z98.82
infibulation N90.813
intestinal bypass Z98.0
jejunostomy Z93.4
laryngectomy Z90.02

Status (post) - *continued*
lapsed immunization schedule Z28.3
lymphaticus E32.8
malignancy
castrate resistant prostate Z19.2
hormone resistant Z19.2
hormone sensitive Z19.1
marmoratus G80.3
mastectomy (unilateral) (bilateral) Z90.1-
military deployment status (current) Z56.82
in theater or in support of military war,
peacekeeping and humanitarian
operations Z56.82
nephrectomy (unilateral) (bilateral) Z90.5
nephrostomy Z93.6
obesity surgery Z98.84
oophorectomy
bilateral Z90.722
unilateral Z90.721
organ replacement
by artificial or mechanical device or prosthesis of
artery Z95.828
bladder Z96.0
blood vessel Z95.828
breast Z97.8
eye globe Z97.0
heart Z95.812
valve Z95.2
intestine Z97.8
joint Z96.60
hip — *see* Presence, hip joint implant
knee — *see* Presence, knee joint implant
specified site NEC Z96.698
kidney Z97.8
larynx Z96.3
lens Z96.1
limbs — *see* Presence, artificial, limb
liver Z97.8
lung Z97.8
pancreas Z97.8
by organ transplant (heterologous)
(homologous) — *see* Transplant
pacemaker
brain Z96.89
cardiac Z95.0
specified NEC Z96.89
pancreatectomy Z90.410
complete Z90.410
partial Z90.411
total Z90.410
physical restraint Z78.1
pneumonectomy (complete) (partial) Z90.2
pneumothorax, therapeutic Z98.3
postcommotio cerebri F07.81
postoperative (postprocedural) NEC Z98.890
breast implant Z98.82
dental Z98.818
crown Z98.811
fillings Z98.811
restoration Z98.811
sealant Z98.810
specified NEC Z98.818
uterine scar Z98.891
pneumothorax, therapeutic Z98.3
postpartum (routine follow-up) Z39.2
care immediately after delivery Z39.0
postsurgical (postprocedural) NEC Z98.890
pneumothorax, therapeutic Z98.3
pregnancy, incidental Z33.1
prosthesis coronary angioplasty Z95.5
pseudophakia Z96.1
renal dialysis (hemodialysis) (peritoneal) Z99.2
retained foreign body — *see* Retained, foreign body
fragments (type of)
reversed jejunal transposition (for bypass) Z98.0
salpingo-oophorectomy
bilateral Z90.722
unilateral Z90.721
sex reassignment surgery status Z87.890
shunt
arteriovenous (for dialysis) Z99.2
cerebrospinal fluid Z98.2
ventricular (communicating) (for drainage) Z98.2
splenectomy Z90.81
thymicolymphaticus E32.8
thymicus E32.8
thymolymphaticus E32.8
thyroidectomy (hypothyroidism) E89.0
tooth (teeth) extraction — *see also* Absence, teeth,
acquired K08.409
tPA (rtPA) administration in a different facility
within the last 24 hours prior to admission to
current facility Z92.82

Status (post) - *continued*
tracheostomy Z93.0
transplant — *see* Transplant
organ removed Z98.85
tubal ligation Z98.51
underimmunization Z28.3
ureterostomy Z93.6
urethrostomy Z93.6
vagina, artificial Z93.8
vasectomy Z98.52
wheelchair confinement Z99.3
Stealing
child problem F91.8
in company with others Z72.810
pathological (compulsive) F63.2
Steam burn — *see* Burn
Steatocystoma multiplex L72.2
Steatohepatitis (nonalcoholic) (NASH) K75.81
Steatoma L72.3
eyelid (cystic) — *see* Dermatosis, eyelid
infected — *see* Hordeolum
Steatorrhea (chronic) K90.9
with lacteal obstruction K90.2
idiopathic (adult) (infantile) K90.9
pancreatic K90.3
primary K90.0
tropical K90.1
Steatosis E88.89
heart — *see* Degeneration, myocardial
kidney N28.89
liver NEC K76.0
Steele-Richardson-Olszewski disease or
syndrome G23.1
Steinbrocker's syndrome G90.8
Steinert's disease G71.11
Stein-Leventhal syndrome E28.2
Stein's syndrome E28.2
STEMI — *see also* - Infarct, myocardium, ST
elevation I21.3
Stenocardia I20.8
Stenocephaly Q75.8
Stenosis, stenotic (cicatricial) — *see also* Stricture
ampulla of Vater K83.1
anus, anal (canal) (sphincter) K62.4
and rectum K62.4
congenital Q42.3
with fistula Q42.2
aorta (ascending) (supraventricular)
(congenital) Q25.1
arteriosclerotic I70.0
calcified I70.0
supravalvular Q25.3
aortic (valve) I35.0
with insufficiency I35.2
congenital Q23.0
rheumatic I06.0
with
incompetency, insufficiency or
regurgitation I06.2
with mitral (valve) disease I08.0
with tricuspid (valve) disease I08.3
mitral (valve) disease I08.0
with tricuspid (valve) disease I08.3
tricuspid (valve) disease I08.2
with mitral (valve) disease I08.3
specified cause NEC I35.0
syphilitic A52.03
aqueduct of Sylvius (congenital) Q03.0
with spina bifida — *see* Spina bifida, by site, with
hydrocephalus
acquired G91.1
artery NEC — *see also* Arteriosclerosis I77.1
celiac I77.4
cerebral — *see* Occlusion, artery, cerebral
extremities — *see* Arteriosclerosis, extremities
precerebral — *see* Occlusion, artery, precerebral
pulmonary (congenital) Q25.6
acquired I28.8
renal I70.1
stent
coronary T82.855
peripheral T82.856
bile duct (common) (hepatic) K83.1
congenital Q44.3
bladder-neck (acquired) N32.0
congenital Q64.31
brain G93.89
bronchus J98.09
congenital Q32.3
syphilitic A52.72
cardia (stomach) K22.2
congenital Q39.3
cardiovascular — *see* Disease, cardiovascular

Stenosis, stenotic (cicatricial) - continued
 caudal M48.08
 cervix, cervical (canal) N88.2
  congenital Q51.828
  in pregnancy or childbirth — see Pregnancy,
   complicated by, abnormal cervix
 colon — see also Obstruction, intestine
  congenital Q42.9
   specified NEC Q42.8
 colostomy K94.03
 common (bile) duct K83.1
  congenital Q44.3
 coronary (artery) — see Disease, heart, ischemic,
  atherosclerotic
 cystic duct — see Obstruction, gallbladder
 due to presence of device, implant or graft —
  see also Complications, by site and type, specified
  NEC T85.858
  arterial graft NEC T82.858
  breast (implant) T85.858
  catheter T85.858
   dialysis (renal) T82.858
    intraperitoneal T85.858
   infusion NEC T82.858
    spinal (epidural) (subdural) T85.850
   urinary (indwelling) T83.85
  fixation, internal (orthopedic) NEC T84.85
  gastrointestinal (bile duct) (esophagus) T85.858
  genital NEC T83.85
  heart NEC T82.857
  joint prosthesis T84.85
  ocular (corneal graft) (orbital implant)
   NEC T85.858
  orthopedic NEC T84.85
  specified NEC T85.858
  urinary NEC T83.85
  vascular NEC T82.858
  ventricular intracranial shunt T85.850
 duodenum K31.5
  congenital Q41.0
 ejaculatory duct NEC N50.89
 endocervical os — see Stenosis, cervix
 enterostomy K94.13
 esophagus K22.2
  congenital Q39.3
  syphilitic A52.79
   congenital A50.59 [K23]
 eustachian tube — see Obstruction, eustachian tube
 external ear canal (acquired) H61.30-
  congenital Q16.1
  due to
   inflammation H61.32-
   trauma H61.31-
  postprocedural H95.81-
  specified cause NEC H61.39-
 gallbladder — see Obstruction, gallbladder
 glottis J38.6
 heart valve (congenital) Q24.8
  aortic Q23.0
  mitral Q23.2
  pulmonary Q22.1
  tricuspid Q22.4
 hepatic duct K83.1
 hymen N89.6
 hypertrophic subaortic (idiopathic) I42.1
 ileum K56.69
  congenital Q41.2
 infundibulum cardia Q24.3
 intervertebral foramina — see also Lesion,
  biomechanical, specified NEC
  connective tissue M99.79
   abdomen M99.79
   cervical region M99.71
   cervicothoracic M99.71
   head region M99.70
   lumbar region M99.73
   lumbosacral M99.73
   occipitocervical M99.70
   sacral region M99.74
   sacrococcygeal M99.74
   sacroiliac M99.74
   specified NEC M99.79
   thoracic region M99.72
   thoracolumbar M99.72
  disc M99.79
   abdomen M99.79
   cervical region M99.71
   cervicothoracic M99.71
   head region M99.70
   lower extremity M99.76
   lumbar region M99.73
   lumbosacral M99.73
   occipitocervical M99.70

Stenosis, stenotic (cicatricial) - continued
 intervertebral foramina - continued
  disc - continued
   pelvic M99.75
   rib cage M99.78
   sacral region M99.74
   sacrococcygeal M99.74
   sacroiliac M99.74
   specified NEC M99.79
   thoracic region M99.72
   thoracolumbar M99.72
   upper extremity M99.77
  osseous M99.69
   abdomen M99.69
   cervical region M99.61
   cervicothoracic M99.61
   head region M99.60
   lower extremity M99.66
   lumbar region M99.63
   lumbosacral M99.63
   occipitocervical M99.60
   pelvic M99.65
   rib cage M99.68
   sacral region M99.64
   sacrococcygeal M99.64
   sacroiliac M99.64
   specified NEC M99.69
   thoracic region M99.62
   thoracolumbar M99.62
   upper extremity M99.67
  subluxation — see Stenosis, intervertebral
   foramina, osseous
 intestine — see also Obstruction, intestine
  congenital (small) Q41.9
   large Q42.9
    specified NEC Q42.8
   specified NEC Q41.8
  jejunum K56.69
   congenital Q41.1
 lacrimal (passage)
  canaliculi H04.54-
  congenital Q10.5
  duct H04.55-
  punctum H04.56-
  sac H04.57-
 lacrimonasal duct — see Stenosis, lacrimal, duct
  congenital Q10.5
 larynx J38.6
  congenital NEC Q31.8
   subglottic Q31.1
  syphilitic A52.73
   congenital A50.59 [J99]
 mitral (chronic) (inactive) (valve) I05.0
  with
   aortic valve disease I08.0
   incompetency, insufficiency or regurgitation I05.2
  active or acute I01.1
   with rheumatic or Sydenham's chorea I02.0
  congenital Q23.2
  specified cause, except rheumatic I34.2
  syphilitic A52.03
 myocardium, myocardial — see also Degeneration,
  myocardial
  hypertrophic subaortic (idiopathic) I42.1
 nares (anterior) (posterior) J34.89
  congenital Q30.0
 nasal duct — see also Stenosis, lacrimal, duct
  congenital Q10.5
 nasolacrimal duct — see also Stenosis, lacrimal,
  duct
  congenital Q10.5
 neural canal — see also Lesion, biomechanical,
  specified NEC
  connective tissue M99.49
   abdomen M99.49
   cervical region M99.41
   cervicothoracic M99.41
   head region M99.40
   lower extremity M99.46
   lumbar region M99.43
   lumbosacral M99.43
   occipitocervical M99.40
   pelvic M99.45
   rib cage M99.48
   sacral region M99.44
   sacrococcygeal M99.44
   sacroiliac M99.44
   specified NEC M99.49
   thoracic region M99.42
   thoracolumbar M99.42
   upper extremity M99.47
  intervertebral disc M99.59
   abdomen M99.59

Stenosis, stenotic (cicatricial) - continued
 neural canal - continued
  intervertebral disc - continued
   cervical region M99.51
   cervicothoracic M99.51
   head region M99.50
   lower extremity M99.56
   lumbar region M99.53
   lumbosacral M99.53
   occipitocervical M99.50
   pelvic M99.55
   rib cage M99.58
   sacral region M99.54
   sacrococcygeal M99.54
   sacroiliac M99.54
   specified NEC M99.59
   thoracic region M99.52
   thoracolumbar M99.52
   upper extremity M99.57
  osseous M99.39
   abdomen M99.39
   cervical region M99.31
   cervicothoracic M99.31
   head region M99.30
   lower extremity M99.36
   lumbar region M99.33
   lumbosacral M99.33
   pelvic M99.35
   rib cage M99.38
   occipitocervical M99.30
   sacral region M99.34
   sacrococcygeal M99.34
   sacroiliac M99.34
   specified NEC M99.39
   thoracic region M99.32
   thoracolumbar M99.32
   upper extremity M99.37
  subluxation M99.29
   cervical region M99.21
   cervicothoracic M99.21
   head region M99.20
   lower extremity M99.26
   lumbar region M99.23
   lumbosacral M99.23
   occipitocervical M99.20
   pelvic M99.25
   rib cage M99.28
   sacral region M99.24
   sacrococcygeal M99.24
   sacroiliac M99.24
   specified NEC M99.29
   thoracic region M99.22
   thoracolumbar M99.22
   upper extremity M99.27
 organ or site, congenital NEC — see Atresia, by site
 papilla of Vater K83.1
 pulmonary (artery) (congenital) Q25.6
  with ventricular septal defect, transposition of
   aorta, and hypertrophy of right ventricle Q21.3
  acquired I28.8
  in tetralogy of Fallot Q21.3
  infundibular Q24.3
  subvalvular Q24.3
  supravalvular Q25.6
  valve I37.0
   with insufficiency I37.2
   congenital Q22.1
   rheumatic I09.89
    with aortic, mitral or tricuspid (valve)
     disease I08.8
  vein, acquired I28.8
  vessel NEC I28.8
 pulmonic (congenital) Q22.1
  infundibular Q24.3
  subvalvular Q24.3
 pylorus (hypertrophic) (acquired) K31.1
  adult K31.1
  congenital Q40.0
  infantile Q40.0
 rectum (sphincter) — see Stricture, rectum
 renal artery I70.1
  congenital Q27.1
 salivary duct (any) K11.8
 sphincter of Oddi K83.1
 spinal M48.00
  cervical region M48.02
  cervicothoracic region M48.03
  lumbar region M48.06
  lumbosacral region M48.07
  occipito-atlanto-axial region M48.01
  sacrococcygeal region M48.08
  thoracic region M48.04
  thoracolumbar region M48.05

Stenosis, stenotic (cicatricial) - *continued*
stent
  vascular
    end stent
      adjacent to stent — *see* Arteriosclerosis
      within the stent
        coronary T82.855
        peripheral T82.856
    in stent
      coronary vessel T82.855
      peripheral vessel T82.856
stomach, hourglass K31.2
subaortic (congenital) Q24.4
  hypertrophic (idiopathic) I42.1
subglottic J38.6
  congenital Q31.1
  postprocedural J95.5
trachea J39.8
  congenital Q32.1
  syphilitic A52.73
  tuberculous NEC A15.5
tracheostomy J95.03
tricuspid (valve) I07.0
  with
    aortic (valve) disease I08.2
    incompetency, insufficiency or regurgitation I07.2
      with aortic (valve) disease I08.2
        with mitral (valve) disease I08.3
    mitral (valve) disease I08.1
      with aortic (valve) disease I08.3
  congenital Q22.4
  nonrheumatic I36.0
    with insufficiency I36.2
tubal N97.1
ureter — *see* Atresia, ureter
ureteropelvic junction, congenital Q62.11
ureterovesical orifice, congenital Q62.12
urethra (valve) — *see also* Stricture, urethra
  congenital Q64.32
urinary meatus, congenital Q64.33
vagina N89.5
  congenital Q52.4
  in pregnancy — *see* Pregnancy, complicated by, abnormal vagina
    causing obstructed labor O65.5
valve (cardiac) (heart) — *see also* Endocarditis I38
  congenital Q24.8
    aortic Q23.0
    mitral Q23.2
    pulmonary Q22.1
    tricuspid Q22.4
vena cava (inferior) (superior) I87.1
  congenital Q26.0
vesicourethral orifice Q64.31
vulva N90.5
Stent jail T82.897
Stercolith (impaction) K56.41
  appendix K38.1
Stercoraceous, stercoral ulcer K63.3
  anus or rectum K62.6
Stereotypies NEC F98.4
Sterility — *see* Infertility
Sterilization — *see* Encounter (for), sterilization
Sternalgia — *see* Angina
Sternopagus Q89.4
Sternum bifidum Q76.7
Steroid
effects (adverse) (adrenocortical) (iatrogenic)
  cushingoid E24.2
    correct substance properly administered — *see* Table of Drugs and Chemicals, by drug, adverse effect
    overdose or wrong substance given or taken — *see* Table of Drugs and Chemicals, by drug, poisoning
  diabetes — *see* category E09
    correct substance properly administered — *see* Table of Drugs and Chemicals, by drug, adverse effect
    overdose or wrong substance given or taken — *see* Table of Drugs and Chemicals, by drug, poisoning
  fever R50.2
  insufficiency E27.3
    correct substance properly administered — *see* Table of Drugs and Chemicals, by drug, adverse effect
    overdose or wrong substance given or taken — *see* Table of Drugs and Chemicals, by drug, poisoning
  responder H40.04-
Stevens-Johnson disease or syndrome L51.1
  toxic epidermal necrolysis overlap L51.3

Stewart-Morel syndrome M85.2
Sticker's disease B08.3
Sticky eye — *see* Conjunctivitis, acute, mucopurulent
Stieda's disease — *see* Bursitis, tibial collateral
Stiff neck — *see* Torticollis
Stiff-man syndrome G25.82
Stiffness, joint NEC M25.60-
  ankle M25.67-
  ankylosis — *see* Ankylosis, joint
  contracture — *see* Contraction, joint
  elbow M25.62-
  foot M25.67-
  hand M25.64-
  hip M25.65-
  knee M25.66-
  shoulder M25.61-
  wrist M25.63-
Stigmata congenital syphilis A50.59
Stillbirth P95
Still-Felty syndrome — *see* Felty's syndrome
Still's disease or syndrome (juvenile) M08.20
  adult-onset M06.1
  ankle M08.27-
  elbow M08.22-
  foot joint M08.27-
  hand joint M08.24-
  hip M08.25-
  knee M08.26-
  multiple site M08.29
  shoulder M08.21-
  vertebra M08.28
  wrist M08.23-
Stimulation, ovary E28.1
Sting (venomous)
  (with allergic or anaphylactic shock) — *see* Table of Drugs and Chemicals, by animal or substance, poisoning
Stippled epiphyses Q78.8
Stitch
  abscess T81.48
  burst (in operation wound) — *see* Disruption, wound, operation
Stokes' disease E05.00
  with thyroid storm E05.01
Stokes-Adams disease or syndrome I45.9
Stokvis (-Talma) **disease** D74.8
Stoma malfunction
  colostomy K94.03
  enterostomy K94.13
  gastrostomy K94.23
  ileostomy K94.13
  tracheostomy J95.03
Stomach — *see* condition
Stomatitis (denture) (ulcerative) K12.1
  angular K13.0
    due to dietary or vitamin deficiency E53.0
  aphthous K12.0
  bovine B08.61
  candidal B37.0
  catarrhal K12.1
  diphtheritic A36.89
  due to
    dietary deficiency E53.0
    thrush B37.0
    vitamin deficiency
      B group NEC E53.9
      B2 (riboflavin) E53.0
  epidemic B08.8
  epizootic B08.8
  follicular K12.1
  gangrenous A69.0
  Geotrichum B48.3
  herpesviral, herpetic B00.2
  herpetiformis K12.0
  malignant K12.1
  membranous acute K12.1
  monilial B37.0
  mycotic B37.0
  necrotizing ulcerative A69.0
  parasitic B37.0
  septic K12.1
  spirochetal A69.1
  suppurative (acute) K12.2
  ulceromembranous A69.1
  vesicular K12.1
    with exanthem (enteroviral) B08.4
    virus disease A93.8
  Vincent's A69.1
Stomatocytosis D58.8
Stomatomycosis B37.0
Stomatorrhagia K13.79
Stone (s) — *see also* Calculus
  bladder (diverticulum) N21.0

Stone (s) - *continued*
  cystine E72.09
  heart syndrome I50.1
  kidney N20.0
  prostate N42.0
  pulpal (dental) K04.2
  renal N20.0
  salivary gland or duct (any) K11.5
  urethra (impacted) N21.1
  urinary (duct) (impacted) (passage) N20.9
    bladder (diverticulum) N21.0
    lower tract N21.9
    specified NEC N21.8
  xanthine E79.8 *[N22]*
Stonecutter's lung J62.8
Stonemason's asthma, disease, lung or pneumoconiosis J62.8
Stoppage
  heart — *see* Arrest, cardiac
  urine — *see* Retention, urine
Storm, thyroid — *see* Thyrotoxicosis
Strabismus (congenital) (nonparalytic) H50.9
  concomitant H50.40
    convergent — *see* Strabismus, convergent concomitant
    divergent — *see* Strabismus, divergent concomitant
  convergent concomitant H50.00
    accommodative component H50.43
    alternating H50.05
      with
        A pattern H50.06
        specified nonconcomitances NEC H50.08
        V pattern H50.07
    monocular H50.01-
      with
        A pattern H50.02-
        specified nonconcomitances NEC H50.04-
        V pattern H50.03-
      intermittent H50.31-
        alternating H50.32
  cyclotropia H50.41
  divergent concomitant H50.10
    alternating H50.15
      with
        A pattern H50.16
        specified noncomitances NEC H50.18
        V pattern H50.17
    monocular H50.11-
      with
        A pattern H50.12-
        specified noncomitances NEC H50.14-
        V pattern H50.13-
      intermittent H50.33
        alternating H50.34
  Duane's syndrome H50.81-
  due to adhesions, scars H50.69
  heterophoria H50.50
    alternating H50.55
    cyclophoria H50.54
    esophoria H50.51
    exophoria H50.52
    vertical H50.53
  heterotropia H50.40
    intermittent H50.30
  hypertropia H50.2-
  hypotropia — *see* Hypertropia
  latent H50.50
  mechanical H50.60
    Brown's sheath syndrome H50.61-
    specified type NEC H50.69
  monofixation syndrome H50.42
  paralytic H49.9
    abducens nerve H49.2-
    fourth nerve H49.1-
    Kearns-Sayre syndrome H49.81-
    ophthalmoplegia (external)
      progressive H49.4-
        with pigmentary retinopathy H49.81-
      total H49.3-
    sixth nerve H49.2-
    specified type NEC H49.88-
    third nerve H49.0-
    trochlear nerve H49.1-
  specified type NEC H50.89
  vertical H50.2-
Strain
  back S39.012
  cervical S16.1
  eye NEC — *see* Disturbance, vision, subjective
  heart — *see* Disease, heart
  low back S39.012
  mental NOS Z73.3
    work-related Z56.6

Strain - *continued*
muscle (tendon) — *see* Injury, muscle, by site, strain
neck S16.1
postural — *see also* Disorder, soft tissue, due to use
physical NOS Z73.3
work-related Z56.6
psychological NEC Z73.3
tendon — *see* Injury, muscle, by site, strain
Straining, on urination R39.16
Strand, vitreous — *see* Opacity, vitreous, membranes and strands
Strangulation, strangulated — *see also* Asphyxia, traumatic
appendix K38.8
bladder-neck N32.0
bowel or colon K56.2
food or foreign body — *see* Foreign body, by site
hemorrhoids — *see* Hemorrhoids, with complication
hernia — *see also* Hernia, by site, with obstruction
with gangrene — *see* Hernia, by site, with gangrene
intestine (large) (small) K56.2
with hernia — *see also* Hernia, by site, with obstruction
with gangrene — *see* Hernia, by site, with gangrene
mesentery K56.2
mucus — *see* Asphyxia, mucus
omentum K56.2
organ or site, congenital NEC — *see* Atresia, by site
ovary — *see* Torsion, ovary
penis N48.89
foreign body T19.4
rupture — *see* Hernia, by site, with obstruction
stomach due to hernia — *see also* Hernia, by site, with obstruction
with gangrene — *see* Hernia, by site, with gangrene
vesicourethral orifice N32.0
Strangury R30.0
Straw itch B88.0
Strawberry
gallbladder K82.4
mark Q82.5
tongue (red) (white) K14.3
Streak (s)
macula, angioid H35.33
ovarian Q50.32
Strephosymbolia F81.0
secondary to organic lesion R48.8
Streptobacillary fever A25.1
Streptobacillosis A25.1
Streptobacillus moniliformis A25.1
Streptococcus, streptococcal — *see also* condition
as cause of disease classified elsewhere B95.5
group
A, as cause of disease classified elsewhere B95.0
B, as cause of disease classified elsewhere B95.1
D, as cause of disease classified elsewhere B95.2
pneumoniae, as cause of disease classified elsewhere B95.3
specified NEC, as cause of disease classified elsewhere B95.4
Streptomycosis B47.1
Streptotrichosis A48.8
Stress F43.9
family — *see* Disruption, family
fetal P84
complicating pregnancy O77.9
due to drug administration O77.1
mental NEC Z73.3
work-related Z56.6
physical NEC Z73.3
work-related Z56.6
polycythemia D75.1
reaction — *see also* Reaction, stress F43.9
work schedule Z56.3
Stretching, nerve — *see* Injury, nerve
Striae albicantes, atrophicae or distensae
(cutis) L90.6
Stricture — *see also* Stenosis
ampulla of Vater K83.1
anus (sphincter) K62.4
congenital Q42.3
with fistula Q42.2
infantile Q42.3
with fistula Q42.2
aorta (ascending) (congenital) Q25.1
arteriosclerotic I70.0
calcified I70.0
supravalvular, congenital Q25.3
aortic (valve) — *see* Stenosis, aortic
aqueduct of Sylvius (congenital) Q03.0

Stricture - *continued*
aqueduct of Sylvius (congenital) - *continued*
with spina bifida — *see* Spina bifida, by site, with hydrocephalus
acquired G91.1
artery I77.1
basilar — *see* Occlusion, artery, basilar
carotid — *see* Occlusion, artery, carotid
celiac I77.4
congenital (peripheral) Q27.8
cerebral Q28.3
coronary Q24.5
digestive system Q27.8
lower limb Q27.8
retinal Q14.1
specified site NEC Q27.8
umbilical Q27.0
upper limb Q27.8
coronary — *see* Disease, heart, ischemic, atherosclerotic
congenital Q24.5
precerebral — *see* Occlusion, artery, precerebral
pulmonary (congenital) Q25.6
acquired I28.8
renal I70.1
vertebral — *see* Occlusion, artery, vertebral
auditory canal (external) (congenital)
acquired — *see* Stenosis, external ear canal
bile duct (common) (hepatic) K83.1
congenital Q44.3
postoperative K91.89
bladder N32.89
neck N32.0
bowel — *see* Obstruction, intestine
brain G93.89
bronchus J98.09
congenital Q32.3
syphilitic A52.72
cardia (stomach) K22.2
congenital Q39.3
cardiac — *see also* Disease, heart
orifice (stomach) K22.2
cecum — *see* Obstruction, intestine
cervix, cervical (canal) N88.2
congenital Q51.828
in pregnancy — *see* Pregnancy, complicated by, abnormal cervix
causing obstructed labor O65.5
colon — *see also* Obstruction, intestine
congenital Q42.9
specified NEC Q42.8
colostomy K94.03
common (bile) duct K83.1
coronary (artery) — *see* Disease, heart, ischemic, atherosclerotic
cystic duct — *see* Obstruction, gallbladder
digestive organs NEC, congenital Q45.8
duodenum K31.5
congenital Q41.0
ear canal (external) (congenital) Q16.1
acquired — *see* Stricture, auditory canal, acquired
ejaculatory duct N50.89
enterostomy K94.13
esophagus K22.2
congenital Q39.3
syphilitic A52.79
congenital A50.59 *[K23]*
eustachian tube — *see also* Obstruction, eustachian tube
congenital Q17.8
fallopian tube N97.1
gonococcal A54.24
tuberculous A18.17
gallbladder — *see* Obstruction, gallbladder
glottis J38.6
heart — *see also* Disease, heart
valve — *see also* Endocarditis I38
aortic Q23.0
mitral Q23.4
pulmonary Q22.1
tricuspid Q22.4
hepatic duct K83.1
hourglass, of stomach K31.2
hymen N89.6
hypopharynx J39.2
ileum K56.69
congenital Q41.2
intestine — *see also* Obstruction, intestine
congenital (small) Q41.9
large Q42.9
specified NEC Q42.8
specified NEC Q41.8
ischemic K55.1

Stricture - *continued*
jejunum K56.69
congenital Q41.1
lacrimal passages — *see also* Stenosis, lacrimal
congenital Q10.5
larynx J38.6
congenital NEC Q31.8
subglottic Q31.1
syphilitic A52.73
congenital A50.59 *[J99]*
meatus
ear (congenital) Q16.1
acquired — *see* Stricture, auditory canal, acquired
osseous (ear) (congenital) Q16.1
acquired — *see* Stricture, auditory canal, acquired
urinarius — *see also* Stricture, urethra
congenital Q64.33
mitral (valve) — *see* Stenosis, mitral
myocardium, myocardial I51.5
hypertrophic subaortic (idiopathic) I42.1
nares (anterior) (posterior) J34.89
congenital Q30.0
nasal duct — *see also* Stenosis, lacrimal, duct
congenital Q10.5
nasolacrimal duct — *see also* Stenosis, lacrimal, duct
congenital Q10.5
nasopharynx J39.2
syphilitic A52.73
nose J34.89
congenital Q30.0
nostril (anterior) (posterior) J34.89
congenital Q30.0
syphilitic A52.73
congenital A50.59 *[J99]*
organ or site, congenital NEC — *see* Atresia, by site
os uteri — *see* Stricture, cervix
osseous meatus (ear) (congenital) Q16.1
acquired — *see* Stricture, auditory canal, acquired
oviduct — *see* Stricture, fallopian tube
pelviureteric junction (congenital) Q62.11
acquired, with hydronephrosis N13.0
penis, by foreign body T19.4
pharynx J39.2
prostate N42.89
pulmonary, pulmonic
artery (congenital) Q25.6
acquired I28.8
noncongenital I28.8
infundibulum (congenital) Q24.3
valve I37.0
congenital Q22.1
vein, acquired I28.8
vessel NEC I28.8
punctum lacrimale — *see also* Stenosis, lacrimal, punctum
congenital Q10.5
pylorus (hypertrophic) K31.1
adult K31.1
congenital Q40.0
infantile Q40.0
rectosigmoid K56.69
rectum (sphincter) K62.4
congenital Q42.1
with fistula Q42.0
due to
chlamydial lymphogranuloma A55
irradiation K91.89
lymphogranuloma venereum A55
gonococcal A54.6
inflammatory (chlamydial) A55
syphilitic A52.74
tuberculous A18.32
renal artery I70.1
congenital Q27.1
salivary duct or gland (any) K11.8
sigmoid (flexure) — *see* Obstruction, intestine
spermatic cord N50.89
stoma (following) (of)
colostomy K94.03
enterostomy K94.13
gastrostomy K94.23
ileostomy K94.13
tracheostomy J95.03
stomach K31.89
congenital Q40.2
hourglass K31.2
subaortic Q24.4
hypertrophic (acquired) (idiopathic) I42.1
subglottic J38.6
syphilitic NEC A52.79
trachea J39.8
congenital Q32.1

Stricture - *continued*
trachea - *continued*
syphilitic A52.73
tuberculous NEC A15.5
tracheostomy J95.03
tricuspid (valve) — *see* Stenosis, tricuspid
tunica vaginalis N50.89
ureter (postoperative) N13.5
with
hydronephrosis N13.1
with infection N13.6
pyelonephritis (chronic) N11.1
congenital — *see* Atresia, ureter
tuberculous A18.11
ureteropelvic junction (congenital) Q62.11
acquired, with hydronephrosis N13.0
ureterovesical orifice N13.5
with infection N13.6
urethra (organic) (spasmodic) N35.9
associated with schistosomiasis B65.0 [N37]
congenital Q64.39
valvular (posterior) Q64.2
due to
infection — *see* Stricture, urethra, postinfective
trauma — *see* Stricture, urethra, post-traumatic
gonococcal, gonorrheal A54.01
infective NEC — *see* Stricture, urethra, postinfective
late effect (sequelae) of injury — *see* Stricture, urethra, post-traumatic
postcatheterization — *see* Stricture, urethra, postprocedural
postinfective NEC
female N35.12
male N35.119
anterior urethra N35.114
bulbous urethra N35.112
meatal N35.111
membranous urethra N35.113
postobstetric N35.021
postoperative — *see* Stricture, urethra, postprocedural
postprocedural
female N99.12
male N99.114
anterior bulbous urethra N99.113
bulbous urethra N99.111
fossa navicularis N99.115
meatal N99.110
membranous urethra N99.112
post-traumatic
female N35.028
due to childbirth N35.021
male N35.014
anterior urethra N35.013
bulbous urethra N35.011
meatal N35.010
membranous urethra N35.012
sequela (late effect) of
childbirth N35.021
injury — *see* Stricture, urethra, post-traumatic
specified cause NEC N35.8
syphilitic A52.76
traumatic — *see* Stricture, urethra, post-traumatic
valvular (posterior) , congenital Q64.2
urinary meatus — *see* Stricture, urethra
uterus, uterine (synechiae) N85.6
os (external) (internal) — *see* Stricture, cervix
vagina (outlet) — *see* Stenosis, vagina
valve (cardiac) (heart) — *see also* Endocarditis
congenital
aortic Q23.0
mitral Q23.2
pulmonary Q22.1
tricuspid Q22.4
vas deferens N50.89
congenital Q55.4
vein I87.1
vena cava (inferior) (superior) NEC I87.1
congenital Q26.0
vesicourethral orifice N32.0
congenital Q64.31
vulva (acquired) N90.5
Stridor R06.1
congenital (larynx) P28.89
Stridulous — *see* condition
Stroke (apoplectic) (brain) (embolic) (ischemic) (paralytic) (thrombotic) I63.9
epileptic — *see* Epilepsy
heat T67.0
in evolution I63.9
intraoperative
during cardiac surgery I97.810

Stroke (apoplectic) (brain) (embolic) (ischemic) (paralytic) (thrombotic) - *continued*
intraoperative - *continued*
during other surgery I97.811
lightning — *see* Lightning
meaning
cerebral hemorrhage - code to Hemorrhage, intracranial
cerebral infarction - code to Infarction, cerebral
postprocedural
following cardiac surgery I97.820
following other surgery I97.821
unspecified (NOS) I63.9
Stromatosis, endometrial D39.0
Strongyloidiasis, strongyloidosis B78.9
cutaneous B78.1
disseminated B78.7
intestinal B78.0
Strophulus pruriginosus L28.2
Struck by lightning — *see* Lightning
Struma — *see also* Goiter
Hashimoto E06.3
lymphomatosa E06.3
nodosa (simplex) E04.9
endemic E01.2
multinodular E01.1
multinodular E04.2
iodine-deficiency related E01.1
toxic or with hyperthyroidism E05.20
with thyroid storm E05.21
multinodular E05.20
with thyroid storm E05.21
uninodular E05.10
with thyroid storm E05.11
toxicosa E05.20
with thyroid storm E05.21
multinodular E05.20
with thyroid storm E05.21
uninodular E05.10
with thyroid storm E05.11
uninodular E04.1
ovarii D27.-
Riedel's E06.5
Strumipriva cachexia E03.4
Strümpell-Marie spine — *see* Spondylitis, ankylosing
Strümpell-Westphal pseudosclerosis E83.01
Stuart deficiency disease (factor X) D68.2
Stuart-Prower factor deficiency (factor X) D68.2
Student's elbow — *see* Bursitis, elbow, olecranon
Stump — *see* Amputation
Stunting, nutritional E45
Stupor (catatonic) R40.1
depressive (single episode) F32.89
recurrent episode F33.8
dissociative F44.2
manic F30.2
manic-depressive F31.89
psychogenic (anergic) F44.2
reaction to exceptional stress (transient) F43.0
Sturge (-Weber) (-Dimitri) (-Kalischer)
disease or syndrome Q85.8
Stuttering F80.81
adult onset F98.5
childhood onset F80.81
following cerebrovascular disease — *see* Disorder, fluency. following cerebrovascular disease
in conditions classified elsewhere R47.82
Sty, stye (external) (internal) (meibomian) (zeisian) — *see* Hordeolum
Subacidity, gastric K31.89
psychogenic F45.8
Subacute — *see* condition
Subarachnoid — *see* condition
Subcortical — *see* condition
Subcostal syndrome, nerve compression — *see* Mononeuropathy, upper limb, specified site NEC
Subcutaneous, subcuticular — *see* condition
Subdural — *see* condition
Subendocardium — *see* condition
Subependymoma
specified site — *see* Neoplasm, uncertain behavior, by site
unspecified site D43.2
Suberosis J67.3
Subglossitis — *see* Glossitis
Subhemophilia D66
Subinvolution
breast (postlactational) (postpuerperal) N64.89
puerperal O90.89
uterus (chronic) (nonpuerperal) N85.3
puerperal O90.89
Sublingual — *see* condition

Sublinguitis — *see* Sialoadenitis
Subluxatable hip Q65.6
Subluxation — *see also* Dislocation
acromioclavicular S43.11-
ankle S93.0-
atlantoaxial, recurrent M43.4
with myelopathy M43.3
carpometacarpal (joint) NEC S63.05-
thumb S63.04-
complex, vertebral — *see* Complex, subluxation
congenital — *see also* Malposition, congenital
hip — *see* Dislocation, hip, congenital, partial
joint (excluding hip)
lower limb Q68.8
shoulder Q68.8
upper limb Q68.8
elbow (traumatic) S53.10-
anterior S53.11-
lateral S53.14-
medial S53.13-
posterior S53.12-
specified type NEC S53.19-
finger S63.20-
index S63.20-
interphalangeal S63.22-
distal S63.24-
index S63.24-
little S63.24-
middle S63.24-
ring S63.24-
index S63.22-
little S63.22-
middle S63.22-
proximal S63.23-
index S63.23-
little S63.23-
middle S63.23-
ring S63.23-
little S63.22-
little S63.20-
metacarpophalangeal S63.21-
index S63.21-
little S63.21-
middle S63.21-
ring S63.21-
middle S63.20-
ring S63.20-
foot S93.30-
specified site NEC S93.33-
tarsal joint S93.31-
tarsometatarsal joint S93.32-
toe — *see* Subluxation, toe
hip S73.00-
anterior S73.03-
obturator S73.02-
central S73.04-
posterior S73.01-
interphalangeal (joint)
finger S63.22-
distal joint S63.24-
index S63.24-
little S63.24-
middle S63.24-
ring S63.24-
index S63.22-
little S63.22-
middle S63.22-
proximal joint S63.23-
index S63.23-
little S63.23-
middle S63.23-
ring S63.23-
ring S63.22-
thumb S63.12-
distal joint S63.14-
proximal joint S63.13-
toe S93.13-
great S93.13-
lesser S93.13-
joint prosthesis — *see* Complications, joint prosthesis, mechanical, displacement, by site
knee S83.10-
cap — *see* Subluxation, patella
patella — *see* Subluxation, patella
proximal tibia
anteriorly S83.11-
laterally S83.14-
medially S83.13-
posteriorly S83.12-
specified type NEC S83.19-
lens — *see* Dislocation, lens, partial
ligament, traumatic — *see* Sprain, by site
metacarpal (bone)

Subluxation - *continued*
  metacarpal (bone) - *continued*
    proximal end S63.06-
  metacarpophalangeal (joint)
    finger S63.21-
      index S63.21-
      little S63.21-
      middle S63.21-
      ring S63.21-
      thumb S63.11-
  metatarsophalangeal joint S93.14-
    great toe S93.14-
    lesser toe S93.14-
  midcarpal (joint) S63.03-
  patella S83.00-
    lateral S83.01-
    recurrent (nontraumatic) — *see* Dislocation,
      patella, recurrent, incomplete
    specified type NEC S83.09-
  pathological — *see* Dislocation, pathological
  radial head S53.00-
    anterior S53.01-
    nursemaid's elbow S53.03-
    posterior S53.02-
    specified type NEC S53.09-
  radiocarpal (joint) S63.02-
  radioulnar (joint)
    distal S63.01-
    proximal — *see* Subluxation, elbow
  shoulder
    congenital Q68.8
    girdle S43.30-
      scapula S43.31-
      specified site NEC S43.39-
    traumatic S43.00-
      anterior S43.01-
      inferior S43.03-
      posterior S43.02-
      specified type NEC S43.08-
  sternoclavicular (joint) S43.20-
    anterior S43.21-
    posterior S43.22-
  symphysis (pubis)
  thumb S63.103
    interphalangeal joint — *see* Subluxation,
      interphalangeal (joint), thumb
    metacarpophalangeal joint — *see* Subluxation,
      metacarpophalangeal (joint), thumb
  toe (s) S93.10-
    great S93.10-
      interphalangeal joint S93.13-
      metatarsophalangeal joint S93.14-
    interphalangeal joint S93.13-
    lesser S93.10-
      interphalangeal joint S93.13-
      metatarsophalangeal joint S93.14-
      metatarsophalangeal joint S93.149
  ulnohumeral joint — *see* Subluxation, elbow
  vertebral
    recurrent NEC — *see* subcategory M43.5
    traumatic
      cervical S13.100
        atlantoaxial joint S13.120
        atlantooccipital joint S13.110
        atloidooccipital joint S13.110
        joint between
          C0 and C1 S13.110
          C1 and C2 S13.120
          C2 and C3 S13.130
          C3 and C4 S13.140
          C4 and C5 S13.150
          C5and C6 S13.160
          C6and C7 S13.170
          C7and T1 S13.180
        occipitoatloid joint S13.110
      lumbar S33.100
        joint between
          L1and L2 S33.110
          L2and L3 S33.120
          L3 and L4 S33.130
          L4and L5 S33.140
      thoracic S23.100
        joint between
          T1and T2 S23.110
          T2and T3 S23.120
          T3 and T4 S23.122
          T4 and T5 S23.130
          T5 and T6 S23.132
          T6 and T7 S23.140
          T7 and T8 S23.142
          T8 and T9 S23.150
          T9 and T10 S23.152
          T10 and T11 S23.160

Subluxation - *continued*
  vertebral - *continued*
    traumatic - *continued*
      thoracic - *continued*
        joint between - *continued*
          T11 and T12 S23.162
          T12 and L1 S23.170
    ulna
      distal end S63.07-
      proximal end — *see* Subluxation, elbow
    wrist (carpal bone) S63.00-
      carpometacarpal joint — *see* Subluxation,
        carpometacarpal (joint)
      distal radioulnar joint — *see* Subluxation,
        radioulnar (joint), distal
      metacarpal bone, proximal — *see* Subluxation,
        metacarpal (bone), proximal end
      midcarpal — *see* Subluxation, midcarpal (joint)
      radiocarpal joint — *see* Subluxation, radiocarpal
        (joint)
      recurrent — *see* Dislocation, recurrent, wrist
      specified site NEC S63.09-
      ulna — *see* Subluxation, ulna, distal end
Submaxillary — *see* condition
Submersion (fatal) (nonfatal) T75.1
Submucous — *see* condition
Subnormal, subnormality
  accommodation (old age) H52.4
  mental — *see* Disability, intellectual
  temperature (accidental) T68
Subphrenic — *see* condition
Subscapular nerve — *see* condition
Subseptus uterus Q51.2
Subsiding appendicitis K36
Substance (other psychoactive) **-induced**
  anxiety disorder F19.980
  bipolar and related disorder F19.94
  delirium F19.921
  depressive disorder F19.94
  major neurocognitive disorder F19.97
  mild neurocognitive disorder F19.988
  obsessive-compulsive and related disorder F19.988
  psychotic disorder F19.959
  sexual dysfunction F19.981
  sleep disorder F19.982
Substernal thyroid E04.9
  congenital Q89.2
Substitution disorder F44.9
Subtentorial — *see* condition
Subthyroidism (acquired) — *see*
  also Hypothyroidism
  congenital E03.1
Succenturiate placenta O43.19-
Sucking thumb, child (excessive) F98.8
Sudamen, sudamina L74.1
Sudanese kala-azar B55.0
Sudden
  heart failure — *see* Failure, heart
  hearing loss — *see* Deafness, sudden
Sudeck's atrophy, disease, or syndrome — *see*
  Algoneurodystrophy
Suffocation — *see* Asphyxia, traumatic
Sugar
  blood
    high (transient) R73.9
    low (transient) E16.2
  in urine R81
Suicide, suicidal (attempted) T14.91
  by poisoning — *see* Table of Drugs and Chemicals
  history of (personal) Z91.5
    in family Z81.8
  ideation — *see* Ideation, suicidal
  risk
    meaning personal history of attempted
      suicide Z91.5
    meaning suicidal ideation — *see* Ideation, suicidal
  tendencies
    meaning personal history of attempted
      suicide Z91.5
    meaning suicidal ideation — *see* Ideation, suicidal
  trauma — *see* nature of injury by site
Suipestifer infection — *see* Infection, salmonella
Sulfhemoglobinemia, sulphemoglobinemia
  (acquired) (with methemoglobinemia) D74.8
Sumatran mite fever A75.3
Summer — *see* condition
Sunburn L55.9
  due to
    tanning bed (acute) L56.8
      chronic L57.8
    ultraviolet radiation (acute) L56.8
      chronic L57.8
  first degree L55.0

Sunburn - *continued*
  second degree L55.1
  third degree L55.2
SUNCT
  (short lasting unilateral neuralgiform headache with
    conjunctival injection and tearing) G44.059
  intractable G44.051
  not intractable G44.059
Sunken acetabulum — *see* Derangement, joint,
  specified type NEC, hip
Sunstroke T67.0
Superfecundation — *see* Pregnancy, multiple
Superfetation — *see* Pregnancy, multiple
Superinvolution (uterus) N85.8
Supernumerary (congenital)
  aortic cusps Q23.8
  auditory ossicles Q16.3
  bone Q79.8
  breast Q83.1
  carpal bones Q74.0
  cusps, heart valve NEC Q24.8
    aortic Q23.8
    mitral Q23.2
    pulmonary Q22.3
  digit (s) Q69.9
  ear (lobule) Q17.0
  fallopian tube Q50.6
  finger Q69.0
  hymen Q52.4
  kidney Q63.0
  lacrimonasal duct Q10.6
  lobule (ear) Q17.0
  mitral cusps Q23.2
  muscle Q79.8
  nipple (s) Q83.3
  organ or site not listed — *see* Accessory
  ossicles, auditory Q16.3
  ovary Q50.31
  oviduct Q50.6
  pulmonary, pulmonic cusps Q22.3
  rib Q76.6
    cervical or first (syndrome) Q76.5
  roots (of teeth) K00.2
  spleen Q89.09
  tarsal bones Q74.2
  teeth K00.1
  testis Q55.29
  thumb Q69.1
  toe Q69.2
  uterus Q51.2
  vagina Q52.1
  vertebra Q76.49
Supervision (of)
  contraceptive — *see* Prescription, contraceptives
  dietary (for) Z71.3
    allergy (food) Z71.3
    colitis Z71.3
    diabetes mellitus Z71.3
    food allergy or intolerance Z71.3
    gastritis Z71.3
    hypercholesterolemia Z71.3
    hypoglycemia Z71.3
    intolerance (food) Z71.3
    obesity Z71.3
    specified NEC Z71.3
  healthy infant or child Z76.2
    foundling Z76.1
  high-risk pregnancy — *see* Pregnancy, complicated
    by, high, risk
  lactation Z39.1
  pregnancy — *see* Pregnancy, supervision of
Supplemental teeth K00.1
Suppression
  binocular vision H53.34
  lactation O92.5
  menstruation N94.89
  ovarian secretion E28.39
  renal N28.9
  urine, urinary secretion R34
Suppuration, suppurative — *see also* condition
  accessory sinus (chronic) — *see* Sinusitis
  adrenal gland
  antrum (chronic) — *see* Sinusitis, maxillary
  bladder — *see* Cystitis
  brain G06.0
    sequelae G09
  breast N61.1
    puerperal, postpartum or gestational — *see*
      Mastitis, obstetric, purulent
  dental periosteum M27.3
  ear (middle) — *see also* Otitis, media
    external NEC — *see* Otitis, externa, infective
    internal — *see* subcategory H83.0

Suppuration, suppurative - *continued*
ethmoidal (chronic) (sinus) — *see* Sinusitis, ethmoidal
fallopian tube — *see* Salpingo-oophoritis
frontal (chronic) (sinus) — *see* Sinusitis, frontal
gallbladder (acute) K81.0
gum K05.20
generalized — *see* Peridontitis, aggressive, generalized
localized — *see* Peridontitis, aggressive, localized
intracranial G06.0
joint — *see* Arthritis, pyogenic or pyemic
labyrinthine — *see* subcategory H83.0
lung — *see* Abscess, lung
mammary gland N61.1
puerperal, postpartum O91.12
associated with lactation O91.13
maxilla, maxillary M27.2
sinus (chronic) — *see* Sinusitis, maxillary
muscle — *see* Myositis, infective
nasal sinus (chronic) — *see* Sinusitis
pancreas, acute — *see also* Pancreatitis, acute K85.80
parotid gland — *see* Sialoadenitis
pelvis, pelvic
female — *see* Disease, pelvis, inflammatory
male K65.0
pericranial — *see* Osteomyelitis
salivary duct or gland (any) — *see* Sialoadenitis
sinus (accessory) (chronic) (nasal) — *see* Sinusitis
sphenoidal sinus (chronic) — *see* Sinusitis, sphenoidal
thymus (gland) E32.1
thyroid (gland) E06.0
tonsil — *see* Tonsillitis
uterus — *see* Endometritis
Supraeruption of tooth (teeth) M26.34
Supraglottitis J04.30
with obstruction J04.31
Suprarenal (gland) — *see* condition
Suprascapular nerve — *see* condition
Suprasellar — *see* condition
Surfer's knots or nodules S89.8-
Surgical
emphysema T81.82
procedures, complication or misadventure — *see* Complications, surgical procedures
shock T81.10
Surveillance (of) (for) — *see also* Observation
alcohol abuse Z71.41
contraceptive — *see* Prescription, contraceptives
dietary Z71.3
drug abuse Z71.51
Susceptibility to disease, genetic Z15.89
malignant neoplasm Z15.09
breast Z15.01
endometrium Z15.04
ovary Z15.02
prostate Z15.03
specified NEC Z15.09
multiple endocrine neoplasia Z15.81
Suspected condition, ruled out — *see also* Observation, suspected
amniotic cavity and membrane Z03.71
cervical shortening Z03.75
fetal anomaly Z03.73
fetal growth Z03.74
maternal and fetal conditions NEC Z03.79
newborn — *see also* Observation, newborn, suspected condition ruled out Z05.9
oligohydramnios Z03.71
placental problem Z03.72
polyhydramnios Z03.71
Suspended uterus
in pregnancy or childbirth — *see* Pregnancy, complicated by, abnormal uterus
Sutton's nevus D22.9
Suture
burst (in operation wound) T81.31
external operation wound T81.31
internal operation wound T81.32
inadvertently left in operation wound — *see* Foreign body, accidentally left during a procedure
removal Z48.02
Swab inadvertently left in operation wound — *see* Foreign body, accidentally left during a procedure
Swallowed, swallowing
difficulty — *see* Dysphagia
foreign body — *see* Foreign body, alimentary tract
Swan-neck deformity (finger) — *see* Deformity, finger, swan-neck
Swearing, compulsive F42.8
in Gilles de la Tourette's syndrome F95.2

Sweat, sweats
fetid L75.0
night R61
Sweating, excessive R61
Sweeley-Klionsky disease E75.21
Sweet's disease or dermatosis L98.2
Swelling (of) R60.9
abdomen, abdominal (not referable to any particular organ) — *see* Mass, abdominal
ankle — *see* Effusion, joint, ankle
arm M79.89
forearm M79.89
breast N63
Calabar B74.3
cervical gland R59.0
chest, localized R22.2
ear H93.8-
extremity (lower) (upper) — *see* Disorder, soft tissue, specified type NEC
finger M79.89
foot M79.89
glands R59.9
generalized R59.1
localized R59.0
hand M79.89
head (localized) R22.0
inflammatory — *see* Inflammation
intra-abdominal — *see* Mass, abdominal
joint — *see* Effusion, joint
leg M79.89
lower M79.89
limb — *see* Disorder, soft tissue, specified type NEC
localized (skin) R22.9
chest R22.2
head R22.0
limb
lower — *see* Mass, localized, limb, lower
upper — *see* Mass, localized, limb, upper
neck R22.1
trunk R22.2
neck (localized) R22.1
pelvic — *see* Mass, abdominal
scrotum N50.89
splenic — *see* Splenomegaly
testis N50.89
toe M79.89
umbilical R19.09
wandering, due to Gnathostoma (spinigerum) B83.1
white — *see* Tuberculosis, arthritis
Swift (-Feer) **disease**
overdose or wrong substance given or taken — *see* Table of Drugs and Chemicals, by drug, poisoning
Swimmer's
cramp T75.1
ear H60.33-
itch B65.3
Swimming in the head R42
Swollen — *see* Swelling
Swyer syndrome Q99.1
Sycosis L73.8
barbae (not parasitic) L73.8
contagiosa (mycotic) B35.0
lupoides L73.8
mycotic B35.0
parasitic B35.0
vulgaris L73.8
Sydenham's chorea — *see* Chorea, Sydenham's
Sylvatic yellow fever A95.0
Sylvest's disease B33.0
Symblepharon H11.23-
congenital Q10.3
Symond's syndrome G93.2
Sympathetic — *see* condition
Sympatheticotonia G90.8
Sympathicoblastoma
specified site — *see* Neoplasm, malignant, by site
unspecified site C74.90
Sympathogonioma — *see* Sympathicoblastoma
Symphalangy (fingers) (toes) Q70.9
Symptoms NEC R68.89
breast NEC N64.59
development NEC R63.8
factitious, self-induced — *see* Disorder, factitious
genital organs, female R10.2
involving
abdomen NEC R19.8
appearance NEC R46.89
awareness R41.9
altered mental status R41.82
amnesia — *see* Amnesia
borderline intellectual functioning R41.83
coma — *see* Coma
disorientation R41.0

Symptoms NEC - *continued*
involving - *continued*
awareness - *continued*
neurologic neglect syndrome R41.4
senile cognitive decline R41.81
specified symptom NEC R41.89
behavior NEC R46.89
cardiovascular system NEC R09.89
chest NEC R09.89
circulatory system NEC R09.89
cognitive functions R41.9
altered mental status R41.82
amnesia — *see* Amnesia
borderline intellectual functioning R41.83
coma — *see* Coma
disorientation R41.0
neurologic neglect syndrome R41.4
senile cognitive decline R41.89
specified symptom NEC R41.89
development NEC R62.50
digestive system NEC R19.8
emotional state NEC R45.89
emotional lability R45.86
food and fluid intake R63.8
general perceptions and sensations R44.9
specified NEC R44.8
musculoskeletal system R29.91
specified NEC R29.898
nervous system R29.90
specified NEC R29.818
pelvis NEC R19.8
respiratory system NEC R09.89
skin and integument R23.9
urinary system R39.9
menopausal N95.1
metabolism NEC R63.8
neurotic F48.8
of infancy R68.19
pelvis NEC, female R10.2
skin and integument NEC R23.9
subcutaneous tissue NEC R23.9
Sympus Q74.2
Syncephalus Q89.4
Synchondrosis
abnormal (congenital) Q78.8
ischiopubic M91.0
Synchysis (scintillans) (senile) (vitreous body) H43.89
Syncope (near) (pre-) R55
anginosa I20.8
bradycardia R00.1
cardiac R55
carotid sinus G90.01
due to spinal (lumbar) puncture G97.1
heart R55
heat T67.1
laryngeal R05
psychogenic F48.8
tussive R05
vasoconstriction R55
vasodepressor R55
vasomotor R55
vasovagal R55
Syndactylism, syndactyly Q70.9
complex (with synostosis)
fingers Q70.0-
toes Q70.2-
simple (without synostosis)
fingers Q70.1-
toes Q70.3-
Syndrome — *see also* Disease
5q minus NOS D46.C
48,XXXX Q97.1
49,XXXXX Q97.1
abdominal
acute R10.0
muscle deficiency Q79.4
abnormal innervation H02.519
left H02.516
lower H02.515
upper H02.514
right H02.513
lower H02.512
upper H02.511
abstinence, neonatal P96.1
acid pulmonary aspiration, obstetric O74.0
acquired immunodeficiency — *see* Human, immunodeficiency virus (HIV) disease
acute abdominal R10.0
acute respiratory distress (adult) (child) J80
idiopathic J84.114
Adair-Dighton Q78.0
Adams-Stokes (-Morgagni) I45.9

Syndrome - *continued*
adiposogenital E23.6
adrenal
  hemorrhage (meningococcal) A39.1
  meningococcic A39.1
adrenocortical — *see* Cushing's, syndrome
adrenogenital E25.9
  congenital, associated with enzyme
    deficiency E25.0
afferent loop NEC K91.89
Alagille's Q44.7
alcohol withdrawal (without convulsions) — *see*
  Dependence, alcohol, with, withdrawal
Alder's D72.0
Aldrich (-Wiskott) D82.0
alien hand R41.4
Alport Q87.81
alveolar hypoventilation E66.2
alveolocapillary block J84.10
amnesic, amnestic (confabulatory) (due to) — *see*
  Disorder, amnesic
amyostatic (Wilson's disease) E83.01
androgen insensitivity E34.50
  complete E34.51
  partial E34.52
androgen resistance — *see also* Syndrome, androgen
  insensitivity E34.50
Angelman Q93.5
anginal — *see* Angina
ankyloglossia superior Q38.1
anterior
  chest wall R07.89
  cord G83.82
  spinal artery G95.19
    compression M47.019
      cervical region M47.012
      cervicothoracic region M47.013
      lumbar region M47.016
      occipito-atlanto-axial region M47.011
      thoracic region M47.014
      thoracolumbar region M47.015
  tibial M76.81-
antibody deficiency D80.9
  agammaglobulinemic D80.1
    hereditary D80.0
  congenital D80.0
  hypogammaglobulinemic D80.1
    hereditary D80.0
anticardiolipin (-antibody) D68.61
antiphospholipid (-antibody) D68.61
aortic
  arch M31.4
  bifurcation I74.09
aortomesenteric duodenum occlusion K31.5
apical ballooning (transient left ventricular) I51.81
arcuate ligament I77.4
argentaffin, argintaffinoma E34.0
Arnold-Chiari — *see* Arnold-Chiari disease
Arrillaga-Ayerza I27.0
arterial tortuosity Q87.82
arteriovenous steal T82.898-
Asherman's N85.6
aspiration, of newborn — *see* Aspiration, by
  substance, with pneumonia
  meconium P24.01
ataxia-telangiectasia G11.3
auriculotemporal G50.8
autoerythrocyte sensitization (Gardner-
  Diamond) D69.2
autoimmune polyglandular E31.0
autoimmune lymphoproliferative [ALPS] D89.82
autoinflammatory M04.9
  specified type NEC M04.8
autosomal — *see* Abnormal, autosomes
Avellis' G46.8
Ayerza (-Arrillaga) I27.0
Babinski-Nageotte G83.89
Bakwin-Krida Q78.5
bare lymphocyte D81.6
Barré-Guillain G61.0
Barré-Liéou M53.0
Barrett's — *see* Barrett's, esophagus
Barsony-Polgar K22.4
Barsony-Teschendorf K22.4
Barth E78.71
Bartter's E26.81
basal cell nevus Q87.89
Basedow's E05.00
  with thyroid storm E05.01
basilar artery G45.0
Batten-Steinert G71.11
battered

Syndrome - *continued*
battered - *continued*
  baby or child — *see* Maltreatment, child, physical
    abuse
  spouse — *see* Maltreatment, adult, physical abuse
Beals Q87.40
Beau's I51.5
Beck's I65.8
Benedikt's G46.3
Béquez César (-Steinbrinck-Chédiak-
  Higashi) E70.330
Bernhardt-Roth — *see* Meralgia paresthetica
Bernheim's I50.9
big spleen D73.1
bilateral polycystic ovarian E28.2
Bing-Horton's — *see* Horton's headache
Birt-Hogg-Dube syndrome Q87.89
Björck (-Thorsen) E34.0
black
  lung J60
  widow spider bite — *see* Toxicity, venom, spider,
    black widow
Blackfan-Diamond D61.01
Blau M04.8
blind loop K90.2
  congenital Q43.8
  postsurgical K91.2
blue sclera Q78.0
blue toe I75.02-
Boder-Sedgewick G11.3
Boerhaave's K22.3
Borjeson Forssman Lehmann Q89.8
Bouillaud's I01.9
Bourneville (-Pringle) Q85.1
Bouveret (-Hoffman) I47.9
brachial plexus G54.0
bradycardia-tachycardia I49.5
brain (nonpsychotic) F09
  with psychosis, psychotic reaction F09
  acute or subacute — *see* Delirium
  congenital — *see* Disability, intellectual
  organic F09
    post-traumatic (nonpsychotic) F07.81
      psychotic F09
  personality change F07.0
  postcontusional F07.81
  post-traumatic, nonpsychotic F07.81
  psycho-organic F09
  psychotic F06.8
brain stem stroke G46.3
Brandt's (acrodermatitis enteropathica) E83.2
broad ligament laceration N83.8
Brock's J98.11
bronze baby P83.8
Brown-Sequard G83.81
bubbly lung P27.0
Buchem's M85.2
Budd-Chiari I82.0
bulbar (progressive) G12.22
Bürger-Grütz E78.3
Burke's K86.89
Burnett's (milk-alkali) E83.52
burning feet E53.9
Bywaters' T79.5
Call-Fleming I67.841
carbohydrate-deficient glycoprotein (CDGS) E77.8
carcinogenic thrombophlebitis I82.1
carcinoid E34.0
cardiac asthma I50.1
cardiacos negros I27.0
cardiofaciocutaneous Q87.89
cardiopulmonary-obesity E66.2
cardiorenal — *see* Hypertension, cardiorenal
cardiorespiratory distress (idiopathic) ,
  newborn P22.0
cardiovascular renal — *see* Hypertension,
  cardiorenal
carotid
  artery (hemispheric) (internal) G45.1
  body G90.01
  sinus G90.01
carpal tunnel G56.0-
Cassidy (-Scholte) E34.0
cat cry Q93.4
cat eye Q92.8
cauda equina G83.4
causalgia — *see* Causalgia
celiac K90.0
  artery compression I77.4
  axis I77.4
central pain G89.0
cerebellar
  hereditary G11.9

Syndrome - *continued*
cerebellar - *continued*
  stroke G46.4
cerebellomedullary malformation — *see* Spina
  bifida
cerebral
  artery
    anterior G46.1
    middle G46.0
    posterior G46.2
  gigantism E22.0
cervical (root) M53.1
  disc — *see* Disorder, disc, cervical, with neuritis
  fusion Q76.1
  posterior, sympathicus M53.0
  rib Q76.5
  sympathetic paralysis G90.2
cervicobrachial (diffuse) M53.1
cervicocranial M53.0
cervicodorsal outlet G54.2
cervicothoracic outlet G54.0
Céstan (-Raymond) I65.8
Charcot's (angina cruris) (intermittent
  claudication) I73.9
Charcot-Weiss-Baker G90.09
CHARGE Q89.8
Chédiak-Higashi (-Steinbrinck) E70.330
chest wall R07.1
Chiari's (hepatic vein thrombosis) I82.0
Chilaiditi's Q43.3
child maltreatment — *see* Maltreatment, child
chondrocostal junction M94.0
chondroectodermal dysplasia Q77.6
chromosome 4 short arm deletion Q93.3
chromosome 5 short arm deletion Q93.4
chronic
  infantile neurological, cutaneous and articular
    (CINCA) M04.2
  pain G89.4
  personality F68.8
Clarke-Hadfield K86.89
Clerambault's automatism G93.89
Clouston's (hidrotic ectodermal dysplasia) Q82.4
clumsiness, clumsy child F82
cluster headache G44.009
  intractable G44.001
  not intractable G44.009
Coffin-Lowry Q89.8
cold injury (newborn) P80.0
combined immunity deficiency D81.9
compartment (deep) (posterior) (traumatic) T79.A0
  abdomen T79.A3
  lower extremity (hip, buttock, thigh, leg, foot,
    toes) T79.A2
  nontraumatic
    abdomen M79.A3
    lower extremity (hip, buttock, thigh, leg, foot,
      toes) M79.A2-
    specified site NEC M79.A9
    upper extremity (shoulder, arm, forearm, wrist,
      hand, fingers) M79.A1-
  postprocedural — *see* Syndrome, compartment,
    nontraumatic
  specified site NEC T79.A9
  upper extremity (shoulder, arm, forearm, wrist,
    hand, fingers) T79.A1
complex regional pain — *see* Syndrome, pain,
  complex regional
compression T79.5
  anterior spinal — *see* Syndrome, anterior, spinal
    artery, compression
  cauda equina G83.4
  celiac artery I77.4
  vertebral artery M47.029
    occipito-atlanto-axial region M47.021
    cervical region M47.022
concussion F07.81
congenital
  affecting multiple systems NEC Q87.89
  central alveolar hypoventilation G47.35
  facial diplegia Q87.0
  muscular hypertrophy-cerebral Q87.89
  oculo-auriculovertebral Q87.0
  oculofacial diplegia (Moebius) Q87.0
  rubella (manifest) P35.0
congestion-fibrosis (pelvic) , female N94.89
congestive dysmenorrhea N94.6
Conn's E26.01
connective tissue M35.9
  overlap NEC M35.1
conus medullaris G95.81
cord
  anterior G83.82

Syndrome - *continued*
cord - *continued*
  posterior G83.83
coronary
  acute NEC I24.9
  insufficiency or intermediate I20.0
  slow flow I20.8
Costen's (complex) M26.69
costochondral junction M94.0
costoclavicular G54.0
costovertebral E22.0
Cowden Q85.8
craniovertebral M53.0
Creutzfeldt-Jakob — *see* Creutzfeldt-Jakob disease
  or syndrome
cri-du-chat Q93.4
crib death R99
cricopharyngeal — *see* Dysphagia
croup J05.0
CRPS I — *see* Syndrome, pain, complex regional I
crush T79.5
cubital tunnel — *see* Lesion, nerve, ulnar
Curschmann (-Batten) (-Steinert) G71.11
Cushing's E24.9
  alcohol-induced E24.4
  due to
    alcohol
    drugs E24.2
    ectopic ACTH E24.3
    overproduction of pituitary ACTH E24.0
  drug-induced E24.2
  overdose or wrong substance given or taken — *see*
    Table of Drugs and Chemicals, by drug,
    poisoning
  pituitary-dependent E24.0
  specified type NEC E24.8
cryopyrin-associated periodic M04.2
cryptophthalmos Q87.0
cystic duct stump K91.5
Dana-Putnam D51.0
Danbolt (-Cross) (acrodermatitis
  enteropathica) E83.2
Dandy-Walker Q03.1
  with spina bifida Q07.01
Danlos' Q79.6
defibrination — *see also* Fibrinolysis
  with
    antepartum hemorrhage — *see* Hemorrhage,
      antepartum, with coagulation defect
    intrapartum hemorrhage — *see* Hemorrhage,
      complicating, delivery
  newborn P60
  postpartum O72.3
Degos' I77.89
Déjérine-Roussy G89.0
delayed sleep phase G47.21
demyelinating G37.9
dependence — *see* F10-F19 with fourth character .2
depersonalization (-derealization) F48.1
De Quervain E34.51
de Toni-Fanconi (-Debré) E72.09
  with cystinosis E72.04
diabetes mellitus-hypertension-nephrosis — *see*
  Diabetes, nephrosis
diabetes mellitus in newborn infant P70.2
diabetes-nephrosis — *see* Diabetes, nephrosis
diabetic amyotrophy — *see* Diabetes, amyotrophy
dialysis associated steal T82.898-
Diamond-Blackfan D61.01
Diamond-Gardener D69.2
DIC (diffuse or disseminated intravascular
  coagulopathy) D65
di George's D82.1
Dighton's Q78.0
disequilibrium E87.8
Döhle body-panmyelopathic D72.0
dorsolateral medullary G46.4
double athetosis G80.3
Down — *see also* Down syndrome Q90.9
Dresbach's (elliptocytosis) D58.1
Dressler's (postmyocardial infarction) I24.1
  postcardiotomy I97.0
drug withdrawal, infant of dependent mother P96.1
dry eye H04.12-
due to abnormality
  chromosomal Q99.9
    sex
      female phenotype Q97.9
      male phenotype Q98.9
      specified NEC Q99.8
dumping (postgastrectomy) K91.1
  nonsurgical K31.89
Dupré's (meningism) R29.1

Syndrome - *continued*
dysmetabolic X E88.81
dyspraxia, developmental F82
Eagle-Barrett Q79.4
Eaton-Lambert — *see* Syndrome, Lambert-Eaton
Ebstein's Q22.5
ectopic ACTH E24.3
eczema-thrombocytopenia D82.0
Eddowes' Q78.0
effort (psychogenic) F45.8
Eisenmenger's I27.89
Ehlers-Danlos Q79.6
Ekman's Q78.0
electric feet E53.8
Ellis-van Creveld Q77.6
empty nest Z60.0
endocrine-hypertensive E27.0
entrapment — *see* Neuropathy, entrapment
eosinophilia-myalgia M35.8
epileptic — *see also* Epilepsy, by type
  absence G40.A09
    intractable G40.A19
      with status epilepticus G40.A11
      without status epilepticus G40.A19
    not intractable G40.A09
      with status epilepticus G40.A01
      without status epilepticus G40.A09
Erdheim-Chester (ECD) E88.89
Erdheim's E22.0
erythrocyte fragmentation D59.4
Evans D69.41
exhaustion F48.8
extrapyramidal G25.9
  specified NEC G25.89
eye retraction — *see* Strabismus
eyelid-malar-mandible Q87.0
Faber's D50.9
facial pain, paroxysmal G50.0
Fallot's Q21.3
familial cold autoinflammatory M04.2
familial eczema-thrombocytopenia (Wiskott-
  Aldrich) D82.0
Fanconi (-de Toni) (-Debré) E72.09
  with cystinosis E72.04
Fanconi's (anemia) (congenital
  pancytopenia) D61.09
fatigue
  chronic R53.82
  psychogenic F48.8
faulty bowel habit K59.39
Feil-Klippel (brevicollis) Q76.1
Felty's — *see* Felty's syndrome
fertile eunuch E23.0
fetal
  alcohol (dysmorphic) Q86.0
  hydantoin Q86.1
Fiedler's I40.1
first arch Q87.0
fish odor E72.8
Fisher's G61.0
Fitzhugh-Curtis
  due to
    Chlamydia trachomatis A74.81
    Neisseria gonorrhorea (gonococcal
      peritonitis) A54.85
Fitz's — *see also* Pancreatitis, acute K85.80
Flajani (-Basedow) E05.00
  with thyroid storm E05.01
flatback — *see* Flatback syndrome
floppy
  baby P94.2
  iris (intraoperative) (IFIS) H21.81
  mitral valve I34.1
flush E34.0
Foix-Alajouanine G95.19
Fong's Q87.2
food protein-induced enterocolitis K52.21
foramen magnum G93.5
Foster-Kennedy H47.14-
Foville's (peduncular) G46.3
fragile X Q99.2
Franceschetti Q75.4
Frey's
  auriculotemporal G50.8
  hyperhidrosis L74.52
Friderichsen-Waterhouse A39.1
Froin's G95.89
frontal lobe F07.0
Fukuhara E88.49
functional
  bowel K59.9
  prepubertal castrate E29.1
Gaisböck's D75.1

Syndrome - *continued*
ganglion (basal ganglia brain) G25.9
  geniculi G51.1
Gardner-Diamond D69.2
gastroesophageal
  junction K22.0
  laceration-hemorrhage K22.6
gastrojejunal loop obstruction K91.89
Gee-Herter-Heubner K90.0
Gelineau's G47.419
  with cataplexy G47.411
genito-anorectal A55
Gerstmann-Sträussler-Scheinker (GSS) A81.82
Gianotti-Crosti L44.4
giant platelet (Bernard-Soulier) D69.1
Gilles de la Tourette's F95.2
goiter-deafness E07.1
Goldberg Q89.8
Goldberg-Maxwell E34.51
Good's D83.8
Gopalan' (burning feet) E53.8
Gorlin's Q87.89
Gougerot-Blum L81.7
Gouley's I31.1
Gower's R55
gray or grey (newborn) P93.0
  platelet D69.1
Gubler-Millard G46.3
Guillain-Barré (-Strohl) G61.0
gustatory sweating G50.8
Hadfield-Clarke K86.89
hair tourniquet — *see* Constriction, external, by site
Hamman's J98.19
hand-foot L27.1
hand-shoulder G90.8
hantavirus (cardio) -pulmonary (HPS)
  (HCPS) B33.4
happy puppet Q93.5
Harada's H30.81-
Hayem-Faber D50.9
headache NEC G44.89
  complicated NEC G44.59
Heberden's I20.8
Hedinger's E34.0
Hegglin's D72.0
HELLP (hemolysis, elevated liver enzymes and low
  platelet count) O14.2-
  complicating
    childbirth O14.24
    puerperium O14.25
hemolytic-uremic D59.3
hemophagocytic, infection-associated D76.2
Henoch-Schönlein D69.0
hepatic flexure K59.8
hepatopulmonary K76.81
hepatorenal K76.7
  following delivery O90.4
  postoperative or postprocedural K91.83
  postpartum, puerperal O90.4
hepatourologic K76.7
Herter (-Gee) (nontropical sprue) K90.0
Heubner-Herter K90.0
Heyd's K76.7
Hilger's G90.09
histamine-like (fish poisoning) — *see* Poisoning,
  fish
histiocytic D76.3
histiocytosis NEC D76.3
HIV infection, acute B20
Hoffmann-Werdnig G12.0
Hollander-Simons E88.1
Hoppe-Goldflam G70.00
  with exacerbation (acute) G70.01
  in crisis G70.01
Horner's G90.2
hungry bone E83.81
hunterian glossitis D51.0
Hutchinson's triad A50.53
hyperabduction G54.0
hyperammonemia-hyperornithinemia-
  homocitrullinemia E72.4
hypereosinophilic (idiopathic) D72.1
hyperimmunoglobulin D M04.1
hyperimmunoglobulin E (IgE) D82.4
hyperkalemic E87.5
hyperkinetic — *see* Hyperkinesia
hypermobility M35.7
hypernatremia E87.0
hyperosmolarity E87.0
hyperperfusion G97.82
hypersplenic D73.1
hypertransfusion, newborn P61.1
hyperventilation F45.8

Syndrome - *continued*
hypervicosity (of serum)
  polycythemic D75.1
  sclerothymic D58.8
hypoglycemic (familial) (neonatal) E16.2
hypokalemic E87.6
hyponatremic E87.1
hypopituitarism E23.0
hypoplastic left-heart Q23.4
hypopotassemia E87.6
hyposmolality E87.1
hypotension, maternal O26.5-
hypothenar hammer I73.89
hypoventilation, obesity (OHS) E66.2
ICF (intravascular coagulation-fibrinolysis) D65
idiopathic
  cardiorespiratory distress, newborn P22.0
  nephrotic (infantile) N04.9
iliotibial band M76.3-
immobility, immobilization (paraplegic) M62.3
immune reconstitution D89.3
immune reconstitution inflammatory [IRIS] D89.3
immunity deficiency, combined D81.9
immunodeficiency
  acquired — *see* Human, immunodeficiency virus
    (HIV) disease
  combined D81.9
impending coronary I20.0
impingement, shoulder M75.4-
inappropriate secretion of antidiuretic
    hormone E22.2
infant
  of diabetic mother P70.1
  gestational diabetes P70.0
infantilism (pituitary) E23.0
inferior vena cava I87.1
inspissated bile (newborn) P59.1
institutional (childhood) F94.2
insufficient sleep F51.12
intermediate coronary (artery) I20.0
interspinous ligament — *see* Spondylopathy,
    specified NEC
intestinal
  carcinoid E34.0
  knot K56.2
intravascular coagulation-fibrinolysis (ICF) D65
iodine-deficiency, congenital E00.9
  type
    mixed E00.2
    myxedematous E00.1
    neurological E00.0
IRDS (idiopathic respiratory distress,
    newborn) P22.0
irritable
  bowel K58.9
    with
      constipation K58.1
      diarrhea K58.0
    mixed K58.2
    psychogenic F45.8
    specified NEC K58.8
  heart (psychogenic) F45.8
  weakness F48.8
ischemic
  bowel (transient) K55.9
    chronic K55.1
    due to mesenteric artery insufficiency K55.1
  steal T82.898
IVC (intravascular coagulopathy) D65
Ivemark's Q89.01
Jaccoud's — *see* Arthropathy, postrheumatic,
    chronic
Jackson's G83.89
Jakob-Creutzfeldt — *see* Creutzfeldt-Jakob disease
    or syndrome
jaw-winking Q07.8
Jervell-Lange-Nielsen I45.81
jet lag G47.25
Job's D71
Joseph-Diamond-Blackfan D61.01
jugular foramen G52.7
Kabuki Q89.8
Kanner's (autism) F84.0
Kartagener's Q89.3
Kelly's D50.1
Kimmelstiel-Wilson — *see* Diabetes, specified type,
    with Kimmelstiel-Wilson disease
Klein (e) -Levine G47.13
Klippel-Feil (brevicollis) Q76.1
Köhler-Pellegrini-Steida — *see* Bursitis, tibial
    collateral
König's K59.8
Korsakoff (-Wernicke) (nonalcoholic) F04

Syndrome - *continued*
Korsakoff (-Wernicke) (nonalcoholic) - *continued*
  alcoholic F10.26
Kostmann's D70.0
Krabbe's congenital muscle hypoplasia Q79.8
labyrinthine — *see* subcategory H83.2
lacunar NEC G46.7
Lambert-Eaton G70.80
  in
    neoplastic disease G73.1
    specified disease NEC G70.81
Landau-Kleffner — *see* Epilepsy, specified NEC
Larsen's Q74.8
lateral
  cutaneous nerve of thigh G57.1-
  medullary G46.4
Launois' E22.0
lazy
  leukocyte D70.8
  posture M62.3
Lemiere I80.8
Lennox-Gastaut G40.812
  intractable G40.814
    with status epilepticus G40.813
    without status epilepticus G40.814
  not intractable G40.812
    with status epilepticus G40.811
    without status epilepticus G40.812
lenticular, progressive E83.01
Leopold-Levi's E05.90
Lev's I44.2
Li-Fraumeni Z15.01
Lichtheim's D51.0
Lightwood's N25.89
Lignac (de Toni) (-Fanconi) (-Debré) E72.09
  with cystinosis E72.04
Likoff's I20.8
limbic epilepsy personality F07.0
liver-kidney K76.7
lobotomy F07.0
Loffler's J82
long arm 18 or 21 deletion Q93.89
long QT I45.81
Louis-Barré G11.3
low
  atmospheric pressure T70.29
  back M54.5
  output (cardiac) I50.9
lower radicular, newborn (birth injury) P14.8
Luetscher's (dehydration) E86.0
Lupus anticoagulant D68.62
Lutembacher's Q21.1
macrophage activation D76.1
  due to infection D76.2
magnesium-deficiency R29.0
Majeed M04.8
Mal de Debarquement R42
malabsorption K90.9
  postsurgical K91.2
malformation, congenital, due to
  alcohol Q86.0
  exogenous cause NEC Q86.8
  hydantoin Q86.1
  warfarin Q86.2
malignant
  carcinoid E34.0
  neuroleptic G21.0
Mallory-Weiss K22.6
mandibulofacial dysostosis Q75.4
manic-depressive — *see* Disorder, bipolar
maple-syrup-urine E71.0
Marable's I77.4
Marfan's Q87.40
  with
    cardiovascular manifestations Q87.418
      aortic dilation Q87.410
    ocular manifestations Q87.42
    skeletal manifestations Q87.43
Marie's (acromegaly) E22.0
mast cell activation — *see* Activation, mast cell
maternal hypotension — *see* Syndrome,
    hypotension, maternal
May (-Hegglin) D72.0
McArdle (-Schmidt) (-Pearson) E74.04
McQuarrie's E16.2
meconium plug (newborn) P76.0
median arcuate ligament I77.4
Meekeren-Ehlers-Danlos Q79.6
megavitamin-B6 E67.2
Meige G24.4
MELAS E88.41
Mendelson's O74.0

Syndrome - *continued*
MERRF (myoclonic epilepsy associated with ragged
    -red fibers) E88.42
mesenteric
  artery (superior) K55.1
  vascular insufficiency K55.1
metabolic E88.81
metastatic carcinoid E34.0
micrognathia-glossoptosis Q87.0
midbrain NEC G93.89
middle lobe (lung) J98.19
middle radicular G54.0
migraine — *see also* Migraine G43.909-
Mikulicz' K11.8
milk-alkali E83.52
Millard-Gubler G46.3
Miller-Dieker Q93.88
Miller-Fisher G61.0
Minkowski-Chauffard D58.0
Mirizzi's K83.1
MNGIE (Mitochondrial Neurogastrointestinal
    Encephalopathy) E88.49
Möbius, ophthalmoplegic migraine — *see* Migraine,
    ophthalmoplegic
monofixation H50.42
Morel-Moore M85.2
Morel-Morgagni M85.2
Morgagni (-Morel) (-Stewart) M85.2
Morgagni-Adams-Stokes I45.9
Muckle-Wells M04.2
mucocutaneous lymph node (acute febrile)
    (MCLS) M30.3
multiple endocrine neoplasia (MEN) — *see*
    Neoplasia, endocrine, multiple (MEN)
multiple operations — *see* Disorder, factitious
Mounier-Kuhn Q32.4
  with bronchiectasis J47.9
    with
      exacerbation (acute) J47.1
      lower respiratory infection J47.0
  acquired J98.09
    with bronchiectasis J47.9
      with
        exacerbation (acute) J47.1
        lower respiratory infection J47.0
myasthenic G70.9
  in
    diabetes mellitus — *see* Diabetes, amyotrophy
    endocrine disease NEC E34.9 *[G73.3]*
    neoplastic disease — *see*
      also Neoplasm D49.9 *[G73.3]*
    thyrotoxicosis (hyperthyroidism) E05.90 *[G73.3]*
      with thyroid storm E05.91 *[G73.3]*
myelodysplastic D46.9
  with
    5q deletion D46.C
    isolated del (5q) chromosomal
      abnormality D46.C
  lesions, low grade D46.20
  specified NEC D46.Z
myelopathic pain G89.0
myeloproliferative (chronic) D47.1
myofascial pain M79.1
Naffziger's G54.0
nail patella Q87.2
NARP (Neuropathy, Ataxia and Retinitis
    pigmentosa) E88.49
neonatal abstinence P96.1
nephritic — *see also* Nephritis
  with edema — *see* Nephrosis
  acute N00.9
  chronic N03.9
  rapidly progressive N01.9
nephrotic (congenital) — *see also* Nephrosis N04.9
  with
    dense deposit disease N04.6
    diffuse
      crescentic glomerulonephritis N04.7
      endocapillary proliferative
        glomerulonephritis N04.4
      membranous glomerulonephritis N04.2
      mesangial proliferative
        glomerulonephritis N04.3
      mesangiocapillary glomerulonephritis N04.5
    focal and segmental glomerular lesions N04.1
    minor glomerular abnormality N04.0
    specified morphological changes NEC N04.8
  diabetic — *see* Diabetes, nephrosis
neurologic neglect R41.4
Nezelof's D81.4
Nonne-Milroy-Meige Q82.0
Nothnagel's vasomotor acroparesthesia I73.89
obesity hypoventilation (OHS) E66.2

Syndrome - *continued*
oculomotor H51.9
ophthalmoplegia-cerebellar ataxia — *see*
  Strabismus, paralytic, third nerve
oral allergy T78.1
oral-facial-digital Q87.0
organic
  affective F06.30
  amnesic (not alcohol- or drug-induced) F04
  brain F09
  depressive F06.31
  hallucinosis F06.0
  personality F07.0
Ormond's N13.5
oro-facial-digital Q87.0
os trigonum Q68.8
Osler-Weber-Rendu I78.0
osteoporosis-osteomalacia M83.8
Osterreicher-Turner Q87.2
otolith — *see* subcategory H81.8
oto-palatal-digital Q87.0
outlet (thoracic) G54.0
ovary
  polycystic E28.2
  resistant E28.39
  sclerocystic E28.2
Owren's D68.2
Paget-Schroetter I82.890
pain — *see also* Pain
  complex regional I G90.50
    lower limb G90.52-
      specified site NEC G90.59
    upper limb G90.51-
  complex regional II — *see* Causalgia
painful
  bruising D69.2
  feet E53.8
  prostate N42.81
paralysis agitans — *see* Parkinsonism
paralytic G83.9
  specified NEC G83.89
Parinaud's H51.0
parkinsonian — *see* Parkinsonism
Parkinson's — *see* Parkinsonism
paroxysmal facial pain G50.0
Parry's E05.00
  with thyroid storm E05.01
Parsonage (-Aldren) -Turner G54.5
patella clunk M25.86-
Paterson (-Brown) (-Kelly) D50.1
pectoral girdle I77.89
pectoralis minor I77.89
Pelger-Huet D72.0
pellagra-cerebellar ataxia-renal
  aminoaciduria E72.02
pellagroid E52
Pellegrini-Stieda — *see* Bursitis, tibial collateral
pelvic congestion-fibrosis, female N94.89
penta X Q97.1
peptic ulcer — *see* Ulcer, peptic
perabduction I77.89
periodic fever M04.1
periodic fever, aphthous stomatitis, pharyngitis, and
  adenopathy [PFAPA] M04.8
periodic headache, in adults and children — *see*
  Headache, periodic syndromes in adults and
  children
periurethral fibrosis N13.5
phantom limb (without pain) G54.7
  with pain G54.6
pharyngeal pouch D82.1
Pick's — *see* Disease, Pick's
Pickwickian E66.2
PIE (pulmonary infiltration with eosinophilia) J82
pigmentary pallidal degeneration
  (progressive) G23.0
pineal E34.8
pituitary E22.0
plantar fascia M72.2
placental transfusion — *see* Pregnancy, complicated
  by, placental transfusion syndromes
plateau iris (post-iridectomy)
  (postprocedural) H21.82
Plummer-Vinson D50.1
pluricarential of infancy E40
plurideficiency E40
pluriglandular (compensatory) E31.8
  autoimmune E31.0
pneumatic hammer T75.21
polyangiitis overlap M30.8
polycarential of infancy E40
polyglandular E31.8
  autoimmune E31.0

Syndrome - *continued*
polysplenia Q89.09
pontine NEC G93.89
popliteal
  artery entrapment I77.89
  web Q87.89
postcardiac injury
  postcardiotomy I97.0
  postmyocardial infarction I24.1
postcardiotomy I97.0
post chemoembolization - code to associated
  conditions
postcholecystectomy K91.5
postcommissurotomy I97.0
postconcussional F07.81
postcontusional F07.81
postencephalitic F07.89
posterior
  cervical sympathetic M53.0
  cord G83.83
  fossa compression G93.5
  reversible encephalopathy (PRES) I67.83
postgastrectomy (dumping) K91.1
postgastric surgery K91.1
postinfarction I24.1
postlaminectomy NEC M96.1
postleukotomy F07.0
postmastectomy lymphedema I97.2
postmyocardial infarction I24.1
postoperative NEC T81.9
  blind loop K90.2
postpartum panhypopituitary (Sheehan) E23.0
postpolio (myelitic) G14
postthrombotic I87.009
  with
    inflammation I87.02-
      with ulcer I87.03-
    specified complication NEC I87.09-
    ulcer I87.01-
      with inflammation I87.03-
  asymptomatic I87.00-
postvagotomy K91.1
postvalvulotomy I97.0
postviral NEC G93.3
  fatigue G93.3
Potain's K31.0
potassium intoxication E87.5
precerebral artery (multiple) (bilateral) G45.2
preinfarction I20.0
preleukemic D46.9
premature senility E34.8
premenstrual dysphoric F32.89
premenstrual tension N94.3
Prinzmetal-Massumi R07.1
prune belly Q79.4
pseudocarpal tunnel (sublimis) — *see* Syndrome,
  carpal tunnel
pseudoparalytica G70.00
  with exacerbation (acute) G70.01
  in crisis G70.01
pseudo -Turner's Q87.1
psycho-organic (nonpsychotic severity) F07.9
  acute or subacute F05
  depressive type F06.31
  hallucinatory type F06.0
  nonpsychotic severity F07.0
  specified NEC F07.89
pulmonary
  arteriosclerosis I27.0
  dysmaturity (Wilson-Mikity) P27.0
  hypoperfusion (idiopathic) P22.0
  renal (hemorrhagic) (Goodpasture's) M31.0
pure
  motor lacunar G46.5
  sensory lacunar G46.6
Putnam-Dana D51.0
pyogenic arthritis, pyoderma gangrenosum, and acne
  [PAPA] M04.8
pyramidopallidonigral G20
pyriformis — *see* Lesion, nerve, sciatic
QT interval prolongation I45.81
radicular NEC — *see* Radiculopathy
  upper limbs, newborn (birth injury) P14.3
rapid time-zone change G47.25
Rasmussen G04.81
Raymond (-Céstan) I65.8
Raynaud's I73.00
  with gangrene I73.01
RDS (respiratory distress syndrome, newborn) P22.0
reactive airways dysfunction J68.3
Refsum's G60.1
Reifenstein E34.52

Syndrome - *continued*
renal glomerulohyalinosis-diabetic — *see* Diabetes,
  nephrosis
Rendu-Osler-Weber I78.0
residual ovary N99.83
resistant ovary E28.39
respiratory
  distress
    acute J80
    adult J80
    child J80
    idiopathic J84.114
    newborn (idiopathic) (type I) P22.0
    type II P22.1
restless legs G25.81
retinoblastoma (familial) C69.2
retroperitoneal fibrosis N13.5
retroviral seroconversion (acute) Z21
Reye's G93.7
Richter — *see* Leukemia, chronic lymphocytic, B-
  cell type
Ridley's I50.1
right
  heart, hypoplastic Q22.6
  ventricular obstruction — *see* Failure, heart,
    congestive
Romano-Ward (prolonged QT interval) I45.81
rotator cuff, shoulder — *see also* Tear, rotator
  cuff M75.10-
Rotes Quérol — *see* Hyperostosis, ankylosing
Roth — *see* Meralgia paresthetica
rubella (congenital) P35.0
Ruvalcaba-Myhre-Smith E71.440
Rytand-Lipsitch I44.2
salt
  depletion E87.1
    due to heat NEC T67.8
      causing heat exhaustion or prostration T67.4
  low E87.1
salt-losing N28.89
Scaglietti-Dagnini E22.0
scalenus anticus (anterior) G54.0
scapulocostal — *see* Mononeuropathy, upper limb,
  specified site NEC
scapuloperoneal G71.0
schizophrenic, of childhood NEC F84.5
Schnitzler D47.2
Scholte's E34.0
Schroeder's E27.0
Schüller-Christian C96.5
Schwachman's — *see* Syndrome, Shwachman's
Schwartz (-Jampel) G71.13
Schwartz-Bartter E22.2
scimitar Q26.8
sclerocystic ovary E28.2
Seitelberger's G31.89
septicemic adrenal hemorrhage A39.1
seroconversion, retroviral (acute) Z21
serous meningitis G93.2
severe acute respiratory (SARS) J12.81
shaken infant T74.4
shock (traumatic) T79.4
  kidney N17.0
    following crush injury T79.5
  toxic A48.3
shock-lung J80
Shone's - code to specific anomalies
short
  bowel K91.2
  rib Q77.2
shoulder-hand — *see* Algoneurodystrophy
Shwachman's D70.4
sicca — *see* Sicca syndrome
sick
  cell E87.1
  sinus I49.5
sick-euthyroid E07.81
sideropenic D50.1
Siemens' ectodermal dysplasia Q82.4
Silfversköld's Q78.9
Simons' E88.1
sinus tarsi M25.57-
sinusitis-bronchiectasis-situs inversus Q89.3
Sipple's E31.22
sirenomelia Q87.2
Slocumb's E27.0
slow flow, coronary I20.8
Sluder's G44.89
Smith-Magenis Q93.88
Sneddon-Wilkinson L13.1
Soto's Q87.3
South African cardiomyopathy I42.8
spasmodic

Syndrome - *continued*
  spasmodic - *continued*
    upward movement, eyes H51.8
    winking F95.8
  Spen's I45.9
  splenic
    agenesis Q89.01
    flexure K59.8
    neutropenia D73.81
  Spurway's Q78.0
  staphylococcal scalded skin L00
  steal
    arteriovenous T82.898-
    ischemic T82.898-
    subclavian G45.8
  Stein-Leventhal E28.2
  Stein's E28.2
  Stevens-Johnson syndrome L51.1
    toxic epidermal necrolysis overlap L51.3
  Stewart-Morel M85.2
  Stickler Q89.8
  stiff baby Q89.8
  stiff man G25.82
  Still-Felty — *see* Felty's syndrome
  Stokes (-Adams) I45.9
  stone heart I50.1
  straight back, congenital Q76.49
  subclavian steal G45.8
  subcoracoid-pectoralis minor G54.0
  subcostal nerve compression I77.89
  subphrenic interposition Q43.3
  superior
    cerebellar artery I63.8
    mesenteric artery K55.1
    semi-circular canal dehiscence H83.8X-
    vena cava I87.1
  supine hypotensive (maternal) — *see* Syndrome, hypotension, maternal
  suprarenal cortical E27.0
  supraspinatus — *see also* Tear, rotator cuff M75.10-
  Susac G93.49
  swallowed blood P78.2
  sweat retention L74.0
  Swyer Q99.1
  Symond's G93.2
  sympathetic
    cervical paralysis G90.2
    pelvic, female N94.89
  systemic inflammatory response (SIRS) , of non-infectious origin (without organ dysfunction) R65.10
    with acute organ dysfunction R65.11
  tachycardia-bradycardia I49.5
  takotsubo I51.81
  TAR (thrombocytopenia with absent radius) Q87.2
  tarsal tunnel G57.5-
  teething K00.7
  tegmental G93.89
  telangiectasic-pigmentation-cataract Q82.8
  temporal pyramidal apex — *see* Otitis, media, suppurative, acute
  temporomandibular joint-pain-dysfunction M26.62-
  Terry's H44.2-
  testicular feminization — *see also* Syndrome, androgen insensitivity E34.51
  thalamic pain (hyperesthetic) G89.0
  thoracic outlet (compression) G54.0
  Thorson-Björck E34.0
  thrombocytopenia with absent radius (TAR) Q87.2
  thyroid-adrenocortical insufficiency E31.0
  tibial
    anterior M76.81-
    posterior M76.82-
  Tietze's M94.0
  time-zone (rapid) G47.25
  Toni-Fanconi E72.09
    with cystinosis E72.04
  Touraine's Q79.8
  tourniquet — *see* Constriction, external, by site
  toxic shock A48.3
  transient left ventricular apical ballooning I51.81
  traumatic vasospastic T75.22
  Treacher Collins Q75.4
  triple X, female Q97.0
  trisomy Q92.9
    13 Q91.7
      meiotic nondisjunction Q91.4
      mitotic nondisjunction Q91.5
      mosaicism Q91.5
      translocation Q91.6
    18 Q91.3
      meiotic nondisjunction Q91.0
      mitotic nondisjunction Q91.1

Syndrome - *continued*
  trisomy - *continued*
    18 - *continued*
      mosaicism Q91.1
      translocation Q91.2
    20 (q) (p) Q92.8
    21 Q90.9
      meiotic nondisjunction Q90.0
      mitotic nondisjunction Q90.1
      mosaicism Q90.1
      translocation Q90.2
    22 Q92.8
  tropical wet feet T69.0-
  Trousseau's I82.1
  tumor lysis (following antineoplastic chemotherapy) (spontaneous) NEC E88.3
  tumor necrosis factor receptor associated periodic (TRAPS) M04.1
  Twiddler's (due to)
    automatic implantable defibrillator T82.198
    cardiac pacemaker T82.198
  Unverricht (-Lundborg) — *see* Epilepsy, generalized, idiopathic
  upward gaze H51.8
  uremia, chronic — *see also* Disease, kidney, chronic N18.9
  urethral N34.3
  urethro-oculo-articular — *see* Reiter's disease
  urohepatic K76.7
  vago-hypoglossal G52.7
  vascular NEC in cerebrovascular disease G46.8
  vasoconstriction, reversible cerebrovascular I67.841
  vasomotor I73.9
  vasospastic (traumatic) T75.22
  vasovagal R55
  van Buchem's M85.2
  van der Hoeve's Q78.0
  VATER Q87.2
  velo-cardio-facial Q93.81
  vena cava (inferior) (superior) (obstruction) I87.1
  vertebral
    artery G45.0
    compression — *see* Syndrome, anterior, spinal artery, compression
    steal G45.0
  vertebro-basilar artery G45.0
  vertebrogenic (pain) M54.89
  vertiginous — *see* Disorder, vestibular function
  Vinson-Plummer D50.1
  virus B34.9
  visceral larva migrans B83.0
  visual disorientation H53.8
  vitamin B6 deficiency E53.1
  vitreal corneal H59.01-
  vitreous (touch) H59.01-
  Vogt-Koyanagi H20.82-
  Volkmann's T79.6
  von Schroetter's I82.890
  von Willebrand (-Jürgen) D68.0
  Waldenström-Kjellberg D50.1
  Wallenberg's G46.3
  water retention E87.79
  Waterhouse (-Friderichsen) A39.1
  Weber-Gubler G46.3
  Weber-Leyden G46.3
  Weber's G46.3
  Wegener's M31.30
    with
      kidney involvement M31.31
      lung involvement M31.30
        with kidney involvement M31.31
  Weingarten's (tropical eosinophilia) J82
  Weiss-Baker G90.09
  Werdnig-Hoffman G12.0
  Wermer's E31.21
  Werner's E34.8
  Wernicke-Korsakoff (nonalcoholic) F04
    alcoholic F10.26
  West's — *see* Epilepsy, spasms
  Westphal-Strümpell E83.01
  wet
    feet (maceration) (tropical) T69.0-
    lung, newborn P22.1
  whiplash S13.4
  whistling face Q87.0
  Wilkie's K55.1
  Wilkinson-Sneddon L13.1
  Willebrand (-Jürgens) D68.0
  Wilson's (hepatolenticular degeneration) E83.01
  Wiskott-Aldrich D82.0
  withdrawal — *see* Withdrawal, state
    drug
      infant of dependent mother P96.1

Syndrome - *continued*
  withdrawal - *continued*
    drug - *continued*
      therapeutic use, newborn P96.2
  Woakes' (ethmoiditis) J33.1
  Wright's (hyperabduction) I77.89
  X I20.9
  XXXX Q97.1
  XXXXX Q97.1
  XXXXY Q98.1
  XXY Q98.0
  yellow nail L60.5
  Zahorsky's B08.5
  Zellweger syndrome E71.510
  Zellweger-like syndrome E71.541
Synechia (anterior) (iris) (posterior) (pupil) — *see also* Adhesions, iris
  intra-uterine (traumatic) N85.6
Synesthesia R20.8
Syngamiasis, syngamosis B83.3
Synodontia K00.2
Synorchidism, synorchism Q55.1
Synostosis (congenital) Q78.8
  astragalo-scaphoid Q74.2
  radioulnar Q74.0
Synovial sarcoma — *see* Neoplasm, connective tissue, malignant
Synovioma (malignant) — *see also* Neoplasm, connective tissue, malignant
  benign — *see* Neoplasm, connective tissue, benign
Synoviosarcoma — *see* Neoplasm, connective tissue, malignant
Synovitis — *see also* Tenosynovitis M65.9
  crepitant
    hand M70.0-
    wrist M70.03-
  gonococcal A54.49
  gouty — *see* Gout
  in (due to)
    crystals M65.8-
    gonorrhea A54.49
    syphilis (late) A52.78
    use, overuse, pressure — *see* Disorder, soft tissue, due to use
  infective NEC — *see* Tenosynovitis, infective NEC
  specified NEC — *see* Tenosynovitis, specified type NEC
  syphilitic A52.78
    congenital (early) A50.02
  toxic — *see* Synovitis, transient
  transient M67.3-
    ankle M67.37-
    elbow M67.32-
    foot joint M67.37-
    hand joint M67.34-
    hip M67.35-
    knee M67.36-
    multiple site M67.39
    pelvic region M67.35-
    shoulder M67.31-
    specified joint NEC M67.38
    wrist M67.33-
  traumatic, current — *see* Sprain
  tuberculous — *see* Tuberculosis, synovitis
  villonodular (pigmented) M12.2-
    ankle M12.27-
    elbow M12.22-
    foot joint M12.27-
    hand joint M12.24-
    hip M12.25-
    knee M12.26-
    multiple site M12.29
    pelvic region M12.25-
    shoulder M12.21-
    specified joint NEC M12.28
    vertebrae M12.28
    wrist M12.23-
Syphilid A51.39
  congenital A50.06
  newborn A50.06
  tubercular (late) A52.79
Syphilis, syphilitic (acquired) A53.9
  abdomen (late) A52.79
  acoustic nerve A52.15
  adenopathy (secondary) A51.49
  adrenal (gland) (with cortical hypofunction) A52.79
  age under 2 years NOS — *see also* Syphilis, congenital, early
    acquired A51.9
  alopecia (secondary) A51.32
  anemia (late) A52.79 [D63.8]
  aneurysm (aorta) (ruptured) A52.01
    central nervous system A52.05

Syphilis, syphilitic (acquired) - *continued*
aneurysm (aorta) (ruptured) - *continued*
  congenital A50.54 *[I79.0]*
anus (late) A52.74
  primary A51.1
  secondary A51.39
aorta (arch) (abdominal) (thoracic) A52.02
  aneurysm A52.01
aortic (insufficiency) (regurgitation)
    (stenosis) A52.03
  aneurysm A52.01
arachnoid (adhesive) (cerebral) (spinal) A52.13
asymptomatic — *see* Syphilis, latent
ataxia (locomotor) A52.11
atrophoderma maculatum A51.39
auricular fibrillation A52.06
bladder (late) A52.76
bone A52.77
  secondary A51.46
brain A52.17
breast (late) A52.79
bronchus (late) A52.72
bubo (primary) A51.0
bulbar palsy A52.19
bursa (late) A52.78
cardiac decompensation A52.06
cardiovascular A52.00
central nervous system (late) (recurrent) (relapse)
    (tertiary) A52.3
  with
    ataxia A52.11
    general paralysis A52.17
      juvenile A50.45
    paresis (general) A52.17
      juvenile A50.45
    tabes (dorsalis) A52.11
      juvenile A50.45
    taboparesis A52.17
      juvenile A50.45
  aneurysm A52.05
  congenital A50.40
    juvenile A50.40
  remission in (sustained) A52.3
  serology doubtful, negative, or positive A52.3
  specified nature or site NEC A52.19
  vascular A52.05
cerebral A52.17
  meningovascular A52.13
  nerves (multiple palsies) A52.15
  sclerosis A52.17
  thrombosis A52.05
cerebrospinal (tabetic type) A52.12
cerebrovascular A52.05
cervix (late) A52.76
chancre (multiple) A51.0
  extragenital A51.2
  Rollet's A51.0
Charcot's joint A52.16
chorioretinitis A51.43
  congenital A50.01
  late A52.71
  prenatal A50.01
choroiditis — *see* Syphilitic chorioretinitis
choroidoretinitis — *see* Syphilitic chorioretinitis
ciliary body (secondary) A51.43
  late A52.71
colon (late) A52.74
combined spinal sclerosis A52.11
condyloma (latum) A51.31
congenital A50.9
  with
    paresis (general) A50.45
    tabes (dorsalis) A50.45
    taboparesis A50.45
  chorioretinitis, choroiditis A50.01 *[H32]*
  early, or less than 2 years after birth NEC A50.2
    with manifestations — *see* Syphilis, congenital,
      early, symptomatic
    latent (without manifestations) A50.1
      negative spinal fluid test A50.1
      serology positive A50.1
    symptomatic A50.09
      cutaneous A50.06
      mucocutaneous A50.07
      oculopathy A50.01
      osteochondropathy A50.02
      pharyngitis A50.03
      pneumonia A50.04
      rhinitis A50.05
      visceral A50.08
    interstitial keratitis A50.31
    juvenile neurosyphilis A50.45
    late, or 2 years or more after birth NEC A50.7

Syphilis, syphilitic (acquired) - *continued*
congenital - *continued*
  late, or 2 years or more after birth NEC - *continued*
    chorioretinitis, choroiditis A50.32
    interstitial keratitis A50.31
    juvenile neurosyphilis A50.45
    latent (without manifestations) A50.6
      negative spinal fluid test A50.6
      serology positive A50.6
    symptomatic or with manifestations NEC A50.59
      arthropathy A50.55
      cardiovascular A50.54
      Clutton's joints A50.51
      Hutchinson's teeth A50.52
      Hutchinson's triad A50.53
      osteochondropathy A50.56
      saddle nose A50.57
conjugal A53.9
  tabes A52.11
conjunctiva (late) A52.71
contact Z20.2
cord bladder A52.19
cornea, late A52.71
coronary (artery) (sclerosis) A52.06
coryza, congenital A50.05
cranial nerve A52.15
  multiple palsies A52.15
cutaneous — *see* Syphilis, skin
dacryocystitis (late) A52.71
degeneration, spinal cord A52.12
dementia paralytica A52.17
  juvenilis A50.45
destruction of bone A52.77
dilatation, aorta A52.01
due to blood transfusion A53.9
dura mater A52.13
ear A52.79
  inner A52.79
    nerve (eighth) A52.15
    neurorecurrence A52.15
early A51.9
  cardiovascular A52.00
  central nervous system A52.3
  latent (without manifestations) (less than 2 years
      after infection) A51.5
    negative spinal fluid test A51.5
    serological relapse after treatment A51.5
    serology positive A51.5
  relapse (treated, untreated) A51.9
  skin A51.39
  symptomatic A51.9
    extragenital chancre A51.2
    primary, except extragenital chancre A51.0
    secondary — *see also* Syphilis, secondary A51.39
      relapse (treated, untreated) A51.49
  ulcer A51.39
eighth nerve (neuritis) A52.15
endemic A65
endocarditis A52.03
  aortic A52.03
  pulmonary A52.03
epididymis (late) A52.76
epiglottis (late) A52.73
epiphysitis (congenital) (early) A50.02
episcleritis (late) A52.71
esophagus A52.79
eustachian tube A52.73
exposure to Z20.2
eye A52.71
eyelid (late) (with gumma) A52.71
fallopian tube (late) A52.76
fracture A52.77
gallbladder (late) A52.74
gastric (polyposis) (late) A52.74
general A53.9
  paralysis A52.17
    juvenile A50.45
  genital (primary) A51.0
glaucoma A52.71
gumma NEC A52.79
  cardiovascular system A52.00
  central nervous system A52.3
  congenital A50.59
heart (block) (decompensation) (disease)
    (failure) A52.06 *[I52]*
  valve NEC A52.03
hemianesthesia A52.19
hemianopsia A52.71
hemiparesis A52.17
hemiplegia A52.17
hepatic artery A52.09
hepatis A52.74
hepatomegaly, congenital A50.08

Syphilis, syphilitic (acquired) - *continued*
hereditaria tarda — *see* Syphilis, congenital, late
hereditary — *see* Syphilis, congenital
Hutchinson's teeth A50.52
hyalitis A52.71
inactive — *see* Syphilis, latent
infantum — *see* Syphilis, congenital
inherited — *see* Syphilis, congenital
internal ear A52.79
intestine (late) A52.74
iris, iritis (secondary) A51.43
  late A52.71
joint (late) A52.77
keratitis (congenital) (interstitial) (late) A50.31
kidney (late) A52.75
lacrimal passages (late) A52.71
larynx (late) A52.73
late A52.9
  cardiovascular A52.00
  central nervous system A52.3
  kidney A52.75
  latent or 2 years or more after infection (without
    manifestations) A52.8
    negative spinal fluid test A52.8
    serology positive A52.8
  paresis A52.17
  specified site NEC A52.79
  symptomatic or with manifestations A52.79
  tabes A52.11
latent A53.0
  with signs or symptoms - code by site and stage
    under Syphilis
  central nervous system A52.2
  date of infection unspecified A53.0
  early, or less than 2 years after infection A51.5
  follow-up of latent syphilis A53.0
    date of infection unspecified A53.0
    late, or 2 years or more after infection A52.8
  late, or 2 years or more after infection A52.8
  positive serology (only finding) A53.0
    date of infection unspecified A53.0
    early, or less than 2 years after infection A51.5
    late, or 2 years or more after infection A52.8
lens (late) A52.71
leukoderma A51.39
  late A52.79
lienitis A52.79
lip A51.39
  chancre (primary) A51.2
  late A52.79
Lissauer's paralysis A52.17
liver A52.74
locomotor ataxia A52.11
lung A52.72
lymph gland (early) (secondary) A51.49
  late A52.79
lymphadenitis (secondary) A51.49
macular atrophy of skin A51.39
  striated A52.79
mediastinum (late) A52.73
meninges (adhesive) (brain) (spinal cord) A52.13
meningitis A52.13
  acute (secondary) A51.41
  congenital A50.41
meningoencephalitis A52.14
meningovascular A52.13
  congenital A50.41
mesarteritis A52.09
  brain A52.04
middle ear A52.77
mitral stenosis A52.03
monoplegia A52.17
mouth (secondary) A51.39
  late A52.79
mucocutaneous (secondary) A51.39
  late A52.79
mucous
  membrane (secondary) A51.39
    late A52.79
  patches A51.39
    congenital A50.07
mulberry molars A50.52
muscle A52.78
myocardium A52.06
nasal sinus (late) A52.73
neonatorum — *see* Syphilis, congenital
nephrotic syndrome (secondary) A51.44
nerve palsy (any cranial nerve) A52.15
  multiple A52.15
nervous system, central A52.3
neuritis A52.15
  acoustic A52.15
neurorecidive of retina A52.19

Syphilis, syphilitic (acquired) - *continued*
  neuroretinitis A52.19
  newborn — *see* Syphilis, congenital
  nodular superficial (late) A52.79
  nonvenereal A65
  nose (late) A52.73
    saddle back deformity A50.57
  occlusive arterial disease A52.09
  oculopathy A52.71
  ophthalmic (late) A52.71
  optic nerve (atrophy) (neuritis) (papilla) A52.15
  orbit (late) A52.71
  organic A53.9
  osseous (late) A52.77
  osteochondritis (congenital)
    (early) A50.02 *[M90.80]*
  osteoporosis A52.77
  ovary (late) A52.76
  oviduct (late) A52.76
  palate (late) A52.79
  pancreas (late) A52.74
  paralysis A52.17
    general A52.17
      juvenile A50.45
  paresis (general) A52.17
    juvenile A50.45
  paresthesia A52.19
  Parkinson's disease or syndrome A52.19
  paroxysmal tachycardia A52.06
  pemphigus (congenital) A50.06
  penis (chancre) A51.0
    late A52.76
  pericardium A52.06
  perichondritis, larynx (late) A52.73
  periosteum (late) A52.77
    congenital (early) A50.02 *[M90.80]*
    early (secondary) A51.46
  peripheral nerve A52.79
  petrous bone (late) A52.77
  pharynx (late) A52.73
    secondary A51.39
  pituitary (gland) (late) A52.79
  pleura (late) A52.73
  pneumonia, white A50.04
  pontine lesion A52.17
  portal vein A52.09
  primary A51.0
    anal A51.1
    and secondary — *see* Syphilis, secondary
    central nervous system A52.3
    extragenital chancre NEC A51.2
    fingers A51.2
    genital A51.0
    lip A51.2
    specified site NEC A51.2
    tonsils A51.2
  prostate (late) A52.76
  ptosis (eyelid) A52.71
  pulmonary (late) A52.72
    artery A52.09
  pyelonephritis (late) A52.75
  recently acquired, symptomatic A51.9
  rectum (late) A52.74
  respiratory tract (late) A52.73
  retina, late A52.71
  retrobulbar neuritis A52.15
  salpingitis A52.76
  sclera (late) A52.71
  sclerosis
    cerebral A52.17
    coronary A52.06
    multiple A52.11
  scotoma (central) A52.71
  scrotum (late) A52.76
  secondary (and primary) A51.49
    adenopathy A51.49
    anus A51.39
    bone A51.46
    chorioretinitis, choroiditis A51.43
    hepatitis A51.45
    liver A51.45
    lymphadenitis A51.49
    meningitis (acute) A51.41
    mouth A51.39
    mucous membranes A51.39
    periosteum, periostitis A51.46
    pharynx A51.39
    relapse (treated, untreated) A51.49
    skin A51.39
    specified form NEC A51.49
    tonsil A51.39
    ulcer A51.39
    viscera NEC A51.49

Syphilis, syphilitic (acquired) - *continued*
  secondary (and primary) - *continued*
    vulva A51.39
    seminal vesicle (late) A52.76
    seronegative with signs or symptoms - code by site
      and stage under Syphilis
    seropositive
      with signs or symptoms - code by site and stage
        under Syphilis
      follow-up of latent syphilis — *see* Syphilis, latent
      only finding — *see* Syphilis, latent
    seventh nerve (paralysis) A52.15
    sinus, sinusitis (late) A52.73
    skeletal system A52.77
    skin (with ulceration) (early) (secondary) A51.39
      late or tertiary A52.79
    small intestine A52.74
    spastic spinal paralysis A52.17
    spermatic cord (late) A52.76
    spinal (cord) A52.12
    spleen A52.79
    splenomegaly A52.79
    spondylitis A52.77
    staphyloma A52.71
    stigmata (congenital) A50.59
    stomach A52.74
    synovium A52.78
    tabes dorsalis (late) A52.11
      juvenile A50.45
    tabetic type A52.11
      juvenile A50.45
    taboparesis A52.17
      juvenile A50.45
    tachycardia A52.06
    tendon (late) A52.78
    tertiary A52.9
      with symptoms NEC A52.79
      cardiovascular A52.00
      central nervous system A52.3
      multiple NEC A52.79
      specified site NEC A52.79
    testis A52.76
    thorax A52.73
    throat A52.73
    thymus (gland) (late) A52.79
    thyroid (late) A52.79
    tongue (late) A52.79
    tonsil (lingual) (late) A52.73
      primary A51.2
      secondary A51.39
    trachea (late) A52.73
    tunica vaginalis (late) A52.76
    ulcer (any site) (early) (secondary) A51.39
      late A52.79
      perforating A52.79
        foot A52.11
    urethra (late) A52.76
    urogenital (late) A52.76
    uterus (late) A52.76
    uveal tract (secondary) A51.43
      late A52.71
    uveitis (secondary) A51.43
      late A52.71
    uvula (late) (perforated) A52.79
    vagina A51.0
      late A52.76
    valvulitis NEC A52.03
    vascular A52.00
      brain (cerebral) A52.05
    ventriculi A52.74
    vesicae urinariae (late) A52.76
    viscera (abdominal) (late) A52.74
      secondary A51.49
    vitreous (opacities) (late) A52.71
      hemorrhage A52.71
    vulva A51.0
      late A52.76
      secondary A51.39
Syphiloma A52.79
  cardiovascular system A52.00
  central nervous system A52.3
  circulatory system A52.00
  congenital A50.59
Syphilophobia F45.29
Syringadenoma — *see also* Neoplasm, skin, benign
  papillary — *see* Neoplasm, skin, benign
Syringobulbia G95.0
Syringocystadenoma — *see* Neoplasm, skin, benign
  papillary — *see* Neoplasm, skin, benign
Syringoma — *see also* Neoplasm, skin, benign
  chondroid — *see* Neoplasm, skin, benign
Syringomyelia G95.0
Syringomyelitis — *see* Encephalitis

Syringomyelocele — *see* Spina bifida
Syringopontia G95.0
System, systemic — *see also* condition
  disease, combined — *see* Degeneration, combined
  inflammatory response syndrome (SIRS) of non-
    infectious origin (without organ
    dysfunction) R65.10
    with acute organ dysfunction R65.11
  lupus erythematosus M32.9
    inhibitor present D68.62

T

Tabacism, tabacosis, tabagism — *see*
  also Poisoning, tobacco
  meaning dependence (without remission) F17.200
    with
      disorder F17.299
      remission F17.211
      specified disorder NEC F17.298
      withdrawal F17.203
Tabardillo A75.9
  flea-borne A75.2
  louse-borne A75.0
Tabes, tabetic A52.10
  with
    central nervous system syphilis A52.10
    Charcot's joint A52.16
    cord bladder A52.19
    crisis, viscera (any) A52.19
    paralysis, general A52.17
    paresis (general) A52.17
    perforating ulcer (foot) A52.19
  arthropathy (Charcot) A52.16
  bladder A52.19
  bone A52.11
  cerebrospinal A52.12
  congenital A50.45
  conjugal A52.10
  dorsalis A52.11
    juvenile A50.49
  juvenile A50.49
  latent A52.19
  mesenterica A18.39
  paralysis, insane, general A52.17
  spasmodic A52.17
  syphilis (cerebrospinal) A52.12
Taboparalysis A52.17
Taboparesis (remission) A52.17
  juvenile A50.45
TAC (trigeminal autonomic cephalgia) **NEC** G44.099
  intractable G44.091
  not intractable G44.099
Tache noir S60.22-
Tachyalimentation K91.2
Tachyarrhythmia, tachyrhythmia — *see*
  Tachycardia
Tachycardia R00.0
  atrial (paroxysmal) I47.1
  auricular I47.1
  AV nodal re-entry (re-entrant) I47.1
  junctional (paroxysmal) I47.1
  newborn P29.11
  nodal (paroxysmal) I47.1
  non-paroxysmal AV nodal I45.89
  paroxysmal (sustained) (nonsustained) I47.9
    with sinus bradycardia I49.5
    atrial (PAT) I47.1
    atrioventricular (AV) (re-entrant) I47.1
      psychogenic F54
    junctional I47.1
      ectopic I47.1
    nodal I47.1
    psychogenic (atrial) (supraventricular)
      (ventricular) F54
    supraventricular (sustained) I47.1
      psychogenic F54
    ventricular I47.2
      psychogenic F54
  psychogenic F45.8
  sick sinus I49.5
  sinoauricular NOS R00.0
    paroxysmal I47.1
  sinus [sinusal] NOS R00.0
    paroxysmal I47.1
  supraventricular I47.1
  ventricular (paroxysmal) (sustained) I47.2
    psychogenic F54
Tachygastria K31.89
Tachypnea R06.82
  hysterical F45.8
  newborn (idiopathic) (transitory) P22.1
  psychogenic F45.8
  transitory, of newborn P22.1

TACO (transfusion associated circulatory overload) E87.71
Taenia (infection) (infestation) B68.9
  diminuta B71.0
  echinococcal infestation B67.90
  mediocanellata B68.1
  nana B71.0
  saginata B68.1
  solium (intestinal form) B68.0
    larval form — *see* Cysticercosis
Taeniasis (intestine) — *see* Taenia
Tag (hypertrophied skin) (infected) L91.8
  adenoid J35.8
  anus K64.4
  hemorrhoidal K64.4
  hymen N89.8
  perineal N90.89
  preauricular Q17.0
  sentinel K64.4
  skin L91.8
    accessory (congenital) Q82.8
    anus K64.4
    congenital Q82.8
    preauricular Q17.0
  tonsil J35.8
  urethra, urethral N36.8
  vulva N90.89
Tahyna fever B33.8
Takahara's disease E80.3
Takayasu's disease or syndrome M31.4
Talcosis (pulmonary) J62.0
Talipes (congenital) Q66.89
  acquired, planus — *see* Deformity, limb, flat foot
  asymmetric Q66.89
  calcaneovalgus Q66.4
  calcaneovarus Q66.1
  calcaneus Q66.89
  cavus Q66.7
  equinovalgus Q66.6
  equinovarus Q66.0
  equinus Q66.89
  percavus Q66.7
  planovalgus Q66.6
  planus (acquired) (any degree) — *see also* Deformity, limb, flat foot
    congenital Q66.5-
    due to rickets (sequelae) E64.3
  valgus Q66.6
  varus Q66.3
Tall stature, constitutional E34.4
Talma's disease M62.89
Talon noir S90.3-
  hand S60.22-
  heel S90.3-
  toe S90.1-
Tamponade, heart I31.4
Tanapox (virus disease) B08.71
Tangier disease E78.6
Tantrum, child problem F91.8
Tapeworm (infection) (infestation) — *see* Infestation, tapeworm
Tapia's syndrome G52.7
TAR (thrombocytopenia with absent radius) **syndrome** Q87.2
Tarral-Besnier disease L44.0
Tarsal tunnel syndrome — *see* Syndrome, tarsal tunnel
Tarsalgia — *see* Pain, limb, lower
Tarsitis (eyelid) H01.8
  syphilitic A52.71
  tuberculous A18.4
Tartar (teeth) (dental calculus) K03.6
Tattoo (mark) L81.8
Tauri's disease E74.09
Taurodontism K00.2
Taussig-Bing syndrome Q20.1
Taybi's syndrome Q87.2
Tay-Sachs amaurotic familial idiocy or disease E75.02
TBI (traumatic brain injury) S06.9
Teacher's node or nodule J38.2
Tear, torn (traumatic) — *see also* Laceration
  with abortion — *see* Abortion
  annular fibrosis M51.35
  anus, anal (sphincter) S31.831
    complicating delivery
      with third degree perineal laceration — *see also* Delivery, complicated, by, laceration, perineum, third degree O70.20
        with mucosa O70.3
      without third degree perineal laceration O70.4
  nontraumatic (healed) (old) K62.81

Tear, torn (traumatic) - *continued*
  articular cartilage, old — *see* Derangement, joint, articular cartilage, by site
  bladder
    with ectopic or molar pregnancy O08.6
    following ectopic or molar pregnancy O08.6
    obstetrical O71.5
    traumatic — *see* Injury, bladder
  bowel
    with ectopic or molar pregnancy O08.6
    following ectopic or molar pregnancy O08.6
    obstetrical trauma O71.5
  broad ligament
    with ectopic or molar pregnancy O08.6
    following ectopic or molar pregnancy O08.6
    obstetrical trauma O71.6
  bucket handle (knee) (meniscus) — *see* Tear, meniscus
  capsule, joint — *see* Sprain
  cartilage — *see also* Sprain
    articular, old — *see* Derangement, joint, articular cartilage, by site
  cervix
    with ectopic or molar pregnancy O08.6
    following ectopic or molar pregnancy O08.6
    obstetrical trauma (current) O71.3
    old N88.1
    traumatic — *see* Injury, uterus
  dural G97.41
    nontraumatic G96.11
  internal organ — *see* Injury, by site
  knee cartilage
    articular (current) S83.3-
    old — *see* Derangement, knee, meniscus, due to old tear
  ligament — *see* Sprain
  meniscus (knee) (current injury) S83.209
    bucket-handle S83.20-
    lateral
      bucket-handle S83.25-
      complex S83.27-
      peripheral S83.26-
      specified type NEC S83.28-
    medial
      bucket-handle S83.21-
      complex S83.23-
      peripheral S83.22-
      specified type NEC S83.24-
    old — *see* Derangement, knee, meniscus, due to old tear
    site other than knee - code as Sprain
    specified type NEC S83.20-
  muscle — *see* Strain
  pelvic
    floor, complicating delivery O70.1
    organ NEC, obstetrical trauma O71.5
      with ectopic or molar pregnancy O08.6
      following ectopic or molar pregnancy O08.6
  perineal, secondary O90.1
  periurethral tissue, obstetrical trauma O71.82
    with ectopic or molar pregnancy O08.6
    following ectopic or molar pregnancy O08.6
  rectovaginal septum — *see* Laceration, vagina
  retina, retinal (without detachment)
    (horseshoe) — *see also* Break, retina, horseshoe
    with detachment — *see* Detachment, retina, with retinal, break
  rotator cuff (nontraumatic) M75.10-
    complete M75.12-
    incomplete M75.11-
    traumatic S46.01-
      capsule S43.42-
  semilunar cartilage, knee — *see* Tear, meniscus
  supraspinatus (complete) (incomplete) (nontraumatic) — *see also* Tear, rotator cuff M75.10-
  tendon — *see* Strain
  tentorial, at birth P10.4
  umbilical cord
    complicating delivery O69.89
  urethra
    with ectopic or molar pregnancy O08.6
    following ectopic or molar pregnancy O08.6
    obstetrical trauma O71.5
  uterus — *see* Injury, uterus
  vagina — *see* Laceration, vagina
  vessel, from catheter — *see* Puncture, accidental complicating surgery
  vulva, complicating delivery O70.0
Tear-stone — *see* Dacryolith
Teeth — *see also* condition
  grinding
    psychogenic F45.8

Teeth - *continued*
  grinding - *continued*
    sleep related G47.63
Teething (syndrome) K00.7
Telangiectasia, telangiectasis (verrucous) I78.1
  ataxic (cerebellar) (Louis-Bar) G11.3
  familial I78.0
  hemorrhagic, hereditary (congenital) (senile) I78.0
  hereditary, hemorrhagic (congenital) (senile) I78.0
  juxtafoveal H35.07-
  macular H35.07-
  parafoveal H35.07-
  retinal (idiopathic) (juxtafoveal) (macular) (parafoveal) H35.07-
  spider I78.1
Telephone scatologia F65.89
Telescoped bowel or intestine K56.1
  congenital Q43.8
Temperature
  body, high (of unknown origin) R50.9
  cold, trauma from T69.9
    newborn P80.0
    specified effect NEC T69.8
Temple — *see* condition
Temporal — *see* condition
Temporomandibular joint pain-dysfunction syndrome M26.62-
Temporosphenoidal — *see* condition
Tendency
  bleeding — *see* Defect, coagulation
  suicide
    meaning personal history of attempted suicide Z91.5
    meaning suicidal ideation — *see* Ideation, suicidal
  to fall R29.6
Tenderness, abdominal R10.819
  epigastric R10.816
  generalized R10.817
  left lower quadrant R10.814
  left upper quadrant R10.812
  periumbilic R10.815
  right lower quadrant R10.813
  right upper quadrant R10.811
  rebound R10.829
    epigastric R10.826
    generalized R10.827
    left lower quadrant R10.824
    left upper quadrant R10.822
    periumbilic R10.825
    right lower quadrant R10.823
    right upper quadrant R10.821
Tendinitis, tendonitis — *see also* Enthesopathy
  Achilles M76.6-
  adhesive — *see* Tenosynovitis, specified type NEC
    shoulder — *see* Capsulitis, adhesive
  bicipital M75.2-
  calcific M65.2-
    ankle M65.27-
    foot M65.27-
    forearm M65.23-
    hand M65.24-
    lower leg M65.26-
    multiple sites M65.29
    pelvic region M65.25-
    shoulder M75.3-
    specified site NEC M65.28
    thigh M65.25-
    upper arm M65.22-
  due to use, overuse, pressure — *see also* Disorder, soft tissue, due to use
    specified NEC — *see* Disorder, soft tissue, due to use, specified NEC
  gluteal M76.0-
  patellar M76.5-
  peroneal M76.7-
  psoas M76.1-
  tibial (posterior) M76.82-
    anterior M76.81-
  trochanteric — *see* Bursitis, hip, trochanteric
Tendon — *see* condition
Tendosynovitis — *see* Tenosynovitis
Tenesmus (rectal) R19.8
  vesical R30.1
Tennis elbow — *see* Epicondylitis, lateral
Tenonitis — *see also* Tenosynovitis
  eye (capsule) H05.04-
Tenontosynovitis — *see* Tenosynovitis
Tenontothecitis — *see* Tenosynovitis
Tenophyte — *see* Disorder, synovium, specified type NEC
Tenosynovitis — *see also* Synovitis M65.9
  adhesive — *see* Tenosynovitis, specified type NEC
    shoulder — *see* Capsulitis, adhesive

Tenosynovitis - *continued*
  bicipital (calcifying) — *see* Tendinitis, bicipital
  gonococcal A54.49
  in (due to)
    crystals M65.8-
    gonorrhea A54.49
    syphilis (late) A52.78
    use, overuse, pressure — *see also* Disorder, soft
      tissue, due to use
      specified NEC — *see* Disorder, soft tissue, due to
        use, specified NEC
  infective NEC M65.1-
    ankle M65.17-
    foot M65.17-
    forearm M65.13-
    hand M65.14-
    lower leg M65.16-
    multiple sites M65.19
    pelvic region M65.15-
    shoulder region M65.11-
    specified site NEC M65.18
    thigh M65.15-
    upper arm M65.12-
  radial styloid M65.4
  shoulder region M65.81-
    adhesive — *see* Capsulitis, adhesive
  specified type NEC M65.88
    ankle M65.87-
    foot M65.87-
    forearm M65.83-
    hand M65.84-
    lower leg M65.86-
    multiple sites M65.89
    pelvic region M65.85-
    shoulder region M65.81-
    specified site NEC M65.88
    thigh M65.85-
    upper arm M65.82-
  tuberculous — *see* Tuberculosis, tenosynovitis
Tenovaginitis — *see* Tenosynovitis
Tension
  arterial, high — *see also* Hypertension
    without diagnosis of hypertension R03.0
  headache G44.209
    intractable G44.201
    not intractable G44.209
  nervous R45.0
  pneumothorax J93.0
  premenstrual N94.3
  state (mental) F48.9
Tentorium — *see* condition
Teratencephalus Q89.8
Teratism Q89.7
Teratoblastoma (malignant) — *see* Neoplasm,
  malignant, by site
Teratocarcinoma — *see also* Neoplasm, malignant,
  by site
  liver C22.7
Teratoma (solid) — *see also* Neoplasm, uncertain
  behavior, by site
  with embryonal carcinoma, mixed — *see* Neoplasm,
    malignant, by site
  with malignant transformation — *see* Neoplasm,
    malignant, by site
  adult (cystic) — *see* Neoplasm, benign, by site
  benign — *see* Neoplasm, benign, by site
  combined with choriocarcinoma — *see* Neoplasm,
    malignant, by site
  cystic (adult) — *see* Neoplasm, benign, by site
  differentiated — *see* Neoplasm, benign, by site
  embryonal — *see also* Neoplasm, malignant, by site
    liver C22.7
  immature — *see* Neoplasm, malignant, by site
    liver C22.7
    adult, benign, cystic, differentiated type or
      mature D13.4
  malignant — *see also* Neoplasm, malignant, by site
    anaplastic — *see* Neoplasm, malignant, by site
    intermediate — *see* Neoplasm, malignant, by site
      specified site — *see* Neoplasm, malignant, by site
      unspecified site C62.90
    undifferentiated — *see* Neoplasm, malignant, by
      site
  mature — *see* Neoplasm, uncertain behavior, by site
  malignant — *see* Neoplasm, by site, malignant, by
    site
  ovary D27.-
    embryonal, immature or malignant C56-
  solid — *see* Neoplasm, uncertain behavior, by site
  testis C62.9-
    adult, benign, cystic, differentiated type or
      mature D29.2-
    scrotal C62.1-

Teratoma (solid) - *continued*
  testis - *continued*
    undescended C62.0-
Termination
  anomalous — *see also* Malposition, congenital
    right pulmonary vein Q26.3
  pregnancy, elective Z33.2
Ternidens diminutus infestation B81.8
Ternidensiasis B81.8
Terror (s) **night** (child) F51.4
Terrorism, victim of Z65.4
Terry's syndrome H44.2-
Tertiary — *see* condition
Test, tests, testing (for)
  adequacy (for dialysis)
    hemodialysis Z49.31
    peritoneal Z49.32
  blood pressure Z01.30
    abnormal reading — *see* Blood, pressure
  blood-alcohol Z04.8
    positive — *see* Findings, abnormal, in blood
  blood-drug Z04.8
    positive — *see* Findings, abnormal, in blood
  blood typing Z01.83
    Rh typing Z01.83
  cardiac pulse generator (battery) Z45.010
  fertility Z31.41
  genetic
    disease carrier status for procreative management
      female Z31.430
      male Z31.440
    male partner of patient with recurrent pregnancy
      loss Z31.441
    procreative management NEC
      female Z31.438
      male Z31.448
  hearing Z01.10
    with abnormal findings NEC Z01.118
  HIV (human immunodeficiency virus)
    nonconclusive (in infants) R75
    positive Z21
    seropositive Z21
  immunity status Z01.84
  intelligence NEC Z01.89
  laboratory (as part of a general medical
    examination) Z00.00
    with abnormal finding Z00.01
    for medicolegal reason NEC Z04.8
  male partner of patient with recurrent pregnancy
    loss Z31.441
  Mantoux (for tuberculosis) Z11.1
    abnormal result R76.11
  pregnancy, positive first pregnancy — *see*
    Pregnancy, normal, first
  procreative Z31.49
    fertility Z31.41
  skin, diagnostic
    allergy Z01.82
      special screening examination — *see* Screening,
        by name of disease
    Mantoux Z11.1
    tuberculin Z11.1
    specified NEC Z01.89
    tuberculin Z11.1
      abnormal result R76.11
  vision Z01.00
    with abnormal findings Z01.01
  Wassermann Z11.3
    positive — *see* Serology for syphilis, positive
Testicle, testicular, testis — *see also* condition
  feminization syndrome — *see also* Syndrome,
    androgen insensitivity E34.51
  migrans Q55.29
Tetanus, tetanic (cephalic) (convulsions) A35
  with
    abortion A34
    ectopic or molar pregnancy O08.0
  following ectopic or molar pregnancy O08.0
  inoculation reaction (due to serum) — *see*
    Complications, vaccination
  neonatorum A33
  obstetrical A34
  puerperal, postpartum, childbirth A34
Tetany (due to) R29.0
  alkalosis E87.3
  associated with rickets E55.0
  convulsions R29.0
    hysterical F44.5
  functional (hysterical) F44.5
  hyperkinetic R29.0
    hysterical F44.5
  hyperpnea R06.4
    hysterical F44.5

Tetany (due to) - *continued*
  hyperpnea - *continued*
    psychogenic F45.8
  hyperventilation — *see also* Hyperventilation R06.4
    hysterical F44.5
  neonatal (without calcium or magnesium
    deficiency) P71.3
  parathyroid (gland) E20.9
  parathyroprival E89.2
  post- (para) thyroidectomy E89.2
  postoperative E89.2
  pseudotetany R29.0
  psychogenic (conversion reaction) F44.5
Tetralogy of Fallot Q21.3
Tetraplegia (chronic) — *see*
  also Quadriplegia G82.50
Thailand hemorrhagic fever A91
Thalassanemia — *see* Thalassemia
Thalassemia (anemia) (disease) D56.9
  with other hemoglobinopathy D56.8
  alpha (major) (severe) (triple gene defect) D56.0
    minor D56.3
    silent carrier D56.3
    trait D56.3
  beta (severe) D56.1
    homozygous D56.1
    major D56.1
    minor D56.3
    trait D56.3
  delta-beta (homozygous) D56.2
    minor D56.3
    trait D56.3
  dominant D56.8
  hemoglobin
    C D56.8
    E-beta D56.5
  intermedia D56.1
  major D56.1
  minor D56.3
  mixed D56.8
  sickle-cell — *see* Disease, sickle-cell, thalassemia
  specified type NEC D56.8
  trait D56.3
  variants D56.8
Thanatophoric dwarfism or short stature Q77.1
Thaysen-Gee disease (nontropical sprue) K90.0
Thaysen's disease K90.0
Thecoma D27-
  luteinized D27-
  malignant C56-
Thelarche, premature E30.8
Thelaziasis B83.8
Thelitis N61.0
  puerperal, postpartum or gestational — *see*
    Infection, nipple
Therapeutic — *see* condition
Therapy
  drug, long-term (current) (prophylactic)
    agents affecting estrogen receptors and estrogen
      levels NEC Z79.818
    anastrozole (Arimidex) Z79.811
    antibiotics Z79.2
      short-term use - omit code
    anticoagulants Z79.01
    anti-inflammatory Z79.1
    antiplatelet Z79.02
    antithrombotics Z79.02
    aromatase inhibitors Z79.811
    aspirin Z79.82
    birth control pill or patch Z79.3
    bisphosphonates Z79.83
    contraceptive, oral Z79.3
    drug, specified NEC Z79.899
    estrogen receptor downregulators Z79.818
    Evista Z79.810
    exemestane (Aromasin) Z79.811
    Fareston Z79.810
    fulvestrant (Faslodex) Z79.818
    gonadotropin-releasing hormone (GnRH)
      agonist Z79.818
    goserelin acetate (Zoladex) Z79.818
    hormone replacement (postmenopausal) Z79.890
    insulin Z79.4
    letrozole (Femara) Z79.811
    leuprolide acetate (leuprorelin) (Lupron) Z79.818
    megestrol acetate (Megace) Z79.818
    methadone
      for pain management Z79.891
      maintenance therapy F11.20
    Nolvadex Z79.810
    opiate analgesic Z79.891
    oral contraceptive Z79.3
    raloxifene (Evista) Z79.810

Therapy - *continued*
drug, long-term (current) (prophylactic) - *continued*
selective estrogen receptor modulators
(SERMs) Z79.810
short term - omit code
steroids
inhaled Z79.51
systemic Z79.52
tamoxifen (Nolvadex) Z79.810
toremifene (Fareston) Z79.810
Thermic — *see* condition
Thermography (abnormal) — *see also* Abnormal,
diagnostic imaging R93.8
breast R92.8
Thermoplegia T67.0
Thesaurismosis, glycogen — *see* Disease, glycogen
storage
Thiamin deficiency E51.9
specified NEC E51.8
Thiaminic deficiency with beriberi E51.11
Thibierge-Weissenbach syndrome — *see* Sclerosis,
systemic
Thickening
bone — *see* Hypertrophy, bone
breast N64.59
endometrium R93.8
epidermal L85.9
specified NEC L85.8
hymen N89.6
larynx J38.7
nail L60.2
congenital Q84.5
periosteal — *see* Hypertrophy, bone
pleura J92.9
with asbestos J92.0
skin R23.4
subepiglottic J38.7
tongue K14.8
valve, heart — *see* Endocarditis
Thigh — *see* condition
Thinning vertebra — *see* Spondylopathy, specified
NEC
Thirst, excessive R63.1
due to deprivation of water T73.1
Thomsen disease G71.12
Thoracic — *see also* condition
kidney Q63.2
outlet syndrome G54.0
Thoracogastroschisis (congenital) Q79.8
Thoracopagus Q89.4
Thorax — *see* condition
Thorn's syndrome N28.89
Thorson-Björck syndrome E34.0
Threadworm (infection) (infestation) B80
Threatened
abortion O20.0
with subsequent abortion O03.9
job loss, anxiety concerning Z56.2
labor (without delivery) O47.9
at or after 37 completed weeks of gestation O47.1
before 37 completed weeks of gestation O47.0-
loss of job, anxiety concerning Z56.2
miscarriage O20.0
unemployment, anxiety concerning Z56.2
Three-day fever A93.1
Threshers' lung J67.0
Thrix annulata (congenital) Q84.1
Throat — *see* condition
Thrombasthenia (Glanzmann) (hemorrhagic)
(hereditary) D69.1
Thromboangiitis I73.1
obliterans (general) I73.1
cerebral I67.89
vessels
brain I67.89
spinal cord I67.89
Thromboarteritis — *see* Arteritis
Thromboasthenia (Glanzmann) (hemorrhagic)
(hereditary) D69.1
Thrombocytasthenia (Glanzmann) D69.1
Thrombocythemia (essential) (hemorrhagic)
(idiopathic) (primary) D47.3
Thrombocytopathy (dystrophic)
(granulopenic) D69.1
Thrombocytopenia, thrombocytopenic D69.6
with absent radius (TAR) Q87.2
congenital D69.42
dilutional D69.59
due to
drugs D69.59
extracorporeal circulation of blood D69.59
(massive) blood transfusion D69.59
platelet alloimmunization D69.59

Thrombocytopenia, thrombocytopenic - *continued*
essential D69.3
heparin induced (HIT) D75.82
hereditary D69.42
idiopathic D69.3
neonatal, transitory P61.0
due to
exchange transfusion P61.0
idiopathic maternal thrombocytopenia P61.0
isoimmunization P61.0
primary NEC D69.49
idiopathic D69.3
puerperal, postpartum O72.3
secondary D69.59
transient neonatal P61.0
Thrombocytosis, essential D47.3
primary D47.3
Thromboembolism — *see* Embolism
Thrombopathy (Bernard-Soulier) D69.1
constitutional D68.0
Willebrand-Jurgens D68.0
Thrombopenia — *see* Thrombocytopenia
Thrombophilia D68.59
primary NEC D68.59
secondary NEC D68.69
specified NEC D68.69
Thrombophlebitis I80.9
antepartum O22.2-
deep O22.3-
superficial O22.2-
cavernous (venous) sinus G08
complicating pregnancy O22.5-
nonpyogenic I67.6
cerebral (sinus) (vein) G08
nonpyogenic I67.6
sequelae G09
due to implanted device — *see* Complications, by
site and type, specified NEC
during or resulting from a procedure NEC T81.72
femoral vein (superficial) I80.1-
femoropopliteal vein I80.0-
hepatic (vein) I80.8
idiopathic, recurrent I82.1
iliofemoral I80.1-
intracranial venous sinus (any) G08
nonpyogenic I67.6
sequelae G09
intraspinal venous sinuses and veins G08
nonpyogenic G95.19
lateral (venous) sinus G08
nonpyogenic I67.6
leg I80.299
superficial I80.0-
longitudinal (venous) sinus G08
nonpyogenic I67.6
lower extremity I80.299
migrans, migrating I82.1
pelvic
with ectopic or molar pregnancy O08.0
following ectopic or molar pregnancy O08.0
puerperal O87.1
popliteal vein — *see* Phlebitis, leg, deep, popliteal
portal (vein) K75.1
postoperative T81.72
pregnancy — *see* Thrombophlebitis, antepartum
puerperal, postpartum, childbirth O87.0
deep O87.1
pelvic O87.1
septic O86.81
superficial O87.0
saphenous (greater) (lesser) I80.0-
sinus (intracranial) G08
nonpyogenic I67.6
specified site NEC I80.8
tibial vein I80.23-
Thrombosis, thrombotic (bland) (multiple)
(progressive) (silent) (vessel) I82.90
anal K64.5
antepartum — *see* Thrombophlebitis, antepartum
aorta, aortic I74.10
abdominal I74.09
saddle I74.01
bifurcation I74.09
saddle I74.01
specified site NEC I74.19
terminal I74.09
thoracic I74.11
valve — *see* Endocarditis, aortic
apoplexy I63.3-
artery, arteries (postinfectional) I74.9
auditory, internal — *see* Occlusion, artery,
precerebral, specified NEC
basilar — *see* Occlusion, artery, basilar

Thrombosis, thrombotic (bland) (multiple)
(progressive) (silent) (vessel) - *continued*
artery, arteries (postinfectional) - *continued*
carotid (common) (internal) — *see* Occlusion,
artery, carotid
cerebellar (anterior inferior) (posterior inferior)
(superior) — *see* Occlusion, artery, cerebellar
cerebral — *see* Occlusion, artery, cerebral
choroidal (anterior) — *see* Occlusion, artery,
cerebral, specified NEC
communicating, posterior — *see* Occlusion, artery,
cerebral, specified NEC
coronary — *see also* Infarct, myocardium
not resulting in infarction I24.0
hepatic I74.8
hypophyseal — *see* Occlusion, artery, cerebral,
specified NEC
iliac I74.5
limb I74.4
lower I74.3
upper I74.2
meningeal, anterior or posterior — *see* Occlusion,
artery, cerebral, specified NEC
mesenteric (with gangrene) — *see also* Infarct,
intestine K55.069
ophthalmic — *see* Occlusion, artery, retina
pontine — *see* Occlusion, artery, cerebral,
specified NEC
precerebral — *see* Occlusion, artery, precerebral
pulmonary (iatrogenic) — *see* Embolism,
pulmonary
renal N28.0
retinal — *see* Occlusion, artery, retina
spinal, anterior or posterior G95.11
traumatic NEC T14.8
vertebral — *see* Occlusion, artery, vertebral
atrium, auricular — *see also* Infarct, myocardium
following acute myocardial infarction (current
complication) I23.6
not resulting in infarction I51.3
basilar (artery) — *see* Occlusion, artery, basilar
brain (artery) (stem) — *see also* Occlusion, artery,
cerebral
due to syphilis A52.05
puerperal O99.43
sinus — *see* Thrombosis, intracranial venous sinus
capillary I78.8
cardiac — *see also* Infarct, myocardium
not resulting in infarction I51.3
valve — *see* Endocarditis
carotid (artery) (common) (internal) — *see*
Occlusion, artery, carotid
cavernous (venous) sinus — *see* Thrombosis,
intracranial venous sinus
cerebellar artery (anterior inferior) (posterior
inferior) (superior) I66.3
cerebral (artery) — *see* Occlusion, artery, cerebral
cerebrovenous sinus — *see also* Thrombosis,
intracranial venous sinus
puerperium O87.3
chronic I82.91
coronary (artery) (vein) — *see also* Infarct,
myocardium
not resulting in infarction I24.0
corpus cavernosum N48.89
cortical I66.9
deep — *see* Embolism, vein, lower extremity
due to device, implant or graft — *see*
also Complications, by site and type, specified
NEC T85.868
arterial graft NEC T82.868
breast (implant) T85.868
catheter NEC T85.868
dialysis (renal) T82.868
intraperitoneal T85.868
infusion NEC T82.868
spinal (epidural) (subdural) T85.860
urinary (indwelling) T83.86
electronic (electrode) (pulse generator) (stimulator)
bone T84.86
cardiac T82.867
nervous system (brain) (peripheral nerve)
(spinal) T85.860
urinary T83.86
fixation, internal (orthopedic) NEC T84.86
gastrointestinal (bile duct) (esophagus) T85.868
genital NEC T83.86
heart T82.867
joint prosthesis T84.86
ocular (corneal graft) (orbital implant)
NEC T85.868
orthopedic NEC T84.86
specified NEC T85.868

Thrombosis, thrombotic (bland) (multiple) (progressive) (silent) (vessel) - *continued*
  due to device, implant or graft - *continued*
    urinary NEC T83.86
    vascular NEC T82.868
    ventricular intracranial shunt T85.860
  during the puerperium — *see* Thrombosis, puerperal
  endocardial — *see also* Infarct, myocardium
    not resulting in infarction I51.3
  eye — *see* Occlusion, retina
  genital organ
    female NEC N94.89
      pregnancy — *see* Thrombophlebitis, antepartum
    male N50.1
  gestational — *see* Phlebopathy, gestational
  heart (chamber) — *see also* Infarct, myocardium
    not resulting in infarction I51.3
  hepatic (vein) I82.0
    artery I74.8
  history (of) Z86.718
  intestine (with gangrene) — *see also* Infarct, intestine K55.069
  intracardiac NEC (apical) (atrial) (auricular) (ventricular) (old) I51.3
  intracranial (arterial) I66.9
    venous sinus (any) G08
      nonpyogenic origin I67.6
      puerperium O87.3
  intramural — *see also* Infarct, myocardium
    not resulting in infarction I51.3
  intraspinal venous sinuses and veins G08
    nonpyogenic G95.19
  kidney (artery) N28.0
  lateral (venous) sinus — *see* Thrombosis, intracranial venous sinus
  leg — *see* Thrombosis, vein, lower extremity
    arterial I74.3
  liver (venous) I82.0
    artery I74.8
    portal vein I81
  longitudinal (venous) sinus — *see* Thrombosis, intracranial venous sinus
  lower limb — *see* Thrombosis, vein, lower extremity
  lung (iatrogenic) (postoperative) — *see* Embolism, pulmonary
  meninges (brain) (arterial) I66.8
  mesenteric (artery) (with gangrene) — *see also* Infarct, intestine K55.069
    vein (inferior) (superior) I81
  mitral I34.8
  mural — *see also* Infarct, myocardium
    due to syphilis A52.06
    not resulting in infarction I51.3
  omentum (with gangrene) — *see also* Infarct, intestine K55.069
  ophthalmic — *see* Occlusion, retina
  pampiniform plexus (male) N50.1
  parietal — *see also* Infarct, myocardium
    not resulting in infarction I24.0
  penis, superficial vein N48.81
  perianal venous K64.5
  peripheral arteries I74.4
    upper I74.2
  personal history (of) Z86.718
  portal I81
    due to syphilis A52.09
  precerebral artery — *see* Occlusion, artery, precerebral
  puerperal, postpartum O87.0
    brain (artery) O99.43
      venous (sinus) O87.3
    cardiac O99.43
    cerebral (artery) O99.43
      venous (sinus) O87.3
    superficial O87.0
  pulmonary (artery) (iatrogenic) (postoperative) (vein) — *see* Embolism, pulmonary
  renal (artery) N28.0
    vein I82.3
  resulting from presence of device, implant or graft — *see* Complications, by site and type, specified NEC
  retina, retinal — *see* Occlusion, retina
  scrotum N50.1
  seminal vesicle N50.1
  sigmoid (venous) sinus — *see* Thrombosis, intracranial venous sinus
  sinus, intracranial (any) — *see* Thrombosis, intracranial venous sinus
  specified site NEC I82.890
    chronic I82.891
  spermatic cord N50.1
  spinal cord (arterial) G95.11

Thrombosis, thrombotic (bland) (multiple) (progressive) (silent) (vessel) - *continued*
  spinal cord (arterial) - *continued*
    due to syphilis A52.09
    pyogenic origin G06.1
  spleen, splenic D73.5
    artery I74.8
  testis N50.1
  tumor — *see* Neoplasm, unspecified behavior, by site
  traumatic NEC T14.8
  tricuspid I07.8
  tunica vaginalis N50.1
  umbilical cord (vessels) , complicating delivery O69.5
  vas deferens N50.1
  vein (acute) I82.90
    antecubital I82.61-
      chronic I82.71-
    axillary I82.A1-
      chronic I82.A2-
    basilic I82.61-
      chronic I82.71-
    brachial I82.62-
      chronic I82.72-
    brachiocephalic (innominate) I82.290
      chronic I82.291
    cerebral, nonpyogenic I67.6
    cephalic I82.61-
      chronic I82.71-
    chronic I82.91
    deep (DVT) I82.40-
      calf I82.4Z-
        chronic I82.5Z-
      lower leg I82.4Z-
        chronic I82.5Z-
      thigh I82.4Y-
        chronic I82.5Y-
      upper leg I82.4Y
        chronic I82.5y--
    femoral I82.41-
      chronic I82.51-
    iliac (iliofemoral) I82.42-
      chronic I82.52-
    innominate I82.290
      chronic I82.291
    internal jugular I82.C1-
      chronic I82.C2-
    lower extremity
      deep I82.40-
        chronic I82.50-
        specified NEC I82.49-
          chronic NEC I82.59-
      distal
        deep I82.4Z-
      proximal
        deep I82.4Y-
          chronic I82.5Y-
      superficial I82.81-
    perianal K64.5
    popliteal I82.43-
      chronic I82.53-
    radial I82.62-
      chronic I82.72-
    renal I82.3
    saphenous (greater) (lesser) I82.81-
    specified NEC I82.890
      chronic NEC I82.891
    subclavian I82.B1-
      chronic I82.B2-
    thoracic NEC I82.290
      chronic I82.291
    tibial I82.44-
      chronic I82.54-
    ulnar I82.62-
      chronic I82.72-
    upper extremity I82.60-
      chronic I82.70-
      deep I82.62-
        chronic I82.72-
      superficial I82.61-
        chronic I82.71-
  vena cava
    inferior I82.220
      chronic I82.221
    superior I82.210
      chronic I82.211
  venous, perianal K64.5
  ventricle — *see also* Infarct, myocardium
    following acute myocardial infarction (current complication) I23.6
    not resulting in infarction I24.0
Thrombus — *see* Thrombosis

Thrush — *see also* Candidiasis
  oral B37.0
  newborn P37.5
  vaginal B37.3
Thumb — *see also* condition
  sucking (child problem) F98.8
Thymitis E32.8
Thymoma (benign) D15.0
  malignant C37
Thymus, thymic (gland) — *see* condition
Thyrocele — *see* Goiter
Thyroglossal — *see also* condition
  cyst Q89.2
  duct, persistent Q89.2
Thyroid (gland) (body) — *see also* condition
  hormone resistance E07.89
  lingual Q89.2
  nodule (cystic) (nontoxic) (single) E04.1
Thyroiditis E06.9
  acute (nonsuppurative) (pyogenic) (suppurative) E06.0
  autoimmune E06.3
  chronic (nonspecific) (sclerosing) E06.5
    with thyrotoxicosis, transient E06.2
    fibrous E06.5
    lymphadenoid E06.3
    lymphocytic E06.3
    lymphoid E06.3
  de Quervain's E06.1
  drug-induced E06.4
  fibrous (chronic) E06.5
  giant-cell (follicular) E06.1
  granulomatous (de Quervain) (subacute) E06.1
  Hashimoto's (struma lymphomatosa) E06.3
  iatrogenic E06.4
  ligneous E06.5
  lymphocytic (chronic) E06.3
  lymphoid E06.3
  lymphomatous E06.3
  nonsuppurative E06.1
  postpartum, puerperal O90.5
  pseudotuberculous E06.1
  pyogenic E06.0
  radiation E06.4
  Riedel's E06.5
  subacute (granulomatous) E06.1
  suppurative E06.0
  tuberculous A18.81
  viral E06.1
  woody E06.5
Thyrolingual duct, persistent Q89.2
Thyromegaly E01.0
Thyrotoxic
  crisis — *see* Thyrotoxicosis
  heart disease or failure — *see also* Thyrotoxicosis E05.90 *[143]*
    with thyroid storm E05.91 *[143]*
  storm — *see* Thyrotoxicosis
Thyrotoxicosis (recurrent) E05.90
  with
    goiter (diffuse) E05.00
      with thyroid storm E05.01
      adenomatous uninodular E05.10
        with thyroid storm E05.11
      multinodular E05.20
        with thyroid storm E05.21
      nodular E05.20
        with thyroid storm E05.21
      uninodular E05.10
        with thyroid storm E05.11
    infiltrative
      dermopathy E05.00
        with thyroid storm E05.01
      ophthalmopathy E05.00
        with thyroid storm E05.01
    single thyroid nodule E05.10
      with thyroid storm E05.11
    thyroid storm E05.91
  due to
    ectopic thyroid nodule or tissue E05.30
      with thyroid storm E05.31
    ingestion of (excessive) thyroid material E05.40
      with thyroid storm E05.41
    overproduction of thyroid-stimulating hormone E05.80
      with thyroid storm E05.81
    specified cause NEC E05.80
      with thyroid storm E05.81
  factitia E05.40
    with thyroid storm E05.41
  heart E05.90 *[143]*
    with thyroid storm E05.91 *[143]*
  failure E05.90 *[143]*

Thyrotoxicosis (recurrent) - *continued*
neonatal (transient) P72.1
transient with chronic thyroiditis E06.2
Tibia vara — *see* Osteochondrosis, juvenile, tibia
Tic (disorder) F95.9
breathing F95.8
child problem F95.0
compulsive F95.1
de la Tourette F95.2
degenerative (generalized) (localized) G25.69
facial G25.69
disorder
chronic
motor F95.1
vocal F95.1
combined vocal and multiple motor F95.2
transient F95.0
douloureux G50.0
atypical G50.1
postherpetic, postzoster B02.22
drug-induced G25.61
eyelid F95.8
habit F95.9
chronic F95.1
transient of childhood F95.0
lid, transient of childhood F95.0
motor-verbal F95.2
occupational F48.8
orbicularis F95.8
transient of childhood F95.0
organic origin G25.69
provisional F95.0
postchoreic G25.69
psychogenic, compulsive F95.1
salaam R25.8
spasm (motor or vocal) F95.9
chronic F95.1
transient of childhood F95.0
specified NEC F95.8
Tick-borne — *see* condition
Tietze's disease or syndrome M94.0
Tight, tightness
anus K62.89
chest R07.89
fascia (lata) M62.89
foreskin (congenital) N47.1
hymen, hymenal ring N89.6
introitus (acquired) (congenital) N89.6
rectal sphincter K62.89
tendon — *see* Short, tendon
urethral sphincter N35.9
Tilting vertebra — *see* Dorsopathy, deforming, specified NEC
Timidity, child F93.8
Tinea (intersecta) (tarsi) B35.9
amiantacea L44.8
asbestina B35.0
barbae B35.0
beard B35.0
black dot B35.0
blanca B36.2
capitis B35.0
corporis B35.4
cruris B35.6
flava B36.0
foot B35.3
furfuracea B36.0
imbricata (Tokelau) B35.5
kerion B35.0
manuum B35.2
microsporic — *see* Dermatophytosis
nigra B36.1
nodosa — *see* Piedra
pedis B35.3
scalp B35.0
specified site NEC B35.8
sycosis B35.0
tonsurans B35.0
trichophytic — *see* Dermatophytosis
unguium B35.1
versicolor B36.0
Tingling sensation (skin) R20.2
Tin-miner's lung J63.5
Tinnitus NOS H93.1-
audible H93.1-
aurium H93.1-
pulsatile H93.A-
subjective H93.1-
Tipped tooth (teeth) M26.33
Tipping
pelvis M95.5
with disproportion (fetopelvic) O33.0
causing obstructed labor O65.0

Tipping - *continued*
tooth (teeth) , fully erupted M26.33
Tiredness R53.83
Tissue — *see* condition
Tobacco (nicotine)
abuse — *see* Tobacco, use
dependence — *see* Dependence, drug, nicotine
harmful use Z72.0
heart — *see* Tobacco, toxic effect
maternal use, affecting newborn P04.2
toxic effect — *see* Table of Drugs and Chemicals, by substance, poisoning
chewing tobacco — *see* Table of Drugs and Chemicals, by substance, poisoning
cigarettes — *see* Table of Drugs and Chemicals, by substance, poisoning
use Z72.0
complicating
childbirth O99.334
pregnancy O99.33-
puerperium O99.335
counseling and surveillance Z71.6
history Z87.891
withdrawal state — *see also* Dependence, drug, nicotine F17.203
Tocopherol deficiency E56.0
Todd's
cirrhosis K74.3
paralysis (postepileptic) (transitory) G83.84
Toe — *see* condition
Toilet, artificial opening — *see* Attention to, artificial, opening
Tokelau (ringworm) B35.5
Tollwut — *see* Rabies
Tommaselli's disease R31.9
correct substance properly administered — *see* Table of Drugs and Chemicals, by drug, adverse effect
overdose or wrong substance given or taken — *see* Table of Drugs and Chemicals, by drug, poisoning
Tongue — *see also* condition
tie Q38.1
Tonic pupil — *see* Anomaly, pupil, function, tonic pupil
Toni-Fanconi syndrome (cystinosis) E72.09
with cystinosis E72.04
Tonsil — *see* condition
Tonsillitis (acute) (catarrhal) (croupous) (follicular) (gangrenous) (infective) (lacunar) (lingual) (malignant) (membranous) (parenchymatous) (phlegmonous) (pseudomembranous) (purulent) (septic) (subacute) (suppurative) (toxic) (ulcerative) (vesicular) (viral) J03.90
chronic J35.01
with adenoiditis J35.03
diphtheritic A36.0
hypertrophic J35.01
with adenoiditis J35.03
recurrent J03.91
specified organism NEC J03.80
recurrent J03.81
staphylococcal J03.80
recurrent J03.81
streptococcal J03.00
recurrent J03.01
tuberculous A15.8
Vincent's A69.1
Tooth, teeth — *see* condition
Toothache K08.89
Topagnosis R20.8
Tophi — *see* Gout, chronic
TORCH infection — *see* Infection, congenital without active infection P00.2
Torn — *see* Tear
Tornwaldt's cyst or disease J39.2
Torsion
accessory tube — *see* Torsion, fallopian tube
adnexa (female) — *see* Torsion, fallopian tube
aorta, acquired I77.1
appendix epididymis N44.04
appendix testis N44.03
bile duct (common) (hepatic) K83.8
congenital Q44.5
bowel, colon or intestine K56.2
cervix — *see* Malposition, uterus
cystic duct K82.8
dystonia — *see* Dystonia, torsion
epididymis (appendix) N44.04
fallopian tube N83.52-
with ovary N83.53
gallbladder K82.8
congenital Q44.1
hydatid of Morgagni
female N83.52-

Torsion - *continued*
hydatid of Morgagni - *continued*
male N44.03
kidney (pedicle) (leading to infarction) N28.0
Meckel's diverticulum (congenital) Q43.0
malignant — *see* Table of Neoplasms, small intestine, malignant
mesentery K56.2
omentum K56.2
organ or site, congenital NEC — *see* Anomaly, by site
ovary (pedicle) N83.51-
with fallopian tube N83.53
congenital Q50.2
oviduct — *see* Torsion, fallopian tube
penis (acquired) N48.82
congenital Q55.63
spasm — *see* Dystonia, torsion
spermatic cord N44.02
extravaginal N44.01
intravaginal N44.02
spleen D73.5
testis, testicle N44.00
appendix N44.03
tibia — *see* Deformity, limb, specified type NEC, lower leg
uterus — *see* Malposition, uterus
Torticollis (intermittent) (spastic) M43.6
congenital (sternomastoid) Q68.0
due to birth injury P15.8
hysterical F44.4
ocular R29.891
psychogenic F45.8
conversion reaction F44.4
rheumatic M43.6
rheumatoid M06.88
spasmodic G24.3
traumatic, current S13.4
Tortipelvis G24.1
Tortuous
aortic arch Q25.46
artery I77.1
organ or site, congenital NEC — *see* Distortion
retinal vessel, congenital Q14.1
ureter N13.8
urethra N36.8
vein — *see* Varix
Torture, victim of Z65.4
Torula, torular (histolytica) (infection) — *see* Cryptococcosis
Torulosis — *see* Cryptococcosis
Torus (mandibularis) (palatinus) M27.0
fracture — *see* Fracture, by site, torus
Touraine's syndrome Q79.8
Tourette's syndrome F95.2
Tourniquet syndrome — *see* Constriction, external, by site
Tower skull Q75.0
with exophthalmos Q87.0
Toxemia R68.89
bacterial — *see* Sepsis
burn — *see* Burn
eclamptic (with pre-existing hypertension) — *see* Eclampsia
erysipelatous — *see* Erysipelas
fatigue R68.89
food — *see* Poisoning, food
gastrointestinal K52.1
intestinal K52.1
kidney — *see* Uremia
malarial — *see* Malaria
myocardial — *see* Myocarditis, toxic
of pregnancy — *see* Pre-eclampsia
pre-eclamptic — *see* Pre-eclampsia
small intestine K52.1
staphylococcal, due to food A05.0
stasis R68.89
uremic — *see* Uremia
urinary — *see* Uremia
Toxemica cerebropathia psychica (nonalcoholic) F04
alcoholic — *see* Alcohol, amnestic disorder
Toxic (poisoning) — *see also* condition T65.91
effect — *see* Table of Drugs and Chemicals, by substance, poisoning
shock syndrome A48.3
thyroid (gland) — *see* Thyrotoxicosis
Toxicemia — *see* Toxemia
Toxicity — *see* Table of Drugs and Chemicals, by substance, poisoning
fava bean D55.0
food, noxious — *see* Poisoning, food

Toxicity - *continued*
from drug or nonmedicinal substance — *see* Table of Drugs and Chemicals, by drug
Toxicosis — *see also* Toxemia
capillary, hemorrhagic D69.0
Toxinfection, gastrointestinal K52.1
Toxocariasis B83.0
Toxoplasma, toxoplasmosis (acquired) B58.9
with
hepatitis B58.1
meningoencephalitis B58.2
ocular involvement B58.00
other organ involvement B58.89
pneumonia, pneumonitis B58.3
congenital (acute) (subacute) (chronic) P37.1
maternal, manifest toxoplasmosis in infant (acute) (subacute) (chronic) P37.1
tPA (rtPA)
administation in a different facility within the last 24 hours prior to admission to current facility Z92.82
Trabeculation, bladder N32.89
Trachea — *see* condition
Tracheitis (catarrhal) (infantile) (membranous) (plastic) (septal) (suppurative) (viral) J04.10
with
bronchitis (15 years of age and above) J40
acute or subacute — *see* Bronchitis, acute
chronic J42
tuberculous NEC A15.5
under 15 years of age J20.9
laryngitis (acute) J04.2
chronic J37.1
tuberculous NEC A15.5
acute J04.10
with obstruction J04.11
chronic J42
with
bronchitis (chronic) J42
laryngitis (chronic) J37.1
diphtheritic (membranous) A36.89
due to external agent — *see* Inflammation, respiratory, upper, due to
syphilitic A52.73
tuberculous A15.5
Trachelitis (nonvenereal) — *see* Cervicitis
Tracheobronchial — *see* condition
Tracheobronchitis (15 years of age and above) — *see also* Bronchitis
due to
Bordetella bronchiseptica A37.80
with pneumonia A37.81
Francisella tularensis A21.8
Tracheobronchomegaly Q32.4
with bronchiectasis J47.9
with
exacerbation (acute) J47.1
lower respiratory infection J47.0
acquired J98.09
with bronchiectasis J47.9
with
exacerbation (acute) J47.1
lower respiratory infection J47.0
Tracheobronchopneumonitis — *see* Pneumonia, broncho-
Tracheocele (external) (internal) J39.8
congenital Q32.1
Tracheomalacia J39.8
congenital Q32.0
Tracheopharyngitis (acute) J06.9
chronic J42
due to external agent — *see* Inflammation, respiratory, upper, due to
Tracheostenosis J39.8
Tracheostomy
complication — *see* Complication, tracheostomy
status Z93.0
attention to Z43.0
malfunctioning J95.03
Trachoma, trachomatous A71.9
active (stage) A71.1
contraction of conjunctiva A71.1
dubium A71.0
initial (stage) A71.0
healed or sequelae B94.0
pannus A71.1
Türck's J37.0
Traction, vitreomacular H43.82-
Train sickness T75.3
Trait (s)
Hb-S D57.3
hemoglobin
abnormal NEC D58.2

Trait (s) - *continued*
hemoglobin - *continued*
abnormal NEC - *continued*
with thalassemia D56.3
C — *see* Disease, hemoglobin C
S (Hb-S) D57.3
Lepore D56.3
personality, accentuated Z73.1
sickle-cell D57.3
with elliptocytosis or spherocytosis D57.3
type A personality Z73.1
Tramp Z59.0
Trance R41.89
hysterical F44.89
Transaminasemia R74.0
Transection
abdomen (partial) S38.3
aorta (incomplete) — *see also* Injury, aorta
complete — *see* Injury, aorta, laceration, major
carotid artery (incomplete) — *see also* Injury, blood vessel, carotid, laceration
complete — *see* Injury, blood vessel, carotid, laceration, major
celiac artery (incomplete) S35.211
branch (incomplete) S35.291
complete S35.292
complete S35.212
innominate
artery (incomplete) — *see also* Injury, blood vessel, thoracic, innominate, artery, laceration
complete — *see* Injury, blood vessel, thoracic, innominate, artery, laceration, major
vein (incomplete) — *see also* Injury, blood vessel, thoracic, innominate, vein, laceration
complete — *see* Injury, blood vessel, thoracic, innominate, vein, laceration, major
jugular vein (external) (incomplete) — *see also* Injury, blood vessel, jugular vein, laceration
complete — *see* Injury, blood vessel, jugular vein, laceration, major
internal (incomplete) — *see also* Injury, blood vessel, jugular vein, internal, laceration
complete — *see* Injury, blood vessel, jugular vein, internal, laceration, major
mesenteric artery (incomplete) — *see also* Injury, mesenteric, artery, laceration
complete — *see* Injury, mesenteric artery, laceration, major
pulmonary vessel (incomplete) — *see also* Injury, blood vessel, thoracic, pulmonary, laceration
complete — *see* Injury, blood vessel, thoracic, pulmonary, laceration, major
subclavian — *see* Transection, innominate
vena cava (incomplete) — *see also* Injury, vena cava
complete — *see* Injury, vena cava, laceration, major
vertebral artery (incomplete) — *see also* Injury, blood vessel, vertebral, laceration
complete — *see* Injury, blood vessel, vertebral, laceration, major
Transfusion
associated (red blood cell)
hemochromatosis E83.111
blood
ABO incompatible — *see* Complication(s), transfusion, incompatibility reaction, ABO
minor blood group (Duffy) (E) (K (ell)) (Kidd) (Lewis) (M) (N) (P) (S) T80.89
reaction or complication — *see* Complications, transfusion
fetomaternal (mother) — *see* Pregnancy, complicated by, placenta, transfusion syndrome
maternofetal (mother) — *see* Pregnancy, complicated by, placenta, transfusion syndrome
placental (syndrome) (mother) — *see* Pregnancy, complicated by, placenta, transfusion syndrome
reaction (adverse) — *see* Complications, transfusion
related acute lung injury (TRALI) J95.84
twin-to-twin — *see* Pregnancy, complicated by, placenta, transfusion syndrome, fetus to fetus
Transient (meaning homeless) — *see also* condition Z59.0
Translocation
balanced autosomal Q95.9
in normal individual Q95.0
chromosomes NEC Q99.8
balanced and insertion in normal individual Q95.0
Down syndrome Q90.2
trisomy
13 Q91.6
18 Q91.2
21 Q90.2
Translucency, iris — *see* Degeneration, iris

Transmission of chemical substances through the placenta — *see* Absorption, chemical, through placenta
Transparency, lung, unilateral J43.0
Transplant (ed) (status) Z94.9
awaiting organ Z76.82
bone Z94.6
marrow Z94.81
candidate Z76.82
complication — *see* Complication, transplant
cornea Z94.7
heart Z94.1
and lung (s) Z94.3
valve Z95.2
prosthetic Z95.2
specified NEC Z95.4
xenogenic Z95.3
intestine Z94.82
kidney Z94.0
liver Z94.4
lung (s) Z94.2
and heart Z94.3
organ (failure) (infection) (rejection) Z94.9
removal status Z98.85
pancreas Z94.83
skin Z94.5
social Z60.3
specified organ or tissue NEC Z94.89
stem cells Z94.84
tissue Z94.9
Transplants, ovarian, endometrial N80.1
Transposed — *see* Transposition
Transposition (congenital) — *see also* Malposition, congenital
abdominal viscera Q89.3
aorta (dextra) Q20.3
appendix Q43.8
colon Q43.8
corrected Q20.5
great vessels (complete) (partial) Q20.3
heart Q24.0
with complete transposition of viscera Q89.3
intestine (large) (small) Q43.8
reversed jejunal (for bypass) (status) Z98.0
scrotum Q55.23
stomach Q40.2
with general transposition of viscera Q89.3
tooth, teeth, fully erupted M26.30
vessels, great (complete) (partial) Q20.3
viscera (abdominal) (thoracic) Q89.3
Transsexualism F64.0
Transverse — *see also* condition
arrest (deep) , in labor O64.0
lie (mother) O32.2
causing obstructed labor O64.8
Transvestism, transvestitism (dual-role) F64.1
fetishistic F65.1
Trapped placenta (with hemorrhage) O72.0
without hemorrhage O73.0
TRAPS (tumor necrosis factor receptor associated periodic syndrome) M04.1
Trauma, traumatism — *see also* Injury
acoustic — *see* subcategory H83.3
birth — *see* Birth, injury
complicating ectopic or molar pregnancy O08.6
during delivery O71.9
following ectopic or molar pregnancy O08.6
obstetric O71.9
specified NEC O71.89
occlusal
primary K08.81
secondary K08.82
Traumatic — *see also* condition
brain injury S06.9
Treacher Collins syndrome Q75.4
Treitz's hernia — *see* Hernia, abdomen, specified site NEC
Trematode infestation — *see* Infestation, fluke
Trematodiasis — *see* Infestation, fluke
Trembling paralysis — *see* Parkinsonism
Tremor (s) R25.1
drug induced G25.1
essential (benign) G25.0
familial G25.0
hereditary G25.0
hysterical F44.4
intention G25.2
medication induced postural G25.1
mercurial — *see* subcategory T56.1
Parkinson's — *see* Parkinsonism
psychogenic (conversion reaction) F44.4
senilis R54

Tremor (s) - *continued*
  specified type NEC G25.2
Trench
  fever A79.0
  foot — *see* Immersion, foot
  mouth A69.1
Treponema pallidum infection — *see* Syphilis
Treponematosis
  due to
    T. pallidum — *see* Syphilis
    T. pertenue — *see* Yaws
Triad
  Hutchinson's (congenital syphilis) A50.53
  Kartagener's Q89.3
  Saint's — *see* Hernia, diaphragm
Trichiasis (eyelid) H02.059
  with entropion — *see* Entropion
  left H02.056
    lower H02.055
    upper H02.054
  right H02.053
    lower H02.052
    upper H02.051
Trichinella spiralis (infection) (infestation) B75
Trichinellosis, trichiniasis, trichinelliasis,
trichinosis B75
  with muscle disorder B75 *[M63.80]*
    ankle B75 *[M63.87-]*
    foot B75 *[M63.87-]*
    forearm B75 *[M63.83-]*
    hand B75 *[M63.84-]*
    lower leg B75 *[M63.86-]*
    multiple sites B75 *[M63.89]*
    pelvic region B75 *[M63.85-]*
    shoulder region B75 *[M63.81-]*
    specified site NEC B75 *[M63.88]*
    thigh B75 *[M63.85-]*
    upper arm B75 *[M63.82-]*
Trichobezoar T18.9
  intestine T18.3
  stomach T18.2
Trichocephaliasis, trichocephalosis B79
Trichocephalus infestation B79
Trichoclasis L67.8
Trichoepithelioma — *see also* Neoplasm, skin,
  benign
    malignant — *see* Neoplasm, skin, malignant
Trichofolliculoma — *see* Neoplasm, skin, benign
Tricholemmoma — *see* Neoplasm, skin, benign
Trichomoniasis A59.9
  bladder A59.03
  cervix A59.09
  intestinal A07.8
  prostate A59.02
  seminal vesicles A59.09
  specified site NEC A59.8
  urethra A59.03
  urogenitalis A59.00
  vagina A59.01
  vulva A59.01
Trichomycosis
  axillaris A48.8
  nodosa, nodularis B36.8
Trichonodosis L67.8
Trichophytid, trichophyton infection — *see*
  Dermatophytosis
Trichophytobezoar T18.9
  intestine T18.3
  stomach T18.2
Trichophytosis — *see* Dermatophytosis
Trichoptilosis L67.8
Trichorrhexis (nodosa) (invaginata) L67.0
Trichosis axillaris A48.8
Trichosporosis nodosa B36.2
Trichostasis spinulosa (congenital) Q84.1
Trichostrongyliasis, trichostrongylosis
  (small intestine) B81.2
Trichostrongylus infection B81.2
Trichotillomania F63.3
Trichromat, trichromatopsia, anomalous
  (congenital) H53.55
Trichuriasis B79
Trichuris trichiura (infection) (infestation) (any
  site) B79
Tricuspid (valve) — *see* condition
Trifid — *see also* Accessory
  kidney (pelvis) Q63.8
  tongue Q38.3
Trigeminal neuralgia — *see* Neuralgia, trigeminal
Trigeminy R00.8
Trigger finger (acquired) M65.30
  congenital Q74.0
  index finger M65.32-

Trigger finger (acquired) - *continued*
  little finger M65.35-
  middle finger M65.33-
  ring finger M65.34-
  thumb M65.31-
Trigonitis (bladder) (chronic)
  (pseudomembranous) N30.30
  with hematuria N30.31
Trigonocephaly Q75.0
Trilocular heart — *see* Cor triloculare
Trimethylaminuria E72.52
Tripartite placenta O43.19-
Triphalangeal thumb Q74.0
Triple — *see also* Accessory
  kidneys Q63.0
  uteri Q51.818
  X, female Q97.0
Triplegia G83.89
  congenital G80.8
Triplet (newborn) — *see also* Newborn, triplet
  complicating pregnancy — *see* Pregnancy, triplet
Triplication — *see* Accessory
Triploidy Q92.7
Trismus R25.2
  neonatorum A33
  newborn A33
Trisomy (syndrome) Q92.9
  autosomes Q92.9
  chromosome specified NEC Q92.8
    partial Q92.2
      due to unbalanced translocation Q92.5
    whole (nonsex chromosome)
      meiotic nondisjunction Q92.0
      mitotic nondisjunction Q92.1
      mosaicism Q92.1
    specified NEC Q92.8
  due to
    dicentrics — *see* Extra, marker chromosomes
    extra rings — *see* Extra, marker chromosomes
    isochromosomes — *see* Extra, marker
      chromosomes
  specified NEC Q92.8
  whole chromosome Q92.9
    meiotic nondisjunction Q92.0
    mitotic nondisjunction Q92.1
    mosaicism Q92.1
    partial Q92.9
    specified NEC Q92.8
  13 (partial) Q91.7
    meiotic nondisjunction Q91.4
    mitotic nondisjunction Q91.5
    mosaicism Q91.5
    translocation Q91.6
  18 (partial) Q91.3
    meiotic nondisjunction Q91.0
    mitotic nondisjunction Q91.1
    mosaicism Q91.1
    translocation Q91.2
  20 Q92.8
  21 (partial) Q90.9
    meiotic nondisjunction Q90.0
    mitotic nondisjunction Q90.1
    mosaicism Q90.1
    translocation Q90.2
  22 Q92.8
Tritanomaly, tritanopia H53.55
Trombiculosis, trombiculiasis, trombidiosis B88.0
Trophedema (congenital) (hereditary) Q82.0
Trophoblastic disease — *see also* Mole,
  hydatidiform O01.9
Tropholymphedema Q82.0
Trophoneurosis NEC G96.8
  disseminated M34.9
Tropical — *see* condition
Trouble — *see also* Disease
  heart — *see* Disease, heart
  kidney — *see* Disease, renal
  nervous R45.0
  sinus — *see* Sinusitis
Trousseau's syndrome (thrombophlebitis
  migrans) I82.1
Truancy, childhood
  from school Z72.810
Truncus
  arteriosus (persistent) Q20.0
  communis Q20.0
Trunk — *see* condition
Trypanosomiasis
  African B56.9
    by Trypanosoma brucei
      gambiense B56.0
      rhodesiense B56.1
    American — *see* Chagas' disease

Trypanosomiasis - *continued*
  Brazilian — *see* Chagas' disease
  by Trypanosoma
    brucei gambiense B56.0
    brucei rhodesiense B56.1
    cruzi — *see* Chagas' disease
  gambiensis, Gambian B56.0
  rhodesiensis, Rhodesian B56.1
  South American — *see* Chagas' disease
  where
    African trypanosomiasis is prevalent B56.9
    Chagas' disease is prevalent B57.2
T-shaped incisors K00.2
Tsutsugamushi (disease) (fever) A75.3
Tube, tubal, tubular — *see* condition
Tubercle — *see also* Tuberculosis
  brain, solitary A17.81
  Darwin's Q17.8
  Ghon, primary infection A15.7
Tuberculid, tuberculide (indurating, subcutaneous)
  (lichenoid) (miliary) (papulonecrotic) (primary)
  (skin) A18.4
Tuberculoma — *see also* Tuberculosis
  brain A17.81
  meninges (cerebral) (spinal) A17.1
  spinal cord A17.81
Tuberculosis, tubercular, tuberculous (calcification)
  (calcified) (caseous) (chromogenic acid-fast bacilli)
  (degeneration) (fibrocaseous) (fistula) (interstitial)
  (isolated circumscribed lesions) (necrosis)
  (parenchymatous) (ulcerative) A15.9
  with pneumoconiosis (any condition in J60-J64) J65
  abdomen (lymph gland) A18.39
  abscess (respiratory) A15.9
    bone A18.03
      hip A18.02
      knee A18.02
      sacrum A18.01
      specified site NEC A18.03
      spinal A18.01
      vertebra A18.01
    brain A17.81
    breast A18.89
    Cowper's gland A18.15
    dura (mater) (cerebral) (spinal) A17.81
    epidural (cerebral) (spinal) A17.81
    female pelvis A18.17
    frontal sinus A15.8
    genital organs NEC A18.10
    genitourinary A18.10
    gland (lymphatic) — *see* Tuberculosis, lymph
      gland
    hip A18.02
    intestine A18.32
    ischiorectal A18.32
    joint NEC A18.02
      hip A18.02
      knee A18.02
      specified NEC A18.02
      vertebral A18.01
    kidney A18.11
    knee A18.02
    latent R76.11
    lumbar (spine) A18.01
    lung — *see* Tuberculosis, pulmonary
    meninges (cerebral) (spinal) A17.0
    muscle A18.09
    perianal (fistula) A18.32
    perinephritic A18.11
    perirectal A18.32
    rectum A18.32
    retropharyngeal A15.8
    sacrum A18.01
    scrofulous A18.2
    scrotum A18.15
    skin (primary) A18.4
    spinal cord A17.81
    spine or vertebra (column) A18.01
    subdiaphragmatic A18.31
    testis A18.15
    urinary A18.13
    uterus A18.17
  accessory sinus — *see* Tuberculosis, sinus
  Addison's disease A18.7
  adenitis — *see* Tuberculosis, lymph gland
  adenoids A15.8
  adenopathy — *see* Tuberculosis, lymph gland
  adherent pericardium A18.84
  adnexa (uteri) A18.17
  adrenal (capsule) (gland) A18.7
  alimentary canal A18.32
  anemia A18.89
  ankle (joint) (bone) A18.02

Tuberculosis, tubercular, tuberculous (calcification) (calcified) (caseous) (chromogenic acid-fast bacilli) (degeneration) (fibrocaseous) (fistula) (interstitial) (isolated circumscribed lesions) (necrosis) (parenchymatous) (ulcerative) - *continued*
- anus A18.32
- apex, apical — *see* Tuberculosis, pulmonary
- appendicitis, appendix A18.32
- arachnoid A17.0
- artery, arteritis A18.89
  - cerebral A18.89
- arthritis (chronic) (synovial) A18.02
  - spine or vertebra (column) A18.01
- articular — *see* Tuberculosis, joint
- ascites A18.31
- asthma — *see* Tuberculosis, pulmonary
- axilla, axillary (gland) A18.2
- bladder A18.12
- bone A18.03
  - hip A18.02
  - knee A18.02
  - limb NEC A18.03
  - sacrum A18.01
  - spine or vertebral column A18.01
- bowel (miliary) A18.32
- brain A17.81
- breast A18.89
- broad ligament A18.17
- bronchi, bronchial, bronchus A15.5
  - ectasia, ectasis (bronchiectasis) — *see* Tuberculosis, pulmonary
  - fistula A15.5
    - primary (progressive) A15.7
  - gland or node A15.4
    - primary (progressive) A15.7
  - lymph gland or node A15.4
    - primary (progressive) A15.7
- bronchiectasis — *see* Tuberculosis, pulmonary
- bronchitis A15.5
- bronchopleural A15.6
- bronchopneumonia, bronchopneumonic — *see* Tuberculosis, pulmonary
- bronchorrhagia A15.5
- bronchotracheal A15.5
- bronze disease A18.7
- buccal cavity A18.83
- bulbourethral gland A18.15
- bursa A18.09
- cachexia A15.9
- cardiomyopathy A18.84
- caries — *see* Tuberculosis, bone
- cartilage A18.02
  - intervertebral A18.01
- catarrhal — *see* Tuberculosis, respiratory
- cecum A18.32
- cellulitis (primary) A18.4
- cerebellum A17.81
- cerebral, cerebrum A17.81
- cerebrospinal A17.81
  - meninges A17.0
- cervical (lymph gland or node) A18.2
- cervicitis, cervix (uteri) A18.16
- chest — *see* Tuberculosis, respiratory
- chorioretinitis A18.53
- choroid, choroiditis A18.53
- ciliary body A18.54
- colitis A18.32
- collier's J65
- colliquativa (primary) A18.4
- colon A18.32
- complex, primary A15.7
- congenital P37.0
- conjunctiva A18.59
- connective tissue (systemic) A18.89
- contact Z20.1
- cornea (ulcer) A18.52
- Cowper's gland A18.15
- coxae A18.02
- coxalgia A18.02
- cul-de-sac of Douglas A18.17
- curvature, spine A18.01
- cutis (colliquativa) (primary) A18.4
- cyst, ovary A18.18
- cystitis A18.12
- dactylitis A18.03
- diarrhea A18.32
- diffuse — *see* Tuberculosis, miliary
- digestive tract A18.32
- disseminated — *see* Tuberculosis, miliary
- duodenum A18.32
- dura (mater) (cerebral) (spinal) A17.0
  - abscess (cerebral) (spinal) A17.81
- dysentery A18.32

Tuberculosis, tubercular, tuberculous (calcification) (calcified) (caseous) (chromogenic acid-fast bacilli) (degeneration) (fibrocaseous) (fistula) (interstitial) (isolated circumscribed lesions) (necrosis) (parenchymatous) (ulcerative) - *continued*
- ear (inner) (middle) A18.6
  - bone A18.03
  - external (primary) A18.4
  - skin (primary) A18.4
- elbow A18.02
- emphysema — *see* Tuberculosis, pulmonary
- empyema A15.6
- encephalitis A17.82
- endarteritis A18.89
- endocarditis A18.84
  - aortic A18.84
  - mitral A18.84
  - pulmonary A18.84
  - tricuspid A18.84
- endocrine glands NEC A18.82
- endometrium A18.17
- enteric, enterica, enteritis A18.32
- enterocolitis A18.32
- epididymis, epididymitis A18.15
- epidural abscess (cerebral) (spinal) A17.81
- epiglottis A15.5
- episcleritis A18.51
- erythema (induratum) (nodosum) (primary) A18.4
- esophagus A18.83
- eustachian tube A18.6
- exposure (to) Z20.1
- exudative — *see* Tuberculosis, pulmonary
- eye A18.50
- eyelid (primary) (lupus) A18.4
- fallopian tube (acute) (chronic) A18.17
- fascia A18.09
- fauces A15.8
- female pelvic inflammatory disease A18.17
- finger A18.03
- first infection A15.7
- gallbladder A18.83
- ganglion A18.09
- gastritis A18.83
- gastrocolic fistula A18.32
- gastroenteritis A18.32
- gastrointestinal tract A18.32
- general, generalized — *see* Tuberculosis, miliary
- genital organs A18.10
- genitourinary A18.10
- genu A18.02
- glandula suprarenalis A18.7
- glandular, general A18.2
- glottis A15.5
- grinder's J65
- gum A18.83
- hand A18.03
- heart A18.84
- hematogenous — *see* Tuberculosis, miliary
- hemoptysis — *see* Tuberculosis, pulmonary
- hemorrhage NEC — *see* Tuberculosis, pulmonary
- hemothorax A15.6
- hepatitis A18.83
- hilar lymph nodes A15.4
  - primary (progressive) A15.7
- hip (joint) (disease) (bone) A18.02
- hydropneumothorax A15.6
- hydrothorax A15.6
- hypoadrenalism A18.7
- hypopharynx A15.8
- ileocecal (hyperplastic) A18.32
- ileocolitis A18.32
- ileum A18.32
- iliac spine (superior) A18.03
- immunological findings only A15.7
- indurativa (primary) A18.4
- infantile A15.7
- infection A15.9
  - without clinical manifestations A15.7
- infraclavicular gland A18.2
- inguinal gland A18.2
- inguinalis A18.2
- intestine (any part) A18.32
- iridocyclitis A18.54
- iris, iritis A18.54
- ischiorectal A18.32
- jaw A18.03
- jejunum A18.32
- joint A18.02
  - vertebral A18.01
- keratitis (interstitial) A18.52
- keratoconjunctivitis A18.52
- kidney A18.11
- knee (joint) A18.02

Tuberculosis, tubercular, tuberculous (calcification) (calcified) (caseous) (chromogenic acid-fast bacilli) (degeneration) (fibrocaseous) (fistula) (interstitial) (isolated circumscribed lesions) (necrosis) (parenchymatous) (ulcerative) - *continued*
- kyphosis, kyphoscoliosis A18.01
- laryngitis A15.5
- larynx A15.5
- latent R76.11
- leptomeninges, leptomeningitis (cerebral) (spinal) A17.0
- lichenoides (primary) A18.4
- linguae A18.83
- lip A18.83
- liver A18.83
- lordosis A18.01
- lung — *see* Tuberculosis, pulmonary
- lupus vulgaris A18.4
- lymph gland or node (peripheral) A18.2
  - abdomen A18.39
  - bronchial A15.4
    - primary (progressive) A15.7
  - cervical A18.2
  - hilar A15.4
    - primary (progressive) A15.7
  - intrathoracic A15.4
    - primary (progressive) A15.7
  - mediastinal A15.4
    - primary (progressive) A15.7
  - mesenteric A18.39
  - retroperitoneal A18.39
  - tracheobronchial A15.4
    - primary (progressive) A15.7
- lymphadenitis — *see* Tuberculosis, lymph gland
- lymphangitis — *see* Tuberculosis, lymph gland
- lymphatic (gland) (vessel) — *see* Tuberculosis, lymph gland
- mammary gland A18.89
- marasmus A15.9
- mastoiditis A18.03
- mediastinal lymph gland or node A15.4
  - primary (progressive) A15.7
- mediastinitis A15.8
  - primary (progressive) A15.7
- mediastinum A15.8
  - primary (progressive) A15.7
- medulla A17.81
- melanosis, Addisonian A18.7
- meninges, meningitis (basilar) (cerebral) (cerebrospinal) (spinal) A17.0
- meningoencephalitis A17.82
- mesentery, mesenteric (gland or node) A18.39
- miliary A19.9
  - acute A19.2
    - multiple sites A19.1
    - single specified site A19.0
  - chronic A19.8
  - specified NEC A19.8
- millstone makers' J65
- miner's J65
- molder's J65
- mouth A18.83
- multiple A19.9
  - acute A19.1
  - chronic A19.8
- muscle A18.09
- myelitis A17.82
- myocardium, myocarditis A18.84
- nasal (passage) (sinus) A15.8
- nasopharynx A15.8
- neck gland A18.2
- nephritis A18.11
- nerve (mononeuropathy) A17.83
- nervous system A17.9
- nose (septum) A15.8
- ocular A18.50
- omentum A18.31
- oophoritis (acute) (chronic) A18.17
- optic (nerve trunk) (papilla) A18.59
- orbit A18.59
- orchitis A18.15
- organ, specified NEC A18.89
- osseous — *see* Tuberculosis, bone
- osteitis — *see* Tuberculosis, bone
- osteomyelitis — *see* Tuberculosis, bone
- otitis media A18.6
- ovary, ovaritis (acute) (chronic) A18.17
- oviduct (acute) (chronic) A18.17
- pachymeningitis A17.0
- palate (soft) A18.83
- pancreas A18.83
- papulonecrotic (a) (primary) A18.4
- parathyroid glands A18.82

Tuberculosis, tubercular, tuberculous (calcification) (calcified) (caseous) (chromogenic acid-fast bacilli) (degeneration) (fibrocaseous) (fistula) (interstitial) (isolated circumscribed lesions) (necrosis) (parenchymatous) (ulcerative) - *continued*
 paronychia (primary) A18.4
 parotid gland or region A18.83
 pelvis (bony) A18.03
 penis A18.15
 peribronchitis A15.5
 pericardium, pericarditis A18.84
 perichondritis, larynx A15.5
 periostitis — *see* Tuberculosis, bone
 perirectal fistula A18.32
 peritoneum NEC A18.31
 peritonitis A18.31
 pharynx, pharyngitis A15.8
 phlyctenulosis (keratoconjunctivitis) A18.52
 phthisis NEC — *see* Tuberculosis, pulmonary
 pituitary gland A18.82
 pleura, pleural, pleurisy, pleuritis (fibrinous) (obliterative) (purulent) (simple plastic) (with effusion) A15.6
  primary (progressive) A15.7
 pneumonia, pneumonic — *see* Tuberculosis, pulmonary
 pneumothorax (spontaneous) (tense valvular) — *see* Tuberculosis, pulmonary
 polyneuropathy A17.89
 polyserositis A19.9
  acute A19.1
  chronic A19.8
 potter's J65
 prepuce A18.15
 primary (complex) A15.7
 proctitis A18.32
 prostate, prostatitis A18.14
 pulmonalis — *see* Tuberculosis, pulmonary
 pulmonary (cavitated) (fibrotic) (infiltrative) (nodular) A15.0
  childhood type or first infection A15.7
  primary (complex) A15.7
 pyelitis A18.11
 pyelonephritis A18.11
 pyemia — *see* Tuberculosis, miliary
 pyonephrosis A18.11
 pyopneumothorax A15.6
 pyothorax A15.6
 rectum (fistula) (with abscess) A18.32
 reinfection stage — *see* Tuberculosis, pulmonary
 renal A18.11
 renis A18.11
 respiratory A15.9
  primary A15.7
  specified site NEC A15.8
 retina, retinitis A18.53
 retroperitoneal (lymph gland or node) A18.39
 rheumatism NEC A18.09
 rhinitis A15.8
 sacroiliac (joint) A18.01
 sacrum A18.01
 salivary gland A18.83
 salpingitis (acute) (chronic) A18.17
 sandblaster's J65
 sclera A18.51
 scoliosis A18.01
 scrofulous A18.2
 scrotum A18.15
 seminal tract or vesicle A18.15
 senile A15.9
 septic — *see* Tuberculosis, miliary
 shoulder (joint) A18.02
  blade A18.03
 sigmoid A18.32
 sinus (any nasal) A15.8
  bone A18.03
  epididymis A18.15
 skeletal NEC A18.03
 skin (any site) (primary) A18.4
 small intestine A18.32
 soft palate A18.83
 spermatic cord A18.15
 spine, spinal (column) A18.01
  cord A17.81
  medulla A17.81
  membrane A17.0
  meninges A17.0
 spleen, splenitis A18.85
 spondylitis A18.01
 sternoclavicular joint A18.02
 stomach A18.83
 stonemason's J65
 subcutaneous tissue (cellular) (primary) A18.4

Tuberculosis, tubercular, tuberculous (calcification) (calcified) (caseous) (chromogenic acid-fast bacilli) (degeneration) (fibrocaseous) (fistula) (interstitial) (isolated circumscribed lesions) (necrosis) (parenchymatous) (ulcerative) - *continued*
 subcutis (primary) A18.4
 subdeltoid bursa A18.83
 submaxillary (region) A18.83
 supraclavicular gland A18.2
 suprarenal (capsule) (gland) A18.7
 swelling, joint (see also category M01) — *see also* Tuberculosis, joint A18.02
 symphysis pubis A18.02
 synovitis A18.09
  articular A18.02
  spine or vertebra A18.01
 systemic — *see* Tuberculosis, miliary
 tarsitis A18.4
 tendon (sheath) — *see* Tuberculosis, tenosynovitis
 tenosynovitis A18.09
  spine or vertebra A18.01
 testis A18.15
 throat A15.8
 thymus gland A18.82
 thyroid gland A18.81
 tongue A18.83
 tonsil, tonsillitis A15.8
 trachea, tracheal A15.5
  lymph gland or node A15.4
   primary (progressive) A15.7
 tracheobronchial A15.5
  lymph gland or node A15.4
   primary (progressive) A15.7
 tubal (acute) (chronic) A18.17
 tunica vaginalis A18.15
 ulcer (skin) (primary) A18.4
  bowel or intestine A18.32
  specified NEC - code under Tuberculosis, by site
 unspecified site A15.9
 ureter A18.11
 urethra, urethral (gland) A18.13
 urinary organ or tract A18.13
 uterus A18.17
 uveal tract A18.54
 uvula A18.83
 vagina A18.18
 vas deferens A18.15
 verruca, verrucosa (cutis) (primary) A18.4
 vertebra (column) A18.01
 vesiculitis A18.15
 vulva A18.18
 wrist (joint) A18.02
Tuberculum
 Carabelli — *see* Note at K00.2
 occlusal — *see* Note at K00.2
 paramolare K00.2
Tuberosity, enitre maxillary M26.07
Tuberous sclerosis (brain) Q85.1
Tubo-ovarian — *see* condition
Tuboplasty, after previous sterilization Z31.0
 aftercare Z31.42
Tubotympanitis, catarrhal (chronic) — *see* Otitis, media, nonsuppurative, chronic, serous
Tularemia A21.9
 with
  conjunctivitis A21.1
  pneumonia A21.2
 abdominal A21.3
 bronchopneumonic A21.2
 conjunctivitis A21.1
 cryptogenic A21.3
 enteric A21.3
 gastrointestinal A21.3
 generalized A21.7
 ingestion A21.3
 intestinal A21.3
 oculoglandular A21.1
 ophthalmic A21.1
 pneumonia (any) , pneumonic A21.2
 pulmonary A21.2
 sepsis A21.7
 specified NEC A21.8
 typhoidal A21.7
 ulceroglandular A21.0
Tularensis conjunctivitis A21.1
Tumefaction — *see also* Swelling
 liver — *see* Hypertrophy, liver
Tumor — *see also* Neoplasm, unspecified behavior, by site
 acinar cell — *see* Neoplasm, uncertain behavior, by site
 acinic cell — *see* Neoplasm, uncertain behavior, by site

Tumor - *continued*
 adenocarcinoid — *see* Neoplasm, malignant, by site
 adenomatoid — *see also* Neoplasm, benign, by site
  odontogenic — *see* Cyst, calcifying odontogenic
 adnexal (skin) — *see* Neoplasm, skin, benign, by site
 adrenal
  cortical (benign) D35.0-
   malignant C74.0-
  rest — *see* Neoplasm, benign, by site
 alpha-cell
  malignant
   pancreas C25.4
   specified site NEC — *see* Neoplasm, malignant, by site
   unspecified site C25.4
  pancreas D13.7
  specified site NEC — *see* Neoplasm, benign, by site
  unspecified site D13.7
 aneurysmal — *see* Aneurysm
 aortic body D44.7
  malignant C75.5
 Askin's — *see* Neoplasm, connective tissue, malignant
 basal cell — *see also* Neoplasm, skin, uncertain behavior D48.5
 Bednar — *see* Neoplasm, skin, malignant
 benign (unclassified) — *see* Neoplasm, benign, by site
 beta-cell
  malignant
   pancreas C25.4
   specified site NEC — *see* Neoplasm, malignant, by site
   unspecified site C25.4
  pancreas D13.7
  specified site NEC — *see* Neoplasm, benign, by site
  unspecified site D13.7
 Brenner D27.9
  borderline malignancy D39.1-
  malignant C56-
  proliferating D39.1-
 bronchial alveolar, intravascular D38.1
 Brooke's — *see* Neoplasm, skin, benign
 brown fat — *see* Lipoma
 Burkitt — *see* Lymphoma, Burkitt
 calcifying epithelial odontogenic — *see* Cyst, calcifying odontogenic
 carcinoid
  benign D3A.00
   appendix D3A.020
   ascending colon D3A.022
   bronchus (lung) D3A.090
   cecum D3A.021
   colon D3A.029
   descending colon D3A.024
   duodenum D3A.010
   foregut NOS D3A.094
   hindgut NOS D3A.096
   ileum D3A.012
   jejunum D3A.011
   kidney D3A.093
   large intestine D3A.029
   lung (bronchus) D3A.090
   midgut NOS D3A.095
   rectum D3A.026
   sigmoid colon D3A.025
   small intestine D3A.019
   specified NEC D3A.098
   stomach D3A.092
   thymus D3A.091
   transverse colon D3A.023
  malignant C7A.00
   appendix C7A.020
   ascending colon C7A.022
   bronchus (lung) C7A.090
   cecum C7A.021
   colon C7A.029
   descending colon C7A.024
   duodenum C7A.010
   foregut NOS C7A.094
   hindgut NOS C7A.096
   ileum C7A.012
   jejunum C7A.011
   kidney C7A.093
   large intestine C7A.029
   lung (bronchus) C7A.090
   midgut NOS C7A.095
   rectum C7A.026
   sigmoid colon C7A.025
   small intestine C7A.019

Tumor - *continued*
 carcinoid - *continued*
  malignant - *continued*
   specified NEC C7A.098
   stomach C7A.092
   thymus C7A.091
   transverse colon C7A.023
  mesentary metastasis C7B.04
  secondary C7B.00
   bone C7B.03
   distant lymph nodes C7B.01
   liver C7B.02
   peritoneum C7B.04
   specified NEC C7B.09
 carotid body D44.6
  malignant C75.4
 cells — *see also* Neoplasm, unspecified behavior, by site
  benign — *see* Neoplasm, benign, by site
  malignant — *see* Neoplasm, malignant, by site
  uncertain whether benign or malignant — *see* Neoplasm, uncertain behavior, by site
 cervix, in pregnancy or childbirth — *see* Pregnancy, complicated by, tumor, cervix
 chondromatous giant cell — *see* Neoplasm, bone, benign
 chromaffin — *see also* Neoplasm, benign, by site
  malignant — *see* Neoplasm, malignant, by site
 Cock's peculiar L72.3
 Codman's — *see* Neoplasm, bone, benign
 dentigerous, mixed — *see* Cyst, calcifying odontogenic
 dermoid — *see* Neoplasm, benign, by site
  with malignant transformation C56-
 desmoid (extra-abdominal) — *see also* Neoplasm, connective tissue, uncertain behavior
  abdominal — *see* Neoplasm, connective tissue, uncertain behavior
 embolus — *see* Neoplasm, secondary, by site
 embryonal (mixed) — *see also* Neoplasm, uncertain behavior, by site
  liver C22.7
 endodermal sinus
  specified site — *see* Neoplasm, malignant, by site
  unspecified site
   female C56.-
   male C62.90
 epithelial
  benign — *see* Neoplasm, benign, by site
  malignant — *see* Neoplasm, malignant, by site
 Ewing's — *see* Neoplasm, bone, malignant, by site
 fatty — *see* Lipoma
 fibroid — *see* Leiomyoma
 G cell
  malignant
   pancreas C25.4
   specified site NEC — *see* Neoplasm, malignant, by site
   unspecified site C25.4
  specified site — *see* Neoplasm, uncertain behavior, by site
  unspecified site D37.8
 germ cell — *see also* Neoplasm, malignant, by site
  mixed — *see* Neoplasm, malignant, by site
 ghost cell, odontogenic — *see* Cyst, calcifying odontogenic
 giant cell — *see also* Neoplasm, uncertain behavior, by site
  bone D48.0
   malignant — *see* Neoplasm, bone, malignant
  chondromatous — *see* Neoplasm, bone, benign
  malignant — *see* Neoplasm, malignant, by site
  soft parts — *see* Neoplasm, connective tissue, uncertain behavior
   malignant — *see* Neoplasm, connective tissue, malignant
 glomus D18.00
  intra-abdominal D18.03
  intracranial D18.02
  jugulare D44.7
   malignant C75.5
  skin D18.01
  specified site NEC D18.09
 gonadal stromal — *see* Neoplasm, uncertain behavior, by site
 granular cell — *see also* Neoplasm, connective tissue, benign
  malignant — *see* Neoplasm, connective tissue, malignant
 granulosa cell D39.1-
  juvenile D39.1-
  malignant C56-
 granulosa cell-theca cell D39.1-

Tumor - *continued*
 granulosa cell-theca cell - *continued*
  malignant C56-
 Grawitz's C64-
 hemorrhoidal — *see* Hemorrhoids
 hilar cell D27-
 hilus cell D27-
 Hurthle cell (benign) D34
  malignant C73
 hydatid — *see* Echinococcus
 hypernephroid — *see also* Neoplasm, uncertain behavior, by site
 interstitial cell — *see also* Neoplasm, uncertain behavior, by site
  benign — *see* Neoplasm, benign, by site
  malignant — *see* Neoplasm, malignant, by site
 intravascular bronchial alveolar D38.1
 islet cell — *see* Neoplasm, benign, by site
  malignant — *see* Neoplasm, malignant, by site
   pancreas C25.4
   specified site NEC — *see* Neoplasm, malignant, by site
   unspecified site C25.4
  pancreas D13.7
  specified site NEC — *see* Neoplasm, benign, by site
  unspecified site D13.7
 juxtaglomerular D41.0-
 Klatskin's C24.0
 Krukenberg's C79.6-
 Leydig cell — *see* Neoplasm, uncertain behavior, by site
  benign — *see* Neoplasm, benign, by site
   specified site — *see* Neoplasm, benign, by site
   unspecified site
    female D27.9
    male D29.20
  malignant — *see* Neoplasm, malignant, by site
   specified site — *see* Neoplasm, malignant, by site
   unspecified site
    female C56.9
    male C62.90
  specified site — *see* Neoplasm, uncertain behavior, by site
  unspecified site
   female D39.10
   male D40.10
 lipid cell, ovary D27-
 lipoid cell, ovary D27-
 malignant — *see also* Neoplasm, malignant, by site C80.1
  fusiform cell (type) C80.1
  giant cell (type) C80.1
  localized, plasma cell — *see* Plasmacytoma, solitary
  mixed NEC C80.1
  small cell (type) C80.1
  spindle cell (type) C80.1
  unclassified C80.1
 mast cell D47.0
  malignant C96.2
 melanotic, neuroectodermal — *see* Neoplasm, benign, by site
 Merkel cell — *see* Carcinoma, Merkel cell
 mesenchymal
  malignant — *see* Neoplasm, connective tissue, malignant
  mixed — *see* Neoplasm, connective tissue, uncertain behavior
 mesodermal, mixed — *see also* Neoplasm, malignant, by site
  liver C22.4
 mesonephric — *see also* Neoplasm, uncertain behavior, by site
  malignant — *see* Neoplasm, malignant, by site
 metastatic
  from specified site — *see* Neoplasm, malignant, by site
  of specified site — *see* Neoplasm, malignant, by site
  to specified site — *see* Neoplasm, secondary, by site
 mixed NEC — *see also* Neoplasm, benign, by site
  malignant — *see* Neoplasm, malignant, by site
 mucinous of low malignant potential
  specified site — *see* Neoplasm, malignant, by site
  unspecified site C56.9
 mucocarcinoid
  specified site — *see* Neoplasm, malignant, by site
  unspecified site C18.1
 mucoepidermoid — *see* Neoplasm, uncertain behavior, by site
 Müllerian, mixed

Tumor - *continued*
 Müllerian, mixed - *continued*
  specified site — *see* Neoplasm, malignant, by site
  unspecified site C54.9
 myoepithelial — *see* Neoplasm, benign, by site
 neuroectodermal (peripheral) — *see* Neoplasm, malignant, by site
  primitive
   specified site — *see* Neoplasm, malignant, by site
   unspecified site C71.9
 neuroendocrine D3A.8
  malignant poorly differentiated C7A.1
  secondary NEC C7B.8
  specified NEC C7A.8
 neurogenic olfactory C30.0
 nonencapsulated sclerosing C73
 odontogenic (adenomatoid) (benign) (calcifying epithelial) (keratocystic) (squamous) — *see* Cyst, calcifying odontogenic
  malignant C41.1
   upper jaw (bone) C41.0
 ovarian stromal D39.1-
 ovary, in pregnancy — *see* Pregnancy, complicated by
 pacinian — *see* Neoplasm, skin, benign
 Pancoast's — *see* Pancoast's syndrome
 papillary — *see also* Papilloma
  cystic D37.9
  mucinous of low malignant potential C56-
   specified site — *see* Neoplasm, malignant, by site
   unspecified site C56.9
  serous of low malignant potential
   specified site — *see* Neoplasm, malignant, by site
   unspecified site C56.9
 pelvic, in pregnancy or childbirth — *see* Pregnancy, complicated by
 phantom F45.8
 phyllodes D48.6-
  benign D24-
  malignant — *see* Neoplasm, breast, malignant
 Pindborg — *see* Cyst, calcifying odontogenic
 placental site trophoblastic D39.2
 plasma cell (malignant) (localized) — *see* Plasmacytoma, solitary
 polyvesicular vitelline
  specified site — *see* Neoplasm, malignant, by site
  unspecified site
   female C56.9
   male C62.90
 Pott's puffy — *see* Osteomyelitis, specified NEC
 Rathke's pouch D44.3
 retinal anlage — *see* Neoplasm, benign, by site
 salivary gland type, mixed — *see* Neoplasm, salivary gland, benign
  malignant — *see* Neoplasm, salivary gland, malignant
 Sampson's N80.1
 Schmincke's — *see* Neoplasm, nasopharynx, malignant
 sclerosing stromal D27-
 sebaceous — *see* Cyst, sebaceous
 secondary — *see* Neoplasm, secondary, by site
  carcinoid C7B.00
   bone C7B.03
   distant lymph nodes C7B.01
   liver C7B.02
   peritoneum C7B.04
   specified NEC C7B.09
  neuroendocrine NEC C7B.8
 serous of low malignant potential
  specified site — *see* Neoplasm, malignant, by site
  unspecified site C56.9
 Sertoli cell — *see* Neoplasm, benign, by site
  with lipid storage
   specified site — *see* Neoplasm, benign, by site
   unspecified site
    female D27.9
    male D29.20
  specified site — *see* Neoplasm, benign, by site
  unspecified site
   female D27.9
   male D29.20
 Sertoli-Leydig cell — *see* Neoplasm, benign, by site
  specified site — *see* Neoplasm, benign, by site
  unspecified site
   female D27.9
   male D29.20
 sex cord (-stromal) — *see* Neoplasm, uncertain behavior, by site
  with annular tubules D39.1-
 skin appendage — *see* Neoplasm, skin, benign
 smooth muscle — *see* Neoplasm, connective tissue, uncertain behavior

Tumor - *continued*
  soft tissue
    benign — *see* Neoplasm, connective tissue, benign
    malignant — *see* Neoplasm, connective tissue, malignant
  sternomastoid (congenital) Q68.0
  stromal
    endometrial D39.0
    gastric D48.1
      benign D21.4
      malignant C16.9
      uncertain behavior D48.1
    gastrointestinal C49.A-
      benign D21.4
      esophagus C49.A1
      large intestine C49.A4
      malignant C49.A0
        colon C49.A4
        duodenum C49.A3
        esophagus C49.A1
        ileum C49.A3
        jejunum C49.A3
        Meckel diverticulum C49.A3
        large intestine C49.A4
        omentum C49.A9
        peritoneum C49.A9
        rectum C49.A5
        small intestine C49.A3
        specified site NEC C49.A9
        stomach C49.A2
      large intestine C49.A4
      rectum C49.A5
      small intestine C49.A3
      specified site NEC C49.A9
      stomach C49.A2
      uncertain behavior D48.1
    intestine
      benign D21.4
      malignant
        large C49.A4
        small C49.A3
      uncertain behavior D48.1
    ovarian D39.1-
    stomach C49.A2
      benign D21.4
      malignant C49.A2
      uncertain behavior D48.1
  testicular D40.10
  sweat gland — *see also* Neoplasm, skin, uncertain behavior
    benign — *see* Neoplasm, skin, benign
    malignant — *see* Neoplasm, skin, malignant
  syphilitic, brain A52.17
  testicular stromal D40.1-
  theca cell D27.-
  theca cell-granulosa cell D39.1-
  Triton, malignant — *see* Neoplasm, nerve, malignant
  trophoblastic, placental site D39.2
  turban D23.4
  uterus (body) , in pregnancy or childbirth — *see* Pregnancy, complicated by, tumor, uterus
  vagina, in pregnancy or childbirth — *see* Pregnancy, complicated by
  varicose — *see* Varix
  von Recklinghausen's — *see* Neurofibromatosis
  vulva or perineum, in pregnancy or childbirth — *see* Pregnancy, complicated by
    causing obstructed labor O65.5
  Warthin's — *see* Neoplasm, salivary gland, benign
  Wilms' C64-
  yolk sac — *see* Neoplasm, malignant, by site
    specified site — *see* Neoplasm, malignant, by site
    unspecified site
      female C56.9
      male C62.90
Tumor lysis syndrome
  (following antineoplastic chemotherapy) (spontaneous) **NEC** E88.3
Tumorlet — *see* Neoplasm, uncertain behavior, by site
Tungiasis B88.1
Tunica vasculosa lentis Q12.2
Turban tumor D23.4
Türck's trachoma J37.0
Turner-Kieser syndrome Q87.2
Turner-like syndrome Q87.1
Turner's
  hypoplasia (tooth) K00.4
  syndrome Q96.9
    specified NEC Q96.8
  tooth K00.4
Turner-Ullrich syndrome Q96.9

Tussis convulsiva — *see* Whooping cough
Twiddler's syndrome (due to)
  automatic implantable defibrillator T82.198
  cardiac pacemaker T82.198
Twilight state
  epileptic F05
  psychogenic F44.89
Twin (newborn) — *see also* Newborn, twin
  conjoined Q89.4
  pregnancy — *see* Pregnancy, twin, conjoined
Twinning, teeth K00.2
Twist, twisted
  bowel, colon or intestine K56.2
  hair (congenital) Q84.1
  mesentery K56.2
  omentum K56.2
  organ or site, congenital NEC — *see* Anomaly, by site
  ovarian pedicle — *see* Torsion, ovary
Twitching R25.3
Tylosis (acquired) L84
  buccalis K13.29
  linguae K13.29
  palmaris et plantaris (congenital) (inherited) Q82.8
    acquired L85.1
Tympanism R14.0
Tympanites (abdominal) (intestinal) R14.0
Tympanitis — *see* Myringitis
Tympanosclerosis — *see* subcategory H74.0
Tympanum — *see* condition
Tympany
  abdomen R14.0
  chest R09.89
Type A behavior pattern Z73.1
Typhlitis — *see* Appendicitis
Typhoenteritis — *see* Typhoid
Typhoid (abortive) (ambulant) (any site) (clinical) (fever) (hemorrhagic) (infection) (intermittent) (malignant) (rheumatic) (Widal negative) A01.00
  with pneumonia A01.03
  abdominal A01.09
  arthritis A01.04
  carrier (suspected) of Z22.0
  cholecystitis (current) A01.09
  endocarditis A01.02
  heart involvement A01.02
  inoculation reaction — *see* Complications, vaccination
  meningitis A01.01
  mesenteric lymph nodes A01.09
  myocarditis A01.02
  osteomyelitis A01.05
  perichondritis, larynx A01.09
  pneumonia A01.03
  spine A01.05
  specified NEC A01.09
  ulcer (perforating) A01.09
Typhomalaria (fever) — *see* Malaria
Typhomania A01.00
Typhoperitonitis A01.09
Typhus (fever) A75.9
  abdominal, abdominalis — *see* Typhoid
  African tick A77.1
  amarillic A95.9
  brain A75.9 *[G94]*
  cerebral A75.9 *[G94]*
  classical A75.0
  due to Rickettsia
    prowazekii A75.0
      recrudescent A75.1
    tsutsugamushi A75.3
    typhi A75.2
  endemic (flea-borne) A75.2
  epidemic (louse-borne) A75.0
  exanthematic NEC A75.0
  exanthematicus SAI A75.0
    brillii SAI A75.1
    mexicanus SAI A75.2
    typhus murinus A75.2
  flea-borne A75.2
  India tick A77.1
  Kenya (tick) A77.1
  louse-borne A75.0
  Mexican A75.2
  mite-borne A75.3
  murine A75.2
  North Asian tick-borne A77.2
  petechial A75.9
  Queensland tick A77.3
  rat A75.2
  recrudescent A75.1
  recurrens — *see* Fever, relapsing
  Sao Paulo A77.0

Typhus (fever) - *continued*
  scrub (China) (India) (Malaysia) (New Guinea) A75.3
  shop (of Malaysia) A75.2
  Siberian tick A77.2
  tick-borne A77.9
  tropical (mite-borne) A75.3
Tyrosinemia E70.21
  newborn, transitory P74.5
Tyrosinosis E70.21
Tyrosinuria E70.29

U

Uhl's anomaly or disease Q24.8
Ulcer, ulcerated, ulcerating, ulceration, ulcerative
  alveolar process M27.3
  amebic (intestine) A06.1
    skin A06.7
  anastomotic — *see* Ulcer, gastrojejunal
  anorectal K62.6
  antral — *see* Ulcer, stomach
  anus (sphincter) (solitary) K62.6
  aorta — *see* Aneurysm
  aphthous (oral) (recurrent) K12.0
    genital organ (s)
      female N76.6
      male N50.89
  artery I77.2
  atrophic — *see* Ulcer, skin
    decubitus — *see* Ulcer, pressure, by site
  back L98.429
    with
      bone necrosis L98.424
      exposed fat layer L98.422
      muscle necrosis L98.423
      skin breakdown only L98.421
  Barrett's (esophagus) K22.10
    with bleeding K22.11
  bile duct (common) (hepatic) K83.8
  bladder (solitary) (sphincter) NEC N32.89
    bilharzial B65.9 *[N33]*
    in schistosomiasis (bilharzial) B65.9 *[N33]*
    submucosal — *see* Cystitis, interstitial
    tuberculous A18.12
  bleeding K27.4
  bone — *see* Osteomyelitis, specified type NEC
  bowel — *see* Ulcer, intestine
  breast N61.1
  bronchus J98.09
  buccal (cavity) (traumatic) K12.1
  Buruli A31.1
  buttock L98.419
    with
      bone necrosis L98.414
      exposed fat layer L98.412
      muscle necrosis L98.413
      skin breakdown only L98.411
  cancerous — *see* Neoplasm, malignant, by site
  cardia K22.10
    with bleeding K22.11
  cardioesophageal (peptic) K22.10
    with bleeding K22.11
  cecum — *see* Ulcer, intestine
  cervix (uteri) (decubitus) (trophic) N86
    with cervicitis N72
  chancroidal A57
  chiclero B55.1
  chronic (cause unknown) — *see* Ulcer, skin
  Cochin-China B55.1
  colon — *see* Ulcer, intestine
  conjunctiva H10.89
  cornea H16.00-
    with hypopyon H16.03-
    central H16.01-
    dendritic (herpes simplex) B00.52
    marginal H16.04-
    Mooren's H16.05-
    mycotic H16.06-
    perforated H16.07-
    ring H16.02-
    tuberculous (phlyctenular) A18.52
  corpus cavernosum (chronic) N48.5
  crural — *see* Ulcer, lower limb
  Curling's — *see* Ulcer, peptic, acute
  Cushing's — *see* Ulcer, peptic, acute
  cystic duct K82.8
  cystitis (interstitial) — *see* Cystitis, interstitial
  decubitus — *see* Ulcer, pressure, by site
  dendritic, cornea (herpes simplex) B00.52
  diabetes, diabetic — *see* Diabetes, ulcer
  Dieulafoy's K25.0
  due to
    infection NEC — *see* Ulcer, skin

Ulcer, ulcerated, ulcerating, ulceration, ulcerative - *continued*
- due to - *continued*
  - radiation NEC L59.8
  - trophic disturbance (any region) — *see* Ulcer, skin
  - X-ray L58.1
- duodenum, duodenal (eroded) (peptic) K26.9
  - with
    - hemorrhage K26.4
      - and perforation K26.6
    - perforation K26.5
  - acute K26.3
    - with
      - hemorrhage K26.0
        - and perforation K26.2
      - perforation K26.1
  - chronic K26.7
    - with
      - hemorrhage K26.4
        - and perforation K26.6
      - perforation K26.5
- dysenteric A09
- elusive — *see* Cystitis, interstitial
- endocarditis (acute) (chronic) (subacute) I28.8
- epiglottis J38.7
- esophagus (peptic) K22.10
  - with bleeding K22.11
  - due to
    - aspirin K22.10
      - with bleeding K22.11
    - gastrointestinal reflux disease K21.0
    - ingestion of chemical or medicament K22.10
      - with bleeding K22.11
    - fungal K22.10
      - with bleeding K22.11
    - infective K22.10
      - with bleeding K22.11
  - varicose — *see* Varix, esophagus
- eyelid (region) H01.8
- fauces J39.2
- Fenwick (-Hunner) (solitary) — *see* Cystitis, interstitial
- fistulous — *see* Ulcer, skin
- foot (indolent) (trophic) — *see* Ulcer, lower limb
- frambesial, initial A66.0
- frenum (tongue) K14.0
- gallbladder or duct K82.8
- gangrenous — *see* Gangrene
- gastric — *see* Ulcer, stomach
- gastrocolic — *see* Ulcer, gastrojejunal
- gastroduodenal — *see* Ulcer, peptic
- gastroesophageal — *see* Ulcer, stomach
- gastrointestinal — *see* Ulcer, gastrojejunal
- gastrojejunal (peptic) K28.9
  - with
    - hemorrhage K28.4
      - and perforation K28.6
    - perforation K28.5
  - acute K28.3
    - with
      - hemorrhage K28.0
        - and perforation K28.2
      - perforation K28.1
  - chronic K28.7
    - with
      - hemorrhage K28.4
        - and perforation K28.6
      - perforation K28.5
- gastrojejunocolic — *see* Ulcer, gastrojejunal
- gingiva K06.8
- gingivitis K05.10
  - nonplaque induced K05.11
  - plaque induced K05.10
- glottis J38.7
- granuloma of pudenda A58
- gum K06.8
- gumma, due to yaws A66.4
- heel — *see* Ulcer, lower limb
- hemorrhoid — *see also* Hemorrhoids, by degree K64.8
- Hunner's — *see* Cystitis, interstitial
- hypopharynx J39.2
- hypopyon (chronic) (subacute) — *see* Ulcer, cornea, with hypopyon
- hypostaticum — *see* Ulcer, varicose
- ileum — *see* Ulcer, intestine
- intestine, intestinal K63.3
  - with perforation K63.1
  - amebic A06.1
  - duodenal — *see* Ulcer, duodenum
  - granulocytopenic (with hemorrhage) — *see* Neutropenia
  - marginal — *see* Ulcer, gastrojejunal

Ulcer, ulcerated, ulcerating, ulceration, ulcerative - *continued*
- intestine, intestinal - *continued*
  - perforating K63.1
    - newborn P78.0
  - primary, small intestine K63.3
  - rectum K62.6
  - stercoraceous, stercoral K63.3
  - tuberculous A18.32
  - typhoid (fever) — *see* Typhoid
  - varicose I86.8
- jejunum, jejunal — *see* Ulcer, gastrojejunal
- keratitis — *see* Ulcer, cornea
- knee — *see* Ulcer, lower limb
- labium (majus) (minus) N76.6
- laryngitis — *see* Laryngitis
- larynx (aphthous) (contact) J38.7
  - diphtheritic A36.2
- leg — *see* Ulcer, lower limb
- lip K13.0
- Lipschütz's N76.6
- lower limb (atrophic) (chronic) (neurogenic) (perforating) (pyogenic) (trophic) (tropical) L97.909
  - with
    - bone necrosis L97.904
    - exposed fat layer L97.902
    - muscle necrosis L97.903
    - skin breakdown only L97.901
  - ankle L97.309
    - with
      - bone necrosis L97.304
      - exposed fat layer L97.302
      - muscle necrosis L97.303
      - skin breakdown only L97.301
    - left L97.329
      - with
        - bone necrosis L97.324
        - exposed fat layer L97.322
        - muscle necrosis L97.323
        - skin breakdown only L97.321
    - right L97.319
      - with
        - bone necrosis L97.314
        - exposed fat layer L97.312
        - muscle necrosis L97.313
        - skin breakdown only L97.311
  - calf L97.209
    - with
      - bone necrosis L97.204
      - exposed fat layer L97.202
      - muscle necrosis L97.203
      - skin breakdown only L97.201
    - left L97.229
      - with
        - bone necrosis L97.224
        - exposed fat layer L97.222
        - muscle necrosis L97.223
        - skin breakdown only L97.221
    - right L97.219
      - with
        - bone necrosis L97.214
        - exposed fat layer L97.212
        - muscle necrosis L97.213
        - skin breakdown only L97.211
  - decubitus — *see* Ulcer, pressure, by site
  - foot specified NEC L97.509
    - with
      - bone necrosis L97.504
      - exposed fat layer L97.502
      - muscle necrosis L97.503
      - skin breakdown only L97.501
    - left L97.529
      - with
        - bone necrosis L97.524
        - exposed fat layer L97.522
        - muscle necrosis L97.523
        - skin breakdown only L97.521
    - right L97.519
      - with
        - bone necrosis L97.514
        - exposed fat layer L97.512
        - muscle necrosis L97.513
        - skin breakdown only L97.511
  - heel L97.409
    - with
      - bone necrosis L97.404
      - exposed fat layer L97.402
      - muscle necrosis L97.403
      - skin breakdown only L97.401
    - left L97.429
      - with
        - bone necrosis L97.424

Ulcer, ulcerated, ulcerating, ulceration, ulcerative - *continued*
- lower limb (atrophic) (chronic) (neurogenic) (perforating) (pyogenic) (trophic) (tropical) - *continued*
  - heel - *continued*
    - left - *continued*
      - with - *continued*
        - exposed fat layer L97.422
        - muscle necrosis L97.423
        - skin breakdown only L97.421
    - right L97.419
      - with
        - bone necrosis L97.414
        - exposed fat layer L97.412
        - muscle necrosis L97.413
        - skin breakdown only L97.411
  - left L97.929
    - with
      - bone necrosis L97.924
      - exposed fat layer L97.922
      - muscle necrosis L97.923
      - skin breakdown only L97.921
  - lower leg NOS L97.909
    - with
      - bone necrosis L97.904
      - exposed fat layer L97.902
      - muscle necrosis L97.903
      - skin breakdown only L97.901
    - left L97.929
      - with
        - bone necrosis L97.924
        - exposed fat layer L97.922
        - muscle necrosis L97.923
        - skin breakdown only L97.921
    - right L97.919
      - with
        - bone necrosis L97.914
        - exposed fat layer L97.912
        - muscle necrosis L97.913
        - skin breakdown only L97.911
  - specified site NEC L97.809
    - with
      - bone necrosis L97.804
      - exposed fat layer L97.802
      - muscle necrosis L97.803
      - skin breakdown only L97.801
    - left L97.829
      - with
        - bone necrosis L97.824
        - exposed fat layer L97.822
        - muscle necrosis L97.823
        - skin breakdown only L97.821
    - right L97.819
      - with
        - bone necrosis L97.814
        - exposed fat layer L97.812
        - muscle necrosis L97.813
        - skin breakdown only L97.811
  - midfoot L97.409
    - with
      - bone necrosis L97.404
      - exposed fat layer L97.402
      - muscle necrosis L97.403
      - skin breakdown only L97.401
    - left L97.429
      - with
        - bone necrosis L97.424
        - exposed fat layer L97.422
        - muscle necrosis L97.423
        - skin breakdown only L97.421
    - right L97.419
      - with
        - bone necrosis L97.414
        - exposed fat layer L97.412
        - muscle necrosis L97.413
        - skin breakdown only L97.411
  - right L97.919
    - with
      - bone necrosis L97.914
      - exposed fat layer L97.912
      - muscle necrosis L97.913
      - skin breakdown only L97.911
  - thigh L97.109
    - with
      - bone necrosis L97.104
      - exposed fat layer L97.102
      - muscle necrosis L97.103
      - skin breakdown only L97.101
    - left L97.129
      - with
        - bone necrosis L97.124
        - exposed fat layer L97.122

Ulcer, ulcerated, ulcerating, ulceration, ulcerative - *continued*
- lower limb (atrophic) (chronic) (neurogenic) (perforating) (pyogenic) (trophic) (tropical) - *continued*
  - thigh - *continued*
    - left - *continued*
      - with - *continued*
        - muscle necrosis L97.123
        - skin breakdown only L97.121
      - right L97.119
        - with
          - bone necrosis L97.114
          - exposed fat layer L97.112
          - muscle necrosis L97.113
          - skin breakdown only L97.111
  - toe L97.509
    - with
      - bone necrosis L97.504
      - exposed fat layer L97.502
      - muscle necrosis L97.503
      - skin breakdown only L97.501
    - left L97.529
      - with
        - bone necrosis L97.524
        - exposed fat layer L97.522
        - muscle necrosis L97.523
        - skin breakdown only L97.521
    - right L97.519
      - with
        - bone necrosis L97.514
        - exposed fat layer L97.512
        - muscle necrosis L97.513
        - skin breakdown only L97.511
  - leprous A30.1
  - syphilitic A52.19
  - varicose — *see* Varix, leg, with, ulcer
  - luetic — *see* Ulcer, syphilitic
- lung J98.4
  - tuberculous — *see* Tuberculosis, pulmonary
- malignant — *see* Neoplasm, malignant, by site
- marginal NEC — *see* Ulcer, gastrojejunal
- meatus (urinarius) N34.2
- Meckel's diverticulum Q43.0
  - malignant — *see* Table of Neoplasms, small intestine, malignant
- Meleney's (chronic undermining) — *see* Ulcer, skin
- Mooren's (cornea) — *see* Ulcer, cornea, Mooren's
- mycobacterial (skin) A31.1
- nasopharynx J39.2
- neck, uterus N86
- neurogenic NEC — *see* Ulcer, skin
- nose, nasal (passage) (infective) (septum) J34.0
  - skin — *see* Ulcer, skin
  - spirochetal A69.8
  - varicose (bleeding) I86.8
- oral mucosa (traumatic) K12.1
- palate (soft) K12.1
- penis (chronic) N48.5
- peptic (site unspecified) K27.9
  - with
    - hemorrhage K27.4
      - and perforation K27.6
    - perforation K27.5
  - acute K27.3
    - with
      - hemorrhage K27.0
        - and perforation K27.2
      - perforation K27.1
  - chronic K27.7
    - with
      - hemorrhage K27.4
        - and perforation K27.6
      - perforation K27.5
  - esophagus K22.10
    - with bleeding K22.11
  - newborn P78.82
  - perforating K27.5
- skin — *see* Ulcer, skin
- peritonsillar J35.8
- phagedenic (tropical) — *see* Ulcer, skin
- pharynx J39.2
- phlebitis — *see* Phlebitis
- plaster — *see* Ulcer, pressure, by site
- popliteal space — *see* Ulcer, lower limb
- postpyloric — *see* Ulcer, duodenum
- prepuce N47.7
- prepyloric — *see* Ulcer, stomach
- pressure (pressure area) L89.9-
  - ankle L89.5-
  - back L89.1-
  - buttock L89.3-
  - coccyx L89.15-

Ulcer, ulcerated, ulcerating, ulceration, ulcerative - *continued*
- pressure (pressure area) - *continued*
  - contiguous site of back, buttock, hip L89.4-
  - elbow L89.0-
  - face L89.81-
  - head L89.81-
  - heel L89.6-
  - hip L89.2-
  - sacral region (tailbone) L89.15-
  - specified site NEC L89.89-
  - stage 1 (healing) (pre-ulcer skin changes limited to persistent focal edema)
    - ankle L89.5-
    - back L89.1-
    - buttock L89.3-
    - coccyx L89.15-
    - contiguous site of back, buttock, hip L89.4-
    - elbow L89.0-
    - face L89.81-
    - head L89.81-
    - heel L89.6-
    - hip L89.2-
    - sacral region (tailbone) L89.15-
    - specified site NEC L89.89-
  - stage 2 (healing) (abrasion, blister, partial thickness skin loss involving epidermis and/or dermis)
    - ankle L89.5-
    - back L89.1-
    - buttock L89.3-
    - coccyx L89.15-
    - contiguous site of back, buttock, hip L89.4-
    - elbow L89.0-
    - face L89.81-
    - head L89.81-
    - heel L89.6-
    - hip L89.2-
    - sacral region (tailbone) L89.15-
    - specified site NEC L89.89-
  - stage 3 (healing) (full thickness skin loss involving damage or necrosis of subcutaneous tissue)
    - ankle L89.5-
    - back L89.1-
    - buttock L89.3-
    - coccyx L89.15-
    - contiguous site of back, buttock, hip L89.4-
    - elbow L89.0-
    - face L89.81-
    - head L89.81-
    - heel L89.6-
    - hip L89.2-
    - sacral region (tailbone) L89.15-
    - specified site NEC L89.89-
  - stage 4 (healing) (necrosis of soft tissues through to underlying muscle, tendon, or bone)
    - ankle L89.5-
    - back L89.1-
    - buttock L89.3-
    - coccyx L89.15-
    - contiguous site of back, buttock, hip L89.4-
    - elbow L89.0-
    - face L89.81-
    - head L89.81-
    - heel L89.6-
    - hip L89.2-
    - sacral region (tailbone) L89.15-
    - specified site NEC L89.89-
  - unspecified stage
    - ankle L89.5-
    - back L89.1-
    - buttock L89.3-
    - coccyx L89.15-
    - contiguous site of back, buttock, hip L89.4-
    - elbow L89.0-
    - face L89.81-
    - head L89.81-
    - heel L89.6-
    - hip L89.2-
    - sacral region (tailbone) L89.15-
    - specified site NEC L89.89-
  - unstageable
    - ankle L89.5-
    - back L89.1-
    - buttock L89.3-
    - coccyx L89.15-
    - contiguous site of back, buttock, hip L89.4-
    - elbow L89.0-
    - face L89.81-
    - head L89.81-
    - heel L89.6-
    - hip L89.2-
    - sacral region (tailbone) L89.15-
    - specified site NEC L89.89-

Ulcer, ulcerated, ulcerating, ulceration, ulcerative - *continued*
- primary of intestine K63.3
  - with perforation K63.1
- prostate N41.9
- pyloric — *see* Ulcer, stomach
- rectosigmoid K63.3
  - with perforation K63.1
- rectum (sphincter) (solitary) K62.6
  - stercoraceous, stercoral K62.6
- retina — *see* Inflammation, chorioretinal
- rodent — *see also* Neoplasm, skin, malignant
- sclera — *see* Scleritis
- scrofulous (tuberculous) A18.2
- scrotum N50.89
  - tuberculous A18.15
  - varicose I86.1
- seminal vesicle N50.89
- sigmoid — *see* Ulcer, intestine
- skin (atrophic) (chronic) (neurogenic) (non-healing) (perforating) (pyogenic) (trophic) (tropical) L98.499
  - with gangrene — *see* Gangrene
  - amebic A06.7
  - back — *see* Ulcer, back
  - buttock — *see* Ulcer, buttock
  - decubitus — *see* Ulcer, pressure
  - lower limb — *see* Ulcer, lower limb
  - mycobacterial A31.1
  - specified site NEC L98.499
    - with
      - bone necrosis L98.494
      - exposed fat layer L98.492
      - muscle necrosis L98.493
      - skin breakdown only L98.491
  - tuberculous (primary) A18.4
  - varicose — *see* Ulcer, varicose
- sloughing — *see* Ulcer, skin
- solitary, anus or rectum (sphincter) K62.6
- sore throat J02.9
  - streptococcal J02.0
- spermatic cord N50.89
- spine (tuberculous) A18.01
- stasis (venous) — *see* Varix, leg, with, ulcer
  - without varicose veins I87.2
- stercoraceous, stercoral K63.3
  - with perforation K63.1
  - anus or rectum K62.6
- stoma, stomal — *see* Ulcer, gastrojejunal
- stomach (eroded) (peptic) (round) K25.9
  - with
    - hemorrhage K25.4
      - and perforation K25.6
    - perforation K25.5
  - acute K25.3
    - with
      - hemorrhage K25.0
        - and perforation K25.2
      - perforation K25.1
  - chronic K25.7
    - with
      - hemorrhage K25.4
        - and perforation K25.6
      - perforation K25.5
- stomal — *see* Ulcer, gastrojejunal
- stomatitis K12.1
- stress — *see* Ulcer, peptic
- strumous (tuberculous) A18.2
- submucosal, bladder — *see* Cystitis, interstitial
- syphilitic (any site) (early) (secondary) A51.39
  - late A52.79
  - perforating A52.79
    - foot A52.11
- testis N50.89
- thigh — *see* Ulcer, lower limb
- throat J39.2
  - diphtheritic A36.0
- toe — *see* Ulcer, lower limb
- tongue (traumatic) K14.0
- tonsil J35.8
  - diphtheritic A36.0
- trachea J39.8
- trophic — *see* Ulcer, skin
- tropical — *see* Ulcer, skin
- tuberculous — *see* Tuberculosis, ulcer
- tunica vaginalis N50.89
- turbinate J34.89
- typhoid (perforating) — *see* Typhoid
- unspecified site — *see* Ulcer, skin
- urethra (meatus) — *see* Urethritis
- uterus N85.8
  - cervix N86
    - with cervicitis N72

Ulcer, ulcerated, ulcerating, ulceration, ulcerative - *continued*
  uterus - *continued*
    neck N86
      with cervicitis N72
    vagina N76.5
      in Behçet's disease M35.2 *[N77.0]*
      pessary N89.8
    valve, heart I33.0
    varicose (lower limb, any part) — *see also* Varix, leg, with, ulcer
      broad ligament I86.2
      esophagus — *see* Varix, esophagus
      inflamed or infected — *see* Varix, leg, with ulcer, with inflammation
      nasal septum I86.8
      perineum I86.3
      scrotum I86.1
      specified site NEC I86.8
      sublingual I86.0
      vulva I86.3
    vas deferens N50.89
    vulva (acute) (infectional) N76.6
      in (due to)
        Behçet's disease M35.2 *[N77.0]*
        herpesviral (herpes simplex) infection A60.04
        tuberculosis A18.18
    vulvobuccal, recurring N76.6
    X-ray L58.1
    yaws A66.4
Ulcerosa scarlatina A38.8
Ulcus — *see also* Ulcer
  cutis tuberculosum A18.4
  duodeni — *see* Ulcer, duodenum
  durum (syphilitic) A51.0
    extragenital A51.2
  gastrojejunale — *see* Ulcer, gastrojejunal
  hypostaticum — *see* Ulcer, varicose
  molle (cutis) (skin) A57
  serpens corneae — *see* Ulcer, cornea, central
  ventriculi — *see* Ulcer, stomach
Ulegyria Q04.8
Ulerythema
  ophryogenes, congenital Q84.2
  sycosiforme L73.8
Ullrich (-Bonnevie) (-Turner) **syndrome** — *see also* Turner's syndrome Q87.1
Ullrich-Feichtiger syndrome Q87.0
Ulnar — *see* condition
Ulorrhagia, ulorrhea K06.8
Umbilicus, umbilical — *see* condition
Unacceptable
  contours of tooth K08.54
  morphology of tooth K08.54
Unavailability (of)
  bed at medical facility Z75.1
  health service-related agencies Z75.4
  medical facilities (at) Z75.3
    due to
      investigation by social service agency Z75.2
      lack of services at home Z75.0
      remoteness from facility Z75.3
      waiting list Z75.1
    home Z75.0
    outpatient clinic Z75.3
  schooling Z55.1
  social service agencies Z75.4
Uncinaria americana infestation B76.1
Uncinariasis B76.9
Uncongenial work Z56.5
Unconscious (ness) — *see* Coma
Under observation — *see* Observation
Underachievement in school Z55.3
Underdevelopment — *see also* Undeveloped
  nose Q30.1
  sexual E30.0
Underdosing — *see also* Table of Drugs and Chemicals, categories T36-T50, with final character 6 Z91.14
  intentional NEC Z91.128
    due to financial hardship of patient Z91.120
  unintentional NEC Z91.138
    due to patient's age related debility Z91.130
Underfeeding, newborn P92.3
Underfill, endodontic M27.53
Underimmunization status Z28.3
Undernourishment — *see* Malnutrition
Undernutrition — *see* Malnutrition
Underweight R63.6
  for gestational age — *see* Light for dates
Underwood's disease P83.0
Undescended — *see also* Malposition, congenital
  cecum Q43.3

Undescended - *continued*
  colon Q43.3
  testicle — *see* Cryptorchid
Undeveloped, undevelopment — *see also* Hypoplasia
  brain (congenital) Q02
  cerebral (congenital) Q02
  heart Q24.8
  lung Q33.6
  testis E29.1
  uterus E30.0
Undiagnosed (disease) R69
Undulant fever — *see* Brucellosis
Unemployment, anxiety concerning Z56.0
  threatened Z56.2
Unequal length (acquired) (limb) — *see also* Deformity, limb, unequal length
  leg — *see also* Deformity, limb, unequal length
    congenital Q72.9-
Unextracted dental root K08.3
Unguis incarnatus L60.0
Unhappiness R45.2
Unicornate uterus Q51.4
Unilateral — *see also* condition
  development, breast N64.89
  organ or site, congenital NEC — *see* Agenesis, by site
Unilocular heart Q20.8
Union, abnormal — *see also* Fusion
  larynx and trachea Q34.8
Universal mesentery Q43.3
Unrepairable overhanging of dental restorative materials K08.52
Unsatisfactory
  restoration of tooth K08.50
    specified NEC K08.59
  sample of cytologic smear
    anus R85.615
    cervix R87.615
    vagina R87.625
  surroundings Z59.1
  work Z56.5
Unsoundness of mind — *see* Psychosis
Unstable
  back NEC — *see* Instability, joint, spine
  hip (congenital) Q65.6
    acquired — *see* Derangement, joint, specified type NEC, hip
  joint — *see* Instability, joint
    secondary to removal of joint prosthesis M96.89
  lie (mother) O32.0
  lumbosacral joint (congenital)
    acquired — *see* subcategory M53.2
  sacroiliac — *see* subcategory M53.2
  spine NEC — *see* Instability, joint, spine
Unsteadiness on feet R26.81
Untruthfulness, child problem F91.8
Unverricht (-Lundborg) **disease or epilepsy** — *see* Epilepsy, generalized, idiopathic
Unwanted pregnancy Z64.0
Upbringing, institutional Z62.22
  away from parents NEC Z62.29
  in care of non-parental family member Z62.21
  in foster care Z62.21
  in orphanage or group home Z62.22
  in welfare custody Z62.21
Upper respiratory — *see* condition
Upset
  gastric K30
  gastrointestinal K30
    psychogenic F45.8
  intestinal (large) (small) K59.9
    psychogenic F45.8
  menstruation N93.9
  mental F48.9
  stomach K30
    psychogenic F45.8
Urachus — *see also* condition
  patent or persistent Q64.4
Urbach-Oppenheim disease (necrobiosis lipoidica diabeticorum) — *see* E08-E13 with .620
Urbach's lipoid proteinosis E78.89
Urbach-Wiethe disease E78.89
Urban yellow fever A95.1
Urea
  blood, high — *see* Uremia
  cycle metabolism disorder — *see* Disorder, urea cycle metabolism
Uremia, uremic N19
  with
    ectopic or molar pregnancy O08.4
    polyneuropathy N18.9 *[G63]*

Uremia, uremic - *continued*
  chronic — *see also* Disease, kidney, chronic N18.9
    due to hypertension — *see* Hypertensive, kidney
  complicating
    ectopic or molar pregnancy O08.4
  congenital P96.0
  extrarenal R39.2
  following ectopic or molar pregnancy O08.4
  newborn P96.0
  prerenal R39.2
Ureter, ureteral — *see* condition
Ureteralgia N23
Ureterectasis — *see* Hydroureter
Ureteritis N28.89
  cystica N28.86
  due to calculus N20.1
    with calculus, kidney N20.2
      with hydronephrosis N13.2
  gonococcal (acute) (chronic) A54.21
  nonspecific N28.89
Ureterocele N28.89
  congenital (orthotopic) Q62.31
  ectopic Q62.32
Ureterolith, ureterolithiasis — *see* Calculus, ureter
Ureterostomy
  attention to Z43.6
  status Z93.6
Urethra, urethral — *see* condition
Urethralgia R39.89
Urethritis (anterior) (posterior) N34.2
  calculous N21.1
  candidal B37.41
  chlamydial A56.01
  diplococcal (gonococcal) A54.01
    with abscess (accessory gland) (periurethral) A54.1
  gonococcal A54.01
    with abscess (accessory gland) (periurethral) A54.1
  nongonococcal N34.1
    Reiter's — *see* Reiter's disease
  nonspecific N34.1
  nonvenereal N34.1
  postmenopausal N34.2
  puerperal O86.22
  Reiter's — *see* Reiter's disease
  specified NEC N34.2
  trichomonal or due to Trichomonas (vaginalis) A59.03
Urethrocele N81.0
  with
    cystocele — *see* Cystocele
    prolapse of uterus — *see* Prolapse, uterus
Urethrolithiasis (with colic or infection) N21.1
Urethrorectal — *see* condition
Urethrorrhagia N36.8
Urethrorrhea R36.9
Urethrostomy
  attention to Z43.6
  status Z93.6
Urethrotrigonitis — *see* Trigonitis
Urethrovaginal — *see* condition
Urgency
  fecal R15.2
  hypertensive — *see* Hypertension
  urinary R39.15
Urhidrosis, uridrosis L74.8
Uric acid in blood (increased) E79.0
Uricacidemia (asymptomatic) E79.0
Uricemia (asymptomatic) E79.0
Uricosuria R82.99
Urinary — *see* condition
Urination
  frequent R35.0
  painful R30.9
Urine
  blood in — *see* Hematuria
  discharge, excessive R35.8
  enuresis, nonorganic origin F98.0
  extravasation R39.0
  frequency R35.0
  incontinence R32
    nonorganic origin F98.0
  intermittent stream R39.198
  pus in N39.0
  retention or stasis R33.9
    organic R33.8
      drug-induced R33.0
    psychogenic F45.8
  secretion
    deficient R34
    excessive R35.8
    frequency R35.0
  stream
    intermittent R39.198

Urine - *continued*
  stream - *continued*
    slowing R39.198
    splitting R39.13
    weak R39.12
Urinemia — *see* Uremia
Urinoma, urethra N36.8
Uroarthritis, infectious (Reiter's) — *see* Reiter's disease
Urodialysis R34
Urolithiasis — *see* Calculus, urinary
Uronephrosis — *see* Hydronephrosis
Uropathy N39.9
  obstructive N13.9
    specified NEC N13.8
  reflux N13.9
    specified NEC N13.8
  vesicoureteral reflux-associated — *see* Reflux, vesicoureteral
Urosepsis - code to condition
Urticaria L50.9
  with angioneurotic edema T78.3
    hereditary D84.1
  allergic L50.0
  cholinergic L50.5
  chronic L50.8
  cold, familial L50.2
  contact L50.6
  dermatographic L50.3
  due to
    cold or heat L50.2
    drugs L50.0
    food L50.0
    inhalants L50.0
    plants L50.6
  serum — *see also* Reaction, serum T80.69
  factitial L50.3
  familial cold M04.2
  giant T78.3
    hereditary D84.1
  gigantea T78.3
  idiopathic L50.1
  larynx T78.3
    hereditary D84.1
  neonatorum P83.8
  nonallergic L50.1
  papulosa (Hebra) L28.2
  pigmentosa Q82.2
  recurrent periodic L50.8
  serum — *see also* Reaction, serum T80.69
  solar L56.3
  specified type NEC L50.8
  thermal (cold) (heat) L50.2
  vibratory L50.4
  xanthelasmoidea Q82.2
Use (of)
  alcohol Z72.89
    with
      intoxication F10.929
      sleep disorder F10.982
    harmful — *see* Abuse, alcohol
  amphetamines — *see* Use, stimulant NEC
  caffeine — *see* Use, stimulant NEC
  cannabis F12.90
    with
      anxiety disorder F12.980
      intoxication F12.929
        with
          delirium F12.921
          perceptual disturbance F12.922
        uncomplicated F12.920
      other specified disorder F12.988
      psychosis F12.959
        delusions F12.950
        hallucinations F12.951
      unspecified disorder F12.99
  cocaine F14.90
    with
      anxiety disorder F14.980
      intoxication F14.929
        with
          delirium F14.921
          perceptual disturbance F14.922
        uncomplicated F14.920
      other specified disorder F14.988
      psychosis F14.959
        delusions F14.950
        hallucinations F14.951
      sexual dysfunction F14.981
      sleep disorder F14.982
      unspecified disorder F14.99
    harmful — *see* Abuse, drug, cocaine
  drug (s) NEC F19.90

Use (of) - *continued*
  drug (s) NEC - *continued*
    with sleep disorder F19.982
    harmful — *see* Abuse, drug, by type
  hallucinogen NEC F16.90
    with
      anxiety disorder F16.980
      intoxication F16.929
        with
          delirium F16.921
        uncomplicated F16.920
      mood disorder F16.94
      other specified disorder F16.988
      perception disorder (flashbacks) F16.983
      psychosis F16.959
        delusions F16.950
        hallucinations F16.951
      unspecified disorder F16.99
    harmful — *see* Abuse, drug, hallucinogen NEC
  inhalants F18.90
    with
      anxiety disorder F18.980
      intoxication F18.929
        with delirium F18.921
        uncomplicated F18.920
      mood disorder F18.94
      other specified disorder F18.988
      persisting dementia F18.97
      psychosis F18.959
        delusions F18.950
        hallucinations F18.951
      unspecified disorder F18.99
    harmful — *see* Abuse, drug, inhalant
  methadone — *see* Use, opioid
  nonprescribed drugs F19.90
    harmful — *see* Abuse, non-psychoactive substance
  opioid F11.90
    with
      disorder F11.99
        mood F11.94
        sleep F11.982
        specified type NEC F11.988
      intoxication F11.929
        with
          delirium F11.921
          perceptual disturbance F11.922
        uncomplicated F11.920
      withdrawal F11.93
    harmful — *see* Abuse, drug, opioid
  patent medicines F19.90
    harmful — *see* Abuse, non-psychoactive substance
  psychoactive drug NEC F19.90
    with
      anxiety disorder F19.980
      intoxication F19.929
        with
          delirium F19.921
          perceptual disturbance F19.922
        uncomplicated F19.920
      mood disorder F19.94
      other specified disorder F19.988
      persisting
        amnestic disorder F19.96
        dementia F19.97
      psychosis F19.959
        delusions F19.950
        hallucinations F19.951
      sexual dysfunction F19.981
      sleep disorder F19.982
      unspecified disorder F19.99
      withdrawal F19.939
        with
          delirium F19.931
          perceptual disturbance F19.932
        uncomplicated F19.930
    harmful — *see* Abuse, drug NEC, psychoactive NEC
  sedative, hypnotic, or anxiolytic F13.90
    with
      anxiety disorder F13.980
      intoxication F13.929
        with
          delirium F13.921
        uncomplicated F13.920
      other specified disorder F13.988
      persisting
        amnestic disorder F13.96
        dementia F13.97
      psychosis F13.959
        delusions F13.950
        hallucinations F13.951
      sexual dysfunction F13.981
      sleep disorder F13.982

Use (of) - *continued*
  sedative, hypnotic, or anxiolytic - *continued*
    with - *continued*
      unspecified disorder F13.99
    harmful — *see* Abuse, drug, sedative, hypnotic, or anxiolytic
  stimulant NEC F15.90
    with
      anxiety disorder F15.980
      intoxication F15.929
        with
          delirium F15.921
          perceptual disturbance F15.922
        uncomplicated F15.920
      mood disorder F15.94
      other specified disorder F15.988
      psychosis F15.959
        delusions F15.950
        hallucinations F15.951
      sexual dysfunction F15.981
      sleep disorder F15.982
      unspecified disorder F15.99
      withdrawal F15.93
    harmful — *see* Abuse, drug, stimulant NEC
  tobacco Z72.0
    with dependence — *see* Dependence, drug, nicotine
  volatile solvents — *see also* Use, inhalant F18.90
    harmful — *see* Abuse, drug, inhalant
Usher-Senear disease or syndrome L10.4
Uta B55.1
Uteromegaly N85.2
Uterovaginal — *see* condition
Uterovesical — *see* condition
Uveal — *see* condition
Uveitis (anterior) — *see also* Iridocyclitis
  acute — *see* Iridocyclitis, acute
  chronic — *see* Iridocyclitis, chronic
  due to toxoplasmosis (acquired) B58.09
    congenital P37.1
  granulomatous — *see* Iridocyclitis, chronic
  heterochromic — *see* Cyclitis, Fuchs' heterochromic
  lens-induced — *see* Iridocyclitis, lens-induced
  posterior — *see* Chorioretinitis
  sympathetic H44.13-
  syphilitic (secondary) A51.43
    congenital (early) A50.01
    late A52.71
  tuberculous A18.54
Uveoencephalitis — *see* Inflammation, chorioretinal
Uveokeratitis — *see* Iridocyclitis
Uveoparotitis D86.89
Uvula — *see* condition
Uvulitis (acute) (catarrhal) (chronic) (membranous) (suppurative) (ulcerative) K12.2

V

Vaccination (prophylactic)
  complication or reaction — *see* Complications, vaccination
  delayed Z28.9
  encounter for Z23
  not done — *see* Immunization, not done, because (of)
Vaccinia (generalized) (localized) T88.1
  congenital P35.8
  without vaccination B08.011
Vacuum, in sinus (accessory) (nasal) J34.89
Vagabond, vagabondage Z59.0
Vagabond's disease B85.1
Vagina, vaginal — *see* condition
Vaginalitis (tunica) (testis) N49.1
Vaginismus (reflex) N94.2
  functional F52.5
  nonorganic F52.5
  psychogenic F52.5
  secondary N94.2
Vaginitis (acute) (circumscribed) (diffuse) (emphysematous) (nonvenereal) (ulcerative) N76.0
  with ectopic or molar pregnancy O08.0
  amebic A06.82
  atrophic, postmenopausal N95.2
  bacterial N76.0
  blennorrhagic (gonococcal) A54.02
  candidal B37.3
  chlamydial A56.02
  chronic N76.1
  due to Trichomonas (vaginalis) A59.01
  following ectopic or molar pregnancy O08.0
  gonococcal A54.02
    with abscess (accessory gland) (periurethral) A54.1
  granuloma A58
  in (due to)

Vaginitis (acute) (circumscribed) (diffuse) (emphysematous) (nonvenereal) (ulcerative) - *continued*
  in (due to) - *continued*
    candidiasis B37.3
    herpesviral (herpes simplex) infection A60.04
    pinworm infection B80 *[N77.1]*
    monilial B37.3
    mycotic (candidal) B37.3
    postmenopausal atrophic N95.2
    puerperal (postpartum) O86.13
    senile (atrophic) N95.2
    subacute or chronic N76.1
    syphilitic (early) A51.0
      late A52.76
    trichomonal A59.01
    tuberculous A18.18
Vaginosis — *see* Vaginitis
Vagotonia G52.2
Vagrancy Z59.0
VAIN — *see* Neoplasia, intraepithelial, vagina
Vallecula — *see* condition
Valley fever B38.0
Valsuani's disease — *see* Anemia, obstetric
Valve, valvular (formation) — *see also* condition
  cerebral ventricle (communicating) in situ Z98.2
  cervix, internal os Q51.828
  congenital NEC — *see* Atresia, by site
  ureter (pelvic junction) (vesical orifice) Q62.39
  urethra (congenital) (posterior) Q64.2
Valvulitis (chronic) — *see* Endocarditis
Valvulopathy — *see* Endocarditis
Van Bogaert's leukoencephalopathy (sclerosing) (subacute) A81.1
Van Bogaert-Scherer-Epstein disease or syndrome E75.5
Van Buchem's syndrome M85.2
Van Creveld-von Gierke disease E74.01
Van der Hoeve (-de Kleyn) **syndrome** Q78.0
Van der Woude's syndrome Q38.0
Van Neck's disease or osteochondrosis M91.0
Vanishing lung J44.9
Vapor asphyxia or suffocation T59.9
  specified agent — *see* Table of Drugs and Chemicals
Variance, lethal ball, prosthetic heart valve T82.09
Variants, thalassemic D56.8
Variations in hair color L67.1
Varicella B01.9
  with
    complications NEC B01.89
    encephalitis B01.11
    encephalomyelitis B01.11
    meningitis B01.0
    myelitis B01.12
    pneumonia B01.2
  congenital P35.8
Varices — *see* Varix
Varicocele (scrotum) (thrombosed) I86.1
  ovary I86.2
  perineum I86.3
  spermatic cord (ulcerated) I86.1
Varicose
  aneurysm (ruptured) I77.0
  dermatitis — *see* Varix, leg, with, inflammation
  eczema — *see* Varix, leg, with, inflammation
  phlebitis — *see* Varix, with, inflammation
  tumor — *see* Varix
  ulcer (lower limb, any part) — *see also* Varix, leg, with, ulcer
    anus — *see also* Hemorrhoids K64.8
    esophagus — *see* Varix, esophagus
    inflamed or infected — *see* Varix, leg, with ulcer, with inflammation
    nasal septum I86.8
    perineum I86.3
    scrotum I86.1
    specified site NEC I86.8
  vein — *see* Varix
  vessel — *see* Varix, leg
Varicosis, varicosities, varicosity — *see* Varix
Variola (major) (minor) B03
Varioloid B03
Varix (lower limb) (ruptured) I83.90
  with
    edema I83.899
    inflammation I83.10
      with ulcer (venous) I83.209
    pain I83.819
    specified complication NEC I83.899
    stasis dermatitis I83.10
      with ulcer (venous) I83.209
    swelling I83.899
    ulcer I83.009

Varix (lower limb) (ruptured) - *continued*
  with - *continued*
    ulcer - *continued*
      with inflammation I83.209
    aneurysmal I77.0
    asymptomatic I83.9-
    bladder I86.2
    broad ligament I86.2
  complicating
    childbirth (lower extremity) O87.4
      anus or rectum O87.2
      genital (vagina, vulva or perineum) O87.8
    pregnancy (lower extremity) O22.0-
      anus or rectum O22.4-
      genital (vagina, vulva or perineum) O22.1-
    puerperium (lower extremity) O87.4
      anus or rectum O87.2
      genital (vagina, vulva, perineum) O87.8
  congenital (any site) Q27.8
  esophagus (idiopathic) (primary) (ulcerated) I85.00
    bleeding I85.01
    congenital Q27.8
    in (due to)
      alcoholic liver disease I85.10
        bleeding I85.11
      cirrhosis of liver I85.10
        bleeding I85.11
      portal hypertension I85.10
        bleeding I85.11
      schistosomiasis I85.10
        bleeding I85.11
      toxic liver disease I85.10
        bleeding I85.11
    secondary I85.10
      bleeding I85.11
  gastric I86.4
  inflamed or infected I83.10
    ulcerated I83.209
  labia (majora) I86.3
  leg (asymptomatic) I83.90
    with
      edema I83.899
      inflammation I83.10
        with ulcer — *see* Varix, leg, with, ulcer, with inflammation by site
      pain I83.819
      specified complication NEC I83.899
      swelling I83.899
      ulcer I83.009
        with inflammation I83.209
        ankle I83.003
          with inflammation I83.203
        calf I83.002
          with inflammation I83.202
        foot NEC I83.005
          with inflammation I83.205
        heel I83.004
          with inflammation I83.204
        lower leg NEC I83.008
          with inflammation I83.208
        midfoot I83.004
          with inflammation I83.204
        thigh I83.001
          with inflammation I83.201
    bilateral (asymptomatic) I83.93
      with
        edema I83.893
        pain I83.813
        specified complication NEC I83.893
        swelling I83.893
        ulcer I83.009
          with inflammation I83.209
    left (asymptomatic) I83.92
      with
        edema I83.892
        pain I83.812
        specified complication NEC I83.892
        swelling I83.892
        inflammation I83.12
          with ulcer — *see* Varix, leg, with, ulcer, with inflammation by site
        ulcer I83.029
          with inflammation I83.229
          ankle I83.023
            with inflammation I83.223
          calf I83.022
            with inflammation I83.222
          foot NEC I83.025
            with inflammation I83.225
          heel I83.024
            with inflammation I83.224
          lower leg NEC I83.028
            with inflammation I83.228

Varix (lower limb) (ruptured) - *continued*
  leg (asymptomatic) - *continued*
    left (asymptomatic) - *continued*
      with - *continued*
        ulcer - *continued*
          midfoot I83.024
            with inflammation I83.224
          thigh I83.021
            with inflammation I83.221
    right (asymptomatic) I83.91
      with
        edema I83.891
        pain I83.811
        specified complication NEC I83.891
        swelling I83.891
        inflammation I83.11
          with ulcer — *see* Varix, leg, with, ulcer, with inflammation by site
        ulcer I83.019
          with inflammation I83.219
          ankle I83.013
            with inflammation I83.213
          calf I83.012
            with inflammation I83.212
          foot NEC I83.015
            with inflammation I83.215
          heel I83.014
            with inflammation I83.214
          lower leg NEC I83.018
            with inflammation I83.218
          midfoot I83.014
            with inflammation I83.214
          thigh I83.011
            with inflammation I83.211
  nasal septum I86.8
  orbit I86.8
    congenital Q27.8
  ovary I86.2
  papillary I78.1
  pelvis I86.2
  perineum I86.3
  pharynx I86.8
  placenta O43.89-
  renal papilla I86.8
  retina H35.09
  scrotum (ulcerated) I86.1
  sigmoid colon I86.8
  specified site NEC I86.8
  spinal (cord) (vessels) I86.8
  spleen, splenic (vein) (with phlebolith) I86.8
  stomach I86.4
  sublingual I86.0
  ulcerated I83.009
    inflamed or infected I83.209
  uterine ligament I86.2
  vagina I86.8
  vocal cord I86.8
  vulva I86.3
Vas deferens — *see* condition
Vas deferentitis N49.1
Vasa previa O69.4
  hemorrhage from, affecting newborn P50.0
Vascular — *see also* condition
  loop on optic papilla Q14.2
  spasm I73.9
  spider I78.1
Vascularization, cornea — *see* Neovascularization, cornea
Vasculitis I77.6
  allergic D69.0
  cryoglobulinemic D89.1
  disseminated I77.6
  hypocomplementemic M31.8
  kidney I77.89
  livedoid L95.0
  nodular L95.8
  retina H35.06-
  rheumatic — *see* Fever, rheumatic
  rheumatoid — *see* Rheumatoid, vasculitis
  skin (limited to) L95.9
    specified NEC L95.8
Vasculopathy, necrotizing M31.9
  cardiac allograft T86.290
  specified NEC M31.8
Vasitis (nodosa) N49.1
  tuberculous A18.15
Vasodilation I73.9
Vasomotor — *see* condition
Vasoplasty, after previous sterilization Z31.0
  aftercare Z31.42
Vasospasm (vasoconstriction) I73.9
  cerebral (cerebrovascular) (artery) I67.848
    reversible I67.841

Vasospasm (vasoconstriction) - *continued*
coronary I20.1
nerve
arm — *see* Mononeuropathy, upper limb
brachial plexus G54.0
cervical plexus G54.2
leg — *see* Mononeuropathy, lower limb
peripheral NOS I73.9
retina (artery) — *see* Occlusion, artery, retina
Vasospastic — *see* condition
Vasovagal attack (paroxysmal) R55
psychogenic F45.8
VATER syndrome Q87.2
Vater's ampulla — *see* condition
Vegetation, vegetative
adenoid (nasal fossa) J35.8
endocarditis (acute) (any valve) (subacute) I33.0
heart (mycotic) (valve) I33.0
Veil
Jackson's Q43.3
Vein, venous — *see* condition
Veldt sore — *see* Ulcer, skin
Velpeau's hernia — *see* Hernia, femoral
Venereal
bubo A55
disease A64
granuloma inguinale A58
lymphogranuloma (Durand-Nicolas-Favre) A55
Venofibrosis I87.8
Venom, venomous — *see* Table of Drugs and Chemicals, by animal or substance, poisoning
Venous — *see* condition
Ventilator lung, newborn P27.8
Ventral — *see* condition
Ventricle, ventricular — *see also* condition
escape I49.3
inversion Q20.5
Ventriculitis (cerebral) — *see also* Encephalitis G04.90
Ventriculostomy status Z98.2
Vernet's syndrome G52.7
Verneuil's disease (syphilitic bursitis) A52.78
Verruca (due to HPV) (filiformis) (simplex) (viral) (vulgaris) B07.9
acuminata A63.0
necrogenica (primary) (tuberculosa) A18.4
plana B07.8
plantaris B07.0
seborrheica L82.1
inflamed L82.0
senile (seborrheic) L82.1
inflamed L82.0
tuberculosa (primary) A18.4
venereal A63.0
Verrucosities — *see* Verruca
Verruga peruana, peruviana A44.1
Version
with extraction
cervix — *see* Malposition, uterus
uterus (postinfectional) (postpartal, old) — *see* Malposition, uterus
Vertebra, vertebral — *see* condition
Vertical talus (congenital) Q66.80
left foot Q66.82
right foot Q66.81
Vertigo R42
auditory — *see* Vertigo, aural
aural H81.31-
benign paroxysmal (positional) H81.1-
central (origin) H81.4-
cerebral H81.4-
Dix and Hallpike (epidemic) — *see* Neuronitis, vestibular
due to infrasound T75.23
epidemic A88.1
Dix and Hallpike — *see* Neuronitis, vestibular
Pedersen's — *see* Neuronitis, vestibular
vestibular neuronitis — *see* Neuronitis, vestibular
hysterical F44.89
infrasound T75.23
labyrinthine — *see* subcategory H81.0
laryngeal R05
malignant positional H81.4-
Ménière's — *see* subcategory H81.0
menopausal N95.1
otogenic — *see* Vertigo, aural
paroxysmal positional, benign — *see* Vertigo, benign paroxysmal
Pedersen's (epidemic) — *see* Neuronitis, vestibular
peripheral NEC H81.39-
positional
benign paroxysmal — *see* Vertigo, benign paroxysmal

Vertigo - *continued*
positional - *continued*
malignant H81.4-
Very-low-density-lipoprotein-type (VLDL) **hyperlipoproteinemia** E78.1
Vesania — *see* Psychosis
Vesical — *see* condition
Vesicle
cutaneous R23.8
seminal — *see* condition
skin R23.8
Vesicocolic — *see* condition
Vesicoperineal — *see* condition
Vesicorectal — *see* condition
Vesicourethrorectal — *see* condition
Vesicovaginal — *see* condition
Vesicular — *see* condition
Vesiculitis (seminal) N49.0
amebic A06.82
gonorrheal (acute) (chronic) A54.23
trichomonal A59.09
tuberculous A18.15
Vestibulitis (ear) (*see also* subcategory) H83.0
nose (external) J34.89
vulvar N94.810
Vestibulopathy , acute peripheral (recurrent) — *see* Neuronitis, vestibular
Vestige, vestigial — *see also* Persistence
branchial Q18.0
structures in vitreous Q14.0
Vibration
adverse effects T75.20
pneumatic hammer syndrome T75.21
specified effect NEC T75.29
vasospastic syndrome T75.22
vertigo from infrasound T75.23
exposure (occupational) Z57.7
vertigo T75.23
Vibriosis A28.9
Victim (of)
crime Z65.4
disaster Z65.5
terrorism Z65.4
torture Z65.4
war Z65.5
Vidal's disease L28.0
Villaret's syndrome G52.7
Villous — *see* condition
VIN — *see* Neoplasia, intraepithelial, vulva
Vincent's infection (angina) (gingivitis) A69.1
stomatitis NEC A69.1
Vinson-Plummer syndrome D50.1
Violence, physical R45.6
Viosterol deficiency — *see* Deficiency, calciferol
Vipoma — *see* Neoplasm, malignant, by site
Viremia B34.9
Virilism (adrenal) E25.9
congenital E25.0
Virilization (female) (suprarenal) E25.9
congenital E25.0
isosexual E28.2
Virulent bubo A57
Virus, viral — *see also* condition
as cause of disease classified elsewhere B97.89
cytomegalovirus B25.9
human immunodeficiency (HIV) — *see* Human, immunodeficiency virus (HIV) disease
infection — *see* Infection, virus
specified NEC B34.8
swine influenza (viruses that normally cause infections in pigs) — *see also* Influenza, due to, identified novel influenza A virus J09.X2
West Nile (fever) A92.30
with
complications NEC A92.39
cranial nerve disorders A92.32
encephalitis A92.31
encephalomyelitis A92.31
neurologic manifestation NEC A92.32
optic neuritis A92.32
polyradiculitis A92.32
Viscera, visceral — *see* condition
Visceroptosis K63.4
Visible peristalsis R19.2
Vision, visual
binocular, suppression H53.34
blurred, blurring H53.8
hysterical F44.6
defect, defective NEC H54.7
disorientation (syndrome) H53.8
disturbance H53.9
hysterical F44.6
double H53.2

Vision, visual - *continued*
examination Z01.00
with abnormal findings Z01.01
field, limitation (defect) — *see* Defect, visual field
hallucinations R44.1
halos H53.19
loss — *see* Loss, vision
sudden — *see* Disturbance, vision, subjective, loss, sudden
low (both eyes) — *see* Low, vision
perception, simultaneous without fusion H53.33
Vitality, lack or want of R53.83
newborn P96.89
Vitamin deficiency — *see* Deficiency, vitamin
Vitelline duct, persistent Q43.0
Vitiligo L80
eyelid H02.739
left H02.736
lower H02.735
upper H02.734
right H02.733
lower H02.732
upper H02.731
pinta A67.2
vulva N90.89
Vitreal corneal syndrome H59.01-
Vitreoretinopathy, proliferative — *see also* Retinopathy, proliferative
with retinal detachment — *see* Detachment, retina, traction
Vitreous — *see also* condition
touch syndrome — *see* Complication, postprocedural, following cataract surgery
Vocal cord — *see* condition
Vogt-Koyanagi syndrome H20.82-
Vogt's disease or syndrome G80.3
Vogt-Spielmeyer amaurotic idiocy or disease E75.4
Voice
change R49.9
specified NEC R49.8
loss — *see* Aphonia
Volhynian fever A79.0
Volkmann's ischemic contracture or paralysis (complicating trauma) T79.6
Volvulus (bowel) (colon) (intestine) K56.2
with perforation K56.2
congenital Q43.8
duodenum K31.5
fallopian tube — *see* Torsion, fallopian tube
oviduct — *see* Torsion, fallopian tube
stomach (due to absence of gastrocolic ligament) K31.89
Vomiting R11.10
with nausea R11.2
asphyxia — *see* Foreign body, by site, causing asphyxia, gastric contents
bilious (cause unknown) R11.14
in newborn P92.01
following gastro-intestinal surgery K91.0
blood — *see* Hematemesis
causing asphyxia, choking, or suffocation — *see* Foreign body, by site
cyclical G43.A0
with refractory migraine G43.A1
intractable G43.A1
not intractable G43.A0
psychogenic F50.89
without refractory migraine G43.A0
fecal mater R11.13
following gastrointestinal surgery K91.0
psychogenic F50.89
functional K31.89
hysterical F50.89
nervous F50.89
neurotic F50.89
newborn NEC P92.09
bilious P92.01
periodic R11.10
psychogenic F50.89
projectile R11.12
psychogenic F50.89
uremic — *see* Uremia
without nausea R11.11
Vomito negro — *see* Fever, yellow
Von Bezold's abscess — *see* Mastoiditis, acute
Von Economo-Cruchet disease A85.8
Von Eulenburg's disease G71.19
Von Gierke's disease E74.01
Von Hippel (-Lindau) **disease or syndrome** Q85.8
Von Jaksch's anemia or disease D64.89
Von Recklinghausen
disease (neurofibromatosis) Q85.01
bones E21.0

Von Schroetter's syndrome I82.890
Von Willebrand (-Jurgens) (-Minot)
  disease or syndrome D68.0
Von Zumbusch's disease L40.1
Voyeurism F65.3
Vrolik's disease Q78.0
Vulva — *see* condition
Vulvismus N94.2
Vulvitis (acute) (allergic) (atrophic) (hypertrophic)
  (intertriginous) (senile) N76.2
  with ectopic or molar pregnancy O08.0
  adhesive, congenital Q52.79
  blennorrhagic (gonococcal) A54.02
  candidal B37.3
  chlamydial A56.02
  due to Haemophilus ducreyi A57
  following ectopic or molar pregnancy O08.0
  gonococcal A54.02
    with abscess (accessory gland) (periurethral) A54.1
  herpesviral A60.04
  leukoplakic N90.4
  monilial B37.3
  puerperal (postpartum) O86.19
  subacute or chronic N76.3
  syphilitic (early) A51.0
    late A52.76
  trichomonal A59.01
  tuberculous A18.18
Vulvodynia N94.819
  specified NEC N94.818
Vulvorectal — *see* condition
Vulvovaginitis (acute) — *see* Vaginitis

W

Waiting list, person on Z75.1
  for organ transplant Z76.82
  undergoing social agency investigation Z75.2
Waldenström
  hypergammaglobulinemia D89.0
  syndrome or macroglobulinemia C88.0
Waldenström-Kjellberg syndrome D50.1
Walking
  difficulty R26.2
    psychogenic F44.4
  sleep F51.3
    hysterical F44.89
Wall, abdominal — *see* condition
Wallenberg's disease or syndrome G46.3
Wallgren's disease I87.8
Wandering
  gallbladder, congenital Q44.1
  in diseases classified elsewhere Z91.83
  kidney, congenital Q63.8
  organ or site, congenital NEC — *see* Malposition,
    congenital, by site
  pacemaker (heart) I49.8
  spleen D73.89
War neurosis F48.8
Wart (due to HPV) (filiform) (infectious)
  (viral) B07.9
  anogenital region (venereal) A63.0
  common B07.8
  external genital organs (venereal) A63.0
  flat B07.8
  Hassal-Henle's (of cornea) H18.49
  Peruvian A44.1
  plantar B07.0
  prosector (tuberculous) A18.4
  seborrheic L82.1
    inflamed L82.0
  senile (seborrheic) L82.1
    inflamed L82.0
  tuberculous A18.4
  venereal A63.0
Warthin's tumor — *see* Neoplasm, salivary gland,
  benign
Wassilieff's disease A27.0
Wasting
  disease R64
    due to malnutrition E41
  extreme (due to malnutrition) E41
  muscle NEC — *see* Atrophy, muscle
Water
  clefts (senile cataract) — *see* Cataract, senile,
    incipient
  deprivation of T73.1
  intoxication E87.79
  itch B76.9
  lack of T73.1
  loading E87.70
  on
    brain — *see* Hydrocephalus
    chest J94.8

Water - *continued*
  poisoning E87.79
Waterbrash R12
Waterhouse (-Friderichsen) **syndrome or disease**
  (meningococcal) A39.1
Water-losing nephritis N25.89
Watermelon stomach K31.819
  with hemorrhage K31.811
  without hemorrhage K31.819
Watsoniasis B66.8
Wax in ear — *see* Impaction, cerumen
Weak, weakening, weakness (generalized) R53.1
  arches (acquired) — *see also* Deformity, limb, flat
    foot
  bladder (sphincter) R32
  facial R29.810
    following
      cerebrovascular disease I69.992
        cerebral infarction I69.392
        intracerebral hemorrhage I69.192
        nontraumatic intracranial hemorrhage
          NEC I69.292
        specified disease NEC I69.892
        stroke I69.392
        subarachnoid hemorrhage I69.092
  foot (double) — *see* Weak, arches
  heart, cardiac — *see* Failure, heart
  mind F70
  muscle M62.81
  myocardium — *see* Failure, heart
  newborn P96.89
  pelvic fundus N81.89
  pubocervical tissue N81.82
  senile R54
  rectovaginal tissue N81.83
  urinary stream R39.12
  valvular — *see* Endocarditis
Wear, worn (with normal or routine use)
  articular bearing surface of internal joint
    prosthesis — *see* Complications, joint prosthesis,
    mechanical, wear of articular bearing surfaces, by
    site
  device, implant or graft — *see* Complications, by
    site, mechanical complication
  tooth, teeth (approximal) (hard tissues)
    (interproximal) (occlusal) K03.0
Weather, weathered
  effects of
    cold T69.9
      specified effect NEC T69.8
    hot — *see* Heat
  skin L57.8
Weaver's syndrome Q87.3
Web, webbed (congenital)
  duodenal Q43.8
  esophagus Q39.4
  fingers Q70.1-
  larynx (glottic) (subglottic) Q31.0
  neck (pterygium colli) Q18.3
  Paterson-Kelly D50.1
  popliteal syndrome Q87.89
  toes Q70.3-
Weber-Christian disease M35.6
Weber-Cockayne syndrome (epidermolysis
  bullosa) Q81.8
Weber-Gubler syndrome G46.3
Weber-Leyden syndrome G46.3
Weber-Osler syndrome I78.0
Weber's paralysis or syndrome G46.3
Wedge-shaped or wedging vertebra — *see*
  Collapse, vertebra NEC
Wegener's granulomatosis or syndrome M31.30
  with
    kidney involvement M31.31
    lung involvement M31.30
      with kidney involvement M31.31
Wegner's disease A50.02
Weight
  1000-2499 grams at birth (low) — *see* Low,
    birthweight
  999 grams or less at birth (extremely low) — *see*
    Low, birthweight, extreme
  and length below 10th percentile for gestational
    age P05.1-
  below but length above 10th percentile for
    gestational age P05.0-
  gain (abnormal) (excessive) R63.5
    in pregnancy — *see* Pregnancy, complicated by,
      excessive weight gain
    low — *see* Pregnancy, complicated by,
      insufficient, weight gain
  loss (abnormal) (cause unknown) R63.4
Weightlessness (effect of) T75.82

Weil (l) -Marchesani syndrome Q87.1
Weil's disease A27.0
Weingarten's syndrome J82
Weir Mitchell's disease I73.81
Weiss-Baker syndrome G90.09
Wells' disease L98.3
Wen — *see* Cyst, sebaceous
Wenckebach's block or phenomenon I44.1
Werdnig-Hoffmann syndrome (muscular
  atrophy) G12.0
Werlhof's disease D69.3
Wermer's disease or syndrome E31.21
Werner-His disease A79.0
Werner's disease or syndrome E34.8
Wernicke-Korsakoff's syndrome or psychosis
  (alcoholic) F10.96
  with dependence F10.26
  drug-induced
    due to drug abuse — *see* Abuse, drug, by type,
      with amnestic disorder
    due to drug dependence — *see* Dependence, drug,
      by type, with amnestic disorder
  nonalcoholic F04
Wernicke-Posadas disease B38.9
Wernicke's
  developmental aphasia F80.2
  disease or syndrome E51.2
  encephalopathy E51.2
  polioencephalitis, superior E51.2
West African fever B50.8
Westphal-Strümpell syndrome E83.01
West's syndrome — *see* Epilepsy, spasms
Wet
  feet, tropical (maceration) (syndrome) — *see*
    Immersion, foot
  lung (syndrome) , newborn P22.1
Wharton's duct — *see* condition
Wheal — *see* Urticaria
Wheezing R06.2
Whiplash injury S13.4
Whipple's disease (*see also*
  subcategory M14.8-) K90.81
Whipworm (disease) (infection) (infestation) B79
Whistling face Q87.0
White — *see also* condition
  kidney, small N03.9
  leg, puerperal, postpartum, childbirth O87.1
  mouth B37.0
  patches of mouth K13.29
  spot lesions, teeth
    chewing surface K02.51
    pit and fissure surface K02.51
    smooth surface K02.61
Whitehead L70.0
Whitlow — *see also* Cellulitis, digit
  with lymphangitis — *see* Lymphangitis, acute, digit
  herpesviral B00.89
Whitmore's disease or fever — *see* Melioidosis
Whooping cough A37.90
  with pneumonia A37.91
  due to Bordetella
    bronchiseptica A37.81
    parapertussis A37.11
    pertussis A37.01
  specified organism NEC A37.81
  due to
    Bordetella
      bronchiseptica A37.80
        with pneumonia A37.81
      parapertussis A37.10
        with pneumonia A37.11
      pertussis A37.00
        with pneumonia A37.01
    specified NEC A37.80
      with pneumonia A37.81
Wichman's asthma J38.5
Wide cranial sutures, newborn P96.3
Widening aorta — *see* Ectasia, aorta
  with aneurysm — *see* Aneurysm, aorta
Wilkie's disease or syndrome K55.1
Wilkinson-Sneddon disease or syndrome L13.1
Willebrand (-Jürgens) **thrombopathy** D68.0
Willige-Hunt disease or syndrome G23.1
Wilms' tumor C64-
Wilson-Mikity syndrome P27.0
Wilson's
  disease or syndrome E83.01
  hepatolenticular degeneration E83.01
  lichen ruber L43.9
Window — *see also* Imperfect, closure
  aorticopulmonary Q21.4
Winter — *see* condition
Wiskott-Aldrich syndrome D82.0

Withdrawal state — *see also* Dependence, drug by type, with withdrawal
alcohol
   with perceptual disturbances F10.232
   without perceptual disturbances F10.239
caffeine F15.93
cannabis F12.288
newborn
   correct therapeutic substance properly administered P96.2
   infant of dependent mother P96.1
   therapeutic substance, neonatal P96.2
Witts' anemia D50.8
Witzelsucht F07.0
Woakes' ethmoiditis or syndrome J33.1
Wolff-Hirschorn syndrome Q93.3
Wolff-Parkinson-White syndrome I45.6
Wolhynian fever A79.0
Wolman's disease E75.5
Wood lung or pneumonitis J67.8
Woolly, wooly hair (congenital) (nevus) Q84.1
Woolsorter's disease A22.1
Word
blindness (congenital) (developmental) F81.0
deafness (congenital) (developmental) H93.25
Worm (s) (infection) (infestation) — *see also* Infestation, helminth
guinea B72
in intestine NEC B82.0
Worm-eaten soles A66.3
Worn out — *see* Exhaustion
cardiac
   defibrillator (with synchronous cardiace pacemaker) Z45.02
   pacemaker
      battery Z45.010
      lead Z45.018
device, implant or graft — *see* Complications, by site, mechanical
Worried well Z71.1
Worries R45.82
Wound, open
abdomen, abdominal
   wall S31.109
      with penetration into peritoneal cavity S31.609
      bite — *see* Bite, abdomen, wall
      epigastric region S31.102
         with penetration into peritoneal cavity S31.602
         bite — *see* Bite, abdomen, wall, epigastric region
         laceration — *see* Laceration, abdomen, wall, epigastric region
         puncture — *see* Puncture, abdomen, wall, epigastric region
      laceration — *see* Laceration, abdomen, wall
      left
         lower quadrant S31.104
            with penetration into peritoneal cavity S31.604
            bite — *see* Bite, abdomen, wall, left, lower quadrant
            laceration — *see* Laceration, abdomen, wall, left, lower quadrant
            puncture — *see* Puncture, abdomen, wall, left, lower quadrant
         upper quadrant S31.101
            with penetration into peritoneal cavity S31.601
            bite — *see* Bite, abdomen, wall, left, upper quadrant
            laceration — *see* Laceration, abdomen, wall, left, upper quadrant
            puncture — *see* Puncture, abdomen, wall, left, upper quadrant
      periumbilic region S31.105
         with penetration into peritoneal cavity S31.605
         bite — *see* Bite, abdomen, wall, periumbilic region
         laceration — *see* Laceration, abdomen, wall, periumbilic region
         puncture — *see* Puncture, abdomen, wall, periumbilic region
      puncture — *see* Puncture, abdomen, wall
      right
         lower quadrant S31.103
            with penetration into peritoneal cavity S31.603
            bite — *see* Bite, abdomen, wall, right, lower quadrant
            laceration — *see* Laceration, abdomen, wall, right, lower quadrant
            puncture — *see* Puncture, abdomen, wall, right, lower quadrant
         upper quadrant S31.100
            with penetration into peritoneal cavity S31.600

Wound, open - *continued*
abdomen, abdominal - *continued*
   wall - *continued*
      right - *continued*
         upper quadrant - *continued*
            bite — *see* Bite, abdomen, wall, right, upper quadrant
            laceration — *see* Laceration, abdomen, wall, right, upper quadrant
            puncture — *see* Puncture, abdomen, wall, right, upper quadrant
alveolar (process) — *see* Wound, open, oral cavity
ankle S91.00-
   bite — *see* Bite, ankle
   laceration — *see* Laceration, ankle
   puncture — *see* Puncture, ankle
antecubital space — *see* Wound, open, elbow
anterior chamber, eye — *see* Wound, open, ocular
anus S31.839
   bite S31.835
   laceration — *see* Laceration, anus
   puncture — *see* Puncture, anus
arm (upper) S41.10-
   with amputation — *see* Amputation, traumatic, arm
   bite — *see* Bite, arm
   forearm — *see* Wound, open, forearm
   laceration — *see* Laceration, arm
   puncture — *see* Puncture, arm
auditory canal (external) (meatus) — *see* Wound, open, ear
auricle, ear — *see* Wound, open, ear
axilla — *see* Wound, open, arm
back — *see also* Wound, open, thorax, back
   lower S31.000
      with penetration into retroperitoneal space S31.001
      bite — *see* Bite, back, lower
      laceration — *see* Laceration, back, lower
      puncture — *see* Puncture, back, lower
bite — *see* Bite
blood vessel — *see* Injury, blood vessel
breast S21.00-
   with amputation — *see* Amputation, traumatic, breast
   bite — *see* Bite, breast
   laceration — *see* Laceration, breast
   puncture — *see* Puncture, breast
buttock S31.809
   bite — *see* Bite, buttock
   laceration — *see* Laceration, buttock
   left S31.829
   puncture — *see* Puncture, buttock
   right S31.819
calf — *see* Wound, open, leg
canaliculus lacrimalis — *see* Wound, open, eyelid
canthus, eye — *see* Wound, open, eyelid
cervical esophagus S11.20
   bite S11.25
   laceration — *see* Laceration, esophagus, traumatic, cervical
   puncture — *see* Puncture, cervical esophagus
cheek (external) S01.40-
   bite — *see* Bite, cheek
   laceration — *see* Laceration, cheek
   puncture — *see* Puncture, cheek
   internal — *see* Wound, open, oral cavity
chest wall — *see* Wound, open, thorax
chin — *see* Wound, open, head, specified site NEC
choroid — *see* Wound, open, ocular
ciliary body (eye) — *see* Wound, open, ocular
clitoris S31.40
   with amputation — *see* Amputation, traumatic, clitoris
   bite S31.45
   laceration — *see* Laceration, vulva
   puncture — *see* Puncture, vulva
conjunctiva — *see* Wound, open, ocular
cornea — *see* Wound, open, ocular
costal region — *see* Wound, open, thorax
Descemet's membrane — *see* Wound, open, ocular
digit (s)
   foot — *see* Wound, open, toe
   hand — *see* Wound, open, finger
ear (canal) (external) S01.30-
   with amputation — *see* Amputation, traumatic, ear
   bite — *see* Bite, ear
   laceration — *see* Laceration, ear
   puncture — *see* Puncture, ear
   drum S09.2-
elbow S51.00-
   bite — *see* Bite, elbow
   laceration — *see* Laceration, elbow

Wound, open - *continued*
elbow - *continued*
   puncture — *see* Puncture, elbow
epididymis — *see* Wound, open, testis
epigastric region S31.102
   with penetration into peritoneal cavity S31.602
   bite — *see* Bite, abdomen, wall, epigastric region
   laceration — *see* Laceration, abdomen, wall, epigastric region
   puncture — *see* Puncture, abdomen, wall, epigastric region
epiglottis — *see* Wound, open, neck, specified site NEC
esophagus (thoracic) S27.819
   cervical — *see* Wound, open, cervical esophagus
   laceration S27.813
   specified type NEC S27.818
eye — *see* Wound, open, ocular
eyeball — *see* Wound, open, ocular
eyebrow — *see* Wound, open, eyelid
eyelid S01.10-
   bite — *see* Bite, eyelid
   laceration — *see* Laceration, eyelid
   puncture — *see* Puncture, eyelid
face NEC — *see* Wound, open, head, specified site NEC
finger (s) S61.209
   with
      amputation — *see* Amputation, traumatic, finger
      damage to nail S61.309
   bite — *see* Bite, finger
   index S61.208
      with
         damage to nail S61.308
      left S61.201
         with
            damage to nail S61.301
      right S61.200
         with
            damage to nail S61.300
   laceration — *see* Laceration, finger
   little S61.208
      with
         damage to nail S61.308
      left S61.207
         with damage to nail S61.307
      right S61.206
         with damage to nail S61.306
   middle S61.208
      with
         damage to nail S61.308
      left S61.203
         with damage to nail S61.303
      right S61.202
         with damage to nail S61.302
   puncture — *see* Puncture, finger
   ring S61.208
      with
         damage to nail S61.308
      left S61.205
         with damage to nail S61.305
      right S61.204
         with damage to nail S61.304
flank — *see* Wound, open, abdomen, wall
foot (except toe (s) alone) S91.30-
   with amputation — *see* Amputation, traumatic, foot
   bite — *see* Bite, foot
   laceration — *see* Laceration, foot
   puncture — *see* Puncture, foot
   toe — *see* Wound, open, toe
forearm S51.80-
   with
      amputation — *see* Amputation, traumatic, forearm
   bite — *see* Bite, forearm
   elbow only — *see* Wound, open, elbow
   laceration — *see* Laceration, forearm
   puncture — *see* Puncture, forearm
forehead — *see* Wound, open, head, specified site NEC
genital organs, external
   with amputation — *see* Amputation, traumatic, genital organs
   bite — *see* Bite, genital organ
   female S31.502
      vagina S31.40
      vulva S31.40
   laceration — *see* Laceration, genital organ
   male S31.501
      penis S31.20
      scrotum S31.30
      testes S31.30

Wound, open - *continued*
  genital organs, external - *continued*
    puncture — *see* Puncture, genital organ
  globe (eye) — *see* Wound, open, ocular
  groin — *see* Wound, open, abdomen, wall
  gum — *see* Wound, open, oral cavity
  hand S61.40-
    with
      amputation — *see* Amputation, traumatic, hand
    bite — *see* Bite, hand
    finger (s) — *see* Wound, open, finger
    laceration — *see* Laceration, hand
    puncture — *see* Puncture, hand
    thumb — *see* Wound, open, thumb
  head S01.90
    bite — *see* Bite, head
    cheek — *see* Wound, open, cheek
    ear — *see* Wound, open, ear
    eyelid — *see* Wound, open, eyelid
    laceration — *see* Laceration, head
    lip — *see* Wound, open, lip
    nose S01.20
    oral cavity — *see* Wound, open, oral cavity
    puncture — *see* Puncture, head
    scalp — *see* Wound, open, scalp
    specified site NEC S01.80
    temporomandibular area — *see* Wound, open, cheek
  heel — *see* Wound, open, foot
  hip S71.00-
    with amputation — *see* Amputation, traumatic, hip
    bite — *see* Bite, hip
    laceration — *see* Laceration, hip
    puncture — *see* Puncture, hip
  hymen S31.40
    bite — *see* Bite, vulva
    laceration — *see* Laceration, vagina
    puncture — *see* Puncture, vagina
  hypochondrium S31.109
    bite — *see* Bite, hypochondrium
    laceration — *see* Laceration, hypochondrium
    puncture — *see* Puncture, hypochondrium
  hypogastric region S31.109
    bite — *see* Bite, hypogastric region
    laceration — *see* Laceration, hypogastric region
    puncture — *see* Puncture, hypogastric region
  iliac (region) — *see* Wound, open, inguinal region
  inguinal region S31.109
    bite — *see* Bite, abdomen, wall, lower quadrant
    laceration — *see* Laceration, inguinal region
    puncture — *see* Puncture, inguinal region
  instep — *see* Wound, open, foot
  interscapular region — *see* Wound, open, thorax, back
  intraocular — *see* Wound, open, ocular
  iris — *see* Wound, open, ocular
  jaw — *see* Wound, open, head, specified site NEC
  knee S81.00-
    bite — *see* Bite, knee
    laceration — *see* Laceration, knee
    puncture — *see* Puncture, knee
  labium (majus) (minus) — *see* Wound, open, vulva
  laceration — *see* Laceration, by site
  lacrimal duct — *see* Wound, open, eyelid
  larynx S11.019
    bite — *see* Bite, larynx
    laceration — *see* Laceration, larynx
    puncture — *see* Puncture, larynx
  left
    lower quadrant S31.104
      with penetration into peritoneal cavity S31.604
      bite — *see* Bite, abdomen, wall, left, lower quadrant
      laceration — *see* Laceration, abdomen, wall, left, lower quadrant
      puncture — *see* Puncture, abdomen, wall, left, lower quadrant
    upper quadrant S31.101
      with penetration into peritoneal cavity S31.601
      bite — *see* Bite, abdomen, wall, left, upper quadrant
      laceration — *see* Laceration, abdomen, wall, left, upper quadrant
      puncture — *see* Puncture, abdomen, wall, left, upper quadrant
  leg (lower) S81.80-
    with amputation — *see* Amputation, traumatic, leg
    ankle — *see* Wound, open, ankle
    bite — *see* Bite, leg
    foot — *see* Wound, open, foot
    knee — *see* Wound, open, knee
    laceration — *see* Laceration, leg
    puncture — *see* Puncture, leg

Wound, open - *continued*
  leg (lower) - *continued*
    toe — *see* Wound, open, toe
    upper — *see* Wound, open, thigh
  lip S01.501
    bite — *see* Bite, lip
    laceration — *see* Laceration, lip
    puncture — *see* Puncture, lip
  loin S31.109
    bite — *see* Bite, abdomen, wall
    laceration — *see* Laceration, loin
    puncture — *see* Puncture, loin
  lower back — *see* Wound, open, back, lower
  lumbar region — *see* Wound, open, back, lower
  malar region — *see* Wound, open, head, specified site NEC
  mammary — *see* Wound, open, breast
  mastoid region — *see* Wound, open, head, specified site NEC
  mouth — *see* Wound, open, oral cavity
  nail
    finger — *see* Wound, open, finger, with damage to nail
    toe — *see* Wound, open, toe, with damage to nail
  nape (neck) — *see* Wound, open, neck
  nasal (septum) (sinus) — *see* Wound, open, nose
  nasopharynx — *see* Wound, open, head, specified site NEC
  neck S11.90
    bite — *see* Bite, neck
    involving
      cervical esophagus S11.20
      larynx — *see* Wound, open, larynx
      pharynx S11.20
      thyroid S11.10
      trachea (cervical) S11.029
        bite — *see* Bite, trachea
        laceration S11.021
          with foreign body S11.022
        puncture S11.023
          with foreign body S11.024
    laceration — *see* Laceration, neck
    puncture — *see* Puncture, neck
    specified site NEC S11.80
      specified type NEC S11.89
  nose (septum) (sinus) S01.20
    with amputation — *see* Amputation, traumatic, nose
    bite — *see* Bite, nose
    laceration — *see* Laceration, nose
    puncture — *see* Puncture, nose
  ocular S05.90
    avulsion (traumatic enucleation) S05.7-
    eyeball S05.6-
      with foreign body S05.5-
    eyelid — *see* Wound, open, eyelid
    laceration and rupture S05.3-
      with prolapse or loss of intraocular tissue S05.2-
    orbit (penetrating) (with or without foreign body) S05.4-
    periocular area — *see* Wound, open, eyelid
    specified NEC S05.8X-
  oral cavity S01.502
    bite S01.552
    laceration — *see* Laceration, oral cavity
    puncture — *see* Puncture, oral cavity
  orbit — *see* Wound, open, ocular, orbit
  palate — *see* Wound, open, oral cavity
  palm — *see* Wound, open, hand
  pelvis, pelvic — *see also* Wound, open, back, lower
    girdle — *see* Wound, open, hip
  penetrating — *see* Puncture, by site
  penis S31.20
    with amputation — *see* Amputation, traumatic, penis
    bite S31.25
    laceration — *see* Laceration, penis
    puncture — *see* Puncture, penis
  perineum
    bite — *see* Bite, perineum
    female S31.502
    laceration — *see* Laceration, perineum
    male S31.501
    puncture — *see* Puncture, perineum
  periocular area (with or without lacrimal passages) — *see* Wound, open, eyelid
  periumbilic region S31.105
    with penetration into peritoneal cavity S31.605
    bite — *see* Bite, abdomen, wall, periumbilic region
    laceration — *see* Laceration, abdomen, wall, periumbilic region
    puncture — *see* Puncture, abdomen, wall, periumbilic region

Wound, open - *continued*
  phalanges
    finger — *see* Wound, open, finger
    toe — *see* Wound, open, toe
  pharynx S11.20
  pinna — *see* Wound, open, ear
  popliteal space — *see* Wound, open, knee
  prepuce — *see* Wound, open, penis
  pubic region — *see* Wound, open, back, lower
  pudendum — *see* Wound, open, genital organs, external
  puncture wound — *see* Puncture
  rectovaginal septum — *see* Wound, open, vagina
  right
    lower quadrant S31.103
      with penetration into peritoneal cavity S31.603
      bite — *see* Bite, abdomen, wall, right, lower quadrant
      laceration — *see* Laceration, abdomen, wall, right, lower quadrant
      puncture — *see* Puncture, abdomen, wall, right, lower quadrant
    upper quadrant S31.100
      with penetration into peritoneal cavity S31.600
      bite — *see* Bite, abdomen, wall, right, upper quadrant
      laceration — *see* Laceration, abdomen, wall, right, upper quadrant
      puncture — *see* Puncture, abdomen, wall, right, upper quadrant
  sacral region — *see* Wound, open, back, lower
  sacroiliac region — *see* Wound, open, back, lower
  salivary gland — *see* Wound, open, oral cavity
  scalp S01.00
    bite S01.05
    laceration — *see* Laceration, scalp
    puncture — *see* Puncture, scalp
  scalpel, newborn (birth injury) P15.8
  scapular region — *see* Wound, open, shoulder
  sclera — *see* Wound, open, ocular
  scrotum S31.30
    with amputation — *see* Amputation, traumatic, scrotum
    bite S31.35
    laceration — *see* Laceration, scrotum
    puncture — *see* Puncture, scrotum
  shin — *see* Wound, open, leg
  shoulder S41.00-
    with amputation — *see* Amputation, traumatic, arm
    bite — *see* Bite, shoulder
    laceration — *see* Laceration, shoulder
    puncture — *see* Puncture, shoulder
  skin NOS T14.8
  spermatic cord — *see* Wound, open, testis
  sternal region — *see* Wound, open, thorax, front wall
  submaxillary region — *see* Wound, open, head, specified site NEC
  submental region — *see* Wound, open, head, specified site NEC
  subungual
    finger (s) — *see* Wound, open, finger
    toe (s) — *see* Wound, open, toe
  supraclavicular region — *see* Wound, open, neck, specified site NEC
  temple, temporal region — *see* Wound, open, head, specified site NEC
  temporomandibular area — *see* Wound, open, cheek
  testis S31.30
    with amputation — *see* Amputation, traumatic, testes
    bite S31.35
    laceration — *see* Laceration, testis
    puncture — *see* Puncture, testis
  thigh S71.10-
    with amputation — *see* Amputation, traumatic, hip
    bite — *see* Bite, thigh
    laceration — *see* Laceration, thigh
    puncture — *see* Puncture, thigh
  thorax, thoracic (wall) S21.90
    back S21.20-
      with penetration S21.40
    bite — *see* Bite, thorax
    breast — *see* Wound, open, breast
    front S21.10-
      with penetration S21.30
    laceration — *see* Laceration, thorax
    puncture — *see* Puncture, thorax
  throat — *see* Wound, open, neck
  thumb S61.009
    with
      amputation — *see* Amputation, traumatic, thumb

Wound, open - *continued*
thumb - *continued*
  with - *continued*
    damage to nail S61.109
    bite — *see* Bite, thumb
    laceration — *see* Laceration, thumb
    left S61.002
      with
        damage to nail S61.102
    puncture — *see* Puncture, thumb
    right S61.001
      with
        damage to nail S61.101
thyroid (gland) — *see* Wound, open, neck, thyroid
toe (s) S91.109
  with
    amputation — *see* Amputation, traumatic, toe
    damage to nail S91.209
  bite — *see* Bite, toe
  great S91.103
    with
      damage to nail S91.203
    left S91.102
      with
        damage to nail S91.202
    right S91.101
      with
        damage to nail S91.201
  laceration — *see* Laceration, toe
  lesser S91.106
    with
      damage to nail S91.206
    left S91.105
      with
        damage to nail S91.205
    right S91.104
      with
        damage to nail S91.204
  puncture — *see* Puncture, toe
tongue — *see* Wound, open, oral cavity
trachea (cervical region) — *see* Wound, open, neck, trachea
tunica vaginalis — *see* Wound, open, testis
tympanum, tympanic membrane S09.2-
  laceration — *see* Laceration, ear, drum
  puncture — *see* Puncture, tympanum
umbilical region — *see* Wound, open, abdomen, wall, periumbilic region
uvula — *see* Wound, open, oral cavity
vagina S31.40
  bite S31.45
  laceration — *see* Laceration, vagina
  puncture — *see* Puncture, vagina
vocal cord S11.039
  bite — *see* Bite, vocal cord
  laceration S11.031
    with foreign body S11.032
  puncture S11.033
    with foreign body S11.034
vitreous (humor) — *see* Wound, open, ocular
vulva S31.40
  with amputation — *see* Amputation, traumatic, vulva
  bite S31.45
  laceration — *see* Laceration, vulva
  puncture — *see* Puncture, vulva
wrist S61.50-
  bite — *see* Bite, wrist
  laceration — *see* Laceration, wrist
  puncture — *see* Puncture, wrist
Wound, superficial — *see* Injury — *see also* specified injury type
Wright's syndrome G54.0
Wrist — *see* condition
Wrong drug (by accident) (given in error) — *see* Table of Drugs and Chemicals, by drug, poisoning
Wry neck — *see* Torticollis
Wuchereria (bancrofti) **infestation** B74.0
Wuchereriasis B74.0
Wuchernde Struma Langhans C73

X

Xanthelasma (eyelid) (palpebrarum) H02.60
left H02.66
  lower H02.65
  upper H02.64
right H02.63
  lower H02.62
  upper H02.61
Xanthelasmatosis (essential) E78.2
Xanthinuria, hereditary E79.8
Xanthoastrocytoma
specified site — *see* Neoplasm, malignant, by site

Xanthoastrocytoma - *continued*
unspecified site C71.9
Xanthofibroma — *see* Neoplasm, connective tissue, benign
Xanthogranuloma D76.3
Xanthoma (s) **, xanthomatosis** (primary) (familial) (hereditary) E75.5
with
  hyperlipoproteinemia
    Type I E78.3
    Type III E78.2
    Type IV E78.1
    Type V E78.3
bone (generalisata) C96.5
cerebrotendinous E75.5
cutaneotendinous E75.5
disseminatum (skin) E78.2
eruptive E78.2
hypercholesterinemic E78.00
hypercholesterolemic E78.00
hyperlipidemic E78.5
joint E75.5
multiple (skin) E78.2
tendon (sheath) E75.5
tubo-eruptive E78.2
tuberosum E78.2
tuberous E78.2
verrucous, oral mucosa K13.4
Xanthosis R23.8
Xenophobia F40.10
Xeroderma — *see also* Ichthyosis
acquired L85.0
eyelid H01.149
  left H01.146
    lower H01.145
    upper H01.144
  right H01.143
    lower H01.142
    upper H01.141
pigmentosum Q82.1
vitamin A deficiency E50.8
Xerophthalmia (vitamin A deficiency) E50.7
unrelated to vitamin A deficiency — *see* Keratoconjunctivitis
Xerosis
conjunctiva H11.14-
  with Bitot's spots — *see also* Pigmentation, conjunctiva
    vitamin A deficiency E50.1
  vitamin A deficiency E50.0
cornea H18.89-
  with ulceration — *see* Ulcer, cornea
  vitamin A deficiency E50.3
  vitamin A deficiency E50.2
cutis L85.3
skin L85.3
Xerostomia K11.7
Xiphopagus Q89.4
XO syndrome Q96.9
X-ray (of)
abnormal findings — *see* Abnormal, diagnostic imaging
breast (mammogram) (routine) Z12.31
chest
  routine (as part of a general medical examination) Z00.00
    with abnormal findings Z00.01
routine (as part of a general medical examination) Z00.00
  with abnormal findings Z00.01
XXXXY syndrome Q98.1
XXY syndrome Q98.0

Y

Yaba pox (virus disease) B08.72
Yatapoxvirus B08.70
specified NEC B08.79
Yawning R06.89
psychogenic F45.8
Yaws A66.9
bone lesions A66.6
butter A66.1
chancre A66.0
cutaneous, less than five years after infection A66.2
early (cutaneous) (macular) (maculopapular) (micropapular) (papular) A66.2
  frambeside A66.2
  skin lesions NEC A66.2
eyelid A66.2
ganglion A66.6
gangosis, gangosa A66.5
gumma, gummata A66.4
  bone A66.6

Yaws - *continued*
gummatous
  frambeside A66.4
  osteitis A66.6
  periostitis A66.6
hydrarthrosis (*see also* subcategory M14.8-) A66.6
hyperkeratosis (early) (late) A66.3
initial lesions A66.0
joint lesions (*see also* subcategory M14.8-) A66.6
juxta-articular nodules A66.7
late nodular (ulcerated) A66.4
latent (without clinical manifestations) (with positive serology) A66.8
mother A66.0
mucosal A66.7
multiple papillomata A66.1
nodular, late (ulcerated) A66.4
osteitis A66.6
papilloma, plantar or palmar A66.1
periostitis (hypertrophic) A66.6
specified NEC A66.7
ulcers A66.4
wet crab A66.1
Yeast infection — *see also* Candidiasis B37.9
Yellow
atrophy (liver) — *see* Failure, hepatic
fever — *see* Fever, yellow
jack — *see* Fever, yellow
jaundice — *see* Jaundice
nail syndrome L60.5
Yersiniosis — *see also* Infection, Yersinia
extraintestinal A28.2
intestinal A04.6

Z

Zahorsky's syndrome (herpangina) B08.5
Zellweger's syndrome Q87.89
Zenker's diverticulum (esophagus) K22.5
Ziehen-Oppenheim disease G24.1
Zieve's syndrome K70.0
Zika NOS A92.5
Zinc
deficiency, dietary E60
metabolism disorder E83.2
Zollinger-Ellison syndrome E16.4
Zona — *see* Herpes, zoster
Zoophobia F40.218
Zoster (herpes) — *see* Herpes, zoster
Zygomycosis B46.9
specified NEC B46.8
Zymotic — *see* condition

Substance	Poisoning, Accidental (unintentional)	Poisoning, Intentional self-harm	Poisoning, Assault	Poisoning, Undetermined	Adverse effect	Underdosing
1-propanol	T51.3X1-	T51.3X2-	T51.3X3-	T51.3X4-	-	-
2-propanol	T51.2X1-	T51.2X2-	T51.2X3-	T51.2X4-	-	-
2,4-D (dichlorophen-oxyacetic acid)	T60.3X1-	T60.3X2-	T60.3X3-	T60.3X4-	-	-
2,4-toluene diisocyanate	T65.0X1-	T65.0X2-	T65.0X3-	T65.0X4-	-	-
2,4,5-T (trichloro-phenoxyacetic acid)	T60.1X1-	T60.1X2-	T60.1X3-	T60.1X4-	-	-
14-hydroxydihydro-morphinone	T40.2X1-	T40.2X2-	T40.2X3-	T40.2X4-	T40.2X5-	T40.2X6-
ABOB	T37.5X1-	T37.5X2-	T37.5X3-	T37.5X4-	T37.5X5-	T37.5X6-
Abrine	T62.2X1-	T62.2X2-	T62.2X3-	T62.2X4-	-	-
Abrus (seed)	T62.2X1-	T62.2X2-	T62.2X3-	T62.2X4-	-	-
Absinthe	T51.0X1-	T51.0X2-	T51.0X3-	T51.0X4-	-	-
beverage	T51.0X1-	T51.0X2-	T51.0X3-	T51.0X4-	-	-
Acaricide	T60.8X1-	T60.8X2-	T60.8X3-	T60.8X4-	-	-
Acebutolol	T44.7X1-	T44.7X2-	T44.7X3-	T44.7X4-	T44.7X5-	T44.7X6-
Acecarbromal	T42.6X1-	T42.6X2-	T42.6X3-	T42.6X4-	T42.6X5-	T42.6X6-
Aceclidine	T44.1X1-	T44.1X2-	T44.1X3-	T44.1X4-	T44.1X5-	T44.1X6-
Acedapsone	T37.0X1-	T37.0X2-	T37.0X3-	T37.0X4-	T37.0X5-	T37.0X6-
Acefylline piperazine	T48.6X1-	T48.6X2-	T48.6X3-	T48.6X4-	T48.6X5-	T48.6X6-
Acemorphan	T40.2X1-	T40.2X2-	T40.2X3-	T40.2X4-	T40.2X5-	T40.2X6-
Acenocoumarin	T45.511-	T45.512-	T45.513-	T45.514-	T45.515-	T45.516-
Acenocoumarol	T45.511-	T45.512-	T45.513-	T45.514-	T45.515-	T45.516-
Acepifylline	T48.6X1-	T48.6X2-	T48.6X3-	T48.6X4-	T48.6X5-	T48.6X6-
Acepromazine	T43.3X1-	T43.3X2-	T43.3X3-	T43.3X4-	T43.3X5-	T43.3X6-
Acesulfamethoxypyridazine	T37.0X1-	T37.0X2-	T37.0X3-	T37.0X4-	T37.0X5-	T37.0X6-
Acetal	T52.8X1-	T52.8X2-	T52.8X3-	T52.8X4-	-	-
Acetaldehyde (vapor)	T52.8X1-	T52.8X2-	T52.8X3-	T52.8X4-	-	-
liquid	T65.891-	T65.892-	T65.893-	T65.894-	-	-
P-Acetamidophenol	T39.1X1-	T39.1X2-	T39.1X3-	T39.1X4-	T39.1X5-	T39.1X6-
Acetaminophen	T39.1X1-	T39.1X2-	T39.1X3-	T39.1X4-	T39.1X5-	T39.1X6-
Acetaminosalol	T39.1X1-	T39.1X2-	T39.1X3-	T39.1X4-	T39.1X5-	T39.1X6-
Acetanilide	T39.1X1-	T39.1X2-	T39.1X3-	T39.1X4-	T39.1X5-	T39.1X6-
Acetarsol	T37.3X1-	T37.3X2-	T37.3X3-	T37.3X4-	T37.3X5-	T37.3X6-
Acetazolamide	T50.2X1-	T50.2X2-	T50.2X3-	T50.2X4-	T50.2X5-	T50.2X6-
Acetiamine	T45.2X1-	T45.2X2-	T45.2X3-	T45.2X4-	T45.2X5-	T45.2X6-
Acetic						
acid	T54.2X1-	T54.2X2-	T54.2X3-	T54.2X4-	-	-
with sodium acetate (ointment)	T49.3X1-	T49.3X2-	T49.3X3-	T49.3X4-	T49.3X5-	T49.3X6-
ester (solvent) (vapor)	T52.8X1-	T52.8X2-	T52.8X3-	T52.8X4-	-	-
irrigating solution	T50.3X1-	T50.3X2-	T50.3X3-	T50.3X4-	T50.3X5-	T50.3X6-
medicinal (lotion)	T49.2X1-	T49.2X2-	T49.2X3-	T49.2X4-	T49.2X5-	T49.2X6-
anhydride	T65.891-	T65.892-	T65.893-	T65.894-	-	-
ether (vapor)	T52.8X1-	T52.8X2-	T52.8X3-	T52.8X4-	-	-
Acetohexamide	T38.3X1-	T38.3X2-	T38.3X3-	T38.3X4-	T38.3X5-	T38.3X6-
Acetohydroxamic acid	T50.991-	T50.992-	T50.993-	T50.994-	T50.995-	T50.996-
Acetomenaphthone	T45.7X1-	T45.7X2-	T45.7X3-	T45.7X4-	T45.7X5-	T45.7X6-
Acetomorphine	T40.1X1-	T40.1X2-	T40.1X3-	T40.1X4-	-	-
Acetone (oils)	T52.4X1-	T52.4X2-	T52.4X3-	T52.4X4-	-	-
chlorinated	T52.4X1-	T52.4X2-	T52.4X3-	T52.4X4-	-	-
vapor	T52.4X1-	T52.4X2-	T52.4X3-	T52.4X4-	-	-
Acetonitrile	T52.8X1-	T52.8X2-	T52.8X3-	T52.8X4-	-	-
Acetophenazine	T43.3X1-	T43.3X2-	T43.3X3-	T43.3X4-	T43.3X5-	T43.3X6-
Acetophenetedin	T39.1X1-	T39.1X2-	T39.1X3-	T39.1X4-	T39.1X5-	T39.1X6-
Acetophenone	T52.4X1-	T52.4X2-	T52.4X3-	T52.4X4-	-	-
Acetorphine	T40.2X1-	T40.2X2-	T40.2X3-	T40.2X4-	-	-
Acetosulfone (sodium)	T37.1X1-	T37.1X2-	T37.1X3-	T37.1X4-	T37.1X5-	T37.1X6-
Acetrizoate (sodium)	T50.8X1-	T50.8X2-	T50.8X3-	T50.8X4-	T50.8X5-	T50.8X6-
Acetrizoic acid	T50.8X1-	T50.8X2-	T50.8X3-	T50.8X4-	T50.8X5-	T50.8X6-
Acetyl						
bromide	T53.6X1-	T53.6X2-	T53.6X3-	T53.6X4-	-	-
chloride	T53.6X1-	T53.6X2-	T53.6X3-	T53.6X4-	-	-
Acetylcarbromal	T42.6X1-	T42.6X2-	T42.6X3-	T42.6X4-	T42.6X5-	T42.6X6-
Acetylcholine						
chloride	T44.1X1-	T44.1X2-	T44.1X3-	T44.1X4-	T44.1X5-	T44.1X6-
derivative	T44.1X1-	T44.1X2-	T44.1X3-	T44.1X4-	T44.1X5-	T44.1X6-
Acetylcysteine	T48.4X1-	T48.4X2-	T48.4X3-	T48.4X4-	T48.4X5-	T48.4X6-
Acetyldigitoxin	T46.0X1-	T46.0X2-	T46.0X3-	T46.0X4-	T46.0X5-	T46.0X6-
Acetyldigoxin	T46.0X1-	T46.0X2-	T46.0X3-	T46.0X4-	T46.0X5-	T46.0X6-
Acetyldihydrocodeine	T40.2X1-	T40.2X2-	T40.2X3-	T40.2X4-	-	-
Acetyldihydrocodeinone	T40.2X1-	T40.2X2-	T40.2X3-	T40.2X4-	-	-
Acetylene (gas)	T59.891-	T59.892-	T59.893-	T59.894-	-	-
dichloride	T53.6X1-	T53.6X2-	T53.6X3-	T53.6X4-	-	-
incomplete combustion of	T58.11X-	T58.12X-	T58.13X-	T58.14X-	-	-
industrial	T59.891-	T59.892-	T59.893-	T59.894-	-	-
tetrachloride	T53.6X1-	T53.6X2-	T53.6X3-	T53.6X4-	-	-
vapor	T53.6X1-	T53.6X2-	T53.6X3-	T53.6X4-	-	-

Substance	Poisoning, Accidental (unintentional)	Poisoning, Intentional self-harm	Poisoning, Assault	Poisoning, Undetermined	Adverse effect	Underdosing
Acetylpheneturide	T42.6X1-	T42.6X2-	T42.6X3-	T42.6X4-	T42.6X5-	T42.6X6-
Acetylphenylhydrazine	T39.8X1-	T39.8X2-	T39.8X3-	T39.8X4-	T39.8X5-	T39.8X6-
Acetylsalicylic acid (salts)	T39.011-	T39.012-	T39.013-	T39.014-	T39.015-	T39.016-
enteric coated	T39.011-	T39.012-	T39.013-	T39.014-	T39.015-	T39.016-
Acetylsulfamethoxypyridazine	T37.0X1-	T37.0X2-	T37.0X3-	T37.0X4-	T37.0X5-	T37.0X6-
Achromycin	T36.4X1-	T36.4X2-	T36.4X3-	T36.4X4-	T36.4X5-	T36.4X6-
ophthalmic preparation	T49.5X1-	T49.5X2-	T49.5X3-	T49.5X4-	T49.5X5-	T49.5X6-
topical NEC	T49.0X1-	T49.0X2-	T49.0X3-	T49.0X4-	T49.0X5-	T49.0X6-
Aciclovir	T37.5X1-	T37.5X2-	T37.5X3-	T37.5X4-	T37.5X5-	T37.5X6-
Acid (corrosive) NEC	T54.2X1-	T54.2X2-	T54.2X3-	T54.2X4-	-	-
Acidifying agent NEC	T50.901-	T50.902-	T50.903-	T50.904-	T50.905-	T50.906-
Acipimox	T46.6X1-	T46.6X2-	T46.6X3-	T46.6X4-	T46.6X5-	T46.6X6-
Acitretin	T50.991-	T50.992-	T50.993-	T50.994-	T50.995-	T50.996-
Aclarubicin	T45.1X1-	T45.1X2-	T45.1X3-	T45.1X4-	T45.1X5-	T45.1X6-
Aclatonium napadisilate	T48.1X1-	T48.1X2-	T48.1X3-	T48.1X4-	T48.1X5-	T48.1X6-
Aconite (wild)	T46.991-	T46.992-	T46.993-	T46.994-	T46.995-	T46.996-
Aconitine	T46.991-	T46.992-	T46.993-	T46.994-	T46.995-	T46.996-
Aconitum ferox	T46.991-	T46.992-	T46.993-	T46.994-	T46.995-	T46.996-
Acridine	T65.6X1-	T65.6X2-	T65.6X3-	T65.6X4-	-	-
vapor	T59.891-	T59.892-	T59.893-	T59.894-	-	-
Acriflavine	T37.91X-	T37.92X-	T37.93X-	T37.94X-	T37.95X-	T37.96X-
Acriflavinium chloride	T49.0X1-	T49.0X2-	T49.0X3-	T49.0X4-	T49.0X5-	T49.0X6-
Acrinol	T49.0X1-	T49.0X2-	T49.0X3-	T49.0X4-	T49.0X5-	T49.0X6-
Acrisorcin	T49.0X1-	T49.0X2-	T49.0X3-	T49.0X4-	T49.0X5-	T49.0X6-
Acrivastine	T45.0X1-	T45.0X2-	T45.0X3-	T45.0X4-	T45.0X5-	T45.0X6-
Acrolein (gas)	T59.891-	T59.892-	T59.893-	T59.894-	-	-
liquid	T54.1X1-	T54.1X2-	T54.1X3-	T54.1X4-	-	-
Acrylamide	T65.891-	T65.892-	T65.893-	T65.894-	-	-
Acrylic resin	T49.3X1-	T49.3X2-	T49.3X3-	T49.3X4-	T49.3X5-	T49.3X6-
Acrylonitrile	T65.891-	T65.892-	T65.893-	T65.894-	-	-
Actaea spicata	T62.2X1-	T62.2X2-	T62.2X3-	T62.2X4-	-	-
berry	T62.1X1-	T62.1X2-	T62.1X3-	T62.1X4-	-	-
Acterol	T37.3X1-	T37.3X2-	T37.3X3-	T37.3X4-	T37.3X5-	T37.3X6-
ACTH	T38.811-	T38.812-	T38.813-	T38.814-	T38.815-	T38.816-
Actinomycin C	T45.1X1-	T45.1X2-	T45.1X3-	T45.1X4-	T45.1X5-	T45.1X6-
Actinomycin D	T45.1X1-	T45.1X2-	T45.1X3-	T45.1X4-	T45.1X5-	T45.1X6-
Activated charcoal — see also Charcoal, medicinal	T47.6X1-	T47.6X2-	T47.6X3-	T47.6X4-	T47.6X5-	T47.6X6-
Acyclovir	T37.5X1-	T37.5X2-	T37.5X3-	T37.5X4-	T37.5X5-	T37.5X6-
Adenine	T45.2X1-	T45.2X2-	T45.2X3-	T45.2X4-	T45.2X5-	T45.2X6-
arabinoside	T37.5X1-	T37.5X2-	T37.5X3-	T37.5X4-	T37.5X5-	T37.5X6-
Adenosine (phosphate)	T46.2X1-	T46.2X2-	T46.2X3-	T46.2X4-	T46.2X5-	T46.2X6-
ADH	T38.891-	T38.892-	T38.893-	T38.894-	T38.895-	T38.896-
Adhesive NEC	T65.891-	T65.892-	T65.893-	T65.894-	-	-
Adicillin	T36.0X1-	T36.0X2-	T36.0X3-	T36.0X4-	T36.0X5-	T36.0X6-
Adiphenine	T44.3X1-	T44.3X2-	T44.3X3-	T44.3X4-	T44.3X5-	T44.3X6-
Adipiodone	T50.8X1-	T50.8X2-	T50.8X3-	T50.8X4-	T50.8X5-	T50.8X6-
Adjunct, pharmaceutical	T50.901-	T50.902-	T50.903-	T50.904-	T50.905-	T50.906-
Adrenal (extract, cortex or medulla) (glucocorticoids) (hormones) (mineralocorticoids)	T38.0X1-	T38.0X2-	T38.0X3-	T38.0X4-	T38.0X5-	T38.0X6-
ENT agent	T49.6X1-	T49.6X2-	T49.6X3-	T49.6X4-	T49.6X5-	T49.6X6-
ophthalmic preparation	T49.5X1-	T49.5X2-	T49.5X3-	T49.5X4-	T49.5X5-	T49.5X6-
topical NEC	T49.0X1-	T49.0X2-	T49.0X3-	T49.0X4-	T49.0X5-	T49.0X6-
Adrenaline	T44.5X1-	T44.5X2-	T44.5X3-	T44.5X4-	T44.5X5-	T44.5X6-
Adrenalin — see Adrenaline						
Adrenergic NEC	T44.901-	T44.902-	T44.903-	T44.904-	T44.905-	T44.906-
blocking agent NEC	T44.8X1-	T44.8X2-	T44.8X3-	T44.8X4-	T44.8X5-	T44.8X6-
beta, heart	T44.7X1-	T44.7X2-	T44.7X3-	T44.7X4-	T44.7X5-	T44.7X6-
specified NEC	T44.991-	T44.992-	T44.993-	T44.994-	T44.995-	T44.996-
Adrenochrome						
(mono) semicarbazone	T46.991-	T46.992-	T46.993-	T46.994-	T46.995-	T46.996-
derivative	T46.991-	T46.992-	T46.993-	T46.994-	T46.995-	T46.996-
Adrenocorticotrophic hormone	T38.811-	T38.812-	T38.813-	T38.814-	T38.815-	T38.816-
Adrenocorticotrophin	T38.811-	T38.812-	T38.813-	T38.814-	T38.815-	T38.816-
Adriamycin	T45.1X1-	T45.1X2-	T45.1X3-	T45.1X4-	T45.1X5-	T45.1X6-
Aerosol spray NEC	T65.91X-	T65.92X-	T65.93X-	T65.94X-	-	-
Aerosporin	T36.8X1-	T36.8X2-	T36.8X3-	T36.8X4-	T36.8X5-	T36.8X6-
ENT agent	T49.6X1-	T49.6X2-	T49.6X3-	T49.6X4-	T49.6X5-	T49.6X6-
ophthalmic preparation	T49.5X1-	T49.5X2-	T49.5X3-	T49.5X4-	T49.5X5-	T49.5X6-
topical NEC	T49.0X1-	T49.0X2-	T49.0X3-	T49.0X4-	T49.0X5-	T49.0X6-
Aethusa cynapium	T62.2X1-	T62.2X2-	T62.2X3-	T62.2X4-	-	-
Afghanistan black	T40.7X1-	T40.7X2-	T40.7X3-	T40.7X4-	T40.7X5-	T40.7X6-
Aflatoxin	T64.01X-	T64.02X-	T64.03X-	T64.04X-	-	-
Afloqualone	T42.8X1-	T42.8X2-	T42.8X3-	T42.8X4-	T42.8X5-	T42.8X6-
African boxwood	T62.2X1-	T62.2X2-	T62.2X3-	T62.2X4-	-	-
Agar	T47.4X1-	T47.4X2-	T47.4X3-	T47.4X4-	T47.4X5-	T47.4X6-

Substance	Poisoning, Accidental (unintentional)	Poisoning, Intentional self-harm	Poisoning, Assault	Poisoning, Undetermined	Adverse effect	Underdosing
Agonist						
predominantly						
alpha-adrenoreceptor	T44.4X1-	T44.4X2-	T44.4X3-	T44.4X4-	T44.4X5-	T44.4X6-
beta-adrenoreceptor	T44.5X1-	T44.5X2-	T44.5X3-	T44.5X4-	T44.5X5-	T44.5X6-
Agricultural agent NEC	T65.91X-	T65.92X-	T65.93X-	T65.94X-	-	-
Agrypnal	T42.3X1-	T42.3X2-	T42.3X3-	T42.3X4-	T42.3X5-	T42.3X6-
AHLG	T50.Z11-	T50.Z12-	T50.Z13-	T50.Z14-	T50.Z15-	T50.Z16-
Air contaminant (s), source/type NOS	T65.91X-	T65.92X-	T65.93X-	T65.94X-		
Ajmaline	T46.2X1-	T46.2X2-	T46.2X3-	T46.2X4-	T46.2X5-	T46.2X6-
Akee	T62.1X1-	T62.1X2-	T62.1X3-	T62.1X4-	-	-
Akrinol	T49.0X1-	T49.0X2-	T49.0X3-	T49.0X4-	T49.0X5-	T49.0X6-
Akritoin	T37.8X1-	T37.8X2-	T37.8X3-	T37.8X4-	T37.8X5-	T37.8X6-
Alacepril	T46.4X1-	T46.4X2-	T46.4X3-	T46.4X4-	T46.4X5-	T46.4X6-
Alantolactone	T37.4X1-	T37.4X2-	T37.4X3-	T37.4X4-	T37.4X5-	T37.4X6-
Albamycin	T36.8X1-	T36.8X2-	T36.8X3-	T36.8X4-	T36.8X5-	T36.8X6-
Albendazole	T37.4X1-	T37.4X2-	T37.4X3-	T37.4X4-	T37.4X5-	T37.4X6-
Albumin						
bovine	T45.8X1-	T45.8X2-	T45.8X3-	T45.8X4-	T45.8X5-	T45.8X6-
human serum	T45.8X1-	T45.8X2-	T45.8X3-	T45.8X4-	T45.8X5-	T45.8X6-
salt-poor	T45.8X1-	T45.8X2-	T45.8X3-	T45.8X4-	T45.8X5-	T45.8X6-
normal human serum	T45.8X1-	T45.8X2-	T45.8X3-	T45.8X4-	T45.8X5-	T45.8X6-
Albuterol	T48.6X1-	T48.6X2-	T48.6X3-	T48.6X4-	T48.6X5-	T48.6X6-
Albutoin	T42.0X1-	T42.0X2-	T42.0X3-	T42.0X4-	T42.0X5-	T42.0X6-
Alclometasone	T49.0X1-	T49.0X2-	T49.0X3-	T49.0X4-	T49.0X5-	T49.0X6-
Alcohol	T51.91X-	T51.92X-	T51.93X-	T51.94X-	-	-
absolute	T51.0X1-	T51.0X2-	T51.0X3-	T51.0X4-	-	-
beverage	T51.0X1-	T51.0X2-	T51.0X3-	T51.0X4-	-	-
allyl	T51.8X1-	T51.8X2-	T51.8X3-	T51.8X4-	-	-
amyl	T51.3X1-	T51.3X2-	T51.3X3-	T51.3X4-	-	-
antifreeze	T51.1X1-	T51.1X2-	T51.1X3-	T51.1X4-	-	-
beverage	T51.0X1-	T51.0X2-	T51.0X3-	T51.0X4-	-	-
butyl	T51.3X1-	T51.3X2-	T51.3X3-	T51.3X4-	-	-
dehydrated	T51.0X1-	T51.0X2-	T51.0X3-	T51.0X4-	-	-
beverage	T51.0X1-	T51.0X2-	T51.0X3-	T51.0X4-	-	-
denatured	T51.0X1-	T51.0X2-	T51.0X3-	T51.0X4-	-	-
deterrent NEC	T50.6X1-	T50.6X2-	T50.6X3-	T50.6X4-	T50.6X5-	T50.6X6-
diagnostic (gastric function)	T50.8X1-	T50.8X2-	T50.8X3-	T50.8X4-	T50.8X5-	T50.8X6-
ethyl	T51.0X1-	T51.0X2-	T51.0X3-	T51.0X4-	-	-
beverage	T51.0X1-	T51.0X2-	T51.0X3-	T51.0X4-	-	-
grain	T51.0X1-	T51.0X2-	T51.0X3-	T51.0X4-	-	-
beverage	T51.0X1-	T51.0X2-	T51.0X3-	T51.0X4-	-	-
industrial	T51.0X1-	T51.0X2-	T51.0X3-	T51.0X4-	-	-
isopropyl	T51.2X1-	T51.2X2-	T51.2X3-	T51.2X4-	-	-
methyl	T51.1X1-	T51.1X2-	T51.1X3-	T51.1X4-	-	-
preparation for consumption	T51.0X1-	T51.0X2-	T51.0X3-	T51.0X4-	-	-
propyl	T51.3X1-	T51.3X2-	T51.3X3-	T51.3X4-	-	-
secondary	T51.2X1-	T51.2X2-	T51.2X3-	T51.2X4-	-	-
radiator	T51.1X1-	T51.1X2-	T51.1X3-	T51.1X4-	-	-
rubbing	T51.2X1-	T51.2X2-	T51.2X3-	T51.2X4-	-	-
specified type NEC	T51.8X1-	T51.8X2-	T51.8X3-	T51.8X4-	-	-
surgical	T51.0X1-	T51.0X2-	T51.0X3-	T51.0X4-	-	-
vapor (from any type of Alcohol)	T59.891-	T59.892-	T59.893-	T59.894-	-	-
wood	T51.1X1-	T51.1X2-	T51.1X3-	T51.1X4-	-	-
Alcuronium (chloride)	T48.1X1-	T48.1X2-	T48.1X3-	T48.1X4-	T48.1X5-	T48.1X6-
Aldactone	T50.0X1-	T50.0X2-	T50.0X3-	T50.0X4-	T50.0X5-	T50.0X6-
Aldesulfone sodium	T37.1X1-	T37.1X2-	T37.1X3-	T37.1X4-	T37.1X5-	T37.1X6-
Aldicarb	T60.0X1-	T60.0X2-	T60.0X3-	T60.0X4-	-	-
Aldomet	T46.5X1-	T46.5X2-	T46.5X3-	T46.5X4-	T46.5X5-	T46.5X6-
Aldosterone	T50.0X1-	T50.0X2-	T50.0X3-	T50.0X4-	T50.0X5-	T50.0X6-
Aldrin (dust)	T60.1X1-	T60.1X2-	T60.1X3-	T60.1X4-	-	-
Aleve — see Naproxen						
Alexitol sodium	T47.1X1-	T47.1X2-	T47.1X3-	T47.1X4-	T47.1X5-	T47.1X6-
Alfacalcidol	T45.2X1-	T45.2X2-	T45.2X3-	T45.2X4-	T45.2X5-	T45.2X6-
Alfadolone	T41.1X1-	T41.1X2-	T41.1X3-	T41.1X4-	T41.1X5-	T41.1X6-
Alfaxalone	T41.1X1-	T41.1X2-	T41.1X3-	T41.1X4-	T41.1X5-	T41.1X6-
Alfentanil	T40.4X1-	T40.4X2-	T40.4X3-	T40.4X4-	T40.4X5-	T40.4X6-
Alfuzosin (hydrochloride)	T44.8X1-	T44.8X2-	T44.8X3-	T44.8X4-	T44.8X5-	T44.8X6-
Algae (harmful) (toxin)	T65.821-	T65.822-	T65.823-	T65.824-	-	-
Algeldrate	T47.1X1-	T47.1X2-	T47.1X3-	T47.1X4-	T47.1X5-	T47.1X6-
Algin	T47.8X1-	T47.8X2-	T47.8X3-	T47.8X4-	T47.8X5-	T47.8X6-
Alglucerase	T45.3X1-	T45.3X2-	T45.3X3-	T45.3X4-	T45.3X5-	T45.3X6-
Alidase	T45.3X1-	T45.3X2-	T45.3X3-	T45.3X4-	T45.3X5-	T45.3X6-
Alimemazine	T43.3X1-	T43.3X2-	T43.3X3-	T43.3X4-	T43.3X5-	T43.3X6-
Aliphatic thiocyanates	T65.0X1-	T65.0X2-	T65.0X3-	T65.0X4-	-	-
Alizapride	T45.0X1-	T45.0X2-	T45.0X3-	T45.0X4-	T45.0X5-	T45.0X6-
Alkali (caustic)	T54.3X1-	T54.3X2-	T54.3X3-	T54.3X4-	-	-
Alkaline antiseptic solution (aromatic)	T49.6X1-	T49.6X2-	T49.6X3-	T49.6X4-	T49.6X5-	T49.6X6-
Alkalinizing agents (medicinal)	T50.901-	T50.902-	T50.903-	T50.904-	T50.905-	T50.906-
Alkalizing agent NEC	T50.901-	T50.902-	T50.903-	T50.904-	T50.905-	T50.906-
Alka-seltzer	T39.011-	T39.012-	T39.013-	T39.014-	T39.015-	T39.016-
Alkavervir	T46.5X1-	T46.5X2-	T46.5X3-	T46.5X4-	T46.5X5-	T46.5X6-
Alkonium (bromide)	T49.0X1-	T49.0X2-	T49.0X3-	T49.0X4-	T49.0X5-	T49.0X6-
Alkylating drug NEC	T45.1X1-	T45.1X2-	T45.1X3-	T45.1X4-	T45.1X5-	T45.1X6-
antimyeloproliferative	T45.1X1-	T45.1X2-	T45.1X3-	T45.1X4-	T45.1X5-	T45.1X6-
lymphatic	T45.1X1-	T45.1X2-	T45.1X3-	T45.1X4-	T45.1X5-	T45.1X6-
Alkylisocyanate	T65.0X1-	T65.0X2-	T65.0X3-	T65.0X4-	-	-
Allantoin	T49.4X1-	T49.4X2-	T49.4X3-	T49.4X4-	T49.4X5-	T49.4X6-
Allegron	T43.011-	T43.012-	T43.013-	T43.014-	T43.015-	T43.016-
Allethrin	T49.0X1-	T49.0X2-	T49.0X3-	T49.0X4-	T49.0X5-	T49.0X6-
Allobarbital	T42.3X1-	T42.3X2-	T42.3X3-	T42.3X4-	T42.3X5-	T42.3X6-
Allopurinol	T50.4X1-	T50.4X2-	T50.4X3-	T50.4X4-	T50.4X5-	T50.4X6-
Allyl						
Alcohol	T51.8X1-	T51.8X2-	T51.8X3-	T51.8X4-	-	-
disulfide	T46.6X1-	T46.6X2-	T46.6X3-	T46.6X4-	T46.6X5-	T46.6X6-
Allylestrenol	T38.5X1-	T38.5X2-	T38.5X3-	T38.5X4-	T38.5X5-	T38.5X6-
Allylisopropylacetylurea	T42.6X1-	T42.6X2-	T42.6X3-	T42.6X4-	T42.6X5-	T42.6X6-
Allylisopropylmalonylurea	T42.3X1-	T42.3X2-	T42.3X3-	T42.3X4-	T42.3X5-	T42.3X6-
Allylthiourea	T49.3X1-	T49.3X2-	T49.3X3-	T49.3X4-	T49.3X5-	T49.3X6-
Allyltribromide	T42.6X1-	T42.6X2-	T42.6X3-	T42.6X4-	T42.6X5-	T42.6X6-
Allypropymal	T42.3X1-	T42.3X2-	T42.3X3-	T42.3X4-	T42.3X5-	T42.3X6-
Almagate	T47.1X1-	T47.1X2-	T47.1X3-	T47.1X4-	T47.1X5-	T47.1X6-
Almasilate	T47.1X1-	T47.1X2-	T47.1X3-	T47.1X4-	T47.1X5-	T47.1X6-
Almitrine	T50.7X1-	T50.7X2-	T50.7X3-	T50.7X4-	T50.7X5-	T50.7X6-
Aloes	T47.2X1-	T47.2X2-	T47.2X3-	T47.2X4-	T47.2X5-	T47.2X6-
Aloglutamol	T47.1X1-	T47.1X2-	T47.1X3-	T47.1X4-	T47.1X5-	T47.1X6-
Aloin	T47.2X1-	T47.2X2-	T47.2X3-	T47.2X4-	T47.2X5-	T47.2X6-
Aloxidone	T42.2X1-	T42.2X2-	T42.2X3-	T42.2X4-	T42.2X5-	T42.2X6-
Alpha						
acetyldigoxin	T46.0X1-	T46.0X2-	T46.0X3-	T46.0X4-	T46.0X5-	T46.0X6-
adrenergic blocking drug	T44.6X1-	T44.6X2-	T44.6X3-	T44.6X4-	T44.6X5-	T44.6X6-
amylase	T45.3X1-	T45.3X2-	T45.3X3-	T45.3X4-	T45.3X5-	T45.3X6-
tocoferol (acetate)	T45.2X1-	T45.2X2-	T45.2X3-	T45.2X4-	T45.2X5-	T45.2X6-
tocopherol	T45.2X1-	T45.2X2-	T45.2X3-	T45.2X4-	T45.2X5-	T45.2X6-
Alphadolone	T41.1X1-	T41.1X2-	T41.1X3-	T41.1X4-	T41.1X5-	T41.1X6-
Alphaprodine	T40.4X1-	T40.4X2-	T40.4X3-	T40.4X4-	T40.4X5-	T40.4X6-
Alphaxalone	T41.1X1-	T41.1X2-	T41.1X3-	T41.1X4-	T41.1X5-	T41.1X6-
Alprazolam	T42.4X1-	T42.4X2-	T42.4X3-	T42.4X4-	T42.4X5-	T42.4X6-
Alprenolol	T44.7X1-	T44.7X2-	T44.7X3-	T44.7X4-	T44.7X5-	T44.7X6-
Alprostadil	T46.7X1-	T46.7X2-	T46.7X3-	T46.7X4-	T46.7X5-	T46.7X6-
Alsactide	T38.811-	T38.812-	T38.813-	T38.814-	T38.815-	T38.816-
Alseroxylon	T46.5X1-	T46.5X2-	T46.5X3-	T46.5X4-	T46.5X5-	T46.5X6-
Alteplase	T45.611-	T45.612-	T45.613-	T45.614-	T45.615-	T45.616-
Altizide	T50.2X1-	T50.2X2-	T50.2X3-	T50.2X4-	T50.2X5-	T50.2X6-
Altretamine	T45.1X1-	T45.1X2-	T45.1X3-	T45.1X4-	T45.1X5-	T45.1X6-
Alum (medicinal)	T49.4X1-	T49.4X2-	T49.4X3-	T49.4X4-	T49.4X5-	T49.4X6-
nonmedicinal (ammonium) (potassium)	T56.891-	T56.892-	T56.893-	T56.894-	-	-
Aluminium, aluminum						
acetate	T49.2X1-	T49.2X2-	T49.2X3-	T49.2X4-	T49.2X5-	T49.2X6-
solution	T49.0X1-	T49.0X2-	T49.0X3-	T49.0X4-	T49.0X5-	T49.0X6-
aspirin	T39.011-	T39.012-	T39.013-	T39.014-	T39.015-	T39.016-
bis (acetylsalicylate)	T39.011-	T39.012-	T39.013-	T39.014-	T39.015-	T39.016-
carbonate (gel, basic)	T47.1X1-	T47.1X2-	T47.1X3-	T47.1X4-	T47.1X5-	T47.1X6-
chlorhydroxide-complex	T47.1X1-	T47.1X2-	T47.1X3-	T47.1X4-	T47.1X5-	T47.1X6-
chloride	T49.2X1-	T49.2X2-	T49.2X3-	T49.2X4-	T49.2X5-	T49.2X6-
clofibrate	T46.6X1-	T46.6X2-	T46.6X3-	T46.6X4-	T46.6X5-	T46.6X6-
diacetate	T49.2X1-	T49.2X2-	T49.2X3-	T49.2X4-	T49.2X5-	T49.2X6-
glycinate	T47.1X1-	T47.1X2-	T47.1X3-	T47.1X4-	T47.1X5-	T47.1X6-
hydroxide (gel)	T47.1X1-	T47.1X2-	T47.1X3-	T47.1X4-	T47.1X5-	T47.1X6-
hydroxide-magnesium carb. gel	T47.1X1-	T47.1X2-	T47.1X3-	T47.1X4-	T47.1X5-	T47.1X6-
magnesium silicate	T47.1X1-	T47.1X2-	T47.1X3-	T47.1X4-	T47.1X5-	T47.1X6-
nicotinate	T46.7X1-	T46.7X2-	T46.7X3-	T46.7X4-	T46.7X5-	T46.7X6-
ointment (surgical) (topical)	T49.3X1-	T49.3X2-	T49.3X3-	T49.3X4-	T49.3X5-	T49.3X6-
phosphate	T47.1X1-	T47.1X2-	T47.1X3-	T47.1X4-	T47.1X5-	T47.1X6-
salicylate	T39.091-	T39.092-	T39.093-	T39.094-	T39.095-	T39.096-
silicate	T47.1X1-	T47.1X2-	T47.1X3-	T47.1X4-	T47.1X5-	T47.1X6-
sodium silicate	T47.1X1-	T47.1X2-	T47.1X3-	T47.1X4-	T47.1X5-	T47.1X6-
subacetate	T49.2X1-	T49.2X2-	T49.2X3-	T49.2X4-	T49.2X5-	T49.2X6-
sulfate	T49.0X1-	T49.0X2-	T49.0X3-	T49.0X4-	T49.0X5-	T49.0X6-
tannate	T47.6X1-	T47.6X2-	T47.6X3-	T47.6X4-	T47.6X5-	T47.6X6-
topical NEC	T49.3X1-	T49.3X2-	T49.3X3-	T49.3X4-	T49.3X5-	T49.3X6-
Alurate	T42.3X1-	T42.3X2-	T42.3X3-	T42.3X4-	T42.3X5-	T42.3X6-
Alverine	T44.3X1-	T44.3X2-	T44.3X3-	T44.3X4-	T44.3X5-	T44.3X6-

Substance	Poisoning, Accidental (unintentional)	Poisoning, Intentional self-harm	Poisoning, Assault	Poisoning, Undetermined	Adverse effect	Underdosing
Alvodine	T40.2X1-	T40.2X2-	T40.2X3-	T40.2X4-	T40.2X5-	T40.2X6-
Amanita phalloides	T62.0X1-	T62.0X2-	T62.0X3-	T62.0X4-	-	-
Amanitine	T62.0X1-	T62.0X2-	T62.0X3-	T62.0X4-	-	-
Amantadine	T42.8X1-	T42.8X2-	T42.8X3-	T42.8X4-	T42.8X5-	T42.8X6-
Ambazone	T49.6X1-	T49.6X2-	T49.6X3-	T49.6X4-	T49.6X5-	T49.6X6-
Ambenonium (chloride)	T44.0X1-	T44.0X2-	T44.0X3-	T44.0X4-	T44.0X5-	T44.0X6-
Ambroxol	T48.4X1-	T48.4X2-	T48.4X3-	T48.4X4-	T48.4X5-	T48.4X6-
Ambuphylline	T48.6X1-	T48.6X2-	T48.6X3-	T48.6X4-	T48.6X5-	T48.6X6-
Ambutonium bromide	T44.3X1-	T44.3X2-	T44.3X3-	T44.3X4-	T44.3X5-	T44.3X6-
Amcinonide	T49.0X1-	T49.0X2-	T49.0X3-	T49.0X4-	T49.0X5-	T49.0X6-
Amdinocilline	T36.0X1-	T36.0X2-	T36.0X3-	T36.0X4-	T36.0X5-	T36.0X6-
Ametazole	T50.8X1-	T50.8X2-	T50.8X3-	T50.8X4-	T50.8X5-	T50.8X6-
Amethocaine	T41.3X1-	T41.3X2-	T41.3X3-	T41.3X4-	T41.3X5-	T41.3X6-
regional	T41.3X1-	T41.3X2-	T41.3X3-	T41.3X4-	T41.3X5-	T41.3X6-
spinal	T41.3X1-	T41.3X2-	T41.3X3-	T41.3X4-	T41.3X5-	T41.3X6-
Amethcpterin	T45.1X1-	T45.1X2-	T45.1X3-	T45.1X4-	T45.1X5-	T45.1X6-
Amezinium metilsulfate	T44.991-	T44.992-	T44.993-	T44.994-	T44.995-	T44.996-
Amfebutamone	T43.291-	T43.292-	T43.293-	T43.294-	T43.295-	T43.296-
Amfepramone	T50.5X1-	T50.5X2-	T50.5X3-	T50.5X4-	T50.5X5-	T50.5X6-
Amfetamine	T43.621-	T43.622-	T43.623-	T43.624-	T43.625-	T43.626-
Amfetaminil	T43.621-	T43.622-	T43.623-	T43.624-	T43.625-	T43.626-
Amfomycin	T36.8X1-	T36.8X2-	T36.8X3-	T36.8X4-	T36.8X5-	T36.8X6-
Amidefrine mesilate	T48.5X1-	T48.5X2-	T48.5X3-	T48.5X4-	T48.5X5-	T48.5X6-
Amidone	T40.3X1-	T40.3X2-	T40.3X3-	T40.3X4-	T40.3X5-	T40.3X6-
Amidopyrine	T39.2X1-	T39.2X2-	T39.2X3-	T39.2X4-	T39.2X5-	T39.2X6-
Amidotrizoate	T50.8X1-	T50.8X2-	T50.8X3-	T50.8X4-	T50.8X5-	T50.8X6-
Amiflamine	T43.1X1-	T43.1X2-	T43.1X3-	T43.1X4-	T43.1X5-	T43.1X6-
Amikacin	T36.5X1-	T36.5X2-	T36.5X3-	T36.5X4-	T36.5X5-	T36.5X6-
Amikhelline	T46.3X1-	T46.3X2-	T46.3X3-	T46.3X4-	T46.3X5-	T46.3X6-
Amiloride	T50.2X1-	T50.2X2-	T50.2X3-	T50.2X4-	T50.2X5-	T50.2X6-
Aminacrine	T49.0X1-	T49.0X2-	T49.0X3-	T49.0X4-	T49.0X5-	T49.0X6-
Amineptine	T43.011-	T43.012-	T43.013-	T43.014-	T43.015-	T43.016-
Aminitrozole	T37.3X1-	T37.3X2-	T37.3X3-	T37.3X4-	T37.3X5-	T37.3X6-
Amino acids	T50.3X1-	T50.3X2-	T50.3X3-	T50.3X4-	T50.3X5-	T50.3X6-
Aminoacetic acid (derivatives)	T50.3X1-	T50.3X2-	T50.3X3-	T50.3X4-	T50.3X5-	T50.3X6-
Aminoacridine	T49.0X1-	T49.0X2-	T49.0X3-	T49.0X4-	T49.0X5-	T49.0X6-
Aminobenzoic acid (-p)	T49.3X1-	T49.3X2-	T49.3X3-	T49.3X4-	T49.3X5-	T49.3X6-
4-Aminobutyric acid	T43.8X1-	T43.8X2-	T43.8X3-	T43.8X4-	T43.8X5-	T43.8X6-
Aminocaproic acid	T45.621-	T45.622-	T45.623-	T45.624-	T45.625-	T45.626-
Aminoethylisothiourium	T45.8X1-	T45.8X2-	T45.8X3-	T45.8X4-	T45.8X5-	T45.8X6-
Aminofenazone	T39.2X1-	T39.2X2-	T39.2X3-	T39.2X4-	T39.2X5-	T39.2X6-
Aminoglutethimide	T45.1X1-	T45.1X2-	T45.1X3-	T45.1X4-	T45.1X5-	T45.1X6-
Aminohippuric acid	T50.8X1-	T50.8X2-	T50.8X3-	T50.8X4-	T50.8X5-	T50.8X6-
Aminomethylbenzoic acid	T45.691-	T45.692-	T45.693-	T45.694-	T45.695-	T45.696-
Aminometradine	T50.2X1-	T50.2X2-	T50.2X3-	T50.2X4-	T50.2X5-	T50.2X6-
Aminopentamide	T44.3X1-	T44.3X2-	T44.3X3-	T44.3X4-	T44.3X5-	T44.3X6-
Aminophenazone	T39.2X1-	T39.2X2-	T39.2X3-	T39.2X4-	T39.2X5-	T39.2X6-
Aminophenol	T54.0X1-	T54.0X2-	T54.0X3-	T54.0X4-	-	-
4-Aminophenol derivatives	T39.1X1-	T39.1X2-	T39.1X3-	T39.1X4-	T39.1X5-	T39.1X6-
Aminophenylpyridone	T43.591-	T43.592-	T43.593-	T43.594-	T43.595-	T43.596-
Aminophylline	T48.6X1-	T48.6X2-	T48.6X3-	T48.6X4-	T48.6X5-	T48.6X6-
Aminopterin sodium	T45.1X1-	T45.1X2-	T45.1X3-	T45.1X4-	T45.1X5-	T45.1X6-
Aminopyrine	T39.2X1-	T39.2X2-	T39.2X3-	T39.2X4-	T39.2X5-	T39.2X6-
8-Aminoquinoline drugs	T37.2X1-	T37.2X2-	T37.2X3-	T37.2X4-	T37.2X5-	T37.2X6-
Aminorex	T50.5X1-	T50.5X2-	T50.5X3-	T50.5X4-	T50.5X5-	T50.5X6-
Aminosalicylic acid	T37.1X1-	T37.1X2-	T37.1X3-	T37.1X4-	T37.1X5-	T37.1X6-
Aminosalylum	T37.1X1-	T37.1X2-	T37.1X3-	T37.1X4-	T37.1X5-	T37.1X6-
Amiodarone	T46.2X1-	T46.2X2-	T46.2X3-	T46.2X4-	T46.2X5-	T46.2X6-
Amiphenazole	T50.7X1-	T50.7X2-	T50.7X3-	T50.7X4-	T50.7X5-	T50.7X6-
Amiquinsin	T46.5X1-	T46.5X2-	T46.5X3-	T46.5X4-	T46.5X5-	T46.5X6-
Amisometradine	T50.2X1-	T50.2X2-	T50.2X3-	T50.2X4-	T50.2X5-	T50.2X6-
Amisulpride	T43.591-	T43.592-	T43.593-	T43.594-	T43.595-	T43.596-
Amitriptyline	T43.011-	T43.012-	T43.013-	T43.014-	T43.015-	T43.016-
Amitriptylinoxide	T43.011-	T43.012-	T43.013-	T43.014-	T43.015-	T43.016-
Amlexanox	T48.6X1-	T48.6X2-	T48.6X3-	T48.6X4-	T48.6X5-	T48.6X6-
Ammonia (fumes) (gas) (vapor)	T59.891-	T59.892-	T59.893-	T59.894-	-	-
aromatic spirit	T48.991-	T48.992-	T48.993-	T48.994-	T48.995-	T48.996-
liquid (household)	T54.3X1-	T54.3X2-	T54.3X3-	T54.3X4-	-	-
Ammoniated mercury	T49.0X1-	T49.0X2-	T49.0X3-	T49.0X4-	T49.0X5-	T49.0X6-
Ammonium						
acid tartrate	T49.5X1-	T49.5X2-	T49.5X3-	T49.5X4-	T49.5X5-	T49.5X6-
bromide	T42.6X1-	T42.6X2-	T42.6X3-	T42.6X4-	T42.6X5-	T42.6X6-
carbonate	T54.3X1-	T54.3X2-	T54.3X3-	T54.3X4-	-	-
chloride	T50.991-	T50.992-	T50.993-	T50.994-	T50.995-	T50.996-
expectorant	T48.4X1-	T48.4X2-	T48.4X3-	T48.4X4-	T48.4X5-	T48.4X6-
compounds (household) NEC	T54.3X1-	T54.3X2-	T54.3X3-	T54.3X4-	-	-
fumes (any usage)	T59.891-	T59.892-	T59.893-	T59.894-	-	-
industrial	T54.3X1-	T54.3X2-	T54.3X3-	T54.3X4-	-	-

Substance	Poisoning, Accidental (unintentional)	Poisoning, Intentional self-harm	Poisoning, Assault	Poisoning, Undetermined	Adverse effect	Underdosing
Ammonium - continued						
ichthyosulronate	T49.4X1-	T49.4X2-	T49.4X3-	T49.4X4-	T49.4X5-	T49.4X6-
mandelate	T37.91X-	T37.92X-	T37.93X-	T37.94X-	T37.95X-	T37.96X-
sulfamate	T60.3X1-	T60.3X2-	T60.3X3-	T60.3X4-	-	-
sulfonate resin	T47.8X1-	T47.8X2-	T47.8X3-	T47.8X4-	T47.8X5-	T47.8X6-
Amobarbital (sodium)	T42.3X1-	T42.3X2-	T42.3X3-	T42.3X4-	T42.3X5-	T42.3X6-
Amodiaquine	T37.2X1-	T37.2X2-	T37.2X3-	T37.2X4-	T37.2X5-	T37.2X6-
Amopyroquin (e)	T37.2X1-	T37.2X2-	T37.2X3-	T37.2X4-	T37.2X5-	T37.2X6-
Amoxapine	T43.011-	T43.012-	T43.013-	T43.014-	T43.015-	T43.016-
Amoxicillin	T36.0X1-	T36.0X2-	T36.0X3-	T36.0X4-	T36.0X5-	T36.0X6-
Amperozide	T43.591-	T43.592-	T43.593-	T43.594-	T43.595-	T43.596-
Amphenidone	T43.591-	T43.592-	T43.593-	T43.594-	T43.595-	T43.596-
Amphetamine NEC	T43.621-	T43.622-	T43.623-	T43.624-	T43.625-	T43.626-
Amphomycin	T36.8X1-	T36.8X2-	T36.8X3-	T36.8X4-	T36.8X5-	T36.8X6-
Amphotalide	T37.4X1-	T37.4X2-	T37.4X3-	T37.4X4-	T37.4X5-	T37.4X6-
Amphotericin B	T36.7X1-	T36.7X2-	T36.7X3-	T36.7X4-	T36.7X5-	T36.7X6-
topical	T49.0X1-	T49.0X2-	T49.0X3-	T49.0X4-	T49.0X5-	T49.0X6-
Ampicillin	T36.0X1-	T36.0X2-	T36.0X3-	T36.0X4-	T36.0X5-	T36.0X6-
Amprotropine	T44.3X1-	T44.3X2-	T44.3X3-	T44.3X4-	T44.3X5-	T44.3X6-
Amsacrine	T45.1X1-	T45.1X2-	T45.1X3-	T45.1X4-	T45.1X5-	T45.1X6-
Amygdaline	T62.2X1-	T62.2X2-	T62.2X3-	T62.2X4-	-	-
Amyl						
acetate	T52.8X1-	T52.8X2-	T52.8X3-	T52.8X4-	-	-
vapor	T59.891-	T59.892-	T59.893-	T59.894-	-	-
alcohol	T51.3X1-	T51.3X2-	T51.3X3-	T51.3X4-	-	-
chloride	T53.6X1-	T53.6X2-	T53.6X3-	T53.6X4-	-	-
formate	T52.8X1-	T52.8X2-	T52.8X3-	T52.8X4-	-	-
nitrite	T46.3X1-	T46.3X2-	T46.3X3-	T46.3X4-	T46.3X5-	T46.3X6-
propionate	T65.891-	T65.892-	T65.893-	T65.894-	-	-
Amylase	T47.5X1-	T47.5X2-	T47.5X3-	T47.5X4-	T47.5X5-	T47.5X6-
Amyleine, regional	T41.3X1-	T41.3X2-	T41.3X3-	T41.3X4-	T41.3X5-	T41.3X6-
Amylene						
dichloride	T53.6X1-	T53.6X2-	T53.6X3-	T53.6X4-	-	-
hydrate	T51.3X1-	T51.3X2-	T51.3X3-	T51.3X4-	-	-
Amylmetacresol	T49.6X1-	T49.6X2-	T49.6X3-	T49.6X4-	T49.6X5-	T49.6X6-
Amylobarbitone	T42.3X1-	T42.3X2-	T42.3X3-	T42.3X4-	T42.3X5-	T42.3X6-
Amylocaine, regional	T41.3X1-	T41.3X2-	T41.3X3-	T41.3X4-	T41.3X5-	T41.3X6-
infiltration (subcutaneous)	T41.3X1-	T41.3X2-	T41.3X3-	T41.3X4-	T41.3X5-	T41.3X6-
nerve block (peripheral) (plexus)	T41.3X1-	T41.3X2-	T41.3X3-	T41.3X4-	T41.3X5-	T41.3X6-
spinal	T41.3X1-	T41.3X2-	T41.3X3-	T41.3X4-	T41.3X5-	T41.3X6-
topical (surface)	T41.3X1-	T41.3X2-	T41.3X3-	T41.3X4-	T41.3X5-	T41.3X6-
Amylopectin	T47.6X1-	T47.6X2-	T47.6X3-	T47.6X4-	T47.6X5-	T47.6X6-
Amytal (sodium)	T42.3X1-	T42.3X2-	T42.3X3-	T42.3X4-	T42.3X5-	T42.3X6-
Anabolic steroid	T38.7X1-	T38.7X2-	T38.7X3-	T38.7X4-	T38.7X5-	T38.7X6-
Analeptic NEC	T50.7X1-	T50.7X2-	T50.7X3-	T50.7X4-	T50.7X5-	T50.7X6-
Analgesic	T39.91X-	T39.92X-	T39.93X-	T39.94X-	T39.95X-	T39.96X-
anti-inflammatory NEC	T39.91X-	T39.92X-	T39.93X-	T39.94X-	T39.95X-	T39.96X-
propionic acid derivative	T39.311-	T39.312-	T39.313-	T39.314-	T39.315-	T39.316-
antirheumatic NEC	T39.4X1-	T39.4X2-	T39.4X3-	T39.4X4-	T39.4X5-	T39.4X6-
aromatic NEC	T39.1X1-	T39.1X2-	T39.1X3-	T39.1X4-	T39.1X5-	T39.1X6-
narcotic NEC	T40.601-	T40.602-	T40.603-	T40.604-	T40.605-	T40.606-
combination	T40.601-	T40.602-	T40.603-	T40.604-	T40.605-	T40.606-
obstetric	T40.601-	T40.602-	T40.603-	T40.604-	T40.605-	T40.606-
non-narcotic NEC	T39.91X-	T39.92X-	T39.93X-	T39.94X-	T39.95X-	T39.96X-
combination	T39.91X-	T39.92X-	T39.93X-	T39.94X-	T39.95X-	T39.96X-
pyrazole	T39.2X1-	T39.2X2-	T39.2X3-	T39.2X4-	T39.2X5-	T39.2X6-
specified NEC	T39.8X1-	T39.8X2-	T39.8X3-	T39.8X4-	T39.8X5-	T39.8X6-
Analgin	T39.2X1-	T39.2X2-	T39.2X3-	T39.2X4-	T39.2X5-	T39.2X6-
Anamirta cocculus	T62.1X1-	T62.1X2-	T62.1X3-	T62.1X4-	-	-
Ancillin	T36.0X1-	T36.0X2-	T36.0X3-	T36.0X4-	T36.0X5-	T36.0X6-
Ancrod	T45.691-	T45.692-	T45.693-	T45.694-	T45.695-	T45.696-
Androgen	T38.7X1-	T38.7X2-	T38.7X3-	T38.7X4-	T38.7X5-	T38.7X6-
Androgen-estrogen mixture	T38.7X1-	T38.7X2-	T38.7X3-	T38.7X4-	T38.7X5-	T38.7X6-
Androstalone	T38.7X1-	T38.7X2-	T38.7X3-	T38.7X4-	T38.7X5-	T38.7X6-
Androstanolone	T38.7X1-	T38.7X2-	T38.7X3-	T38.7X4-	T38.7X5-	T38.7X6-
Androsterone	T38.7X1-	T38.7X2-	T38.7X3-	T38.7X4-	T38.7X5-	T38.7X6-
Anemone pulsatilla	T62.2X1-	T62.2X2-	T62.2X3-	T62.2X4-	-	-
Anesthesia						
caudal	T41.3X1-	T41.3X2-	T41.3X3-	T41.3X4-	T41.3X5-	T41.3X6-
endotracheal	T41.0X1-	T41.0X2-	T41.0X3-	T41.0X4-	T41.0X5-	T41.0X6-
epidural	T41.3X1-	T41.3X2-	T41.3X3-	T41.3X4-	T41.3X5-	T41.3X6-
inhalation	T41.0X1-	T41.0X2-	T41.0X3-	T41.0X4-	T41.0X5-	T41.0X6-
local	T41.3X1-	T41.3X2-	T41.3X3-	T41.3X4-	T41.3X5-	T41.3X6-
mucosal	T41.3X1-	T41.3X2-	T41.3X3-	T41.3X4-	T41.3X5-	T41.3X6-
muscle relaxation	T48.1X1-	T48.1X2-	T48.1X3-	T48.1X4-	T48.1X5-	T48.1X6-
nerve blocking	T41.3X1-	T41.3X2-	T41.3X3-	T41.3X4-	T41.3X5-	T41.3X6-
plexus blocking	T41.3X1-	T41.3X2-	T41.3X3-	T41.3X4-	T41.3X5-	T41.3X6-

Substance	Poisoning, Accidental (unintentional)	Poisoning, Intentional self-harm	Poisoning, Assault	Poisoning, Undetermined	Adverse effect	Underdosing
Anesthesia - *continued*						
potentiated	T41.201-	T41.202-	T41.203-	T41.204-	T41.205-	T41.206-
rectal	T41.201-	T41.202-	T41.203-	T41.204-	T41.205-	T41.206-
general	T41.201-	T41.202-	T41.203-	T41.204-	T41.205-	T41.206-
local	T41.3X1-	T41.3X2-	T41.3X3-	T41.3X4-	T41.3X5-	T41.3X6-
regional	T41.3X1-	T41.3X2-	T41.3X3-	T41.3X4-	T41.3X5-	T41.3X6-
surface	T41.3X1-	T41.3X2-	T41.3X3-	T41.3X4-	T41.3X5-	T41.3X6-
Anesthetic NEC — *see also* Anesthesia	T41.41X-	T41.42X-	T41.43X-	T41.44X-	T41.45X-	T41.46X-
with muscle relaxant	T41.201-	T41.202-	T41.203-	T41.204-	T41.205-	T41.206-
general	T41.201-	T41.202-	T41.203-	T41.204-	T41.205-	T41.206-
local	T41.3X1-	T41.3X2-	T41.3X3-	T41.3X4-	T41.3X5-	T41.3X6-
gaseous NEC	T41.0X1-	T41.0X2-	T41.0X3-	T41.0X4-	T41.0X5-	T41.0X6-
general NEC	T41.201-	T41.202-	T41.203-	T41.204-	T41.205-	T41.206-
halogenated hydrocarbon derivatives NEC	T41.0X1-	T41.0X2-	T41.0X3-	T41.0X4-	T41.0X5-	T41.0X6-
infiltration NEC	T41.3X1-	T41.3X2-	T41.3X3-	T41.3X4-	T41.3X5-	T41.3X6-
intravenous NEC	T41.1X1-	T41.1X2-	T41.1X3-	T41.1X4-	T41.1X5-	T41.1X6-
local NEC	T41.3X1-	T41.3X2-	T41.3X3-	T41.3X4-	T41.3X5-	T41.3X6-
rectal	T41.201-	T41.202-	T41.203-	T41.204-	T41.205-	T41.206-
general	T41.201-	T41.202-	T41.203-	T41.204-	T41.205-	T41.206-
local	T41.3X1-	T41.3X2-	T41.3X3-	T41.3X4-	T41.3X5-	T41.3X6-
regional NEC	T41.3X1-	T41.3X2-	T41.3X3-	T41.3X4-	T41.3X5-	T41.3X6-
spinal NEC	T41.3X1-	T41.3X2-	T41.3X3-	T41.3X4-	T41.3X5-	T41.3X6-
thiobarbiturate	T41.1X1-	T41.1X2-	T41.1X3-	T41.1X4-	T41.1X5-	T41.1X6-
topical	T41.3X1-	T41.3X2-	T41.3X3-	T41.3X4-	T41.3X5-	T41.3X6-
Aneurine	T45.2X1-	T45.2X2-	T45.2X3-	T45.2X4-	T45.2X5-	T45.2X6-
Angio-Conray	T50.8X1-	T50.8X2-	T50.8X3-	T50.8X4-	T50.8X5-	T50.8X6-
Angiotensin	T44.5X1-	T44.5X2-	T44.5X3-	T44.5X4-	T44.5X5-	T44.5X6-
Angiotensinamide	T44.991-	T44.992-	T44.993-	T44.994-	T44.995-	T44.996-
Anhydrohydroxy-progesterone	T38.5X1-	T38.5X2-	T38.5X3-	T38.5X4-	T38.5X5-	T38.5X6-
Anhydron	T50.2X1-	T50.2X2-	T50.2X3-	T50.2X4-	T50.2X5-	T50.2X6-
Anileridine	T40.4X1-	T40.4X2-	T40.4X3-	T40.4X4-	T40.4X5-	T40.4X6-
Aniline (dye) (liquid)	T65.3X1-	T65.3X2-	T65.3X3-	T65.3X4-	-	-
analgesic	T39.1X1-	T39.1X2-	T39.1X3-	T39.1X4-	T39.1X5-	T39.1X6-
derivatives, therapeutic NEC	T39.1X1-	T39.1X2-	T39.1X3-	T39.1X4-	T39.1X5-	T39.1X6-
vapor	T65.3X1-	T65.3X2-	T65.3X3-	T65.3X4-	-	-
Aniscoropine	T44.3X1-	T44.3X2-	T44.3X3-	T44.3X4-	T44.3X5-	T44.3X6-
Anise oil	T47.5X1-	T47.5X2-	T47.5X3-	T47.5X4-	T47.5X5-	T47.5X6-
Anisidine	T65.3X1-	T65.3X2-	T65.3X3-	T65.3X4-	-	-
Anisindione	T45.511-	T45.512-	T45.513-	T45.514-	T45.515-	T45.516-
Anisotropine methyl-bromide	T44.3X1-	T44.3X2-	T44.3X3-	T44.3X4-	T44.3X5-	T44.3X6-
Anistreplase	T45.611-	T45.612-	T45.613-	T45.614-	T45.615-	T45.616-
Anorexiant (central)	T50.5X1-	T50.5X2-	T50.5X3-	T50.5X4-	T50.5X5-	T50.5X6-
Anorexic agents	T50.5X1-	T50.5X2-	T50.5X3-	T50.5X4-	T50.5X5-	T50.5X6-
Ansamycin	T36.6X1-	T36.6X2-	T36.6X3-	T36.6X4-	T36.6X5-	T36.6X6-
Ant (bite) (sting)	T63.421-	T63.422-	T63.423-	T63.424-	-	-
Ant poison — *see* Insecticide						
Antabuse	T50.6X1-	T50.6X2-	T50.6X3-	T50.6X4-	T50.6X5-	T50.6X6-
Antacid NEC	T47.1X1-	T47.1X2-	T47.1X3-	T47.1X4-	T47.1X5-	T47.1X6-
Antagonist						
Aldosterone	T50.0X1-	T50.0X2-	T50.0X3-	T50.0X4-	T50.0X5-	T50.0X6-
alpha-adrenoreceptor	T44.6X1-	T44.6X2-	T44.6X3-	T44.6X4-	T44.6X5-	T44.6X6-
anticoagulant	T45.7X1-	T45.7X2-	T45.7X3-	T45.7X4-	T45.7X5-	T45.7X6-
beta-adrenoreceptor	T44.7X1-	T44.7X2-	T44.7X3-	T44.7X4-	T44.7X5-	T44.7X6-
extrapyramidal NEC	T44.3X1-	T44.3X2-	T44.3X3-	T44.3X4-	T44.3X5-	T44.3X6-
folic acid	T45.1X1-	T45.1X2-	T45.1X3-	T45.1X4-	T45.1X5-	T45.1X6-
H2 receptor	T47.0X1-	T47.0X2-	T47.0X3-	T47.0X4-	T47.0X5-	T47.0X6-
heavy metal	T45.8X1-	T45.8X2-	T45.8X3-	T45.8X4-	T45.8X5-	T45.8X6-
narcotic analgesic	T50.7X1-	T50.7X2-	T50.7X3-	T50.7X4-	T50.7X5-	T50.7X6-
opiate	T50.7X1-	T50.7X2-	T50.7X3-	T50.7X4-	T50.7X5-	T50.7X6-
pyrimidine	T45.1X1-	T45.1X2-	T45.1X3-	T45.1X4-	T45.1X5-	T45.1X6-
serotonin	T46.5X1-	T46.5X2-	T46.5X3-	T46.5X4-	T46.5X5-	T46.5X6-
Antazolin (e)	T45.0X1-	T45.0X2-	T45.0X3-	T45.0X4-	T45.0X5-	T45.0X6-
Anterior pituitary hormone NEC	T38.811-	T38.812-	T38.813-	T38.814-	T38.815-	T38.816-
Anthelmintic NEC	T37.4X1-	T37.4X2-	T37.4X3-	T37.4X4-	T37.4X5-	T37.4X6-
Anthiolimine	T37.4X1-	T37.4X2-	T37.4X3-	T37.4X4-	T37.4X5-	T37.4X6-
Anthralin	T49.4X1-	T49.4X2-	T49.4X3-	T49.4X4-	T49.4X5-	T49.4X6-
Anthramycin	T45.1X1-	T45.1X2-	T45.1X3-	T45.1X4-	T45.1X5-	T45.1X6-
Antiadrenergic NEC	T44.8X1-	T44.8X2-	T44.8X3-	T44.8X4-	T44.8X5-	T44.8X6-
Antiallergic NEC	T45.0X1-	T45.0X2-	T45.0X3-	T45.0X4-	T45.0X5-	T45.0X6-
Anti-anemic (drug) (preparation)	T45.8X1-	T45.8X2-	T45.8X3-	T45.8X4-	T45.8X5-	T45.8X6-
Antiandrogen NEC	T38.6X1-	T38.6X2-	T38.6X3-	T38.6X4-	T38.6X5-	T38.6X6-
Antianxiety drug NEC	T43.501-	T43.502-	T43.503-	T43.504-	T43.505-	T43.506-
Antiaris toxicaria	T65.891-	T65.892-	T65.893-	T65.894-	-	-
Antiarteriosclerotic drug	T46.6X1-	T46.6X2-	T46.6X3-	T46.6X4-	T46.6X5-	T46.6X6-

Substance	Poisoning, Accidental (unintentional)	Poisoning, Intentional self-harm	Poisoning, Assault	Poisoning, Undetermined	Adverse effect	Underdosing
Antiasthmatic drug NEC	T48.6X1-	T48.6X2-	T48.6X3-	T48.6X4-	T48.6X5-	T48.6X6-
Antibiotic NEC	T36.91X-	T36.92X-	T36.93X-	T36.94X-	T36.95X-	T36.96X-
aminoglycoside	T36.5X1-	T36.5X2-	T36.5X3-	T36.5X4-	T36.5X5-	T36.5X6-
anticancer	T45.1X1-	T45.1X2-	T45.1X3-	T45.1X4-	T45.1X5-	T45.1X6-
antifungal	T36.7X1-	T36.7X2-	T36.7X3-	T36.7X4-	T36.7X5-	T36.7X6-
antimycobacterial	T36.5X1-	T36.5X2-	T36.5X3-	T36.5X4-	T36.5X5-	T36.5X6-
antineoplastic	T45.1X1-	T45.1X2-	T45.1X3-	T45.1X4-	T45.1X5-	T45.1X6-
cephalosporin (group)	T36.1X1-	T36.1X2-	T36.1X3-	T36.1X4-	T36.1X5-	T36.1X6-
chloramphenicol (group)	T36.2X1-	T36.2X2-	T36.2X3-	T36.2X4-	T36.2X5-	T36.2X6-
ENT	T49.6X1-	T49.6X2-	T49.6X3-	T49.6X4-	T49.6X5-	T49.6X6-
eye	T49.5X1-	T49.5X2-	T49.5X3-	T49.5X4-	T49.5X5-	T49.5X6-
fungicidal (local)	T49.0X1-	T49.0X2-	T49.0X3-	T49.0X4-	T49.0X5-	T49.0X6-
intestinal	T36.8X1-	T36.8X2-	T36.8X3-	T36.8X4-	T36.8X5-	T36.8X6-
b-lactam NEC	T36.1X1-	T36.1X2-	T36.1X3-	T36.1X4-	T36.1X5-	T36.1X6-
local	T49.0X1-	T49.0X2-	T49.0X3-	T49.0X4-	T49.0X5-	T49.0X6-
macrolides	T36.3X1-	T36.3X2-	T36.3X3-	T36.3X4-	T36.3X5-	T36.3X6-
polypeptide	T36.8X1-	T36.8X2-	T36.8X3-	T36.8X4-	T36.8X5-	T36.8X6-
specified NEC	T36.8X1-	T36.8X2-	T36.8X3-	T36.8X4-	T36.8X5-	T36.8X6-
tetracycline (group)	T36.4X1-	T36.4X2-	T36.4X3-	T36.4X4-	T36.4X5-	T36.4X6-
throat	T49.6X1-	T49.6X2-	T49.6X3-	T49.6X4-	T49.6X5-	T49.6X6-
Anticancer agents NEC	T45.1X1-	T45.1X2-	T45.1X3-	T45.1X4-	T45.1X5-	T45.1X6-
Anticholesterolemic drug NEC	T46.6X1-	T46.6X2-	T46.6X3-	T46.6X4-	T46.6X5-	T46.6X6-
Anticholinergic NEC	T44.3X1-	T44.3X2-	T44.3X3-	T44.3X4-	T44.3X5-	T44.3X6-
Anticholinesterase	T44.0X1-	T44.0X2-	T44.0X3-	T44.0X4-	T44.0X5-	T44.0X6-
organophosphorus	T44.0X1-	T44.0X2-	T44.0X3-	T44.0X4-	T44.0X5-	T44.0X6-
insecticide	T60.0X1-	T60.0X2-	T60.0X3-	T60.0X4-	-	-
nerve gas	T59.891-	T59.892-	T59.893-	T59.894-	-	-
reversible	T44.0X1-	T44.0X2-	T44.0X3-	T44.0X4-	T44.0X5-	T44.0X6-
ophthalmological	T49.5X1-	T49.5X2-	T49.5X3-	T49.5X4-	T49.5X5-	T49.5X6-
Anticoagulant NEC	T45.511-	T45.512-	T45.513-	T45.514-	T45.515-	T45.516-
Antagonist	T45.7X1-	T45.7X2-	T45.7X3-	T45.7X4-	T45.7X5-	T45.7X6-
Anti-common-cold drug NEC	T48.5X1-	T48.5X2-	T48.5X3-	T48.5X4-	T48.5X5-	T48.5X6-
Anticonvulsant	T42.71X-	T42.72X-	T42.73X-	T42.74X-	T42.75X-	T42.76X-
barbiturate	T42.3X1-	T42.3X2-	T42.3X3-	T42.3X4-	T42.3X5-	T42.3X6-
combination (with barbiturate)	T42.3X1-	T42.3X2-	T42.3X3-	T42.3X4-	T42.3X5-	T42.3X6-
hydantoin	T42.0X1-	T42.0X2-	T42.0X3-	T42.0X4-	T42.0X5-	T42.0X6-
hypnotic NEC	T42.6X1-	T42.6X2-	T42.6X3-	T42.6X4-	T42.6X5-	T42.6X6-
oxazolidinedione	T42.2X1-	T42.2X2-	T42.2X3-	T42.2X4-	T42.2X5-	T42.2X6-
pyrimidinedione	T42.6X1-	T42.6X2-	T42.6X3-	T42.6X4-	T42.6X5-	T42.6X6-
specified NEC	T42.6X1-	T42.6X2-	T42.6X3-	T42.6X4-	T42.6X5-	T42.6X6-
succinimide	T42.2X1-	T42.2X2-	T42.2X3-	T42.2X4-	T42.2X5-	T42.2X6-
Anti-D immunoglobulin (human)	T50.Z11-	T50.Z12-	T50.Z13-	T50.Z14-	T50.Z15-	T50.Z16-
Antidepressant	T43.201-	T43.202-	T43.203-	T43.204-	T43.205-	T43.206-
monoamine oxidase inhibitor	T43.1X1-	T43.1X2-	T43.1X3-	T43.1X4-	T43.1X5-	T43.1X6-
selective serotonin norepinephrine reuptake inhibitor	T43.211-	T43.212-	T43.213-	T43.214-	T43.215-	T43.216-
selective serotonin reuptake inhibitor	T43.221-	T43.222-	T43.223-	T43.224-	T43.225-	T43.226-
specified NEC	T43.291-	T43.292-	T43.293-	T43.294-	T43.295-	T43.296-
tetracyclic	T43.021-	T43.022-	T43.023-	T43.024-	T43.025-	T43.026-
triazolopyridine	T43.211-	T43.212-	T43.213-	T43.214-	T43.215-	T43.216-
tricyclic	T43.011-	T43.012-	T43.013-	T43.014-	T43.015-	T43.016-
Antidiabetic NEC	T38.3X1-	T38.3X2-	T38.3X3-	T38.3X4-	T38.3X5-	T38.3X6-
biguanide	T38.3X1-	T38.3X2-	T38.3X3-	T38.3X4-	T38.3X5-	T38.3X6-
and sulfonyl combined	T38.3X1-	T38.3X2-	T38.3X3-	T38.3X4-	T38.3X5-	T38.3X6-
combined	T38.3X1-	T38.3X2-	T38.3X3-	T38.3X4-	T38.3X5-	T38.3X6-
sulfonylurea	T38.3X1-	T38.3X2-	T38.3X3-	T38.3X4-	T38.3X5-	T38.3X6-
Antidiarrheal drug NEC	T47.6X1-	T47.6X2-	T47.6X3-	T47.6X4-	T47.6X5-	T47.6X6-
absorbent	T47.6X1-	T47.6X2-	T47.6X3-	T47.6X4-	T47.6X5-	T47.6X6-
Antidiphtheria serum	T50.Z11-	T50.Z12-	T50.Z13-	T50.Z14-	T50.Z15-	T50.Z16-
Antidiuretic hormone	T38.891-	T38.892-	T38.893-	T38.894-	T38.895-	T38.896-
Antidote NEC	T50.6X1-	T50.6X2-	T50.6X3-	T50.6X4-	T50.6X5-	T50.6X6-
heavy metal	T45.8X1-	T45.8X2-	T45.8X3-	T45.8X4-	T45.8X5-	T45.8X6-
Antidysrhythmic NEC	T46.2X1-	T46.2X2-	T46.2X3-	T46.2X4-	T46.2X5-	T46.2X6-
Antiemetic drug	T45.0X1-	T45.0X2-	T45.0X3-	T45.0X4-	T45.0X5-	T45.0X6-
Antiepilepsy agent	T42.71X-	T42.72X-	T42.73X-	T42.74X-	T42.75X-	T42.76X-
combination	T42.5X1-	T42.5X2-	T42.5X3-	T42.5X4-	T42.5X5-	T42.5X6-
mixed	T42.5X1-	T42.5X2-	T42.5X3-	T42.5X4-	T42.5X5-	T42.5X6-
specified, NEC	T42.6X1-	T42.6X2-	T42.6X3-	T42.6X4-	T42.6X5-	T42.6X6-
Antiestrogen NEC	T38.6X1-	T38.6X2-	T38.6X3-	T38.6X4-	T38.6X5-	T38.6X6-
Antifertility pill	T38.4X1-	T38.4X2-	T38.4X3-	T38.4X4-	T38.4X5-	T38.4X6-
Antifibrinolytic drug	T45.621-	T45.622-	T45.623-	T45.624-	T45.625-	T45.626-
Antifilarial drug	T37.4X1-	T37.4X2-	T37.4X3-	T37.4X4-	T37.4X5-	T37.4X6-
Antiflatulent	T47.5X1-	T47.5X2-	T47.5X3-	T47.5X4-	T47.5X5-	T47.5X6-
Antifreeze	T65.91X-	T65.92X-	T65.93X-	T65.94X-	-	-
alcohol	T51.1X1-	T51.1X2-	T51.1X3-	T51.1X4-	-	-

Substance	Poisoning, Accidental (unintentional)	Poisoning, Intentional self-harm	Poisoning, Assault	Poisoning, Undetermined	Adverse effect	Underdosing
Antifreeze - *continued*						
ethylene glycol	T51.8X1-	T51.8X2-	T51.8X3-	T51.8X4-	-	-
Antifungal						
antibiotic (systemic)	T36.7X1-	T36.7X2-	T36.7X3-	T36.7X4-	T36.7X5-	T36.7X6-
anti-infective NEC	T37.91X-	T37.92X-	T37.93X-	T37.94X-	T37.95X-	T37.96X-
disinfectant, local	T49.0X1-	T49.0X2-	T49.0X3-	T49.0X4-	T49.0X5-	T49.0X6-
nonmedicinal (spray)	T60.3X1-	T60.3X2-	T60.3X3-	T60.3X4-	-	-
topical	T49.0X1-	T49.0X2-	T49.0X3-	T49.0X4-	T49.0X5-	T49.0X6-
Anti-gastric-secretion drug NEC	T47.1X1-	T47.1X2-	T47.1X3-	T47.1X4-	T47.1X5-	T47.1X6-
Antigonadotrophin NEC	T38.6X1-	T38.6X2-	T38.6X3-	T38.6X4-	T38.6X5-	T38.6X6-
Antihallucinogen	T43.501-	T43.502-	T43.503-	T43.504-	T43.505-	T43.506-
Antihelmintics	T37.4X1-	T37.4X2-	T37.4X3-	T37.4X4-	T37.4X5-	T37.4X6-
Antihemophilic						
factor	T45.8X1-	T45.8X2-	T45.8X3-	T45.8X4-	T45.8X5-	T45.8X6-
fraction	T45.8X1-	T45.8X2-	T45.8X3-	T45.8X4-	T45.8X5-	T45.8X6-
globulin concentrate	T45.7X1-	T45.7X2-	T45.7X3-	T45.7X4-	T45.7X5-	T45.7X6-
human plasma	T45.8X1-	T45.8X2-	T45.8X3-	T45.8X4-	T45.8X5-	T45.8X6-
plasma, dried	T45.7X1-	T45.7X2-	T45.7X3-	T45.7X4-	T45.7X5-	T45.7X6-
Antihemorrhoidal preparation	T49.2X1-	T49.2X2-	T49.2X3-	T49.2X4-	T49.2X5-	T49.2X6-
Antiheparin drug	T45.7X1-	T45.7X2-	T45.7X3-	T45.7X4-	T45.7X5-	T45.7X6-
Antihistamine	T45.0X1-	T45.0X2-	T45.0X3-	T45.0X4-	T45.0X5-	T45.0X6-
Antihookworm drug	T37.4X1-	T37.4X2-	T37.4X3-	T37.4X4-	T37.4X5-	T37.4X6-
Anti-human lymphocytic globulin	T50.Z11-	T50.Z12-	T50.Z13-	T50.Z14-	T50.Z15-	T50.Z16-
Antihyperlipidemic drug	T46.6X1-	T46.6X2-	T46.6X3-	T46.6X4-	T46.6X5-	T46.6X6-
Antihypertensive drug NEC	T46.5X1-	T46.5X2-	T46.5X3-	T46.5X4-	T46.5X5-	T46.5X6-
Anti-infective NEC	T37.91X-	T37.92X-	T37.93X-	T37.94X-	T37.95X-	T37.96X-
anthelmintic	T37.4X1-	T37.4X2-	T37.4X3-	T37.4X4-	T37.4X5-	T37.4X6-
antibiotics	T36.91X-	T36.92X-	T36.93X-	T36.94X-	T36.95X-	T36.96X-
specified NEC	T36.8X1-	T36.8X2-	T36.8X3-	T36.8X4-	T36.8X5-	T36.8X6-
antimalarial	T37.2X1-	T37.2X2-	T37.2X3-	T37.2X4-	T37.2X5-	T37.2X6-
antimycobacterial NEC	T37.1X1-	T37.1X2-	T37.1X3-	T37.1X4-	T37.1X5-	T37.1X6-
antibiotics	T36.5X1-	T36.5X2-	T36.5X3-	T36.5X4-	T36.5X5-	T36.5X6-
antiprotozoal NEC	T37.3X1-	T37.3X2-	T37.3X3-	T37.3X4-	T37.3X5-	T37.3X6-
blood	T37.2X1-	T37.2X2-	T37.2X3-	T37.2X4-	T37.2X5-	T37.2X6-
antiviral	T37.5X1-	T37.5X2-	T37.5X3-	T37.5X4-	T37.5X5-	T37.5X6-
arsenical	T37.8X1-	T37.8X2-	T37.8X3-	T37.8X4-	T37.8X5-	T37.8X6-
bismuth, local	T49.0X1-	T49.0X2-	T49.0X3-	T49.0X4-	T49.0X5-	T49.0X6-
ENT	T49.6X1-	T49.6X2-	T49.6X3-	T49.6X4-	T49.6X5-	T49.6X6-
eye NEC	T49.5X1-	T49.5X2-	T49.5X3-	T49.5X4-	T49.5X5-	T49.5X6-
heavy metals NEC	T37.8X1-	T37.8X2-	T37.8X3-	T37.8X4-	T37.8X5-	T37.8X6-
local NEC	T49.0X1-	T49.0X2-	T49.0X3-	T49.0X4-	T49.0X5-	T49.0X6-
specified NEC	T49.0X1-	T49.0X2-	T49.0X3-	T49.0X4-	T49.0X5-	T49.0X6-
mixed	T37.91X-	T37.92X-	T37.93X-	T37.94X-	T37.95X-	T37.96X-
ophthalmic preparation	T49.5X1-	T49.5X2-	T49.5X3-	T49.5X4-	T49.5X5-	T49.5X6-
topical NEC	T49.0X1-	T49.0X2-	T49.0X3-	T49.0X4-	T49.0X5-	T49.0X6-
Anti-inflammatory drug NEC	T39.391-	T39.392-	T39.393-	T39.394-	T39.395-	T39.396-
local	T49.0X1-	T49.0X2-	T49.0X3-	T49.0X4-	T49.0X5-	T49.0X6-
nonsteroidal NEC	T39.391-	T39.392-	T39.393-	T39.394-	T39.395-	T39.396-
propionic acid derivative	T39.311-	T39.312-	T39.313-	T39.314-	T39.315-	T39.316-
specified NEC	T39.391-	T39.392-	T39.393-	T39.394-	T39.395-	T39.396-
Antikaluretic	T50.3X1-	T50.3X2-	T50.3X3-	T50.3X4-	T50.3X5-	T50.3X6-
Antiknock (tetraethyl lead)	T56.0X1-	T56.0X2-	T56.0X3-	T56.0X4-	-	-
Antilipemic drug NEC	T46.6X1-	T46.6X2-	T46.6X3-	T46.6X4-	T46.6X5-	T46.6X6-
Antimalarial	T37.2X1-	T37.2X2-	T37.2X3-	T37.2X4-	T37.2X5-	T37.2X6-
prophylactic NEC	T37.2X1-	T37.2X2-	T37.2X3-	T37.2X4-	T37.2X5-	T37.2X6-
pyrimidine derivative	T37.2X1-	T37.2X2-	T37.2X3-	T37.2X4-	T37.2X5-	T37.2X6-
Antimetabolite	T45.1X1-	T45.1X2-	T45.1X3-	T45.1X4-	T45.1X5-	T45.1X6-
Antimitotic agent	T45.1X1-	T45.1X2-	T45.1X3-	T45.1X4-	T45.1X5-	T45.1X6-
Antimony (compounds) (vapor) **NEC**	T56.891-	T56.892-	T56.893-	T56.894-	-	-
anti-infectives	T37.8X1-	T37.8X2-	T37.8X3-	T37.8X4-	T37.8X5-	T37.8X6-
dimercaptosuccinate	T37.3X1-	T37.3X2-	T37.3X3-	T37.3X4-	T37.3X5-	T37.3X6-
hydride	T56.891-	T56.892-	T56.893-	T56.894-	-	-
pesticide (vapor)	T60.8X1-	T60.8X2-	T60.8X3-	T60.8X4-	-	-
potassium (sodium) tartrate	T37.8X1-	T37.8X2-	T37.8X3-	T37.8X4-	T37.8X5-	T37.8X6-
sodium dimercaptosuccinate	T37.3X1-	T37.3X2-	T37.3X3-	T37.3X4-	T37.3X5-	T37.3X6-
tartrated	T37.8X1-	T37.8X2-	T37.8X3-	T37.8X4-	T37.8X5-	T37.8X6-
Antimuscarinic NEC	T44.3X1-	T44.3X2-	T44.3X3-	T44.3X4-	T44.3X5-	T44.3X6-
Antimycobacterial drug NEC	T37.1X1-	T37.1X2-	T37.1X3-	T37.1X4-	T37.1X5-	T37.1X6-
antibiotics	T36.5X1-	T36.5X2-	T36.5X3-	T36.5X4-	T36.5X5-	T36.5X6-
combination	T37.1X1-	T37.1X2-	T37.1X3-	T37.1X4-	T37.1X5-	T37.1X6-
Antinausea drug	T45.0X1-	T45.0X2-	T45.0X3-	T45.0X4-	T45.0X5-	T45.0X6-
Antinematode drug	T37.4X1-	T37.4X2-	T37.4X3-	T37.4X4-	T37.4X5-	T37.4X6-
Antineoplastic NEC	T45.1X1-	T45.1X2-	T45.1X3-	T45.1X4-	T45.1X5-	T45.1X6-
alkaloidal	T45.1X1-	T45.1X2-	T45.1X3-	T45.1X4-	T45.1X5-	T45.1X6-
antibiotics	T45.1X1-	T45.1X2-	T45.1X3-	T45.1X4-	T45.1X5-	T45.1X6-

Substance	Poisoning, Accidental (unintentional)	Poisoning, Intentional self-harm	Poisoning, Assault	Poisoning, Undetermined	Adverse effect	Underdosing
Antineoplastic NEC - *continued*						
combination	T45.1X1-	T45.1X2-	T45.1X3-	T45.1X4-	T45.1X5-	T45.1X6-
estrogen	T38.5X1-	T38.5X2-	T38.5X3-	T38.5X4-	T38.5X5-	T38.5X6-
steroid	T38.7X1-	T38.7X2-	T38.7X3-	T38.7X4-	T38.7X5-	T38.7X6-
Antiparasitic drug (systemic)	T37.91X-	T37.92X-	T37.93X-	T37.94X-	T37.95X-	T37.96X-
local	T49.0X1-	T49.0X2-	T49.0X3-	T49.0X4-	T49.0X5-	T49.0X6-
specified NEC	T37.8X1-	T37.8X2-	T37.8X3-	T37.8X4-	T37.8X5-	T37.8X6-
Antiparkinsonism drug NEC	T42.8X1-	T42.8X2-	T42.8X3-	T42.8X4-	T42.8X5-	T42.8X6-
Antiperspirant NEC	T49.2X1-	T49.2X2-	T49.2X3-	T49.2X4-	T49.2X5-	T49.2X6-
Antiphlogistic NEC	T39.4X1-	T39.4X2-	T39.4X3-	T39.4X4-	T39.4X5-	T39.4X6-
Antiplatyhelmintic drug	T37.4X1-	T37.4X2-	T37.4X3-	T37.4X4-	T37.4X5-	T37.4X6-
Antiprotozoal drug NEC	T37.3X1-	T37.3X2-	T37.3X3-	T37.3X4-	T37.3X5-	T37.3X6-
blood	T37.2X1-	T37.2X2-	T37.2X3-	T37.2X4-	T37.2X5-	T37.2X6-
local	T49.0X1-	T49.0X2-	T49.0X3-	T49.0X4-	T49.0X5-	T49.0X6-
Antipruritic drug NEC	T49.1X1-	T49.1X2-	T49.1X3-	T49.1X4-	T49.1X5-	T49.1X6-
Antipsychotic drug	T43.501-	T43.502-	T43.503-	T43.504-	T43.505-	T43.506-
specified NEC	T43.591-	T43.592-	T43.593-	T43.594-	T43.595-	T43.596-
Antipyretic	T39.91X-	T39.92X-	T39.93X-	T39.94X-	T39.95X-	T39.96X-
specified NEC	T39.8X1-	T39.8X2-	T39.8X3-	T39.8X4-	T39.8X5-	T39.8X6-
Antipyrine	T39.2X1-	T39.2X2-	T39.2X3-	T39.2X4-	T39.2X5-	T39.2X6-
Antirabies hyperimmune serum	T50.Z11-	T50.Z12-	T50.Z13-	T50.Z14-	T50.Z15-	T50.Z16-
Antirheumatic NEC	T39.4X1-	T39.4X2-	T39.4X3-	T39.4X4-	T39.4X5-	T39.4X6-
Antirigidity drug NEC	T42.8X1-	T42.8X2-	T42.8X3-	T42.8X4-	T42.8X5-	T42.8X6-
Antischistosomal drug	T37.4X1-	T37.4X2-	T37.4X3-	T37.4X4-	T37.4X5-	T37.4X6-
Antiscorpion sera	T50.Z11-	T50.Z12-	T50.Z13-	T50.Z14-	T50.Z15-	T50.Z16-
Antiseborrheics	T49.4X1-	T49.4X2-	T49.4X3-	T49.4X4-	T49.4X5-	T49.4X6-
Antiseptics (external) (medicinal)	T49.0X1-	T49.0X2-	T49.0X3-	T49.0X4-	T49.0X5-	T49.0X6-
Antistine	T45.0X1-	T45.0X2-	T45.0X3-	T45.0X4-	T45.0X5-	T45.0X6-
Antitapeworm drug	T37.4X1-	T37.4X2-	T37.4X3-	T37.4X4-	T37.4X5-	T37.4X6-
Antitetanus immunoglobulin	T50.Z11-	T50.Z12-	T50.Z13-	T50.Z14-	T50.Z15-	T50.Z16-
Antithyroid drug NEC	T38.2X1-	T38.2X2-	T38.2X3-	T38.2X4-	T38.2X5-	T38.2X6-
Antitoxin	T50.Z11-	T50.Z12-	T50.Z13-	T50.Z14-	T50.Z15-	T50.Z16-
diphtheria	T50.Z11-	T50.Z12-	T50.Z13-	T50.Z14-	T50.Z15-	T50.Z16-
gas gangrene	T50.Z11-	T50.Z12-	T50.Z13-	T50.Z14-	T50.Z15-	T50.Z16-
tetanus	T50.Z11-	T50.Z12-	T50.Z13-	T50.Z14-	T50.Z15-	T50.Z16-
Antitrichomonal drug	T37.3X1-	T37.3X2-	T37.3X3-	T37.3X4-	T37.3X5-	T37.3X6-
Antituberculars	T37.1X1-	T37.1X2-	T37.1X3-	T37.1X4-	T37.1X5-	T37.1X6-
antibiotics	T36.5X1-	T36.5X2-	T36.5X3-	T36.5X4-	T36.5X5-	T36.5X6-
Antitussive NEC	T48.3X1-	T48.3X2-	T48.3X3-	T48.3X4-	T48.3X5-	T48.3X6-
codeine mixture	T40.2X1-	T40.2X2-	T40.2X3-	T40.2X4-	T40.2X5-	T40.2X6-
opiate	T40.2X1-	T40.2X2-	T40.2X3-	T40.2X4-	T40.2X5-	T40.2X6-
Antivaricose drug	T46.8X1-	T46.8X2-	T46.8X3-	T46.8X4-	T46.8X5-	T46.8X6-
Antivenin, antivenom (sera)	T50.Z11-	T50.Z12-	T50.Z13-	T50.Z14-	T50.Z15-	T50.Z16-
crotaline	T50.Z11-	T50.Z12-	T50.Z13-	T50.Z14-	T50.Z15-	T50.Z16-
spider bite	T50.Z11-	T50.Z12-	T50.Z13-	T50.Z14-	T50.Z15-	T50.Z16-
Antivertigo drug	T45.0X1-	T45.0X2-	T45.0X3-	T45.0X4-	T45.0X5-	T45.0X6-
Antiviral drug NEC	T37.5X1-	T37.5X2-	T37.5X3-	T37.5X4-	T37.5X5-	T37.5X6-
eye	T49.5X1-	T49.5X2-	T49.5X3-	T49.5X4-	T49.5X5-	T49.5X6-
Antiwhipworm drug	T37.4X1-	T37.4X2-	T37.4X3-	T37.4X4-	T37.4X5-	T37.4X6-
Antrol — *see also* by specific chemical substance	T60.91X-	T60.92X-	T60.93X-	T60.94X-	-	-
fungicide	T60.91X-	T60.92X-	T60.93X-	T60.94X-	-	-
ANTU (alpha naphthylthiourea)	T60.4X1-	T60.4X2-	T60.4X3-	T60.4X4-	-	-
Apalcillin	T36.0X1-	T36.0X2-	T36.0X3-	T36.0X4-	T36.0X5-	T36.0X6-
APC	T48.5X1-	T48.5X2-	T48.5X3-	T48.5X4-	T48.5X5-	T48.5X6-
Aplonidine	T44.4X1-	T44.4X2-	T44.4X3-	T44.4X4-	T44.4X5-	T44.4X6-
Apomorphine	T47.7X1-	T47.7X2-	T47.7X3-	T47.7X4-	T47.7X5-	T47.7X6-
Appetite depressants, central	T50.5X1-	T50.5X2-	T50.5X3-	T50.5X4-	T50.5X5-	T50.5X6-
Apraclonidine (hydrochloride)	T44.4X1-	T44.4X2-	T44.4X3-	T44.4X4-	T44.4X5-	T44.4X6-
Apresoline	T46.5X1-	T46.5X2-	T46.5X3-	T46.5X4-	T46.5X5-	T46.5X6-
Aprindine	T46.2X1-	T46.2X2-	T46.2X3-	T46.2X4-	T46.2X5-	T46.2X6-
Aprobarbital	T42.3X1-	T42.3X2-	T42.3X3-	T42.3X4-	T42.3X5-	T42.3X6-
Apronalide	T42.6X1-	T42.6X2-	T42.6X3-	T42.6X4-	T42.6X5-	T42.6X6-
Aprotinin	T45.621-	T45.622-	T45.623-	T45.624-	T45.625-	T45.626-
Aptocaine	T41.3X1-	T41.3X2-	T41.3X3-	T41.3X4-	T41.3X5-	T41.3X6-
Aqua fortis	T54.2X1-	T54.2X2-	T54.2X3-	T54.2X4-	-	-
Ara-A	T37.5X1-	T37.5X2-	T37.5X3-	T37.5X4-	T37.5X5-	T37.5X6-
Ara-C	T45.1X1-	T45.1X2-	T45.1X3-	T45.1X4-	T45.1X5-	T45.1X6-
Arachis oil	T49.3X1-	T49.3X2-	T49.3X3-	T49.3X4-	T49.3X5-	T49.3X6-
cathartic	T47.4X1-	T47.4X2-	T47.4X3-	T47.4X4-	T47.4X5-	T47.4X6-
Aralen	T37.2X1-	T37.2X2-	T37.2X3-	T37.2X4-	T37.2X5-	T37.2X6-
Arecoline	T44.1X1-	T44.1X2-	T44.1X3-	T44.1X4-	T44.1X5-	T44.1X6-
Arginine	T50.991-	T50.992-	T50.993-	T50.994-	T50.995-	T50.996-
glutamate	T50.991-	T50.992-	T50.993-	T50.994-	T50.995-	T50.996-
Argyrol	T49.0X1-	T49.0X2-	T49.0X3-	T49.0X4-	T49.0X5-	T49.0X6-
ENT agent	T49.6X1-	T49.6X2-	T49.6X3-	T49.6X4-	T49.6X5-	T49.6X6-

Substance	Poisoning, Accidental (unintentional)	Poisoning, Intentional self-harm	Poisoning, Assault	Poisoning, Undetermined	Adverse effect	Underdosing
Argyrol - *continued*						
ophthalmic preparation	T49.5X1-	T49.5X2-	T49.5X3-	T49.5X4-	T49.5X5-	T49.5X6-
Aristocort	T38.0X1-	T38.0X2-	T38.0X3-	T38.0X4-	T38.0X5-	T38.0X6-
ENT agent	T49.6X1-	T49.6X2-	T49.6X3-	T49.6X4-	T49.6X5-	T49.6X6-
ophthalmic preparation	T49.5X1-	T49.5X2-	T49.5X3-	T49.5X4-	T49.5X5-	T49.5X6-
topical NEC	T49.0X1-	T49.0X2-	T49.0X3-	T49.0X4-	T49.0X5-	T49.0X6-
Aromatics, corrosive	T54.1X1-	T54.1X2-	T54.1X3-	T54.1X4-	-	-
disinfectants	T54.1X1-	T54.1X2-	T54.1X3-	T54.1X4-	-	-
Arsenate of lead	T57.0X1-	T57.0X2-	T57.0X3-	T57.0X4-	-	-
herbicide	T57.0X1-	T57.0X2-	T57.0X3-	T57.0X4-	-	-
Arsenic, arsenicals (compounds) (dust) (vapor) NEC	T57.0X1-	T57.0X2-	T57.0X3-	T57.0X4-	-	-
anti-infectives	T37.8X1-	T37.8X2-	T37.8X3-	T37.8X4-	T37.8X5-	T37.8X6-
pesticide (dust) (fumes)	T57.0X1-	T57.0X2-	T57.0X3-	T57.0X4-	-	-
Arsine (gas)	T57.0X1-	T57.0X2-	T57.0X3-	T57.0X4-	-	-
Arsphenamine (silver)	T37.8X1-	T37.8X2-	T37.8X3-	T37.8X4-	T37.8X5-	T37.8X6-
Arsthinol	T37.3X1-	T37.3X2-	T37.3X3-	T37.3X4-	T37.3X5-	T37.3X6-
Artane	T44.3X1-	T44.3X2-	T44.3X3-	T44.3X4-	T44.3X5-	T44.3X6-
Arthropod (venomous) **NEC**	T63.481-	T63.482-	T63.483-	T63.484-	-	-
Articaine	T41.3X1-	T41.3X2-	T41.3X3-	T41.3X4-	T41.3X5-	T41.3X6-
Asbestos	T57.8X1-	T57.8X2-	T57.8X3-	T57.8X4-	-	-
Ascaridole	T37.4X1-	T37.4X2-	T37.4X3-	T37.4X4-	T37.4X5-	T37.4X6-
Ascorbic acid	T45.2X1-	T45.2X2-	T45.2X3-	T45.2X4-	T45.2X5-	T45.2X6-
Asiaticoside	T49.0X1-	T49.0X2-	T49.0X3-	T49.0X4-	T49.0X5-	T49.0X6-
Asparaginase	T45.1X1-	T45.1X2-	T45.1X3-	T45.1X4-	T45.1X5-	T45.1X6-
Aspidium (oleoresin)	T37.4X1-	T37.4X2-	T37.4X3-	T37.4X4-	T37.4X5-	T37.4X6-
Aspirin (aluminum) (soluble)	T39.011-	T39.012-	T39.013-	T39.014-	T39.015-	T39.016-
Aspoxicillin	T36.0X1-	T36.0X2-	T36.0X3-	T36.0X4-	T36.0X5-	T36.0X6-
Astemizole	T45.0X1-	T45.0X2-	T45.0X3-	T45.0X4-	T45.0X5-	T45.0X6-
Astringent (local)	T49.2X1-	T49.2X2-	T49.2X3-	T49.2X4-	T49.2X5-	T49.2X6-
specified NEC	T49.2X1-	T49.2X2-	T49.2X3-	T49.2X4-	T49.2X5-	T49.2X6-
Astromicin	T36.5X1-	T36.5X2-	T36.5X3-	T36.5X4-	T36.5X5-	T36.5X6-
Ataractic drug NEC	T43.501-	T43.502-	T43.503-	T43.504-	T43.505-	T43.506-
Atenolol	T44.7X1-	T44.7X2-	T44.7X3-	T44.7X4-	T44.7X5-	T44.7X6-
Atonia drug, intestinal	T47.4X1-	T47.4X2-	T47.4X3-	T47.4X4-	T47.4X5-	T47.4X6-
Atophan	T50.4X1-	T50.4X2-	T50.4X3-	T50.4X4-	T50.4X5-	T50.4X6-
Atracurium besilate	T48.1X1-	T48.1X2-	T48.1X3-	T48.1X4-	T48.1X5-	T48.1X6-
Atropine	T44.3X1-	T44.3X2-	T44.3X3-	T44.3X4-	T44.3X5-	T44.3X6-
derivative	T44.3X1-	T44.3X2-	T44.3X3-	T44.3X4-	T44.3X5-	T44.3X6-
methonitrate	T44.3X1-	T44.3X2-	T44.3X3-	T44.3X4-	T44.3X5-	T44.3X6-
Attapulgite	T47.6X1-	T47.6X2-	T47.6X3-	T47.6X4-	T47.6X5-	T47.6X6-
Auramine	T65.891-	T65.892-	T65.893-	T65.894-	-	-
dye	T65.6X1-	T65.6X2-	T65.6X3-	T65.6X4-	-	-
fungicide	T60.3X1-	T60.3X2-	T60.3X3-	T60.3X4-	-	-
Auranofin	T39.4X1-	T39.4X2-	T39.4X3-	T39.4X4-	T39.4X5-	T39.4X6-
Aurantiin	T46.991-	T46.992-	T46.993-	T46.994-	T46.995-	T46.996-
Aureomycin	T36.4X1-	T36.4X2-	T36.4X3-	T36.4X4-	T36.4X5-	T36.4X6-
ophthalmic preparation	T49.5X1-	T49.5X2-	T49.5X3-	T49.5X4-	T49.5X5-	T49.5X6-
topical NEC	T49.0X1-	T49.0X2-	T49.0X3-	T49.0X4-	T49.0X5-	T49.0X6-
Aurothioglucose	T39.4X1-	T39.4X2-	T39.4X3-	T39.4X4-	T39.4X5-	T39.4X6-
Aurothioglycanide	T39.4X1-	T39.4X2-	T39.4X3-	T39.4X4-	T39.4X5-	T39.4X6-
Aurothiomalate sodium	T39.4X1-	T39.4X2-	T39.4X3-	T39.4X4-	T39.4X5-	T39.4X6-
Aurotioprol	T39.4X1-	T39.4X2-	T39.4X3-	T39.4X4-	T39.4X5-	T39.4X6-
Automobile fuel	T52.0X1-	T52.0X2-	T52.0X3-	T52.0X4-	-	-
Autonomic nervous system agent NEC	T44.901-	T44.902-	T44.903-	T44.904-	T44.905-	T44.906-
Avlosulfon	T37.1X1-	T37.1X2-	T37.1X3-	T37.1X4-	T37.1X5-	T37.1X6-
Avomine	T42.6X1-	T42.6X2-	T42.6X3-	T42.6X4-	T42.6X5-	T42.6X6-
Axerophthol	T45.2X1-	T45.2X2-	T45.2X3-	T45.2X4-	T45.2X5-	T45.2X6-
Azacitidine	T45.1X1-	T45.1X2-	T45.1X3-	T45.1X4-	T45.1X5-	T45.1X6-
Azacyclonol	T43.591-	T43.592-	T43.593-	T43.594-	T43.595-	T43.596-
Azadirachta	T60.2X1-	T60.2X2-	T60.2X3-	T60.2X4-	-	-
Azanidazole	T37.3X1-	T37.3X2-	T37.3X3-	T37.3X4-	T37.3X5-	T37.3X6-
Azapetine	T46.7X1-	T46.7X2-	T46.7X3-	T46.7X4-	T46.7X5-	T46.7X6-
Azapropazone	T39.2X1-	T39.2X2-	T39.2X3-	T39.2X4-	T39.2X5-	T39.2X6-
Azaribine	T45.1X1-	T45.1X2-	T45.1X3-	T45.1X4-	T45.1X5-	T45.1X6-
Azaserine	T45.1X1-	T45.1X2-	T45.1X3-	T45.1X4-	T45.1X5-	T45.1X6-
Azatadine	T45.0X1-	T45.0X2-	T45.0X3-	T45.0X4-	T45.0X5-	T45.0X6-
Azatepa	T45.1X1-	T45.1X2-	T45.1X3-	T45.1X4-	T45.1X5-	T45.1X6-
Azathioprine	T45.1X1-	T45.1X2-	T45.1X3-	T45.1X4-	T45.1X5-	T45.1X6-
Azelaic acid	T49.0X1-	T49.0X2-	T49.0X3-	T49.0X4-	T49.0X5-	T49.0X6-
Azelastine	T45.0X1-	T45.0X2-	T45.0X3-	T45.0X4-	T45.0X5-	T45.0X6-
Azidocillin	T36.0X1-	T36.0X2-	T36.0X3-	T36.0X4-	T36.0X5-	T36.0X6-
Azidothymidine	T37.5X1-	T37.5X2-	T37.5X3-	T37.5X4-	T37.5X5-	T37.5X6-
Azinphos (ethyl) (methyl)	T60.0X1-	T60.0X2-	T60.0X3-	T60.0X4-	-	-
Aziridine (chelating)	T54.1X1-	T54.1X2-	T54.1X3-	T54.1X4-	-	-
Azithromycin	T36.3X1-	T36.3X2-	T36.3X3-	T36.3X4-	T36.3X5-	T36.3X6-

Substance	Poisoning, Accidental (unintentional)	Poisoning, Intentional self-harm	Poisoning, Assault	Poisoning, Undetermined	Adverse effect	Underdosing
Azlocillin	T36.0X1-	T36.0X2-	T36.0X3-	T36.0X4-	T36.0X5-	T36.0X6-
Azobenzene smoke	T65.3X1-	T65.3X2-	T65.3X3-	T65.3X4-	-	-
acaricide	T60.8X1-	T60.8X2-	T60.8X3-	T60.8X4-	-	-
Azosulfamide	T37.0X1-	T37.0X2-	T37.0X3-	T37.0X4-	T37.0X5-	T37.0X6-
AZT	T37.5X1-	T37.5X2-	T37.5X3-	T37.5X4-	T37.5X5-	T37.5X6-
Aztreonam	T36.1X1-	T36.1X2-	T36.1X3-	T36.1X4-	T36.1X5-	T36.1X6-
Azulfidine	T37.0X1-	T37.0X2-	T37.0X3-	T37.0X4-	T37.0X5-	T37.0X6-
Azuresin	T50.8X1-	T50.8X2-	T50.8X3-	T50.8X4-	T50.8X5-	T50.8X6-
Bacampicillin	T36.0X1-	T36.0X2-	T36.0X3-	T36.0X4-	T36.0X5-	T36.0X6-
Bacillus						
lactobacillus	T47.8X1-	T47.8X2-	T47.8X3-	T47.8X4-	T47.8X5-	T47.8X6-
subtilis	T47.6X1-	T47.6X2-	T47.6X3-	T47.6X4-	T47.6X5-	T47.6X6-
Bacimycin	T49.0X1-	T49.0X2-	T49.0X3-	T49.0X4-	T49.0X5-	T49.0X6-
ophthalmic preparation	T49.5X1-	T49.5X2-	T49.5X3-	T49.5X4-	T49.5X5-	T49.5X6-
Bacitracin zinc	T49.0X1-	T49.0X2-	T49.0X3-	T49.0X4-	T49.0X5-	T49.0X6-
with neomycin	T49.0X1-	T49.0X2-	T49.0X3-	T49.0X4-	T49.0X5-	T49.0X6-
ENT agent	T49.6X1-	T49.6X2-	T49.6X3-	T49.6X4-	T49.6X5-	T49.6X6-
ophthalmic preparation	T49.5X1-	T49.5X2-	T49.5X3-	T49.5X4-	T49.5X5-	T49.5X6-
topical NEC	T49.0X1-	T49.0X2-	T49.0X3-	T49.0X4-	T49.0X5-	T49.0X6-
Baclofen	T42.8X1-	T42.8X2-	T42.8X3-	T42.8X4-	T42.8X5-	T42.8X6-
Baking soda	T50.991-	T50.992-	T50.993-	T50.994-	T50.995-	T50.996-
BAL	T45.8X1-	T45.8X2-	T45.8X3-	T45.8X4-	T45.8X5-	T45.8X6-
Bambuterol	T48.6X1-	T48.6X2-	T48.6X3-	T48.6X4-	T48.6X5-	T48.6X6-
Bamethan (sulfate)	T46.7X1-	T46.7X2-	T46.7X3-	T46.7X4-	T46.7X5-	T46.7X6-
Bamifylline	T48.6X1-	T48.6X2-	T48.6X3-	T48.6X4-	T48.6X5-	T48.6X6-
Bamipine	T45.0X1-	T45.0X2-	T45.0X3-	T45.0X4-	T45.0X5-	T45.0X6-
Baneberry — *see* Actaea spicata						
Banewort — *see* Belladonna						
Barbenyl	T42.3X1-	T42.3X2-	T42.3X3-	T42.3X4-	T42.3X5-	T42.3X6-
Barbexaclone	T42.6X1-	T42.6X2-	T42.6X3-	T42.6X4-	T42.6X5-	T42.6X6-
Barbital	T42.3X1-	T42.3X2-	T42.3X3-	T42.3X4-	T42.3X5-	T42.3X6-
sodium	T42.3X1-	T42.3X2-	T42.3X3-	T42.3X4-	T42.3X5-	T42.3X6-
Barbitone	T42.3X1-	T42.3X2-	T42.3X3-	T42.3X4-	T42.3X5-	T42.3X6-
Barbiturate NEC	T42.3X1-	T42.3X2-	T42.3X3-	T42.3X4-	T42.3X5-	T42.3X6-
with tranquilizer	T42.3X1-	T42.3X2-	T42.3X3-	T42.3X4-	T42.3X5-	T42.3X6-
anesthetic (intravenous)	T41.1X1-	T41.1X2-	T41.1X3-	T41.1X4-	T41.1X5-	T41.1X6-
Barium (carbonate) (chloride) (sulfite)	T57.8X1-	T57.8X2-	T57.8X3-	T57.8X4-	-	-
diagnostic agent	T50.8X1-	T50.8X2-	T50.8X3-	T50.8X4-	T50.8X5-	T50.8X6-
pesticide	T60.4X1-	T60.4X2-	T60.4X3-	T60.4X4-	-	-
rodenticide	T60.4X1-	T60.4X2-	T60.4X3-	T60.4X4-	-	-
sulfate (medicinal)	T50.8X1-	T50.8X2-	T50.8X3-	T50.8X4-	T50.8X5-	T50.8X6-
Barrier cream	T49.3X1-	T49.3X2-	T49.3X3-	T49.3X4-	T49.3X5-	T49.3X6-
Basic fuchsin	T49.0X1-	T49.0X2-	T49.0X3-	T49.0X4-	T49.0X5-	T49.0X6-
Battery acid or fluid	T54.2X1-	T54.2X2-	T54.2X3-	T54.2X4-	-	-
Bay rum	T51.8X1-	T51.8X2-	T51.8X3-	T51.8X4-	-	-
BCG (vaccine)	T50.A91-	T50.A92-	T50.A93-	T50.A94-	T50.A95-	T50.A96-
BCNU	T45.1X1-	T45.1X2-	T45.1X3-	T45.1X4-	T45.1X5-	T45.1X6-
Bearsfoot	T62.2X1-	T62.2X2-	T62.2X3-	T62.2X4-	-	-
Beclamide	T42.6X1-	T42.6X2-	T42.6X3-	T42.6X4-	T42.6X5-	T42.6X6-
Beclomethasone	T44.5X1-	T44.5X2-	T44.5X3-	T44.5X4-	T44.5X5-	T44.5X6-
Bee (sting) (venom)	T63.441-	T63.442-	T63.443-	T63.444-	-	-
Befunolol	T49.5X1-	T49.5X2-	T49.5X3-	T49.5X4-	T49.5X5-	T49.5X6-
Bekanamycin	T36.5X1-	T36.5X2-	T36.5X3-	T36.5X4-	T36.5X5-	T36.5X6-
Belladonna — *see also* Nightshade						
alkaloids	T44.3X1-	T44.3X2-	T44.3X3-	T44.3X4-	T44.3X5-	T44.3X6-
extract	T44.3X1-	T44.3X2-	T44.3X3-	T44.3X4-	T44.3X5-	T44.3X6-
herb	T44.3X1-	T44.3X2-	T44.3X3-	T44.3X4-	T44.3X5-	T44.3X6-
Bemegride	T50.7X1-	T50.7X2-	T50.7X3-	T50.7X4-	T50.7X5-	T50.7X6-
Benactyzine	T44.3X1-	T44.3X2-	T44.3X3-	T44.3X4-	T44.3X5-	T44.3X6-
Benadryl	T45.0X1-	T45.0X2-	T45.0X3-	T45.0X4-	T45.0X5-	T45.0X6-
Benaprizine	T44.3X1-	T44.3X2-	T44.3X3-	T44.3X4-	T44.3X5-	T44.3X6-
Benazepril	T46.4X1-	T46.4X2-	T46.4X3-	T46.4X4-	T46.4X5-	T46.4X6-
Bencyclane	T46.7X1-	T46.7X2-	T46.7X3-	T46.7X4-	T46.7X5-	T46.7X6-
Bendazol	T46.3X1-	T46.3X2-	T46.3X3-	T46.3X4-	T46.3X5-	T46.3X6-
Bendrofluazide	T50.2X1-	T50.2X2-	T50.2X3-	T50.2X4-	T50.2X5-	T50.2X6-
Bendroflumethiazide	T50.2X1-	T50.2X2-	T50.2X3-	T50.2X4-	T50.2X5-	T50.2X6-
Benemid	T50.4X1-	T50.4X2-	T50.4X3-	T50.4X4-	T50.4X5-	T50.4X6-
Benethamine penicillin	T36.0X1-	T36.0X2-	T36.0X3-	T36.0X4-	T36.0X5-	T36.0X6-
Benexate	T47.1X1-	T47.1X2-	T47.1X3-	T47.1X4-	T47.1X5-	T47.1X6-
Benfluorex	T46.6X1-	T46.6X2-	T46.6X3-	T46.6X4-	T46.6X5-	T46.6X6-
Benfotiamine	T45.2X1-	T45.2X2-	T45.2X3-	T45.2X4-	T45.2X5-	T45.2X6-
Benisone	T49.0X1-	T49.0X2-	T49.0X3-	T49.0X4-	T49.0X5-	T49.0X6-
Benomyl	T60.0X1-	T60.0X2-	T60.0X3-	T60.0X4-	-	-
Benoquin	T49.8X1-	T49.8X2-	T49.8X3-	T49.8X4-	T49.8X5-	T49.8X6-
Benoxinate	T41.3X1-	T41.3X2-	T41.3X3-	T41.3X4-	T41.3X5-	T41.3X6-

Substance	Poisoning, Accidental (unintentional)	Poisoning, Intentional self-harm	Poisoning, Assault	Poisoning, Undetermined	Adverse effect	Underdosing
Benperidol	T43.4X1-	T43.4X2-	T43.4X3-	T43.4X4-	T43.4X5-	T43.4X6-
Benproperine	T48.3X1-	T48.3X2-	T48.3X3-	T48.3X4-	T48.3X5-	T48.3X6-
Benserazide	T42.8X1-	T42.8X2-	T42.8X3-	T42.8X4-	T42.8X5-	T42.8X6-
Bentazepam	T42.4X1-	T42.4X2-	T42.4X3-	T42.4X4-	T42.4X5-	T42.4X6-
Bentiromide	T50.8X1-	T50.8X2-	T50.8X3-	T50.8X4-	T50.8X5-	T50.8X6-
Bentonite	T49.3X1-	T49.3X2-	T49.3X3-	T49.3X4-	T49.3X5-	T49.3X6-
Benzalbutyramide	T46.6X1-	T46.6X2-	T46.6X3-	T46.6X4-	T46.6X5-	T46.6X6-
Benzalkonium (chloride)	T49.0X1-	T49.0X2-	T49.0X3-	T49.0X4-	T49.0X5-	T49.0X6-
ophthalmic preparation	T49.5X1-	T49.5X2-	T49.5X3-	T49.5X4-	T49.5X5-	T49.5X6-
Benzamidosalicylate (calcium)	T37.1X1-	T37.1X2-	T37.1X3-	T37.1X4-	T37.1X5-	T37.1X6-
Benzamine	T41.3X1-	T41.3X2-	T41.3X3-	T41.3X4-	T41.3X5-	T41.3X6-
lactate	T49.1X1-	T49.1X2-	T49.1X3-	T49.1X4-	T49.1X5-	T49.1X6-
Benzamphetamine	T50.5X1-	T50.5X2-	T50.5X3-	T50.5X4-	T50.5X5-	T50.5X6-
Benzapril hydrochloride	T46.5X1-	T46.5X2-	T46.5X3-	T46.5X4-	T46.5X5-	T46.5X6-
Benzathine benzylpenicillin	T36.8X1-	T36.8X2-	T36.8X3-	T36.8X4-	T36.8X5-	T36.8X6-
Benzathine penicillin	T36.0X1-	T36.0X2-	T36.0X3-	T36.0X4-	T36.0X5-	T36.0X6-
Benzatropine	T42.8X1-	T42.8X2-	T42.8X3-	T42.8X4-	T42.8X5-	T42.8X6-
Benzbromarone	T50.4X1-	T50.4X2-	T50.4X3-	T50.4X4-	T50.4X5-	T50.4X6-
Benzcarbimine	T45.1X1-	T45.1X2-	T45.1X3-	T45.1X4-	T45.1X5-	T45.1X6-
Benzedrex	T44.991-	T44.992-	T44.993-	T44.994-	T44.995-	T44.996-
Benzedrine (amphetamine)	T43.621-	T43.622-	T43.623-	T43.624-	T43.625-	T43.626-
Benzenamine	T65.3X1-	T65.3X2-	T65.3X3-	T65.3X4-	-	-
Benzene	T52.1X1-	T52.1X2-	T52.1X3-	T52.1X4-	-	-
homologues (acetyl) (dimethyl) (methyl) (solvent)	T52.2X1-	T52.2X2-	T52.2X3-	T52.2X4-	-	-
Benzethonium (chloride)	T49.0X1-	T49.0X2-	T49.0X3-	T49.0X4-	T49.0X5-	T49.0X6-
Benzfetamine	T50.5X1-	T50.5X2-	T50.5X3-	T50.5X4-	T50.5X5-	T50.5X6-
Benzhexol	T44.3X1-	T44.3X2-	T44.3X3-	T44.3X4-	T44.3X5-	T44.3X6-
Benzhydramine (chloride)	T45.0X1-	T45.0X2-	T45.0X3-	T45.0X4-	T45.0X5-	T45.0X6-
Benzidine	T65.891-	T65.892-	T65.893-	T65.894-	-	-
Benzilonium bromide	T44.3X1-	T44.3X2-	T44.3X3-	T44.3X4-	T44.3X5-	T44.3X6-
Benzimidazole	T60.3X1-	T60.3X2-	T60.3X3-	T60.3X4-	-	-
Benzin (e) — see Ligroin						
Benziodarone	T46.3X1-	T46.3X2-	T46.3X3-	T46.3X4-	T46.3X5-	T46.3X6-
Benznidazole	T37.3X1-	T37.3X2-	T37.3X3-	T37.3X4-	T37.3X5-	T37.3X6-
Benzocaine	T41.3X1-	T41.3X2-	T41.3X3-	T41.3X4-	T41.3X5-	T41.3X6-
Benzodiapin	T42.4X1-	T42.4X2-	T42.4X3-	T42.4X4-	T42.4X5-	T42.4X6-
Benzodiazepine NEC	T42.4X1-	T42.4X2-	T42.4X3-	T42.4X4-	T42.4X5-	T42.4X6-
Benzoic acid	T49.0X1-	T49.0X2-	T49.0X3-	T49.0X4-	T49.0X5-	T49.0X6-
with salicylic acid	T49.0X1-	T49.0X2-	T49.0X3-	T49.0X4-	T49.0X5-	T49.0X6-
Benzoin (tincture)	T48.5X1-	T48.5X2-	T48.5X3-	T48.5X4-	T48.5X5-	T48.5X6-
Benzol (benzene)	T52.1X1-	T52.1X2-	T52.1X3-	T52.1X4-	-	-
vapor	T52.0X1-	T52.0X2-	T52.0X3-	T52.0X4-	-	-
Benzomorphan	T40.2X1-	T40.2X2-	T40.2X3-	T40.2X4-	T40.2X5-	T40.2X6-
Benzonatate	T48.3X1-	T48.3X2-	T48.3X3-	T48.3X4-	T48.3X5-	T48.3X6-
Benzophenones	T49.3X1-	T49.3X2-	T49.3X3-	T49.3X4-	T49.3X5-	T49.3X6-
Benzopyrone	T46.991-	T46.992-	T46.993-	T46.994-	T46.995-	T46.996-
Benzothiadiazides	T50.2X1-	T50.2X2-	T50.2X3-	T50.2X4-	T50.2X5-	T50.2X6-
Benzoxonium chloride	T49.0X1-	T49.0X2-	T49.0X3-	T49.0X4-	T49.0X5-	T49.0X6-
Benzoyl peroxide	T49.0X1-	T49.0X2-	T49.0X3-	T49.0X4-	T49.0X5-	T49.0X6-
Benzoylpas calcium	T37.1X1-	T37.1X2-	T37.1X3-	T37.1X4-	T37.1X5-	T37.1X6-
Benzperidin	T43.591-	T43.592-	T43.593-	T43.594-	T43.595-	T43.596-
Benzperidol	T43.591-	T43.592-	T43.593-	T43.594-	T43.595-	T43.596-
Benzphetamine	T50.5X1-	T50.5X2-	T50.5X3-	T50.5X4-	T50.5X5-	T50.5X6-
Benzpyrinium bromide	T44.1X1-	T44.1X2-	T44.1X3-	T44.1X4-	T44.1X5-	T44.1X6-
Benzquinamide	T45.0X1-	T45.0X2-	T45.0X3-	T45.0X4-	T45.0X5-	T45.0X6-
Benzthiazide	T50.2X1-	T50.2X2-	T50.2X3-	T50.2X4-	T50.2X5-	T50.2X6-
Benztropine						
anticholinergic	T44.3X1-	T44.3X2-	T44.3X3-	T44.3X4-	T44.3X5-	T44.3X6-
antiparkinson	T42.8X1-	T42.8X2-	T42.8X3-	T42.8X4-	T42.8X5-	T42.8X6-
Benzydamine	T49.0X1-	T49.0X2-	T49.0X3-	T49.0X4-	T49.0X5-	T49.0X6-
Benzyl						
acetate	T52.8X1-	T52.8X2-	T52.8X3-	T52.8X4-	-	-
alcohol	T49.0X1-	T49.0X2-	T49.0X3-	T49.0X4-	T49.0X5-	T49.0X6-
benzoate	T49.0X1-	T49.0X2-	T49.0X3-	T49.0X4-	T49.0X5-	T49.0X6-
Benzoic acid	T49.0X1-	T49.0X2-	T49.0X3-	T49.0X4-	T49.0X5-	T49.0X6-
morphine	T40.2X1-	T40.2X2-	T40.2X3-	T40.2X4-	-	-
nicotinate	T46.6X1-	T46.6X2-	T46.6X3-	T46.6X4-	T46.6X5-	T46.6X6-
penicillin	T36.0X1-	T36.0X2-	T36.0X3-	T36.0X4-	T36.0X5-	T36.0X6-
Benzylhydrochlorthia-zide	T50.2X1-	T50.2X2-	T50.2X3-	T50.2X4-	T50.2X5-	T50.2X6-
Benzylpenicillin	T36.0X1-	T36.0X2-	T36.0X3-	T36.0X4-	T36.0X5-	T36.0X6-
Benzylthiouracil	T38.2X1-	T38.2X2-	T38.2X3-	T38.2X4-	T38.2X5-	T38.2X6-
Bephenium hydroxy-naphthoate	T37.4X1-	T37.4X2-	T37.4X3-	T37.4X4-	T37.4X5-	T37.4X6-
Bepridil	T46.1X1-	T46.1X2-	T46.1X3-	T46.1X4-	T46.1X5-	T46.1X6-
Bergamot oil	T65.891-	T65.892-	T65.893-	T65.894-	-	-
Bergapten	T50.991-	T50.992-	T50.993-	T50.994-	T50.995-	T50.996-
Berries, poisonous	T62.1X1-	T62.1X2-	T62.1X3-	T62.1X4-	-	-

Substance	Poisoning, Accidental (unintentional)	Poisoning, Intentional self-harm	Poisoning, Assault	Poisoning, Undetermined	Adverse effect	Underdosing
Beryllium (compounds)	T56.7X1-	T56.7X2-	T56.7X3-	T56.7X4-	-	-
b-acetyldigoxin	T46.0X1-	T46.0X2-	T46.0X3-	T46.0X4-	T46.0X5-	T46.0X6-
beta adrenergic blocking agent, heart	T44.7X1-	T44.7X2-	T44.7X3-	T44.7X4-	T44.7X5-	T44.7X6-
b-benzalbutyramide	T46.6X1-	T46.6X2-	T46.6X3-	T46.6X4-	T46.6X5-	T46.6X6-
Betacarotene	T45.2X1-	T45.2X2-	T45.2X3-	T45.2X4-	T45.2X5-	T45.2X6-
b-eucaine	T49.1X1-	T49.1X2-	T49.1X3-	T49.1X4-	T49.1X5-	T49.1X6-
Beta-Chlor	T42.6X1-	T42.6X2-	T42.6X3-	T42.6X4-	T42.6X5-	T42.6X6-
b-galactosidase	T47.5X1-	T47.5X2-	T47.5X3-	T47.5X4-	T47.5X5-	T47.5X6-
Betahistine	T46.7X1-	T46.7X2-	T46.7X3-	T46.7X4-	T46.7X5-	T46.7X6-
Betaine	T47.5X1-	T47.5X2-	T47.5X3-	T47.5X4-	T47.5X5-	T47.5X6-
Betamethasone	T49.0X1-	T49.0X2-	T49.0X3-	T49.0X4-	T49.0X5-	T49.0X6-
topical	T49.0X1-	T49.0X2-	T49.0X3-	T49.0X4-	T49.0X5-	T49.0X6-
Betamicin	T36.8X1-	T36.8X2-	T36.8X3-	T36.8X4-	T36.8X5-	T36.8X6-
Betanidine	T46.5X1-	T46.5X2-	T46.5X3-	T46.5X4-	T46.5X5-	T46.5X6-
b-sitosterol (s)	T46.6X1-	T46.6X2-	T46.6X3-	T46.6X4-	T46.6X5-	T46.6X6-
Betaxolol	T44.7X1-	T44.7X2-	T44.7X3-	T44.7X4-	T44.7X5-	T44.7X6-
Betazole	T50.8X1-	T50.8X2-	T50.8X3-	T50.8X4-	T50.8X5-	T50.8X6-
Bethanechol	T44.1X1-	T44.1X2-	T44.1X3-	T44.1X4-	T44.1X5-	T44.1X6-
chloride	T44.1X1-	T44.1X2-	T44.1X3-	T44.1X4-	T44.1X5-	T44.1X6-
Bethanidine	T46.5X1-	T46.5X2-	T46.5X3-	T46.5X4-	T46.5X5-	T46.5X6-
Betoxycaine	T41.3X1-	T41.3X2-	T41.3X3-	T41.3X4-	T41.3X5-	T41.3X6-
Betula oil	T49.3X1-	T49.3X2-	T49.3X3-	T49.3X4-	T49.3X5-	T49.3X6-
Bevantolol	T44.7X1-	T44.7X2-	T44.7X3-	T44.7X4-	T44.7X5-	T44.7X6-
Bevonium metilsulfate	T44.3X1-	T44.3X2-	T44.3X3-	T44.3X4-	T44.3X5-	T44.3X6-
Bezafibrate	T46.6X1-	T46.6X2-	T46.6X3-	T46.6X4-	T46.6X5-	T46.6X6-
Bezitramide	T40.4X1-	T40.4X2-	T40.4X3-	T40.4X4-	T40.4X5-	T40.4X6-
BHA	T50.991-	T50.992-	T50.993-	T50.994-	T50.995-	T50.996-
Bhang	T40.7X1-	T40.7X2-	T40.7X3-	T40.7X4-	T40.7X5-	T40.7X6-
BHC (medicinal)	T49.0X1-	T49.0X2-	T49.0X3-	T49.0X4-	T49.0X5-	T49.0X6-
nonmedicinal (vapor)	T53.6X1-	T53.6X2-	T53.6X3-	T53.6X4-	-	-
Bialamicol	T37.3X1-	T37.3X2-	T37.3X3-	T37.3X4-	T37.3X5-	T37.3X6-
Bibenzonium bromide	T48.3X1-	T48.3X2-	T48.3X3-	T48.3X4-	T48.3X5-	T48.3X6-
Bibrocathol	T49.5X1-	T49.5X2-	T49.5X3-	T49.5X4-	T49.5X5-	T49.5X6-
Bichloride of mercury — see Mercury, chloride						
Bichromates (calcium) (potassium) (sodium) (crystals)	T57.8X1-	T57.8X2-	T57.8X3-	T57.8X4-	-	-
fumes	T56.2X1-	T56.2X2-	T56.2X3-	T56.2X4-	-	-
Biclotymol	T49.6X1-	T49.6X2-	T49.6X3-	T49.6X4-	T49.6X5-	T49.6X6-
Bicucculine	T50.7X1-	T50.7X2-	T50.7X3-	T50.7X4-	T50.7X5-	T50.7X6-
Bifemelane	T43.291-	T43.292-	T43.293-	T43.294-	T43.295-	T43.296-
Biguanide derivatives, oral	T38.3X1-	T38.3X2-	T38.3X3-	T38.3X4-	T38.3X5-	T38.3X6-
Bile salts	T47.5X1-	T47.5X2-	T47.5X3-	T47.5X4-	T47.5X5-	T47.5X6-
Biligrafin	T50.8X1-	T50.8X2-	T50.8X3-	T50.8X4-	T50.8X5-	T50.8X6-
Bilopaque	T50.8X1-	T50.8X2-	T50.8X3-	T50.8X4-	T50.8X5-	T50.8X6-
Binifibrate	T46.6X1-	T46.6X2-	T46.6X3-	T46.6X4-	T46.6X5-	T46.6X6-
Binitrobenzol	T65.3X1-	T65.3X2-	T65.3X3-	T65.3X4-	-	-
Bioflavonoid (s)	T46.991-	T46.992-	T46.993-	T46.994-	T46.995-	T46.996-
Biological substance NEC	T50.901-	T50.902-	T50.903-	T50.904-	T50.905-	T50.906-
Biotin	T45.2X1-	T45.2X2-	T45.2X3-	T45.2X4-	T45.2X5-	T45.2X6-
Biperiden	T44.3X1-	T44.3X2-	T44.3X3-	T44.3X4-	T44.3X5-	T44.3X6-
Bisacodyl	T47.2X1-	T47.2X2-	T47.2X3-	T47.2X4-	T47.2X5-	T47.2X6-
Bisbentiamine	T45.2X1-	T45.2X2-	T45.2X3-	T45.2X4-	T45.2X5-	T45.2X6-
Bisbutiamine	T45.2X1-	T45.2X2-	T45.2X3-	T45.2X4-	T45.2X5-	T45.2X6-
Bisdequalinium (salts) (diacetate)	T49.6X1-	T49.6X2-	T49.6X3-	T49.6X4-	T49.6X5-	T49.6X6-
Bishydroxycoumarin	T45.511-	T45.512-	T45.513-	T45.514-	T45.515-	T45.516-
Bismarsen	T37.8X1-	T37.8X2-	T37.8X3-	T37.8X4-	T37.8X5-	T37.8X6-
Bismuth salts	T47.6X1-	T47.6X2-	T47.6X3-	T47.6X4-	T47.6X5-	T47.6X6-
aluminate	T47.1X1-	T47.1X2-	T47.1X3-	T47.1X4-	T47.1X5-	T47.1X6-
anti-infectives	T37.8X1-	T37.8X2-	T37.8X3-	T37.8X4-	T37.8X5-	T37.8X6-
formic iodide	T49.0X1-	T49.0X2-	T49.0X3-	T49.0X4-	T49.0X5-	T49.0X6-
glycolylarsenate	T49.0X1-	T49.0X2-	T49.0X3-	T49.0X4-	T49.0X5-	T49.0X6-
nonmedicinal (compounds) NEC	T65.91X-	T65.92X-	T65.93X-	T65.94X-	-	-
subcarbonate	T47.6X1-	T47.6X2-	T47.6X3-	T47.6X4-	T47.6X5-	T47.6X6-
subsalicylate	T37.8X1-	T37.8X2-	T37.8X3-	T37.8X4-	T37.8X5-	T37.8X6-
sulfarsphenamine	T37.8X1-	T37.8X2-	T37.8X3-	T37.8X4-	T37.8X5-	T37.8X6-
Bisoprolol	T44.7X1-	T44.7X2-	T44.7X3-	T44.7X4-	T44.7X5-	T44.7X6-
Bisoxatin	T47.2X1-	T47.2X2-	T47.2X3-	T47.2X4-	T47.2X5-	T47.2X6-
Bisulepin (hydrochloride)	T45.0X1-	T45.0X2-	T45.0X3-	T45.0X4-	T45.0X5-	T45.0X6-
Bithionol	T37.8X1-	T37.8X2-	T37.8X3-	T37.8X4-	T37.8X5-	T37.8X6-
anthelminthic	T37.4X1-	T37.4X2-	T37.4X3-	T37.4X4-	T37.4X5-	T37.4X6-
Bitolterol	T48.6X1-	T48.6X2-	T48.6X3-	T48.6X4-	T48.6X5-	T48.6X6-
Bitoscanate	T37.4X1-	T37.4X2-	T37.4X3-	T37.4X4-	T37.4X5-	T37.4X6-
Bitter almond oil	T62.8X1-	T62.8X2-	T62.8X3-	T62.8X4-	-	-
Bittersweet	T62.2X1-	T62.2X2-	T62.2X3-	T62.2X4-	-	-

Substance	Poisoning, Accidental (unintentional)	Poisoning, Intentional self-harm	Poisoning, Assault	Poisoning, Undetermined	Adverse effect	Underdosing
Black						
flag	T60.91X-	T60.92X-	T60.93X-	T60.94X-	-	-
henbane	T62.2X1-	T62.2X2-	T62.2X3-	T62.2X4-	-	-
leaf (40)	T60.91X-	T60.92X-	T60.93X-	T60.94X-	-	-
widow spider (bite)	T63.311-	T63.312-	T63.313-	T63.314-	-	-
antivenin	T50.Z11-	T50.Z12-	T50.Z13-	T50.Z14-	T50.Z15-	T50.Z16-
Blast furnace gas (carbon monoxide from)	T58.8X1-	T58.8X2-	T58.8X3-	T58.8X4-	-	-
Bleach	T54.91X-	T54.92X-	T54.93X-	T54.94X-	-	-
Bleaching agent (medicinal)	T49.4X1-	T49.4X2-	T49.4X3-	T49.4X4-	T49.4X5-	T49.4X6-
Bleomycin	T45.1X1-	T45.1X2-	T45.1X3-	T45.1X4-	T45.1X5-	T45.1X6-
Blockain	T41.3X1-	T41.3X2-	T41.3X3-	T41.3X4-	T41.3X5-	T41.3X6-
infiltration (subcutaneous)	T41.3X1-	T41.3X2-	T41.3X3-	T41.3X4-	T41.3X5-	T41.3X6-
nerve block (peripheral) (plexus)	T41.3X1-	T41.3X2-	T41.3X3-	T41.3X4-	T41.3X5-	T41.3X6-
topical (surface)	T41.3X1-	T41.3X2-	T41.3X3-	T41.3X4-	T41.3X5-	T41.3X6-
Blockers, calcium channel	T46.1X1-	T46.1X2-	T46.1X3-	T46.1X4-	T46.1X5-	T46.1X6-
Blood (derivatives) (natural) (plasma) (whole)	T45.8X1-	T45.8X2-	T45.8X3-	T45.8X4-	T45.8X5-	T45.8X6-
dried	T45.8X1-	T45.8X2-	T45.8X3-	T45.8X4-	T45.8X5-	T45.8X6-
drug affecting NEC	T45.91X-	T45.92X-	T45.93X-	T45.94X-	T45.95X-	T45.96X-
expander NEC	T45.8X1-	T45.8X2-	T45.8X3-	T45.8X4-	T45.8X5-	T45.8X6-
fraction NEC	T45.8X1-	T45.8X2-	T45.8X3-	T45.8X4-	T45.8X5-	T45.8X6-
substitute (macromolecular)	T45.8X1-	T45.8X2-	T45.8X3-	T45.8X4-	T45.8X5-	T45.8X6-
Blue velvet	T40.2X1-	T40.2X2-	T40.2X3-	T40.2X4-	-	-
Bone meal	T62.8X1-	T62.8X2-	T62.8X3-	T62.8X4-	-	-
Bonine	T45.0X1-	T45.0X2-	T45.0X3-	T45.0X4-	T45.0X5-	T45.0X6-
Bopindolol	T44.7X1-	T44.7X2-	T44.7X3-	T44.7X4-	T44.7X5-	T44.7X6-
Boracic acid	T49.0X1-	T49.0X2-	T49.0X3-	T49.0X4-	T49.0X5-	T49.0X6-
ENT agent	T49.6X1-	T49.6X2-	T49.6X3-	T49.6X4-	T49.6X5-	T49.6X6-
ophthalmic preparation	T49.5X1-	T49.5X2-	T49.5X3-	T49.5X4-	T49.5X5-	T49.5X6-
Borane complex	T57.8X1-	T57.8X2-	T57.8X3-	T57.8X4-	-	-
Borate (s)	T57.8X1-	T57.8X2-	T57.8X3-	T57.8X4-	-	-
buffer	T50.991-	T50.992-	T50.993-	T50.994-	T50.995-	T50.996-
cleanser	T54.91X-	T54.92X-	T54.93X-	T54.94X-	-	-
sodium	T57.8X1-	T57.8X2-	T57.8X3-	T57.8X4-	-	-
Borax (cleanser)	T54.91X-	T54.92X-	T54.93X-	T54.94X-	-	-
Bordeaux mixture	T60.3X1-	T60.3X2-	T60.3X3-	T60.3X4-	-	-
Boric acid	T49.0X1-	T49.0X2-	T49.0X3-	T49.0X4-	T49.0X5-	T49.0X6-
ENT agent	T49.6X1-	T49.6X2-	T49.6X3-	T49.6X4-	T49.6X5-	T49.6X6-
ophthalmic preparation	T49.5X1-	T49.5X2-	T49.5X3-	T49.5X4-	T49.5X5-	T49.5X6-
Bornaprine	T44.3X1-	T44.3X2-	T44.3X3-	T44.3X4-	T44.3X5-	T44.3X6-
Boron	T57.8X1-	T57.8X2-	T57.8X3-	T57.8X4-	-	-
hydride NEC	T57.8X1-	T57.8X2-	T57.8X3-	T57.8X4-	-	-
fumes or gas	T57.8X1-	T57.8X2-	T57.8X3-	T57.8X4-	-	-
trifluoride	T59.891-	T59.892-	T59.893-	T59.894-	-	-
Botox	T48.291-	T48.292-	T48.293-	T48.294-	T48.295-	T48.296-
Botulinus anti-toxin (type A, B)	T50.Z11-	T50.Z12-	T50.Z13-	T50.Z14-	T50.Z15-	T50.Z16-
Brake fluid vapor	T59.891-	T59.892-	T59.893-	T59.894-	-	-
Brallobarbital	T42.3X1-	T42.3X2-	T42.3X3-	T42.3X4-	T42.3X5-	T42.3X6-
Bran (wheat)	T47.4X1-	T47.4X2-	T47.4X3-	T47.4X4-	T47.4X5-	T47.4X6-
Brass (fumes)	T56.891-	T56.892-	T56.893-	T56.894-	-	-
Brasso	T52.0X1-	T52.0X2-	T52.0X3-	T52.0X4-	-	-
Bretylium tosilate	T46.2X1-	T46.2X2-	T46.2X3-	T46.2X4-	T46.2X5-	T46.2X6-
Brevital (sodium)	T41.1X1-	T41.1X2-	T41.1X3-	T41.1X4-	T41.1X5-	T41.1X6-
Brinase	T45.3X1-	T45.3X2-	T45.3X3-	T45.3X4-	T45.3X5-	T45.3X6-
British antilewisite	T45.8X1-	T45.8X2-	T45.8X3-	T45.8X4-	T45.8X5-	T45.8X6-
Brodifacoum	T60.4X1-	T60.4X2-	T60.4X3-	T60.4X4-	-	-
Bromal (hydrate)	T42.6X1-	T42.6X2-	T42.6X3-	T42.6X4-	T42.6X5-	T42.6X6-
Bromazepam	T42.4X1-	T42.4X2-	T42.4X3-	T42.4X4-	T42.4X5-	T42.4X6-
Bromazine	T45.0X1-	T45.0X2-	T45.0X3-	T45.0X4-	T45.0X5-	T45.0X6-
Brombenzylcyanide	T59.3X1-	T59.3X2-	T59.3X3-	T59.3X4-	-	-
Bromelains	T45.3X1-	T45.3X2-	T45.3X3-	T45.3X4-	T45.3X5-	T45.3X6-
Bromethalin	T60.4X1-	T60.4X2-	T60.4X3-	T60.4X4-	-	-
Bromhexine	T48.4X1-	T48.4X2-	T48.4X3-	T48.4X4-	T48.4X5-	T48.4X6-
Bromide salts	T42.6X1-	T42.6X2-	T42.6X3-	T42.6X4-	T42.6X5-	T42.6X6-
Bromindione	T45.511-	T45.512-	T45.513-	T45.514-	T45.515-	T45.516-
Bromine						
compounds (medicinal)	T42.6X1-	T42.6X2-	T42.6X3-	T42.6X4-	T42.6X5-	T42.6X6-
sedative	T42.6X1-	T42.6X2-	T42.6X3-	T42.6X4-	T42.6X5-	T42.6X6-
vapor	T59.891-	T59.892-	T59.893-	T59.894-	-	-
Bromisoval	T42.6X1-	T42.6X2-	T42.6X3-	T42.6X4-	T42.6X5-	T42.6X6-
Bromisovalum	T42.6X1-	T42.6X2-	T42.6X3-	T42.6X4-	T42.6X5-	T42.6X6-
Bromobenzylcyanide	T59.3X1-	T59.3X2-	T59.3X3-	T59.3X4-	-	-
Bromochlorosalicylani-lide	T49.0X1-	T49.0X2-	T49.0X3-	T49.0X4-	T49.0X5-	T49.0X6-
Bromocriptine	T42.8X1-	T42.8X2-	T42.8X3-	T42.8X4-	T42.8X5-	T42.8X6-
Bromodiphenhydramine	T45.0X1-	T45.0X2-	T45.0X3-	T45.0X4-	T45.0X5-	T45.0X6-
Bromoform	T42.6X1-	T42.6X2-	T42.6X3-	T42.6X4-	T42.6X5-	T42.6X6-

Substance	Poisoning, Accidental (unintentional)	Poisoning, Intentional self-harm	Poisoning, Assault	Poisoning, Undetermined	Adverse effect	Underdosing
Bromophenol blue reagent	T50.991-	T50.992-	T50.993-	T50.994-	T50.995-	T50.996-
Bromopride	T47.8X1-	T47.8X2-	T47.8X3-	T47.8X4-	T47.8X5-	T47.8X6-
Bromosalicylchloranitide	T49.0X1-	T49.0X2-	T49.0X3-	T49.0X4-	T49.0X5-	T49.0X6-
Bromosalicylhydroxamic acid	T37.1X1-	T37.1X2-	T37.1X3-	T37.1X4-	T37.1X5-	T37.1X6-
Bromo-seltzer	T39.1X1-	T39.1X2-	T39.1X3-	T39.1X4-	T39.1X5-	T39.1X6-
Bromoxynil	T60.3X1-	T60.3X2-	T60.3X3-	T60.3X4-	-	-
Bromperidol	T43.4X1-	T43.4X2-	T43.4X3-	T43.4X4-	T43.4X5-	T43.4X6-
Brompheniramine	T45.0X1-	T45.0X2-	T45.0X3-	T45.0X4-	T45.0X5-	T45.0X6-
Bromsulfophthalein	T50.8X1-	T50.8X2-	T50.8X3-	T50.8X4-	T50.8X5-	T50.8X6-
Bromural	T42.6X1-	T42.6X2-	T42.6X3-	T42.6X4-	T42.6X5-	T42.6X6-
Bromvaletone	T42.6X1-	T42.6X2-	T42.6X3-	T42.6X4-	T42.6X5-	T42.6X6-
Bronchodilator NEC	T48.6X1-	T48.6X2-	T48.6X3-	T48.6X4-	T48.6X5-	T48.6X6-
Brotizolam	T42.4X1-	T42.4X2-	T42.4X3-	T42.4X4-	T42.4X5-	T42.4X6-
Brovincamine	T46.7X1-	T46.7X2-	T46.7X3-	T46.7X4-	T46.7X5-	T46.7X6-
Brown recluse spider (bite) (venom)	T63.331-	T63.332-	T63.333-	T63.334-	-	-
Brown spider (bite) (venom)	T63.391-	T63.392-	T63.393-	T63.394-	-	-
Broxaterol	T48.6X1-	T48.6X2-	T48.6X3-	T48.6X4-	T48.6X5-	T48.6X6-
Broxuridine	T45.1X1-	T45.1X2-	T45.1X3-	T45.1X4-	T45.1X5-	T45.1X6-
Broxyquinoline	T37.8X1-	T37.8X2-	T37.8X3-	T37.8X4-	T37.8X5-	T37.8X6-
Bruceine	T48.291-	T48.292-	T48.293-	T48.294-	T48.295-	T48.296-
Brucia	T62.2X1-	T62.2X2-	T62.2X3-	T62.2X4-	-	-
Brucine	T65.1X1-	T65.1X2-	T65.1X3-	T65.1X4-	-	-
Brunswick green — see Copper						
Bruten — see Ibuprofen						
Bryonia	T47.2X1-	T47.2X2-	T47.2X3-	T47.2X4-	T47.2X5-	T47.2X6-
Buclizine	T45.0X1-	T45.0X2-	T45.0X3-	T45.0X4-	T45.0X5-	T45.0X6-
Buclosamide	T49.0X1-	T49.0X2-	T49.0X3-	T49.0X4-	T49.0X5-	T49.0X6-
Budesonide	T44.5X1-	T44.5X2-	T44.5X3-	T44.5X4-	T44.5X5-	T44.5X6-
Budralazine	T46.5X1-	T46.5X2-	T46.5X3-	T46.5X4-	T46.5X5-	T46.5X6-
Bufferin	T39.011-	T39.012-	T39.013-	T39.014-	T39.015-	T39.016-
Buflomedil	T46.7X1-	T46.7X2-	T46.7X3-	T46.7X4-	T46.7X5-	T46.7X6-
Buformin	T38.3X1-	T38.3X2-	T38.3X3-	T38.3X4-	T38.3X5-	T38.3X6-
Bufotenine	T40.991-	T40.992-	T40.993-	T40.994-	-	-
Bufrolin	T48.6X1-	T48.6X2-	T48.6X3-	T48.6X4-	T48.6X5-	T48.6X6-
Bufylline	T48.6X1-	T48.6X2-	T48.6X3-	T48.6X4-	T48.6X5-	T48.6X6-
Bulk filler	T50.5X1-	T50.5X2-	T50.5X3-	T50.5X4-	T50.5X5-	T50.5X6-
cathartic	T47.4X1-	T47.4X2-	T47.4X3-	T47.4X4-	T47.4X5-	T47.4X6-
Bumetanide	T50.1X1-	T50.1X2-	T50.1X3-	T50.1X4-	T50.1X5-	T50.1X6-
Bunaftine	T46.2X1-	T46.2X2-	T46.2X3-	T46.2X4-	T46.2X5-	T46.2X6-
Bunamiodyl	T50.8X1-	T50.8X2-	T50.8X3-	T50.8X4-	T50.8X5-	T50.8X6-
Bunazosin	T44.6X1-	T44.6X2-	T44.6X3-	T44.6X4-	T44.6X5-	T44.6X6-
Bunitrolol	T44.7X1-	T44.7X2-	T44.7X3-	T44.7X4-	T44.7X5-	T44.7X6-
Buphenine	T46.7X1-	T46.7X2-	T46.7X3-	T46.7X4-	T46.7X5-	T46.7X6-
Bupivacaine	T41.3X1-	T41.3X2-	T41.3X3-	T41.3X4-	T41.3X5-	T41.3X6-
infiltration (subcutaneous)	T41.3X1-	T41.3X2-	T41.3X3-	T41.3X4-	T41.3X5-	T41.3X6-
nerve block (peripheral) (plexus)	T41.3X1-	T41.3X2-	T41.3X3-	T41.3X4-	T41.3X5-	T41.3X6-
spinal	T41.3X1-	T41.3X2-	T41.3X3-	T41.3X4-	T41.3X5-	T41.3X6-
Bupranolol	T44.7X1-	T44.7X2-	T44.7X3-	T44.7X4-	T44.7X5-	T44.7X6-
Buprenorphine	T40.4X1-	T40.4X2-	T40.4X3-	T40.4X4-	T40.4X5-	T40.4X6-
Bupropion	T43.291-	T43.292-	T43.293-	T43.294-	T43.295-	T43.296-
Burimamide	T47.1X1-	T47.1X2-	T47.1X3-	T47.1X4-	T47.1X5-	T47.1X6-
Buserelin	T38.891-	T38.892-	T38.893-	T38.894-	T38.895-	T38.896-
Buspirone	T43.591-	T43.592-	T43.593-	T43.594-	T43.595-	T43.596-
Busulfan, busulphan	T45.1X1-	T45.1X2-	T45.1X3-	T45.1X4-	T45.1X5-	T45.1X6-
Butabarbital (sodium)	T42.3X1-	T42.3X2-	T42.3X3-	T42.3X4-	T42.3X5-	T42.3X6-
Butabarbitone	T42.3X1-	T42.3X2-	T42.3X3-	T42.3X4-	T42.3X5-	T42.3X6-
Butabarpal	T42.3X1-	T42.3X2-	T42.3X3-	T42.3X4-	T42.3X5-	T42.3X6-
Butacaine	T41.3X1-	T41.3X2-	T41.3X3-	T41.3X4-	T41.3X5-	T41.3X6-
Butalamine	T46.7X1-	T46.7X2-	T46.7X3-	T46.7X4-	T46.7X5-	T46.7X6-
Butalbital	T42.3X1-	T42.3X2-	T42.3X3-	T42.3X4-	T42.3X5-	T42.3X6-
Butallylonal	T42.3X1-	T42.3X2-	T42.3X3-	T42.3X4-	T42.3X5-	T42.3X6-
Butamben	T41.3X1-	T41.3X2-	T41.3X3-	T41.3X4-	T41.3X5-	T41.3X6-
Butamirate	T48.3X1-	T48.3X2-	T48.3X3-	T48.3X4-	T48.3X5-	T48.3X6-
Butane (distributed in mobile container)	T59.891-	T59.892-	T59.893-	T59.894-	-	-
distributed through pipes	T59.891-	T59.892-	T59.893-	T59.894-	-	-
incomplete combustion	T58.11X-	T58.12X-	T58.13X-	T58.14X-	-	-
Butanilicaine	T41.3X1-	T41.3X2-	T41.3X3-	T41.3X4-	T41.3X5-	T41.3X6-
Butanol	T51.3X1-	T51.3X2-	T51.3X3-	T51.3X4-	-	-
Butanone, 2-butanone	T52.4X1-	T52.4X2-	T52.4X3-	T52.4X4-	-	-
Butantrone	T49.4X1-	T49.4X2-	T49.4X3-	T49.4X4-	T49.4X5-	T49.4X6-
Butaperazine	T43.3X1-	T43.3X2-	T43.3X3-	T43.3X4-	T43.3X5-	T43.3X6-
Butazolidin	T39.2X1-	T39.2X2-	T39.2X3-	T39.2X4-	T39.2X5-	T39.2X6-
Butetamate	T48.6X1-	T48.6X2-	T48.6X3-	T48.6X4-	T48.6X5-	T48.6X6-
Butethal	T42.3X1-	T42.3X2-	T42.3X3-	T42.3X4-	T42.3X5-	T42.3X6-

Substance	Poisoning, Accidental (unintentional)	Poisoning, Intentional self-harm	Poisoning, Assault	Poisoning, Undetermined	Adverse effect	Underdosing
Butethamate	T44.3X1-	T44.3X2-	T44.3X3-	T44.3X4-	T44.3X5-	T44.3X6-
Buthalitone (sodium)	T41.1X1-	T41.1X2-	T41.1X3-	T41.1X4-	T41.1X5-	T41.1X6-
Butisol (sodium)	T42.3X1-	T42.3X2-	T42.3X3-	T42.3X4-	T42.3X5-	T42.3X6-
Butizide	T50.2X1-	T50.2X2-	T50.2X3-	T50.2X4-	T50.2X5-	T50.2X6-
Butobarbital	T42.3X1-	T42.3X2-	T42.3X3-	T42.3X4-	T42.3X5-	T42.3X6-
sodium	T42.3X1-	T42.3X2-	T42.3X3-	T42.3X4-	T42.3X5-	T42.3X6-
Butobarbitone	T42.3X1-	T42.3X2-	T42.3X3-	T42.3X4-	T42.3X5-	T42.3X6-
Butoconazole (nitrate)	T49.0X1-	T49.0X2-	T49.0X3-	T49.0X4-	T49.0X5-	T49.0X6-
Butorphanol	T40.4X1-	T40.4X2-	T40.4X3-	T40.4X4-	T40.4X5-	T40.4X6-
Butriptyline	T43.011-	T43.012-	T43.013-	T43.014-	T43.015-	T43.016-
Butropium bromide	T44.3X1-	T44.3X2-	T44.3X3-	T44.3X4-	T44.3X5-	T44.3X6-
Butter of antimony — see Antimony						
Buttercups	T62.2X1-	T62.2X2-	T62.2X3-	T62.2X4-	-	-
Butyl						
acetate (secondary)	T52.8X1-	T52.8X2-	T52.8X3-	T52.8X4-	-	-
alcohol	T51.3X1-	T51.3X2-	T51.3X3-	T51.3X4-	-	-
aminobenzoate	T41.3X1-	T41.3X2-	T41.3X3-	T41.3X4-	T41.3X5-	T41.3X6-
butyrate	T52.8X1-	T52.8X2-	T52.8X3-	T52.8X4-	-	-
carbinol	T51.3X1-	T51.3X2-	T51.3X3-	T51.3X4-	-	-
carbitol	T52.3X1-	T52.3X2-	T52.3X3-	T52.3X4-	-	-
cellosolve	T52.3X1-	T52.3X2-	T52.3X3-	T52.3X4-	-	-
chloral (hydrate)	T42.6X1-	T42.6X2-	T42.6X3-	T42.6X4-	T42.6X5-	T42.6X6-
formate	T52.8X1-	T52.8X2-	T52.8X3-	T52.8X4-	-	-
lactate	T52.8X1-	T52.8X2-	T52.8X3-	T52.8X4-	-	-
propionate	T52.8X1-	T52.8X2-	T52.8X3-	T52.8X4-	-	-
scopolamine bromide	T44.3X1-	T44.3X2-	T44.3X3-	T44.3X4-	T44.3X5-	T44.3X6-
thiobarbital sodium	T41.1X1-	T41.1X2-	T41.1X3-	T41.1X4-	T41.1X5-	T41.1X6-
Butylated hydroxy-anisole	T50.991-	T50.992-	T50.993-	T50.994-	T50.995-	T50.996-
Butylchloral hydrate	T42.6X1-	T42.6X2-	T42.6X3-	T42.6X4-	T42.6X5-	T42.6X6-
Butyltoluene	T52.2X1-	T52.2X2-	T52.2X3-	T52.2X4-	-	-
Butyn	T41.3X1-	T41.3X2-	T41.3X3-	T41.3X4-	T41.3X5-	T41.3X6-
Butyrophenone (-based tranquilizers)	T43.4X1-	T43.4X2-	T43.4X3-	T43.4X4-	T43.4X5-	T43.4X6-
Cabergoline	T42.8X1-	T42.8X2-	T42.8X3-	T42.8X4-	T42.8X5-	T42.8X6-
Cacodyl, cacodylic acid	T57.0X1-	T57.0X2-	T57.0X3-	T57.0X4-	-	-
Cactinomycin	T45.1X1-	T45.1X2-	T45.1X3-	T45.1X4-	T45.1X5-	T45.1X6-
Cade oil	T49.4X1-	T49.4X2-	T49.4X3-	T49.4X4-	T49.4X5-	T49.4X6-
Cadexomer iodine	T49.0X1-	T49.0X2-	T49.0X3-	T49.0X4-	T49.0X5-	T49.0X6-
Cadmium (chloride) (fumes) (oxide)	T56.3X1-	T56.3X2-	T56.3X3-	T56.3X4-	-	-
sulfide (medicinal) NEC	T49.4X1-	T49.4X2-	T49.4X3-	T49.4X4-	T49.4X5-	T49.4X6-
Cadralazine	T46.5X1-	T46.5X2-	T46.5X3-	T46.5X4-	T46.5X5-	T46.5X6-
Caffeine	T43.611-	T43.612-	T43.613-	T43.614-	T43.615-	T43.616-
Calabar bean	T62.2X1-	T62.2X2-	T62.2X3-	T62.2X4-	-	-
Caladium seguinum	T62.2X1-	T62.2X2-	T62.2X3-	T62.2X4-	-	-
Calamine (lotion)	T49.3X1-	T49.3X2-	T49.3X3-	T49.3X4-	T49.3X5-	T49.3X6-
Calcifediol	T45.2X1-	T45.2X2-	T45.2X3-	T45.2X4-	T45.2X5-	T45.2X6-
Calciferol	T45.2X1-	T45.2X2-	T45.2X3-	T45.2X4-	T45.2X5-	T45.2X6-
Calcitonin	T50.991-	T50.992-	T50.993-	T50.994-	T50.995-	T50.996-
Calcitriol	T45.2X1-	T45.2X2-	T45.2X3-	T45.2X4-	T45.2X5-	T45.2X6-
Calcium	T50.3X1-	T50.3X2-	T50.3X3-	T50.3X4-	T50.3X5-	T50.3X6-
actylsalicylate	T39.011-	T39.012-	T39.013-	T39.014-	T39.015-	T39.016-
benzamidosalicylate	T37.1X1-	T37.1X2-	T37.1X3-	T37.1X4-	T37.1X5-	T37.1X6-
bromide	T42.6X1-	T42.6X2-	T42.6X3-	T42.6X4-	T42.6X5-	T42.6X6-
bromolactobionate	T42.6X1-	T42.6X2-	T42.6X3-	T42.6X4-	T42.6X5-	T42.6X6-
carbaspirin	T39.011-	T39.012-	T39.013-	T39.014-	T39.015-	T39.016-
carbimide	T50.6X1-	T50.6X2-	T50.6X3-	T50.6X4-	T50.6X5-	T50.6X6-
carbonate	T47.1X1-	T47.1X2-	T47.1X3-	T47.1X4-	T47.1X5-	T47.1X6-
chloride	T50.991-	T50.992-	T50.993-	T50.994-	T50.995-	T50.996-
anhydrous	T50.991-	T50.992-	T50.993-	T50.994-	T50.995-	T50.996-
cyanide	T57.8X1-	T57.8X2-	T57.8X3-	T57.8X4-	-	-
dioctyl sulfosuccinate	T47.4X1-	T47.4X2-	T47.4X3-	T47.4X4-	T47.4X5-	T47.4X6-
disodium edathamil	T45.8X1-	T45.8X2-	T45.8X3-	T45.8X4-	T45.8X5-	T45.8X6-
disodium edetate	T45.8X1-	T45.8X2-	T45.8X3-	T45.8X4-	T45.8X5-	T45.8X6-
dobesilate	T46.991-	T46.992-	T46.993-	T46.994-	T46.995-	T46.996-
EDTA	T45.8X1-	T45.8X2-	T45.8X3-	T45.8X4-	T45.8X5-	T45.8X6-
ferrous citrate	T45.4X1-	T45.4X2-	T45.4X3-	T45.4X4-	T45.4X5-	T45.4X6-
folinate	T45.8X1-	T45.8X2-	T45.8X3-	T45.8X4-	T45.8X5-	T45.8X6-
glubionate	T50.3X1-	T50.3X2-	T50.3X3-	T50.3X4-	T50.3X5-	T50.3X6-
gluconate	T50.3X1-	T50.3X2-	T50.3X3-	T50.3X4-	T50.3X5-	T50.3X6-
gluconogalactogluc-onate	T50.3X1-	T50.3X2-	T50.3X3-	T50.3X4-	T50.3X5-	T50.3X6-
hydrate, hydroxide	T54.3X1-	T54.3X2-	T54.3X3-	T54.3X4-	-	-
hypochlorite	T54.3X1-	T54.3X2-	T54.3X3-	T54.3X4-	-	-
iodide	T48.4X1-	T48.4X2-	T48.4X3-	T48.4X4-	T48.4X5-	T48.4X6-
ipodate	T50.8X1-	T50.8X2-	T50.8X3-	T50.8X4-	T50.8X5-	T50.8X6-
lactate	T50.3X1-	T50.3X2-	T50.3X3-	T50.3X4-	T50.3X5-	T50.3X6-
leucovorin	T45.8X1-	T45.8X2-	T45.8X3-	T45.8X4-	T45.8X5-	T45.8X6-

Substance	Poisoning, Accidental (unintentional)	Poisoning, Intentional self-harm	Poisoning, Assault	Poisoning, Undetermined	Adverse effect	Underdosing
Calcium - continued						
mandelate	T37.91X-	T37.92X-	T37.93X-	T37.94X-	T37.95X-	T37.96X-
oxide	T54.3X1-	T54.3X2-	T54.3X3-	T54.3X4-	-	-
pantothenate	T45.2X1-	T45.2X2-	T45.2X3-	T45.2X4-	T45.2X5-	T45.2X6-
phosphate	T50.3X1-	T50.3X2-	T50.3X3-	T50.3X4-	T50.3X5-	T50.3X6-
salicylate	T39.091-	T39.092-	T39.093-	T39.094-	T39.095-	T39.096-
salts	T50.3X1-	T50.3X2-	T50.3X3-	T50.3X4-	T50.3X5-	T50.3X6-
Calculus-dissolving drug	T50.991-	T50.992-	T50.993-	T50.994-	T50.995-	T50.996-
Calomel	T49.0X1-	T49.0X2-	T49.0X3-	T49.0X4-	T49.0X5-	T49.0X6-
Caloric agent	T50.3X1-	T50.3X2-	T50.3X3-	T50.3X4-	T50.3X5-	T50.3X6-
Calusterone	T38.7X1-	T38.7X2-	T38.7X3-	T38.7X4-	T38.7X5-	T38.7X6-
Camazepam	T42.4X1-	T42.4X2-	T42.4X3-	T42.4X4-	T42.4X5-	T42.4X6-
Camomile	T49.0X1-	T49.0X2-	T49.0X3-	T49.0X4-	T49.0X5-	T49.0X6-
Camoquin	T37.2X1-	T37.2X2-	T37.2X3-	T37.2X4-	T37.2X5-	T37.2X6-
Camphor						
insecticide	T60.2X1-	T60.2X2-	T60.2X3-	T60.2X4-	-	-
medicinal	T49.8X1-	T49.8X2-	T49.8X3-	T49.8X4-	T49.8X5-	T49.8X6-
Camylofin	T44.3X1-	T44.3X2-	T44.3X3-	T44.3X4-	T44.3X5-	T44.3X6-
Cancer chemotherapy drug regimen	T45.1X1-	T45.1X2-	T45.1X3-	T45.1X4-	T45.1X5-	T45.1X6-
Candeptin	T49.0X1-	T49.0X2-	T49.0X3-	T49.0X4-	T49.0X5-	T49.0X6-
Candicidin	T49.0X1-	T49.0X2-	T49.0X3-	T49.0X4-	T49.0X5-	T49.0X6-
Cannabinol	T40.7X1-	T40.7X2-	T40.7X3-	T40.7X4-	T40.7X5-	T40.7X6-
Cannabis (derivatives)	T40.7X1-	T40.7X2-	T40.7X3-	T40.7X4-	T40.7X5-	T40.7X6-
Canned heat	T51.1X1-	T51.1X2-	T51.1X3-	T51.1X4-	-	-
Canrenoic acid	T50.0X1-	T50.0X2-	T50.0X3-	T50.0X4-	T50.0X5-	T50.0X6-
Canrenone	T50.0X1-	T50.0X2-	T50.0X3-	T50.0X4-	T50.0X5-	T50.0X6-
Cantharides, cantharidin, cantharis	T49.8X1-	T49.8X2-	T49.8X3-	T49.8X4-	T49.8X5-	T49.8X6-
Canthaxanthin	T50.991-	T50.992-	T50.993-	T50.994-	T50.995-	T50.996-
Capillary-active drug NEC	T46.901-	T46.902-	T46.903-	T46.904-	T46.905-	T46.906-
Capreomycin	T36.8X1-	T36.8X2-	T36.8X3-	T36.8X4-	T36.8X5-	T36.8X6-
Capsicum	T49.4X1-	T49.4X2-	T49.4X3-	T49.4X4-	T49.4X5-	T49.4X6-
Captafol	T60.3X1-	T60.3X2-	T60.3X3-	T60.3X4-	-	-
Captan	T60.3X1-	T60.3X2-	T60.3X3-	T60.3X4-	-	-
Captodiame, captodiamine	T43.591-	T43.592-	T43.593-	T43.594-	T43.595-	T43.596-
Captopril	T46.4X1-	T46.4X2-	T46.4X3-	T46.4X4-	T46.4X5-	T46.4X6-
Caramiphen	T44.3X1-	T44.3X2-	T44.3X3-	T44.3X4-	T44.3X5-	T44.3X6-
Carazolol	T44.7X1-	T44.7X2-	T44.7X3-	T44.7X4-	T44.7X5-	T44.7X6-
Carbachol	T44.1X1-	T44.1X2-	T44.1X3-	T44.1X4-	T44.1X5-	T44.1X6-
Carbacrylamine (resin)	T50.3X1-	T50.3X2-	T50.3X3-	T50.3X4-	T50.3X5-	T50.3X6-
Carbamate (insecticide)	T60.0X1-	T60.0X2-	T60.0X3-	T60.0X4-	-	-
Carbamate (sedative)	T42.6X1-	T42.6X2-	T42.6X3-	T42.6X4-	T42.6X5-	T42.6X6-
herbicide	T60.0X1-	T60.0X2-	T60.0X3-	T60.0X4-	-	-
insecticide	T60.0X1-	T60.0X2-	T60.0X3-	T60.0X4-	-	-
Carbamazepine	T42.1X1-	T42.1X2-	T42.1X3-	T42.1X4-	T42.1X5-	T42.1X6-
Carbamide	T47.3X1-	T47.3X2-	T47.3X3-	T47.3X4-	T47.3X5-	T47.3X6-
peroxide	T49.0X1-	T49.0X2-	T49.0X3-	T49.0X4-	T49.0X5-	T49.0X6-
topical	T49.8X1-	T49.8X2-	T49.8X3-	T49.8X4-	T49.8X5-	T49.8X6-
Carbamylcholine chloride	T44.1X1-	T44.1X2-	T44.1X3-	T44.1X4-	T44.1X5-	T44.1X6-
Carbaril	T60.0X1-	T60.0X2-	T60.0X3-	T60.0X4-	-	-
Carbarsone	T37.3X1-	T37.3X2-	T37.3X3-	T37.3X4-	T37.3X5-	T37.3X6-
Carbaryl	T60.0X1-	T60.0X2-	T60.0X3-	T60.0X4-	-	-
Carbaspirin	T39.011-	T39.012-	T39.013-	T39.014-	T39.015-	T39.016-
Carbazochrome (salicylate) (sodium sulfonate)	T49.4X1-	T49.4X2-	T49.4X3-	T49.4X4-	T49.4X5-	T49.4X6-
Carbenicillin	T36.0X1-	T36.0X2-	T36.0X3-	T36.0X4-	T36.0X5-	T36.0X6-
Carbenoxolone	T47.1X1-	T47.1X2-	T47.1X3-	T47.1X4-	T47.1X5-	T47.1X6-
Carbetapentane	T48.3X1-	T48.3X2-	T48.3X3-	T48.3X4-	T48.3X5-	T48.3X6-
Carbethyl salicylate	T39.091-	T39.092-	T39.093-	T39.094-	T39.095-	T39.096-
Carbidopa (with levodopa)	T42.8X1-	T42.8X2-	T42.8X3-	T42.8X4-	T42.8X5-	T42.8X6-
Carbimazole	T38.2X1-	T38.2X2-	T38.2X3-	T38.2X4-	T38.2X5-	T38.2X6-
Carbinol	T51.1X1-	T51.1X2-	T51.1X3-	T51.1X4-	-	-
Carbinoxamine	T45.0X1-	T45.0X2-	T45.0X3-	T45.0X4-	T45.0X5-	T45.0X6-
Carbiphene	T39.8X1-	T39.8X2-	T39.8X3-	T39.8X4-	T39.8X5-	T39.8X6-
Carbitol	T52.3X1-	T52.3X2-	T52.3X3-	T52.3X4-	-	-
Carbo medicinalis	T47.6X1-	T47.6X2-	T47.6X3-	T47.6X4-	T47.6X5-	T47.6X6-
Carbocaine	T41.3X1-	T41.3X2-	T41.3X3-	T41.3X4-	T41.3X5-	T41.3X6-
infiltration (subcutaneous)	T41.3X1-	T41.3X2-	T41.3X3-	T41.3X4-	T41.3X5-	T41.3X6-
nerve block (peripheral) (plexus)	T41.3X1-	T41.3X2-	T41.3X3-	T41.3X4-	T41.3X5-	T41.3X6-
topical (surface)	T41.3X1-	T41.3X2-	T41.3X3-	T41.3X4-	T41.3X5-	T41.3X6-
Carbocisteine	T48.4X1-	T48.4X2-	T48.4X3-	T48.4X4-	T48.4X5-	T48.4X6-
Carbocromen	T46.3X1-	T46.3X2-	T46.3X3-	T46.3X4-	T46.3X5-	T46.3X6-
Carbol fuchsin	T49.0X1-	T49.0X2-	T49.0X3-	T49.0X4-	T49.0X5-	T49.0X6-
Carbolic acid — see also Phenol	T54.0X1-	T54.0X2-	T54.0X3-	T54.0X4-	-	-
Carbolonium (bromide)	T48.1X1-	T48.1X2-	T48.1X3-	T48.1X4-	T48.1X5-	T48.1X6-
Carbomycin	T36.8X1-	T36.8X2-	T36.8X3-	T36.8X4-	T36.8X5-	T36.8X6-

Substance	Poisoning, Accidental (unintentional)	Poisoning, Intentional self-harm	Poisoning, Assault	Poisoning, Undetermined	Adverse effect	Underdosing
Carbon						
bisulfide (liquid)	T65.4X1-	T65.4X2-	T65.4X3-	T65.4X4-	-	-
vapor	T65.4X1-	T65.4X2-	T65.4X3-	T65.4X4-	-	-
dioxide (gas)	T59.7X1-	T59.7X2-	T59.7X3-	T59.7X4-	-	-
medicinal	T41.5X1-	T41.5X2-	T41.5X3-	T41.5X4-	T41.5X5-	T41.5X6-
nonmedicinal	T59.7X1-	T59.7X2-	T59.7X3-	T59.7X4-	-	-
snow	T49.4X1-	T49.4X2-	T49.4X3-	T49.4X4-	T49.4X5-	T49.4X6-
disulfide (liquid)	T65.4X1-	T65.4X2-	T65.4X3-	T65.4X4-	-	-
vapor	T65.4X1-	T65.4X2-	T65.4X3-	T65.4X4-	-	-
monoxide (from incomplete combustion)	T58.91X-	T58.92X-	T58.93X-	T58.94X-	-	-
blast furnace gas	T58.8X1-	T58.8X2-	T58.8X3-	T58.8X4-	-	-
butane (distributed in mobile container)	T58.11X-	T58.12X-	T58.13X-	T58.14X-	-	-
distributed through pipes	T58.11X-	T58.12X-	T58.13X-	T58.14X-	-	-
charcoal fumes	T58.2X1-	T58.2X2-	T58.2X3-	T58.2X4-	-	-
coal	T58.2X1-	T58.2X2-	T58.2X3-	T58.2X4-	-	-
coke (in domestic stoves, fireplaces)	T58.2X1-	T58.2X2-	T58.2X3-	T58.2X4-	-	-
gas (piped)	T58.11X-	T58.12X-	T58.13X-	T58.14X-	-	-
solid (in domestic stoves, fireplaces)	T58.2X1-	T58.2X2-	T58.2X3-	T58.2X4-	-	-
exhaust gas (motor) not in transit	T58.01X-	T58.02X-	T58.03X-	T58.04X-	-	-
combustion engine, any not in watercraft	T58.01X-	T58.02X-	T58.03X-	T58.04X-	-	-
farm tractor, not in transit	T58.01X-	T58.02X-	T58.03X-	T58.04X-	-	-
gas engine	T58.01X-	T58.02X-	T58.03X-	T58.04X-	-	-
motor pump	T58.01X-	T58.02X-	T58.03X-	T58.04X-	-	-
motor vehicle, not in transit	T58.01X-	T58.02X-	T58.03X-	T58.04X-	-	-
fuel (in domestic use)	T58.2X1-	T58.2X2-	T58.2X3-	T58.2X4-	-	-
gas (piped)	T58.11X-	T58.12X-	T58.13X-	T58.14X-	-	-
in mobile container	T58.11X-	T58.12X-	T58.13X-	T58.14X-	-	-
piped (natural)	T58.11X-	T58.12X-	T58.13X-	T58.14X-	-	-
utility	T58.11X-	T58.12X-	T58.13X-	T58.14X-	-	-
in mobile container	T58.11X-	T58.12X-	T58.13X-	T58.14X-	-	-
illuminating gas	T58.11X-	T58.12X-	T58.13X-	T58.14X-	-	-
industrial fuels or gases, any	T58.8X1-	T58.8X2-	T58.8X3-	T58.8X4-	-	-
kerosene (in domestic stoves, fireplaces)	T58.2X1-	T58.2X2-	T58.2X3-	T58.2X4-	-	-
kiln gas or vapor	T58.8X1-	T58.8X2-	T58.8X3-	T58.8X4-	-	-
motor exhaust gas, not in transit	T58.01X-	T58.02X-	T58.03X-	T58.04X-	-	-
piped gas (manufactured) (natural)	T58.11X-	T58.12X-	T58.13X-	T58.14X-	-	-
producer gas	T58.8X1-	T58.8X2-	T58.8X3-	T58.8X4-	-	-
propane (distributed in mobile container)	T58.11X-	T58.12X-	T58.13X-	T58.14X-	-	-
distributed through pipes	T58.11X-	T58.12X-	T58.13X-	T58.14X-	-	-
specified source NEC	T58.8X1-	T58.8X2-	T58.8X3-	T58.8X4-	-	-
stove gas	T58.11X-	T58.12X-	T58.13X-	T58.14X-	-	-
piped	T58.11X-	T58.12X-	T58.13X-	T58.14X-	-	-
utility gas	T58.11X-	T58.12X-	T58.13X-	T58.14X-	-	-
piped	T58.11X-	T58.12X-	T58.13X-	T58.14X-	-	-
water gas	T58.11X-	T58.12X-	T58.13X-	T58.14X-	-	-
wood (in domestic stoves, fireplaces)	T58.2X1-	T58.2X2-	T58.2X3-	T58.2X4-	-	-
tetrachloride (vapor) NEC	T53.0X1-	T53.0X2-	T53.0X3-	T53.0X4-	-	-
liquid (cleansing agent) NEC	T53.0X1-	T53.0X2-	T53.0X3-	T53.0X4-	-	-
solvent	T53.0X1-	T53.0X2-	T53.0X3-	T53.0X4-	-	-
Carbonic acid gas	T59.7X1-	T59.7X2-	T59.7X3-	T59.7X4-	-	-
anhydrase inhibitor NEC	T50.2X1-	T50.2X2-	T50.2X3-	T50.2X4-	T50.2X5-	T50.2X6-
Carbophenothion	T60.0X1-	T60.0X2-	T60.0X3-	T60.0X4-	-	-
Carboplatin	T45.1X1-	T45.1X2-	T45.1X3-	T45.1X4-	T45.1X5-	T45.1X6-
Carboprost	T48.0X1-	T48.0X2-	T48.0X3-	T48.0X4-	T48.0X5-	T48.0X6-
Carboquone	T45.1X1-	T45.1X2-	T45.1X3-	T45.1X4-	T45.1X5-	T45.1X6-
Carbowax	T49.3X1-	T49.3X2-	T49.3X3-	T49.3X4-	T49.3X5-	T49.3X6-
Carboxymethyl-cellulose	T47.4X1-	T47.4X2-	T47.4X3-	T47.4X4-	T47.4X5-	T47.4X6-
S-Carboxymethyl-cysteine	T48.4X1-	T48.4X2-	T48.4X3-	T48.4X4-	T48.4X5-	T48.4X6-
Carbrital	T42.3X1-	T42.3X2-	T42.3X3-	T42.3X4-	T42.3X5-	T42.3X6-
Carbromal	T42.6X1-	T42.6X2-	T42.6X3-	T42.6X4-	T42.6X5-	T42.6X6-
Carbutamide	T38.3X1-	T38.3X2-	T38.3X3-	T38.3X4-	T38.3X5-	T38.3X6-
Carbuterol	T48.6X1-	T48.6X2-	T48.6X3-	T48.6X4-	T48.6X5-	T48.6X6-
Cardiac						
depressants	T46.2X1-	T46.2X2-	T46.2X3-	T46.2X4-	T46.2X5-	T46.2X6-
rhythm regulator	T46.2X1-	T46.2X2-	T46.2X3-	T46.2X4-	T46.2X5-	T46.2X6-
specified NEC	T46.2X1-	T46.2X2-	T46.2X3-	T46.2X4-	T46.2X5-	T46.2X6-
Cardiografin	T50.8X1-	T50.8X2-	T50.8X3-	T50.8X4-	T50.8X5-	T50.8X6-
Cardio-green	T50.8X1-	T50.8X2-	T50.8X3-	T50.8X4-	T50.8X5-	T50.8X6-

Substance	Poisoning, Accidental (unintentional)	Poisoning, Intentional self-harm	Poisoning, Assault	Poisoning, Undetermined	Adverse effect	Underdosing
Cardiotonic (glycoside) **NEC**	T46.0X1-	T46.0X2-	T46.0X3-	T46.0X4-	T46.0X5-	T46.0X6-
Cardiovascular drug NEC	T46.901-	T46.902-	T46.903-	T46.904-	T46.905-	T46.906-
Cardrase	T50.2X1-	T50.2X2-	T50.2X3-	T50.2X4-	T50.2X5-	T50.2X6-
Carfecillin	T36.0X1-	T36.0X2-	T36.0X3-	T36.0X4-	T36.0X5-	T36.0X6-
Carfenazine	T43.3X1-	T43.3X2-	T43.3X3-	T43.3X4-	T43.3X5-	T43.3X6-
Carfusin	T49.0X1-	T49.0X2-	T49.0X3-	T49.0X4-	T49.0X5-	T49.0X6-
Carindacillin	T36.0X1-	T36.0X2-	T36.0X3-	T36.0X4-	T36.0X5-	T36.0X6-
Carisoprodol	T42.8X1-	T42.8X2-	T42.8X3-	T42.8X4-	T42.8X5-	T42.8X6-
Carmellose	T47.4X1-	T47.4X2-	T47.4X3-	T47.4X4-	T47.4X5-	T47.4X6-
Carminative	T47.5X1-	T47.5X2-	T47.5X3-	T47.5X4-	T47.5X5-	T47.5X6-
Carmofur	T45.1X1-	T45.1X2-	T45.1X3-	T45.1X4-	T45.1X5-	T45.1X6-
Carmustine	T45.1X1-	T45.1X2-	T45.1X3-	T45.1X4-	T45.1X5-	T45.1X6-
Carotene	T45.2X1-	T45.2X2-	T45.2X3-	T45.2X4-	T45.2X5-	T45.2X6-
Carphenazine	T43.3X1-	T43.3X2-	T43.3X3-	T43.3X4-	T43.3X5-	T43.3X6-
Carpipramine	T42.4X1-	T42.4X2-	T42.4X3-	T42.4X4-	T42.4X5-	T42.4X6-
Carprofen	T39.311-	T39.312-	T39.313-	T39.314-	T39.315-	T39.316-
Carpronium chloride	T44.3X1-	T44.3X2-	T44.3X3-	T44.3X4-	T44.3X5-	T44.3X6-
Carrageenan	T47.8X1-	T47.8X2-	T47.8X3-	T47.8X4-	T47.8X5-	T47.8X6-
Carteolol	T44.7X1-	T44.7X2-	T44.7X3-	T44.7X4-	T44.7X5-	T44.7X6-
Carter's Little Pills	T47.2X1-	T47.2X2-	T47.2X3-	T47.2X4-	T47.2X5-	T47.2X6-
Cascara (sagrada)	T47.2X1-	T47.2X2-	T47.2X3-	T47.2X4-	T47.2X5-	T47.2X6-
Cassava	T62.2X1-	T62.2X2-	T62.2X3-	T62.2X4-	-	-
Castellani's paint	T49.0X1-	T49.0X2-	T49.0X3-	T49.0X4-	T49.0X5-	T49.0X6-
Castor						
bean	T62.2X1-	T62.2X2-	T62.2X3-	T62.2X4-	-	-
oil	T47.2X1-	T47.2X2-	T47.2X3-	T47.2X4-	T47.2X5-	T47.2X6-
Catalase	T45.3X1-	T45.3X2-	T45.3X3-	T45.3X4-	T45.3X5-	T45.3X6-
Caterpillar (sting)	T63.431-	T63.432-	T63.433-	T63.434-	-	-
Catha (edulis) (tea)	T43.691-	T43.692-	T43.693-	T43.694-	-	-
Cathartic NEC	T47.4X1-	T47.4X2-	T47.4X3-	T47.4X4-	T47.4X5-	T47.4X6-
anthacene derivative	T47.2X1-	T47.2X2-	T47.2X3-	T47.2X4-	T47.2X5-	T47.2X6-
bulk	T47.4X1-	T47.4X2-	T47.4X3-	T47.4X4-	T47.4X5-	T47.4X6-
contact	T47.2X1-	T47.2X2-	T47.2X3-	T47.2X4-	T47.2X5-	T47.2X6-
emollient NEC	T47.4X1-	T47.4X2-	T47.4X3-	T47.4X4-	T47.4X5-	T47.4X6-
irritant NEC	T47.2X1-	T47.2X2-	T47.2X3-	T47.2X4-	T47.2X5-	T47.2X6-
mucilage	T47.4X1-	T47.4X2-	T47.4X3-	T47.4X4-	T47.4X5-	T47.4X6-
saline	T47.3X1-	T47.3X2-	T47.3X3-	T47.3X4-	T47.3X5-	T47.3X6-
vegetable	T47.2X1-	T47.2X2-	T47.2X3-	T47.2X4-	T47.2X5-	T47.2X6-
Cathine	T50.5X1-	T50.5X2-	T50.5X3-	T50.5X4-	T50.5X5-	T50.5X6-
Cathomycin	T36.8X1-	T36.8X2-	T36.8X3-	T36.8X4-	T36.8X5-	T36.8X6-
Cation exchange resin	T50.3X1-	T50.3X2-	T50.3X3-	T50.3X4-	T50.3X5-	T50.3X6-
Caustic (s) **NEC**	T54.91X-	T54.92X-	T54.93X-	T54.94X-	-	-
alkali	T54.3X1-	T54.3X2-	T54.3X3-	T54.3X4-	-	-
hydroxide	T54.3X1-	T54.3X2-	T54.3X3-	T54.3X4-	-	-
potash	T54.3X1-	T54.3X2-	T54.3X3-	T54.3X4-	-	-
soda	T54.3X1-	T54.3X2-	T54.3X3-	T54.3X4-	-	-
specified NEC	T54.91X-	T54.92X-	T54.93X-	T54.94X-	-	-
Ceepryn	T49.0X1-	T49.0X2-	T49.0X3-	T49.0X4-	T49.0X5-	T49.0X6-
ENT agent	T49.6X1-	T49.6X2-	T49.6X3-	T49.6X4-	T49.6X5-	T49.6X6-
lozenges	T49.6X1-	T49.6X2-	T49.6X3-	T49.6X4-	T49.6X5-	T49.6X6-
Cefacetrile	T36.1X1-	T36.1X2-	T36.1X3-	T36.1X4-	T36.1X5-	T36.1X6-
Cefaclor	T36.1X1-	T36.1X2-	T36.1X3-	T36.1X4-	T36.1X5-	T36.1X6-
Cefadroxil	T36.1X1-	T36.1X2-	T36.1X3-	T36.1X4-	T36.1X5-	T36.1X6-
Cefalexin	T36.1X1-	T36.1X2-	T36.1X3-	T36.1X4-	T36.1X5-	T36.1X6-
Cefaloglycin	T36.1X1-	T36.1X2-	T36.1X3-	T36.1X4-	T36.1X5-	T36.1X6-
Cefaloridine	T36.1X1-	T36.1X2-	T36.1X3-	T36.1X4-	T36.1X5-	T36.1X6-
Cefalosporins	T36.1X1-	T36.1X2-	T36.1X3-	T36.1X4-	T36.1X5-	T36.1X6-
Cefalotin	T36.1X1-	T36.1X2-	T36.1X3-	T36.1X4-	T36.1X5-	T36.1X6-
Cefamandole	T36.1X1-	T36.1X2-	T36.1X3-	T36.1X4-	T36.1X5-	T36.1X6-
Cefamycin antibiotic	T36.1X1-	T36.1X2-	T36.1X3-	T36.1X4-	T36.1X5-	T36.1X6-
Cefapirin	T36.1X1-	T36.1X2-	T36.1X3-	T36.1X4-	T36.1X5-	T36.1X6-
Cefatrizine	T36.1X1-	T36.1X2-	T36.1X3-	T36.1X4-	T36.1X5-	T36.1X6-
Cefazedone	T36.1X1-	T36.1X2-	T36.1X3-	T36.1X4-	T36.1X5-	T36.1X6-
Cefazolin	T36.1X1-	T36.1X2-	T36.1X3-	T36.1X4-	T36.1X5-	T36.1X6-
Cefbuperazone	T36.1X1-	T36.1X2-	T36.1X3-	T36.1X4-	T36.1X5-	T36.1X6-
Cefetamet	T36.1X1-	T36.1X2-	T36.1X3-	T36.1X4-	T36.1X5-	T36.1X6-
Cefixime	T36.1X1-	T36.1X2-	T36.1X3-	T36.1X4-	T36.1X5-	T36.1X6-
Cefmenoxime	T36.1X1-	T36.1X2-	T36.1X3-	T36.1X4-	T36.1X5-	T36.1X6-
Cefmetazole	T36.1X1-	T36.1X2-	T36.1X3-	T36.1X4-	T36.1X5-	T36.1X6-
Cefminox	T36.1X1-	T36.1X2-	T36.1X3-	T36.1X4-	T36.1X5-	T36.1X6-
Cefonicid	T36.1X1-	T36.1X2-	T36.1X3-	T36.1X4-	T36.1X5-	T36.1X6-
Cefoperazone	T36.1X1-	T36.1X2-	T36.1X3-	T36.1X4-	T36.1X5-	T36.1X6-
Ceforanide	T36.1X1-	T36.1X2-	T36.1X3-	T36.1X4-	T36.1X5-	T36.1X6-
Cefotaxime	T36.1X1-	T36.1X2-	T36.1X3-	T36.1X4-	T36.1X5-	T36.1X6-
Cefotetan	T36.1X1-	T36.1X2-	T36.1X3-	T36.1X4-	T36.1X5-	T36.1X6-
Cefotiam	T36.1X1-	T36.1X2-	T36.1X3-	T36.1X4-	T36.1X5-	T36.1X6-
Cefoxitin	T36.1X1-	T36.1X2-	T36.1X3-	T36.1X4-	T36.1X5-	T36.1X6-
Cefpimizole	T36.1X1-	T36.1X2-	T36.1X3-	T36.1X4-	T36.1X5-	T36.1X6-

Substance	Poisoning, Accidental (unintentional)	Poisoning, Intentional self-harm	Poisoning, Assault	Poisoning, Undetermined	Adverse effect	Underdosing
Cefpiramide	T36.1X1-	T36.1X2-	T36.1X3-	T36.1X4-	T36.1X5-	T36.1X6-
Cefradine	T36.1X1-	T36.1X2-	T36.1X3-	T36.1X4-	T36.1X5-	T36.1X6-
Cefroxadine	T36.1X1-	T36.1X2-	T36.1X3-	T36.1X4-	T36.1X5-	T36.1X6-
Cefsulodin	T36.1X1-	T36.1X2-	T36.1X3-	T36.1X4-	T36.1X5-	T36.1X6-
Ceftazidime	T36.1X1-	T36.1X2-	T36.1X3-	T36.1X4-	T36.1X5-	T36.1X6-
Cefteram	T36.1X1-	T36.1X2-	T36.1X3-	T36.1X4-	T36.1X5-	T36.1X6-
Ceftezole	T36.1X1-	T36.1X2-	T36.1X3-	T36.1X4-	T36.1X5-	T36.1X6-
Ceftizoxime	T36.1X1-	T36.1X2-	T36.1X3-	T36.1X4-	T36.1X5-	T36.1X6-
Ceftriaxone	T36.1X1-	T36.1X2-	T36.1X3-	T36.1X4-	T36.1X5-	T36.1X6-
Cefuroxime	T36.1X1-	T36.1X2-	T36.1X3-	T36.1X4-	T36.1X5-	T36.1X6-
Cefuzonam	T36.1X1-	T36.1X2-	T36.1X3-	T36.1X4-	T36.1X5-	T36.1X6-
Celestone	T38.0X1-	T38.0X2-	T38.0X3-	T38.0X4-	T38.0X5-	T38.0X6-
topical	T49.0X1-	T49.0X2-	T49.0X3-	T49.0X4-	T49.0X5-	T49.0X6-
Celiprolol	T44.7X1-	T44.7X2-	T44.7X3-	T44.7X4-	T44.7X5-	T44.7X6-
Cell stimulants and proliferants	T49.8X1-	T49.8X2-	T49.8X3-	T49.8X4-	T49.8X5-	T49.8X6-
Cellosolve	T52.91X-	T52.92X-	T52.93X-	T52.94X-	-	-
Cellulose						
cathartic	T47.4X1-	T47.4X2-	T47.4X3-	T47.4X4-	T47.4X5-	T47.4X6-
hydroxyethyl	T47.4X1-	T47.4X2-	T47.4X3-	T47.4X4-	T47.4X5-	T47.4X6-
nitrates (topical)	T49.3X1-	T49.3X2-	T49.3X3-	T49.3X4-	T49.3X5-	T49.3X6-
oxidized	T49.4X1-	T49.4X2-	T49.4X3-	T49.4X4-	T49.4X5-	T49.4X6-
Centipede (bite)	T63.411-	T63.412-	T63.413-	T63.414-	-	-
Central nervous system						
depressants	T42.71X-	T42.72X-	T42.73X-	T42.74X-	T42.75X-	T42.76X-
anesthetic (general) NEC	T41.201-	T41.202-	T41.203-	T41.204-	T41.205-	T41.206-
gases NEC	T41.0X1-	T41.0X2-	T41.0X3-	T41.0X4-	T41.0X5-	T41.0X6-
intravenous	T41.1X1-	T41.1X2-	T41.1X3-	T41.1X4-	T41.1X5-	T41.1X6-
barbiturates	T42.3X1-	T42.3X2-	T42.3X3-	T42.3X4-	T42.3X5-	T42.3X6-
benzodiazepines	T42.4X1-	T42.4X2-	T42.4X3-	T42.4X4-	T42.4X5-	T42.4X6-
bromides	T42.6X1-	T42.6X2-	T42.6X3-	T42.6X4-	T42.6X5-	T42.6X6-
cannabis sativa	T40.7X1-	T40.7X2-	T40.7X3-	T40.7X4-	T40.7X5-	T40.7X6-
chloral hydrate	T42.6X1-	T42.6X2-	T42.6X3-	T42.6X4-	T42.6X5-	T42.6X6-
ethanol	T51.0X1-	T51.0X2-	T51.0X3-	T51.0X4-	-	-
hallucinogenics	T40.901-	T40.902-	T40.903-	T40.904-	T40.905-	T40.906-
hypnotics	T42.71X-	T42.72X-	T42.73X-	T42.74X-	T42.75X-	T42.76X-
specified NEC	T42.6X1-	T42.6X2-	T42.6X3-	T42.6X4-	T42.6X5-	T42.6X6-
muscle relaxants	T42.8X1-	T42.8X2-	T42.8X3-	T42.8X4-	T42.8X5-	T42.8X6-
paraldehyde	T42.6X1-	T42.6X2-	T42.6X3-	T42.6X4-	T42.6X5-	T42.6X6-
sedatives; sedative-hypnotics	T42.71X-	T42.72X-	T42.73X-	T42.74X-	T42.75X-	T42.76X-
mixed NEC	T42.6X1-	T42.6X2-	T42.6X3-	T42.6X4-	T42.6X5-	T42.6X6-
specified NEC	T42.6X1-	T42.6X2-	T42.6X3-	T42.6X4-	T42.6X5-	T42.6X6-
muscle-tone depressants	T42.8X1-	T42.8X2-	T42.8X3-	T42.8X4-	T42.8X5-	T42.8X6-
stimulants	T43.601-	T43.602-	T43.603-	T43.604-	T43.605-	T43.606-
amphetamines	T43.621-	T43.622-	T43.623-	T43.624-	T43.625-	T43.626-
analeptics	T50.7X1-	T50.7X2-	T50.7X3-	T50.7X4-	T50.7X5-	T50.7X6-
antidepressants	T43.201-	T43.202-	T43.203-	T43.204-	T43.205-	T43.206-
opiate antagonists	T50.7X1-	T50.7X2-	T50.7X3-	T50.7X4-	T50.7X5-	T50.7X6-
specified NEC	T43.691-	T43.692-	T43.693-	T43.694-	T43.695-	T43.696-
Cephalexin	T36.1X1-	T36.1X2-	T36.1X3-	T36.1X4-	T36.1X5-	T36.1X6-
Cephaloglycin	T36.1X1-	T36.1X2-	T36.1X3-	T36.1X4-	T36.1X5-	T36.1X6-
Cephaloridine	T36.1X1-	T36.1X2-	T36.1X3-	T36.1X4-	T36.1X5-	T36.1X6-
Cephalosporins	T36.1X1-	T36.1X2-	T36.1X3-	T36.1X4-	T36.1X5-	T36.1X6-
N (adicillin)	T36.0X1-	T36.0X2-	T36.0X3-	T36.0X4-	T36.0X5-	T36.0X6-
Cephalothin	T36.1X1-	T36.1X2-	T36.1X3-	T36.1X4-	T36.1X5-	T36.1X6-
Cephalotin	T36.1X1-	T36.1X2-	T36.1X3-	T36.1X4-	T36.1X5-	T36.1X6-
Cephradine	T36.1X1-	T36.1X2-	T36.1X3-	T36.1X4-	T36.1X5-	T36.1X6-
Cerbera (odallam)	T62.2X1-	T62.2X2-	T62.2X3-	T62.2X4-	-	-
Cerberin	T46.0X1-	T46.0X2-	T46.0X3-	T46.0X4-	T46.0X5-	T46.0X6-
Cerebral stimulants	T43.601-	T43.602-	T43.603-	T43.604-	T43.605-	T43.606-
psychotherapeutic	T43.601-	T43.602-	T43.603-	T43.604-	T43.605-	T43.606-
specified NEC	T43.691-	T43.692-	T43.693-	T43.694-	T43.695-	T43.696-
Cerium oxalate	T45.0X1-	T45.0X2-	T45.0X3-	T45.0X4-	T45.0X5-	T45.0X6-
Cerous oxalate	T45.0X1-	T45.0X2-	T45.0X3-	T45.0X4-	T45.0X5-	T45.0X6-
Ceruletide	T50.8X1-	T50.8X2-	T50.8X3-	T50.8X4-	T50.8X5-	T50.8X6-
Cetalkonium (chloride)	T49.0X1-	T49.0X2-	T49.0X3-	T49.0X4-	T49.0X5-	T49.0X6-
Cethexonium chloride	T49.0X1-	T49.0X2-	T49.0X3-	T49.0X4-	T49.0X5-	T49.0X6-
Cetiedil	T46.7X1-	T46.7X2-	T46.7X3-	T46.7X4-	T46.7X5-	T46.7X6-
Cetirizine	T45.0X1-	T45.0X2-	T45.0X3-	T45.0X4-	T45.0X5-	T45.0X6-
Cetomacrogol	T50.991-	T50.992-	T50.993-	T50.994-	T50.995-	T50.996-
Cetotiamine	T45.2X1-	T45.2X2-	T45.2X3-	T45.2X4-	T45.2X5-	T45.2X6-
Cetoxime	T45.0X1-	T45.0X2-	T45.0X3-	T45.0X4-	T45.0X5-	T45.0X6-
Cetraxate	T47.1X1-	T47.1X2-	T47.1X3-	T47.1X4-	T47.1X5-	T47.1X6-
Cetrimide	T49.0X1-	T49.0X2-	T49.0X3-	T49.0X4-	T49.0X5-	T49.0X6-
Cetrimonium (bromide)	T49.0X1-	T49.0X2-	T49.0X3-	T49.0X4-	T49.0X5-	T49.0X6-
Cetylpyridinium chloride	T49.0X1-	T49.0X2-	T49.0X3-	T49.0X4-	T49.0X5-	T49.0X6-
ENT agent	T49.6X1-	T49.6X2-	T49.6X3-	T49.6X4-	T49.6X5-	T49.6X6-
lozenges	T49.6X1-	T49.6X2-	T49.6X3-	T49.6X4-	T49.6X5-	T49.6X6-

Substance	Poisoning, Accidental (unintentional)	Poisoning, Intentional self-harm	Poisoning, Assault	Poisoning, Undetermined	Adverse effect	Underdosing
Cevadilla — see Sabadilla						
Cevitamic acid	T45.2X1-	T45.2X2-	T45.2X3-	T45.2X4-	T45.2X5-	T45.2X6-
Chalk, precipitated	T47.1X1-	T47.1X2-	T47.1X3-	T47.1X4-	T47.1X5-	T47.1X6-
Chamomile	T49.0X1-	T49.0X2-	T49.0X3-	T49.0X4-	T49.0X5-	T49.0X6-
Ch'an su	T46.0X1-	T46.0X2-	T46.0X3-	T46.0X4-	T46.0X5-	T46.0X6-
Charcoal	T47.6X1-	T47.6X2-	T47.6X3-	T47.6X4-	T47.6X5-	T47.6X6-
activated — see also Charcoal, medicinal	T47.6X1-	T47.6X2-	T47.6X3-	T47.6X4-	T47.6X5-	T47.6X6-
fumes (Carbon monoxide)	T58.2X1-	T58.2X2-	T58.2X3-	T58.2X4-	-	-
industrial	T58.8X1-	T58.8X2-	T58.8X3-	T58.8X4-	-	-
medicinal (activated)	T47.6X1-	T47.6X2-	T47.6X3-	T47.6X4-	T47.6X5-	T47.6X6-
antidiarrheal	T47.6X1-	T47.6X2-	T47.6X3-	T47.6X4-	T47.6X5-	T47.6X6-
poison control	T47.8X1-	T47.8X2-	T47.8X3-	T47.8X4-	T47.8X5-	T47.8X6-
specified use other than for diarrhea	T47.8X1-	T47.8X2-	T47.8X3-	T47.8X4-	T47.8X5-	T47.8X6-
topical	T49.8X1-	T49.8X2-	T49.8X3-	T49.8X4-	T49.8X5-	T49.8X6-
Chaulmosulfone	T37.1X1-	T37.1X2-	T37.1X3-	T37.1X4-	T37.1X5-	T37.1X6-
Chelating agent NEC	T50.6X1-	T50.6X2-	T50.6X3-	T50.6X4-	T50.6X5-	T50.6X6-
Chelidonium majus	T62.2X1-	T62.2X2-	T62.2X3-	T62.2X4-	-	-
Chemical substance NEC	T65.91X-	T65.92X-	T65.93X-	T65.94X-	-	-
Chenodeoxycholic acid	T47.5X1-	T47.5X2-	T47.5X3-	T47.5X4-	T47.5X5-	T47.5X6-
Chenodiol	T47.5X1-	T47.5X2-	T47.5X3-	T47.5X4-	T47.5X5-	T47.5X6-
Chenopodium	T37.4X1-	T37.4X2-	T37.4X3-	T37.4X4-	T37.4X5-	T37.4X6-
Cherry laurel	T62.2X1-	T62.2X2-	T62.2X3-	T62.2X4-	-	-
Chinidin (e)	T46.2X1-	T46.2X2-	T46.2X3-	T46.2X4-	T46.2X5-	T46.2X6-
Chiniofon	T37.8X1-	T37.8X2-	T37.8X3-	T37.8X4-	T37.8X5-	T37.8X6-
Chlophedianol	T48.3X1-	T48.3X2-	T48.3X3-	T48.3X4-	T48.3X5-	T48.3X6-
Chloral	T42.6X1-	T42.6X2-	T42.6X3-	T42.6X4-	T42.6X5-	T42.6X6-
derivative	T42.6X1-	T42.6X2-	T42.6X3-	T42.6X4-	T42.6X5-	T42.6X6-
hydrate	T42.6X1-	T42.6X2-	T42.6X3-	T42.6X4-	T42.6X5-	T42.6X6-
Chloralamide	T42.6X1-	T42.6X2-	T42.6X3-	T42.6X4-	T42.6X5-	T42.6X6-
Chloralodol	T42.6X1-	T42.6X2-	T42.6X3-	T42.6X4-	T42.6X5-	T42.6X6-
Chloralose	T60.4X1-	T60.4X2-	T60.4X3-	T60.4X4-	-	-
Chlorambucil	T45.1X1-	T45.1X2-	T45.1X3-	T45.1X4-	T45.1X5-	T45.1X6-
Chloramine	T57.8X1-	T57.8X2-	T57.8X3-	T57.8X4-	-	-
T	T49.0X1-	T49.0X2-	T49.0X3-	T49.0X4-	T49.0X5-	T49.0X6-
topical	T49.0X1-	T49.0X2-	T49.0X3-	T49.0X4-	T49.0X5-	T49.0X6-
Chloramphenicol	T36.2X1-	T36.2X2-	T36.2X3-	T36.2X4-	T36.2X5-	T36.2X6-
ENT agent	T49.6X1-	T49.6X2-	T49.6X3-	T49.6X4-	T49.6X5-	T49.6X6-
ophthalmic preparation	T49.5X1-	T49.5X2-	T49.5X3-	T49.5X4-	T49.5X5-	T49.5X6-
topical NEC	T49.0X1-	T49.0X2-	T49.0X3-	T49.0X4-	T49.0X5-	T49.0X6-
Chlorate (potassium) (sodium) NEC	T60.3X1-	T60.3X2-	T60.3X3-	T60.3X4-	-	-
herbicide	T60.3X1-	T60.3X2-	T60.3X3-	T60.3X4-	-	-
Chlorazanil	T50.2X1-	T50.2X2-	T50.2X3-	T50.2X4-	T50.2X5-	T50.2X6-
Chlorbenzene, chlorbenzol	T53.7X1-	T53.7X2-	T53.7X3-	T53.7X4-	-	-
Chlorbenzoxamine	T44.3X1-	T44.3X2-	T44.3X3-	T44.3X4-	T44.3X5-	T44.3X6-
Chlorbutol	T42.6X1-	T42.6X2-	T42.6X3-	T42.6X4-	T42.6X5-	T42.6X6-
Chlorcyclizine	T45.0X1-	T45.0X2-	T45.0X3-	T45.0X4-	T45.0X5-	T45.0X6-
Chlordan (e) (dust)	T60.1X1-	T60.1X2-	T60.1X3-	T60.1X4-	-	-
Chlordantoin	T49.0X1-	T49.0X2-	T49.0X3-	T49.0X4-	T49.0X5-	T49.0X6-
Chlordiazepoxide	T42.4X1-	T42.4X2-	T42.4X3-	T42.4X4-	T42.4X5-	T42.4X6-
Chlordiethyl benzamide	T49.3X1-	T49.3X2-	T49.3X3-	T49.3X4-	T49.3X5-	T49.3X6-
Chloresium	T49.8X1-	T49.8X2-	T49.8X3-	T49.8X4-	T49.8X5-	T49.8X6-
Chlorethiazol	T42.6X1-	T42.6X2-	T42.6X3-	T42.6X4-	T42.6X5-	T42.6X6-
Chlorethyl — see Ethyl chloride						
Chloretone	T42.6X1-	T42.6X2-	T42.6X3-	T42.6X4-	T42.6X5-	T42.6X6-
Chlorex	T53.6X1-	T53.6X2-	T53.6X3-	T53.6X4-	-	-
insecticide	T60.1X1-	T60.1X2-	T60.1X3-	T60.1X4-	-	-
Chlorfenvinphos	T60.0X1-	T60.0X2-	T60.0X3-	T60.0X4-	-	-
Chlorhexadol	T42.6X1-	T42.6X2-	T42.6X3-	T42.6X4-	T42.6X5-	T42.6X6-
Chlorhexamide	T45.1X1-	T45.1X2-	T45.1X3-	T45.1X4-	T45.1X5-	T45.1X6-
Chlorhexidine	T49.0X1-	T49.0X2-	T49.0X3-	T49.0X4-	T49.0X5-	T49.0X6-
Chlorhydroxyquinolin	T49.0X1-	T49.0X2-	T49.0X3-	T49.0X4-	T49.0X5-	T49.0X6-
Chloride of lime (bleach)	T54.3X1-	T54.3X2-	T54.3X3-	T54.3X4-	-	-
Chlorimipramine	T43.011-	T43.012-	T43.013-	T43.014-	T43.015-	T43.016-
Chlorinated						
camphene	T53.6X1-	T53.6X2-	T53.6X3-	T53.6X4-	-	-
diphenyl	T53.7X1-	T53.7X2-	T53.7X3-	T53.7X4-	-	-
hydrocarbons NEC	T53.91X-	T53.92X-	T53.93X-	T53.94X-	-	-
solvents	T53.91X-	T53.92X-	T53.93X-	T53.94X-	-	-
lime (bleach)	T54.3X1-	T54.3X2-	T54.3X3-	T54.3X4-	-	-
and boric acid solution	T49.0X1-	T49.0X2-	T49.0X3-	T49.0X4-	T49.0X5-	T49.0X6-
naphthalene (insecticide)	T60.1X1-	T60.1X2-	T60.1X3-	T60.1X4-	-	-
industrial (non-pesticide)	T53.7X1-	T53.7X2-	T53.7X3-	T53.7X4-	-	-
pesticide NEC	T60.8X1-	T60.8X2-	T60.8X3-	T60.8X4-	-	-
soda — see also sodium hypochlorite						

Chlorinated — Cilazapril *(side tab)*

Table of Drugs and Chemicals *(side tab)*

Substance	Poisoning, Accidental (unintentional)	Poisoning, Intentional self-harm	Poisoning, Assault	Poisoning, Undetermined	Adverse effect	Underdosing
Chlorinated - *continued*						
solution	T49.0X1-	T49.0X2-	T49.0X3-	T49.0X4-	T49.0X5-	T49.0X6-
Chlorine (fumes) (gas)	T59.4X1-	T59.4X2-	T59.4X3-	T59.4X4-	-	-
bleach	T54.3X1-	T54.3X2-	T54.3X3-	T54.3X4-	-	-
compound gas NEC	T59.4X1-	T59.4X2-	T59.4X3-	T59.4X4-	-	-
disinfectant	T59.4X1-	T59.4X2-	T59.4X3-	T59.4X4-	-	-
releasing agents NEC	T59.4X1-	T59.4X2-	T59.4X3-	T59.4X4-	-	-
Chlorisondamine chloride	T46.991-	T46.992-	T46.993-	T46.994-	T46.995-	T46.996-
Chlormadinone	T38.5X1-	T38.5X2-	T38.5X3-	T38.5X4-	T38.5X5-	T38.5X6-
Chlormephos	T60.0X1-	T60.0X2-	T60.0X3-	T60.0X4-		
Chlormerodrin	T50.2X1-	T50.2X2-	T50.2X3-	T50.2X4-	T50.2X5-	T50.2X6-
Chlormethiazole	T42.6X1-	T42.6X2-	T42.6X3-	T42.6X4-	T42.6X5-	T42.6X6-
Chlormethine	T45.1X1-	T45.1X2-	T45.1X3-	T45.1X4-	T45.1X5-	T45.1X6-
Chlormethylenecycline	T36.4X1-	T36.4X2-	T36.4X3-	T36.4X4-	T36.4X5-	T36.4X6-
Chlormezanone	T42.6X1-	T42.6X2-	T42.6X3-	T42.6X4-	T42.6X5-	T42.6X6-
Chloroacetic acid	T60.3X1-	T60.3X2-	T60.3X3-	T60.3X4-	-	-
Chloroacetone	T59.3X1-	T59.3X2-	T59.3X3-	T59.3X4-	-	-
Chloroacetophenone	T59.3X1-	T59.3X2-	T59.3X3-	T59.3X4-	-	-
Chloroaniline	T53.7X1-	T53.7X2-	T53.7X3-	T53.7X4-	-	-
Chlorobenzene, chlorobenzol	T53.7X1-	T53.7X2-	T53.7X3-	T53.7X4-	-	-
Chlorobromomethane (fire extinguisher)	T53.6X1-	T53.6X2-	T53.6X3-	T53.6X4-	-	-
Chlorobutanol	T49.0X1-	T49.0X2-	T49.0X3-	T49.0X4-	T49.0X5-	T49.0X6-
Chlorocresol	T49.0X1-	T49.0X2-	T49.0X3-	T49.0X4-	T49.0X5-	T49.0X6-
Chlorodehydro-methyltestosterone	T38.7X1-	T38.7X2-	T38.7X3-	T38.7X4-	T38.7X5-	T38.7X6-
Chlorodinitrobenzene	T53.7X1-	T53.7X2-	T53.7X3-	T53.7X4-	-	-
dust or vapor	T53.7X1-	T53.7X2-	T53.7X3-	T53.7X4-	-	-
Chlorodiphenyl	T53.7X1-	T53.7X2-	T53.7X3-	T53.7X4-	-	-
Chloroethane — *see* Ethyl chloride						
Chloroethylene	T53.6X1-	T53.6X2-	T53.6X3-	T53.6X4-	-	-
Chlorofluorocarbons	T53.5X1-	T53.5X2-	T53.5X3-	T53.5X4-	-	-
Chloroform (fumes) (vapor)	T53.1X1-	T53.1X2-	T53.1X3-	T53.1X4-	-	-
anesthetic	T41.0X1-	T41.0X2-	T41.0X3-	T41.0X4-	T41.0X5-	T41.0X6-
solvent	T53.1X1-	T53.1X2-	T53.1X3-	T53.1X4-	-	-
water, concentrated	T41.0X1-	T41.0X2-	T41.0X3-	T41.0X4-	T41.0X5-	T41.0X6-
Chloroguanide	T37.2X1-	T37.2X2-	T37.2X3-	T37.2X4-	T37.2X5-	T37.2X6-
Chloromycetin	T36.2X1-	T36.2X2-	T36.2X3-	T36.2X4-	T36.2X5-	T36.2X6-
ENT agent	T49.6X1-	T49.6X2-	T49.6X3-	T49.6X4-	T49.6X5-	T49.6X6-
ophthalmic preparation	T49.5X1-	T49.5X2-	T49.5X3-	T49.5X4-	T49.5X5-	T49.5X6-
otic solution	T49.6X1-	T49.6X2-	T49.6X3-	T49.6X4-	T49.6X5-	T49.6X6-
topical NEC	T49.0X1-	T49.0X2-	T49.0X3-	T49.0X4-	T49.0X5-	T49.0X6-
Chloronitrobenzene	T53.7X1-	T53.7X2-	T53.7X3-	T53.7X4-	-	-
dust or vapor	T53.7X1-	T53.7X2-	T53.7X3-	T53.7X4-	-	-
Chlorophacinone	T60.4X1-	T60.4X2-	T60.4X3-	T60.4X4-	-	-
Chlorophenol	T53.7X1-	T53.7X2-	T53.7X3-	T53.7X4-	-	-
Chlorophenothane	T60.1X1-	T60.1X2-	T60.1X3-	T60.1X4-	-	-
Chlorophyll	T50.991-	T50.992-	T50.993-	T50.994-	T50.995-	T50.996-
Chloropicrin (fumes)	T53.6X1-	T53.6X2-	T53.6X3-	T53.6X4-	-	-
fumigant	T60.8X1-	T60.8X2-	T60.8X3-	T60.8X4-	-	-
fungicide	T60.3X1-	T60.3X2-	T60.3X3-	T60.3X4-	-	-
pesticide	T60.8X1-	T60.8X2-	T60.8X3-	T60.8X4-	-	-
Chloroprocaine	T41.3X1-	T41.3X2-	T41.3X3-	T41.3X4-	T41.3X5-	T41.3X6-
infiltration (subcutaneous)	T41.3X1-	T41.3X2-	T41.3X3-	T41.3X4-	T41.3X5-	T41.3X6-
nerve block (peripheral) (plexus)	T41.3X1-	T41.3X2-	T41.3X3-	T41.3X4-	T41.3X5-	T41.3X6-
spinal	T41.3X1-	T41.3X2-	T41.3X3-	T41.3X4-	T41.3X5-	T41.3X6-
Chloroptic	T49.5X1-	T49.5X2-	T49.5X3-	T49.5X4-	T49.5X5-	T49.5X6-
Chloropurine	T45.1X1-	T45.1X2-	T45.1X3-	T45.1X4-	T45.1X5-	T45.1X6-
Chloropyramine	T45.0X1-	T45.0X2-	T45.0X3-	T45.0X4-	T45.0X5-	T45.0X6-
Chloropyrifos	T60.0X1-	T60.0X2-	T60.0X3-	T60.0X4-	-	-
Chloropyrilene	T45.0X1-	T45.0X2-	T45.0X3-	T45.0X4-	T45.0X5-	T45.0X6-
Chloroquine	T37.2X1-	T37.2X2-	T37.2X3-	T37.2X4-	T37.2X5-	T37.2X6-
Chlorothalonil	T60.3X1-	T60.3X2-	T60.3X3-	T60.3X4-	-	-
Chlorothen	T45.0X1-	T45.0X2-	T45.0X3-	T45.0X4-	T45.0X5-	T45.0X6-
Chlorothiazide	T50.2X1-	T50.2X2-	T50.2X3-	T50.2X4-	T50.2X5-	T50.2X6-
Chlorothymol	T49.4X1-	T49.4X2-	T49.4X3-	T49.4X4-	T49.4X5-	T49.4X6-
Chlorotrianisene	T38.5X1-	T38.5X2-	T38.5X3-	T38.5X4-	T38.5X5-	T38.5X6-
Chlorovinyldichloro-arsine, not in war	T57.0X1-	T57.0X2-	T57.0X3-	T57.0X4-	-	-
Chloroxine	T49.4X1-	T49.4X2-	T49.4X3-	T49.4X4-	T49.4X5-	T49.4X6-
Chloroxylenol	T49.0X1-	T49.0X2-	T49.0X3-	T49.0X4-	T49.0X5-	T49.0X6-
Chlorphenamine	T45.0X1-	T45.0X2-	T45.0X3-	T45.0X4-	T45.0X5-	T45.0X6-
Chlorphenesin	T42.8X1-	T42.8X2-	T42.8X3-	T42.8X4-	T42.8X5-	T42.8X6-
topical (antifungal)	T49.0X1-	T49.0X2-	T49.0X3-	T49.0X4-	T49.0X5-	T49.0X6-
Chlorpheniramine	T45.0X1-	T45.0X2-	T45.0X3-	T45.0X4-	T45.0X5-	T45.0X6-
Chlorphenoxamine	T45.0X1-	T45.0X2-	T45.0X3-	T45.0X4-	T45.0X5-	T45.0X6-

Substance	Poisoning, Accidental (unintentional)	Poisoning, Intentional self-harm	Poisoning, Assault	Poisoning, Undetermined	Adverse effect	Underdosing
Chlorphentermine	T50.5X1-	T50.5X2-	T50.5X3-	T50.5X4-	T50.5X5-	T50.5X6-
Chlorprocaine — *see* Chloroprocaine						
Chlorproguanil	T37.2X1-	T37.2X2-	T37.2X3-	T37.2X4-	T37.2X5-	T37.2X6-
Chlorpromazine	T43.3X1-	T43.3X2-	T43.3X3-	T43.3X4-	T43.3X5-	T43.3X6-
Chlorpropamide	T38.3X1-	T38.3X2-	T38.3X3-	T38.3X4-	T38.3X5-	T38.3X6-
Chlorprothixene	T43.4X1-	T43.4X2-	T43.4X3-	T43.4X4-	T43.4X5-	T43.4X6-
Chlorquinaldol	T49.0X1-	T49.0X2-	T49.0X3-	T49.0X4-	T49.0X5-	T49.0X6-
Chlorquinol	T49.0X1-	T49.0X2-	T49.0X3-	T49.0X4-	T49.0X5-	T49.0X6-
Chlortalidone	T50.2X1-	T50.2X2-	T50.2X3-	T50.2X4-	T50.2X5-	T50.2X6-
Chlortetracycline	T36.4X1-	T36.4X2-	T36.4X3-	T36.4X4-	T36.4X5-	T36.4X6-
Chlorthalidone	T50.2X1-	T50.2X2-	T50.2X3-	T50.2X4-	T50.2X5-	T50.2X6-
Chlorthiophos	T60.0X1-	T60.0X2-	T60.0X3-	T60.0X4-	-	-
Chlortrianisene	T38.5X1-	T38.5X2-	T38.5X3-	T38.5X4-	T38.5X5-	T38.5X6-
Chlor-Trimeton	T45.0X1-	T45.0X2-	T45.0X3-	T45.0X4-	T45.0X5-	T45.0X6-
Chlorthion	T60.0X1-	T60.0X2-	T60.0X3-	T60.0X4-	-	-
Chlorzoxazone	T42.8X1-	T42.8X2-	T42.8X3-	T42.8X4-	T42.8X5-	T42.8X6-
Choke damp	T59.7X1-	T59.7X2-	T59.7X3-	T59.7X4-		
Cholagogues	T47.5X1-	T47.5X2-	T47.5X3-	T47.5X4-	T47.5X5-	T47.5X6-
Cholebrine	T50.8X1-	T50.8X2-	T50.8X3-	T50.8X4-	T50.8X5-	T50.8X6-
Cholecalciferol	T45.2X1-	T45.2X2-	T45.2X3-	T45.2X4-	T45.2X5-	T45.2X6-
Cholecystokinin	T50.8X1-	T50.8X2-	T50.8X3-	T50.8X4-	T50.8X5-	T50.8X6-
Cholera vaccine	T50.A91-	T50.A92-	T50.A93-	T50.A94-	T50.A95-	T50.A96-
Choleretic	T47.5X1-	T47.5X2-	T47.5X3-	T47.5X4-	T47.5X5-	T47.5X6-
Cholesterol-lowering agents	T46.6X1-	T46.6X2-	T46.6X3-	T46.6X4-	T46.6X5-	T46.6X6-
Cholestyramine (resin)	T46.6X1-	T46.6X2-	T46.6X3-	T46.6X4-	T46.6X5-	T46.6X6-
Cholic acid	T47.5X1-	T47.5X2-	T47.5X3-	T47.5X4-	T47.5X5-	T47.5X6-
Choline	T48.6X1-	T48.6X2-	T48.6X3-	T48.6X4-	T48.6X5-	T48.6X6-
chloride	T50.991-	T50.992-	T50.993-	T50.994-	T50.995-	T50.996-
dihydrogen citrate	T50.991-	T50.992-	T50.993-	T50.994-	T50.995-	T50.996-
salicylate	T39.091-	T39.092-	T39.093-	T39.094-	T39.095-	T39.096-
theophyllinate	T48.6X1-	T48.6X2-	T48.6X3-	T48.6X4-	T48.6X5-	T48.6X6-
Cholinergic (drug) **NEC**	T44.1X1-	T44.1X2-	T44.1X3-	T44.1X4-	T44.1X5-	T44.1X6-
muscle tone enhancer	T44.1X1-	T44.1X2-	T44.1X3-	T44.1X4-	T44.1X5-	T44.1X6-
organophosphorus	T44.0X1-	T44.0X2-	T44.0X3-	T44.0X4-	T44.0X5-	T44.0X6-
insecticide	T60.0X1-	T60.0X2-	T60.0X3-	T60.0X4-	-	-
nerve gas	T59.891-	T59.892-	T59.893-	T59.894-		
trimethyl ammonium propanediol	T44.1X1-	T44.1X2-	T44.1X3-	T44.1X4-	T44.1X5-	T44.1X6-
Cholinesterase reactivator	T50.6X1-	T50.6X2-	T50.6X3-	T50.6X4-	T50.6X5-	T50.6X6-
Cholografin	T50.8X1-	T50.8X2-	T50.8X3-	T50.8X4-	T50.8X5-	T50.8X6-
Chorionic gonadotropin	T38.891-	T38.892-	T38.893-	T38.894-	T38.895-	T38.896-
Chromate	T56.2X1-	T56.2X2-	T56.2X3-	T56.2X4-	-	-
dust or mist	T56.2X1-	T56.2X2-	T56.2X3-	T56.2X4-	-	-
lead — *see also* lead	T56.0X1-	T56.0X2-	T56.0X3-	T56.0X4-	-	-
paint	T56.0X1-	T56.0X2-	T56.0X3-	T56.0X4-	-	-
Chromic						
acid	T56.2X1-	T56.2X2-	T56.2X3-	T56.2X4-	-	-
dust or mist	T56.2X1-	T56.2X2-	T56.2X3-	T56.2X4-	-	-
phosphate 32P	T45.1X1-	T45.1X2-	T45.1X3-	T45.1X4-	T45.1X5-	T45.1X6-
Chromium	T56.2X1-	T56.2X2-	T56.2X3-	T56.2X4-	-	-
compounds — *see* Chromate						
sesquioxide	T50.8X1-	T50.8X2-	T50.8X3-	T50.8X4-	T50.8X5-	T50.8X6-
Chromomycin A3	T45.1X1-	T45.1X2-	T45.1X3-	T45.1X4-	T45.1X5-	T45.1X6-
Chromonar	T46.3X1-	T46.3X2-	T46.3X3-	T46.3X4-	T46.3X5-	T46.3X6-
Chromyl chloride	T56.2X1-	T56.2X2-	T56.2X3-	T56.2X4-	-	-
Chrysarobin	T49.4X1-	T49.4X2-	T49.4X3-	T49.4X4-	T49.4X5-	T49.4X6-
Chrysazin	T47.2X1-	T47.2X2-	T47.2X3-	T47.2X4-	T47.2X5-	T47.2X6-
Chymar	T45.3X1-	T45.3X2-	T45.3X3-	T45.3X4-	T45.3X5-	T45.3X6-
ophthalmic preparation	T49.5X1-	T49.5X2-	T49.5X3-	T49.5X4-	T49.5X5-	T49.5X6-
Chymopapain	T45.3X1-	T45.3X2-	T45.3X3-	T45.3X4-	T45.3X5-	T45.3X6-
Chymotrypsin	T45.3X1-	T45.3X2-	T45.3X3-	T45.3X4-	T45.3X5-	T45.3X6-
ophthalmic preparation	T49.5X1-	T49.5X2-	T49.5X3-	T49.5X4-	T49.5X5-	T49.5X6-
Cianidanol	T50.991-	T50.992-	T50.993-	T50.994-	T50.995-	T50.996-
Cianopramine	T43.011-	T43.012-	T43.013-	T43.014-	T43.015-	T43.016-
Cibenzoline	T46.2X1-	T46.2X2-	T46.2X3-	T46.2X4-	T46.2X5-	T46.2X6-
Ciclacillin	T36.0X1-	T36.0X2-	T36.0X3-	T36.0X4-	T36.0X5-	T36.0X6-
Ciclobarbital — *see* Hexobarbital						
Ciclonicate	T46.7X1-	T46.7X2-	T46.7X3-	T46.7X4-	T46.7X5-	T46.7X6-
Ciclopirox (olamine)	T49.0X1-	T49.0X2-	T49.0X3-	T49.0X4-	T49.0X5-	T49.0X6-
Ciclosporin	T45.1X1-	T45.1X2-	T45.1X3-	T45.1X4-	T45.1X5-	T45.1X6-
Cicuta maculata or virosa	T62.2X1-	T62.2X2-	T62.2X3-	T62.2X4-	-	-
Cicutoxin	T62.2X1-	T62.2X2-	T62.2X3-	T62.2X4-	-	-
Cigarette lighter fluid	T52.0X1-	T52.0X2-	T52.0X3-	T52.0X4-	-	-
Cigarettes (tobacco)	T65.221-	T65.222-	T65.223-	T65.224-	-	-
Ciguatoxin	T61.01X-	T61.02X-	T61.03X-	T61.04X-	-	-
Cilazapril	T46.4X1-	T46.4X2-	T46.4X3-	T46.4X4-	T46.4X5-	T46.4X6-

Substance	Poisoning, Accidental (unintentional)	Poisoning, Intentional self-harm	Poisoning, Assault	Poisoning, Undetermined	Adverse effect	Underdosing
Cimetidine	T47.0X1-	T47.0X2-	T47.0X3-	T47.0X4-	T47.0X5-	T47.0X6-
Cimetropium bromide	T44.3X1-	T44.3X2-	T44.3X3-	T44.3X4-	T44.3X5-	T44.3X6-
Cinchocaine	T41.3X1-	T41.3X2-	T41.3X3-	T41.3X4-	T41.3X5-	T41.3X6-
topical (surface)	T41.3X1-	T41.3X2-	T41.3X3-	T41.3X4-	T41.3X5-	T41.3X6-
Cinchona	T37.2X1-	T37.2X2-	T37.2X3-	T37.2X4-	T37.2X5-	T37.2X6-
Cinchonine alkaloids	T37.2X1-	T37.2X2-	T37.2X3-	T37.2X4-	T37.2X5-	T37.2X6-
Cinchophen	T50.4X1-	T50.4X2-	T50.4X3-	T50.4X4-	T50.4X5-	T50.4X6-
Cinepazide	T46.7X1-	T46.7X2-	T46.7X3-	T46.7X4-	T46.7X5-	T46.7X6-
Cinnamedrine	T48.5X1-	T48.5X2-	T48.5X3-	T48.5X4-	T48.5X5-	T48.5X6-
Cinnarizine	T45.0X1-	T45.0X2-	T45.0X3-	T45.0X4-	T45.0X5-	T45.0X6-
Cinoxacin	T37.8X1-	T37.8X2-	T37.8X3-	T37.8X4-	T37.8X5-	T37.8X6-
Ciprofibrate	T46.6X1-	T46.6X2-	T46.6X3-	T46.6X4-	T46.6X5-	T46.6X6-
Ciprofloxacin	T36.8X1-	T36.8X2-	T36.8X3-	T36.8X4-	T36.8X5-	T36.8X6-
Cisapride	T47.8X1-	T47.8X2-	T47.8X3-	T47.8X4-	T47.8X5-	T47.8X6-
Cisplatin	T45.1X1-	T45.1X2-	T45.1X3-	T45.1X4-	T45.1X5-	T45.1X6-
Citalopram	T43.221-	T43.222-	T43.223-	T43.224-	T43.225-	T43.226-
Citanest	T41.3X1-	T41.3X2-	T41.3X3-	T41.3X4-	T41.3X5-	T41.3X6-
infiltration (subcutaneous)	T41.3X1-	T41.3X2-	T41.3X3-	T41.3X4-	T41.3X5-	T41.3X6-
nerve block (peripheral) (plexus)	T41.3X1-	T41.3X2-	T41.3X3-	T41.3X4-	T41.3X5-	T41.3X6-
Citric acid	T47.5X1-	T47.5X2-	T47.5X3-	T47.5X4-	T47.5X5-	T47.5X6-
Citrovorum (factor)	T45.8X1-	T45.8X2-	T45.8X3-	T45.8X4-	T45.8X5-	T45.8X6-
Claviceps purpurea	T62.2X1-	T62.2X2-	T62.2X3-	T62.2X4-	-	-
Clavulanic acid	T36.1X1-	T36.1X2-	T36.1X3-	T36.1X4-	T36.1X5-	T36.1X6-
Cleaner, cleansing agent, type not specified	T65.891-	T65.892-	T65.893-	T65.894-	-	-
of paint or varnish	T52.91X-	T52.92X-	T52.93X-	T52.94X-	-	-
specified type NEC	T65.891-	T65.892-	T65.893-	T65.894-	-	-
Clebopride	T47.8X1-	T47.8X2-	T47.8X3-	T47.8X4-	T47.8X5-	T47.8X6-
Clefamide	T37.3X1-	T37.3X2-	T37.3X3-	T37.3X4-	T37.3X5-	T37.3X6-
Clemastine	T45.0X1-	T45.0X2-	T45.0X3-	T45.0X4-	T45.0X5-	T45.0X6-
Clematis vitalba	T62.2X1-	T62.2X2-	T62.2X3-	T62.2X4-	-	-
Clemizole	T45.0X1-	T45.0X2-	T45.0X3-	T45.0X4-	T45.0X5-	T45.0X6-
penicillin	T36.0X1-	T36.0X2-	T36.0X3-	T36.0X4-	T36.0X5-	T36.0X6-
Clenbuterol	T48.6X1-	T48.6X2-	T48.6X3-	T48.6X4-	T48.6X5-	T48.6X6-
Clidinium bromide	T44.3X1-	T44.3X2-	T44.3X3-	T44.3X4-	T44.3X5-	T44.3X6-
Clindamycin	T36.8X1-	T36.8X2-	T36.8X3-	T36.8X4-	T36.8X5-	T36.8X6-
Clinofibrate	T46.6X1-	T46.6X2-	T46.6X3-	T46.6X4-	T46.6X5-	T46.6X6-
Clioquinol	T37.8X1-	T37.8X2-	T37.8X3-	T37.8X4-	T37.8X5-	T37.8X6-
Cliradon	T40.2X1-	T40.2X2-	T40.2X3-	T40.2X4-	-	-
Clobazam	T42.4X1-	T42.4X2-	T42.4X3-	T42.4X4-	T42.4X5-	T42.4X6-
Clobenzorex	T50.5X1-	T50.5X2-	T50.5X3-	T50.5X4-	T50.5X5-	T50.5X6-
Clobetasol	T49.0X1-	T49.0X2-	T49.0X3-	T49.0X4-	T49.0X5-	T49.0X6-
Clobetasone	T49.0X1-	T49.0X2-	T49.0X3-	T49.0X4-	T49.0X5-	T49.0X6-
Clobutinol	T48.3X1-	T48.3X2-	T48.3X3-	T48.3X4-	T48.3X5-	T48.3X6-
Clocortolone	T38.0X1-	T38.0X2-	T38.0X3-	T38.0X4-	T38.0X5-	T38.0X6-
Clodantoin	T49.0X1-	T49.0X2-	T49.0X3-	T49.0X4-	T49.0X5-	T49.0X6-
Clodronic acid	T50.991-	T50.992-	T50.993-	T50.994-	T50.995-	T50.996-
Clofazimine	T37.1X1-	T37.1X2-	T37.1X3-	T37.1X4-	T37.1X5-	T37.1X6-
Clofedanol	T48.3X1-	T48.3X2-	T48.3X3-	T48.3X4-	T48.3X5-	T48.3X6-
Clofenamide	T50.2X1-	T50.2X2-	T50.2X3-	T50.2X4-	T50.2X5-	T50.2X6-
Clofenotane	T49.0X1-	T49.0X2-	T49.0X3-	T49.0X4-	T49.0X5-	T49.0X6-
Clofezone	T39.2X1-	T39.2X2-	T39.2X3-	T39.2X4-	T39.2X5-	T39.2X6-
Clofibrate	T46.6X1-	T46.6X2-	T46.6X3-	T46.6X4-	T46.6X5-	T46.6X6-
Clofibride	T46.6X1-	T46.6X2-	T46.6X3-	T46.6X4-	T46.6X5-	T46.6X6-
Cloforex	T50.5X1-	T50.5X2-	T50.5X3-	T50.5X4-	T50.5X5-	T50.5X6-
Clomethiazole	T42.6X1-	T42.6X2-	T42.6X3-	T42.6X4-	T42.6X5-	T42.6X6-
Clometocillin	T36.0X1-	T36.0X2-	T36.0X3-	T36.0X4-	T36.0X5-	T36.0X6-
Clomifene	T38.5X1-	T38.5X2-	T38.5X3-	T38.5X4-	T38.5X5-	T38.5X6-
Clomiphene	T38.5X1-	T38.5X2-	T38.5X3-	T38.5X4-	T38.5X5-	T38.5X6-
Clomipramine	T43.011-	T43.012-	T43.013-	T43.014-	T43.015-	T43.016-
Clomocycline	T36.4X1-	T36.4X2-	T36.4X3-	T36.4X4-	T36.4X5-	T36.4X6-
Clonazepam	T42.4X1-	T42.4X2-	T42.4X3-	T42.4X4-	T42.4X5-	T42.4X6-
Clonidine	T46.5X1-	T46.5X2-	T46.5X3-	T46.5X4-	T46.5X5-	T46.5X6-
Clonixin	T39.8X1-	T39.8X2-	T39.8X3-	T39.8X4-	T39.8X5-	T39.8X6-
Clopamide	T50.2X1-	T50.2X2-	T50.2X3-	T50.2X4-	T50.2X5-	T50.2X6-
Clopenthixol	T43.4X1-	T43.4X2-	T43.4X3-	T43.4X4-	T43.4X5-	T43.4X6-
Cloperastine	T48.3X1-	T48.3X2-	T48.3X3-	T48.3X4-	T48.3X5-	T48.3X6-
Clophedianol	T48.3X1-	T48.3X2-	T48.3X3-	T48.3X4-	T48.3X5-	T48.3X6-
Cloponone	T36.2X1-	T36.2X2-	T36.2X3-	T36.2X4-	T36.2X5-	T36.2X6-
Cloprednol	T38.0X1-	T38.0X2-	T38.0X3-	T38.0X4-	T38.0X5-	T38.0X6-
Cloral betaine	T42.6X1-	T42.6X2-	T42.6X3-	T42.6X4-	T42.6X5-	T42.6X6-
Cloramfenicol	T36.2X1-	T36.2X2-	T36.2X3-	T36.2X4-	T36.2X5-	T36.2X6-
Clorazepate (dipotassium)	T42.4X1-	T42.4X2-	T42.4X3-	T42.4X4-	T42.4X5-	T42.4X6-
Clorexolone	T50.2X1-	T50.2X2-	T50.2X3-	T50.2X4-	T50.2X5-	T50.2X6-
Clorfenamine	T45.0X1-	T45.0X2-	T45.0X3-	T45.0X4-	T45.0X5-	T45.0X6-
Clorgiline	T43.1X1-	T43.1X2-	T43.1X3-	T43.1X4-	T43.1X5-	T43.1X6-
Clorotepine	T44.3X1-	T44.3X2-	T44.3X3-	T44.3X4-	T44.3X5-	T44.3X6-

Substance	Poisoning, Accidental (unintentional)	Poisoning, Intentional self-harm	Poisoning, Assault	Poisoning, Undetermined	Adverse effect	Underdosing
Clorox (bleach)	T54.91X-	T54.92X-	T54.93X-	T54.94X-	-	-
Clorprenaline	T48.6X1-	T48.6X2-	T48.6X3-	T48.6X4-	T48.6X5-	T48.6X6-
Clortermine	T50.5X1-	T50.5X2-	T50.5X3-	T50.5X4-	T50.5X5-	T50.5X6-
Clotiapine	T43.591-	T43.592-	T43.593-	T43.594-	T43.595-	T43.596-
Clotiazepam	T42.4X1-	T42.4X2-	T42.4X3-	T42.4X4-	T42.4X5-	T42.4X6-
Clotibric acid	T46.6X1-	T46.6X2-	T46.6X3-	T46.6X4-	T46.6X5-	T46.6X6-
Clotrimazole	T49.0X1-	T49.0X2-	T49.0X3-	T49.0X4-	T49.0X5-	T49.0X6-
Cloxacillin	T36.0X1-	T36.0X2-	T36.0X3-	T36.0X4-	T36.0X5-	T36.0X6-
Cloxazolam	T42.4X1-	T42.4X2-	T42.4X3-	T42.4X4-	T42.4X5-	T42.4X6-
Cloxiquine	T49.0X1-	T49.0X2-	T49.0X3-	T49.0X4-	T49.0X5-	T49.0X6-
Clozapine	T42.4X1-	T42.4X2-	T42.4X3-	T42.4X4-	T42.4X5-	T42.4X6-
Coagulant NEC	T45.7X1-	T45.7X2-	T45.7X3-	T45.7X4-	T45.7X5-	T45.7X6-
Coal (carbon monoxide from — see also Carbon, monoxide, coal	T58.2X1-	T58.2X2-	T58.2X3-	T58.2X4-	-	-
oil — see Kerosene						
tar	T49.1X1-	T49.1X2-	T49.1X3-	T49.1X4-	T49.1X5-	T49.1X6-
fumes	T59.891-	T59.892-	T59.893-	T59.894-	-	-
medicinal (ointment)	T49.4X1-	T49.4X2-	T49.4X3-	T49.4X4-	T49.4X5-	T49.4X6-
analgesics NEC	T39.2X1-	T39.2X2-	T39.2X3-	T39.2X4-	T39.2X5-	T39.2X6-
naphtha (solvent)	T52.0X1-	T52.0X2-	T52.0X3-	T52.0X4-	-	-
Cobalamine	T45.2X1-	T45.2X2-	T45.2X3-	T45.2X4-	T45.2X5-	T45.2X6-
Cobalt (nonmedicinal) (fumes) (industrial)	T56.891-	T56.892-	T56.893-	T56.894-	-	-
medicinal (trace) (chloride)	T45.8X1-	T45.8X2-	T45.8X3-	T45.8X4-	T45.8X5-	T45.8X6-
Cobra (venom)	T63.041-	T63.042-	T63.043-	T63.044-	-	-
Coca (leaf)	T40.5X1-	T40.5X2-	T40.5X3-	T40.5X4-	T40.5X5-	T40.5X6-
Cocaine	T40.5X1-	T40.5X2-	T40.5X3-	T40.5X4-	T40.5X5-	T40.5X6-
topical anesthetic	T41.3X1-	T41.3X2-	T41.3X3-	T41.3X4-	T41.3X5-	T41.3X6-
Cocarboxylase	T45.3X1-	T45.3X2-	T45.3X3-	T45.3X4-	T45.3X5-	T45.3X6-
Coccidioidin	T50.8X1-	T50.8X2-	T50.8X3-	T50.8X4-	T50.8X5-	T50.8X6-
Cocculus indicus	T62.1X1-	T62.1X2-	T62.1X3-	T62.1X4-	-	-
Cochineal	T65.6X1-	T65.6X2-	T65.6X3-	T65.6X4-	-	-
medicinal products	T50.991-	T50.992-	T50.993-	T50.994-	T50.995-	T50.996-
Codeine	T40.2X1-	T40.2X2-	T40.2X3-	T40.2X4-	T40.2X5-	T40.2X6-
Cod-liver oil	T45.2X1-	T45.2X2-	T45.2X3-	T45.2X4-	T45.2X5-	T45.2X6-
Coenzyme A	T50.991-	T50.992-	T50.993-	T50.994-	T50.995-	T50.996-
Coffee	T62.8X1-	T62.8X2-	T62.8X3-	T62.8X4-	-	-
Cogalactoiso-merase	T50.991-	T50.992-	T50.993-	T50.994-	T50.995-	T50.996-
Cogentin	T44.3X1-	T44.3X2-	T44.3X3-	T44.3X4-	T44.3X5-	T44.3X6-
Coke fumes or gas (carbon monoxide)	T58.2X1-	T58.2X2-	T58.2X3-	T58.2X4-	-	-
industrial use	T58.8X1-	T58.8X2-	T58.8X3-	T58.8X4-	-	-
Colace	T47.4X1-	T47.4X2-	T47.4X3-	T47.4X4-	T47.4X5-	T47.4X6-
Colaspase	T45.1X1-	T45.1X2-	T45.1X3-	T45.1X4-	T45.1X5-	T45.1X6-
Colchicine	T50.4X1-	T50.4X2-	T50.4X3-	T50.4X4-	T50.4X5-	T50.4X6-
Colchicum	T62.2X1-	T62.2X2-	T62.2X3-	T62.2X4-	-	-
Cold cream	T49.3X1-	T49.3X2-	T49.3X3-	T49.3X4-	T49.3X5-	T49.3X6-
Colecalciferol	T45.2X1-	T45.2X2-	T45.2X3-	T45.2X4-	T45.2X5-	T45.2X6-
Colestipol	T46.6X1-	T46.6X2-	T46.6X3-	T46.6X4-	T46.6X5-	T46.6X6-
Colestyramine	T46.6X1-	T46.6X2-	T46.6X3-	T46.6X4-	T46.6X5-	T46.6X6-
Colimycin	T36.8X1-	T36.8X2-	T36.8X3-	T36.8X4-	T36.8X5-	T36.8X6-
Colistimethate	T36.8X1-	T36.8X2-	T36.8X3-	T36.8X4-	T36.8X5-	T36.8X6-
Colistin	T36.8X1-	T36.8X2-	T36.8X3-	T36.8X4-	T36.8X5-	T36.8X6-
sulfate (eye preparation)	T49.5X1-	T49.5X2-	T49.5X3-	T49.5X4-	T49.5X5-	T49.5X6-
Collagen	T50.991-	T50.992-	T50.993-	T50.994-	T50.995-	T50.996-
Collagenase	T49.4X1-	T49.4X2-	T49.4X3-	T49.4X4-	T49.4X5-	T49.4X6-
Collodion	T49.3X1-	T49.3X2-	T49.3X3-	T49.3X4-	T49.3X5-	T49.3X6-
Colocynth	T47.2X1-	T47.2X2-	T47.2X3-	T47.2X4-	T47.2X5-	T47.2X6-
Colophony adhesive	T49.3X1-	T49.3X2-	T49.3X3-	T49.3X4-	T49.3X5-	T49.3X6-
Colorant — see also Dye	T50.991-	T50.992-	T50.993-	T50.994-	T50.995-	T50.996-
Coloring matter — see Dye(s)						
Combustion gas (after combustion) — see Carbon, monoxide						
prior to combustion	T59.891-	T59.892-	T59.893-	T59.894-	-	-
Compazine	T43.3X1-	T43.3X2-	T43.3X3-	T43.3X4-	T43.3X5-	T43.3X6-
Compound						
42 (warfarin)	T60.4X1-	T60.4X2-	T60.4X3-	T60.4X4-	-	-
269 (endrin)	T60.1X1-	T60.1X2-	T60.1X3-	T60.1X4-	-	-
497 (dieldrin)	T60.1X1-	T60.1X2-	T60.1X3-	T60.1X4-	-	-
1080 (sodium fluoroacetate)	T60.4X1-	T60.4X2-	T60.4X3-	T60.4X4-	-	-
3422 (parathion)	T60.0X1-	T60.0X2-	T60.0X3-	T60.0X4-	-	-
3911 (phorate)	T60.0X1-	T60.0X2-	T60.0X3-	T60.0X4-	-	-
3956 (toxaphene)	T60.1X1-	T60.1X2-	T60.1X3-	T60.1X4-	-	-
4049 (malathion)	T60.0X1-	T60.0X2-	T60.0X3-	T60.0X4-	-	-
4069 (malathion)	T60.0X1-	T60.0X2-	T60.0X3-	T60.0X4-	-	-
4124 (dicapthon)	T60.0X1-	T60.0X2-	T60.0X3-	T60.0X4-	-	-

Substance	Poisoning, Accidental (unintentional)	Poisoning, Intentional self-harm	Poisoning, Assault	Poisoning, Undetermined	Adverse effect	Underdosing
Compound - *continued*						
E (cortisone)	T38.0X1-	T38.0X2-	T38.0X3-	T38.0X4-	T38.0X5-	T38.0X6-
F (hydrocortisone)	T38.0X1-	T38.0X2-	T38.0X3-	T38.0X4-	T38.0X5-	T38.0X6-
Congener, anabolic	T38.7X1-	T38.7X2-	T38.7X3-	T38.7X4-	T38.7X5-	T38.7X6-
Congo red	T50.8X1-	T50.8X2-	T50.8X3-	T50.8X4-	T50.8X5-	T50.8X6-
Coniine, conine	T62.2X1-	T62.2X2-	T62.2X3-	T62.2X4-	-	-
Conium (maculatum)	T62.2X1-	T62.2X2-	T62.2X3-	T62.2X4-	-	-
Conjugated estrogenic substances	T38.5X1-	T38.5X2-	T38.5X3-	T38.5X4-	T38.5X5-	T38.5X6-
Contac	T48.5X1-	T48.5X2-	T48.5X3-	T48.5X4-	T48.5X5-	T48.5X6-
Contact lens solution	T49.5X1-	T49.5X2-	T49.5X3-	T49.5X4-	T49.5X5-	T49.5X6-
Contraceptive (oral)	T38.4X1-	T38.4X2-	T38.4X3-	T38.4X4-	T38.4X5-	T38.4X6-
vaginal	T49.8X1-	T49.8X2-	T49.8X3-	T49.8X4-	T49.8X5-	T49.8X6-
Contrast medium, radiography	T50.8X1-	T50.8X2-	T50.8X3-	T50.8X4-	T50.8X5-	T50.8X6-
Convallaria glycosides	T46.0X1-	T46.0X2-	T46.0X3-	T46.0X4-	T46.0X5-	T46.0X6-
Convallaria majalis	T62.2X1-	T62.2X2-	T62.2X3-	T62.2X4-	-	-
berry	T62.1X1-	T62.1X2-	T62.1X3-	T62.1X4-	-	-
Copper (dust) (fumes) (nonmedicinal) **NEC**	T56.4X1-	T56.4X2-	T56.4X3-	T56.4X4-	-	-
arsenate, arsenite	T57.0X1-	T57.0X2-	T57.0X3-	T57.0X4-	-	-
insecticide	T60.2X1-	T60.2X2-	T60.2X3-	T60.2X4-	-	-
emetic	T47.7X1-	T47.7X2-	T47.7X3-	T47.7X4-	T47.7X5-	T47.7X6-
fungicide	T60.3X1-	T60.3X2-	T60.3X3-	T60.3X4-	-	-
gluconate	T49.0X1-	T49.0X2-	T49.0X3-	T49.0X4-	T49.0X5-	T49.0X6-
insecticide	T60.2X1-	T60.2X2-	T60.2X3-	T60.2X4-	-	-
medicinal (trace)	T45.8X1-	T45.8X2-	T45.8X3-	T45.8X4-	T45.8X5-	T45.8X6-
oleate	T49.0X1-	T49.0X2-	T49.0X3-	T49.0X4-	T49.0X5-	T49.0X6-
sulfate	T56.4X1-	T56.4X2-	T56.4X3-	T56.4X4-	-	-
cupric	T56.4X1-	T56.4X2-	T56.4X3-	T56.4X4-	-	-
fungicide	T60.3X1-	T60.3X2-	T60.3X3-	T60.3X4-	-	-
medicinal						
ear	T49.6X1-	T49.6X2-	T49.6X3-	T49.6X4-	T49.6X5-	T49.6X6-
emetic	T47.7X1-	T47.7X2-	T47.7X3-	T47.7X4-	T47.7X5-	T47.7X6-
eye	T49.5X1-	T49.5X2-	T49.5X3-	T49.5X4-	T49.5X5-	T49.5X6-
cuprous	T56.4X1-	T56.4X2-	T56.4X3-	T56.4X4-	-	-
fungicide	T60.3X1-	T60.3X2-	T60.3X3-	T60.3X4-	-	-
medicinal						
ear	T49.6X1-	T49.6X2-	T49.6X3-	T49.6X4-	T49.6X5-	T49.6X6-
emetic	T47.7X1-	T47.7X2-	T47.7X3-	T47.7X4-	T47.7X5-	T47.7X6-
eye	T49.5X1-	T49.5X2-	T49.5X3-	T49.5X4-	T49.5X5-	T49.5X6-
Copperhead snake (bite) (venom)	T63.061-	T63.062-	T63.063-	T63.064-	-	-
Coral (sting)	T63.691-	T63.692-	T63.693-	T63.694-	-	-
snake (bite) (venom)	T63.021-	T63.022-	T63.023-	T63.024-	-	-
Corbadrine	T49.6X1-	T49.6X2-	T49.6X3-	T49.6X4-	T49.6X5-	T49.6X6-
Cordite	T65.891-	T65.892-	T65.893-	T65.894-	-	-
vapor	T59.891-	T59.892-	T59.893-	T59.894-	-	-
Cordran	T49.0X1-	T49.0X2-	T49.0X3-	T49.0X4-	T49.0X5-	T49.0X6-
Corn cures	T49.4X1-	T49.4X2-	T49.4X3-	T49.4X4-	T49.4X5-	T49.4X6-
Corn starch	T49.3X1-	T49.3X2-	T49.3X3-	T49.3X4-	T49.3X5-	T49.3X6-
Cornhusker's lotion	T49.3X1-	T49.3X2-	T49.3X3-	T49.3X4-	T49.3X5-	T49.3X6-
Coronary vasodilator NEC	T46.3X1-	T46.3X2-	T46.3X3-	T46.3X4-	T46.3X5-	T46.3X6-
Corrosive NEC	T54.91X1-	T54.92X-	T54.93X-	T54.94X-	-	-
acid NEC	T54.2X1-	T54.2X2-	T54.2X3-	T54.2X4-	-	-
aromatics	T54.1X1-	T54.1X2-	T54.1X3-	T54.1X4-	-	-
disinfectant	T54.1X1-	T54.1X2-	T54.1X3-	T54.1X4-	-	-
fumes NEC	T54.91X-	T54.92X-	T54.93X-	T54.94X-	-	-
specified NEC	T54.91X-	T54.92X-	T54.93X-	T54.94X-	-	-
sublimate	T56.1X1-	T56.1X2-	T56.1X3-	T56.1X4-	-	-
Cortate	T38.0X1-	T38.0X2-	T38.0X3-	T38.0X4-	T38.0X5-	T38.0X6-
Cort-Dome	T38.0X1-	T38.0X2-	T38.0X3-	T38.0X4-	T38.0X5-	T38.0X6-
ENT agent	T49.6X1-	T49.6X2-	T49.6X3-	T49.6X4-	T49.6X5-	T49.6X6-
ophthalmic preparation	T49.5X1-	T49.5X2-	T49.5X3-	T49.5X4-	T49.5X5-	T49.5X6-
topical NEC	T49.0X1-	T49.0X2-	T49.0X3-	T49.0X4-	T49.0X5-	T49.0X6-
Cortef	T38.0X1-	T38.0X2-	T38.0X3-	T38.0X4-	T38.0X5-	T38.0X6-
ENT agent	T49.6X1-	T49.6X2-	T49.6X3-	T49.6X4-	T49.6X5-	T49.6X6-
ophthalmic preparation	T49.5X1-	T49.5X2-	T49.5X3-	T49.5X4-	T49.5X5-	T49.5X6-
topical NEC	T49.0X1-	T49.0X2-	T49.0X3-	T49.0X4-	T49.0X5-	T49.0X6-
Corticosteroid	T38.0X1-	T38.0X2-	T38.0X3-	T38.0X4-	T38.0X5-	T38.0X6-
ENT agent	T49.6X1-	T49.6X2-	T49.6X3-	T49.6X4-	T49.6X5-	T49.6X6-
mineral	T50.0X1-	T50.0X2-	T50.0X3-	T50.0X4-	T50.0X5-	T50.0X6-
ophthalmic	T49.5X1-	T49.5X2-	T49.5X3-	T49.5X4-	T49.5X5-	T49.5X6-
topical NEC	T49.0X1-	T49.0X2-	T49.0X3-	T49.0X4-	T49.0X5-	T49.0X6-
Corticotropin	T38.811-	T38.812-	T38.813-	T38.814-	T38.815-	T38.816-
Cortisol	T49.0X1-	T49.0X2-	T49.0X3-	T49.0X4-	T49.0X5-	T49.0X6-
ENT agent	T49.6X1-	T49.6X2-	T49.6X3-	T49.6X4-	T49.6X5-	T49.6X6-
ophthalmic preparation	T49.5X1-	T49.5X2-	T49.5X3-	T49.5X4-	T49.5X5-	T49.5X6-
topical NEC	T49.0X1-	T49.0X2-	T49.0X3-	T49.0X4-	T49.0X5-	T49.0X6-

Substance	Poisoning, Accidental (unintentional)	Poisoning, Intentional self-harm	Poisoning, Assault	Poisoning, Undetermined	Adverse effect	Underdosing
Cortisone (acetate)	T38.0X1-	T38.0X2-	T38.0X3-	T38.0X4-	T38.0X5-	T38.0X6-
ENT agent	T49.6X1-	T49.6X2-	T49.6X3-	T49.6X4-	T49.6X5-	T49.6X6-
ophthalmic preparation	T49.5X1-	T49.5X2-	T49.5X3-	T49.5X4-	T49.5X5-	T49.5X6-
topical NEC	T49.0X1-	T49.0X2-	T49.0X3-	T49.0X4-	T49.0X5-	T49.0X6-
Cortivazol	T38.0X1-	T38.0X2-	T38.0X3-	T38.0X4-	T38.0X5-	T38.0X6-
Cortogen	T38.0X1-	T38.0X2-	T38.0X3-	T38.0X4-	T38.0X5-	T38.0X6-
ENT agent	T49.6X1-	T49.6X2-	T49.6X3-	T49.6X4-	T49.6X5-	T49.6X6-
ophthalmic preparation	T49.5X1-	T49.5X2-	T49.5X3-	T49.5X4-	T49.5X5-	T49.5X6-
Cortone	T38.0X1-	T38.0X2-	T38.0X3-	T38.0X4-	T38.0X5-	T38.0X6-
ENT agent	T49.6X1-	T49.6X2-	T49.6X3-	T49.6X4-	T49.6X5-	T49.6X6-
ophthalmic preparation	T49.5X1-	T49.5X2-	T49.5X3-	T49.5X4-	T49.5X5-	T49.5X6-
Cortril	T38.0X1-	T38.0X2-	T38.0X3-	T38.0X4-	T38.0X5-	T38.0X6-
ENT agent	T49.6X1-	T49.6X2-	T49.6X3-	T49.6X4-	T49.6X5-	T49.6X6-
ophthalmic preparation	T49.5X1-	T49.5X2-	T49.5X3-	T49.5X4-	T49.5X5-	T49.5X6-
topical NEC	T49.0X1-	T49.0X2-	T49.0X3-	T49.0X4-	T49.0X5-	T49.0X6-
Corynebacterium parvum	T45.1X1-	T45.1X2-	T45.1X3-	T45.1X4-	T45.1X5-	T45.1X6-
Cosmetic preparation	T49.8X1-	T49.8X2-	T49.8X3-	T49.8X4-	T49.8X5-	T49.8X6-
Cosmetics	T49.8X1-	T49.8X2-	T49.8X3-	T49.8X4-	T49.8X5-	T49.8X6-
Cosyntropin	T38.811-	T38.812-	T38.813-	T38.814-	T38.815-	T38.816-
Cotarnine	T45.7X1-	T45.7X2-	T45.7X3-	T45.7X4-	T45.7X5-	T45.7X6-
Co-trimoxazole	T36.8X1-	T36.8X2-	T36.8X3-	T36.8X4-	T36.8X5-	T36.8X6-
Cottonseed oil	T49.3X1-	T49.3X2-	T49.3X3-	T49.3X4-	T49.3X5-	T49.3X6-
Cough mixture (syrup)	T48.4X1-	T48.4X2-	T48.4X3-	T48.4X4-	T48.4X5-	T48.4X6-
containing opiates	T40.2X1-	T40.2X2-	T40.2X3-	T40.2X4-	T40.2X5-	T40.2X6-
expectorants	T48.4X1-	T48.4X2-	T48.4X3-	T48.4X4-	T48.4X5-	T48.4X6-
Coumadin	T45.511-	T45.512-	T45.513-	T45.514-	T45.515-	T45.516-
rodenticide	T60.4X1-	T60.4X2-	T60.4X3-	T60.4X4-	-	-
Coumaphos	T60.0X1-	T60.0X2-	T60.0X3-	T60.0X4-	-	-
Coumarin	T45.511-	T45.512-	T45.513-	T45.514-	T45.515-	T45.516-
Coumetarol	T45.511-	T45.512-	T45.513-	T45.514-	T45.515-	T45.516-
Cowbane	T62.2X1-	T62.2X2-	T62.2X3-	T62.2X4-	-	-
Cozyme	T45.2X1-	T45.2X2-	T45.2X3-	T45.2X4-	T45.2X5-	T45.2X6-
Crack	T40.5X1-	T40.5X2-	T40.5X3-	T40.5X4-	-	-
Crataegus extract	T46.0X1-	T46.0X2-	T46.0X3-	T46.0X4-	T46.0X5-	T46.0X6-
Creolin	T54.1X1-	T54.1X2-	T54.1X3-	T54.1X4-	-	-
disinfectant	T54.1X1-	T54.1X2-	T54.1X3-	T54.1X4-	-	-
Creosol (compound)	T49.0X1-	T49.0X2-	T49.0X3-	T49.0X4-	T49.0X5-	T49.0X6-
Creosote (coal tar) (beechwood)	T49.0X1-	T49.0X2-	T49.0X3-	T49.0X4-	T49.0X5-	T49.0X6-
medicinal (expectorant)	T48.4X1-	T48.4X2-	T48.4X3-	T48.4X4-	T48.4X5-	T48.4X6-
syrup	T48.4X1-	T48.4X2-	T48.4X3-	T48.4X4-	T48.4X5-	T48.4X6-
Cresol (s)	T49.0X1-	T49.0X2-	T49.0X3-	T49.0X4-	T49.0X5-	T49.0X6-
and soap solution	T49.0X1-	T49.0X2-	T49.0X3-	T49.0X4-	T49.0X5-	T49.0X6-
Cresyl acetate	T49.0X1-	T49.0X2-	T49.0X3-	T49.0X4-	T49.0X5-	T49.0X6-
Cresylic acid	T49.0X1-	T49.0X2-	T49.0X3-	T49.0X4-	T49.0X5-	T49.0X6-
Crimidine	T60.4X1-	T60.4X2-	T60.4X3-	T60.4X4-	-	-
Croconazole	T37.8X1-	T37.8X2-	T37.8X3-	T37.8X4-	T37.8X5-	T37.8X6-
Cromoglicic acid	T48.6X1-	T48.6X2-	T48.6X3-	T48.6X4-	T48.6X5-	T48.6X6-
Cromolyn	T48.6X1-	T48.6X2-	T48.6X3-	T48.6X4-	T48.6X5-	T48.6X6-
Cromonar	T46.3X1-	T46.3X2-	T46.3X3-	T46.3X4-	T46.3X5-	T46.3X6-
Cropropamide	T39.8X1-	T39.8X2-	T39.8X3-	T39.8X4-	T39.8X5-	T39.8X6-
with crotethamide	T50.7X1-	T50.7X2-	T50.7X3-	T50.7X4-	T50.7X5-	T50.7X6-
Crotamiton	T49.0X1-	T49.0X2-	T49.0X3-	T49.0X4-	T49.0X5-	T49.0X6-
Crotethamide	T39.8X1-	T39.8X2-	T39.8X3-	T39.8X4-	T39.8X5-	T39.8X6-
with cropropamide	T50.7X1-	T50.7X2-	T50.7X3-	T50.7X4-	T50.7X5-	T50.7X6-
Croton (oil)	T47.2X1-	T47.2X2-	T47.2X3-	T47.2X4-	T47.2X5-	T47.2X6-
chloral	T42.6X1-	T42.6X2-	T42.6X3-	T42.6X4-	T42.6X5-	T42.6X6-
Crude oil	T52.0X1-	T52.0X2-	T52.0X3-	T52.0X4-	-	-
Cryogenine	T39.8X1-	T39.8X2-	T39.8X3-	T39.8X4-	T39.8X5-	T39.8X6-
Cryolite (vapor)	T60.1X1-	T60.1X2-	T60.1X3-	T60.1X4-	-	-
insecticide	T60.1X1-	T60.1X2-	T60.1X3-	T60.1X4-	-	-
Cryptenamine (tannates)	T46.5X1-	T46.5X2-	T46.5X3-	T46.5X4-	T46.5X5-	T46.5X6-
Crystal violet	T49.0X1-	T49.0X2-	T49.0X3-	T49.0X4-	T49.0X5-	T49.0X6-
Cuckoopint	T62.2X1-	T62.2X2-	T62.2X3-	T62.2X4-	-	-
Cumetharol	T45.511-	T45.512-	T45.513-	T45.514-	T45.515-	T45.516-
Cupric						
acetate	T60.3X1-	T60.3X2-	T60.3X3-	T60.3X4-	-	-
acetoarsenite	T57.0X1-	T57.0X2-	T57.0X3-	T57.0X4-	-	-
arsenate	T57.0X1-	T57.0X2-	T57.0X3-	T57.0X4-	-	-
gluconate	T49.0X1-	T49.0X2-	T49.0X3-	T49.0X4-	T49.0X5-	T49.0X6-
oleate	T49.0X1-	T49.0X2-	T49.0X3-	T49.0X4-	T49.0X5-	T49.0X6-
sulfate	T56.4X1-	T56.4X2-	T56.4X3-	T56.4X4-	-	-
Cuprous sulfate — *see also* Copper sulfate	T56.4X1-	T56.4X2-	T56.4X3-	T56.4X4-	-	-
Curare, curarine	T48.1X1-	T48.1X2-	T48.1X3-	T48.1X4-	T48.1X5-	T48.1X6-
Cyamemazine	T43.3X1-	T43.3X2-	T43.3X3-	T43.3X4-	T43.3X5-	T43.3X6-
Cyamopsis tetragono-loba	T46.6X1-	T46.6X2-	T46.6X3-	T46.6X4-	T46.6X5-	T46.6X6-
Cyanacetyl hydrazide	T37.1X1-	T37.1X2-	T37.1X3-	T37.1X4-	T37.1X5-	T37.1X6-

Substance	Poisoning, Accidental (unintentional)	Poisoning, Intentional self-harm	Poisoning, Assault	Poisoning, Undetermined	Adverse effect	Underdosing
Cyanic acid (gas)	T59.891-	T59.892-	T59.893-	T59.894-	-	-
Cyanide (s) (compounds) (potassium) (sodium) NEC	T65.0X1-	T65.0X2-	T65.0X3-	T65.0X4-	-	-
dust or gas (inhalation) NEC	T57.3X1-	T57.3X2-	T57.3X3-	T57.3X4-	-	-
fumigant	T65.0X1-	T65.0X2-	T65.0X3-	T65.0X4-	-	-
hydrogen	T57.3X1-	T57.3X2-	T57.3X3-	T57.3X4-	-	-
mercuric — see Mercury						
pesticide (dust) (fumes)	T65.0X1-	T65.0X2-	T65.0X3-	T65.0X4-	-	-
Cyanoacrylate adhesive	T49.3X1-	T49.3X2-	T49.3X3-	T49.3X4-	T49.3X5-	T49.3X6-
Cyanocobalamin	T45.8X1-	T45.8X2-	T45.8X3-	T45.8X4-	T45.8X5-	T45.8X6-
Cyanogen (chloride) (gas) NEC	T59.891-	T59.892-	T59.893-	T59.894-		
Cyclacillin	T36.0X1-	T36.0X2-	T36.0X3-	T36.0X4-	T36.0X5-	T36.0X6-
Cyclaine	T41.3X1-	T41.3X2-	T41.3X3-	T41.3X4-	T41.3X5-	T41.3X6-
Cyclamate	T50.991-	T50.992-	T50.993-	T50.994-	T50.995-	T50.996-
Cyclamen europaeum	T62.2X1-	T62.2X2-	T62.2X3-	T62.2X4-	-	-
Cyclandelate	T46.7X1-	T46.7X2-	T46.7X3-	T46.7X4-	T46.7X5-	T46.7X6-
Cyclazocine	T50.7X1-	T50.7X2-	T50.7X3-	T50.7X4-	T50.7X5-	T50.7X6-
Cyclizine	T45.0X1-	T45.0X2-	T45.0X3-	T45.0X4-	T45.0X5-	T45.0X6-
Cyclobarbital	T42.3X1-	T42.3X2-	T42.3X3-	T42.3X4-	T42.3X5-	T42.3X6-
Cyclobarbitone	T42.3X1-	T42.3X2-	T42.3X3-	T42.3X4-	T42.3X5-	T42.3X6-
Cyclobenzaprine	T48.1X1-	T48.1X2-	T48.1X3-	T48.1X4-	T48.1X5-	T48.1X6-
Cyclodrine	T44.3X1-	T44.3X2-	T44.3X3-	T44.3X4-	T44.3X5-	T44.3X6-
Cycloguanil embonate	T37.2X1-	T37.2X2-	T37.2X3-	T37.2X4-	T37.2X5-	T37.2X6-
Cyclohexane	T52.8X1-	T52.8X2-	T52.8X3-	T52.8X4-	-	-
Cyclohexanol	T51.8X1-	T51.8X2-	T51.8X3-	T51.8X4-	-	-
Cyclohexanone	T52.4X1-	T52.4X2-	T52.4X3-	T52.4X4-	-	-
Cycloheximide	T60.3X1-	T60.3X2-	T60.3X3-	T60.3X4-	-	-
Cyclohexyl acetate	T52.8X1-	T52.8X2-	T52.8X3-	T52.8X4-	-	-
Cycloleucin	T45.1X1-	T45.1X2-	T45.1X3-	T45.1X4-	T45.1X5-	T45.1X6-
Cyclomethycaine	T41.3X1-	T41.3X2-	T41.3X3-	T41.3X4-	T41.3X5-	T41.3X6-
Cyclopentamine	T44.4X1-	T44.4X2-	T44.4X3-	T44.4X4-	T44.4X5-	T44.4X6-
Cyclopenthiazide	T50.2X1-	T50.2X2-	T50.2X3-	T50.2X4-	T50.2X5-	T50.2X6-
Cyclopentolate	T44.3X1-	T44.3X2-	T44.3X3-	T44.3X4-	T44.3X5-	T44.3X6-
Cyclophosphamide	T45.1X1-	T45.1X2-	T45.1X3-	T45.1X4-	T45.1X5-	T45.1X6-
Cycloplegic drug	T49.5X1-	T49.5X2-	T49.5X3-	T49.5X4-	T49.5X5-	T49.5X6-
Cyclopropane	T41.291-	T41.292-	T41.293-	T41.294-	T41.295-	T41.296-
Cyclopyrabital	T39.8X1-	T39.8X2-	T39.8X3-	T39.8X4-	T39.8X5-	T39.8X6-
Cycloserine	T37.1X1-	T37.1X2-	T37.1X3-	T37.1X4-	T37.1X5-	T37.1X6-
Cyclosporin	T45.1X1-	T45.1X2-	T45.1X3-	T45.1X4-	T45.1X5-	T45.1X6-
Cyclothiazide	T50.2X1-	T50.2X2-	T50.2X3-	T50.2X4-	T50.2X5-	T50.2X6-
Cycrimine	T44.3X1-	T44.3X2-	T44.3X3-	T44.3X4-	T44.3X5-	T44.3X6-
Cyhalothrin	T60.1X1-	T60.1X2-	T60.1X3-	T60.1X4-	-	-
Cymarin	T46.0X1-	T46.0X2-	T46.0X3-	T46.0X4-	T46.0X5-	T46.0X6-
Cypermethrin	T60.1X1-	T60.1X2-	T60.1X3-	T60.1X4-	-	-
Cyphenothrin	T60.2X1-	T60.2X2-	T60.2X3-	T60.2X4-	-	-
Cyproheptadine	T45.0X1-	T45.0X2-	T45.0X3-	T45.0X4-	T45.0X5-	T45.0X6-
Cyproterone	T38.6X1-	T38.6X2-	T38.6X3-	T38.6X4-	T38.6X5-	T38.6X6-
Cysteamine	T50.6X1-	T50.6X2-	T50.6X3-	T50.6X4-	T50.6X5-	T50.6X6-
Cytarabine	T45.1X1-	T45.1X2-	T45.1X3-	T45.1X4-	T45.1X5-	T45.1X6-
Cytisus						
laburnum	T62.2X1-	T62.2X2-	T62.2X3-	T62.2X4-	-	-
scoparius	T62.2X1-	T62.2X2-	T62.2X3-	T62.2X4-	-	-
Cytochrome C	T47.5X1-	T47.5X2-	T47.5X3-	T47.5X4-	T47.5X5-	T47.5X6-
Cytomel	T38.1X1-	T38.1X2-	T38.1X3-	T38.1X4-	T38.1X5-	T38.1X6-
Cytosine arabinoside	T45.1X1-	T45.1X2-	T45.1X3-	T45.1X4-	T45.1X5-	T45.1X6-
Cytoxan	T45.1X1-	T45.1X2-	T45.1X3-	T45.1X4-	T45.1X5-	T45.1X6-
Cytozyme	T45.7X1-	T45.7X2-	T45.7X3-	T45.7X4-	T45.7X5-	T45.7X6-
2,4-D	T60.3X1-	T60.3X2-	T60.3X3-	T60.3X4-		
Dacarbazine	T45.1X1-	T45.1X2-	T45.1X3-	T45.1X4-	T45.1X5-	T45.1X6-
Dactinomycin	T45.1X1-	T45.1X2-	T45.1X3-	T45.1X4-	T45.1X5-	T45.1X6-
DADPS	T37.1X1-	T37.1X2-	T37.1X3-	T37.1X4-	T37.1X5-	T37.1X6-
Dakin's solution	T49.0X1-	T49.0X2-	T49.0X3-	T49.0X4-	T49.0X5-	T49.0X6-
Dalapon (sodium)	T60.3X1-	T60.3X2-	T60.3X3-	T60.3X4-		
Dalmane	T42.4X1-	T42.4X2-	T42.4X3-	T42.4X4-	T42.4X5-	T42.4X6-
Danazol	T38.6X1-	T38.6X2-	T38.6X3-	T38.6X4-	T38.6X5-	T38.6X6-
Danilone	T45.511-	T45.512-	T45.513-	T45.514-	T45.515-	T45.516-
Danthron	T47.2X1-	T47.2X2-	T47.2X3-	T47.2X4-	T47.2X5-	T47.2X6-
Dantrolene	T42.8X1-	T42.8X2-	T42.8X3-	T42.8X4-	T42.8X5-	T42.8X6-
Dantron	T47.2X1-	T47.2X2-	T47.2X3-	T47.2X4-	T47.2X5-	T47.2X6-
Daphne (gnidium) (mezereum)	T62.2X1-	T62.2X2-	T62.2X3-	T62.2X4-	-	-
berry	T62.1X1-	T62.1X2-	T62.1X3-	T62.1X4-	-	-
Dapsone	T37.1X1-	T37.1X2-	T37.1X3-	T37.1X4-	T37.1X5-	T37.1X6-
Daraprim	T37.2X1-	T37.2X2-	T37.2X3-	T37.2X4-	T37.2X5-	T37.2X6-
Darnel	T62.2X1-	T62.2X2-	T62.2X3-	T62.2X4-	-	-
Darvon	T39.8X1-	T39.8X2-	T39.8X3-	T39.8X4-	T39.8X5-	T39.8X6-
Daunomycin	T45.1X1-	T45.1X2-	T45.1X3-	T45.1X4-	T45.1X5-	T45.1X6-
Daunorubicin	T45.1X1-	T45.1X2-	T45.1X3-	T45.1X4-	T45.1X5-	T45.1X6-
DBI	T38.3X1-	T38.3X2-	T38.3X3-	T38.3X4-	T38.3X5-	T38.3X6-

Substance	Poisoning, Accidental (unintentional)	Poisoning, Intentional self-harm	Poisoning, Assault	Poisoning, Undetermined	Adverse effect	Underdosing
D-Con	T60.91X-	T60.92X-	T60.93X-	T60.94X-	-	-
insecticide	T60.2X1-	T60.2X2-	T60.2X3-	T60.2X4-	-	-
rodenticide	T60.4X1-	T60.4X2-	T60.4X3-	T60.4X4-	-	-
DDAVP	T38.891-	T38.892-	T38.893-	T38.894-	T38.895-	T38.896-
DDE (bis (chlorophenyl) -dichloroethylene)	T60.2X1-	T60.2X2-	T60.2X3-	T60.2X4-	-	-
DDS	T37.1X1-	T37.1X2-	T37.1X3-	T37.1X4-	T37.1X5-	T37.1X6-
DDT (dust)	T60.1X1-	T60.1X2-	T60.1X3-	T60.1X4-	-	-
Deadly nightshade — see also Belladonna	T62.2X1-	T62.2X2-	T62.2X3-	T62.2X4-		
berry	T62.1X1-	T62.1X2-	T62.1X3-	T62.1X4-	-	-
Deamino-D-arginine vasopressin	T38.891-	T38.892-	T38.893-	T38.894-	T38.895-	T38.896-
Deanol (aceglumate)	T50.991-	T50.992-	T50.993-	T50.994-	T50.995-	T50.996-
Debrisoquine	T46.5X1-	T46.5X2-	T46.5X3-	T46.5X4-	T46.5X5-	T46.5X6-
Decaborane	T57.8X1-	T57.8X2-	T57.8X3-	T57.8X4-	-	-
fumes	T59.891-	T59.892-	T59.893-	T59.894-	-	-
Decadron	T38.0X1-	T38.0X2-	T38.0X3-	T38.0X4-	T38.0X5-	T38.0X6-
ENT agent	T49.6X1-	T49.6X2-	T49.6X3-	T49.6X4-	T49.6X5-	T49.6X6-
ophthalmic preparation	T49.5X1-	T49.5X2-	T49.5X3-	T49.5X4-	T49.5X5-	T49.5X6-
topical NEC	T49.0X1-	T49.0X2-	T49.0X3-	T49.0X4-	T49.0X5-	T49.0X6-
Decahydronaphthalene	T52.8X1-	T52.8X2-	T52.8X3-	T52.8X4-	-	-
Decalin	T52.8X1-	T52.8X2-	T52.8X3-	T52.8X4-	-	-
Decamethonium (bromide)	T48.1X1-	T48.1X2-	T48.1X3-	T48.1X4-	T48.1X5-	T48.1X6-
Decholin	T47.5X1-	T47.5X2-	T47.5X3-	T47.5X4-	T47.5X5-	T47.5X6-
Declomycin	T36.4X1-	T36.4X2-	T36.4X3-	T36.4X4-	T36.4X5-	T36.4X6-
Decongestant, nasal (mucosa)	T48.5X1-	T48.5X2-	T48.5X3-	T48.5X4-	T48.5X5-	T48.5X6-
combination	T48.5X1-	T48.5X2-	T48.5X3-	T48.5X4-	T48.5X5-	T48.5X6-
Deet	T60.8X1-	T60.8X2-	T60.8X3-	T60.8X4-	-	-
Deferoxamine	T45.8X1-	T45.8X2-	T45.8X3-	T45.8X4-	T45.8X5-	T45.8X6-
Deflazacort	T38.0X1-	T38.0X2-	T38.0X3-	T38.0X4-	T38.0X5-	T38.0X6-
Deglycyrrhizinized extract of licorice	T48.4X1-	T48.4X2-	T48.4X3-	T48.4X4-	T48.4X5-	T48.4X6-
Dehydrocholic acid	T47.5X1-	T47.5X2-	T47.5X3-	T47.5X4-	T47.5X5-	T47.5X6-
Dehydroemetine	T37.3X1-	T37.3X2-	T37.3X3-	T37.3X4-	T37.3X5-	T37.3X6-
Dekalin	T52.8X1-	T52.8X2-	T52.8X3-	T52.8X4-	-	-
Delalutin	T38.5X1-	T38.5X2-	T38.5X3-	T38.5X4-	T38.5X5-	T38.5X6-
Delorazepam	T42.4X1-	T42.4X2-	T42.4X3-	T42.4X4-	T42.4X5-	T42.4X6-
Delphinium	T62.2X1-	T62.2X2-	T62.2X3-	T62.2X4-	-	-
Deltamethrin	T60.1X1-	T60.1X2-	T60.1X3-	T60.1X4-	-	-
Deltasone	T38.0X1-	T38.0X2-	T38.0X3-	T38.0X4-	T38.0X5-	T38.0X6-
Delta	T38.0X1-	T38.0X2-	T38.0X3-	T38.0X4-	T38.0X5-	T38.0X6-
Delvinal	T42.3X1-	T42.3X2-	T42.3X3-	T42.3X4-	T42.3X5-	T42.3X6-
Demecarium (bromide)	T49.5X1-	T49.5X2-	T49.5X3-	T49.5X4-	T49.5X5-	T49.5X6-
Demeclocycline	T36.4X1-	T36.4X2-	T36.4X3-	T36.4X4-	T36.4X5-	T36.4X6-
Demecolcine	T45.1X1-	T45.1X2-	T45.1X3-	T45.1X4-	T45.1X5-	T45.1X6-
Demegestone	T38.5X1-	T38.5X2-	T38.5X3-	T38.5X4-	T38.5X5-	T38.5X6-
Demelanizing agents	T49.8X1-	T49.8X2-	T49.8X3-	T49.8X4-	T49.8X5-	T49.8X6-
Demephion -O and -S	T60.0X1-	T60.0X2-	T60.0X3-	T60.0X4-	-	-
Demerol	T40.2X1-	T40.2X2-	T40.2X3-	T40.2X4-	T40.2X5-	T40.2X6-
Demethylchlortetracycline	T36.4X1-	T36.4X2-	T36.4X3-	T36.4X4-	T36.4X5-	T36.4X6-
Demethyltetracycline	T36.4X1-	T36.4X2-	T36.4X3-	T36.4X4-	T36.4X5-	T36.4X6-
Demeton -O and -S	T60.0X1-	T60.0X2-	T60.0X3-	T60.0X4-	-	-
Demulcent (external)	T49.3X1-	T49.3X2-	T49.3X3-	T49.3X4-	T49.3X5-	T49.3X6-
specified NEC	T49.3X1-	T49.3X2-	T49.3X3-	T49.3X4-	T49.3X5-	T49.3X6-
Demulen	T38.4X1-	T38.4X2-	T38.4X3-	T38.4X4-	T38.4X5-	T38.4X6-
Denatured alcohol	T51.0X1-	T51.0X2-	T51.0X3-	T51.0X4-	-	-
Dendrid	T49.5X1-	T49.5X2-	T49.5X3-	T49.5X4-	T49.5X5-	T49.5X6-
Dental drug, topical application NEC	T49.7X1-	T49.7X2-	T49.7X3-	T49.7X4-	T49.7X5-	T49.7X6-
Dentifrice	T49.7X1-	T49.7X2-	T49.7X3-	T49.7X4-	T49.7X5-	T49.7X6-
Deodorant spray (feminine hygiene)	T49.8X1-	T49.8X2-	T49.8X3-	T49.8X4-	T49.8X5-	T49.8X6-
Deoxycortone	T50.0X1-	T50.0X2-	T50.0X3-	T50.0X4-	T50.0X5-	T50.0X6-
2-Deoxy-5-fluorouridine	T45.1X1-	T45.1X2-	T45.1X3-	T45.1X4-	T45.1X5-	T45.1X6-
5-Deoxy-5-fluorouridine	T45.1X1-	T45.1X2-	T45.1X3-	T45.1X4-	T45.1X5-	T45.1X6-
Deoxyribonuclease (pancreatic)	T45.3X1-	T45.3X2-	T45.3X3-	T45.3X4-	T45.3X5-	T45.3X6-
Depilatory	T49.4X1-	T49.4X2-	T49.4X3-	T49.4X4-	T49.4X5-	T49.4X6-
Deprenalin	T42.8X1-	T42.8X2-	T42.8X3-	T42.8X4-	T42.8X5-	T42.8X6-
Deprenyl	T42.8X1-	T42.8X2-	T42.8X3-	T42.8X4-	T42.8X5-	T42.8X6-
Depressant, appetite	T50.5X1-	T50.5X2-	T50.5X3-	T50.5X4-	T50.5X5-	T50.5X6-
Depressant						
appetite (central)	T50.5X1-	T50.5X2-	T50.5X3-	T50.5X4-	T50.5X5-	T50.5X6-
cardiac	T46.2X1-	T46.2X2-	T46.2X3-	T46.2X4-	T46.2X5-	T46.2X6-
central nervous system (anesthetic) — see also Central nervous system, depressants	T42.71X-	T42.72X-	T42.73X-	T42.74X-	T42.75X-	T42.76X-

Substance	Poisoning, Accidental (unintentional)	Poisoning, Intentional self-harm	Poisoning, Assault	Poisoning, Undetermined	Adverse effect	Underdosing
Depressant - *continued*						
general anesthetic	T41.201-	T41.202-	T41.203-	T41.204-	T41.205-	T41.206-
muscle tone	T42.8X1-	T42.8X2-	T42.8X3-	T42.8X4-	T42.8X5-	T42.8X6-
muscle tone, central	T42.8X1-	T42.8X2-	T42.8X3-	T42.8X4-	T42.8X5-	T42.8X6-
psychotherapeutic	T43.501-	T43.502-	T43.503-	T43.504-	T43.505-	T43.506-
Deptropine	T45.0X1-	T45.0X2-	T45.0X3-	T45.0X4-	T45.0X5-	T45.0X6-
Dequalinium (chloride)	T49.0X1-	T49.0X2-	T49.0X3-	T49.0X4-	T49.0X5-	T49.0X6-
Derris root	T60.2X1-	T60.2X2-	T60.2X3-	T60.2X4-	-	-
Deserpidine	T46.5X1-	T46.5X2-	T46.5X3-	T46.5X4-	T46.5X5-	T46.5X6-
Desferrioxamine	T45.8X1-	T45.8X2-	T45.8X3-	T45.8X4-	T45.8X5-	T45.8X6-
Desipramine	T43.011-	T43.012-	T43.013-	T43.014-	T43.015-	T43.016-
Deslanoside	T46.0X1-	T46.0X2-	T46.0X3-	T46.0X4-	T46.0X5-	T46.0X6-
Desloughing agent	T49.4X1-	T49.4X2-	T49.4X3-	T49.4X4-	T49.4X5-	T49.4X6-
Desmethylimipramine	T43.011-	T43.012-	T43.013-	T43.014-	T43.015-	T43.016-
Desmopressin	T38.891-	T38.892-	T38.893-	T38.894-	T38.895-	T38.896-
Desocodeine	T40.2X1-	T40.2X2-	T40.2X3-	T40.2X4-	T40.2X5-	T40.2X6-
Desogestrel	T38.5X1-	T38.5X2-	T38.5X3-	T38.5X4-	T38.5X5-	T38.5X6-
Desomorphine	T40.2X1-	T40.2X2-	T40.2X3-	T40.2X4-	-	-
Desonide	T49.0X1-	T49.0X2-	T49.0X3-	T49.0X4-	T49.0X5-	T49.0X6-
Desoximetasone	T49.0X1-	T49.0X2-	T49.0X3-	T49.0X4-	T49.0X5-	T49.0X6-
Desoxycorticosteroid	T50.0X1-	T50.0X2-	T50.0X3-	T50.0X4-	T50.0X5-	T50.0X6-
Desoxycortone	T50.0X1-	T50.0X2-	T50.0X3-	T50.0X4-	T50.0X5-	T50.0X6-
Desoxyephedrine	T43.621-	T43.622-	T43.623-	T43.624-	T43.625-	T43.626-
Detaxtran	T46.6X1-	T46.6X2-	T46.6X3-	T46.6X4-	T46.6X5-	T46.6X6-
Detergent	T49.2X1-	T49.2X2-	T49.2X3-	T49.2X4-	T49.2X5-	T49.2X6-
external medication	T49.2X1-	T49.2X2-	T49.2X3-	T49.2X4-	T49.2X5-	T49.2X6-
local	T49.2X1-	T49.2X2-	T49.2X3-	T49.2X4-	T49.2X5-	T49.2X6-
medicinal	T49.2X1-	T49.2X2-	T49.2X3-	T49.2X4-	T49.2X5-	T49.2X6-
nonmedicinal	T55.1X1-	T55.1X2-	T55.1X3-	T55.1X4-	-	-
specified NEC	T55.1X1-	T55.1X2-	T55.1X3-	T55.1X4-	-	-
Deterrent, alcohol	T50.6X1-	T50.6X2-	T50.6X3-	T50.6X4-	T50.6X5-	T50.6X6-
Detoxifying agent	T50.6X1-	T50.6X2-	T50.6X3-	T50.6X4-	T50.6X5-	T50.6X6-
Detrothyronine	T38.1X1-	T38.1X2-	T38.1X3-	T38.1X4-	T38.1X5-	T38.1X6-
Dettol (external medication)	T49.0X1-	T49.0X2-	T49.0X3-	T49.0X4-	T49.0X5-	T49.0X6-
Dexamethasone	T38.0X1-	T38.0X2-	T38.0X3-	T38.0X4-	T38.0X5-	T38.0X6-
ENT agent	T49.6X1-	T49.6X2-	T49.6X3-	T49.6X4-	T49.6X5-	T49.6X6-
ophthalmic preparation	T49.5X1-	T49.5X2-	T49.5X3-	T49.5X4-	T49.5X5-	T49.5X6-
topical NEC	T49.0X1-	T49.0X2-	T49.0X3-	T49.0X4-	T49.0X5-	T49.0X6-
Dexamfetamine	T43.621-	T43.622-	T43.623-	T43.624-	T43.625-	T43.626-
Dexamphetamine	T43.621-	T43.622-	T43.623-	T43.624-	T43.625-	T43.626-
Dexbrompheniramine	T45.0X1-	T45.0X2-	T45.0X3-	T45.0X4-	T45.0X5-	T45.0X6-
Dexchlorpheniramine	T45.0X1-	T45.0X2-	T45.0X3-	T45.0X4-	T45.0X5-	T45.0X6-
Dexedrine	T43.621-	T43.622-	T43.623-	T43.624-	T43.625-	T43.626-
Dexetimide	T44.3X1-	T44.3X2-	T44.3X3-	T44.3X4-	T44.3X5-	T44.3X6-
Dexfenfluramine	T50.5X1-	T50.5X2-	T50.5X3-	T50.5X4-	T50.5X5-	T50.5X6-
Dexpanthenol	T45.2X1-	T45.2X2-	T45.2X3-	T45.2X4-	T45.2X5-	T45.2X6-
Dextran (40) (70) (150)	T45.8X1-	T45.8X2-	T45.8X3-	T45.8X4-	T45.8X5-	T45.8X6-
Dextriferron	T45.4X1-	T45.4X2-	T45.4X3-	T45.4X4-	T45.4X5-	T45.4X6-
Dextro calcium pantothenate	T45.2X1-	T45.2X2-	T45.2X3-	T45.2X4-	T45.2X5-	T45.2X6-
Dextro pantothenyl alcohol	T45.2X1-	T45.2X2-	T45.2X3-	T45.2X4-	T45.2X5-	T45.2X6-
Dextroamphetamine	T43.621-	T43.622-	T43.623-	T43.624-	T43.625-	T43.626-
Dextromethorphan	T48.3X1-	T48.3X2-	T48.3X3-	T48.3X4-	T48.3X5-	T48.3X6-
Dextromoramide	T40.4X1-	T40.4X2-	T40.4X3-	T40.4X4-	-	-
topical	T49.8X1-	T49.8X2-	T49.8X3-	T49.8X4-	T49.8X5-	T49.8X6-
Dextropropoxyphene	T40.4X1-	T40.4X2-	T40.4X3-	T40.4X4-	T40.4X5-	T40.4X6-
Dextrorphan	T40.2X1-	T40.2X2-	T40.2X3-	T40.2X4-	T40.2X5-	T40.2X6-
Dextrose	T50.3X1-	T50.3X2-	T50.3X3-	T50.3X4-	T50.3X5-	T50.3X6-
concentrated solution, intravenous	T46.8X1-	T46.8X2-	T46.8X3-	T46.8X4-	T46.8X5-	T46.8X6-
Dextrothyroxin	T38.1X1-	T38.1X2-	T38.1X3-	T38.1X4-	T38.1X5-	T38.1X6-
Dextrothyroxine sodium	T38.1X1-	T38.1X2-	T38.1X3-	T38.1X4-	T38.1X5-	T38.1X6-
DFP	T44.0X1-	T44.0X2-	T44.0X3-	T44.0X4-	T44.0X5-	T44.0X6-
DHE	T37.3X1-	T37.3X2-	T37.3X3-	T37.3X4-	T37.3X5-	T37.3X6-
45	T46.5X1-	T46.5X2-	T46.5X3-	T46.5X4-	T46.5X5-	T46.5X6-
Diabinese	T38.3X1-	T38.3X2-	T38.3X3-	T38.3X4-	T38.3X5-	T38.3X6-
Diacetone alcohol	T52.4X1-	T52.4X2-	T52.4X3-	T52.4X4-	-	-
Diacetyl monoxime	T50.991-	T50.992-	T50.993-	T50.994-	-	-
Diacetylmorphine	T40.1X1-	T40.1X2-	T40.1X3-	T40.1X4-	-	-
Diachylon plaster	T49.4X1-	T49.4X2-	T49.4X3-	T49.4X4-	T49.4X5-	T49.4X6-
Diaethylstilboestrolum	T38.5X1-	T38.5X2-	T38.5X3-	T38.5X4-	T38.5X5-	T38.5X6-
Diagnostic agent NEC	T50.8X1-	T50.8X2-	T50.8X3-	T50.8X4-	T50.8X5-	T50.8X6-
Dial (soap)	T49.2X1-	T49.2X2-	T49.2X3-	T49.2X4-	T49.2X5-	T49.2X6-
sedative	T42.3X1-	T42.3X2-	T42.3X3-	T42.3X4-	T42.3X5-	T42.3X6-
Dialkyl carbonate	T52.91X-	T52.92X-	T52.93X-	T52.94X-	-	-
Diallylbarbituric acid	T42.3X1-	T42.3X2-	T42.3X3-	T42.3X4-	T42.3X5-	T42.3X6-
Diallymal	T42.3X1-	T42.3X2-	T42.3X3-	T42.3X4-	T42.3X5-	T42.3X6-
Dialysis solution (intraperitoneal)	T50.3X1-	T50.3X2-	T50.3X3-	T50.3X4-	T50.3X5-	T50.3X6-

Substance	Poisoning, Accidental (unintentional)	Poisoning, Intentional self-harm	Poisoning, Assault	Poisoning, Undetermined	Adverse effect	Underdosing
Diaminodiphenylsulfone	T37.1X1-	T37.1X2-	T37.1X3-	T37.1X4-	T37.1X5-	T37.1X6-
Diamorphine	T40.1X1-	T40.1X2-	T40.1X3-	T40.1X4-	-	-
Diamox	T50.2X1-	T50.2X2-	T50.2X3-	T50.2X4-	T50.2X5-	T50.2X6-
Diamthazole	T49.0X1-	T49.0X2-	T49.0X3-	T49.0X4-	T49.0X5-	T49.0X6-
Dianthone	T47.2X1-	T47.2X2-	T47.2X3-	T47.2X4-	T47.2X5-	T47.2X6-
Diaphenylsulfone	T37.0X1-	T37.0X2-	T37.0X3-	T37.0X4-	T37.0X5-	T37.0X6-
Diasone (sodium)	T37.1X1-	T37.1X2-	T37.1X3-	T37.1X4-	T37.1X5-	T37.1X6-
Diastase	T47.5X1-	T47.5X2-	T47.5X3-	T47.5X4-	T47.5X5-	T47.5X6-
Diatrizoate	T50.8X1-	T50.8X2-	T50.8X3-	T50.8X4-	T50.8X5-	T50.8X6-
Diazepam	T42.4X1-	T42.4X2-	T42.4X3-	T42.4X4-	T42.4X5-	T42.4X6-
Diazinon	T60.0X1-	T60.0X2-	T60.0X3-	T60.0X4-	-	-
Diazomethane (gas)	T59.891-	T59.892-	T59.893-	T59.894-	-	-
Diazoxide	T46.5X1-	T46.5X2-	T46.5X3-	T46.5X4-	T46.5X5-	T46.5X6-
Dibekacin	T36.5X1-	T36.5X2-	T36.5X3-	T36.5X4-	T36.5X5-	T36.5X6-
Dibenamine	T44.6X1-	T44.6X2-	T44.6X3-	T44.6X4-	T44.6X5-	T44.6X6-
Dibenzepin	T43.011-	T43.012-	T43.013-	T43.014-	T43.015-	T43.016-
Dibenzheptropine	T45.0X1-	T45.0X2-	T45.0X3-	T45.0X4-	T45.0X5-	T45.0X6-
Dibenzyline	T44.6X1-	T44.6X2-	T44.6X3-	T44.6X4-	T44.6X5-	T44.6X6-
Diborane (gas)	T59.891-	T59.892-	T59.893-	T59.894-	-	-
Dibromochloropropane	T60.8X1-	T60.8X2-	T60.8X3-	T60.8X4-	-	-
Dibromodulcitol	T45.1X1-	T45.1X2-	T45.1X3-	T45.1X4-	T45.1X5-	T45.1X6-
Dibromoethane	T53.6X1-	T53.6X2-	T53.6X3-	T53.6X4-	-	-
Dibromomannitol	T45.1X1-	T45.1X2-	T45.1X3-	T45.1X4-	T45.1X5-	T45.1X6-
Dibromopropamidine isethionate	T49.0X1-	T49.0X2-	T49.0X3-	T49.0X4-	T49.0X5-	T49.0X6-
Dibrompropamidine	T49.0X1-	T49.0X2-	T49.0X3-	T49.0X4-	T49.0X5-	T49.0X6-
Dibucaine	T41.3X1-	T41.3X2-	T41.3X3-	T41.3X4-	T41.3X5-	T41.3X6-
topical (surface)	T41.3X1-	T41.3X2-	T41.3X3-	T41.3X4-	T41.3X5-	T41.3X6-
Dibunate sodium	T48.3X1-	T48.3X2-	T48.3X3-	T48.3X4-	T48.3X5-	T48.3X6-
Dibutoline sulfate	T44.3X1-	T44.3X2-	T44.3X3-	T44.3X4-	T44.3X5-	T44.3X6-
Dicamba	T60.3X1-	T60.3X2-	T60.3X3-	T60.3X4-	-	-
Dicapthon	T60.0X1-	T60.0X2-	T60.0X3-	T60.0X4-	-	-
Dichlobenil	T60.3X1-	T60.3X2-	T60.3X3-	T60.3X4-	-	-
Dichlone	T60.3X1-	T60.3X2-	T60.3X3-	T60.3X4-	-	-
Dichloralphenozone	T42.6X1-	T42.6X2-	T42.6X3-	T42.6X4-	T42.6X5-	T42.6X6-
Dichlorbenzidine	T65.3X1-	T65.3X2-	T65.3X3-	T65.3X4-	-	-
Dichlorhydrin	T52.8X1-	T52.8X2-	T52.8X3-	T52.8X4-	-	-
Dichlorhydroxyquinoline	T37.8X1-	T37.8X2-	T37.8X3-	T37.8X4-	T37.8X5-	T37.8X6-
Dichlorobenzene	T53.7X1-	T53.7X2-	T53.7X3-	T53.7X4-	-	-
Dichlorobenzyl alcohol	T49.6X1-	T49.6X2-	T49.6X3-	T49.6X4-	T49.6X5-	T49.6X6-
Dichlorodifluoromethane	T53.5X1-	T53.5X2-	T53.5X3-	T53.5X4-	-	-
Dichloroethane	T52.8X1-	T52.8X2-	T52.8X3-	T52.8X4-	-	-
Sym-Dichloroethyl ether	T53.6X1-	T53.6X2-	T53.6X3-	T53.6X4-	-	-
Dichloroethyl sulfide, not in war	T59.891-	T59.892-	T59.893-	T59.894-	-	-
Dichloroethylene	T53.6X1-	T53.6X2-	T53.6X3-	T53.6X4-	-	-
Dichloroformoxine, not in war	T59.891-	T59.892-	T59.893-	T59.894-	-	-
Dichlorohydrin, alpha-dichlorohydrin	T52.8X1-	T52.8X2-	T52.8X3-	T52.8X4-	-	-
Dichloromethane (solvent)	T53.4X1-	T53.4X2-	T53.4X3-	T53.4X4-	-	-
vapor	T53.4X1-	T53.4X2-	T53.4X3-	T53.4X4-	-	-
Dichloronaphthoquinone	T60.3X1-	T60.3X2-	T60.3X3-	T60.3X4-	-	-
Dichlorophen	T37.4X1-	T37.4X2-	T37.4X3-	T37.4X4-	T37.4X5-	T37.4X6-
2,4-Dichlorophenoxyacetic acid	T60.3X1-	T60.3X2-	T60.3X3-	T60.3X4-	-	-
Dichloropropene	T60.3X1-	T60.3X2-	T60.3X3-	T60.3X4-	-	-
Dichloropropionic acid	T60.3X1-	T60.3X2-	T60.3X3-	T60.3X4-	-	-
Dichlorphenamide	T50.2X1-	T50.2X2-	T50.2X3-	T50.2X4-	T50.2X5-	T50.2X6-
Dichlorvos	T60.0X1-	T60.0X2-	T60.0X3-	T60.0X4-	-	-
Diclofenac	T39.391-	T39.392-	T39.393-	T39.394-	T39.395-	T39.396-
Diclofenamide	T50.2X1-	T50.2X2-	T50.2X3-	T50.2X4-	T50.2X5-	T50.2X6-
Diclofensine	T43.291-	T43.292-	T43.293-	T43.294-	T43.295-	T43.296-
Diclonixine	T39.8X1-	T39.8X2-	T39.8X3-	T39.8X4-	T39.8X5-	T39.8X6-
Dicloxacillin	T36.0X1-	T36.0X2-	T36.0X3-	T36.0X4-	T36.0X5-	T36.0X6-
Dicophane	T49.0X1-	T49.0X2-	T49.0X3-	T49.0X4-	T49.0X5-	T49.0X6-
Dicoumarol, dicoumarin, dicumarol	T45.511-	T45.512-	T45.513-	T45.514-	T45.515-	T45.516-
Dicrotophos	T60.0X1-	T60.0X2-	T60.0X3-	T60.0X4-	-	-
Dicyanogen (gas)	T65.0X1-	T65.0X2-	T65.0X3-	T65.0X4-	-	-
Dicyclomine	T44.3X1-	T44.3X2-	T44.3X3-	T44.3X4-	T44.3X5-	T44.3X6-
Dicycloverine	T44.3X1-	T44.3X2-	T44.3X3-	T44.3X4-	T44.3X5-	T44.3X6-
Dideoxycytidine	T37.5X1-	T37.5X2-	T37.5X3-	T37.5X4-	T37.5X5-	T37.5X6-
Dideoxyinosine	T37.5X1-	T37.5X2-	T37.5X3-	T37.5X4-	T37.5X5-	T37.5X6-
Dieldrin (vapor)	T60.1X1-	T60.1X2-	T60.1X3-	T60.1X4-	-	-
Diemal	T42.3X1-	T42.3X2-	T42.3X3-	T42.3X4-	T42.3X5-	T42.3X6-
Dienestrol	T38.5X1-	T38.5X2-	T38.5X3-	T38.5X4-	T38.5X5-	T38.5X6-
Dienoestrol	T38.5X1-	T38.5X2-	T38.5X3-	T38.5X4-	T38.5X5-	T38.5X6-
Dietetic drug NEC	T50.901-	T50.902-	T50.903-	T50.904-	T50.905-	T50.906-

Substance	Poisoning, Accidental (unintentional)	Poisoning, Intentional self-harm	Poisoning, Assault	Poisoning, Undetermined	Adverse effect	Underdosing
Diethazine	T42.8X1-	T42.8X2-	T42.8X3-	T42.8X4-	T42.8X5-	T42.8X6-
Diethyl						
barbituric acid	T42.3X1-	T42.3X2-	T42.3X3-	T42.3X4-	T42.3X5-	T42.3X6-
carbamazine	T37.4X1-	T37.4X2-	T37.4X3-	T37.4X4-	T37.4X5-	T37.4X6-
carbinol	T51.3X1-	T51.3X2-	T51.3X3-	T51.3X4-	-	-
carbonate	T52.8X1-	T52.8X2-	T52.8X3-	T52.8X4-	-	-
ether (vapor) — see also ether	T41.0X1-	T41.0X2-	T41.0X3-	T41.0X4-	T41.0X5-	T41.0X6-
oxide	T52.8X1-	T52.8X2-	T52.8X3-	T52.8X4-	-	-
propion	T50.5X1-	T50.5X2-	T50.5X3-	T50.5X4-	T50.5X5-	T50.5X6-
stilbestrol	T38.5X1-	T38.5X2-	T38.5X3-	T38.5X4-	T38.5X5-	T38.5X6-
toluamide (nonmedicinal)	T60.8X1-	T60.8X2-	T60.8X3-	T60.8X4-		
medicinal	T49.3X1-	T49.3X2-	T49.3X3-	T49.3X4-	T49.3X5-	T49.3X6-
Diethylcarbamazine	T37.4X1-	T37.4X2-	T37.4X3-	T37.4X4-	T37.4X5-	T37.4X6-
Diethylene						
dioxide	T52.8X1-	T52.8X2-	T52.8X3-	T52.8X4-	-	-
glycol (monoacetate) (monobutyl ether) (monoethyl ether)	T52.3X1-	T52.3X2-	T52.3X3-	T52.3X4-	-	-
Diethylhexylphthalate	T65.891-	T65.892-	T65.893-	T65.894-	-	-
Diethylpropion	T50.5X1-	T50.5X2-	T50.5X3-	T50.5X4-	T50.5X5-	T50.5X6-
Diethylstilbestrol	T38.5X1-	T38.5X2-	T38.5X3-	T38.5X4-	T38.5X5-	T38.5X6-
Diethylstilboestrol	T38.5X1-	T38.5X2-	T38.5X3-	T38.5X4-	T38.5X5-	T38.5X6-
Diethylsulfone-diethylmethane	T42.6X1-	T42.6X2-	T42.6X3-	T42.6X4-	T42.6X5-	T42.6X6-
Diethyltoluamide	T49.0X1-	T49.0X2-	T49.0X3-	T49.0X4-	T49.0X5-	T49.0X6-
Diethyltryptamine (DET)	T40.991-	T40.992-	T40.993-	T40.994-	-	-
Difebarbamate	T42.3X1-	T42.3X2-	T42.3X3-	T42.3X4-	T42.3X5-	T42.3X6-
Difencloxazine	T40.2X1-	T40.2X2-	T40.2X3-	T40.2X4-	T40.2X5-	T40.2X6-
Difenidol	T45.0X1-	T45.0X2-	T45.0X3-	T45.0X4-	T45.0X5-	T45.0X6-
Difenoxin	T47.6X1-	T47.6X2-	T47.6X3-	T47.6X4-	T47.6X5-	T47.6X6-
Difetarsone	T37.3X1-	T37.3X2-	T37.3X3-	T37.3X4-	T37.3X5-	T37.3X6-
Diffusin	T45.3X1-	T45.3X2-	T45.3X3-	T45.3X4-	T45.3X5-	T45.3X6-
Diflorasone	T49.0X1-	T49.0X2-	T49.0X3-	T49.0X4-	T49.0X5-	T49.0X6-
Diflos	T44.0X1-	T44.0X2-	T44.0X3-	T44.0X4-	T44.0X5-	T44.0X6-
Diflubenzuron	T60.1X1-	T60.1X2-	T60.1X3-	T60.1X4-		
Diflucortolone	T49.0X1-	T49.0X2-	T49.0X3-	T49.0X4-	T49.0X5-	T49.0X6-
Diflunisal	T39.091-	T39.092-	T39.093-	T39.094-	T39.095-	T39.096-
Difluoromethyldopa	T42.8X1-	T42.8X2-	T42.8X3-	T42.8X4-	T42.8X5-	T42.8X6-
Difluorophate	T44.0X1-	T44.0X2-	T44.0X3-	T44.0X4-	T44.0X5-	T44.0X6-
Digestant NEC	T47.5X1-	T47.5X2-	T47.5X3-	T47.5X4-	T47.5X5-	T47.5X6-
Digitalin (e)	T46.0X1-	T46.0X2-	T46.0X3-	T46.0X4-	T46.0X5-	T46.0X6-
Digitalis (leaf) (glycoside)	T46.0X1-	T46.0X2-	T46.0X3-	T46.0X4-	T46.0X5-	T46.0X6-
lanata	T46.0X1-	T46.0X2-	T46.0X3-	T46.0X4-	T46.0X5-	T46.0X6-
purpurea	T46.0X1-	T46.0X2-	T46.0X3-	T46.0X4-	T46.0X5-	T46.0X6-
Digitoxin	T46.0X1-	T46.0X2-	T46.0X3-	T46.0X4-	T46.0X5-	T46.0X6-
Digitoxose	T46.0X1-	T46.0X2-	T46.0X3-	T46.0X4-	T46.0X5-	T46.0X6-
Digoxin	T46.0X1-	T46.0X2-	T46.0X3-	T46.0X4-	T46.0X5-	T46.0X6-
Digoxine	T46.0X1-	T46.0X2-	T46.0X3-	T46.0X4-	T46.0X5-	T46.0X6-
Dihydralazine	T46.5X1-	T46.5X2-	T46.5X3-	T46.5X4-	T46.5X5-	T46.5X6-
Dihydrazine	T46.5X1-	T46.5X2-	T46.5X3-	T46.5X4-	T46.5X5-	T46.5X6-
Dihydrocodeine	T40.2X1-	T40.2X2-	T40.2X3-	T40.2X4-	T40.2X5-	T40.2X6-
Dihydrocodeinone	T40.2X1-	T40.2X2-	T40.2X3-	T40.2X4-	T40.2X5-	T40.2X6-
Dihydroergocornine	T46.7X1-	T46.7X2-	T46.7X3-	T46.7X4-	T46.7X5-	T46.7X6-
Dihydroergocristine (mesilate)	T46.7X1-	T46.7X2-	T46.7X3-	T46.7X4-	T46.7X5-	T46.7X6-
Dihydroergokryptine	T46.7X1-	T46.7X2-	T46.7X3-	T46.7X4-	T46.7X5-	T46.7X6-
Dihydroergotamine	T46.5X1-	T46.5X2-	T46.5X3-	T46.5X4-	T46.5X5-	T46.5X6-
Dihydroergotoxine	T46.7X1-	T46.7X2-	T46.7X3-	T46.7X4-	T46.7X5-	T46.7X6-
mesilate	T46.7X1-	T46.7X2-	T46.7X3-	T46.7X4-	T46.7X5-	T46.7X6-
Dihydrohydroxycodeinone	T40.2X1-	T40.2X2-	T40.2X3-	T40.2X4-	T40.2X5-	T40.2X6-
Dihydrohydroxymorphinone	T40.2X1-	T40.2X2-	T40.2X3-	T40.2X4-	T40.2X5-	T40.2X6-
Dihydroisocodeine	T40.2X1-	T40.2X2-	T40.2X3-	T40.2X4-	T40.2X5-	T40.2X6-
Dihydromorphine	T40.2X1-	T40.2X2-	T40.2X3-	T40.2X4-	-	-
Dihydromorphinone	T40.2X1-	T40.2X2-	T40.2X3-	T40.2X4-		T40.2X6-
Dihydrostreptomycin	T36.5X1-	T36.5X2-	T36.5X3-	T36.5X4-	T36.5X5-	T36.5X6-
Dihydrotachysterol	T45.2X1-	T45.2X2-	T45.2X3-	T45.2X4-	T45.2X5-	T45.2X6-
Dihydroxyaluminum aminoacetate	T47.1X1-	T47.1X2-	T47.1X3-	T47.1X4-	T47.1X5-	T47.1X6-
Dihydroxyaluminum sodium carbonate	T47.1X1-	T47.1X2-	T47.1X3-	T47.1X4-	T47.1X5-	T47.1X6-
Dihydroxyanthraquinone	T47.2X1-	T47.2X2-	T47.2X3-	T47.2X4-	T47.2X5-	T47.2X6-
Dihydroxycodeinone	T40.2X1-	T40.2X2-	T40.2X3-	T40.2X4-	T40.2X5-	T40.2X6-
Dihydroxypropyl theophylline	T50.2X1-	T50.2X2-	T50.2X3-	T50.2X4-	T50.2X5-	T50.2X6-
Diiodohydroxyquin	T37.8X1-	T37.8X2-	T37.8X3-	T37.8X4-	T37.8X5-	T37.8X6-
topical	T49.0X1-	T49.0X2-	T49.0X3-	T49.0X4-	T49.0X5-	T49.0X6-
Diiodohydroxyquinoline	T37.8X1-	T37.8X2-	T37.8X3-	T37.8X4-	T37.8X5-	T37.8X6-
Diiodotyrosine	T38.2X1-	T38.2X2-	T38.2X3-	T38.2X4-	T38.2X5-	T38.2X6-
Diisopromine	T44.3X1-	T44.3X2-	T44.3X3-	T44.3X4-	T44.3X5-	T44.3X6-
Diisopropylamine	T46.3X1-	T46.3X2-	T46.3X3-	T46.3X4-	T46.3X5-	T46.3X6-

Substance	Poisoning, Accidental (unintentional)	Poisoning, Intentional self-harm	Poisoning, Assault	Poisoning, Undetermined	Adverse effect	Underdosing
Diisopropylfluorophos-phonate	T44.0X1-	T44.0X2-	T44.0X3-	T44.0X4-	T44.0X5-	T44.0X6-
Dilantin	T42.0X1-	T42.0X2-	T42.0X3-	T42.0X4-	T42.0X5-	T42.0X6-
Dilaudid	T40.2X1-	T40.2X2-	T40.2X3-	T40.2X4-	T40.2X5-	T40.2X6-
Dilazep	T46.3X1-	T46.3X2-	T46.3X3-	T46.3X4-	T46.3X5-	T46.3X6-
Dill	T47.5X1-	T47.5X2-	T47.5X3-	T47.5X4-	T47.5X5-	T47.5X6-
Diloxanide	T37.3X1-	T37.3X2-	T37.3X3-	T37.3X4-	T37.3X5-	T37.3X6-
Diltiazem	T46.1X1-	T46.1X2-	T46.1X3-	T46.1X4-	T46.1X5-	T46.1X6-
Dimazole	T49.0X1-	T49.0X2-	T49.0X3-	T49.0X4-	T49.0X5-	T49.0X6-
Dimefline	T50.7X1-	T50.7X2-	T50.7X3-	T50.7X4-	T50.7X5-	T50.7X6-
Dimefox	T60.0X1-	T60.0X2-	T60.0X3-	T60.0X4-	-	-
Dimemorfan	T48.3X1-	T48.3X2-	T48.3X3-	T48.3X4-	T48.3X5-	T48.3X6-
Dimenhydrinate	T45.0X1-	T45.0X2-	T45.0X3-	T45.0X4-	T45.0X5-	T45.0X6-
Dimercaprol (British anti-lewisite)	T45.8X1-	T45.8X2-	T45.8X3-	T45.8X4-	T45.8X5-	T45.8X6-
Dimercaptopropanol	T45.8X1-	T45.8X2-	T45.8X3-	T45.8X4-	T45.8X5-	T45.8X6-
Dimestrol	T38.5X1-	T38.5X2-	T38.5X3-	T38.5X4-	T38.5X5-	T38.5X6-
Dimetane	T45.0X1-	T45.0X2-	T45.0X3-	T45.0X4-	T45.0X5-	T45.0X6-
Dimethicone	T47.1X1-	T47.1X2-	T47.1X3-	T47.1X4-	T47.1X5-	T47.1X6-
Dimethindene	T45.0X1-	T45.0X2-	T45.0X3-	T45.0X4-	T45.0X5-	T45.0X6-
Dimethisoquin	T49.1X1-	T49.1X2-	T49.1X3-	T49.1X4-	T49.1X5-	T49.1X6-
Dimethisterone	T38.5X1-	T38.5X2-	T38.5X3-	T38.5X4-	T38.5X5-	T38.5X6-
Dimethoate	T60.0X1-	T60.0X2-	T60.0X3-	T60.0X4-	-	-
Dimethocaine	T41.3X1-	T41.3X2-	T41.3X3-	T41.3X4-	T41.3X5-	T41.3X6-
Dimethoxanate	T48.3X1-	T48.3X2-	T48.3X3-	T48.3X4-	T48.3X5-	T48.3X6-
Dimethyl						
arsine, arsinic acid	T57.0X1-	T57.0X2-	T57.0X3-	T57.0X4-	-	-
carbinol	T51.2X1-	T51.2X2-	T51.2X3-	T51.2X4-	-	-
carbonate	T52.8X1-	T52.8X2-	T52.8X3-	T52.8X4-	-	-
diguanide	T38.3X1-	T38.3X2-	T38.3X3-	T38.3X4-	T38.3X5-	T38.3X6-
ketone	T52.4X1-	T52.4X2-	T52.4X3-	T52.4X4-	-	-
vapor	T52.4X1-	T52.4X2-	T52.4X3-	T52.4X4-		
meperidine	T40.2X1-	T40.2X2-	T40.2X3-	T40.2X4-	T40.2X5-	T40.2X6-
parathion	T60.0X1-	T60.0X2-	T60.0X3-	T60.0X4-	-	-
phthlate	T49.3X1-	T49.3X2-	T49.3X3-	T49.3X4-	T49.3X5-	T49.3X6-
polysiloxane	T47.8X1-	T47.8X2-	T47.8X3-	T47.8X4-	T47.8X5-	T47.8X6-
sulfate (fumes)	T59.891-	T59.892-	T59.893-	T59.894-	-	-
liquid	T65.891-	T65.892-	T65.893-	T65.894-	-	-
sulfoxide (nonmedicinal)	T52.8X1-	T52.8X2-	T52.8X3-	T52.8X4-		
medicinal	T49.4X1-	T49.4X2-	T49.4X3-	T49.4X4-	T49.4X5-	T49.4X6-
tryptamine	T40.991-	T40.992-	T40.993-	T40.994-	-	-
tubocurarine	T48.1X1-	T48.1X2-	T48.1X3-	T48.1X4-	T48.1X5-	T48.1X6-
Dimethylamine sulfate	T49.4X1-	T49.4X2-	T49.4X3-	T49.4X4-	T49.4X5-	T49.4X6-
Dimethylformamide	T52.8X1-	T52.8X2-	T52.8X3-	T52.8X4-		
Dimethyltubocurarinium chloride	T48.1X1-	T48.1X2-	T48.1X3-	T48.1X4-	T48.1X5-	T48.1X6-
Dimeticone	T47.1X1-	T47.1X2-	T47.1X3-	T47.1X4-	T47.1X5-	T47.1X6-
Dimetilan	T60.0X1-	T60.0X2-	T60.0X3-	T60.0X4-	-	-
Dimetindene	T45.0X1-	T45.0X2-	T45.0X3-	T45.0X4-	T45.0X5-	T45.0X6-
Dimetotiazine	T43.3X1-	T43.3X2-	T43.3X3-	T43.3X4-	T43.3X5-	T43.3X6-
Dimorpholamine	T50.7X1-	T50.7X2-	T50.7X3-	T50.7X4-	T50.7X5-	T50.7X6-
Dimoxyline	T46.3X1-	T46.3X2-	T46.3X3-	T46.3X4-	T46.3X5-	T46.3X6-
Dinitrobenzene	T65.3X1-	T65.3X2-	T65.3X3-	T65.3X4-		
vapor	T59.891-	T59.892-	T59.893-	T59.894-	-	-
Dinitrobenzol	T65.3X1-	T65.3X2-	T65.3X3-	T65.3X4-		
vapor	T59.891-	T59.892-	T59.893-	T59.894-	-	-
Dinitrobutylphenol	T65.3X1-	T65.3X2-	T65.3X3-	T65.3X4-		
Dinitro (-ortho-) cresol (pesticide) (spray)	T65.3X1-	T65.3X2-	T65.3X3-	T65.3X4-		
Dinitrocyclohexylphenol	T65.3X1-	T65.3X2-	T65.3X3-	T65.3X4-		-
Dinitrophenol	T65.3X1-	T65.3X2-	T65.3X3-	T65.3X4-		
Dinoprost	T48.0X1-	T48.0X2-	T48.0X3-	T48.0X4-	T48.0X5-	T48.0X6-
Dinoprostone	T48.0X1-	T48.0X2-	T48.0X3-	T48.0X4-	T48.0X5-	T48.0X6-
Dinoseb	T60.3X1-	T60.3X2-	T60.3X3-	T60.3X4-		
Dioctyl sulfosuccinate (calcium) (sodium)	T47.4X1-	T47.4X2-	T47.4X3-	T47.4X4-	T47.4X5-	T47.4X6-
Diodone	T50.8X1-	T50.8X2-	T50.8X3-	T50.8X4-	T50.8X5-	T50.8X6-
Diodoquin	T37.8X1-	T37.8X2-	T37.8X3-	T37.8X4-	T37.8X5-	T37.8X6-
Dionin	T40.2X1-	T40.2X2-	T40.2X3-	T40.2X4-	T40.2X5-	T40.2X6-
Diosmin	T46.991-	T46.992-	T46.993-	T46.994-	T46.995-	T46.996-
Dioxane	T52.8X1-	T52.8X2-	T52.8X3-	T52.8X4-	-	-
Dioxathion	T60.0X1-	T60.0X2-	T60.0X3-	T60.0X4-	-	-
Dioxin	T53.7X1-	T53.7X2-	T53.7X3-	T53.7X4-	-	-
Dioxopromethazine	T43.3X1-	T43.3X2-	T43.3X3-	T43.3X4-	T43.3X5-	T43.3X6-
Dioxyline	T46.3X1-	T46.3X2-	T46.3X3-	T46.3X4-	T46.3X5-	T46.3X6-
Dipentene	T52.8X1-	T52.8X2-	T52.8X3-	T52.8X4-	-	-
Diperodon	T41.3X1-	T41.3X2-	T41.3X3-	T41.3X4-	T41.3X5-	T41.3X6-
Diphacinone	T60.4X1-	T60.4X2-	T60.4X3-	T60.4X4-	-	-

Diphemanil — Elaterium

Substance	Poisoning, Accidental (unintentional)	Poisoning, Intentional self-harm	Poisoning, Assault	Poisoning, Undetermined	Adverse effect	Underdosing
Diphemanil	T44.3X1-	T44.3X2-	T44.3X3-	T44.3X4-	T44.3X5-	T44.3X6-
metilsulfate	T44.3X1-	T44.3X2-	T44.3X3-	T44.3X4-	T44.3X5-	T44.3X6-
Diphenadione	T45.511-	T45.512-	T45.513-	T45.514-	T45.515-	T45.516-
rodenticide	T60.4X1-	T60.4X2-	T60.4X3-	T60.4X4-	-	-
Diphenhydramine	T45.0X1-	T45.0X2-	T45.0X3-	T45.0X4-	T45.0X5-	T45.0X6-
Diphenidol	T45.0X1-	T45.0X2-	T45.0X3-	T45.0X4-	T45.0X5-	T45.0X6-
Diphenoxylate	T47.6X1-	T47.6X2-	T47.6X3-	T47.6X4-	T47.6X5-	T47.6X6-
Diphenylamine	T65.3X1-	T65.3X2-	T65.3X3-	T65.3X4-	-	-
Diphenylbutazone	T39.2X1-	T39.2X2-	T39.2X3-	T39.2X4-	T39.2X5-	T39.2X6-
Diphenylchloroarsine, not in war	T57.0X1-	T57.0X2-	T57.0X3-	T57.0X4-	-	-
Diphenylhydantoin	T42.0X1-	T42.0X2-	T42.0X3-	T42.0X4-	T42.0X5-	T42.0X6-
Diphenylmethane dye	T52.1X1-	T52.1X2-	T52.1X3-	T52.1X4-	-	-
Diphenylpyraline	T45.0X1-	T45.0X2-	T45.0X3-	T45.0X4-	T45.0X5-	T45.0X6-
Diphtheria						
antitoxin	T50.Z11-	T50.Z12-	T50.Z13-	T50.Z14-	T50.Z15-	T50.Z16-
toxoid	T50.A91-	T50.A92-	T50.A93-	T50.A94-	T50.A95-	T50.A96-
with tetanus toxoid	T50.A21-	T50.A22-	T50.A23-	T50.A24-	T50.A25-	T50.A26-
with pertussis component	T50.A11-	T50.A12-	T50.A13-	T50.A14-	T50.A15-	T50.A16-
vaccine	T50.A91-	T50.A92-	T50.A93-	T50.A94-	T50.A95-	T50.A96-
combination						
including pertussis	T50.A11-	T50.A12-	T50.A13-	T50.A14-	T50.A15-	T50.A16-
without pertussis	T50.A21-	T50.A22-	T50.A23-	T50.A24-	T50.A25-	T50.A26-
Diphylline	T50.2X1-	T50.2X2-	T50.2X3-	T50.2X4-	T50.2X5-	T50.2X6-
Dipipanone	T40.4X1-	T40.4X2-	T40.4X3-	T40.4X4-	-	-
Dipivefrine	T49.5X1-	T49.5X2-	T49.5X3-	T49.5X4-	T49.5X5-	T49.5X6-
Diplovax	T50.B91-	T50.B92-	T50.B93-	T50.B94-	T50.B95-	T50.B96-
Diprophylline	T50.2X1-	T50.2X2-	T50.2X3-	T50.2X4-	T50.2X5-	T50.2X6-
Dipropyline	T48.291-	T48.292-	T48.293-	T48.294-	T48.295-	T48.296-
Dipyridamole	T46.3X1-	T46.3X2-	T46.3X3-	T46.3X4-	T46.3X5-	T46.3X6-
Dipyrone	T39.2X1-	T39.2X2-	T39.2X3-	T39.2X4-	T39.2X5-	T39.2X6-
Diquat (dibromide)	T60.3X1-	T60.3X2-	T60.3X3-	T60.3X4-	-	-
Disinfectant	T65.891-	T65.892-	T65.893-	T65.894-	-	-
alkaline	T54.3X1-	T54.3X2-	T54.3X3-	T54.3X4-	-	-
aromatic	T54.1X1-	T54.1X2-	T54.1X3-	T54.1X4-	-	-
intestinal	T37.8X1-	T37.8X2-	T37.8X3-	T37.8X4-	T37.8X5-	T37.8X6-
Disipal	T42.8X1-	T42.8X2-	T42.8X3-	T42.8X4-	T42.8X5-	T42.8X6-
Disodium edetate	T50.6X1-	T50.6X2-	T50.6X3-	T50.6X4-	T50.6X5-	T50.6X6-
Disoprofol	T41.291-	T41.292-	T41.293-	T41.294-	T41.295-	T41.296-
Disopyramide	T46.2X1-	T46.2X2-	T46.2X3-	T46.2X4-	T46.2X5-	T46.2X6-
Distigmine (bromide)	T44.0X1-	T44.0X2-	T44.0X3-	T44.0X4-	T44.0X5-	T44.0X6-
Disulfamide	T50.2X1-	T50.2X2-	T50.2X3-	T50.2X4-	T50.2X5-	T50.2X6-
Disulfanilamide	T37.0X1-	T37.0X2-	T37.0X3-	T37.0X4-	T37.0X5-	T37.0X6-
Disulfiram	T50.6X1-	T50.6X2-	T50.6X3-	T50.6X4-	T50.6X5-	T50.6X6-
Disulfoton	T60.0X1-	T60.0X2-	T60.0X3-	T60.0X4-	-	-
Dithiazanine iodide	T37.4X1-	T37.4X2-	T37.4X3-	T37.4X4-	T37.4X5-	T37.4X6-
Dithiocarbamate	T60.0X1-	T60.0X2-	T60.0X3-	T60.0X4-	-	-
Dithranol	T49.4X1-	T49.4X2-	T49.4X3-	T49.4X4-	T49.4X5-	T49.4X6-
Diucardin	T50.2X1-	T50.2X2-	T50.2X3-	T50.2X4-	T50.2X5-	T50.2X6-
Diupres	T50.2X1-	T50.2X2-	T50.2X3-	T50.2X4-	T50.2X5-	T50.2X6-
Diuretic NEC	T50.2X1-	T50.2X2-	T50.2X3-	T50.2X4-	T50.2X5-	T50.2X6-
benzothiadiazine	T50.2X1-	T50.2X2-	T50.2X3-	T50.2X4-	T50.2X5-	T50.2X6-
carbonic acid anhydrase inhibitors	T50.2X1-	T50.2X2-	T50.2X3-	T50.2X4-	T50.2X5-	T50.2X6-
furfuryl NEC	T50.2X1-	T50.2X2-	T50.2X3-	T50.2X4-	T50.2X5-	T50.2X6-
loop (high-ceiling)	T50.1X1-	T50.1X2-	T50.1X3-	T50.1X4-	T50.1X5-	T50.1X6-
mercurial NEC	T50.2X1-	T50.2X2-	T50.2X3-	T50.2X4-	T50.2X5-	T50.2X6-
osmotic	T50.2X1-	T50.2X2-	T50.2X3-	T50.2X4-	T50.2X5-	T50.2X6-
purine NEC	T50.2X1-	T50.2X2-	T50.2X3-	T50.2X4-	T50.2X5-	T50.2X6-
saluretic NEC	T50.2X1-	T50.2X2-	T50.2X3-	T50.2X4-	T50.2X5-	T50.2X6-
sulfonamide	T50.2X1-	T50.2X2-	T50.2X3-	T50.2X4-	T50.2X5-	T50.2X6-
thiazide NEC	T50.2X1-	T50.2X2-	T50.2X3-	T50.2X4-	T50.2X5-	T50.2X6-
xanthine	T50.2X1-	T50.2X2-	T50.2X3-	T50.2X4-	T50.2X5-	T50.2X6-
Diurgin	T50.2X1-	T50.2X2-	T50.2X3-	T50.2X4-	T50.2X5-	T50.2X6-
Diuril	T50.2X1-	T50.2X2-	T50.2X3-	T50.2X4-	T50.2X5-	T50.2X6-
Diuron	T60.3X1-	T60.3X2-	T60.3X3-	T60.3X4-	-	-
Divalproex	T42.6X1-	T42.6X2-	T42.6X3-	T42.6X4-	T42.6X5-	T42.6X6-
Divinyl ether	T41.0X1-	T41.0X2-	T41.0X3-	T41.0X4-	T41.0X5-	T41.0X6-
Dixanthogen	T49.0X1-	T49.0X2-	T49.0X3-	T49.0X4-	T49.0X5-	T49.0X6-
Dixyrazine	T43.3X1-	T43.3X2-	T43.3X3-	T43.3X4-	T43.3X5-	T43.3X6-
D-lysergic acid diethylamide	T40.8X1-	T40.8X2-	T40.8X3-	T40.8X4-	-	-
DMCT	T36.4X1-	T36.4X2-	T36.4X3-	T36.4X4-	T36.4X5-	T36.4X6-
DMSO — see Dimethyl sulfoxide						
DNBP	T60.3X1-	T60.3X2-	T60.3X3-	T60.3X4-	-	-
DNOC	T65.3X1-	T65.3X2-	T65.3X3-	T65.3X4-	-	-
Dobutamine	T44.5X1-	T44.5X2-	T44.5X3-	T44.5X4-	T44.5X5-	T44.5X6-
DOCA	T38.0X1-	T38.0X2-	T38.0X3-	T38.0X4-	T38.0X5-	T38.0X6-
Docusate sodium	T47.4X1-	T47.4X2-	T47.4X3-	T47.4X4-	T47.4X5-	T47.4X6-

Substance	Poisoning, Accidental (unintentional)	Poisoning, Intentional self-harm	Poisoning, Assault	Poisoning, Undetermined	Adverse effect	Underdosing
Dodicin	T49.0X1-	T49.0X2-	T49.0X3-	T49.0X4-	T49.0X5-	T49.0X6-
Dofamium chloride	T49.0X1-	T49.0X2-	T49.0X3-	T49.0X4-	T49.0X5-	T49.0X6-
Dolophine	T40.3X1-	T40.3X2-	T40.3X3-	T40.3X4-	T40.3X5-	T40.3X6-
Doloxene	T39.8X1-	T39.8X2-	T39.8X3-	T39.8X4-	T39.8X5-	T39.8X6-
Domestic gas (after combustion) — see Gas, utility						
prior to combustion	T59.891-	T59.892-	T59.893-	T59.894-	-	-
Domiodol	T48.4X1-	T48.4X2-	T48.4X3-	T48.4X4-	T48.4X5-	T48.4X6-
Domiphen (bromide)	T49.0X1-	T49.0X2-	T49.0X3-	T49.0X4-	T49.0X5-	T49.0X6-
Domperidone	T45.0X1-	T45.0X2-	T45.0X3-	T45.0X4-	T45.0X5-	T45.0X6-
Dopa	T42.8X1-	T42.8X2-	T42.8X3-	T42.8X4-	T42.8X5-	T42.8X6-
Dopamine	T44.991-	T44.992-	T44.993-	T44.994-	T44.995-	T44.996-
Doriden	T42.6X1-	T42.6X2-	T42.6X3-	T42.6X4-	T42.6X5-	T42.6X6-
Dormiral	T42.3X1-	T42.3X2-	T42.3X3-	T42.3X4-	T42.3X5-	T42.3X6-
Dormison	T42.6X1-	T42.6X2-	T42.6X3-	T42.6X4-	T42.6X5-	T42.6X6-
Dornase	T48.4X1-	T48.4X2-	T48.4X3-	T48.4X4-	T48.4X5-	T48.4X6-
Dorsacaine	T41.3X1-	T41.3X2-	T41.3X3-	T41.3X4-	T41.3X5-	T41.3X6-
Dosulepin	T43.011-	T43.012-	T43.013-	T43.014-	T43.015-	T43.016-
Dothiepin	T43.011-	T43.012-	T43.013-	T43.015-	T43.015-	T43.016-
Doxantrazole	T48.6X1-	T48.6X2-	T48.6X3-	T48.6X4-	T48.6X5-	T48.6X6-
Doxapram	T50.7X1-	T50.7X2-	T50.7X3-	T50.7X4-	T50.7X5-	T50.7X6-
Doxazosin	T44.6X1-	T44.6X2-	T44.6X3-	T44.6X4-	T44.6X5-	T44.6X6-
Doxepin	T43.011-	T43.012-	T43.013-	T43.014-	T43.015-	T43.016-
Doxifluridine	T45.1X1-	T45.1X2-	T45.1X3-	T45.1X4-	T45.1X5-	T45.1X6-
Doxorubicin	T45.1X1-	T45.1X2-	T45.1X3-	T45.1X4-	T45.1X5-	T45.1X6-
Doxycycline	T36.4X1-	T36.4X2-	T36.4X3-	T36.4X4-	T36.4X5-	T36.4X6-
Doxylamine	T45.0X1-	T45.0X2-	T45.0X3-	T45.0X4-	T45.0X5-	T45.0X6-
Dramamine	T45.0X1-	T45.0X2-	T45.0X3-	T45.0X4-	T45.0X5-	T45.0X6-
Drano (drain cleaner)	T54.3X1-	T54.3X2-	T54.3X3-	T54.3X4-	-	-
Dressing, live pulp	T49.7X1-	T49.7X2-	T49.7X3-	T49.7X4-	T49.7X5-	T49.7X6-
Drocode	T40.2X1-	T40.2X2-	T40.2X3-	T40.2X4-	T40.2X5-	T40.2X6-
Dromoran	T40.2X1-	T40.2X2-	T40.2X3-	T40.2X4-	T40.2X5-	T40.2X6-
Dromostanolone	T38.7X1-	T38.7X2-	T38.7X3-	T38.7X4-	T38.7X5-	T38.7X6-
Dronabinol	T40.7X1-	T40.7X2-	T40.7X3-	T40.7X4-	T40.7X5-	T40.7X6-
Droperidol	T43.591-	T43.592-	T43.593-	T43.594-	T43.595-	T43.596-
Dropropizine	T48.3X1-	T48.3X2-	T48.3X3-	T48.3X4-	T48.3X5-	T48.3X6-
Drostanolone	T38.7X1-	T38.7X2-	T38.7X3-	T38.7X4-	T38.7X5-	T38.7X6-
Drotaverine	T44.3X1-	T44.3X2-	T44.3X3-	T44.3X4-	T44.3X5-	T44.3X6-
Drotrecogin alfa	T45.511-	T45.512-	T45.513-	T45.514-	T45.515-	T45.516-
Drug NEC	T50.901-	T50.902-	T50.903-	T50.904-	T50.905-	T50.906-
specified NEC	T50.991-	T50.992-	T50.993-	T50.994-	T50.995-	T50.996-
DTIC	T45.1X1-	T45.1X2-	T45.1X3-	T45.1X4-	T45.1X5-	T45.1X6-
Duboisine	T44.3X1-	T44.3X2-	T44.3X3-	T44.3X4-	T44.3X5-	T44.3X6-
Dulcolax	T47.2X1-	T47.2X2-	T47.2X3-	T47.2X4-	T47.2X5-	T47.2X6-
Duponol (C) (EP)	T49.2X1-	T49.2X2-	T49.2X3-	T49.2X4-	T49.2X5-	T49.2X6-
Durabolin	T38.7X1-	T38.7X2-	T38.7X3-	T38.7X4-	T38.7X5-	T38.7X6-
Dyclone	T41.3X1-	T41.3X2-	T41.3X3-	T41.3X4-	T41.3X5-	T41.3X6-
Dyclonine	T41.3X1-	T41.3X2-	T41.3X3-	T41.3X4-	T41.3X5-	T41.3X6-
Dydrogesterone	T38.5X1-	T38.5X2-	T38.5X3-	T38.5X4-	T38.5X5-	T38.5X6-
Dye NEC	T65.6X1-	T65.6X2-	T65.6X3-	T65.6X4-	-	-
antiseptic	T49.0X1-	T49.0X2-	T49.0X3-	T49.0X4-	T49.0X5-	T49.0X6-
diagnostic agents	T50.8X1-	T50.8X2-	T50.8X3-	T50.8X4-	T50.8X5-	T50.8X6-
pharmaceutical NEC	T50.901-	T50.902-	T50.903-	T50.904-	T50.905-	T50.906-
Dyflos	T44.0X1-	T44.0X2-	T44.0X3-	T44.0X4-	T44.0X5-	T44.0X6-
Dymelor	T38.3X1-	T38.3X2-	T38.3X3-	T38.3X4-	T38.3X5-	T38.3X6-
Dynamite	T65.3X1-	T65.3X2-	T65.3X3-	T65.3X4-	-	-
fumes	T59.891-	T59.892-	T59.893-	T59.894-	-	-
Dyphylline	T44.3X1-	T44.3X2-	T44.3X3-	T44.3X4-	T44.3X5-	T44.3X6-
Ear drug NEC	T49.6X1-	T49.6X2-	T49.6X3-	T49.6X4-	T49.6X5-	T49.6X6-
Ear preparations	T49.6X1-	T49.6X2-	T49.6X3-	T49.6X4-	T49.6X5-	T49.6X6-
Echothiophate, echothiopate, echothiopate	T49.5X1-	T49.5X2-	T49.5X3-	T49.5X4-	T49.5X5-	T49.5X6-
Econazole	T49.0X1-	T49.0X2-	T49.0X3-	T49.0X4-	T49.0X5-	T49.0X6-
Ecothiopate iodide	T49.5X1-	T49.5X2-	T49.5X3-	T49.5X4-	T49.5X5-	T49.5X6-
Ecstasy	T43.621-	T43.622-	T43.623-	T43.624-	T43.625-	T43.626-
Ectylurea	T42.6X1-	T42.6X2-	T42.6X3-	T42.6X4-	T42.6X5-	T42.6X6-
Edathamil disodium	T45.8X1-	T45.8X2-	T45.8X3-	T45.8X4-	T45.8X5-	T45.8X6-
Edecrin	T50.1X1-	T50.1X2-	T50.1X3-	T50.1X4-	T50.1X5-	T50.1X6-
Edetate, disodium (calcium)	T45.8X1-	T45.8X2-	T45.8X3-	T45.8X4-	T45.8X5-	T45.8X6-
Edoxudine	T49.5X1-	T49.5X2-	T49.5X3-	T49.5X4-	T49.5X5-	T49.5X6-
Edrophonium	T44.0X1-	T44.0X2-	T44.0X3-	T44.0X4-	T44.0X5-	T44.0X6-
chloride	T44.0X1-	T44.0X2-	T44.0X3-	T44.0X4-	T44.0X5-	T44.0X6-
EDTA	T50.6X1-	T50.6X2-	T50.6X3-	T50.6X4-	T50.6X5-	T50.6X6-
Eflornithine	T37.2X1-	T37.2X2-	T37.2X3-	T37.2X4-	T37.2X5-	T37.2X6-
Efloxate	T46.3X1-	T46.3X2-	T46.3X3-	T46.3X4-	T46.3X5-	T46.3X6-
Elase	T49.8X1-	T49.8X2-	T49.8X3-	T49.8X4-	T49.8X5-	T49.8X6-
Elastase	T47.5X1-	T47.5X2-	T47.5X3-	T47.5X4-	T47.5X5-	T47.5X6-
Elaterium	T47.2X1-	T47.2X2-	T47.2X3-	T47.2X4-	T47.2X5-	T47.2X6-

Substance	Poisoning, Accidental (unintentional)	Poisoning, Intentional self-harm	Poisoning, Assault	Poisoning, Undetermined	Adverse effect	Underdosing
Elcatonin	T50.991-	T50.992-	T50.993-	T50.994-	T50.995-	T50.996-
Elder	T62.2X1-	T62.2X2-	T62.2X3-	T62.2X4-	-	-
berry, (unripe)	T62.1X1-	T62.1X2-	T62.1X3-	T62.1X4-	-	-
Electrolyte balance drug	T50.3X1-	T50.3X2-	T50.3X3-	T50.3X4-	T50.3X5-	T50.3X6-
Electrolytes NEC	T50.3X1-	T50.3X2-	T50.3X3-	T50.3X4-	T50.3X5-	T50.3X6-
Electrolytic agent NEC	T50.3X1-	T50.3X2-	T50.3X3-	T50.3X4-	T50.3X5-	T50.3X6-
Elemental diet	T50.901-	T50.902-	T50.903-	T50.904-	T50.905-	T50.906-
Elliptinium acetate	T45.1X1-	T45.1X2-	T45.1X3-	T45.1X4-	T45.1X5-	T45.1X6-
Embramine	T45.0X1-	T45.0X2-	T45.0X3-	T45.0X4-	T45.0X5-	T45.0X6-
Emepronium (salts)	T44.3X1-	T44.3X2-	T44.3X3-	T44.3X4-	T44.3X5-	T44.3X6-
bromide	T44.3X1-	T44.3X2-	T44.3X3-	T44.3X4-	T44.3X5-	T44.3X6-
Emetic NEC	T47.7X1-	T47.7X2-	T47.7X3-	T47.7X4-	T47.7X5-	T47.7X6-
Emetine	T37.3X1-	T37.3X2-	T37.3X3-	T37.3X4-	T37.3X5-	T37.3X6-
Emollient NEC	T49.3X1-	T49.3X2-	T49.3X3-	T49.3X4-	T49.3X5-	T49.3X6-
Emorfazone	T39.8X1-	T39.8X2-	T39.8X3-	T39.8X4-	T39.8X5-	T39.8X6-
Emylcamate	T43.591-	T43.592-	T43.593-	T43.594-	T43.595-	T43.596-
Enalapril	T46.4X1-	T46.4X2-	T46.4X3-	T46.4X4-	T46.4X5-	T46.4X6-
Enalaprilat	T46.4X1-	T46.4X2-	T46.4X3-	T46.4X4-	T46.4X5-	T46.4X6-
Encainide	T46.2X1-	T46.2X2-	T46.2X3-	T46.2X4-	T46.2X5-	T46.2X6-
Endocaine	T41.3X1-	T41.3X2-	T41.3X3-	T41.3X4-	T41.3X5-	T41.3X6-
Endosulfan	T60.2X1-	T60.2X2-	T60.2X3-	T60.2X4-	-	-
Endothall	T60.3X1-	T60.3X2-	T60.3X3-	T60.3X4-	-	-
Endralazine	T46.5X1-	T46.5X2-	T46.5X3-	T46.5X4-	T46.5X5-	T46.5X6-
Endrin	T60.1X1-	T60.1X2-	T60.1X3-	T60.1X4-	-	-
Enflurane	T41.0X1-	T41.0X2-	T41.0X3-	T41.0X4-	T41.0X5-	T41.0X6-
Enhexymal	T42.3X1-	T42.3X2-	T42.3X3-	T42.3X4-	T42.3X5-	T42.3X6-
Enocitabine	T45.1X1-	T45.1X2-	T45.1X3-	T45.1X4-	T45.1X5-	T45.1X6-
Enovid	T38.4X1-	T38.4X2-	T38.4X3-	T38.4X4-	T38.4X5-	T38.4X6-
Enoxacin	T36.8X1-	T36.8X2-	T36.8X3-	T36.8X4-	T36.8X5-	T36.8X6-
Enoxaparin (sodium)	T45.511-	T45.512-	T45.513-	T45.514-	T45.515-	T45.516-
Enpiprazole	T43.591-	T43.592-	T43.593-	T43.594-	T43.595-	T43.596-
Enprofylline	T48.6X1-	T48.6X2-	T48.6X3-	T48.6X4-	T48.6X5-	T48.6X6-
Enprostil	T47.1X1-	T47.1X2-	T47.1X3-	T47.1X4-	T47.1X5-	T47.1X6-
ENT preparations (anti-infectives)	T49.6X1-	T49.6X2-	T49.6X3-	T49.6X4-	T49.6X5-	T49.6X6-
Enterogastrone	T38.891-	T38.892-	T38.893-	T38.894-	T38.895-	T38.896-
Enviomycin	T36.8X1-	T36.8X2-	T36.8X3-	T36.8X4-	T36.8X5-	T36.8X6-
Enzodase	T45.3X1-	T45.3X2-	T45.3X3-	T45.3X4-	T45.3X5-	T45.3X6-
Enzyme NEC	T45.3X1-	T45.3X2-	T45.3X3-	T45.3X4-	T45.3X5-	T45.3X6-
depolymerizing	T49.8X1-	T49.8X2-	T49.8X3-	T49.8X4-	T49.8X5-	T49.8X6-
fibrolytic	T45.3X1-	T45.3X2-	T45.3X3-	T45.3X4-	T45.3X5-	T45.3X6-
gastric	T47.5X1-	T47.5X2-	T47.5X3-	T47.5X4-	T47.5X5-	T47.5X6-
intestinal	T47.5X1-	T47.5X2-	T47.5X3-	T47.5X4-	T47.5X5-	T47.5X6-
local action	T49.4X1-	T49.4X2-	T49.4X3-	T49.4X4-	T49.4X5-	T49.4X6-
proteolytic	T49.4X1-	T49.4X2-	T49.4X3-	T49.4X4-	T49.4X5-	T49.4X6-
thrombolytic	T45.3X1-	T45.3X2-	T45.3X3-	T45.3X4-	T45.3X5-	T45.3X6-
EPAB	T41.3X1-	T41.3X2-	T41.3X3-	T41.3X4-	T41.3X5-	T41.3X6-
Epanutin	T42.0X1-	T42.0X2-	T42.0X3-	T42.0X4-	T42.0X5-	T42.0X6-
Ephedra	T44.991-	T44.992-	T44.993-	T44.994-	T44.995-	T44.996-
Ephedrine	T44.991-	T44.992-	T44.993-	T44.994-	T44.995-	T44.996-
Epichlorhydrin, epichlorohydrin	T52.8X1-	T52.8X2-	T52.8X3-	T52.8X4-	-	-
Epicillin	T36.0X1-	T36.0X2-	T36.0X3-	T36.0X4-	T36.0X5-	T36.0X6-
Epiestriol	T38.5X1-	T38.5X2-	T38.5X3-	T38.5X4-	T38.5X5-	T38.5X6-
Epilim — see Sodium valproate						
Epimestrol	T38.5X1-	T38.5X2-	T38.5X3-	T38.5X4-	T38.5X5-	T38.5X6-
Epinephrine	T44.5X1-	T44.5X2-	T44.5X3-	T44.5X4-	T44.5X5-	T44.5X6-
Epirubicin	T45.1X1-	T45.1X2-	T45.1X3-	T45.1X4-	T45.1X5-	T45.1X6-
Epitiostanol	T38.7X1-	T38.7X2-	T38.7X3-	T38.7X4-	T38.7X5-	T38.7X6-
Epitizide	T50.2X1-	T50.2X2-	T50.2X3-	T50.2X4-	T50.2X5-	T50.2X6-
EPN	T60.0X1-	T60.0X2-	T60.0X3-	T60.0X4-	-	-
EPO	T45.8X1-	T45.8X2-	T45.8X3-	T45.8X4-	T45.8X5-	T45.8X6-
Epoetin alpha	T45.8X1-	T45.8X2-	T45.8X3-	T45.8X4-	T45.8X5-	T45.8X6-
Epomediol	T50.991-	T50.992-	T50.993-	T50.994-	T50.995-	T50.996-
Epoprostenol	T45.521-	T45.522-	T45.523-	T45.524-	T45.525-	T45.526-
Epoxy resin	T65.891-	T65.892-	T65.893-	T65.894-	-	-
Eprazinone	T48.4X1-	T48.4X2-	T48.4X3-	T48.4X4-	T48.4X5-	T48.4X6-
Epsilon amino-caproic acid	T45.621-	T45.622-	T45.623-	T45.624-	T45.625-	T45.626-
Epsom salt	T47.3X1-	T47.3X2-	T47.3X3-	T47.3X4-	T47.3X5-	T47.3X6-
Eptazocine	T40.4X1-	T40.4X2-	T40.4X3-	T40.4X4-	T40.4X5-	T40.4X6-
Equanil	T43.591-	T43.592-	T43.593-	T43.594-	T43.595-	T43.596-
Equisetum	T62.2X1-	T62.2X2-	T62.2X3-	T62.2X4-	-	-
diuretic	T50.2X1-	T50.2X2-	T50.2X3-	T50.2X4-	T50.2X5-	T50.2X6-
Ergobasine	T48.0X1-	T48.0X2-	T48.0X3-	T48.0X4-	T48.0X5-	T48.0X6-
Ergocalciferol	T45.2X1-	T45.2X2-	T45.2X3-	T45.2X4-	T45.2X5-	T45.2X6-
Ergoloid mesylates	T46.7X1-	T46.7X2-	T46.7X3-	T46.7X4-	T46.7X5-	T46.7X6-
Ergometrine	T48.0X1-	T48.0X2-	T48.0X3-	T48.0X4-	T48.0X5-	T48.0X6-
Ergonovine	T48.0X1-	T48.0X2-	T48.0X3-	T48.0X4-	T48.0X5-	T48.0X6-
Ergot NEC	T64.81X-	T64.82X-	T64.83X-	T64.84X-	-	-
derivative	T48.0X1-	T48.0X2-	T48.0X3-	T48.0X4-	T48.0X5-	T48.0X6-
medicinal (alkaloids)	T48.0X1-	T48.0X2-	T48.0X3-	T48.0X4-	T48.0X5-	T48.0X6-
prepared	T48.0X1-	T48.0X2-	T48.0X3-	T48.0X4-	T48.0X5-	T48.0X6-
Ergotamine	T46.5X1-	T46.5X2-	T46.5X3-	T46.5X4-	T46.5X5-	T46.5X6-
Ergotocine	T48.0X1-	T48.0X2-	T48.0X3-	T48.0X4-	T48.0X5-	T48.0X6-
Ergotrate	T48.0X1-	T48.0X2-	T48.0X3-	T48.0X4-	T48.0X5-	T48.0X6-
Eritrityl tetranitrate	T46.3X1-	T46.3X2-	T46.3X3-	T46.3X4-	T46.3X5-	T46.3X6-
Erythrityl tetranitrate	T46.3X1-	T46.3X2-	T46.3X3-	T46.3X4-	T46.3X5-	T46.3X6-
Erythrol tetranitrate	T46.3X1-	T46.3X2-	T46.3X3-	T46.3X4-	T46.3X5-	T46.3X6-
Erythromycin (salts)	T36.3X1-	T36.3X2-	T36.3X3-	T36.3X4-	T36.3X5-	T36.3X6-
ophthalmic preparation	T49.5X1-	T49.5X2-	T49.5X3-	T49.5X4-	T49.5X5-	T49.5X6-
topical NEC	T49.0X1-	T49.0X2-	T49.0X3-	T49.0X4-	T49.0X5-	T49.0X6-
Erythropoietin	T45.8X1-	T45.8X2-	T45.8X3-	T45.8X4-	T45.8X5-	T45.8X6-
human	T45.8X1-	T45.8X2-	T45.8X3-	T45.8X4-	T45.8X5-	T45.8X6-
Escin	T46.991-	T46.992-	T46.993-	T46.994-	T46.995-	T46.996-
Esculin	T45.2X1-	T45.2X2-	T45.2X3-	T45.2X4-	T45.2X5-	T45.2X6-
Esculoside	T45.2X1-	T45.2X2-	T45.2X3-	T45.2X4-	T45.2X5-	T45.2X6-
ESDT (ether-soluble tar distillate)	T49.1X1-	T49.1X2-	T49.1X3-	T49.1X4-	T49.1X5-	T49.1X6-
Eserine	T49.5X1-	T49.5X2-	T49.5X3-	T49.5X4-	T49.5X5-	T49.5X6-
Esflurbiprofen	T39.311-	T39.312-	T39.313-	T39.314-	T39.315-	T39.316-
Eskabarb	T42.3X1-	T42.3X2-	T42.3X3-	T42.3X4-	T42.3X5-	T42.3X6-
Eskalith	T43.8X1-	T43.8X2-	T43.8X3-	T43.8X4-	T43.8X5-	T43.8X6-
Esmolol	T44.7X1-	T44.7X2-	T44.7X3-	T44.7X4-	T44.7X5-	T44.7X6-
Estanozolol	T38.7X1-	T38.7X2-	T38.7X3-	T38.7X4-	T38.7X5-	T38.7X6-
Estazolam	T42.4X1-	T42.4X2-	T42.4X3-	T42.4X4-	T42.4X5-	T42.4X6-
Estradiol	T38.5X1-	T38.5X2-	T38.5X3-	T38.5X4-	T38.5X5-	T38.5X6-
with testosterone	T38.7X1-	T38.7X2-	T38.7X3-	T38.7X4-	T38.7X5-	T38.7X6-
benzoate	T38.5X1-	T38.5X2-	T38.5X3-	T38.5X4-	T38.5X5-	T38.5X6-
Estramustine	T45.1X1-	T45.1X2-	T45.1X3-	T45.1X4-	T45.1X5-	T45.1X6-
Estriol	T38.5X1-	T38.5X2-	T38.5X3-	T38.5X4-	T38.5X5-	T38.5X6-
Estrogen	T38.5X1-	T38.5X2-	T38.5X3-	T38.5X4-	T38.5X5-	T38.5X6-
with progesterone	T38.5X1-	T38.5X2-	T38.5X3-	T38.5X4-	T38.5X5-	T38.5X6-
conjugated	T38.5X1-	T38.5X2-	T38.5X3-	T38.5X4-	T38.5X5-	T38.5X6-
Estrone	T38.5X1-	T38.5X2-	T38.5X3-	T38.5X4-	T38.5X5-	T38.5X6-
Estropipate	T38.5X1-	T38.5X2-	T38.5X3-	T38.5X4-	T38.5X5-	T38.5X6-
Etacrynate sodium	T50.1X1-	T50.1X2-	T50.1X3-	T50.1X4-	T50.1X5-	T50.1X6-
Etacrynic acid	T50.1X1-	T50.1X2-	T50.1X3-	T50.1X4-	T50.1X5-	T50.1X6-
Etafedrine	T48.6X1-	T48.6X2-	T48.6X3-	T48.6X4-	T48.6X5-	T48.6X6-
Etafenone	T46.3X1-	T46.3X2-	T46.3X3-	T46.3X4-	T46.3X5-	T46.3X6-
Etambutol	T37.1X1-	T37.1X2-	T37.1X3-	T37.1X4-	T37.1X5-	T37.1X6-
Etamiphyllin	T48.6X1-	T48.6X2-	T48.6X3-	T48.6X4-	T48.6X5-	T48.6X6-
Etamivan	T50.7X1-	T50.7X2-	T50.7X3-	T50.7X4-	T50.7X5-	T50.7X6-
Etamsylate	T45.7X1-	T45.7X2-	T45.7X3-	T45.7X4-	T45.7X5-	T45.7X6-
Etebenecid	T50.4X1-	T50.4X2-	T50.4X3-	T50.4X4-	T50.4X5-	T50.4X6-
Ethacridine	T49.0X1-	T49.0X2-	T49.0X3-	T49.0X4-	T49.0X5-	T49.0X6-
Ethacrynic acid	T50.1X1-	T50.1X2-	T50.1X3-	T50.1X4-	T50.1X5-	T50.1X6-
Ethadione	T42.2X1-	T42.2X2-	T42.2X3-	T42.2X4-	T42.2X5-	T42.2X6-
Ethambutol	T37.1X1-	T37.1X2-	T37.1X3-	T37.1X4-	T37.1X5-	T37.1X6-
Ethamide	T50.2X1-	T50.2X2-	T50.2X3-	T50.2X4-	T50.2X5-	T50.2X6-
Ethamivan	T50.7X1-	T50.7X2-	T50.7X3-	T50.7X4-	T50.7X5-	T50.7X6-
Ethamsylate	T45.7X1-	T45.7X2-	T45.7X3-	T45.7X4-	T45.7X5-	T45.7X6-
Ethanol	T51.0X1-	T51.0X2-	T51.0X3-	T51.0X4-	-	-
beverage	T51.0X1-	T51.0X2-	T51.0X3-	T51.0X4-	-	-
Ethanolamine oleate	T46.8X1-	T46.8X2-	T46.8X3-	T46.8X4-	T46.8X5-	T46.8X6-
Ethaverine	T44.3X1-	T44.3X2-	T44.3X3-	T44.3X4-	T44.3X5-	T44.3X6-
Ethchlorvynol	T42.6X1-	T42.6X2-	T42.6X3-	T42.6X4-	T42.6X5-	T42.6X6-
Ethebenecid	T50.4X1-	T50.4X2-	T50.4X3-	T50.4X4-	T50.4X5-	T50.4X6-
Ether (vapor)	T41.0X1-	T41.0X2-	T41.0X3-	T41.0X4-	T41.0X5-	T41.0X6-
anesthetic	T41.0X1-	T41.0X2-	T41.0X3-	T41.0X4-	T41.0X5-	T41.0X6-
divinyl	T41.0X1-	T41.0X2-	T41.0X3-	T41.0X4-	T41.0X5-	T41.0X6-
ethyl (medicinal)	T41.0X1-	T41.0X2-	T41.0X3-	T41.0X4-	T41.0X5-	T41.0X6-
nonmedicinal	T52.8X1-	T52.8X2-	T52.8X3-	T52.8X4-	-	-
petroleum — see Ligroin						
solvent	T52.8X1-	T52.8X2-	T52.8X3-	T52.8X4-	-	-
Ethiazide	T50.2X1-	T50.2X2-	T50.2X3-	T50.2X4-	T50.2X5-	T50.2X6-
Ethidium chloride (vapor)	T59.891-	T59.892-	T59.893-	T59.894-	-	-
Ethinamate	T42.6X1-	T42.6X2-	T42.6X3-	T42.6X4-	T42.6X5-	T42.6X6-
Ethinylestradiol, ethinyloestradiol	T38.5X1-	T38.5X2-	T38.5X3-	T38.5X4-	T38.5X5-	T38.5X6-
with						
levonorgestrel	T38.4X1-	T38.4X2-	T38.4X3-	T38.4X4-	T38.4X5-	T38.4X6-
norethisterone	T38.4X1-	T38.4X2-	T38.4X3-	T38.4X4-	T38.4X5-	T38.4X6-
Ethiodized oil (131 I)	T50.8X1-	T50.8X2-	T50.8X3-	T50.8X4-	T50.8X5-	T50.8X6-
Ethion	T60.0X1-	T60.0X2-	T60.0X3-	T60.0X4-	-	-
Ethionamide	T37.1X1-	T37.1X2-	T37.1X3-	T37.1X4-	T37.1X5-	T37.1X6-
Ethioniamide	T37.1X1-	T37.1X2-	T37.1X3-	T37.1X4-	T37.1X5-	T37.1X6-

Table of Drugs and Chemicals (left margin, vertical)

Ethisterone — Fecal softener (left margin, vertical)

Substance	Poisoning, Accidental (unintentional)	Poisoning, Intentional self-harm	Poisoning, Assault	Poisoning, Undetermined	Adverse effect	Underdosing
Ethisterone	T38.5X1-	T38.5X2-	T38.5X3-	T38.5X4-	T38.5X5-	T38.5X6-
Ethobral	T42.3X1-	T42.3X2-	T42.3X3-	T42.3X4-	T42.3X5-	T42.3X6-
Ethocaine (infiltration) (topical)	T41.3X1-	T41.3X2-	T41.3X3-	T41.3X4-	T41.3X5-	T41.3X6-
nerve block (peripheral) (plexus)	T41.3X1-	T41.3X2-	T41.3X3-	T41.3X4-	T41.3X5-	T41.3X6-
spinal	T41.3X1-	T41.3X2-	T41.3X3-	T41.3X4-	T41.3X5-	T41.3X6-
Ethoheptazine	T40.4X1-	T40.4X2-	T40.4X3-	T40.4X4-	T40.4X5-	T40.4X6-
Ethopropazine	T44.3X1-	T44.3X2-	T44.3X3-	T44.3X4-	T44.3X5-	T44.3X6-
Ethosuximide	T42.2X1-	T42.2X2-	T42.2X3-	T42.2X4-	T42.2X5-	T42.2X6-
Ethotoin	T42.0X1-	T42.0X2-	T42.0X3-	T42.0X4-	T42.0X5-	T42.0X6-
Ethoxazene	T37.91X-	T37.92X-	T37.93X-	T37.94X-	T37.95X-	T37.96X-
Ethoxazorutoside	T46.991-	T46.992-	T46.993-	T46.994-	T46.995-	T46.996-
2-Ethoxyethanol	T52.3X1-	T52.3X2-	T52.3X3-	T52.3X4-	-	-
Ethoxzolamide	T50.2X1-	T50.2X2-	T50.2X3-	T50.2X4-	T50.2X5-	T50.2X6-
Ethyl						
acetate	T52.8X1-	T52.8X2-	T52.8X3-	T52.8X4-	-	-
alcohol	T51.0X1-	T51.0X2-	T51.0X3-	T51.0X4-	-	-
beverage	T51.0X1-	T51.0X2-	T51.0X3-	T51.0X4-	-	-
aldehyde (vapor)	T59.891-	T59.892-	T59.893-	T59.894-	-	-
liquid	T52.8X1-	T52.8X2-	T52.8X3-	T52.8X4-	-	-
aminobenzoate	T41.3X1-	T41.3X2-	T41.3X3-	T41.3X4-	T41.3X5-	T41.3X6-
aminophenothiazine	T43.3X1-	T43.3X2-	T43.3X3-	T43.3X4-	T43.3X5-	T43.3X6-
benzoate	T52.8X1-	T52.8X2-	T52.8X3-	T52.8X4-	-	-
biscoumacetate	T45.511-	T45.512-	T45.513-	T45.514-	T45.515-	T45.516-
bromide (anesthetic)	T41.0X1-	T41.0X2-	T41.0X3-	T41.0X4-	T41.0X5-	T41.0X6-
carbamate	T45.1X1-	T45.1X2-	T45.1X3-	T45.1X4-	T45.1X5-	T45.1X6-
carbinol	T51.3X1-	T51.3X2-	T51.3X3-	T51.3X4-	-	-
carbonate	T52.8X1-	T52.8X2-	T52.8X3-	T52.8X4-	-	-
chaulmoograte	T37.1X1-	T37.1X2-	T37.1X3-	T37.1X4-	T37.1X5-	T37.1X6-
chloride (anesthetic)	T41.0X1-	T41.0X2-	T41.0X3-	T41.0X4-	T41.0X5-	T41.0X6-
anesthetic (local)	T41.3X1-	T41.3X2-	T41.3X3-	T41.3X4-	T41.3X5-	T41.3X6-
inhaled	T41.0X1-	T41.0X2-	T41.0X3-	T41.0X4-	T41.0X5-	T41.0X6-
local	T49.4X1-	T49.4X2-	T49.4X3-	T49.4X4-	T49.4X5-	T49.4X6-
solvent	T53.6X1-	T53.6X2-	T53.6X3-	T53.6X4-	-	-
dibunate	T48.3X1-	T48.3X2-	T48.3X3-	T48.3X4-	T48.3X5-	T48.3X6-
dichloroarsine (vapor)	T57.0X1-	T57.0X2-	T57.0X3-	T57.0X4-	-	-
estranol	T38.7X1-	T38.7X2-	T38.7X3-	T38.7X4-	T38.7X5-	T38.7X6-
ether — *see also* ether	T52.8X1-	T52.8X2-	T52.8X3-	T52.8X4-	-	-
formate NEC (solvent)	T52.0X1-	T52.0X2-	T52.0X3-	T52.0X4-	-	-
fumarate	T49.4X1-	T49.4X2-	T49.4X3-	T49.4X4-	T49.4X5-	T49.4X6-
hydroxyisobutyrate NEC (solvent)	T52.8X1-	T52.8X2-	T52.8X3-	T52.8X4-	-	-
iodoacetate	T59.3X1-	T59.3X2-	T59.3X3-	T59.3X4-	-	-
lactate NEC (solvent)	T52.8X1-	T52.8X2-	T52.8X3-	T52.8X4-	-	-
loflazepate	T42.4X1-	T42.4X2-	T42.4X3-	T42.4X4-	T42.4X5-	T42.4X6-
mercuric chloride	T56.1X1-	T56.1X2-	T56.1X3-	T56.1X4-	-	-
methylcarbinol	T51.8X1-	T51.8X2-	T51.8X3-	T51.8X4-	-	-
morphine	T40.2X1-	T40.2X2-	T40.2X3-	T40.2X4-	T40.2X5-	T40.2X6-
noradrenaline	T48.6X1-	T48.6X2-	T48.6X3-	T48.6X4-	T48.6X5-	T48.6X6-
oxybutyrate NEC (solvent)	T52.8X1-	T52.8X2-	T52.8X3-	T52.8X4-	-	-
Ethylene (gas)	T59.891-	T59.892-	T59.893-	T59.894-	-	-
anesthetic (general)	T41.0X1-	T41.0X2-	T41.0X3-	T41.0X4-	T41.0X5-	T41.0X6-
chlorohydrin	T52.8X1-	T52.8X2-	T52.8X3-	T52.8X4-	-	-
vapor	T53.6X1-	T53.6X2-	T53.6X3-	T53.6X4-	-	-
dichloride	T52.8X1-	T52.8X2-	T52.8X3-	T52.8X4-	-	-
vapor	T53.6X1-	T53.6X2-	T53.6X3-	T53.6X4-	-	-
dinitrate	T52.3X1-	T52.3X2-	T52.3X3-	T52.3X4-	-	-
glycol (s)	T52.8X1-	T52.8X2-	T52.8X3-	T52.8X4-	-	-
dinitrate	T52.3X1-	T52.3X2-	T52.3X3-	T52.3X4-	-	-
monobutyl ether	T52.3X1-	T52.3X2-	T52.3X3-	T52.3X4-	-	-
imine	T54.1X1-	T54.1X2-	T54.1X3-	T54.1X4-	-	-
oxide (fumigant) (nonmedicinal)	T59.891-	T59.892-	T59.893-	T59.894-	-	-
medicinal	T49.0X1-	T49.0X2-	T49.0X3-	T49.0X4-	T49.0X5-	T49.0X6-
Ethylenediamine theophylline	T48.6X1-	T48.6X2-	T48.6X3-	T48.6X4-	T48.6X5-	T48.6X6-
Ethylenediaminetetra-acetic acid	T50.6X1-	T50.6X2-	T50.6X3-	T50.6X4-	T50.6X5-	T50.6X6-
Ethylenedinitrilotetra-acetate	T50.6X1-	T50.6X2-	T50.6X3-	T50.6X4-	T50.6X5-	T50.6X6-
Ethylestrenol	T38.7X1-	T38.7X2-	T38.7X3-	T38.7X4-	T38.7X5-	T38.7X6-
Ethylhydroxycellulose	T47.4X1-	T47.4X2-	T47.4X3-	T47.4X4-	T47.4X5-	T47.4X6-
Ethylidene						
chloride NEC	T53.6X1-	T53.6X2-	T53.6X3-	T53.6X4-	-	-
diacetate	T60.3X1-	T60.3X2-	T60.3X3-	T60.3X4-	-	-
dicoumarin	T45.511-	T45.512-	T45.513-	T45.514-	T45.515-	T45.516-
dicoumarol	T45.511-	T45.512-	T45.513-	T45.514-	T45.515-	T45.516-
diethyl ether	T52.0X1-	T52.0X2-	T52.0X3-	T52.0X4-	-	-
Ethylmorphine	T40.2X1-	T40.2X2-	T40.2X3-	T40.2X4-	T40.2X5-	T40.2X6-
Ethylnorepinephrine	T48.6X1-	T48.6X2-	T48.6X3-	T48.6X4-	T48.6X5-	T48.6X6-

Substance	Poisoning, Accidental (unintentional)	Poisoning, Intentional self-harm	Poisoning, Assault	Poisoning, Undetermined	Adverse effect	Underdosing
Ethylparachlorophen-oxyisobutyrate	T46.6X1-	T46.6X2-	T46.6X3-	T46.6X4-	T46.6X5-	T46.6X6-
Ethynodiol	T38.4X1-	T38.4X2-	T38.4X3-	T38.4X4-	T38.4X5-	T38.4X6-
with mestranol diacetate	T38.4X1-	T38.4X2-	T38.4X3-	T38.4X4-	T38.4X5-	T38.4X6-
Etidocaine	T41.3X1-	T41.3X2-	T41.3X3-	T41.3X4-	T41.3X5-	T41.3X6-
infiltration (subcutaneous)	T41.3X1-	T41.3X2-	T41.3X3-	T41.3X4-	T41.3X5-	T41.3X6-
nerve (peripheral) (plexus)	T41.3X1-	T41.3X2-	T41.3X3-	T41.3X4-	T41.3X5-	T41.3X6-
Etidronate	T50.991-	T50.992-	T50.993-	T50.994-	T50.995-	T50.996-
Etidronic acid (disodium salt)	T50.991-	T50.992-	T50.993-	T50.994-	T50.995-	T50.996-
Etifoxine	T42.6X1-	T42.6X2-	T42.6X3-	T42.6X4-	T42.6X5-	T42.6X6-
Etilefrine	T44.4X1-	T44.4X2-	T44.4X3-	T44.4X4-	T44.4X5-	T44.4X6-
Etilfen	T42.3X1-	T42.3X2-	T42.3X3-	T42.3X4-	T42.3X5-	T42.3X6-
Etinodiol	T38.4X1-	T38.4X2-	T38.4X3-	T38.4X4-	T38.4X5-	T38.4X6-
Etiroxate	T46.6X1-	T46.6X2-	T46.6X3-	T46.6X4-	T46.6X5-	T46.6X6-
Etizolam	T42.4X1-	T42.4X2-	T42.4X3-	T42.4X4-	T42.4X5-	T42.4X6-
Etodolac	T39.391-	T39.392-	T39.393-	T39.394-	T39.395-	T39.396-
Etofamide	T37.3X1-	T37.3X2-	T37.3X3-	T37.3X4-	T37.3X5-	T37.3X6-
Etofibrate	T46.6X1-	T46.6X2-	T46.6X3-	T46.6X4-	T46.6X5-	T46.6X6-
Etofylline	T46.7X1-	T46.7X2-	T46.7X3-	T46.7X4-	T46.7X5-	T46.7X6-
clofibrate	T46.6X1-	T46.6X2-	T46.6X3-	T46.6X4-	T46.6X5-	T46.6X6-
Etoglucid	T45.1X1-	T45.1X2-	T45.1X3-	T45.1X4-	T45.1X5-	T45.1X6-
Etomidate	T41.1X1-	T41.1X2-	T41.1X3-	T41.1X4-	T41.1X5-	T41.1X6-
Etomide	T39.8X1-	T39.8X2-	T39.8X3-	T39.8X4-	T39.8X5-	T39.8X6-
Etomidoline	T44.3X1-	T44.3X2-	T44.3X3-	T44.3X4-	T44.3X5-	T44.3X6-
Etoposide	T45.1X1-	T45.1X2-	T45.1X3-	T45.1X4-	T45.1X5-	T45.1X6-
Etorphine	T40.2X1-	T40.2X2-	T40.2X3-	T40.2X4-	T40.2X5-	T40.2X6-
Etoval	T42.3X1-	T42.3X2-	T42.3X3-	T42.3X4-	T42.3X5-	T42.3X6-
Etozolin	T50.1X1-	T50.1X2-	T50.1X3-	T50.1X4-	T50.1X5-	T50.1X6-
Etretinate	T50.991-	T50.992-	T50.993-	T50.994-	T50.995-	T50.996-
Etryptamine	T43.691-	T43.692-	T43.693-	T43.694-	T43.695-	T43.696-
Etybenzatropine	T44.3X1-	T44.3X2-	T44.3X3-	T44.3X4-	T44.3X5-	T44.3X6-
Etynodiol	T38.4X1-	T38.4X2-	T38.4X3-	T38.4X4-	T38.4X5-	T38.4X6-
Eucaine	T41.3X1-	T41.3X2-	T41.3X3-	T41.3X4-	T41.3X5-	T41.3X6-
Eucalyptus oil	T49.7X1-	T49.7X2-	T49.7X3-	T49.7X4-	T49.7X5-	T49.7X6-
Eucatropine	T49.5X1-	T49.5X2-	T49.5X3-	T49.5X4-	T49.5X5-	T49.5X6-
Eucodal	T40.2X1-	T40.2X2-	T40.2X3-	T40.2X4-	T40.2X5-	T40.2X6-
Euneryl	T42.3X1-	T42.3X2-	T42.3X3-	T42.3X4-	T42.3X5-	T42.3X6-
Euphthalmine	T44.3X1-	T44.3X2-	T44.3X3-	T44.3X4-	T44.3X5-	T44.3X6-
Eurax	T49.0X1-	T49.0X2-	T49.0X3-	T49.0X4-	T49.0X5-	T49.0X6-
Euresol	T49.4X1-	T49.4X2-	T49.4X3-	T49.4X4-	T49.4X5-	T49.4X6-
Euthroid	T38.1X1-	T38.1X2-	T38.1X3-	T38.1X4-	T38.1X5-	T38.1X6-
Evans blue	T50.8X1-	T50.8X2-	T50.8X3-	T50.8X4-	T50.8X5-	T50.8X6-
Evipal	T42.3X1-	T42.3X2-	T42.3X3-	T42.3X4-	T42.3X5-	T42.3X6-
sodium	T41.1X1-	T41.1X2-	T41.1X3-	T41.1X4-	T41.1X5-	T41.1X6-
Evipan	T42.3X1-	T42.3X2-	T42.3X3-	T42.3X4-	T42.3X5-	T42.3X6-
sodium	T41.1X1-	T41.1X2-	T41.1X3-	T41.1X4-	T41.1X5-	T41.1X6-
Exalamide	T49.0X1-	T49.0X2-	T49.0X3-	T49.0X4-	T49.0X5-	T49.0X6-
Exalgin	T39.1X1-	T39.1X2-	T39.1X3-	T39.1X4-	T39.1X5-	T39.1X6-
Excipients, pharmaceutical	T50.901-	T50.902-	T50.903-	T50.904-	T50.905-	T50.906-
Exhaust gas (engine) (motor vehicle)	T58.01X-	T58.02X-	T58.03X-	T58.04X-	-	-
Ex-Lax (phenolphthalein)	T47.2X1-	T47.2X2-	T47.2X3-	T47.2X4-	T47.2X5-	T47.2X6-
Expectorant NEC	T48.4X1-	T48.4X2-	T48.4X3-	T48.4X4-	T48.4X5-	T48.4X6-
Extended insulin zinc suspension	T38.3X1-	T38.3X2-	T38.3X3-	T38.3X4-	T38.3X5-	T38.3X6-
External medications (skin) (mucous membrane)	T49.91X-	T49.92X-	T49.93X-	T49.94X-	T49.95X-	T49.96X-
dental agent	T49.7X1-	T49.7X2-	T49.7X3-	T49.7X4-	T49.7X5-	T49.7X6-
ENT agent	T49.6X1-	T49.6X2-	T49.6X3-	T49.6X4-	T49.6X5-	T49.6X6-
ophthalmic preparation	T49.5X1-	T49.5X2-	T49.5X3-	T49.5X4-	T49.5X5-	T49.5X6-
specified NEC	T49.8X1-	T49.8X2-	T49.8X3-	T49.8X4-	T49.8X5-	T49.8X6-
Extrapyramidal antagonist NEC	T44.3X1-	T44.3X2-	T44.3X3-	T44.3X4-	T44.3X5-	T44.3X6-
Eye agents (anti-infective)	T49.5X1-	T49.5X2-	T49.5X3-	T49.5X4-	T49.5X5-	T49.5X6-
Eye drug NEC	T49.5X1-	T49.5X2-	T49.5X3-	T49.5X4-	T49.5X5-	T49.5X6-
FAC (fluorouracil + doxorubicin + cyclophosphamide)	T45.1X1-	T45.1X2-	T45.1X3-	T45.1X4-	T45.1X5-	T45.1X6-
Factor						
I (fibrinogen)	T45.8X1-	T45.8X2-	T45.8X3-	T45.8X4-	T45.8X5-	T45.8X6-
III (thromboplastin)	T45.8X1-	T45.8X2-	T45.8X3-	T45.8X4-	T45.8X5-	T45.8X6-
VIII (antihemophilic Factor) (concentrate)	T45.8X1-	T45.8X2-	T45.8X3-	T45.8X4-	T45.8X5-	T45.8X6-
IX complex	T45.7X1-	T45.7X2-	T45.7X3-	T45.7X4-	T45.7X5-	T45.7X6-
human	T45.8X1-	T45.8X2-	T45.8X3-	T45.8X4-	T45.8X5-	T45.8X6-
Famotidine	T47.0X1-	T47.0X2-	T47.0X3-	T47.0X4-	T47.0X5-	T47.0X6-
Fat suspension, intravenous	T50.991-	T50.992-	T50.993-	T50.994-	T50.995-	T50.996-
Fazadinium bromide	T48.1X1-	T48.1X2-	T48.1X3-	T48.1X4-	T48.1X5-	T48.1X6-
Febarbamate	T42.3X1-	T42.3X2-	T42.3X3-	T42.3X4-	T42.3X5-	T42.3X6-
Fecal softener	T47.4X1-	T47.4X2-	T47.4X3-	T47.4X4-	T47.4X5-	T47.4X6-

Substance	Poisoning, Accidental (unintentional)	Poisoning, Intentional self-harm	Poisoning, Assault	Poisoning, Undetermined	Adverse effect	Underdosing
Fedrilate	T48.3X1-	T48.3X2-	T48.3X3-	T48.3X4-	T48.3X5-	T48.3X6-
Felodipine	T46.1X1-	T46.1X2-	T46.1X3-	T46.1X4-	T46.1X5-	T46.1X6-
Felypressin	T38.891-	T38.892-	T38.893-	T38.894-	T38.895-	T38.896-
Femoxetine	T43.221-	T43.222-	T43.223-	T43.224-	T43.225-	T43.226-
Fenalcomine	T46.3X1-	T46.3X2-	T46.3X3-	T46.3X4-	T46.3X5-	T46.3X6-
Fenamisal	T37.1X1-	T37.1X2-	T37.1X3-	T37.1X4-	T37.1X5-	T37.1X6-
Fenazone	T39.2X1-	T39.2X2-	T39.2X3-	T39.2X4-	T39.2X5-	T39.2X6-
Fenbendazole	T37.4X1-	T37.4X2-	T37.4X3-	T37.4X4-	T37.4X5-	T37.4X6-
Fenbutrazate	T50.5X1-	T50.5X2-	T50.5X3-	T50.5X4-	T50.5X5-	T50.5X6-
Fencamfamine	T43.691-	T43.692-	T43.693-	T43.694-	T43.695-	T43.696-
Fendiline	T46.1X1-	T46.1X2-	T46.1X3-	T46.1X4-	T46.1X5-	T46.1X6-
Fenetylline	T43.691-	T43.692-	T43.693-	T43.694-	T43.695-	T43.696-
Fenflumizole	T39.391-	T39.392-	T39.393-	T39.394-	T39.395-	T39.396-
Fenfluramine	T50.5X1-	T50.5X2-	T50.5X3-	T50.5X4-	T50.5X5-	T50.5X6-
Fenobarbital	T42.3X1-	T42.3X2-	T42.3X3-	T42.3X4-	T42.3X5-	T42.3X6-
Fenofibrate	T46.6X1-	T46.6X2-	T46.6X3-	T46.6X4-	T46.6X5-	T46.6X6-
Fenoprofen	T39.311-	T39.312-	T39.313-	T39.314-	T39.315-	T39.316-
Fenoterol	T48.6X1-	T48.6X2-	T48.6X3-	T48.6X4-	T48.6X5-	T48.6X6-
Fenoverine	T44.3X1-	T44.3X2-	T44.3X3-	T44.3X4-	T44.3X5-	T44.3X6-
Fenoxazoline	T48.5X1-	T48.5X2-	T48.5X3-	T48.5X4-	T48.5X5-	T48.5X6-
Fenproporex	T50.5X1-	T50.5X2-	T50.5X3-	T50.5X4-	T50.5X5-	T50.5X6-
Fenquizone	T50.2X1-	T50.2X2-	T50.2X3-	T50.2X4-	T50.2X5-	T50.2X6-
Fentanyl	T40.4X1-	T40.4X2-	T40.4X3-	T40.4X4-	T40.4X5-	T40.4X6-
Fentazin	T43.3X1-	T43.3X2-	T43.3X3-	T43.3X4-	T43.3X5-	T43.3X6-
Fenthion	T60.0X1-	T60.0X2-	T60.0X3-	T60.0X4-	-	-
Fenticlor	T49.0X1-	T49.0X2-	T49.0X3-	T49.0X4-	T49.0X5-	T49.0X6-
Fenylbutazone	T39.2X1-	T39.2X2-	T39.2X3-	T39.2X4-	T39.2X5-	T39.2X6-
Feprazone	T39.2X1-	T39.2X2-	T39.2X3-	T39.2X4-	T39.2X5-	T39.2X6-
Fer de lance (bite) (venom)	T63.061-	T63.062-	T63.063-	T63.064-	-	-
Ferric — see also Iron						
chloride	T45.4X1-	T45.4X2-	T45.4X3-	T45.4X4-	T45.4X5-	T45.4X6-
citrate	T45.4X1-	T45.4X2-	T45.4X3-	T45.4X4-	T45.4X5-	T45.4X6-
hydroxide						
colloidal	T45.4X1-	T45.4X2-	T45.4X3-	T45.4X4-	T45.4X5-	T45.4X6-
polymaltose	T45.4X1-	T45.4X2-	T45.4X3-	T45.4X4-	T45.4X5-	T45.4X6-
pyrophosphate	T45.4X1-	T45.4X2-	T45.4X3-	T45.4X4-	T45.4X5-	T45.4X6-
Ferritin	T45.4X1-	T45.4X2-	T45.4X3-	T45.4X4-	T45.4X5-	T45.4X6-
Ferrocholinate	T45.4X1-	T45.4X2-	T45.4X3-	T45.4X4-	T45.4X5-	T45.4X6-
Ferrodextrane	T45.4X1-	T45.4X2-	T45.4X3-	T45.4X4-	T45.4X5-	T45.4X6-
Ferropolimaler	T45.4X1-	T45.4X2-	T45.4X3-	T45.4X4-	T45.4X5-	T45.4X6-
Ferrous — see also Iron						
phosphate	T45.4X1-	T45.4X2-	T45.4X3-	T45.4X4-	T45.4X5-	T45.4X6-
salt	T45.4X1-	T45.4X2-	T45.4X3-	T45.4X4-	T45.4X5-	T45.4X6-
with folic acid	T45.4X1-	T45.4X2-	T45.4X3-	T45.4X4-	T45.4X5-	T45.4X6-
Ferrous fumarate, gluconate, lactate, salt NEC, sulfate (medicinal)	T45.4X1-	T45.4X2-	T45.4X3-	T45.4X4-	T45.4X5-	T45.4X6-
Ferrovanadium (fumes)	T59.891-	T59.892-	T59.893-	T59.894-	-	-
Ferrum — see Iron						
Fertilizers NEC	T65.891-	T65.892-	T65.893-	T65.894-	-	-
with herbicide mixture	T60.3X1-	T60.3X2-	T60.3X3-	T60.3X4-	-	-
Fetoxilate	T47.6X1-	T47.6X2-	T47.6X3-	T47.6X4-	T47.6X5-	T47.6X6-
Fiber, dietary	T47.4X1-	T47.4X2-	T47.4X3-	T47.4X4-	T47.4X5-	T47.4X6-
Fiberglass	T65.831-	T65.832-	T65.833-	T65.834-	-	-
Fibrinogen (human)	T45.8X1-	T45.8X2-	T45.8X3-	T45.8X4-	T45.8X5-	T45.8X6-
Fibrinolysin (human)	T45.691-	T45.692-	T45.693-	T45.694-	T45.695-	T45.696-
Fibrinolysis						
affecting drug	T45.601-	T45.602-	T45.603-	T45.604-	T45.605-	T45.606-
inhibitor NEC	T45.621-	T45.622-	T45.623-	T45.624-	T45.625-	T45.626-
Fibrinolytic drug	T45.611-	T45.612-	T45.613-	T45.614-	T45.615-	T45.616-
Filix mas	T37.4X1-	T37.4X2-	T37.4X3-	T37.4X4-	T37.4X5-	T37.4X6-
Filtering cream	T49.3X1-	T49.3X2-	T49.3X3-	T49.3X4-	T49.3X5-	T49.3X6-
Fiorinal	T39.011-	T39.012-	T39.013-	T39.014-	T39.015-	T39.016-
Firedamp	T59.891-	T59.892-	T59.893-	T59.894-	-	-
Fish, noxious, nonbacterial	T61.91X-	T61.92X-	T61.93X-	T61.94X-	-	-
ciguatera	T61.01X-	T61.02X-	T61.03X-	T61.04X-	-	-
scombroid	T61.11X-	T61.12X-	T61.13X-	T61.14X-	-	-
shell	T61.781-	T61.782-	T61.783-	T61.784-	-	-
specified NEC	T61.771-	T61.772-	T61.773-	T61.774-	-	-
Flagyl	T37.3X1-	T37.3X2-	T37.3X3-	T37.3X4-	T37.3X5-	T37.3X6-
Flavine adenine dinucleotide	T45.2X1-	T45.2X2-	T45.2X3-	T45.2X4-	T45.2X5-	T45.2X6-
Flavodic acid	T46.991-	T46.992-	T46.993-	T46.994-	T46.995-	T46.996-
Flavoxate	T44.3X1-	T44.3X2-	T44.3X3-	T44.3X4-	T44.3X5-	T44.3X6-
Flaxedil	T48.1X1-	T48.1X2-	T48.1X3-	T48.1X4-	T48.1X5-	T48.1X6-
Flaxseed (medicinal)	T49.3X1-	T49.3X2-	T49.3X3-	T49.3X4-	T49.3X5-	T49.3X6-
Flecainide	T46.2X1-	T46.2X2-	T46.2X3-	T46.2X4-	T46.2X5-	T46.2X6-
Fleroxacin	T36.8X1-	T36.8X2-	T36.8X3-	T36.8X4-	T36.8X5-	T36.8X6-
Floctafenine	T39.8X1-	T39.8X2-	T39.8X3-	T39.8X4-	T39.8X5-	T39.8X6-

Substance	Poisoning, Accidental (unintentional)	Poisoning, Intentional self-harm	Poisoning, Assault	Poisoning, Undetermined	Adverse effect	Underdosing
Flomax	T44.6X1-	T44.6X2-	T44.6X3-	T44.6X4-	T44.6X5-	T44.6X6-
Flomoxef	T36.1X1-	T36.1X2-	T36.1X3-	T36.1X4-	T36.1X5-	T36.1X6-
Flopropione	T44.3X1-	T44.3X2-	T44.3X3-	T44.3X4-	T44.3X5-	T44.3X6-
Florantyrone	T47.5X1-	T47.5X2-	T47.5X3-	T47.5X4-	T47.5X5-	T47.5X6-
Floraquin	T37.8X1-	T37.8X2-	T37.8X3-	T37.8X4-	T37.8X5-	T37.8X6-
Florinef	T38.0X1-	T38.0X2-	T38.0X3-	T38.0X4-	T38.0X5-	T38.0X6-
ENT agent	T49.6X1-	T49.6X2-	T49.6X3-	T49.6X4-	T49.6X5-	T49.6X6-
ophthalmic preparation	T49.5X1-	T49.5X2-	T49.5X3-	T49.5X4-	T49.5X5-	T49.5X6-
topical NEC	T49.0X1-	T49.0X2-	T49.0X3-	T49.0X4-	T49.0X5-	T49.0X6-
Flowers of sulfur	T49.4X1-	T49.4X2-	T49.4X3-	T49.4X4-	T49.4X5-	T49.4X6-
Floxuridine	T45.1X1-	T45.1X2-	T45.1X3-	T45.1X4-	T45.1X5-	T45.1X6-
Fluanisone	T43.4X1-	T43.4X2-	T43.4X3-	T43.4X4-	T43.4X5-	T43.4X6-
Flubendazole	T37.4X1-	T37.4X2-	T37.4X3-	T37.4X4-	T37.4X5-	T37.4X6-
Fluclorolone acetonide	T49.0X1-	T49.0X2-	T49.0X3-	T49.0X4-	T49.0X5-	T49.0X6-
Flucloxacillin	T36.0X1-	T36.0X2-	T36.0X3-	T36.0X4-	T36.0X5-	T36.0X6-
Fluconazole	T37.8X1-	T37.8X2-	T37.8X3-	T37.8X4-	T37.8X5-	T37.8X6-
Flucytosine	T37.8X1-	T37.8X2-	T37.8X3-	T37.8X4-	T37.8X5-	T37.8X6-
Fludeoxyglucose (18F)	T50.8X1-	T50.8X2-	T50.8X3-	T50.8X4-	T50.8X5-	T50.8X6-
Fludiazepam	T42.4X1-	T42.4X2-	T42.4X3-	T42.4X4-	T42.4X5-	T42.4X6-
Fludrocortisone	T50.0X1-	T50.0X2-	T50.0X3-	T50.0X4-	T50.0X5-	T50.0X6-
ENT agent	T49.6X1-	T49.6X2-	T49.6X3-	T49.6X4-	T49.6X5-	T49.6X6-
ophthalmic preparation	T49.5X1-	T49.5X2-	T49.5X3-	T49.5X4-	T49.5X5-	T49.5X6-
topical NEC	T49.0X1-	T49.0X2-	T49.0X3-	T49.0X4-	T49.0X5-	T49.0X6-
Fludroxycortide	T49.0X1-	T49.0X2-	T49.0X3-	T49.0X4-	T49.0X5-	T49.0X6-
Flufenamic acid	T39.391-	T39.392-	T39.393-	T39.394-	T39.395-	T39.396-
Fluindione	T45.511-	T45.512-	T45.513-	T45.514-	T45.515-	T45.516-
Flumequine	T37.8X1-	T37.8X2-	T37.8X3-	T37.8X4-	T37.8X5-	T37.8X6-
Flumethasone	T49.0X1-	T49.0X2-	T49.0X3-	T49.0X4-	T49.0X5-	T49.0X6-
Flumethiazide	T50.2X1-	T50.2X2-	T50.2X3-	T50.2X4-	T50.2X5-	T50.2X6-
Flumidin	T37.5X1-	T37.5X2-	T37.5X3-	T37.5X4-	T37.5X5-	T37.5X6-
Flunarizine	T46.7X1-	T46.7X2-	T46.7X3-	T46.7X4-	T46.7X5-	T46.7X6-
Flunidazole	T37.8X1-	T37.8X2-	T37.8X3-	T37.8X4-	T37.8X5-	T37.8X6-
Flunisolide	T48.6X1-	T48.6X2-	T48.6X3-	T48.6X4-	T48.6X5-	T48.6X6-
Flunitrazepam	T42.4X1-	T42.4X2-	T42.4X3-	T42.4X4-	T42.4X5-	T42.4X6-
Fluocinolone (acetonide)	T49.0X1-	T49.0X2-	T49.0X3-	T49.0X4-	T49.0X5-	T49.0X6-
Fluocinonide	T49.0X1-	T49.0X2-	T49.0X3-	T49.0X4-	T49.0X5-	T49.0X6-
Fluocortin (butyl)	T49.0X1-	T49.0X2-	T49.0X3-	T49.0X4-	T49.0X5-	T49.0X6-
Fluocortolone	T49.0X1-	T49.0X2-	T49.0X3-	T49.0X4-	T49.0X5-	T49.0X6-
Fluohydrocortisone	T38.0X1-	T38.0X2-	T38.0X3-	T38.0X4-	T38.0X5-	T38.0X6-
ENT agent	T49.6X1-	T49.6X2-	T49.6X3-	T49.6X4-	T49.6X5-	T49.6X6-
ophthalmic preparation	T49.5X1-	T49.5X2-	T49.5X3-	T49.5X4-	T49.5X5-	T49.5X6-
topical NEC	T49.0X1-	T49.0X2-	T49.0X3-	T49.0X4-	T49.0X5-	T49.0X6-
Fluonid	T49.0X1-	T49.0X2-	T49.0X3-	T49.0X4-	T49.0X5-	T49.0X6-
Fluopromazine	T43.3X1-	T43.3X2-	T43.3X3-	T43.3X4-	T43.3X5-	T43.3X6-
Fluoracetate	T60.8X1-	T60.8X2-	T60.8X3-	T60.8X4-	-	-
Fluorescein	T50.8X1-	T50.8X2-	T50.8X3-	T50.8X4-	T50.8X5-	T50.8X6-
Fluorhydrocortisone	T50.0X1-	T50.0X2-	T50.0X3-	T50.0X4-	T50.0X5-	T50.0X6-
Fluoride (nonmedicinal) (pesticide) (sodium) NEC	T60.8X1-	T60.8X2-	T60.8X3-	T60.8X4-	-	-
hydrogen — see Hydrofluoric acid						
medicinal NEC	T50.991-	T50.992-	T50.993-	T50.994-	T50.995-	T50.996-
dental use	T49.7X1-	T49.7X2-	T49.7X3-	T49.7X4-	T49.7X5-	T49.7X6-
not pesticide NEC	T54.91X-	T54.92X-	T54.93X-	T54.94X-	-	-
stannous	T49.7X1-	T49.7X2-	T49.7X3-	T49.7X4-	T49.7X5-	T49.7X6-
Fluorinated corticosteroids	T38.0X1-	T38.0X2-	T38.0X3-	T38.0X4-	T38.0X5-	T38.0X6-
Fluorine (gas)	T59.5X1-	T59.5X2-	T59.5X3-	T59.5X4-	-	-
salt — see Fluoride(s)						
Fluoristan	T49.7X1-	T49.7X2-	T49.7X3-	T49.7X4-	T49.7X5-	T49.7X6-
Fluormetholone	T49.0X1-	T49.0X2-	T49.0X3-	T49.0X4-	T49.0X5-	T49.0X6-
Fluoroacetate	T60.8X1-	T60.8X2-	T60.8X3-	T60.8X4-	-	-
Fluorocarbon monomer	T53.6X1-	T53.6X2-	T53.6X3-	T53.6X4-	-	-
Fluorocytosine	T37.8X1-	T37.8X2-	T37.8X3-	T37.8X4-	T37.8X5-	T37.8X6-
Fluorodeoxyuridine	T45.1X1-	T45.1X2-	T45.1X3-	T45.1X4-	T45.1X5-	T45.1X6-
Fluorometholone	T49.0X1-	T49.0X2-	T49.0X3-	T49.0X4-	T49.0X5-	T49.0X6-
ophthalmic preparation	T49.5X1-	T49.5X2-	T49.5X3-	T49.5X4-	T49.5X5-	T49.5X6-
Fluorophosphate insecticide	T60.0X1-	T60.0X2-	T60.0X3-	T60.0X4-	-	-
Fluorosol	T46.3X1-	T46.3X2-	T46.3X3-	T46.3X4-	T46.3X5-	T46.3X6-
Fluorouracil	T45.1X1-	T45.1X2-	T45.1X3-	T45.1X4-	T45.1X5-	T45.1X6-
Fluorphenylalanine	T49.5X1-	T49.5X2-	T49.5X3-	T49.5X4-	T49.5X5-	T49.5X6-
Fluothane	T41.0X1-	T41.0X2-	T41.0X3-	T41.0X4-	T41.0X5-	T41.0X6-
Fluoxetine	T43.221-	T43.222-	T43.223-	T43.224-	T43.225-	T43.226-
Fluoxymesterone	T38.7X1-	T38.7X2-	T38.7X3-	T38.7X4-	T38.7X5-	T38.7X6-
Flupenthixol	T43.4X1-	T43.4X2-	T43.4X3-	T43.4X4-	T43.4X5-	T43.4X6-
Flupentixol	T43.4X1-	T43.4X2-	T43.4X3-	T43.4X4-	T43.4X5-	T43.4X6-
Fluphenazine	T43.3X1-	T43.3X2-	T43.3X3-	T43.3X4-	T43.3X5-	T43.3X6-
Fluprednidene	T49.0X1-	T49.0X2-	T49.0X3-	T49.0X4-	T49.0X5-	T49.0X6-
Fluprednisolone	T38.0X1-	T38.0X2-	T38.0X3-	T38.0X4-	T38.0X5-	T38.0X6-

Left margin: Table of Drugs and Chemicals — Fluradoline — Garamycin

Substance	Poisoning, Accidental (unintentional)	Poisoning, Intentional self-harm	Poisoning, Assault	Poisoning, Undetermined	Adverse effect	Underdosing
Fluradoline	T39.8X1-	T39.8X2-	T39.8X3-	T39.8X4-	T39.8X5-	T39.8X6-
Flurandrenolide	T49.0X1-	T49.0X2-	T49.0X3-	T49.0X4-	T49.0X5-	T49.0X6-
Flurandrenolone	T49.0X1-	T49.0X2-	T49.0X3-	T49.0X4-	T49.0X5-	T49.0X6-
Flurazepam	T42.4X1-	T42.4X2-	T42.4X3-	T42.4X4-	T42.4X5-	T42.4X6-
Flurbiprofen	T39.311-	T39.312-	T39.313-	T39.314-	T39.315-	T39.316-
Flurobate	T49.0X1-	T49.0X2-	T49.0X3-	T49.0X4-	T49.0X5-	T49.0X6-
Fluroxene	T41.0X1-	T41.0X2-	T41.0X3-	T41.0X4-	T41.0X5-	T41.0X6-
Fluspirilene	T43.591-	T43.592-	T43.593-	T43.594-	T43.595-	T43.596-
Flutamide	T38.6X1-	T38.6X2-	T38.6X3-	T38.6X4-	T38.6X5-	T38.6X6-
Flutazolam	T42.4X1-	T42.4X2-	T42.4X3-	T42.4X4-	T42.4X5-	T42.4X6-
Fluticasone propionate	T49.1X1-	T49.1X2-	T49.1X3-	T49.1X4-	T49.1X5-	T49.1X6-
Flutoprazepam	T42.4X1-	T42.4X2-	T42.4X3-	T42.4X4-	T42.4X5-	T42.4X6-
Flutropium bromide	T48.6X1-	T48.6X2-	T48.6X3-	T48.6X4-	T48.6X5-	T48.6X6-
Fluvoxamine	T43.221-	T43.222-	T43.223-	T43.224-	T43.225-	T43.226-
Folacin	T45.8X1-	T45.8X2-	T45.8X3-	T45.8X4-	T45.8X5-	T45.8X6-
Folic acid	T45.8X1-	T45.8X2-	T45.8X3-	T45.8X4-	T45.8X5-	T45.8X6-
with ferrous salt	T45.2X1-	T45.2X2-	T45.2X3-	T45.2X4-	T45.2X5-	T45.2X6-
antagonist	T45.1X1-	T45.1X2-	T45.1X3-	T45.1X4-	T45.1X5-	T45.1X6-
Folinic acid	T45.8X1-	T45.8X2-	T45.8X3-	T45.8X4-	T45.8X5-	T45.8X6-
Folium stramoniae	T48.6X1-	T48.6X2-	T48.6X3-	T48.6X4-	T48.6X5-	T48.6X6-
Follicle-stimulating hormone, human	T38.811-	T38.812-	T38.813-	T38.814-	T38.815-	T38.816-
Folpet	T60.3X1-	T60.3X2-	T60.3X3-	T60.3X4-	-	-
Fominoben	T48.3X1-	T48.3X2-	T48.3X3-	T48.3X4-	T48.3X5-	T48.3X6-
Food, foodstuffs, noxious, nonbacterial, NEC	T62.91X-	T62.92X-	T62.93X-	T62.94X-	-	-
berries	T62.1X1-	T62.1X2-	T62.1X3-	T62.1X4-	-	-
fish — see also Fish	T61.91X-	T61.92X-	T61.93X-	T61.94X-	-	-
mushrooms	T62.0X1-	T62.0X2-	T62.0X3-	T62.0X4-	-	-
plants	T62.2X1-	T62.2X2-	T62.2X3-	T62.2X4-	-	-
seafood	T61.91X-	T61.92X-	T61.93X-	T61.94X-	-	-
specified NEC	T61.8X1-	T61.8X2-	T61.8X3-	T61.8X4-	-	-
seeds	T62.2X1-	T62.2X2-	T62.2X3-	T62.2X4-	-	-
shellfish	T61.781-	T61.782-	T61.783-	T61.784-	-	-
specified NEC	T62.8X1-	T62.8X2-	T62.8X3-	T62.8X4-	-	-
Fool's parsley	T62.2X1-	T62.2X2-	T62.2X3-	T62.2X4-	-	-
Formaldehyde (solution), gas or vapor	T59.2X1-	T59.2X2-	T59.2X3-	T59.2X4-	-	-
fungicide	T60.3X1-	T60.3X2-	T60.3X3-	T60.3X4-	-	-
Formalin	T59.2X1-	T59.2X2-	T59.2X3-	T59.2X4-	-	-
fungicide	T60.3X1-	T60.3X2-	T60.3X3-	T60.3X4-	-	-
vapor	T59.2X1-	T59.2X2-	T59.2X3-	T59.2X4-	-	-
Formic acid	T54.2X1-	T54.2X2-	T54.2X3-	T54.2X4-	-	-
vapor	T59.891-	T59.892-	T59.893-	T59.894-	-	-
Foscarnet sodium	T37.5X1-	T37.5X2-	T37.5X3-	T37.5X4-	T37.5X5-	T37.5X6-
Fosfestrol	T38.5X1-	T38.5X2-	T38.5X3-	T38.5X4-	T38.5X5-	T38.5X6-
Fosfomycin	T36.8X1-	T36.8X2-	T36.8X3-	T36.8X4-	T36.8X5-	T36.8X6-
Fosfonet sodium	T37.5X1-	T37.5X2-	T37.5X3-	T37.5X4-	T37.5X5-	T37.5X6-
Fosinopril	T46.4X1-	T46.4X2-	T46.4X3-	T46.4X4-	T46.4X5-	T46.4X6-
sodium	T46.4X1-	T46.4X2-	T46.4X3-	T46.4X4-	T46.4X5-	T46.4X6-
Fowler's solution	T57.0X1-	T57.0X2-	T57.0X3-	T57.0X4-	-	-
Foxglove	T62.2X1-	T62.2X2-	T62.2X3-	T62.2X4-	-	-
Framycetin	T36.5X1-	T36.5X2-	T36.5X3-	T36.5X4-	T36.5X5-	T36.5X6-
Frangula	T47.2X1-	T47.2X2-	T47.2X3-	T47.2X4-	T47.2X5-	T47.2X6-
extract	T47.2X1-	T47.2X2-	T47.2X3-	T47.2X4-	T47.2X5-	T47.2X6-
Frei antigen	T50.8X1-	T50.8X2-	T50.8X3-	T50.8X4-	T50.8X5-	T50.8X6-
Freon	T53.5X1-	T53.5X2-	T53.5X3-	T53.5X4-	-	-
Fructose	T50.3X1-	T50.3X2-	T50.3X3-	T50.3X4-	T50.3X5-	T50.3X6-
Frusemide	T50.1X1-	T50.1X2-	T50.1X3-	T50.1X4-	T50.1X5-	T50.1X6-
FSH	T38.811-	T38.812-	T38.813-	T38.814-	T38.815-	T38.816-
Ftorafur	T45.1X1-	T45.1X2-	T45.1X3-	T45.1X4-	T45.1X5-	T45.1X6-
Fuel						
automobile	T52.0X1-	T52.0X2-	T52.0X3-	T52.0X4-	-	-
exhaust gas, not in transit	T58.01X-	T58.02X-	T58.03X-	T58.04X-	-	-
vapor NEC	T52.0X1-	T52.0X2-	T52.0X3-	T52.0X4-	-	-
gas (domestic use) — see also Carbon, monoxide, fuel, utility	T59.891-	T59.892-	T59.893-	T59.894-	-	-
utility	T59.891-	T59.892-	T59.893-	T59.894-	-	-
in mobile container	T59.891-	T59.892-	T59.893-	T59.894-	-	-
incomplete combustion of — see Carbon, monoxide, fuel, utility						
piped (natural)	T59.891-	T59.892-	T59.893-	T59.894-	-	-
industrial, incomplete combustion	T58.8X1-	T58.8X2-	T58.8X3-	T58.8X4-	-	-
Fugillin	T36.8X1-	T36.8X2-	T36.8X3-	T36.8X4-	T36.8X5-	T36.8X6-
Fulminate of mercury	T56.1X1-	T56.1X2-	T56.1X3-	T56.1X4-	-	-
Fulvicin	T36.7X1-	T36.7X2-	T36.7X3-	T36.7X4-	T36.7X5-	T36.7X6-
Fumadil	T36.8X1-	T36.8X2-	T36.8X3-	T36.8X4-	T36.8X5-	T36.8X6-

Substance	Poisoning, Accidental (unintentional)	Poisoning, Intentional self-harm	Poisoning, Assault	Poisoning, Undetermined	Adverse effect	Underdosing
Fumagillin	T36.8X1-	T36.8X2-	T36.8X3-	T36.8X4-	T36.8X5-	T36.8X6-
Fumaric acid	T49.4X1-	T49.4X2-	T49.4X3-	T49.4X4-	T49.4X5-	T49.4X6-
Fumes (from)	T59.91X-	T59.92X-	T59.93X-	T59.94X-	-	-
carbon monoxide — see Carbon, monoxide						
charcoal (domestic use) — see Charcoal, fumes						
chloroform — see Chloroform						
coke (in domestic stoves, fireplaces) — see Coke fumes						
corrosive NEC	T54.91X-	T54.92X-	T54.93X-	T54.94X-	-	-
ether — see ether						
freons	T53.5X1-	T53.5X2-	T53.5X3-	T53.5X4-	-	-
hydrocarbons	T59.891-	T59.892-	T59.893-	T59.894-	-	-
petroleum (liquefied)	T59.891-	T59.892-	T59.893-	T59.894-	-	-
distributed through pipes (pure or mixed with air)	T59.891-	T59.892-	T59.893-	T59.894-	-	-
lead — see lead						
metal — see Metals, or the specified metal						
nitrogen dioxide	T59.0X1-	T59.0X2-	T59.0X3-	T59.0X4-	-	-
pesticides — see Pesticides						
petroleum (liquefied)	T59.891-	T59.892-	T59.893-	T59.894-	-	-
distributed through pipes (pure or mixed with air)	T59.891-	T59.892-	T59.893-	T59.894-	-	-
polyester	T59.891-	T59.892-	T59.893-	T59.894-	-	-
specified source NEC — see also substance specified	T59.891-	T59.892-	T59.893-	T59.894-	-	-
sulfur dioxide	T59.1X1-	T59.1X2-	T59.1X3-	T59.1X4-	-	-
Fumigant NEC	T60.91X-	T60.92X-	T60.93X-	T60.94X-	-	-
Fungi, noxious, used as food	T62.0X1-	T62.0X2-	T62.0X3-	T62.0X4-	-	-
Fungicide NEC (nonmedicinal)	T60.3X1-	T60.3X2-	T60.3X3-	T60.3X4-	-	-
Fungizone	T36.7X1-	T36.7X2-	T36.7X3-	T36.7X4-	T36.7X5-	T36.7X6-
topical	T49.0X1-	T49.0X2-	T49.0X3-	T49.0X4-	T49.0X5-	T49.0X6-
Furacin	T49.0X1-	T49.0X2-	T49.0X3-	T49.0X4-	T49.0X5-	T49.0X6-
Furadantin	T37.91X-	T37.92X-	T37.93X-	T37.94X-	T37.95X-	T37.96X-
Furazolidone	T37.8X1-	T37.8X2-	T37.8X3-	T37.8X4-	T37.8X5-	T37.8X6-
Furazolium chloride	T49.0X1-	T49.0X2-	T49.0X3-	T49.0X4-	T49.0X5-	T49.0X6-
Furfural	T52.8X1-	T52.8X2-	T52.8X3-	T52.8X4-	-	-
Furnace (coal burning) (domestic), gas from	T58.2X1-	T58.2X2-	T58.2X3-	T58.2X4-	-	-
industrial	T58.8X1-	T58.8X2-	T58.8X3-	T58.8X4-	-	-
Furniture polish	T65.891-	T65.892-	T65.893-	T65.894-	-	-
Furosemide	T50.1X1-	T50.1X2-	T50.1X3-	T50.1X4-	T50.1X5-	T50.1X6-
Furoxone	T37.91X-	T37.92X-	T37.93X-	T37.94X-	T37.95X-	T37.96X-
Fursultiamine	T45.2X1-	T45.2X2-	T45.2X3-	T45.2X4-	T45.2X5-	T45.2X6-
Fusafungine	T36.8X1-	T36.8X2-	T36.8X3-	T36.8X4-	T36.8X5-	T36.8X6-
Fusel oil (any) (amyl) (butyl) (propyl), vapor	T51.3X1-	T51.3X2-	T51.3X3-	T51.3X4-		
Fusidate (ethanolamine) (sodium)	T36.8X1-	T36.8X2-	T36.8X3-	T36.8X4-	T36.8X5-	T36.8X6-
Fusidic acid	T36.8X1-	T36.8X2-	T36.8X3-	T36.8X4-	T36.8X5-	T36.8X6-
Fytic acid, nonasodium	T50.6X1-	T50.6X2-	T50.6X3-	T50.6X4-	T50.6X5-	T50.6X6-
GABA	T43.8X1-	T43.8X2-	T43.8X3-	T43.8X4-	T43.8X5-	T43.8X6-
Gadopentetic acid	T50.8X1-	T50.8X2-	T50.8X3-	T50.8X4-	T50.8X5-	T50.8X6-
Galactose	T50.3X1-	T50.3X2-	T50.3X3-	T50.3X4-	T50.3X5-	T50.3X6-
b-Galactosidase	T47.5X1-	T47.5X2-	T47.5X3-	T47.5X4-	T47.5X5-	T47.5X6-
Galantamine	T44.0X1-	T44.0X2-	T44.0X3-	T44.0X4-	T44.0X5-	T44.0X6-
Gallamine (triethiodide)	T48.1X1-	T48.1X2-	T48.1X3-	T48.1X4-	T48.1X5-	T48.1X6-
Gallium citrate	T50.991-	T50.992-	T50.993-	T50.994-	T50.995-	T50.996-
Gallopamil	T46.1X1-	T46.1X2-	T46.1X3-	T46.1X4-	T46.1X5-	T46.1X6-
Gamboge	T47.2X1-	T47.2X2-	T47.2X3-	T47.2X4-	T47.2X5-	T47.2X6-
Gamimune	T50.Z11-	T50.Z12-	T50.Z13-	T50.Z14-	T50.Z15-	T50.Z16-
Gamma globulin	T50.Z11-	T50.Z12-	T50.Z13-	T50.Z14-	T50.Z15-	T50.Z16-
Gamma-aminobutyric acid	T43.8X1-	T43.8X2-	T43.8X3-	T43.8X4-	T43.8X5-	T43.8X6-
Gamma-benzene hexachloride (medicinal)	T49.0X1-	T49.0X2-	T49.0X3-	T49.0X4-	T49.0X5-	T49.0X6-
nonmedicinal, vapor	T53.6X1-	T53.6X2-	T53.6X3-	T53.6X4-	-	-
Gamma-BHC (medicinal) — see also Gamma-benzene hexachloride	T49.0X1-	T49.0X2-	T49.0X3-	T49.0X4-	T49.0X5-	T49.0X6-
Gamulin	T50.Z11-	T50.Z12-	T50.Z13-	T50.Z14-	T50.Z15-	T50.Z16-
Ganciclovir (sodium)	T37.5X1-	T37.5X2-	T37.5X3-	T37.5X4-	T37.5X5-	T37.5X6-
Ganglionic blocking drug NEC	T44.2X1-	T44.2X2-	T44.2X3-	T44.2X4-	T44.2X5-	T44.2X6-
specified NEC	T44.2X1-	T44.2X2-	T44.2X3-	T44.2X4-	T44.2X5-	T44.2X6-
Ganja	T40.7X1-	T40.7X2-	T40.7X3-	T40.7X4-	T40.7X5-	T40.7X6-
Garamycin	T36.5X1-	T36.5X2-	T36.5X3-	T36.5X4-	T36.5X5-	T36.5X6-
ophthalmic preparation	T49.5X1-	T49.5X2-	T49.5X3-	T49.5X4-	T49.5X5-	T49.5X6-
topical NEC	T49.0X1-	T49.0X2-	T49.0X3-	T49.0X4-	T49.0X5-	T49.0X6-

Substance	Poisoning, Accidental (unintentional)	Poisoning, Intentional self-harm	Poisoning, Assault	Poisoning, Undetermined	Adverse effect	Underdosing
Gardenal	T42.3X1-	T42.3X2-	T42.3X3-	T42.3X4-	T42.3X5-	T42.3X6-
Gardepanyl	T42.3X1-	T42.3X2-	T42.3X3-	T42.3X4-	T42.3X5-	T42.3X6-
Gas	T59.91X-	T59.92X-	T59.93X-	T59.94X-	-	-
acetylene	T59.891-	T59.892-	T59.893-	T59.894-	-	-
incomplete combustion of	T58.11X-	T58.12X-	T58.13X-	T58.14X-	-	-
air contaminants, source or type not specified	T59.91X-	T59.92X-	T59.93X-	T59.94X-	-	-
anesthetic	T41.0X1-	T41.0X2-	T41.0X3-	T41.0X4-	T41.0X5-	T41.0X6-
blast furnace	T58.8X1-	T58.8X2-	T58.8X3-	T58.8X4-	-	-
butane — see butane						
carbon monoxide — see Carbon, monoxide						
chlorine	T59.4X1-	T59.4X2-	T59.4X3-	T59.4X4-	-	-
coal	T58.2X1-	T58.2X2-	T58.2X3-	T58.2X4-	-	-
cyanide	T57.3X1-	T57.3X2-	T57.3X3-	T57.3X4-	-	-
dicyanogen	T65.0X1-	T65.0X2-	T65.0X3-	T65.0X4-	-	-
domestic — see Domestic gas						
exhaust	T58.01X-	T58.02X-	T58.03X-	T58.04X-	-	-
from utility (for cooking, heating, or lighting) (after combustion) — see Carbon, monoxide, fuel, utility						
prior to combustion	T59.891-	T59.892-	T59.893-	T59.894-	-	-
from wood- or coal-burning stove or fireplace	T58.2X1-	T58.2X2-	T58.2X3-	T58.2X4-	-	-
fuel (domestic use) (after combustion) — see also Carbon, monoxide, fuel						
industrial use	T58.8X1-	T58.8X2-	T58.8X3-	T58.8X4-	-	-
prior to combustion	T59.891-	T59.892-	T59.893-	T59.894-	-	-
utility	T59.891-	T59.892-	T59.893-	T59.894-	-	-
in mobile container	T59.891-	T59.892-	T59.893-	T59.894-	-	-
incomplete combustion of — see Carbon, monoxide, fuel, utility						
piped (natural)	T59.891-	T59.892-	T59.893-	T59.894-	-	-
garage	T58.01X-	T58.02X-	T58.03X-	T58.04X-	-	-
hydrocarbon NEC	T59.891-	T59.892-	T59.893-	T59.894-	-	-
incomplete combustion of — see Carbon, monoxide, fuel, utility						
liquefied — see butane						
piped	T59.891-	T59.892-	T59.893-	T59.894-	-	-
hydrocyanic acid	T65.0X1-	T65.0X2-	T65.0X3-	T65.0X4-	-	-
illuminating (after combustion)	T58.11X-	T58.12X-	T58.13X-	T58.14X-	-	-
prior to combustion	T59.891-	T59.892-	T59.893-	T59.894-	-	-
incomplete combustion, any — see Carbon, monoxide						
kiln	T58.8X1-	T58.8X2-	T58.8X3-	T58.8X4-	-	-
lacrimogenic	T59.3X1-	T59.3X2-	T59.3X3-	T59.3X4-	-	-
liquefied petroleum — see butane						
marsh	T59.891-	T59.892-	T59.893-	T59.894-	-	-
motor exhaust, not in transit	T58.01X-	T58.02X-	T58.03X-	T58.04X-	-	-
mustard, not in war	T59.891-	T59.892-	T59.893-	T59.894-	-	-
natural	T59.891-	T59.892-	T59.893-	T59.894-	-	-
nerve, not in war	T59.91X-	T59.92X-	T59.93X-	T59.94X-	-	-
oil	T52.0X1-	T52.0X2-	T52.0X3-	T52.0X4-	-	-
petroleum (liquefied) (distributed in mobile containers)	T59.891-	T59.892-	T59.893-	T59.894-	-	-
piped (pure or mixed with air)	T59.891-	T59.892-	T59.893-	T59.894-	-	-
piped (manufactured) (natural) NEC	T59.891-	T59.892-	T59.893-	T59.894-	-	-
producer	T58.8X1-	T58.8X2-	T58.8X3-	T58.8X4-	-	-
propane — see propane						
refrigerant (chlorofluoro-carbon)	T53.5X1-	T53.5X2-	T53.5X3-	T53.5X4-	-	-
not chlorofluoro-carbon	T59.891-	T59.892-	T59.893-	T59.894-	-	-
sewer	T59.91X-	T59.92X-	T59.93X-	T59.94X-	-	-
specified source NEC	T59.91X-	T59.92X-	T59.93X-	T59.94X-	-	-
stove (after combustion)	T58.11X-	T58.12X-	T58.13X-	T58.14X-	-	-
prior to combustion	T59.891-	T59.892-	T59.893-	T59.894-	-	-
tear	T59.3X1-	T59.3X2-	T59.3X3-	T59.3X4-	-	-
therapeutic	T41.5X1-	T41.5X2-	T41.5X3-	T41.5X4-	T41.5X5-	T41.5X6-
utility (for cooking, heating, or lighting) (piped) NEC	T59.891-	T59.892-	T59.893-	T59.894-	-	-
in mobile container	T59.891-	T59.892-	T59.893-	T59.894-	-	-

Substance	Poisoning, Accidental (unintentional)	Poisoning, Intentional self-harm	Poisoning, Assault	Poisoning, Undetermined	Adverse effect	Underdosing
Gas - continued						
incomplete combustion of — see Carbon, monoxide, fuel, utility						
piped (natural)	T59.891-	T59.892-	T59.893-	T59.894-	-	-
water	T58.11X-	T58.12X-	T58.13X-	T58.14X-	-	-
incomplete combustion of — see Carbon, monoxide, fuel, utility						
Gaseous substance — see Gas						
Gasoline	T52.0X1-	T52.0X2-	T52.0X3-	T52.0X4-	-	-
vapor	T52.0X1-	T52.0X2-	T52.0X3-	T52.0X4-	-	-
Gastric enzymes	T47.5X1-	T47.5X2-	T47.5X3-	T47.5X4-	T47.5X5-	T47.5X6-
Gastrografin	T50.8X1-	T50.8X2-	T50.8X3-	T50.8X4-	T50.8X5-	T50.8X6-
Gastrointestinal drug	T47.91X-	T47.92X-	T47.93X-	T47.94X-	T47.95X-	T47.96X-
biological	T47.8X1-	T47.8X2-	T47.8X3-	T47.8X4-	T47.8X5-	T47.8X6-
specified NEC	T47.8X1-	T47.8X2-	T47.8X3-	T47.8X4-	T47.8X5-	T47.8X6-
Gaultheria procumbens	T62.2X1-	T62.2X2-	T62.2X3-	T62.2X4-	-	-
Gefarnate	T44.3X1-	T44.3X2-	T44.3X3-	T44.3X4-	T44.3X5-	T44.3X6-
Gelatin (intravenous)	T45.8X1-	T45.8X2-	T45.8X3-	T45.8X4-	T45.8X5-	T45.8X6-
absorbable (sponge)	T45.7X1-	T45.7X2-	T45.7X3-	T45.7X4-	T45.7X5-	T45.7X6-
Gelfilm	T49.8X1-	T49.8X2-	T49.8X3-	T49.8X4-	T49.8X5-	T49.8X6-
Gelfoam	T45.7X1-	T45.7X2-	T45.7X3-	T45.7X4-	T45.7X5-	T45.7X6-
Gelsemine	T50.991-	T50.992-	T50.993-	T50.994-	T50.995-	T50.996-
Gelsemium (sempervirens)	T62.2X1-	T62.2X2-	T62.2X3-	T62.2X4-	-	-
Gemeprost	T48.0X1-	T48.0X2-	T48.0X3-	T48.0X4-	T48.0X5-	T48.0X6-
Gemfibrozil	T46.6X1-	T46.6X2-	T46.6X3-	T46.6X4-	T46.6X5-	T46.6X6-
Gemonil	T42.3X1-	T42.3X2-	T42.3X3-	T42.3X4-	T42.3X5-	T42.3X6-
Gentamicin	T36.5X1-	T36.5X2-	T36.5X3-	T36.5X4-	T36.5X5-	T36.5X6-
ophthalmic preparation	T49.5X1-	T49.5X2-	T49.5X3-	T49.5X4-	T49.5X5-	T49.5X6-
topical NEC	T49.0X1-	T49.0X2-	T49.0X3-	T49.0X4-	T49.0X5-	T49.0X6-
Gentian	T47.5X1-	T47.5X2-	T47.5X3-	T47.5X4-	T47.5X5-	T47.5X6-
violet	T49.0X1-	T49.0X2-	T49.0X3-	T49.0X4-	T49.0X5-	T49.0X6-
Gepefrine	T44.4X1-	T44.4X2-	T44.4X3-	T44.4X4-	T44.4X5-	T44.4X6-
Gestonorone caproate	T38.5X1-	T38.5X2-	T38.5X3-	T38.5X4-	T38.5X5-	T38.5X6-
Gexane	T49.0X1-	T49.0X2-	T49.0X3-	T49.0X4-	T49.0X5-	T49.0X6-
Gila monster (venom)	T63.111-	T63.112-	T63.113-	T63.114-	-	-
Ginger	T47.5X1-	T47.5X2-	T47.5X3-	T47.5X4-	T47.5X5-	T47.5X6-
Jamaica — see Jamaica, ginger						
Gitalin	T46.0X1-	T46.0X2-	T46.0X3-	T46.0X4-	T46.0X5-	T46.0X6-
amorphous	T46.0X1-	T46.0X2-	T46.0X3-	T46.0X4-	T46.0X5-	T46.0X6-
Gitaloxin	T46.0X1-	T46.0X2-	T46.0X3-	T46.0X4-	T46.0X5-	T46.0X6-
Gitoxin	T46.0X1-	T46.0X2-	T46.0X3-	T46.0X4-	T46.0X5-	T46.0X6-
Glafenine	T39.8X1-	T39.8X2-	T39.8X3-	T39.8X4-	T39.8X5-	T39.8X6-
Glandular extract (medicinal) NEC	T50.Z91-	T50.Z92-	T50.Z93-	T50.Z94-	T50.Z95-	T50.Z96-
Glaucarubin	T37.3X1-	T37.3X2-	T37.3X3-	T37.3X4-	T37.3X5-	T37.3X6-
Glibenclamide	T38.3X1-	T38.3X2-	T38.3X3-	T38.3X4-	T38.3X5-	T38.3X6-
Glibornuride	T38.3X1-	T38.3X2-	T38.3X3-	T38.3X4-	T38.3X5-	T38.3X6-
Gliclazide	T38.3X1-	T38.3X2-	T38.3X3-	T38.3X4-	T38.3X5-	T38.3X6-
Glimidine	T38.3X1-	T38.3X2-	T38.3X3-	T38.3X4-	T38.3X5-	T38.3X6-
Glipizide	T38.3X1-	T38.3X2-	T38.3X3-	T38.3X4-	T38.3X5-	T38.3X6-
Gliquidone	T38.3X1-	T38.3X2-	T38.3X3-	T38.3X4-	T38.3X5-	T38.3X6-
Glisolamide	T38.3X1-	T38.3X2-	T38.3X3-	T38.3X4-	T38.3X5-	T38.3X6-
Glisoxepide	T38.3X1-	T38.3X2-	T38.3X3-	T38.3X4-	T38.3X5-	T38.3X6-
Globin zinc insulin	T38.3X1-	T38.3X2-	T38.3X3-	T38.3X4-	T38.3X5-	T38.3X6-
Globulin						
antilymphocytic	T50.Z11-	T50.Z12-	T50.Z13-	T50.Z14-	T50.Z15-	T50.Z16-
antirhesus	T50.Z11-	T50.Z12-	T50.Z13-	T50.Z14-	T50.Z15-	T50.Z16-
antivenin	T50.Z11-	T50.Z12-	T50.Z13-	T50.Z14-	T50.Z15-	T50.Z16-
antiviral	T50.Z11-	T50.Z12-	T50.Z13-	T50.Z14-	T50.Z15-	T50.Z16-
Glucagon	T38.3X1-	T38.3X2-	T38.3X3-	T38.3X4-	T38.3X5-	T38.3X6-
Glucocorticoids	T38.0X1-	T38.0X2-	T38.0X3-	T38.0X4-	T38.0X5-	T38.0X6-
Glucocorticosteroid	T38.0X1-	T38.0X2-	T38.0X3-	T38.0X4-	T38.0X5-	T38.0X6-
Gluconic acid	T50.991-	T50.992-	T50.993-	T50.994-	T50.995-	T50.996-
Glucosamine sulfate	T39.4X1-	T39.4X2-	T39.4X3-	T39.4X4-	T39.4X5-	T39.4X6-
Glucose	T50.3X1-	T50.3X2-	T50.3X3-	T50.3X4-	T50.3X5-	T50.3X6-
with sodium chloride	T50.3X1-	T50.3X2-	T50.3X3-	T50.3X4-	T50.3X5-	T50.3X6-
Glucosulfone sodium	T37.1X1-	T37.1X2-	T37.1X3-	T37.1X4-	T37.1X5-	T37.1X6-
Glucurolactone	T47.8X1-	T47.8X2-	T47.8X3-	T47.8X4-	T47.8X5-	T47.8X6-
Glue NEC	T52.8X1-	T52.8X2-	T52.8X3-	T52.8X4-	-	-
Glutamic acid	T47.5X1-	T47.5X2-	T47.5X3-	T47.5X4-	T47.5X5-	T47.5X6-
Glutaral (medicinal)	T49.0X1-	T49.0X2-	T49.0X3-	T49.0X4-	T49.0X5-	T49.0X6-
nonmedicinal	T65.891-	T65.892-	T65.893-	T65.894-	-	-
Glutaraldehyde (nonmedicinal)	T65.891-	T65.892-	T65.893-	T65.894-	-	-
medicinal	T49.0X1-	T49.0X2-	T49.0X3-	T49.0X4-	T49.0X5-	T49.0X6-

Substance	Poisoning, Accidental (unintentional)	Poisoning, Intentional self-harm	Poisoning, Assault	Poisoning, Undetermined	Adverse effect	Underdosing
Glutathione	T50.6X1-	T50.6X2-	T50.6X3-	T50.6X4-	T50.6X5-	T50.6X6-
Glutethimide	T42.6X1-	T42.6X2-	T42.6X3-	T42.6X4-	T42.6X5-	T42.6X6-
Glyburide	T38.3X1-	T38.3X2-	T38.3X3-	T38.3X4-	T38.3X5-	T38.3X6-
Glycerin	T47.4X1-	T47.4X2-	T47.4X3-	T47.4X4-	T47.4X5-	T47.4X6-
Glycerol	T47.4X1-	T47.4X2-	T47.4X3-	T47.4X4-	T47.4X5-	T47.4X6-
borax	T49.6X1-	T49.6X2-	T49.6X3-	T49.6X4-	T49.6X5-	T49.6X6-
intravenous	T50.3X1-	T50.3X2-	T50.3X3-	T50.3X4-	T50.3X5-	T50.3X6-
iodinated	T48.4X1-	T48.4X2-	T48.4X3-	T48.4X4-	T48.4X5-	T48.4X6-
Glycerophosphate	T50.991-	T50.992-	T50.993-	T50.994-	T50.995-	T50.996-
Glyceryl						
gualacolate	T48.4X1-	T48.4X2-	T48.4X3-	T48.4X4-	T48.4X5-	T48.4X6-
nitrate	T46.3X1-	T46.3X2-	T46.3X3-	T46.3X4-	T46.3X5-	T46.3X6-
triacetate (topical)	T49.0X1-	T49.0X2-	T49.0X3-	T49.0X4-	T49.0X5-	T49.0X6-
trinitrate	T46.3X1-	T46.3X2-	T46.3X3-	T46.3X4-	T46.3X5-	T46.3X6-
Glycine	T50.3X1-	T50.3X2-	T50.3X3-	T50.3X4-	T50.3X5-	T50.3X6-
Glyclopyramide	T38.3X1-	T38.3X2-	T38.3X3-	T38.3X4-	T38.3X5-	T38.3X6-
Glycobiarsol	T37.3X1-	T37.3X2-	T37.3X3-	T37.3X4-	T37.3X5-	T37.3X6-
Glycols (ether)	T52.3X1-	T52.3X2-	T52.3X3-	T52.3X4-	-	-
Glyconiazide	T37.1X1-	T37.1X2-	T37.1X3-	T37.1X4-	T37.1X5-	T37.1X6-
Glycopyrrolate	T44.3X1-	T44.3X2-	T44.3X3-	T44.3X4-	T44.3X5-	T44.3X6-
Glycopyrronium	T44.3X1-	T44.3X2-	T44.3X3-	T44.3X4-	T44.3X5-	T44.3X6-
bromide	T44.3X1-	T44.3X2-	T44.3X3-	T44.3X4-	T44.3X5-	T44.3X6-
Glycoside, cardiac (stimulant)	T46.0X1-	T46.0X2-	T46.0X3-	T46.0X4-	T46.0X5-	T46.0X6-
Glycyclamide	T38.3X1-	T38.3X2-	T38.3X3-	T38.3X4-	T38.3X5-	T38.3X6-
Glycyrrhiza extract	T48.4X1-	T48.4X2-	T48.4X3-	T48.4X4-	T48.4X5-	T48.4X6-
Glycyrrhizic acid	T48.4X1-	T48.4X2-	T48.4X3-	T48.4X4-	T48.4X5-	T48.4X6-
Glycyrrhizinate potassium	T48.4X1-	T48.4X2-	T48.4X3-	T48.4X4-	T48.4X5-	T48.4X6-
Glymidine sodium	T38.3X1-	T38.3X2-	T38.3X3-	T38.3X4-	T38.3X5-	T38.3X6-
Glyphosate	T60.3X1-	T60.3X2-	T60.3X3-	T60.3X4-	-	-
Glyphylline	T48.6X1-	T48.6X2-	T48.6X3-	T48.6X4-	T48.6X5-	T48.6X6-
Gold						
colloidal (I98Au)	T45.1X1-	T45.1X2-	T45.1X3-	T45.1X4-	T45.1X5-	T45.1X6-
salts	T39.4X1-	T39.4X2-	T39.4X3-	T39.4X4-	T39.4X5-	T39.4X6-
Golden sulfide of antimony	T56.891-	T56.892-	T56.893-	T56.894-	-	-
Goldylocks	T62.2X1-	T62.2X2-	T62.2X3-	T62.2X4-	-	-
Gonadal tissue extract	T38.901-	T38.902-	T38.903-	T38.904-	T38.905-	T38.906-
female	T38.5X1-	T38.5X2-	T38.5X3-	T38.5X4-	T38.5X5-	T38.5X6-
male	T38.7X1-	T38.7X2-	T38.7X3-	T38.7X4-	T38.7X5-	T38.7X6-
Gonadorelin	T38.891-	T38.892-	T38.893-	T38.894-	T38.895-	T38.896-
Gonadotropin	T38.891-	T38.892-	T38.893-	T38.894-	T38.895-	T38.896-
chorionic	T38.891-	T38.892-	T38.893-	T38.894-	T38.895-	T38.896-
pituitary	T38.811-	T38.812-	T38.813-	T38.814-	T38.815-	T38.816-
Goserelin	T45.1X1-	T45.1X2-	T45.1X3-	T45.1X4-	T45.1X5-	T45.1X6-
Grain alcohol	T51.0X1-	T51.0X2-	T51.0X3-	T51.0X4-	-	-
Gramicidin	T49.0X1-	T49.0X2-	T49.0X3-	T49.0X4-	T49.0X5-	T49.0X6-
Granisetron	T45.0X1-	T45.0X2-	T45.0X3-	T45.0X4-	T45.0X5-	T45.0X6-
Gratiola officinalis	T62.2X1-	T62.2X2-	T62.2X3-	T62.2X4-	-	-
Grease	T65.891-	T65.892-	T65.893-	T65.894-	-	-
Green hellebore	T62.2X1-	T62.2X2-	T62.2X3-	T62.2X4-	-	-
Green soap	T49.2X1-	T49.2X2-	T49.2X3-	T49.2X4-	T49.2X5-	T49.2X6-
Grifulvin	T36.7X1-	T36.7X2-	T36.7X3-	T36.7X4-	T36.7X5-	T36.7X6-
Griseofulvin	T36.7X1-	T36.7X2-	T36.7X3-	T36.7X4-	T36.7X5-	T36.7X6-
Growth hormone	T38.811-	T38.812-	T38.813-	T38.814-	T38.815-	T38.816-
Guaiac reagent	T50.991-	T50.992-	T50.993-	T50.994-	T50.995-	T50.996-
Guaiacol derivatives	T48.4X1-	T48.4X2-	T48.4X3-	T48.4X4-	T48.4X5-	T48.4X6-
Guaifenesin	T48.4X1-	T48.4X2-	T48.4X3-	T48.4X4-	T48.4X5-	T48.4X6-
Guaimesal	T48.4X1-	T48.4X2-	T48.4X3-	T48.4X4-	T48.4X5-	T48.4X6-
Guaiphenesin	T48.4X1-	T48.4X2-	T48.4X3-	T48.4X4-	T48.4X5-	T48.4X6-
Guamecycline	T36.4X1-	T36.4X2-	T36.4X3-	T36.4X4-	T36.4X5-	T36.4X6-
Guanabenz	T46.5X1-	T46.5X2-	T46.5X3-	T46.5X4-	T46.5X5-	T46.5X6-
Guanacline	T46.5X1-	T46.5X2-	T46.5X3-	T46.5X4-	T46.5X5-	T46.5X6-
Guanadrel	T46.5X1-	T46.5X2-	T46.5X3-	T46.5X4-	T46.5X5-	T46.5X6-
Guanatol	T37.2X1-	T37.2X2-	T37.2X3-	T37.2X4-	T37.2X5-	T37.2X6-
Guanethidine	T46.5X1-	T46.5X2-	T46.5X3-	T46.5X4-	T46.5X5-	T46.5X6-
Guanfacine	T46.5X1-	T46.5X2-	T46.5X3-	T46.5X4-	T46.5X5-	T46.5X6-
Guano	T65.891-	T65.892-	T65.893-	T65.894-	-	-
Guanochlor	T46.5X1-	T46.5X2-	T46.5X3-	T46.5X4-	T46.5X5-	T46.5X6-
Guanoclor	T46.5X1-	T46.5X2-	T46.5X3-	T46.5X4-	T46.5X5-	T46.5X6-
Guanoctine	T46.5X1-	T46.5X2-	T46.5X3-	T46.5X4-	T46.5X5-	T46.5X6-
Guanoxabenz	T46.5X1-	T46.5X2-	T46.5X3-	T46.5X4-	T46.5X5-	T46.5X6-
Guanoxan	T46.5X1-	T46.5X2-	T46.5X3-	T46.5X4-	T46.5X5-	T46.5X6-
Guar gum (medicinal)	T46.6X1-	T46.6X2-	T46.6X3-	T46.6X4-	T46.6X5-	T46.6X6-
Hachimycin	T36.7X1-	T36.7X2-	T36.7X3-	T36.7X4-	T36.7X5-	T36.7X6-
Hair						
dye	T49.4X1-	T49.4X2-	T49.4X3-	T49.4X4-	T49.4X5-	T49.4X6-
preparation NEC	T49.4X1-	T49.4X2-	T49.4X3-	T49.4X4-	T49.4X5-	T49.4X6-
Halazepam	T42.4X1-	T42.4X2-	T42.4X3-	T42.4X4-	T42.4X5-	T42.4X6-
Halcinolone	T49.0X1-	T49.0X2-	T49.0X3-	T49.0X4-	T49.0X5-	T49.0X6-
Halcinonide	T49.0X1-	T49.0X2-	T49.0X3-	T49.0X4-	T49.0X5-	T49.0X6-
Halethazole	T49.0X1-	T49.0X2-	T49.0X3-	T49.0X4-	T49.0X5-	T49.0X6-
Hallucinogen NEC	T40.901-	T40.902-	T40.903-	T40.904-	T40.905-	T40.906-
Halofantrine	T37.2X1-	T37.2X2-	T37.2X3-	T37.2X4-	T37.2X5-	T37.2X6-
Halofenate	T46.6X1-	T46.6X2-	T46.6X3-	T46.6X4-	T46.6X5-	T46.6X6-
Halometasone	T49.0X1-	T49.0X2-	T49.0X3-	T49.0X4-	T49.0X5-	T49.0X6-
Haloperidol	T43.4X1-	T43.4X2-	T43.4X3-	T43.4X4-	T43.4X5-	T43.4X6-
Haloprogin	T49.0X1-	T49.0X2-	T49.0X3-	T49.0X4-	T49.0X5-	T49.0X6-
Halotex	T49.0X1-	T49.0X2-	T49.0X3-	T49.0X4-	T49.0X5-	T49.0X6-
Halothane	T41.0X1-	T41.0X2-	T41.0X3-	T41.0X4-	T41.0X5-	T41.0X6-
Haloxazolam	T42.4X1-	T42.4X2-	T42.4X3-	T42.4X4-	T42.4X5-	T42.4X6-
Halquinols	T49.0X1-	T49.0X2-	T49.0X3-	T49.0X4-	T49.0X5-	T49.0X6-
Hamamelis	T49.2X1-	T49.2X2-	T49.2X3-	T49.2X4-	T49.2X5-	T49.2X6-
Haptendextran	T45.8X1-	T45.8X2-	T45.8X3-	T45.8X4-	T45.8X5-	T45.8X6-
Harmonyl	T46.5X1-	T46.5X2-	T46.5X3-	T46.5X4-	T46.5X5-	T46.5X6-
Hartmann's solution	T50.3X1-	T50.3X2-	T50.3X3-	T50.3X4-	T50.3X5-	T50.3X6-
Hashish	T40.7X1-	T40.7X2-	T40.7X3-	T40.7X4-	T40.7X5-	T40.7X6-
Hawaiian Woodrose seeds	T40.991-	T40.992-	T40.993-	T40.994-	-	-
HCB	T60.3X1-	T60.3X2-	T60.3X3-	T60.3X4-	-	-
HCH	T53.6X1-	T53.6X2-	T53.6X3-	T53.6X4-	-	-
medicinal	T49.0X1-	T49.0X2-	T49.0X3-	T49.0X4-	T49.0X5-	T49.0X6-
HCN	T57.3X1-	T57.3X2-	T57.3X3-	T57.3X4-	-	-
Headache cures, drugs, powders NEC	T50.901-	T50.902-	T50.903-	T50.904-	T50.905-	T50.906-
Heavenly Blue (morning glory)	T40.991-	T40.992-	T40.993-	T40.994-	-	-
Heavy metal antidote	T45.8X1-	T45.8X2-	T45.8X3-	T45.8X4-	T45.8X5-	T45.8X6-
Hedaquinium	T49.0X1-	T49.0X2-	T49.0X3-	T49.0X4-	T49.0X5-	T49.0X6-
Hedge hyssop	T62.2X1-	T62.2X2-	T62.2X3-	T62.2X4-	-	-
Heet	T49.8X1-	T49.8X2-	T49.8X3-	T49.8X4-	T49.8X5-	T49.8X6-
Helenin	T37.4X1-	T37.4X2-	T37.4X3-	T37.4X4-	T37.4X5-	T37.4X6-
Helium (nonmedicinal) NEC	T59.891-	T59.892-	T59.893-	T59.894-	-	-
medicinal	T48.991-	T48.992-	T48.993-	T48.994-	T48.995-	T48.996-
Hellebore (black) (green) (white)	T62.2X1-	T62.2X2-	T62.2X3-	T62.2X4-	-	-
Hematin	T45.8X1-	T45.8X2-	T45.8X3-	T45.8X4-	T45.8X5-	T45.8X6-
Hematinic preparation	T45.8X1-	T45.8X2-	T45.8X3-	T45.8X4-	T45.8X5-	T45.8X6-
Hematological agent	T45.91X-	T45.92X-	T45.93X-	T45.94X-	T45.95X-	T45.96X-
specified NEC	T45.8X1-	T45.8X2-	T45.8X3-	T45.8X4-	T45.8X5-	T45.8X6-
Hemlock	T62.2X1-	T62.2X2-	T62.2X3-	T62.2X4-	-	-
Hemostatic	T45.621-	T45.622-	T45.623-	T45.624-	T45.625-	T45.626-
drug, systemic	T45.621-	T45.622-	T45.623-	T45.624-	T45.625-	T45.626-
Hemostyptic	T49.4X1-	T49.4X2-	T49.4X3-	T49.4X4-	T49.4X5-	T49.4X6-
Henbane	T62.2X1-	T62.2X2-	T62.2X3-	T62.2X4-	-	-
Heparin (sodium)	T45.511-	T45.512-	T45.513-	T45.514-	T45.515-	T45.516-
action reverser	T45.7X1-	T45.7X2-	T45.7X3-	T45.7X4-	T45.7X5-	T45.7X6-
Heparin-fraction	T45.511-	T45.512-	T45.513-	T45.514-	T45.515-	T45.516-
Heparinoid (systemic)	T45.511-	T45.512-	T45.513-	T45.514-	T45.515-	T45.516-
Hepatic secretion stimulant	T47.8X1-	T47.8X2-	T47.8X3-	T47.8X4-	T47.8X5-	T47.8X6-
Hepatitis B						
immune globulin	T50.Z11-	T50.Z12-	T50.Z13-	T50.Z14-	T50.Z15-	T50.Z16-
vaccine	T50.B91-	T50.B92-	T50.B93-	T50.B94-	T50.B95-	T50.B96-
Hepronicate	T46.7X1-	T46.7X2-	T46.7X3-	T46.7X4-	T46.7X5-	T46.7X6-
Heptabarb	T42.3X1-	T42.3X2-	T42.3X3-	T42.3X4-	T42.3X5-	T42.3X6-
Heptabarbital	T42.3X1-	T42.3X2-	T42.3X3-	T42.3X4-	T42.3X5-	T42.3X6-
Heptabarbitone	T42.3X1-	T42.3X2-	T42.3X3-	T42.3X4-	T42.3X5-	T42.3X6-
Heptachlor	T60.1X1-	T60.1X2-	T60.1X3-	T60.1X4-	-	-
Heptalgin	T40.2X1-	T40.2X2-	T40.2X3-	T40.2X4-	T40.2X5-	T40.2X6-
Heptaminol	T46.3X1-	T46.3X2-	T46.3X3-	T46.3X4-	T46.3X5-	T46.3X6-
Herbicide NEC	T60.3X1-	T60.3X2-	T60.3X3-	T60.3X4-	-	-
Heroin	T40.1X1-	T40.1X2-	T40.1X3-	T40.1X4-	-	-
Herplex	T49.5X1-	T49.5X2-	T49.5X3-	T49.5X4-	T49.5X5-	T49.5X6-
HES	T45.8X1-	T45.8X2-	T45.8X3-	T45.8X4-	T45.8X5-	T45.8X6-
Hesperidin	T46.991-	T46.992-	T46.993-	T46.994-	T46.995-	T46.996-
Hetacillin	T36.0X1-	T36.0X2-	T36.0X3-	T36.0X4-	T36.0X5-	T36.0X6-
Hetastarch	T45.8X1-	T45.8X2-	T45.8X3-	T45.8X4-	T45.8X5-	T45.8X6-
HETP	T60.0X1-	T60.0X2-	T60.0X3-	T60.0X4-	-	-
Hexachlorobenzene (vapor)	T60.3X1-	T60.3X2-	T60.3X3-	T60.3X4-	-	-
Hexachlorocyclohexane	T53.6X1-	T53.6X2-	T53.6X3-	T53.6X4-	-	-
Hexachlorophene	T49.0X1-	T49.0X2-	T49.0X3-	T49.0X4-	T49.0X5-	T49.0X6-
Hexadiline	T46.3X1-	T46.3X2-	T46.3X3-	T46.3X4-	T46.3X5-	T46.3X6-
Hexadimethrine (bromide)	T45.7X1-	T45.7X2-	T45.7X3-	T45.7X4-	T45.7X5-	T45.7X6-
Hexadylamine	T46.3X1-	T46.3X2-	T46.3X3-	T46.3X4-	T46.3X5-	T46.3X6-
Hexaethyl tetraphos-phate	T60.0X1-	T60.0X2-	T60.0X3-	T60.0X4-	-	-
Hexafluorenium bromide	T48.1X1-	T48.1X2-	T48.1X3-	T48.1X4-	T48.1X5-	T48.1X6-
Hexafl</uronium (bromide)	T48.1X1-	T48.1X2-	T48.1X3-	T48.1X4-	T48.1X5-	T48.1X6-
Hexa-germ	T49.2X1-	T49.2X2-	T49.2X3-	T49.2X4-	T49.2X5-	T49.2X6-
Hexahydrobenzol	T52.8X1-	T52.8X2-	T52.8X3-	T52.8X4-	-	-

Substance	Poisoning, Accidental (unintentional)	Poisoning, Intentional self-harm	Poisoning, Assault	Poisoning, Undetermined	Adverse effect	Underdosing
Hexahydrocresol (s)	T51.8X1-	T51.8X2-	T51.8X3-	T51.8X4-	-	-
arsenide	T57.0X1-	T57.0X2-	T57.0X3-	T57.0X4-	-	-
arseniurated	T57.0X1-	T57.0X2-	T57.0X3-	T57.0X4-	-	-
cyanide	T57.3X1-	T57.3X2-	T57.3X3-	T57.3X4-	-	-
gas	T59.891-	T59.892-	T59.893-	T59.894-	-	-
Fluoride (liquid)	T57.8X1-	T57.8X2-	T57.8X3-	T57.8X4-	-	-
vapor	T59.891-	T59.892-	T59.893-	T59.894-	-	-
phophorated	T60.0X1-	T60.0X2-	T60.0X3-	T60.0X4-	-	-
sulfate	T57.8X1-	T57.8X2-	T57.8X3-	T57.8X4-	-	-
sulfide (gas)	T59.6X1-	T59.6X2-	T59.6X3-	T59.6X4-	-	-
arseniurated	T57.0X1-	T57.0X2-	T57.0X3-	T57.0X4-	-	-
sulfurated	T57.8X1-	T57.8X2-	T57.8X3-	T57.8X4-	-	-
Hexahydrophenol	T51.8X1-	T51.8X2-	T51.8X3-	T51.8X4-	-	-
Hexalen	T51.8X1-	T51.8X2-	T51.8X3-	T51.8X4-	-	-
Hexamethonium bromide	T44.2X1-	T44.2X2-	T44.2X3-	T44.2X4-	T44.2X5-	T44.2X6-
Hexamethylene	T52.8X1-	T52.8X2-	T52.8X3-	T52.8X4-	-	-
Hexamethylmelamine	T45.1X1-	T45.1X2-	T45.1X3-	T45.1X4-	T45.1X5-	T45.1X6-
Hexamidine	T49.0X1-	T49.0X2-	T49.0X3-	T49.0X4-	T49.0X5-	T49.0X6-
Hexamine (mandelate)	T37.8X1-	T37.8X2-	T37.8X3-	T37.8X4-	T37.8X5-	T37.8X6-
Hexanone, 2-hexanone	T52.4X1-	T52.4X2-	T52.4X3-	T52.4X4-		
Hexanuorenium	T48.1X1-	T48.1X2-	T48.1X3-	T48.1X4-	T48.1X5-	T48.1X6-
Hexapropymate	T42.6X1-	T42.6X2-	T42.6X3-	T42.6X4-	T42.6X5-	T42.6X6-
Hexasonium iodide	T44.3X1-	T44.3X2-	T44.3X3-	T44.3X4-	T44.3X5-	T44.3X6-
Hexcarbacholine bromide	T48.1X1-	T48.1X2-	T48.1X3-	T48.1X4-	T48.1X5-	T48.1X6-
Hexemal	T42.3X1-	T42.3X2-	T42.3X3-	T42.3X4-	T42.3X5-	T42.3X6-
Hexestrol	T38.5X1-	T38.5X2-	T38.5X3-	T38.5X4-	T38.5X5-	T38.5X6-
Hexethal (sodium)	T42.3X1-	T42.3X2-	T42.3X3-	T42.3X4-	T42.3X5-	T42.3X6-
Hexetidine	T37.8X1-	T37.8X2-	T37.8X3-	T37.8X4-	T37.8X5-	T37.8X6-
Hexobarbital	T42.3X1-	T42.3X2-	T42.3X3-	T42.3X4-	T42.3X5-	T42.3X6-
rectal	T41.291-	T41.292-	T41.293-	T41.294-	T41.295-	T41.296-
sodium	T41.1X1-	T41.1X2-	T41.1X3-	T41.1X4-	T41.1X5-	T41.1X6-
Hexobendine	T46.3X1-	T46.3X2-	T46.3X3-	T46.3X4-	T46.3X5-	T46.3X6-
Hexocyclium	T44.3X1-	T44.3X2-	T44.3X3-	T44.3X4-	T44.3X5-	T44.3X6-
metilsulfate	T44.3X1-	T44.3X2-	T44.3X3-	T44.3X4-	T44.3X5-	T44.3X6-
Hexoestrol	T38.5X1-	T38.5X2-	T38.5X3-	T38.5X4-	T38.5X5-	T38.5X6-
Hexone	T52.4X1-	T52.4X2-	T52.4X3-	T52.4X4-		
Hexoprenaline	T48.6X1-	T48.6X2-	T48.6X3-	T48.6X4-	T48.6X5-	T48.6X6-
Hexylcaine	T41.3X1-	T41.3X2-	T41.3X3-	T41.3X4-	T41.3X5-	T41.3X6-
Hexylresorcinol	T52.2X1-	T52.2X2-	T52.2X3-	T52.2X4-		
HGH (human growth hormone)	T38.811-	T38.812-	T38.813-	T38.814-	T38.815-	T38.816-
Hinkle's pills	T47.2X1-	T47.2X2-	T47.2X3-	T47.2X4-	T47.2X5-	T47.2X6-
Histalog	T50.8X1-	T50.8X2-	T50.8X3-	T50.8X4-	T50.8X5-	T50.8X6-
Histamine (phosphate)	T50.8X1-	T50.8X2-	T50.8X3-	T50.8X4-	T50.8X5-	T50.8X6-
Histoplasmin	T50.8X1-	T50.8X2-	T50.8X3-	T50.8X4-	T50.8X5-	T50.8X6-
Holly berries	T62.2X1-	T62.2X2-	T62.2X3-	T62.2X4-		
Homatropine	T44.3X1-	T44.3X2-	T44.3X3-	T44.3X4-	T44.3X5-	T44.3X6-
methylbromide	T44.3X1-	T44.3X2-	T44.3X3-	T44.3X4-	T44.3X5-	T44.3X6-
Homochlorcyclizine	T45.0X1-	T45.0X2-	T45.0X3-	T45.0X4-	T45.0X5-	T45.0X6-
Homosalate	T49.3X1-	T49.3X2-	T49.3X3-	T49.3X4-	T49.3X5-	T49.3X6-
Homo-tet	T50.Z11-	T50.Z12-	T50.Z13-	T50.Z14-	T50.Z15-	T50.Z16-
Hormone	T38.801-	T38.802-	T38.803-	T38.804-	T38.805-	T38.806-
adrenal cortical steroids	T38.0X1-	T38.0X2-	T38.0X3-	T38.0X4-	T38.0X5-	T38.0X6-
androgenic	T38.7X1-	T38.7X2-	T38.7X3-	T38.7X4-	T38.7X5-	T38.7X6-
anterior pituitary NEC	T38.811-	T38.812-	T38.813-	T38.814-	T38.815-	T38.816-
antidiabetic agents	T38.3X1-	T38.3X2-	T38.3X3-	T38.3X4-	T38.3X5-	T38.3X6-
antidiuretic	T38.891-	T38.892-	T38.893-	T38.894-	T38.895-	T38.896-
cancer therapy	T45.1X1-	T45.1X2-	T45.1X3-	T45.1X4-	T45.1X5-	T45.1X6-
follicle stimulating	T38.811-	T38.812-	T38.813-	T38.814-	T38.815-	T38.816-
gonadotropic	T38.891-	T38.892-	T38.893-	T38.894-	T38.895-	T38.896-
pituitary	T38.811-	T38.812-	T38.813-	T38.814-	T38.815-	T38.816-
growth	T38.811-	T38.812-	T38.813-	T38.814-	T38.815-	T38.816-
luteinizing	T38.811-	T38.812-	T38.813-	T38.814-	T38.815-	T38.816-
ovarian	T38.5X1-	T38.5X2-	T38.5X3-	T38.5X4-	T38.5X5-	T38.5X6-
oxytocic	T48.0X1-	T48.0X2-	T48.0X3-	T48.0X4-	T48.0X5-	T48.0X6-
parathyroid (derivatives)	T50.991-	T50.992-	T50.993-	T50.994-	T50.995-	T50.996-
pituitary (posterior) NEC	T38.891-	T38.892-	T38.893-	T38.894-	T38.895-	T38.896-
anterior	T38.811-	T38.812-	T38.813-	T38.814-	T38.815-	T38.816-
specified, NEC	T38.891-	T38.892-	T38.893-	T38.894-	T38.895-	T38.896-
thyroid	T38.1X1-	T38.1X2-	T38.1X3-	T38.1X4-	T38.1X5-	T38.1X6-
Hornet (sting)	T63.451-	T63.452-	T63.453-	T63.454-	-	-
Horse anti-human lymphocytic serum	T50.Z11-	T50.Z12-	T50.Z13-	T50.Z14-	T50.Z15-	T50.Z16-
Horticulture agent NEC	T65.91X-	T65.92X-	T65.93X-	T65.94X-	-	-
with pesticide	T60.91X-	T60.92X-	T60.93X-	T60.94X-	-	-
Human						
albumin	T45.8X1-	T45.8X2-	T45.8X3-	T45.8X4-	T45.8X5-	T45.8X6-
growth hormone (HGH)	T38.811-	T38.812-	T38.813-	T38.814-	T38.815-	T38.816-
immune serum	T50.Z11-	T50.Z12-	T50.Z13-	T50.Z14-	T50.Z15-	T50.Z16-

Substance	Poisoning, Accidental (unintentional)	Poisoning, Intentional self-harm	Poisoning, Assault	Poisoning, Undetermined	Adverse effect	Underdosing
Hyaluronidase	T45.3X1-	T45.3X2-	T45.3X3-	T45.3X4-	T45.3X5-	T45.3X6-
Hyazyme	T45.3X1-	T45.3X2-	T45.3X3-	T45.3X4-	T45.3X5-	T45.3X6-
Hycodan	T40.2X1-	T40.2X2-	T40.2X3-	T40.2X4-	T40.2X5-	T40.2X6-
Hydantoin derivative NEC	T42.0X1-	T42.0X2-	T42.0X3-	T42.0X4-	T42.0X5-	T42.0X6-
Hydeltra	T38.0X1-	T38.0X2-	T38.0X3-	T38.0X4-	T38.0X5-	T38.0X6-
Hydergine	T44.6X1-	T44.6X2-	T44.6X3-	T44.6X4-	T44.6X5-	T44.6X6-
Hydrabamine penicillin	T36.0X1-	T36.0X2-	T36.0X3-	T36.0X4-	T36.0X5-	T36.0X6-
Hydralazine	T46.5X1-	T46.5X2-	T46.5X3-	T46.5X4-	T46.5X5-	T46.5X6-
Hydrargaphen	T49.0X1-	T49.0X2-	T49.0X3-	T49.0X4-	T49.0X5-	T49.0X6-
Hydrargyri amino-chloridum	T49.0X1-	T49.0X2-	T49.0X3-	T49.0X4-	T49.0X5-	T49.0X6-
Hydrastine	T48.291-	T48.292-	T48.293-	T48.294-	T48.295-	T48.296-
Hydrazine	T54.1X1-	T54.1X2-	T54.1X3-	T54.1X4-	-	-
monoamine oxidase inhibitors	T43.1X1-	T43.1X2-	T43.1X3-	T43.1X4-	T43.1X5-	T43.1X6-
Hydrazoic acid, azides	T54.2X1-	T54.2X2-	T54.2X3-	T54.2X4-	-	-
Hydriodic acid	T48.4X1-	T48.4X2-	T48.4X3-	T48.4X4-	T48.4X5-	T48.4X6-
Hydrocarbon gas	T59.891-	T59.892-	T59.893-	T59.894-	-	-
incomplete combustion of — *see* Carbon, monoxide, fuel, utility						
liquefied (mobile container)	T59.891-	T59.892-	T59.893-	T59.894-	-	-
piped (natural)	T59.891-	T59.892-	T59.893-	T59.894-	-	-
Hydrochloric acid (liquid)	T54.2X1-	T54.2X2-	T54.2X3-	T54.2X4-		
medicinal (digestant)	T47.5X1-	T47.5X2-	T47.5X3-	T47.5X4-	T47.5X5-	T47.5X6-
vapor	T59.891-	T59.892-	T59.893-	T59.894-	-	-
Hydrochlorothiazide	T50.2X1-	T50.2X2-	T50.2X3-	T50.2X4-	T50.2X5-	T50.2X6-
Hydrocodone	T40.2X1-	T40.2X2-	T40.2X3-	T40.2X4-	T40.2X5-	T40.2X6-
Hydrocortisone (derivatives)	T38.0X1-	T38.0X2-	T38.0X3-	T38.0X4-	T38.0X5-	T38.0X6-
aceponate	T49.0X1-	T49.0X2-	T49.0X3-	T49.0X4-	T49.0X5-	T49.0X6-
ENT agent	T49.6X1-	T49.6X2-	T49.6X3-	T49.6X4-	T49.6X5-	T49.6X6-
ophthalmic preparation	T49.5X1-	T49.5X2-	T49.5X3-	T49.5X4-	T49.5X5-	T49.5X6-
topical NEC	T49.0X1-	T49.0X2-	T49.0X3-	T49.0X4-	T49.0X5-	T49.0X6-
Hydrocortone	T38.0X1-	T38.0X2-	T38.0X3-	T38.0X4-	T38.0X5-	T38.0X6-
ENT agent	T49.6X1-	T49.6X2-	T49.6X3-	T49.6X4-	T49.6X5-	T49.6X6-
ophthalmic preparation	T49.5X1-	T49.5X2-	T49.5X3-	T49.5X4-	T49.5X5-	T49.5X6-
topical NEC	T49.0X1-	T49.0X2-	T49.0X3-	T49.0X4-	T49.0X5-	T49.0X6-
Hydrocyanic acid (liquid)	T57.3X1-	T57.3X2-	T57.3X3-	T57.3X4-	-	-
gas	T65.0X1-	T65.0X2-	T65.0X3-	T65.0X4-	-	-
Hydroflumethiazide	T50.2X1-	T50.2X2-	T50.2X3-	T50.2X4-	T50.2X5-	T50.2X6-
Hydrofluoric acid (liquid)	T54.2X1-	T54.2X2-	T54.2X3-	T54.2X4-		
vapor	T59.891-	T59.892-	T59.893-	T59.894-	-	-
Hydrogen	T59.891-	T59.892-	T59.893-	T59.894-	-	-
arsenide	T57.0X1-	T57.0X2-	T57.0X3-	T57.0X4-	-	-
arseniureted	T57.0X1-	T57.0X2-	T57.0X3-	T57.0X4-	-	-
chloride	T57.8X1-	T57.8X2-	T57.8X3-	T57.8X4-	-	-
cyanide (salts)	T57.3X1-	T57.3X2-	T57.3X3-	T57.3X4-	-	-
gas	T57.3X1-	T57.3X2-	T57.3X3-	T57.3X4-	-	-
Fluoride	T59.5X1-	T59.5X2-	T59.5X3-	T59.5X4-	-	-
vapor	T59.5X1-	T59.5X2-	T59.5X3-	T59.5X4-	-	-
peroxide	T49.0X1-	T49.0X2-	T49.0X3-	T49.0X4-	T49.0X5-	T49.0X6-
phosphureted	T57.1X1-	T57.1X2-	T57.1X3-	T57.1X4-	-	-
sulfide	T59.6X1-	T59.6X2-	T59.6X3-	T59.6X4-	-	-
arseniureted	T57.0X1-	T57.0X2-	T57.0X3-	T57.0X4-	-	-
sulfureted	T59.6X1-	T59.6X2-	T59.6X3-	T59.6X4-	-	-
Hydromethylpyridine	T46.7X1-	T46.7X2-	T46.7X3-	T46.7X4-	T46.7X5-	T46.7X6-
Hydromorphinol	T40.2X1-	T40.2X2-	T40.2X3-	T40.2X4-		
Hydromorphinone	T40.2X1-	T40.2X2-	T40.2X3-	T40.2X4-	T40.2X5-	T40.2X6-
Hydromorphone	T40.2X1-	T40.2X2-	T40.2X3-	T40.2X4-	T40.2X5-	T40.2X6-
Hydromox	T50.2X1-	T50.2X2-	T50.2X3-	T50.2X4-	T50.2X5-	T50.2X6-
Hydrophilic lotion	T49.3X1-	T49.3X2-	T49.3X3-	T49.3X4-	T49.3X5-	T49.3X6-
Hydroquinidine	T46.2X1-	T46.2X2-	T46.2X3-	T46.2X4-	T46.2X5-	T46.2X6-
Hydroquinone	T52.2X1-	T52.2X2-	T52.2X3-	T52.2X4-	-	-
vapor	T59.891-	T59.892-	T59.893-	T59.894-	-	-
Hydrosulfuric acid (gas)	T59.6X1-	T59.6X2-	T59.6X3-	T59.6X4-	-	-
Hydrotalcite	T47.1X1-	T47.1X2-	T47.1X3-	T47.1X4-	T47.1X5-	T47.1X6-
Hydrous wool fat	T49.3X1-	T49.3X2-	T49.3X3-	T49.3X4-	T49.3X5-	T49.3X6-
Hydroxide, caustic	T54.3X1-	T54.3X2-	T54.3X3-	T54.3X4-		
Hydroxocobalamin	T45.8X1-	T45.8X2-	T45.8X3-	T45.8X4-	T45.8X5-	T45.8X6-
Hydroxyamphetamine	T49.5X1-	T49.5X2-	T49.5X3-	T49.5X4-	T49.5X5-	T49.5X6-
Hydroxycarbamide	T45.1X1-	T45.1X2-	T45.1X3-	T45.1X4-	T45.1X5-	T45.1X6-
Hydroxychloroquine	T37.8X1-	T37.8X2-	T37.8X3-	T37.8X4-	T37.8X5-	T37.8X6-
Hydroxydihydrocodeinone	T40.2X1-	T40.2X2-	T40.2X3-	T40.2X4-	T40.2X5-	T40.2X6-
Hydroxyestrone	T38.5X1-	T38.5X2-	T38.5X3-	T38.5X4-	T38.5X5-	T38.5X6-
Hydroxyethyl starch	T45.8X1-	T45.8X2-	T45.8X3-	T45.8X4-	T45.8X5-	T45.8X6-
Hydroxymethylpenta-none	T52.4X1-	T52.4X2-	T52.4X3-	T52.4X4-		
Hydroxyphenamate	T43.591-	T43.592-	T43.593-	T43.594-	T43.595-	T43.596-
Hydroxyphenylbutazone	T39.2X1-	T39.2X2-	T39.2X3-	T39.2X4-	T39.2X5-	T39.2X6-
Hydroxyprogesterone	T38.5X1-	T38.5X2-	T38.5X3-	T38.5X4-	T38.5X5-	T38.5X6-
caproate	T38.5X1-	T38.5X2-	T38.5X3-	T38.5X4-	T38.5X5-	T38.5X6-

Substance	Poisoning, Accidental (unintentional)	Poisoning, Intentional self-harm	Poisoning, Assault	Poisoning, Undetermined	Adverse effect	Underdosing
Hydroxyquinoline (derivatives) NEC	T37.8X1-	T37.8X2-	T37.8X3-	T37.8X4-	T37.8X5-	T37.8X6-
Hydroxystilbamidine	T37.3X1-	T37.3X2-	T37.3X3-	T37.3X4-	T37.3X5-	T37.3X6-
Hydroxytoluene (nonmedicinal)	T54.0X1-	T54.0X2-	T54.0X3-	T54.0X4-	-	-
medicinal	T49.0X1-	T49.0X2-	T49.0X3-	T49.0X4-	T49.0X5-	T49.0X6-
Hydroxyurea	T45.1X1-	T45.1X2-	T45.1X3-	T45.1X4-	T45.1X5-	T45.1X6-
Hydroxyzine	T43.591-	T43.592-	T43.593-	T43.594-	T43.595-	T43.596-
Hyoscine	T44.3X1-	T44.3X2-	T44.3X3-	T44.3X4-	T44.3X5-	T44.3X6-
Hyoscyamine	T44.3X1-	T44.3X2-	T44.3X3-	T44.3X4-	T44.3X5-	T44.3X6-
Hyoscyamus	T44.3X1-	T44.3X2-	T44.3X3-	T44.3X4-	T44.3X5-	T44.3X6-
dry extract	T44.3X1-	T44.3X2-	T44.3X3-	T44.3X4-	T44.3X5-	T44.3X6-
Hypaque	T50.8X1-	T50.8X2-	T50.8X3-	T50.8X4-	T50.8X5-	T50.8X6-
Hypertussis	T50.Z11-	T50.Z12-	T50.Z13-	T50.Z14-	T50.Z15-	T50.Z16-
Hypnotic	T42.71X-	T42.72X-	T42.73X-	T42.74X-	T42.75X-	T42.76X-
anticonvulsant	T42.71X-	T42.72X-	T42.73X-	T42.74X-	T42.75X-	T42.76X-
specified NEC	T42.6X1-	T42.6X2-	T42.6X3-	T42.6X4-	T42.6X5-	T42.6X6-
Hypochlorite	T49.0X1-	T49.0X2-	T49.0X3-	T49.0X4-	T49.0X5-	T49.0X6-
Hypophysis, posterior	T38.891-	T38.892-	T38.893-	T38.894-	T38.895-	T38.896-
Hypotensive NEC	T46.5X1-	T46.5X2-	T46.5X3-	T46.5X4-	T46.5X5-	T46.5X6-
Hypromellose	T49.5X1-	T49.5X2-	T49.5X3-	T49.5X4-	T49.5X5-	T49.5X6-
Ibacitabine	T37.5X1-	T37.5X2-	T37.5X3-	T37.5X4-	T37.5X5-	T37.5X6-
Ibopamine	T44.991-	T44.992-	T44.993-	T44.994-	T44.995-	T44.996-
Ibufenac	T39.311-	T39.312-	T39.313-	T39.314-	T39.315-	T39.316-
Ibuprofen	T39.311-	T39.312-	T39.313-	T39.314-	T39.315-	T39.316-
Ibuproxam	T39.311-	T39.312-	T39.313-	T39.314-	T39.315-	T39.316-
Ibuterol	T48.6X1-	T48.6X2-	T48.6X3-	T48.6X4-	T48.6X5-	T48.6X6-
Ichthammol	T49.0X1-	T49.0X2-	T49.0X3-	T49.0X4-	T49.0X5-	T49.0X6-
Ichthyol	T49.4X1-	T49.4X2-	T49.4X3-	T49.4X4-	T49.4X5-	T49.4X6-
Idarubicin	T45.1X1-	T45.1X2-	T45.1X3-	T45.1X4-	T45.1X5-	T45.1X6-
Idrocilamide	T42.8X1-	T42.8X2-	T42.8X3-	T42.8X4-	T42.8X5-	T42.8X6-
Ifenprodil	T46.7X1-	T46.7X2-	T46.7X3-	T46.7X4-	T46.7X5-	T46.7X6-
Ifosfamide	T45.1X1-	T45.1X2-	T45.1X3-	T45.1X4-	T45.1X5-	T45.1X6-
Iletin	T38.3X1-	T38.3X2-	T38.3X3-	T38.3X4-	T38.3X5-	T38.3X6-
Ilex	T62.2X1-	T62.2X2-	T62.2X3-	T62.2X4-	-	-
Illuminating gas (after combustion)	T58.11X-	T58.12X-	T58.13X-	T58.14X-	-	-
prior to combustion	T59.891-	T59.892-	T59.893-	T59.894-	-	-
Ilopan	T45.2X1-	T45.2X2-	T45.2X3-	T45.2X4-	T45.2X5-	T45.2X6-
Iloprost	T46.7X1-	T46.7X2-	T46.7X3-	T46.7X4-	T46.7X5-	T46.7X6-
Ilotycin	T36.3X1-	T36.3X2-	T36.3X3-	T36.3X4-	T36.3X5-	T36.3X6-
ophthalmic preparation	T49.5X1-	T49.5X2-	T49.5X3-	T49.5X4-	T49.5X5-	T49.5X6-
topical NEC	T49.0X1-	T49.0X2-	T49.0X3-	T49.0X4-	T49.0X5-	T49.0X6-
Imidazole-4-carboxamide	T45.1X1-	T45.1X2-	T45.1X3-	T45.1X4-	T45.1X5-	T45.1X6-
Imipenem	T36.0X1-	T36.0X2-	T36.0X3-	T36.0X4-	T36.0X5-	T36.0X6-
Imipramine	T43.011-	T43.012-	T43.013-	T43.014-	T43.015-	T43.016-
Iminostilbene	T42.1X1-	T42.1X2-	T42.1X3-	T42.1X4-	T42.1X5-	T42.1X6-
Immu-G	T50.Z11-	T50.Z12-	T50.Z13-	T50.Z14-	T50.Z15-	T50.Z16-
Immuglobin	T50.Z11-	T50.Z12-	T50.Z13-	T50.Z14-	T50.Z15-	T50.Z16-
Immune						
globulin	T50.Z11-	T50.Z12-	T50.Z13-	T50.Z14-	T50.Z15-	T50.Z16-
serum globulin	T50.Z11-	T50.Z12-	T50.Z13-	T50.Z14-	T50.Z15-	T50.Z16-
Immunoglobin human (intravenous) (normal)	T50.Z11-	T50.Z12-	T50.Z13-	T50.Z14-	T50.Z15-	T50.Z16-
unmodified	T50.Z11-	T50.Z12-	T50.Z13-	T50.Z14-	T50.Z15-	T50.Z16-
Immunosuppressive drug	T45.1X1-	T45.1X2-	T45.1X3-	T45.1X4-	T45.1X5-	T45.1X6-
Immu-tetanus	T50.Z11-	T50.Z12-	T50.Z13-	T50.Z14-	T50.Z15-	T50.Z16-
Indalpine	T43.221-	T43.222-	T43.223-	T43.224-	T43.225-	T43.226-
Indanazoline	T48.5X1-	T48.5X2-	T48.5X3-	T48.5X4-	T48.5X5-	T48.5X6-
Indandione (derivatives)	T45.511-	T45.512-	T45.513-	T45.514-	T45.515-	T45.516-
Indapamide	T46.5X1-	T46.5X2-	T46.5X3-	T46.5X4-	T46.5X5-	T46.5X6-
Indendione (derivatives)	T45.511-	T45.512-	T45.513-	T45.514-	T45.515-	T45.516-
Indenolol	T44.7X1-	T44.7X2-	T44.7X3-	T44.7X4-	T44.7X5-	T44.7X6-
Inderal	T44.7X1-	T44.7X2-	T44.7X3-	T44.7X4-	T44.7X5-	T44.7X6-
Indian						
hemp	T40.7X1-	T40.7X2-	T40.7X3-	T40.7X4-	T40.7X5-	T40.7X6-
tobacco	T62.2X1-	T62.2X2-	T62.2X3-	T62.2X4-	-	-
Indigo carmine	T50.8X1-	T50.8X2-	T50.8X3-	T50.8X4-	T50.8X5-	T50.8X6-
Indobufen	T45.521-	T45.522-	T45.523-	T45.524-	T45.525-	T45.526-
Indocin	T39.2X1-	T39.2X2-	T39.2X3-	T39.2X4-	T39.2X5-	T39.2X6-
Indocyanine green	T50.8X1-	T50.8X2-	T50.8X3-	T50.8X4-	T50.8X5-	T50.8X6-
Indometacin	T39.391-	T39.392-	T39.393-	T39.394-	T39.395-	T39.396-
Indomethacin	T39.391-	T39.392-	T39.393-	T39.394-	T39.395-	T39.396-
farnesil	T39.4X1-	T39.4X2-	T39.4X3-	T39.4X4-	T39.4X5-	T39.4X6-
Indoramin	T44.6X1-	T44.6X2-	T44.6X3-	T44.6X4-	T44.6X5-	T44.6X6-
Industrial						
alcohol	T51.0X1-	T51.0X2-	T51.0X3-	T51.0X4-	-	-
fumes	T59.891-	T59.892-	T59.893-	T59.894-	-	-
solvents (fumes) (vapors)	T52.91X-	T52.92X-	T52.93X-	T52.94X-	-	-

Substance	Poisoning, Accidental (unintentional)	Poisoning, Intentional self-harm	Poisoning, Assault	Poisoning, Undetermined	Adverse effect	Underdosing
Influenza vaccine	T50.B91-	T50.B92-	T50.B93-	T50.B94-	T50.B95-	T50.B96-
Ingested substance NEC	T65.91X-	T65.92X-	T65.93X-	T65.94X-	-	-
INH	T37.1X1-	T37.1X2-	T37.1X3-	T37.1X4-	T37.1X5-	T37.1X6-
Inhalation, gas (noxious) — see Gas						
Inhibitor						
angiotensin-converting enzyme	T46.4X1-	T46.4X2-	T46.4X3-	T46.4X4-	T46.4X5-	T46.4X6-
carbonic anhydrase	T50.2X1-	T50.2X2-	T50.2X3-	T50.2X4-	T50.2X5-	T50.2X6-
fibrinolysis	T45.621-	T45.622-	T45.623-	T45.624-	T45.625-	T45.626-
monoamine oxidase NEC	T43.1X1-	T43.1X2-	T43.1X3-	T43.1X4-	T43.1X5-	T43.1X6-
hydrazine	T43.1X1-	T43.1X2-	T43.1X3-	T43.1X4-	T43.1X5-	T43.1X6-
postsynaptic	T43.8X1-	T43.8X2-	T43.8X3-	T43.8X4-	T43.8X5-	T43.8X6-
prothrombin synthesis	T45.511-	T45.512-	T45.513-	T45.514-	T45.515-	T45.516-
Ink	T65.891-	T65.892-	T65.893-	T65.894-	-	-
Inorganic substance NEC	T57.91X-	T57.92X-	T57.93X-	T57.94X-	-	-
Inosine pranobex	T37.5X1-	T37.5X2-	T37.5X3-	T37.5X4-	T37.5X5-	T37.5X6-
Inositol	T50.991-	T50.992-	T50.993-	T50.994-	T50.995-	T50.996-
nicotinate	T46.7X1-	T46.7X2-	T46.7X3-	T46.7X4-	T46.7X5-	T46.7X6-
Inproquone	T45.1X1-	T45.1X2-	T45.1X3-	T45.1X4-	T45.1X5-	T45.1X6-
Insect (sting) , venomous	T63.481-	T63.482-	T63.483-	T63.484-	-	-
ant	T63.421-	T63.422-	T63.423-	T63.424-	-	-
bee	T63.441-	T63.442-	T63.443-	T63.444-	-	-
caterpillar	T63.431-	T63.432-	T63.433-	T63.434-	-	-
hornet	T63.451-	T63.452-	T63.453-	T63.454-	-	-
wasp	T63.461-	T63.462-	T63.463-	T63.464-	-	-
Insecticide NEC	T60.91X-	T60.92X-	T60.93X-	T60.94X-	-	-
carbamate	T60.0X1-	T60.0X2-	T60.0X3-	T60.0X4-	-	-
chlorinated	T60.1X1-	T60.1X2-	T60.1X3-	T60.1X4-	-	-
mixed	T60.91X-	T60.92X-	T60.93X-	T60.94X-	-	-
organochlorine	T60.1X1-	T60.1X2-	T60.1X3-	T60.1X4-	-	-
organophosphorus	T60.0X1-	T60.0X2-	T60.0X3-	T60.0X4-	-	-
Insular tissue extract	T38.3X1-	T38.3X2-	T38.3X3-	T38.3X4-	T38.3X5-	T38.3X6-
Insulin (amorphous) (globin) (isophane) (Lente) (NPH) (Semilente) (Ultralente)						
defalan	T38.3X1-	T38.3X2-	T38.3X3-	T38.3X4-	T38.3X5-	T38.3X6-
human	T38.3X1-	T38.3X2-	T38.3X3-	T38.3X4-	T38.3X5-	T38.3X6-
injection, soluble	T38.3X1-	T38.3X2-	T38.3X3-	T38.3X4-	T38.3X5-	T38.3X6-
biphasic	T38.3X1-	T38.3X2-	T38.3X3-	T38.3X4-	T38.3X5-	T38.3X6-
intermediate acting	T38.3X1-	T38.3X2-	T38.3X3-	T38.3X4-	T38.3X5-	T38.3X6-
protamine zinc	T38.3X1-	T38.3X2-	T38.3X3-	T38.3X4-	T38.3X5-	T38.3X6-
slow acting	T38.3X1-	T38.3X2-	T38.3X3-	T38.3X4-	T38.3X5-	T38.3X6-
zinc						
protamine injection	T38.3X1-	T38.3X2-	T38.3X3-	T38.3X4-	T38.3X5-	T38.3X6-
suspension (amorphous) (crystalline)	T38.3X1-	T38.3X2-	T38.3X3-	T38.3X4-	T38.3X5-	T38.3X6-
Interferon (alpha) (beta) (gamma)	T37.5X1-	T37.5X2-	T37.5X3-	T37.5X4-	T37.5X5-	T37.5X6-
Intestinal motility control drug	T47.6X1-	T47.6X2-	T47.6X3-	T47.6X4-	T47.6X5-	T47.6X6-
biological	T47.8X1-	T47.8X2-	T47.8X3-	T47.8X4-	T47.8X5-	T47.8X6-
Intranarcon	T41.1X1-	T41.1X2-	T41.1X3-	T41.1X4-	T41.1X5-	T41.1X6-
Intravenous						
amino acids	T50.991-	T50.992-	T50.993-	T50.994-	T50.995-	T50.996-
fat suspension	T50.991-	T50.992-	T50.993-	T50.994-	T50.995-	T50.996-
Inulin	T50.8X1-	T50.8X2-	T50.8X3-	T50.8X4-	T50.8X5-	T50.8X6-
Invert sugar	T50.3X1-	T50.3X2-	T50.3X3-	T50.3X4-	T50.3X5-	T50.3X6-
Inza — see Naproxen						
Iobenzamic acid	T50.8X1-	T50.8X2-	T50.8X3-	T50.8X4-	T50.8X5-	T50.8X6-
Iocarmic acid	T50.8X1-	T50.8X2-	T50.8X3-	T50.8X4-	T50.8X5-	T50.8X6-
Iocetamic acid	T50.8X1-	T50.8X2-	T50.8X3-	T50.8X4-	T50.8X5-	T50.8X6-
Iodamide	T50.8X1-	T50.8X2-	T50.8X3-	T50.8X4-	T50.8X5-	T50.8X6-
Iodide NEC — see also Iodine	T49.0X1-	T49.0X2-	T49.0X3-	T49.0X4-	T49.0X5-	T49.0X6-
mercury (ointment)	T49.0X1-	T49.0X2-	T49.0X3-	T49.0X4-	T49.0X5-	T49.0X6-
methylate	T49.0X1-	T49.0X2-	T49.0X3-	T49.0X4-	T49.0X5-	T49.0X6-
potassium (expectorant) NEC	T48.4X1-	T48.4X2-	T48.4X3-	T48.4X4-	T48.4X5-	T48.4X6-
Iodinated						
contrast medium	T50.8X1-	T50.8X2-	T50.8X3-	T50.8X4-	T50.8X5-	T50.8X6-
glycerol	T48.4X1-	T48.4X2-	T48.4X3-	T48.4X4-	T48.4X5-	T48.4X6-
human serum albumin (131I)	T50.8X1-	T50.8X2-	T50.8X3-	T50.8X4-	T50.8X5-	T50.8X6-
Iodine (antiseptic, external) (tincture) NEC	T49.0X1-	T49.0X2-	T49.0X3-	T49.0X4-	T49.0X5-	T49.0X6-
125 — see also Radiation sickness, and Exposure to radioactivce isotopes	T50.8X1-	T50.8X2-	T50.8X3-	T50.8X4-	T50.8X5-	T50.8X6-
therapeutic	T50.991-	T50.992-	T50.993-	T50.994-	T50.995-	T50.996-
131 — see also Radiation sickness, and Exposure to radioactivce isotopes	T50.8X1-	T50.8X2-	T50.8X3-	T50.8X4-	T50.8X5-	T50.8X6-
therapeutic	T38.2X1-	T38.2X2-	T38.2X3-	T38.2X4-	T38.2X5-	T38.2X6-

Substance	Poisoning, Accidental (unintentional)	Poisoning, Intentional self-harm	Poisoning, Assault	Poisoning, Undetermined	Adverse effect	Underdosing
Iodine NEC - *continued*						
diagnostic	T50.8X1-	T50.8X2-	T50.8X3-	T50.8X4-	T50.8X5-	T50.8X6-
for thyroid conditions (antithyroid)	T38.2X1-	T38.2X2-	T38.2X3-	T38.2X4-	T38.2X5-	T38.2X6-
solution	T49.0X1-	T49.0X2-	T49.0X3-	T49.0X4-	T49.0X5-	T49.0X6-
vapor	T59.891-	T59.892-	T59.893-	T59.894-	-	-
Iodipamide	T50.8X1-	T50.8X2-	T50.8X3-	T50.8X4-	T50.8X5-	T50.8X6-
Iodized (poppy seed) **oil**	T50.8X1-	T50.8X2-	T50.8X3-	T50.8X4-	T50.8X5-	T50.8X6-
Iodobismitol	T37.8X1-	T37.8X2-	T37.8X3-	T37.8X4-	T37.8X5-	T37.8X6-
Iodochlorhydroxyquin	T37.8X1-	T37.8X2-	T37.8X3-	T37.8X4-	T37.8X5-	T37.8X6-
topical	T49.0X1-	T49.0X2-	T49.0X3-	T49.0X4-	T49.0X5-	T49.0X6-
Iodochlorhydroxyquinoline	T37.8X1-	T37.8X2-	T37.8X3-	T37.8X4-	T37.8X5-	T37.8X6-
Iodocholesterol (131I)	T50.8X1-	T50.8X2-	T50.8X3-	T50.8X4-	T50.8X5-	T50.8X6-
Iodoform	T49.0X1-	T49.0X2-	T49.0X3-	T49.0X4-	T49.0X5-	T49.0X6-
Iodohippuric acid	T50.8X1-	T50.8X2-	T50.8X3-	T50.8X4-	T50.8X5-	T50.8X6-
Iodopanoic acid	T50.8X1-	T50.8X2-	T50.8X3-	T50.8X4-	T50.8X5-	T50.8X6-
Iodophthalein (sodium)	T50.8X1-	T50.8X2-	T50.8X3-	T50.8X4-	T50.8X5-	T50.8X6-
Iodopyracet	T50.8X1-	T50.8X2-	T50.8X3-	T50.8X4-	T50.8X5-	T50.8X6-
Iodoquinol	T37.8X1-	T37.8X2-	T37.8X3-	T37.8X4-	T37.8X5-	T37.8X6-
Iodoxamic acid	T50.8X1-	T50.8X2-	T50.8X3-	T50.8X4-	T50.8X5-	T50.8X6-
Iofendylate	T50.8X1-	T50.8X2-	T50.8X3-	T50.8X4-	T50.8X5-	T50.8X6-
Ioglycamic acid	T50.8X1-	T50.8X2-	T50.8X3-	T50.8X4-	T50.8X5-	T50.8X6-
Iohexol	T50.8X1-	T50.8X2-	T50.8X3-	T50.8X4-	T50.8X5-	T50.8X6-
Ion exchange resin						
anion	T47.8X1-	T47.8X2-	T47.8X3-	T47.8X4-	T47.8X5-	T47.8X6-
cation	T50.3X1-	T50.3X2-	T50.3X3-	T50.3X4-	T50.3X5-	T50.3X6-
cholestyramine	T46.6X1-	T46.6X2-	T46.6X3-	T46.6X4-	T46.6X5-	T46.6X6-
intestinal	T47.8X1-	T47.8X2-	T47.8X3-	T47.8X4-	T47.8X5-	T47.8X6-
Iopamidol	T50.8X1-	T50.8X2-	T50.8X3-	T50.8X4-	T50.8X5-	T50.8X6-
Iopanoic acid	T50.8X1-	T50.8X2-	T50.8X3-	T50.8X4-	T50.8X5-	T50.8X6-
Iophenoic acid	T50.8X1-	T50.8X2-	T50.8X3-	T50.8X4-	T50.8X5-	T50.8X6-
Iopodate, sodium	T50.8X1-	T50.8X2-	T50.8X3-	T50.8X4-	T50.8X5-	T50.8X6-
Iopodic acid	T50.8X1-	T50.8X2-	T50.8X3-	T50.8X4-	T50.8X5-	T50.8X6-
Iopromide	T50.8X1-	T50.8X2-	T50.8X3-	T50.8X4-	T50.8X5-	T50.8X6-
Iopydol	T50.8X1-	T50.8X2-	T50.8X3-	T50.8X4-	T50.8X5-	T50.8X6-
Iotalamic acid	T50.8X1-	T50.8X2-	T50.8X3-	T50.8X4-	T50.8X5-	T50.8X6-
Iothalamate	T50.8X1-	T50.8X2-	T50.8X3-	T50.8X4-	T50.8X5-	T50.8X6-
Iothiouracil	T38.2X1-	T38.2X2-	T38.2X3-	T38.2X4-	T38.2X5-	T38.2X6-
Iotrol	T50.8X1-	T50.8X2-	T50.8X3-	T50.8X4-	T50.8X5-	T50.8X6-
Iotrolan	T50.8X1-	T50.8X2-	T50.8X3-	T50.8X4-	T50.8X5-	T50.8X6-
Iotroxate	T50.8X1-	T50.8X2-	T50.8X3-	T50.8X4-	T50.8X5-	T50.8X6-
Iotroxic acid	T50.8X1-	T50.8X2-	T50.8X3-	T50.8X4-	T50.8X5-	T50.8X6-
Ioversol	T50.8X1-	T50.8X2-	T50.8X3-	T50.8X4-	T50.8X5-	T50.8X6-
Ioxaglate	T50.8X1-	T50.8X2-	T50.8X3-	T50.8X4-	T50.8X5-	T50.8X6-
Ioxaglic acid	T50.8X1-	T50.8X2-	T50.8X3-	T50.8X4-	T50.8X5-	T50.8X6-
Ioxitalamic acid	T50.8X1-	T50.8X2-	T50.8X3-	T50.8X4-	T50.8X5-	T50.8X6-
Ipecac	T47.7X1-	T47.7X2-	T47.7X3-	T47.7X4-	T47.7X5-	T47.7X6-
Ipecacuanha	T48.4X1-	T48.4X2-	T48.4X3-	T48.4X4-	T48.4X5-	T48.4X6-
Ipodate, calcium	T50.8X1-	T50.8X2-	T50.8X3-	T50.8X4-	T50.8X5-	T50.8X6-
Ipral	T42.3X1-	T42.3X2-	T42.3X3-	T42.3X4-	T42.3X5-	T42.3X6-
Ipratropium (bromide)	T48.6X1-	T48.6X2-	T48.6X3-	T48.6X4-	T48.6X5-	T48.6X6-
Ipriflavone	T46.3X1-	T46.3X2-	T46.3X3-	T46.3X4-	T46.3X5-	T46.3X6-
Iprindole	T43.011-	T43.012-	T43.013-	T43.014-	T43.015-	T43.016-
Iproclozide	T43.1X1-	T43.1X2-	T43.1X3-	T43.1X4-	T43.1X5-	T43.1X6-
Iprofenin	T50.8X1-	T50.8X2-	T50.8X3-	T50.8X4-	T50.8X5-	T50.8X6-
Iproheptine	T49.2X1-	T49.2X2-	T49.2X3-	T49.2X4-	T49.2X5-	T49.2X6-
Iproniazid	T43.1X1-	T43.1X2-	T43.1X3-	T43.1X4-	T43.1X5-	T43.1X6-
Iproplatin	T45.1X1-	T45.1X2-	T45.1X3-	T45.1X4-	T45.1X5-	T45.1X6-
Iproveratril	T46.1X1-	T46.1X2-	T46.1X3-	T46.1X4-	T46.1X5-	T46.1X6-
Iron (compounds) (medicinal) **NEC**	T45.4X1-	T45.4X2-	T45.4X3-	T45.4X4-	T45.4X5-	T45.4X6-
ammonium	T45.4X1-	T45.4X2-	T45.4X3-	T45.4X4-	T45.4X5-	T45.4X6-
dextran injection	T45.4X1-	T45.4X2-	T45.4X3-	T45.4X4-	T45.4X5-	T45.4X6-
nonmedicinal	T56.891-	T56.892-	T56.893-	T56.894-	-	-
salts	T45.4X1-	T45.4X2-	T45.4X3-	T45.4X4-	T45.4X5-	T45.4X6-
sorbitex	T45.4X1-	T45.4X2-	T45.4X3-	T45.4X4-	T45.4X5-	T45.4X6-
sorbitol citric acid complex	T45.4X1-	T45.4X2-	T45.4X3-	T45.4X4-	T45.4X5-	T45.4X6-
Irrigating fluid (vaginal)	T49.8X1-	T49.8X2-	T49.8X3-	T49.8X4-	T49.8X5-	T49.8X6-
eye	T49.5X1-	T49.5X2-	T49.5X3-	T49.5X4-	T49.5X5-	T49.5X6-
Isepamicin	T36.5X1-	T36.5X2-	T36.5X3-	T36.5X4-	T36.5X5-	T36.5X6-
Isoaminile (citrate)	T48.3X1-	T48.3X2-	T48.3X3-	T48.3X4-	T48.3X5-	T48.3X6-
Isoamyl nitrite	T46.3X1-	T46.3X2-	T46.3X3-	T46.3X4-	T46.3X5-	T46.3X6-
Isobenzan	T60.1X1-	T60.1X2-	T60.1X3-	T60.1X4-	-	-
Isobutyl acetate	T52.8X1-	T52.8X2-	T52.8X3-	T52.8X4-	-	-
Isocarboxazid	T43.1X1-	T43.1X2-	T43.1X3-	T43.1X4-	T43.1X5-	T43.1X6-
Isoconazole	T49.0X1-	T49.0X2-	T49.0X3-	T49.0X4-	T49.0X5-	T49.0X6-
Isocyanate	T65.0X1-	T65.0X2-	T65.0X3-	T65.0X4-	-	-
Isoephedrine	T44.991-	T44.992-	T44.993-	T44.994-	T44.995-	T44.996-

Substance	Poisoning, Accidental (unintentional)	Poisoning, Intentional self-harm	Poisoning, Assault	Poisoning, Undetermined	Adverse effect	Underdosing
Isoetarine	T48.6X1-	T48.6X2-	T48.6X3-	T48.6X4-	T48.6X5-	T48.6X6-
Isoethadione	T42.2X1-	T42.2X2-	T42.2X3-	T42.2X4-	T42.2X5-	T42.2X6-
Isoetharine	T44.5X1-	T44.5X2-	T44.5X3-	T44.5X4-	T44.5X5-	T44.5X6-
Isoflurane	T41.0X1-	T41.0X2-	T41.0X3-	T41.0X4-	T41.0X5-	T41.0X6-
Isoflurophate	T44.0X1-	T44.0X2-	T44.0X3-	T44.0X4-	T44.0X5-	T44.0X6-
Isomaltose, ferric complex	T45.4X1-	T45.4X2-	T45.4X3-	T45.4X4-	T45.4X5-	T45.4X6-
Isometheptene	T44.3X1-	T44.3X2-	T44.3X3-	T44.3X4-	T44.3X5-	T44.3X6-
Isoniazid	T37.1X1-	T37.1X2-	T37.1X3-	T37.1X4-	T37.1X5-	T37.1X6-
with						
rifampicin	T36.6X1-	T36.6X2-	T36.6X3-	T36.6X4-	T36.6X5-	T36.6X6-
thioacetazone	T37.1X1-	T37.1X2-	T37.1X3-	T37.1X4-	T37.1X5-	T37.1X6-
Isonicotinic acid hydrazide	T37.1X1-	T37.1X2-	T37.1X3-	T37.1X4-	T37.1X5-	T37.1X6-
Isonipecaine	T40.4X1-	T40.4X2-	T40.4X3-	T40.4X4-	T40.4X5-	T40.4X6-
Isopentaquine	T37.2X1-	T37.2X2-	T37.2X3-	T37.2X4-	T37.2X5-	T37.2X6-
Isophane insulin	T38.3X1-	T38.3X2-	T38.3X3-	T38.3X4-	T38.3X5-	T38.3X6-
Isophorone	T65.891-	T65.892-	T65.893-	T65.894-	-	-
Isophosphamide	T45.1X1-	T45.1X2-	T45.1X3-	T45.1X4-	T45.1X5-	T45.1X6-
Isopregnenone	T38.5X1-	T38.5X2-	T38.5X3-	T38.5X4-	T38.5X5-	T38.5X6-
Isoprenaline	T48.6X1-	T48.6X2-	T48.6X3-	T48.6X4-	T48.6X5-	T48.6X6-
Isopromethazine	T43.3X1-	T43.3X2-	T43.3X3-	T43.3X4-	T43.3X5-	T43.3X6-
Isopropamide	T44.3X1-	T44.3X2-	T44.3X3-	T44.3X4-	T44.3X5-	T44.3X6-
iodide	T44.3X1-	T44.3X2-	T44.3X3-	T44.3X4-	T44.3X5-	T44.3X6-
Isopropanol	T51.2X1-	T51.2X2-	T51.2X3-	T51.2X4-	-	-
Isopropyl						
acetate	T52.8X1-	T52.8X2-	T52.8X3-	T52.8X4-	-	-
alcohol	T51.2X1-	T51.2X2-	T51.2X3-	T51.2X4-	-	-
medicinal	T49.4X1-	T49.4X2-	T49.4X3-	T49.4X4-	T49.4X5-	T49.4X6-
ether	T52.8X1-	T52.8X2-	T52.8X3-	T52.8X4-	-	-
Isopropylaminophenazone	T39.2X1-	T39.2X2-	T39.2X3-	T39.2X4-	T39.2X5-	T39.2X6-
Isoproterenol	T48.6X1-	T48.6X2-	T48.6X3-	T48.6X4-	T48.6X5-	T48.6X6-
Isosorbide dinitrate	T46.3X1-	T46.3X2-	T46.3X3-	T46.3X4-	T46.3X5-	T46.3X6-
Isothipendyl	T45.0X1-	T45.0X2-	T45.0X3-	T45.0X4-	T45.0X5-	T45.0X6-
Isotretinoin	T50.991-	T50.992-	T50.993-	T50.994-	T50.995-	T50.996-
Isoxazolyl penicillin	T36.0X1-	T36.0X2-	T36.0X3-	T36.0X4-	T36.0X5-	T36.0X6-
Isoxicam	T39.391-	T39.392-	T39.393-	T39.394-	T39.395-	T39.396-
Isoxsuprine	T46.7X1-	T46.7X2-	T46.7X3-	T46.7X4-	T46.7X5-	T46.7X6-
Ispagula	T47.4X1-	T47.4X2-	T47.4X3-	T47.4X4-	T47.4X5-	T47.4X6-
husk	T47.4X1-	T47.4X2-	T47.4X3-	T47.4X4-	T47.4X5-	T47.4X6-
Isradipine	T46.1X1-	T46.1X2-	T46.1X3-	T46.1X4-	T46.1X5-	T46.1X6-
I-thyroxine sodium	T38.1X1-	T38.1X2-	T38.1X3-	T38.1X4-	T38.1X5-	T38.1X6-
Itraconazole	T37.8X1-	T37.8X2-	T37.8X3-	T37.8X4-	T37.8X5-	T37.8X6-
Itramin tosilate	T46.3X1-	T46.3X2-	T46.3X3-	T46.3X4-	T46.3X5-	T46.3X6-
Ivermectin	T37.4X1-	T37.4X2-	T37.4X3-	T37.4X4-	T37.4X5-	T37.4X6-
Izoniazid	T37.1X1-	T37.1X2-	T37.1X3-	T37.1X4-	T37.1X5-	T37.1X6-
with thioacetazone	T37.1X1-	T37.1X2-	T37.1X3-	T37.1X4-	T37.1X5-	T37.1X6-
Jalap	T47.2X1-	T47.2X2-	T47.2X3-	T47.2X4-	T47.2X5-	T47.2X6-
Jamaica						
dogwood (bark)	T39.8X1-	T39.8X2-	T39.8X3-	T39.8X4-	T39.8X5-	T39.8X6-
ginger	T65.891-	T65.892-	T65.893-	T65.894-	-	-
root	T62.2X1-	T62.2X2-	T62.2X3-	T62.2X4-	-	-
Jatropha	T62.2X1-	T62.2X2-	T62.2X3-	T62.2X4-	-	-
curcas	T62.2X1-	T62.2X2-	T62.2X3-	T62.2X4-	-	-
Jectofer	T45.4X1-	T45.4X2-	T45.4X3-	T45.4X4-	T45.4X5-	T45.4X6-
Jellyfish (sting)	T63.621-	T63.622-	T63.623-	T63.624-	-	-
Jequirity (bean)	T62.2X1-	T62.2X2-	T62.2X3-	T62.2X4-	-	-
Jimson weed (stramonium)	T62.2X1-	T62.2X2-	T62.2X3-	T62.2X4-	-	-
seeds	T62.2X1-	T62.2X2-	T62.2X3-	T62.2X4-	-	-
Josamycin	T36.3X1-	T36.3X2-	T36.3X3-	T36.3X4-	T36.3X5-	T36.3X6-
Juniper tar	T49.1X1-	T49.1X2-	T49.1X3-	T49.1X4-	T49.1X5-	T49.1X6-
Kallidinogenase	T46.7X1-	T46.7X2-	T46.7X3-	T46.7X4-	T46.7X5-	T46.7X6-
Kallikrein	T46.7X1-	T46.7X2-	T46.7X3-	T46.7X4-	T46.7X5-	T46.7X6-
Kanamycin	T36.5X1-	T36.5X2-	T36.5X3-	T36.5X4-	T36.5X5-	T36.5X6-
Kantrex	T36.5X1-	T36.5X2-	T36.5X3-	T36.5X4-	T36.5X5-	T36.5X6-
Kaolin	T47.6X1-	T47.6X2-	T47.6X3-	T47.6X4-	T47.6X5-	T47.6X6-
light	T47.6X1-	T47.6X2-	T47.6X3-	T47.6X4-	T47.6X5-	T47.6X6-
Karaya (gum)	T47.4X1-	T47.4X2-	T47.4X3-	T47.4X4-	T47.4X5-	T47.4X6-
Kebuzone	T39.2X1-	T39.2X2-	T39.2X3-	T39.2X4-	T39.2X5-	T39.2X6-
Kelevan	T60.1X1-	T60.1X2-	T60.1X3-	T60.1X4-	-	-
Kemithal	T41.1X1-	T41.1X2-	T41.1X3-	T41.1X4-	T41.1X5-	T41.1X6-
Kenacort	T38.0X1-	T38.0X2-	T38.0X3-	T38.0X4-	T38.0X5-	T38.0X6-
Keratolytic drug NEC	T49.4X1-	T49.4X2-	T49.4X3-	T49.4X4-	T49.4X5-	T49.4X6-
anthracene	T49.4X1-	T49.4X2-	T49.4X3-	T49.4X4-	T49.4X5-	T49.4X6-
Keratoplastic NEC	T49.4X1-	T49.4X2-	T49.4X3-	T49.4X4-	T49.4X5-	T49.4X6-
Kerosene, kerosine (fuel) (solvent) **NEC**	T52.0X1-	T52.0X2-	T52.0X3-	T52.0X4-	-	-
insecticide	T52.0X1-	T52.0X2-	T52.0X3-	T52.0X4-	-	-
vapor	T52.0X1-	T52.0X2-	T52.0X3-	T52.0X4-	-	-
Ketamine	T41.291-	T41.292-	T41.293-	T41.294-	T41.295-	T41.296-

Table of Drugs and Chemicals — left: **Ketazolam — Lincomycin** (vertical)

Substance	Poisoning, Accidental (unintentional)	Poisoning, Intentional self-harm	Poisoning, Assault	Poisoning, Undetermined	Adverse effect	Underdosing
Ketazolam	T42.4X1-	T42.4X2-	T42.4X3-	T42.4X4-	T42.4X5-	T42.4X6-
Ketazon	T39.2X1-	T39.2X2-	T39.2X3-	T39.2X4-	T39.2X5-	T39.2X6-
Ketobemidone	T40.4X1-	T40.4X2-	T40.4X3-	T40.4X4-	-	-
Ketoconazole	T49.0X1-	T49.0X2-	T49.0X3-	T49.0X4-	T49.0X5-	T49.0X6-
Ketols	T52.4X1-	T52.4X2-	T52.4X3-	T52.4X4-	-	-
Ketone oils	T52.4X1-	T52.4X2-	T52.4X3-	T52.4X4-	-	-
Ketoprofen	T39.311-	T39.312-	T39.313-	T39.314-	T39.315-	T39.316-
Ketorolac	T39.8X1-	T39.8X2-	T39.8X3-	T39.8X4-	T39.8X5-	T39.8X6-
Ketotifen	T45.0X1-	T45.0X2-	T45.0X3-	T45.0X4-	T45.0X5-	T45.0X6-
Khat	T43.691-	T43.692-	T43.693-	T43.694-	-	-
Khellin	T46.3X1-	T46.3X2-	T46.3X3-	T46.3X4-	T46.3X5-	T46.3X6-
Khelloside	T46.3X1-	T46.3X2-	T46.3X3-	T46.3X4-	T46.3X5-	T46.3X6-
Kiln gas or vapor (carbon monoxide)	T58.8X1-	T58.8X2-	T58.8X3-	T58.8X4-		
Kitasamycin	T36.3X1-	T36.3X2-	T36.3X3-	T36.3X4-	T36.3X5-	T36.3X6-
Konsyl	T47.4X1-	T47.4X2-	T47.4X3-	T47.4X4-	T47.4X5-	T47.4X6-
Kosam seed	T62.2X1-	T62.2X2-	T62.2X3-	T62.2X4-	-	-
Krait (venom)	T63.091-	T63.092-	T63.093-	T63.094-	-	-
Kwell (insecticide)	T60.1X1-	T60.1X2-	T60.1X3-	T60.1X4-	-	-
anti-infective (topical)	T49.0X1-	T49.0X2-	T49.0X3-	T49.0X4-	T49.0X5-	T49.0X6-
Labetalol	T44.8X1-	T44.8X2-	T44.8X3-	T44.8X4-	T44.8X5-	T44.8X6-
Laburnum (seeds)	T62.2X1-	T62.2X2-	T62.2X3-	T62.2X4-	-	-
leaves	T62.2X1-	T62.2X2-	T62.2X3-	T62.2X4-	-	-
Lachesine	T49.5X1-	T49.5X2-	T49.5X3-	T49.5X4-	T49.5X5-	T49.5X6-
Lacidipine	T46.5X1-	T46.5X2-	T46.5X3-	T46.5X4-	T46.5X5-	T46.5X6-
Lacquer	T65.6X1-	T65.6X2-	T65.6X3-	T65.6X4-	-	-
Lacrimogenic gas	T59.3X1-	T59.3X2-	T59.3X3-	T59.3X4-	-	-
Lactated potassic saline	T50.3X1-	T50.3X2-	T50.3X3-	T50.3X4-	T50.3X5-	T50.3X6-
Lactic acid	T49.8X1-	T49.8X2-	T49.8X3-	T49.8X4-	T49.8X5-	T49.8X6-
Lactobacillus						
acidophilus	T47.6X1-	T47.6X2-	T47.6X3-	T47.6X4-	T47.6X5-	T47.6X6-
compound	T47.6X1-	T47.6X2-	T47.6X3-	T47.6X4-	T47.6X5-	T47.6X6-
bifidus, lyophilized	T47.6X1-	T47.6X2-	T47.6X3-	T47.6X4-	T47.6X5-	T47.6X6-
bulgaricus	T47.6X1-	T47.6X2-	T47.6X3-	T47.6X4-	T47.6X5-	T47.6X6-
sporogenes	T47.6X1-	T47.6X2-	T47.6X3-	T47.6X4-	T47.6X5-	T47.6X6-
Lactoflavin	T45.2X1-	T45.2X2-	T45.2X3-	T45.2X4-	T45.2X5-	T45.2X6-
Lactose (as excipient)	T50.901-	T50.902-	T50.903-	T50.904-	T50.905-	T50.906-
Lactuca (virosa) (extract)	T42.6X1-	T42.6X2-	T42.6X3-	T42.6X4-	T42.6X5-	T42.6X6-
Lactucarium	T42.6X1-	T42.6X2-	T42.6X3-	T42.6X4-	T42.6X5-	T42.6X6-
Lactulose	T47.3X1-	T47.3X2-	T47.3X3-	T47.3X4-	T47.3X5-	T47.3X6-
Laevo — see Levo-						
Lanatosides	T46.0X1-	T46.0X2-	T46.0X3-	T46.0X4-	T46.0X5-	T46.0X6-
Lanolin	T49.3X1-	T49.3X2-	T49.3X3-	T49.3X4-	T49.3X5-	T49.3X6-
Largactil	T43.3X1-	T43.3X2-	T43.3X3-	T43.3X4-	T43.3X5-	T43.3X6-
Larkspur	T62.2X1-	T62.2X2-	T62.2X3-	T62.2X4-	-	-
Laroxyl	T43.011-	T43.012-	T43.013-	T43.014-	T43.015-	T43.016-
Lasix	T50.1X1-	T50.1X2-	T50.1X3-	T50.1X4-	T50.1X5-	T50.1X6-
Lassar's paste	T49.4X1-	T49.4X2-	T49.4X3-	T49.4X4-	T49.4X5-	T49.4X6-
Latamoxef	T36.1X1-	T36.1X2-	T36.1X3-	T36.1X4-	T36.1X5-	T36.1X6-
Latex	T65.811-	T65.812-	T65.813-	T65.814-	-	-
Lathyrus (seed)	T62.2X1-	T62.2X2-	T62.2X3-	T62.2X4-	-	-
Laudanum	T40.0X1-	T40.0X2-	T40.0X3-	T40.0X4-	T40.0X5-	T40.0X6-
Laudexium	T48.1X1-	T48.1X2-	T48.1X3-	T48.1X4-	T48.1X5-	T48.1X6-
Laughing gas	T41.0X1-	T41.0X2-	T41.0X3-	T41.0X4-	T41.0X5-	T41.0X6-
Laurel, black or cherry	T62.2X1-	T62.2X2-	T62.2X3-	T62.2X4-	-	-
Laurolinium	T49.0X1-	T49.0X2-	T49.0X3-	T49.0X4-	T49.0X5-	T49.0X6-
Lauryl sulfoacetate	T49.2X1-	T49.2X2-	T49.2X3-	T49.2X4-	T49.2X5-	T49.2X6-
Laxative NEC	T47.4X1-	T47.4X2-	T47.4X3-	T47.4X4-	T47.4X5-	T47.4X6-
osmotic	T47.3X1-	T47.3X2-	T47.3X3-	T47.3X4-	T47.3X5-	T47.3X6-
saline	T47.3X1-	T47.3X2-	T47.3X3-	T47.3X4-	T47.3X5-	T47.3X6-
stimulant	T47.2X1-	T47.2X2-	T47.2X3-	T47.2X4-	T47.2X5-	T47.2X6-
L-dopa	T42.8X1-	T42.8X2-	T42.8X3-	T42.8X4-	T42.8X5-	T42.8X6-
Lead (dust) (fumes) (vapor) NEC	T56.0X1-	T56.0X2-	T56.0X3-	T56.0X4-	-	-
acetate	T49.2X1-	T49.2X2-	T49.2X3-	T49.2X4-	T49.2X5-	T49.2X6-
alkyl (fuel additive)	T56.0X1-	T56.0X2-	T56.0X3-	T56.0X4-	-	-
anti-infectives	T37.8X1-	T37.8X2-	T37.8X3-	T37.8X4-	T37.8X5-	T37.8X6-
antiknock compound (tetraethyl)	T56.0X1-	T56.0X2-	T56.0X3-	T56.0X4-	-	-
arsenate, arsenite (dust) (herbicide) (insecticide) (vapor)	T57.0X1-	T57.0X2-	T57.0X3-	T57.0X4-	-	-
carbonate	T56.0X1-	T56.0X2-	T56.0X3-	T56.0X4-	-	-
paint	T56.0X1-	T56.0X2-	T56.0X3-	T56.0X4-	-	-
chromate	T56.0X1-	T56.0X2-	T56.0X3-	T56.0X4-	-	-
paint	T56.0X1-	T56.0X2-	T56.0X3-	T56.0X4-	-	-
dioxide	T56.0X1-	T56.0X2-	T56.0X3-	T56.0X4-	-	-
inorganic	T56.0X1-	T56.0X2-	T56.0X3-	T56.0X4-	-	-

Substance	Poisoning, Accidental (unintentional)	Poisoning, Intentional self-harm	Poisoning, Assault	Poisoning, Undetermined	Adverse effect	Underdosing
Lead NEC - *continued*						
iodide	T56.0X1-	T56.0X2-	T56.0X3-	T56.0X4-	-	-
pigment (paint)	T56.0X1-	T56.0X2-	T56.0X3-	T56.0X4-	-	-
monoxide (dust)	T56.0X1-	T56.0X2-	T56.0X3-	T56.0X4-	-	-
paint	T56.0X1-	T56.0X2-	T56.0X3-	T56.0X4-	-	-
organic	T56.0X1-	T56.0X2-	T56.0X3-	T56.0X4-	-	-
oxide	T56.0X1-	T56.0X2-	T56.0X3-	T56.0X4-	-	-
paint	T56.0X1-	T56.0X2-	T56.0X3-	T56.0X4-	-	-
paint	T56.0X1-	T56.0X2-	T56.0X3-	T56.0X4-	-	-
salts	T56.0X1-	T56.0X2-	T56.0X3-	T56.0X4-	-	-
specified compound NEC	T56.0X1-	T56.0X2-	T56.0X3-	T56.0X4-	-	-
tetra-ethyl	T56.0X1-	T56.0X2-	T56.0X3-	T56.0X4-	-	-
Lebanese red	T40.7X1-	T40.7X2-	T40.7X3-	T40.7X4-	T40.7X5-	T40.7X6-
Lefetamine	T39.8X1-	T39.8X2-	T39.8X3-	T39.8X4-	T39.8X5-	T39.8X6-
Lenperone	T43.4X1-	T43.4X2-	T43.4X3-	T43.4X4-	T43.4X5-	T43.4X6-
Lente lietin (insulin)	T38.3X1-	T38.3X2-	T38.3X3-	T38.3X4-	T38.3X5-	T38.3X6-
Leptazol	T50.7X1-	T50.7X2-	T50.7X3-	T50.7X4-	T50.7X5-	T50.7X6-
Leptophos	T60.0X1-	T60.0X2-	T60.0X3-	T60.0X4-	-	-
Leritine	T40.2X1-	T40.2X2-	T40.2X3-	T40.2X4-	T40.2X5-	T40.2X6-
Letosteine	T48.4X1-	T48.4X2-	T48.4X3-	T48.4X4-	T48.4X5-	T48.4X6-
Letter	T38.1X1-	T38.1X2-	T38.1X3-	T38.1X4-	T38.1X5-	T38.1X6-
Lettuce opium	T42.6X1-	T42.6X2-	T42.6X3-	T42.6X4-	T42.6X5-	T42.6X6-
Leucinocaine	T41.3X1-	T41.3X2-	T41.3X3-	T41.3X4-	T41.3X5-	T41.3X6-
Leucocianidol	T46.991-	T46.992-	T46.993-	T46.994-	T46.995-	T46.996-
Leucovorin (factor)	T45.8X1-	T45.8X2-	T45.8X3-	T45.8X4-	T45.8X5-	T45.8X6-
Leukeran	T45.1X1-	T45.1X2-	T45.1X3-	T45.1X4-	T45.1X5-	T45.1X6-
Leuprolide	T38.891-	T38.892-	T38.893-	T38.894-	T38.895-	T38.896-
Levalbuterol	T48.6X1-	T48.6X2-	T48.6X3-	T48.6X4-	T48.6X5-	T48.6X6-
Levallorphan	T50.7X1-	T50.7X2-	T50.7X3-	T50.7X4-	T50.7X5-	T50.7X6-
Levamisole	T37.4X1-	T37.4X2-	T37.4X3-	T37.4X4-	T37.4X5-	T37.4X6-
Levanil	T42.6X1-	T42.6X2-	T42.6X3-	T42.6X4-	T42.6X5-	T42.6X6-
Levarterenol	T44.4X1-	T44.4X2-	T44.4X3-	T44.4X4-	T44.4X5-	T44.4X6-
Levdropropizine	T48.3X1-	T48.3X2-	T48.3X3-	T48.3X4-	T48.3X5-	T48.3X6-
Levobunolol	T49.5X1-	T49.5X2-	T49.5X3-	T49.5X4-	T49.5X5-	T49.5X6-
Levocabastine (hydrochloride)	T45.0X1-	T45.0X2-	T45.0X3-	T45.0X4-	T45.0X5-	T45.0X6-
Levocarnitine	T50.991-	T50.992-	T50.993-	T50.994-	T50.995-	T50.996-
Levodopa	T42.8X1-	T42.8X2-	T42.8X3-	T42.8X4-	T42.8X5-	T42.8X6-
with carbidopa	T42.8X1-	T42.8X2-	T42.8X3-	T42.8X4-	T42.8X5-	T42.8X6-
Levo-dromoran	T40.2X1-	T40.2X2-	T40.2X3-	T40.2X4-	T40.2X5-	T40.2X6-
Levoglutamide	T50.991-	T50.992-	T50.993-	T50.994-	T50.995-	T50.996-
Levoid	T38.1X1-	T38.1X2-	T38.1X3-	T38.1X4-	T38.1X5-	T38.1X6-
Levo-iso-methadone	T40.3X1-	T40.3X2-	T40.3X3-	T40.3X4-	T40.3X5-	T40.3X6-
Levomepromazine	T43.3X1-	T43.3X2-	T43.3X3-	T43.3X4-	T43.3X5-	T43.3X6-
Levonordefrin	T49.6X1-	T49.6X2-	T49.6X3-	T49.6X4-	T49.6X5-	T49.6X6-
Levonorgestrel	T38.4X1-	T38.4X2-	T38.4X3-	T38.4X4-	T38.4X5-	T38.4X6-
with ethinylestradiol	T38.5X1-	T38.5X2-	T38.5X3-	T38.5X4-	T38.5X5-	T38.5X6-
Levopromazine	T43.3X1-	T43.3X2-	T43.3X3-	T43.3X4-	T43.3X5-	T43.3X6-
Levoprome	T42.6X1-	T42.6X2-	T42.6X3-	T42.6X4-	T42.6X5-	T42.6X6-
Levopropoxyphene	T40.4X1-	T40.4X2-	T40.4X3-	T40.4X4-	T40.4X5-	T40.4X6-
Levopropylhexedrine	T50.5X1-	T50.5X2-	T50.5X3-	T50.5X4-	T50.5X5-	T50.5X6-
Levoproxyphylline	T48.6X1-	T48.6X2-	T48.6X3-	T48.6X4-	T48.6X5-	T48.6X6-
Levorphanol	T40.4X1-	T40.4X2-	T40.4X3-	T40.4X4-	T40.4X5-	T40.4X6-
Levothyroxine	T38.1X1-	T38.1X2-	T38.1X3-	T38.1X4-	T38.1X5-	T38.1X6-
sodium	T38.1X1-	T38.1X2-	T38.1X3-	T38.1X4-	T38.1X5-	T38.1X6-
Levsin	T44.3X1-	T44.3X2-	T44.3X3-	T44.3X4-	T44.3X5-	T44.3X6-
Levulose	T50.3X1-	T50.3X2-	T50.3X3-	T50.3X4-	T50.3X5-	T50.3X6-
Lewisite (gas) , not in war	T57.0X1-	T57.0X2-	T57.0X3-	T57.0X4-	-	-
Librium	T42.4X1-	T42.4X2-	T42.4X3-	T42.4X4-	T42.4X5-	T42.4X6-
Lidex	T49.0X1-	T49.0X2-	T49.0X3-	T49.0X4-	T49.0X5-	T49.0X6-
Lidocaine	T41.3X1-	T41.3X2-	T41.3X3-	T41.3X4-	T41.3X5-	T41.3X6-
regional	T41.3X1-	T41.3X2-	T41.3X3-	T41.3X4-	T41.3X5-	T41.3X6-
spinal	T41.3X1-	T41.3X2-	T41.3X3-	T41.3X4-	T41.3X5-	T41.3X6-
Lidofenin	T50.8X1-	T50.8X2-	T50.8X3-	T50.8X4-	T50.8X5-	T50.8X6-
Lidoflazine	T46.1X1-	T46.1X2-	T46.1X3-	T46.1X4-	T46.1X5-	T46.1X6-
Lighter fluid	T52.0X1-	T52.0X2-	T52.0X3-	T52.0X4-	-	-
Lignin hemicellulose	T47.6X1-	T47.6X2-	T47.6X3-	T47.6X4-	T47.6X5-	T47.6X6-
Lignocaine	T41.3X1-	T41.3X2-	T41.3X3-	T41.3X4-	T41.3X5-	T41.3X6-
regional	T41.3X1-	T41.3X2-	T41.3X3-	T41.3X4-	T41.3X5-	T41.3X6-
spinal	T41.3X1-	T41.3X2-	T41.3X3-	T41.3X4-	T41.3X5-	T41.3X6-
Ligroin (e) (solvent)	T52.0X1-	T52.0X2-	T52.0X3-	T52.0X4-	-	-
vapor	T59.891-	T59.892-	T59.893-	T59.894-	-	-
Ligustrum vulgare	T62.2X1-	T62.2X2-	T62.2X3-	T62.2X4-	-	-
Lily of the valley	T62.2X1-	T62.2X2-	T62.2X3-	T62.2X4-	-	-
Lime (chloride)	T54.3X1-	T54.3X2-	T54.3X3-	T54.3X4-	-	-
Limonene	T52.8X1-	T52.8X2-	T52.8X3-	T52.8X4-	-	-
Lincomycin	T36.8X1-	T36.8X2-	T36.8X3-	T36.8X4-	T36.8X5-	T36.8X6-

Substance	Poisoning, Accidental (unintentional)	Poisoning, Intentional self-harm	Poisoning, Assault	Poisoning, Undetermined	Adverse effect	Underdosing
Lindane (insecticide) (nonmedicinal) (vapor)	T53.6X1-	T53.6X2-	T53.6X3-	T53.6X4-	-	-
medicinal	T49.0X1-	T49.0X2-	T49.0X3-	T49.0X4-	T49.0X5-	T49.0X6-
Liniments NEC	T49.91X-	T49.92X-	T49.93X-	T49.94X-	T49.95X-	T49.96X-
Linoleic acid	T46.6X1-	T46.6X2-	T46.6X3-	T46.6X4-	T46.6X5-	T46.6X6-
Linolenic acid	T46.6X1-	T46.6X2-	T46.6X3-	T46.6X4-	T46.6X5-	T46.6X6-
Linseed	T47.4X1-	T47.4X2-	T47.4X3-	T47.4X4-	T47.4X5-	T47.4X6-
Liothyronine	T38.1X1-	T38.1X2-	T38.1X3-	T38.1X4-	T38.1X5-	T38.1X6-
Liotrix	T38.1X1-	T38.1X2-	T38.1X3-	T38.1X4-	T38.1X5-	T38.1X6-
Lipancreatin	T47.5X1-	T47.5X2-	T47.5X3-	T47.5X4-	T47.5X5-	T47.5X6-
Lipo-alprostadil	T46.7X1-	T46.7X2-	T46.7X3-	T46.7X4-	T46.7X5-	T46.7X6-
Lipo-Lutin	T38.5X1-	T38.5X2-	T38.5X3-	T38.5X4-	T38.5X5-	T38.5X6-
Lipotropic drug NEC	T50.901-	T50.902-	T50.903-	T50.904-	T50.905-	T50.906-
Liquefied petroleum gases	T59.891-	T59.892-	T59.893-	T59.894-	-	-
piped (pure or mixed with air)	T59.891-	T59.892-	T59.893-	T59.894-	-	-
Liquid						
paraffin	T47.4X1-	T47.4X2-	T47.4X3-	T47.4X4-	T47.4X5-	T47.4X6-
petrolatum	T47.4X1-	T47.4X2-	T47.4X3-	T47.4X4-	T47.4X5-	T47.4X6-
topical	T49.3X1-	T49.3X2-	T49.3X3-	T49.3X4-	T49.3X5-	T49.3X6-
specified NEC	T65.891-	T65.892-	T65.893-	T65.894-	-	-
substance	T65.91X-	T65.92X-	T65.93X-	T65.94X-	-	-
Liquor creosolis compositus	T65.891-	T65.892-	T65.893-	T65.894-	-	-
Liquorice	T48.4X1-	T48.4X2-	T48.4X3-	T48.4X4-	T48.4X5-	T48.4X6-
extract	T47.8X1-	T47.8X2-	T47.8X3-	T47.8X4-	T47.8X5-	T47.8X6-
Lisinopril	T46.4X1-	T46.4X2-	T46.4X3-	T46.4X4-	T46.4X5-	T46.4X6-
Lisuride	T42.8X1-	T42.8X2-	T42.8X3-	T42.8X4-	T42.8X5-	T42.8X6-
Lithane	T43.8X1-	T43.8X2-	T43.8X3-	T43.8X4-	T43.8X5-	T43.8X6-
Lithium	T56.891-	T56.892-	T56.893-	T56.894-	-	-
gluconate	T43.591-	T43.592-	T43.593-	T43.594-	T43.595-	T43.596-
salts (carbonate)	T43.591-	T43.592-	T43.593-	T43.594-	T43.595-	T43.596-
Lithonate	T43.8X1-	T43.8X2-	T43.8X3-	T43.8X4-	T43.8X5-	T43.8X6-
Liver						
extract	T45.8X1-	T45.8X2-	T45.8X3-	T45.8X4-	T45.8X5-	T45.8X6-
for parenteral use	T45.8X1-	T45.8X2-	T45.8X3-	T45.8X4-	T45.8X5-	T45.8X6-
fraction 1	T45.8X1-	T45.8X2-	T45.8X3-	T45.8X4-	T45.8X5-	T45.8X6-
hydrolysate	T45.8X1-	T45.8X2-	T45.8X3-	T45.8X4-	T45.8X5-	T45.8X6-
Lizard (bite) (venom)	T63.121-	T63.122-	T63.123-	T63.124-	-	-
LMD	T45.8X1-	T45.8X2-	T45.8X3-	T45.8X4-	T45.8X5-	T45.8X6-
Lobelia	T62.2X1-	T62.2X2-	T62.2X3-	T62.2X4-	-	-
Lobeline	T50.7X1-	T50.7X2-	T50.7X3-	T50.7X4-	T50.7X5-	T50.7X6-
Local action drug NEC	T49.8X1-	T49.8X2-	T49.8X3-	T49.8X4-	T49.8X5-	T49.8X6-
Locorten	T49.0X1-	T49.0X2-	T49.0X3-	T49.0X4-	T49.0X5-	T49.0X6-
Lofepramine	T43.011-	T43.012-	T43.013-	T43.014-	T43.015-	T43.016-
Lolium temulentum	T62.2X1-	T62.2X2-	T62.2X3-	T62.2X4-	-	-
Lomotil	T47.6X1-	T47.6X2-	T47.6X3-	T47.6X4-	T47.6X5-	T47.6X6-
Lomustine	T45.1X1-	T45.1X2-	T45.1X3-	T45.1X4-	T45.1X5-	T45.1X6-
Lonidamine	T45.1X1-	T45.1X2-	T45.1X3-	T45.1X4-	T45.1X5-	T45.1X6-
Loperamide	T47.6X1-	T47.6X2-	T47.6X3-	T47.6X4-	T47.6X5-	T47.6X6-
Loprazolam	T42.4X1-	T42.4X2-	T42.4X3-	T42.4X4-	T42.4X5-	T42.4X6-
Lorajmine	T46.2X1-	T46.2X2-	T46.2X3-	T46.2X4-	T46.2X5-	T46.2X6-
Loratidine	T45.0X1-	T45.0X2-	T45.0X3-	T45.0X4-	T45.0X5-	T45.0X6-
Lorazepam	T42.4X1-	T42.4X2-	T42.4X3-	T42.4X4-	T42.4X5-	T42.4X6-
Lorcainide	T46.2X1-	T46.2X2-	T46.2X3-	T46.2X4-	T46.2X5-	T46.2X6-
Lormetazepam	T42.4X1-	T42.4X2-	T42.4X3-	T42.4X4-	T42.4X5-	T42.4X6-
Lotions NEC	T49.91X-	T49.92X-	T49.93X-	T49.94X-	T49.95X-	T49.96X-
Lotusate	T42.3X1-	T42.3X2-	T42.3X3-	T42.3X4-	T42.3X5-	T42.3X6-
Lovastatin	T46.6X1-	T46.6X2-	T46.6X3-	T46.6X4-	T46.6X5-	T46.6X6-
Lowila	T49.2X1-	T49.2X2-	T49.2X3-	T49.2X4-	T49.2X5-	T49.2X6-
Loxapine	T43.591-	T43.592-	T43.593-	T43.594-	T43.595-	T43.596-
Lozenges (throat)	T49.6X1-	T49.6X2-	T49.6X3-	T49.6X4-	T49.6X5-	T49.6X6-
LSD	T40.8X1-	T40.8X2-	T40.8X3-	T40.8X4-	-	-
L-Tryptophan — see amino acid						
Lubricant, eye	T49.5X1-	T49.5X2-	T49.5X3-	T49.5X4-	T49.5X5-	T49.5X6-
Lubricating oil NEC	T52.0X1-	T52.0X2-	T52.0X3-	T52.0X4-	-	-
Lucanthone	T37.4X1-	T37.4X2-	T37.4X3-	T37.4X4-	T37.4X5-	T37.4X6-
Luminal	T42.3X1-	T42.3X2-	T42.3X3-	T42.3X4-	T42.3X5-	T42.3X6-
Lung irritant (gas) NEC	T59.91X-	T59.92X-	T59.93X-	T59.94X-	-	-
Luteinizing hormone	T38.811-	T38.812-	T38.813-	T38.814-	T38.815-	T38.816-
Lutocylol	T38.5X1-	T38.5X2-	T38.5X3-	T38.5X4-	T38.5X5-	T38.5X6-
Lutromone	T38.5X1-	T38.5X2-	T38.5X3-	T38.5X4-	T38.5X5-	T38.5X6-
Lututrin	T48.291-	T48.292-	T48.293-	T48.294-	T48.295-	T48.296-
Lye (concentrated)	T54.3X1-	T54.3X2-	T54.3X3-	T54.3X4-	-	-
Lygranum (skin test)	T50.8X1-	T50.8X2-	T50.8X3-	T50.8X4-	T50.8X5-	T50.8X6-
Lymecycline	T36.4X1-	T36.4X2-	T36.4X3-	T36.4X4-	T36.4X5-	T36.4X6-
Lymphogranuloma venereum antigen	T50.8X1-	T50.8X2-	T50.8X3-	T50.8X4-	T50.8X5-	T50.8X6-
Lynestrenol	T38.4X1-	T38.4X2-	T38.4X3-	T38.4X4-	T38.4X5-	T38.4X6-

Substance	Poisoning, Accidental (unintentional)	Poisoning, Intentional self-harm	Poisoning, Assault	Poisoning, Undetermined	Adverse effect	Underdosing
Lyovac Sodium Edecrin	T50.1X1-	T50.1X2-	T50.1X3-	T50.1X4-	T50.1X5-	T50.1X6-
Lypressin	T38.891-	T38.892-	T38.893-	T38.894-	T38.895-	T38.896-
Lysergic acid diethylamide	T40.8X1-	T40.8X2-	T40.8X3-	T40.8X4-	-	-
Lysergide	T40.8X1-	T40.8X2-	T40.8X3-	T40.8X4-	-	-
Lysine vasopressin	T38.891-	T38.892-	T38.893-	T38.894-	T38.895-	T38.896-
Lysol	T54.1X1-	T54.1X2-	T54.1X3-	T54.1X4-	-	-
Lysozyme	T49.0X1-	T49.0X2-	T49.0X3-	T49.0X4-	T49.0X5-	T49.0X6-
Lytta (vitatta)	T49.8X1-	T49.8X2-	T49.8X3-	T49.8X4-	T49.8X5-	T49.8X6-
Mace	T59.3X1-	T59.3X2-	T59.3X3-	T59.3X4-	-	-
Macrogol	T50.991-	T50.992-	T50.993-	T50.994-	T50.995-	T50.996-
Macrolide						
anabolic drug	T38.7X1-	T38.7X2-	T38.7X3-	T38.7X4-	T38.7X5-	T38.7X6-
antibiotic	T36.3X1-	T36.3X2-	T36.3X3-	T36.3X4-	T36.3X5-	T36.3X6-
Mafenide	T49.0X1-	T49.0X2-	T49.0X3-	T49.0X4-	T49.0X5-	T49.0X6-
Magaldrate	T47.1X1-	T47.1X2-	T47.1X3-	T47.1X4-	T47.1X5-	T47.1X6-
Magic mushroom	T40.991-	T40.992-	T40.993-	T40.994-	-	-
Magnamycin	T36.8X1-	T36.8X2-	T36.8X3-	T36.8X4-	T36.8X5-	T36.8X6-
Magnesia magma	T47.1X1-	T47.1X2-	T47.1X3-	T47.1X4-	T47.1X5-	T47.1X6-
Magnesium NEC	T56.891-	T56.892-	T56.893-	T56.894-	-	-
carbonate	T47.1X1-	T47.1X2-	T47.1X3-	T47.1X4-	T47.1X5-	T47.1X6-
citrate	T47.4X1-	T47.4X2-	T47.4X3-	T47.4X4-	T47.4X5-	T47.4X6-
hydroxide	T47.1X1-	T47.1X2-	T47.1X3-	T47.1X4-	T47.1X5-	T47.1X6-
oxide	T47.1X1-	T47.1X2-	T47.1X3-	T47.1X4-	T47.1X5-	T47.1X6-
peroxide	T49.0X1-	T49.0X2-	T49.0X3-	T49.0X4-	T49.0X5-	T49.0X6-
salicylate	T39.091-	T39.092-	T39.093-	T39.094-	T39.095-	T39.096-
silicofluoride	T50.3X1-	T50.3X2-	T50.3X3-	T50.3X4-	T50.3X5-	T50.3X6-
sulfate	T47.4X1-	T47.4X2-	T47.4X3-	T47.4X4-	T47.4X5-	T47.4X6-
thiosulfate	T45.0X1-	T45.0X2-	T45.0X3-	T45.0X4-	T45.0X5-	T45.0X6-
trisilicate	T47.1X1-	T47.1X2-	T47.1X3-	T47.1X4-	T47.1X5-	T47.1X6-
Malathion (medicinal)	T49.0X1-	T49.0X2-	T49.0X3-	T49.0X4-	T49.0X5-	T49.0X6-
insecticide	T60.0X1-	T60.0X2-	T60.0X3-	T60.0X4-	-	-
Male fern extract	T37.4X1-	T37.4X2-	T37.4X3-	T37.4X4-	T37.4X5-	T37.4X6-
M-AMSA	T45.1X1-	T45.1X2-	T45.1X3-	T45.1X4-	T45.1X5-	T45.1X6-
Mandelic acid	T37.8X1-	T37.8X2-	T37.8X3-	T37.8X4-	T37.8X5-	T37.8X6-
Manganese (dioxide) (salts)	T57.2X1-	T57.2X2-	T57.2X3-	T57.2X4-	-	-
medicinal	T50.991-	T50.992-	T50.993-	T50.994-	T50.995-	T50.996-
Mannitol	T47.3X1-	T47.3X2-	T47.3X3-	T47.3X4-	T47.3X5-	T47.3X6-
hexanitrate	T46.3X1-	T46.3X2-	T46.3X3-	T46.3X4-	T46.3X5-	T46.3X6-
Mannomustine	T45.1X1-	T45.1X2-	T45.1X3-	T45.1X4-	T45.1X5-	T45.1X6-
MAO inhibitors	T43.1X1-	T43.1X2-	T43.1X3-	T43.1X4-	T43.1X5-	T43.1X6-
Mapharsen	T37.8X1-	T37.8X2-	T37.8X3-	T37.8X4-	T37.8X5-	T37.8X6-
Maphenide	T49.0X1-	T49.0X2-	T49.0X3-	T49.0X4-	T49.0X5-	T49.0X6-
Maprotiline	T43.021-	T43.022-	T43.023-	T43.024-	T43.025-	T43.026-
Marcaine	T41.3X1-	T41.3X2-	T41.3X3-	T41.3X4-	T41.3X5-	T41.3X6-
infiltration (subcutaneous)	T41.3X1-	T41.3X2-	T41.3X3-	T41.3X4-	T41.3X5-	T41.3X6-
nerve block (peripheral) (plexus)	T41.3X1-	T41.3X2-	T41.3X3-	T41.3X4-	T41.3X5-	T41.3X6-
Marezine	T45.0X1-	T45.0X2-	T45.0X3-	T45.0X4-	T45.0X5-	T45.0X6-
Marihuana	T40.7X1-	T40.7X2-	T40.7X3-	T40.7X4-	T40.7X5-	T40.7X6-
Marijuana	T40.7X1-	T40.7X2-	T40.7X3-	T40.7X4-	T40.7X5-	T40.7X6-
Marine (sting)	T63.691-	T63.692-	T63.693-	T63.694-	-	-
animals (sting)	T63.691-	T63.692-	T63.693-	T63.694-	-	-
plants (sting)	T63.711-	T63.712-	T63.713-	T63.714-	-	-
Marplan	T43.1X1-	T43.1X2-	T43.1X3-	T43.1X4-	T43.1X5-	T43.1X6-
Marsh gas	T59.891-	T59.892-	T59.893-	T59.894-	-	-
Marsilid	T43.1X1-	T43.1X2-	T43.1X3-	T43.1X4-	T43.1X5-	T43.1X6-
Matulane	T45.1X1-	T45.1X2-	T45.1X3-	T45.1X4-	T45.1X5-	T45.1X6-
Mazindol	T50.5X1-	T50.5X2-	T50.5X3-	T50.5X4-	T50.5X5-	T50.5X6-
MCPA	T60.3X1-	T60.3X2-	T60.3X3-	T60.3X4-	-	-
MDMA	T43.621-	T43.622-	T43.623-	T43.624-	T43.625-	T43.626-
Meadow saffron	T62.2X1-	T62.2X2-	T62.2X3-	T62.2X4-	-	-
Measles virus vaccine (attenuated)	T50.B91-	T50.B92-	T50.B93-	T50.B94-	T50.B95-	T50.B96-
Meat, noxious	T62.8X1-	T62.8X2-	T62.8X3-	T62.8X4-	-	-
Meballymal	T42.3X1-	T42.3X2-	T42.3X3-	T42.3X4-	T42.3X5-	T42.3X6-
Mebanazine	T43.1X1-	T43.1X2-	T43.1X3-	T43.1X4-	T43.1X5-	T43.1X6-
Mebaral	T42.3X1-	T42.3X2-	T42.3X3-	T42.3X4-	T42.3X5-	T42.3X6-
Mebendazole	T37.4X1-	T37.4X2-	T37.4X3-	T37.4X4-	T37.4X5-	T37.4X6-
Mebeverine	T44.3X1-	T44.3X2-	T44.3X3-	T44.3X4-	T44.3X5-	T44.3X6-
Mebhydrolin	T45.0X1-	T45.0X2-	T45.0X3-	T45.0X4-	T45.0X5-	T45.0X6-
Mebumal	T42.3X1-	T42.3X2-	T42.3X3-	T42.3X4-	T42.3X5-	T42.3X6-
Mebutamate	T43.591-	T43.592-	T43.593-	T43.594-	T43.595-	T43.596-
Mecamylamine	T44.2X1-	T44.2X2-	T44.2X3-	T44.2X4-	T44.2X5-	T44.2X6-
Mechlorethamine	T45.1X1-	T45.1X2-	T45.1X3-	T45.1X4-	T45.1X5-	T45.1X6-
Mecillinam	T36.0X1-	T36.0X2-	T36.0X3-	T36.0X4-	T36.0X5-	T36.0X6-
Meclizine (hydrochloride)	T45.0X1-	T45.0X2-	T45.0X3-	T45.0X4-	T45.0X5-	T45.0X6-
Meclocycline	T36.4X1-	T36.4X2-	T36.4X3-	T36.4X4-	T36.4X5-	T36.4X6-
Meclofenamate	T39.391-	T39.392-	T39.393-	T39.394-	T39.395-	T39.396-

Substance	Poisoning, Accidental (unintentional)	Poisoning, Intentional self-harm	Poisoning, Assault	Poisoning, Undetermined	Adverse effect	Underdosing
Meclofenamic acid	T39.391-	T39.392-	T39.393-	T39.394-	T39.395-	T39.396-
Meclofenoxate	T43.691-	T43.692-	T43.693-	T43.694-	T43.395-	T43.696-
Meclozine	T45.0X1-	T45.0X2-	T45.0X3-	T45.0X4-	T45.0X5-	T45.0X6-
Mecobalamin	T45.8X1-	T45.8X2-	T45.8X3-	T45.8X4-	T45.8X5-	T45.8X6-
Mecoprop	T60.3X1-	T60.3X2-	T60.3X3-	T60.3X4-	-	-
Mecrilate	T49.3X1-	T49.3X2-	T49.3X3-	T49.3X4-	T49.3X5-	T49.3X6-
Mecysteine	T48.4X1-	T48.4X2-	T48.4X3-	T48.4X4-	T48.4X5-	T48.4X6-
Medazepam	T42.4X1-	T42.4X2-	T42.4X3-	T42.4X4-	T42.4X5-	T42.4X6-
Medicament NEC	T50.901-	T50.902-	T50.903-	T50.904-	T50.905-	T50.906-
Medinal	T42.3X1-	T42.3X2-	T42.3X3-	T42.3X4-	T42.3X5-	T42.3X6-
Medomin	T42.3X1-	T42.3X2-	T42.3X3-	T42.3X4-	T42.3X5-	T42.3X6-
Medrogestone	T38.5X1-	T38.5X2-	T38.5X3-	T38.5X4-	T38.5X5-	T38.5X6-
Medroxalol	T44.8X1-	T44.8X2-	T44.8X3-	T44.8X4-	T44.8X5-	T44.8X6-
Medroxyprogesterone acetate (depot)	T38.5X1-	T38.5X2-	T38.5X3-	T38.5X4-	T38.5X5-	T38.5X6-
Medrysone	T49.0X1-	T49.0X2-	T49.0X3-	T49.0X4-	T49.0X5-	T49.0X6-
Mefenamic acid	T39.391-	T39.392-	T39.393-	T39.394-	T39.395-	T39.396-
Mefenorex	T50.5X1-	T50.5X2-	T50.5X3-	T50.5X4-	T50.5X5-	T50.5X6-
Mefloquine	T37.2X1-	T37.2X2-	T37.2X3-	T37.2X4-	T37.2X5-	T37.2X6-
Mefruside	T50.2X1-	T50.2X2-	T50.2X3-	T50.2X4-	T50.2X5-	T50.2X6-
Megahallucinogen	T40.901-	T40.902-	T40.903-	T40.904-	T40.905-	T40.906-
Megestrol	T38.5X1-	T38.5X2-	T38.5X3-	T38.5X4-	T38.5X5-	T38.5X6-
Meglumine						
antimoniate	T37.8X1-	T37.8X2-	T37.8X3-	T37.8X4-	T37.8X5-	T37.8X6-
diatrizoate	T50.8X1-	T50.8X2-	T50.8X3-	T50.8X4-	T50.8X5-	T50.8X6-
iodipamide	T50.8X1-	T50.8X2-	T50.8X3-	T50.8X4-	T50.8X5-	T50.8X6-
iotroxate	T50.8X1-	T50.8X2-	T50.8X3-	T50.8X4-	T50.8X5-	T50.8X6-
MEK (methyl ethyl ketone)	T52.4X1-	T52.4X2-	T52.4X3-	T52.4X4-	-	-
Meladinin	T49.3X1-	T49.3X2-	T49.3X3-	T49.3X4-	T49.3X5-	T49.3X6-
Meladrazine	T44.3X1-	T44.3X2-	T44.3X3-	T44.3X4-	T44.3X5-	T44.3X6-
Melaleuca alternifolia oil	T49.0X1-	T49.0X2-	T49.0X3-	T49.0X4-	T49.0X5-	T49.0X6-
Melanizing agents	T49.3X1-	T49.3X2-	T49.3X3-	T49.3X4-	T49.3X5-	T49.3X6-
Melanocyte-stimulating hormone	T38.891-	T38.892-	T38.893-	T38.894-	T38.895-	T38.896-
Melarsonyl potassium	T37.3X1-	T37.3X2-	T37.3X3-	T37.3X4-	T37.3X5-	T37.3X6-
Melarsoprol	T37.3X1-	T37.3X2-	T37.3X3-	T37.3X4-	T37.3X5-	T37.3X6-
Melia azedarach	T62.2X1-	T62.2X2-	T62.2X3-	T62.2X4-	-	-
Melitracen	T43.011-	T43.012-	T43.013-	T43.014-	T43.015-	T43.016-
Mellaril	T43.3X1-	T43.3X2-	T43.3X3-	T43.3X4-	T43.3X5-	T43.3X6-
Meloxine	T49.3X1-	T49.3X2-	T49.3X3-	T49.3X4-	T49.3X5-	T49.3X6-
Melperone	T43.4X1-	T43.4X2-	T43.4X3-	T43.4X4-	T43.4X5-	T43.4X6-
Melphalan	T45.1X1-	T45.1X2-	T45.1X3-	T45.1X4-	T45.1X5-	T45.1X6-
Memantine	T43.8X1-	T43.8X2-	T43.8X3-	T43.8X4-	T43.8X5-	T43.8X6-
Menadiol	T45.7X1-	T45.7X2-	T45.7X3-	T45.7X4-	T45.7X5-	T45.7X6-
sodium sulfate	T45.7X1-	T45.7X2-	T45.7X3-	T45.7X4-	T45.7X5-	T45.7X6-
Menadione	T45.7X1-	T45.7X2-	T45.7X3-	T45.7X4-	T45.7X5-	T45.7X6-
sodium bisulfite	T45.7X1-	T45.7X2-	T45.7X3-	T45.7X4-	T45.7X5-	T45.7X6-
Menaphthone	T45.7X1-	T45.7X2-	T45.7X3-	T45.7X4-	T45.7X5-	T45.7X6-
Menaquinone	T45.7X1-	T45.7X2-	T45.7X3-	T45.7X4-	T45.7X5-	T45.7X6-
Menatetrenone	T45.7X1-	T45.7X2-	T45.7X3-	T45.7X4-	T45.7X5-	T45.7X6-
Meningococcal vaccine	T50.A91-	T50.A92-	T50.A93-	T50.A94-	T50.A95-	T50.A96-
Menningovax (-AC) (-C)	T50.A91-	T50.A92-	T50.A93-	T50.A94-	T50.A95-	T50.A96-
Menotropins	T38.811-	T38.812-	T38.813-	T38.814-	T38.815-	T38.816-
Menthol	T48.5X1-	T48.5X2-	T48.5X3-	T48.5X4-	T48.5X5-	T48.5X6-
Mepacrine	T37.2X1-	T37.2X2-	T37.2X3-	T37.2X4-	T37.2X5-	T37.2X6-
Meparfynol	T42.6X1-	T42.6X2-	T42.6X3-	T42.6X4-	T42.6X5-	T42.6X6-
Mepartricin	T36.7X1-	T36.7X2-	T36.7X3-	T36.7X4-	T36.7X5-	T36.7X6-
Mepazine	T43.3X1-	T43.3X2-	T43.3X3-	T43.3X4-	T43.3X5-	T43.3X6-
Mepenzolate	T44.3X1-	T44.3X2-	T44.3X3-	T44.3X4-	T44.3X5-	T44.3X6-
bromide	T44.3X1-	T44.3X2-	T44.3X3-	T44.3X4-	T44.3X5-	T44.3X6-
Meperidine	T40.4X1-	T40.4X2-	T40.4X3-	T40.4X4-	T40.4X5-	T40.4X6-
Mephebarbital	T42.3X1-	T42.3X2-	T42.3X3-	T42.3X4-	T42.3X5-	T42.3X6-
Mephenamin (e)	T42.8X1-	T42.8X2-	T42.8X3-	T42.8X4-	T42.8X5-	T42.8X6-
Mephenesin	T42.8X1-	T42.8X2-	T42.8X3-	T42.8X4-	T42.8X5-	T42.8X6-
Mephenhydramine	T45.0X1-	T45.0X2-	T45.0X3-	T45.0X4-	T45.0X5-	T45.0X6-
Mephenoxalone	T42.8X1-	T42.8X2-	T42.8X3-	T42.8X4-	T42.8X5-	T42.8X6-
Mephentermine	T44.991-	T44.992-	T44.993-	T44.994-	T44.995-	T44.996-
Mephenytoin	T42.0X1-	T42.0X2-	T42.0X3-	T42.0X4-	T42.0X5-	T42.0X6-
with phenobarbital	T42.3X1-	T42.3X2-	T42.3X3-	T42.3X4-	T42.3X5-	T42.3X6-
Mephobarbital	T42.3X1-	T42.3X2-	T42.3X3-	T42.3X4-	T42.3X5-	T42.3X6-
Mephosfolan	T60.0X1-	T60.0X2-	T60.0X3-	T60.0X4-	-	-
Mepindolol	T44.7X1-	T44.7X2-	T44.7X3-	T44.7X4-	T44.7X5-	T44.7X6-
Mepiperphenidol	T44.3X1-	T44.3X2-	T44.3X3-	T44.3X4-	T44.3X5-	T44.3X6-
Mepitiostane	T38.7X1-	T38.7X2-	T38.7X3-	T38.7X4-	T38.7X5-	T38.7X6-
Mepivacaine	T41.3X1-	T41.3X2-	T41.3X3-	T41.3X4-	T41.3X5-	T41.3X6-
epidural	T41.3X1-	T41.3X2-	T41.3X3-	T41.3X4-	T41.3X5-	T41.3X6-
Meprednisone	T38.0X1-	T38.0X2-	T38.0X3-	T38.0X4-	T38.0X5-	T38.0X6-
Meprobam	T43.591-	T43.592-	T43.593-	T43.594-	T43.595-	T43.596-

Substance	Poisoning, Accidental (unintentional)	Poisoning, Intentional self-harm	Poisoning, Assault	Poisoning, Undetermined	Adverse effect	Underdosing
Meprobamate	T43.591-	T43.592-	T43.593-	T43.594-	T43.595-	T43.596-
Meproscillarin	T46.0X1-	T46.0X2-	T46.0X3-	T46.0X4-	T46.0X5-	T46.0X6-
Meprylcaine	T41.3X1-	T41.3X2-	T41.3X3-	T41.3X4-	T41.3X5-	T41.3X6-
Meptazinol	T39.8X1-	T39.8X2-	T39.8X3-	T39.8X4-	T39.8X5-	T39.8X6-
Mepyramine	T45.0X1-	T45.0X2-	T45.0X3-	T45.0X4-	T45.0X5-	T45.0X6-
Mequitazine	T43.3X1-	T43.3X2-	T43.3X3-	T43.3X4-	T43.3X5-	T43.3X6-
Meralluride	T50.2X1-	T50.2X2-	T50.2X3-	T50.2X4-	T50.2X5-	T50.2X6-
Merbaphen	T50.2X1-	T50.2X2-	T50.2X3-	T50.2X4-	T50.2X5-	T50.2X6-
Merbromin	T49.0X1-	T49.0X2-	T49.0X3-	T49.0X4-	T49.0X5-	T49.0X6-
Mercaptobenzothiazole salts	T49.0X1-	T49.0X2-	T49.0X3-	T49.0X4-	T49.0X5-	T49.0X6-
Mercaptomerin	T50.2X1-	T50.2X2-	T50.2X3-	T50.2X4-	T50.2X5-	T50.2X6-
Mercaptopurine	T45.1X1-	T45.1X2-	T45.1X3-	T45.1X4-	T45.1X5-	T45.1X6-
Mercumatilin	T50.2X1-	T50.2X2-	T50.2X3-	T50.2X4-	T50.2X5-	T50.2X6-
Mercuramide	T50.2X1-	T50.2X2-	T50.2X3-	T50.2X4-	T50.2X5-	T50.2X6-
Mercurochrome	T49.0X1-	T49.0X2-	T49.0X3-	T49.0X4-	T49.0X5-	T49.0X6-
Mercurophylline	T50.2X1-	T50.2X2-	T50.2X3-	T50.2X4-	T50.2X5-	T50.2X6-
Mercury, mercurial, mercuric, mercurous (compounds) (cyanide) (fumes) (nonmedicinal) (vapor) NEC	T56.1X1-	T56.1X2-	T56.1X3-	T56.1X4-		
ammoniated	T49.0X1-	T49.0X2-	T49.0X3-	T49.0X4-	T49.0X5-	T49.0X6-
anti-infective						
local	T49.0X1-	T49.0X2-	T49.0X3-	T49.0X4-	T49.0X5-	T49.0X6-
systemic	T37.8X1-	T37.8X2-	T37.8X3-	T37.8X4-	T37.8X5-	T37.8X6-
topical	T49.0X1-	T49.0X2-	T49.0X3-	T49.0X4-	T49.0X5-	T49.0X6-
chloride (ammoniated)	T49.0X1-	T49.0X2-	T49.0X3-	T49.0X4-	T49.0X5-	T49.0X6-
fungicide	T56.1X1-	T56.1X2-	T56.1X3-	T56.1X4-	-	-
diuretic NEC	T50.2X1-	T50.2X2-	T50.2X3-	T50.2X4-	T50.2X5-	T50.2X6-
fungicide	T56.1X1-	T56.1X2-	T56.1X3-	T56.1X4-	-	-
organic (fungicide)	T56.1X1-	T56.1X2-	T56.1X3-	T56.1X4-	-	-
oxide, yellow	T49.0X1-	T49.0X2-	T49.0X3-	T49.0X4-	T49.0X5-	T49.0X6-
Mersalyl	T50.2X1-	T50.2X2-	T50.2X3-	T50.2X4-	T50.2X5-	T50.2X6-
Merthiolate	T49.0X1-	T49.0X2-	T49.0X3-	T49.0X4-	T49.0X5-	T49.0X6-
ophthalmic preparation	T49.5X1-	T49.5X2-	T49.5X3-	T49.5X4-	T49.5X5-	T49.5X6-
Meruvax	T50.B91-	T50.B92-	T50.B93-	T50.B94-	T50.B95-	T50.B96-
Mesalazine	T47.8X1-	T47.8X2-	T47.8X3-	T47.8X4-	T47.8X5-	T47.8X6-
Mescal buttons	T40.991-	T40.992-	T40.993-	T40.994-	-	-
Mescaline	T40.991-	T40.992-	T40.993-	T40.994-	-	-
Mesna	T48.4X1-	T48.4X2-	T48.4X3-	T48.4X4-	T48.4X5-	T48.4X6-
Mesoglycan	T46.6X1-	T46.6X2-	T46.6X3-	T46.6X4-	T46.6X5-	T46.6X6-
Mesoridazine	T43.3X1-	T43.3X2-	T43.3X3-	T43.3X4-	T43.3X5-	T43.3X6-
Mestanolone	T38.7X1-	T38.7X2-	T38.7X3-	T38.7X4-	T38.7X5-	T38.7X6-
Mesterolone	T38.7X1-	T38.7X2-	T38.7X3-	T38.7X4-	T38.7X5-	T38.7X6-
Mestranol	T38.5X1-	T38.5X2-	T38.5X3-	T38.5X4-	T38.5X5-	T38.5X6-
Mesulergine	T42.8X1-	T42.8X2-	T42.8X3-	T42.8X4-	T42.8X5-	T42.8X6-
Mesulfen	T49.0X1-	T49.0X2-	T49.0X3-	T49.0X4-	T49.0X5-	T49.0X6-
Mesuximide	T42.2X1-	T42.2X2-	T42.2X3-	T42.2X4-	T42.2X5-	T42.2X6-
Metabutethamine	T41.3X1-	T41.3X2-	T41.3X3-	T41.3X4-	T41.3X5-	T41.3X6-
Metactesylacetate	T49.0X1-	T49.0X2-	T49.0X3-	T49.0X4-	T49.0X5-	T49.0X6-
Metacycline	T36.4X1-	T36.4X2-	T36.4X3-	T36.4X4-	T36.4X5-	T36.4X6-
Metaldehyde (snail killer) NEC	T60.8X1-	T60.8X2-	T60.8X3-	T60.8X4-	-	-
Metals (heavy) (nonmedicinal)	T56.91X-	T56.92X-	T56.93X-	T56.94X-	-	-
dust, fumes, or vapor NEC	T56.91X-	T56.92X-	T56.93X-	T56.94X-	-	-
light NEC	T56.91X-	T56.92X-	T56.93X-	T56.94X-	-	-
dust, fumes, or vapor NEC	T56.91X-	T56.92X-	T56.93X-	T56.94X-	-	-
specified NEC	T56.891-	T56.892-	T56.893-	T56.894-	-	-
thallium	T56.811-	T56.812-	T56.813-	T56.814-	-	-
Metamfetamine	T43.621-	T43.622-	T43.623-	T43.624-	T43.625-	T43.626-
Metamizole sodium	T39.2X1-	T39.2X2-	T39.2X3-	T39.2X4-	T39.2X5-	T39.2X6-
Metampicillin	T36.0X1-	T36.0X2-	T36.0X3-	T36.0X4-	T36.0X5-	T36.0X6-
Metamucil	T47.4X1-	T47.4X2-	T47.4X3-	T47.4X4-	T47.4X5-	T47.4X6-
Metandienone	T38.7X1-	T38.7X2-	T38.7X3-	T38.7X4-	T38.7X5-	T38.7X6-
Metandrostenolone	T38.7X1-	T38.7X2-	T38.7X3-	T38.7X4-	T38.7X5-	T38.7X6-
Metaphen	T49.0X1-	T49.0X2-	T49.0X3-	T49.0X4-	T49.0X5-	T49.0X6-
Metaphos	T60.0X1-	T60.0X2-	T60.0X3-	T60.0X4-	-	-
Metapramine	T43.011-	T43.012-	T43.013-	T43.014-	T43.015-	T43.016-
Metaproterenol	T48.291-	T48.292-	T48.293-	T48.294-	T48.295-	T48.296-
Metaraminol	T44.4X1-	T44.4X2-	T44.4X3-	T44.4X4-	T44.4X5-	T44.4X6-
Metaxalone	T42.8X1-	T42.8X2-	T42.8X3-	T42.8X4-	T42.8X5-	T42.8X6-
Metenolone	T38.7X1-	T38.7X2-	T38.7X3-	T38.7X4-	T38.7X5-	T38.7X6-
Metergoline	T42.8X1-	T42.8X2-	T42.8X3-	T42.8X4-	T42.8X5-	T42.8X6-
Metescufylline	T46.991-	T46.992-	T46.993-	T46.994-	T46.995-	T46.996-
Metetoin	T42.0X1-	T42.0X2-	T42.0X3-	T42.0X4-	T42.0X5-	T42.0X6-
Metformin	T38.3X1-	T38.3X2-	T38.3X3-	T38.3X4-	T38.3X5-	T38.3X6-
Methacholine	T44.1X1-	T44.1X2-	T44.1X3-	T44.1X4-	T44.1X5-	T44.1X6-
Methacycline	T36.4X1-	T36.4X2-	T36.4X3-	T36.4X4-	T36.4X5-	T36.4X6-
Methadone	T40.3X1-	T40.3X2-	T40.3X3-	T40.3X4-	T40.3X5-	T40.3X6-
Methallenestril	T38.5X1-	T38.5X2-	T38.5X3-	T38.5X4-	T38.5X5-	T38.5X6-

Substance	Poisoning, Accidental (unintentional)	Poisoning, Intentional self-harm	Poisoning, Assault	Poisoning, Undetermined	Adverse effect	Underdosing
Methallenoestril	T38.5X1-	T38.5X2-	T38.5X3-	T38.5X4-	T38.5X5-	T38.5X6-
Methamphetamine	T43.621-	T43.622-	T43.623-	T43.624-	T43.625-	T43.626-
Methampyrone	T39.2X1-	T39.2X2-	T39.2X3-	T39.2X4-	T39.2X5-	T39.2X6-
Methandienone	T38.7X1-	T38.7X2-	T38.7X3-	T38.7X4-	T38.7X5-	T38.7X6-
Methandriol	T38.7X1-	T38.7X2-	T38.7X3-	T38.7X4-	T38.7X5-	T38.7X6-
Methandrostenolone	T38.7X1-	T38.7X2-	T38.7X3-	T38.7X4-	T38.7X5-	T38.7X6-
Methane	T59.891-	T59.892-	T59.893-	T59.894-	-	-
Methanethiol	T59.891-	T59.892-	T59.893-	T59.894-	-	-
Methaniazide	T37.1X1-	T37.1X2-	T37.1X3-	T37.1X4-	T37.1X5-	T37.1X6-
Methanol (vapor)	T51.1X1-	T51.1X2-	T51.1X3-	T51.1X4-	-	-
Methantheline	T44.3X1-	T44.3X2-	T44.3X3-	T44.3X4-	T44.3X5-	T44.3X6-
Methanthelinium bromide	T44.3X1-	T44.3X2-	T44.3X3-	T44.3X4-	T44.3X5-	T44.3X6-
Methaphenilene	T45.0X1-	T45.0X2-	T45.0X3-	T45.0X4-	T45.0X5-	T45.0X6-
Methapyrilene	T45.0X1-	T45.0X2-	T45.0X3-	T45.0X4-	T45.0X5-	T45.0X6-
Methaqualone (compound)	T42.6X1-	T42.6X2-	T42.6X3-	T42.6X4-	T42.6X5-	T42.6X6-
Metharbital	T42.3X1-	T42.3X2-	T42.3X3-	T42.3X4-	T42.3X5-	T42.3X6-
Methazolamide	T50.2X1-	T50.2X2-	T50.2X3-	T50.2X4-	T50.2X5-	T50.2X6-
Methdilazine	T43.3X1-	T43.3X2-	T43.3X3-	T43.3X4-	T43.3X5-	T43.3X6-
Methedrine	T43.621-	T43.622-	T43.623-	T43.624-	T43.625-	T43.626-
Methenamine (mandelate)	T37.8X1-	T37.8X2-	T37.8X3-	T37.8X4-	T37.8X5-	T37.8X6-
Methenolone	T38.7X1-	T38.7X2-	T38.7X3-	T38.7X4-	T38.7X5-	T38.7X6-
Methergine	T48.0X1-	T48.0X2-	T48.0X3-	T48.0X4-	T48.0X5-	T48.0X6-
Methetoin	T42.0X1-	T42.0X2-	T42.0X3-	T42.0X4-	T42.0X5-	T42.0X6-
Methiacil	T38.2X1-	T38.2X2-	T38.2X3-	T38.2X4-	T38.2X5-	T38.2X6-
Methicillin	T36.0X1-	T36.0X2-	T36.0X3-	T36.0X4-	T36.0X5-	T36.0X6-
Methimazole	T38.2X1-	T38.2X2-	T38.2X3-	T38.2X4-	T38.2X5-	T38.2X6-
Methiodal sodium	T50.8X1-	T50.8X2-	T50.8X3-	T50.8X4-	T50.8X5-	T50.8X6-
Methionine	T50.991-	T50.992-	T50.993-	T50.994-	T50.995-	T50.996-
Methisazone	T37.5X1-	T37.5X2-	T37.5X3-	T37.5X4-	T37.5X5-	T37.5X6-
Methisoprinol	T37.5X1-	T37.5X2-	T37.5X3-	T37.5X4-	T37.5X5-	T37.5X6-
Methitural	T42.3X1-	T42.3X2-	T42.3X3-	T42.3X4-	T42.3X5-	T42.3X6-
Methixene	T44.3X1-	T44.3X2-	T44.3X3-	T44.3X4-	T44.3X5-	T44.3X6-
Methobarbital, methobarbitone	T42.3X1-	T42.3X2-	T42.3X3-	T42.3X4-	T42.3X5-	T42.3X6-
Methocarbamol	T42.8X1-	T42.8X2-	T42.8X3-	T42.8X4-	T42.8X5-	T42.8X6-
skeletal muscle relaxant	T48.1X1-	T48.1X2-	T48.1X3-	T48.1X4-	T48.1X5-	T48.1X6-
Methohexital	T41.1X1-	T41.1X2-	T41.1X3-	T41.1X4-	T41.1X5-	T41.1X6-
Methohexitone	T41.1X1-	T41.1X2-	T41.1X3-	T41.1X4-	T41.1X5-	T41.1X6-
Methoin	T42.0X1-	T42.0X2-	T42.0X3-	T42.0X4-	T42.0X5-	T42.0X6-
Methopholine	T39.8X1-	T39.8X2-	T39.8X3-	T39.8X4-	T39.8X5-	T39.8X6-
Methopromazine	T43.3X1-	T43.3X2-	T43.3X3-	T43.3X4-	T43.3X5-	T43.3X6-
Methorate	T48.3X1-	T48.3X2-	T48.3X3-	T48.3X4-	T48.3X5-	T48.3X6-
Methoserpidine	T46.5X1-	T46.5X2-	T46.5X3-	T46.5X4-	T46.5X5-	T46.5X6-
Methotrexate	T45.1X1-	T45.1X2-	T45.1X3-	T45.1X4-	T45.1X5-	T45.1X6-
Methotrimeprazine	T43.3X1-	T43.3X2-	T43.3X3-	T43.3X4-	T43.3X5-	T43.3X6-
Methoxa-Dome	T49.3X1-	T49.3X2-	T49.3X3-	T49.3X4-	T49.3X5-	T49.3X6-
Methoxamine	T44.4X1-	T44.4X2-	T44.4X3-	T44.4X4-	T44.4X5-	T44.4X6-
Methoxsalen	T50.991-	T50.992-	T50.993-	T50.994-	T50.995-	T50.996-
Methoxyaniline	T65.3X1-	T65.3X2-	T65.3X3-	T65.3X4-	-	-
Methoxybenzyl penicillin	T36.0X1-	T36.0X2-	T36.0X3-	T36.0X4-	T36.0X5-	T36.0X6-
Methoxychlor	T53.7X1-	T53.7X2-	T53.7X3-	T53.7X4-	-	-
Methoxy-DDT	T53.7X1-	T53.7X2-	T53.7X3-	T53.7X4-	-	-
2-Methoxyethanol	T52.3X1-	T52.3X2-	T52.3X3-	T52.3X4-	-	-
Methoxyflurane	T41.0X1-	T41.0X2-	T41.0X3-	T41.0X4-	T41.0X5-	T41.0X6-
Methoxyphenamine	T48.6X1-	T48.6X2-	T48.6X3-	T48.6X4-	T48.6X5-	T48.6X6-
Methoxypromazine	T43.3X1-	T43.3X2-	T43.3X3-	T43.3X4-	T43.3X5-	T43.3X6-
5-Methoxypsoralen (5-MOP)	T50.991-	T50.992-	T50.993-	T50.994-	T50.995-	T50.996-
8-Methoxypsoralen (8-MOP)	T50.991-	T50.992-	T50.993-	T50.994-	T50.995-	T50.996-
Methscopolamine bromide	T44.3X1-	T44.3X2-	T44.3X3-	T44.3X4-	T44.3X5-	T44.3X6-
Methsuximide	T42.2X1-	T42.2X2-	T42.2X3-	T42.2X4-	T42.2X5-	T42.2X6-
Methyclothiazide	T50.2X1-	T50.2X2-	T50.2X3-	T50.2X4-	T50.2X5-	T50.2X6-
Methyl						
acetate	T52.4X1-	T52.4X2-	T52.4X3-	T52.4X4-	-	-
acetone	T52.4X1-	T52.4X2-	T52.4X3-	T52.4X4-	-	-
acrylate	T65.891-	T65.892-	T65.893-	T65.894-	-	-
alcohol	T51.1X1-	T51.1X2-	T51.1X3-	T51.1X4-	-	-
aminophenol	T65.3X1-	T65.3X2-	T65.3X3-	T65.3X4-	-	-
amphetamine	T43.621-	T43.622-	T43.623-	T43.624-	T43.625-	T43.626-
androstanolone	T38.7X1-	T38.7X2-	T38.7X3-	T38.7X4-	T38.7X5-	T38.7X6-
atropine	T44.3X1-	T44.3X2-	T44.3X3-	T44.3X4-	T44.3X5-	T44.3X6-
benzene	T52.2X1-	T52.2X2-	T52.2X3-	T52.2X4-	-	-
benzoate	T52.8X1-	T52.8X2-	T52.8X3-	T52.8X4-	-	-
benzol	T52.2X1-	T52.2X2-	T52.2X3-	T52.2X4-	-	-
bromide (gas)	T59.891-	T59.892-	T59.893-	T59.894-	-	-
fumigant	T60.8X1-	T60.8X2-	T60.8X3-	T60.8X4-	-	-
butanol	T51.3X1-	T51.3X2-	T51.3X3-	T51.3X4-	-	-
carbinol	T51.1X1-	T51.1X2-	T51.1X3-	T51.1X4-	-	-
carbonate	T52.8X1-	T52.8X2-	T52.8X3-	T52.8X4-	-	-

Substance	Poisoning, Accidental (unintentional)	Poisoning, Intentional self-harm	Poisoning, Assault	Poisoning, Undetermined	Adverse effect	Underdosing
Methyl - continued						
CCNU	T45.1X1-	T45.1X2-	T45.1X3-	T45.1X4-	T45.1X5-	T45.1X6-
cellosolve	T52.91X-	T52.92X-	T52.93X-	T52.94X-	-	-
cellulose	T47.4X1-	T47.4X2-	T47.4X3-	T47.4X4-	T47.4X5-	T47.4X6-
chloride (gas)	T59.891-	T59.892-	T59.893-	T59.894-	-	-
chloroformate	T59.3X1-	T59.3X2-	T59.3X3-	T59.3X4-	-	-
cyclohexane	T52.8X1-	T52.8X2-	T52.8X3-	T52.8X4-	-	-
cyclohexanol	T51.8X1-	T51.8X2-	T51.8X3-	T51.8X4-	-	-
cyclohexanone	T52.8X1-	T52.8X2-	T52.8X3-	T52.8X4-	-	-
cyclohexyl acetate	T52.8X1-	T52.8X2-	T52.8X3-	T52.8X4-	-	-
demeton	T60.0X1-	T60.0X2-	T60.0X3-	T60.0X4-	-	-
dihydromorphinone	T40.2X1-	T40.2X2-	T40.2X3-	T40.2X4-	T40.2X5-	T40.2X6-
ergometrine	T48.0X1-	T48.0X2-	T48.0X3-	T48.0X4-	T48.0X5-	T48.0X6-
ergonovine	T48.0X1-	T48.0X2-	T48.0X3-	T48.0X4-	T48.0X5-	T48.0X6-
ethyl ketone	T52.4X1-	T52.4X2-	T52.4X3-	T52.4X4-	-	-
glucamine antimonate	T37.8X1-	T37.8X2-	T37.8X3-	T37.8X4-	T37.8X5-	T37.8X6-
hydrazine	T65.891-	T65.892-	T65.893-	T65.894-	-	-
iodide	T65.891-	T65.892-	T65.893-	T65.894-	-	-
isobutyl ketone	T52.4X1-	T52.4X2-	T52.4X3-	T52.4X4-	-	-
isothiocyanate	T60.3X1-	T60.3X2-	T60.3X3-	T60.3X4-	-	-
mercaptan	T59.891-	T59.892-	T59.893-	T59.894-	-	-
morphine NEC	T40.2X1-	T40.2X2-	T40.2X3-	T40.2X4-	T40.2X5-	T40.2X6-
nicotinate	T49.4X1-	T49.4X2-	T49.4X3-	T49.4X4-	T49.4X5-	T49.4X6-
paraben	T49.0X1-	T49.0X2-	T49.0X3-	T49.0X4-	T49.0X5-	T49.0X6-
parafynol	T42.6X1-	T42.6X2-	T42.6X3-	T42.6X4-	T42.6X5-	T42.6X6-
parathion	T60.0X1-	T60.0X2-	T60.0X3-	T60.0X4-	-	-
peridol	T43.4X1-	T43.4X2-	T43.4X3-	T43.4X4-	T43.4X5-	T43.4X6-
phenidate	T43.631-	T43.632-	T43.633-	T43.634-	T43.635-	T43.636-
prednisolone	T38.0X1-	T38.0X2-	T38.0X3-	T38.0X4-	T38.0X5-	T38.0X6-
ENT agent	T49.6X1-	T49.6X2-	T49.6X3-	T49.6X4-	T49.6X5-	T49.6X6-
ophthalmic preparation	T49.5X1-	T49.5X2-	T49.5X3-	T49.5X4-	T49.5X5-	T49.5X6-
topical NEC	T49.0X1-	T49.0X2-	T49.0X3-	T49.0X4-	T49.0X5-	T49.0X6-
propylcarbinol	T51.3X1-	T51.3X2-	T51.3X3-	T51.3X4-	-	-
rosaniline NEC	T49.0X1-	T49.0X2-	T49.0X3-	T49.0X4-	T49.0X5-	T49.0X6-
salicylate	T49.2X1-	T49.2X2-	T49.2X3-	T49.2X4-	T49.2X5-	T49.2X6-
sulfate (fumes)	T59.891-	T59.892-	T59.893-	T59.894-	-	-
liquid	T52.8X1-	T52.8X2-	T52.8X3-	T52.8X4-	-	-
sulfonal	T42.6X1-	T42.6X2-	T42.6X3-	T42.6X4-	T42.6X5-	T42.6X6-
testosterone	T38.7X1-	T38.7X2-	T38.7X3-	T38.7X4-	T38.7X5-	T38.7X6-
thiouracil	T38.2X1-	T38.2X2-	T38.2X3-	T38.2X4-	T38.2X5-	T38.2X6-
Methylamphetamine	T43.621-	T43.622-	T43.623-	T43.624-	T43.625-	T43.626-
Methylated spirit	T51.1X1-	T51.1X2-	T51.1X3-	T51.1X4-	-	-
Methylatropine nitrate	T44.3X1-	T44.3X2-	T44.3X3-	T44.3X4-	T44.3X5-	T44.3X6-
Methylbenactyzium bromide	T44.3X1-	T44.3X2-	T44.3X3-	T44.3X4-	T44.3X5-	T44.3X6-
Methylbenzethonium chloride	T49.0X1-	T49.0X2-	T49.0X3-	T49.0X4-	T49.0X5-	T49.0X6-
Methylcellulose	T47.4X1-	T47.4X2-	T47.4X3-	T47.4X4-	T47.4X5-	T47.4X6-
laxative	T47.4X1-	T47.4X2-	T47.4X3-	T47.4X4-	T47.4X5-	T47.4X6-
Methylchlorophenoxy-acetic acid	T60.3X1-	T60.3X2-	T60.3X3-	T60.3X4-	-	-
Methyldopa	T46.5X1-	T46.5X2-	T46.5X3-	T46.5X4-	T46.5X5-	T46.5X6-
Methyldopate	T46.5X1-	T46.5X2-	T46.5X3-	T46.5X4-	T46.5X5-	T46.5X6-
Methylene						
blue	T50.6X1-	T50.6X2-	T50.6X3-	T50.6X4-	T50.6X5-	T50.6X6-
chloride or dichloride (solvent) NEC	T53.4X1-	T53.4X2-	T53.4X3-	T53.4X4-	-	-
Methylenedioxyamphetamine	T43.621-	T43.622-	T43.623-	T43.624-	T43.625-	T43.626-
Methylenedioxymethamphetamine	T43.621-	T43.622-	T43.623-	T43.624-	T43.625-	T43.626-
Methylergometrine	T48.0X1-	T48.0X2-	T48.0X3-	T48.0X4-	T48.0X5-	T48.0X6-
Methylergonovine	T48.0X1-	T48.0X2-	T48.0X3-	T48.0X4-	T48.0X5-	T48.0X6-
Methylestrenolone	T38.5X1-	T38.5X2-	T38.5X3-	T38.5X4-	T38.5X5-	T38.5X6-
Methylethyl cellulose	T50.991-	T50.992-	T50.993-	T50.994-	T50.995-	T50.996-
Methylhexabital	T42.3X1-	T42.3X2-	T42.3X3-	T42.3X4-	T42.3X5-	T42.3X6-
Methylmorphine	T40.2X1-	T40.2X2-	T40.2X3-	T40.2X4-	T40.2X5-	T40.2X6-
Methylparaben (ophthalmic)	T49.5X1-	T49.5X2-	T49.5X3-	T49.5X4-	T49.5X5-	T49.5X6-
Methylparafynol	T42.6X1-	T42.6X2-	T42.6X3-	T42.6X4-	T42.6X5-	T42.6X6-
Methylpentynol, methylpenthynol	T42.6X1-	T42.6X2-	T42.6X3-	T42.6X4-	T42.6X5-	T42.6X6-
Methylphenidate	T43.631-	T43.632-	T43.633-	T43.634-	T43.635-	T43.636-
Methylphenobarbital	T42.3X1-	T42.3X2-	T42.3X3-	T42.3X4-	T42.3X5-	T42.3X6-
Methylpolysiloxane	T47.1X1-	T47.1X2-	T47.1X3-	T47.1X4-	T47.1X5-	T47.1X6-
Methylprednisolone — see Methyl, prednisolone						
Methylrosaniline	T49.0X1-	T49.0X2-	T49.0X3-	T49.0X4-	T49.0X5-	T49.0X6-
Methylrosanilinium chloride	T49.0X1-	T49.0X2-	T49.0X3-	T49.0X4-	T49.0X5-	T49.0X6-
Methyltestosterone	T38.7X1-	T38.7X2-	T38.7X3-	T38.7X4-	T38.7X5-	T38.7X6-
Methylthionine chloride	T50.6X1-	T50.6X2-	T50.6X3-	T50.6X4-	T50.6X5-	T50.6X6-
Methylthioninium chloride	T50.6X1-	T50.6X2-	T50.6X3-	T50.6X4-	T50.6X5-	T50.6X6-
Methylthiouracil	T38.2X1-	T38.2X2-	T38.2X3-	T38.2X4-	T38.2X5-	T38.2X6-

Substance	Poisoning, Accidental (unintentional)	Poisoning, Intentional self-harm	Poisoning, Assault	Poisoning, Undetermined	Adverse effect	Underdosing
Methyprylon	T42.6X1-	T42.6X2-	T42.6X3-	T42.6X4-	T42.6X5-	T42.6X6-
Methysergide	T46.5X1-	T46.5X2-	T46.5X3-	T46.5X4-	T46.5X5-	T46.5X6-
Metiamide	T47.1X1-	T47.1X2-	T47.1X3-	T47.1X4-	T47.1X5-	T47.1X6-
Meticillin	T36.0X1-	T36.0X2-	T36.0X3-	T36.0X4-	T36.0X5-	T36.0X6-
Meticrane	T50.2X1-	T50.2X2-	T50.2X3-	T50.2X4-	T50.2X5-	T50.2X6-
Metildigoxin	T46.0X1-	T46.0X2-	T46.0X3-	T46.0X4-	T46.0X5-	T46.0X6-
Metipranolol	T49.5X1-	T49.5X2-	T49.5X3-	T49.5X4-	T49.5X5-	T49.5X6-
Metirosine	T46.5X1-	T46.5X2-	T46.5X3-	T46.5X4-	T46.5X5-	T46.5X6-
Metisazone	T37.5X1-	T37.5X2-	T37.5X3-	T37.5X4-	T37.5X5-	T37.5X6-
Metixene	T44.3X1-	T44.3X2-	T44.3X3-	T44.3X4-	T44.3X5-	T44.3X6-
Metizoline	T48.5X1-	T48.5X2-	T48.5X3-	T48.5X4-	T48.5X5-	T48.5X6-
Metoclopramide	T45.0X1-	T45.0X2-	T45.0X3-	T45.0X4-	T45.0X5-	T45.0X6-
Metofenazate	T43.3X1-	T43.3X2-	T43.3X3-	T43.3X4-	T43.3X5-	T43.3X6-
Metofoline	T39.8X1-	T39.8X2-	T39.8X3-	T39.8X4-	T39.8X5-	T39.8X6-
Metolazone	T50.2X1-	T50.2X2-	T50.2X3-	T50.2X4-	T50.2X5-	T50.2X6-
Metopon	T40.2X1-	T40.2X2-	T40.2X3-	T40.2X4-	T40.2X5-	T40.2X6-
Metoprine	T45.1X1-	T45.1X2-	T45.1X3-	T45.1X4-	T45.1X5-	T45.1X6-
Metoprolol	T44.7X1-	T44.7X2-	T44.7X3-	T44.7X4-	T44.7X5-	T44.7X6-
Metrifonate	T60.0X1-	T60.0X2-	T60.0X3-	T60.0X4-	-	-
Metrizamide	T50.8X1-	T50.8X2-	T50.8X3-	T50.8X4-	T50.8X5-	T50.8X6-
Metrizoic acid	T50.8X1-	T50.8X2-	T50.8X3-	T50.8X4-	T50.8X5-	T50.8X6-
Metronidazole	T37.8X1-	T37.8X2-	T37.8X3-	T37.8X4-	T37.8X5-	T37.8X6-
Metycaine	T41.3X1-	T41.3X2-	T41.3X3-	T41.3X4-	T41.3X5-	T41.3X6-
infiltration (subcutaneous)	T41.3X1-	T41.3X2-	T41.3X3-	T41.3X4-	T41.3X5-	T41.3X6-
nerve block (peripheral) (plexus)	T41.3X1-	T41.3X2-	T41.3X3-	T41.3X4-	T41.3X5-	T41.3X6-
topical (surface)	T41.3X1-	T41.3X2-	T41.3X3-	T41.3X4-	T41.3X5-	T41.3X6-
Metyrapone	T50.8X1-	T50.8X2-	T50.8X3-	T50.8X4-	T50.8X5-	T50.8X6-
Mevinphos	T60.0X1-	T60.0X2-	T60.0X3-	T60.0X4-	-	-
Mexazolam	T42.4X1-	T42.4X2-	T42.4X3-	T42.4X4-	T42.4X5-	T42.4X6-
Mexenone	T49.3X1-	T49.3X2-	T49.3X3-	T49.3X4-	T49.3X5-	T49.3X6-
Mexiletine	T46.2X1-	T46.2X2-	T46.2X3-	T46.2X4-	T46.2X5-	T46.2X6-
Mezereon	T62.2X1-	T62.2X2-	T62.2X3-	T62.2X4-	-	-
berries	T62.1X1-	T62.1X2-	T62.1X3-	T62.1X4-	-	-
Mezlocillin	T36.0X1-	T36.0X2-	T36.0X3-	T36.0X4-	T36.0X5-	T36.0X6-
Mianserin	T43.021-	T43.022-	T43.023-	T43.024-	T43.025-	T43.026-
Micatin	T49.0X1-	T49.0X2-	T49.0X3-	T49.0X4-	T49.0X5-	T49.0X6-
Miconazole	T49.0X1-	T49.0X2-	T49.0X3-	T49.0X4-	T49.0X5-	T49.0X6-
Micronomicin	T36.5X1-	T36.5X2-	T36.5X3-	T36.5X4-	T36.5X5-	T36.5X6-
Midazolam	T42.4X1-	T42.4X2-	T42.4X3-	T42.4X4-	T42.4X5-	T42.4X6-
Midecamycin	T36.3X1-	T36.3X2-	T36.3X3-	T36.3X4-	T36.3X5-	T36.3X6-
Mifepristone	T38.6X1-	T38.6X2-	T38.6X3-	T38.6X4-	T38.6X5-	T38.6X6-
Milk of magnesia	T47.1X1-	T47.1X2-	T47.1X3-	T47.1X4-	T47.1X5-	T47.1X6-
Millipede (tropical) (venomous)	T63.411-	T63.412-	T63.413-	T63.414-		
Miltown	T43.591-	T43.592-	T43.593-	T43.594-	T43.595-	T43.596-
Milverine	T44.3X1-	T44.3X2-	T44.3X3-	T44.3X4-	T44.3X5-	T44.3X6-
Minaprine	T43.291-	T43.292-	T43.293-	T43.294-	T43.295-	T43.296-
Minaxolone	T41.291-	T41.292-	T41.293-	T41.294-	T41.295-	T41.296-
Mineral						
acids	T54.2X1-	T54.2X2-	T54.2X3-	T54.2X4-	-	-
oil (laxative) (medicinal)	T47.4X1-	T47.4X2-	T47.4X3-	T47.4X4-	T47.4X5-	T47.4X6-
emulsion	T47.2X1-	T47.2X2-	T47.2X3-	T47.2X4-	T47.2X5-	T47.2X6-
nonmedicinal	T52.0X1-	T52.0X2-	T52.0X3-	T52.0X4-	-	-
topical	T49.3X1-	T49.3X2-	T49.3X3-	T49.3X4-	T49.3X5-	T49.3X6-
salt NEC	T50.3X1-	T50.3X2-	T50.3X3-	T50.3X4-	T50.3X5-	T50.3X6-
spirits	T52.0X1-	T52.0X2-	T52.0X3-	T52.0X4-	-	-
Mineralocorticosteroid	T50.0X1-	T50.0X2-	T50.0X3-	T50.0X4-	T50.0X5-	T50.0X6-
Minocycline	T36.4X1-	T36.4X2-	T36.4X3-	T36.4X4-	T36.4X5-	T36.4X6-
Minoxidil	T46.7X1-	T46.7X2-	T46.7X3-	T46.7X4-	T46.7X5-	T46.7X6-
Miokamycin	T36.3X1-	T36.3X2-	T36.3X3-	T36.3X4-	T36.3X5-	T36.3X6-
Miotic drug	T49.5X1-	T49.5X2-	T49.5X3-	T49.5X4-	T49.5X5-	T49.5X6-
Mipafox	T60.0X1-	T60.0X2-	T60.0X3-	T60.0X4-	-	-
Mirex	T60.1X1-	T60.1X2-	T60.1X3-	T60.1X4-	-	-
Mirtazapine	T43.021-	T43.022-	T43.023-	T43.024-	T43.025-	T43.026-
Misonidazole	T37.3X1-	T37.3X2-	T37.3X3-	T37.3X4-	T37.3X5-	T37.3X6-
Misoprostol	T47.1X1-	T47.1X2-	T47.1X3-	T47.1X4-	T47.1X5-	T47.1X6-
Mithramycin	T45.1X1-	T45.1X2-	T45.1X3-	T45.1X4-	T45.1X5-	T45.1X6-
Mitobronitol	T45.1X1-	T45.1X2-	T45.1X3-	T45.1X4-	T45.1X5-	T45.1X6-
Mitoguazone	T45.1X1-	T45.1X2-	T45.1X3-	T45.1X4-	T45.1X5-	T45.1X6-
Mitolactol	T45.1X1-	T45.1X2-	T45.1X3-	T45.1X4-	T45.1X5-	T45.1X6-
Mitomycin	T45.1X1-	T45.1X2-	T45.1X3-	T45.1X4-	T45.1X5-	T45.1X6-
Mitopodozide	T45.1X1-	T45.1X2-	T45.1X3-	T45.1X4-	T45.1X5-	T45.1X6-
Mitotane	T45.1X1-	T45.1X2-	T45.1X3-	T45.1X4-	T45.1X5-	T45.1X6-
Mitoxantrone	T45.1X1-	T45.1X2-	T45.1X3-	T45.1X4-	T45.1X5-	T45.1X6-
Mivacurium chloride	T48.1X1-	T48.1X2-	T48.1X3-	T48.1X4-	T48.1X5-	T48.1X6-
Miyari bacteria	T47.6X1-	T47.6X2-	T47.6X3-	T47.6X4-	T47.6X5-	T47.6X6-
Moclobemide	T43.1X1-	T43.1X2-	T43.1X3-	T43.1X4-	T43.1X5-	T43.1X6-
Moderil	T46.5X1-	T46.5X2-	T46.5X3-	T46.5X4-	T46.5X5-	T46.5X6-

Substance	Poisoning, Accidental (unintentional)	Poisoning, Intentional self-harm	Poisoning, Assault	Poisoning, Undetermined	Adverse effect	Underdosing
Mofebutazone	T39.2X1-	T39.2X2-	T39.2X3-	T39.2X4-	T39.2X5-	T39.2X6-
Mogadon — see Nitrazepam						
Molindone	T43.591-	T43.592-	T43.593-	T43.594-	T43.595-	T43.596-
Molsidomine	T46.3X1-	T46.3X2-	T46.3X3-	T46.3X4-	T46.3X5-	T46.3X6-
Mometasone	T49.0X1-	T49.0X2-	T49.0X3-	T49.0X4-	T49.0X5-	T49.0X6-
Monistat	T49.0X1-	T49.0X2-	T49.0X3-	T49.0X4-	T49.0X5-	T49.0X6-
Monkshood	T62.2X1-	T62.2X2-	T62.2X3-	T62.2X4-	-	-
Monoamine oxidase inhibitor NEC	T43.1X1-	T43.1X2-	T43.1X3-	T43.1X4-	T43.1X5-	T43.1X6-
hydrazine	T43.1X1-	T43.1X2-	T43.1X3-	T43.1X4-	T43.1X5-	T43.1X6-
Monobenzone	T49.4X1-	T49.4X2-	T49.4X3-	T49.4X4-	T49.4X5-	T49.4X6-
Monochloroacetic acid	T60.3X1-	T60.3X2-	T60.3X3-	T60.3X4-	-	-
Monochlorobenzene	T53.7X1-	T53.7X2-	T53.7X3-	T53.7X4-	-	-
Monoethanolamine	T46.8X1-	T46.8X2-	T46.8X3-	T46.8X4-	T46.8X5-	T46.8X6-
oleate	T46.8X1-	T46.8X2-	T46.8X3-	T46.8X4-	T46.8X5-	T46.8X6-
Monooctanoin	T50.991-	T50.992-	T50.993-	T50.994-	T50.995-	T50.996-
Monophenylbutazone	T39.2X1-	T39.2X2-	T39.2X3-	T39.2X4-	T39.2X5-	T39.2X6-
Monosodium glutamate	T65.891-	T65.892-	T65.893-	T65.894-	-	-
Monosulfiram	T49.0X1-	T49.0X2-	T49.0X3-	T49.0X4-	T49.0X5-	T49.0X6-
Monoxide, carbon — see Carbon, monoxide						
Monoxidine hydrochloride	T46.1X1-	T46.1X2-	T46.1X3-	T46.1X4-	T46.1X5-	T46.1X6-
Monuron	T60.3X1-	T60.3X2-	T60.3X3-	T60.3X4-	-	-
Moperone	T43.4X1-	T43.4X2-	T43.4X3-	T43.4X4-	T43.4X5-	T43.4X6-
Mopidamol	T45.1X1-	T45.1X2-	T45.1X3-	T45.1X4-	T45.1X5-	T45.1X6-
MOPP (mechloreth-amine + vincristine + prednisone + procarba-zine)	T45.1X1-	T45.1X2-	T45.1X3-	T45.1X4-	T45.1X5-	T45.1X6-
Morfin	T40.2X1-	T40.2X2-	T40.2X3-	T40.2X4-	T40.2X5-	T40.2X6-
Morinamide	T37.1X1-	T37.1X2-	T37.1X3-	T37.1X4-	T37.1X5-	T37.1X6-
Morning glory seeds	T40.991-	T40.992-	T40.993-	T40.994-		
Moroxydine	T37.5X1-	T37.5X2-	T37.5X3-	T37.5X4-	T37.5X5-	T37.5X6-
Morphazinamide	T37.1X1-	T37.1X2-	T37.1X3-	T37.1X4-	T37.1X5-	T37.1X6-
Morphine	T40.2X1-	T40.2X2-	T40.2X3-	T40.2X4-	T40.2X5-	T40.2X6-
antagonist	T50.7X1-	T50.7X2-	T50.7X3-	T50.7X4-	T50.7X5-	T50.7X6-
Morpholinylethylmorphine	T40.2X1-	T40.2X2-	T40.2X3-	T40.2X4-		
Morsuximide	T42.2X1-	T42.2X2-	T42.2X3-	T42.2X4-	T42.2X5-	T42.2X6-
Mosapramine	T43.591-	T43.592-	T43.593-	T43.594-	T43.595-	T43.596-
Moth balls — see also Pesticides	T60.2X1-	T60.2X2-	T60.2X3-	T60.2X4-		
naphthalene	T60.2X1-	T60.2X2-	T60.2X3-	T60.2X4-		
paradichlorobenzene	T60.1X1-	T60.1X2-	T60.1X3-	T60.1X4-		
Motor exhaust gas	T58.01X-	T58.02X-	T58.03X-	T58.04X-		
Mouthwash (antiseptic) (zinc chloride)	T49.6X1-	T49.6X2-	T49.6X3-	T49.6X4-	T49.6X5-	T49.6X6-
Moxastine	T45.0X1-	T45.0X2-	T45.0X3-	T45.0X4-	T45.0X5-	T45.0X6-
Moxaverine	T44.3X1-	T44.3X2-	T44.3X3-	T44.3X4-	T44.3X5-	T44.3X6-
Moxisylyte	T46.7X1-	T46.7X2-	T46.7X3-	T46.7X4-	T46.7X5-	T46.7X6-
Mucilage, plant	T47.4X1-	T47.4X2-	T47.4X3-	T47.4X4-	T47.4X5-	T47.4X6-
Mucolytic drug	T48.4X1-	T48.4X2-	T48.4X3-	T48.4X4-	T48.4X5-	T48.4X6-
Mucomyst	T48.4X1-	T48.4X2-	T48.4X3-	T48.4X4-	T48.4X5-	T48.4X6-
Mucous membrane agents (external)	T49.91X-	T49.92X-	T49.93X-	T49.94X-	T49.95X-	T49.96X-
specified NEC	T49.8X1-	T49.8X2-	T49.8X3-	T49.8X4-	T49.8X5-	T49.8X6-
Mumps						
immune globulin (human)	T50.Z11-	T50.Z12-	T50.Z13-	T50.Z14-	T50.Z15-	T50.Z16-
skin test antigen	T50.8X1-	T50.8X2-	T50.8X3-	T50.8X4-	T50.8X5-	T50.8X6-
vaccine	T50.B91-	T50.B92-	T50.B93-	T50.B94-	T50.B95-	T50.B96-
Mumpsvax	T50.B91-	T50.B92-	T50.B93-	T50.B94-	T50.B95-	T50.B96-
Mupirocin	T49.0X1-	T49.0X2-	T49.0X3-	T49.0X4-	T49.0X5-	T49.0X6-
Muriatic acid — see Hydrochloric acid						
Muromonab-CD3	T45.1X1-	T45.1X2-	T45.1X3-	T45.1X4-	T45.1X5-	T45.1X6-
Muscle-action drug NEC	T48.201-	T48.202-	T48.203-	T48.204-	T48.205-	T48.206-
Muscle affecting agents NEC	T48.201-	T48.202-	T48.203-	T48.204-	T48.205-	T48.206-
oxytocic	T48.0X1-	T48.0X2-	T48.0X3-	T48.0X4-	T48.0X5-	T48.0X6-
relaxants	T48.201-	T48.202-	T48.203-	T48.204-	T48.205-	T48.206-
central nervous system	T42.8X1-	T42.8X2-	T42.8X3-	T42.8X4-	T42.8X5-	T42.8X6-
skeletal	T48.1X1-	T48.1X2-	T48.1X3-	T48.1X4-	T48.1X5-	T48.1X6-
smooth	T44.3X1-	T44.3X2-	T44.3X3-	T44.3X4-	T44.3X5-	T44.3X6-
Muscle relaxant — see Relaxant, muscle						
Muscle-tone depressant, central NEC	T42.8X1-	T42.8X2-	T42.8X3-	T42.8X4-	T42.8X5-	T42.8X6-
specified NEC	T42.8X1-	T42.8X2-	T42.8X3-	T42.8X4-	T42.8X5-	T42.8X6-
Mushroom, noxious	T62.0X1-	T62.0X2-	T62.0X3-	T62.0X4-	-	-
Mussel, noxious	T61.781-	T61.782-	T61.783-	T61.784-	-	-
Mustard (emetic)	T47.7X1-	T47.7X2-	T47.7X3-	T47.7X4-	T47.7X5-	T47.7X6-
black	T47.7X1-	T47.7X2-	T47.7X3-	T47.7X4-	T47.7X5-	T47.7X6-

Substance	Poisoning, Accidental (unintentional)	Poisoning, Intentional self-harm	Poisoning, Assault	Poisoning, Undetermined	Adverse effect	Underdosing
Mustard - *continued*						
gas, not in war	T59.91X-	T59.92X-	T59.93X-	T59.94X-	-	-
nitrogen	T45.1X1-	T45.1X2-	T45.1X3-	T45.1X4-	T45.1X5-	T45.1X6-
Mustine	T45.1X1-	T45.1X2-	T45.1X3-	T45.1X4-	T45.1X5-	T45.1X6-
M-vac	T45.1X1-	T45.1X2-	T45.1X3-	T45.1X4-	T45.1X5-	T45.1X6-
Mycifradin	T36.5X1-	T36.5X2-	T36.5X3-	T36.5X4-	T36.5X5-	T36.5X6-
topical	T49.0X1-	T49.0X2-	T49.0X3-	T49.0X4-	T49.0X5-	T49.0X6-
Mycitracin	T36.8X1-	T36.8X2-	T36.8X3-	T36.8X4-	T36.8X5-	T36.8X6-
ophthalmic preparation	T49.5X1-	T49.5X2-	T49.5X3-	T49.5X4-	T49.5X5-	T49.5X6-
Mycostatin	T36.7X1-	T36.7X2-	T36.7X3-	T36.7X4-	T36.7X5-	T36.7X6-
topical	T49.0X1-	T49.0X2-	T49.0X3-	T49.0X4-	T49.0X5-	T49.0X6-
Mycotoxins	T64.81X-	T64.82X-	T64.83X-	T64.84X-	-	-
aflatoxin	T64.01X-	T64.02X-	T64.03X-	T64.04X-	-	-
specified NEC	T64.81X-	T64.82X-	T64.83X-	T64.84X-	-	-
Mydriacyl	T44.3X1-	T44.3X2-	T44.3X3-	T44.3X4-	T44.3X5-	T44.3X6-
Mydriatic drug	T49.5X1-	T49.5X2-	T49.5X3-	T49.5X4-	T49.5X5-	T49.5X6-
Myelobromal	T45.1X1-	T45.1X2-	T45.1X3-	T45.1X4-	T45.1X5-	T45.1X6-
Myleran	T45.1X1-	T45.1X2-	T45.1X3-	T45.1X4-	T45.1X5-	T45.1X6-
Myochrysin (e)	T39.2X1-	T39.2X2-	T39.2X3-	T39.2X4-	T39.2X5-	T39.2X6-
Myoneural blocking agents	T48.1X1-	T48.1X2-	T48.1X3-	T48.1X4-	T48.1X5-	T48.1X6-
Myralact	T49.0X1-	T49.0X2-	T49.0X3-	T49.0X4-	T49.0X5-	T49.0X6-
Myristica fragrans	T62.2X1-	T62.2X2-	T62.2X3-	T62.2X4-	-	-
Myristicin	T65.891-	T65.892-	T65.893-	T65.894-	-	-
Mysoline	T42.3X1-	T42.3X2-	T42.3X3-	T42.3X4-	T42.3X5-	T42.3X6-
Nabilone	T40.7X1-	T40.7X2-	T40.7X3-	T40.7X4-	T40.7X5-	T40.7X6-
Nabumetone	T39.391-	T39.392-	T39.393-	T39.394-	T39.395-	T39.396-
Nadolol	T44.7X1-	T44.7X2-	T44.7X3-	T44.7X4-	T44.7X5-	T44.7X6-
Nafcillin	T36.0X1-	T36.0X2-	T36.0X3-	T36.0X4-	T36.0X5-	T36.0X6-
Nafoxidine	T38.6X1-	T38.6X2-	T38.6X3-	T38.6X4-	T38.6X5-	T38.6X6-
Naftazone	T46.991-	T46.992-	T46.993-	T46.994-	T46.995-	T46.996-
Naftidrofuryl (oxalate)	T46.7X1-	T46.7X2-	T46.7X3-	T46.7X4-	T46.7X5-	T46.7X6-
Naftifine	T49.0X1-	T49.0X2-	T49.0X3-	T49.0X4-	T49.0X5-	T49.0X6-
Nail polish remover	T52.0X1-	T52.92X-	T52.93X-	T52.94X-	-	-
Nalbuphine	T40.4X1-	T40.4X2-	T40.4X3-	T40.4X4-	T40.4X5-	T40.4X6-
Naled	T60.0X1-	T60.0X2-	T60.0X3-	T60.0X4-	-	-
Nalidixic acid	T37.8X1-	T37.8X2-	T37.8X3-	T37.8X4-	T37.8X5-	T37.8X6-
Nalorphine	T50.7X1-	T50.7X2-	T50.7X3-	T50.7X4-	T50.7X5-	T50.7X6-
Naloxone	T50.7X1-	T50.7X2-	T50.7X3-	T50.7X4-	T50.7X5-	T50.7X6-
Naltrexone	T50.7X1-	T50.7X2-	T50.7X3-	T50.7X4-	T50.7X5-	T50.7X6-
Namenda	T43.8X1-	T43.8X2-	T43.8X3-	T43.8X4-	T43.8X5-	T43.8X6-
Nandrolone	T38.7X1-	T38.7X2-	T38.7X3-	T38.7X4-	T38.7X5-	T38.7X6-
Naphazoline	T48.5X1-	T48.5X2-	T48.5X3-	T48.5X4-	T48.5X5-	T48.5X6-
Naphtha (painters') (petroleum)	T52.0X1-	T52.0X2-	T52.0X3-	T52.0X4-	-	-
solvent	T52.0X1-	T52.0X2-	T52.0X3-	T52.0X4-	-	-
vapor	T52.0X1-	T52.0X2-	T52.0X3-	T52.0X4-	-	-
Naphthalene (non-chlorinated)	T60.2X1-	T60.2X2-	T60.2X3-	T60.2X4-	-	-
chlorinated	T60.1X1-	T60.1X2-	T60.1X3-	T60.1X4-	-	-
vapor	T60.1X1-	T60.1X2-	T60.1X3-	T60.1X4-	-	-
insecticide or moth repellent	T60.2X1-	T60.2X2-	T60.2X3-	T60.2X4-	-	-
chlorinated	T60.1X1-	T60.1X2-	T60.1X3-	T60.1X4-	-	-
vapor	T60.2X1-	T60.2X2-	T60.2X3-	T60.2X4-	-	-
chlorinated	T60.1X1-	T60.1X2-	T60.1X3-	T60.1X4-	-	-
Naphthol	T65.891-	T65.892-	T65.893-	T65.894-	-	-
Naphthylamine	T65.891-	T65.892-	T65.893-	T65.894-	-	-
Naphthylthiourea (ANTU)	T60.4X1-	T60.4X2-	T60.4X3-	T60.4X4-	-	-
Naprosyn — *see* Naproxen						
Naproxen	T39.311-	T39.312-	T39.313-	T39.314-	T39.315-	T39.316-
Narcotic (drug)	T40.601-	T40.602-	T40.603-	T40.604-	T40.605-	T40.606-
analgesic NEC	T40.601-	T40.602-	T40.603-	T40.604-	T40.605-	T40.606-
antagonist	T50.7X1-	T50.7X2-	T50.7X3-	T50.7X4-	T50.7X5-	T50.7X6-
specified NEC	T40.691-	T40.692-	T40.693-	T40.694-	T40.695-	T40.696-
synthetic	T40.4X1-	T40.4X2-	T40.4X3-	T40.4X4-	T40.4X5-	T40.4X6-
Narcotine	T48.3X1-	T48.3X2-	T48.3X3-	T48.3X4-	T48.3X5-	T48.3X6-
Nardil	T43.1X1-	T43.1X2-	T43.1X3-	T43.1X4-	T43.1X5-	T43.1X6-
Nasal drug NEC	T49.6X1-	T49.6X2-	T49.6X3-	T49.6X4-	T49.6X5-	T49.6X6-
Natamycin	T49.0X1-	T49.0X2-	T49.0X3-	T49.0X4-	T49.0X5-	T49.0X6-
Natrium cyanide — *see* Cyanide(s)						
Natural						
blood (product)	T45.8X1-	T45.8X2-	T45.8X3-	T45.8X4-	T45.8X5-	T45.8X6-
gas (piped)	T59.891-	T59.892-	T59.893-	T59.894-	-	-
incomplete combustion	T58.11X-	T58.12X-	T58.13X-	T58.14X-	-	-
Nealbarbital	T42.3X1-	T42.3X2-	T42.3X3-	T42.3X4-	T42.3X5-	T42.3X6-
Nectadon	T48.3X1-	T48.3X2-	T48.3X3-	T48.3X4-	T48.3X5-	T48.3X6-
Nedocromil	T48.6X1-	T48.6X2-	T48.6X3-	T48.6X4-	T48.6X5-	T48.6X6-
Nefopam	T39.8X1-	T39.8X2-	T39.8X3-	T39.8X4-	T39.8X5-	T39.8X6-
Nematocyst (sting)	T63.691-	T63.692-	T63.693-	T63.694-	-	-
Nembutal	T42.3X1-	T42.3X2-	T42.3X3-	T42.3X4-	T42.3X5-	T42.3X6-

Substance	Poisoning, Accidental (unintentional)	Poisoning, Intentional self-harm	Poisoning, Assault	Poisoning, Undetermined	Adverse effect	Underdosing
Nemonapride	T43.591-	T43.592-	T43.593-	T43.594-	T43.595-	T43.596-
Neoarsphenamine	T37.8X1-	T37.8X2-	T37.8X3-	T37.8X4-	T37.8X5-	T37.8X6-
Neocinchophen	T50.4X1-	T50.4X2-	T50.4X3-	T50.4X4-	T50.4X5-	T50.4X6-
Neomycin (derivatives)	T36.5X1-	T36.5X2-	T36.5X3-	T36.5X4-	T36.5X5-	T36.5X6-
with						
bacitracin	T49.0X1-	T49.0X2-	T49.0X3-	T49.0X4-	T49.0X5-	T49.0X6-
neostigmine	T44.0X1-	T44.0X2-	T44.0X3-	T44.0X4-	T44.0X5-	T44.0X6-
ENT agent	T49.6X1-	T49.6X2-	T49.6X3-	T49.6X4-	T49.6X5-	T49.6X6-
ophthalmic preparation	T49.5X1-	T49.5X2-	T49.5X3-	T49.5X4-	T49.5X5-	T49.5X6-
topical NEC	T49.0X1-	T49.0X2-	T49.0X3-	T49.0X4-	T49.0X5-	T49.0X6-
Neonal	T42.3X1-	T42.3X2-	T42.3X3-	T42.3X4-	T42.3X5-	T42.3X6-
Neoprontosil	T37.0X1-	T37.0X2-	T37.0X3-	T37.0X4-	T37.0X5-	T37.0X6-
Neosalvarsan	T37.8X1-	T37.8X2-	T37.8X3-	T37.8X4-	T37.8X5-	T37.8X6-
Neosilversalvarsan	T37.8X1-	T37.8X2-	T37.8X3-	T37.8X4-	T37.8X5-	T37.8X6-
Neosporin	T36.8X1-	T36.8X2-	T36.8X3-	T36.8X4-	T36.8X5-	T36.8X6-
ENT agent	T49.6X1-	T49.6X2-	T49.6X3-	T49.6X4-	T49.6X5-	T49.6X6-
opthalmic preparation	T49.5X1-	T49.5X2-	T49.5X3-	T49.5X4-	T49.5X5-	T49.5X6-
topical NEC	T49.0X1-	T49.0X2-	T49.0X3-	T49.0X4-	T49.0X5-	T49.0X6-
Neostigmine bromide	T44.0X1-	T44.0X2-	T44.0X3-	T44.0X4-	T44.0X5-	T44.0X6-
Neraval	T42.3X1-	T42.3X2-	T42.3X3-	T42.3X4-	T42.3X5-	T42.3X6-
Neravan	T42.3X1-	T42.3X2-	T42.3X3-	T42.3X4-	T42.3X5-	T42.3X6-
Nerium oleander	T62.2X1-	T62.2X2-	T62.2X3-	T62.2X4-	-	-
Nerve gas, not in war	T59.91X-	T59.92X-	T59.93X-	T59.94X-	-	-
Nesacaine	T41.3X1-	T41.3X2-	T41.3X3-	T41.3X4-	T41.3X5-	T41.3X6-
infiltration (subcutaneous)	T41.3X1-	T41.3X2-	T41.3X3-	T41.3X4-	T41.3X5-	T41.3X6-
nerve block (peripheral) (plexus)	T41.3X1-	T41.3X2-	T41.3X3-	T41.3X4-	T41.3X5-	T41.3X6-
Netilmicin	T36.5X1-	T36.5X2-	T36.5X3-	T36.5X4-	T36.5X5-	T36.5X6-
Neurobarb	T42.3X1-	T42.3X2-	T42.3X3-	T42.3X4-	T42.3X5-	T42.3X6-
Neuroleptic drug NEC	T43.501-	T43.502-	T43.503-	T43.504-	T43.505-	T43.506-
Neuromuscular blocking drug	T48.1X1-	T48.1X2-	T48.1X3-	T48.1X4-	T48.1X5-	T48.1X6-
Neutral insulin injection	T38.3X1-	T38.3X2-	T38.3X3-	T38.3X4-	T38.3X5-	T38.3X6-
Neutral spirits	T51.0X1-	T51.0X2-	T51.0X3-	T51.0X4-	-	-
beverage	T51.0X1-	T51.0X2-	T51.0X3-	T51.0X4-	-	-
Niacin	T46.7X1-	T46.7X2-	T46.7X3-	T46.7X4-	T46.7X5-	T46.7X6-
Niacinamide	T45.2X1-	T45.2X2-	T45.2X3-	T45.2X4-	T45.2X5-	T45.2X6-
Nialamide	T43.1X1-	T43.1X2-	T43.1X3-	T43.1X4-	T43.1X5-	T43.1X6-
Niaprazine	T42.6X1-	T42.6X2-	T42.6X3-	T42.6X4-	T42.6X5-	T42.6X6-
Nicametate	T46.7X1-	T46.7X2-	T46.7X3-	T46.7X4-	T46.7X5-	T46.7X6-
Nicardipine	T46.1X1-	T46.1X2-	T46.1X3-	T46.1X4-	T46.1X5-	T46.1X6-
Nicergoline	T46.7X1-	T46.7X2-	T46.7X3-	T46.7X4-	T46.7X5-	T46.7X6-
Nickel (carbonyl) (tetra-carbonyl) (fumes) (vapor)	T56.891-	T56.892-	T56.893-	T56.894-	-	-
Nickelocene	T56.891-	T56.892-	T56.893-	T56.894-	-	-
Niclosamide	T37.4X1-	T37.4X2-	T37.4X3-	T37.4X4-	T37.4X5-	T37.4X6-
Nicofuranose	T46.7X1-	T46.7X2-	T46.7X3-	T46.7X4-	T46.7X5-	T46.7X6-
Nicomorphine	T40.2X1-	T40.2X2-	T40.2X3-	T40.2X4-	-	-
Nicorandil	T46.3X1-	T46.3X2-	T46.3X3-	T46.3X4-	T46.3X5-	T46.3X6-
Nicotiana (plant)	T62.2X1-	T62.2X2-	T62.2X3-	T62.2X4-	-	-
Nicotinamide	T45.2X1-	T45.2X2-	T45.2X3-	T45.2X4-	T45.2X5-	T45.2X6-
Nicotine (insecticide) (spray) (sulfate) NEC	T60.2X1-	T60.2X2-	T60.2X3-	T60.2X4-	-	-
from tobacco	T65.291-	T65.292-	T65.293-	T65.294-	-	-
cigarettes	T65.221-	T65.222-	T65.223-	T65.224-	-	-
not insecticide	T65.291-	T65.292-	T65.293-	T65.294-	-	-
Nicotinic acid	T46.7X1-	T46.7X2-	T46.7X3-	T46.7X4-	T46.7X5-	T46.7X6-
Nicotinyl alcohol	T46.7X1-	T46.7X2-	T46.7X3-	T46.7X4-	T46.7X5-	T46.7X6-
Nicoumalone	T45.511-	T45.512-	T45.513-	T45.514-	T45.515-	T45.516-
Nifedipine	T46.1X1-	T46.1X2-	T46.1X3-	T46.1X4-	T46.1X5-	T46.1X6-
Nifenazone	T39.2X1-	T39.2X2-	T39.2X3-	T39.2X4-	T39.2X5-	T39.2X6-
Nifuraldezone	T37.91X-	T37.92X-	T37.93X-	T37.94X-	T37.95X-	T37.96X-
Nifuratel	T37.8X1-	T37.8X2-	T37.8X3-	T37.8X4-	T37.8X5-	T37.8X6-
Nifurtimox	T37.3X1-	T37.3X2-	T37.3X3-	T37.3X4-	T37.3X5-	T37.3X6-
Nifurtoinol	T37.8X1-	T37.8X2-	T37.8X3-	T37.8X4-	T37.8X5-	T37.8X6-
Nightshade, deadly (solanum — *see also* Belladonna	T62.2X1-	T62.2X2-	T62.2X3-	T62.2X4-	-	-
berry	T62.1X1-	T62.1X2-	T62.1X3-	T62.1X4-	-	-
Nikethamide	T50.7X1-	T50.7X2-	T50.7X3-	T50.7X4-	T50.7X5-	T50.7X6-
Nilstat	T36.7X1-	T36.7X2-	T36.7X3-	T36.7X4-	T36.7X5-	T36.7X6-
topical	T49.0X1-	T49.0X2-	T49.0X3-	T49.0X4-	T49.0X5-	T49.0X6-
Nilutamide	T38.6X1-	T38.6X2-	T38.6X3-	T38.6X4-	T38.6X5-	T38.6X6-
Nimesulide	T39.391-	T39.392-	T39.393-	T39.394-	T39.395-	T39.396-
Nimetazepam	T42.4X1-	T42.4X2-	T42.4X3-	T42.4X4-	T42.4X5-	T42.4X6-
Nimodipine	T46.1X1-	T46.1X2-	T46.1X3-	T46.1X4-	T46.1X5-	T46.1X6-
Nimorazole	T37.3X1-	T37.3X2-	T37.3X3-	T37.3X4-	T37.3X5-	T37.3X6-
Nimustine	T45.1X1-	T45.1X2-	T45.1X3-	T45.1X4-	T45.1X5-	T45.1X6-
Niridazole	T37.4X1-	T37.4X2-	T37.4X3-	T37.4X4-	T37.4X5-	T37.4X6-

Substance	Poisoning, Accidental (unintentional)	Poisoning, Intentional self-harm	Poisoning, Assault	Poisoning, Undetermined	Adverse effect	Underdosing
Nisentil	T40.2X1-	T40.2X2-	T40.2X3-	T40.2X4-	T40.2X5-	T40.2X6-
Nisoldipine	T46.1X1-	T46.1X2-	T46.1X3-	T46.1X4-	T46.1X5-	T46.1X6-
Nitramine	T65.3X1-	T65.3X2-	T65.3X3-	T65.3X4-	-	-
Nitrate, organic	T46.3X1-	T46.3X2-	T46.3X3-	T46.3X4-	T46.3X5-	T46.3X6-
Nitrazepam	T42.4X1-	T42.4X2-	T42.4X3-	T42.4X4-	T42.4X5-	T42.4X6-
Nitrefazole	T50.6X1-	T50.6X2-	T50.6X3-	T50.6X4-	T50.6X5-	T50.6X6-
Nitrendipine	T46.1X1-	T46.1X2-	T46.1X3-	T46.1X4-	T46.1X5-	T46.1X6-
Nitric						
acid (liquid)	T54.2X1-	T54.2X2-	T54.2X3-	T54.2X4-	-	-
vapor	T59.891-	T59.892-	T59.893-	T59.894-	-	-
oxide (gas)	T59.0X1-	T59.0X2-	T59.0X3-	T59.0X4-	-	-
Nitrimidazine	T37.3X1-	T37.3X2-	T37.3X3-	T37.3X4-	T37.3X5-	T37.3X6-
Nitrite, amyl (medicinal) (vapor)	T46.3X1-	T46.3X2-	T46.3X3-	T46.3X4-	T46.3X5-	T46.3X6-
Nitroaniline	T65.3X1-	T65.3X2-	T65.3X3-	T65.3X4-	-	-
vapor	T59.891-	T59.892-	T59.893-	T59.894-	-	-
Nitrobenzene, nitrobenzol	T65.3X1-	T65.3X2-	T65.3X3-	T65.3X4-	-	-
vapor	T65.3X1-	T65.3X2-	T65.3X3-	T65.3X4-	-	-
Nitrocellulose	T65.891-	T65.892-	T65.893-	T65.894-	-	-
lacquer	T65.891-	T65.892-	T65.893-	T65.894-	-	-
Nitrodiphenyl	T65.3X1-	T65.3X2-	T65.3X3-	T65.3X4-	-	-
Nitrofural	T49.0X1-	T49.0X2-	T49.0X3-	T49.0X4-	T49.0X5-	T49.0X6-
Nitrofurantoin	T37.8X1-	T37.8X2-	T37.8X3-	T37.8X4-	T37.8X5-	T37.8X6-
Nitrofurazone	T49.0X1-	T49.0X2-	T49.0X3-	T49.0X4-	T49.0X5-	T49.0X6-
Nitrogen	T59.0X1-	T59.0X2-	T59.0X3-	T59.0X4-	-	-
mustard	T45.1X1-	T45.1X2-	T45.1X3-	T45.1X4-	T45.1X5-	T45.1X6-
Nitroglycerin, nitro-glycerol (medicinal)	T46.3X1-	T46.3X2-	T46.3X3-	T46.3X4-	T46.3X5-	T46.3X6-
nonmedicinal	T65.5X1-	T65.5X2-	T65.5X3-	T65.5X4-	-	-
fumes	T65.5X1-	T65.5X2-	T65.5X3-	T65.5X4-	-	-
Nitroglycol	T52.3X1-	T52.3X2-	T52.3X3-	T52.3X4-	-	-
Nitrohydrochloric acid	T54.2X1-	T54.2X2-	T54.2X3-	T54.2X4-	-	-
Nitromersol	T49.0X1-	T49.0X2-	T49.0X3-	T49.0X4-	T49.0X5-	T49.0X6-
Nitronaphthalene	T65.891-	T65.892-	T65.893-	T65.894-	-	-
Nitrophenol	T54.0X1-	T54.0X2-	T54.0X3-	T54.0X4-	-	-
Nitropropane	T52.8X1-	T52.8X2-	T52.8X3-	T52.8X4-	-	-
Nitroprusside	T46.5X1-	T46.5X2-	T46.5X3-	T46.5X4-	T46.5X5-	T46.5X6-
Nitrosodimethylamine	T65.3X1-	T65.3X2-	T65.3X3-	T65.3X4-	-	-
Nitrothiazol	T37.4X1-	T37.4X2-	T37.4X3-	T37.4X4-	T37.4X5-	T37.4X6-
Nitrotoluene, nitrotoluol	T65.3X1-	T65.3X2-	T65.3X3-	T65.3X4-	-	-
vapor	T65.3X1-	T65.3X2-	T65.3X3-	T65.3X4-	-	-
Nitrous						
acid (liquid)	T54.2X1-	T54.2X2-	T54.2X3-	T54.2X4-	-	-
fumes	T59.891-	T59.892-	T59.893-	T59.894-	-	-
ether spirit	T46.3X1-	T46.3X2-	T46.3X3-	T46.3X4-	T46.3X5-	T46.3X6-
oxide	T41.0X1-	T41.0X2-	T41.0X3-	T41.0X4-	T41.0X5-	T41.0X6-
Nitroxoline	T37.8X1-	T37.8X2-	T37.8X3-	T37.8X4-	T37.8X5-	T37.8X6-
Nitrozone	T49.0X1-	T49.0X2-	T49.0X3-	T49.0X4-	T49.0X5-	T49.0X6-
Nizatidine	T47.0X1-	T47.0X2-	T47.0X3-	T47.0X4-	T47.0X5-	T47.0X6-
Nizofenone	T43.8X1-	T43.8X2-	T43.8X3-	T43.8X4-	T43.8X5-	T43.8X6-
Noctec	T42.6X1-	T42.6X2-	T42.6X3-	T42.6X4-	T42.6X5-	T42.6X6-
Noludar	T42.6X1-	T42.6X2-	T42.6X3-	T42.6X4-	T42.6X5-	T42.6X6-
Nomegestrol	T38.5X1-	T38.5X2-	T38.5X3-	T38.5X4-	T38.5X5-	T38.5X6-
Nomifensine	T43.291-	T43.292-	T43.293-	T43.294-	T43.295-	T43.296-
Nonoxinol	T49.8X1-	T49.8X2-	T49.8X3-	T49.8X4-	T49.8X5-	T49.8X6-
Nonylphenoxy (polyethoxy-ethanol)	T49.8X1-	T49.8X2-	T49.8X3-	T49.8X4-	T49.8X5-	T49.8X6-
Noptil	T42.3X1-	T42.3X2-	T42.3X3-	T42.3X4-	T42.3X5-	T42.3X6-
Noradrenaline	T44.4X1-	T44.4X2-	T44.4X3-	T44.4X4-	T44.4X5-	T44.4X6-
Noramidopyrine	T39.2X1-	T39.2X2-	T39.2X3-	T39.2X4-	T39.2X5-	T39.2X6-
methanesulfonate sodium	T39.2X1-	T39.2X2-	T39.2X3-	T39.2X4-	T39.2X5-	T39.2X6-
Norbormide	T60.4X1-	T60.4X2-	T60.4X3-	T60.4X4-	-	-
Nordazepam	T42.4X1-	T42.4X2-	T42.4X3-	T42.4X4-	T42.4X5-	T42.4X6-
Norepinephrine	T44.4X1-	T44.4X2-	T44.4X3-	T44.4X4-	T44.4X5-	T44.4X6-
Norethandrolone	T38.7X1-	T38.7X2-	T38.7X3-	T38.7X4-	T38.7X5-	T38.7X6-
Norethindrone	T38.4X1-	T38.4X2-	T38.4X3-	T38.4X4-	T38.4X5-	T38.4X6-
Norethisterone (acetate) (enantate)	T38.4X1-	T38.4X2-	T38.4X3-	T38.4X4-	T38.4X5-	T38.4X6-
with ethinylestradiol	T38.5X1-	T38.5X2-	T38.5X3-	T38.5X4-	T38.5X5-	T38.5X6-
Noretynodrel	T38.5X1-	T38.5X2-	T38.5X3-	T38.5X4-	T38.5X5-	T38.5X6-
Norfenefrine	T44.4X1-	T44.4X2-	T44.4X3-	T44.4X4-	T44.4X5-	T44.4X6-
Norfloxacin	T36.8X1-	T36.8X2-	T36.8X3-	T36.8X4-	T36.8X5-	T36.8X6-
Norgestrel	T38.4X1-	T38.4X2-	T38.4X3-	T38.4X4-	T38.4X5-	T38.4X6-
Norgestrienone	T38.4X1-	T38.4X2-	T38.4X3-	T38.4X4-	T38.4X5-	T38.4X6-
Norlestrin	T38.4X1-	T38.4X2-	T38.4X3-	T38.4X4-	T38.4X5-	T38.4X6-
Norlutin	T38.4X1-	T38.4X2-	T38.4X3-	T38.4X4-	T38.4X5-	T38.4X6-
Normal serum albumin (human) **, salt-poor**	T45.8X1-	T45.8X2-	T45.8X3-	T45.8X4-	T45.8X5-	T45.8X6-
Normethandrone	T38.5X1-	T38.5X2-	T38.5X3-	T38.5X4-	T38.5X5-	T38.5X6-

Substance	Poisoning, Accidental (unintentional)	Poisoning, Intentional self-harm	Poisoning, Assault	Poisoning, Undetermined	Adverse effect	Underdosing
Normison — *see* Benzodiazepines						
Normorphine	T40.2X1-	T40.2X2-	T40.2X3-	T40.2X4-	-	-
Norpseudoephedrine	T50.5X1-	T50.5X2-	T50.5X3-	T50.5X4-	T50.5X5-	T50.5X6-
Nortestosterone (furanpropionate)	T38.7X1-	T38.7X2-	T38.7X3-	T38.7X4-	T38.7X5-	T38.7X6-
Nortriptyline	T43.011-	T43.012-	T43.013-	T43.014-	T43.015-	T43.016-
Noscapine	T48.3X1-	T48.3X2-	T48.3X3-	T48.3X4-	T48.3X5-	T48.3X6-
Nose preparations	T49.6X1-	T49.6X2-	T49.6X3-	T49.6X4-	T49.6X5-	T49.6X6-
Novobiocin	T36.5X1-	T36.5X2-	T36.5X3-	T36.5X4-	T36.5X5-	T36.5X6-
Novocain (infiltration) (topical)	T41.3X1-	T41.3X2-	T41.3X3-	T41.3X4-	T41.3X5-	T41.3X6-
nerve block (peripheral) (plexus)	T41.3X1-	T41.3X2-	T41.3X3-	T41.3X4-	T41.3X5-	T41.3X6-
spinal	T41.3X1-	T41.3X2-	T41.3X3-	T41.3X4-	T41.3X5-	T41.3X6-
Noxious foodstuff	T62.91X-	T62.92X-	T62.93X-	T62.94X-	-	-
specified NEC	T62.8X1-	T62.8X2-	T62.8X3-	T62.8X4-	-	-
Noxiptiline	T43.011-	T43.012-	T43.013-	T43.014-	T43.015-	T43.016-
Noxytiolin	T49.0X1-	T49.0X2-	T49.0X3-	T49.0X4-	T49.0X5-	T49.0X6-
NPH Iletin (insulin)	T38.3X1-	T38.3X2-	T38.3X3-	T38.3X4-	T38.3X5-	T38.3X6-
Numorphan	T40.2X1-	T40.2X2-	T40.2X3-	T40.2X4-	T40.2X5-	T40.2X6-
Nunol	T42.3X1-	T42.3X2-	T42.3X3-	T42.3X4-	T42.3X5-	T42.3X6-
Nupercaine (spinal anesthetic)	T41.3X1-	T41.3X2-	T41.3X3-	T41.3X4-	T41.3X5-	T41.3X6-
topical (surface)	T41.3X1-	T41.3X2-	T41.3X3-	T41.3X4-	T41.3X5-	T41.3X6-
Nutmeg oil (liniment)	T49.3X1-	T49.3X2-	T49.3X3-	T49.3X4-	T49.3X5-	T49.3X6-
Nutritional supplement	T50.901-	T50.902-	T50.903-	T50.904-	T50.905-	T50.906-
Nux vomica	T65.1X1-	T65.1X2-	T65.1X3-	T65.1X4-	-	-
Nydrazid	T37.1X1-	T37.1X2-	T37.1X3-	T37.1X4-	T37.1X5-	T37.1X6-
Nylidrin	T46.7X1-	T46.7X2-	T46.7X3-	T46.7X4-	T46.7X5-	T46.7X6-
Nystatin	T36.7X1-	T36.7X2-	T36.7X3-	T36.7X4-	T36.7X5-	T36.7X6-
topical	T49.0X1-	T49.0X2-	T49.0X3-	T49.0X4-	T49.0X5-	T49.0X6-
Nytol	T45.0X1-	T45.0X2-	T45.0X3-	T45.0X4-	T45.0X5-	T45.0X6-
Obidoxime chloride	T50.6X1-	T50.6X2-	T50.6X3-	T50.6X4-	T50.6X5-	T50.6X6-
Octafonium (chloride)	T49.3X1-	T49.3X2-	T49.3X3-	T49.3X4-	T49.3X5-	T49.3X6-
Octamethyl pyrophos-phoramide	T60.0X1-	T60.0X2-	T60.0X3-	T60.0X4-	-	-
Octanoin	T50.991-	T50.992-	T50.993-	T50.994-	T50.995-	T50.996-
Octatropine methyl-bromide	T44.3X1-	T44.3X2-	T44.3X3-	T44.3X4-	T44.3X5-	T44.3X6-
Octotiamine	T45.2X1-	T45.2X2-	T45.2X3-	T45.2X4-	T45.2X5-	T45.2X6-
Octoxinol (9)	T49.8X1-	T49.8X2-	T49.8X3-	T49.8X4-	T49.8X5-	T49.8X6-
Octreotide	T38.991-	T38.992-	T38.993-	T38.994-	T38.995-	T38.996-
Octyl nitrite	T46.3X1-	T46.3X2-	T46.3X3-	T46.3X4-	T46.3X5-	T46.3X6-
Oestradiol	T38.5X1-	T38.5X2-	T38.5X3-	T38.5X4-	T38.5X5-	T38.5X6-
Oestriol	T38.5X1-	T38.5X2-	T38.5X3-	T38.5X4-	T38.5X5-	T38.5X6-
Oestrogen	T38.5X1-	T38.5X2-	T38.5X3-	T38.5X4-	T38.5X5-	T38.5X6-
Oestrone	T38.5X1-	T38.5X2-	T38.5X3-	T38.5X4-	T38.5X5-	T38.5X6-
Ofloxacin	T36.8X1-	T36.8X2-	T36.8X3-	T36.8X4-	T36.8X5-	T36.8X6-
Oil (of)	T65.891-	T65.892-	T65.893-	T65.894-	-	-
bitter almond	T62.8X1-	T62.8X2-	T62.8X3-	T62.8X4-	-	-
cloves	T49.7X1-	T49.7X2-	T49.7X3-	T49.7X4-	T49.7X5-	T49.7X6-
colors	T65.6X1-	T65.6X2-	T65.6X3-	T65.6X4-	-	-
fumes	T59.891-	T59.892-	T59.893-	T59.894-	-	-
lubricating	T52.0X1-	T52.0X2-	T52.0X3-	T52.0X4-	-	-
Niobe	T52.8X1-	T52.8X2-	T52.8X3-	T52.8X4-	-	-
vitriol (liquid)	T54.2X1-	T54.2X2-	T54.2X3-	T54.2X4-	-	-
fumes	T54.2X1-	T54.2X2-	T54.2X3-	T54.2X4-	-	-
wintergreen (bitter) NEC	T49.3X1-	T49.3X2-	T49.3X3-	T49.3X4-	T49.3X5-	T49.3X6-
Oily preparation (for skin)	T49.3X1-	T49.3X2-	T49.3X3-	T49.3X4-	T49.3X5-	T49.3X6-
Ointment NEC	T49.3X1-	T49.3X2-	T49.3X3-	T49.3X4-	T49.3X5-	T49.3X6-
Olanzapine	T43.591-	T43.592-	T43.593-	T43.594-	T43.595-	T43.596-
Oleander	T62.2X1-	T62.2X2-	T62.2X3-	T62.2X4-	-	-
Oleandomycin	T36.3X1-	T36.3X2-	T36.3X3-	T36.3X4-	T36.3X5-	T36.3X6-
Oleandrin	T46.0X1-	T46.0X2-	T46.0X3-	T46.0X4-	T46.0X5-	T46.0X6-
Oleic acid	T46.6X1-	T46.6X2-	T46.6X3-	T46.6X4-	T46.6X5-	T46.6X6-
Oleovitamin A	T45.2X1-	T45.2X2-	T45.2X3-	T45.2X4-	T45.2X5-	T45.2X6-
Oleum ricini	T47.2X1-	T47.2X2-	T47.2X3-	T47.2X4-	T47.2X5-	T47.2X6-
Olive oil (medicinal) **NEC**	T47.4X1-	T47.4X2-	T47.4X3-	T47.4X4-	T47.4X5-	T47.4X6-
Olivomycin	T45.1X1-	T45.1X2-	T45.1X3-	T45.1X4-	T45.1X5-	T45.1X6-
Olsalazine	T47.8X1-	T47.8X2-	T47.8X3-	T47.8X4-	T47.8X5-	T47.8X6-
Omeprazole	T47.1X1-	T47.1X2-	T47.1X3-	T47.1X4-	T47.1X5-	T47.1X6-
OMPA	T60.0X1-	T60.0X2-	T60.0X3-	T60.0X4-	-	-
Oncovin	T45.1X1-	T45.1X2-	T45.1X3-	T45.1X4-	T45.1X5-	T45.1X6-
Ondansetron	T45.0X1-	T45.0X2-	T45.0X3-	T45.0X4-	T45.0X5-	T45.0X6-
Ophthaine	T41.3X1-	T41.3X2-	T41.3X3-	T41.3X4-	T41.3X5-	T41.3X6-
Ophthetic	T41.3X1-	T41.3X2-	T41.3X3-	T41.3X4-	T41.3X5-	T41.3X6-
Opiate NEC	T40.601-	T40.602-	T40.603-	T40.604-	T40.605-	T40.606-
antagonists	T50.7X1-	T50.7X2-	T50.7X3-	T50.7X4-	T50.7X5-	T50.7X6-
Opioid NEC	T40.2X1-	T40.2X2-	T40.2X3-	T40.2X4-	T40.2X5-	T40.2X6-
Opipramol	T43.011-	T43.012-	T43.013-	T43.014-	T43.015-	T43.016-

Substance	Poisoning, Accidental (unintentional)	Poisoning, Intentional self-harm	Poisoning, Assault	Poisoning, Undetermined	Adverse effect	Underdosing
Opium alkaloids (total)	T40.0X1-	T40.0X2-	T40.0X3-	T40.0X4-	T40.0X5-	T40.0X6-
standardized powdered	T40.0X1-	T40.0X2-	T40.0X3-	T40.0X4-	T40.0X5-	T40.0X6-
tincture (camphorated)	T40.0X1-	T40.0X2-	T40.0X3-	T40.0X4-	T40.0X5-	T40.0X6-
Oracon	T38.4X1-	T38.4X2-	T38.4X3-	T38.4X4-	T38.4X5-	T38.4X6-
Oragrafin	T50.8X1-	T50.8X2-	T50.8X3-	T50.8X4-	T50.8X5-	T50.8X6-
Oral contraceptives	T38.4X1-	T38.4X2-	T38.4X3-	T38.4X4-	T38.4X5-	T38.4X6-
Oral rehydration salts	T50.3X1-	T50.3X2-	T50.3X3-	T50.3X4-	T50.3X5-	T50.3X6-
Orazamide	T50.991-	T50.992-	T50.993-	T50.994-	T50.995-	T50.996-
Orciprenaline	T48.291-	T48.292-	T48.293-	T48.294-	T48.295-	T48.296-
Organidin	T48.4X1-	T48.4X2-	T48.4X3-	T48.4X4-	T48.4X5-	T48.4X6-
Organonitrate NEC	T46.3X1-	T46.3X2-	T46.3X3-	T46.3X4-	T46.3X5-	T46.3X6-
Organophosphates	T60.0X1-	T60.0X2-	T60.0X3-	T60.0X4-	-	-
Orimune	T50.B91-	T50.B92-	T50.B93-	T50.B94-	T50.B95-	T50.B96-
Orinase	T38.3X1-	T38.3X2-	T38.3X3-	T38.3X4-	T38.3X5-	T38.3X6-
Ormeloxifene	T38.6X1-	T38.6X2-	T38.6X3-	T38.6X4-	T38.6X5-	T38.6X6-
Ornidazole	T37.3X1-	T37.3X2-	T37.3X3-	T37.3X4-	T37.3X5-	T37.3X6-
Ornithine aspartate	T50.991-	T50.992-	T50.993-	T50.994-	T50.995-	T50.996-
Ornoprostil	T47.1X1-	T47.1X2-	T47.1X3-	T47.1X4-	T47.1X5-	T47.1X6-
Orphenadrine (hydrochloride)	T42.8X1-	T42.8X2-	T42.8X3-	T42.8X4-	T42.8X5-	T42.8X6-
Ortal (sodium)	T42.3X1-	T42.3X2-	T42.3X3-	T42.3X4-	T42.3X5-	T42.3X6-
Orthoboric acid	T49.0X1-	T49.0X2-	T49.0X3-	T49.0X4-	T49.0X5-	T49.0X6-
ENT agent	T49.6X1-	T49.6X2-	T49.6X3-	T49.6X4-	T49.6X5-	T49.6X6-
ophthalmic preparation	T49.5X1-	T49.5X2-	T49.5X3-	T49.5X4-	T49.5X5-	T49.5X6-
Orthocaine	T41.3X1-	T41.3X2-	T41.3X3-	T41.3X4-	T41.3X5-	T41.3X6-
Orthodichlorobenzene	T53.7X1-	T53.7X2-	T53.7X3-	T53.7X4-	-	-
Ortho-Novum	T38.4X1-	T38.4X2-	T38.4X3-	T38.4X4-	T38.4X5-	T38.4X6-
Orthotolidine (reagent)	T54.2X1-	T54.2X2-	T54.2X3-	T54.2X4-	-	-
Osmic acid (liquid)	T54.2X1-	T54.2X2-	T54.2X3-	T54.2X4-	-	-
fumes	T54.2X1-	T54.2X2-	T54.2X3-	T54.2X4-	-	-
Osmotic diuretics	T50.2X1-	T50.2X2-	T50.2X3-	T50.2X4-	T50.2X5-	T50.2X6-
Otilonium bromide	T44.3X1-	T44.3X2-	T44.3X3-	T44.3X4-	T44.3X5-	T44.3X6-
Otorhinolaryngological drug NEC	T49.6X1-	T49.6X2-	T49.6X3-	T49.6X4-	T49.6X5-	T49.6X6-
Ouabain (e)	T46.0X1-	T46.0X2-	T46.0X3-	T46.0X4-	T46.0X5-	T46.0X6-
Ovarian						
hormone	T38.5X1-	T38.5X2-	T38.5X3-	T38.5X4-	T38.5X5-	T38.5X6-
stimulant	T38.5X1-	T38.5X2-	T38.5X3-	T38.5X4-	T38.5X5-	T38.5X6-
Ovral	T38.4X1-	T38.4X2-	T38.4X3-	T38.4X4-	T38.4X5-	T38.4X6-
Ovulen	T38.4X1-	T38.4X2-	T38.4X3-	T38.4X4-	T38.4X5-	T38.4X6-
Oxacillin	T36.0X1-	T36.0X2-	T36.0X3-	T36.0X4-	T36.0X5-	T36.0X6-
Oxalic acid	T54.2X1-	T54.2X2-	T54.2X3-	T54.2X4-	-	-
ammonium salt	T50.991-	T50.992-	T50.993-	T50.994-	T50.995-	T50.996-
Oxamniquine	T37.4X1-	T37.4X2-	T37.4X3-	T37.4X4-	T37.4X5-	T37.4X6-
Oxanamide	T43.591-	T43.592-	T43.593-	T43.594-	T43.595-	T43.596-
Oxandrolone	T38.7X1-	T38.7X2-	T38.7X3-	T38.7X4-	T38.7X5-	T38.7X6-
Oxantel	T37.4X1-	T37.4X2-	T37.4X3-	T37.4X4-	T37.4X5-	T37.4X6-
Oxapium iodide	T44.3X1-	T44.3X2-	T44.3X3-	T44.3X4-	T44.3X5-	T44.3X6-
Oxaprotiline	T43.021-	T43.022-	T43.023-	T43.024-	T43.025-	T43.026-
Oxaprozin	T39.311-	T39.312-	T39.313-	T39.314-	T39.315-	T39.316-
Oxatomide	T45.0X1-	T45.0X2-	T45.0X3-	T45.0X4-	T45.0X5-	T45.0X6-
Oxazepam	T42.4X1-	T42.4X2-	T42.4X3-	T42.4X4-	T42.4X5-	T42.4X6-
Oxazimedrine	T50.5X1-	T50.5X2-	T50.5X3-	T50.5X4-	T50.5X5-	T50.5X6-
Oxazolam	T42.4X1-	T42.4X2-	T42.4X3-	T42.4X4-	T42.4X5-	T42.4X6-
Oxazolidine derivatives	T42.2X1-	T42.2X2-	T42.2X3-	T42.2X4-	T42.2X5-	T42.2X6-
Oxazolidinedione (derivative)	T42.2X1-	T42.2X2-	T42.2X3-	T42.2X4-	T42.2X5-	T42.2X6-
Ox bile extract	T47.5X1-	T47.5X2-	T47.5X3-	T47.5X4-	T47.5X5-	T47.5X6-
Oxcarbazepine	T42.1X1-	T42.1X2-	T42.1X3-	T42.1X4-	T42.1X5-	T42.1X6-
Oxedrine	T44.4X1-	T44.4X2-	T44.4X3-	T44.4X4-	T44.4X5-	T44.4X6-
Oxeladin (citrate)	T48.3X1-	T48.3X2-	T48.3X3-	T48.3X4-	T48.3X5-	T48.3X6-
Oxendolone	T38.5X1-	T38.5X2-	T38.5X3-	T38.5X4-	T38.5X5-	T38.5X6-
Oxetacaine	T41.3X1-	T41.3X2-	T41.3X3-	T41.3X4-	T41.3X5-	T41.3X6-
Oxethazine	T41.3X1-	T41.3X2-	T41.3X3-	T41.3X4-	T41.3X5-	T41.3X6-
Oxetorone	T39.8X1-	T39.8X2-	T39.8X3-	T39.8X4-	T39.8X5-	T39.8X6-
Oxiconazole	T49.0X1-	T49.0X2-	T49.0X3-	T49.0X4-	T49.0X5-	T49.0X6-
Oxidizing agent NEC	T54.91X-	T54.92X-	T54.93X-	T54.94X-	-	-
Oxipurinol	T50.4X1-	T50.4X2-	T50.4X3-	T50.4X4-	T50.4X5-	T50.4X6-
Oxitriptan	T43.291-	T43.292-	T43.293-	T43.294-	T43.295-	T43.296-
Oxitropium bromide	T48.6X1-	T48.6X2-	T48.6X3-	T48.6X4-	T48.6X5-	T48.6X6-
Oxodipine	T46.1X1-	T46.1X2-	T46.1X3-	T46.1X4-	T46.1X5-	T46.1X6-
Oxolamine	T48.3X1-	T48.3X2-	T48.3X3-	T48.3X4-	T48.3X5-	T48.3X6-
Oxolinic acid	T37.8X1-	T37.8X2-	T37.8X3-	T37.8X4-	T37.8X5-	T37.8X6-
Oxomemazine	T43.3X1-	T43.3X2-	T43.3X3-	T43.3X4-	T43.3X5-	T43.3X6-
Oxophenarsine	T37.3X1-	T37.3X2-	T37.3X3-	T37.3X4-	T37.3X5-	T37.3X6-
Oxprenolol	T44.7X1-	T44.7X2-	T44.7X3-	T44.7X4-	T44.7X5-	T44.7X6-
Oxsoralen	T49.3X1-	T49.3X2-	T49.3X3-	T49.3X4-	T49.3X5-	T49.3X6-
Oxtriphylline	T48.6X1-	T48.6X2-	T48.6X3-	T48.6X4-	T48.6X5-	T48.6X6-
Oxybate sodium	T41.291-	T41.292-	T41.293-	T41.294-	T41.295-	T41.296-
Oxybuprocaine	T41.3X1-	T41.3X2-	T41.3X3-	T41.3X4-	T41.3X5-	T41.3X6-

Substance	Poisoning, Accidental (unintentional)	Poisoning, Intentional self-harm	Poisoning, Assault	Poisoning, Undetermined	Adverse effect	Underdosing
Oxybutynin	T44.3X1-	T44.3X2-	T44.3X3-	T44.3X4-	T44.3X5-	T44.3X6-
Oxychlorosene	T49.0X1-	T49.0X2-	T49.0X3-	T49.0X4-	T49.0X5-	T49.0X6-
Oxycodone	T40.2X1-	T40.2X2-	T40.2X3-	T40.2X4-	T40.2X5-	T40.2X6-
Oxyfedrine	T46.3X1-	T46.3X2-	T46.3X3-	T46.3X4-	T46.3X5-	T46.3X6-
Oxygen	T41.5X1-	T41.5X2-	T41.5X3-	T41.5X4-	T41.5X5-	T41.5X6-
Oxylone	T49.0X1-	T49.0X2-	T49.0X3-	T49.0X4-	T49.0X5-	T49.0X6-
ophthalmic preparation	T49.5X1-	T49.5X2-	T49.5X3-	T49.5X4-	T49.5X5-	T49.5X6-
Oxymesterone	T38.7X1-	T38.7X2-	T38.7X3-	T38.7X4-	T38.7X5-	T38.7X6-
Oxymetazoline	T48.5X1-	T48.5X2-	T48.5X3-	T48.5X4-	T48.5X5-	T48.5X6-
Oxymetholone	T38.7X1-	T38.7X2-	T38.7X3-	T38.7X4-	T38.7X5-	T38.7X6-
Oxymorphone	T40.2X1-	T40.2X2-	T40.2X3-	T40.2X4-	T40.2X5-	T40.2X6-
Oxypertine	T43.591-	T43.592-	T43.593-	T43.594-	T43.595-	T43.596-
Oxyphenbutazone	T39.2X1-	T39.2X2-	T39.2X3-	T39.2X4-	T39.2X5-	T39.2X6-
Oxyphencyclimine	T44.3X1-	T44.3X2-	T44.3X3-	T44.3X4-	T44.3X5-	T44.3X6-
Oxyphenisatine	T47.2X1-	T47.2X2-	T47.2X3-	T47.2X4-	T47.2X5-	T47.2X6-
Oxyphenonium bromide	T44.3X1-	T44.3X2-	T44.3X3-	T44.3X4-	T44.3X5-	T44.3X6-
Oxypolygelatin	T45.8X1-	T45.8X2-	T45.8X3-	T45.8X4-	T45.8X5-	T45.8X6-
Oxyquinoline (derivatives)	T37.8X1-	T37.8X2-	T37.8X3-	T37.8X4-	T37.8X5-	T37.8X6-
Oxytetracycline	T36.4X1-	T36.4X2-	T36.4X3-	T36.4X4-	T36.4X5-	T36.4X6-
Oxytocic drug NEC	T48.0X1-	T48.0X2-	T48.0X3-	T48.0X4-	T48.0X5-	T48.0X6-
Oxytocin (synthetic)	T48.0X1-	T48.0X2-	T48.0X3-	T48.0X4-	T48.0X5-	T48.0X6-
Ozone	T59.891-	T59.892-	T59.893-	T59.894-	-	-
PABA	T49.3X1-	T49.3X2-	T49.3X3-	T49.3X4-	T49.3X5-	T49.3X6-
Packed red cells	T45.8X1-	T45.8X2-	T45.8X3-	T45.8X4-	T45.8X5-	T45.8X6-
Padimate	T49.3X1-	T49.3X2-	T49.3X3-	T49.3X4-	T49.3X5-	T49.3X6-
Paint NEC	T65.6X1-	T65.6X2-	T65.6X3-	T65.6X4-	-	-
cleaner	T52.91X-	T52.92X-	T52.93X-	T52.94X-	-	-
fumes NEC	T59.891-	T59.892-	T59.893-	T59.894-	-	-
lead (fumes)	T56.0X1-	T56.0X2-	T56.0X3-	T56.0X4-	-	-
solvent NEC	T52.8X1-	T52.8X2-	T52.8X3-	T52.8X4-	-	-
stripper	T52.8X1-	T52.8X2-	T52.8X3-	T52.8X4-	-	-
Palfium	T40.2X1-	T40.2X2-	T40.2X3-	T40.2X4-	-	-
Palm kernel oil	T50.991-	T50.992-	T50.993-	T50.994-	T50.995-	T50.996-
Paludrine	T37.2X1-	T37.2X2-	T37.2X3-	T37.2X4-	T37.2X5-	T37.2X6-
PAM (pralidoxime)	T50.6X1-	T50.6X2-	T50.6X3-	T50.6X4-	T50.6X5-	T50.6X6-
Pamaquine (naphthoute)	T37.2X1-	T37.2X2-	T37.2X3-	T37.2X4-	T37.2X5-	T37.2X6-
Panadol	T39.1X1-	T39.1X2-	T39.1X3-	T39.1X4-	T39.1X5-	T39.1X6-
Pancreatic						
digestive secretion stimulant	T47.8X1-	T47.8X2-	T47.8X3-	T47.8X4-	T47.8X5-	T47.8X6-
dornase	T45.3X1-	T45.3X2-	T45.3X3-	T45.3X4-	T45.3X5-	T45.3X6-
Pancreatin	T47.5X1-	T47.5X2-	T47.5X3-	T47.5X4-	T47.5X5-	T47.5X6-
Pancrelipase	T47.5X1-	T47.5X2-	T47.5X3-	T47.5X4-	T47.5X5-	T47.5X6-
Pancuronium (bromide)	T48.1X1-	T48.1X2-	T48.1X3-	T48.1X4-	T48.1X5-	T48.1X6-
Pangamic acid	T45.2X1-	T45.2X2-	T45.2X3-	T45.2X4-	T45.2X5-	T45.2X6-
Panthenol	T45.2X1-	T45.2X2-	T45.2X3-	T45.2X4-	T45.2X5-	T45.2X6-
topical	T49.8X1-	T49.8X2-	T49.8X3-	T49.8X4-	T49.8X5-	T49.8X6-
Pantopon	T40.0X1-	T40.0X2-	T40.0X3-	T40.0X4-	T40.0X5-	T40.0X6-
Pantothenic acid	T45.2X1-	T45.2X2-	T45.2X3-	T45.2X4-	T45.2X5-	T45.2X6-
Panwarfin	T45.511-	T45.512-	T45.513-	T45.514-	T45.515-	T45.516-
Papain	T47.5X1-	T47.5X2-	T47.5X3-	T47.5X4-	T47.5X5-	T47.5X6-
digestant	T47.5X1-	T47.5X2-	T47.5X3-	T47.5X4-	T47.5X5-	T47.5X6-
Papaveretum	T40.0X1-	T40.0X2-	T40.0X3-	T40.0X4-	T40.0X5-	T40.0X6-
Papaverine	T44.3X1-	T44.3X2-	T44.3X3-	T44.3X4-	T44.3X5-	T44.3X6-
Para-acetamidophenol	T39.1X1-	T39.1X2-	T39.1X3-	T39.1X4-	T39.1X5-	T39.1X6-
Para-aminobenzoic acid	T49.3X1-	T49.3X2-	T49.3X3-	T49.3X4-	T49.3X5-	T49.3X6-
Para-aminophenol derivatives	T39.1X1-	T39.1X2-	T39.1X3-	T39.1X4-	T39.1X5-	T39.1X6-
Para-aminosalicylic acid	T37.1X1-	T37.1X2-	T37.1X3-	T37.1X4-	T37.1X5-	T37.1X6-
Paracetaldehyde	T42.6X1-	T42.6X2-	T42.6X3-	T42.6X4-	T42.6X5-	T42.6X6-
Paracetamol	T39.1X1-	T39.1X2-	T39.1X3-	T39.1X4-	T39.1X5-	T39.1X6-
Parachlorophenol (camphorated)	T49.0X1-	T49.0X2-	T49.0X3-	T49.0X4-	T49.0X5-	T49.0X6-
Paracodin	T40.2X1-	T40.2X2-	T40.2X3-	T40.2X4-	T40.2X5-	T40.2X6-
Paradione	T42.2X1-	T42.2X2-	T42.2X3-	T42.2X4-	T42.2X5-	T42.2X6-
Paraffin (s) (wax)	T52.0X1-	T52.0X2-	T52.0X3-	T52.0X4-	-	-
liquid (medicinal)	T47.4X1-	T47.4X2-	T47.4X3-	T47.4X4-	T47.4X5-	T47.4X6-
nonmedicinal	T52.0X1-	T52.0X2-	T52.0X3-	T52.0X4-	-	-
Paraformaldehyde	T60.3X1-	T60.3X2-	T60.3X3-	T60.3X4-	-	-
Paraldehyde	T42.6X1-	T42.6X2-	T42.6X3-	T42.6X4-	T42.6X5-	T42.6X6-
Paramethadione	T42.2X1-	T42.2X2-	T42.2X3-	T42.2X4-	T42.2X5-	T42.2X6-
Paramethasone	T38.0X1-	T38.0X2-	T38.0X3-	T38.0X4-	T38.0X5-	T38.0X6-
acetate	T49.0X1-	T49.0X2-	T49.0X3-	T49.0X4-	T49.0X5-	T49.0X6-
Paraoxon	T60.0X1-	T60.0X2-	T60.0X3-	T60.0X4-	-	-
Paraquat	T60.3X1-	T60.3X2-	T60.3X3-	T60.3X4-	-	-
Parasympatholytic NEC	T44.3X1-	T44.3X2-	T44.3X3-	T44.3X4-	T44.3X5-	T44.3X6-
Parasympathomimetic drug NEC	T44.1X1-	T44.1X2-	T44.1X3-	T44.1X4-	T44.1X5-	T44.1X6-
Parathion	T60.0X1-	T60.0X2-	T60.0X3-	T60.0X4-	-	-
Parathormone	T50.991-	T50.992-	T50.993-	T50.994-	T50.995-	T50.996-

Substance	Poisoning, Accidental (unintentional)	Poisoning, Intentional self-harm	Poisoning, Assault	Poisoning, Undetermined	Adverse effect	Underdosing
Parathyroid extract	T50.991-	T50.992-	T50.993-	T50.994-	T50.995-	T50.996-
Paratyphoid vaccine	T50.A91-	T50.A92-	T50.A93-	T50.A94-	T50.A95-	T50.A96-
Paredrine	T44.4X1-	T44.4X2-	T44.4X3-	T44.4X4-	T44.4X5-	T44.4X6-
Paregoric	T40.0X1-	T40.0X2-	T40.0X3-	T40.0X4-	T40.0X5-	T40.0X6-
Pargyline	T46.5X1-	T46.5X2-	T46.5X3-	T46.5X4-	T46.5X5-	T46.5X6-
Paris green	T57.0X1-	T57.0X2-	T57.0X3-	T57.0X4-	-	-
insecticide	T57.0X1-	T57.0X2-	T57.0X3-	T57.0X4-	-	-
Parnate	T43.1X1-	T43.1X2-	T43.1X3-	T43.1X4-	T43.1X5-	T43.1X6-
Paromomycin	T36.5X1-	T36.5X2-	T36.5X3-	T36.5X4-	T36.5X5-	T36.5X6-
Paroxypropione	T45.1X1-	T45.1X2-	T45.1X3-	T45.1X4-	T45.1X5-	T45.1X6-
Parzone	T40.2X1-	T40.2X2-	T40.2X3-	T40.2X4-	T40.2X5-	T40.2X6-
PAS	T37.1X1-	T37.1X2-	T37.1X3-	T37.1X4-	T37.1X5-	T37.1X6-
Pasiniazid	T37.1X1-	T37.1X2-	T37.1X3-	T37.1X4-	T37.1X5-	T37.1X6-
PBB (polybrominated biphenyls)	T65.891-	T65.892-	T65.893-	T65.894-	-	-
PCB	T65.891-	T65.892-	T65.893-	T65.894-	-	-
PCP						
meaning pentachlorophenol	T60.1X1-	T60.1X2-	T60.1X3-	T60.1X4-	-	-
fungicide	T60.3X1-	T60.3X2-	T60.3X3-	T60.3X4-	-	-
herbicide	T60.3X1-	T60.3X2-	T60.3X3-	T60.3X4-	-	-
insecticide	T60.1X1-	T60.1X2-	T60.1X3-	T60.1X4-	-	-
meaning phencyclidine	T40.991-	T40.992-	T40.993-	T40.994-	-	-
Peach kernel oil (emulsion)	T47.4X1-	T47.4X2-	T47.4X3-	T47.4X4-	T47.4X5-	T47.4X6-
Peanut oil (emulsion) NEC	T47.4X1-	T47.4X2-	T47.4X3-	T47.4X4-	T47.4X5-	T47.4X6-
topical	T49.3X1-	T49.3X2-	T49.3X3-	T49.3X4-	T49.3X5-	T49.3X6-
Pearly Gates (morning glory seeds)	T40.991-	T40.992-	T40.993-	T40.994-	-	-
Pecazine	T43.3X1-	T43.3X2-	T43.3X3-	T43.3X4-	T43.3X5-	T43.3X6-
Pectin	T47.6X1-	T47.6X2-	T47.6X3-	T47.6X4-	T47.6X5-	T47.6X6-
Pefloxacin	T37.8X1-	T37.8X2-	T37.8X3-	T37.8X4-	T37.8X5-	T37.8X6-
Pegademase, bovine	T50.Z91-	T50.Z92-	T50.Z93-	T50.Z94-	T50.Z95-	T50.Z96-
Pelletierine tannate	T37.4X1-	T37.4X2-	T37.4X3-	T37.4X4-	T37.4X5-	T37.4X6-
Pemirolast (potassium)	T48.6X1-	T48.6X2-	T48.6X3-	T48.6X4-	T48.6X5-	T48.6X6-
Pemoline	T50.7X1-	T50.7X2-	T50.7X3-	T50.7X4-	T50.7X5-	T50.7X6-
Pempidine	T44.2X1-	T44.2X2-	T44.2X3-	T44.2X4-	T44.2X5-	T44.2X6-
Penamecillin	T36.0X1-	T36.0X2-	T36.0X3-	T36.0X4-	T36.0X5-	T36.0X6-
Penbutolol	T44.7X1-	T44.7X2-	T44.7X3-	T44.7X4-	T44.7X5-	T44.7X6-
Penethamate	T36.0X1-	T36.0X2-	T36.0X3-	T36.0X4-	T36.0X5-	T36.0X6-
Penfluridol	T43.591-	T43.592-	T43.593-	T43.594-	T43.595-	T43.596-
Penflutizide	T50.2X1-	T50.2X2-	T50.2X3-	T50.2X4-	T50.2X5-	T50.2X6-
Pengitoxin	T46.0X1-	T46.0X2-	T46.0X3-	T46.0X4-	T46.0X5-	T46.0X6-
Penicillamine	T50.6X1-	T50.6X2-	T50.6X3-	T50.6X4-	T50.6X5-	T50.6X6-
Penicillin (any)	T36.0X1-	T36.0X2-	T36.0X3-	T36.0X4-	T36.0X5-	T36.0X6-
Penicillinase	T45.3X1-	T45.3X2-	T45.3X3-	T45.3X4-	T45.3X5-	T45.3X6-
Penicilloyl polylysine	T50.8X1-	T50.8X2-	T50.8X3-	T50.8X4-	T50.8X5-	T50.8X6-
Penimepicycline	T36.4X1-	T36.4X2-	T36.4X3-	T36.4X4-	T36.4X5-	T36.4X6-
Pentachloroethane	T53.6X1-	T53.6X2-	T53.6X3-	T53.6X4-	-	-
Pentachloronaphthalene	T53.7X1-	T53.7X2-	T53.7X3-	T53.7X4-	-	-
Pentachlorophenol (pesticide)	T60.1X1-	T60.1X2-	T60.1X3-	T60.1X4-	-	-
fungicide	T60.3X1-	T60.3X2-	T60.3X3-	T60.3X4-	-	-
herbicide	T60.3X1-	T60.3X2-	T60.3X3-	T60.3X4-	-	-
insecticide	T60.1X1-	T60.1X2-	T60.1X3-	T60.1X4-	-	-
Pentaerythritol	T46.3X1-	T46.3X2-	T46.3X3-	T46.3X4-	T46.3X5-	T46.3X6-
chloral	T42.6X1-	T42.6X2-	T42.6X3-	T42.6X4-	T42.6X5-	T42.6X6-
tetranitrate NEC	T46.3X1-	T46.3X2-	T46.3X3-	T46.3X4-	T46.3X5-	T46.3X6-
Pentaerythrityl tetranitrate	T46.3X1-	T46.3X2-	T46.3X3-	T46.3X4-	T46.3X5-	T46.3X6-
Pentagastrin	T50.8X1-	T50.8X2-	T50.8X3-	T50.8X4-	T50.8X5-	T50.8X6-
Pentalin	T53.6X1-	T53.6X2-	T53.6X3-	T53.6X4-	-	-
Pentamethonium bromide	T44.2X1-	T44.2X2-	T44.2X3-	T44.2X4-	T44.2X5-	T44.2X6-
Pentamidine	T37.3X1-	T37.3X2-	T37.3X3-	T37.3X4-	T37.3X5-	T37.3X6-
Pentanol	T51.3X1-	T51.3X2-	T51.3X3-	T51.3X4-	-	-
Pentapyrrolinium (bitartrate)	T44.2X1-	T44.2X2-	T44.2X3-	T44.2X4-	T44.2X5-	T44.2X6-
Pentaquine	T37.2X1-	T37.2X2-	T37.2X3-	T37.2X4-	T37.2X5-	T37.2X6-
Pentazocine	T40.4X1-	T40.4X2-	T40.4X3-	T40.4X4-	T40.4X5-	T40.4X6-
Pentetrazole	T50.7X1-	T50.7X2-	T50.7X3-	T50.7X4-	T50.7X5-	T50.7X6-
Penthienate bromide	T44.3X1-	T44.3X2-	T44.3X3-	T44.3X4-	T44.3X5-	T44.3X6-
Pentifylline	T46.7X1-	T46.7X2-	T46.7X3-	T46.7X4-	T46.7X5-	T46.7X6-
Pentobarbital	T42.3X1-	T42.3X2-	T42.3X3-	T42.3X4-	T42.3X5-	T42.3X6-
sodium	T42.3X1-	T42.3X2-	T42.3X3-	T42.3X4-	T42.3X5-	T42.3X6-
Pentobarbitone	T42.3X1-	T42.3X2-	T42.3X3-	T42.3X4-	T42.3X5-	T42.3X6-
Pentolonium tartrate	T44.2X1-	T44.2X2-	T44.2X3-	T44.2X4-	T44.2X5-	T44.2X6-
Pentosan polysulfate (sodium)	T39.8X1-	T39.8X2-	T39.8X3-	T39.8X4-	T39.8X5-	T39.8X6-
Pentostatin	T45.1X1-	T45.1X2-	T45.1X3-	T45.1X4-	T45.1X5-	T45.1X6-
Pentothal	T41.1X1-	T41.1X2-	T41.1X3-	T41.1X4-	T41.1X5-	T41.1X6-
Pentoxifylline	T46.7X1-	T46.7X2-	T46.7X3-	T46.7X4-	T46.7X5-	T46.7X6-
Pentoxyverine	T48.3X1-	T48.3X2-	T48.3X3-	T48.3X4-	T48.3X5-	T48.3X6-
Pentrinat	T46.3X1-	T46.3X2-	T46.3X3-	T46.3X4-	T46.3X5-	T46.3X6-
Pentylenetetrazole	T50.7X1-	T50.7X2-	T50.7X3-	T50.7X4-	T50.7X5-	T50.7X6-
Pentylsalicylamide	T37.1X1-	T37.1X2-	T37.1X3-	T37.1X4-	T37.1X5-	T37.1X6-

Substance	Poisoning, Accidental (unintentional)	Poisoning, Intentional self-harm	Poisoning, Assault	Poisoning, Undetermined	Adverse effect	Underdosing
Pentymal	T42.3X1-	T42.3X2-	T42.3X3-	T42.3X4-	T42.3X5-	T42.3X6-
Peplomycin	T45.1X1-	T45.1X2-	T45.1X3-	T45.1X4-	T45.1X5-	T45.1X6-
Peppermint (oil)	T47.5X1-	T47.5X2-	T47.5X3-	T47.5X4-	T47.5X5-	T47.5X6-
Pepsin	T47.5X1-	T47.5X2-	T47.5X3-	T47.5X4-	T47.5X5-	T47.5X6-
digestant	T47.5X1-	T47.5X2-	T47.5X3-	T47.5X4-	T47.5X5-	T47.5X6-
Pepstatin	T47.1X1-	T47.1X2-	T47.1X3-	T47.1X4-	T47.1X5-	T47.1X6-
Peptavlon	T50.8X1-	T50.8X2-	T50.8X3-	T50.8X4-	T50.8X5-	T50.8X6-
Perazine	T43.3X1-	T43.3X2-	T43.3X3-	T43.3X4-	T43.3X5-	T43.3X6-
Percaine (spinal)	T41.3X1-	T41.3X2-	T41.3X3-	T41.3X4-	T41.3X5-	T41.3X6-
topical (surface)	T41.3X1-	T41.3X2-	T41.3X3-	T41.3X4-	T41.3X5-	T41.3X6-
Perchloroethylene	T53.3X1-	T53.3X2-	T53.3X3-	T53.3X4-	-	-
medicinal	T37.4X1-	T37.4X2-	T37.4X3-	T37.4X4-	T37.4X5-	T37.4X6-
vapor	T53.3X1-	T53.3X2-	T53.3X3-	T53.3X4-	-	-
Percodan	T40.2X1-	T40.2X2-	T40.2X3-	T40.2X4-	T40.2X5-	T40.2X6-
Percogesic — see also acetaminophen	T45.0X1-	T45.0X2-	T45.0X3-	T45.0X4-	T45.0X5-	T45.0X6-
Percorten	T38.0X1-	T38.0X2-	T38.0X3-	T38.0X4-	T38.0X5-	T38.0X6-
Pergolide	T42.8X1-	T42.8X2-	T42.8X3-	T42.8X4-	T42.8X5-	T42.8X6-
Pergonal	T38.811-	T38.812-	T38.813-	T38.814-	T38.815-	T38.816-
Perhexilene	T46.3X1-	T46.3X2-	T46.3X3-	T46.3X4-	T46.3X5-	T46.3X6-
Perhexiline (maleate)	T46.3X1-	T46.3X2-	T46.3X3-	T46.3X4-	T46.3X5-	T46.3X6-
Periactin	T45.0X1-	T45.0X2-	T45.0X3-	T45.0X4-	T45.0X5-	T45.0X6-
Periciazine	T43.3X1-	T43.3X2-	T43.3X3-	T43.3X4-	T43.3X5-	T43.3X6-
Periclor	T42.6X1-	T42.6X2-	T42.6X3-	T42.6X4-	T42.6X5-	T42.6X6-
Perindopril	T46.4X1-	T46.4X2-	T46.4X3-	T46.4X4-	T46.4X5-	T46.4X6-
Perisoxal	T39.8X1-	T39.8X2-	T39.8X3-	T39.8X4-	T39.8X5-	T39.8X6-
Peritoneal dialysis solution	T50.3X1-	T50.3X2-	T50.3X3-	T50.3X4-	T50.3X5-	T50.3X6-
Peritrate	T46.3X1-	T46.3X2-	T46.3X3-	T46.3X4-	T46.3X5-	T46.3X6-
Perlapine	T42.4X1-	T42.4X2-	T42.4X3-	T42.4X4-	T42.4X5-	T42.4X6-
Permanganate	T65.891-	T65.892-	T65.893-	T65.894-	-	-
Permethrin	T60.1X1-	T60.1X2-	T60.1X3-	T60.1X4-	-	-
Pernocton	T42.3X1-	T42.3X2-	T42.3X3-	T42.3X4-	T42.3X5-	T42.3X6-
Pernoston	T42.3X1-	T42.3X2-	T42.3X3-	T42.3X4-	T42.3X5-	T42.3X6-
Peronine	T40.2X1-	T40.2X2-	T40.2X3-	T40.2X4-	-	-
Perphenazine	T43.3X1-	T43.3X2-	T43.3X3-	T43.3X4-	T43.3X5-	T43.3X6-
Pertofrane	T43.011-	T43.012-	T43.013-	T43.014-	T43.015-	T43.016-
Pertussis						
immune serum (human)	T50.Z11-	T50.Z12-	T50.Z13-	T50.Z14-	T50.Z15-	T50.Z16-
vaccine (with diphtheria toxoid) (with tetanus toxoid)	T50.A11-	T50.A12-	T50.A13-	T50.A14-	T50.A15-	T50.A16-
Peruvian balsam	T49.0X1-	T49.0X2-	T49.0X3-	T49.0X4-	T49.0X5-	T49.0X6-
Peruvoside	T46.0X1-	T46.0X2-	T46.0X3-	T46.0X4-	T46.0X5-	T46.0X6-
Pesticide (dust) (fumes) (vapor) NEC	T60.91X-	T60.92X-	T60.93X-	T60.94X-	-	-
arsenic	T57.0X1-	T57.0X2-	T57.0X3-	T57.0X4-	-	-
chlorinated	T60.1X1-	T60.1X2-	T60.1X3-	T60.1X4-	-	-
cyanide	T65.0X1-	T65.0X2-	T65.0X3-	T65.0X4-	-	-
kerosene	T52.0X1-	T52.0X2-	T52.0X3-	T52.0X4-	-	-
mixture (of compounds)	T60.91X-	T60.92X-	T60.93X-	T60.94X-	-	-
naphthalene	T60.2X1-	T60.2X2-	T60.2X3-	T60.2X4-	-	-
organochlorine (compounds)	T60.1X1-	T60.1X2-	T60.1X3-	T60.1X4-	-	-
petroleum (distillate) (products) NEC	T60.8X1-	T60.8X2-	T60.8X3-	T60.8X4-	-	-
specified ingredient NEC	T60.8X1-	T60.8X2-	T60.8X3-	T60.8X4-	-	-
strychnine	T65.1X1-	T65.1X2-	T65.1X3-	T65.1X4-	-	-
thallium	T60.4X1-	T60.4X2-	T60.4X3-	T60.4X4-	-	-
Pethidine	T40.4X1-	T40.4X2-	T40.4X3-	T40.4X4-	T40.4X5-	T40.4X6-
Petrichloral	T42.6X1-	T42.6X2-	T42.6X3-	T42.6X4-	T42.6X5-	T42.6X6-
Petrol	T52.0X1-	T52.0X2-	T52.0X3-	T52.0X4-	-	
vapor	T52.0X1-	T52.0X2-	T52.0X3-	T52.0X4-	-	
Petrolatum	T49.3X1-	T49.3X2-	T49.3X3-	T49.3X4-	T49.3X5-	T49.3X6-
hydrophilic	T49.3X1-	T49.3X2-	T49.3X3-	T49.3X4-	T49.3X5-	T49.3X6-
liquid	T47.4X1-	T47.4X2-	T47.4X3-	T47.4X4-	T47.4X5-	T47.4X6-
topical	T49.3X1-	T49.3X2-	T49.3X3-	T49.3X4-	T49.3X5-	T49.3X6-
nonmedicinal	T52.0X1-	T52.0X2-	T52.0X3-	T52.0X4-	-	
red veterinary	T49.3X1-	T49.3X2-	T49.3X3-	T49.3X4-	T49.3X5-	T49.3X6-
white	T49.3X1-	T49.3X2-	T49.3X3-	T49.3X4-	T49.3X5-	T49.3X6-
Petroleum (products) NEC	T52.0X1-	T52.0X2-	T52.0X3-	T52.0X4-	-	
benzine (s) — see Ligroin						
ether — see Ligroin						
jelly — see Petrolatum						
naphtha — see Ligroin						
pesticide	T60.8X1-	T60.8X2-	T60.8X3-	T60.8X4-	-	
solids	T52.0X1-	T52.0X2-	T52.0X3-	T52.0X4-	-	
solvents	T52.0X1-	T52.0X2-	T52.0X3-	T52.0X4-	-	
vapor	T52.0X1-	T52.0X2-	T52.0X3-	T52.0X4-	-	
Peyote	T40.991-	T40.992-	T40.993-	T40.994-	-	
Phanodorm, phanodorn	T42.3X1-	T42.3X2-	T42.3X3-	T42.3X4-	T42.3X5-	T42.3X6-

Substance	Poisoning, Accidental (unintentional)	Poisoning, Intentional self-harm	Poisoning, Assault	Poisoning, Undetermined	Adverse effect	Underdosing
Phanquinone	T37.3X1-	T37.3X2-	T37.3X3-	T37.3X4-	T37.3X5-	T37.3X6-
Phanquone	T37.3X1-	T37.3X2-	T37.3X3-	T37.3X4-	T37.3X5-	T37.3X6-
Pharmaceutical						
adjunct NEC	T50.901-	T50.902-	T50.903-	T50.904-	T50.905-	T50.906-
excipient NEC	T50.901-	T50.902-	T50.903-	T50.904-	T50.905-	T50.906-
sweetener	T50.901-	T50.902-	T50.903-	T50.904-	T50.905-	T50.906-
viscous agent	T50.901-	T50.902-	T50.903-	T50.904-	T50.905-	T50.906-
Phemitone	T42.3X1-	T42.3X2-	T42.3X3-	T42.3X4-	T42.3X5-	T42.3X6-
Phenacaine	T41.3X1-	T41.3X2-	T41.3X3-	T41.3X4-	T41.3X5-	T41.3X6-
Phenacemide	T42.6X1-	T42.6X2-	T42.6X3-	T42.6X4-	T42.6X5-	T42.6X6-
Phenacetin	T39.1X1-	T39.1X2-	T39.1X3-	T39.1X4-	T39.1X5-	T39.1X6-
Phenadoxone	T40.2X1-	T40.2X2-	T40.2X3-	T40.2X4-	-	-
Phenaglycodol	T43.591-	T43.592-	T43.593-	T43.594-	T43.595-	T43.596-
Phenantoin	T42.0X1-	T42.0X2-	T42.0X3-	T42.0X4-	T42.0X5-	T42.0X6-
Phenaphthazine reagent	T50.991-	T50.992-	T50.993-	T50.994-	T50.995-	T50.996-
Phenazocine	T40.4X1-	T40.4X2-	T40.4X3-	T40.4X4-	T40.4X5-	T40.4X6-
Phenazone	T39.2X1-	T39.2X2-	T39.2X3-	T39.2X4-	T39.2X5-	T39.2X6-
Phenazopyridine	T39.8X1-	T39.8X2-	T39.8X3-	T39.8X4-	T39.8X5-	T39.8X6-
Phenbenicillin	T36.0X1-	T36.0X2-	T36.0X3-	T36.0X4-	T36.0X5-	T36.0X6-
Phenbutrazate	T50.5X1-	T50.5X2-	T50.5X3-	T50.5X4-	T50.5X5-	T50.5X6-
Phencyclidine	T40.991-	T40.992-	T40.993-	T40.994-	T40.995-	T40.996-
Phendimetrazine	T50.5X1-	T50.5X2-	T50.5X3-	T50.5X4-	T50.5X5-	T50.5X6-
Phenelzine	T43.1X1-	T43.1X2-	T43.1X3-	T43.1X4-	T43.1X5-	T43.1X6-
Phenemal	T42.3X1-	T42.3X2-	T42.3X3-	T42.3X4-	T42.3X5-	T42.3X6-
Phenergan	T42.6X1-	T42.6X2-	T42.6X3-	T42.6X4-	T42.6X5-	T42.6X6-
Pheneticillin	T36.0X1-	T36.0X2-	T36.0X3-	T36.0X4-	T36.0X5-	T36.0X6-
Pheneturide	T42.6X1-	T42.6X2-	T42.6X3-	T42.6X4-	T42.6X5-	T42.6X6-
Phenformin	T38.3X1-	T38.3X2-	T38.3X3-	T38.3X4-	T38.3X5-	T38.3X6-
Phenglutarimide	T44.3X1-	T44.3X2-	T44.3X3-	T44.3X4-	T44.3X5-	T44.3X6-
Phenicarbazide	T39.8X1-	T39.8X2-	T39.8X3-	T39.8X4-	T39.8X5-	T39.8X6-
Phenindamine	T45.0X1-	T45.0X2-	T45.0X3-	T45.0X4-	T45.0X5-	T45.0X6-
Phenindione	T45.511-	T45.512-	T45.513-	T45.514-	T45.515-	T45.516-
Pheniprazine	T43.1X1-	T43.1X2-	T43.1X3-	T43.1X4-	T43.1X5-	T43.1X6-
Pheniramine	T45.0X1-	T45.0X2-	T45.0X3-	T45.0X4-	T45.0X5-	T45.0X6-
Phenisatin	T47.2X1-	T47.2X2-	T47.2X3-	T47.2X4-	T47.2X5-	T47.2X6-
Phenmetrazine	T50.5X1-	T50.5X2-	T50.5X3-	T50.5X4-	T50.5X5-	T50.5X6-
Phenobal	T42.3X1-	T42.3X2-	T42.3X3-	T42.3X4-	T42.3X5-	T42.3X6-
Phenobarbital	T42.3X1-	T42.3X2-	T42.3X3-	T42.3X4-	T42.3X5-	T42.3X6-
with						
mephenytoin	T42.3X1-	T42.3X2-	T42.3X3-	T42.3X4-	T42.3X5-	T42.3X6-
phenytoin	T42.3X1-	T42.3X2-	T42.3X3-	T42.3X4-	T42.3X5-	T42.3X6-
sodium	T42.3X1-	T42.3X2-	T42.3X3-	T42.3X4-	T42.3X5-	T42.3X6-
Phenobarbitone	T42.3X1-	T42.3X2-	T42.3X3-	T42.3X4-	T42.3X5-	T42.3X6-
Phenobutiodil	T50.8X1-	T50.8X2-	T50.8X3-	T50.8X4-	T50.8X5-	T50.8X6-
Phenoctide	T49.0X1-	T49.0X2-	T49.0X3-	T49.0X4-	T49.0X5-	T49.0X6-
Phenol	T49.0X1-	T49.0X2-	T49.0X3-	T49.0X4-	T49.0X5-	T49.0X6-
disinfectant	T54.0X1-	T54.0X2-	T54.0X3-	T54.0X4-	-	-
in oil injection	T46.8X1-	T46.8X2-	T46.8X3-	T46.8X4-	T46.8X5-	T46.8X6-
medicinal	T49.1X1-	T49.1X2-	T49.1X3-	T49.1X4-	T49.1X5-	T49.1X6-
nonmedicinal NEC	T54.0X1-	T54.0X2-	T54.0X3-	T54.0X4-	-	-
pesticide	T60.8X1-	T60.8X2-	T60.8X3-	T60.8X4-	-	-
red	T50.8X1-	T50.8X2-	T50.8X3-	T50.8X4-	T50.8X5-	T50.8X6-
Phenolic preparation	T49.1X1-	T49.1X2-	T49.1X3-	T49.1X4-	T49.1X5-	T49.1X6-
Phenolphthalein	T47.2X1-	T47.2X2-	T47.2X3-	T47.2X4-	T47.2X5-	T47.2X6-
Phenolsulfonphthalein	T50.8X1-	T50.8X2-	T50.8X3-	T50.8X4-	T50.8X5-	T50.8X6-
Phenomorphan	T40.2X1-	T40.2X2-	T40.2X3-	T40.2X4-	-	-
Phenonyl	T42.3X1-	T42.3X2-	T42.3X3-	T42.3X4-	T42.3X5-	T42.3X6-
Phenoperidine	T40.4X1-	T40.4X2-	T40.4X3-	T40.4X4-	-	-
Phenopyrazone	T46.991-	T46.992-	T46.993-	T46.994-	T46.995-	T46.996-
Phenoquin	T50.4X1-	T50.4X2-	T50.4X3-	T50.4X4-	T50.4X5-	T50.4X6-
Phenothiazine (psychotropic) NEC	T43.3X1-	T43.3X2-	T43.3X3-	T43.3X4-	T43.3X5-	T43.3X6-
insecticide	T60.2X1-	T60.2X2-	T60.2X3-	T60.2X4-	-	-
Phenothrin	T49.0X1-	T49.0X2-	T49.0X3-	T49.0X4-	T49.0X5-	T49.0X6-
Phenoxybenzamine	T46.7X1-	T46.7X2-	T46.7X3-	T46.7X4-	T46.7X5-	T46.7X6-
Phenoxyethanol	T49.0X1-	T49.0X2-	T49.0X3-	T49.0X4-	T49.0X5-	T49.0X6-
Phenoxymethyl penicillin	T36.0X1-	T36.0X2-	T36.0X3-	T36.0X4-	T36.0X5-	T36.0X6-
Phenprobamate	T42.8X1-	T42.8X2-	T42.8X3-	T42.8X4-	T42.8X5-	T42.8X6-
Phenprocoumon	T45.511-	T45.512-	T45.513-	T45.514-	T45.515-	T45.516-
Phensuximide	T42.2X1-	T42.2X2-	T42.2X3-	T42.2X4-	T42.2X5-	T42.2X6-
Phentermine	T50.5X1-	T50.5X2-	T50.5X3-	T50.5X4-	T50.5X5-	T50.5X6-
Phenthicillin	T36.0X1-	T36.0X2-	T36.0X3-	T36.0X4-	T36.0X5-	T36.0X6-
Phentolamine	T46.7X1-	T46.7X2-	T46.7X3-	T46.7X4-	T46.7X5-	T46.7X6-
Phenyl						
butazone	T39.2X1-	T39.2X2-	T39.2X3-	T39.2X4-	T39.2X5-	T39.2X6-
enediamine	T65.3X1-	T65.3X2-	T65.3X3-	T65.3X4-	-	-
hydrazine	T65.3X1-	T65.3X2-	T65.3X3-	T65.3X4-	-	-
antineoplastic	T45.1X1-	T45.1X2-	T45.1X3-	T45.1X4-	T45.1X5-	T45.1X6-

Substance	Poisoning, Accidental (unintentional)	Poisoning, Intentional self-harm	Poisoning, Assault	Poisoning, Undetermined	Adverse effect	Underdosing
Phenyl - *continued*						
mercuric compounds — *see* Mercury						
salicylate	T49.3X1-	T49.3X2-	T49.3X3-	T49.3X4-	T49.3X5-	T49.3X6-
Phenylalanine mustard	T45.1X1-	T45.1X2-	T45.1X3-	T45.1X4-	T45.1X5-	T45.1X6-
Phenylbutazone	T39.2X1-	T39.2X2-	T39.2X3-	T39.2X4-	T39.2X5-	T39.2X6-
Phenylenediamine	T65.3X1-	T65.3X2-	T65.3X3-	T65.3X4-	-	-
Phenylephrine	T44.4X1-	T44.4X2-	T44.4X3-	T44.4X4-	T44.4X5-	T44.4X6-
Phenylethylbiguanide	T38.3X1-	T38.3X2-	T38.3X3-	T38.3X4-	T38.3X5-	T38.3X6-
Phenylmercuric						
acetate	T49.0X1-	T49.0X2-	T49.0X3-	T49.0X4-	T49.0X5-	T49.0X6-
borate	T49.0X1-	T49.0X2-	T49.0X3-	T49.0X4-	T49.0X5-	T49.0X6-
nitrate	T49.0X1-	T49.0X2-	T49.0X3-	T49.0X4-	T49.0X5-	T49.0X6-
Phenylmethylbarbitone	T42.3X1-	T42.3X2-	T42.3X3-	T42.3X4-	T42.3X5-	T42.3X6-
Phenylpropanol	T47.5X1-	T47.5X2-	T47.5X3-	T47.5X4-	T47.5X5-	T47.5X6-
Phenylpropanolamine	T44.991-	T44.992-	T44.993-	T44.994-	T44.995-	T44.996-
Phenylsulfthion	T60.0X1-	T60.0X2-	T60.0X3-	T60.0X4-	-	-
Phenyltoloxamine	T45.0X1-	T45.0X2-	T45.0X3-	T45.0X4-	T45.0X5-	T45.0X6-
Phenyramidol, phenyramidon	T39.8X1-	T39.8X2-	T39.8X3-	T39.8X4-	T39.8X5-	T39.8X6-
Phenytoin	T42.0X1-	T42.0X2-	T42.0X3-	T42.0X4-	T42.0X5-	T42.0X6-
with Phenobarbital	T42.3X1-	T42.3X2-	T42.3X3-	T42.3X4-	T42.3X5-	T42.3X6-
pHisoHex	T49.2X1-	T49.2X2-	T49.2X3-	T49.2X4-	T49.2X5-	T49.2X6-
Pholcodine	T48.3X1-	T48.3X2-	T48.3X3-	T48.3X4-	T48.3X5-	T48.3X6-
Pholedrine	T46.991-	T46.992-	T46.993-	T46.994-	T46.995-	T46.996-
Phorate	T60.0X1-	T60.0X2-	T60.0X3-	T60.0X4-	-	-
Phosdrin	T60.0X1-	T60.0X2-	T60.0X3-	T60.0X4-	-	-
Phosfolan	T60.0X1-	T60.0X2-	T60.0X3-	T60.0X4-	-	-
Phosgene (gas)	T59.891-	T59.892-	T59.893-	T59.894-	-	-
Phosphamidon	T60.0X1-	T60.0X2-	T60.0X3-	T60.0X4-	-	-
Phosphate	T65.891-	T65.892-	T65.893-	T65.894-	-	-
laxative	T47.4X1-	T47.4X2-	T47.4X3-	T47.4X4-	T47.4X5-	T47.4X6-
organic	T60.0X1-	T60.0X2-	T60.0X3-	T60.0X4-	-	-
solvent	T52.91X-	T52.92X-	T52.93X-	T52.94X-	-	-
tricresyl	T65.891-	T65.892-	T65.893-	T65.894-	-	-
Phosphine	T57.1X1-	T57.1X2-	T57.1X3-	T57.1X4-	-	-
fumigant	T57.1X1-	T57.1X2-	T57.1X3-	T57.1X4-	-	-
Phospholine	T49.5X1-	T49.5X2-	T49.5X3-	T49.5X4-	T49.5X5-	T49.5X6-
Phosphoric acid	T54.2X1-	T54.2X2-	T54.2X3-	T54.2X4-	-	-
Phosphorus (compound) NEC	T57.1X1-	T57.1X2-	T57.1X3-	T57.1X4-	-	-
pesticide	T60.0X1-	T60.0X2-	T60.0X3-	T60.0X4-	-	-
Phthalates	T65.891-	T65.892-	T65.893-	T65.894-	-	-
Phthalic anhydride	T65.891-	T65.892-	T65.893-	T65.894-	-	-
Phthalimidoglutarimide	T42.6X1-	T42.6X2-	T42.6X3-	T42.6X4-	T42.6X5-	T42.6X6-
Phthalylsulfathiazole	T37.0X1-	T37.0X2-	T37.0X3-	T37.0X4-	T37.0X5-	T37.0X6-
Phylloquinone	T45.7X1-	T45.7X2-	T45.7X3-	T45.7X4-	T45.7X5-	T45.7X6-
Physeptone	T40.3X1-	T40.3X2-	T40.3X3-	T40.3X4-	T40.3X5-	T40.3X6-
Physostigma venenosum	T62.2X1-	T62.2X2-	T62.2X3-	T62.2X4-	-	-
Physostigmine	T49.5X1-	T49.5X2-	T49.5X3-	T49.5X4-	T49.5X5-	T49.5X6-
Phytolacca decandra	T62.2X1-	T62.2X2-	T62.2X3-	T62.2X4-	-	-
berries	T62.1X1-	T62.1X2-	T62.1X3-	T62.1X4-	-	-
Phytomenadione	T45.7X1-	T45.7X2-	T45.7X3-	T45.7X4-	T45.7X5-	T45.7X6-
Phytonadione	T45.7X1-	T45.7X2-	T45.7X3-	T45.7X4-	T45.7X5-	T45.7X6-
Picoperine	T48.3X1-	T48.3X2-	T48.3X3-	T48.3X4-	T48.3X5-	T48.3X6-
Picosulfate (sodium)	T47.2X1-	T47.2X2-	T47.2X3-	T47.2X4-	T47.2X5-	T47.2X6-
Picric (acid)	T54.2X1-	T54.2X2-	T54.2X3-	T54.2X4-	-	-
Picrotoxin	T50.7X1-	T50.7X2-	T50.7X3-	T50.7X4-	T50.7X5-	T50.7X6-
Piketoprofen	T49.0X1-	T49.0X2-	T49.0X3-	T49.0X4-	T49.0X5-	T49.0X6-
Pilocarpine	T44.1X1-	T44.1X2-	T44.1X3-	T44.1X4-	T44.1X5-	T44.1X6-
Pilocarpus (jaborandi) extract	T44.1X1-	T44.1X2-	T44.1X3-	T44.1X4-	T44.1X5-	T44.1X6-
Pilsicainide (hydrochloride)	T46.2X1-	T46.2X2-	T46.2X3-	T46.2X4-	T46.2X5-	T46.2X6-
Pimaricin	T36.7X1-	T36.7X2-	T36.7X3-	T36.7X4-	T36.7X5-	T36.7X6-
Pimeclone	T50.7X1-	T50.7X2-	T50.7X3-	T50.7X4-	T50.7X5-	T50.7X6-
Pimelic ketone	T52.8X1-	T52.8X2-	T52.8X3-	T52.8X4-	-	-
Pimethixene	T45.0X1-	T45.0X2-	T45.0X3-	T45.0X4-	T45.0X5-	T45.0X6-
Piminodine	T40.2X1-	T40.2X2-	T40.2X3-	T40.2X4-	T40.2X5-	T40.2X6-
Pimozide	T43.591-	T43.592-	T43.593-	T43.594-	T43.595-	T43.596-
Pinacidil	T46.5X1-	T46.5X2-	T46.5X3-	T46.5X4-	T46.5X5-	T46.5X6-
Pinaverium bromide	T44.3X1-	T44.3X2-	T44.3X3-	T44.3X4-	T44.3X5-	T44.3X6-
Pinazepam	T42.4X1-	T42.4X2-	T42.4X3-	T42.4X4-	T42.4X5-	T42.4X6-
Pindolol	T44.7X1-	T44.7X2-	T44.7X3-	T44.7X4-	T44.7X5-	T44.7X6-
Pindone	T60.4X1-	T60.4X2-	T60.4X3-	T60.4X4-	-	-
Pine oil (disinfectant)	T65.891-	T65.892-	T65.893-	T65.894-	-	-
Pinkroot	T37.4X1-	T37.4X2-	T37.4X3-	T37.4X4-	T37.4X5-	T37.4X6-
Pipadone	T40.2X1-	T40.2X2-	T40.2X3-	T40.2X4-	-	-
Pipamazine	T45.0X1-	T45.0X2-	T45.0X3-	T45.0X4-	T45.0X5-	T45.0X6-
Pipamperone	T43.4X1-	T43.4X2-	T43.4X3-	T43.4X4-	T43.4X5-	T43.4X6-
Pipazetate	T48.3X1-	T48.3X2-	T48.3X3-	T48.3X4-	T48.3X5-	T48.3X6-
Pipemidic acid	T37.8X1-	T37.8X2-	T37.8X3-	T37.8X4-	T37.8X5-	T37.8X6-

Table of Drugs and Chemicals — Pipenzolate bromide — Pramoxine

Substance	Poisoning, Accidental (unintentional)	Poisoning, Intentional self-harm	Poisoning, Assault	Poisoning, Undetermined	Adverse effect	Underdosing
Pipenzolate bromide	T44.3X1-	T44.3X2-	T44.3X3-	T44.3X4-	T44.3X5-	T44.3X6-
Piperacetazine	T43.3X1-	T43.3X2-	T43.3X3-	T43.3X4-	T43.3X5-	T43.3X6-
Piperacillin	T36.0X1-	T36.0X2-	T36.0X3-	T36.0X4-	T36.0X5-	T36.0X6-
Piperazine	T37.4X1-	T37.4X2-	T37.4X3-	T37.4X4-	T37.4X5-	T37.4X6-
estrone sulfate	T38.5X1-	T38.5X2-	T38.5X3-	T38.5X4-	T38.5X5-	T38.5X6-
Piper cubeba	T62.2X1-	T62.2X2-	T62.2X3-	T62.2X4-	-	-
Piperidione	T48.3X1-	T48.3X2-	T48.3X3-	T48.3X4-	T48.3X5-	T48.3X6-
Piperidolate	T44.3X1-	T44.3X2-	T44.3X3-	T44.3X4-	T44.3X5-	T44.3X6-
Piperocaine	T41.3X1-	T41.3X2-	T41.3X3-	T41.3X4-	T41.3X5-	T41.3X6-
infiltration (subcutaneous)	T41.3X1-	T41.3X2-	T41.3X3-	T41.3X4-	T41.3X5-	T41.3X6-
nerve block (peripheral) (plexus)	T41.3X1-	T41.3X2-	T41.3X3-	T41.3X4-	T41.3X5-	T41.3X6-
topical (surface)	T41.3X1-	T41.3X2-	T41.3X3-	T41.3X4-	T41.3X5-	T41.3X6-
Piperonyl butoxide	T60.8X1-	T60.8X2-	T60.8X3-	T60.8X4-	-	-
Pipethanate	T44.3X1-	T44.3X2-	T44.3X3-	T44.3X4-	T44.3X5-	T44.3X6-
Pipobroman	T45.1X1-	T45.1X2-	T45.1X3-	T45.1X4-	T45.1X5-	T45.1X6-
Pipotiazine	T43.3X1-	T43.3X2-	T43.3X3-	T43.3X4-	T43.3X5-	T43.3X6-
Pipoxizine	T45.0X1-	T45.0X2-	T45.0X3-	T45.0X4-	T45.0X5-	T45.0X6-
Pipradrol	T43.691-	T43.692-	T43.693-	T43.694-	T43.695-	T43.696-
Piprinhydrinate	T45.0X1-	T45.0X2-	T45.0X3-	T45.0X4-	T45.0X5-	T45.0X6-
Pirarubicin	T45.1X1-	T45.1X2-	T45.1X3-	T45.1X4-	T45.1X5-	T45.1X6-
Pirazinamide	T37.1X1-	T37.1X2-	T37.1X3-	T37.1X4-	T37.1X5-	T37.1X6-
Pirbuterol	T48.6X1-	T48.6X2-	T48.6X3-	T48.6X4-	T48.6X5-	T48.6X6-
Pirenzepine	T47.1X1-	T47.1X2-	T47.1X3-	T47.1X4-	T47.1X5-	T47.1X6-
Piretanide	T50.1X1-	T50.1X2-	T50.1X3-	T50.1X4-	T50.1X5-	T50.1X6-
Piribedil	T42.8X1-	T42.8X2-	T42.8X3-	T42.8X4-	T42.8X5-	T42.8X6-
Piridoxilate	T46.3X1-	T46.3X2-	T46.3X3-	T46.3X4-	T46.3X5-	T46.3X6-
Piritramide	T40.4X1-	T40.4X2-	T40.4X3-	T40.4X4-	-	-
Piromidic acid	T37.8X1-	T37.8X2-	T37.8X3-	T37.8X4-	T37.8X5-	T37.8X6-
Piroxicam	T39.391-	T39.392-	T39.393-	T39.394-	T39.395-	T39.396-
beta-cyclodextrin complex	T39.8X1-	T39.8X2-	T39.8X3-	T39.8X4-	T39.8X5-	T39.8X6-
Pirozadil	T46.6X1-	T46.6X2-	T46.6X3-	T46.6X4-	T46.6X5-	T46.6X6-
Piscidia (bark) (erythrina)	T39.8X1-	T39.8X2-	T39.8X3-	T39.8X4-	T39.8X5-	T39.8X6-
Pitch	T65.891-	T65.892-	T65.893-	T65.894-	-	-
Pitkin's solution	T41.3X1-	T41.3X2-	T41.3X3-	T41.3X4-	T41.3X5-	T41.3X6-
Pitocin	T48.0X1-	T48.0X2-	T48.0X3-	T48.0X4-	T48.0X5-	T48.0X6-
Pitressin (tannate)	T38.891-	T38.892-	T38.893-	T38.894-	T38.895-	T38.896-
Pituitary extracts (posterior)	T38.891-	T38.892-	T38.893-	T38.894-	T38.895-	T38.896-
anterior	T38.811-	T38.812-	T38.813-	T38.814-	T38.815-	T38.816-
Pituitrin	T38.891-	T38.892-	T38.893-	T38.894-	T38.895-	T38.896-
Pivampicillin	T36.0X1-	T36.0X2-	T36.0X3-	T36.0X4-	T36.0X5-	T36.0X6-
Pivmecillinam	T36.0X1-	T36.0X2-	T36.0X3-	T36.0X4-	T36.0X5-	T36.0X6-
Placental hormone	T38.891-	T38.892-	T38.893-	T38.894-	T38.895-	T38.896-
Placidyl	T42.6X1-	T42.6X2-	T42.6X3-	T42.6X4-	T42.6X5-	T42.6X6-
Plague vaccine	T50.A91-	T50.A92-	T50.A93-	T50.A94-	T50.A95-	T50.A96-
Plant						
food or fertilizer NEC	T65.891-	T65.892-	T65.893-	T65.894-	-	-
containing herbicide	T60.3X1-	T60.3X2-	T60.3X3-	T60.3X4-	-	-
noxious, used as food	T62.2X1-	T62.2X2-	T62.2X3-	T62.2X4-	-	-
berries	T62.1X1-	T62.1X2-	T62.1X3-	T62.1X4-	-	-
seeds	T62.2X1-	T62.2X2-	T62.2X3-	T62.2X4-	-	-
specified type NEC	T62.2X1-	T62.2X2-	T62.2X3-	T62.2X4-	-	-
Plasma	T45.8X1-	T45.8X2-	T45.8X3-	T45.8X4-	T45.8X5-	T45.8X6-
expander NEC	T45.8X1-	T45.8X2-	T45.8X3-	T45.8X4-	T45.8X5-	T45.8X6-
protein fraction (human)	T45.8X1-	T45.8X2-	T45.8X3-	T45.8X4-	T45.8X5-	T45.8X6-
Plasmanate	T45.8X1-	T45.8X2-	T45.8X3-	T45.8X4-	T45.8X5-	T45.8X6-
Plasminogen (tissue) activator	T45.611-	T45.612-	T45.613-	T45.614-	T45.615-	T45.616-
Plaster dressing	T49.3X1-	T49.3X2-	T49.3X3-	T49.3X4-	T49.3X5-	T49.3X6-
Plastic dressing	T49.3X1-	T49.3X2-	T49.3X3-	T49.3X4-	T49.3X5-	T49.3X6-
Plegicil	T43.3X1-	T43.3X2-	T43.3X3-	T43.3X4-	T43.3X5-	T43.3X6-
Plicamycin	T45.1X1-	T45.1X2-	T45.1X3-	T45.1X4-	T45.1X5-	T45.1X6-
Podophyllotoxin	T49.8X1-	T49.8X2-	T49.8X3-	T49.8X4-	T49.8X5-	T49.8X6-
Podophyllum (resin)	T49.4X1-	T49.4X2-	T49.4X3-	T49.4X4-	T49.4X5-	T49.4X6-
Poison NEC	T65.91X-	T65.92X-	T65.93X-	T65.94X-	-	-
Poisonous berries	T62.1X1-	T62.1X2-	T62.1X3-	T62.1X4-	-	-
Pokeweed (any part)	T62.2X1-	T62.2X2-	T62.2X3-	T62.2X4-	-	-
Poldine metilsulfate	T44.3X1-	T44.3X2-	T44.3X3-	T44.3X4-	T44.3X5-	T44.3X6-
Polidexide (sulfate)	T46.6X1-	T46.6X2-	T46.6X3-	T46.6X4-	T46.6X5-	T46.6X6-
Polidocanol	T46.8X1-	T46.8X2-	T46.8X3-	T46.8X4-	T46.8X5-	T46.8X6-
Poliomyelitis vaccine	T50.B91-	T50.B92-	T50.B93-	T50.B94-	T50.B95-	T50.B96-
Polish (car) (floor) (furni-ture) (metal) (porcelain) (silver)	T65.891-	T65.892-	T65.893-	T65.894-	-	-
abrasive	T65.891-	T65.892-	T65.893-	T65.894-	-	-
porcelain	T65.891-	T65.892-	T65.893-	T65.894-	-	-
Poloxalkol	T47.4X1-	T47.4X2-	T47.4X3-	T47.4X4-	T47.4X5-	T47.4X6-
Poloxamer	T47.4X1-	T47.4X2-	T47.4X3-	T47.4X4-	T47.4X5-	T47.4X6-
Polyaminostyrene resins	T50.3X1-	T50.3X2-	T50.3X3-	T50.3X4-	T50.3X5-	T50.3X6-
Polycarbophil	T47.4X1-	T47.4X2-	T47.4X3-	T47.4X4-	T47.4X5-	T47.4X6-

Substance	Poisoning, Accidental (unintentional)	Poisoning, Intentional self-harm	Poisoning, Assault	Poisoning, Undetermined	Adverse effect	Underdosing
Polychlorinated biphenyl	T65.891-	T65.892-	T65.893-	T65.894-	-	-
Polycycline	T36.4X1-	T36.4X2-	T36.4X3-	T36.4X4-	T36.4X5-	T36.4X6-
Polyester fumes	T59.891-	T59.892-	T59.893-	T59.894-	-	-
Polyester resin hardener	T52.91X-	T52.92X-	T52.93X-	T52.94X-	-	-
fumes	T59.891-	T59.892-	T59.893-	T59.894-	-	-
Polyestradiol phosphate	T38.5X1-	T38.5X2-	T38.5X3-	T38.5X4-	T38.5X5-	T38.5X6-
Polyethanolamine alkyl sulfate	T49.2X1-	T49.2X2-	T49.2X3-	T49.2X4-	T49.2X5-	T49.2X6-
Polyethylene adhesive	T49.3X1-	T49.3X2-	T49.3X3-	T49.3X4-	T49.3X5-	T49.3X6-
Polyferose	T45.4X1-	T45.4X2-	T45.4X3-	T45.4X4-	T45.4X5-	T45.4X6-
Polygeline	T45.8X1-	T45.8X2-	T45.8X3-	T45.8X4-	T45.8X5-	T45.8X6-
Polymyxin	T36.8X1-	T36.8X2-	T36.8X3-	T36.8X4-	T36.8X5-	T36.8X6-
B	T36.8X1-	T36.8X2-	T36.8X3-	T36.8X4-	T36.8X5-	T36.8X6-
ENT agent	T49.6X1-	T49.6X2-	T49.6X3-	T49.6X4-	T49.6X5-	T49.6X6-
ophthalmic preparation	T49.5X1-	T49.5X2-	T49.5X3-	T49.5X4-	T49.5X5-	T49.5X6-
topical NEC	T49.0X1-	T49.0X2-	T49.0X3-	T49.0X4-	T49.0X5-	T49.0X6-
E sulfate (eye preparation)	T49.5X1-	T49.5X2-	T49.5X3-	T49.5X4-	T49.5X5-	T49.5X6-
Polynoxylin	T49.0X1-	T49.0X2-	T49.0X3-	T49.0X4-	T49.0X5-	T49.0X6-
Polyoestradiol phosphate	T38.5X1-	T38.5X2-	T38.5X3-	T38.5X4-	T38.5X5-	T38.5X6-
Polyoxymethyleneurea	T49.0X1-	T49.0X2-	T49.0X3-	T49.0X4-	T49.0X5-	T49.0X6-
Polysilane	T47.8X1-	T47.8X2-	T47.8X3-	T47.8X4-	T47.8X5-	T47.8X6-
Polytetrafluoroethylene (inhaled)	T59.891-	T59.892-	T59.893-	T59.894-	-	-
Polythiazide	T50.2X1-	T50.2X2-	T50.2X3-	T50.2X4-	T50.2X5-	T50.2X6-
Polyvidone	T45.8X1-	T45.8X2-	T45.8X3-	T45.8X4-	T45.8X5-	T45.8X6-
Polyvinylpyrrolidone	T45.8X1-	T45.8X2-	T45.8X3-	T45.8X4-	T45.8X5-	T45.8X6-
Pontocaine (hydrochloride) (infiltration) (topical)	T41.3X1-	T41.3X2-	T41.3X3-	T41.3X4-	T41.3X5-	T41.3X6-
nerve block (peripheral) (plexus)	T41.3X1-	T41.3X2-	T41.3X3-	T41.3X4-	T41.3X5-	T41.3X6-
spinal	T41.3X1-	T41.3X2-	T41.3X3-	T41.3X4-	T41.3X5-	T41.3X6-
Porfiromycin	T45.1X1-	T45.1X2-	T45.1X3-	T45.1X4-	T45.1X5-	T45.1X6-
Posterior pituitary hormone NEC	T38.891-	T38.892-	T38.893-	T38.894-	T38.895-	T38.896-
Pot	T40.7X1-	T40.7X2-	T40.7X3-	T40.7X4-	T40.7X5-	T40.7X6-
Potash (caustic)	T54.3X1-	T54.3X2-	T54.3X3-	T54.3X4-	-	-
Potassic saline injection (lactated)	T50.3X1-	T50.3X2-	T50.3X3-	T50.3X4-	T50.3X5-	T50.3X6-
Potassium (salts) NEC	T50.3X1-	T50.3X2-	T50.3X3-	T50.3X4-	T50.3X5-	T50.3X6-
aminobenzoate	T45.8X1-	T45.8X2-	T45.8X3-	T45.8X4-	T45.8X5-	T45.8X6-
aminosalicylate	T37.1X1-	T37.1X2-	T37.1X3-	T37.1X4-	T37.1X5-	T37.1X6-
antimony ' tartrate'	T37.8X1-	T37.8X2-	T37.8X3-	T37.8X4-	T37.8X5-	T37.8X6-
arsenite (solution)	T57.0X1-	T57.0X2-	T57.0X3-	T57.0X4-	-	-
bichromate	T56.2X1-	T56.2X2-	T56.2X3-	T56.2X4-	-	-
bisulfate	T47.3X1-	T47.3X2-	T47.3X3-	T47.3X4-	T47.3X5-	T47.3X6-
bromide	T42.6X1-	T42.6X2-	T42.6X3-	T42.6X4-	T42.6X5-	T42.6X6-
canrenoate	T50.0X1-	T50.0X2-	T50.0X3-	T50.0X4-	T50.0X5-	T50.0X6-
carbonate	T54.3X1-	T54.3X2-	T54.3X3-	T54.3X4-	-	-
chlorate NEC	T65.891-	T65.892-	T65.893-	T65.894-	-	-
chloride	T50.3X1-	T50.3X2-	T50.3X3-	T50.3X4-	T50.3X5-	T50.3X6-
citrate	T50.991-	T50.992-	T50.993-	T50.994-	T50.995-	T50.996-
cyanide	T65.0X1-	T65.0X2-	T65.0X3-	T65.0X4-	-	-
ferric hexacyanoferrate (medicinal)	T50.6X1-	T50.6X2-	T50.6X3-	T50.6X4-	T50.6X5-	T50.6X6-
nonmedicinal	T65.891-	T65.892-	T65.893-	T65.894-	-	-
Fluoride	T57.8X1-	T57.8X2-	T57.8X3-	T57.8X4-	-	-
glucaldrate	T47.1X1-	T47.1X2-	T47.1X3-	T47.1X4-	T47.1X5-	T47.1X6-
hydroxide	T54.3X1-	T54.3X2-	T54.3X3-	T54.3X4-	-	-
iodate	T49.0X1-	T49.0X2-	T49.0X3-	T49.0X4-	T49.0X5-	T49.0X6-
iodide	T48.4X1-	T48.4X2-	T48.4X3-	T48.4X4-	T48.4X5-	T48.4X6-
nitrate	T57.8X1-	T57.8X2-	T57.8X3-	T57.8X4-	-	-
oxalate	T65.891-	T65.892-	T65.893-	T65.894-	-	-
perchlorate (nonmedicinal) NEC	T65.891-	T65.892-	T65.893-	T65.894-	-	-
antithyroid	T38.2X1-	T38.2X2-	T38.2X3-	T38.2X4-	T38.2X5-	T38.2X6-
medicinal	T38.2X1-	T38.2X2-	T38.2X3-	T38.2X4-	T38.2X5-	T38.2X6-
Permanganate (nonmedicinal)	T65.891-	T65.892-	T65.893-	T65.894-	-	-
medicinal	T49.0X1-	T49.0X2-	T49.0X3-	T49.0X4-	T49.0X5-	T49.0X6-
sulfate	T47.2X1-	T47.2X2-	T47.2X3-	T47.2X4-	T47.2X5-	T47.2X6-
Potassium-removing resin	T50.3X1-	T50.3X2-	T50.3X3-	T50.3X4-	T50.3X5-	T50.3X6-
Potassium-retaining drug	T50.3X1-	T50.3X2-	T50.3X3-	T50.3X4-	T50.3X5-	T50.3X6-
Povidone	T45.8X1-	T45.8X2-	T45.8X3-	T45.8X4-	T45.8X5-	T45.8X6-
iodine	T49.0X1-	T49.0X2-	T49.0X3-	T49.0X4-	T49.0X5-	T49.0X6-
Practolol	T44.7X1-	T44.7X2-	T44.7X3-	T44.7X4-	T44.7X5-	T44.7X6-
Prajmalium bitartrate	T46.2X1-	T46.2X2-	T46.2X3-	T46.2X4-	T46.2X5-	T46.2X6-
Pralidoxime (iodide)	T50.6X1-	T50.6X2-	T50.6X3-	T50.6X4-	T50.6X5-	T50.6X6-
chloride	T50.6X1-	T50.6X2-	T50.6X3-	T50.6X4-	T50.6X5-	T50.6X6-
Pramiverine	T44.3X1-	T44.3X2-	T44.3X3-	T44.3X4-	T44.3X5-	T44.3X6-
Pramocaine	T49.1X1-	T49.1X2-	T49.1X3-	T49.1X4-	T49.1X5-	T49.1X6-
Pramoxine	T49.1X1-	T49.1X2-	T49.1X3-	T49.1X4-	T49.1X5-	T49.1X6-

Substance	Poisoning, Accidental (unintentional)	Poisoning, Intentional self-harm	Poisoning, Assault	Poisoning, Undetermined	Adverse effect	Underdosing
Prasterone	T38.7X1-	T38.7X2-	T38.7X3-	T38.7X4-	T38.7X5-	T38.7X6-
Pravastatin	T46.6X1-	T46.6X2-	T46.6X3-	T46.6X4-	T46.6X5-	T46.6X6-
Prazepam	T42.4X1-	T42.4X2-	T42.4X3-	T42.4X4-	T42.4X5-	T42.4X6-
Praziquantel	T37.4X1-	T37.4X2-	T37.4X3-	T37.4X4-	T37.4X5-	T37.4X6-
Prazitone	T43.291-	T43.292-	T43.293-	T43.294-	T43.295-	T43.296-
Prazosin	T44.6X1-	T44.6X2-	T44.6X3-	T44.6X4-	T44.6X5-	T44.6X6-
Prednicarbate	T49.0X1-	T49.0X2-	T49.0X3-	T49.0X4-	T49.0X5-	T49.0X6-
Prednimustine	T45.1X1-	T45.1X2-	T45.1X3-	T45.1X4-	T45.1X5-	T45.1X6-
Prednisolone	T38.0X1-	T38.0X2-	T38.0X3-	T38.0X4-	T38.0X5-	T38.0X6-
ENT agent	T49.6X1-	T49.6X2-	T49.6X3-	T49.6X4-	T49.6X5-	T49.6X6-
ophthalmic preparation	T49.5X1-	T49.5X2-	T49.5X3-	T49.5X4-	T49.5X5-	T49.5X6-
steaglate	T49.0X1-	T49.0X2-	T49.0X3-	T49.0X4-	T49.0X5-	T49.0X6-
topical NEC	T49.0X1-	T49.0X2-	T49.0X3-	T49.0X4-	T49.0X5-	T49.0X6-
Prednisone	T38.0X1-	T38.0X2-	T38.0X3-	T38.0X4-	T38.0X5-	T38.0X6-
Prednylidene	T38.0X1-	T38.0X2-	T38.0X3-	T38.0X4-	T38.0X5-	T38.0X6-
Pregnandiol	T38.5X1-	T38.5X2-	T38.5X3-	T38.5X4-	T38.5X5-	T38.5X6-
Pregneninolone	T38.5X1-	T38.5X2-	T38.5X3-	T38.5X4-	T38.5X5-	T38.5X6-
Preludin	T43.691-	T43.692-	T43.693-	T43.694-	T43.695-	T43.696-
Premarin	T38.5X1-	T38.5X2-	T38.5X3-	T38.5X4-	T38.5X5-	T38.5X6-
Premedication anesthetic	T41.201-	T41.202-	T41.203-	T41.204-	T41.205-	T41.206-
Prenalterol	T44.5X1-	T44.5X2-	T44.5X3-	T44.5X4-	T44.5X5-	T44.5X6-
Prenoxdiazine	T48.3X1-	T48.3X2-	T48.3X3-	T48.3X4-	T48.3X5-	T48.3X6-
Prenylamine	T46.3X1-	T46.3X2-	T46.3X3-	T46.3X4-	T46.3X5-	T46.3X6-
Preparation H	T49.8X1-	T49.8X2-	T49.8X3-	T49.8X4-	T49.8X5-	T49.8X6-
Preparation, local	T49.4X1-	T49.4X2-	T49.4X3-	T49.4X4-	T49.4X5-	T49.4X6-
Preservative (nonmedicinal)	T65.891-	T65.892-	T65.893-	T65.894-	-	-
medicinal	T50.901-	T50.902-	T50.903-	T50.904-	T50.905-	T50.906-
wood	T60.91X-	T60.92X-	T60.93X-	T60.94X-	-	-
Prethcamide	T50.7X1-	T50.7X2-	T50.7X3-	T50.7X4-	T50.7X5-	T50.7X6-
Pride of China	T62.2X1-	T62.2X2-	T62.2X3-	T62.2X4-	-	-
Pridinol	T44.3X1-	T44.3X2-	T44.3X3-	T44.3X4-	T44.3X5-	T44.3X6-
Prifinium bromide	T44.3X1-	T44.3X2-	T44.3X3-	T44.3X4-	T44.3X5-	T44.3X6-
Prilocaine	T41.3X1-	T41.3X2-	T41.3X3-	T41.3X4-	T41.3X5-	T41.3X6-
infiltration (subcutaneous)	T41.3X1-	T41.3X2-	T41.3X3-	T41.3X4-	T41.3X5-	T41.3X6-
nerve block (peripheral) (plexus)	T41.3X1-	T41.3X2-	T41.3X3-	T41.3X4-	T41.3X5-	T41.3X6-
regional	T41.3X1-	T41.3X2-	T41.3X3-	T41.3X4-	T41.3X5-	T41.3X6-
Primaquine	T37.2X1-	T37.2X2-	T37.2X3-	T37.2X4-	T37.2X5-	T37.2X6-
Primidone	T42.6X1-	T42.6X2-	T42.6X3-	T42.6X4-	T42.6X5-	T42.6X6-
Primula (veris)	T62.2X1-	T62.2X2-	T62.2X3-	T62.2X4-	-	-
Prinadol	T40.2X1-	T40.2X2-	T40.2X3-	T40.2X4-	T40.2X5-	T40.2X6-
Priscol, Priscoline	T44.6X1-	T44.6X2-	T44.6X3-	T44.6X4-	T44.6X5-	T44.6X6-
Pristinamycin	T36.3X1-	T36.3X2-	T36.3X3-	T36.3X4-	T36.3X5-	T36.3X6-
Privet	T62.2X1-	T62.2X2-	T62.2X3-	T62.2X4-	-	-
berries	T62.1X1-	T62.1X2-	T62.1X3-	T62.1X4-	-	-
Privine	T44.4X1-	T44.4X2-	T44.4X3-	T44.4X4-	T44.4X5-	T44.4X6-
Pro-Banthine	T44.3X1-	T44.3X2-	T44.3X3-	T44.3X4-	T44.3X5-	T44.3X6-
Probarbital	T42.3X1-	T42.3X2-	T42.3X3-	T42.3X4-	T42.3X5-	T42.3X6-
Probenecid	T50.4X1-	T50.4X2-	T50.4X3-	T50.4X4-	T50.4X5-	T50.4X6-
Probucol	T46.6X1-	T46.6X2-	T46.6X3-	T46.6X4-	T46.6X5-	T46.6X6-
Procainamide	T46.2X1-	T46.2X2-	T46.2X3-	T46.2X4-	T46.2X5-	T46.2X6-
Procaine	T41.3X1-	T41.3X2-	T41.3X3-	T41.3X4-	T41.3X5-	T41.3X6-
benzylpenicillin	T36.0X1-	T36.0X2-	T36.0X3-	T36.0X4-	T36.0X5-	T36.0X6-
nerve block (periphreal) (plexus)	T41.3X1-	T41.3X2-	T41.3X3-	T41.3X4-	T41.3X5-	T41.3X6-
penicillin G	T36.0X1-	T36.0X2-	T36.0X3-	T36.0X4-	T36.0X5-	T36.0X6-
regional	T41.3X1-	T41.3X2-	T41.3X3-	T41.3X4-	T41.3X5-	T41.3X6-
spinal	T41.3X1-	T41.3X2-	T41.3X3-	T41.3X4-	T41.3X5-	T41.3X6-
Procalmidol	T43.591-	T43.592-	T43.593-	T43.594-	T43.595-	T43.596-
Procarbazine	T45.1X1-	T45.1X2-	T45.1X3-	T45.1X4-	T45.1X5-	T45.1X6-
Procaterol	T44.5X1-	T44.5X2-	T44.5X3-	T44.5X4-	T44.5X5-	T44.5X6-
Prochlorperazine	T43.3X1-	T43.3X2-	T43.3X3-	T43.3X4-	T43.3X5-	T43.3X6-
Procyclidine	T44.3X1-	T44.3X2-	T44.3X3-	T44.3X4-	T44.3X5-	T44.3X6-
Producer gas	T58.8X1-	T58.8X2-	T58.8X3-	T58.8X4-	-	-
Profadol	T40.4X1-	T40.4X2-	T40.4X3-	T40.4X4-	T40.4X5-	T40.4X6-
Profenamine	T44.3X1-	T44.3X2-	T44.3X3-	T44.3X4-	T44.3X5-	T44.3X6-
Profenil	T44.3X1-	T44.3X2-	T44.3X3-	T44.3X4-	T44.3X5-	T44.3X6-
Proflavine	T49.0X1-	T49.0X2-	T49.0X3-	T49.0X4-	T49.0X5-	T49.0X6-
Progabide	T42.6X1-	T42.6X2-	T42.6X3-	T42.6X4-	T42.6X5-	T42.6X6-
Progesterone	T38.5X1-	T38.5X2-	T38.5X3-	T38.5X4-	T38.5X5-	T38.5X6-
Progestin	T38.5X1-	T38.5X2-	T38.5X3-	T38.5X4-	T38.5X5-	T38.5X6-
oral contraceptive	T38.4X1-	T38.4X2-	T38.4X3-	T38.4X4-	T38.4X5-	T38.4X6-
Progestogen NEC	T38.5X1-	T38.5X2-	T38.5X3-	T38.5X4-	T38.5X5-	T38.5X6-
Progestone	T38.5X1-	T38.5X2-	T38.5X3-	T38.5X4-	T38.5X5-	T38.5X6-
Proglumide	T47.1X1-	T47.1X2-	T47.1X3-	T47.1X4-	T47.1X5-	T47.1X6-
Proguanil	T37.2X1-	T37.2X2-	T37.2X3-	T37.2X4-	T37.2X5-	T37.2X6-
Prolactin	T38.811-	T38.812-	T38.813-	T38.814-	T38.815-	T38.816-
Prolintane	T43.691-	T43.692-	T43.693-	T43.694-	T43.695-	T43.696-

Substance	Poisoning, Accidental (unintentional)	Poisoning, Intentional self-harm	Poisoning, Assault	Poisoning, Undetermined	Adverse effect	Underdosing
Proloid	T38.1X1-	T38.1X2-	T38.1X3-	T38.1X4-	T38.1X5-	T38.1X6-
Proluton	T38.5X1-	T38.5X2-	T38.5X3-	T38.5X4-	T38.5X5-	T38.5X6-
Promacetin	T37.1X1-	T37.1X2-	T37.1X3-	T37.1X4-	T37.1X5-	T37.1X6-
Promazine	T43.3X1-	T43.3X2-	T43.3X3-	T43.3X4-	T43.3X5-	T43.3X6-
Promedol	T40.2X1-	T40.2X2-	T40.2X3-	T40.2X4-	-	-
Promegestone	T38.5X1-	T38.5X2-	T38.5X3-	T38.5X4-	T38.5X5-	T38.5X6-
Promethazine (teoclate)	T43.3X1-	T43.3X2-	T43.3X3-	T43.3X4-	T43.3X5-	T43.3X6-
Promin	T37.1X1-	T37.1X2-	T37.1X3-	T37.1X4-	T37.1X5-	T37.1X6-
Pronase	T45.3X1-	T45.3X2-	T45.3X3-	T45.3X4-	T45.3X5-	T45.3X6-
Pronestyl (hydrochloride)	T46.2X1-	T46.2X2-	T46.2X3-	T46.2X4-	T46.2X5-	T46.2X6-
Pronetalol	T44.7X1-	T44.7X2-	T44.7X3-	T44.7X4-	T44.7X5-	T44.7X6-
Prontosil	T37.0X1-	T37.0X2-	T37.0X3-	T37.0X4-	T37.0X5-	T37.0X6-
Propachlor	T60.3X1-	T60.3X2-	T60.3X3-	T60.3X4-	-	-
Propafenone	T46.2X1-	T46.2X2-	T46.2X3-	T46.2X4-	T46.2X5-	T46.2X6-
Propallylonal	T42.3X1-	T42.3X2-	T42.3X3-	T42.3X4-	T42.3X5-	T42.3X6-
Propamidine	T49.0X1-	T49.0X2-	T49.0X3-	T49.0X4-	T49.0X5-	T49.0X6-
Propane (distributed in mobile container)	T59.891-	T59.892-	T59.893-	T59.894-	-	-
distributed through pipes	T59.891-	T59.892-	T59.893-	T59.894-	-	-
incomplete combustion	T58.11X-	T58.12X-	T58.13X-	T58.14X-	-	-
Propanidid	T41.291-	T41.292-	T41.293-	T41.294-	T41.295-	T41.296-
Propanil	T60.3X1-	T60.3X2-	T60.3X3-	T60.3X4-	-	-
1-Propanol	T51.3X1-	T51.3X2-	T51.3X3-	T51.3X4-	-	-
2-Propanol	T51.2X1-	T51.2X2-	T51.2X3-	T51.2X4-	-	-
Propantheline	T44.3X1-	T44.3X2-	T44.3X3-	T44.3X4-	T44.3X5-	T44.3X6-
bromide	T44.3X1-	T44.3X2-	T44.3X3-	T44.3X4-	T44.3X5-	T44.3X6-
Proparacaine	T41.3X1-	T41.3X2-	T41.3X3-	T41.3X4-	T41.3X5-	T41.3X6-
Propatylnitrate	T46.3X1-	T46.3X2-	T46.3X3-	T46.3X4-	T46.3X5-	T46.3X6-
Propicillin	T36.0X1-	T36.0X2-	T36.0X3-	T36.0X4-	T36.0X5-	T36.0X6-
Propiolactone	T49.0X1-	T49.0X2-	T49.0X3-	T49.0X4-	T49.0X5-	T49.0X6-
Propiomazine	T45.0X1-	T45.0X2-	T45.0X3-	T45.0X4-	T45.0X5-	T45.0X6-
Propionaldehyde (medicinal)	T42.6X1-	T42.6X2-	T42.6X3-	T42.6X4-	T42.6X5-	T42.6X6-
Propionate (calcium) (sodium)	T49.0X1-	T49.0X2-	T49.0X3-	T49.0X4-	T49.0X5-	T49.0X6-
Propion gel	T49.0X1-	T49.0X2-	T49.0X3-	T49.0X4-	T49.0X5-	T49.0X6-
Propitocaine	T41.3X1-	T41.3X2-	T41.3X3-	T41.3X4-	T41.3X5-	T41.3X6-
infiltration (subcutaneous)	T41.3X1-	T41.3X2-	T41.3X3-	T41.3X4-	T41.3X5-	T41.3X6-
nerve block (peripheral) (plexus)	T41.3X1-	T41.3X2-	T41.3X3-	T41.3X4-	T41.3X5-	T41.3X6-
Propofol	T41.291-	T41.292-	T41.293-	T41.294-	T41.295-	T41.296-
Propoxur	T60.0X1-	T60.0X2-	T60.0X3-	T60.0X4-	-	-
Propoxycaine	T41.3X1-	T41.3X2-	T41.3X3-	T41.3X4-	T41.3X5-	T41.3X6-
infiltration (subcutaneous)	T41.3X1-	T41.3X2-	T41.3X3-	T41.3X4-	T41.3X5-	T41.3X6-
nerve block (peripheral) (plexus)	T41.3X1-	T41.3X2-	T41.3X3-	T41.3X4-	T41.3X5-	T41.3X6-
topical (surface)	T41.3X1-	T41.3X2-	T41.3X3-	T41.3X4-	T41.3X5-	T41.3X6-
Propoxyphene	T40.4X1-	T40.4X2-	T40.4X3-	T40.4X4-	T40.4X5-	T40.4X6-
Propranolol	T44.7X1-	T44.7X2-	T44.7X3-	T44.7X4-	T44.7X5-	T44.7X6-
Propyl						
alcohol	T51.3X1-	T51.3X2-	T51.3X3-	T51.3X4-	-	-
carbinol	T51.3X1-	T51.3X2-	T51.3X3-	T51.3X4-	-	-
hexadrine	T44.4X1-	T44.4X2-	T44.4X3-	T44.4X4-	T44.4X5-	T44.4X6-
iodone	T50.8X1-	T50.8X2-	T50.8X3-	T50.8X4-	T50.8X5-	T50.8X6-
thiouracil	T38.2X1-	T38.2X2-	T38.2X3-	T38.2X4-	T38.2X5-	T38.2X6-
Propylaminopheno-thiazine	T43.3X1-	T43.3X2-	T43.3X3-	T43.3X4-	T43.3X5-	T43.3X6-
Propylene	T59.891-	T59.892-	T59.893-	T59.894-	-	-
Propylhexedrine	T48.5X1-	T48.5X2-	T48.5X3-	T48.5X4-	T48.5X5-	T48.5X6-
Propyliodone	T50.8X1-	T50.8X2-	T50.8X3-	T50.8X4-	T50.8X5-	T50.8X6-
Propylparaben (ophthalmic)	T49.5X1-	T49.5X2-	T49.5X3-	T49.5X4-	T49.5X5-	T49.5X6-
Propylthiouracil	T38.2X1-	T38.2X2-	T38.2X3-	T38.2X4-	T38.2X5-	T38.2X6-
Propyphenazone	T39.2X1-	T39.2X2-	T39.2X3-	T39.2X4-	T39.2X5-	T39.2X6-
Proquazone	T39.391-	T39.392-	T39.393-	T39.394-	T39.395-	T39.396-
Proscillaridin	T46.0X1-	T46.0X2-	T46.0X3-	T46.0X4-	T46.0X5-	T46.0X6-
Prostacyclin	T45.521-	T45.522-	T45.523-	T45.524-	T45.525-	T45.526-
Prostaglandin (I2)	T45.521-	T45.522-	T45.523-	T45.524-	T45.525-	T45.526-
E1	T46.7X1-	T46.7X2-	T46.7X3-	T46.7X4-	T46.7X5-	T46.7X6-
E2	T48.0X1-	T48.0X2-	T48.0X3-	T48.0X4-	T48.0X5-	T48.0X6-
F2 alpha	T48.0X1-	T48.0X2-	T48.0X3-	T48.0X4-	T48.0X5-	T48.0X6-
Prostigmin	T44.0X1-	T44.0X2-	T44.0X3-	T44.0X4-	T44.0X5-	T44.0X6-
Prosultiamine	T45.2X1-	T45.2X2-	T45.2X3-	T45.2X4-	T45.2X5-	T45.2X6-
Protamine sulfate	T45.7X1-	T45.7X2-	T45.7X3-	T45.7X4-	T45.7X5-	T45.7X6-
zinc insulin	T38.3X1-	T38.3X2-	T38.3X3-	T38.3X4-	T38.3X5-	T38.3X6-
Protease	T47.5X1-	T47.5X2-	T47.5X3-	T47.5X4-	T47.5X5-	T47.5X6-
Protectant, skin NEC	T49.3X1-	T49.3X2-	T49.3X3-	T49.3X4-	T49.3X5-	T49.3X6-
Protein hydrolysate	T50.991-	T50.992-	T50.993-	T50.994-	T50.995-	T50.996-
Prothiaden — see Dothiepin hydrochloride						
Prothionamide	T37.1X1-	T37.1X2-	T37.1X3-	T37.1X4-	T37.1X5-	T37.1X6-
Prothipendyl	T43.591-	T43.592-	T43.593-	T43.594-	T43.595-	T43.596-

Substance	Poisoning, Accidental (unintentional)	Poisoning, Intentional self-harm	Poisoning, Assault	Poisoning, Undetermined	Adverse effect	Underdosing
Prothoate	T60.0X1-	T60.0X2-	T60.0X3-	T60.0X4-	-	-
Prothrombin						
activator	T45.7X1-	T45.7X2-	T45.7X3-	T45.7X4-	T45.7X5-	T45.7X6-
synthesis inhibitor	T45.511-	T45.512-	T45.513-	T45.514-	T45.515-	T45.516-
Protionamide	T37.1X1-	T37.1X2-	T37.1X3-	T37.1X4-	T37.1X5-	T37.1X6-
Protirelin	T38.891-	T38.892-	T38.893-	T38.894-	T38.895-	T38.896-
Protokylol	T48.6X1-	T48.6X2-	T48.6X3-	T48.6X4-	T48.6X5-	T48.6X6-
Protopam	T50.6X1-	T50.6X2-	T50.6X3-	T50.6X4-	T50.6X5-	T50.6X6-
Protoveratrine (s) (A) (B)	T46.5X1-	T46.5X2-	T46.5X3-	T46.5X4-	T46.5X5-	T46.5X6-
Protriptyline	T43.011-	T43.012-	T43.013-	T43.014-	T43.015-	T43.016-
Provera	T38.5X1-	T38.5X2-	T38.5X3-	T38.5X4-	T38.5X5-	T38.5X6-
Provitamin A	T45.2X1-	T45.2X2-	T45.2X3-	T45.2X4-	T45.2X5-	T45.2X6-
Proxibarbal	T42.3X1-	T42.3X2-	T42.3X3-	T42.3X4-	T42.3X5-	T42.3X6-
Proxymetacaine	T41.3X1-	T41.3X2-	T41.3X3-	T41.3X4-	T41.3X5-	T41.3X6-
Proxyphylline	T48.6X1-	T48.6X2-	T48.6X3-	T48.6X4-	T48.6X5-	T48.6X6-
Prozac — *see* Fluoxetine hydrochloride						
Prunus						
laurocerasus	T62.2X1-	T62.2X2-	T62.2X3-	T62.2X4-	-	-
virginiana	T62.2X1-	T62.2X2-	T62.2X3-	T62.2X4-	-	-
Prussian blue						
commercial	T65.891-	T65.892-	T65.893-	T65.894-	-	-
therapeutic	T50.6X1-	T50.6X2-	T50.6X3-	T50.6X4-	T50.6X5-	T50.6X6-
Prussic acid	T65.0X1-	T65.0X2-	T65.0X3-	T65.0X4-	-	-
vapor	T57.3X1-	T57.3X2-	T57.3X3-	T57.3X4-	-	-
Pseudoephedrine	T44.991-	T44.992-	T44.993-	T44.994-	T44.995-	T44.996-
Psilocin	T40.991-	T40.992-	T40.993-	T40.994-	-	-
Psilocybin	T40.991-	T40.992-	T40.993-	T40.994-	-	-
Psilocybine	T40.991-	T40.992-	T40.993-	T40.994-	-	-
Psoralene (nonmedicinal)	T65.891-	T65.892-	T65.893-	T65.894-	-	-
Psoralens (medicinal)	T50.991-	T50.992-	T50.993-	T50.994-	T50.995-	T50.996-
PSP (phenolsulfonphthalein)	T50.8X1-	T50.8X2-	T50.8X3-	T50.8X4-	T50.8X5-	T50.8X6-
Psychodysleptic drug NEC	T40.901-	T40.902-	T40.903-	T40.904-	T40.905-	T40.906-
Psychostimulant	T43.601-	T43.602-	T43.603-	T43.604-	T43.605-	T43.606-
amphetamine	T43.621-	T43.622-	T43.623-	T43.624-	T43.625-	T43.626-
caffeine	T43.611-	T43.612-	T43.613-	T43.614-	T43.615-	T43.616-
methylphenidate	T43.631-	T43.632-	T43.633-	T43.634-	T43.635-	T43.636-
specified NEC	T43.691-	T43.692-	T43.693-	T43.694-	T43.695-	T43.696-
Psychotherapeutic drug NEC	T43.91X-	T43.92X-	T43.93X-	T43.94X-	T43.95X-	T43.96X-
antidepressants — *see also* Antidepressant	T43.201-	T43.202-	T43.203-	T43.204-	T43.205-	T43.206-
specified NEC	T43.8X1-	T43.8X2-	T43.8X3-	T43.8X4-	T43.8X5-	T43.8X6-
tranquilizers NEC	T43.501-	T43.502-	T43.503-	T43.504-	T43.505-	T43.506-
Psychotomimetic agents	T40.901-	T40.902-	T40.903-	T40.904-	T40.905-	T40.906-
Psychotropic drug NEC	T43.91X-	T43.92X-	T43.93X-	T43.94X-	T43.95X-	T43.96X-
specified NEC	T43.8X1-	T43.8X2-	T43.8X3-	T43.8X4-	T43.8X5-	T43.8X6-
Psyllium hydrophilic mucilloid	T47.4X1-	T47.4X2-	T47.4X3-	T47.4X4-	T47.4X5-	T47.4X6-
Pteroylglutamic acid	T45.8X1-	T45.8X2-	T45.8X3-	T45.8X4-	T45.8X5-	T45.8X6-
Pteroyltriglutamate	T45.1X1-	T45.1X2-	T45.1X3-	T45.1X4-	T45.1X5-	T45.1X6-
PTFE — *see* Polytetrafluoroethylene						
Pulp						
devitalizing paste	T49.7X1-	T49.7X2-	T49.7X3-	T49.7X4-	T49.7X5-	T49.7X6-
dressing	T49.7X1-	T49.7X2-	T49.7X3-	T49.7X4-	T49.7X5-	T49.7X6-
Pulsatilla	T62.2X1-	T62.2X2-	T62.2X3-	T62.2X4-	-	-
Pumpkin seed extract	T37.4X1-	T37.4X2-	T37.4X3-	T37.4X4-	T37.4X5-	T37.4X6-
Purex (bleach)	T54.91X-	T54.92X-	T54.93X-	T54.94X-	-	-
Purgative NEC — *see also* Cathartic	T47.4X1-	T47.4X2-	T47.4X3-	T47.4X4-	T47.4X5-	T47.4X6-
Purine analogue (antineoplastic)	T45.1X1-	T45.1X2-	T45.1X3-	T45.1X4-	T45.1X5-	T45.1X6-
Purine diuretics	T50.2X1-	T50.2X2-	T50.2X3-	T50.2X4-	T50.2X5-	T50.2X6-
Purinethol	T45.1X1-	T45.1X2-	T45.1X3-	T45.1X4-	T45.1X5-	T45.1X6-
PVP	T45.8X1-	T45.8X2-	T45.8X3-	T45.8X4-	T45.8X5-	T45.8X6-
Pyrabital	T39.8X1-	T39.8X2-	T39.8X3-	T39.8X4-	T39.8X5-	T39.8X6-
Pyramidon	T39.2X1-	T39.2X2-	T39.2X3-	T39.2X4-	T39.2X5-	T39.2X6-
Pyrantel	T37.4X1-	T37.4X2-	T37.4X3-	T37.4X4-	T37.4X5-	T37.4X6-
Pyrathiazine	T45.0X1-	T45.0X2-	T45.0X3-	T45.0X4-	T45.0X5-	T45.0X6-
Pyrazinamide	T37.1X1-	T37.1X2-	T37.1X3-	T37.1X4-	T37.1X5-	T37.1X6-
Pyrazinoic acid (amide)	T37.1X1-	T37.1X2-	T37.1X3-	T37.1X4-	T37.1X5-	T37.1X6-
Pyrazole (derivatives)	T39.2X1-	T39.2X2-	T39.2X3-	T39.2X4-	T39.2X5-	T39.2X6-
Pyrazolone analgesic NEC	T39.2X1-	T39.2X2-	T39.2X3-	T39.2X4-	T39.2X5-	T39.2X6-
Pyrethrin, pyrethrum (nonmedicinal)	T60.2X1-	T60.2X2-	T60.2X3-	T60.2X4-	-	-
Pyrethrum extract	T49.0X1-	T49.0X2-	T49.0X3-	T49.0X4-	T49.0X5-	T49.0X6-
Pyribenzamine	T45.0X1-	T45.0X2-	T45.0X3-	T45.0X4-	T45.0X5-	T45.0X6-
Pyridine	T52.8X1-	T52.8X2-	T52.8X3-	T52.8X4-	-	-
aldoxime methiodide	T50.6X1-	T50.6X2-	T50.6X3-	T50.6X4-	T50.6X5-	T50.6X6-
aldoxime methyl chloride	T50.6X1-	T50.6X2-	T50.6X3-	T50.6X4-	T50.6X5-	T50.6X6-
Pyridine - *continued*						
vapor	T59.891-	T59.892-	T59.893-	T59.894-	-	-
Pyridium	T39.8X1-	T39.8X2-	T39.8X3-	T39.8X4-	T39.8X5-	T39.8X6-
Pyridostigmine bromide	T44.0X1-	T44.0X2-	T44.0X3-	T44.0X4-	T44.0X5-	T44.0X6-
Pyridoxal phosphate	T45.2X1-	T45.2X2-	T45.2X3-	T45.2X4-	T45.2X5-	T45.2X6-
Pyridoxine	T45.2X1-	T45.2X2-	T45.2X3-	T45.2X4-	T45.2X5-	T45.2X6-
Pyrilamine	T45.0X1-	T45.0X2-	T45.0X3-	T45.0X4-	T45.0X5-	T45.0X6-
Pyrimethamine	T37.2X1-	T37.2X2-	T37.2X3-	T37.2X4-	T37.2X5-	T37.2X6-
with sulfadoxine	T37.2X1-	T37.2X2-	T37.2X3-	T37.2X4-	T37.2X5-	T37.2X6-
Pyrimidine antagonist	T45.1X1-	T45.1X2-	T45.1X3-	T45.1X4-	T45.1X5-	T45.1X6-
Pyriminil	T60.4X1-	T60.4X2-	T60.4X3-	T60.4X4-	-	-
Pyrithione zinc	T49.4X1-	T49.4X2-	T49.4X3-	T49.4X4-	T49.4X5-	T49.4X6-
Pyrithyldione	T42.6X1-	T42.6X2-	T42.6X3-	T42.6X4-	T42.6X5-	T42.6X6-
Pyrogallic acid	T49.0X1-	T49.0X2-	T49.0X3-	T49.0X4-	T49.0X5-	T49.0X6-
Pyrogallol	T49.0X1-	T49.0X2-	T49.0X3-	T49.0X4-	T49.0X5-	T49.0X6-
Pyroxylin	T49.3X1-	T49.3X2-	T49.3X3-	T49.3X4-	T49.3X5-	T49.3X6-
Pyrrobutamine	T45.0X1-	T45.0X2-	T45.0X3-	T45.0X4-	T45.0X5-	T45.0X6-
Pyrrolizidine alkaloids	T62.8X1-	T62.8X2-	T62.8X3-	T62.8X4-	-	-
Pyrvinium chloride	T37.4X1-	T37.4X2-	T37.4X3-	T37.4X4-	T37.4X5-	T37.4X6-
PZI	T38.3X1-	T38.3X2-	T38.3X3-	T38.3X4-	T38.3X5-	T38.3X6-
Quaalude	T42.6X1-	T42.6X2-	T42.6X3-	T42.6X4-	T42.6X5-	T42.6X6-
Quarternary ammonium						
anti-infective	T49.0X1-	T49.0X2-	T49.0X3-	T49.0X4-	T49.0X5-	T49.0X6-
ganglion blocking	T44.2X1-	T44.2X2-	T44.2X3-	T44.2X4-	T44.2X5-	T44.2X6-
parasympatholytic	T44.3X1-	T44.3X2-	T44.3X3-	T44.3X4-	T44.3X5-	T44.3X6-
Quazepam	T42.4X1-	T42.4X2-	T42.4X3-	T42.4X4-	T42.4X5-	T42.4X6-
Quicklime	T54.3X1-	T54.3X2-	T54.3X3-	T54.3X4-	-	-
Quillaja extract	T48.4X1-	T48.4X2-	T48.4X3-	T48.4X4-	T48.4X5-	T48.4X6-
Quinacrine	T37.2X1-	T37.2X2-	T37.2X3-	T37.2X4-	T37.2X5-	T37.2X6-
Quinaglute	T46.2X1-	T46.2X2-	T46.2X3-	T46.2X4-	T46.2X5-	T46.2X6-
Quinalbarbital	T42.3X1-	T42.3X2-	T42.3X3-	T42.3X4-	T42.3X5-	T42.3X6-
Quinalbarbitone sodium	T42.3X1-	T42.3X2-	T42.3X3-	T42.3X4-	T42.3X5-	T42.3X6-
Quinalphos	T60.0X1-	T60.0X2-	T60.0X3-	T60.0X4-	-	-
Quinapril	T46.4X1-	T46.4X2-	T46.4X3-	T46.4X4-	T46.4X5-	T46.4X6-
Quinestradiol	T38.5X1-	T38.5X2-	T38.5X3-	T38.5X4-	T38.5X5-	T38.5X6-
Quinestradol	T38.5X1-	T38.5X2-	T38.5X3-	T38.5X4-	T38.5X5-	T38.5X6-
Quinestrol	T38.5X1-	T38.5X2-	T38.5X3-	T38.5X4-	T38.5X5-	T38.5X6-
Quinethazone	T50.2X1-	T50.2X2-	T50.2X3-	T50.2X4-	T50.2X5-	T50.2X6-
Quingestanol	T38.4X1-	T38.4X2-	T38.4X3-	T38.4X4-	T38.4X5-	T38.4X6-
Quinidine	T46.2X1-	T46.2X2-	T46.2X3-	T46.2X4-	T46.2X5-	T46.2X6-
Quinine	T37.2X1-	T37.2X2-	T37.2X3-	T37.2X4-	T37.2X5-	T37.2X6-
Quiniobine	T37.8X1-	T37.8X2-	T37.8X3-	T37.8X4-	T37.8X5-	T37.8X6-
Quinisocaine	T49.1X1-	T49.1X2-	T49.1X3-	T49.1X4-	T49.1X5-	T49.1X6-
Quinocide	T37.2X1-	T37.2X2-	T37.2X3-	T37.2X4-	T37.2X5-	T37.2X6-
Quinoline (derivatives) **NEC**	T37.8X1-	T37.8X2-	T37.8X3-	T37.8X4-	T37.8X5-	T37.8X6-
Quinupramine	T43.011-	T43.012-	T43.013-	T43.014-	T43.015-	T43.016-
Quotane	T41.3X1-	T41.3X2-	T41.3X3-	T41.3X4-	T41.3X5-	T41.3X6-
Rabies						
immune globulin (human)	T50.Z11-	T50.Z12-	T50.Z13-	T50.Z14-	T50.Z15-	T50.Z16-
vaccine	T50.B91-	T50.B92-	T50.B93-	T50.B94-	T50.B95-	T50.B96-
Racemoramide	T40.2X1-	T40.2X2-	T40.2X3-	T40.2X4-	-	-
Racemorphan	T40.2X1-	T40.2X2-	T40.2X3-	T40.2X4-	T40.2X5-	T40.2X6-
Racepinefrin	T44.5X1-	T44.5X2-	T44.5X3-	T44.5X4-	T44.5X5-	T44.5X6-
Raclopride	T43.591-	T43.592-	T43.593-	T43.594-	T43.595-	T43.596-
Radiator alcohol	T51.1X1-	T51.1X2-	T51.1X3-	T51.1X4-	-	-
Radioactive drug NEC	T50.8X1-	T50.8X2-	T50.8X3-	T50.8X4-	T50.8X5-	T50.8X6-
Radio-opaque (drugs) (materials)	T50.8X1-	T50.8X2-	T50.8X3-	T50.8X4-	T50.8X5-	T50.8X6-
Ramifenazone	T39.2X1-	T39.2X2-	T39.2X3-	T39.2X4-	T39.2X5-	T39.2X6-
Ramipril	T46.4X1-	T46.4X2-	T46.4X3-	T46.4X4-	T46.4X5-	T46.4X6-
Ranitidine	T47.0X1-	T47.0X2-	T47.0X3-	T47.0X4-	T47.0X5-	T47.0X6-
Ranunculus	T62.2X1-	T62.2X2-	T62.2X3-	T62.2X4-	-	-
Rat poison NEC	T60.4X1-	T60.4X2-	T60.4X3-	T60.4X4-	-	-
Rattlesnake (venom)	T63.011-	T63.012-	T63.013-	T63.014-	-	-
Raubasine	T46.7X1-	T46.7X2-	T46.7X3-	T46.7X4-	T46.7X5-	T46.7X6-
Raudixin	T46.5X1-	T46.5X2-	T46.5X3-	T46.5X4-	T46.5X5-	T46.5X6-
Rautensin	T46.5X1-	T46.5X2-	T46.5X3-	T46.5X4-	T46.5X5-	T46.5X6-
Rautina	T46.5X1-	T46.5X2-	T46.5X3-	T46.5X4-	T46.5X5-	T46.5X6-
Rautotal	T46.5X1-	T46.5X2-	T46.5X3-	T46.5X4-	T46.5X5-	T46.5X6-
Rauwiloid	T46.5X1-	T46.5X2-	T46.5X3-	T46.5X4-	T46.5X5-	T46.5X6-
Rauwoldin	T46.5X1-	T46.5X2-	T46.5X3-	T46.5X4-	T46.5X5-	T46.5X6-
Rauwolfia (alkaloids)	T46.5X1-	T46.5X2-	T46.5X3-	T46.5X4-	T46.5X5-	T46.5X6-
Razoxane	T45.1X1-	T45.1X2-	T45.1X3-	T45.1X4-	T45.1X5-	T45.1X6-
Realgar	T57.0X1-	T57.0X2-	T57.0X3-	T57.0X4-	-	-
Recombinant (R) — *see* specific protein						
Red blood cells, packed	T45.8X1-	T45.8X2-	T45.8X3-	T45.8X4-	T45.8X5-	T45.8X6-
Red squill (scilliroside)	T60.4X1-	T60.4X2-	T60.4X3-	T60.4X4-	-	-

Substance	Poisoning, Accidental (unintentional)	Poisoning, Intentional self-harm	Poisoning, Assault	Poisoning, Undetermined	Adverse effect	Underdosing
Reducing agent, industrial NEC	T65.891-	T65.892-	T65.893-	T65.894-	-	-
Refrigerant gas (chlorofluoro-carbon)	T53.5X1-	T53.5X2-	T53.5X3-	T53.5X4-	-	-
not chlorofluoro-carbon	T59.891-	T59.892-	T59.893-	T59.894-	-	-
Regroton	T50.2X1-	T50.2X2-	T50.2X3-	T50.2X4-	T50.2X5-	T50.2X6-
Rehydration salts (oral)	T50.3X1-	T50.3X2-	T50.3X3-	T50.3X4-	T50.3X5-	T50.3X6-
Rela	T42.8X1-	T42.8X2-	T42.8X3-	T42.8X4-	T42.8X5-	T42.8X6-
Relaxant, muscle						
anesthetic	T48.1X1-	T48.1X2-	T48.1X3-	T48.1X4-	T48.1X5-	T48.1X6-
central nervous system	T42.8X1-	T42.8X2-	T42.8X3-	T42.8X4-	T42.8X5-	T42.8X6-
skeletal NEC	T48.1X1-	T48.1X2-	T48.1X3-	T48.1X4-	T48.1X5-	T48.1X6-
smooth NEC	T44.3X1-	T44.3X2-	T44.3X3-	T44.3X4-	T44.3X5-	T44.3X6-
Remoxipride	T43.591-	T43.592-	T43.593-	T43.594-	T43.595-	T43.596-
Renese	T50.2X1-	T50.2X2-	T50.2X3-	T50.2X4-	T50.2X5-	T50.2X6-
Renografin	T50.8X1-	T50.8X2-	T50.8X3-	T50.8X4-	T50.8X5-	T50.8X6-
Replacement solution	T50.3X1-	T50.3X2-	T50.3X3-	T50.3X4-	T50.3X5-	T50.3X6-
Reproterol	T48.6X1-	T48.6X2-	T48.6X3-	T48.6X4-	T48.6X5-	T48.6X6-
Rescinnamine	T46.5X1-	T46.5X2-	T46.5X3-	T46.5X4-	T46.5X5-	T46.5X6-
Reserpin (e)	T46.5X1-	T46.5X2-	T46.5X3-	T46.5X4-	T46.5X5-	T46.5X6-
Resorcin, resorcinol (nonmedicinal)	T65.891-	T65.892-	T65.893-	T65.894-		
medicinal	T49.4X1-	T49.4X2-	T49.4X3-	T49.4X4-	T49.4X5-	T49.4X6-
Respaire	T48.4X1-	T48.4X2-	T48.4X3-	T48.4X4-	T48.4X5-	T48.4X6-
Respiratory drug NEC	T48.901-	T48.902-	T48.903-	T48.904-	T48.905-	T48.906-
antiasthmatic NEC	T48.6X1-	T48.6X2-	T48.6X3-	T48.6X4-	T48.6X5-	T48.6X6-
anti-common-cold NEC	T48.5X1-	T48.5X2-	T48.5X3-	T48.5X4-	T48.5X5-	T48.5X6-
expectorant NEC	T48.4X1-	T48.4X2-	T48.4X3-	T48.4X4-	T48.4X5-	T48.4X6-
stimulant	T48.901-	T48.902-	T48.903-	T48.904-	T48.905-	T48.906-
Retinoic acid	T49.0X1-	T49.0X2-	T49.0X3-	T49.0X4-	T49.0X5-	T49.0X6-
Retinol	T45.2X1-	T45.2X2-	T45.2X3-	T45.2X4-	T45.2X5-	T45.2X6-
Rh (D) immune globulin (human)	T50.Z11-	T50.Z12-	T50.Z13-	T50.Z14-	T50.Z15-	T50.Z16-
Rhodine	T39.011-	T39.012-	T39.013-	T39.014-	T39.015-	T39.016-
RhoGAM	T50.Z11-	T50.Z12-	T50.Z13-	T50.Z14-	T50.Z15-	T50.Z16-
Rhubarb						
dry extract	T47.2X1-	T47.2X2-	T47.2X3-	T47.2X4-	T47.2X5-	T47.2X6-
tincture, compound	T47.2X1-	T47.2X2-	T47.2X3-	T47.2X4-	T47.2X5-	T47.2X6-
Ribavirin	T37.5X1-	T37.5X2-	T37.5X3-	T37.5X4-	T37.5X5-	T37.5X6-
Riboflavin	T45.2X1-	T45.2X2-	T45.2X3-	T45.2X4-	T45.2X5-	T45.2X6-
Ribostamycin	T36.5X1-	T36.5X2-	T36.5X3-	T36.5X4-	T36.5X5-	T36.5X6-
Ricin	T62.2X1-	T62.2X2-	T62.2X3-	T62.2X4-	-	-
Ricinus communis	T62.2X1-	T62.2X2-	T62.2X3-	T62.2X4-	-	-
Rickettsial vaccine NEC	T50.A91-	T50.A92-	T50.A93-	T50.A94-	T50.A95-	T50.A96-
Rifabutin	T36.6X1-	T36.6X2-	T36.6X3-	T36.6X4-	T36.6X5-	T36.6X6-
Rifamide	T36.6X1-	T36.6X2-	T36.6X3-	T36.6X4-	T36.6X5-	T36.6X6-
Rifampicin	T36.6X1-	T36.6X2-	T36.6X3-	T36.6X4-	T36.6X5-	T36.6X6-
with isoniazid	T37.1X1-	T37.1X2-	T37.1X3-	T37.1X4-	T37.1X5-	T37.1X6-
Rifampin	T36.6X1-	T36.6X2-	T36.6X3-	T36.6X4-	T36.6X5-	T36.6X6-
Rifamycin	T36.6X1-	T36.6X2-	T36.6X3-	T36.6X4-	T36.6X5-	T36.6X6-
Rifaximin	T36.6X1-	T36.6X2-	T36.6X3-	T36.6X4-	T36.6X5-	T36.6X6-
Rimantadine	T37.5X1-	T37.5X2-	T37.5X3-	T37.5X4-	T37.5X5-	T37.5X6-
Rimazolium metilsulfate	T39.8X1-	T39.8X2-	T39.8X3-	T39.8X4-	T39.8X5-	T39.8X6-
Rimifon	T37.1X1-	T37.1X2-	T37.1X3-	T37.1X4-	T37.1X5-	T37.1X6-
Rimiterol	T48.6X1-	T48.6X2-	T48.6X3-	T48.6X4-	T48.6X5-	T48.6X6-
Ringer (lactate) solution	T50.3X1-	T50.3X2-	T50.3X3-	T50.3X4-	T50.3X5-	T50.3X6-
Ristocetin	T36.8X1-	T36.8X2-	T36.8X3-	T36.8X4-	T36.8X5-	T36.8X6-
Ritalin	T43.631-	T43.632-	T43.633-	T43.634-	T43.635-	T43.636-
Ritodrine	T44.5X1-	T44.5X2-	T44.5X3-	T44.5X4-	T44.5X5-	T44.5X6-
Roach killer — see Insecticide						
Rociverine	T44.3X1-	T44.3X2-	T44.3X3-	T44.3X4-	T44.3X5-	T44.3X6-
Rocky Mountain spotted fever vaccine	T50.A91-	T50.A92-	T50.A93-	T50.A94-	T50.A95-	T50.A96-
Rodenticide NEC	T60.4X1-	T60.4X2-	T60.4X3-	T60.4X4-	-	-
Rohypnol	T42.4X1-	T42.4X2-	T42.4X3-	T42.4X4-	T42.4X5-	T42.4X6-
Rokitamycin	T36.3X1-	T36.3X2-	T36.3X3-	T36.3X4-	T36.3X5-	T36.3X6-
Rolaids	T47.1X1-	T47.1X2-	T47.1X3-	T47.1X4-	T47.1X5-	T47.1X6-
Rolitetracycline	T36.4X1-	T36.4X2-	T36.4X3-	T36.4X4-	T36.4X5-	T36.4X6-
Romilar	T48.3X1-	T48.3X2-	T48.3X3-	T48.3X4-	T48.3X5-	T48.3X6-
Ronifibrate	T46.6X1-	T46.6X2-	T46.6X3-	T46.6X4-	T46.6X5-	T46.6X6-
Rosaprostol	T47.1X1-	T47.1X2-	T47.1X3-	T47.1X4-	T47.1X5-	T47.1X6-
Rose bengal sodium (131I)	T50.8X1-	T50.8X2-	T50.8X3-	T50.8X4-	T50.8X5-	T50.8X6-
Rose water ointment	T49.3X1-	T49.3X2-	T49.3X3-	T49.3X4-	T49.3X5-	T49.3X6-
Rosoxacin	T37.8X1-	T37.8X2-	T37.8X3-	T37.8X4-	T37.8X5-	T37.8X6-
Rotenone	T60.2X1-	T60.2X2-	T60.2X3-	T60.2X4-	-	-
Rotoxamine	T45.0X1-	T45.0X2-	T45.0X3-	T45.0X4-	T45.0X5-	T45.0X6-
Rough-on-rats	T60.4X1-	T60.4X2-	T60.4X3-	T60.4X4-	-	-
Roxatidine	T47.0X1-	T47.0X2-	T47.0X3-	T47.0X4-	T47.0X5-	T47.0X6-

Substance	Poisoning, Accidental (unintentional)	Poisoning, Intentional self-harm	Poisoning, Assault	Poisoning, Undetermined	Adverse effect	Underdosing
Roxithromycin	T36.3X1-	T36.3X2-	T36.3X3-	T36.3X4-	T36.3X5-	T36.3X6-
Rt-PA	T45.611-	T45.612-	T45.613-	T45.614-	T45.615-	T45.616-
Rubbing alcohol	T51.2X1-	T51.2X2-	T51.2X3-	T51.2X4-	-	-
Rubefacient	T49.4X1-	T49.4X2-	T49.4X3-	T49.4X4-	T49.4X5-	T49.4X6-
Rubella vaccine	T50.B91-	T50.B92-	T50.B93-	T50.B94-	T50.B95-	T50.B96-
Rubeola vaccine	T50.B91-	T50.B92-	T50.B93-	T50.B94-	T50.B95-	T50.B96-
Rubidium chloride Rb82	T50.8X1-	T50.8X2-	T50.8X3-	T50.8X4-	T50.8X5-	T50.8X6-
Rubidomycin	T45.1X1-	T45.1X2-	T45.1X3-	T45.1X4-	T45.1X5-	T45.1X6-
Rue	T62.2X1-	T62.2X2-	T62.2X3-	T62.2X4-	-	-
Rufocromomycin	T45.1X1-	T45.1X2-	T45.1X3-	T45.1X4-	T45.1X5-	T45.1X6-
Russel's viper venin	T45.7X1-	T45.7X2-	T45.7X3-	T45.7X4-	T45.7X5-	T45.7X6-
Ruta (graveolens)	T62.2X1-	T62.2X2-	T62.2X3-	T62.2X4-	-	-
Rutinum	T46.991-	T46.992-	T46.993-	T46.994-	T46.995-	T46.996-
Rutoside	T46.991-	T46.992-	T46.993-	T46.994-	T46.995-	T46.996-
Sabadilla (plant)	T62.2X1-	T62.2X2-	T62.2X3-	T62.2X4-	-	-
pesticide	T60.2X1-	T60.2X2-	T60.2X3-	T60.2X4-	-	-
Saccharated iron oxide	T45.8X1-	T45.8X2-	T45.8X3-	T45.8X4-	T45.8X5-	T45.8X6-
Saccharin	T50.901-	T50.902-	T50.903-	T50.904-	T50.905-	T50.906-
Saccharomyces boulardii	T47.6X1-	T47.6X2-	T47.6X3-	T47.6X4-	T47.6X5-	T47.6X6-
Safflower oil	T46.6X1-	T46.6X2-	T46.6X3-	T46.6X4-	T46.6X5-	T46.6X6-
Safrazine	T43.1X1-	T43.1X2-	T43.1X3-	T43.1X4-	T43.1X5-	T43.1X6-
Salazosulfapyridine	T37.0X1-	T37.0X2-	T37.0X3-	T37.0X4-	T37.0X5-	T37.0X6-
Salbutamol	T48.6X1-	T48.6X2-	T48.6X3-	T48.6X4-	T48.6X5-	T48.6X6-
Salicylamide	T39.091-	T39.092-	T39.093-	T39.094-	T39.095-	T39.096-
Salicylate NEC	T39.091-	T39.092-	T39.093-	T39.094-	T39.095-	T39.096-
methyl	T49.3X1-	T49.3X2-	T49.3X3-	T49.3X4-	T49.3X5-	T49.3X6-
theobromine calcium	T50.2X1-	T50.2X2-	T50.2X3-	T50.2X4-	T50.2X5-	T50.2X6-
Salicylazosulfapyridine	T37.0X1-	T37.0X2-	T37.0X3-	T37.0X4-	T37.0X5-	T37.0X6-
Salicylhydroxamic acid	T49.0X1-	T49.0X2-	T49.0X3-	T49.0X4-	T49.0X5-	T49.0X6-
Salicylic acid	T49.4X1-	T49.4X2-	T49.4X3-	T49.4X4-	T49.4X5-	T49.4X6-
with benzoic acid	T49.4X1-	T49.4X2-	T49.4X3-	T49.4X4-	T49.4X5-	T49.4X6-
congeners	T39.091-	T39.092-	T39.093-	T39.094-	T39.095-	T39.096-
derivative	T39.091-	T39.092-	T39.093-	T39.094-	T39.095-	T39.096-
salts	T39.091-	T39.092-	T39.093-	T39.094-	T39.095-	T39.096-
Salinazid	T37.1X1-	T37.1X2-	T37.1X3-	T37.1X4-	T37.1X5-	T37.1X6-
Salmeterol	T48.6X1-	T48.6X2-	T48.6X3-	T48.6X4-	T48.6X5-	T48.6X6-
Salol	T49.3X1-	T49.3X2-	T49.3X3-	T49.3X4-	T49.3X5-	T49.3X6-
Salsalate	T39.091-	T39.092-	T39.093-	T39.094-	T39.095-	T39.096-
Salt substitute	T50.901-	T50.902-	T50.903-	T50.904-	T50.905-	T50.906-
Salt-replacing drug	T50.901-	T50.902-	T50.903-	T50.904-	T50.905-	T50.906-
Salt-retaining mineralocorticoid	T50.0X1-	T50.0X2-	T50.0X3-	T50.0X4-	T50.0X5-	T50.0X6-
Saluretic NEC	T50.2X1-	T50.2X2-	T50.2X3-	T50.2X4-	T50.2X5-	T50.2X6-
Saluron	T50.2X1-	T50.2X2-	T50.2X3-	T50.2X4-	T50.2X5-	T50.2X6-
Salvarsan 606 (neosilver) (silver)	T37.8X1-	T37.8X2-	T37.8X3-	T37.8X4-	T37.8X5-	T37.8X6-
Sambucus canadensis	T62.2X1-	T62.2X2-	T62.2X3-	T62.2X4-	-	-
berry	T62.1X1-	T62.1X2-	T62.1X3-	T62.1X4-	-	-
Sandril	T46.5X1-	T46.5X2-	T46.5X3-	T46.5X4-	T46.5X5-	T46.5X6-
Sanguinaria canadensis	T62.2X1-	T62.2X2-	T62.2X3-	T62.2X4-	-	-
Saniflush (cleaner)	T54.2X1-	T54.2X2-	T54.2X3-	T54.2X4-	-	-
Santonin	T37.4X1-	T37.4X2-	T37.4X3-	T37.4X4-	T37.4X5-	T37.4X6-
Santyl	T49.8X1-	T49.8X2-	T49.8X3-	T49.8X4-	T49.8X5-	T49.8X6-
Saralasin	T46.5X1-	T46.5X2-	T46.5X3-	T46.5X4-	T46.5X5-	T46.5X6-
Sarcolysin	T45.1X1-	T45.1X2-	T45.1X3-	T45.1X4-	T45.1X5-	T45.1X6-
Sarkomycin	T45.1X1-	T45.1X2-	T45.1X3-	T45.1X4-	T45.1X5-	T45.1X6-
Saroten	T43.011-	T43.012-	T43.013-	T43.014-	T43.015-	T43.016-
Saturnine — see Lead						
Savin (oil)	T49.4X1-	T49.4X2-	T49.4X3-	T49.4X4-	T49.4X5-	T49.4X6-
Scammony	T47.2X1-	T47.2X2-	T47.2X3-	T47.2X4-	T47.2X5-	T47.2X6-
Scarlet red	T49.8X1-	T49.8X2-	T49.8X3-	T49.8X4-	T49.8X5-	T49.8X6-
Scheele's green	T57.0X1-	T57.0X2-	T57.0X3-	T57.0X4-	-	-
insecticide	T57.0X1-	T57.0X2-	T57.0X3-	T57.0X4-	-	-
Schizontozide (blood) (tissue)	T37.2X1-	T37.2X2-	T37.2X3-	T37.2X4-	T37.2X5-	T37.2X6-
Schradan	T60.0X1-	T60.0X2-	T60.0X3-	T60.0X4-	-	-
Schweinfurth green	T57.0X1-	T57.0X2-	T57.0X3-	T57.0X4-	-	-
insecticide	T57.0X1-	T57.0X2-	T57.0X3-	T57.0X4-	-	-
Scilla, rat poison	T60.4X1-	T60.4X2-	T60.4X3-	T60.4X4-	-	-
Scillaren	T60.4X1-	T60.4X2-	T60.4X3-	T60.4X4-	-	-
Sclerosing agent	T46.8X1-	T46.8X2-	T46.8X3-	T46.8X4-	T46.8X5-	T46.8X6-
Scombrotoxin	T61.11X-	T61.12X-	T61.13X-	T61.14X-	-	-
Scopolamine	T44.3X1-	T44.3X2-	T44.3X3-	T44.3X4-	T44.3X5-	T44.3X6-
Scopolia extract	T44.3X1-	T44.3X2-	T44.3X3-	T44.3X4-	T44.3X5-	T44.3X6-
Scouring powder	T65.891-	T65.892-	T65.893-	T65.894-	-	-
Sea						
anemone (sting)	T63.631-	T63.632-	T63.633-	T63.634-	-	-
cucumber (sting)	T63.691-	T63.692-	T63.693-	T63.694-	-	-
snake (bite) (venom)	T63.091-	T63.092-	T63.093-	T63.094-	-	-

Substance	Poisoning, Accidental (unintentional)	Poisoning, Intentional self-harm	Poisoning, Assault	Poisoning, Undetermined	Adverse effect	Underdosing
Sea - *continued*						
urchin spine (puncture)	T63.691-	T63.692-	T63.693-	T63.694-	-	-
Seafood	T61.91X-	T61.92X-	T61.93X-	T61.94X-	-	-
specified NEC	T61.8X1-	T61.8X2-	T61.8X3-	T61.8X4-	-	-
Secbutabarbital	T42.3X1-	T42.3X2-	T42.3X3-	T42.3X4-	T42.3X5-	T42.3X6-
Secbutabarbitone	T42.3X1-	T42.3X2-	T42.3X3-	T42.3X4-	T42.3X5-	T42.3X6-
Secnidazole	T37.3X1-	T37.3X2-	T37.3X3-	T37.3X4-	T37.3X5-	T37.3X6-
Secobarbital	T42.3X1-	T42.3X2-	T42.3X3-	T42.3X4-	T42.3X5-	T42.3X6-
Seconal	T42.3X1-	T42.3X2-	T42.3X3-	T42.3X4-	T42.3X5-	T42.3X6-
Secretin	T50.8X1-	T50.8X2-	T50.8X3-	T50.8X4-	T50.8X5-	T50.8X6-
Sedative NEC	T42.71X-	T42.72X-	T42.73X-	T42.74X-	T42.75X-	T42.76X-
mixed NEC	T42.6X1-	T42.6X2-	T42.6X3-	T42.6X4-	T42.6X5-	T42.6X6-
Sedormid	T42.6X1-	T42.6X2-	T42.6X3-	T42.6X4-	T42.6X5-	T42.6X6-
Seed disinfectant or dressing	T60.8X1-	T60.8X2-	T60.8X3-	T60.8X4-	-	-
Seeds (poisonous)	T62.2X1-	T62.2X2-	T62.2X3-	T62.2X4-	-	-
Selegiline	T42.8X1-	T42.8X2-	T42.8X3-	T42.8X4-	T42.8X5-	T42.8X6-
Selenium NEC	T56.891-	T56.892-	T56.893-	T56.894-	-	-
disulfide or sulfide	T49.4X1-	T49.4X2-	T49.4X3-	T49.4X4-	T49.4X5-	T49.4X6-
fumes	T59.891-	T59.892-	T59.893-	T59.894-	-	-
sulfide	T49.4X1-	T49.4X2-	T49.4X3-	T49.4X4-	T49.4X5-	T49.4X6-
Selenomethionine (75Se)	T50.8X1-	T50.8X2-	T50.8X3-	T50.8X4-	T50.8X5-	T50.8X6-
Selsun	T49.4X1-	T49.4X2-	T49.4X3-	T49.4X4-	T49.4X5-	T49.4X6-
Semustine	T45.1X1-	T45.1X2-	T45.1X3-	T45.1X4-	T45.1X5-	T45.1X6-
Senega syrup	T48.4X1-	T48.4X2-	T48.4X3-	T48.4X4-	T48.4X5-	T48.4X6-
Senna	T47.2X1-	T47.2X2-	T47.2X3-	T47.2X4-	T47.2X5-	T47.2X6-
Sennoside A+B	T47.2X1-	T47.2X2-	T47.2X3-	T47.2X4-	T47.2X5-	T47.2X6-
Septisol	T49.2X1-	T49.2X2-	T49.2X3-	T49.2X4-	T49.2X5-	T49.2X6-
Seractide	T38.811-	T38.812-	T38.813-	T38.814-	T38.815-	T38.816-
Serax	T42.4X1-	T42.4X2-	T42.4X3-	T42.4X4-	T42.4X5-	T42.4X6-
Serenesil	T42.6X1-	T42.6X2-	T42.6X3-	T42.6X4-	T42.6X5-	T42.6X6-
Serenium (hydrochloride)	T37.91X-	T37.92X-	T37.93X-	T37.94X-	T37.95X-	T37.96X-
Serepax — *see* Oxazepam						
Sermorelin	T38.891-	T38.892-	T38.893-	T38.894-	T38.895-	T38.896-
Sernyl	T41.1X1-	T41.1X2-	T41.1X3-	T41.1X4-	T41.1X5-	T41.1X6-
Serotonin	T50.991-	T50.992-	T50.993-	T50.994-	T50.995-	T50.996-
Serpasil	T46.5X1-	T46.5X2-	T46.5X3-	T46.5X4-	T46.5X5-	T46.5X6-
Serrapeptase	T45.3X1-	T45.3X2-	T45.3X3-	T45.3X4-	T45.3X5-	T45.3X6-
Serum						
antibotulinus	T50.Z11-	T50.Z12-	T50.Z13-	T50.Z14-	T50.Z15-	T50.Z16-
anticytotoxic	T50.Z11-	T50.Z12-	T50.Z13-	T50.Z14-	T50.Z15-	T50.Z16-
antidiphtheria	T50.Z11-	T50.Z12-	T50.Z13-	T50.Z14-	T50.Z15-	T50.Z16-
antimeningococcus	T50.Z11-	T50.Z12-	T50.Z13-	T50.Z14-	T50.Z15-	T50.Z16-
anti-Rh	T50.Z11-	T50.Z12-	T50.Z13-	T50.Z14-	T50.Z15-	T50.Z16-
anti-snake-bite	T50.Z11-	T50.Z12-	T50.Z13-	T50.Z14-	T50.Z15-	T50.Z16-
antitetanic	T50.Z11-	T50.Z12-	T50.Z13-	T50.Z14-	T50.Z15-	T50.Z16-
antitoxic	T50.Z11-	T50.Z12-	T50.Z13-	T50.Z14-	T50.Z15-	T50.Z16-
complement (inhibitor)	T45.8X1-	T45.8X2-	T45.8X3-	T45.8X4-	T45.8X5-	T45.8X6-
convalescent	T50.Z11-	T50.Z12-	T50.Z13-	T50.Z14-	T50.Z15-	T50.Z16-
hemolytic complement	T45.8X1-	T45.8X2-	T45.8X3-	T45.8X4-	T45.8X5-	T45.8X6-
immune (human)	T50.Z11-	T50.Z12-	T50.Z13-	T50.Z14-	T50.Z15-	T50.Z16-
protective NEC	T50.Z11-	T50.Z12-	T50.Z13-	T50.Z14-	T50.Z15-	T50.Z16-
Setastine	T45.0X1-	T45.0X2-	T45.0X3-	T45.0X4-	T45.0X5-	T45.0X6-
Setoperone	T43.591-	T43.592-	T43.593-	T43.594-	T43.595-	T43.596-
Sewer gas	T59.91X-	T59.92X-	T59.93X-	T59.94X-	-	-
Shampoo	T55.0X1-	T55.0X2-	T55.0X3-	T55.0X4-	-	-
Shellfish, noxious, nonbacterial	T61.781-	T61.782-	T61.783-	T61.784-	-	-
Sildenafil	T46.7X1-	T46.7X2-	T46.7X3-	T46.7X4-	T46.7X5-	T46.7X6-
Silibinin	T50.991-	T50.992-	T50.993-	T50.994-	T50.995-	T50.996-
Silicone NEC	T65.891-	T65.892-	T65.893-	T65.894-	-	-
medicinal	T49.3X1-	T49.3X2-	T49.3X3-	T49.3X4-	T49.3X5-	T49.3X6-
Silvadene	T49.0X1-	T49.0X2-	T49.0X3-	T49.0X4-	T49.0X5-	T49.0X6-
Silver	T49.0X1-	T49.0X2-	T49.0X3-	T49.0X4-	T49.0X5-	T49.0X6-
anti-infectives	T49.0X1-	T49.0X2-	T49.0X3-	T49.0X4-	T49.0X5-	T49.0X6-
arsphenamine	T37.8X1-	T37.8X2-	T37.8X3-	T37.8X4-	T37.8X5-	T37.8X6-
colloidal	T49.0X1-	T49.0X2-	T49.0X3-	T49.0X4-	T49.0X5-	T49.0X6-
nitrate	T49.0X1-	T49.0X2-	T49.0X3-	T49.0X4-	T49.0X5-	T49.0X6-
ophthalmic preparation	T49.5X1-	T49.5X2-	T49.5X3-	T49.5X4-	T49.5X5-	T49.5X6-
toughened (keratolytic)	T49.4X1-	T49.4X2-	T49.4X3-	T49.4X4-	T49.4X5-	T49.4X6-
nonmedicinal (dust)	T56.891-	T56.892-	T56.893-	T56.894-	-	-
protein	T49.5X1-	T49.5X2-	T49.5X3-	T49.5X4-	T49.5X5-	T49.5X6-
salvarsan	T37.8X1-	T37.8X2-	T37.8X3-	T37.8X4-	T37.8X5-	T37.8X6-
sulfadiazine	T49.4X1-	T49.4X2-	T49.4X3-	T49.4X4-	T49.4X5-	T49.4X6-
Silymarin	T50.991-	T50.992-	T50.993-	T50.994-	T50.995-	T50.996-
Simaldrate	T47.1X1-	T47.1X2-	T47.1X3-	T47.1X4-	T47.1X5-	T47.1X6-
Simazine	T60.3X1-	T60.3X2-	T60.3X3-	T60.3X4-	-	-
Simethicone	T47.1X1-	T47.1X2-	T47.1X3-	T47.1X4-	T47.1X5-	T47.1X6-
Simfibrate	T46.6X1-	T46.6X2-	T46.6X3-	T46.6X4-	T46.6X5-	T46.6X6-

Substance	Poisoning, Accidental (unintentional)	Poisoning, Intentional self-harm	Poisoning, Assault	Poisoning, Undetermined	Adverse effect	Underdosing
Simvastatin	T46.6X1-	T46.6X2-	T46.6X3-	T46.6X4-	T46.6X5-	T46.6X6-
Sincalide	T50.8X1-	T50.8X2-	T50.8X3-	T50.8X4-	T50.8X5-	T50.8X6-
Sinequan	T43.011-	T43.012-	T43.013-	T43.014-	T43.015-	T43.016-
Singoserp	T46.5X1-	T46.5X2-	T46.5X3-	T46.5X4-	T46.5X5-	T46.5X6-
Sintrom	T45.511-	T45.512-	T45.513-	T45.514-	T45.515-	T45.516-
Sisomicin	T36.5X1-	T36.5X2-	T36.5X3-	T36.5X4-	T36.5X5-	T36.5X6-
Sitosterols	T46.6X1-	T46.6X2-	T46.6X3-	T46.6X4-	T46.6X5-	T46.6X6-
Skeletal muscle relaxants	T48.1X1-	T48.1X2-	T48.1X3-	T48.1X4-	T48.1X5-	T48.1X6-
Skin						
agents (external)	T49.91X-	T49.92X-	T49.93X-	T49.94X-	T49.95X-	T49.96X-
specified NEC	T49.8X1-	T49.8X2-	T49.8X3-	T49.8X4-	T49.8X5-	T49.8X6-
test antigen	T50.8X1-	T50.8X2-	T50.8X3-	T50.8X4-	T50.8X5-	T50.8X6-
Sleep-eze	T45.0X1-	T45.0X2-	T45.0X3-	T45.0X4-	T45.0X5-	T45.0X6-
Sleeping draught, pill	T42.71X-	T42.72X-	T42.73X-	T42.74X-	T42.75X-	T42.76X-
Smallpox vaccine	T50.B11-	T50.B12-	T50.B13-	T50.B14-	T50.B15-	T50.B16-
Smelter fumes NEC	T56.91X-	T56.92X-	T56.93X-	T56.94X-	-	-
Smog	T59.1X1-	T59.1X2-	T59.1X3-	T59.1X4-	-	-
Smoke NEC	T59.811-	T59.812-	T59.813-	T59.814-	-	-
Smooth muscle relaxant	T44.3X1-	T44.3X2-	T44.3X3-	T44.3X4-	T44.3X5-	T44.3X6-
Snail killer NEC	T60.8X1-	T60.8X2-	T60.8X3-	T60.8X4-	-	-
Snake venom or bite	T63.001-	T63.002-	T63.003-	T63.004-	-	-
hemocoagulase	T45.7X1-	T45.7X2-	T45.7X3-	T45.7X4-	T45.7X5-	T45.7X6-
Snuff	T65.211-	T65.212-	T65.213-	T65.214-	-	-
Soap (powder) (product)	T55.0X1-	T55.0X2-	T55.0X3-	T55.0X4-	-	-
enema	T47.4X1-	T47.4X2-	T47.4X3-	T47.4X4-	T47.4X5-	T47.4X6-
medicinal, soft	T49.2X1-	T49.2X2-	T49.2X3-	T49.2X4-	T49.2X5-	T49.2X6-
superfatted	T49.2X1-	T49.2X2-	T49.2X3-	T49.2X4-	T49.2X5-	T49.2X6-
Sobrerol	T48.4X1-	T48.4X2-	T48.4X3-	T48.4X4-	T48.4X5-	T48.4X6-
Soda (caustic)	T54.3X1-	T54.3X2-	T54.3X3-	T54.3X4-	-	-
bicarb	T47.1X1-	T47.1X2-	T47.1X3-	T47.1X4-	T47.1X5-	T47.1X6-
chlorinated — *see* Sodium, hypochlorite						
Sodium						
acetosulfone	T37.1X1-	T37.1X2-	T37.1X3-	T37.1X4-	T37.1X5-	T37.1X6-
acetrizoate	T50.8X1-	T50.8X2-	T50.8X3-	T50.8X4-	T50.8X5-	T50.8X6-
acid phosphate	T50.3X1-	T50.3X2-	T50.3X3-	T50.3X4-	T50.3X5-	T50.3X6-
alginate	T47.8X1-	T47.8X2-	T47.8X3-	T47.8X4-	T47.8X5-	T47.8X6-
amidotrizoate	T50.8X1-	T50.8X2-	T50.8X3-	T50.8X4-	T50.8X5-	T50.8X6-
aminopterin	T45.1X1-	T45.1X2-	T45.1X3-	T45.1X4-	T45.1X5-	T45.1X6-
amylosulfate	T47.8X1-	T47.8X2-	T47.8X3-	T47.8X4-	T47.8X5-	T47.8X6-
amytal	T42.3X1-	T42.3X2-	T42.3X3-	T42.3X4-	T42.3X5-	T42.3X6-
antimony gluconate	T37.3X1-	T37.3X2-	T37.3X3-	T37.3X4-	T37.3X5-	T37.3X6-
arsenate	T57.0X1-	T57.0X2-	T57.0X3-	T57.0X4-	-	-
aurothiomalate	T39.4X1-	T39.4X2-	T39.4X3-	T39.4X4-	T39.4X5-	T39.4X6-
aurothiosulfate	T39.4X1-	T39.4X2-	T39.4X3-	T39.4X4-	T39.4X5-	T39.4X6-
barbiturate	T42.3X1-	T42.3X2-	T42.3X3-	T42.3X4-	T42.3X5-	T42.3X6-
basic phosphate	T47.4X1-	T47.4X2-	T47.4X3-	T47.4X4-	T47.4X5-	T47.4X6-
bicarbonate	T47.1X1-	T47.1X2-	T47.1X3-	T47.1X4-	T47.1X5-	T47.1X6-
bichromate	T57.8X1-	T57.8X2-	T57.8X3-	T57.8X4-	-	-
biphosphate	T50.3X1-	T50.3X2-	T50.3X3-	T50.3X4-	T50.3X5-	T50.3X6-
bisulfate	T65.891-	T65.892-	T65.893-	T65.894-	-	-
borate						
cleanser	T57.8X1-	T57.8X2-	T57.8X3-	T57.8X4-	-	-
eye	T49.5X1-	T49.5X2-	T49.5X3-	T49.5X4-	T49.5X5-	T49.5X6-
therapeutic	T49.8X1-	T49.8X2-	T49.8X3-	T49.8X4-	T49.8X5-	T49.8X6-
bromide	T42.6X1-	T42.6X2-	T42.6X3-	T42.6X4-	T42.6X5-	T42.6X6-
cacodylate (nonmedicinal) NEC	T50.8X1-	T50.8X2-	T50.8X3-	T50.8X4-	T50.8X5-	T50.8X6-
anti-infective	T37.8X1-	T37.8X2-	T37.8X3-	T37.8X4-	T37.8X5-	T37.8X6-
herbicide	T60.3X1-	T60.3X2-	T60.3X3-	T60.3X4-	-	-
calcium edetate	T45.8X1-	T45.8X2-	T45.8X3-	T45.8X4-	T45.8X5-	T45.8X6-
carbonate NEC	T54.3X1-	T54.3X2-	T54.3X3-	T54.3X4-	-	-
chlorate NEC	T65.891-	T65.892-	T65.893-	T65.894-	-	-
herbicide	T54.91X-	T54.92X-	T54.93X-	T54.94X-	-	-
chloride	T50.3X1-	T50.3X2-	T50.3X3-	T50.3X4-	T50.3X5-	T50.3X6-
with glucose	T50.3X1-	T50.3X2-	T50.3X3-	T50.3X4-	T50.3X5-	T50.3X6-
chromate	T65.891-	T65.892-	T65.893-	T65.894-	-	-
citrate	T50.991-	T50.992-	T50.993-	T50.994-	T50.995-	T50.996-
cromoglicate	T48.6X1-	T48.6X2-	T48.6X3-	T48.6X4-	T48.6X5-	T48.6X6-
cyanide	T65.0X1-	T65.0X2-	T65.0X3-	T65.0X4-	-	-
cyclamate	T50.3X1-	T50.3X2-	T50.3X3-	T50.3X4-	T50.3X5-	T50.3X6-
dehydrocholate	T45.8X1-	T45.8X2-	T45.8X3-	T45.8X4-	T45.8X5-	T45.8X6-
diatrizoate	T50.8X1-	T50.8X2-	T50.8X3-	T50.8X4-	T50.8X5-	T50.8X6-
dibunate	T48.4X1-	T48.4X2-	T48.4X3-	T48.4X4-	T48.4X5-	T48.4X6-
dioctyl sulfosuccinate	T47.4X1-	T47.4X2-	T47.4X3-	T47.4X4-	T47.4X5-	T47.4X6-
dipantoyl ferrate	T45.8X1-	T45.8X2-	T45.8X3-	T45.8X4-	T45.8X5-	T45.8X6-
edetate	T45.8X1-	T45.8X2-	T45.8X3-	T45.8X4-	T45.8X5-	T45.8X6-
ethacrynate	T50.1X1-	T50.1X2-	T50.1X3-	T50.1X4-	T50.1X5-	T50.1X6-

Substance	Poisoning, Accidental (unintentional)	Poisoning, Intentional self-harm	Poisoning, Assault	Poisoning, Undetermined	Adverse effect	Underdosing
Sodium - *continued*						
feredetate	T45.8X1-	T45.8X2-	T45.8X3-	T45.8X4-	T45.8X5-	T45.8X6-
Fluoride — *see* Fluoride						
fluoroacetate (dust) (pesticide)	T60.4X1-	T60.4X2-	T60.4X3-	T60.4X4-	-	-
free salt	T50.3X1-	T50.3X2-	T50.3X3-	T50.3X4-	T50.3X5-	T50.3X6-
fusidate	T36.8X1-	T36.8X2-	T36.8X3-	T36.8X4-	T36.8X5-	T36.8X6-
glucaldrate	T47.1X1-	T47.1X2-	T47.1X3-	T47.1X4-	T47.1X5-	T47.1X6-
glucosulfone	T37.1X1-	T37.1X2-	T37.1X3-	T37.1X4-	T37.1X5-	T37.1X6-
glutamate	T45.8X1-	T45.8X2-	T45.8X3-	T45.8X4-	T45.8X5-	T45.8X6-
hydrogen carbonate	T50.3X1-	T50.3X2-	T50.3X3-	T50.3X4-	T50.3X5-	T50.3X6-
hydroxide	T54.3X1-	T54.3X2-	T54.3X3-	T54.3X4-	-	-
hypochlorite (bleach) NEC	T54.3X1-	T54.3X2-	T54.3X3-	T54.3X4-	-	-
disinfectant	T54.3X1-	T54.3X2-	T54.3X3-	T54.3X4-	-	-
medicinal (anti-infective) (external)	T49.0X1-	T49.0X2-	T49.0X3-	T49.0X4-	T49.0X5-	T49.0X6-
vapor	T54.3X1-	T54.3X2-	T54.3X3-	T54.3X4-	-	-
hyposulfite	T49.0X1-	T49.0X2-	T49.0X3-	T49.0X4-	T49.0X5-	T49.0X6-
indigotin disulfonate	T50.8X1-	T50.8X2-	T50.8X3-	T50.8X4-	T50.8X5-	T50.8X6-
iodide	T50.991-	T50.992-	T50.993-	T50.994-	T50.995-	T50.996-
I-131	T50.8X1-	T50.8X2-	T50.8X3-	T50.8X4-	T50.8X5-	T50.8X6-
therapeutic	T38.2X1-	T38.2X2-	T38.2X3-	T38.2X4-	T38.2X5-	T38.2X6-
iodohippurate (131I)	T50.8X1-	T50.8X2-	T50.8X3-	T50.8X4-	T50.8X5-	T50.8X6-
iopodate	T50.8X1-	T50.8X2-	T50.8X3-	T50.8X4-	T50.8X5-	T50.8X6-
iothalamate	T50.8X1-	T50.8X2-	T50.8X3-	T50.8X4-	T50.8X5-	T50.8X6-
iron edetate	T45.4X1-	T45.4X2-	T45.4X3-	T45.4X4-	T45.4X5-	T45.4X6-
lactate (compound solution)	T45.8X1-	T45.8X2-	T45.8X3-	T45.8X4-	T45.8X5-	T45.8X6-
lauryl (sulfate)	T49.2X1-	T49.2X2-	T49.2X3-	T49.2X4-	T49.2X5-	T49.2X6-
L-triiodothyronine	T38.1X1-	T38.1X2-	T38.1X3-	T38.1X4-	T38.1X5-	T38.1X6-
magnesium citrate	T50.991-	T50.992-	T50.993-	T50.994-	T50.995-	T50.996-
mersalate	T50.2X1-	T50.2X2-	T50.2X3-	T50.2X4-	T50.2X5-	T50.2X6-
metasilicate	T65.891-	T65.892-	T65.893-	T65.894-	-	-
metrizoate	T50.8X1-	T50.8X2-	T50.8X3-	T50.8X4-	T50.8X5-	T50.8X6-
monofluoroacetate (pesticide)	T60.1X1-	T60.1X2-	T60.1X3-	T60.1X4-	-	-
morrhuate	T46.8X1-	T46.8X2-	T46.8X3-	T46.8X4-	T46.8X5-	T46.8X6-
nafcillin	T36.0X1-	T36.0X2-	T36.0X3-	T36.0X4-	T36.0X5-	T36.0X6-
nitrate (oxidizing agent)	T65.891-	T65.892-	T65.893-	T65.894-	-	-
nitrite	T50.6X1-	T50.6X2-	T50.6X3-	T50.6X4-	T50.6X5-	T50.6X6-
nitroferricyanide	T46.5X1-	T46.5X2-	T46.5X3-	T46.5X4-	T46.5X5-	T46.5X6-
nitroprusside	T46.5X1-	T46.5X2-	T46.5X3-	T46.5X4-	T46.5X5-	T46.5X6-
oxalate	T65.891-	T65.892-	T65.893-	T65.894-	-	-
oxide/peroxide	T65.891-	T65.892-	T65.893-	T65.894-	-	-
oxybate	T41.291-	T41.292-	T41.293-	T41.294-	T41.295-	T41.296-
para-aminohippurate	T50.8X1-	T50.8X2-	T50.8X3-	T50.8X4-	T50.8X5-	T50.8X6-
perborate (nonmedicinal) NEC	T65.891-	T65.892-	T65.893-	T65.894-	-	-
medicinal	T49.0X1-	T49.0X2-	T49.0X3-	T49.0X4-	T49.0X5-	T49.0X6-
soap	T55.0X1-	T55.0X2-	T55.0X3-	T55.0X4-	-	-
percarbonate — *see* Sodium, perborate						
pertechnetate Tc99m	T50.8X1-	T50.8X2-	T50.8X3-	T50.8X4-	T50.8X5-	T50.8X6-
phosphate						
cellulose	T45.8X1-	T45.8X2-	T45.8X3-	T45.8X4-	T45.8X5-	T45.8X6-
dibasic	T47.2X1-	T47.2X2-	T47.2X3-	T47.2X4-	T47.2X5-	T47.2X6-
monobasic	T47.2X1-	T47.2X2-	T47.2X3-	T47.2X4-	T47.2X5-	T47.2X6-
phytate	T50.6X1-	T50.6X2-	T50.6X3-	T50.6X4-	T50.6X5-	T50.6X6-
picosulfate	T47.2X1-	T47.2X2-	T47.2X3-	T47.2X4-	T47.2X5-	T47.2X6-
polyhydroxyaluminium monocarbonate	T47.1X1-	T47.1X2-	T47.1X3-	T47.1X4-	T47.1X5-	T47.1X6-
polystyrene sulfonate	T50.3X1-	T50.3X2-	T50.3X3-	T50.3X4-	T50.3X5-	T50.3X6-
propionate	T49.0X1-	T49.0X2-	T49.0X3-	T49.0X4-	T49.0X5-	T49.0X6-
propyl hydroxybenzoate	T50.991-	T50.992-	T50.993-	T50.994-	T50.995-	T50.996-
psylliate	T46.8X1-	T46.8X2-	T46.8X3-	T46.8X4-	T46.8X5-	T46.8X6-
removing resins	T50.3X1-	T50.3X2-	T50.3X3-	T50.3X4-	T50.3X5-	T50.3X6-
salicylate	T39.091-	T39.092-	T39.093-	T39.094-	T39.095-	T39.096-
salt NEC	T50.3X1-	T50.3X2-	T50.3X3-	T50.3X4-	T50.3X5-	T50.3X6-
selenate	T60.2X1-	T60.2X2-	T60.2X3-	T60.2X4-	-	-
stibogluconate	T37.3X1-	T37.3X2-	T37.3X3-	T37.3X4-	T37.3X5-	T37.3X6-
sulfate	T47.4X1-	T47.4X2-	T47.4X3-	T47.4X4-	T47.4X5-	T47.4X6-
sulfoxone	T37.1X1-	T37.1X2-	T37.1X3-	T37.1X4-	T37.1X5-	T37.1X6-
tetradecyl sulfate	T46.8X1-	T46.8X2-	T46.8X3-	T46.8X4-	T46.8X5-	T46.8X6-
thiopental	T41.1X1-	T41.1X2-	T41.1X3-	T41.1X4-	T41.1X5-	T41.1X6-
thiosalicylate	T39.091-	T39.092-	T39.093-	T39.094-	T39.095-	T39.096-
thiosulfate	T50.6X1-	T50.6X2-	T50.6X3-	T50.6X4-	T50.6X5-	T50.6X6-
tolbutamide	T38.3X1-	T38.3X2-	T38.3X3-	T38.3X4-	T38.3X5-	T38.3X6-
(L) -triiodothyronine	T38.1X1-	T38.1X2-	T38.1X3-	T38.1X4-	T38.1X5-	T38.1X6-
tyropanoate	T50.8X1-	T50.8X2-	T50.8X3-	T50.8X4-	T50.8X5-	T50.8X6-
valproate	T42.6X1-	T42.6X2-	T42.6X3-	T42.6X4-	T42.6X5-	T42.6X6-
versenate	T50.6X1-	T50.6X2-	T50.6X3-	T50.6X4-	T50.6X5-	T50.6X6-
Sodium-free salt	T50.901-	T50.902-	T50.903-	T50.904-	T50.905-	T50.906-

Substance	Poisoning, Accidental (unintentional)	Poisoning, Intentional self-harm	Poisoning, Assault	Poisoning, Undetermined	Adverse effect	Underdosing
Sodium-removing resin	T50.3X1-	T50.3X2-	T50.3X3-	T50.3X4-	T50.3X5-	T50.3X6-
Soft soap	T55.0X1-	T55.0X2-	T55.0X3-	T55.0X4-	-	-
Solanine	T62.2X1-	T62.2X2-	T62.2X3-	T62.2X4-	-	-
berries	T62.1X1-	T62.1X2-	T62.1X3-	T62.1X4-	-	-
Solanum dulcamara	T62.2X1-	T62.2X2-	T62.2X3-	T62.2X4-	-	-
berries	T62.1X1-	T62.1X2-	T62.1X3-	T62.1X4-	-	-
Solapsone	T37.1X1-	T37.1X2-	T37.1X3-	T37.1X4-	T37.1X5-	T37.1X6-
Solar lotion	T49.3X1-	T49.3X2-	T49.3X3-	T49.3X4-	T49.3X5-	T49.3X6-
Solasulfone	T37.1X1-	T37.1X2-	T37.1X3-	T37.1X4-	T37.1X5-	T37.1X6-
Soldering fluid	T65.891-	T65.892-	T65.893-	T65.894-		
Solid substance	T65.91X-	T65.92X-	T65.93X-	T65.94X-	-	-
specified NEC	T65.891-	T65.892-	T65.893-	T65.894-	-	-
Solvent, industrial NEC	T52.91X-	T52.92X-	T52.93X-	T52.94X-	-	-
naphtha	T52.0X1-	T52.0X2-	T52.0X3-	T52.0X4-	-	-
petroleum	T52.0X1-	T52.0X2-	T52.0X3-	T52.0X4-	-	-
specified NEC	T52.8X1-	T52.8X2-	T52.8X3-	T52.8X4-	-	-
Soma	T42.8X1-	T42.8X2-	T42.8X3-	T42.8X4-	T42.8X5-	T42.8X6-
Somatorelin	T38.891-	T38.892-	T38.893-	T38.894-	T38.895-	T38.896-
Somatostatin	T38.991-	T38.992-	T38.993-	T38.994-	T38.995-	T38.996-
Somatotropin	T38.811-	T38.812-	T38.813-	T38.814-	T38.815-	T38.816-
Somatrem	T38.811-	T38.812-	T38.813-	T38.814-	T38.815-	T38.816-
Somatropin	T38.811-	T38.812-	T38.813-	T38.814-	T38.815-	T38.816-
Sominex	T45.0X1-	T45.0X2-	T45.0X3-	T45.0X4-	T45.0X5-	T45.0X6-
Somnos	T42.6X1-	T42.6X2-	T42.6X3-	T42.6X4-	T42.6X5-	T42.6X6-
Somonal	T42.3X1-	T42.3X2-	T42.3X3-	T42.3X4-	T42.3X5-	T42.3X6-
Soneryl	T42.3X1-	T42.3X2-	T42.3X3-	T42.3X4-	T42.3X5-	T42.3X6-
Soothing syrup	T50.901-	T50.902-	T50.903-	T50.904-	T50.905-	T50.906-
Sopor	T42.6X1-	T42.6X2-	T42.6X3-	T42.6X4-	T42.6X5-	T42.6X6-
Soporific	T42.71X-	T42.72X-	T42.73X-	T42.74X-	T42.75X-	T42.76X-
Soporific drug	T42.71X-	T42.72X-	T42.73X-	T42.74X-	T42.75X-	T42.76X-
specified type NEC	T42.6X1-	T42.6X2-	T42.6X3-	T42.6X4-	T42.6X5-	T42.6X6-
Sorbide nitrate	T46.3X1-	T46.3X2-	T46.3X3-	T46.3X4-	T46.3X5-	T46.3X6-
Sorbitol	T47.4X1-	T47.4X2-	T47.4X3-	T47.4X4-	T47.4X5-	T47.4X6-
Sotalol	T44.7X1-	T44.7X2-	T44.7X3-	T44.7X4-	T44.7X5-	T44.7X6-
Sotradecol	T46.8X1-	T46.8X2-	T46.8X3-	T46.8X4-	T46.8X5-	T46.8X6-
Soysterol	T46.6X1-	T46.6X2-	T46.6X3-	T46.6X4-	T46.6X5-	T46.6X6-
Spacoline	T44.3X1-	T44.3X2-	T44.3X3-	T44.3X4-	T44.3X5-	T44.3X6-
Spanish fly	T49.8X1-	T49.8X2-	T49.8X3-	T49.8X4-	T49.8X5-	T49.8X6-
Sparine	T43.3X1-	T43.3X2-	T43.3X3-	T43.3X4-	T43.3X5-	T43.3X6-
Sparteine	T48.0X1-	T48.0X2-	T48.0X3-	T48.0X4-	T48.0X5-	T48.0X6-
Spasmolytic						
anticholinergics	T44.3X1-	T44.3X2-	T44.3X3-	T44.3X4-	T44.3X5-	T44.3X6-
autonomic	T44.3X1-	T44.3X2-	T44.3X3-	T44.3X4-	T44.3X5-	T44.3X6-
bronchial NEC	T48.6X1-	T48.6X2-	T48.6X3-	T48.6X4-	T48.6X5-	T48.6X6-
quaternary ammonium	T44.3X1-	T44.3X2-	T44.3X3-	T44.3X4-	T44.3X5-	T44.3X6-
skeletal muscle NEC	T48.1X1-	T48.1X2-	T48.1X3-	T48.1X4-	T48.1X5-	T48.1X6-
Spectinomycin	T36.5X1-	T36.5X2-	T36.5X3-	T36.5X4-	T36.5X5-	T36.5X6-
Speed	T43.621-	T43.622-	T43.623-	T43.624-	T43.625-	T43.626-
Spermicide	T49.8X1-	T49.8X2-	T49.8X3-	T49.8X4-	T49.8X5-	T49.8X6-
Spider (bite) (venom)	T63.391-	T63.392-	T63.393-	T63.394-	-	-
antivenin	T50.Z11-	T50.Z12-	T50.Z13-	T50.Z14-	T50.Z15-	T50.Z16-
Spigelia (root)	T37.4X1-	T37.4X2-	T37.4X3-	T37.4X4-	T37.4X5-	T37.4X6-
Spindle inactivator	T50.4X1-	T50.4X2-	T50.4X3-	T50.4X4-	T50.4X5-	T50.4X6-
Spiperone	T43.4X1-	T43.4X2-	T43.4X3-	T43.4X4-	T43.4X5-	T43.4X6-
Spiramycin	T36.3X1-	T36.3X2-	T36.3X3-	T36.3X4-	T36.3X5-	T36.3X6-
Spirapril	T46.4X1-	T46.4X2-	T46.4X3-	T46.4X4-	T46.4X5-	T46.4X6-
Spirilene	T43.591-	T43.592-	T43.593-	T43.594-	T43.595-	T43.596-
Spirit (s) (neutral) **NEC**	T51.0X1-	T51.0X2-	T51.0X3-	T51.0X4-	-	-
beverage	T51.0X1-	T51.0X2-	T51.0X3-	T51.0X4-	-	-
industrial	T51.0X1-	T51.0X2-	T51.0X3-	T51.0X4-	-	-
mineral	T52.0X1-	T52.0X2-	T52.0X3-	T52.0X4-	-	-
of salt — *see* Hydrochloric acid						
surgical	T51.0X1-	T51.0X2-	T51.0X3-	T51.0X4-	-	-
Spironolactone	T50.0X1-	T50.0X2-	T50.0X3-	T50.0X4-	T50.0X5-	T50.0X6-
Spiroperidol	T43.4X1-	T43.4X2-	T43.4X3-	T43.4X4-	T43.4X5-	T43.4X6-
Sponge, absorbable (gelatin)	T45.7X1-	T45.7X2-	T45.7X3-	T45.7X4-	T45.7X5-	T45.7X6-
Sporostacin	T49.0X1-	T49.0X2-	T49.0X3-	T49.0X4-	T49.0X5-	T49.0X6-
Spray (aerosol)	T65.91X-	T65.92X-	T65.93X-	T65.94X-		
cosmetic	T65.891-	T65.892-	T65.893-	T65.894-	-	-
medicinal NEC	T50.901-	T50.902-	T50.903-	T50.904-	T50.905-	T50.906-
pesticides — *see* Pesticides						
specified content — *see* specific substance						
Spurge flax	T62.2X1-	T62.2X2-	T62.2X3-	T62.2X4-	-	-
Spurges	T62.2X1-	T62.2X2-	T62.2X3-	T62.2X4-	-	-
Sputum viscosity-lowering drug	T48.4X1-	T48.4X2-	T48.4X3-	T48.4X4-	T48.4X5-	T48.4X6-

Table of Drugs and Chemicals

Sodium — Sputum viscosity-lowering drug

Substance	Poisoning, Accidental (unintentional)	Poisoning, Intentional self-harm	Poisoning, Assault	Poisoning, Undetermined	Adverse effect	Underdosing
Squill	T46.0X1-	T46.0X2-	T46.0X3-	T46.0X4-	T46.0X5-	T46.0X6-
rat poison	T60.4X1-	T60.4X2-	T60.4X3-	T60.4X4-	-	-
Squirting cucumber (cathartic)	T47.2X1-	T47.2X2-	T47.2X3-	T47.2X4-	T47.2X5-	T47.2X6-
Stains	T65.6X1-	T65.6X2-	T65.6X3-	T65.6X4-	-	-
Stannous fluoride	T49.7X1-	T49.7X2-	T49.7X3-	T49.7X4-	T49.7X5-	T49.7X6-
Stanolone	T38.7X1-	T38.7X2-	T38.7X3-	T38.7X4-	T38.7X5-	T38.7X6-
Stanozolol	T38.7X1-	T38.7X2-	T38.7X3-	T38.7X4-	T38.7X5-	T38.7X6-
Staphisagria or stavesacre (pediculicide)	T49.0X1-	T49.0X2-	T49.0X3-	T49.0X4-	T49.0X5-	T49.0X6-
Starch	T50.901-	T50.902-	T50.903-	T50.904-	T50.905-	T50.906-
Stelazine	T43.3X1-	T43.3X2-	T43.3X3-	T43.3X4-	T43.3X5-	T43.3X6-
Stemetil	T43.3X1-	T43.3X2-	T43.3X3-	T43.3X4-	T43.3X5-	T43.3X6-
Stepronin	T48.4X1-	T48.4X2-	T48.4X3-	T48.4X4-	T48.4X5-	T48.4X6-
Sterculia	T47.4X1-	T47.4X2-	T47.4X3-	T47.4X4-	T47.4X5-	T47.4X6-
Sternutator gas	T59.891-	T59.892-	T59.893-	T59.894-		
Steroid	T38.0X1-	T38.0X2-	T38.0X3-	T38.0X4-	T38.0X5-	T38.0X6-
anabolic	T38.7X1-	T38.7X2-	T38.7X3-	T38.7X4-	T38.7X5-	T38.7X6-
androgenic	T38.7X1-	T38.7X2-	T38.7X3-	T38.7X4-	T38.7X5-	T38.7X6-
antineoplastic, hormone	T38.7X1-	T38.7X2-	T38.7X3-	T38.7X4-	T38.7X5-	T38.7X6-
estrogen	T38.5X1-	T38.5X2-	T38.5X3-	T38.5X4-	T38.5X5-	T38.5X6-
ENT agent	T49.6X1-	T49.6X2-	T49.6X3-	T49.6X4-	T49.6X5-	T49.6X6-
ophthalmic preparation	T49.5X1-	T49.5X2-	T49.5X3-	T49.5X4-	T49.5X5-	T49.5X6-
topical NEC	T49.0X1-	T49.0X2-	T49.0X3-	T49.0X4-	T49.0X5-	T49.0X6-
Stibine	T56.891-	T56.892-	T56.893-	T56.894-	-	-
Stibogluconate	T37.3X1-	T37.3X2-	T37.3X3-	T37.3X4-	T37.3X5-	T37.3X6-
Stibophen	T37.4X1-	T37.4X2-	T37.4X3-	T37.4X4-	T37.4X5-	T37.4X6-
Stilbamidine (isetionate)	T37.3X1-	T37.3X2-	T37.3X3-	T37.3X4-	T37.3X5-	T37.3X6-
Stilbestrol	T38.5X1-	T38.5X2-	T38.5X3-	T38.5X4-	T38.5X5-	T38.5X6-
Stilboestrol	T38.5X1-	T38.5X2-	T38.5X3-	T38.5X4-	T38.5X5-	T38.5X6-
Stimulant						
central nervous system — *see also* Psychostimulant	T43.601-	T43.602-	T43.603-	T43.604-	T43.605-	T43.606-
analeptics	T50.7X1-	T50.7X2-	T50.7X3-	T50.7X4-	T50.7X5-	T50.7X6-
opiate antagonist	T50.7X1-	T50.7X2-	T50.7X3-	T50.7X4-	T50.7X5-	T50.7X6-
psychotherapeutic NEC — *see also* Psychotherapeutic drug	T43.601-	T43.602-	T43.603-	T43.604-	T43.605-	T43.606-
specified NEC	T43.691-	T43.692-	T43.693-	T43.694-	T43.695-	T43.696-
respiratory	T48.901-	T48.902-	T48.903-	T48.904-	T48.905-	T48.906-
Stone-dissolving drug	T50.901-	T50.902-	T50.903-	T50.904-	T50.905-	T50.906-
Storage battery (cells) (acid)	T54.2X1-	T54.2X2-	T54.2X3-	T54.2X4-	-	-
Stovaine	T41.3X1-	T41.3X2-	T41.3X3-	T41.3X4-	T41.3X5-	T41.3X6-
infiltration (subcutaneous)	T41.3X1-	T41.3X2-	T41.3X3-	T41.3X4-	T41.3X5-	T41.3X6-
nerve block (peripheral) (plexus)	T41.3X1-	T41.3X2-	T41.3X3-	T41.3X4-	T41.3X5-	T41.3X6-
spinal	T41.3X1-	T41.3X2-	T41.3X3-	T41.3X4-	T41.3X5-	T41.3X6-
topical (surface)	T41.3X1-	T41.3X2-	T41.3X3-	T41.3X4-	T41.3X5-	T41.3X6-
Stovarsal	T37.8X1-	T37.8X2-	T37.8X3-	T37.8X4-	T37.8X5-	T37.8X6-
Stove gas — *see* Gas, stove						
Stoxil	T49.5X1-	T49.5X2-	T49.5X3-	T49.5X4-	T49.5X5-	T49.5X6-
Stramonium	T48.6X1-	T48.6X2-	T48.6X3-	T48.6X4-	T48.6X5-	T48.6X6-
natural state	T62.2X1-	T62.2X2-	T62.2X3-	T62.2X4-	-	-
Streptodornase	T45.3X1-	T45.3X2-	T45.3X3-	T45.3X4-	T45.3X5-	T45.3X6-
Streptoduocin	T36.5X1-	T36.5X2-	T36.5X3-	T36.5X4-	T36.5X5-	T36.5X6-
Streptokinase	T45.611-	T45.612-	T45.613-	T45.614-	T45.615-	T45.616-
Streptomycin (derivative)	T36.5X1-	T36.5X2-	T36.5X3-	T36.5X4-	T36.5X5-	T36.5X6-
Streptonivicin	T36.5X1-	T36.5X2-	T36.5X3-	T36.5X4-	T36.5X5-	T36.5X6-
Streptovarycin	T36.5X1-	T36.5X2-	T36.5X3-	T36.5X4-	T36.5X5-	T36.5X6-
Streptozocin	T45.1X1-	T45.1X2-	T45.1X3-	T45.1X4-	T45.1X5-	T45.1X6-
Streptozotocin	T45.1X1-	T45.1X2-	T45.1X3-	T45.1X4-	T45.1X5-	T45.1X6-
Stripper (paint) (solvent)	T52.8X1-	T52.8X2-	T52.8X3-	T52.8X4-	-	-
Strobane	T60.1X1-	T60.1X2-	T60.1X3-	T60.1X4-	-	-
Strofantina	T46.0X1-	T46.0X2-	T46.0X3-	T46.0X4-	T46.0X5-	T46.0X6-
Strophanthin (g) (k)	T46.0X1-	T46.0X2-	T46.0X3-	T46.0X4-	T46.0X5-	T46.0X6-
Strophanthus	T46.0X1-	T46.0X2-	T46.0X3-	T46.0X4-	T46.0X5-	T46.0X6-
Strophantin	T46.0X1-	T46.0X2-	T46.0X3-	T46.0X4-	T46.0X5-	T46.0X6-
Strophantin-g	T46.0X1-	T46.0X2-	T46.0X3-	T46.0X4-	T46.0X5-	T46.0X6-
Strychnine (nonmedicinal) (pesticide) (salts)	T65.1X1-	T65.1X2-	T65.1X3-	T65.1X4-	-	-
medicinal	T48.291-	T48.292-	T48.293-	T48.294-	T48.295-	T48.296-
Strychnos (ignatii) — *see* Strychnine						
Styramate	T42.8X1-	T42.8X2-	T42.8X3-	T42.8X4-	T42.8X5-	T42.8X6-
Styrene	T65.891-	T65.892-	T65.893-	T65.894-	-	-
Succinimide, antiepileptic or anticonvulsant	T42.2X1-	T42.2X2-	T42.2X3-	T42.2X4-	T42.2X5-	T42.2X6-
mercuric — *see* Mercury						
Succinylcholine	T48.1X1-	T48.1X2-	T48.1X3-	T48.1X4-	T48.1X5-	T48.1X6-
Succinylsulfathiazole	T37.0X1-	T37.0X2-	T37.0X3-	T37.0X4-	T37.0X5-	T37.0X6-

Substance	Poisoning, Accidental (unintentional)	Poisoning, Intentional self-harm	Poisoning, Assault	Poisoning, Undetermined	Adverse effect	Underdosing
Sucralfate	T47.1X1-	T47.1X2-	T47.1X3-	T47.1X4-	T47.1X5-	T47.1X6-
Sucrose	T50.3X1-	T50.3X2-	T50.3X3-	T50.3X4-	T50.3X5-	T50.3X6-
Sufentanil	T40.4X1-	T40.4X2-	T40.4X3-	T40.4X4-	T40.4X5-	T40.4X6-
Sulbactam	T36.0X1-	T36.0X2-	T36.0X3-	T36.0X4-	T36.0X5-	T36.0X6-
Sulbenicillin	T36.0X1-	T36.0X2-	T36.0X3-	T36.0X4-	T36.0X5-	T36.0X6-
Sulbentine	T49.0X1-	T49.0X2-	T49.0X3-	T49.0X4-	T49.0X5-	T49.0X6-
Sulfacetamide	T49.0X1-	T49.0X2-	T49.0X3-	T49.0X4-	T49.0X5-	T49.0X6-
ophthalmic preparation	T49.5X1-	T49.5X2-	T49.5X3-	T49.5X4-	T49.5X5-	T49.5X6-
Sulfachlorpyridazine	T37.0X1-	T37.0X2-	T37.0X3-	T37.0X4-	T37.0X5-	T37.0X6-
Sulfacitine	T37.0X1-	T37.0X2-	T37.0X3-	T37.0X4-	T37.0X5-	T37.0X6-
Sulfadiasulfone sodium	T37.0X1-	T37.0X2-	T37.0X3-	T37.0X4-	T37.0X5-	T37.0X6-
Sulfadiazine	T37.0X1-	T37.0X2-	T37.0X3-	T37.0X4-	T37.0X5-	T37.0X6-
silver (topical)	T49.0X1-	T49.0X2-	T49.0X3-	T49.0X4-	T49.0X5-	T49.0X6-
Sulfadimethoxine	T37.0X1-	T37.0X2-	T37.0X3-	T37.0X4-	T37.0X5-	T37.0X6-
Sulfadimidine	T37.0X1-	T37.0X2-	T37.0X3-	T37.0X4-	T37.0X5-	T37.0X6-
Sulfadoxine	T37.0X1-	T37.0X2-	T37.0X3-	T37.0X4-	T37.0X5-	T37.0X6-
with pyrimethamine	T37.2X1-	T37.2X2-	T37.2X3-	T37.2X4-	T37.2X5-	T37.2X6-
Sulfaethidole	T37.0X1-	T37.0X2-	T37.0X3-	T37.0X4-	T37.0X5-	T37.0X6-
Sulfafurazole	T37.0X1-	T37.0X2-	T37.0X3-	T37.0X4-	T37.0X5-	T37.0X6-
Sulfaguanidine	T37.0X1-	T37.0X2-	T37.0X3-	T37.0X4-	T37.0X5-	T37.0X6-
Sulfalene	T37.0X1-	T37.0X2-	T37.0X3-	T37.0X4-	T37.0X5-	T37.0X6-
Sulfaloxate	T37.0X1-	T37.0X2-	T37.0X3-	T37.0X4-	T37.0X5-	T37.0X6-
Sulfaloxic acid	T37.0X1-	T37.0X2-	T37.0X3-	T37.0X4-	T37.0X5-	T37.0X6-
Sulfamazone	T39.2X1-	T39.2X2-	T39.2X3-	T39.2X4-	T39.2X5-	T39.2X6-
Sulfamerazine	T37.0X1-	T37.0X2-	T37.0X3-	T37.0X4-	T37.0X5-	T37.0X6-
Sulfameter	T37.0X1-	T37.0X2-	T37.0X3-	T37.0X4-	T37.0X5-	T37.0X6-
Sulfamethazine	T37.0X1-	T37.0X2-	T37.0X3-	T37.0X4-	T37.0X5-	T37.0X6-
Sulfamethizole	T37.0X1-	T37.0X2-	T37.0X3-	T37.0X4-	T37.0X5-	T37.0X6-
Sulfamethoxazole	T37.0X1-	T37.0X2-	T37.0X3-	T37.0X4-	T37.0X5-	T37.0X6-
with trimethoprim	T36.8X1-	T36.8X2-	T36.8X3-	T36.8X4-	T36.8X5-	T36.8X6-
Sulfamethoxydiazine	T37.0X1-	T37.0X2-	T37.0X3-	T37.0X4-	T37.0X5-	T37.0X6-
Sulfamethoxypyridazine	T37.0X1-	T37.0X2-	T37.0X3-	T37.0X4-	T37.0X5-	T37.0X6-
Sulfamethylthiazole	T37.0X1-	T37.0X2-	T37.0X3-	T37.0X4-	T37.0X5-	T37.0X6-
Sulfametoxydiazine	T37.0X1-	T37.0X2-	T37.0X3-	T37.0X4-	T37.0X5-	T37.0X6-
Sulfamidopyrine	T39.2X1-	T39.2X2-	T39.2X3-	T39.2X4-	T39.2X5-	T39.2X6-
Sulfamonomethoxine	T37.0X1-	T37.0X2-	T37.0X3-	T37.0X4-	T37.0X5-	T37.0X6-
Sulfamoxole	T37.0X1-	T37.0X2-	T37.0X3-	T37.0X4-	T37.0X5-	T37.0X6-
Sulfamylon	T49.0X1-	T49.0X2-	T49.0X3-	T49.0X4-	T49.0X5-	T49.0X6-
Sulfan blue (diagnostic dye)	T50.8X1-	T50.8X2-	T50.8X3-	T50.8X4-	T50.8X5-	T50.8X6-
Sulfanilamide	T37.0X1-	T37.0X2-	T37.0X3-	T37.0X4-	T37.0X5-	T37.0X6-
Sulfanilylguanidine	T37.0X1-	T37.0X2-	T37.0X3-	T37.0X4-	T37.0X5-	T37.0X6-
Sulfaperin	T37.0X1-	T37.0X2-	T37.0X3-	T37.0X4-	T37.0X5-	T37.0X6-
Sulfaphenazole	T37.0X1-	T37.0X2-	T37.0X3-	T37.0X4-	T37.0X5-	T37.0X6-
Sulfaphenylthiazole	T37.0X1-	T37.0X2-	T37.0X3-	T37.0X4-	T37.0X5-	T37.0X6-
Sulfaproxyline	T37.0X1-	T37.0X2-	T37.0X3-	T37.0X4-	T37.0X5-	T37.0X6-
Sulfapyridine	T37.0X1-	T37.0X2-	T37.0X3-	T37.0X4-	T37.0X5-	T37.0X6-
Sulfapyrimidine	T37.0X1-	T37.0X2-	T37.0X3-	T37.0X4-	T37.0X5-	T37.0X6-
Sulfarsphenamine	T37.8X1-	T37.8X2-	T37.8X3-	T37.8X4-	T37.8X5-	T37.8X6-
Sulfasalazine	T37.0X1-	T37.0X2-	T37.0X3-	T37.0X4-	T37.0X5-	T37.0X6-
Sulfasuxidine	T37.0X1-	T37.0X2-	T37.0X3-	T37.0X4-	T37.0X5-	T37.0X6-
Sulfasymazine	T37.0X1-	T37.0X2-	T37.0X3-	T37.0X4-	T37.0X5-	T37.0X6-
Sulfated amylopectin	T47.8X1-	T47.8X2-	T47.8X3-	T47.8X4-	T47.8X5-	T47.8X6-
Sulfathiazole	T37.0X1-	T37.0X2-	T37.0X3-	T37.0X4-	T37.0X5-	T37.0X6-
Sulfatostearate	T49.2X1-	T49.2X2-	T49.2X3-	T49.2X4-	T49.2X5-	T49.2X6-
Sulfinpyrazone	T50.4X1-	T50.4X2-	T50.4X3-	T50.4X4-	T50.4X5-	T50.4X6-
Sulfiram	T49.0X1-	T49.0X2-	T49.0X3-	T49.0X4-	T49.0X5-	T49.0X6-
Sulfisomidine	T37.0X1-	T37.0X2-	T37.0X3-	T37.0X4-	T37.0X5-	T37.0X6-
Sulfisoxazole	T37.0X1-	T37.0X2-	T37.0X3-	T37.0X4-	T37.0X5-	T37.0X6-
ophthalmic preparation	T49.5X1-	T49.5X2-	T49.5X3-	T49.5X4-	T49.5X5-	T49.5X6-
Sulfobromophthalein (sodium)	T50.8X1-	T50.8X2-	T50.8X3-	T50.8X4-	T50.8X5-	T50.8X6-
Sulfobromphthalein	T50.8X1-	T50.8X2-	T50.8X3-	T50.8X4-	T50.8X5-	T50.8X6-
Sulfogaiacol	T48.4X1-	T48.4X2-	T48.4X3-	T48.4X4-	T48.4X5-	T48.4X6-
Sulfomyxin	T36.8X1-	T36.8X2-	T36.8X3-	T36.8X4-	T36.8X5-	T36.8X6-
Sulfonal	T42.6X1-	T42.6X2-	T42.6X3-	T42.6X4-	T42.6X5-	T42.6X6-
Sulfonamide NEC	T37.0X1-	T37.0X2-	T37.0X3-	T37.0X4-	T37.0X5-	T37.0X6-
eye	T49.5X1-	T49.5X2-	T49.5X3-	T49.5X4-	T49.5X5-	T49.5X6-
Sulfonazide	T37.1X1-	T37.1X2-	T37.1X3-	T37.1X4-	T37.1X5-	T37.1X6-
Sulfones	T37.1X1-	T37.1X2-	T37.1X3-	T37.1X4-	T37.1X5-	T37.1X6-
Sulfonethylmethane	T42.6X1-	T42.6X2-	T42.6X3-	T42.6X4-	T42.6X5-	T42.6X6-
Sulfonmethane	T42.6X1-	T42.6X2-	T42.6X3-	T42.6X4-	T42.6X5-	T42.6X6-
Sulfonphthal, sulfonphthol	T50.8X1-	T50.8X2-	T50.8X3-	T50.8X4-	T50.8X5-	T50.8X6-
Sulfonylurea derivatives, oral	T38.3X1-	T38.3X2-	T38.3X3-	T38.3X4-	T38.3X5-	T38.3X6-
Sulforidazine	T43.3X1-	T43.3X2-	T43.3X3-	T43.3X4-	T43.3X5-	T43.3X6-
Sulfoxone	T37.1X1-	T37.1X2-	T37.1X3-	T37.1X4-	T37.1X5-	T37.1X6-
Sulfur, sulfurated, sulfuric, sulfurous, sulfuryl (compounds NEC) (medicinal)	T49.4X1-	T49.4X2-	T49.4X3-	T49.4X4-	T49.4X5-	T49.4X6-
acid	T54.2X1-	T54.2X2-	T54.2X3-	T54.2X4-	-	-

Substance	Poisoning, Accidental (unintentional)	Poisoning, Intentional self-harm	Poisoning, Assault	Poisoning, Undetermined	Adverse effect	Underdosing
Sulfur, sulfurated, sulfuric, sulfurous, sulfuryl - *continued*						
dioxide (gas)	T59.1X1-	T59.1X2-	T59.1X3-	T59.1X4-	-	-
ether — *see* Ether(s)						
hydrogen	T59.6X1-	T59.6X2-	T59.6X3-	T59.6X4-	-	-
medicinal (keratolytic) (ointment) NEC	T49.4X1-	T49.4X2-	T49.4X3-	T49.4X4-	T49.4X5-	T49.4X6-
ointment	T49.0X1-	T49.0X2-	T49.0X3-	T49.0X4-	T49.0X5-	T49.0X6-
pesticide (vapor)	T60.91X-	T60.92X-	T60.93X-	T60.94X-	-	-
vapor NEC	T59.891-	T59.892-	T59.893-	T59.894-	-	-
Sulfuric acid	T54.2X1-	T54.2X2-	T54.2X3-	T54.2X4-	-	-
Sulglicotide	T47.1X1-	T47.1X2-	T47.1X3-	T47.1X4-	T47.1X5-	T47.1X6-
Sulindac	T39.391-	T39.392-	T39.393-	T39.394-	T39.395-	T39.396-
Sulisatin	T47.2X1-	T47.2X2-	T47.2X3-	T47.2X4-	T47.2X5-	T47.2X6-
Sulisobenzone	T49.3X1-	T49.3X2-	T49.3X3-	T49.3X4-	T49.3X5-	T49.3X6-
Sulkowitch's reagent	T50.8X1-	T50.8X2-	T50.8X3-	T50.8X4-	T50.8X5-	T50.8X6-
Sulmetozine	T44.3X1-	T44.3X2-	T44.3X3-	T44.3X4-	T44.3X5-	T44.3X6-
Suloctidil	T46.7X1-	T46.7X2-	T46.7X3-	T46.7X4-	T46.7X5-	T46.7X6-
Sulph- — *see also* Sulf-						
Sulphadiazine	T37.0X1-	T37.0X2-	T37.0X3-	T37.0X4-	T37.0X5-	T37.0X6-
Sulphadimethoxine	T37.0X1-	T37.0X2-	T37.0X3-	T37.0X4-	T37.0X5-	T37.0X6-
Sulphadimidine	T37.0X1-	T37.0X2-	T37.0X3-	T37.0X4-	T37.0X5-	T37.0X6-
Sulphadione	T37.1X1-	T37.1X2-	T37.1X3-	T37.1X4-	T37.1X5-	T37.1X6-
Sulphafurazole	T37.0X1-	T37.0X2-	T37.0X3-	T37.0X4-	T37.0X5-	T37.0X6-
Sulphamethizole	T37.0X1-	T37.0X2-	T37.0X3-	T37.0X4-	T37.0X5-	T37.0X6-
Sulphamethoxazole	T37.0X1-	T37.0X2-	T37.0X3-	T37.0X4-	T37.0X5-	T37.0X6-
Sulphan blue	T50.8X1-	T50.8X2-	T50.8X3-	T50.8X4-	T50.8X5-	T50.8X6-
Sulphaphenazole	T37.0X1-	T37.0X2-	T37.0X3-	T37.0X4-	T37.0X5-	T37.0X6-
Sulphapyridine	T37.0X1-	T37.0X2-	T37.0X3-	T37.0X4-	T37.0X5-	T37.0X6-
Sulphasalazine	T37.0X1-	T37.0X2-	T37.0X3-	T37.0X4-	T37.0X5-	T37.0X6-
Sulphinpyrazone	T50.4X1-	T50.4X2-	T50.4X3-	T50.4X4-	T50.4X5-	T50.4X6-
Sulpiride	T43.591-	T43.592-	T43.593-	T43.594-	T43.595-	T43.596-
Sulprostone	T48.0X1-	T48.0X2-	T48.0X3-	T48.0X4-	T48.0X5-	T48.0X6-
Sulpyrine	T39.2X1-	T39.2X2-	T39.2X3-	T39.2X4-	T39.2X5-	T39.2X6-
Sultamicillin	T36.0X1-	T36.0X2-	T36.0X3-	T36.0X4-	T36.0X5-	T36.0X6-
Sulthiame	T42.6X1-	T42.6X2-	T42.6X3-	T42.6X4-	T42.6X5-	T42.6X6-
Sultiame	T42.6X1-	T42.6X2-	T42.6X3-	T42.6X4-	T42.6X5-	T42.6X6-
Sultopride	T43.591-	T43.592-	T43.593-	T43.594-	T43.595-	T43.596-
Sumatriptan	T39.8X1-	T39.8X2-	T39.8X3-	T39.8X4-	T39.8X5-	T39.8X6-
Sunflower seed oil	T46.6X1-	T46.6X2-	T46.6X3-	T46.6X4-	T46.6X5-	T46.6X6-
Superinone	T48.4X1-	T48.4X2-	T48.4X3-	T48.4X4-	T48.4X5-	T48.4X6-
Suprofen	T39.311-	T39.312-	T39.313-	T39.314-	T39.315-	T39.316-
Suramin (sodium)	T37.4X1-	T37.4X2-	T37.4X3-	T37.4X4-	T37.4X5-	T37.4X6-
Surfacaine	T41.3X1-	T41.3X2-	T41.3X3-	T41.3X4-	T41.3X5-	T41.3X6-
Surital	T41.1X1-	T41.1X2-	T41.1X3-	T41.1X4-	T41.1X5-	T41.1X6-
Sutilains	T45.3X1-	T45.3X2-	T45.3X3-	T45.3X4-	T45.3X5-	T45.3X6-
Suxamethonium (chloride)	T48.1X1-	T48.1X2-	T48.1X3-	T48.1X4-	T48.1X5-	T48.1X6-
Suxethonium (chloride)	T48.1X1-	T48.1X2-	T48.1X3-	T48.1X4-	T48.1X5-	T48.1X6-
Suxibuzone	T39.2X1-	T39.2X2-	T39.2X3-	T39.2X4-	T39.2X5-	T39.2X6-
Sweet niter spirit	T46.3X1-	T46.3X2-	T46.3X3-	T46.3X4-	T46.3X5-	T46.3X6-
Sweet oil (birch)	T49.3X1-	T49.3X2-	T49.3X3-	T49.3X4-	T49.3X5-	T49.3X6-
Sweetener	T50.901-	T50.902-	T50.903-	T50.904-	T50.905-	T50.906-
Sym-dichloroethyl ether	T53.6X1-	T53.6X2-	T53.6X3-	T53.6X4-	-	-
Sympatholytic NEC	T44.8X1-	T44.8X2-	T44.8X3-	T44.8X4-	T44.8X5-	T44.8X6-
haloalkylamine	T44.8X1-	T44.8X2-	T44.8X3-	T44.8X4-	T44.8X5-	T44.8X6-
Sympathomimetic NEC	T44.901-	T44.902-	T44.903-	T44.904-	T44.905-	T44.906-
anti-common-cold	T48.5X1-	T48.5X2-	T48.5X3-	T48.5X4-	T48.5X5-	T48.5X6-
bronchodilator	T48.6X1-	T48.6X2-	T48.6X3-	T48.6X4-	T48.6X5-	T48.6X6-
specified NEC	T44.991-	T44.992-	T44.993-	T44.994-	T44.995-	T44.996-
Synagis	T50.B91-	T50.B92-	T50.B93-	T50.B94-	T50.B95-	T50.B96-
Synalar	T49.0X1-	T49.0X2-	T49.0X3-	T49.0X4-	T49.0X5-	T49.0X6-
Synthroid	T38.1X1-	T38.1X2-	T38.1X3-	T38.1X4-	T38.1X5-	T38.1X6-
Syntocinon	T48.0X1-	T48.0X2-	T48.0X3-	T48.0X4-	T48.0X5-	T48.0X6-
Syrosingopine	T46.5X1-	T46.5X2-	T46.5X3-	T46.5X4-	T46.5X5-	T46.5X6-
Systemic drug	T45.91X-	T45.92X-	T45.93X-	T45.94X-	T45.95X-	T45.96X-
specified NEC	T45.8X1-	T45.8X2-	T45.8X3-	T45.8X4-	T45.8X5-	T45.8X6-
2,4,5-T	T60.3X1-	T60.3X2-	T60.3X3-	T60.3X4-	-	-
Tablets — *see also* specified substance	T50.901-	T50.902-	T50.903-	T50.904-	T50.905-	T50.906-
Tace	T38.5X1-	T38.5X2-	T38.5X3-	T38.5X4-	T38.5X5-	T38.5X6-
Tacrine	T44.0X1-	T44.0X2-	T44.0X3-	T44.0X4-	T44.0X5-	T44.0X6-
Tadalafil	T46.7X1-	T46.7X2-	T46.7X3-	T46.7X4-	T46.7X5-	T46.7X6-
Talampicillin	T36.0X1-	T36.0X2-	T36.0X3-	T36.0X4-	T36.0X5-	T36.0X6-
Talbutal	T42.3X1-	T42.3X2-	T42.3X3-	T42.3X4-	T42.3X5-	T42.3X6-
Talc powder	T49.3X1-	T49.3X2-	T49.3X3-	T49.3X4-	T49.3X5-	T49.3X6-
Talcum	T49.3X1-	T49.3X2-	T49.3X3-	T49.3X4-	T49.3X5-	T49.3X6-
Taleranol	T38.6X1-	T38.6X2-	T38.6X3-	T38.6X4-	T38.6X5-	T38.6X6-
Tamoxifen	T38.6X1-	T38.6X2-	T38.6X3-	T38.6X4-	T38.6X5-	T38.6X6-

Substance	Poisoning, Accidental (unintentional)	Poisoning, Intentional self-harm	Poisoning, Assault	Poisoning, Undetermined	Adverse effect	Underdosing
Tamsulosin	T44.6X1-	T44.6X2-	T44.6X3-	T44.6X4-	T44.6X5-	T44.6X6-
Tandearil, tanderil	T39.2X1-	T39.2X2-	T39.2X3-	T39.2X4-	T39.2X5-	T39.2X6-
Tannic acid	T49.2X1-	T49.2X2-	T49.2X3-	T49.2X4-	T49.2X5-	T49.2X6-
medicinal (astringent)	T49.2X1-	T49.2X2-	T49.2X3-	T49.2X4-	T49.2X5-	T49.2X6-
Tannin — *see* Tannic acid						
Tansy	T62.2X1-	T62.2X2-	T62.2X3-	T62.2X4-	-	-
TAO	T36.3X1-	T36.3X2-	T36.3X3-	T36.3X4-	T36.3X5-	T36.3X6-
Tapazole	T38.2X1-	T38.2X2-	T38.2X3-	T38.2X4-	T38.2X5-	T38.2X6-
Tar NEC	T52.0X1-	T52.0X2-	T52.0X3-	T52.0X4-	-	-
camphor	T60.1X1-	T60.1X2-	T60.1X3-	T60.1X4-	-	-
distillate	T49.1X1-	T49.1X2-	T49.1X3-	T49.1X4-	T49.1X5-	T49.1X6-
fumes	T59.891-	T59.892-	T59.893-	T59.894-	-	-
medicinal	T49.1X1-	T49.1X2-	T49.1X3-	T49.1X4-	T49.1X5-	T49.1X6-
ointment	T49.1X1-	T49.1X2-	T49.1X3-	T49.1X4-	T49.1X5-	T49.1X6-
Taractan	T43.591-	T43.592-	T43.593-	T43.594-	T43.595-	T43.596-
Tarantula (venomous)	T63.321-	T63.322-	T63.323-	T63.324-	-	-
Tartar emetic	T37.8X1-	T37.8X2-	T37.8X3-	T37.8X4-	T37.8X5-	T37.8X6-
Tartaric acid	T65.891-	T65.892-	T65.893-	T65.894-	-	-
Tartrate, laxative	T47.4X1-	T47.4X2-	T47.4X3-	T47.4X4-	T47.4X5-	T47.4X6-
Tartrated antimony (anti-infective)	T37.8X1-	T37.8X2-	T37.8X3-	T37.8X4-	T37.8X5-	T37.8X6-
Tauromustine	T45.1X1-	T45.1X2-	T45.1X3-	T45.1X4-	T45.1X5-	T45.1X6-
TCA — *see* Trichloroacetic acid						
TCDD	T53.7X1-	T53.7X2-	T53.7X3-	T53.7X4-	-	-
TDI (vapor)	T65.0X1-	T65.0X2-	T65.0X3-	T65.0X4-	-	-
Tear						
gas	T59.3X1-	T59.3X2-	T59.3X3-	T59.3X4-	-	-
solution	T49.5X1-	T49.5X2-	T49.5X3-	T49.5X4-	T49.5X5-	T49.5X6-
Teclothiazide	T50.2X1-	T50.2X2-	T50.2X3-	T50.2X4-	T50.2X5-	T50.2X6-
Teclozan	T37.3X1-	T37.3X2-	T37.3X3-	T37.3X4-	T37.3X5-	T37.3X6-
Tegafur	T45.1X1-	T45.1X2-	T45.1X3-	T45.1X4-	T45.1X5-	T45.1X6-
Tegretol	T42.1X1-	T42.1X2-	T42.1X3-	T42.1X4-	T42.1X5-	T42.1X6-
Teicoplanin	T36.8X1-	T36.8X2-	T36.8X3-	T36.8X4-	T36.8X5-	T36.8X6-
Telepaque	T50.8X1-	T50.8X2-	T50.8X3-	T50.8X4-	T50.8X5-	T50.8X6-
Tellurium	T56.891-	T56.892-	T56.893-	T56.894-	-	-
fumes	T56.891-	T56.892-	T56.893-	T56.894-	-	-
TEM	T45.1X1-	T45.1X2-	T45.1X3-	T45.1X4-	T45.1X5-	T45.1X6-
Temazepam	T42.4X1-	T42.4X2-	T42.4X3-	T42.4X4-	T42.4X5-	T42.4X6-
Temocillin	T36.0X1-	T36.0X2-	T36.0X3-	T36.0X4-	T36.0X5-	T36.0X6-
Tenamfetamine	T43.621-	T43.622-	T43.623-	T43.624-	T43.625-	T43.626-
Teniposide	T45.1X1-	T45.1X2-	T45.1X3-	T45.1X4-	T45.1X5-	T45.1X6-
Tenitramine	T46.3X1-	T46.3X2-	T46.3X3-	T46.3X4-	T46.3X5-	T46.3X6-
Tenoglicin	T48.4X1-	T48.4X2-	T48.4X3-	T48.4X4-	T48.4X5-	T48.4X6-
Tenonitrozole	T37.3X1-	T37.3X2-	T37.3X3-	T37.3X4-	T37.3X5-	T37.3X6-
Tenoxicam	T39.391-	T39.392-	T39.393-	T39.394-	T39.395-	T39.396-
TEPA	T45.1X1-	T45.1X2-	T45.1X3-	T45.1X4-	T45.1X5-	T45.1X6-
TEPP	T60.0X1-	T60.0X2-	T60.0X3-	T60.0X4-	-	-
Teprotide	T46.5X1-	T46.5X2-	T46.5X3-	T46.5X4-	T46.5X5-	T46.5X6-
Terazosin	T44.6X1-	T44.6X2-	T44.6X3-	T44.6X4-	T44.6X5-	T44.6X6-
Terbufos	T60.0X1-	T60.0X2-	T60.0X3-	T60.0X4-	-	-
Terbutaline	T48.6X1-	T48.6X2-	T48.6X3-	T48.6X4-	T48.6X5-	T48.6X6-
Terconazole	T49.0X1-	T49.0X2-	T49.0X3-	T49.0X4-	T49.0X5-	T49.0X6-
Terfenadine	T45.0X1-	T45.0X2-	T45.0X3-	T45.0X4-	T45.0X5-	T45.0X6-
Teriparatide (acetate)	T50.991-	T50.992-	T50.993-	T50.994-	T50.995-	T50.996-
Terizidone	T37.1X1-	T37.1X2-	T37.1X3-	T37.1X4-	T37.1X5-	T37.1X6-
Terlipressin	T38.891-	T38.892-	T38.893-	T38.894-	T38.895-	T38.896-
Terodiline	T46.3X1-	T46.3X2-	T46.3X3-	T46.3X4-	T46.3X5-	T46.3X6-
Teroxalene	T37.4X1-	T37.4X2-	T37.4X3-	T37.4X4-	T37.4X5-	T37.4X6-
Terpin (cis) **hydrate**	T48.4X1-	T48.4X2-	T48.4X3-	T48.4X4-	T48.4X5-	T48.4X6-
Terramycin	T36.4X1-	T36.4X2-	T36.4X3-	T36.4X4-	T36.4X5-	T36.4X6-
Tertatolol	T44.7X1-	T44.7X2-	T44.7X3-	T44.7X4-	T44.7X5-	T44.7X6-
Tessalon	T48.3X1-	T48.3X2-	T48.3X3-	T48.3X4-	T48.3X5-	T48.3X6-
Testolactone	T38.7X1-	T38.7X2-	T38.7X3-	T38.7X4-	T38.7X5-	T38.7X6-
Testosterone	T38.7X1-	T38.7X2-	T38.7X3-	T38.7X4-	T38.7X5-	T38.7X6-
Tetanus toxoid or vaccine	T50.A91-	T50.A92-	T50.A93-	T50.A94-	T50.A95-	T50.A96-
antitoxin	T50.Z11-	T50.Z12-	T50.Z13-	T50.Z14-	T50.Z15-	T50.Z16-
immune globulin (human)	T50.Z11-	T50.Z12-	T50.Z13-	T50.Z14-	T50.Z15-	T50.Z16-
toxoid	T50.A91-	T50.A92-	T50.A93-	T50.A94-	T50.A95-	T50.A96-
with diphtheria toxoid	T50.A21-	T50.A22-	T50.A23-	T50.A24-	T50.A25-	T50.A26-
with pertussis	T50.A11-	T50.A12-	T50.A13-	T50.A14-	T50.A15-	T50.A16-
Tetrabenazine	T43.591-	T43.592-	T43.593-	T43.594-	T43.595-	T43.596-
Tetracaine	T41.3X1-	T41.3X2-	T41.3X3-	T41.3X4-	T41.3X5-	T41.3X6-
nerve block (peripheral) (plexus)	T41.3X1-	T41.3X2-	T41.3X3-	T41.3X4-	T41.3X5-	T41.3X6-
regional	T41.3X1-	T41.3X2-	T41.3X3-	T41.3X4-	T41.3X5-	T41.3X6-
spinal	T41.3X1-	T41.3X2-	T41.3X3-	T41.3X4-	T41.3X5-	T41.3X6-
Tetrachlorethylene — *see* Tetrachloroethylene						

Substance	Poisoning, Accidental (unintentional)	Poisoning, Intentional self-harm	Poisoning, Assault	Poisoning, Undetermined	Adverse effect	Underdosing
Tetrachlormethiazide	T50.2X1-	T50.2X2-	T50.2X3-	T50.2X4-	T50.2X5-	T50.2X6-
2,3,7,8-Tetrachlorodibenzo-p-dioxin	T53.7X1-	T53.7X2-	T53.7X3-	T53.7X4-	-	-
Tetrachloroethane	T53.6X1-	T53.6X2-	T53.6X3-	T53.6X4-	-	-
vapor	T53.6X1-	T53.6X2-	T53.6X3-	T53.6X4-	-	-
paint or varnish	T53.6X1-	T53.6X2-	T53.6X3-	T53.6X4-	-	-
Tetrachloroethylene (liquid)	T53.3X1-	T53.3X2-	T53.3X3-	T53.3X4-	-	-
medicinal	T37.4X1-	T37.4X2-	T37.4X3-	T37.4X4-	T37.4X5-	T37.4X6-
vapor	T53.3X1-	T53.3X2-	T53.3X3-	T53.3X4-	-	-
Tetrachloromethane — see Carbon tetrachloride						
Tetracosactide	T38.811-	T38.812-	T38.813-	T38.814-	T38.815-	T38.816-
Tetracosactrin	T38.811-	T38.812-	T38.813-	T38.814-	T38.815-	T38.816-
Tetracycline	T36.4X1-	T36.4X2-	T36.4X3-	T36.4X4-	T36.4X5-	T36.4X6-
ophthalmic preparation	T49.5X1-	T49.5X2-	T49.5X3-	T49.5X4-	T49.5X5-	T49.5X6-
topical NEC	T49.0X1-	T49.0X2-	T49.0X3-	T49.0X4-	T49.0X5-	T49.0X6-
Tetradifon	T60.8X1-	T60.8X2-	T60.8X3-	T60.8X4-	-	-
Tetradotoxin	T61.771-	T61.772-	T61.773-	T61.774-	-	-
Tetraethyl						
lead	T56.0X1-	T56.0X2-	T56.0X3-	T56.0X4-	-	-
pyrophosphate	T60.0X1-	T60.0X2-	T60.0X3-	T60.0X4-	-	-
Tetraethylammonium chloride	T44.2X1-	T44.2X2-	T44.2X3-	T44.2X4-	T44.2X5-	T44.2X6-
Tetraethylthiuram disulfide	T50.6X1-	T50.6X2-	T50.6X3-	T50.6X4-	T50.6X5-	T50.6X6-
Tetrahydroaminoacridine	T44.0X1-	T44.0X2-	T44.0X3-	T44.0X4-	T44.0X5-	T44.0X6-
Tetrahydrocannabinol	T40.7X1-	T40.7X2-	T40.7X3-	T40.7X4-	T40.7X5-	T40.7X6-
Tetrahydrofuran	T52.8X1-	T52.8X2-	T52.8X3-	T52.8X4-	-	-
Tetrahydronaphthalene	T52.8X1-	T52.8X2-	T52.8X3-	T52.8X4-	-	-
Tetrahydrozoline	T49.5X1-	T49.5X2-	T49.5X3-	T49.5X4-	T49.5X5-	T49.5X6-
Tetralin	T52.8X1-	T52.8X2-	T52.8X3-	T52.8X4-	-	-
Tetramethrin	T60.2X1-	T60.2X2-	T60.2X3-	T60.2X4-	-	-
Tetramethylthiuram (disulfide) NEC	T60.3X1-	T60.3X2-	T60.3X3-	T60.3X4-	-	-
medicinal	T49.0X1-	T49.0X2-	T49.0X3-	T49.0X4-	T49.0X5-	T49.0X6-
Tetramisole	T37.4X1-	T37.4X2-	T37.4X3-	T37.4X4-	T37.4X5-	T37.4X6-
Tetranicotinoyl fructose	T46.7X1-	T46.7X2-	T46.7X3-	T46.7X4-	T46.7X5-	T46.7X6-
Tetrazepam	T42.4X1-	T42.4X2-	T42.4X3-	T42.4X4-	T42.4X5-	T42.4X6-
Tetronal	T42.6X1-	T42.6X2-	T42.6X3-	T42.6X4-	T42.6X5-	T42.6X6-
Tetryl	T65.3X1-	T65.3X2-	T65.3X3-	T65.3X4-	-	-
Tetrylammonium chloride	T44.2X1-	T44.2X2-	T44.2X3-	T44.2X4-	T44.2X5-	T44.2X6-
Tetryzoline	T49.5X1-	T49.5X2-	T49.5X3-	T49.5X4-	T49.5X5-	T49.5X6-
Thalidomide	T45.1X1-	T45.1X2-	T45.1X3-	T45.1X4-	T45.1X5-	T45.1X6-
Thallium (compounds) (dust) NEC	T56.811-	T56.812-	T56.813-	T56.814-	-	-
pesticide	T60.4X1-	T60.4X2-	T60.4X3-	T60.4X4-	-	-
THC	T40.7X1-	T40.7X2-	T40.7X3-	T40.7X4-	T40.7X5-	T40.7X6-
Thebacon	T48.3X1-	T48.3X2-	T48.3X3-	T48.3X4-	T48.3X5-	T48.3X6-
Thebaine	T40.2X1-	T40.2X2-	T40.2X3-	T40.2X4-	T40.2X5-	T40.2X6-
Thenoic acid	T49.6X1-	T49.6X2-	T49.6X3-	T49.6X4-	T49.6X5-	T49.6X6-
Thenyldiamine	T45.0X1-	T45.0X2-	T45.0X3-	T45.0X4-	T45.0X5-	T45.0X6-
Theobromine (calcium salicylate)	T48.6X1-	T48.6X2-	T48.6X3-	T48.6X4-	T48.6X5-	T48.6X6-
sodium salicylate	T48.6X1-	T48.6X2-	T48.6X3-	T48.6X4-	T48.6X5-	T48.6X6-
Theophyllamine	T48.6X1-	T48.6X2-	T48.6X3-	T48.6X4-	T48.6X5-	T48.6X6-
Theophylline	T48.6X1-	T48.6X2-	T48.6X3-	T48.6X4-	T48.6X5-	T48.6X6-
aminobenzoic acid	T48.6X1-	T48.6X2-	T48.6X3-	T48.6X4-	T48.6X5-	T48.6X6-
ethylenediamine	T48.6X1-	T48.6X2-	T48.6X3-	T48.6X4-	T48.6X5-	T48.6X6-
piperazine p-amino-benzoate	T48.6X1-	T48.6X2-	T48.6X3-	T48.6X4-	T48.6X5-	T48.6X6-
Thiabendazole	T37.4X1-	T37.4X2-	T37.4X3-	T37.4X4-	T37.4X5-	T37.4X6-
Thialbarbital	T41.1X1-	T41.1X2-	T41.1X3-	T41.1X4-	T41.1X5-	T41.1X6-
Thiamazole	T38.2X1-	T38.2X2-	T38.2X3-	T38.2X4-	T38.2X5-	T38.2X6-
Thiambutosine	T37.1X1-	T37.1X2-	T37.1X3-	T37.1X4-	T37.1X5-	T37.1X6-
Thiamine	T45.2X1-	T45.2X2-	T45.2X3-	T45.2X4-	T45.2X5-	T45.2X6-
Thiamphenicol	T36.2X1-	T36.2X2-	T36.2X3-	T36.2X4-	T36.2X5-	T36.2X6-
Thiamylal	T41.1X1-	T41.1X2-	T41.1X3-	T41.1X4-	T41.1X5-	T41.1X6-
sodium	T41.1X1-	T41.1X2-	T41.1X3-	T41.1X4-	T41.1X5-	T41.1X6-
Thiazesim	T43.291-	T43.292-	T43.293-	T43.294-	T43.295-	T43.296-
Thiazides (diuretics)	T50.2X1-	T50.2X2-	T50.2X3-	T50.2X4-	T50.2X5-	T50.2X6-
Thiazinamium metilsulfate	T43.3X1-	T43.3X2-	T43.3X3-	T43.3X4-	T43.3X5-	T43.3X6-
Thiethylperazine	T43.3X1-	T43.3X2-	T43.3X3-	T43.3X4-	T43.3X5-	T43.3X6-
Thimerosal	T49.0X1-	T49.0X2-	T49.0X3-	T49.0X4-	T49.0X5-	T49.0X6-
ophthalmic preparation	T49.5X1-	T49.5X2-	T49.5X3-	T49.5X4-	T49.5X5-	T49.5X6-
Thioacetazone	T37.1X1-	T37.1X2-	T37.1X3-	T37.1X4-	T37.1X5-	T37.1X6-
with isoniazid	T37.1X1-	T37.1X2-	T37.1X3-	T37.1X4-	T37.1X5-	T37.1X6-
Thiobarbital sodium	T41.1X1-	T41.1X2-	T41.1X3-	T41.1X4-	T41.1X5-	T41.1X6-
Thiobarbiturate anesthetic	T41.1X1-	T41.1X2-	T41.1X3-	T41.1X4-	T41.1X5-	T41.1X6-
Thiobismol	T37.8X1-	T37.8X2-	T37.8X3-	T37.8X4-	T37.8X5-	T37.8X6-
Thiobutabarbital sodium	T41.1X1-	T41.1X2-	T41.1X3-	T41.1X4-	T41.1X5-	T41.1X6-
Thiocarbamate (insecticide)	T60.0X1-	T60.0X2-	T60.0X3-	T60.0X4-	-	-
Thiocarbamide	T38.2X1-	T38.2X2-	T38.2X3-	T38.2X4-	T38.2X5-	T38.2X6-
Thiocarbarsone	T37.8X1-	T37.8X2-	T37.8X3-	T37.8X4-	T37.8X5-	T37.8X6-
Thiocarlide	T37.1X1-	T37.1X2-	T37.1X3-	T37.1X4-	T37.1X5-	T37.1X6-
Thioctamide	T50.991-	T50.992-	T50.993-	T50.994-	T50.995-	T50.996-
Thioctic acid	T50.991-	T50.992-	T50.993-	T50.994-	T50.995-	T50.996-
Thiofos	T60.0X1-	T60.0X2-	T60.0X3-	T60.0X4-	-	-
Thioglycolate	T49.4X1-	T49.4X2-	T49.4X3-	T49.4X4-	T49.4X5-	T49.4X6-
Thioglycolic acid	T65.891-	T65.892-	T65.893-	T65.894-	-	-
Thioguanine	T45.1X1-	T45.1X2-	T45.1X3-	T45.1X4-	T45.1X5-	T45.1X6-
Thiomercaptomerin	T50.2X1-	T50.2X2-	T50.2X3-	T50.2X4-	T50.2X5-	T50.2X6-
Thiomerin	T50.2X1-	T50.2X2-	T50.2X3-	T50.2X4-	T50.2X5-	T50.2X6-
Thiomersal	T49.0X1-	T49.0X2-	T49.0X3-	T49.0X4-	T49.0X5-	T49.0X6-
Thionazin	T60.0X1-	T60.0X2-	T60.0X3-	T60.0X4-	-	-
Thiopental (sodium)	T41.1X1-	T41.1X2-	T41.1X3-	T41.1X4-	T41.1X5-	T41.1X6-
Thiopentone (sodium)	T41.1X1-	T41.1X2-	T41.1X3-	T41.1X4-	T41.1X5-	T41.1X6-
Thiopropazate	T43.3X1-	T43.3X2-	T43.3X3-	T43.3X4-	T43.3X5-	T43.3X6-
Thioproperazine	T43.3X1-	T43.3X2-	T43.3X3-	T43.3X4-	T43.3X5-	T43.3X6-
Thioridazine	T43.3X1-	T43.3X2-	T43.3X3-	T43.3X4-	T43.3X5-	T43.3X6-
Thiosinamine	T49.3X1-	T49.3X2-	T49.3X3-	T49.3X4-	T49.3X5-	T49.3X6-
Thiotepa	T45.1X1-	T45.1X2-	T45.1X3-	T45.1X4-	T45.1X5-	T45.1X6-
Thiothixene	T43.4X1-	T43.4X2-	T43.4X3-	T43.4X4-	T43.4X5-	T43.4X6-
Thiouracil (benzyl) (methyl) (propyl)	T38.2X1-	T38.2X2-	T38.2X3-	T38.2X4-	T38.2X5-	T38.2X6-
Thiourea	T38.2X1-	T38.2X2-	T38.2X3-	T38.2X4-	T38.2X5-	T38.2X6-
Thiphenamil	T44.3X1-	T44.3X2-	T44.3X3-	T44.3X4-	T44.3X5-	T44.3X6-
Thiram	T60.3X1-	T60.3X2-	T60.3X3-	T60.3X4-	-	-
medicinal	T49.2X1-	T49.2X2-	T49.2X3-	T49.2X4-	T49.2X5-	T49.2X6-
Thonzylamine (systemic)	T45.0X1-	T45.0X2-	T45.0X3-	T45.0X4-	T45.0X5-	T45.0X6-
mucosal decongestant	T48.5X1-	T48.5X2-	T48.5X3-	T48.5X4-	T48.5X5-	T48.5X6-
Thorazine	T43.3X1-	T43.3X2-	T43.3X3-	T43.3X4-	T43.3X5-	T43.3X6-
Thorium dioxide suspension	T50.8X1-	T50.8X2-	T50.8X3-	T50.8X4-	T50.8X5-	T50.8X6-
Thornapple	T62.2X1-	T62.2X2-	T62.2X3-	T62.2X4-	-	-
Throat drug NEC	T49.6X1-	T49.6X2-	T49.6X3-	T49.6X4-	T49.6X5-	T49.6X6-
Thrombin	T45.7X1-	T45.7X2-	T45.7X3-	T45.7X4-	T45.7X5-	T45.7X6-
Thrombolysin	T45.611-	T45.612-	T45.613-	T45.614-	T45.615-	T45.616-
Thromboplastin	T45.7X1-	T45.7X2-	T45.7X3-	T45.7X4-	T45.7X5-	T45.7X6-
Thurfyl nicotinate	T46.7X1-	T46.7X2-	T46.7X3-	T46.7X4-	T46.7X5-	T46.7X6-
Thymol	T49.0X1-	T49.0X2-	T49.0X3-	T49.0X4-	T49.0X5-	T49.0X6-
Thymopentin	T37.5X1-	T37.5X2-	T37.5X3-	T37.5X4-	T37.5X5-	T37.5X6-
Thymoxamine	T46.7X1-	T46.7X2-	T46.7X3-	T46.7X4-	T46.7X5-	T46.7X6-
Thymus extract	T38.891-	T38.892-	T38.893-	T38.894-	T38.895-	T38.896-
Thyreotrophic hormone	T38.811-	T38.812-	T38.813-	T38.814-	T38.815-	T38.816-
Thyroglobulin	T38.1X1-	T38.1X2-	T38.1X3-	T38.1X4-	T38.1X5-	T38.1X6-
Thyroid (hormone)	T38.1X1-	T38.1X2-	T38.1X3-	T38.1X4-	T38.1X5-	T38.1X6-
Thyrolar	T38.1X1-	T38.1X2-	T38.1X3-	T38.1X4-	T38.1X5-	T38.1X6-
Thyrotrophin	T38.811-	T38.812-	T38.813-	T38.814-	T38.815-	T38.816-
Thyrotropic hormone	T38.811-	T38.812-	T38.813-	T38.814-	T38.815-	T38.816-
Thyroxine	T38.1X1-	T38.1X2-	T38.1X3-	T38.1X4-	T38.1X5-	T38.1X6-
Tiabendazole	T37.4X1-	T37.4X2-	T37.4X3-	T37.4X4-	T37.4X5-	T37.4X6-
Tiamizide	T50.2X1-	T50.2X2-	T50.2X3-	T50.2X4-	T50.2X5-	T50.2X6-
Tianeptine	T43.291-	T43.292-	T43.293-	T43.294-	T43.295-	T43.296-
Tiapamil	T46.1X1-	T46.1X2-	T46.1X3-	T46.1X4-	T46.1X5-	T46.1X6-
Tiapride	T43.591-	T43.592-	T43.593-	T43.594-	T43.595-	T43.596-
Tiaprofenic acid	T39.311-	T39.312-	T39.313-	T39.314-	T39.315-	T39.316-
Tiaramide	T39.8X1-	T39.8X2-	T39.8X3-	T39.8X4-	T39.8X5-	T39.8X6-
Ticarcillin	T36.0X1-	T36.0X2-	T36.0X3-	T36.0X4-	T36.0X5-	T36.0X6-
Ticlatone	T49.0X1-	T49.0X2-	T49.0X3-	T49.0X4-	T49.0X5-	T49.0X6-
Ticlopidine	T45.521-	T45.522-	T45.523-	T45.524-	T45.525-	T45.526-
Ticrynafen	T50.1X1-	T50.1X2-	T50.1X3-	T50.1X4-	T50.1X5-	T50.1X6-
Tidiacic	T50.991-	T50.992-	T50.993-	T50.994-	T50.995-	T50.996-
Tiemonium	T44.3X1-	T44.3X2-	T44.3X3-	T44.3X4-	T44.3X5-	T44.3X6-
iodide	T44.3X1-	T44.3X2-	T44.3X3-	T44.3X4-	T44.3X5-	T44.3X6-
Tienilic acid	T50.1X1-	T50.1X2-	T50.1X3-	T50.1X4-	T50.1X5-	T50.1X6-
Tifenamil	T44.3X1-	T44.3X2-	T44.3X3-	T44.3X4-	T44.3X5-	T44.3X6-
Tigan	T45.0X1-	T45.0X2-	T45.0X3-	T45.0X4-	T45.0X5-	T45.0X6-
Tigloidine	T44.3X1-	T44.3X2-	T44.3X3-	T44.3X4-	T44.3X5-	T44.3X6-
Tilactase	T47.5X1-	T47.5X2-	T47.5X3-	T47.5X4-	T47.5X5-	T47.5X6-
Tiletamine	T41.291-	T41.292-	T41.293-	T41.294-	T41.295-	T41.296-
Tilidine	T40.4X1-	T40.4X2-	T40.4X3-	T40.4X4-	-	-
Timepidium bromide	T44.3X1-	T44.3X2-	T44.3X3-	T44.3X4-	T44.3X5-	T44.3X6-
Timiperone	T43.4X1-	T43.4X2-	T43.4X3-	T43.4X4-	T43.4X5-	T43.4X6-
Timolol	T44.7X1-	T44.7X2-	T44.7X3-	T44.7X4-	T44.7X5-	T44.7X6-
Tin (chloride) (dust) (oxide) NEC	T56.6X1-	T56.6X2-	T56.6X3-	T56.6X4-	-	-
anti-infectives	T37.8X1-	T37.8X2-	T37.8X3-	T37.8X4-	T37.8X5-	T37.8X6-
Tincture, iodine — see Iodine						
Tindal	T43.3X1-	T43.3X2-	T43.3X3-	T43.3X4-	T43.3X5-	T43.3X6-
Tinidazole	T37.3X1-	T37.3X2-	T37.3X3-	T37.3X4-	T37.3X5-	T37.3X6-
Tinoridine	T39.8X1-	T39.8X2-	T39.8X3-	T39.8X4-	T39.8X5-	T39.8X6-

Substance	Poisoning, Accidental (unintentional)	Poisoning, Intentional self-harm	Poisoning, Assault	Poisoning, Undetermined	Adverse effect	Underdosing
Tiocarlide	T37.1X1-	T37.1X2-	T37.1X3-	T37.1X4-	T37.1X5-	T37.1X6-
Tioclomarol	T45.511-	T45.512-	T45.513-	T45.514-	T45.515-	T45.516-
Tioconazole	T49.0X1-	T49.0X2-	T49.0X3-	T49.0X4-	T49.0X5-	T49.0X6-
Tioguanine	T45.1X1-	T45.1X2-	T45.1X3-	T45.1X4-	T45.1X5-	T45.1X6-
Tiopronin	T50.991-	T50.992-	T50.993-	T50.994-	T50.995-	T50.996-
Tiotixene	T43.4X1-	T43.4X2-	T43.4X3-	T43.4X4-	T43.4X5-	T43.4X6-
Tioxolone	T49.4X1-	T49.4X2-	T49.4X3-	T49.4X4-	T49.4X5-	T49.4X6-
Tipepidine	T48.3X1-	T48.3X2-	T48.3X3-	T48.3X4-	T48.3X5-	T48.3X6-
Tiquizium bromide	T44.3X1-	T44.3X2-	T44.3X3-	T44.3X4-	T44.3X5-	T44.3X6-
Tiratricol	T38.1X1-	T38.1X2-	T38.1X3-	T38.1X4-	T38.1X5-	T38.1X6-
Tisopurine	T50.4X1-	T50.4X2-	T50.4X3-	T50.4X4-	T50.4X5-	T50.4X6-
Titanium (compounds) (vapor)	T56.891-	T56.892-	T56.893-	T56.894-	-	-
dioxide	T49.3X1-	T49.3X2-	T49.3X3-	T49.3X4-	T49.3X5-	T49.3X6-
ointment	T49.3X1-	T49.3X2-	T49.3X3-	T49.3X4-	T49.3X5-	T49.3X6-
oxide	T49.3X1-	T49.3X2-	T49.3X3-	T49.3X4-	T49.3X5-	T49.3X6-
tetrachloride	T56.891-	T56.892-	T56.893-	T56.894-	-	-
Titanocene	T56.891-	T56.892-	T56.893-	T56.894-	-	-
Titroid	T38.1X1-	T38.1X2-	T38.1X3-	T38.1X4-	T38.1X5-	T38.1X6-
Tizanidine	T42.8X1-	T42.8X2-	T42.8X3-	T42.8X4-	T42.8X5-	T42.8X6-
TMTD	T60.3X1-	T60.3X2-	T60.3X3-	T60.3X4-	-	-
TNT (fumes)	T65.3X1-	T65.3X2-	T65.3X3-	T65.3X4-	-	-
Toadstool	T62.0X1-	T62.0X2-	T62.0X3-	T62.0X4-	-	-
Tobacco NEC	T65.291-	T65.292-	T65.293-	T65.294-	-	-
cigarettes	T65.221-	T65.222-	T65.223-	T65.224-	-	-
Indian	T62.2X1-	T62.2X2-	T62.2X3-	T62.2X4-	-	-
smoke, second-hand	T65.221-	T65.222-	T65.223-	T65.224-	-	-
Tobramycin	T36.5X1-	T36.5X2-	T36.5X3-	T36.5X4-	T36.5X5-	T36.5X6-
Tocainide	T46.2X1-	T46.2X2-	T46.2X3-	T46.2X4-	T46.2X5-	T46.2X6-
Tocoferol	T45.2X1-	T45.2X2-	T45.2X3-	T45.2X4-	T45.2X5-	T45.2X6-
Tocopherol	T45.2X1-	T45.2X2-	T45.2X3-	T45.2X4-	T45.2X5-	T45.2X6-
acetate	T45.2X1-	T45.2X2-	T45.2X3-	T45.2X4-	T45.2X5-	T45.2X6-
Tocosamine	T48.0X1-	T48.0X2-	T48.0X3-	T48.0X4-	T48.0X5-	T48.0X6-
Todralazine	T46.5X1-	T46.5X2-	T46.5X3-	T46.5X4-	T46.5X5-	T46.5X6-
Tofisopam	T42.4X1-	T42.4X2-	T42.4X3-	T42.4X4-	T42.4X5-	T42.4X6-
Tofranil	T43.011-	T43.012-	T43.013-	T43.014-	T43.015-	T43.016-
Toilet deodorizer	T65.891-	T65.892-	T65.893-	T65.894-	-	-
Tolamolol	T44.7X1-	T44.7X2-	T44.7X3-	T44.7X4-	T44.7X5-	T44.7X6-
Tolazamide	T38.3X1-	T38.3X2-	T38.3X3-	T38.3X4-	T38.3X5-	T38.3X6-
Tolazoline	T46.7X1-	T46.7X2-	T46.7X3-	T46.7X4-	T46.7X5-	T46.7X6-
Tolbutamide (sodium)	T38.3X1-	T38.3X2-	T38.3X3-	T38.3X4-	T38.3X5-	T38.3X6-
Tolciclate	T49.0X1-	T49.0X2-	T49.0X3-	T49.0X4-	T49.0X5-	T49.0X6-
Tolmetin	T39.391-	T39.392-	T39.393-	T39.394-	T39.395-	T39.396-
Tolnaftate	T49.0X1-	T49.0X2-	T49.0X3-	T49.0X4-	T49.0X5-	T49.0X6-
Tolonidine	T46.5X1-	T46.5X2-	T46.5X3-	T46.5X4-	T46.5X5-	T46.5X6-
Toloxatone	T42.6X1-	T42.6X2-	T42.6X3-	T42.6X4-	T42.6X5-	T42.6X6-
Tolperisone	T44.3X1-	T44.3X2-	T44.3X3-	T44.3X4-	T44.3X5-	T44.3X6-
Tolserol	T42.8X1-	T42.8X2-	T42.8X3-	T42.8X4-	T42.8X5-	T42.8X6-
Toluene (liquid)	T52.2X1-	T52.2X2-	T52.2X3-	T52.2X4-	-	-
diisocyanate	T65.0X1-	T65.0X2-	T65.0X3-	T65.0X4-	-	-
Toluidine	T65.891-	T65.892-	T65.893-	T65.894-	-	-
vapor	T59.891-	T59.892-	T59.893-	T59.894-	-	-
Toluol (liquid)	T52.2X1-	T52.2X2-	T52.2X3-	T52.2X4-	-	-
vapor	T52.2X1-	T52.2X2-	T52.2X3-	T52.2X4-	-	-
Toluylenediamine	T65.3X1-	T65.3X2-	T65.3X3-	T65.3X4-	-	-
Tolylene-2,4-diisocyanate	T65.0X1-	T65.0X2-	T65.0X3-	T65.0X4-	-	-
Tonic NEC	T50.901-	T50.902-	T50.903-	T50.904-	T50.905-	T50.906-
Topical action drug NEC	T49.91X-	T49.92X-	T49.93X-	T49.94X-	T49.95X-	T49.96X-
ear, nose or throat	T49.6X1-	T49.6X2-	T49.6X3-	T49.6X4-	T49.6X5-	T49.6X6-
eye	T49.5X1-	T49.5X2-	T49.5X3-	T49.5X4-	T49.5X5-	T49.5X6-
skin	T49.91X-	T49.92X-	T49.93X-	T49.94X-	T49.95X-	T49.96X-
specified NEC	T49.8X1-	T49.8X2-	T49.8X3-	T49.8X4-	T49.8X5-	T49.8X6-
Toquizine	T44.3X1-	T44.3X2-	T44.3X3-	T44.3X4-	T44.3X5-	T44.3X6-
Toremifene	T38.6X1-	T38.6X2-	T38.6X3-	T38.6X4-	T38.6X5-	T38.6X6-
Tosylchloramide sodium	T49.8X1-	T49.8X2-	T49.8X3-	T49.8X4-	T49.8X5-	T49.8X6-
Toxaphene (dust) (spray)	T60.1X1-	T60.1X2-	T60.1X3-	T60.1X4-	-	-
Toxin, diphtheria (Schick Test)	T50.8X1-	T50.8X2-	T50.8X3-	T50.8X4-	T50.8X5-	T50.8X6-
Toxoid						
combined	T50.A21-	T50.A22-	T50.A23-	T50.A24-	T50.A25-	T50.A26-
diphtheria	T50.A91-	T50.A92-	T50.A93-	T50.A94-	T50.A95-	T50.A96-
tetanus	T50.A91-	T50.A92-	T50.A93-	T50.A94-	T50.A95-	T50.A96-
Trace element NEC	T45.8X1-	T45.8X2-	T45.8X3-	T45.8X4-	T45.8X5-	T45.8X6-
Tractor fuel NEC	T52.0X1-	T52.0X2-	T52.0X3-	T52.0X4-	-	-
Tragacanth	T50.991-	T50.992-	T50.993-	T50.994-	T50.995-	T50.996-
Tramadol	T40.4X1-	T40.4X2-	T40.4X3-	T40.4X4-	T40.4X5-	T40.4X6-
Tramazoline	T48.5X1-	T48.5X2-	T48.5X3-	T48.5X4-	T48.5X5-	T48.5X6-
Tranexamic acid	T45.621-	T45.622-	T45.623-	T45.624-	T45.625-	T45.626-
Tranilast	T45.0X1-	T45.0X2-	T45.0X3-	T45.0X4-	T45.0X5-	T45.0X6-

Substance	Poisoning, Accidental (unintentional)	Poisoning, Intentional self-harm	Poisoning, Assault	Poisoning, Undetermined	Adverse effect	Underdosing
Tranquilizer NEC	T43.501-	T43.502-	T43.503-	T43.504-	T43.505-	T43.506-
with hypnotic or sedative	T42.6X1-	T42.6X2-	T42.6X3-	T42.6X4-	T42.6X5-	T42.6X6-
benzodiazepine NEC	T42.4X1-	T42.4X2-	T42.4X3-	T42.4X4-	T42.4X5-	T42.4X6-
butyrophenone NEC	T43.4X1-	T43.4X2-	T43.4X3-	T43.4X4-	T43.4X5-	T43.4X6-
carbamate	T43.591-	T43.592-	T43.593-	T43.594-	T43.595-	T43.596-
dimethylamine	T43.3X1-	T43.3X2-	T43.3X3-	T43.3X4-	T43.3X5-	T43.3X6-
ethylamine	T43.3X1-	T43.3X2-	T43.3X3-	T43.3X4-	T43.3X5-	T43.3X6-
hydroxyzine	T43.591-	T43.592-	T43.593-	T43.594-	T43.595-	T43.596-
major NEC	T43.501-	T43.502-	T43.503-	T43.504-	T43.505-	T43.506-
penothiazine NEC	T43.3X1-	T43.3X2-	T43.3X3-	T43.3X4-	T43.3X5-	T43.3X6-
phenothiazine-based	T43.3X1-	T43.3X2-	T43.3X3-	T43.3X4-	T43.3X5-	T43.3X6-
piperazine NEC	T43.3X1-	T43.3X2-	T43.3X3-	T43.3X4-	T43.3X5-	T43.3X6-
piperidine	T43.3X1-	T43.3X2-	T43.3X3-	T43.3X4-	T43.3X5-	T43.3X6-
propylamine	T43.3X1-	T43.3X2-	T43.3X3-	T43.3X4-	T43.3X5-	T43.3X6-
specified NEC	T43.591-	T43.592-	T43.593-	T43.594-	T43.595-	T43.596-
thioxanthene NEC	T43.591-	T43.592-	T43.593-	T43.594-	T43.595-	T43.596-
Tranxene	T42.4X1-	T42.4X2-	T42.4X3-	T42.4X4-	T42.4X5-	T42.4X6-
Tranylcypromine	T43.1X1-	T43.1X2-	T43.1X3-	T43.1X4-	T43.1X5-	T43.1X6-
Trapidil	T46.3X1-	T46.3X2-	T46.3X3-	T46.3X4-	T46.3X5-	T46.3X6-
Trasentine	T44.3X1-	T44.3X2-	T44.3X3-	T44.3X4-	T44.3X5-	T44.3X6-
Travert	T50.3X1-	T50.3X2-	T50.3X3-	T50.3X4-	T50.3X5-	T50.3X6-
Trazodone	T43.211-	T43.212-	T43.213-	T43.214-	T43.215-	T43.216-
Trecator	T37.1X1-	T37.1X2-	T37.1X3-	T37.1X4-	T37.1X5-	T37.1X6-
Treosulfan	T45.1X1-	T45.1X2-	T45.1X3-	T45.1X4-	T45.1X5-	T45.1X6-
Tretamine	T45.1X1-	T45.1X2-	T45.1X3-	T45.1X4-	T45.1X5-	T45.1X6-
Tretinoin	T49.0X1-	T49.0X2-	T49.0X3-	T49.0X4-	T49.0X5-	T49.0X6-
Tretoquinol	T48.6X1-	T48.6X2-	T48.6X3-	T48.6X4-	T48.6X5-	T48.6X6-
Triacetin	T49.0X1-	T49.0X2-	T49.0X3-	T49.0X4-	T49.0X5-	T49.0X6-
Triacetoxyanthracene	T49.4X1-	T49.4X2-	T49.4X3-	T49.4X4-	T49.4X5-	T49.4X6-
Triacetyloleandomycin	T36.3X1-	T36.3X2-	T36.3X3-	T36.3X4-	T36.3X5-	T36.3X6-
Triamcinolone	T49.0X1-	T49.0X2-	T49.0X3-	T49.0X4-	T49.0X5-	T49.0X6-
ENT agent	T49.6X1-	T49.6X2-	T49.6X3-	T49.6X4-	T49.6X5-	T49.6X6-
hexacetonide	T49.0X1-	T49.0X2-	T49.0X3-	T49.0X4-	T49.0X5-	T49.0X6-
ophthalmic preparation	T49.5X1-	T49.5X2-	T49.5X3-	T49.5X4-	T49.5X5-	T49.5X6-
topical NEC	T49.0X1-	T49.0X2-	T49.0X3-	T49.0X4-	T49.0X5-	T49.0X6-
Triampyzine	T44.3X1-	T44.3X2-	T44.3X3-	T44.3X4-	T44.3X5-	T44.3X6-
Triamterene	T50.2X1-	T50.2X2-	T50.2X3-	T50.2X4-	T50.2X5-	T50.2X6-
Triazine (herbicide)	T60.3X1-	T60.3X2-	T60.3X3-	T60.3X4-	-	-
Triaziquone	T45.1X1-	T45.1X2-	T45.1X3-	T45.1X4-	T45.1X5-	T45.1X6-
Triazolam	T42.4X1-	T42.4X2-	T42.4X3-	T42.4X4-	T42.4X5-	T42.4X6-
Triazole (herbicide)	T60.3X1-	T60.3X2-	T60.3X3-	T60.3X4-	-	-
Tribenoside	T46.991-	T46.992-	T46.993-	T46.994-	T46.995-	T46.996-
Tribromacetaldehyde	T42.6X1-	T42.6X2-	T42.6X3-	T42.6X4-	T42.6X5-	T42.6X6-
Tribromoethanol, rectal	T41.291-	T41.292-	T41.293-	T41.294-	T41.295-	T41.296-
Tribromomethane	T42.6X1-	T42.6X2-	T42.6X3-	T42.6X4-	T42.6X5-	T42.6X6-
Trichlorethane	T53.2X1-	T53.2X2-	T53.2X3-	T53.2X4-	-	-
Trichlorethylene	T53.2X1-	T53.2X2-	T53.2X3-	T53.2X4-	-	-
Trichlorfon	T60.0X1-	T60.0X2-	T60.0X3-	T60.0X4-	-	-
Trichlormethiazide	T50.2X1-	T50.2X2-	T50.2X3-	T50.2X4-	T50.2X5-	T50.2X6-
Trichlormethine	T45.1X1-	T45.1X2-	T45.1X3-	T45.1X4-	T45.1X5-	T45.1X6-
Trichloroacetic acid, Trichloracetic acid	T54.2X1-	T54.2X2-	T54.2X3-	T54.2X4-	-	-
medicinal	T49.4X1-	T49.4X2-	T49.4X3-	T49.4X4-	T49.4X5-	T49.4X6-
Trichloroethane	T53.2X1-	T53.2X2-	T53.2X3-	T53.2X4-	-	-
Trichloroethanol	T42.6X1-	T42.6X2-	T42.6X3-	T42.6X4-	T42.6X5-	T42.6X6-
Trichloroethyl phosphate	T42.6X1-	T42.6X2-	T42.6X3-	T42.6X4-	T42.6X5-	T42.6X6-
Trichloroethylene (liquid) (vapor)	T53.2X1-	T53.2X2-	T53.2X3-	T53.2X4-		
anesthetic (gas)	T41.0X1-	T41.0X2-	T41.0X3-	T41.0X4-	T41.0X5-	T41.0X6-
vapor NEC	T53.2X1-	T53.2X2-	T53.2X3-	T53.2X4-	-	-
Trichlorofluoromethane NEC	T53.5X1-	T53.5X2-	T53.5X3-	T53.5X4-	-	-
Trichloronate	T60.0X1-	T60.0X2-	T60.0X3-	T60.0X4-	-	-
2,4,5-Trichlorophen-oxyacetic acid	T60.3X1-	T60.3X2-	T60.3X3-	T60.3X4-	-	-
Trichloropropane	T53.6X1-	T53.6X2-	T53.6X3-	T53.6X4-	-	-
Trichlorotriethylamine	T45.1X1-	T45.1X2-	T45.1X3-	T45.1X4-	T45.1X5-	T45.1X6-
Trichomonacides NEC	T37.3X1-	T37.3X2-	T37.3X3-	T37.3X4-	T37.3X5-	T37.3X6-
Trichomycin	T36.7X1-	T36.7X2-	T36.7X3-	T36.7X4-	T36.7X5-	T36.7X6-
Triclobisonium chloride	T49.0X1-	T49.0X2-	T49.0X3-	T49.0X4-	T49.0X5-	T49.0X6-
Triclocarban	T49.0X1-	T49.0X2-	T49.0X3-	T49.0X4-	T49.0X5-	T49.0X6-
Triclofos	T42.6X1-	T42.6X2-	T42.6X3-	T42.6X4-	T42.6X5-	T42.6X6-
Triclosan	T49.0X1-	T49.0X2-	T49.0X3-	T49.0X4-	T49.0X5-	T49.0X6-
Tricresyl phosphate	T65.891-	T65.892-	T65.893-	T65.894-	-	-
solvent	T52.91X-	T52.92X-	T52.93X-	T52.94X-	-	-
Tricyclamol chloride	T44.3X1-	T44.3X2-	T44.3X3-	T44.3X4-	T44.3X5-	T44.3X6-
Tridesilon	T49.0X1-	T49.0X2-	T49.0X3-	T49.0X4-	T49.0X5-	T49.0X6-
Tridihexethyl iodide	T44.3X1-	T44.3X2-	T44.3X3-	T44.3X4-	T44.3X5-	T44.3X6-
Tridione	T42.2X1-	T42.2X2-	T42.2X3-	T42.2X4-	T42.2X5-	T42.2X6-

Substance	Poisoning, Accidental (unintentional)	Poisoning, Intentional self-harm	Poisoning, Assault	Poisoning, Undetermined	Adverse effect	Underdosing
Trientine	T45.8X1-	T45.8X2-	T45.8X3-	T45.8X4-	T45.8X5-	T45.8X6-
Triethanolamine NEC	T54.3X1-	T54.3X2-	T54.3X3-	T54.3X4-	-	-
detergent	T54.3X1-	T54.3X2-	T54.3X3-	T54.3X4-	-	-
trinitrate (biphosphate)	T46.3X1-	T46.3X2-	T46.3X3-	T46.3X4-	T46.3X5-	T46.3X6-
Triethanomelamine	T45.1X1-	T45.1X2-	T45.1X3-	T45.1X4-	T45.1X5-	T45.1X6-
Triethylenemelamine	T45.1X1-	T45.1X2-	T45.1X3-	T45.1X4-	T45.1X5-	T45.1X6-
Triethylenephosphoramide	T45.1X1-	T45.1X2-	T45.1X3-	T45.1X4-	T45.1X5-	T45.1X6-
Triethylenethiophosphoramide	T45.1X1-	T45.1X2-	T45.1X3-	T45.1X4-	T45.1X5-	T45.1X6-
Trifluoperazine	T43.3X1-	T43.3X2-	T43.3X3-	T43.3X4-	T43.3X5-	T43.3X6-
Trifluoroethyl vinyl ether	T41.0X1-	T41.0X2-	T41.0X3-	T41.0X4-	T41.0X5-	T41.0X6-
Trifluperidol	T43.4X1-	T43.4X2-	T43.4X3-	T43.4X4-	T43.4X5-	T43.4X6-
Triflupromazine	T43.3X1-	T43.3X2-	T43.3X3-	T43.3X4-	T43.3X5-	T43.3X6-
Trifluridine	T37.5X1-	T37.5X2-	T37.5X3-	T37.5X4-	T37.5X5-	T37.5X6-
Triflusal	T45.521-	T45.522-	T45.523-	T45.524-	T45.525-	T45.526-
Trihexyphenidyl	T44.3X1-	T44.3X2-	T44.3X3-	T44.3X4-	T44.3X5-	T44.3X6-
Triiodothyronine	T38.1X1-	T38.1X2-	T38.1X3-	T38.1X4-	T38.1X5-	T38.1X6-
Trilene	T41.0X1-	T41.0X2-	T41.0X3-	T41.0X4-	T41.0X5-	T41.0X6-
Trilostane	T38.991-	T38.992-	T38.993-	T38.994-	T38.995-	T38.996-
Trimebutine	T44.3X1-	T44.3X2-	T44.3X3-	T44.3X4-	T44.3X5-	T44.3X6-
Trimecaine	T41.3X1-	T41.3X2-	T41.3X3-	T41.3X4-	T41.3X5-	T41.3X6-
Trimeprazine (tartrate)	T44.3X1-	T44.3X2-	T44.3X3-	T44.3X4-	T44.3X5-	T44.3X6-
Trimetaphan camsilate	T44.2X1-	T44.2X2-	T44.2X3-	T44.2X4-	T44.2X5-	T44.2X6-
Trimetazidine	T46.7X1-	T46.7X2-	T46.7X3-	T46.7X4-	T46.7X5-	T46.7X6-
Trimethadione	T42.2X1-	T42.2X2-	T42.2X3-	T42.2X4-	T42.2X5-	T42.2X6-
Trimethaphan	T44.2X1-	T44.2X2-	T44.2X3-	T44.2X4-	T44.2X5-	T44.2X6-
Trimethidinium	T44.2X1-	T44.2X2-	T44.2X3-	T44.2X4-	T44.2X5-	T44.2X6-
Trimethobenzamide	T45.0X1-	T45.0X2-	T45.0X3-	T45.0X4-	T45.0X5-	T45.0X6-
Trimethoprim	T37.8X1-	T37.8X2-	T37.8X3-	T37.8X4-	T37.8X5-	T37.8X6-
with sulfamethoxazole	T36.8X1-	T36.8X2-	T36.8X3-	T36.8X4-	T36.8X5-	T36.8X6-
Trimethylcarbinol	T51.3X1-	T51.3X2-	T51.3X3-	T51.3X4-	-	-
Trimethylpsoralen	T49.3X1-	T49.3X2-	T49.3X3-	T49.3X4-	T49.3X5-	T49.3X6-
Trimeton	T45.0X1-	T45.0X2-	T45.0X3-	T45.0X4-	T45.0X5-	T45.0X6-
Trimetrexate	T45.1X1-	T45.1X2-	T45.1X3-	T45.1X4-	T45.1X5-	T45.1X6-
Trimipramine	T43.011-	T43.012-	T43.013-	T43.014-	T43.015-	T43.016-
Trimustine	T45.1X1-	T45.1X2-	T45.1X3-	T45.1X4-	T45.1X5-	T45.1X6-
Trinitrine	T46.3X1-	T46.3X2-	T46.3X3-	T46.3X4-	T46.3X5-	T46.3X6-
Trinitrobenzol	T65.3X1-	T65.3X2-	T65.3X3-	T65.3X4-	-	-
Trinitrophenol	T65.3X1-	T65.3X2-	T65.3X3-	T65.3X4-	-	-
Trinitrotoluene (fumes)	T65.3X1-	T65.3X2-	T65.3X3-	T65.3X4-	-	-
Trional	T42.6X1-	T42.6X2-	T42.6X3-	T42.6X4-	T42.6X5-	T42.6X6-
Triorthocresyl phosphate	T65.891-	T65.892-	T65.893-	T65.894-	-	-
Trioxide of arsenic	T57.0X1-	T57.0X2-	T57.0X3-	T57.0X4-	-	-
Trioxysalen	T49.4X1-	T49.4X2-	T49.4X3-	T49.4X4-	T49.4X5-	T49.4X6-
Tripamide	T50.2X1-	T50.2X2-	T50.2X3-	T50.2X4-	T50.2X5-	T50.2X6-
Triparanol	T46.6X1-	T46.6X2-	T46.6X3-	T46.6X4-	T46.6X5-	T46.6X6-
Tripelennamine	T45.0X1-	T45.0X2-	T45.0X3-	T45.0X4-	T45.0X5-	T45.0X6-
Triperiden	T44.3X1-	T44.3X2-	T44.3X3-	T44.3X4-	T44.3X5-	T44.3X6-
Triperidol	T43.4X1-	T43.4X2-	T43.4X3-	T43.4X4-	T43.4X5-	T43.4X6-
Triphenylphosphate	T65.891-	T65.892-	T65.893-	T65.894-	-	-
Triple						
bromides	T42.6X1-	T42.6X2-	T42.6X3-	T42.6X4-	T42.6X5-	T42.6X6-
carbonate	T47.1X1-	T47.1X2-	T47.1X3-	T47.1X4-	T47.1X5-	T47.1X6-
vaccine						
DPT	T50.A11-	T50.A12-	T50.A13-	T50.A14-	T50.A15-	T50.A16-
including pertussis	T50.A11-	T50.A12-	T50.A13-	T50.A14-	T50.A15-	T50.A16-
MMR	T50.B91-	T50.B92-	T50.B93-	T50.B94-	T50.B95-	T50.B96-
Triprolidine	T45.0X1-	T45.0X2-	T45.0X3-	T45.0X4-	T45.0X5-	T45.0X6-
Trisodium hydrogen edetate	T50.6X1-	T50.6X2-	T50.6X3-	T50.6X4-	T50.6X5-	T50.6X6-
Trisoralen	T49.3X1-	T49.3X2-	T49.3X3-	T49.3X4-	T49.3X5-	T49.3X6-
Trisulfapyrimidines	T37.0X1-	T37.0X2-	T37.0X3-	T37.0X4-	T37.0X5-	T37.0X6-
Trithiozine	T44.3X1-	T44.3X2-	T44.3X3-	T44.3X4-	T44.3X5-	T44.3X6-
Tritiozine	T44.3X1-	T44.3X2-	T44.3X3-	T44.3X4-	T44.3X5-	T44.3X6-
Tritoqualine	T45.0X1-	T45.0X2-	T45.0X3-	T45.0X4-	T45.0X5-	T45.0X6-
Trofosfamide	T45.1X1-	T45.1X2-	T45.1X3-	T45.1X4-	T45.1X5-	T45.1X6-
Troleandomycin	T36.3X1-	T36.3X2-	T36.3X3-	T36.3X4-	T36.3X5-	T36.3X6-
Trolnitrate (phosphate)	T46.3X1-	T46.3X2-	T46.3X3-	T46.3X4-	T46.3X5-	T46.3X6-
Tromantadine	T37.5X1-	T37.5X2-	T37.5X3-	T37.5X4-	T37.5X5-	T37.5X6-
Trometamol	T50.2X1-	T50.2X2-	T50.2X3-	T50.2X4-	T50.2X5-	T50.2X6-
Tromethamine	T50.2X1-	T50.2X2-	T50.2X3-	T50.2X4-	T50.2X5-	T50.2X6-
Tronothane	T41.3X1-	T41.3X2-	T41.3X3-	T41.3X4-	T41.3X5-	T41.3X6-
Tropacine	T44.3X1-	T44.3X2-	T44.3X3-	T44.3X4-	T44.3X5-	T44.3X6-
Tropatepine	T44.3X1-	T44.3X2-	T44.3X3-	T44.3X4-	T44.3X5-	T44.3X6-
Tropicamide	T44.3X1-	T44.3X2-	T44.3X3-	T44.3X4-	T44.3X5-	T44.3X6-
Trospium chloride	T44.3X1-	T44.3X2-	T44.3X3-	T44.3X4-	T44.3X5-	T44.3X6-
Troxerutin	T46.991-	T46.992-	T46.993-	T46.994-	T46.995-	T46.996-
Troxidone	T42.2X1-	T42.2X2-	T42.2X3-	T42.2X4-	T42.2X5-	T42.2X6-
Tryparsamide	T37.3X1-	T37.3X2-	T37.3X3-	T37.3X4-	T37.3X5-	T37.3X6-

Substance	Poisoning, Accidental (unintentional)	Poisoning, Intentional self-harm	Poisoning, Assault	Poisoning, Undetermined	Adverse effect	Underdosing
Trypsin	T45.3X1-	T45.3X2-	T45.3X3-	T45.3X4-	T45.3X5-	T45.3X6-
Tryptizol	T43.011-	T43.012-	T43.013-	T43.014-	T43.015-	T43.016-
TSH	T38.811-	T38.812-	T38.813-	T38.814-	T38.815-	T38.816-
Tuaminoheptane	T48.5X1-	T48.5X2-	T48.5X3-	T48.5X4-	T48.5X5-	T48.5X6-
Tuberculin, purified protein derivative (PPD)	T50.8X1-	T50.8X2-	T50.8X3-	T50.8X4-	T50.8X5-	T50.8X6-
Tubocurare	T48.1X1-	T48.1X2-	T48.1X3-	T48.1X4-	T48.1X5-	T48.1X6-
Tubocurarine (chloride)	T48.1X1-	T48.1X2-	T48.1X3-	T48.1X4-	T48.1X5-	T48.1X6-
Tulobuterol	T48.6X1-	T48.6X2-	T48.6X3-	T48.6X4-	T48.6X5-	T48.6X6-
Turpentine (spirits of)	T52.8X1-	T52.8X2-	T52.8X3-	T52.8X4-	-	-
vapor	T52.8X1-	T52.8X2-	T52.8X3-	T52.8X4-	-	-
Tybamate	T43.591-	T43.592-	T43.593-	T43.594-	T43.595-	T43.596-
Tyloxapol	T48.4X1-	T48.4X2-	T48.4X3-	T48.4X4-	T48.4X5-	T48.4X6-
Tymazoline	T48.5X1-	T48.5X2-	T48.5X3-	T48.5X4-	T48.5X5-	T48.5X6-
Typhoid-paratyphoid vaccine	T50.A91-	T50.A92-	T50.A93-	T50.A94-	T50.A95-	T50.A96-
Typhus vaccine	T50.A91-	T50.A92-	T50.A93-	T50.A94-	T50.A95-	T50.A96-
Tyropanoate	T50.8X1-	T50.8X2-	T50.8X3-	T50.8X4-	T50.8X5-	T50.8X6-
Tyrothricin	T49.6X1-	T49.6X2-	T49.6X3-	T49.6X4-	T49.6X5-	T49.6X6-
ENT agent	T49.6X1-	T49.6X2-	T49.6X3-	T49.6X4-	T49.6X5-	T49.6X6-
ophthalmic preparation	T49.5X1-	T49.5X2-	T49.5X3-	T49.5X4-	T49.5X5-	T49.5X6-
Ufenamate	T39.391-	T39.392-	T39.393-	T39.394-	T39.395-	T39.396-
Ultraviolet light protectant	T49.3X1-	T49.3X2-	T49.3X3-	T49.3X4-	T49.3X5-	T49.3X6-
Undecenoic acid	T49.0X1-	T49.0X2-	T49.0X3-	T49.0X4-	T49.0X5-	T49.0X6-
Undecoylium	T49.0X1-	T49.0X2-	T49.0X3-	T49.0X4-	T49.0X5-	T49.0X6-
Undecylenic acid (derivatives)	T49.0X1-	T49.0X2-	T49.0X3-	T49.0X4-	T49.0X5-	T49.0X6-
Unna's boot	T49.3X1-	T49.3X2-	T49.3X3-	T49.3X4-	T49.3X5-	T49.3X6-
Unsaturated fatty acid	T46.6X1-	T46.6X2-	T46.6X3-	T46.6X4-	T46.6X5-	T46.6X6-
Uracil mustard	T45.1X1-	T45.1X2-	T45.1X3-	T45.1X4-	T45.1X5-	T45.1X6-
Uramustine	T45.1X1-	T45.1X2-	T45.1X3-	T45.1X4-	T45.1X5-	T45.1X6-
Urapidil	T46.5X1-	T46.5X2-	T46.5X3-	T46.5X4-	T46.5X5-	T46.5X6-
Urari	T48.1X1-	T48.1X2-	T48.1X3-	T48.1X4-	T48.1X5-	T48.1X6-
Urate oxidase	T50.4X1-	T50.4X2-	T50.4X3-	T50.4X4-	T50.4X5-	T50.4X6-
Urea	T47.3X1-	T47.3X2-	T47.3X3-	T47.3X4-	T47.3X5-	T47.3X6-
peroxide	T49.0X1-	T49.0X2-	T49.0X3-	T49.0X4-	T49.0X5-	T49.0X6-
stibamine	T37.4X1-	T37.4X2-	T37.4X3-	T37.4X4-	T37.4X5-	T37.4X6-
topical	T49.8X1-	T49.8X2-	T49.8X3-	T49.8X4-	T49.8X5-	T49.8X6-
Urethane	T45.1X1-	T45.1X2-	T45.1X3-	T45.1X4-	T45.1X5-	T45.1X6-
Urginea (maritima) (scilla) — see Squill						
Uric acid metabolism drug NEC	T50.4X1-	T50.4X2-	T50.4X3-	T50.4X4-	T50.4X5-	T50.4X6-
Uricosuric agent	T50.4X1-	T50.4X2-	T50.4X3-	T50.4X4-	T50.4X5-	T50.4X6-
Urinary anti-infective	T37.8X1-	T37.8X2-	T37.8X3-	T37.8X4-	T37.8X5-	T37.8X6-
Urofollitropin	T38.811-	T38.812-	T38.813-	T38.814-	T38.815-	T38.816-
Urokinase	T45.611-	T45.612-	T45.613-	T45.614-	T45.615-	T45.616-
Urokon	T50.8X1-	T50.8X2-	T50.8X3-	T50.8X4-	T50.8X5-	T50.8X6-
Ursodeoxycholic acid	T50.991-	T50.992-	T50.993-	T50.994-	T50.995-	T50.996-
Ursodiol	T50.991-	T50.992-	T50.993-	T50.994-	T50.995-	T50.996-
Urtica	T62.2X1-	T62.2X2-	T62.2X3-	T62.2X4-	-	-
Utility gas — see Gas, utility						
Vaccine NEC	T50.Z91-	T50.Z92-	T50.Z93-	T50.Z94-	T50.Z95-	T50.Z96-
antineoplastic	T50.Z91-	T50.Z92-	T50.Z93-	T50.Z94-	T50.Z95-	T50.Z96-
bacterial NEC	T50.A91-	T50.A92-	T50.A93-	T50.A94-	T50.A95-	T50.A96-
with						
other bacterial component	T50.A21-	T50.A22-	T50.A23-	T50.A24-	T50.A25-	T50.A26-
pertussis component	T50.A11-	T50.A12-	T50.A13-	T50.A14-	T50.A15-	T50.A16-
viral-rickettsial component	T50.A21-	T50.A22-	T50.A23-	T50.A24-	T50.A25-	T50.A26-
mixed NEC	T50.A21-	T50.A22-	T50.A23-	T50.A24-	T50.A25-	T50.A26-
BCG	T50.A91-	T50.A92-	T50.A93-	T50.A94-	T50.A95-	T50.A96-
cholera	T50.A91-	T50.A92-	T50.A93-	T50.A94-	T50.A95-	T50.A96-
diphtheria	T50.A91-	T50.A92-	T50.A93-	T50.A94-	T50.A95-	T50.A96-
with tetanus	T50.A21-	T50.A22-	T50.A23-	T50.A24-	T50.A25-	T50.A26-
and pertussis	T50.A11-	T50.A12-	T50.A13-	T50.A14-	T50.A15-	T50.A16-
influenza	T50.B91-	T50.B92-	T50.B93-	T50.B94-	T50.B95-	T50.B96-
measles	T50.B91-	T50.B92-	T50.B93-	T50.B94-	T50.B95-	T50.B96-
with mumps and rubella	T50.B91-	T50.B92-	T50.B93-	T50.B94-	T50.B95-	T50.B96-
meningococcal	T50.A91-	T50.A92-	T50.A93-	T50.A94-	T50.A95-	T50.A96-
mumps	T50.B91-	T50.B92-	T50.B93-	T50.B94-	T50.B95-	T50.B96-
paratyphoid	T50.A91-	T50.A92-	T50.A93-	T50.A94-	T50.A95-	T50.A96-
pertussis	T50.A11-	T50.A12-	T50.A13-	T50.A14-	T50.A15-	T50.A16-
with diphtheria	T50.A11-	T50.A12-	T50.A13-	T50.A14-	T50.A15-	T50.A16-
and tetanus	T50.A11-	T50.A12-	T50.A13-	T50.A14-	T50.A15-	T50.A16-
with other component	T50.A11-	T50.A12-	T50.A13-	T50.A14-	T50.A15-	T50.A16-
plague	T50.A91-	T50.A92-	T50.A93-	T50.A94-	T50.A95-	T50.A96-
poliomyelitis	T50.B91-	T50.B92-	T50.B93-	T50.B94-	T50.B95-	T50.B96-
poliovirus	T50.B91-	T50.B92-	T50.B93-	T50.B94-	T50.B95-	T50.B96-
rabies	T50.B91-	T50.B92-	T50.B93-	T50.B94-	T50.B95-	T50.B96-
respiratory syncytial virus	T50.B91-	T50.B92-	T50.B93-	T50.B94-	T50.B95-	T50.B96-

Substance	Poisoning, Accidental (unintentional)	Poisoning, Intentional self-harm	Poisoning, Assault	Poisoning, Undetermined	Adverse effect	Underdosing
Vaccine NEC - *continued*						
rickettsial NEC	T50.A91-	T50.A92-	T50.A93-	T50.A94-	T50.A95-	T50.A96-
with						
bacterial component	T50.A21-	T50.A22-	T50.A23-	T50.A24-	T50.A25-	T50.A26-
Rocky Mountain spotted fever	T50.A91-	T50.A92-	T50.A93-	T50.A94-	T50.A95-	T50.A96-
rubella	T50.B91-	T50.B92-	T50.B93-	T50.B94-	T50.B95-	T50.B96-
sabin oral	T50.B91-	T50.B92-	T50.B93-	T50.B94-	T50.B95-	T50.B96-
smallpox	T50.B11-	T50.B12-	T50.B13-	T50.B14-	T50.B15-	T50.B16-
TAB	T50.A91-	T50.A92-	T50.A93-	T50.A94-	T50.A95-	T50.A96-
tetanus	T50.A91-	T50.A92-	T50.A93-	T50.A94-	T50.A95-	T50.A96-
typhoid	T50.A91-	T50.A92-	T50.A93-	T50.A94-	T50.A95-	T50.A96-
typhus	T50.A91-	T50.A92-	T50.A93-	T50.A94-	T50.A95-	T50.A96-
viral NEC	T50.B91-	T50.B92-	T50.B93-	T50.B94-	T50.B95-	T50.B96-
yellow fever	T50.B91-	T50.B92-	T50.B93-	T50.B94-	T50.B95-	T50.B96-
Vaccinia immune globulin	T50.Z11-	T50.Z12-	T50.Z13-	T50.Z14-	T50.Z15-	T50.Z16-
Vaginal contraceptives	T49.8X1-	T49.8X2-	T49.8X3-	T49.8X4-	T49.8X5-	T49.8X6-
Valerian						
root	T42.6X1-	T42.6X2-	T42.6X3-	T42.6X4-	T42.6X5-	T42.6X6-
tincture	T42.6X1-	T42.6X2-	T42.6X3-	T42.6X4-	T42.6X5-	T42.6X6-
Valethamate bromide	T44.3X1-	T44.3X2-	T44.3X3-	T44.3X4-	T44.3X5-	T44.3X6-
Valisone	T49.0X1-	T49.0X2-	T49.0X3-	T49.0X4-	T49.0X5-	T49.0X6-
Valium	T42.4X1-	T42.4X2-	T42.4X3-	T42.4X4-	T42.4X5-	T42.4X6-
Valmid	T42.6X1-	T42.6X2-	T42.6X3-	T42.6X4-	T42.6X5-	T42.6X6-
Valnoctamide	T42.6X1-	T42.6X2-	T42.6X3-	T42.6X4-	T42.6X5-	T42.6X6-
Valproate (sodium)	T42.6X1-	T42.6X2-	T42.6X3-	T42.6X4-	T42.6X5-	T42.6X6-
Valproic acid	T42.6X1-	T42.6X2-	T42.6X3-	T42.6X4-	T42.6X5-	T42.6X6-
Valpromide	T42.6X1-	T42.6X2-	T42.6X3-	T42.6X4-	T42.6X5-	T42.6X6-
Vanadium	T56.891-	T56.892-	T56.893-	T56.894-	-	-
Vancomycin	T36.8X1-	T36.8X2-	T36.8X3-	T36.8X4-	T36.8X5-	T36.8X6-
Vapor — *see also* Gas	T59.91X-	T59.92X-	T59.93X-	T59.94X-	-	-
kiln (carbon monoxide)	T58.8X1-	T58.8X2-	T58.8X3-	T58.8X4-	-	-
lead — *see* lead						
specified source NEC	T59.891-	T59.892-	T59.893-	T59.894-	-	-
Vardenafil	T46.7X1-	T46.7X2-	T46.7X3-	T46.7X4-	T46.7X5-	T46.7X6-
Varicose reduction drug	T46.8X1-	T46.8X2-	T46.8X3-	T46.8X4-	T46.8X5-	T46.8X6-
Varnish	T65.4X1-	T65.4X2-	T65.4X3-	T65.4X4-	-	-
cleaner	T52.91X-	T52.92X-	T52.93X-	T52.94X-	-	-
Vaseline	T49.3X1-	T49.3X2-	T49.3X3-	T49.3X4-	T49.3X5-	T49.3X6-
Vasodilan	T46.7X1-	T46.7X2-	T46.7X3-	T46.7X4-	T46.7X5-	T46.7X6-
Vasodilator						
coronary NEC	T46.3X1-	T46.3X2-	T46.3X3-	T46.3X4-	T46.3X5-	T46.3X6-
peripheral NEC	T46.7X1-	T46.7X2-	T46.7X3-	T46.7X4-	T46.7X5-	T46.7X6-
Vasopressin	T38.891-	T38.892-	T38.893-	T38.894-	T38.895-	T38.896-
Vasopressor drugs	T38.891-	T38.892-	T38.893-	T38.894-	T38.895-	T38.896-
Vecuronium bromide	T48.1X1-	T48.1X2-	T48.1X3-	T48.1X4-	T48.1X5-	T48.1X6-
Vegetable extract, astringent	T49.2X1-	T49.2X2-	T49.2X3-	T49.2X4-	T49.2X5-	T49.2X6-
Venlafaxine	T43.211-	T43.212-	T43.213-	T43.214-	T43.215-	T43.216-
Venom, venomous (bite) (sting)	T63.91X-	T63.92X-	T63.93X-	T63.94X-	-	-
amphibian NEC	T63.831-	T63.832-	T63.833-	T63.834-	-	-
animal NEC	T63.891-	T63.892-	T63.893-	T63.894-	-	-
ant	T63.421-	T63.422-	T63.423-	T63.424-	-	-
arthropod NEC	T63.481-	T63.482-	T63.483-	T63.484-	-	-
bee	T63.441-	T63.442-	T63.443-	T63.444-	-	-
centipede	T63.411-	T63.412-	T63.413-	T63.414-	-	-
fish	T63.591-	T63.592-	T63.593-	T63.594-	-	-
frog	T63.811-	T63.812-	T63.813-	T63.814-	-	-
hornet	T63.451-	T63.452-	T63.453-	T63.454-	-	-
insect NEC	T63.481-	T63.482-	T63.483-	T63.484-	-	-
lizard	T63.121-	T63.122-	T63.123-	T63.124-	-	-
marine						
animals	T63.691-	T63.692-	T63.693-	T63.694-	-	-
bluebottle	T63.611-	T63.612-	T63.613-	T63.614-	-	-
jellyfish NEC	T63.621-	T63.622-	T63.623-	T63.624-	-	-
Portugese Man-o-war	T63.611-	T63.612-	T63.613-	T63.614-	-	-
sea anemone	T63.631-	T63.632-	T63.633-	T63.634-	-	-
specified NEC	T63.691-	T63.692-	T63.693-	T63.694-	-	-
fish	T63.591-	T63.592-	T63.593-	T63.594-	-	-
plants	T63.711-	T63.712-	T63.713-	T63.714-	-	-
sting ray	T63.511-	T63.512-	T63.513-	T63.514-	-	-
millipede (tropical)	T63.411-	T63.412-	T63.413-	T63.414-	-	-
plant NEC	T63.791-	T63.792-	T63.793-	T63.794-	-	-
marine	T63.711-	T63.712-	T63.713-	T63.714-	-	-
reptile	T63.191-	T63.192-	T63.193-	T63.194-	-	-
gila monster	T63.111-	T63.112-	T63.113-	T63.114-	-	-
lizard NEC	T63.121-	T63.122-	T63.123-	T63.124-	-	-
scorpion	T63.2X1-	T63.2X2-	T63.2X3-	T63.2X4-	-	-
snake	T63.001-	T63.002-	T63.003-	T63.004-	-	-
African NEC	T63.081-	T63.082-	T63.083-	T63.084-	-	-

Substance	Poisoning, Accidental (unintentional)	Poisoning, Intentional self-harm	Poisoning, Assault	Poisoning, Undetermined	Adverse effect	Underdosing
Venom, venomous - *continued*						
American (North) (South) NEC	T63.061-	T63.062-	T63.063-	T63.064-	-	-
Asian	T63.081-	T63.082-	T63.083-	T63.084-	-	-
Australian	T63.071-	T63.072-	T63.073-	T63.074-	-	-
cobra	T63.041-	T63.042-	T63.043-	T63.044-	-	-
coral snake	T63.021-	T63.022-	T63.023-	T63.024-	-	-
rattlesnake	T63.011-	T63.012-	T63.013-	T63.014-	-	-
specified NEC	T63.091-	T63.092-	T63.093-	T63.094-	-	-
taipan	T63.031-	T63.032-	T63.033-	T63.034-	-	-
specified NEC	T63.891-	T63.892-	T63.893-	T63.894-	-	-
spider	T63.301-	T63.302-	T63.303-	T63.304-	-	-
black widow	T63.311-	T63.312-	T63.313-	T63.314-	-	-
brown recluse	T63.331-	T63.332-	T63.333-	T63.334-	-	-
specified NEC	T63.391-	T63.392-	T63.393-	T63.394-	-	-
tarantula	T63.321-	T63.322-	T63.323-	T63.324-	-	-
sting ray	T63.511-	T63.512-	T63.513-	T63.514-	-	-
toad	T63.821-	T63.822-	T63.823-	T63.824-	-	-
wasp	T63.461-	T63.462-	T63.463-	T63.464-	-	-
Venous sclerosing drug NEC	T46.8X1-	T46.8X2-	T46.8X4-	T46.8X4-	T46.8X5-	T46.8X6-
Ventolin — *see* Albuterol						
Veramon	T42.3X1-	T42.3X2-	T42.3X3-	T42.3X4-	T42.3X5-	T42.3X6-
Verapamil	T46.1X1-	T46.1X2-	T46.1X3-	T46.1X4-	T46.1X5-	T46.1X6-
Veratrine	T46.5X1-	T46.5X2-	T46.5X3-	T46.5X4-	T46.5X5-	T46.5X6-
Veratrum						
album	T62.2X1-	T62.2X2-	T62.2X3-	T62.2X4-	-	-
alkaloids	T46.5X1-	T46.5X2-	T46.5X3-	T46.5X4-	T46.5X5-	T46.5X6-
viride	T62.2X1-	T62.2X2-	T62.2X3-	T62.2X4-	-	-
Verdigris	T60.3X1-	T60.3X2-	T60.3X3-	T60.3X4-	-	-
Veronal	T42.3X1-	T42.3X2-	T42.3X3-	T42.3X4-	T42.3X5-	T42.3X6-
Veroxil	T37.4X1-	T37.4X2-	T37.4X3-	T37.4X4-	T37.4X5-	T37.4X6-
Versenate	T50.6X1-	T50.6X2-	T50.6X3-	T50.6X4-	T50.6X5-	T50.6X6-
Versidyne	T39.8X1-	T39.8X2-	T39.8X3-	T39.8X4-	T39.8X5-	T39.8X6-
Vetrabutine	T48.0X1-	T48.0X2-	T48.0X3-	T48.0X4-	T48.0X5-	T48.0X6-
Vidarabine	T37.5X1-	T37.5X2-	T37.5X3-	T37.5X4-	T37.5X5-	T37.5X6-
Vienna						
green	T57.0X1-	T57.0X2-	T57.0X3-	T57.0X4-	-	-
insecticide	T60.2X1-	T60.2X2-	T60.2X3-	T60.2X4-	-	-
red	T57.0X1-	T57.0X2-	T57.0X3-	T57.0X4-	-	-
pharmaceutical dye	T50.991-	T50.992-	T50.993-	T50.994-	T50.995-	T50.996-
Vigabatrin	T42.6X1-	T42.6X2-	T42.6X3-	T42.6X4-	T42.6X5-	T42.6X6-
Viloxazine	T43.291-	T43.292-	T43.293-	T43.294-	T43.295-	T43.296-
Viminol	T39.8X1-	T39.8X2-	T39.8X3-	T39.8X4-	T39.8X5-	T39.8X6-
Vinbarbital, vinbarbitone	T42.3X1-	T42.3X2-	T42.3X3-	T42.3X4-	T42.3X5-	T42.3X6-
Vinblastine	T45.1X1-	T45.1X2-	T45.1X3-	T45.1X4-	T45.1X5-	T45.1X6-
Vinburnine	T46.7X1-	T46.7X2-	T46.7X3-	T46.7X4-	T46.7X5-	T46.7X6-
Vincamine	T45.1X1-	T45.1X2-	T45.1X3-	T45.1X4-	T45.1X5-	T45.1X6-
Vincristine	T45.1X1-	T45.1X2-	T45.1X3-	T45.1X4-	T45.1X5-	T45.1X6-
Vindesine	T45.1X1-	T45.1X2-	T45.1X3-	T45.1X4-	T45.1X5-	T45.1X6-
Vinesthene, vinethene	T41.0X1-	T41.0X2-	T41.0X3-	T41.0X4-	T41.0X5-	T41.0X6-
Vinorelbine tartrate	T45.1X1-	T45.1X2-	T45.1X3-	T45.1X4-	T45.1X5-	T45.1X6-
Vinpocetine	T46.7X1-	T46.7X2-	T46.7X3-	T46.7X4-	T46.7X5-	T46.7X6-
Vinyl						
acetate	T65.891-	T65.892-	T65.893-	T65.894-	-	-
bital	T42.3X1-	T42.3X2-	T42.3X3-	T42.3X4-	T42.3X5-	T42.3X6-
bromide	T65.891-	T65.892-	T65.893-	T65.894-	-	-
chloride	T59.891-	T59.892-	T59.893-	T59.894-	-	-
ether	T41.0X1-	T41.0X2-	T41.0X3-	T41.0X4-	T41.0X5-	T41.0X6-
Vinylbital	T42.3X1-	T42.3X2-	T42.3X3-	T42.3X4-	T42.3X5-	T42.3X6-
Vinylidene chloride	T65.891-	T65.892-	T65.893-	T65.894-	-	-
Vioform	T37.8X1-	T37.8X2-	T37.8X3-	T37.8X4-	T37.8X5-	T37.8X6-
topical	T49.0X1-	T49.0X2-	T49.0X3-	T49.0X4-	T49.0X5-	T49.0X6-
Viomycin	T36.8X1-	T36.8X2-	T36.8X3-	T36.8X4-	T36.8X5-	T36.8X6-
Viosterol	T45.2X1-	T45.2X2-	T45.2X3-	T45.2X4-	T45.2X5-	T45.2X6-
Viper (venom)	T63.091-	T63.092-	T63.093-	T63.094-	-	-
Viprynium	T37.4X1-	T37.4X2-	T37.4X3-	T37.4X4-	T37.4X5-	T37.4X6-
Viquidil	T46.7X1-	T46.7X2-	T46.7X3-	T46.7X4-	T46.7X5-	T46.7X6-
Viral vaccine NEC	T50.B91-	T50.B92-	T50.B93-	T50.B94-	T50.B95-	T50.B96-
Virginiamycin	T36.8X1-	T36.8X2-	T36.8X3-	T36.8X4-	T36.8X5-	T36.8X6-
Virugon	T37.5X1-	T37.5X2-	T37.5X3-	T37.5X4-	T37.5X5-	T37.5X6-
Viscous agent	T50.901-	T50.902-	T50.903-	T50.904-	T50.905-	T50.906-
Visine	T49.5X1-	T49.5X2-	T49.5X3-	T49.5X4-	T49.5X5-	T49.5X6-
Visnadine	T46.3X1-	T46.3X2-	T46.3X3-	T46.3X4-	T46.3X5-	T46.3X6-
Vitamin NEC	T45.2X1-	T45.2X2-	T45.2X3-	T45.2X4-	T45.2X5-	T45.2X6-
A	T45.2X1-	T45.2X2-	T45.2X3-	T45.2X4-	T45.2X5-	T45.2X6-
B NEC	T45.2X1-	T45.2X2-	T45.2X3-	T45.2X4-	T45.2X5-	T45.2X6-
nicotinic acid	T46.7X1-	T46.7X2-	T46.7X3-	T46.7X4-	T46.7X5-	T46.7X6-
B1	T45.2X1-	T45.2X2-	T45.2X3-	T45.2X4-	T45.2X5-	T45.2X6-

Substance	Poisoning, Accidental (unintentional)	Poisoning, Intentional self-harm	Poisoning, Assault	Poisoning, Undetermined	Adverse effect	Underdosing
Vitamin NEC - *continued*						
B2	T45.2X1-	T45.2X2-	T45.2X3-	T45.2X4-	T45.2X5-	T45.2X6-
B6	T45.2X1-	T45.2X2-	T45.2X3-	T45.2X4-	T45.2X5-	T45.2X6-
B12	T45.2X1-	T45.2X2-	T45.2X3-	T45.2X4-	T45.2X5-	T45.2X6-
B15	T45.2X1-	T45.2X2-	T45.2X3-	T45.2X4-	T45.2X5-	T45.2X6-
C	T45.2X1-	T45.2X2-	T45.2X3-	T45.2X4-	T45.2X5-	T45.2X6-
D	T45.2X1-	T45.2X2-	T45.2X3-	T45.2X4-	T45.2X5-	T45.2X6-
D2	T45.2X1-	T45.2X2-	T45.2X3-	T45.2X4-	T45.2X5-	T45.2X6-
D3	T45.2X1-	T45.2X2-	T45.2X3-	T45.2X4-	T45.2X5-	T45.2X6-
E	T45.2X1-	T45.2X2-	T45.2X3-	T45.2X4-	T45.2X5-	T45.2X6-
E acetate	T45.2X1-	T45.2X2-	T45.2X3-	T45.2X4-	T45.2X5-	T45.2X6-
hematopoietic	T45.8X1-	T45.8X2-	T45.8X3-	T45.8X4-	T45.8X5-	T45.8X6-
K NEC	T45.7X1-	T45.7X2-	T45.7X3-	T45.7X4-	T45.7X5-	T45.7X6-
K1	T45.7X1-	T45.7X2-	T45.7X3-	T45.7X4-	T45.7X5-	T45.7X6-
K2	T45.7X1-	T45.7X2-	T45.7X3-	T45.7X4-	T45.7X5-	T45.7X6-
PP	T45.2X1-	T45.2X2-	T45.2X3-	T45.2X4-	T45.2X5-	T45.2X6-
ulceroprotectant	T47.1X1-	T47.1X2-	T47.1X3-	T47.1X4-	T47.1X5-	T47.1X6-
Vleminckx's solution	T49.4X1-	T49.4X2-	T49.4X3-	T49.4X4-	T49.4X5-	T49.4X6-
Voltaren — *see* Diclofenac						
sodium						
Warfarin	T45.511-	T45.512-	T45.513-	T45.514-	T45.515-	T45.516-
rodenticide	T60.4X1-	T60.4X2-	T60.4X3-	T60.4X4-	-	-
sodium	T60.4X1-	T60.4X2-	T60.4X3-	T60.4X4-	-	-
Wasp (sting)	T63.461-	T63.462-	T63.463-	T63.464-	-	-
Water						
balance drug	T50.3X1-	T50.3X2-	T50.3X3-	T50.3X4-	T50.3X5-	T50.3X6-
distilled	T50.3X1-	T50.3X2-	T50.3X3-	T50.3X4-	T50.3X5-	T50.3X6-
gas — *see* Gas, water						
incomplete combustion						
of — *see* Carbon, monoxide,						
fuel, utility						
hemlock	T62.2X1-	T62.2X2-	T62.2X3-	T62.2X4-	-	-
moccasin (venom)	T63.061-	T63.062-	T63.063-	T63.064-	-	-
purified	T50.3X1-	T50.3X2-	T50.3X3-	T50.3X4-	T50.3X5-	T50.3X6-
Wax (paraffin) (petroleum)	T52.0X1-	T52.0X2-	T52.0X3-	T52.0X4-	-	-
automobile	T65.891-	T65.892-	T65.893-	T65.894-	-	-
floor	T52.0X1-	T52.0X2-	T52.0X3-	T52.0X4-	-	-
Weed killers NEC	T60.3X1-	T60.3X2-	T60.3X3-	T60.3X4-	-	-
Welldorm	T42.6X1-	T42.6X2-	T42.6X3-	T42.6X4-	T42.6X5-	T42.6X6-
White						
arsenic	T57.0X1-	T57.0X2-	T57.0X3-	T57.0X4-	-	-
hellebore	T62.2X1-	T62.2X2-	T62.2X3-	T62.2X4-	-	-
lotion (keratolytic)	T49.4X1-	T49.4X2-	T49.4X3-	T49.4X4-	T49.4X5-	T49.4X6-
spirit	T52.0X1-	T52.0X2-	T52.0X3-	T52.0X4-	-	-
Whitewash	T65.891-	T65.892-	T65.893-	T65.894-	-	-
Whole blood (human)	T45.8X1-	T45.8X2-	T45.8X3-	T45.8X4-	T45.8X5-	T45.8X6-
Wild						
black cherry	T62.2X1-	T62.2X2-	T62.2X3-	T62.2X4-	-	-
poisonous plants NEC	T62.2X1-	T62.2X2-	T62.2X3-	T62.2X4-	-	-
Window cleaning fluid	T65.891-	T65.892-	T65.893-	T65.894-	-	-
Wintergreen (oil)	T49.3X1-	T49.3X2-	T49.3X3-	T49.3X4-	T49.3X5-	T49.3X6-
Wisterine	T62.2X1-	T62.2X2-	T62.2X3-	T62.2X4-	-	-
Witch hazel	T49.2X1-	T49.2X2-	T49.2X3-	T49.2X4-	T49.2X5-	T49.2X6-
Wood alcohol or spirit	T51.1X1-	T51.1X2-	T51.1X3-	T51.1X4-	-	-
Wool fat (hydrous)	T49.3X1-	T49.3X2-	T49.3X3-	T49.3X4-	T49.3X5-	T49.3X6-
Woorali	T48.1X1-	T48.1X2-	T48.1X3-	T48.1X4-	T48.1X5-	T48.1X6-
Wormseed, American	T37.4X1-	T37.4X2-	T37.4X3-	T37.4X4-	T37.4X5-	T37.4X6-
Xamoterol	T44.5X1-	T44.5X2-	T44.5X3-	T44.5X4-	T44.5X5-	T44.5X6-
Xanthine diuretics	T50.2X1-	T50.2X2-	T50.2X3-	T50.2X4-	T50.2X5-	T50.2X6-
Xanthinol nicotinate	T46.7X1-	T46.7X2-	T46.7X3-	T46.7X4-	T46.7X5-	T46.7X6-
Xanthotoxin	T49.3X1-	T49.3X2-	T49.3X3-	T49.3X4-	T49.3X5-	T49.3X6-
Xantinol nicotinate	T46.7X1-	T46.7X2-	T46.7X3-	T46.7X4-	T46.7X5-	T46.7X6-
Xantocillin	T36.0X1-	T36.0X2-	T36.0X3-	T36.0X4-	T36.0X5-	T36.0X6-
Xenon (127Xe) (133Xe)	T50.8X1-	T50.8X2-	T50.8X3-	T50.8X4-	T50.8X5-	T50.8X6-
Xenysalate	T49.4X1-	T49.4X2-	T49.4X3-	T49.4X4-	T49.4X5-	T49.4X6-
Xibornol	T37.8X1-	T37.8X2-	T37.8X3-	T37.8X4-	T37.8X5-	T37.8X6-
Xigris	T45.511-	T45.512-	T45.513-	T45.514-	T45.515-	T45.516-
Xipamide	T50.2X1-	T50.2X2-	T50.2X3-	T50.2X4-	T50.2X5-	T50.2X6-
Xylene (vapor)	T52.2X1-	T52.2X2-	T52.2X3-	T52.2X4-	-	-
Xylocaine (infiltration) (topical)	T41.3X1-	T41.3X2-	T41.3X3-	T41.3X4-	T41.3X5-	T41.3X6-
nerve block (peripheral) (plexus)	T41.3X1-	T41.3X2-	T41.3X3-	T41.3X4-	T41.3X5-	T41.3X6-
spinal	T41.3X1-	T41.3X2-	T41.3X3-	T41.3X4-	T41.3X5-	T41.3X6-
Xylol (vapor)	T52.2X1-	T52.2X2-	T52.2X3-	T52.2X4-	-	-
Xylometazoline	T48.5X1-	T48.5X2-	T48.5X3-	T48.5X4-	T48.5X5-	T48.5X6-
Yeast	T45.2X1-	T45.2X2-	T45.2X3-	T45.2X4-	T45.2X5-	T45.2X6-
dried	T45.2X1-	T45.2X2-	T45.2X3-	T45.2X4-	T45.2X5-	T45.2X6-

Substance	Poisoning, Accidental (unintentional)	Poisoning, Intentional self-harm	Poisoning, Assault	Poisoning, Undetermined	Adverse effect	Underdosing
Yellow						
fever vaccine	T50.B91-	T50.B92-	T50.B93-	T50.B94-	T50.B95-	T50.B96-
jasmine	T62.2X1-	T62.2X2-	T62.2X3-	T62.2X4-	-	-
phenolphthalein	T47.2X1-	T47.2X2-	T47.2X3-	T47.2X4-	T47.2X5-	T47.2X6-
Yew	T62.2X1-	T62.2X2-	T62.2X3-	T62.2X4-	-	-
Yohimbic acid	T40.991-	T40.992-	T40.993-	T40.994-	T40.995-	T40.996-
Zactane	T39.8X1-	T39.8X2-	T39.8X3-	T39.8X4-	T39.8X5-	T39.8X6-
Zalcitabine	T37.5X1-	T37.5X2-	T37.5X3-	T37.5X4-	T37.5X5-	T37.5X6-
Zaroxolyn	T50.2X1-	T50.2X2-	T50.2X3-	T50.2X4-	T50.2X5-	T50.2X6-
Zephiran (topical)	T49.0X1-	T49.0X2-	T49.0X3-	T49.0X4-	T49.0X5-	T49.0X6-
ophthalmic preparation	T49.5X1-	T49.5X2-	T49.5X3-	T49.5X4-	T49.5X5-	T49.5X6-
Zeranol	T38.7X1-	T38.7X2-	T38.7X3-	T38.7X4-	T38.7X5-	T38.7X6-
Zerone	T51.1X1-	T51.1X2-	T51.1X3-	T51.1X4-	-	-
Zidovudine	T37.5X1-	T37.5X2-	T37.5X3-	T37.5X4-	T37.5X5-	T37.5X6-
Zimeldine	T43.221-	T43.222-	T43.223-	T43.224-	T43.225-	T43.226-
Zinc (compounds) (fumes) (vapor) NEC	T56.5X1-	T56.5X2-	T56.5X3-	T56.5X4-	-	-
anti-infectives	T49.0X1-	T49.0X2-	T49.0X3-	T49.0X4-	T49.0X5-	T49.0X6-
antivaricose	T46.8X1-	T46.8X2-	T46.8X3-	T46.8X4-	T46.8X5-	T46.8X6-
bacitracin	T49.0X1-	T49.0X2-	T49.0X3-	T49.0X4-	T49.0X5-	T49.0X6-
chloride (mouthwash)	T49.6X1-	T49.6X2-	T49.6X3-	T49.6X4-	T49.6X5-	T49.6X6-
chromate	T56.5X1-	T56.5X2-	T56.5X3-	T56.5X4-	-	-
gelatin	T49.3X1-	T49.3X2-	T49.3X3-	T49.3X4-	T49.3X5-	T49.3X6-
oxide	T49.3X1-	T49.3X2-	T49.3X3-	T49.3X4-	T49.3X5-	T49.3X6-
plaster	T49.3X1-	T49.3X2-	T49.3X3-	T49.3X4-	T49.3X5-	T49.3X6-
peroxide	T49.0X1-	T49.0X2-	T49.0X3-	T49.0X4-	T49.0X5-	T49.0X6-
pesticides	T56.5X1-	T56.5X2-	T56.5X3-	T56.5X4-	-	-
phosphide	T60.4X1-	T60.4X2-	T60.4X3-	T60.4X4-	-	-
pyrithionate	T49.4X1-	T49.4X2-	T49.4X3-	T49.4X4-	T49.4X5-	T49.4X6-
stearate	T49.3X1-	T49.3X2-	T49.3X3-	T49.3X4-	T49.3X5-	T49.3X6-
sulfate	T49.5X1-	T49.5X2-	T49.5X3-	T49.5X4-	T49.5X5-	T49.5X6-
ENT agent	T49.6X1-	T49.6X2-	T49.6X3-	T49.6X4-	T49.6X5-	T49.6X6-
ophthalmic solution	T49.5X1-	T49.5X2-	T49.5X3-	T49.5X4-	T49.5X5-	T49.5X6-
topical NEC	T49.0X1-	T49.0X2-	T49.0X3-	T49.0X4-	T49.0X5-	T49.0X6-
undecylenate	T49.0X1-	T49.0X2-	T49.0X3-	T49.0X4-	T49.0X5-	T49.0X6-
Zineb	T60.0X1-	T60.0X2-	T60.0X3-	T60.0X4-	-	-
Zinostatin	T45.1X1-	T45.1X2-	T45.1X3-	T45.1X4-	T45.1X5-	T45.1X6-
Zipeprol	T48.3X1-	T48.3X2-	T48.3X3-	T48.3X4-	T48.3X5-	T48.3X6-
Zofenopril	T46.4X1-	T46.4X2-	T46.4X3-	T46.4X4-	T46.4X5-	T46.4X6-
Zolpidem	T42.6X1-	T42.6X2-	T42.6X3-	T42.6X4-	T42.6X5-	T42.6X6-
Zomepirac	T39.391-	T39.392-	T39.393-	T39.394-	T39.395-	T39.396-
Zopiclone	T42.6X1-	T42.6X2-	T42.6X3-	T42.6X4-	T42.6X5-	T42.6X6-
Zorubicin	T45.1X1-	T45.1X2-	T45.1X3-	T45.1X4-	T45.1X5-	T45.1X6-
Zotepine	T43.591-	T43.592-	T43.593-	T43.594-	T43.595-	T43.596-
Zovant	T45.511-	T45.512-	T45.513-	T45.514-	T45.515-	T45.516-
Zoxazolamine	T42.8X1-	T42.8X2-	T42.8X3-	T42.8X4-	T42.8X5-	T42.8X6-
Zuclopenthixol	T43.4X1-	T43.4X2-	T43.4X3-	T43.4X4-	T43.4X5-	T43.4X6-
Zygadenus (venenosus)	T62.2X1-	T62.2X2-	T62.2X3-	T62.2X4-	-	-
Zyprexa	T43.591-	T43.592-	T43.593-	T43.594-	T43.595-	T43.596-

Accident (to) - *continued*
 transport (involving injury to) - *continued*
  aircraft NEC - *continued*
   occupant injured (in) - *continued*
    powered craft accident - *continued*
     spacecraft - *continued*
      forced landing V95.42
      specified type NEC V95.49
     specified craft NEC V95.8
     ultralight V95.10
      collision V95.13
      crash V95.11
      explosion V95.15
      fire V95.14
      forced landing V95.12
      specified type NEC V95.19
     specified accident NEC V97.0
     while boarding or alighting V97.1
    person (injured by)
     falling from, in or on aircraft V97.0
     machinery on aircraft V97.89
     on ground with aircraft involvement V97.39
     rotating propeller V97.32
     struck by object falling from aircraft V97.31
     sucked into aircraft jet V97.33
     while boarding or alighting aircraft V97.1
   airport (battery-powered) passenger vehicle — *see*
    Accident, transport, industrial vehicle occupant
   all-terrain vehicle occupant (nontraffic) V86.99
    driver V86.59
    dune buggy — *see* Accident, transport, dune
     buggy occupant
    hanger-on V86.79
    passenger V86.69
    snowmobile — *see* Accident, transport,
     snowmobile occupant
    traffic V86.39
     driver V86.09
     hanger-on V86.29
     passenger V86.19
    while boarding or alighting V86.49
   ambulance occupant (traffic) V86.31
    driver V86.01
    hanger-on V86.21
    nontraffic V86.91
     driver V86.51
     hanger-on V86.71
     passenger V86.61
    passenger V86.11
    while boarding or alighting V86.41
   animal-drawn vehicle occupant (in) V80.929
    collision (with)
     animal V80.12
      being ridden V80.711
     animal-drawn vehicle V80.721
     bus V80.42
     car V80.42
     fixed or stationary object V80.82
     military vehicle V80.920
     nonmotor vehicle V80.791
     pedal cycle V80.22
     pedestrian V80.12
     pickup V80.42
     railway train or vehicle V80.62
     specified motor vehicle NEC V80.52
     streetcar V80.731
     truck V80.42
     two- or three-wheeled motor vehicle V80.32
     van V80.42
    noncollision V80.02
    specified circumstance NEC V80.928
   animal-rider V80.919
    collision (with)
     animal V80.11
      being ridden V80.710
     animal-drawn vehicle V80.720
     bus V80.41
     car V80.41
     fixed or stationary object V80.81
     military vehicle V80.910
     nonmotor vehicle V80.790
     pedal cycle V80.21
     pedestrian V80.11
     pickup V80.41
     railway train or vehicle V80.61
     specified motor vehicle NEC V80.51
     streetcar V80.730
     truck V80.41
     two- or three-wheeled motor vehicle V80.31
     van V80.41
    noncollision V80.018
     specified as horse rider V80.010
    specified circumstance NEC V80.918

Accident (to) - *continued*
 transport (involving injury to) - *continued*
  armored car — *see* Accident, transport, truck
   occupant
  battery-powered truck (baggage) (mail) — *see*
   Accident, transport, industrial vehicle occupant
  bus occupant V79.9
   collision (with)
    animal (traffic) V70.9
     being ridden (traffic) V76.9
      nontraffic V76.3
      while boarding or alighting V76.4
     nontraffic V70.3
     while boarding or alighting V70.4
    animal-drawn vehicle (traffic) V76.9
     nontraffic V76.3
     while boarding or alighting V76.4
    bus (traffic) V74.9
     nontraffic V74.3
     while boarding or alighting V74.4
    car (traffic) V73.9
     nontraffic V73.3
     while boarding or alighting V73.4
    motor vehicle NOS (traffic) V79.60
     nontraffic V79.20
     specified type NEC (traffic) V79.69
      nontraffic V79.29
    pedal cycle (traffic) V71.9
     nontraffic V71.3
     while boarding or alighting V71.4
    pickup truck (traffic) V73.9
     nontraffic V73.3
     while boarding or alighting V73.4
    railway vehicle (traffic) V75.9
     nontraffic V75.3
     while boarding or alighting V75.4
    specified vehicle NEC (traffic) V76.9
     nontraffic V76.3
     while boarding or alighting V76.4
    stationary object (traffic) V77.9
     nontraffic V77.3
     while boarding or alighting V77.4
    streetcar (traffic) V76.9
     nontraffic V76.3
     while boarding or alighting V76.4
    three wheeled motor vehicle (traffic) V72.9
     nontraffic V72.3
     while boarding or alighting V72.4
    truck (traffic) V74.9
     nontraffic V74.3
     while boarding or alighting V74.4
    two wheeled motor vehicle (traffic) V72.9
     nontraffic V72.3
     while boarding or alighting V72.4
    van (traffic) V73.9
     nontraffic V73.3
     while boarding or alighting V73.4
   driver
    collision (with)
     animal (traffic) V70.5
      being ridden (traffic) V76.5
       nontraffic V76.0
      nontraffic V70.0
     animal-drawn vehicle (traffic) V76.5
      nontraffic V76.0
     bus (traffic) V74.5
      nontraffic V74.0
     car (traffic) V73.5
      nontraffic V73.0
     motor vehicle NOS (traffic) V79.40
      nontraffic V79.00
      specified type NEC (traffic) V79.49
       nontraffic V79.09
     pedal cycle (traffic) V71.5
      nontraffic V71.0
     pickup truck (traffic) V73.5
      nontraffic V73.0
     railway vehicle (traffic) V75.5
      nontraffic V75.0
     specified vehicle NEC (traffic) V76.5
      nontraffic V76.0
     stationary object (traffic) V77.5
      nontraffic V77.0
     streetcar (traffic) V76.5
      nontraffic V76.0
     three wheeled motor vehicle (traffic) V72.5
      nontraffic V72.0
     truck (traffic) V74.5
      nontraffic V74.0
     two wheeled motor vehicle (traffic) V72.5
      nontraffic V72.0
     van (traffic) V73.5
      nontraffic V73.0

Accident (to) - *continued*
 transport (involving injury to) - *continued*
  bus occupant - *continued*
   driver - *continued*
     noncollision accident (traffic) V78.5
      nontraffic V78.0
     noncollision accident (traffic) V78.9
      nontraffic V78.3
     while boarding or alighting V78.4
    nontraffic V79.3
   hanger-on
    collision (with)
     animal (traffic) V70.7
      being ridden (traffic) V76.7
       nontraffic V76.2
      nontraffic V70.2
     animal-drawn vehicle (traffic) V76.7
      nontraffic V76.2
     bus (traffic) V74.7
      nontraffic V74.2
     car (traffic) V73.7
      nontraffic V73.2
     pedal cycle (traffic) V71.7
      nontraffic V71.2
     pickup truck (traffic) V73.7
      nontraffic V73.2
     railway vehicle (traffic) V75.7
      nontraffic V75.2
     specified vehicle NEC (traffic) V76.7
      nontraffic V76.2
     stationary object (traffic) V77.7
      nontraffic V77.2
     streetcar (traffic) V76.7
      nontraffic V76.2
     three wheeled motor vehicle (traffic) V72.7
      nontraffic V72.2
     truck (traffic) V74.7
      nontraffic V74.2
     two wheeled motor vehicle (traffic) V72.7
      nontraffic V72.2
     van (traffic) V73.7
      nontraffic V73.2
    noncollision accident (traffic) V78.7
     nontraffic V78.2
   passenger
    collision (with)
     animal (traffic) V70.6
      being ridden (traffic) V76.6
       nontraffic V76.1
      nontraffic V70.1
     animal-drawn vehicle (traffic) V76.6
      nontraffic V76.1
     bus (traffic) V74.6
      nontraffic V74.1
     car (traffic) V73.6
      nontraffic V73.1
     motor vehicle NOS (traffic) V79.50
      nontraffic V79.10
      specified type NEC (traffic) V79.59
       nontraffic V79.19
     pedal cycle (traffic) V71.6
      nontraffic V71.1
     pickup truck (traffic) V73.6
      nontraffic V73.1
     railway vehicle (traffic) V75.6
      nontraffic V75.1
     specified vehicle NEC (traffic) V76.6
      nontraffic V76.1
     stationary object (traffic) V77.6
      nontraffic V77.1
     streetcar (traffic) V76.6
      nontraffic V76.1
     three wheeled motor vehicle (traffic) V72.6
      nontraffic V72.1
     truck (traffic) V74.6
      nontraffic V74.1
     two wheeled motor vehicle (traffic) V72.6
      nontraffic V72.1
     van (traffic) V73.6
      nontraffic V73.1
    noncollision accident (traffic) V78.6
     nontraffic V78.1
   specified type NEC V79.88
   military vehicle V79.81
  cable car, not on rails V98.0
   on rails — *see* Accident, transport, streetcar
    occupant
  car occupant V49.9
   ambulance occupant — *see* Accident, transport,
    ambulance occupant
   collision (with)
    animal (traffic) V40.9
     being ridden (traffic) V46.9

Accident (to) - *continued*
  transport (involving injury to) - *continued*
    car occupant - *continued*
      collision (with) - *continued*
        animal (traffic) - *continued*
          being ridden (traffic) - *continued*
            nontraffic V46.3
            while boarding or alighting V46.4
          nontraffic V40.3
          while boarding or alighting V40.4
        animal-drawn vehicle (traffic) V46.9
          nontraffic V46.3
          while boarding or alighting V46.4
        bus (traffic) V44.9
          nontraffic V44.3
          while boarding or alighting V44.4
        car (traffic) V43.92
          nontraffic V43.32
          while boarding or alighting V43.42
        motor vehicle NOS (traffic) V49.60
          nontraffic V49.20
          specified type NEC (traffic) V49.69
            nontraffic V49.29
        pedal cycle (traffic) V41.9
          nontraffic V41.3
          while boarding or alighting V41.4
        pickup truck (traffic) V43.93
          nontraffic V43.33
          while boarding or alighting V43.43
        railway vehicle (traffic) V45.9
          nontraffic V45.3
          while boarding or alighting V45.4
        specified vehicle NEC (traffic) V46.9
          nontraffic V46.3
          while boarding or alighting V46.4
        sport utility vehicle (traffic) V43.91
          nontraffic V43.31
          while boarding or alighting V43.41
        stationary object (traffic) V47.92
          nontraffic V47.32
          while boarding or alighting V47.4
        streetcar (traffic) V46.9
          nontraffic V46.3
          while boarding or alighting V46.4
        three wheeled motor vehicle (traffic) V42.9
          nontraffic V42.3
          while boarding or alighting V42.4
        truck (traffic) V44.9
          nontraffic V44.3
          while boarding or alighting V44.4
        two wheeled motor vehicle (traffic) V42.9
          nontraffic V42.3
          while boarding or alighting V42.4
        van (traffic) V43.94
          nontraffic V43.34
          while boarding or alighting V43.44
      driver
        collision (with)
          animal (traffic) V40.5
            being ridden (traffic) V46.5
              nontraffic V46.0
            nontraffic V40.0
          animal-drawn vehicle (traffic) V46.5
            nontraffic V46.0
          bus (traffic) V44.5
            nontraffic V44.0
          car (traffic) V43.52
            nontraffic V43.02
          motor vehicle NOS (traffic) V49.40
            nontraffic V49.00
            specified type NEC (traffic) V49.49
              nontraffic V49.09
          pedal cycle (traffic) V41.5
            nontraffic V41.0
          pickup truck (traffic) V43.53
            nontraffic V43.03
          railway vehicle (traffic) V45.5
            nontraffic V45.0
          specified vehicle NEC (traffic) V46.5
            nontraffic V46.0
          sport utility vehicle (traffic) V43.51
            nontraffic V43.01
          stationary object (traffic) V47.52
            nontraffic V47.02
          streetcar (traffic) V46.5
            nontraffic V46.0
          three wheeled motor vehicle (traffic) V42.5
            nontraffic V42.0
          truck (traffic) V44.5
            nontraffic V44.0
          two wheeled motor vehicle (traffic) V42.5
            nontraffic V42.0
          van (traffic) V43.54

Accident (to) - *continued*
  transport (involving injury to) - *continued*
    car occupant - *continued*
      driver - *continued*
        collision (with) - *continued*
          van (traffic) - *continued*
            nontraffic V43.04
          noncollision accident (traffic) V48.5
            nontraffic V48.0
        noncollision accident (traffic) V48.9
          nontraffic V48.3
          while boarding or alighting V48.4
        nontraffic V49.3
      hanger-on
        collision (with)
          animal (traffic) V40.7
            being ridden (traffic) V46.7
              nontraffic V46.2
            nontraffic V40.2
          animal-drawn vehicle (traffic) V46.7
            nontraffic V46.2
          bus (traffic) V44.7
            nontraffic V44.2
          car (traffic) V43.72
            nontraffic V43.22
          pedal cycle (traffic) V41.7
            nontraffic V41.2
          pickup truck (traffic) V43.73
            nontraffic V43.23
          railway vehicle (traffic) V45.7
            nontraffic V45.2
          specified vehicle NEC (traffic) V46.7
            nontraffic V46.2
          sport utility vehicle (traffic) V43.71
            nontraffic V43.21
          stationary object (traffic) V47.7
            nontraffic V47.2
          streetcar (traffic) V46.7
            nontraffic V46.2
          three wheeled motor vehicle (traffic) V42.7
            nontraffic V42.2
          truck (traffic) V44.7
            nontraffic V44.2
          two wheeled motor vehicle (traffic) V42.7
            nontraffic V42.2
          van (traffic) V43.74
            nontraffic V43.24
        noncollision accident (traffic) V48.7
          nontraffic V48.2
      passenger
        collision (with)
          animal (traffic) V40.6
            being ridden (traffic) V46.6
              nontraffic V46.1
            nontraffic V40.1
          animal-drawn vehicle (traffic) V46.6
            nontraffic V46.1
          bus (traffic) V44.6
            nontraffic V44.1
          car (traffic) V43.62
            nontraffic V43.12
          motor vehicle NOS (traffic) V49.50
            nontraffic V49.10
            specified type NEC (traffic) V49.59
              nontraffic V49.19
          pedal cycle (traffic) V41.6
            nontraffic V41.1
          pickup truck (traffic) V43.63
            nontraffic V43.13
          railway vehicle (traffic) V45.6
            nontraffic V45.1
          specified vehicle NEC (traffic) V46.6
            nontraffic V46.1
          sport utility vehicle (traffic) V43.61
            nontraffic V43.11
          stationary object (traffic) V47.62
            nontraffic V47.12
          streetcar (traffic) V46.6
            nontraffic V46.1
          three wheeled motor vehicle (traffic) V42.6
            nontraffic V42.1
          truck (traffic) V44.6
            nontraffic V44.1
          two wheeled motor vehicle (traffic) V42.6
            nontraffic V42.1
          van (traffic) V43.64
            nontraffic V43.14
        noncollision accident (traffic) V48.6
          nontraffic V48.1
        specified type NEC V49.88
        military vehicle V49.81
      coal car — *see* Accident, transport, industrial vehicle occupant

Accident (to) - *continued*
  transport (involving injury to) - *continued*
    construction vehicle occupant (nontraffic) V85.9
      driver V85.5
      hanger-on V85.7
      passenger V85.6
      traffic V85.3
        driver V85.0
        hanger-on V85.2
        passenger V85.1
      while boarding or alighting V85.4
    dirt bike rider — *see* Accident, transport, all-terrain vehicle occupant
    due to cataclysm — *see* Forces of nature, by type
    dune buggy occupant (nontraffic) V86.93
      driver V86.53
      hanger-on V86.73
      passenger V86.63
      traffic V86.33
        driver V86.03
        hanger-on V86.23
        passenger V86.13
      while boarding or alighting V86.43
    forklift — *see* Accident, transport, industrial vehicle occupant
    go cart — *see* Accident, transport, all-terrain vehicle occupant
    golf cart — *see* Accident, transport, all-terrain vehicle occupant
    heavy transport vehicle occupant — *see* Accident, transport, truck occupant
    ice yacht V98.2
    industrial vehicle occupant (nontraffic) V83.9
      driver V83.5
      hanger-on V83.7
      passenger V83.6
      traffic V83.3
        driver V83.0
        hanger-on V83.2
        passenger V83.1
      while boarding or alighting V83.4
    interurban electric car — *see* Accident, transport, streetcar
    land yacht V98.1
    logging car — *see* Accident, transport, industrial vehicle occupant
    military vehicle occupant (traffic) V86.34
      driver V86.04
      hanger-on V86.24
      nontraffic V86.94
        driver V86.54
        hanger-on V86.74
        passenger V86.64
      passenger V86.14
      while boarding or alighting V86.44
    mine tram — *see* Accident, transport, industrial vehicle occupant
    motorcoach — *see* Accident, transport, bus occupant
    motorcyclist V29.9
      collision (with)
        animal (traffic) V20.9
          being ridden (traffic) V26.9
            nontraffic V26.2
            while boarding or alighting V26.3
          nontraffic V20.2
          while boarding or alighting V20.3
        animal-drawn vehicle (traffic) V26.9
          nontraffic V26.2
          while boarding or alighting V26.3
        bus (traffic) V24.9
          nontraffic V24.2
          while boarding or alighting V24.3
        car (traffic) V23.9
          nontraffic V23.2
          while boarding or alighting V23.3
        motor vehicle NOS (traffic) V29.60
          nontraffic V29.20
          specified type NEC (traffic) V29.69
            nontraffic V29.29
        pedal cycle (traffic) V21.9
          nontraffic V21.2
          while boarding or alighting V21.3
        pickup truck (traffic) V23.9
          nontraffic V23.2
          while boarding or alighting V23.3
        railway vehicle (traffic) V25.9
          nontraffic V25.2
          while boarding or alighting V25.3
        specified vehicle NEC (traffic) V26.9
          nontraffic V26.2
          while boarding or alighting V26.3
        stationary object (traffic) V27.9

Accident (to) - *continued*
transport (involving injury to) - *continued*
motorcyclist - *continued*
collision (with) - *continued*
stationary object (traffic) - *continued*
nontraffic V27.2
while boarding or alighting V27.3
streetcar (traffic) V26.9
nontraffic V26.2
while boarding or alighting V26.3
three wheeled motor vehicle (traffic) V22.9
nontraffic V22.2
while boarding or alighting V22.3
truck (traffic) V24.9
nontraffic V24.2
while boarding or alighting V24.3
two wheeled motor vehicle (traffic) V22.9
nontraffic V22.2
while boarding or alighting V22.3
van (traffic) V23.9
nontraffic V23.2
while boarding or alighting V23.3
driver
collision (with)
animal (traffic) V20.4
being ridden (traffic) V26.4
nontraffic V26.0
nontraffic V20.0
animal-drawn vehicle (traffic) V26.4
nontraffic V26.0
bus (traffic) V24.4
nontraffic V24.0
car (traffic) V23.4
nontraffic V23.0
motor vehicle NOS (traffic) V29.40
nontraffic V29.00
specified type NEC (traffic) V29.49
nontraffic V29.09
pedal cycle (traffic) V21.4
nontraffic V21.0
pickup truck (traffic) V23.4
nontraffic V23.0
railway vehicle (traffic) V25.4
nontraffic V25.0
specified vehicle NEC (traffic) V26.4
nontraffic V26.0
stationary object (traffic) V27.4
nontraffic V27.0
streetcar (traffic) V26.4
nontraffic V26.0
three wheeled motor vehicle (traffic) V22.4
nontraffic V22.0
truck (traffic) V24.4
nontraffic V24.0
two wheeled motor vehicle (traffic) V22.4
nontraffic V22.0
van (traffic) V23.4
nontraffic V23.0
noncollision accident (traffic) V28.4
nontraffic V28.0
noncollision accident (traffic) V28.9
nontraffic V28.2
while boarding or alighting V28.3
nontraffic V29.3
passenger
collision (with)
animal (traffic) V20.5
being ridden (traffic) V26.5
nontraffic V26.1
nontraffic V20.1
animal-drawn vehicle (traffic) V26.5
nontraffic V26.1
bus (traffic) V24.5
nontraffic V24.1
car (traffic) V23.5
nontraffic V23.1
motor vehicle NOS (traffic) V29.50
nontraffic V29.10
specified type NEC (traffic) V29.59
nontraffic V29.19
pedal cycle (traffic) V21.5
nontraffic V21.1
pickup truck (traffic) V23.5
nontraffic V23.1
railway vehicle (traffic) V25.5
nontraffic V25.1
specified vehicle NEC (traffic) V26.5
nontraffic V26.1
stationary object (traffic) V27.5
nontraffic V27.1
streetcar (traffic) V26.5
nontraffic V26.1
three wheeled motor vehicle (traffic) V22.5

Accident (to) - *continued*
transport (involving injury to) - *continued*
motorcyclist - *continued*
passenger - *continued*
collision (with) - *continued*
three wheeled motor vehicle (traffic) - *continued*
nontraffic V22.1
truck (traffic) V24.5
nontraffic V24.1
two wheeled motor vehicle (traffic) V22.5
nontraffic V22.1
van (traffic) V23.5
nontraffic V23.1
noncollision accident (traffic) V28.5
nontraffic V28.1
specified type NEC V29.88
military vehicle V29.81
motor vehicle NEC occupant (traffic) V89.2
occupant (of)
aircraft (powered) V95.9
fixed wing
commercial — *see* Accident, transport, aircraft, occupant, powered, fixed wing, commercial
private — *see* Accident, transport, aircraft, occupant, powered, fixed wing, private
nonpowered V96.9
specified NEC V95.8
airport battery-powered vehicle — *see* Accident, transport, industrial vehicle occupant
all-terrain vehicle (ATV) — *see* Accident, transport, all-terrain vehicle occupant
animal-drawn vehicle — *see* Accident, transport, animal-drawn vehicle occupant
automobile — *see* Accident, transport, car occupant
balloon V96.00
battery-powered vehicle — *see* Accident, transport, industrial vehicle occupant
bicycle — *see* Accident, transport, pedal cyclist
motorized — *see* Accident, transport, motorcycle rider
boat NEC — *see* Accident, watercraft
bulldozer — *see* Accident, transport, construction vehicle occupant
bus — *see* Accident, transport, bus occupant
cable car (on rails) — *see also* Accident, transport, streetcar occupant
not on rails V98.0
car — *see also* Accident, transport, car occupant
cable (on rails) — *see also* Accident, transport, streetcar occupant
not on rails V98.0
coach — *see* Accident, transport, bus occupant
coal-car — *see* Accident, transport, industrial vehicle occupant
digger — *see* Accident, transport, construction vehicle occupant
dump truck — *see* Accident, transport, construction vehicle occupant
earth-leveler — *see* Accident, transport, construction vehicle occupant
farm machinery (self-propelled) — *see* Accident, transport, agricultural vehicle occupant
forklift — *see* Accident, transport, industrial vehicle occupant
glider (unpowered) V96.20
hang V96.10
powered (microlight) (ultralight) — *see* Accident, transport, aircraft, occupant, powered, glider
glider (unpowered) NEC V96.20
hang-glider V96.10
harvester — *see* Accident, transport, agricultural vehicle occupant
heavy (transport) vehicle — *see* Accident, transport, truck occupant
helicopter — *see* Accident, transport, aircraft, occupant, helicopter
ice-yacht V98.2
kite (carrying person) V96.8
land-yacht V98.1
logging car — *see* Accident, transport, industrial vehicle occupant
mechanical shovel — *see* Accident, transport, construction vehicle occupant
microlight — *see* Accident, transport, aircraft, occupant, powered, glider
minibus — *see* Accident, transport, pickup truck occupant
minivan — *see* Accident, transport, pickup truck occupant

Accident (to) - *continued*
transport (involving injury to) - *continued*
occupant (of) - *continued*
moped — *see* Accident, transport, motorcycle
motor scooter — *see* Accident, transport, motorcycle
motorcycle (with sidecar) — *see* Accident, transport, motorcycle
pedal cycle — *see also* Accident, transport, pedal cyclist
pick-up (truck) — *see* Accident, transport, pickup truck occupant
railway (train) (vehicle) (subterranean) (elevated) — *see* Accident, transport, railway vehicle occupant
rickshaw — *see* Accident, transport, pedal cycle
motorized — *see* Accident, transport, three-wheeled motor vehicle
pedal driven — *see* Accident, transport, pedal cyclist
road-roller — *see* Accident, transport, construction vehicle occupant
ship NOS V94.9
ski-lift (chair) (gondola) V98.3
snowmobile — *see* Accident, transport, snowmobile occupant
spacecraft, spaceship — *see* Accident, transport, aircraft, occupant, spacecraft
sport utility vehicle — *see* Accident, transport, pickup truck occupant
streetcar (interurban) (operating on public street or highway) — *see* Accident, transport, streetcar occupant
SUV — *see* Accident, transport, pickup truck occupant
téléférique V98.0
three-wheeled vehicle (motorized) — *see also* Accident, transport, three-wheeled motor vehicle occupant
nonmotorized — *see* Accident, transport, pedal cycle
tractor (farm) (and trailer) — *see* Accident, transport, agricultural vehicle occupant
train — *see* Accident, transport, railway vehicle occupant
tram — *see* Accident, transport, streetcar occupant
in mine or quarry — *see* Accident, transport, industrial vehicle occupant
tricycle — *see* Accident, transport, pedal cycle
motorized — *see* Accident, transport, three-wheeled motor vehicle
trolley — *see* Accident, transport, streetcar occupant
in mine or quarry — *see* Accident, transport, industrial vehicle occupant
tub, in mine or quarry — *see* Accident, transport, industrial vehicle occupant
ultralight — *see* Accident, transport, aircraft, occupant, powered, glider
van — *see* Accident, transport, van occupant
vehicle NEC V89.9
heavy transport — *see* Accident, transport, truck occupant
motor (traffic) NEC V89.2
nontraffic NEC V89.0
watercraft NOS V94.9
causing drowning — *see* Drowning, resulting from accident to boat
parachutist V97.29
after accident to aircraft — *see* Accident, transport, aircraft
entangled in object V97.21
injured on landing V97.22
pedal cyclist V19.9
collision (with)
animal (traffic) V10.9
being ridden (traffic) V16.9
nontraffic V16.2
nontraffic V10.2
while boarding or alighting V10.3
animal-drawn vehicle (traffic) V16.9
nontraffic V16.2
while boarding or alighting V16.3
bus (traffic) V14.9
nontraffic V14.2
while boarding or alighting V14.3
car (traffic) V13.9
nontraffic V13.2
while boarding or alighting V13.3
motor vehicle NOS (traffic) V19.60
nontraffic V19.20

Accident (to) - *continued*
  transport (involving injury to) - *continued*
    pedal cyclist - *continued*
      collision (with) - *continued*
        motor vehicle NOS (traffic) - *continued*
          specified type NEC (traffic) V19.69
          nontraffic V19.29
        pedal cycle (traffic) V11.9
          nontraffic V11.2
          while boarding or alighting V11.3
        pickup truck (traffic) V13.9
          nontraffic V13.2
          while boarding or alighting V13.3
        railway vehicle (traffic) V15.9
          nontraffic V15.2
          while boarding or alighting V15.3
        specified vehicle NEC (traffic) V16.9
          nontraffic V16.2
          while boarding or alighting V16.3
        stationary object (traffic) V17.9
          nontraffic V17.2
          while boarding or alighting V17.3
        streetcar (traffic) V16.9
          nontraffic V16.2
          while boarding or alighting V16.3
        three wheeled motor vehicle (traffic) V12.9
          nontraffic V12.2
          while boarding or alighting V12.3
        truck (traffic) V14.9
          nontraffic V14.2
          while boarding or alighting V14.3
        two wheeled motor vehicle (traffic) V12.9
          nontraffic V12.2
          while boarding or alighting V12.3
        van (traffic) V13.9
          nontraffic V13.2
          while boarding or alighting V13.3
      driver
        collision (with)
          animal (traffic) V10.4
            being ridden (traffic) V16.4
              nontraffic V16.0
            nontraffic V10.0
          animal-drawn vehicle (traffic) V16.4
            nontraffic V16.0
          bus (traffic) V14.4
            nontraffic V14.0
          car (traffic) V13.4
            nontraffic V13.0
          motor vehicle NOS (traffic) V19.40
            nontraffic V19.00
            specified type NEC (traffic) V19.49
              nontraffic V19.09
          pedal cycle (traffic) V11.4
            nontraffic V11.0
          pickup truck (traffic) V13.4
            nontraffic V13.0
          railway vehicle (traffic) V15.4
            nontraffic V15.0
          specified vehicle NEC (traffic) V16.4
            nontraffic V16.0
          stationary object (traffic) V17.4
            nontraffic V17.0
          streetcar (traffic) V16.4
            nontraffic V16.0
          three wheeled motor vehicle (traffic) V12.4
            nontraffic V12.0
          truck (traffic) V14.4
            nontraffic V14.0
          two wheeled motor vehicle (traffic) V12.4
            nontraffic V12.0
          van (traffic) V13.4
            nontraffic V13.0
        noncollision accident (traffic) V18.4
          nontraffic V18.0
      noncollision accident (traffic) V18.9
        nontraffic V18.2
        while boarding or alighting V18.3
      nontraffic V19.3
      passenger
        collision (with)
          animal (traffic) V10.5
            being ridden (traffic) V16.5
              nontraffic V16.1
            nontraffic V10.1
          animal-drawn vehicle (traffic) V16.5
            nontraffic V16.1
          bus (traffic) V14.5
            nontraffic V14.1
          car (traffic) V13.5
            nontraffic V13.1
          motor vehicle NOS (traffic) V19.50
            nontraffic V19.10

Accident (to) - *continued*
  transport (involving injury to) - *continued*
    pedal cyclist - *continued*
      passenger - *continued*
        collision (with) - *continued*
          motor vehicle NOS (traffic) - *continued*
            specified type NEC (traffic) V19.59
            nontraffic V19.19
          pedal cycle (traffic) V11.5
            nontraffic V11.1
          pickup truck (traffic) V13.5
            nontraffic V13.1
          railway vehicle (traffic) V15.5
            nontraffic V15.1
          specified vehicle NEC (traffic) V16.5
            nontraffic V16.1
          stationary object (traffic) V17.5
            nontraffic V17.1
          streetcar (traffic) V16.5
            nontraffic V16.1
          three wheeled motor vehicle (traffic) V12.5
            nontraffic V12.1
          truck (traffic) V14.5
            nontraffic V14.1
          two wheeled motor vehicle (traffic) V12.5
            nontraffic V12.1
          van (traffic) V13.5
            nontraffic V13.1
        noncollision accident (traffic) V18.5
          nontraffic V18.1
      specified type NEC V19.88
      military vehicle V19.81
    pedestrian
      conveyance (occupant) V09.9
        babystroller V00.828
          collision (with) V09.9
            animal being ridden or animal drawn
              vehicle V06.99
              nontraffic V06.09
              traffic V06.19
            bus or heavy transport V04.99
              nontraffic V04.09
              traffic V04.19
            car V03.99
              nontraffic V03.09
              traffic V03.19
            pedal cycle V01.99
              nontraffic V01.09
              traffic V01.19
            pick-up truck or van V03.99
              nontraffic V03.09
              traffic V03.19
            railway (train) (vehicle) V05.99
              nontraffic V05.09
              traffic V05.19
            streetcar V06.99
              nontraffic V06.09
              traffic V06.19
            stationary object V00.822
            two- or three-wheeled motor vehicle V02.99
              nontraffic V02.09
              traffic V02.19
            vehicle V09.9
              animal-drawn V06.99
                nontraffic V06.09
                traffic V06.19
              motor
                nontraffic V09.00
                traffic V09.20
          fall V00.821
          nontraffic V09.1
            involving motor vehicle NEC V09.00
          traffic V09.3
            involving motor vehicle NEC V09.20
        flat-bottomed NEC V00.388
          collision (with) V09.9
            animal being ridden or animal drawn
              vehicle V06.99
              nontraffic V06.09
              traffic V06.19
            bus or heavy transport V04.99
              nontraffic V04.09
              traffic V04.19
            car V03.99
              nontraffic V03.09
              traffic V03.19
            pedal cycle V01.99
              nontraffic V01.09
              traffic V01.19
            pick-up truck or van V03.99
              nontraffic V03.09
              traffic V03.19
            railway (train) (vehicle) V05.99

Accident (to) - *continued*
  transport (involving injury to) - *continued*
    pedestrian - *continued*
      conveyance (occupant) - *continued*
        flat-bottomed NEC - *continued*
          collision (with) - *continued*
            railway (train) (vehicle) - *continued*
              nontraffic V05.09
              traffic V05.19
            stationary object V00.382
            streetcar V06.99
              nontraffic V06.09
              traffic V06.19
            two- or three-wheeled motor vehicle V02.99
              nontraffic V02.09
              traffic V02.19
            vehicle V09.9
              animal-drawn V06.99
                nontraffic V06.09
                traffic V06.19
              motor
                nontraffic V09.00
                traffic V09.20
          fall V00.381
          nontraffic V09.1
            involving motor vehicle NEC V09.00
          snow
            board — *see* Accident, transport, pedestrian,
              conveyance, snow board
            ski- — *see* Accident, transport, pedestrian,
              conveyance, skis (snow)
          traffic V09.3
            involving motor vehicle NEC V09.20
        gliding type NEC V00.288
          collision (with) V09.9
            animal being ridden or animal drawn
              vehicle V06.99
              nontraffic V06.09
              traffic V06.19
            bus or heavy transport V04.99
              nontraffic V04.09
              traffic V04.19
            car V03.99
              nontraffic V03.09
              traffic V03.19
            pedal cycle V01.99
              nontraffic V01.09
              traffic V01.19
            pick-up truck or van V03.99
              nontraffic V03.09
              traffic V03.19
            railway (train) (vehicle) V05.99
              nontraffic V05.09
              traffic V05.19
            stationary object V00.282
            streetcar V06.99
              nontraffic V06.09
              traffic V06.19
            two- or three-wheeled motor vehicle V02.99
              nontraffic V02.09
              traffic V02.19
            vehicle V09.9
              animal-drawn V06.99
                nontraffic V06.09
                traffic V06.19
              motor
                nontraffic V09.00
                traffic V09.20
          fall V00.281
          heelies — *see* Accident, transport, pedestrian,
            conveyance, heelies
          ice skate — *see* Accident, transport,
            pedestrian, conveyance, ice skate
          nontraffic V09.1
            involving motor vehicle NEC V09.00
          sled — *see* Accident, transport, pedestrian,
            conveyance, sled
          traffic V09.3
            involving motor vehicle NEC V09.20
          wheelies — *see* Accident, transport,
            pedestrian, conveyance, heelies
        heelies V00.158
          colliding with stationary object V00.152
          fall V00.151
        ice skates V00.218
          collision (with) V09.9
            animal being ridden or animal drawn
              vehicle V06.99
              nontraffic V06.09
              traffic V06.19
            bus or heavy transport V04.99
              nontraffic V04.09
              traffic V04.19

Accident (to) - *continued*
  transport (involving injury to) - *continued*
    pedestrian - *continued*
      conveyance (occupant) - *continued*
        skis (snow) - *continued*
          collision (with) - *continued*
            car V03.99
              nontraffic V03.09
              traffic V03.19
            pedal cycle V01.99
              nontraffic V01.09
              traffic V01.19
            pick-up truck or van V03.99
              nontraffic V03.09
              traffic V03.19
            railway (train) (vehicle) V05.99
              nontraffic V05.09
              traffic V05.19
            streetcar V06.99
              nontraffic V06.09
              traffic V06.19
            stationary object V00.322
            two- or three-wheeled motor vehicle V02.99
              nontraffic V02.09
              traffic V02.19
            vehicle V09.9
              animal-drawn V06.99
                nontraffic V06.09
                traffic V06.19
              motor
                nontraffic V09.00
                traffic V09.20
          fall V00.321
          nontraffic V09.1
            involving motor vehicle NEC V09.00
          traffic V09.3
            involving motor vehicle NEC V09.20
         snow board V00.318
          collision (with) V09.9
            animal being ridden or animal drawn
              vehicle V06.99
              nontraffic V06.09
              traffic V06.19
            bus or heavy transport V04.99
              nontraffic V04.09
              traffic V04.19
            car V03.99
              nontraffic V03.09
              traffic V03.19
            pedal cycle V01.99
              nontraffic V01.09
              traffic V01.19
            pick-up truck or van V03.99
              nontraffic V03.09
              traffic V03.19
            railway (train) (vehicle) V05.99
              nontraffic V05.09
              traffic V05.19
            streetcar V06.99
              nontraffic V06.09
              traffic V06.19
            stationary object V00.312
            two- or three-wheeled motor vehicle V02.99
              nontraffic V02.09
              traffic V02.19
            vehicle V09.9
              animal-drawn V06.99
                nontraffic V06.09
                traffic V06.19
              motor
                nontraffic V09.00
                traffic V09.20
          fall V00.311
          nontraffic V09.1
            involving motor vehicle NEC V09.00
          traffic V09.3
            involving motor vehicle NEC V09.20
         specified type NEC V00.898
          collision (with) V09.9
            animal being ridden or animal drawn
              vehicle V06.99
              nontraffic V06.09
              traffic V06.19
            bus or heavy transport V04.99
              nontraffic V04.09
              traffic V04.19
            car V03.99
              nontraffic V03.09
              traffic V03.19
            pedal cycle V01.99
              nontraffic V01.09
              traffic V01.19
            pick-up truck or van V03.99

Accident (to) - *continued*
  transport (involving injury to) - *continued*
    pedestrian - *continued*
      conveyance (occupant) - *continued*
        specified type NEC - *continued*
          collision (with) - *continued*
            pick-up truck or van - *continued*
              nontraffic V03.09
              traffic V03.19
            railway (train) (vehicle) V05.99
              nontraffic V05.09
              traffic V05.19
            streetcar V06.99
              nontraffic V06.09
              traffic V06.19
            stationary object V00.892
            two- or three-wheeled motor vehicle V02.99
              nontraffic V02.09
              traffic V02.19
            vehicle V09.9
              animal-drawn V06.99
                nontraffic V06.09
                traffic V06.19
              motor
                nontraffic V09.00
                traffic V09.20
          fall V00.891
          nontraffic V09.1
            involving motor vehicle NEC V09.00
          traffic V09.3
            involving motor vehicle NEC V09.20
         traffic V09.3
           involving motor vehicle V09.20
            military V09.21
            specified type NEC V09.29
        wheelchair (powered) V00.818
          collision (with) V09.9
            animal being ridden or animal drawn
              vehicle V06.99
              nontraffic V06.09
              traffic V06.19
            bus or heavy transport V04.99
              nontraffic V04.09
              traffic V04.19
            car V03.99
              nontraffic V03.09
              traffic V03.19
            pedal cycle V01.99
              nontraffic V01.09
              traffic V01.19
            pick-up truck or van V03.99
              nontraffic V03.09
              traffic V03.19
            railway (train) (vehicle) V05.99
              nontraffic V05.09
              traffic V05.19
            streetcar V06.99
              nontraffic V06.09
              traffic V06.19
            stationary object V00.812
            two- or three-wheeled motor vehicle V02.99
              nontraffic V02.09
              traffic V02.19
            vehicle V09.9
              animal-drawn V06.99
                nontraffic V06.09
                traffic V06.19
              motor
                nontraffic V09.00
                traffic V09.20
          fall V00.811
          nontraffic V09.1
            involving motor vehicle NEC V09.00
          traffic V09.3
            involving motor vehicle NEC V09.20
         wheeled shoe V00.158
          colliding with stationary object V00.152
          fall V00.151
      on foot — *see also* Accident, pedestrian
        collision (with)
          animal being ridden or animal drawn
            vehicle V06.90
            nontraffic V06.00
            traffic V06.10
          bus or heavy transport V04.90
            nontraffic V04.00
            traffic V04.10
          car V03.90
            nontraffic V03.00
            traffic V03.10
          pedal cycle V01.90
            nontraffic V01.00
            traffic V01.10

Accident (to) - *continued*
  transport (involving injury to) - *continued*
    pedestrian - *continued*
      on foot - *continued*
        collision (with) - *continued*
          pick-up truck or van V03.90
            nontraffic V03.00
            traffic V03.10
          railway (train) (vehicle) V05.90
            nontraffic V05.00
            traffic V05.10
          streetcar V06.90
            nontraffic V06.00
            traffic V06.10
          two- or three-wheeled motor vehicle V02.90
            nontraffic V02.00
            traffic V02.10
          vehicle V09.9
            animal-drawn V06.90
              nontraffic V06.00
              traffic V06.10
            motor
              nontraffic V09.00
              traffic V09.20
         nontraffic V09.1
          involving motor vehicle V09.00
            military V09.01
            specified type NEC V09.09
        traffic V09.3
         involving motor vehicle V09.20
           military V09.21
           specified type NEC V09.29
    person NEC (unknown way or transportation) V99
      collision (between)
        bus (with)
          heavy transport vehicle (traffic) V87.5
          nontraffic V88.5
        car (with)
          nontraffic V88.5
          bus (traffic) V87.3
          nontraffic V88.3
          heavy transport vehicle (traffic) V87.4
          nontraffic V88.4
          pick-up truck or van (traffic) V87.2
          nontraffic V88.2
          train or railway vehicle (traffic) V87.6
          nontraffic V88.6
          two-or three-wheeled motor vehicle
            (traffic) V87.0
          nontraffic V88.0
        motor vehicle (traffic) NEC V87.7
          nontraffic V88.7
        two-or three-wheeled vehicle (with) (traffic)
          motor vehicle NEC V87.1
          nontraffic V88.1
        nonmotor vehicle (collision) (noncollision)
          (traffic) V87.9
          nontraffic V88.9
    pickup truck occupant V59.9
      collision (with)
        animal (traffic) V50.9
          being ridden (traffic) V56.9
           nontraffic V56.3
           while boarding or alighting V56.4
          nontraffic V50.3
          while boarding or alighting V50.4
        animal-drawn vehicle (traffic) V56.9
          nontraffic V56.3
          while boarding or alighting V56.4
        bus (traffic) V54.9
          nontraffic V54.3
          while boarding or alighting V54.4
        car (traffic) V53.9
          nontraffic V53.3
          while boarding or alighting V53.4
        motor vehicle NOS (traffic) V59.60
          nontraffic V59.20
          specified type NEC (traffic) V59.69
          nontraffic V59.29
        pedal cycle (traffic) V51.9
          nontraffic V51.3
          while boarding or alighting V51.4
        pickup truck (traffic) V53.9
          nontraffic V53.3
          while boarding or alighting V53.4
        railway vehicle (traffic) V55.9
          nontraffic V55.3
          while boarding or alighting V55.4
        specified vehicle NEC (traffic) V56.9
          nontraffic V56.3
          while boarding or alighting V56.4
        stationary object (traffic) V57.9
          nontraffic V57.3

Accident (to) - *continued*
transport (involving injury to) - *continued*
  pickup truck occupant - *continued*
    collision (with) - *continued*
      stationary object (traffic) - *continued*
        while boarding or alighting V57.4
      streetcar (traffic) V56.9
        nontraffic V56.3
        while boarding or alighting V56.4
      three wheeled motor vehicle (traffic) V52.9
        nontraffic V52.3
        while boarding or alighting V52.4
      truck (traffic) V54.9
        nontraffic V54.3
        while boarding or alighting V54.4
      two wheeled motor vehicle (traffic) V52.9
        nontraffic V52.3
        while boarding or alighting V52.4
      van (traffic) V53.9
        nontraffic V53.3
        while boarding or alighting V53.4
    driver
      collision (with)
        animal (traffic) V50.5
          being ridden (traffic) V56.5
            nontraffic V56.0
          nontraffic V50.0
        animal-drawn vehicle (traffic) V56.5
          nontraffic V56.0
        bus (traffic) V54.5
          nontraffic V54.0
        car (traffic) V53.5
          nontraffic V53.0
        motor vehicle NOS (traffic) V59.40
          nontraffic V59.00
          specified type NEC (traffic) V59.49
            nontraffic V59.09
        pedal cycle (traffic) V51.5
          nontraffic V51.0
        pickup truck (traffic) V53.5
          nontraffic V53.0
        railway vehicle (traffic) V55.5
          nontraffic V55.0
        specified vehicle NEC (traffic) V56.5
          nontraffic V56.0
        stationary object (traffic) V57.5
          nontraffic V57.0
        streetcar (traffic) V56.5
          nontraffic V56.0
        three wheeled motor vehicle (traffic) V52.5
          nontraffic V52.0
        truck (traffic) V54.5
          nontraffic V54.0
        two wheeled motor vehicle (traffic) V52.5
          nontraffic V52.0
        van (traffic) V53.5
          nontraffic V53.0
      noncollision accident (traffic) V58.5
        nontraffic V58.0
    noncollision accident (traffic) V58.9
      nontraffic V58.3
      while boarding or alighting V58.4
    nontraffic V59.3
    hanger-on
      collision (with)
        animal (traffic) V50.7
          being ridden (traffic) V56.7
            nontraffic V56.2
          nontraffic V50.2
        animal-drawn vehicle (traffic) V56.7
          nontraffic V56.2
        bus (traffic) V54.7
          nontraffic V54.2
        car (traffic) V53.7
          nontraffic V53.2
        pedal cycle (traffic) V51.7
          nontraffic V51.2
        pickup truck (traffic) V53.7
          nontraffic V53.2
        railway vehicle (traffic) V55.7
          nontraffic V55.2
        specified vehicle NEC (traffic) V56.7
          nontraffic V56.2
        stationary object (traffic) V57.7
          nontraffic V57.2
        streetcar (traffic) V56.7
          nontraffic V56.2
        three wheeled motor vehicle (traffic) V52.7
          nontraffic V52.2
        truck (traffic) V54.7
          nontraffic V54.2
        two wheeled motor vehicle (traffic) V52.7
          nontraffic V52.2

Accident (to) - *continued*
transport (involving injury to) - *continued*
  pickup truck occupant - *continued*
    hanger-on - *continued*
      collision (with) - *continued*
        van (traffic) V53.7
          nontraffic V53.2
      noncollision accident (traffic) V58.7
        nontraffic V58.2
    passenger
      collision (with)
        animal (traffic) V50.6
          being ridden (traffic) V56.6
            nontraffic V56.1
          nontraffic V50.1
        animal-drawn vehicle (traffic) V56.6
          nontraffic V56.1
        bus (traffic) V54.6
          nontraffic V54.1
        car (traffic) V53.6
          nontraffic V53.1
        motor vehicle NOS (traffic) V59.50
          nontraffic V59.10
          specified type NEC (traffic) V59.59
            nontraffic V59.19
        pedal cycle (traffic) V51.6
          nontraffic V51.1
        pickup truck (traffic) V53.6
          nontraffic V53.1
        railway vehicle (traffic) V55.6
          nontraffic V55.1
        specified vehicle NEC (traffic) V56.6
          nontraffic V56.1
        stationary object (traffic) V57.6
          nontraffic V57.1
        streetcar (traffic) V56.6
          nontraffic V56.1
        three wheeled motor vehicle (traffic) V52.6
          nontraffic V52.1
        truck (traffic) V54.6
          nontraffic V54.1
        two wheeled motor vehicle (traffic) V52.6
          nontraffic V52.1
        van (traffic) V53.6
          nontraffic V53.1
      noncollision accident (traffic) V58.6
        nontraffic V58.1
    specified type NEC V59.88
    military vehicle V59.81
  quarry truck — *see* Accident, transport, industrial
    vehicle occupant
  race car — *see* Accident, transport, motor vehicle
    NEC occupant
  railway vehicle occupant V81.9
    collision (with) V81.3
      motor vehicle (non-military) (traffic) V81.1
        military V81.83
        nontraffic V81.0
      rolling stock V81.2
      specified object NEC V81.3
    during derailment V81.7
      with antecedent collision — *see* Accident,
        transport, railway vehicle occupant, collision
    explosion V81.81
    fall (in railway vehicle) V81.5
      during derailment V81.7
        with antecedent collision — *see* Accident,
          transport, railway vehicle occupant,
          collision
      from railway vehicle V81.6
        during derailment V81.7
          with antecedent collision — *see* Accident,
            transport, railway vehicle occupant,
            collision
      while boarding or alighting V81.4
    fire V81.81
    object falling onto train V81.82
    specified type NEC V81.89
    while boarding or alighting V81.4
  ski lift V98.3
  snowmobile occupant (nontraffic) V86.92
    driver V86.52
    hanger-on V86.72
    passenger V86.62
    traffic V86.32
      driver V86.02
      hanger-on V86.22
      passenger V86.12
    while boarding or alighting V86.42
  specified NEC V98.8
  sport utility vehicle occupant — *see also* Accident,
    transport, pickup truck occupant
  streetcar occupant V82.9

Accident (to) - *continued*
transport (involving injury to) - *continued*
  streetcar occupant - *continued*
    collision (with) V82.3
      motor vehicle (traffic) V82.1
        nontraffic V82.0
      rolling stock V82.2
    during derailment V82.7
      with antecedent collision — *see* Accident,
        transport, streetcar occupant, collision
    fall (in streetcar) V82.5
      during derailment V82.7
        with antecedent collision — *see* Accident,
        transport, streetcar occupant, collision
      from streetcar V82.6
        during derailment V82.7
          with antecedent collision — *see* Accident,
          transport, streetcar occupant, collision
        while boarding or alighting V82.4
      while boarding or alighting V82.4
    specified type NEC V82.8
    while boarding or alighting V82.4
  three-wheeled motor vehicle occupant V39.9
    collision (with)
      animal (traffic) V30.9
        being ridden (traffic) V36.9
          nontraffic V36.3
          while boarding or alighting V36.4
        nontraffic V30.3
        while boarding or alighting V30.4
      animal-drawn vehicle (traffic) V36.9
        nontraffic V36.3
        while boarding or alighting V36.4
      bus (traffic) V34.9
        nontraffic V34.3
        while boarding or alighting V34.4
      car (traffic) V33.9
        nontraffic V33.3
        while boarding or alighting V33.4
      motor vehicle NOS (traffic) V39.60
        nontraffic V39.20
        specified type NEC (traffic) V39.69
          nontraffic V39.29
      pedal cycle (traffic) V31.9
        nontraffic V31.3
        while boarding or alighting V31.4
      pickup truck (traffic) V33.9
        nontraffic V33.3
        while boarding or alighting V33.4
      railway vehicle (traffic) V35.9
        nontraffic V35.3
        while boarding or alighting V35.4
      specified vehicle NEC (traffic) V36.9
        nontraffic V36.3
        while boarding or alighting V36.4
      stationary object (traffic) V37.9
        nontraffic V37.3
        while boarding or alighting V37.4
      streetcar (traffic) V36.9
        nontraffic V36.3
        while boarding or alighting V36.4
      three wheeled motor vehicle (traffic) V32.9
        nontraffic V32.3
        while boarding or alighting V32.4
      truck (traffic) V34.9
        nontraffic V34.3
        while boarding or alighting V34.4
      two wheeled motor vehicle (traffic) V32.9
        nontraffic V32.3
        while boarding or alighting V32.4
      van (traffic) V33.9
        nontraffic V33.3
        while boarding or alighting V33.4
    driver
      collision (with)
        animal (traffic) V30.5
          being ridden (traffic) V36.5
            nontraffic V36.0
          nontraffic V30.0
        animal-drawn vehicle (traffic) V36.5
          nontraffic V36.0
        bus (traffic) V34.5
          nontraffic V34.0
        car (traffic) V33.5
          nontraffic V33.0
        motor vehicle NOS (traffic) V39.40
          nontraffic V39.00
          specified type NEC (traffic) V39.49
            nontraffic V39.09
        pedal cycle (traffic) V31.5
          nontraffic V31.0
        pickup truck (traffic) V33.5
          nontraffic V33.0

Accident (to) - *continued*
  transport (involving injury to) - *continued*
    three-wheeled motor vehicle occupant - *continued*
      driver - *continued*
        collision (with) - *continued*
          railway vehicle (traffic) V35.5
            nontraffic V35.0
          specified vehicle NEC (traffic) V36.5
            nontraffic V36.0
          stationary object (traffic) V37.5
            nontraffic V37.0
          streetcar (traffic) V36.5
            nontraffic V36.0
          three wheeled motor vehicle (traffic) V32.5
            nontraffic V32.0
          truck (traffic) V34.5
            nontraffic V34.0
          two wheeled motor vehicle (traffic) V32.5
            nontraffic V32.0
          van (traffic) V33.5
            nontraffic V33.0
        noncollision accident (traffic) V38.5
          nontraffic V38.0
        noncollision accident (traffic) V38.9
          nontraffic V38.3
        while boarding or alighting V38.4
        nontraffic V39.3
      hanger-on
        collision (with)
          animal (traffic) V30.7
            being ridden (traffic) V36.7
              nontraffic V36.2
            nontraffic V30.2
          animal-drawn vehicle (traffic) V36.7
            nontraffic V36.2
          bus (traffic) V34.7
            nontraffic V34.2
          car (traffic) V33.7
            nontraffic V33.2
          pedal cycle (traffic) V31.7
            nontraffic V31.2
          pickup truck (traffic) V33.7
            nontraffic V33.2
          railway vehicle (traffic) V35.7
            nontraffic V35.2
          specified vehicle NEC (traffic) V36.7
            nontraffic V36.2
          stationary object (traffic) V37.7
            nontraffic V37.2
          streetcar (traffic) V36.7
            nontraffic V36.2
          three wheeled motor vehicle (traffic) V32.7
            nontraffic V32.2
          truck (traffic) V34.7
            nontraffic V34.2
          two wheeled motor vehicle (traffic) V32.7
            nontraffic V32.2
          van (traffic) V33.7
            nontraffic V33.2
        noncollision accident (traffic) V38.7
          nontraffic V38.2
      passenger
        collision (with)
          animal (traffic) V30.6
            being ridden (traffic) V36.6
              nontraffic V36.1
            nontraffic V30.1
          animal-drawn vehicle (traffic) V36.6
            nontraffic V36.1
          bus (traffic) V34.6
            nontraffic V34.1
          car (traffic) V33.6
            nontraffic V33.1
          motor vehicle NOS (traffic) V39.50
            nontraffic V39.10
            specified type NEC (traffic) V39.59
              nontraffic V39.19
          pedal cycle (traffic) V31.6
            nontraffic V31.1
          pickup truck (traffic) V33.6
            nontraffic V33.1
          railway vehicle (traffic) V35.6
            nontraffic V35.1
          specified vehicle NEC (traffic) V36.6
            nontraffic V36.1
          stationary object (traffic) V37.6
            nontraffic V37.1
          streetcar (traffic) V36.6
            nontraffic V36.1
          three wheeled motor vehicle (traffic) V32.6
            nontraffic V32.1
          truck (traffic) V34.6
            nontraffic V34.1

Accident (to) - *continued*
  transport (involving injury to) - *continued*
    three-wheeled motor vehicle occupant - *continued*
      passenger - *continued*
        collision (with) - *continued*
          two wheeled motor vehicle (traffic) V32.6
            nontraffic V32.1
          van (traffic) V33.6
            nontraffic V33.1
        noncollision accident (traffic) V38.6
          nontraffic V38.1
      specified type NEC V39.89
        military vehicle V39.81
    tractor (farm) (and trailer) — *see* Accident, transport, agricultural vehicle occupant
    tram — *see* Accident, transport, streetcar
      in mine or quarry — *see* Accident, transport, industrial vehicle occupant
    trolley — *see* Accident, transport, streetcar
      in mine or quarry — *see* Accident, transport, industrial vehicle occupant
    truck (heavy) occupant V69.9
      collision (with)
        animal (traffic) V60.9
          being ridden (traffic) V66.9
            nontraffic V66.3
            while boarding or alighting V66.4
          nontraffic V60.3
            while boarding or alighting V60.4
        animal-drawn vehicle (traffic) V66.9
          nontraffic V66.3
          while boarding or alighting V66.4
        bus (traffic) V64.9
          nontraffic V64.3
          while boarding or alighting V64.4
        car (traffic) V63.9
          nontraffic V63.3
          while boarding or alighting V63.4
        motor vehicle NOS (traffic) V69.60
          nontraffic V69.20
          specified type NEC (traffic) V69.69
            nontraffic V69.29
        pedal cycle (traffic) V61.9
          nontraffic V61.3
          while boarding or alighting V61.4
        pickup truck (traffic) V63.9
          nontraffic V63.3
          while boarding or alighting V63.4
        railway vehicle (traffic) V65.9
          nontraffic V65.3
          while boarding or alighting V65.4
        specified vehicle NEC (traffic) V66.9
          nontraffic V66.3
          while boarding or alighting V66.4
        stationary object (traffic) V67.9
          nontraffic V67.3
          while boarding or alighting V67.4
        streetcar (traffic) V66.9
          nontraffic V66.3
          while boarding or alighting V66.4
        three wheeled motor vehicle (traffic) V62.9
          nontraffic V62.3
          while boarding or alighting V62.4
        truck (traffic) V64.9
          nontraffic V64.3
          while boarding or alighting V64.4
        two wheeled motor vehicle (traffic) V62.9
          nontraffic V62.3
          while boarding or alighting V62.4
        van (traffic) V63.9
          nontraffic V63.3
          while boarding or alighting V63.4
      driver
        collision (with)
          animal (traffic) V60.5
            being ridden (traffic) V66.5
              nontraffic V66.0
            nontraffic V60.0
          animal-drawn vehicle (traffic) V66.5
            nontraffic V66.0
          bus (traffic) V64.5
            nontraffic V64.0
          car (traffic) V63.5
            nontraffic V63.0
          motor vehicle NOS (traffic) V69.40
            nontraffic V69.00
            specified type NEC (traffic) V69.49
              nontraffic V69.09
          pedal cycle (traffic) V61.5
            nontraffic V61.0
          pickup truck (traffic) V63.5
            nontraffic V63.0
          railway vehicle (traffic) V65.5

Accident (to) - *continued*
  transport (involving injury to) - *continued*
    truck (heavy) occupant - *continued*
      driver - *continued*
        collision (with) - *continued*
          railway vehicle (traffic) - *continued*
            nontraffic V65.0
          specified vehicle NEC (traffic) V66.5
            nontraffic V66.0
          stationary object (traffic) V67.5
            nontraffic V67.0
          streetcar (traffic) V66.5
            nontraffic V66.0
          three wheeled motor vehicle (traffic) V62.5
            nontraffic V62.0
          truck (traffic) V64.5
            nontraffic V64.0
          two wheeled motor vehicle (traffic) V62.5
            nontraffic V62.0
          van (traffic) V63.5
            nontraffic V63.0
        noncollision accident (traffic) V68.5
          nontraffic V68.0
      dump — *see* Accident, transport, construction vehicle occupant
      hanger-on
        collision (with)
          animal (traffic) V60.7
            being ridden (traffic) V66.7
              nontraffic V66.2
            nontraffic V60.2
          animal-drawn vehicle (traffic) V66.7
            nontraffic V66.2
          bus (traffic) V64.7
            nontraffic V64.2
          car (traffic) V63.7
            nontraffic V63.2
          pedal cycle (traffic) V61.7
            nontraffic V61.2
          pickup truck (traffic) V63.7
            nontraffic V63.2
          railway vehicle (traffic) V65.7
            nontraffic V65.2
          specified vehicle NEC (traffic) V66.7
            nontraffic V66.2
          stationary object (traffic) V67.7
            nontraffic V67.2
          streetcar (traffic) V66.7
            nontraffic V66.2
          three wheeled motor vehicle (traffic) V62.7
            nontraffic V62.2
          truck (traffic) V64.7
            nontraffic V64.2
          two wheeled motor vehicle (traffic) V62.7
            nontraffic V62.2
          van (traffic) V63.7
            nontraffic V63.2
        noncollision accident (traffic) V68.7
          nontraffic V68.2
      noncollision accident (traffic) V68.9
        nontraffic V68.3
        while boarding or alighting V68.4
      nontraffic V69.3
      passenger
        collision (with)
          animal (traffic) V60.6
            being ridden (traffic) V66.6
              nontraffic V66.1
            nontraffic V60.1
          animal-drawn vehicle (traffic) V66.6
            nontraffic V66.1
          bus (traffic) V64.6
            nontraffic V64.1
          car (traffic) V63.6
            nontraffic V63.1
          motor vehicle NOS (traffic) V69.50
            nontraffic V69.10
            specified type NEC (traffic) V69.59
              nontraffic V69.19
          pedal cycle (traffic) V61.6
            nontraffic V61.1
          pickup truck (traffic) V63.6
            nontraffic V63.1
          railway vehicle (traffic) V65.6
            nontraffic V65.1
          specified vehicle NEC (traffic) V66.6
            nontraffic V66.1
          stationary object (traffic) V67.6
            nontraffic V67.1
          streetcar (traffic) V66.6
            nontraffic V66.1
          three wheeled motor vehicle (traffic) V62.6
            nontraffic V62.1

Accident (to) - *continued*
transport (involving injury to) - *continued*
truck (heavy) occupant - *continued*
passenger - *continued*
collision (with) - *continued*
truck (traffic) V64.6
nontraffic V64.1
two wheeled motor vehicle (traffic) V62.6
nontraffic V62.1
van (traffic) V63.6
nontraffic V63.1
noncollision accident (traffic) V68.6
nontraffic V68.1
pickup — *see* Accident, transport, pickup truck occupant
specified type NEC V69.88
military vehicle V69.81
van occupant V59.9
collision (with)
animal (traffic) V50.9
being ridden (traffic) V56.9
nontraffic V56.3
while boarding or alighting V56.4
nontraffic V50.3
while boarding or alighting V50.4
animal-drawn vehicle (traffic) V56.9
nontraffic V56.3
while boarding or alighting V56.4
bus (traffic) V54.9
nontraffic V54.3
while boarding or alighting V54.4
car (traffic) V53.9
nontraffic V53.3
while boarding or alighting V53.4
motor vehicle NOS (traffic) V59.60
nontraffic V59.20
specified type NEC (traffic) V59.69
nontraffic V59.29
pedal cycle (traffic) V51.9
nontraffic V51.3
while boarding or alighting V51.4
pickup truck (traffic) V53.9
nontraffic V53.3
while boarding or alighting V53.4
railway vehicle (traffic) V55.9
nontraffic V55.3
while boarding or alighting V55.4
specified vehicle NEC (traffic) V56.9
nontraffic V56.3
while boarding or alighting V56.4
stationary object (traffic) V57.9
nontraffic V57.3
while boarding or alighting V57.4
streetcar (traffic) V56.9
nontraffic V56.3
while boarding or alighting V56.4
three wheeled motor vehicle (traffic) V52.9
nontraffic V52.3
while boarding or alighting V52.4
truck (traffic) V54.9
nontraffic V54.3
while boarding or alighting V54.4
two wheeled motor vehicle (traffic) V52.9
nontraffic V52.3
while boarding or alighting V52.4
van (traffic) V53.9
nontraffic V53.3
while boarding or alighting V53.4
driver
collision (with)
animal (traffic) V50.5
being ridden (traffic) V56.5
nontraffic V56.0
nontraffic V50.0
animal-drawn vehicle (traffic) V56.5
nontraffic V56.0
bus (traffic) V54.5
nontraffic V54.0
car (traffic) V53.5
nontraffic V53.0
motor vehicle NOS (traffic) V59.40
nontraffic V59.00
specified type NEC (traffic) V59.49
nontraffic V59.09
pedal cycle (traffic) V51.5
nontraffic V51.0
pickup truck (traffic) V53.5
nontraffic V53.0
railway vehicle (traffic) V55.5
nontraffic V55.0
specified vehicle NEC (traffic) V56.5
nontraffic V56.0
stationary object (traffic) V57.5

Accident (to) - *continued*
transport (involving injury to) - *continued*
van occupant - *continued*
driver - *continued*
collision (with) - *continued*
stationary object (traffic) - *continued*
nontraffic V57.0
streetcar (traffic) V56.5
nontraffic V56.0
three wheeled motor vehicle (traffic) V52.5
nontraffic V52.0
truck (traffic) V54.5
nontraffic V54.0
two wheeled motor vehicle (traffic) V52.5
nontraffic V52.0
van (traffic) V53.5
nontraffic V53.0
noncollision accident (traffic) V58.5
nontraffic V58.0
noncollision accident (traffic) V58.9
nontraffic V58.3
while boarding or alighting V58.4
nontraffic V59.3
hanger-on
collision (with)
animal (traffic) V50.7
being ridden (traffic) V56.7
nontraffic V56.2
nontraffic V50.2
animal-drawn vehicle (traffic) V56.7
nontraffic V56.2
bus (traffic) V54.7
nontraffic V54.2
car (traffic) V53.7
nontraffic V53.2
pedal cycle (traffic) V51.7
nontraffic V51.2
pickup truck (traffic) V53.7
nontraffic V53.2
railway vehicle (traffic) V55.7
nontraffic V55.2
specified vehicle NEC (traffic) V56.7
nontraffic V56.2
stationary object (traffic) V57.7
nontraffic V57.2
streetcar (traffic) V56.7
nontraffic V56.2
three wheeled motor vehicle (traffic) V52.7
nontraffic V52.2
truck (traffic) V54.7
nontraffic V54.2
two wheeled motor vehicle (traffic) V52.7
nontraffic V52.2
van (traffic) V53.7
nontraffic V53.2
noncollision accident (traffic) V58.7
nontraffic V58.2
passenger
collision (with)
animal (traffic) V50.6
being ridden (traffic) V56.6
nontraffic V56.1
nontraffic V50.1
animal-drawn vehicle (traffic) V56.6
nontraffic V56.1
bus (traffic) V54.6
nontraffic V54.1
car (traffic) V53.6
nontraffic V53.1
motor vehicle NOS (traffic) V59.50
nontraffic V59.10
specified type NEC (traffic) V59.59
nontraffic V59.19
pedal cycle (traffic) V51.6
nontraffic V51.1
pickup truck (traffic) V53.6
nontraffic V53.1
railway vehicle (traffic) V55.6
nontraffic V55.1
specified vehicle NEC (traffic) V56.6
nontraffic V56.1
stationary object (traffic) V57.6
nontraffic V57.1
streetcar (traffic) V56.6
nontraffic V56.1
three wheeled motor vehicle (traffic) V52.6
nontraffic V52.1
truck (traffic) V54.6
nontraffic V54.1
two wheeled motor vehicle (traffic) V52.6
nontraffic V52.1
van (traffic) V53.6
nontraffic V53.1

Accident (to) - *continued*
transport (involving injury to) - *continued*
van occupant - *continued*
passenger - *continued*
noncollision accident (traffic) V58.6
nontraffic V58.1
specified type NEC V59.88
military vehicle V59.81
watercraft occupant — *see* Accident, watercraft
vehicle NEC V89.9
animal-drawn NEC — *see* Accident, transport, animal-drawn vehicle occupant
special
agricultural — *see* Accident, transport, agricultural vehicle occupant
construction — *see* Accident, transport, construction vehicle occupant
industrial — *see* Accident, transport, industrial vehicle occupant
three-wheeled NEC (motorized) — *see* Accident, transport, three-wheeled motor vehicle occupant
watercraft V94.9
causing
drowning — *see* Drowning, due to, accident to, watercraft
injury NEC V91.89
crushed between craft and object V91.19
powered craft V91.13
ferry boat V91.11
fishing boat V91.12
jetskis V91.13
liner V91.11
merchant ship V91.10
passenger ship V91.11
unpowered craft V91.18
canoe V91.15
inflatable V91.16
kayak V91.15
sailboat V91.14
surf-board V91.18
windsurfer V91.18
fall on board V91.29
powered craft V91.23
ferry boat V91.21
fishing boat V91.22
jetskis V91.23
liner V91.21
merchant ship V91.20
passenger ship V91.21
unpowered craft
canoe V91.25
inflatable V91.26
kayak V91.25
sailboat V91.24
fire on board causing burn V91.09
powered craft V91.03
ferry boat V91.01
fishing boat V91.02
jetskis V91.03
liner V91.01
merchant ship V91.00
passenger ship V91.01
unpowered craft V91.08
canoe V91.05
inflatable V91.06
kayak V91.05
sailboat V91.04
surf-board V91.08
water skis V91.07
windsurfer V91.08
hit by falling object V91.39
powered craft V91.33
ferry boat V91.31
fishing boat V91.32
jetskis V91.33
liner V91.31
merchant ship V91.30
passenger ship V91.31
unpowered craft V91.38
canoe V91.35
inflatable V91.36
kayak V91.35
sailboat V91.34
surf-board V91.38
water skis V91.37
windsurfer V91.38
specified type NEC V91.89
powered craft V91.83
ferry boat V91.81
fishing boat V91.82
jetskis V91.83
liner V91.81

Accident (to) - *continued*
  watercraft - *continued*
    causing - *continued*
      injury NEC - *continued*
        specified type NEC - *continued*
          powered craft - *continued*
            merchant ship V91.80
            passenger ship V91.81
          unpowered craft V91.88
            canoe V91.85
            inflatable V91.86
            kayak V91.85
            sailboat V91.84
            surf-board V91.88
            water skis V91.87
            windsurfer V91.88
      due to, caused by cataclysm — *see* Forces of
          nature, by type
      military NEC V94.818
        with civilian watercraft V94.810
        civilian in water injured by V94.811
      nonpowered, struck by
        nonpowered vessel V94.22
        powered vessel V94.21
      specified type NEC V94.89
      striking swimmer
        powered V94.11
        unpowered V94.12
Acid throwing (assault) Y08.89
Activity (involving) (of victim at time of event) Y93.9
  aerobic and step exercise (class) Y93.A3
  alpine skiing Y93.23
  animal care NEC Y93.K9
  arts and handcrafts NEC Y93.D9
  athletics NEC Y93.79
  athletics played as a team or group NEC Y93.69
  athletics played individually NEC Y93.59
  baking Y93.G3
  ballet Y93.41
  barbells Y93.B3
  BASE (Building, Antenna, Span, Earth)
      jumping Y93.33
  baseball Y93.64
  basketball Y93.67
  bathing (personal) Y93.E1
  beach volleyball Y93.68
  bike riding Y93.55
  blackout game Y93.85
  boogie boarding Y93.18
  bowling Y93.54
  boxing Y93.71
  brass instrument playing Y93.J4
  building construction Y93.H3
  bungee jumping Y93.34
  calisthenics Y93.A2
  canoeing (in calm and turbulent water) Y93.16
  capture the flag Y93.6A
  cardiorespiratory exercise NEC Y93.A9
  caregiving (providing) NEC Y93.F9
    bathing Y93.F1
    lifting Y93.F2
  cellular
    communication device Y93.C2
    telephone Y93.C2
  challenge course Y93.A5
  cheerleading Y93.45
  choking game Y93.85
  circuit training Y93.A4
  cleaning
    floor Y93.E5
  climbing NEC Y93.39
    mountain Y93.31
    rock Y93.31
    wall Y93.31
  clothing care and maintenance NEC Y93.E9
  combatives Y93.75
  computer
    keyboarding Y93.C1
    technology NEC Y93.C9
  confidence course Y93.A5
  construction (building) Y93.H3
  cooking and baking Y93.G3
  cool down exercises Y93.A2
  cricket Y93.69
  crocheting Y93.D1
  cross country skiing Y93.24
  dancing (all types) Y93.41
  digging
    dirt Y93.H1
  dirt digging Y93.H1
  dishwashing Y93.G1
  diving (platform) (springboard) Y93.12
    underwater Y93.15

Activity (involving) (of victim at time of event) -
continued
  dodge ball Y93.6A
  downhill skiing Y93.23
  drum playing Y93.J2
  dumbbells Y93.B3
  electronic
    devices NEC Y93.C9
      hand held interactive Y93.C2
    game playing (using) (with)
      interactive device Y93.C2
      keyboard or other stationary device Y93.C1
  elliptical machine Y93.A1
  exercise (s)
    machines ((primarily) for)
      cardiorespiratory conditioning Y93.A1
      muscle strengthening Y93.B1
    muscle strengthening (non-machine) NEC Y93.B9
  external motion NEC Y93.I9
    rollercoaster Y93.I1
  fainting game Y93.85
  field hockey Y93.65
  figure skating (pairs) (singles) Y93.21
  flag football Y93.62
  floor mopping and cleaning Y93.E5
  food preparation and clean up Y93.G1
  football (American) NOS Y93.61
    flag Y93.62
    tackle Y93.61
    touch Y93.62
  four square Y93.6A
  free weights Y93.B3
  frisbee (ultimate) Y93.74
  furniture
    building Y93.D3
    finishing Y93.D3
    repair Y93.D3
  game playing (electronic)
    using keyboard or other stationary device Y93.C1
    using interactive device Y93.C2
  gardening Y93.H2
  golf Y93.53
  grass drills Y93.A6
  grilling and smoking food Y93.G2
  grooming and shearing an animal Y93.K3
  guerilla drills Y93.A6
  gymnastics (rhythmic) Y93.43
  handball Y93.73
  handcrafts NEC Y93.D9
  hand held interactive electronic device Y93.C2
  hang gliding Y93.35
  hiking (on level or elevated terrain) Y93.01
  hockey (ice) Y93.22
    field Y93.65
  horseback riding Y93.52
  household (interior) maintenance NEC Y93.E9
  ice NEC Y93.29
    dancing Y93.21
    hockey Y93.22
    skating Y93.21
  inline roller skating Y93.51
  ironing Y93.E4
  judo Y93.75
  jumping (off) NEC Y93.39
    BASE (Building, Antenna, Span, Earth) Y93.33
    bungee Y93.34
    jacks Y93.A2
    rope Y93.56
  jumping jacks Y93.A2
  jumping rope Y93.56
  karate Y93.75
  kayaking (in calm and turbulent water) Y93.16
  keyboarding (computer) Y93.C1
  kickball Y93.6A
  knitting Y93.D1
  lacrosse Y93.65
  land maintenance NEC Y93.H9
  landscaping Y93.H2
  laundry Y93.E2
  machines (exercise)
    primarily for cardiorespiratory
        conditioning Y93.A1
    primarily for muscle strengthening Y93.B1
  maintenance
    exterior building NEC Y93.H9
    household (interior) NEC Y93.E9
    land Y93.H9
    property Y93.H9
  marching (on level or elevated terrain) Y93.01
  martial arts Y93.75
  microwave oven Y93.G3
  milking an animal Y93.K2
  mopping (floor) Y93.E5

Activity (involving) (of victim at time of event) -
continued
  mountain climbing Y93.31
  muscle strengthening
    exercises (non-machine) NEC Y93.B9
    machines Y93.B1
  musical keyboard (electronic) playing Y93.J1
  nordic skiing Y93.24
  obstacle course Y93.A5
  oven (microwave) Y93.G3
  packing up and unpacking in moving to a new
      residence Y93.E6
  parasailing Y93.19
  pass out game Y93.85
  percussion instrument playing NEC Y93.J2
  personal
    bathing and showering Y93.E1
    hygiene NEC Y93.E8
    showering Y93.E1
  physical games generally associated with school
      recess, summer camp and children Y93.6A
  physical training NEC Y93.A9
  piano playing Y93.J1
  pilates Y93.B4
  platform diving Y93.12
  playing musical instrument
    brass instrument Y93.J4
    drum Y93.J2
    musical keyboard (electronic) Y93.J1
    percussion instrument NEC Y93.J2
    piano Y93.J1
    string instrument Y93.J3
    winds instrument Y93.J4
  property maintenance
    exterior NEC Y93.H9
    interior NEC Y93.E9
  pruning (garden and lawn) Y93.H2
  pull-ups Y93.B2
  push-ups Y93.B2
  racquetball Y93.73
  rafting (in calm and turbulent water) Y93.16
  raking (leaves) Y93.H1
  rappelling Y93.32
  refereeing a sports activity Y93.81
  residential relocation Y93.E6
  rhythmic gymnastics Y93.43
  rhythmic movement NEC Y93.49
  riding
    horseback Y93.52
    rollercoaster Y93.I1
  rock climbing Y93.31
  rollercoaster riding Y93.I1
  roller skating (inline) Y93.51
  rough housing and horseplay Y93.83
  rowing (in calm and turbulent water) Y93.16
  rugby Y93.63
  running Y93.02
  SCUBA diving Y93.15
  sewing Y93.D2
  shoveling Y93.H1
    dirt Y93.H1
    snow Y93.H1
  showering (personal) Y93.E1
  sit-ups Y93.B2
  skateboarding Y93.51
  skating (ice) Y93.21
    roller Y93.51
  skiing (alpine) (downhill) Y93.23
    cross country Y93.24
    nordic Y93.24
    water Y93.17
  sledding (snow) Y93.23
  sleeping (sleep) Y93.84
  smoking and grilling food Y93.G2
  snorkeling Y93.15
  snow NEC Y93.29
    boarding Y93.23
    shoveling Y93.H1
    sledding Y93.23
    tubing Y93.23
  soccer Y93.66
  softball Y93.64
  specified NEC Y93.89
  spectator at an event Y93.82
  sports NEC Y93.79
    sports played as a team or group NEC Y93.69
    sports played individually NEC Y93.59
  springboard diving Y93.12
  squash Y93.73
  stationary bike Y93.A1
  step (stepping) exercise (class) Y93.A3
  stepper machine Y93.A1
  stove Y93.G3

Activity (involving) (of victim at time of event) - *continued*
  string instrument playing Y93.J3
  surfing Y93.18
    wind Y93.18
  swimming Y93.11
  tackle football Y93.61
  tap dancing Y93.41
  tennis Y93.73
  tobogganing Y93.23
  touch football Y93.62
  track and field events (non-running) Y93.57
    running Y93.02
  trampoline Y93.44
  treadmill Y93.A1
  trimming shrubs Y93.H2
  tubing (in calm and turbulent water) Y93.16
    snow Y93.23
  ultimate frisbee Y93.74
  underwater diving Y93.15
  unpacking in moving to a new residence Y93.E6
  use of stove, oven and microwave oven Y93.G3
  vacuuming Y93.E3
  volleyball (beach) (court) Y93.68
  wake boarding Y93.17
  walking an animal Y93.K1
  walking (on level or elevated terrain) Y93.01
    an animal Y93.K1
  wall climbing Y93.31
  warm up and cool down exercises Y93.A2
  water NEC Y93.19
    aerobics Y93.14
    craft NEC Y93.19
    exercise Y93.14
    polo Y93.13
    skiing Y93.17
    sliding Y93.18
    survival training and testing Y93.19
  weeding (garden and lawn) Y93.H2
  wind instrument playing Y93.J4
  windsurfing Y93.18
  wrestling Y93.72
  yoga Y93.42
Adverse effect of drugs — *see* Table of Drugs and Chemicals
Aerosinusitis - — *see* Air, pressure
After-effect, late — *see* Sequelae
Air
  blast in war operations — *see* War operations, air blast
  pressure
    change, rapid
      during
        ascent W94.29
          while (in) (surfacing from)
            aircraft W94.23
            deep water diving W94.21
            underground W94.22
        descent W94.39
          in
            aircraft W94.31
            water W94.32
    high, prolonged W94.0
    low, prolonged W94.12
      due to residence or long visit at high altitude W94.11
Alpine sickness W94.11
Altitude sickness W94.11
Anaphylactic shock, anaphylaxis — *see* Table of Drugs and Chemicals
Andes disease W94.11
Arachnidism, arachnoidism X58
Arson (with intent to injure or kill) X97
Asphyxia, asphyxiation
  by
    food (bone) (seed) — *see* categories T17 and T18
    gas — *see also* Table of Drugs and Chemicals
      legal
        execution — *see* Legal, intervention, gas
        intervention — *see* Legal, intervention, gas
  from
    fire — *see also* Exposure, fire
      in war operations — *see* War operations, fire
    ignition — *see* Ignition
    vomitus T17.81
  in war operations — *see* War operations, restriction of airway
Aspiration
  food (any type) (into respiratory tract) (with asphyxia, obstruction respiratory tract, suffocation) — *see* categories T17 and T18
  foreign body — *see* Foreign body, aspiration

Aspiration - *continued*
  vomitus (with asphyxia, obstruction respiratory tract, suffocation) T17.81
Assassination (attempt) — *see* Assault
Assault (homicidal) (by) (in) Y09
  arson X97
  bite (of human being) Y04.1
  bodily force Y04.8
    bite Y04.1
    bumping into Y04.2
    sexual — *see* subcategories T74.0, T76.0
    unarmed fight Y04.0
  bomb X96.9
    antipersonnel X96.0
    fertilizer X96.3
    gasoline X96.1
    letter X96.2
    petrol X96.1
    pipe X96.3
    specified NEC X96.8
  brawl (hand) (fists) (foot) (unarmed) Y04.0
  burning, burns (by fire) NEC X97
    acid Y08.89
    caustic, corrosive substance Y08.89
    chemical from swallowing caustic, corrosive substance — *see* Table of Drugs and Chemicals
    cigarette (s) X97
    hot object X98.9
      fluid NEC X98.2
      household appliance X98.3
      specified NEC X98.8
      steam X98.0
      tap water X98.1
      vapors X98.0
    scalding — *see* Assault, burning
    steam X98.0
    vitriol Y08.89
  caustic, corrosive substance (gas) Y08.89
  crashing of
    aircraft Y08.81
    motor vehicle Y03.8
      pushed in front of Y02.0
      run over Y03.0
      specified NEC Y03.8
  cutting or piercing instrument X99.9
    dagger X99.2
    glass X99.0
    knife X99.1
    specified NEC X99.8
    sword X99.2
  dagger X99.2
  drowning (in) X92.9
    bathtub X92.0
    natural water X92.3
    specified NEC X92.8
    swimming pool X92.1
      following fall X92.2
  dynamite X96.8
  explosive (s) (material) X96.9
  fight (hand) (fists) (foot) (unarmed) Y04.0
    with weapon — *see* Assault, by type of weapon
  fire X97
  firearm X95.9
    airgun X95.01
    handgun X93
    hunting rifle X94.1
    larger X94.9
      specified NEC X94.8
    machine gun X94.2
    shotgun X94.0
    specified NEC X95.8
  gunshot (wound) NEC — *see* Assault, firearm, by type
  incendiary device X97
  injury Y09
    to child due to criminal abortion attempt NEC Y08.89
  knife X99.1
  late effect of — *see* X92-Y08 with 7th character S
  placing before moving object NEC Y02.8
    motor vehicle Y02.0
  poisoning — *see* categories T36-T65 with 7th character S
  puncture, any part of body — *see* Assault, cutting or piercing instrument
  pushing
    before moving object NEC Y02.8
      motor vehicle Y02.0
      subway train Y02.1
      train Y02.1
    from high place Y01
  rape T74.2-
  scalding — *see* Assault, burning

Assault (homicidal) (by) (in) - *continued*
  sequelae of — *see* X92-Y08 with 7th character S
  sexual (by bodily force) T74.2-
  shooting — *see* Assault, firearm
  specified means NEC Y08.89
  stab, any part of body — *see* Assault, cutting or piercing instrument
  steam X98.0
  striking against
    other person Y04.2
    sports equipment Y08.09
      baseball bat Y08.02
      hockey stick Y08.01
  struck by
    sports equipment Y08.09
      baseball bat Y08.02
      hockey stick Y08.01
  submersion — *see* Assault, drowning
  violence Y09
  weapon Y09
    blunt Y00
    cutting or piercing — *see* Assault, cutting or piercing instrument
    firearm — *see* Assault, firearm
  wound Y09
    cutting — *see* Assault, cutting or piercing instrument
    gunshot — *see* Assault, firearm
    knife X99.1
    piercing — *see* Assault, cutting or piercing instrument
    puncture — *see* Assault, cutting or piercing instrument
    stab — *see* Assault, cutting or piercing instrument
Attack by mammals NEC W55.89
Avalanche — *see* Landslide
Aviator's disease - — *see* Air, pressure

B

Barotitis, barodontalgia, barosinusitis, barotrauma (otitic) (sinus) - — *see* Air, pressure
Battered (baby) (child) (person) (syndrome) X58
Bayonet wound W26.1
  in
    legal intervention — *see* Legal, intervention, sharp object, bayonet
    war operations — *see* War operations, combat
  stated as undetermined whether accidental or intentional Y28.8
  suicide (attempt) X78.2
Bean in nose — *see* categories T17 and T18
Bed set on fire NEC — *see* Exposure, fire, uncontrolled, building, bed
Beheading (by guillotine)
  homicide X99.9
  legal execution — *see* Legal, intervention
Bending, injury in (prolonged) (static) X50.1
Bends - — *see* Air, pressure, change
Bite, bitten by
  alligator W58.01
  arthropod (nonvenomous) NEC W57
  bull W55.21
  cat W55.01
  cow W55.21
  crocodile W58.11
  dog W54.0
  goat W55.31
  hoof stock NEC W55.31
  horse W55.11
  human being (accidentally) W50.3
    with intent to injure or kill Y04.1
    as, or caused by, a crowd or human stampede (with fall) W52
    assault Y04.1
    homicide (attempt) Y04.1
    in
      fight Y04.1
  insect (nonvenomous) W57
  lizard (nonvenomous) W59.01
  mammal NEC W55.81
    marine W56.31
  marine animal (nonvenomous) W56.81
  millipede W57
  moray eel W56.51
  mouse W53.01
  person (s) (accidentally) W50.3
    with intent to injure or kill Y04.1
    as, or caused by, a crowd or human stampede (with fall) W52
    assault Y04.1
    homicide (attempt) Y04.1
    in
      fight Y04.1

Bite, bitten by - *continued*
pig W55.41
raccoon W55.51
rat W53.11
reptile W59.81
lizard W59.01
snake W59.11
turtle W59.21
terrestrial W59.81
rodent W53.81
mouse W53.01
rat W53.11
specified NEC W53.81
squirrel W53.21
shark W56.41
sheep W55.31
snake (nonvenomous) W59.11
spider (nonvenomous) W57
squirrel W53.21
Blast (air) **in war operations** — *see* War operations, blast
Blizzard X37.2
Blood alcohol level Y90.9
less than 20mg/100ml Y90.0
presence in blood, level not specified Y90.9
20-39mg/100ml Y90.1
40-59mg/100ml Y90.2
60-79mg/100ml Y90.3
80-99mg/100ml Y90.4
100-119mg/100ml Y90.5
120-199mg/100ml Y90.6
200-239mg/100ml Y90.7
Blow X58
by law-enforcing agent, police (on duty) — *see* Legal, intervention, manhandling
blunt object — *see* Legal, intervention, blunt object
Blowing up — *see* Explosion
Brawl (hand) (fists) (foot) Y04.0
Breakage (accidental) (part of)
ladder (causing fall) W11
scaffolding (causing fall) W12
Broken
glass, contact with — *see* Contact, with, glass
power line (causing electric shock) W85
Bumping against, into (accidentally)
object NEC W22.8
with fall — *see* Fall, due to, bumping against, object
caused by crowd or human stampede (with fall) W52
sports equipment W21.9
person (s) W51
with fall W03
due to ice or snow W00.0
assault Y04.2
caused by, a crowd or human stampede (with fall) W52
homicide (attempt) Y04.2
sports equipment W21.9
Burn, burned, burning (accidental) (by) (from) (on)
acid NEC — *see* Table of Drugs and Chemicals
bed linen — *see* Exposure, fire, uncontrolled, in building, bed
blowtorch X08.8
with ignition of clothing NEC X06.2
nightwear X05
bonfire, campfire (controlled) — *see also* Exposure, fire, controlled, not in building
uncontrolled — *see* Exposure, fire, uncontrolled, not in building
candle X08.8
with ignition of clothing NEC X06.2
nightwear X05
caustic liquid, substance (external) (internal) NEC — *see* Table of Drugs and Chemicals
chemical (external) (internal) — *see also* Table of Drugs and Chemicals
in war operations — *see* War operations. fire
cigar (s) or cigarette (s) X08.8
with ignition of clothing NEC X06.2
nightwear X05
clothes, clothing NEC (from controlled fire) X06.2
with conflagration — *see* Exposure, fire, uncontrolled, building
not in building or structure — *see* Exposure, fire, uncontrolled, not in building
cooker (hot) X15.8
stated as undetermined whether accidental or intentional Y27.3
suicide (attempt) X77.3
electric blanket X16
engine (hot) X17
fire, flames — *see* Exposure, fire

Burn, burned, burning (accidental) (by) (from) (on) - *continued*
flare, Very pistol — *see* Discharge, firearm NEC
heat
from appliance (electrical) (household) X15.8
cooker X15.8
hotplate X15.2
kettle X15.8
light bulb X15.8
saucepan X15.3
skillet X15.3
stove X15.0
stated as undetermined whether accidental or intentional Y27.3
suicide (attempt) X77.3
toaster X15.1
in local application or packing during medical or surgical procedure Y63.5
heating
appliance, radiator or pipe X16
homicide (attempt) — *see* Assault, burning
hot
air X14.1
cooker X15.8
drink X10.0
engine X17
fat X10.2
fluid NEC X12
food X10.1
gases X14.1
heating appliance X16
household appliance NEC X15.8
kettle X15.8
liquid NEC X12
machinery X17
metal (molten) (liquid) NEC X18
object (not producing fire or flames) NEC X19
oil (cooking) X10.2
pipe (s) X16
radiator X16
saucepan (glass) (metal) X15.3
stove (kitchen) X15.0
substance NEC X19
caustic or corrosive NEC — *see* Table of Drugs and Chemicals
toaster X15.1
tool X17
vapor X13.1
water (tap) — *see* Contact, with, hot, tap water
hotplate X15.2
suicide (attempt) X77.3
ignition — *see* Ignition
in war operations — *see* War operations, fire
inflicted by other person X97
by hot objects, hot vapor, and steam — *see* Assault, burning, hot object
internal, from swallowed caustic, corrosive liquid, substance — *see* Table of Drugs and Chemicals
iron (hot) X15.8
stated as undetermined whether accidental or intentional Y27.3
suicide (attempt) X77.3
kettle (hot) X15.8
stated as undetermined whether accidental or intentional Y27.3
suicide (attempt) X77.3
lamp (flame) X08.8
with ignition of clothing NEC X06.2
nightwear X05
lighter (cigar) (cigarette) X08.8
with ignition of clothing NEC X06.2
nightwear X05
lightning — *see* subcategory T75.0
causing fire — *see* Exposure, fire
liquid (boiling) (hot) NEC X12
stated as undetermined whether accidental or intentional Y27.2
suicide (attempt) X77.2
local application of externally applied substance in medical or surgical care Y63.5
on board watercraft
due to
accident to watercraft V91.09
powered craft V91.03
ferry boat V91.01
fishing boat V91.02
jetskis V91.03
liner V91.01
merchant ship V91.00
passenger ship V91.01
unpowered craft V91.08
canoe V91.05
inflatable V91.06

Burn, burned, burning (accidental) (by) (from) (on) - *continued*
on board watercraft - *continued*
due to - *continued*
accident to watercraft - *continued*
unpowered craft - *continued*
kayak V91.05
sailboat V91.04
surf-board V91.08
water skis V91.07
windsurfer V91.08
fire on board V93.09
ferry boat V93.01
fishing boat V93.02
jetskis V93.03
liner V93.01
merchant ship V93.00
passenger ship V93.01
powered craft NEC V93.03
sailboat V93.04
specified heat source NEC on board V93.19
ferry boat V93.11
fishing boat V93.12
jetskis V93.13
liner V93.11
merchant ship V93.10
passenger ship V93.11
powered craft NEC V93.13
sailboat V93.14
machinery (hot) X17
matches X08.8
with ignition of clothing NEC X06.2
nightwear X05
mattress — *see* Exposure, fire, uncontrolled, building, bed
medicament, externally applied Y63.5
metal (hot) (liquid) (molten) NEC X18
nightwear (nightclothes, nightdress, gown, pajamas, robe) X05
object (hot) NEC X19
pipe (hot) X16
smoking X08.8
with ignition of clothing NEC X06.2
nightwear X05
powder — *see* Powder burn
radiator (hot) X16
saucepan (hot) (glass) (metal) X15.3
stated as undetermined whether accidental or intentional Y27.3
suicide (attempt) X77.3
self-inflicted X76
stated as undetermined whether accidental or intentional Y26
steam X13.1
pipe X16
stated as undetermined whether accidental or intentional Y27.8
stated as undetermined whether accidental or intentional Y27.0
suicide (attempt) X77.0
stove (hot) (kitchen) X15.0
stated as undetermined whether accidental or intentional Y27.3
suicide (attempt) X77.3
substance (hot) NEC X19
boiling X12
stated as undetermined whether accidental or intentional Y27.2
suicide (attempt) X77.2
molten (metal) X18
suicide (attempt) NEC X76
hot
household appliance X77.3
object X77.9
stated as undetermined whether accidental or intentional Y27.0
therapeutic misadventure
heat in local application or packing during medical or surgical procedure Y63.5
overdose of radiation Y63.2
toaster (hot) X15.1
stated as undetermined whether accidental or intentional Y27.3
suicide (attempt) X77.3
tool (hot) X17
torch, welding X08.8
with ignition of clothing NEC X06.2
nightwear X05
trash fire (controlled) — *see* Exposure, fire, controlled, not in building
uncontrolled — *see* Exposure, fire, uncontrolled, not in building
vapor (hot) X13.1

Burn, burned, burning (accidental) (by) (from) (on) - *continued*
  vapor (hot) - *continued*
    stated as undetermined whether accidental or intentional Y27.0
    suicide (attempt) X77.0
  Very pistol — *see* Discharge, firearm NEC
Butted by animal W55.82
  bull W55.22
  cow W55.22
  goat W55.32
  horse W55.12
  pig W55.42
  sheep W55.32

C

Caisson disease - — *see* Air, pressure, change
Campfire (exposure to) (controlled) — *see also* Exposure, fire, controlled, not in building
  uncontrolled — *see* Exposure, fire, uncontrolled, not in building
Capital punishment (any means) — *see* Legal, intervention
Car sickness T75.3
Casualty (not due to war) **NEC** X58
  war — *see* War operations
Cat
  bite W55.01
  scratch W55.03
Cataclysm, cataclysmic (any injury) **NEC** — *see* Forces of nature
Catching fire — *see* Exposure, fire
Caught
  between
    folding object W23.0
    objects (moving) (stationary and moving) W23.0
      and machinery — *see* Contact, with, by type of machine
      stationary W23.1
    sliding door and door frame W23.0
  by, in
    machinery (moving parts of) — *see* Contact, with, by type of machine
    washing-machine wringer W23.0
  under packing crate (due to losing grip) W23.1
Cave-in caused by cataclysmic earth surface movement or eruption — *see* Landslide
Change (s) in air pressure - — *see* Air, pressure, change
Choked, choking (on) (any object except food or vomitus)
  food (bone) (seed) — *see* categories T17 and T18
  vomitus T17.81-
Civil insurrection — *see* War operations
Cloudburst (any injury) X37.8
Cold, exposure to (accidental) (excessive) (extreme) (natural) (place) **NEC** — *see* Exposure, cold
Collapse
  building W20.1
    burning (uncontrolled fire) X00.2
  dam or man-made structure (causing earth movement) X36.0
  machinery — *see* Contact, with, by type of machine
  structure W20.1
    burning (uncontrolled fire) X00.2
Collision (accidental) **NEC** — *see also* Accident, transport V89.9
  pedestrian W51
    with fall W03
      due to ice or snow W00.0
      involving pedestrian conveyance — *see* Accident, transport, pedestrian, conveyance
    and
      crowd or human stampede (with fall) W52
      object W22.8
        with fall — *see* Fall, due to, bumping against, object
  person (s) — *see* Collision, pedestrian
  transport vehicle NEC V89.9
    and
      avalanche, fallen or not moving — *see* Accident, transport
        falling or moving — *see* Landslide
      landslide, fallen or not moving — *see* Accident, transport
        falling or moving — *see* Landslide
    due to cataclysm — *see* Forces of nature, by type
  intentional, purposeful suicide (attempt) — *see* Suicide, collision
Combustion, spontaneous — *see* Ignition
Complication (delayed) **of or following** (medical or surgical procedure) Y84.9
  with misadventure — *see* Misadventure

Complication (delayed) **of or following** (medical or surgical procedure) - *continued*
  amputation of limb (s) Y83.5
  anastomosis (arteriovenous) (blood vessel) (gastrojejunal) (tendon) (natural or artificial material) Y83.2
  aspiration (of fluid) Y84.4
    tissue Y84.8
  biopsy Y84.8
  blood
    sampling Y84.7
    transfusion
      procedure Y84.8
  bypass Y83.2
  catheterization (urinary) Y84.6
    cardiac Y84.0
  colostomy Y83.3
  cystostomy Y83.3
  dialysis (kidney) Y84.1
  drug — *see* Table of Drugs and Chemicals
  due to misadventure — *see* Misadventure
  duodenostomy Y83.3
  electroshock therapy Y84.3
  external stoma, creation of Y83.3
  formation of external stoma Y83.3
  gastrostomy Y83.3
  graft Y83.2
  hypothermia (medically-induced) Y84.8
  implant, implantation (of)
    artificial
      internal device (cardiac pacemaker) (electrodes in brain) (heart valve prosthesis) (orthopedic) Y83.1
    material or tissue (for anastomosis or bypass) Y83.2
      with creation of external stoma Y83.3
    natural tissues (for anastomosis or bypass) Y83.2
      with creation of external stoma Y83.3
  infusion
    procedure Y84.8
  injection — *see* Table of Drugs and Chemicals
    procedure Y84.8
  insertion of gastric or duodenal sound Y84.5
  insulin-shock therapy Y84.3
  paracentesis (abdominal) (thoracic) (aspirative) Y84.4
  procedures other than surgical operation — *see* Complication of or following, by type of procedure
  radiological procedure or therapy Y84.2
  removal of organ (partial) (total) NEC Y83.6
  sampling
    blood Y84.7
    fluid NEC Y84.4
    tissue Y84.8
  shock therapy Y84.3
  surgical operation NEC — *see also* Complication of or following, by type of operation Y83.9
    reconstructive NEC Y83.4
      with
        anastomosis, bypass or graft Y83.2
        formation of external stoma Y83.3
    specified NEC Y83.8
  transfusion — *see also* Table of Drugs and Chemicals
    procedure Y84.8
  transplant, transplantation (heart) (kidney) (liver) (whole organ, any) Y83.0
    partial organ Y83.4
  ureterostomy Y83.3
  vaccination — *see also* Table of Drugs and Chemicals
    procedure Y84.8
Compression
  divers' squeeze - — *see* Air, pressure, change
  trachea by
    food (lodged in esophagus) — *see* categories T17 and T18
    vomitus (lodged in esophagus) T17.81-
Conflagration — *see* Exposure, fire, uncontrolled
Constriction (external)
  hair W49.01
  jewelry W49.04
  ring W49.04
  rubber band W49.03
  specified item NEC W49.09
  string W49.02
  thread W49.02
Contact (accidental)
  with
    abrasive wheel (metalworking) W31.1
    alligator W58.09
      bite W58.01

Contact (accidental) - *continued*
  with - *continued*
    alligator - *continued*
      crushing W58.03
      strike W58.02
    amphibian W62.9
      frog W62.0
      toad W62.1
    animal (nonvenomous) NEC W64
      marine W56.89
        bite W56.81
        dolphin — *see* Contact, with, dolphin
        fish NEC — *see* Contact, with, fish
        mammal — *see* Contact, with, mammal, marine
        orca — *see* Contact, with, orca
        sea lion — *see* Contact, with, sea lion
        shark — *see* Contact, with, shark
      strike W56.82
    animate mechanical force NEC W64
    arrow W21.89
      not thrown, projected or falling W45.8
    arthropods (nonvenomous) W57
    axe W27.0
    band-saw (industrial) W31.2
    bayonet — *see* Bayonet wound
    bee (s) X58
    bench-saw (industrial) W31.2
    bird W61.99
      bite W61.91
      chicken — *see* Contact, with, chicken
      duck — *see* Contact, with, duck
      goose — *see* Contact, with, goose
      macaw — *see* Contact, with, macaw
      parrot — *see* Contact, with, parrot
      psittacine — *see* Contact, with, psittacine
      strike W61.92
      turkey — *see* Contact, with, turkey
    blender W29.0
    boiling water X12
      stated as undetermined whether accidental or intentional Y27.2
      suicide (attempt) X77.2
    bore, earth-drilling or mining (land) (seabed) W31.0
    buffalo — *see* Contact, with, hoof stock NEC
    bull W55.29
      bite W55.21
      gored W55.22
      strike W55.22
    bumper cars W31.81
    camel — *see* Contact, with, hoof stock NEC
    can
      lid W26.8
      opener W27.4
        powered W29.0
    cat W55.09
      bite W55.01
      scratch W55.03
    caterpillar (venomous) X58
    centipede (venomous) X58
    chain
      hoist W24.0
        agricultural operations W30.89
      saw W29.3
    chicken W61.39
      peck W61.33
      strike W61.32
    chisel W27.0
    circular saw W31.2
    cobra X58
    combine (harvester) W30.0
    conveyer belt W24.1
    cooker (hot) X15.8
      stated as undetermined whether accidental or intentional Y27.3
      suicide (attempt) X77.3
    coral X58
    cotton gin W31.82
    cow W55.29
      bite W55.21
      strike W55.22
    crane W24.0
      agricultural operations W30.89
    crocodile W58.19
      bite W58.11
      crushing W58.13
      strike W58.12
    dagger W26.1
      stated as undetermined whether accidental or intentional Y28.2
      suicide (attempt) X78.2
    dairy equipment W31.82
    dart W21.89

Contact (accidental) - *continued*
  with - *continued*
    dart - *continued*
      not thrown, projected or falling W45.8
    deer — *see* Contact, with, hoof stock NEC
    derrick W24.0
      agricultural operations W30.89
        hay W30.2
    dog W54.8
      bite W54.0
      strike W54.1
    dolphin W56.09
      bite W56.01
      strike W56.02
    donkey — *see* Contact, with, hoof stock NEC
    drill (powered) W29.8
      earth (land) (seabed) W31.0
      nonpowered W27.8
    drive belt W24.0
      agricultural operations W30.89
    dry ice — *see* Exposure, cold, man-made
    dryer (clothes) (powered) (spin) W29.2
    duck W61.69
      bite W61.61
      strike W61.62
    earth (-)
      drilling machine (industrial) W31.0
      scraping machine in stationary use W31.83
    edge of stiff paper W26.2
    electric
      beater W29.0
      blanket X16
      fan W29.2
        commercial W31.82
      knife W29.1
      mixer W29.0
    elevator (building) W24.0
      agricultural operations W30.89
        grain W30.3
    engine (s), hot NEC X17
    excavating machine W31.0
    farm machine W30.9
    feces — *see* Contact, with, by type of animal
    fer de lance X58
    fish W56.59
      bite W56.51
      shark — *see* Contact, with, shark
      strike W56.52
    flying horses W31.81
    forging (metalworking) machine W31.1
    fork W27.4
    forklift (truck) W24.0
      agricultural operations W30.89
    frog W62.0
    garden
      cultivator (powered) W29.3
        riding W30.89
      fork W27.1
    gas turbine W31.3
    Gila monster X58
    giraffe — *see* Contact, with, hoof stock NEC
    glass (sharp) (broken) W25
      with subsequent fall W18.02
      assault X99.0
      due to fall — *see* Fall, by type
      stated as undetermined whether accidental or
        intentional Y28.0
      suicide (attempt) X78.0
    goat W55.39
      bite W55.31
      strike W55.32
    goose W61.59
      bite W61.51
      strike W61.52
    hand
      saw W27.0
      tool (not powered) NEC W27.8
        powered W29.8
    harvester W30.0
    hay-derrick W30.2
    heat NEC X19
      from appliance (electrical) (household) — *see*
        Contact, with, hot, household appliance
      heating appliance X16
    heating
      appliance (hot) X16
      pad (electric) X16
    hedge-trimmer (powered) W29.3
    hoe W27.1
    hoist (chain) (shaft) NEC W24.0
      agricultural W30.89
    hoof stock NEC W55.39
      bite W55.31

Contact (accidental) - *continued*
  with - *continued*
    hoof stock NEC - *continued*
      strike W55.32
    hornet (s) X58
    horse W55.19
      bite W55.11
      strike W55.12
    hot
      air X14.1
        inhalation X14.0
      cooker X15.8
      drinks X10.0
      engine X17
      fats X10.2
      fluids NEC X12
        assault X98.2
        suicide (attempt) X77.2
        undetermined whether accidental or
          intentional Y27.2
      food X10.1
      gases X14.1
        inhalation X14.0
      heating appliance X16
      household appliance X15.8
        assault X98.3
        cooker X15.8
        hotplate X15.2
        kettle X15.8
        light bulb X15.8
        object NEC X19
          assault X98.8
          stated as undetermined whether accidental or
            intentional Y27.9
          suicide (attempt) X77.8
        saucepan X15.3
        skillet X15.3
        stove X15.0
        stated as undetermined whether accidental or
          intentional Y27.3
        suicide (attempt) X77.3
        toaster X15.1
      kettle X15.8
      light bulb X15.8
      liquid NEC — *see also* Burn X12
        drinks X10.0
        stated as undetermined whether accidental or
          intentional Y27.2
        suicide (attempt) X77.2
        tap water X11.8
          stated as undetermined whether accidental or
            intentional Y27.1
          suicide (attempt) X77.1
      machinery X17
      metal (molten) (liquid) NEC X18
      object (not producing fire or flames) NEC X19
      oil (cooking) X10.2
      pipe X16
      plate X15.2
      radiator X16
      saucepan (glass) (metal) X15.3
      skillet X15.3
      stove (kitchen) X15.0
      substance NEC X19
      tap-water X11.8
        assault X98.1
        heated on stove X12
          stated as undetermined whether accidental or
            intentional Y27.2
          suicide (attempt) X77.2
        in bathtub X11.0
        running X11.1
        stated as undetermined whether accidental or
          intentional Y27.1
        suicide (attempt) X77.1
      toaster X15.1
      tool X17
      vapors X13.1
        inhalation X13.0
      water (tap) X11.8
        boiling X12
          stated as undetermined whether accidental or
            intentional Y27.2
          suicide (attempt) X77.2
        heated on stove X12
          stated as undetermined whether accidental or
            intentional Y27.2
          suicide (attempt) X77.2
        in bathtub X11.0
        running X11.1
        stated as undetermined whether accidental or
          intentional Y27.1
        suicide (attempt) X77.1

Contact (accidental) - *continued*
  with - *continued*
    hotplate X15.2
    ice-pick W27.4
    insect (nonvenomous) NEC W57
    kettle (hot) X15.8
    knife W26.0
      assault X99.1
      electric W29.1
      stated as undetermined whether accidental or
        intentional Y28.1
      suicide (attempt) X78.1
    lathe (metalworking) W31.1
      turnings W45.8
      woodworking W31.2
    lawnmower (powered) (ridden) W28
      causing electrocution W86.8
        suicide (attempt) X83.1
      unpowered W27.1
    lift, lifting (devices) W24.0
      agricultural operations W30.89
      shaft W24.0
    liquefied gas — *see* Exposure, cold, man-made
    liquid air, hydrogen, nitrogen — *see* Exposure,
      cold, man-made
    lizard (nonvenomous) W59.09
      bite W59.01
      strike W59.02
    llama — *see* Contact, with, hoof stock NEC
    macaw W61.19
      bite W61.11
      strike W61.12
    machine, machinery W31.9
      abrasive wheel W31.1
      agricultural including animal-powered W30.9
        combine harvester W30.0
        grain storage elevator W30.3
        hay derrick W30.2
        power take-off device W30.1
        reaper W30.0
        specified NEC W30.89
        thresher W30.0
        transport vehicle, stationary W30.81
      band saw W31.2
      bench saw W31.2
      circular saw W31.2
      commercial NEC W31.82
      drilling, metal (industrial) W31.1
      earth-drilling W31.0
      earthmoving or scraping W31.89
      excavating W31.89
      forging machine W31.1
      gas turbine W31.3
      hot X17
      internal combustion engine W31.3
      land drill W31.0
      lathe W31.1
      lifting (devices) W24.0
      metal drill W31.1
      metalworking (industrial) W31.1
      milling, metal W31.1
      mining W31.0
      molding W31.2
      overhead plane W31.2
      power press, metal W31.1
      prime mover W31.3
      printing W31.89
      radial saw W31.2
      recreational W31.81
      roller-coaster W31.81
      rolling mill, metal W31.1
      sander W31.2
      seabed drill W31.0
      shaft
        hoist W31.0
        lift W31.0
      specified NEC W31.89
      spinning W31.89
      steam engine W31.3
      transmission W24.1
      undercutter W31.0
      water driven turbine W31.3
      weaving W31.89
      woodworking or forming (industrial) W31.2
    mammal (feces) (urine) W55.89
      bull — *see* Contact, with, bull
      cat — *see* Contact, with, cat
      cow — *see* Contact, with, cow
      goat — *see* Contact, with, goat
      hoof stock — *see* Contact, with, hoof stock
      horse — *see* Contact, with, horse
    marine W56.39
      dolphin — *see* Contact, with, dolphin

Contact (accidental) - *continued*
with - *continued*
mammal (feces) (urine) - *continued*
marine - *continued*
orca — *see* Contact, with, orca
sea lion — *see* Contact, with, sea lion
specified NEC W56.39
bite W56.31
strike W56.32
pig — *see* Contact, with, pig
raccoon — *see* Contact, with, raccoon
rodent — *see* Contact, with, rodent
sheep — *see* Contact, with, sheep
specified NEC W55.89
bite W55.81
strike W55.82
marine
animal W56.89
bite W56.81
dolphin — *see* Contact, with, dolphin
fish NEC — *see* Contact, with, fish
mammal — *see* Contact, with, mammal, marine
orca — *see* Contact, with, orca
sea lion — *see* Contact, with, sea lion
shark — *see* Contact, with, shark
strike W56.82
meat
grinder (domestic) W29.0
industrial W31.82
nonpowered W27.4
slicer (domestic) W29.0
industrial W31.82
merry go round W31.81
metal, hot (liquid) (molten) NEC X18
millipede W57
nail W45.0
gun W29.4
needle (sewing) W27.3
hypodermic W46.0
contaminated W46.1
object (blunt) NEC
hot NEC X19
legal intervention — *see* Legal, intervention, blunt object
sharp NEC W45.8
inflicted by other person NEC W45.8
stated as
intentional homicide (attempt) — *see* Assault, cutting or piercing instrument
legal intervention — *see* Legal, intervention, sharp object
self-inflicted X78.9
orca W56.29
bite W56.21
strike W56.22
overhead plane W31.2
paper (as sharp object) W26.2
paper-cutter W27.5
parrot W61.09
bite W61.01
strike W61.02
pig W55.49
bite W55.41
strike W55.42
pipe, hot X16
pitchfork W27.1
plane (metal) (wood) W27.0
overhead W31.2
plant thorns, spines, sharp leaves or other mechanisms W60
powered
garden cultivator W29.3
household appliance, implement, or machine W29.8
saw (industrial) W31.2
hand W29.8
printing machine W31.89
psittacine bird W61.29
bite W61.21
macaw — *see* Contact, with, macaw
parrot — *see* Contact, with, parrot
strike W61.22
pulley (block) (transmission) W24.0
agricultural operations W30.89
raccoon W55.59
bite W55.51
strike W55.52
radial-saw (industrial) W31.2
radiator (hot) X16
rake W27.1
rattlesnake X58
reaper W30.0
reptile W59.89

Contact (accidental) - *continued*
with - *continued*
reptile - *continued*
lizard — *see* Contact, with, lizard
snake — *see* Contact, with, snake
specified NEC W59.89
bite W59.81
crushing W59.83
strike W59.82
turtle — *see* Contact, with, turtle
rivet gun (powered) W29.4
road scraper — *see* Accident, transport, construction vehicle
rodent (feces) (urine) W53.89
bite W53.81
mouse W53.09
bite W53.01
rat W53.19
bite W53.11
specified NEC W53.89
bite W53.81
squirrel W53.29
bite W53.21
roller coaster W31.81
rope NEC W24.0
agricultural operations W30.89
saliva — *see* Contact, with, by type of animal
sander W29.8
industrial W31.2
saucepan (hot) (glass) (metal) X15.3
saw W27.0
band (industrial) W31.2
bench (industrial) W31.2
chain W29.3
hand W27.0
sawing machine, metal W31.1
scissors W27.2
scorpion X58
screwdriver W27.0
powered W29.8
sea
anemone, cucumber or urchin (spine) X58
lion W56.19
bite W56.11
strike W56.12
serpent — *see* Contact, with, snake, by type
sewing-machine (electric) (powered) W29.2
not powered W27.8
shaft (hoist) (lift) (transmission) NEC W24.0
agricultural W30.89
shark W56.49
bite W56.41
strike W56.42
sharp object (s) W26.9
specified NEC W26.8
shears (hand) W27.2
powered (industrial) W31.1
domestic W29.2
sheep W55.39
bite W55.31
strike W55.32
shovel W27.8
steam — *see* Accident, transport, construction vehicle
snake (nonvenomous) W59.19
bite W59.11
crushing W59.13
strike W59.12
spade W27.1
spider (venomous) X58
spin-drier W29.2
spinning machine W31.89
splinter W45.8
sports equipment W21.9
staple gun (powered) W29.8
steam X13.1
engine W31.3
inhalation X13.0
pipe X16
shovel W31.89
stove (hot) (kitchen) X15.0
substance, hot NEC X19
molten (metal) X18
sword W26.1
assault X99.2
stated as undetermined whether accidental or intentional Y28.2
suicide (attempt) X78.2
tarantula X58
thresher W30.0
tin can lid W26.8
toad W62.1
toaster (hot) X15.1

Contact (accidental) - *continued*
with - *continued*
tool W27.8
hand (not powered) W27.8
auger W27.0
axe W27.0
can opener W27.4
chisel W27.0
fork W27.4
garden W27.1
handsaw W27.0
hoe W27.1
ice-pick W27.4
kitchen utensil W27.4
manual
lawn mower W27.1
sewing machine W27.8
meat grinder W27.4
needle (sewing) W27.3
hypodermic W46.0
contaminated W46.1
paper cutter W27.5
pitchfork W27.1
rake W27.1
scissors W27.2
screwdriver W27.0
specified NEC W27.8
workbench W27.0
hot X17
powered W29.8
blender W29.0
commercial W31.82
can opener W29.0
commercial W31.82
chainsaw W29.3
clothes dryer W29.2
commercial W31.82
dishwasher W29.2
commercial W31.82
edger W29.3
electric fan W29.2
commercial W31.82
electric knife W29.1
food processor W29.0
commercial W31.82
garbage disposal W29.0
commercial W31.82
garden tool W29.3
hedge trimmer W29.3
ice maker W29.0
commercial W31.82
kitchen appliance W29.0
commercial W31.82
lawn mower W28
meat grinder W29.0
commercial W31.82
mixer W29.0
commercial W31.82
rototiller W29.3
sewing machine W29.2
commercial W31.82
washing machine W29.2
commercial W31.82
transmission device (belt, cable, chain, gear, pinion, shaft) W24.1
agricultural operations W30.89
turbine (gas) (water-driven) W31.3
turkey W61.49
peck W61.43
strike W61.42
turtle (nonvenomous) W59.29
bite W59.21
strike W59.22
terrestrial W59.89
bite W59.81
crushing W59.83
strike W59.82
under-cutter W31.0
urine — *see* Contact, with, by type of animal
vehicle
agricultural use (transport) — *see* Accident, transport, agricultural vehicle
not on public highway W30.81
industrial use (transport) — *see* Accident, transport, industrial vehicle
not on public highway W31.83
off-road use (transport) — *see* Accident, transport, all-terrain or off-road vehicle
not on public highway W31.83
special construction use (transport) — *see* Accident, transport, construction vehicle
not on public highway W31.83
venomous

Contact (accidental) - *continued*
  with - *continued*
    venomous - *continued*
      animal X58
      arthropods X58
      lizard X58
      marine animal NEC X58
      marine plant NEC X58
      millipedes (tropical) X58
      plant (s) X58
      snake X58
      spider X58
      viper X58
      washing-machine (powered) W29.2
      wasp X58
      weaving-machine W31.89
      winch W24.0
        agricultural operations W30.89
      wire NEC W24.0
        agricultural operations W30.89
      wood slivers W45.8
      yellow jacket X58
      zebra — *see* Contact, with, hoof stock NEC
    pressure X50.9
    stress X50.9
Coup de soleil X32
Crash
  aircraft (in transit) (powered) V95.9
    balloon V96.01
    fixed wing NEC (private) V95.21
      commercial V95.31
    glider V96.21
      hang V96.11
      powered V95.11
    helicopter V95.01
    in war operations — *see* War operations, destruction of aircraft
    microlight V95.11
    nonpowered V96.9
      specified NEC V96.8
    powered NEC V95.8
    stated as
      homicide (attempt) Y08.81
      suicide (attempt) X83.0
    ultralight V95.11
  spacecraft V95.41
  transport vehicle NEC — *see also* Accident, transport V89.9
    homicide (attempt) Y03.8
    motor NEC (traffic) V89.2
      homicide (attempt) Y03.8
      suicide (attempt) — *see* Suicide, collision
Cruelty (mental) (physical) (sexual) X58
Crushed (accidentally) X58
  between objects (moving) (stationary and moving) W23.0
    stationary W23.1
  by
    alligator W58.03
    avalanche NEC — *see* Landslide
    cave-in W20.0
      caused by cataclysmic earth surface movement — *see* Landslide
    crocodile W58.13
    crowd or human stampede W52
    falling
      aircraft V97.39
        in war operations — *see* War operations, destruction of aircraft
      earth, material W20.0
        caused by cataclysmic earth surface movement — *see* Landslide
      object NEC W20.8
    landslide NEC — *see* Landslide
    lizard (nonvenomous) W59.09
    machinery — *see* Contact, with, by type of machine
    reptile NEC W59.89
    snake (nonvenomous) W59.13
  in
    machinery — *see* Contact, with, by type of machine
Cut, cutting (any part of body) (accidental) — *see also* Contact, with, by object or machine
  during medical or surgical treatment as misadventure — *see* Index to Diseases and Injuries, Complications
  homicide (attempt) — *see* Assault, cutting or piercing instrument
  inflicted by other person — *see* Assault, cutting or piercing instrument
  legal
    execution — *see* Legal, intervention

Cut, cutting (any part of body) (accidental) - *continued*
  legal - *continued*
    intervention — *see* Legal, intervention, sharp object
  machine NEC — *see also* Contact, with, by type of machine W31.9
  self-inflicted — *see* Suicide, cutting or piercing instrument
  suicide (attempt) — *see* Suicide, cutting or piercing instrument
Cyclone (any injury) X37.1

D

Decapitation (accidental circumstances) **NEC** X58
  homicide X99.9
  legal execution — *see* Legal, intervention
Dehydration from lack of water X58
Deprivation X58
Derailment (accidental)
  railway (rolling stock) (train) (vehicle) (without antecedent collision) V81.7
    with antecedent collision — *see* Accident, transport, railway vehicle occupant
  streetcar (without antecedent collision) V82.7
    with antecedent collision — *see* Accident, transport, streetcar occupant
Descent
  parachute (voluntary) (without accident to aircraft) V97.29
    due to accident to aircraft — *see* Accident, transport, aircraft
Desertion X58
Destitution X58
Disability, late effect or sequela of injury — *see* Sequelae
Discharge (accidental)
  airgun W34.010
    assault X95.01
    homicide (attempt) X95.01
    stated as undetermined whether accidental or intentional Y24.0
    suicide (attempt) X74.01
  BB gun — *see* Discharge, airgun
  firearm (accidental) W34.00
    assault X95.9
    handgun (pistol) (revolver) W32.0
      assault X93
      homicide (attempt) X93
      legal intervention — *see* Legal, intervention, firearm, handgun
      stated as undetermined whether accidental or intentional Y22
      suicide (attempt) X72
    homicide (attempt) X95.9
    hunting rifle W33.02
      assault X94.1
      homicide (attempt) X94.1
      legal intervention
        injuring
          bystander Y35.032
          law enforcement personnel Y35.031
          suspect Y35.033
      stated as undetermined whether accidental or intentional Y23.1
      suicide (attempt) X73.1
    larger W33.00
      assault X94.9
      homicide (attempt) X94.9
      hunting rifle — *see* Discharge, firearm, hunting rifle
      legal intervention — *see* Legal, intervention, firearm by type of firearm
      machine gun — *see* Discharge, firearm, machine gun
      shotgun — *see* Discharge, firearm, shotgun
    specified NEC W33.09
      assault X94.8
      homicide (attempt) X94.8
      legal intervention
        injuring
          bystander Y35.092
          law enforcement personnel Y35.091
          suspect Y35.093
      stated as undetermined whether accidental or intentional Y23.8
      suicide (attempt) X73.8
    stated as undetermined whether accidental or intentional Y23.9
    suicide (attempt) X73.9
    legal intervention
      injuring
        bystander Y35.002

Discharge (accidental) - *continued*
  firearm (accidental) - *continued*
    legal intervention - *continued*
      injuring - *continued*
        law enforcement personnel Y35.001
        suspect Y35.03
      using rubber bullet
        injuring
          bystander Y35.042
          law enforcement personnel Y35.041
          suspect Y35.043
    machine gun W33.03
      assault X94.2
      homicide (attempt) X94.2
      legal intervention — *see* Legal, intervention, firearm, machine gun
      stated as undetermined whether accidental or intentional Y23.3
      suicide (attempt) X73.2
    pellet gun — *see* Discharge, airgun
    shotgun W33.01
      assault X94.0
      homicide (attempt) X94.0
      legal intervention — *see* Legal, intervention, firearm, specified NEC
      stated as undetermined whether accidental or intentional Y23.0
      suicide (attempt) X73.0
    specified NEC W34.09
      assault X95.8
      homicide (attempt) X95.8
      legal intervention — *see* Legal, intervention, firearm, specified NEC
      stated as undetermined whether accidental or intentional Y24.8
      suicide (attempt) X74.8
    stated as undetermined whether accidental or intentional Y24.9
    suicide (attempt) X74.9
    Very pistol W34.09
      assault X95.8
      homicide (attempt) X95.8
      stated as undetermined whether accidental or intentional Y24.8
      suicide (attempt) X74.8
  firework (s) W39
    stated as undetermined whether accidental or intentional Y25
  gas-operated gun NEC W34.018
    airgun — *see* Discharge, airgun
    assault X95.09
    homicide (attempt) X95.09
    paintball gun — *see* Discharge, paintball gun
    stated as undetermined whether accidental or intentional Y24.8
    suicide (attempt) X74.09
  gun NEC — *see also* Discharge, firearm NEC
    air — *see* Discharge, airgun
    BB — *see* Discharge, airgun
    for single hand use — *see* Discharge, firearm, handgun
    hand — *see* Discharge, firearm, handgun
    machine — *see* Discharge, firearm, machine gun
    other specified — *see* Discharge, firearm NEC
    paintball — *see* Discharge, paintball gun
    pellet — *see* Discharge, airgun
  handgun — *see* Discharge, firearm, handgun
  machine gun — *see* Discharge, firearm, machine gun
  paintball gun W34.011
    assault X95.02
    homicide (attempt) X95.02
    stated as undetermined whether accidental or intentional Y24.8
    suicide (attempt) X74.02
  pistol — *see* Discharge, firearm, handgun
    flare — *see* Discharge, firearm, Very pistol
    pellet — *see* Discharge, airgun
    Very — *see* Discharge, firearm, Very pistol
  revolver — *see* Discharge, firearm, handgun
  rifle (hunting) — *see* Discharge, firearm, hunting rifle
  shotgun — *see* Discharge, firearm, shotgun
  spring-operated gun NEC W34.018
    assault X95.09
    homicide (attempt) X95.09
    stated as undetermined whether accidental or intentional Y24.8
    suicide (attempt) X74.09
Disease
  Andes W94.11
  aviator's - — *see* Air, pressure
  range W94.11

Diver's disease, palsy, paralysis, squeeze - — *see*
Air, pressure
Diving (into water) — *see* Accident, diving
Dog bite W54.0
Dragged by transport vehicle NEC — *see also* Accident, transport V09.9
Drinking poison (accidental) — *see* Table of Drugs and Chemicals
Dropped (accidentally) **while being carried or supported by other person** W04
Drowning (accidental) W74
assault X92.9
due to
accident (to)
machinery — *see* Contact, with, by type of machine
watercraft V90.89
burning V90.29
powered V90.23
merchant ship V90.20
passenger ship V90.21
fishing boat V90.22
jetskis V90.23
unpowered V90.28
canoe V90.25
inflatable V90.26
kayak V90.25
sailboat V90.24
water skis V90.27
crushed V90.39
powered V90.33
merchant ship V90.30
passenger ship V90.31
fishing boat V90.32
jetskis V90.33
unpowered V90.38
canoe V90.35
inflatable V90.36
kayak V90.35
sailboat V90.34
water skis V90.37
overturning V90.09
powered V90.03
merchant ship V90.00
passenger ship V90.01
fishing boat V90.02
jetskis V90.03
unpowered V90.08
canoe V90.05
inflatable V90.06
kayak V90.05
sailboat V90.04
sinking V90.19
powered V90.13
merchant ship V90.10
passenger ship V90.11
fishing boat V90.12
jetskis V90.13
unpowered V90.18
canoe V90.15
inflatable V90.16
kayak V90.15
sailboat V90.14
specified type NEC V90.89
powered V90.83
merchant ship V90.80
passenger ship V90.81
fishing boat V90.82
jetskis V90.83
unpowered V90.88
canoe V90.85
inflatable V90.86
kayak V90.85
sailboat V90.84
water skis V90.87
avalanche — *see* Landslide
cataclysmic
earth surface movement NEC — *see* Forces of nature, earth movement
storm — *see* Forces of nature, cataclysmic storm
cloudburst X37.8
cyclone X37.1
fall overboard (from) V92.09
powered craft V92.03
ferry boat V92.01
liner V92.01
merchant ship V92.00
passenger ship V92.01
fishing boat V92.02
jetskis V92.03
unpowered craft V92.08
canoe V92.05
inflatable V92.06

Drowning (accidental) - *continued*
due to - *continued*
fall overboard (from) - *continued*
unpowered craft - *continued*
kayak V92.05
sailboat V92.04
surf-board V92.08
water skis V92.07
windsurfer V92.08
resulting from
accident to watercraft — *see* Drowning, due to, accident to, watercraft
being washed overboard (from) V92.29
powered craft V92.23
ferry boat V92.21
liner V92.21
merchant ship V92.20
passenger ship V92.21
fishing boat V92.22
jetskis V92.23
unpowered craft V92.28
canoe V92.25
inflatable V92.26
kayak V92.25
sailboat V92.24
surf-board V92.28
water skis V92.27
windsurfer V92.28
motion of watercraft V92.19
powered craft V92.13
ferry boat V92.11
liner V92.11
merchant ship V92.10
passenger ship V92.11
fishing boat V92.12
jetskis V92.13
unpowered craft
canoe V92.15
inflatable V92.16
kayak V92.15
sailboat V92.14
hurricane X37.0
jumping into water from watercraft (involved in accident) — *see also* Drowning, due to, accident to, watercraft
without accident to or on watercraft W16.711
tidal wave NEC — *see* Forces of nature, tidal wave
torrential rain X37.8
following
fall
into
bathtub W16.211
bucket W16.221
fountain — *see* Drowning, following, fall, into, water, specified NEC
quarry — *see* Drowning, following, fall, into, water, specified NEC
reservoir — *see* Drowning, following, fall, into, water, specified NEC
swimming-pool W16.011
striking
bottom W16.021
wall W16.031
stated as undetermined whether accidental or intentional Y21.3
suicide (attempt) X71.2
water NOS W16.41
natural (lake) (open sea) (river) (stream) (pond) W16.111
striking
bottom W16.121
side W16.131
specified NEC W16.311
striking
bottom W16.321
wall W16.331
overboard NEC — *see* Drowning, due to, fall overboard
jump or dive
from boat W16.711
striking bottom W16.721
into
fountain — *see* Drowning, following, jump or dive, into, water, specified NEC
quarry — *see* Drowning, following, jump or dive, into, water, specified NEC
reservoir — *see* Drowning, following, jump or dive, into, water, specified NEC
swimming-pool W16.511
striking
bottom W16.521
wall W16.531
suicide (attempt) X71.2

Drowning (accidental) - *continued*
following - *continued*
jump or dive - *continued*
into - *continued*
water NOS W16.91
natural (lake) (open sea) (river) (stream) (pond) W16.611
specified NEC W16.811
striking
bottom W16.821
wall W16.831
striking bottom W16.621
homicide (attempt) X92.9
in
bathtub (accidental) W65
assault X92.0
following fall W16.211
stated as undetermined whether accidental or intentional Y21.1
stated as undetermined whether accidental or intentional Y21.0
suicide (attempt) X71.0
lake — *see* Drowning, in, natural water
natural water (lake) (open sea) (river) (stream) (pond) W69
assault X92.3
following
dive or jump W16.611
striking bottom W16.621
fall W16.111
striking
bottom W16.121
side W16.131
stated as undetermined whether accidental or intentional Y21.4
suicide (attempt) X71.3
quarry — *see* Drowning, in, specified place NEC
quenching tank — *see* Drowning, in, specified place NEC
reservoir — *see* Drowning, in, specified place NEC
river — *see* Drowning, in, natural water
sea — *see* Drowning, in, natural water
specified place NEC W73
assault X92.8
following
dive or jump W16.811
striking
bottom W16.821
wall W16.831
fall W16.311
striking
bottom W16.321
wall W16.331
stated as undetermined whether accidental or intentional Y21.8
suicide (attempt) X71.8
stream — *see* Drowning, in, natural water
swimming-pool W67
assault X92.1
following fall X92.2
following
dive or jump W16.511
striking
bottom W16.521
wall W16.531
fall W16.011
striking
bottom W16.021
wall W16.031
stated as undetermined whether accidental or intentional Y21.2
following fall Y21.3
suicide (attempt) X71.1
following fall X71.2
war operations — *see* War operations, restriction of airway
resulting from accident to watercraftCsee Drowning, due to, accident, watercraft
self-inflicted X71.9
stated as undetermined whether accidental or intentional Y21.9
suicide (attempt) X71.9

E

Earth falling (on) W20.0
caused by cataclysmic earth surface movement or eruption — *see* Landslide
Earth (surface) **movement NEC** — *see* Forces of nature, earth movement
Earthquake (any injury) X34
Effect (s) (adverse) **of**
air pressure (any) - —— *see* Air, pressure
cold, excessive (exposure to) — *see* Exposure, cold

Effect (s) (adverse) **of** - *continued*
heat (excessive) — *see* Heat
hot place (weather) — *see* Heat
insolation X30
late — *see* Sequelae
motion — *see* Motion
nuclear explosion or weapon in war
operations — *see* War operations, nuclear
weapon
radiation — *see* Radiation
travel — *see* Travel
Electric shock (accidental) (by) (in) — *see* Exposure,
electric current
Electrocution (accidental) — *see* Exposure, electric
current
Endotracheal tube wrongly placed during
anesthetic procedure
Entanglement
in
bed linen, causing suffocation — *see* category T71
wheel of pedal cycle V19.88
Entry of foreign body or material — *see* Foreign
body
Environmental pollution related condition- see Z57
Execution, legal (any method) — *see* Legal,
intervention
Exhaustion
cold — *see* Exposure, cold
due to excessive exertion — *see*
also Overexertion X50.9
heat — *see* Heat
Explosion (accidental) (of) (with secondary
fire) W40.9
acetylene W40.1
aerosol can W36.1
air tank (compressed) (in machinery) W36.2
aircraft (in transit) (powered) NEC V95.9
balloon V96.05
fixed wing NEC (private) V95.25
commercial V95.35
glider V96.25
hang V96.15
powered V95.15
helicopter V95.05
in war operations — *see* War operations,
destruction of aircraft
microlight V95.15
nonpowered V96.9
specified NEC V96.8
powered NEC V95.8
stated as
homicide (attempt) Y03.8
suicide (attempt) X83.0
ultralight V95.15
anesthetic gas in operating room W40.1
antipersonnel bomb W40.8
assault X96.0
homicide (attempt) X96.0
suicide (attempt) X75
assault X96.9
bicycle tire W37.0
blasting (cap) (materials) W40.0
boiler (machinery) , not on transport vehicle W35
on watercraft — *see* Explosion, in, watercraft
butane W40.1
caused by other person X96.9
coal gas W40.1
detonator W40.0
dump (munitions) W40.8
dynamite W40.0
in
assault X96.8
homicide (attempt) X96.8
legal intervention
injuring
bystander Y35.112
law enforcement personnel Y35.111
suspect Y35.113
suicide (attempt) X75
explosive (material) W40.9
gas W40.1
in blasting operation W40.0
specified NEC W40.8
in
assault X96.8
homicide (attempt) X96.8
legal intervention
injuring
bystander Y35.192
law enforcement personnel Y35.191
suspect Y35.193
suicide (attempt) X75
factory (munitions) W40.8

Explosion (accidental) (of) (with secondary fire) -
continued
fertilizer bomb W40.8
assault X96.3
homicide (attempt) X96.3
suicide (attempt) X75
firearm (parts) NEC W34.19
airgun W34.110
BB gun W34.110
gas, air or spring-operated gun NEC W34.118
handgun W32.1
hunting rifle W33.12
larger firearm W33.10
specified NEC W33.19
machine gun W33.13
paintball gun W34.111
pellet gun W34.110
shotgun W33.11
Very pistol [flare] W34.19
fire-damp W40.1
fireworks W39
gas (coal) (explosive) W40.1
cylinder W36.9
aerosol can W36.1
air tank W36.2
pressurized W36.3
specified NEC W36.8
gasoline (fumes) (tank) not in moving motor
vehicle W40.1
bomb W40.8
assault X96.1
homicide (attempt) X96.1
suicide (attempt) X75
in motor vehicle — *see* Accident, transport, by
type of vehicle
grain store W40.8
grenade W40.8
in
assault X96.8
homicide (attempt) X96.8
legal intervention
injuring
bystander Y35.192
law enforcement personnel Y35.191
suspect Y35.193
suicide (attempt) X75
handgun (parts) — *see* Explosion, firearm, hangun
(parts)
homicide (attempt) X96.9
antipersonnel bomb — *see* Explosion,
antipersonnel bomb
fertilizer bomb — *see* Explosion, fertilizer bomb
gasoline bomb — *see* Explosion, gasoline bomb
letter bomb — *see* Explosion, letter bomb
pipe bomb — *see* Explosion, pipe bomb
specified NEC X96.8
hose, pressurized W37.8
hot water heater, tank (in machinery) W35
on watercraft — *see* Explosion, in, watercraft
in, on
dump W40.8
factory W40.8
mine (of explosive gases) NEC W40.1
watercraft V93.59
powered craft V93.53
ferry boat V93.51
fishing boat V93.52
jetskis V93.53
liner V93.51
merchant ship V93.50
passenger ship V93.51
sailboat V93.54
letter bomb W40.8
assault X96.2
homicide (attempt) X96.2
suicide (attempt) X75
machinery — *see also* Contact, with, by type of
machine
on board watercraft — *see* Explosion, in,
watercraft
pressure vessel — *see* Explosion, by type of vessel
methane W40.1
mine W40.1
missile NEC W40.8
mortar bomb W40.8
in
assault X96.8
homicide (attempt) X96.8
legal intervention
injuring
bystander Y35.192
law enforcement personnel Y35.191
suspect Y35.193

Explosion (accidental) (of) (with secondary fire) -
continued
mortar bomb - *continued*
in - *continued*
suicide (attempt) X75
munitions (dump) (factory) W40.8
pipe, pressurized W37.8
bomb W40.8
assault X96.4
homicide (attempt) X96.4
suicide (attempt) X75
pressure, pressurized
cooker W38
gas tank (in machinery) W36.3
hose W37.8
pipe W37.8
specified device NEC W38
tire W37.8
bicycle W37.0
vessel (in machinery) W38
propane W40.1
self-inflicted X75
shell (artillery) NEC W40.8
during war operations — *see* War operations,
explosion
in
legal intervention
injuring
bystander Y35.122
law enforcement personnel Y35.121
suspect Y35.123
war — *see* War operations, explosion
spacecraft V95.45
steam or water lines (in machinery) W37.8
stove W40.9
stated as undetermined whether accidental or
intentional Y25
suicide (attempt) X75
tire, pressurized W37.8
bicycle W37.0
undetermined whether accidental or intentional Y25
vehicle tire NEC W37.8
bicycle W37.0
war operations — *see* War operations, explosion
Exposure (to) X58
air pressure change — *see* Air, pressure
cold (accidental) (excessive) (extreme) (natural)
(place) X31
assault Y08.89
due to
man-made conditions W93.8
dry ice (contact) W93.01
inhalation W93.02
liquid air (contact) (hydrogen)
(nitrogen) W93.11
inhalation W93.12
refrigeration unit (deep freeze) W93.2
suicide (attempt) X83.2
weather (conditions) X31
homicide (attempt) Y08.89
self-inflicted X83.2
due to abandonment or neglect X58
electric current W86.8
appliance (faulty) W86.8
domestic W86.0
caused by other person Y08.89
conductor (faulty) W86.1
control apparatus (faulty) W86.1
electric power generating plant, distribution
station W86.1
electroshock gun — *see* Exposure, electric current,
taser
high-voltage cable W85
homicide (attempt) Y08.89
legal execution — *see* Legal, intervention,
specified means NEC
lightning — *see* subcategory T75.0
live rail W86.8
misadventure in medical or surgical procedure in
electroshock therapy Y63.4
motor (electric) (faulty) W86.8
domestic W86.0
self-inflicted X83.1
specified NEC W86.8
domestic W86.0
stun gun — *see* Exposure, electric current, taser
suicide (attempt) X83.1
taser W86.8
assault Y08.89
legal intervention — *see* category Y35
self-harm (intentional) X83.8
undetermined intent Y33
third rail W86.8

Fall, falling (accidental) - *continued*
earth (with asphyxia or suffocation (by pressure)
) — *see* Earth, falling
from, off, out of
aircraft NEC (with accident to aircraft NEC) V97.0
while boarding or alighting V97.1
balcony W13.0
bed W06
boat, ship, watercraft NEC (with drowning or
submersion) — *see* Drowning, due to, fall
overboard
with hitting bottom or object V94.0
bridge W13.1
building W13.9
burning (uncontrolled fire) X00.3
cavity W17.2
chair W07
cherry picker W17.89
cliff W15
dock W17.4
embankment W17.81
escalator W10.0
flagpole W13.8
furniture NEC W08
grocery cart W17.82
haystack W17.89
high place NEC W17.89
stated as undetermined whether accidental or
intentional Y30
hole W17.2
incline W10.2
ladder W11
lifting device W17.89
machine, machinery — *see also* Contact, with, by
type of machine
not in operation W17.89
manhole W17.1
mobile elevated work platform [MEWP] W17.89
motorized mobility scooter W05.2
one level to another NEC W17.89
intentional, purposeful, suicide (attempt) X80
stated as undetermined whether accidental or
intentional Y30
pit W17.2
playground equipment W09.8
jungle gym W09.2
slide W09.0
swing W09.1
quarry W17.89
railing W13.9
ramp W10.2
roof W13.2
scaffolding W12
scooter (nonmotorized) W05.1
motorized mobility W05.2
sky lift W17.89
stairs, steps W10.9
curb W10.1
due to ice or snow W00.1
escalator W10.0
incline W10.2
ramp W10.2
sidewalk curb W10.1
specified NEC W10.8
stepladder W11
storm drain W17.1
streetcar NEC V82.6
with antecedent collision — *see* Accident,
transport, streetcar occupant
while boarding or alighting V82.4
structure NEC W13.8
burning (uncontrolled fire) X00.3
table W08
toilet W18.11
with subsequent striking against object W18.12
train NEC V81.6
during derailment (without antecedent
collision) V81.7
with antecedent collision — *see* Accident,
transport, railway vehicle occupant
while boarding or alighting V81.4
transport vehicle after collision — *see* Accident,
transport, by type of vehicle, collision
tree W14
vehicle (in motion) NEC — *see also* Accident,
transport V89.9
motor NEC — *see also* Accident, transport,
occupant, by type of vehicle V87.8
stationary W17.89
while boarding or alighting — *see* Accident,
transport, by type of vehicle, while boarding
or alighting
viaduct W13.8

Fall, falling (accidental) - *continued*
from, off, out of - *continued*
wall W13.8
watercraft — *see also* Drowning, due to, fall
overboard
with hitting bottom or object V94.0
well W17.0
wheelchair, non-moving W05.0
powered — *see* Accident, transport, pedestrian,
conveyance occupant, specified type NEC
window W13.4
in, on
aircraft NEC V97.0
with accident to aircraft V97.0
while boarding or alighting V97.1
bathtub (empty) W18.2
filled W16.212
causing drowning W16.211
escalator W10.0
incline W10.2
ladder W11
machine, machinery — *see* Contact, with, by type
of machine
object, edged, pointed or sharp (with cut) — *see*
Fall, by type
playground equipment W09.8
jungle gym W09.2
slide W09.0
swing W09.1
ramp W10.2
scaffolding W12
shower W18.2
causing drowning W16.211
staircase, stairs, steps W10.9
curb W10.1
due to ice or snow W00.1
escalator W10.0
incline W10.2
specified NEC W10.8
streetcar (without antecedent collision) V82.5
with antecedent collision — *see* Accident,
transport, streetcar occupant
while boarding or alighting V82.4
train (without antecedent collision) V81.5
with antecedent collision — *see* Accident,
transport, railway vehicle occupant
during derailment (without antecedent
collision) V81.7
with antecedent collision — *see* Accident,
transport, railway vehicle occupant
while boarding or alighting V81.4
transport vehicle after collision — *see* Accident,
transport, by type of vehicle, collision
watercraft V93.39
due to
accident to craft V91.29
powered craft V91.23
ferry boat V91.21
fishing boat V91.22
jetskis V91.23
liner V91.21
merchant ship V91.20
passenger ship V91.21
unpowered craft
canoe V91.25
inflatable V91.26
kayak V91.25
sailboat V91.24
powered craft V93.33
ferry boat V93.31
fishing boat V93.32
jetskis V93.33
liner V93.31
merchant ship V93.30
passenger ship V93.31
unpowered craft V93.38
canoe V93.35
inflatable V93.36
kayak V93.35
sailboat V93.34
surf-board V93.38
windsurfer V93.38
into
cavity W17.2
dock W17.4
fire — *see* Exposure, fire, by type
haystack W17.89
hole W17.2
lake — *see* Fall, into, water
manhole W17.1
moving part of machinery — *see* Contact, with, by
type of machine
ocean — *see* Fall, into, water

Fall, falling (accidental) - *continued*
into - *continued*
opening in surface NEC W17.89
pit W17.2
pond — *see* Fall, into, water
quarry W17.89
river — *see* Fall, into, water
shaft W17.89
storm drain W17.1
stream — *see* Fall, into, water
swimming pool — *see also* Fall, into, water, in,
swimming pool
empty W17.3
tank W17.89
water W16.42
causing drowning W16.41
from watercraft — *see* Drowning, due to, fall
overboard
hitting diving board W21.4
in
bathtub W16.212
causing drowning W16.211
bucket W16.222
causing drowning W16.221
natural body of water W16.112
causing drowning W16.111
striking
bottom W16.122
causing drowning W16.121
side W16.132
causing drowning W16.131
specified water NEC W16.312
causing drowning W16.311
striking
bottom W16.322
causing drowning W16.321
wall W16.332
causing drowning W16.331
swimming pool W16.012
causing drowning W16.011
striking
bottom W16.022
causing drowning W16.021
wall W16.032
causing drowning W16.031
utility bucket W16.222
causing drowning W16.221
well W17.0
involving
bed W06
chair W07
furniture NEC W08
glass — *see* Fall, by type
playground equipment W09.8
jungle gym W09.2
slide W09.0
swing W09.1
roller blades — *see* Accident, transport, pedestrian,
conveyance
skateboard (s) — *see* Accident, transport,
pedestrian, conveyance
skates (ice) (in line) (roller) — *see* Accident,
transport, pedestrian, conveyance
skis — *see* Accident, transport, pedestrian,
conveyance
table W08
wheelchair, non-moving W05.0
powered — *see* Accident, transport, pedestrian,
conveyance, specified type NEC
object — *see* Struck by, object, falling
off
toilet W18.11
with subsequent striking against object W18.12
on same level W18.30
due to
specified NEC W18.39
stepping on an object W18.31
out of
bed W06
building NEC W13.8
chair W07
furniture NEC W08
wheelchair, non-moving W05.0
powered — *see* Accident, transport, pedestrian,
conveyance, specified type NEC
window W13.4
over
animal W01.0
cliff W15
embankment W17.81
small object W01.0
rock W20.8
same level W18.30

Fall, falling (accidental) - *continued*
same level - *continued*
from
being crushed, pushed, or stepped on by a crowd or human stampede W52
collision, pushing, shoving, by or with other person W03
slipping, stumbling, tripping W01.0
involving ice or snow W00.0
involving skates (ice) (roller), skateboard, skis — *see* Accident, transport, pedestrian, conveyance
snowslide (avalanche) — *see* Landslide
stone W20.8
structure W20.1
burning (uncontrolled fire) X00.3
through
bridge W13.1
floor W13.3
roof W13.2
wall W13.8
window W13.4
timber W20.8
tree (caused by lightning) W20.8
while being carried or supported by other person(s) W04
Fallen on by
animal (not being ridden) NEC W55.89
Felo-de-se — *see* Suicide
Fight (hand) (fists) (foot) — *see* Assault, fight
Fire (accidental) — *see* Exposure, fire
Firearm discharge — *see* Discharge, firearm
Fireball effects from nuclear explosion in war operations — *see* War operations, nuclear weapons
Fireworks (explosion) W39
Flash burns from explosion — *see* Explosion
Flood (any injury) (caused by) X38
collapse of man-made structure causing earth movement X36.0
tidal wave — *see* Forces of nature, tidal wave
Food (any type) **in**
air passages (with asphyxia, obstruction, or suffocation) — *see* categories T17 and T18
alimentary tract causing asphyxia (due to compression of trachea) — *see* categories T17 and T18
Forces of nature X39.8
avalanche X36.1
causing transport accident — *see* Accident, transport, by type of vehicle
blizzard X37.2
cataclysmic storm X37.9
with flood X38
blizzard X37.2
cloudburst X37.8
cyclone X37.1
dust storm X37.3
hurricane X37.0
specified storm NEC X37.8
storm surge X37.0
tornado X37.1
twister X37.1
typhoon X37.0
cloudburst X37.8
cold (natural) X31
cyclone X37.1
dam collapse causing earth movement X36.0
dust storm X37.3
earth movement X36.1
earthquake X34
caused by dam or structure collapse X36.0
earthquake X34
flood (caused by) X38
dam collapse X36.0
tidal wave — *see* Forces of nature, tidal wave
heat (natural) X30
hurricane X37.0
landslide X36.1
causing transport accident — *see* Accident, transport, by type of vehicle
lightning — *see* subcategory T75.0
causing fire — *see* Exposure, fire
mudslide X36.1
causing transport accident — *see* Accident, transport, by type of vehicle
radiation (natural) X39.08
radon X39.01
radon X39.01
specified force NEC X39.8
storm surge X37.0
structure collapse causing earth movement X36.0
sunlight X32

Forces of nature - *continued*
tidal wave X37.41
due to
earthquake X37.41
landslide X37.43
storm X37.42
volcanic eruption X37.41
tornado X37.1
tsunami X37.41
twister X37.1
typhoon X37.0
volcanic eruption X35
Foreign body
aspiration — *see* Index to Diseases and Injuries, Foreign body, respiratory tract
embedded in skin W45
entering through skin W45.8
can lid W26.8
nail W45.0
paper W26.2
specified NEC W45.8
splinter W45.8
Forest fire (exposure to) — *see* Exposure, fire, uncontrolled, not in building
Found injured X58
from exposure (to) — *see* Exposure
on
highway, road (way), street V89.9
railway right of way V81.9
Fracture (circumstances unknown or unspecified) X58
due to specified cause NEC X58
Freezing — *see* Exposure, cold
Frostbite X31
due to man-made conditions — *see* Exposure, cold, man-made
Frozen — *see* Exposure, cold

G

Gored by bull W55.22
Gunshot wound W34.00

H

Hailstones, injured by X39.8
Hanged herself or himself — *see* Hanging, self-inflicted
Hanging (accidental) (*see also* category T71)
legal execution — *see* Legal, intervention, specified means NEC
Heat (effects of) (excessive) X30
due to
man-made conditions W92
on board watercraft V93.29
fishing boat V93.22
merchant ship V93.20
passenger ship V93.21
sailboat V93.24
specified powered craft NEC V93.23
weather (conditions) X30
from
electric heating apparatus causing burning X16
nuclear explosion in war operations — *see* War operations, nuclear weapons
inappropriate in local application or packing in medical or surgical procedure Y63.5
Hemorrhage
delayed following medical or surgical treatment without mention of misadventure — *see* Index to Diseases and Injuries, Complication(s)
during medical or surgical treatment as misadventure — *see* Index to Diseases and Injuries, Complication(s)
High
altitude (effects) - — *see* Air, pressure, low
level of radioactivity, effects — *see* Radiation
pressure (effects) - — *see* Air, pressure, high
temperature, effects — *see* Heat
Hit, hitting (accidental) **by** — *see* Struck by
Hitting against — *see* Striking against
Homicide (attempt) (justifiable) — *see* Assault
Hot
place, effects — *see also* Heat
weather, effects X30
House fire (uncontrolled) — *see* Exposure, fire, uncontrolled, building
Humidity, causing problem X39.8
Hunger X58
Hurricane (any injury) X37.0
Hypobarism, hypobaropathy - — *see* Air, pressure, low

I

Ictus
caloris — *see also* Heat

Ictus - *continued*
solaris X30
Ignition (accidental) — *see also* Exposure, fire X08.8
anesthetic gas in operating room W40.1
apparel X06.2
from highly flammable material X04
nightwear X05
bed linen (sheets) (spreads) (pillows) (mattress) — *see* Exposure, fire, uncontrolled, building, bed
benzine X04
clothes, clothing NEC (from controlled fire) X06.2
from
highly flammable material X04
ether X04
in operating room W40.1
explosive material — *see* Explosion
gasoline X04
jewelry (plastic) (any) X06.0
kerosene X04
material
explosive — *see* Explosion
highly flammable with secondary explosion X04
nightwear X05
paraffin X04
petrol X04
Immersion (accidental) — *see also* Drowning
hand or foot due to cold (excessive) X31
Implantation of quills of porcupine W55.89
Inanition (from) (hunger) X58
thirst X58
Inappropriate operation performed
correct operation on wrong side or body part (wrong side) (wrong site) Y65.53
operation intended for another patient done on wrong patient Y65.52
wrong operation performed on correct patient Y65.51
Inattention after, at birth (homicidal intent) (infanticidal intent) X58
Incident, adverse
device
anesthesiology Y70.8
accessory Y70.2
diagnostic Y70.0
miscellaneous Y70.8
monitoring Y70.0
prosthetic Y70.2
rehabilitative Y70.1
surgical Y70.3
therapeutic Y70.1
cardiovascular Y71.8
accessory Y71.2
diagnostic Y71.0
miscellaneous Y71.8
monitoring Y71.0
prosthetic Y71.2
rehabilitative Y71.1
surgical Y71.3
therapeutic Y71.1
gastroenterology Y73.8
accessory Y73.2
diagnostic Y73.0
miscellaneous Y73.8
monitoring Y73.0
prosthetic Y73.2
rehabilitative Y73.1
surgical Y73.3
therapeutic Y73.1
general
hospital Y74.8
accessory Y74.2
diagnostic Y74.0
miscellaneous Y74.8
monitoring Y74.0
prosthetic Y74.2
rehabilitative Y74.1
surgical Y74.3
therapeutic Y74.1
surgical Y81.8
accessory Y81.2
diagnostic Y81.0
miscellaneous Y81.8
monitoring Y81.0
prosthetic Y81.2
rehabilitative Y81.1
surgical Y81.3
therapeutic Y81.1
gynecological Y76.8
accessory Y76.2
diagnostic Y76.0
miscellaneous Y76.8
monitoring Y76.0

Incident, adverse - *continued*
 device - *continued*
 gynecological - *continued*
 prosthetic Y76.2
 rehabilitative Y76.1
 surgical Y76.3
 therapeutic Y76.1
 medical Y82.9
 specified type NEC Y82.8
 neurological Y75.8
 accessory Y75.2
 diagnostic Y75.0
 miscellaneous Y75.8
 monitoring Y75.0
 prosthetic Y75.2
 rehabilitative Y75.1
 surgical Y75.3
 therapeutic Y75.1
 obstetrical Y76.8
 accessory Y76.2
 diagnostic Y76.0
 miscellaneous Y76.8
 monitoring Y76.0
 prosthetic Y76.2
 rehabilitative Y76.1
 surgical Y76.3
 therapeutic Y76.1
 ophthalmic Y77.8
 accessory Y77.2
 diagnostic Y77.0
 miscellaneous Y77.8
 monitoring Y77.0
 prosthetic Y77.2
 rehabilitative Y77.1
 surgical Y77.3
 therapeutic Y77.1
 orthopedic Y79.8
 accessory Y79.2
 diagnostic Y79.0
 miscellaneous Y79.8
 monitoring Y79.0
 prosthetic Y79.2
 rehabilitative Y79.1
 surgical Y79.3
 therapeutic Y79.1
 otorhinolaryngological Y72.8
 accessory Y72.2
 diagnostic Y72.0
 miscellaneous Y72.8
 monitoring Y72.0
 prosthetic Y72.2
 rehabilitative Y72.1
 surgical Y72.3
 therapeutic Y72.1
 personal use Y74.8
 accessory Y74.2
 diagnostic Y74.0
 miscellaneous Y74.8
 monitoring Y74.0
 prosthetic Y74.2
 rehabilitative Y74.1
 surgical Y74.3
 therapeutic Y74.1
 physical medicine Y80.8
 accessory Y80.2
 diagnostic Y80.0
 miscellaneous Y80.8
 monitoring Y80.0
 prosthetic Y80.2
 rehabilitative Y80.1
 surgical Y80.3
 therapeutic Y80.1
 plastic surgical Y81.8
 accessory Y81.2
 diagnostic Y81.0
 miscellaneous Y81.8
 monitoring Y81.0
 prosthetic Y81.2
 rehabilitative Y81.1
 surgical Y81.3
 therapeutic Y81.1
 radiological Y78.8
 accessory Y78.2
 diagnostic Y78.0
 miscellaneous Y78.8
 monitoring Y78.0
 prosthetic Y78.2
 rehabilitative Y78.1
 surgical Y78.3
 therapeutic Y78.1
 urology Y73.8
 accessory Y73.2
 diagnostic Y73.0

Incident, adverse - *continued*
 device - *continued*
 urology - *continued*
 miscellaneous Y73.8
 monitoring Y73.0
 prosthetic Y73.2
 rehabilitative Y73.1
 surgical Y73.3
 therapeutic Y73.1
Incineration (accidental) — *see* Exposure, fire
Infanticide — *see* Assault
Infrasound waves (causing injury) W49.9
Ingestion
 foreign body (causing injury) (with
 obstruction) — *see* Foreign body, alimentary
 canal
 poisonous
 plant (s) X58
 substance NEC — *see* Table of Drugs and
 Chemicals
Inhalation
 excessively cold substance, man-made — *see*
 Exposure, cold, man-made
 food (any type) (into respiratory tract) (with
 asphyxia, obstruction respiratory tract,
 suffocation) — *see* categories T17 and T18
 foreign body — *see* Foreign body, aspiration
 gastric contents (with asphyxia, obstruction
 respiratory passage, suffocation) T17.81-
 hot air or gases X14.0
 liquid air, hydrogen, nitrogen W93.12
 suicide (attempt) X83.2
 steam X13.0
 assault X98.0
 stated as undetermined whether accidental or
 intentional Y27.0
 suicide (attempt) X77.0
 toxic gas — *see* Table of Drugs and Chemicals
 vomitus (with asphyxia, obstruction respiratory
 passage, suffocation) T17.81-
Injury, injured (accidental (ly)) **NOS** X58
 by, caused by, from
 assault — *see* Assault
 law-enforcing agent, police, in course of legal
 intervention — *see* Legal intervention
 suicide (attempt) X83.8
 due to, in
 civil insurrection — *see* War operations
 fight — *see also* Assault, fight Y04.0
 war operations — *see* War operations
 homicide — *see also* Assault Y09
 inflicted (by)
 in course of arrest (attempted) , suppression of
 disturbance, maintenance of order, by law-
 enforcing agents — *see* Legal intervention
 other person
 stated as
 accidental X58
 intentional, homicide (attempt) — *see* Assault
 undetermined whether accidental or
 intentional Y33
 purposely (inflicted) by other person (s) — *see*
 Assault
 self-inflicted X83.8
 stated as accidental X58
 specified cause NEC X58
 undetermined whether accidental or intentional Y33
Insolation, effects X30
Insufficient nourishment X58
Interruption of respiration (by)
 food (lodged in esophagus) — *see* categories T17
 and T18
 vomitus (lodged in esophagus) T17.81-
Intervention, legal — *see* Legal intervention
Intoxication
 drug — *see* Table of Drugs and Chemicals
 poison — *see* Table of Drugs and Chemicals

J

Jammed (accidentally)
 between objects (moving) (stationary and
 moving) W23.0
 stationary W23.1
Jumped, jumping
 before moving object NEC X81.8
 motor vehicle X81.0
 subway train X81.1
 train X81.1
 undetermined whether accidental or
 intentional Y31
 from
 boat (into water) voluntarily, without accident (to
 or on boat) W16.712

Jumped, jumping - *continued*
 from - *continued*
 boat (into water) voluntarily, without accident (to
 or on boat) - *continued*
 with
 accident to or on boat — *see* Accident,
 watercraft
 drowning or submersion W16.711
 suicide (attempt) X71.3
 striking bottom W16.722
 causing drowning W16.721
 building — *see also* Jumped, from, high
 place W13.9
 burning (uncontrolled fire) X00.5
 high place NEC W17.89
 suicide (attempt) X80
 undetermined whether accidental or
 intentional Y30
 structure — *see also* Jumped, from, high
 place W13.9
 burning (uncontrolled fire) X00.5
 into water W16.92
 causing drowning W16.91
 from, off watercraft — *see* Jumped, from, boat
 in
 natural body W16.612
 causing drowning W16.611
 striking bottom W16.622
 causing drowning W16.621
 specified place NEC W16.812
 causing drowning W16.811
 striking
 bottom W16.822
 causing drowning W16.821
 wall W16.832
 causing drowning W16.831
 swimming pool W16.512
 causing drowning W16.511
 striking
 bottom W16.522
 causing drowning W16.521
 wall W16.532
 causing drowning W16.531
 suicide (attempt) X71.3

K

Kicked by
 animal NEC W55.82
 person (s) (accidentally) W50.1
 with intent to injure or kill Y04.0
 as, or caused by, a crowd or human stampede (with
 fall) W52
 assault Y04.0
 homicide (attempt) Y04.0
 in
 fight Y04.0
 legal intervention
 injuring
 bystander Y35.812
 law enforcement personnel Y35.811
 suspect Y35.813
Kicking
 against
 object W22.8
 sports equipment W21.9
 stationary W22.09
 sports equipment W21.89
 person — *see* Striking against, person
 sports equipment W21.9
 carpet stretcher with knee X50.3
Killed, killing (accidentally) **NOS** — *see
 also* Injury X58
 in
 action — *see* War operations
 brawl, fight (hand) (fists) (foot) Y04.0
 by weapon — *see also* Assault
 cutting, piercing — *see* Assault, cutting or
 piercing instrument
 firearm — *see* Discharge, firearm, by type,
 homicide
 self
 stated as
 accident NOS X58
 suicide — *see* Suicide
 undetermined whether accidental or
 intentional Y33
Kneeling (prolonged) (static) X50.1
Knocked down (accidentally) (by) **NOS** X58
 animal (not being ridden) NEC — *see also* Struck
 by, by type of animal
 crowd or human stampede W52
 person W51
 in brawl, fight Y04.0

Knocked down (accidentally) (by) **NOS** - *continued*
transport vehicle NEC — *see also* Accident,
transport V09.9

L

Laceration NEC — *see* Injury
Lack of
care (helpless person) (infant) (newborn) X58
food except as result of abandonment or neglect X58
due to abandonment or neglect X58
water except as result of transport accident X58
due to transport accident — *see* Accident,
transport, by type
helpless person, infant, newborn X58
Landslide (falling on transport vehicle) X36.1
caused by collapse of man-made structure X36.0
Late effect — *see* Sequelae
Legal
execution (any method) — *see* Legal, intervention
intervention (by)
baton — *see* Legal, intervention, blunt object,
baton
bayonet — *see* Legal, intervention, sharp object,
bayonet
blow — *see* Legal, intervention, manhandling
blunt object
baton
injuring
bystander Y35.312
law enforcement personnel Y35.311
suspect Y35.313
injuring
bystander Y35.302
law enforcement personnel Y35.301
suspect Y35.303
specified NEC
injuring
bystander Y35.392
law enforcement personnel Y35.391
suspect Y35.393
stave
injuring
bystander Y35.392
law enforcement personnel Y35.391
suspect Y35.393
bomb — *see* Legal, intervention, explosive
cutting or piercing instrument — *see* Legal,
intervention, sharp object
dynamite — *see* Legal, intervention, explosive,
dynamite
explosive (s)
dynamite
injuring
bystander Y35.112
law enforcement personnel Y35.111
suspect Y35.113
grenade
injuring
bystander Y35.192
law enforcement personnel Y35.191
suspect Y35.193
injuring
bystander Y35.102
law enforcement personnel Y35.101
suspect Y35.103
mortar bomb
injuring
bystander Y35.192
law enforcement personnel Y35.191
suspect Y35.193
shell
injuring
bystander Y35.122
law enforcement personnel Y35.121
suspect Y35.123
specified NEC
injuring
bystander Y35.192
law enforcement personnel Y35.191
suspect Y35.193
firearm (s) (discharge)
handgun
injuring
bystander Y35.022
law enforcement personnel Y35.021
suspect Y35.023
injuring
bystander Y35.002
law enforcement personnel Y35.001
suspect Y35.003
machine gun
injuring
bystander Y35.012

Legal - *continued*
intervention (by) - *continued*
firearm (s) (discharge) - *continued*
machine gun - *continued*
injuring - *continued*
law enforcement personnel Y35.011
suspect Y35.013
rifle pellet
injuring
bystander Y35.032
law enforcement personnel Y35.031
suspect Y35.033
rubber bullet
injuring
bystander Y35.042
law enforcement personnel Y35.041
suspect Y35.043
shotgun — *see* Legal, intervention, firearm,
specified NEC
specified NEC
injuring
bystander Y35.092
law enforcement personnel Y35.091
suspect Y35.093
gas (asphyxiation) (poisoning)
injuring
bystander Y35.202
law enforcement personnel Y35.201
suspect Y35.203
specified NEC
injuring
bystander Y35.292
law enforcement personnel Y35.291
suspect Y35.293
tear gas
injuring
bystander Y35.212
law enforcement personnel Y35.211
suspect Y35.213
grenade — *see* Legal, intervention, explosive,
grenade
injuring
bystander Y35.92
law enforcement personnel Y35.91
suspect Y35.93
late effect (of) — *see* with 7th character S Y35
manhandling
injuring
bystander Y35.812
law enforcement personnel Y35.811
suspect Y35.813
sequelae (of) — *see* with 7th character S Y35
sharp objects
bayonet
injuring
bystander Y35.412
law enforcement personnel Y35.411
suspect Y35.413
injuring
bystander Y35.402
law enforcement personnel Y35.401
suspect Y35.403
specified NEC
injuring
bystander Y35.492
law enforcement personnel Y35.491
suspect Y35.493
specified means NEC
injuring
bystander Y35.892
law enforcement personnel Y35.891
suspect Y35.893
stabbing — *see* Legal, intervention, sharp object
stave — *see* Legal, intervention, blunt object, stave
tear gas — *see* Legal, intervention, gas, tear gas
truncheon — *see* Legal, intervention, blunt object,
stave
Lifting — *see also* Overexertion
heavy objects X50.0
weights X50.0
Lightning (shock) (stroke) (struck by) — *see*
subcategory T75.0
causing fire — *see* Exposure, fire
Loss of control (transport vehicle) **NEC** — *see*
Accident, transport
Lost at sea NOS — *see* Drowning, due to, fall
overboard
Low
pressure (effects) - — *see* Air, pressure, low
temperature (effects) — *see* Exposure, cold
**Lying before train, vehicle or other moving
object** X81.8
subway train X81.1

Lying before train, vehicle or other moving object -
continued
train X81.1
undetermined whether accidental or intentional Y31
Lynching — *see* Assault

M

Malfunction (mechanism or component) (of)
firearm W34.10
airgun W34.110
BB gun W34.110
gas, air or spring-operated gun NEC W34.118
handgun W32.1
hunting rifle W33.12
larger firearm W33.10
specified NEC W33.19
machine gun W33.13
paintball gun W34.111
pellet gun W34.110
shotgun W33.11
specified NEC W34.19
Very pistol [flare] W34.19
handgun — *see* Malfunction, firearm, handgun
Maltreatment — *see* Perpetrator
Mangled (accidentally) **NOS** X58
Manhandling (in brawl, fight) Y04.0
legal intervention — *see* Legal, intervention,
manhandling
Manslaughter (nonaccidental) — *see* Assault
Mauled by animal NEC W55.89
Medical procedure, complication of (delayed or as
an abnormal reaction without mention of
misadventure) — *see* Complication of or
following, by specified type of procedure
due to or as a result of misadventure — *see*
Misadventure
Melting (due to fire) — *see also* Exposure, fire
apparel NEC X06.3
clothes, clothing NEC X06.3
nightwear X05
fittings or furniture (burning building) (uncontrolled
fire) X00.8
nightwear X05
plastic jewelry X06.1
Mental cruelty X58
Military operations (injuries to military and civilians
occuring during peacetime on military property
and during routine military exercises and
operations) (by) (from) (involving) Y37.90-
air blast Y37.20-
aircraft
destruction — *see* Military operations, destruction
of aircraft
airway restriction — *see* Military operations,
restriction of airways
asphyxiation — *see* Military operations, restriction
of airways
biological weapons Y37.6X-
blast Y37.20-
blast fragments Y37.20-
blast wave Y37.20-
blast wind Y37.20-
bomb Y37.20-
dirty Y37.50-
gasoline Y37.31-
incendiary Y37.31-
petrol Y37.31-
bullet Y37.43-
incendiary Y37.32-
rubber Y37.41-
chemical weapons Y37.7X-
combat
hand to hand (unarmed) combat Y37.44-
using blunt or piercing object Y37.45-
conflagration — *see* Military operations, fire
conventional warfare NEC Y37.49-
depth-charge Y37.01-
destruction of aircraft Y37.10-
due to
air to air missile Y37.11-
collision with other aircraft Y37.12-
detonation (accidental) of onboard munitions and
explosives Y37.14-
enemy fire or explosives Y37.11-
explosive placed on aircraft Y37.11-
onboard fire Y37.13-
rocket propelled grenade [RPG] Y37.11-
small arms fire Y37.11-
surface to air missile Y37.11-
specified NEC Y37.19-
detonation (accidental) of
onboard marine weapons Y37.05-
own munitions or munitions launch device Y37.24-

Military operations
(injuries to military and civilians occuring during
peacetime on military property and during routine
military exercises and operations) (by) (from)
(involving) - *continued*
  dirty bomb Y37.50-
  explosion (of) Y37.20-
    aerial bomb Y37.21-
    bomb NOS — *see also* Military operations,
      bomb(s) Y37.20-
    own munitions or munitions launch device
      (accidental) Y37.24-
    fragments Y37.20-
    grenade Y37.29-
    guided missile Y37.22-
    improvised explosive device [IED] (person-borne)
      (roadside) (vehicle-borne) Y37.23-
    land mine Y37.29-
    marine mine (at sea) (in harbor) Y37.02-
    marine weapon Y37.00-
      specified NEC Y37.09-
    sea-based artillery shell Y37.03-
    specified NEC Y37.29-
    torpedo Y37.04-
  fire Y37.30-
    specified NEC Y37.39-
  firearms
    discharge Y37.43-
    pellets Y37.42-
  flamethrower Y37.33-
  fragments (from) (of)
    improvised explosive device [IED] (person-borne)
      (roadside) (vehicle-borne) Y37.26-
    munitions Y37.25-
    specified NEC Y37.29-
    weapons Y37.27-
  friendly fire Y37.92-
  hand to hand (unarmed) combat Y37.44-
  hot substances — *see* Military operations, fire
  incendiary bullet Y37.32-
  nuclear weapon (effects of) Y37.50-
    acute radiation exposure Y37.54-
    blast pressure Y37.51-
    direct blast Y37.51-
    direct heat Y37.53-
    fallout exposure Y37.54-
    fireball Y37.53-
    indirect blast (struck or crushed by blast debris)
      (being thrown by blast) Y37.52-
    ionizing radiation (immediate exposure) Y37.54-
    nuclear radiation Y37.54-
    radiation
      ionizing (immediate exposure) Y37.54-
        nuclear Y37.54-
        thermal Y37.53-
      specified NEC Y37.59-
      secondary effects Y37.54-
      thermal radiation Y37.53-
  restriction of air (airway)
    intentional Y37.46-
    unintentional Y37.47-
  rubber bullets Y37.41-
  shrapnel NOS Y37.29-
  suffocation — *see* Military operations, restriction of
    airways
  unconventional warfare NEC Y37.7X-
  underwater blast NOS Y37.00-
  warfare
    conventional NEC Y37.49-
    unconventional NEC Y37.7X-
  weapons
    biological weapons Y37.6X-
    chemical Y37.7X-
    nuclear (effects of) Y37.50-
      acute radiation exposure Y37.54-
      blast pressure Y37.51-
      direct blast Y37.51-
      direct heat Y37.53-
      fallout exposure Y37.54-
      fireball Y37.53-
      indirect blast (struck or crushed by blast debris)
        (being thrown by blast) Y37.52-
      radiation
        ionizing (immediate exposure) Y37.54-
          nuclear Y37.54-
          thermal Y37.53-
        secondary effects Y37.54-
        specified NEC Y37.59-
    of mass destruction [WMD] Y37.91-
  weapon of mass destruction [WMD] Y37.91-

Misadventure (s) **to patient** (s) **during surgical or**
  medical care Y69
  contaminated medical or biological substance
    (blood, drug, fluid) Y64.9
    administered (by) NEC Y64.9
      immunization Y64.1
      infusion Y64.0
      injection Y64.1
      specified means NEC Y64.8
      transfusion Y64.0
      vaccination Y64.1
  excessive amount of blood or other fluid during
    transfusion or infusion Y63.0
  failure
    in dosage Y63.9
      electroshock therapy Y63.4
      inappropriate temperature (too hot or too cold) in
        local application and packing Y63.5
      infusion
        excessive amount of fluid Y63.0
        incorrect dilution of fluid Y63.1
      insulin-shock therapy Y63.4
      nonadministration of necessary drug or biological
        substance Y63.6
      overdose — *see* Table of Drugs and Chemicals
        radiation, in therapy Y63.2
      radiation
        overdose Y63.2
      specified procedure NEC Y63.8
      transfusion
        excessive amount of blood Y63.0
    mechanical, of instrument or apparatus (any)
      (during any procedure) Y65.8
    sterile precautions (during procedure) Y62.9
      aspiration of fluid or tissue (by puncture or
        catheterization, except heart) Y62.6
      biopsy (except needle aspiration) Y62.8
        needle (aspirating) Y62.6
      blood sampling Y62.6
      catheterization Y62.6
        heart Y62.5
      dialysis (kidney) Y62.2
      endoscopic examination Y62.4
      enema Y62.8
      immunization Y62.3
      infusion Y62.1
      injection Y62.3
      needle biopsy Y62.6
      paracentesis (abdominal) (thoracic) Y62.6
      perfusion Y62.2
      puncture (lumbar) Y62.6
      removal of catheter or packing Y62.8
      specified procedure NEC Y62.8
      surgical operation Y62.0
      transfusion Y62.1
      vaccination Y62.3
    suture or ligature during surgical procedure Y65.2
    to introduce or to remove tube or instrument — *see*
      Failure, to
  hemorrhage — *see* Index to Diseases and Injuries,
    Complication(s)
  inadvertent exposure of patient to radiation Y63.3
  inappropriate
    operation performed — *see* Inappropriate operation
      performed
    temperature (too hot or too cold) in local
      application or packing Y63.5
  infusion — *see also* Misadventure, by type,
    infusion Y69
    excessive amount of fluid Y63.0
    incorrect dilution of fluid Y63.1
    wrong fluid Y65.1
  mismatched blood in transfusion Y65.0
  nonadministration of necessary drug or biological
    substance Y63.6
  overdose — *see* Table of Drugs and Chemicals
    radiation (in therapy) Y63.2
  perforation — *see* Index to Diseases and Injuries,
    Complication(s)
  performance of inappropriate operation — *see*
    Inappropriate operation performed
  puncture — *see* Index to Diseases and Injuries,
    Complication(s)
  specified type NEC Y65.8
    failure
      suture or ligature during surgical operation Y65.2
      to introduce or to remove tube or
        instrument — *see* Failure, to
    infusion of wrong fluid Y65.1
    performance of inappropriate operation — *see*
      Inappropriate operation performed
    transfusion of mismatched blood Y65.0
    wrong

Misadventure (s) **to patient** (s)
  during surgical or medical care - *continued*
    specified type NEC - *continued*
      wrong - *continued*
        fluid in infusion Y65.1
        placement of endotracheal tube during anesthetic
          procedure Y65.3
    transfusion — *see* Misadventure, by type,
      transfusion
      excessive amount of blood Y63.0
      mismatched blood Y65.0
    wrong
      drug given in error — *see* Table of Drugs and
        Chemicals
      fluid in infusion Y65.1
      placement of endotracheal tube during anesthetic
        procedure Y65.3
Mismatched blood in transfusion Y65.0
Motion sickness T75.3
Mountain sickness W94.11
Mudslide (of cataclysmic nature) — *see* Landslide
Murder (attempt) — *see* Assault

N

Nail
  contact with W45.0
    gun W29.4
  embedded in skin W45.0
Neglect (criminal) (homicidal intent) X58
Noise (causing injury) (pollution) W42.9
  supersonic W42.0
Nonadministration (of)
  drug or biological substance (necessary) Y63.6
  surgical and medical care Y66
Nosocomial condition Y95

O

Object
  falling
    from, in, on, hitting
      machinery — *see* Contact, with, by type of
        machine
  set in motion by
    accidental explosion or rupture of pressure
      vessel W38
    firearm — *see* Discharge, firearm, by type
    machine (ry) — *see* Contact, with, by type of
      machine
Overdose (drug) — *see* Table of Drugs and
  Chemicals
  radiation Y63.2
Overexertion X50.9
  from
    prolonged static or awkward postures X50.1
    repetitive movements X50.3
    specified strenuous movements or postures
      NEC X50.9
    strenuous movement or load X50.0
Overexposure (accidental) (to)
  cold — *see also* Exposure, cold X31
    due to man-made conditions — *see* Exposure, cold,
      man-made
  heat — *see also* Heat X30
  radiation — *see* Radiation
  radioactivity W88.0
  sun (sunburn) X32
  weather NEC — *see* Forces of nature
  wind NEC — *see* Forces of nature
Overheated — *see* Heat
Overturning (accidental)
  machinery — *see* Contact, with, by type of machine
  transport vehicle NEC — *see also* Accident,
    transport V89.9
  watercraft (causing drowning, submersion) — *see*
    also Drowning, due to, accident to, watercraft,
    overturning
    causing injury except drowning or
      submersion — *see* Accident, watercraft,
      causing, injury NEC

P

Parachute descent (voluntary) (without accident to
  aircraft) V97.29
  due to accident to aircraft — *see* Accident, transport,
    aircraft
Pecked by bird W61.99
**Perforation during medical or surgical treatment
  as misadventure** — *see* Index to Diseases and
  Injuries, Complication(s)
**Perpetrator, perpetration, of assault, maltreatment
  and neglect** (by) Y07.9
  boyfriend Y07.03
  brother Y07.410
    stepbrother Y07.435

Perpetrator, perpetration, of assault, maltreatment and neglect (by) - *continued*
coach Y07.53
cousin
  female Y07.491
  male Y07.490
daycare provider Y07.519
  at-home
    adult care Y07.512
    childcare Y07.510
  care center
    adult care Y07.513
    childcare Y07.511
family member NEC Y07.499
father Y07.11
  adoptive Y07.13
  foster Y07.420
  stepfather Y07.430
foster father Y07.420
foster mother Y07.421
girl friend Y07.04
healthcare provider Y07.529
  mental health Y07.521
  specified NEC Y07.528
husband Y07.01
instructor Y07.53
mother Y07.12
  adoptive Y07.14
  foster Y07.421
  stepmother Y07.433
nonfamily member Y07.50
  specified NEC Y07.59
nurse Y07.528
occupational therapist Y07.528
partner of parent
  female Y07.434
  male Y07.432
physical therapist Y07.528
sister Y07.411
speech therapist Y07.528
stepbrother Y07.435
stepfather Y07.430
stepmother Y07.433
stepsister Y07.436
teacher Y07.53
wife Y07.02
Piercing — *see* Contact, with, by type of object or machine
Pinched
  between objects (moving) (stationary and moving) W23.0
  stationary W23.1
Pinned under machine (ry) — *see* Contact, with, by type of machine
Place of occurrence Y92.9
abandoned house Y92.89
airplane Y92.813
airport Y92.520
ambulatory health services establishment NEC Y92.538
ambulatory surgery center Y92.530
amusement park Y92.831
apartment (co-op) — *see* Place of occurrence, residence, apartment
assembly hall Y92.29
bank Y92.510
barn Y92.71
baseball field Y92.320
basketball court Y92.310
beach Y92.832
boarding house — *see* Place of occurrence, residence, boarding house
boat Y92.814
bowling alley Y92.39
bridge Y92.89
building under construction Y92.61
bus Y92.811
  station Y92.521
cafe Y92.511
campsite Y92.833
campus — *see* Place of occurrence, school
canal Y92.89
car Y92.810
casino Y92.59
children's home — *see* Place of occurrence, residence, institutional, orphanage
church Y92.22
cinema Y92.26
clubhouse Y92.29
coal pit Y92.64
college (community) Y92.214
condominium — *see* Place of occurrence, residence, apartment

Place of occurrence - *continued*
construction area — *see* Place of occurrence, industrial and construction area
convalescent home — *see* Place of occurrence, residence, institutional, nursing home
court-house Y92.240
cricket ground Y92.328
cultural building Y92.258
  art gallery Y92.250
  museum Y92.251
  music hall Y92.252
  opera house Y92.253
  specified NEC Y92.258
  theater Y92.254
dancehall Y92.252
day nursery Y92.210
dentist office Y92.531
derelict house Y92.89
desert Y92.820
dock NOS Y92.89
dockyard Y92.62
doctor's office Y92.531
dormitory — *see* Place of occurrence, residence, institutional, school dormitory
dry dock Y92.62
factory (building) (premises) Y92.63
farm (land under cultivation) (outbuildings) Y92.79
  barn Y92.71
  chicken coop Y92.72
  field Y92.73
  hen house Y92.72
  house — *see* Place of occurrence, residence, house
  orchard Y92.74
  specified NEC Y92.79
football field Y92.321
forest Y92.821
freeway Y92.411
gallery Y92.250
garage (commercial) Y92.59
  boarding house Y92.044
  military base Y92.135
  mobile home Y92.025
  nursing home Y92.124
  orphanage Y92.114
  private house Y92.015
  reform school Y92.155
gas station Y92.524
gasworks Y92.69
golf course Y92.39
gravel pit Y92.64
grocery Y92.512
gymnasium Y92.39
handball court Y92.318
harbor Y92.89
harness racing course Y92.39
healthcare provider office Y92.531
highway (interstate) Y92.411
hill Y92.828
hockey rink Y92.330
home — *see* Place of occurrence, residence
hospice — *see* Place of occurrence, residence, institutional, nursing home
hospital Y92.239
  cafeteria Y92.233
  corridor Y92.232
  operating room Y92.234
  patient
    bathroom Y92.231
    room Y92.230
  specified NEC Y92.238
hotel Y92.59
house — *see also* Place of occurrence, residence
  abandoned Y92.89
  under construction Y92.61
industrial and construction area (yard) Y92.69
  building under construction Y92.61
  dock Y92.62
  dry dock Y92.62
  factory Y92.63
  gasworks Y92.69
  mine Y92.64
  oil rig Y92.65
  pit Y92.64
  power station Y92.69
  shipyard Y92.62
  specified NEC Y92.69
  tunnel under construction Y92.69
  workshop Y92.69
kindergarten Y92.211
lacrosse field Y92.328
lake Y92.828
library Y92.241
mall Y92.59

Place of occurrence - *continued*
market Y92.512
marsh Y92.828
military
  base — *see* Place of occurrence, residence, institutional, military base
  training ground Y92.84
mine Y92.64
mosque Y92.22
motel Y92.59
motorway (interstate) Y92.411
mountain Y92.828
movie-house Y92.26
museum Y92.251
music-hall Y92.252
not applicable Y92.9
nuclear power station Y92.69
nursing home — *see* Place of occurrence, residence, institutional, nursing home
office building Y92.59
offshore installation Y92.65
oil rig Y92.65
old people's home — *see* Place of occurrence, residence, institutional, specified NEC
opera-house Y92.253
orphanage — *see* Place of occurrence, residence, institutional, orphanage
outpatient surgery center Y92.530
park (public) Y92.830
  amusement Y92.831
parking garage Y92.89
  lot Y92.481
pavement Y92.480
physician office Y92.531
polo field Y92.328
pond Y92.828
post office Y92.242
power station Y92.69
prairie Y92.828
prison — *see* Place of occurrence, residence, institutional, prison
public
  administration building Y92.248
    city hall Y92.243
    courthouse Y92.240
    library Y92.241
    post office Y92.242
    specified NEC Y92.248
  building NEC Y92.29
  hall Y92.29
  place NOS Y92.89
race course Y92.39
radio station Y92.59
railway line (bridge) Y92.85
ranch (outbuildings) — *see* Place of occurrence, farm
recreation area Y92.838
  amusement park Y92.831
  beach Y92.832
  campsite Y92.833
  park (public) Y92.830
  seashore Y92.832
  specified NEC Y92.838
religious institution Y92.22
reform school - — *see* Place of occurrence, residence, institutional, reform school
residence (non-institutional) (private) Y92.009
  apartment Y92.039
    bathroom Y92.031
    bedroom Y92.032
    kitchen Y92.030
    specified NEC Y92.038
  bathroom Y92.002
  bedroom Y92.003
  boarding house Y92.049
    bathroom Y92.041
    bedroom Y92.042
    driveway Y92.043
    garage Y92.044
    garden Y92.046
    kitchen Y92.040
    specified NEC Y92.048
    swimming pool Y92.045
    yard Y92.046
  dining room Y92.001
  garden Y92.007
  home Y92.009
  house, single family Y92.019
    bathroom Y92.012
    bedroom Y92.013
    dining room Y92.011
    driveway Y92.014
    garage Y92.015

Place of occurrence - *continued*
  residence (non-institutional) (private) - *continued*
    house, single family - *continued*
      garden Y92.017
      kitchen Y92.010
      specified NEC Y92.018
      swimming pool Y92.016
      yard Y92.017
    institutional Y92.10
      children's home — *see* Place of occurrence, residence, institutional, orphanage
      hospice — *see* Place of occurrence, residence, institutional, nursing home
      military base Y92.139
        barracks Y92.133
        garage Y92.135
        garden Y92.137
        kitchen Y92.130
        mess hall Y92.131
        specified NEC Y92.138
        swimming pool Y92.136
        yard Y92.137
      nursing home Y92.129
        bathroom Y92.121
        bedroom Y92.122
        driveway Y92.123
        garage Y92.124
        garden Y92.126
        kitchen Y92.120
        specified NEC Y92.128
        swimming pool Y92.125
        yard Y92.126
      orphanage Y92.119
        bathroom Y92.111
        bedroom Y92.112
        driveway Y92.113
        garage Y92.114
        garden Y92.116
        kitchen Y92.110
        specified NEC Y92.118
        swimming pool Y92.115
        yard Y92.116
      prison Y92.149
        bathroom Y92.142
        cell Y92.143
        courtyard Y92.147
        dining room Y92.141
        kitchen Y92.140
        specified NEC Y92.148
        swimming pool Y92.146
      reform school Y92.159
        bathroom Y92.152
        bedroom Y92.153
        dining room Y92.151
        driveway Y92.154
        garage Y92.155
        garden Y92.157
        kitchen Y92.150
        specified NEC Y92.158
        swimming pool Y92.156
        yard Y92.157
      school dormitory Y92.169
        bathroom Y92.162
        bedroom Y92.163
        dining room Y92.161
        kitchen Y92.160
        specified NEC Y92.168
      specified NEC Y92.199
        bathroom Y92.192
        bedroom Y92.193
        dining room Y92.191
        driveway Y92.194
        garage Y92.195
        garden Y92.197
        kitchen Y92.190
        specified NEC Y92.198
        swimming pool Y92.196
        yard Y92.197
    kitchen Y92.000
    mobile home Y92.029
      bathroom Y92.022
      bedroom Y92.023
      dining room Y92.021
      driveway Y92.024
      garage Y92.025
      garden Y92.027
      kitchen Y92.020
      specified NEC Y92.028
      swimming pool Y92.026
      yard Y92.027
    specified place in residence NEC Y92.008
    specified residence type NEC Y92.099
      bathroom Y92.091

Place of occurrence - *continued*
  residence (non-institutional) (private) - *continued*
    specified residence type NEC - *continued*
      bedroom Y92.092
      driveway Y92.093
      garage Y92.094
      garden Y92.096
      kitchen Y92.090
      specified NEC Y92.098
      swimming pool Y92.095
      yard Y92.096
  restaurant Y92.511
  riding school Y92.39
  river Y92.828
  road Y92.488
  rodeo ring Y92.39
  rugby field Y92.328
  same day surgery center Y92.530
  sand pit Y92.64
  school (private) (public) (state) Y92.219
    college Y92.214
    daycare center Y92.210
    elementary school Y92.211
    high school Y92.213
    kindergarten Y92.211
    middle school Y92.212
    specified NEC Y92.218
    trace school Y92.215
    university Y92.214
    vocational school Y92.215
  sea (shore) Y92.832
  senior citizen center Y92.29
  service area
    airport Y92.520
    bus station Y92.521
    gas station Y92.524
    highway rest stop Y92.523
    railway station Y92.522
  shipyard Y92.62
  shop (commercial) Y92.513
  sidewalk Y92.480
  silo Y92.79
  skating rink (roller) Y92.331
    ice Y92.330
  slaughter house Y92.86
  soccer field Y92.322
  specified place NEC Y92.89
  sports area Y92.39
    athletic
      court Y92.318
        basketball Y92.310
        specified NEC Y92.318
        squash Y92.311
        tennis Y92.312
      field Y92.328
        baseball Y92.320
        cricket ground Y92.328
        football Y92.321
        hockey Y92.328
        soccer Y92.322
        specified NEC Y92.328
    golf course Y92.39
    gymnasium Y92.39
    riding school Y92.39
    skating rink (roller) Y92.331
      ice Y92.330
    stadium Y92.39
    swimming pool Y92.34
  squash court Y92.311
  stadium Y92.39
  steeplechasing course Y92.39
  store Y92.512
  stream Y92.828
  street and highway Y92.410
    bike path Y92.482
    freeway Y92.411
    highway ramp Y92.415
    interstate highway Y92.411
    local residential or business street Y92.414
    motorway Y92.411
    parkway Y92.412
    parking lot Y92.481
    sidewalk Y92.480
    specified NEC Y92.488
    state road Y92.413
  subway car Y92.816
  supermarket Y92.512
  swamp Y92.828
  swimming pool (public) Y92.34
    private (at) Y92.095
      boarding house Y92.045
      military base Y92.136
      mobile home Y92.026

Place of occurrence - *continued*
  swimming pool (public) - *continued*
    private (at) - *continued*
      nursing home Y92.125
      orphanage Y92.115
      prison Y92.146
      reform school Y92.156
      single family residence Y92.016
  synagogue Y92.22
  television station Y92.59
  tennis court Y92.312
  theater Y92.254
  trade area Y92.59
    bank Y92.510
    cafe Y92.511
    casino Y92.59
    garage Y92.59
    hotel Y92.59
    market Y92.512
    office building Y92.59
    radio station Y92.59
    restaurant Y92.511
    shop Y92.513
    shopping mall Y92.59
    store Y92.512
    supermarket Y92.512
    television station Y92.59
    warehouse Y92.59
  trailer park, residential — *see* Place of occurrence, residence, mobile home
  trailer site NOS Y92.89
  train Y92.815
    station Y92.522
  truck Y92.812
  tunnel under construction Y92.69
  urgent (health) care center Y92.532
  university Y92.214
  vehicle (transport) Y92.818
    airplane Y92.813
    boat Y92.814
    bus Y92.811
    car Y92.810
    specified NEC Y92.818
    subway car Y92.816
    train Y92.815
    truck Y92.812
  warehouse Y92.59
  water reservoir Y92.89
  wilderness area Y92.828
    desert Y92.820
    forest Y92.821
    marsh Y92.828
    mountain Y92.828
    prairie Y92.828
    specified NEC Y92.828
    swamp Y92.828
  workshop Y92.69
  yard, private Y92.096
    boarding house Y92.046
    single family house Y92.017
    mobile home Y92.027
  youth center Y92.29
  zoo (zoological garden) Y92.834
Plumbism — *see* Table of Drugs and Chemicals, lead
Poisoning (accidental) (by) — *see also* Table of Drugs and Chemicals
  by plant, thorns, spines, sharp leaves or other mechanisms NEC X58
  carbon monoxide
    generated by
      motor vehicle — *see* Accident, transport
      watercraft (in transit) (not in transit) V93.89
        ferry boat V93.81
        fishing boat V93.82
        jet skis V93.83
        liner V93.81
        merchant ship V93.80
        passenger ship V93.81
        powered craft NEC V93.83
  caused by injection of poisons into skin by plant thorns, spines, sharp leaves X58
  marine or sea plants (venomous) X58
  exhaust gas
    generated by
      motor vehicle — *see* Accident, transport
      watercraft (in transit) (not in transit) V93.89
        ferry boat V93.81
        fishing boat V93.82
        jet skis V93.83
        liner V93.81
        merchant ship V93.80
        passenger ship V93.81
        powered craft NEC V93.83

Poisoning (accidental) (by) - *continued*
fumes or smoke due to
explosion — *see also* Explosion W40.9
fire — *see* Exposure, fire
ignition — *see* Ignition
gas
in legal intervention — *see* Legal, intervention, gas
legal execution — *see* Legal, intervention, gas
in war operations — *see* War operations
legal
execution — *see* Legal, intervention, gas
intervention
by gas — *see* Legal, intervention, gas
other specified means — *see* Legal, intervention, specified means NEC
Powder burn (by) (from)
airgun W34.110
BB gun W34.110
firearm NEC W34.19
gas, air or spring-operated gun NEC W34.118
handgun W32.1
hunting rifle W33.12
larger firearm W33.10
specified NEC W33.19
machine gun W33.13
paintball gun W34.111
pellet gun W34.110
shotgun W33.11
Very pistol [flare] W34.19
Premature cessation (of) **surgical and medical care** Y66
Privation (food) (water) X58
Procedure (operation)
correct, on wrong side or body part (wrong side) (wrong site) Y65.53
intended for another patient done on wrong patient Y65.52
performed on patient not scheduled for surgery Y65.52
performed on wrong patient Y65.52
wrong, performed on correct patient Y65.51
Prolonged
sitting in transport vehicle — *see* Travel, by type of vehicle
stay in
high altitude as cause of anoxia, barodontalgia, barotitis or hypoxia W94.11
weightless environment X52
Pulling, excessive — *see also* Overexertion X50.9
Puncture, puncturing — *see also* Contact, with, by type of object or machine
by
plant thorns, spines, sharp leaves or other mechanisms NEC W60
during medical or surgical treatment as misadventure — *see* Index to Diseases and Injuries, Complication(s)
Pushed, pushing (accidental) (injury in)
by other person (s) (accidental) W51
with fall W03
due to ice or snow W00.0
as, or caused by, a crowd or human stampede (with fall) W52
before moving object NEC Y02.8
motor vehicle Y02.0
subway train Y02.1
train Y02.1
from
high place NEC
in accidental circumstances W17.89
stated as
intentional, homicide (attempt) Y01
undetermined whether accidental or intentional Y30
transport vehicle NEC — *see also* Accident, transport V89.9
stated as
intentional, homicide (attempt) Y08.89
overexertion X50.9

R

Radiation (exposure to)
arc lamps W89.0
atomic power plant (malfunction) NEC W88.1
complication of or abnormal reaction to medical radiotherapy Y84.2
electromagnetic, ionizing W88.0
gamma rays W88.1
in
war operations (from or following nuclear explosion) — *see* War operations
inadvertent exposure of patient (receiving test or therapy) Y63.3

Radiation (exposure to) - *continued*
infrared (heaters and lamps) W90.1
excessive heat from W92
ionized, ionizing (particles, artificially accelerated)
radioisotopes W88.1
specified NEC W88.8
x-rays W88.0
isotopes, radioactive — *see* Radiation, radioactive isotopes
laser (s) W90.2
in war operations — *see* War operations
misadventure in medical care Y63.2
light sources (man-made visible and ultraviolet) W89.9
natural X32
specified NEC W89.8
tanning bed W89.1
welding light W89.0
man-made visible light W89.9
specified NEC W89.8
tanning bed W89.1
welding light W89.0
microwave W90.8
misadventure in medical or surgical procedure Y63.2
natural NEC X39.08
radon X39.01
overdose (in medical or surgical procedure) Y63.2
radar W90.0
radioactive isotopes (any) W88.1
atomic power plant malfunction W88.1
misadventure in medical or surgical treatment Y63.2
radiofrequency W90.0
radium NEC W88.1
sun X32
ultraviolet (light) (man-made) W89.9
natural X32
specified NEC W89.8
tanning bed W89.1
welding light W89.0
welding arc, torch, or light W89.0
excessive heat from W92
x-rays (hard) (soft) W88.0
Range disease W94.11
Rape (attempted) T74.2-
Rat bite W53.11
Reaching (prolonged) (static) X50.1
Reaction, abnormal to medical procedure — *see also* Complication of or following, by type of procedure Y84.9
with misadventure — *see* Misadventure
biologicals — *see* Table of Drugs and Chemicals
drugs — *see* Table of Drugs and Chemicals
vaccine — *see* Table of Drugs and Chemicals
Recoil
airgun W34.110
BB gun W34.110
firearm NEC W34.19
gas, air or spring-operated gun NEC W34.118
handgun W32.1
hunting rifle W33.12
larger firearm W33.10
specified NEC W33.19
machine gun W33.13
paintball gun W34.111
pellet W34.110
shotgun W33.11
Very pistol [flare] W34.19
Reduction in
atmospheric pressure - — *see* Air, pressure, change
Rock falling on or hitting (accidentally) (person) W20.8
in cave-in W20.0
Run over (accidentally) (by)
animal (not being ridden) NEC W55.89
machinery — *see* Contact, with, by specified type of machine
transport vehicle NEC — *see also* Accident, transport V09.9
intentional homicide (attempt) Y03.0
motor NEC V09.20
intentional homicide (attempt) Y03.0
Running
before moving object X81.8
motor vehicle X81.0
Running off, away
animal (being ridden) — *see also* Accident, transport V80.918
not being ridden W55.89
animal-drawn vehicle NEC — *see also* Accident, transport V80.928
highway, road (way) , street

Running off, away - *continued*
highway, road (way) , street - *continued*
transport vehicle NEC — *see also* Accident, transport V89.9
Rupture pressurized devices — *see* Explosion, by type of device

S

Saturnism — *see* Table of Drugs and Chemicals, lead
Scald, scalding (accidental) (by) (from) (in) X19
air (hot) X14.1
gases (hot) X14.1
homicide (attempt) — *see* Assault, burning, hot object
inflicted by other person
stated as intentional, homicide (attempt) — *see* Assault, burning, hot object
liquid (boiling) (hot) NEC X12
stated as undetermined whether accidental or intentional Y27.2
suicide (attempt) X77.2
local application of externally applied substance in medical or surgical care Y63.5
metal (molten) (liquid) (hot) NEC X18
self-inflicted X77.9
stated as undetermined whether accidental or intentional Y27.8
steam X13.1
assault X98.0
stated as undetermined whether accidental or intentional Y27.0
suicide (attempt) X77.0
suicide (attempt) X77.9
vapor (hot) X13.1
assault X98.0
stated as undetermined whether accidental or intentional Y27.0
suicide (attempt) X77.0
Scratched by
cat W55.03
person (s) (accidentally) W50.4
with intent to injure or kill Y04.0
as, or caused by, a crowd or human stampede (with fall) W52
assault Y04.0
homicide (attempt) Y04.0
in
fight Y04.0
legal intervention
injuring
bystander Y35.892
law enforcement personnel Y35.891
suspect Y35.893
Seasickness T75.3
Self-harm NEC — *see also* External cause by type, undetermined whether accidental or intentional
intentional — *see* Suicide
poisoning NEC — *see* Table of drugs and biologicals, accident
Self-inflicted (injury) **NEC** — *see also* External cause by type, undetermined whether accidental or intentional
intentional — *see* Suicide
poisoning NEC — *see* Table of drugs and biologicals, accident
Sequelae (of)
accident NEC — *see* W00-X58 with 7th character S
assault (homicidal) (any means) — *see* X92-Y08 with 7th character S
homicide, attempt (any means) — *see* X92-Y08 with 7th character S
injury undetermined whether accidentally or purposely inflicted — *see* Y21-Y33 with 7th character S
intentional self-harm (classifiable to X71 -X83) — *see* X71-X83 with 7th character S
legal intervention — *see* with 7th character S Y35
motor vehicle accident — *see* V00-V99 with 7th character S
suicide, attempt (any means) — *see* X71-X83 with 7th character S
transport accident — *see* V00-V99 with 7th character S
war operations — *see* War operations
Shock
electric — *see* Exposure, electric current
from electric appliance (any) (faulty) W86.8
domestic W86.0
suicide (attempt) X83.1
Shooting, shot (accidental (ly)) — *see also* Discharge, firearm, by type
herself or himself — *see* Discharge, firearm by type, self-inflicted

Shooting, shot (accidental (ly)) - *continued*
  homicide (attempt) — *see* Discharge, firearm by type, homicide
  in war operations — *see* War operations
  inflicted by other person — *see* Discharge, firearm by type, homicide
    accidental — *see* Discharge, firearm, by type of firearm
  legal
    execution — *see* Legal, intervention, firearm
    intervention — *see* Legal, intervention, firearm
  self-inflicted — *see* Discharge, firearm by type, suicide
    accidental — *see* Discharge, firearm, by type of firearm
  suicide (attempt) — *see* Discharge, firearm by type, suicide
Shoving (accidentally) **by other person** — *see* Pushed, by other person
Sickness
  alpine W94.11
  motion — *see* Motion
  mountain W94.11
Sinking (accidental)
  watercraft (causing drowning, submersion) — *see also* Drowning, due to, accident to, watercraft, sinking
    causing injury except drowning or submersion — *see* Accident, watercraft, causing, injury NEC
Siriasis X32
Sitting (prolonged) (static) X50.1
Slashed wrists — *see* Cut, self-inflicted
Slipping (accidental) (on same level) (with fall) W01.0
  on
    ice W00.0
      with skates — *see* Accident, transport, pedestrian, conveyance
    mud W01.0
    oil W01.0
    snow W00.0
      with skis — *see* Accident, transport, pedestrian, conveyance
    surface (slippery) (wet) NEC W01.0
  without fall W18.40
    due to
      specified NEC W18.49
      stepping from one level to another W18.43
      stepping into hole or opening W18.42
      stepping on object W18.41
Sliver, wood, contact with W45.8
Smoldering (due to fire) — *see* Exposure, fire
Sodomy (attempted) **by force** T74.2-
Sound waves (causing injury) W42.9
  supersonic W42.0
Splinter, contact with W45.8
Stab, stabbing — *see* Cut
Standing (prolonged) (static) X50.1
Starvation X58
Status of external cause Y99.9
  child assisting in compensated work for family Y99.8
  civilian activity done for financial or other compensation Y99.0
  civilian activity done for income or pay Y99.0
  family member assisting in compensated work for other family member Y99.8
  hobby not done for income Y99.8
  leisure activity Y99.8
  military activity Y99.1
  off-duty activity of military personnel Y99.8
  recreation or sport not for income or while a student Y99.8
  specified NEC Y99.8
  student activity Y99.8
  volunteer activity Y99.2
Stepped on
  by
    animal (not being ridden) NEC W55.89
    crowd or human stampede W52
    person W50.0
Stepping on
  object W22.8
    with fall W18.31
      sports equipment W21.9
    stationary W22.09
      sports equipment W21.89
  person W51
    by crowd or human stampede W52
    sports equipment W21.9
Sting
  arthropod, nonvenomous W57

Sting - *continued*
  insect, nonvenomous W57
Storm (cataclysmic) — *see* Forces of nature, cataclysmic storm
Straining, excessive — *see also* Overexertion X50.9
Strangling — *see* Strangulation
Strangulation (accidental) — *see* category T71
Strenuous movements — *see also* Overexertion X50.9
Striking against
  airbag (automobile) W22.10
    driver side W22.11
    front passenger side W22.12
    specified NEC W22.19
  bottom when
    diving or jumping into water (in) W16.822
      causing drowning W16.821
      from boat W16.722
        causing drowning W16.721
      natural body W16.622
        causing drowning W16.821
      swimming pool W16.522
        causing drowning W16.521
    falling into water (in) W16.322
      causing drowning W16.321
      fountain — *see* Striking against, bottom when, falling into water, specified NEC
      natural body W16.122
        causing drowning W16.121
      reservoir — *see* Striking against, bottom when, falling into water, specified NEC
      specified NEC W16.322
        causing drowning W16.321
      swimming pool W16.022
        causing drowning W16.021
  diving board (swimming-pool) W21.4
  object W22.8
    with
      drowning or submersion — *see* Drowning
      fall — *see* Fall, due to, bumping against, object
    caused by crowd or human stampede (with fall) W52
    furniture W22.03
    lamppost W22.02
    sports equipment W21.9
    stationary W22.09
      sports equipment W21.89
    wall W22.01
  person (s) W51
    with fall W03
      due to ice or snow W00.0
    as, or caused by, a crowd or human stampede (with fall) W52
    assault Y04.2
    homicide (attempt) Y04.2
  sports equipment W21.9
  wall (when) W22.01
    diving or jumping into water (in) W16.832
      causing drowning W16.831
      swimming pool W16.532
        causing drowning W16.531
    falling into water (in) W16.332
      causing drowning W16.331
      fountain — *see* Striking against, wall when, falling into water, specified NEC
      natural body W16.132
        causing drowning W16.131
      reservoir — *see* Striking against, wall when, falling into water, specified NEC
      specified NEC W16.332
        causing drowning W16.331
      swimming pool W16.032
        causing drowning W16.031
    swimming pool (when) W22.042
      causing drowning W22.041
      diving or jumping into water W16.532
        causing drowning W16.531
      falling into water W16.032
        causing drowning W16.031
Struck (accidentally) **by**
  airbag (automobile) W22.10
    driver side W22.11
    front passenger side W22.12
    specified NEC W22.19
  alligator W58.02
  animal (not being ridden) NEC W55.89
  avalanche — *see* Landslide
  ball (hit) (thrown) W21.00
    assault Y08.09
    baseball W21.03
    basketball W21.05
    golf ball W21.04
    football W21.01

Struck (accidentally) **by** - *continued*
  ball (hit) (thrown) - *continued*
    soccer W21.02
    softball W21.07
    specified NEC W21.09
    volleyball W21.06
  bat or racquet
    baseball bat W21.11
      assault Y08.02
    golf club W21.13
      assault Y08.09
    specified NEC W21.19
      assault Y08.09
    tennis racquet W21.12
      assault Y08.09
  bullet — *see also* Discharge, firearm by type
    in war operations — *see* War operations
  crocodile W58.12
  dog W54.1
  flare, Very pistol — *see* Discharge, firearm NEC
  hailstones X39.8
  hockey (ice)
    field
      puck W21.221
      stick W21.211
    puck W21.220
    stick W21.210
      assault Y08.01
  landslide — *see* Landslide
  law-enforcement agent (on duty) — *see* Legal, intervention, manhandling
    with blunt object — *see* Legal, intervention, blunt object
  lightning — *see* subcategory T75.0
    causing fire — *see* Exposure, fire
  machine — *see* Contact, with, by type of machine
  mammal NEC W55.89
    marine W56.32
  marine animal W56.82
  missile
    firearm — *see* Discharge, firearm by type
    in war operations — *see* War operations, missile
  object W22.8
    blunt W22.8
      assault Y00
      suicide (attempt) X79
      undetermined whether accidental or intentional Y29
    falling W20.8
      from, in, on
        building W20.1
          burning (uncontrolled fire) X00.4
        cataclysmic
          earth surface movement NEC — *see* Landslide
          storm — *see* Forces of nature, cataclysmic storm
        cave-in W20.0
        earthquake X34
        machine (in operation) — *see* Contact, with, by type of machine
        structure W20.1
          burning X00.4
        transport vehicle (in motion) — *see* Accident, transport, by type of vehicle
        watercraft V93.49
          due to
            accident to craft V91.39
              powered craft V91.33
                ferry boat V91.31
                fishing boat V91.32
                jetskis V91.33
                liner V91.31
                merchant ship V91.30
                passenger ship V91.31
             unpowered craft V91.38
                canoe V91.35
                inflatable V91.36
                kayak V91.35
                sailboat V91.34
                surf-board V91.38
                windsurfer V91.38
            powered craft V93.43
              ferry boat V93.41
              fishing boat V93.42
              jetskis V93.43
              liner V93.41
              merchant ship V93.40
              passenger ship V93.41
            unpowered craft V93.48
              sailboat V93.44
              surf-board V93.48
              windsurfer V93.48
  moving NEC W20.8

Struck (accidentally) **by** - *continued*
object - *continued*
  projected W20.8
    assault Y00
    in sports W21.9
      assault Y08.09
      ball W21.00
        baseball W21.03
        basketball W21.05
        football W21.01
        golf ball W21.04
        soccer W21.02
        softball W21.07
        specified NEC W21.09
        volleyball W21.06
      bat or racquet
        baseball bat W21.11
          assault Y08.02
        golf club W21.13
          assault Y08.09
        specified NEC W21.19
          assault Y08.09
        tennis racquet W21.12
          assault Y08.09
      hockey (ice)
        field
          puck W21.221
          stick W21.211
        puck W21.220
        stick W21.210
          assault Y08.01
      specified NEC W21.89
  set in motion by explosion — *see* Explosion
  thrown W20.8
    assault Y00
    in sports W21.9
      assault Y08.09
      ball W21.00
        baseball W21.03
        basketball W21.05
        football W21.01
        golf ball W21.04
        soccer W21.02
        soft ball W21.07
        specified NEC W21.09
        volleyball W21.06
      bat or racquet
        baseball bat W21.11
          assault Y08.02
        golf club W21.13
          assault Y08.09
        specified NEC W21.19
          assault Y08.09
        tennis racquet W21.12
          assault Y08.09
      hockey (ice)
        field
          puck W21.221
          stick W21.211
        puck W21.220
        stick W21.210
          assault Y08.01
      specified NEC W21.89
other person (s) W50.0
  with
    blunt object W22.8
    intentional, homicide (attempt) Y00
    sports equipment W21.9
    undetermined whether accidental or
      intentional Y29
  fall W03
    due to ice or snow W00.0
  as, or caused by, a crowd or human stampede (with
    fall) W52
  assault Y04.2
  homicide (attempt) Y04.2
  in legal intervention
    injuring
      bystander Y35.812
      law enforcement personnel Y35.811
      suspect Y35.813
  sports equipment W21.9
  police (on duty) — *see* Legal, intervention,
    manhandling
    with blunt object — *see* Legal, intervention, blunt
      object
  sports equipment W21.9
    assault Y08.09
    ball W21.00
      baseball W21.03
      basketball W21.05
      football W21.01
      golf ball W21.04

Struck (accidentally) **by** - *continued*
  sports equipment - *continued*
    ball - *continued*
      soccer W21.02
      soft ball W21.07
      specified NEC W21.09
      volleyball W21.06
    bat or racquet
      baseball bat W21.11
        assault Y08.02
      golf club W21.13
        assault Y08.09
      specified NEC W21.19
      tennis racquet W21.12
        assault Y08.09
    cleats (shoe) W21.31
    foot wear NEC W21.39
    football helmet W21.81
    hockey (ice)
      field
        puck W21.221
        stick W21.211
      puck W21.220
      stick W21.210
        assault Y08.01
    skate blades W21.32
    specified NEC W21.89
      assault Y08.09
  thunderbolt — *see* subcategory T75.0
    causing fire — *see* Exposure, fire
  transport vehicle NEC — *see also* Accident,
    transport V09.9
    intentional, homicide (attempt) Y03.0
    motor NEC — *see also* Accident, transport V09.20
      homicide Y03.0
  vehicle (transport) NEC — *see* Accident, transport,
    by type of vehicle
    stationary (falling from jack, hydraulic lift,
      ramp) W20.8
Stumbling
  over
    animal NEC W01.0
      with fall W18.09
    carpet, rug or (small) object W22.8
      with fall W18.09
    person W51
      with fall W03
        due to ice or snow W00.0
  without fall W18.40
    due to
      specified NEC W18.49
      stepping from one level to another W18.43
      stepping into hole or opening W18.42
      stepping on object W18.41
Submersion (accidental) — *see* Drowning
Suffocation (accidental) (by external means) (by
  pressure) (mechanical) (*see also* category T71)
  due to, by
    avalanche — *see* Landslide
    explosion — *see* Explosion
    fire — *see* Exposure, fire
    food, any type (aspiration) (ingestion)
      (inhalation) — *see* categories T17 and T18
    ignition — *see* Ignition
    landslide — *see* Landslide
    machine (ry) — *see* Contact, with, by type of
      machine
    vomitus (aspiration) (inhalation) T17.81-
  in
    burning building X00.8
Suicide, suicidal (attempted) (by) X83.8
  blunt object X79
  burning, burns X76
    hot object X77.9
      fluid NEC X77.2
      household appliance X77.3
      specified NEC X77.8
      steam X77.0
      tap water X77.1
      vapors X77.0
  caustic substance — *see* Table of Drugs and
    Chemicals
  cold, extreme X83.2
  collision of motor vehicle with
    motor vehicle X82.0
    specified NEC X82.8
    train X82.1
    tree X82.2
  crashing of aircraft X83.0
  cut (any part of body) X78.9
  cutting or piercing instrument X78.9
    dagger X78.2
    glass X78.0

Suicide, suicidal (attempted) (by) - *continued*
  cutting or piercing instrument - *continued*
    knife X78.1
    specified NEC X78.8
    sword X78.2
  drowning (in) X71.9
    bathtub X71.0
    natural water X71.3
    specified NEC X71.8
    swimming pool X71.1
      following fall X71.2
  electrocution X83.1
  explosive (s) (material) X75
  fire, flames X76
  firearm X74.9
    airgun X74.01
    handgun X72
    hunting rifle X73.1
    larger X73.9
      specified NEC X73.8
    machine gun X73.2
    shotgun X73.0
    specified NEC X74.8
  hanging X83.8
  hot object — *see* Suicide, burning, hot object
  jumping
    before moving object X81.8
      motor vehicle X81.0
      subway train X81.1
      train X81.1
    from high place X80
  late effect of attempt — *see* X71-X83 with 7th
    character S
  lying before moving object, train, vehicle X81.8
  poisoning — *see* Table of Drugs and Chemicals
  puncture (any part of body) — *see* Suicide, cutting
    or piercing instrument
  scald — *see* Suicide, burning, hot object
  sequelae of attempt — *see* X71-X83 with 7th
    character S
  sharp object (any) — *see* Suicide, cutting or piercing
    instrument
  shooting — *see* Suicide, firearm
  specified means NEC X83.8
  stab (any part of body) — *see* Suicide, cutting or
    piercing instrument
  steam, hot vapors X77.0
  strangulation X83.8
  submersion — *see* Suicide, drowning
  suffocation X83.8
  wound NEC X83.8
Sunstroke X32
Supersonic waves (causing injury) W42.0
Surgical procedure, complication of (delayed or as
  an abnormal reaction without mention of
  misadventure) — *see also* Complication of or
  following, by type of procedure
  due to or as a result of misadventure — *see*
    Misadventure
Swallowed, swallowing
  foreign body — *see* Foreign body, alimentary canal
  poison — *see* Table of Drugs and Chemicals
  substance
    caustic or corrosive — *see* Table of Drugs and
      Chemicals
    poisonous — *see* Table of Drugs and Chemicals

T

Tackle in sport W03
Terrorism (involving) Y38.80
  biological weapons Y38.6X-
  chemical weapons Y38.7X-
  conflagration Y38.3X-
  drowning and submersion Y38.89-
  explosion Y38.2X-
    destruction of aircraft Y38.1X-
    marine weapons Y38.0X-
  fire Y38.3X-
  firearms Y38.4X-
  hot substances Y38.3X-
  lasers Y38.89-
  nuclear weapons Y38.5X-
  piercing or stabbing instruments Y38.89-
  secondary effects Y38.9X-
  specified method NEC Y38.89-
  suicide bomber Y38.81-
Thirst X58
Threat to breathing
  aspiration — *see* Aspiration
  due to cave-in, falling earth or substance NEC — *see*
    category T71

Thrown (accidentally)
  against part (any) of or object in transport vehicle (in
    motion) NEC — *see also* Accident, transport
  from
    high place, homicide (attempt) Y01
    machinery — *see* Contact, with, by type of
      machine
    transport vehicle NEC — *see also* Accident,
      transport V89.9
    off — *see* Thrown, from
Thunderbolt — *see* subcategory T75.0
  causing fire — *see* Exposure, fire
Tidal wave (any injury) **NEC** — *see* Forces of nature,
  tidal wave
Took
  overdose (drug) — *see* Table of Drugs and
    Chemicals
  poison — *see* Table of Drugs and Chemicals
Tornado (any injury) X37.1
Torrential rain (any injury) X37.8
Torture X58
Trampled by animal NEC W55.89
Trapped (accidentally)
  between objects (moving) (stationary and
    moving) — *see* Caught
  by part (any) of
    motorcycle V29.88
    pedal cycle V19.88
    transport vehicle NEC — *see also* Accident,
      transport V89.9
Travel (effects) (sickness) T75.3
Tree falling on or hitting (accidentally)
  (person) W20.8
Tripping
  over
    animal W01.0
      with fall W01.0
    carpet, rug or (small) object W22.8
      with fall W18.09
    person W51
      with fall W03
        due to ice or snow W00.0
    without fall W18.40
    due to
      specified NEC W18.49
      stepping from one level to another W18.43
      stepping into hole or opening W18.42
      stepping on object W18.41
Twisted by person (s) (accidentally) W50.2
  with intent to injure or kill Y04.0
  as, or caused by, a crowd or human stampede (with
    fall) W52
  assault Y04.0
  homicide (attempt) Y04.0
  in
    fight Y04.0
  legal intervention — *see* Legal, intervention,
    manhandling
Twisting (prolonged) (static) X50.1

U

Underdosing of necessary drugs, medicaments or
  biological substances Y63.6
Undetermined intent (contact) (exposure) -
  automobile collision Y32
  blunt object Y29
  drowning (submersion) (in) Y21.9
    bathtub Y21.0
      after fall Y21.1
    natural water (lake) (ocean) (pond) (river)
      (stream) Y21.4
    specified place NEC Y21.8
    swimming pool Y21.2
      after fall Y21.3
  explosive material Y25
  fall, jump or push from high place Y30
  falling, lying or running before moving object Y31
  fire Y26
  firearm discharge Y24.9
    airgun (BB) (pellet) Y24.0
    handgun (pistol) (revolver) Y22
    hunting rifle Y23.1
    larger Y23.9
      hunting rifle Y23.1
      machine gun Y23.3
      military Y23.2
      shotgun Y23.0
      specified type NEC Y23.8
    machine gun Y23.3
    military Y23.2
    shotgun Y23.0
    specified type NEC Y24.8
    Very pistol Y24.8

Undetermined intent (contact) (exposure) -
continued
  hot object Y27.9
    fluid NEC Y27.2
    household appliance Y27.3
    specified object NEC Y27.8
    steam Y27.0
    tap water Y27.1
    vapor Y27.0
  jump, fall or push from high place Y30
  lying, falling or running before moving object Y31
  motor vehicle crash Y32
  push, fall or jump from high place Y30
  running, falling or lying before moving object Y31
  sharp object Y28.9
    dagger Y28.2
    glass Y28.0
    knife Y28.1
    specified object NEC Y28.8
    sword Y28.2
  smoke Y26
  specified event NEC Y33
Use of hand as hammer X50.3

V

Vibration (causing injury) W49.9
Victim (of)
  avalanche — *see* Landslide
  earth movements NEC — *see* Forces of nature, earth
    movement
  earthquake X34
  flood — *see* Flood
  landslide — *see* Landslide
  lightning — *see* subcategory T75.0
    causing fire — *see* Exposure, fire
  storm (cataclysmic) NEC — *see* Forces of nature,
    cataclysmic storm
  volcanic eruption X35
Volcanic eruption (any injury) X35
Vomitus, gastric contents in air passages (with
  asphyxia, obstruction or suffocation) T17.81-

W

Walked into stationary object (any) W22.09
  furniture W22.03
  lamppost W22.02
  wall W22.01
War operations (injuries to military personnel and
  civilians during war, civil insurrection and
  peacekeeping missions) (by) (from)
  (involving) Y36.90
  after cessation of hostilities Y36.89-
    explosion (of)
      bomb placed during war operations Y36.82-
      mine placed during war operations Y36.81-
      specified NEC Y36.88-
  air blast Y36.20-
  aircraft
    destruction — *see* War operations, destruction of
      aircraft
  airway restriction — *see* War operations, restriction
    of airways
  asphyxiation — *see* War operations, restriction of
    airways
  biological weapons Y36.6X-
  blast Y36.20-
  blast fragments Y36.20-
  blast wave Y36.20-
  blast wind Y36.20-
  bomb Y36.20-
    dirty Y36.50-
    gasoline Y36.31-
    incendiary Y36.31-
    petrol Y36.31-
  bullet Y36.43-
    incendiary Y36.32-
    rubber Y36.41-
  chemical weapons Y36.7X-
  combat
    hand to hand (unarmed) combat Y36.44-
    using blunt or piercing object Y36.45-
  conflagration — *see* War operations, fire
  conventional warfare NEC Y36.49-
  depth-charge Y36.01-
  destruction of aircraft Y36.10-
    due to
      air to air missile Y36.11-
      collision with other aircraft Y36.12-
      detonation (accidental) of onboard munitions and
        explosives Y36.14-
      enemy fire or explosives Y36.11-
      explosive placed on aircraft Y36.11-
      onboard fire Y36.13-
      rocket propelled grenade [RPG] Y36.11-

War operations
  (injuries to military personnel and civilians during
  war, civil insurrection and peacekeeping missions)
  (by) (from) (involving) - *continued*
  destruction of aircraft - *continued*
    due to - *continued*
      small arms fire Y36.11-
        surface to air missile Y36.11-
      specified NEC Y36.19-
  detonation (accidental) of
    onboard marine weapons Y36.05-
    own munitions or munitions launch device Y36.24-
  dirty bomb Y36.50-
  explosion (of) Y36.20-
    after cessation of hostilities
      bomb placed during war operations Y36.82-
      mine placed during war operations Y36.81-
    aerial bomb Y36.21-
    bomb NOS — *see also* War operations,
      bomb(s) Y36.20-
    own munitions or munitions launch device
      (accidental) Y36.24-
    fragments Y36.20-
    grenade Y36.29-
    guided missile Y36.22-
    improvised explosive device [IED] (person-borne)
      (roadside) (vehicle-borne) Y36.23-
    land mine Y36.29-
    marine mine (at sea) (in harbor) Y36.02-
    marine weapon Y36.00-
      specified NEC Y36.09-
    sea-based artillery shell Y36.03-
    specified NEC Y36.29-
    torpedo Y36.04-
  fire Y36.30-
    specified NEC Y36.39-
  firearms
    discharge Y36.43-
    pellets Y36.42-
  flamethrower Y36.33-
  fragments (from) (of)
    improvised explosive device [IED] (person-borne)
      (roadside) (vehicle-borne) Y36.26-
    munitions Y36.25-
    specified NEC Y36.29-
    weapons Y36.27-
  friendly fire Y36.92
  hand to hand (unarmed) combat Y36.44-
  hot substances — *see* War operations, fire
  incendiary bullet Y36.32-
  nuclear weapon (effects of) Y36.50-
    acute radiation exposure Y36.54-
    blast pressure Y36.51-
    direct blast Y36.51-
    direct heat Y36.53-
    fallout exposure Y36.54-
    fireball Y36.53-
    indirect blast (struck or crushed by blast debris)
      (being thrown by blast) Y36.52-
    ionizing radiation (immediate exposure) Y36.54-
    nuclear radiation Y36.54-
    radiation
      ionizing (immediate exposure) Y36.54-
      nuclear Y36.54-
      thermal Y36.53-
    specified NEC Y36.59-
    secondary effects Y36.54-
    thermal radiation Y36.53-
  restriction of air (airway)
    intentional Y36.46-
    unintentional Y36.47-
  rubber bullets Y36.41-
  shrapnel NOS Y36.29-
  suffocation — *see* War operations, restriction of
    airways
  unconventional warfare NEC Y36.7X-
  underwater blast NOS Y36.00-
  warfare
    conventional NEC Y36.49-
    unconventional NEC Y36.7X-
  weapons
    biological weapons Y36.6X-
    chemical Y36.7X-
    nuclear (effects of) Y36.50-
      acute radiation exposure Y36.54-
      blast pressure Y36.51-
      direct blast Y36.51-
      direct heat Y36.53-
      fallout exposure Y36.54-
      fireball Y36.53-
      indirect blast (struck or crushed by blast debris)
        (being thrown by blast) Y36.52-
      radiation

War operations (injuries to military personnel and civilians during war, civil insurrection and peacekeeping missions) (by) (from) (involving) - *continued*
  weapons - *continued*
    nuclear (effects of) - *continued*
      radiation - *continued*
        ionizing (immediate exposure) Y36.54-
        nuclear Y36.54-
        thermal Y36.53-
      secondary effects Y36.54-
      specified NEC Y36.59-
    of mass destruction [WMD] Y36.91
  weapon of mass destruction [WMD] Y36.91
Washed
  away by flood — *see* Flood
  off road by storm (transport vehicle) — *see* Forces of nature, cataclysmic storm
Weather exposure NEC — *see* Forces of nature
Weightlessness (causing injury) (effects of) (in spacecraft, real or simulated) X52
Work related condition Y99.0
Wound (accidental) **NEC** — *see also* Injury X58
  battle — *see also* War operations Y36.90
  gunshot — *see* Discharge, firearm by type
Wreck transport vehicle NEC — *see also* Accident, transport V89.9
Wrong
  device implanted into correct surgical site Y65.51
  fluid in infusion Y65.1
  procedure (operation) on correct patient Y65.51
  patient, procedure performed on Y65.52

CHAPTER 1: CERTAIN INFECTIOUS AND PARASITIC DISEASES (A00-B99)

INCLUDES diseases generally recognized as communicable or transmissible

Use additional code to identify resistance to antimicrobial drugs (Z16.-)

EXCLUDES 1 *certain localized infections - see body system-related chapters*

EXCLUDES 2 *carrier or suspected carrier of infectious disease (Z22.-)*
infectious and parasitic diseases complicating pregnancy, childbirth and the puerperium (O98.-)
infectious and parasitic diseases specific to the perinatal period (P35-P39)
influenza and other acute respiratory infections (J00-J22)

This chapter contains the following blocks:

A00-A09	Intestinal infectious diseases
A15-A19	Tuberculosis
A20-A28	Certain zoonotic bacterial diseases
A30-A49	Other bacterial diseases
A50-A64	Infections with a predominantly sexual mode of transmission
A65-A69	Other spirochetal diseases
A70-A74	Other diseases caused by chlamydiae
A75-A79	Rickettsioses
A80-A89	Viral and prion infections of the central nervous system
A90-A99	Arthropod-borne viral fevers and viral hemorrhagic fevers
B00-B09	Viral infections characterized by skin and mucous membrane lesions
B10	Other human herpesviruses
B15-B19	Viral hepatitis
B20	Human immunodeficiency virus [HIV] disease
B25-B34	Other viral diseases
B35-B49	Mycoses
B50-B64	Protozoal diseases
B65-B83	Helminthiases
B85-B89	Pediculosis, acariasis and other infestations
B90-B94	Sequelae of infectious and parasitic diseases
B95-B97	Bacterial and viral infectious agents
B99	Other infectious diseases

Intestinal infectious diseases (A00-A09)

A00 Cholera

A00.0 Cholera due to Vibrio cholerae 01, biovar cholerae
Classical cholera

A00.1 Cholera due to Vibrio cholerae 01, biovar eltor
Cholera eltor

A00.9 Cholera, unspecified

A01 Typhoid and paratyphoid fevers

A01.0 Typhoid fever
Infection due to Salmonella typhi

A01.00 Typhoid fever, unspecified

A01.01 Typhoid meningitis

A01.02 Typhoid fever with heart involvement
Typhoid endocarditis
Typhoid myocarditis

A01.03 Typhoid pneumonia

A01.04 Typhoid arthritis

A01.05 Typhoid osteomyelitis

A01.09 Typhoid fever with other complications

A01.1 Paratyphoid fever A

A01.2 Paratyphoid fever B

A01.3 Paratyphoid fever C

A01.4 Paratyphoid fever, unspecified
Infection due to Salmonella paratyphi NOS

A02 Other salmonella infections

INCLUDES infection or foodborne intoxication due to any Salmonella species other than S. typhi and S. paratyphi

A02.0 Salmonella enteritis
Salmonellosis

A02.1 Salmonella sepsis

A02.2 Localized salmonella infections

A02.20 Localized salmonella infection, unspecified

A02.21 Salmonella meningitis

A02.22 Salmonella pneumonia

A02.23 Salmonella arthritis

CODING TIP ✓ Salmonella arthritis is a reactive arthritis. Code A02.23 indicates the arthritis and its cause. Do not assign an additional code for arthritis.

A02.24 Salmonella osteomyelitis

A02.25 Salmonella pyelonephritis
Salmonella tubulo-interstitial nephropathy

A02.29 Salmonella with other localized infection

A02.8 Other specified salmonella infections

A02.9 Salmonella infection, unspecified

A03 Shigellosis

A03.0 Shigellosis due to Shigella dysenteriae
Group A shigellosis [Shiga-Kruse dysentery]

A03.1 Shigellosis due to Shigella flexneri
Group B shigellosis

A03.2 Shigellosis due to Shigella boydii
Group C shigellosis

A03.3 Shigellosis due to Shigella sonnei
Group D shigellosis

A03.8 Other shigellosis

A03.9 Shigellosis, unspecified
Bacillary dysentery NOS

A04 Other bacterial intestinal infections

EXCLUDES 1 *bacterial foodborne intoxications, NEC (A05.-)*
tuberculous enteritis (A18.32)

A04.0 Enteropathogenic Escherichia coli infection

A04.1 Enterotoxigenic Escherichia coli infection

A04.2 Enteroinvasive Escherichia coli infection

A04.3 Enterohemorrhagic Escherichia coli infection

A04.4 Other intestinal Escherichia coli infections
Escherichia coli enteritis NOS

A04.5 Campylobacter enteritis

A04.6 Enteritis due to Yersinia enterocolitica

EXCLUDES 1 *extraintestinal yersiniosis (A28.2)*

CODING TIP ✓ Arthropathy associated with Yersinia requires an additional code from M02.-.

A04.7 Enterocolitis due to Clostridium difficile
Foodborne intoxication by Clostridium difficile
Pseudomembraneous colitis

A04.8 Other specified bacterial intestinal infections

A04.9 Bacterial intestinal infection, unspecified
Bacterial enteritis NOS

A05 Other bacterial foodborne intoxications, not elsewhere classified

EXCLUDES 1 *Clostridium difficile foodborne intoxication and infection (A04.7)*
Escherichia coli infection (A04.0-A04.4)
listeriosis (A32.-)
salmonella foodborne intoxication and infection (A02.-)
toxic effect of noxious foodstuffs (T61-T62)

A05.0 Foodborne staphylococcal intoxication

A05.1 Botulism food poisoning
Botulism NOS
Classical foodborne intoxication due to Clostridium botulinum

EXCLUDES 1 *infant botulism (A48.51)*
wound botulism (A48.52)

● New ▲ Revised *Manifestation* 🔢 Digit Indicators ▤ Laterality Ⓐ Adult (15+ years) Ⓜ Maternity (12-55 years) Ⓝ Newborn Ⓟ Pediatric (0-17 years) ♂ Male ♀ Female
✖ ~~Deleted~~ Unspecified ✚ Additional code

DEFINITION Muscle-paralyzing disease caused by ingesting the neurotoxins produced by the bacteria Clostridium botulinum.

Botulism food poisoning

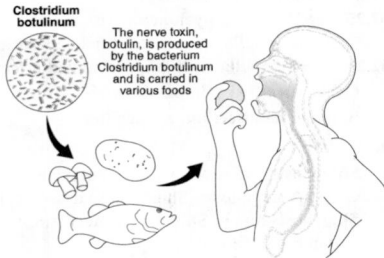

Symptoms include double vision, blurred vision, drooping eyelids, slurred speech, difficulty swallowing, dry mouth, and muscle weakness

Giardiasis (lambliasis)

Symptoms may include diarrhea, gas and bloating, abdominal cramps, nausea, loss of appetite, and fatigue

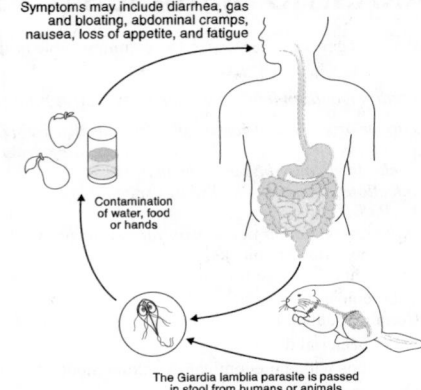

The Giardia lamblia parasite is passed in stool from humans or animals

A05.2	**Foodborne Clostridium perfringens [Clostridium welchii] intoxication**
	Enteritis necroticans
	Pig-bel
A05.3	**Foodborne Vibrio parahaemolyticus intoxication**
A05.4	**Foodborne Bacillus cereus intoxication**
A05.5	**Foodborne Vibrio vulnificus intoxication**
A05.8	**Other specified bacterial foodborne intoxications**
A05.9	**Bacterial foodborne intoxication, unspecified**

A06 Amebiasis

INCLUDES infection due to Entamoeba histolytica

EXCLUDES 1 other protozoal intestinal diseases (A07.-)

EXCLUDES 2 acanthamebiasis (B60.1-)
Naegleriasis (B60.2)

A06.0	**Acute amebic dysentery**
	Acute amebiasis
	Intestinal amebiasis NOS
A06.1	**Chronic intestinal amebiasis**
A06.2	**Amebic nondysenteric colitis**
A06.3	**Ameboma of intestine**
	Ameboma NOS
A06.4	**Amebic liver abscess**
	Hepatic amebiasis
A06.5	**Amebic lung abscess**
	Amebic abscess of lung (and liver)
A06.6	**Amebic brain abscess**
	Amebic abscess of brain (and liver) (and lung)
A06.7	**Cutaneous amebiasis**

A06.8 Amebic infection of other sites

	A06.81	**Amebic cystitis**
	A06.82	**Other amebic genitourinary infections**
		Amebic balanitis
		Amebic vesiculitis
		Amebic vulvovaginitis
	A06.89	**Other amebic infections**
		Amebic appendicitis
		Amebic splenic abscess

A06.9	**Amebiasis, unspecified**

A07 Other protozoal intestinal diseases

A07.0	**Balantidiasis**
	Balantidial dysentery
A07.1	**Giardiasis [lambliasis]**

A07.2	**Cryptosporidiosis**
A07.3	**Isosporiasis**
	Infection due to Isospora belli and Isospora hominis
	Intestinal coccidiosis
	Isosporosis
A07.4	**Cyclosporiasis**
A07.8	**Other specified protozoal intestinal diseases**
	Intestinal microsporidiosis
	Intestinal trichomoniasis
	Sarcocystosis
	Sarcosporidiosis

Other specified protozoal intestinal diseases

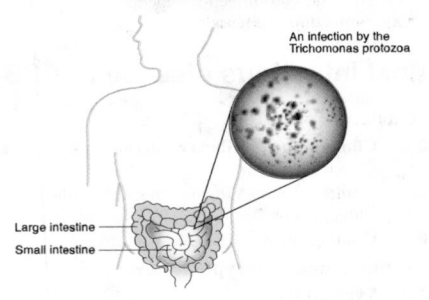

An infection by the Trichomonas protozoa

Large intestine
Small intestine

A07.9	**Protozoal intestinal disease, unspecified**
	Flagellate diarrhea
	Protozoal colitis
	Protozoal diarrhea
	Protozoal dysentery

A08 Viral and other specified intestinal infections

EXCLUDES 1 influenza with involvement of gastrointestinal tract (J09.X3, J10.2, J11.2)

A08.0	**Rotaviral enteritis**

A08.1 Acute gastroenteropathy due to Norwalk agent and other small round viruses

	A08.11	**Acute gastroenteropathy due to Norwalk agent**
		Acute gastroenteropathy due to Norovirus
		Acute gastroenteropathy due to Norwalk-like agent
	A08.19	**Acute gastroenteropathy due to other small round viruses**
		Acute gastroenteropathy due to small round virus [SRV] NOS

A08.2	**Adenoviral enteritis**

A08.3 Other viral enteritis

	A08.31	**Calicivirus enteritis**
	A08.32	**Astrovirus enteritis**
	A08.39	**Other viral enteritis**
		Coxsackie virus enteritis
		Echovirus enteritis
		Enterovirus enteritis NEC
		Torovirus enteritis

● New   ▲ Revised   *Manifestation*   🔳- 🔳 Digit Indicators   ⊟ Laterality   ⚠ Adult (15+ years)   Ⓜ Maternity (12-55 years)   Ⓝ Newborn   Ⓟ Pediatric (0-17 years)   ♂ Male   ♀ Female
✖ Deleted   Unspecified   + Additional code

446   © 2017 DecisionHealth   2017 ICD-10-CM Expert for Physicians

A08.4 **Viral intestinal infection, unspecified**
Viral enteritis NOS
Viral gastroenteritis NOS
Viral gastroenteropathy NOS

A08.8 **Other specified intestinal infections**

A09 **Infectious gastroenteritis and colitis, unspecified**
Infectious colitis NOS
Infectious enteritis NOS
Infectious gastroenteritis NOS

> **EXCLUDES 1** *colitis NOS (K52.9)*
> *diarrhea NOS (R19.7)*
> *enteritis NOS (K52.9)*
> *gastroenteritis NOS (K52.9)*
> *noninfective gastroenteritis and colitis,*
> *unspecified (K52.9)*

Tuberculosis (A15-A19)

INCLUDES infections due to Mycobacterium tuberculosis and
Mycobacterium bovis

EXCLUDES 1 *congenital tuberculosis (P37.0)*
nonspecific reaction to test for tuberculosis without active
tuberculosis (R76.1-)
pneumoconiosis associated with tuberculosis, any type in A15
(J65)
positive PPD (R76.11)
positive tuberculin skin test without active tuberculosis (R76.11)
sequelae of tuberculosis (B90.-)
silicotuberculosis (J65)

CODING TIP ✓ Codes from A15-A19 should not be assigned to report a
positive PPD (Mantoux) test. A positive PPD (Mantoux) skin test without
active tuberculosis should be coded to R76.11.

A15 **Respiratory tuberculosis**

A15.0 **Tuberculosis of lung**
Tuberculous bronchiectasis
Tuberculous fibrosis of lung
Tuberculous pneumonia
Tuberculous pneumothorax

A15.4 **Tuberculosis of intrathoracic lymph nodes**
Tuberculosis of hilar lymph nodes
Tuberculosis of mediastinal lymph nodes
Tuberculosis of tracheobronchial lymph nodes

> **EXCLUDES 1** *tuberculosis specified as primary (A15.7)*

A15.5 **Tuberculosis of larynx, trachea and bronchus**
Tuberculosis of bronchus
Tuberculosis of glottis
Tuberculosis of larynx
Tuberculosis of trachea

A15.6 **Tuberculous pleurisy**
Tuberculosis of pleura Tuberculous empyema

> **EXCLUDES 1** *primary respiratory tuberculosis (A15.7)*

A15.7 **Primary respiratory tuberculosis**

A15.8 **Other respiratory tuberculosis**
Mediastinal tuberculosis
Nasopharyngeal tuberculosis
Tuberculosis of nose
Tuberculosis of sinus [any nasal]

A15.9 **Respiratory tuberculosis unspecified**

A17 **Tuberculosis of nervous system**

A17.0 **Tuberculous meningitis**
Tuberculosis of meninges (cerebral)(spinal)
Tuberculous leptomeningitis

> **EXCLUDES 1** *tuberculous meningoencephalitis (A17.82)*

A17.1 **Meningeal tuberculoma**
Tuberculoma of meninges (cerebral) (spinal)

> **EXCLUDES 2** *tuberculoma of brain and spinal cord*
> *(A17.81)*

A17.8 **Other tuberculosis of nervous system**

A17.81 **Tuberculoma of brain and spinal cord**
Tuberculous abscess of brain and spinal cord

A17.82 **Tuberculous meningoencephalitis**
Tuberculous myelitis

A17.83 **Tuberculous neuritis**
Tuberculous mononeuropathy

A17.89 **Other tuberculosis of nervous system**
Tuberculous polyneuropathy

A17.9 **Tuberculosis of nervous system, unspecified**

A18 **Tuberculosis of other organs**

A18.0 **Tuberculosis of bones and joints**

A18.01 **Tuberculosis of spine**
Pott's disease or curvature of spine
Tuberculous arthritis
Tuberculous osteomyelitis of spine
Tuberculous spondylitis

A18.02 **Tuberculous arthritis of other joints**
Tuberculosis of hip (joint)
Tuberculosis of knee (joint)

A18.03 **Tuberculosis of other bones**
Tuberculous mastoiditis
Tuberculous osteomyelitis

A18.09 **Other musculoskeletal tuberculosis**
Tuberculous myositis
Tuberculous synovitis
Tuberculous tenosynovitis

A18.1 **Tuberculosis of genitourinary system** ♀

A18.10 **Tuberculosis of genitourinary system, unspecified**

A18.11 **Tuberculosis of kidney and ureter**

A18.12 **Tuberculosis of bladder**

A18.13 **Tuberculosis of other urinary organs**
Tuberculous urethritis

A18.14 **Tuberculosis of prostate** ♂ Ⓐ

A18.15 **Tuberculosis of other male genital organs** ♂

A18.16 **Tuberculosis of cervix** ♀

A18.17 **Tuberculous female pelvic inflammatory disease** ♀
Tuberculous endometritis
Tuberculous oophoritis and salpingitis

A18.18 **Tuberculosis of other female genital organs** ♀
Tuberculous ulceration of vulva

A18.2 **Tuberculous peripheral lymphadenopathy**
Tuberculous adenitis

> **EXCLUDES 2** *tuberculosis of bronchial and mediastinal*
> *lymph nodes (A15.4)*
> *tuberculosis of mesenteric and*
> *retroperitoneal lymph nodes (A18.39)*
> *tuberculous tracheobronchial adenopathy*
> *(A15.4)*

A18.3 **Tuberculosis of intestines, peritoneum and mesenteric glands**

A18.31 **Tuberculous peritonitis**
Tuberculous ascites

A18.32 **Tuberculous enteritis**
Tuberculosis of anus and rectum
Tuberculosis of intestine (large) (small)

A18.39 **Retroperitoneal tuberculosis**
Tuberculosis of mesenteric glands
Tuberculosis of retroperitoneal (lymph glands)

A18.4 **Tuberculosis of skin and subcutaneous tissue**
Erythema induratum, tuberculous
Lupus excedens
Lupus vulgaris NOS
Lupus vulgaris of eyelid
Scrofuloderma
Tuberculosis of external ear

> **EXCLUDES 2** *lupus erythematosus (L93.-)*
> *lupus NOS (M32.9)*
> *systemic (M32.-)*

A18.5 **Tuberculosis of eye**

> **EXCLUDES 2** *lupus vulgaris of eyelid (A18.4)*

A18.50 **Tuberculosis of eye, unspecified**

A18.51 **Tuberculous episcleritis**

A18.52 **Tuberculous keratitis**
Tuberculous interstitial keratitis
Tuberculous keratoconjunctivitis (interstitial)
(phlyctenular)

A18.53 **Tuberculous chorioretinitis**

A18.54 **Tuberculous iridocyclitis**

A18.59 **Other tuberculosis of eye**
Tuberculous conjunctivitis

A18.6 **Tuberculosis of (inner) (middle) ear**
Tuberculous otitis media

> **EXCLUDES 2** *tuberculosis of external ear (A18.4)*
> *tuberculous mastoiditis (A18.03)*

A18.7 **Tuberculosis of adrenal glands**
Tuberculous Addison's disease

A18.8 **Tuberculosis of other specified organs**

A18.81 **Tuberculosis of thyroid gland**

● New   ▲ Revised   *Manifestation*   ❹-❼ Digit Indicators   ▣ Laterality   Ⓐ Adult (15+ years)   Ⓜ Maternity (12-55 years)   Ⓝ Newborn   Ⓟ Pediatric (0-17 years)   ♂ Male   ♀ Female
✖ Deleted   Unspecified   + Additional code

A18.82 **Tuberculosis of other endocrine glands**
Tuberculosis of pituitary gland
Tuberculosis of thymus gland

A18.83 **Tuberculosis of digestive tract organs, not elsewhere classified**
EXCLUDES 1 *tuberculosis of intestine (A18.32)*

A18.84 **Tuberculosis of heart**
Tuberculous cardiomyopathy
Tuberculous endocarditis
Tuberculous myocarditis
Tuberculous pericarditis

A18.85 **Tuberculosis of spleen**
A18.89 **Tuberculosis of other sites**
Tuberculosis of muscle
Tuberculous cerebral arteritis

A19 **Miliary tuberculosis**
INCLUDES disseminated tuberculosis
generalized tuberculosis
tuberculous polyserositis

A19.0 **Acute miliary tuberculosis of a single specified site**
A19.1 **Acute miliary tuberculosis of multiple sites**
A19.2 **Acute miliary tuberculosis, unspecified**
A19.8 **Other miliary tuberculosis**
A19.9 **Miliary tuberculosis, unspecified**

Certain zoonotic bacterial diseases (A20-A28)

A20 **Plague**
INCLUDES infection due to Yersinia pestis

A20.0 **Bubonic plague**
DEFINITION Infection with the Yersinia pestis bacillus, transmitted via flea, tick, and lice bites and by contact with infected persons or materials, causing severe inflammation and death of skin cells.

A20.1 **Cellulocutaneous plague**
A20.2 **Pneumonic plague**
DEFINITION Rapidly progressive, often fatal plague pneumonia caused by direct inhalation of bacteria with severe cough producing frothy, bloody, mucoid sputum.

A20.3 **Plague meningitis**
A20.7 **Septicemic plague**
DEFINITION High-density bloodstream infection in acute bubonic plague; may cause death before the appearance of buboes or pulmonary manifestations.

A20.8 **Other forms of plague**
Abortive plague
Asymptomatic plague
Pestis minor

A20.9 **Plague, unspecified**

A21 **Tularemia**
INCLUDES deer-fly fever
infection due to Francisella tularensis
rabbit fever

A21.0 **Ulceroglandular tularemia**
A21.1 **Oculoglandular tularemia**
Ophthalmic tularemia
A21.2 **Pulmonary tularemia**
A21.3 **Gastrointestinal tularemia**
Abdominal tularemia
A21.7 **Generalized tularemia**
A21.8 **Other forms of tularemia**
A21.9 **Tularemia, unspecified**

A22 **Anthrax**
INCLUDES infection due to Bacillus anthracis

A22.0 **Cutaneous anthrax**
Malignant carbuncle
Malignant pustule
A22.1 **Pulmonary anthrax**
Inhalation anthrax
Ragpicker's disease
Woolsorter's disease
A22.2 **Gastrointestinal anthrax**
A22.7 **Anthrax sepsis**
A22.8 **Other forms of anthrax**
Anthrax meningitis

A22.9 **Anthrax, unspecified**
A23 **Brucellosis**
INCLUDES Malta fever
Mediterranean fever
undulant fever
A23.0 **Brucellosis due to Brucella melitensis**
A23.1 **Brucellosis due to Brucella abortus**
A23.2 **Brucellosis due to Brucella suis**
A23.3 **Brucellosis due to Brucella canis**
A23.8 **Other brucellosis**
A23.9 **Brucellosis, unspecified**
A24 **Glanders and melioidosis**
A24.0 **Glanders**
Infection due to Pseudomonas mallei
Malleus
A24.1 **Acute and fulminating melioidosis**
Melioidosis pneumonia
Melioidosis sepsis
A24.2 **Subacute and chronic melioidosis**
A24.3 **Other melioidosis**
A24.9 **Melioidosis, unspecified**
Infection due to Pseudomonas pseudomallei NOS
Whitmore's disease
A25 **Rat-bite fevers**
A25.0 **Spirillosis**
Sodoku
A25.1 **Streptobacillosis**
Epidemic arthritic erythema
Haverhill fever
Streptobacillary rat-bite fever
A25.9 **Rat-bite fever, unspecified**
A26 **Erysipeloid**
A26.0 **Cutaneous erysipeloid**
Erythema migrans
A26.7 **Erysipelothrix sepsis**
A26.8 **Other forms of erysipeloid**
A26.9 **Erysipeloid, unspecified**
A27 **Leptospirosis**
A27.0 **Leptospirosis icterohemorrhagica**
Leptospiral or spirochetal jaundice (hemorrhagic)
Weil's disease
A27.8 **Other forms of leptospirosis**
A27.81 **Aseptic meningitis in leptospirosis**
A27.89 **Other forms of leptospirosis**
A27.9 **Leptospirosis, unspecified**
A28 **Other zoonotic bacterial diseases, not elsewhere classified**
A28.0 **Pasteurellosis**
A28.1 **Cat-scratch disease**
Cat-scratch fever
A28.2 **Extraintestinal yersiniosis**
EXCLUDES 1 *enteritis due to Yersinia enterocolitica (A04.6)*
plague (A20.-)
A28.8 **Other specified zoonotic bacterial diseases, not elsewhere classified**
A28.9 **Zoonotic bacterial disease, unspecified**

Other bacterial diseases (A30-A49)

A30 **Leprosy [Hansen's disease]**
INCLUDES infection due to Mycobacterium leprae
EXCLUDES 1 *sequelae of leprosy (B92)*
CODING TIP Arthropathy associated with Leprosy requires an additional code from M01.-.
A30.0 **Indeterminate leprosy**
I leprosy
A30.1 **Tuberculoid leprosy**
TT leprosy
A30.2 **Borderline tuberculoid leprosy**
BT leprosy
A30.3 **Borderline leprosy**
BB leprosy
A30.4 **Borderline lepromatous leprosy**
BL leprosy

A30.5 **Lepromatous leprosy**
LL leprosy

A30.8 **Other forms of leprosy**

A30.9 **Leprosy, unspecified**

A31 Infection due to other mycobacteria

> **EXCLUDES 2** *leprosy (A30.-)*
> *tuberculosis (A15-A19)*

A31.0 **Pulmonary mycobacterial infection**
Infection due to Mycobacterium avium
Infection due to Mycobacterium intracellulare [Battey bacillus]
Infection due to Mycobacterium kansasii

A31.1 **Cutaneous mycobacterial infection**
Buruli ulcer
Infection due to Mycobacterium marinum
Infection due to Mycobacterium ulcerans

A31.2 **Disseminated mycobacterium avium-intracellulare complex (DMAC)**
MAC sepsis

A31.8 **Other mycobacterial infections**

A31.9 **Mycobacterial infection, unspecified**
Atypical mycobacterial infection NOS
Mycobacteriosis NOS

A32 Listeriosis

> **INCLUDES** listerial foodborne infection
> **EXCLUDES 1** *neonatal (disseminated) listeriosis (P37.2)*

A32.0 **Cutaneous listeriosis**

A32.1 **Listerial meningitis and meningoencephalitis**

A32.11 **Listerial meningitis**

A32.12 **Listerial meningoencephalitis**

A32.7 **Listerial sepsis**

A32.8 **Other forms of listeriosis**

A32.81 **Oculoglandular listeriosis**

A32.82 **Listerial endocarditis**

A32.89 **Other forms of listeriosis**
Listerial cerebral arteritis

A32.9 **Listeriosis, unspecified**

A33 **Tetanus neonatorum** N

A34 **Obstetrical tetanus** ♀ Ⓜ

A35 **Other tetanus**
Tetanus NOS

> **EXCLUDES 1** *obstetrical tetanus (A34)*
> *tetanus neonatorum (A33)*

> **DEFINITION** Potentially fatal disease due to the neurotoxin of Clostridium tetani, entering the body through contaminated wound, burn, or ulcer; causes muscular contractions, hyperreflexia, lockjaw, respiratory spasm, seizures, and paralysis.

A36 Diphtheria

A36.0 **Pharyngeal diphtheria**
Diphtheritic membranous angina
Tonsillar diphtheria

> **DEFINITION** An acute infectious disease usually confined to the upper respiratory tract, caused by toxigenic strains of Corynebacterium dipththeriae, and acquired by contact with an infected person or carrier of the disease.

A36.1 **Nasopharyngeal diphtheria**

A36.2 **Laryngeal diphtheria**
Diphtheritic laryngotracheitis

A36.3 **Cutaneous diphtheria**

> **EXCLUDES 2** *erythrasma (L08.1)*

A36.8 **Other diphtheria**

A36.81 **Diphtheritic cardiomyopathy**
Diphtheritic myocarditis

A36.82 **Diphtheritic radiculomyelitis**

A36.83 **Diphtheritic polyneuritis**

A36.84 **Diphtheritic tubulo-interstitial nephropathy**

A36.85 **Diphtheritic cystitis**

A36.86 **Diphtheritic conjunctivitis**

A36.89 **Other diphtheritic complications**
Diphtheritic peritonitis

A36.9 **Diphtheria, unspecified**

A37 Whooping cough

A37.0 **Whooping cough due to Bordetella pertussis**

> **DEFINITION** Infectious disease caused by Bordetella pertussis, marked by inflammation of mucous membranes and cough, ending in a prolonged crowing or whooping respiration.

A37.00 **Whooping cough due to Bordetella pertussis without pneumonia**

A37.01 **Whooping cough due to Bordetella pertussis with pneumonia**

A37.1 **Whooping cough due to Bordetella parapertussis**

A37.10 **Whooping cough due to Bordetella parapertussis without pneumonia**

A37.11 **Whooping cough due to Bordetella parapertussis with pneumonia**

A37.8 **Whooping cough due to other Bordetella species**

A37.80 **Whooping cough due to other Bordetella species without pneumonia**

A37.81 **Whooping cough due to other Bordetella species with pneumonia**

A37.9 **Whooping cough, unspecified species**

A37.90 **Whooping cough, unspecified species without pneumonia**

A37.91 **Whooping cough, unspecified species with pneumonia**

A38 Scarlet fever

> **INCLUDES** scarlatina
> **EXCLUDES 2** *streptococcal sore throat (J02.0)*

A38.0 **Scarlet fever with otitis media**

> **DEFINITION** Infection with group A beta-hemolytic streptococcal bacteria causing sore throat, fever, and rough, bright red "sandpaper" rash over most of the body.

A38.1 **Scarlet fever with myocarditis**

A38.8 **Scarlet fever with other complications**

A38.9 **Scarlet fever, uncomplicated**
Scarlet fever, NOS

A39 Meningococcal infection

A39.0 **Meningococcal meningitis**

> **DEFINITION** Inflammation of the membranes (meninges) around the brain or spinal cord causing fever, headache, stiff neck, muscle aches, and skin rashes.

A39.1 **Waterhouse-Friderichsen syndrome**
Meningococcal hemorrhagic adrenalitis
Meningococcic adrenal syndrome

> **DEFINITION** Syndrome associated with meningococcal meningitis, marked by sudden fever, purple skin discoloration, and hemorrhage into the adrenal glands with cardiovascular collapse.

A39.2 **Acute meningococcemia**

A39.3 **Chronic meningococcemia**

A39.4 **Meningococcemia, unspecified**

A39.5 **Meningococcal heart disease**

A39.50 **Meningococcal carditis, unspecified**

A39.51 **Meningococcal endocarditis**

A39.52 **Meningococcal myocarditis**

A39.53 **Meningococcal pericarditis**

A39.8 **Other meningococcal infections**

A39.81 **Meningococcal encephalitis**

A39.82 **Meningococcal retrobulbar neuritis**

A39.83 **Meningococcal arthritis**

A39.84 **Postmeningococcal arthritis**

A39.89 **Other meningococcal infections**
Meningococcal conjunctivitis

A39.9 **Meningococcal infection, unspecified**
Meningococcal disease NOS

▲ ▣ A40   Streptococcal sepsis

Code first:
- postprocedural streptococcal sepsis (T81.4-)
- streptococcal sepsis during labor (O75.3)
- streptococcal sepsis following abortion or ectopic or molar pregnancy (O03-O07, O08.0)
- streptococcal sepsis following immunization (T88.0)
- streptococcal sepsis following infusion, transfusion or therapeutic injection (T80.2-)

EXCLUDES 1 *neonatal (P36.0-P36.1)*
puerperal sepsis (O85)
sepsis due to Streptococcus, group D (A41.81)

GUIDELINES   Section I.C.1.d.1)(a)(i-iii)

Negative or inconclusive blood cultures do not preclude a diagnosis of sepsis in patients with clinical evidence of the condition, however, the provider should be queried.

The term urosepsis is a nonspecific term. It is not to be considered synonymous with sepsis. It has no default code in the Alphabetic Index. Should a provider use this term, he/she must be queried for clarification.

If a patient has sepsis and associated acute organ dysfunction or multiple organ dysfunction (MOD), follow the instructions for coding severe sepsis.

GUIDELINES   Section I.C.1.d.1)(a)(iv)

If a patient has sepsis and an acute organ dysfunction, but the medical record documentation indicates that the acute organ dysfunction is related to a medical condition other than the sepsis, do not assign a code from subcategory R65.2, Severe sepsis. An acute organ dysfunction must be associated with the sepsis in order to assign the severe sepsis code. If the documentation is not clear as to whether an acute organ dysfunction is related to the sepsis or another medical condition, query the provider.

GUIDELINES   Section I.C.15.k

Code O85, Puerperal sepsis, should be assigned with a secondary code to identify the causal organism (e.g., for a bacterial infection, assign a code from category B95-B96, Bacterial infections in conditions classified elsewhere). A code from category A40, Streptococcal sepsis, or A41, Other sepsis, should not be used for puerperal sepsis. If applicable, use additional codes to identify severe sepsis (R65.2-) and any associated acute organ dysfunction.

CODING TIP ✓   Do not assign a code from A40-A41 to indicate a bacterial infection in conditions classified elsewhere, e.g., a localized infection. Codes classified in A40-A41 are used to indicate systemic infection.

CODING TIP ✓   Severe sepsis is defined as sepsis resulting in organ dysfunction. If sepsis is associated with organ dysfunction or failure, add R65.2 to indicate severe sepsis. Additional codes are used to identify associated organ dysfunction.

A40.0   Sepsis due to streptococcus, group A

A40.1   Sepsis due to streptococcus, group B

A40.3   Sepsis due to Streptococcus pneumoniae
Pneumococcal sepsis

A40.8   Other streptococcal sepsis

A40.9   Streptococcal sepsis, unspecified

▲ ▣ A41   Other sepsis

Code first:
- postprocedural sepsis (T81.4-)
- sepsis during labor (O75.3)
- sepsis following abortion, ectopic or molar pregnancy (O03-O07, O08.0)
- sepsis following immunization (T88.0)
- sepsis following infusion, transfusion or therapeutic injection (T80.2-)

EXCLUDES 1 *bacteremia NOS (R78.81)*
neonatal (P36.-)
puerperal sepsis (O85)
streptococcal sepsis (A40.-)

EXCLUDES 2 *sepsis (due to) (in) actinomycotic (A42.7)*
sepsis (due to) (in) anthrax (A22.7)
sepsis (due to) (in) candidal (B37.7)
sepsis (due to) (in) Erysipelothrix (A26.7)
sepsis (due to) (in) extraintestinal yersiniosis (A28.2)
sepsis (due to) (in) gonococcal (A54.86)
sepsis (due to) (in) herpesviral (B00.7)
sepsis (due to) (in) listerial (A32.7)
sepsis (due to) (in) melioidosis (A24.1)
sepsis (due to) (in) meningococcal (A39.2-A39.4)
sepsis (due to) (in) plague (A20.7)
sepsis (due to) (in) tularemia (A21.7)
toxic shock syndrome (A48.3)

GUIDELINES   Section I.C.1.d.1)(a)

For a diagnosis of sepsis, assign the appropriate code for the underlying systemic infection. If the type of infection or causal organism is not further specified, assign code A41.9, Sepsis, unspecified organism. A code from subcategory R65.2, Severe sepsis, should not be assigned unless severe sepsis or an associated acute organ dysfunction is documented.

GUIDELINES   Section I.C.1.d.1)(b)

The coding of severe sepsis requires a minimum of two codes: first a code for the underlying systemic infection, followed by a code from subcategory R65.2, Severe sepsis. If the causal organism is not documented, assign code A41.9, Sepsis, unspecified organism, for the infection. Additional code(s) for the associated acute organ dysfunction are also required. Due to the complex nature of severe sepsis, some cases may require querying the provider prior to assignment of the codes.

GUIDELINES   Section I.C.15.k

Code O85, Puerperal sepsis, should be assigned with a secondary code to identify the causal organism (e.g., for a bacterial infection, assign a code from category B95-B96, Bacterial infections in conditions classified elsewhere). A code from category A40, Streptococcal sepsis, or A41, Other sepsis, should not be used for puerperal sepsis. If applicable, use additional codes to identify severe sepsis (R65.2-) and any associated acute organ dysfunction.

CODING TIP ✓   Do not assign a code from A40-A41 to indicate a bacterial infection in conditions classified elsewhere, e.g., a localized infection. Codes classified in A40-A41 are used to indicate systemic infection.

CODING TIP ✓   Severe sepsis is defined as sepsis resulting in organ dysfunction. If sepsis is associated with organ dysfunction or failure, add R65.2 to indicate severe sepsis. Additional codes are used to identify associated organ dysfunction.

▤ A41.0   Sepsis due to Staphylococcus aureus

A41.01   Sepsis due to Methicillin susceptible Staphylococcus aureus
MSSA sepsis
Staphylococcus aureus sepsis NOS

A41.02   Sepsis due to Methicillin resistant Staphylococcus aureus

---

● New   ▲ Revised   *Manifestation*   ▣-▢ Digit Indicators   ▤ Laterality   ▲ Adult (15+ years)   ▨ Maternity (12-55 years)   ▨ Newborn   ▣ Pediatric (0-17 years)   ♂ Male   ♀ Female
✖ Deleted   Unspecified   + Additional code

450   © 2017 DecisionHealth   2017 ICD-10-CM Expert for Physicians

A40 — A41.02

GUIDELINES Section I.C.1.e.1)(a). When a patient is diagnosed with an infection that is due to methicillin resistant Staphylococcus aureus (MRSA), and that infection has a combination code that includes the causal organism (e.g., sepsis, pneumonia) assign the appropriate combination code for the condition (e.g., code A41.02 ...). Do not assign code B95.62, Methicillin resistant Staphylococcus aureus infection as the cause of diseases classified elsewhere, as an additional code because the combination code includes the type of infection and the MRSA organism.

A41.1 **Sepsis due to other specified staphylococcus**
Coagulase negative staphylococcus sepsis

A41.2 **Sepsis due to unspecified staphylococcus**

A41.3 **Sepsis due to Hemophilus influenzae**

A41.4 **Sepsis due to anaerobes**
EXCLUDES 1 *gas gangrene (A48.0)*

⑤ A41.5 **Sepsis due to other Gram-negative organisms**

A41.50 **Gram-negative sepsis, unspecified**
Gram-negative sepsis NOS

A41.51 **Sepsis due to Escherichia coli [E. coli]**

A41.52 **Sepsis due to Pseudomonas**
Pseudomonas aeroginosa

A41.53 **Sepsis due to Serratia**

A41.59 **Other Gram-negative sepsis**

⑤ A41.8 **Other specified sepsis**

A41.81 **Sepsis due to Enterococcus**

A41.89 **Other specified sepsis**

A41.9 **Sepsis, unspecified organism**
Septicemia NOS

④ A42 **Actinomycosis**
EXCLUDES 1 *actinomycetoma (B47.1)*

A42.0 **Pulmonary actinomycosis**

A42.1 **Abdominal actinomycosis**

A42.2 **Cervicofacial actinomycosis**

A42.7 **Actinomycotic sepsis**

⑤ A42.8 **Other forms of actinomycosis**

A42.81 **Actinomycotic meningitis**

A42.82 **Actinomycotic encephalitis**

A42.89 **Other forms of actinomycosis**

A42.9 **Actinomycosis, unspecified**

④ A43 **Nocardiosis**

A43.0 **Pulmonary nocardiosis**

A43.1 **Cutaneous nocardiosis**

A43.8 **Other forms of nocardiosis**

A43.9 **Nocardiosis, unspecified**

④ A44 **Bartonellosis**

A44.0 **Systemic bartonellosis**
Oroya fever

A44.1 **Cutaneous and mucocutaneous bartonellosis**
Verruga peruana

A44.8 **Other forms of bartonellosis**

A44.9 **Bartonellosis, unspecified**

A46 **Erysipelas**
EXCLUDES 1 *postpartum or puerperal erysipelas (O86.89)*

DEFINITION Superficial cellulitis with dermal lymphatic involvement, commonly caused by group A beta-hemolytic streptococci; presents with shiny, raised, indurated, tender lesions with distinct margins, commonly on the legs and face.

④ A48 **Other bacterial diseases, not elsewhere classified**
EXCLUDES 1 *actinomycetoma (B47.1)*

A48.0 **Gas gangrene**
Clostridial cellulitis
Clostridial myonecrosis

A48.1 **Legionnaires' disease**

A48.2 **Nonpneumonic Legionnaires' disease [Pontiac fever]**

+ A48.3 **Toxic shock syndrome**
Use additional code to identify the organism (B95, B96)
EXCLUDES 1 *endotoxic shock NOS (R57.8)*
sepsis NOS (A41.9)

A48.4 **Brazilian purpuric fever**
Systemic Hemophilus aegyptius infection

⑤ A48.5 **Other specified botulism**
Non-foodborne intoxication due to toxins of Clostridium botulinum [C. botulinum]
EXCLUDES 1 *food poisoning due to toxins of Clostridium botulinum (A05.1)*

A48.51 **Infant botulism**

+ A48.52 **Wound botulism**
Non-foodborne botulism NOS
Use additional code for associated wound
DEFINITION Wound infection with Clostridium botulinum producing neurological effects of severe hypotonia and paralysis without gastrointestinal symptoms of food poisoning.

A48.8 **Other specified bacterial diseases**

④ A49 **Bacterial infection of unspecified site**
EXCLUDES 1 *bacterial agents as the cause of diseases classified elsewhere (B95-B96)*
chlamydial infection NOS (A74.9)
meningococcal infection NOS (A39.9)
rickettsial infection NOS (A79.9)
spirochetal infection NOS (A69.9)

⑤ A49.0 **Staphylococcal infection, unspecified site**

A49.01 **Methicillin susceptible Staphylococcus aureus infection, unspecified site**
Methicillin susceptible Staphylococcus aureus (MSSA) infection
Staphylococcus aureus infection NOS

A49.02 **Methicillin resistant Staphylococcus aureus infection, unspecified site**
Methicillin resistant Staphylococcus aureus (MRSA) infection

A49.1 **Streptococcal infection, unspecified site**

A49.2 **Hemophilus influenzae infection, unspecified site**

A49.3 **Mycoplasma infection, unspecified site**

A49.8 **Other bacterial infections of unspecified site**

A49.9 **Bacterial infection, unspecified**
EXCLUDES 1 *bacteremia NOS (R78.81)*

Infections with a predominantly sexual mode of transmission (A50-A64)

EXCLUDES 1 *human immunodeficiency virus [HIV] disease (B20)*
nonspecific and nongonococcal urethritis (N34.1)
Reiter's disease (M02.3-)

④ A50 **Congenital syphilis**

⑤ A50.0 **Early congenital syphilis, symptomatic**
Any congenital syphilitic condition specified as early or manifest less than two years after birth.

A50.01 **Early congenital syphilitic oculopathy**

A50.02 **Early congenital syphilitic osteochondropathy**

A50.03 **Early congenital syphilitic pharyngitis**
Early congenital syphilitic laryngitis

A50.04 **Early congenital syphilitic pneumonia**

A50.05 **Early congenital syphilitic rhinitis**

A50.06 **Early cutaneous congenital syphilis**

A50.07 **Early mucocutaneous congenital syphilis**

A50.08 **Early visceral congenital syphilis**

A50.09 **Other early congenital syphilis, symptomatic**

A50.1 **Early congenital syphilis, latent**
Congenital syphilis without clinical manifestations, with positive serological reaction and negative spinal fluid test, less than two years after birth.

A50.2 **Early congenital syphilis, unspecified**
Congenital syphilis NOS less than two years after birth.

⑤ A50.3 **Late congenital syphilitic oculopathy**
EXCLUDES 1 *Hutchinson's triad (A50.53)*

A50.30 **Late congenital syphilitic oculopathy, unspecified**

A50.31 **Late congenital syphilitic interstitial keratitis**

A50.32 **Late congenital syphilitic chorioretinitis**

A50.39 **Other late congenital syphilitic oculopathy**

⑤ + A50.4 **Late congenital neurosyphilis [juvenile neurosyphilis]**
Use additional code to identify any associated mental disorder
EXCLUDES 1 *Hutchinson's triad (A50.53)*

● New ▲ Revised *Manifestation* ④-⑦ Digit Indicators ▤ Laterality Ⓐ Adult (15+ years) Ⓜ Maternity (12-55 years) Ⓝ Newborn Ⓟ Pediatric (0-17 years) ♂ Male ♀ Female
✖ Deleted Unspecified + Additional code

2017 ICD-10-CM Expert for Physicians

© 2017 DecisionHealth

451

A41.02 — A50.4

+ **A50.40**   **Late congenital neurosyphilis, unspecified**
          Juvenile neurosyphilis NOS
+ **A50.41**   **Late congenital syphilitic meningitis**
+ **A50.42**   **Late congenital syphilitic encephalitis**
+ **A50.43**   **Late congenital syphilitic polyneuropathy**
+ **A50.44**   **Late congenital syphilitic optic nerve atrophy**
+ **A50.45**   **Juvenile general paresis**
          Dementia paralytica juvenilis
          Juvenile tabetoparetic neurosyphilis
+ **A50.49**   **Other late congenital neurosyphilis**
          Juvenile tabes dorsalis
⑤ **A50.5**   **Other late congenital syphilis, symptomatic**
          Any congenital syphilitic condition specified as late or
             manifest two years or more after birth.
   A50.51   **Clutton's joints**
   A50.52   **Hutchinson's teeth**
   A50.53   **Hutchinson's triad**
   A50.54   **Late congenital cardiovascular syphilis**
   A50.55   **Late congenital syphilitic arthropathy**
   A50.56   **Late congenital syphilitic osteochondropathy**
   A50.57   **Syphilitic saddle nose**
   A50.59   **Other late congenital syphilis, symptomatic**
   A50.6   **Late congenital syphilis, latent**
          Congenital syphilis without clinical manifestations, with
             positive serological reaction and negative spinal fluid test,
             two years or more after birth.
   A50.7   **Late congenital syphilis, unspecified**
          Congenital syphilis NOS two years or more after birth.
   A50.9   **Congenital syphilis, unspecified**

④ **A51**   **Early syphilis**
   A51.0   **Primary genital syphilis**
          Syphilitic chancre NOS
   A51.1   **Primary anal syphilis**
   A51.2   **Primary syphilis of other sites**
⑤ **A51.3**   **Secondary syphilis of skin and mucous membranes**
   A51.31   **Condyloma latum**
   A51.32   **Syphilitic alopecia**
   A51.39   **Other secondary syphilis of skin**
          Syphilitic leukoderma
          Syphilitic mucous patch
          EXCLUDES 1   *late syphilitic leukoderma (A52.79)*
⑤ **A51.4**   **Other secondary syphilis**
   A51.41   **Secondary syphilitic meningitis**
   A51.42   **Secondary syphilitic female pelvic disease**   ♀
   A51.43   **Secondary syphilitic oculopathy**
          Secondary syphilitic chorioretinitis
          Secondary syphilitic iridocyclitis, iritis
          Secondary syphilitic uveitis
   A51.44   **Secondary syphilitic nephritis**
   A51.45   **Secondary syphilitic hepatitis**
   A51.46   **Secondary syphilitic osteopathy**
   A51.49   **Other secondary syphilitic conditions**
          Secondary syphilitic lymphadenopathy
          Secondary syphilitic myositis
   A51.5   **Early syphilis, latent**
          Syphilis (acquired) without clinical manifestations, with
             positive serological reaction and negative spinal fluid test,
             less than two years after infection.
   A51.9   **Early syphilis, unspecified**

④ **A52**   **Late syphilis**
⑤ **A52.0**   **Cardiovascular and cerebrovascular syphilis**
   A52.00   **Cardiovascular syphilis, unspecified**
   A52.01   **Syphilitic aneurysm of aorta**
   A52.02   **Syphilitic aortitis**
   A52.03   **Syphilitic endocarditis**
          Syphilitic aortic valve incompetence or stenosis
          Syphilitic mitral valve stenosis
          Syphilitic pulmonary valve regurgitation
   A52.04   **Syphilitic cerebral arteritis**
   A52.05   **Other cerebrovascular syphilis**
          Syphilitic cerebral aneurysm (ruptured) (non-ruptured)
          Syphilitic cerebral thrombosis

   A52.06   **Other syphilitic heart involvement**
          Syphilitic coronary artery disease
          Syphilitic myocarditis
          Syphilitic pericarditis
   A52.09   **Other cardiovascular syphilis**
⑤ **A52.1**   **Symptomatic neurosyphilis**
   A52.10   **Symptomatic neurosyphilis, unspecified**
   A52.11   **Tabes dorsalis**
          Locomotor ataxia (progressive)
          Tabetic neurosyphilis
   A52.12   **Other cerebrospinal syphilis**
   A52.13   **Late syphilitic meningitis**
   A52.14   **Late syphilitic encephalitis**
   A52.15   **Late syphilitic neuropathy**
          Late syphilitic acoustic neuritis
          Late syphilitic optic (nerve) atrophy
          Late syphilitic polyneuropathy
          Late syphilitic retrobulbar neuritis
   A52.16   **Charcôt's arthropathy (tabetic)**
   A52.17   **General paresis**
          Dementia paralytica
   A52.19   **Other symptomatic neurosyphilis**
          Syphilitic parkinsonism
   A52.2   **Asymptomatic neurosyphilis**
   A52.3   **Neurosyphilis, unspecified**
          Gumma (syphilitic)
          Syphilis (late)
          Syphiloma
⑤ **A52.7**   **Other symptomatic late syphilis**
   A52.71   **Late syphilitic oculopathy**
          Late syphilitic chorioretinitis
          Late syphilitic episcleritis
   A52.72   **Syphilis of lung and bronchus**
   A52.73   **Symptomatic late syphilis of other respiratory organs**
   A52.74   **Syphilis of liver and other viscera**
          Late syphilitic peritonitis
   A52.75   **Syphilis of kidney and ureter**
          Syphilitic glomerular disease
   A52.76   **Other genitourinary symptomatic late syphilis**
          Late syphilitic female pelvic inflammatory disease
   A52.77   **Syphilis of bone and joint**
   A52.78   **Syphilis of other musculoskeletal tissue**
          Late syphilitic bursitis
          Syphilis [stage unspecified] of bursa
          Syphilis [stage unspecified] of muscle
          Syphilis [stage unspecified] of synovium
          Syphilis [stage unspecified] of tendon
   A52.79   **Other symptomatic late syphilis**
          Late syphilitic leukoderma
          Syphilis of adrenal gland
          Syphilis of pituitary gland
          Syphilis of thyroid gland
          Syphilitic splenomegaly
          EXCLUDES 1   *syphilitic leukoderma (secondary)*
                        (A51.39)
   A52.8   **Late syphilis, latent**
          Syphilis (acquired) without clinical manifestations, with
             positive serological reaction and negative spinal fluid test,
             two years or more after infection
   A52.9   **Late syphilis, unspecified**
④ **A53**   **Other and unspecified syphilis**
   A53.0   **Latent syphilis, unspecified as early or late**
          Latent syphilis NOS
          Positive serological reaction for syphilis
   A53.9   **Syphilis, unspecified**
          Infection due to Treponema pallidum NOS
          Syphilis (acquired) NOS
          EXCLUDES 1   *syphilis NOS under two years of age*
                        (A50.2)
④ **A54**   **Gonococcal infection**
⑤ **A54.0**   **Gonococcal infection of lower genitourinary tract without periurethral or accessory gland abscess**
          EXCLUDES 1   *gonococcal infection with genitourinary*
                        gland abscess (A54.1)
                        gonococcal infection with periurethral
                        abscess (A54.1)
   A54.00   **Gonococcal infection of lower genitourinary tract, unspecified**
   A54.01   **Gonococcal cystitis and urethritis, unspecified**

● New   ▲ Revised   *Manifestation*   ④-⑦ Digit Indicators   ⊟ Laterality   Ⓐ Adult   Ⓜ Maternity   Ⓝ Newborn   Ⓟ Pediatric   ♂ Male   ♀ Female
✖ Deleted   Unspecified   + Additional code   (15+ years)   (12-55 years)   (0-17 years)

A54.02   **Gonococcal vulvovaginitis, unspecified** ♀

A54.03   **Gonococcal cervicitis, unspecified** ♀

A54.09   **Other gonococcal infection of lower genitourinary tract**

A54.1   **Gonococcal infection of lower genitourinary tract with periurethral and accessory gland abscess**
Gonococcal Bartholin's gland abscess

⑤ A54.2   **Gonococcal pelviperitonitis and other gonococcal genitourinary infection**

A54.21   **Gonococcal infection of kidney and ureter**

A54.22   **Gonococcal prostatitis** ♂

A54.23   **Gonococcal infection of other male genital organs** ♂
Gonococcal epididymitis
Gonococcal orchitis

A54.24   **Gonococcal female pelvic inflammatory disease** ♀
Gonococcal pelviperitonitis
EXCLUDES 1   *gonococcal peritonitis (A54.85)*

A54.29   **Other gonococcal genitourinary infections**

⑤ A54.3   **Gonococcal infection of eye**

A54.30   **Gonococcal infection of eye, unspecified**

A54.31   **Gonococcal conjunctivitis**
Ophthalmia neonatorum due to gonococcus

A54.32   **Gonococcal iridocyclitis**

A54.33   **Gonococcal keratitis**

A54.39   **Other gonococcal eye infection**
Gonococcal endophthalmia

⑤ A54.4   **Gonococcal infection of musculoskeletal system**

A54.40   **Gonococcal infection of musculoskeletal system, unspecified**

A54.41   **Gonococcal spondylopathy**

A54.42   **Gonococcal arthritis**
EXCLUDES 2   *gonococcal infection of spine (A54.41)*

A54.43   **Gonococcal osteomyelitis**
EXCLUDES 2   *gonococcal infection of spine (A54.41)*

A54.49   **Gonococcal infection of other musculoskeletal tissue**
Gonococcal bursitis
Gonococcal myositis
Gonococcal synovitis
Gonococcal tenosynovitis

A54.5   **Gonococcal pharyngitis**

A54.6   **Gonococcal infection of anus and rectum**

⑤ A54.8   **Other gonococcal infections**

A54.81   **Gonococcal meningitis**

A54.82   **Gonococcal brain abscess**

A54.83   **Gonococcal heart infection**
Gonococcal endocarditis
Gonococcal myocarditis
Gonococcal pericarditis

A54.84   **Gonococcal pneumonia**

A54.85   **Gonococcal peritonitis**
EXCLUDES 1   *gonococcal pelviperitonitis (A54.24)*

A54.86   **Gonococcal sepsis**

A54.89   **Other gonococcal infections**
Gonococcal keratoderma
Gonococcal lymphadenitis

A54.9   **Gonococcal infection, unspecified**

A55   **Chlamydial lymphogranuloma (venereum)**
Climatic or tropical bubo
Durand-Nicolas-Favre disease
Esthiomene
Lymphogranuloma inguinale
DEFINITION   Sexually transmitted infection by Chlamydia trachomatis, seen in warm climates; presents with primary cutaneous or mucosal lesion at infection site and acute unilateral or bilateral lymphadenopathy.

④ A56   **Other sexually transmitted chlamydial diseases**
INCLUDES   sexually transmitted diseases due to Chlamydia trachomatis
EXCLUDES 1   *neonatal chlamydial conjunctivitis (P39.1)*
neonatal chlamydial pneumonia (P23.1)
EXCLUDES 2   *chlamydial lymphogranuloma (A55)*
conditions classified to A74.-

⑤ A56.0   **Chlamydial infection of lower genitourinary tract**

A56.00   **Chlamydial infection of lower genitourinary tract, unspecified**

A56.01   **Chlamydial cystitis and urethritis**

A56.02   **Chlamydial vulvovaginitis** ♀

A56.09   **Other chlamydial infection of lower genitourinary tract**
Chlamydial cervicitis

⑤ A56.1   **Chlamydial infection of pelviperitoneum and other genitourinary organs**

A56.11   **Chlamydial female pelvic inflammatory disease** ♀

A56.19   **Other chlamydial genitourinary infection**
Chlamydial epididymitis
Chlamydial orchitis

A56.2   **Chlamydial infection of genitourinary tract, unspecified**

A56.3   **Chlamydial infection of anus and rectum**

A56.4   **Chlamydial infection of pharynx**

A56.8   **Sexually transmitted chlamydial infection of other sites**

A57   **Chancroid**
Ulcus molle
DEFINITION   Sexually transmitted disease, characterized by a painful, primary ulcer, usually on the external genitalia.

A58   **Granuloma inguinale**
Donovanosis

④ A59   **Trichomoniasis**
EXCLUDES 2   *intestinal trichomoniasis (A07.8)*

⑤ A59.0   **Urogenital trichomoniasis**

A59.00   **Urogenital trichomoniasis, unspecified**
Fluor (vaginalis) due to Trichomonas
Leukorrhea (vaginalis) due to Trichomonas

A59.01   **Trichomonal vulvovaginitis** ♀
DEFINITION   Sexually transmitted disease caused by the protozoan Trichomonas vaginalis infecting the vagina and external female genitalia.

A59.02   **Trichomonal prostatitis** ♂

A59.03   **Trichomonal cystitis and urethritis**

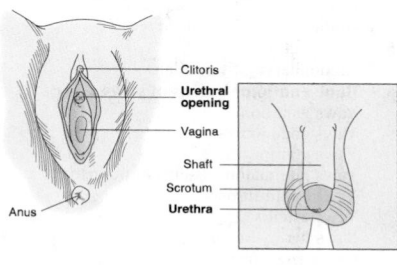

Trichomonal cystitis and urethritis
A sexually transmitted disease caused by the protozoan
Trichomonas vaginalis infecting the urethra

A59.09   **Other urogenital trichomoniasis**
Trichomonas cervicitis

A59.8   **Trichomoniasis of other sites**

A59.9   **Trichomoniasis, unspecified**

④ A60   **Anogenital herpesviral [herpes simplex] infections**

⑤ A60.0   **Herpesviral infection of genitalia and urogenital tract**

A60.00   **Herpesviral infection of urogenital system, unspecified**

A60.01   **Herpesviral infection of penis** ♂

A60.02   **Herpesviral infection of other male genital organs** ♂

A60.03   **Herpesviral cervicitis** ♀

A60.04   **Herpesviral vulvovaginitis** ♀
Herpesviral [herpes simplex] ulceration
Herpesviral [herpes simplex] vaginitis
Herpesviral [herpes simplex] vulvitis

A60.09   **Herpesviral infection of other urogenital tract**

A60.1   **Herpesviral infection of perianal skin and rectum**

A60.9   **Anogenital herpesviral infection, unspecified**

④ A63   **Other predominantly sexually transmitted diseases, not elsewhere classified**
EXCLUDES 2   *molluscum contagiosum (B08.1)*
papilloma of cervix (D26.0)

A63.0   **Anogenital (venereal) warts**
Anogenital warts due to (human) papillomavirus [HPV]
Condyloma acuminatum

DEFINITION A wartlike growth on the skin or mucous membrane, in the area of the anus or external genitalia.

A63.8   **Other specified predominantly sexually transmitted diseases**

A64   **Unspecified sexually transmitted disease**

Other spirochetal diseases (A65-A69)

EXCLUDES 2   *leptospirosis (A27.-)*
                  syphilis (A50-A53)

A65   **Nonvenereal syphilis**
      Bejel
      Endemic syphilis
      Njovera

4 A66   **Yaws**
      INCLUDES   bouba
                      frambesia (tropica)
                      pian

A66.0   **Initial lesions of yaws**
      Chancre of yaws
      Frambesia, initial or primary
      Initial frambesial ulcer
      Mother yaw

A66.1   **Multiple papillomata and wet crab yaws**
      Frambesioma
      Pianoma
      Plantar or palmar papilloma of yaws

A66.2   **Other early skin lesions of yaws**
      Cutaneous yaws, less than five years after infection
      Early yaws
         (cutaneous)(macular)(maculopapular)(micropapular)(papular)
      Frambeside of early yaws

A66.3   **Hyperkeratosis of yaws**
      Ghoul hand
      Hyperkeratosis, palmar or plantar (early) (late) due to yaws
      Worm-eaten soles

A66.4   **Gummata and ulcers of yaws**
      Gummatous frambeside
      Nodular late yaws (ulcerated)

A66.5   **Gangosa**
      Rhinopharyngitis mutilans

A66.6   **Bone and joint lesions of yaws**
      Yaws ganglion
      Yaws goundou
      Yaws gumma, bone
      Yaws gummatous osteitis or periostitis
      Yaws hydrarthrosis
      Yaws osteitis
      Yaws periostitis (hypertrophic)

A66.7   **Other manifestations of yaws**
      Juxta-articular nodules of yaws
      Mucosal yaws

A66.8   **Latent yaws**
      Yaws without clinical manifestations, with positive serology

A66.9   **Yaws, unspecified**

4 A67   **Pinta [carate]**

A67.0   **Primary lesions of pinta**
      Chancre (primary) of pinta
      Papule (primary) of pinta

A67.1   **Intermediate lesions of pinta**
      Erythematous plaques of pinta
      Hyperchromic lesions of pinta
      Hyperkeratosis of pinta
      Pintids

A67.2   **Late lesions of pinta**
      Achromic skin lesions of pinta
      Cicatricial skin lesions of pinta
      Dyschromic skin lesions of pinta

A67.3   **Mixed lesions of pinta**
      Achromic with hyperchromic skin lesions of pinta [carate]

A67.9   **Pinta, unspecified**

4 A68   **Relapsing fevers**
      INCLUDES   recurrent fever
      EXCLUDES 2   *Lyme disease (A69.2-)*

A68.0   **Louse-borne relapsing fever**
      Relapsing fever due to Borrelia recurrentis

A68.1   **Tick-borne relapsing fever**
      Relapsing fever due to any Borrelia species other than Borrelia recurrentis

A68.9   **Relapsing fever, unspecified**

4 A69   **Other spirochetal infections**

A69.0   **Necrotizing ulcerative stomatitis**
      Cancrum oris
      Fusospirochetal gangrene
      Noma
      Stomatitis gangrenosa

A69.1   **Other Vincent's infections**
      Fusospirochetal pharyngitis
      Necrotizing ulcerative (acute) gingivitis
      Necrotizing ulcerative (acute) gingivostomatitis
      Spirochetal stomatitis
      Trench mouth
      Vincent's angina
      Vincent's gingivitis

5 A69.2   **Lyme disease**
      Erythema chronicum migrans due to Borrelia burgdorferi
      DEFINITION   Tick-transmitted infection caused by Borrelia burgdorferi, manifesting with erythema chronicum migrans, myalgia, arthritis of the large joints, and nervous and cardiovascular system involvement.

A69.20   **Lyme disease, unspecified**

Lyme disease

Borrelia burgdorferi bacteria is transmitted through the bite of a tick

A69.21   **Meningitis due to Lyme disease**

A69.22   **Other neurologic disorders in Lyme disease**
      Cranial neuritis
      Meningoencephalitis
      Polyneuropathy

A69.23   **Arthritis due to Lyme disease**

A69.29   **Other conditions associated with Lyme disease**
      Myopericarditis due to Lyme disease

A69.8   **Other specified spirochetal infections**

A69.9   **Spirochetal infection, unspecified**

Other diseases caused by chlamydiae (A70-A74)

EXCLUDES 1   *sexually transmitted chlamydial diseases (A55-A56)*

A70   **Chlamydia psittaci infections**
      Ornithosis
      Parrot fever
      Psittacosis

4 A71   **Trachoma**
      EXCLUDES 1   *sequelae of trachoma (B94.0)*

A71.0   **Initial stage of trachoma**
      Trachoma dubium

A71.1   **Active stage of trachoma**
      Granular conjunctivitis (trachomatous)
      Trachomatous follicular conjunctivitis
      Trachomatous pannus

A71.9   **Trachoma, unspecified**

4 A74   **Other diseases caused by chlamydiae**
      EXCLUDES 1   *neonatal chlamydial conjunctivitis (P39.1)*
                   neonatal chlamydial pneumonia (P23.1)
                   Reiter's disease (M02.3-)
                   sexually transmitted chlamydial diseases (A55-A56)
      EXCLUDES 2   *chlamydial pneumonia (J16.0)*

● New   ▲ Revised   *Manifestation*   **4 - 7** Digit Indicators   ⊟ Laterality   Ⓐ Adult (15+ years)   Ⓜ Maternity (12-55 years)   Ⓝ Newborn   Ⓟ Pediatric (0-17 years)   ♂ Male   ♀ Female
✖ Deleted   Unspecified   + Additional code

454   © 2017 DecisionHealth   2017 ICD-10-CM Expert for Physicians

A74.0   **Chlamydial conjunctivitis**
        Paratrachoma
⑤ A74.8   **Other chlamydial diseases**
    A74.81   **Chlamydial peritonitis**
    A74.89   **Other chlamydial diseases**
A74.9   **Chlamydial infection, unspecified**
        Chlamydiosis NOS

Rickettsioses (A75-A79)

④ A75   **Typhus fever**
    EXCLUDES 1   *rickettsiosis due to Ehrlichia sennetsu (A79.81)*

A75.0   **Epidemic louse-borne typhus fever due to Rickettsia prowazekii**
        Classical typhus (fever)
        Epidemic (louse-borne) typhus
A75.1   **Recrudescent typhus [Brill's disease]**
        Brill-Zinsser disease
A75.2   **Typhus fever due to Rickettsia typhi**
        Murine (flea-borne) typhus
A75.3   **Typhus fever due to Rickettsia tsutsugamushi**
        Scrub (mite-borne) typhus
        Tsutsugamushi fever
A75.9   **Typhus fever, unspecified**
        Typhus (fever) NOS

④ A77   **Spotted fever [tick-borne rickettsioses]**
A77.0   **Spotted fever due to Rickettsia rickettsii**
        Rocky Mountain spotted fever
        Sao Paulo fever
A77.1   **Spotted fever due to Rickettsia conorii**
        African tick typhus
        Boutonneuse fever
        India tick typhus
        Kenya tick typhus
        Marseilles fever
        Mediterranean tick fever
A77.2   **Spotted fever due to Rickettsia siberica**
        North Asian tick fever
        Siberian tick typhus
A77.3   **Spotted fever due to Rickettsia australis**
        Queensland tick typhus
⑤ A77.4   **Ehrlichiosis**
    EXCLUDES 1   *Rickettsiosis due to Ehrlichia sennetsu (A79.81)*
    A77.40   **Ehrlichiosis, unspecified**
    A77.41   **Ehrlichiosis chafeensis [E. chafeensis]**
    A77.49   **Other ehrlichiosis**
A77.8   **Other spotted fevers**
A77.9   **Spotted fever, unspecified**
        Tick-borne typhus NOS

A78   **Q fever**
        Infection due to Coxiella burnetii
        Nine Mile fever
        Quadrilateral fever
④ A79   **Other rickettsioses**
A79.0   **Trench fever**
        Quintan fever
        Wolhynian fever
A79.1   **Rickettsialpox due to Rickettsia akari**
        Kew Garden fever
        Vesicular rickettsiosis
⑤ A79.8   **Other specified rickettsioses**
    A79.81   **Rickettsiosis due to Ehrlichia sennetsu**
    A79.89   **Other specified rickettsioses**
A79.9   **Rickettsiosis, unspecified**
        Rickettsial infection NOS

Viral and prion infections of the central nervous system (A80-A89)

EXCLUDES 1   *postpolio syndrome (G14)*
            sequelae of poliomyelitis (B91)
            sequelae of viral encephalitis (B94.1)
④ A80   **Acute poliomyelitis**

CODING TIP ✓   Do not assign a code from category A80 to indicate sequela of poliomyelitis or post polio syndrome. A80- codes are used to report acute, active poliomyelitis only. Use B91 for sequelae of polio, see G14 for post polio syndrome as documented by the physician.

A80.0   **Acute paralytic poliomyelitis, vaccine-associated**
A80.1   **Acute paralytic poliomyelitis, wild virus, imported**
A80.2   **Acute paralytic poliomyelitis, wild virus, indigenous**
⑤ A80.3   **Acute paralytic poliomyelitis, other and unspecified**
    A80.30   **Acute paralytic poliomyelitis, unspecified**
    A80.39   **Other acute paralytic poliomyelitis**
A80.4   **Acute nonparalytic poliomyelitis**
A80.9   **Acute poliomyelitis, unspecified**
④+ A81   **Atypical virus infections of central nervous system**
    INCLUDES   diseases of the central nervous system caused by prions
    Use additional code to identify:
    dementia with behavioral disturbance (F02.81)
    dementia without behavioral disturbance (F02.80)
⑤+ A81.0   **Creutzfeldt-Jakob disease**
    DEFINITION   Degenerative neural disease caused by a prion (an infectious protein); presents with loss of muscular control, balance, and memory, twitching movements, nervousness and agitation, changes in personality, and dementia.
    + A81.00   **Creutzfeldt-Jakob disease, unspecified**
            Jakob-Creutzfeldt disease, unspecified
    + A81.01   **Variant Creutzfeldt-Jakob disease**
            vCJD
            DEFINITION   Rare, transmissible form of fatal Jakob-Creutzfeldt disease, affecting younger people with a longer duration, causing spongiform degeneration of the brain with unusual psychiatric and sensory symptoms.
    + A81.09   **Other Creutzfeldt-Jakob disease**
            CJD
            Familial Creutzfeldt-Jakob disease
            Iatrogenic Creutzfeldt-Jakob disease
            Sporadic Creutzfeldt-Jakob disease
            Subacute spongiform encephalopathy (with dementia)
+ A81.1   **Subacute sclerosing panencephalitis**
        Dawson's inclusion body encephalitis
        Van Bogaert's sclerosing leukoencephalopathy
+ A81.2   **Progressive multifocal leukoencephalopathy**
        Multifocal leukoencephalopathy NOS
⑤+ A81.8   **Other atypical virus infections of central nervous system**
    + A81.81   **Kuru**
    + A81.82   **Gerstmann-Sträussler-Scheinker syndrome**
            GSS syndrome
            DEFINITION   Extremely rare, inherited, fatal disease of the brain that progresses slowly, causing lack of muscle coordination, unsteady gait, dementia, slurred speech, spasticity, and coma before death.
    + A81.83   **Fatal familial insomnia**
            FFI
            DEFINITION   Very rare, inherited brain disease caused by prion protein mutation from soluble to insoluble, resulting in plaques forming in the thalamus, causing insomnia that progresses to dementia, unresponsiveness, and death.
    + A81.89   **Other atypical virus infections of central nervous system**
+ A81.9   **Atypical virus infection of central nervous system, unspecified**
        Prion diseases of the central nervous system NOS
④ A82   **Rabies**
A82.0   **Sylvatic rabies**
A82.1   **Urban rabies**
A82.9   **Rabies, unspecified**
④ A83   **Mosquito-borne viral encephalitis**
    INCLUDES   mosquito-borne viral meningoencephalitis
    EXCLUDES 2   *Venezuelan equine encephalitis (A92.2)*
                West Nile fever (A92.3-)
                West Nile virus (A92.3-)

A83.0   **Japanese encephalitis**
A83.1   **Western equine encephalitis**
A83.2   **Eastern equine encephalitis**
A83.3   **St Louis encephalitis**
A83.4   **Australian encephalitis**
       Kunjin virus disease
A83.5   **California encephalitis**
       California meningoencephalitis
       La Crosse encephalitis
A83.6   **Rocio virus disease**
A83.8   **Other mosquito-borne viral encephalitis**
A83.9   **Mosquito-borne viral encephalitis, unspecified**

A84   **Tick-borne viral encephalitis**
    INCLUDES   tick-borne viral meningoencephalitis
A84.0   **Far Eastern tick-borne encephalitis [Russian spring-summer encephalitis]**
A84.1   **Central European tick-borne encephalitis**
A84.8   **Other tick-borne viral encephalitis**
       Louping ill
       Powassan virus disease
A84.9   **Tick-borne viral encephalitis, unspecified**

A85   **Other viral encephalitis, not elsewhere classified**
    INCLUDES   specified viral encephalomyelitis NEC
             specified viral meningoencephalitis NEC
    EXCLUDES 1   *benign myalgic encephalomyelitis (G93.3)*
           encephalitis due to cytomegalovirus (B25.8)
           encephalitis due to herpesvirus NEC (B10.0-)
           encephalitis due to herpesvirus [herpes simplex] (B00.4)
           encephalitis due to measles virus (B05.0)
           encephalitis due to mumps virus (B26.2)
           encephalitis due to poliomyelitis virus (A80.-)
           encephalitis due to zoster (B02.0)
           lymphocytic choriomeningitis (A87.2)
A85.0   **Enteroviral encephalitis**
       Enteroviral encephalomyelitis
A85.1   **Adenoviral encephalitis**
       Adenoviral meningoencephalitis
A85.2   **Arthropod-borne viral encephalitis, unspecified**
    EXCLUDES 1   *West nile virus with encephalitis (A92.31)*
A85.8   **Other specified viral encephalitis**
       Encephalitis lethargica
       Von Economo-Cruchet disease

A86   **Unspecified viral encephalitis**
       Viral encephalomyelitis NOS
       Viral meningoencephalitis NOS

A87   **Viral meningitis**
    EXCLUDES 1   *meningitis due to herpesvirus [herpes simplex] (B00.3)*
           meningitis due to herpesvirus [herpes simplex] (B00.3)
           meningitis due to measles virus (B05.1)
           meningitis due to mumps virus (B26.1)
           meningitis due to poliomyelitis virus (A80.-)
           meningitis due to zoster (B02.1)
A87.0   **Enteroviral meningitis**
       Coxsackievirus meningitis
       Echovirus meningitis
A87.1   **Adenoviral meningitis**
A87.2   **Lymphocytic choriomeningitis**
       Lymphocytic meningoencephalitis
A87.8   **Other viral meningitis**
A87.9   **Viral meningitis, unspecified**

A88   **Other viral infections of central nervous system, not elsewhere classified**
    EXCLUDES 1   *viral encephalitis NOS (A86)*
           viral meningitis NOS (A87.9)
A88.0   **Enteroviral exanthematous fever [Boston exanthem]**
A88.1   **Epidemic vertigo**
A88.8   **Other specified viral infections of central nervous system**
A89   **Unspecified viral infection of central nervous system**

Arthropod-borne viral fevers and viral hemorrhagic fevers (A90-A99)

A90   **Dengue fever [classical dengue]**
    EXCLUDES 1   *dengue hemorrhagic fever (A91)*

A91   **Dengue hemorrhagic fever**
A92   **Other mosquito-borne viral fevers**
    EXCLUDES 1   *Ross River disease (B33.1)*
A92.0   **Chikungunya virus disease**
       Chikungunya (hemorrhagic) fever
A92.1   **O'nyong-nyong fever**
A92.2   **Venezuelan equine fever**
       Venezuelan equine encephalitis
       Venezuelan equine encephalomyelitis virus disease
A92.3   **West Nile virus infection**
       West Nile fever

West Nile virus infection

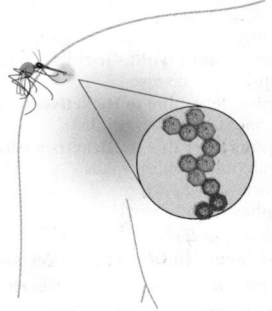

A92.30   **West Nile virus infection, unspecified**
       West Nile fever NOS
       West Nile fever without complications
       West Nile virus NOS
A92.31   **West Nile virus infection with encephalitis**
       West Nile encephalitis
       West Nile encephalomyelitis
+ A92.32   **West Nile virus infection with other neurologic manifestation**
       Use additional code to specify the neurologic manifestation
+ A92.39   **West Nile virus infection with other complications**
       Use additional code to specify the other conditions
• A92.4   **Rift Valley fever**
• A92.5   **Zika virus disease**
       Zika virus fever
       Zika virus infection
       Zika NOS
A92.8   **Other specified mosquito-borne viral fevers**
A92.9   **Mosquito-borne viral fever, unspecified**

A93   **Other arthropod-borne viral fevers, not elsewhere classified**
A93.0   **Oropouche virus disease**
       Oropouche fever
A93.1   **Sandfly fever**
       Pappataci fever
       Phlebotomus fever
A93.2   **Colorado tick fever**
A93.8   **Other specified arthropod-borne viral fevers**
       Piry virus disease
       Vesicular stomatitis virus disease [Indiana fever]

A94   **Unspecified arthropod-borne viral fever**
       Arboviral fever NOS
       Arbovirus infection NOS
A95   **Yellow fever**
A95.0   **Sylvatic yellow fever**
       Jungle yellow fever
A95.1   **Urban yellow fever**
A95.9   **Yellow fever, unspecified**

A96   **Arenaviral hemorrhagic fever**
A96.0   **Junin hemorrhagic fever**
       Argentinian hemorrhagic fever
A96.1   **Machupo hemorrhagic fever**
       Bolivian hemorrhagic fever
A96.2   **Lassa fever**
A96.8   **Other arenaviral hemorrhagic fevers**
A96.9   **Arenaviral hemorrhagic fever, unspecified**

• New   ▲ Revised   *Manifestation*   4-7 Digit Indicators   Laterality   Adult (15+ years)   Maternity (12-55 years)   Newborn   Pediatric (0-17 years)   ♂ Male   ♀ Female
✖ Deleted   Unspecified   + Additional code

456   © 2017 DecisionHealth   2017 ICD-10-CM Expert for Physicians

▣ **A98** **Other viral hemorrhagic fevers, not elsewhere classified**

> **EXCLUDES 1** *chikungunya hemorrhagic fever (A92.0)*
> *dengue hemorrhagic fever (A91)*

A98.0 **Crimean-Congo hemorrhagic fever**
Central Asian hemorrhagic fever

A98.1 **Omsk hemorrhagic fever**

A98.2 **Kyasanur Forest disease**

A98.3 **Marburg virus disease**

A98.4 **Ebola virus disease**

A98.5 **Hemorrhagic fever with renal syndrome**
Epidemic hemorrhagic fever
Korean hemorrhagic fever
Russian hemorrhagic fever
Hantaan virus disease
Hantavirus disease with renal manifestations
Nephropathia epidemica
Songo fever

> **EXCLUDES 1** *hantavirus (cardio) -pulmonary syndrome (B33.4)*

A98.8 **Other specified viral hemorrhagic fevers**

A99 **Unspecified viral hemorrhagic fever**

Viral infections characterized by skin and mucous membrane lesions (B00-B09)

▣ **B00** **Herpesviral [herpes simplex] infections**

> **EXCLUDES 1** *congenital herpesviral infections (P35.2)*

> **EXCLUDES 2** *anogenital herpesviral infection (A60.-)*
> *gammaherpesviral mononucleosis (B27.0-)*
> *herpangina (B08.5)*

> **CODING TIP ✓** Conditions classified to B00 are due to herpes simplex virus, and conditions stated as due to herpes zoster virus (such as shingles) should not be coded using codes from B00-. Category B02- includes infections due to herpes zoster virus.

B00.0 **Eczema herpeticum**
Kaposi's varicelliform eruption

> **DEFINITION** Potentially fatal infection with the herpes simplex virus at the site of an existing skin condition, often atopic dermatitis, causing severe rash, fever, and fatigue.

B00.1 **Herpesviral vesicular dermatitis**
Herpes simplex facialis
Herpes simplex labialis
Herpes simplex otitis externa
Vesicular dermatitis of ear
Vesicular dermatitis of lip

B00.2 **Herpesviral gingivostomatitis and pharyngotonsillitis**
Herpesviral pharyngitis

B00.3 **Herpesviral meningitis**

B00.4 **Herpesviral encephalitis**
Herpesviral meningoencephalitis
Simian B disease

> **EXCLUDES 1** *herpesviral encephalitis due to herpesvirus 6 and 7 (B10.01, B10.09)*
> *non-simplex herpesviral encephalitis (B10.0-)*

▤ **B00.5** **Herpesviral ocular disease**

B00.50 **Herpesviral ocular disease, unspecified**

B00.51 **Herpesviral iridocyclitis**
Herpesviral iritis
Herpesviral uveitis, anterior

B00.52 **Herpesviral keratitis**
Herpesviral keratoconjunctivitis

B00.53 **Herpesviral conjunctivitis**

B00.59 **Other herpesviral disease of eye**
Herpesviral dermatitis of eyelid

B00.7 **Disseminated herpesviral disease**
Herpesviral sepsis

▤ **B00.8** **Other forms of herpesviral infections**

B00.81 **Herpesviral hepatitis**

B00.82 **Herpes simplex myelitis**

B00.89 **Other herpesviral infection**
Herpesviral whitlow

> **DEFINITION** Viral infection that results in a painful, blistery eruption on one of the digits.

B00.9 **Herpesviral infection, unspecified**
Herpes simplex infection NOS

▣ **B01** **Varicella [chickenpox]**

B01.0 **Varicella meningitis**

▤ **B01.1** **Varicella encephalitis, myelitis and encephalomyelitis**
Postchickenpox encephalitis, myelitis and encephalomyelitis

B01.11 **Varicella encephalitis and encephalomyelitis**
Postchickenpox encephalitis and encephalomyelitis

B01.12 **Varicella myelitis**
Postchickenpox myelitis

B01.2 **Varicella pneumonia**

▤ **B01.8** **Varicella with other complications**

B01.81 **Varicella keratitis**

B01.89 **Other varicella complications**

B01.9 **Varicella without complication**
Varicella NOS

▣ **B02** **Zoster [herpes zoster]**

> **INCLUDES** shingles
> zona

Zoster (herpes zoster)

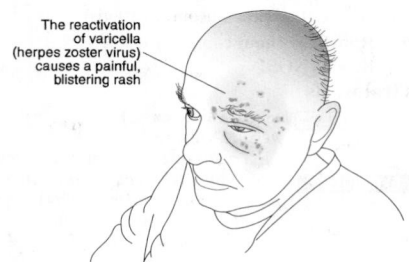

The reactivation of varicella (herpes zoster virus) causes a painful, blistering rash

B02.0 **Zoster encephalitis**
Zoster meningoencephalitis

B02.1 **Zoster meningitis**

▤ **B02.2** **Zoster with other nervous system involvement**

B02.21 **Postherpetic geniculate ganglionitis**

B02.22 **Postherpetic trigeminal neuralgia**

B02.23 **Postherpetic polyneuropathy**

B02.24 **Postherpetic myelitis**
Herpes zoster myelitis

B02.29 **Other postherpetic nervous system involvement**
Postherpetic radiculopathy

▤ **B02.3** **Zoster ocular disease**

B02.30 **Zoster ocular disease, unspecified**

B02.31 **Zoster conjunctivitis**

B02.32 **Zoster iridocyclitis**

B02.33 **Zoster keratitis**
Herpes zoster keratoconjunctivitis

B02.34 **Zoster scleritis**

B02.39 **Other herpes zoster eye disease**
Zoster blepharitis

B02.7 **Disseminated zoster**

B02.8 **Zoster with other complications**
Herpes zoster otitis externa

B02.9 **Zoster without complications**
Zoster NOS

B03 **Smallpox**
Note: In 1980 the 33rd World Health Assembly declared that smallpox had been eradicated.
The classification is maintained for surveillance purposes.

B04 **Monkeypox**

▣ **B05** **Measles**

> **INCLUDES** morbilli

> **EXCLUDES 1** *subacute sclerosing panencephalitis (A81.1)*

B05.0 **Measles complicated by encephalitis**
Postmeasles encephalitis

● New ▲ Revised *Manifestation* ▣-▨ Digit Indicators ⊟ Laterality Ⓐ Adult (15+ years) Ⓜ Maternity (12-55 years) Ⓝ Newborn Ⓟ Pediatric (0-17 years) ♂ Male ♀ Female
✖ Deleted Unspecified + Additional code

2017 ICD-10-CM Expert for Physicians

© 2017 DecisionHealth

457

B05.1   **Measles complicated by meningitis**
Postmeasles meningitis

B05.2   **Measles complicated by pneumonia**
Postmeasles pneumonia

B05.3   **Measles complicated by otitis media**
Postmeasles otitis media

B05.4   **Measles with intestinal complications**

⑤ **B05.8**   **Measles with other complications**

   B05.81   **Measles keratitis and keratoconjunctivitis**

   B05.89   **Other measles complications**

B05.9   **Measles without complication**
Measles NOS

④ **B06**   **Rubella [German measles]**

   EXCLUDES 1   *congenital rubella (P35.0)*

⑤ **B06.0**   **Rubella with neurological complications**

   B06.00   **Rubella with neurological complication, unspecified**

   B06.01   **Rubella encephalitis**
Rubella meningoencephalitis

   B06.02   **Rubella meningitis**

   B06.09   **Other neurological complications of rubella**

⑤ **B06.8**   **Rubella with other complications**

   B06.81   **Rubella pneumonia**

   B06.82   **Rubella arthritis**

   B06.89   **Other rubella complications**

B06.9   **Rubella without complication**
Rubella NOS

④ **B07**   **Viral warts**

   INCLUDES   verruca simplex
verruca vulgaris
viral warts due to human papillomavirus

   EXCLUDES 2   *anogenital (venereal) warts (A63.0)*
papilloma of bladder (D41.4)
papilloma of cervix (D26.0)
papilloma larynx (D14.1)

B07.0   **Plantar wart**
Verruca plantaris

   DEFINITION   Noncancerous skin growths on the soles of the feet, often under pressure points, caused by the human papilloma virus that enters through tiny cuts or cracks in the skin.

B07.8   **Other viral warts**
Common wart
Flat wart
Verruca plana

B07.9   **Viral wart, unspecified**

④ **B08**   **Other viral infections characterized by skin and mucous membrane lesions, not elsewhere classified**

   EXCLUDES 1   *vesicular stomatitis virus disease (A93.8)*

⑤ **B08.0**   **Other orthopoxvirus infections**

   EXCLUDES 2   *monkeypox (B04)*

⑥ **B08.01**   **Cowpox and vaccinia not from vaccine**

   B08.010   **Cowpox**

   B08.011   **Vaccinia not from vaccine**

     EXCLUDES 1   *vaccinia (from vaccination) (generalized) (T88.1)*

   B08.02   **Orf virus disease**
Contagious pustular dermatitis
Ecthyma contagiosum

     DEFINITION   Skin disease closely related to smallpox, manifesting with localized, small, red, fluid-filled pustules that scab and heal, providing immunity to smallpox.

   B08.03   **Pseudocowpox [milker's node]**

   B08.04   **Paravaccinia, unspecified**

   B08.09   **Other orthopoxvirus infections**
Orthopoxvirus infection NOS

B08.1   **Molluscum contagiosum**

⑤ **B08.2**   **Exanthema subitum [sixth disease]**
Roseola infantum

   B08.20   **Exanthema subitum [sixth disease], unspecified**
Roseola infantum, unspecified

   DEFINITION   Common childhood herpes viral illness of mild upper respiratory symptoms, swollen glands, high fever lasting 3-7 days ending abruptly, followed by a rash.

   B08.21   **Exanthema subitum [sixth disease] due to human herpesvirus 6**
Roseola infantum due to human herpesvirus 6

   B08.22   **Exanthema subitum [sixth disease] due to human herpesvirus 7**
Roseola infantum due to human herpesvirus 7

   B08.3   **Erythema infectiosum [fifth disease]**

     DEFINITION   A mild infectious disease occurring mainly in early childhood, marked by a rosy-red rash on the cheeks, often spreading to the trunk and limbs. Fever and arthritis may also be present.

   B08.4   **Enteroviral vesicular stomatitis with exanthem**
Hand, foot and mouth disease

   B08.5   **Enteroviral vesicular pharyngitis**
Herpangina

⑤ **B08.6**   **Parapoxvirus infections**

   B08.60   **Parapoxvirus infection, unspecified**

   B08.61   **Bovine stomatitis**

   B08.62   **Sealpox**

   B08.69   **Other parapoxvirus infections**

⑤ **B08.7**   **Yatapoxvirus infections**

   B08.70   **Yatapoxvirus infection, unspecified**

   B08.71   **Tanapox virus disease**

   B08.72   **Yaba pox virus disease**
Yaba monkey tumor disease

   B08.79   **Other yatapoxvirus infections**

   B08.8   **Other specified viral infections characterized by skin and mucous membrane lesions**
Enteroviral lymphonodular pharyngitis
Foot-and-mouth disease
Poxvirus NEC

B09   **Unspecified viral infection characterized by skin and mucous membrane lesions**
Viral enanthema NOS
Viral exanthema NOS

Other human herpesviruses (B10)

④ **B10**   **Other human herpesviruses**

   EXCLUDES 2   *cytomegalovirus (B25.9)*
Epstein-Barr virus (B27.0-)
herpes NOS (B00.9)
herpes simplex (B00.-)
herpes zoster (B02.-)
human herpesvirus NOS (B00.-)
human herpesvirus 1 and 2 (B00.-)
human herpesvirus 3 (B01.-, B02.-)
human herpesvirus 4 (B27.0-)
human herpesvirus 5 (B25.-)
varicella (B01.-)
zoster (B02.-)

⑤ **B10.0**   **Other human herpesvirus encephalitis**

   EXCLUDES 2   *herpes encephalitis NOS (B00.4)*
herpes simplex encephalitis (B00.4)
human herpesvirus encephalitis (B00.4)
simian B herpes virus encephalitis (B00.4)

   B10.01   **Human herpesvirus 6 encephalitis**

   B10.09   **Other human herpesvirus encephalitis**
Human herpesvirus 7 encephalitis

⑤ **B10.8**   **Other human herpesvirus infection**

   B10.81   **Human herpesvirus 6 infection**

   B10.82   **Human herpesvirus 7 infection**

   B10.89   **Other human herpesvirus infection**
Human herpesvirus 8 infection
Kaposi's sarcoma-associated herpesvirus infection

Viral hepatitis (B15-B19)

   EXCLUDES 1   *sequelae of viral hepatitis (B94.2)*

   EXCLUDES 2   *cytomegaloviral hepatitis (B25.1)*
herpesviral [herpes simplex] hepatitis (B00.81)

● New   ▲ Revised   *Manifestation*   ④-⑦ Digit Indicators   ▤ Laterality   Ⓐ Adult (15+ years)   Ⓜ Maternity (12-55 years)   Ⓝ Newborn   Ⓟ Pediatric (0-17 years)   ♂ Male   ♀ Female

✖ Deleted   Unspecified   + Additional code

458   © 2017 DecisionHealth   2017 ICD-10-CM Expert for Physicians

CODING TIP ✓ When viral hepatitis is also documented as a confirmed diagnosis in a patient with any diagnosis classifiable to K74.-, the appropriate code from B15-B19 should also be assigned.

⬛ **B15   Acute hepatitis A**

B15.0   Hepatitis A with hepatic coma

B15.9   Hepatitis A without hepatic coma
Hepatitis A (acute)(viral) NOS

⬛ **B16   Acute hepatitis B**

B16.0   Acute hepatitis B with delta-agent with hepatic coma

B16.1   Acute hepatitis B with delta-agent without hepatic coma

B16.2   Acute hepatitis B without delta-agent with hepatic coma

B16.9   Acute hepatitis B without delta-agent and without hepatic coma
Hepatitis B (acute) (viral) NOS

⬛ **B17   Other acute viral hepatitis**

B17.0   Acute delta-(super) infection of hepatitis B carrier

◫ **B17.1   Acute hepatitis C**

B17.10   Acute hepatitis C without hepatic coma
Acute hepatitis C NOS

B17.11   Acute hepatitis C with hepatic coma

B17.2   Acute hepatitis E

B17.8   Other specified acute viral hepatitis
Hepatitis non-A non-B (acute) (viral) NEC

▲ **B17.9   Acute viral hepatitis, unspecified**
Acute hepatitis NOS
Acute infectious hepatitis NOS

▲ ⬛ **B18   Chronic viral hepatitis**

INCLUDES Carrier of viral hepatitis

B18.0   Chronic viral hepatitis B with delta-agent

▲ **B18.1   Chronic viral hepatitis B without delta-agent**
Carrier of viral hepatitis B
Chronic (viral) hepatitis B

▲ **B18.2   Chronic viral hepatitis C**
Carrier of viral hepatitis C

▲ **B18.8   Other chronic viral hepatitis**
Carrier of other viral hepatitis

▲ **B18.9   Chronic viral hepatitis, unspecified**
Carrier of unspecified viral hepatitis

⬛ **B19   Unspecified viral hepatitis**

B19.0   Unspecified viral hepatitis with hepatic coma

◫ **B19.1   Unspecified viral hepatitis B**

B19.10   Unspecified viral hepatitis B without hepatic coma
Unspecified viral hepatitis B NOS

B19.11   Unspecified viral hepatitis B with hepatic coma

◫ **B19.2   Unspecified viral hepatitis C**

B19.20   Unspecified viral hepatitis C without hepatic coma
Viral hepatitis C NOS

B19.21   Unspecified viral hepatitis C with hepatic coma

B19.9   Unspecified viral hepatitis without hepatic coma
Viral hepatitis NOS

Human immunodeficiency virus [HIV] disease (B20)

+ B20   Human immunodeficiency virus [HIV] disease

INCLUDES acquired immune deficiency syndrome [AIDS]
AIDS-related complex [ARC]
HIV infection, symptomatic

Code first:
Human immunodeficiency virus [HIV] disease complicating pregnancy, childbirth and the puerperium, if applicable (O98.7-)

Use additional code(s) to identify all manifestations of HIV infection

EXCLUDES 1 *asymptomatic human immunodeficiency virus [HIV] infection status (Z21)*
exposure to HIV virus (Z20.6)
inconclusive serologic evidence of HIV (R75)

GUIDELINES Section I.C.1.a.1)
Code only confirmed cases of HIV infection/illness: This [guideline] is an exception to the hospital inpatient guideline Section II, H. In this context, "confirmation" does not require documentation of positive serology or culture for HIV; the provider's diagnostic statement that the patient is HIV positive, or has an HIV-related illness is sufficient. B20, Human immunideficiency virus (HIV) disease should be assigned.

GUIDELINES Section I.C.1.a.2)(a)
If a patient is admitted for an HIV-related condition, the principal diagnosis should be B20, Human immunodeficiency virus [HIV] disease followed by additional diagnosis codes for all reported HIV-related conditions.

GUIDELINES Section I.C.1.a.2)(b)
If a patient with HIV disease is admitted for an unrelated condition (such as a traumatic injury), the code for the unrelated condition (e.g., the nature of injury code) should be the principal diagnosis. Other diagnoses would be B20 followed by additional diagnosis codes for all reported HIV-related conditions.

GUIDELINES Section I.C.1.a.2)(c)
Whether the patient is newly diagnosed or has had previous admissions/encounters for HIV conditions is irrelevant to the sequencing decision.

GUIDELINES Section I.C.1.a.2)(e)
Patients with inconclusive HIV serology, but no definitive diagnosis or manifestations of the illness, may be assigned code R75, Inconclusive laboratory evidence of human immunodeficiency virus [HIV].

GUIDELINES Section I.C.1.a.2)(f)
Patients previously diagnosed with any HIV illness (B20) should never be assigned to R75 or Z21, Asymptomatic human immunodeficiency virus [HIV] infection status.

Other viral diseases (B25-B34)

⬛ **B25   Cytomegaloviral disease**

EXCLUDES 1 *congenital cytomegalovirus infection (P35.1)*
cytomegaloviral mononucleosis (B27.1-)

B25.0   Cytomegaloviral pneumonitis

B25.1   Cytomegaloviral hepatitis

B25.2   Cytomegaloviral pancreatitis

B25.8   Other cytomegaloviral diseases
Cytomegaloviral encephalitis

B25.9   Cytomegaloviral disease, unspecified

⬛ **B26   Mumps**

INCLUDES epidemic parotitis
infectious parotitis

B26.0   Mumps orchitis   ♂

B26.1   Mumps meningitis

B26.2   Mumps encephalitis

B26.3   Mumps pancreatitis

◫ **B26.8   Mumps with other complications**

B26.81   Mumps hepatitis

B26.82   Mumps myocarditis

B26.83   Mumps nephritis

B26.84   Mumps polyneuropathy

B26.85   Mumps arthritis

B26.89   Other mumps complications

B26.9   Mumps without complication
Mumps NOS
Mumps parotitis NOS

⬛ **B27   Infectious mononucleosis**

INCLUDES glandular fever
monocytic angina
Pfeiffer's disease

◫ **B27.0   Gammaherpesviral mononucleosis**
Mononucleosis due to Epstein-Barr virus

B27.00   Gammaherpesviral mononucleosis without complication

B27.01   Gammaherpesviral mononucleosis with polyneuropathy

B27.02   Gammaherpesviral mononucleosis with meningitis

B27.09   Gammaherpesviral mononucleosis with other complications
Hepatomegaly in gammaherpesviral mononucleosis

● New ▲ Revised *Manifestation* ⬛-◨ Digit Indicators ⊟ Laterality Ⓐ Adult (15+ years) Ⓜ Maternity (12-55 years) Ⓝ Newborn Ⓟ Pediatric (0-17 years) ♂ Male ♀ Female
✖ Deleted Unspecified + Additional code

2017 ICD-10-CM Expert for Physicians   © 2017 DecisionHealth   459

S **B27.1   Cytomegaloviral mononucleosis**
    B27.10   Cytomegaloviral mononucleosis without complications
    B27.11   Cytomegaloviral mononucleosis with polyneuropathy
    B27.12   Cytomegaloviral mononucleosis with meningitis
    B27.19   Cytomegaloviral mononucleosis with other complication
      Hepatomegaly in cytomegaloviral mononucleosis

S **B27.8   Other infectious mononucleosis**
    B27.80   Other infectious mononucleosis without complication
    B27.81   Other infectious mononucleosis with polyneuropathy
    B27.82   Other infectious mononucleosis with meningitis
    B27.89   Other infectious mononucleosis with other complication
      Hepatomegaly in other infectious mononucleosis

S **B27.9   Infectious mononucleosis, unspecified**
    B27.90   Infectious mononucleosis, unspecified without complication
    B27.91   Infectious mononucleosis, unspecified with polyneuropathy
    B27.92   Infectious mononucleosis, unspecified with meningitis
    B27.99   Infectious mononucleosis, unspecified with other complication
      Hepatomegaly in unspecified infectious mononucleosis

4 **B30   Viral conjunctivitis**
    EXCLUDES 1   *herpesviral [herpes simplex] ocular disease (B00.5)*
      ocular zoster (B02.3)
    B30.0   Keratoconjunctivitis due to adenovirus
      Epidemic keratoconjunctivitis
      Shipyard eye
    B30.1   Conjunctivitis due to adenovirus
      Acute adenoviral follicular conjunctivitis
      Swimming-pool conjunctivitis
    B30.2   Viral pharyngoconjunctivitis
    B30.3   Acute epidemic hemorrhagic conjunctivitis (enteroviral)
      Conjunctivitis due to coxsackievirus 24
      Conjunctivitis due to enterovirus 70
      Hemorrhagic conjunctivitis (acute)(epidemic)
    B30.8   Other viral conjunctivitis
      Newcastle conjunctivitis
    B30.9   Viral conjunctivitis, unspecified

4 **B33   Other viral diseases, not elsewhere classified**
    B33.0   Epidemic myalgia
      Bornholm disease
    B33.1   Ross River disease
      Epidemic polyarthritis and exanthema
      Ross River fever
  S **B33.2   Viral carditis**
      Coxsackie (virus) carditis
    B33.20   Viral carditis, unspecified
    B33.21   Viral endocarditis
    B33.22   Viral myocarditis
    B33.23   Viral pericarditis
    B33.24   Viral cardiomyopathy
    B33.3   Retrovirus infections, not elsewhere classified
      Retrovirus infection NOS
+ **B33.4   Hantavirus (cardio)-pulmonary syndrome [HPS] [HCPS]**
      Hantavirus disease with pulmonary manifestations
      Sin nombre virus disease
      Use additional code to identify any associated acute kidney failure (N17.9)
      EXCLUDES 1   *hantavirus disease with renal manifestations (A98.5)*
        hemorrhagic fever with renal manifestations (A98.5)
    B33.8   Other specified viral diseases
      EXCLUDES 1   *anogenital human papillomavirus infection (A63.0)*
        viral warts due to human papillomavirus infection (B07)

4 **B34   Viral infection of unspecified site**
    EXCLUDES 1   *anogenital human papillomavirus infection (A63.0)*
      cytomegaloviral disease NOS (B25.9)
      herpesvirus [herpes simplex] infection NOS (B00.9)
      retrovirus infection NOS (B33.3)
      viral agents as the cause of diseases classified elsewhere (B97.-)
      viral warts due to human papillomavirus infection (B07)
    B34.0   Adenovirus infection, unspecified
    B34.1   Enterovirus infection, unspecified
      Coxsackievirus infection NOS
      Echovirus infection NOS
    B34.2   Coronavirus infection, unspecified
      EXCLUDES 1   *pneumonia due to SARS-associated coronavirus (J12.81)*
    B34.3   Parvovirus infection, unspecified
    B34.4   Papovavirus infection, unspecified
    B34.8   Other viral infections of unspecified site
    B34.9   Viral infection, unspecified
      Viremia NOS

Mycoses (B35-B49)

EXCLUDES 2   *hypersensitivity pneumonitis due to organic dust (J67.-)*
    mycosis fungoides (C84.0-)

4 **B35   Dermatophytosis**
    INCLUDES   favus
      infections due to species of Epidermophyton, Micro-sporum and Trichophyton
      tinea, any type except those in B36.-
    B35.0   Tinea barbae and tinea capitis
      Beard ringworm
      Kerion
      Scalp ringworm
      Sycosis, mycotic
      DEFINITION   Superficial fungal infections of the skin of bearded parts of the face and neck, and the scalp.
    B35.1   Tinea unguium
      Dermatophytic onychia
      Dermatophytosis of nail
      Onychomycosis
      Ringworm of nails
      DEFINITION   Fungal infection of the nails, first the surface, lateral and distal edges, and later, the part beneath the nail plate.
    B35.2   Tinea manuum
      Dermatophytosis of hand
      Hand ringworm
    B35.3   Tinea pedis
      Athlete's foot
      Dermatophytosis of foot
      Foot ringworm
    B35.4   Tinea corporis
      Ringworm of the body
    B35.5   Tinea imbricata
      Tokelau
      DEFINITION   A fungal infection which affects skin with few or no hair follicles, typically seen in humid climates. The early lesion is annular with a circle of scales at the outside boundary.
    B35.6   Tinea cruris
      Dhobi itch
      Groin ringworm
      Jock itch
      DEFINITION   Fungal infection of the groin commonly known as jock itch.
    B35.8   Other dermatophytoses
      Disseminated dermatophytosis
      Granulomatous dermatophytosis
    B35.9   Dermatophytosis, unspecified
      Ringworm NOS

4 **B36   Other superficial mycoses**
    B36.0   Pityriasis versicolor
      Tinea flava
      Tinea versicolor

● New   ▲ Revised   *Manifestation*   4-7 Digit Indicators   ⊟ Laterality   Ⓐ Adult (15+ years)   Ⓜ Maternity (12-55 years)   Ⓝ Newborn   Ⓟ Pediatric (0-17 years)   ♂ Male   ♀ Female
✖ Deleted   Unspecified   + Additional code

B36.1 **Tinea nigra**
Keratomycosis nigricans palmaris
Microsporosis nigra
Pityriasis nigra

DEFINITION A minor fungal infection having dark lesions with the appearance of spattered silver nitrate on the skin.

B36.2 **White piedra**
Tinea blanca

DEFINITION A fungal disease of hair covered skin, marked by pale patches and bald spot where the infection occurred.

B36.3 **Black piedra**
B36.8 **Other specified superficial mycoses**
B36.9 **Superficial mycosis, unspecified**

▟ **B37** **Candidiasis**

INCLUDES candidosis
moniliasis

EXCLUDES 1 *neonatal candidiasis (P37.5)*

B37.0 **Candidal stomatitis**
Oral thrush

DEFINITION Fungal infection located in the mouth.

Candidal stomatitis
Candidiasis of the mouth (thrush)

Fungus infection caused by Candida

B37.1 **Pulmonary candidiasis**
Candidal bronchitis
Candidal pneumonia

B37.2 **Candidiasis of skin and nail**
Candidal onychia
Candidal paronychia

EXCLUDES 2 *diaper dermatitis (L22)*

B37.3 **Candidiasis of vulva and vagina** ♀
Candidal vulvovaginitis
Monilial vulvovaginitis
Vaginal thrush

▤ **B37.4** **Candidiasis of other urogenital sites**

B37.41 **Candidal cystitis and urethritis**

CODING TIP ✓ B37.41 is a combination code that includes both the infection of the urinary tract and candida as the infectious cause. No additional codes should be assigned for urinary infection.

B37.42 **Candidal balanitis**
B37.49 **Other urogenital candidiasis**
Candidal pyelonephritis

B37.5 **Candidal meningitis**
B37.6 **Candidal endocarditis**
B37.7 **Candidal sepsis**
Disseminated candidiasis
Systemic candidiasis
AHA: 4Q 2014, 46

▤ **B37.8** **Candidiasis of other sites**

B37.81 **Candidal esophagitis**

DEFINITION Fungal infection of the esophagus, usually occurring in patients with immunocompromised states.

B37.82 **Candidal enteritis**
Candidal proctitis
B37.83 **Candidal cheilitis**
B37.84 **Candidal otitis externa**

B37.89 **Other sites of candidiasis**
Candidal osteomyelitis
B37.9 **Candidiasis, unspecified**
Thrush NOS

▟ **B38** **Coccidioidomycosis**

Primary coccidioidomycosis (pulmonary)
A respiratory disease caused by inhaling the fungus Coccidioides immitis

Lung

B38.0 **Acute pulmonary coccidioidomycosis**
B38.1 **Chronic pulmonary coccidioidomycosis**
B38.2 **Pulmonary coccidioidomycosis, unspecified**
B38.3 **Cutaneous coccidioidomycosis**
B38.4 **Coccidioidomycosis meningitis**
B38.7 **Disseminated coccidioidomycosis**
Generalized coccidioidomycosis

▤ **B38.8** **Other forms of coccidioidomycosis**

B38.81 **Prostatic coccidioidomycosis** ♂
B38.89 **Other forms of coccidioidomycosis**
B38.9 **Coccidioidomycosis, unspecified**

▟+ **B39** **Histoplasmosis**
Code first:
associated AIDS (B20)
Use additional code for any associated manifestations, such as:
endocarditis (I39)
meningitis (G02)
pericarditis (I32)
retinititis (H32)

+ **B39.0** **Acute pulmonary histoplasmosis capsulati**
+ **B39.1** **Chronic pulmonary histoplasmosis capsulati**
+ **B39.2** **Pulmonary histoplasmosis capsulati, unspecified**
+ **B39.3** **Disseminated histoplasmosis capsulati**
Generalized histoplasmosis capsulati
+ **B39.4** **Histoplasmosis capsulati, unspecified**
American histoplasmosis
+ **B39.5** **Histoplasmosis duboisii**
African histoplasmosis
+ **B39.9** **Histoplasmosis, unspecified**

▟ **B40** **Blastomycosis**

EXCLUDES 1 *Brazilian blastomycosis (B41.-)*
keloidal blastomycosis (B48.0)

B40.0 **Acute pulmonary blastomycosis**
B40.1 **Chronic pulmonary blastomycosis**
B40.2 **Pulmonary blastomycosis, unspecified**
B40.3 **Cutaneous blastomycosis**
B40.7 **Disseminated blastomycosis**
Generalized blastomycosis

▤ **B40.8** **Other forms of blastomycosis**

B40.81 **Blastomycotic meningoencephalitis**
Meningomyelitis due to blastomycosis
B40.89 **Other forms of blastomycosis**
B40.9 **Blastomycosis, unspecified**

▟ **B41** **Paracoccidioidomycosis**

INCLUDES Brazilian blastomycosis
Lutz' disease

B41.0 **Pulmonary paracoccidioidomycosis**
B41.7 **Disseminated paracoccidioidomycosis**
Generalized paracoccidioidomycosis
B41.8 **Other forms of paracoccidioidomycosis**
B41.9 **Paracoccidioidomycosis, unspecified**

▟ **B42** **Sporotrichosis**

B42.0 **Pulmonary sporotrichosis**

● New   ▲ Revised   *Manifestation*   ▟-▰ Digit Indicators   ▤ Laterality   Ⓐ Adult (15+ years)   Ⓜ Maternity (12-55 years)   Ⓝ Newborn   Ⓟ Pediatric (0-17 years)   ♂ Male   ♀ Female
✖ Deleted   Unspecified   + Additional code

2017 ICD-10-CM Expert for Physicians   © 2017 DecisionHealth   461

B42.1 **Lymphocutaneous sporotrichosis**
B42.7 **Disseminated sporotrichosis**
Generalized sporotrichosis
§ B42.8 **Other forms of sporotrichosis**
B42.81 **Cerebral sporotrichosis**
Meningitis due to sporotrichosis
B42.82 **Sporotrichosis arthritis**
B42.89 **Other forms of sporotrichosis**
B42.9 **Sporotrichosis, unspecified**

⊞ B43 **Chromomycosis and pheomycotic abscess**
B43.0 **Cutaneous chromomycosis**
Dermatitis verrucosa
B43.1 **Pheomycotic brain abscess**
Cerebral chromomycosis
B43.2 **Subcutaneous pheomycotic abscess and cyst**
B43.8 **Other forms of chromomycosis**
B43.9 **Chromomycosis, unspecified**

⊞ B44 **Aspergillosis**
| INCLUDES | aspergilloma |

B44.0 **Invasive pulmonary aspergillosis**
B44.1 **Other pulmonary aspergillosis**
B44.2 **Tonsillar aspergillosis**
B44.7 **Disseminated aspergillosis**
Generalized aspergillosis
§ B44.8 **Other forms of aspergillosis**
B44.81 **Allergic bronchopulmonary aspergillosis**
B44.89 **Other forms of aspergillosis**
B44.9 **Aspergillosis, unspecified**

⊞ B45 **Cryptococcosis**
B45.0 **Pulmonary cryptococcosis**
| DEFINITION | Yeastlike fungus infection, by cryptococcus neoformans, commonly occurring in the soil, which infects via the lungs and may spread to the brain and meninges.

B45.1 **Cerebral cryptococcosis**
Cryptococcal meningitis
Cryptococcosis meningocerebralis
| DEFINITION | Infection of the brain and/or its surrounding tissues causing hydrocephalus and intracerebral cysts due to infection with cryptococcus fungus.

B45.2 **Cutaneous cryptococcosis**
B45.3 **Osseous cryptococcosis**
B45.7 **Disseminated cryptococcosis**
Generalized cryptococcosis
B45.8 **Other forms of cryptococcosis**
B45.9 **Cryptococcosis, unspecified**

⊞ B46 **Zygomycosis**
B46.0 **Pulmonary mucormycosis**
B46.1 **Rhinocerebral mucormycosis**
B46.2 **Gastrointestinal mucormycosis**
B46.3 **Cutaneous mucormycosis**
Subcutaneous mucormycosis
B46.4 **Disseminated mucormycosis**
Generalized mucormycosis
B46.5 **Mucormycosis, unspecified**
B46.8 **Other zygomycoses**
Entomophthoromycosis
B46.9 **Zygomycosis, unspecified**
Phycomycosis NOS

⊞ B47 **Mycetoma**
B47.0 **Eumycetoma**
Madura foot, mycotic
Maduromycosis
B47.1 **Actinomycetoma**
B47.9 **Mycetoma, unspecified**
Madura foot NOS
| DEFINITION | Chronic infection involving the feet, characterized by formation of localized lesions, with swelling and multiple draining sinuses.

⊞ B48 **Other mycoses, not elsewhere classified**
B48.0 **Lobomycosis**
Keloidal blastomycosis
Lobo's disease

| DEFINITION | A fungal infection of the skin caused by Lobo loboi and characterized by keloidal nodular lesions occurring on the face, ears, and extremities.

B48.1 **Rhinosporidiosis**
B48.2 **Allescheriasis**
Infection due to Pseudallescheria boydii
| EXCLUDES 1 | *eumycetoma (B47.0)*

B48.3 **Geotrichosis**
Geotrichum stomatitis
B48.4 **Penicillosis**
B48.8 **Other specified mycoses**
Adiaspiromycosis
Infection of tissue and organs by Alternaria
Infection of tissue and organs by Drechslera
Infection of tissue and organs by Fusarium
Infection of tissue and organs by saprophytic fungi NEC
AHA: 4Q 2014, 46
AHA: 2Q 2014, 13

B49 **Unspecified mycosis**
Fungemia NOS

Protozoal diseases (B50-B64)

| EXCLUDES 1 | *amebiasis (A06.-)*
other protozoal intestinal diseases (A07.-)

⊞ B50 **Plasmodium falciparum malaria**
| INCLUDES | mixed infections of Plasmodium falciparum with any other Plasmodium species

B50.0 **Plasmodium falciparum malaria with cerebral complications**
Cerebral malaria NOS
B50.8 **Other severe and complicated Plasmodium falciparum malaria**
Severe or complicated Plasmodium falciparum malaria NOS
B50.9 **Plasmodium falciparum malaria, unspecified**

⊞ B51 **Plasmodium vivax malaria**
| INCLUDES | mixed infections of Plasmodium vivax with other Plasmodium species, except Plasmodium falciparum
| EXCLUDES 1 | *plasmodium vivav with Plasmodium falciparum (B50.-)*

B51.0 **Plasmodium vivax malaria with rupture of spleen**
B51.8 **Plasmodium vivax malaria with other complications**
B51.9 **Plasmodium vivax malaria without complication**
Plasmodium vivax malaria NOS

⊞ B52 **Plasmodium malariae malaria**
| INCLUDES | mixed infections of Plasmodium malariae with other Plasmodium species, except Plasmodium falciparum and Plasmodium vivax
| EXCLUDES 1 | *Plasmodium falciparum (B50.-)*
Plasmodium vivax (B51.-)

B52.0 **Plasmodium malariae malaria with nephropathy**
B52.8 **Plasmodium malariae malaria with other complications**
B52.9 **Plasmodium malariae malaria without complication**
Plasmodium malariae malaria NOS

⊞ B53 **Other specified malaria**
B53.0 **Plasmodium ovale malaria**
| EXCLUDES 1 | *Plasmodium ovale with Plasmodium falciparum (B50.-)*
Plasmodium ovale with Plasmodium malariae (B52.-)
Plasmodium ovale with Plasmodium vivax (B51.-)

B53.1 **Malaria due to simian plasmodia**
| EXCLUDES 1 | *Malaria due to simian plasmodia with Plasmodium falciparum (B50.-)*
Malaria due to simian plasmodia with Plasmodium malariae (B52.-)
Malaria due to simian plasmodia with Plasmodium ovale (B53.0)
Malaria due to simian plasmodia with Plasmodium vivax (B51.-)

B53.8 **Other malaria, not elsewhere classified**

B54   Unspecified malaria

Malaria

Parasites are released when mosquito feeds

Stages in liver

Liver cell

Parasites are released into bloodstream and enter red blood cells

Some parasites reach the sexual stage and are ingested by a mosquito where they reproduce in the insect's gut

Parasites multiply in red blood cells

Red blood cell ruptures and spreads more parasites

B55   Leishmaniasis

B55.0   Visceral leishmaniasis
Kala-azar
Post-kala-azar dermal leishmaniasis

B55.1   Cutaneous leishmaniasis

B55.2   Mucocutaneous leishmaniasis

B55.9   Leishmaniasis, unspecified

B56   African trypanosomiasis

B56.0   Gambiense trypanosomiasis
Infection due to Trypanosoma brucei gambiense
West African sleeping sickness

B56.1   Rhodesiense trypanosomiasis
East African sleeping sickness
Infection due to Trypanosoma brucei rhodesiense

B56.9   African trypanosomiasis, unspecified
Sleeping sickness NOS

B57   Chagas' disease

INCLUDES   American trypanosomiasis
infection due to Trypanosoma cruzi

B57.0   Acute Chagas' disease with heart involvement
Acute Chagas' disease with myocarditis

B57.1   Acute Chagas' disease without heart involvement
Acute Chagas' disease NOS

B57.2   Chagas' disease (chronic) with heart involvement
American trypanosomiasis NOS
Chagas' disease (chronic) NOS
Chagas' disease (chronic) with myocarditis
Trypanosomiasis NOS

B57.3   Chagas' disease (chronic) with digestive system involvement

B57.30   Chagas' disease with digestive system involvement, unspecified

B57.31   Megaesophagus in Chagas' disease

B57.32   Megacolon in Chagas' disease

B57.39   Other digestive system involvement in Chagas' disease

B57.4   Chagas' disease (chronic) with nervous system involvement

B57.40   Chagas' disease with nervous system involvement, unspecified

B57.41   Meningitis in Chagas' disease

B57.42   Meningoencephalitis in Chagas' disease

B57.49   Other nervous system involvement in Chagas' disease

B57.5   Chagas' disease (chronic) with other organ involvement

B58   Toxoplasmosis

INCLUDES   infection due to Toxoplasma gondii

EXCLUDES 1   congenital toxoplasmosis (P37.1)

B58.0   Toxoplasma oculopathy

B58.00   Toxoplasma oculopathy, unspecified

B58.01   Toxoplasma chorioretinitis

B58.09   Other toxoplasma oculopathy
Toxoplasma uveitis

B58.1   Toxoplasma hepatitis

B58.2   Toxoplasma meningoencephalitis

B58.3   Pulmonary toxoplasmosis

B58.8   Toxoplasmosis with other organ involvement

B58.81   Toxoplasma myocarditis

B58.82   Toxoplasma myositis

B58.83   Toxoplasma tubulo-interstitial nephropathy
Toxoplasma pyelonephritis

B58.89   Toxoplasmosis with other organ involvement

B58.9   Toxoplasmosis, unspecified

B59   Pneumocystosis
Pneumonia due to Pneumocystis carinii
Pneumonia due to Pneumocystis jiroveci

B60   Other protozoal diseases, not elsewhere classified

EXCLUDES 1   cryptosporidiosis (A07.2)
intestinal microsporidiosis (A07.8)
isosporiasis (A07.3)

B60.0   Babesiosis
Piroplasmosis

B60.1   Acanthamebiasis

B60.10   Acanthamebiasis, unspecified

B60.11   Meningoencephalitis due to Acanthamoeba (culbertsoni)

B60.12   Conjunctivitis due to Acanthamoeba

B60.13   Keratoconjunctivitis due to Acanthamoeba

B60.19   Other acanthamebic disease

B60.2   Naegleriasis
Primary amebic meningoencephalitis

B60.8   Other specified protozoal diseases
Microsporidiosis

B64   Unspecified protozoal disease

Helminthiases (B65-B83)

B65   Schistosomiasis [bilharziasis]

INCLUDES   snail fever

B65.0   Schistosomiasis due to Schistosoma haematobium [urinary schistosomiasis]

B65.1   Schistosomiasis due to Schistosoma mansoni [intestinal schistosomiasis]

B65.2   Schistosomiasis due to Schistosoma japonicum
Asiatic schistosomiasis

B65.3   Cercarial dermatitis
Swimmer's itch

DEFINITION   An itching inflammation of the skin due to penetration of larval forms of schistosomes (parasitic worms), occurring in bathers of infested waters.

B65.8   Other schistosomiasis
Infection due to Schistosoma intercalatum
Infection due to Schistosoma mattheei
Infection due to Schistosoma mekongi

B65.9   Schistosomiasis, unspecified

B66   Other fluke infections

B66.0   Opisthorchiasis
Infection due to cat liver fluke
Infection due to Opisthorchis (felineus)(viverrini)

B66.1   Clonorchiasis
Chinese liver fluke disease
Infection due to Clonorchis sinensis
Oriental liver fluke disease

B66.2   Dicroceliasis
Infection due to Dicrocoelium dendriticum
Lancet fluke infection

B66.3   Fascioliasis
Infection due to Fasciola gigantica
Infection due to Fasciola hepatica
Infection due to Fasciola indica
Sheep liver fluke disease

B66.4   Paragonimiasis
Infection due to Paragonimus species
Lung fluke disease
Pulmonary distomiasis

B66.5   Fasciolopsiasis
Infection due to Fasciolopsis buski
Intestinal distomiasis

B66.8   Other specified fluke infections
Echinostomiasis
Heterophyiasis
Metagonimiasis
Nanophyetiasis
Watsoniasis

● New   ▲ Revised   *Manifestation*   ◢-◪ Digit Indicators   ⊟ Laterality   Ⓐ Adult (15+ years)   Ⓜ Maternity (12-55 years)   Ⓝ Newborn (0-17 years)   Ⓟ Pediatric (0-17 years)   ♂ Male   ♀ Female
✖ Deleted   Unspecified   + Additional code

2017 ICD-10-CM Expert for Physicians

© 2017 DecisionHealth   463

B66.9 **Fluke infection, unspecified**

☑ **B67 Echinococcosis**

> INCLUDES hydatidosis

B67.0 **Echinococcus granulosus infection of liver**

> DEFINITION A genus of parasitic tapeworm passed from dogs. The larvae form large cysts in the liver, causing serious and sometimes fatal disease.

B67.1 **Echinococcus granulosus infection of lung**

B67.2 **Echinococcus granulosus infection of bone**

☑ B67.3 **Echinococcus granulosus infection, other and multiple sites**

B67.31 **Echinococcus granulosus infection, thyroid gland**

B67.32 **Echinococcus granulosus infection, multiple sites**

B67.39 **Echinococcus granulosus infection, other sites**

B67.4 **Echinococcus granulosus infection, unspecified**
Dog tapeworm (infection)

B67.5 **Echinococcus multilocularis infection of liver**

☑ B67.6 **Echinococcus multilocularis infection, other and multiple sites**

B67.61 **Echinococcus multilocularis infection, multiple sites**

B67.69 **Echinococcus multilocularis infection, other sites**

B67.7 **Echinococcus multilocularis infection, unspecified**

B67.8 **Echinococcosis, unspecified, of liver**

☑ B67.9 **Echinococcosis, other and unspecified**

B67.90 **Echinococcosis, unspecified**
Echinococcosis NOS

B67.99 **Other echinococcosis**

☑ **B68 Taeniasis**

> EXCLUDES 1 *cysticercosis (B69.-)*

B68.0 **Taenia solium taeniasis**
Pork tapeworm (infection)

B68.1 **Taenia saginata taeniasis**
Beef tapeworm (infection)
Infection due to adult tapeworm Taenia saginata

B68.9 **Taeniasis, unspecified**

☑ **B69 Cysticercosis**

> INCLUDES cysticerciasis infection due to larval form of Taenia solium

B69.0 **Cysticercosis of central nervous system**

B69.1 **Cysticercosis of eye**

☑ B69.8 **Cysticercosis of other sites**

B69.81 **Myositis in cysticercosis**

B69.89 **Cysticercosis of other sites**

B69.9 **Cysticercosis, unspecified**

> DEFINITION Infection caused by the pork tapeworm when its larvae enter the body and form cysts.

☑ **B70 Diphyllobothriasis and sparganosis**

B70.0 **Diphyllobothriasis**
Diphyllobothrium (adult) (latum) (pacificum) infection
Fish tapeworm (infection)

> EXCLUDES 2 *larval diphyllobothriasis (B70.1)*

B70.1 **Sparganosis**
Infection due to Sparganum (mansoni) (proliferum)
Infection due to Spirometra larva
Larval diphyllobothriasis
Spirometrosis

☑ **B71 Other cestode infections**

B71.0 **Hymenolepiasis**
Dwarf tapeworm infection
Rat tapeworm (infection)

B71.1 **Dipylidiasis**

B71.8 **Other specified cestode infections**
Coenurosis

B71.9 **Cestode infection, unspecified**
Tapeworm (infection) NOS

B72 Dracunculiasis

> INCLUDES guinea worm infection
> infection due to Dracunculus medinensis

☑ **B73 Onchocerciasis**

> INCLUDES onchocerca volvulus infection
> onchocercosis
> river blindness

☑ B73.0 **Onchocerciasis with eye disease**

B73.00 **Onchocerciasis with eye involvement, unspecified**

B73.01 **Onchocerciasis with endophthalmitis**

B73.02 **Onchocerciasis with glaucoma**

B73.09 **Onchocerciasis with other eye involvement**
Infestation of eyelid due to onchocerciasis

B73.1 **Onchocerciasis without eye disease**

☑ **B74 Filariasis**

> EXCLUDES 2 *onchocerciasis (B73)*
> *tropical (pulmonary) eosinophilia NOS (J82)*

B74.0 **Filariasis due to Wuchereria bancrofti**
Bancroftian elephantiasis
Bancroftian filariasis

B74.1 **Filariasis due to Brugia malayi**

B74.2 **Filariasis due to Brugia timori**

B74.3 **Loiasis**
Calabar swelling
Eyeworm disease of Africa
Loa loa infection

B74.4 **Mansonelliasis**
Infection due to Mansonella ozzardi
Infection due to Mansonella perstans
Infection due to Mansonella streptocerca

B74.8 **Other filariases**
Dirofilariasis

B74.9 **Filariasis, unspecified**

B75 Trichinellosis

> INCLUDES infection due to Trichinella species
> trichiniasis

☑ **B76 Hookworm diseases**

> INCLUDES uncinariasis

B76.0 **Ancylostomiasis**
Infection due to Ancylostoma species

B76.1 **Necatoriasis**
Infection due to Necator americanus

B76.8 **Other hookworm diseases**

B76.9 **Hookworm disease, unspecified**
Cutaneous larva migrans NOS

☑ **B77 Ascariasis**

> INCLUDES ascaridiasis
> roundworm infection

B77.0 **Ascariasis with intestinal complications**

☑ B77.8 **Ascariasis with other complications**

B77.81 **Ascariasis pneumonia**

B77.89 **Ascariasis with other complications**

B77.9 **Ascariasis, unspecified**

☑ **B78 Strongyloidiasis**

> EXCLUDES 1 *trichostrongyliasis (B81.2)*

B78.0 **Intestinal strongyloidiasis**

B78.1 **Cutaneous strongyloidiasis**

B78.7 **Disseminated strongyloidiasis**

B78.9 **Strongyloidiasis, unspecified**

B79 Trichuriasis

> INCLUDES trichocephaliasis
> whipworm (disease) (infection)

B80 Enterobiasis

> INCLUDES oxyuriasis
> pinworm infection
> threadworm infection

☑ **B81 Other intestinal helminthiases, not elsewhere classified**

> EXCLUDES 1 *angiostrongyliasis due to Parastrongylus cantonensis (B83.2)*

B81.0 **Anisakiasis**
Infection due to Anisakis larva

B81.1 **Intestinal capillariasis**
Capillariasis NOS
Infection due to Capillaria philippinensis

> EXCLUDES 2 *hepatic capillariasis (B83.8)*

B81.2 **Trichostrongyliasis**

B81.3 **Intestinal angiostrongyliasis**
Angiostrongyliasis due to Parastrongylus costaricensis

B81.4 **Mixed intestinal helminthiases**
Infection due to intestinal helminths classified to more than one of the categories B65.0-B81.3 and B81.8
Mixed helminthiasis NOS

B81.8 **Other specified intestinal helminthiases**
Infection due to Oesophagostomum species [esophagostomiasis]
Infection due to Ternidens diminutus [ternidensiasis]

● New ▲ Revised *Manifestation* ☑-☑ Digit Indicators ▤ Laterality Ⓐ Adult (15+ years) Ⓜ Maternity (12-55 years) Ⓝ Newborn Ⓟ Pediatric (0-17 years) ♂ Male ♀ Female
✖ ~~Deleted~~ Unspecified ✚ Additional code

⊞ **B82**   **Unspecified intestinal parasitism**
- **B82.0**   **Intestinal helminthiasis, unspecified**
- **B82.9**   **Intestinal parasitism, unspecified**

⊞ **B83**   **Other helminthiases**
> **EXCLUDES 1**   *capillariasis NOS (B81.1)*
>
> **EXCLUDES 2**   *intestinal capillariasis (B81.1)*

- **B83.0**   **Visceral larva migrans**
  Toxocariasis
- **B83.1**   **Gnathostomiasis**
  Wandering swelling
- **B83.2**   **Angiostrongyliasis due to Parastrongylus cantonensis**
  Eosinophilic meningoencephalitis due to Parastrongylus cantonensis
  > **EXCLUDES 2**   *intestinal angiostrongyliasis (B81.3)*
- **B83.3**   **Syngamiasis**
  Syngamosis
- **B83.4**   **Internal hirudiniasis**
  > **EXCLUDES 2**   *external hirudiniasis (B88.3)*
- **B83.8**   **Other specified helminthiases**
  Acanthocephaliasis
  Gongylonemiasis
  Hepatic capillariasis
  Metastrongyliasis
  Thelaziasis
- **B83.9**   **Helminthiasis, unspecified**
  Worms NOS
  > **EXCLUDES 1**   *intestinal helminthiasis NOS (B82.0)*

Pediculosis, acariasis and other infestations (B85-B89)

⊞ **B85**   **Pediculosis and phthiriasis**
- **B85.0**   **Pediculosis due to Pediculus humanus capitis**
  Head-louse infestation
- **B85.1**   **Pediculosis due to Pediculus humanus corporis**
  Body-louse infestation
- **B85.2**   **Pediculosis, unspecified**
- **B85.3**   **Phthiriasis**
  Infestation by crab-louse
  Infestation by Phthirus pubis
- **B85.4**   **Mixed pediculosis and phthiriasis**
  Infestation classifiable to more than one of the categories B85.0-B85.3

B86   **Scabies**
Sarcoptic itch

⊞ **B87**   **Myiasis**
> **INCLUDES**   infestation by larva of flies

- **B87.0**   **Cutaneous myiasis**
  Creeping myiasis
  > **DEFINITION**   Infestation by the fly larvae of the genus Oestrus causing inflamed furuncles where the larvae are maturing beneath the skin.
- **B87.1**   **Wound myiasis**
  Traumatic myiasis
- **B87.2**   **Ocular myiasis**
- **B87.3**   **Nasopharyngeal myiasis**
  Laryngeal myiasis
- **B87.4**   **Aural myiasis**
- ⑤ **B87.8**   **Myiasis of other sites**
  - **B87.81**   **Genitourinary myiasis**
  - **B87.82**   **Intestinal myiasis**
  - **B87.89**   **Myiasis of other sites**
- **B87.9**   **Myiasis, unspecified**

⊞ **B88**   **Other infestations**
- **B88.0**   **Other acariasis**
  Acarine dermatitis
  Dermatitis due to Demodex species
  Dermatitis due to Dermanyssus gallinae
  Dermatitis due to Liponyssoides sanguineus
  Trombiculosis
  > **EXCLUDES 2**   *scabies (B86)*
- **B88.1**   **Tungiasis [sandflea infestation]**
- **B88.2**   **Other arthropod infestations**
  Scarabiasis

- **B88.3**   **External hirudiniasis**
  Leech infestation NOS
  > **EXCLUDES 2**   *internal hirudiniasis (B83.4)*
- **B88.8**   **Other specified infestations**
  Ichthyoparasitism due to Vandellia cirrhosa
  Linguatulosis
  Porocephaliasis
- **B88.9**   **Infestation, unspecified**
  Infestation (skin) NOS
  Infestation by mites NOS
  Skin parasites NOS

B89   **Unspecified parasitic disease**

Sequelae of infectious and parasitic diseases (B90-B94)

Note: Categories B90-B94 are to be used to indicate conditions in categories A00-B89 as the cause of sequelae, which are themselves classified elsewhere. The 'sequelae' include conditions specified as such; they also include residuals of diseases classifiable to the above categories if there is evidence that the disease itself is no longer present. Codes from these categories are not to be used for chronic infections. Code chronic current infections to active infectious disease as appropriate.

Code first:
> condition resulting from (sequela) the infectious or parasitic disease

⊞ **B90**   **Sequelae of tuberculosis**
> **CODING TIP ✓**   Conditions classified here are specifically reportable as sequelae or late effects of tuberculosis. The active disease is no longer present. Acute tuberculosis should be coded to A15-A19.

- **B90.0**   **Sequelae of central nervous system tuberculosis**
- **B90.1**   **Sequelae of genitourinary tuberculosis**
- **B90.2**   **Sequelae of tuberculosis of bones and joints**
- **B90.8**   **Sequelae of tuberculosis of other organs**
  > **EXCLUDES 2**   *sequelae of respiratory tuberculosis (B90.9)*
- **B90.9**   **Sequelae of respiratory and unspecified tuberculosis**
  Sequelae of tuberculosis NOS

B91   **Sequelae of poliomyelitis**
> **EXCLUDES 1**   *postpolio syndrome (G14)*

> **CODING TIP ✓**   Conditions classified here are specifically reportable as sequelae of poliomyelitis. Acute poliomyelitis should be coded to A80. When postpolio syndrome is specified, report code G14 rather than B91.

B92   **Sequelae of leprosy**

⊞ **B94**   **Sequelae of other and unspecified infectious and parasitic diseases**
- **B94.0**   **Sequelae of trachoma**
- **B94.1**   **Sequelae of viral encephalitis**
- **B94.2**   **Sequelae of viral hepatitis**
- **B94.8**   **Sequelae of other specified infectious and parasitic diseases**
- **B94.9**   **Sequelae of unspecified infectious and parasitic disease**

Bacterial and viral infectious agents (B95-B97)

Note: These categories are provided for use as supplementary or additional codes to identify the infectious agent(s) in diseases classified elsewhere.

> **GUIDELINES**   Section I.C.1.b
> Certain infections are classified in chapters other than Chapter 1 and no organism is identified as part of the infection code. In these instances, it is necessary to use an additional code from Chapter 1 to identify the organism. A code from category B95, Streptococcus, Staphylococcus, and Enterococcus as the cause of diseases classified to other chapters, B96, Other bacterial agents as the cause of diseases classified to other chapters, or B97, Viral agents as the cause of diseases classified to other chapters, is to be used as an additional code to identify the organism. An instructional note will be found at the infection code advising that an additional organism code is required.
>
> **Section I.C.1.c**
> Many bacterial infections are resistant to current antibiotics. It is necessary to identify all infections documented as antibiotic resistant. Assign a code from category Z16, Resistance to antimicrobial drugs, following the infection code only if the infection code does not identify drug resistance.

● New   ▲ Revised   *Manifestation*   ④-⑦ Digit Indicators   ⊟ Laterality   🅐 Adult (15+ years)   Ⓜ Maternity (12-55 years)   🅝 Newborn   🅟 Pediatric (0-17 years)   ♂ Male   ♀ Female

✖ Deleted   Unspecified   + Additional code

2017 ICD-10-CM Expert for Physicians   © 2017 DecisionHealth   465

CODING TIP ✓ Conditions classified here are specifically reportable as additional codes to identify infectious agents in diseases classified elsewhere. Do not assign codes from B95-B97 without a code for the underlying disease process first.

◢ B95   Streptococcus, Staphylococcus, and Enterococcus as the cause of diseases classified elsewhere

B95.0   Streptococcus, group A, as the cause of diseases classified elsewhere

B95.1   Streptococcus, group B, as the cause of diseases classified elsewhere

B95.2   Enterococcus as the cause of diseases classified elsewhere

B95.3   Streptococcus pneumoniae as the cause of diseases classified elsewhere

B95.4   Other streptococcus as the cause of diseases classified elsewhere

B95.5   Unspecified streptococcus as the cause of diseases classified elsewhere

⑤ B95.6   Staphylococcus aureus as the cause of diseases classified elsewhere

B95.61   Methicillin susceptible Staphylococcus aureus infection as the cause of diseases classified elsewhere
Methicillin susceptible Staphylococcus aureus (MSSA) infection as the cause of diseases classified elsewhere
Staphylococcus aureus infection NOS as the cause of diseases classified elsewhere

B95.62   Methicillin resistant Staphylococcus aureus infection as the cause of diseases classified elsewhere
Methicillin resistant staphylococcus aureus (MRSA) infection as the cause of diseases classified elsewhere

GUIDELINES   Section I.C.1.e.1)
Selection and sequencing of MRSA codes:

(a) Combination codes for MRSA infection.
When a patient is diagnosed with an infection that is due to MRSA, and that infection has a combination code that includes the causal organism (e.g., sepsis, pneumonia) assign the appropriate combination code for the condition (e.g., code A41.02, Sepsis due to Methicillin resistant Staphylococcus aureus or code J15.212, Pneumonia due to Methicillin resistant Staphylococcus aureus). Do not assign code B95.62, Methicillin resistant Staphylococcus aureus infection as the cause of diseases classified elsewhere, as an additional code because the combination code includes the type of infection and the MRSA organism. Do not assign a code from subcategory Z16.11, Resistance to penicillins, as an additional diagnosis.

(b) Other codes for MRSA infection. When there is documentation of a current infection (e.g., wound infection, stitch abscess, urinary tract infection) due to MRSA, and that infection does not have a combination code that includes the causal organism, assign the appropriate code to identify the condition along with code B95.62, Methicillin resistant Staphylococcus aureus infection as the cause of diseases classified elsewhere for the MRSA infection. Do not assign a code from subcategory Z16.11, Resistance to penicillins.
AHA: 1Q 2016, 12-13

B95.7   Other staphylococcus as the cause of diseases classified elsewhere
CODING TIP ✓ Use this code when another Staph is identified, such as Staphyloccus epidermidis.

B95.8   Unspecified staphylococcus as the cause of diseases classified elsewhere

◢ B96   Other bacterial agents as the cause of diseases classified elsewhere

B96.0   Mycoplasma pneumoniae [M. pneumoniae] as the cause of diseases classified elsewhere
Pleuro-pneumonia-like-organism [PPLO]

B96.1   Klebsiella pneumoniae [K. pneumoniae] as the cause of diseases classified elsewhere

⑤ B96.2   Escherichia coli [E. coli] as the cause of diseases classified elsewhere

B96.20   Unspecified Escherichia coli [E. coli] as the cause of diseases classified elsewhere
Escherichia coli [E. coli] NOS

B96.21   Shiga toxin-producing Escherichia coli [E. coli] (STEC) O157 as the cause of diseases classified elsewhere
E. coli O157:H- (nonmotile) with confirmation of Shiga toxin
E. coli O157 with confirmation of Shiga toxin when H antigen is unknown, or is not H7
O157:H7 Escherichia coli [E.coli] with or without confirmation of Shiga toxin-production
Shiga toxin-producing Escherichia coli [E.coli] O157:H7 with or without confirmation of Shiga toxin-production
STEC O157:H7 with or without confirmation of Shiga toxin-production

B96.22   Other specified Shiga toxin-producing Escherichia coli [E. coli] (STEC) as the cause of diseases classified elsewhere
Non-O157 Shiga toxin-producing Escherichia coli [E.coli]
Non-O157 Shiga toxin-producing Escherichia coli [E.coli] with known O group

B96.23   Unspecified Shiga toxin-producing Escherichia coli [E. coli] (STEC) as the cause of diseases classified elsewhere
Shiga toxin-producing Escherichia coli [E. coli] with unspecified O group
STEC NOS

B96.29   Other Escherichia coli [E. coli] as the cause of diseases classified elsewhere
Non-Shiga toxin-producing E. coli

B96.3   Hemophilus influenzae [H. influenzae] as the cause of diseases classified elsewhere

B96.4   Proteus (mirabilis) (morganii) as the cause of diseases classified elsewhere

B96.5   Pseudomonas (aeruginosa) (mallei) (pseudomallei) as the cause of diseases classified elsewhere
AHA: 1Q 2015, 18

B96.6   Bacteroides fragilis [B. fragilis] as the cause of diseases classified elsewhere

B96.7   Clostridium perfringens [C. perfringens] as the cause of diseases classified elsewhere

⑤ B96.8   Other specified bacterial agents as the cause of diseases classified elsewhere

B96.81   Helicobacter pylori [H. pylori] as the cause of diseases classified elsewhere
DEFINITION Common gastric pathogen causing dyspepsia, gastritis, peptic ulcer disease, gastric adenocarcinoma, and gastric lymphoma.

B96.82   Vibrio vulnificus as the cause of diseases classified elsewhere

B96.89   Other specified bacterial agents as the cause of diseases classified elsewhere

◢ B97   Viral agents as the cause of diseases classified elsewhere

B97.0   Adenovirus as the cause of diseases classified elsewhere

⑤ B97.1   Enterovirus as the cause of diseases classified elsewhere

B97.10   Unspecified enterovirus as the cause of diseases classified elsewhere

B97.11   Coxsackievirus as the cause of diseases classified elsewhere

B97.12   Echovirus as the cause of diseases classified elsewhere
DEFINITION A group of DNA-containing viruses that affect the tissue linings of the respiratory tract, eyes, intestines, and urinary tract. There are approximately 50 serotypes.

B97.19   Other enterovirus as the cause of diseases classified elsewhere

⑤ B97.2   Coronavirus as the cause of diseases classified elsewhere

B97.21   SARS-associated coronavirus as the cause of diseases classified elsewhere
EXCLUDES 1 *pneumonia due to SARS-associated coronavirus (J12.81)*

B97.29   Other coronavirus as the cause of diseases classified elsewhere

⑤ B97.3   Retrovirus as the cause of diseases classified elsewhere
EXCLUDES 1 *Human immunodeficiency virus [HIV] disease (B20)*

● New   ▲ Revised   *Manifestation*   ◪-◪ Digit Indicators   ⊟ Laterality   Ⓐ Adult (15+ years)   Ⓜ Maternity (12-55 years)   Ⓝ Newborn   Ⓟ Pediatric (0-17 years)   ♂ Male   ♀ Female
✖ ~~Deleted~~   Unspecified   ＋ Additional code

466   © 2017 DecisionHealth   2017 ICD-10-CM Expert for Physicians

B95 — B97.3

B97.30   Unspecified retrovirus as the cause of diseases classified elsewhere

B97.31   Lentivirus as the cause of diseases classified elsewhere

B97.32   Oncovirus as the cause of diseases classified elsewhere

B97.33   Human T-cell lymphotrophic virus, type I [HTLV-I] as the cause of diseases classified elsewhere

B97.34   Human T-cell lymphotrophic virus, type II [HTLV-II] as the cause of diseases classified elsewhere

B97.35   Human immunodeficiency virus, type 2 [HIV 2] as the cause of diseases classified elsewhere

B97.39   Other retrovirus as the cause of diseases classified elsewhere

B97.4   Respiratory syncytial virus as the cause of diseases classified elsewhere

B97.5   Reovirus as the cause of diseases classified elsewhere

B97.6   Parvovirus as the cause of diseases classified elsewhere

B97.7   Papillomavirus as the cause of diseases classified elsewhere

⑤ B97.8   Other viral agents as the cause of diseases classified elsewhere

B97.81   Human metapneumovirus as the cause of diseases classified elsewhere

B97.89   Other viral agents as the cause of diseases classified elsewhere

Other infectious diseases (B99)

④ B99   Other and unspecified infectious diseases

B99.8   Other infectious disease

B99.9   Unspecified infectious disease

● New   ▲ Revised   *Manifestation*   ④-⑦ Digit Indicators   ⊟ Laterality   Ⓐ Adult (15+ years)   Ⓜ Maternity (12-55 years)   Ⓝ Newborn   Ⓟ Pediatric (0-17 years)   ♂ Male   ♀ Female
✖ Deleted   Unspecified   + Additional code

2017 ICD-10-CM Expert for Physicians

© 2017 DecisionHealth   467

CHAPTER 2: NEOPLASMS (C00-D49)

Note: Functional activity
All neoplasms are classified in this chapter, whether they are functionally active or not. An additional code from Chapter 4 may be used, to identify functional activity associated with any neoplasm.
Morphology [Histology]
Chapter 2 classifies neoplasms primarily by site (topography), with broad groupings for behavior, malignant, in situ, benign, etc. The Table of Neoplasms should be used to identify the correct topography code. In a few cases, such as for malignant melanoma and certain neuroendocrine tumors, the morphology (histologic type) is included in the category and codes.
Primary malignant neoplasms overlapping site boundaries
A primary malignant neoplasm that overlaps two or more contiguous (next to each other) sites should be classified to the subcategory/code .8 ('overlapping lesion'), unless the combination is specifically indexed elsewhere. For multiple neoplasms of the same site that are not contiguous, such as tumors in different quadrants of the same breast, codes for each site should be assigned.
Malignant neoplasm of ectopic tissue
Malignant neoplasms of ectopic tissue are to be coded to the site mentioned, e.g., ectopic pancreatic malignant neoplasms are coded to pancreas, unspecified (C25.9).

GUIDELINES   Section I.C.2
Chapter 2 of the ICD-10-CM contains the codes for most benign and all malignant neoplasms. Certain benign neoplasms, such as prostatic adenomas, may be found in the specific body system chapters. To properly code a neoplasm it is necessary to determine from the record if the neoplasm is benign, in-situ, malignant, or of uncertain histologic behavior. If malignant, any secondary (metastatic) sites should also be determined.

GUIDELINES   Section I.C.2
The neoplasm table in the Alphabetic Index should be referenced first. However, if the histological term is documented, that term should be referenced first, rather than going immediately to the Neoplasm Table, in order to determine which column in the Neoplasm Table is appropriate. For example, if the documentation indicates "adenoma," refer to the term in the Alphabetic Index to review the entries under this term and the instructional note to "see also neoplasm, by site, benign." The table provides the proper code based on the type of neoplasm and the site.
This chapter contains the following blocks:

C00-C14	Malignant neoplasms of lip, oral cavity and pharynx
C15-C26	Malignant neoplasms of digestive organs
C30-C39	Malignant neoplasms of respiratory and intrathoracic organs
C40-C41	Malignant neoplasms of bone and articular cartilage
C43-C44	Melanoma and other malignant neoplasms of skin
C45-C49	Malignant neoplasms of mesothelial and soft tissue
C50	Malignant neoplasms of breast
C51-C58	Malignant neoplasms of female genital organs
C60-C63	Malignant neoplasms of male genital organs
C64-C68	Malignant neoplasms of urinary tract
C69-C72	Malignant neoplasms of eye, brain and other parts of central nervous system
C73-C75	Malignant neoplasms of thyroid and other endocrine glands
C7A	Malignant neuroendocrine tumors
C7B	Secondary neuroendocrine tumors
C76-C80	Malignant neoplasms of ill-defined, other secondary and unspecified sites
C81-C96	Malignant neoplasms of lymphoid, hematopoietic and related tissue
D00-D09	In situ neoplasms
D10-D36	Benign neoplasms, except benign neuroendocrine tumors
D3A	Benign neuroendocrine tumors
D37-D48	Neoplasms of uncertain behavior, polycythemia vera and myelodysplastic syndromes
D49	Neoplasms of unspecified behavior

Malignant neoplasms (C00-C96)

Malignant neoplasms, stated or presumed to be primary (of specified sites), and certain specified histologies, except neuroendocrine, and of lymphoid, hematopoietic and related tissue (C00-C75)

Malignant neoplasms of lip, oral cavity and pharynx (C00-C14)

CODING TIP ✓   Codes classifiable to C00-C14 include active cancer. History of cancer to the lip, pharynx, or oral cavity should be coded to Z85.81-.

▲ ⁴ + **C00**   **Malignant neoplasm of lip**
Use additional code to identify:
   alcohol abuse and dependence (F10.-)
   history of tobacco dependence (Z87.891)
   tobacco dependence (F17.-)
   tobacco use (Z72.0)
   EXCLUDES 1   *malignant melanoma of lip (C43.0)*
      Merkel cell carcinoma of lip (C4A.0)
      other and unspecified malignant neoplasm of skin of lip (C44.0-)

+ **C00.0**   **Malignant neoplasm of external upper lip**
   Malignant neoplasm of lipstick area of upper lip
   Malignant neoplasm of upper lip NOS
   Malignant neoplasm of vermilion border of upper lip

+ **C00.1**   **Malignant neoplasm of external lower lip**
   Malignant neoplasm of lower lip NOS
   Malignant neoplasm of lipstick area of lower lip
   Malignant neoplasm of vermilion border of lower lip

+ **C00.2**   **Malignant neoplasm of external lip, unspecified**
   Malignant neoplasm of vermilion border of lip NOS

+ **C00.3**   **Malignant neoplasm of upper lip, inner aspect**
   Malignant neoplasm of buccal aspect of upper lip
   Malignant neoplasm of frenulum of upper lip
   Malignant neoplasm of mucosa of upper lip
   Malignant neoplasm of oral aspect of upper lip

+ **C00.4**   **Malignant neoplasm of lower lip, inner aspect**
   Malignant neoplasm of buccal aspect of lower lip
   Malignant neoplasm of frenulum of lower lip
   Malignant neoplasm of mucosa of lower lip
   Malignant neoplasm of oral aspect of lower lip

+ **C00.5**   **Malignant neoplasm of lip, unspecified, inner aspect**
   Malignant neoplasm of buccal aspect of lip, unspecified
   Malignant neoplasm of frenulum of lip, unspecified
   Malignant neoplasm of mucosa of lip, unspecified
   Malignant neoplasm of oral aspect of lip, unspecified

+ **C00.6**   **Malignant neoplasm of commissure of lip, unspecified**

+ **C00.8**   **Malignant neoplasm of overlapping sites of lip**

+ **C00.9**   **Malignant neoplasm of lip, unspecified**

▲ + **C01**   **Malignant neoplasm of base of tongue**
   Malignant neoplasm of dorsal surface of base of tongue
   Malignant neoplasm of fixed part of tongue NOS
   Malignant neoplasm of posterior third of tongue
   Use additional code to identify:
   alcohol abuse and dependence (F10.-)
   history of tobacco dependence (Z87.891)
   tobacco dependence (F17.-)
   tobacco use (Z72.0)

▲ ⁴ + **C02**   **Malignant neoplasm of other and unspecified parts of tongue**
   Use additional code to identify:
   alcohol abuse and dependence (F10.-)
   history of tobacco dependence (Z87.891)
   tobacco dependence (F17.-)
   tobacco use (Z72.0)

+ **C02.0**   **Malignant neoplasm of dorsal surface of tongue**
   Malignant neoplasm of anterior two-thirds of tongue, dorsal surface
   EXCLUDES 2   *malignant neoplasm of dorsal surface of base of tongue (C01)*

● New   ▲ Revised   *Manifestation*   ⁴-⁷ Digit Indicators   ⊟ Laterality   Ⓐ Adult (15+ years)   Ⓜ Maternity (12-55 years)   Ⓝ Newborn   Ⓟ Pediatric (0-17 years)   ♂ Male   ♀ Female
✖ Deleted   Unspecified   + Additional code

+ C02.1 Malignant neoplasm of border of tongue
Malignant neoplasm of tip of tongue

+ C02.2 Malignant neoplasm of ventral surface of tongue
Malignant neoplasm of anterior two-thirds of tongue, ventral surface
Malignant neoplasm of frenulum linguae

+ C02.3 Malignant neoplasm of anterior two-thirds of tongue, part unspecified
Malignant neoplasm of middle third of tongue NOS
Malignant neoplasm of mobile part of tongue NOS

+ C02.4 Malignant neoplasm of lingual tonsil
EXCLUDES 2 *malignant neoplasm of tonsil NOS (C09.9)*

+ C02.8 Malignant neoplasm of overlapping sites of tongue
Malignant neoplasm of two or more contiguous sites of tongue

+ C02.9 Malignant neoplasm of tongue, unspecified

▲ ▣ **+ C03 Malignant neoplasm of gum**
INCLUDES malignant neoplasm of alveolar (ridge) mucosa
malignant neoplasm of gingiva
Use additional code to identify:
alcohol abuse and dependence (F10.-)
history of tobacco dependence (Z87.891)
tobacco dependence (F17.-)
tobacco use (Z72.0)
EXCLUDES 2 *malignant odontogenic neoplasms (C41.0-C41.1)*

+ C03.0 Malignant neoplasm of upper gum
+ C03.1 Malignant neoplasm of lower gum
+ C03.9 Malignant neoplasm of gum, unspecified

▲ ▣ **+ C04 Malignant neoplasm of floor of mouth**
Use additional code to identify:
alcohol abuse and dependence (F10.-)
history of tobacco dependence (Z87.891)
tobacco dependence (F17.-)
tobacco use (Z72.0)

+ C04.0 Malignant neoplasm of anterior floor of mouth
Malignant neoplasm of anterior to the premolar-canine junction

+ C04.1 Malignant neoplasm of lateral floor of mouth
+ C04.8 Malignant neoplasm of overlapping sites of floor of mouth
+ C04.9 Malignant neoplasm of floor of mouth, unspecified

▲ ▣ **+ C05 Malignant neoplasm of palate**
Use additional code to identify:
alcohol abuse and dependence (F10.-)
history of tobacco dependence (Z87.891)
tobacco dependence (F17.-)
tobacco use (Z72.0)
EXCLUDES 1 *Kaposi's sarcoma of palate (C46.2)*

+ C05.0 Malignant neoplasm of hard palate
+ C05.1 Malignant neoplasm of soft palate
EXCLUDES 2 *malignant neoplasm of nasopharyngeal surface of soft palate (C11.3)*

+ C05.2 Malignant neoplasm of uvula
+ C05.8 Malignant neoplasm of overlapping sites of palate
+ C05.9 Malignant neoplasm of palate, unspecified
Malignant neoplasm of roof of mouth

▲ ▣ **+ C06 Malignant neoplasm of other and unspecified parts of mouth**
Use additional code to identify:
alcohol abuse and dependence (F10.-)
history of tobacco dependence (Z87.891)
tobacco dependence (F17.-)
tobacco use (Z72.0)

+ C06.0 Malignant neoplasm of cheek mucosa
Malignant neoplasm of buccal mucosa NOS
Malignant neoplasm of internal cheek

+ C06.1 Malignant neoplasm of vestibule of mouth
Malignant neoplasm of buccal sulcus (upper) (lower)
Malignant neoplasm of labial sulcus (upper) (lower)

+ C06.2 Malignant neoplasm of retromolar area
▣ **+ C06.8 Malignant neoplasm of overlapping sites of other and unspecified parts of mouth**
+ C06.80 Malignant neoplasm of overlapping sites of unspecified parts of mouth

+ C06.89 Malignant neoplasm of overlapping sites of other parts of mouth
'book leaf' neoplasm [ventral surface of tongue and floor of mouth]

+ C06.9 Malignant neoplasm of mouth, unspecified
Malignant neoplasm of minor salivary gland, unspecified site
Malignant neoplasm of oral cavity NOS

▲ **+ C07 Malignant neoplasm of parotid gland**
Use additional code to identify:
alcohol abuse and dependence (F10.-)
exposure to environmental tobacco smoke (Z77.22)
exposure to tobacco smoke in the perinatal period (P96.81)
history of tobacco dependence (Z87.891)
occupational exposure to environmental tobacco smoke (Z57.31)
tobacco dependence (F17.-)
tobacco use (Z72.0)

▲ ▣ **+ C08 Malignant neoplasm of other and unspecified major salivary glands**
INCLUDES malignant neoplasm of salivary ducts
Use additional code to identify:
alcohol abuse and dependence (F10.-)
exposure to environmental tobacco smoke (Z77.22)
exposure to tobacco smoke in the perinatal period (P96.81)
history of tobacco dependence (Z87.891)
occupational exposure to environmental tobacco smoke (Z57.31)
tobacco dependence (F17.-)
tobacco use (Z72.0)
EXCLUDES 1 *malignant neoplasms of specified minor salivary glands which are classified according to their anatomical location*
EXCLUDES 2 *malignant neoplasms of minor salivary glands NOS (C06.9)*
malignant neoplasm of parotid gland (C07)

+ C08.0 Malignant neoplasm of submandibular gland
Malignant neoplasm of submaxillary gland

+ C08.1 Malignant neoplasm of sublingual gland
+ C08.9 Malignant neoplasm of major salivary gland, unspecified
Malignant neoplasm of salivary gland (major) NOS

▲ ▣ **+ C09 Malignant neoplasm of tonsil**
Use additional code to identify:
alcohol abuse and dependence (F10.-)
exposure to environmental tobacco smoke (Z77.22)
exposure to tobacco smoke in the perinatal period (P96.81)
history of tobacco dependence (Z87.891)
occupational exposure to environmental tobacco smoke (Z57.31)
tobacco dependence (F17.-)
tobacco use (Z72.0)
EXCLUDES 2 *malignant neoplasm of lingual tonsil (C02.4)*
malignant neoplasm of pharyngeal tonsil (C11.1)

+ C09.0 Malignant neoplasm of tonsillar fossa
+ C09.1 Malignant neoplasm of tonsillar pillar (anterior) (posterior)
+ C09.8 Malignant neoplasm of overlapping sites of tonsil
+ C09.9 Malignant neoplasm of tonsil, unspecified
Malignant neoplasm of tonsil NOS
Malignant neoplasm of faucial tonsils
Malignant neoplasm of palatine tonsils

▲ ▣ **+ C10 Malignant neoplasm of oropharynx**
Use additional code to identify:
alcohol abuse and dependence (F10.-)
exposure to environmental tobacco smoke (Z77.22)
exposure to tobacco smoke in the perinatal period (P96.81)
history of tobacco dependence (Z87.891)
occupational exposure to environmental tobacco smoke (Z57.31)
tobacco dependence (F17.-)
tobacco use (Z72.0)
EXCLUDES 2 *malignant neoplasm of tonsil (C09.-)*

+ C10.0 Malignant neoplasm of vallecula
+ C10.1 Malignant neoplasm of anterior surface of epiglottis
Malignant neoplasm of epiglottis, free border [margin]
Malignant neoplasm of glossoepiglottic fold(s)
EXCLUDES 2 *malignant neoplasm of epiglottis (suprahyoid portion) NOS (C32.1)*

+ C10.2 Malignant neoplasm of lateral wall of oropharynx

● New   ▲ Revised   *Manifestation*   ▣ - ▣ Digit Indicators   ▤ Laterality   ▣ Adult (15+ years)   ▣ Maternity (12-55 years)   ▣ Newborn   ▣ Pediatric (0-17 years)   ♂ Male   ♀ Female
✖ Deleted   Unspecified   + Additional code

+ **C10.3**   **Malignant neoplasm of posterior wall of oropharynx**

+ **C10.4**   **Malignant neoplasm of branchial cleft**
Malignant neoplasm of branchial cyst [site of neoplasm]

+ **C10.8**   **Malignant neoplasm of overlapping sites of oropharynx**
Malignant neoplasm of junctional region of oropharynx

+ **C10.9**   **Malignant neoplasm of oropharynx, unspecified**

▲ ◳+ **C11**   **Malignant neoplasm of nasopharynx**
Use additional code to identify:
exposure to environmental tobacco smoke (Z77.22)
exposure to tobacco smoke in the perinatal period (P96.81)
history of tobacco dependence (Z87.891)
occupational exposure to environmental tobacco smoke (Z57.31)
tobacco dependence (F17.-)
tobacco use (Z72.0)

+ **C11.0**   **Malignant neoplasm of superior wall of nasopharynx**
Malignant neoplasm of roof of nasopharynx

+ **C11.1**   **Malignant neoplasm of posterior wall of nasopharynx**
Malignant neoplasm of adenoid
Malignant neoplasm of pharyngeal tonsil

+ **C11.2**   **Malignant neoplasm of lateral wall of nasopharynx**
Malignant neoplasm of fossa of Rosenmüller
Malignant neoplasm of opening of auditory tube
Malignant neoplasm of pharyngeal recess

+ **C11.3**   **Malignant neoplasm of anterior wall of nasopharynx**
Malignant neoplasm of floor of nasopharynx
Malignant neoplasm of nasopharyngeal (anterior) (posterior) surface of soft palate
Malignant neoplasm of posterior margin of nasal choana
Malignant neoplasm of posterior margin of nasal septum

+ **C11.8**   **Malignant neoplasm of overlapping sites of nasopharynx**

+ **C11.9**   **Malignant neoplasm of nasopharynx, unspecified**
Malignant neoplasm of nasopharyngeal wall NOS

▲+ **C12**   **Malignant neoplasm of pyriform sinus**
Malignant neoplasm of pyriform fossa
Use additional code to identify:
exposure to environmental tobacco smoke (Z77.22)
exposure to tobacco smoke in the perinatal period (P96.81)
history of tobacco dependence (Z87.891)
occupational exposure to environmental tobacco smoke (Z57.31)
tobacco dependence (F17.-)
tobacco use (Z72.0)

▲ ◳+ **C13**   **Malignant neoplasm of hypopharynx**
Use additional code to identify:
exposure to environmental tobacco smoke (Z77.22)
exposure to tobacco smoke in the perinatal period (P96.81)
history of tobacco dependence (Z87.891)
occupational exposure to environmental tobacco smoke (Z57.31)
tobacco dependence (F17.-)
tobacco use (Z72.0)

     EXCLUDES 2   *malignant neoplasm of pyriform sinus (C12)*

+ **C13.0**   **Malignant neoplasm of postcricoid region**

+ **C13.1**   **Malignant neoplasm of aryepiglottic fold, hypopharyngeal aspect**
Malignant neoplasm of aryepiglottic fold, marginal zone
Malignant neoplasm of aryepiglottic fold NOS
Malignant neoplasm of interarytenoid fold, marginal zone
Malignant neoplasm of interarytenoid fold NOS

     EXCLUDES 2   *malignant neoplasm of aryepiglottic fold or interarytenoid fold, laryngeal aspect (C32.1)*

+ **C13.2**   **Malignant neoplasm of posterior wall of hypopharynx**

+ **C13.8**   **Malignant neoplasm of overlapping sites of hypopharynx**

+ **C13.9**   **Malignant neoplasm of hypopharynx, unspecified**
Malignant neoplasm of hypopharyngeal wall NOS

▲ ◳+ **C14**   **Malignant neoplasm of other and ill-defined sites in the lip, oral cavity and pharynx**
Use additional code to identify:
alcohol abuse and dependence (F10.-)
exposure to environmental tobacco smoke (Z77.22)
exposure to tobacco smoke in the perinatal period (P96.81)
history of tobacco dependence (Z87.891)
occupational exposure to environmental tobacco smoke (Z57.31)
tobacco dependence (F17.-)
tobacco use (Z72.0)

     EXCLUDES 1   *malignant neoplasm of oral cavity NOS (C06.9)*

+ **C14.0**   **Malignant neoplasm of pharynx, unspecified**

+ **C14.2**   **Malignant neoplasm of Waldeyer's ring**

+ **C14.8**   **Malignant neoplasm of overlapping sites of lip, oral cavity and pharynx**
Primary malignant neoplasm of two or more contiguous sites of lip, oral cavity and pharynx

     EXCLUDES 1   *'book leaf' neoplasm [ventral surface of tongue and floor of mouth] (C06.89)*

Malignant neoplasms of digestive organs (C15-C26)

   EXCLUDES 1   *Kaposi's sarcoma of gastrointestinal sites (C46.4)*

   EXCLUDES 2   *gastrointestinal stromal tumors (C49.A-)*

   CODING TIP ✓   Codes classifiable to C15-C26 include active cancer. History of cancer to digestive organs should be coded to Z85.0-.

◳+ **C15**   **Malignant neoplasm of esophagus**
Use additional code to identify:
alcohol abuse and dependence (F10.-)

+ **C15.3**   **Malignant neoplasm of upper third of esophagus**

+ **C15.4**   **Malignant neoplasm of middle third of esophagus**

+ **C15.5**   **Malignant neoplasm of lower third of esophagus**

     EXCLUDES 1   *malignant neoplasm of cardio-esophageal junction (C16.0)*

+ **C15.8**   **Malignant neoplasm of overlapping sites of esophagus**

+ **C15.9**   **Malignant neoplasm of esophagus, unspecified**

◳+ **C16**   **Malignant neoplasm of stomach**
Use additional code to identify:
alcohol abuse and dependence (F10.-)

     EXCLUDES 2   *malignant carcinoid tumor of the stomach (C7A.092)*

+ **C16.0**   **Malignant neoplasm of cardia**
Malignant neoplasm of cardiac orifice
Malignant neoplasm of cardio-esophageal junction
Malignant neoplasm of esophagus and stomach
Malignant neoplasm of gastro-esophageal junction

+ **C16.1**   **Malignant neoplasm of fundus of stomach**

+ **C16.2**   **Malignant neoplasm of body of stomach**

+ **C16.3**   **Malignant neoplasm of pyloric antrum**
Malignant neoplasm of gastric antrum

+ **C16.4**   **Malignant neoplasm of pylorus**
Malignant neoplasm of prepylorus
Malignant neoplasm of pyloric canal

+ **C16.5**   **Malignant neoplasm of lesser curvature of stomach, unspecified**
Malignant neoplasm of lesser curvature of stomach, not classifiable to C16.1-C16.4

+ **C16.6**   **Malignant neoplasm of greater curvature of stomach, unspecified**
Malignant neoplasm of greater curvature of stomach, not classifiable to C16.0-C16.4

+ **C16.8**   **Malignant neoplasm of overlapping sites of stomach**

+ **C16.9**   **Malignant neoplasm of stomach, unspecified**
Gastric cancer NOS

◳ **C17**   **Malignant neoplasm of small intestine**

     EXCLUDES 1   *malignant carcinoid tumors of the small intestine (C7A.01)*

C17.0   **Malignant neoplasm of duodenum**

C17.1   **Malignant neoplasm of jejunum**

C17.2   **Malignant neoplasm of ileum**

     EXCLUDES 1   *malignant neoplasm of ileocecal valve (C18.0)*

C17.3   **Meckel's diverticulum, malignant**

     EXCLUDES 1   *Meckel's diverticulum, congenital (Q43.0)*

C17.8   **Malignant neoplasm of overlapping sites of small intestine**

C17.9   **Malignant neoplasm of small intestine, unspecified**

◳ **C18**   **Malignant neoplasm of colon**

     EXCLUDES 1   *malignant carcinoid tumors of the colon (C7A.02-)*

C18.0   **Malignant neoplasm of cecum**
Malignant neoplasm of ileocecal valve

C18.1   **Malignant neoplasm of appendix**

C18.2   **Malignant neoplasm of ascending colon**

C18.3   **Malignant neoplasm of hepatic flexure**

C18.4   **Malignant neoplasm of transverse colon**

C18.5   **Malignant neoplasm of splenic flexure**

● New   ▲ Revised   *Manifestation*   ◳-◷ Digit Indicators   ▤ Laterality   ▲ Adult (15+ years)   Ⓜ Maternity (12-55 years)   Ⓝ Newborn   Ⓟ Pediatric (0-17 years)   ♂ Male   ♀ Female
✖ Deleted   Unspecified   + Additional code

2017 ICD-10-CM Expert for Physicians

© 2017 DecisionHealth   471

C10.3 — C18.5

Neoplasms

	C18.6	**Malignant neoplasm of descending colon**
	C18.7	**Malignant neoplasm of sigmoid colon**

C18.6 | **Malignant neoplasm of descending colon**
C18.7 | **Malignant neoplasm of sigmoid colon**
Malignant neoplasm of sigmoid (flexure)

EXCLUDES 1 *malignant neoplasm of rectosigmoid junction (C19)*

C18.8 | **Malignant neoplasm of overlapping sites of colon**
C18.9 | **Malignant neoplasm of colon, unspecified**
Malignant neoplasm of large intestine NOS

C19 | **Malignant neoplasm of rectosigmoid junction**
Malignant neoplasm of colon with rectum
Malignant neoplasm of rectosigmoid (colon)

EXCLUDES 1 *malignant carcinoid tumors of the colon (C7A.02-)*

C20 | **Malignant neoplasm of rectum**
Malignant neoplasm of rectal ampulla

EXCLUDES 1 *malignant carcinoid tumor of the rectum (C7A.026)*

C21 | **Malignant neoplasm of anus and anal canal**

EXCLUDES 2 *malignant carcinoid tumors of the colon (C7A.02-)*
malignant melanoma of anal margin (C43.51)
malignant melanoma of anal skin (C43.51)
malignant melanoma of perianal skin (C43.51)
other and unspecified malignant neoplasm of anal margin (C44.500, C44.510, C44.520, C44.590)
other and unspecified malignant neoplasm of anal skin (C44.500, C44.510, C44.520, C44.590)
other and unspecified malignant neoplasm of perianal skin (C44.500, C44.510, C44.520, C44.590)

C21.0 | **Malignant neoplasm of anus, unspecified**
C21.1 | **Malignant neoplasm of anal canal**
Malignant neoplasm of anal sphincter
C21.2 | **Malignant neoplasm of cloacogenic zone**
C21.8 | **Malignant neoplasm of overlapping sites of rectum, anus and anal canal**
Malignant neoplasm of anorectal junction
Malignant neoplasm of anorectum
Primary malignant neoplasm of two or more contiguous sites of rectum, anus and anal canal

+ C22 | **Malignant neoplasm of liver and intrahepatic bile ducts**
Use additional code to identify:
alcohol abuse and dependence (F10.-)
hepatitis B (B16.-, B18.0-B18.1)
hepatitis C (B17.1-, B18.2)

EXCLUDES 1 *malignant neoplasm of biliary tract NOS (C24.9)*
secondary malignant neoplasm of liver and intrahepatic bile duct (C78.7)

+ C22.0 | **Liver cell carcinoma**
Hepatocellular carcinoma
Hepatoma
AHA: 1Q 2016, 18-19
+ C22.1 | **Intrahepatic bile duct carcinoma**
Cholangiocarcinoma
EXCLUDES 1 *malignant neoplasm of hepatic duct (C24.0)*
+ C22.2 | **Hepatoblastoma**
+ C22.3 | **Angiosarcoma of liver**
Kupffer cell sarcoma
+ C22.4 | **Other sarcomas of liver**
+ C22.7 | **Other specified carcinomas of liver**
+ C22.8 | **Malignant neoplasm of liver, primary, unspecified as to type**
+ C22.9 | **Malignant neoplasm of liver, not specified as primary or secondary**
C23 | **Malignant neoplasm of gallbladder**
C24 | **Malignant neoplasm of other and unspecified parts of biliary tract**
EXCLUDES 1 *malignant neoplasm of intrahepatic bile duct (C22.1)*
C24.0 | **Malignant neoplasm of extrahepatic bile duct**
Malignant neoplasm of biliary duct or passage NOS
Malignant neoplasm of common bile duct
Malignant neoplasm of cystic duct
Malignant neoplasm of hepatic duct
C24.1 | **Malignant neoplasm of ampulla of Vater**

C24.8 | **Malignant neoplasm of overlapping sites of biliary tract**
Malignant neoplasm involving both intrahepatic and extrahepatic bile ducts
Primary malignant neoplasm of two or more contiguous sites of biliary tract
C24.9 | **Malignant neoplasm of biliary tract, unspecified**

▲ ▣ + **C25** | **Malignant neoplasm of pancreas**
Code also:
exocrine pancreatic insufficiency (K86.81)
Use additional code to identify:
alcohol abuse and dependence (F10.-)

+ C25.0 | **Malignant neoplasm of head of pancreas**
+ C25.1 | **Malignant neoplasm of body of pancreas**
+ C25.2 | **Malignant neoplasm of tail of pancreas**
+ C25.3 | **Malignant neoplasm of pancreatic duct**
+ C25.4 | **Malignant neoplasm of endocrine pancreas**
Malignant neoplasm of islets of Langerhans
Use additional code to identify any functional activity.
+ C25.7 | **Malignant neoplasm of other parts of pancreas**
Malignant neoplasm of neck of pancreas
+ C25.8 | **Malignant neoplasm of overlapping sites of pancreas**
+ C25.9 | **Malignant neoplasm of pancreas, unspecified**

▣ **C26** | **Malignant neoplasm of other and ill-defined digestive organs**
EXCLUDES 1 *malignant neoplasm of peritoneum and retroperitoneum (C48.-)*
C26.0 | **Malignant neoplasm of intestinal tract, part unspecified**
Malignant neoplasm of intestine NOS
C26.1 | **Malignant neoplasm of spleen**
EXCLUDES 1 *Hodgkin lymphoma (C81.-)*
non-Hodgkin lymphoma (C82-C85)
C26.9 | **Malignant neoplasm of ill-defined sites within the digestive system**
Malignant neoplasm of alimentary canal or tract NOS
Malignant neoplasm of gastrointestinal tract NOS
EXCLUDES 1 *malignant neoplasm of abdominal NOS (C76.2)*
malignant neoplasm of intra-abdominal NOS (C76.2)

Malignant neoplasms of respiratory and intrathoracic organs (C30-C39)

INCLUDES malignant neoplasm of middle ear
EXCLUDES 1 *mesothelioma (C45.-)*

CODING TIP ✓ Codes classifiable to C30-C39 include active cancer. History of cancer to respiratory system and other intrathoracic organs should be coded using codes from Z85.1- and Z85.2-.

▣ **C30** | **Malignant neoplasm of nasal cavity and middle ear**
C30.0 | **Malignant neoplasm of nasal cavity**
Malignant neoplasm of cartilage of nose
Malignant neoplasm of nasal concha
Malignant neoplasm of internal nose
Malignant neoplasm of septum of nose
Malignant neoplasm of vestibule of nose
EXCLUDES 1 *malignant neoplasm of nasal bone (C41.0)*
malignant neoplasm of nose NOS (C76.0)
malignant neoplasm of olfactory bulb (C72.2-)
malignant neoplasm of posterior margin of nasal septum and choana (C11.3)
malignant melanoma of skin of nose (C43.31)
malignant neoplasm of turbinates (C41.0)
other and unspecified malignant neoplasm of skin of nose C44.301, C44.311, C44.321, C44.391)

● New ▲ Revised *Manifestation* ▣-▣ Digit Indicators ▤ Laterality ⒶAdult (15+ years) ⓂMaternity (12-55 years) ⓃNewborn ⓅPediatric (0-17 years) ♂Male ♀Female
✖ Deleted Unspecified + Additional code

472 © 2017 DecisionHealth 2017 ICD-10-CM Expert for Physicians

C18.6 — C30.0

C30.1 **Malignant neoplasm of middle ear**
Malignant neoplasm of antrum tympanicum
Malignant neoplasm of auditory tube
Malignant neoplasm of eustachian tube
Malignant neoplasm of inner ear
Malignant neoplasm of mastoid air cells
Malignant neoplasm of tympanic cavity

> **EXCLUDES 1** *malignant neoplasm of auricular canal (external) (C43.2-,C44.2-)*
> *malignant neoplasm of bone of ear (meatus) (C41.0)*
> *malignant neoplasm of cartilage of ear (C49.0)*
> *malignant melanoma of skin of (external) ear (C43.2-)*
> *other and unspecified malignant neoplasm of skin of (external) ear (C44.2-)*

C31 **Malignant neoplasm of accessory sinuses**

C31.0 **Malignant neoplasm of maxillary sinus**
Malignant neoplasm of antrum (Highmore) (maxillary)

C31.1 **Malignant neoplasm of ethmoidal sinus**

C31.2 **Malignant neoplasm of frontal sinus**

C31.3 **Malignant neoplasm of sphenoid sinus**

C31.8 **Malignant neoplasm of overlapping sites of accessory sinuses**

C31.9 **Malignant neoplasm of accessory sinus, unspecified**

C32 **Malignant neoplasm of larynx**
Use additional code to identify:
alcohol abuse and dependence (F10.-)
exposure to environmental tobacco smoke (Z77.22)
exposure to tobacco smoke in the perinatal period (P96.81)
history of tobacco dependence (Z87.891)
occupational exposure to environmental tobacco smoke (Z57.31)
tobacco dependence (F17.-)
tobacco use (Z72.0)

+ C32.0 **Malignant neoplasm of glottis**
Malignant neoplasm of intrinsic larynx
Malignant neoplasm of laryngeal commissure (anterior)(posterior)
Malignant neoplasm of vocal cord (true) NOS

+ C32.1 **Malignant neoplasm of supraglottis**
Malignant neoplasm of aryepiglottic fold or interarytenoid fold, laryngeal aspect
Malignant neoplasm of epiglottis (suprahyoid portion) NOS
Malignant neoplasm of extrinsic larynx
Malignant neoplasm of false vocal cord
Malignant neoplasm of posterior (laryngeal) surface of epiglottis
Malignant neoplasm of ventricular bands

> **EXCLUDES 2** *malignant neoplasm of anterior surface of epiglottis (C10.1)*
> *malignant neoplasm of aryepiglottic fold or interarytenoid fold, hypopharyngeal aspect (C13.1)*
> *malignant neoplasm of aryepiglottic fold or interarytenoid fold, marginal zone (C13.1)*
> *malignant neoplasm of aryepiglottic fold or interarytenoid fold NOS (C13.1)*

+ C32.2 **Malignant neoplasm of subglottis**

+ C32.3 **Malignant neoplasm of laryngeal cartilage**

+ C32.8 **Malignant neoplasm of overlapping sites of larynx**

+ C32.9 **Malignant neoplasm of larynx, unspecified**

▲ + C33 **Malignant neoplasm of trachea**
Use additional code to identify:
exposure to environmental tobacco smoke (Z77.22)
exposure to tobacco smoke in the perinatal period (P96.81)
history of tobacco dependence (Z87.891)
occupational exposure to environmental tobacco smoke (Z57.31)
tobacco dependence (F17.-)
tobacco use (Z72.0)

▲ + C34 **Malignant neoplasm of bronchus and lung**
Use additional code to identify:
exposure to environmental tobacco smoke (Z77.22)
exposure to tobacco smoke in the perinatal period (P96.81)
history of tobacco dependence (Z87.891)
occupational exposure to environmental tobacco smoke (Z57.31)
tobacco dependence (F17.-)
tobacco use (Z72.0)

> **EXCLUDES 1** *Kaposi's sarcoma of lung (C46.5-)*
> *malignant carcinoid tumor of the bronchus and lung (C7A.090)*

+ C34.0 **Malignant neoplasm of main bronchus**
Malignant neoplasm of carina
Malignant neoplasm of hilus (of lung)

+ C34.00 **Malignant neoplasm of unspecified main bronchus**

+ C34.01 **Malignant neoplasm of right main bronchus**

+ C34.02 **Malignant neoplasm of left main bronchus**

+ C34.1 **Malignant neoplasm of upper lobe, bronchus or lung**

+ C34.10 **Malignant neoplasm of upper lobe, unspecified bronchus or lung**

+ C34.11 **Malignant neoplasm of upper lobe, right bronchus or lung**

+ C34.12 **Malignant neoplasm of upper lobe, left bronchus or lung**

+ C34.2 **Malignant neoplasm of middle lobe, bronchus or lung**

+ C34.3 **Malignant neoplasm of lower lobe, bronchus or lung**

+ C34.30 **Malignant neoplasm of lower lobe, unspecified bronchus or lung**

+ C34.31 **Malignant neoplasm of lower lobe, right bronchus or lung**

+ C34.32 **Malignant neoplasm of lower lobe, left bronchus or lung**

+ C34.8 **Malignant neoplasm of overlapping sites of bronchus and lung**

+ C34.80 **Malignant neoplasm of overlapping sites of unspecified bronchus and lung**

+ C34.81 **Malignant neoplasm of overlapping sites of right bronchus and lung**

+ C34.82 **Malignant neoplasm of overlapping sites of left bronchus and lung**

+ C34.9 **Malignant neoplasm of unspecified part of bronchus or lung**

+ C34.90 **Malignant neoplasm of unspecified part of unspecified bronchus or lung**
Lung cancer NOS
AHA: 2Q 2014, 10

+ C34.91 **Malignant neoplasm of unspecified part of right bronchus or lung**

+ C34.92 **Malignant neoplasm of unspecified part of left bronchus or lung**

C37 **Malignant neoplasm of thymus**

> **EXCLUDES 1** *malignant carcinoid tumor of the thymus (C7A.091)*

C38 **Malignant neoplasm of heart, mediastinum and pleura**

> **EXCLUDES 1** *mesothelioma (C45.-)*

C38.0 **Malignant neoplasm of heart**
Malignant neoplasm of pericardium

> **EXCLUDES 1** *malignant neoplasm of great vessels (C49.3)*

C38.1 **Malignant neoplasm of anterior mediastinum**

C38.2 **Malignant neoplasm of posterior mediastinum**

C38.3 **Malignant neoplasm of mediastinum, part unspecified**

C38.4 **Malignant neoplasm of pleura**

C38.8 **Malignant neoplasm of overlapping sites of heart, mediastinum and pleura**

▲ + C39 **Malignant neoplasm of other and ill-defined sites in the respiratory system and intrathoracic organs**
Use additional code to identify:
exposure to environmental tobacco smoke (Z77.22)
exposure to tobacco smoke in the perinatal period (P96.81)
history of tobacco dependence (Z87.891)
occupational exposure to environmental tobacco smoke (Z57.31)
tobacco dependence (F17.-)
tobacco use (Z72.0)

> **EXCLUDES 1** *intrathoracic malignant neoplasm NOS (C76.1)*
> *thoracic malignant neoplasm NOS (C76.1)*

● New   ▲ Revised   *Manifestation*   �4-7 Digit Indicators   ▤ Laterality   Ⓐ Adult (15+ years)   Ⓜ Maternity (12-55 years)   Ⓝ Newborn   Ⓟ Pediatric (0-17 years)   ♂ Male   ♀ Female
✖ Deleted   Unspecified   + Additional code

+ C39.0   **Malignant neoplasm of upper respiratory tract, part unspecified**

+ C39.9   **Malignant neoplasm of lower respiratory tract, part unspecified**
     Malignant neoplasm of respiratory tract NOS

Malignant neoplasms of bone and articular cartilage (C40-C41)

INCLUDES   malignant neoplasm of cartilage (articular) (joint)
     malignant neoplasm of periosteum

EXCLUDES 1   *malignant neoplasm of bone marrow NOS (C96.9)*
     malignant neoplasm of synovia (C49.-)

CODING TIP ✓   Codes classifiable to C40-C41 include active cancer. History of cancer to bone or soft tissue should be coded to Z85.83-.

4+ C40   **Malignant neoplasm of bone and articular cartilage of limbs**
     Use additional code to identify major osseous defect, if applicable (M89.7-)

5+ C40.0   **Malignant neoplasm of scapula and long bones of upper limb**

6+ C40.00   **Malignant neoplasm of scapula and long bones of unspecified upper limb**

6+ C40.01   **Malignant neoplasm of scapula and long bones of right upper limb**

6+ C40.02   **Malignant neoplasm of scapula and long bones of left upper limb**

5+ C40.1   **Malignant neoplasm of short bones of upper limb**

6+ C40.10   **Malignant neoplasm of short bones of unspecified upper limb**

6+ C40.11   **Malignant neoplasm of short bones of right upper limb**

6+ C40.12   **Malignant neoplasm of short bones of left upper limb**

5+ C40.2   **Malignant neoplasm of long bones of lower limb**

6+ C40.20   **Malignant neoplasm of long bones of unspecified lower limb**

6+ C40.21   **Malignant neoplasm of long bones of right lower limb**

6+ C40.22   **Malignant neoplasm of long bones of left lower limb**

5+ C40.3   **Malignant neoplasm of short bones of lower limb**

6+ C40.30   **Malignant neoplasm of short bones of unspecified lower limb**

6+ C40.31   **Malignant neoplasm of short bones of right lower limb**

6+ C40.32   **Malignant neoplasm of short bones of left lower limb**

5+ C40.8   **Malignant neoplasm of overlapping sites of bone and articular cartilage of limb**

6+ C40.80   **Malignant neoplasm of overlapping sites of bone and articular cartilage of unspecified limb**

6+ C40.81   **Malignant neoplasm of overlapping sites of bone and articular cartilage of right limb**

6+ C40.82   **Malignant neoplasm of overlapping sites of bone and articular cartilage of left limb**

5+ C40.9   **Malignant neoplasm of unspecified bones and articular cartilage of limb**

6+ C40.90   **Malignant neoplasm of unspecified bones and articular cartilage of unspecified limb**

6+ C40.91   **Malignant neoplasm of unspecified bones and articular cartilage of right limb**

6+ C40.92   **Malignant neoplasm of unspecified bones and articular cartilage of left limb**

4 C41   **Malignant neoplasm of bone and articular cartilage of other and unspecified sites**

EXCLUDES 1   *malignant neoplasm of bones of limbs (C40.-)*
     malignant neoplasm of cartilage of ear (C49.0)
     malignant neoplasm of cartilage of eyelid (C49.0)
     malignant neoplasm of cartilage of larynx (C32.3)
     malignant neoplasm of cartilage of limbs (C40.-)
     malignant neoplasm of cartilage of nose (C30.0)

C41.0   **Malignant neoplasm of bones of skull and face**
     Malignant neoplasm of maxilla (superior)
     Malignant neoplasm of orbital bone

EXCLUDES 2   *carcinoma, any type except intraosseous or odontogenic of:*
     maxillary sinus (C31.0)
     upper jaw (C03.0)
     malignant neoplasm of jaw bone (lower) (C41.1)

C41.1   **Malignant neoplasm of mandible**
     Malignant neoplasm of inferior maxilla
     Malignant neoplasm of lower jaw bone

EXCLUDES 2   *carcinoma, any type except intraosseous or odontogenic of:*
     jaw NOS (C03.9)
     lower (C03.1)
     malignant neoplasm of upper jaw bone (C41.0)

C41.2   **Malignant neoplasm of vertebral column**

EXCLUDES 1   *malignant neoplasm of sacrum and coccyx (C41.4)*

C41.3   **Malignant neoplasm of ribs, sternum and clavicle**

C41.4   **Malignant neoplasm of pelvic bones, sacrum and coccyx**

C41.9   **Malignant neoplasm of bone and articular cartilage, unspecified**

Melanoma and other malignant neoplasms of skin (C43-C44)

CODING TIP ✓   Codes classifiable to C43-C44 include active cancer. History of cancer to skin should be coded to Z85.82-.

4 C43   **Malignant melanoma of skin**

EXCLUDES 1   *melanoma in situ (D03.-)*

EXCLUDES 2   *malignant melanoma of skin of genital organs (C51-C52, C60.-, C63.-)*
     Merkel cell carcinoma (C4A.-)
     sites other than skin-code to malignant neoplasm of the site

Malignant melanoma of skin

Malignant melanoma

C43.0   **Malignant melanoma of lip**

EXCLUDES 1   *malignant neoplasm of vermilion border of lip (C00.0-C00.2)*

5 C43.1   **Malignant melanoma of eyelid, including canthus**

6 C43.10   **Malignant melanoma of unspecified eyelid, including canthus**

6 C43.11   **Malignant melanoma of right eyelid, including canthus**

6 C43.12   **Malignant melanoma of left eyelid, including canthus**

5 C43.2   **Malignant melanoma of ear and external auricular canal**

6 C43.20   **Malignant melanoma of unspecified ear and external auricular canal**

6 C43.21   **Malignant melanoma of right ear and external auricular canal**

6 C43.22   **Malignant melanoma of left ear and external auricular canal**

5 C43.3   **Malignant melanoma of other and unspecified parts of face**

C43.30   **Malignant melanoma of unspecified part of face**

C43.31   **Malignant melanoma of nose**

C43.39   **Malignant melanoma of other parts of face**

● New   ▲ Revised   *Manifestation*   **4- 7** Digit Indicators   ▤ Laterality   Ⓐ Adult (15+ years)   Ⓜ Maternity (12-55 years)   Ⓝ Newborn   Ⓟ Pediatric (0-17 years)   ♂ Male   ♀ Female

✖ Deleted   Unspecified   + Additional code

474   © 2017 DecisionHealth   2017 ICD-10-CM Expert for Physicians

C39.0 — C43.39

C43.4 Malignant melanoma of scalp and neck

C43.5 Malignant melanoma of trunk

> EXCLUDES 2 *malignant neoplasm of anus NOS (C21.0)*
> *malignant neoplasm of scrotum (C63.2)*

C43.51 Malignant melanoma of anal skin
Malignant melanoma of anal margin
Malignant melanoma of perianal skin

C43.52 Malignant melanoma of skin of breast

C43.59 Malignant melanoma of other part of trunk

C43.6 Malignant melanoma of upper limb, including shoulder

C43.60 Malignant melanoma of unspecified upper limb, including shoulder

C43.61 Malignant melanoma of right upper limb, including shoulder

C43.62 Malignant melanoma of left upper limb, including shoulder

C43.7 Malignant melanoma of lower limb, including hip

C43.70 Malignant melanoma of unspecified lower limb, including hip

C43.71 Malignant melanoma of right lower limb, including hip

C43.72 Malignant melanoma of left lower limb, including hip

C43.8 Malignant melanoma of overlapping sites of skin

C43.9 Malignant melanoma of skin, unspecified
Malignant melanoma of unspecified site of skin
Melanoma (malignant) NOS

C4A Merkel cell carcinoma

C4A.0 Merkel cell carcinoma of lip

> EXCLUDES 1 *malignant neoplasm of vermilion border of lip (C00.0-C00.2)*

C4A.1 Merkel cell carcinoma of eyelid, including canthus

C4A.10 Merkel cell carcinoma of unspecified eyelid, including canthus

C4A.11 Merkel cell carcinoma of right eyelid, including canthus

C4A.12 Merkel cell carcinoma of left eyelid, including canthus

C4A.2 Merkel cell carcinoma of ear and external auricular canal

C4A.20 Merkel cell carcinoma of unspecified ear and external auricular canal

C4A.21 Merkel cell carcinoma of right ear and external auricular canal

C4A.22 Merkel cell carcinoma of left ear and external auricular canal

C4A.3 Merkel cell carcinoma of other and unspecified parts of face

C4A.30 Merkel cell carcinoma of unspecified part of face

C4A.31 Merkel cell carcinoma of nose

C4A.39 Merkel cell carcinoma of other parts of face

C4A.4 Merkel cell carcinoma of scalp and neck

C4A.5 Merkel cell carcinoma of trunk

> EXCLUDES 2 *malignant neoplasm of anus NOS (C21.0)*
> *malignant neoplasm of scrotum (C63.2)*

C4A.51 Merkel cell carcinoma of anal skin
Merkel cell carcinoma of anal margin
Merkel cell carcinoma of perianal skin

C4A.52 Merkel cell carcinoma of skin of breast

C4A.59 Merkel cell carcinoma of other part of trunk

C4A.6 Merkel cell carcinoma of upper limb, including shoulder

C4A.60 Merkel cell carcinoma of unspecified upper limb, including shoulder

C4A.61 Merkel cell carcinoma of right upper limb, including shoulder

C4A.62 Merkel cell carcinoma of left upper limb, including shoulder

C4A.7 Merkel cell carcinoma of lower limb, including hip

C4A.70 Merkel cell carcinoma of unspecified lower limb, including hip

C4A.71 Merkel cell carcinoma of right lower limb, including hip

C4A.72 Merkel cell carcinoma of left lower limb, including hip

C4A.8 Merkel cell carcinoma of overlapping sites

C4A.9 Merkel cell carcinoma, unspecified
Merkel cell carcinoma of unspecified site
Merkel cell carcinoma NOS

C44 Other and unspecified malignant neoplasm of skin

> INCLUDES malignant neoplasm of sebaceous glands
> malignant neoplasm of sweat glands
> EXCLUDES 1 *Kaposi's sarcoma of skin (C46.0)*
> *malignant melanoma of skin (C43.-)*
> *malignant neoplasm of skin of genital organs (C51-C52, C60.-, C63.2)*
> *Merkel cell carcinoma (C4A.-)*

C44.0 Other and unspecified malignant neoplasm of skin of lip

> EXCLUDES 1 *malignant neoplasm of lip (C00.-)*

C44.00 Unspecified malignant neoplasm of skin of lip

C44.01 Basal cell carcinoma of skin of lip

C44.02 Squamous cell carcinoma of skin of lip

C44.09 Other specified malignant neoplasm of skin of lip

C44.1 Other and unspecified malignant neoplasm of skin of eyelid, including canthus

> EXCLUDES 1 *connective tissue of eyelid (C49.0)*

C44.10 Unspecified malignant neoplasm of skin of eyelid, including canthus

C44.101 Unspecified malignant neoplasm of skin of unspecified eyelid, including canthus

C44.102 Unspecified malignant neoplasm of skin of right eyelid, including canthus

C44.109 Unspecified malignant neoplasm of skin of left eyelid, including canthus

C44.11 Basal cell carcinoma of skin of eyelid, including canthus

C44.111 Basal cell carcinoma of skin of unspecified eyelid, including canthus

C44.112 Basal cell carcinoma of skin of right eyelid, including canthus

C44.119 Basal cell carcinoma of skin of left eyelid, including canthus

C44.12 Squamous cell carcinoma of skin of eyelid, including canthus

C44.121 Squamous cell carcinoma of skin of unspecified eyelid, including canthus

C44.122 Squamous cell carcinoma of skin of right eyelid, including canthus

C44.129 Squamous cell carcinoma of skin of left eyelid, including canthus

C44.19 Other specified malignant neoplasm of skin of eyelid, including canthus

C44.191 Other specified malignant neoplasm of skin of unspecified eyelid, including canthus

C44.192 Other specified malignant neoplasm of skin of right eyelid, including canthus

C44.199 Other specified malignant neoplasm of skin of left eyelid, including canthus

C44.2 Other and unspecified malignant neoplasm of skin of ear and external auricular canal

> EXCLUDES 1 *connective tissue of ear (C49.0)*

C44.20 Unspecified malignant neoplasm of skin of ear and external auricular canal

C44.201 Unspecified malignant neoplasm of skin of unspecified ear and external auricular canal

C44.202 Unspecified malignant neoplasm of skin of right ear and external auricular canal

C44.209 Unspecified malignant neoplasm of skin of left ear and external auricular canal

C44.21 Basal cell carcinoma of skin of ear and external auricular canal

C44.211 Basal cell carcinoma of skin of unspecified ear and external auricular canal

C44.212 Basal cell carcinoma of skin of right ear and external auricular canal

C44.219 Basal cell carcinoma of skin of left ear and external auricular canal

C44.22 Squamous cell carcinoma of skin of ear and external auricular canal

C44.221 Squamous cell carcinoma of skin of unspecified ear and external auricular canal

C44.222 Squamous cell carcinoma of skin of right ear and external auricular canal

C44.229 Squamous cell carcinoma of skin of left ear and external auricular canal

---

● New ▲ Revised *Manifestation* 4-7 Digit Indicators ▣ Laterality ▢ Adult (15+ years) ▢ Maternity (12-55 years) ▢ Newborn ▢ Pediatric (0-17 years) ♂ Male ♀ Female
✖ Deleted Unspecified ✚ Additional code

Ⓖ **C44.29** Other specified malignant neoplasm of skin of ear and external auricular canal

⊟ **C44.291** Other specified malignant neoplasm of skin of unspecified ear and external auricular canal

⊟ **C44.292** Other specified malignant neoplasm of skin of right ear and external auricular canal

⊟ **C44.299** Other specified malignant neoplasm of skin of left ear and external auricular canal

Ⓢ **C44.3** Other and unspecified malignant neoplasm of skin of other and unspecified parts of face

Ⓖ **C44.30** Unspecified malignant neoplasm of skin of other and unspecified parts of face

C44.300 Unspecified malignant neoplasm of skin of unspecified part of face

C44.301 Unspecified malignant neoplasm of skin of nose

C44.309 Unspecified malignant neoplasm of skin of other parts of face

Ⓖ **C44.31** Basal cell carcinoma of skin of other and unspecified parts of face

C44.310 Basal cell carcinoma of skin of unspecified parts of face

C44.311 Basal cell carcinoma of skin of nose

C44.319 Basal cell carcinoma of skin of other parts of face

Ⓖ **C44.32** Squamous cell carcinoma of skin of other and unspecified parts of face

C44.320 Squamous cell carcinoma of skin of unspecified parts of face

C44.321 Squamous cell carcinoma of skin of nose

C44.329 Squamous cell carcinoma of skin of other parts of face

Ⓖ **C44.39** Other specified malignant neoplasm of skin of other and unspecified parts of face

C44.390 Other specified malignant neoplasm of skin of unspecified parts of face

C44.391 Other specified malignant neoplasm of skin of nose

C44.399 Other specified malignant neoplasm of skin of other parts of face

Ⓢ **C44.4** Other and unspecified malignant neoplasm of skin of scalp and neck

C44.40 Unspecified malignant neoplasm of skin of scalp and neck

C44.41 Basal cell carcinoma of skin of scalp and neck

C44.42 Squamous cell carcinoma of skin of scalp and neck

C44.49 Other specified malignant neoplasm of skin of scalp and neck

Ⓢ **C44.5** Other and unspecified malignant neoplasm of skin of trunk

EXCLUDES 1 anus NOS (C21.0)
scrotum (C63.2)

Ⓖ **C44.50** Unspecified malignant neoplasm of skin of trunk

C44.500 Unspecified malignant neoplasm of anal skin
Unspecified malignant neoplasm of anal margin
Unspecified malignant neoplasm of perianal skin

C44.501 Unspecified malignant neoplasm of skin of breast

C44.509 Unspecified malignant neoplasm of skin of other part of trunk

Ⓖ **C44.51** Basal cell carcinoma of skin of trunk

C44.510 Basal cell carcinoma of anal skin
Basal cell carcinoma of anal margin
Basal cell carcinoma of perianal skin

C44.511 Basal cell carcinoma of skin of breast

C44.519 Basal cell carcinoma of skin of other part of trunk

Ⓖ **C44.52** Squamous cell carcinoma of skin of trunk

C44.520 Squamous cell carcinoma of anal skin
Squamous cell carcinoma of anal margin
Squamous cell carcinoma of perianal skin

C44.521 Squamous cell carcinoma of skin of breast

C44.529 Squamous cell carcinoma of skin of other part of trunk

Ⓖ **C44.59** Other specified malignant neoplasm of skin of trunk

C44.590 Other specified malignant neoplasm of anal skin
Other specified malignant neoplasm of anal margin
Other specified malignant neoplasm of perianal skin

C44.591 Other specified malignant neoplasm of skin of breast

C44.599 Other specified malignant neoplasm of skin of other part of trunk

Ⓢ **C44.6** Other and unspecified malignant neoplasm of skin of upper limb, including shoulder

Ⓖ **C44.60** Unspecified malignant neoplasm of skin of upper limb, including shoulder

⊟ **C44.601** Unspecified malignant neoplasm of skin of unspecified upper limb, including shoulder

⊟ **C44.602** Unspecified malignant neoplasm of skin of right upper limb, including shoulder

⊟ **C44.609** Unspecified malignant neoplasm of skin of left upper limb, including shoulder

Ⓖ **C44.61** Basal cell carcinoma of skin of upper limb, including shoulder

⊟ **C44.611** Basal cell carcinoma of skin of unspecified upper limb, including shoulder

⊟ **C44.612** Basal cell carcinoma of skin of right upper limb, including shoulder

⊟ **C44.619** Basal cell carcinoma of skin of left upper limb, including shoulder

Ⓖ **C44.62** Squamous cell carcinoma of skin of upper limb, including shoulder

⊟ **C44.621** Squamous cell carcinoma of skin of unspecified upper limb, including shoulder

⊟ **C44.622** Squamous cell carcinoma of skin of right upper limb, including shoulder

⊟ **C44.629** Squamous cell carcinoma of skin of left upper limb, including shoulder

Ⓖ **C44.69** Other specified malignant neoplasm of skin of upper limb, including shoulder

⊟ **C44.691** Other specified malignant neoplasm of skin of unspecified upper limb, including shoulder

⊟ **C44.692** Other specified malignant neoplasm of skin of right upper limb, including shoulder

⊟ **C44.699** Other specified malignant neoplasm of skin of left upper limb, including shoulder

Ⓢ **C44.7** Other and unspecified malignant neoplasm of skin of lower limb, including hip

Ⓖ **C44.70** Unspecified malignant neoplasm of skin of lower limb, including hip

⊟ **C44.701** Unspecified malignant neoplasm of skin of unspecified lower limb, including hip

⊟ **C44.702** Unspecified malignant neoplasm of skin of right lower limb, including hip

⊟ **C44.709** Unspecified malignant neoplasm of skin of left lower limb, including hip

Ⓖ **C44.71** Basal cell carcinoma of skin of lower limb, including hip

⊟ **C44.711** Basal cell carcinoma of skin of unspecified lower limb, including hip

⊟ **C44.712** Basal cell carcinoma of skin of right lower limb, including hip

⊟ **C44.719** Basal cell carcinoma of skin of left lower limb, including hip

Ⓖ **C44.72** Squamous cell carcinoma of skin of lower limb, including hip

⊟ **C44.721** Squamous cell carcinoma of skin of unspecified lower limb, including hip

⊟ **C44.722** Squamous cell carcinoma of skin of right lower limb, including hip

⊟ **C44.729** Squamous cell carcinoma of skin of left lower limb, including hip

Ⓖ **C44.79** Other specified malignant neoplasm of skin of lower limb, including hip

⊟ **C44.791** Other specified malignant neoplasm of skin of unspecified lower limb, including hip

⊟ **C44.792** Other specified malignant neoplasm of skin of right lower limb, including hip

⊟ **C44.799** Other specified malignant neoplasm of skin of left lower limb, including hip

Ⓢ **C44.8** Other and unspecified malignant neoplasm of overlapping sites of skin

C44.80   Unspecified malignant neoplasm of overlapping sites of skin

C44.81   Basal cell carcinoma of overlapping sites of skin

C44.82   Squamous cell carcinoma of overlapping sites of skin

C44.89   Other specified malignant neoplasm of overlapping sites of skin

🔲 C44.9   **Other and unspecified malignant neoplasm of skin, unspecified**

C44.90   Unspecified malignant neoplasm of skin, unspecified
Malignant neoplasm of unspecified site of skin

C44.91   Basal cell carcinoma of skin, unspecified

C44.92   Squamous cell carcinoma of skin, unspecified

C44.99   Other specified malignant neoplasm of skin, unspecified

Malignant neoplasms of mesothelial and soft tissue (C45-C49)

CODING TIP ✓   Codes classifiable to C45-C49 include active cancer. History of cancer to soft tissue should be coded to Z85.83-.

🔟 **C45**   **Mesothelioma**

C45.0   **Mesothelioma of pleura**
      EXCLUDES 1   *other malignant neoplasm of pleura (C38.4)*

C45.1   **Mesothelioma of peritoneum**
Mesothelioma of cul-de-sac
Mesothelioma of mesentery
Mesothelioma of mesocolon
Mesothelioma of omentum
Mesothelioma of peritoneum (parietal) (pelvic)
      EXCLUDES 1   *other malignant neoplasm of soft tissue of peritoneum (C48.-)*

C45.2   **Mesothelioma of pericardium**
      EXCLUDES 1   *other malignant neoplasm of pericardium (C38.0)*

C45.7   **Mesothelioma of other sites**

C45.9   **Mesothelioma, unspecified**

🔟 **C46**   **Kaposi's sarcoma**
Code first:
any human immunodeficiency virus [HIV] disease (B20)

C46.0   **Kaposi's sarcoma of skin**

C46.1   **Kaposi's sarcoma of soft tissue**
Kaposi's sarcoma of blood vessel
Kaposi's sarcoma of connective tissue
Kaposi's sarcoma of fascia
Kaposi's sarcoma of ligament
Kaposi's sarcoma of lymphatic(s) NEC
Kaposi's sarcoma of muscle
      EXCLUDES 2   *Kaposi's sarcoma of lymph glands and nodes (C46.3)*

C46.2   **Kaposi's sarcoma of palate**

C46.3   **Kaposi's sarcoma of lymph nodes**

C46.4   **Kaposi's sarcoma of gastrointestinal sites**

🔲 C46.5   **Kaposi's sarcoma of lung**

🔲 C46.50   **Kaposi's sarcoma of unspecified lung**

🔲 C46.51   **Kaposi's sarcoma of right lung**

🔲 C46.52   **Kaposi's sarcoma of left lung**

C46.7   **Kaposi's sarcoma of other sites**

C46.9   **Kaposi's sarcoma, unspecified**
Kaposi's sarcoma of unspecified site

🔟 **C47**   **Malignant neoplasm of peripheral nerves and autonomic nervous system**
      INCLUDES   malignant neoplasm of sympathetic and parasympathetic nerves and ganglia
      EXCLUDES 1   *Kaposi's sarcoma of soft tissue (C46.1)*

C47.0   **Malignant neoplasm of peripheral nerves of head, face and neck**
      EXCLUDES 1   *malignant neoplasm of peripheral nerves of orbit (C69.6-)*

🔲 C47.1   **Malignant neoplasm of peripheral nerves of upper limb, including shoulder**

🔲 C47.10   **Malignant neoplasm of peripheral nerves of unspecified upper limb, including shoulder**

🔲 C47.11   **Malignant neoplasm of peripheral nerves of right upper limb, including shoulder**

🔲 C47.12   **Malignant neoplasm of peripheral nerves of left upper limb, including shoulder**

🔲 C47.2   **Malignant neoplasm of peripheral nerves of lower limb, including hip**

🔲 C47.20   **Malignant neoplasm of peripheral nerves of unspecified lower limb, including hip**

🔲 C47.21   **Malignant neoplasm of peripheral nerves of right lower limb, including hip**

🔲 C47.22   **Malignant neoplasm of peripheral nerves of left lower limb, including hip**

C47.3   **Malignant neoplasm of peripheral nerves of thorax**

C47.4   **Malignant neoplasm of peripheral nerves of abdomen**

C47.5   **Malignant neoplasm of peripheral nerves of pelvis**

C47.6   **Malignant neoplasm of peripheral nerves of trunk, unspecified**
Malignant neoplasm of peripheral nerves of unspecified part of trunk

C47.8   **Malignant neoplasm of overlapping sites of peripheral nerves and autonomic nervous system**

C47.9   **Malignant neoplasm of peripheral nerves and autonomic nervous system, unspecified**
Malignant neoplasm of unspecified site of peripheral nerves and autonomic nervous system

🔟 **C48**   **Malignant neoplasm of retroperitoneum and peritoneum**
      EXCLUDES 1   *Kaposi's sarcoma of connective tissue (C46.1)*
mesothelioma (C45.-)

C48.0   **Malignant neoplasm of retroperitoneum**

C48.1   **Malignant neoplasm of specified parts of peritoneum**
Malignant neoplasm of cul-de-sac
Malignant neoplasm of mesentery
Malignant neoplasm of mesocolon
Malignant neoplasm of omentum
Malignant neoplasm of parietal peritoneum
Malignant neoplasm of pelvic peritoneum

C48.2   **Malignant neoplasm of peritoneum, unspecified**

C48.8   **Malignant neoplasm of overlapping sites of retroperitoneum and peritoneum**

🔟 **C49**   **Malignant neoplasm of other connective and soft tissue**
      INCLUDES   malignant neoplasm of blood vessel
malignant neoplasm of bursa
malignant neoplasm of cartilage
malignant neoplasm of fascia
malignant neoplasm of fat
malignant neoplasm of ligament, except uterine
malignant neoplasm of lymphatic vessel
malignant neoplasm of muscle
malignant neoplasm of synovia
malignant neoplasm of tendon (sheath)
      EXCLUDES 1   *malignant neoplasm of cartilage (of):*
articular (C40-C41)
larynx (C32.3)
nose (C30.0)
malignant neoplasm of connective tissue of breast (C50.-)
      EXCLUDES 2   *Kaposi's sarcoma of soft tissue (C46.1)*
malignant neoplasm of heart (C38.0)
malignant neoplasm of peripheral nerves and autonomic nervous system (C47.-)
malignant neoplasm of peritoneum (C48.2)
malignant neoplasm of retroperitoneum (C48.0)
malignant neoplasm of uterine ligament (C57.3)
mesothelioma (C45.-)

C49.0   **Malignant neoplasm of connective and soft tissue of head, face and neck**
Malignant neoplasm of connective tissue of ear
Malignant neoplasm of connective tissue of eyelid
      EXCLUDES 1   *connective tissue of orbit (C69.6-)*

🔲 C49.1   **Malignant neoplasm of connective and soft tissue of upper limb, including shoulder**

🔲 C49.10   **Malignant neoplasm of connective and soft tissue of unspecified upper limb, including shoulder**

🔲 C49.11   **Malignant neoplasm of connective and soft tissue of right upper limb, including shoulder**

🔲 C49.12   **Malignant neoplasm of connective and soft tissue of left upper limb, including shoulder**

🔲 C49.2   **Malignant neoplasm of connective and soft tissue of lower limb, including hip**

🔲 C49.20   **Malignant neoplasm of connective and soft tissue of unspecified lower limb, including hip**

🔲 C49.21   **Malignant neoplasm of connective and soft tissue of right lower limb, including hip**

● New   ▲ Revised   *Manifestation*   🔟-🔢 Digit Indicators   🔲 Laterality   🅰 Adult (15+ years)   🅼 Maternity (12-55 years)   🅽 Newborn   🅿 Pediatric (0-17 years)   ♂ Male   ♀ Female
✖ Deleted   Unspecified   + Additional code

⊟ C49.22	Malignant neoplasm of connective and soft tissue of left lower limb, including hip		

C49.3 **Malignant neoplasm of connective and soft tissue of thorax**
Malignant neoplasm of axilla
Malignant neoplasm of diaphragm
Malignant neoplasm of great vessels
EXCLUDES 1 *malignant neoplasm of breast (C50.-)*
malignant neoplasm of heart (C38.0)
malignant neoplasm of mediastinum (C38.1-C38.3)
malignant neoplasm of thymus (C37)
AHA: 3Q 2015, 19

C49.4 **Malignant neoplasm of connective and soft tissue of abdomen**
Malignant neoplasm of abdominal wall
Malignant neoplasm of hypochondrium

C49.5 **Malignant neoplasm of connective and soft tissue of pelvis**
Malignant neoplasm of buttock
Malignant neoplasm of groin
Malignant neoplasm of perineum

C49.6 **Malignant neoplasm of connective and soft tissue of trunk, unspecified**
Malignant neoplasm of back NOS

C49.8 **Malignant neoplasm of overlapping sites of connective and soft tissue**
Primary malignant neoplasm of two or more contiguous sites of connective and soft tissue

C49.9 **Malignant neoplasm of connective and soft tissue, unspecified**

● ⑤ C49.A **Gastrointestinal stromal tumor**
● C49.A0 **Gastrointestinal stromal tumor, unspecified site**
● C49.A1 **Gastrointestinal stromal tumor of esophagus**
● C49.A2 **Gastrointestinal stromal tumor of stomach**
● C49.A3 **Gastrointestinal stromal tumor of small intestine**
● C49.A4 **Gastrointestinal stromal tumor of large intestine**
● C49.A5 **Gastrointestinal stromal tumor of rectum**
● C49.A9 **Gastrointestinal stromal tumor of other sites**

Malignant neoplasms of breast (C50)

CODING TIP ✓ Code C50 indicates active cancer. History of cancer to the breast should be coded to Z85.3. Add a Z79.81- code for treatment agents affecting estrogen receptors and estrogen levels.

④ + C50 **Malignant neoplasm of breast**
INCLUDES connective tissue of breast
Paget's disease of breast
Paget's disease of nipple
Use additional code to identify estrogen receptor status (Z17.0, Z17.1)
EXCLUDES 1 *skin of breast (C44.501, C44.511, C44.521, C44.591)*

⑤ + C50.0 **Malignant neoplasm of nipple and areola**
⑥ + C50.01 **Malignant neoplasm of nipple and areola, female**
⊟ + C50.011 **Malignant neoplasm of nipple and areola, right female breast** ♀
⊟ + C50.012 **Malignant neoplasm of nipple and areola, left female breast** ♀
⊟ + C50.019 **Malignant neoplasm of nipple and areola, unspecified female breast** ♀

⑥ + C50.02 **Malignant neoplasm of nipple and areola, male**
⊟ + C50.021 **Malignant neoplasm of nipple and areola, right male breast** ♂
⊟ + C50.022 **Malignant neoplasm of nipple and areola, left male breast** ♂
⊟ + C50.029 **Malignant neoplasm of nipple and areola, unspecified male breast** ♂

⑤ + C50.1 **Malignant neoplasm of central portion of breast**
⑥ + C50.11 **Malignant neoplasm of central portion of breast, female**
⊟ + C50.111 **Malignant neoplasm of central portion of right female breast** ♀
⊟ + C50.112 **Malignant neoplasm of central portion of left female breast** ♀
⊟ + C50.119 **Malignant neoplasm of central portion of unspecified female breast** ♀

⑥ + C50.12 **Malignant neoplasm of central portion of breast, male**

⊟ + C50.121 **Malignant neoplasm of central portion of right male breast** ♂
⊟ + C50.122 **Malignant neoplasm of central portion of left male breast** ♂
⊟ + C50.129 **Malignant neoplasm of central portion of unspecified male breast** ♂

⑤ + C50.2 **Malignant neoplasm of upper-inner quadrant of breast**
⑥ + C50.21 **Malignant neoplasm of upper-inner quadrant of breast, female**
⊟ + C50.211 **Malignant neoplasm of upper-inner quadrant of right female breast** ♀
⊟ + C50.212 **Malignant neoplasm of upper-inner quadrant of left female breast** ♀
⊟ + C50.219 **Malignant neoplasm of upper-inner quadrant of unspecified female breast** ♀

⑥ + C50.22 **Malignant neoplasm of upper-inner quadrant of breast, male**
⊟ + C50.221 **Malignant neoplasm of upper-inner quadrant of right male breast** ♂
⊟ + C50.222 **Malignant neoplasm of upper-inner quadrant of left male breast** ♂
⊟ + C50.229 **Malignant neoplasm of upper-inner quadrant of unspecified male breast** ♂

⑤ + C50.3 **Malignant neoplasm of lower-inner quadrant of breast**
⑥ + C50.31 **Malignant neoplasm of lower-inner quadrant of breast, female**
⊟ + C50.311 **Malignant neoplasm of lower-inner quadrant of right female breast** ♀
⊟ + C50.312 **Malignant neoplasm of lower-inner quadrant of left female breast** ♀
⊟ + C50.319 **Malignant neoplasm of lower-inner quadrant of unspecified female breast** ♀

⑥ + C50.32 **Malignant neoplasm of lower-inner quadrant of breast, male**
⊟ + C50.321 **Malignant neoplasm of lower-inner quadrant of right male breast** ♂
⊟ + C50.322 **Malignant neoplasm of lower-inner quadrant of left male breast** ♂
⊟ + C50.329 **Malignant neoplasm of lower-inner quadrant of unspecified male breast** ♂

⑤ + C50.4 **Malignant neoplasm of upper-outer quadrant of breast**
⑥ + C50.41 **Malignant neoplasm of upper-outer quadrant of breast, female**
⊟ + C50.411 **Malignant neoplasm of upper-outer quadrant of right female breast** ♀
⊟ + C50.412 **Malignant neoplasm of upper-outer quadrant of left female breast** ♀
⊟ + C50.419 **Malignant neoplasm of upper-outer quadrant of unspecified female breast** ♀

⑥ + C50.42 **Malignant neoplasm of upper-outer quadrant of breast, male**
⊟ + C50.421 **Malignant neoplasm of upper-outer quadrant of right male breast** ♂
⊟ + C50.422 **Malignant neoplasm of upper-outer quadrant of left male breast** ♂
⊟ + C50.429 **Malignant neoplasm of upper-outer quadrant of unspecified male breast** ♂

⑤ + C50.5 **Malignant neoplasm of lower-outer quadrant of breast**
⑥ + C50.51 **Malignant neoplasm of lower-outer quadrant of breast, female**
⊟ + C50.511 **Malignant neoplasm of lower-outer quadrant of right female breast** ♀
⊟ + C50.512 **Malignant neoplasm of lower-outer quadrant of left female breast** ♀
⊟ + C50.519 **Malignant neoplasm of lower-outer quadrant of unspecified female breast** ♀

⑥ + C50.52 **Malignant neoplasm of lower-outer quadrant of breast, male**
⊟ + C50.521 **Malignant neoplasm of lower-outer quadrant of right male breast** ♂
⊟ + C50.522 **Malignant neoplasm of lower-outer quadrant of left male breast** ♂
⊟ + C50.529 **Malignant neoplasm of lower-outer quadrant of unspecified male breast** ♂

⑤ + C50.6 **Malignant neoplasm of axillary tail of breast**
⑥ + C50.61 **Malignant neoplasm of axillary tail of breast, female**

● New ▲ Revised *Manifestation* ④- ⑦ Digit Indicators ⊟ Laterality △ Adult (15+ years) Ⓜ Maternity (12-55 years) ℕ Newborn ℙ Pediatric (0-17 years) ♂ Male ♀ Female
✖ Deleted Unspecified + Additional code

⊟+ **C50.611** Malignant neoplasm of axillary tail of right female breast ♀

⊟+ **C50.612** Malignant neoplasm of axillary tail of left female breast ♀

⊟+ **C50.619** Malignant neoplasm of axillary tail of unspecified female breast ♀

⑥+ **C50.62** Malignant neoplasm of axillary tail of breast, male

⊟+ **C50.621** Malignant neoplasm of axillary tail of right male breast ♂

⊟+ **C50.622** Malignant neoplasm of axillary tail of left male breast ♂

⊟+ **C50.629** Malignant neoplasm of axillary tail of unspecified male breast ♂

⑥+ **C50.8** Malignant neoplasm of overlapping sites of breast

⑥+ **C50.81** Malignant neoplasm of overlapping sites of breast, female

⊟+ **C50.811** Malignant neoplasm of overlapping sites of right female breast ♀

⊟+ **C50.812** Malignant neoplasm of overlapping sites of left female breast ♀

⊟+ **C50.819** Malignant neoplasm of overlapping sites of unspecified female breast ♀

⑥+ **C50.82** Malignant neoplasm of overlapping sites of breast, male

⊟+ **C50.821** Malignant neoplasm of overlapping sites of right male breast ♂

⊟+ **C50.822** Malignant neoplasm of overlapping sites of left male breast ♂

⊟+ **C50.829** Malignant neoplasm of overlapping sites of unspecified male breast ♂

⑥+ **C50.9** Malignant neoplasm of breast of unspecified site

⑥+ **C50.91** Malignant neoplasm of breast of unspecified site, female

⊟+ **C50.911** Malignant neoplasm of unspecified site of right female breast ♀

⊟+ **C50.912** Malignant neoplasm of unspecified site of left female breast ♀

⊟+ **C50.919** Malignant neoplasm of unspecified site of unspecified female breast ♀

⑥+ **C50.92** Malignant neoplasm of breast of unspecified site, male

⊟+ **C50.921** Malignant neoplasm of unspecified site of right male breast ♂

⊟+ **C50.922** Malignant neoplasm of unspecified site of left male breast ♂

⊟+ **C50.929** Malignant neoplasm of unspecified site of unspecified male breast ♂

Malignant neoplasms of female genital organs (C51-C58)

| INCLUDES | malignant neoplasm of skin of female genital organs |

CODING TIP✓ Categories C51-C58 indicate active cancer. See Z85.40-Z85.44 for personal history of primary malignancy of female genital organs and Z85.45-Z85.49 for personal history of primary malignancy of male genital organs.

④ **C51** Malignant neoplasm of vulva

| EXCLUDES 1 | *carcinoma in situ of vulva (D07.1)* |

C51.0 Malignant neoplasm of labium majus ♀
Malignant neoplasm of Bartholin's [greater vestibular] gland

C51.1 Malignant neoplasm of labium minus ♀

C51.2 Malignant neoplasm of clitoris ♀

C51.8 Malignant neoplasm of overlapping sites of vulva ♀

C51.9 Malignant neoplasm of vulva, unspecified ♀
Malignant neoplasm of external female genitalia NOS
Malignant neoplasm of pudendum

C52 Malignant neoplasm of vagina ♀

| EXCLUDES 1 | *carcinoma in situ of vagina (D07.2)* |

④ **C53** Malignant neoplasm of cervix uteri ♀

| EXCLUDES 1 | *carcinoma in situ of cervix uteri (D06.-)* |

C53.0 Malignant neoplasm of endocervix ♀

C53.1 Malignant neoplasm of exocervix ♀

C53.8 Malignant neoplasm of overlapping sites of cervix uteri ♀

C53.9 Malignant neoplasm of cervix uteri, unspecified ♀

④ **C54** Malignant neoplasm of corpus uteri

C54.0 Malignant neoplasm of isthmus uteri
Malignant neoplasm of lower uterine segment

C54.1 Malignant neoplasm of endometrium ♀

C54.2 Malignant neoplasm of myometrium ♀

C54.3 Malignant neoplasm of fundus uteri ♀

C54.8 Malignant neoplasm of overlapping sites of corpus uteri ♀

C54.9 Malignant neoplasm of corpus uteri, unspecified ♀

C55 Malignant neoplasm of uterus, part unspecified ♀

④+ **C56** Malignant neoplasm of ovary
Use additional code to identify any functional activity

⊟+ **C56.1** Malignant neoplasm of right ovary ♀

⊟+ **C56.2** Malignant neoplasm of left ovary ♀

⊟+ **C56.9** Malignant neoplasm of unspecified ovary ♀

④ **C57** Malignant neoplasm of other and unspecified female genital organs

⑤ **C57.0** Malignant neoplasm of fallopian tube
Malignant neoplasm of oviduct
Malignant neoplasm of uterine tube

⊟ **C57.00** Malignant neoplasm of unspecified fallopian tube ♀

⊟ **C57.01** Malignant neoplasm of right fallopian tube ♀

⊟ **C57.02** Malignant neoplasm of left fallopian tube ♀

⑤ **C57.1** Malignant neoplasm of broad ligament

⊟ **C57.10** Malignant neoplasm of unspecified broad ligament ♀

⊟ **C57.11** Malignant neoplasm of right broad ligament ♀

⊟ **C57.12** Malignant neoplasm of left broad ligament ♀

⑤ **C57.2** Malignant neoplasm of round ligament

⊟ **C57.20** Malignant neoplasm of unspecified round ligament ♀

⊟ **C57.21** Malignant neoplasm of right round ligament ♀

⊟ **C57.22** Malignant neoplasm of left round ligament ♀

C57.3 Malignant neoplasm of parametrium ♀
Malignant neoplasm of uterine ligament NOS

C57.4 Malignant neoplasm of uterine adnexa, unspecified ♀

C57.7 Malignant neoplasm of other specified female genital organs ♀
Malignant neoplasm of wolffian body or duct

C57.8 Malignant neoplasm of overlapping sites of female genital organs ♀
Primary malignant neoplasm of two or more contiguous sites of the female genital organs whose point of origin cannot be determined
Primary tubo-ovarian malignant neoplasm whose point of origin cannot be determined
Primary utero-ovarian malignant neoplasm whose point of origin cannot be determined

C57.9 Malignant neoplasm of female genital organ, unspecified ♀
Malignant neoplasm of female genitourinary tract NOS

C58 Malignant neoplasm of placenta ♀

| INCLUDES | choriocarcinoma NOS
chorionepithelioma NOS |

| EXCLUDES 1 | *chorioadenoma (destruens) (D39.2)*
hydatidiform mole NOS (O01.9)
invasive hydatidiform mole (D39.2)
male choriocarcinoma NOS (C62.9-)
malignant hydatidiform mole (D39.2) |

Malignant neoplasms of male genital organs (C60-C63)

| INCLUDES | malignant neoplasm of skin of male genital organs |

CODING TIP✓ Codes classifiable to C60-C63 include active cancer. History of cancer to the male genital organs should be coded to Z85.4-.

④ **C60** Malignant neoplasm of penis

C60.0 Malignant neoplasm of prepuce ♂
Malignant neoplasm of foreskin

C60.1 Malignant neoplasm of glans penis ♂

C60.2 Malignant neoplasm of body of penis ♂
Malignant neoplasm of corpus cavernosum

C60.8 Malignant neoplasm of overlapping sites of penis ♂

● New ▲ Revised *Manifestation* ④-❼ Digit Indicators ⊟ Laterality 🄰 Adult (15+ years) 🄼 Maternity (12-55 years) 🄽 Newborn 🄿 Pediatric (0-17 years) ♂ Male ♀ Female
✖ Deleted Unspecified + Additional code

2017 ICD-10-CM Expert for Physicians

© 2017 DecisionHealth

479

Neoplasms

C50.611 — C60.8

C60.9 Malignant neoplasm of penis, unspecified ♂
Malignant neoplasm of skin of penis NOS

+ C61 Malignant neoplasm of prostate ♂
Use additional code to identify:
hormone sensitivity status (Z19.1-Z19.2)
rising PSA following treatment for malignant neoplasm of
prostate (R97.21)
EXCLUDES 1 *malignant neoplasm of seminal vesicle (C63.7)*

4 + C62 Malignant neoplasm of testis
Use additional code to identify any functional activity

5 + C62.0 Malignant neoplasm of undescended testis
Malignant neoplasm of ectopic testis
Malignant neoplasm of retained testis

+ C62.00 Malignant neoplasm of unspecified undescended ♂
testis

+ C62.01 Malignant neoplasm of undescended right testis ♂

+ C62.02 Malignant neoplasm of undescended left testis ♂

5 + C62.1 Malignant neoplasm of descended testis
Malignant neoplasm of scrotal testis

+ C62.10 Malignant neoplasm of unspecified descended ♂
testis

+ C62.11 Malignant neoplasm of descended right testis ♂

+ C62.12 Malignant neoplasm of descended left testis ♂

5 + C62.9 Malignant neoplasm of testis, unspecified whether
descended or undescended

+ C62.90 Malignant neoplasm of unspecified testis, ♂
unspecified whether descended or undescended
Malignant neoplasm of testis NOS

+ C62.91 Malignant neoplasm of right testis, unspecified ♂
whether descended or undescended

+ C62.92 Malignant neoplasm of left testis, unspecified ♂
whether descended or undescended

4 C63 Malignant neoplasm of other and unspecified male
genital organs

5 C63.0 Malignant neoplasm of epididymis

C63.00 Malignant neoplasm of unspecified epididymis ♂

C63.01 Malignant neoplasm of right epididymis ♂

C63.02 Malignant neoplasm of left epididymis ♂

5 C63.1 Malignant neoplasm of spermatic cord

C63.10 Malignant neoplasm of unspecified spermatic ♂
cord

C63.11 Malignant neoplasm of right spermatic cord ♂

C63.12 Malignant neoplasm of left spermatic cord ♂

C63.2 Malignant neoplasm of scrotum ♂
Malignant neoplasm of skin of scrotum

C63.7 Malignant neoplasm of other specified male genital ♂
organs
Malignant neoplasm of seminal vesicle
Malignant neoplasm of tunica vaginalis

C63.8 Malignant neoplasm of overlapping sites of male ♂
genital organs
Primary malignant neoplasm of two or more contiguous sites
of male genital organs whose point of origin cannot be
determined

C63.9 Malignant neoplasm of male genital organ, unspecified ♂
Malignant neoplasm of male genitourinary tract NOS

Malignant neoplasms of urinary tract
(C64-C68)

CODING TIP ✓ Codes classifiable to C64-C68 include active cancer.
History of cancer to the urinary tract should be coded to Z85.5-.

4 C64 Malignant neoplasm of kidney, except renal pelvis
EXCLUDES 1 *malignant carcinoid tumor of the kidney*
(C7A.093)
malignant neoplasm of renal calyces (C65.-)
malignant neoplasm of renal pelvis (C65.-)

C64.1 Malignant neoplasm of right kidney, except renal pelvis

C64.2 Malignant neoplasm of left kidney, except renal pelvis

C64.9 Malignant neoplasm of unspecified kidney, except renal
pelvis

4 C65 Malignant neoplasm of renal pelvis
INCLUDES malignant neoplasm of pelviureteric junction
malignant neoplasm of renal calyces

C65.1 Malignant neoplasm of right renal pelvis

C65.2 Malignant neoplasm of left renal pelvis

C65.9 Malignant neoplasm of unspecified renal pelvis

4 C66 Malignant neoplasm of ureter
EXCLUDES 1 *malignant neoplasm of ureteric orifice of bladder*
(C67.6)

C66.1 Malignant neoplasm of right ureter

C66.2 Malignant neoplasm of left ureter

C66.9 Malignant neoplasm of unspecified ureter

4 C67 Malignant neoplasm of bladder

C67.0 Malignant neoplasm of trigone of bladder

C67.1 Malignant neoplasm of dome of bladder

C67.2 Malignant neoplasm of lateral wall of bladder

C67.3 Malignant neoplasm of anterior wall of bladder

C67.4 Malignant neoplasm of posterior wall of bladder

C67.5 Malignant neoplasm of bladder neck
Malignant neoplasm of internal urethral orifice

C67.6 Malignant neoplasm of ureteric orifice

C67.7 Malignant neoplasm of urachus

C67.8 Malignant neoplasm of overlapping sites of bladder

C67.9 Malignant neoplasm of bladder, unspecified
AHA: 1Q 2016, 19

4 C68 Malignant neoplasm of other and unspecified urinary
organs
EXCLUDES 1 *malignant neoplasm of female genitourinary tract*
NOS (C57.9)
malignant neoplasm of male genitourinary tract
NOS (C63.9)

C68.0 Malignant neoplasm of urethra
EXCLUDES 1 *malignant neoplasm of urethral orifice of*
bladder (C67.5)

C68.1 Malignant neoplasm of paraurethral glands

C68.8 Malignant neoplasm of overlapping sites of urinary
organs
Primary malignant neoplasm of two or more contiguous sites
of urinary organs whose point of origin cannot be
determined

C68.9 Malignant neoplasm of urinary organ, unspecified
Malignant neoplasm of urinary system NOS

Malignant neoplasms of eye, brain and other
parts of central nervous system (C69-C72)

CODING TIP ✓ Codes classifiable to C69-C72 include active cancer.
History of cancer to eye, brain, or other area of nervous system should be
coded to Z85.84-.

4 C69 Malignant neoplasm of eye and adnexa
EXCLUDES 1 *malignant neoplasm of connective tissue of eyelid*
(C49.0)
malignant neoplasm of eyelid (skin) (C43.1-,
C44.1-)
malignant neoplasm of optic nerve (C72.3-)

5 C69.0 Malignant neoplasm of conjunctiva

C69.00 Malignant neoplasm of unspecified conjunctiva

C69.01 Malignant neoplasm of right conjunctiva

C69.02 Malignant neoplasm of left conjunctiva

5 C69.1 Malignant neoplasm of cornea

C69.10 Malignant neoplasm of unspecified cornea

C69.11 Malignant neoplasm of right cornea

C69.12 Malignant neoplasm of left cornea

5 C69.2 Malignant neoplasm of retina
EXCLUDES 1 *dark area on retina (D49.81)*
neoplasm of unspecified behavior of retina
and choroid (D49.81)
retinal freckle (D49.81)

C69.20 Malignant neoplasm of unspecified retina

C69.21 Malignant neoplasm of right retina

C69.22 Malignant neoplasm of left retina

5 C69.3 Malignant neoplasm of choroid

C69.30 Malignant neoplasm of unspecified choroid

C69.31 Malignant neoplasm of right choroid

C69.32 Malignant neoplasm of left choroid

5 C69.4 Malignant neoplasm of ciliary body

C69.40 Malignant neoplasm of unspecified ciliary body

C69.41 Malignant neoplasm of right ciliary body

C69.42 Malignant neoplasm of left ciliary body

● New ▲ Revised *Manifestation* 4-7 Digit Indicators ⊟ Laterality A Adult (15+ years) M Maternity (12-55 years) N Newborn P Pediatric (0-17 years) ♂ Male ♀ Female
✖ Deleted Unspecified + Additional code

480 © 2017 DecisionHealth 2017 ICD-10-CM Expert for Physicians

⊟ **C69.5** **Malignant neoplasm of lacrimal gland and duct**
Malignant neoplasm of lacrimal sac
Malignant neoplasm of nasolacrimal duct

⊟ **C69.50** **Malignant neoplasm of unspecified lacrimal gland and duct**

⊟ **C69.51** **Malignant neoplasm of right lacrimal gland and duct**

⊟ **C69.52** **Malignant neoplasm of left lacrimal gland and duct**

⊟ **C69.6** **Malignant neoplasm of orbit**
Malignant neoplasm of connective tissue of orbit
Malignant neoplasm of extraocular muscle
Malignant neoplasm of peripheral nerves of orbit
Malignant neoplasm of retrobulbar tissue
Malignant neoplasm of retro-ocular tissue

> **EXCLUDES 1** *malignant neoplasm of orbital bone (C41.0)*

⊟ **C69.60** **Malignant neoplasm of unspecified orbit**

⊟ **C69.61** **Malignant neoplasm of right orbit**

⊟ **C69.62** **Malignant neoplasm of left orbit**

⊟ **C69.8** **Malignant neoplasm of overlapping sites of eye and adnexa**

⊟ **C69.80** **Malignant neoplasm of overlapping sites of unspecified eye and adnexa**

⊟ **C69.81** **Malignant neoplasm of overlapping sites of right eye and adnexa**

⊟ **C69.82** **Malignant neoplasm of overlapping sites of left eye and adnexa**

⊟ **C69.9** **Malignant neoplasm of unspecified site of eye**
Malignant neoplasm of eyeball

⊟ **C69.90** **Malignant neoplasm of unspecified site of unspecified eye**

⊟ **C69.91** **Malignant neoplasm of unspecified site of right eye**

⊟ **C69.92** **Malignant neoplasm of unspecified site of left eye**

C70 **Malignant neoplasm of meninges**

C70.0 **Malignant neoplasm of cerebral meninges**

C70.1 **Malignant neoplasm of spinal meninges**

C70.9 **Malignant neoplasm of meninges, unspecified**

C71 **Malignant neoplasm of brain**

> **EXCLUDES 1** *malignant neoplasm of cranial nerves (C72.2-C72.5)*
> *retrobulbar malignant neoplasm (C69.6-)*

C71.0 **Malignant neoplasm of cerebrum, except lobes and ventricles**
Malignant neoplasm of supratentorial NOS

C71.1 **Malignant neoplasm of frontal lobe**

C71.2 **Malignant neoplasm of temporal lobe**

C71.3 **Malignant neoplasm of parietal lobe**

C71.4 **Malignant neoplasm of occipital lobe**

C71.5 **Malignant neoplasm of cerebral ventricle**

> **EXCLUDES 1** *malignant neoplasm of fourth cerebral ventricle (C71.7)*

C71.6 **Malignant neoplasm of cerebellum**

C71.7 **Malignant neoplasm of brain stem**
Malignant neoplasm of fourth cerebral ventricle
Infratentorial malignant neoplasm NOS

C71.8 **Malignant neoplasm of overlapping sites of brain**

C71.9 **Malignant neoplasm of brain, unspecified**
AHA: 3Q 2014, 4

C72 **Malignant neoplasm of spinal cord, cranial nerves and other parts of central nervous system**

> **EXCLUDES 1** *malignant neoplasm of meninges (C70.-)*
> *malignant neoplasm of peripheral nerves and autonomic nervous system (C47.-)*

C72.0 **Malignant neoplasm of spinal cord**

C72.1 **Malignant neoplasm of cauda equina**

⊟ **C72.2** **Malignant neoplasm of olfactory nerve**
Malignant neoplasm of olfactory bulb

⊟ **C72.20** **Malignant neoplasm of unspecified olfactory nerve**

⊟ **C72.21** **Malignant neoplasm of right olfactory nerve**

⊟ **C72.22** **Malignant neoplasm of left olfactory nerve**

⊟ **C72.3** **Malignant neoplasm of optic nerve**

⊟ **C72.30** **Malignant neoplasm of unspecified optic nerve**

⊟ **C72.31** **Malignant neoplasm of right optic nerve**

⊟ **C72.32** **Malignant neoplasm of left optic nerve**

⊟ **C72.4** **Malignant neoplasm of acoustic nerve**

⊟ **C72.40** **Malignant neoplasm of unspecified acoustic nerve**

⊟ **C72.41** **Malignant neoplasm of right acoustic nerve**

⊟ **C72.42** **Malignant neoplasm of left acoustic nerve**

⊟ **C72.5** **Malignant neoplasm of other and unspecified cranial nerves**

C72.50 **Malignant neoplasm of unspecified cranial nerve**
Malignant neoplasm of cranial nerve NOS

C72.59 **Malignant neoplasm of other cranial nerves**

C72.9 **Malignant neoplasm of central nervous system, unspecified**
Malignant neoplasm of unspecified site of central nervous system
Malignant neoplasm of nervous system NOS

Malignant neoplasms of thyroid and other endocrine glands (C73-C75)

> **CODING TIP** ✓ Codes classifiable to C73-C75 include active cancer. History of cancer to endocrine glands should be coded to Z85.85-.

+ C73 **Malignant neoplasm of thyroid gland**
Use additional code to identify any functional activity

C74 **Malignant neoplasm of adrenal gland**

⊟ **C74.0** **Malignant neoplasm of cortex of adrenal gland**

⊟ **C74.00** **Malignant neoplasm of cortex of unspecified adrenal gland**

⊟ **C74.01** **Malignant neoplasm of cortex of right adrenal gland**

⊟ **C74.02** **Malignant neoplasm of cortex of left adrenal gland**

⊟ **C74.1** **Malignant neoplasm of medulla of adrenal gland**

⊟ **C74.10** **Malignant neoplasm of medulla of unspecified adrenal gland**

⊟ **C74.11** **Malignant neoplasm of medulla of right adrenal gland**

⊟ **C74.12** **Malignant neoplasm of medulla of left adrenal gland**

⊟ **C74.9** **Malignant neoplasm of unspecified part of adrenal gland**

⊟ **C74.90** **Malignant neoplasm of unspecified part of unspecified adrenal gland**

⊟ **C74.91** **Malignant neoplasm of unspecified part of right adrenal gland**

⊟ **C74.92** **Malignant neoplasm of unspecified part of left adrenal gland**

C75 **Malignant neoplasm of other endocrine glands and related structures**

> **EXCLUDES 1** *malignant carcinoid tumors (C7A.0-)*
> *malignant neoplasm of adrenal gland (C74.-)*
> *malignant neoplasm of endocrine pancreas (C25.4)*
> *malignant neoplasm of islets of Langerhans (C25.4)*
> *malignant neoplasm of ovary (C56.-)*
> *malignant neoplasm of testis (C62.-)*
> *malignant neoplasm of thymus (C37)*
> *malignant neoplasm of thyroid gland (C73)*
> *malignant neuroendocrine tumors (C7A.-)*

C75.0 **Malignant neoplasm of parathyroid gland**

C75.1 **Malignant neoplasm of pituitary gland**

C75.2 **Malignant neoplasm of craniopharyngeal duct**

C75.3 **Malignant neoplasm of pineal gland**

C75.4 **Malignant neoplasm of carotid body**

C75.5 **Malignant neoplasm of aortic body and other paraganglia**

C75.8 **Malignant neoplasm with pluriglandular involvement, unspecified**

C75.9 **Malignant neoplasm of endocrine gland, unspecified**

Malignant neuroendocrine tumors (C7A)

+ C7A **Malignant neuroendocrine tumors**
Code also:
any associated multiple endocrine neoplasia [MEN] syndromes (E31.2-)
Use additional code to identify any associated endocrine syndrome, such as:
carcinoid syndrome (E34.0)

> **EXCLUDES 2** *malignant pancreatic islet cell tumors (C25.4)*
> *Merkel cell carcinoma (C4A.-)*

● New ▲ Revised *Manifestation* / Unspecified ◀-▼ Digit Indicators / + Additional code ⊟ Laterality Ⓐ Adult (15+ years) Ⓜ Maternity (12-55 years) Ⓝ Newborn Ⓟ Pediatric (0-17 years) ♂ Male ♀ Female
✖ Deleted

Neoplasms

CODING TIP ✓ Codes Classifiable to C7A- include primary neuroendocrine tumors, which are considered active malignant carcinoid tumors. Neoplasms that have been previously excised or eratidated and have no further treatment directed at that site should have a code from category Z85- for the anatomical location and not a code from C7A-.

⑤+ C7A.0　Malignant carcinoid tumors
　+ C7A.00　　Malignant carcinoid tumor of unspecified site
　⑥+ C7A.01　Malignant carcinoid tumors of the small intestine
　　+ C7A.010　Malignant carcinoid tumor of the duodenum
　　+ C7A.011　Malignant carcinoid tumor of the jejunum
　　+ C7A.012　Malignant carcinoid tumor of the ileum
　　+ C7A.019　Malignant carcinoid tumor of the small intestine, unspecified portion
　⑥+ C7A.02　Malignant carcinoid tumors of the appendix, large intestine, and rectum
　　+ C7A.020　Malignant carcinoid tumor of the appendix
　　+ C7A.021　Malignant carcinoid tumor of the cecum
　　+ C7A.022　Malignant carcinoid tumor of the ascending colon
　　+ C7A.023　Malignant carcinoid tumor of the transverse colon
　　+ C7A.024　Malignant carcinoid tumor of the descending colon
　　+ C7A.025　Malignant carcinoid tumor of the sigmoid colon
　　+ C7A.026　Malignant carcinoid tumor of the rectum
　　+ C7A.029　Malignant carcinoid tumor of the large intestine, unspecified portion
　　　　　Malignant carcinoid tumor of the colon NOS
　⑥+ C7A.09　Malignant carcinoid tumors of other sites
　　+ C7A.090　Malignant carcinoid tumor of the bronchus and lung
　　+ C7A.091　Malignant carcinoid tumor of the thymus
　　+ C7A.092　Malignant carcinoid tumor of the stomach
　　+ C7A.093　Malignant carcinoid tumor of the kidney
　▲+ C7A.094　Malignant carcinoid tumor of the foregut, unspecified
　▲+ C7A.095　Malignant carcinoid tumor of the midgut, unspecified
　▲+ C7A.096　Malignant carcinoid tumor of the hindgut, unspecified
　　+ C7A.098　Malignant carcinoid tumors of other sites
+ C7A.1　Malignant poorly differentiated neuroendocrine tumors
　　Malignant poorly differentiated neuroendocrine tumor NOS
　　Malignant poorly differentiated neuroendocrine carcinoma, any site
　　High grade neuroendocrine carcinoma, any site
+ C7A.8　Other malignant neuroendocrine tumors

Secondary neuroendocrine tumors (C7B)

④+ C7B　Secondary neuroendocrine tumors
　Use additional code to identify any functional activity
　CODING TIP ✓ Codes Classifiable to C7B- include secondary (metastases) neuroendocrine tumors, which are considered active malignant carcinoid tumors. Neoplasms that have been previously excised or eratidated and have no further treatment directed at that site should have a code from Z85- for the anatomical location and not a code from C7B-.

⑤+ C7B.0　Secondary carcinoid tumors
　+ C7B.00　Secondary carcinoid tumors, unspecified site
　+ C7B.01　Secondary carcinoid tumors of distant lymph nodes
　+ C7B.02　Secondary carcinoid tumors of liver
　+ C7B.03　Secondary carcinoid tumors of bone
　+ C7B.04　Secondary carcinoid tumors of peritoneum
　　　　　Mesentary metastasis of carcinoid tumor
　+ C7B.09　Secondary carcinoid tumors of other sites
+ C7B.1　Secondary Merkel cell carcinoma
　　Merkel cell carcinoma nodal presentation
　　Merkel cell carcinoma visceral metastatic presentation
+ C7B.8　Other secondary neuroendocrine tumors

Malignant neoplasms of ill-defined, other secondary and unspecified sites (C76-C80)

④ C76　Malignant neoplasm of other and ill-defined sites
　EXCLUDES 1　*malignant neoplasm of female genitourinary tract NOS (C57.9)*
　　　malignant neoplasm of male genitourinary tract NOS (C63.9)
　　　malignant neoplasm of lymphoid, hematopoietic and related tissue (C81-C96)
　　　malignant neoplasm of skin (C44.-)
　　　malignant neoplasm of unspecified site NOS (C80.1)
　C76.0　Malignant neoplasm of head, face and neck
　　　Malignant neoplasm of cheek NOS
　　　Malignant neoplasm of nose NOS
　C76.1　Malignant neoplasm of thorax
　　　Intrathoracic malignant neoplasm NOS
　　　Malignant neoplasm of axilla NOS
　　　Thoracic malignant neoplasm NOS
　C76.2　Malignant neoplasm of abdomen
　C76.3　Malignant neoplasm of pelvis
　　　Malignant neoplasm of groin NOS
　　　Malignant neoplasm of sites overlapping systems within the pelvis
　　　Rectovaginal (septum) malignant neoplasm
　　　Rectovesical (septum) malignant neoplasm
　⑤ C76.4　Malignant neoplasm of upper limb
　　⊟ C76.40　Malignant neoplasm of unspecified upper limb
　　⊟ C76.41　Malignant neoplasm of right upper limb
　　⊟ C76.42　Malignant neoplasm of left upper limb
　⑤ C76.5　Malignant neoplasm of lower limb
　　⊟ C76.50　Malignant neoplasm of unspecified lower limb
　　⊟ C76.51　Malignant neoplasm of right lower limb
　　⊟ C76.52　Malignant neoplasm of left lower limb
　C76.8　Malignant neoplasm of other specified ill-defined sites
　　　Malignant neoplasm of overlapping ill-defined sites
④ C77　Secondary and unspecified malignant neoplasm of lymph nodes
　EXCLUDES 1　*malignant neoplasm of lymph nodes, specified as primary (C81-C86, C88, C96.-)*
　　　mesentary metastasis of carcinoid tumor (C7B.04)
　　　secondary carcinoid tumors of distant lymph nodes (C7B.01)

　CODING TIP ✓ Codes classifiable to C77- include neoplasms specified as secondary active neoplasms of lymph nodes. Primary neoplasms of lymphatic tissue should not be coded using codes from C77-. Neoplasms that have been previously excised or eradicated and have no further treatment directed at that site should have a code from category Z85- and not a code from C77-.

　C77.0　Secondary and unspecified malignant neoplasm of lymph nodes of head, face and neck
　　　Secondary and unspecified malignant neoplasm of supraclavicular lymph nodes
　C77.1　Secondary and unspecified malignant neoplasm of intrathoracic lymph nodes
　C77.2　Secondary and unspecified malignant neoplasm of intra-abdominal lymph nodes
　C77.3　Secondary and unspecified malignant neoplasm of axilla and upper limb lymph nodes
　　　Secondary and unspecified malignant neoplasm of pectoral lymph nodes
　C77.4　Secondary and unspecified malignant neoplasm of inguinal and lower limb lymph nodes
　C77.5　Secondary and unspecified malignant neoplasm of intrapelvic lymph nodes
　C77.8　Secondary and unspecified malignant neoplasm of lymph nodes of multiple regions
　C77.9　Secondary and unspecified malignant neoplasm of lymph node, unspecified

● New　▲ Revised　*Manifestation*　④-⑦ Digit Indicators　⊟ Laterality　Ⓐ Adult (15+ years)　Ⓜ Maternity (12-55 years)　Ⓝ Newborn　Ⓟ Pediatric (0-17 years)　♂ Male　♀ Female
✖ ~~Deleted~~　Unspecified　+ Additional code

▲ ◢ C78   **Secondary malignant neoplasm of respiratory and digestive organs**

> **EXCLUDES 1** *secondary carcinoid tumors of liver (C7B.02)*
> *secondary carcinoid tumors of peritoneum (C7B.04)*
>
> **EXCLUDES 2** *lymph node metastases (C77.0)*

> **CODING TIP ✓**   Codes classifiable to C78- include neoplasms specified as secondary active neoplasms. Primary neoplasms should not be coded using codes from C78-. Neoplasms that have been previously excised or eratidated and have no further treatment directed at that site should have a code from category Z85- for the anatomical location and not a code from C78-.

◢ C78.0   Secondary malignant neoplasm of lung
- ▤ C78.00   Secondary malignant neoplasm of unspecified lung
- ▤ C78.01   Secondary malignant neoplasm of right lung
- ▤ C78.02   Secondary malignant neoplasm of left lung

C78.1   Secondary malignant neoplasm of mediastinum

C78.2   Secondary malignant neoplasm of pleura

◢ C78.3   Secondary malignant neoplasm of other and unspecified respiratory organs
- C78.30   Secondary malignant neoplasm of unspecified respiratory organ
- C78.39   Secondary malignant neoplasm of other respiratory organs

C78.4   Secondary malignant neoplasm of small intestine

C78.5   Secondary malignant neoplasm of large intestine and rectum

C78.6   Secondary malignant neoplasm of retroperitoneum and peritoneum

C78.7   Secondary malignant neoplasm of liver and intrahepatic bile duct

◢ C78.8   Secondary malignant neoplasm of other and unspecified digestive organs
- C78.80   Secondary malignant neoplasm of unspecified digestive organ
- ▲ C78.89   Secondary malignant neoplasm of other digestive organs
  Code also:
  exocrine pancreatic insufficiency (K86.81)

▲ ◢ C79   **Secondary malignant neoplasm of other and unspecified sites**

> **EXCLUDES 1** *secondary carcinoid tumors (C7B.-)*
> *secondary neuroendocrine tumors (C7B.-)*
>
> **EXCLUDES 2** *lymph node metastases (C77.0)*

> **CODING TIP ✓**   Codes classifiable to C79- include neoplasms specified as secondary active neoplasms. Primary neoplasms should not be coded using codes from C78-. Neoplasms that have been previously excised or eratidated and have no further treatment directed at that site should have a code from category Z85- for the anatomical location and not a code from C79-.

◢ C79.0   Secondary malignant neoplasm of kidney and renal pelvis
- ▤ C79.00   Secondary malignant neoplasm of unspecified kidney and renal pelvis
- ▤ C79.01   Secondary malignant neoplasm of right kidney and renal pelvis
- ▤ C79.02   Secondary malignant neoplasm of left kidney and renal pelvis

◢ C79.1   Secondary malignant neoplasm of bladder and other and unspecified urinary organs
- C79.10   Secondary malignant neoplasm of unspecified urinary organs
- C79.11   Secondary malignant neoplasm of bladder
- C79.19   Secondary malignant neoplasm of other urinary organs

C79.2   Secondary malignant neoplasm of skin

> **EXCLUDES 1** *secondary Merkel cell carcinoma (C7B.1)*

◢ C79.3   Secondary malignant neoplasm of brain and cerebral meninges
- C79.31   Secondary malignant neoplasm of brain
- C79.32   Secondary malignant neoplasm of cerebral meninges

◢ C79.4   Secondary malignant neoplasm of other and unspecified parts of nervous system
- C79.40   Secondary malignant neoplasm of unspecified part of nervous system

C79.49   Secondary malignant neoplasm of other parts of nervous system

◢ C79.5   Secondary malignant neoplasm of bone and bone marrow

> **EXCLUDES 1** *secondary carcinoid tumors of bone (C7B.03)*

C79.51   Secondary malignant neoplasm of bone
C79.52   Secondary malignant neoplasm of bone marrow

◢ C79.6   Secondary malignant neoplasm of ovary
- ▤ C79.60   Secondary malignant neoplasm of unspecified ovary   ♀
- ▤ C79.61   Secondary malignant neoplasm of right ovary   ♀
- ▤ C79.62   Secondary malignant neoplasm of left ovary   ♀

◢ C79.7   Secondary malignant neoplasm of adrenal gland
- ▤ C79.70   Secondary malignant neoplasm of unspecified adrenal gland
- ▤ C79.71   Secondary malignant neoplasm of right adrenal gland
- ▤ C79.72   Secondary malignant neoplasm of left adrenal gland

◢ C79.8   Secondary malignant neoplasm of other specified sites
C79.81   Secondary malignant neoplasm of breast
C79.82   Secondary malignant neoplasm of genital organs
C79.89   Secondary malignant neoplasm of other specified sites

C79.9   Secondary malignant neoplasm of unspecified site
Metastatic cancer NOS
Metastatic disease NOS

> **EXCLUDES 1** *carcinomatosis NOS (C80.0)*
> *generalized cancer NOS (C80.0)*
> *malignant (primary) neoplasm of unspecified site (C80.1)*

◢ C80   **Malignant neoplasm without specification of site**

> **EXCLUDES 1** *malignant carcinoid tumor of unspecified site (C7A.00)*
> *malignant neoplasm of specified multiple sites-code to each site*

C80.0   Disseminated malignant neoplasm, unspecified
Carcinomatosis NOS
Generalized cancer, unspecified site (primary) (secondary)
Generalized malignancy, unspecified site (primary) (secondary)

> **GUIDELINES**   Section I.C.2.j
> Code C80.0 is for use only in those cases where the patient has advanced metastatic disease and no known primary or secondary sites are specified. It should not be used in place of assigning codes for the primary site and all known secondary sites.

C80.1   Malignant (primary) neoplasm, unspecified
Cancer NOS
Cancer unspecified site (primary)
Carcinoma unspecified site (primary)
Malignancy unspecified site (primary)

> **EXCLUDES 1** *secondary malignant neoplasm of unspecified site (C79.9)*

> **GUIDELINES**   Section I.C.2.k
> Code C80.1 equates to Cancer, unspecified. This code should only be used when no determination can be made as to the primary site of a malignancy. This code should rarely be used in the inpatient setting.

> **CODING TIP ✓**   When coding a secondary site of the cancer and the primary site is unknown, C80.1 should be added for unknown primary site. A biopsy-proven malignancy for which a primary site cannot be found constitutes 0.5% to 7% of all cancer patients.

+ C80.2   Malignant neoplasm associated with transplanted organ
Code first:
complication of transplanted organ (T86.-)
Use additional code to identify the specific malignancy

> **GUIDELINES**   Section I.C.2.r
> A malignant neoplasm of a transplanted organ should be coded as a transplant complication. Assign first the appropriate code from category T86.-, Complications of transplanted organs and tissue, followed by code C80.2. Use an additional code for the specific malignancy.

● New   ▲ Revised   *Manifestation*   ◢-◪ Digit Indicators   ▤ Laterality   Ⓐ Adult (15+ years)   Ⓜ Maternity (12-55 years)   Ⓝ Newborn   Ⓟ Pediatric (0-17 years)   ♂ Male   ♀ Female
✖ Deleted   Unspecified   + Additional code

CODING TIP ✓ When coding malignancy associated with any transplanted organ, C80.2 must be assigned, but must be preceeded by the appropriate code from T86- (Complications of transplanted organs and tissue), and should be followed by the appropriate code for the specific neoplasm identified.

Malignant neoplasms of lymphoid, hematopoietic and related tissue (C81-C96)

EXCLUDES 2 *Kaposi's sarcoma of lymph nodes (C46.3)*
secondary and unspecified neoplasm of lymph nodes (C77.-)
secondary neoplasm of bone marrow (C79.52)
secondary neoplasm of spleen (C78.89)

CODING TIP ✓ Codes classifiable to C81-C96 include active malignancy of lymphoid, hematopeotic and related tissues. Secondary neoplastic disease of lymph tissue should not be coded using codes from C81-C96.

◢ C81   Hodgkin lymphoma

EXCLUDES 1 *personal history of Hodgkin lymphoma (Z85.71)*

⑤ C81.0   Nodular lymphocyte predominant Hodgkin lymphoma

C81.00   Nodular lymphocyte predominant Hodgkin lymphoma, unspecified site

C81.01   Nodular lymphocyte predominant Hodgkin lymphoma, lymph nodes of head, face, and neck

C81.02   Nodular lymphocyte predominant Hodgkin lymphoma, intrathoracic lymph nodes

C81.03   Nodular lymphocyte predominant Hodgkin lymphoma, intra-abdominal lymph nodes

C81.04   Nodular lymphocyte predominant Hodgkin lymphoma, lymph nodes of axilla and upper limb

C81.05   Nodular lymphocyte predominant Hodgkin lymphoma, lymph nodes of inguinal region and lower limb

C81.06   Nodular lymphocyte predominant Hodgkin lymphoma, intrapelvic lymph nodes

C81.07   Nodular lymphocyte predominant Hodgkin lymphoma, spleen

C81.08   Nodular lymphocyte predominant Hodgkin lymphoma, lymph nodes of multiple sites

C81.09   Nodular lymphocyte predominant Hodgkin lymphoma, extranodal and solid organ sites

▲ ⑤ C81.1   Nodular sclerosis Hodgkin lymphoma
Nodular sclerosis classical Hodgkin lymphoma

▲ C81.10   Nodular sclerosis Hodgkin lymphoma, unspecified site

▲ C81.11   Nodular sclerosis Hodgkin lymphoma, lymph nodes of head, face, and neck

▲ C81.12   Nodular sclerosis Hodgkin lymphoma, intrathoracic lymph nodes

▲ C81.13   Nodular sclerosis Hodgkin lymphoma, intra-abdominal lymph nodes

▲ C81.14   Nodular sclerosis Hodgkin lymphoma, lymph nodes of axilla and upper limb

▲ C81.15   Nodular sclerosis Hodgkin lymphoma, lymph nodes of inguinal region and lower limb

▲ C81.16   Nodular sclerosis Hodgkin lymphoma, intrapelvic lymph nodes

▲ C81.17   Nodular sclerosis Hodgkin lymphoma, spleen

▲ C81.18   Nodular sclerosis Hodgkin lymphoma, lymph nodes of multiple sites

▲ C81.19   Nodular sclerosis Hodgkin lymphoma, extranodal and solid organ sites

▲ ⑤ C81.2   Mixed cellularity Hodgkin lymphoma
Mixed cellularity classical Hodgkin lymphoma

▲ C81.20   Mixed cellularity Hodgkin lymphoma, unspecified site

▲ C81.21   Mixed cellularity Hodgkin lymphoma, lymph nodes of head, face, and neck

▲ C81.22   Mixed cellularity Hodgkin lymphoma, intrathoracic lymph nodes

▲ C81.23   Mixed cellularity Hodgkin lymphoma, intra-abdominal lymph nodes

▲ C81.24   Mixed cellularity Hodgkin lymphoma, lymph nodes of axilla and upper limb

▲ C81.25   Mixed cellularity Hodgkin lymphoma, lymph nodes of inguinal region and lower limb

▲ C81.26   Mixed cellularity Hodgkin lymphoma, intrapelvic lymph nodes

▲ C81.27   Mixed cellularity Hodgkin lymphoma, spleen

▲ C81.28   Mixed cellularity Hodgkin lymphoma, lymph nodes of multiple sites

▲ C81.29   Mixed cellularity Hodgkin lymphoma, extranodal and solid organ sites

▲ ⑤ C81.3   Lymphocyte depleted Hodgkin lymphoma
Lymphocyte depleted classical Hodgkin lymphoma

▲ C81.30   Lymphocyte depleted Hodgkin lymphoma, unspecified site

▲ C81.31   Lymphocyte depleted Hodgkin lymphoma, lymph nodes of head, face, and neck

▲ C81.32   Lymphocyte depleted Hodgkin lymphoma, intrathoracic lymph nodes

▲ C81.33   Lymphocyte depleted Hodgkin lymphoma, intra-abdominal lymph nodes

▲ C81.34   Lymphocyte depleted Hodgkin lymphoma, lymph nodes of axilla and upper limb

▲ C81.35   Lymphocyte depleted Hodgkin lymphoma, lymph nodes of inguinal region and lower limb

▲ C81.36   Lymphocyte depleted Hodgkin lymphoma, intrapelvic lymph nodes

▲ C81.37   Lymphocyte depleted Hodgkin lymphoma, spleen

▲ C81.38   Lymphocyte depleted Hodgkin lymphoma, lymph nodes of multiple sites

▲ C81.39   Lymphocyte depleted Hodgkin lymphoma, extranodal and solid organ sites

▲ ⑤ C81.4   Lymphocyte-rich Hodgkin lymphoma
Lymphocyte-rich classical Hodgkin lymphoma

EXCLUDES 1 *nodular lymphocyte predominant Hodgkin lymphoma (C81.0-)*

▲ C81.40   Lymphocyte-rich Hodgkin lymphoma, unspecified site

▲ C81.41   Lymphocyte-rich Hodgkin lymphoma, lymph nodes of head, face, and neck

▲ C81.42   Lymphocyte-rich Hodgkin lymphoma, intrathoracic lymph nodes

▲ C81.43   Lymphocyte-rich Hodgkin lymphoma, intra-abdominal lymph nodes

▲ C81.44   Lymphocyte-rich Hodgkin lymphoma, lymph nodes of axilla and upper limb

▲ C81.45   Lymphocyte-rich Hodgkin lymphoma, lymph nodes of inguinal region and lower limb

▲ C81.46   Lymphocyte-rich Hodgkin lymphoma, intrapelvic lymph nodes

▲ C81.47   Lymphocyte-rich Hodgkin lymphoma, spleen

▲ C81.48   Lymphocyte-rich Hodgkin lymphoma, lymph nodes of multiple sites

▲ C81.49   Lymphocyte-rich Hodgkin lymphoma, extranodal and solid organ sites

▲ ⑤ C81.7   Other Hodgkin lymphoma
Classical Hodgkin lymphoma NOS
Other classical Hodgkin lymphoma

▲ C81.70   Other Hodgkin lymphoma, unspecified site

▲ C81.71   Other Hodgkin lymphoma, lymph nodes of head, face, and neck

▲ C81.72   Other Hodgkin lymphoma, intrathoracic lymph nodes

▲ C81.73   Other Hodgkin lymphoma, intra-abdominal lymph nodes

▲ C81.74   Other Hodgkin lymphoma, lymph nodes of axilla and upper limb

▲ C81.75   Other Hodgkin lymphoma, lymph nodes of inguinal region and lower limb

▲ C81.76   Other Hodgkin lymphoma, intrapelvic lymph nodes

▲ C81.77   Other Hodgkin lymphoma, spleen

▲ C81.78   Other Hodgkin lymphoma, lymph nodes of multiple sites

▲ C81.79   Other Hodgkin lymphoma, extranodal and solid organ sites

⑤ C81.9   Hodgkin lymphoma, unspecified

C81.90   Hodgkin lymphoma, unspecified, unspecified site

C81.91   Hodgkin lymphoma, unspecified, lymph nodes of head, face, and neck

C81.92   Hodgkin lymphoma, unspecified, intrathoracic lymph nodes

C81.93   Hodgkin lymphoma, unspecified, intra-abdominal lymph nodes

C81.94   Hodgkin lymphoma, unspecified, lymph nodes of axilla and upper limb

● New   ▲ Revised   *Manifestation*   ◢-◪ Digit Indicators   ▤ Laterality   Ⓐ Adult (15+ years)   Ⓜ Maternity (12-55 years)   Ⓝ Newborn   Ⓟ Pediatric (0-17 years)   ♂ Male   ♀ Female

✖ Deleted   Unspecified   + Additional code

484   © 2017 DecisionHealth   2017 ICD-10-CM Expert for Physicians

C80.2 — C81.94

C81.95	Hodgkin lymphoma, unspecified, lymph nodes of inguinal region and lower limb
C81.96	Hodgkin lymphoma, unspecified, intrapelvic lymph nodes
C81.97	Hodgkin lymphoma, unspecified, spleen
C81.98	Hodgkin lymphoma, unspecified, lymph nodes of multiple sites
C81.99	Hodgkin lymphoma, unspecified, extranodal and solid organ sites

④ **C82 Follicular lymphoma**

INCLUDES   follicular lymphoma with or without diffuse areas

EXCLUDES 1   *mature T/NK-cell lymphomas (C84.-)*
personal history of non-Hodgkin lymphoma (Z85.72)

⑤ **C82.0   Follicular lymphoma grade I**

C82.00	Follicular lymphoma grade I, unspecified site
C82.01	Follicular lymphoma grade I, lymph nodes of head, face, and neck
C82.02	Follicular lymphoma grade I, intrathoracic lymph nodes
C82.03	Follicular lymphoma grade I, intra-abdominal lymph nodes
C82.04	Follicular lymphoma grade I, lymph nodes of axilla and upper limb
C82.05	Follicular lymphoma grade I, lymph nodes of inguinal region and lower limb
C82.06	Follicular lymphoma grade I, intrapelvic lymph nodes
C82.07	Follicular lymphoma grade I, spleen
C82.08	Follicular lymphoma grade I, lymph nodes of multiple sites
C82.09	Follicular lymphoma grade I, extranodal and solid organ sites

⑤ **C82.1   Follicular lymphoma grade II**

C82.10	Follicular lymphoma grade II, unspecified site
C82.11	Follicular lymphoma grade II, lymph nodes of head, face, and neck
C82.12	Follicular lymphoma grade II, intrathoracic lymph nodes
C82.13	Follicular lymphoma grade II, intra-abdominal lymph nodes
C82.14	Follicular lymphoma grade II, lymph nodes of axilla and upper limb
C82.15	Follicular lymphoma grade II, lymph nodes of inguinal region and lower limb
C82.16	Follicular lymphoma grade II, intrapelvic lymph nodes
C82.17	Follicular lymphoma grade II, spleen
C82.18	Follicular lymphoma grade II, lymph nodes of multiple sites
C82.19	Follicular lymphoma grade II, extranodal and solid organ sites

⑤ **C82.2   Follicular lymphoma grade III, unspecified**

C82.20	Follicular lymphoma grade III, unspecified, unspecified site
C82.21	Follicular lymphoma grade III, unspecified, lymph nodes of head, face, and neck
C82.22	Follicular lymphoma grade III, unspecified, intrathoracic lymph nodes
C82.23	Follicular lymphoma grade III, unspecified, intra-abdominal lymph nodes
C82.24	Follicular lymphoma grade III, unspecified, lymph nodes of axilla and upper limb
C82.25	Follicular lymphoma grade III, unspecified, lymph nodes of inguinal region and lower limb
C82.26	Follicular lymphoma grade III, unspecified, intrapelvic lymph nodes
C82.27	Follicular lymphoma grade III, unspecified, spleen
C82.28	Follicular lymphoma grade III, unspecified, lymph nodes of multiple sites
C82.29	Follicular lymphoma grade III, unspecified, extranodal and solid organ sites

⑤ **C82.3   Follicular lymphoma grade IIIa**

C82.30	Follicular lymphoma grade IIIa, unspecified site
C82.31	Follicular lymphoma grade IIIa, lymph nodes of head, face, and neck
C82.32	Follicular lymphoma grade IIIa, intrathoracic lymph nodes
C82.33	Follicular lymphoma grade IIIa, intra-abdominal lymph nodes
C82.34	Follicular lymphoma grade IIIa, lymph nodes of axilla and upper limb
C82.35	Follicular lymphoma grade IIIa, lymph nodes of inguinal region and lower limb
C82.36	Follicular lymphoma grade IIIa, intrapelvic lymph nodes
C82.37	Follicular lymphoma grade IIIa, spleen
C82.38	Follicular lymphoma grade IIIa, lymph nodes of multiple sites
C82.39	Follicular lymphoma grade IIIa, extranodal and solid organ sites

⑤ **C82.4   Follicular lymphoma grade IIIb**

C82.40	Follicular lymphoma grade IIIb, unspecified site
C82.41	Follicular lymphoma grade IIIb, lymph nodes of head, face, and neck
C82.42	Follicular lymphoma grade IIIb, intrathoracic lymph nodes
C82.43	Follicular lymphoma grade IIIb, intra-abdominal lymph nodes
C82.44	Follicular lymphoma grade IIIb, lymph nodes of axilla and upper limb
C82.45	Follicular lymphoma grade IIIb, lymph nodes of inguinal region and lower limb
C82.46	Follicular lymphoma grade IIIb, intrapelvic lymph nodes
C82.47	Follicular lymphoma grade IIIb, spleen
C82.48	Follicular lymphoma grade IIIb, lymph nodes of multiple sites
C82.49	Follicular lymphoma grade IIIb, extranodal and solid organ sites

⑤ **C82.5   Diffuse follicle center lymphoma**

C82.50	Diffuse follicle center lymphoma, unspecified site
C82.51	Diffuse follicle center lymphoma, lymph nodes of head, face, and neck
C82.52	Diffuse follicle center lymphoma, intrathoracic lymph nodes
C82.53	Diffuse follicle center lymphoma, intra-abdominal lymph nodes
C82.54	Diffuse follicle center lymphoma, lymph nodes of axilla and upper limb
C82.55	Diffuse follicle center lymphoma, lymph nodes of inguinal region and lower limb
C82.56	Diffuse follicle center lymphoma, intrapelvic lymph nodes
C82.57	Diffuse follicle center lymphoma, spleen
C82.58	Diffuse follicle center lymphoma, lymph nodes of multiple sites
C82.59	Diffuse follicle center lymphoma, extranodal and solid organ sites

⑤ **C82.6   Cutaneous follicle center lymphoma**

C82.60	Cutaneous follicle center lymphoma, unspecified site
C82.61	Cutaneous follicle center lymphoma, lymph nodes of head, face, and neck
C82.62	Cutaneous follicle center lymphoma, intrathoracic lymph nodes
C82.63	Cutaneous follicle center lymphoma, intra-abdominal lymph nodes
C82.64	Cutaneous follicle center lymphoma, lymph nodes of axilla and upper limb
C82.65	Cutaneous follicle center lymphoma, lymph nodes of inguinal region and lower limb
C82.66	Cutaneous follicle center lymphoma, intrapelvic lymph nodes
C82.67	Cutaneous follicle center lymphoma, spleen
C82.68	Cutaneous follicle center lymphoma, lymph nodes of multiple sites
C82.69	Cutaneous follicle center lymphoma, extranodal and solid organ sites

⑤ **C82.8   Other types of follicular lymphoma**

C82.80	Other types of follicular lymphoma, unspecified site
C82.81	Other types of follicular lymphoma, lymph nodes of head, face, and neck
C82.82	Other types of follicular lymphoma, intrathoracic lymph nodes

---

● New   ▲ Revised   *Manifestation*   ④-⑦ Digit Indicators   ⊟ Laterality   Ⓐ Adult (15+ years)   Ⓜ Maternity (12-55 years)   Ⓝ Newborn   Ⓟ Pediatric (0-17 years)   ♂ Male   ♀ Female
✖ Deleted   Unspecified   ✚ Additional code

C82.83   Other types of follicular lymphoma, intra-abdominal lymph nodes

C82.84   Other types of follicular lymphoma, lymph nodes of axilla and upper limb

C82.85   Other types of follicular lymphoma, lymph nodes of inguinal region and lower limb

C82.86   Other types of follicular lymphoma, intrapelvic lymph nodes

C82.87   Other types of follicular lymphoma, spleen

C82.88   Other types of follicular lymphoma, lymph nodes of multiple sites

C82.89   Other types of follicular lymphoma, extranodal and solid organ sites

⑤ **C82.9**   **Follicular lymphoma, unspecified**

C82.90   Follicular lymphoma, unspecified, unspecified site

C82.91   Follicular lymphoma, unspecified, lymph nodes of head, face, and neck

C82.92   Follicular lymphoma, unspecified, intrathoracic lymph nodes

C82.93   Follicular lymphoma, unspecified, intra-abdominal lymph nodes

C82.94   Follicular lymphoma, unspecified, lymph nodes of axilla and upper limb

C82.95   Follicular lymphoma, unspecified, lymph nodes of inguinal region and lower limb

C82.96   Follicular lymphoma, unspecified, intrapelvic lymph nodes

C82.97   Follicular lymphoma, unspecified, spleen

C82.98   Follicular lymphoma, unspecified, lymph nodes of multiple sites

C82.99   Follicular lymphoma, unspecified, extranodal and solid organ sites

④ **C83**   **Non-follicular lymphoma**

> **EXCLUDES 1**   *personal history of non-Hodgkin lymphoma (Z85.72)*

⑤ **C83.0**   **Small cell B-cell lymphoma**

Lymphoplasmacytic lymphoma
Nodal marginal zone lymphoma
Non-leukemic variant of B-CLL
Splenic marginal zone lymphoma

> **EXCLUDES 1**   *chronic lymphocytic leukemia (C91.1)*
> *mature T/NK-cell lymphomas (C84.-)*
> *Waldenström macroglobulinemia (C88.0)*

> **DEFINITION**   Uncommon, low-grade, slow-growing B-cell non-Hodgkin's lymphoma involving the marginal, patchy area of the lymph node outside the mantle zone; not very responsive to traditional therapy.

C83.00   Small cell B-cell lymphoma, unspecified site

C83.01   Small cell B-cell lymphoma, lymph nodes of head, face, and neck

C83.02   Small cell B-cell lymphoma, intrathoracic lymph nodes

C83.03   Small cell B-cell lymphoma, intra-abdominal lymph nodes

C83.04   Small cell B-cell lymphoma, lymph nodes of axilla and upper limb

C83.05   Small cell B-cell lymphoma, lymph nodes of inguinal region and lower limb

C83.06   Small cell B-cell lymphoma, intrapelvic lymph nodes

C83.07   Small cell B-cell lymphoma, spleen

C83.08   Small cell B-cell lymphoma, lymph nodes of multiple sites

C83.09   Small cell B-cell lymphoma, extranodal and solid organ sites

⑤ **C83.1**   **Mantle cell lymphoma**

Centrocytic lymphoma
Malignant lymphomatous polyposis

C83.10   Mantle cell lymphoma, unspecified site

C83.11   Mantle cell lymphoma, lymph nodes of head, face, and neck

C83.12   Mantle cell lymphoma, intrathoracic lymph nodes

C83.13   Mantle cell lymphoma, intra-abdominal lymph nodes

C83.14   Mantle cell lymphoma, lymph nodes of axilla and upper limb

C83.15   Mantle cell lymphoma, lymph nodes of inguinal region and lower limb

C83.16   Mantle cell lymphoma, intrapelvic lymph nodes

C83.17   Mantle cell lymphoma, spleen

C83.18   Mantle cell lymphoma, lymph nodes of multiple sites

C83.19   Mantle cell lymphoma, extranodal and solid organ sites

⑤ **C83.3**   **Diffuse large B-cell lymphoma**

Anaplastic diffuse large B-cell lymphoma
CD30-positive diffuse large B-cell lymphoma
Centroblastic diffuse large B-cell lymphoma
Diffuse large B-cell lymphoma, subtype not specified
Immunoblastic diffuse large B-cell lymphoma
Plasmablastic diffuse large B-cell lymphoma
Diffuse large B-cell lymphoma, subtype not specified
T-cell rich diffuse large B-cell lymphoma

> **EXCLUDES 1**   *mediastinal (thymic) large B-cell lymphoma (C85.2-)*
> *mature T/NK-cell lymphomas (C84.-)*

C83.30   Diffuse large B-cell lymphoma, unspecified site

C83.31   Diffuse large B-cell lymphoma, lymph nodes of head, face, and neck

C83.32   Diffuse large B-cell lymphoma, intrathoracic lymph nodes

C83.33   Diffuse large B-cell lymphoma, intra-abdominal lymph nodes

C83.34   Diffuse large B-cell lymphoma, lymph nodes of axilla and upper limb

C83.35   Diffuse large B-cell lymphoma, lymph nodes of inguinal region and lower limb

C83.36   Diffuse large B-cell lymphoma, intrapelvic lymph nodes

C83.37   Diffuse large B-cell lymphoma, spleen

C83.38   Diffuse large B-cell lymphoma, lymph nodes of multiple sites

C83.39   Diffuse large B-cell lymphoma, extranodal and solid organ sites

⑤ **C83.5**   **Lymphoblastic (diffuse) lymphoma**

B-precursor lymphoma
Lymphoblastic B-cell lymphoma
Lymphoblastic lymphoma NOS
Lymphoblastic T-cell lymphoma
T-precursor lymphoma

C83.50   Lymphoblastic (diffuse) lymphoma, unspecified site

C83.51   Lymphoblastic (diffuse) lymphoma, lymph nodes of head, face, and neck

C83.52   Lymphoblastic (diffuse) lymphoma, intrathoracic lymph nodes

C83.53   Lymphoblastic (diffuse) lymphoma, intra-abdominal lymph nodes

C83.54   Lymphoblastic (diffuse) lymphoma, lymph nodes of axilla and upper limb

C83.55   Lymphoblastic (diffuse) lymphoma, lymph nodes of inguinal region and lower limb

C83.56   Lymphoblastic (diffuse) lymphoma, intrapelvic lymph nodes

C83.57   Lymphoblastic (diffuse) lymphoma, spleen

C83.58   Lymphoblastic (diffuse) lymphoma, lymph nodes of multiple sites

C83.59   Lymphoblastic (diffuse) lymphoma, extranodal and solid organ sites

⑤ **C83.7**   **Burkitt lymphoma**

Atypical Burkitt lymphoma
Burkitt-like lymphoma

> **EXCLUDES 1**   *mature B-cell leukemia Burkitt type (C91.A-)*

C83.70   Burkitt lymphoma, unspecified site

C83.71   Burkitt lymphoma, lymph nodes of head, face, and neck

C83.72   Burkitt lymphoma, intrathoracic lymph nodes

C83.73   Burkitt lymphoma, intra-abdominal lymph nodes

C83.74   Burkitt lymphoma, lymph nodes of axilla and upper limb

C83.75   Burkitt lymphoma, lymph nodes of inguinal region and lower limb

C83.76   Burkitt lymphoma, intrapelvic lymph nodes

C83.77   Burkitt lymphoma, spleen

C83.78   Burkitt lymphoma, lymph nodes of multiple sites

C83.79   Burkitt lymphoma, extranodal and solid organ sites

● New   ▲ Revised   *Manifestation*   ④-⑦ Digit Indicators   ⊟ Laterality   Ⓐ Adult (15+ years)   Ⓜ Maternity (12-55 years)   Ⓝ Newborn   Ⓟ Pediatric (0-17 years)   ♂ Male   ♀ Female

✖ Deleted   Unspecified   + Additional code

⑤ C83.8   Other non-follicular lymphoma
Intravascular large B-cell lymphoma
Lymphoid granulomatosis
Primary effusion B-cell lymphoma

> **EXCLUDES 1** *mediastinal (thymic) large B-cell lymphoma (C85.2-)*
> *T-cell rich B-cell lymphoma (C83.3-)*

- **C83.80**   Other non-follicular lymphoma, unspecified site
- **C83.81**   Other non-follicular lymphoma, lymph nodes of head, face, and neck
- **C83.82**   Other non-follicular lymphoma, intrathoracic lymph nodes
- **C83.83**   Other non-follicular lymphoma, intra-abdominal lymph nodes
- **C83.84**   Other non-follicular lymphoma, lymph nodes of axilla and upper limb
- **C83.85**   Other non-follicular lymphoma, lymph nodes of inguinal region and lower limb
- **C83.86**   Other non-follicular lymphoma, intrapelvic lymph nodes
- **C83.87**   Other non-follicular lymphoma, spleen
- **C83.88**   Other non-follicular lymphoma, lymph nodes of multiple sites
- **C83.89**   Other non-follicular lymphoma, extranodal and solid organ sites

⑤ C83.9   Non-follicular (diffuse) lymphoma, unspecified

- **C83.90**   Non-follicular (diffuse) lymphoma, unspecified, unspecified site
- **C83.91**   Non-follicular (diffuse) lymphoma, unspecified, lymph nodes of head, face, and neck
- **C83.92**   Non-follicular (diffuse) lymphoma, unspecified, intrathoracic lymph nodes
- **C83.93**   Non-follicular (diffuse) lymphoma, unspecified, intra-abdominal lymph nodes
- **C83.94**   Non-follicular (diffuse) lymphoma, unspecified, lymph nodes of axilla and upper limb
- **C83.95**   Non-follicular (diffuse) lymphoma, unspecified, lymph nodes of inguinal region and lower limb
- **C83.96**   Non-follicular (diffuse) lymphoma, unspecified, intrapelvic lymph nodes
- **C83.97**   Non-follicular (diffuse) lymphoma, unspecified, spleen
- **C83.98**   Non-follicular (diffuse) lymphoma, unspecified, lymph nodes of multiple sites
- **C83.99**   Non-follicular (diffuse) lymphoma, unspecified, extranodal and solid organ sites

④ C84   Mature T/NK-cell lymphomas

> **EXCLUDES 1** *personal history of non-Hodgkin lymphoma (Z85.72)*

⑤ C84.0   Mycosis fungoides

> **EXCLUDES 1** *peripheral T-cell lymphoma, not classified (C84.4-)*

> **DEFINITION** A rare, progressive form of slow-growing cutaneous T-cell lymphoma associated with a chromosome abnormality that evolves into a generalized, high grade, aggressive systemic form of lymphoma.

- **C84.00**   Mycosis fungoides, unspecified site
- **C84.01**   Mycosis fungoides, lymph nodes of head, face, and neck
- **C84.02**   Mycosis fungoides, intrathoracic lymph nodes
- **C84.03**   Mycosis fungoides, intra-abdominal lymph nodes
- **C84.04**   Mycosis fungoides, lymph nodes of axilla and upper limb
- **C84.05**   Mycosis fungoides, lymph nodes of inguinal region and lower limb
- **C84.06**   Mycosis fungoides, intrapelvic lymph nodes
- **C84.07**   Mycosis fungoides, spleen
- **C84.08**   Mycosis fungoides, lymph nodes of multiple sites
- **C84.09**   Mycosis fungoides, extranodal and solid organ sites

⑤ C84.1   Sézary disease

- **C84.10**   Sézary disease, unspecified site
- **C84.11**   Sézary disease, lymph nodes of head, face, and neck
- **C84.12**   Sézary disease, intrathoracic lymph nodes
- **C84.13**   Sézary disease, intra-abdominal lymph nodes
- **C84.14**   Sézary disease, lymph nodes of axilla and upper limb
- **C84.15**   Sézary disease, lymph nodes of inguinal region and lower limb
- **C84.16**   Sézary disease, intrapelvic lymph nodes
- **C84.17**   Sézary disease, spleen
- **C84.18**   Sézary disease, lymph nodes of multiple sites
- **C84.19**   Sézary disease, extranodal and solid organ sites

⑤ C84.4   Peripheral T-cell lymphoma, not classified
Lennert's lymphoma
Lymphoepithelioid lymphoma
Mature T-cell lymphoma, not elsewhere classified

> **DEFINITION** Aggressive, non-Hodgkin's lymphoma derived from mature neoplastic T-cell lymphocytes that have moved to other tissue, causing site-related symptoms and generalized lymphadenopathy.

- **C84.40**   Peripheral T-cell lymphoma, not classified, unspecified site
- **C84.41**   Peripheral T-cell lymphoma, not classified, lymph nodes of head, face, and neck
- **C84.42**   Peripheral T-cell lymphoma, not classified, intrathoracic lymph nodes
- **C84.43**   Peripheral T-cell lymphoma, not classified, intra-abdominal lymph nodes
- **C84.44**   Peripheral T-cell lymphoma, not classified, lymph nodes of axilla and upper limb
- **C84.45**   Peripheral T-cell lymphoma, not classified, lymph nodes of inguinal region and lower limb
- **C84.46**   Peripheral T-cell lymphoma, not classified, intrapelvic lymph nodes
- **C84.47**   Peripheral T-cell lymphoma, not classified, spleen
- **C84.48**   Peripheral T-cell lymphoma, not classified, lymph nodes of multiple sites
- **C84.49**   Peripheral T-cell lymphoma, not classified, extranodal and solid organ sites

⑤ C84.6   Anaplastic large cell lymphoma, ALK-positive
Anaplastic large cell lymphoma, CD30-positive

- **C84.60**   Anaplastic large cell lymphoma, ALK-positive, unspecified site
- **C84.61**   Anaplastic large cell lymphoma, ALK-positive, lymph nodes of head, face, and neck
- **C84.62**   Anaplastic large cell lymphoma, ALK-positive, intrathoracic lymph nodes
- **C84.63**   Anaplastic large cell lymphoma, ALK-positive, intra-abdominal lymph nodes
- **C84.64**   Anaplastic large cell lymphoma, ALK-positive, lymph nodes of axilla and upper limb
- **C84.65**   Anaplastic large cell lymphoma, ALK-positive, lymph nodes of inguinal region and lower limb
- **C84.66**   Anaplastic large cell lymphoma, ALK-positive, intrapelvic lymph nodes
- **C84.67**   Anaplastic large cell lymphoma, ALK-positive, spleen
- **C84.68**   Anaplastic large cell lymphoma, ALK-positive, lymph nodes of multiple sites
- **C84.69**   Anaplastic large cell lymphoma, ALK-positive, extranodal and solid organ sites

⑤ C84.7   Anaplastic large cell lymphoma, ALK-negative

> **EXCLUDES 1** *primary cutaneous CD30-positive T-cell proliferations (C86.6-)*

- **C84.70**   Anaplastic large cell lymphoma, ALK-negative, unspecified site
- **C84.71**   Anaplastic large cell lymphoma, ALK-negative, lymph nodes of head, face, and neck
- **C84.72**   Anaplastic large cell lymphoma, ALK-negative, intrathoracic lymph nodes
- **C84.73**   Anaplastic large cell lymphoma, ALK-negative, intra-abdominal lymph nodes
- **C84.74**   Anaplastic large cell lymphoma, ALK-negative, lymph nodes of axilla and upper limb
- **C84.75**   Anaplastic large cell lymphoma, ALK-negative, lymph nodes of inguinal region and lower limb
- **C84.76**   Anaplastic large cell lymphoma, ALK-negative, intrapelvic lymph nodes
- **C84.77**   Anaplastic large cell lymphoma, ALK-negative, spleen
- **C84.78**   Anaplastic large cell lymphoma, ALK-negative, lymph nodes of multiple sites
- **C84.79**   Anaplastic large cell lymphoma, ALK-negative, extranodal and solid organ sites

⑤ C84.A   Cutaneous T-cell lymphoma, unspecified

| ● New | ▲ Revised | *Manifestation* | ④-⑦ Digit Indicators | ▤ Laterality | Ⓐ Adult (15+ years) | Ⓜ Maternity (12-55 years) | Ⓝ Newborn | Ⓟ Pediatric (0-17 years) | ♂ Male | ♀ Female |
| ✖ Deleted | | Unspecified | + Additional code | | | | | | | |

2017 ICD-10-CM Expert for Physicians   © 2017 DecisionHealth   487

C84.A0 **Cutaneous T-cell lymphoma, unspecified, unspecified site**

C84.A1 **Cutaneous T-cell lymphoma, unspecified lymph nodes of head, face, and neck**

C84.A2 **Cutaneous T-cell lymphoma, unspecified, intrathoracic lymph nodes**

C84.A3 **Cutaneous T-cell lymphoma, unspecified, intra-abdominal lymph nodes**

C84.A4 **Cutaneous T-cell lymphoma, unspecified, lymph nodes of axilla and upper limb**

C84.A5 **Cutaneous T-cell lymphoma, unspecified, lymph nodes of inguinal region and lower limb**

C84.A6 **Cutaneous T-cell lymphoma, unspecified, intrapelvic lymph nodes**

C84.A7 **Cutaneous T-cell lymphoma, unspecified, spleen**

C84.A8 **Cutaneous T-cell lymphoma, unspecified, lymph nodes of multiple sites**

C84.A9 **Cutaneous T-cell lymphoma, unspecified, extranodal and solid organ sites**

⑤ **C84.Z** **Other mature T/NK-cell lymphomas**

Note: If T-cell lineage or involvement is mentioned in conjunction with a specific lymphoma, code to the more specific description.

> **EXCLUDES 1** *angioimmunoblastic T-cell lymphoma (C86.5)*
> *blastic NK-cell lymphoma (C86.4)*
> *enteropathy-type T-cell lymphoma (C86.2)*
> *extranodal NK-cell lymphoma, nasal type (C86.0)*
> *hepatosplenic T-cell lymphoma (C86.1)*
> *primary cutaneous CD30-positive T-cell proliferations (C86.6)*
> *subcutaneous panniculitis-like T-cell lymphoma (C86.3)*
> *T-cell leukemia (C91.1-)*

C84.Z0 **Other mature T/NK-cell lymphomas, unspecified site**

C84.Z1 **Other mature T/NK-cell lymphomas, lymph nodes of head, face, and neck**

C84.Z2 **Other mature T/NK-cell lymphomas, intrathoracic lymph nodes**

C84.Z3 **Other mature T/NK-cell lymphomas, intra-abdominal lymph nodes**

C84.Z4 **Other mature T/NK-cell lymphomas, lymph nodes of axilla and upper limb**

C84.Z5 **Other mature T/NK-cell lymphomas, lymph nodes of inguinal region and lower limb**

C84.Z6 **Other mature T/NK-cell lymphomas, intrapelvic lymph nodes**

C84.Z7 **Other mature T/NK-cell lymphomas, spleen**

C84.Z8 **Other mature T/NK-cell lymphomas, lymph nodes of multiple sites**

C84.Z9 **Other mature T/NK-cell lymphomas, extranodal and solid organ sites**

⑤ **C84.9** **Mature T/NK-cell lymphomas, unspecified**

NK/T cell lymphoma NOS

> **EXCLUDES 1** *mature T-cell lymphoma, not elsewhere classified (C84.4-)*

C84.90 **Mature T/NK-cell lymphomas, unspecified, unspecified site**

C84.91 **Mature T/NK-cell lymphomas, unspecified, lymph nodes of head, face, and neck**

C84.92 **Mature T/NK-cell lymphomas, unspecified, intrathoracic lymph nodes**

C84.93 **Mature T/NK-cell lymphomas, unspecified, intra-abdominal lymph nodes**

C84.94 **Mature T/NK-cell lymphomas, unspecified, lymph nodes of axilla and upper limb**

C84.95 **Mature T/NK-cell lymphomas, unspecified, lymph nodes of inguinal region and lower limb**

C84.96 **Mature T/NK-cell lymphomas, unspecified, intrapelvic lymph nodes**

C84.97 **Mature T/NK-cell lymphomas, unspecified, spleen**

C84.98 **Mature T/NK-cell lymphomas, unspecified, lymph nodes of multiple sites**

C84.99 **Mature T/NK-cell lymphomas, unspecified, extranodal and solid organ sites**

④ **C85** **Other specified and unspecified types of non-Hodgkin lymphoma**

> **EXCLUDES 1** *other specified types of T/NK-cell lymphoma (C86.-)*
> *personal history of non-Hodgkin lymphoma (Z85.72)*

⑤ **C85.1** **Unspecified B-cell lymphoma**

Note: If B-cell lineage or involvement is mentioned in conjunction with a specific lymphoma, code to the more specific description.

C85.10 **Unspecified B-cell lymphoma, unspecified site**

C85.11 **Unspecified B-cell lymphoma, lymph nodes of head, face, and neck**

C85.12 **Unspecified B-cell lymphoma, intrathoracic lymph nodes**

C85.13 **Unspecified B-cell lymphoma, intra-abdominal lymph nodes**

C85.14 **Unspecified B-cell lymphoma, lymph nodes of axilla and upper limb**

C85.15 **Unspecified B-cell lymphoma, lymph nodes of inguinal region and lower limb**

C85.16 **Unspecified B-cell lymphoma, intrapelvic lymph nodes**

C85.17 **Unspecified B-cell lymphoma, spleen**

C85.18 **Unspecified B-cell lymphoma, lymph nodes of multiple sites**

C85.19 **Unspecified B-cell lymphoma, extranodal and solid organ sites**

⑤ **C85.2** **Mediastinal (thymic) large B-cell lymphoma**

C85.20 **Mediastinal (thymic) large B-cell lymphoma, unspecified site**

C85.21 **Mediastinal (thymic) large B-cell lymphoma, lymph nodes of head, face, and neck**

C85.22 **Mediastinal (thymic) large B-cell lymphoma, intrathoracic lymph nodes**

C85.23 **Mediastinal (thymic) large B-cell lymphoma, intra-abdominal lymph nodes**

C85.24 **Mediastinal (thymic) large B-cell lymphoma, lymph nodes of axilla and upper limb**

C85.25 **Mediastinal (thymic) large B-cell lymphoma, lymph nodes of inguinal region and lower limb**

C85.26 **Mediastinal (thymic) large B-cell lymphoma, intrapelvic lymph nodes**

C85.27 **Mediastinal (thymic) large B-cell lymphoma, spleen**

C85.28 **Mediastinal (thymic) large B-cell lymphoma, lymph nodes of multiple sites**

C85.29 **Mediastinal (thymic) large B-cell lymphoma, extranodal and solid organ sites**

⑤ **C85.8** **Other specified types of non-Hodgkin lymphoma**

C85.80 **Other specified types of non-Hodgkin lymphoma, unspecified site**

C85.81 **Other specified types of non-Hodgkin lymphoma, lymph nodes of head, face, and neck**

C85.82 **Other specified types of non-Hodgkin lymphoma, intrathoracic lymph nodes**

C85.83 **Other specified types of non-Hodgkin lymphoma, intra-abdominal lymph nodes**

C85.84 **Other specified types of non-Hodgkin lymphoma, lymph nodes of axilla and upper limb**

C85.85 **Other specified types of non-Hodgkin lymphoma, lymph nodes of inguinal region and lower limb**

C85.86 **Other specified types of non-Hodgkin lymphoma, intrapelvic lymph nodes**

C85.87 **Other specified types of non-Hodgkin lymphoma, spleen**

C85.88 **Other specified types of non-Hodgkin lymphoma, lymph nodes of multiple sites**

C85.89 **Other specified types of non-Hodgkin lymphoma, extranodal and solid organ sites**

⑤ **C85.9** **Non-Hodgkin lymphoma, unspecified**

Lymphoma NOS
Malignant lymphoma NOS
Non-Hodgkin lymphoma NOS

C85.90 **Non-Hodgkin lymphoma, unspecified, unspecified site**

C85.91 **Non-Hodgkin lymphoma, unspecified, lymph nodes of head, face, and neck**

● New ▲ Revised *Manifestation* ④-⑦ Digit Indicators ▱ Laterality Ⓐ Adult (15+ years) Ⓜ Maternity (12-55 years) Ⓝ Newborn Ⓟ Pediatric (0-17 years) ♂ Male ♀ Female
✖ Deleted Unspecified + Additional code

488   © 2017 DecisionHealth   2017 ICD-10-CM Expert for Physicians

C84.A0 — C85.91

C85.92 Non-Hodgkin lymphoma, unspecified, intrathoracic lymph nodes

C85.93 Non-Hodgkin lymphoma, unspecified, intra-abdominal lymph nodes

C85.94 Non-Hodgkin lymphoma, unspecified, lymph nodes of axilla and upper limb

C85.95 Non-Hodgkin lymphoma, unspecified, lymph nodes of inguinal region and lower limb

C85.96 Non-Hodgkin lymphoma, unspecified, intrapelvic lymph nodes

C85.97 Non-Hodgkin lymphoma, unspecified, spleen

C85.98 Non-Hodgkin lymphoma, unspecified, lymph nodes of multiple sites

C85.99 Non-Hodgkin lymphoma, unspecified, extranodal and solid organ sites

C86 Other specified types of T/NK-cell lymphoma
  EXCLUDES 1 *anaplastic large cell lymphoma, ALK negative (C84.7-)*
   anaplastic large cell lymphoma, ALK positive (C84.6-)
   mature T/NK-cell lymphomas (C84.-)
   other specified types of non-Hodgkin lymphoma (C85.8-)

C86.0 Extranodal NK/T-cell lymphoma, nasal type

C86.1 Hepatosplenic T-cell lymphoma
  Alpha-beta and gamma delta types

C86.2 Enteropathy-type (intestinal) T-cell lymphoma
  Enteropathy associated T-cell lymphoma

C86.3 Subcutaneous panniculitis-like T-cell lymphoma

C86.4 Blastic NK-cell lymphoma

C86.5 Angioimmunoblastic T-cell lymphoma
  Angioimmunoblastic lymphadenopathy with dysproteinemia (AILD)

C86.6 Primary cutaneous CD30-positive T-cell proliferations
  Lymphomatoid papulosis
  Primary cutaneous anaplastic large cell lymphoma
  Primary cutaneous CD30-positive large T-cell lymphoma

C88 Malignant immunoproliferative diseases and certain other B-cell lymphomas
  EXCLUDES 1 *B-cell lymphoma, unspecified (C85.1-)*
   personal history of other malignant neoplasms of lymphoid, hematopoietic and related tissues (Z85.79)

C88.0 Waldenström macroglobulinemia
  Lymphoplasmacytic lymphoma with IgM-production
  Macroglobulinemia (idiopathic) (primary)
  EXCLUDES 1 *small cell B-cell lymphoma (C83.0)*

C88.2 Heavy chain disease
  Franklin disease
  Gamma heavy chain disease
  Mu heavy chain disease

C88.3 Immunoproliferative small intestinal disease
  Alpha heavy chain disease
  Mediterranean lymphoma

C88.4 Extranodal marginal zone B-cell lymphoma of mucosa-associated lymphoid tissue [MALT-lymphoma]
  Lymphoma of skin-associated lymphoid tissue [SALT-lymphoma]
  Lymphoma of bronchial-associated lymphoid tissue [BALT-lymphoma]
  EXCLUDES 1 *high malignant (diffuse large B-cell) lymphoma (C83.3-)*

C88.8 Other malignant immunoproliferative diseases

C88.9 Malignant immunoproliferative disease, unspecified
  Immunoproliferative disease NOS

C90 Multiple myeloma and malignant plasma cell neoplasms
  EXCLUDES 1 *personal history of other malignant neoplasms of lymphoid, hematopoietic and related tissues (Z85.79)*

GUIDELINES Section I.C.2.n

The categories for leukemia [C91 - C95], and category C90, Multiple myeloma and malignant plasma cell neoplasms, have codes indicating whether or not the leukemia has achieved remission. There are also codes Z85.6, Personal history of leukemia, and Z85.79, Personal history of other malignant neoplasms of lymphoid, hematopoietic and related tissues. If the documentation is unclear, as to whether the leukemia has achieved remission, the provider should be queried.

CODING TIP ✓ Terms such as "in remission" and "in relapse" must be specified by the physician in order to indicate assignment of a code specifying these terms. If the physician has not specified one of these terms, select the code for "not having achieved remission."

C90.0 Multiple myeloma
  Kahler's disease
  Medullary plasmacytoma
  Myelomatosis
  Plasma cell myeloma
  EXCLUDES 1 *solitary myeloma (C90.3-)*
   solitary plasmactyoma (C90.3-)

C90.00 Multiple myeloma not having achieved remission
  Multiple myeloma with failed remission
  Multiple myeloma NOS

Multiple myeloma

A type of cancer characterized by excessive numbers of malignant plasma cells in the bone marrow

C90.01 Multiple myeloma in remission

C90.02 Multiple myeloma in relapse

C90.1 Plasma cell leukemia
  Plasmacytic leukemia

C90.10 Plasma cell leukemia not having achieved remission
  Plasma cell leukemia with failed remission
  Plasma cell leukemia NOS

C90.11 Plasma cell leukemia in remission

C90.12 Plasma cell leukemia in relapse

C90.2 Extramedullary plasmacytoma

C90.20 Extramedullary plasmacytoma not having achieved remission
  Extramedullary plasmacytoma with failed remission
  Extramedullary plasmacytoma NOS

C90.21 Extramedullary plasmacytoma in remission

C90.22 Extramedullary plasmacytoma in relapse

C90.3 Solitary plasmacytoma
  Localized malignant plasma cell tumor NOS
  Plasmacytoma NOS
  Solitary myeloma

C90.30 Solitary plasmacytoma not having achieved remission
  Solitary plasmacytoma with failed remission
  Solitary plasmacytoma NOS

C90.31 Solitary plasmacytoma in remission

C90.32 Solitary plasmacytoma in relapse

C91 Lymphoid leukemia
  EXCLUDES 1 *personal history of leukemia (Z85.6)*

● New ▲ Revised *Manifestation* / Unspecified 4 - 7 Digit Indicators / + Additional code ⊟ Laterality Ⓐ Adult (15+ years) Ⓜ Maternity (12-55 years) Ⓝ Newborn Ⓟ Pediatric (0-17 years) ♂ Male ♀ Female
✖ Deleted

CODING TIP ✓ Terms such as "in remission" and "in relapse" must be specified by the physician in order to indicate assignment of a code specifying these terms. If the physician has not specified one of these terms, select the code for "not having achieved remission."

🅢 **C91.0   Acute lymphoblastic leukemia [ALL]**
　　　　　Note: Code C91.0 should only be used for T-cell and B-cell precursor leukemia

　　C91.00   Acute lymphoblastic leukemia not having achieved remission
　　　　　Acute lymphoblastic leukemia with failed remission
　　　　　Acute lymphoblastic leukemia NOS
　　C91.01   Acute lymphoblastic leukemia, in remission
　　C91.02   Acute lymphoblastic leukemia, in relapse

🅢 **C91.1   Chronic lymphocytic leukemia of B-cell type**
　　　　　Lymphoplasmacytic leukemia
　　　　　Richter syndrome
　　　　　EXCLUDES 1 *lymphoplasmacytic lymphoma (C83.0-)*

　　C91.10   Chronic lymphocytic leukemia of B-cell type not having achieved remission
　　　　　Chronic lymphocytic leukemia of B-cell type with failed remission
　　　　　Chronic lymphocytic leukemia of B-cell type NOS
　　C91.11   Chronic lymphocytic leukemia of B-cell type in remission
　　C91.12   Chronic lymphocytic leukemia of B-cell type in relapse

🅢 **C91.3   Prolymphocytic leukemia of B-cell type**
　　C91.30   Prolymphocytic leukemia of B-cell type not having achieved remission
　　　　　Prolymphocytic leukemia of B-cell type with failed remission
　　　　　Prolymphocytic leukemia of B-cell type NOS
　　C91.31   Prolymphocytic leukemia of B-cell type, in remission
　　C91.32   Prolymphocytic leukemia of B-cell type, in relapse

🅢 **C91.4   Hairy cell leukemia**
　　　　　Leukemic reticuloendotheliosis
　　C91.40   Hairy cell leukemia not having achieved remission
　　　　　Hairy cell leukemia with failed remission
　　　　　Hairy cell leukemia NOS
　　C91.41   Hairy cell leukemia, in remission
　　C91.42   Hairy cell leukemia, in relapse

🅢 **C91.5   Adult T-cell lymphoma/leukemia (HTLV-1-associated)**
　　　　　Acute variant of adult T-cell lymphoma/leukemia (HTLV-1-associated)
　　　　　Chronic variant of adult T-cell lymphoma/leukemia (HTLV-1-associated)
　　　　　Lymphomatoid variant of adult T-cell lymphoma/leukemia (HTLV-1-associated)
　　　　　Smouldering variant of adult T-cell lymphoma/leukemia (HTLV-1-associated)
　　C91.50   Adult T-cell lymphoma/leukemia (HTLV-1-associated) not having achieved remission   Ⓐ
　　　　　Adult T-cell lymphoma/leukemia (HTLV-1-associated) with failed remission
　　　　　Adult T-cell lymphoma/leukemia (HTLV-1-associated) NOS
　　C91.51   Adult T-cell lymphoma/leukemia (HTLV-1-associated), in remission   Ⓐ
　　C91.52   Adult T-cell lymphoma/leukemia (HTLV-1-associated), in relapse   Ⓐ

🅢 **C91.6   Prolymphocytic leukemia of T-cell type**
　　C91.60   Prolymphocytic leukemia of T-cell type not having achieved remission
　　　　　Prolymphocytic leukemia of T-cell type with failed remission
　　　　　Prolymphocytic leukemia of T-cell type NOS
　　C91.61   Prolymphocytic leukemia of T-cell type, in remission
　　C91.62   Prolymphocytic leukemia of T-cell type, in relapse

🅢 **C91.A   Mature B-cell leukemia Burkitt-type**
　　　　　EXCLUDES 1 *Burkitt lymphoma (C83.7-)*

　　C91.A0   Mature B-cell leukemia Burkitt-type not having achieved remission
　　　　　Mature B-cell leukemia Burkitt-type with failed remission
　　　　　Mature B-cell leukemia Burkitt-type NOS
　　C91.A1   Mature B-cell leukemia Burkitt-type, in remission
　　C91.A2   Mature B-cell leukemia Burkitt-type, in relapse

🅢 **C91.Z   Other lymphoid leukemia**
　　　　　T-cell large granular lymphocytic leukemia (associated with rheumatoid arthritis)
　　C91.Z0   Other lymphoid leukemia not having achieved remission
　　　　　Other lymphoid leukemia with failed remission
　　　　　Other lymphoid leukemia NOS
　　C91.Z1   Other lymphoid leukemia, in remission
　　C91.Z2   Other lymphoid leukemia, in relapse

🅢 **C91.9   Lymphoid leukemia, unspecified**
　　C91.90   Lymphoid leukemia, unspecified not having achieved remission
　　　　　Lymphoid leukemia with failed remission
　　　　　Lymphoid leukemia NOS
　　C91.91   Lymphoid leukemia, unspecified, in remission
　　C91.92   Lymphoid leukemia, unspecified, in relapse

④ **C92   Myeloid leukemia**
　　INCLUDES   granulocytic leukemia
　　　　　　　myelogenous leukemia
　　EXCLUDES 1 *personal history of leukemia (Z85.6)*

CODING TIP ✓ Terms such as "in remission" and "in relapse" must be specified by the physician in order to indicate assignment of a code specifying these terms. If the physician has not specified one of these terms, select the code for "not having achieved remission."

🅢 **C92.0   Acute myeloblastic leukemia**
　　　　　Acute myeloblastic leukemia, minimal differentiation
　　　　　Acute myeloblastic leukemia (with maturation)
　　　　　Acute myeloblastic leukemia 1/ETO
　　　　　Acute myeloblastic leukemia M0
　　　　　Acute myeloblastic leukemia M1
　　　　　Acute myeloblastic leukemia M2
　　　　　Acute myeloblastic leukemia with t(8;21)
　　　　　Acute myeloblastic leukemia (without a FAB classification) NOS
　　　　　Refractory anemia with excess blasts in transformation [RAEB T]
　　　　　EXCLUDES 1 *acute exacerbation of chronic myeloid leukemia (C92.10)*
　　　　　　　　　refractory anemia with excess of blasts not in transformation (D46.2-)

　　C92.00   Acute myeloblastic leukemia, not having achieved remission
　　　　　Acute myeloblastic leukemia with failed remission
　　　　　Acute myeloblastic leukemia NOS
　　C92.01   Acute myeloblastic leukemia, in remission
　　C92.02   Acute myeloblastic leukemia, in relapse

🅢 **C92.1   Chronic myeloid leukemia, BCR/ABL-positive**
　　　　　Chronic myelogenous leukemia, Philadelphia chromosome (Ph1) positive
　　　　　Chronic myelogenous leukemia, t(9;22) (q34;q11)
　　　　　Chronic myelogenous leukemia with crisis of blast cells
　　　　　EXCLUDES 1 *atypical chronic myeloid leukemia BCR/ABL-negative (C92.2-)*
　　　　　　　　　chronic myelomonocytic leukemia (C93.1-)
　　　　　　　　　chronic myeloproliferative disease (D47.1)

　　C92.10   Chronic myeloid leukemia, BCR/ABL-positive, not having achieved remission
　　　　　Chronic myeloid leukemia, BCR/ABL-positive with failed remission
　　　　　Chronic myeloid leukemia, BCR/ABL-positive NOS
　　C92.11   Chronic myeloid leukemia, BCR/ABL-positive, in remission
　　C92.12   Chronic myeloid leukemia, BCR/ABL-positive, in relapse

🅢 **C92.2   Atypical chronic myeloid leukemia, BCR/ABL-negative**
　　C92.20   Atypical chronic myeloid leukemia, BCR/ABL-negative, not having achieved remission
　　　　　Atypical chronic myeloid leukemia, BCR/ABL-negative with failed remission
　　　　　Atypical chronic myeloid leukemia, BCR/ABL-negative NOS
　　C92.21   Atypical chronic myeloid leukemia, BCR/ABL-negative, in remission
　　C92.22   Atypical chronic myeloid leukemia, BCR/ABL-negative, in relapse

🅢 **C92.3   Myeloid sarcoma**
　　　　　A malignant tumor of immature myeloid cells
　　　　　Chloroma
　　　　　Granulocytic sarcoma

● New　▲ Revised　*Manifestation*　④-⑦ Digit Indicators　⊟ Laterality　Ⓐ Adult (15+ years)　Ⓜ Maternity (12-55 years)　Ⓝ Newborn　Ⓟ Pediatric (0-17 years)　♂ Male　♀ Female
✖ Deleted　Unspecified　+ Additional code

C92.30   **Myeloid sarcoma, not having achieved remission**
Myeloid sarcoma with failed remission
Myeloid sarcoma NOS
C92.31   **Myeloid sarcoma, in remission**
C92.32   **Myeloid sarcoma, in relapse**

⑤ **C92.4**   **Acute promyelocytic leukemia**
AML M3
AML Me with t(15;17) and variants
C92.40   **Acute promyelocytic leukemia, not having achieved remission**
Acute promyelocytic leukemia with failed remission
Acute promyelocytic leukemia NOS
C92.41   **Acute promyelocytic leukemia, in remission**
C92.42   **Acute promyelocytic leukemia, in relapse**

⑤ **C92.5**   **Acute myelomonocytic leukemia**
AML M4
AML M4 Eo with inv(16) or t(16;16)
C92.50   **Acute myelomonocytic leukemia, not having achieved remission**
Acute myelomonocytic leukemia with failed remission
Acute myelomonocytic leukemia NOS
C92.51   **Acute myelomonocytic leukemia, in remission**
C92.52   **Acute myelomonocytic leukemia, in relapse**

⑤ **C92.6**   **Acute myeloid leukemia with 11q23-abnormality**
Acute myeloid leukemia with variation of MLL-gene
C92.60   **Acute myeloid leukemia with 11q23-abnormality not having achieved remission**
Acute myeloid leukemia with 11q23-abnormality with failed remission
Acute myeloid leukemia with 11q23-abnormality NOS
C92.61   **Acute myeloid leukemia with 11q23-abnormality in remission**
C92.62   **Acute myeloid leukemia with 11q23-abnormality in relapse**

⑤ **C92.A**   **Acute myeloid leukemia with multilineage dysplasia**
Acute myeloid leukemia with dysplasia of remaining hematopoesis and/or myelodysplastic disease in its history
C92.A0   **Acute myeloid leukemia with multilineage dysplasia, not having achieved remission**
Acute myeloid leukemia with multilineage dysplasia with failed remission
Acute myeloid leukemia with multilineage dysplasia NOS
C92.A1   **Acute myeloid leukemia with multilineage dysplasia, in remission**
C92.A2   **Acute myeloid leukemia with multilineage dysplasia, in relapse**

⑤ **C92.Z**   **Other myeloid leukemia**
C92.Z0   **Other myeloid leukemia not having achieved remission**
Myeloid leukemia NEC with failed remission
Myeloid leukemia NEC
C92.Z1   **Other myeloid leukemia, in remission**
C92.Z2   **Other myeloid leukemia, in relapse**

⑤ **C92.9**   **Myeloid leukemia, unspecified**
C92.90   **Myeloid leukemia, unspecified, not having achieved remission**
Myeloid leukemia, unspecified with failed remission
Myeloid leukemia, unspecified NOS
C92.91   **Myeloid leukemia, unspecified in remission**
C92.92   **Myeloid leukemia, unspecified in relapse**

④ **C93**   **Monocytic leukemia**
INCLUDES   monocytoid leukemia
EXCLUDES 1   *personal history of leukemia (Z85.6)*
CODING TIP ✓   Terms such as "in remission" and "in relapse" must be specified by the physician in order to indicate assignment of a code specifying these terms. If the physician has not specified one of these terms, select the code for "not having achieved remission."

⑤ **C93.0**   **Acute monoblastic/monocytic leukemia**
AML M5
AML M5a
AML M5b
C93.00   **Acute monoblastic/monocytic leukemia, not having achieved remission**
Acute monoblastic/monocytic leukemia with failed remission
Acute monoblastic/monocytic leukemia NOS
C93.01   **Acute monoblastic/monocytic leukemia, in remission**

C93.02   **Acute monoblastic/monocytic leukemia, in relapse**

⑤ **C93.1**   **Chronic myelomonocytic leukemia**
Chronic monocytic leukemia
CMML-1
CMML-2
CMML with eosinophilia
C93.10   **Chronic myelomonocytic leukemia not having achieved remission**
Chronic myelomonocytic leukemia with failed remission
Chronic myelomonocytic leukemia NOS
C93.11   **Chronic myelomonocytic leukemia, in remission**
C93.12   **Chronic myelomonocytic leukemia, in relapse**

⑤ **C93.3**   **Juvenile myelomonocytic leukemia**
C93.30   **Juvenile myelomonocytic leukemia, not having achieved remission**   Ⓟ
Juvenile myelomonocytic leukemia with failed remission
Juvenile myelomonocytic leukemia NOS
C93.31   **Juvenile myelomonocytic leukemia, in remission**   Ⓟ
C93.32   **Juvenile myelomonocytic leukemia, in relapse**   Ⓟ

⑤ **C93.Z**   **Other monocytic leukemia**
C93.Z0   **Other monocytic leukemia, not having achieved remission**
Other monocytic leukemia NOS
C93.Z1   **Other monocytic leukemia, in remission**
C93.Z2   **Other monocytic leukemia, in relapse**

⑤ **C93.9**   **Monocytic leukemia, unspecified**
C93.90   **Monocytic leukemia, unspecified, not having achieved remission**
Monocytic leukemia, unspecified with failed remission
Monocytic leukemia, unspecified NOS
C93.91   **Monocytic leukemia, unspecified in remission**
C93.92   **Monocytic leukemia, unspecified in relapse**

④ **C94**   **Other leukemias of specified cell type**
EXCLUDES 1   *leukemic reticuloendotheliosis (C91.4-)*
myelodysplastic syndromes (D46.-)
personal history of leukemia (Z85.6)
plasma cell leukemia (C90.1-)
CODING TIP ✓   Terms such as "in remission" and "in relapse" must be specified by the physician in order to indicate assignment of a code specifying these terms. If the physician has not specified one of these terms, select the code for "not having achieved remission."

⑤ **C94.0**   **Acute erythroid leukemia**
Acute myeloid leukemia M6(a)(b)
Erythroleukemia
C94.00   **Acute erythroid leukemia, not having achieved remission**
Acute erythroid leukemia with failed remission
Acute erythroid leukemia NOS
C94.01   **Acute erythroid leukemia, in remission**
C94.02   **Acute erythroid leukemia, in relapse**

⑤ **C94.2**   **Acute megakaryoblastic leukemia**
Acute myeloid leukemia M7
Acute megakaryocytic leukemia
▲ **C94.20**   **Acute megakaryoblastic leukemia not having achieved remission**
Acute megakaryoblastic leukemia with failed remission
Acute megakaryoblastic leukemia NOS
C94.21   **Acute megakaryoblastic leukemia, in remission**
C94.22   **Acute megakaryoblastic leukemia, in relapse**

⑤ **C94.3**   **Mast cell leukemia**
C94.30   **Mast cell leukemia not having achieved remission**
Mast cell leukemia with failed remission
Mast cell leukemia NOS
C94.31   **Mast cell leukemia, in remission**
C94.32   **Mast cell leukemia, in relapse**

⑤ **C94.4**   **Acute panmyelosis with myelofibrosis**
Acute myelofibrosis
EXCLUDES 1   *myelofibrosis NOS (D75.81)*
secondary myelofibrosis NOS (D75.81)
C94.40   **Acute panmyelosis with myelofibrosis not having achieved remission**
Acute myelofibrosis NOS
Acute panmyelosis with myelofibrosis with failed remission
Acute panmyelosis NOS
C94.41   **Acute panmyelosis with myelofibrosis, in remission**

● New   ▲ Revised   *Manifestation*   ④-⑦ Digit Indicators   ⊟ Laterality   Ⓐ Adult (15+ years)   Ⓜ Maternity (12-55 years)   Ⓝ Newborn   Ⓟ Pediatric (0-17 years)   ♂ Male   ♀ Female
✖ Deleted   Unspecified   + Additional code

Neoplasms

C94.42   Acute panmyelosis with myelofibrosis, in relapse
C94.6   **Myelodysplastic disease, not classified**
    Myeloproliferative disease, not classified
⑤ C94.8   **Other specified leukemias**
    Aggressive NK-cell leukemia
    Acute basophilic leukemia
C94.80   **Other specified leukemias not having achieved remission**
    Other specified leukemia with failed remission
    Other specified leukemias NOS
C94.81   **Other specified leukemias, in remission**
C94.82   **Other specified leukemias, in relapse**

④ **C95**   **Leukemia of unspecified cell type**

> **EXCLUDES 1**   *personal history of leukemia (Z85.6)*

> **CODING TIP ✓**   Terms such as "in remission" and "in relapse" must be specified by the physician in order to indicate assignment of a code specifying these terms. If the physician has not specified one of these terms, select the code for "not having achieved remission."

Leukemia of unspecified cell type

Leukemia begins in a cell in the bone marrow. The cell undergoes a leukemic change and it multiplies into many cells. The leukemia cells grow and survive better than normal cells and eventually crowd out the normal cells.

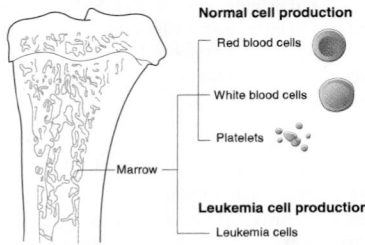

Normal cell production
— Red blood cells
— White blood cells
— Platelets
Marrow
Leukemia cell production
— Leukemia cells

⑤ C95.0   **Acute leukemia of unspecified cell type**
    Acute bilineal leukemia
    Acute mixed lineage leukemia
    Biphenotypic acute leukemia
    Stem cell leukemia of unclear lineage

> **EXCLUDES 1**   *acute exacerbation of unspecified chronic leukemia (C95.10)*

C95.00   **Acute leukemia of unspecified cell type not having achieved remission**
    Acute leukemia of unspecified cell type with failed remission
    Acute leukemia NOS
C95.01   **Acute leukemia of unspecified cell type, in remission**
C95.02   **Acute leukemia of unspecified cell type, in relapse**

⑤ C95.1   **Chronic leukemia of unspecified cell type**
C95.10   **Chronic leukemia of unspecified cell type not having achieved remission**
    Chronic leukemia of unspecified cell type with failed remission
    Chronic leukemia NOS
C95.11   **Chronic leukemia of unspecified cell type, in remission**
C95.12   **Chronic leukemia of unspecified cell type, in relapse**

⑤ C95.9   **Leukemia, unspecified**
C95.90   **Leukemia, unspecified not having achieved remission**
    Leukemia, unspecified with failed remission
    Leukemia NOS
C95.91   **Leukemia, unspecified, in remission**
C95.92   **Leukemia, unspecified, in relapse**

④ **C96**   **Other and unspecified malignant neoplasms of lymphoid, hematopoietic and related tissue**

> **EXCLUDES 1**   *personal history of other malignant neoplasms of lymphoid, hematopoietic and related tissues (Z85.79)*

C96.0   **Multifocal and multisystemic (disseminated) Langerhans-cell histiocytosis**
    Histiocytosis X, multisystemic
    Letterer-Siwe disease

> **EXCLUDES 1**   *adult pulmonary Langerhans cell histiocytosis (J84.82)*
> *multifocal and unisystemic Langerhans-cell histiocytosis (C96.5)*
> *unifocal Langerhans-cell histiocytosis (C96.6)*

C96.2   **Malignant mast cell tumor**
    Aggressive systemic mastocytosis
    Mast cell sarcoma

> **EXCLUDES 1**   *indolent mastocytosis (D47.0)*
> *mast cell leukemia (C94.30)*
> *mastocytosis (congenital) (cutaneous) (Q82.2)*

C96.4   **Sarcoma of dendritic cells (accessory cells)**
    Follicular dendritic cell sarcoma
    Interdigitating dendritic cell sarcoma
    Langerhans cell sarcoma

C96.5   **Multifocal and unisystemic Langerhans-cell histiocytosis**
    Hand-Schüller-Christian disease
    Histiocytosis X, multifocal

> **EXCLUDES 1**   *multifocal and multisystemic (disseminated) Langerhans-cell histiocytosis (C96.0)*
> *unifocal Langerhans-cell histiocytosis (C96.6)*

C96.6   **Unifocal Langerhans-cell histiocytosis**
    Eosinophilic granuloma
    Histiocytosis X, unifocal
    Histiocytosis X NOS
    Langerhans-cell histiocytosis NOS

> **EXCLUDES 1**   *multifocal and multisysemic (disseminated) Langerhans-cell histiocytosis (C96.0)*
> *multifocal and unisystemic Langerhans-cell histiocytosis (C96.5)*

C96.A   **Histiocytic sarcoma**
    Malignant histiocytosis
C96.Z   **Other specified malignant neoplasms of lymphoid, hematopoietic and related tissue**
C96.9   **Malignant neoplasm of lymphoid, hematopoietic and related tissue, unspecified**

In situ neoplasms (D00-D09)

> **INCLUDES**   Bowen's disease
> erythroplasia
> grade III intraepithelial neoplasia
> Queyrat's erythroplasia

> **CODING TIP ✓**   Carcinomas in situ are defined as cancer that has stayed in place in the specific location of origin and not spread to any neighboring tissue. The physician must specifically state "in situ" in order to indicate the correct assignment of any D00-D09 codes. Do not assign a code from D00-D09 unless the physician has specifically defined the malignancy as "in situ" or pre-cancerous.

④ **D00**   **Carcinoma in situ of oral cavity, esophagus and stomach**

> **EXCLUDES 1**   *melanoma in situ (D03.-)*

▲ ⑤ ✚ **D00.0**   **Carcinoma in situ of lip, oral cavity and pharynx**
    Use additional code to identify:
    exposure to environmental tobacco smoke (Z77.22)
    exposure to tobacco smoke in the perinatal period (P96.81)
    history of tobacco dependence (Z87.891)
    occupational exposure to environmental tobacco smoke (Z57.31)
    tobacco dependence (F17.-)
    tobacco use (Z72.0)

> **EXCLUDES 1**   *carcinoma in situ of aryepiglottic fold or interarytenoid fold, laryngeal aspect (D02.0)*
> *carcinoma in situ of epiglottis NOS (D02.0)*
> *carcinoma in situ of epiglottis suprahyoid portion (D02.0)*
> *carcinoma in situ of skin of lip (D03.0, D04.0)*

✚ D00.00   **Carcinoma in situ of oral cavity, unspecified site**
✚ D00.01   **Carcinoma in situ of labial mucosa and vermilion border**
✚ D00.02   **Carcinoma in situ of buccal mucosa**

● New   ▲ Revised   *Manifestation*   ④-⑦ Digit Indicators   ▤ Laterality   Ⓐ Adult (15+ years)   Ⓜ Maternity (12-55 years)   Ⓝ Newborn   Ⓟ Pediatric (0-17 years)   ♂ Male   ♀ Female
✖ ~~Deleted~~   Unspecified   ✚ Additional code

492   © 2017 DecisionHealth   2017 ICD-10-CM Expert for Physicians

+ D00.03 Carcinoma in situ of gingiva and edentulous alveolar ridge

+ D00.04 Carcinoma in situ of soft palate

+ D00.05 Carcinoma in situ of hard palate

+ D00.06 Carcinoma in situ of floor of mouth

+ D00.07 Carcinoma in situ of tongue

+ D00.08 Carcinoma in situ of pharynx
Carcinoma in situ of aryepiglottic fold NOS
Carcinoma in situ of hypopharyngeal aspect of aryepiglottic fold
Carcinoma in situ of marginal zone of aryepiglottic fold

D00.1 Carcinoma in situ of esophagus

D00.2 Carcinoma in situ of stomach

⬜ D01 Carcinoma in situ of other and unspecified digestive organs

> **EXCLUDES 1**   *melanoma in situ (D03.-)*

D01.0 Carcinoma in situ of colon

> **EXCLUDES 1**   *carcinoma in situ of rectosigmoid junction (D01.1)*

D01.1 Carcinoma in situ of rectosigmoid junction

D01.2 Carcinoma in situ of rectum

▲ D01.3 Carcinoma in situ of anus and anal canal
Anal intraepithelial neoplasia III [AIN III]
Severe dysplasia of anus

> **EXCLUDES 1**   *anal intraepithelial neoplasia I and II [AIN I and AIN II] (K62.82)*
> *carcinoma in situ of anal margin (D04.5)*
> *carcinoma in situ of anal skin (D04.5)*
> *carcinoma in situ of perianal skin (D04.5)*

⑤ D01.4 Carcinoma in situ of other and unspecified parts of intestine

> **EXCLUDES 1**   *carcinoma in situ of ampulla of Vater (D01.5)*

D01.40 Carcinoma in situ of unspecified part of intestine

D01.49 Carcinoma in situ of other parts of intestine

D01.5 Carcinoma in situ of liver, gallbladder and bile ducts
Carcinoma in situ of ampulla of Vater

D01.7 Carcinoma in situ of other specified digestive organs
Carcinoma in situ of pancreas

D01.9 Carcinoma in situ of digestive organ, unspecified

▲ ⬜ + D02 Carcinoma in situ of middle ear and respiratory system
Use additional code to identify:
exposure to environmental tobacco smoke (Z77.22)
exposure to tobacco smoke in the perinatal period (P96.81)
history of tobacco dependence (Z87.891)
occupational exposure to environmental tobacco smoke (Z57.31)
tobacco dependence (F17.-)
tobacco use (Z72.0)

> **EXCLUDES 1**   *melanoma in situ (D03.-)*

+ D02.0 Carcinoma in situ of larynx
Carcinoma in situ of aryepiglottic fold or interarytenoid fold, laryngeal aspect
Carcinoma in situ of epiglottis (suprahyoid portion)

> **EXCLUDES 1**   *carcinoma in situ of aryepiglottic fold or interarytenoid fold NOS (D00.08)*
> *carcinoma in situ of hypopharyngeal aspect (D00.08)*
> *carcinoma in situ of marginal zone (D00.08)*

+ D02.1 Carcinoma in situ of trachea

⑤ + D02.2 Carcinoma in situ of bronchus and lung

⊟ + D02.20 Carcinoma in situ of unspecified bronchus and lung

⊟ + D02.21 Carcinoma in situ of right bronchus and lung

⊟ + D02.22 Carcinoma in situ of left bronchus and lung

+ D02.3 Carcinoma in situ of other parts of respiratory system
Carcinoma in situ of accessory sinuses
Carcinoma in situ of middle ear
Carcinoma in situ of nasal cavities

> **EXCLUDES 1**   *carcinoma in situ of ear (external) (skin) (D04.2-)*
> *carcinoma in situ of nose NOS D09.8*
> *carcinoma in situ of skin of nose (D04.3)*

+ D02.4 Carcinoma in situ of respiratory system, unspecified

⬜ D03 Melanoma in situ

D03.0 Melanoma in situ of lip

⑤ D03.1 Melanoma in situ of eyelid, including canthus

⊟ D03.10 Melanoma in situ of unspecified eyelid, including canthus

⊟ D03.11 Melanoma in situ of right eyelid, including canthus

⊟ D03.12 Melanoma in situ of left eyelid, including canthus

⑤ D03.2 Melanoma in situ of ear and external auricular canal

⊟ D03.20 Melanoma in situ of unspecified ear and external auricular canal

⊟ D03.21 Melanoma in situ of right ear and external auricular canal

⊟ D03.22 Melanoma in situ of left ear and external auricular canal

⑤ D03.3 Melanoma in situ of other and unspecified parts of face

D03.30 Melanoma in situ of unspecified part of face

D03.39 Melanoma in situ of other parts of face

D03.4 Melanoma in situ of scalp and neck

⑤ D03.5 Melanoma in situ of trunk

D03.51 Melanoma in situ of anal skin
Melanoma in situ of anal margin
Melanoma in situ of perianal skin

D03.52 Melanoma in situ of breast (skin) (soft tissue)

D03.59 Melanoma in situ of other part of trunk

⑤ D03.6 Melanoma in situ of upper limb, including shoulder

⊟ D03.60 Melanoma in situ of unspecified upper limb, including shoulder

⊟ D03.61 Melanoma in situ of right upper limb, including shoulder

⊟ D03.62 Melanoma in situ of left upper limb, including shoulder

⑤ D03.7 Melanoma in situ of lower limb, including hip

⊟ D03.70 Melanoma in situ of unspecified lower limb, including hip

⊟ D03.71 Melanoma in situ of right lower limb, including hip

⊟ D03.72 Melanoma in situ of left lower limb, including hip

D03.8 Melanoma in situ of other sites
Melanoma in situ of scrotum

> **EXCLUDES 1**   *carcinoma in situ of scrotum (D07.61)*

D03.9 Melanoma in situ, unspecified

⬜ D04 Carcinoma in situ of skin

> **EXCLUDES 1**   *erythroplasia of Queyrat (penis) NOS (D07.4)*
> *melanoma in situ (D03.-)*

D04.0 Carcinoma in situ of skin of lip

> **EXCLUDES 1**   *carcinoma in situ of vermilion border of lip (D00.01)*

⑤ D04.1 Carcinoma in situ of skin of eyelid, including canthus

⊟ D04.10 Carcinoma in situ of skin of unspecified eyelid, including canthus

---

Carcinoma in situ of skin; eyelid

Early stage of skin cancer that is confined to the epidermis and has not invaded the deeper tissue of the dermis

---

⊟ D04.11 Carcinoma in situ of skin of right eyelid, including canthus

⊟ D04.12 Carcinoma in situ of skin of left eyelid, including canthus

⑤ D04.2 Carcinoma in situ of skin of ear and external auricular canal

⊟ D04.20 Carcinoma in situ of skin of unspecified ear and external auricular canal

⊟ D04.21 Carcinoma in situ of skin of right ear and external auricular canal

---

● New   ▲ Revised   *Manifestation*   ⬜-⑦ Digit Indicators   ⊟ Laterality   Ⓐ Adult (15+ years)   Ⓜ Maternity (12-55 years)   Ⓝ Newborn   Ⓟ Pediatric (0-17 years)   ♂ Male   ♀ Female
✖ ~~Deleted~~   Unspecified   + Additional code

Neoplasms

- ⊟ **D04.22**   Carcinoma in situ of skin of left ear and external auricular canal
- ⑤ **D04.3**   Carcinoma in situ of skin of other and unspecified parts of face
  - **D04.30**   Carcinoma in situ of skin of unspecified part of face
  - **D04.39**   Carcinoma in situ of skin of other parts of face
- **D04.4**   Carcinoma in situ of skin of scalp and neck
- **D04.5**   Carcinoma in situ of skin of trunk
  - Carcinoma in situ of anal margin
  - Carcinoma in situ of anal skin
  - Carcinoma in situ of perianal skin
  - Carcinoma in situ of skin of breast
  - **EXCLUDES 1**   *carcinoma in situ of anus NOS (D01.3)*
    - *carcinoma in situ of scrotum (D07.61)*
    - *carcinoma in situ of skin of genital organs (D07.-)*
- ⑤ **D04.6**   Carcinoma in situ of skin of upper limb, including shoulder
  - ⊟ **D04.60**   Carcinoma in situ of skin of unspecified upper limb, including shoulder
  - ⊟ **D04.61**   Carcinoma in situ of skin of right upper limb, including shoulder
  - ⊟ **D04.62**   Carcinoma in situ of skin of left upper limb, including shoulder
- ⑤ **D04.7**   Carcinoma in situ of skin of lower limb, including hip
  - ⊟ **D04.70**   Carcinoma in situ of skin of unspecified lower limb, including hip
  - ⊟ **D04.71**   Carcinoma in situ of skin of right lower limb, including hip
  - ⊟ **D04.72**   Carcinoma in situ of skin of left lower limb, including hip
- **D04.8**   Carcinoma in situ of skin of other sites
- **D04.9**   Carcinoma in situ of skin, unspecified
- ④ **D05**   Carcinoma in situ of breast
  - **EXCLUDES 1**   *carcinoma in situ of skin of breast (D04.5)*
    - *melanoma in situ of breast (skin) (D03.5)*
    - *Paget's disease of breast or nipple (C50.-)*
  - ⑤ **D05.0**   Lobular carcinoma in situ of breast
    - ⊟ **D05.00**   Lobular carcinoma in situ of unspecified breast
    - ⊟ **D05.01**   Lobular carcinoma in situ of right breast
    - ⊟ **D05.02**   Lobular carcinoma in situ of left breast
  - ⑤ **D05.1**   Intraductal carcinoma in situ of breast
    - ⊟ **D05.10**   Intraductal carcinoma in situ of unspecified breast
    - ⊟ **D05.11**   Intraductal carcinoma in situ of right breast
    - ⊟ **D05.12**   Intraductal carcinoma in situ of left breast
  - ⑤ **D05.8**   Other specified type of carcinoma in situ of breast
    - ⊟ **D05.80**   Other specified type of carcinoma in situ of unspecified breast
    - ⊟ **D05.81**   Other specified type of carcinoma in situ of right breast
    - ⊟ **D05.82**   Other specified type of carcinoma in situ of left breast
  - ⑤ **D05.9**   Unspecified type of carcinoma in situ of breast
    - ⊟ **D05.90**   Unspecified type of carcinoma in situ of unspecified breast
    - ⊟ **D05.91**   Unspecified type of carcinoma in situ of right breast
    - ⊟ **D05.92**   Unspecified type of carcinoma in situ of left breast
- ④ **D06**   Carcinoma in situ of cervix uteri
  - **INCLUDES**   cervical adenocarcinoma in situ
    - cervical intraepithelial glandular neoplasia
    - cervical intraepithelial neoplasia III [CIN III]
    - severe dysplasia of cervix uteri
  - **EXCLUDES 1**   *cervical intraepithelial neoplasia II [CIN II] (N87.1)*
    - *cytologic evidence of malignancy of cervix without histologic confirmation (R87.614)*
    - *high grade squamous intraepithelial lesion (HGSIL) of cervix (R87.613)*
    - *melanoma in situ of cervix (D03.5)*
    - *moderate cervical dysplasia (N87.1)*
  - **D06.0**   Carcinoma in situ of endocervix   ♀
  - **D06.1**   Carcinoma in situ of exocervix   ♀
  - **D06.7**   Carcinoma in situ of other parts of cervix   ♀
  - **D06.9**   Carcinoma in situ of cervix, unspecified   ♀

- ④ **D07**   Carcinoma in situ of other and unspecified genital organs
  - **EXCLUDES 1**   *melanoma in situ of trunk (D03.5)*
  - **D07.0**   Carcinoma in situ of endometrium   ♀
  - **D07.1**   Carcinoma in situ of vulva   ♀
    - Severe dysplasia of vulva
    - Vulvar intraepithelial neoplasia III [VIN III]
    - **EXCLUDES 1**   *moderate dysplasia of vulva (N90.1)*
      - *vulvar intraepithelial neoplasia II [VIN II] (N90.1)*
  - **D07.2**   Carcinoma in situ of vagina   ♀
    - Severe dysplasia of vagina
    - Vaginal intraepithelial neoplasia III [VAIN III]
    - **EXCLUDES 1**   *moderate dysplasia of vagina (N89.1)*
      - *vaginal intraepithelial neoplasia II [VIN II] (N89.1)*
  - ⑤ **D07.3**   Carcinoma in situ of other and unspecified female genital organs
    - **D07.30**   Carcinoma in situ of unspecified female genital organs   ♀
    - **D07.39**   Carcinoma in situ of other female genital organs   ♀
  - **D07.4**   Carcinoma in situ of penis   ♂
    - Erythroplasia of Queyrat NOS
  - ▲ **D07.5**   Carcinoma in situ of prostate   ♂
    - Prostatic intraepithelial neoplasia III (PIN III)
    - Severe dysplasia of prostate
    - **EXCLUDES 1**   *dysplasia (mild) (moderate) of prostate (N42.3-)*
      - *prostatic intraepithelial neoplasia II [PIN II] (N42.3-)*
  - ⑤ **D07.6**   Carcinoma in situ of other and unspecified male genital organs
    - **D07.60**   Carcinoma in situ of unspecified male genital organs   ♂
    - **D07.61**   Carcinoma in situ of scrotum   ♂
    - **D07.69**   Carcinoma in situ of other male genital organs   ♂
- ④ **D09**   Carcinoma in situ of other and unspecified sites
  - **EXCLUDES 1**   *melanoma in situ (D03.-)*
  - **D09.0**   Carcinoma in situ of bladder
  - ⑤ **D09.1**   Carcinoma in situ of other and unspecified urinary organs
    - **D09.10**   Carcinoma in situ of unspecified urinary organ
    - **D09.19**   Carcinoma in situ of other urinary organs
  - ⑤ **D09.2**   Carcinoma in situ of eye
    - **EXCLUDES 1**   *carcinoma in situ of skin of eyelid (D04.1-)*
    - ⊟ **D09.20**   Carcinoma in situ of unspecified eye
    - ⊟ **D09.21**   Carcinoma in situ of right eye
    - ⊟ **D09.22**   Carcinoma in situ of left eye
  - **D09.3**   Carcinoma in situ of thyroid and other endocrine glands
    - **EXCLUDES 1**   *carcinoma in situ of endocrine pancreas (D01.7)*
      - *carcinoma in situ of ovary (D07.39)*
      - *carcinoma in situ of testis (D07.69)*
  - **D09.8**   Carcinoma in situ of other specified sites
  - **D09.9**   Carcinoma in situ, unspecified

Benign neoplasms, except benign neuroendocrine tumors (D10-D36)

- ④ **D10**   Benign neoplasm of mouth and pharynx
  - **D10.0**   Benign neoplasm of lip
    - Benign neoplasm of lip (frenulum) (inner aspect) (mucosa) (vermilion border)
    - **EXCLUDES 1**   *benign neoplasm of skin of lip (D22.0, D23.0)*
  - **D10.1**   Benign neoplasm of tongue
    - Benign neoplasm of lingual tonsil
  - **D10.2**   Benign neoplasm of floor of mouth
  - ▲ ⑤ **D10.3**   Benign neoplasm of other and unspecified parts of mouth
    - **D10.30**   Benign neoplasm of unspecified part of mouth

---

● New   ▲ Revised   *Manifestation*   ④-⑦ Digit Indicators   ⊟ Laterality   Ⓐ Adult (15+ years)   Ⓜ Maternity (12-55 years)   Ⓝ Newborn   Ⓟ Pediatric (0-17 years)   ♂ Male   ♀ Female

✖ Deleted   Unspecified   + Additional code

494   © 2017 DecisionHealth   2017 ICD-10-CM Expert for Physicians

D10.39 Benign neoplasm of other parts of mouth
Benign neoplasm of minor salivary gland NOS
> EXCLUDES 1   *benign odontogenic neoplasms*
> *(D16.4-D16.5)*
> *benign neoplasm of mucosa of lip*
> *(D10.0)*
> *benign neoplasm of nasopharyngeal*
> *surface of soft palate (D10.6)*

D10.4 Benign neoplasm of tonsil
Benign neoplasm of tonsil (faucial) (palatine)
> EXCLUDES 1   *benign neoplasm of lingual tonsil (D10.1)*
> *benign neoplasm of pharyngeal tonsil*
> *(D10.6)*
> *benign neoplasm of tonsillar fossa (D10.5)*
> *benign neoplasm of tonsillar pillars (D10.5)*

D10.5 Benign neoplasm of other parts of oropharynx
Benign neoplasm of epiglottis, anterior aspect
Benign neoplasm of tonsillar fossa
Benign neoplasm of tonsillar pillars
Benign neoplasm of vallecula
> EXCLUDES 1   *benign neoplasm of epiglottis NOS (D14.1)*
> *benign neoplasm of epiglottis, suprahyoid*
> *portion (D14.1)*

D10.6 Benign neoplasm of nasopharynx
Benign neoplasm of pharyngeal tonsil
Benign neoplasm of posterior margin of septum and choanae

D10.7 Benign neoplasm of hypopharynx

D10.9 Benign neoplasm of pharynx, unspecified

D11 Benign neoplasm of major salivary glands
> EXCLUDES 1   *benign neoplasms of specified minor salivary*
> *glands which are classified according to their*
> *anatomical location*
> *benign neoplasms of minor salivary glands NOS*
> *(D10.39)*

D11.0 Benign neoplasm of parotid gland

D11.7 Benign neoplasm of other major salivary glands
Benign neoplasm of sublingual salivary gland
Benign neoplasm of submandibular salivary gland

D11.9 Benign neoplasm of major salivary gland, unspecified

D12 Benign neoplasm of colon, rectum, anus and anal canal
> EXCLUDES 1   *benign carcinoid tumors of the large intestine,*
> *and rectum (D3A.02-)*

> CODING TIP ✓   Adenomatous polyps are coded to D12.
> Hyperplastic polyps are coded to K63.5.

D12.0 Benign neoplasm of cecum
Benign neoplasm of ileocecal valve

D12.1 Benign neoplasm of appendix
> EXCLUDES 1   *benign carcinoid tumor of the appendix*
> *(D3A.020)*

D12.2 Benign neoplasm of ascending colon

D12.3 Benign neoplasm of transverse colon
Benign neoplasm of hepatic flexure
Benign neoplasm of splenic flexure

D12.4 Benign neoplasm of descending colon
AHA: 2Q 2015, 14

D12.5 Benign neoplasm of sigmoid colon

D12.6 Benign neoplasm of colon, unspecified
Adenomatosis of colon
Benign neoplasm of large intestine NOS
Polyposis (hereditary) of colon
> EXCLUDES 1   *inflammatory polyp of colon (K51.4-)*
> *polyp of colon NOS (K63.5)*

D12.7 Benign neoplasm of rectosigmoid junction

D12.8 Benign neoplasm of rectum
> EXCLUDES 1   *benign carcinoid tumor of the rectum*
> *(D3A.026)*

D12.9 Benign neoplasm of anus and anal canal
Benign neoplasm of anus NOS
> EXCLUDES 1   *benign neoplasm of anal margin*
> *(D22.5, D23.5)*
> *benign neoplasm of anal skin*
> *(D22.5, D23.5)*
> *benign neoplasm of perianal skin*
> *(D22.5, D23.5)*

D13 Benign neoplasm of other and ill-defined parts of digestive system
> EXCLUDES 1   *benign stromal tumors of digestive system*
> *(D21.4)*

D13.0 Benign neoplasm of esophagus

D13.1 Benign neoplasm of stomach
> EXCLUDES 1   *benign carcinoid tumor of the stomach*
> *(D3A.092)*

D13.2 Benign neoplasm of duodenum
> EXCLUDES 1   *benign carcinoid tumor of the duodenum*
> *(D3A.010)*

D13.3 Benign neoplasm of other and unspecified parts of small intestine
> EXCLUDES 1   *benign carcinoid tumors of the small*
> *intestine (D3A.01-)*
> *benign carcinoid tumor of ileocecal valve (D12.0)*

D13.30 Benign neoplasm of unspecified part of small intestine

D13.39 Benign neoplasm of other parts of small intestine

D13.4 Benign neoplasm of liver
Benign neoplasm of intrahepatic bile ducts

D13.5 Benign neoplasm of extrahepatic bile ducts

D13.6 Benign neoplasm of pancreas
> EXCLUDES 1   *benign neoplasm of endocrine pancreas*
> *(D13.7)*

+ D13.7 Benign neoplasm of endocrine pancreas
Islet cell tumor
Benign neoplasm of islets of Langerhans
Use additional code to identify any functional activity.

D13.9 Benign neoplasm of ill-defined sites within the digestive system
Benign neoplasm of digestive system NOS
Benign neoplasm of intestine NOS
Benign neoplasm of spleen

D14 Benign neoplasm of middle ear and respiratory system

D14.0 Benign neoplasm of middle ear, nasal cavity and accessory sinuses
Benign neoplasm of cartilage of nose
> EXCLUDES 1   *benign neoplasm of auricular canal*
> *(external) (D22.2-, D23.2-)*
> *benign neoplasm of bone of ear (D16.4)*
> *benign neoplasm of bone of nose (D16.4)*
> *benign neoplasm of cartilage of ear (D21.0)*
> *benign neoplasm of ear (external) (skin)*
> *(D22.2-, D23.2-)*
> *benign neoplasm of nose NOS (D36.7)*
> *benign neoplasm of skin of nose*
> *(D22.39, D23.39)*
> *benign neoplasm of olfactory bulb (D33.3)*
> *benign neoplasm of posterior margin of*
> *septum and choanae (D10.6)*
> *polyp of accessory sinus (J33.8)*
> *polyp of ear (middle) (H74.4)*
> *polyp of nasal (cavity) (J33.-)*

D14.1 Benign neoplasm of larynx
Adenomatous polyp of larynx
Benign neoplasm of epiglottis (suprahyoid portion)
> EXCLUDES 1   *benign neoplasm of epiglottis, anterior*
> *aspect (D10.5)*
> *polyp (nonadenomatous) of vocal cord or*
> *larynx (J38.1)*

D14.2 Benign neoplasm of trachea

D14.3 Benign neoplasm of bronchus and lung
> EXCLUDES 1   *benign carcinoid tumor of the bronchus and*
> *lung (D3A.090)*

D14.30 Benign neoplasm of unspecified bronchus and lung

D14.31 Benign neoplasm of right bronchus and lung

D14.32 Benign neoplasm of left bronchus and lung

D14.4 Benign neoplasm of respiratory system, unspecified

D15 Benign neoplasm of other and unspecified intrathoracic organs
> EXCLUDES 1   *benign neoplasm of mesothelial tissue (D19.-)*

D15.0 Benign neoplasm of thymus
> EXCLUDES 1   *benign carcinoid tumor of the thymus*
> *(D3A.091)*

D15.1 Benign neoplasm of heart
> EXCLUDES 1   *benign neoplasm of great vessels (D21.3)*

D15.2 Benign neoplasm of mediastinum

D15.7 Benign neoplasm of other specified intrathoracic organs

D15.9 Benign neoplasm of intrathoracic organ, unspecified

● New   ▲ Revised   *Manifestation*   ◪-◿ Digit Indicators   ⊟ Laterality   Ⓐ Adult (15+ years)   Ⓜ Maternity (12-55 years)   Ⓝ Newborn   Ⓟ Pediatric (0-17 years)   ♂ Male   ♀ Female
✖ Deleted   Unspecified   + Additional code

⬣ D16   Benign neoplasm of bone and articular cartilage

> EXCLUDES 1   *benign neoplasm of connective tissue of ear (D21.0)*
> *benign neoplasm of connective tissue of eyelid (D21.0)*
> *benign neoplasm of connective tissue of larynx (D14.1)*
> *benign neoplasm of connective tissue of nose (D14.0)*
> *benign neoplasm of synovia (D21.-)*

⑤ D16.0   Benign neoplasm of scapula and long bones of upper limb

   ▤ D16.00   Benign neoplasm of scapula and long bones of unspecified upper limb

   ▤ D16.01   Benign neoplasm of scapula and long bones of right upper limb

   ▤ D16.02   Benign neoplasm of scapula and long bones of left upper limb

⑤ D16.1   Benign neoplasm of short bones of upper limb

   ▤ D16.10   Benign neoplasm of short bones of unspecified upper limb

   ▤ D16.11   Benign neoplasm of short bones of right upper limb

   ▤ D16.12   Benign neoplasm of short bones of left upper limb

⑤ D16.2   Benign neoplasm of long bones of lower limb

   ▤ D16.20   Benign neoplasm of long bones of unspecified lower limb

   ▤ D16.21   Benign neoplasm of long bones of right lower limb

   ▤ D16.22   Benign neoplasm of long bones of left lower limb

⑤ D16.3   Benign neoplasm of short bones of lower limb

   ▤ D16.30   Benign neoplasm of short bones of unspecified lower limb

   ▤ D16.31   Benign neoplasm of short bones of right lower limb

   ▤ D16.32   Benign neoplasm of short bones of left lower limb

▲ D16.4   Benign neoplasm of bones of skull and face
Benign neoplasm of maxilla (superior)
Benign neoplasm of orbital bone
Keratocyst of maxilla
Keratocystic odontogenic tumor of maxilla

> EXCLUDES 2   *benign neoplasm of lower jaw bone (D16.5)*

D16.5   Benign neoplasm of lower jaw bone
Keratocyst of mandible
Keratocystic odontogenic tumor of mandible

D16.6   Benign neoplasm of vertebral column

> EXCLUDES 1   *benign neoplasm of sacrum and coccyx (D16.8)*

D16.7   Benign neoplasm of ribs, sternum and clavicle

D16.8   Benign neoplasm of pelvic bones, sacrum and coccyx

D16.9   Benign neoplasm of bone and articular cartilage, unspecified

⬣ D17   Benign lipomatous neoplasm

D17.0   Benign lipomatous neoplasm of skin and subcutaneous tissue of head, face and neck

D17.1   Benign lipomatous neoplasm of skin and subcutaneous tissue of trunk

⑤ D17.2   Benign lipomatous neoplasm of skin and subcutaneous tissue of limb

   ▤ D17.20   Benign lipomatous neoplasm of skin and subcutaneous tissue of unspecified limb

   ▤ D17.21   Benign lipomatous neoplasm of skin and subcutaneous tissue of right arm

   ▤ D17.22   Benign lipomatous neoplasm of skin and subcutaneous tissue of left arm

   ▤ D17.23   Benign lipomatous neoplasm of skin and subcutaneous tissue of right leg

   ▤ D17.24   Benign lipomatous neoplasm of skin and subcutaneous tissue of left leg

⑤ D17.3   Benign lipomatous neoplasm of skin and subcutaneous tissue of other and unspecified sites

   D17.30   Benign lipomatous neoplasm of skin and subcutaneous tissue of unspecified sites

   D17.39   Benign lipomatous neoplasm of skin and subcutaneous tissue of other sites

D17.4   Benign lipomatous neoplasm of intrathoracic organs

D17.5   Benign lipomatous neoplasm of intra-abdominal organs

> EXCLUDES 1   *benign lipomatous neoplasm of peritoneum and retroperitoneum (D17.79)*

D17.6   Benign lipomatous neoplasm of spermatic cord   ♂

⑤ D17.7   Benign lipomatous neoplasm of other sites

   D17.71   Benign lipomatous neoplasm of kidney

D17.72   Benign lipomatous neoplasm of other genitourinary organ

D17.79   Benign lipomatous neoplasm of other sites
Benign lipomatous neoplasm of peritoneum
Benign lipomatous neoplasm of retroperitoneum

D17.9   Benign lipomatous neoplasm, unspecified
Lipoma NOS

Benign lipomatous neoplasm

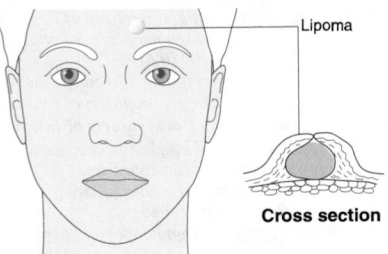

Lipoma

Cross section

⬣ D18   Hemangioma and lymphangioma, any site

> EXCLUDES 1   *benign neoplasm of glomus jugulare (D35.6)*
> *blue or pigmented nevus (D22.-)*
> *nevus NOS (D22.-)*
> *vascular nevus (Q82.5)*

⑤ D18.0   Hemangioma
Angioma NOS
Cavernous nevus

   D18.00   Hemangioma unspecified site

   D18.01   Hemangioma of skin and subcutaneous tissue

   D18.02   Hemangioma of intracranial structures

   D18.03   Hemangioma of intra-abdominal structures

   D18.09   Hemangioma of other sites

D18.1   Lymphangioma, any site

⬣ D19   Benign neoplasm of mesothelial tissue

D19.0   Benign neoplasm of mesothelial tissue of pleura

D19.1   Benign neoplasm of mesothelial tissue of peritoneum

D19.7   Benign neoplasm of mesothelial tissue of other sites

D19.9   Benign neoplasm of mesothelial tissue, unspecified
Benign mesothelioma NOS

⬣ D20   Benign neoplasm of soft tissue of retroperitoneum and peritoneum

> EXCLUDES 1   *benign lipomatous neoplasm of peritoneum and retroperitoneum (D17.79)*
> *benign neoplasm of mesothelial tissue (D19.-)*

D20.0   Benign neoplasm of soft tissue of retroperitoneum

D20.1   Benign neoplasm of soft tissue of peritoneum

● New   ▲ Revised   *Manifestation*   ⬣-⬣ Digit Indicators   ▤ Laterality   Ⓐ Adult (15+ years)   Ⓜ Maternity (12-55 years)   Ⓝ Newborn   Ⓟ Pediatric (0-17 years)   ♂ Male   ♀ Female

✖ Deleted   Unspecified   + Additional code

496   © 2017 DecisionHealth   2017 ICD-10-CM Expert for Physicians

D16 — D20.1

⁴ D21 Other benign neoplasms of connective and other soft tissue

INCLUDES
benign neoplasm of blood vessel
benign neoplasm of bursa
benign neoplasm of cartilage
benign neoplasm of fascia
benign neoplasm of fat
benign neoplasm of ligament, except uterine
benign neoplasm of lymphatic channel
benign neoplasm of muscle
benign neoplasm of synovia
benign neoplasm of tendon (sheath)
benign stromal tumors

EXCLUDES 1
benign neoplasm of articular cartilage (D16.-)
benign neoplasm of cartilage of larynx (D14.1)
benign neoplasm of cartilage of nose (D14.0)
benign neoplasm of connective tissue of breast (D24.-)
benign neoplasm of peripheral nerves and autonomic nervous system (D36.1-)
benign neoplasm of peritoneum (D20.1)
benign neoplasm of retroperitoneum (D20.0)
benign neoplasm of uterine ligament, any (D28.2)
benign neoplasm of vascular tissue (D18.-)
hemangioma (D18.0-)
lipomatous neoplasm (D17.-)
lymphangioma (D18.1)
uterine leiomyoma (D25.-)

D21.0 Benign neoplasm of connective and other soft tissue of head, face and neck
Benign neoplasm of connective tissue of ear
Benign neoplasm of connective tissue of eyelid
EXCLUDES 1 *benign neoplasm of connective tissue of orbit (D31.6-)*

⁵ D21.1 Benign neoplasm of connective and other soft tissue of upper limb, including shoulder
- **D21.10** Benign neoplasm of connective and other soft tissue of unspecified upper limb, including shoulder
- **D21.11** Benign neoplasm of connective and other soft tissue of right upper limb, including shoulder
- **D21.12** Benign neoplasm of connective and other soft tissue of left upper limb, including shoulder

⁵ D21.2 Benign neoplasm of connective and other soft tissue of lower limb, including hip
- **D21.20** Benign neoplasm of connective and other soft tissue of unspecified lower limb, including hip
- **D21.21** Benign neoplasm of connective and other soft tissue of right lower limb, including hip
- **D21.22** Benign neoplasm of connective and other soft tissue of left lower limb, including hip

D21.3 Benign neoplasm of connective and other soft tissue of thorax
Benign neoplasm of axilla
Benign neoplasm of diaphragm
Benign neoplasm of great vessels
EXCLUDES 1 *benign neoplasm of heart (D15.1)*
benign neoplasm of mediastinum (D15.2)
benign neoplasm of thymus (D15.0)

D21.4 Benign neoplasm of connective and other soft tissue of abdomen
Benign stromal tumors of abdomen

D21.5 Benign neoplasm of connective and other soft tissue of pelvis
EXCLUDES 1 *benign neoplasm of any uterine ligament (D28.2)*
uterine leiomyoma (D25.-)

D21.6 Benign neoplasm of connective and other soft tissue of trunk, unspecified
Benign neoplasm of back NOS

D21.9 Benign neoplasm of connective and other soft tissue, unspecified

⁴ D22 Melanocytic nevi
INCLUDES
atypical nevus
blue hairy pigmented nevus
nevus NOS

D22.0 Melanocytic nevi of lip

⁵ D22.1 Melanocytic nevi of eyelid, including canthus
- **D22.10** Melanocytic nevi of unspecified eyelid, including canthus
- **D22.11** Melanocytic nevi of right eyelid, including canthus
- **D22.12** Melanocytic nevi of left eyelid, including canthus

⁵ D22.2 Melanocytic nevi of ear and external auricular canal
- **D22.20** Melanocytic nevi of unspecified ear and external auricular canal
- **D22.21** Melanocytic nevi of right ear and external auricular canal
- **D22.22** Melanocytic nevi of left ear and external auricular canal

⁵ D22.3 Melanocytic nevi of other and unspecified parts of face
- **D22.30** Melanocytic nevi of unspecified part of face
- **D22.39** Melanocytic nevi of other parts of face

D22.4 Melanocytic nevi of scalp and neck

D22.5 Melanocytic nevi of trunk
Melanocytic nevi of anal margin
Melanocytic nevi of anal skin
Melanocytic nevi of perianal skin
Melanocytic nevi of skin of breast

⁵ D22.6 Melanocytic nevi of upper limb, including shoulder
- **D22.60** Melanocytic nevi of unspecified upper limb, including shoulder
- **D22.61** Melanocytic nevi of right upper limb, including shoulder
- **D22.62** Melanocytic nevi of left upper limb, including shoulder

⁵ D22.7 Melanocytic nevi of lower limb, including hip
- **D22.70** Melanocytic nevi of unspecified lower limb, including hip
- **D22.71** Melanocytic nevi of right lower limb, including hip
- **D22.72** Melanocytic nevi of left lower limb, including hip

D22.9 Melanocytic nevi, unspecified

⁴ D23 Other benign neoplasms of skin
INCLUDES
benign neoplasm of hair follicles
benign neoplasm of sebaceous glands
benign neoplasm of sweat glands
EXCLUDES 1 *benign lipomatous neoplasms of skin (D17.0-D17.3)*
melanocytic nevi (D22.-)

D23.0 Other benign neoplasm of skin of lip
EXCLUDES 1 *benign neoplasm of vermilion border of lip (D10.0)*

⁵ D23.1 Other benign neoplasm of skin of eyelid, including canthus
- **D23.10** Other benign neoplasm of skin of unspecified eyelid, including canthus
- **D23.11** Other benign neoplasm of skin of right eyelid, including canthus
- **D23.12** Other benign neoplasm of skin of left eyelid, including canthus

⁵ D23.2 Other benign neoplasm of skin of ear and external auricular canal
- **D23.20** Other benign neoplasm of skin of unspecified ear and external auricular canal
- **D23.21** Other benign neoplasm of skin of right ear and external auricular canal
- **D23.22** Other benign neoplasm of skin of left ear and external auricular canal

⁵ D23.3 Other benign neoplasm of skin of other and unspecified parts of face
- **D23.30** Other benign neoplasm of skin of unspecified part of face
- **D23.39** Other benign neoplasm of skin of other parts of face

D23.4 Other benign neoplasm of skin of scalp and neck

D23.5 Other benign neoplasm of skin of trunk
Other benign neoplasm of anal margin
Other benign neoplasm of anal skin
Other benign neoplasm of perianal skin
Other benign neoplasm of skin of breast
EXCLUDES 1 *benign neoplasm of anus NOS (D12.9)*

⁵ D23.6 Other benign neoplasm of skin of upper limb, including shoulder
- **D23.60** Other benign neoplasm of skin of unspecified upper limb, including shoulder
- **D23.61** Other benign neoplasm of skin of right upper limb, including shoulder
- **D23.62** Other benign neoplasm of skin of left upper limb, including shoulder

⁵ D23.7 Other benign neoplasm of skin of lower limb, including hip

● New ▲ Revised *Manifestation* ④-⑦ Digit Indicators Laterality Ⓐ Adult (15+ years) Ⓜ Maternity (12-55 years) Ⓝ Newborn Ⓟ Pediatric (0-17 years) ♂ Male ♀ Female
✖ Deleted Unspecified + Additional code

2017 ICD-10-CM Expert for Physicians   © 2017 DecisionHealth   497

D21 — D23.7

⊟ D23.70	Other benign neoplasm of skin of unspecified lower limb, including hip	
⊟ D23.71	Other benign neoplasm of skin of right lower limb, including hip	
⊟ D23.72	Other benign neoplasm of skin of left lower limb, including hip	
D23.9	Other benign neoplasm of skin, unspecified	

⊿ D24   Benign neoplasm of breast

INCLUDES   benign neoplasm of connective tissue of breast
benign neoplasm of soft parts of breast
fibroadenoma of breast

EXCLUDES 2   *adenofibrosis of breast (N60.2)*
benign cyst of breast (N60.-)
benign mammary dysplasia (N60.-)
benign neoplasm of skin of breast (D22.5, D23.5)
fibrocystic disease of breast (N60.-)

⊟ D24.1	Benign neoplasm of right breast	
⊟ D24.2	Benign neoplasm of left breast	
⊟ D24.9	Benign neoplasm of unspecified breast	

⊿ D25   Leiomyoma of uterus

INCLUDES   uterine fibroid
uterine fibromyoma
uterine myoma

D25.0	Submucous leiomyoma of uterus	♀
D25.1	Intramural leiomyoma of uterus	♀
	Interstitial leiomyoma of uterus	
D25.2	Subserosal leiomyoma of uterus	♀
	Subperitoneal leiomyoma of uterus	
D25.9	Leiomyoma of uterus, unspecified	♀

⊿ D26   Other benign neoplasms of uterus

D26.0	Other benign neoplasm of cervix uteri	♀
D26.1	Other benign neoplasm of corpus uteri	♀
D26.7	Other benign neoplasm of other parts of uterus	♀
D26.9	Other benign neoplasm of uterus, unspecified	♀

▲ ⊿ + D27   Benign neoplasm of ovary

Use additional code to identify any functional activity.

EXCLUDES 2   *corpus albicans cyst (N83.2-)*
corpus luteum cyst (N83.1-)
endometrial cyst (N80.1)
follicular (atretic) cyst (N83.0-)
graafian follicle cyst (N83.0-)
ovarian cyst NEC (N83.2-)
ovarian retention cyst (N83.2-)

⊟ + D27.0	Benign neoplasm of right ovary	♀
⊟ + D27.1	Benign neoplasm of left ovary	♀
⊟ + D27.9	Benign neoplasm of unspecified ovary	♀

⊿ D28   Benign neoplasm of other and unspecified female genital organs

INCLUDES   adenomatous polyp
benign neoplasm of skin of female genital organs
benign teratoma

EXCLUDES 1   *epoophoron cyst (Q50.5)*
fimbrial cyst (Q50.4)
Gartner's duct cyst (Q52.4)
parovarian cyst (Q50.5)

D28.0	Benign neoplasm of vulva	♀
D28.1	Benign neoplasm of vagina	♀
D28.2	Benign neoplasm of uterine tubes and ligaments	♀
	Benign neoplasm of fallopian tube	
	Benign neoplasm of uterine ligament (broad) (round)	
D28.7	Benign neoplasm of other specified female genital organs	♀
D28.9	Benign neoplasm of female genital organ, unspecified	♀

⊿ D29   Benign neoplasm of male genital organs

INCLUDES   benign neoplasm of skin of male genital organs

D29.0	Benign neoplasm of penis	♂
D29.1	Benign neoplasm of prostate	♂

EXCLUDES 1   *enlarged prostate (N40.-)*

⑤ + D29.2   Benign neoplasm of testis

Use additional code to identify any functional activity.

⊟ + D29.20	Benign neoplasm of unspecified testis	♂
⊟ + D29.21	Benign neoplasm of right testis	♂
⊟ + D29.22	Benign neoplasm of left testis	♂
⑤ D29.3	Benign neoplasm of epididymis	
⊟ D29.30	Benign neoplasm of unspecified epididymis	♂

⊟ D29.31	Benign neoplasm of right epididymis	♂
⊟ D29.32	Benign neoplasm of left epididymis	♂
D29.4	Benign neoplasm of scrotum	
	Benign neoplasm of skin of scrotum	
D29.8	Benign neoplasm of other specified male genital organs	♂
	Benign neoplasm of seminal vesicle	
	Benign neoplasm of spermatic cord	
	Benign neoplasm of tunica vaginalis	
D29.9	Benign neoplasm of male genital organ, unspecified	♂

⊿ D30   Benign neoplasm of urinary organs

⑤ D30.0   Benign neoplasm of kidney

EXCLUDES 1   *benign carcinoid tumor of the kidney (D3A.093)*
benign neoplasm of renal calyces (D30.1-)
benign neoplasm of renal pelvis (D30.1-)

⊟ D30.00	Benign neoplasm of unspecified kidney	
⊟ D30.01	Benign neoplasm of right kidney	
⊟ D30.02	Benign neoplasm of left kidney	

⑤ D30.1   Benign neoplasm of renal pelvis

⊟ D30.10	Benign neoplasm of unspecified renal pelvis	
⊟ D30.11	Benign neoplasm of right renal pelvis	
⊟ D30.12	Benign neoplasm of left renal pelvis	

⑤ D30.2   Benign neoplasm of ureter

EXCLUDES 1   *benign neoplasm of ureteric orifice of bladder (D30.3)*

⊟ D30.20	Benign neoplasm of unspecified ureter	
⊟ D30.21	Benign neoplasm of right ureter	
⊟ D30.22	Benign neoplasm of left ureter	
D30.3	Benign neoplasm of bladder	
	Benign neoplasm of ureteric orifice of bladder	
	Benign neoplasm of urethral orifice of bladder	
D30.4	Benign neoplasm of urethra	

EXCLUDES 1   *benign neoplasm of urethral orifice of bladder (D30.3)*

D30.8	Benign neoplasm of other specified urinary organs	
	Benign neoplasm of paraurethral glands	
D30.9	Benign neoplasm of urinary organ, unspecified	
	Benign neoplasm of urinary system NOS	

⊿ D31   Benign neoplasm of eye and adnexa

EXCLUDES 1   *benign neoplasm of connective tissue of eyelid (D21.0)*
benign neoplasm of optic nerve (D33.3)
benign neoplasm of skin of eyelid (D22.1-, D23.1-)

⑤ D31.0   Benign neoplasm of conjunctiva

⊟ D31.00	Benign neoplasm of unspecified conjunctiva	
⊟ D31.01	Benign neoplasm of right conjunctiva	
⊟ D31.02	Benign neoplasm of left conjunctiva	

⑤ D31.1   Benign neoplasm of cornea

⊟ D31.10	Benign neoplasm of unspecified cornea	
⊟ D31.11	Benign neoplasm of right cornea	
⊟ D31.12	Benign neoplasm of left cornea	

⑤ D31.2   Benign neoplasm of retina

EXCLUDES 1   *dark area on retina (D49.81)*
hemangioma of retina (D49.81)
neoplasm of unspecified behavior of retina and choroid (D49.81)
retinal freckle (D49.81)

⊟ D31.20	Benign neoplasm of unspecified retina	
⊟ D31.21	Benign neoplasm of right retina	
⊟ D31.22	Benign neoplasm of left retina	

⑤ D31.3   Benign neoplasm of choroid

⊟ D31.30	Benign neoplasm of unspecified choroid	
⊟ D31.31	Benign neoplasm of right choroid	
⊟ D31.32	Benign neoplasm of left choroid	

⑤ D31.4   Benign neoplasm of ciliary body

⊟ D31.40	Benign neoplasm of unspecified ciliary body	
⊟ D31.41	Benign neoplasm of right ciliary body	
⊟ D31.42	Benign neoplasm of left ciliary body	

⑤ D31.5   Benign neoplasm of lacrimal gland and duct

Benign neoplasm of lacrimal sac
Benign neoplasm of nasolacrimal duct

⊟ D31.50	Benign neoplasm of unspecified lacrimal gland and duct	

● New	▲ Revised	*Manifestation*	⊿-⑦ Digit Indicators	⊟ Laterality	Ⓐ Adult (15+ years)	Ⓜ Maternity (12-55 years)	Ⓝ Newborn	Ⓟ Pediatric (0-17 years)	♂ Male	♀ Female
✖ Deleted		Unspecified	+ Additional code		

☐ **D31.51** **Benign neoplasm of right lacrimal gland and duct**
☐ **D31.52** **Benign neoplasm of left lacrimal gland and duct**
☐ **D31.6** **Benign neoplasm of unspecified site of orbit**
Benign neoplasm of connective tissue of orbit
Benign neoplasm of extraocular muscle
Benign neoplasm of peripheral nerves of orbit
Benign neoplasm of retrobulbar tissue
Benign neoplasm of retro-ocular tissue
EXCLUDES 1 *benign neoplasm of orbital bone (D16.4)*

☐ **D31.60** **Benign neoplasm of unspecified site of unspecified orbit**
☐ **D31.61** **Benign neoplasm of unspecified site of right orbit**
☐ **D31.62** **Benign neoplasm of unspecified site of left orbit**
☐ **D31.9** **Benign neoplasm of unspecified part of eye**
Benign neoplasm of eyeball
☐ **D31.90** **Benign neoplasm of unspecified part of unspecified eye**
☐ **D31.91** **Benign neoplasm of unspecified part of right eye**
☐ **D31.92** **Benign neoplasm of unspecified part of left eye**
4 **D32** **Benign neoplasm of meninges**
D32.0 **Benign neoplasm of cerebral meninges**
D32.1 **Benign neoplasm of spinal meninges**
D32.9 **Benign neoplasm of meninges, unspecified**
Meningioma NOS
4 **D33** **Benign neoplasm of brain and other parts of central nervous system**
EXCLUDES 1 *angioma (D18.0-)*
benign neoplasm of meninges (D32.-)
benign neoplasm of peripheral nerves and
autonomic nervous system (D36.1-)
hemangioma (D18.0-)
neurofibromatosis (Q85.0-)
retro-ocular benign neoplasm (D31.6-)

D33.0 **Benign neoplasm of brain, supratentorial**
Benign neoplasm of cerebral ventricle
Benign neoplasm of cerebrum
Benign neoplasm of frontal lobe
Benign neoplasm of occipital lobe
Benign neoplasm of parietal lobe
Benign neoplasm of temporal lobe
EXCLUDES 1 *benign neoplasm of fourth ventricle (D33.1)*

D33.1 **Benign neoplasm of brain, infratentorial**
Benign neoplasm of brain stem
Benign neoplasm of cerebellum
Benign neoplasm of fourth ventricle
D33.2 **Benign neoplasm of brain, unspecified**
D33.3 **Benign neoplasm of cranial nerves**
Benign neoplasm of olfactory bulb
D33.4 **Benign neoplasm of spinal cord**
D33.7 **Benign neoplasm of other specified parts of central nervous system**
D33.9 **Benign neoplasm of central nervous system, unspecified**
Benign neoplasm of nervous system (central) NOS
+ **D34** **Benign neoplasm of thyroid gland**
Use additional code to identify any functional activity
4 + **D35** **Benign neoplasm of other and unspecified endocrine glands**
Use additional code to identify any functional activity
EXCLUDES 1 *benign neoplasm of endocrine pancreas (D13.7)*
benign neoplasm of ovary (D27.-)
benign neoplasm of testis (D29.2.-)
benign neoplasm of thymus (D15.0)
☐ + **D35.0** **Benign neoplasm of adrenal gland**
☐ + **D35.00** **Benign neoplasm of unspecified adrenal gland**
☐ + **D35.01** **Benign neoplasm of right adrenal gland**
☐ + **D35.02** **Benign neoplasm of left adrenal gland**
+ **D35.1** **Benign neoplasm of parathyroid gland**
+ **D35.2** **Benign neoplasm of pituitary gland**
AHA: 3Q 2014, 22
+ **D35.3** **Benign neoplasm of craniopharyngeal duct**
+ **D35.4** **Benign neoplasm of pineal gland**
+ **D35.5** **Benign neoplasm of carotid body**
+ **D35.6** **Benign neoplasm of aortic body and other paraganglia**
Benign tumor of glomus jugulare
+ **D35.7** **Benign neoplasm of other specified endocrine glands**

+ **D35.9** **Benign neoplasm of endocrine gland, unspecified**
Benign neoplasm of unspecified endocrine gland
4 **D36** **Benign neoplasm of other and unspecified sites**
D36.0 **Benign neoplasm of lymph nodes**
EXCLUDES 1 *lymphangioma (D18.1)*
☐ **D36.1** **Benign neoplasm of peripheral nerves and autonomic nervous system**
EXCLUDES 1 *benign neoplasm of peripheral nerves of*
orbit (D31.6-)
neurofibromatosis (Q85.0-)
D36.10 **Benign neoplasm of peripheral nerves and autonomic nervous system, unspecified**
D36.11 **Benign neoplasm of peripheral nerves and autonomic nervous system of face, head, and neck**
D36.12 **Benign neoplasm of peripheral nerves and autonomic nervous system, upper limb, including shoulder**
D36.13 **Benign neoplasm of peripheral nerves and autonomic nervous system of lower limb, including hip**
D36.14 **Benign neoplasm of peripheral nerves and autonomic nervous system of thorax**
D36.15 **Benign neoplasm of peripheral nerves and autonomic nervous system of abdomen**
D36.16 **Benign neoplasm of peripheral nerves and autonomic nervous system of pelvis**
D36.17 **Benign neoplasm of peripheral nerves and autonomic nervous system of trunk, unspecified**

D36.7 **Benign neoplasm of other specified sites**
Benign neoplasm of nose NOS
D36.9 **Benign neoplasm, unspecified site**

Benign neuroendocrine tumors (D3A)

4 + **D3A** **Benign neuroendocrine tumors**
Code also:
any associated multiple endocrine neoplasia [MEN] syndromes (E31.2-)
Use additional code to identify any associated endocrine
syndrome, such as:
carcinoid syndrome (E34.0)
EXCLUDES 2 *benign pancreatic islet cell tumors (D13.7)*

☐ + **D3A.0** **Benign carcinoid tumors**
+ **D3A.00** **Benign carcinoid tumor of unspecified site**
Carcinoid tumor NOS
☐ + **D3A.01** **Benign carcinoid tumors of the small intestine**
+ **D3A.010** **Benign carcinoid tumor of the duodenum**
+ **D3A.011** **Benign carcinoid tumor of the jejunum**
+ **D3A.012** **Benign carcinoid tumor of the ileum**
+ **D3A.019** **Benign carcinoid tumor of the small intestine, unspecified portion**
☐ + **D3A.02** **Benign carcinoid tumors of the appendix, large intestine, and rectum**
+ **D3A.020** **Benign carcinoid tumor of the appendix**
+ **D3A.021** **Benign carcinoid tumor of the cecum**
+ **D3A.022** **Benign carcinoid tumor of the ascending colon**
+ **D3A.023** **Benign carcinoid tumor of the transverse colon**
+ **D3A.024** **Benign carcinoid tumor of the descending colon**
+ **D3A.025** **Benign carcinoid tumor of the sigmoid colon**
+ **D3A.026** **Benign carcinoid tumor of the rectum**
+ **D3A.029** **Benign carcinoid tumor of the large intestine, unspecified portion**
Benign carcinoid tumor of the colon NOS
☐ + **D3A.09** **Benign carcinoid tumors of other sites**
+ **D3A.090** **Benign carcinoid tumor of the bronchus and lung**
+ **D3A.091** **Benign carcinoid tumor of the thymus**
+ **D3A.092** **Benign carcinoid tumor of the stomach**
+ **D3A.093** **Benign carcinoid tumor of the kidney**
▲ + **D3A.094** **Benign carcinoid tumor of the foregut, unspecified**
▲ + **D3A.095** **Benign carcinoid tumor of the midgut, unspecified**

● New ▲ Revised *Manifestation* 4-7 Digit Indicators ☐ Laterality A Adult (15+ years) M Maternity (12-55 years) N Newborn P Pediatric (0-17 years) ♂ Male ♀ Female
✖ Deleted Unspecified + Additional code

2017 ICD-10-CM Expert for Physicians

© 2017 DecisionHealth

499

D31.51 — D3A.095

Neoplasms

▲ + **D3A.096** **Benign carcinoid tumor of the hindgut, unspecified**

+ **D3A.098** **Benign carcinoid tumors of other sites**

+ **D3A.8** **Other benign neuroendocrine tumors**
Neuroendocrine tumor NOS

Neoplasms of uncertain behavior, polycythemia vera and myelodysplastic syndromes (D37-D48)

Note: Categories D37-D44, and D48 classify by site neoplasms of uncertain behavior, i.e., histologic confirmation whether the neoplasm is malignant or benign cannot be made.

EXCLUDES 1 *neoplasms of unspecified behavior (D49.-)*

CODING TIP ✓ Codes classifiable to D37-D48 include tumors specifically reported as those of "uncertain behavior." This term is a specific diagnostic statement that must be reported by the physician in order to support assignment of any code from D37-D48, as these tumors include lesions whose behavior cannot be predicted.

D37 **Neoplasm of uncertain behavior of oral cavity and digestive organs**

EXCLUDES 1 *stromal tumors of uncertain behavior of digestive system (D48.1)*

D37.0 **Neoplasm of uncertain behavior of lip, oral cavity and pharynx**

EXCLUDES 1 *neoplasm of uncertain behavior of aryepiglottic fold or interarytenoid fold, laryngeal aspect (D38.0)*
neoplasm of uncertain behavior of epiglottis NOS (D38.0)
neoplasm of uncertain behavior of skin of lip (D48.5)
neoplasm of uncertain behavior of suprahyoid portion of epiglottis (D38.0)

D37.01 **Neoplasm of uncertain behavior of lip**
Neoplasm of uncertain behavior of vermilion border of lip

D37.02 **Neoplasm of uncertain behavior of tongue**

D37.03 **Neoplasm of uncertain behavior of the major salivary glands**

D37.030 **Neoplasm of uncertain behavior of the parotid salivary glands**

D37.031 **Neoplasm of uncertain behavior of the sublingual salivary glands**

D37.032 **Neoplasm of uncertain behavior of the submandibular salivary glands**

D37.039 **Neoplasm of uncertain behavior of the major salivary glands, unspecified**

D37.04 **Neoplasm of uncertain behavior of the minor salivary glands**
Neoplasm of uncertain behavior of submucosal salivary glands of lip
Neoplasm of uncertain behavior of submucosal salivary glands of cheek
Neoplasm of uncertain behavior of submucosal salivary glands of hard palate
Neoplasm of uncertain behavior of submucosal salivary glands of soft palate

D37.05 **Neoplasm of uncertain behavior of pharynx**
Neoplasm of uncertain behavior of aryepiglottic fold of pharynx NOS
Neoplasm of uncertain behavior of hypopharyngeal aspect of aryepiglottic fold of pharynx
Neoplasm of uncertain behavior of marginal zone of aryepiglottic fold of pharynx

D37.09 **Neoplasm of uncertain behavior of other specified sites of the oral cavity**

D37.1 **Neoplasm of uncertain behavior of stomach**

D37.2 **Neoplasm of uncertain behavior of small intestine**

D37.3 **Neoplasm of uncertain behavior of appendix**

D37.4 **Neoplasm of uncertain behavior of colon**

D37.5 **Neoplasm of uncertain behavior of rectum**
Neoplasm of uncertain behavior of rectosigmoid junction

D37.6 **Neoplasm of uncertain behavior of liver, gallbladder and bile ducts**
Neoplasm of uncertain behavior of ampulla of Vater

D37.8 **Neoplasm of uncertain behavior of other specified digestive organs**
Neoplasm of uncertain behavior of anal canal
Neoplasm of uncertain behavior of anal sphincter
Neoplasm of uncertain behavior of anus NOS
Neoplasm of uncertain behavior of esophagus
Neoplasm of uncertain behavior of intestine NOS
Neoplasm of uncertain behavior of pancreas

EXCLUDES 1 *neoplasm of uncertain behavior of anal margin (D48.5)*
neoplasm of uncertain behavior of anal skin (D48.5)
neoplasm of uncertain behavior of perianal skin (D48.5)

D37.9 **Neoplasm of uncertain behavior of digestive organ, unspecified**

D38 **Neoplasm of uncertain behavior of middle ear and respiratory and intrathoracic organs**

EXCLUDES 1 *neoplasm of uncertain behavior of heart (D48.7)*

D38.0 **Neoplasm of uncertain behavior of larynx**
Neoplasm of uncertain behavior of aryepiglottic fold or interarytenoid fold, laryngeal aspect
Neoplasm of uncertain behavior of epiglottis (suprahyoid portion)

EXCLUDES 1 *neoplasm of uncertain behavior of aryepiglottic fold or interarytenoid fold NOS (D37.05)*
neoplasm of uncertain behavior of hypopharyngeal aspect of aryepiglottic fold (D37.05)
neoplasm of uncertain behavior of marginal zone of aryepiglottic fold (D37.05)

D38.1 **Neoplasm of uncertain behavior of trachea, bronchus and lung**

D38.2 **Neoplasm of uncertain behavior of pleura**

D38.3 **Neoplasm of uncertain behavior of mediastinum**

D38.4 **Neoplasm of uncertain behavior of thymus**

D38.5 **Neoplasm of uncertain behavior of other respiratory organs**
Neoplasm of uncertain behavior of accessory sinuses
Neoplasm of uncertain behavior of cartilage of nose
Neoplasm of uncertain behavior of middle ear
Neoplasm of uncertain behavior of nasal cavities

EXCLUDES 1 *neoplasm of uncertain behavior of ear (external) (skin) (D48.5)*
neoplasm of uncertain behavior of nose NOS (D48.7)
neoplasm of uncertain behavior of skin of nose (D48.5)

D38.6 **Neoplasm of uncertain behavior of respiratory organ, unspecified**

D39 **Neoplasm of uncertain behavior of female genital organs**

D39.0 **Neoplasm of uncertain behavior of uterus** ♀

+ **D39.1** **Neoplasm of uncertain behavior of ovary** ♀
Use additional code to identify any functional activity.

+ **D39.10** **Neoplasm of uncertain behavior of unspecified ovary** ♀

+ **D39.11** **Neoplasm of uncertain behavior of right ovary** ♀

+ **D39.12** **Neoplasm of uncertain behavior of left ovary** ♀

D39.2 **Neoplasm of uncertain behavior of placenta** ♀
Chorioadenoma destruens
Invasive hydatidiform mole
Malignant hydatidiform mole

EXCLUDES 1 *hydatidiform mole NOS (O01.9)*

D39.8 **Neoplasm of uncertain behavior of other specified female genital organs** ♀
Neoplasm of uncertain behavior of skin of female genital organs

D39.9 **Neoplasm of uncertain behavior of female genital organ, unspecified** ♀

D40 **Neoplasm of uncertain behavior of male genital organs**

D40.0 **Neoplasm of uncertain behavior of prostate** ♂

D40.1 **Neoplasm of uncertain behavior of testis** ♂

D40.10 **Neoplasm of uncertain behavior of unspecified testis** ♂

D40.11 **Neoplasm of uncertain behavior of right testis** ♂

D40.12 **Neoplasm of uncertain behavior of left testis** ♂

● New ▲ Revised *Manifestation* 🔢-🔢 Digit Indicators ▣ Laterality Ⓐ Adult (15+ years) Ⓜ Maternity (12-55 years) Ⓝ Newborn Ⓟ Pediatric (0-17 years) ♂ Male ♀ Female
✖ Deleted Unspecified + Additional code

D40.8 Neoplasm of uncertain behavior of other specified male ♂ genital organs
Neoplasm of uncertain behavior of skin of male genital organs

D40.9 Neoplasm of uncertain behavior of male genital organ, ♂ unspecified

D41 Neoplasm of uncertain behavior of urinary organs

D41.0 Neoplasm of uncertain behavior of kidney
> EXCLUDES 1 *neoplasm of uncertain behavior of renal pelvis (D41.1-)*

D41.00 Neoplasm of uncertain behavior of unspecified kidney

D41.01 Neoplasm of uncertain behavior of right kidney

D41.02 Neoplasm of uncertain behavior of left kidney

D41.1 Neoplasm of uncertain behavior of renal pelvis

D41.10 Neoplasm of uncertain behavior of unspecified renal pelvis

D41.11 Neoplasm of uncertain behavior of right renal pelvis

D41.12 Neoplasm of uncertain behavior of left renal pelvis

D41.2 Neoplasm of uncertain behavior of ureter

D41.20 Neoplasm of uncertain behavior of unspecified ureter

D41.21 Neoplasm of uncertain behavior of right ureter

D41.22 Neoplasm of uncertain behavior of left ureter

D41.3 Neoplasm of uncertain behavior of urethra

D41.4 Neoplasm of uncertain behavior of bladder

D41.8 Neoplasm of uncertain behavior of other specified urinary organs

D41.9 Neoplasm of uncertain behavior of unspecified urinary organ

D42 Neoplasm of uncertain behavior of meninges

D42.0 Neoplasm of uncertain behavior of cerebral meninges

D42.1 Neoplasm of uncertain behavior of spinal meninges

D42.9 Neoplasm of uncertain behavior of meninges, unspecified

D43 Neoplasm of uncertain behavior of brain and central nervous system
> EXCLUDES 1 *neoplasm of uncertain behavior of peripheral nerves and autonomic nervous system (D48.2)*

D43.0 Neoplasm of uncertain behavior of brain, supratentorial
Neoplasm of uncertain behavior of cerebral ventricle
Neoplasm of uncertain behavior of cerebrum
Neoplasm of uncertain behavior of frontal lobe
Neoplasm of uncertain behavior of occipital lobe
Neoplasm of uncertain behavior of parietal lobe
Neoplasm of uncertain behavior of temporal lobe
> EXCLUDES 1 *neoplasm of uncertain behavior of fourth ventricle (D43.1)*

D43.1 Neoplasm of uncertain behavior of brain, infratentorial
Neoplasm of uncertain behavior of brain stem
Neoplasm of uncertain behavior of cerebellum
Neoplasm of uncertain behavior of fourth ventricle

D43.2 Neoplasm of uncertain behavior of brain, unspecified

D43.3 Neoplasm of uncertain behavior of cranial nerves

D43.4 Neoplasm of uncertain behavior of spinal cord

D43.8 Neoplasm of uncertain behavior of other specified parts of central nervous system

D43.9 Neoplasm of uncertain behavior of central nervous system, unspecified
Neoplasm of uncertain behavior of nervous system (central) NOS

D44 Neoplasm of uncertain behavior of endocrine glands
> EXCLUDES 1 *multiple endocrine adenomatosis (E31.2-)*
> *multiple endocrine neoplasia (E31.2-)*
> *neoplasm of uncertain behavior of endocrine pancreas (D37.8)*
> *neoplasm of uncertain behavior of ovary (D39.1-)*
> *neoplasm of uncertain behavior of testis (D40.1-)*
> *neoplasm of uncertain behavior of thymus (D38.4)*

D44.0 Neoplasm of uncertain behavior of thyroid gland

D44.1 Neoplasm of uncertain behavior of adrenal gland
Use additional code to identify any functional activity.

D44.10 Neoplasm of uncertain behavior of unspecified adrenal gland

D44.11 Neoplasm of uncertain behavior of right adrenal gland

D44.12 Neoplasm of uncertain behavior of left adrenal gland

D44.2 Neoplasm of uncertain behavior of parathyroid gland

D44.3 Neoplasm of uncertain behavior of pituitary gland
Use additional code to identify any functional activity.

D44.4 Neoplasm of uncertain behavior of craniopharyngeal duct

D44.5 Neoplasm of uncertain behavior of pineal gland

D44.6 Neoplasm of uncertain behavior of carotid body

D44.7 Neoplasm of uncertain behavior of aortic body and other paraganglia

D44.9 Neoplasm of uncertain behavior of unspecified endocrine gland

D45 Polycythemia vera
> EXCLUDES 1 *familial polycythemia (D75.0)*
> *secondary polycythemia (D75.1)*

D46 Myelodysplastic syndromes
Use additional code for adverse effect, if applicable, to identify drug (T36-T50 with fifth or sixth character 5)
> EXCLUDES 2 *drug-induced aplastic anemia (D61.1)*

D46.0 Refractory anemia without ring sideroblasts, so stated
Refractory anemia without sideroblasts, without excess of blasts

D46.1 Refractory anemia with ring sideroblasts
RARS

D46.2 Refractory anemia with excess of blasts [RAEB]

D46.20 Refractory anemia with excess of blasts, unspecified
RAEB NOS

D46.21 Refractory anemia with excess of blasts 1
RAEB 1

D46.22 Refractory anemia with excess of blasts 2
RAEB 2

D46.A Refractory cytopenia with multilineage dysplasia

D46.B Refractory cytopenia with multilineage dysplasia and ring sideroblasts
RCMD RS

D46.C Myelodysplastic syndrome with isolated del(5q) chromosomal abnormality
Myelodysplastic syndrome with 5q deletion
5q minus syndrome NOS

D46.4 Refractory anemia, unspecified

D46.Z Other myelodysplastic syndromes
> EXCLUDES 1 *chronic myelomonocytic leukemia (C93.1-)*

D46.9 Myelodysplastic syndrome, unspecified
Myelodysplasia NOS

D47 Other neoplasms of uncertain behavior of lymphoid, hematopoietic and related tissue

D47.0 Histiocytic and mast cell tumors of uncertain behavior
Indolent systemic mastocytosis
Mast cell tumor NOS
Mastocytoma NOS
> EXCLUDES 1 *malignant mast cell tumor (C96.2)*
> *mastocytosis (congenital) (cutaneous) (Q82.2)*

D47.1 Chronic myeloproliferative disease
Chronic neutrophilic leukemia
Myeloproliferative disease, unspecified
> EXCLUDES 1 *atypical chronic myeloid leukemia BCR/ABL-negative (C92.2-)*
> *chronic myeloid leukemia BCR/ABL-positive (C92.1-)*
> *myelofibrosis NOS (D75.81)*
> *myelophthisic anemia (D61.82)*
> *myelophthisis (D61.82)*
> *secondary myelofibrosis NOS (D75.81)*

D47.2 Monoclonal gammopathy
Monoclonal gammopathy of undetermined significance [MGUS]

D47.3 Essential (hemorrhagic) thrombocythemia
Essential thrombocytosis
Idiopathic hemorrhagic thrombocythemia
> DEFINITION Rare myeloproliferative disorder characterized by uncontrolled over-production of blood platelet precursor cells, leading to splenomegaly, hemorrhaging from the intestines, gums, or nose, and blood vessel thrombosis.

● New ▲ Revised *Manifestation* ◰-◷ Digit Indicators ▤ Laterality Ⓐ Adult (15+ years) Ⓜ Maternity (12-55 years) Ⓝ Newborn Ⓟ Pediatric (0-17 years) ♂ Male ♀ Female
✖ Deleted Unspecified + Additional code

2017 ICD-10-CM Expert for Physicians

© 2017 DecisionHealth 501

D47.4   Osteomyelofibrosis
Chronic idiopathic myelofibrosis
Myelofibrosis (idiopathic) (with myeloid metaplasia)
Myelosclerosis (megakaryocytic) with myeloid metaplasia
Secondary myelofibrosis in myeloproliferative disease
> **EXCLUDES 1** *acute myelofibrosis (C94.4-)*

⑤ D47.Z   Other specified neoplasms of uncertain behavior of lymphoid, hematopoietic and related tissue

D47.Z1   Post-transplant lymphoproliferative disorder (PTLD)
Code first:
complications of transplanted organs and tissue (T86.-)

● D47.Z2   Castleman disease
Code also:
if applicable human herpesvirus 8 infection (B10.89)
> **EXCLUDES 2** *Kaposi's sarcoma (C46-)*

D47.Z9   Other specified neoplasms of uncertain behavior of lymphoid, hematopoietic and related tissue
Histiocytic tumors of uncertain behavior

D47.9   Neoplasm of uncertain behavior of lymphoid, hematopoietic and related tissue, unspecified
Lymphoproliferative disease NOS

④ D48   Neoplasm of uncertain behavior of other and unspecified sites
> **EXCLUDES 1** *neurofibromatosis (nonmalignant) (Q85.0-)*

D48.0   Neoplasm of uncertain behavior of bone and articular cartilage
> **EXCLUDES 1** *neoplasm of uncertain behavior of cartilage of ear (D48.1)*
> *neoplasm of uncertain behavior of cartilage of larynx (D38.0)*
> *neoplasm of uncertain behavior of cartilage of nose (D38.5)*
> *neoplasm of uncertain behavior of connective tissue of eyelid (D48.1)*
> *neoplasm of uncertain behavior of synovia (D48.1)*

D48.1   Neoplasm of uncertain behavior of connective and other soft tissue
Neoplasm of uncertain behavior of connective tissue of ear
Neoplasm of uncertain behavior of connective tissue of eyelid
Stromal tumors of uncertain behavior of digestive system
> **EXCLUDES 1** *neoplasm of uncertain behavior of articular cartilage (D48.0)*
> *neoplasm of uncertain behavior of cartilage of larynx (D38.0)*
> *neoplasm of uncertain behavior of cartilage of nose (D38.5)*
> *neoplasm of uncertain behavior of connective tissue of breast (D48.6-)*

D48.2   Neoplasm of uncertain behavior of peripheral nerves and autonomic nervous system
> **EXCLUDES 1** *neoplasm of uncertain behavior of peripheral nerves of orbit (D48.7)*

D48.3   Neoplasm of uncertain behavior of retroperitoneum
D48.4   Neoplasm of uncertain behavior of peritoneum
D48.5   Neoplasm of uncertain behavior of skin
Neoplasm of uncertain behavior of anal margin
Neoplasm of uncertain behavior of anal skin
Neoplasm of uncertain behavior of perianal skin
Neoplasm of uncertain behavior of skin of breast
> **EXCLUDES 1** *neoplasm of uncertain behavior of anus NOS (D37.8)*
> *neoplasm of uncertain behavior of skin of genital organs (D39.8, D40.8)*
> *neoplasm of uncertain behavior of vermilion border of lip (D37.0)*

⑤ D48.6   Neoplasm of uncertain behavior of breast
Neoplasm of uncertain behavior of connective tissue of breast
Cystosarcoma phyllodes
> **EXCLUDES 1** *neoplasm of uncertain behavior of skin of breast (D48.5)*

▣ D48.60   Neoplasm of uncertain behavior of unspecified breast
▣ D48.61   Neoplasm of uncertain behavior of right breast
▣ D48.62   Neoplasm of uncertain behavior of left breast

D48.7   Neoplasm of uncertain behavior of other specified sites
Neoplasm of uncertain behavior of eye
Neoplasm of uncertain behavior of heart
Neoplasm of uncertain behavior of peripheral nerves of orbit
> **EXCLUDES 1** *neoplasm of uncertain behavior of connective tissue (D48.1)*
> *neoplasm of uncertain behavior of skin of eyelid (D48.5)*

D48.9   Neoplasm of uncertain behavior, unspecified

Neoplasms of unspecified behavior (D49)

④ D49   Neoplasms of unspecified behavior
Note: Category D49 classifies by site neoplasms of unspecified morphology and behavior. The term 'mass', unless otherwise stated, is not to be regarded as a neoplastic growth.
> **INCLUDES** 'growth' NOS
> neoplasm NOS
> new growth NOS
> tumor NOS
> **EXCLUDES 1** *neoplasms of uncertain behavior (D37-D44, D48)*

> **CODING TIP ✓** Codes classifiable to D49 include tumors that have not been defined as malignant or benign. Unspecified behavior is a specific diagnostic criteria that must be indicated in the documentation. It is not equivalent to NEC/NOS.

D49.0   Neoplasm of unspecified behavior of digestive system
> **EXCLUDES 1** *neoplasm of unspecified behavior of margin of anus (D49.2)*
> *neoplasm of unspecified behavior of perianal skin (D49.2)*
> *neoplasm of unspecified behavior of skin of anus (D49.2)*

D49.1   Neoplasm of unspecified behavior of respiratory system
▲ D49.2   Neoplasm of unspecified behavior of bone, soft tissue, and skin
> **EXCLUDES 1** *neoplasm of unspecified behavior of anal canal (D49.0)*
> *neoplasm of unspecified behavior of anus NOS (D49.0)*
> *neoplasm of unspecified behavior of bone marrow (D49.89)*
> *neoplasm of unspecified behavior of cartilage of larynx (D49.1)*
> *neoplasm of unspecified behavior of cartilage of nose (D49.1)*
> *neoplasm of unspecified behavior of connective tissue of breast (D49.3)*
> *neoplasm of unspecified behavior of skin of genital organs (D49.59)*
> *neoplasm of unspecified behavior of vermilion border of lip (D49.0)*

D49.3   Neoplasm of unspecified behavior of breast
> **EXCLUDES 1** *neoplasm of unspecified behavior of skin of breast (D49.2)*

D49.4   Neoplasm of unspecified behavior of bladder
▲ ⑤ D49.5   Neoplasm of unspecified behavior of other genitourinary organs

● ⑥ D49.51   Neoplasm of unspecified behavior of kidney
● ▣ D49.511   Neoplasm of unspecified behavior of right kidney
● ▣ D49.512   Neoplasm of unspecified behavior of left kidney
● ▣ D49.519   Neoplasm of unspecified behavior of unspecified kidney
● D49.59   Neoplasm of unspecified behavior of other genitourinary organ

D49.6   Neoplasm of unspecified behavior of brain
> **EXCLUDES 1** *neoplasm of unspecified behavior of cerebral meninges (D49.7)*
> *neoplasm of unspecified behavior of cranial nerves (D49.7)*

D49.7   Neoplasm of unspecified behavior of endocrine glands and other parts of nervous system
> **EXCLUDES 1** *neoplasm of unspecified behavior of peripheral, sympathetic, and parasympathetic nerves and ganglia (D49.2)*

● New   ▲ Revised   *Manifestation*   ④-⑦ Digit Indicators   ▣ Laterality   Ⓐ Adult (15+ years)   Ⓜ Maternity (12-55 years)   Ⓝ Newborn   Ⓟ Pediatric (0-17 years)   ♂ Male   ♀ Female
✖ ̶D̶e̶l̶e̶t̶e̶d̶   Unspecified   + Additional code

502   © 2017 DecisionHealth   2017 ICD-10-CM Expert for Physicians

D47.4 — D49.7

⑤ **D49.8** **Neoplasm of unspecified behavior of other specified sites**

    EXCLUDES 1   *neoplasm of unspecified behavior of eyelid (skin) (D49.2)*
            neoplasm of unspecified behavior of eyelid cartilage (D49.2)
            neoplasm of unspecified behavior of great vessels (D49.2)
            neoplasm of unspecified behavior of optic nerve (D49.7)

    D49.81 **Neoplasm of unspecified behavior of retina and choroid**

         Dark area on retina
         Retinal freckle

    D49.89 **Neoplasm of unspecified behavior of other specified sites**

D49.9 **Neoplasm of unspecified behavior of unspecified site**

● New   ▲ Revised   *Manifestation*   ④-⑦ Digit Indicators   ⊟ Laterality   Ⓐ Adult (15+ years)   Ⓜ Maternity (12-55 years)   Ⓝ Newborn   Ⓟ Pediatric (0-17 years)   ♂ Male   ♀ Female

✖ Deleted   Unspecified   + Additional code

2017 ICD-10-CM Expert for Physicians   © 2017 DecisionHealth   503

CHAPTER 3: DISEASES OF THE BLOOD AND BLOOD-FORMING ORGANS AND CERTAIN DISORDERS INVOLVING THE IMMUNE MECHANISM (D50-D89)

EXCLUDES 2
autoimmune disease (systemic) NOS (M35.9)
certain conditions originating in the perinatal period (P00-P96)
complications of pregnancy, childbirth and the puerperium (O00-O9A)
congenital malformations, deformations and chromosomal abnormalities (Q00-Q99)
endocrine, nutritional and metabolic diseases (E00-E88)
human immunodeficiency virus [HIV] disease (B20)
injury, poisoning and certain other consequences of external causes (S00-T88)
neoplasms (C00-D49)
symptoms, signs and abnormal clinical and laboratory findings, not elsewhere classified (R00-R94)

This chapter contains the following blocks:

D50-D53	Nutritional anemias
D55-D59	Hemolytic anemias
D60-D64	Aplastic and other anemias and other bone marrow failure syndromes
D65-D69	Coagulation defects, purpura and other hemorrhagic conditions
D70-D77	Other disorders of blood and blood-forming organs
D78	Intraoperative and postprocedural complications of the spleen
D80-D89	Certain disorders involving the immune mechanism

Nutritional anemias (D50-D53)

D50 Iron deficiency anemia

INCLUDES asiderotic anemia
hypochromic anemia

CODING TIP ✓ Do not assign codes from category D50 when the record only reports "iron deficiency" but does not specifically state "iron deficiency anemia" or "anemia due to iron deficiency." Iron deficiency (without anemia) should be coded to E61.1.

D50.0 Iron deficiency anemia secondary to blood loss (chronic)
Posthemorrhagic anemia (chronic)

EXCLUDES 1 *acute posthemorrhagic anemia (D62)*
congenital anemia from fetal blood loss (P61.3)

CODING TIP ✓ The term "chronic" is a non-essential modifier in the code title for iron deficiency anemia secondary to blood loss (chronic). When the record specifies posthemorrhagic anemia (not specified as acute), D50.0 should be assigned. No time period is specifically required for the condition.

DEFINITION Iron depletion from sustained RBC loss in long-term bleeding, often from an ulcerous lesion, causing decreased hemoglobin and insufficient tissue oxygenation.

D50.1 Sideropenic dysphagia
Kelly-Paterson syndrome
Plummer-Vinson syndrome

D50.8 Other iron deficiency anemias
Iron deficiency anemia due to inadequate dietary iron intake

CODING TIP ✓ Code D50.8 should be used to report anemia due to dietary iron deficiency.

D50.9 Iron deficiency anemia, unspecified

CODING TIP ✓ When the record specifies only "hypochromic anemia" with no cause provided, report code D50.9.

DEFINITION Insufficient stores of iron in the body causing decreased hemoglobin and a reduction in red blood cell oxygen carrying capacity.

D51 Vitamin B12 deficiency anemia

EXCLUDES 1 *vitamin B12 deficiency (E53.8)*

CODING TIP ✓ Do not assign codes from category D51 when the record only reports "vitamin B12 deficiency" but does not specifically state "vitamin B12 deficiency anemia" or "anemia due to vitamin B12 deficiency." A deficiency (without anemia) should be coded to E53.8.

Vitamin B12 deficiency anemia

Deficiency of Vitamin B12 in diet. Symptoms include loss of appetite, diarrhea, numbness and tingling in the hands and/or feet, pale skin color, and a soreness in the mouth and/or tongue

Meat, fish, dairy products, and eggs are the best sources of Vitamin B12

D51.0 Vitamin B12 deficiency anemia due to intrinsic factor deficiency
Addison anemia
Biermer anemia
Pernicious (congenital) anemia
Congenital intrinsic factor deficiency

DEFINITION Anemia due to underlying Vitamin B12 malabsorption caused by inadequate production of intrinsic factor in the gastric mucosa.

D51.1 Vitamin B12 deficiency anemia due to selective vitamin B12 malabsorption with proteinuria
Imerslund (Gräsbeck) syndrome
Megaloblastic hereditary anemia

D51.2 Transcobalamin II deficiency

D51.3 Other dietary vitamin B12 deficiency anemia
Vegan anemia

D51.8 Other vitamin B12 deficiency anemias

D51.9 Vitamin B12 deficiency anemia, unspecified

D52 Folate deficiency anemia

EXCLUDES 1 *folate deficiency without anemia (E53.8)*

DEFINITION Lack of folic acid causing large, immature, misshapen red blood cells, called megaloblasts, to form in the bone marrow.

D52.0 Dietary folate deficiency anemia
Nutritional megaloblastic anemia

+ D52.1 Drug-induced folate deficiency anemia
Use additional code for adverse effect, if applicable, to identify drug (T36-T50 with fifth or sixth character 5)

D52.8 Other folate deficiency anemias

D52.9 Folate deficiency anemia, unspecified
Folic acid deficiency anemia NOS

D53 Other nutritional anemias

INCLUDES megaloblastic anemia unresponsive to vitamin B12 or folate therapy

D53.0 Protein deficiency anemia
Amino-acid deficiency anemia
Orotaciduric anemia

EXCLUDES 1 *Lesch-Nyhan syndrome (E79.1)*

D53.1 Other megaloblastic anemias, not elsewhere classified
Megaloblastic anemia NOS

EXCLUDES 1 *Di Guglielmo's disease (C94.0)*

D53.2 Scorbutic anemia

EXCLUDES 1 *scurvy (E54)*

D53.8 Other specified nutritional anemias
Anemia associated with deficiency of copper
Anemia associated with deficiency of molybdenum
Anemia associated with deficiency of zinc

EXCLUDES 1 *nutritional deficiencies without anemia, such as:*
copper deficiency NOS (E61.0)
molybdenum deficiency NOS (E61.5)
zinc deficiency NOS (E60)

D53.9 Nutritional anemia, unspecified
Simple chronic anemia

EXCLUDES 1 *anemia NOS (D64.9)*

Hemolytic anemias (D55-D59)

◪ D55   **Anemia due to enzyme disorders**
> **EXCLUDES 1**   *drug-induced enzyme deficiency anemia (D59.2)*

D55.0   **Anemia due to glucose-6-phosphate dehydrogenase [G6PD] deficiency**
Favism
G6PD deficiency anemia

D55.1   **Anemia due to other disorders of glutathione metabolism**
Anemia (due to) enzyme deficiencies, except G6PD, related to the hexose monophosphate [HMP] shunt pathway
Anemia (due to) hemolytic nonspherocytic (hereditary), type I
> **DEFINITION**   Anemia resulting from damage or destruction of RBCs in high numbers due to insufficient glutathione, a tripeptide used by RBCs to protect against oxidative damage.

D55.2   **Anemia due to disorders of glycolytic enzymes**
Hemolytic nonspherocytic (hereditary) anemia, type II
Hexokinase deficiency anemia
Pyruvate kinase [PK] deficiency anemia
Triose-phosphate isomerase deficiency anemia
> **EXCLUDES 1**   *disorders of glycolysis not associated with anemia (E74.8)*

D55.3   **Anemia due to disorders of nucleotide metabolism**
D55.8   **Other anemias due to enzyme disorders**
D55.9   **Anemia due to enzyme disorder, unspecified**

◪ D56   **Thalassemia**
> **EXCLUDES 1**   *sickle-cell thalassemia (D57.4-)*

✚ D56.0   **Alpha thalassemia**
Alpha thalassemia major
Hemoglobin H Constant Spring
Hemoglobin H disease
Hydrops fetalis due to alpha thalassemia
Severe alpha thalassemia
Triple gene defect alpha thalassemia
Use additional code, if applicable, for hydrops fetalis due to alpha thalassemia (P56.99)
> **EXCLUDES 1**   *alpha thalassemia trait or minor (D56.3)*
> *asymptomatic alpha thalassemia (D56.3)*
> *hydrops fetalis due to isoimmunization (P56.0)*
> *hydrops fetalis not due to immune hemolysis (P83.2)*

> **DEFINITION**   Hemoglobinopathy caused by genetic decrease in alpha globin chain formation needed for normal hemoglobin A (2 alpha and 2 beta chains), forming unstable hemoglobin and leading to RBC breakage.

D56.1   **Beta thalassemia**
Beta thalassemia major
Cooley's anemia
Homozygous beta thalassemia
Severe beta thalassemia
Thalassemia intermedia
Thalassemia major
> **EXCLUDES 1**   *beta thalassemia minor (D56.3)*
> *beta thalassemia trait (D56.3)*
> *delta-beta thalassemia (D56.2)*
> *hemoglobin E-beta thalassemia (D56.5)*
> *sickle-cell beta thalassemia (D57.4-)*

> **DEFINITION**   Hemoglobinopathy caused by genetic decrease in beta globin chain formation needed for normal hemoglobin A (2 alpha and 2 beta chains), leaving insoluble alpha chain aggregates that interfere with RBC production, maturation, and membrane function.

D56.2   **Delta-beta thalassemia**
Homozygous delta-beta thalassemia
> **EXCLUDES 1**   *delta-beta thalassemia minor (D56.3)*
> *delta-beta thalassemia trait (D56.3)*

D56.3   **Thalassemia minor**
Alpha thalassemia minor
Alpha thalassemia silent carrier
Alpha thalassemia trait
Beta thalassemia minor
Beta thalassemia trait
Delta-beta thalassemia minor
Delta-beta thalassemia trait
Thalassemia trait NOS
> **EXCLUDES 1**   *alpha thalassemia (D56.0)*
> *beta thalassemia (D56.1)*
> *delta-beta thalassemia (D56.2)*
> *hemoglobin E-beta thalassemia (D56.5)*
> *sickle-cell trait (D57.3)*

> **DEFINITION**   Alpha, beta, and delta-beta hemoglobinopathies caused by small gene mutations resulting in mild signs and symptoms of anemia, or asymptomatic trait or silent carrier forms.

D56.4   **Hereditary persistence of fetal hemoglobin [HPFH]**
D56.5   **Hemoglobin E-beta thalassemia**
> **EXCLUDES 1**   *beta thalassemia (D56.1)*
> *beta thalassemia minor (D56.3)*
> *beta thalassemia trait (D56.3)*
> *delta-beta thalassemia (D56.2)*
> *delta-beta thalassemia trait (D56.3)*
> *hemoglobin E disease (D58.2)*
> *other hemoglobinopathies (D58.2)*
> *sickle-cell beta thalassemia (D57.4-)*

> **DEFINITION**   Hemoglobinopathy caused by variations in beta globin chain formation, producing unstable hemoglobin E and causing microcytic anemia, poor growth, splenomegaly, and heart failure.

D56.8   **Other thalassemias**
Dominant thalassemia
Hemoglobin C thalassemia
Mixed thalassemia
Thalassemia with other hemoglobinopathy
> **EXCLUDES 1**   *hemoglobin C disease (D58.2)*
> *hemoglobin E disease (D58.2)*
> *other hemoglobinopathies (D58.2)*
> *sickle-cell anemia (D57.-)*
> *sickle-cell thalassemia (D57.4)*

D56.9   **Thalassemia, unspecified**
Mediterranean anemia (with other hemoglobinopathy)
> **DEFINITION**   Inherited blood disease causing disruption in the normal production of hemoglobin and a high rate of red blood cell destruction.

◪ ✚ D57   **Sickle-cell disorders**
Use additional code for any associated fever (R50.81)
> **EXCLUDES 1**   *other hemoglobinopathies (D58.-)*

◖ ✚ D57.0   **Hb-SS disease with crisis**
Sickle-cell disease NOS with crisis
Hb-SS disease with vasoocclusive pain

    ✚ D57.00   **Hb-SS disease with crisis, unspecified**
> **DEFINITION**   Hereditary disease in which RBCs contain abnormal hemoglobin S, making them elongated and crescent-shaped. The fragile, sickled cells become blocked in tiny blood vessels and break apart, causing vaso-occlusive pain.

    ✚ D57.01   **Hb-SS disease with acute chest syndrome**
> **DEFINITION**   Life-threatening complication of sickle-cell disease in which blood clots form in the tiny blood vessels of the lungs with repeated episodes of bleeding from the alveoli and hemosiderin buildup.

    ✚ D57.02   **Hb-SS disease with splenic sequestration**
> **CODING TIP ✓**   Sickle cell with splenic sequestration crisis occurs when the sickle red blood cells block the blood vessels inside the spleen, preventing blood from leaving the spleen and causing splenomegaly and anemia. In Hb-SS disease a sickle cell gene "S" is inherited from each parent. Commonly called sickle cell anemia, this is the most severe form.

● New   ▲ Revised   *Manifestation*   ◪-◿ Digit Indicators   ▭ Laterality   Ⓐ Adult (15+ years)   Ⓜ Maternity (12-55 years)   Ⓝ Newborn   Ⓟ Pediatric (0-17 years)   ♂ Male   ♀ Female
✖ Deleted   Unspecified   ✚ Additional code

DEFINITION Life-threatening complication of sickle-cell disease in which sickled cells become trapped in the spleen, causing acute swelling, high fever, intense abdominal pain, jaundice, leukocytosis, and tissue infarction.

+ D57.1 **Sickle-cell disease without crisis**
Hb-SS disease without crisis
Sickle-cell anemia NOS
Sickle-cell disease NOS
Sickle-cell disorder NOS

DEFINITION Chronic, hereditary disease in which red blood cells contain abnormal hemoglobin S and are stiff and misshapen like a crescent, inhibiting blood flow through small blood vessels.

Sickle-cell disease without crisis

Normal red blood cells
Cells are compact and flexible, enabling them to squeeze through small capillaries

Sickled red blood cells
Cells are stiff and angular, causing them to become stuck in small capillaries

⑤+ D57.2 **Sickle-cell/Hb-C disease**
Hb-SC disease
Hb-S/Hb-C disease
+ D57.20 Sickle-cell/Hb-C disease without crisis
⑥+ D57.21 Sickle-cell/Hb-C disease with crisis
+ D57.211 Sickle-cell/Hb-C disease with acute chest syndrome
+ D57.212 Sickle-cell/Hb-C disease with splenic sequestration

CODING TIP ✓ Sickle cell with splenic sequestration crisis occurs when the sickle red blood cells block the blood vessels inside the spleen, preventing blood from leaving the spleen and causing splenomegaly and anemia. In Hb-C disease a sickle cell "S" gene is inhereted from one parent and a gene for abnormal hemoglobin "C" is inherited from the other parent. This is usually a milder form of SCD.

+ D57.219 **Sickle-cell/Hb-C disease with crisis, unspecified**
Sickle-cell/Hb-C disease with crisis NOS
+ D57.3 **Sickle-cell trait**
Hb-S trait
Heterozygous hemoglobin S

CODING TIP ✓ When a patient is reported only to have sickle cell "trait" but no sickle cell disease is stated, report only D57.3. A person who carries the sickle cell trait rarely exhibits any disease symptoms, but can pass the gene on.

DEFINITION Condition in which a person carries one gene for normal hemoglobin and one for abnormal hemoglobin S that sickles red blood cells, producing only mild anemia or remaining asymptomatic.

⑤+ D57.4 **Sickle-cell thalassemia**
Sickle-cell beta thalassemia
Thalassemia Hb-S disease

CODING TIP ✓ Sickle cell thalassemia is a form of sickle cell disease that affects the production of hemoglobin in red blood cells, resulting in a reduction or absence of normal hemoglobin.

+ D57.40 **Sickle-cell thalassemia without crisis**
Microdrepanocytosis
Sickle-cell thalassemia NOS

DEFINITION Inherited form of anemia, occurring mainly among people of Mediterranean descent, caused by faulty synthesis of part of the hemoglobin molecule.

⑥+ D57.41 **Sickle-cell thalassemia with crisis**
Sickle-cell thalassemia with vasoocclusive pain
+ D57.411 **Sickle-cell thalassemia with acute chest syndrome**
+ D57.412 **Sickle-cell thalassemia with splenic sequestration**
+ D57.419 **Sickle-cell thalassemia with crisis, unspecified**
Sickle-cell thalassemia with crisis NOS
⑤+ D57.8 **Other sickle-cell disorders**
Hb-SD disease
Hb-SE disease
+ D57.80 **Other sickle-cell disorders without crisis**
⑥+ D57.81 **Other sickle-cell disorders with crisis**
+ D57.811 **Other sickle-cell disorders with acute chest syndrome**
+ D57.812 **Other sickle-cell disorders with splenic sequestration**
+ D57.819 **Other sickle-cell disorders with crisis, unspecified**
Other sickle-cell disorders with crisis NOS
④ D58 **Other hereditary hemolytic anemias**
EXCLUDES 1 *hemolytic anemia of the newborn (P55.-)*

D58.0 **Hereditary spherocytosis**
Acholuric (familial) jaundice
Congenital (spherocytic) hemolytic icterus
Minkowski-Chauffard syndrome
DEFINITION Congenital form of spherocytosis with hemolytic anemia, abnormal fragility of erythrocytes, jaundice, and splenomegaly.

D58.1 **Hereditary elliptocytosis**
Elliptocytosis (congenital)
Ovalocytosis (congenital) (hereditary)
D58.2 **Other hemoglobinopathies**
Abnormal hemoglobin NOS
Congenital Heinz body anemia
Hb-C disease
Hb-D disease
Hb-E disease
Hemoglobinopathy NOS
Unstable hemoglobin hemolytic disease
EXCLUDES 1 *familial polycythemia (D75.0)*
Hb-M disease (D74.0)
hemoglobin E-beta thalassemia (D56.5)
hereditary persistence of fetal hemoglobin [HPFH] (D56.4)
high-altitude polycythemia (D75.1)
methemoglobinemia (D74.-)
other hemoglobinopathies with thalassemia (D56.8)
D58.8 **Other specified hereditary hemolytic anemias**
Stomatocytosis
D58.9 **Hereditary hemolytic anemia, unspecified**
④ D59 **Acquired hemolytic anemia**
+ D59.0 **Drug-induced autoimmune hemolytic anemia**
Use additional code for adverse effect, if applicable, to identify drug (T36-T50 with fifth or sixth character 5)
D59.1 **Other autoimmune hemolytic anemias**
Autoimmune hemolytic disease (cold type) (warm type)
Chronic cold hemagglutinin disease
Cold agglutinin disease
Cold agglutinin hemoglobinuria
Cold type (secondary) (symptomatic) hemolytic anemia
Warm type (secondary) (symptomatic) hemolytic anemia
EXCLUDES 1 *Evans syndrome (D69.41)*
hemolytic disease of newborn (P55.-)
paroxysmal cold hemoglobinuria (D59.6)
+ D59.2 **Drug-induced nonautoimmune hemolytic anemia**
Drug-induced enzyme deficiency anemia
Use additional code for adverse effect, if applicable, to identify drug (T36-T50 with fifth or sixth character 5)

● New ▲ Revised *Manifestation* ④-⑦ Digit Indicators ⊟Laterality Ⓐ Adult (15+ years) Ⓜ Maternity (12-55 years) Ⓝ Newborn Ⓟ Pediatric (0-17 years) ♂ Male ♀Female
✖ Deleted Unspecified + Additional code
2017 ICD-10-CM Expert for Physicians

© 2017 DecisionHealth

507

Diseases of the Blood and Blood-forming Organs and Certain Disorders Involving the Immune Mechanism *(left margin)*

+ D59.3 Hemolytic-uremic syndrome
Use additional code to identify associated:
E. coli infection (B96.2-)
Pneumococcal pneumonia (J13)
Shigella dysenteriae (A03.9)

DEFINITION Condition in which platelets become clogged in narrow renal blood vessels, leading to the destruction of red blood cells and kidney failure. Symptoms include severe abdominal pain, diarrhea, nausea, and vomiting.

D59.4 Other nonautoimmune hemolytic anemias
Mechanical hemolytic anemia
Microangiopathic hemolytic anemia
Toxic hemolytic anemia

D59.5 Paroxysmal nocturnal hemoglobinuria [Marchiafava-Micheli]
EXCLUDES 1 *hemoglobinuria NOS (R82.3)*

+ D59.6 Hemoglobinuria due to hemolysis from other external causes
Hemoglobinuria from exertion
March hemoglobinuria
Paroxysmal cold hemoglobinuria
Use additional code (Chapter 20) to identify external cause
EXCLUDES 1 *hemoglobinuria NOS (R82.3)*

CODING TIP ✓ Hemoglobinuria is a condition where excess hemoglobin is found in high concentrations in the urine. Code D59.6 only when the hemoglobinuria is stated as due to hemolysis related to a specific other cause (the hemolysis of red blood cells due to another specific cause or condition is resulting in the hemoglobinuria). An external cause code (from Chapter 20) should be assigned to identify the external cause.

D59.8 Other acquired hemolytic anemias
D59.9 Acquired hemolytic anemia, unspecified
Idiopathic hemolytic anemia, chronic

Aplastic and other anemias and other bone marrow failure syndromes (D60-D64)

D60 Acquired pure red cell aplasia [erythroblastopenia]
INCLUDES red cell aplasia (acquired) (adult) (with thymoma)
EXCLUDES 1 *congenital red cell aplasia (D61.01)*

D60.0 Chronic acquired pure red cell aplasia
DEFINITION Decline of RBC precursor cells in the bone marrow until nearly absent while WBC precursors are present at normal levels; causes normochromic, normoblastic anemia.

D60.1 Transient acquired pure red cell aplasia
D60.8 Other acquired pure red cell aplasias
D60.9 Acquired pure red cell aplasia, unspecified

D61 Other aplastic anemias and other bone marrow failure syndromes
EXCLUDES 1 *neutropenia (D70.-)*

D61.0 Constitutional aplastic anemia
D61.01 Constitutional (pure) red blood cell aplasia
Blackfan-Diamond syndrome
Congenital (pure) red cell aplasia
Familial hypoplastic anemia
Primary (pure) red cell aplasia
Red cell (pure) aplasia of infants
EXCLUDES 1 *acquired red cell aplasia (D60.9)*

D61.09 Other constitutional aplastic anemia
Fanconi's anemia
Pancytopenia with malformations

+ D61.1 Drug-induced aplastic anemia
Use additional code for adverse effect, if applicable, to identify drug (T36-T50 with fifth or sixth character 5)
CODING TIP ✓ When the record specifies only "anemia due to antineoplastic chemotherapy" but does not specify it as aplastic anemia due to the antineoplastic chemotherapy, report code D64.81.

D61.2 Aplastic anemia due to other external agents
Code first:
, if applicable, toxic effects of substances chiefly nonmedicinal as to source (T51-T65)

D61.3 Idiopathic aplastic anemia
D61.8 Other specified aplastic anemias and other bone marrow failure syndromes
▲ D61.81 Pancytopenia
EXCLUDES 1 *pancytopenia (due to) (with) aplastic anemia (D61.9)*
pancytopenia (due to) (with) bone marrow infiltration (D61.82)
pancytopenia (due to) (with) congenital (pure) red cell aplasia (D61.01)
pancytopenia (due to) (with) hairy cell leukemia (C91.4-)
pancytopenia (due to) (with) human immunodeficiency virus disease (B20.-)
pancytopenia (due to) (with) leukoerythroblastic anemia (D61.82)
pancytopenia (due to) (with) myeloproliferative disease (D47.1)
EXCLUDES 2 *pancytopenia (due to) (with) myelodysplastic syndromes (D46.-)*
DEFINITION Decreased count of all elements in the blood: red blood cells, white blood cells, and platelets.

D61.810 Antineoplastic chemotherapy induced pancytopenia
EXCLUDES 2 *aplastic anemia due to antineoplastic chemotherapy (D61.1)*

D61.811 Other drug-induced pancytopenia
EXCLUDES 2 *aplastic anemia due to drugs (D61.1)*

D61.818 Other pancytopenia
D61.82 Myelophthisis
Leukoerythroblastic anemia
Myelophthisic anemia
Panmyelophthisis
Code also the underlying disorder, such as:
malignant neoplasm of breast (C50.-)
tuberculosis (A15.-)
EXCLUDES 1 *idiopathic myelofibrosis (D47.1)*
myelofibrosis NOS (D75.81)
myelofibrosis with myeloid metaplasia (D47.4)
primary myelofibrosis (D47.1)
secondary myelofibrosis (D75.81)
DEFINITION Replacement of hemopoietic tissue in the bone marrow by abnormal infiltrates, usually fibrotic tissue or malignant tumors, suppressing bone marrow function.

D61.89 Other specified aplastic anemias and other bone marrow failure syndromes
D61.9 Aplastic anemia, unspecified
Hypoplastic anemia NOS
Medullary hypoplasia

D62 Acute posthemorrhagic anemia
EXCLUDES 1 *anemia due to chronic blood loss (D50.0)*
blood loss anemia NOS (D50.0)
congenital anemia from fetal blood loss (P61.3)
CODING TIP ✓ Do not assign D62 when the clinical record documentation specifies only "blood loss anemia" or "chronic blood loss anemia." Code D62 should only be used when posthemorrhagic anemia is specified as acute.

D63 Anemia in chronic diseases classified elsewhere
D63.0 Anemia in neoplastic disease
Code first:
neoplasm (C00-D49)
EXCLUDES 1 *anemia due to antineoplastic chemotherapy (D64.81)*
aplastic anemia due to antineoplastic chemotherapy (D61.1)
GUIDELINES Section 1.C.2.c.1
When admission/encounter is for management of an anemia associated with the malignancy, and the treatment is only for anemia, the appropriate code for the malignancy is sequenced as the principal or first-listed diagnosis followed by the appropriate code for the anemia (such as code D63.0, Anemia in neoplastic disease).

● New   ▲ Revised   *Manifestation*   ▣-▢ Digit Indicators   ▤ Laterality   Adult (15+ years)   Maternity (12-55 years)   Newborn   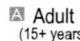 Pediatric (0-17 years)   ♂ Male   ♀ Female
✖ Deleted   Unspecified   + Additional code

508   © 2017 DecisionHealth   2017 ICD-10-CM Expert for Physicians

D59.3 — D63.0 *(left margin)*

CODING TIP ✓ When a patient is admitted for anemia due to neoplastic disease (D63.0), a code for the appropriate neoplasm must be first assigned, regardless of whether the focus of care is the neoplastic disease or the anemia.

D63.1 Anemia in chronic kidney disease
Erythropoietin resistant anemia (EPO resistant anemia)
Code first:
underlying chronic kidney disease (CKD) (N18.-)

CODING TIP ✓ Only assign D63.1 when a diagnostic statement specifically indicates a relationship between anemia and chronic kidney disease, using terms such as "due to," "with," or "related to." Do not assign D63.1 when the record only indicates anemia and chronic kidney disease.

D63.8 *Anemia in other chronic diseases classified elsewhere*
Code first underlying disease, such as:
diphyllobothriasis (B70.0)
hookworm disease (B76.0-B76.9)
hypothyroidism (E00.0-E03.9)
malaria (B50.0-B54)
symptomatic late syphilis (A52.79)
tuberculosis (A18.89)

◢ D64 Other anemias
EXCLUDES 1 *refractory anemia (D46.-)*
refractory anemia with excess blasts in transformation [RAEB T] (C92.0-)

D64.0 Hereditary sideroblastic anemia
Sex-linked hypochromic sideroblastic anemia
DEFINITION Group of blood disorders in which the bone marrow's ability to produce normal red blood cells is impaired and sideroblasts, or deformed red blood cells, are present in the bloodstream.

D64.1 Secondary sideroblastic anemia due to disease
Code first:
underlying disease

✚ D64.2 Secondary sideroblastic anemia due to drugs and toxins
Code first:
poisoning due to drug or toxin, if applicable (T36-T65 with fifth or sixth character 1-4 or 6)
Use additional code for adverse effect, if applicable, to identify drug (T36-T50 with fifth or sixth character 5)

D64.3 Other sideroblastic anemias
Sideroblastic anemia NOS
Pyridoxine-responsive sideroblastic anemia NEC

D64.4 Congenital dyserythropoietic anemia
Dyshematopoietic anemia (congenital)
EXCLUDES 1 *Blackfan-Diamond syndrome (D61.01)*
Di Guglielmo's disease (C94.0)

CODING TIP ✓ Congenital dyserythropoietic anemia is defined as a congenital condition resulting in immature red blood cells that are unusually shaped and cannot develop into functional mature cells, leading to a shortage of healthy red blood cells. These patients also frequently have thrombocytopenia, which should be additionally coded if present.

◲ D64.8 Other specified anemias
▲ D64.81 Anemia due to antineoplastic chemotherapy
Antineoplastic chemotherapy induced anemia
EXCLUDES 1 *aplastic anemia due to antineoplastic chemotherapy (D61.1)*
EXCLUDES 2 *anemia in neoplastic disease (D63.0)*

GUIDELINES Section I.C.2.c.2)
When the admission/encounter is for management of an anemia associated with an adverse effect of the administration of chemotherapy or immunotherapy and the only treatment is for the anemia, the anemia code is sequenced first followed by the appropriate codes for the neoplasm and the adverse effect (T45.1X5, Adverse effect of antineoplastic and immunosuppressive drugs).

GUIDELINES Section I.C.2.c.2)
When the admission/encounter is for management of an anemia associated with an adverse effect of the administration of chemotherapy or immunotherapy and the only treatment is for the anemia, the anemia code is sequenced first followed by the appropriate codes for the neoplasm and the adverse effect (T45.1X5, Adverse effect of antineoplastic and immunosuppressive drugs).

When the admission/encounter is for management of an anemia associated with an adverse effect of radiotherapy, the anemia code should be sequenced first, followed by the appropriate neoplasm code and code Y84.2, radiological procedure and radiotherapy as the cause of abnormal reaction of the patient, or of later complication, without mention of misadventure at the time of the procedure.

CODING TIP ✓ Do not assign D64.81 to indicate aplastic anemia due to antineoplastic chemotherapy. If the diagnostic statements specifically report aplastic anemia due to antineoplastic chemotherapy, assign D61.1.

CODING TIP ✓ Do not assign D64.81 to indicate anemia due to neoplastic disease. Anemia due neoplastic disease should be coded to D63.0. D64.81 is for the management of anemia due to chemotherapy. Reference the guidelines for sequencing information since anemia secondary to chemotherapy is different than anemia due to neoplasm.
AHA: 4Q 2014, 22

D64.89 Other specified anemias
Infantile pseudoleukemia

D64.9 Anemia, unspecified

Coagulation defects, purpura and other hemorrhagic conditions (D65-D69)

CODING TIP ✓ Do not use codes from D65-69 to indicate a prolonged bleeding time due to taking an anticoagulant. These codes are for hemophilias.

D65 Disseminated intravascular coagulation [defibrination syndrome]
Afibrinogenemia, acquired
Consumption coagulopathy
Diffuse or disseminated intravascular coagulation [DIC]
Fibrinolytic hemorrhage, acquired
Fibrinolytic purpura
Purpura fulminans
EXCLUDES 1 *disseminated intravascular coagulation (complicating) :*
abortion or ectopic or molar pregnancy (O00-O07, O08.1)
in newborn (P60)
pregnancy, childbirth and the puerperium (O45.0, O46.0, O67.0, O72.3)
DEFINITION Bleeding disorder characterized by an abnormal reduction in the elements involved in blood clotting; marked by profuse hemorrhaging in the late stages.

D66 Hereditary factor VIII deficiency
Classical hemophilia
Deficiency factor VIII (with functional defect)
Hemophilia NOS
Hemophilia A
EXCLUDES 1 *factor VIII deficiency with vascular defect (D68.0)*

● New ▲ Revised *Manifestation* ◲-◸ Digit Indicators ◲ Laterality ◮ Adult (15+ years) ◲ Maternity (12-55 years) ◲ Newborn ◲ Pediatric (0-17 years) ♂ Male ♀ Female
✖ ̶D̶e̶l̶e̶t̶e̶d̶ Unspecified ✚ Additional code

2017 ICD-10-CM Expert for Physicians

© 2017 DecisionHealth 509

DEFINITION Most common form of hemophilia, referred to as classic hemophilia or hemophilia A; characterized by profuse bleeding from injuries, as well as bleeding from the joints, muscles, digestive tract, and brain.

Congenital factor VIII disorder
(Also known as hemophilia A or classic hemophilia)

Characterized by an increased tendency to bleeding, bleeding from the joints, muscles, digestive tract and brain, and large bruises of the skin

Factor VIII, one of the proteins needed to form blood clots, is missing or reduced

D67   Hereditary factor IX deficiency
Christmas disease
Factor IX deficiency (with functional defect)
Hemophilia B
Plasma thromboplastin component [PTC] deficiency

DEFINITION A clotting disorder of blood, caused by hereditary deficiency of factor IX.

⑷ D68   Other coagulation defects
EXCLUDES 1 *abnormal coagulation profile (R79.1)*
coagulation defects complicating abortion or ectopic or molar pregnancy (O00-O07, O08.1)
coagulation defects complicating pregnancy, childbirth and the puerperium (O45.0, O46.0, O67.0, O72.3)

D68.0   Von Willebrand's disease
Angiohemophilia
Factor VIII deficiency with vascular defect
Vascular hemophilia
EXCLUDES 1 *capillary fragility (hereditary) (D69.8)*
factor VIII deficiency NOS (D66)
factor VIII deficiency with functional defect (D66)

D68.1   Hereditary factor XI deficiency
Hemophilia C
Plasma thromboplastin antecedent [PTA] deficiency
Rosenthal's disease

D68.2   Hereditary deficiency of other clotting factors
AC globulin deficiency
Congenital afibrinogenemia
Deficiency of factor I [fibrinogen]
Deficiency of factor II [prothrombin]
Deficiency of factor V [labile]
Deficiency of factor VII [stable]
Deficiency of factor X [Stuart-Prower]
Deficiency of factor XII [Hageman]
Deficiency of factor XIII [fibrin stabilizing]
Dysfibrinogenemia (congenital)
Hypoproconvertinemia
Owren's disease
Proaccelerin deficiency

⑸ D68.3   Hemorrhagic disorder due to circulating anticoagulants
⑹ D68.31   Hemorrhagic disorder due to intrinsic circulating anticoagulants, antibodies, or inhibitors
D68.311   Acquired hemophilia
Autoimmune hemophilia
Autoimmune inhibitors to clotting factors
Secondary hemophilia

D68.312   Antiphospholipid antibody with hemorrhagic disorder
Lupus anticoagulant (LAC) with hemorrhagic disorder
Systemic lupus erythematosus [SLE] inhibitor with hemorrhagic disorder
EXCLUDES 1 *antiphospholipid antibody, finding without diagnosis (R76.0)*
antiphospholipid antibody syndrome (D68.61)
antiphospholipid antibody with hypercoagulable state (D68.61)
lupus anticoagulant (LAC) finding without diagnosis (R76.0)
lupus anticoagulant (LAC) with hypercoagulable state (D68.62)
systemic lupus erythematosus [SLE] inhibitor finding without diagnosis (R76.0)
systemic lupus erythematosus [SLE] inhibitor with hypercoagulable state (D68.62)

D68.318   Other hemorrhagic disorder due to intrinsic circulating anticoagulants, antibodies, or inhibitors
Antithromboplastinemia
Antithromboplastinogenemia
Hemorrhagic disorder due to intrinsic increase in antithrombin
Hemorrhagic disorder due to intrinsic increase in anti-VIIIa
Hemorrhagic disorder due to intrinsic increase in anti-IXa
Hemorrhagic disorder due to intrinsic increase in anti-XIa

✚ D68.32   Hemorrhagic disorder due to extrinsic circulating anticoagulants
Drug-induced hemorrhagic disorder
Hemorrhagic disorder due to increase in anti-IIa
Hemorrhagic disorder due to increase in anti-Xa
Hyperheparinemia
Use additional code for adverse effect, if applicable, to identify drug (T45.515, T45.525)
AHA: 1Q 2016, 14

D68.4   Acquired coagulation factor deficiency
Deficiency of coagulation factor due to liver disease
Deficiency of coagulation factor due to vitamin K deficiency
EXCLUDES 1 *vitamin K deficiency of newborn (P53)*

⑸ D68.5   Primary thrombophilia
Primary hypercoagulable states
EXCLUDES 1 *antiphospholipid syndrome (D68.61)*
lupus anticoagulant (D68.62)
secondary activated protein C resistance (D68.69)
secondary antiphospholipid antibody syndrome (D68.69)
secondary lupus anticoagulant with hypercoagulable state (D68.69)
secondary systemic lupus erythematosus [SLE] inhibitor with hypercoagulable state (D68.69)
systemic lupus erythematosus [SLE] inhibitor finding without diagnosis (R76.0)
systemic lupus erythematosus [SLE] inhibitor with hemorrhagic disorder (D68.312)
thrombotic thrombocytopenic purpura (M31.1)

DEFINITION Abnormal development of blood clots in arteries or veins.

D68.51   Activated protein C resistance
Factor V Leiden mutation
D68.52   Prothrombin gene mutation
D68.59   Other primary thrombophilia
Antithrombin III deficiency
Hypercoagulable state NOS
Primary hypercoagulable state NEC
Primary thrombophilia NEC
Protein C deficiency
Protein S deficiency
Thrombophilia NOS

● New   ▲ Revised   *Manifestation*   ⑷-⑺ Digit Indicators   ▤ Laterality   Ⓐ Adult (15+ years)   Ⓜ Maternity (12-55 years)   Ⓝ Newborn   Ⓟ Pediatric (0-17 years)   ♂ Male   ♀ Female
✖ Deleted   Unspecified   ✚ Additional code

510   © 2017 DecisionHealth   2017 ICD-10-CM Expert for Physicians

⑤ D68.6 **Other thrombophilia**
Other hypercoagulable states
> **EXCLUDES 1** *diffuse or disseminated intravascular coagulation [DIC] (D65)*
> *heparin induced thrombocytopenia (HIT) (D75.82)*
> *hyperhomocysteinemia (E72.11)*

D68.61 **Antiphospholipid syndrome**
Anticardiolipin syndrome
Antiphospholipid antibody syndrome
> **EXCLUDES 1** *anti-phospholipid antibody, finding without diagnosis (R76.0)*
> *anti-phospholipid antibody with hemorrhagic disorder (D68.312)*
> *lupus anticoagulant syndrome (D68.62)*

▲ D68.62 **Lupus anticoagulant syndrome**
Lupus anticoagulant
Presence of systemic lupus erythematosus [SLE] inhibitor
> **EXCLUDES 1** *anticardiolipin syndrome (D68.61)*
> *antiphospholipid syndrome (D68.61)*
> *lupus anticoagulant (LAC) finding without diagnosis (R76.0)*
> *lupus anticoagulant (LAC) with hemorrhagic disorder (D68.312)*

D68.69 **Other thrombophilia**
Hypercoagulable states NEC
Secondary hypercoagulable state NOS

D68.8 **Other specified coagulation defects**
> **EXCLUDES 1** *hemorrhagic disease of newborn (P53)*

D68.9 **Coagulation defect, unspecified**

④ D69 **Purpura and other hemorrhagic conditions**
> **EXCLUDES 1** *benign hypergammaglobulinemic purpura (D89.0)*
> *cryoglobulinemic purpura (D89.1)*
> *essential (hemorrhagic) thrombocythemia (D47.3)*
> *hemorrhagic thrombocythemia (D47.3)*
> *purpura fulminans (D65)*
> *thrombotic thrombocytopenic purpura (M31.1)*
> *Waldenström hypergammaglobulinemic purpura (D89.0)*

D69.0 **Allergic purpura**
Allergic vasculitis
Nonthrombocytopenic hemorrhagic purpura
Nonthrombocytopenic idiopathic purpura
Purpura anaphylactoid
Purpura Henoch(-Schönlein)
Purpura rheumatica
Vascular purpura
> **EXCLUDES 1** *thrombocytopenic hemorrhagic purpura (D69.3)*

> **DEFINITION** Allergic reaction causing hemorrhaging of the skin and mucous membranes; produces purple discolorations on the skin surface.

Allergic purpura

Purple discoloration caused by hemorrhaging

D69.1 **Qualitative platelet defects**
Bernard-Soulier [giant platelet] syndrome
Glanzmann's disease
Grey platelet syndrome
Thromboasthenia (hemorrhagic) (hereditary)
Thrombocytopathy
> **EXCLUDES 1** *von Willebrand's disease (D68.0)*

D69.2 **Other nonthrombocytopenic purpura**
Purpura NOS
Purpura simplex
Senile purpura

D69.3 **Immune thrombocytopenic purpura**
Hemorrhagic (thrombocytopenic) purpura
Idiopathic thrombocytopenic purpura
Tidal platelet dysgenesis

⑤ D69.4 **Other primary thrombocytopenia**
> **EXCLUDES 1** *transient neonatal thrombocytopenia (P61.0)*
> *Wiskott-Aldrich syndrome (D82.0)*

D69.41 **Evans syndrome**
D69.42 **Congenital and hereditary thrombocytopenia purpura**
Congenital thrombocytopenia
Hereditary thrombocytopenia
Code first congenital or hereditary disorder, such as: thrombocytopenia with absent radius (TAR syndrome) (Q87.2)

D69.49 **Other primary thrombocytopenia**
Megakaryocytic hypoplasia
Primary thrombocytopenia NOS

⑤ D69.5 **Secondary thrombocytopenia**
> **EXCLUDES 1** *heparin induced thrombocytopenia (HIT) (D75.82)*
> *transient thrombocytopenia of newborn (P61.0)*

> **DEFINITION** Uncommon but life-threatening adverse reaction in which arterial or venous thrombotic complications develop that can lead to pulmonary embolism, amputation, stroke, or acute myocardial infarction.

D69.51 **Posttransfusion purpura**
Posttransfusion purpura from whole blood (fresh) or blood products
PTP

D69.59 **Other secondary thrombocytopenia**
AHA: 4Q 2014, 22

D69.6 **Thrombocytopenia, unspecified**

D69.8 **Other specified hemorrhagic conditions**
Capillary fragility (hereditary)
Vascular pseudohemophilia

D69.9 **Hemorrhagic condition, unspecified**

Other disorders of blood and blood-forming organs (D70-D77)

④ + D70 **Neutropenia**
> **INCLUDES** agranulocytosis
> decreased absolute neurophile count (ANC)

Use additional code for any associated:
fever (R50.81)
mucositis (J34.81, K12.3-, K92.81, N76.81)
> **EXCLUDES 1** *neutropenic splenomegaly (D73.81)*
> *transient neonatal neutropenia (P61.5)*

+ D70.0 **Congenital agranulocytosis**
Congenital neutropenia
Infantile genetic agranulocytosis
Kostmann's disease

+ D70.1 **Agranulocytosis secondary to cancer chemotherapy**
Code also:
underlying neoplasm
Use additional code for adverse effect, if applicable, to identify drug (T45.1X5)
AHA: 4Q 2014, 22

+ D70.2 **Other drug-induced agranulocytosis**
Use additional code for adverse effect, if applicable, to identify drug (T36-T50 with fifth or sixth character 5)

+ D70.3 **Neutropenia due to infection**

+ D70.4 **Cyclic neutropenia**
Cyclic hematopoiesis
Periodic neutropenia

+ D70.8 **Other neutropenia**

+ D70.9 **Neutropenia, unspecified**

● New   ▲ Revised   *Manifestation*   ④-⑦ Digit Indicators   ⊟ Laterality   Ⓐ Adult (15+ years)   Ⓜ Maternity (12-55 years)   Ⓝ Newborn   Ⓟ Pediatric (0-17 years)   ♂ Male   ♀ Female
✖ Deleted   Unspecified   + Additional code

2017 ICD-10-CM Expert for Physicians   © 2017 DecisionHealth   511

D71   **Functional disorders of polymorphonuclear neutrophils**
Cell membrane receptor complex [CR3] defect
Chronic (childhood) granulomatous disease
Congenital dysphagocytosis
Progressive septic granulomatosis

◢ D72   **Other disorders of white blood cells**

   EXCLUDES 1   *basophilia (D72.824)*
                    immunity disorders (D80-D89)
                    neutropenia (D70)
                    preleukemia (syndrome) (D46.9)

   D72.0   **Genetic anomalies of leukocytes**
         Alder (granulation) (granulocyte) anomaly
         Alder syndrome
         Hereditary leukocytic hypersegmentation
         Hereditary leukocytic hyposegmentation
         Hereditary leukomelanopathy
         May-Hegglin (granulation) (granulocyte) anomaly
         May-Hegglin syndrome
         Pelger-Huët (granulation) (granulocyte) anomaly
         Pelger-Huët syndrome

       EXCLUDES 1   *Chédiak (-Steinbrinck) -Higashi syndrome (E70.330)*

   D72.1   **Eosinophilia**
         Allergic eosinophilia
         Hereditary eosinophilia

       EXCLUDES 1   *Löffler's syndrome (J82)*
                        pulmonary eosinophilia (J82)

Eosinophilia
Elevated number of eosinophils in the bloodstream

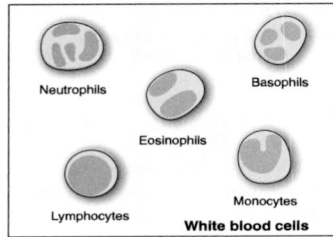

Neutrophils   Basophils
Eosinophils
Lymphocytes   Monocytes
White blood cells

◢ D72.8   **Other specified disorders of white blood cells**
       EXCLUDES 1   *leukemia (C91-C95)*

   ◢ D72.81   **Decreased white blood cell count**
            EXCLUDES 1   *neutropenia (D70.-)*

     D72.810   **Lymphocytopenia**
            Decreased lymphocytes

     D72.818   **Other decreased white blood cell count**
            Basophilic leukopenia
            Eosinophilic leukopenia
            Monocytopenia
            Other decreased leukocytes
            Plasmacytopenia

     D72.819   **Decreased white blood cell count, unspecified**
            Decreased leukocytes, unspecified
            Leukocytopenia, unspecified
            Leukopenia
            EXCLUDES 1   *malignant leukopenia (D70.9)*

   ◢ D72.82   **Elevated white blood cell count**
            EXCLUDES 1   *eosinophilia (D72.1)*

     D72.820   **Lymphocytosis (symptomatic)**
            Elevated lymphocytes

     D72.821   **Monocytosis (symptomatic)**
            EXCLUDES 1   *infectious mononucleosis (B27.-)*

     D72.822   **Plasmacytosis**

     D72.823   **Leukemoid reaction**
            Basophilic leukemoid reaction
            Leukemoid reaction NOS
            Lymphocytic leukemoid reaction
            Monocytic leukemoid reaction
            Myelocytic leukemoid reaction
            Neutrophilic leukemoid reaction

DEFINITION   A state of circulating blood presenting a clinical picture resembling or indistinguishable from leukemia due to a condition such as infection, bone marrow compromise, liver failure, and inflammatory disorders.

   D72.824   **Basophilia**
            DEFINITION   Abnormally increased number of basophils in the blood, which release histamine and serotonin upon stimulation.

   D72.825   **Bandemia**
         Bandemia without diagnosis of specific infection
         EXCLUDES 1   *confirmed infection - code to infection*
                    leukemia (C91.-, C92.-, C93.-, C94.-, C95.-)

         DEFINITION   Nonspecific elevated count of immature white blood cells when other white blood cell counts are normal.

   D72.828   **Other elevated white blood cell count**

   D72.829   **Elevated white blood cell count, unspecified**
         Elevated leukocytes, unspecified
         Leukocytosis, unspecified

   D72.89   **Other specified disorders of white blood cells**
         Abnormality of white blood cells NEC

   D72.9   **Disorder of white blood cells, unspecified**
         Abnormal leukocyte differential NOS

◢ D73   **Diseases of spleen**

   D73.0   **Hyposplenism**
         Atrophy of spleen
       EXCLUDES 1   *asplenia (congenital) (Q89.01)*
                    postsurgical absence of spleen (Z90.81)

   D73.1   **Hypersplenism**
       EXCLUDES 1   *neutropenic splenomegaly (D73.81)*
                    primary splenic neutropenia (D73.81)
                    splenitis, splenomegaly in late syphilis (A52.79)
                    splenitis, splenomegaly in tuberculosis (A18.85)
                    splenomegaly NOS (R16.1)
                    splenomegaly congenital (Q89.0)

   D73.2   **Chronic congestive splenomegaly**

   D73.3   **Abscess of spleen**

   D73.4   **Cyst of spleen**

   D73.5   **Infarction of spleen**
         Splenic rupture, nontraumatic
         Torsion of spleen
       EXCLUDES 1   *rupture of spleen due to Plasmodium vivax malaria (B51.0)*
                    traumatic rupture of spleen (S36.03-)

   ◢ D73.8   **Other diseases of spleen**

     D73.81   **Neutropenic splenomegaly**
            Werner-Schultz disease

     D73.89   **Other diseases of spleen**
            Fibrosis of spleen NOS
            Perisplenitis
            Splenitis NOS

   D73.9   **Disease of spleen, unspecified**

◢ D74   **Methemoglobinemia**

   D74.0   **Congenital methemoglobinemia**
         Congenital NADH-methemoglobin reductase deficiency
         Hemoglobin-M [Hb-M] disease
         Methemoglobinemia, hereditary

   D74.8   **Other methemoglobinemias**
         Acquired methemoglobinemia (with sulfhemoglobinemia)
         Toxic methemoglobinemia

   D74.9   **Methemoglobinemia, unspecified**
       DEFINITION   Presence of a higher than normal level of methemoglobin, a form of hemoglobin that does not bind oxygen, in the blood. When its concentration is elevated in red blood cells, anemia and hypoxia may occur.

● New   ▲ Revised   *Manifestation*   **◢-◤** Digit Indicators   ▭ Laterality   Ⓐ Adult (15+ years)   Ⓜ Maternity (12-55 years)   Ⓝ Newborn   Ⓟ Pediatric (0-17 years)   ♂ Male   ♀ Female

✖ Deleted   Unspecified   + Additional code

512   © 2017 DecisionHealth   2017 ICD-10-CM Expert for Physicians

◪ D75 Other and unspecified diseases of blood and blood-forming organs

EXCLUDES 2 *acute lymphadenitis (L04.-)*
chronic lymphadenitis (I88.1)
enlarged lymph nodes (R59.-)
hypergammaglobulinemia NOS (D89.2)
lymphadenitis NOS (I88.9)
mesenteric lymphadenitis (acute) (chronic) (I88.0)

D75.0 Familial erythrocytosis
Benign polycythemia
Familial polycythemia
EXCLUDES 1 *hereditary ovalocytosis (D58.1)*

D75.1 Secondary polycythemia
Acquired polycythemia
Emotional polycythemia
Erythrocytosis NOS
Hypoxemic polycythemia
Nephrogenous polycythemia
Polycythemia due to erythropoietin
Polycythemia due to fall in plasma volume
Polycythemia due to high altitude
Polycythemia due to stress
Polycythemia NOS
Relative polycythemia
EXCLUDES 1 *polycythemia neonatorum (P61.1)*
polycythemia vera (D45)

◰ D75.8 Other specified diseases of blood and blood-forming organs

✚ D75.81 Myelofibrosis
Myelofibrosis NOS
Secondary myelofibrosis NOS
Code first the underlying disorder, such as:
malignant neoplasm of breast (C50.-)
Use additional code, if applicable, for associated therapy-related myelodysplastic syndrome (D46.-)
Use additional code for adverse effect, if applicable, to identify drug (T45.1X5)
EXCLUDES 1 *acute myelofibrosis (C94.4-)*
idiopathic myelofibrosis (D47.1)
leukoerythroblastic anemia (D61.82)
myelofibrosis with myeloid metaplasia (D47.4)
myelophthisic anemia (D61.82)
myelophthisis (D61.82)
primary myelofibrosis (D47.1)

D75.82 Heparin induced thrombocytopenia (HIT)
D75.89 Other specified diseases of blood and blood-forming organs

D75.9 Disease of blood and blood-forming organs, unspecified

▲ ◪ D76 Other specified diseases with participation of lymphoreticular and reticulohistiocytic tissue

EXCLUDES 1 *(Abt-) Letterer-Siwe disease (C96.0)*
eosinophilic granuloma (C96.6)
Hand-Schüller-Christian disease (C96.5)
histiocytic medullary reticulosis (C96.9)
histiocytic sarcoma (C96.A)
histiocytosis X, multifocal (C96.5)
histiocytosis X, unifocal (C96.6)
Langerhans-cell histiocytosis, multifocal (C96.5)
Langerhans-cell histiocytosis NOS (C96.6)
Langerhans-cell histiocytosis, unifocal (C96.6)
leukemic reticuloendotheliosis (C91.4-)
lipomelanotic reticulosis (I89.8)
malignant histiocytosis (C96.A)
malignant reticulosis (C86.0)
nonlipid reticuloendotheliosis (C96.0)

D76.1 Hemophagocytic lymphohistiocytosis
Familial hemophagocytic reticulosis
Histiocytoses of mononuclear phagocytes

✚ D76.2 Hemophagocytic syndrome, infection-associated
Use additional code to identify infectious agent or disease.

D76.3 Other histiocytosis syndromes
Reticulohistiocytoma (giant-cell)
Sinus histiocytosis with massive lymphadenopathy
Xanthogranuloma

D77 *Other disorders of blood and blood-forming organs in diseases classified elsewhere*

Code first underlying disease, such as:
amyloidosis (E85.-)
congenital early syphilis (A50.0)
echinococcosis (B67.0-B67.9)
malaria (B50.0-B54)
schistosomiasis [bilharziasis] (B65.0-B65.9)
vitamin C deficiency (E54)
EXCLUDES 1 *rupture of spleen due to Plasmodium vivax malaria (B51.0)*
splenitis, splenomegaly in late syphilis (A52.79)
splenitis, splenomegaly in tuberculosis (A18.85)

Intraoperative and postprocedural complications of the spleen (D78)

CODING TIP ✓ Conditions classifiable to D78- are classifiable as intraoperative and postprocedural complications. These conditions should only be assigned when diagnostic statements clearly indicate that the condition is a complication of a procedure.

◪ D78 Intraoperative and postprocedural complications of the spleen

◰ D78.0 Intraoperative hemorrhage and hematoma of the spleen complicating a procedure
EXCLUDES 1 *intraoperative hemorrhage and hematoma of the spleen due to accidental puncture or laceration during a procedure (D78.1-)*

D78.01 Intraoperative hemorrhage and hematoma of the spleen complicating a procedure on the spleen
D78.02 Intraoperative hemorrhage and hematoma of the spleen complicating other procedure

◰ D78.1 Accidental puncture and laceration of the spleen during a procedure
D78.11 Accidental puncture and laceration of the spleen during a procedure on the spleen
D78.12 Accidental puncture and laceration of the spleen during other procedure

▲ ◰ D78.2 Postprocedural hemorrhage of the spleen following a procedure
▲ D78.21 Postprocedural hemorrhage of the spleen following a procedure on the spleen
▲ D78.22 Postprocedural hemorrhage of the spleen following other procedure

● ◰ D78.3 Postprocedural hematoma and seroma of the spleen following a procedure
● D78.31 Postprocedural hematoma of the spleen following a procedure on the spleen
● D78.32 Postprocedural hematoma of the spleen following other procedure
● D78.33 Postprocedural seroma of the spleen following a procedure on the spleen
● D78.34 Postprocedural seroma of the spleen following other procedure

◰ ✚ D78.8 Other intraoperative and postprocedural complications of the spleen
Use additional code, if applicable, to further specify disorder
✚ D78.81 Other intraoperative complications of the spleen
✚ D78.89 Other postprocedural complications of the spleen

Certain disorders involving the immune mechanism (D80-D89)

INCLUDES defects in the complement system
immunodeficiency disorders, except human immunodeficiency virus [HIV] disease
sarcoidosis
EXCLUDES 1 *autoimmune disease (systemic) NOS (M35.9)*
functional disorders of polymorphonuclear neutrophils (D71)
human immunodeficiency virus [HIV] disease (B20)

◪ D80 Immunodeficiency with predominantly antibody defects

D80.0 Hereditary hypogammaglobulinemia
Autosomal recessive agammaglobulinemia (Swiss type)
X-linked agammaglobulinemia [Bruton] (with growth hormone deficiency)

D80.1 **Nonfamilial hypogammaglobulinemia**
Agammaglobulinemia with immunoglobulin-bearing B-lymphocytes
Common variable agammaglobulinemia [CVAgamma]
Hypogammaglobulinemia NOS
> **DEFINITION** Loss of the body's ability to respond to infection because of a lack of immunoglobulins (antibodies) in the blood.

D80.2 **Selective deficiency of immunoglobulin A [IgA]**

D80.3 **Selective deficiency of immunoglobulin G [IgG] subclasses**

D80.4 **Selective deficiency of immunoglobulin M [IgM]**

D80.5 **Immunodeficiency with increased immunoglobulin M [IgM]**

D80.6 **Antibody deficiency with near-normal immunoglobulins or with hyperimmunoglobulinemia**

D80.7 **Transient hypogammaglobulinemia of infancy**   N

D80.8 **Other immunodeficiencies with predominantly antibody defects**
Kappa light chain deficiency

D80.9 **Immunodeficiency with predominantly antibody defects, unspecified**

D81 **Combined immunodeficiencies**
> **EXCLUDES 1** *autosomal recessive agammaglobulinemia (Swiss type) (D80.0)*

D81.0 **Severe combined immunodeficiency [SCID] with reticular dysgenesis**

D81.1 **Severe combined immunodeficiency [SCID] with low T- and B-cell numbers**

D81.2 **Severe combined immunodeficiency [SCID] with low or normal B-cell numbers**

D81.3 **Adenosine deaminase [ADA] deficiency**

D81.4 **Nezelof's syndrome**

D81.5 **Purine nucleoside phosphorylase [PNP] deficiency**

D81.6 **Major histocompatibility complex class I deficiency**
Bare lymphocyte syndrome

D81.7 **Major histocompatibility complex class II deficiency**

D81.8 **Other combined immunodeficiencies**

D81.81 **Biotin-dependent carboxylase deficiency**
Multiple carboxylase deficiency
> **EXCLUDES 1** *biotin-dependent carboxylase deficiency due to dietary deficiency of biotin (E53.8)*

D81.810 **Biotinidase deficiency**

D81.818 **Other biotin-dependent carboxylase deficiency**
Holocarboxylase synthetase deficiency
Other multiple carboxylase deficiency

D81.819 **Biotin-dependent carboxylase deficiency, unspecified**
Multiple carboxylase deficiency, unspecified

D81.89 **Other combined immunodeficiencies**

D81.9 **Combined immunodeficiency, unspecified**
Severe combined immunodeficiency disorder [SCID] NOS

D82 **Immunodeficiency associated with other major defects**
> **EXCLUDES 1** *ataxia telangiectasia [Louis-Bar] (G11.3)*

D82.0 **Wiskott-Aldrich syndrome**
Immunodeficiency with thrombocytopenia and eczema
> **DEFINITION** X-linked immunodeficiency syndrome presenting with eczema, thrombocytopenia, and recurrent pyogenic infection.

D82.1 **Di George's syndrome**
Pharyngeal pouch syndrome
Thymic alymphoplasia
Thymic aplasia or hypoplasia with immunodeficiency
> **DEFINITION** Congenital disorder with hypoplasia or aplasia of the thymus and parathyroid glands; associated with congenital heart defects, great vessel anomalies, esophageal atresia, and abnormal facial structure.

D82.2 **Immunodeficiency with short-limbed stature**

D82.3 **Immunodeficiency following hereditary defective response to Epstein-Barr virus**
X-linked lymphoproliferative disease

D82.4 **Hyperimmunoglobulin E [IgE] syndrome**

> **CODING TIP ✓** Patients with Hyperimmunoglobulin E [IgE] Syndrome have a lifelong condition characterized by elevated IgE levels, which may also be referred to as "Job Syndrome." These patients are highly prone to problematic skin conditions such as eczema, skin lesions and infections (abscesses), sinus infections, and other respiratory infections, which should be additionally coded when present.

D82.8 **Immunodeficiency associated with other specified major defects**

D82.9 **Immunodeficiency associated with major defect, unspecified**

D83 **Common variable immunodeficiency**

D83.0 **Common variable immunodeficiency with predominant abnormalities of B-cell numbers and function**

D83.1 **Common variable immunodeficiency with predominant immunoregulatory T-cell disorders**

D83.2 **Common variable immunodeficiency with autoantibodies to B- or T-cells**

D83.8 **Other common variable immunodeficiencies**

D83.9 **Common variable immunodeficiency, unspecified**

D84 **Other immunodeficiencies**

D84.0 **Lymphocyte function antigen-1 [LFA-1] defect**

D84.1 **Defects in the complement system**
C1 esterase inhibitor [C1-INH] deficiency

D84.8 **Other specified immunodeficiencies**

D84.9 **Immunodeficiency, unspecified**

D86 **Sarcoidosis**

D86.0 **Sarcoidosis of lung**

D86.1 **Sarcoidosis of lymph nodes**

D86.2 **Sarcoidosis of lung with sarcoidosis of lymph nodes**

D86.3 **Sarcoidosis of skin**

D86.8 **Sarcoidosis of other sites**

D86.81 **Sarcoid meningitis**

D86.82 **Multiple cranial nerve palsies in sarcoidosis**

D86.83 **Sarcoid iridocyclitis**

D86.84 **Sarcoid pyelonephritis**
Tubulo-interstitial nephropathy in sarcoidosis

D86.85 **Sarcoid myocarditis**

D86.86 **Sarcoid arthropathy**
Polyarthritis in sarcoidosis

D86.87 **Sarcoid myositis**

D86.89 **Sarcoidosis of other sites**
Hepatic granuloma
Uveoparotid fever [Heerfordt]

D86.9 **Sarcoidosis, unspecified**

D89 **Other disorders involving the immune mechanism, not elsewhere classified**
> **EXCLUDES 1** *hyperglobulinemia NOS (R77.1)*
> *monoclonal gammopathy (of undetermined significance) (D47.2)*
> **EXCLUDES 2** *transplant failure and rejection (T86.-)*

D89.0 **Polyclonal hypergammaglobulinemia**
Benign hypergammaglobulinemic purpura
Polyclonal gammopathy NOS

D89.1 **Cryoglobulinemia**
Cryoglobulinemic purpura
Cryoglobulinemic vasculitis
Essential cryoglobulinemia
Idiopathic cryoglobulinemia
Mixed cryoglobulinemia
Primary cryoglobulinemia
Secondary cryoglobulinemia

D89.2 **Hypergammaglobulinemia, unspecified**

+ D89.3 **Immune reconstitution syndrome**
Immune reconstitution inflammatory syndrome [IRIS]
Use additional code for adverse effect, if applicable, to identify drug (T36-T50 with fifth or sixth character 5)

● D89.4 **Mast cell activation syndrome and related disorders**
> **EXCLUDES 1** *aggressive systemic mastocytosis (C96.2)*
> *cutaneous mastocytosis (Q82.2)*
> *indolent systemic mastocytosis (D47.0)*
> *malignant mastocytoma (C96.2)*
> *mast cell leukemia (C94.3-)*
> *mastocytoma (D47.0)*
> *systemic mastocytosis associated with a clonal hematologic non-mast cell lineage disease (SM-AHNMD) (D47.0)*

● New   ▲ Revised   *Manifestation*   🔟-🔢 Digit Indicators   ⬒ Laterality   🅐 Adult (15+ years)   Ⓜ Maternity (12-55 years)   🅝 Newborn   🅟 Pediatric (0-17 years)   ♂ Male   ♀ Female
✖ Deleted   Unspecified   + Additional code

● **D89.40**   **Mast cell activation, unspecified**

Mast cell activation disorder, unspecified
Mast cell activation syndrome, NOS

● **D89.41**   **Monoclonal mast cell activation syndrome**

● **D89.42**   **Idiopathic mast cell activation syndrome**

● **D89.43**   **Secondary mast cell activation**

Secondary mast cell activation syndrome
Code also:
    underlying etiology, if known

● **D89.49**   **Other mast cell activation disorder**

Other mast cell activation syndrome

⑤ **D89.8**   **Other specified disorders involving the immune mechanism, not elsewhere classified**

⑥ ✚ **D89.81**   **Graft-versus-host disease**

Code first underlying cause, such as:
    complications of transplanted organs and tissue
      (T86.-)
    complications of blood transfusion (T80.89)
Use additional code to identify associated
manifestations, such as:
    desquamative dermatitis (L30.8)
    diarrhea (R19.7)
    elevated bilirubin (R17)
    hair loss (L65.9)

CODING TIP ✓   Code D89.81 may only be assigned when the provider specifically indicates this condition. Development of complicating disease, such as ESRD or neoplasm in a transplanted organ should not be assumed to indicate graft versus host disease.

✚ **D89.810**   **Acute graft-versus-host disease**

✚ **D89.811**   **Chronic graft-versus-host disease**

✚ **D89.812**   **Acute on chronic graft-versus-host disease**

✚ **D89.813**   **Graft-versus-host disease, unspecified**

D89.82   **Autoimmune lymphoproliferative syndrome [ALPS]**

D89.89   **Other specified disorders involving the immune mechanism, not elsewhere classified**

EXCLUDES 1   *human immunodeficiency virus disease (B20)*

D89.9   **Disorder involving the immune mechanism, unspecified**

Immune disease NOS
AHA: 3Q 2015, 22

● New   ▲ Revised   *Manifestation*   ④-⑦ Digit Indicators   ⊟ Laterality   Ⓐ Adult (15+ years)   Ⓜ Maternity (12-55 years)   Ⓝ Newborn   Ⓟ Pediatric (0-17 years)   ♂ Male   ♀ Female

✖ Deleted   Unspecified   ✚ Additional code

2017 ICD-10-CM Expert for Physicians   © 2017 DecisionHealth   515

CHAPTER 4: ENDOCRINE, NUTRITIONAL AND METABOLIC DISEASES (E00-E89)

Note: All neoplasms, whether functionally active or not, are classified in Chapter 2. Appropriate codes in this chapter (i.e. E05.8, E07.0, E16-E31, E34.-) may be used as additional codes to indicate either functional activity by neoplasms and ectopic endocrine tissue or hyperfunction and hypofunction of endocrine glands associated with neoplasms and other conditions classified elsewhere.

EXCLUDES 1   *transitory endocrine and metabolic disorders specific to newborn (P70-P74)*

This chapter contains the following blocks:

E00-E07	Disorders of thyroid gland
E08-E13	Diabetes mellitus
E15-E16	Other disorders of glucose regulation and pancreatic internal secretion
E20-E35	Disorders of other endocrine glands
E36	Intraoperative complications of endocrine system
E40-E46	Malnutrition
E50-E64	Other nutritional deficiencies
E65-E68	Overweight, obesity and other hyperalimentation
E70-E88	Metabolic disorders
E89	Postprocedural endocrine and metabolic complications and disorders, not elsewhere classified

Disorders of thyroid gland (E00-E07)

⁴⁺ E00   Congenital iodine-deficiency syndrome

Use additional code (F70-F79) to identify associated intellectual disabilities.

EXCLUDES 1   *subclinical iodine-deficiency hypothyroidism (E02)*

CODING TIP ✓   Congenital iodine-deficiency syndrome is a congenital disorder often referred to as "cretinism." Congenital iodine-deficiency syndrome results from a thyroid hormone deficiency during fetal development and marked in childhood by dwarfed stature, mental retardation, dystrophy of the bones, and a low basal metabolism.

CODING TIP ✓   Do not assign a code from E00 to identify any condition that it is not reported as "congenital" (present from birth).

⁺ E00.0   Congenital iodine-deficiency syndrome, neurological type
Endemic cretinism, neurological type

DEFINITION   Underactive thyroid gland present at birth with inadequate hormone production and slowed metabolic processes. Untreated, it can cause brain damage, mental retardation, and developmental delays.

⁺ E00.1   Congenital iodine-deficiency syndrome, myxedematous type
Endemic hypothyroid cretinism
Endemic cretinism, myxedematous type

⁺ E00.2   Congenital iodine-deficiency syndrome, mixed type
Endemic cretinism, mixed type

⁺ E00.9   Congenital iodine-deficiency syndrome, unspecified
Congenital iodine-deficiency hypothyroidism NOS
Endemic cretinism NOS

⁴ E01   Iodine-deficiency related thyroid disorders and allied conditions

EXCLUDES 1   *congenital iodine-deficiency syndrome (E00.-)*
subclinical iodine-deficiency hypothyroidism (E02)

E01.0   Iodine-deficiency related diffuse (endemic) goiter

E01.1   Iodine-deficiency related multinodular (endemic) goiter
Iodine-deficiency related nodular goiter

E01.2   Iodine-deficiency related (endemic) goiter, unspecified
Endemic goiter NOS

E01.8   Other iodine-deficiency related thyroid disorders and allied conditions
Acquired iodine-deficiency hypothyroidism NOS

E02   Subclinical iodine-deficiency hypothyroidism

DEFINITION   Early stage of hypothyroidism marked by increased TSH levels and normal free thyroxin T4 levels; occurs when the body requires additional TSH in order to produce enough thyroxin, and developing into overt hypothyroidism in a few years.

⁴ E03   Other hypothyroidism

EXCLUDES 1   *iodine-deficiency related hypothyroidism (E00-E02)*
postprocedural hypothyroidism (E89.0)

Other hypothyroidism

Normal   Hypothyroidism

Thyroid

Normal thyroid   Insufficient thyroid
hormone production   hormone production

E03.0   Congenital hypothyroidism with diffuse goiter
Congenital parenchymatous goiter (nontoxic)
Congenital goiter (nontoxic) NOS

EXCLUDES 1   *transitory congenital goiter with normal function (P72.0)*

DEFINITION   Abnormal hormone production or blocked TSH receptors in the fetus causing underactive thyroid with diffuse enlargement at birth, tracheal compression, difficulty breathing, and dysphagia.

E03.1   Congenital hypothyroidism without goiter
Aplasia of thyroid (with myxedema)
Congenital atrophy of thyroid
Congenital hypothyroidism NOS

⁺ E03.2   Hypothyroidism due to medicaments and other exogenous substances
Code first:
poisoning due to drug or toxin, if applicable (T36-T65 with fifth or sixth character 1-4 or 6)
Use additional code for adverse effect, if applicable, to identify drug (T36-T50 with fifth or sixth character 5)

E03.3   Postinfectious hypothyroidism

DEFINITION   Damage to normal thyroid function from a previous infection, resulting in tiredness, weight gain, constipation, cold intolerance, dry skin, slowed mental function, and depression.

E03.4   Atrophy of thyroid (acquired)

EXCLUDES 1   *congenital atrophy of thyroid (E03.1)*

DEFINITION   Abnormally small thyroid due to tissue degeneration and wasting; the gland becomes nonviable or severely reduced in function.

E03.5   Myxedema coma

DEFINITION   Fully symptomatic hypothyroid disease manifesting with coma in a seriously decompensated state, mostly in the elderly, accompanied by hypothermia, hypoventilation with hypoxia, hypercapnia, hyponatremia, and bradycardia.

E03.8   Other specified hypothyroidism

E03.9   Hypothyroidism, unspecified
Myxedema NOS

DEFINITION   Failure of the thyroid gland to produce enough hormone to maintain the body's metabolism, causing fatigue, weight gain, muscle aches and cramps, cold intolerance, memory loss, and depression.

⁴ E04   Other nontoxic goiter

EXCLUDES 1   *congenital goiter (NOS) (diffuse) (parenchymatous) (E03.0)*
iodine-deficiency related goiter (E00-E02)

E04.0   Nontoxic diffuse goiter
Diffuse (colloid) nontoxic goiter
Simple nontoxic goiter

DEFINITION   Generalized, simple, painless thyroid enlargement without impairment of glandular function due to an overload of thyroid-stimulating hormone (TSH) from the pituitary gland.

E04.1   Nontoxic single thyroid nodule
Colloid nodule (cystic) (thyroid)
Nontoxic uninodular goiter
Thyroid (cystic) nodule NOS

● New   ▲ Revised   *Manifestation*   ④-⑦ Digit Indicators   ⊟ Laterality   Ⓐ Adult (15+ years)   Ⓜ Maternity (12-55 years)   Ⓝ Newborn   Ⓟ Pediatric (0-17 years)   ♂ Male   ♀ Female
✖ ~~Deleted~~   Unspecified   ⁺ Additional code

DEFINITION A simple, painless, cyst-like node or singular goiter on the thyroid that is not impairing the normal glandular function.

E04.2 **Nontoxic multinodular goiter**
Cystic goiter NOS
Multinodular (cystic) goiter NOS
DEFINITION Multiple hard knobs, or cysts, in the thyroid detected by palpation but not impairing function or causing disease.

E04.8 **Other specified nontoxic goiter**

E04.9 **Nontoxic goiter, unspecified**
Goiter NOS
Nodular goiter (nontoxic) NOS

④ **E05** **Thyrotoxicosis [hyperthyroidism]**
EXCLUDES 1 *chronic thyroiditis with transient thyrotoxicosis (E06.2)*
neonatal thyrotoxicosis (P72.1)

CODING TIP ✓ Thyrotoxicosis is another term for hyperthyroidism and these terms may frequently be used interchangeably in clinical records. Unspecified hyperthyroidism should be coded to E05.9-.

CODING TIP ✓ Codes from category E05 are combination codes that indicate the presence or absence of thyrotoxic crisis or storm. A thyrotoxic crisis (also called "thyroid storm") is a condition that may occur among individuals with hyperthyroidism and is marked by tachycardia, fever, and hypertension, which may or may not result in congestive heart failure and/or shock. Thyrotoxic crisis should only be coded when specified by the physician and cannot be assumed based upon other symptoms alone.

⑤ **E05.0** **Thyrotoxicosis with diffuse goiter**
Exophthalmic or toxic goiter NOS
Graves' disease
Toxic diffuse goiter
DEFINITION Thyrotropin receptor antibody production that mimics the pituitary's normal regulatory hormone, overriding it and increasing thyroid hormone production, marked by enlarged thyroid and bulging eyes.

E05.00 **Thyrotoxicosis with diffuse goiter without thyrotoxic crisis or storm**
DEFINITION Hyperthyroid conditions with excessive hormone production and speeding up of body functions; increased heart rate and blood pressure, excessive sweating, hand tremors, nervousness and anxiety, insomnia, and weight loss with increased appetite.

E05.01 **Thyrotoxicosis with diffuse goiter with thyrotoxic crisis or storm**
DEFINITION Severe, sudden worsening of hyperthyroid conditions from injury, stress, or gland removal that can lead to coma and death, manifesting with tachycardia, arrhythmia, vomiting, high fever, diarrhea, and dehydration.

⑤ **E05.1** **Thyrotoxicosis with toxic single thyroid nodule**
Thyrotoxicosis with toxic uninodular goiter

E05.10 **Thyrotoxicosis with toxic single thyroid nodule without thyrotoxic crisis or storm**

E05.11 **Thyrotoxicosis with toxic single thyroid nodule with thyrotoxic crisis or storm**

⑤ **E05.2** **Thyrotoxicosis with toxic multinodular goiter**
Toxic nodular goiter NOS

E05.20 **Thyrotoxicosis with toxic multinodular goiter without thyrotoxic crisis or storm**

E05.21 **Thyrotoxicosis with toxic multinodular goiter with thyrotoxic crisis or storm**

⑤ **E05.3** **Thyrotoxicosis from ectopic thyroid tissue**

E05.30 **Thyrotoxicosis from ectopic thyroid tissue without thyrotoxic crisis or storm**

E05.31 **Thyrotoxicosis from ectopic thyroid tissue with thyrotoxic crisis or storm**

⑤ **E05.4** **Thyrotoxicosis factitia**

CODING TIP ✓ Thyrotoxicosis factitia is a condition of higher than normal thyroid hormones (T3 and T4) resulting from excess ingestion of thyroid hormone (medication). The condition may be iatrogenic (adverse effect resulting from taking prescription correctly) or due to intentional ingestion of excess medication (poisoning). The cause of the condition should be identified and the coder should follow guidelines for coding of adverse effects and poisoning when assigning a code from E05.4-.

E05.40 **Thyrotoxicosis factitia without thyrotoxic crisis or storm**

E05.41 **Thyrotoxicosis factitia with thyrotoxic crisis or storm**

⑤ **E05.8** **Other thyrotoxicosis**
Overproduction of thyroid-stimulating hormone

E05.80 **Other thyrotoxicosis without thyrotoxic crisis or storm**

E05.81 **Other thyrotoxicosis with thyrotoxic crisis or storm**

⑤ **E05.9** **Thyrotoxicosis, unspecified**
Hyperthyroidism NOS

E05.90 **Thyrotoxicosis, unspecified without thyrotoxic crisis or storm**

E05.91 **Thyrotoxicosis, unspecified with thyrotoxic crisis or storm**

④ **E06** **Thyroiditis**
EXCLUDES 1 *postpartum thyroiditis (O90.5)*

CODING TIP ✓ Thyroiditis is a condition marked by inflammation of the thyroid (may or may not be infectious in nature), and should not be confused with hyperthyroidism. Various forms of thyroiditis may result in either hyper- or hypothyroidism.

✚ **E06.0** **Acute thyroiditis**
Abscess of thyroid
Pyogenic thyroiditis
Suppurative thyroiditis
Use additional code (B95-B97) to identify infectious agent.
DEFINITION Painful infection of the thyroid gland, often with abscess and pus formation.

Acute thyroiditis

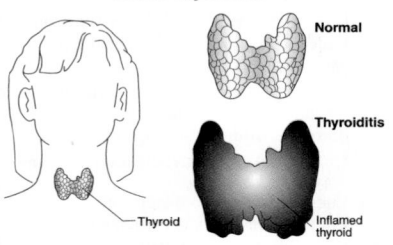

E06.1 **Subacute thyroiditis**
de Quervain thyroiditis
Giant-cell thyroiditis
Granulomatous thyroiditis
Nonsuppurative thyroiditis
Viral thyroiditis
EXCLUDES 1 *autoimmune thyroiditis (E06.3)*

DEFINITION Thyroid inflammation often resulting from another disease, such as mumps or flu, presenting with fever, radiating neck pain, and hyperthyroidism symptoms than can last months.

E06.2 **Chronic thyroiditis with transient thyrotoxicosis**
EXCLUDES 1 *autoimmune thyroiditis (E06.3)*

E06.3 **Autoimmune thyroiditis**
Hashimoto's thyroiditis
Hashitoxicosis (transient)
Lymphadenoid goiter
Lymphocytic thyroiditis
Struma lymphomatosa
DEFINITION Autoimmune inflammation of the thyroid with lymphocyte infiltration that presents with painless thyroid enlargement and hypothyroid symptoms.

● New   ▲ Revised   *Manifestation*   ④-⑦ Digit Indicators   ▯ Laterality   Ⓐ Adult (15+ years)   Ⓜ Maternity (12-55 years)   Ⓝ Newborn   Ⓟ Pediatric (0-17 years)   ♂ Male   ♀ Female
✖ Deleted   Unspecified   ✚ Additional code

518   © 2017 DecisionHealth   2017 ICD-10-CM Expert for Physicians

+ E06.4　**Drug-induced thyroiditis**
Use additional code for adverse effect, if applicable, to identify drug (T36-T50 with fifth or sixth character 5)

CODING TIP ✓　Drug-induced thyroiditis should only be coded when clinical record documentation clearly indicates thyroiditis (inflammation of the thyroid), resulting from the administration of a specific drug or chemical. The causative drug or chemical should be identified and the coder should follow guidelines for coding of adverse effects and poisoning when assigning a code from E06.4.

DEFINITION　Iatrogenic inflammation of the thyroid due to taking certain medications, such as lithium, or an overdose of iodine.

E06.5　**Other chronic thyroiditis**
Chronic fibrous thyroiditis
Chronic thyroiditis NOS
Ligneous thyroiditis
Riedel thyroiditis

E06.9　**Thyroiditis, unspecified**

DEFINITION　Inflammation of the thyroid with noticeable swelling, often on one side, possibly inducing symptoms of hyper- or hypothyroidism, from unspecified causation or acuity.

4 E07　**Other disorders of thyroid**

E07.0　**Hypersecretion of calcitonin**
C-cell hyperplasia of thyroid
Hypersecretion of thyrocalcitonin

E07.1　**Dyshormogenetic goiter**
Familial dyshormogenetic goiter
Pendred's syndrome
EXCLUDES 1　*transitory congenital goiter with normal function (P72.0)*

5 E07.8　**Other specified disorders of thyroid**

E07.81　**Sick-euthyroid syndrome**
Euthyroid sick-syndrome
DEFINITION　Condition in which thyroid hormone levels are off due to a non-thyroid related problem.

E07.89　**Other specified disorders of thyroid**
Abnormality of thyroid-binding globulin
Hemorrhage of thyroid
Infarction of thyroid

E07.9　**Disorder of thyroid, unspecified**

Diabetes mellitus (E08-E13)

GUIDELINES　Section I.C.4.a.1)-3)
The diabetes mellitus codes are combination codes that include the type of diabetes mellitus, the body system affected, and the complications affecting that body system. As many codes within a particular category as are necessary to describe all of the complications of the disease may be used. They should be sequenced based on the reason for a particular encounter. Assign as many codes from categories E08 – E13 as needed to identify all of the associated conditions that the patient has.

The age of a patient is not the sole determining factor, though most type 1 diabetics develop the condition before reaching puberty. For this reason type 1 diabetes mellitus is also referred to as juvenile diabetes.

If the type of diabetes mellitus is not documented in the medical record the default is E11.-, Type 2 diabetes mellitus.

If the documentation in a medical record does not indicate the type of diabetes but does indicate that the patient uses insulin, code E11, Type 2 diabetes mellitus, should be assigned. Code Z79.4 ... should also be assigned to indicate that the patient uses insulin. Code Z79.4 should not be assigned if insulin is given temporarily to bring a type 2 patient's blood sugar under control during an encounter.

GUIDELINES　Section I.C.4.a.6)
Codes under categories E08, Diabetes mellitus due to underlying condition, E09, Drug or chemical induced diabetes mellitus, and E13, Other specified diabetes mellitus, identify complications/manifestations associated with secondary diabetes mellitus. Secondary diabetes is always caused by another condition or event (e.g., cystic fibrosis, malignant neoplasm of pancreas, pancreatectomy, adverse effect of drug, or poisoning).

CODING TIP ✓　Codes for diabetes mellitus do not identify controlled vs uncontrolled. When hyperglycemia, uncontrolled, poorly controlled, or out of control, is documented, diabetes with hyperglycemia should be coded. The clinical record should support the hyperglycemia.

CODING TIP ✓　Codes E08-E13 are combination codes that generally do not require a second code unless specified by the code specific guidelines. Specifically, when coding diabetes with an ulcer or diabetic chronic kidney disease, a second code is required. A second code to identify gastroparesis (K31.84) may be assigned when coding diabetic gastroparesis.

CODING TIP ✓　Reference the alphabetical index to review conditions that the classification assumes are related to diabetes. All manifestations/complications listed under the word 'with' in the index are presumed related unless the physician specified a different cause in documentation.

▲ 4 + E08　**Diabetes mellitus due to underlying condition**
Code first the underlying condition, such as:
congenital rubella (P35.0)
Cushing's syndrome (E24.-)
cystic fibrosis (E84.-)
malignant neoplasm (C00-C96)
malnutrition (E40-E46)
pancreatitis and other diseases of the pancreas (K85-K86.-)
Use additional code to identify control using:
insulin (Z79.4)
oral antidiabetic drugs (Z79.84)
oral hypoglycemic drugs (Z79.84)
EXCLUDES 1　*drug or chemical induced diabetes mellitus (E09.-)*
gestational diabetes (O24.4-)
neonatal diabetes mellitus (P70.2)
postpancreatectomy diabetes mellitus (E13.-)
postprocedural diabetes mellitus (E13.-)
secondary diabetes mellitus NEC (E13.-)
type 1 diabetes mellitus (E10.-)
type 2 diabetes mellitus (E11.-)

GUIDELINES　Section I.C.4.a.6)
Codes under categories E08, Diabetes mellitus due to underlying condition, E09, Drug or chemical induced diabetes mellitus, and E13, Other specified diabetes mellitus, identify complications/manifestations associated with secondary diabetes mellitus. Secondary diabetes is always caused by another condition or event (e.g., cystic fibrosis, malignant neoplasm of pancreas, pancreatectomy, adverse effect of drug, or poisoning).

CODING TIP ✓　When coding diabetes mellitus due to an underlying condition, the underlying condition and relationship to diabetes should be specified by the provider. This category does not include unspecified secondary diabetes, postprocedural/postpancreatectomy diabetes, or diabetes due to the effects of drugs or chemicals.

CODING TIP ✓　When assigning any diabetes code from E08, E09, E11, or E13, an additional Z code (Z79.4) to identify insulin use must also be assigned if the patient requires insulin (including sliding scale insulin). Do not assign an additional code to identify insulin use that is temporary.

5 + E08.0　**Diabetes mellitus due to underlying condition with hyperosmolarity**

+ E08.00　**Diabetes mellitus due to underlying condition with hyperosmolarity without nonketotic hyperglycemic-hyperosmolar coma (NKHHC)**

+ E08.01　**Diabetes mellitus due to underlying condition with hyperosmolarity with coma**

5 + E08.1　**Diabetes mellitus due to underlying condition with ketoacidosis**

+ E08.10　**Diabetes mellitus due to underlying condition with ketoacidosis without coma**

+ E08.11　**Diabetes mellitus due to underlying condition with ketoacidosis with coma**

5 + E08.2　**Diabetes mellitus due to underlying condition with kidney complications**

+ E08.21　**Diabetes mellitus due to underlying condition with diabetic nephropathy**
Diabetes mellitus due to underlying condition with intercapillary glomerulosclerosis
Diabetes mellitus due to underlying condition with intracapillary glomerulonephrosis
Diabetes mellitus due to underlying condition with Kimmelstiel-Wilson disease

● New　▲ Revised　*Manifestation*　4-7 Digit Indicators　⊟ Laterality　A Adult (15+ years)　M Maternity (12-55 years)　N Newborn　P Pediatric (0-17 years)　♂ Male　♀ Female
✖ Deleted　Unspecified　+ Additional code

2017 ICD-10-CM Expert for Physicians　　　　　© 2017 DecisionHealth　　　519

+ E08.22   Diabetes mellitus due to underlying condition with diabetic chronic kidney disease
Use additional code to identify stage of chronic kidney disease (N18.1-N18.6)

> **CODING TIP ✓**   When diabetic CKD and hypertension are documented, sequence the appropriate category of diabetes with CKD (E--.22) and the appropriate hypertension code (I12 or I13) prior to N18. The hypertension or the diabetes may be sequenced first depending on the focus of care.

> **CODING TIP ✓**   Assign an additional code from N18- to indicate the stage of CKD. When diabetic nephropathy and CKD are documented, code diabetic CKD, not nephropathy.

+ E08.29   Diabetes mellitus due to underlying condition with other diabetic kidney complication
Renal tubular degeneration in diabetes mellitus due to underlying condition

⑤ + E08.3   Diabetes mellitus due to underlying condition with ophthalmic complications

> **CODING TIP ✓**   When coding diabetes with ophthalmic manifestations, review the clinical record and plan of care to ensure that the functional impact of visual impairments is reported.

⑥ + E08.31   Diabetes mellitus due to underlying condition with unspecified diabetic retinopathy

+ E08.311   Diabetes mellitus due to underlying condition with unspecified diabetic retinopathy with macular edema

+ E08.319   Diabetes mellitus due to underlying condition with unspecified diabetic retinopathy without macular edema

▲ ⑥ + E08.32   Diabetes mellitus due to underlying condition with mild nonproliferative diabetic retinopathy
Diabetes mellitus due to underlying condition with nonproliferative diabetic retinopathy NOS

One of the following 7th characters is to be assigned to codes in subcategory E08.32 to designate laterality of the disease:
1   right eye
2   left eye
3   bilateral
9   unspecified eye

⑦ ⊟ + E08.321-   Diabetes mellitus due to underlying condition with mild nonproliferative diabetic retinopathy with macular edema

⑦ ⊟ + E08.329-   Diabetes mellitus due to underlying condition with mild nonproliferative diabetic retinopathy without macular edema

▲ ⑥ + E08.33   Diabetes mellitus due to underlying condition with moderate nonproliferative diabetic retinopathy

One of the following 7th characters is to be assigned to codes in subcategory E08.33 to designate laterality of the disease:
1   right eye
2   left eye
3   bilateral
9   unspecified eye

⑦ ⊟ + E08.331-   Diabetes mellitus due to underlying condition with moderate nonproliferative diabetic retinopathy with macular edema

⑦ ⊟ + E08.339-   Diabetes mellitus due to underlying condition with moderate nonproliferative diabetic retinopathy without macular edema

▲ ⑥ + E08.34   Diabetes mellitus due to underlying condition with severe nonproliferative diabetic retinopathy

One of the following 7th characters is to be assigned to codes in subcategory E08.34 to designate laterality of the disease:
1   right eye
2   left eye
3   bilateral
9   unspecified eye

⑦ ⊟ + E08.341-   Diabetes mellitus due to underlying condition with severe nonproliferative diabetic retinopathy with macular edema

⑦ ⊟ + E08.349-   Diabetes mellitus due to underlying condition with severe nonproliferative diabetic retinopathy without macular edema

▲ ⑥ + E08.35   Diabetes mellitus due to underlying condition with proliferative diabetic retinopathy

One of the following 7th characters is to be assigned to codes in subcategory E08.35 to designate laterality of the disease:
1   right eye
2   left eye
3   bilateral
9   unspecified eye

⑦ ⊟ + E08.351-   Diabetes mellitus due to underlying condition with proliferative diabetic retinopathy with macular edema

● ⑦ ⊟ + E08.352-   Diabetes mellitus due to underlying condition with proliferative diabetic retinopathy with traction retinal detachment involving the macula

● ⑦ ⊟ + E08.353-   Diabetes mellitus due to underlying condition with proliferative diabetic retinopathy with traction retinal detachment not involving the macula

● ⑦ ⊟ + E08.354-   Diabetes mellitus due to underlying condition with proliferative diabetic retinopathy with combined traction retinal detachment and rhegmatogenous retinal detachment

● ⑦ ⊟ + E08.355-   Diabetes mellitus due to underlying condition with stable proliferative diabetic retinopathy

⑦ ⊟ + E08.359-   Diabetes mellitus due to underlying condition with proliferative diabetic retinopathy without macular edema

+ E08.36   Diabetes mellitus due to underlying condition with diabetic cataract

● ⑦ ⊟ + E08.37X-   Diabetes mellitus due to underlying condition with diabetic macular edema, resolved following treatment

One of the following 7th characters is to be assigned to code E08.37 to designate laterality of the disease:
1   right eye
2   left eye
3   bilateral
9   unspecified eye

+ E08.39   Diabetes mellitus due to underlying condition with other diabetic ophthalmic complication
Use additional code to identify manifestation, such as: diabetic glaucoma (H40-H42)

> **CODING TIP ✓**   When a diagnosis of diabetes mellitus due to an underlying condition with diabetic glaucoma is reported, assign E08.39. The most common type of diabetic glaucoma is open angle glaucoma coded with H40.1-.

⑤ + E08.4   Diabetes mellitus due to underlying condition with neurological complications

> **CODING TIP ✓**   When coding diabetes with neurological complications, the physician must indicate a clear relationship between the diabetes and neurologic condition. Diabetes due to an underlying condition with loss of protective sensation or diabetic peripheral neuropathy should be coded to E08.42.

+ E08.40   Diabetes mellitus due to underlying condition with diabetic neuropathy, unspecified

+ E08.41   Diabetes mellitus due to underlying condition with diabetic mononeuropathy

+ E08.42   Diabetes mellitus due to underlying condition with diabetic polyneuropathy
Diabetes mellitus due to underlying condition with diabetic neuralgia

+ E08.43   Diabetes mellitus due to underlying condition with diabetic autonomic (poly)neuropathy
Diabetes mellitus due to underlying condition with diabetic gastroparesis
AHA: 4Q 2013, 115

+ E08.44   Diabetes mellitus due to underlying condition with diabetic amyotrophy

+ E08.49   Diabetes mellitus due to underlying condition with other diabetic neurological complication

● New   ▲ Revised   *Manifestation* / Unspecified   ④-⑦ Digit Indicators   ⊟ Laterality   Ⓐ Adult (15+ years)   Ⓜ Maternity (12-55 years)   Ⓝ Newborn   Ⓟ Pediatric (0-17 years)   ♂ Male   ♀ Female
✖ Deleted   + Additional code

520   © 2017 DecisionHealth   2017 ICD-10-CM Expert for Physicians

⑤ + **E08.5** **Diabetes mellitus due to underlying condition with circulatory complications**

+ **E08.51** **Diabetes mellitus due to underlying condition with diabetic peripheral angiopathy without gangrene**

+ **E08.52** **Diabetes mellitus due to underlying condition with diabetic peripheral angiopathy with gangrene**
Diabetes mellitus due to underlying condition with diabetic gangrene

+ **E08.59** **Diabetes mellitus due to underlying condition with other circulatory complications**

⑥ + **E08.6** **Diabetes mellitus due to underlying condition with other specified complications**

⑥ + **E08.61** **Diabetes mellitus due to underlying condition with diabetic arthropathy**

+ **E08.610** **Diabetes mellitus due to underlying condition with diabetic neuropathic arthropathy**
Diabetes mellitus due to underlying condition with Charcôt's joints

+ **E08.618** **Diabetes mellitus due to underlying condition with other diabetic arthropathy**

⑥ + **E08.62** **Diabetes mellitus due to underlying condition with skin complications**

+ **E08.620** **Diabetes mellitus due to underlying condition with diabetic dermatitis**
Diabetes mellitus due to underlying condition with diabetic necrobiosis lipoidica

+ **E08.621** **Diabetes mellitus due to underlying condition with foot ulcer**
Use additional code to identify site of ulcer (L97.4-, L97.5-)

+ **E08.622** **Diabetes mellitus due to underlying condition with other skin ulcer**
Use additional code to identify site of ulcer (L97.1-L97.9, L98.41-L98.49)

+ **E08.628** **Diabetes mellitus due to underlying condition with other skin complications**

⑥ + **E08.63** **Diabetes mellitus due to underlying condition with oral complications**

+ **E08.630** **Diabetes mellitus due to underlying condition with periodontal disease**

+ **E08.638** **Diabetes mellitus due to underlying condition with other oral complications**

⑥ + **E08.64** **Diabetes mellitus due to underlying condition with hypoglycemia**

+ **E08.641** **Diabetes mellitus due to underlying condition with hypoglycemia with coma**

+ **E08.649** **Diabetes mellitus due to underlying condition with hypoglycemia without coma**

CODING TIP ✓ If encephalopathy is due to hypoglycemia, use G93.41 as an additional code.

+ **E08.65** **Diabetes mellitus due to underlying condition with hyperglycemia**

+ **E08.69** **Diabetes mellitus due to underlying condition with other specified complication**
Use additional code to identify complication

CODING TIP ✓ When osteomyelitis is specified as due to diabetes mellitus due to an underlying condition, code first the underlying condition, and assign code E08.69, followed by the appropriate code to specify the type and location of the osteomyelitis. ICD-10 does not allow for an assumed relationship between diabetes and osteomyelitis.

+ **E08.8** **Diabetes mellitus due to underlying condition with unspecified complications**

+ **E08.9** **Diabetes mellitus due to underlying condition without complications**

▲ ④ + **E09** **Drug or chemical induced diabetes mellitus**
Code first:
poisoning due to drug or toxin, if applicable (T36-T65 with fifth or sixth character 1-4 or 6)
Use additional code for adverse effect, if applicable, to identify drug (T36-T50 with fifth or sixth character 5)
Use additional code to identify control using:
insulin (Z79.4)
oral antidiabetic drugs (Z79.84)
oral hypoglycemic drugs (Z79.84)

EXCLUDES 1 *diabetes mellitus due to underlying condition (E08.-)*
gestational diabetes (O24.4-)
neonatal diabetes mellitus (P70.2)
postpancreatectomy diabetes mellitus (E13.-)
postprocedural diabetes mellitus (E13.-)
secondary diabetes mellitus NEC (E13.-)
type 1 diabetes mellitus (E10.-)
type 2 diabetes mellitus (E11.-)

GUIDELINES **Section I.C.4.a**
The diabetes mellitus codes are combination codes that include the type of diabetes mellitus, the body system affected, and the complications affecting that body system. As many codes within a particular category as are necessary to describe all of the complications of the disease may be used. They should be sequenced based on the reason for a particular encounter. Assign as many codes from categories E08 — E13 as needed to identify all of the associated conditions that the patient has.

GUIDELINES **Section I.C.4.a.6)**
Codes under categories E08, Diabetes mellitus due to underlying condition, E09, Drug or chemical induced diabetes mellitus, and E13, Other specified diabetes mellitus, identify complications/manifestations associated with secondary diabetes mellitus. Secondary diabetes is always caused by another condition or event (e.g., cystic fibrosis, malignant neoplasm of pancreas, pancreatectomy, adverse effect of drug, or poisoning).

CODING TIP ✓ When assigning any diabetes code from E08, E09, E11, or E13, an additional Z code (Z79.4) to identify insulin use must also be assigned if the patient requires insulin (including sliding scale insulin). Do not assign an additional code to identify insulin use that is temporary.

⑤ + **E09.0** **Drug or chemical induced diabetes mellitus with hyperosmolarity**

+ **E09.00** **Drug or chemical induced diabetes mellitus with hyperosmolarity without nonketotic hyperglycemic-hyperosmolar coma (NKHHC)**

+ **E09.01** **Drug or chemical induced diabetes mellitus with hyperosmolarity with coma**

⑤ + **E09.1** **Drug or chemical induced diabetes mellitus with ketoacidosis**

+ **E09.10** **Drug or chemical induced diabetes mellitus with ketoacidosis without coma**

+ **E09.11** **Drug or chemical induced diabetes mellitus with ketoacidosis with coma**

⑤ + **E09.2** **Drug or chemical induced diabetes mellitus with kidney complications**

+ **E09.21** **Drug or chemical induced diabetes mellitus with diabetic nephropathy**
Drug or chemical induced diabetes mellitus with intercapillary glomerulosclerosis
Drug or chemical induced diabetes mellitus with intracapillary glomerulonephrosis
Drug or chemical induced diabetes mellitus with Kimmelstiel-Wilson disease

+ **E09.22** **Drug or chemical induced diabetes mellitus with diabetic chronic kidney disease**
Use additional code to identify stage of chronic kidney disease (N18.1-N18.6)

CODING TIP ✓ When diabetic CKD and hypertension are documented, sequence the appropriate category of diabetes with CKD (E--.22) and the appropriate hypertension code (I12 or I13) prior to N18. The hypertension or the diabetes may be sequenced first depending on the focus of care.

● New   ▲ Revised   *Manifestation*   ④-⑦ Digit Indicators   ⊟ Laterality   Ⓐ Adult (15+ years)   Ⓜ Maternity (12-55 years)   Ⓝ Newborn   Ⓟ Pediatric (0-17 years)   ♂ Male   ♀ Female
✖ Deleted   Unspecified   + Additional code

CODING TIP ✓ Assign an additional code from N18- to indicate the stage of CKD. When diabetic nephropathy and CKD are documented, code diabetic CKD, not nephropathy.

+ E09.29 Drug or chemical induced diabetes mellitus with other diabetic kidney complication
Drug or chemical induced diabetes mellitus with renal tubular degeneration

⑤+ E09.3 Drug or chemical induced diabetes mellitus with ophthalmic complications

CODING TIP ✓ When coding diabetes with ophthalmic manifestations, review the clinical record and plan of care to ensure that the functional impact of visual impairments is reported.

⑥+ E09.31 Drug or chemical induced diabetes mellitus with unspecified diabetic retinopathy

+ E09.311 Drug or chemical induced diabetes mellitus with unspecified diabetic retinopathy with macular edema

+ E09.319 Drug or chemical induced diabetes mellitus with unspecified diabetic retinopathy without macular edema

▲⑥+ E09.32 Drug or chemical induced diabetes mellitus with mild nonproliferative diabetic retinopathy
Drug or chemical induced diabetes mellitus with nonproliferative diabetic retinopathy NOS

One of the following 7th characters is to be assigned to codes in subcategory E09.32 to designate laterality of the disease:
1   right eye
2   left eye
3   bilateral
9   unspecified eye

🗷⊟+ E09.321- Drug or chemical induced diabetes mellitus with mild nonproliferative diabetic retinopathy with macular edema

🗷⊟+ E09.329- Drug or chemical induced diabetes mellitus with mild nonproliferative diabetic retinopathy without macular edema

▲⑥+ E09.33 Drug or chemical induced diabetes mellitus with moderate nonproliferative diabetic retinopathy

One of the following 7th characters is to be assigned to codes in subcategory E09.33 to designate laterality of the disease:
1   right eye
2   left eye
3   bilateral
9   unspecified eye

🗷⊟+ E09.331- Drug or chemical induced diabetes mellitus with moderate nonproliferative diabetic retinopathy with macular edema

🗷⊟+ E09.339- Drug or chemical induced diabetes mellitus with moderate nonproliferative diabetic retinopathy without macular edema

▲⑥+ E09.34 Drug or chemical induced diabetes mellitus with severe nonproliferative diabetic retinopathy

One of the following 7th characters is to be assigned to codes in subcategory E09.34 to designate laterality of the disease:
1   right eye
2   left eye
3   bilateral
9   unspecified eye

🗷⊟+ E09.341- Drug or chemical induced diabetes mellitus with severe nonproliferative diabetic retinopathy with macular edema

🗷⊟+ E09.349- Drug or chemical induced diabetes mellitus with severe nonproliferative diabetic retinopathy without macular edema

▲⑥+ E09.35 Drug or chemical induced diabetes mellitus with proliferative diabetic retinopathy

One of the following 7th characters is to be assigned to codes in subcategory E09.35 to designate laterality of the disease:
1   right eye
2   left eye
3   bilateral
9   unspecified eye

🗷⊟+ E09.351- Drug or chemical induced diabetes mellitus with proliferative diabetic retinopathy with macular edema

●🗷⊟+ E09.352- Drug or chemical induced diabetes mellitus with proliferative diabetic retinopathy with traction retinal detachment involving the macula

●🗷⊟+ E09.353- Drug or chemical induced diabetes mellitus with proliferative diabetic retinopathy with traction retinal detachment not involving the macula

●🗷⊟+ E09.354- Drug or chemical induced diabetes mellitus with proliferative diabetic retinopathy with combined traction retinal detachment and rhegmatogenous retinal detachment

●🗷⊟+ E09.355- Drug or chemical induced diabetes mellitus with stable proliferative diabetic retinopathy

🗷⊟+ E09.359- Drug or chemical induced diabetes mellitus with proliferative diabetic retinopathy without macular edema

+ E09.36 Drug or chemical induced diabetes mellitus with diabetic cataract

●🗷⊟+ E09.37X- Drug or chemical induced diabetes mellitus with diabetic macular edema, resolved following treatment

One of the following 7th characters is to be assigned to code E09.37 to designate laterality of the disease:
1   right eye
2   left eye
3   bilateral
9   unspecified eye

+ E09.39 Drug or chemical induced diabetes mellitus with other diabetic ophthalmic complication
Use additional code to identify manifestation, such as: diabetic glaucoma (H40-H42)

CODING TIP ✓ When a diagnosis of drug or chemical induced diabetes mellitus with diabetic glaucoma is reported, assign E09.39. The most common type of diabetic glaucoma is open angle glaucoma coded with H40.1-.

⑤+ E09.4 Drug or chemical induced diabetes mellitus with neurological complications

CODING TIP ✓ When coding diabetes with neurological complications, the physician must indicate a clear relationship between the diabetes and neurologic condition. Drug or chemical induced diabetes mellitus with loss of protective sensation or diabetic peripheral neuropathy should be coded to E09.42.

+ E09.40 Drug or chemical induced diabetes mellitus with neurological complications with diabetic neuropathy, unspecified

+ E09.41 Drug or chemical induced diabetes mellitus with neurological complications with diabetic mononeuropathy

+ E09.42 Drug or chemical induced diabetes mellitus with neurological complications with diabetic polyneuropathy
Drug or chemical induced diabetes mellitus with diabetic neuralgia

+ E09.43 Drug or chemical induced diabetes mellitus with neurological complications with diabetic autonomic (poly)neuropathy
Drug or chemical induced diabetes mellitus with diabetic gastroparesis
AHA: 4Q 2013, 115

+ E09.44 Drug or chemical induced diabetes mellitus with neurological complications with diabetic amyotrophy

● New ▲ Revised *Manifestation* ④-🗷 Digit Indicators ⊟ Laterality 🅐 Adult (15+ years) Ⓜ Maternity (12-55 years) Ⓝ Newborn 🅟 Pediatric (0-17 years) ♂ Male ♀ Female
✖ Deleted Unspecified + Additional code

522   © 2017 DecisionHealth   2017 ICD-10-CM Expert for Physicians

+ E09.49 **Drug or chemical induced diabetes mellitus with neurological complications with other diabetic neurological complication**

⑤ + E09.5 **Drug or chemical induced diabetes mellitus with circulatory complications**

+ E09.51 **Drug or chemical induced diabetes mellitus with diabetic peripheral angiopathy without gangrene**

+ E09.52 **Drug or chemical induced diabetes mellitus with diabetic peripheral angiopathy with gangrene**
Drug or chemical induced diabetes mellitus with diabetic gangrene

+ E09.59 **Drug or chemical induced diabetes mellitus with other circulatory complications**

⑤ + E09.6 **Drug or chemical induced diabetes mellitus with other specified complications**

⑥ + E09.61 **Drug or chemical induced diabetes mellitus with diabetic arthropathy**

+ E09.610 **Drug or chemical induced diabetes mellitus with diabetic neuropathic arthropathy**
Drug or chemical induced diabetes mellitus with Charcôt's joints

+ E09.618 **Drug or chemical induced diabetes mellitus with other diabetic arthropathy**

⑥ + E09.62 **Drug or chemical induced diabetes mellitus with skin complications**

+ E09.620 **Drug or chemical induced diabetes mellitus with diabetic dermatitis**
Drug or chemical induced diabetes mellitus with diabetic necrobiosis lipoidica

+ E09.621 **Drug or chemical induced diabetes mellitus with foot ulcer**
Use additional code to identify site of ulcer (L97.4-, L97.5-)

+ E09.622 **Drug or chemical induced diabetes mellitus with other skin ulcer**
Use additional code to identify site of ulcer (L97.1-L97.9, L98.41-L98.49)

+ E09.628 **Drug or chemical induced diabetes mellitus with other skin complications**

⑥ + E09.63 **Drug or chemical induced diabetes mellitus with oral complications**

+ E09.630 **Drug or chemical induced diabetes mellitus with periodontal disease**

+ E09.638 **Drug or chemical induced diabetes mellitus with other oral complications**

⑥ + E09.64 **Drug or chemical induced diabetes mellitus with hypoglycemia**

+ E09.641 **Drug or chemical induced diabetes mellitus with hypoglycemia with coma**

+ E09.649 **Drug or chemical induced diabetes mellitus with hypoglycemia without coma**
CODING TIP ✓ If encephalopathy is due to hypoglycemia, use G93.41 as an additional code.

+ E09.65 **Drug or chemical induced diabetes mellitus with hyperglycemia**

+ E09.69 **Drug or chemical induced diabetes mellitus with other specified complication**
Use additional code to identify complication
CODING TIP ✓ When osteomyelitis is specified as due to drug or chemical induced diabetes mellitus, code first any applicable poisoning by the causative drug or toxin, and assign code E09.69, or assign code E09.69, followed by the appropriate code to identify an adverse effect by the drug, and then assign the appropriate code to specify the type and location of the osteomyelitis. ICD-10 does not allow for an assumed relationship between diabetes and osteomyelitis.

+ E09.8 **Drug or chemical induced diabetes mellitus with unspecified complications**

+ E09.9 **Drug or chemical induced diabetes mellitus without complications**

④ E10 **Type 1 diabetes mellitus**
INCLUDES brittle diabetes (mellitus)
diabetes (mellitus) due to autoimmune process
diabetes (mellitus) due to immune mediated pancreatic islet beta-cell destruction
idiopathic diabetes (mellitus)
juvenile onset diabetes (mellitus)
ketosis-prone diabetes (mellitus)
EXCLUDES 1 *diabetes mellitus due to underlying condition (E08.-)*
drug or chemical induced diabetes mellitus (E09.-)
gestational diabetes (O24.4-)
hyperglycemia NOS (R73.9)
neonatal diabetes mellitus (P70.2)
postpancreatectomy diabetes mellitus (E13.-)
postprocedural diabetes mellitus (E13.-)
secondary diabetes mellitus NEC (E13.-)
type 2 diabetes mellitus (E11.-)
GUIDELINES Section I.C.4.a.1)
The age of a patient is not the sole determining factor, though most type 1 diabetics develop the condition before reaching puberty. For this reason type 1 diabetes mellitus is also referred to as juvenile diabetes.

⑤ E10.1 **Type 1 diabetes mellitus with ketoacidosis**
DEFINITION Diabetic complication characterized by hyperglycemia, hyperketonemia, and metabolic acidosis; often presents with nausea, vomiting, and abdominal pain; may progress to cerebral edema or lead to coma and/or death.

E10.10 **Type 1 diabetes mellitus with ketoacidosis without coma**
AHA: 3Q 2013, 20

E10.11 **Type 1 diabetes mellitus with ketoacidosis with coma**

⑤ E10.2 **Type 1 diabetes mellitus with kidney complications**

E10.21 **Type 1 diabetes mellitus with diabetic nephropathy**
Type 1 diabetes mellitus with intercapillary glomerulosclerosis
Type 1 diabetes mellitus with intracapillary glomerulonephrosis
Type 1 diabetes mellitus with Kimmelstiel-Wilson disease

+ E10.22 **Type 1 diabetes mellitus with diabetic chronic kidney disease**
Use additional code to identify stage of chronic kidney disease (N18.1-N18.6)
CODING TIP ✓ When diabetic CKD and hypertension are documented, sequence the appropriate category of diabetes with CKD (E--.22) and the appropriate hypertension code (I12 or I13) prior to N18. The hypertension or the diabetes may be sequenced first depending on the focus of care.
CODING TIP ✓ Assign an additional code from N18- to indicate the stage of CKD. When diabetic nephropathy and CKD are documented, code diabetic CKD, not nephropathy.

E10.29 **Type 1 diabetes mellitus with other diabetic kidney complication**
Type 1 diabetes mellitus with renal tubular degeneration
AHA: 1Q 2016, 13

⑤ E10.3 **Type 1 diabetes mellitus with ophthalmic complications**
CODING TIP ✓ When coding diabetes with ophthalmic manifestations, review the clinical record and plan of care to ensure that the functional impact of visual impairments is reported.

⑥ E10.31 **Type 1 diabetes mellitus with unspecified diabetic retinopathy**

E10.311 **Type 1 diabetes mellitus with unspecified diabetic retinopathy with macular edema**

E10.319 **Type 1 diabetes mellitus with unspecified diabetic retinopathy without macular edema**

● New   ▲ Revised   *Manifestation*   ④-⑦ Digit Indicators   ⊟ Laterality   Ⓐ Adult (15+ years)   Ⓜ Maternity (12-55 years)   Ⓝ Newborn   Ⓟ Pediatric (0-17 years)   ♂ Male   ♀ Female
✖ ~~Deleted~~   Unspecified   + Additional code

▲ ⑥ **E10.32**   **Type 1 diabetes mellitus with mild nonproliferative diabetic retinopathy**
Type 1 diabetes mellitus with nonproliferative diabetic retinopathy NOS

One of the following 7th characters is to be assigned to codes in subcategory E10.32 to designate laterality of the disease:
1   right eye
2   left eye
3   bilateral
9   unspecified eye

⑦ ⊟ **E10.321-**   **Type 1 diabetes mellitus with mild nonproliferative diabetic retinopathy with macular edema**

⑦ ⊟ **E10.329-**   **Type 1 diabetes mellitus with mild nonproliferative diabetic retinopathy without macular edema**

▲ ⑥ **E10.33**   **Type 1 diabetes mellitus with moderate nonproliferative diabetic retinopathy**

One of the following 7th characters is to be assigned to codes in subcategory E10.33 to designate laterality of the disease:
1   right eye
2   left eye
3   bilateral
9   unspecified eye

⑦ ⊟ **E10.331-**   **Type 1 diabetes mellitus with moderate nonproliferative diabetic retinopathy with macular edema**

⑦ ⊟ **E10.339-**   **Type 1 diabetes mellitus with moderate nonproliferative diabetic retinopathy without macular edema**

▲ ⑥ **E10.34**   **Type 1 diabetes mellitus with severe nonproliferative diabetic retinopathy**

One of the following 7th characters is to be assigned to codes in subcategory E10.34 to designate laterality of the disease:
1   right eye
2   left eye
3   bilateral
9   unspecified eye

⑦ ⊟ **E10.341-**   **Type 1 diabetes mellitus with severe nonproliferative diabetic retinopathy with macular edema**

⑦ ⊟ **E10.349-**   **Type 1 diabetes mellitus with severe nonproliferative diabetic retinopathy without macular edema**

▲ ⑥ **E10.35**   **Type 1 diabetes mellitus with proliferative diabetic retinopathy**

One of the following 7th characters is to be assigned to codes in subcategory E10.35 to designate laterality of the disease:
1   right eye
2   left eye
3   bilateral
9   unspecified eye

⑦ ⊟ **E10.351-**   **Type 1 diabetes mellitus with proliferative diabetic retinopathy with macular edema**

● ⑦ ⊟ **E10.352-**   **Type 1 diabetes mellitus with proliferative diabetic retinopathy with traction retinal detachment involving the macula**

● ⑦ ⊟ **E10.353-**   **Type 1 diabetes mellitus with proliferative diabetic retinopathy with traction retinal detachment not involving the macula**

● ⑦ ⊟ **E10.354-**   **Type 1 diabetes mellitus with proliferative diabetic retinopathy with combined traction retinal detachment and rhegmatogenous retinal detachment**

● ⑦ ⊟ **E10.355-**   **Type 1 diabetes mellitus with stable proliferative diabetic retinopathy**

⑦ ⊟ **E10.359-**   **Type 1 diabetes mellitus with proliferative diabetic retinopathy without macular edema**

E10.36   **Type 1 diabetes mellitus with diabetic cataract**

● ⑦ ⊟ **E10.37X-**   **Type 1 diabetes mellitus with diabetic macular edema, resolved following treatment**

One of the following 7th characters is to be assigned to code E10.37 to designate laterality of the disease:
1   right eye
2   left eye
3   bilateral
9   unspecified eye

+ **E10.39**   **Type 1 diabetes mellitus with other diabetic ophthalmic complication**
Use additional code to identify manifestation, such as: diabetic glaucoma (H40-H42)

CODING TIP ✓   When a diagnosis of type 1 diabetes mellitus with diabetic glaucoma is reported, assign E10.39. The most common type of diabetic glaucoma is open angle glaucoma coded with H40.1-.

⑤ **E10.4**   **Type 1 diabetes mellitus with neurological complications**

CODING TIP ✓   When coding diabetes with neurological complications, the physician must indicate a clear relationship between the diabetes and neurologic condition. Type 1 diabetes with loss of protective sensation or diabetic peripheral neuropathy should be coded to E10.42.

E10.40   **Type 1 diabetes mellitus with diabetic neuropathy, unspecified**

E10.41   **Type 1 diabetes mellitus with diabetic mononeuropathy**

E10.42   **Type 1 diabetes mellitus with diabetic polyneuropathy**
Type 1 diabetes mellitus with diabetic neuralgia

E10.43   **Type 1 diabetes mellitus with diabetic autonomic (poly)neuropathy**
Type 1 diabetes mellitus with diabetic gastroparesis
AHA: 4Q 2013, 115

E10.44   **Type 1 diabetes mellitus with diabetic amyotrophy**

E10.49   **Type 1 diabetes mellitus with other diabetic neurological complication**

⑤ **E10.5**   **Type 1 diabetes mellitus with circulatory complications**

E10.51   **Type 1 diabetes mellitus with diabetic peripheral angiopathy without gangrene**

E10.52   **Type 1 diabetes mellitus with diabetic peripheral angiopathy with gangrene**
Type 1 diabetes mellitus with diabetic gangrene

E10.59   **Type 1 diabetes mellitus with other circulatory complications**

⑤ **E10.6**   **Type 1 diabetes mellitus with other specified complications**

⑥ **E10.61**   **Type 1 diabetes mellitus with diabetic arthropathy**

E10.610   **Type 1 diabetes mellitus with diabetic neuropathic arthropathy**
Type 1 diabetes mellitus with Charcôt's joints

E10.618   **Type 1 diabetes mellitus with other diabetic arthropathy**

⑥ **E10.62**   **Type 1 diabetes mellitus with skin complications**

E10.620   **Type 1 diabetes mellitus with diabetic dermatitis**
Type 1 diabetes mellitus with diabetic necrobiosis lipoidica

+ **E10.621**   **Type 1 diabetes mellitus with foot ulcer**
Use additional code to identify site of ulcer (L97.4-, L97.5-)

+ **E10.622**   **Type 1 diabetes mellitus with other skin ulcer**
Use additional code to identify site of ulcer (L97.1-L97.9, L98.41-L98.49)

E10.628   **Type 1 diabetes mellitus with other skin complications**

⑥ **E10.63**   **Type 1 diabetes mellitus with oral complications**

E10.630   **Type 1 diabetes mellitus with periodontal disease**

E10.638   **Type 1 diabetes mellitus with other oral complications**

⑥ **E10.64**   **Type 1 diabetes mellitus with hypoglycemia**

E10.641   **Type 1 diabetes mellitus with hypoglycemia with coma**

E10.649   **Type 1 diabetes mellitus with hypoglycemia without coma**

● New   ▲ Revised   *Manifestation*   ④-⑦ Digit Indicators   ⊟ Laterality   Ⓐ Adult (15+ years)   Ⓜ Maternity (12-55 years)   Ⓝ Newborn   Ⓟ Pediatric (0-17 years)   ♂ Male   ♀ Female
✖ ~~Deleted~~   Unspecified   + Additional code

524   © 2017 DecisionHealth   2017 ICD-10-CM Expert for Physicians

CODING TIP ✓ If encephalopathy is due to hypoglycemia, use G93.41 as an additional code.

AHA: 1Q 2016, 13

E10.65 Type 1 diabetes mellitus with hyperglycemia

+ **E10.69** Type 1 diabetes mellitus with other specified complication

Use additional code to identify complication

CODING TIP ✓ When osteomyelitis is specified as due to type 1 diabetes mellitus, assign code E10.69, followed by the appropriate code to specify the type and location of the osteomyelitis. ICD-10 does not allow for an assumed relationship between diabetes and osteomyelitis.

E10.8 Type 1 diabetes mellitus with unspecified complications

E10.9 Type 1 diabetes mellitus without complications

▲ ▣ + **E11** Type 2 diabetes mellitus

INCLUDES diabetes (mellitus) due to insulin secretory defect
diabetes NOS
insulin resistant diabetes (mellitus)

Use additional code to identify control using:
insulin (Z79.4)
oral antidiabetic drugs (Z79.84)
oral hypoglycemic drugs (Z79.84)

EXCLUDES 1 *diabetes mellitus due to underlying condition (E08.-)*
drug or chemical induced diabetes mellitus (E09.-)
gestational diabetes (O24.4-)
neonatal diabetes mellitus (P70.2)
postpancreatectomy diabetes mellitus (E13.-)
postprocedural diabetes mellitus (E13.-)
secondary diabetes mellitus NEC (E13.-)
type 1 diabetes mellitus (E10.-)

GUIDELINES Section I.C.4.a.2)-3)
If the type of diabetes mellitus is not documented in the medical record the default is E11.-, Type 2 diabetes mellitus. If the documentation in a medical record does not indicate the type of diabetes but does indicate that the patient uses insulin, code E11, Type 2 diabetes mellitus, should be assigned. Code Z79.4 should also be assigned to indicate that the patient uses insulin. Code Z79.4 should not be assigned if insulin is given temporarily to bring a type 2 patient's blood sugar under control during an encounter.

CODING TIP ✓ When assigning any diabetes code from E08, E09, E11, or E13, an additional Z code (Z79.4) to identify insulin use must also be assigned if the patient requires insulin (including sliding scale insulin). Do not assign an additional code to identify insulin use that is temporary.

▣ + **E11.0** Type 2 diabetes mellitus with hyperosmolarity

DEFINITION Metabolic diabetic emergency presenting with altered consciousness varying from confusion or disorientation to coma, with extreme dehydration, and high blood concentrations of sugar and sodium.

+ **E11.00** Type 2 diabetes mellitus with hyperosmolarity without nonketotic hyperglycemic-hyperosmolar coma (NKHHC)

+ **E11.01** Type 2 diabetes mellitus with hyperosmolarity with coma

▣ + **E11.2** Type 2 diabetes mellitus with kidney complications

+ **E11.21** Type 2 diabetes mellitus with diabetic nephropathy
Type 2 diabetes mellitus with intercapillary glomerulosclerosis
Type 2 diabetes mellitus with intracapillary glomerulonephrosis
Type 2 diabetes mellitus with Kimmelstiel-Wilson disease

+ **E11.22** Type 2 diabetes mellitus with diabetic chronic kidney disease
Use additional code to identify stage of chronic kidney disease (N18.1-N18.6)

CODING TIP ✓ When diabetic CKD and hypertension are documented, sequence the appropriate category of diabetes with CKD (E--.22) and the appropriate hypertension code (I12 or I13) prior to N18. The hypertension or the diabetes may be sequenced first depending on the focus of care.

CODING TIP ✓ Assign an additional code from N18- to indicate the stage of CKD. When diabetic nephropathy and CKD are documented, code diabetic CKD, not nephropathy.

AHA: 2Q 2016, 36
AHA: 1Q 2016, 12-13

+ **E11.29** Type 2 diabetes mellitus with other diabetic kidney complication
Type 2 diabetes mellitus with renal tubular degeneration

▣ + **E11.3** Type 2 diabetes mellitus with ophthalmic complications

CODING TIP ✓ When coding diabetes with ophthalmic manifestations, review the clinical record and plan of care to ensure that the functional impact of visual impairments is reported.

▣ + **E11.31** Type 2 diabetes mellitus with unspecified diabetic retinopathy

+ **E11.311** Type 2 diabetes mellitus with unspecified diabetic retinopathy with macular edema

+ **E11.319** Type 2 diabetes mellitus with unspecified diabetic retinopathy without macular edema

AHA: 3Q 2013, 20

▲ ▣ + **E11.32** Type 2 diabetes mellitus with mild nonproliferative diabetic retinopathy
Type 2 diabetes mellitus with nonproliferative diabetic retinopathy NOS

One of the following 7th characters is to be assigned to codes in subcategory E11.32 to designate laterality of the disease:
1   right eye
2   left eye
3   bilateral
9   unspecified eye

▼ ▣ + **E11.321-** Type 2 diabetes mellitus with mild nonproliferative diabetic retinopathy with macular edema

▼ ▣ + **E11.329-** Type 2 diabetes mellitus with mild nonproliferative diabetic retinopathy without macular edema

▲ ▣ + **E11.33** Type 2 diabetes mellitus with moderate nonproliferative diabetic retinopathy

One of the following 7th characters is to be assigned to codes in subcategory E11.33 to designate laterality of the disease:
1   right eye
2   left eye
3   bilateral
9   unspecified eye

▼ ▣ + **E11.331-** Type 2 diabetes mellitus with moderate nonproliferative diabetic retinopathy with macular edema

▼ ▣ + **E11.339-** Type 2 diabetes mellitus with moderate nonproliferative diabetic retinopathy without macular edema

▲ ▣ + **E11.34** Type 2 diabetes mellitus with severe nonproliferative diabetic retinopathy

One of the following 7th characters is to be assigned to codes in subcategory E11.34 to designate laterality of the disease:
1   right eye
2   left eye
3   bilateral
9   unspecified eye

▼ ▣ + **E11.341-** Type 2 diabetes mellitus with severe nonproliferative diabetic retinopathy with macular edema

▼ ▣ + **E11.349-** Type 2 diabetes mellitus with severe nonproliferative diabetic retinopathy without macular edema

● New ▲ Revised *Manifestation* ▣-▣ Digit Indicators ▣ Laterality ▣ Adult (15+ years) ▣ Maternity (12-55 years) ▣ Newborn ▣ Pediatric (0-17 years) ♂ Male ♀ Female
✖ Deleted Unspecified + Additional code

2017 ICD-10-CM Expert for Physicians   © 2017 DecisionHealth   525

▲ 6 + E11.35   **Type 2 diabetes mellitus with proliferative diabetic retinopathy**

One of the following 7th characters is to be assigned to codes in subcategory E11.35 to designate laterality of the disease:
1   right eye
2   left eye
3   bilateral
9   unspecified eye

7 ▤ + E11.351-   **Type 2 diabetes mellitus with proliferative diabetic retinopathy with macular edema**

● 7 ▤ + E11.352-   **Type 2 diabetes mellitus with proliferative diabetic retinopathy with traction retinal detachment involving the macula**

● 7 ▤ + E11.353-   **Type 2 diabetes mellitus with proliferative diabetic retinopathy with traction retinal detachment not involving the macula**

● 7 ▤ + E11.354-   **Type 2 diabetes mellitus with proliferative diabetic retinopathy with combined traction retinal detachment and rhegmatogenous retinal detachment**

● 7 ▤ + E11.355-   **Type 2 diabetes mellitus with stable proliferative diabetic retinopathy**

7 ▤ + E11.359-   **Type 2 diabetes mellitus with proliferative diabetic retinopathy without macular edema**

+ E11.36   **Type 2 diabetes mellitus with diabetic cataract**
AHA: 2Q 2016, 36

● 7 ▤ + E11.37X-   **Type 2 diabetes mellitus with diabetic macular edema, resolved following treatment**

One of the following 7th characters is to be assigned to code E11.37 to designate laterality of the disease:
1   right eye
2   left eye
3   bilateral
9   unspecified eye

+ E11.39   **Type 2 diabetes mellitus with other diabetic ophthalmic complication**
Use additional code to identify manifestation, such as: diabetic glaucoma (H40-H42)

CODING TIP ✓ When a diagnosis of type 2 or unspecified diabetes mellitus with diabetic glaucoma is reported, assign E11.39. The most common type of diabetic glaucoma is open angle glaucoma coded with H40.1-.

5 + E11.4   **Type 2 diabetes mellitus with neurological complications**

CODING TIP ✓ When coding diabetes with neurological complications, the physician must indicate a clear relationship between the diabetes and neurologic condition. Type 2 or unspecified diabetes with loss of protective sensation or diabetic peripheral neuropathy with loss of protective sensation should be coded to E11.42.

+ E11.40   **Type 2 diabetes mellitus with diabetic neuropathy, unspecified**
AHA: 4Q 2013, 129

+ E11.41   **Type 2 diabetes mellitus with diabetic mononeuropathy**

+ E11.42   **Type 2 diabetes mellitus with diabetic polyneuropathy**
Type 2 diabetes mellitus with diabetic neuralgia
AHA: 1Q 2016, 12-13

+ E11.43   **Type 2 diabetes mellitus with diabetic autonomic (poly)neuropathy**
Type 2 diabetes mellitus with diabetic gastroparesis
AHA: 2Q 2016, 36
AHA: 4Q 2013, 115

+ E11.44   **Type 2 diabetes mellitus with diabetic amyotrophy**
AHA: 2Q 2016, 36

+ E11.49   **Type 2 diabetes mellitus with other diabetic neurological complication**

5 + E11.5   **Type 2 diabetes mellitus with circulatory complications**

+ E11.51   **Type 2 diabetes mellitus with diabetic peripheral angiopathy without gangrene**

+ E11.52   **Type 2 diabetes mellitus with diabetic peripheral angiopathy with gangrene**
Type 2 diabetes mellitus with diabetic gangrene

+ E11.59   **Type 2 diabetes mellitus with other circulatory complications**

5 + E11.6   **Type 2 diabetes mellitus with other specified complications**

6 + E11.61   **Type 2 diabetes mellitus with diabetic arthropathy**

+ E11.610   **Type 2 diabetes mellitus with diabetic neuropathic arthropathy**
Type 2 diabetes mellitus with Charcôt's joints
AHA: 2Q 2016, 36

+ E11.618   **Type 2 diabetes mellitus with other diabetic arthropathy**
AHA: 2Q 2016, 36

6 + E11.62   **Type 2 diabetes mellitus with skin complications**

+ E11.620   **Type 2 diabetes mellitus with diabetic dermatitis**
Type 2 diabetes mellitus with diabetic necrobiosis lipoidica

+ E11.621   **Type 2 diabetes mellitus with foot ulcer**
Use additional code to identify site of ulcer (L97.4-, L97.5-)
AHA: 1Q 2016, 12-13

+ E11.622   **Type 2 diabetes mellitus with other skin ulcer**
Use additional code to identify site of ulcer (L97.1-L97.9, L98.41-L98.49)

+ E11.628   **Type 2 diabetes mellitus with other skin complications**

6 + E11.63   **Type 2 diabetes mellitus with oral complications**

+ E11.630   **Type 2 diabetes mellitus with periodontal disease**

+ E11.638   **Type 2 diabetes mellitus with other oral complications**

6 + E11.64   **Type 2 diabetes mellitus with hypoglycemia**

+ E11.641   **Type 2 diabetes mellitus with hypoglycemia with coma**

+ E11.649   **Type 2 diabetes mellitus with hypoglycemia without coma**

CODING TIP ✓ If encephalopathy is due to hypoglycemia, use G93.41 as an additional code.
AHA: 3Q 2015, 21

+ E11.65   **Type 2 diabetes mellitus with hyperglycemia**
AHA: 3Q 2013, 20

+ E11.69   **Type 2 diabetes mellitus with other specified complication**
Use additional code to identify complication

CODING TIP ✓ When osteomyelitis is specified as due to type 2 or unspecified diabetes mellitus, assign code E11.69, followed by the appropriate code to specify the type and location of the osteomyelitis. ICD-10 does not allow for an assumed relationship between diabetes and osteomyelitis.

+ E11.8   **Type 2 diabetes mellitus with unspecified complications**

+ E11.9   **Type 2 diabetes mellitus without complications**

DEFINITION Underproduction or underutilization of insulin; presents with abnormally high blood sugar (glucose) levels, resulting in impaired carbohydrate and fat metabolism.
AHA: 2Q 2016, 36
AHA: 4Q 2013, 128

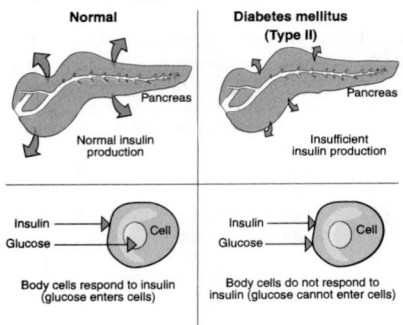

Type 2 diabetes mellitus without complications

Normal	Diabetes mellitus (Type II)
Pancreas	Pancreas
Normal insulin production	Insufficient insulin production
Insulin → Glucose → Cell	Insulin → Glucose → Cell
Body cells respond to insulin (glucose enters cells)	Body cells do not respond to insulin (glucose cannot enter cells)

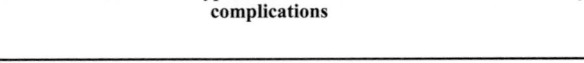

● New   ▲ Revised   *Manifestation*   4-7 Digit Indicators   ▤ Laterality   Ⓐ Adult (15+ years)   Ⓜ Maternity (12-55 years)   Ⓝ Newborn   Ⓟ Pediatric (0-17 years)   ♂ Male   ♀ Female
✖ Deleted   Unspecified   + Additional code

526   © 2017 DecisionHealth   2017 ICD-10-CM Expert for Physicians

▲ ◢ + **E13** **Other specified diabetes mellitus**

> **INCLUDES** diabetes mellitus due to genetic defects of beta-cell function
> diabetes mellitus due to genetic defects in insulin action
> postpancreatectomy diabetes mellitus
> postprocedural diabetes mellitus
> secondary diabetes mellitus NEC

Use additional code to identify control using:
insulin (Z79.4)
oral antidiabetic drugs (Z79.84)
oral hypoglycemic drugs (Z79.84)

> **EXCLUDES 1** *diabetes (mellitus) due to autoimmune process (E10.-)*
> *diabetes (mellitus) due to immune mediated pancreatic islet beta-cell destruction (E10.-)*
> *diabetes mellitus due to underlying condition (E08.-)*
> *drug or chemical induced diabetes mellitus (E09.-)*
> *gestational diabetes (O24.4-)*
> *neonatal diabetes mellitus (P70.2)*
> *type 1 diabetes mellitus (E10.-)*
> *type 2 diabetes mellitus (E11.-)*

> **GUIDELINES** **Section I.C.4.a.6)**
> Codes under categories E08, Diabetes mellitus due to underlying condition, E09, Drug or chemical induced diabetes mellitus, and E13, Other specified diabetes mellitus, identify complications/manifestations associated with secondary diabetes mellitus. Secondary diabetes is always caused by another condition or event (e.g., cystic fibrosis, malignant neoplasm of pancreas, pancreatectomy, adverse effect of drug, or poisoning).

> **CODING TIP ✓** When assigning any diabetes code from E08, E09, E11, or E13, an additional Z code (Z79.4) to identify insulin use must also be assigned if the patient requires insulin (including sliding scale insulin). Do not assign an additional code to identify insulin use that is temporary.

> **CODING TIP ✓** When diabetes is specified as due to surgical removal of the pancreas (causing a lack of insulin), proper sequencing requires the coder to assign first code E89.1 Postprocedural hypoinsulinemia, followed by the appropriate code from category E13, as well as a code for acquired absence of pancreas (Z90.41-), and insulin use (Z79.4).

⑤ + **E13.0** **Other specified diabetes mellitus with hyperosmolarity**

+ **E13.00** **Other specified diabetes mellitus with hyperosmolarity without nonketotic hyperglycemic-hyperosmolar coma (NKHHC)**

+ **E13.01** **Other specified diabetes mellitus with hyperosmolarity with coma**

⑤ + **E13.1** **Other specified diabetes mellitus with ketoacidosis**

+ **E13.10** **Other specified diabetes mellitus with ketoacidosis without coma**

> **CODING TIP ✓** Until a specific code is released for Type II diabetes with ketoacidosis, use E13.10.
> AHA: 2Q 2016, 10
> AHA: 1Q 2013, 26

+ **E13.11** **Other specified diabetes mellitus with ketoacidosis with coma**

⑤ + **E13.2** **Other specified diabetes mellitus with kidney complications**

+ **E13.21** **Other specified diabetes mellitus with diabetic nephropathy**
> Other specified diabetes mellitus with intercapillary glomerulosclerosis
> Other specified diabetes mellitus with intracapillary glomerulonephrosis
> Other specified diabetes mellitus with Kimmelstiel-Wilson disease

+ **E13.22** **Other specified diabetes mellitus with diabetic chronic kidney disease**
> *Use additional code to identify stage of chronic kidney disease (N18.1-N18.6)*

> **CODING TIP ✓** When diabetic CKD and hypertension are documented, sequence the appropriate category of diabetes with CKD (E--.22) and the appropriate hypertension code (I12 or I13) prior to N18. The hypertension or the diabetes may be sequenced first depending on the focus of care.

> **CODING TIP ✓** Assign an additional code from N18- to indicate the stage of CKD. When diabetic nephropathy and CKD are documented, code diabetic CKD, not nephropathy.

+ **E13.29** **Other specified diabetes mellitus with other diabetic kidney complication**
> Other specified diabetes mellitus with renal tubular degeneration

⑤ + **E13.3** **Other specified diabetes mellitus with ophthalmic complications**

⑥ + **E13.31** **Other specified diabetes mellitus with unspecified diabetic retinopathy**

+ **E13.311** **Other specified diabetes mellitus with unspecified diabetic retinopathy with macular edema**

+ **E13.319** **Other specified diabetes mellitus with unspecified diabetic retinopathy without macular edema**

▲ ⑥ + **E13.32** **Other specified diabetes mellitus with mild nonproliferative diabetic retinopathy**
> Other specified diabetes mellitus with nonproliferative diabetic retinopathy NOS

> One of the following 7th characters is to be assigned to codes in subcategory E13.32 to designate laterality of the disease:
> 1   right eye
> 2   left eye
> 3   bilateral
> 9   unspecified eye

⑦◳ + **E13.321-** **Other specified diabetes mellitus with mild nonproliferative diabetic retinopathy with macular edema**

⑦◳ + **E13.329-** **Other specified diabetes mellitus with mild nonproliferative diabetic retinopathy without macular edema**

▲ ⑥ + **E13.33** **Other specified diabetes mellitus with moderate nonproliferative diabetic retinopathy**

> One of the following 7th characters is to be assigned to codes in subcategory E13.33 to designate laterality of the disease:
> 1   right eye
> 2   left eye
> 3   bilateral
> 9   unspecified eye

⑦◳ + **E13.331-** **Other specified diabetes mellitus with moderate nonproliferative diabetic retinopathy with macular edema**

⑦◳ + **E13.339-** **Other specified diabetes mellitus with moderate nonproliferative diabetic retinopathy without macular edema**

▲ ⑥ + **E13.34** **Other specified diabetes mellitus with severe nonproliferative diabetic retinopathy**

> One of the following 7th characters is to be assigned to codes in subcategory E13.34 to designate laterality of the disease:
> 1   right eye
> 2   left eye
> 3   bilateral
> 9   unspecified eye

⑦◳ + **E13.341-** **Other specified diabetes mellitus with severe nonproliferative diabetic retinopathy with macular edema**

⑦◳ + **E13.349-** **Other specified diabetes mellitus with severe nonproliferative diabetic retinopathy without macular edema**

● New   ▲ Revised   *Manifestation*   ◢-⑦ Digit Indicators   ⊟ Laterality   Ⓐ Adult (15+ years)   Ⓜ Maternity (12-55 years)   Ⓝ Newborn (0-17 years)   Ⓟ Pediatric   ♂ Male   ♀ Female
✖ Deleted   Unspecified   + Additional code

2017 ICD-10-CM Expert for Physicians

© 2017 DecisionHealth   527

▲ 🖪 + **E13.35**   **Other specified diabetes mellitus with proliferative diabetic retinopathy**

One of the following 7th characters is to be assigned to codes in subcategory E13.35 to designate laterality of the disease:
1   right eye
2   left eye
3   bilateral
9   unspecified eye

🗗🗏 + **E13.351-**   **Other specified diabetes mellitus with proliferative diabetic retinopathy with macular edema**

● 🗗🗏 + **E13.352-**   **Other specified diabetes mellitus with proliferative diabetic retinopathy with traction retinal detachment involving the macula**

● 🗗🗏 + **E13.353-**   **Other specified diabetes mellitus with proliferative diabetic retinopathy with traction retinal detachment not involving the macula**

● 🗗🗏 + **E13.354-**   **Other specified diabetes mellitus with proliferative diabetic retinopathy with combined traction retinal detachment and rhegmatogenous retinal detachment**

● 🗗🗏 + **E13.355-**   **Other specified diabetes mellitus with stable proliferative diabetic retinopathy**

🗗🗏 + **E13.359-**   **Other specified diabetes mellitus with proliferative diabetic retinopathy without macular edema**

+ **E13.36**   **Other specified diabetes mellitus with diabetic cataract**

● 🗗🗏 + **E13.37X-**   **Other specified diabetes mellitus with diabetic macular edema, resolved following treatment**

One of the following 7th characters is to be assigned to code E13.37 to designate laterality of the disease:
1   right eye
2   left eye
3   bilateral
9   unspecified eye

+ **E13.39**   **Other specified diabetes mellitus with other diabetic ophthalmic complication**
Use additional code to identify manifestation, such as: diabetic glaucoma (H40-H42)
CODING TIP ✓   When a diagnosis of other specified diabetes mellitus with diabetic glaucoma is reported, assign code E13.39. The most common type of diabetic glaucoma is open angle glaucoma coded with H40.-1.

🖪 + **E13.4**   **Other specified diabetes mellitus with neurological complications**
CODING TIP ✓   When coding diabetes with neurological complications, the physician must indicate a clear relationship between the diabetes and neurologic condition. Other specified diabetes with loss of protective sensation or diabetic peripheral neuropathy should be coded to E13.42.

+ **E13.40**   **Other specified diabetes mellitus with diabetic neuropathy, unspecified**

+ **E13.41**   **Other specified diabetes mellitus with diabetic mononeuropathy**

+ **E13.42**   **Other specified diabetes mellitus with diabetic polyneuropathy**
Other specified diabetes mellitus with diabetic neuralgia

+ **E13.43**   **Other specified diabetes mellitus with diabetic autonomic (poly)neuropathy**
Other specified diabetes mellitus with diabetic gastroparesis
AHA: 4Q 2013, 115

+ **E13.44**   **Other specified diabetes mellitus with diabetic amyotrophy**

+ **E13.49**   **Other specified diabetes mellitus with other diabetic neurological complication**

🖪 + **E13.5**   **Other specified diabetes mellitus with circulatory complications**

+ **E13.51**   **Other specified diabetes mellitus with diabetic peripheral angiopathy without gangrene**

+ **E13.52**   **Other specified diabetes mellitus with diabetic peripheral angiopathy with gangrene**
Other specified diabetes mellitus with diabetic gangrene

+ **E13.59**   **Other specified diabetes mellitus with other circulatory complications**

🖪 + **E13.6**   **Other specified diabetes mellitus with other specified complications**

🖪 + **E13.61**   **Other specified diabetes mellitus with diabetic arthropathy**

+ **E13.610**   **Other specified diabetes mellitus with diabetic neuropathic arthropathy**
Other specified diabetes mellitus with Charcôt's joints

+ **E13.618**   **Other specified diabetes mellitus with other diabetic arthropathy**

🖪 + **E13.62**   **Other specified diabetes mellitus with skin complications**

+ **E13.620**   **Other specified diabetes mellitus with diabetic dermatitis**
Other specified diabetes mellitus with diabetic necrobiosis lipoidica

+ **E13.621**   **Other specified diabetes mellitus with foot ulcer**
Use additional code to identify site of ulcer (L97.4-, L97.5-)

+ **E13.622**   **Other specified diabetes mellitus with other skin ulcer**
Use additional code to identify site of ulcer (L97.1-L97.9, L98.41-L98.49)

+ **E13.628**   **Other specified diabetes mellitus with other skin complications**

🖪 + **E13.63**   **Other specified diabetes mellitus with oral complications**

+ **E13.630**   **Other specified diabetes mellitus with periodontal disease**

+ **E13.638**   **Other specified diabetes mellitus with other oral complications**

🖪 + **E13.64**   **Other specified diabetes mellitus with hypoglycemia**

+ **E13.641**   **Other specified diabetes mellitus with hypoglycemia with coma**

+ **E13.649**   **Other specified diabetes mellitus with hypoglycemia without coma**
CODING TIP ✓   If encephalopathy is due to hypoglycemia, use G93.41 as an additional code.

+ **E13.65**   **Other specified diabetes mellitus with hyperglycemia**

+ **E13.69**   **Other specified diabetes mellitus with other specified complication**
Use additional code to identify complication
CODING TIP ✓   When osteomyelitis is specified as due to other specified diabetes mellitus, assign code E13.69, followed by the appropriate code to specify the type and location of the osteomyelitis. ICD-10 does not allow for an assumed relationship between diabetes and osteomyelitis.

+ **E13.8**   **Other specified diabetes mellitus with unspecified complications**

+ **E13.9**   **Other specified diabetes mellitus without complications**

Other disorders of glucose regulation and pancreatic internal secretion (E15-E16)

E15   **Nondiabetic hypoglycemic coma**
INCLUDES   drug-induced insulin coma in nondiabetic
hyperinsulinism with hypoglycemic coma
hypoglycemic coma NOS

🔳 **E16**   **Other disorders of pancreatic internal secretion**

▲ + **E16.0**   **Drug-induced hypoglycemia without coma**
Use additional code for adverse effect, if applicable, to identify drug (T36-T50 with fifth or sixth character 5)
EXCLUDES 1   *diabetes with hypoglycemia without coma (E09.692)*

▲ **E16.1**   **Other hypoglycemia**
Functional hyperinsulinism
Functional nonhyperinsulinemic hypoglycemia
Hyperinsulinism NOS
Hyperplasia of pancreatic islet beta cells NOS
EXCLUDES 1   *diabetes with hypoglycemia (E08.649, E10.649, E11.649, E13.649)*
hypoglycemia in infant of diabetic mother (P70.1)
neonatal hypoglycemia (P70.4)

● New   ▲ Revised   *Manifestation*   🔳-🗗 Digit Indicators   🗏 Laterality   🅰 Adult (15+ years)   Ⓜ Maternity (12-55 years)   Ⓝ Newborn   🅿 Pediatric (0-17 years)   ♂ Male   ♀ Female
✖ Deleted   Unspecified   + Additional code

CODING TIP ✓ Do not assign E16.1 to report hypoglycemia in a patient with a known diagnosis of diabetes, including post-procedural hypoinsulinemia.

▲ **E16.2 Hypoglycemia, unspecified**

EXCLUDES 1 *diabetes with hypoglycemia (E08.649, E10.649, E11.649, E13.649)*

DEFINITION Condition in which blood sugar levels are too low for normal functioning, manifesting as weakness, trembling, hunger, headache, irritability, racing heartbeat, confusion, even convulsions or coma.

E16.3 Increased secretion of glucagon
Hyperplasia of pancreatic endocrine cells with glucagon excess

E16.4 Increased secretion of gastrin
Hypergastrinemia
Hyperplasia of pancreatic endocrine cells with gastrin excess
Zollinger-Ellison syndrome

E16.8 Other specified disorders of pancreatic internal secretion
Increased secretion from endocrine pancreas of growth hormone-releasing hormone
Increased secretion from endocrine pancreas of pancreatic polypeptide
Increased secretion from endocrine pancreas of somatostatin
Increased secretion from endocrine pancreas of vasoactive-intestinal polypeptide

E16.9 Disorder of pancreatic internal secretion, unspecified
Islet-cell hyperplasia NOS
Pancreatic endocrine cell hyperplasia NOS

Disorders of other endocrine glands (E20-E35)

EXCLUDES 1 *galactorrhea (N64.3)*
gynecomastia (N62)

◢ **E20 Hypoparathyroidism**

EXCLUDES 1 *Di George's syndrome (D82.1)*
postprocedural hypoparathyroidism (E89.2)
tetany NOS (R29.0)
transitory neonatal hypoparathyroidism (P71.4)

DEFINITION Reduced production of parathyroid hormone causing tingling of the hands, fingers, and mouth, muscle cramps, and possibly convulsions.

E20.0 Idiopathic hypoparathyroidism

E20.1 Pseudohypoparathyroidism

CODING TIP ✓ Patients with pseudohypoparathyroidism produce adequate levels of PTH, but are resistant to its effects due to a genetic abnormality. These patients typically exhibit low blood calcium and elevated phosphorus, which are characteristic of hypoparathyroidism and should not be separately coded.

DEFINITION Condition of hypoparathyroidism symptoms manifesting due to an inadequate response to the parathyroid hormone, rather than an insufficient amount of the hormone.

E20.8 Other hypoparathyroidism

E20.9 Hypoparathyroidism, unspecified
Parathyroid tetany

◢ **E21 Hyperparathyroidism and other disorders of parathyroid gland**

EXCLUDES 1 *adult osteomalacia (M83.-)*
ectopic hyperparathyroidism (E34.2)
familial hypocalciuric hypercalcemia (E83.52)
hungry bone syndrome (E83.81)
infantile and juvenile osteomalacia (E55.0)

E21.0 Primary hyperparathyroidism
Hyperplasia of parathyroid
Osteitis fibrosa cystica generalisata [von Recklinghausen's disease of bone]

DEFINITION Excessive production of parathyroid hormone, usually caused by hyperplasia of the gland itself, causing decreased calcium levels in bones.

E21.1 Secondary hyperparathyroidism, not elsewhere classified

EXCLUDES 1 *secondary hyperparathyroidism of renal origin (N25.81)*

CODING TIP ✓ Do not assign E21.1 if the causative mechanism of the diagnosed secondary hyperparathyroid disease is of renal (kidney) origin. E21.1 should only be assigned when the hyperparathyroidism is not reported as primary and has a clear cause reported as not of renal origin.

E21.2 Other hyperparathyroidism
Tertiary hyperparathyroidism

EXCLUDES 1 *familial hypocalciuric hypercalcemia (E83.52)*

E21.3 Hyperparathyroidism, unspecified

E21.4 Other specified disorders of parathyroid gland

E21.5 Disorder of parathyroid gland, unspecified

◢ **E22 Hyperfunction of pituitary gland**

EXCLUDES 1 *Cushing's syndrome (E24.-)*
Nelson's syndrome (E24.1)
overproduction of ACTH not associated with Cushing's disease (E27.0)
overproduction of pituitary ACTH (E24.0)
overproduction of thyroid-stimulating hormone (E05.8-)

E22.0 Acromegaly and pituitary gigantism
Overproduction of growth hormone

EXCLUDES 1 *constitutional gigantism (E34.4)*
constitutional tall stature (E34.4)
increased secretion from endocrine pancreas of growth hormone-releasing hormone (E16.8)

DEFINITION Acromegaly: Abnormally large growth of the hands, feet and facial features due to the production of too much growth hormone in adults by the pituitary gland.

✚ **E22.1 Hyperprolactinemia**
Use additional code for adverse effect, if applicable, to identify drug (T36-T50 with fifth or sixth character 5)

E22.2 Syndrome of inappropriate secretion of antidiuretic hormone

E22.8 Other hyperfunction of pituitary gland
Central precocious puberty

E22.9 Hyperfunction of pituitary gland, unspecified

◢ **E23 Hypofunction and other disorders of the pituitary gland**

INCLUDES the listed conditions whether the disorder is in the pituitary or the hypothalamus

EXCLUDES 1 *postprocedural hypopituitarism (E89.3)*

E23.0 Hypopituitarism
Fertile eunuch syndrome
Hypogonadotropic hypogonadism
Idiopathic growth hormone deficiency
Isolated deficiency of gonadotropin
Isolated deficiency of growth hormone
Isolated deficiency of pituitary hormone
Kallmann's syndrome
Lorain-Levi short stature
Necrosis of pituitary gland (postpartum)
Panhypopituitarism
Pituitary cachexia
Pituitary insufficiency NOS
Pituitary short stature
Sheehan's syndrome
Simmonds' disease

DEFINITION A type of dwarfism with retention of infantile characteristics, due to undersecretion of growth hormone and gonadotropin deficiency.

✚ **E23.1 Drug-induced hypopituitarism**
Use additional code for adverse effect, if applicable, to identify drug (T36-T50 with fifth or sixth character 5)

E23.2 Diabetes insipidus

EXCLUDES 1 *nephrogenic diabetes insipidus (N25.1)*

DEFINITION Insufficient vasopressin production/secretion of antidiuretic hormone (ADH) resulting in intense thirst and excretion of large amounts of urine.

E23.3 Hypothalamic dysfunction, not elsewhere classified

EXCLUDES 1 *Prader-Willi syndrome (Q87.1)*
Russell-Silver syndrome (Q87.1)

E23.6 Other disorders of pituitary gland
Abscess of pituitary
Adiposogenital dystrophy

● New　▲ Revised　*Manifestation*　◢-◿ Digit Indicators　⬓ Laterality　Ⓐ Adult (15+ years)　Ⓜ Maternity (12-55 years)　Ⓝ Newborn　Ⓟ Pediatric (0-17 years)　♂ Male　♀ Female
✖ Deleted　Unspecified　✚ Additional code

E23.7 **Disorder of pituitary gland, unspecified**

⬛ E24 **Cushing's syndrome**

> **EXCLUDES 1** *congenital adrenal hyperplasia (E25.0)*

> **CODING TIP ✓** When Cushing's syndrome is stated as the cause of diabetes mellitus in the patient, assign the appropriate code for Cushing's syndrome, followed by the appropriate code from category E08 for diabetes mellitus due to an underlying condition.

E24.0 **Pituitary-dependent Cushing's disease**
Overproduction of pituitary ACTH
Pituitary-dependent hypercorticalism

E24.1 **Nelson's syndrome**

+ E24.2 **Drug-induced Cushing's syndrome**
Use additional code for adverse effect, if applicable, to identify drug (T36-T50 with fifth or sixth character 5)

> **CODING TIP ✓** Code E24.2 should only be assigned when documentation clearly indicates a relationship between Cushing's syndrome and a drug or chemical as the underlying cause. Assign a code from T36-T50 to indicate the drug and adverse effect.

E24.3 **Ectopic ACTH syndrome**

E24.4 **Alcohol-induced pseudo-Cushing's syndrome**

E24.8 **Other Cushing's syndrome**

E24.9 **Cushing's syndrome, unspecified**

> **DEFINITION** Disorder caused by prolonged exposure of body tissues to high levels of cortisol, presenting with upper body obesity, thinning arms and legs, brittle bones, severe fatigue, weakness, high blood pressure, and high blood sugar.

⬛ E25 **Adrenogenital disorders**

> **INCLUDES** adrenogenital syndromes, virilizing or feminizing, whether acquired or due to adrenal hyperplasia consequent on inborn enzyme defects in hormone synthesis
> Female adrenal pseudohermaphroditism
> Female heterosexual precocious pseudopuberty
> Male isosexual precocious pseudopuberty
> Male macrogenitosomia praecox
> Male sexual precocity with adrenal hyperplasia
> Male virilization (female)

> **EXCLUDES 1** *indeterminate sex and pseudohermaphroditism (Q56)*
> *chromosomal abnormalities (Q90-Q99)*

E25.0 **Congenital adrenogenital disorders associated with enzyme deficiency**
Congenital adrenal hyperplasia
21-Hydroxylase deficiency
Salt-losing congenital adrenal hyperplasia

+ E25.8 **Other adrenogenital disorders**
Idiopathic adrenogenital disorder
Use additional code for adverse effect, if applicable, to identify drug (T36-T50 with fifth or sixth character 5)

E25.9 **Adrenogenital disorder, unspecified**
Adrenogenital syndrome NOS

⬛ E26 **Hyperaldosteronism**

⑤ E26.0 **Primary hyperaldosteronism**

> **DEFINITION** Excessive aldosterone production; typically presents with loss of potassium, muscular weakness, and elevated blood pressure.

E26.01 **Conn's syndrome**
Code also:
adrenal adenoma (D35.0-)

> **DEFINITION** Excess secretion of aldosterone due to an adrenocortical adenoma, causing hypokalemia, alkalosis, muscular weakness, polyuria, polydipsia, and hypertension.

E26.02 **Glucocorticoid-remediable aldosteronism**
Familial aldosteronism type I

E26.09 **Other primary hyperaldosteronism**
Primary aldosteronism due to adrenal hyperplasia (bilateral)

E26.1 **Secondary hyperaldosteronism**

⑤ E26.8 **Other hyperaldosteronism**

E26.81 **Bartter's syndrome**

> **DEFINITION** Group of symptoms caused by the kidneys' inability to reabsorb potassium, also known as urinary potassium wasting; causes renal cell enlargement, alkalosis, hyperaldosteronism, cramping, constipation, urinary frequency, and weakness.

E26.89 **Other hyperaldosteronism**

E26.9 **Hyperaldosteronism, unspecified**
Aldosteronism NOS
Hyperaldosteronism NOS

⬛ E27 **Other disorders of adrenal gland**

E27.0 **Other adrenocortical overactivity**
Overproduction of ACTH, not associated with Cushing's disease
Premature adrenarche

> **EXCLUDES 1** *Cushing's syndrome (E24.-)*

E27.1 **Primary adrenocortical insufficiency**
Addison's disease
Autoimmune adrenalitis

> **EXCLUDES 1** *Addison only phenotype adrenoleukodystrophy (E71.528)*
> *amyloidosis (E85.-)*
> *tuberculous Addison's disease (A18.7)*
> *Waterhouse-Friderichsen syndrome (A39.1)*

E27.2 **Addisonian crisis**
Adrenal crisis
Adrenocortical crisis

> **CODING TIP ✓** Do not assign E27.2 to indicate Addison's disease. Code E27.2 indicates Addisonian crisis, a severe and life threatening condition that may occur in individuals with Addison's disease or other conditions resulting in severely elevated cortisol levels. Addison's disease in the absence of crisis should be coded to E27.1.

> **DEFINITION** Low levels of the glucocorticoid hormone, cortisol, secreted by the adrenal glands and responsible for regulating blood pressure, cardiovascular function, inflammatory response, insulin effects, and metabolism.

+ E27.3 **Drug-induced adrenocortical insufficiency**
Use additional code for adverse effect, if applicable, to identify drug (T36-T50 with fifth or sixth character 5)

> **CODING TIP ✓** Code E27.3 should only be assigned when documentation clearly indicates a relationship between adrenocortical insufficiency and a drug or chemical as the underlying cause. Assign a code from T36-T50 following E27.3 to indicate the drug and adverse effect.

⑤ E27.4 **Other and unspecified adrenocortical insufficiency**

> **EXCLUDES 1** *adrenoleukodystrophy [Addison-Schilder] (E71.528)*
> *Waterhouse-Friderichsen syndrome (A39.1)*

E27.40 **Unspecified adrenocortical insufficiency**
Adrenocortical insufficiency NOS
Hypoaldosteronism

E27.49 **Other adrenocortical insufficiency**
Adrenal hemorrhage
Adrenal infarction

E27.5 **Adrenomedullary hyperfunction**
Adrenomedullary hyperplasia
Catecholamine hypersecretion

> **DEFINITION** Overproduction of adrenaline hormones by the adrenal medulla, causing heart disease, high blood pressure, and related problems.

E27.8 **Other specified disorders of adrenal gland**
Abnormality of cortisol-binding globulin

E27.9 **Disorder of adrenal gland, unspecified**

⬛ E28 **Ovarian dysfunction**

> **EXCLUDES 1** *isolated gonadotropin deficiency (E23.0)*
> *postprocedural ovarian failure (E89.4-)*

+ E28.0 **Estrogen excess** ♀
Use additional code for adverse effect, if applicable, to identify drug (T36-T50 with fifth or sixth character 5)

+ E28.1 **Androgen excess** ♀
Hypersecretion of ovarian androgens
Use additional code for adverse effect, if applicable, to identify drug (T36-T50 with fifth or sixth character 5)

● New   ▲ Revised   *Manifestation*   🔢-🔢 Digit Indicators   ▱ Laterality   🅰 Adult (15+ years)   Ⓜ Maternity (12-55 years)   Ⓝ Newborn   🅿 Pediatric (0-17 years)   ♂ Male   ♀ Female
✖ ~~Deleted~~   Unspecified   + Additional code

E28.2   Polycystic ovarian syndrome   ♀
Sclerocystic ovary syndrome
Stein-Leventhal syndrome

CODING TIP ✓   Polycystic ovarian syndrome (PCOS) is associated with increased risk for a number of other endocrine disorders, including insulin resistance, hypothyroidism, and obesity. When present, these other diagnoses should also be reported.

DEFINITION   Syndrome in which the ovaries produce too many androgens, causing ovarian cysts and interfering with the menstrual cycle; results in missed, heavy, or irregular periods, infertility, abdominal discomfort, acne, weight gain, and uterine bleeding.

⑤ E28.3   Primary ovarian failure
EXCLUDES 1   pure gonadal dysgenesis (Q99.1)
Turner's syndrome (Q96.-)

⑥ E28.31   Premature menopause

E28.310   Symptomatic premature menopause   ♀
Symptoms such as flushing, sleeplessness, headache, lack of concentration, associated with premature menopause

E28.319   Asymptomatic premature menopause   ♀
Premature menopause NOS

E28.39   Other primary ovarian failure   ♀
Decreased estrogen
Resistant ovary syndrome

E28.8   Other ovarian dysfunction   ♀
Ovarian hyperfunction NOS
EXCLUDES 1   postprocedural ovarian failure (E89.4-)

E28.9   Ovarian dysfunction, unspecified   ♀

▲ ④ E29   Testicular dysfunction
EXCLUDES 1   androgen insensitivity syndrome (E34.5-)
azoospermia or oligospermia NOS (N46.0-N46.1)
isolated gonadotropin deficiency (E23.0)
Klinefelter's syndrome (Q98.0-Q98.1, Q98.4)

E29.0   Testicular hyperfunction   ♂
Hypersecretion of testicular hormones
DEFINITION   Excessive testosterone production, often due to an active tumor on the testicle. Commonly presents with increased muscle and bone growth in children and increased secondary sex characteristics.

**Testicular hyperfunction
unspecified protein calorie**

The secretion of too much testosterone into the body

Vas deferens
Bladder
Spermatic cord
Penis
Epididymis
Testicles producing sperm and testosterone

✚ E29.1   Testicular hypofunction   ♂
Defective biosynthesis of testicular androgen NOS
5-delta-Reductase deficiency (with male pseudohermaphroditism)
Testicular hypogonadism NOS
Use additional code for adverse effect, if applicable, to identify drug (T36-T50 with fifth or sixth character 5)
EXCLUDES 1   postprocedural testicular hypofunction (E89.5)
DEFINITION   Underdevelopment of all the genital tissues with decreased functional activities of the gonads.

E29.8   Other testicular dysfunction   ♂
E29.9   Testicular dysfunction, unspecified   ♂

④ E30   Disorders of puberty, not elsewhere classified
E30.0   Delayed puberty
Constitutional delay of puberty
Delayed sexual development

E30.1   Precocious puberty   Ⓟ
Precocious menstruation
EXCLUDES 1   Albright (-McCune) (-Sternberg) syndrome (Q78.1)
central precocious puberty (E22.8)
congenital adrenal hyperplasia (E25.0)
female heterosexual precocious pseudopuberty (E25.-)
male isosexual precocious pseudopuberty (E25.-)

E30.8   Other disorders of puberty   Ⓟ
Premature thelarche

E30.9   Disorder of puberty, unspecified

④ E31   Polyglandular dysfunction
EXCLUDES 1   ataxia telangiectasia [Louis-Bar] (G11.3)
dystrophia myotonica [Steinert] (G71.11)
pseudohypoparathyroidism (E20.1)

E31.0   Autoimmune polyglandular failure
Schmidt's syndrome
DEFINITION   Schmidt's syndrome: hypofunction of more than one endocrine gland in different combinations, including the thyroid, adrenals, gonads, parathyroid, and pancreas; occurs primarily in adult females.

E31.1   Polyglandular hyperfunction
EXCLUDES 1   multiple endocrine adenomatosis (E31.2-)
multiple endocrine neoplasia (E31.2-)

⑤ E31.2   Multiple endocrine neoplasia [MEN] syndromes
Multiple endocrine adenomatosis
Code also:
any associated malignancies and other conditions associated with the syndromes
CODING TIP ✓   MEN syndromes are distinct, inherited autosomal disorders, which may present in conjunction with endocrine tumors.

E31.20   Multiple endocrine neoplasia [MEN] syndrome, unspecified
Multiple endocrine adenomatosis NOS
Multiple endocrine neoplasia [MEN] syndrome NOS

E31.21   Multiple endocrine neoplasia [MEN] type I
Wermer's syndrome
DEFINITION   Hyperplasia or tumors of the parathyroid, pancreatic islet cells, and pituitary gland; causes oversecretion of hormones, kidney stones, infertility, and severe peptic ulcers.

E31.22   Multiple endocrine neoplasia [MEN] type IIA
Sipple's syndrome
DEFINITION   Triad of thyroid medullary carcinoma, adrenal gland tumor, and parathyroid hyperplasia.

E31.23   Multiple endocrine neoplasia [MEN] type IIB
E31.8   Other polyglandular dysfunction
E31.9   Polyglandular dysfunction, unspecified

④ E32   Diseases of thymus
EXCLUDES 1   aplasia or hypoplasia of thymus with immunodeficiency (D82.1)
myasthenia gravis (G70.0)

E32.0   Persistent hyperplasia of thymus
Hypertrophy of thymus

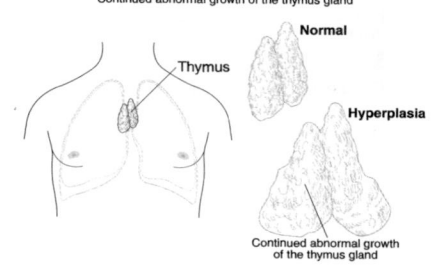

Persistent hyperplasia of thymus
Continued abnormal growth of the thymus gland

Normal
Thymus
Hyperplasia
Continued abnormal growth of the thymus gland

E32.1   Abscess of thymus

● New   ▲ Revised   *Manifestation*   ④-❼ Digit Indicators   ▤ Laterality   Ⓐ Adult (15+ years)   Ⓜ Maternity (12-55 years)   Ⓝ Newborn   Ⓟ Pediatric (0-17 years)   ♂ Male   ♀ Female
✖ Deleted   Unspecified   ✚ Additional code

Endocrine, Nutritional and Metabolic Diseases

E32.8   Other diseases of thymus
> **EXCLUDES 1**   *aplasia or hypoplasia with immunodeficiency (D82.1)*
> *thymoma (D15.0)*

E32.9   Disease of thymus, unspecified

◢ E34   Other endocrine disorders
> **EXCLUDES 1**   *pseudohypoparathyroidism (E20.1)*

E34.0   Carcinoid syndrome
Note: May be used as an additional code to identify functional activity associated with a carcinoid tumor.

CODING TIP ✓   Carcinoid syndrome is a specific syndrome causing a variety of symptoms in patients with advanced stage malignant carcinoid tumors. When coding carcinoid syndrome, the specific type and location of the carcinoid tumor should be identified and additionally coded by assigning the appropriate code(s) from category C7A and/or C7B.

DEFINITION   Condition in which cancerous cells secrete hormones into the bloodstream causing chemical imbalances in the body with symptoms of periodic flushing, diarrhea, abdominal pain, and high blood pressure.

E34.1   Other hypersecretion of intestinal hormones

E34.2   Ectopic hormone secretion, not elsewhere classified
> **EXCLUDES 1**   *ectopic ACTH syndrome (E24.3)*

DEFINITION   Condition that occurs when a glandular tumor metastasizes, moving from its original location to another area of the body, and continues to secrete hormones.

E34.3   Short stature due to endocrine disorder
Constitutional short stature
Laron-type short stature
> **EXCLUDES 1**   *achondroplastic short stature (Q77.4)*
> *hypochondroplastic short stature (Q77.4)*
> *nutritional short stature (E45)*
> *pituitary short stature (E23.0)*
> *progeria (E34.8)*
> *renal short stature (N25.0)*
> *Russell-Silver syndrome (Q87.1)*
> *short-limbed stature with immunodeficiency (D82.2)*
> *short stature in specific dysmorphic syndromes - code to syndrome - see Alphabetical Index*
> *short stature NOS (R62.52)*

E34.4   Constitutional tall stature
Constitutional gigantism

⑤ E34.5   Androgen insensitivity syndrome
DEFINITION   Defects in androgen action causing feminization of external genitalia, abnormal sexual development, infertility, and pseudohermaphroditism in males.

E34.50   Androgen insensitivity syndrome, unspecified
Androgen insensitivity NOS

E34.51   Complete androgen insensitivity syndrome
Complete androgen insensitivity
de Quervain syndrome
Goldberg-Maxwell syndrome

E34.52   Partial androgen insensitivity syndrome
Partial androgen insensitivity
Reifenstein syndrome

E34.8   Other specified endocrine disorders
Pineal gland dysfunction
Progeria
> **EXCLUDES 2**   *pseudohypoparathyroidism (E20.1)*

E34.9   Endocrine disorder, unspecified
Endocrine disturbance NOS
Hormone disturbance NOS

+ E35   *Disorders of endocrine glands in diseases classified elsewhere*
Code first underlying disease, such as:
late congenital syphilis of thymus gland [Dubois disease] (A50.5)
Use additional code , if applicable, to identify:
sequelae of tuberculosis of other organs (B90.8)
> **EXCLUDES 1**   *Echinococcus granulosus infection of thyroid gland (B67.3)*
> *meningococcal hemorrhagic adrenalitis (A39.1)*
> *syphilis of endocrine gland (A52.79)*
> *tuberculosis of adrenal gland, except calcification (A18.7)*
> *tuberculosis of endocrine gland NEC (A18.82)*
> *tuberculosis of thyroid gland (A18.81)*
> *Waterhouse-Friderichsen syndrome (A39.1)*

Intraoperative complications of endocrine system (E36)

CODING TIP ✓   Codes classifiable to E36 are complication codes (intraoperative complications) and should only be coded when the physician specifically indicates a relationship between the operative procedure and the specific complication. If no relationship between the condition suspected to be a complication and the operative procedure is stated, the provider may be queried to clarify if the condition is classifiable as a complication.

◢ E36   Intraoperative complications of endocrine system
> **EXCLUDES 2**   *postprocedural endocrine and metabolic complications and disorders, not elsewhere classified (E89.-)*

⑤ E36.0   Intraoperative hemorrhage and hematoma of an endocrine system organ or structure complicating a procedure
> **EXCLUDES 1**   *intraoperative hemorrhage and hematoma of an endocrine system organ or structure due to accidental puncture or laceration during a procedure (E36.1-)*

E36.01   Intraoperative hemorrhage and hematoma of an endocrine system organ or structure complicating an endocrine system procedure

E36.02   Intraoperative hemorrhage and hematoma of an endocrine system organ or structure complicating other procedure

⑤ E36.1   Accidental puncture and laceration of an endocrine system organ or structure during a procedure

E36.11   Accidental puncture and laceration of an endocrine system organ or structure during an endocrine system procedure

E36.12   Accidental puncture and laceration of an endocrine system organ or structure during other procedure

+ E36.8   Other intraoperative complications of endocrine system
Use additional code, if applicable, to further specify disorder

Malnutrition (E40-E46)

> **EXCLUDES 1**   *intestinal malabsorption (K90.-)*
> *sequelae of protein-calorie malnutrition (E64.0)*
> **EXCLUDES 2**   *nutritional anemias (D50-D53)*
> *starvation (T73.0)*

CODING TIP ✓   Malnutrition is defined as insufficient, excessive or imbalanced nutrient consumption. Not all patients experiencing malnutrition will present with inadequate intake or low body weight/BMI. The specific type of malnutrition (such as severe, moderate, Kwashiorkor, etc.) must be indicated by the patient's provider and cannot be assumed. When documentation only states "malnutrition," assign E46.

E40   Kwashiorkor
Severe malnutrition with nutritional edema with dyspigmentation of skin and hair
> **EXCLUDES 1**   *marasmic kwashiorkor (E42)*

E41   Nutritional marasmus
Severe malnutrition with marasmus
> **EXCLUDES 1**   *marasmic kwashiorkor (E42)*

DEFINITION   Chronic wasting of body tissues, especially in young children, commonly due to prolonged dietary deficiency of protein and calories.

● New   ▲ Revised   *Manifestation*   ◨-◲ Digit Indicators   ▤ Laterality   Ⓐ Adult (15+ years)   Ⓜ Maternity (12-55 years)   Ⓝ Newborn   Ⓟ Pediatric (0-17 years)   ♂ Male   ♀ Female
✖ Deleted   Unspecified   + Additional code

532   © 2017 DecisionHealth   2017 ICD-10-CM Expert for Physicians

E42 **Marasmic kwashiorkor**
Intermediate form severe protein-calorie malnutrition
Severe protein-calorie malnutrition with signs of both kwashiorkor and marasmus

E43 **Unspecified severe protein-calorie malnutrition**
Starvation edema

4️⃣ **E44** **Protein-calorie malnutrition of moderate and mild degree**

E44.0 **Moderate protein-calorie malnutrition**

E44.1 **Mild protein-calorie malnutrition**

E45 **Retarded development following protein-calorie malnutrition**
Nutritional short stature
Nutritional stunting
Physical retardation due to malnutrition

E46 **Unspecified protein-calorie malnutrition**
Malnutrition NOS
Protein-calorie imbalance NOS
EXCLUDES 1 *nutritional deficiency NOS (E63.9)*

Malnutrition

Other nutritional deficiencies (E50-E64)

EXCLUDES 2 *nutritional anemias (D50-D53)*

CODING TIP ✓ Do not use codes from E50-E64 to indicate anemia due to a nutritional deficiency. When a patient has a specific diagnosis of anemia due to a nutritional deficiency, assign the appropriate specified code from Chapter 3.

4️⃣ **E50** **Vitamin A deficiency**
EXCLUDES 1 *sequelae of vitamin A deficiency (E64.1)*

E50.0 **Vitamin A deficiency with conjunctival xerosis**
DEFINITION Vitamin A deficiency with dryness of the membrane that lines eyelids and covers the exposed surface of the sclera.

E50.1 **Vitamin A deficiency with Bitot's spot and conjunctival xerosis**
Bitot's spot in the young child
DEFINITION Vitamin A deficiency with superficial spots of keratinized epithelium on the conjunctiva, accompanied by dryness.

E50.2 **Vitamin A deficiency with corneal xerosis**

E50.3 **Vitamin A deficiency with corneal ulceration and xerosis**

E50.4 **Vitamin A deficiency with keratomalacia**
DEFINITION Vitamin A deficiency with softening of the corneas that may lead to corneal infection or rupture.

E50.5 **Vitamin A deficiency with night blindness**

E50.6 **Vitamin A deficiency with xerophthalmic scars of cornea**

E50.7 **Other ocular manifestations of vitamin A deficiency**
Xerophthalmia NOS

E50.8 **Other manifestations of vitamin A deficiency**
Follicular keratosis
Xeroderma

E50.9 **Vitamin A deficiency, unspecified**
Hypovitaminosis A NOS

Vitamin A deficiency

Foods providing body with Vitamin A

Body does not take in a sufficient amount of Vitamin A or does not absorb Vitamin A properly. The most common symptoms include dry eyes and eye inflammation.

4️⃣ **E51** **Thiamine deficiency**
EXCLUDES 1 *sequelae of thiamine deficiency (E64.8)*

5️⃣ **E51.1** **Beriberi**
DEFINITION Severe Vitamin B1 (thiamine) deficiency causing nerve, heart, and/or brain abnormalities.

E51.11 **Dry beriberi**
Beriberi NOS
Beriberi with polyneuropathy

E51.12 **Wet beriberi**
Beriberi with cardiovascular manifestations
Cardiovascular beriberi
Shoshin disease

E51.2 **Wernicke's encephalopathy**

E51.8 **Other manifestations of thiamine deficiency**

E51.9 **Thiamine deficiency, unspecified**

E52 **Niacin deficiency [pellagra]**
Niacin (-tryptophan) deficiency
Nicotinamide deficiency
Pellagra (alcoholic)
EXCLUDES 1 *sequelae of niacin deficiency (E64.8)*

DEFINITION Niacin and amino acid tryptophan deficiency affecting the skin, digestive tract, and brain.

4️⃣ **E53** **Deficiency of other B group vitamins**
EXCLUDES 1 *sequelae of vitamin B deficiency (E64.8)*

E53.0 **Riboflavin deficiency**
Ariboflavinosis
Vitamin B2 deficiency
DEFINITION Riboflavin deficiency causing dry throat and nasal passages, mouth sores, magenta-colored tongue, and overproduction of oil on the skin.

E53.1 **Pyridoxine deficiency**
Vitamin B6 deficiency
EXCLUDES 1 *pyridoxine-responsive sideroblastic anemia (D64.3)*

E53.8 **Deficiency of other specified B group vitamins**
Biotin deficiency
Cyanocobalamin deficiency
Folate deficiency
Folic acid deficiency
Pantothenic acid deficiency
Vitamin B12 deficiency
EXCLUDES 1 *folate deficiency anemia (D52.-)*
vitamin B12 deficiency anemia (D51.-)

E53.9 **Vitamin B deficiency, unspecified**

E54 **Ascorbic acid deficiency**
Deficiency of vitamin C
Scurvy
EXCLUDES 1 *scorbutic anemia (D53.2)*
sequelae of vitamin C deficiency (E64.2)

DEFINITION Condition known as scurvy caused by deficiency of ascorbic acid (vitamin C) and marked by weakness, anemia, spongy gums, and mucocutaneous hemorrhages.

4️⃣ **E55** **Vitamin D deficiency**
EXCLUDES 1 *adult osteomalacia (M83.-)*
osteoporosis (M80.-)
sequelae of rickets (E64.3)

● New ▲ Revised *Manifestation* 4️⃣-7️⃣ Digit Indicators ▤ Laterality 🅰 Adult (15+ years) 🅼 Maternity (12-55 years) 🅽 Newborn 🅿 Pediatric (0-17 years) ♂ Male ♀ Female
✖ ~~Deleted~~ Unspecified + Additional code

2017 ICD-10-CM Expert for Physicians

© 2017 DecisionHealth

533

E55.0   Rickets, active
Infantile osteomalacia
Juvenile osteomalacia
> **EXCLUDES 1**   *celiac rickets (K90.0)*
> *Crohn's rickets (K50.-)*
> *hereditary vitamin D-dependent rickets (E83.32)*
> *inactive rickets (E64.3)*
> *renal rickets (N25.0)*
> *sequelae of rickets (E64.3)*
> *vitamin D-resistant rickets (E83.31)*

> **DEFINITION**   Childhood disease caused by a lack of vitamin D, resulting in soft, spongy bones and bone pain as well as skeletal deformities (e.g., bowlegs, scoliosis), distortion of the rib cage, and oddly-shaped skull.

E55.9   Vitamin D deficiency, unspecified
Avitaminosis D

▣ E56   Other vitamin deficiencies
> **EXCLUDES 1**   *sequelae of other vitamin deficiencies (E64.8)*

E56.0   Deficiency of vitamin E

E56.1   Deficiency of vitamin K
> **EXCLUDES 1**   *deficiency of coagulation factor due to vitamin K deficiency (D68.4)*
> *vitamin K deficiency of newborn (P53)*

E56.8   Deficiency of other vitamins

E56.9   Vitamin deficiency, unspecified

E58   Dietary calcium deficiency
> **EXCLUDES 1**   *disorders of calcium metabolism (E83.5-)*
> *sequelae of calcium deficiency (E64.8)*

E59   Dietary selenium deficiency
Keshan disease
> **EXCLUDES 1**   *sequelae of selenium deficiency (E64.8)*

E60   Dietary zinc deficiency

▣ + E61   Deficiency of other nutrient elements
Use additional code for adverse effect, if applicable, to identify drug (T36-T50 with fifth or sixth character 5)
> **EXCLUDES 1**   *disorders of mineral metabolism (E83.-)*
> *iodine deficiency related thyroid disorders (E00-E02)*
> *sequelae of malnutrition and other nutritional deficiencies (E64.-)*

+ E61.0   Copper deficiency

+ E61.1   Iron deficiency
> **EXCLUDES 1**   *iron deficiency anemia (D50.-)*

+ E61.2   Magnesium deficiency

+ E61.3   Manganese deficiency

+ E61.4   Chromium deficiency

+ E61.5   Molybdenum deficiency

+ E61.6   Vanadium deficiency

+ E61.7   Deficiency of multiple nutrient elements

+ E61.8   Deficiency of other specified nutrient elements

+ E61.9   Deficiency of nutrient element, unspecified

▣ E63   Other nutritional deficiencies
> **EXCLUDES 1**   *dehydration (E86.0)*
> *failure to thrive, adult (R62.7)*
> *failure to thrive, child (R62.51)*
> *feeding problems in newborn (P92.-)*
> *sequelae of malnutrition and other nutritional deficiencies (E64.-)*

E63.0   Essential fatty acid [EFA] deficiency

E63.1   Imbalance of constituents of food intake

E63.8   Other specified nutritional deficiencies

E63.9   Nutritional deficiency, unspecified

▣ E64   Sequelae of malnutrition and other nutritional deficiencies
Note: This category is to be used to indicate conditions in categories E43, E44, E46, E50-E63 as the cause of sequelae, which are themselves classified elsewhere. The 'sequelae' include conditions specified as such; they also include the late effects of diseases classifiable to the above categories if the disease itself is no longer present
Code first:
> condition resulting from (sequela) of malnutrition and other nutritional deficiencies

E64.0   Sequelae of protein-calorie malnutrition
> **EXCLUDES 2**   *retarded development following protein-calorie malnutrition (E45)*

E64.1   Sequelae of vitamin A deficiency

E64.2   Sequelae of vitamin C deficiency

E64.3   Sequelae of rickets

E64.8   Sequelae of other nutritional deficiencies

E64.9   Sequelae of unspecified nutritional deficiency

Overweight, obesity and other hyperalimentation (E65-E68)

E65   Localized adiposity
Fat pad

▣ + E66   Overweight and obesity
Code first:
> obesity complicating pregnancy, childbirth and the puerperium, if applicable (O99.21-)
Use additional code to identify body mass index (BMI), if known (Z68.-)
> **EXCLUDES 1**   *adiposogenital dystrophy (E23.6)*
> *lipomatosis NOS (E88.2)*
> *lipomatosis dolorosa [Dercum] (E88.2)*
> *Prader-Willi syndrome (Q87.1)*

> **CODING TIP ✓**   When assigning a code for any overweight, obesity, or morbid obesity, physician documentation indicating obesity as a diagnosis is required. If suspected, but not present, the coder may query the provider to obtain confirmation of the condition, but may not code obesity without confirmation from the provider. BMI Z68.- may be calculated and coded based upon documentation from other clinicians and calculated BMI may be coded alone without a diagnosis of obesity. BMI may only be reported as secondary code.

▣ + E66.0   Obesity due to excess calories
> **DEFINITION**   Increased body weight with excessive accumulation of fat caused by overeating and/or a sedentary lifestyle.

+ E66.01   Morbid (severe) obesity due to excess calories
> **EXCLUDES 1**   *morbid (severe) obesity with alveolar hypoventilation (E66.2)*

> **CODING TIP ✓**   Note that the alphabetical index refers to this code for morbid obesity. This code is used when morbid obesity is documented.

+ E66.09   Other obesity due to excess calories

+ E66.1   Drug-induced obesity
Use additional code for adverse effect, if applicable, to identify drug (T36-T50 with fifth or sixth character 5)
> **CODING TIP ✓**   This code should only be assigned when documentation clearly indicates a relationship between obesity and a drug or chemical as the underlying cause. Assign a code from T36-T50 following E66.1 to indicate the drug and adverse effect.

▲ + E66.2   Morbid (severe) obesity with alveolar hypoventilation
Obesity hypoventilation syndrome (OHS)
Pickwickian syndrome

+ E66.3   Overweight

+ E66.8   Other obesity

+ E66.9   Obesity, unspecified
Obesity NOS
AHA: 4Q 2013, 129

▣ E67   Other hyperalimentation
> **EXCLUDES 1**   *hyperalimentation NOS (R63.2)*
> *sequelae of hyperalimentation (E68)*

E67.0   Hypervitaminosis A

E67.1   Hypercarotinemia
> **DEFINITION**   Elevated carotene levels in the blood from excessive ingestion of carotenoids or the inability to convert carotenoids to vitamin A; often presents with yellowing of the skin.

E67.2   Megavitamin-B6 syndrome

E67.3   Hypervitaminosis D

E67.8   Other specified hyperalimentation

E68   Sequelae of hyperalimentation
Code first:
> condition resulting from (sequela) of hyperalimentation

Metabolic disorders (E70-E88)

EXCLUDES 1 *androgen insensitivity syndrome (E34.5-)*
congenital adrenal hyperplasia (E25.0)
Ehlers-Danlos syndrome (Q79.6)
hemolytic anemias attributable to enzyme disorders (D55.-)
Marfan's syndrome (Q87.4)
5-alpha-reductase deficiency (E29.1)

E70   Disorders of aromatic amino-acid metabolism

E70.0   Classical phenylketonuria

DEFINITION Inherited metabolic disorder caused by an enzyme deficiency resulting in accumulation of phenylalanine and its metabolites in the blood with excess excretion in the urine; causes mental retardation, seizures, eczema, and abnormal body odor.

E70.1   Other hyperphenylalaninemias

E70.2   Disorders of tyrosine metabolism

EXCLUDES 1 *transitory tyrosinemia of newborn (P74.5)*

E70.20   Disorder of tyrosine metabolism, unspecified

E70.21   Tyrosinemia
Hypertyrosinemia

E70.29   Other disorders of tyrosine metabolism
Alkaptonuria
Ochronosis

E70.3   Albinism

E70.30   Albinism, unspecified

E70.31   Ocular albinism

E70.310   X-linked ocular albinism

E70.311   Autosomal recessive ocular albinism

E70.318   Other ocular albinism

E70.319   Ocular albinism, unspecified

E70.32   Oculocutaneous albinism

EXCLUDES 1 *Chediak-Higashi syndrome (E70.330)*
Hermansky-Pudlak syndrome (E70.331)

E70.320   Tyrosinase negative oculocutaneous albinism
Albinism I
Oculocutaneous albinism ty-neg

E70.321   Tyrosinase positive oculocutaneous albinism
Albinism II
Oculocutaneous albinism ty-pos

E70.328   Other oculocutaneous albinism
Cross syndrome

E70.329   Oculocutaneous albinism, unspecified

E70.33   Albinism with hematologic abnormality

E70.330   Chediak-Higashi syndrome

E70.331   Hermansky-Pudlak syndrome

E70.338   Other albinism with hematologic abnormality

E70.339   Albinism with hematologic abnormality, unspecified

E70.39   Other specified albinism
Piebaldism

E70.4   Disorders of histidine metabolism

E70.40   Disorders of histidine metabolism, unspecified

E70.41   Histidinemia

E70.49   Other disorders of histidine metabolism

E70.5   Disorders of tryptophan metabolism

E70.8   Other disorders of aromatic amino-acid metabolism

E70.9   Disorder of aromatic amino-acid metabolism, unspecified

E71   Disorders of branched-chain amino-acid metabolism and fatty-acid metabolism

E71.0   Maple-syrup-urine disease

E71.1   Other disorders of branched-chain amino-acid metabolism

E71.11   Branched-chain organic acidurias

E71.110   Isovaleric acidemia

E71.111   3-methylglutaconic aciduria

E71.118   Other branched-chain organic acidurias

E71.12   Disorders of propionate metabolism

E71.120   Methylmalonic acidemia

E71.121   Propionic acidemia

E71.128   Other disorders of propionate metabolism

E71.19   Other disorders of branched-chain amino-acid metabolism
Hyperleucine-isoleucinemia
Hypervalinemia

E71.2   Disorder of branched-chain amino-acid metabolism, unspecified

E71.3   Disorders of fatty-acid metabolism

EXCLUDES 1 *peroxisomal disorders (E71.5)*
Refsum's disease (G60.1)
Schilder's disease (G37.0)

EXCLUDES 2 *carnitine deficiency due to inborn error of metabolism (E71.42)*

E71.30   Disorder of fatty-acid metabolism, unspecified

E71.31   Disorders of fatty-acid oxidation

E71.310   Long chain/very long chain acyl CoA dehydrogenase deficiency
LCAD
VLCAD

E71.311   Medium chain acyl CoA dehydrogenase deficiency
MCAD

E71.312   Short chain acyl CoA dehydrogenase deficiency
SCAD

E71.313   Glutaric aciduria type II
Glutaric aciduria type II A
Glutaric aciduria type II B
Glutaric aciduria type II C

EXCLUDES 1 *glutaric aciduria (type 1) NOS (E72.3)*

E71.314   Muscle carnitine palmitoyltransferase deficiency

E71.318   Other disorders of fatty-acid oxidation

E71.32   Disorders of ketone metabolism

E71.39   Other disorders of fatty-acid metabolism

E71.4   Disorders of carnitine metabolism

EXCLUDES 1 *Muscle carnitine palmitoyltransferase deficiency (E71.314)*

E71.40   Disorder of carnitine metabolism, unspecified

E71.41   Primary carnitine deficiency

E71.42   Carnitine deficiency due to inborn errors of metabolism
Code also:
associated inborn error or metabolism

E71.43   Iatrogenic carnitine deficiency
Carnitine deficiency due to hemodialysis
Carnitine deficiency due to Valproic acid therapy

E71.44   Other secondary carnitine deficiency

E71.440   Ruvalcaba-Myhre-Smith syndrome

E71.448   Other secondary carnitine deficiency

E71.5   Peroxisomal disorders

EXCLUDES 1 *Schilder's disease (G37.0)*

E71.50   Peroxisomal disorder, unspecified

E71.51   Disorders of peroxisome biogenesis
Group 1 peroxisomal disorders

EXCLUDES 1 *Refsum's disease (G60.1)*

E71.510   Zellweger syndrome

E71.511   Neonatal adrenoleukodystrophy N

EXCLUDES 1 *X-linked adrenoleukodystrophy (E71.42-)*

E71.518   Other disorders of peroxisome biogenesis

E71.52   X-linked adrenoleukodystrophy

E71.520   Childhood cerebral X-linked adrenoleukodystrophy

E71.521   Adolescent X-linked adrenoleukodystrophy

E71.522   Adrenomyeloneuropathy

E71.528   Other X-linked adrenoleukodystrophy
Addison only phenotype adrenoleukodystrophy
Addison-Schilder adrenoleukodystrophy

E71.529   X-linked adrenoleukodystrophy, unspecified type

E71.53   Other group 2 peroxisomal disorders

E71.54   Other peroxisomal disorders

E71.540   Rhizomelic chondrodysplasia punctata

EXCLUDES 1 *chondrodysplasia punctata NOS (Q77.3)*

E71.541   Zellweger-like syndrome

E71.542   Other group 3 peroxisomal disorders

E71.548   Other peroxisomal disorders

● New   ▲ Revised   *Manifestation*   🔲-🔢 Digit Indicators   ▤ Laterality   🅰 Adult (15+ years)   🅜 Maternity (12-55 years)   🅝 Newborn   🅟 Pediatric (0-17 years)   ♂ Male   ♀ Female
✖ Deleted   Unspecified   + Additional code

2017 ICD-10-CM Expert for Physicians

© 2017 DecisionHealth   535

E70 — E71.548

4 **E72   Other disorders of amino-acid metabolism**

> EXCLUDES 1   *disorders of:*
> *aromatic amino-acid metabolism (E70.-)*
> *branched-chain amino-acid metabolism*
> *(E71.0-E71.2)*
> *fatty-acid metabolism (E71.3)*
> *purine and pyrimidine metabolism (E79.-)*
> *gout (M1A.-, M10.-)*

5 **E72.0   Disorders of amino-acid transport**

> EXCLUDES 1   *disorders of tryptophan metabolism (E70.5)*

E72.00   Disorders of amino-acid transport, unspecified

E72.01   Cystinuria

E72.02   Hartnup's disease

+ **E72.03   Lowe's syndrome**
Use additional code for associated glaucoma (H42)

E72.04   Cystinosis
Fanconi (-de Toni) (-Debré) syndrome with cystinosis

> EXCLUDES 1   *Fanconi (-de Toni) (-Debré)*
> *syndrome without cystinosis*
> *(E72.09)*

E72.09   Other disorders of amino-acid transport
Fanconi (-de Toni) (-Debré) syndrome, unspecified

5 **E72.1   Disorders of sulfur-bearing amino-acid metabolism**

> EXCLUDES 1   *cystinosis (E72.04)*
> *cystinuria (E72.01)*
> *transcobalamin II deficiency (D51.2)*

E72.10   Disorders of sulfur-bearing amino-acid metabolism, unspecified

E72.11   Homocystinuria
Cystathionine synthase deficiency

E72.12   Methylenetetrahydrofolate reductase deficiency

E72.19   Other disorders of sulfur-bearing amino-acid metabolism
Cystathioninuria
Methioninemia
Sulfite oxidase deficiency

5 **E72.2   Disorders of urea cycle metabolism**

> EXCLUDES 1   *disorders of ornithine metabolism (E72.4)*

E72.20   Disorder of urea cycle metabolism, unspecified
Hyperammonemia

> EXCLUDES 1   *hyperammonemia- hyperornithinemia-*
> *homocitrullinemia syndrome E72.4*
> *transient hyperammonemia of newborn*
> *(P74.6)*

E72.21   Argininemia

E72.22   Arginosuccinic aciduria

E72.23   Citrullinemia

E72.29   Other disorders of urea cycle metabolism

E72.3   Disorders of lysine and hydroxylysine metabolism
Glutaric aciduria NOS
Glutaric aciduria (type I)
Hydroxylysinemia
Hyperlysinemia

> EXCLUDES 1   *glutaric aciduria type II (E71.313)*
> *Refsum's disease (G60.1)*
> *Zellweger syndrome (E71.510)*

E72.4   Disorders of ornithine metabolism
Hyperammonemia-Hyperornithinemia-Homocitrullinemia
syndrome
Ornithinemia (types I, II)
Ornithine transcarbamylase deficiency

> EXCLUDES 1   *hereditary choroidal dystrophy (H31.2-)*

5 **E72.5   Disorders of glycine metabolism**

E72.50   Disorder of glycine metabolism, unspecified

E72.51   Non-ketotic hyperglycinemia

E72.52   Trimethylaminuria

E72.53   Hyperoxaluria
Oxalosis
Oxaluria

E72.59   Other disorders of glycine metabolism
D-glycericacidemia
Hyperhydroxyprolinemia
Hyperprolinemia (types I, II)
Sarcosinemia

E72.8   Other specified disorders of amino-acid metabolism
Disorders of beta-amino-acid metabolism
Disorders of gamma-glutamyl cycle

E72.9   Disorder of amino-acid metabolism, unspecified

4 **E73   Lactose intolerance**

E73.0   Congenital lactase deficiency

E73.1   Secondary lactase deficiency

E73.8   Other lactose intolerance

E73.9   Lactose intolerance, unspecified

4 **E74   Other disorders of carbohydrate metabolism**

> EXCLUDES 1   *diabetes mellitus (E08-E13)*
> *hypoglycemia NOS (E16.2)*
> *increased secretion of glucagon (E16.3)*
> *mucopolysaccharidosis (E76.0-E76.3)*

5 **E74.0   Glycogen storage disease**

E74.00   Glycogen storage disease, unspecified

E74.01   von Gierke disease
Type I glycogen storage disease

E74.02   Pompe disease
Cardiac glycogenosis
Type II glycogen storage disease

> CODING TIP ✓   Pompe disease is also called type
> II glycogen storage disease and is a congenital
> disease caused by a metabolic error in which the
> body deposits an abnormally high amount of
> glycogen in the kidneys and liver. The disease
> produces symptoms such as hypoglycemia (low
> blood sugar) and hyperlipemia (an excess of lipid
> molecules in the blood, which can lead to
> problems such as clogged arteries and heart
> attacks).

E74.03   Cori disease
Forbes disease
Type III glycogen storage disease

E74.04   McArdle disease
Type V glycogen storage disease

E74.09   Other glycogen storage disease
Andersen disease
Hers disease
Tauri disease
Glycogen storage disease, types 0, IV, VI-XI
Liver phosphorylase deficiency
Muscle phosphofructokinase deficiency

5 **E74.1   Disorders of fructose metabolism**

> EXCLUDES 1   *muscle phosphofructokinase deficiency*
> *(E74.09)*

E74.10   Disorder of fructose metabolism, unspecified

E74.11   Essential fructosuria
Fructokinase deficiency

E74.12   Hereditary fructose intolerance
Fructosemia

E74.19   Other disorders of fructose metabolism
Fructose-1, 6-diphosphatase deficiency

5 **E74.2   Disorders of galactose metabolism**

E74.20   Disorders of galactose metabolism, unspecified

E74.21   Galactosemia

E74.29   Other disorders of galactose metabolism
Galactokinase deficiency

5 **E74.3   Other disorders of intestinal carbohydrate absorption**

> EXCLUDES 2   *lactose intolerance (E73.-)*

E74.31   Sucrase-isomaltase deficiency

E74.39   Other disorders of intestinal carbohydrate absorption
Disorder of intestinal carbohydrate absorption NOS
Glucose-galactose malabsorption
Sucrase deficiency

E74.4   Disorders of pyruvate metabolism and gluconeogenesis
Deficiency of phosphoenolpyruvate carboxykinase
Deficiency of pyruvate carboxylase
Deficiency of pyruvate dehydrogenase

> EXCLUDES 1   *disorders of pyruvate metabolism and*
> *gluconeogenesis with anemia (D55.-)*
> *Leigh's syndrome (G31.82)*

E74.8   Other specified disorders of carbohydrate metabolism
Essential pentosuria
Renal glycosuria

> DEFINITION   Excess glucose in the urine with normal
> levels in the blood, due to renal tubules' inability to
> reabsorb glucose completely.

E74.9   Disorder of carbohydrate metabolism, unspecified

● New   ▲ Revised   *Manifestation*   4-7 Digit Indicators   ⊟ Laterality   A Adult (15+ years)   M Maternity (12-55 years)   N Newborn   P Pediatric (0-17 years)   ♂ Male   ♀ Female

✖ ~~Deleted~~   Unspecified   + Additional code

4 E75   Disorders of sphingolipid metabolism and other lipid storage disorders

> EXCLUDES 1   *mucolipidosis, types I-III (E77.0-E77.1)*
> *Refsum's disease (G60.1)*

5 E75.0   GM2 gangliosidosis

E75.00   **GM2 gangliosidosis, unspecified**

E75.01   **Sandhoff disease**

E75.02   **Tay-Sachs disease**

E75.09   **Other GM2 gangliosidosis**
Adult GM2 gangliosidosis
Juvenile GM2 gangliosidosis

5 E75.1   Other and unspecified gangliosidosis

E75.10   **Unspecified gangliosidosis**
Gangliosidosis NOS

E75.11   **Mucolipidosis IV**

E75.19   **Other gangliosidosis**
GM1 gangliosidosis
GM3 gangliosidosis

5 E75.2   Other sphingolipidosis

> EXCLUDES 1   *adrenoleukodystrophy [Addison-Schilder] (E71.528)*

E75.21   **Fabry (-Anderson) disease**

E75.22   **Gaucher disease**

E75.23   **Krabbe disease**

6 E75.24   Niemann-Pick disease

E75.240   **Niemann-Pick disease type A**

E75.241   **Niemann-Pick disease type B**

E75.242   **Niemann-Pick disease type C**

E75.243   **Niemann-Pick disease type D**

E75.248   **Other Niemann-Pick disease**

E75.249   **Niemann-Pick disease, unspecified**

E75.25   **Metachromatic leukodystrophy**

E75.29   **Other sphingolipidosis**
Farber's syndrome
Sulfatase deficiency
Sulfatide lipidosis

E75.3   **Sphingolipidosis, unspecified**

E75.4   **Neuronal ceroid lipofuscinosis**
Batten disease
Bielschowsky-Jansky disease
Kufs disease
Spielmeyer-Vogt disease

E75.5   **Other lipid storage disorders**
Cerebrotendinous cholesterosis [van Bogaert-Scherer-Epstein]
Wolman's disease

E75.6   **Lipid storage disorder, unspecified**

4 E76   Disorders of glycosaminoglycan metabolism

5 E76.0   Mucopolysaccharidosis, type I

E76.01   **Hurler's syndrome**

E76.02   **Hurler-Scheie syndrome**

E76.03   **Scheie's syndrome**

E76.1   **Mucopolysaccharidosis, type II**
Hunter's syndrome

5 E76.2   Other mucopolysaccharidoses

6 E76.21   Morquio mucopolysaccharidoses

E76.210   **Morquio A mucopolysaccharidoses**
Classic Morquio syndrome
Morquio syndrome A
Mucopolysaccharidosis, type IVA

E76.211   **Morquio B mucopolysaccharidoses**
Morquio-like mucopolysaccharidoses
Morquio-like syndrome
Morquio syndrome B
Mucopolysaccharidosis, type IVB

E76.219   **Morquio mucopolysaccharidoses, unspecified**
Morquio syndrome
Mucopolysaccharidosis, type IV

E76.22   **Sanfilippo mucopolysaccharidoses**
Mucopolysaccharidosis, type III (A) (B) (C) (D)
Sanfilippo A syndrome
Sanfilippo B syndrome
Sanfilippo C syndrome
Sanfilippo D syndrome

E76.29   **Other mucopolysaccharidoses**
beta-Glucuronidase deficiency
Maroteaux-Lamy (mild) (severe) syndrome
Mucopolysaccharidosis, types VI, VII

E76.3   **Mucopolysaccharidosis, unspecified**

E76.8   **Other disorders of glucosaminoglycan metabolism**

E76.9   **Glucosaminoglycan metabolism disorder, unspecified**

4 E77   Disorders of glycoprotein metabolism

E77.0   **Defects in post-translational modification of lysosomal enzymes**
Mucolipidosis II [I-cell disease]
Mucolipidosis III [pseudo-Hurler polydystrophy]

E77.1   **Defects in glycoprotein degradation**
Aspartylglucosaminuria
Fucosidosis
Mannosidosis
Sialidosis [mucolipidosis I]

E77.8   **Other disorders of glycoprotein metabolism**

E77.9   **Disorder of glycoprotein metabolism, unspecified**

4 E78   Disorders of lipoprotein metabolism and other lipidemias

> EXCLUDES 1   *sphingolipidosis (E75.0-E75.3)*

▲ 5 E78.0   Pure hypercholesterolemia

● E78.00   **Pure hypercholesterolemia, unspecified**
Fredrickson's hyperlipoproteinemia, type IIa
Hyperbetalipoproteinemia
Low-density-lipoprotein-type [LDL] hyperlipoproteinemia

● E78.01   **Familial hypercholesterolemia**

E78.1   **Pure hyperglyceridemia**
Elevated fasting triglycerides
Endogenous hyperglyceridemia
Fredrickson's hyperlipoproteinemia, type IV
Hyperlipidemia, group B
Hyperprebetalipoproteinemia
Very-low-density-lipoprotein-type [VLDL] hyperlipoproteinemia

E78.2   **Mixed hyperlipidemia**
Broad- or floating-betalipoproteinemia
Combined hyperlipidemia NOS
Elevated cholesterol with elevated triglycerides NEC
Fredrickson's hyperlipoproteinemia, type IIb or III
Hyperbetalipoproteinemia with prebetalipoproteinemia
Hypercholesteremia with endogenous hyperglyceridemia
Hyperlipidemia, group C
Tubo-eruptive xanthoma
Xanthoma tuberosum

> EXCLUDES 1   *cerebrotendinous cholesterosis [van Bogaert-Scherer- Epstein] (E75.5)*
> *familial combined hyperlipidemia (E78.4)*

E78.3   **Hyperchylomicronemia**
Chylomicron retention disease
Fredrickson's hyperlipoproteinemia, type I or V
Hyperlipidemia, group D
Mixed hyperglyceridemia

E78.4   **Other hyperlipidemia**
Familial combined hyperlipidemia

> DEFINITION   An excess of lipids or fats in the blood.

E78.5   **Hyperlipidemia, unspecified**

Normal   Hyperlipidemia

Artery
Lipids
Increased lipids (fat) in bloodstream

E78.6   **Lipoprotein deficiency**
Abetalipoproteinemia
Depressed HDL cholesterol
High-density lipoprotein deficiency
Hypoalphalipoproteinemia
Hypobetalipoproteinemia (familial)
Lecithin cholesterol acyltransferase deficiency
Tangier disease

5 E78.7   Disorders of bile acid and cholesterol metabolism

> EXCLUDES 1   *Niemann-Pick disease type C (E75.242)*

E78.70   **Disorder of bile acid and cholesterol metabolism, unspecified**

E78.71   **Barth syndrome**

● New   ▲ Revised   *Manifestation*   4-7 Digit Indicators   ▯ Laterality   A Adult (15+ years)   M Maternity (12-55 years)   N Newborn   P Pediatric (0-17 years)   ♂ Male   ♀ Female
✖ Deleted   Unspecified   + Additional code

E78.72 **Smith-Lemli-Opitz syndrome**

E78.79 **Other disorders of bile acid and cholesterol metabolism**

⑤ E78.8 **Other disorders of lipoprotein metabolism**

E78.81 **Lipoid dermatoarthritis**

E78.89 **Other lipoprotein metabolism disorders**

E78.9 **Disorder of lipoprotein metabolism, unspecified**

⓸ E79 **Disorders of purine and pyrimidine metabolism**

> EXCLUDES 1 *Ataxia-telangiectasia (Q87.1)*
> *Bloom's syndrome (Q82.8)*
> *Cockayne's syndrome (Q87.1)*
> *calculus of kidney (N20.0)*
> *combined immunodeficiency disorders (D81.-)*
> *Fanconi's anemia (D61.09)*
> *gout (M1A.-, M10.-)*
> *orotaciduric anemia (D53.0)*
> *progeria (E34.8)*
> *Werner's syndrome (E34.8)*
> *xeroderma pigmentosum (Q82.1)*

E79.0 **Hyperuricemia without signs of inflammatory arthritis and tophaceous disease**
Asymptomatic hyperuricemia

E79.1 **Lesch-Nyhan syndrome**
HGPRT deficiency

E79.2 **Myoadenylate deaminase deficiency**

E79.8 **Other disorders of purine and pyrimidine metabolism**
Hereditary xanthinuria

E79.9 **Disorder of purine and pyrimidine metabolism, unspecified**

⓸ E80 **Disorders of porphyrin and bilirubin metabolism**

> INCLUDES defects of catalase and peroxidase

E80.0 **Hereditary erythropoietic porphyria**
Congenital erythropoietic porphyria
Erythropoietic protoporphyria

E80.1 **Porphyria cutanea tarda**

⑤ E80.2 **Other and unspecified porphyria**

E80.20 **Unspecified porphyria**
Porphyria NOS

E80.21 **Acute intermittent (hepatic) porphyria**

E80.29 **Other porphyria**
Hereditary coproporphyria

E80.3 **Defects of catalase and peroxidase**
Acatalasia [Takahara]

E80.4 **Gilbert syndrome**

> DEFINITION A harmless inborn error of bilirubin metabolism from an abnormal liver enzyme causing a benign elevation of unconjugated bilirubin with no liver damage or hematologic abnormalities.

E80.5 **Crigler-Najjar syndrome**

E80.6 **Other disorders of bilirubin metabolism**
Dubin-Johnson syndrome
Rotor's syndrome

E80.7 **Disorder of bilirubin metabolism, unspecified**

⓸ E83 **Disorders of mineral metabolism**

> EXCLUDES 1 *dietary mineral deficiency (E58-E61)*
> *parathyroid disorders (E20-E21)*
> *vitamin D deficiency (E55.-)*

⑤ E83.0 **Disorders of copper metabolism**

E83.00 **Disorder of copper metabolism, unspecified**

E83.01 **Wilson's disease**
Code also:
associated Kayser Fleischer ring (H18.04-)

E83.09 **Other disorders of copper metabolism**
Menkes' (kinky hair) (steely hair) disease

⑤ E83.1 **Disorders of iron metabolism**

> EXCLUDES 1 *iron deficiency anemia (D50.-)*
> *sideroblastic anemia (D64.0-D64.3)*

E83.10 **Disorder of iron metabolism, unspecified**

⑥ E83.11 **Hemochromatosis**

E83.110 **Hereditary hemochromatosis**
Bronzed diabetes
Pigmentary cirrhosis (of liver)
Primary (hereditary) hemochromatosis

> DEFINITION A genetic problem causing the body to store too much iron, resulting in liver swelling, skin bronzing, and development of diabetes, arthritis, and organ failure.

E83.111 **Hemochromatosis due to repeated red blood cell transfusions**
Iron overload due to repeated red blood cell transfusions
Transfusion (red blood cell) associated hemochromatosis

E83.118 **Other hemochromatosis**

E83.119 **Hemochromatosis, unspecified**

✚ E83.19 **Other disorders of iron metabolism**
Use additional code, if applicable, for idiopathic pulmonary hemosiderosis (J84.03)

E83.2 **Disorders of zinc metabolism**
Acrodermatitis enteropathica

⑤ E83.3 **Disorders of phosphorus metabolism and phosphatases**

> EXCLUDES 1 *adult osteomalacia (M83.-)*
> *osteoporosis (M80.-)*

E83.30 **Disorder of phosphorus metabolism, unspecified**

E83.31 **Familial hypophosphatemia**
Vitamin D-resistant osteomalacia
Vitamin D-resistant rickets

> EXCLUDES 1 *vitamin D-deficiency rickets (E55.0)*

E83.32 **Hereditary vitamin D-dependent rickets (type 1) (type 2)**
25-hydroxyvitamin D 1-alpha-hydroxylase deficiency
Pseudovitamin D deficiency
Vitamin D receptor defect

E83.39 **Other disorders of phosphorus metabolism**
Acid phosphatase deficiency
Hypophosphatasia

⑤ E83.4 **Disorders of magnesium metabolism**

E83.40 **Disorders of magnesium metabolism, unspecified**

E83.41 **Hypermagnesemia**

E83.42 **Hypomagnesemia**

E83.49 **Other disorders of magnesium metabolism**

⑤ E83.5 **Disorders of calcium metabolism**

> EXCLUDES 1 *chondrocalcinosis (M11.1-M11.2)*
> *hungry bone syndrome (E83.81)*
> *hyperparathyroidism (E21.0-E21.3)*

E83.50 **Unspecified disorder of calcium metabolism**

E83.51 **Hypocalcemia**

> DEFINITION Reduced calcium levels in the blood causing hyperactive deep tendon reflexes, Chvostek's sign, muscle and abdominal cramps, and carpopedal spasm.

E83.52 **Hypercalcemia**
Familial hypocalciuric hypercalcemia

> DEFINITION Excess calcium levels in the blood causing fatigue, muscle weakness, depression, anorexia, nausea, and constipation.

E83.59 **Other disorders of calcium metabolism**
Idiopathic hypercalciuria

⑤ E83.8 **Other disorders of mineral metabolism**

E83.81 **Hungry bone syndrome**

> DEFINITION Low levels of calcium due to elevated parathyroid hormone levels or thyrotoxicosis that later return to normal or lower levels after treatment, causing bones to hoard calcium, resulting in increased bone density.

E83.89 **Other disorders of mineral metabolism**

E83.9 **Disorder of mineral metabolism, unspecified**

▲ ⓸ E84 **Cystic fibrosis**

> INCLUDES mucoviscidosis

Code also:
exocrine pancreatic insufficiency (K86.81)

> CODING TIP ✓ When reporting a E84 code, do not use an additional code for other disease of the lung. Chronic lung disease with bronchiectasis is an integral part of the cystic fibrosis and is not reported separately. However, an infection, such as pneumonia, should be coded separately. A patient with both pulmonary manifestations and gastrointestinal manifestations is coded with E84.0 and E84.1. Other manifestations (E84.8) include diabetes (E08) and right ventricular hypertrophy (I51.7).

+ E84.0 Cystic fibrosis with pulmonary manifestations
Use additional code to identify any infectious organism
present, such as:
Pseudomonas (B96.5)

⑤ E84.1 Cystic fibrosis with intestinal manifestations
E84.11 Meconium ileus in cystic fibrosis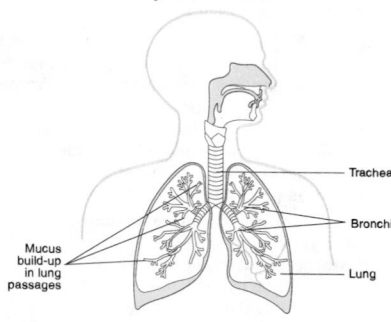
EXCLUDES 1 *meconium ileus not due to cystic*
fibrosis (P76.0)
E84.19 Cystic fibrosis with other intestinal manifestations
Distal intestinal obstruction syndrome
E84.8 Cystic fibrosis with other manifestations
E84.9 Cystic fibrosis, unspecified

DEFINITION Defective gene causing overproduction
of mucous that builds up in lung passages, resulting in
life-threatening respiratory problems.

Cystic fibrosis

Trachea

Bronchi

Mucus
build-up
in lung
passages

Lung

④ E85 Amyloidosis
EXCLUDES 1 *Alzheimer's disease (G30.0-)*

▲ E85.0 Non-neuropathic heredofamilial amyloidosis
Hereditary amyloid nephropathy
E85.1 Neuropathic heredofamilial amyloidosis
Amyloid polyneuropathy (Portuguese)
AHA: 4Q 2012, 99-100

E85.2 Heredofamilial amyloidosis, unspecified
E85.3 Secondary systemic amyloidosis
Hemodialysis-associated amyloidosis
E85.4 Organ-limited amyloidosis
Localized amyloidosis
E85.8 Other amyloidosis
E85.9 Amyloidosis, unspecified

DEFINITION Abnormal accumulation of amyloid-like
proteins in tissues.

▲ ④ + E86 Volume depletion
Use additional code(s) for any associated disorders of electrolyte
and acid-base balance (E87.-)
EXCLUDES 1 *dehydration of newborn (P74.1)*
hypovolemic shock NOS (R57.1)
postprocedural hypovolemic shock (T81.19)
traumatic hypovolemic shock (T79.4)

+ E86.0 Dehydration
GUIDELINES Section I.C.2.c.3)
When the admission/encounter is for management of
dehydration due to the malignancy and only the
dehydration is being treated (intravenous rehydration),
the dehydration is sequenced first, followed by the
code(s) for the malignancy.
AHA: 1Q 2014, 7

+ E86.1 Hypovolemia
Depletion of volume of plasma
DEFINITION Abnormal decrease in the total volume
of circulating blood with a corresponding loss of sodium
electrolytes.

+ E86.9 Volume depletion, unspecified
④ E87 Other disorders of fluid, electrolyte and acid-base
balance
EXCLUDES 1 *diabetes insipidus (E23.2)*
electrolyte imbalance associated with
hyperemesis gravidarum (O21.1)
electrolyte imbalance following ectopic or molar
pregnancy (O08.5)
familial periodic paralysis (G72.3)

E87.0 Hyperosmolality and hypernatremia
Sodium [Na] excess
Sodium [Na] overload
AHA: 1Q 2014, 7
E87.1 Hypo-osmolality and hyponatremia
Sodium [Na] deficiency
EXCLUDES 1 *syndrome of inappropriate secretion of*
antidiuretic hormone (E22.2)
AHA: 1Q 2014, 7
E87.2 Acidosis
Acidosis NOS
Lactic acidosis
Metabolic acidosis
Respiratory acidosis
EXCLUDES 1 *diabetic acidosis - see categories E08-E10,*
E13 with ketoacidosis
DEFINITION An abnormal increase in the acidity of
body fluids, caused either by accumulation of acids or
by depletion of bicarbonates.
E87.3 Alkalosis
Alkalosis NOS
Metabolic alkalosis
Respiratory alkalosis
E87.4 Mixed disorder of acid-base balance
E87.5 Hyperkalemia
Potassium [K] excess
Potassium [K] overload
DEFINITION An abnormally high concentration of
potassium ions in the blood.

Hyperkalemia

Excessive amount of
potassium in blood stream

E87.6 Hypokalemia
Potassium [K] deficiency
DEFINITION Low potassium level in the blood
causing neuromuscular disorders ranging from
weakness to paralysis, electrocardiographic
abnormalities, renal disease, and gastrointestinal
disorders.
⑤ E87.7 Fluid overload
EXCLUDES 1 *edema NOS (R60.9)*
fluid retention (R60.9)
DEFINITION High infusion rates or transfusion
volumes not processed effectively by the recipient,
causing circulatory system overload marked by acute
respiratory distress.
E87.70 Fluid overload, unspecified
E87.71 Transfusion associated circulatory overload
Fluid overload due to transfusion (blood) (blood
components)
TACO
E87.79 Other fluid overload
E87.8 Other disorders of electrolyte and fluid balance, not
elsewhere classified
Electrolyte imbalance NOS
Hyperchloremia
Hypochloremia
④ + E88 Other and unspecified metabolic disorders
Use additional codes for associated conditions
EXCLUDES 1 *histiocytosis X (chronic) (C96.6)*

⑤ + E88.0 Disorders of plasma-protein metabolism, not elsewhere
classified
EXCLUDES 1 *disorder of lipoprotein metabolism (E78.-)*
monoclonal gammopathy
(of undetermined significance) (D47.2)
polyclonal hypergammaglobulinemia
(D89.0)
Waldenström macroglobulinemia (C88.0)

● New ▲ Revised *Manifestation* ④- ⑦ Digit Indicators ⊟ Laterality Ⓐ Adult (15+ years) Ⓜ Maternity (12-55 years) Ⓝ Newborn Ⓟ Pediatric (0-17 years) ♂ Male ♀ Female
✖ Deleted Unspecified + Additional code

2017 ICD-10-CM Expert for Physicians

© 2017 decisionHealth

539

+ E88.01 **Alpha-1-antitrypsin deficiency**
AAT deficiency

+ E88.09 **Other disorders of plasma-protein metabolism, not elsewhere classified**
Bisalbuminemia

+ E88.1 **Lipodystrophy, not elsewhere classified**
Lipodystrophy NOS
EXCLUDES 1 *Whipple's disease (K90.81)*
DEFINITION Defective fat metabolism resulting in abnormal or degenerative subcutaneous fat deposits that appear as lumps or dents under the skin.

+ E88.2 **Lipomatosis, not elsewhere classified**
Lipomatosis NOS
Lipomatosis (Check) dolorosa [Dercum]

+ E88.3 **Tumor lysis syndrome**
Tumor lysis syndrome (spontaneous)
Tumor lysis syndrome following antineoplastic drug chemotherapy
Use additional code for adverse effect, if applicable, to identify drug (T45.1X5)

⑤+ E88.4 **Mitochondrial metabolism disorders**
EXCLUDES 1 *disorders of pyruvate metabolism (E74.4)*
Kearns-Sayre syndrome (H49.81)
Leber's disease (H47.22)
Leigh's encephalopathy (G31.82)
Mitochondrial myopathy, NEC (G71.3)
Reye's syndrome (G93.7)

+ E88.40 **Mitochondrial metabolism disorder, unspecified**

+ E88.41 **MELAS syndrome**
Mitochondrial myopathy, encephalopathy, lactic acidosis and stroke-like episodes

▲+ E88.42 **MERRF syndrome**
Myoclonic epilepsy associated with ragged-red fibers
Code also:
progressive myoclonic epilepsy (G40.3-)

+ E88.49 **Other mitochondrial metabolism disorders**

⑤+ E88.8 **Other specified metabolic disorders**

+ E88.81 **Metabolic syndrome**
Dysmetabolic syndrome X
Use additional codes for associated manifestations, such as:
obesity (E66.-)
CODING TIP ✓ Metabolic Syndrome (also called Dysmetabolic syndrome X) involves a cluster of symptoms placing individuals at risk for development of a number of disease processes. Manifestations of metabolic syndrome confirmed by the physician, such as obesity (and BMI as calculated by the clinical record documentation) should additionally be coded following E88.81.

+ E88.89 **Other specified metabolic disorders**
Launois-Bensaude adenolipomatosis
EXCLUDES 1 *adult pulmonary Langerhans cell histiocytosis (J84.82)*

+ E88.9 **Metabolic disorder, unspecified**

Postprocedural endocrine and metabolic complications and disorders, not elsewhere classified (E89)

CODING TIP ✓ Conditions classifiable to E89 are classifiable as postprocedural complications. These conditions should only be assigned when diagnostic statements clearly indicate that the condition is a complication of a procedure.

④ E89 **Postprocedural endocrine and metabolic complications and disorders, not elsewhere classified**
EXCLUDES 2 *intraoperative complications of endocrine system organ or structure (E36.0-, E36.1-, E36.8)*

E89.0 **Postprocedural hypothyroidism**
Postirradiation hypothyroidism
Postsurgical hypothyroidism
DEFINITION Underactive thyroid gland due to surgery or radiation, causing an inadequate production of thyroid hormone and a slowing of metabolic processes.

+ E89.1 **Postprocedural hypoinsulinemia**
Postpancreatectomy hyperglycemia
Postsurgical hypoinsulinemia
Use additional code, if applicable, to identify:
acquired absence of pancreas (Z90.41-)
diabetes mellitus (postpancreatectomy) (postprocedural) (E13.-)
insulin use (Z79.4)
EXCLUDES 1 *transient postprocedural hyperglycemia (R73.9)*
transient postprocedural hypoglycemia (E16.2)
GUIDELINES Section I.C.4.a.6)(b)(i)
For postpancreatectomy diabetes mellitus (lack of insulin due to the surgical removal of all or part of the pancreas), assign code E89.1, Postprocedural hypoinsulinemia. Assign a code from category E13 and a code from subcategory Z90.41-, Acquired absence of pancreas, as additional codes.
CODING TIP ✓ Because the pancreas is the organ that produces insulin, the removal of even a portion of the pancreas can produce diabetic-like symptoms. If manifestations are produced because of the hyperglycemia and lack of insulin, add the codes for manifestations after the E89.1 code with the appropriate E13 code(s). Also add the acquired absence of pancreas (Z90.41-) and use of insulin (Z79.4).

E89.2 **Postprocedural hypoparathyroidism**
Parathyroprival tetany

E89.3 **Postprocedural hypopituitarism**
Postirradiation hypopituitarism

⑤ E89.4 **Postprocedural ovarian failure**

E89.40 **Asymptomatic postprocedural ovarian failure** ♀
Postprocedural ovarian failure NOS

E89.41 **Symptomatic postprocedural ovarian failure** ♀
Symptoms such as flushing, sleeplessness, headache, lack of concentration, associated with postprocedural menopause

E89.5 **Postprocedural testicular hypofunction** ♂

E89.6 **Postprocedural adrenocortical (-medullary) hypofunction**

⑤ E89.8 **Other postprocedural endocrine and metabolic complications and disorders**

▲ ⑥ E89.81 **Postprocedural hemorrhage of an endocrine system organ or structure following a procedure**

▲ E89.810 **Postprocedural hemorrhage of an endocrine system organ or structure following an endocrine system procedure**

▲ E89.811 **Postprocedural hemorrhage of an endocrine system organ or structure following other procedure**

● ⑥ E89.82 **Postprocedural hematoma and seroma of an endocrine system organ or structure**

● E89.820 **Postprocedural hematoma of an endocrine system organ or structure following an endocrine system procedure**

● E89.821 **Postprocedural hematoma of an endocrine system organ or structure following other procedure**

● E89.822 **Postprocedural seroma of an endocrine system organ or structure following an endocrine system procedure**

● E89.823 **Postprocedural seroma of an endocrine system organ or structure following other procedure**

+ E89.89 **Other postprocedural endocrine and metabolic complications and disorders**
Use additional code, if applicable, to further specify disorder

---

CHAPTER 5: MENTAL, BEHAVIORAL AND NEURODEVELOPMENTAL DISORDERS (F01-F99)

INCLUDES disorders of psychological development

EXCLUDES 2 *symptoms, signs and abnormal clinical laboratory findings, not elsewhere classified (R00-R99)*

This chapter contains the following blocks:

F01-F09	Mental disorders due to known physiological conditions
F10-F19	Mental and behavioral disorders due to psychoactive substance use
F20-F29	Schizophrenia, schizotypal, delusional, and other non-mood psychotic disorders
F30-F39	Mood [affective] disorders
F40-F48	Anxiety, dissociative, stress-related, somatoform and other nonpsychotic mental disorders
F50-F59	Behavioral syndromes associated with physiological disturbances and physical factors
F60-F69	Disorders of adult personality and behavior
F70-F79	Intellectual disabilities
F80-F89	Pervasive and specific developmental disorders
F90-F98	Behavioral and emotional disorders with onset usually occurring in childhood and adolescence
F99	Unspecified mental disorder

Mental disorders due to known physiological conditions (F01-F09)

Note: This block comprises a range of mental disorders grouped together on the basis of their having in common a demonstrable etiology in cerebral disease, brain injury, or other insult leading to cerebral dysfunction. The dysfunction may be primary, as in diseases, injuries, and insults that affect the brain directly and selectively; or secondary, as in systemic diseases and disorders that attack the brain only as one of the multiple organs or systems of the body that are involved.

CODING TIP ✓ Conditions classifiable here are specifically reportable as due to an underlying cause or condition.

◘ F01   Vascular dementia

Vascular dementia as a result of infarction of the brain due to vascular disease, including hypertensive cerebrovascular disease.

INCLUDES arteriosclerotic dementia

Code first:
the underlying physiological condition or sequelae of cerebrovascular disease.

⑤ F01.5   Vascular dementia

CODING TIP ✓ Vascular dementia must be specified by the physician and may also be reported as "multi-infarct dementia." In this case it should be coded as a sequelae of cerebrovascular accident (stroke). This type of dementia also may be related to other cerebral vascular disorders including vascular hypertension and cerebral atherosclerosis.

▲ F01.50   Vascular dementia without behavioral disturbance   Ⓐ

Major neurocognitive disorder without behavioral disturbance

▲ + F01.51   Vascular dementia with behavioral disturbance   Ⓐ

Major neurocognitive disorder due to vascular disease, with behavioral disturbance
Major neurocognitive disorder with aggressive behavior
Major neurocognitive disorder with combative behavior
Major neurocognitive disorder with violent behavior
Vascular dementia with aggressive behavior
Vascular dementia with combative behavior
Vascular dementia with violent behavior
Use additional code, if applicable, to identify wandering in vascular dementia (Z91.83)

▲ ◘ F02   Dementia in other diseases classified elsewhere

INCLUDES Major neurocognitive disorder in other diseases classified elsewhere

Code first the underlying physiological condition, such as:
Alzheimer's (G30.-)
cerebral lipidosis (E75.4)
Creutzfeldt-Jakob disease (A81.0-)
dementia with Lewy bodies (G31.83)
dementia with Parkinsonism (G31.83)
epilepsy and recurrent seizures (G40.-)
frontotemporal dementia (G31.09)
hepatolenticular degeneration (E83.0)
human immunodeficiency virus [HIV] disease (B20)
Huntington's disease (G10)
hypercalcemia (E83.52)
hypothyroidism, acquired (E00-E03.-)
intoxications (T36-T65)
Jakob-Creutzfeldt disease (A81.0-)
multiple sclerosis (G35)
neurosyphilis (A52.17)
niacin deficiency [pellagra] (E52)
Parkinson's disease (G20)
Pick's disease (G31.01)
polyarteritis nodosa (M30.0)
prion disease (A81.9)
systemic lupus erythematosus (M32.-)
traumatic brain injury (S06.-)
trypanosomiasis (B56.-, B57.-)
vitamin B deficiency (E53.8)

EXCLUDES 2 *dementia in alcohol and psychoactive substance disorders (F10-F19, with .17, .27, .97)*
vascular dementia (F01.5-)

⑤ F02.8   Dementia in other diseases classified elsewhere

CODING TIP ✓ Codes F02.80 and F02.81 are manifestation only codes and should be used only to report dementia in an etiology/manifestation pairing. An F02.8- code should never be used alone and inappropriate use of these codes may result in claims edits. Always code the etiology first, followed by the appropriate F02.8- code to specify dementia with or without behavioral disturbance. The physician must provide a diagnosis of dementia.

▲ F02.80   *Dementia in other diseases classified elsewhere without behavioral disturbance*

Dementia in other diseases classified elsewhere NOS
Major neurocognitive disorder in other diseases classified elsewhere
AHA: 2Q 2016, 6

▲ + F02.81   *Dementia in other diseases classified elsewhere with behavioral disturbance*

Dementia in other diseases classified elsewhere with aggressive behavior
Dementia in other diseases classified elsewhere with combative behavior
Dementia in other diseases classified elsewhere with violent behavior
Major neurocognitive disorder in other diseases classified elsewhere with aggressive behavior
Major neurocognitive disorder in other diseases classified elsewhere with combative behavior
Major neurocognitive disorder in other diseases classified elsewhere with violent behavior
Use additional code, if applicable, to identify wandering in dementia in conditions classified elsewhere (Z91.83)

◘ F03   Unspecified dementia

Presenile dementia NOS
Presenile psychosis NOS
Primary degenerative dementia NOS
Senile dementia NOS
Senile dementia depressed or paranoid type
Senile psychosis NOS

EXCLUDES 1 *senility NOS (R41.81)*

EXCLUDES 2 *mild memory disturbance due to known physiological condition (F06.8)*
senile dementia with delirium or acute confusional state (F05)

DEFINITION Loss of cognitive and intellectual functions, such as impaired memory, judgment, and intellect, without impaired perception or consciousness.

⑤ F03.9   Unspecified dementia

● New   ▲ Revised   *Manifestation*   ◘-⑦ Digit Indicators   ▤ Laterality   Ⓐ Adult (15+ years)   Ⓜ Maternity (12-55 years)   Ⓝ Newborn   Ⓟ Pediatric (0-17 years)   ♂ Male   ♀ Female
✖ Deleted   Unspecified   + Additional code

2017 ICD-10-CM Expert for Physicians

© 2017 DecisionHealth   541

F01 — F03.9

Mental, Behavioral and Neurodevelopmental Disorders

CODING TIP✓ Codes F03.90 and F03.91 are to be used for dementia that is not specified as due to another condition, and is reported as unspecified, senile psychosis, senile dementia (may also state depressed or paranoid type), primary degenerative dementia, or presenile dementia/psychosis. Do not confuse these conditions with organic brain disease or senility NOS. Senility NOS should not be coded with an F03.9- code (see excludes 1 notes) as this is less specific. When senile dementia is specified, the appropriate F03.9- code should be used.

F03.90   **Unspecified dementia without behavioral disturbance**   Ⓐ
Dementia NOS
AHA: 4Q 2012, 92

+ F03.91   **Unspecified dementia with behavioral disturbance**   Ⓐ
Unspecified dementia with aggressive behavior
Unspecified dementia with combative behavior
Unspecified dementia with violent behavior
Use additional code, if applicable, to identify wandering in unspecified dementia (Z91.83)

F04   **Amnestic disorder due to known physiological condition**
Korsakov's psychosis or syndrome, nonalcoholic
Code first:
the underlying physiological condition
EXCLUDES 1   *amnesia NOS (R41.3)*
anterograde amnesia (R41.1)
dissociative amnesia (F44.0)
retrograde amnesia (R41.2)
EXCLUDES 2   *alcohol-induced or unspecified Korsakov's syndrome (F10.26, F10.96)*
Korsakov's syndrome induced by other psychoactive substances (F13.26, F13.96, F19.16, F19.26, F19.96)

F05   **Delirium due to known physiological condition**
Acute or subacute brain syndrome
Acute or subacute confusional state (nonalcoholic)
Acute or subacute infective psychosis
Acute or subacute organic reaction
Acute or subacute psycho-organic syndrome
Delirium of mixed etiology
Delirium superimposed on dementia
Sundowning
Code first:
the underlying physiological condition
EXCLUDES 1   *delirium NOS (R41.0)*
EXCLUDES 2   *delirium tremens alcohol-induced or unspecified (F10.231, F10.921)*

CODING TIP✓ Patients with dementia may also have delirium or sundowning. When appropriate, add F05 when dementia is coded.

◪ F06   **Other mental disorders due to known physiological condition**
INCLUDES   mental disorders due to endocrine disorder
mental disorders due to exogenous hormone
mental disorders due to exogenous toxic substance
mental disorders due to primary cerebral disease
mental disorders due to somatic illness
mental disorders due to systemic disease affecting the brain
Code first:
the underlying physiological condition
EXCLUDES 1   *unspecified dementia (F03)*
EXCLUDES 2   *delirium due to known physiological condition (F05)*
dementia as classified in F01-F02
other mental disorders associated with alcohol and other psychoactive substances (F10-F19)

F06.0   **Psychotic disorder with hallucinations due to known physiological condition**
Organic hallucinatory state (nonalcoholic)
EXCLUDES 2   *hallucinations and perceptual disturbance induced by alcohol and other psychoactive substances (F10-F19 with .151, .251, .951)*
schizophrenia (F20.-)

▲ F06.1   **Catatonic disorder due to known physiological condition**
Catatonia associated with another mental disorder
Catatonia NOS
EXCLUDES 1   *catatonic stupor (R40.1)*
stupor NOS (R40.1)
EXCLUDES 2   *catatonic schizophrenia (F20.2)*
dissociative stupor (F44.2)

F06.2   **Psychotic disorder with delusions due to known physiological condition**
Paranoid and paranoid-hallucinatory organic states
Schizophrenia-like psychosis in epilepsy
EXCLUDES 2   *alcohol and drug-induced psychotic disorder (F10-F19 with .150, .250, .950)*
brief psychotic disorder (F23)
delusional disorder (F22)
schizophrenia (F20.-)

Ⓢ F06.3   **Mood disorder due to known physiological condition**
EXCLUDES 2   *mood disorders due to alcohol and other psychoactive substances (F10-F19 with .14, .24, .94)*
mood disorders, not due to known physiological condition or unspecified (F30-F39)

F06.30   **Mood disorder due to known physiological condition, unspecified**

F06.31   **Mood disorder due to known physiological condition with depressive features**

F06.32   **Mood disorder due to known physiological condition with major depressive-like episode**

F06.33   **Mood disorder due to known physiological condition with manic features**

F06.34   **Mood disorder due to known physiological condition with mixed features**

F06.4   **Anxiety disorder due to known physiological condition**
EXCLUDES 2   *anxiety disorders due to alcohol and other psychoactive substances (F10-F19 with .180, .280, .980)*
anxiety disorders, not due to known physiological condition or unspecified (F40.-, F41.-)

F06.8   **Other specified mental disorders due to known physiological condition**
Epileptic psychosis NOS
Organic dissociative disorder
Organic emotionally labile [asthenic] disorder

◪ F07   **Personality and behavioral disorders due to known physiological condition**
Code first:
the underlying physiological condition

F07.0   **Personality change due to known physiological condition**
Frontal lobe syndrome
Limbic epilepsy personality syndrome
Lobotomy syndrome
Organic personality disorder
Organic pseudopsychopathic personality
Organic pseudoretarded personality
Postleucotomy syndrome
Code first:
underlying physiological condition
EXCLUDES 1   *mild cognitive impairment (G31.84)*
postconcussional syndrome (F07.81)
postencephalitic syndrome (F07.89)
signs and symptoms involving emotional state (R45.-)
EXCLUDES 2   *specific personality disorder (F60.-)*

DEFINITION   Frontal lobe syndrome: Damage to the frontal lobe of the brain, typically manifesting as apathy, a lack of planning, emotional bluntness, the absence of abstract thought and attention, and judgment changes.

Ⓢ F07.8   **Other personality and behavioral disorders due to known physiological condition**

+ F07.81   **Postconcussional syndrome**
Postcontusional syndrome (encephalopathy)
Post-traumatic brain syndrome, nonpsychotic
Use additional code to identify associated post-traumatic headache, if applicable (G44.3-)
EXCLUDES 1   *current concussion (brain) (S06.0-)*
postencephalitic syndrome (F07.89)

● New   ▲ Revised   *Manifestation*   ◪-◪ Digit Indicators   Ⓔ Laterality   Ⓐ Adult (15+ years)   Ⓜ Maternity (12-55 years)   Ⓝ Newborn   Ⓟ Pediatric (0-17 years)   ♂ Male   ♀ Female
✖ Deleted   Unspecified   + Additional code

CODING TIP ✓ Code F07.81 should not be used for the patient who has a current concussion (see the Excludes 1 notes). Postconcussional syndrome is a complex disorder resulting from traumatic brain injury and is not associated with the severity of the initial injury. No documented loss of consciousness with the initial injury is necessary for a diagnosis of postconcussional syndrome, but the physicals must specify this disorder.

DEFINITION Symptoms such as headache, amnesia, and lack of concentration due to a severe blow to the skull.

F07.89   **Other personality and behavioral disorders due to known physiological condition**
Postencephalitic syndrome
Right hemispheric organic affective disorder

F07.9   **Unspecified personality and behavioral disorder due to known physiological condition**
Organic psychosyndrome

F09   **Unspecified mental disorder due to known physiological condition**
Mental disorder NOS due to known physiological condition
Organic brain syndrome NOS
Organic mental disorder NOS
Organic psychosis NOS
Symptomatic psychosis NOS
Code first:
   the underlying physiological condition
EXCLUDES 1 *psychosis NOS (F29)*

Mental and behavioral disorders due to psychoactive substance use (F10-F19)

GUIDELINES Section I.C.5.b.1)-3)
Selection of codes for "in remission" for categories F10-F19, Mental and behavioral disorders due to psychoactive substance use (categories F10-F19 with -.21), requires the provider's clinical judgment. The appropriate codes for "in remission" are assigned only on the basis of provider documentation (as defined in the Official Guidelines for Coding and Reporting).

When the provider documentation refers to use, abuse and dependence of the same substance (e.g. alcohol, opioid, cannabis, etc.), only one code should be assigned to identify the pattern of use based on the following hierarchy:
• If both use and abuse are documented, assign only the code for abuse
• If both abuse and dependence are documented, assign only the code for dependence
• If use, abuse and dependence are all documented, assign only the code for dependence
• If both use and dependence are documented, assign only the code for dependence.

As with all other diagnoses, the codes for psychoactive substance use (F10.9-, F11.9-, F12.9-, F13.9-, F14.9-, F15.9-, F16.9-) should only be assigned based on provider documentation and when they meet the definition of a reportable diagnosis (see Section III, Reporting Additional Diagnoses). The codes are to be used only when the psychoactive substance use is associated with a mental or behavioral disorder, and such a relationship is documented by the provider.

GUIDELINES Section I.C.5.c.2) When the provider documentation refers to use, abuse and dependence of the same substance (e.g. alcohol, opioid, cannabis, etc.), only one code should be assigned to identify the pattern of use based on the following hierarchy: • If both use and abuse are documented, assign only the code for abuse • If both abuse and dependence are documented, assign only the code for dependence • If use, abuse and dependence are all documented, assign only the code for dependence • If both use and dependence are documented, assign only the code for dependence.

GUIDELINES Section I.C.5.c.3) As with all other diagnoses, the codes for psychoactive substance use (F10.9-, F11.9-, F12.9-, F13.9-, F14.9-, F15.9-, F16.9-) should only be assigned based on provider documentation and when they meet the definition of a reportable diagnosis (see Section III, Reporting Additional Diagnoses). The codes are to be used only when the psychoactive substance use is associated with a mental or behavioral disorder, and such a relationship is documented by the provider.

CODING TIP ✓ When coding disorders due to psychoactive use, abuse, and dependence, refer to provider documentation to determine the appropriate code selection for either use, abuse, or dependence. Only one code should be used to specify use, abuse, or dependence on a substance, even when documentation uses multiple terms to refer to use, abuse, and/or dependence on a substance. Coders should refer to the appropriate hierarchy to determine code selection. When both use and abuse are specified, abuse should be coded. When use and dependence are specified, dependence should be coded. When abuse and dependence are specified, dependence should be coded. When use, abuse, and dependence are specified, dependence should be coded. When coding tobacco use, do not use a code from F10-F19. The code for tobacco use is located in Chapter 21: Factors Influencing Health Status and Contact with Health Services (Z72.0).

④ **+ F10**   **Alcohol related disorders**
     Use additional code for blood alcohol level, if applicable (Y90.-)

⑤ **+ F10.1**   **Alcohol abuse**
   EXCLUDES 1 *alcohol dependence (F10.2-)*
               alcohol use, unspecified (F10.9-)

▲ **+ F10.10**   **Alcohol abuse, uncomplicated**
Alcohol use disorder, mild

⑥ **+ F10.12**   **Alcohol abuse with intoxication**
   + F10.120   **Alcohol abuse with intoxication, uncomplicated**
   + F10.121   **Alcohol abuse with intoxication delirium**
   + F10.129   **Alcohol abuse with intoxication, unspecified**

▲ **+ F10.14**   **Alcohol abuse with alcohol-induced mood disorder**
Alcohol use disorder, mild, with alcohol-induced bipolar or related disorder
Alcohol use disorder, mild, with alcohol-induced depressive disorder

⑥ **+ F10.15**   **Alcohol abuse with alcohol-induced psychotic disorder**
   + F10.150   **Alcohol abuse with alcohol-induced psychotic disorder with delusions**
   + F10.151   **Alcohol abuse with alcohol-induced psychotic disorder with hallucinations**
   + F10.159   **Alcohol abuse with alcohol-induced psychotic disorder, unspecified**

⑥ **+ F10.18**   **Alcohol abuse with other alcohol-induced disorders**
   + F10.180   **Alcohol abuse with alcohol-induced anxiety disorder**
   + F10.181   **Alcohol abuse with alcohol-induced sexual dysfunction**
   + F10.182   **Alcohol abuse with alcohol-induced sleep disorder**
   + F10.188   **Alcohol abuse with other alcohol-induced disorder**

   + F10.19   **Alcohol abuse with unspecified alcohol-induced disorder**

⑤ **+ F10.2**   **Alcohol dependence**
   EXCLUDES 1 *alcohol abuse (F10.1-)*
               alcohol use, unspecified (F10.9-)
   EXCLUDES 2 *toxic effect of alcohol (T51.0-)*

▲ **+ F10.20**   **Alcohol dependence, uncomplicated**
Alcohol use disorder, moderate
Alcohol use disorder, severe

   + F10.21   **Alcohol dependence, in remission**

▲ ⑥ **+ F10.22**   **Alcohol dependence with intoxication**
Acute drunkenness (in alcoholism)
   EXCLUDES 2 *alcohol dependence with withdrawal (F10.23-)*
   + F10.220   **Alcohol dependence with intoxication, uncomplicated**
   + F10.221   **Alcohol dependence with intoxication delirium**
   + F10.229   **Alcohol dependence with intoxication, unspecified**

▲ ⑥ **+ F10.23**   **Alcohol dependence with withdrawal**
   EXCLUDES 2 *Alcohol dependence with intoxication (F10.22-)*
   + F10.230   **Alcohol dependence with withdrawal, uncomplicated**
   + F10.231   **Alcohol dependence with withdrawal delirium**
     DEFINITION Delirium occurring when an alcoholic is denied alcohol for a significant period of time.

● New   ▲ Revised   *Manifestation*   ④-⑦ Digit Indicators   ⊟ Laterality   Ⓐ Adult (15+ years)   Ⓜ Maternity (12-55 years)   Ⓝ Newborn   Ⓟ Pediatric (0-17 years)   ♂ Male   ♀ Female
✖ Deleted   Unspecified   + Additional code

+ F10.232 Alcohol dependence with withdrawal with perceptual disturbance

+ F10.239 Alcohol dependence with withdrawal, unspecified

AHA: 2Q 2015, 15

▲ + F10.24 Alcohol dependence with alcohol-induced mood disorder

Alcohol use disorder, moderate, with alcohol-induced bipolar or related disorder

Alcohol use disorder, moderate, with alcohol-induced depressive disorder

Alcohol use disorder, severe, with alcohol-induced bipolar or related disorder

Alcohol use disorder, severe, with alcohol-induced depressive disorder

⑥ + F10.25 Alcohol dependence with alcohol-induced psychotic disorder

+ F10.250 Alcohol dependence with alcohol-induced psychotic disorder with delusions

+ F10.251 Alcohol dependence with alcohol-induced psychotic disorder with hallucinations

+ F10.259 Alcohol dependence with alcohol-induced psychotic disorder, unspecified

▲ + F10.26 Alcohol dependence with alcohol-induced persisting amnestic disorder

Alcohol use disorder, moderate, with alcohol-induced major neurocognitive disorder, amnestic-confabulatory type

Alcohol use disorder, severe, with alcohol-induced major neurocognitive disorder, amnestic-confabulatory type

▲ + F10.27 Alcohol dependence with alcohol-induced persisting dementia

Alcohol use disorder, moderate, with alcohol-induced major neurocognitive disorder, nonamnestic-confabulatory type

Alcohol use disorder, severe, with alcohol-induced major neurocognitive disorder, nonamnestic-confabulatory type

DEFINITION Lasting state of dementia due to chronic alcoholism.

⑥ + F10.28 Alcohol dependence with other alcohol-induced disorders

+ F10.280 Alcohol dependence with alcohol-induced anxiety disorder

+ F10.281 Alcohol dependence with alcohol-induced sexual dysfunction

+ F10.282 Alcohol dependence with alcohol-induced sleep disorder

▲ + F10.288 Alcohol dependence with other alcohol-induced disorder

Alcohol use disorder, moderate, with alcohol-induced mild neurocognitive disorder

Alcohol use disorder, severe, with alcohol-induced mild neurocognitive disorder

+ F10.29 Alcohol dependence with unspecified alcohol-induced disorder

⑤ + F10.9 Alcohol use, unspecified

EXCLUDES 1 alcohol abuse (F10.1-)
alcohol dependence (F10.2-)

⑥ + F10.92 Alcohol use, unspecified with intoxication

+ F10.920 Alcohol use, unspecified with intoxication, uncomplicated

+ F10.921 Alcohol use, unspecified with intoxication delirium

+ F10.929 Alcohol use, unspecified with intoxication, unspecified

▲ + F10.94 Alcohol use, unspecified with alcohol-induced mood disorder

Alcohol induced bipolar or related disorder, without use disorder

Alcohol induced depressive disorder, without use disorder

⑥ + F10.95 Alcohol use, unspecified with alcohol-induced psychotic disorder

+ F10.950 Alcohol use, unspecified with alcohol-induced psychotic disorder with delusions

+ F10.951 Alcohol use, unspecified with alcohol-induced psychotic disorder with hallucinations

▲ + F10.959 Alcohol use, unspecified with alcohol-induced psychotic disorder, unspecified

Alcohol-induced psychotic disorder without use disorder

▲ + F10.96 Alcohol use, unspecified with alcohol-induced persisting amnestic disorder

Alcohol-induced major neurocognitive disorder, amnestic-confabulatory type, without use disorder

▲ + F10.97 Alcohol use, unspecified with alcohol-induced persisting dementia

Alcohol-induced major neurocognitive disorder, nonamnestic-confabulatory type, without use disorder

⑥ + F10.98 Alcohol use, unspecified with other alcohol-induced disorders

▲ + F10.980 Alcohol use, unspecified with alcohol-induced anxiety disorder

Alcohol induced anxiety disorder, without use disorder

▲ + F10.981 Alcohol use, unspecified with alcohol-induced sexual dysfunction

Alcohol induced sexual dysfunction, without use disorder

▲ + F10.982 Alcohol use, unspecified with alcohol-induced sleep disorder

Alcohol induced sleep disorder, without use disorder

DEFINITION Disruption of normal sleep patterns due to the consumption of alcohol.

▲ + F10.988 Alcohol use, unspecified with other alcohol-induced disorder

Alcohol induced mild neurocognitive disorder, without use disorder

+ F10.99 Alcohol use, unspecified with unspecified alcohol-induced disorder

④ F11   Opioid related disorders

⑤ F11.1   Opioid abuse

EXCLUDES 1 opioid dependence (F11.2-)
opioid use, unspecified (F11.9-)

▲ F11.10 Opioid abuse, uncomplicated

Opioid use disorder, mild

⑥ F11.12 Opioid abuse with intoxication

F11.120 Opioid abuse with intoxication, uncomplicated

F11.121 Opioid abuse with intoxication delirium

F11.122 Opioid abuse with intoxication with perceptual disturbance

F11.129 Opioid abuse with intoxication, unspecified

▲ F11.14 Opioid abuse with opioid-induced mood disorder

Opioid use disorder, mild, with opioid-induced depressive disorder

⑥ F11.15 Opioid abuse with opioid-induced psychotic disorder

F11.150 Opioid abuse with opioid-induced psychotic disorder with delusions

F11.151 Opioid abuse with opioid-induced psychotic disorder with hallucinations

F11.159 Opioid abuse with opioid-induced psychotic disorder, unspecified

⑥ F11.18 Opioid abuse with other opioid-induced disorder

F11.181 Opioid abuse with opioid-induced sexual dysfunction

F11.182 Opioid abuse with opioid-induced sleep disorder

F11.188 Opioid abuse with other opioid-induced disorder

F11.19 Opioid abuse with unspecified opioid-induced disorder

⑤ F11.2   Opioid dependence

EXCLUDES 1 opioid abuse (F11.1-)
opioid use, unspecified (F11.9-)

EXCLUDES 2 opioid poisoning (T40.0-T40.2-)

▲ F11.20 Opioid dependence, uncomplicated

Opioid use disorder, moderate

Opioid use disorder, severe

F11.21 Opioid dependence, in remission

⑥ F11.22 Opioid dependence with intoxication

EXCLUDES 1 opioid dependence with withdrawal (F11.23)

F11.220 Opioid dependence with intoxication, uncomplicated

● New   ▲ Revised   *Manifestation*   ④-⑦ Digit Indicators   ⊟ Laterality   Ⓐ Adult (15+ years)   Ⓜ Maternity (12-55 years)   Ⓝ Newborn   Ⓟ Pediatric (0-17 years)   ♂ Male   ♀ Female

✖ Deleted   Unspecified   + Additional code

544   © 2017 DecisionHealth   2017 ICD-10-CM Expert for Physicians

F11.221   Opioid dependence with intoxication delirium

F11.222   Opioid dependence with intoxication with perceptual disturbance

F11.229   Opioid dependence with intoxication, unspecified

F11.23   **Opioid dependence with withdrawal**

> **EXCLUDES 1**   *opioid dependence with intoxication (F11.22-)*

▲ F11.24   **Opioid dependence with opioid-induced mood disorder**

Opioid use disorder, moderate, with opioid induced depressive disorder

G F11.25   **Opioid dependence with opioid-induced psychotic disorder**

F11.250   Opioid dependence with opioid-induced psychotic disorder with delusions

F11.251   Opioid dependence with opioid-induced psychotic disorder with hallucinations

F11.259   Opioid dependence with opioid-induced psychotic disorder, unspecified

G F11.28   **Opioid dependence with other opioid-induced disorder**

F11.281   Opioid dependence with opioid-induced sexual dysfunction

F11.282   Opioid dependence with opioid-induced sleep disorder

F11.288   Opioid dependence with other opioid-induced disorder

F11.29   **Opioid dependence with unspecified opioid-induced disorder**

S F11.9   **Opioid use, unspecified**

> **EXCLUDES 1**   *opioid abuse (F11.1-)*
> *opioid dependence (F11.2-)*

F11.90   **Opioid use, unspecified, uncomplicated**

G F11.92   **Opioid use, unspecified with intoxication**

> **EXCLUDES 1**   *opioid use, unspecified with withdrawal (F11.93)*

F11.920   Opioid use, unspecified with intoxication, uncomplicated

▲ F11.921   Opioid use, unspecified with intoxication delirium

Opioid-induced delirium

F11.922   Opioid use, unspecified with intoxication with perceptual disturbance

F11.929   Opioid use, unspecified with intoxication, unspecified

F11.93   **Opioid use, unspecified with withdrawal**

> **EXCLUDES 1**   *opioid use, unspecified with intoxication (F11.92-)*

▲ F11.94   **Opioid use, unspecified with opioid-induced mood disorder**

Opioid induced depressive disorder, without use disorder

G F11.95   **Opioid use, unspecified with opioid-induced psychotic disorder**

F11.950   Opioid use, unspecified with opioid-induced psychotic disorder with delusions

F11.951   Opioid use, unspecified with opioid-induced psychotic disorder with hallucinations

F11.959   Opioid use, unspecified with opioid-induced psychotic disorder, unspecified

G F11.98   **Opioid use, unspecified with other specified opioid-induced disorder**

▲ F11.981   Opioid use, unspecified with opioid-induced sexual dysfunction

Opioid induced sexual dysfunction, without use disorder

▲ F11.982   Opioid use, unspecified with opioid-induced sleep disorder

Opioid induced sleep disorder, without use disorder

▲ F11.988   Opioid use, unspecified with other opioid-induced disorder

Opioid induced anxiety disorder, without use disorder

F11.99   **Opioid use, unspecified with unspecified opioid-induced disorder**

4 **F12**   **Cannabis related disorders**

> **INCLUDES**   marijuana

S F12.1   **Cannabis abuse**

> **EXCLUDES 1**   *cannabis dependence (F12.2-)*
> *cannabis use, unspecified (F12.9-)*

▲ F12.10   **Cannabis abuse, uncomplicated**

Cannabis use disorder, mild

G F12.12   **Cannabis abuse with intoxication**

F12.120   Cannabis abuse with intoxication, uncomplicated

F12.121   Cannabis abuse with intoxication delirium

F12.122   Cannabis abuse with intoxication with perceptual disturbance

F12.129   Cannabis abuse with intoxication, unspecified

G F12.15   **Cannabis abuse with psychotic disorder**

F12.150   Cannabis abuse with psychotic disorder with delusions

F12.151   Cannabis abuse with psychotic disorder with hallucinations

F12.159   Cannabis abuse with psychotic disorder, unspecified

G F12.18   **Cannabis abuse with other cannabis-induced disorder**

F12.180   Cannabis abuse with cannabis-induced anxiety disorder

▲ F12.188   Cannabis abuse with other cannabis-induced disorder

Cannabis use disorder, mild, with cannabis-induced sleep disorder

F12.19   **Cannabis abuse with unspecified cannabis-induced disorder**

S F12.2   **Cannabis dependence**

> **EXCLUDES 1**   *cannabis abuse (F12.1-)*
> *cannabis use, unspecified (F12.9-)*
> **EXCLUDES 2**   *cannabis poisoning (T40.7-)*

▲ F12.20   **Cannabis dependence, uncomplicated**

Cannabis use disorder, moderate
Cannabis use disorder, severe

F12.21   **Cannabis dependence, in remission**

G F12.22   **Cannabis dependence with intoxication**

F12.220   Cannabis dependence with intoxication, uncomplicated

F12.221   Cannabis dependence with intoxication delirium

F12.222   Cannabis dependence with intoxication with perceptual disturbance

F12.229   Cannabis dependence with intoxication, unspecified

G F12.25   **Cannabis dependence with psychotic disorder**

F12.250   Cannabis dependence with psychotic disorder with delusions

F12.251   Cannabis dependence with psychotic disorder with hallucinations

F12.259   Cannabis dependence with psychotic disorder, unspecified

G F12.28   **Cannabis dependence with other cannabis-induced disorder**

F12.280   Cannabis dependence with cannabis-induced anxiety disorder

▲ F12.288   Cannabis dependence with other cannabis-induced disorder

Cannabis use disorder, moderate, with cannabis-induced sleep disorder
Cannabis use disorder, severe, with cannabis-induced sleep disorder
Cannabis withdrawal

F12.29   **Cannabis dependence with unspecified cannabis-induced disorder**

S F12.9   **Cannabis use, unspecified**

> **EXCLUDES 1**   *cannabis abuse (F12.1-)*
> *cannabis dependence (F12.2-)*

F12.90   **Cannabis use, unspecified, uncomplicated**

G F12.92   **Cannabis use, unspecified with intoxication**

F12.920   Cannabis use, unspecified with intoxication, uncomplicated

F12.921   Cannabis use, unspecified with intoxication delirium

F12.922   Cannabis use, unspecified with intoxication with perceptual disturbance

F12.929   Cannabis use, unspecified with intoxication, unspecified

● New   ▲ Revised   *Manifestation*   4-7 Digit Indicators   ▤ Laterality   ▣ Adult (15+ years)   ▣ Maternity (12-55 years)   ▣ Newborn   ▣ Pediatric (0-17 years)   ♂ Male   ♀ Female
✖ Deleted   Unspecified   + Additional code

2017 ICD-10-CM Expert for Physicians   © 2017 DecisionHealth   545

⑤ F12.95   **Cannabis use, unspecified with psychotic disorder**

F12.950   **Cannabis use, unspecified with psychotic disorder with delusions**

F12.951   **Cannabis use, unspecified with psychotic disorder with hallucinations**

▲ **F12.959**   **Cannabis use, unspecified with psychotic disorder, unspecified**
Cannabis induced psychotic disorder, without use disorder

⑤ F12.98   **Cannabis use, unspecified with other cannabis-induced disorder**

▲ **F12.980**   **Cannabis use, unspecified with anxiety disorder**
Cannabis induced anxiety disorder, without use disorder

▲ **F12.988**   **Cannabis use, unspecified with other cannabis-induced disorder**
Cannabis induced sleep disorder, without use disorder

F12.99   **Cannabis use, unspecified with unspecified cannabis-induced disorder**

④ F13   **Sedative, hypnotic, or anxiolytic related disorders**

⑤ F13.1   **Sedative, hypnotic or anxiolytic-related abuse**

> **EXCLUDES 1**   *sedative, hypnotic or anxiolytic-related dependence (F13.2-)*
> *sedative, hypnotic, or anxiolytic use, unspecified (F13.9-)*

▲ **F13.10**   **Sedative, hypnotic or anxiolytic abuse, uncomplicated**
Sedative, hypnotic, or anxiolytic use disorder, mild

⑥ F13.12   **Sedative, hypnotic or anxiolytic abuse with intoxication**

F13.120   **Sedative, hypnotic or anxiolytic abuse with intoxication, uncomplicated**

F13.121   **Sedative, hypnotic or anxiolytic abuse with intoxication delirium**

F13.129   **Sedative, hypnotic or anxiolytic abuse with intoxication, unspecified**

▲ **F13.14**   **Sedative, hypnotic or anxiolytic abuse with sedative, hypnotic or anxiolytic-induced mood disorder**
Sedative, hypnotic, or anxiolytic use disorder, mild, with sedative, hypnotic, or anxiolytic induced bipolar or related disorder
Sedative, hypnotic, or anxiolytic use disorder, mild, with sedative, hypnotic, or anxiolytic induced depressive disorder

⑥ F13.15   **Sedative, hypnotic or anxiolytic abuse with sedative, hypnotic or anxiolytic-induced psychotic disorder**

F13.150   **Sedative, hypnotic or anxiolytic abuse with sedative, hypnotic or anxiolytic-induced psychotic disorder with delusions**

F13.151   **Sedative, hypnotic or anxiolytic abuse with sedative, hypnotic or anxiolytic-induced psychotic disorder with hallucinations**

F13.159   **Sedative, hypnotic or anxiolytic abuse with sedative, hypnotic or anxiolytic-induced psychotic disorder, unspecified**

⑥ F13.18   **Sedative, hypnotic or anxiolytic abuse with other sedative, hypnotic or anxiolytic-induced disorders**

F13.180   **Sedative, hypnotic or anxiolytic abuse with sedative, hypnotic or anxiolytic-induced anxiety disorder**

F13.181   **Sedative, hypnotic or anxiolytic abuse with sedative, hypnotic or anxiolytic-induced sexual dysfunction**

F13.182   **Sedative, hypnotic or anxiolytic abuse with sedative, hypnotic or anxiolytic-induced sleep disorder**

F13.188   **Sedative, hypnotic or anxiolytic abuse with other sedative, hypnotic or anxiolytic-induced disorder**

F13.19   **Sedative, hypnotic or anxiolytic abuse with unspecified sedative, hypnotic or anxiolytic-induced disorder**

⑤ F13.2   **Sedative, hypnotic or anxiolytic-related dependence**

> **EXCLUDES 1**   *sedative, hypnotic or anxiolytic-related abuse (F13.1-)*
> *sedative, hypnotic, or anxiolytic use, unspecified (F13.9-)*
>
> **EXCLUDES 2**   *sedative, hypnotic, or anxiolytic poisoning (T42.-)*

F13.20   **Sedative, hypnotic or anxiolytic dependence, uncomplicated**

F13.21   **Sedative, hypnotic or anxiolytic dependence, in remission**

⑥ F13.22   **Sedative, hypnotic or anxiolytic dependence with intoxication**

> **EXCLUDES 1**   *sedative, hypnotic or anxiolytic dependence with withdrawal (F13.23-)*

F13.220   **Sedative, hypnotic or anxiolytic dependence with intoxication, uncomplicated**

F13.221   **Sedative, hypnotic or anxiolytic dependence with intoxication delirium**

F13.229   **Sedative, hypnotic or anxiolytic dependence with intoxication, unspecified**

▲ **⑥ F13.23**   **Sedative, hypnotic or anxiolytic dependence with withdrawal**
Sedative, hypnotic, or anxiolytic use disorder, moderate
Sedative, hypnotic, or anxiolytic use disorder, severe

> **EXCLUDES 1**   *sedative, hypnotic or anxiolytic dependence with intoxication (F13.22-)*
>
> **DEFINITION**   Curtailed drug use, resulting in physical or psychological symptoms lasting hours to weeks, commonly featuring headache, anxiety, depression, chills, sweats, and tremors.

F13.230   **Sedative, hypnotic or anxiolytic dependence with withdrawal, uncomplicated**

F13.231   **Sedative, hypnotic or anxiolytic dependence with withdrawal delirium**

▲ **F13.232**   **Sedative, hypnotic or anxiolytic dependence with withdrawal with perceptual disturbance**
Sedative, hypnotic, or anxiolytic withdrawal with perceptual disturbances

▲ **F13.239**   **Sedative, hypnotic or anxiolytic dependence with withdrawal, unspecified**
Sedative, hypnotic, or anxiolytic withdrawal without perceptual disturbances

▲ **F13.24**   **Sedative, hypnotic or anxiolytic dependence with sedative, hypnotic or anxiolytic-induced mood disorder**
Sedative, hypnotic, or anxiolytic use disorder, moderate, with sedative, hypnotic, or anxiolytic induced bipolar or related disorder
Sedative, hypnotic, or anxiolytic use disorder, moderate, with sedative, hypnotic, or anxiolytic induced depressive disorder
Sedative, hypnotic, or anxiolytic use disorder, severe, with sedative, hypnotic, or anxiolytic-induced bipolar or related disorder
Sedative, hypnotic, or anxiolytic use disorder, severe, with sedative, hypnotic, or anxiolytic induced depressive disorder

⑥ F13.25   **Sedative, hypnotic or anxiolytic dependence with sedative, hypnotic or anxiolytic-induced psychotic disorder**

F13.250   **Sedative, hypnotic or anxiolytic dependence with sedative, hypnotic or anxiolytic-induced psychotic disorder with delusions**

F13.251   **Sedative, hypnotic or anxiolytic dependence with sedative, hypnotic or anxiolytic-induced psychotic disorder with hallucinations**

F13.259   **Sedative, hypnotic or anxiolytic dependence with sedative, hypnotic or anxiolytic-induced psychotic disorder, unspecified**

F13.26   **Sedative, hypnotic or anxiolytic dependence with sedative, hypnotic or anxiolytic-induced persisting amnestic disorder**

▲ **F13.27**   **Sedative, hypnotic or anxiolytic dependence with sedative, hypnotic or anxiolytic-induced persisting dementia**
Sedative, hypnotic, or anxiolytic use disorder, moderate, with sedative, hypnotic, or anxiolytic induced major neurocognitive disorder
Sedative, hypnotic, or anxiolytic use disorder, severe, with sedative, hypnotic, or anxiolytic-induced major neurocognitive disorder

⑥ F13.28   **Sedative, hypnotic or anxiolytic dependence with other sedative, hypnotic or anxiolytic-induced disorders**

● New   ▲ Revised   *Manifestation*   ④-⑦ Digit Indicators   ☐ Laterality   Ⓐ Adult (15+ years)   Ⓜ Maternity (12-55 years)   Ⓝ Newborn   Ⓟ Pediatric (0-17 years)   ♂ Male   ♀ Female
✖ Deleted   Unspecified   + Additional code

546   © 2017 DecisionHealth   2017 ICD-10-CM Expert for Physicians

F13.280 Sedative, hypnotic or anxiolytic dependence with sedative, hypnotic or anxiolytic-induced anxiety disorder

F13.281 Sedative, hypnotic or anxiolytic dependence with sedative, hypnotic or anxiolytic-induced sexual dysfunction

F13.282 Sedative, hypnotic or anxiolytic dependence with sedative, hypnotic or anxiolytic-induced sleep disorder

▲ F13.288 Sedative, hypnotic or anxiolytic dependence with other sedative, hypnotic or anxiolytic-induced disorder

Sedative, hypnotic, or anxiolytic use disorder, moderate, with sedative, hypnotic, or anxiolytic induced mild neurocognitive disorder
Sedative, hypnotic, or anxiolytic use disorder, severe, with sedative, hypnotic, or anxiolytic induced mild neurocognitive disorder

F13.29 Sedative, hypnotic or anxiolytic dependence with unspecified sedative, hypnotic or anxiolytic-induced disorder

F13.9 Sedative, hypnotic or anxiolytic-related use, unspecified
EXCLUDES 1 sedative, hypnotic or anxiolytic-related abuse (F13.1-)
sedative, hypnotic or anxiolytic-related dependence (F13.2-)

F13.90 Sedative, hypnotic, or anxiolytic use, unspecified, uncomplicated

F13.92 Sedative, hypnotic or anxiolytic use, unspecified with intoxication
EXCLUDES 1 sedative, hypnotic or anxiolytic use, unspecified with withdrawal (F13.93-)

F13.920 Sedative, hypnotic or anxiolytic use, unspecified with intoxication, uncomplicated

▲ F13.921 Sedative, hypnotic or anxiolytic use, unspecified with intoxication delirium

Sedative, hypnotic, or anxiolytic-induced delirium

F13.929 Sedative, hypnotic or anxiolytic use, unspecified with intoxication, unspecified

F13.93 Sedative, hypnotic or anxiolytic use, unspecified with withdrawal
EXCLUDES 1 sedative, hypnotic or anxiolytic use, unspecified with intoxication (F13.92-)

F13.930 Sedative, hypnotic or anxiolytic use, unspecified with withdrawal, uncomplicated

F13.931 Sedative, hypnotic or anxiolytic use, unspecified with withdrawal delirium

F13.932 Sedative, hypnotic or anxiolytic use, unspecified with withdrawal with perceptual disturbances

F13.939 Sedative, hypnotic or anxiolytic use, unspecified with withdrawal, unspecified

▲ F13.94 Sedative, hypnotic or anxiolytic use, unspecified with sedative, hypnotic or anxiolytic-induced mood disorder

Sedative, hypnotic, or anxiolytic-induced bipolar or related disorder, without use disorder
Sedative, hypnotic, or anxiolytic-induced depressive disorder, without use disorder

F13.95 Sedative, hypnotic or anxiolytic use, unspecified with sedative, hypnotic or anxiolytic-induced psychotic disorder

F13.950 Sedative, hypnotic or anxiolytic use, unspecified with sedative, hypnotic or anxiolytic-induced psychotic disorder with delusions

F13.951 Sedative, hypnotic or anxiolytic use, unspecified with sedative, hypnotic or anxiolytic-induced psychotic disorder with hallucinations

▲ F13.959 Sedative, hypnotic or anxiolytic use, unspecified with sedative, hypnotic or anxiolytic-induced psychotic disorder, unspecified

Sedative, hypnotic, or anxiolytic induced psychotic disorder, without use disorder

F13.96 Sedative, hypnotic or anxiolytic use, unspecified with sedative, hypnotic or anxiolytic-induced persisting amnestic disorder

▲ F13.97 Sedative, hypnotic or anxiolytic use, unspecified with sedative, hypnotic or anxiolytic-induced persisting dementia

Sedative, hypnotic, or anxiolytic induced major neurocognitive disorder, without use disorder

F13.98 Sedative, hypnotic or anxiolytic use, unspecified with other sedative, hypnotic or anxiolytic-induced disorders

▲ F13.980 Sedative, hypnotic or anxiolytic use, unspecified with sedative, hypnotic or anxiolytic-induced anxiety disorder

Sedative, hypnotic, or anxiolytic induced anxiety disorder, without use disorder

▲ F13.981 Sedative, hypnotic or anxiolytic use, unspecified with sedative, hypnotic or anxiolytic-induced sexual dysfunction

Sedative, hypnotic, or anxiolytic induced sexual dysfunction disorder, without use disorder

▲ F13.982 Sedative, hypnotic or anxiolytic use, unspecified with sedative, hypnotic or anxiolytic-induced sleep disorder

Sedative, hypnotic, or anxiolytic induced sleep disorder, without use disorder

▲ F13.988 Sedative, hypnotic or anxiolytic use, unspecified with other sedative, hypnotic or anxiolytic-induced disorder

Sedative, hypnotic, or anxiolytic induced mild neurocognitive disorder

F13.99 Sedative, hypnotic or anxiolytic use, unspecified with unspecified sedative, hypnotic or anxiolytic-induced disorder

F14 Cocaine related disorders
EXCLUDES 2 other stimulant-related disorders (F15.-)

F14.1 Cocaine abuse
EXCLUDES 1 cocaine dependence (F14.2-)
cocaine use, unspecified (F14.9-)

▲ F14.10 Cocaine abuse, uncomplicated
Cocaine use disorder, mild

F14.12 Cocaine abuse with intoxication

F14.120 Cocaine abuse with intoxication, uncomplicated
F14.121 Cocaine abuse with intoxication with delirium
F14.122 Cocaine abuse with intoxication with perceptual disturbance
F14.129 Cocaine abuse with intoxication, unspecified

▲ F14.14 Cocaine abuse with cocaine-induced mood disorder
Cocaine use disorder, mild, with cocaine-induced bipolar or related disorder
Cocaine use disorder, mild, with cocaine-induced depressive disorder

F14.15 Cocaine abuse with cocaine-induced psychotic disorder

F14.150 Cocaine abuse with cocaine-induced psychotic disorder with delusions
F14.151 Cocaine abuse with cocaine-induced psychotic disorder with hallucinations
F14.159 Cocaine abuse with cocaine-induced psychotic disorder, unspecified

F14.18 Cocaine abuse with other cocaine-induced disorder

F14.180 Cocaine abuse with cocaine-induced anxiety disorder
F14.181 Cocaine abuse with cocaine-induced sexual dysfunction
F14.182 Cocaine abuse with cocaine-induced sleep disorder
▲ F14.188 Cocaine abuse with other cocaine-induced disorder
Cocaine use disorder, mild, with cocaine-induced obsessive compulsive or related disorder

F14.19 Cocaine abuse with unspecified cocaine-induced disorder

F14.2 Cocaine dependence
EXCLUDES 1 cocaine abuse (F14.1-)
cocaine use, unspecified (F14.9-)
EXCLUDES 2 cocaine poisoning (T40.5-)

▲ F14.20 Cocaine dependence, uncomplicated
Cocaine use disorder, moderate
Cocaine use disorder, severe

F14.21 Cocaine dependence, in remission

⑥ **F14.22 Cocaine dependence with intoxication**
> **EXCLUDES 1** *cocaine dependence with withdrawal (F14.23)*

F14.220 Cocaine dependence with intoxication, uncomplicated

F14.221 Cocaine dependence with intoxication delirium

F14.222 Cocaine dependence with intoxication with perceptual disturbance

F14.229 Cocaine dependence with intoxication, unspecified

F14.23 Cocaine dependence with withdrawal
> **EXCLUDES 1** *cocaine dependence with intoxication (F14.22-)*

▲ **F14.24 Cocaine dependence with cocaine-induced mood disorder**
Cocaine use disorder, moderate, with cocaine-induced bipolar or related disorder
Cocaine use disorder, moderate, with cocaine-induced depressive disorder
Cocaine use disorder, severe, with cocaine-induced bipolar or related disorder
Cocaine use disorder, severe, with cocaine-induced depressive disorder

⑥ **F14.25 Cocaine dependence with cocaine-induced psychotic disorder**

F14.250 Cocaine dependence with cocaine-induced psychotic disorder with delusions

F14.251 Cocaine dependence with cocaine-induced psychotic disorder with hallucinations

F14.259 Cocaine dependence with cocaine-induced psychotic disorder, unspecified

⑥ **F14.28 Cocaine dependence with other cocaine-induced disorder**

F14.280 Cocaine dependence with cocaine-induced anxiety disorder

F14.281 Cocaine dependence with cocaine-induced sexual dysfunction

F14.282 Cocaine dependence with cocaine-induced sleep disorder

▲ **F14.288 Cocaine dependence with other cocaine-induced disorder**
Cocaine use disorder, moderate, with cocaine-induced obsessive compulsive or related disorder
Cocaine use disorder, severe, with cocaine-induced obsessive compulsive or related disorder

F14.29 Cocaine dependence with unspecified cocaine-induced disorder

⑤ **F14.9 Cocaine use, unspecified**
> **EXCLUDES 1** *cocaine abuse (F14.1-)*
> *cocaine dependence (F14.2-)*

F14.90 Cocaine use, unspecified, uncomplicated

⑥ **F14.92 Cocaine use, unspecified with intoxication**

F14.920 Cocaine use, unspecified with intoxication, uncomplicated

F14.921 Cocaine use, unspecified with intoxication delirium

F14.922 Cocaine use, unspecified with intoxication with perceptual disturbance

F14.929 Cocaine use, unspecified with intoxication, unspecified

▲ **F14.94 Cocaine use, unspecified with cocaine-induced mood disorder**
Cocaine induced bipolar or related disorder, without use disorder
Cocaine induced depressive disorder, without use disorder

⑥ **F14.95 Cocaine use, unspecified with cocaine-induced psychotic disorder**

F14.950 Cocaine use, unspecified with cocaine-induced psychotic disorder with delusions

F14.951 Cocaine use, unspecified with cocaine-induced psychotic disorder with hallucinations

▲ **F14.959 Cocaine use, unspecified with cocaine-induced psychotic disorder, unspecified**
Cocaine induced psychotic disorder, without use disorder

⑥ **F14.98 Cocaine use, unspecified with other specified cocaine-induced disorder**

▲ **F14.980 Cocaine use, unspecified with cocaine-induced anxiety disorder**
Cocaine induced anxiety disorder, without use disorder

▲ **F14.981 Cocaine use, unspecified with cocaine-induced sexual dysfunction**
Cocaine induced sexual dysfunction, without use disorder

▲ **F14.982 Cocaine use, unspecified with cocaine-induced sleep disorder**
Cocaine induced sleep disorder, without use disorder

▲ **F14.988 Cocaine use, unspecified with other cocaine-induced disorder**
Cocaine induced obsessive compulsive or related disorder

F14.99 Cocaine use, unspecified with unspecified cocaine-induced disorder

④ **F15 Other stimulant related disorders**
> **INCLUDES** amphetamine-related disorders
> caffeine
> **EXCLUDES 2** *cocaine-related disorders (F14.-)*
> **CODING TIP ✓** Use this category of codes for methamphetamines and "bath salts" abuse and dependence.

⑤ **F15.1 Other stimulant abuse**
> **EXCLUDES 1** *other stimulant dependence (F15.2-)*
> *other stimulant use, unspecified (F15.9-)*

▲ **F15.10 Other stimulant abuse, uncomplicated**
Amphetamine type substance use disorder, mild
Other or unspecified stimulant use disorder, mild

⑥ **F15.12 Other stimulant abuse with intoxication**

F15.120 Other stimulant abuse with intoxication, uncomplicated

F15.121 Other stimulant abuse with intoxication delirium

▲ **F15.122 Other stimulant abuse with intoxication with perceptual disturbance**
Amphetamine or other stimulant use disorder, mild, with amphetamine or other stimulant intoxication, with perceptual disturbances

▲ **F15.129 Other stimulant abuse with intoxication, unspecified**
Amphetamine or other stimulant use disorder, mild, with amphetamine or other stimulant intoxication, without perceptual disturbances

▲ **F15.14 Other stimulant abuse with stimulant-induced mood disorder**
Amphetamine or other stimulant use disorder, mild, with amphetamine or other stimulant induced bipolar or related disorder
Amphetamine or other stimulant use disorder, mild, with amphetamine or other stimulant induced depressive disorder

⑥ **F15.15 Other stimulant abuse with stimulant-induced psychotic disorder**

F15.150 Other stimulant abuse with stimulant-induced psychotic disorder with delusions

F15.151 Other stimulant abuse with stimulant-induced psychotic disorder with hallucinations

F15.159 Other stimulant abuse with stimulant-induced psychotic disorder, unspecified

⑥ **F15.18 Other stimulant abuse with other stimulant-induced disorder**

F15.180 Other stimulant abuse with stimulant-induced anxiety disorder

F15.181 Other stimulant abuse with stimulant-induced sexual dysfunction

F15.182 Other stimulant abuse with stimulant-induced sleep disorder

▲ **F15.188 Other stimulant abuse with other stimulant-induced disorder**
Amphetamine or other stimulant use disorder, mild, with amphetamine or other stimulant induced obsessive-compulsive or related disorder

F15.19 Other stimulant abuse with unspecified stimulant-induced disorder

⑤ **F15.2 Other stimulant dependence**
> **EXCLUDES 1** *other stimulant abuse (F15.1-)*
> *other stimulant use, unspecified (F15.9-)*

● New   ▲ Revised   *Manifestation*   ④-⑦ Digit Indicators   ⊟ Laterality   🅐 Adult (15+ years)   Ⓜ Maternity (12-55 years)   Ⓝ Newborn   🅟 Pediatric (0-17 years)   ♂ Male   ♀ Female
✖ Deleted   Unspecified   + Additional code

▲ **F15.20** **Other stimulant dependence, uncomplicated**
Amphetamine type substance use disorder, moderate
Amphetamine type substance use disorder, severe
Other or unspecified stimulant use disorder, moderate
Other or unspecified stimulant use disorder, severe

F15.21 **Other stimulant dependence, in remission**

⑤ **F15.22** **Other stimulant dependence with intoxication**
EXCLUDES 1 *other stimulant dependence with withdrawal (F15.23)*

F15.220 **Other stimulant dependence with intoxication, uncomplicated**

F15.221 **Other stimulant dependence with intoxication delirium**

▲ **F15.222** **Other stimulant dependence with intoxication with perceptual disturbance**
Amphetamine or other stimulant use disorder, moderate, with amphetamine or other stimulant intoxication, with perceptual disturbances
Amphetamine or other stimulant use disorder, severe, with amphetamine or other stimulant intoxication, with perceptual disturbances

▲ **F15.229** **Other stimulant dependence with intoxication, unspecified**
Amphetamine or other stimulant use disorder, moderate, with amphetamine or other stimulant intoxication, without perceptual disturbances
Amphetamine or other stimulant use disorder, severe, with amphetamine or other stimulant intoxication, without perceptual disturbances

▲ **F15.23** **Other stimulant dependence with withdrawal**
Amphetamine or other stimulant withdrawal
EXCLUDES 1 *other stimulant dependence with intoxication (F15.22-)*

▲ **F15.24** **Other stimulant dependence with stimulant-induced mood disorder**
Amphetamine or other stimulant use disorder, moderate, with amphetamine or other stimulant-induced bipolar or related disorder
Amphetamine or other stimulant use disorder, moderate, with amphetamine or other stimulant induced depressive disorder
Amphetamine or other stimulant use disorder, severe, with amphetamine or other stimulant-induced bipolar or related disorder
Amphetamine or other stimulant use disorder, severe, with amphetamine or other stimulant-induced depressive disorder

⑤ **F15.25** **Other stimulant dependence with stimulant-induced psychotic disorder**

F15.250 **Other stimulant dependence with stimulant-induced psychotic disorder with delusions**

F15.251 **Other stimulant dependence with stimulant-induced psychotic disorder with hallucinations**

F15.259 **Other stimulant dependence with stimulant-induced psychotic disorder, unspecified**

⑤ **F15.28** **Other stimulant dependence with other stimulant-induced disorder**

F15.280 **Other stimulant dependence with stimulant-induced anxiety disorder**

F15.281 **Other stimulant dependence with stimulant-induced sexual dysfunction**

F15.282 **Other stimulant dependence with stimulant-induced sleep disorder**

▲ **F15.288** **Other stimulant dependence with other stimulant-induced disorder**
Amphetamine or other stimulant use disorder, moderate, with amphetamine or other stimulant induced obsessive compulsive or related disorder
Amphetamine or other stimulant use disorder, severe, with amphetamine or other stimulant induced obsessive compulsive or related disorder

F15.29 **Other stimulant dependence with unspecified stimulant-induced disorder**

⑤ **F15.9** **Other stimulant use, unspecified**
EXCLUDES 1 *other stimulant abuse (F15.1-)*
other stimulant dependence (F15.2-)

F15.90 **Other stimulant use, unspecified, uncomplicated**

⑤ **F15.92** **Other stimulant use, unspecified with intoxication**
EXCLUDES 1 *other stimulant use, unspecified with withdrawal (F15.93)*

F15.920 **Other stimulant use, unspecified with intoxication, uncomplicated**

▲ **F15.921** **Other stimulant use, unspecified with intoxication delirium**
Amphetamine or other stimulant-induced delirium

F15.922 **Other stimulant use, unspecified with intoxication with perceptual disturbance**

▲ **F15.929** **Other stimulant use, unspecified with intoxication, unspecified**
Caffeine intoxication

▲ **F15.93** **Other stimulant use, unspecified with withdrawal**
Caffeine withdrawal
EXCLUDES 1 *other stimulant use, unspecified with intoxication (F15.92-)*

▲ **F15.94** **Other stimulant use, unspecified with stimulant-induced mood disorder**
Amphetamine or other stimulant-induced bipolar or related disorder, without use disorder
Amphetamine or other stimulant-induced depressive disorder, without use disorder

⑤ **F15.95** **Other stimulant use, unspecified with stimulant-induced psychotic disorder**

F15.950 **Other stimulant use, unspecified with stimulant-induced psychotic disorder with delusions**

F15.951 **Other stimulant use, unspecified with stimulant-induced psychotic disorder with hallucinations**

▲ **F15.959** **Other stimulant use, unspecified with stimulant-induced psychotic disorder, unspecified**
Amphetamine or other stimulant-induced induced psychotic disorder, without use disorder

⑤ **F15.98** **Other stimulant use, unspecified with other stimulant-induced disorder**

▲ **F15.980** **Other stimulant use, unspecified with stimulant-induced anxiety disorder**
Amphetamine or other stimulant-induced anxiety disorder, without use disorder
Caffeine induced anxiety disorder, without use disorder

▲ **F15.981** **Other stimulant use, unspecified with stimulant-induced sexual dysfunction**
Amphetamine or other stimulant-induced sexual dysfunction, without use disorder

▲ **F15.982** **Other stimulant use, unspecified with stimulant-induced sleep disorder**
Amphetamine or other stimulant-induced sleep disorder, without use disorder
Caffeine induced sleep disorder, without use disorder

▲ **F15.988** **Other stimulant use, unspecified with other stimulant-induced disorder**
Amphetamine or other stimulant-induced obsessive compulsive or related disorder, without use disorder

F15.99 **Other stimulant use, unspecified with unspecified stimulant-induced disorder**

④ **F16** **Hallucinogen related disorders**
INCLUDES ecstasy
PCP
phencyclidine

⑤ **F16.1** **Hallucinogen abuse**
EXCLUDES 1 *hallucinogen dependence (F16.2-)*
hallucinogen use, unspecified (F16.9-)

▲ **F16.10** **Hallucinogen abuse, uncomplicated**
Other hallucinogen use disorder, mild
Phencyclidine use disorder, mild

⑤ **F16.12** **Hallucinogen abuse with intoxication**

F16.120 **Hallucinogen abuse with intoxication, uncomplicated**

F16.121 **Hallucinogen abuse with intoxication with delirium**

F16.122 **Hallucinogen abuse with intoxication with perceptual disturbance**

F16.129 **Hallucinogen abuse with intoxication, unspecified**

● New ▲ Revised *Manifestation* ④-⑦ Digit Indicators ⊟ Laterality Ⓐ Adult (15+ years) Ⓜ Maternity (12-55 years) Ⓝ Newborn Ⓟ Pediatric (0-17 years) ♂ Male ♀ Female
✖ Deleted Unspecified + Additional code

Mental, Behavioral and Neurodevelopmental Disorders

▲ **F16.14**   **Hallucinogen abuse with hallucinogen-induced mood disorder**
Other hallucinogen use disorder, mild, with other hallucinogen induced bipolar or related disorder
Other hallucinogen use disorder, mild, with other hallucinogen induced depressive disorder
Phencyclidine use disorder, mild, with phencyclidine induced bipolar or related disorder
Phencyclidine use disorder, mild, with phencyclidine induced depressive disorder

⑥ **F16.15**   **Hallucinogen abuse with hallucinogen-induced psychotic disorder**

   F16.150   Hallucinogen abuse with hallucinogen-induced psychotic disorder with delusions

   F16.151   Hallucinogen abuse with hallucinogen-induced psychotic disorder with hallucinations

   F16.159   Hallucinogen abuse with hallucinogen-induced psychotic disorder, unspecified

⑥ **F16.18**   **Hallucinogen abuse with other hallucinogen-induced disorder**

   F16.180   Hallucinogen abuse with hallucinogen-induced anxiety disorder

   F16.183   Hallucinogen abuse with hallucinogen persisting perception disorder (flashbacks)

   F16.188   Hallucinogen abuse with other hallucinogen-induced disorder

   F16.19   **Hallucinogen abuse with unspecified hallucinogen-induced disorder**

⑤ **F16.2**   **Hallucinogen dependence**
EXCLUDES 1   *hallucinogen abuse (F16.1-)*
hallucinogen use, unspecified (F16.9-)

▲ **F16.20**   **Hallucinogen dependence, uncomplicated**
Other hallucinogen use disorder, moderate
Other hallucinogen use disorder, severe
Phencyclidine use disorder, moderate
Phencyclidine use disorder, severe

   F16.21   **Hallucinogen dependence, in remission**

⑥ **F16.22**   **Hallucinogen dependence with intoxication**

   F16.220   Hallucinogen dependence with intoxication, uncomplicated

   F16.221   Hallucinogen dependence with intoxication with delirium

   F16.229   Hallucinogen dependence with intoxication, unspecified

▲ **F16.24**   **Hallucinogen dependence with hallucinogen-induced mood disorder**
Other hallucinogen use disorder, moderate, with other hallucinogen induced bipolar or related disorder
Other hallucinogen use disorder, moderate, with other hallucinogen induced depressive disorder
Other hallucinogen use disorder, severe, with other hallucinogen-induced bipolar or related disorder
Other hallucinogen use disorder, severe, with other hallucinogen-induced depressive disorder
Phencyclidine use disorder, moderate, with phencyclidine induced bipolar or related disorder
Phencyclidine use disorder, moderate, with phencyclidine induced depressive disorder
Phencyclidine use disorder, severe, with phencyclidine induced bipolar or related disorder
Phencyclidine use disorder, severe, with phencyclidine-induced depressive disorder

⑥ **F16.25**   **Hallucinogen dependence with hallucinogen-induced psychotic disorder**

   F16.250   Hallucinogen dependence with hallucinogen-induced psychotic disorder with delusions

   F16.251   Hallucinogen dependence with hallucinogen-induced psychotic disorder with hallucinations

   F16.259   Hallucinogen dependence with hallucinogen-induced psychotic disorder, unspecified

⑥ **F16.28**   **Hallucinogen dependence with other hallucinogen-induced disorder**

   F16.280   Hallucinogen dependence with hallucinogen-induced anxiety disorder

   F16.283   Hallucinogen dependence with hallucinogen persisting perception disorder (flashbacks)

   F16.288   Hallucinogen dependence with other hallucinogen-induced disorder

   F16.29   **Hallucinogen dependence with unspecified hallucinogen-induced disorder**

⑤ **F16.9**   **Hallucinogen use, unspecified**
EXCLUDES 1   *hallucinogen abuse (F16.1-)*
hallucinogen dependence (F16.2-)

   F16.90   **Hallucinogen use, unspecified, uncomplicated**

⑥ **F16.92**   **Hallucinogen use, unspecified with intoxication**

   F16.920   Hallucinogen use, unspecified with intoxication, uncomplicated

▲ **F16.921**   Hallucinogen use, unspecified with intoxication with delirium
Other hallucinogen intoxication delirium

   F16.929   Hallucinogen use, unspecified with intoxication, unspecified

▲ **F16.94**   **Hallucinogen use, unspecified with hallucinogen-induced mood disorder**
Other hallucinogen induced bipolar or related disorder, without use disorder
Other hallucinogen induced depressive disorder, without use disorder
Phencyclidine induced bipolar or related disorder, without use disorder
Phencyclidine induced depressive disorder, without use disorder

⑥ **F16.95**   **Hallucinogen use, unspecified with hallucinogen-induced psychotic disorder**

   F16.950   Hallucinogen use, unspecified with hallucinogen-induced psychotic disorder with delusions

   F16.951   Hallucinogen use, unspecified with hallucinogen-induced psychotic disorder with hallucinations

▲ **F16.959**   Hallucinogen use, unspecified with hallucinogen-induced psychotic disorder, unspecified
Other hallucinogen induced psychotic disorder, without use disorder
Phencyclidine induced psychotic disorder, without use disorder

⑥ **F16.98**   **Hallucinogen use, unspecified with other specified hallucinogen-induced disorder**

▲ **F16.980**   Hallucinogen use, unspecified with hallucinogen-induced anxiety disorder
Other hallucinogen-induced anxiety disorder, without use disorder
Phencyclidine induced anxiety disorder, without use disorder

   F16.983   Hallucinogen use, unspecified with hallucinogen persisting perception disorder (flashbacks)

   F16.988   Hallucinogen use, unspecified with other hallucinogen-induced disorder

   F16.99   **Hallucinogen use, unspecified with unspecified hallucinogen-induced disorder**

④ **F17**   **Nicotine dependence**
EXCLUDES 1   *history of tobacco dependence (Z87.891)*
tobacco use NOS (Z72.0)
EXCLUDES 2   *tobacco use (smoking) during pregnancy, childbirth and the puerperium (O99.33-)*
toxic effect of nicotine (T65.2-)

⑤ **F17.2**   **Nicotine dependence**
CODING TIP ✓   Use the appropriate code to specify nicotine product when known. ICD-10 codes provide for greater specificity, allowing the coder to specify dependence on a specific nicotine product.

⑥ **F17.20**   **Nicotine dependence, unspecified**

▲ **F17.200**   Nicotine dependence, unspecified, uncomplicated
Tobacco use disorder, mild
Tobacco use disorder, moderate
Tobacco use disorder, severe
CODING TIP ✓   Use code F17.200 if the physician documents "smoker" or tobacco/nicotine dependence.
AHA: 1Q 2016, 36-37
AHA: 4Q 2013, 108

   F17.201   Nicotine dependence, unspecified, in remission

▲ **F17.203**   Nicotine dependence unspecified, with withdrawal
Tobacco withdrawal

● New   ▲ Revised   *Manifestation*   ④-⑦ Digit Indicators   ▤ Laterality   ▣ Adult (15+ years)   Ⓜ Maternity (12-55 years)   Ⓝ Newborn   ▣ Pediatric (0-17 years)   ♂ Male   ♀ Female
✖ Deleted   Unspecified   + Additional code

550   © 2017 DecisionHealth   2017 ICD-10-CM Expert for Physicians

F17.208   Nicotine dependence, unspecified, with other nicotine-induced disorders

F17.209   Nicotine dependence, unspecified, with unspecified nicotine-induced disorders

🅖 F17.21   Nicotine dependence, cigarettes

F17.210   Nicotine dependence, cigarettes, uncomplicated

CODING TIP ✓   Do not use code F17.210 to report tobacco use. The provider/physician must specify tobacco dependence.
AHA: 4Q 2013, 109

F17.211   Nicotine dependence, cigarettes, in remission

CODING TIP ✓   Do not use code F17.211 to report a history of tobacco use in a patient who has discontinued the use of cigarettes/quit smoking. History of smoking should be coded to Z87.891.

F17.213   Nicotine dependence, cigarettes, with withdrawal

F17.218   Nicotine dependence, cigarettes, with other nicotine-induced disorders
AHA: 4Q 2013, 109

F17.219   Nicotine dependence, cigarettes, with unspecified nicotine-induced disorders

🅖 F17.22   Nicotine dependence, chewing tobacco

F17.220   Nicotine dependence, chewing tobacco, uncomplicated

F17.221   Nicotine dependence, chewing tobacco, in remission

F17.223   Nicotine dependence, chewing tobacco, with withdrawal

F17.228   Nicotine dependence, chewing tobacco, with other nicotine-induced disorders

F17.229   Nicotine dependence, chewing tobacco, with unspecified nicotine-induced disorders

🅖 F17.29   Nicotine dependence, other tobacco product

F17.290   Nicotine dependence, other tobacco product, uncomplicated

F17.291   Nicotine dependence, other tobacco product, in remission

F17.293   Nicotine dependence, other tobacco product, with withdrawal

F17.298   Nicotine dependence, other tobacco product, with other nicotine-induced disorders

F17.299   Nicotine dependence, other tobacco product, with unspecified nicotine-induced disorders

🄸 **F18   Inhalant related disorders**

INCLUDES   volatile solvents

🅂 F18.1   Inhalant abuse

EXCLUDES 1   *inhalant dependence (F18.2-)*
inhalant use, unspecified (F18.9-)

▲ F18.10   Inhalant abuse, uncomplicated
Inhalant use disorder, mild

🅖 F18.12   Inhalant abuse with intoxication

F18.120   Inhalant abuse with intoxication, uncomplicated

F18.121   Inhalant abuse with intoxication delirium

F18.129   Inhalant abuse with intoxication, unspecified

▲ F18.14   Inhalant abuse with inhalant-induced mood disorder
Inhalant use disorder, mild, with inhalant induced depressive disorder

🅖 F18.15   Inhalant abuse with inhalant-induced psychotic disorder

F18.150   Inhalant abuse with inhalant-induced psychotic disorder with delusions

F18.151   Inhalant abuse with inhalant-induced psychotic disorder with hallucinations

F18.159   Inhalant abuse with inhalant-induced psychotic disorder, unspecified

▲ F18.17   Inhalant abuse with inhalant-induced dementia
Inhalant use disorder, mild, with inhalant induced major neurocognitive disorder

🅖 F18.18   Inhalant abuse with other inhalant-induced disorders

F18.180   Inhalant abuse with inhalant-induced anxiety disorder

▲ F18.188   Inhalant abuse with other inhalant-induced disorder
Inhalant use disorder, mild, with inhalant induced mild neurocognitive disorder

F18.19   Inhalant abuse with unspecified inhalant-induced disorder

🅂 F18.2   Inhalant dependence

EXCLUDES 1   *inhalant abuse (F18.1-)*
inhalant use, unspecified (F18.9-)

▲ F18.20   Inhalant dependence, uncomplicated
Inhalant use disorder, moderate
Inhalant use disorder, severe

F18.21   Inhalant dependence, in remission

🅖 F18.22   Inhalant dependence with intoxication

F18.220   Inhalant dependence with intoxication, uncomplicated

F18.221   Inhalant dependence with intoxication delirium

F18.229   Inhalant dependence with intoxication, unspecified

▲ F18.24   Inhalant dependence with inhalant-induced mood disorder
Inhalant use disorder, moderate, with inhalant induced depressive disorder
Inhalant use disorder, severe, with inhalant induced depressive disorder

🅖 F18.25   Inhalant dependence with inhalant-induced psychotic disorder

F18.250   Inhalant dependence with inhalant-induced psychotic disorder with delusions

F18.251   Inhalant dependence with inhalant-induced psychotic disorder with hallucinations

F18.259   Inhalant dependence with inhalant-induced psychotic disorder, unspecified

▲ F18.27   Inhalant dependence with inhalant-induced dementia
Inhalant use disorder, moderate, with inhalant induced major neurocognitive disorder
Inhalant use disorder, severe, with inhalant induced major neurocognitive disorder

🅖 F18.28   Inhalant dependence with other inhalant-induced disorders

F18.280   Inhalant dependence with inhalant-induced anxiety disorder

▲ F18.288   Inhalant dependence with other inhalant-induced disorder
Inhalant use disorder, moderate, with inhalant-induced mild neurocognitive disorder
Inhalant use disorder, severe, with inhalant-induced mild neurocognitive disorder

F18.29   Inhalant dependence with unspecified inhalant-induced disorder

🅂 F18.9   Inhalant use, unspecified

EXCLUDES 1   *inhalant abuse (F18.1-)*
inhalant dependence (F18.2-)

F18.90   Inhalant use, unspecified, uncomplicated

🅖 F18.92   Inhalant use, unspecified with intoxication

F18.920   Inhalant use, unspecified with intoxication, uncomplicated

F18.921   Inhalant use, unspecified with intoxication with delirium

F18.929   Inhalant use, unspecified with intoxication, unspecified

▲ F18.94   Inhalant use, unspecified with inhalant-induced mood disorder
Inhalant induced depressive disorder

🅖 F18.95   Inhalant use, unspecified with inhalant-induced psychotic disorder

F18.950   Inhalant use, unspecified with inhalant-induced psychotic disorder with delusions

F18.951   Inhalant use, unspecified with inhalant-induced psychotic disorder with hallucinations

F18.959   Inhalant use, unspecified with inhalant-induced psychotic disorder, unspecified

▲ F18.97   Inhalant use, unspecified with inhalant-induced persisting dementia
Inhalant-induced major neurocognitive disorder

🅖 F18.98   Inhalant use, unspecified with other inhalant-induced disorders

F18.980   Inhalant use, unspecified with inhalant-induced anxiety disorder

---

● New   ▲ Revised   *Manifestation*   🄸-🄼 Digit Indicators   ⬄ Laterality   🄰 Adult (15+ years)   🄼 Maternity (12-55 years)   🄽 Newborn   🄿 Pediatric (0-17 years)   ♂ Male   ♀ Female
✖ Deleted   Unspecified   + Additional code

Mental, Behavioral and Neurodevelopmental Disorders

▲ **F18.988**   **Inhalant use, unspecified with other inhalant-induced disorder**
Inhalant-induced mild neurocognitive disorder

F18.99   **Inhalant use, unspecified with unspecified inhalant-induced disorder**

▣ **F19**   **Other psychoactive substance related disorders**
INCLUDES   polysubstance drug use (indiscriminate drug use)

⑤ **F19.1**   **Other psychoactive substance abuse**
EXCLUDES 1   *other psychoactive substance dependence (F19.2-)*
other psychoactive substance use, unspecified (F19.9-)

▲ **F19.10**   **Other psychoactive substance abuse, uncomplicated**
Other (or unknown) substance use disorder, mild

⑥ **F19.12**   **Other psychoactive substance abuse with intoxication**

F19.120   **Other psychoactive substance abuse with intoxication, uncomplicated**

F19.121   **Other psychoactive substance abuse with intoxication delirium**

F19.122   **Other psychoactive substance abuse with intoxication with perceptual disturbances**

F19.129   **Other psychoactive substance abuse with intoxication, unspecified**

▲ **F19.14**   **Other psychoactive substance abuse with psychoactive substance-induced mood disorder**
Other (or unknown) substance use disorder, mild, with other (or unknown) substance-induced bipolar or related disorder
Other (or unknown) substance use disorder, mild, with other (or unknown) substance-induced depressive disorder

⑥ **F19.15**   **Other psychoactive substance abuse with psychoactive substance-induced psychotic disorder**

F19.150   **Other psychoactive substance abuse with psychoactive substance-induced psychotic disorder with delusions**

F19.151   **Other psychoactive substance abuse with psychoactive substance-induced psychotic disorder with hallucinations**

F19.159   **Other psychoactive substance abuse with psychoactive substance-induced psychotic disorder, unspecified**

F19.16   **Other psychoactive substance abuse with psychoactive substance-induced persisting amnestic disorder**

▲ **F19.17**   **Other psychoactive substance abuse with psychoactive substance-induced persisting dementia**
Other (or unknown) substance use disorder, mild, with other (or unknown) substance-induced major neurocognitive disorder

⑥ **F19.18**   **Other psychoactive substance abuse with other psychoactive substance-induced disorders**

F19.180   **Other psychoactive substance abuse with psychoactive substance-induced anxiety disorder**

F19.181   **Other psychoactive substance abuse with psychoactive substance-induced sexual dysfunction**

F19.182   **Other psychoactive substance abuse with psychoactive substance-induced sleep disorder**

▲ **F19.188**   **Other psychoactive substance abuse with other psychoactive substance-induced disorder**
Other (or unknown) substance use disorder, mild, with other (or unknown) substance induced mild neurocognitive disorder
Other (or unknown) substance use disorder, mild, with other (or unknown) substance induced obsessive-compulsive or related disorder

F19.19   **Other psychoactive substance abuse with unspecified psychoactive substance-induced disorder**

⑤ **F19.2**   **Other psychoactive substance dependence**
EXCLUDES 1   *other psychoactive substance abuse (F19.1-)*
other psychoactive substance use, unspecified (F19.9-)

▲ **F19.20**   **Other psychoactive substance dependence, uncomplicated**
Other (or unknown) substance use disorder, moderate
Other (or unknown) substance use disorder, severe

F19.21   **Other psychoactive substance dependence, in remission**

⑥ **F19.22**   **Other psychoactive substance dependence with intoxication**
EXCLUDES 1   *other psychoactive substance dependence with withdrawal (F19.23-)*

F19.220   **Other psychoactive substance dependence with intoxication, uncomplicated**

F19.221   **Other psychoactive substance dependence with intoxication delirium**

F19.222   **Other psychoactive substance dependence with intoxication with perceptual disturbance**

F19.229   **Other psychoactive substance dependence with intoxication, unspecified**

⑥ **F19.23**   **Other psychoactive substance dependence with withdrawal**
EXCLUDES 1   *other psychoactive substance dependence with intoxication (F19.22-)*

F19.230   **Other psychoactive substance dependence with withdrawal, uncomplicated**

F19.231   **Other psychoactive substance dependence with withdrawal delirium**

F19.232   **Other psychoactive substance dependence with withdrawal with perceptual disturbance**

F19.239   **Other psychoactive substance dependence with withdrawal, unspecified**

▲ **F19.24**   **Other psychoactive substance dependence with psychoactive substance-induced mood disorder**
Other (or unknown) substance use disorder, moderate, with other (or unknown) substance induced bipolar or related disorder
Other (or unknown) substance use disorder, moderate, with other (or unknown) substance induced depressive disorder
Other (or unknown) substance use disorder, severe, with other (or unknown) substance induced bipolar or related disorder
Other (or unknown) substance use disorder, severe, with other (or unknown) substance induced depressive disorder

⑥ **F19.25**   **Other psychoactive substance dependence with psychoactive substance-induced psychotic disorder**

F19.250   **Other psychoactive substance dependence with psychoactive substance-induced psychotic disorder with delusions**

F19.251   **Other psychoactive substance dependence with psychoactive substance-induced psychotic disorder with hallucinations**

F19.259   **Other psychoactive substance dependence with psychoactive substance-induced psychotic disorder, unspecified**

F19.26   **Other psychoactive substance dependence with psychoactive substance-induced persisting amnestic disorder**

▲ **F19.27**   **Other psychoactive substance dependence with psychoactive substance-induced persisting dementia**
Other (or unknown) substance use disorder, moderate, with other (or unknown) substance induced major neurocognitive disorder
Other (or unknown) substance use disorder, severe, with other (or unknown) substance induced major neurocognitive disorder

⑥ **F19.28**   **Other psychoactive substance dependence with other psychoactive substance-induced disorders**

F19.280   **Other psychoactive substance dependence with psychoactive substance-induced anxiety disorder**

F19.281   **Other psychoactive substance dependence with psychoactive substance-induced sexual dysfunction**

F19.282   **Other psychoactive substance dependence with psychoactive substance-induced sleep disorder**

● New   ▲ Revised   *Manifestation*   ❹-❼ Digit Indicators   ▤ Laterality   ▨ Adult (15+ years)   ▥ Maternity (12-55 years)   ▧ Newborn   ▣ Pediatric (0-17 years)   ♂ Male   ♀ Female
✖ Deleted   Unspecified   + Additional code

552   © 2017 DecisionHealth   2017 ICD-10-CM Expert for Physicians

▲ **F19.288** **Other psychoactive substance dependence with other psychoactive substance-induced disorder**
Other (or unknown) substance use disorder, moderate, with other (or unknown) substance induced mild neurocognitive disorder
Other (or unknown) substance use disorder, severe, with other (or unknown) substance induced mild neurocognitive disorder
Other (or unknown) substance use disorder, moderate, with other (or unknown) substance induced obsessive compulsive or related disorder
Other (or unknown) substance use disorder, severe, with other (or unknown) substance induced obsessive-compulsive or related disorder

F19.29 **Other psychoactive substance dependence with unspecified psychoactive substance-induced disorder**

⑤ **F19.9** **Other psychoactive substance use, unspecified**
EXCLUDES 1 other psychoactive substance abuse (F19.1-)
other psychoactive substance dependence (F19.2-)

F19.90 **Other psychoactive substance use, unspecified, uncomplicated**

⑥ **F19.92** **Other psychoactive substance use, unspecified with intoxication**
EXCLUDES 1 other psychoactive substance use, unspecified with withdrawal (F19.93)

F19.920 **Other psychoactive substance use, unspecified with intoxication, uncomplicated**

▲ **F19.921** **Other psychoactive substance use, unspecified with intoxication with delirium**
Other (or unknown) substance-induced delirium

F19.922 **Other psychoactive substance use, unspecified with intoxication with perceptual disturbance**

F19.929 **Other psychoactive substance use, unspecified with intoxication, unspecified**

⑥ **F19.93** **Other psychoactive substance use, unspecified with withdrawal**
EXCLUDES 1 other psychoactive substance use, unspecified with intoxication (F19.92-)

F19.930 **Other psychoactive substance use, unspecified with withdrawal, uncomplicated**

F19.931 **Other psychoactive substance use, unspecified with withdrawal delirium**

F19.932 **Other psychoactive substance use, unspecified with withdrawal with perceptual disturbance**

F19.939 **Other psychoactive substance use, unspecified with withdrawal, unspecified**

▲ **F19.94** **Other psychoactive substance use, unspecified with psychoactive substance-induced mood disorder**
Other (or unknown) substance-induced bipolar or related disorder, without use disorder
Other (or unknown) substance-induced depressive disorder, without use disorder

⑥ **F19.95** **Other psychoactive substance use, unspecified with psychoactive substance-induced psychotic disorder**

F19.950 **Other psychoactive substance use, unspecified with psychoactive substance-induced psychotic disorder with delusions**

F19.951 **Other psychoactive substance use, unspecified with psychoactive substance-induced psychotic disorder with hallucinations**

▲ **F19.959** **Other psychoactive substance use, unspecified with psychoactive substance-induced psychotic disorder, unspecified**
Other or unknown substance-induced psychotic disorder, without use disorder

F19.96 **Other psychoactive substance use, unspecified with psychoactive substance-induced persisting amnestic disorder**

▲ **F19.97** **Other psychoactive substance use, unspecified with psychoactive substance-induced persisting dementia**
Other (or unknown) substance-induced major neurocognitive disorder, without use disorder

⑥ **F19.98** **Other psychoactive substance use, unspecified with other psychoactive substance-induced disorders**

▲ **F19.980** **Other psychoactive substance use, unspecified with psychoactive substance-induced anxiety disorder**
Other (or unknown) substance-induced anxiety disorder, without use disorder

▲ **F19.981** **Other psychoactive substance use, unspecified with psychoactive substance-induced sexual dysfunction**
Other (or unknown) substance-induced sexual dysfunction, without use disorder

▲ **F19.982** **Other psychoactive substance use, unspecified with psychoactive substance-induced sleep disorder**
Other (or unknown) substance-induced sleep disorder, without use disorder

▲ **F19.988** **Other psychoactive substance use, unspecified with other psychoactive substance-induced disorder**
Other (or unknown) substance-induced mild neurocognitive disorder, without use disorder
Other (or unknown) substance-induced obsessive-compulsive or relateddisorder, without use disorder

F19.99 **Other psychoactive substance use, unspecified with unspecified psychoactive substance-induced disorder**

Schizophrenia, schizotypal, delusional, and other non-mood psychotic disorders (F20-F29)

④ **F20** **Schizophrenia**
EXCLUDES 1 brief psychotic disorder (F23)
cyclic schizophrenia (F25.0)
mood [affective] disorders with psychotic symptoms (F30.2, F31.2, F31.5, F31.64, F32.3, F33.3)
schizoaffective disorder (F25.-)
schizophrenic reaction NOS (F23)
EXCLUDES 2 schizophrenic reaction in:
alcoholism (F10.15-, F10.25-, F10.95-)
brain disease (F06.2)
epilepsy (F06.2)
psychoactive drug use (F11-F19 with .15, .25, .95)
schizotypal disorder (F21)

F20.0 **Paranoid schizophrenia**
Paraphrenic schizophrenia
EXCLUDES 1 involutional paranoid state (F22)
paranoia (F22)
DEFINITION Schizophrenia marked by displays of megalomania, delusions of persecution and/or grandeur, hallucinations, and aggressive behavior.

F20.1 **Disorganized schizophrenia**
Hebephrenic schizophrenia
Hebephrenia

F20.2 **Catatonic schizophrenia**
Schizophrenic catalepsy
Schizophrenic catatonia
Schizophrenic flexibilitas cerea
EXCLUDES 1 catatonic stupor (R40.1)

▲ **F20.3** **Undifferentiated schizophrenia**
Atypical schizophrenia
EXCLUDES 1 acute schizophrenia-like psychotic disorder (F23)
EXCLUDES 2 post-schizophrenic depression (F32.89)

F20.5 **Residual schizophrenia**
Restzustand (schizophrenic)
Schizophrenic residual state

⑤ **F20.8** **Other schizophrenia**

F20.81 **Schizophreniform disorder**
Schizophreniform psychosis NOS

F20.89 **Other schizophrenia**
Cenesthopathic schizophrenia
Simple schizophrenia

F20.9 **Schizophrenia, unspecified**

● New ▲ Revised *Manifestation* ④-⑦ Digit Indicators ⊟ Laterality Ⓐ Adult (15+ years) Ⓜ Maternity (12-55 years) Ⓝ Newborn Ⓟ Pediatric (0-17 years) ♂ Male ♀ Female
✖ Deleted Unspecified + Additional code

2017 ICD-10-CM Expert for Physicians

© 2017 DecisionHealth   553

F21 **Schizotypal disorder**
Borderline schizophrenia
Latent schizophrenia
Latent schizophrenic reaction
Prepsychotic schizophrenia
Prodromal schizophrenia
Pseudoneurotic schizophrenia
Pseudopsychopathic schizophrenia
Schizotypal personality disorder

EXCLUDES 2 *Asperger's syndrome (F84.5)*
schizoid personality disorder (F60.1)

CODING TIP ✓ Do not use code F21 when Schizophrenia or Schizoaffective disorder is specified by the physician. Schizotypal disorder is a personality disorder characterized by behaviors that impact interpersonal relationships, appearance, and often exacerbate depressive and/or anxious symptoms.

F22 **Delusional disorders**
Delusional dysmorphophobia
Involutional paranoid state
Paranoia
Paranoia querulans
Paranoid psychosis
Paranoid state
Paraphrenia (late)
Sensitiver Beziehungswahn

EXCLUDES 1 *mood [affective] disorders with psychotic symptoms*
(F30.2, F31.2, F31.5, F31.64, F32.3, F33.3)
paranoid schizophrenia (F20.0)

EXCLUDES 2 *paranoid personality disorder (F60.0)*
paranoid psychosis, psychogenic (F23)
paranoid reaction (F23)

DEFINITION Paranoia: Extreme, irrational distrust of others.

F23 **Brief psychotic disorder**
Paranoid reaction
Psychogenic paranoid psychosis

EXCLUDES 2 *mood [affective] disorders with psychotic symptoms*
(F30.2, F31.2, F31.5, F31.64, F32.3, F33.3)

F24 **Shared psychotic disorder**
Folie à deux
Induced paranoid disorder
Induced psychotic disorder

F25 **Schizoaffective disorders**

EXCLUDES 1 *mood [affective] disorders with psychotic symptoms*
(F30.2, F31.2, F31.5, F31.64, F32.3, F33.3)
schizophrenia (F20.-)

CODING TIP ✓ Do not use F25.- codes when schizophrenia is specified by the physician. Schizoaffective disorder is diagnosed in patients who do not meet the criteria for either schizophrenia or bipolar disorder but often demonstrate characteristics of both disorders.

F25.0 **Schizoaffective disorder, bipolar type**
Cyclic schizophrenia
Schizoaffective disorder, manic type
Schizoaffective disorder, mixed type
Schizoaffective psychosis, bipolar type
Schizophreniform psychosis, manic type

F25.1 **Schizoaffective disorder, depressive type**
Schizoaffective psychosis, depressive type
Schizophreniform psychosis, depressive type

F25.8 **Other schizoaffective disorders**

F25.9 **Schizoaffective disorder, unspecified**
Schizoaffective psychosis NOS

F28 **Other psychotic disorder not due to a substance or known physiological condition**
Chronic hallucinatory psychosis

F29 **Unspecified psychosis not due to a substance or known physiological condition**
Psychosis NOS

EXCLUDES 1 *mental disorder NOS (F99)*
unspecified mental disorder due to known physiological condition (F09)

Mood [affective] disorders (F30-F39)

F30 **Manic episode**

INCLUDES bipolar disorder, single manic episode
mixed affective episode

EXCLUDES 1 *bipolar disorder (F31.-)*
major depressive disorder, single episode (F32.-)
major depressive disorder, recurrent (F33.-)

F30.1 **Manic episode without psychotic symptoms**

F30.10 **Manic episode without psychotic symptoms, unspecified**

F30.11 **Manic episode without psychotic symptoms, mild**

F30.12 **Manic episode without psychotic symptoms, moderate**

F30.13 **Manic episode, severe, without psychotic symptoms**

F30.2 **Manic episode, severe with psychotic symptoms**
Manic stupor
Mania with mood-congruent psychotic symptoms
Mania with mood-incongruent psychotic symptoms

F30.3 **Manic episode in partial remission**

F30.4 **Manic episode in full remission**

F30.8 **Other manic episodes**
Hypomania

F30.9 **Manic episode, unspecified**
Mania NOS

F31 **Bipolar disorder**

INCLUDES manic-depressive illness
manic-depressive psychosis
manic-depressive reaction

EXCLUDES 1 *bipolar disorder, single manic episode (F30.-)*
major depressive disorder, single episode (F32.-)
major depressive disorder, recurrent (F33.-)

EXCLUDES 2 *cyclothymia (F34.0)*

CODING TIP ✓ When assigning a code for bipolar disorder, no additional code for depression or depressive disorder should be assigned if the patient is also reported to have depression and/or depressive symptoms. Individuals with bipolar disorder may have alternating periods of emotional highs and lows reported as cyclothymic features. When cyclothymic features are additionally reported by the physician, cyclothymia (F34.0) should be additionally coded.

F31.0 **Bipolar disorder, current episode hypomanic**

F31.1 **Bipolar disorder, current episode manic without psychotic features**

F31.10 **Bipolar disorder, current episode manic without psychotic features, unspecified**

F31.11 **Bipolar disorder, current episode manic without psychotic features, mild**

F31.12 **Bipolar disorder, current episode manic without psychotic features, moderate**

F31.13 **Bipolar disorder, current episode manic without psychotic features, severe**

F31.2 **Bipolar disorder, current episode manic severe with psychotic features**
Bipolar disorder, current episode manic with mood-congruent psychotic symptoms
Bipolar disorder, current episode manic with mood-incongruent psychotic symptoms

F31.3 **Bipolar disorder, current episode depressed, mild or moderate severity**

F31.30 **Bipolar disorder, current episode depressed, mild or moderate severity, unspecified**

F31.31 **Bipolar disorder, current episode depressed, mild**

F31.32 **Bipolar disorder, current episode depressed, moderate**

F31.4 **Bipolar disorder, current episode depressed, severe, without psychotic features**

CODING TIP ✓ Unlike ICD-9, in ICD-10, depression documented as with anxiety is not coded to dysthymic disorder. When physician documentation reports depression with anxiety, use F41.8, Other specified anxiety disorders.

F31.5 **Bipolar disorder, current episode depressed, severe, with psychotic features**
Bipolar disorder, current episode depressed with mood-incongruent psychotic symptoms
Bipolar disorder, current episode depressed with mood-congruent psychotic symptoms

---

● New   ▲ Revised   *Manifestation*   **4-7** Digit Indicators   ▤ Laterality   ▣ Adult (15+ years)   ▣ Maternity (12-55 years)   ▣ Newborn   ▣ Pediatric (0-17 years)   ♂ Male   ♀ Female
✖ Deleted   Unspecified   + Additional code

⑤ **F31.6** **Bipolar disorder, current episode mixed**

F31.60 **Bipolar disorder, current episode mixed, unspecified**

F31.61 **Bipolar disorder, current episode mixed, mild**

F31.62 **Bipolar disorder, current episode mixed, moderate**

F31.63 **Bipolar disorder, current episode mixed, severe, without psychotic features**

F31.64 **Bipolar disorder, current episode mixed, severe, with psychotic features**
Bipolar disorder, current episode mixed with mood-congruent psychotic symptoms
Bipolar disorder, current episode mixed with mood-incongruent psychotic symptoms

⑤ **F31.7** **Bipolar disorder, currently in remission**

F31.70 **Bipolar disorder, currently in remission, most recent episode unspecified**

F31.71 **Bipolar disorder, in partial remission, most recent episode hypomanic**

F31.72 **Bipolar disorder, in full remission, most recent episode hypomanic**

F31.73 **Bipolar disorder, in partial remission, most recent episode manic**

F31.74 **Bipolar disorder, in full remission, most recent episode manic**

F31.75 **Bipolar disorder, in partial remission, most recent episode depressed**

F31.76 **Bipolar disorder, in full remission, most recent episode depressed**

F31.77 **Bipolar disorder, in partial remission, most recent episode mixed**

F31.78 **Bipolar disorder, in full remission, most recent episode mixed**

⑤ **F31.8** **Other bipolar disorders**

F31.81 **Bipolar II disorder**

F31.89 **Other bipolar disorder**
Recurrent manic episodes NOS

F31.9 **Bipolar disorder, unspecified**

④ **F32** **Major depressive disorder, single episode**

> **INCLUDES** single episode of agitated depression
> single episode of depressive reaction
> single episode of major depression
> single episode of psychogenic depression
> single episode of reactive depression
> single episode of vital depression

> **EXCLUDES 1** *bipolar disorder (F31.-)*
> *manic episode (F30.-)*
> *recurrent depressive disorder (F33.-)*

> **EXCLUDES 2** *adjustment disorder (F43.2)*

F32.0 **Major depressive disorder, single episode, mild**

F32.1 **Major depressive disorder, single episode, moderate**

F32.2 **Major depressive disorder, single episode, severe without psychotic features**

F32.3 **Major depressive disorder, single episode, severe with psychotic features**
Single episode of major depression with mood-congruent psychotic symptoms
Single episode of major depression with mood-incongruent psychotic symptoms
Single episode of major depression with psychotic symptoms
Single episode of psychogenic depressive psychosis
Single episode of psychotic depression
Single episode of reactive depressive psychosis

F32.4 **Major depressive disorder, single episode, in partial remission**

F32.5 **Major depressive disorder, single episode, in full remission**

▲ ⑤ **F32.8** **Other depressive episodes**

● **F32.81** **Premenstrual dysphoric disorder**

> **EXCLUDES 1** *premenstrual tension syndrome (N94.3)*

● **F32.89** **Other specified depressive episodes**
Atypical depression
Post-schizophrenic depression
Single episode of 'masked' depression NOS

F32.9 **Major depressive disorder, single episode, unspecified**
Depression NOS
Depressive disorder NOS
Major depression NOS

> **CODING TIP ✓** **Documentation:** Unspecified and chronic depression should be coded to F32.9. A physician must provide confirmation of the diagnosis of depression in order to assign this code and it should not be assigned based upon the presence of symptoms alone.
> AHA: 4Q 2013, 107, 108

④ **F33** **Major depressive disorder, recurrent**

> **INCLUDES** recurrent episodes of depressive reaction
> recurrent episodes of endogenous depression
> recurrent episodes of major depression
> recurrent episodes of psychogenic depression
> recurrent episodes of reactive depression
> recurrent episodes of seasonal depressive disorder
> recurrent episodes of vital depression

> **EXCLUDES 1** *bipolar disorder (F31.-)*
> *manic episode (F30.-)*

F33.0 **Major depressive disorder, recurrent, mild**

F33.1 **Major depressive disorder, recurrent, moderate**

F33.2 **Major depressive disorder, recurrent severe without psychotic features**

F33.3 **Major depressive disorder, recurrent, severe with psychotic symptoms**
Endogenous depression with psychotic symptoms
Recurrent severe episodes of major depression with mood-congruent psychotic symptoms
Recurrent severe episodes of major depression with mood-incongruent psychotic symptoms
Recurrent severe episodes of major depression with psychotic symptoms
Recurrent severe episodes of psychogenic depressive psychosis
Recurrent severe episodes of psychotic depression
Recurrent severe episodes of reactive depressive psychosis

⑤ **F33.4** **Major depressive disorder, recurrent, in remission**

F33.40 **Major depressive disorder, recurrent, in remission, unspecified**

F33.41 **Major depressive disorder, recurrent, in partial remission**

F33.42 **Major depressive disorder, recurrent, in full remission**

F33.8 **Other recurrent depressive disorders**
Recurrent brief depressive episodes

F33.9 **Major depressive disorder, recurrent, unspecified**
Monopolar depression NOS

④ **F34** **Persistent mood [affective] disorders**

F34.0 **Cyclothymic disorder**
Affective personality disorder
Cycloid personality
Cyclothymia
Cyclothymic personality

> **DEFINITION** Mild mood swings between elevated mood and mild depression.

▲ **F34.1** **Dysthymic disorder**
Depressive neurosis
Depressive personality disorder
Dysthymia
Neurotic depression
Persistent anxiety depression
Persistent depressive disorder

> **EXCLUDES 2** *anxiety depression (mild or not persistent) (F41.8)*

⑤ **F34.8** **Other persistent mood [affective] disorders**

● **F34.81** **Disruptive mood dysregulation disorder**

● **F34.89** **Other specified persistent mood disorders**

F34.9 **Persistent mood [affective] disorder, unspecified**

F39 **Unspecified mood [affective] disorder**
Affective psychosis NOS

Anxiety, dissociative, stress-related, somatoform and other nonpsychotic mental disorders (F40-F48)

④ **F40** **Phobic anxiety disorders**

⑤ **F40.0** **Agoraphobia**

F40.00 **Agoraphobia, unspecified**

Mental, Behavioral and Neurodevelopmental Disorders

F40.01   **Agoraphobia with panic disorder**
Panic disorder with agoraphobia
> **EXCLUDES 1**   *panic disorder without agoraphobia (F41.0)*

> **DEFINITION**   Fear of open spaces or crowds, traveling, or leaving a safe place, accompanied by panic attacks.

F40.02   **Agoraphobia without panic disorder**

⑤ F40.1   **Social phobias**
Anthropophobia
Social anxiety disorder of childhood
Social neurosis
> **DEFINITION**   Intense fear of appearing in public, especially in situations where one is the center of attention.

F40.10   **Social phobia, unspecified**

F40.11   **Social phobia, generalized**

⑤ F40.2   **Specific (isolated) phobias**
> **EXCLUDES 2**   *dysmorphophobia (nondelusional) (F45.22)*
> *nosophobia (F45.22)*

⑥ F40.21   **Animal type phobia**
F40.210   **Arachnophobia**
Fear of spiders
F40.218   **Other animal type phobia**

⑥ F40.22   **Natural environment type phobia**
F40.220   **Fear of thunderstorms**
F40.228   **Other natural environment type phobia**

⑥ F40.23   **Blood, injection, injury type phobia**
F40.230   **Fear of blood**
F40.231   **Fear of injections and transfusions**
F40.232   **Fear of other medical care**
F40.233   **Fear of injury**

⑥ F40.24   **Situational type phobia**
F40.240   **Claustrophobia**
F40.241   **Acrophobia**
F40.242   **Fear of bridges**
F40.243   **Fear of flying**
F40.248   **Other situational type phobia**

⑥ F40.29   **Other specified phobia**
F40.290   **Androphobia**
Fear of men
F40.291   **Gynephobia**
Fear of women
F40.298   **Other specified phobia**

F40.8   **Other phobic anxiety disorders**
Phobic anxiety disorder of childhood

F40.9   **Phobic anxiety disorder, unspecified**
Phobia NOS
Phobic state NOS

◧ F41   **Other anxiety disorders**
> **EXCLUDES 2**   *anxiety in:*
> *acute stress reaction (F43.0)*
> *transient adjustment reaction (F43.2)*
> *neurasthenia (F48.8)*
> *psychophysiologic disorders (F45.-)*
> *separation anxiety (F93.0)*

F41.0   **Panic disorder [episodic paroxysmal anxiety] without agoraphobia**
Panic attack
Panic state
> **EXCLUDES 1**   *panic disorder with agoraphobia (F40.01)*

> **DEFINITION**   Unexplained bouts of intense fear or anxiety, accompanied by physiological symptoms of elevated heart rate, sweating, trembling, dizziness, and dyspnea.

F41.1   **Generalized anxiety disorder**
Anxiety neurosis
Anxiety reaction
Anxiety state
Overanxious disorder
> **EXCLUDES 2**   *neurasthenia (F48.8)*

> **DEFINITION**   Persistent, uncontrollable worry about aspects of a person's life; diagnosed when symptoms last longer than six months, with anxiety present on the majority of days in that time.

F41.3   **Other mixed anxiety disorders**

F41.8   **Other specified anxiety disorders**
Anxiety depression (mild or not persistent)
Anxiety hysteria
Mixed anxiety and depressive disorder
> **CODING TIP ✓**   **Documentation:** When physician documentation specifies depression with anxiety, F41.8 should be assigned. The term "with" is considered a relational term and is interpreted to mean "associated with" or "due to."

F41.9   **Anxiety disorder, unspecified**
Anxiety NOS

▲ ◧ F42   **Obsessive-compulsive disorder**
> **EXCLUDES 2**   *obsessive-compulsive personality (disorder) (F60.5)*
> *obsessive-compulsive symptoms occurring in depression (F32-F33)*
> *obsessive-compulsive symptoms occurring in schizophrenia (F20.-)*

> **DEFINITION**   Recurrent obsessions of thought or action that are time-consuming or disruptive to daily life and can produce anxiety or distress.

● F42.2   **Mixed obsessional thoughts and acts**

● F42.3   **Hoarding disorder**

● F42.4   **Excoriation (skin-picking) disorder**
> **EXCLUDES 1**   *factitial dermatitis (L98.1)*
> *other specified behavioral and emotional disorders with onset usually occurring in early childhood and adolescence (F98.8)*

● F42.8   **Other obsessive-compulsive disorder**
Anancastic neurosis
Obsessive-compulsive neurosis

● F42.9   **Obsessive-compulsive disorder, unspecified**

◧ F43   **Reaction to severe stress, and adjustment disorders**

F43.0   **Acute stress reaction**
Acute crisis reaction
Acute reaction to stress
Combat and operational stress reaction
Combat fatigue
Crisis state
Psychic shock

⑤ F43.1   **Post-traumatic stress disorder (PTSD)**
Traumatic neurosis
> **DEFINITION**   Chronic stressful response to traumatic events such as combat, rape, physical assault, and natural disasters with sudden, powerful memories (flashbacks) of the event, anxiety, and panic.

F43.10   **Post-traumatic stress disorder, unspecified**
F43.11   **Post-traumatic stress disorder, acute**
F43.12   **Post-traumatic stress disorder, chronic**

⑤ F43.2   **Adjustment disorders**
Culture shock
Grief reaction
Hospitalism in children
> **EXCLUDES 2**   *separation anxiety disorder of childhood (F93.0)*

F43.20   **Adjustment disorder, unspecified**

F43.21   **Adjustment disorder with depressed mood**
> **CODING TIP ✓**   Complicated bereavement of any nature is coded to F43.21. Bereavement (uncomplicated) due to loss of a family member only is coded Z63.4.

> **DEFINITION**   Prolonged depressive state as a reaction to an event or change in the patient's life.
AHA: 1Q 2014, 25

F43.22   **Adjustment disorder with anxiety**
F43.23   **Adjustment disorder with mixed anxiety and depressed mood**
F43.24   **Adjustment disorder with disturbance of conduct**
F43.25   **Adjustment disorder with mixed disturbance of emotions and conduct**
F43.29   **Adjustment disorder with other symptoms**

▲ F43.8   **Other reactions to severe stress**
Other specified trauma and stressor-related disorder

● New   ▲ Revised   *Manifestation*   ◧-◪ Digit Indicators   ▤ Laterality   ◭ **Adult** (15+ years)   ◩ **Maternity** (12-55 years)   ◪ **Newborn**   ◪ **Pediatric** (0-17 years)   ♂ **Male**   ♀ **Female**
✖ Deleted   Unspecified   + Additional code

▲ **F43.9**   **Reaction to severe stress, unspecified**
Trauma and stressor-related disorder, NOS

◁ **F44**   **Dissociative and conversion disorders**

INCLUDES	conversion hysteria
	conversion reaction
	hysteria
	hysterical psychosis

EXCLUDES 2	*malingering [conscious simulation] (Z76.5)*

▲ **F44.0**   **Dissociative amnesia**

EXCLUDES 1	*amnesia NOS (R41.3)*
	anterograde amnesia (R41.1)
	dissociative amnesia with dissociative fugue (F44.1)
	retrograde amnesia (R41.2)

EXCLUDES 2	*alcohol-or other psychoactive substance-induced amnestic disorder (F10, F13, F19 with .26, .96)*
	amnestic disorder due to known physiological condition (F04)
	postictal amnesia in epilepsy (G40.-)

DEFINITION	Psychological trauma causing temporary forgetting of personal information and inability to perform complex tasks, like driving or cooking.

▲ **F44.1**   **Dissociative fugue**
Dissociative amnesia with dissociative fugue

EXCLUDES 2	*postictal fugue in epilepsy (G40.-)*

DEFINITION	Disorder occurring in response to a severe, recent stressor, in which the patient invents a new personality and becomes unable to remember his/her previous identity, lasting days or months.

F44.2   **Dissociative stupor**

EXCLUDES 1	*catatonic stupor (R40.1)*
	stupor NOS (R40.1)

EXCLUDES 2	*catatonic disorder due to known physiological condition (F06.1)*
	depressive stupor (F32, F33)
	manic stupor (F30, F31)

F44.4   **Conversion disorder with motor symptom or deficit**
Dissociative motor disorders
Psychogenic aphonia
Psychogenic dysphonia

F44.5   **Conversion disorder with seizures or convulsions**
Dissociative convulsions

F44.6   **Conversion disorder with sensory symptom or deficit**
Dissociative anesthesia and sensory loss
Psychogenic deafness

F44.7   **Conversion disorder with mixed symptom presentation**

⑤ **F44.8**   **Other dissociative and conversion disorders**

    F44.81   **Dissociative identity disorder**
        Multiple personality disorder

    F44.89   **Other dissociative and conversion disorders**
        Ganser's syndrome
        Psychogenic confusion
        Psychogenic twilight state
        Trance and possession disorders

F44.9   **Dissociative and conversion disorder, unspecified**
Dissociative disorder NOS

◁ **F45**   **Somatoform disorders**

EXCLUDES 2	*dissociative and conversion disorders (F44.-)*
	factitious disorders (F68.1-)
	hair-plucking (F63.3)
	lalling (F80.0)
	lisping (F80.0)
	malingering [conscious simulation] (Z76.5)
	nail-biting (F98.8)
	psychological or behavioral factors associated with disorders or diseases classified elsewhere (F54)
	sexual dysfunction, not due to a substance or known physiological condition (F52.-)
	thumb-sucking (F98.8)
	tic disorders (in childhood and adolescence) (F95.-)
	Tourette's syndrome (F95.2)
	trichotillomania (F63.3)

F45.0   **Somatization disorder**
Briquet's disorder
Multiple psychosomatic disorder

▲ **F45.1**   **Undifferentiated somatoform disorder**
Somatic symptom disorder
Undifferentiated psychosomatic disorder

⑤ **F45.2**   **Hypochondriacal disorders**

EXCLUDES 2	*delusional dysmorphophobia (F22)*
	fixed delusions about bodily functions or shape (F22)

DEFINITION	Chronic worry about nonexistent illnesses that one believes one may have.

    F45.20   **Hypochondriacal disorder, unspecified**

▲   **F45.21**   **Hypochondriasis**
        Hypochondriacal neurosis
        Illness anxiety disorder

    F45.22   **Body dysmorphic disorder**
        Dysmorphophobia (nondelusional)
        Nosophobia

    F45.29   **Other hypochondriacal disorders**

⑤ **F45.4**   **Pain disorders related to psychological factors**

EXCLUDES 1	*pain NOS (R52)*

    F45.41   **Pain disorder exclusively related to psychological factors**
        Somatoform pain disorder (persistent)

GUIDELINES	Section I.C.5.a

Assign code F45.41 for pain that is exclusively related to psychological disorders. As indicated by the Excludes 1 note under category G89, a code from category G89 should not be assigned with code F45.41.

CODING TIP ✓	Do not use F45.41 to report somatoform disorder not related to pain, chronic pain syndrome, or psychological factors related to chroninot relain disorders (G89.-, F45.42).

    F45.42   **Pain disorder with related psychological factors**
        Code also:
          associated acute or chronic pain (G89.-)

GUIDELINES	Section I.C.5.a

Code F45.42 should be used with a code from category G89, Pain, not elsewhere classified, if there is documentation of a psychological component for a patient with acute or chronic pain.

CODING TIP ✓	When the clinical record specifies that the patient has a pain disorder with related psychological factors, this code should be assigned with an additional code from G89.-.

F45.8   **Other somatoform disorders**
Psychogenic dysmenorrhea
Psychogenic dysphagia, including 'globus hystericus'
Psychogenic pruritus
Psychogenic torticollis
Somatoform autonomic dysfunction
Teeth grinding

EXCLUDES 1	*sleep related teeth grinding (G47.63)*

F45.9   **Somatoform disorder, unspecified**
Psychosomatic disorder NOS

◁ **F48**   **Other nonpsychotic mental disorders**

F48.1   **Depersonalization-derealization syndrome**

F48.2   **Pseudobulbar affect**
Involuntary emotional expression disorder
Code first underlying cause, if known, such as:
   amyotrophic lateral sclerosis (G12.21)
   multiple sclerosis (G35)
   sequelae of cerebrovascular disease (I69.-)
   sequelae of traumatic intracranial injury (S06.-)

F48.8   **Other specified nonpsychotic mental disorders**
Dhat syndrome
Neurasthenia
Occupational neurosis, including writer's cramp
Psychasthenia
Psychasthenic neurosis
Psychogenic syncope

F48.9   **Nonpsychotic mental disorder, unspecified**
Neurosis NOS

● New   ▲ Revised   *Manifestation*   ◁-☑ Digit Indicators   ⊟ Laterality   🅰 Adult (15+ years)   Ⓜ Maternity (12-55 years)   ℕ Newborn   ℙ Pediatric (0-17 years)   ♂ Male   ♀ Female
✖ Deleted   Unspecified   + Additional code

Behavioral syndromes associated with physiological disturbances and physical factors (F50-F59)

◢ F50   Eating disorders
EXCLUDES 1   *anorexia NOS (R63.0)*
feeding difficulties (R63.3)
polyphagia (R63.2)
EXCLUDES 2   *feeding disorder in infancy or childhood (F98.2-)*

▲ ⑤ F50.0   Anorexia nervosa
EXCLUDES 1   *loss of appetite (R63.0)*
psychogenic loss of appetite (F50.89)

CODING TIP ✓   This code can be assigned only if specified as "anorexia nervosa," which is differentiated from simple anorexia (loss of appetite) due to psychological features, including intense fear of weight gain, body image distortions, and a refusal to maintain normal body weight.

F50.00   **Anorexia nervosa, unspecified**

F50.01   **Anorexia nervosa, restricting type**

F50.02   **Anorexia nervosa, binge eating/purging type**
EXCLUDES 1   *bulimia nervosa (F50.2)*

F50.2   Bulimia nervosa
Bulimia NOS
Hyperorexia nervosa
EXCLUDES 1   *anorexia nervosa, binge eating/purging type (F50.02)*

DEFINITION   Repetitive episodes of binge eating followed by excessive measures to avoid gaining weight, such as self-induced vomiting and extreme exercising.

▲ ⑤ F50.8   Other eating disorders
EXCLUDES 2   *pica of infancy and childhood (F98.3)*

● F50.81   **Binge eating disorder**

● F50.89   **Other specified eating disorder**
Pica in adults
Psychogenic loss of appetite

F50.9   Eating disorder, unspecified
Atypical anorexia nervosa
Atypical bulimia nervosa

◢ F51   Sleep disorders not due to a substance or known physiological condition
EXCLUDES 2   *organic sleep disorders (G47.-)*

⑤ F51.0   Insomnia not due to a substance or known physiological condition
EXCLUDES 2   *alcohol related insomnia (F10.182, F10.282, F10.982)*
drug-related insomnia (F11.182, F11.282, F11.982, F13.182, F13.282, F13.982, F14.182, F14.282, F14.982, F15.182, F15.282, F15.982, F19.182, F19.282, F19.982)
insomnia NOS (G47.0-)
insomnia due to known physiological condition (G47.0-)
organic insomnia (G47.0-)
sleep deprivation (Z72.820)

F51.01   **Primary insomnia**
Idiopathic insomnia

F51.02   **Adjustment insomnia**

F51.03   **Paradoxical insomnia**

F51.04   **Psychophysiologic insomnia**

F51.05   **Insomnia due to other mental disorder**
Code also:
associated mental disorder

F51.09   **Other insomnia not due to a substance or known physiological condition**

⑤ F51.1   Hypersomnia not due to a substance or known physiological condition
EXCLUDES 2   *alcohol related hypersomnia (F10.182, F10.282, F10.982)*
drug-related hypersomnia (F11.182, F11.282, F11.982, F13.182, F13.282, F13.982, F14.182, F14.282, F14.982, F15.182, F15.282, F15.982, F19.182, F19.282, F19.982)
hypersomnia NOS (G47.10)
hypersomnia due to known physiological condition (G47.10)
idiopathic hypersomnia (G47.11, G47.12)
narcolepsy (G47.4-)

F51.11   **Primary hypersomnia**

F51.12   **Insufficient sleep syndrome**
EXCLUDES 1   *sleep deprivation (Z72.820)*

F51.13   **Hypersomnia due to other mental disorder**
Code also:
associated mental disorder

F51.19   **Other hypersomnia not due to a substance or known physiological condition**

F51.3   Sleepwalking [somnambulism]

F51.4   Sleep terrors [night terrors]

F51.5   Nightmare disorder
Dream anxiety disorder

F51.8   Other sleep disorders not due to a substance or known physiological condition

F51.9   Sleep disorder not due to a substance or known physiological condition, unspecified
Emotional sleep disorder NOS

◢ F52   Sexual dysfunction not due to a substance or known physiological condition
EXCLUDES 2   *Dhat syndrome (F48.8)*

▲ F52.0   Hypoactive sexual desire disorder
Lack or loss of sexual desire
Sexual anhedonia
EXCLUDES 1   *decreased libido (R68.82)*

DEFINITION   Markedly decreased sexual desire.

F52.1   Sexual aversion disorder
Sexual aversion and lack of sexual enjoyment

▲ ⑤ F52.2   Sexual arousal disorders
Failure of genital response

F52.21   **Male erectile disorder**   ♂
Psychogenic impotence
EXCLUDES 1   *impotence of organic origin (N52.-)*
impotence NOS (N52.-)

F52.22   **Female sexual arousal disorder**   ♀

⑤ F52.3   Orgasmic disorder
Inhibited orgasm
Psychogenic anorgasmy

F52.31   **Female orgasmic disorder**   ♀

▲ F52.32   **Male orgasmic disorder**   ♂
Delayed ejaculation

F52.4   Premature ejaculation   ♂

F52.5   Vaginismus not due to a substance or known physiological condition   ♀
Psychogenic vaginismus
EXCLUDES 2   *vaginismus (due to a known physiological condition) (N94.2)*

▲ F52.6   Dyspareunia not due to a substance or known physiological condition   ♀
Genito-pelvic pain penetration disorder
Psychogenic dyspareunia
EXCLUDES 2   *dyspareunia (due to a known physiological condition) (N94.1-)*

F52.8   Other sexual dysfunction not due to a substance or known physiological condition
Excessive sexual drive
Nymphomania
Satyriasis

F52.9   Unspecified sexual dysfunction not due to a substance or known physiological condition
Sexual dysfunction NOS

● New   ▲ Revised   *Manifestation*   ◢-◪ Digit Indicators   ⊟ Laterality   Ⓐ Adult (15+ years)   Ⓜ Maternity (12-55 years)   Ⓝ Newborn   Ⓟ Pediatric (0-17 years)   ♂ Male   ♀ Female
✖ Deleted̶   Unspecified   + Additional code

F53 **Puerperal psychosis** ♀
Postpartum depression
> **EXCLUDES 1** *mood disorders with psychotic features (F30.2, F31.2, F31.5, F31.64, F32.3, F33.3)*
> *postpartum dysphoria (O90.6)*
> *psychosis in schizophrenia, schizotypal, delusional, and other psychotic disorders (F20-F29)*

F54 **Psychological and behavioral factors associated with disorders or diseases classified elsewhere**
Psychological factors affecting physical conditions
Code first the associated physical disorder, such as:
asthma (J45.-)
dermatitis (L23-L25)
gastric ulcer (K25.-)
mucous colitis (K58.-)
ulcerative colitis (K51.-)
urticaria (L50.-)
> **EXCLUDES 2** *tension-type headache (G44.2)*

> **CODING TIP ✓** Assign code F54 when a psychological condition causes exacerbation of a specific physical condition, such as asthma or ulcers. This code may not be used alone and documentation should specify that the psychological condition has caused exacerbation of the physical state. Code the physical condition first, followed by F54.

⬛ F55 **Abuse of non-psychoactive substances**
> **EXCLUDES 2** *abuse of psychoactive substances (F10-F19)*

F55.0 Abuse of antacids
F55.1 Abuse of herbal or folk remedies
F55.2 Abuse of laxatives
F55.3 Abuse of steroids or hormones
F55.4 Abuse of vitamins
F55.8 Abuse of other non-psychoactive substances

F59 **Unspecified behavioral syndromes associated with physiological disturbances and physical factors**
Psychogenic physiological dysfunction NOS
> **CODING TIP ✓** Do not use F59 to report psychosomatic disorder. Psychosomatic disorder has a specific code and should be coded to F45.9

Disorders of adult personality and behavior (F60-F69)

⬛ F60 **Specific personality disorders**
F60.0 **Paranoid personality disorder**
Expansive paranoid personality (disorder)
Fanatic personality (disorder)
Querulant personality (disorder)
Paranoid personality (disorder)
Sensitive paranoid personality (disorder)
> **EXCLUDES 2** *paranoia (F22)*
> *paranoia querulans (F22)*
> *paranoid psychosis (F22)*
> *paranoid schizophrenia (F20.0)*
> *paranoid state (F22)*

F60.1 **Schizoid personality disorder**
> **EXCLUDES 2** *Asperger's syndrome (F84.5)*
> *delusional disorder (F22)*
> *schizoid disorder of childhood (F84.5)*
> *schizophrenia (F20.-)*
> *schizotypal disorder (F21)*

F60.2 **Antisocial personality disorder**
Amoral personality (disorder)
Asocial personality (disorder)
Dissocial personality disorder
Psychopathic personality (disorder)
Sociopathic personality (disorder)
> **EXCLUDES 1** *conduct disorders (F91.-)*
> **EXCLUDES 2** *borderline personality disorder (F60.3)*

F60.3 **Borderline personality disorder**
Aggressive personality (disorder)
Emotionally unstable personality disorder
Explosive personality (disorder)
> **EXCLUDES 2** *antisocial personality disorder (F60.2)*

> **DEFINITION** Disorder in which a person is quick to anger, aggressive, abnormally emotional, and argumentative.

F60.4 **Histrionic personality disorder**
Hysterical personality (disorder)
Psychoinfantile personality (disorder)

▲ F60.5 **Obsessive-compulsive personality disorder**
Anankastic personality (disorder)
Compulsive personality (disorder)
Obsessional personality (disorder)
> **EXCLUDES 2** *obsessive-compulsive disorder (F42-)*

F60.6 **Avoidant personality disorder**
Anxious personality disorder

F60.7 **Dependent personality disorder**
Asthenic personality (disorder)
Inadequate personality (disorder)
Passive personality (disorder)

⑤ F60.8 **Other specific personality disorders**
F60.81 **Narcissistic personality disorder**
F60.89 **Other specific personality disorders**
Eccentric personality disorder
'Haltlose' type personality disorder
Immature personality disorder
Passive-aggressive personality disorder
Psychoneurotic personality disorder
Self-defeating personality disorder

F60.9 **Personality disorder, unspecified**
Character disorder NOS
Character neurosis NOS
Pathological personality NOS

⬛ F63 **Impulse disorders**
> **EXCLUDES 2** *habitual excessive use of alcohol or psychoactive substances (F10-F19)*
> *impulse disorders involving sexual behavior (F65.-)*

F63.0 **Pathological gambling**
Compulsive gambling
> **EXCLUDES 1** *gambling and betting NOS (Z72.6)*
> **EXCLUDES 2** *excessive gambling by manic patients (F30, F31)*
> *gambling in antisocial personality disorder (F60.2)*

F63.1 **Pyromania**
Pathological fire-setting
> **EXCLUDES 2** *fire-setting (by) (in):*
> *adult with antisocial personality disorder (F60.2)*
> *alcohol or psychoactive substance intoxication (F10-F19)*
> *conduct disorders (F91.-)*
> *mental disorders due to known physiological condition (F01-F09)*
> *schizophrenia (F20.-)*

> **DEFINITION** Uncontrollable impulse to set fires.

F63.2 **Kleptomania**
Pathological stealing
> **EXCLUDES 1** *shoplifting as the reason for observation for suspected mental disorder (Z03.8)*
> **EXCLUDES 2** *depressive disorder with stealing (F31-F33)*
> *stealing due to underlying mental condition-code to mental condition*
> *stealing in mental disorders due to known physiological condition (F01-F09)*

> **DEFINITION** Irresistible impulse to steal.

F63.3 **Trichotillomania**
Hair plucking
> **EXCLUDES 2** *other stereotyped movement disorder (F98.4)*

⑤ F63.8 **Other impulse disorders**
F63.81 **Intermittent explosive disorder**
F63.89 **Other impulse disorders**
F63.9 **Impulse disorder, unspecified**
Impulse control disorder NOS

⬛ F64 **Gender identity disorders**
● F64.0 **Transsexualism**
Gender identity disorder in adolescence and adulthood
Gender dysphoria in adolescents and adults

● New ▲ Revised *Manifestation* ⬛-⑦ Digit Indicators ▤ Laterality Ⓐ Adult (15+ years) Ⓜ Maternity (12-55 years) Ⓝ Newborn Ⓟ Pediatric (0-17 years) ♂ Male ♀ Female
✖ Deleted Unspecified + Additional code

2017 ICD-10-CM Expert for Physicians

© 2017 DecisionHealth

559

F53 — F64.0

▲ + **F64.1**　**Dual role transvestism**
Use additional code to identify sex reassignment status (Z87.890)
EXCLUDES 1　*gender identity disorder in childhood (F64.2)*
EXCLUDES 2　*fetishistic transvestism (F65.1)*

▲ **F64.2**　**Gender identity disorder of childhood**
Gender dysphoria in children
EXCLUDES 1　*gender identity disorder in adolescence and adulthood (F64.0)*
EXCLUDES 2　*sexual maturation disorder (F66)*

F64.8　**Other gender identity disorders**

F64.9　**Gender identity disorder, unspecified**
Gender-role disorder NOS

☑ **F65**　**Paraphilias**

F65.0　**Fetishism**

F65.1　**Transvestic fetishism**
Fetishistic transvestism

F65.2　**Exhibitionism**
DEFINITION　Compulsion to expose genitals in public.

F65.3　**Voyeurism**
DEFINITION　Uncontrollable compulsion to covertly observe others who are nude or engaged in sexual activity.

F65.4　**Pedophilia**

☑ **F65.5**　**Sadomasochism**

F65.50　**Sadomasochism, unspecified**

F65.51　**Sexual masochism**
DEFINITION　Psychosexual disorder marked by the need to be humiliated or hurt to achieve sexual gratification.

F65.52　**Sexual sadism**
DEFINITION　Psychosexual disorder marked by the need to humiliate or injure others to achieve sexual gratification.

☑ **F65.8**　**Other paraphilias**

F65.81　**Frotteurism**

F65.89　**Other paraphilias**
Necrophilia
DEFINITION　Sexual attraction to corpses.

F65.9　**Paraphilia, unspecified**
Sexual deviation NOS

F66　**Other sexual disorders**
Sexual maturation disorder
Sexual relationship disorder

☑ **F68**　**Other disorders of adult personality and behavior**

☑ **F68.1**　**Factitious disorder**
Compensation neurosis
Elaboration of physical symptoms for psychological reasons
Hospital hopper syndrome
Münchausen's syndrome
Peregrinating patient
EXCLUDES 2　*factitial dermatitis (L98.1)*
person feigning illness (with obvious motivation) (Z76.5)

F68.10　**Factitious disorder, unspecified**

F68.11　**Factitious disorder with predominantly psychological signs and symptoms**

F68.12　**Factitious disorder with predominantly physical signs and symptoms**

F68.13　**Factitious disorder with combined psychological and physical signs and symptoms**

F68.8　**Other specified disorders of adult personality and behavior**

F69　**Unspecified disorder of adult personality and behavior**　🅰

Intellectual Disabilities (F70-F79)

Code first:
　any associated physical or developmental disorders
EXCLUDES 1　*borderline intellectual functioning, IQ above 70 to 84 (R41.83)*

CODING TIP ✓　When IQ is specified, use the appropriate code from F70-F79 to specify level of intellectual disability based upon reported IQ. When developmental delays or disorders are additionally noted in a patient with Intellectual disability, these should be coded first.

F70　**Mild intellectual disabilities**
IQ level 50-55 to approximately 70
Mild mental subnormality

F71　**Moderate intellectual disabilities**
IQ level 35-40 to 50-55
Moderate mental subnormality

F72　**Severe intellectual disabilities**
IQ 20-25 to 35-40
Severe mental subnormality

F73　**Profound intellectual disabilities**
IQ level below 20-25
Profound mental subnormality

F78　**Other intellectual disabilities**

F79　**Unspecified intellectual disabilities**
Mental deficiency NOS
Mental subnormality NOS

Pervasive and specific developmental disorders (F80-F89)

CODING TIP ✓　Disorders coded to categories F80-F89 should be specified as related to a developmental origin.

☑ **F80**　**Specific developmental disorders of speech and language**

▲ **F80.0**　**Phonological disorder**
Dyslalia
Functional speech articulation disorder
Lalling
Lisping
Phonological developmental disorder
Speech articulation developmental disorder
Speech-sound disorder
EXCLUDES 1　*speech articulation impairment due to aphasia NOS (R47.01)*
speech articulation impairment due to apraxia (R48.2)
EXCLUDES 2　*speech articulation impairment due to hearing loss (F80.4)*
speech articulation impairment due to intellectual disabilities (F70-F79)
speech articulation impairment with expressive language developmental disorder (F80.1)
speech articulation impairment with mixed receptive expressive language developmental disorder (F80.2)
CODING TIP ✓　Code any additional speech articulation disorders in addition, when applicable.

F80.1　**Expressive language disorder**
Developmental dysphasia or aphasia, expressive type
EXCLUDES 1　*mixed receptive-expressive language disorder (F80.2)*
dysphasia and aphasia NOS (R47.-)
EXCLUDES 2　*acquired aphasia with epilepsy [Landau-Kleffner] (G40.80-)*
selective mutism (F94.0)
intellectual disabilities (F70-F79)
pervasive developmental disorders (F84.-)
CODING TIP ✓　Language disorders should not be coded here unless specified as related to a developmental cause.

● New　▲ Revised　*Manifestation*　☑-☑ Digit Indicators　⊟ Laterality　🅰 Adult (15+ years)　Ⓜ Maternity (12-55 years)　Ⓝ Newborn　Ⓟ Pediatric (0-17 years)　♂ Male　♀ Female
✖ ~~Deleted~~　Unspecified　+ Additional code

560　　© 2017 DecisionHealth　　　　　　　　　　　　　　2017 ICD-10-CM Expert for Physicians

F80.2   Mixed receptive-expressive language disorder
Developmental dysphasia or aphasia, receptive type
Developmental Wernicke's aphasia

> **EXCLUDES 1**   *central auditory processing disorder (H93.25)*
> *dysphasia or aphasia NOS (R47.-)*
> *expressive language disorder (F80.1)*
> *expressive type dysphasia or aphasia (F80.1)*
> *word deafness (H93.25)*

> **EXCLUDES 2**   *acquired aphasia with epilepsy [Landau-Kleffner] (G40.80-)*
> *pervasive developmental disorders (F84.-)*
> *selective mutism (F94.0)*
> *intellectual disabilities (F70-F79)*

> **DEFINITION**   Problems comprehending as well as expressing verbal language.

F80.4   Speech and language development delay due to hearing loss
Code also:
type of hearing loss (H90.-, H91.-)

F80.8   Other developmental disorders of speech and language

F80.81   Childhood onset fluency disorder
Cluttering NOS
Stuttering NOS

> **EXCLUDES 1**   *adult onset fluency disorder (F98.5)*
> *fluency disorder in conditions classified elsewhere (R47.82)*
> *fluency disorder (stuttering) following cerebrovascular disease (I69. with final characters -23)*

● F80.82   Social pragmatic communication disorder

> **EXCLUDES 1**   *Asperger's syndrome (F84.5)*
> *autistic disorder (F84.0)*

F80.89   Other developmental disorders of speech and language

F80.9   Developmental disorder of speech and language, unspecified
Communication disorder NOS
Language disorder NOS

F81   Specific developmental disorders of scholastic skills

F81.0   Specific reading disorder
'Backward reading'
Developmental dyslexia
Specific reading retardation

> **EXCLUDES 1**   *alexia NOS (R48.0)*
> *dyslexia NOS (R48.0)*

F81.2   Mathematics disorder
Developmental acalculia
Developmental arithmetical disorder
Developmental Gerstmann's syndrome

> **EXCLUDES 1**   *acalculia NOS (R48.8)*

> **EXCLUDES 2**   *arithmetical difficulties associated with a reading disorder (F81.0)*
> *arithmetical difficulties associated with a spelling disorder (F81.81)*
> *arithmetical difficulties due to inadequate teaching (Z55.8)*

F81.8   Other developmental disorders of scholastic skills

F81.81   Disorder of written expression
Specific spelling disorder

F81.89   Other developmental disorders of scholastic skills

F81.9   Developmental disorder of scholastic skills, unspecified
Knowledge acquisition disability NOS
Learning disability NOS
Learning disorder NOS

F82   Specific developmental disorder of motor function
Clumsy child syndrome
Developmental coordination disorder
Developmental dyspraxia

> **EXCLUDES 1**   *abnormalities of gait and mobility (R26.-)*
> *lack of coordination (R27.-)*

> **EXCLUDES 2**   *lack of coordination secondary to intellectual disabilities (F70-F79)*

● + F84   Pervasive developmental disorders
Use additional code to identify any associated medical condition and intellectual disabilities.

▲ + F84.0   Autistic disorder
Autism spectrum disorder
Infantile autism
Infantile psychosis
Kanner's syndrome

> **EXCLUDES 1**   *Asperger's syndrome (F84.5)*

> **DEFINITION**   Neurological disorder appearing at a young age that impairs social development and communication skills, and resulting in abnormal behavior that varies in degree of severity and ability to function.

+ F84.2   Rett's syndrome

> **EXCLUDES 1**   *Asperger's syndrome (F84.5)*
> *Autistic disorder (F84.0)*
> *Other childhood disintegrative disorder (F84.3)*

+ F84.3   Other childhood disintegrative disorder
Dementia infantilis
Disintegrative psychosis
Heller's syndrome
Symbiotic psychosis
Use additional code to identify any associated neurological condition.

> **EXCLUDES 1**   *Asperger's syndrome (F84.5)*
> *Autistic disorder (F84.0)*
> *Rett's syndrome (F84.2)*

+ F84.5   Asperger's syndrome
Asperger's disorder
Autistic psychopathy
Schizoid disorder of childhood

+ F84.8   Other pervasive developmental disorders
Overactive disorder associated with intellectual disabilities and stereotyped movements

+ F84.9   Pervasive developmental disorder, unspecified
Atypical autism

▲ F88   Other disorders of psychological development
Developmental agnosia
Global developmental delay
Other specified neurodevelopmental disorder

▲ F89   Unspecified disorder of psychological development
Developmental disorder NOS
Neurodevelopmental disorder NOS

Behavioral and emotional disorders with onset usually occurring in childhood and adolescence (F90-F98)

Note: Codes within categories F90-F98 may be used regardless of the age of a patient. These disorders generally have onset within the childhood or adolescent years, but may continue throughout life or not be diagnosed until adulthood

> **CODING TIP ✓**   Disorders classified to categories F90-F98 are frequently diagnosed in childhood and adolescence. However, a diagnosis may be made at any time during an individual's lifetime and may still be reported here when the diagnosis criteria are applicable.

F90   Attention-deficit hyperactivity disorders

> **INCLUDES**   attention deficit disorder with hyperactivity
> attention deficit syndrome with hyperactivity

> **EXCLUDES 2**   *anxiety disorders (F40.-, F41.-)*
> *mood [affective] disorders (F30-F39)*
> *pervasive developmental disorders (F84.-)*
> *schizophrenia (F20.-)*

F90.0   Attention-deficit hyperactivity disorder, predominantly inattentive type

F90.1   Attention-deficit hyperactivity disorder, predominantly hyperactive type

F90.2   Attention-deficit hyperactivity disorder, combined type

F90.8   Attention-deficit hyperactivity disorder, other type

F90.9   Attention-deficit hyperactivity disorder, unspecified type
Attention-deficit hyperactivity disorder of childhood or adolescence NOS
Attention-deficit hyperactivity disorder NOS

● New ▲ Revised *Manifestation* **◐-◼** Digit Indicators ⊟ Laterality Ⓐ Adult (15+ years) Ⓜ Maternity (12-55 years) Ⓝ Newborn Ⓟ Pediatric (0-17 years) ♂ Male ♀ Female
✖ Deleted Unspecified + Additional code

F91   Conduct disorders

> **EXCLUDES 1** *antisocial behavior (Z72.81-)*
> *antisocial personality disorder (F60.2)*
>
> **EXCLUDES 2** *conduct problems associated with attention-deficit hyperactivity disorder (F90.-)*
> *mood [affective] disorders (F30-F39)*
> *pervasive developmental disorders (F84.-)*
> *schizophrenia (F20.-)*

F91.0   Conduct disorder confined to family context

F91.1   Conduct disorder, childhood-onset type
Unsocialized conduct disorder
Conduct disorder, solitary aggressive type
Unsocialized aggressive disorder

F91.2   Conduct disorder, adolescent-onset type
Socialized conduct disorder
Conduct disorder, group type

F91.3   Oppositional defiant disorder

▲ **F91.8   Other conduct disorders**
Other specified conduct disorder
Other specified disruptive disorder

▲ **F91.9   Conduct disorder, unspecified**
Behavioral disorder NOS
Conduct disorder NOS
Disruptive behavior disorder NOS
Disruptive disorder NOS

F93   Emotional disorders with onset specific to childhood

F93.0   Separation anxiety disorder of childhood   [P]

> **EXCLUDES 2** *mood [affective] disorders (F30-F39)*
> *nonpsychotic mental disorders (F40-F48)*
> *phobic anxiety disorder of childhood (F40.8)*
> *social phobia (F40.1)*

> **DEFINITION**   Abnormal anxiety when separated from a parent, guardian, or usual environment.

F93.8   Other childhood emotional disorders   [P]
Identity disorder

> **EXCLUDES 2** *gender identity disorder of childhood (F64.2)*

F93.9   Childhood emotional disorder, unspecified   [P]

F94   Disorders of social functioning with onset specific to childhood and adolescence

F94.0   Selective mutism
Elective mutism

> **EXCLUDES 2** *pervasive developmental disorders (F84.-)*
> *schizophrenia (F20.-)*
> *specific developmental disorders of speech and language (F80.-)*
> *transient mutism as part of separation anxiety in young children (F93.0)*

+ **F94.1   Reactive attachment disorder of childhood**   [P]
Use additional code to identify any associated failure to thrive or growth retardation

> **EXCLUDES 1** *disinhibited attachment disorder of childhood (F94.2)*
> *normal variation in pattern of selective attachment*
>
> **EXCLUDES 2** *Asperger's syndrome (F84.5)*
> *maltreatment syndromes (T74.-)*
> *sexual or physical abuse in childhood, resulting in psychosocial problems (Z62.81-)*

F94.2   Disinhibited attachment disorder of childhood   [P]
Affectionless psychopathy
Institutional syndrome

> **EXCLUDES 1** *reactive attachment disorder of childhood (F94.1)*
>
> **EXCLUDES 2** *Asperger's syndrome (F84.5)*
> *attention-deficit hyperactivity disorders (F90.-)*
> *hospitalism in children (F43.2-)*

F94.8   Other childhood disorders of social functioning   [P]

F94.9   Childhood disorder of social functioning, unspecified   [P]

F95   Tic disorder

▲ **F95.0   Transient tic disorder**
Provisional tic disorder

F95.1   Chronic motor or vocal tic disorder

F95.2   Tourette's disorder
Combined vocal and multiple motor tic disorder [de la Tourette]
Tourette's syndrome

F95.8   Other tic disorders

F95.9   Tic disorder, unspecified
Tic NOS

▲ **F98   Other behavioral and emotional disorders with onset usually occurring in childhood and adolescence**

> **EXCLUDES 2** *breath-holding spells (R06.89)*
> *gender identity disorder of childhood (F64.2)*
> *Kleine-Levin syndrome (G47.13)*
> *obsessive-compulsive disorder (F42-)*
> *sleep disorders not due to a substance or known physiological condition (F51.-)*

F98.0   Enuresis not due to a substance or known physiological condition
Enuresis (primary) (secondary) of nonorganic origin
Functional enuresis
Psychogenic enuresis
Urinary incontinence of nonorganic origin

> **EXCLUDES 1** *enuresis NOS (R32)*

+ **F98.1   Encopresis not due to a substance or known physiological condition**
Functional encopresis
Incontinence of feces of nonorganic origin
Psychogenic encopresis
Use additional code to identify the cause of any coexisting constipation.

> **EXCLUDES 1** *encopresis NOS (R15.-)*

F98.2   Other feeding disorders of infancy and childhood

> **EXCLUDES 1** *feeding difficulties (R63.3)*
>
> **EXCLUDES 2** *anorexia nervosa and other eating disorders (F50.-)*
> *feeding problems of newborn (P92.-)*
> *pica of infancy or childhood (F98.3)*

F98.21   Rumination disorder of infancy   [P]

F98.29   Other feeding disorders of infancy and early childhood   [P]

F98.3   Pica of infancy and childhood   [P]

> **DEFINITION**   Compulsion to eat inedible substances, such as dirt or rocks.

▲ **F98.4   Stereotyped movement disorders**
Stereotype/habit disorder

> **EXCLUDES 1** *abnormal involuntary movements (R25.-)*
>
> **EXCLUDES 2** *compulsions in obsessive-compulsive disorder (F42-)*
> *hair plucking (F63.3)*
> *movement disorders of organic origin (G20-G25)*
> *nail-biting (F98.8)*
> *nose-picking (F98.8)*
> *stereotypies that are part of a broader psychiatric condition (F01-F95)*
> *thumb-sucking (F98.8)*
> *tic disorders (F95.-)*
> *trichotillomania (F63.3)*

F98.5   Adult onset fluency disorder

> **EXCLUDES 1** *childhood onset fluency disorder (F80.81)*
> *dysphasia (R47.02)*
> *fluency disorder in conditions classified elsewhere (R47.82)*
> *fluency disorder (stuttering) following cerebrovascular disease (I69. with final characters -23)*
> *tic disorders (F95.-)*

> **CODING TIP ✓**   This code is used for post-childhood onset of stuttering symptoms secondary to emotional stress or trauma. Do not assign F98.5 to report fluency disorder as a sequelae of cerebral vascular disease or another cause, or to identify dysphasia.

> **DEFINITION**   Normal flow of speech disrupted by repeated sounds or pauses.

F98.8   Other specified behavioral and emotional disorders with onset usually occurring in childhood and adolescence   [P]
Excessive masturbation
Nail-biting
Nose-picking
Thumb-sucking

F98.9   Unspecified behavioral and emotional disorders with onset usually occurring in childhood and adolescence   [P]

| ● New | ▲ Revised | *Manifestation* | ◳-◸ Digit Indicators | ▭ Laterality | Ⓐ Adult (15+ years) | Ⓜ Maternity (12-55 years) | Ⓝ Newborn | ℙ Pediatric (0-17 years) | ♂ Male | ♀ Female |
| ✖ ~~Deleted~~ | | Unspecified | + Additional code | | | | | | | |

Mental, Behavioral and Neurodevelopmental Disorders

Unspecified mental disorder (F99)

F99 **Mental disorder, not otherwise specified**

Mental illness NOS

> **EXCLUDES 1** *unspecified mental disorder due to known physiological condition (F09)*

> **CODING TIP ✓** Use F99 only when the clinical documentation from the provider reports mental illness but does not specify anything further.

● New   ▲ Revised   *Manifestation*   ➍-➐ Digit Indicators   ▣ Laterality   Ⓐ Adult (15+ years)   Ⓜ Maternity (12-55 years)   Ⓝ Newborn   Ⓟ Pediatric (0-17 years)   ♂ Male   ♀ Female
✖ Deleted   Unspecified   ✚ Additional code

CHAPTER 6: DISEASES OF THE NERVOUS SYSTEM (G00-G99)

EXCLUDES 2   *certain conditions originating in the perinatal period (P04-P96)*
certain infectious and parasitic diseases (A00-B99)
complications of pregnancy, childbirth and the puerperium (O00-O9A)
congenital malformations, deformations, and chromosomal abnormalities (Q00-Q99)
endocrine, nutritional and metabolic diseases (E00-E88)
injury, poisoning and certain other consequences of external causes (S00-T88)
neoplasms (C00-D49)
symptoms, signs and abnormal clinical and laboratory findings, not elsewhere classified (R00-R94)

This chapter contains the following blocks:

G00-G09	Inflammatory diseases of the central nervous system
G10-G14	Systemic atrophies primarily affecting the central nervous system
G20-G26	Extrapyramidal and movement disorders
G30-G32	Other degenerative diseases of the nervous system
G35-G37	Demyelinating diseases of the central nervous system
G40-G47	Episodic and paroxysmal disorders
G50-G59	Nerve, nerve root and plexus disorders
G60-G65	Polyneuropathies and other disorders of the peripheral nervous system
G70-G73	Diseases of myoneural junction and muscle
G80-G83	Cerebral palsy and other paralytic syndromes
G89-G99	Other disorders of the nervous system

Inflammatory diseases of the central nervous system (G00-G09)

CODING TIP ✓   If the central nervous system infection (CNS) is resolved but has a potential for reoccurence, use Z86.61, personal history of CNS infections. If the CNS infection is resolved, but the patient suffers neurological deficits, code the residual deficit followed by the sequela code G09.

⊿ G00   Bacterial meningitis, not elsewhere classified

INCLUDES   bacterial arachnoiditis
bacterial leptomeningitis
bacterial meningitis
bacterial pachymeningitis

EXCLUDES 1   *bacterial:*
meningoencephalitis (G04.2)
meningomyelitis (G04.2)

Diseases of the nervous system

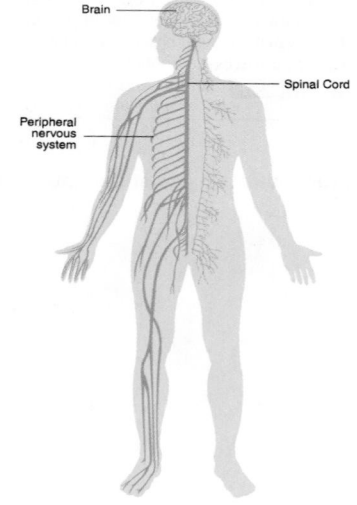

Brain

Spinal Cord

Peripheral nervous system

G00.0   Hemophilus meningitis
Meningitis due to Hemophilus influenzae

DEFINITION   Bacterial infection of the tissues (meninges) surrounding the brain and spinal cord, causing fever, headache, vomiting, malaise, and stiff neck and may progress to confusion, stupor, convulsions, coma, and death.

▲ G00.1   Pneumococcal meningitis
Meningtitis due to Streptococcal pneumoniae

+ G00.2   Streptococcal meningitis
Use additional code to further identify organism (B95.0-B95.5)

+ G00.3   Staphylococcal meningitis
Use additional code to further identify organism (B95.61-B95.8)

Staphylococcal meningitis

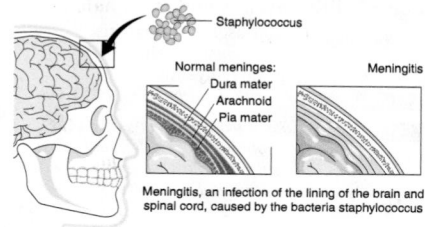

Staphylococcus

Normal meninges:
Dura mater
Arachnoid
Pia mater

Meningitis

Meningitis, an infection of the lining of the brain and spinal cord, caused by the bacteria staphylococcus

+ G00.8   Other bacterial meningitis
Meningitis due to Escherichia coli
Meningitis due to Friedländer's bacillus
Meningitis due to Klebsiella
Use additional code to further identify organism (B96.-)

G00.9   Bacterial meningitis, unspecified
Meningitis due to gram-negative bacteria, unspecified
Purulent meningitis NOS
Pyogenic meningitis NOS
Suppurative meningitis NOS

G01   *Meningitis in bacterial diseases classified elsewhere*
Code first:
underlying disease

EXCLUDES 1   *meningitis (in) :*
gonococcal (A54.81)
leptospirosis (A27.81)
listeriosis (A32.11)
Lyme disease (A69.21)
meningococcal (A39.0)
neurosyphilis (A52.13)
tuberculosis (A17.0)
meningoencephalitis and meningomyelitis in bacterial diseases classified elsewhere (G05)

G02   *Meningitis in other infectious and parasitic diseases classified elsewhere*
Code first underlying disease, such as:
African trypanosomiasis (B56.-)
poliovirus infection (A80.-)

EXCLUDES 1   *candidal meningitis (B37.5)*
coccidioidomycosis meningitis (B38.4)
cryptococcal meningitis (B45.1)
herpesviral [herpes simplex] meningitis (B00.3)
infectious mononucleosis complicated by meningitis (B27.- with fourth character 2)
measles complicated by meningitis (B05.1)
meningoencephalitis and meningomyelitis in other infectious and parasitic diseases classified elsewhere (G05)
mumps meningitis (B26.1)
rubella meningitis (B06.02)
varicella [chickenpox] meningitis (B01.0)
zoster meningitis (B02.1)

⊿ G03   Meningitis due to other and unspecified causes

INCLUDES   arachnoiditis NOS
leptomeningitis NOS
meningitis NOS
pachymeningitis NOS

EXCLUDES 1   *meningoencephalitis (G04.-)*
meningomyelitis (G04.-)

● New   ▲ Revised   *Manifestation*   ⊿-◪ Digit Indicators   ▤ Laterality   ☖ Adult (15+ years)   ☒ Maternity (12-55 years)   ☒ Newborn   ▣ Pediatric (0-17 years)   ♂ Male   ♀ Female
✖ Deleted   Unspecified   + Additional code

G03.0 **Nonpyogenic meningitis**
Aseptic meningitis
Nonbacterial meningitis

G03.1 **Chronic meningitis**

G03.2 **Benign recurrent meningitis [Mollaret]**

CODING TIP ✓ Do not confuse chronic meningitis with benign recurrent Mollaret's type meningitis. Mollaret's meningitis is a rare disorder characterized by a recurrent, mild, and aseptic inflammation of the meninges due to an unknown cause.

G03.8 **Meningitis due to other specified causes**

G03.9 **Meningitis, unspecified**
Arachnoiditis (spinal) NOS

CODING TIP ✓ Meningitis that is not specified as acute, chronic, or due to a specified cause should be coded to G03.9.

4 G04 **Encephalitis, myelitis and encephalomyelitis**

INCLUDES acute ascending myelitis
meningoencephalitis
meningomyelitis

EXCLUDES 1 *encephalopathy NOS (G93.40)*

EXCLUDES 2 *acute transverse myelitis (G37.3-)*
alcoholic encephalopathy (G31.2)
benign myalgic encephalomyelitis (G93.3)
multiple sclerosis (G35)
subacute necrotizing myelitis (G37.4)
toxic encephalitis (G92)
toxic encephalopathy (G92)

5 G04.0 **Acute disseminated encephalitis and encephalomyelitis (ADEM)**

EXCLUDES 1 *acute necrotizing hemorrhagic encephalopathy (G04.3-)*
other noninfectious acute disseminated encephalomyelitis (noninfectious ADEM) (G04.81)

G04.00 **Acute disseminated encephalitis and encephalomyelitis, unspecified**

G04.01 **Postinfectious acute disseminated encephalitis and encephalomyelitis (postinfectious ADEM)**

EXCLUDES 1 *post chickenpox encephalitis (B01.1)*
post measles encephalitis (B05.0)
post measles myelitis (B05.1)

+ G04.02 **Postimmunization acute disseminated encephalitis, myelitis and encephalomyelitis**
Encephalitis, post immunization
Encephalomyelitis, post immunization
Use additional code to identify the vaccine (T50.A-, T50.B-, T50.Z-)

CODING TIP ✓ G04.02 should be assigned for encephalitis, myelitis, and encephalomyelitis that is reported to be caused by the administration of vaccines. An additional code is needed to identify the vaccine.

G04.1 **Tropical spastic paraplegia**

G04.2 **Bacterial meningoencephalitis and meningomyelitis, not elsewhere classified**

5 G04.3 **Acute necrotizing hemorrhagic encephalopathy**

EXCLUDES 1 *acute disseminated encephalitis and encephalomyelitis (G04.0-)*

G04.30 **Acute necrotizing hemorrhagic encephalopathy, unspecified**

G04.31 **Postinfectious acute necrotizing hemorrhagic encephalopathy**

+ G04.32 **Postimmunization acute necrotizing hemorrhagic encephalopathy**
Use additional code to identify the vaccine (T50.A-, T50.B-, T50.Z-)

G04.39 **Other acute necrotizing hemorrhagic encephalopathy**
Code also:
underlying etiology, if applicable

5 G04.8 **Other encephalitis, myelitis and encephalomyelitis**
Code also:
any associated seizure (G40.-, R56.9)

G04.81 **Other encephalitis and encephalomyelitis**
Noninfectious acute disseminated encephalomyelitis (noninfectious ADEM)

G04.89 **Other myelitis**

5 G04.9 **Encephalitis, myelitis and encephalomyelitis, unspecified**

G04.90 **Encephalitis and encephalomyelitis, unspecified**
Ventriculitis (cerebral) NOS

G04.91 **Myelitis, unspecified**

4 G05 **Encephalitis, myelitis and encephalomyelitis in diseases classified elsewhere**
Code first underlying disease, such as:
human immunodeficiency virus [HIV] disease (B20)
poliovirus (A80.-)
suppurative otitis media (H66.01-H66.4)
trichinellosis (B75)

EXCLUDES 1 *adenoviral encephalitis, myelitis and encephalomyelitis (A85.1)*
congenital toxoplasmosis encephalitis, myelitis and encephalomyelitis (P37.1)
cytomegaloviral encephalitis, myelitis and encephalomyelitis (B25.8)
encephalitis, myelitis and encephalomyelitis (in) measles (B05.0)
encephalitis, myelitis and encephalomyelitis (in) systemic lupus erythematosus (M32.19)
enteroviral encephalitis, myelitis and encephalomyelitis (A85.0)
eosinophilic meningoencephalitis (B83.2)
herpesviral [herpes simplex] encephalitis, myelitis and encephalomyelitis (B00.4)
listerial encephalitis, myelitis and encephalomyelitis (A32.12)
meningococcal encephalitis, myelitis and encephalomyelitis (A39.81)
mumps encephalitis, myelitis and encephalomyelitis (B26.2)
postchickenpox encephalitis, myelitis and encephalomyelitis (B01.1-)
rubella encephalitis, myelitis and encephalomyelitis (B06.01)
toxoplasmosis encephalitis, myelitis and encephalomyelitis (B58.2)
zoster encephalitis, myelitis and encephalomyelitis (B02.0)

G05.3 *Encephalitis and encephalomyelitis in diseases classified elsewhere*
Meningoencephalitis in diseases classified elsewhere

G05.4 *Myelitis in diseases classified elsewhere*
Meningomyelitis in diseases classified elsewhere

4 + G06 **Intracranial and intraspinal abscess and granuloma**
Use additional code (B95-B97) to identify infectious agent.

+ G06.0 **Intracranial abscess and granuloma**
Brain [any part] abscess (embolic)
Cerebellar abscess (embolic)
Cerebral abscess (embolic)
Intracranial epidural abscess or granuloma
Intracranial extradural abscess or granuloma
Intracranial subdural abscess or granuloma
Otogenic abscess (embolic)

EXCLUDES 1 *tuberculous intracranial abscess and granuloma (A17.81)*

Intracranial abscess and granuloma

566   © 2017 DecisionHealth

● New   ▲ Revised   *Manifestation*   4 - 7 Digit Indicators   ▣ Laterality   A Adult (15+ years)   M Maternity (12-55 years)   N Newborn   P Pediatric (0-17 years)   ♂ Male   ♀ Female
✖ Deleted   Unspecified   + Additional code

2017 ICD-10-CM Expert for Physicians

+ G06.1 Intraspinal abscess and granuloma
Abscess (embolic) of spinal cord [any part]
Intraspinal epidural abscess or granuloma
Intraspinal extradural abscess or granuloma
Intraspinal subdural abscess or granuloma
> **EXCLUDES 1** *tuberculous intraspinal abscess and granuloma (A17.81)*

+ G06.2 Extradural and subdural abscess, unspecified

G07 *Intracranial and intraspinal abscess and granuloma in diseases classified elsewhere*
Code first underlying disease, such as:
schistosomiasis granuloma of brain (B65.-)
> **EXCLUDES 1** *abscess of brain:*
> *amebic (A06.6)*
> *chromomycotic (B43.1)*
> *gonococcal (A54.82)*
> *tuberculous (A17.81)*
> *tuberculoma of meninges (A17.1)*

G08 Intracranial and intraspinal phlebitis and thrombophlebitis
Septic embolism of intracranial or intraspinal venous sinuses and veins
Septic endophlebitis of intracranial or intraspinal venous sinuses and veins
Septic phlebitis of intracranial or intraspinal venous sinuses and veins
Septic thrombophlebitis of intracranial or intraspinal venous sinuses and veins
Septic thrombosis of intracranial or intraspinal venous sinuses and veins
> **EXCLUDES 1** *intracranial phlebitis and thrombophlebitis complicating:*
> *abortion, ectopic or molar pregnancy (O00-O07, O08.7)*
> *pregnancy, childbirth and the puerperium (O22.5, O87.3)*
> *nonpyogenic intracranial phlebitis and thrombophlebitis (I67.6)*
> **EXCLUDES 2** *intracranial phlebitis and thrombophlebitis complicating nonpyogenic intraspinal phlebitis and thrombophlebitis (G95.1)*
> **DEFINITION** Inflammation and/or blood clot formation in a large vein or channel for venous blood circulation in the brain or spine.

G09 Sequelae of inflammatory diseases of central nervous system
Note: Category G09 is to be used to indicate conditions whose primary classification is to G00-G08 as the cause of sequelae, themselves classifiable elsewhere. The 'sequelae' include conditions specified as residuals.
Code first:
condition resulting from (sequela) of inflammatory diseases of central nervous system

Systemic atrophies primarily affecting the central nervous system (G10-G14)

G10 Huntington's disease
Huntington's chorea
Huntington's dementia
> **CODING TIP ✓** Huntington's disease is a progressive neurological disorder that includes dementia and mental deterioration as part of its progressive course. An additional code (F02-) should be assigned to identify dementia with or without behavioral disturbance.
> **DEFINITION** A genetic, degenerative disorder of the neurons of the brain, characterized by progressive difficulty with physical and mental tasks until death occurs.

◢ G11 Hereditary ataxia
> **EXCLUDES 2** *cerebral palsy (G80.-)*
> *hereditary and idiopathic neuropathy (G60.-)*
> *metabolic disorders (E70-E88)*
> **CODING TIP ✓** **Documentation:** When assigning a code from category G11.-, the coder should review the record in full and assign the most specific code. Coders should not, however, assign codes for early vs. late onset or a hereditary vs. congenital condition unless specifically reported as confirmed by the patient's physician in the record.

G11.0 Congenital nonprogressive ataxia
G11.1 Early-onset cerebellar ataxia
Early-onset cerebellar ataxia with essential tremor
Early-onset cerebellar ataxia with myoclonus [Hunt's ataxia]
Early-onset cerebellar ataxia with retained tendon reflexes
Friedreich's ataxia (autosomal recessive)
X-linked recessive spinocerebellar ataxia
G11.2 Late-onset cerebellar ataxia Ⓐ
G11.3 Cerebellar ataxia with defective DNA repair
Ataxia telangiectasia [Louis-Bar]
> **EXCLUDES 2** *Cockayne's syndrome (Q87.1)*
> *other disorders of purine and pyrimidine metabolism (E79.-)*
> *xeroderma pigmentosum (Q82.1)*
G11.4 Hereditary spastic paraplegia
> **DEFINITION** Hereditary disorder characterized by lower-limb spasticity and near total loss of joint flexibility while the upper limbs remain unaffected.
G11.8 Other hereditary ataxias
G11.9 Hereditary ataxia, unspecified
Hereditary cerebellar ataxia NOS
Hereditary cerebellar degeneration
Hereditary cerebellar disease
Hereditary cerebellar syndrome

◢ G12 Spinal muscular atrophy and related syndromes
G12.0 Infantile spinal muscular atrophy, type I [Werdnig-Hoffman]
G12.1 Other inherited spinal muscular atrophy
Adult form spinal muscular atrophy
Childhood form, type II spinal muscular atrophy
Distal spinal muscular atrophy
Juvenile form, type III spinal muscular atrophy [Kugelberg-Welander]
Progressive bulbar palsy of childhood [Fazio-Londe]
Scapuloperoneal form spinal muscular atrophy
◢ G12.2 Motor neuron disease
G12.20 Motor neuron disease, unspecified
G12.21 Amyotrophic lateral sclerosis Ⓐ
Progressive spinal muscle atrophy

Amyotrophic lateral sclerosis (ALS)

Also known as Lou Gehrig's Disease, ALS is caused by the degeneration and death of motor neurons in the spinal cord and brain

Normal spinal neuron   Diseased spinal neuron

Affected nerve fiber

Normal nerve fiber

Normal skeletal muscle   Wasted skeletal muscle

G12.22 Progressive bulbar palsy
G12.29 Other motor neuron disease
Familial motor neuron disease
Primary lateral sclerosis
G12.8 Other spinal muscular atrophies and related syndromes
G12.9 Spinal muscular atrophy, unspecified
◢ G13 Systemic atrophies primarily affecting central nervous system in diseases classified elsewhere
G13.0 *Paraneoplastic neuromyopathy and neuropathy*
Carcinomatous neuromyopathy
Sensorial paraneoplastic neuropathy [Denny Brown]
Code first:
underlying neoplasm (C00-D49)
G13.1 *Other systemic atrophy primarily affecting central nervous system in neoplastic disease*
Paraneoplastic limbic encephalopathy
Code first:
underlying neoplasm (C00-D49)
G13.2 *Systemic atrophy primarily affecting the central nervous system in myxedema*
Code first underlying disease, such as:
hypothyroidism (E03.-)
myxedematous congenital iodine deficiency (E00.1)

● New ▲ Revised *Manifestation* ◢-◢ Digit Indicators ⊟ Laterality Ⓐ Adult (15+ years) Ⓜ Maternity (12-55 years) Ⓝ Newborn Ⓟ Pediatric (0-17 years) ♂ Male ♀ Female
✖ Deleted Unspecified + Additional code

G13.8 *Systemic atrophy primarily affecting central nervous system in other diseases classified elsewhere*
Code first:
underlying disease

G14 **Postpolio syndrome**
| INCLUDES | postpolio myelitic syndrome

| EXCLUDES 1 | *sequelae of poliomyelitis (B91)*

| CODING TIP ✓ | Post Polio Syndrome is differentiated from sequelae of poliomyelitis or residual deficits related to resolved poliomyelitis. When the record only specifies residual deficits related to resolved poliomyelitis, but does not specify post polio syndrome, coders should assign B91, Sequelae of poliomyelitis.

Extrapyramidal and movement disorders (G20-G26)

G20 **Parkinson's disease**
Hemiparkinsonism
Idiopathic Parkinsonism or Parkinson's disease
Paralysis agitans
Parkinsonism or Parkinson's disease NOS
Primary Parkinsonism or Parkinson's disease
| EXCLUDES 1 | *dementia with Parkinsonism (G31.83)*

| CODING TIP ✓ | When a patient is reported to have Parkinson's disease with related dementia, assign G20 followed by a code from category F02.8-, Dementia in diseases classified elsewhere. The physician must report the dementia as related to the Parkinson's disease in order to code the dementia as a manifestation.

| CODING TIP ✓ | Parkinsonism disorders are representative of multiple primary and secondary disorders that result in Parkinsonian traits, but not all patients with Parkinsonism disorders have Parkinson's disease. Only when the physician specifies Parkinson's disease should G20 be coded. Do not assign code G20 for a patient with a Parkinsonism disorder.
AHA: 2Q 2016, 7

◢ G21 **Secondary parkinsonism**
| EXCLUDES 1 | *dementia with Parkinsonism (G31.83)*
Huntington's disease (G10)
Shy-Drager syndrome (G90.3)
syphilitic Parkinsonism (A52.19)

+ G21.0 **Malignant neuroleptic syndrome**
Use additional code for adverse effect, if applicable, to identify drug (T43.3X5, T43.4X5, T43.505, T43.595)
| EXCLUDES 1 | *neuroleptic induced parkinsonism (G21.11)*

⑤ G21.1 **Other drug-induced secondary parkinsonism**
| CODING TIP ✓ | Drug induced parkinsonism is considered an adverse effect of a drug. The causative relationship must be stated by the physician. Assign an additional code to identify the drug.

+ G21.11 **Neuroleptic induced parkinsonism**
Use additional code for adverse effect, if applicable, to identify drug (T43.3X5, T43.4X5, T43.505, T43.595)
| EXCLUDES 1 | *malignant neuroleptic syndrome (G21.0)*

+ G21.19 **Other drug induced secondary parkinsonism**
Use additional code for adverse effect, if applicable, to identify drug (T36-T50 with fifth or sixth character 5)

G21.2 **Secondary parkinsonism due to other external agents**
Code first:
(T51-T65) to identify external agent

G21.3 **Postencephalitic parkinsonism**
G21.4 **Vascular parkinsonism**
G21.8 **Other secondary parkinsonism**
G21.9 **Secondary parkinsonism, unspecified**

◢ G23 **Other degenerative diseases of basal ganglia**
| EXCLUDES 2 | *multi-system degeneration of the autonomic nervous system (G90.3)*

G23.0 **Hallervorden-Spatz disease**
Pigmentary pallidal degeneration
G23.1 **Progressive supranuclear ophthalmoplegia [Steele-Richardson-Olszewski]**
Progressive supranuclear palsy
G23.2 **Striatonigral degeneration**

G23.8 **Other specified degenerative diseases of basal ganglia**
Calcification of basal ganglia
G23.9 **Degenerative disease of basal ganglia, unspecified**

◢ G24 **Dystonia**
| INCLUDES | dyskinesia
| EXCLUDES 2 | *athetoid cerebral palsy (G80.3)*

| CODING TIP ✓ | Dystonias may be specified to congenital or acquired, primary or secondary, and may be anatomically specific. When coding dystonias, the coder should attempt to obtain specific information regarding the origin of the dystonia and the specific type of movement disorder so that the most specific code may be assigned.

⑤ + G24.0 **Drug induced dystonia**
Use additional code code for adverse effect, if applicable, to identify drug (T36-T50 with fifth or sixth character 5)

+ G24.01 **Drug induced subacute dyskinesia**
Drug induced blepharospasm
Drug induced orofacial dyskinesia
Neuroleptic induced tardive dyskinesia
Tardive dyskinesia
| CODING TIP ✓ | Tardive dyskinesia due to use of medications, also referred to as lingual-facial-buccal dyskinesia, which presents as uncontrollable movements of the mouth, tongue, jaw, and cheeks, should be coded using G24.01 followed by the appropriate code to identify the drug causing the dyskinesia. This effect is commonly found following the use of neuroleptic medications.

| DEFINITION | Involuntary repetitive movements of facial, buccal, oral, and cervical muscles, induced by long-term use of antipsychotic agent, sometimes persisting after withdrawal of the agent.

+ G24.02 **Drug induced acute dystonia**
Acute dystonic reaction to drugs
Neuroleptic induced acute dystonia
+ G24.09 **Other drug induced dystonia**
G24.1 **Genetic torsion dystonia**
Dystonia deformans progressiva
Dystonia musculorum deformans
Familial torsion dystonia
Idiopathic familial dystonia
Idiopathic (torsion) dystonia NOS
(Schwalbe-) Ziehen-Oppenheim disease
G24.2 **Idiopathic nonfamilial dystonia**
G24.3 **Spasmodic torticollis**
| EXCLUDES 1 | *congenital torticollis (Q68.0)*
hysterical torticollis (F44.4)
ocular torticollis (R29.891)
psychogenic torticollis (F45.8)
torticollis NOS (M43.6)
traumatic recurrent torticollis (S13.4)

| DEFINITION | Contractions of the neck muscles causing contortion, pain, and abnormal head posture.

G24.4 **Idiopathic orofacial dystonia**
Orofacial dyskinesia
| EXCLUDES 1 | *drug induced orofacial dyskinesia (G24.01)*

G24.5 **Blepharospasm**
| EXCLUDES 1 | *drug induced blepharospasm (G24.01)*

| DEFINITION | Spasm of the orbicularis oculi muscle, causing uncontrolled winking or blinking.

G24.8 **Other dystonia**
Acquired torsion dystonia NOS
G24.9 **Dystonia, unspecified**
Dyskinesia NOS

◢ G25 **Other extrapyramidal and movement disorders**
| EXCLUDES 2 | *sleep related movement disorders (G47.6-)*

G25.0 **Essential tremor**
Familial tremor
| EXCLUDES 1 | *tremor NOS (R25.1)*

| CODING TIP ✓ | Do not assign G25.0 to report unspecified tremors or tremors in a patient with a confirmed diagnosis of Parkinson's disease.

+ G25.1 **Drug-induced tremor**
Use additional code for adverse effect, if applicable, to identify drug (T36-T50 with fifth or sixth character 5)

● New   ▲ Revised   *Manifestation*   ◢-⑦ Digit Indicators   ▣ Laterality   Ⓐ Adult (15+ years)   Ⓜ Maternity (12-55 years)   Ⓝ Newborn   Ⓟ Pediatric (0-17 years)   ♂ Male   ♀ Female
✖ Deleted   Unspecified   + Additional code

568   © 2017 DecisionHealth   2017 ICD-10-CM Expert for Physicians

G25.2 **Other specified forms of tremor**
Intention tremor

✛ **G25.3** **Myoclonus**
Drug-induced myoclonus
Palatal myoclonus
Use additional code for adverse effect, if applicable, to identify drug (T36-T50 with fifth or sixth character 5)
EXCLUDES 1 *facial myokymia (G51.4)*
myoclonic epilepsy (G40.-)
CODING TIP ✓ Myoclonus is also reported as muscle twitching and is often a symptom of a more specific disease process. When the specific disease process is known, code the underlying disease. If myoclonus is related to the adverse effect of a medication, use an additional code to identify the drug. This code should not be assigned for myoclonic epilepsy or seizures.
DEFINITION Spontaneous contractions of a muscle or group of muscles as a part of a disease process, drug side effect, or abnormal physiological response.

✛ **G25.4** **Drug-induced chorea**
Use additional code for adverse effect, if applicable, to identify drug (T36-T50 with fifth or sixth character 5)

G25.5 **Other chorea**
Chorea NOS
EXCLUDES 1 *chorea NOS with heart involvement (I02.0)*
Huntington's chorea (G10)
rheumatic chorea (I02.-)
Sydenham's chorea (I02.-)

⑤ **G25.6** **Drug induced tics and other tics of organic origin**
✛ **G25.61** **Drug induced tics**
Use additional code for adverse effect, if applicable, to identify drug (T36-T50 with fifth or sixth character 5)
G25.69 **Other tics of organic origin**
EXCLUDES 1 *habit spasm (F95.9)*
tic NOS (F95.9)
Tourette's syndrome (F95.2)

⑤✛ **G25.7** **Other and unspecified drug induced movement disorders**
Use additional code for adverse effect, if applicable, to identify drug (T36-T50 with fifth or sixth character 5)
✛ **G25.70** **Drug induced movement disorder, unspecified**
✛ **G25.71** **Drug induced akathisia**
Drug induced acathisia
Neuroleptic induced acute akathisia
CODING TIP ✓ Akathisia is a syndrome characterized by a restless inability to maintain stillness or to "sit still" and is frequently induced by the use of various medications, including antipsychotics. When caused by the effect of a drug, an additional code should be assigned to identify the drug.
✛ **G25.79** **Other drug induced movement disorders**
⑤ **G25.8** **Other specified extrapyramidal and movement disorders**
G25.81 **Restless legs syndrome**
DEFINITION Irresistible urge to move legs, particularly when sitting or lying down, with leg sensations such as creeping, crawling, itching, tugging, tightening, or pulling alleviated upon movement.
G25.82 **Stiff-man syndrome**
DEFINITION Progressive fluctuating rigidity of axial and limb muscles in the absence of any signs of cerebral and/or spinal cord disease.
G25.83 **Benign shuddering attacks**
G25.89 **Other specified extrapyramidal and movement disorders**
G25.9 **Extrapyramidal and movement disorder, unspecified**

G26 **Extrapyramidal and movement disorders in diseases classified elsewhere**
Code first:
underlying disease

Other degenerative diseases of the nervous system (G30-G32)

④✛ **G30** **Alzheimer's disease**
INCLUDES Alzheimer's dementia senile and presenile forms
Use additional code to identify:
delirium, if applicable (F05)
dementia with behavioral disturbance (F02.81)
dementia without behavioral disturbance (F02.80)
EXCLUDES 1 *senile degeneration of brain NEC (G31.1)*
senile dementia NOS (F03)
senility NOS (R41.81)
CODING TIP ✓ **Documentation:** Alzheimer's disease is a particular neurological condition and must be specifically confirmed by a physician. Early onset Alzheimer's is defined as diagnosis prior to the age of 65, however the designation of early and late onset must be documented by, or confirmed with, the patient's physician and may not be assumed. Query the physician if the information is not readily available and, if unable to make a determination, assign code G30.9 for Alzheimer's disease, unspecified.
DEFINITION Progressive degenerative disease of the brain of unknown cause with diffuse atrophy throughout the cerebral cortex; it initially presents with slight memory disturbance or personality changes that progressively deteriorate to profound memory loss and dementia.
✛ **G30.0** **Alzheimer's disease with early onset**
CODING TIP ✓ Early onset Alzheimer's is very uncommon and is diagnosed prior to the age of 65. Coders may not assume a diagnosis of early onset Alzheimer's disease, but must have confirmed evidence of this from the patient's physician in order to assign the diagnosis appropriately.
✛ **G30.1** **Alzheimer's disease with late onset** Ⓐ
CODING TIP ✓ Late onset Alzheimer's is the most common type and presents with symptoms after the age of 65. Coders may not assume a diagnosis of Late onset Alzheimer's disease, but must have confirmed evidence of this from the patient's physician in order to assign the diagnosis appropriately.
✛ **G30.8** **Other Alzheimer's disease**
✛ **G30.9** **Alzheimer's disease, unspecified**
AHA: 2Q 2016, 6
AHA: 4Q 2012, 95

④✛ **G31** **Other degenerative diseases of nervous system, not elsewhere classified**
Use additional code to identify:
dementia with behavioral disturbance (F02.81)
dementia without behavioral disturbance (F02.80)
EXCLUDES 2 *Reye's syndrome (G93.7)*
⑤✛ **G31.0** **Frontotemporal dementia**
✛ **G31.01** **Pick's disease**
Primary progressive aphasia
Progressive isolated aphasia
DEFINITION Rare, progressive, degenerative disease of the brain, similar to Alzheimer's disease but with cortical atrophy confined to the frontal and temporal lobes.
✛ **G31.09** **Other frontotemporal dementia**
Frontal dementia
✛ **G31.1** **Senile degeneration of brain, not elsewhere classified**
EXCLUDES 1 *Alzheimer's disease (G30.-)*
senility NOS (R41.81)
✛ **G31.2** **Degeneration of nervous system due to alcohol**
Alcoholic cerebellar ataxia
Alcoholic cerebellar degeneration
Alcoholic cerebral degeneration
Alcoholic encephalopathy
Dysfunction of the autonomic nervous system due to alcohol
Code also:
associated alcoholism (F10.-)

● New ▲ Revised *Manifestation* ④-⑦ Digit Indicators ⊟ Laterality Ⓐ Adult (15+ years) Ⓜ Maternity (12-55 years) Ⓝ Newborn Ⓟ Pediatric (0-17 years) ♂ Male ♀ Female
✖ Deleted Unspecified ✛ Additional code

2017 ICD-10-CM Expert for Physicians

© 2017 DecisionHealth 569

G25.2 — G31.2

CODING TIP ✓ Cerebellar ataxia, encephalopathy, cerebellar degeneration, and autonomic dysfunction/degeneration, when specified as due to alcohol, should be coded to G31.2. Also assign the appropriate F10.- code to identify alcohol dependence/alcoholism, and, when applicable, a code to specify dementia (with or without behavior disturbance) as a manifestation (F02.8-).

⑤ + **G31.8** **Other specified degenerative diseases of nervous system**

+ **G31.81** **Alpers disease**
Grey-matter degeneration

+ **G31.82** **Leigh's disease**
Subacute necrotizing encephalopathy

+ **G31.83** **Dementia with Lewy bodies**
Dementia with Parkinsonism
Lewy body dementia
Lewy body disease

▲ + **G31.84** **Mild cognitive impairment, so stated**

EXCLUDES 1 *age related cognitive decline (R41.81)*
altered mental status (R41.82)
cerebral degeneration (G31.9)
change in mental status (R41.82)
cognitive deficits following (sequelae of) cerebral hemorrhage or infarction (I69.01-, I69.11-, I69.21-, I69.31-, I69.81-, I69.91-)
cognitive impairment due to intracranial or head injury (S06.-)
dementia (F01.-, F02.-, F03)
mild memory disturbance (F06.8)
neurologic neglect syndrome (R41.4)
personality change, nonpsychotic (F68.8)

DEFINITION Impairment in memory or other specific cognitive function, beyond what is normally seen at a given age, but with function remaining relatively intact in the other cognitive domains.

+ **G31.85** **Corticobasal degeneration**

+ **G31.89** **Other specified degenerative diseases of nervous system**

+ **G31.9** **Degenerative disease of nervous system, unspecified**

④ **G32** **Other degenerative disorders of nervous system in diseases classified elsewhere**

G32.0 *Subacute combined degeneration of spinal cord in diseases classified elsewhere*
Dana-Putnam syndrome
Sclerosis of spinal cord (combined) (dorsolateral) (posterolateral)
Code first underlying disease, such as:
anemia (D51.9)
dietary (D51.3)
pernicious (D51.0)
vitamin B12 deficiency (E53.8)

EXCLUDES 1 *syphilitic combined degeneration of spinal cord (A52.11)*

⑤ **G32.8** **Other specified degenerative disorders of nervous system in diseases classified elsewhere**
Code first underlying disease, such as:
amyloidosis cerebral degeneration (E85.-)
cerebral degeneration (due to) hypothyroidism (E00.0-E03.9)
cerebral degeneration (due to) neoplasm (C00-D49)
cerebral degeneration (due to) vitamin B deficiency, except thiamine (E52-E53.-)

EXCLUDES 1 *superior hemorrhagic polioencephalitis [Wernicke's encephalopathy] (E51.2)*

G32.81 *Cerebellar ataxia in diseases classified elsewhere*
Code first underlying disease, such as:
celiac disease (with gluten ataxia) (K90.0)
cerebellar ataxia (in) neoplastic disease (paraneoplastic cerebellar degeneration) (C00-D49)
non-celiac gluten ataxia (M35.9)

EXCLUDES 1 *systemic atrophy primarily affecting the central nervous system in alcoholic cerebellar ataxia (G31.2)*
systemic atrophy primarily affecting the central nervous system in myxedema (G13.2)

G32.89 *Other specified degenerative disorders of nervous system in diseases classified elsewhere*
Degenerative encephalopathy in diseases classified elsewhere

Demyelinating diseases of the central nervous system (G35-G37)

G35 **Multiple sclerosis**
Disseminated multiple sclerosis
Generalized multiple sclerosis
Multiple sclerosis NOS
Multiple sclerosis of brain stem
Multiple sclerosis of cord

Multiple sclerosis (MS)

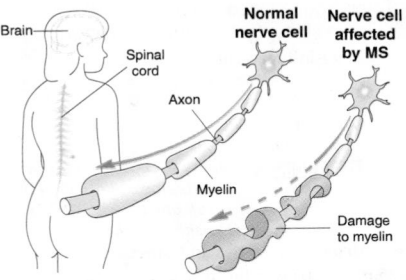

④ **G36** **Other acute disseminated demyelination**

EXCLUDES 1 *postinfectious encephalitis and encephalomyelitis NOS (G04.01)*

G36.0 **Neuromyelitis optica [Devic]**
Demyelination in optic neuritis
EXCLUDES 1 *optic neuritis NOS (H46)*

G36.1 **Acute and subacute hemorrhagic leukoencephalitis [Hurst]**

G36.8 **Other specified acute disseminated demyelination**

G36.9 **Acute disseminated demyelination, unspecified**

④ **G37** **Other demyelinating diseases of central nervous system**

G37.0 **Diffuse sclerosis of central nervous system**
Periaxial encephalitis
Schilder's disease
EXCLUDES 1 *X linked adrenoleukodystrophy (E71.52-)*

G37.1 **Central demyelination of corpus callosum**

G37.2 **Central pontine myelinolysis**

G37.3 **Acute transverse myelitis in demyelinating disease of central nervous system**
Acute transverse myelitis NOS
Acute transverse myelopathy
EXCLUDES 1 *multiple sclerosis (G35)*
neuromyelitis optica [Devic] (G36.0)

DEFINITION Spinal cord disorder with inflammatory lesions across the entire width of one level; numbness, back pain, weakness, sensory loss, motor and sphincter deficits, loss of bladder and bowel control appear quickly and progress to paraplegia.

G37.4 **Subacute necrotizing myelitis of central nervous system**

G37.5 **Concentric sclerosis [Balo] of central nervous system**

G37.8 **Other specified demyelinating diseases of central nervous system**

G37.9 **Demyelinating disease of central nervous system, unspecified**

● New   ▲ Revised   *Manifestation*   ④-⑦ Digit Indicators   ▱ Laterality   ◭ Adult (15+ years)   Ⓜ Maternity (12-55 years)   Ⓝ Newborn   Ⓟ Pediatric (0-17 years)   ♂ Male   ♀ Female
✖ Deleted   Unspecified   + Additional code

570   © 2017 DecisionHealth

2017 ICD-10-CM Expert for Physicians

Episodic and paroxysmal disorders (G40-G47)

▲ �4 **G40** **Epilepsy and recurrent seizures**

Note: the following terms are to be considered equivalent to intractable: pharmacoresistant (pharmacologically resistant), treatment resistant, refractory (medically) and poorly controlled

EXCLUDES 1 *conversion disorder with seizures (F44.5)*
convulsions NOS (R56.9)
post traumatic seizures (R56.1)
seizure (convulsive) NOS (R56.9)
seizure of newborn (P90)

EXCLUDES 2 *hippocampal sclerosis (G93.81)*
mesial temporal sclerosis (G93.81)
temporal sclerosis (G93.81)
Todd's paralysis (G83.84)

CODING TIP ✓ When coding epileptic syndromes, coders should note that seizure(s)/epileptic disorders noted by the physician as treatment- or medication-resistant, refractory, or poorly controlled should be coded to intractable. Coders should not assign R56.9, Unspecified convulsions, for patients experiencing seizure disorders or recurrent seizures. Recurrent seizures and unspecified seizure disorders, when not reported as intractable, should be coded to G40.909.

⑤ **G40.0** **Localization-related (focal) (partial) idiopathic epilepsy and epileptic syndromes with seizures of localized onset**
Benign childhood epilepsy with centrotemporal EEG spikes
Childhood epilepsy with occipital EEG paroxysms

EXCLUDES 1 *adult onset localization-related epilepsy (G40.1-, G40.2-)*

⑥ **G40.00** **Localization-related (focal) (partial) idiopathic epilepsy and epileptic syndromes with seizures of localized onset, not intractable**
Localization-related (focal) (partial) idiopathic epilepsy and epileptic syndromes with seizures of localized onset without intractability

G40.001 **Localization-related (focal) (partial) idiopathic epilepsy and epileptic syndromes with seizures of localized onset, not intractable, with status epilepticus**

G40.009 **Localization-related (focal) (partial) idiopathic epilepsy and epileptic syndromes with seizures of localized onset, not intractable, without status epilepticus**
Localization-related (focal) (partial) idiopathic epilepsy and epileptic syndromes with seizures of localized onset NOS

⑥ **G40.01** **Localization-related (focal) (partial) idiopathic epilepsy and epileptic syndromes with seizures of localized onset, intractable**

G40.011 **Localization-related (focal) (partial) idiopathic epilepsy and epileptic syndromes with seizures of localized onset, intractable, with status epilepticus**

G40.019 **Localization-related (focal) (partial) idiopathic epilepsy and epileptic syndromes with seizures of localized onset, intractable, without status epilepticus**

⑤ **G40.1** **Localization-related (focal) (partial) symptomatic epilepsy and epileptic syndromes with simple partial seizures**
Attacks without alteration of consciousness
Epilepsia partialis continua [Kozhevnikof]
Simple partial seizures developing into secondarily generalized seizures

⑥ **G40.10** **Localization-related (focal) (partial) symptomatic epilepsy and epileptic syndromes with simple partial seizures, not intractable**
Localization-related (focal) (partial) symptomatic epilepsy and epileptic syndromes with simple partial seizures without intractability

G40.101 **Localization-related (focal) (partial) symptomatic epilepsy and epileptic syndromes with simple partial seizures, not intractable, with status epilepticus**

G40.109 **Localization-related (focal) (partial) symptomatic epilepsy and epileptic syndromes with simple partial seizures, not intractable, without status epilepticus**
Localization-related (focal) (partial) symptomatic epilepsy and epileptic syndromes with simple partial seizures NOS

⑥ **G40.11** **Localization-related (focal) (partial) symptomatic epilepsy and epileptic syndromes with simple partial seizures, intractable**

G40.111 **Localization-related (focal) (partial) symptomatic epilepsy and epileptic syndromes with simple partial seizures, intractable, with status epilepticus**

G40.119 **Localization-related (focal) (partial) symptomatic epilepsy and epileptic syndromes with simple partial seizures, intractable, without status epilepticus**

⑤ **G40.2** **Localization-related (focal) (partial) symptomatic epilepsy and epileptic syndromes with complex partial seizures**
Attacks with alteration of consciousness, often with automatisms
Complex partial seizures developing into secondarily generalized seizures

⑥ **G40.20** **Localization-related (focal) (partial) symptomatic epilepsy and epileptic syndromes with complex partial seizures, not intractable**
Localization-related (focal) (partial) symptomatic epilepsy and epileptic syndromes with complex partial seizures without intractability

G40.201 **Localization-related (focal) (partial) symptomatic epilepsy and epileptic syndromes with complex partial seizures, not intractable, with status epilepticus**

G40.209 **Localization-related (focal) (partial) symptomatic epilepsy and epileptic syndromes with complex partial seizures, not intractable, without status epilepticus**
Localization-related (focal) (partial) symptomatic epilepsy and epileptic syndromes with complex partial seizures NOS

⑥ **G40.21** **Localization-related (focal) (partial) symptomatic epilepsy and epileptic syndromes with complex partial seizures, intractable**

G40.211 **Localization-related (focal) (partial) symptomatic epilepsy and epileptic syndromes with complex partial seizures, intractable, with status epilepticus**

G40.219 **Localization-related (focal) (partial) symptomatic epilepsy and epileptic syndromes with complex partial seizures, intractable, without status epilepticus**

⑤ **G40.3** **Generalized idiopathic epilepsy and epileptic syndromes**
Code also:
MERRF syndrome, if applicable (E88.42)

⑥ **G40.30** **Generalized idiopathic epilepsy and epileptic syndromes, not intractable**
Generalized idiopathic epilepsy and epileptic syndromes without intractability

G40.301 **Generalized idiopathic epilepsy and epileptic syndromes, not intractable, with status epilepticus**

G40.309 **Generalized idiopathic epilepsy and epileptic syndromes, not intractable, without status epilepticus**
Generalized idiopathic epilepsy and epileptic syndromes NOS

⑥ **G40.31** **Generalized idiopathic epilepsy and epileptic syndromes, intractable**

G40.311 **Generalized idiopathic epilepsy and epileptic syndromes, intractable, with status epilepticus**

G40.319 **Generalized idiopathic epilepsy and epileptic syndromes, intractable, without status epilepticus**

⑤ **G40.A** **Absence epileptic syndrome**
Childhood absence epilepsy [pyknolepsy]
Juvenile absence epilepsy
Absence epileptic syndrome, NOS

⑥ **G40.A0** **Absence epileptic syndrome, not intractable**

G40.A01 **Absence epileptic syndrome, not intractable, with status epilepticus**

G40.A09 **Absence epileptic syndrome, not intractable, without status epilepticus**

⑥ **G40.A1** **Absence epileptic syndrome, intractable**

G40.A11 **Absence epileptic syndrome, intractable, with status epilepticus**

G40.A19 **Absence epileptic syndrome, intractable, without status epilepticus**

● New   ▲ Revised   *Manifestation*   ◄-☑ Digit Indicators   ▤ Laterality   ▲ Adult (15+ years)   Ⓜ Maternity (12-55 years)   Ⓝ Newborn   ▣ Pediatric (0-17 years)   ♂ Male   ♀ Female
✖ Deleted   Unspecified   + Additional code

Diseases of the Nervous System

⑤ G40.B   Juvenile myoclonic epilepsy [impulsive petit mal]

⑥ G40.B0   Juvenile myoclonic epilepsy, not intractable

G40.B01   Juvenile myoclonic epilepsy, not intractable, with status epilepticus

G40.B09   Juvenile myoclonic epilepsy, not intractable, without status epilepticus

⑥ G40.B1   Juvenile myoclonic epilepsy, intractable

G40.B11   Juvenile myoclonic epilepsy, intractable, with status epilepticus

G40.B19   Juvenile myoclonic epilepsy, intractable, without status epilepticus

⑤ G40.4   Other generalized epilepsy and epileptic syndromes

Epilepsy with grand mal seizures on awakening
Epilepsy with myoclonic absences
Epilepsy with myoclonic-astatic seizures
Grand mal seizure NOS
Nonspecific atonic epileptic seizures
Nonspecific clonic epileptic seizures
Nonspecific myoclonic epileptic seizures
Nonspecific tonic epileptic seizures
Nonspecific tonic-clonic epileptic seizures
Symptomatic early myoclonic encephalopathy

⑥ G40.40   Other generalized epilepsy and epileptic syndromes, not intractable

Other generalized epilepsy and epileptic syndromes without intractability
Other generalized epilepsy and epileptic syndromes NOS

G40.401   Other generalized epilepsy and epileptic syndromes, not intractable, with status epilepticus

G40.409   Other generalized epilepsy and epileptic syndromes, not intractable, without status epilepticus

⑥ G40.41   Other generalized epilepsy and epileptic syndromes, intractable

G40.411   Other generalized epilepsy and epileptic syndromes, intractable, with status epilepticus

G40.419   Other generalized epilepsy and epileptic syndromes, intractable, without status epilepticus

⑤ ✚ G40.5   Epileptic seizures related to external causes

Epileptic seizures related to alcohol
Epileptic seizures related to drugs
Epileptic seizures related to hormonal changes
Epileptic seizures related to sleep deprivation
Epileptic seizures related to stress
Code also:
, if applicable, associated epilepsy and recurrent seizures (G40.-)
Use additional code for adverse effect, if applicable, to identify drug (T36-T50 with fifth or sixth character 5)

⑥ ✚ G40.50   Epileptic seizures related to external causes, not intractable

✚ G40.501   Epileptic seizures related to external causes, not intractable, with status epilepticus

✚ G40.509   Epileptic seizures related to external causes, not intractable, without status epilepticus

Epileptic seizures related to external causes, NOS

⑤ G40.8   Other epilepsy and recurrent seizures

Epilepsies and epileptic syndromes undetermined as to whether they are focal or generalized
Landau-Kleffner syndrome

⑥ G40.80   Other epilepsy

G40.801   Other epilepsy, not intractable, with status epilepticus

Other epilepsy without intractability with status epilepticus

G40.802   Other epilepsy, not intractable, without status epilepticus

Other epilepsy NOS
Other epilepsy without intractability without status epilepticus

G40.803   Other epilepsy, intractable, with status epilepticus

G40.804   Other epilepsy, intractable, without status epilepticus

⑥ G40.81   Lennox-Gastaut syndrome

G40.811   Lennox-Gastaut syndrome, not intractable, with status epilepticus

G40.812   Lennox-Gastaut syndrome, not intractable, without status epilepticus

G40.813   Lennox-Gastaut syndrome, intractable, with status epilepticus

G40.814   Lennox-Gastaut syndrome, intractable, without status epilepticus

⑥ G40.82   Epileptic spasms

Infantile spasms
Salaam attacks
West's syndrome

G40.821   Epileptic spasms, not intractable, with status epilepticus

G40.822   Epileptic spasms, not intractable, without status epilepticus

G40.823   Epileptic spasms, intractable, with status epilepticus

G40.824   Epileptic spasms, intractable, without status epilepticus

G40.89   Other seizures

EXCLUDES 1   *post traumatic seizures (R56.1)*
recurrent seizures NOS (G40.909)
seizure NOS (R56.9)

⑤ G40.9   Epilepsy, unspecified

⑥ G40.90   Epilepsy, unspecified, not intractable

Epilepsy, unspecified, without intractability

G40.901   Epilepsy, unspecified, not intractable, with status epilepticus

G40.909   Epilepsy, unspecified, not intractable, without status epilepticus

Epilepsy NOS
Epileptic convulsions NOS
Epileptic fits NOS
Epileptic seizures NOS
Recurrent seizures NOS
Seizure disorder NOS

CODING TIP ✓   Recurrent seizures and unspecified seizure disorders, when not identified as intractable, should be reported using this code. Do not assign R56.9, Unspecified convulsions, to report a diagnosis of recurrent seizures or seizure disorder.

⑥ G40.91   Epilepsy, unspecified, intractable

Intractable seizure disorder NOS

G40.911   Epilepsy, unspecified, intractable, with status epilepticus

G40.919   Epilepsy, unspecified, intractable, without status epilepticus

④ ✚ G43   Migraine

Note: the following terms are to be considered equivalent to intractable: pharmacoresistant (pharmacologically resistant), treatment resistant, refractory (medically) and poorly controlled
Use additional code for adverse effect, if applicable, to identify drug (T36-T50 with fifth or sixth character 5)

EXCLUDES 1   *headache NOS (R51)*
lower half migraine (G44.00)
EXCLUDES 2   *headache syndromes (G44.-)*

⑤ ✚ G43.0   Migraine without aura

Common migraine

EXCLUDES 1   *chronic migraine without aura (G43.7-)*

⑥ ✚ G43.00   Migraine without aura, not intractable

Migraine without aura without mention of refractory migraine

✚ G43.001   Migraine without aura, not intractable, with status migrainosus

✚ G43.009   Migraine without aura, not intractable, without status migrainosus

Migraine without aura NOS

⑥ ✚ G43.01   Migraine without aura, intractable

Migraine without aura with refractory migraine

✚ G43.011   Migraine without aura, intractable, with status migrainosus

✚ G43.019   Migraine without aura, intractable, without status migrainosus

● New   ▲ Revised   *Manifestation*   ④-⑦ Digit Indicators   ⊟ Laterality   Ⓐ Adult (15+ years)   Ⓜ Maternity (12-55 years)   Ⓝ Newborn   Ⓟ Pediatric (0-17 years)   ♂ Male   ♀ Female
✖ Deleted   Unspecified   ✚ Additional code

⑥＋ G43.1   Migraine with aura
Basilar migraine
Classical migraine
Migraine equivalents
Migraine preceded or accompanied by transient focal
   neurological phenomena
Migraine triggered seizures
Migraine with acute-onset aura
Migraine with aura without headache (migraine equivalents)
Migraine with prolonged aura
Migraine with typical aura
Retinal migraine
Code also:
   any associated seizure (G40.-, R56.9)
   EXCLUDES 1   *persistent migraine aura (G43.5-, G43.6-)*

⑥＋ G43.10   Migraine with aura, not intractable
Migraine with aura without mention of refractory
   migraine

＋ G43.101   Migraine with aura, not intractable, with status migrainosus

＋ G43.109   Migraine with aura, not intractable, without status migrainosus
Migraine with aura NOS

⑥＋ G43.11   Migraine with aura, intractable
Migraine with aura with refractory migraine

＋ G43.111   Migraine with aura, intractable, with status migrainosus

＋ G43.119   Migraine with aura, intractable, without status migrainosus

⑥＋ G43.4   Hemiplegic migraine
Familial migraine
Sporadic migraine

⑥＋ G43.40   Hemiplegic migraine, not intractable
Hemiplegic migraine without refractory migraine

＋ G43.401   Hemiplegic migraine, not intractable, with status migrainosus

＋ G43.409   Hemiplegic migraine, not intractable, without status migrainosus
Hemiplegic migraine NOS

⑥＋ G43.41   Hemiplegic migraine, intractable
Hemiplegic migraine with refractory migraine

＋ G43.411   Hemiplegic migraine, intractable, with status migrainosus

＋ G43.419   Hemiplegic migraine, intractable, without status migrainosus

⑥＋ G43.5   Persistent migraine aura without cerebral infarction

⑥＋ G43.50   Persistent migraine aura without cerebral infarction, not intractable
Persistent migraine aura without cerebral infarction,
   without refractory migraine

＋ G43.501   Persistent migraine aura without cerebral infarction, not intractable, with status migrainosus

＋ G43.509   Persistent migraine aura without cerebral infarction, not intractable, without status migrainosus
Persistent migraine aura NOS

⑥＋ G43.51   Persistent migraine aura without cerebral infarction, intractable
Persistent migraine aura without cerebral infarction,
   with refractory migraine

＋ G43.511   Persistent migraine aura without cerebral infarction, intractable, with status migrainosus

＋ G43.519   Persistent migraine aura without cerebral infarction, intractable, without status migrainosus

⑥＋ G43.6   Persistent migraine aura with cerebral infarction
Code also:
   the type of cerebral infarction (I63.-)

⑥＋ G43.60   Persistent migraine aura with cerebral infarction, not intractable
Persistent migraine aura with cerebral infarction,
   without refractory migraine

＋ G43.601   Persistent migraine aura with cerebral infarction, not intractable, with status migrainosus

＋ G43.609   Persistent migraine aura with cerebral infarction, not intractable, without status migrainosus

⑥＋ G43.61   Persistent migraine aura with cerebral infarction, intractable
Persistent migraine aura with cerebral infarction, with
   refractory migraine

＋ G43.611   Persistent migraine aura with cerebral infarction, intractable, with status migrainosus

＋ G43.619   Persistent migraine aura with cerebral infarction, intractable, without status migrainosus

⑥＋ G43.7   Chronic migraine without aura
Transformed migraine
   EXCLUDES 1   *migraine without aura (G43.0-)*

⑥＋ G43.70   Chronic migraine without aura, not intractable
Chronic migraine without aura, without refractory
   migraine

＋ G43.701   Chronic migraine without aura, not intractable, with status migrainosus

＋ G43.709   Chronic migraine without aura, not intractable, without status migrainosus
Chronic migraine without aura NOS

⑥＋ G43.71   Chronic migraine without aura, intractable
Chronic migraine without aura, with refractory
   migraine

＋ G43.711   Chronic migraine without aura, intractable, with status migrainosus

＋ G43.719   Chronic migraine without aura, intractable, without status migrainosus

⑥＋ G43.A   Cyclical vomiting

＋ G43.A0   Cyclical vomiting, not intractable
Cyclical vomiting, without refractory migraine

＋ G43.A1   Cyclical vomiting, intractable
Cyclical vomiting, with refractory migraine

⑥＋ G43.B   Ophthalmoplegic migraine

＋ G43.B0   Ophthalmoplegic migraine, not intractable
Ophthalmoplegic migraine, without refractory migraine

＋ G43.B1   Ophthalmoplegic migraine, intractable
Ophthalmoplegic migraine, with refractory migraine

⑥＋ G43.C   Periodic headache syndromes in child or adult

＋ G43.C0   Periodic headache syndromes in child or adult, not intractable
Periodic headache syndromes in child or adult, without
   refractory migraine

＋ G43.C1   Periodic headache syndromes in child or adult, intractable
Periodic headache syndromes in child or adult, with
   refractory migraine

⑥＋ G43.D   Abdominal migraine

＋ G43.D0   Abdominal migraine, not intractable
Abdominal migraine, without refractory migraine

＋ G43.D1   Abdominal migraine, intractable
Abdominal migraine, with refractory migraine

⑥＋ G43.8   Other migraine

⑥＋ G43.80   Other migraine, not intractable
Other migraine, without refractory migraine

＋ G43.801   Other migraine, not intractable, with status migrainosus

＋ G43.809   Other migraine, not intractable, without status migrainosus

⑥＋ G43.81   Other migraine, intractable
Other migraine, with refractory migraine

＋ G43.811   Other migraine, intractable, with status migrainosus

＋ G43.819   Other migraine, intractable, without status migrainosus

⑥＋ G43.82   Menstrual migraine, not intractable
Menstrual headache, not intractable
Menstrual migraine, without refractory migraine
Menstrually related migraine, not intractable
Pre-menstrual headache, not intractable
Pre-menstrual migraine, not intractable
Pure menstrual migraine, not intractable
Code also:
   associated premenstrual tension syndrome (N94.3)

＋ G43.821   Menstrual migraine, not intractable, with status migrainosus ♀

＋ G43.829   Menstrual migraine, not intractable, without status migrainosus ♀
Menstrual migraine NOS

● New   ▲ Revised   *Manifestation*   ④-⑦ Digit Indicators   ⊟ Laterality   Ⓐ Adult (15+ years)   Ⓜ Maternity (12-55 years)   Ⓝ Newborn   ⓅPediatric (0-17 years)   ♂ Male   ♀ Female
✕ Deleted   Unspecified   ＋ Additional code

2017 ICD-10-CM Expert for Physicians

© 2017 DecisionHealth   573

⑥✚ G43.83   Menstrual migraine, intractable
Menstrual headache, intractable
Menstrual migraine, with refractory migraine
Menstrually related migraine, intractable
Pre-menstrual headache, intractable
Pre-menstrual migraine, intractable
Pure menstrual migraine, intractable
Code also:
  associated premenstrual tension syndrome (N94.3)

**✚ G43.831   Menstrual migraine, intractable, with status ♀
                migrainosus**
**✚ G43.839   Menstrual migraine, intractable, without ♀
                status migrainosus**

⑤✚ G43.9   Migraine, unspecified

⑥✚ G43.90   Migraine, unspecified, not intractable
Migraine, unspecified, without refractory migraine

**✚ G43.901   Migraine, unspecified, not intractable, with
                status migrainosus**
Status migrainosus NOS

**✚ G43.909   Migraine, unspecified, not intractable, without
                status migrainosus**
Migraine NOS

⑥✚ G43.91   Migraine, unspecified, intractable
Migraine, unspecified, with refractory migraine

**✚ G43.911   Migraine, unspecified, intractable, with status
                migrainosus**
**✚ G43.919   Migraine, unspecified, intractable, without
                status migrainosus**

④ G44   Other headache syndromes
EXCLUDES 1	headache NOS (R51)
EXCLUDES 2	atypical facial pain (G50.1)
	headache due to lumbar puncture (G97.1)
	migraines (G43.-)
	trigeminal neuralgia (G50.0)

**⑤ G44.0   Cluster headaches and other trigeminal autonomic
            cephalgias (TAC)**

⑥ G44.00   Cluster headache syndrome, unspecified
Ciliary neuralgia
Cluster headache NOS
Histamine cephalgia
Lower half migraine
Migrainous neuralgia

**G44.001   Cluster headache syndrome, unspecified,
              intractable**
**G44.009   Cluster headache syndrome, unspecified, not
              intractable**
Cluster headache syndrome NOS

⑥ G44.01   Episodic cluster headache
DEFINITION   Distinctive headache marked by
excruciating, searing pain that develops quickly
without warning on one side and occurs in
frequent attacks lasting from 15 minutes to 3
hours, in cyclical patterns of up to 12 weeks,
followed by remission periods.

G44.011   Episodic cluster headache, intractable
G44.019   Episodic cluster headache, not intractable
Episodic cluster headache NOS

⑥ G44.02   Chronic cluster headache
G44.021   Chronic cluster headache, intractable
G44.029   Chronic cluster headache, not intractable
Chronic cluster headache NOS

⑥ G44.03   Episodic paroxysmal hemicrania
Paroxysmal hemicrania NOS
DEFINITION   Rare headache with severe
throbbing or boring pain in the eye or temple on
one side and accompanying autonomic responses;
occurring in frequent, daily attacks with relatively
long headache-free periods.

G44.031   Episodic paroxysmal hemicrania, intractable
**G44.039   Episodic paroxysmal hemicrania, not
              intractable**
Episodic paroxysmal hemicrania NOS

⑥ G44.04   Chronic paroxysmal hemicrania
G44.041   Chronic paroxysmal hemicrania, intractable
G44.049   Chronic paroxysmal hemicrania, not intractable
Chronic paroxysmal hemicrania NOS

**⑥ G44.05   Short lasting unilateral neuralgiform headache with
            conjunctival injection and tearing (SUNCT)**

**G44.051   Short lasting unilateral neuralgiform headache
              with conjunctival injection and tearing
              (SUNCT), intractable**
**G44.059   Short lasting unilateral neuralgiform headache
              with conjunctival injection and tearing
              (SUNCT), not intractable**
Short lasting unilateral neuralgiform headache with
conjunctival injection and tearing (SUNCT)
NOS

⑥ G44.09   Other trigeminal autonomic cephalgias (TAC)
**G44.091   Other trigeminal autonomic cephalgias (TAC),
              intractable**
**G44.099   Other trigeminal autonomic cephalgias (TAC),
              not intractable**

G44.1   Vascular headache, not elsewhere classified
EXCLUDES 2	cluster headache (G44.0)
	complicated headache syndromes (G44.5-)
	drug-induced headache (G44.4-)
	migraine (G43.-)
	other specified headache syndromes (G44.8-)
	post-traumatic headache (G44.3-)
	tension-type headache (G44.2-)

⑤ G44.2   Tension-type headache

⑥ G44.20   Tension-type headache, unspecified
DEFINITION   Common, muscular contraction
headaches, that produce a mild to moderate, dull,
achy tightening pain over the forehead and sides
like a band encircling the head or pain at the back
of the neck or base of the skull.

G44.201   Tension-type headache, unspecified, intractable
**G44.209   Tension-type headache, unspecified, not
              intractable**
Tension headache NOS

⑥ G44.21   Episodic tension-type headache
G44.211   Episodic tension-type headache, intractable
G44.219   Episodic tension-type headache, not intractable
Episodic tension-type headache NOS

⑥ G44.22   Chronic tension-type headache
G44.221   Chronic tension-type headache, intractable
G44.229   Chronic tension-type headache, not intractable
Chronic tension-type headache NOS

⑤ G44.3   Post-traumatic headache

⑥ G44.30   Post-traumatic headache, unspecified
DEFINITION   Headache as a result of head
trauma or injury, with frequency and severity
diminishing over time; symptoms such as
insomnia, concentration problems, personality
changes, and dizziness often accompany the
headache.

**G44.301   Post-traumatic headache, unspecified,
              intractable**
**G44.309   Post-traumatic headache, unspecified, not
              intractable**
Post-traumatic headache NOS

⑥ G44.31   Acute post-traumatic headache
G44.311   Acute post-traumatic headache, intractable
G44.319   Acute post-traumatic headache, not intractable
Acute post-traumatic headache NOS

⑥ G44.32   Chronic post-traumatic headache
G44.321   Chronic post-traumatic headache, intractable
**G44.329   Chronic post-traumatic headache, not
              intractable**
Chronic post-traumatic headache NOS

⑤✚ G44.4   Drug-induced headache, not elsewhere classified
Medication overuse headache
*Use additional code for adverse effect, if applicable, to
identify drug (T36-T50 with fifth or sixth character 5)*
DEFINITION   Most common type of chronic daily
headache caused by overuse of migraine-abortive ergot
alkaloids and analgesic drugs.

**✚ G44.40   Drug-induced headache, not elsewhere classified, not
              intractable**
**✚ G44.41   Drug-induced headache, not elsewhere classified,
              intractable**

⑤ G44.5   Complicated headache syndromes

● New   ▲ Revised   *Manifestation*   ④-⑦ Digit Indicators   ⊟ Laterality   ⬛ Adult (15+ years)   ⬛ Maternity (12-55 years)   ⬛ Newborn   ⬛ Pediatric (0-17 years)   ♂ Male   ♀ Female
✖ Deleted   Unspecified   ✚ Additional code

574   © 2017 DecisionHealth   2017 ICD-10-CM Expert for Physicians

G44.51   **Hemicrania continua**

G44.52   **New daily persistent headache (NDPH)**

G44.53   **Primary thunderclap headache**

> **DEFINITION**   Dramatic, sudden, severe headache coming without warning, peaking within 60 seconds, then fading over several hours; sometimes signaling a potentially life-threatening condition, such as a ruptured cerebral aneurysm or subarachnoid hemorrhage.

G44.59   **Other complicated headache syndrome**

⑤ G44.8   **Other specified headache syndromes**

G44.81   **Hypnic headache**

> **DEFINITION**   Relatively rare headache connected to REM sleep, marked by being awakened with intense throbbing or dull type pain through the head, accompanied by nausea, and lasting about an hour.

G44.82   **Headache associated with sexual activity**
Orgasmic headache
Preorgasmic headache

G44.83   **Primary cough headache**

> **DEFINITION**   Headache triggered by bouts of coughing or physically straining movements, such as laughing or sneezing, often described as sharp, stabbing, or splitting on both sides of the head and back of the skull.

G44.84   **Primary exertional headache**

G44.85   **Primary stabbing headache**

G44.89   **Other headache syndrome**

④ G45   **Transient cerebral ischemic attacks and related syndromes**

> **EXCLUDES 1**   neonatal cerebral ischemia (P91.0)
> transient retinal artery occlusion (H34.0-)

G45.0   **Vertebro-basilar artery syndrome**

> **DEFINITION**   Obstruction of the vertebral or basilar artery temporarily blocking blood flow to the brain, causing vertigo, diplopia, nystagmus, and muscle weakness.

G45.1   **Carotid artery syndrome (hemispheric)**   Ⓐ

G45.2   **Multiple and bilateral precerebral artery syndromes**   Ⓐ

G45.3   **Amaurosis fugax**

> **CODING TIP ✓**   Amaurosis fugax is a sudden loss of vision in one eye related to impaired carotid blood flow and impaired retinal blood supply and is generally temporary. The condition may signal pending stroke and should not be confused with blindness. Coders should not code blindness in a patient with this condition.

G45.4   **Transient global amnesia**

> **EXCLUDES 1**   amnesia NOS (R41.3)

G45.8   **Other transient cerebral ischemic attacks and related syndromes**   Ⓐ

G45.9   **Transient cerebral ischemic attack, unspecified**   Ⓐ
Spasm of cerebral artery
TIA
Transient cerebral ischemia NOS

> **CODING TIP ✓**   There is no code to report sequelae of a TIA, as these are considered to be "transient" and should not cause residual effects. If residual effects are noted, the coder should query the physician to determine if the patient experienced a CVA. A history of TIA (or CVA) with no residual neurological deficits may be coded to Z86.73, Personal history of transient ischemic attack, and cerebral infarction, without residual deficits.

④ G46   **Vascular syndromes of brain in cerebrovascular diseases**
Code first:
underlying cerebrovascular disease (I60-I69)

> **CODING TIP ✓**   Conditions classified to G46.- include syndromes occurring as a result of specific types of cerebral vascular disease and cerebral vascular accidents (CVA). When a syndrome classifiable to G46.- occurs as a residual of a non-traumatic CVA, assign the appropriate I69 code to indicate sequelae of cerebrovascular disease. These syndromes may be coded as "other sequelae" of CVAs and should then be coded following the appropriate I69 code with the 6th character '8.'

G46.0   **Middle cerebral artery syndrome**   Ⓐ

G46.1   **Anterior cerebral artery syndrome**   Ⓐ

G46.2   **Posterior cerebral artery syndrome**   Ⓐ

G46.3   **Brain stem stroke syndrome**
Benedikt syndrome
Claude syndrome
Foville syndrome
Millard-Gubler syndrome
Wallenberg syndrome
Weber syndrome

G46.4   **Cerebellar stroke syndrome**

G46.5   **Pure motor lacunar syndrome**

G46.6   **Pure sensory lacunar syndrome**

G46.7   **Other lacunar syndromes**

G46.8   **Other vascular syndromes of brain in cerebrovascular diseases**

④ G47   **Sleep disorders**

> **EXCLUDES 2**   nightmares (F51.5)
> nonorganic sleep disorders (F51.-)
> sleep terrors (F51.4)
> sleepwalking (F51.3)

⑤ G47.0   **Insomnia**

> **EXCLUDES 2**   alcohol related insomnia
> (F10.182, F10.282, F10.982)
> drug-related insomnia
> (F11.182, F11.282, F11.982, F13.182,
> F13.282, F13.982, F14.182, F14.282,
> F14.982, F15.182, F15.282, F15.982,
> F19.182, F19.282, F19.982)
> idiopathic insomnia (F51.01)
> insomnia due to a mental disorder (F51.05)
> insomnia not due to a substance or known
> physiological condition (F51.0-)
> nonorganic insomnia (F51.0-)
> primary insomnia (F51.01)
> sleep apnea (G47.3-)

G47.00   **Insomnia, unspecified**
Insomnia NOS

G47.01   **Insomnia due to medical condition**
Code also:
associated medical condition

G47.09   **Other insomnia**

⑤ G47.1   **Hypersomnia**

> **EXCLUDES 2**   alcohol-related hypersomnia
> (F10.182, F10.282, F10.982)
> drug-related hypersomnia
> (F11.182, F11.282, F11.982, F13.182,
> F13.282, F13.982, F14.182, F14.282,
> F14.982, F15.182, F15.282, F15.982,
> F19.182, F19.282, F19.982)
> hypersomnia due to a mental disorder
> (F51.13)
> hypersomnia not due to a substance or
> known physiological condition (F51.1-)
> primary hypersomnia (F51.11)
> sleep apnea (G47.3-)

G47.10   **Hypersomnia, unspecified**
Hypersomnia NOS

G47.11   **Idiopathic hypersomnia with long sleep time**
Idiopathic hypersomnia NOS

G47.12   **Idiopathic hypersomnia without long sleep time**

G47.13   **Recurrent hypersomnia**
Kleine-Levin syndrome
Menstrual related hypersomnia

G47.14   **Hypersomnia due to medical condition**
Code also:
associated medical condition

G47.19   **Other hypersomnia**

⑤ G47.2   **Circadian rhythm sleep disorders**
Disorders of the sleep wake schedule
Inversion of nyctohemeral rhythm
Inversion of sleep rhythm

G47.20   **Circadian rhythm sleep disorder, unspecified type**
Sleep wake schedule disorder NOS

G47.21   **Circadian rhythm sleep disorder, delayed sleep phase type**
Delayed sleep phase syndrome

G47.22   **Circadian rhythm sleep disorder, advanced sleep phase type**

● New   ▲ Revised   *Manifestation*   ④-⑦ Digit Indicators   ▣ Laterality   Ⓐ Adult (15+ years)   Ⓜ Maternity (12-55 years)   Ⓝ Newborn   Ⓟ Pediatric (0-17 years)   ♂ Male   ♀ Female
✖ Deleted   Unspecified   + Additional code

G47.23 Circadian rhythm sleep disorder, irregular sleep wake type
Irregular sleep-wake pattern

G47.24 Circadian rhythm sleep disorder, free running type

G47.25 Circadian rhythm sleep disorder, jet lag type

G47.26 Circadian rhythm sleep disorder, shift work type

G47.27 Circadian rhythm sleep disorder in conditions classified elsewhere
Code first:
underlying condition

G47.29 Other circadian rhythm sleep disorder

⑤ **G47.3 Sleep apnea**
Code also:
any associated underlying condition
EXCLUDES 1   *apnea NOS (R06.81)*
Cheyne-Stokes breathing (R06.3)
pickwickian syndrome (E66.2)
sleep apnea of newborn (P28.3)

G47.30 Sleep apnea, unspecified
Sleep apnea NOS

G47.31 Primary central sleep apnea

G47.32 High altitude periodic breathing

G47.33 Obstructive sleep apnea (adult) (pediatric)
EXCLUDES 1   *obstructive sleep apnea of newborn (P28.3)*

G47.34 Idiopathic sleep related nonobstructive alveolar hypoventilation
Sleep related hypoxia

G47.35 Congenital central alveolar hypoventilation syndrome

G47.36 Sleep related hypoventilation in conditions classified elsewhere
Sleep related hypoxemia in conditions classified elsewhere
Code first:
underlying condition

G47.37 Central sleep apnea in conditions classified elsewhere
Code first:
underlying condition

G47.39 Other sleep apnea

⑤ **G47.4 Narcolepsy and cataplexy**

⑥ **G47.41 Narcolepsy**

G47.411 Narcolepsy with cataplexy

G47.419 Narcolepsy without cataplexy
Narcolepsy NOS

⑥ **G47.42 Narcolepsy in conditions classified elsewhere**
Code first:
underlying condition

G47.421 Narcolepsy in conditions classified elsewhere with cataplexy

G47.429 Narcolepsy in conditions classified elsewhere without cataplexy

⑤ **G47.5 Parasomnia**
EXCLUDES 1   *alcohol induced parasomnia (F10.182, F10.282, F10.982)*
drug induced parasomnia (F11.182, F11.282, F11.982, F13.182, F13.282, F13.982, F14.182, F14.282, F14.982, F15.182, F15.282, F15.982, F19.182, F19.282, F19.982)
parasomnia not due to a substance or known physiological condition (F51.8)

G47.50 Parasomnia, unspecified
Parasomnia NOS

G47.51 Confusional arousals

G47.52 REM sleep behavior disorder

G47.53 Recurrent isolated sleep paralysis

G47.54 Parasomnia in conditions classified elsewhere
Code first:
underlying condition

G47.59 Other parasomnia

⑤ **G47.6 Sleep related movement disorders**
EXCLUDES 2   *restless legs syndrome (G25.81)*

G47.61 Periodic limb movement disorder
Periodic limb movement disorder
DEFINITION   Involuntary limb movement or jerking during or just before sleep.

G47.62 Sleep related leg cramps

G47.63 Sleep related bruxism
EXCLUDES 1   *psychogenic bruxism (F45.8)*
DEFINITION   Grinding the teeth during sleep.

G47.69 Other sleep related movement disorders

G47.8 Other sleep disorders

G47.9 Sleep disorder, unspecified
Sleep disorder NOS

Nerve, nerve root and plexus disorders (G50-G59)

EXCLUDES 1   *current traumatic nerve, nerve root and plexus disorders - see Injury, nerve by body region*
neuralgia NOS (M79.2)
neuritis NOS (M79.2)
peripheral neuritis in pregnancy (O26.82-)
radiculitis NOS (M54.1-)

CODING TIP ✓   When coding neuralgias and neuropathy, coders should be cautious to understand the definitions of the terms neuralgia, neuritis, and neuropathy. Neuritis is an inflammation of the nerve. Neuritis should not be coded here unless specifically noted in the includes notes for the specific code selected. Neuralgia indicates nerve pain, which may or may not be the result of neuritis or other disease or damage to the nerve, such as in phantom limb pain/syndrome (with pain). Neuropathy indicates neuropathic pain related to damaged and diseased nerve pathways.

④ **G50 Disorders of trigeminal nerve**
INCLUDES   disorders of 5th cranial nerve

G50.0 Trigeminal neuralgia
Syndrome of paroxysmal facial pain
Tic douloureux

G50.1 Atypical facial pain

G50.8 Other disorders of trigeminal nerve

G50.9 Disorder of trigeminal nerve, unspecified

④ **G51 Facial nerve disorders**
INCLUDES   disorders of 7th cranial nerve

G51.0 Bell's palsy
Facial palsy
DEFINITION   Temporary, unilateral facial muscle weakness or paralysis resulting from damage or trauma to one of the paired facial nerves.

G51.1 Geniculate ganglionitis
EXCLUDES 1   *postherpetic geniculate ganglionitis (B02.21)*
DEFINITION   Inflammation of the facial nerve ganglion.

G51.2 Melkersson's syndrome
Melkersson-Rosenthal syndrome

G51.3 Clonic hemifacial spasm

G51.4 Facial myokymia

G51.8 Other disorders of facial nerve

G51.9 Disorder of facial nerve, unspecified

④ **G52 Disorders of other cranial nerves**
EXCLUDES 2   *disorders of acoustic [8th] nerve (H93.3)*
disorders of optic [2nd] nerve (H46, H47.0)
paralytic strabismus due to nerve palsy (H49.0-H49.2)

G52.0 Disorders of olfactory nerve
Disorders of 1st cranial nerve

G52.1 Disorders of glossopharyngeal nerve
Disorder of 9th cranial nerve
Glossopharyngeal neuralgia

G52.2 Disorders of vagus nerve
Disorders of pneumogastric [10th] nerve

G52.3 Disorders of hypoglossal nerve
Disorders of 12th cranial nerve

G52.7 Disorders of multiple cranial nerves
Polyneuritis cranialis

G52.8 Disorders of other specified cranial nerves

G52.9 Cranial nerve disorder, unspecified

● New   ▲ Revised   *Manifestation*   ④-⑦ Digit Indicators   ⊟ Laterality   Ⓐ Adult (15+ years)   Ⓜ Maternity (12-55 years)   Ⓝ Newborn   Ⓟ Pediatric (0-17 years)   ♂ Male   ♀ Female
✖ Deleted   Unspecified   + Additional code

G53   *Cranial nerve disorders in diseases classified elsewhere*

Code first underlying disease, such as:
neoplasm (C00-D49)

> **EXCLUDES 1**   *multiple cranial nerve palsy in sarcoidosis
(D86.82)*
> *multiple cranial nerve palsy in syphilis (A52.15)*
> *postherpetic geniculate ganglionitis (B02.21)*
> *postherpetic trigeminal neuralgia (B02.22)*

4 G54   **Nerve root and plexus disorders**

> **EXCLUDES 1**   *current traumatic nerve root and plexus disorders
- see nerve injury by body region*
> *intervertebral disc disorders (M50-M51)*
> *neuralgia or neuritis NOS (M79.2)*
> *neuritis or radiculitis brachial NOS (M54.13)*
> *neuritis or radiculitis lumbar NOS (M54.16)*
> *neuritis or radiculitis lumbosacral NOS
(M54.17)*
> *neuritis or radiculitis thoracic NOS (M54.14)*
> *radiculitis NOS (M54.10)*
> *radiculopathy NOS (M54.10)*
> *spondylosis (M47.-)*

G54.0   **Brachial plexus disorders**
Thoracic outlet syndrome

G54.1   **Lumbosacral plexus disorders**

G54.2   **Cervical root disorders, not elsewhere classified**

G54.3   **Thoracic root disorders, not elsewhere classified**

G54.4   **Lumbosacral root disorders, not elsewhere classified**

G54.5   **Neuralgic amyotrophy**
Parsonage-Aldren-Turner syndrome
Shoulder-girdle neuritis

> **EXCLUDES 1**   *neuralgic amyotrophy in diabetes mellitus
(E08-E13 with .44)*

> **CODING TIP ✓**   Do not assign code G54.5 for diabetic
amyotrophy. Diabetes with amyotrophy should be coded
with the appropriate combination code to specify the
type of diabetes and the neuralgic amyotrophy
manifestation (E08-E13 with 4th and 5th character .44)

G54.6   **Phantom limb syndrome with pain**

G54.7   **Phantom limb syndrome without pain**
Phantom limb syndrome NOS

G54.8   **Other nerve root and plexus disorders**

G54.9   **Nerve root and plexus disorder, unspecified**

G55   *Nerve root and plexus compressions in diseases
classified elsewhere*

Code first underlying disease, such as:
neoplasm (C00-D49)

> **EXCLUDES 1**   *nerve root compression (due to) (in) ankylosing
spondylitis (M45.-)*
> *nerve root compression (due to) (in)
dorsopathies (M53.-, M54.-)*
> *nerve root compression (due to) (in)
intervertebral disc disorders (M50.1.-, M51.1.-
)*
> *nerve root compression (due to) (in)
spondylopathies (M46.-, M48.-)*
> *nerve root compression (due to) (in) spondylosis
(M47.0-M47.2.-)*

4 G56   **Mononeuropathies of upper limb**

> **EXCLUDES 1**   *current traumatic nerve disorder - see nerve
injury by body region*

> **CODING TIP ✓**   Complex Regional Pain Syndromes (CRPS
Type I or II or unspecified) are no longer classified and
coded to causalgias and mononeuropathies. When CRPS
Type I, Type II or unspecified is reported, it should be coded
to the appropriate G90.5- code.

5 G56.0   **Carpal tunnel syndrome**

> **DEFINITION**   Pain, burning, tingling and/or numbness
in the fingers and hand, often extending to the elbow,
due to compression of the median nerve within the
carpal tunnel.

☐ G56.00   **Carpal tunnel syndrome, unspecified upper limb**

☐ G56.01   **Carpal tunnel syndrome, right upper limb**

☐ G56.02   **Carpal tunnel syndrome, left upper limb**

●☐ G56.03   **Carpal tunnel syndrome, bilateral upper limbs**

5 G56.1   **Other lesions of median nerve**

☐ G56.10   **Other lesions of median nerve, unspecified upper
limb**

☐ G56.11   **Other lesions of median nerve, right upper limb**

☐ G56.12   **Other lesions of median nerve, left upper limb**

●☐ G56.13   **Other lesions of median nerve, bilateral upper limbs**

5 G56.2   **Lesion of ulnar nerve**
Tardy ulnar nerve palsy

☐ G56.20   **Lesion of ulnar nerve, unspecified upper limb**

☐ G56.21   **Lesion of ulnar nerve, right upper limb**

☐ G56.22   **Lesion of ulnar nerve, left upper limb**

●☐ G56.23   **Lesion of ulnar nerve, bilateral upper limbs**

5 G56.3   **Lesion of radial nerve**

☐ G56.30   **Lesion of radial nerve, unspecified upper limb**

☐ G56.31   **Lesion of radial nerve, right upper limb**

☐ G56.32   **Lesion of radial nerve, left upper limb**

●☐ G56.33   **Lesion of radial nerve, bilateral upper limbs**

5 G56.4   **Causalgia of upper limb**
Complex regional pain syndrome II of upper limb

> **EXCLUDES 1**   *complex regional pain syndrome I of lower
limb (G90.52-)*
> *complex regional pain syndrome I of upper
limb (G90.51-)*
> *complex regional pain syndrome II of lower
limb (G57.7-)*
> *reflex sympathetic dystrophy of lower limb
(G90.52-)*
> *reflex sympathetic dystrophy of upper limb
(G90.51-)*

> **DEFINITION**   A burning pain in the arm along the
course of a peripheral nerve usually associated with
skin changes.

☐ G56.40   **Causalgia of unspecified upper limb**

☐ G56.41   **Causalgia of right upper limb**

☐ G56.42   **Causalgia of left upper limb**

●☐ G56.43   **Causalgia of bilateral upper limbs**

5 G56.8   **Other specified mononeuropathies of upper limb**
Interdigital neuroma of upper limb

☐ G56.80   **Other specified mononeuropathies of unspecified
upper limb**

☐ G56.81   **Other specified mononeuropathies of right upper
limb**

☐ G56.82   **Other specified mononeuropathies of left upper limb**

●☐ G56.83   **Other specified mononeuropathies of bilateral upper
limbs**

5 G56.9   **Unspecified mononeuropathy of upper limb**

☐ G56.90   **Unspecified mononeuropathy of unspecified upper
limb**

☐ G56.91   **Unspecified mononeuropathy of right upper limb**

☐ G56.92   **Unspecified mononeuropathy of left upper limb**

●☐ G56.93   **Unspecified mononeuropathy of bilateral upper
limbs**

4 G57   **Mononeuropathies of lower limb**

> **EXCLUDES 1**   *current traumatic nerve disorder - see nerve
injury by body region*

5 G57.0   **Lesion of sciatic nerve**

> **EXCLUDES 1**   *sciatica NOS (M54.3-)*

> **EXCLUDES 2**   *sciatica attributed to intervertebral disc
disorder (M51.1.-)*

☐ G57.00   **Lesion of sciatic nerve, unspecified lower limb**

☐ G57.01   **Lesion of sciatic nerve, right lower limb**

☐ G57.02   **Lesion of sciatic nerve, left lower limb**

●☐ G57.03   **Lesion of sciatic nerve, bilateral lower limbs**

5 G57.1   **Meralgia paresthetica**
Lateral cutaneous nerve of thigh syndrome

☐ G57.10   **Meralgia paresthetica, unspecified lower limb**

☐ G57.11   **Meralgia paresthetica, right lower limb**

☐ G57.12   **Meralgia paresthetica, left lower limb**

●☐ G57.13   **Meralgia paresthetica, bilateral lower limbs**

5 G57.2   **Lesion of femoral nerve**

☐ G57.20   **Lesion of femoral nerve, unspecified lower limb**

☐ G57.21   **Lesion of femoral nerve, right lower limb**

☐ G57.22   **Lesion of femoral nerve, left lower limb**

●☐ G57.23   **Lesion of femoral nerve, bilateral lower limbs**

5 G57.3   **Lesion of lateral popliteal nerve**
Peroneal nerve palsy

☐ G57.30   **Lesion of lateral popliteal nerve, unspecified lower
limb**

● New   ▲ Revised   *Manifestation*   4-7 Digit Indicators   ☐ Laterality   🅐 Adult (15+ years)   🅜 Maternity (12-55 years)   🅝 Newborn   🅟 Pediatric (0-17 years)   ♂ Male   ♀ Female

Unspecified   + Additional code

✗ Deleted

2017 ICD-10-CM Expert for Physicians

© 2017 DecisionHealth

577

☐ G57.31   Lesion of lateral popliteal nerve, right lower limb
☐ G57.32   Lesion of lateral popliteal nerve, left lower limb
● ☐ G57.33   Lesion of lateral popliteal nerve, bilateral lower limbs
⑤ G57.4   Lesion of medial popliteal nerve
☐ G57.40   **Lesion of medial popliteal nerve, unspecified lower limb**
☐ G57.41   **Lesion of medial popliteal nerve, right lower limb**
☐ G57.42   **Lesion of medial popliteal nerve, left lower limb**
● ☐ G57.43   **Lesion of medial popliteal nerve, bilateral lower limbs**
⑤ G57.5   Tarsal tunnel syndrome
   DEFINITION   Pain, burning, tingling, and/or numbness of the sole of the foot, often extending to the ankle, due to compression of the posterior tibial nerve or plantar nerves within the tarsal tunnel.
☐ G57.50   **Tarsal tunnel syndrome, unspecified lower limb**
☐ G57.51   **Tarsal tunnel syndrome, right lower limb**
☐ G57.52   **Tarsal tunnel syndrome, left lower limb**
● ☐ G57.53   **Tarsal tunnel syndrome, bilateral lower limbs**
⑤ G57.6   Lesion of plantar nerve
   Morton's metatarsalgia
   DEFINITION   Thickening of tissue that surrounds the digital nerve leading to the toes. Most frequently develops between the third and fourth toes, usually in response to irritation, trauma or excessive pressure.
☐ G57.60   **Lesion of plantar nerve, unspecified lower limb**
☐ G57.61   **Lesion of plantar nerve, right lower limb**
☐ G57.62   **Lesion of plantar nerve, left lower limb**
● ☐ G57.63   **Lesion of plantar nerve, bilateral lower limbs**
⑤ G57.7   Causalgia of lower limb
   Complex regional pain syndrome II of lower limb
   EXCLUDES 1   *complex regional pain syndrome I of lower limb (G90.52-)*
   complex regional pain syndrome I of upper limb (G90.51-)
   complex regional pain syndrome II of upper limb (G56.4-)
   reflex sympathetic dystrophy of lower limb (G90.52-)
   reflex sympathetic dystrophy of upper limb (G90.51-)
☐ G57.70   **Causalgia of unspecified lower limb**
☐ G57.71   **Causalgia of right lower limb**
☐ G57.72   **Causalgia of left lower limb**
● ☐ G57.73   **Causalgia of bilateral lower limbs**
⑤ G57.8   Other specified mononeuropathies of lower limb
   Interdigital neuroma of lower limb
☐ G57.80   **Other specified mononeuropathies of unspecified lower limb**
☐ G57.81   **Other specified mononeuropathies of right lower limb**
☐ G57.82   **Other specified mononeuropathies of left lower limb**
● ☐ G57.83   **Other specified mononeuropathies of bilateral lower limbs**
⑤ G57.9   Unspecified mononeuropathy of lower limb
☐ G57.90   **Unspecified mononeuropathy of unspecified lower limb**
☐ G57.91   **Unspecified mononeuropathy of right lower limb**
☐ G57.92   **Unspecified mononeuropathy of left lower limb**
● ☐ G57.93   **Unspecified mononeuropathy of bilateral lower limbs**
④ **G58**   **Other mononeuropathies**
   G58.0   **Intercostal neuropathy**
   G58.7   **Mononeuritis multiplex**
   G58.8   **Other specified mononeuropathies**
   G58.9   **Mononeuropathy, unspecified**
   G59   **Mononeuropathy in diseases classified elsewhere**
      Code first:
      underlying disease
   EXCLUDES 1   *diabetic mononeuropathy (E08-E13 with .41)*
   syphilitic nerve paralysis (A52.19)
   syphilitic neuritis (A52.15)
   tuberculous mononeuropathy (A17.83)

Polyneuropathies and other disorders of the peripheral nervous system (G60-G65)

EXCLUDES 1   *neuralgia NOS (M79.2)*
neuritis NOS (M79.2)
peripheral neuritis in pregnancy (O26.82-)
radiculitis NOS (M54.10)

④ **G60**   **Hereditary and idiopathic neuropathy**
   G60.0   **Hereditary motor and sensory neuropathy**
      Charcot-Marie-Tooth disease
      Déjérine-Sottas disease
      Hereditary motor and sensory neuropathy, types I-IV
      Hypertrophic neuropathy of infancy
      Peroneal muscular atrophy (axonal type) (hypertrophic type)
      Roussy-Levy syndrome
   G60.1   **Refsum's disease**
      Infantile Refsum disease
   G60.2   **Neuropathy in association with hereditary ataxia**
   G60.3   **Idiopathic progressive neuropathy**
   G60.8   **Other hereditary and idiopathic neuropathies**
      Dominantly inherited sensory neuropathy
      Morvan's disease
      Nelaton's syndrome
      Recessively inherited sensory neuropathy
   G60.9   **Hereditary and idiopathic neuropathy, unspecified**

④ **G61**   **Inflammatory polyneuropathy**
   CODING TIP ✓   When an inflammatory neuropathy is reported as unresolved, assign the appropriate code from G61.-. If inflammatory neuropathy is documented as resolved but residual neurologic deficits remain as sequelae, assign the appropriate code from category G65.-, Sequelae of inflammatory and toxic polyneuropathies.
   G61.0   **Guillain-Barre syndrome**
      Acute (post-)infective polyneuritis
      Miller Fisher Syndrome
      CODING TIP ✓   When Guillain-Barre syndrome is reported as unresolved, assign code G61.0. If a Guillain-Barre syndrome is documented as resolved but residual neurologic deficits remain as sequelae, assign code G65.0, Sequelae of Guillain-Barre syndrome (code first the residual defects when coding G65.0). Acute inflammatory demyelinating polyneuropathy is included in this code.
      DEFINITION   Disorder that causes the body's immune system to attack the nerves; paralysis begins at the feet and progresses upwards through the legs and torso to the arms and face.
      AHA: 2Q 2014, 4

Guillain-Barre syndrome (GBS)

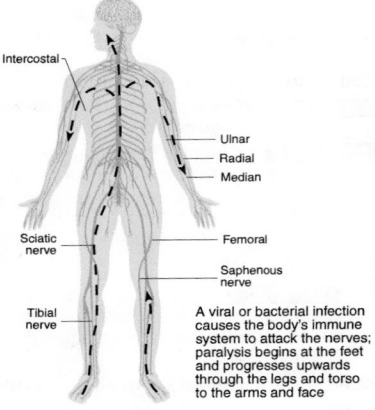

Intercostal

Ulnar
Radial
Median

Sciatic nerve

Femoral

Saphenous nerve

Tibial nerve

A viral or bacterial infection causes the body's immune system to attack the nerves; paralysis begins at the feet and progresses upwards through the legs and torso to the arms and face

✚ G61.1   **Serum neuropathy**
   Use additional code for adverse effect, if applicable, to identify serum (T50.-)
⑤ G61.8   **Other inflammatory polyneuropathies**
   G61.81   **Chronic inflammatory demyelinating polyneuritis**

● **G61.82** **Multifocal motor neuropathy**
MMN
G61.89 **Other inflammatory polyneuropathies**
G61.9 **Inflammatory polyneuropathy, unspecified**

◢ **G62** **Other and unspecified polyneuropathies**

✛ **G62.0** **Drug-induced polyneuropathy**
Use additional code for adverse effect, if applicable, to
identify drug (T36-T50 with fifth or sixth character 5)

CODING TIP ✓ Assign G62.0 when the polyneuropathy is specifically reported by the physician as related to the use of a drug. An additional code should be assigned to identify the drug.

G62.1 **Alcoholic polyneuropathy**

CODING TIP ✓ Assign G62.1 when the physician specifically reports that the polyneuropathy results from alcohol use. The coder should also code any history of or current use of alcohol.

DEFINITION Loss of nerve function due to damage from prolonged, excessive alcohol consumption; commonly presents with numbness, weakness, and burning in the feet.

G62.2 **Polyneuropathy due to other toxic agents**
Code first:
(T51-T65) to identify toxic agent

◢ **G62.8** **Other specified polyneuropathies**

G62.81 **Critical illness polyneuropathy**
Acute motor neuropathy

✛ **G62.82** **Radiation-induced polyneuropathy**
Use additional external cause code (W88-W90, X39.0-)
to identify cause

G62.89 **Other specified polyneuropathies**
AHA: 2Q 2016, 11

G62.9 **Polyneuropathy, unspecified**
Neuropathy NOS

G63 *Polyneuropathy in diseases classified elsewhere*
Code first underlying disease, such as:
amyloidosis (E85.-)
endocrine disease, except diabetes
(E00-E07, E15-E16, E20-E34)
metabolic diseases (E70-E88)
neoplasm (C00-D49)
nutritional deficiency (E40-E64)

EXCLUDES 1 *polyneuropathy (in) :*
diabetes mellitus (E08-E13 with .42)
diphtheria (A36.83)
infectious mononucleosis (B27.0-B27.9 with 1)
Lyme disease (A69.22)
mumps (B26.84)
postherpetic (B02.23)
rheumatoid arthritis (M05.33)
scleroderma (M34.83)
systemic lupus erythematosus (M32.19)

CODING TIP ✓ Do not assign code G63 for diabetic polyneuropathy. Diabetes with polyneuropathy should be coded with the appropriate combination code to specify the type of diabetes and the polyneuropathy manifestation.

CODING TIP ✓ Code G63 is a manifestation code and must be sequenced following the code for the underlying disease process identified as the etiological cause for the polyneuropathy.
AHA: 4Q 2012, 99-100

G64 **Other disorders of peripheral nervous system**
Disorder of peripheral nervous system NOS

◢ **G65** **Sequelae of inflammatory and toxic polyneuropathies**
Code first:
condition resulting from (sequela) of inflammatory and toxic polyneuropathies
G65.0 **Sequelae of Guillain-Barré syndrome**
G65.1 **Sequelae of other inflammatory polyneuropathy**
G65.2 **Sequelae of toxic polyneuropathy**

Diseases of myoneural junction and muscle (G70-G73)

◢ **G70** **Myasthenia gravis and other myoneural disorders**
EXCLUDES 1 *botulism (A05.1, A48.51-A48.52)*
transient neonatal myasthenia gravis (P94.0)

◙ **G70.0** **Myasthenia gravis**

CODING TIP ✓ When myasthenia gravis is not documented as with or without exacerbation (no exacerbation is specified), assign code G70.00, without (acute) exacerbation.

G70.00 **Myasthenia gravis without (acute) exacerbation**
Myasthenia gravis NOS
G70.01 **Myasthenia gravis with (acute) exacerbation**
Myasthenia gravis in crisis
G70.1 **Toxic myoneural disorders**
Code first:
(T51-T65) to identify toxic agent
G70.2 **Congenital and developmental myasthenia**
◙ **G70.8** **Other specified myoneural disorders**
G70.80 **Lambert-Eaton syndrome, unspecified**
Lambert-Eaton syndrome NOS
G70.81 **Lambert-Eaton syndrome in disease classified elsewhere**
Code first:
underlying disease
EXCLUDES 1 *Lambert-Eaton syndrome in neoplastic disease (G73.1)*
G70.89 **Other specified myoneural disorders**
G70.9 **Myoneural disorder, unspecified**

◢ **G71** **Primary disorders of muscles**
EXCLUDES 2 *arthrogryposis multiplex congenita (Q74.3)*
metabolic disorders (E70-E88)
myositis (M60.-)

G71.0 **Muscular dystrophy**
Autosomal recessive, childhood type, muscular dystrophy resembling Duchenne or Becker muscular dystrophy
Benign [Becker] muscular dystrophy
Benign scapuloperoneal muscular dystrophy with early contractures [Emery-Dreifuss]
Congenital muscular dystrophy NOS
Congenital muscular dystrophy with specific morphological abnormalities of the muscle fiber
Distal muscular dystrophy
Facioscapulohumeral muscular dystrophy
Limb-girdle muscular dystrophy
Ocular muscular dystrophy
Oculopharyngeal muscular dystrophy
Scapuloperoneal muscular dystrophy
Severe [Duchenne] muscular dystrophy

◙ **G71.1** **Myotonic disorders**
G71.11 **Myotonic muscular dystrophy**
Dystrophia myotonica [Steinert]
Myotonia atrophica
Myotonic dystrophy
Proximal myotonic myopathy (PROMM)
Steinert disease
G71.12 **Myotonia congenita**
Acetazolamide responsive myotonia congenita
Dominant myotonia congenita [Thomsen disease]
Myotonia levior
Recessive myotonia congenita [Becker disease]
G71.13 **Myotonic chondrodystrophy**
Chondrodystrophic myotonia
Congenital myotonic chondrodystrophy
Schwartz-Jampel disease

DEFINITION Muscle disorder of late infancy with distinctive signs: mask-like face with small features, short stature or dwarfism, limited joint mobility, hip dysplasia, and generalized myotonia with hypertrophied diaphragmatic muscles. Death usually occurs due to respiratory compromise.

✛ **G71.14** **Drug induced myotonia**
Use additional code for adverse effect, if applicable, to
identify drug (T36-T50 with fifth or sixth character 5)
G71.19 **Other specified myotonic disorders**
Myotonia fluctuans
Myotonia permanens
Neuromyotonia [Isaacs]
Paramyotonia congenita (of von Eulenburg)
Pseudomyotonia
Symptomatic myotonia

● New ▲ Revised *Manifestation* ◢-◼ Digit Indicators ▱ Laterality Ⓐ Adult (15+ years) Ⓜ Maternity (12-55 years) Ⓝ Newborn Ⓟ Pediatric (0-17 years) ♂ Male ♀ Female
✖ Deleted Unspecified ✛ Additional code

2017 ICD-10-CM Expert for Physicians

© 2017 DecisionHealth

579

G71.2 **Congenital myopathies**
Central core disease
Fiber-type disproportion
Minicore disease
Multicore disease
Myotubular (centronuclear) myopathy
Nemaline myopathy
EXCLUDES 1 *arthrogryposis multiplex congenita (Q74.3)*

G71.3 **Mitochondrial myopathy, not elsewhere classified**
EXCLUDES 1 *Kearns-Sayre syndrome (H49.81)*
Leber's disease (H47.21)
Leigh's encephalopathy (G31.82)
mitochondrial metabolism disorders
    (E88.4.-)
Reye's syndrome (G93.7)

G71.8 **Other primary disorders of muscles**

G71.9 **Primary disorder of muscle, unspecified**
Hereditary myopathy NOS

◢ G72 **Other and unspecified myopathies**
EXCLUDES 1 *arthrogryposis multiplex congenita (Q74.3)*
dermatopolymyositis (M33.-)
ischemic infarction of muscle (M62.2-)
myositis (M60.-)
polymyositis (M33.2.-)

+ G72.0 **Drug-induced myopathy**
Use additional code for adverse effect, if applicable, to
    identify drug (T36-T50 with fifth or sixth character 5)

+ G72.1 **Alcoholic myopathy**
Use additional code to identify alcoholism (F10.-)

G72.2 **Myopathy due to other toxic agents**
Code first:
    (T51-T65) to identify toxic agent

G72.3 **Periodic paralysis**
Familial periodic paralysis
Hyperkalemic periodic paralysis (familial)
Hypokalemic periodic paralysis (familial)
Myotonic periodic paralysis (familial)
Normokalemic paralysis (familial)
Potassium sensitive periodic paralysis
EXCLUDES 1 *paramyotonia congenita (of von Eulenburg)*
    (G71.19)

⑤ G72.4 **Inflammatory and immune myopathies, not elsewhere classified**
G72.41 **Inclusion body myositis [IBM]**
G72.49 **Other inflammatory and immune myopathies, not elsewhere classified**
Inflammatory myopathy NOS

⑤ G72.8 **Other specified myopathies**
G72.81 **Critical illness myopathy**
Acute necrotizing myopathy
Acute quadriplegic myopathy
Intensive care (ICU) myopathy
Myopathy of critical illness
G72.89 **Other specified myopathies**

G72.9 **Myopathy, unspecified**

◢ G73 **Disorders of myoneural junction and muscle in diseases classified elsewhere**
G73.1 **Lambert-Eaton syndrome in neoplastic disease**
Code first:
    underlying neoplasm (C00-D49)
EXCLUDES 1 *Lambert-Eaton syndrome not associated*
    with neoplasm (G70.80-G70.81)

G73.3 *Myasthenic syndromes in other diseases classified elsewhere*
Code first underlying disease, such as:
    neoplasm (C00-D49)
    thyrotoxicosis (E05.-)

G73.7 *Myopathy in diseases classified elsewhere*
Code first underlying disease, such as:
    hyperparathyroidism (E21.0, E21.3)
    hypoparathyroidism (E20.-)
    glycogen storage disease (E74.0)
    lipid storage disorders (E75.-)
EXCLUDES 1 *myopathy in:*
    rheumatoid arthritis (M05.32)
    sarcoidosis (D86.87)
    scleroderma (M34.82)
    sicca syndrome [Sjögren] (M35.03)
    systemic lupus erythematosus (M32.19)

Cerebral palsy and other paralytic syndromes (G80-G83)

GUIDELINES   Section I.C.6.a
Codes from category G81, Hemiplegia and hemiparesis, and subcategories, G83.1, Monoplegia of lower limb, G83.2, Monoplegia of upper limb, and G83.3, Monoplegia, unspecified, identify whether the dominant or nondominant side is affected. Should the affected side be documented, but not specified as dominant or nondominant, and the classification system does not indicate a default, code selection is as follows:
• For ambidextrous patients, the default should be dominant.
• If the left side is affected, the default is non-dominant.
• If the right side is affected, the default is dominant.

CODING TIP ✓   When coding cerebral palsy and other paralytic syndromes, the dominance rule stated in the guidelines applies. Coders should note that there is no option to code unspecified side since dominant side may be assumed in ICD-10.

◢ G80 **Cerebral palsy**
EXCLUDES 1 *hereditary spastic paraplegia (G11.4)*

G80.0 **Spastic quadriplegic cerebral palsy**
Congenital spastic paralysis (cerebral)
DEFINITION   Palsy presenting with spastic paralysis of all four limbs from early brain damage.

G80.1 **Spastic diplegic cerebral palsy**
Spastic cerebral palsy NOS

G80.2 **Spastic hemiplegic cerebral palsy**
DEFINITION   Palsy affecting the limbs on either the left or the right side (e.g., the right arm and right leg).

G80.3 **Athetoid cerebral palsy**
Double athetosis (syndrome)
Dyskinetic cerebral palsy
Dystonic cerebral palsy
Vogt disease
DEFINITION   Permanent, nonprogressive, motor disorder caused by brain damage usually occurring shortly before, during, or after birth and characterized by uncontrolled, writhing movements of the hands, feet, arms, or legs.

G80.4 **Ataxic cerebral palsy**

G80.8 **Other cerebral palsy**
Mixed cerebral palsy syndromes

G80.9 **Cerebral palsy, unspecified**
Cerebral palsy NOS

◢ G81 **Hemiplegia and hemiparesis**
Note: This category is to be used only when hemiplegia (complete)(incomplete) is reported without further specification, or is stated to be old or longstanding but of unspecified cause. The category is also for use in multiple coding to identify these types of hemiplegia resulting from any cause.
EXCLUDES 1 *congenital cerebral palsy (G80.-)*
hemiplegia and hemiparesis due to sequela of
    cerebrovascular disease
    (I69.05-, I69.15-, I69.25-, I69.35-, I69.85-,
    I69.95-)

CODING TIP ✓   When paraplegia, hemiplegia, hemiparesis, or another paralytic state results from a brain or spinal cord injury, code the paralysis/paresis followed by the code for the spinal injury with the 7th character "S" to report sequelae of the injury.
AHA: 4Q 2012, 106

⑤ G81.0 **Flaccid hemiplegia**
◱ G81.00 **Flaccid hemiplegia affecting unspecified side**
◱ G81.01 **Flaccid hemiplegia affecting right dominant side**
◱ G81.02 **Flaccid hemiplegia affecting left dominant side**
◱ G81.03 **Flaccid hemiplegia affecting right nondominant side**
◱ G81.04 **Flaccid hemiplegia affecting left nondominant side**
⑤ G81.1 **Spastic hemiplegia**
◱ G81.10 **Spastic hemiplegia affecting unspecified side**
◱ G81.11 **Spastic hemiplegia affecting right dominant side**
◱ G81.12 **Spastic hemiplegia affecting left dominant side**
◱ G81.13 **Spastic hemiplegia affecting right nondominant side**
◱ G81.14 **Spastic hemiplegia affecting left nondominant side**
⑤ G81.9 **Hemiplegia, unspecified**

● New   ▲ Revised   *Manifestation*   ◱-◸ Digit Indicators   ⊟ Laterality   🅰 Adult   🅼 Maternity   🅽 Newborn   🅿 Pediatric   ♂ Male   ♀ Female
✖ Deleted   Unspecified   + Additional code   (15+ years)   (12-55 years)   (0-17 years)

🔲 **G81.90** Hemiplegia, unspecified affecting unspecified side

🔲 **G81.91** Hemiplegia, unspecified affecting right dominant side

🔲 **G81.92** Hemiplegia, unspecified affecting left dominant side

🔲 **G81.93** Hemiplegia, unspecified affecting right nondominant side

🔲 **G81.94** Hemiplegia, unspecified affecting left nondominant side

AHA: 1Q 2015, 26

◤ **G82** **Paraplegia (paraparesis) and quadriplegia (quadriparesis)**

Note: This category is to be used only when the listed conditions are reported without further specification, or are stated to be old or longstanding but of unspecified cause. The category is also for use in multiple coding to identify these conditions resulting from any cause

EXCLUDES 1 *congenital cerebral palsy (G80.-)*
functional quadriplegia (R53.2)
hysterical paralysis (F44.4)

CODING TIP ✓ When paraplegia, hemiplegia, hemiparesis, or another paralytic state results from a brain or spinal cord injury, code the paralysis/paresis followed by the code for the spinal injury with the 7th character "S" to report sequelae of the injury.

⑤ **G82.2** **Paraplegia**

Paralysis of both lower limbs NOS
Paraparesis (lower) NOS
Paraplegia (lower) NOS

G82.20 Paraplegia, unspecified
G82.21 Paraplegia, complete
G82.22 Paraplegia, incomplete

⑤ **G82.5** **Quadriplegia**

G82.50 Quadriplegia, unspecified
G82.51 Quadriplegia, C1-C4 complete
G82.52 Quadriplegia, C1-C4 incomplete
G82.53 Quadriplegia, C5-C7 complete
G82.54 Quadriplegia, C5-C7 incomplete

◤ **G83** **Other paralytic syndromes**

Note: This category is to be used only when the listed conditions are reported without further specification, or are stated to be old or longstanding but of unspecified cause. The category is also for use in multiple coding to identify these conditions resulting from any cause.

INCLUDES paralysis (complete) (incomplete), except as in G80-G82

CODING TIP ✓ When paraplegia, hemiplegia, hemiparesis, or another paralytic state results from a brain or spinal cord injury, code the paralysis/paresis followed by the code for the spinal injury with the 7th character "S" to report sequelae of the injury.

G83.0 **Diplegia of upper limbs**

Diplegia (upper)
Paralysis of both upper limbs

⑤ **G83.1** **Monoplegia of lower limb**

Paralysis of lower limb

EXCLUDES 1 *monoplegia of lower limbs due to sequela of cerebrovascular disease (I69.04-, I69.14-, I69.24-, I69.34-, I69.84-, I69.94-)*

AHA: 4Q 2012, 106

🔲 **G83.10** Monoplegia of lower limb affecting unspecified side

🔲 **G83.11** Monoplegia of lower limb affecting right dominant side

🔲 **G83.12** Monoplegia of lower limb affecting left dominant side

🔲 **G83.13** Monoplegia of lower limb affecting right nondominant side

🔲 **G83.14** Monoplegia of lower limb affecting left nondominant side

⑤ **G83.2** **Monoplegia of upper limb**

Paralysis of upper limb

EXCLUDES 1 *monoplegia of upper limbs due to sequela of cerebrovascular disease (I69.03-, I69.13-, I69.23-, I69.33-, I69.83-, I69.93-)*

AHA: 4Q 2012, 106

🔲 **G83.20** Monoplegia of upper limb affecting unspecified side

🔲 **G83.21** Monoplegia of upper limb affecting right dominant side

🔲 **G83.22** Monoplegia of upper limb affecting left dominant side

🔲 **G83.23** Monoplegia of upper limb affecting right nondominant side

🔲 **G83.24** Monoplegia of upper limb affecting left nondominant side

⑤ **G83.3** **Monoplegia, unspecified**

AHA: 4Q 2012, 106

🔲 **G83.30** Monoplegia, unspecified affecting unspecified side

🔲 **G83.31** Monoplegia, unspecified affecting right dominant side

🔲 **G83.32** Monoplegia, unspecified affecting left dominant side

🔲 **G83.33** Monoplegia, unspecified affecting right nondominant side

🔲 **G83.34** Monoplegia, unspecified affecting left nondominant side

G83.4 **Cauda equina syndrome**

Neurogenic bladder due to cauda equina syndrome

EXCLUDES 1 *cord bladder NOS (G95.89)*
neurogenic bladder NOS (N31.9)

CODING TIP ✓ Assign G83.4 only when the physician specifically reports cauda equina syndrome. This code includes neurogenic bladder and no additional code for neurogenic bladder should be assigned when present.

DEFINITION Emergent condition due to compression of spinal nerve roots causing dull aching pain in the perineum, bladder, and sacrum with associated paresthesia, bladder dysfunction, and/or paralysis.

G83.5 **Locked-in state**

⑤ **G83.8** **Other specified paralytic syndromes**

EXCLUDES 1 *paralytic syndromes due to current spinal cord injury-code to spinal cord injury (S14, S24, S34)*

G83.81 Brown-Séquard syndrome
G83.82 Anterior cord syndrome
G83.83 Posterior cord syndrome
G83.84 Todd's paralysis (postepileptic)
G83.89 Other specified paralytic syndromes

G83.9 **Paralytic syndrome, unspecified**

● New ▲ Revised *Manifestation* �4-7 Digit Indicators 🔲 Laterality ⒶAdult (15+ years) Ⓜ Maternity (12-55 years) Ⓝ Newborn �Ⓟ Pediatric (0-17 years) ♂ Male ♀ Female

✖ Deleted Unspecified + Additional code

2017 ICD-10-CM Expert for Physicians

© 2017 DecisionHealth

581

Other disorders of the nervous system (G89-G99)

▲ ◢ **G89   Pain, not elsewhere classified**
Code also:
  related psychological factors associated with pain (F45.42)
  EXCLUDES 1   *generalized pain NOS (R52)*
  pain disorders exclusively related to psychological factors (F45.41)
  pain NOS (R52)
  EXCLUDES 2   *atypical face pain (G50.1)*
  headache syndromes (G44.-)
  localized pain, unspecified type - code to pain by site, such as:
  abdomen pain (R10.-)
  back pain (M54.9)
  breast pain (N64.4)
  chest pain (R07.1-R07.9)
  ear pain (H92.0-)
  eye pain (H57.1)
  headache (R51)
  joint pain (M25.5-)
  limb pain (M79.6-)
  lumbar region pain (M54.5)
  painful urination (R30.9)
  pelvic and perineal pain (R10.2)
  shoulder pain (M25.51-)
  spine pain (M54.-)
  throat pain (R07.0)
  tongue pain (K14.6)
  tooth pain (K08.8)
  renal colic (N23)
  migraines (G43.-)
  myalgia (M79.1)
  pain from prosthetic devices, implants, and grafts (T82.84, T83.84, T84.84, T85.84-)
  phantom limb syndrome with pain (G54.6)
  vulvar vestibulitis (N94.810)
  vulvodynia (N94.81-)

GUIDELINES   Section I.C.5.a
Assign code F45.41 for pain that is exclusively related to psychological disorders. As indicated by the Excludes 1 note under category G89, a code from category G89 should not be assigned with code F45.41. Code F45.42, Pain disorders with related psychological factors, should be used with a code from category G89 if there is documentation of a psychological component for a patient with acute or chronic pain.

GUIDELINES   Section I.C.6.b.1)
Codes in category G89 may be used in conjunction with codes from other categories and chapters to provide more detail about acute or chronic pain and neoplasm-related pain, unless otherwise indicated below. If the pain is not specified as acute or chronic, postthoracotomy, postprocedural, or neoplasm-related, do not assign codes from category G89. A code from category G89 should not be assigned if the underlying (definitive) diagnosis is known, unless the reason for the encounter is pain control/management and not management of the underlying condition.

When an admission or encounter is for a procedure aimed at treating the underlying condition (e.g., spinal fusion, kyphoplasty), a code for the underlying condition (e.g., vertebral fracture, spinal stenosis) should be assigned as the principal diagnosis. No code from category G89 should be assigned.

CODING TIP ✓   Documentation: Pain disorders should be coded only when specified by the physician and when the plan of care specifically addresses pain with interventions and goals to address the pain as a focus of care.

G89.0   Central pain syndrome
  Déjérine-Roussy syndrome
  Myelopathic pain syndrome
  Thalamic pain syndrome (hyperesthetic)

GUIDELINES   Section I.C.6.b.6)
Central pain syndrome (G89.0) and chronic pain syndrome (G89.4) are different than the term "chronic pain," and therefore codes should only be used when the provider has specifically documented this condition.

CODING TIP ✓   Do not code G89.0 unless the physician specifies central pain syndrome. Use G89.0 if: 1) Traumatic or brain-related damage to the central nervous system (e.g. damage from stroke, MS, tumors, epilepsy, Parkinson's); 2) The character and extent of the pain is partly related to a variety of causes; 3) Treatment includes pain medications. It also might be appropriate for patients on antidepressants and anticonvulsants.

⑤ **G89.1   Acute pain, not elsewhere classified**
G89.11   Acute pain due to trauma
G89.12   Acute post-thoracotomy pain
  Post-thoracotomy pain NOS

GUIDELINES   Section I.C.6.b.3)(a)-(b)
The provider's documentation should be used to guide the coding of postoperative pain. The default for post-thoracotomy and other postoperative pain not specified as acute or chronic is the code for the acute form. Routine or expected postoperative pain immediately after surgery should not be coded.

(a) Postoperative pain not associated with a specific postoperative complication is assigned to the appropriate postoperative pain code in category G89.

(b) Postoperative pain associated with specific postoperative complication (such as painful wire sutures) is assigned to the appropriate code(s) found in Chapter 19, Injury, poisoning, and certain other consequences of external causes. If appropriate, use additional code(s) from category G89 to identify acute or chronic pain (G89.18 or G89.28).

G89.18   Other acute postprocedural pain
  Postoperative pain NOS
  Postprocedural pain NOS

CODING TIP ✓   G89.18 is the default code for post-operative/post-procedural pain when not specified as acute or chronic. G89.18 should not be coded in all patients who experience pain following a procedure. It is expected that some pain would be experienced following a procedure.

⑤ **G89.2   Chronic pain, not elsewhere classified**
  EXCLUDES 1   *causalgia, lower limb (G57.7-)*
  causalgia, upper limb (G56.4-)
  central pain syndrome (G89.0)
  chronic pain syndrome (G89.4)
  complex regional pain syndrome II, lower limb (G57.7-)
  complex regional pain syndrome II, upper limb (G56.4-)
  neoplasm related chronic pain (G89.3)
  reflex sympathetic dystrophy (G90.5-)

GUIDELINES   Section I.C.6.b.4)
Chronic pain is classified to subcategory G89.2. There is no time frame defining when pain becomes chronic pain. The provider's documentation should be used to guide use of these codes.

CODING TIP ✓   No specific time frame is required in order to code chronic pain

G89.21   Chronic pain due to trauma
G89.22   Chronic post-thoracotomy pain
G89.28   Other chronic postprocedural pain
  Other chronic postoperative pain

CODING TIP ✓   Unspecified post-procedural pain should not be coded to G89.28. When not specified as acute or chronic, post-procedural/post-operative pain should be coded to G89.18, Other acute postprocedural pain. G89.28 should not be coded in all patients who experience pain following a procedure. It is expected that some pain would be experienced following a procedure.

G89.29   Other chronic pain

● New   ▲ Revised   *Manifestation*   ◢-❼ Digit Indicators   ▭ Laterality   Ⓐ Adult (15+ years)   Ⓜ Maternity (12-55 years)   Ⓝ Newborn   Ⓟ Pediatric (0-17 years)   ♂ Male   ♀ Female
✖ Deleted   Unspecified   + Additional code

582   © 2017 DecisionHealth   2017 ICD-10-CM Expert for Physicians

G89.3 **Neoplasm related pain (acute) (chronic)**
Cancer associated pain
Pain due to malignancy (primary) (secondary)
Tumor associated pain

> **GUIDELINES** Section I.C.6.b.5)
> Code G89.3 is assigned to pain documented as being related, associated or due to cancer, primary or secondary malignancy, or tumor. This code is assigned regardless of whether the pain is acute or chronic. This code may be assigned as the principal or first listed code when the stated reason for the admission/encounter is documented as pain control/pain management. The underlying neoplasm should be reported as an additional diagnosis.
>
> When the reason for the admission/encounter is management of the neoplasm and the pain associated with the neoplasm is also documented, code G89.3 may be assigned as an additional diagnosis. It is not necessary to assign an additional code for the site of the pain.

> **CODING TIP** ✓ When pain is known to be associated with a known neoplasm and the plan of care will include interventions to address the pain, first code the neoplasm, then follow with code G89.3.

G89.4 **Chronic pain syndrome**
Chronic pain associated with significant psychosocial dysfunction

> **GUIDELINES** Section I.C.6.b.6)
> Central pain syndrome (G89.0) and chronic pain syndrome (G89.4) are different than the term "chronic pain," and therefore codes should only be used when the provider has specifically documented this condition.

> **CODING TIP** ✓ Do not confuse chronic pain syndrome with chronic pain (unspecified). Chronic pain syndrome is a specifically diagnosed condition that must be reported by the patient's physician and includes a cycle of psychological and physical components.

◢ G90 **Disorders of autonomic nervous system**

> **EXCLUDES 1** dysfunction of the autonomic nervous system due to alcohol (G31.2)

◳ G90.0 **Idiopathic peripheral autonomic neuropathy**

G90.01 **Carotid sinus syncope**
Carotid sinus syndrome

> **DEFINITION** Exaggerated response to carotid sinus baroreceptor stimulation causing bradycardia, hypotension, and dizziness.

G90.09 **Other idiopathic peripheral autonomic neuropathy**
Idiopathic peripheral autonomic neuropathy NOS

> **CODING TIP** ✓ Do not assign G90.09 for polyneuropathy or unspecified peripheral neuropathy. G90.09 is assigned to specify peripheral autonomic neuropathy, a condition that impairs nervous system function between the autonomic nervous system and the brain, resulting in autonomic dysregulation.

G90.1 **Familial dysautonomia [Riley-Day]**

G90.2 **Horner's syndrome**
Bernard(-Horner) syndrome
Cervical sympathetic dystrophy or paralysis

G90.3 **Multi-system degeneration of the autonomic nervous system**
Neurogenic orthostatic hypotension [Shy-Drager]

> **EXCLUDES 1** orthostatic hypotension NOS (I95.1)

+ G90.4 **Autonomic dysreflexia**
Use additional code to identify the cause, such as:
fecal impaction (K56.41)
pressure ulcer (pressure area) (L89.-)
urinary tract infection (N39.0)

◳ G90.5 **Complex regional pain syndrome I (CRPS I)**
Reflex sympathetic dystrophy

> **EXCLUDES 1** *causalgia of lower limb (G57.7-)*
> *causalgia of upper limb (G56.4-)*
> *complex regional pain syndrome II of lower limb (G57.7-)*
> *complex regional pain syndrome II of upper limb (G56.4-)*

G90.50 **Complex regional pain syndrome I, unspecified**

◉ G90.51 **Complex regional pain syndrome I of upper limb**

◻ G90.511 **Complex regional pain syndrome I of right upper limb**

◻ G90.512 **Complex regional pain syndrome I of left upper limb**

◻ G90.513 **Complex regional pain syndrome I of upper limb, bilateral**

◻ G90.519 **Complex regional pain syndrome I of unspecified upper limb**

◉ G90.52 **Complex regional pain syndrome I of lower limb**

◻ G90.521 **Complex regional pain syndrome I of right lower limb**

◻ G90.522 **Complex regional pain syndrome I of left lower limb**

◻ G90.523 **Complex regional pain syndrome I of lower limb, bilateral**

◻ G90.529 **Complex regional pain syndrome I of unspecified lower limb**

G90.59 **Complex regional pain syndrome I of other specified site**

G90.8 **Other disorders of autonomic nervous system**

G90.9 **Disorder of the autonomic nervous system, unspecified**

◢ G91 **Hydrocephalus**

> **INCLUDES** acquired hydrocephalus

> **EXCLUDES 1** *Arnold-Chiari syndrome with hydrocephalus (Q07.-)*
> *congenital hydrocephalus (Q03.-)*
> *spina bifida with hydrocephalus (Q05.-)*

G91.0 **Communicating hydrocephalus**
Secondary normal pressure hydrocephalus

G91.1 **Obstructive hydrocephalus**

G91.2 **(Idiopathic) normal pressure hydrocephalus**
Normal pressure hydrocephalus NOS

> **DEFINITION** Disruption of normal cerebrospinal fluid circulation and gradual ventricular enlargement without known cause resulting in abnormal gait, cognitive impairment, and urinary incontinence.

G91.3 **Post-traumatic hydrocephalus, unspecified**

G91.4 *Hydrocephalus in diseases classified elsewhere*
Code first underlying condition, such as:
congenital syphilis (A50.4-)
neoplasm (C00-D49)

> **EXCLUDES 1** *hydrocephalus due to congenital toxoplasmosis (P37.1)*

AHA: 3Q 2014, 4

G91.8 **Other hydrocephalus**

G91.9 **Hydrocephalus, unspecified**

G92 **Toxic encephalopathy**
Toxic encephalitis
Toxic metabolic encephalopathy
Code first:
(T51-T65) to identify toxic agent

Toxic encephalopathy

Brain tissue degeneration due to toxic substance

Exposure to toxic substance

Brain

◢ G93 **Other disorders of brain**

G93.0 **Cerebral cysts**
Arachnoid cyst
Porencephalic cyst, acquired

> **EXCLUDES 1** *acquired periventricular cysts of newborn (P91.1)*
> *congenital cerebral cysts (Q04.6)*

● New   ▲ Revised   *Manifestation*   ◢-◻ Digit Indicators   ▣ Laterality   ▣ Adult (15+ years)   Ⓜ Maternity (12-55 years)   Ⓝ Newborn   Ⓟ Pediatric (0-17 years)   ♂ Male   ♀ Female
✖ Deleted   Unspecified   + Additional code

G93.1   **Anoxic brain damage, not elsewhere classified**

> **EXCLUDES 1**   *cerebral anoxia due to anesthesia during labor and delivery (O74.3)*
> *cerebral anoxia due to anesthesia during the puerperium (O89.2)*
> *neonatal anoxia (P84)*

> **CODING TIP ✓**   When the anoxic brain damage is noted as a sequelae of an injury, a code from Chapter 19, Injury, Poisoning and Certain other consequences of External Causes, should be additionally assigned (with a 7th character 'S')

G93.2   **Benign intracranial hypertension**

> **EXCLUDES 1**   *hypertensive encephalopathy (I67.4)*

G93.3   **Postviral fatigue syndrome**
Benign myalgic encephalomyelitis

> **EXCLUDES 1**   *chronic fatigue syndrome NOS (R53.82)*

⑤ G93.4   **Other and unspecified encephalopathy**

> **EXCLUDES 1**   *alcoholic encephalopathy (G31.2)*
> *encephalopathy in diseases classified elsewhere (G94)*
> *hypertensive encephalopathy (I67.4)*
> *toxic (metabolic) encephalopathy (G92)*

G93.40   **Encephalopathy, unspecified**

Encephalopathy

Any disease or disorder of the brain that alters brain function or structure

G93.41   **Metabolic encephalopathy**
Septic encephalopathy

> **DEFINITION**   Neuropsychiatric disturbances due to metabolic brain disease, commonly caused by hypoxia, ischemia, hypoglycemia, or diseases of other organs.
> AHA: 3Q 2015, 21

G93.49   **Other encephalopathy**
Encephalopathy NEC

G93.5   **Compression of brain**
Arnold-Chiari type 1 compression of brain
Compression of brain (stem)
Herniation of brain (stem)

> **EXCLUDES 1**   *diffuse traumatic compression of brain (S06.2-)*
> *focal traumatic compression of brain (S06.3-)*

G93.6   **Cerebral edema**

> **EXCLUDES 1**   *cerebral edema due to birth injury (P11.0)*
> *traumatic cerebral edema (S06.1-)*

G93.7   **Reye's syndrome**   [P]
Code first:
    (T39.0-) , if salicylates-induced

> **DEFINITION**   Rare, acute, sometimes fatal childhood disease with recurrent vomiting, elevated serum transaminase levels and liver changes, then acute brain swelling, consciousness disturbances and seizures.

⑤ G93.8   **Other specified disorders of brain**

G93.81   **Temporal sclerosis**
Hippocampal sclerosis
Mesial temporal sclerosis

G93.82   **Brain death**

G93.89   **Other specified disorders of brain**
Postradiation encephalopathy

G93.9   **Disorder of brain, unspecified**

G94   *Other disorders of brain in diseases classified elsewhere*
Code first:
    underlying disease

> **EXCLUDES 1**   *encephalopathy in congenital syphilis (A50.49)*
> *encephalopathy in influenza (J09.X9, J10.81, J11.81)*
> *encephalopathy in syphilis (A52.19)*
> *hydrocephalus in diseases classified elsewhere (G91.4)*

◀ G95   **Other and unspecified diseases of spinal cord**

> **EXCLUDES 2**   *myelitis (G04.-)*

G95.0   **Syringomyelia and syringobulbia**

> **DEFINITION**   Cyst formation within the spinal cord resulting from trauma, hemorrhage, meningitis, tumor, or Chiari 1 malformation. The growing cyst destroys the cord's center, causing neurologic deficits that progress to greater degrees when not treated surgically.

⑤ G95.1   **Vascular myelopathies**

> **EXCLUDES 2**   *intraspinal phlebitis and thrombophlebitis, except non-pyogenic (G08)*

G95.11   **Acute infarction of spinal cord (embolic) (nonembolic)**
Anoxia of spinal cord
Arterial thrombosis of spinal cord

G95.19   **Other vascular myelopathies**
Edema of spinal cord
Hematomyelia
Nonpyogenic intraspinal phlebitis and thrombophlebitis
Subacute necrotic myelopathy

⑤ G95.2   **Other and unspecified cord compression**

G95.20   **Unspecified cord compression**

G95.29   **Other cord compression**

⑤ G95.8   **Other specified diseases of spinal cord**

> **EXCLUDES 1**   *neurogenic bladder NOS (N31.9)*
> *neurogenic bladder due to cauda equina syndrome (G83.4)*
> *neuromuscular dysfunction of bladder without spinal cord lesion (N31.-)*

G95.81   **Conus medullaris syndrome**

G95.89   **Other specified diseases of spinal cord**
Cord bladder NOS
Drug-induced myelopathy
Radiation-induced myelopathy

> **EXCLUDES 1**   *myelopathy NOS (G95.9)*

G95.9   **Disease of spinal cord, unspecified**
Myelopathy NOS

◀ G96   **Other disorders of central nervous system**

G96.0   **Cerebrospinal fluid leak**

> **EXCLUDES 1**   *cerebrospinal fluid leak from spinal puncture (G97.0)*

⑤ G96.1   **Disorders of meninges, not elsewhere classified**

G96.11   **Dural tear**

> **EXCLUDES 1**   *accidental puncture or laceration of dura during a procedure (G97.41)*

> AHA: 4Q 2014, 24

G96.12   **Meningeal adhesions (cerebral) (spinal)**

G96.19   **Other disorders of meninges, not elsewhere classified**

G96.8   **Other specified disorders of central nervous system**

G96.9   **Disorder of central nervous system, unspecified**

◀ G97   **Intraoperative and postprocedural complications and disorders of nervous system, not elsewhere classified**

> **EXCLUDES 2**   *intraoperative and postprocedural cerebrovascular infarction (I97.81-, I97.82-)*

> **CODING TIP ✓**   Documentation: Do not assign any code for intraoperative and postprocedural complications and disorders of the nervous system without specific documentation from the patient's physician providing a specific relationship between the complication and the procedure.

G97.0   **Cerebrospinal fluid leak from spinal puncture**

G97.1   **Other reaction to spinal and lumbar puncture**
Headache due to lumbar puncture

G97.2   **Intracranial hypotension following ventricular shunting**

● New   ▲ Revised   *Manifestation*   ❹-❼ Digit Indicators   ▤ Laterality   Ⓐ Adult (15+ years)   Ⓜ Maternity (12-55 years)   Ⓝ Newborn   Ⓟ Pediatric (0-17 years)   ♂ Male   ♀ Female
✖ Deleted   Unspecified   ✚ Additional code

584   © 2017 DecisionHealth   2017 ICD-10-CM Expert for Physicians

⑤ **G97.3 Intraoperative hemorrhage and hematoma of a nervous system organ or structure complicating a procedure**
　　EXCLUDES 1 *intraoperative hemorrhage and hematoma of a nervous system organ or structure due to accidental puncture and laceration during a procedure (G97.4-)*

G97.31 Intraoperative hemorrhage and hematoma of a nervous system organ or structure complicating a nervous system procedure

G97.32 Intraoperative hemorrhage and hematoma of a nervous system organ or structure complicating other procedure

⑤ **G97.4 Accidental puncture and laceration of a nervous system organ or structure during a procedure**

G97.41 Accidental puncture or laceration of dura during a procedure
Incidental (inadvertent) durotomy
AHA: 4Q 2014, 24

G97.48 Accidental puncture and laceration of other nervous system organ or structure during a nervous system procedure

G97.49 Accidental puncture and laceration of other nervous system organ or structure during other procedure

▲⑤ **G97.5 Postprocedural hemorrhage of a nervous system organ or structure following a procedure**

▲ **G97.51 Postprocedural hemorrhage of a nervous system organ or structure following a nervous system procedure**

▲ **G97.52 Postprocedural hemorrhage of a nervous system organ or structure following other procedure**

●⑤ **G97.6 Postprocedural hematoma and seroma of a nervous system organ or structure following a procedure**

● **G97.61 Postprocedural hematoma of a nervous system organ or structure following a nervous system procedure**

● **G97.62 Postprocedural hematoma of a nervous system organ or structure following other procedure**

● **G97.63 Postprocedural seroma of a nervous system organ or structure following a nervous system procedure**

● **G97.64 Postprocedural seroma of a nervous system organ or structure following other procedure**

⑤➕ **G97.8 Other intraoperative and postprocedural complications and disorders of nervous system**
Use additional code to further specify disorder

➕ **G97.81 Other intraoperative complications of nervous system**

➕ **G97.82 Other postprocedural complications and disorders of nervous system**

④ **G98 Other disorders of nervous system not elsewhere classified**
　　INCLUDES nervous system disorder NOS

G98.0 Neurogenic arthritis, not elsewhere classified
Nonsyphilitic neurogenic arthropathy NEC
Nonsyphilitic neurogenic spondylopathy NEC
　　EXCLUDES 1 *spondylopathy (in) :*
syringomyelia and syringobulbia (G95.0)
tabes dorsalis (A52.11)

G98.8 Other disorders of nervous system
Nervous system disorder NOS

④ **G99 Other disorders of nervous system in diseases classified elsewhere**

G99.0 *Autonomic neuropathy in diseases classified elsewhere*
Code first underlying disease, such as:
amyloidosis (E85.-)
gout (M1A.-, M10.-)
hyperthyroidism (E05.-)
　　EXCLUDES 1 *diabetic autonomic neuropathy (E08-E13 with .43)*

G99.2 *Myelopathy in diseases classified elsewhere*
Code first underlying disease, such as:
neoplasm (C00-D49)
　　EXCLUDES 1 *myelopathy in:*
intervertebral disease (M50.0-, M51.0-)
spondylosis (M47.0-, M47.1-)

G99.8 *Other specified disorders of nervous system in diseases classified elsewhere*
Code first underlying disorder, such as:
amyloidosis (E85.-)
avitaminosis (E56.9)
　　EXCLUDES 1 *nervous system involvement in:*
cysticercosis (B69.0)
rubella (B06.0-)
syphilis (A52.1-)

CHAPTER 7: DISEASES OF THE EYE AND ADNEXA (H00-H59)

Note: Use an external cause code following the code for the eye condition, if applicable, to identify the cause of the eye condition

EXCLUDES 2 *certain conditions originating in the perinatal period (P04-P96)*
certain infectious and parasitic diseases (A00-B99)
complications of pregnancy, childbirth and the puerperium (O00-O9A)
congenital malformations, deformations, and chromosomal abnormalities (Q00-Q99)
diabetes mellitus related eye conditions (E09.3-, E10.3-, E11.3-, E13.3-)
endocrine, nutritional and metabolic diseases (E00-E88)
injury (trauma) of eye and orbit (S05.-)
injury, poisoning and certain other consequences of external causes (S00-T88)
neoplasms (C00-D49)
symptoms, signs and abnormal clinical and laboratory findings, not elsewhere classified (R00-R94)
syphilis related eye disorders (A50.01, A50.3-, A51.43, A52.71)

This chapter contains the following blocks:
H00-H05	Disorders of eyelid, lacrimal system and orbit
H10-H11	Disorders of conjunctiva
H15-H22	Disorders of sclera, cornea, iris and ciliary body
H25-H28	Disorders of lens
H30-H36	Disorders of choroid and retina
H40-H42	Glaucoma
H43-H44	Disorders of vitreous body and globe
H46-H47	Disorders of optic nerve and visual pathways
H49-H52	Disorders of ocular muscles, binocular movement, accommodation and refraction
H53-H54	Visual disturbances and blindness
H55-H57	Other disorders of eye and adnexa
H59	Intraoperative and postprocedural complications and disorders of eye and adnexa, not elsewhere classified

Disorders of eyelid, lacrimal system and orbit (H00-H05)

EXCLUDES 2 *open wound of eyelid (S01.1-)*
superficial injury of eyelid (S00.1-, S00.2-)

4 **H00** **Hordeolum and chalazion**

Diseases of the eye and adnexa

Swelling

Cornea

Accumulation of liquid

5 **H00.0** **Hordeolum (externum) (internum) of eyelid**

6 **H00.01** **Hordeolum externum**
Hordeolum NOS
Stye
DEFINITION Staph infection of an oil gland in an eyelash follicle.

☐ H00.011 **Hordeolum externum right upper eyelid**
☐ H00.012 **Hordeolum externum right lower eyelid**
☐ H00.013 **Hordeolum externum right eye, unspecified eyelid**
☐ H00.014 **Hordeolum externum left upper eyelid**
☐ H00.015 **Hordeolum externum left lower eyelid**
☐ H00.016 **Hordeolum externum left eye, unspecified eyelid**
☐ H00.019 **Hordeolum externum unspecified eye, unspecified eyelid**

6 **H00.02** **Hordeolum internum**
Infection of meibomian gland
☐ H00.021 **Hordeolum internum right upper eyelid**

☐ H00.022 **Hordeolum internum right lower eyelid**
☐ H00.023 **Hordeolum internum right eye, unspecified eyelid**
☐ H00.024 **Hordeolum internum left upper eyelid**
☐ H00.025 **Hordeolum internum left lower eyelid**
☐ H00.026 **Hordeolum internum left eye, unspecified eyelid**
☐ H00.029 **Hordeolum internum unspecified eye, unspecified eyelid**

6 **H00.03** **Abscess of eyelid**
Furuncle of eyelid
☐ H00.031 **Abscess of right upper eyelid**
☐ H00.032 **Abscess of right lower eyelid**
☐ H00.033 **Abscess of eyelid right eye, unspecified eyelid**
☐ H00.034 **Abscess of left upper eyelid**
☐ H00.035 **Abscess of left lower eyelid**
☐ H00.036 **Abscess of eyelid left eye, unspecified eyelid**
☐ H00.039 **Abscess of eyelid unspecified eye, unspecified eyelid**

5 **H00.1** **Chalazion**
Meibomian (gland) cyst
EXCLUDES 2 *infected meibomian gland (H00.02-)*
DEFINITION Cyst of the tarsal (eyelid) gland.
☐ H00.11 **Chalazion right upper eyelid**
☐ H00.12 **Chalazion right lower eyelid**
☐ H00.13 **Chalazion right eye, unspecified eyelid**
☐ H00.14 **Chalazion left upper eyelid**
☐ H00.15 **Chalazion left lower eyelid**
☐ H00.16 **Chalazion left eye, unspecified eyelid**
☐ H00.19 **Chalazion unspecified eye, unspecified eyelid**

4 **H01** **Other inflammation of eyelid**

5 **H01.0** **Blepharitis**
EXCLUDES 1 *blepharoconjunctivitis (H10.5-)*

6 **H01.00** **Unspecified blepharitis**
DEFINITION An inflammation of the eyelids or lid margins.
☐ H01.001 **Unspecified blepharitis right upper eyelid**
☐ H01.002 **Unspecified blepharitis right lower eyelid**
☐ H01.003 **Unspecified blepharitis right eye, unspecified eyelid**
☐ H01.004 **Unspecified blepharitis left upper eyelid**
☐ H01.005 **Unspecified blepharitis left lower eyelid**
☐ H01.006 **Unspecified blepharitis left eye, unspecified eyelid**
☐ H01.009 **Unspecified blepharitis unspecified eye, unspecified eyelid**

6 **H01.01** **Ulcerative blepharitis**
☐ H01.011 **Ulcerative blepharitis right upper eyelid**
☐ H01.012 **Ulcerative blepharitis right lower eyelid**
☐ H01.013 **Ulcerative blepharitis right eye, unspecified eyelid**
☐ H01.014 **Ulcerative blepharitis left upper eyelid**
☐ H01.015 **Ulcerative blepharitis left lower eyelid**
☐ H01.016 **Ulcerative blepharitis left eye, unspecified eyelid**
☐ H01.019 **Ulcerative blepharitis unspecified eye, unspecified eyelid**

6 **H01.02** **Squamous blepharitis**
☐ H01.021 **Squamous blepharitis right upper eyelid**
☐ H01.022 **Squamous blepharitis right lower eyelid**
☐ H01.023 **Squamous blepharitis right eye, unspecified eyelid**
☐ H01.024 **Squamous blepharitis left upper eyelid**
☐ H01.025 **Squamous blepharitis left lower eyelid**
☐ H01.026 **Squamous blepharitis left eye, unspecified eyelid**
☐ H01.029 **Squamous blepharitis unspecified eye, unspecified eyelid**

5 **H01.1** **Noninfectious dermatoses of eyelid**

● New ▲ Revised *Manifestation* 4-7 Digit Indicators ☐ Laterality A Adult (15+ years) M Maternity (12-55 years) N Newborn P Pediatric (0-17 years) ♂ Male ♀ Female
✖ Deleted Unspecified + Additional code
2017 ICD-10-CM Expert for Physicians

© 2017 DecisionHealth 587

Diseases of the Eye and Adnexa

⑥ **H01.11** **Allergic dermatitis of eyelid**
Contact dermatitis of eyelid

☐ **H01.111** **Allergic dermatitis of right upper eyelid**

☐ **H01.112** **Allergic dermatitis of right lower eyelid**

☐ **H01.113** **Allergic dermatitis of right eye, unspecified eyelid**

☐ **H01.114** **Allergic dermatitis of left upper eyelid**

☐ **H01.115** **Allergic dermatitis of left lower eyelid**

☐ **H01.116** **Allergic dermatitis of left eye, unspecified eyelid**

☐ **H01.119** **Allergic dermatitis of unspecified eye, unspecified eyelid**

⑥ **H01.12** **Discoid lupus erythematosus of eyelid**

☐ **H01.121** **Discoid lupus erythematosus of right upper eyelid**

☐ **H01.122** **Discoid lupus erythematosus of right lower eyelid**

☐ **H01.123** **Discoid lupus erythematosus of right eye, unspecified eyelid**

☐ **H01.124** **Discoid lupus erythematosus of left upper eyelid**

☐ **H01.125** **Discoid lupus erythematosus of left lower eyelid**

☐ **H01.126** **Discoid lupus erythematosus of left eye, unspecified eyelid**

☐ **H01.129** **Discoid lupus erythematosus of unspecified eye, unspecified eyelid**

⑥ **H01.13** **Eczematous dermatitis of eyelid**

☐ **H01.131** **Eczematous dermatitis of right upper eyelid**

☐ **H01.132** **Eczematous dermatitis of right lower eyelid**

☐ **H01.133** **Eczematous dermatitis of right eye, unspecified eyelid**

☐ **H01.134** **Eczematous dermatitis of left upper eyelid**

☐ **H01.135** **Eczematous dermatitis of left lower eyelid**

☐ **H01.136** **Eczematous dermatitis of left eye, unspecified eyelid**

☐ **H01.139** **Eczematous dermatitis of unspecified eye, unspecified eyelid**

⑥ **H01.14** **Xeroderma of eyelid**

☐ **H01.141** **Xeroderma of right upper eyelid**

☐ **H01.142** **Xeroderma of right lower eyelid**

☐ **H01.143** **Xeroderma of right eye, unspecified eyelid**

☐ **H01.144** **Xeroderma of left upper eyelid**

☐ **H01.145** **Xeroderma of left lower eyelid**

☐ **H01.146** **Xeroderma of left eye, unspecified eyelid**

☐ **H01.149** **Xeroderma of unspecified eye, unspecified eyelid**

H01.8 **Other specified inflammations of eyelid**

H01.9 **Unspecified inflammation of eyelid**
Inflammation of eyelid NOS

④ **H02** **Other disorders of eyelid**

EXCLUDES 1 *congenital malformations of eyelid (Q10.0-Q10.3)*

⑤ **H02.0** **Entropion and trichiasis of eyelid**

⑥ **H02.00** **Unspecified entropion of eyelid**

DEFINITION Inward curling of the eyelid margin, usually the bottom, so the lashes irritate the surface of the eyeball.

☐ **H02.001** **Unspecified entropion of right upper eyelid**

☐ **H02.002** **Unspecified entropion of right lower eyelid**

☐ **H02.003** **Unspecified entropion of right eye, unspecified eyelid**

☐ **H02.004** **Unspecified entropion of left upper eyelid**

☐ **H02.005** **Unspecified entropion of left lower eyelid**

☐ **H02.006** **Unspecified entropion of left eye, unspecified eyelid**

☐ **H02.009** **Unspecified entropion of unspecified eye, unspecified eyelid**

⑥ **H02.01** **Cicatricial entropion of eyelid**

☐ **H02.011** **Cicatricial entropion of right upper eyelid**

☐ **H02.012** **Cicatricial entropion of right lower eyelid**

☐ **H02.013** **Cicatricial entropion of right eye, unspecified eyelid**

☐ **H02.014** **Cicatricial entropion of left upper eyelid**

☐ **H02.015** **Cicatricial entropion of left lower eyelid**

☐ **H02.016** **Cicatricial entropion of left eye, unspecified eyelid**

☐ **H02.019** **Cicatricial entropion of unspecified eye, unspecified eyelid**

⑥ **H02.02** **Mechanical entropion of eyelid**

☐ **H02.021** **Mechanical entropion of right upper eyelid**

☐ **H02.022** **Mechanical entropion of right lower eyelid**

☐ **H02.023** **Mechanical entropion of right eye, unspecified eyelid**

☐ **H02.024** **Mechanical entropion of left upper eyelid**

☐ **H02.025** **Mechanical entropion of left lower eyelid**

☐ **H02.026** **Mechanical entropion of left eye, unspecified eyelid**

☐ **H02.029** **Mechanical entropion of unspecified eye, unspecified eyelid**

⑥ **H02.03** **Senile entropion of eyelid**

☐ **H02.031** **Senile entropion of right upper eyelid** Ⓐ

☐ **H02.032** **Senile entropion of right lower eyelid** Ⓐ

☐ **H02.033** **Senile entropion of right eye, unspecified eyelid** Ⓐ

☐ **H02.034** **Senile entropion of left upper eyelid** Ⓐ

☐ **H02.035** **Senile entropion of left lower eyelid** Ⓐ

☐ **H02.036** **Senile entropion of left eye, unspecified eyelid** Ⓐ

☐ **H02.039** **Senile entropion of unspecified eye, unspecified eyelid** Ⓐ

⑥ **H02.04** **Spastic entropion of eyelid**

☐ **H02.041** **Spastic entropion of right upper eyelid**

☐ **H02.042** **Spastic entropion of right lower eyelid**

☐ **H02.043** **Spastic entropion of right eye, unspecified eyelid**

☐ **H02.044** **Spastic entropion of left upper eyelid**

☐ **H02.045** **Spastic entropion of left lower eyelid**

☐ **H02.046** **Spastic entropion of left eye, unspecified eyelid**

☐ **H02.049** **Spastic entropion of unspecified eye, unspecified eyelid**

⑥ **H02.05** **Trichiasis without entropian**

☐ **H02.051** **Trichiasis without entropian right upper eyelid**

☐ **H02.052** **Trichiasis without entropian right lower eyelid**

☐ **H02.053** **Trichiasis without entropian right eye, unspecified eyelid**

☐ **H02.054** **Trichiasis without entropian left upper eyelid**

☐ **H02.055** **Trichiasis without entropian left lower eyelid**

☐ **H02.056** **Trichiasis without entropian left eye, unspecified eyelid**

☐ **H02.059** **Trichiasis without entropian unspecified eye, unspecified eyelid**

⑤ **H02.1** **Ectropion of eyelid**

⑥ **H02.10** **Unspecified ectropion of eyelid**

DEFINITION Outward curling of the eyelid away from the eye, usually the lower, exposing the inner surface and causing irritation, dryness, pain and possible conjunctivitis and keratitis.

☐ **H02.101** **Unspecified ectropion of right upper eyelid**

☐ **H02.102** **Unspecified ectropion of right lower eyelid**

☐ **H02.103** **Unspecified ectropion of right eye, unspecified eyelid**

☐ **H02.104** **Unspecified ectropion of left upper eyelid**

☐ **H02.105** **Unspecified ectropion of left lower eyelid**

☐ **H02.106** **Unspecified ectropion of left eye, unspecified eyelid**

☐ **H02.109** **Unspecified ectropion of unspecified eye, unspecified eyelid**

⑥ **H02.11** **Cicatricial ectropion of eyelid**

☐ **H02.111** **Cicatricial ectropion of right upper eyelid**

☐ **H02.112** **Cicatricial ectropion of right lower eyelid**

☐ **H02.113** **Cicatricial ectropion of right eye, unspecified eyelid**

☐ **H02.114** **Cicatricial ectropion of left upper eyelid**

● New ▲ Revised *Manifestation* ④-⑦ Digit Indicators ☐ Laterality Ⓐ Adult (15+ years) Ⓜ Maternity (12-55 years) Ⓝ Newborn Ⓟ Pediatric (0-17 years) ♂ Male ♀ Female
✖ Deleted Unspecified + Additional code

588   © 2017 DecisionHealth   2017 ICD-10-CM Expert for Physicians

H02.115   Cicatricial ectropion of left lower eyelid

H02.116   Cicatricial ectropion of left eye, unspecified eyelid

H02.119   Cicatricial ectropion of unspecified eye, unspecified eyelid

◯ **H02.12**   Mechanical ectropion of eyelid

H02.121   Mechanical ectropion of right upper eyelid

H02.122   Mechanical ectropion of right lower eyelid

H02.123   Mechanical ectropion of right eye, unspecified eyelid

H02.124   Mechanical ectropion of left upper eyelid

H02.125   Mechanical ectropion of left lower eyelid

H02.126   Mechanical ectropion of left eye, unspecified eyelid

H02.129   Mechanical ectropion of unspecified eye, unspecified eyelid

◯ **H02.13**   Senile ectropion of eyelid

H02.131   Senile ectropion of right upper eyelid   Ⓐ

H02.132   Senile ectropion of right lower eyelid   Ⓐ

H02.133   Senile ectropion of right eye, unspecified eyelid   Ⓐ

H02.134   Senile ectropion of left upper eyelid   Ⓐ

H02.135   Senile ectropion of left lower eyelid   Ⓐ

H02.136   Senile ectropion of left eye, unspecified eyelid   Ⓐ

H02.139   Senile ectropion of unspecified eye, unspecified eyelid   Ⓐ

◯ **H02.14**   Spastic ectropion of eyelid

H02.141   Spastic ectropion of right upper eyelid

H02.142   Spastic ectropion of right lower eyelid

H02.143   Spastic ectropion of right eye, unspecified eyelid

H02.144   Spastic ectropion of left upper eyelid

H02.145   Spastic ectropion of left lower eyelid

H02.146   Spastic ectropion of left eye, unspecified eyelid

H02.149   Spastic ectropion of unspecified eye, unspecified eyelid

Ⓢ **H02.2**   Lagophthalmos

◯ **H02.20**   Unspecified lagophthalmos

H02.201   Unspecified lagophthalmos right upper eyelid

H02.202   Unspecified lagophthalmos right lower eyelid

H02.203   Unspecified lagophthalmos right eye, unspecified eyelid

H02.204   Unspecified lagophthalmos left upper eyelid

H02.205   Unspecified lagophthalmos left lower eyelid

H02.206   Unspecified lagophthalmos left eye, unspecified eyelid

H02.209   Unspecified lagophthalmos unspecified eye, unspecified eyelid

◯ **H02.21**   Cicatricial lagophthalmos

DEFINITION   Inability to completely close the eye due to the presence of scar tissue.

H02.211   Cicatricial lagophthalmos right upper eyelid

H02.212   Cicatricial lagophthalmos right lower eyelid

H02.213   Cicatricial lagophthalmos right eye, unspecified eyelid

H02.214   Cicatricial lagophthalmos left upper eyelid

H02.215   Cicatricial lagophthalmos left lower eyelid

H02.216   Cicatricial lagophthalmos left eye, unspecified eyelid

H02.219   Cicatricial lagophthalmos unspecified eye, unspecified eyelid

◯ **H02.22**   Mechanical lagophthalmos

H02.221   Mechanical lagophthalmos right upper eyelid

H02.222   Mechanical lagophthalmos right lower eyelid

H02.223   Mechanical lagophthalmos right eye, unspecified eyelid

H02.224   Mechanical lagophthalmos left upper eyelid

H02.225   Mechanical lagophthalmos left lower eyelid

H02.226   Mechanical lagophthalmos left eye, unspecified eyelid

H02.229   Mechanical lagophthalmos unspecified eye, unspecified eyelid

◯ **H02.23**   Paralytic lagophthalmos

H02.231   Paralytic lagophthalmos right upper eyelid

H02.232   Paralytic lagophthalmos right lower eyelid

H02.233   Paralytic lagophthalmos right eye, unspecified eyelid

H02.234   Paralytic lagophthalmos left upper eyelid

H02.235   Paralytic lagophthalmos left lower eyelid

H02.236   Paralytic lagophthalmos left eye, unspecified eyelid

H02.239   Paralytic lagophthalmos unspecified eye, unspecified eyelid

Ⓢ **H02.3**   Blepharochalasis

Pseudoptosis

DEFINITION   Sagging of the skin of the eyelid. In the upper eyelid, the skin sags over the eye obstructing vision; usually due to changes in elastin and collagen, affecting the skin's elasticity.

H02.30   Blepharochalasis unspecified eye, unspecified eyelid

H02.31   Blepharochalasis right upper eyelid

H02.32   Blepharochalasis right lower eyelid

H02.33   Blepharochalasis right eye, unspecified eyelid

H02.34   Blepharochalasis left upper eyelid

H02.35   Blepharochalasis left lower eyelid

H02.36   Blepharochalasis left eye, unspecified eyelid

Ⓢ **H02.4**   Ptosis of eyelid

◯ **H02.40**   Unspecified ptosis of eyelid

H02.401   Unspecified ptosis of right eyelid

H02.402   Unspecified ptosis of left eyelid

H02.403   Unspecified ptosis of bilateral eyelids

H02.409   Unspecified ptosis of unspecified eyelid

◯ **H02.41**   Mechanical ptosis of eyelid

H02.411   Mechanical ptosis of right eyelid

H02.412   Mechanical ptosis of left eyelid

H02.413   Mechanical ptosis of bilateral eyelids

H02.419   Mechanical ptosis of unspecified eyelid

◯ **H02.42**   Myogenic ptosis of eyelid

H02.421   Myogenic ptosis of right eyelid

H02.422   Myogenic ptosis of left eyelid

H02.423   Myogenic ptosis of bilateral eyelids

H02.429   Myogenic ptosis of unspecified eyelid

◯ **H02.43**   Paralytic ptosis of eyelid

Neurogenic ptosis of eyelid

H02.431   Paralytic ptosis of right eyelid

H02.432   Paralytic ptosis of left eyelid

H02.433   Paralytic ptosis of bilateral eyelids

H02.439   Paralytic ptosis unspecified eyelid

Ⓢ **H02.5**   Other disorders affecting eyelid function

EXCLUDES 2   blepharospasm (G24.5)
organic tic (G25.69)
psychogenic tic (F95.-)

◯ **H02.51**   Abnormal innervation syndrome

H02.511   Abnormal innervation syndrome right upper eyelid

H02.512   Abnormal innervation syndrome right lower eyelid

H02.513   Abnormal innervation syndrome right eye, unspecified eyelid

H02.514   Abnormal innervation syndrome left upper eyelid

H02.515   Abnormal innervation syndrome left lower eyelid

H02.516   Abnormal innervation syndrome left eye, unspecified eyelid

H02.519   Abnormal innervation syndrome unspecified eye, unspecified eyelid

◯ **H02.52**   Blepharophimosis

Ankyloblepharon

● New   ▲ Revised   *Manifestation*   ④-⑦ Digit Indicators   ▱ Laterality   Ⓐ Adult (15+ years)   Ⓜ Maternity (12-55 years)   Ⓝ Newborn   Ⓟ Pediatric (0-17 years)   ♂ Male   ♀ Female

✖ ~~Deleted~~   Unspecified   + Additional code

DEFINITION Hereditary disorder in which the palpebral fissures (space between the eyelids) is narrowed, giving the appearance of continually squinting.

- H02.521 **Blepharophimosis right upper eyelid**
- H02.522 **Blepharophimosis right lower eyelid**
- H02.523 **Blepharophimosis right eye, unspecified eyelid**
- H02.524 **Blepharophimosis left upper eyelid**
- H02.525 **Blepharophimosis left lower eyelid**
- H02.526 **Blepharophimosis left eye, unspecified eyelid**
- H02.529 **Blepharophimosis unspecified eye, unspecified lid**

⑥ H02.53 **Eyelid retraction**
Eyelid lag
- H02.531 **Eyelid retraction right upper eyelid**
- H02.532 **Eyelid retraction right lower eyelid**
- H02.533 **Eyelid retraction right eye, unspecified eyelid**
- H02.534 **Eyelid retraction left upper eyelid**
- H02.535 **Eyelid retraction left lower eyelid**
- H02.536 **Eyelid retraction left eye, unspecified eyelid**
- H02.539 **Eyelid retraction unspecified eye, unspecified lid**

H02.59 **Other disorders affecting eyelid function**
Deficient blink reflex
Sensory disorders

⑤ H02.6 **Xanthelasma of eyelid**
- H02.60 **Xanthelasma of unspecified eye, unspecified eyelid**
- H02.61 **Xanthelasma of right upper eyelid**
- H02.62 **Xanthelasma of right lower eyelid**
- H02.63 **Xanthelasma of right eye, unspecified eyelid**
- H02.64 **Xanthelasma of left upper eyelid**
- H02.65 **Xanthelasma of left lower eyelid**
- H02.66 **Xanthelasma of left eye, unspecified eyelid**

⑤ H02.7 **Other and unspecified degenerative disorders of eyelid and periocular area**
H02.70 **Unspecified degenerative disorders of eyelid and periocular area**

⑥ H02.71 **Chloasma of eyelid and periocular area**
Dyspigmentation of eyelid
Hyperpigmentation of eyelid
- H02.711 **Chloasma of right upper eyelid and periocular area**
- H02.712 **Chloasma of right lower eyelid and periocular area**
- H02.713 **Chloasma of right eye, unspecified eyelid and periocular area**
- H02.714 **Chloasma of left upper eyelid and periocular area**
- H02.715 **Chloasma of left lower eyelid and periocular area**
- H02.716 **Chloasma of left eye, unspecified eyelid and periocular area**
- H02.719 **Chloasma of unspecified eye, unspecified eyelid and periocular area**

⑥ H02.72 **Madarosis of eyelid and periocular area**
Hypotrichosis of eyelid
- H02.721 **Madarosis of right upper eyelid and periocular area**
- H02.722 **Madarosis of right lower eyelid and periocular area**
- H02.723 **Madarosis of right eye, unspecified eyelid and periocular area**
- H02.724 **Madarosis of left upper eyelid and periocular area**
- H02.725 **Madarosis of left lower eyelid and periocular area**
- H02.726 **Madarosis of left eye, unspecified eyelid and periocular area**
- H02.729 **Madarosis of unspecified eye, unspecified eyelid and periocular area**

⑥ H02.73 **Vitiligo of eyelid and periocular area**
Hypopigmentation of eyelid

- H02.731 **Vitiligo of right upper eyelid and periocular area**
- H02.732 **Vitiligo of right lower eyelid and periocular area**
- H02.733 **Vitiligo of right eye, unspecified eyelid and periocular area**
- H02.734 **Vitiligo of left upper eyelid and periocular area**
- H02.735 **Vitiligo of left lower eyelid and periocular area**
- H02.736 **Vitiligo of left eye, unspecified eyelid and periocular area**
- H02.739 **Vitiligo of unspecified eye, unspecified eyelid and periocular area**

H02.79 **Other degenerative disorders of eyelid and periocular area**

⑤ H02.8 **Other specified disorders of eyelid**

⑥✚ H02.81 **Retained foreign body in eyelid**
Use additional code to identify the type of retained foreign body (Z18.-)
EXCLUDES 1 *laceration of eyelid with foreign body (S01.12-)*
retained intraocular foreign body (H44.6-, H44.7-)
superficial foreign body of eyelid and periocular area (S00.25-)
- ✚ H02.811 **Retained foreign body in right upper eyelid**
- ✚ H02.812 **Retained foreign body in right lower eyelid**
- ✚ H02.813 **Retained foreign body in right eye, unspecified eyelid**
- ✚ H02.814 **Retained foreign body in left upper eyelid**
- ✚ H02.815 **Retained foreign body in left lower eyelid**
- ✚ H02.816 **Retained foreign body in left eye, unspecified eyelid**
- ✚ H02.819 **Retained foreign body in unspecified eye, unspecified eyelid**

⑥ H02.82 **Cysts of eyelid**
Sebaceous cyst of eyelid
- H02.821 **Cysts of right upper eyelid**
- H02.822 **Cysts of right lower eyelid**
- H02.823 **Cysts of right eye, unspecified eyelid**
- H02.824 **Cysts of left upper eyelid**
- H02.825 **Cysts of left lower eyelid**
- H02.826 **Cysts of left eye, unspecified eyelid**
- H02.829 **Cysts of unspecified eye, unspecified eyelid**

⑥ H02.83 **Dermatochalasis of eyelid**
- H02.831 **Dermatochalasis of right upper eyelid**
- H02.832 **Dermatochalasis of right lower eyelid**
- H02.833 **Dermatochalasis of right eye, unspecified eyelid**
- H02.834 **Dermatochalasis of left upper eyelid**
- H02.835 **Dermatochalasis of left lower eyelid**
- H02.836 **Dermatochalasis of left eye, unspecified eyelid**
- H02.839 **Dermatochalasis of unspecified eye, unspecified eyelid**

⑥ H02.84 **Edema of eyelid**
Hyperemia of eyelid
- H02.841 **Edema of right upper eyelid**
- H02.842 **Edema of right lower eyelid**
- H02.843 **Edema of right eye, unspecified eyelid**
- H02.844 **Edema of left upper eyelid**
- H02.845 **Edema of left lower eyelid**
- H02.846 **Edema of left eye, unspecified eyelid**
- H02.849 **Edema of unspecified eye, unspecified eyelid**

⑥ H02.85 **Elephantiasis of eyelid**
- H02.851 **Elephantiasis of right upper eyelid**
- H02.852 **Elephantiasis of right lower eyelid**
- H02.853 **Elephantiasis of right eye, unspecified eyelid**
- H02.854 **Elephantiasis of left upper eyelid**
- H02.855 **Elephantiasis of left lower eyelid**
- H02.856 **Elephantiasis of left eye, unspecified eyelid**
- H02.859 **Elephantiasis of unspecified eye, unspecified eyelid**

⑥ H02.86 **Hypertrichosis of eyelid**

● New ▲ Revised *Manifestation* ④-❼ Digit Indicators ▣ Laterality 🅐 Adult (15+ years) 🅜 Maternity (12-55 years) 🅝 Newborn 🄿 Pediatric (0-17 years) ♂ Male ♀ Female
✖ Deleted Unspecified ✚ Additional code

590   © 2017 DecisionHealth   2017 ICD-10-CM Expert for Physicians

⊟ H02.861   Hypertrichosis of right upper eyelid

⊟ H02.862   Hypertrichosis of right lower eyelid

⊟ H02.863   Hypertrichosis of right eye, unspecified eyelid

⊟ H02.864   Hypertrichosis of left upper eyelid

⊟ H02.865   Hypertrichosis of left lower eyelid

⊟ H02.866   Hypertrichosis of left eye, unspecified eyelid

⊟ H02.869   Hypertrichosis of unspecified eye, unspecified eyelid

Ⓖ H02.87   Vascular anomalies of eyelid

⊟ H02.871   Vascular anomalies of right upper eyelid

⊟ H02.872   Vascular anomalies of right lower eyelid

⊟ H02.873   Vascular anomalies of right eye, unspecified eyelid

⊟ H02.874   Vascular anomalies of left upper eyelid

⊟ H02.875   Vascular anomalies of left lower eyelid

⊟ H02.876   Vascular anomalies of left eye, unspecified eyelid

⊟ H02.879   Vascular anomalies of unspecified eye, unspecified eyelid

H02.89   Other specified disorders of eyelid
Hemorrhage of eyelid

H02.9   Unspecified disorder of eyelid
Disorder of eyelid NOS

Ⓐ H04   Disorders of lacrimal system

EXCLUDES 1   *congenital malformations of lacrimal system (Q10.4-Q10.6)*

Ⓢ H04.0   Dacryoadenitis

Ⓖ H04.00   Unspecified dacryoadenitis

DEFINITION   Inflammation of the lacrimal gland.

⊟ H04.001   Unspecified dacryoadenitis, right lacrimal gland

⊟ H04.002   Unspecified dacryoadenitis, left lacrimal gland

⊟ H04.003   Unspecified dacryoadenitis, bilateral lacrimal glands

⊟ H04.009   Unspecified dacryoadenitis, unspecified lacrimal gland

Ⓖ H04.01   Acute dacryoadenitis

⊟ H04.011   Acute dacryoadenitis, right lacrimal gland

⊟ H04.012   Acute dacryoadenitis, left lacrimal gland

⊟ H04.013   Acute dacryoadenitis, bilateral lacrimal glands

⊟ H04.019   Acute dacryoadenitis, unspecified lacrimal gland

Ⓖ H04.02   Chronic dacryoadenitis

⊟ H04.021   Chronic dacryoadenitis, right lacrimal gland

⊟ H04.022   Chronic dacryoadenitis, left lacrimal gland

⊟ H04.023   Chronic dacryoadenitis, bilateral lacrimal gland

⊟ H04.029   Chronic dacryoadenitis, unspecified lacrimal gland

Ⓖ H04.03   Chronic enlargement of lacrimal gland

⊟ H04.031   Chronic enlargement of right lacrimal gland

⊟ H04.032   Chronic enlargement of left lacrimal gland

⊟ H04.033   Chronic enlargement of bilateral lacrimal glands

⊟ H04.039   Chronic enlargement of unspecified lacrimal gland

Ⓢ H04.1   Other disorders of lacrimal gland

Ⓖ H04.11   Dacryops

⊟ H04.111   Dacryops of right lacrimal gland

⊟ H04.112   Dacryops of left lacrimal gland

⊟ H04.113   Dacryops of bilateral lacrimal glands

⊟ H04.119   Dacryops of unspecified lacrimal gland

Ⓖ H04.12   Dry eye syndrome
Tear film insufficiency, NOS

⊟ H04.121   Dry eye syndrome of right lacrimal gland

⊟ H04.122   Dry eye syndrome of left lacrimal gland

⊟ H04.123   Dry eye syndrome of bilateral lacrimal glands

⊟ H04.129   Dry eye syndrome of unspecified lacrimal gland

Ⓖ H04.13   Lacrimal cyst
Lacrimal cystic degeneration

⊟ H04.131   Lacrimal cyst, right lacrimal gland

⊟ H04.132   Lacrimal cyst, left lacrimal gland

⊟ H04.133   Lacrimal cyst, bilateral lacrimal glands

⊟ H04.139   Lacrimal cyst, unspecified lacrimal gland

Ⓖ H04.14   Primary lacrimal gland atrophy

DEFINITION   Wasting of the lacrimal glands causing severe dryness with decreased tear production.

⊟ H04.141   Primary lacrimal gland atrophy, right lacrimal gland

⊟ H04.142   Primary lacrimal gland atrophy, left lacrimal gland

⊟ H04.143   Primary lacrimal gland atrophy, bilateral lacrimal glands

⊟ H04.149   Primary lacrimal gland atrophy, unspecified lacrimal gland

Ⓖ H04.15   Secondary lacrimal gland atrophy

⊟ H04.151   Secondary lacrimal gland atrophy, right lacrimal gland

⊟ H04.152   Secondary lacrimal gland atrophy, left lacrimal gland

⊟ H04.153   Secondary lacrimal gland atrophy, bilateral lacrimal glands

⊟ H04.159   Secondary lacrimal gland atrophy, unspecified lacrimal gland

Ⓖ H04.16   Lacrimal gland dislocation

DEFINITION   Lacrimal gland separated from the tear ducts, preventing tears from passing normally to the eye.

⊟ H04.161   Lacrimal gland dislocation, right lacrimal gland

⊟ H04.162   Lacrimal gland dislocation, left lacrimal gland

⊟ H04.163   Lacrimal gland dislocation, bilateral lacrimal glands

⊟ H04.169   Lacrimal gland dislocation, unspecified lacrimal gland

H04.19   Other specified disorders of lacrimal gland

Ⓢ H04.2   Epiphora

Ⓖ H04.20   Unspecified epiphora

⊟ H04.201   Unspecified epiphora, right lacrimal gland

⊟ H04.202   Unspecified epiphora, left lacrimal gland

⊟ H04.203   Unspecified epiphora, bilateral lacrimal glands

⊟ H04.209   Unspecified epiphora, unspecified lacrimal gland

Ⓖ H04.21   Epiphora due to excess lacrimation

⊟ H04.211   Epiphora due to excess lacrimation, right lacrimal gland

⊟ H04.212   Epiphora due to excess lacrimation, left lacrimal gland

⊟ H04.213   Epiphora due to excess lacrimation, bilateral lacrimal glands

⊟ H04.219   Epiphora due to excess lacrimation, unspecified lacrimal gland

Ⓖ H04.22   Epiphora due to insufficient drainage

⊟ H04.221   Epiphora due to insufficient drainage, right lacrimal gland

⊟ H04.222   Epiphora due to insufficient drainage, left lacrimal gland

⊟ H04.223   Epiphora due to insufficient drainage, bilateral lacrimal glands

⊟ H04.229   Epiphora due to insufficient drainage, unspecified lacrimal gland

Ⓢ H04.3   Acute and unspecified inflammation of lacrimal passages

EXCLUDES 1   *neonatal dacryocystitis (P39.1)*

Ⓖ H04.30   Unspecified dacryocystitis

DEFINITION   Inflammation of the lacrimal sac in the eye causing obstruction of the tube draining tears into the nose.

⊟ H04.301   Unspecified dacryocystitis of right lacrimal passage

⊟ H04.302   Unspecified dacryocystitis of left lacrimal passage

⊟ H04.303   Unspecified dacryocystitis of bilateral lacrimal passages

● New   ▲ Revised   *Manifestation*   ◢-☷ Digit Indicators   ⊟ Laterality   Ⓐ Adult (15+ years)   Ⓜ Maternity (12-55 years)   Ⓝ Newborn   Ⓟ Pediatric (0-17 years)   ♂ Male   ♀ Female
✖ Deleted   Unspecified   + Additional code

2017 ICD-10-CM Expert for Physicians

© 2017 DecisionHealth   591

H02.861 — H04.303

⊟ **H04.309**   **Unspecified dacryocystitis of unspecified lacrimal passage**

Ⓖ **H04.31**   Phlegmonous dacryocystitis

⊟ **H04.311**   **Phlegmonous dacryocystitis of right lacrimal passage**

⊟ **H04.312**   **Phlegmonous dacryocystitis of left lacrimal passage**

⊟ **H04.313**   **Phlegmonous dacryocystitis of bilateral lacrimal passages**

⊟ **H04.319**   **Phlegmonous dacryocystitis of unspecified lacrimal passage**

Ⓖ **H04.32**   Acute dacryocystitis

Acute dacryopericystitis

> **DEFINITION**   Sudden, severe inflammation of the tear sac, usually due to blockage of the tear ducts.

⊟ **H04.321**   **Acute dacryocystitis of right lacrimal passage**

⊟ **H04.322**   **Acute dacryocystitis of left lacrimal passage**

⊟ **H04.323**   **Acute dacryocystitis of bilateral lacrimal passages**

⊟ **H04.329**   **Acute dacryocystitis of unspecified lacrimal passage**

Ⓖ **H04.33**   Acute lacrimal canaliculitis

> **DEFINITION**   Sudden, severe inflammation of the lacrimal passages or tear ducts.

⊟ **H04.331**   **Acute lacrimal canaliculitis of right lacrimal passage**

⊟ **H04.332**   **Acute lacrimal canaliculitis of left lacrimal passage**

⊟ **H04.333**   **Acute lacrimal canaliculitis of bilateral lacrimal passages**

⊟ **H04.339**   **Acute lacrimal canaliculitis of unspecified lacrimal passage**

⑤ **H04.4**   **Chronic inflammation of lacrimal passages**

Ⓖ **H04.41**   **Chronic dacryocystitis**

⊟ **H04.411**   **Chronic dacryocystitis of right lacrimal passage**

⊟ **H04.412**   **Chronic dacryocystitis of left lacrimal passage**

⊟ **H04.413**   **Chronic dacryocystitis of bilateral lacrimal passages**

⊟ **H04.419**   **Chronic dacryocystitis of unspecified lacrimal passage**

Ⓖ **H04.42**   **Chronic lacrimal canaliculitis**

⊟ **H04.421**   **Chronic lacrimal canaliculitis of right lacrimal passage**

⊟ **H04.422**   **Chronic lacrimal canaliculitis of left lacrimal passage**

⊟ **H04.423**   **Chronic lacrimal canaliculitis of bilateral lacrimal passages**

⊟ **H04.429**   **Chronic lacrimal canaliculitis of unspecified lacrimal passage**

Ⓖ **H04.43**   Chronic lacrimal mucocele

> **DEFINITION**   Inflammation of the lacrimal system in which the tear ducts, and then the eyes, become filled with mucous.

⊟ **H04.431**   **Chronic lacrimal mucocele of right lacrimal passage**

⊟ **H04.432**   **Chronic lacrimal mucocele of left lacrimal passage**

⊟ **H04.433**   **Chronic lacrimal mucocele of bilateral lacrimal passages**

⊟ **H04.439**   **Chronic lacrimal mucocele of unspecified lacrimal passage**

⑤ **H04.5**   **Stenosis and insufficiency of lacrimal passages**

Ⓖ **H04.51**   **Dacryolith**

⊟ **H04.511**   **Dacryolith of right lacrimal passage**

⊟ **H04.512**   **Dacryolith of left lacrimal passage**

⊟ **H04.513**   **Dacryolith of bilateral lacrimal passages**

⊟ **H04.519**   **Dacryolith of unspecified lacrimal passage**

Ⓖ **H04.52**   Eversion of lacrimal punctum

> **DEFINITION**   Tear duct exit turned away from the eye, causing tears to flow directly onto the face instead of moistening the eyeball.

⊟ **H04.521**   **Eversion of right lacrimal punctum**

⊟ **H04.522**   **Eversion of left lacrimal punctum**

⊟ **H04.523**   **Eversion of bilateral lacrimal punctum**

⊟ **H04.529**   **Eversion of unspecified lacrimal punctum**

Ⓖ **H04.53**   Neonatal obstruction of nasolacrimal duct

> **EXCLUDES 1**   *congenital stenosis and stricture of lacrimal duct (Q10.5)*

⊟ **H04.531**   **Neonatal obstruction of right nasolacrimal duct** Ⓝ

⊟ **H04.532**   **Neonatal obstruction of left nasolacrimal duct** Ⓝ

⊟ **H04.533**   **Neonatal obstruction of bilateral nasolacrimal duct** Ⓝ

⊟ **H04.539**   **Neonatal obstruction of unspecified nasolacrimal duct** Ⓝ

Ⓖ **H04.54**   Stenosis of lacrimal canaliculi

⊟ **H04.541**   **Stenosis of right lacrimal canaliculi**

⊟ **H04.542**   **Stenosis of left lacrimal canaliculi**

⊟ **H04.543**   **Stenosis of bilateral lacrimal canaliculi**

⊟ **H04.549**   **Stenosis of unspecified lacrimal canaliculi**

Ⓖ **H04.55**   Acquired stenosis of nasolacrimal duct

⊟ **H04.551**   **Acquired stenosis of right nasolacrimal duct**

⊟ **H04.552**   **Acquired stenosis of left nasolacrimal duct**

⊟ **H04.553**   **Acquired stenosis of bilateral nasolacrimal duct**

⊟ **H04.559**   **Acquired stenosis of unspecified nasolacrimal duct**

Ⓖ **H04.56**   Stenosis of lacrimal punctum

⊟ **H04.561**   **Stenosis of right lacrimal punctum**

⊟ **H04.562**   **Stenosis of left lacrimal punctum**

⊟ **H04.563**   **Stenosis of bilateral lacrimal punctum**

⊟ **H04.569**   **Stenosis of unspecified lacrimal punctum**

Ⓖ **H04.57**   Stenosis of lacrimal sac

⊟ **H04.571**   **Stenosis of right lacrimal sac**

⊟ **H04.572**   **Stenosis of left lacrimal sac**

⊟ **H04.573**   **Stenosis of bilateral lacrimal sac**

⊟ **H04.579**   **Stenosis of unspecified lacrimal sac**

⑤ **H04.6**   **Other changes of lacrimal passages**

Ⓖ **H04.61**   **Lacrimal fistula**

⊟ **H04.611**   **Lacrimal fistula right lacrimal passage**

⊟ **H04.612**   **Lacrimal fistula left lacrimal passage**

⊟ **H04.613**   **Lacrimal fistula bilateral lacrimal passages**

⊟ **H04.619**   **Lacrimal fistula unspecified lacrimal passage**

H04.69   **Other changes of lacrimal passages**

⑤ **H04.8**   **Other disorders of lacrimal system**

Ⓖ **H04.81**   **Granuloma of lacrimal passages**

⊟ **H04.811**   **Granuloma of right lacrimal passage**

⊟ **H04.812**   **Granuloma of left lacrimal passage**

⊟ **H04.813**   **Granuloma of bilateral lacrimal passages**

⊟ **H04.819**   **Granuloma of unspecified lacrimal passage**

H04.89   **Other disorders of lacrimal system**

H04.9   **Disorder of lacrimal system, unspecified**

④ **H05**   **Disorders of orbit**

> **EXCLUDES 1**   *congenital malformation of orbit (Q10.7)*

⑤ **H05.0**   **Acute inflammation of orbit**

H05.00   **Unspecified acute inflammation of orbit**

Ⓖ **H05.01**   **Cellulitis of orbit**

Abscess of orbit

⊟ **H05.011**   **Cellulitis of right orbit**

⊟ **H05.012**   **Cellulitis of left orbit**

⊟ **H05.013**   **Cellulitis of bilateral orbits**

⊟ **H05.019**   **Cellulitis of unspecified orbit**

Ⓖ **H05.02**   **Osteomyelitis of orbit**

⊟ **H05.021**   **Osteomyelitis of right orbit**

⊟ **H05.022**   **Osteomyelitis of left orbit**

⊟ **H05.023**   **Osteomyelitis of bilateral orbits**

⊟ **H05.029**   **Osteomyelitis of unspecified orbit**

Ⓖ **H05.03**   **Periostitis of orbit**

⊟ **H05.031**   **Periostitis of right orbit**

⊟ **H05.032**   **Periostitis of left orbit**

● New   ▲ Revised   *Manifestation*   ④-❼ Digit Indicators   ⊟ Laterality   Ⓐ Adult (15+ years)   Ⓜ Maternity (12-55 years)   Ⓝ Newborn   Ⓟ Pediatric (0-17 years)   ♂ Male   ♀ Female

✖ Deleted   Unspecified   + Additional code

592   © 2017 DecisionHealth   2017 ICD-10-CM Expert for Physicians

☐ H05.033 **Periostitis of bilateral orbits**
☐ H05.039 **Periostitis of unspecified orbit**
ⓖ H05.04 **Tenonitis of orbit**
☐ H05.041 **Tenonitis of right orbit**
☐ H05.042 **Tenonitis of left orbit**
☐ H05.043 **Tenonitis of bilateral orbits**
☐ H05.049 **Tenonitis of unspecified orbit**
ⓢ H05.1 **Chronic inflammatory disorders of orbit**
H05.10 **Unspecified chronic inflammatory disorders of orbit**
ⓖ H05.11 **Granuloma of orbit**
Pseudotumor (inflammatory) of orbit
☐ H05.111 **Granuloma of right orbit**
☐ H05.112 **Granuloma of left orbit**
☐ H05.113 **Granuloma of bilateral orbits**
☐ H05.119 **Granuloma of unspecified orbit**
ⓖ H05.12 **Orbital myositis**
DEFINITION Inflammation of one of the muscles that moves the eyeball.
☐ H05.121 **Orbital myositis, right orbit**
☐ H05.122 **Orbital myositis, left orbit**
☐ H05.123 **Orbital myositis, bilateral**
☐ H05.129 **Orbital myositis, unspecified orbit**
ⓢ H05.2 **Exophthalmic conditions**
H05.20 **Unspecified exophthalmos**
ⓖ H05.21 **Displacement (lateral) of globe**
DEFINITION Condition in which the eyeball is situated towards the side of the head, away from the nose.
☐ H05.211 **Displacement (lateral) of globe, right eye**
☐ H05.212 **Displacement (lateral) of globe, left eye**
☐ H05.213 **Displacement (lateral) of globe, bilateral**
☐ H05.219 **Displacement (lateral) of globe, unspecified eye**
ⓖ H05.22 **Edema of orbit**
Orbital congestion
☐ H05.221 **Edema of right orbit**
☐ H05.222 **Edema of left orbit**
☐ H05.223 **Edema of bilateral orbit**
☐ H05.229 **Edema of unspecified orbit**
ⓖ H05.23 **Hemorrhage of orbit**
☐ H05.231 **Hemorrhage of right orbit**
☐ H05.232 **Hemorrhage of left orbit**
☐ H05.233 **Hemorrhage of bilateral orbit**
☐ H05.239 **Hemorrhage of unspecified orbit**
ⓖ H05.24 **Constant exophthalmos**
☐ H05.241 **Constant exophthalmos, right eye**
☐ H05.242 **Constant exophthalmos, left eye**
☐ H05.243 **Constant exophthalmos, bilateral**
☐ H05.249 **Constant exophthalmos, unspecified eye**
ⓖ H05.25 **Intermittent exophthalmos**
☐ H05.251 **Intermittent exophthalmos, right eye**
☐ H05.252 **Intermittent exophthalmos, left eye**
☐ H05.253 **Intermittent exophthalmos, bilateral**
☐ H05.259 **Intermittent exophthalmos, unspecified eye**
ⓖ H05.26 **Pulsating exophthalmos**
☐ H05.261 **Pulsating exophthalmos, right eye**
☐ H05.262 **Pulsating exophthalmos, left eye**
☐ H05.263 **Pulsating exophthalmos, bilateral**
☐ H05.269 **Pulsating exophthalmos, unspecified eye**
ⓢ H05.3 **Deformity of orbit**
EXCLUDES 1 *congenital deformity of orbit (Q10.7)*
hypertelorism (Q75.2)
H05.30 **Unspecified deformity of orbit**
ⓖ H05.31 **Atrophy of orbit**
☐ H05.311 **Atrophy of right orbit**
☐ H05.312 **Atrophy of left orbit**
☐ H05.313 **Atrophy of bilateral orbit**
☐ H05.319 **Atrophy of unspecified orbit**

ⓖ H05.32 **Deformity of orbit due to bone disease**
Code also:
associated bone disease
☐ H05.321 **Deformity of right orbit due to bone disease**
☐ H05.322 **Deformity of left orbit due to bone disease**
☐ H05.323 **Deformity of bilateral orbits due to bone disease**
☐ H05.329 **Deformity of unspecified orbit due to bone disease**
ⓖ H05.33 **Deformity of orbit due to trauma or surgery**
☐ H05.331 **Deformity of right orbit due to trauma or surgery**
☐ H05.332 **Deformity of left orbit due to trauma or surgery**
☐ H05.333 **Deformity of bilateral orbits due to trauma or surgery**
☐ H05.339 **Deformity of unspecified orbit due to trauma or surgery**
ⓖ H05.34 **Enlargement of orbit**
☐ H05.341 **Enlargement of right orbit**
☐ H05.342 **Enlargement of left orbit**
☐ H05.343 **Enlargement of bilateral orbits**
☐ H05.349 **Enlargement of unspecified orbit**
ⓖ H05.35 **Exostosis of orbit**
DEFINITION Abnormal bone growth of the eye socket; can impair vision and prevent the eye from moving properly.
☐ H05.351 **Exostosis of right orbit**
☐ H05.352 **Exostosis of left orbit**
☐ H05.353 **Exostosis of bilateral orbits**
☐ H05.359 **Exostosis of unspecified orbit**
ⓢ H05.4 **Enophthalmos**
ⓖ H05.40 **Unspecified enophthalmos**
DEFINITION Condition in which the eye is recessed abnormally deep within the eye socket.
☐ H05.401 **Unspecified enophthalmos, right eye**
☐ H05.402 **Unspecified enophthalmos, left eye**
☐ H05.403 **Unspecified enophthalmos, bilateral**
☐ H05.409 **Unspecified enophthalmos, unspecified eye**
ⓖ H05.41 **Enophthalmos due to atrophy of orbital tissue**
☐ H05.411 **Enophthalmos due to atrophy of orbital tissue, right eye**
☐ H05.412 **Enophthalmos due to atrophy of orbital tissue, left eye**
☐ H05.413 **Enophthalmos due to atrophy of orbital tissue, bilateral**
☐ H05.419 **Enophthalmos due to atrophy of orbital tissue, unspecified eye**
ⓖ H05.42 **Enophthalmos due to trauma or surgery**
☐ H05.421 **Enophthalmos due to trauma or surgery, right eye**
☐ H05.422 **Enophthalmos due to trauma or surgery, left eye**
☐ H05.423 **Enophthalmos due to trauma or surgery, bilateral**
☐ H05.429 **Enophthalmos due to trauma or surgery, unspecified eye**
ⓢ✛ H05.5 **Retained (old) foreign body following penetrating wound of orbit**
Retrobulbar foreign body
Use additional code to identify the type of retained foreign body (Z18.-)
EXCLUDES 1 *current penetrating wound of orbit (S05.4-)*
EXCLUDES 2 *retained foreign body of eyelid (H02.81-)*
retained intraocular foreign body (H44.6-, H44.7-)
☐✛ H05.50 **Retained (old) foreign body following penetrating wound of unspecified orbit**
☐✛ H05.51 **Retained (old) foreign body following penetrating wound of right orbit**
☐✛ H05.52 **Retained (old) foreign body following penetrating wound of left orbit**
☐✛ H05.53 **Retained (old) foreign body following penetrating wound of bilateral orbits**
ⓢ H05.8 **Other disorders of orbit**

● New ▲ Revised *Manifestation* ❹-❼ Digit Indicators ☐ Laterality Ⓐ Adult (15+ years) Ⓜ Maternity (12-55 years) Ⓝ Newborn Ⓟ Pediatric (0-17 years) ♂ Male ♀ Female
✖ Deleted Unspecified ✛ Additional code

2017 ICD-10-CM Expert for Physicians

© 2017 DecisionHealth

593

H05.033 — H05.8

Diseases of the Eye and Adnexa

H05.81 — H10.81

⑥ **H05.81**   **Cyst of orbit**
Encephalocele of orbit
- ▣ **H05.811**   **Cyst of right orbit**
- ▣ **H05.812**   **Cyst of left orbit**
- ▣ **H05.813**   **Cyst of bilateral orbits**
- ▣ **H05.819**   **Cyst of unspecified orbit**

⑥ **H05.82**   **Myopathy of extraocular muscles**
- ▣ **H05.821**   **Myopathy of extraocular muscles, right orbit**
- ▣ **H05.822**   **Myopathy of extraocular muscles, left orbit**
- ▣ **H05.823**   **Myopathy of extraocular muscles, bilateral**
- ▣ **H05.829**   **Myopathy of extraocular muscles, unspecified orbit**

H05.89   **Other disorders of orbit**

H05.9   **Unspecified disorder of orbit**

Disorders of conjunctiva (H10-H11)

④ **H10**   **Conjunctivitis**
> **EXCLUDES 1**   *keratoconjunctivitis (H16.2-)*

> **CODING TIP** ✓   Consider codes from H10 when an infectious organism is not identified and the documentation only supports a clinical picture of conjunctivitis. If a certain bacterial or viral cause is known, a code from the Infectious and parasitic disease chapter may be more appropriate.

⑤ **H10.0**   **Mucopurulent conjunctivitis**

⑥ **H10.01**   **Acute follicular conjunctivitis**
- ▣ **H10.011**   **Acute follicular conjunctivitis, right eye**
- ▣ **H10.012**   **Acute follicular conjunctivitis, left eye**
- ▣ **H10.013**   **Acute follicular conjunctivitis, bilateral**
- ▣ **H10.019**   **Acute follicular conjunctivitis, unspecified eye**

⑥ **H10.02**   **Other mucopurulent conjunctivitis**
> **CODING TIP** ✓   Subcategory H10.02 is commonly referred to as pink eye.

> **DEFINITION**   Inflammation of the conjunctiva with the production of mucous and pus.
- ▣ **H10.021**   **Other mucopurulent conjunctivitis, right eye**
- ▣ **H10.022**   **Other mucopurulent conjunctivitis, left eye**
- ▣ **H10.023**   **Other mucopurulent conjunctivitis, bilateral**
- ▣ **H10.029**   **Other mucopurulent conjunctivitis, unspecified eye**

⑤ **H10.1**   **Acute atopic conjunctivitis**
Acute papillary conjunctivitis
> **DEFINITION**   Sudden, severe case of conjunctivitis caused by allergies.
- ▣ **H10.10**   **Acute atopic conjunctivitis, unspecified eye**
- ▣ **H10.11**   **Acute atopic conjunctivitis, right eye**
- ▣ **H10.12**   **Acute atopic conjunctivitis, left eye**
- ▣ **H10.13**   **Acute atopic conjunctivitis, bilateral**

⑤ **H10.2**   **Other acute conjunctivitis**
> **CODING TIP** ✓   Consider subcategory H10.2 when light or noxious chemicals cause conjunctivitis.

⑥ **H10.21**   **Acute toxic conjunctivitis**
Acute chemical conjunctivitis
Code first:
(T51-T65) to identify chemical and intent
> **EXCLUDES 1**   *burn and corrosion of eye and adnexa (T26.-)*
- ▣ **H10.211**   **Acute toxic conjunctivitis, right eye**
- ▣ **H10.212**   **Acute toxic conjunctivitis, left eye**
- ▣ **H10.213**   **Acute toxic conjunctivitis, bilateral**
- ▣ **H10.219**   **Acute toxic conjunctivitis, unspecified eye**

⑥ **H10.22**   **Pseudomembranous conjunctivitis**
- ▣ **H10.221**   **Pseudomembranous conjunctivitis, right eye**
- ▣ **H10.222**   **Pseudomembranous conjunctivitis, left eye**
- ▣ **H10.223**   **Pseudomembranous conjunctivitis, bilateral**
- ▣ **H10.229**   **Pseudomembranous conjunctivitis, unspecified eye**

⑥ **H10.23**   **Serous conjunctivitis, except viral**
> **EXCLUDES 1**   *viral conjunctivitis (B30.-)*

- ▣ **H10.231**   **Serous conjunctivitis, except viral, right eye**
- ▣ **H10.232**   **Serous conjunctivitis, except viral, left eye**
- ▣ **H10.233**   **Serous conjunctivitis, except viral, bilateral**
- ▣ **H10.239**   **Serous conjunctivitis, except viral, unspecified eye**

⑤ **H10.3**   **Unspecified acute conjunctivitis**
> **EXCLUDES 1**   *ophthalmia neonatorum NOS (P39.1)*
- ▣ **H10.30**   **Unspecified acute conjunctivitis, unspecified eye**
- ▣ **H10.31**   **Unspecified acute conjunctivitis, right eye**
- ▣ **H10.32**   **Unspecified acute conjunctivitis, left eye**
- ▣ **H10.33**   **Unspecified acute conjunctivitis, bilateral**

⑤ **H10.4**   **Chronic conjunctivitis**

⑥ **H10.40**   **Unspecified chronic conjunctivitis**
- ▣ **H10.401**   **Unspecified chronic conjunctivitis, right eye**
- ▣ **H10.402**   **Unspecified chronic conjunctivitis, left eye**
- ▣ **H10.403**   **Unspecified chronic conjunctivitis, bilateral**
- ▣ **H10.409**   **Unspecified chronic conjunctivitis, unspecified eye**

⑥ **H10.41**   **Chronic giant papillary conjunctivitis**
- ▣ **H10.411**   **Chronic giant papillary conjunctivitis, right eye**
- ▣ **H10.412**   **Chronic giant papillary conjunctivitis, left eye**
- ▣ **H10.413**   **Chronic giant papillary conjunctivitis, bilateral**
- ▣ **H10.419**   **Chronic giant papillary conjunctivitis, unspecified eye**

⑥ **H10.42**   **Simple chronic conjunctivitis**
- ▣ **H10.421**   **Simple chronic conjunctivitis, right eye**
- ▣ **H10.422**   **Simple chronic conjunctivitis, left eye**
- ▣ **H10.423**   **Simple chronic conjunctivitis, bilateral**
- ▣ **H10.429**   **Simple chronic conjunctivitis, unspecified eye**

⑥ **H10.43**   **Chronic follicular conjunctivitis**
- ▣ **H10.431**   **Chronic follicular conjunctivitis, right eye**
- ▣ **H10.432**   **Chronic follicular conjunctivitis, left eye**
- ▣ **H10.433**   **Chronic follicular conjunctivitis, bilateral**
- ▣ **H10.439**   **Chronic follicular conjunctivitis, unspecified eye**

H10.44   **Vernal conjunctivitis**
> **EXCLUDES 1**   *vernal keratoconjunctivitis with limbar and corneal involvement (H16.26-)*

> **DEFINITION**   Seasonal inflammation of the conjunctiva due to an allergic reaction to pollen, mold, or another seasonal factor.

H10.45   **Other chronic allergic conjunctivitis**

⑤ **H10.5**   **Blepharoconjunctivitis**

⑥ **H10.50**   **Unspecified blepharoconjunctivitis**
- ▣ **H10.501**   **Unspecified blepharoconjunctivitis, right eye**
- ▣ **H10.502**   **Unspecified blepharoconjunctivitis, left eye**
- ▣ **H10.503**   **Unspecified blepharoconjunctivitis, bilateral**
- ▣ **H10.509**   **Unspecified blepharoconjunctivitis, unspecified eye**

⑥ **H10.51**   **Ligneous conjunctivitis**
- ▣ **H10.511**   **Ligneous conjunctivitis, right eye**
- ▣ **H10.512**   **Ligneous conjunctivitis, left eye**
- ▣ **H10.513**   **Ligneous conjunctivitis, bilateral**
- ▣ **H10.519**   **Ligneous conjunctivitis, unspecified eye**

⑥ **H10.52**   **Angular blepharoconjunctivitis**
- ▣ **H10.521**   **Angular blepharoconjunctivitis, right eye**
- ▣ **H10.522**   **Angular blepharoconjunctivitis, left eye**
- ▣ **H10.523**   **Angular blepharoconjunctivitis, bilateral**
- ▣ **H10.529**   **Angular blepharoconjunctivitis, unspecified eye**

⑥ **H10.53**   **Contact blepharoconjunctivitis**
- ▣ **H10.531**   **Contact blepharoconjunctivitis, right eye**
- ▣ **H10.532**   **Contact blepharoconjunctivitis, left eye**
- ▣ **H10.533**   **Contact blepharoconjunctivitis, bilateral**
- ▣ **H10.539**   **Contact blepharoconjunctivitis, unspecified eye**

⑤ **H10.8**   **Other conjunctivitis**

⑥ **H10.81**   **Pingueculitis**
> **EXCLUDES 1**   *pinguecula (H11.15-)*

● New   ▲ Revised   *Manifestation*   ④-⑦ Digit Indicators   ▣ Laterality   🅰 Adult (15+ years)   🅼 Maternity (12-55 years)   🅽 Newborn   🅿 Pediatric (0-17 years)   ♂ Male   ♀ Female
✖ ~~Deleted~~   Unspecified   ✚ Additional code

DEFINITION Yellowish, raised areas of limbal conjunctival tissue, usually seen with chronic sun exposure, that become acutely vascularized, irritated, and inflamed.

- ⊟ H10.811   **Pingueculitis, right eye**
- ⊟ H10.812   **Pingueculitis, left eye**
- ⊟ H10.813   **Pingueculitis, bilateral**
- ⊟ H10.819   **Pingueculitis, unspecified eye**
-    H10.89   **Other conjunctivitis**
-    H10.9   **Unspecified conjunctivitis**

⬜ **H11   Other disorders of conjunctiva**

    EXCLUDES 1   *keratoconjunctivitis (H16.2-)*

⬜ **H11.0   Pterygium of eye**

    EXCLUDES 1   *pseudopterygium (H11.81-)*

⬜ **H11.00   Unspecified pterygium of eye**

    DEFINITION   Raised, wedge-shaped overgrowth of the conjunctiva onto the cornea of the eye.

- ⊟ H11.001   **Unspecified pterygium of right eye**
- ⊟ H11.002   **Unspecified pterygium of left eye**
- ⊟ H11.003   **Unspecified pterygium of eye, bilateral**
- ⊟ H11.009   **Unspecified pterygium of unspecified eye**

⬜ **H11.01   Amyloid pterygium**

- ⊟ H11.011   **Amyloid pterygium of right eye**
- ⊟ H11.012   **Amyloid pterygium of left eye**
- ⊟ H11.013   **Amyloid pterygium of eye, bilateral**
- ⊟ H11.019   **Amyloid pterygium of unspecified eye**

⬜ **H11.02   Central pterygium of eye**

- ⊟ H11.021   **Central pterygium of right eye**
- ⊟ H11.022   **Central pterygium of left eye**
- ⊟ H11.023   **Central pterygium of eye, bilateral**
- ⊟ H11.029   **Central pterygium of unspecified eye**

⬜ **H11.03   Double pterygium of eye**

- ⊟ H11.031   **Double pterygium of right eye**
- ⊟ H11.032   **Double pterygium of left eye**
- ⊟ H11.033   **Double pterygium of eye, bilateral**
- ⊟ H11.039   **Double pterygium of unspecified eye**

⬜ **H11.04   Peripheral pterygium of eye, stationary**

- ⊟ H11.041   **Peripheral pterygium, stationary, right eye**
- ⊟ H11.042   **Peripheral pterygium, stationary, left eye**
- ⊟ H11.043   **Peripheral pterygium, stationary, bilateral**
- ⊟ H11.049   **Peripheral pterygium, stationary, unspecified eye**

⬜ **H11.05   Peripheral pterygium of eye, progressive**

- ⊟ H11.051   **Peripheral pterygium, progressive, right eye**
- ⊟ H11.052   **Peripheral pterygium, progressive, left eye**
- ⊟ H11.053   **Peripheral pterygium, progressive, bilateral**
- ⊟ H11.059   **Peripheral pterygium, progressive, unspecified eye**

⬜ **H11.06   Recurrent pterygium of eye**

- ⊟ H11.061   **Recurrent pterygium of right eye**
- ⊟ H11.062   **Recurrent pterygium of left eye**
- ⊟ H11.063   **Recurrent pterygium of eye, bilateral**
- ⊟ H11.069   **Recurrent pterygium of unspecified eye**

⬜ **H11.1   Conjunctival degenerations and deposits**

    EXCLUDES 2   *pseudopterygium (H11.81)*

-    H11.10   **Unspecified conjunctival degenerations**

⬜ **H11.11   Conjunctival deposits**

- ⊟ H11.111   **Conjunctival deposits, right eye**
- ⊟ H11.112   **Conjunctival deposits, left eye**
- ⊟ H11.113   **Conjunctival deposits, bilateral**
- ⊟ H11.119   **Conjunctival deposits, unspecified eye**

⬜ **H11.12   Conjunctival concretions**

    DEFINITION   Yellow-white granules or cysts which form just beneath the conjunctiva, wearing it away and causing the sensation of a foreign body in the eye.

- ⊟ H11.121   **Conjunctival concretions, right eye**

- ⊟ H11.122   **Conjunctival concretions, left eye**
- ⊟ H11.123   **Conjunctival concretions, bilateral**
- ⊟ H11.129   **Conjunctival concretions, unspecified eye**

⬜ **H11.13   Conjunctival pigmentations**

    Conjunctival argyrosis [argyria]

- ⊟ H11.131   **Conjunctival pigmentations, right eye**
- ⊟ H11.132   **Conjunctival pigmentations, left eye**
- ⊟ H11.133   **Conjunctival pigmentations, bilateral**
- ⊟ H11.139   **Conjunctival pigmentations, unspecified eye**

⬜ **H11.14   Conjunctival xerosis, unspecified**

    EXCLUDES 1   *xerosis of conjunctiva due to vitamin A deficiency (E50.0, E50.1)*

- ⊟ H11.141   **Conjunctival xerosis, unspecified, right eye**
- ⊟ H11.142   **Conjunctival xerosis, unspecified, left eye**
- ⊟ H11.143   **Conjunctival xerosis, unspecified, bilateral**
- ⊟ H11.149   **Conjunctival xerosis, unspecified, unspecified eye**

⬜ **H11.15   Pinguecula**

    EXCLUDES 1   *pingueculitis (H10.81-)*

    DEFINITION   Small, nonmalignant, yellowish growth on the conjunctiva often asymptomatic and requiring no treatment but may cause irritation.

- ⊟ H11.151   **Pinguecula, right eye**
- ⊟ H11.152   **Pinguecula, left eye**
- ⊟ H11.153   **Pinguecula, bilateral**
- ⊟ H11.159   **Pinguecula, unspecified eye**

⬜ **H11.2   Conjunctival scars**

⬜ **H11.21   Conjunctival adhesions and strands (localized)**

- ⊟ H11.211   **Conjunctival adhesions and strands (localized), right eye**
- ⊟ H11.212   **Conjunctival adhesions and strands (localized), left eye**
- ⊟ H11.213   **Conjunctival adhesions and strands (localized), bilateral**
- ⊟ H11.219   **Conjunctival adhesions and strands (localized), unspecified eye**

⬜ **H11.22   Conjunctival granuloma**

- ⊟ H11.221   **Conjunctival granuloma, right eye**
- ⊟ H11.222   **Conjunctival granuloma, left eye**
- ⊟ H11.223   **Conjunctival granuloma, bilateral**
- ⊟ H11.229   **Conjunctival granuloma, unspecified**

⬜ **H11.23   Symblepharon**

    DEFINITION   Conjunctiva of the eyelid that has adhered to the eye, sometimes over the cornea, requiring surgical removal.

- ⊟ H11.231   **Symblepharon, right eye**
- ⊟ H11.232   **Symblepharon, left eye**
- ⊟ H11.233   **Symblepharon, bilateral**
- ⊟ H11.239   **Symblepharon, unspecified eye**

⬜ **H11.24   Scarring of conjunctiva**

- ⊟ H11.241   **Scarring of conjunctiva, right eye**
- ⊟ H11.242   **Scarring of conjunctiva, left eye**
- ⊟ H11.243   **Scarring of conjunctiva, bilateral**
- ⊟ H11.249   **Scarring of conjunctiva, unspecified eye**

⬜ **H11.3   Conjunctival hemorrhage**

    Subconjunctival hemorrhage

- ⊟ H11.30   **Conjunctival hemorrhage, unspecified eye**
- ⊟ H11.31   **Conjunctival hemorrhage, right eye**
- ⊟ H11.32   **Conjunctival hemorrhage, left eye**
- ⊟ H11.33   **Conjunctival hemorrhage, bilateral**

⬜ **H11.4   Other conjunctival vascular disorders and cysts**

⬜ **H11.41   Vascular abnormalities of conjunctiva**

    Conjunctival aneurysm

- ⊟ H11.411   **Vascular abnormalities of conjunctiva, right eye**
- ⊟ H11.412   **Vascular abnormalities of conjunctiva, left eye**
- ⊟ H11.413   **Vascular abnormalities of conjunctiva, bilateral**
- ⊟ H11.419   **Vascular abnormalities of conjunctiva, unspecified eye**

⬜ **H11.42   Conjunctival edema**

- ⊟ H11.421   **Conjunctival edema, right eye**
- ⊟ H11.422   **Conjunctival edema, left eye**
- ⊟ H11.423   **Conjunctival edema, bilateral**
- ⊟ H11.429   **Conjunctival edema, unspecified eye**

● New   ▲ Revised   *Manifestation*   ◳-◱ Digit Indicators   ⊟ Laterality   Ⓐ Adult (15+ years)   Ⓜ Maternity (12-55 years)   Ⓝ Newborn   Ⓟ Pediatric (0-17 years)   ♂ Male   ♀ Female

✖ Deleted   Unspecified   + Additional code

H11.43 Conjunctival hyperemia
- H11.431 Conjunctival hyperemia, right eye
- H11.432 Conjunctival hyperemia, left eye
- H11.433 Conjunctival hyperemia, bilateral
- H11.439 Conjunctival hyperemia, unspecified eye

H11.44 Conjunctival cysts
- H11.441 Conjunctival cysts, right eye
- H11.442 Conjunctival cysts, left eye
- H11.443 Conjunctival cysts, bilateral
- H11.449 Conjunctival cysts, unspecified eye

H11.8 Other specified disorders of conjunctiva
H11.81 Pseudopterygium of conjunctiva
- H11.811 Pseudopterygium of conjunctiva, right eye
- H11.812 Pseudopterygium of conjunctiva, left eye
- H11.813 Pseudopterygium of conjunctiva, bilateral
- H11.819 Pseudopterygium of conjunctiva, unspecified eye

H11.82 Conjunctivochalasis

DEFINITION Loosening of the conjunctiva's attachment to the eye, causing wrinkling, dryness, and a tendency to trap particles in the folds, causing chronic inflammation.

- H11.821 Conjunctivochalasis, right eye
- H11.822 Conjunctivochalasis, left eye
- H11.823 Conjunctivochalasis, bilateral
- H11.829 Conjunctivochalasis, unspecified eye

H11.89 Other specified disorders of conjunctiva
H11.9 Unspecified disorder of conjunctiva

Disorders of sclera, cornea, iris and ciliary body (H15-H22)

H15 Disorders of sclera
H15.0 Scleritis
H15.00 Unspecified scleritis
- H15.001 Unspecified scleritis, right eye
- H15.002 Unspecified scleritis, left eye
- H15.003 Unspecified scleritis, bilateral
- H15.009 Unspecified scleritis, unspecified eye

H15.01 Anterior scleritis
- H15.011 Anterior scleritis, right eye
- H15.012 Anterior scleritis, left eye
- H15.013 Anterior scleritis, bilateral
- H15.019 Anterior scleritis, unspecified eye

H15.02 Brawny scleritis

DEFINITION Severe inflammation of the sclera affecting the border between the sclera and the cornea.

- H15.021 Brawny scleritis, right eye
- H15.022 Brawny scleritis, left eye
- H15.023 Brawny scleritis, bilateral
- H15.029 Brawny scleritis, unspecified eye

H15.03 Posterior scleritis
Sclerotenonitis
- H15.031 Posterior scleritis, right eye
- H15.032 Posterior scleritis, left eye
- H15.033 Posterior scleritis, bilateral
- H15.039 Posterior scleritis, unspecified eye

H15.04 Scleritis with corneal involvement
- H15.041 Scleritis with corneal involvement, right eye
- H15.042 Scleritis with corneal involvement, left eye
- H15.043 Scleritis with corneal involvement, bilateral
- H15.049 Scleritis with corneal involvement, unspecified eye

H15.05 Scleromalacia perforans
- H15.051 Scleromalacia perforans, right eye
- H15.052 Scleromalacia perforans, left eye
- H15.053 Scleromalacia perforans, bilateral
- H15.059 Scleromalacia perforans, unspecified eye

H15.09 Other scleritis
Scleral abscess
- H15.091 Other scleritis, right eye
- H15.092 Other scleritis, left eye
- H15.093 Other scleritis, bilateral
- H15.099 Other scleritis, unspecified eye

H15.1 Episcleritis
H15.10 Unspecified episcleritis
- H15.101 Unspecified episcleritis, right eye
- H15.102 Unspecified episcleritis, left eye
- H15.103 Unspecified episcleritis, bilateral
- H15.109 Unspecified episcleritis, unspecified eye

H15.11 Episcleritis periodica fugax

DEFINITION Periodic attacks of inflammation of the sclera; typically of rapid onset and short duration.

- H15.111 Episcleritis periodica fugax, right eye
- H15.112 Episcleritis periodica fugax, left eye
- H15.113 Episcleritis periodica fugax, bilateral
- H15.119 Episcleritis periodica fugax, unspecified eye

H15.12 Nodular episcleritis
- H15.121 Nodular episcleritis, right eye
- H15.122 Nodular episcleritis, left eye
- H15.123 Nodular episcleritis, bilateral
- H15.129 Nodular episcleritis, unspecified eye

H15.8 Other disorders of sclera

EXCLUDES 2 blue sclera (Q13.5)
degenerative myopia (H44.2-)

H15.81 Equatorial staphyloma
- H15.811 Equatorial staphyloma, right eye
- H15.812 Equatorial staphyloma, left eye
- H15.813 Equatorial staphyloma, bilateral
- H15.819 Equatorial staphyloma, unspecified eye

H15.82 Localized anterior staphyloma
- H15.821 Localized anterior staphyloma, right eye
- H15.822 Localized anterior staphyloma, left eye
- H15.823 Localized anterior staphyloma, bilateral
- H15.829 Localized anterior staphyloma, unspecified eye

H15.83 Staphyloma posticum
- H15.831 Staphyloma posticum, right eye
- H15.832 Staphyloma posticum, left eye
- H15.833 Staphyloma posticum, bilateral
- H15.839 Staphyloma posticum, unspecified eye

H15.84 Scleral ectasia

DEFINITION Contents of the eyeball protrude through an abnormally thin section of the sclera.

- H15.841 Scleral ectasia, right eye
- H15.842 Scleral ectasia, left eye
- H15.843 Scleral ectasia, bilateral
- H15.849 Scleral ectasia, unspecified eye

H15.85 Ring staphyloma
- H15.851 Ring staphyloma, right eye
- H15.852 Ring staphyloma, left eye
- H15.853 Ring staphyloma, bilateral
- H15.859 Ring staphyloma, unspecified eye

H15.89 Other disorders of sclera
H15.9 Unspecified disorder of sclera

H16 Keratitis
H16.0 Corneal ulcer
H16.00 Unspecified corneal ulcer
- H16.001 Unspecified corneal ulcer, right eye
- H16.002 Unspecified corneal ulcer, left eye
- H16.003 Unspecified corneal ulcer, bilateral
- H16.009 Unspecified corneal ulcer, unspecified eye

H16.01 Central corneal ulcer
- H16.011 Central corneal ulcer, right eye
- H16.012 Central corneal ulcer, left eye
- H16.013 Central corneal ulcer, bilateral
- H16.019 Central corneal ulcer, unspecified eye

H16.02 Ring corneal ulcer

● New   ▲ Revised   *Manifestation*   4-7 Digit Indicators   ⊟ Laterality   Ⓐ Adult (15+ years)   Ⓜ Maternity (12-55 years)   Ⓝ Newborn   Ⓟ Pediatric (0-17 years)   ♂ Male   ♀ Female
✖ Deleted   Unspecified   + Additional code

596   © 2017 DecisionHealth   2017 ICD-10-CM Expert for Physicians

DEFINITION Ring of ulceration encircling the entire edge of the cornea.

- H16.021 **Ring corneal ulcer, right eye**
- H16.022 **Ring corneal ulcer, left eye**
- H16.023 **Ring corneal ulcer, bilateral**
- H16.029 **Ring corneal ulcer, unspecified eye**

H16.03 Corneal ulcer with hypopyon

- H16.031 **Corneal ulcer with hypopyon, right eye**
- H16.032 **Corneal ulcer with hypopyon, left eye**
- H16.033 **Corneal ulcer with hypopyon, bilateral**
- H16.039 **Corneal ulcer with hypopyon, unspecified eye**

H16.04 Marginal corneal ulcer

- H16.041 **Marginal corneal ulcer, right eye**
- H16.042 **Marginal corneal ulcer, left eye**
- H16.043 **Marginal corneal ulcer, bilateral**
- H16.049 **Marginal corneal ulcer, unspecified eye**

H16.05 Mooren's corneal ulcer

- H16.051 **Mooren's corneal ulcer, right eye**
- H16.052 **Mooren's corneal ulcer, left eye**
- H16.053 **Mooren's corneal ulcer, bilateral**
- H16.059 **Mooren's corneal ulcer, unspecified eye**

H16.06 Mycotic corneal ulcer

DEFINITION Corneal ulcer caused by a fungal infection.

- H16.061 **Mycotic corneal ulcer, right eye**
- H16.062 **Mycotic corneal ulcer, left eye**
- H16.063 **Mycotic corneal ulcer, bilateral**
- H16.069 **Mycotic corneal ulcer, unspecified eye**

H16.07 Perforated corneal ulcer

Perforated corneal ulcer

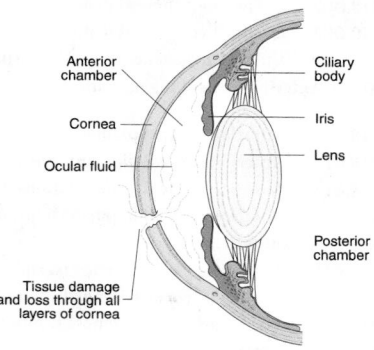

Anterior chamber
Cornea
Ocular fluid
Ciliary body
Iris
Lens
Posterior chamber
Tissue damage and loss through all layers of cornea

- H16.071 **Perforated corneal ulcer, right eye**
- H16.072 **Perforated corneal ulcer, left eye**
- H16.073 **Perforated corneal ulcer, bilateral**
- H16.079 **Perforated corneal ulcer, unspecified eye**

H16.1 Other and unspecified superficial keratitis without conjunctivitis

H16.10 Unspecified superficial keratitis

- H16.101 **Unspecified superficial keratitis, right eye**
- H16.102 **Unspecified superficial keratitis, left eye**
- H16.103 **Unspecified superficial keratitis, bilateral**
- H16.109 **Unspecified superficial keratitis, unspecified eye**

H16.11 Macular keratitis
Areolar keratitis
Nummular keratitis
Stellate keratitis
Striate keratitis

- H16.111 **Macular keratitis, right eye**
- H16.112 **Macular keratitis, left eye**
- H16.113 **Macular keratitis, bilateral**
- H16.119 **Macular keratitis, unspecified eye**

H16.12 Filamentary keratitis

DEFINITION Keratitis with twisted filaments of mucoid material on the surface of the cornea.

- H16.121 **Filamentary keratitis, right eye**
- H16.122 **Filamentary keratitis, left eye**
- H16.123 **Filamentary keratitis, bilateral**
- H16.129 **Filamentary keratitis, unspecified eye**

H16.13 Photokeratitis
Snow blindness
Welders keratitis

DEFINITION Painful, inflamed cornea that develops due to over-exposure to ultraviolet light.

- H16.131 **Photokeratitis, right eye**
- H16.132 **Photokeratitis, left eye**
- H16.133 **Photokeratitis, bilateral**
- H16.139 **Photokeratitis, unspecified eye**

H16.14 Punctate keratitis

- H16.141 **Punctate keratitis, right eye**
- H16.142 **Punctate keratitis, left eye**
- H16.143 **Punctate keratitis, bilateral**
- H16.149 **Punctate keratitis, unspecified eye**

H16.2 Keratoconjunctivitis

DEFINITION Inflammation of both the cornea and the conjunctiva; presents with burning, bloodshot, watery eyes sensitive to bright light, blurred vision, and a sensation of something in the eye.

H16.20 Unspecified keratoconjunctivitis
Superficial keratitis with conjunctivitis NOS

- H16.201 **Unspecified keratoconjunctivitis, right eye**
- H16.202 **Unspecified keratoconjunctivitis, left eye**
- H16.203 **Unspecified keratoconjunctivitis, bilateral**
- H16.209 **Unspecified keratoconjunctivitis, unspecified eye**

H16.21 Exposure keratoconjunctivitis

DEFINITION Dryness and inflammation of the cornea and conjunctiva caused by the failure of the eyelid to completely close during sleep and/or blinking.

- H16.211 **Exposure keratoconjunctivitis, right eye**
- H16.212 **Exposure keratoconjunctivitis, left eye**
- H16.213 **Exposure keratoconjunctivitis, bilateral**
- H16.219 **Exposure keratoconjunctivitis, unspecified eye**

H16.22 Keratoconjunctivitis sicca, not specified as Sjögren's

EXCLUDES 1 *Sjögren's syndrome (M35.01)*

- H16.221 **Keratoconjunctivitis sicca, not specified as Sjögren's, right eye**
- H16.222 **Keratoconjunctivitis sicca, not specified as Sjögren's, left eye**
- H16.223 **Keratoconjunctivitis sicca, not specified as Sjögren's, bilateral**
- H16.229 **Keratoconjunctivitis sicca, not specified as Sjögren's, unspecified eye**

H16.23 Neurotrophic keratoconjunctivitis

- H16.231 **Neurotrophic keratoconjunctivitis, right eye**
- H16.232 **Neurotrophic keratoconjunctivitis, left eye**
- H16.233 **Neurotrophic keratoconjunctivitis, bilateral**
- H16.239 **Neurotrophic keratoconjunctivitis, unspecified eye**

H16.24 Ophthalmia nodosa

- H16.241 **Ophthalmia nodosa, right eye**
- H16.242 **Ophthalmia nodosa, left eye**
- H16.243 **Ophthalmia nodosa, bilateral**
- H16.249 **Ophthalmia nodosa, unspecified eye**

H16.25 Phlyctenular keratoconjunctivitis

- H16.251 **Phlyctenular keratoconjunctivitis, right eye**
- H16.252 **Phlyctenular keratoconjunctivitis, left eye**
- H16.253 **Phlyctenular keratoconjunctivitis, bilateral**
- H16.259 **Phlyctenular keratoconjunctivitis, unspecified eye**

H16.26 Vernal keratoconjunctivitis, with limbar and corneal involvement

EXCLUDES 1 *vernal conjunctivitis without limbar and corneal involvement (H10.44)*

● New ▲ Revised *Manifestation* ❹-❼ Digit Indicators ⊟ Laterality Ⓐ Adult (15+ years) Ⓜ Maternity (12-55 years) Ⓝ Newborn Ⓟ Pediatric (0-17 years) ♂ Male ♀ Female
✖ Deleted Unspecified + Additional code

⊟ H16.261 Vernal keratoconjunctivitis, with limbar and corneal involvement, right eye

⊟ H16.262 Vernal keratoconjunctivitis, with limbar and corneal involvement, left eye

⊟ H16.263 Vernal keratoconjunctivitis, with limbar and corneal involvement, bilateral

⊟ H16.269 Vernal keratoconjunctivitis, with limbar and corneal involvement, unspecified eye

☑ H16.29 Other keratoconjunctivitis

⊟ H16.291 Other keratoconjunctivitis, right eye

⊟ H16.292 Other keratoconjunctivitis, left eye

⊟ H16.293 Other keratoconjunctivitis, bilateral

⊟ H16.299 Other keratoconjunctivitis, unspecified eye

☑ H16.3 Interstitial and deep keratitis

☑ H16.30 Unspecified interstitial keratitis

⊟ H16.301 Unspecified interstitial keratitis, right eye

⊟ H16.302 Unspecified interstitial keratitis, left eye

⊟ H16.303 Unspecified interstitial keratitis, bilateral

⊟ H16.309 Unspecified interstitial keratitis, unspecified eye

☑ H16.31 Corneal abscess

⊟ H16.311 Corneal abscess, right eye

⊟ H16.312 Corneal abscess, left eye

⊟ H16.313 Corneal abscess, bilateral

⊟ H16.319 Corneal abscess, unspecified eye

☑ H16.32 Diffuse interstitial keratitis
Cogan's syndrome
DEFINITION Rare disorder characterized by recurrent inflammation of the cornea with episodes of dizziness and hearing loss that can lead to blindness and deafness if left untreated.

⊟ H16.321 Diffuse interstitial keratitis, right eye

⊟ H16.322 Diffuse interstitial keratitis, left eye

⊟ H16.323 Diffuse interstitial keratitis, bilateral

⊟ H16.329 Diffuse interstitial keratitis, unspecified eye

☑ H16.33 Sclerosing keratitis

⊟ H16.331 Sclerosing keratitis, right eye

⊟ H16.332 Sclerosing keratitis, left eye

⊟ H16.333 Sclerosing keratitis, bilateral

⊟ H16.339 Sclerosing keratitis, unspecified eye

☑ H16.39 Other interstitial and deep keratitis

⊟ H16.391 Other interstitial and deep keratitis, right eye

⊟ H16.392 Other interstitial and deep keratitis, left eye

⊟ H16.393 Other interstitial and deep keratitis, bilateral

⊟ H16.399 Other interstitial and deep keratitis, unspecified eye

☑ H16.4 Corneal neovascularization

☑ H16.40 Unspecified corneal neovascularization

⊟ H16.401 Unspecified corneal neovascularization, right eye

⊟ H16.402 Unspecified corneal neovascularization, left eye

⊟ H16.403 Unspecified corneal neovascularization, bilateral

⊟ H16.409 Unspecified corneal neovascularization, unspecified eye

☑ H16.41 Ghost vessels (corneal)

⊟ H16.411 Ghost vessels (corneal), right eye

⊟ H16.412 Ghost vessels (corneal), left eye

⊟ H16.413 Ghost vessels (corneal), bilateral

⊟ H16.419 Ghost vessels (corneal), unspecified eye

☑ H16.42 Pannus (corneal)

⊟ H16.421 Pannus (corneal), right eye

⊟ H16.422 Pannus (corneal), left eye

⊟ H16.423 Pannus (corneal), bilateral

⊟ H16.429 Pannus (corneal), unspecified eye

☑ H16.43 Localized vascularization of cornea

⊟ H16.431 Localized vascularization of cornea, right eye

⊟ H16.432 Localized vascularization of cornea, left eye

⊟ H16.433 Localized vascularization of cornea, bilateral

⊟ H16.439 Localized vascularization of cornea, unspecified eye

☑ H16.44 Deep vascularization of cornea

⊟ H16.441 Deep vascularization of cornea, right eye

⊟ H16.442 Deep vascularization of cornea, left eye

⊟ H16.443 Deep vascularization of cornea, bilateral

⊟ H16.449 Deep vascularization of cornea, unspecified eye

H16.8 Other keratitis

H16.9 Unspecified keratitis

☑ H17 Corneal scars and opacities

☑ H17.0 Adherent leukoma

⊟ H17.00 Adherent leukoma, unspecified eye

⊟ H17.01 Adherent leukoma, right eye

⊟ H17.02 Adherent leukoma, left eye

⊟ H17.03 Adherent leukoma, bilateral

☑ H17.1 Central corneal opacity

⊟ H17.10 Central corneal opacity, unspecified eye

⊟ H17.11 Central corneal opacity, right eye

⊟ H17.12 Central corneal opacity, left eye

⊟ H17.13 Central corneal opacity, bilateral

☑ H17.8 Other corneal scars and opacities

☑ H17.81 Minor opacity of cornea
Corneal nebula

⊟ H17.811 Minor opacity of cornea, right eye

⊟ H17.812 Minor opacity of cornea, left eye

⊟ H17.813 Minor opacity of cornea, bilateral

⊟ H17.819 Minor opacity of cornea, unspecified eye

☑ H17.82 Peripheral opacity of cornea

⊟ H17.821 Peripheral opacity of cornea, right eye

⊟ H17.822 Peripheral opacity of cornea, left eye

⊟ H17.823 Peripheral opacity of cornea, bilateral

⊟ H17.829 Peripheral opacity of cornea, unspecified eye

H17.89 Other corneal scars and opacities

H17.9 Unspecified corneal scar and opacity

☑ H18 Other disorders of cornea

☑ H18.0 Corneal pigmentations and deposits

☑ H18.00 Unspecified corneal deposit

⊟ H18.001 Unspecified corneal deposit, right eye

⊟ H18.002 Unspecified corneal deposit, left eye

⊟ H18.003 Unspecified corneal deposit, bilateral

⊟ H18.009 Unspecified corneal deposit, unspecified eye

☑ H18.01 Anterior corneal pigmentations
Staehli's line

⊟ H18.011 Anterior corneal pigmentations, right eye

⊟ H18.012 Anterior corneal pigmentations, left eye

⊟ H18.013 Anterior corneal pigmentations, bilateral

⊟ H18.019 Anterior corneal pigmentations, unspecified eye

☑ H18.02 Argentous corneal deposits

⊟ H18.021 Argentous corneal deposits, right eye

⊟ H18.022 Argentous corneal deposits, left eye

⊟ H18.023 Argentous corneal deposits, bilateral

⊟ H18.029 Argentous corneal deposits, unspecified eye

☑ H18.03 Corneal deposits in metabolic disorders
Code also:
associated metabolic disorder

⊟ H18.031 Corneal deposits in metabolic disorders, right eye

⊟ H18.032 Corneal deposits in metabolic disorders, left eye

⊟ H18.033 Corneal deposits in metabolic disorders, bilateral

⊟ H18.039 Corneal deposits in metabolic disorders, unspecified eye

☑ H18.04 Kayser-Fleischer ring
Code also:
associated Wilson's disease (E83.01)
DEFINITION Gray-green or brownish ring of copper deposits on the exterior of the cornea that grow slowly inward; often seen with liver disorders.

⊟ H18.041 Kayser-Fleischer ring, right eye

⊟ H18.042 Kayser-Fleischer ring, left eye

⊟ H18.043 Kayser-Fleischer ring, bilateral

⊟ H18.049 Kayser-Fleischer ring, unspecified eye

☑ H18.05 Posterior corneal pigmentations
Krukenberg's spindle

⊟ H18.051 Posterior corneal pigmentations, right eye

● New ▲ Revised *Manifestation* ☑-☑ Digit Indicators ⊟ Laterality Ⓐ Adult (15+ years) Ⓜ Maternity (12-55 years) Ⓝ Newborn Ⓟ Pediatric (0-17 years) ♂ Male ♀ Female
✖ Deleted Unspecified + Additional code

598   © 2017 DecisionHealth   2017 ICD-10-CM Expert for Physicians

H18.052   Posterior corneal pigmentations, left eye
H18.053   Posterior corneal pigmentations, bilateral
H18.059   Posterior corneal pigmentations, unspecified eye

Ⓖ H18.06   Stromal corneal pigmentations
Hematocornea
H18.061   Stromal corneal pigmentations, right eye
H18.062   Stromal corneal pigmentations, left eye
H18.063   Stromal corneal pigmentations, bilateral
H18.069   Stromal corneal pigmentations, unspecified eye

Ⓢ H18.1   Bullous keratopathy
H18.10   Bullous keratopathy, unspecified eye
H18.11   Bullous keratopathy, right eye
H18.12   Bullous keratopathy, left eye
H18.13   Bullous keratopathy, bilateral

Ⓢ H18.2   Other and unspecified corneal edema
H18.20   Unspecified corneal edema
Ⓖ H18.21   Corneal edema secondary to contact lens
EXCLUDES 2   *other corneal disorders due to contact lens (H18.82-)*
H18.211   Corneal edema secondary to contact lens, right eye
H18.212   Corneal edema secondary to contact lens, left eye
H18.213   Corneal edema secondary to contact lens, bilateral
H18.219   Corneal edema secondary to contact lens, unspecified eye

Ⓖ H18.22   Idiopathic corneal edema
H18.221   Idiopathic corneal edema, right eye
H18.222   Idiopathic corneal edema, left eye
H18.223   Idiopathic corneal edema, bilateral
H18.229   Idiopathic corneal edema, unspecified eye

Ⓖ H18.23   Secondary corneal edema
H18.231   Secondary corneal edema, right eye
H18.232   Secondary corneal edema, left eye
H18.233   Secondary corneal edema, bilateral
H18.239   Secondary corneal edema, unspecified eye

Ⓢ H18.3   Changes of corneal membranes
H18.30   Unspecified corneal membrane change
Ⓖ H18.31   Folds and rupture in Bowman's membrane
H18.311   Folds and rupture in Bowman's membrane, right eye
H18.312   Folds and rupture in Bowman's membrane, left eye
H18.313   Folds and rupture in Bowman's membrane, bilateral
H18.319   Folds and rupture in Bowman's membrane, unspecified eye

Ⓖ H18.32   Folds in Descemet's membrane
DEFINITION   Fold in the membrane between the innermost layer of the cornea and the stroma (strong, supportive layer), affecting vision and preventing the flow of nutrients out of the cornea.
H18.321   Folds in Descemet's membrane, right eye
H18.322   Folds in Descemet's membrane, left eye
H18.323   Folds in Descemet's membrane, bilateral
H18.329   Folds in Descemet's membrane, unspecified eye

Ⓖ H18.33   Rupture in Descemet's membrane
H18.331   Rupture in Descemet's membrane, right eye
H18.332   Rupture in Descemet's membrane, left eye
H18.333   Rupture in Descemet's membrane, bilateral
H18.339   Rupture in Descemet's membrane, unspecified eye

Ⓢ H18.4   Corneal degeneration
EXCLUDES 1   *Mooren's ulcer (H16.0-)*
recurrent erosion of cornea (H18.83-)
H18.40   Unspecified corneal degeneration
Ⓖ H18.41   Arcus senilis
Senile corneal changes
H18.411   Arcus senilis, right eye
H18.412   Arcus senilis, left eye
H18.413   Arcus senilis, bilateral
H18.419   Arcus senilis, unspecified eye

Ⓖ H18.42   Band keratopathy
DEFINITION   Degeneration of the cornea in which calcium deposits are laid in horizontal band-like layers, obscuring the patient's vision.
H18.421   Band keratopathy, right eye
H18.422   Band keratopathy, left eye
H18.423   Band keratopathy, bilateral
H18.429   Band keratopathy, unspecified eye
H18.43   Other calcerous corneal degeneration
Ⓖ H18.44   Keratomalacia
EXCLUDES 1   *keratomalacia due to vitamin A deficiency (E50.4)*
H18.441   Keratomalacia, right eye
H18.442   Keratomalacia, left eye
H18.443   Keratomalacia, bilateral
H18.449   Keratomalacia, unspecified eye
Ⓖ H18.45   Nodular corneal degeneration
H18.451   Nodular corneal degeneration, right eye
H18.452   Nodular corneal degeneration, left eye
H18.453   Nodular corneal degeneration, bilateral
H18.459   Nodular corneal degeneration, unspecified eye
Ⓖ H18.46   Peripheral corneal degeneration
H18.461   Peripheral corneal degeneration, right eye
H18.462   Peripheral corneal degeneration, left eye
H18.463   Peripheral corneal degeneration, bilateral
H18.469   Peripheral corneal degeneration, unspecified eye
H18.49   Other corneal degeneration

Ⓢ H18.5   Hereditary corneal dystrophies
H18.50   Unspecified hereditary corneal dystrophies
H18.51   Endothelial corneal dystrophy
Fuchs' dystrophy
H18.52   Epithelial (juvenile) corneal dystrophy
DEFINITION   Multiple lesions on the outermost layer of the cornea occurring in the early years, which gradually grow together and obscure vision.
H18.53   Granular corneal dystrophy
H18.54   Lattice corneal dystrophy
H18.55   Macular corneal dystrophy
H18.59   Other hereditary corneal dystrophies

Ⓢ H18.6   Keratoconus
Ⓖ H18.60   Keratoconus, unspecified
H18.601   Keratoconus, unspecified, right eye
H18.602   Keratoconus, unspecified, left eye
H18.603   Keratoconus, unspecified, bilateral
H18.609   Keratoconus, unspecified, unspecified eye
Ⓖ H18.61   Keratoconus, stable
H18.611   Keratoconus, stable, right eye
H18.612   Keratoconus, stable, left eye
H18.613   Keratoconus, stable, bilateral
H18.619   Keratoconus, stable, unspecified eye
Ⓖ H18.62   Keratoconus, unstable
Acute hydrops
H18.621   Keratoconus, unstable, right eye
H18.622   Keratoconus, unstable, left eye
H18.623   Keratoconus, unstable, bilateral
H18.629   Keratoconus, unstable, unspecified eye

Ⓢ H18.7   Other and unspecified corneal deformities
EXCLUDES 1   *congenital malformations of cornea (Q13.3-Q13.4)*
H18.70   Unspecified corneal deformity
Ⓖ H18.71   Corneal ectasia
H18.711   Corneal ectasia, right eye
H18.712   Corneal ectasia, left eye
H18.713   Corneal ectasia, bilateral
H18.719   Corneal ectasia, unspecified eye
Ⓖ H18.72   Corneal staphyloma
H18.721   Corneal staphyloma, right eye
H18.722   Corneal staphyloma, left eye
H18.723   Corneal staphyloma, bilateral
H18.729   Corneal staphyloma, unspecified eye
Ⓖ H18.73   Descemetocele
H18.731   Descemetocele, right eye

● New   ▲ Revised   *Manifestation*   Unspecified   ❹-❼ Digit Indicators   + Additional code   ▤ Laterality   🅰 Adult (15+ years)   Ⓜ Maternity (12-55 years)   Ⓝ Newborn   🅿 Pediatric (0-17 years)   ♂ Male   ♀ Female
✖ Deleted

2017 ICD-10-CM Expert for Physicians

© 2017 DecisionHealth   599

H18.052 — H18.731

Diseases of the Eye and Adnexa

H18.732 — H21.1X1

⊟ H18.732   Descemetocele, left eye
⊟ H18.733   Descemetocele, bilateral
⊟ H18.739   Descemetocele, unspecified eye
⑥ H18.79   Other corneal deformities
⊟ H18.791   Other corneal deformities, right eye
⊟ H18.792   Other corneal deformities, left eye
⊟ H18.793   Other corneal deformities, bilateral
⊟ H18.799   Other corneal deformities, unspecified eye
⑤ H18.8   Other specified disorders of cornea
⑥ H18.81   Anesthesia and hypoesthesia of cornea
      DEFINITION   Decreased or complete loss of corneal sensitivity to pain and irritation.
⊟ H18.811   Anesthesia and hypoesthesia of cornea, right eye
⊟ H18.812   Anesthesia and hypoesthesia of cornea, left eye
⊟ H18.813   Anesthesia and hypoesthesia of cornea, bilateral
⊟ H18.819   Anesthesia and hypoesthesia of cornea, unspecified eye
⑥ H18.82   Corneal disorder due to contact lens
      EXCLUDES 2   *corneal edema due to contact lens (H18.21-)*
⊟ H18.821   Corneal disorder due to contact lens, right eye
⊟ H18.822   Corneal disorder due to contact lens, left eye
⊟ H18.823   Corneal disorder due to contact lens, bilateral
⊟ H18.829   Corneal disorder due to contact lens, unspecified eye
⑥ H18.83   Recurrent erosion of cornea
⊟ H18.831   Recurrent erosion of cornea, right eye
⊟ H18.832   Recurrent erosion of cornea, left eye
⊟ H18.833   Recurrent erosion of cornea, bilateral
⊟ H18.839   Recurrent erosion of cornea, unspecified eye
⑥ H18.89   Other specified disorders of cornea
⊟ H18.891   Other specified disorders of cornea, right eye
⊟ H18.892   Other specified disorders of cornea, left eye
⊟ H18.893   Other specified disorders of cornea, bilateral
⊟ H18.899   Other specified disorders of cornea, unspecified eye

H18.9   Unspecified disorder of cornea

④ H20   Iridocyclitis
⑤ H20.0   Acute and subacute iridocyclitis
      Acute anterior uveitis
      Acute cyclitis
      Acute iritis
      Subacute anterior uveitis
      Subacute cyclitis
      Subacute iritis
      EXCLUDES 1   *iridocyclitis, iritis, uveitis (due to) (in) diabetes mellitus (E08-E13 with .39)*
      iridocyclitis, iritis, uveitis (due to) (in) diphtheria (A36.89)
      iridocyclitis, iritis, uveitis (due to) (in) gonococcal (A54.32)
      iridocyclitis, iritis, uveitis (due to) (in) herpes (simplex) (B00.51)
      iridocyclitis, iritis, uveitis (due to) (in) herpes zoster (B02.32)
      iridocyclitis, iritis, uveitis (due to) (in) late congenital syphilis (A50.39)
      iridocyclitis, iritis, uveitis (due to) (in) late syphilis (A52.71)
      iridocyclitis, iritis, uveitis (due to) (in) sarcoidosis (D86.83)
      iridocyclitis, iritis, uveitis (due to) (in) syphilis (A51.43)
      iridocyclitis, iritis, uveitis (due to) (in) toxoplasmosis (B58.09)
      iridocyclitis, iritis, uveitis (due to) (in) tuberculosis (A18.54)
H20.00   Unspecified acute and subacute iridocyclitis
⑥ H20.01   Primary iridocyclitis
⊟ H20.011   Primary iridocyclitis, right eye
⊟ H20.012   Primary iridocyclitis, left eye
⊟ H20.013   Primary iridocyclitis, bilateral
⊟ H20.019   Primary iridocyclitis, unspecified eye
⑥ H20.02   Recurrent acute iridocyclitis
⊟ H20.021   Recurrent acute iridocyclitis, right eye

⊟ H20.022   Recurrent acute iridocyclitis, left eye
⊟ H20.023   Recurrent acute iridocyclitis, bilateral
⊟ H20.029   Recurrent acute iridocyclitis, unspecified eye
⑥ H20.03   Secondary infectious iridocyclitis
⊟ H20.031   Secondary infectious iridocyclitis, right eye
⊟ H20.032   Secondary infectious iridocyclitis, left eye
⊟ H20.033   Secondary infectious iridocyclitis, bilateral
⊟ H20.039   Secondary infectious iridocyclitis, unspecified eye
⑥ H20.04   Secondary noninfectious iridocyclitis
⊟ H20.041   Secondary noninfectious iridocyclitis, right eye
⊟ H20.042   Secondary noninfectious iridocyclitis, left eye
⊟ H20.043   Secondary noninfectious iridocyclitis, bilateral
⊟ H20.049   Secondary noninfectious iridocyclitis, unspecified eye
⑥ H20.05   Hypopyon
      DEFINITION   Accumulation of pus in the anterior chamber of the eye between the cornea and the iris and lens.
⊟ H20.051   Hypopyon, right eye
⊟ H20.052   Hypopyon, left eye
⊟ H20.053   Hypopyon, bilateral
⊟ H20.059   Hypopyon, unspecified eye
⑤➕ H20.1   Chronic iridocyclitis
      Use additional code for any associated cataract (H26.21-)
      EXCLUDES 2   *posterior cyclitis (H30.2-)*
⊟➕ H20.10   Chronic iridocyclitis, unspecified eye
⊟➕ H20.11   Chronic iridocyclitis, right eye
⊟➕ H20.12   Chronic iridocyclitis, left eye
⊟➕ H20.13   Chronic iridocyclitis, bilateral
⑤ H20.2   Lens-induced iridocyclitis
⊟ H20.20   Lens-induced iridocyclitis, unspecified eye
⊟ H20.21   Lens-induced iridocyclitis, right eye
⊟ H20.22   Lens-induced iridocyclitis, left eye
⊟ H20.23   Lens-induced iridocyclitis, bilateral
⑤ H20.8   Other iridocyclitis
      EXCLUDES 2   *glaucomatocyclitis crises (H40.4-)*
      posterior cyclitis (H30.2-)
      sympathetic uveitis (H44.13-)
⑥ H20.81   Fuchs' heterochromic cyclitis
⊟ H20.811   Fuchs' heterochromic cyclitis, right eye
⊟ H20.812   Fuchs' heterochromic cyclitis, left eye
⊟ H20.813   Fuchs' heterochromic cyclitis, bilateral
⊟ H20.819   Fuchs' heterochromic cyclitis, unspecified eye
⑥ H20.82   Vogt-Koyanagi syndrome
⊟ H20.821   Vogt-Koyanagi syndrome, right eye
⊟ H20.822   Vogt-Koyanagi syndrome, left eye
⊟ H20.823   Vogt-Koyanagi syndrome, bilateral
⊟ H20.829   Vogt-Koyanagi syndrome, unspecified eye
H20.9   Unspecified iridocyclitis
      Uveitis NOS
④ H21   Other disorders of iris and ciliary body
      EXCLUDES 2   *sympathetic uveitis (H44.1-)*
⑤ H21.0   Hyphema
      EXCLUDES 1   *traumatic hyphema (S05.1-)*
      DEFINITION   Bleeding in the iris that pools in the bottom of the cornea causing vision to be extremely blurred.
⊟ H21.00   Hyphema, unspecified eye
⊟ H21.01   Hyphema, right eye
⊟ H21.02   Hyphema, left eye
⊟ H21.03   Hyphema, bilateral
⑤ H21.1   Other vascular disorders of iris and ciliary body
      Neovascularization of iris or ciliary body
      Rubeosis iridis
      Rubeosis of iris
⑥ H21.1X   Other vascular disorders of iris and ciliary body
⊟ H21.1X1   Other vascular disorders of iris and ciliary body, right eye

● New   ▲ Revised   *Manifestation*   ④-➐ Digit Indicators   ⊟ Laterality   Ⓐ Adult (15+ years)   Ⓜ Maternity (12-55 years)   Ⓝ Newborn   Ⓟ Pediatric (0-17 years)   ♂ Male   ♀ Female
✖ Deleted   Unspecified   ➕ Additional code

600   © 2017 DecisionHealth   2017 ICD-10-CM Expert for Physicians

⊟ H21.1X2   Other vascular disorders of iris and ciliary body, left eye
⊟ H21.1X3   Other vascular disorders of iris and ciliary body, bilateral
⊟ H21.1X9   Other vascular disorders of iris and ciliary body, unspecified eye

⑤ H21.2   Degeneration of iris and ciliary body
  ⑥ H21.21   Degeneration of chamber angle
    ⊟ H21.211   Degeneration of chamber angle, right eye
    ⊟ H21.212   Degeneration of chamber angle, left eye
    ⊟ H21.213   Degeneration of chamber angle, bilateral
    ⊟ H21.219   Degeneration of chamber angle, unspecified eye
  ⑥ H21.22   Degeneration of ciliary body
    ⊟ H21.221   Degeneration of ciliary body, right eye
    ⊟ H21.222   Degeneration of ciliary body, left eye
    ⊟ H21.223   Degeneration of ciliary body, bilateral
    ⊟ H21.229   Degeneration of ciliary body, unspecified eye
  ⑥ H21.23   Degeneration of iris (pigmentary)
    Translucency of iris

    DEFINITION   Fading of the pigmentation (color) of the iris, allowing light to seep in rather than being blocked; presents with light-sensitivity and blurred vision.

    ⊟ H21.231   Degeneration of iris (pigmentary), right eye
    ⊟ H21.232   Degeneration of iris (pigmentary), left eye
    ⊟ H21.233   Degeneration of iris (pigmentary), bilateral
    ⊟ H21.239   Degeneration of iris (pigmentary), unspecified eye
  ⑥ H21.24   Degeneration of pupillary margin
    ⊟ H21.241   Degeneration of pupillary margin, right eye
    ⊟ H21.242   Degeneration of pupillary margin, left eye
    ⊟ H21.243   Degeneration of pupillary margin, bilateral
    ⊟ H21.249   Degeneration of pupillary margin, unspecified eye
  ⑥ H21.25   Iridoschisis
    ⊟ H21.251   Iridoschisis, right eye
    ⊟ H21.252   Iridoschisis, left eye
    ⊟ H21.253   Iridoschisis, bilateral
    ⊟ H21.259   Iridoschisis, unspecified eye
  ⑥ H21.26   Iris atrophy (essential) (progressive)
    ⊟ H21.261   Iris atrophy (essential) (progressive), right eye
    ⊟ H21.262   Iris atrophy (essential) (progressive), left eye
    ⊟ H21.263   Iris atrophy (essential) (progressive), bilateral
    ⊟ H21.269   Iris atrophy (essential) (progressive), unspecified eye
  ⑥ H21.27   Miotic pupillary cyst

    DEFINITION   Fluid-filled pockets in the iris at the pupil's edge, causing the iris to contract and interfering with vision when light is less than optimal.

    ⊟ H21.271   Miotic pupillary cyst, right eye
    ⊟ H21.272   Miotic pupillary cyst, left eye
    ⊟ H21.273   Miotic pupillary cyst, bilateral
    ⊟ H21.279   Miotic pupillary cyst, unspecified eye
  H21.29   Other iris atrophy
⑤ H21.3   Cyst of iris, ciliary body and anterior chamber

  EXCLUDES 2   miotic pupillary cyst (H21.27-)

  ⑥ H21.30   Idiopathic cysts of iris, ciliary body or anterior chamber
    Cyst of iris, ciliary body or anterior chamber NOS
    ⊟ H21.301   Idiopathic cysts of iris, ciliary body or anterior chamber, right eye
    ⊟ H21.302   Idiopathic cysts of iris, ciliary body or anterior chamber, left eye
    ⊟ H21.303   Idiopathic cysts of iris, ciliary body or anterior chamber, bilateral
    ⊟ H21.309   Idiopathic cysts of iris, ciliary body or anterior chamber, unspecified eye
  ⑥ H21.31   Exudative cysts of iris or anterior chamber
    ⊟ H21.311   Exudative cysts of iris or anterior chamber, right eye
    ⊟ H21.312   Exudative cysts of iris or anterior chamber, left eye
    ⊟ H21.313   Exudative cysts of iris or anterior chamber, bilateral

    ⊟ H21.319   Exudative cysts of iris or anterior chamber, unspecified eye
  ⑥ H21.32   Implantation cysts of iris, ciliary body or anterior chamber
    ⊟ H21.321   Implantation cysts of iris, ciliary body or anterior chamber, right eye
    ⊟ H21.322   Implantation cysts of iris, ciliary body or anterior chamber, left eye
    ⊟ H21.323   Implantation cysts of iris, ciliary body or anterior chamber, bilateral
    ⊟ H21.329   Implantation cysts of iris, ciliary body or anterior chamber, unspecified eye
  ⑥ H21.33   Parasitic cyst of iris, ciliary body or anterior chamber
    ⊟ H21.331   Parasitic cyst of iris, ciliary body or anterior chamber, right eye
    ⊟ H21.332   Parasitic cyst of iris, ciliary body or anterior chamber, left eye
    ⊟ H21.333   Parasitic cyst of iris, ciliary body or anterior chamber, bilateral
    ⊟ H21.339   Parasitic cyst of iris, ciliary body or anterior chamber, unspecified eye
  ⑥ H21.34   Primary cyst of pars plana
    ⊟ H21.341   Primary cyst of pars plana, right eye
    ⊟ H21.342   Primary cyst of pars plana, left eye
    ⊟ H21.343   Primary cyst of pars plana, bilateral
    ⊟ H21.349   Primary cyst of pars plana, unspecified eye
  ⑥ H21.35   Exudative cyst of pars plana
    ⊟ H21.351   Exudative cyst of pars plana, right eye
    ⊟ H21.352   Exudative cyst of pars plana, left eye
    ⊟ H21.353   Exudative cyst of pars plana, bilateral
    ⊟ H21.359   Exudative cyst of pars plana, unspecified eye
⑤ H21.4   Pupillary membranes
  Iris bombé
  Pupillary occlusion
  Pupillary seclusion

  EXCLUDES 1   congenital pupillary membranes (Q13.8)

  ⊟ H21.40   Pupillary membranes, unspecified eye
  ⊟ H21.41   Pupillary membranes, right eye
  ⊟ H21.42   Pupillary membranes, left eye
  ⊟ H21.43   Pupillary membranes, bilateral
⑤ H21.5   Other and unspecified adhesions and disruptions of iris and ciliary body

  EXCLUDES 1   corectopia (Q13.2)

  ⑥ H21.50   Unspecified adhesions of iris
    Synechia (iris) NOS
    ⊟ H21.501   Unspecified adhesions of iris, right eye
    ⊟ H21.502   Unspecified adhesions of iris, left eye
    ⊟ H21.503   Unspecified adhesions of iris, bilateral
    ⊟ H21.509   Unspecified adhesions of iris and ciliary body, unspecified eye
  ⑥ H21.51   Anterior synechiae (iris)
    ⊟ H21.511   Anterior synechiae (iris), right eye
    ⊟ H21.512   Anterior synechiae (iris), left eye
    ⊟ H21.513   Anterior synechiae (iris), bilateral
    ⊟ H21.519   Anterior synechiae (iris), unspecified eye
  ⑥ H21.52   Goniosynechiae

    DEFINITION   Adhesion of the iris to the posterior surface of the cornea, in the angle of the anterior chamber of the eye.

    ⊟ H21.521   Goniosynechiae, right eye
    ⊟ H21.522   Goniosynechiae, left eye
    ⊟ H21.523   Goniosynechiae, bilateral
    ⊟ H21.529   Goniosynechiae, unspecified eye
  ⑥ H21.53   Iridodialysis

    DEFINITION   Separation or loosening of the iris from its root at the ciliary body, usually from trauma or surgical accident.

    ⊟ H21.531   Iridodialysis, right eye
    ⊟ H21.532   Iridodialysis, left eye
    ⊟ H21.533   Iridodialysis, bilateral
    ⊟ H21.539   Iridodialysis, unspecified eye
  ⑥ H21.54   Posterior synechiae (iris)

● New   ▲ Revised   *Manifestation*   ❹-❼ Digit Indicators   ⊟ Laterality   Ⓐ Adult (15+ years)   Ⓜ Maternity (12-55 years)   Ⓝ Newborn   Ⓟ Pediatric (0-17 years)   ♂ Male   ♀ Female
✖ Deleted   Unspecified   + Additional code

Diseases of the Eye and Adnexa

DEFINITION Adhesion where the lens and the iris grow together, preventing the iris from dilating and contracting properly.

  ☐ **H21.541**   Posterior synechiae (iris), right eye
  ☐ **H21.542**   Posterior synechiae (iris), left eye
  ☐ **H21.543**   Posterior synechiae (iris), bilateral
  ☐ **H21.549**   Posterior synechiae (iris), unspecified eye
 G H21.55   Recession of chamber angle
  ☐ **H21.551**   Recession of chamber angle, right eye
  ☐ **H21.552**   Recession of chamber angle, left eye
  ☐ **H21.553**   Recession of chamber angle, bilateral
  ☐ **H21.559**   Recession of chamber angle, unspecified eye
 G H21.56   **Pupillary abnormalities**
        Deformed pupil
        Ectopic pupil
        Rupture of sphincter, pupil
        EXCLUDES 1 *congenital deformity of pupil (Q13.2-)*
  ☐ **H21.561**   Pupillary abnormality, right eye
  ☐ **H21.562**   Pupillary abnormality, left eye
  ☐ **H21.563**   Pupillary abnormality, bilateral
  ☐ **H21.569**   Pupillary abnormality, unspecified eye
 S H21.8   **Other specified disorders of iris and ciliary body**
  ✛ H21.81   **Floppy iris syndrome**
        Intraoperative floppy iris syndrome (IFIS)
        Use additional code for adverse effect, if applicable, to identify drug (T36-T50 with fifth or sixth character 5)
        DEFINITION Syndrome occurring in one who has taken alpha-blockers; a dilated iris does not stay dilated, causing potentially injurious surgical complications.
  H21.82   Plateau iris syndrome (post-iridectomy) (postprocedural)
  H21.89   Other specified disorders of iris and ciliary body
 H21.9   Unspecified disorder of iris and ciliary body
H22   ***Disorders of iris and ciliary body in diseases classified elsewhere***
    Code first underlying disease, such as:
      gout (M1A.-, M10.-)
      leprosy (A30.-)
      parasitic disease (B89)

Disorders of lens (H25-H28)

▣ H25   **Age-related cataract**
    Senile cataract
    EXCLUDES 2 *capsular glaucoma with pseudoexfoliation of lens (H40.1-)*
 S H25.0   **Age-related incipient cataract**
  G H25.01   **Cortical age-related cataract**
   ☐ **H25.011**   Cortical age-related cataract, right eye Ⓐ
   ☐ **H25.012**   Cortical age-related cataract, left eye Ⓐ
   ☐ **H25.013**   Cortical age-related cataract, bilateral Ⓐ
   ☐ **H25.019**   Cortical age-related cataract, unspecified eye Ⓐ
  G H25.03   **Anterior subcapsular polar age-related cataract**
   ☐ **H25.031**   Anterior subcapsular polar age-related cataract, right eye Ⓐ
   ☐ **H25.032**   Anterior subcapsular polar age-related cataract, left eye Ⓐ
   ☐ **H25.033**   Anterior subcapsular polar age-related cataract, bilateral Ⓐ
   ☐ **H25.039**   Anterior subcapsular polar age-related cataract, unspecified eye Ⓐ
  G H25.04   **Posterior subcapsular polar age-related cataract**
   ☐ **H25.041**   Posterior subcapsular polar age-related cataract, right eye Ⓐ
   ☐ **H25.042**   Posterior subcapsular polar age-related cataract, left eye Ⓐ
   ☐ **H25.043**   Posterior subcapsular polar age-related cataract, bilateral Ⓐ
   ☐ **H25.049**   Posterior subcapsular polar age-related cataract, unspecified eye Ⓐ
  G H25.09   **Other age-related incipient cataract**
      Coronary age-related cataract
      Punctate age-related cataract
      Water clefts

   ☐ **H25.091**   Other age-related incipient cataract, right eye Ⓐ
   ☐ **H25.092**   Other age-related incipient cataract, left eye Ⓐ
   ☐ **H25.093**   Other age-related incipient cataract, bilateral Ⓐ
   ☐ **H25.099**   Other age-related incipient cataract, unspecified eye Ⓐ
 S H25.1   **Age-related nuclear cataract**
    Cataracta brunescens
    Nuclear sclerosis cataract
  ☐ **H25.10**   **Age-related nuclear cataract, unspecified eye** Ⓐ
  ☐ **H25.11**   **Age-related nuclear cataract, right eye** Ⓐ
  ☐ **H25.12**   **Age-related nuclear cataract, left eye** Ⓐ
      AHA: 1Q 2016, 32-33
  ☐ **H25.13**   **Age-related nuclear cataract, bilateral** Ⓐ
      AHA: 1Q 2016, 32-33
 S H25.2   **Age-related cataract, morgagnian type**
    Age-related hypermature cataract
  ☐ **H25.20**   Age-related cataract, morgagnian type, unspecified eye Ⓐ
  ☐ **H25.21**   Age-related cataract, morgagnian type, right eye Ⓐ
  ☐ **H25.22**   Age-related cataract, morgagnian type, left eye Ⓐ
  ☐ **H25.23**   Age-related cataract, morgagnian type, bilateral Ⓐ
 S H25.8   **Other age-related cataract**
  G H25.81   **Combined forms of age-related cataract**
   ☐ **H25.811**   Combined forms of age-related cataract, right eye Ⓐ
   ☐ **H25.812**   Combined forms of age-related cataract, left eye Ⓐ
   ☐ **H25.813**   Combined forms of age-related cataract, bilateral Ⓐ
   ☐ **H25.819**   Combined forms of age-related cataract, unspecified eye Ⓐ
  H25.89   Other age-related cataract Ⓐ
  H25.9   Unspecified age-related cataract Ⓐ
▣ H26   **Other cataract**
    EXCLUDES 1 *congenital cataract (Q12.0)*
    DEFINITION Partial or complete clouding on or in the lens or lens capsule of the eye, obscuring vision.
 S H26.0   **Infantile and juvenile cataract**
  G H26.00   **Unspecified infantile and juvenile cataract**
   ☐ **H26.001**   Unspecified infantile and juvenile cataract, right eye Ⓟ
   ☐ **H26.002**   Unspecified infantile and juvenile cataract, left eye Ⓟ
   ☐ **H26.003**   Unspecified infantile and juvenile cataract, bilateral Ⓟ
   ☐ **H26.009**   Unspecified infantile and juvenile cataract, unspecified eye Ⓟ
  G H26.01   **Infantile and juvenile cortical, lamellar, or zonular cataract**
   ☐ **H26.011**   Infantile and juvenile cortical, lamellar, or zonular cataract, right eye Ⓟ
   ☐ **H26.012**   Infantile and juvenile cortical, lamellar, or zonular cataract, left eye Ⓟ
   ☐ **H26.013**   Infantile and juvenile cortical, lamellar, or zonular cataract, bilateral Ⓟ
   ☐ **H26.019**   Infantile and juvenile cortical, lamellar, or zonular cataract, unspecified eye Ⓟ
  G H26.03   **Infantile and juvenile nuclear cataract**
   ☐ **H26.031**   Infantile and juvenile nuclear cataract, right eye Ⓟ
   ☐ **H26.032**   Infantile and juvenile nuclear cataract, left eye Ⓟ
   ☐ **H26.033**   Infantile and juvenile nuclear cataract, bilateral Ⓟ
   ☐ **H26.039**   Infantile and juvenile nuclear cataract, unspecified eye Ⓟ
  G H26.04   **Anterior subcapsular polar infantile and juvenile cataract**
   ☐ **H26.041**   Anterior subcapsular polar infantile and juvenile cataract, right eye Ⓟ
   ☐ **H26.042**   Anterior subcapsular polar infantile and juvenile cataract, left eye Ⓟ
   ☐ **H26.043**   Anterior subcapsular polar infantile and juvenile cataract, bilateral Ⓟ

● New   ▲ Revised   *Manifestation*   �४-Ⴗ Digit Indicators   ☐ Laterality   Ⓐ Adult (15+ years)   Ⓜ Maternity (12-55 years)   Ⓝ Newborn   Ⓟ Pediatric (0-17 years)   ♂ Male   ♀ Female
✖ Deleted   Unspecified   ✛ Additional code

602   © 2017 DecisionHealth   2017 ICD-10-CM Expert for Physicians

H21.54 — H26.043

    H26.049   **Anterior subcapsular polar infantile and juvenile cataract, unspecified eye** P

H26.05   **Posterior subcapsular polar infantile and juvenile cataract**

    H26.051   **Posterior subcapsular polar infantile and juvenile cataract, right eye** P

    H26.052   **Posterior subcapsular polar infantile and juvenile cataract, left eye** P

    H26.053   **Posterior subcapsular polar infantile and juvenile cataract, bilateral** P

    H26.059   **Posterior subcapsular polar infantile and juvenile cataract, unspecified eye** P

H26.06   **Combined forms of infantile and juvenile cataract**

    H26.061   **Combined forms of infantile and juvenile cataract, right eye** P

    H26.062   **Combined forms of infantile and juvenile cataract, left eye** P

    H26.063   **Combined forms of infantile and juvenile cataract, bilateral** P

    H26.069   **Combined forms of infantile and juvenile cataract, unspecified eye** P

H26.09   **Other infantile and juvenile cataract** P

+ H26.1   **Traumatic cataract**
   Use additional code (Chapter 20) to identify external cause

+ H26.10   **Unspecified traumatic cataract**

   + H26.101   **Unspecified traumatic cataract, right eye**

   + H26.102   **Unspecified traumatic cataract, left eye**

   + H26.103   **Unspecified traumatic cataract, bilateral**

   + H26.109   **Unspecified traumatic cataract, unspecified eye**

+ H26.11   **Localized traumatic opacities**

   + H26.111   **Localized traumatic opacities, right eye**

   + H26.112   **Localized traumatic opacities, left eye**

   + H26.113   **Localized traumatic opacities, bilateral**

   + H26.119   **Localized traumatic opacities, unspecified eye**

+ H26.12   **Partially resolved traumatic cataract**

   + H26.121   **Partially resolved traumatic cataract, right eye**

   + H26.122   **Partially resolved traumatic cataract, left eye**

   + H26.123   **Partially resolved traumatic cataract, bilateral**

   + H26.129   **Partially resolved traumatic cataract, unspecified eye**

+ H26.13   **Total traumatic cataract**

   + H26.131   **Total traumatic cataract, right eye**

   + H26.132   **Total traumatic cataract, left eye**

   + H26.133   **Total traumatic cataract, bilateral**

   + H26.139   **Total traumatic cataract, unspecified eye**

H26.2   **Complicated cataract**

H26.20   **Unspecified complicated cataract**
   Cataracta complicata NOS

H26.21   **Cataract with neovascularization**
   Code also associated condition, such as:
     chronic iridocyclitis (H20.1-)

   H26.211   **Cataract with neovascularization, right eye**

   H26.212   **Cataract with neovascularization, left eye**

   H26.213   **Cataract with neovascularization, bilateral**

   H26.219   **Cataract with neovascularization, unspecified eye**

H26.22   **Cataract secondary to ocular disorders (degenerative) (inflammatory)**
   Code also:
     associated ocular disorder

   H26.221   **Cataract secondary to ocular disorders (degenerative) (inflammatory), right eye**

   H26.222   **Cataract secondary to ocular disorders (degenerative) (inflammatory), left eye**

   H26.223   **Cataract secondary to ocular disorders (degenerative) (inflammatory), bilateral**

   H26.229   **Cataract secondary to ocular disorders (degenerative) (inflammatory), unspecified eye**

H26.23   **Glaucomatous flecks (subcapsular)**
   Code first:
     underlying glaucoma (H40-H42)

   H26.231   **Glaucomatous flecks (subcapsular), right eye**

   H26.232   **Glaucomatous flecks (subcapsular), left eye**

   H26.233   **Glaucomatous flecks (subcapsular), bilateral**

   H26.239   **Glaucomatous flecks (subcapsular), unspecified eye**

+ H26.3   **Drug-induced cataract**
   Toxic cataract
   Use additional code for adverse effect, if applicable, to identify drug (T36-T50 with fifth or sixth character 5)

   DEFINITION   Cataract caused by exposure to a drug or other toxic substance, such as a miotic, antimiotic, corticosteroid, metal, nitro compound, or substituted hydrocarbon.

   + H26.30   **Drug-induced cataract, unspecified eye**

   + H26.31   **Drug-induced cataract, right eye**

   + H26.32   **Drug-induced cataract, left eye**

   + H26.33   **Drug-induced cataract, bilateral**

H26.4   **Secondary cataract**

   H26.40   **Unspecified secondary cataract**

H26.41   **Soemmering's ring**

   DEFINITION   Doughnut-shaped remnant of lens behind the pupil, occurring after cataract surgery or secondary to trauma.

   H26.411   **Soemmering's ring, right eye**

   H26.412   **Soemmering's ring, left eye**

   H26.413   **Soemmering's ring, bilateral**

   H26.419   **Soemmering's ring, unspecified eye**

H26.49   **Other secondary cataract**

   H26.491   **Other secondary cataract, right eye**

   H26.492   **Other secondary cataract, left eye**

   H26.493   **Other secondary cataract, bilateral**

   H26.499   **Other secondary cataract, unspecified eye**

H26.8   **Other specified cataract**

H26.9   **Unspecified cataract**

H27   **Other disorders of lens**

   EXCLUDES 1   *congenital lens malformations (Q12.-)*
     mechanical complications of intraocular lens implant (T85.2)
     pseudophakia (Z96.1)

H27.0   **Aphakia**
   Acquired absence of lens
   Acquired aphakia
   Aphakia due to trauma

   EXCLUDES 1   *cataract extraction status (Z98.4-)*
     congenital absence of lens (Q12.3)
     congenital aphakia (Q12.3)

   DEFINITION   Absence of the crystalline lens of the eye.

   H27.00   **Aphakia, unspecified eye**

   H27.01   **Aphakia, right eye**

   H27.02   **Aphakia, left eye**

   H27.03   **Aphakia, bilateral**

H27.1   **Dislocation of lens**

   H27.10   **Unspecified dislocation of lens**

H27.11   **Subluxation of lens**

   H27.111   **Subluxation of lens, right eye**

   H27.112   **Subluxation of lens, left eye**

   H27.113   **Subluxation of lens, bilateral**

   H27.119   **Subluxation of lens, unspecified eye**

H27.12   **Anterior dislocation of lens**

   H27.121   **Anterior dislocation of lens, right eye**

   H27.122   **Anterior dislocation of lens, left eye**

   H27.123   **Anterior dislocation of lens, bilateral**

   H27.129   **Anterior dislocation of lens, unspecified eye**

H27.13   **Posterior dislocation of lens**

   H27.131   **Posterior dislocation of lens, right eye**

   H27.132   **Posterior dislocation of lens, left eye**

   H27.133   **Posterior dislocation of lens, bilateral**

   H27.139   **Posterior dislocation of lens, unspecified eye**

H27.8   **Other specified disorders of lens**

H27.9   **Unspecified disorder of lens**

H28 *Cataract in diseases classified elsewhere*

Code first underlying disease, such as:
hypoparathyroidism (E20.-)
myotonia (G71.1-)
myxedema (E03.-)
protein-calorie malnutrition (E40-E46)

EXCLUDES 1 *cataract in diabetes mellitus (E08.36, E09.36, E10.36, E11.36, E13.36)*

Disorders of choroid and retina (H30-H36)

H30 Chorioretinal inflammation

H30.0 Focal chorioretinal inflammation
Focal chorioretinitis
Focal choroiditis
Focal retinitis
Focal retinochoroiditis

H30.00 Unspecified focal chorioretinal inflammation
Focal chorioretinitis NOS
Focal choroiditis NOS
Focal retinitis NOS
Focal retinochoroiditis NOS

H30.001 Unspecified focal chorioretinal inflammation, right eye

H30.002 Unspecified focal chorioretinal inflammation, left eye

H30.003 Unspecified focal chorioretinal inflammation, bilateral

H30.009 Unspecified focal chorioretinal inflammation, unspecified eye

H30.01 Focal chorioretinal inflammation, juxtapapillary

H30.011 Focal chorioretinal inflammation, juxtapapillary, right eye

H30.012 Focal chorioretinal inflammation, juxtapapillary, left eye

H30.013 Focal chorioretinal inflammation, juxtapapillary, bilateral

H30.019 Focal chorioretinal inflammation, juxtapapillary, unspecified eye

H30.02 Focal chorioretinal inflammation of posterior pole

H30.021 Focal chorioretinal inflammation of posterior pole, right eye

H30.022 Focal chorioretinal inflammation of posterior pole, left eye

H30.023 Focal chorioretinal inflammation of posterior pole, bilateral

H30.029 Focal chorioretinal inflammation of posterior pole, unspecified eye

H30.03 Focal chorioretinal inflammation, peripheral

H30.031 Focal chorioretinal inflammation, peripheral, right eye

H30.032 Focal chorioretinal inflammation, peripheral, left eye

H30.033 Focal chorioretinal inflammation, peripheral, bilateral

H30.039 Focal chorioretinal inflammation, peripheral, unspecified eye

H30.04 Focal chorioretinal inflammation, macular or paramacular

H30.041 Focal chorioretinal inflammation, macular or paramacular, right eye

H30.042 Focal chorioretinal inflammation, macular or paramacular, left eye

H30.043 Focal chorioretinal inflammation, macular or paramacular, bilateral

H30.049 Focal chorioretinal inflammation, macular or paramacular, unspecified eye

H30.1 Disseminated chorioretinal inflammation
Disseminated chorioretinitis
Disseminated choroiditis
Disseminated retinitis
Disseminated retinochoroiditis

EXCLUDES 2 *exudative retinopathy (H35.02-)*

H30.10 Unspecified disseminated chorioretinal inflammation
Disseminated chorioretinitis NOS
Disseminated choroiditis NOS
Disseminated retinitis NOS
Disseminated retinochoroiditis NOS

H30.101 Unspecified disseminated chorioretinal inflammation, right eye

H30.102 Unspecified disseminated chorioretinal inflammation, left eye

H30.103 Unspecified disseminated chorioretinal inflammation, bilateral

H30.109 Unspecified disseminated chorioretinal inflammation, unspecified eye

H30.11 Disseminated chorioretinal inflammation of posterior pole

H30.111 Disseminated chorioretinal inflammation of posterior pole, right eye

H30.112 Disseminated chorioretinal inflammation of posterior pole, left eye

H30.113 Disseminated chorioretinal inflammation of posterior pole, bilateral

H30.119 Disseminated chorioretinal inflammation of posterior pole, unspecified eye

H30.12 Disseminated chorioretinal inflammation, peripheral

H30.121 Disseminated chorioretinal inflammation, peripheral right eye

H30.122 Disseminated chorioretinal inflammation, peripheral, left eye

H30.123 Disseminated chorioretinal inflammation, peripheral, bilateral

H30.129 Disseminated chorioretinal inflammation, peripheral, unspecified eye

H30.13 Disseminated chorioretinal inflammation, generalized

H30.131 Disseminated chorioretinal inflammation, generalized, right eye

H30.132 Disseminated chorioretinal inflammation, generalized, left eye

H30.133 Disseminated chorioretinal inflammation, generalized, bilateral

H30.139 Disseminated chorioretinal inflammation, generalized, unspecified eye

H30.14 Acute posterior multifocal placoid pigment epitheliopathy

H30.141 Acute posterior multifocal placoid pigment epitheliopathy, right eye

H30.142 Acute posterior multifocal placoid pigment epitheliopathy, left eye

H30.143 Acute posterior multifocal placoid pigment epitheliopathy, bilateral

H30.149 Acute posterior multifocal placoid pigment epitheliopathy, unspecified eye

H30.2 Posterior cyclitis
Pars planitis

DEFINITION Inflammation of the peripheral retina and the ciliary body, the hair-like structures that hold the lens of the eye in place.

H30.20 Posterior cyclitis, unspecified eye

H30.21 Posterior cyclitis, right eye

H30.22 Posterior cyclitis, left eye

H30.23 Posterior cyclitis, bilateral

H30.8 Other chorioretinal inflammations

H30.81 Harada's disease

H30.811 Harada's disease, right eye

H30.812 Harada's disease, left eye

H30.813 Harada's disease, bilateral

H30.819 Harada's disease, unspecified eye

H30.89 Other chorioretinal inflammations

H30.891 Other chorioretinal inflammations, right eye

H30.892 Other chorioretinal inflammations, left eye

H30.893 Other chorioretinal inflammations, bilateral

H30.899 Other chorioretinal inflammations, unspecified eye

● New ▲ Revised *Manifestation* ❹-❼ Digit Indicators ▱ Laterality A Adult (15+ years) M Maternity (12-55 years) N Newborn P Pediatric (0-17 years) ♂ Male ♀ Female
✖ Deleted Unspecified ✚ Additional code

⑤ **H30.9** **Unspecified chorioretinal inflammation**
Chorioretinitis NOS
Choroiditis NOS
Neuroretinitis NOS
Retinitis NOS
Retinochoroiditis NOS

□ **H30.90** **Unspecified chorioretinal inflammation, unspecified eye**

□ **H30.91** **Unspecified chorioretinal inflammation, right eye**

□ **H30.92** **Unspecified chorioretinal inflammation, left eye**

□ **H30.93** **Unspecified chorioretinal inflammation, bilateral**

④ **H31** **Other disorders of choroid**

⑤ **H31.0** **Chorioretinal scars**

EXCLUDES 2 *postsurgical chorioretinal scars (H59.81-)*

⑥ **H31.00** **Unspecified chorioretinal scars**

□ **H31.001** **Unspecified chorioretinal scars, right eye**

□ **H31.002** **Unspecified chorioretinal scars, left eye**

□ **H31.003** **Unspecified chorioretinal scars, bilateral**

□ **H31.009** **Unspecified chorioretinal scars, unspecified eye**

⑥ **H31.01** **Macula scars of posterior pole (postinflammatory) (post-traumatic)**

EXCLUDES 1 *postprocedural chorioretinal scar (H59.81-)*

□ **H31.011** **Macula scars of posterior pole (postinflammatory) (post-traumatic), right eye**

□ **H31.012** **Macula scars of posterior pole (postinflammatory) (post-traumatic), left eye**

□ **H31.013** **Macula scars of posterior pole (postinflammatory) (post-traumatic), bilateral**

□ **H31.019** **Macula scars of posterior pole (postinflammatory) (post-traumatic), unspecified eye**

⑥ **H31.02** **Solar retinopathy**

DEFINITION Scar on the retina resulting from solar radiation.

□ **H31.021** **Solar retinopathy, right eye**

□ **H31.022** **Solar retinopathy, left eye**

□ **H31.023** **Solar retinopathy, bilateral**

□ **H31.029** **Solar retinopathy, unspecified eye**

⑥ **H31.09** **Other chorioretinal scars**

□ **H31.091** **Other chorioretinal scars, right eye**

□ **H31.092** **Other chorioretinal scars, left eye**

□ **H31.093** **Other chorioretinal scars, bilateral**

□ **H31.099** **Other chorioretinal scars, unspecified eye**

⑤ **H31.1** **Choroidal degeneration**

EXCLUDES 2 *angioid streaks of macula (H35.33)*

⑥ **H31.10** **Unspecified choroidal degeneration**
Choroidal sclerosis NOS

□ **H31.101** **Choroidal degeneration, unspecified, right eye**

□ **H31.102** **Choroidal degeneration, unspecified, left eye**

□ **H31.103** **Choroidal degeneration, unspecified, bilateral**

□ **H31.109** **Choroidal degeneration, unspecified, unspecified eye**

⑥ **H31.11** **Age-related choroidal atrophy**

□ **H31.111** **Age-related choroidal atrophy, right eye** Ⓐ

□ **H31.112** **Age-related choroidal atrophy, left eye** Ⓐ

□ **H31.113** **Age-related choroidal atrophy, bilateral** Ⓐ

□ **H31.119** **Age-related choroidal atrophy, unspecified eye** Ⓐ

⑥ **H31.12** **Diffuse secondary atrophy of choroid**

□ **H31.121** **Diffuse secondary atrophy of choroid, right eye**

□ **H31.122** **Diffuse secondary atrophy of choroid, left eye**

□ **H31.123** **Diffuse secondary atrophy of choroid, bilateral**

□ **H31.129** **Diffuse secondary atrophy of choroid, unspecified eye**

⑤ **H31.2** **Hereditary choroidal dystrophy**

EXCLUDES 2 *hyperornithinemia (E72.4)*
ornithinemia (E72.4)

H31.20 **Hereditary choroidal dystrophy, unspecified**

H31.21 **Choroideremia**

H31.22 **Choroidal dystrophy (central areolar) (generalized) (peripapillary)**

H31.23 **Gyrate atrophy, choroid**

H31.29 **Other hereditary choroidal dystrophy**

⑤ **H31.3** **Choroidal hemorrhage and rupture**

⑥ **H31.30** **Unspecified choroidal hemorrhage**

□ **H31.301** **Unspecified choroidal hemorrhage, right eye**

□ **H31.302** **Unspecified choroidal hemorrhage, left eye**

□ **H31.303** **Unspecified choroidal hemorrhage, bilateral**

□ **H31.309** **Unspecified choroidal hemorrhage, unspecified eye**

⑥ **H31.31** **Expulsive choroidal hemorrhage**

□ **H31.311** **Expulsive choroidal hemorrhage, right eye**

□ **H31.312** **Expulsive choroidal hemorrhage, left eye**

□ **H31.313** **Expulsive choroidal hemorrhage, bilateral**

□ **H31.319** **Expulsive choroidal hemorrhage, unspecified eye**

⑥ **H31.32** **Choroidal rupture**

□ **H31.321** **Choroidal rupture, right eye**

□ **H31.322** **Choroidal rupture, left eye**

□ **H31.323** **Choroidal rupture, bilateral**

□ **H31.329** **Choroidal rupture, unspecified eye**

⑤ **H31.4** **Choroidal detachment**

⑥ **H31.40** **Unspecified choroidal detachment**

□ **H31.401** **Unspecified choroidal detachment, right eye**

□ **H31.402** **Unspecified choroidal detachment, left eye**

□ **H31.403** **Unspecified choroidal detachment, bilateral**

□ **H31.409** **Unspecified choroidal detachment, unspecified eye**

⑥ **H31.41** **Hemorrhagic choroidal detachment**

□ **H31.411** **Hemorrhagic choroidal detachment, right eye**

□ **H31.412** **Hemorrhagic choroidal detachment, left eye**

□ **H31.413** **Hemorrhagic choroidal detachment, bilateral**

□ **H31.419** **Hemorrhagic choroidal detachment, unspecified eye**

⑥ **H31.42** **Serous choroidal detachment**

□ **H31.421** **Serous choroidal detachment, right eye**

□ **H31.422** **Serous choroidal detachment, left eye**

□ **H31.423** **Serous choroidal detachment, bilateral**

□ **H31.429** **Serous choroidal detachment, unspecified eye**

H31.8 **Other specified disorders of choroid**

H31.9 **Unspecified disorder of choroid**

H32 *Chorioretinal disorders in diseases classified elsewhere*
Code first underlying disease, such as:
congenital toxoplasmosis (P37.1)
histoplasmosis (B39.-)
leprosy (A30.-)

EXCLUDES 1 *chorioretinitis (in) :*
toxoplasmosis (acquired) (B58.01)
tuberculosis (A18.53)

④ **H33** **Retinal detachments and breaks**

EXCLUDES 1 *detachment of retinal pigment epithelium (H35.72-, H35.73-)*

DEFINITION Condition in which the retina separates from its underlying layer of cells in the back of the eye, resulting in a decrease in the visual field or blindness.

⑤ **H33.0** **Retinal detachment with retinal break**
Rhegmatogenous retinal detachment

EXCLUDES 1 *serous retinal detachment (without retinal break) (H33.2-)*

⑥ **H33.00** **Unspecified retinal detachment with retinal break**

□ **H33.001** **Unspecified retinal detachment with retinal break, right eye**

□ **H33.002** **Unspecified retinal detachment with retinal break, left eye**

□ **H33.003** **Unspecified retinal detachment with retinal break, bilateral**

□ **H33.009** **Unspecified retinal detachment with retinal break, unspecified eye**

⑥ **H33.01** **Retinal detachment with single break**

□ **H33.011** **Retinal detachment with single break, right eye**

□ **H33.012** **Retinal detachment with single break, left eye**

□ **H33.013** **Retinal detachment with single break, bilateral**

● New   ▲ Revised   *Manifestation*   ④-⑦ Digit Indicators   □ Laterality   Ⓐ Adult (15+ years)   Ⓜ Maternity (12-55 years)   Ⓝ Newborn   Ⓟ Pediatric (0-17 years)   ♂ Male   ♀ Female
✖ Deleted   Unspecified   + Additional code

2017 ICD-10-CM Expert for Physicians

© 2017 DecisionHealth

605

Diseases of the Eye and Adnexa

H33.019 — H34.819-

⊟ H33.019   **Retinal detachment with single break, unspecified eye**

Ⓖ H33.02   **Retinal detachment with multiple breaks**

⊟ H33.021   **Retinal detachment with multiple breaks, right eye**

⊟ H33.022   **Retinal detachment with multiple breaks, left eye**

⊟ H33.023   **Retinal detachment with multiple breaks, bilateral**

⊟ H33.029   **Retinal detachment with multiple breaks, unspecified eye**

Ⓖ H33.03   **Retinal detachment with giant retinal tear**

⊟ H33.031   **Retinal detachment with giant retinal tear, right eye**

⊟ H33.032   **Retinal detachment with giant retinal tear, left eye**

⊟ H33.033   **Retinal detachment with giant retinal tear, bilateral**

⊟ H33.039   **Retinal detachment with giant retinal tear, unspecified eye**

Ⓖ H33.04   **Retinal detachment with retinal dialysis**

⊟ H33.041   **Retinal detachment with retinal dialysis, right eye**

⊟ H33.042   **Retinal detachment with retinal dialysis, left eye**

⊟ H33.043   **Retinal detachment with retinal dialysis, bilateral**

⊟ H33.049   **Retinal detachment with retinal dialysis, unspecified eye**

Ⓖ H33.05   **Total retinal detachment**

⊟ H33.051   **Total retinal detachment, right eye**

⊟ H33.052   **Total retinal detachment, left eye**

⊟ H33.053   **Total retinal detachment, bilateral**

⊟ H33.059   **Total retinal detachment, unspecified eye**

Ⓢ H33.1   **Retinoschisis and retinal cysts**

> **EXCLUDES 1**   *congenital retinoschisis (Q14.1)*
> *microcystoid degeneration of retina (H35.42-)*

Ⓖ H33.10   **Unspecified retinoschisis**

⊟ H33.101   **Unspecified retinoschisis, right eye**

⊟ H33.102   **Unspecified retinoschisis, left eye**

⊟ H33.103   **Unspecified retinoschisis, bilateral**

⊟ H33.109   **Unspecified retinoschisis, unspecified eye**

Ⓖ H33.11   **Cyst of ora serrata**

⊟ H33.111   **Cyst of ora serrata, right eye**

⊟ H33.112   **Cyst of ora serrata, left eye**

⊟ H33.113   **Cyst of ora serrata, bilateral**

⊟ H33.119   **Cyst of ora serrata, unspecified eye**

Ⓖ H33.12   **Parasitic cyst of retina**

⊟ H33.121   **Parasitic cyst of retina, right eye**

⊟ H33.122   **Parasitic cyst of retina, left eye**

⊟ H33.123   **Parasitic cyst of retina, bilateral**

⊟ H33.129   **Parasitic cyst of retina, unspecified eye**

Ⓖ H33.19   **Other retinoschisis and retinal cysts**
Pseudocyst of retina

⊟ H33.191   **Other retinoschisis and retinal cysts, right eye**

⊟ H33.192   **Other retinoschisis and retinal cysts, left eye**

⊟ H33.193   **Other retinoschisis and retinal cysts, bilateral**

⊟ H33.199   **Other retinoschisis and retinal cysts, unspecified eye**

Ⓢ H33.2   **Serous retinal detachment**
Retinal detachment NOS
Retinal detachment without retinal break

> **EXCLUDES 1**   *central serous chorioretinopathy (H35.71-)*

⊟ H33.20   **Serous retinal detachment, unspecified eye**

⊟ H33.21   **Serous retinal detachment, right eye**

⊟ H33.22   **Serous retinal detachment, left eye**

⊟ H33.23   **Serous retinal detachment, bilateral**

Ⓢ H33.3   **Retinal breaks without detachment**

> **EXCLUDES 1**   *chorioretinal scars after surgery for detachment (H59.81-)*
> *peripheral retinal degeneration without break (H35.4-)*

Ⓖ H33.30   **Unspecified retinal break**

⊟ H33.301   **Unspecified retinal break, right eye**

⊟ H33.302   **Unspecified retinal break, left eye**

⊟ H33.303   **Unspecified retinal break, bilateral**

⊟ H33.309   **Unspecified retinal break, unspecified eye**

Ⓖ H33.31   **Horseshoe tear of retina without detachment**
Operculum of retina without detachment

⊟ H33.311   **Horseshoe tear of retina without detachment, right eye**

⊟ H33.312   **Horseshoe tear of retina without detachment, left eye**

⊟ H33.313   **Horseshoe tear of retina without detachment, bilateral**

⊟ H33.319   **Horseshoe tear of retina without detachment, unspecified eye**

Ⓖ H33.32   **Round hole of retina without detachment**

⊟ H33.321   **Round hole, right eye**

⊟ H33.322   **Round hole, left eye**

⊟ H33.323   **Round hole, bilateral**

⊟ H33.329   **Round hole, unspecified eye**

Ⓖ H33.33   **Multiple defects of retina without detachment**

⊟ H33.331   **Multiple defects of retina without detachment, right eye**

⊟ H33.332   **Multiple defects of retina without detachment, left eye**

⊟ H33.333   **Multiple defects of retina without detachment, bilateral**

⊟ H33.339   **Multiple defects of retina without detachment, unspecified eye**

Ⓢ H33.4   **Traction detachment of retina**
Proliferative vitreo-retinopathy with retinal detachment

⊟ H33.40   **Traction detachment of retina, unspecified eye**

⊟ H33.41   **Traction detachment of retina, right eye**

⊟ H33.42   **Traction detachment of retina, left eye**

⊟ H33.43   **Traction detachment of retina, bilateral**

H33.8   **Other retinal detachments**

Ⓐ H34   **Retinal vascular occlusions**

> **EXCLUDES 1**   *amaurosis fugax (G45.3)*

Ⓢ H34.0   **Transient retinal artery occlusion**

⊟ H34.00   **Transient retinal artery occlusion, unspecified eye**

⊟ H34.01   **Transient retinal artery occlusion, right eye**

⊟ H34.02   **Transient retinal artery occlusion, left eye**

⊟ H34.03   **Transient retinal artery occlusion, bilateral**

Ⓢ H34.1   **Central retinal artery occlusion**

⊟ H34.10   **Central retinal artery occlusion, unspecified eye**

⊟ H34.11   **Central retinal artery occlusion, right eye**

⊟ H34.12   **Central retinal artery occlusion, left eye**

⊟ H34.13   **Central retinal artery occlusion, bilateral**

Ⓢ H34.2   **Other retinal artery occlusions**

Ⓖ H34.21   **Partial retinal artery occlusion**
Hollenhorst's plaque
Retinal microembolism

⊟ H34.211   **Partial retinal artery occlusion, right eye**

⊟ H34.212   **Partial retinal artery occlusion, left eye**

⊟ H34.213   **Partial retinal artery occlusion, bilateral**

⊟ H34.219   **Partial retinal artery occlusion, unspecified eye**

Ⓖ H34.23   **Retinal artery branch occlusion**

⊟ H34.231   **Retinal artery branch occlusion, right eye**

⊟ H34.232   **Retinal artery branch occlusion, left eye**

⊟ H34.233   **Retinal artery branch occlusion, bilateral**

⊟ H34.239   **Retinal artery branch occlusion, unspecified eye**

Ⓢ H34.8   **Other retinal vascular occlusions**

▲ Ⓖ H34.81   **Central retinal vein occlusion**

> One of the following 7th characters is to be assigned to codes in subcategory H34.81 to designate the severity of the occlusion:
> 0   with macular edema
> 1   with retinal neovascularization
> 2   stable

7️⃣⊟ H34.811-   **Central retinal vein occlusion, right eye**

7️⃣⊟ H34.812-   **Central retinal vein occlusion, left eye**

7️⃣⊟ H34.813-   **Central retinal vein occlusion, bilateral**

7️⃣⊟ H34.819-   **Central retinal vein occlusion, unspecified eye**

● New   ▲ Revised   *Manifestation*   4-7 Digit Indicators   ⊟ Laterality   Ⓐ Adult (15+ years)   Ⓜ Maternity (12-55 years)   Ⓝ Newborn   Ⓟ Pediatric (0-17 years)   ♂ Male   ♀ Female
✖ Deleted   Unspecified   + Additional code

606   © 2017 DecisionHealth   2017 ICD-10-CM Expert for Physicians

⑥ **H34.82** **Venous engorgement**
Incipient retinal vein occlusion
Partial retinal vein occlusion
⊟ H34.821 **Venous engorgement, right eye**
⊟ H34.822 **Venous engorgement, left eye**
⊟ H34.823 **Venous engorgement, bilateral**
⊟ H34.829 **Venous engorgement, unspecified eye**
▲ ⑥ **H34.83** **Tributary (branch) retinal vein occlusion**

One of the following 7th characters is to be assigned to codes in subcategory H34.83 to designate the severity of the occlusion:
0   with macular edema
1   with retinal neovascularization
2   stable

7 ⊟ H34.831- **Tributary (branch) retinal vein occlusion, right eye**
7 ⊟ H34.832- **Tributary (branch) retinal vein occlusion, left eye**
7 ⊟ H34.833- **Tributary (branch) retinal vein occlusion, bilateral**
7 ⊟ H34.839- **Tributary (branch) retinal vein occlusion, unspecified eye**
H34.9 **Unspecified retinal vascular occlusion**
④ **H35** **Other retinal disorders**

EXCLUDES 2 *diabetic retinal disorders (E08.311-E08.359, E09.311-E09.359, E10.311-E10.359, E11.311-E11.359, E13.311-E13.359)*

⑤ **H35.0** **Background retinopathy and retinal vascular changes**
Code also:
    any associated hypertension (I10.-)

GUIDELINES **Section I.C.9.a.5)**
Subcategory H35.0, Background retinopathy and retinal vascular changes, should be used with a code from category I10-I15, Hypertensive disease to include the systemic hypertension. The sequencing is based on the reason for the encounter.

H35.00 **Unspecified background retinopathy**
⑥ **H35.01** **Changes in retinal vascular appearance**
Retinal vascular sheathing
⊟ H35.011 **Changes in retinal vascular appearance, right eye**
⊟ H35.012 **Changes in retinal vascular appearance, left eye**
⊟ H35.013 **Changes in retinal vascular appearance, bilateral**
⊟ H35.019 **Changes in retinal vascular appearance, unspecified eye**
⑥ **H35.02** **Exudative retinopathy**
Coats retinopathy
⊟ H35.021 **Exudative retinopathy, right eye**
⊟ H35.022 **Exudative retinopathy, left eye**
⊟ H35.023 **Exudative retinopathy, bilateral**
⊟ H35.029 **Exudative retinopathy, unspecified eye**
⑥ **H35.03** **Hypertensive retinopathy**
⊟ H35.031 **Hypertensive retinopathy, right eye**
⊟ H35.032 **Hypertensive retinopathy, left eye**
⊟ H35.033 **Hypertensive retinopathy, bilateral**
⊟ H35.039 **Hypertensive retinopathy, unspecified eye**
⑥ **H35.04** **Retinal micro-aneurysms, unspecified**
⊟ H35.041 **Retinal micro-aneurysms, unspecified, right eye**
⊟ H35.042 **Retinal micro-aneurysms, unspecified, left eye**
⊟ H35.043 **Retinal micro-aneurysms, unspecified, bilateral**
⊟ H35.049 **Retinal micro-aneurysms, unspecified, unspecified eye**
⑥ **H35.05** **Retinal neovascularization, unspecified**
⊟ H35.051 **Retinal neovascularization, unspecified, right eye**
⊟ H35.052 **Retinal neovascularization, unspecified, left eye**
⊟ H35.053 **Retinal neovascularization, unspecified, bilateral**
⊟ H35.059 **Retinal neovascularization, unspecified, unspecified eye**

⑥ **H35.06** **Retinal vasculitis**
Eales disease
Retinal perivasculitis
⊟ H35.061 **Retinal vasculitis, right eye**
⊟ H35.062 **Retinal vasculitis, left eye**
⊟ H35.063 **Retinal vasculitis, bilateral**
⊟ H35.069 **Retinal vasculitis, unspecified eye**
⑥ **H35.07** **Retinal telangiectasis**
⊟ H35.071 **Retinal telangiectasis, right eye**
⊟ H35.072 **Retinal telangiectasis, left eye**
⊟ H35.073 **Retinal telangiectasis, bilateral**
⊟ H35.079 **Retinal telangiectasis, unspecified eye**
H35.09 **Other intraretinal microvascular abnormalities**
Retinal varices
⑤ **H35.1** **Retinopathy of prematurity**
⑥ **H35.10** **Retinopathy of prematurity, unspecified**
Retinopathy of prematurity NOS
⊟ H35.101 **Retinopathy of prematurity, unspecified, right eye**
⊟ H35.102 **Retinopathy of prematurity, unspecified, left eye**
⊟ H35.103 **Retinopathy of prematurity, unspecified, bilateral**
⊟ H35.109 **Retinopathy of prematurity, unspecified, unspecified eye**
⑥ **H35.11** **Retinopathy of prematurity, stage 0**
⊟ H35.111 **Retinopathy of prematurity, stage 0, right eye**
⊟ H35.112 **Retinopathy of prematurity, stage 0, left eye**
⊟ H35.113 **Retinopathy of prematurity, stage 0, bilateral**
⊟ H35.119 **Retinopathy of prematurity, stage 0, unspecified eye**
⑥ **H35.12** **Retinopathy of prematurity, stage 1**
⊟ H35.121 **Retinopathy of prematurity, stage 1, right eye**
⊟ H35.122 **Retinopathy of prematurity, stage 1, left eye**
⊟ H35.123 **Retinopathy of prematurity, stage 1, bilateral**
⊟ H35.129 **Retinopathy of prematurity, stage 1, unspecified eye**
⑥ **H35.13** **Retinopathy of prematurity, stage 2**
⊟ H35.131 **Retinopathy of prematurity, stage 2, right eye**
⊟ H35.132 **Retinopathy of prematurity, stage 2, left eye**
⊟ H35.133 **Retinopathy of prematurity, stage 2, bilateral**
⊟ H35.139 **Retinopathy of prematurity, stage 2, unspecified eye**
⑥ **H35.14** **Retinopathy of prematurity, stage 3**
⊟ H35.141 **Retinopathy of prematurity, stage 3, right eye**
⊟ H35.142 **Retinopathy of prematurity, stage 3, left eye**
⊟ H35.143 **Retinopathy of prematurity, stage 3, bilateral**
⊟ H35.149 **Retinopathy of prematurity, stage 3, unspecified eye**
⑥ **H35.15** **Retinopathy of prematurity, stage 4**
⊟ H35.151 **Retinopathy of prematurity, stage 4, right eye**
⊟ H35.152 **Retinopathy of prematurity, stage 4, left eye**
⊟ H35.153 **Retinopathy of prematurity, stage 4, bilateral**
⊟ H35.159 **Retinopathy of prematurity, stage 4, unspecified eye**
⑥ **H35.16** **Retinopathy of prematurity, stage 5**
⊟ H35.161 **Retinopathy of prematurity, stage 5, right eye**
⊟ H35.162 **Retinopathy of prematurity, stage 5, left eye**
⊟ H35.163 **Retinopathy of prematurity, stage 5, bilateral**
⊟ H35.169 **Retinopathy of prematurity, stage 5, unspecified eye**
⑥ **H35.17** **Retrolental fibroplasia**
⊟ H35.171 **Retrolental fibroplasia, right eye**
⊟ H35.172 **Retrolental fibroplasia, left eye**
⊟ H35.173 **Retrolental fibroplasia, bilateral**
⊟ H35.179 **Retrolental fibroplasia, unspecified eye**
⑤ **H35.2** **Other non-diabetic proliferative retinopathy**
Proliferative vitreo-retinopathy
EXCLUDES 1 *proliferative vitreo-retinopathy with retinal detachment (H33.4-)*
⊟ **H35.20** **Other non-diabetic proliferative retinopathy, unspecified eye**

● New   ▲ Revised   *Manifestation*   4-7 Digit Indicators   ⊟ Laterality   Ⓐ Adult (15+ years)   Ⓜ Maternity (12-55 years)   Ⓝ Newborn   Ⓟ Pediatric (0-17 years)   ♂ Male   ♀ Female
✖ Deleted   Unspecified   + Additional code

Diseases of the Eye and Adnexa

H35.21 — H35.60

⊟ **H35.21**   **Other non-diabetic proliferative retinopathy, right eye**

⊟ **H35.22**   **Other non-diabetic proliferative retinopathy, left eye**

⊟ **H35.23**   **Other non-diabetic proliferative retinopathy, bilateral**

⑤ **H35.3**   **Degeneration of macula and posterior pole**

H35.30   **Unspecified macular degeneration**   Ⓐ
Age-related macular degeneration

▲ⓖ **H35.31**   **Nonexudative age-related macular degeneration**
Atrophic age-related macular degeneration
Dry age-related macular degeneration

One of the following 7th characters is to be assigned to codes in subcategory H35.31 to designate the stage of the disease:
0   stage unspecified
1   early dry stage
2   intermediate dry stage
3   advanced atrophic without subfoveal involvement
4   advanced atrophic with subfoveal involvement

●⑦⊟ **H35.311-**   **Nonexudative age-related macular degeneration, right eye**   Ⓐ

●⑦⊟ **H35.312-**   **Nonexudative age-related macular degeneration, left eye**   Ⓐ

●⑦⊟ **H35.313-**   **Nonexudative age-related macular degeneration, bilateral**   Ⓐ

●⑦⊟ **H35.319-**   **Nonexudative age-related macular degeneration, unspecified eye**   Ⓐ

▲ⓖ **H35.32**   **Exudative age-related macular degeneration**
Wet age-related macular degeneration

One of the following 7th characters is to be assigned to codes in subcategory H35.32 to designate the stage of the disease:
0   stage unspecified
1   with active choroidal neovascularization
2   with inactive choroidal neovascularization
3   with inactive scar

●⑦⊟ **H35.321-**   **Exudative age-related macular degeneration, right eye**   Ⓐ

●⑦⊟ **H35.322-**   **Exudative age-related macular degeneration, left eye**   Ⓐ

●⑦⊟ **H35.323-**   **Exudative age-related macular degeneration, bilateral**   Ⓐ

●⑦⊟ **H35.329-**   **Exudative age-related macular degeneration, unspecified eye**   Ⓐ

H35.33   **Angioid streaks of macula**

ⓖ **H35.34**   **Macular cyst, hole, or pseudohole**

⊟ **H35.341**   **Macular cyst, hole, or pseudohole, right eye**

⊟ **H35.342**   **Macular cyst, hole, or pseudohole, left eye**

⊟ **H35.343**   **Macular cyst, hole, or pseudohole, bilateral**

⊟ **H35.349**   **Macular cyst, hole, or pseudohole, unspecified eye**

ⓖ **H35.35**   **Cystoid macular degeneration**

EXCLUDES 1   *cystoid macular edema following cataract surgery (H59.03-)*

⊟ **H35.351**   **Cystoid macular degeneration, right eye**

⊟ **H35.352**   **Cystoid macular degeneration, left eye**

⊟ **H35.353**   **Cystoid macular degeneration, bilateral**

⊟ **H35.359**   **Cystoid macular degeneration, unspecified eye**

ⓖ **H35.36**   **Drusen (degenerative) of macula**

DEFINITION   Small, bright deposits or accumulations of material seen in the retina and/or optic disc that are associated with a variety of eye diseases including macular degeneration, hereditary retinal degeneration, and loss of peripheral vision.

⊟ **H35.361**   **Drusen (degenerative) of macula, right eye**

⊟ **H35.362**   **Drusen (degenerative) of macula, left eye**

⊟ **H35.363**   **Drusen (degenerative) of macula, bilateral**

⊟ **H35.369**   **Drusen (degenerative) of macula, unspecified eye**

ⓖ **H35.37**   **Puckering of macula**

⊟ **H35.371**   **Puckering of macula, right eye**

⊟ **H35.372**   **Puckering of macula, left eye**

⊟ **H35.373**   **Puckering of macula, bilateral**

⊟ **H35.379**   **Puckering of macula, unspecified eye**

ⓖ✚ **H35.38**   **Toxic maculopathy**
Code first:
poisoning due to drug or toxin, if applicable (T36-T65 with fifth or sixth character 1-4 or 6)
Use additional code for adverse effect, if applicable, to identify drug (T36-T50 with fifth or sixth character 5)

⊟✚ **H35.381**   **Toxic maculopathy, right eye**

⊟✚ **H35.382**   **Toxic maculopathy, left eye**

⊟✚ **H35.383**   **Toxic maculopathy, bilateral**

⊟✚ **H35.389**   **Toxic maculopathy, unspecified eye**

⑤ **H35.4**   **Peripheral retinal degeneration**

EXCLUDES 1   *hereditary retinal degeneration (dystrophy) (H35.5-)*
peripheral retinal degeneration with retinal break (H33.3-)

H35.40   **Unspecified peripheral retinal degeneration**

ⓖ **H35.41**   **Lattice degeneration of retina**
Palisade degeneration of retina

⊟ **H35.411**   **Lattice degeneration of retina, right eye**

⊟ **H35.412**   **Lattice degeneration of retina, left eye**

⊟ **H35.413**   **Lattice degeneration of retina, bilateral**

⊟ **H35.419**   **Lattice degeneration of retina, unspecified eye**

ⓖ **H35.42**   **Microcystoid degeneration of retina**

⊟ **H35.421**   **Microcystoid degeneration of retina, right eye**

⊟ **H35.422**   **Microcystoid degeneration of retina, left eye**

⊟ **H35.423**   **Microcystoid degeneration of retina, bilateral**

⊟ **H35.429**   **Microcystoid degeneration of retina, unspecified eye**

ⓖ **H35.43**   **Paving stone degeneration of retina**

⊟ **H35.431**   **Paving stone degeneration of retina, right eye**

⊟ **H35.432**   **Paving stone degeneration of retina, left eye**

⊟ **H35.433**   **Paving stone degeneration of retina, bilateral**

⊟ **H35.439**   **Paving stone degeneration of retina, unspecified eye**

ⓖ **H35.44**   **Age-related reticular degeneration of retina**

⊟ **H35.441**   **Age-related reticular degeneration of retina, right eye**   Ⓐ

⊟ **H35.442**   **Age-related reticular degeneration of retina, left eye**   Ⓐ

⊟ **H35.443**   **Age-related reticular degeneration of retina, bilateral**   Ⓐ

⊟ **H35.449**   **Age-related reticular degeneration of retina, unspecified eye**   Ⓐ

ⓖ **H35.45**   **Secondary pigmentary degeneration**

⊟ **H35.451**   **Secondary pigmentary degeneration, right eye**

⊟ **H35.452**   **Secondary pigmentary degeneration, left eye**

⊟ **H35.453**   **Secondary pigmentary degeneration, bilateral**

⊟ **H35.459**   **Secondary pigmentary degeneration, unspecified eye**

ⓖ **H35.46**   **Secondary vitreoretinal degeneration**

⊟ **H35.461**   **Secondary vitreoretinal degeneration, right eye**

⊟ **H35.462**   **Secondary vitreoretinal degeneration, left eye**

⊟ **H35.463**   **Secondary vitreoretinal degeneration, bilateral**

⊟ **H35.469**   **Secondary vitreoretinal degeneration, unspecified eye**

⑤ **H35.5**   **Hereditary retinal dystrophy**

EXCLUDES 1   *dystrophies primarily involving Bruch's membrane (H31.1-)*

H35.50   **Unspecified hereditary retinal dystrophy**

H35.51   **Vitreoretinal dystrophy**

H35.52   **Pigmentary retinal dystrophy**
Albipunctate retinal dystrophy
Retinitis pigmentosa
Tapetoretinal dystrophy

H35.53   **Other dystrophies primarily involving the sensory retina**
Stargardt's disease

DEFINITION   Stargardt's disease: genetic condition causing degeneration of the macula, occurring by age 20, with rapid loss of visual acuity and abnormal pigmentation of the macula.

H35.54   **Dystrophies primarily involving the retinal pigment epithelium**
Vitelliform retinal dystrophy

⑤ **H35.6**   **Retinal hemorrhage**

⊟ **H35.60**   **Retinal hemorrhage, unspecified eye**

● New   ▲ Revised   *Manifestation*   ④-⑦ Digit Indicators   ⊟ Laterality   Ⓐ Adult (15+ years)   Ⓜ Maternity (12-55 years)   Ⓝ Newborn   Ⓟ Pediatric (0-17 years)   ♂ Male   ♀ Female

✖ ~~Deleted~~   Unspecified   ✚ Additional code

608   © 2017 DecisionHealth

2017 ICD-10-CM Expert for Physicians

☐ **H35.61** Retinal hemorrhage, right eye
☐ **H35.62** Retinal hemorrhage, left eye
☐ **H35.63** Retinal hemorrhage, bilateral
⑤ **H35.7** Separation of retinal layers

> **EXCLUDES 1** *retinal detachment (serous) (H33.2-)*
> *rhegmatogenous retinal detachment (H33.0-)*

H35.70 Unspecified separation of retinal layers
⑥ **H35.71** Central serous chorioretinopathy

> **DEFINITION** Fluid seepage from the choroid into the retina, causing the retinal layers to fill and separate from each other.

☐ **H35.711** Central serous chorioretinopathy, right eye
☐ **H35.712** Central serous chorioretinopathy, left eye
☐ **H35.713** Central serous chorioretinopathy, bilateral
☐ **H35.719** Central serous chorioretinopathy, unspecified eye
⑥ **H35.72** Serous detachment of retinal pigment epithelium
☐ **H35.721** Serous detachment of retinal pigment epithelium, right eye
☐ **H35.722** Serous detachment of retinal pigment epithelium, left eye
☐ **H35.723** Serous detachment of retinal pigment epithelium, bilateral
☐ **H35.729** Serous detachment of retinal pigment epithelium, unspecified eye
⑥ **H35.73** Hemorrhagic detachment of retinal pigment epithelium
☐ **H35.731** Hemorrhagic detachment of retinal pigment epithelium, right eye
☐ **H35.732** Hemorrhagic detachment of retinal pigment epithelium, left eye
☐ **H35.733** Hemorrhagic detachment of retinal pigment epithelium, bilateral
☐ **H35.739** Hemorrhagic detachment of retinal pigment epithelium, unspecified eye
⑤ **H35.8** Other specified retinal disorders

> **EXCLUDES 2** *retinal hemorrhage (H35.6-)*

H35.81 Retinal edema
Retinal cotton wool spots
H35.82 Retinal ischemia
H35.89 Other specified retinal disorders
H35.9 Unspecified retinal disorder
H36 *Retinal disorders in diseases classified elsewhere*
Code first underlying disease, such as:
lipid storage disorders (E75.-)
sickle-cell disorders (D57.-)

> **EXCLUDES 1** *arteriosclerotic retinopathy (H35.0-)*
> *diabetic retinopathy*
> *(E08.3-, E09.3-, E10.3-, E11.3-, E13.3-)*

Glaucoma (H40-H42)

④ **H40** Glaucoma

> **EXCLUDES 1** *absolute glaucoma (H44.51-)*
> *congenital glaucoma (Q15.0)*
> *traumatic glaucoma due to birth injury (P15.3)*

> **GUIDELINES** Section I.C.7.a.1)
> Assign as many codes from category H40, Glaucoma, as needed to identify the type of glaucoma, the affected eye, and the glaucoma stage.

> **GUIDELINES** Section I.C.7.a.2)-3)
> When a patient has bilateral glaucoma and both eyes are documented as being the same type and stage, and there is a code for bilateral glaucoma, report only the code for the type of glaucoma, bilateral, with the seventh character for the stage.
> When a patient has bilateral glaucoma and each eye is documented as having a different type or stage, and the classification distinguishes laterality, assign the appropriate code for each eye rather than the code for bilateral glaucoma.

⑤ **H40.0** Glaucoma suspect

> **DEFINITION** Increase in intraocular pressure causing pathologic changes in the optic disk and defects in the field of vision.

⑥ **H40.00** Preglaucoma, unspecified

☐ **H40.001** Preglaucoma, unspecified, right eye
☐ **H40.002** Preglaucoma, unspecified, left eye
☐ **H40.003** Preglaucoma, unspecified, bilateral
☐ **H40.009** Preglaucoma, unspecified, unspecified eye
⑥ **H40.01** Open angle with borderline findings, low risk
Open angle, low risk
☐ **H40.011** Open angle with borderline findings, low risk, right eye
☐ **H40.012** Open angle with borderline findings, low risk, left eye
☐ **H40.013** Open angle with borderline findings, low risk, bilateral
☐ **H40.019** Open angle with borderline findings, low risk, unspecified eye
⑥ **H40.02** Open angle with borderline findings, high risk
Open angle, high risk
☐ **H40.021** Open angle with borderline findings, high risk, right eye
☐ **H40.022** Open angle with borderline findings, high risk, left eye
☐ **H40.023** Open angle with borderline findings, high risk, bilateral
☐ **H40.029** Open angle with borderline findings, high risk, unspecified eye
⑥ **H40.03** Anatomical narrow angle
Primary angle closure suspect
☐ **H40.031** Anatomical narrow angle, right eye
☐ **H40.032** Anatomical narrow angle, left eye
☐ **H40.033** Anatomical narrow angle, bilateral
☐ **H40.039** Anatomical narrow angle, unspecified eye
⑥ **H40.04** Steroid responder
☐ **H40.041** Steroid responder, right eye
☐ **H40.042** Steroid responder, left eye
☐ **H40.043** Steroid responder, bilateral
☐ **H40.049** Steroid responder, unspecified eye
⑥ **H40.05** Ocular hypertension
☐ **H40.051** Ocular hypertension, right eye
☐ **H40.052** Ocular hypertension, left eye
☐ **H40.053** Ocular hypertension, bilateral
☐ **H40.059** Ocular hypertension, unspecified eye
⑥ **H40.06** Primary angle closure without glaucoma damage
☐ **H40.061** Primary angle closure without glaucoma damage, right eye
☐ **H40.062** Primary angle closure without glaucoma damage, left eye
☐ **H40.063** Primary angle closure without glaucoma damage, bilateral
☐ **H40.069** Primary angle closure without glaucoma damage, unspecified eye
⑤ **H40.1** Open-angle glaucoma

Open-angle glaucoma
An increase in fluid pressure in the eye resulting from the outflow of ocular fluid being blocked

Canal of Schlemm (obstructed)
Trabecular meshwork
Iris
Anterior chamber
Chamber angle (open)
Ciliary body
Lens

● New ▲ Revised *Manifestation* ④-⑦ Digit Indicators ☐ Laterality Ⓐ Adult (15+ years) Ⓜ Maternity (12-55 years) Ⓝ Newborn Ⓟ Pediatric (0-17 years) ♂ Male ♀ Female
✖ Deleted Unspecified + Additional code

2017 ICD-10-CM Expert for Physicians

© 2017 DecisionHealth 609

☑ H40.10X-   Unspecified open-angle glaucoma

One of the following 7th characters is to be assigned to code H40.10 to designate the stage of glaucoma
0   stage unspecified
1   mild stage
2   moderate stage
3   severe stage
4   indeterminate stage

GUIDELINES   Section I.C.7.a
When a patient has bilateral glaucoma and both eyes are documented as being the same type and stage, and the classification does not provide a code for bilateral glaucoma (i.e., subcategories H40.10, H40.11 and H40.20), report only one code for the type of glaucoma with the appropriate seventh character for the stage.

When a patient has bilateral glaucoma and each eye is documented as having a different type, and the classification does not distinguish laterality (i.e., subcategories H40.10, H40.11 and H40.20), assign one code for each type of glaucoma with the appropriate seventh character for the stage.

When a patient has bilateral glaucoma and each eye is documented as having the same type, but different stage, and the classification does not distinguish laterality (i.e., subcategories H40.10, H40.11 and H40.20), assign a code for the type of glaucoma for each eye with the seventh character for the specific glaucoma stage documented for each eye.

▲ ⑥ H40.11   Primary open-angle glaucoma
Chronic simple glaucoma

One of the following 7th characters is to be assigned to each code in subcategory H40.11 to designate the stage of glaucoma
0   stage unspecified
1   mild stage
2   moderate stage
3   severe stage
4   indeterminate stage

GUIDELINES   Section I.C.7.a
When a patient has bilateral glaucoma and both eyes are documented as being the same type and stage, and the classification does not provide a code for bilateral glaucoma (i.e., subcategories H40.10, H40.11 and H40.20), report only one code for the type of glaucoma with the appropriate seventh character for the stage.

When a patient has bilateral glaucoma and each eye is documented as having a different type, and the classification does not distinguish laterality (i.e., subcategories H40.10, H40.11 and H40.20), assign one code for each type of glaucoma with the appropriate seventh character for the stage.

When a patient has bilateral glaucoma and each eye is documented as having the same type, but different stage, and the classification does not distinguish laterality (i.e., subcategories H40.10, H40.11 and H40.20), assign a code for the type of glaucoma for each eye with the seventh character for the specific glaucoma stage documented for each eye.

● ☑ ⊟ H40.111-   Primary open-angle glaucoma, right eye
● ☑ ⊟ H40.112-   Primary open-angle glaucoma, left eye
● ☑ ⊟ H40.113-   Primary open-angle glaucoma, bilateral
● ☑ ⊟ H40.119-   Primary open-angle glaucoma, unspecified eye

⑥ H40.12   Low-tension glaucoma

One of the following 7th characters is to be assigned to each code in subcategory H40.12 to designate the stage of glaucoma
0   stage unspecified
1   mild stage
2   moderate stage
3   severe stage
4   indeterminate stage

☑ ⊟ H40.121-   Low-tension glaucoma, right eye
☑ ⊟ H40.122-   Low-tension glaucoma, left eye
☑ ⊟ H40.123-   Low-tension glaucoma, bilateral
☑ ⊟ H40.129-   Low-tension glaucoma, unspecified eye

⑥ H40.13   Pigmentary glaucoma

One of the following 7th characters is to be assigned to each code in subcategory H40.13 to designate the stage of glaucoma
0   stage unspecified
1   mild stage
2   moderate stage
3   severe stage
4   indeterminate stage

DEFINITION   Granules of pigment coloring the eye break off and block drainage canals, increasing intraocular pressure.

☑ ⊟ H40.131-   Pigmentary glaucoma, right eye
☑ ⊟ H40.132-   Pigmentary glaucoma, left eye
☑ ⊟ H40.133-   Pigmentary glaucoma, bilateral
☑ ⊟ H40.139-   Pigmentary glaucoma, unspecified eye

⑥ H40.14   Capsular glaucoma with pseudoexfoliation of lens

One of the following 7th characters is to be assigned to each code in subcategory H40.14 to designate the stage of glaucoma
0   stage unspecified
1   mild stage
2   moderate stage
3   severe stage
4   indeterminate stage

☑ ⊟ H40.141-   Capsular glaucoma with pseudoexfoliation of lens, right eye
☑ ⊟ H40.142-   Capsular glaucoma with pseudoexfoliation of lens, left eye
☑ ⊟ H40.143-   Capsular glaucoma with pseudoexfoliation of lens, bilateral
☑ ⊟ H40.149-   Capsular glaucoma with pseudoexfoliation of lens, unspecified eye

⑥ H40.15   Residual stage of open-angle glaucoma
⊟ H40.151   Residual stage of open-angle glaucoma, right eye
⊟ H40.152   Residual stage of open-angle glaucoma, left eye
⊟ H40.153   Residual stage of open-angle glaucoma, bilateral
⊟ H40.159   Residual stage of open-angle glaucoma, unspecified eye

⑤ H40.2   Primary angle-closure glaucoma
EXCLUDES 1   aqueous misdirection (H40.83-)
malignant glaucoma (H40.83-)

☑ H40.20X-   Unspecified primary angle-closure glaucoma

One of the following 7th characters is to be assigned to code H40.20 to designate the stage of glaucoma
0   stage unspecified
1   mild stage
2   moderate stage
3   severe stage
4   indeterminate stage

● New   ▲ Revised   *Manifestation*   ④-☑ Digit Indicators   ⊟ Laterality   Ⓐ Adult (15+ years)   Ⓜ Maternity (12-55 years)   Ⓝ Newborn   Ⓟ Pediatric (0-17 years)   ♂ Male   ♀ Female
✖ Deleted   Unspecified   + Additional code

610   © 2017 DecisionHealth   2017 ICD-10-CM Expert for Physicians

GUIDELINES Section I.C.7.a

When a patient has bilateral glaucoma and both eyes are documented as being the same type and stage, and the classification does not provide a code for bilateral glaucoma (i.e., subcategories H40.10, H40.11 and H40.20), report only one code for the type of glaucoma with the appropriate seventh character for the stage.

When a patient has bilateral glaucoma and each eye is documented as having a different type, and the classification does not distinguish laterality (i.e., subcategories H40.10, H40.11 and H40.20), assign one code for each type of glaucoma with the appropriate seventh character for the stage.

When a patient has bilateral glaucoma and each eye is documented as having the same type, but different stage, and the classification does not distinguish laterality (i.e., subcategories H40.10, H40.11 and H40.20), assign a code for the type of glaucoma for each eye with the seventh character for the specific glaucoma stage documented for each eye.

H40.21 **Acute angle-closure glaucoma**

Acute angle-closure glaucoma attack
Acute angle-closure glaucoma crisis

DEFINITION Severe, sudden increase in intraocular pressure due to a blockage of the chamber angle at the junction of the iris and cornea, preventing normal aqueous fluid drainage and causing rapid loss of vision.

	H40.211	Acute angle-closure glaucoma, right eye
	H40.212	Acute angle-closure glaucoma, left eye
	H40.213	Acute angle-closure glaucoma, bilateral
	H40.219	Acute angle-closure glaucoma, unspecified eye

H40.22 **Chronic angle-closure glaucoma**

Chronic primary angle closure glaucoma

One of the following 7th characters is to be assigned to each code in subcategory H40.22 to designate the stage of glaucoma
0   stage unspecified
1   mild stage
2   moderate stage
3   severe stage
4   indeterminate stage

7	H40.221-	Chronic angle-closure glaucoma, right eye
7	H40.222-	Chronic angle-closure glaucoma, left eye
7	H40.223-	Chronic angle-closure glaucoma, bilateral
7	H40.229-	Chronic angle-closure glaucoma, unspecified eye

H40.23 **Intermittent angle-closure glaucoma**

	H40.231	Intermittent angle-closure glaucoma, right eye
	H40.232	Intermittent angle-closure glaucoma, left eye
	H40.233	Intermittent angle-closure glaucoma, bilateral
	H40.239	Intermittent angle-closure glaucoma, unspecified eye

H40.24 **Residual stage of angle-closure glaucoma**

	H40.241	Residual stage of angle-closure glaucoma, right eye
	H40.242	Residual stage of angle-closure glaucoma, left eye
	H40.243	Residual stage of angle-closure glaucoma, bilateral
	H40.249	Residual stage of angle-closure glaucoma, unspecified eye

H40.3 **Glaucoma secondary to eye trauma**

Code also:
    underlying condition

One of the following 7th characters is to be assigned to each code in subcategory H40.3 to designate the stage of glaucoma
0   stage unspecified
1   mild stage
2   moderate stage
3   severe stage
4   indeterminate stage

7	H40.30X-	**Glaucoma secondary to eye trauma, unspecified eye**
7	H40.31X-	**Glaucoma secondary to eye trauma, right eye**
7	H40.32X-	**Glaucoma secondary to eye trauma, left eye**
7	H40.33X-	**Glaucoma secondary to eye trauma, bilateral**

H40.4 **Glaucoma secondary to eye inflammation**

Code also:
    underlying condition

One of the following 7th characters is to be assigned to each code in subcategory H40.4 to designate the stage of glaucoma
0   stage unspecified
1   mild stage
2   moderate stage
3   severe stage
4   indeterminate stage

7	H40.40X-	**Glaucoma secondary to eye inflammation, unspecified eye**
7	H40.41X-	**Glaucoma secondary to eye inflammation, right eye**
7	H40.42X-	**Glaucoma secondary to eye inflammation, left eye**
7	H40.43X-	**Glaucoma secondary to eye inflammation, bilateral**

H40.5 **Glaucoma secondary to other eye disorders**

Code also:
    underlying eye disorder

One of the following 7th characters is to be assigned to each code in subcategory H40.5 to designate the stage of glaucoma
0   stage unspecified
1   mild stage
2   moderate stage
3   severe stage
4   indeterminate stage

7	H40.50X-	**Glaucoma secondary to other eye disorders, unspecified eye**
7	H40.51X-	**Glaucoma secondary to other eye disorders, right eye**
7	H40.52X-	**Glaucoma secondary to other eye disorders, left eye**
7	H40.53X-	**Glaucoma secondary to other eye disorders, bilateral**

+ H40.6 **Glaucoma secondary to drugs**

Use additional code for adverse effect, if applicable, to identify drug (T36-T50 with fifth or sixth character 5)

One of the following 7th characters is to be assigned to each code in subcategory H40.6 to designate the stage of glaucoma
0   stage unspecified
1   mild stage
2   moderate stage
3   severe stage
4   indeterminate stage

7 +	H40.60X-	**Glaucoma secondary to drugs, unspecified eye**
7 +	H40.61X-	**Glaucoma secondary to drugs, right eye**
7 +	H40.62X-	**Glaucoma secondary to drugs, left eye**
7 +	H40.63X-	**Glaucoma secondary to drugs, bilateral**

H40.8 **Other glaucoma**

H40.81 **Glaucoma with increased episcleral venous pressure**

DEFINITION Blood pressure of the veins in the white of the eye increases as the pressure of intraocular fluid increases.

	H40.811	Glaucoma with increased episcleral venous pressure, right eye
	H40.812	Glaucoma with increased episcleral venous pressure, left eye

---

● New   ▲ Revised   *Manifestation*   **◼-◾ Digit Indicators**   ⊟ Laterality   ◭ Adult (15+ years)   ◹ Maternity (12-55 years)   ◺ Newborn (0-17 years)   ◪ Pediatric (0-17 years)   ♂ Male   ♀ Female
✖ Deleted   Unspecified   + Additional code

Diseases of the Eye and Adnexa

H40.813 — H44.119

⊟ **H40.813** **Glaucoma with increased episcleral venous pressure, bilateral**

⊟ **H40.819** **Glaucoma with increased episcleral venous pressure, unspecified eye**

⑥ **H40.82** **Hypersecretion glaucoma**

> **DEFINITION** Overproduction of ocular fluid rather than insufficient drainage that causes increased intraocular pressure.

⊟ **H40.821** **Hypersecretion glaucoma, right eye**

⊟ **H40.822** **Hypersecretion glaucoma, left eye**

⊟ **H40.823** **Hypersecretion glaucoma, bilateral**

⊟ **H40.829** **Hypersecretion glaucoma, unspecified eye**

⑥ **H40.83** **Aqueous misdirection**

Malignant glaucoma

⊟ **H40.831** **Aqueous misdirection, right eye**

⊟ **H40.832** **Aqueous misdirection, left eye**

⊟ **H40.833** **Aqueous misdirection, bilateral**

⊟ **H40.839** **Aqueous misdirection, unspecified eye**

H40.89 **Other specified glaucoma**

H40.9 **Unspecified glaucoma**

▲ **H42** *Glaucoma in diseases classified elsewhere*

Code first underlying condition, such as:
amyloidosis (E85.-)
aniridia (Q13.1)
Lowe's syndrome (E72.03)
Reiger's anomaly (Q13.81)
specified metabolic disorder (E70-E88)

> **EXCLUDES 1** *glaucoma (in) onchocerciasis (B73.02)*
> *glaucoma (in) syphilis (A52.71)*
> *glaucoma (in) tuberculous (A18.59)*

> **EXCLUDES 2** *glaucoma (in) diabetes mellitus (E08.39, E09.39, E10.39, E11.39, E13.39)*

> **CODING TIP ✓** Do not use this code as a manifestation of diabetes.

Disorders of vitreous body and globe (H43-H44)

④ **H43** **Disorders of vitreous body**

⑤ **H43.0** **Vitreous prolapse**

> **EXCLUDES 1** *vitreous syndrome following cataract surgery (H59.0-)*
> *traumatic vitreous prolapse (S05.2-)*

⊟ **H43.00** **Vitreous prolapse, unspecified eye**

⊟ **H43.01** **Vitreous prolapse, right eye**

⊟ **H43.02** **Vitreous prolapse, left eye**

⊟ **H43.03** **Vitreous prolapse, bilateral**

⑤ **H43.1** **Vitreous hemorrhage**

⊟ **H43.10** **Vitreous hemorrhage, unspecified eye**

⊟ **H43.11** **Vitreous hemorrhage, right eye**

⊟ **H43.12** **Vitreous hemorrhage, left eye**

⊟ **H43.13** **Vitreous hemorrhage, bilateral**

⑤ **H43.2** **Crystalline deposits in vitreous body**

⊟ **H43.20** **Crystalline deposits in vitreous body, unspecified eye**

⊟ **H43.21** **Crystalline deposits in vitreous body, right eye**

⊟ **H43.22** **Crystalline deposits in vitreous body, left eye**

⊟ **H43.23** **Crystalline deposits in vitreous body, bilateral**

⑤ **H43.3** **Other vitreous opacities**

⑥ **H43.31** **Vitreous membranes and strands**

⊟ **H43.311** **Vitreous membranes and strands, right eye**

⊟ **H43.312** **Vitreous membranes and strands, left eye**

⊟ **H43.313** **Vitreous membranes and strands, bilateral**

⊟ **H43.319** **Vitreous membranes and strands, unspecified eye**

⑥ **H43.39** **Other vitreous opacities**

Vitreous floaters

⊟ **H43.391** **Other vitreous opacities, right eye**

⊟ **H43.392** **Other vitreous opacities, left eye**

⊟ **H43.393** **Other vitreous opacities, bilateral**

⊟ **H43.399** **Other vitreous opacities, unspecified eye**

⑤ **H43.8** **Other disorders of vitreous body**

> **EXCLUDES 1** *proliferative vitreo-retinopathy with retinal detachment (H33.4-)*

> **EXCLUDES 2** *vitreous abscess (H44.02-)*

⑥ **H43.81** **Vitreous degeneration**

Vitreous detachment

⊟ **H43.811** **Vitreous degeneration, right eye**

⊟ **H43.812** **Vitreous degeneration, left eye**

⊟ **H43.813** **Vitreous degeneration, bilateral**

⊟ **H43.819** **Vitreous degeneration, unspecified eye**

⑥ **H43.82** **Vitreomacular adhesion**

Vitreomacular traction

⊟ **H43.821** **Vitreomacular adhesion, right eye** Ⓐ

⊟ **H43.822** **Vitreomacular adhesion, left eye** Ⓐ

⊟ **H43.823** **Vitreomacular adhesion, bilateral** Ⓐ

⊟ **H43.829** **Vitreomacular adhesion, unspecified eye** Ⓐ

H43.89 **Other disorders of vitreous body**

H43.9 **Unspecified disorder of vitreous body**

④ **H44** **Disorders of globe**

> **INCLUDES** disorders affecting multiple structures of eye

⑤ **+ H44.0** **Purulent endophthalmitis**

Use additional code to identify organism

> **EXCLUDES 1** *bleb associated endophthalmitis (H59.4-)*

⑥ **+ H44.00** **Unspecified purulent endophthalmitis**

Purulent endophthalmitis

An inflammation of the tissues of the eye resulting in pus formation

Swelling — Cornea — Accumulation of liquid

⊟ **+ H44.001** **Unspecified purulent endophthalmitis, right eye**

⊟ **+ H44.002** **Unspecified purulent endophthalmitis, left eye**

⊟ **+ H44.003** **Unspecified purulent endophthalmitis, bilateral**

⊟ **+ H44.009** **Unspecified purulent endophthalmitis, unspecified eye**

⑥ **+ H44.01** **Panophthalmitis (acute)**

> **DEFINITION** Inflammation affecting all the structures or tissues of the eye.

⊟ **+ H44.011** **Panophthalmitis (acute), right eye**

⊟ **+ H44.012** **Panophthalmitis (acute), left eye**

⊟ **+ H44.013** **Panophthalmitis (acute), bilateral**

⊟ **+ H44.019** **Panophthalmitis (acute), unspecified eye**

⑥ **+ H44.02** **Vitreous abscess (chronic)**

⊟ **+ H44.021** **Vitreous abscess (chronic), right eye**

⊟ **+ H44.022** **Vitreous abscess (chronic), left eye**

⊟ **+ H44.023** **Vitreous abscess (chronic), bilateral**

⊟ **+ H44.029** **Vitreous abscess (chronic), unspecified eye**

⑤ **H44.1** **Other endophthalmitis**

> **EXCLUDES 1** *bleb associated endophthalmitis (H59.4-)*

> **EXCLUDES 2** *ophthalmia nodosa (H16.2-)*

⑥ **H44.11** **Panuveitis**

> **DEFINITION** Inflammation of the entire pigmented layer of the eye (uveal tract).

⊟ **H44.111** **Panuveitis, right eye**

⊟ **H44.112** **Panuveitis, left eye**

⊟ **H44.113** **Panuveitis, bilateral**

⊟ **H44.119** **Panuveitis, unspecified eye**

● New   ▲ Revised   *Manifestation*   ④ - ⑦ Digit Indicators   ⊟ Laterality   Ⓐ Adult (15+ years)   Ⓜ Maternity (12-55 years)   Ⓝ Newborn   Ⓟ Pediatric (0-17 years)   ♂ Male   ♀ Female
✖ Deleted   Unspecified   + Additional code

⑥ **H44.12** Parasitic endophthalmitis, unspecified
◻ **H44.121** Parasitic endophthalmitis, unspecified, right eye
◻ **H44.122** Parasitic endophthalmitis, unspecified, left eye
◻ **H44.123** Parasitic endophthalmitis, unspecified, bilateral
◻ **H44.129** Parasitic endophthalmitis, unspecified, unspecified eye

⑥ **H44.13** Sympathetic uveitis
◻ **H44.131** Sympathetic uveitis, right eye
◻ **H44.132** Sympathetic uveitis, left eye
◻ **H44.133** Sympathetic uveitis, bilateral
◻ **H44.139** Sympathetic uveitis, unspecified eye

H44.19 Other endophthalmitis

⑤ **H44.2** Degenerative myopia
Malignant myopia
◻ **H44.20** Degenerative myopia, unspecified eye
◻ **H44.21** Degenerative myopia, right eye
◻ **H44.22** Degenerative myopia, left eye
◻ **H44.23** Degenerative myopia, bilateral

⑤ **H44.3** Other and unspecified degenerative disorders of globe
H44.30 Unspecified degenerative disorder of globe
⑥ **H44.31** Chalcosis
◻ **H44.311** Chalcosis, right eye
◻ **H44.312** Chalcosis, left eye
◻ **H44.313** Chalcosis, bilateral
◻ **H44.319** Chalcosis, unspecified eye

⑥ **H44.32** Siderosis of eye
◻ **H44.321** Siderosis of eye, right eye
◻ **H44.322** Siderosis of eye, left eye
◻ **H44.323** Siderosis of eye, bilateral
◻ **H44.329** Siderosis of eye, unspecified eye

⑥ **H44.39** Other degenerative disorders of globe
◻ **H44.391** Other degenerative disorders of globe, right eye
◻ **H44.392** Other degenerative disorders of globe, left eye
◻ **H44.393** Other degenerative disorders of globe, bilateral
◻ **H44.399** Other degenerative disorders of globe, unspecified eye

⑤ **H44.4** Hypotony of eye
H44.40 Unspecified hypotony of eye
⑥ **H44.41** Flat anterior chamber hypotony of eye
◻ **H44.411** Flat anterior chamber hypotony of right eye
◻ **H44.412** Flat anterior chamber hypotony of left eye
◻ **H44.413** Flat anterior chamber hypotony of eye, bilateral
◻ **H44.419** Flat anterior chamber hypotony of unspecified eye

⑥ **H44.42** Hypotony of eye due to ocular fistula
◻ **H44.421** Hypotony of right eye due to ocular fistula
◻ **H44.422** Hypotony of left eye due to ocular fistula
◻ **H44.423** Hypotony of eye due to ocular fistula, bilateral
◻ **H44.429** Hypotony of unspecified eye due to ocular fistula

⑥ **H44.43** Hypotony of eye due to other ocular disorders
◻ **H44.431** Hypotony of eye due to other ocular disorders, right eye
◻ **H44.432** Hypotony of eye due to other ocular disorders, left eye
◻ **H44.433** Hypotony of eye due to other ocular disorders, bilateral
◻ **H44.439** Hypotony of eye due to other ocular disorders, unspecified eye

⑥ **H44.44** Primary hypotony of eye
◻ **H44.441** Primary hypotony of right eye
◻ **H44.442** Primary hypotony of left eye
◻ **H44.443** Primary hypotony of eye, bilateral
◻ **H44.449** Primary hypotony of unspecified eye

⑤ **H44.5** Degenerated conditions of globe
H44.50 Unspecified degenerated conditions of globe
⑥ **H44.51** Absolute glaucoma
◻ **H44.511** Absolute glaucoma, right eye
◻ **H44.512** Absolute glaucoma, left eye
◻ **H44.513** Absolute glaucoma, bilateral
◻ **H44.519** Absolute glaucoma, unspecified eye

⑥ **H44.52** Atrophy of globe
Phthisis bulbi
◻ **H44.521** Atrophy of globe, right eye
◻ **H44.522** Atrophy of globe, left eye
◻ **H44.523** Atrophy of globe, bilateral
◻ **H44.529** Atrophy of globe, unspecified eye

⑥ **H44.53** Leucocoria
◻ **H44.531** Leucocoria, right eye
◻ **H44.532** Leucocoria, left eye
◻ **H44.533** Leucocoria, bilateral
◻ **H44.539** Leucocoria, unspecified eye

⑤➕ **H44.6** Retained (old) intraocular foreign body, magnetic
Use additional code to identify magnetic foreign body (Z18.11)
EXCLUDES 1	current intraocular foreign body (S05.-)
EXCLUDES 2	retained foreign body in eyelid (H02.81-)
	retained (old) foreign body following penetrating wound of orbit (H05.5-)
	retained (old) intraocular foreign body, nonmagnetic (H44.7-)

⑥➕ **H44.60** Unspecified retained (old) intraocular foreign body, magnetic
◻➕ **H44.601** Unspecified retained (old) intraocular foreign body, magnetic, right eye
◻➕ **H44.602** Unspecified retained (old) intraocular foreign body, magnetic, left eye
◻➕ **H44.603** Unspecified retained (old) intraocular foreign body, magnetic, bilateral
◻➕ **H44.609** Unspecified retained (old) intraocular foreign body, magnetic, unspecified eye

⑥➕ **H44.61** Retained (old) magnetic foreign body in anterior chamber
◻➕ **H44.611** Retained (old) magnetic foreign body in anterior chamber, right eye
◻➕ **H44.612** Retained (old) magnetic foreign body in anterior chamber, left eye
◻➕ **H44.613** Retained (old) magnetic foreign body in anterior chamber, bilateral
◻➕ **H44.619** Retained (old) magnetic foreign body in anterior chamber, unspecified eye

⑥➕ **H44.62** Retained (old) magnetic foreign body in iris or ciliary body
◻➕ **H44.621** Retained (old) magnetic foreign body in iris or ciliary body, right eye
◻➕ **H44.622** Retained (old) magnetic foreign body in iris or ciliary body, left eye
◻➕ **H44.623** Retained (old) magnetic foreign body in iris or ciliary body, bilateral
◻➕ **H44.629** Retained (old) magnetic foreign body in iris or ciliary body, unspecified eye

⑥➕ **H44.63** Retained (old) magnetic foreign body in lens
◻➕ **H44.631** Retained (old) magnetic foreign body in lens, right eye
◻➕ **H44.632** Retained (old) magnetic foreign body in lens, left eye
◻➕ **H44.633** Retained (old) magnetic foreign body in lens, bilateral
◻➕ **H44.639** Retained (old) magnetic foreign body in lens, unspecified eye

⑥➕ **H44.64** Retained (old) magnetic foreign body in posterior wall of globe
◻➕ **H44.641** Retained (old) magnetic foreign body in posterior wall of globe, right eye
◻➕ **H44.642** Retained (old) magnetic foreign body in posterior wall of globe, left eye
◻➕ **H44.643** Retained (old) magnetic foreign body in posterior wall of globe, bilateral
◻➕ **H44.649** Retained (old) magnetic foreign body in posterior wall of globe, unspecified eye

⑥➕ **H44.65** Retained (old) magnetic foreign body in vitreous body
◻➕ **H44.651** Retained (old) magnetic foreign body in vitreous body, right eye
◻➕ **H44.652** Retained (old) magnetic foreign body in vitreous body, left eye
◻➕ **H44.653** Retained (old) magnetic foreign body in vitreous body, bilateral

● New ▲ Revised *Manifestation* ◪-◻ Digit Indicators ◻ Laterality Ⓐ Adult (15+ years) Ⓜ Maternity (12-55 years) Ⓝ Newborn Ⓟ Pediatric (0-17 years) ♂ Male ♀ Female
✖ Deleted Unspecified + Additional code

2017 ICD-10-CM Expert for Physicians

© 2017 DecisionHealth

613

H44.12 — H44.653

☒ + H44.659   Retained (old) magnetic foreign body in vitreous body, unspecified eye

⑥ + H44.69   Retained (old) intraocular foreign body, magnetic, in other or multiple sites

☒ + H44.691   Retained (old) intraocular foreign body, magnetic, in other or multiple sites, right eye

☒ + H44.692   Retained (old) intraocular foreign body, magnetic, in other or multiple sites, left eye

☒ + H44.693   Retained (old) intraocular foreign body, magnetic, in other or multiple sites, bilateral

☒ + H44.699   Retained (old) intraocular foreign body, magnetic, in other or multiple sites, unspecified eye

☒ + **H44.7   Retained (old) intraocular foreign body, nonmagnetic**
Use additional code to identify nonmagnetic foreign body (Z18.01-Z18.10, Z18.12, Z18.2-Z18.9)

EXCLUDES 1   *current intraocular foreign body (S05.-)*

EXCLUDES 2   *retained foreign body in eyelid (H02.81-)*
retained (old) foreign body following penetrating wound of orbit (H05.5-)
retained (old) intraocular foreign body, magnetic (H44.6-)

⑥ + **H44.70   Unspecified retained (old) intraocular foreign body, nonmagnetic**

☒ + H44.701   Unspecified retained (old) intraocular foreign body, nonmagnetic, right eye

☒ + H44.702   Unspecified retained (old) intraocular foreign body, nonmagnetic, left eye

☒ + H44.703   Unspecified retained (old) intraocular foreign body, nonmagnetic, bilateral

☒ + H44.709   Unspecified retained (old) intraocular foreign body, nonmagnetic, unspecified eye
Retained (old) intraocular foreign body NOS

⑥ + **H44.71   Retained (nonmagnetic) (old) foreign body in anterior chamber**

☒ + H44.711   Retained (nonmagnetic) (old) foreign body in anterior chamber, right eye

☒ + H44.712   Retained (nonmagnetic) (old) foreign body in anterior chamber, left eye

☒ + H44.713   Retained (nonmagnetic) (old) foreign body in anterior chamber, bilateral

☒ + H44.719   Retained (nonmagnetic) (old) foreign body in anterior chamber, unspecified eye

⑥ + **H44.72   Retained (nonmagnetic) (old) foreign body in iris or ciliary body**

☒ + H44.721   Retained (nonmagnetic) (old) foreign body in iris or ciliary body, right eye

☒ + H44.722   Retained (nonmagnetic) (old) foreign body in iris or ciliary body, left eye

☒ + H44.723   Retained (nonmagnetic) (old) foreign body in iris or ciliary body, bilateral

☒ + H44.729   Retained (nonmagnetic) (old) foreign body in iris or ciliary body, unspecified eye

⑥ + **H44.73   Retained (nonmagnetic) (old) foreign body in lens**

☒ + H44.731   Retained (nonmagnetic) (old) foreign body in lens, right eye

☒ + H44.732   Retained (nonmagnetic) (old) foreign body in lens, left eye

☒ + H44.733   Retained (nonmagnetic) (old) foreign body in lens, bilateral

☒ + H44.739   Retained (nonmagnetic) (old) foreign body in lens, unspecified eye

⑥ + **H44.74   Retained (nonmagnetic) (old) foreign body in posterior wall of globe**

☒ + H44.741   Retained (nonmagnetic) (old) foreign body in posterior wall of globe, right eye

☒ + H44.742   Retained (nonmagnetic) (old) foreign body in posterior wall of globe, left eye

☒ + H44.743   Retained (nonmagnetic) (old) foreign body in posterior wall of globe, bilateral

☒ + H44.749   Retained (nonmagnetic) (old) foreign body in posterior wall of globe, unspecified eye

⑥ + **H44.75   Retained (nonmagnetic) (old) foreign body in vitreous body**

☒ + H44.751   Retained (nonmagnetic) (old) foreign body in vitreous body, right eye

☒ + H44.752   Retained (nonmagnetic) (old) foreign body in vitreous body, left eye

☒ + H44.753   Retained (nonmagnetic) (old) foreign body in vitreous body, bilateral

☒ + H44.759   Retained (nonmagnetic) (old) foreign body in vitreous body, unspecified eye

⑥ + **H44.79   Retained (old) intraocular foreign body, nonmagnetic, in other or multiple sites**

☒ + H44.791   Retained (old) intraocular foreign body, nonmagnetic, in other or multiple sites, right eye

☒ + H44.792   Retained (old) intraocular foreign body, nonmagnetic, in other or multiple sites, left eye

☒ + H44.793   Retained (old) intraocular foreign body, nonmagnetic, in other or multiple sites, bilateral

☒ + H44.799   Retained (old) intraocular foreign body, nonmagnetic, in other or multiple sites, unspecified eye

☒ **H44.8   Other disorders of globe**

⑥ **H44.81   Hemophthalmos**

DEFINITION   Accumulation of blood within the eyeball that is not due to a current injury.

☒ H44.811   Hemophthalmos, right eye
☒ H44.812   Hemophthalmos, left eye
☒ H44.813   Hemophthalmos, bilateral
☒ H44.819   Hemophthalmos, unspecified eye

⑥ **H44.82   Luxation of globe**
☒ H44.821   Luxation of globe, right eye
☒ H44.822   Luxation of globe, left eye
☒ H44.823   Luxation of globe, bilateral
☒ H44.829   Luxation of globe, unspecified eye

H44.89   Other disorders of globe
H44.9   Unspecified disorder of globe

Disorders of optic nerve and visual pathways (H46-H47)

☒ **H46   Optic neuritis**
EXCLUDES 2   *ischemic optic neuropathy (H47.01-)*
neuromyelitis optica [Devic] (G36.0)

☒ **H46.0   Optic papillitis**

DEFINITION   Swelling of the optic disc where the optic nerve connects to the retina.

☒ H46.00   Optic papillitis, unspecified eye
☒ H46.01   Optic papillitis, right eye
☒ H46.02   Optic papillitis, left eye
☒ H46.03   Optic papillitis, bilateral

☒ **H46.1   Retrobulbar neuritis**
Retrobulbar neuritis NOS
EXCLUDES 1   *syphilitic retrobulbar neuritis (A52.15)*

DEFINITION   Inflammation of the optic nerve directly behind the eye.

☒ H46.10   Retrobulbar neuritis, unspecified eye
☒ H46.11   Retrobulbar neuritis, right eye
☒ H46.12   Retrobulbar neuritis, left eye
☒ H46.13   Retrobulbar neuritis, bilateral

H46.2   Nutritional optic neuropathy
H46.3   Toxic optic neuropathy
Code first:
(T51-T65) to identify cause

H46.8   Other optic neuritis
H46.9   Unspecified optic neuritis

☒ **H47   Other disorders of optic [2nd] nerve and visual pathways**

☒ **H47.0   Disorders of optic nerve, not elsewhere classified**

⑥ **H47.01   Ischemic optic neuropathy**
☒ H47.011   Ischemic optic neuropathy, right eye
☒ H47.012   Ischemic optic neuropathy, left eye
☒ H47.013   Ischemic optic neuropathy, bilateral
☒ H47.019   Ischemic optic neuropathy, unspecified eye

⑥ **H47.02   Hemorrhage in optic nerve sheath**
☒ H47.021   Hemorrhage in optic nerve sheath, right eye
☒ H47.022   Hemorrhage in optic nerve sheath, left eye
☒ H47.023   Hemorrhage in optic nerve sheath, bilateral

● New   ▲ Revised   *Manifestation*   ❶-❼ Digit Indicators   ☒ Laterality   Ⓐ Adult (15+ years)   Ⓜ Maternity (12-55 years)   Ⓝ Newborn   Ⓟ Pediatric (0-17 years)   ♂ Male   ♀ Female
✖ Deleted   Unspecified   + Additional code

614   © 2017 DecisionHealth   2017 ICD-10-CM Expert for Physicians

☐ **H47.029**   Hemorrhage in optic nerve sheath, unspecified eye

◩ **H47.03**   Optic nerve hypoplasia
- ☐ **H47.031**   Optic nerve hypoplasia, right eye
- ☐ **H47.032**   Optic nerve hypoplasia, left eye
- ☐ **H47.033**   Optic nerve hypoplasia, bilateral
- ☐ **H47.039**   Optic nerve hypoplasia, unspecified eye

◩ **H47.09**   Other disorders of optic nerve, not elsewhere classified
Compression of optic nerve
- ☐ **H47.091**   Other disorders of optic nerve, not elsewhere classified, right eye
- ☐ **H47.092**   Other disorders of optic nerve, not elsewhere classified, left eye
- ☐ **H47.093**   Other disorders of optic nerve, not elsewhere classified, bilateral
- ☐ **H47.099**   Other disorders of optic nerve, not elsewhere classified, unspecified eye

◵ **H47.1**   Papilledema
H47.10   Unspecified papilledema
H47.11   Papilledema associated with increased intracranial pressure

> **DEFINITION**   Swelling of the optic disk (the part of the retina that connects to the optic nerve) caused by increased intracranial pressure.

H47.12   Papilledema associated with decreased ocular pressure
H47.13   Papilledema associated with retinal disorder
◩ **H47.14**   Foster-Kennedy syndrome

> **DEFINITION**   Disease that presents with papilledema in one eye and atrophy of the optic nerve of the other; caused by increased intracranial pressure from a tumor.

- ☐ **H47.141**   Foster-Kennedy syndrome, right eye
- ☐ **H47.142**   Foster-Kennedy syndrome, left eye
- ☐ **H47.143**   Foster-Kennedy syndrome, bilateral
- ☐ **H47.149**   Foster-Kennedy syndrome, unspecified eye

◵ **H47.2**   Optic atrophy
H47.20   Unspecified optic atrophy
◩ **H47.21**   Primary optic atrophy
- ☐ **H47.211**   Primary optic atrophy, right eye
- ☐ **H47.212**   Primary optic atrophy, left eye
- ☐ **H47.213**   Primary optic atrophy, bilateral
- ☐ **H47.219**   Primary optic atrophy, unspecified eye

H47.22   Hereditary optic atrophy
Leber's optic atrophy
◩ **H47.23**   Glaucomatous optic atrophy
- ☐ **H47.231**   Glaucomatous optic atrophy, right eye
- ☐ **H47.232**   Glaucomatous optic atrophy, left eye
- ☐ **H47.233**   Glaucomatous optic atrophy, bilateral
- ☐ **H47.239**   Glaucomatous optic atrophy, unspecified eye

◩ **H47.29**   Other optic atrophy
Temporal pallor of optic disc
- ☐ **H47.291**   Other optic atrophy, right eye
- ☐ **H47.292**   Other optic atrophy, left eye
- ☐ **H47.293**   Other optic atrophy, bilateral
- ☐ **H47.299**   Other optic atrophy, unspecified eye

◵ **H47.3**   Other disorders of optic disc
◩ **H47.31**   Coloboma of optic disc

> **DEFINITION**   Congenital defect of the iris in which there is a gap, hole, or cleft that failed to close; may cause ghost images, blurred or decreased visual activity.

- ☐ **H47.311**   Coloboma of optic disc, right eye
- ☐ **H47.312**   Coloboma of optic disc, left eye
- ☐ **H47.313**   Coloboma of optic disc, bilateral
- ☐ **H47.319**   Coloboma of optic disc, unspecified eye

◩ **H47.32**   Drusen of optic disc
- ☐ **H47.321**   Drusen of optic disc, right eye
- ☐ **H47.322**   Drusen of optic disc, left eye
- ☐ **H47.323**   Drusen of optic disc, bilateral
- ☐ **H47.329**   Drusen of optic disc, unspecified eye

◩ **H47.33**   Pseudopapilledema of optic disc
- ☐ **H47.331**   Pseudopapilledema of optic disc, right eye
- ☐ **H47.332**   Pseudopapilledema of optic disc, left eye
- ☐ **H47.333**   Pseudopapilledema of optic disc, bilateral
- ☐ **H47.339**   Pseudopapilledema of optic disc, unspecified eye

◩ **H47.39**   Other disorders of optic disc
- ☐ **H47.391**   Other disorders of optic disc, right eye
- ☐ **H47.392**   Other disorders of optic disc, left eye
- ☐ **H47.393**   Other disorders of optic disc, bilateral
- ☐ **H47.399**   Other disorders of optic disc, unspecified eye

◵ **H47.4**   Disorders of optic chiasm
Code also:
   underlying condition
H47.41   Disorders of optic chiasm in (due to) inflammatory disorders
H47.42   Disorders of optic chiasm in (due to) neoplasm
H47.43   Disorders of optic chiasm in (due to) vascular disorders
H47.49   Disorders of optic chiasm in (due to) other disorders

◵ **H47.5**   Disorders of other visual pathways
Disorders of optic tracts, geniculate nuclei and optic radiations
Code also:
   underlying condition
◩ **H47.51**   Disorders of visual pathways in (due to) inflammatory disorders
- ☐ **H47.511**   Disorders of visual pathways in (due to) inflammatory disorders, right side
- ☐ **H47.512**   Disorders of visual pathways in (due to) inflammatory disorders, left side
- ☐ **H47.519**   Disorders of visual pathways in (due to) inflammatory disorders, unspecified side

◩ **H47.52**   Disorders of visual pathways in (due to) neoplasm
- ☐ **H47.521**   Disorders of visual pathways in (due to) neoplasm, right side
- ☐ **H47.522**   Disorders of visual pathways in (due to) neoplasm, left side
- ☐ **H47.529**   Disorders of visual pathways in (due to) neoplasm, unspecified side

◩ **H47.53**   Disorders of visual pathways in (due to) vascular disorders
- ☐ **H47.531**   Disorders of visual pathways in (due to) vascular disorders, right side
- ☐ **H47.532**   Disorders of visual pathways in (due to) vascular disorders, left side
- ☐ **H47.539**   Disorders of visual pathways in (due to) vascular disorders, unspecified side

◵ **H47.6**   Disorders of visual cortex
Code also:
   underlying condition

> **EXCLUDES 1**   *injury to visual cortex S04.04*

◩ **H47.61**   Cortical blindness

> **DEFINITION**   Blindness caused by a defect of the brain and not the eyes.

- ☐ **H47.611**   Cortical blindness, right side of brain
- ☐ **H47.612**   Cortical blindness, left side of brain
- ☐ **H47.619**   Cortical blindness, unspecified side of brain

◩ **H47.62**   Disorders of visual cortex in (due to) inflammatory disorders
- ☐ **H47.621**   Disorders of visual cortex in (due to) inflammatory disorders, right side of brain
- ☐ **H47.622**   Disorders of visual cortex in (due to) inflammatory disorders, left side of brain
- ☐ **H47.629**   Disorders of visual cortex in (due to) inflammatory disorders, unspecified side of brain

◩ **H47.63**   Disorders of visual cortex in (due to) neoplasm
- ☐ **H47.631**   Disorders of visual cortex in (due to) neoplasm, right side of brain
- ☐ **H47.632**   Disorders of visual cortex in (due to) neoplasm, left side of brain
- ☐ **H47.639**   Disorders of visual cortex in (due to) neoplasm, unspecified side of brain

◩ **H47.64**   Disorders of visual cortex in (due to) vascular disorders
- ☐ **H47.641**   Disorders of visual cortex in (due to) vascular disorders, right side of brain
- ☐ **H47.642**   Disorders of visual cortex in (due to) vascular disorders, left side of brain

---

● New   ▲ Revised   *Manifestation*   ④-❼ Digit Indicators   ☐ Laterality   🅰 Adult (15+ years)   🅼 Maternity (12-55 years)   🅽 Newborn   🅿 Pediatric (0-17 years)   ♂ Male   ♀ Female
✖ Deleted   Unspecified   + Additional code

⊟ H47.649   Disorders of visual cortex in (due to) vascular disorders, unspecified side of brain

H47.9   Unspecified disorder of visual pathways

Disorders of ocular muscles, binocular movement, accommodation and refraction (H49-H52)

EXCLUDES 2   *nystagmus and other irregular eye movements (H55)*

◪ **H49   Paralytic strabismus**

EXCLUDES 2   *internal ophthalmoplegia (H52.51-)*
internuclear ophthalmoplegia (H51.2-)
progressive supranuclear ophthalmoplegia (G23.1)

⑤ **H49.0   Third [oculomotor] nerve palsy**

⊟ H49.00   **Third [oculomotor] nerve palsy, unspecified eye**

⊟ H49.01   **Third [oculomotor] nerve palsy, right eye**

⊟ H49.02   **Third [oculomotor] nerve palsy, left eye**

⊟ H49.03   **Third [oculomotor] nerve palsy, bilateral**

⑤ **H49.1   Fourth [trochlear] nerve palsy**

⊟ H49.10   **Fourth [trochlear] nerve palsy, unspecified eye**

⊟ H49.11   **Fourth [trochlear] nerve palsy, right eye**

⊟ H49.12   **Fourth [trochlear] nerve palsy, left eye**

⊟ H49.13   **Fourth [trochlear] nerve palsy, bilateral**

⑤ **H49.2   Sixth [abducent] nerve palsy**

⊟ H49.20   **Sixth [abducent] nerve palsy, unspecified eye**

⊟ H49.21   **Sixth [abducent] nerve palsy, right eye**

⊟ H49.22   **Sixth [abducent] nerve palsy, left eye**

⊟ H49.23   **Sixth [abducent] nerve palsy, bilateral**

⑤ **H49.3   Total (external) ophthalmoplegia**

DEFINITION   Paralysis of all of the muscles that move the eye as well as the muscles controlling the diameter of the pupil and shape of the lens.

⊟ H49.30   **Total (external) ophthalmoplegia, unspecified eye**

⊟ H49.31   **Total (external) ophthalmoplegia, right eye**

⊟ H49.32   **Total (external) ophthalmoplegia, left eye**

⊟ H49.33   **Total (external) ophthalmoplegia, bilateral**

⑤ **H49.4   Progressive external ophthalmoplegia**

EXCLUDES 1   *Kearns-Sayre syndrome (H49.81-)*

⊟ H49.40   **Progressive external ophthalmoplegia, unspecified eye**

⊟ H49.41   **Progressive external ophthalmoplegia, right eye**

⊟ H49.42   **Progressive external ophthalmoplegia, left eye**

⊟ H49.43   **Progressive external ophthalmoplegia, bilateral**

⑤ **H49.8   Other paralytic strabismus**

⑥ ✚ **H49.81   Kearns-Sayre syndrome**

Progressive external ophthalmoplegia with pigmentary retinopathy

Use additional code for other manifestation, such as: heart block (I45.9)

⊟ ✚ H49.811   **Kearns-Sayre syndrome, right eye**

⊟ ✚ H49.812   **Kearns-Sayre syndrome, left eye**

⊟ ✚ H49.813   **Kearns-Sayre syndrome, bilateral**

⊟ ✚ H49.819   **Kearns-Sayre syndrome, unspecified eye**

⑥ **H49.88   Other paralytic strabismus**

External ophthalmoplegia NOS

⊟ H49.881   **Other paralytic strabismus, right eye**

⊟ H49.882   **Other paralytic strabismus, left eye**

⊟ H49.883   **Other paralytic strabismus, bilateral**

⊟ H49.889   **Other paralytic strabismus, unspecified eye**

H49.9   **Unspecified paralytic strabismus**

◪ **H50   Other strabismus**

⑤ **H50.0   Esotropia**

Convergent concomitant strabismus

EXCLUDES 1   *intermittent esotropia (H50.31-, H50.32)*

DEFINITION   Deviation of the visual axis of one or both eyes inward toward that of the other eye.

H50.00   **Unspecified esotropia**

⑥ **H50.01   Monocular esotropia**

⊟ H50.011   **Monocular esotropia, right eye**

⊟ H50.012   **Monocular esotropia, left eye**

⑥ **H50.02   Monocular esotropia with A pattern**

⊟ H50.021   **Monocular esotropia with A pattern, right eye**

⊟ H50.022   **Monocular esotropia with A pattern, left eye**

⑥ **H50.03   Monocular esotropia with V pattern**

⊟ H50.031   **Monocular esotropia with V pattern, right eye**

⊟ H50.032   **Monocular esotropia with V pattern, left eye**

⑥ **H50.04   Monocular esotropia with other noncomitancies**

⊟ H50.041   **Monocular esotropia with other noncomitancies, right eye**

⊟ H50.042   **Monocular esotropia with other noncomitancies, left eye**

H50.05   **Alternating esotropia**

H50.06   **Alternating esotropia with A pattern**

H50.07   **Alternating esotropia with V pattern**

H50.08   **Alternating esotropia with other noncomitancies**

⑤ **H50.1   Exotropia**

Divergent concomitant strabismus

EXCLUDES 1   *intermittent exotropia (H50.33-, H50.34)*

DEFINITION   An abnormal alignment of one or both eyes in which one or both eyes deviate outward.

H50.10   **Unspecified exotropia**

Exotropia

A type of strabismus in which one or both eyes turn outwards

Exotropia with V pattern: eye deviates downwards and outwards

Exotropia with A pattern: eye deviates upwards and outwards

⑥ **H50.11   Monocular exotropia**

⊟ H50.111   **Monocular exotropia, right eye**

⊟ H50.112   **Monocular exotropia, left eye**

⑥ **H50.12   Monocular exotropia with A pattern**

⊟ H50.121   **Monocular exotropia with A pattern, right eye**

⊟ H50.122   **Monocular exotropia with A pattern, left eye**

⑥ **H50.13   Monocular exotropia with V pattern**

⊟ H50.131   **Monocular exotropia with V pattern, right eye**

⊟ H50.132   **Monocular exotropia with V pattern, left eye**

⑥ **H50.14   Monocular exotropia with other noncomitancies**

⊟ H50.141   **Monocular exotropia with other noncomitancies, right eye**

⊟ H50.142   **Monocular exotropia with other noncomitancies, left eye**

H50.15   **Alternating exotropia**

H50.16   **Alternating exotropia with A pattern**

H50.17   **Alternating exotropia with V pattern**

H50.18   **Alternating exotropia with other noncomitancies**

⑤ **H50.2   Vertical strabismus**

Hypertropia

⊟ H50.21   **Vertical strabismus, right eye**

⊟ H50.22   **Vertical strabismus, left eye**

⑤ **H50.3   Intermittent heterotropia**

H50.30   **Unspecified intermittent heterotropia**

⑥ **H50.31   Intermittent monocular esotropia**

⊟ H50.311   **Intermittent monocular esotropia, right eye**

⊟ H50.312   **Intermittent monocular esotropia, left eye**

H50.32   **Intermittent alternating esotropia**

⑥ **H50.33   Intermittent monocular exotropia**

⊟ H50.331   **Intermittent monocular exotropia, right eye**

⊟ H50.332   **Intermittent monocular exotropia, left eye**

H50.34   **Intermittent alternating exotropia**

⑤ **H50.4   Other and unspecified heterotropia**

● New   ▲ Revised   *Manifestation*   ◪-🆖 Digit Indicators   ⊟ Laterality   🅐 Adult (15+ years)   🅜 Maternity (12-55 years)   🅝 Newborn   🅟 Pediatric (0-17 years)   ♂ Male   ♀ Female
✖ Deleted   Unspecified   ✚ Additional code

616   © 2017 DecisionHealth   2017 ICD-10-CM Expert for Physicians

H50.40 Unspecified heterotropia
◧ H50.41 Cyclotropia
  ⊟ H50.411 Cyclotropia, right eye
  ⊟ H50.412 Cyclotropia, left eye
  H50.42 Monofixation syndrome
  H50.43 Accommodative component in esotropia
⑤ H50.5 Heterophoria
  H50.50 Unspecified heterophoria
  H50.51 Esophoria
  H50.52 Exophoria
  H50.53 Vertical heterophoria
  H50.54 Cyclophoria
  H50.55 Alternating heterophoria
⑤ H50.6 Mechanical strabismus
  H50.60 Mechanical strabismus, unspecified
◧ H50.61 Brown's sheath syndrome
    DEFINITION Condition in which the muscle that moves the eye upward and inward is too short, impairing eye movement.
  ⊟ H50.611 Brown's sheath syndrome, right eye
  ⊟ H50.612 Brown's sheath syndrome, left eye
  H50.69 Other mechanical strabismus
    Strabismus due to adhesions
    Traumatic limitation of duction of eye muscle
⑤ H50.8 Other specified strabismus
◧ H50.81 Duane's syndrome
    DEFINITION Congenital eye muscle disorder due to cranial nerve dysfunction that inhibits normal rotation of one or both eyes inward and outward, also causing abnormal inward turning with distant viewing and eye retraction when viewing up close.
  ⊟ H50.811 Duane's syndrome, right eye
  ⊟ H50.812 Duane's syndrome, left eye
  H50.89 Other specified strabismus
  H50.9 Unspecified strabismus
◪ H51 Other disorders of binocular movement
  H51.0 Palsy (spasm) of conjugate gaze
⑤ H51.1 Convergence insufficiency and excess
  H51.11 Convergence insufficiency
  H51.12 Convergence excess
    DEFINITION Eyes fail to move in a coordinated fashion when viewing objects up close.
⑤ H51.2 Internuclear ophthalmoplegia
  ⊟ H51.20 Internuclear ophthalmoplegia, unspecified eye
  ⊟ H51.21 Internuclear ophthalmoplegia, right eye
  ⊟ H51.22 Internuclear ophthalmoplegia, left eye
  ⊟ H51.23 Internuclear ophthalmoplegia, bilateral
  H51.8 Other specified disorders of binocular movement
  H51.9 Unspecified disorder of binocular movement
◪ H52 Disorders of refraction and accommodation
⑤ H52.0 Hypermetropia
  ⊟ H52.00 Hypermetropia, unspecified eye
  ⊟ H52.01 Hypermetropia, right eye
  ⊟ H52.02 Hypermetropia, left eye
  ⊟ H52.03 Hypermetropia, bilateral
⑤ H52.1 Myopia
    EXCLUDES 1 degenerative myopia (H44.2-)
  ⊟ H52.10 Myopia, unspecified eye
  ⊟ H52.11 Myopia, right eye
  ⊟ H52.12 Myopia, left eye
  ⊟ H52.13 Myopia, bilateral
⑤ H52.2 Astigmatism
    DEFINITION Condition in which the cornea is not shaped perfectly round, causing light to focus on more than one point of the retina and resulting in blurred vision.
◧ H52.20 Unspecified astigmatism
  ⊟ H52.201 Unspecified astigmatism, right eye
  ⊟ H52.202 Unspecified astigmatism, left eye
  ⊟ H52.203 Unspecified astigmatism, bilateral
  ⊟ H52.209 Unspecified astigmatism, unspecified eye
◧ H52.21 Irregular astigmatism
  ⊟ H52.211 Irregular astigmatism, right eye
  ⊟ H52.212 Irregular astigmatism, left eye
  ⊟ H52.213 Irregular astigmatism, bilateral
  ⊟ H52.219 Irregular astigmatism, unspecified eye
◧ H52.22 Regular astigmatism
  ⊟ H52.221 Regular astigmatism, right eye
  ⊟ H52.222 Regular astigmatism, left eye
  ⊟ H52.223 Regular astigmatism, bilateral
  ⊟ H52.229 Regular astigmatism, unspecified eye
⑤ H52.3 Anisometropia and aniseikonia
  H52.31 Anisometropia
    DEFINITION Each eye has a different refractive power.
  H52.32 Aniseikonia
    DEFINITION One eye sees an object differently in size and shape than the way the other eye sees it.
  H52.4 Presbyopia
    DEFINITION Lens of the eye loses its elasticity due to age, making it more difficult to focus on near points.
⑤ H52.5 Disorders of accommodation
◧ H52.51 Internal ophthalmoplegia (complete) (total)
  ⊟ H52.511 Internal ophthalmoplegia (complete) (total), right eye
  ⊟ H52.512 Internal ophthalmoplegia (complete) (total), left eye
  ⊟ H52.513 Internal ophthalmoplegia (complete) (total), bilateral
  ⊟ H52.519 Internal ophthalmoplegia (complete) (total), unspecified eye
◧ H52.52 Paresis of accommodation
    DEFINITION Paralysis of the ciliary muscles of the eye that results in the loss of visual accommodation.
  ⊟ H52.521 Paresis of accommodation, right eye
  ⊟ H52.522 Paresis of accommodation, left eye
  ⊟ H52.523 Paresis of accommodation, bilateral
  ⊟ H52.529 Paresis of accommodation, unspecified eye
◧ H52.53 Spasm of accommodation
    DEFINITION Abnormal, uncontrolled contraction of the ciliary muscle, usually initially presenting as near-sightedness.
  ⊟ H52.531 Spasm of accommodation, right eye
  ⊟ H52.532 Spasm of accommodation, left eye
  ⊟ H52.533 Spasm of accommodation, bilateral
  ⊟ H52.539 Spasm of accommodation, unspecified eye
  H52.6 Other disorders of refraction
  H52.7 Unspecified disorder of refraction

Visual disturbances and blindness (H53-H54)

◪ H53 Visual disturbances
⑤ H53.0 Amblyopia ex anopsia
    EXCLUDES 1 amblyopia due to vitamin A deficiency (E50.5)
◧ H53.00 Unspecified amblyopia
  ⊟ H53.001 Unspecified amblyopia, right eye
  ⊟ H53.002 Unspecified amblyopia, left eye
  ⊟ H53.003 Unspecified amblyopia, bilateral
  ⊟ H53.009 Unspecified amblyopia, unspecified eye
◧ H53.01 Deprivation amblyopia
  ⊟ H53.011 Deprivation amblyopia, right eye
  ⊟ H53.012 Deprivation amblyopia, left eye
  ⊟ H53.013 Deprivation amblyopia, bilateral
  ⊟ H53.019 Deprivation amblyopia, unspecified eye
◧ H53.02 Refractive amblyopia
  ⊟ H53.021 Refractive amblyopia, right eye
  ⊟ H53.022 Refractive amblyopia, left eye
  ⊟ H53.023 Refractive amblyopia, bilateral

● New   ▲ Revised   *Manifestation*   ◪-◮ Digit Indicators   ⊟ Laterality   Ⓐ Adult (15+ years)   Ⓜ Maternity (12-55 years)   Ⓝ Newborn   Ⓟ Pediatric (0-17 years)   ♂ Male   ♀ Female
✖ Deleted   Unspecified   + Additional code

2017 ICD-10-CM Expert for Physicians   © 2017 DecisionHealth   617

Diseases of the Eye and Adnexa

☐ **H53.029** Refractive amblyopia, unspecified eye

ⓖ **H53.03** Strabismic amblyopia

> **EXCLUDES 1** *strabismus (H50.-)*

☐ **H53.031** Strabismic amblyopia, right eye

☐ **H53.032** Strabismic amblyopia, left eye

☐ **H53.033** Strabismic amblyopia, bilateral

☐ **H53.039** Strabismic amblyopia, unspecified eye

●ⓖ **H53.04** Amblyopia suspect

●☐ **H53.041** Amblyopia suspect, right eye

●☐ **H53.042** Amblyopia suspect, left eye

●☐ **H53.043** Amblyopia suspect, bilateral

●☐ **H53.049** Amblyopia suspect, unspecified eye

ⓢ **H53.1** Subjective visual disturbances

> **EXCLUDES 1** *subjective visual disturbances due to vitamin A deficiency (E50.5)*
> *visual hallucinations (R44.1)*

H53.10 Unspecified subjective visual disturbances

H53.11 Day blindness
Hemeralopia

ⓖ **H53.12** Transient visual loss
Scintillating scotoma

> **EXCLUDES 1** *amaurosis fugax (G45.3-)*
> *transient retinal artery occlusion (H34.0-)*

☐ **H53.121** Transient visual loss, right eye

☐ **H53.122** Transient visual loss, left eye

☐ **H53.123** Transient visual loss, bilateral

☐ **H53.129** Transient visual loss, unspecified eye

ⓖ **H53.13** Sudden visual loss

☐ **H53.131** Sudden visual loss, right eye

☐ **H53.132** Sudden visual loss, left eye

☐ **H53.133** Sudden visual loss, bilateral

☐ **H53.139** Sudden visual loss, unspecified eye

ⓖ **H53.14** Visual discomfort
Asthenopia
Photophobia

☐ **H53.141** Visual discomfort, right eye

☐ **H53.142** Visual discomfort, left eye

☐ **H53.143** Visual discomfort, bilateral

☐ **H53.149** Visual discomfort, unspecified

H53.15 Visual distortions of shape and size
Metamorphopsia

H53.16 Psychophysical visual disturbances

H53.19 Other subjective visual disturbances
Visual halos

> **DEFINITION** Photopsia: sparks or flashes in the field of vision, due to retinal irritation.

H53.2 Diplopia
Double vision

ⓢ **H53.3** Other and unspecified disorders of binocular vision

H53.30 Unspecified disorder of binocular vision

H53.31 Abnormal retinal correspondence

H53.32 Fusion with defective stereopsis

H53.33 Simultaneous visual perception without fusion

> **DEFINITION** Imaging from both eyes reaches the brain and are both processed, but without being merged into a single image; the patient sees two side-by-side images instead of one.

H53.34 Suppression of binocular vision

ⓢ **H53.4** Visual field defects

H53.40 Unspecified visual field defects

ⓖ **H53.41** Scotoma involving central area
Central scotoma

☐ **H53.411** Scotoma involving central area, right eye

☐ **H53.412** Scotoma involving central area, left eye

☐ **H53.413** Scotoma involving central area, bilateral

☐ **H53.419** Scotoma involving central area, unspecified eye

ⓖ **H53.42** Scotoma of blind spot area
Enlarged blind spot

> **DEFINITION** Blind spot (scotoma) in the central five degrees of the patient's vision.

☐ **H53.421** Scotoma of blind spot area, right eye

☐ **H53.422** Scotoma of blind spot area, left eye

☐ **H53.423** Scotoma of blind spot area, bilateral

☐ **H53.429** Scotoma of blind spot area, unspecified eye

ⓖ **H53.43** Sector or arcuate defects
Arcuate scotoma
Bjerrum scotoma

☐ **H53.431** Sector or arcuate defects, right eye

☐ **H53.432** Sector or arcuate defects, left eye

☐ **H53.433** Sector or arcuate defects, bilateral

☐ **H53.439** Sector or arcuate defects, unspecified eye

ⓖ **H53.45** Other localized visual field defect
Peripheral visual field defect
Ring scotoma NOS
Scotoma NOS

☐ **H53.451** Other localized visual field defect, right eye

☐ **H53.452** Other localized visual field defect, left eye

☐ **H53.453** Other localized visual field defect, bilateral

☐ **H53.459** Other localized visual field defect, unspecified eye

ⓖ **H53.46** Homonymous bilateral field defects
Homonymous hemianopia
Homonymous hemianopsia
Quadrant anopia
Quadrant anopsia

☐ **H53.461** Homonymous bilateral field defects, right side

☐ **H53.462** Homonymous bilateral field defects, left side

☐ **H53.469** Homonymous bilateral field defects, unspecified side
Homonymous bilateral field defects NOS

H53.47 Heteronymous bilateral field defects
Heteronymous hemianop(s)ia

ⓖ **H53.48** Generalized contraction of visual field

☐ **H53.481** Generalized contraction of visual field, right eye

☐ **H53.482** Generalized contraction of visual field, left eye

☐ **H53.483** Generalized contraction of visual field, bilateral

☐ **H53.489** Generalized contraction of visual field, unspecified eye

ⓢ **H53.5** Color vision deficiencies
Color blindness

> **EXCLUDES 2** *day blindness (H53.11)*

H53.50 Unspecified color vision deficiencies
Color blindness NOS

H53.51 Achromatopsia

> **DEFINITION** Nonprogressive, hereditary visual disorder and retinal abnormality causing decreased vision, light sensitivity, nystagmus, and complete color blindness.

H53.52 Acquired color vision deficiency

H53.53 Deuteranomaly
Deuteranopia

> **DEFINITION** A deficiency in color perception primarily affecting red-green hues due to deficient pigment sensitive to green wavelengths, a common form of color blindness.

H53.54 Protanomaly
Protanopia

H53.55 Tritanomaly
Tritanopia

> **DEFINITION** A deficiency in color perception characterized by an inability to discern blue and yellow due to an absence of blue-sensitive pigment in the retina.

H53.59 Other color vision deficiencies

ⓢ **H53.6** Night blindness

> **EXCLUDES 1** *night blindness due to vitamin A deficiency (E50.5)*

H53.60 Unspecified night blindness

H53.61 Abnormal dark adaptation curve

H53.62 Acquired night blindness

H53.63 Congenital night blindness

H53.69 Other night blindness

ⓢ **H53.7** Vision sensitivity deficiencies

H53.71 Glare sensitivity

H53.72 Impaired contrast sensitivity

H53.8 Other visual disturbances

H53.9 Unspecified visual disturbance

● New ▲ Revised *Manifestation* ❹-❼ Digit Indicators ☐ Laterality 🄰 Adult (15+ years) Ⓜ Maternity (12-55 years) Ⓝ Newborn Ⓟ Pediatric (0-17 years) ♂ Male ♀ Female
✖ Deleted Unspecified + Additional code

618 © 2017 DecisionHealth

2017 ICD-10-CM Expert for Physicians

H53.029 — H53.9

H54   Blindness and low vision

Note: For definition of visual impairment categories see table below

Code first:

any associated underlying cause of the blindness

EXCLUDES 1 *amaurosis fugax (G45.3)*

CODING TIP ✓ Do not use H54 codes for patients with common refractive errors, e.g. farsightedness, nearsightedness, astigmatism, etc. These codes are to indicate the level of vision for those with other eye conditions such as cataracts, retinopathy, glaucoma, hemianopsia, etc.

H54.0   Blindness, both eyes

Visual impairment categories 3, 4, 5 in both eyes.

CODING TIP ✓ Do not use H54.0 to indicate blindness in the USA. See H54.8.

H54.1   Blindness, one eye, low vision other eye

Visual impairment categories 3, 4, 5 in one eye, with categories 1 or 2 in the other eye.

H54.10   Blindness, one eye, low vision other eye, unspecified eyes

H54.11   Blindness, right eye, low vision left eye

H54.12   Blindness, left eye, low vision right eye

H54.2   Low vision, both eyes

Visual impairment categories 1 or 2 in both eyes.

H54.3   Unqualified visual loss, both eyes

Visual impairment category 9 in both eyes.

H54.4   Blindness, one eye

Visual impairment categories 3, 4, 5 in one eye [normal vision in other eye]

H54.40   Blindness, one eye, unspecified eye

H54.41   Blindness, right eye, normal vision left eye

H54.42   Blindness, left eye, normal vision right eye

H54.5   Low vision, one eye

Visual impairment categories 1 or 2 in one eye [normal vision in other eye].

H54.50   Low vision, one eye, unspecified eye

H54.51   Low vision, right eye, normal vision left eye

H54.52   Low vision, left eye, normal vision right eye

H54.6   Unqualified visual loss, one eye

Visual impairment category 9 in one eye [normal vision in other eye].

H54.60   Unqualified visual loss, one eye, unspecified

H54.61   Unqualified visual loss, right eye, normal vision left eye

H54.62   Unqualified visual loss, left eye, normal vision right eye

H54.7   Unspecified visual loss

Visual impairment category 9 NOS

H54.8   Legal blindness, as defined in USA

Blindness NOS according to USA definition

Note: The table below gives a classification of severity of visual impairment recommended by a WHO Study Group on the Prevention of Blindness, Geneva, 6-10 November 1972.

The term 'low vision' in category H54 comprises categories 1 and 2 of the table, the term 'blindness' categories 3, 4 and 5, and the term 'unqualified visual loss' category 9.

If the extent of the visual field is taken into account, patients with a field no greater than 10 but greater than 5 around central fixation should be placed in category 3 and patients with a field no greater than 5 around central fixation should be placed in category 4, even if the central acuity is not impaired.

EXCLUDES 1 *legal blindness with specification of impairment level (H54.0-H54.7)*

Category of visual impairment	Visual acuity with best possible correction	
	Maximum less than:	Minimum equal to or better than:
1	6/18 3/10(0.3) 20/70	6/60 1/10(0.1) 20/200
2	6/60 1/10(0.1) 20/200	3/60 1/20(0.05) 20/400
3	3/60 1/20(0.05) 20/400	1/60(finger counting at one meter) 1/50(0.02) 5/300(20/1200)
4	1/60(finger counting at one meter) 1/50(0.02) 5/300	Light perception
5	No light perception	
9	Undetermined or unspecified	

CODING TIP ✓ Use this code to indicate blindness in both eyes.

Other disorders of eye and adnexa (H55-H57)

H55   Nystagmus and other irregular eye movements

H55.0   Nystagmus

H55.00   Unspecified nystagmus

H55.01   Congenital nystagmus

H55.02   Latent nystagmus

DEFINITION Involuntary rapid movement of the eyeball occurring only when one eye is covered.

H55.03   Visual deprivation nystagmus

H55.04   Dissociated nystagmus

DEFINITION Involuntary rhythmic movements in both eyes that are dissimilar in direction, extent, and frequency of movement.

H55.09   Other forms of nystagmus

H55.8   Other irregular eye movements

H55.81   Saccadic eye movements

DEFINITION Rapid and involuntary eye movement while changing focus on stationary objects.

H55.89   Other irregular eye movements

H57   Other disorders of eye and adnexa

H57.0   Anomalies of pupillary function

H57.00   Unspecified anomaly of pupillary function

H57.01   Argyll Robertson pupil, atypical

EXCLUDES 1 *syphilitic Argyll Robertson pupil (A52.19)*

H57.02   Anisocoria

DEFINITION Pupils of unequal size.

H57.03   Miosis

DEFINITION Constriction of the pupil.

H57.04   Mydriasis

H57.05   Tonic pupil

H57.051   Tonic pupil, right eye

H57.052   Tonic pupil, left eye

H57.053   Tonic pupil, bilateral

H57.059   Tonic pupil, unspecified eye

H57.09   Other anomalies of pupillary function

H57.1   Ocular pain

H57.10   Ocular pain, unspecified eye

H57.11   Ocular pain, right eye

H57.12   Ocular pain, left eye

H57.13   Ocular pain, bilateral

H57.8   Other specified disorders of eye and adnexa

H57.9   Unspecified disorder of eye and adnexa

● New   ▲ Revised   *Manifestation*   ◄-▶ Digit Indicators   ⊟ Laterality   Ⓐ Adult (15+ years)   Ⓜ Maternity (12-55 years)   Ⓝ Newborn   Ⓟ Pediatric (0-17 years)   ♂ Male   ♀ Female
✖ Deleted   Unspecified   + Additional code

Intraoperative and postprocedural complications and disorders of eye and adnexa, not elsewhere classified (H59)

◢ **H59**   **Intraoperative and postprocedural complications and disorders of eye and adnexa, not elsewhere classified**

 EXCLUDES 1   *mechanical complication of intraocular lens (T85.2)*
mechanical complication of other ocular prosthetic devices, implants and grafts (T85.3)
pseudophakia (Z96.1)
secondary cataracts (H26.4-)

Ⓢ **H59.0**   **Disorders of the eye following cataract surgery**

 Ⓖ **H59.01**   **Keratopathy (bullous aphakic) following cataract surgery**
 Vitreal corneal syndrome
 Vitreous (touch) syndrome

  ⊟ **H59.011**   **Keratopathy (bullous aphakic) following cataract surgery, right eye**

  ⊟ **H59.012**   **Keratopathy (bullous aphakic) following cataract surgery, left eye**

  ⊟ **H59.013**   **Keratopathy (bullous aphakic) following cataract surgery, bilateral**

  ⊟ **H59.019**   **Keratopathy (bullous aphakic) following cataract surgery, unspecified eye**

 Ⓖ **H59.02**   **Cataract (lens) fragments in eye following cataract surgery**

  ⊟ **H59.021**   **Cataract (lens) fragments in eye following cataract surgery, right eye**

  ⊟ **H59.022**   **Cataract (lens) fragments in eye following cataract surgery, left eye**

  ⊟ **H59.023**   **Cataract (lens) fragments in eye following cataract surgery, bilateral**

  ⊟ **H59.029**   **Cataract (lens) fragments in eye following cataract surgery, unspecified eye**

 Ⓖ **H59.03**   **Cystoid macular edema following cataract surgery**

  ⊟ **H59.031**   **Cystoid macular edema following cataract surgery, right eye**

  ⊟ **H59.032**   **Cystoid macular edema following cataract surgery, left eye**

  ⊟ **H59.033**   **Cystoid macular edema following cataract surgery, bilateral**

  ⊟ **H59.039**   **Cystoid macular edema following cataract surgery, unspecified eye**

 Ⓖ **H59.09**   **Other disorders of the eye following cataract surgery**

  ⊟ **H59.091**   **Other disorders of the right eye following cataract surgery**

  ⊟ **H59.092**   **Other disorders of the left eye following cataract surgery**

  ⊟ **H59.093**   **Other disorders of the eye following cataract surgery, bilateral**

  ⊟ **H59.099**   **Other disorders of unspecified eye following cataract surgery**

Ⓢ **H59.1**   **Intraoperative hemorrhage and hematoma of eye and adnexa complicating a procedure**

 EXCLUDES 1   *intraoperative hemorrhage and hematoma of eye and adnexa due to accidental puncture or laceration during a procedure (H59.2-)*

 Ⓖ **H59.11**   **Intraoperative hemorrhage and hematoma of eye and adnexa complicating an ophthalmic procedure**

  ⊟ **H59.111**   **Intraoperative hemorrhage and hematoma of right eye and adnexa complicating an ophthalmic procedure**

  ⊟ **H59.112**   **Intraoperative hemorrhage and hematoma of left eye and adnexa complicating an ophthalmic procedure**

  ⊟ **H59.113**   **Intraoperative hemorrhage and hematoma of eye and adnexa complicating an ophthalmic procedure, bilateral**

  ⊟ **H59.119**   **Intraoperative hemorrhage and hematoma of unspecified eye and adnexa complicating an ophthalmic procedure**

 Ⓖ **H59.12**   **Intraoperative hemorrhage and hematoma of eye and adnexa complicating other procedure**

  ⊟ **H59.121**   **Intraoperative hemorrhage and hematoma of right eye and adnexa complicating other procedure**

  ⊟ **H59.122**   **Intraoperative hemorrhage and hematoma of left eye and adnexa complicating other procedure**

  ⊟ **H59.123**   **Intraoperative hemorrhage and hematoma of eye and adnexa complicating other procedure, bilateral**

  ⊟ **H59.129**   **Intraoperative hemorrhage and hematoma of unspecified eye and adnexa complicating other procedure**

Ⓢ **H59.2**   **Accidental puncture and laceration of eye and adnexa during a procedure**

 Ⓖ **H59.21**   **Accidental puncture and laceration of eye and adnexa during an ophthalmic procedure**

  ⊟ **H59.211**   **Accidental puncture and laceration of right eye and adnexa during an ophthalmic procedure**

  ⊟ **H59.212**   **Accidental puncture and laceration of left eye and adnexa during an ophthalmic procedure**

  ⊟ **H59.213**   **Accidental puncture and laceration of eye and adnexa during an ophthalmic procedure, bilateral**

  ⊟ **H59.219**   **Accidental puncture and laceration of unspecified eye and adnexa during an ophthalmic procedure**

 Ⓖ **H59.22**   **Accidental puncture and laceration of eye and adnexa during other procedure**

  ⊟ **H59.221**   **Accidental puncture and laceration of right eye and adnexa during other procedure**

  ⊟ **H59.222**   **Accidental puncture and laceration of left eye and adnexa during other procedure**

  ⊟ **H59.223**   **Accidental puncture and laceration of eye and adnexa during other procedure, bilateral**

  ⊟ **H59.229**   **Accidental puncture and laceration of unspecified eye and adnexa during other procedure**

▲ Ⓢ **H59.3**   **Postprocedural hemorrhage, hematoma, and seroma of eye and adnexa following a procedure**

 ▲ Ⓖ **H59.31**   **Postprocedural hemorrhage of eye and adnexa following an ophthalmic procedure**

  ▲ ⊟ **H59.311**   **Postprocedural hemorrhage of right eye and adnexa following an ophthalmic procedure**

  ▲ ⊟ **H59.312**   **Postprocedural hemorrhage of left eye and adnexa following an ophthalmic procedure**

  ▲ ⊟ **H59.313**   **Postprocedural hemorrhage of eye and adnexa following an ophthalmic procedure, bilateral**

  ▲ ⊟ **H59.319**   **Postprocedural hemorrhage of unspecified eye and adnexa following an ophthalmic procedure**

 ▲ Ⓖ **H59.32**   **Postprocedural hemorrhage of eye and adnexa following other procedure**

  ▲ ⊟ **H59.321**   **Postprocedural hemorrhage of right eye and adnexa following other procedure**

  ▲ ⊟ **H59.322**   **Postprocedural hemorrhage of left eye and adnexa following other procedure**

  ▲ ⊟ **H59.323**   **Postprocedural hemorrhage of eye and adnexa following other procedure, bilateral**

  ▲ ⊟ **H59.329**   **Postprocedural hemorrhage of unspecified eye and adnexa following other procedure**

 ● Ⓖ **H59.33**   **Postprocedural hematoma of eye and adnexa following an ophthalmic procedure**

  ● ⊟ **H59.331**   **Postprocedural hematoma of right eye and adnexa following an ophthalmic procedure**

  ● ⊟ **H59.332**   **Postprocedural hematoma of left eye and adnexa following an ophthalmic procedure**

  ● ⊟ **H59.333**   **Postprocedural hematoma of eye and adnexa following an ophthalmic procedure, bilateral**

  ● ⊟ **H59.339**   **Postprocedural hematoma of unspecified eye and adnexa following an ophthalmic procedure**

 ● Ⓖ **H59.34**   **Postprocedural hematoma of eye and adnexa following other procedure**

  ● ⊟ **H59.341**   **Postprocedural hematoma of right eye and adnexa following other procedure**

  ● ⊟ **H59.342**   **Postprocedural hematoma of left eye and adnexa following other procedure**

  ● ⊟ **H59.343**   **Postprocedural hematoma of eye and adnexa following other procedure, bilateral**

  ● ⊟ **H59.349**   **Postprocedural hematoma of unspecified eye and adnexa following other procedure**

● New   ▲ Revised   *Manifestation*   ◳-◰ Digit Indicators   ⊟ Laterality   Ⓐ Adult (15+ years)   Ⓜ Maternity (12-55 years)   Ⓝ Newborn   Ⓟ Pediatric (0-17 years)   ♂ Male   ♀ Female
✖ Deleted̶   Unspecified   + Additional code

620   © 2017 DecisionHealth   2017 ICD-10-CM Expert for Physicians

● ⑥ **H59.35**   **Postprocedural seroma of eye and adnexa following an ophthalmic procedure**

  ● ⊟ **H59.351**   Postprocedural seroma of right eye and adnexa following an ophthalmic procedure

  ● ⊟ **H59.352**   Postprocedural seroma of left eye and adnexa following an ophthalmic procedure

  ● ⊟ **H59.353**   Postprocedural seroma of eye and adnexa following an ophthalmic procedure, bilateral

  ● ⊟ **H59.359**   Postprocedural seroma of unspecified eye and adnexa following an ophthalmic procedure

● ⑥ **H59.36**   **Postprocedural seroma of eye and adnexa following other procedure**

  ● ⊟ **H59.361**   Postprocedural seroma of right eye and adnexa following other procedure

  ● ⊟ **H59.362**   Postprocedural seroma of left eye and adnexa following other procedure

  ● ⊟ **H59.363**   Postprocedural seroma of eye and adnexa following other procedure, bilateral

  ● ⊟ **H59.369**   Postprocedural seroma of unspecified eye and adnexa following other procedure

⑤ **H59.4**   **Inflammation (infection) of postprocedural bleb**
   Postprocedural blebitis
   EXCLUDES 1   *filtering (vitreous) bleb after glaucoma surgery status (Z98.83)*

  H59.40   **Inflammation (infection) of postprocedural bleb, unspecified**

  H59.41   **Inflammation (infection) of postprocedural bleb, stage 1**

  H59.42   **Inflammation (infection) of postprocedural bleb, stage 2**

  H59.43   **Inflammation (infection) of postprocedural bleb, stage 3**
   Bleb endophthalmitis

⑤ **H59.8**   **Other intraoperative and postprocedural complications and disorders of eye and adnexa, not elsewhere classified**

  ⑥ **H59.81**   **Chorioretinal scars after surgery for detachment**

   ⊟ **H59.811**   Chorioretinal scars after surgery for detachment, right eye

   ⊟ **H59.812**   Chorioretinal scars after surgery for detachment, left eye

   ⊟ **H59.813**   Chorioretinal scars after surgery for detachment, bilateral

   ⊟ **H59.819**   Chorioretinal scars after surgery for detachment, unspecified eye

  H59.88   **Other intraoperative complications of eye and adnexa, not elsewhere classified**

  H59.89   **Other postprocedural complications and disorders of eye and adnexa, not elsewhere classified**

● New   ▲ Revised   *Manifestation*   ❹-❼ Digit Indicators   ⊟ Laterality   🅰 Adult (15+ years)   🅼 Maternity (12-55 years)   🅽 Newborn   🅿 Pediatric (0-17 years)   ♂ Male   ♀ Female
✖ Deleted   Unspecified   + Additional code

2017 ICD-10-CM Expert for Physicians   © 2017 DecisionHealth   621

CHAPTER 8: DISEASES OF THE EAR AND MASTOID PROCESS (H60-H95)

Note: Use an external cause code following the code for the ear condition, if applicable, to identify the cause of the ear condition

EXCLUDES 2
certain conditions originating in the perinatal period (P04-P96)
certain infectious and parasitic diseases (A00-B99)
complications of pregnancy, childbirth and the puerperium (O00-O9A)
congenital malformations, deformations and chromosomal abnormalities (Q00-Q99)
endocrine, nutritional and metabolic diseases (E00-E88)
injury, poisoning and certain other consequences of external causes (S00-T88)
neoplasms (C00-D49)
symptoms, signs and abnormal clinical and laboratory findings, not elsewhere classified (R00-R94)

This chapter contains the following blocks:
H60-H62	Diseases of external ear
H65-H75	Diseases of middle ear and mastoid
H80-H83	Diseases of inner ear
H90-H94	Other disorders of ear
H95	Intraoperative and postprocedural complications and disorders of ear and mastoid process, not elsewhere classified

Diseases of external ear (H60-H62)

H60 Otitis externa

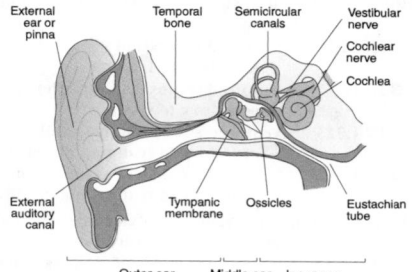

Diseases of Ear and Mastoid Process

Labels: External ear or pinna; Temporal bone; Semicircular canals; Vestibular nerve; Cochlear nerve; Cochlea; External auditory canal; Tympanic membrane; Ossicles; Eustachian tube; Outer ear; Middle ear; Inner ear

H60.0 Abscess of external ear
Boil of external ear
Carbuncle of auricle or external auditory canal
Furuncle of external ear

☐ H60.00 Abscess of external ear, unspecified ear
☐ H60.01 Abscess of right external ear
☐ H60.02 Abscess of left external ear
☐ H60.03 Abscess of external ear, bilateral

H60.1 Cellulitis of external ear
Cellulitis of auricle
Cellulitis of external auditory canal

☐ H60.10 Cellulitis of external ear, unspecified ear
☐ H60.11 Cellulitis of right external ear
☐ H60.12 Cellulitis of left external ear
☐ H60.13 Cellulitis of external ear, bilateral

H60.2 Malignant otitis externa
☐ H60.20 Malignant otitis externa, unspecified ear
☐ H60.21 Malignant otitis externa, right ear
☐ H60.22 Malignant otitis externa, left ear
☐ H60.23 Malignant otitis externa, bilateral

H60.3 Other infective otitis externa
H60.31 Diffuse otitis externa
☐ H60.311 Diffuse otitis externa, right ear
☐ H60.312 Diffuse otitis externa, left ear
☐ H60.313 Diffuse otitis externa, bilateral
☐ H60.319 Diffuse otitis externa, unspecified ear
H60.32 Hemorrhagic otitis externa
☐ H60.321 Hemorrhagic otitis externa, right ear
☐ H60.322 Hemorrhagic otitis externa, left ear
☐ H60.323 Hemorrhagic otitis externa, bilateral
☐ H60.329 Hemorrhagic otitis externa, unspecified ear
H60.33 Swimmer's ear
☐ H60.331 Swimmer's ear, right ear
☐ H60.332 Swimmer's ear, left ear
☐ H60.333 Swimmer's ear, bilateral
☐ H60.339 Swimmer's ear, unspecified ear
H60.39 Other infective otitis externa
☐ H60.391 Other infective otitis externa, right ear
☐ H60.392 Other infective otitis externa, left ear
☐ H60.393 Other infective otitis externa, bilateral
☐ H60.399 Other infective otitis externa, unspecified ear

H60.4 Cholesteatoma of external ear
Keratosis obturans of external ear (canal)
EXCLUDES 2 *cholesteatoma of middle ear (H71.-)*
recurrent cholesteatoma of postmastoidectomy cavity (H95.0-)
☐ H60.40 Cholesteatoma of external ear, unspecified ear
☐ H60.41 Cholesteatoma of right external ear
☐ H60.42 Cholesteatoma of left external ear
☐ H60.43 Cholesteatoma of external ear, bilateral

H60.5 Acute noninfective otitis externa
H60.50 Unspecified acute noninfective otitis externa
Acute otitis externa NOS
☐ H60.501 Unspecified acute noninfective otitis externa, right ear
☐ H60.502 Unspecified acute noninfective otitis externa, left ear
☐ H60.503 Unspecified acute noninfective otitis externa, bilateral
☐ H60.509 Unspecified acute noninfective otitis externa, unspecified ear
H60.51 Acute actinic otitis externa
☐ H60.511 Acute actinic otitis externa, right ear
☐ H60.512 Acute actinic otitis externa, left ear
☐ H60.513 Acute actinic otitis externa, bilateral
☐ H60.519 Acute actinic otitis externa, unspecified ear
H60.52 Acute chemical otitis externa
☐ H60.521 Acute chemical otitis externa, right ear
☐ H60.522 Acute chemical otitis externa, left ear
☐ H60.523 Acute chemical otitis externa, bilateral
☐ H60.529 Acute chemical otitis externa, unspecified ear
H60.53 Acute contact otitis externa
☐ H60.531 Acute contact otitis externa, right ear
☐ H60.532 Acute contact otitis externa, left ear
☐ H60.533 Acute contact otitis externa, bilateral
☐ H60.539 Acute contact otitis externa, unspecified ear
H60.54 Acute eczematoid otitis externa
☐ H60.541 Acute eczematoid otitis externa, right ear
☐ H60.542 Acute eczematoid otitis externa, left ear
☐ H60.543 Acute eczematoid otitis externa, bilateral
☐ H60.549 Acute eczematoid otitis externa, unspecified ear
H60.55 Acute reactive otitis externa
☐ H60.551 Acute reactive otitis externa, right ear
☐ H60.552 Acute reactive otitis externa, left ear
☐ H60.553 Acute reactive otitis externa, bilateral
☐ H60.559 Acute reactive otitis externa, unspecified ear
H60.59 Other noninfective acute otitis externa
☐ H60.591 Other noninfective acute otitis externa, right ear
☐ H60.592 Other noninfective acute otitis externa, left ear
☐ H60.593 Other noninfective acute otitis externa, bilateral
☐ H60.599 Other noninfective acute otitis externa, unspecified ear

H60.6 Unspecified chronic otitis externa
☐ H60.60 Unspecified chronic otitis externa, unspecified ear
☐ H60.61 Unspecified chronic otitis externa, right ear
☐ H60.62 Unspecified chronic otitis externa, left ear

● New ▲ Revised *Manifestation* ◀-▶ Digit Indicators ☐ Laterality Ⓐ Adult (15+ years) Ⓜ Maternity (12-55 years) Ⓝ Newborn Ⓟ Pediatric (0-17 years) ♂ Male ♀ Female
✖ Deleted Unspecified + Additional code

Diseases of the Ear and Mastoid Process

▱ H60.63   Unspecified chronic otitis externa, bilateral

⑤ H60.8   Other otitis externa

  ⑥ H60.8X   Other otitis externa

    ▱ H60.8X1   Other otitis externa, right ear

    ▱ H60.8X2   Other otitis externa, left ear

    ▱ H60.8X3   Other otitis externa, bilateral

    ▱ H60.8X9   Other otitis externa, unspecified ear

⑤ H60.9   Unspecified otitis externa

  ▱ H60.90   Unspecified otitis externa, unspecified ear

  ▱ H60.91   Unspecified otitis externa, right ear

  ▱ H60.92   Unspecified otitis externa, left ear

  ▱ H60.93   Unspecified otitis externa, bilateral

▱ **H61**   **Other disorders of external ear**

  ⑤ H61.0   Chondritis and perichondritis of external ear

    Chondrodermatitis nodularis chronica helicis
    Perichondritis of auricle
    Perichondritis of pinna

    DEFINITION   Inflammation of the cartilage of the outer, visible part of the ear.

  ⑥ H61.00   Unspecified perichondritis of external ear

    ▱ H61.001   Unspecified perichondritis of right external ear

    ▱ H61.002   Unspecified perichondritis of left external ear

    ▱ H61.003   Unspecified perichondritis of external ear, bilateral

    ▱ H61.009   Unspecified perichondritis of external ear, unspecified ear

  ⑥ H61.01   Acute perichondritis of external ear

    ▱ H61.011   Acute perichondritis of right external ear

    ▱ H61.012   Acute perichondritis of left external ear

    ▱ H61.013   Acute perichondritis of external ear, bilateral

    ▱ H61.019   Acute perichondritis of external ear, unspecified ear

  ⑥ H61.02   Chronic perichondritis of external ear

    ▱ H61.021   Chronic perichondritis of right external ear

    ▱ H61.022   Chronic perichondritis of left external ear

    ▱ H61.023   Chronic perichondritis of external ear, bilateral

    ▱ H61.029   Chronic perichondritis of external ear, unspecified ear

  ⑥ H61.03   Chondritis of external ear

    Chondritis of auricle
    Chondritis of pinna

    ▱ H61.031   Chondritis of right external ear

    ▱ H61.032   Chondritis of left external ear

      AHA: 1Q 2015, 18

    ▱ H61.033   Chondritis of external ear, bilateral

    ▱ H61.039   Chondritis of external ear, unspecified ear

  ⑤ H61.1   Noninfective disorders of pinna

    EXCLUDES 2   *cauliflower ear (M95.1-)*
                     gouty tophi of ear (M1A.-)

  ⑥ H61.10   Unspecified noninfective disorders of pinna

    Disorder of pinna NOS

    ▱ H61.101   Unspecified noninfective disorders of pinna, right ear

    ▱ H61.102   Unspecified noninfective disorders of pinna, left ear

    ▱ H61.103   Unspecified noninfective disorders of pinna, bilateral

    ▱ H61.109   Unspecified noninfective disorders of pinna, unspecified ear

  ⑥ H61.11   Acquired deformity of pinna

    Acquired deformity of auricle

    EXCLUDES 2   *cauliflower ear (M95.1-)*

    ▱ H61.111   Acquired deformity of pinna, right ear

    ▱ H61.112   Acquired deformity of pinna, left ear

    ▱ H61.113   Acquired deformity of pinna, bilateral

    ▱ H61.119   Acquired deformity of pinna, unspecified ear

  ⑥ H61.12   Hematoma of pinna

    Hematoma of auricle

    DEFINITION   Swelling filled with blood on the outer ear.

    ▱ H61.121   Hematoma of pinna, right ear

    ▱ H61.122   Hematoma of pinna, left ear

    ▱ H61.123   Hematoma of pinna, bilateral

    ▱ H61.129   Hematoma of pinna, unspecified ear

  ⑥ H61.19   Other noninfective disorders of pinna

    ▱ H61.191   Noninfective disorders of pinna, right ear

    ▱ H61.192   Noninfective disorders of pinna, left ear

    ▱ H61.193   Noninfective disorders of pinna, bilateral

    ▱ H61.199   Noninfective disorders of pinna, unspecified ear

⑤ H61.2   **Impacted cerumen**

  Wax in ear

  DEFINITION   Ear wax blocking the external ear canal.

  ▱ H61.20   Impacted cerumen, unspecified ear

  ▱ H61.21   Impacted cerumen, right ear

  ▱ H61.22   Impacted cerumen, left ear

  ▱ H61.23   Impacted cerumen, bilateral

⑤ H61.3   **Acquired stenosis of external ear canal**

  Collapse of external ear canal

  EXCLUDES 1   *postprocedural stenosis of external ear canal (H95.81-)*

  ⑥ H61.30   Acquired stenosis of external ear canal, unspecified

    ▱ H61.301   Acquired stenosis of right external ear canal, unspecified

    ▱ H61.302   Acquired stenosis of left external ear canal, unspecified

    ▱ H61.303   Acquired stenosis of external ear canal, unspecified, bilateral

    ▱ H61.309   Acquired stenosis of external ear canal, unspecified, unspecified ear

  ⑥ H61.31   Acquired stenosis of external ear canal secondary to trauma

    ▱ H61.311   Acquired stenosis of right external ear canal secondary to trauma

    ▱ H61.312   Acquired stenosis of left external ear canal secondary to trauma

    ▱ H61.313   Acquired stenosis of external ear canal secondary to trauma, bilateral

    ▱ H61.319   Acquired stenosis of external ear canal secondary to trauma, unspecified ear

  ⑥ H61.32   Acquired stenosis of external ear canal secondary to inflammation and infection

    ▱ H61.321   Acquired stenosis of right external ear canal secondary to inflammation and infection

    ▱ H61.322   Acquired stenosis of left external ear canal secondary to inflammation and infection

    ▱ H61.323   Acquired stenosis of external ear canal secondary to inflammation and infection, bilateral

    ▱ H61.329   Acquired stenosis of external ear canal secondary to inflammation and infection, unspecified ear

  ⑥ H61.39   Other acquired stenosis of external ear canal

    ▱ H61.391   Other acquired stenosis of right external ear canal

    ▱ H61.392   Other acquired stenosis of left external ear canal

    ▱ H61.393   Other acquired stenosis of external ear canal, bilateral

    ▱ H61.399   Other acquired stenosis of external ear canal, unspecified ear

⑤ H61.8   **Other specified disorders of external ear**

  ⑥ H61.81   Exostosis of external canal

    DEFINITION   A bony growth covered with cartilage on the outer ear.

    ▱ H61.811   Exostosis of right external canal

    ▱ H61.812   Exostosis of left external canal

    ▱ H61.813   Exostosis of external canal, bilateral

    ▱ H61.819   Exostosis of external canal, unspecified ear

  ⑥ H61.89   Other specified disorders of external ear

    ▱ H61.891   Other specified disorders of right external ear

    ▱ H61.892   Other specified disorders of left external ear

    ▱ H61.893   Other specified disorders of external ear, bilateral

    ▱ H61.899   Other specified disorders of external ear, unspecified ear

⑤ H61.9   **Disorder of external ear, unspecified**

● New   ▲ Revised   *Manifestation*   4-7 Digit Indicators   ▱ Laterality   Ⓐ Adult (15+ years)   Ⓜ Maternity (12-55 years)   Ⓝ Newborn   Ⓟ Pediatric (0-17 years)   ♂ Male   ♀ Female

✖ Deleted   Unspecified   + Additional code

⊟ H61.90   Disorder of external ear, unspecified, unspecified ear

⊟ H61.91   Disorder of right external ear, unspecified

⊟ H61.92   Disorder of left external ear, unspecified

⊟ H61.93   Disorder of external ear, unspecified, bilateral

◢ H62   **Disorders of external ear in diseases classified elsewhere**

⑤ H62.4   Otitis externa in other diseases classified elsewhere
Code first underlying disease, such as:
   erysipelas (A46)
   impetigo (L01.0)

> **EXCLUDES 1**   *otitis externa (in) :*
> *candidiasis (B37.84)*
> *herpes viral [herpes simplex] (B00.1)*
> *herpes zoster (B02.8)*

⊟ H62.40   *Otitis externa in other diseases classified elsewhere, unspecified ear*

⊟ H62.41   *Otitis externa in other diseases classified elsewhere, right ear*

⊟ H62.42   *Otitis externa in other diseases classified elsewhere, left ear*

⊟ H62.43   *Otitis externa in other diseases classified elsewhere, bilateral*

⑤ H62.8   Other disorders of external ear in diseases classified elsewhere
Code first underlying disease, such as:
   gout (M1A.-, M10.-)

⑥ H62.8X   Other disorders of external ear in diseases classified elsewhere

⊟ H62.8X1   Other disorders of right external ear in diseases classified elsewhere

⊟ H62.8X2   Other disorders of left external ear in diseases classified elsewhere

⊟ H62.8X3   Other disorders of external ear in diseases classified elsewhere, bilateral

⊟ H62.8X9   Other disorders of external ear in diseases classified elsewhere, unspecified ear

Diseases of middle ear and mastoid (H65-H75)

▲ ◢ + H65   **Nonsuppurative otitis media**

> **INCLUDES**   nonsuppurative otitis media with myringitis

Use additional code for any associated perforated tympanic membrane (H72.-)
Use additional code to identify:
exposure to environmental tobacco smoke (Z77.22)
exposure to tobacco smoke in the perinatal period (P96.81)
history of tobacco dependence (Z87.891)
occupational exposure to environmental tobacco smoke (Z57.31)
tobacco dependence (F17.-)
tobacco use (Z72.0)

⑤ + H65.0   Acute serous otitis media
Acute and subacute secretory otitis

⊟ + H65.00   Acute serous otitis media, unspecified ear

⊟ + H65.01   Acute serous otitis media, right ear

⊟ + H65.02   Acute serous otitis media, left ear

⊟ + H65.03   Acute serous otitis media, bilateral

⊟ + H65.04   Acute serous otitis media, recurrent, right ear

⊟ + H65.05   Acute serous otitis media, recurrent, left ear

⊟ + H65.06   Acute serous otitis media, recurrent, bilateral

⊟ + H65.07   Acute serous otitis media, recurrent, unspecified ear

⑤ + H65.1   Other acute nonsuppurative otitis media

> **EXCLUDES 1**   *otitic barotrauma (T70.0)*
> *otitis media (acute) NOS (H66.9)*

⑥ + H65.11   Acute and subacute allergic otitis media (mucoid) (sanguinous) (serous)

⊟ + H65.111   Acute and subacute allergic otitis media (mucoid) (sanguinous) (serous), right ear

⊟ + H65.112   Acute and subacute allergic otitis media (mucoid) (sanguinous) (serous), left ear

⊟ + H65.113   Acute and subacute allergic otitis media (mucoid) (sanguinous) (serous), bilateral

⊟ + H65.114   Acute and subacute allergic otitis media (mucoid) (sanguinous) (serous), recurrent, right ear

⊟ + H65.115   Acute and subacute allergic otitis media (mucoid) (sanguinous) (serous), recurrent, left ear

⊟ + H65.116   Acute and subacute allergic otitis media (mucoid) (sanguinous) (serous), recurrent, bilateral

⊟ + H65.117   Acute and subacute allergic otitis media (mucoid) (sanguinous) (serous), recurrent, unspecified ear

⊟ + H65.119   Acute and subacute allergic otitis media (mucoid) (sanguinous) (serous), unspecified ear

⑥ + H65.19   Other acute nonsuppurative otitis media
Acute and subacute mucoid otitis media
Acute and subacute nonsuppurative otitis media NOS
Acute and subacute sanguinous otitis media
Acute and subacute seromucinous otitis media

⊟ + H65.191   Other acute nonsuppurative otitis media, right ear

⊟ + H65.192   Other acute nonsuppurative otitis media, left ear

⊟ + H65.193   Other acute nonsuppurative otitis media, bilateral

⊟ + H65.194   Other acute nonsuppurative otitis media, recurrent, right ear

⊟ + H65.195   Other acute nonsuppurative otitis media, recurrent, left ear

⊟ + H65.196   Other acute nonsuppurative otitis media, recurrent, bilateral

⊟ + H65.197   Other acute nonsuppurative otitis media recurrent, unspecified ear

⊟ + H65.199   Other acute nonsuppurative otitis media, unspecified ear

⑤ + H65.2   Chronic serous otitis media
Chronic tubotympanal catarrh

⊟ + H65.20   Chronic serous otitis media, unspecified ear

⊟ + H65.21   Chronic serous otitis media, right ear

⊟ + H65.22   Chronic serous otitis media, left ear

⊟ + H65.23   Chronic serous otitis media, bilateral

⑤ + H65.3   Chronic mucoid otitis media
Chronic mucinous otitis media
Chronic secretory otitis media
Chronic transudative otitis media
Glue ear

> **EXCLUDES 1**   *adhesive middle ear disease (H74.1)*

> **DEFINITION**   Long-term middle ear infection causing mucous to become trapped in the middle ear.

⊟ + H65.30   Chronic mucoid otitis media, unspecified ear

⊟ + H65.31   Chronic mucoid otitis media, right ear

⊟ + H65.32   Chronic mucoid otitis media, left ear

⊟ + H65.33   Chronic mucoid otitis media, bilateral

⑤ + H65.4   Other chronic nonsuppurative otitis media

⑥ + H65.41   Chronic allergic otitis media

⊟ + H65.411   Chronic allergic otitis media, right ear

⊟ + H65.412   Chronic allergic otitis media, left ear

⊟ + H65.413   Chronic allergic otitis media, bilateral

⊟ + H65.419   Chronic allergic otitis media, unspecified ear

⑥ + H65.49   Other chronic nonsuppurative otitis media
Chronic exudative otitis media
Chronic nonsuppurative otitis media NOS
Chronic otitis media with effusion (nonpurulent)
Chronic seromucinous otitis media

⊟ + H65.491   Other chronic nonsuppurative otitis media, right ear

⊟ + H65.492   Other chronic nonsuppurative otitis media, left ear

⊟ + H65.493   Other chronic nonsuppurative otitis media, bilateral

⊟ + H65.499   Other chronic nonsuppurative otitis media, unspecified ear

---

● New   ▲ Revised   *Manifestation*   ◢-◗ Digit Indicators   ⊟ Laterality   Ⓐ Adult (15+ years)   Ⓜ Maternity (12-55 years)   Ⓝ Newborn   Ⓟ Pediatric (0-17 years)   ♂ Male   ♀ Female
✖ Deleted   Unspecified   + Additional code

2017 ICD-10-CM Expert for Physicians

© 2017 DecisionHealth

625

H61.90 — H65.499

H65.9 Unspecified nonsuppurative otitis media
Allergic otitis media NOS
Catarrhal otitis media NOS
Exudative otitis media NOS
Mucoid otitis media NOS
Otitis media with effusion (nonpurulent) NOS
Secretory otitis media NOS
Seromucinous otitis media NOS
Serous otitis media NOS
Transudative otitis media NOS

H65.90 Unspecified nonsuppurative otitis media, unspecified ear

H65.91 Unspecified nonsuppurative otitis media, right ear

H65.92 Unspecified nonsuppurative otitis media, left ear

H65.93 Unspecified nonsuppurative otitis media, bilateral

▲ H66 Suppurative and unspecified otitis media

INCLUDES suppurative and unspecified otitis media with myringitis
Use additional code to identify:
exposure to environmental tobacco smoke (Z77.22)
exposure to tobacco smoke in the perinatal period (P96.81)
history of tobacco dependence (Z87.891)
occupational exposure to environmental tobacco smoke (Z57.31)
tobacco dependence (F17.-)
tobacco use (Z72.0)

H66.0 Acute suppurative otitis media

H66.00 Acute suppurative otitis media without spontaneous rupture of ear drum

H66.001 Acute suppurative otitis media without spontaneous rupture of ear drum, right ear
AHA: 1Q 2016, 34

H66.002 Acute suppurative otitis media without spontaneous rupture of ear drum, left ear

H66.003 Acute suppurative otitis media without spontaneous rupture of ear drum, bilateral

H66.004 Acute suppurative otitis media without spontaneous rupture of ear drum, recurrent, right ear

H66.005 Acute suppurative otitis media without spontaneous rupture of ear drum, recurrent, left ear

H66.006 Acute suppurative otitis media without spontaneous rupture of ear drum, recurrent, bilateral

H66.007 Acute suppurative otitis media without spontaneous rupture of ear drum, recurrent, unspecified ear

H66.009 Acute suppurative otitis media without spontaneous rupture of ear drum, unspecified ear

H66.01 Acute suppurative otitis media with spontaneous rupture of ear drum

H66.011 Acute suppurative otitis media with spontaneous rupture of ear drum, right ear

H66.012 Acute suppurative otitis media with spontaneous rupture of ear drum, left ear

H66.013 Acute suppurative otitis media with spontaneous rupture of ear drum, bilateral

H66.014 Acute suppurative otitis media with spontaneous rupture of ear drum, recurrent, right ear

H66.015 Acute suppurative otitis media with spontaneous rupture of ear drum, recurrent, left ear

H66.016 Acute suppurative otitis media with spontaneous rupture of ear drum, recurrent, bilateral

H66.017 Acute suppurative otitis media with spontaneous rupture of ear drum, recurrent, unspecified ear

H66.019 Acute suppurative otitis media with spontaneous rupture of ear drum, unspecified ear

H66.1 Chronic tubotympanic suppurative otitis media
Benign chronic suppurative otitis media
Chronic tubotympanic disease
Use additional code for any associated perforated tympanic membrane (H72.-)

H66.10 Chronic tubotympanic suppurative otitis media, unspecified

H66.11 Chronic tubotympanic suppurative otitis media, right ear

H66.12 Chronic tubotympanic suppurative otitis media, left ear

H66.13 Chronic tubotympanic suppurative otitis media, bilateral

H66.2 Chronic atticoantral suppurative otitis media
Chronic atticoantral disease
Use additional code for any associated perforated tympanic membrane (H72.-)

H66.20 Chronic atticoantral suppurative otitis media, unspecified ear

H66.21 Chronic atticoantral suppurative otitis media, right ear

H66.22 Chronic atticoantral suppurative otitis media, left ear

H66.23 Chronic atticoantral suppurative otitis media, bilateral

H66.3 Other chronic suppurative otitis media
Chronic suppurative otitis media NOS
Use additional code for any associated perforated tympanic membrane (H72.-)
EXCLUDES 1 *tuberculous otitis media (A18.6)*

H66.3X Other chronic suppurative otitis media

H66.3X1 Other chronic suppurative otitis media, right ear

H66.3X2 Other chronic suppurative otitis media, left ear

H66.3X3 Other chronic suppurative otitis media, bilateral

H66.3X9 Other chronic suppurative otitis media, unspecified ear

H66.4 Suppurative otitis media, unspecified
Purulent otitis media NOS
Use additional code for any associated perforated tympanic membrane (H72.-)

H66.40 Suppurative otitis media, unspecified, unspecified ear

H66.41 Suppurative otitis media, unspecified, right ear

H66.42 Suppurative otitis media, unspecified, left ear

H66.43 Suppurative otitis media, unspecified, bilateral

H66.9 Otitis media, unspecified
Otitis media NOS
Acute otitis media NOS
Chronic otitis media NOS
Use additional code for any associated perforated tympanic membrane (H72.-)

H66.90 Otitis media, unspecified, unspecified ear

H66.91 Otitis media, unspecified, right ear

H66.92 Otitis media, unspecified, left ear

H66.93 Otitis media, unspecified, bilateral

H67 Otitis media in diseases classified elsewhere
Code first underlying disease, such as:
viral disease NEC (B00-B34)
Use additional code for any associated perforated tympanic membrane (H72.-)
EXCLUDES 1 *otitis media in:*
influenza (J09.X9, J10.83, J11.83)
measles (B05.3)
scarlet fever (A38.0)
tuberculosis (A18.6)

H67.1 *Otitis media in diseases classified elsewhere, right ear*

H67.2 *Otitis media in diseases classified elsewhere, left ear*

H67.3 *Otitis media in diseases classified elsewhere, bilateral*

H67.9 *Otitis media in diseases classified elsewhere, unspecified ear*

H68 Eustachian salpingitis and obstruction

H68.0 Eustachian salpingitis

H68.00 Unspecified Eustachian salpingitis

H68.001 Unspecified Eustachian salpingitis, right ear

H68.002 Unspecified Eustachian salpingitis, left ear

H68.003 Unspecified Eustachian salpingitis, bilateral

H68.009 Unspecified Eustachian salpingitis, unspecified ear

H68.01 Acute Eustachian salpingitis

H68.011   Acute Eustachian salpingitis, right ear
H68.012   Acute Eustachian salpingitis, left ear
H68.013   Acute Eustachian salpingitis, bilateral
H68.019   Acute Eustachian salpingitis, unspecified ear
H68.02   Chronic Eustachian salpingitis
H68.021   Chronic Eustachian salpingitis, right ear
H68.022   Chronic Eustachian salpingitis, left ear
H68.023   Chronic Eustachian salpingitis, bilateral
H68.029   Chronic Eustachian salpingitis, unspecified ear
H68.1   Obstruction of Eustachian tube
Stenosis of Eustachian tube
Stricture of Eustachian tube
H68.10   Unspecified obstruction of Eustachian tube
H68.101   Unspecified obstruction of Eustachian tube, right ear
H68.102   Unspecified obstruction of Eustachian tube, left ear
H68.103   Unspecified obstruction of Eustachian tube, bilateral
H68.109   Unspecified obstruction of Eustachian tube, unspecified ear
H68.11   Osseous obstruction of Eustachian tube
H68.111   Osseous obstruction of Eustachian tube, right ear
H68.112   Osseous obstruction of Eustachian tube, left ear
H68.113   Osseous obstruction of Eustachian tube, bilateral
H68.119   Osseous obstruction of Eustachian tube, unspecified ear
H68.12   Intrinsic cartilagenous obstruction of Eustachian tube
H68.121   Intrinsic cartilagenous obstruction of Eustachian tube, right ear
H68.122   Intrinsic cartilagenous obstruction of Eustachian tube, left ear
H68.123   Intrinsic cartilagenous obstruction of Eustachian tube, bilateral
H68.129   Intrinsic cartilagenous obstruction of Eustachian tube, unspecified ear
H68.13   Extrinsic cartilagenous obstruction of Eustachian tube
Compression of Eustachian tube
H68.131   Extrinsic cartilagenous obstruction of Eustachian tube, right ear
H68.132   Extrinsic cartilagenous obstruction of Eustachian tube, left ear
H68.133   Extrinsic cartilagenous obstruction of Eustachian tube, bilateral
H68.139   Extrinsic cartilagenous obstruction of Eustachian tube, unspecified ear
H69   Other and unspecified disorders of Eustachian tube
H69.0   Patulous Eustachian tube
H69.00   Patulous Eustachian tube, unspecified ear
H69.01   Patulous Eustachian tube, right ear
H69.02   Patulous Eustachian tube, left ear
H69.03   Patulous Eustachian tube, bilateral
H69.8   Other specified disorders of Eustachian tube
H69.80   Other specified disorders of Eustachian tube, unspecified ear
H69.81   Other specified disorders of Eustachian tube, right ear
H69.82   Other specified disorders of Eustachian tube, left ear
H69.83   Other specified disorders of Eustachian tube, bilateral
H69.9   Unspecified Eustachian tube disorder
H69.90   Unspecified Eustachian tube disorder, unspecified ear
H69.91   Unspecified Eustachian tube disorder, right ear
H69.92   Unspecified Eustachian tube disorder, left ear
H69.93   Unspecified Eustachian tube disorder, bilateral
H70   Mastoiditis and related conditions
H70.0   Acute mastoiditis
Abscess of mastoid
Empyema of mastoid

H70.00   Acute mastoiditis without complications
H70.001   Acute mastoiditis without complications, right ear
H70.002   Acute mastoiditis without complications, left ear
H70.003   Acute mastoiditis without complications, bilateral
H70.009   Acute mastoiditis without complications, unspecified ear
H70.01   Subperiosteal abscess of mastoid
H70.011   Subperiosteal abscess of mastoid, right ear
H70.012   Subperiosteal abscess of mastoid, left ear
H70.013   Subperiosteal abscess of mastoid, bilateral
H70.019   Subperiosteal abscess of mastoid, unspecified ear
H70.09   Acute mastoiditis with other complications
H70.091   Acute mastoiditis with other complications, right ear
H70.092   Acute mastoiditis with other complications, left ear
H70.093   Acute mastoiditis with other complications, bilateral
H70.099   Acute mastoiditis with other complications, unspecified ear
H70.1   Chronic mastoiditis
Caries of mastoid
Fistula of mastoid
    EXCLUDES 1   tuberculous mastoiditis (A18.03)
H70.10   Chronic mastoiditis, unspecified ear
H70.11   Chronic mastoiditis, right ear
H70.12   Chronic mastoiditis, left ear
H70.13   Chronic mastoiditis, bilateral
H70.2   Petrositis
Inflammation of petrous bone
H70.20   Unspecified petrositis
    DEFINITION   Inflammation of the dense, hard bone behind the temple protecting the inner ear.
H70.201   Unspecified petrositis, right ear
H70.202   Unspecified petrositis, left ear
H70.203   Unspecified petrositis, bilateral
H70.209   Unspecified petrositis, unspecified ear
H70.21   Acute petrositis
H70.211   Acute petrositis, right ear
H70.212   Acute petrositis, left ear
H70.213   Acute petrositis, bilateral
H70.219   Acute petrositis, unspecified ear
H70.22   Chronic petrositis
H70.221   Chronic petrositis, right ear
H70.222   Chronic petrositis, left ear
H70.223   Chronic petrositis, bilateral
H70.229   Chronic petrositis, unspecified ear
H70.8   Other mastoiditis and related conditions
    EXCLUDES 1   preauricular sinus and cyst (Q18.1)
    sinus, fistula, and cyst of branchial cleft (Q18.0)
H70.81   Postauricular fistula
H70.811   Postauricular fistula, right ear
H70.812   Postauricular fistula, left ear
H70.813   Postauricular fistula, bilateral
H70.819   Postauricular fistula, unspecified ear
H70.89   Other mastoiditis and related conditions
H70.891   Other mastoiditis and related conditions, right ear
H70.892   Other mastoiditis and related conditions, left ear
H70.893   Other mastoiditis and related conditions, bilateral
H70.899   Other mastoiditis and related conditions, unspecified ear
H70.9   Unspecified mastoiditis
H70.90   Unspecified mastoiditis, unspecified ear
H70.91   Unspecified mastoiditis, right ear

● New   ▲ Revised   *Manifestation*   4-7 Digit Indicators   ⊟ Laterality   A Adult (15+ years)   M Maternity (12-55 years)   N Newborn   P Pediatric (0-17 years)   ♂ Male   ♀ Female
✖ Deleted   Unspecified   + Additional code

Diseases of the Ear and Mastoid Process

⊟ **H70.92** Unspecified mastoiditis, left ear

⊟ **H70.93** Unspecified mastoiditis, bilateral

◢ **H71** **Cholesteatoma of middle ear**

> **EXCLUDES 2** *cholesteatoma of external ear (H60.4-)*
> *recurrent cholesteatoma of postmastoidectomy cavity (H95.0-)*

> **DEFINITION** Cyst-like mass filled with cell debris and cholesterol crystals in the middle ear and/or mastoid process that can damage the ossicles, causing deafness, vertigo, and nerve deterioration.

⑤ **H71.0** Cholesteatoma of attic

⊟ **H71.00** Cholesteatoma of attic, unspecified ear

⊟ **H71.01** Cholesteatoma of attic, right ear

⊟ **H71.02** Cholesteatoma of attic, left ear

⊟ **H71.03** Cholesteatoma of attic, bilateral

⑤ **H71.1** Cholesteatoma of tympanum

⊟ **H71.10** Cholesteatoma of tympanum, unspecified ear

⊟ **H71.11** Cholesteatoma of tympanum, right ear

⊟ **H71.12** Cholesteatoma of tympanum, left ear

⊟ **H71.13** Cholesteatoma of tympanum, bilateral

⑤ **H71.2** Cholesteatoma of mastoid

⊟ **H71.20** Cholesteatoma of mastoid, unspecified ear

⊟ **H71.21** Cholesteatoma of mastoid, right ear

⊟ **H71.22** Cholesteatoma of mastoid, left ear

⊟ **H71.23** Cholesteatoma of mastoid, bilateral

⑤ **H71.3** Diffuse cholesteatosis

⊟ **H71.30** Diffuse cholesteatosis, unspecified ear

⊟ **H71.31** Diffuse cholesteatosis, right ear

⊟ **H71.32** Diffuse cholesteatosis, left ear

⊟ **H71.33** Diffuse cholesteatosis, bilateral

⑤ **H71.9** Unspecified cholesteatoma

⊟ **H71.90** Unspecified cholesteatoma, unspecified ear

⊟ **H71.91** Unspecified cholesteatoma, right ear

⊟ **H71.92** Unspecified cholesteatoma, left ear

⊟ **H71.93** Unspecified cholesteatoma, bilateral

◢ **H72** **Perforation of tympanic membrane**

> **INCLUDES** persistent post-traumatic perforation of ear drum
> postinflammatory perforation of ear drum

> Code first:
> any associated otitis media
> (H65.-, H66.1-, H66.2-, H66.3-, H66.4-, H66.9-, H67.-)

> **EXCLUDES 1** *acute suppurative otitis media with rupture of the tympanic membrane (H66.01-)*
> *traumatic rupture of ear drum (S09.2-)*

Perforation of tympanic membrane

Temporal bone
Semicircular canals
Vestibular nerve
Cochlea
The tympanic membrane is perforated
Ossicles
Eustachian tube

Outer ear | Middle ear | Inner ear

⑤ **H72.0** Central perforation of tympanic membrane

⊟ **H72.00** Central perforation of tympanic membrane, unspecified ear

⊟ **H72.01** Central perforation of tympanic membrane, right ear

⊟ **H72.02** Central perforation of tympanic membrane, left ear

⊟ **H72.03** Central perforation of tympanic membrane, bilateral

⑤ **H72.1** Attic perforation of tympanic membrane
Perforation of pars flaccida

⊟ **H72.10** Attic perforation of tympanic membrane, unspecified ear

⊟ **H72.11** Attic perforation of tympanic membrane, right ear

⊟ **H72.12** Attic perforation of tympanic membrane, left ear

⊟ **H72.13** Attic perforation of tympanic membrane, bilateral

⑤ **H72.2** Other marginal perforations of tympanic membrane

⑥ **H72.2X** Other marginal perforations of tympanic membrane

⊟ **H72.2X1** Other marginal perforations of tympanic membrane, right ear

⊟ **H72.2X2** Other marginal perforations of tympanic membrane, left ear

⊟ **H72.2X3** Other marginal perforations of tympanic membrane, bilateral

⊟ **H72.2X9** Other marginal perforations of tympanic membrane, unspecified ear

⑤ **H72.8** Other perforations of tympanic membrane

⑥ **H72.81** Multiple perforations of tympanic membrane

⊟ **H72.811** Multiple perforations of tympanic membrane, right ear

⊟ **H72.812** Multiple perforations of tympanic membrane, left ear

⊟ **H72.813** Multiple perforations of tympanic membrane, bilateral

⊟ **H72.819** Multiple perforations of tympanic membrane, unspecified ear

⑥ **H72.82** Total perforations of tympanic membrane

⊟ **H72.821** Total perforations of tympanic membrane, right ear

⊟ **H72.822** Total perforations of tympanic membrane, left ear

⊟ **H72.823** Total perforations of tympanic membrane, bilateral

⊟ **H72.829** Total perforations of tympanic membrane, unspecified ear

⑤ **H72.9** Unspecified perforation of tympanic membrane

⊟ **H72.90** Unspecified perforation of tympanic membrane, unspecified ear

⊟ **H72.91** Unspecified perforation of tympanic membrane, right ear

⊟ **H72.92** Unspecified perforation of tympanic membrane, left ear

⊟ **H72.93** Unspecified perforation of tympanic membrane, bilateral

◢ **H73** **Other disorders of tympanic membrane**

⑤ **H73.0** Acute myringitis

> **EXCLUDES 1** *acute myringitis with otitis media (H65, H66)*

⑥ **H73.00** Unspecified acute myringitis
Acute tympanitis NOS

⊟ **H73.001** Acute myringitis, right ear

⊟ **H73.002** Acute myringitis, left ear

⊟ **H73.003** Acute myringitis, bilateral

⊟ **H73.009** Acute myringitis, unspecified ear

⑥ **H73.01** Bullous myringitis

> **DEFINITION** Inflammation of the eardrum caused by a virus and characterized by blood-filled blisters.

⊟ **H73.011** Bullous myringitis, right ear

⊟ **H73.012** Bullous myringitis, left ear

⊟ **H73.013** Bullous myringitis, bilateral

⊟ **H73.019** Bullous myringitis, unspecified ear

⑥ **H73.09** Other acute myringitis

⊟ **H73.091** Other acute myringitis, right ear

⊟ **H73.092** Other acute myringitis, left ear

⊟ **H73.093** Other acute myringitis, bilateral

⊟ **H73.099** Other acute myringitis, unspecified ear

⑤ **H73.1** Chronic myringitis
Chronic tympanitis

> **EXCLUDES 1** *chronic myringitis with otitis media (H65, H66)*

⊟ **H73.10** Chronic myringitis, unspecified ear

⊟ **H73.11** Chronic myringitis, right ear

⊟ **H73.12** Chronic myringitis, left ear

⊟ **H73.13** Chronic myringitis, bilateral

● New ▲ Revised *Manifestation* ◢-❼ Digit Indicators ⊟ Laterality Ⓐ Adult (15+ years) Ⓜ Maternity (12-55 years) Ⓝ Newborn Ⓟ Pediatric (0-17 years) ♂ Male ♀ Female
✖ Deleted Unspecified + Additional code

⑤ **H73.2** **Unspecified myringitis**
- ☐ H73.20 Unspecified myringitis, unspecified ear
- ☐ H73.21 Unspecified myringitis, right ear
- ☐ H73.22 Unspecified myringitis, left ear
- ☐ H73.23 Unspecified myringitis, bilateral

⑤ **H73.8** **Other specified disorders of tympanic membrane**
- ⑥ H73.81 Atrophic flaccid tympanic membrane
  > **DEFINITION** Eardrum that has wasted away and lost its tension, resulting in severe hearing loss.
  - ☐ H73.811 Atrophic flaccid tympanic membrane, right ear
  - ☐ H73.812 Atrophic flaccid tympanic membrane, left ear
  - ☐ H73.813 Atrophic flaccid tympanic membrane, bilateral
  - ☐ H73.819 Atrophic flaccid tympanic membrane, unspecified ear
- ⑥ H73.82 Atrophic nonflaccid tympanic membrane
  - ☐ H73.821 Atrophic nonflaccid tympanic membrane, right ear
  - ☐ H73.822 Atrophic nonflaccid tympanic membrane, left ear
  - ☐ H73.823 Atrophic nonflaccid tympanic membrane, bilateral
  - ☐ H73.829 Atrophic nonflaccid tympanic membrane, unspecified ear
- ⑥ H73.89 Other specified disorders of tympanic membrane
  - ☐ H73.891 Other specified disorders of tympanic membrane, right ear
  - ☐ H73.892 Other specified disorders of tympanic membrane, left ear
  - ☐ H73.893 Other specified disorders of tympanic membrane, bilateral
  - ☐ H73.899 Other specified disorders of tympanic membrane, unspecified ear

⑤ **H73.9** **Unspecified disorder of tympanic membrane**
- ☐ H73.90 Unspecified disorder of tympanic membrane, unspecified ear
- ☐ H73.91 Unspecified disorder of tympanic membrane, right ear
- ☐ H73.92 Unspecified disorder of tympanic membrane, left ear
- ☐ H73.93 Unspecified disorder of tympanic membrane, bilateral

④ **H74** **Other disorders of middle ear mastoid**
> **EXCLUDES 2** mastoiditis (H70.-)

⑤ **H74.0** **Tympanosclerosis**
> **DEFINITION** Thickening and hardening of the eardrum, reducing its ability to vibrate and transmit sound.
- ☐ H74.01 Tympanosclerosis, right ear
- ☐ H74.02 Tympanosclerosis, left ear
- ☐ H74.03 Tympanosclerosis, bilateral
- ☐ H74.09 Tympanosclerosis, unspecified ear

⑤ **H74.1** **Adhesive middle ear disease**
Adhesive otitis
> **EXCLUDES 1** glue ear (H65.3-)
- ☐ H74.11 Adhesive right middle ear disease
- ☐ H74.12 Adhesive left middle ear disease
- ☐ H74.13 Adhesive middle ear disease, bilateral
- ☐ H74.19 Adhesive middle ear disease, unspecified ear

⑤ **H74.2** **Discontinuity and dislocation of ear ossicles**
- ☐ H74.20 Discontinuity and dislocation of ear ossicles, unspecified ear
- ☐ H74.21 Discontinuity and dislocation of right ear ossicles
- ☐ H74.22 Discontinuity and dislocation of left ear ossicles
- ☐ H74.23 Discontinuity and dislocation of ear ossicles, bilateral

⑤ **H74.3** **Other acquired abnormalities of ear ossicles**
- ⑥ H74.31 Ankylosis of ear ossicles
  - ☐ H74.311 Ankylosis of ear ossicles, right ear
  - ☐ H74.312 Ankylosis of ear ossicles, left ear
  - ☐ H74.313 Ankylosis of ear ossicles, bilateral
  - ☐ H74.319 Ankylosis of ear ossicles, unspecified ear
- ⑥ H74.32 Partial loss of ear ossicles
  - ☐ H74.321 Partial loss of ear ossicles, right ear
  - ☐ H74.322 Partial loss of ear ossicles, left ear
  - ☐ H74.323 Partial loss of ear ossicles, bilateral
  - ☐ H74.329 Partial loss of ear ossicles, unspecified ear
- ⑥ H74.39 Other acquired abnormalities of ear ossicles
  - ☐ H74.391 Other acquired abnormalities of right ear ossicles
  - ☐ H74.392 Other acquired abnormalities of left ear ossicles
  - ☐ H74.393 Other acquired abnormalities of ear ossicles, bilateral
  - ☐ H74.399 Other acquired abnormalities of ear ossicles, unspecified ear

⑤ **H74.4** **Polyp of middle ear**
- ☐ H74.40 Polyp of middle ear, unspecified ear
- ☐ H74.41 Polyp of right middle ear
- ☐ H74.42 Polyp of left middle ear
- ☐ H74.43 Polyp of middle ear, bilateral

⑤ **H74.8** **Other specified disorders of middle ear and mastoid**
- ⑥ H74.8X Other specified disorders of middle ear and mastoid
  - ☐ H74.8X1 Other specified disorders of right middle ear and mastoid
  - ☐ H74.8X2 Other specified disorders of left middle ear and mastoid
  - ☐ H74.8X3 Other specified disorders of middle ear and mastoid, bilateral
  - ☐ H74.8X9 Other specified disorders of middle ear and mastoid, unspecified ear

⑤ **H74.9** **Unspecified disorder of middle ear and mastoid**
- ☐ H74.90 Unspecified disorder of middle ear and mastoid, unspecified ear
- ☐ H74.91 Unspecified disorder of right middle ear and mastoid
- ☐ H74.92 Unspecified disorder of left middle ear and mastoid
- ☐ H74.93 Unspecified disorder of middle ear and mastoid, bilateral

④ **H75** **Other disorders of middle ear and mastoid in diseases classified elsewhere**
Code first:
underlying disease

⑤ **H75.0** **Mastoiditis in infectious and parasitic diseases classified elsewhere**
> **EXCLUDES 1** mastoiditis (in) :
> syphilis (A52.77)
> tuberculosis (A18.03)
- ☐ H75.00 *Mastoiditis in infectious and parasitic diseases classified elsewhere, unspecified ear*
- ☐ H75.01 *Mastoiditis in infectious and parasitic diseases classified elsewhere, right ear*
- ☐ H75.02 *Mastoiditis in infectious and parasitic diseases classified elsewhere, left ear*
- ☐ H75.03 *Mastoiditis in infectious and parasitic diseases classified elsewhere, bilateral*

⑤ **H75.8** **Other specified disorders of middle ear and mastoid in diseases classified elsewhere**
- ☐ H75.80 Other specified disorders of middle ear and mastoid in diseases classified elsewhere, unspecified ear
- ☐ H75.81 Other specified disorders of right middle ear and mastoid in diseases classified elsewhere
- ☐ H75.82 Other specified disorders of left middle ear and mastoid in diseases classified elsewhere
- ☐ H75.83 Other specified disorders of middle ear and mastoid in diseases classified elsewhere, bilateral

Diseases of inner ear (H80-H83)

④ **H80** **Otosclerosis**
> **INCLUDES** Otospongiosis

⑤ **H80.0** **Otosclerosis involving oval window, nonobliterative**
- ☐ H80.00 Otosclerosis involving oval window, nonobliterative, unspecified ear
- ☐ H80.01 Otosclerosis involving oval window, nonobliterative, right ear
- ☐ H80.02 Otosclerosis involving oval window, nonobliterative, left ear
- ☐ H80.03 Otosclerosis involving oval window, nonobliterative, bilateral

---

● New ▲ Revised *Manifestation* ④-⑦ Digit Indicators ☐ Laterality Ⓐ Adult (15+ years) Ⓜ Maternity (12-55 years) Ⓝ Newborn Ⓟ Pediatric (0-17 years) ♂ Male ♀ Female
✖ Deleted Unspecified + Additional code

H80.1 Otosclerosis involving oval window, obliterative
- **H80.10** Otosclerosis involving oval window, obliterative, unspecified ear
- **H80.11** Otosclerosis involving oval window, obliterative, right ear
- **H80.12** Otosclerosis involving oval window, obliterative, left ear
- **H80.13** Otosclerosis involving oval window, obliterative, bilateral

H80.2 Cochlear otosclerosis
Otosclerosis involving otic capsule
Otosclerosis involving round window

DEFINITION Formation of bony tissue in the cochlea, causing hearing loss.
- **H80.20** Cochlear otosclerosis, unspecified ear
- **H80.21** Cochlear otosclerosis, right ear
- **H80.22** Cochlear otosclerosis, left ear
- **H80.23** Cochlear otosclerosis, bilateral

H80.8 Other otosclerosis
- **H80.80** Other otosclerosis, unspecified ear
- **H80.81** Other otosclerosis, right ear
- **H80.82** Other otosclerosis, left ear
- **H80.83** Other otosclerosis, bilateral

H80.9 Unspecified otosclerosis
- **H80.90** Unspecified otosclerosis, unspecified ear
- **H80.91** Unspecified otosclerosis, right ear
- **H80.92** Unspecified otosclerosis, left ear
- **H80.93** Unspecified otosclerosis, bilateral

H81 Disorders of vestibular function
EXCLUDES 1 epidemic vertigo (A88.1)
vertigo NOS (R42)

H81.0 Ménière's disease
Labyrinthine hydrops
Ménière's syndrome or vertigo

DEFINITION Disorder of the inner ear causing attacks of vertigo, tinnitus, and progressive hearing loss involving all tones.
- **H81.01** Ménière's disease, right ear
- **H81.02** Ménière's disease, left ear
- **H81.03** Ménière's disease, bilateral
- **H81.09** Ménière's disease, unspecified ear

H81.1 Benign paroxysmal vertigo
- **H81.10** Benign paroxysmal vertigo, unspecified ear
- **H81.11** Benign paroxysmal vertigo, right ear
- **H81.12** Benign paroxysmal vertigo, left ear
- **H81.13** Benign paroxysmal vertigo, bilateral

H81.2 Vestibular neuronitis
- **H81.20** Vestibular neuronitis, unspecified ear
- **H81.21** Vestibular neuronitis, right ear
- **H81.22** Vestibular neuronitis, left ear
- **H81.23** Vestibular neuronitis, bilateral

H81.3 Other peripheral vertigo
H81.31 Aural vertigo
- **H81.311** Aural vertigo, right ear
- **H81.312** Aural vertigo, left ear
- **H81.313** Aural vertigo, bilateral
- **H81.319** Aural vertigo, unspecified ear

H81.39 Other peripheral vertigo
Lermoyez' syndrome
Otogenic vertigo
Peripheral vertigo NOS
- **H81.391** Other peripheral vertigo, right ear
- **H81.392** Other peripheral vertigo, left ear
- **H81.393** Other peripheral vertigo, bilateral
- **H81.399** Other peripheral vertigo, unspecified ear

H81.4 Vertigo of central origin
Central positional nystagmus
- **H81.41** Vertigo of central origin, right ear
- **H81.42** Vertigo of central origin, left ear
- **H81.43** Vertigo of central origin, bilateral
- **H81.49** Vertigo of central origin, unspecified ear

H81.8 Other disorders of vestibular function

H81.8X Other disorders of vestibular function
- **H81.8X1** Other disorders of vestibular function, right ear
- **H81.8X2** Other disorders of vestibular function, left ear
- **H81.8X3** Other disorders of vestibular function, bilateral
- **H81.8X9** Other disorders of vestibular function, unspecified ear

H81.9 Unspecified disorder of vestibular function
Vertiginous syndrome NOS
- **H81.90** Unspecified disorder of vestibular function, unspecified ear
- **H81.91** Unspecified disorder of vestibular function, right ear
- **H81.92** Unspecified disorder of vestibular function, left ear
- **H81.93** Unspecified disorder of vestibular function, bilateral

H82 Vertiginous syndromes in diseases classified elsewhere
Code first:
underlying disease
EXCLUDES 1 epidemic vertigo (A88.1)
- **H82.1** Vertiginous syndromes in diseases classified elsewhere, right ear
- **H82.2** Vertiginous syndromes in diseases classified elsewhere, left ear
- **H82.3** Vertiginous syndromes in diseases classified elsewhere, bilateral
- **H82.9** Vertiginous syndromes in diseases classified elsewhere, unspecified ear

H83 Other diseases of inner ear
H83.0 Labyrinthitis
- **H83.01** Labyrinthitis, right ear
- **H83.02** Labyrinthitis, left ear
- **H83.03** Labyrinthitis, bilateral
- **H83.09** Labyrinthitis, unspecified ear

H83.1 Labyrinthine fistula
- **H83.11** Labyrinthine fistula, right ear
- **H83.12** Labyrinthine fistula, left ear
- **H83.13** Labyrinthine fistula, bilateral
- **H83.19** Labyrinthine fistula, unspecified ear

H83.2 Labyrinthine dysfunction
Labyrinthine hypersensitivity
Labyrinthine hypofunction
Labyrinthine loss of function
H83.2X Labyrinthine dysfunction
- **H83.2X1** Labyrinthine dysfunction, right ear
- **H83.2X2** Labyrinthine dysfunction, left ear
- **H83.2X3** Labyrinthine dysfunction, bilateral
- **H83.2X9** Labyrinthine dysfunction, unspecified ear

H83.3 Noise effects on inner ear
Acoustic trauma of inner ear
Noise-induced hearing loss of inner ear
H83.3X Noise effects on inner ear
- **H83.3X1** Noise effects on right inner ear
- **H83.3X2** Noise effects on left inner ear
- **H83.3X3** Noise effects on inner ear, bilateral
- **H83.3X9** Noise effects on inner ear, unspecified ear

H83.8 Other specified diseases of inner ear
H83.8X Other specified diseases of inner ear
- **H83.8X1** Other specified diseases of right inner ear
- **H83.8X2** Other specified diseases of left inner ear
- **H83.8X3** Other specified diseases of inner ear, bilateral
- **H83.8X9** Other specified diseases of inner ear, unspecified ear

H83.9 Unspecified disease of inner ear
- **H83.90** Unspecified disease of inner ear, unspecified ear
- **H83.91** Unspecified disease of right inner ear
- **H83.92** Unspecified disease of left inner ear
- **H83.93** Unspecified disease of inner ear, bilateral

Other disorders of ear (H90-H94)

⁴ **H90** **Conductive and sensorineural hearing loss**

EXCLUDES 1 *deaf nonspeaking NEC (H91.3)*
deafness NOS (H91.9-)
hearing loss NOS (H91.9-)
noise-induced hearing loss (H83.3-)
ototoxic hearing loss (H91.0-)
sudden (idiopathic) hearing loss (H91.2-)

H90.0 Conductive hearing loss, bilateral

⁵ **H90.1** Conductive hearing loss, unilateral with unrestricted hearing on the contralateral side

☐ **H90.11** Conductive hearing loss, unilateral, right ear, with unrestricted hearing on the contralateral side

☐ **H90.12** Conductive hearing loss, unilateral, left ear, with unrestricted hearing on the contralateral side

H90.2 Conductive hearing loss, unspecified
Conductive deafness NOS

DEFINITION Loss of audio acuity caused by transmission interference of sound waves before they can reach the inner ear and the auditory nerve.

H90.3 Sensorineural hearing loss, bilateral

⁵ **H90.4** Sensorineural hearing loss, unilateral with unrestricted hearing on the contralateral side

☐ **H90.41** Sensorineural hearing loss, unilateral, right ear, with unrestricted hearing on the contralateral side

☐ **H90.42** Sensorineural hearing loss, unilateral, left ear, with unrestricted hearing on the contralateral side

H90.5 Unspecified sensorineural hearing loss
Central hearing loss NOS
Congenital deafness NOS
Neural hearing loss NOS
Perceptive hearing loss NOS
Sensorineural deafness NOS
Sensory hearing loss NOS

EXCLUDES 1 *abnormal auditory perception (H93.2-)*
psychogenic deafness (F44.6)

DEFINITION Sensory-nerve based hearing loss caused by a disorder affecting the VIII cranial nerve, the inner ear sensory perception, or the central processing area of the brain.

H90.6 Mixed conductive and sensorineural hearing loss, bilateral
AHA: 2Q 2015, 7

⁵ **H90.7** Mixed conductive and sensorineural hearing loss, unilateral with unrestricted hearing on the contralateral side

☐ **H90.71** Mixed conductive and sensorineural hearing loss, unilateral, right ear, with unrestricted hearing on the contralateral side

☐ **H90.72** Mixed conductive and sensorineural hearing loss, unilateral, left ear, with unrestricted hearing on the contralateral side

H90.8 Mixed conductive and sensorineural hearing loss, unspecified

● ⑤ **H90.A** Conductive and sensorineural hearing loss with restricted hearing on the contralateral side

● ⑥ **H90.A1** Conductive hearing loss, unilateral, with restricted hearing on the contralateral side

● ☐ **H90.A11** Conductive hearing loss, unilateral, right ear with restricted hearing on the contralateral side

● ☐ **H90.A12** Conductive hearing loss, unilateral, left ear with restricted hearing on the contralateral side

● ⑥ **H90.A2** Sensorineural hearing loss, unilateral, with restricted hearing on the contralateral side

● ☐ **H90.A21** Sensorineural hearing loss, unilateral, right ear, with restricted hearing on the contralateral side

● ☐ **H90.A22** Sensorineural hearing loss, unilateral, left ear, with restricted hearing on the contralateral side

● ⑥ **H90.A3** Mixed conductive and sensorineural hearing loss, unilateral with restricted hearing on the contralateral side

● ☐ **H90.A31** Mixed conductive and sensorineural hearing loss, unilateral, right ear with restricted hearing on the contralateral side

● ☐ **H90.A32** Mixed conductive and sensorineural hearing loss, unilateral, left ear with restricted hearing on the contralateral side

⁴ **H91** **Other and unspecified hearing loss**

EXCLUDES 1 *abnormal auditory perception (H93.2-)*
hearing loss as classified in H90.-
impacted cerumen (H61.2-)
noise-induced hearing loss (H83.3-)
psychogenic deafness (F44.6)
transient ischemic deafness (H93.01-)

⑤ + **H91.0** Ototoxic hearing loss
Code first:
poisoning due to drug or toxin, if applicable (T36-T65 with fifth or sixth character 1-4 or 6)
Use additional code for adverse effect, if applicable, to identify drug (T36-T50 with fifth or sixth character 5)

☐ + **H91.01** Ototoxic hearing loss, right ear

☐ + **H91.02** Ototoxic hearing loss, left ear

☐ + **H91.03** Ototoxic hearing loss, bilateral

☐ + **H91.09** Ototoxic hearing loss, unspecified ear

⑤ **H91.1** Presbycusis
Presbyacusia

DEFINITION Gradual hearing loss that normally occurs with age.

☐ **H91.10** Presbycusis, unspecified ear
☐ **H91.11** Presbycusis, right ear
☐ **H91.12** Presbycusis, left ear
☐ **H91.13** Presbycusis, bilateral

⑤ **H91.2** Sudden idiopathic hearing loss
Sudden hearing loss NOS

☐ **H91.20** Sudden idiopathic hearing loss, unspecified ear
☐ **H91.21** Sudden idiopathic hearing loss, right ear
☐ **H91.22** Sudden idiopathic hearing loss, left ear
☐ **H91.23** Sudden idiopathic hearing loss, bilateral

H91.3 Deaf nonspeaking, not elsewhere classified

⑤ **H91.8** Other specified hearing loss

⑥ **H91.8X** Other specified hearing loss

☐ **H91.8X1** Other specified hearing loss, right ear
☐ **H91.8X2** Other specified hearing loss, left ear
☐ **H91.8X3** Other specified hearing loss, bilateral
☐ **H91.8X9** Other specified hearing loss, unspecified ear

⑤ **H91.9** Unspecified hearing loss
Deafness NOS
High frequency deafness
Low frequency deafness

☐ **H91.90** Unspecified hearing loss, unspecified ear
☐ **H91.91** Unspecified hearing loss, right ear
☐ **H91.92** Unspecified hearing loss, left ear
☐ **H91.93** Unspecified hearing loss, bilateral

⁴ **H92** **Otalgia and effusion of ear**

⑤ **H92.0** Otalgia
☐ **H92.01** Otalgia, right ear
☐ **H92.02** Otalgia, left ear
☐ **H92.03** Otalgia, bilateral
☐ **H92.09** Otalgia, unspecified ear

⑤ **H92.1** Otorrhea

EXCLUDES 1 *leakage of cerebrospinal fluid through ear (G96.0)*

DEFINITION Fluid leaking from the ear.

☐ **H92.10** Otorrhea, unspecified ear
☐ **H92.11** Otorrhea, right ear
☐ **H92.12** Otorrhea, left ear
☐ **H92.13** Otorrhea, bilateral

⑤ **H92.2** Otorrhagia

EXCLUDES 1 *traumatic otorrhagia - code to injury*

☐ **H92.20** Otorrhagia, unspecified ear
☐ **H92.21** Otorrhagia, right ear
☐ **H92.22** Otorrhagia, left ear
☐ **H92.23** Otorrhagia, bilateral

⁴ **H93** **Other disorders of ear, not elsewhere classified**

⑤ **H93.0** Degenerative and vascular disorders of ear

EXCLUDES 1 *presbycusis (H91.1)*

Diseases of the Ear and Mastoid Process

⑥ **H93.01**   **Transient ischemic deafness**
> **DEFINITION**   A passing hearing loss that occurs when blood flow to the auditory organs is decreased due to injury or disease.

☒ **H93.011**   Transient ischemic deafness, right ear
☒ **H93.012**   Transient ischemic deafness, left ear
☒ **H93.013**   Transient ischemic deafness, bilateral
☒ **H93.019**   Transient ischemic deafness, unspecified ear

⑥ **H93.09**   **Unspecified degenerative and vascular disorders of ear**

☒ **H93.091**   Unspecified degenerative and vascular disorders of right ear
☒ **H93.092**   Unspecified degenerative and vascular disorders of left ear
☒ **H93.093**   Unspecified degenerative and vascular disorders of ear, bilateral
☒ **H93.099**   Unspecified degenerative and vascular disorders of unspecified ear

⑤ **H93.1**   **Tinnitus**
> **DEFINITION**   Ringing, hissing, roaring or other sound in the ear in the absence of any apparent stimulus.

☒ **H93.11**   Tinnitus, right ear
☒ **H93.12**   Tinnitus, left ear
☒ **H93.13**   Tinnitus, bilateral
☒ **H93.19**   Tinnitus, unspecified ear

● ⑤ **H93.A**   **Pulsatile tinnitus**
● ☒ **H93.A1**   Pulsatile tinnitus, right ear
● ☒ **H93.A2**   Pulsatile tinnitus, left ear
● ☒ **H93.A3**   Pulsatile tinnitus, bilateral
● ☒ **H93.A9**   Pulsatile tinnitus, unspecified ear

⑤ **H93.2**   **Other abnormal auditory perceptions**
> **EXCLUDES 2**   auditory hallucinations (R44.0)

⑥ **H93.21**   **Auditory recruitment**
☒ **H93.211**   Auditory recruitment, right ear
☒ **H93.212**   Auditory recruitment, left ear
☒ **H93.213**   Auditory recruitment, bilateral
☒ **H93.219**   Auditory recruitment, unspecified ear

⑥ **H93.22**   **Diplacusis**
> **DEFINITION**   One sound is heard as two separate sounds at different tones or pitches.

☒ **H93.221**   Diplacusis, right ear
☒ **H93.222**   Diplacusis, left ear
☒ **H93.223**   Diplacusis, bilateral
☒ **H93.229**   Diplacusis, unspecified ear

⑥ **H93.23**   **Hyperacusis**
> **DEFINITION**   Hearing is abnormally heightened; normal sounds seem amplified, even cause ear pain.

☒ **H93.231**   Hyperacusis, right ear
☒ **H93.232**   Hyperacusis, left ear
☒ **H93.233**   Hyperacusis, bilateral
☒ **H93.239**   Hyperacusis, unspecified ear

⑥ **H93.24**   **Temporary auditory threshold shift**
☒ **H93.241**   Temporary auditory threshold shift, right ear
☒ **H93.242**   Temporary auditory threshold shift, left ear
☒ **H93.243**   Temporary auditory threshold shift, bilateral
☒ **H93.249**   Temporary auditory threshold shift, unspecified ear

H93.25   **Central auditory processing disorder**
Congenital auditory imperception
Word deafness
> **EXCLUDES 1**   mixed receptive-expressive language disorder (F80.2)

⑥ **H93.29**   **Other abnormal auditory perceptions**
☒ **H93.291**   Other abnormal auditory perceptions, right ear
☒ **H93.292**   Other abnormal auditory perceptions, left ear
☒ **H93.293**   Other abnormal auditory perceptions, bilateral
☒ **H93.299**   Other abnormal auditory perceptions, unspecified ear

⑤ **H93.3**   **Disorders of acoustic nerve**
Disorder of 8th cranial nerve
> **EXCLUDES 1**   acoustic neuroma (D33.3)
> syphilitic acoustic neuritis (A52.15)

⑥ **H93.3X**   **Disorders of acoustic nerve**
☒ **H93.3X1**   Disorders of right acoustic nerve
☒ **H93.3X2**   Disorders of left acoustic nerve
☒ **H93.3X3**   Disorders of bilateral acoustic nerves
☒ **H93.3X9**   Disorders of unspecified acoustic nerve

⑤ **H93.8**   **Other specified disorders of ear**
⑥ **H93.8X**   **Other specified disorders of ear**
☒ **H93.8X1**   Other specified disorders of right ear
☒ **H93.8X2**   Other specified disorders of left ear
☒ **H93.8X3**   Other specified disorders of ear, bilateral
☒ **H93.8X9**   Other specified disorders of ear, unspecified ear

⑤ **H93.9**   **Unspecified disorder of ear**
☒ **H93.90**   Unspecified disorder of ear, unspecified ear
☒ **H93.91**   Unspecified disorder of right ear
☒ **H93.92**   Unspecified disorder of left ear
☒ **H93.93**   Unspecified disorder of ear, bilateral

④ **H94**   **Other disorders of ear in diseases classified elsewhere**

⑤ **H94.0**   **Acoustic neuritis in infectious and parasitic diseases classified elsewhere**
Code first underlying disease, such as:
parasitic disease (B65-B89)
> **EXCLUDES 1**   acoustic neuritis (in) :
> herpes zoster (B02.29)
> syphilis (A52.15)

☒ **H94.00**   *Acoustic neuritis in infectious and parasitic diseases classified elsewhere, unspecified ear*
☒ **H94.01**   *Acoustic neuritis in infectious and parasitic diseases classified elsewhere, right ear*
☒ **H94.02**   *Acoustic neuritis in infectious and parasitic diseases classified elsewhere, left ear*
☒ **H94.03**   *Acoustic neuritis in infectious and parasitic diseases classified elsewhere, bilateral*

⑤ **H94.8**   **Other specified disorders of ear in diseases classified elsewhere**
Code first underlying disease, such as:
congenital syphilis (A50.0)
> **EXCLUDES 1**   aural myiasis (B87.4)
> syphilitic labyrinthitis (A52.79)

☒ **H94.80**   Other specified disorders of ear in diseases classified elsewhere, unspecified ear
☒ **H94.81**   Other specified disorders of right ear in diseases classified elsewhere
☒ **H94.82**   Other specified disorders of left ear in diseases classified elsewhere
☒ **H94.83**   Other specified disorders of ear in diseases classified elsewhere, bilateral

Intraoperative and postprocedural complications and disorders of ear and mastoid process, not elsewhere classified (H95)

④ **H95**   **Intraoperative and postprocedural complications and disorders of ear and mastoid process, not elsewhere classified**

⑤ **H95.0**   **Recurrent cholesteatoma of postmastoidectomy cavity**
☒ **H95.00**   Recurrent cholesteatoma of postmastoidectomy cavity, unspecified ear
☒ **H95.01**   Recurrent cholesteatoma of postmastoidectomy cavity, right ear
☒ **H95.02**   Recurrent cholesteatoma of postmastoidectomy cavity, left ear
☒ **H95.03**   Recurrent cholesteatoma of postmastoidectomy cavity, bilateral ears

⑤ **H95.1**   **Other disorders of ear and mastoid process following mastoidectomy**
⑥ **H95.11**   **Chronic inflammation of postmastoidectomy cavity**
☒ **H95.111**   Chronic inflammation of postmastoidectomy cavity, right ear
☒ **H95.112**   Chronic inflammation of postmastoidectomy cavity, left ear
☒ **H95.113**   Chronic inflammation of postmastoidectomy cavity, bilateral ears
☒ **H95.119**   Chronic inflammation of postmastoidectomy cavity, unspecified ear

---

● New   ▲ Revised   *Manifestation*   ④-❼ Digit Indicators   ☒ Laterality   Ⓐ Adult (15+ years)   Ⓜ Maternity (12-55 years)   Ⓝ Newborn   Ⓟ Pediatric (0-17 years)   ♂ Male   ♀ Female

✖ ~~Deleted~~   Unspecified   + Additional code

632   © 2017 DecisionHealth   2017 ICD-10-CM Expert for Physicians

H93.01 — H95.119

Ⓖ **H95.12**   Granulation of postmastoidectomy cavity
   ▫ **H95.121**   Granulation of postmastoidectomy cavity, right ear
   ▫ **H95.122**   Granulation of postmastoidectomy cavity, left ear
   ▫ **H95.123**   Granulation of postmastoidectomy cavity, bilateral ears
   ▫ **H95.129**   **Granulation of postmastoidectomy cavity, unspecified ear**

Ⓖ **H95.13**   Mucosal cyst of postmastoidectomy cavity
   ▫ **H95.131**   Mucosal cyst of postmastoidectomy cavity, right ear
   ▫ **H95.132**   Mucosal cyst of postmastoidectomy cavity, left ear
   ▫ **H95.133**   Mucosal cyst of postmastoidectomy cavity, bilateral ears
   ▫ **H95.139**   **Mucosal cyst of postmastoidectomy cavity, unspecified ear**

Ⓖ **H95.19**   Other disorders following mastoidectomy
   ▫ **H95.191**   Other disorders following mastoidectomy, right ear
   ▫ **H95.192**   Other disorders following mastoidectomy, left ear
   ▫ **H95.193**   Other disorders following mastoidectomy, bilateral ears
   ▫ **H95.199**   **Other disorders following mastoidectomy, unspecified ear**

Ⓢ **H95.2**   **Intraoperative hemorrhage and hematoma of ear and mastoid process complicating a procedure**
   EXCLUDES 1   *intraoperative hemorrhage and hematoma of ear and mastoid process due to accidental puncture or laceration during a procedure (H95.3-)*
   H95.21   Intraoperative hemorrhage and hematoma of ear and mastoid process complicating a procedure on the ear and mastoid process
   H95.22   Intraoperative hemorrhage and hematoma of ear and mastoid process complicating other procedure

Ⓢ **H95.3**   **Accidental puncture and laceration of ear and mastoid process during a procedure**
   H95.31   Accidental puncture and laceration of the ear and mastoid process during a procedure on the ear and mastoid process
   H95.32   Accidental puncture and laceration of the ear and mastoid process during other procedure

▲ Ⓢ **H95.4**   **Postprocedural hemorrhage of ear and mastoid process following a procedure**
   ▲ **H95.41**   Postprocedural hemorrhage of ear and mastoid process following a procedure on the ear and mastoid process
   ▲ **H95.42**   Postprocedural hemorrhage of ear and mastoid process following other procedure

● Ⓢ **H95.5**   **Postprocedural hematoma and seroma of ear and mastoid process following a procedure**
   ● **H95.51**   Postprocedural hematoma of ear and mastoid process following a procedure on the ear and mastoid process
   ● **H95.52**   Postprocedural hematoma of ear and mastoid process following other procedure
   ● **H95.53**   Postprocedural seroma of ear and mastoid process following a procedure on the ear and mastoid process
   ● **H95.54**   Postprocedural seroma of ear and mastoid process following other procedure

Ⓢ **H95.8**   **Other intraoperative and postprocedural complications and disorders of the ear and mastoid process, not elsewhere classified**
   EXCLUDES 2   *postprocedural complications and disorders following mastoidectomy (H95.0-, H95.1-)*

Ⓖ **H95.81**   Postprocedural stenosis of external ear canal
   ▫ **H95.811**   Postprocedural stenosis of right external ear canal
   ▫ **H95.812**   Postprocedural stenosis of left external ear canal
   ▫ **H95.813**   Postprocedural stenosis of external ear canal, bilateral
   ▫ **H95.819**   **Postprocedural stenosis of unspecified external ear canal**

➕ **H95.88**   **Other intraoperative complications and disorders of the ear and mastoid process, not elsewhere classified**
   Use additional code , if applicable, to further specify disorder

➕ **H95.89**   **Other postprocedural complications and disorders of the ear and mastoid process, not elsewhere classified**
   Use additional code, if applicable, to further specify disorder

● New   ▲ Revised   *Manifestation*   ❹-❼ Digit Indicators   ▫ Laterality   Ⓐ Adult (15+ years)   Ⓜ Maternity (12-55 years)   Ⓝ Newborn   Ⓟ Pediatric (0-17 years)   ♂ Male   ♀ Female
✖ ~~Deleted~~   Unspecified   ➕ Additional code

2017 ICD-10-CM Expert for Physicians   © 2017 DecisionHealth   633

CHAPTER 9: DISEASES OF THE CIRCULATORY SYSTEM (I00-I99)

EXCLUDES 2 certain conditions originating in the perinatal period (P04-P96)
certain infectious and parasitic diseases (A00-B99)
complications of pregnancy, childbirth and the puerperium (O00-O9A)
congenital malformations, deformations, and chromosomal abnormalities (Q00-Q99)
endocrine, nutritional and metabolic diseases (E00-E88)
injury, poisoning and certain other consequences of external causes (S00-T88)
neoplasms (C00-D49)
symptoms, signs and abnormal clinical and laboratory findings, not elsewhere classified (R00-R94)
systemic connective tissue disorders (M30-M36)
transient cerebral ischemic attacks and related syndromes (G45.-)

This chapter contains the following blocks:

I00-I02 Acute rheumatic fever
I05-I09 Chronic rheumatic heart diseases
I10-I16 Hypertensive diseases
I20-I25 Ischemic heart diseases
I26-I28 Pulmonary heart disease and diseases of pulmonary circulation
I30-I52 Other forms of heart disease
I60-I69 Cerebrovascular diseases
I70-I79 Diseases of arteries, arterioles and capillaries
I80-I89 Diseases of veins, lymphatic vessels and lymph nodes, not elsewhere classified
I95-I99 Other and unspecified disorders of the circulatory system

Acute rheumatic fever (I00-I02)

CODING TIP✓ Pericarditis, endocarditis, and myocarditis are only coded here when specified as "rheumatic." Do not assign a code for acute, chronic, infective, or other non-rheumatic pericarditis, endocarditis, or myocarditis using a code from I00-I02.

I00 **Rheumatic fever without heart involvement**
INCLUDES arthritis, rheumatic, acute or subacute
EXCLUDES 1 rheumatic fever with heart involvement (I01.0 -I01.9)
DEFINITION Delayed, febrile, inflammatory disease resulting about 20 days after streptococcal infection; presents with joint pain, migratory arthritis, skin rash on the trunk and proximal extremities, and nosebleeds; can cause cardiac damage.

I01 **Rheumatic fever with heart involvement**
EXCLUDES 1 chronic diseases of rheumatic origin (I05-I09) unless rheumatic fever is also present or there is evidence of reactivation or activity of the rheumatic process.

I01.0 **Acute rheumatic pericarditis**
Any condition in I00 with pericarditis
Rheumatic pericarditis (acute)
EXCLUDES 1 acute pericarditis not specified as rheumatic (I30.-)

I01.1 **Acute rheumatic endocarditis**
Any condition in I00 with endocarditis or valvulitis
Acute rheumatic valvulitis

I01.2 **Acute rheumatic myocarditis**
Any condition in I00 with myocarditis

I01.8 **Other acute rheumatic heart disease**
Any condition in I00 with other or multiple types of heart involvement
Acute rheumatic pancarditis

I01.9 **Acute rheumatic heart disease, unspecified**
Any condition in I00 with unspecified type of heart involvement
Rheumatic carditis, acute
Rheumatic heart disease, active or acute

I02 **Rheumatic chorea**
INCLUDES Sydenham's chorea
EXCLUDES 1 chorea NOS (G25.5)
Huntington's chorea (G10)

CODING TIP✓ Rheumatic chorea may also be referred to as "St. Vitus Dance" and is more frequently diagnosed in children and adolescents.

I02.0 **Rheumatic chorea with heart involvement**
Chorea NOS with heart involvement
Rheumatic chorea with heart involvement of any type classifiable under I01.-

I02.9 **Rheumatic chorea without heart involvement**
Rheumatic chorea NOS

Chronic rheumatic heart diseases (I05-I09)

CODING TIP✓ Categories I05-I09 include disease of the heart valve(s) specified as rheumatic.

I05 **Rheumatic mitral valve diseases**
INCLUDES conditions classifiable to both I05.0 and I05.2-I05.9, whether specified as rheumatic or not
EXCLUDES 1 mitral valve disease specified as nonrheumatic (I34.-)
mitral valve disease with aortic and/or tricuspid valve involvement (I08.-)

I05.0 **Rheumatic mitral stenosis**
Mitral (valve) obstruction (rheumatic)

I05.1 **Rheumatic mitral insufficiency**
Rheumatic mitral incompetence
Rheumatic mitral regurgitation
EXCLUDES 1 mitral insufficiency not specified as rheumatic (I34.0)

I05.2 **Rheumatic mitral stenosis with insufficiency**
Rheumatic mitral stenosis with incompetence or regurgitation

I05.8 **Other rheumatic mitral valve diseases**
Rheumatic mitral (valve) failure

I05.9 **Rheumatic mitral valve disease, unspecified**
Rheumatic mitral (valve) disorder (chronic) NOS

I06 **Rheumatic aortic valve diseases**
EXCLUDES 1 aortic valve disease not specified as rheumatic (I35.-)
aortic valve disease with mitral and/or tricuspid valve involvement (I08.-)

I06.0 **Rheumatic aortic stenosis**
Rheumatic aortic (valve) obstruction

I06.1 **Rheumatic aortic insufficiency**
Rheumatic aortic incompetence
Rheumatic aortic regurgitation

I06.2 **Rheumatic aortic stenosis with insufficiency**
Rheumatic aortic stenosis with incompetence or regurgitation

I06.8 **Other rheumatic aortic valve diseases**

I06.9 **Rheumatic aortic valve disease, unspecified**
Rheumatic aortic (valve) disease NOS

I07 **Rheumatic tricuspid valve diseases**
INCLUDES rheumatic tricuspid valve diseases specified as rheumatic or unspecified
EXCLUDES 1 tricuspid valve disease specified as nonrheumatic (I36.-)
tricuspid valve disease with aortic and/or mitral valve involvement (I08.-)

I07.0 **Rheumatic tricuspid stenosis**
Tricuspid (valve) stenosis (rheumatic)

I07.1 **Rheumatic tricuspid insufficiency**
Tricuspid (valve) insufficiency (rheumatic)

I07.2 **Rheumatic tricuspid stenosis and insufficiency**

I07.8 **Other rheumatic tricuspid valve diseases**

I07.9 **Rheumatic tricuspid valve disease, unspecified**
Rheumatic tricuspid valve disorder NOS

I08 **Multiple valve diseases**
INCLUDES multiple valve diseases specified as rheumatic or unspecified
EXCLUDES 1 endocarditis, valve unspecified (I38)
multiple valve disease specified a nonrheumatic (I34.-, I35.-, I36.-, I37.-, I38.-, Q22.-, Q23.-, Q24.8-)
rheumatic valve disease NOS (I09.1)

I08.0 **Rheumatic disorders of both mitral and aortic valves**
Involvement of both mitral and aortic valves specified as rheumatic or unspecified

I08.1 **Rheumatic disorders of both mitral and tricuspid valves**

Diseases of the Circulatory System

I08.2   **Rheumatic disorders of both aortic and tricuspid valves**

I08.3   **Combined rheumatic disorders of mitral, aortic and tricuspid valves**

I08.8   **Other rheumatic multiple valve diseases**

I08.9   **Rheumatic multiple valve disease, unspecified**

> **CODING TIP ✓**   When the clinical record reports rheumatic disease of multiple valves, but the affected valves are not specified, assign code I08.9.

▣ I09   **Other rheumatic heart diseases**

I09.0   **Rheumatic myocarditis**

> **EXCLUDES 1**   *myocarditis not specified as rheumatic (I51.4)*

> **DEFINITION**   Chronic inflammation and degeneration of heart muscle due to rheumatic heart disease.

I09.1   **Rheumatic diseases of endocardium, valve unspecified**
Rheumatic endocarditis (chronic)
Rheumatic valvulitis (chronic)

> **EXCLUDES 1**   *endocarditis, valve unspecified (I38)*

I09.2   **Chronic rheumatic pericarditis**
Adherent pericardium, rheumatic
Chronic rheumatic mediastinopericarditis
Chronic rheumatic myopericarditis

> **EXCLUDES 1**   *chronic pericarditis not specified as rheumatic (I31.-)*

▣ I09.8   **Other specified rheumatic heart diseases**

✛ I09.81   **Rheumatic heart failure**
Use additional code to identify type of heart failure (I50.-)

> **DEFINITION**   Severe rheumatic damage to heart valves causing heart failure.

I09.89   **Other specified rheumatic heart diseases**
Rheumatic disease of pulmonary valve

I09.9   **Rheumatic heart disease, unspecified**
Rheumatic carditis

> **EXCLUDES 1**   *rheumatoid carditis (M05.31)*

Hypertensive diseases (I10-I16)

Use additional code to identify:
exposure to environmental tobacco smoke (Z77.22)
history of tobacco dependence (Z87.891)
occupational exposure to environmental tobacco smoke (Z57.31)
tobacco dependence (F17.-)
tobacco use (Z72.0)

> **EXCLUDES 1**   *neonatal hypertension (P29.2)*
> *primary pulmonary hypertension (I27.0)*

> **EXCLUDES 2**   *hypertensive disease complicating pregnancy, childbirth and the puerperium (O10-O11, O13-O16)*

I10   **Essential (primary) hypertension**

> **INCLUDES**   high blood pressure
> hypertension (arterial) (benign) (essential) (malignant) (primary) (systemic)

> **EXCLUDES 1**   *hypertensive disease complicating pregnancy, childbirth and the puerperium (O10-O11, O13-O16)*

> **EXCLUDES 2**   *essential (primary) hypertension involving vessels of brain (I60-I69)*
> *essential (primary) hypertension involving vessels of eye (H35.0-)*

AHA: 4Q 2013, 128

▣ I11   **Hypertensive heart disease**

> **INCLUDES**   any condition in I51.4-I51.9 due to hypertension

> **GUIDELINES**   Section I.C.9.a.1)
> Heart conditions classified to I50.- or I51.4-I51.9, are assigned to category I11, Hypertensive heart disease, when a causal relationship is stated (due to hypertension) or implied (hypertensive). Use an additional code from category I50, Heart failure, to identify the type of heart failure in those patients with heart failure. The same heart conditions (I50.-, I51.4-I51.9) with hypertension, but without a stated causal relationship, are coded separately. Sequence according to the circumstances of the admission/encounter.

> **CODING TIP ✓**   When assigning a code from I11.-, documentation must support a relationship between hypertension and a condition classifiable to I51.4-I51.9. Look for terms such as "due to", "related to", "hypertensive". A physician must confirm the relationship and clinical record documentation must support the relationship.

✛ I11.0   **Hypertensive heart disease with heart failure**
Hypertensive heart failure
Use additional code to identify type of heart failure (I50.-)

I11.9   **Hypertensive heart disease without heart failure**
Hypertensive heart disease NOS

▣ I12   **Hypertensive chronic kidney disease**

> **INCLUDES**   any condition in N18 and N26 - due to hypertension
> arteriosclerosis of kidney
> arteriosclerotic nephritis (chronic) (interstitial)
> hypertensive nephropathy
> nephrosclerosis

> **EXCLUDES 1**   *hypertension due to kidney disease (I15.0, I15.1)*
> *renovascular hypertension (I15.0)*
> *secondary hypertension (I15.-)*

> **EXCLUDES 2**   *acute kidney failure (N17.-)*

> **GUIDELINES**   Section I.C.9.a.2)
> Assign codes from category I12, Hypertensive chronic kidney disease, when both hypertension and a condition classifiable to category N18, Chronic kidney disease (CKD), are present. Unlike hypertension with heart disease, ICD-10-CM presumes a cause-and-effect relationship and classifies chronic kidney disease with hypertension as hypertensive chronic kidney disease.
>
> The appropriate code from category N18 should be used as a secondary code with a code from category I12 to identify the stage of chronic kidney disease.
> *See Section I.C.14. Chronic kidney disease.* If a patient has hypertensive chronic kidney disease and acute renal failure, an additional code for the acute renal failure (category N17) is required.

> **CODING TIP ✓**   A relationship may be assumed between hypertension and any condition classifiable to N18.- or N26.-. This is due to the pathology of hypertension, which impacts renal function, often resulting in kidney dysfunction. The exception to this assumption is when clinical record documentation reports that hypertension has been caused secondary to the kidney dysfunction (renovascular hypertension). When this is the case, the hypertension is secondary to the renal dysfunction and is coded using a code from I15.-

✛ I12.0   **Hypertensive chronic kidney disease with stage 5 chronic kidney disease or end stage renal disease**
Use additional code to identify the stage of chronic kidney disease (N18.5, N18.6)

✛ I12.9   **Hypertensive chronic kidney disease with stage 1 through stage 4 chronic kidney disease, or unspecified chronic kidney disease**
Hypertensive chronic kidney disease NOS
Hypertensive renal disease NOS
Use additional code to identify the stage of chronic kidney disease (N18.1-N18.4, N18.9)

▣ I13   **Hypertensive heart and chronic kidney disease**

> **INCLUDES**   any condition in I11.- with any condition in I12.-
> cardiorenal disease
> cardiovascular renal disease

● New   ▲ Revised   *Manifestation*   ▣-▯ Digit Indicators   ▭ Laterality   Ⓐ Adult (15+ years)   Ⓜ Maternity (12-55 years)   Ⓝ Newborn   Ⓟ Pediatric (0-17 years)   ♂ Male   ♀ Female
✖ Deleted   Unspecified   ✛ Additional code

636   © 2017 DecisionHealth   2017 ICD-10-CM Expert for Physicians

I08.2 — I13

GUIDELINES Section I.C.9.a.3)
The codes in category I13 are combination codes that include hypertension, heart disease and chronic kidney disease. The Includes note at I13 specifies that the conditions included at I11 and I12 are included together in I13. If a patient has hypertension, heart disease and chronic kidney disease then a code from I13 should be used, not individual codes for hypertension, heart disease and chronic kidney disease, or codes from I11 or I12.

Assign codes from combination category I13 when both hypertensive kidney disease and hypertensive heart disease are stated in the diagnosis. Assume a relationship between the hypertension and the chronic kidney disease, whether or not the condition is so designated. If heart failure is present, assign an additional code from category I50 to identify the type of heart failure.

+ I13.0   Hypertensive heart and chronic kidney disease with heart failure and stage 1 through stage 4 chronic kidney disease, or unspecified chronic kidney disease
Use additional code to identify type of heart failure (I50.-)
Use additional code to identify stage of chronic kidney disease (N18.1-N18.4, N18.9)

⑤ I13.1   Hypertensive heart and chronic kidney disease without heart failure

+ I13.10   Hypertensive heart and chronic kidney disease without heart failure, with stage 1 through stage 4 chronic kidney disease, or unspecified chronic kidney disease
Hypertensive heart disease and hypertensive chronic kidney disease NOS
Use additional code to identify the stage of chronic kidney disease (N18.1-N18.4, N18.9)

+ I13.11   Hypertensive heart and chronic kidney disease without heart failure, with stage 5 chronic kidney disease, or end stage renal disease
Use additional code to identify the stage of chronic kidney disease (N18.5, N18.6)

+ I13.2   Hypertensive heart and chronic kidney disease with heart failure and with stage 5 chronic kidney disease, or end stage renal disease
Use additional code to identify type of heart failure (I50.-)
Use additional code to identify the stage of chronic kidney disease (N18.5, N18.6)

◳ I15   Secondary hypertension
Code also:
underlying condition
EXCLUDES 1 *postprocedural hypertension (I97.3)*
EXCLUDES 2 *secondary hypertension involving vessels of brain (I60-I69)*
secondary hypertension involving vessels of eye (H35.0-)

GUIDELINES Section I.C.9.a.6)
Secondary hypertension is due to an underlying condition. Two codes are required: one to identify the underlying etiology and one from category I15 to identify the hypertension. Sequencing of codes is determined by the reason for admission/encounter.

CODING TIP ✓ When hypertension is reported in the clinical record and confirmed by the physician as due to kidney (renal) dysfunction, assign a code from I15.-

I15.0   Renovascular hypertension
CODING TIP ✓ Do not confuse hypertensive chronic kidney disease with renovascular hypertension, a condition in which the kidney dysfunction causes the hypertension. When this is the case, the hypertension is secondary to the renal dysfunction and is coded using I15.0. The two conditions may be coded in either order. An additional code for the underlying condition should also be assigned.

I15.1   Hypertension secondary to other renal disorders
I15.2   Hypertension secondary to endocrine disorders
CODING TIP ✓ Assign I15.2 when hypertension is specified as due to Cushing's syndrome, primary aldosteronism, acromegaly, hypo/hyperthyroidism, or another specified endocrine disorder. Do not assign a code from I10-I13.0 when hypertension is specified as secondary to one of these causes.

I15.8   Other secondary hypertension

I15.9   Secondary hypertension, unspecified
● ◳ I16   Hypertensive crisis
Code also:
any identified hypertensive disease (I10-I15)
● I16.0   Hypertensive urgency
● I16.1   Hypertensive emergency
● I16.9   Hypertensive crisis, unspecified

Ischemic heart diseases (I20-I25)

Use additional code to identify presence of hypertension (I10-I16)
CODING TIP ✓ Always use an additional code to report any diagnosis of hypertension when assigning a code from I20.- to I25.-

▲ ◳ + I20   Angina pectoris
Use additional code to identify:
exposure to environmental tobacco smoke (Z77.22)
history of tobacco dependence (Z87.891)
occupational exposure to environmental tobacco smoke (Z57.31)
tobacco dependence (F17.-)
tobacco use (Z72.0)
EXCLUDES 1 *angina pectoris with atherosclerotic heart disease of native coronary arteries (I25.1-)*
atherosclerosis of coronary artery bypass graft(s) and coronary artery of transplanted heart with angina pectoris (I25.7-)
postinfarction angina (I23.7)

GUIDELINES Section I.C.9.b. ICD-10-CM has combination codes for atherosclerotic heart disease with angina pectoris. The subcategories for these codes are I25.11, Atherosclerotic heart disease of native coronary artery with angina pectoris and I25.7, Atherosclerosis of coronary artery bypass graft(s) and coronary artery of transplanted heart with angina pectoris.
When using one of these combination codes it is not necessary to use an additional code for angina pectoris. A causal relationship can be assumed in a patient with both atherosclerosis and angina pectoris, unless the documentation indicates the angina is due to something other than the atherosclerosis. If a patient with coronary artery disease is admitted due to an acute myocardial infarction (AMI), the AMI should be sequenced before the coronary artery disease.

CODING TIP ✓ Do not assign a code from I20.- for a patient who also has coronary artery disease (CAD)/atherosclerotic heart disease (ASHD). Angina in a patient with CAD/ASHD should be coded to the appropriate I25.11- code.

+ I20.0   Unstable angina   Ⓐ
Accelerated angina
Crescendo angina
De novo effort angina
Intermediate coronary syndrome
Preinfarction syndrome
Worsening effort angina
+ I20.1   Angina pectoris with documented spasm   Ⓐ
Angiospastic angina
Prinzmetal angina
Spasm-induced angina
Variant angina
▲ + I20.8   Other forms of angina pectoris   Ⓐ
Angina equivalent
Angina of effort
Coronary slow flow syndrome
Stenocardia
Stable angina
Use additional code(s) for symptoms associated with angina equivalent
+ I20.9   Angina pectoris, unspecified   Ⓐ
Angina NOS
Anginal syndrome
Cardiac angina
Ischemic chest pain

▲ ◩+ **I21** **ST elevation (STEMI) and non-ST elevation (NSTEMI) myocardial infarction**

INCLUDES cardiac infarction
coronary (artery) embolism
coronary (artery) occlusion
coronary (artery) rupture
coronary (artery) thrombosis
infarction of heart, myocardium, or ventricle
myocardial infarction specified as acute or with a stated duration of 4 weeks (28 days) or less from onset

Use additional code, if applicable, to identify:
exposure to environmental tobacco smoke (Z77.22)
history of tobacco dependence (Z87.891)
occupational exposure to environmental tobacco smoke (Z57.31)
status post administration of tPA (rtPA) in a different facility within the last 24 hours prior to admission to current facility (Z92.82)
tobacco dependence (F17.-)
tobacco use (Z72.0)

EXCLUDES 2 *old myocardial infarction (I25.2)*
postmyocardial infarction syndrome (I24.1)
subsequent myocardial infarction (I22.-)

GUIDELINES **Section I.C.9.b**
If a patient with coronary artery disease is admitted due to an acute myocardial infarction (AMI), the AMI should be sequenced before the coronary artery disease.

GUIDELINES **Section I.C.9.e.1)**
The ICD-10-CM codes for acute myocardial infarction (AMI) identify the site, such as anterolateral wall or true posterior wall. Subcategories I21.0-I21.2 and code I21.3 are used for ST elevation myocardial infarction (STEMI). Code I21.4, Non-ST elevation (NSTEMI) myocardial infarction, is used for non ST elevation myocardial infarction (NSTEMI) and nontransmural MIs.

For encounters occurring while the myocardial infarction is equal to, or less than, four weeks old, including transfers to another acute setting or a postacute setting, and the patient requires continued care for the myocardial infarction, codes from category I21 may continue to be reported. For encounters after the 4 week time frame and the patient is still receiving care related to the myocardial infarction, the appropriate aftercare code should be assigned, rather than a code from category I21. For old or healed myocardial infarctions not requiring further care, code I25.2, Old myocardial infarction, may be assigned.

CODING TIP ✓ When assigning any code from I21.- to report STEMI or NSTEMI, note that ICD-10 coding guidelines only allow assignment of these codes for 4 weeks following the occurrence of the MI. Use I22 codes for any subsequent MI during the same 4 weeks.
AHA: 1Q 2013, 25-26
AHA: 4Q 2012, 97, 103-104

◩+ **I21.0** **ST elevation (STEMI) myocardial infarction of anterior wall**

+ **I21.01** **ST elevation (STEMI) myocardial infarction involving left main coronary artery** A

+ **I21.02** **ST elevation (STEMI) myocardial infarction involving left anterior descending coronary artery** A
ST elevation (STEMI) myocardial infarction involving diagonal coronary artery
AHA: 1Q 2013, 26

+ **I21.09** **ST elevation (STEMI) myocardial infarction involving other coronary artery of anterior wall** A
Acute transmural myocardial infarction of anterior wall
Anteroapical transmural (Q wave) infarction (acute)
Anterolateral transmural (Q wave) infarction (acute)
Anteroseptal transmural (Q wave) infarction (acute)
Transmural (Q wave) infarction (acute) (of) anterior (wall) NOS
AHA: 4Q 2012, 102

◩+ **I21.1** **ST elevation (STEMI) myocardial infarction of inferior wall**

+ **I21.11** **ST elevation (STEMI) myocardial infarction involving right coronary artery** A
Inferoposterior transmural (Q wave) infarction (acute)

+ **I21.19** **ST elevation (STEMI) myocardial infarction involving other coronary artery of inferior wall** A
Acute transmural myocardial infarction of inferior wall
Inferolateral transmural (Q wave) infarction (acute)
Transmural (Q wave) infarction (acute) (of) diaphragmatic wall
Transmural (Q wave) infarction (acute) (of) inferior (wall) NOS

EXCLUDES 2 *ST elevation (STEMI) myocardial infarction involving left circumflex coronary artery (I21.21)*
AHA: 4Q 2012, 97

◩+ **I21.2** **ST elevation (STEMI) myocardial infarction of other sites**

+ **I21.21** **ST elevation (STEMI) myocardial infarction involving left circumflex coronary artery** A
ST elevation (STEMI) myocardial infarction involving oblique marginal coronary artery

+ **I21.29** **ST elevation (STEMI) myocardial infarction involving other sites** A
Acute transmural myocardial infarction of other sites
Apical-lateral transmural (Q wave) infarction (acute)
Basal-lateral transmural (Q wave) infarction (acute)
High lateral transmural (Q wave) infarction (acute)
Lateral (wall) NOS transmural (Q wave) infarction (acute)
Posterior (true) transmural (Q wave) infarction (acute)
Posterobasal transmural (Q wave) infarction (acute)
Posterolateral transmural (Q wave) infarction (acute)
Posteroseptal transmural (Q wave) infarction (acute)
Septal transmural (Q wave) infarction (acute) NOS

+ **I21.3** **ST elevation (STEMI) myocardial infarction of unspecified site** A
Acute transmural myocardial infarction of unspecified site
Myocardial infarction (acute) NOS
Transmural (Q wave) myocardial infarction NOS

GUIDELINES **Section I.C.9.e.2)**
Code I21.3 is the default for unspecified acute myocardial infarction. If only STEMI or transmural MI without the site is documented, assign code I21.3.

+ **I21.4** **Non-ST elevation (NSTEMI) myocardial infarction** A
Acute subendocardial myocardial infarction
Non-Q wave myocardial infarction NOS
Nontransmural myocardial infarction NOS

GUIDELINES **Section I.C.9.e.1)**
Code I21.4 is used for non ST elevation myocardial infarction (NSTEMI) and nontransmural MIs.

GUIDELINES **Section I.C.9.e.3)**
If an AMI is documented as nontransmural or subendocardial, but the site is provided, it is still coded as a subendocardial AMI.
AHA: 2Q 2015, 16

▲ ◩+ **I22** **Subsequent ST elevation (STEMI) and non-ST elevation (NSTEMI) myocardial infarction**

INCLUDES acute myocardial infarction occurring within four weeks (28 days) of a previous acute myocardial infarction, regardless of site
cardiac infarction
coronary (artery) embolism
coronary (artery) occlusion
coronary (artery) rupture
coronary (artery) thrombosis
infarction of heart, myocardium, or ventricle
recurrent myocardial infarction
reinfarction of myocardium
rupture of heart, myocardium, or ventricle

Use additional code, if applicable, to identify:
exposure to environmental tobacco smoke (Z77.22)
history of tobacco dependence (Z87.891)
occupational exposure to environmental tobacco smoke (Z57.31)
status post administration of tPA (rtPA) in a different facility within the last 24 hours prior to admission to current facility (Z92.82)
tobacco dependence (F17.-)
tobacco use (Z72.0)

● New   ▲ Revised   *Manifestation*   ◩-◪ Digit Indicators   ▤ Laterality   ▣ Adult (15+ years)   ▣ Maternity (12-55 years)   ▣ Newborn   ▣ Pediatric (0-17 years)   ♂ Male   ♀ Female
✖ Deleted   Unspecified   + Additional code

638   © 2017 DecisionHealth   2017 ICD-10-CM Expert for Physicians

GUIDELINES Section I.C.9.e.4)
A code from category I22 is to be used when a patient who has suffered an AMI has a new AMI within the 4 week time frame of the initial AMI. A code from category I22 must be used in conjunction with a code from category I21. The sequencing of the I22 and I21 codes depends on the circumstances of the encounter.

CODING TIP✓ When documentation reports an acute STEMI or NSTEMI occurring within 4 weeks following a prior acute STEMI or NSTEMI, a code from I22.- should be assigned. Codes from I22.- may be assigned for 4 weeks following the occurrence of the initial MI. If the time period since the initial MI (STEMI or NSTEMI) has been less than 4 weeks, then both a code for the initial MI (I21.-) and subsequent MI (I22.-) should be used. If the initial MI (STEMI or NSTEMI) occurred more than 4 weeks ago, then codes from I21.- and I22.- should not be assigned.

AHA: 1Q 2013, 25

AHA: 4Q 2012, 97, 103-104

+ **I22.0** **Subsequent ST elevation (STEMI) myocardial infarction of anterior wall**
Subsequent acute transmural myocardial infarction of anterior wall
Subsequent transmural (Q wave) infarction (acute)(of) anterior (wall) NOS
Subsequent anteroapical transmural (Q wave) infarction (acute)
Subsequent anterolateral transmural (Q wave) infarction (acute)
Subsequent anteroseptal transmural (Q wave) infarction (acute)

+ **I22.1** **Subsequent ST elevation (STEMI) myocardial infarction of inferior wall**
Subsequent acute transmural myocardial infarction of inferior wall
Subsequent transmural (Q wave) infarction (acute)(of) diaphragmatic wall
Subsequent transmural (Q wave) infarction (acute)(of) inferior (wall) NOS
Subsequent inferolateral transmural (Q wave) infarction (acute)
Subsequent inferoposterior transmural (Q wave) infarction (acute)
AHA: 4Q 2012, 97, 102, 103-104

+ **I22.2** **Subsequent non-ST elevation (NSTEMI) myocardial infarction**
Subsequent acute subendocardial myocardial infarction
Subsequent non-Q wave myocardial infarction NOS
Subsequent nontransmural myocardial infarction NOS

+ **I22.8** **Subsequent ST elevation (STEMI) myocardial infarction of other sites**
Subsequent acute transmural myocardial infarction of other sites
Subsequent apical-lateral transmural (Q wave) myocardial infarction (acute)
Subsequent basal-lateral transmural (Q wave) myocardial infarction (acute)
Subsequent high lateral transmural (Q wave) myocardial infarction (acute)
Subsequent transmural (Q wave) myocardial infarction (acute)(of) lateral (wall) NOS
Subsequent posterior (true)transmural (Q wave) myocardial infarction (acute)
Subsequent posterobasal transmural (Q wave) myocardial infarction (acute)
Subsequent posterolateral transmural (Q wave) myocardial infarction (acute)
Subsequent posteroseptal transmural (Q wave) myocardial infarction (acute)
Subsequent septal NOS transmural (Q wave) myocardial infarction (acute)

+ **I22.9** **Subsequent ST elevation (STEMI) myocardial infarction of unspecified site**
Subsequent acute myocardial infarction of unspecified site
Subsequent myocardial infarction (acute) NOS

I23 **Certain current complications following ST elevation (STEMI) and non-ST elevation (NSTEMI) myocardial infarction (within the 28 day period)**

CODING TIP✓ When assigning a code from category I23.-, the coder must also assign a code from category I21.- or I22.-, as appropriate, which may only be assigned for the 4 week period following the initial or subsequent STEMI or STEMI. Use of codes from category I23.- is not appropriate after the 4 week period has lapsed.

I23.0 **Hemopericardium as current complication following acute myocardial infarction**
EXCLUDES 1 hemopericardium not specified as current complication following acute myocardial infarction (I31.2)
CODING TIP✓ Documentation: Hemopericardium is frequently documented with cardiac wall rupture, including ventricular rupture, following MI, and results in pooling of blood in the pericardial space, leading to tamponade. This life threatening condition may occur during or shortly after an MI.

I23.1 **Atrial septal defect as current complication following acute myocardial infarction**
EXCLUDES 1 acquired atrial septal defect not specified as current complication following acute myocardial infarction (I51.0)

I23.2 **Ventricular septal defect as current complication following acute myocardial infarction**
EXCLUDES 1 acquired ventricular septal defect not specified as current complication following acute myocardial infarction (I51.0)

I23.3 **Rupture of cardiac wall without hemopericardium as current complication following acute myocardial infarction**

I23.4 **Rupture of chordae tendineae as current complication following acute myocardial infarction**
EXCLUDES 1 rupture of chordae tendineae not specified as current complication following acute myocardial infarction (I51.1)
DEFINITION Tear in the fibrous, cord-like tissue connecting the papillary muscles to the valves, holding the valve flaps in place to prevent their eversion.

I23.5 **Rupture of papillary muscle as current complication following acute myocardial infarction**
EXCLUDES 1 rupture of papillary muscle not specified as current complication following acute myocardial infarction (I51.2)

I23.6 **Thrombosis of atrium, auricular appendage, and ventricle as current complications following acute myocardial infarction**
EXCLUDES 1 thrombosis of atrium, auricular appendage, and ventricle not specified as current complication following acute myocardial infarction (I51.3)

I23.7 **Postinfarction angina**
CODING TIP✓ Post-infarction angina includes a syndrome of ischemic chest pain occurring either at rest or during minimal activity 24 hours or more following an acute MI. It is more common after NSTEMI. Post infarction angina is considered a complication (not simply angina after an MI) and must be documented by the physician. The code is used for only 4 weeks after the initial MI. Once the 4 weeks have passed and the patient continues with angina, I25.118 is used for the ASHD with other specified angina.
AHA: 2Q 2015, 16-17

I23.8 **Other current complications following acute myocardial infarction**

I24 **Other acute ischemic heart diseases**
EXCLUDES 1 angina pectoris (I20.-)
transient myocardial ischemia in newborn (P29.4)

I24.0 **Acute coronary thrombosis not resulting in myocardial infarction**
Acute coronary (artery) (vein) embolism not resulting in myocardial infarction
Acute coronary (artery) (vein) occlusion not resulting in myocardial infarction
Acute coronary (artery) (vein) thromboembolism not resulting in myocardial infarction
EXCLUDES 1 atherosclerotic heart disease (I25.1-)
AHA: 1Q 2013, 24

● New ▲ Revised *Manifestation* ◳-◷ Digit Indicators ⊟ Laterality Ⓐ Adult (15+ years) Ⓜ Maternity (12-55 years) Ⓝ Newborn Ⓟ Pediatric (0-17 years) ♂ Male ♀ Female
✖ Deleted Unspecified + Additional code

2017 ICD-10-CM Expert for Physicians

© 2017 DecisionHealth   639

I22 — I24.0

I24.1   **Dressler's syndrome**   A
            Postmyocardial infarction syndrome
            EXCLUDES 1   *postinfarction angina (I23.7)*

            DEFINITION   Fever, chest pain, pleuritis, and
            pericarditis weeks or months after heart injury caused
            by surgery or myocardial infarction.

I24.8   **Other forms of acute ischemic heart disease**   A

I24.9   **Acute ischemic heart disease, unspecified**   A
            EXCLUDES 1   *ischemic heart disease (chronic) NOS
            (I25.9)*

▲ ④ ✛ **I25**   **Chronic ischemic heart disease**
            Use additional code to identify:
            chronic total occlusion of coronary artery (I25.82)
            exposure to environmental tobacco smoke (Z77.22)
            history of tobacco dependence (Z87.891)
            *occupational exposure to environmental tobacco smoke
               (Z57.31)*
            tobacco dependence (F17.-)
            tobacco use (Z72.0)

            GUIDELINES   Section I.C.9.b
            ICD-10-CM has combination codes for atherosclerotic heart
            disease with angina pectoris. The subcategories for these
            codes are I25.11, Atherosclerotic heart disease of native
            coronary artery with angina pectoris, and I25.7,
            Atherosclerosis of coronary artery bypass graft(s) and
            coronary artery of transplanted heart with angina pectoris.

            When using one of these combination codes it is not
            necessary to use an additional code for angina pectoris. A
            causal relationship can be assumed in a patient with both
            atherosclerosis and angina pectoris, unless the
            documentation indicates the angina is due to something
            other than the atherosclerosis.

            If a patient with coronary artery disease is admitted due to
            an acute myocardial infarction (AMI), the AMI should be
            sequenced before the coronary artery disease.

⑤ ✛ **I25.1**   **Atherosclerotic heart disease of native coronary artery**
            Atherosclerotic cardiovascular disease
            Coronary (artery) atheroma
            Coronary (artery) atherosclerosis
            Coronary (artery) disease
            Coronary (artery) sclerosis
            Use additional code, if applicable, to identify:
            *coronary atherosclerosis due to calcified coronary lesion
               (I25.84)*
            coronary atherosclerosis due to lipid rich plaque (I25.83)
            EXCLUDES 2   *atheroembolism (I75.-)*
                              *atherosclerosis of coronary artery bypass
                              graft(s) and transplanted heart (I25.7-)*

   ✛ **I25.10**   **Atherosclerotic heart disease of native coronary**   A
                   artery without angina pectoris
                   Atherosclerotic heart disease NOS
                   DEFINITION   Clogging of coronary arteries with
                   fatty plaque build-up, restricting blood flow and
                   hardening the arteries.
                   AHA: 2Q 2015, 17
                   AHA: 4Q 2013, 128
                   AHA: 4Q 2012, 92

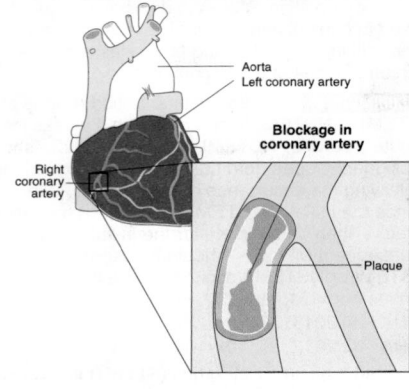

**Atherosclerotic heart disease of native
coronary artery without angina pectoris**

Aorta
Left coronary artery

Blockage in
coronary artery

Right
coronary
artery

Plaque

⑥ ✛ **I25.11**   **Atherosclerotic heart disease of native coronary
                   artery with angina pectoris**
                   CODING TIP ✓   When a patient presents with both
                   coronary artery disease (CAD) / atherosclerotic
                   heart disease and angina, a code from I25.11-
                   should be assigned. If the specific type of angina
                   is not specified in the clinical record, assign code
                   I25.119.

   ✛ **I25.110**   **Atherosclerotic heart disease of native**   A
                    **coronary artery with unstable angina
                    pectoris**
                    EXCLUDES 1   *unstable angina without
                                      atherosclerotic heart disease
                                      (I20.0)*

   ✛ **I25.111**   **Atherosclerotic heart disease of native**   A
                    **coronary artery with angina pectoris with
                    documented spasm**
                    EXCLUDES 1   *angina pectoris with documented
                                      spasm without atherosclerotic
                                      heart disease (I20.1)*

   ✛ **I25.118**   **Atherosclerotic heart disease of native**   A
                    **coronary artery with other forms of angina
                    pectoris**
                    EXCLUDES 1   *other forms of angina pectoris
                                      without atherosclerotic heart
                                      disease (I20.8)*
                    AHA: 2Q 2015, 16-17

   ✛ **I25.119**   **Atherosclerotic heart disease of native**   A
                    **coronary artery with unspecified angina
                    pectoris**
                    Atherosclerotic heart disease with angina NOS
                    Atherosclerotic heart disease with ischemic chest
                    pain
                    EXCLUDES 1   *unspecified angina pectoris
                                      without atherosclerotic heart
                                      disease (I20.9)*

✛ **I25.2**   **Old myocardial infarction**   A
              Healed myocardial infarction
              Past myocardial infarction diagnosed by ECG or other
                 investigation, but currently presenting no symptoms
              GUIDELINES   Section I.C.9.e.1)
              For old or healed myocardial infarctions not requiring
              further care, code I25.2 may be assigned.

✛ **I25.3**   **Aneurysm of heart**
              Mural aneurysm
              Ventricular aneurysm

⑤ ✛ **I25.4**   **Coronary artery aneurysm and dissection**
   ✛ **I25.41**   **Coronary artery aneurysm**
                   Coronary arteriovenous fistula, acquired
                   EXCLUDES 1   *congenital coronary (artery)
                                     aneurysm (Q24.5)*
   ✛ **I25.42**   **Coronary artery dissection**

✛ **I25.5**   **Ischemic cardiomyopathy**
              EXCLUDES 2   *coronary atherosclerosis (I25.1-, I25.7-)*

✛ **I25.6**   **Silent myocardial ischemia**

● New   ▲ Revised   *Manifestation*   ④-⑦ Digit Indicators   ⊟ Laterality   A Adult (15+ years)   M Maternity (12-55 years)   N Newborn   P Pediatric (0-17 years)   ♂ Male   ♀ Female
✖ Deleted   Unspecified   ✛ Additional code

640   © 2017 DecisionHealth   2017 ICD-10-CM Expert for Physicians

B + I25.7 **Atherosclerosis of coronary artery bypass graft(s) and coronary artery of transplanted heart with angina pectoris**
Use additional code, if applicable, to identify:
coronary atherosclerosis due to calcified coronary lesion (I25.84)
coronary atherosclerosis due to lipid rich plaque (I25.83)
> EXCLUDES 1 *atherosclerosis of bypass graft (s) of transplanted heart without angina pectoris (I25.812)*
> *atherosclerosis of coronary artery bypass graft (s) without angina pectoris (I25.810)*
> *atherosclerosis of native coronary artery of transplanted heart without angina pectoris (I25.811)*
> *embolism or thrombus of coronary artery bypass graft (s) (T82.8-)*

6 + I25.70 **Atherosclerosis of coronary artery bypass graft(s), unspecified, with angina pectoris**

+ I25.700 **Atherosclerosis of coronary artery bypass graft(s), unspecified, with unstable angina pectoris** [A]
> EXCLUDES 1 *unstable angina pectoris without atherosclerosis of coronary artery bypass graft (I20.0)*

+ I25.701 **Atherosclerosis of coronary artery bypass graft(s), unspecified, with angina pectoris with documented spasm** [A]
> EXCLUDES 1 *angina pectoris with documented spasm without atherosclerosis of coronary artery bypass graft (I20.1)*

+ I25.708 **Atherosclerosis of coronary artery bypass graft(s), unspecified, with other forms of angina pectoris** [A]
> EXCLUDES 1 *other forms of angina pectoris without atherosclerosis of coronary artery bypass graft (I20.8)*

+ I25.709 **Atherosclerosis of coronary artery bypass graft(s), unspecified, with unspecified angina pectoris** [A]
> EXCLUDES 1 *unspecified angina pectoris without atherosclerosis of coronary artery bypass graft (I20.9)*

6 + I25.71 **Atherosclerosis of autologous vein coronary artery bypass graft(s) with angina pectoris**

+ I25.710 **Atherosclerosis of autologous vein coronary artery bypass graft(s) with unstable angina pectoris** [A]
> EXCLUDES 1 *unstable angina without atherosclerosis of autologous vein coronary artery bypass graft (s) (I20.0)*

+ I25.711 **Atherosclerosis of autologous vein coronary artery bypass graft(s) with angina pectoris with documented spasm** [A]
> EXCLUDES 1 *angina pectoris with documented spasm without atherosclerosis of autologous vein coronary artery bypass graft (s) (I20.1)*

+ I25.718 **Atherosclerosis of autologous vein coronary artery bypass graft(s) with other forms of angina pectoris** [A]
> EXCLUDES 1 *other forms of angina pectoris without atherosclerosis of autologous vein coronary artery bypass graft (s) (I20.8)*

+ I25.719 **Atherosclerosis of autologous vein coronary artery bypass graft(s) with unspecified angina pectoris** [A]
> EXCLUDES 1 *unspecified angina pectoris without atherosclerosis of autologous vein coronary artery bypass graft (s) (I20.9)*

6 + I25.72 **Atherosclerosis of autologous artery coronary artery bypass graft(s) with angina pectoris**
Atherosclerosis of internal mammary artery graft with angina pectoris

+ I25.720 **Atherosclerosis of autologous artery coronary** [A] **artery bypass graft(s) with unstable angina pectoris**
> EXCLUDES 1 *unstable angina without atherosclerosis of autologous artery coronary artery bypass graft (s) (I20.0)*

+ I25.721 **Atherosclerosis of autologous artery coronary** [A] **artery bypass graft(s) with angina pectoris with documented spasm**
> EXCLUDES 1 *angina pectoris with documented spasm without atherosclerosis of autologous artery coronary artery bypass graft (s) (I20.1)*

+ I25.728 **Atherosclerosis of autologous artery coronary** [A] **artery bypass graft(s) with other forms of angina pectoris**
> EXCLUDES 1 *other forms of angina pectoris without atherosclerosis of autologous artery coronary artery bypass graft (s) (I20.8)*

+ I25.729 **Atherosclerosis of autologous artery coronary artery bypass graft(s) with unspecified angina pectoris** [A]
> EXCLUDES 1 *unspecified angina pectoris without atherosclerosis of autologous artery coronary artery bypass graft (s) (I20.9)*

6 + I25.73 **Atherosclerosis of nonautologous biological coronary artery bypass graft(s) with angina pectoris**

+ I25.730 **Atherosclerosis of nonautologous biological** [A] **coronary artery bypass graft(s) with unstable angina pectoris**
> EXCLUDES 1 *unstable angina without atherosclerosis of nonautologous biological coronary artery bypass graft (s) (I20.0)*

+ I25.731 **Atherosclerosis of nonautologous biological** [A] **coronary artery bypass graft(s) with angina pectoris with documented spasm**
> EXCLUDES 1 *angina pectoris with documented spasm without atherosclerosis of nonautologous biological coronary artery bypass graft (s) (I20.1)*

+ I25.738 **Atherosclerosis of nonautologous biological** [A] **coronary artery bypass graft(s) with other forms of angina pectoris**
> EXCLUDES 1 *other forms of angina pectoris without atherosclerosis of nonautologous biological coronary artery bypass graft (s) (I20.8)*

+ I25.739 **Atherosclerosis of nonautologous biological** [A] **coronary artery bypass graft(s) with unspecified angina pectoris**
> EXCLUDES 1 *unspecified angina pectoris without atherosclerosis of nonautologous biological coronary artery bypass graft (s) (I20.9)*

6 + I25.75 **Atherosclerosis of native coronary artery of transplanted heart with angina pectoris**
> EXCLUDES 1 *atherosclerosis of native coronary artery of transplanted heart without angina pectoris (I25.811)*

+ I25.750 **Atherosclerosis of native coronary artery of** [A] **transplanted heart with unstable angina**

+ I25.751 **Atherosclerosis of native coronary artery of** [A] **transplanted heart with angina pectoris with documented spasm**

+ I25.758 **Atherosclerosis of native coronary artery of** [A] **transplanted heart with other forms of angina pectoris**

+ I25.759 **Atherosclerosis of native coronary artery of** [A] **transplanted heart with unspecified angina pectoris**

● New ▲ Revised *Manifestation* 4-7 Digit Indicators ⊟ Laterality [A] Adult (15+ years) [M] Maternity (12-55 years) [N] Newborn [P] Pediatric (0-17 years) ♂ Male ♀ Female
✖ Deleted Unspecified + Additional code

2017 ICD-10-CM Expert for Physicians

© 2017 DecisionHealth

641

Diseases of the Circulatory System

I25.7 — I25.759

⑥+ I25.76   Atherosclerosis of bypass graft of coronary artery of transplanted heart with angina pectoris

> **EXCLUDES 1** *atherosclerosis of bypass graft of coronary artery of transplanted heart without angina pectoris (I25.812)*

  + I25.760   Atherosclerosis of bypass graft of coronary artery of transplanted heart with unstable angina   Ⓐ

  + I25.761   Atherosclerosis of bypass graft of coronary artery of transplanted heart with angina pectoris with documented spasm   Ⓐ

  + I25.768   Atherosclerosis of bypass graft of coronary artery of transplanted heart with other forms of angina pectoris   Ⓐ

  + I25.769   Atherosclerosis of bypass graft of coronary artery of transplanted heart with unspecified angina pectoris   Ⓐ

⑥+ I25.79   Atherosclerosis of other coronary artery bypass graft(s) with angina pectoris

  + I25.790   Atherosclerosis of other coronary artery bypass graft(s) with unstable angina pectoris   Ⓐ

> **EXCLUDES 1** *unstable angina without atherosclerosis of other coronary artery bypass graft (s) (I20.0)*

  + I25.791   Atherosclerosis of other coronary artery bypass graft(s) with angina pectoris with documented spasm   Ⓐ

> **EXCLUDES 1** *angina pectoris with documented spasm without atherosclerosis of other coronary artery bypass graft (s) (I20.1)*

  + I25.798   Atherosclerosis of other coronary artery bypass graft(s) with other forms of angina pectoris   Ⓐ

> **EXCLUDES 1** *other forms of angina pectoris without atherosclerosis of other coronary artery bypass graft (s) (I20.8)*

  + I25.799   Atherosclerosis of other coronary artery bypass graft(s) with unspecified angina pectoris   Ⓐ

> **EXCLUDES 1** *unspecified angina pectoris without atherosclerosis of other coronary artery bypass graft (s) (I20.9)*

⑤+ I25.8   Other forms of chronic ischemic heart disease

  ⑥+ I25.81   Atherosclerosis of other coronary vessels without angina pectoris

Use additional code, if applicable, to identify:
coronary atherosclerosis due to calcified coronary lesion (I25.84)
coronary atherosclerosis due to lipid rich plaque (I25.83)

> **EXCLUDES 1** *atherosclerotic heart disease of native coronary artery without angina pectoris (I25.10)*

  + I25.810   Atherosclerosis of coronary artery bypass graft(s) without angina pectoris   Ⓐ

Atherosclerosis of coronary artery bypass graft NOS

> **EXCLUDES 1** *atherosclerosis of coronary bypass graft (s) with angina pectoris (I25.70-I25.73-, I25.79-)*

  + I25.811   Atherosclerosis of native coronary artery of transplanted heart without angina pectoris   Ⓐ

Atherosclerosis of native coronary artery of transplanted heart NOS

> **EXCLUDES 1** *atherosclerosis of native coronary artery of transplanted heart with angina pectoris (I25.75-)*

  + I25.812   Atherosclerosis of bypass graft of coronary artery of transplanted heart without angina pectoris   Ⓐ

Atherosclerosis of bypass graft of transplanted heart NOS

> **EXCLUDES 1** *atherosclerosis of bypass graft of transplanted heart with angina pectoris (I25.76)*

+ I25.82   Chronic total occlusion of coronary artery

Complete occlusion of coronary artery
Total occlusion of coronary artery
Code first:
  coronary atherosclerosis (I25.1-, I25.7-, I25.81-)

> **EXCLUDES 1** *acute coronary occlusion with myocardial infarction (I21.-, I22.-)*
> *acute coronary occlusion without myocardial infarction (I24.0)*

+ I25.83   Coronary atherosclerosis due to lipid rich plaque   Ⓐ

Code first:
  coronary atherosclerosis (I25.1-, I25.7-, I25.81-)

+ I25.84   Coronary atherosclerosis due to calcified coronary lesion

Coronary atherosclerosis due to severely calcified coronary lesion
Code first:
  coronary atherosclerosis (I25.1-, I25.7-, I25.81-)

+ I25.89   Other forms of chronic ischemic heart disease

+ I25.9   Chronic ischemic heart disease, unspecified

Ischemic heart disease (chronic) NOS

Pulmonary heart disease and diseases of pulmonary circulation (I26-I28)

④ I26   Pulmonary embolism

> **INCLUDES** pulmonary (acute) (artery)(vein) infarction
> pulmonary (acute) (artery)(vein) thromboembolism
> pulmonary (acute) (artery)(vein) thrombosis

> **EXCLUDES 2** *chronic pulmonary embolism (I27.82)*
> *personal history of pulmonary embolism (Z86.711)*
> *pulmonary embolism complicating abortion, ectopic or molar pregnancy (O00-O07, O08.2)*
> *pulmonary embolism complicating pregnancy, childbirth and the puerperium (O88.-)*
> *pulmonary embolism due to trauma (T79.0, T79.1)*
> *pulmonary embolism due to complications of surgical and medical care (T80.0, T81.7-, T82.8-)*
> *septic (non-pulmonary) arterial embolism (I76)*

⑤ I26.0   Pulmonary embolism with acute cor pulmonale

> **CODING TIP ✓** Category I26.0- codes should be assigned only when cor pulmonale is reported as occurring and associated with a pulmonary embolus. Cor pulmonale is a right ventricular dysfunction and failure.

  I26.01   Septic pulmonary embolism with acute cor pulmonale

Code first:
  underlying infection

> **CODING TIP ✓** The term septic pulmonary embolism indicates a pulmonary embolus resulting from embolization of infectious particles which enter the lungs in the pulmonary arterial system. This can occur as a result of infectious DVT, periodontal disease, infected venous catheters, endocarditis, or other systemic infections. This code should only be assigned when the embolus is stated as septic and related to an infectious cause. A second code for the underlying/causative infection must be assigned.

  I26.02   Saddle embolus of pulmonary artery with acute cor pulmonale

  I26.09   Other pulmonary embolism with acute cor pulmonale

Acute cor pulmonale NOS
AHA: 4Q 2014, 22

⑤ I26.9   Pulmonary embolism without acute cor pulmonale

  I26.90   Septic pulmonary embolism without acute cor pulmonale

Code first:
  underlying infection

  I26.92   Saddle embolus of pulmonary artery without acute cor pulmonale

---

● New   ▲ Revised   *Manifestation*   ④-⑦ Digit Indicators   ⊟ Laterality   Ⓐ Adult (15+ years)   Ⓜ Maternity (12-55 years)   Ⓝ Newborn   Ⓟ Pediatric (0-17 years)   ♂ Male   ♀ Female

✖ Deleted   Unspecified   + Additional code

642   © 2017 DecisionHealth   2017 ICD-10-CM Expert for Physicians

I26.99   Other pulmonary embolism without acute cor pulmonale
Acute pulmonary embolism NOS
Pulmonary embolism NOS

◢ I27   **Other pulmonary heart diseases**

I27.0   **Primary pulmonary hypertension**
> **EXCLUDES 1**   *pulmonary hypertension NOS (I27.2)*
> *secondary pulmonary hypertension (I27.2)*

I27.1   **Kyphoscoliotic heart disease**

I27.2   **Other secondary pulmonary hypertension**
Pulmonary hypertension NOS
Code also:
   associated underlying condition
AHA: 2Q 2016, 8
AHA: 4Q 2014, 21, 22

⑤ I27.8   **Other specified pulmonary heart diseases**

I27.81   **Cor pulmonale (chronic)**
Cor pulmonale NOS
> **EXCLUDES 1**   *acute cor pulmonale (I26.0-)*

AHA: 4Q 2014, 21

✛ I27.82   **Chronic pulmonary embolism**
Use additional code, if applicable, for associated long-term (current) use of anticoagulants (Z79.01)
> **EXCLUDES 1**   *personal history of pulmonary embolism (Z86.711)*

I27.89   **Other specified pulmonary heart diseases**
Eisenmenger's complex
Eisenmenger's syndrome
> **EXCLUDES 1**   *Eisenmenger's defect (Q21.8)*

I27.9   **Pulmonary heart disease, unspecified**
Chronic cardiopulmonary disease

◢ I28   **Other diseases of pulmonary vessels**

I28.0   **Arteriovenous fistula of pulmonary vessels**
> **EXCLUDES 1**   *congenital arteriovenous fistula (Q25.72)*

> **DEFINITION**   Abnormal passage between the pulmonary arterial and venous systems, which causes unoxygenated blood to enter systemic circulation.

I28.1   **Aneurysm of pulmonary artery**
> **EXCLUDES 1**   *congenital aneurysm (Q25.79)*
> *congenital arteriovenous aneurysm (Q25.72)*

> **DEFINITION**   Bulging in one portion of the arterial wall that brings blood to the lungs, forming a pouch or sac with the potential for rupture.

I28.8   **Other diseases of pulmonary vessels**
Pulmonary arteritis
Pulmonary endarteritis
Rupture of pulmonary vessels
Stenosis of pulmonary vessels
Stricture of pulmonary vessels

I28.9   **Disease of pulmonary vessels, unspecified**

Other forms of heart disease (I30-I52)

> **CODING TIP ✓**   Pericarditis, endocarditis, myocarditis and valve disorders not specified as rheumatic may be coded here when a more specific code (such as meningococcal pericarditis) is not appropriate.

◢ I30   **Acute pericarditis**
> **INCLUDES**   acute mediastinopericarditis
> acute myopericarditis
> acute pericardial effusion
> acute pleuropericarditis
> acute pneumopericarditis
> **EXCLUDES 1**   *Dressler's syndrome (I24.1)*
> *rheumatic pericarditis (acute) (I01.0)*

I30.0   **Acute nonspecific idiopathic pericarditis**

✛ I30.1   **Infective pericarditis**
Pneumococcal pericarditis
Pneumopyopericardium
Purulent pericarditis
Pyopericarditis
Pyopericardium
Pyopneumopericardium
Staphylococcal pericarditis
Streptococcal pericarditis
Suppurative pericarditis
Viral pericarditis
Use additional code (B95-B97) to identify infectious agent

I30.8   **Other forms of acute pericarditis**

I30.9   **Acute pericarditis, unspecified**

◢ I31   **Other diseases of pericardium**
> **EXCLUDES 1**   *diseases of pericardium specified as rheumatic (I09.2)*
> *postcardiotomy syndrome (I97.0)*
> *traumatic injury to pericardium (S26.-)*

I31.0   **Chronic adhesive pericarditis**
Accretio cordis
Adherent pericardium
Adhesive mediastinopericarditis
> **DEFINITION**   Pericardial inflammation with adhesion between the two pericardial layers or between the pericardium and the heart or neighboring structures.

I31.1   **Chronic constrictive pericarditis**
Concretio cordis
Pericardial calcification

I31.2   **Hemopericardium, not elsewhere classified**
> **EXCLUDES 1**   *hemopericardium as current complication following acute myocardial infarction (I23.0)*

> **DEFINITION**   Bleeding causing the sac around the heart to fill with blood.

I31.3   **Pericardial effusion (noninflammatory)**
Chylopericardium
> **EXCLUDES 1**   *acute pericardial effusion (I30.9)*

I31.4   **Cardiac tamponade**
Code first:
   underlying cause
> **DEFINITION**   Increased pressure on the heart due to fluid in the pericardial sac, impairing ventricular filling action and causing decreased cardiac output.

I31.8   **Other specified diseases of pericardium**
Epicardial plaques
Focal pericardial adhesions

I31.9   **Disease of pericardium, unspecified**
Pericarditis (chronic) NOS

I32   *Pericarditis in diseases classified elsewhere*
Code first:
   underlying disease
> **EXCLUDES 1**   *pericarditis (in) :*
> *coxsackie (virus) (B33.23)*
> *gonococcal (A54.83)*
> *meningococcal (A39.53)*
> *rheumatoid (arthritis) (M05.31)*
> *syphilitic (A52.06)*
> *systemic lupus erythematosus (M32.12)*
> *tuberculosis (A18.84)*

> **DEFINITION**   Inflammation of the membranous sac around the heart occurring with another underlying disease process, causing chest pain, coughing, fatigue, and fever.

◢ I33   **Acute and subacute endocarditis**
> **EXCLUDES 1**   *acute rheumatic endocarditis (I01.1)*
> *endocarditis NOS (I38)*

✛ I33.0   **Acute and subacute infective endocarditis**
Bacterial endocarditis (acute) (subacute)
Infective endocarditis (acute) (subacute) NOS
Endocarditis lenta (acute) (subacute)
Malignant endocarditis (acute) (subacute)
Purulent endocarditis (acute) (subacute)
Septic endocarditis (acute) (subacute)
Ulcerative endocarditis (acute) (subacute)
Vegetative endocarditis (acute) (subacute)
Use additional code (B95-B97) to identify infectious agent

● New   ▲ Revised   *Manifestation*   ◰-◷ Digit Indicators   ⊟ Laterality   Ⓐ Adult (15+ years)   Ⓜ Maternity (12-55 years)   Ⓝ Newborn (0-17 years)   Ⓟ Pediatric   ♂ Male   ♀ Female
✖ Deleted   Unspecified   + Additional code

2017 ICD-10-CM Expert for Physicians   © 2017 DecisionHealth   643

Diseases of the Circulatory System

I33.9   **Acute and subacute endocarditis, unspecified**
Acute endocarditis NOS
Acute myoendocarditis NOS
Acute periendocarditis NOS
Subacute endocarditis NOS
Subacute myoendocarditis NOS
Subacute periendocarditis NOS

4 I34   **Nonrheumatic mitral valve disorders**

EXCLUDES 1   *mitral valve disease (I05.9)*
mitral valve failure (I05.8)
mitral valve stenosis (I05.0)
mitral valve disorder of unspecified cause with diseases of aortic and/or tricuspid valve (s) (I08.-)
mitral valve disorder of unspecified cause with mitral stenosis or obstruction (I05.0)
mitral valve disorder specified as congenital (Q23.2, Q23.3)
mitral valve disorder specified as rheumatic (I05.-)

I34.0   **Nonrheumatic mitral (valve) insufficiency**
Nonrheumatic mitral (valve) incompetence NOS
Nonrheumatic mitral (valve) regurgitation NOS

I34.1   **Nonrheumatic mitral (valve) prolapse**
Floppy nonrheumatic mitral valve syndrome
EXCLUDES 1   *Marfan's syndrome (Q87.4-)*

I34.2   **Nonrheumatic mitral (valve) stenosis**
I34.8   **Other nonrheumatic mitral valve disorders**
I34.9   **Nonrheumatic mitral valve disorder, unspecified**

4 I35   **Nonrheumatic aortic valve disorders**

EXCLUDES 1   *aortic valve disorder of unspecified cause but with diseases of mitral and/or tricuspid valve (s) (I08.-)*
aortic valve disorder specified as congenital (Q23.0, Q23.1)
aortic valve disorder specified as rheumatic (I06.-)
hypertrophic subaortic stenosis (I42.1)

I35.0   **Nonrheumatic aortic (valve) stenosis**

Nonrheumatic aortic (valve) stenosis

Stenosis of aortic valve
Aorta
Aortic valve
Blood is unable to flow freely from the left ventricle to the aorta
Right ventricle
Left ventricle

I35.1   **Nonrheumatic aortic (valve) insufficiency**
Nonrheumatic aortic (valve) incompetence NOS
Nonrheumatic aortic (valve) regurgitation NOS

I35.2   **Nonrheumatic aortic (valve) stenosis with insufficiency**
I35.8   **Other nonrheumatic aortic valve disorders**
I35.9   **Nonrheumatic aortic valve disorder, unspecified**

4 I36   **Nonrheumatic tricuspid valve disorders**

EXCLUDES 1   *tricuspid valve disorders of unspecified cause (I07.-)*
tricuspid valve disorders specified as congenital (Q22.4, Q22.8, Q22.9)
tricuspid valve disorders specified as rheumatic (I07.-)
tricuspid valve disorders with aortic and/or mitral valve involvement (I08.-)

I36.0   **Nonrheumatic tricuspid (valve) stenosis**
I36.1   **Nonrheumatic tricuspid (valve) insufficiency**
Nonrheumatic tricuspid (valve) incompetence
Nonrheumatic tricuspid (valve) regurgitation

I36.2   **Nonrheumatic tricuspid (valve) stenosis with insufficiency**
I36.8   **Other nonrheumatic tricuspid valve disorders**
I36.9   **Nonrheumatic tricuspid valve disorder, unspecified**

4 I37   **Nonrheumatic pulmonary valve disorders**

EXCLUDES 1   *pulmonary valve disorder specified as congenital (Q22.1, Q22.2, Q22.3)*
pulmonary valve disorder specified as rheumatic (I09.89)

I37.0   **Nonrheumatic pulmonary valve stenosis**
I37.1   **Nonrheumatic pulmonary valve insufficiency**
Nonrheumatic pulmonary valve incompetence
Nonrheumatic pulmonary valve regurgitation

I37.2   **Nonrheumatic pulmonary valve stenosis with insufficiency**
I37.8   **Other nonrheumatic pulmonary valve disorders**
I37.9   **Nonrheumatic pulmonary valve disorder, unspecified**

I38   **Endocarditis, valve unspecified**

INCLUDES   endocarditis (chronic) NOS
valvular incompetence NOS
valvular insufficiency NOS
valvular regurgitation NOS
valvular stenosis NOS
valvulitis (chronic) NOS

EXCLUDES 1   *congenital insufficiency of cardiac valve NOS (Q24.8)*
congenital stenosis of cardiac valve NOS (Q24.8)
endocardial fibroelastosis (I42.4)
endocarditis specified as rheumatic (I09.1)

I39   ***Endocarditis and heart valve disorders in diseases classified elsewhere***

Code first underlying disease, such as:
Q fever (A78)
EXCLUDES 1   *endocardial involvement in:*
candidiasis (B37.6)
gonococcal infection (A54.83)
Libman-Sacks disease (M32.11)
listerosis (A32.82)
meningococcal infection (A39.51)
rheumatoid arthritis (M05.31)
syphilis (A52.03)
tuberculosis (A18.84)
typhoid fever (A01.02)

CODING TIP ✓   I39 is a manifestation code and may be used only in conjunction with a code to report the causative underlying disease process.

CODING TIP ✓   **Documentation:** Assign this code only when the clinical record supports a cause and effect relationship between the underlying disease process and the endocarditis/valve disorder.

4 I40   **Acute myocarditis**

INCLUDES   subacute myocarditis
EXCLUDES 1   *acute rheumatic myocarditis (I01.2)*
DEFINITION   Severe inflammation of heart muscle tissue.

+ I40.0   **Infective myocarditis**
Septic myocarditis
Use additional code (B95-B97) to identify infectious agent

I40.1   **Isolated myocarditis**
Fiedler's myocarditis
Giant cell myocarditis
Idiopathic myocarditis

I40.8   **Other acute myocarditis**
I40.9   **Acute myocarditis, unspecified**

I41   ***Myocarditis in diseases classified elsewhere***

Code first underlying disease, such as:
typhus (A75.0-A75.9)
EXCLUDES 1   *myocarditis (in) :*
Chagas' disease (chronic) (B57.2)
acute (B57.0)
coxsackie (virus) infection (B33.22)
diphtheritic (A36.81)
gonococcal (A54.83)
influenzal (J09.X9, J10.82, J11.82)
meningococcal (A39.52)
mumps (B26.82)
rheumatoid arthritis (M05.31)
sarcoid (D86.85)
syphilis (A52.06)
toxoplasmosis (B58.81)
tuberculous (A18.84)

● New   ▲ Revised   *Manifestation*   4-7 Digit Indicators   ⊟ Laterality   A Adult (15+ years)   M Maternity (12-55 years)   N Newborn   P Pediatric (0-17 years)   ♂ Male   ♀ Female
✖ Deleted   Unspecified   + Additional code

644   © 2017 DecisionHealth   2017 ICD-10-CM Expert for Physicians

CODING TIP ✓ I41 is a manifestation code and may be used only in conjunction with a code to report the causative underlying disease process.

CODING TIP ✓ **Documentation:** Assign this code only when the clinical record supports a cause and effect relationship between the underlying disease process and myocarditis.

▲ ◼ **I42   Cardiomyopathy**

INCLUDES   myocardiopathy

Code first:
  pre-existing cardiomyopathy complicating pregnancy and puerperium (O99.4)

EXCLUDES 2   ischemic cardiomyopathy (I25.5)
  peripartum cardiomyopathy (O90.3)
  ventricular hypertrophy (I51.7)

I42.0   **Dilated cardiomyopathy**
  Congestive cardiomyopathy

I42.1   **Obstructive hypertrophic cardiomyopathy**
  Hypertrophic subaortic stenosis (idiopathic)

I42.2   **Other hypertrophic cardiomyopathy**
  Nonobstructive hypertrophic cardiomyopathy

I42.3   **Endomyocardial (eosinophilic) disease**
  Endomyocardial (tropical) fibrosis
  Löffler's endocarditis

I42.4   **Endocardial fibroelastosis**
  Congenital cardiomyopathy
  Elastomyofibrosis

I42.5   **Other restrictive cardiomyopathy**
  Constrictive cardiomyopathy NOS

I42.6   **Alcoholic cardiomyopathy**
  Code also:
    presence of alcoholism (F10.-)
  DEFINITION   Dilated disease of the heart muscle due to alcohol abuse.

+ I42.7   **Cardiomyopathy due to drug and external agent**
  Code first:
    poisoning due to drug or toxin, if applicable (T36-T65 with fifth or sixth character 1-4 or 6)
  Use additional code for adverse effect, if applicable, to identify drug (T36-T50 with fifth or sixth character 5)

I42.8   **Other cardiomyopathies**
I42.9   **Cardiomyopathy, unspecified**
  Cardiomyopathy (primary) (secondary) NOS

I43   *Cardiomyopathy in diseases classified elsewhere*
  Code first underlying disease, such as:
    amyloidosis (E85.-)
    glycogen storage disease (E74.0)
    gout (M10.0-)
    thyrotoxicosis (E05.0-E05.9-)
  EXCLUDES 1   cardiomyopathy (in) :
    coxsackie (virus) (B33.24)
    diphtheria (A36.81)
    sarcoidosis (D86.85)
    tuberculosis (A18.84)

CODING TIP ✓ I43 is a manifestation code and may be used only in conjunction with a code to report the causative underlying disease process.

CODING TIP ✓ **Documentation:** Assign this code only when the clinical record supports a cause and effect relationship between the underlying disease process and cardiomyopathy.

◼ **I44   Atrioventricular and left bundle-branch block**

CODING TIP ✓ When reviewing documentation for heart block, it is important to differentiate heart block degree from heart block type.

I44.0   **Atrioventricular block, first degree**
I44.1   **Atrioventricular block, second degree**
  Atrioventricular block, type I and II
  Möbitz block block, type I and II
  Second degree block, type I and II
  Wenckebach's block

I44.2   **Atrioventricular block, complete**
  Complete heart block NOS
  Third degree block
  DEFINITION   No conduction of electrical impulses occurs between the atria and ventricles, requiring a pacemaker to maintain rhythm.

◼ I44.3   **Other and unspecified atrioventricular block**
  Atrioventricular block NOS
  I44.30   **Unspecified atrioventricular block**
  I44.39   **Other atrioventricular block**
I44.4   **Left anterior fascicular block**
I44.5   **Left posterior fascicular block**
◼ I44.6   **Other and unspecified fascicular block**
  I44.60   **Unspecified fascicular block**
    Left bundle-branch hemiblock NOS
  I44.69   **Other fascicular block**
I44.7   **Left bundle-branch block, unspecified**

◼ **I45   Other conduction disorders**

CODING TIP ✓ When reviewing documentation for heart block, it is important to differentiate heart block degree from heart block type.

I45.0   **Right fascicular block**
◼ I45.1   **Other and unspecified right bundle-branch block**
  I45.10   **Unspecified right bundle-branch block**
    Right bundle-branch block NOS
  I45.19   **Other right bundle-branch block**
I45.2   **Bifascicular block**
I45.3   **Trifascicular block**
I45.4   **Nonspecific intraventricular block**
  Bundle-branch block NOS
  DEFINITION   A condition in which portions of the heart's conduction system are defective and either slow or block the electrical impulses traveling through specialized conduction tissue on the way to the ventricles.
I45.5   **Other specified heart block**
  Sinoatrial block
  Sinoauricular block
  EXCLUDES 1   heart block NOS (I45.9)
I45.6   **Pre-excitation syndrome**
  Accelerated atrioventricular conduction
  Accessory atrioventricular conduction
  Anomalous atrioventricular excitation
  Lown-Ganong-Levine syndrome
  Pre-excitation atrioventricular conduction
  Wolff-Parkinson-White syndrome
◼ I45.8   **Other specified conduction disorders**
  I45.81   **Long QT syndrome**
    DEFINITION   Hereditary defect of the heart's electrical conduction system with an abnormally long gap in the time it takes for the ventricles to contract.
  I45.89   **Other specified conduction disorders**
    Atrioventricular [AV] dissociation
    Interference dissociation
    Isorhythmic dissociation
    Nonparoxysmal AV nodal tachycardia
    AHA: 2Q 2013, 31-32
I45.9   **Conduction disorder, unspecified**
  Heart block NOS
  Stokes-Adams syndrome

◼ **I46   Cardiac arrest**
  EXCLUDES 1   cardiogenic shock (R57.0)
I46.2   **Cardiac arrest due to underlying cardiac condition**
  Code first:
    underlying cardiac condition
I46.8   **Cardiac arrest due to other underlying condition**
  Code first:
    underlying condition
I46.9   **Cardiac arrest, cause unspecified**

◼ **I47   Paroxysmal tachycardia**
  Code first tachycardia complicating:
    abortion or ectopic or molar pregnancy (O00-O07, O08.8)
    obstetric surgery and procedures (O75.4)
  EXCLUDES 1   tachycardia NOS (R00.0)
    sinoauricular tachycardia NOS (R00.0)
    sinus [sinusal] tachycardia NOS (R00.0)

CODING TIP ✓ Do not assign a code from I47.- when only tachycardia is reported in the record and is not specified, or is reported in the record as sinus tachycardia or sinoauricular. When tachycardia is reported as sinus tachycardia or is not specified, report code R00.0 rather than a code from I47.-.

Diseases of the Circulatory System

I47.0 **Re-entry ventricular arrhythmia**
I47.1 **Supraventricular tachycardia**
Atrial (paroxysmal) tachycardia
Atrioventricular [AV] (paroxysmal) tachycardia
Atrioventricular re-entrant (nodal) tachycardia [AVNRT]
  [AVRT]
Junctional (paroxysmal) tachycardia
Nodal (paroxysmal) tachycardia
  DEFINITION Abnormally rapid atrial rhythm occurring from time to time, most often in the young.

I47.2 **Ventricular tachycardia**
  DEFINITION Potentially lethal rapid heart beat initiating in the ventricles marked by three of more consecutive premature beats.
  AHA: 3Q 2013, 23

I47.9 **Paroxysmal tachycardia, unspecified**
Bouveret (-Hoffman) syndrome

I48 **Atrial fibrillation and flutter**
  CODING TIP ✓ When assigning a code for atrial fibrillation or flutter, assign the most specific code according to the diagnostic statements given by the patient's physician.
  DEFINITION Abnormal heart rhythm that occurs in the atria of the heart.

I48.0 **Paroxysmal atrial fibrillation**
I48.1 **Persistent atrial fibrillation**
  CODING TIP ✓ Documentation: Do not assume a diagnosis of persistent atrial fibrillation in a patient who has a longstanding history of atrial fibrillation. This code may be assigned only with a supportive confirmation diagnosis by the physician.

I48.2 **Chronic atrial fibrillation**
Permanent atrial fibrillation
  CODING TIP ✓ Documentation: Do not assume a diagnosis of chronic atrial fibrillation in a patient who has a longstanding history of atrial fibrillation or has simply had atrial fibrillation for a longstanding period of time. This code may only be assigned with a supportive confirmation diagnosis by the physician. Without such a diagnostic statement, an unspecified code (I48.91) must be assigned.
  AHA: 4Q 2013, 128

I48.3 **Typical atrial flutter**
Type I atrial flutter
I48.4 **Atypical atrial flutter**
Type II atrial flutter
I48.9 **Unspecified atrial fibrillation and atrial flutter**
  I48.91 **Unspecified atrial fibrillation**
  I48.92 **Unspecified atrial flutter**

I49 **Other cardiac arrhythmias**
  Code first cardiac arrhythmia complicating:
  abortion or ectopic or molar pregnancy (O00-O07, O08.8)
  obstetric surgery and procedures (O75.4)
  EXCLUDES 1 *bradycardia NOS (R00.1)*
    neonatal dysrhythmia (P29.1-)
    sinoatrial bradycardia (R00.1)
    sinus bradycardia (R00.1)
    vagal bradycardia (R00.1)
I49.0 **Ventricular fibrillation and flutter**
  I49.01 **Ventricular fibrillation**
  I49.02 **Ventricular flutter**
I49.1 **Atrial premature depolarization**
Atrial premature beats
I49.2 **Junctional premature depolarization**
I49.3 **Ventricular premature depolarization**
I49.4 **Other and unspecified premature depolarization**
  I49.40 **Unspecified premature depolarization**
    Premature beats NOS
  I49.49 **Other premature depolarization**
    Ectopic beats
    Extrasystoles
    Extrasystolic arrhythmias
    Premature contractions
I49.5 **Sick sinus syndrome**
Tachycardia-bradycardia syndrome

I49.8 **Other specified cardiac arrhythmias**
Coronary sinus rhythm disorder
Ectopic rhythm disorder
Nodal rhythm disorder
I49.9 **Cardiac arrhythmia, unspecified**
Arrhythmia (cardiac) NOS

▲ **I50** **Heart failure**
  Code first:
  heart failure complicating abortion or ectopic or molar pregnancy (O00-O07, O08.8)
  heart failure due to hypertension (I11.0)
  heart failure due to hypertension with chronic kidney disease (I13.-)
  heart failure following surgery (I97.13-)
  obstetric surgery and procedures (O75.4)
  rheumatic heart failure (I09.81)
  EXCLUDES 1 *neonatal cardiac failure (P29.0)*
  EXCLUDES 2 *cardiac arrest (I46.-)*
  GUIDELINES Section 1.C.9.a.1 When the cause of heart failure is established by the provider as due to HTN, the HTN (I11 category) must be coded first followed by heart failure. The same heart condition with HTN but without provider stated causal relationship are coded separately and sequenced according to the circumstances of the encounter.
  GUIDELINES Section I.C.9.a.1) Heart conditions classified to I50.- or I51.4-I51.9, are assigned to category I11, Hypertensive heart disease, when a causal relationship is stated (due to hypertension) or implied (hypertensive). Use an additional code from category I50, Heart failure, to identify the type of heart failure in those patients with heart failure. The same heart conditions (I50.-, I51.4-I51.9) with hypertension, but without a stated causal relationship, are coded separately. Sequence according to the circumstances of the admission/encounter.
  CODING TIP ✓ The term "congestive" is a non-essential modifier for heart failure codes. When coding heart failure, note the non-essential modifier (congestive) and that no additional code should be used if a patient has both CHF and a more specific form of heart failure, such as diastolic heart failure, for example.
  CODING TIP ✓ When both heart failure and a code from category I11.- will be coded, the heart failure (I50.-) code should immediately follow the code from category I11.-. When both heart failure and a code from category I13.- will be coded, the heart failure (I50.-) code, should immediately follow the code from I13.- and should precede the code from N18.- used to specify kidney disease.

I50.1 **Left ventricular failure**
Cardiac asthma
Edema of lung with heart disease NOS
Edema of lung with heart failure
Left heart failure
Pulmonary edema with heart disease NOS
Pulmonary edema with heart failure
  EXCLUDES 1 *edema of lung without heart disease or heart failure (J81.-)*
    pulmonary edema without heart disease or failure (J81.-)
I50.2 **Systolic (congestive) heart failure**
  EXCLUDES 1 *combined systolic (congestive) and diastolic (congestive) heart failure (I50.4-)*
  DEFINITION Heart muscle fails to contract with adequate force and not enough oxygen-rich blood is pumped to the body.
  I50.20 **Unspecified systolic (congestive) heart failure**
  I50.21 **Acute systolic (congestive) heart failure**
  I50.22 **Chronic systolic (congestive) heart failure**
  I50.23 **Acute on chronic systolic (congestive) heart failure**
    AHA: 2Q 2013, 33
I50.3 **Diastolic (congestive) heart failure**
  EXCLUDES 1 *combined systolic (congestive) and diastolic (congestive) heart failure (I50.4-)*
  DEFINITION Heart muscle contracts normally but ventricles fail to relax properly after contraction, resulting in less blood entering the heart.
  I50.30 **Unspecified diastolic (congestive) heart failure**

● New   ▲ Revised   *Manifestation*   ❹-❼ Digit Indicators   ▣ Laterality   Ⓐ Adult (15+ years)   Ⓜ Maternity (12-55 years)   Ⓝ Newborn   Ⓟ Pediatric (0-17 years)   ♂ Male   ♀ Female
✖ Deleted   Unspecified   + Additional code

I50.31 Acute diastolic (congestive) heart failure

I50.32 Chronic diastolic (congestive) heart failure

I50.33 Acute on chronic diastolic (congestive) heart failure

I50.4 Combined systolic (congestive) and diastolic (congestive) heart failure

> **DEFINITION** Heart fails both to contract and relax properly, resulting in an insufficient amount of blood moving through the circulatory system.

I50.40 Unspecified combined systolic (congestive) and diastolic (congestive) heart failure

I50.41 Acute combined systolic (congestive) and diastolic (congestive) heart failure

I50.42 Chronic combined systolic (congestive) and diastolic (congestive) heart failure

I50.43 Acute on chronic combined systolic (congestive) and diastolic (congestive) heart failure

▲ **I50.9** Heart failure, unspecified

Biventricular (heart) failure NOS
Cardiac, heart or myocardial failure NOS
Congestive heart disease
Congestive heart failure NOS
Right ventricular failure (secondary to left heart failure)

> **EXCLUDES 2** fluid overload (E87.70)

> **CODING TIP✓** Do not assign a code for left heart failure (I50.1) when coding I50.9, as this is assumed. These two codes should never be used together.
> AHA: 2Q 2015, 15
> AHA: 4Q 2014, 21
> AHA: 4Q 2012, 92

I51 Complications and ill-defined descriptions of heart disease

> **EXCLUDES 1** any condition in I51.4-I51.9 due to hypertension (I11.-)
> any condition in I51.4-I51.9 due to hypertension and chronic kidney disease (I13.-)
> heart disease specified as rheumatic (I00-I09)

I51.0 Cardiac septal defect, acquired

Acquired septal atrial defect (old)
Acquired septal auricular defect (old)
Acquired septal ventricular defect (old)

> **EXCLUDES 1** cardiac septal defect as current complication following acute myocardial infarction (I23.1, I23.2)

I51.1 Rupture of chordae tendineae, not elsewhere classified

> **EXCLUDES 1** rupture of chordae tendineae as current complication following acute myocardial infarction (I23.4)

> **DEFINITION** Tear in the fibrous, cord-like tissue connecting the papillary muscles to the valves, holding the valve flaps in place to prevent their eversion.

I51.2 Rupture of papillary muscle, not elsewhere classified

> **EXCLUDES 1** rupture of papillary muscle as current complication following acute myocardial infarction (I23.5)

I51.3 Intracardiac thrombosis, not elsewhere classified

Apical thrombosis (old)
Atrial thrombosis (old)
Auricular thrombosis (old)
Mural thrombosis (old)
Ventricular thrombosis (old)

> **EXCLUDES 1** intracardiac thrombosis as current complication following acute myocardial infarction (I23.6)
> AHA: 1Q 2013, 24

I51.4 Myocarditis, unspecified

Chronic (interstitial) myocarditis
Myocardial fibrosis
Myocarditis NOS

> **EXCLUDES 1** acute or subacute myocarditis (I40.-)

I51.5 Myocardial degeneration

Fatty degeneration of heart or myocardium
Myocardial disease
Senile degeneration of heart or myocardium

> **DEFINITION** Wasting away of the heart muscle.

I51.7 Cardiomegaly

Cardiac dilatation
Cardiac hypertrophy
Ventricular dilatation

I51.8 Other ill-defined heart diseases

I51.81 Takotsubo syndrome

Reversible left ventricular dysfunction following sudden emotional stress
Stress induced cardiomyopathy
Takotsubo cardiomyopathy
Transient left ventricular apical ballooning syndrome

I51.89 Other ill-defined heart diseases

Carditis (acute)(chronic)
Pancarditis (acute)(chronic)

I51.9 Heart disease, unspecified

I52 *Other heart disorders in diseases classified elsewhere*

Code first underlying disease, such as:
congenital syphilis (A50.5)
mucopolysaccharidosis (E76.3)
schistosomiasis (B65.0-B65.9)

> **EXCLUDES 1** heart disease (in):
> gonococcal infection (A54.83)
> meningococcal infection (A39.50)
> rheumatoid arthritis (M05.31)
> syphilis (A52.06)

Cerebrovascular diseases (I60-I69)

Use additional code to identify presence of:
alcohol abuse and dependence (F10.-)
exposure to environmental tobacco smoke (Z77.22)
history of tobacco dependence (Z87.891)
hypertension (I10-I15)
occupational exposure to environmental tobacco smoke (Z57.31)
tobacco dependence (F17.-)
tobacco use (Z72.0)

> **EXCLUDES 1** transient cerebral ischemic attacks and related syndromes (G45.-)
> traumatic intracranial hemorrhage (S06.-)

▲ **I60** Nontraumatic subarachnoid hemorrhage

> **INCLUDES** ruptured cerebral aneurysm
> **EXCLUDES 1** syphilitic ruptured cerebral aneurysm (A52.05)
> **EXCLUDES 2** sequelae of subarachnoid hemorrhage (I69.0-)
> AHA: 4Q 2012, 92

I60.0 Nontraumatic subarachnoid hemorrhage from carotid siphon and bifurcation

I60.00 Nontraumatic subarachnoid hemorrhage from unspecified carotid siphon and bifurcation

I60.01 Nontraumatic subarachnoid hemorrhage from right carotid siphon and bifurcation

I60.02 Nontraumatic subarachnoid hemorrhage from left carotid siphon and bifurcation

I60.1 Nontraumatic subarachnoid hemorrhage from middle cerebral artery

I60.10 Nontraumatic subarachnoid hemorrhage from unspecified middle cerebral artery

I60.11 Nontraumatic subarachnoid hemorrhage from right middle cerebral artery

I60.12 Nontraumatic subarachnoid hemorrhage from left middle cerebral artery

▲ **I60.2** Nontraumatic subarachnoid hemorrhage from anterior communicating artery

✖ ~~I60.20~~ ~~Nontraumatic subarachnoid hemorrhage from unspecified anterior communicating artery~~

✖ ~~I60.21~~ ~~Nontraumatic subarachnoid hemorrhage from right anterior communicating artery~~

✖ ~~I60.22~~ ~~Nontraumatic subarachnoid hemorrhage from left anterior communicating artery~~

I60.3 Nontraumatic subarachnoid hemorrhage from posterior communicating artery

I60.30 Nontraumatic subarachnoid hemorrhage from unspecified posterior communicating artery

I60.31 Nontraumatic subarachnoid hemorrhage from right posterior communicating artery

I60.32 Nontraumatic subarachnoid hemorrhage from left posterior communicating artery

I60.4 Nontraumatic subarachnoid hemorrhage from basilar artery

I60.5 Nontraumatic subarachnoid hemorrhage from vertebral artery

I60.50 Nontraumatic subarachnoid hemorrhage from unspecified vertebral artery

● New ▲ Revised *Manifestation* �4-7 Digit Indicators ⊟ Laterality Ⓐ Adult (15+ years) Ⓜ Maternity (12-55 years) Ⓝ Newborn (0-17 years) Ⓟ Pediatric ♂ Male ♀ Female
✖ ~~Deleted~~ Unspecified + Additional code

2017 ICD-10-CM Expert for Physicians © 2017 DecisionHealth 647

Diseases of the Circulatory System

☐ **I60.51** Nontraumatic subarachnoid hemorrhage from right vertebral artery

☐ **I60.52** Nontraumatic subarachnoid hemorrhage from left vertebral artery

I60.6 Nontraumatic subarachnoid hemorrhage from other intracranial arteries

I60.7 **Nontraumatic subarachnoid hemorrhage from unspecified intracranial artery**
Ruptured (congenital) berry aneurysm
Ruptured (congenital) cerebral aneurysm
Subarachnoid hemorrhage (nontraumatic) from cerebral artery NOS
Subarachnoid hemorrhage (nontraumatic) from communicating artery NOS
EXCLUDES 1 *berry aneurysm, nonruptured (I67.1)*

I60.8 Other nontraumatic subarachnoid hemorrhage
Meningeal hemorrhage
Rupture of cerebral arteriovenous malformation

I60.9 **Nontraumatic subarachnoid hemorrhage, unspecified**

▲ ▣ **I61** **Nontraumatic intracerebral hemorrhage**
EXCLUDES 2 *sequelae of intracerebral hemorrhage (I69.1-)*

I61.0 Nontraumatic intracerebral hemorrhage in hemisphere, subcortical
Deep intracerebral hemorrhage (nontraumatic)

I61.1 Nontraumatic intracerebral hemorrhage in hemisphere, cortical
Cerebral lobe hemorrhage (nontraumatic)
Superficial intracerebral hemorrhage (nontraumatic)

I61.2 **Nontraumatic intracerebral hemorrhage in hemisphere, unspecified**

I61.3 Nontraumatic intracerebral hemorrhage in brain stem

I61.4 Nontraumatic intracerebral hemorrhage in cerebellum

I61.5 Nontraumatic intracerebral hemorrhage, intraventricular

I61.6 Nontraumatic intracerebral hemorrhage, multiple localized

I61.8 Other nontraumatic intracerebral hemorrhage

I61.9 **Nontraumatic intracerebral hemorrhage, unspecified**
AHA: 4Q 2012, 92

▲ ▣ **I62** **Other and unspecified nontraumatic intracranial hemorrhage**
EXCLUDES 2 *sequelae of intracranial hemorrhage (I69.2)*

⑤ **I62.0** **Nontraumatic subdural hemorrhage**

I62.00 **Nontraumatic subdural hemorrhage, unspecified**

I62.01 **Nontraumatic acute subdural hemorrhage**

I62.02 **Nontraumatic subacute subdural hemorrhage**

I62.03 **Nontraumatic chronic subdural hemorrhage**

I62.1 **Nontraumatic extradural hemorrhage**
Nontraumatic epidural hemorrhage

I62.9 **Nontraumatic intracranial hemorrhage, unspecified**
AHA: 4Q 2012, 92

▲ ▣ ✚ **I63** **Cerebral infarction**
INCLUDES occlusion and stenosis of cerebral and precerebral arteries, resulting in cerebral infarction
Use additional code, if applicable, to identify status post administration of tPA (rtPA) in a different facility within the last 24 hours prior to admission to current facility (Z92.82)
Use additional code, if known, to indicate National Institutes of Health Stroke Scale (NIHSS) score (R29.7-)
EXCLUDES 2 *sequelae of cerebral infarction (I69.3-)*
AHA: 4Q 2012, 92

⑤ ✚ **I63.0** **Cerebral infarction due to thrombosis of precerebral arteries**

✚ **I63.00** **Cerebral infarction due to thrombosis of unspecified precerebral artery**

⑥ ✚ **I63.01** **Cerebral infarction due to thrombosis of vertebral artery**

☐ ✚ **I63.011** Cerebral infarction due to thrombosis of right vertebral artery Ⓐ

☐ ✚ **I63.012** Cerebral infarction due to thrombosis of left vertebral artery Ⓐ

● ☐ ✚ **I63.013** Cerebral infarction due to thrombosis of bilateral vertebral arteries

☐ ✚ **I63.019** **Cerebral infarction due to thrombosis of unspecified vertebral artery** Ⓐ

✚ **I63.02** Cerebral infarction due to thrombosis of basilar artery Ⓐ

⑥ ✚ **I63.03** Cerebral infarction due to thrombosis of carotid artery

☐ ✚ **I63.031** Cerebral infarction due to thrombosis of right carotid artery

☐ ✚ **I63.032** Cerebral infarction due to thrombosis of left carotid artery

● ☐ ✚ **I63.033** Cerebral infarction due to thrombosis of bilateral carotid arteries

☐ ✚ **I63.039** **Cerebral infarction due to thrombosis of unspecified carotid artery**

✚ **I63.09** Cerebral infarction due to thrombosis of other precerebral artery

⑤ ✚ **I63.1** Cerebral infarction due to embolism of precerebral arteries

✚ **I63.10** Cerebral infarction due to embolism of unspecified precerebral artery

⑥ ✚ **I63.11** Cerebral infarction due to embolism of vertebral artery

☐ ✚ **I63.111** Cerebral infarction due to embolism of right vertebral artery Ⓐ

☐ ✚ **I63.112** Cerebral infarction due to embolism of left vertebral artery Ⓐ

● ☐ ✚ **I63.113** Cerebral infarction due to embolism of bilateral vertebral arteries

☐ ✚ **I63.119** **Cerebral infarction due to embolism of unspecified vertebral artery** Ⓐ

✚ **I63.12** Cerebral infarction due to embolism of basilar artery Ⓐ

⑥ ✚ **I63.13** Cerebral infarction due to embolism of carotid artery

☐ ✚ **I63.131** Cerebral infarction due to embolism of right carotid artery

☐ ✚ **I63.132** Cerebral infarction due to embolism of left carotid artery

● ☐ ✚ **I63.133** Cerebral infarction due to embolism of bilateral carotid arteries

☐ ✚ **I63.139** **Cerebral infarction due to embolism of unspecified carotid artery**

✚ **I63.19** Cerebral infarction due to embolism of other precerebral artery

⑤ ✚ **I63.2** Cerebral infarction due to unspecified occlusion or stenosis of precerebral arteries

✚ **I63.20** Cerebral infarction due to unspecified occlusion or stenosis of unspecified precerebral arteries

⑥ ✚ **I63.21** Cerebral infarction due to unspecified occlusion or stenosis of vertebral arteries

☐ ✚ **I63.211** Cerebral infarction due to unspecified occlusion or stenosis of right vertebral arteries Ⓐ

☐ ✚ **I63.212** Cerebral infarction due to unspecified occlusion or stenosis of left vertebral arteries Ⓐ

● ☐ ✚ **I63.213** Cerebral infarction due to unspecified occlusion or stenosis of bilateral vertebral arteries

☐ ✚ **I63.219** **Cerebral infarction due to unspecified occlusion or stenosis of unspecified vertebral arteries** Ⓐ

✚ **I63.22** Cerebral infarction due to unspecified occlusion or stenosis of basilar arteries Ⓐ

⑥ ✚ **I63.23** Cerebral infarction due to unspecified occlusion or stenosis of carotid arteries

☐ ✚ **I63.231** Cerebral infarction due to unspecified occlusion or stenosis of right carotid arteries

☐ ✚ **I63.232** Cerebral infarction due to unspecified occlusion or stenosis of left carotid arteries

● ☐ ✚ **I63.233** Cerebral infarction due to unspecified occlusion or stenosis of bilateral carotid arteries

☐ ✚ **I63.239** **Cerebral infarction due to unspecified occlusion or stenosis of unspecified carotid arteries**

✚ **I63.29** Cerebral infarction due to unspecified occlusion or stenosis of other precerebral arteries

⑤ ✚ **I63.3** Cerebral infarction due to thrombosis of cerebral arteries

✚ **I63.30** **Cerebral infarction due to thrombosis of unspecified cerebral artery** Ⓐ

⑥ ✚ **I63.31** Cerebral infarction due to thrombosis of middle cerebral artery

☐ ✚ **I63.311** Cerebral infarction due to thrombosis of right middle cerebral artery Ⓐ

● New   ▲ Revised   *Manifestation*   ▣-▣ Digit Indicators   ☐ Laterality   Ⓐ Adult (15+ years)   Ⓜ Maternity (12-55 years)   Ⓝ Newborn   Ⓟ Pediatric (0-17 years)   ♂ Male   ♀ Female
✖ Deleted   Unspecified   ✚ Additional code

648   © 2017 DecisionHealth   2017 ICD-10-CM Expert for Physicians

☐ + **I63.312** Cerebral infarction due to thrombosis of left middle cerebral artery Ⓐ

● ☐ + **I63.313** Cerebral infarction due to thrombosis of bilateral middle cerebral arteries

☐ + **I63.319** Cerebral infarction due to thrombosis of unspecified middle cerebral artery Ⓐ

Ⓖ + **I63.32** Cerebral infarction due to thrombosis of anterior cerebral artery

☐ + **I63.321** Cerebral infarction due to thrombosis of right anterior cerebral artery Ⓐ

☐ + **I63.322** Cerebral infarction due to thrombosis of left anterior cerebral artery Ⓐ

● ☐ + **I63.323** Cerebral infarction due to thrombosis of bilateral anterior arteries

☐ + **I63.329** Cerebral infarction due to thrombosis of unspecified anterior cerebral artery Ⓐ

Ⓖ + **I63.33** Cerebral infarction due to thrombosis of posterior cerebral artery

☐ + **I63.331** Cerebral infarction due to thrombosis of right posterior cerebral artery Ⓐ

☐ + **I63.332** Cerebral infarction due to thrombosis of left posterior cerebral artery Ⓐ

● ☐ + **I63.333** Cerebral infarction to thrombosis of bilateral posterior arteries

☐ + **I63.339** Cerebral infarction due to thrombosis of unspecified posterior cerebral artery Ⓐ

Ⓖ + **I63.34** Cerebral infarction due to thrombosis of cerebellar artery

☐ + **I63.341** Cerebral infarction due to thrombosis of right cerebellar artery Ⓐ

☐ + **I63.342** Cerebral infarction due to thrombosis of left cerebellar artery Ⓐ

● ☐ + **I63.343** Cerebral infarction to thrombosis of bilateral cerebellar arteries

☐ + **I63.349** Cerebral infarction due to thrombosis of unspecified cerebellar artery Ⓐ

+ **I63.39** Cerebral infarction due to thrombosis of other cerebral artery Ⓐ

Ⓢ + **I63.4** Cerebral infarction due to embolism of cerebral arteries

+ **I63.40** Cerebral infarction due to embolism of unspecified cerebral artery Ⓐ

Ⓖ + **I63.41** Cerebral infarction due to embolism of middle cerebral artery

☐ + **I63.411** Cerebral infarction due to embolism of right middle cerebral artery Ⓐ

☐ + **I63.412** Cerebral infarction due to embolism of left middle cerebral artery Ⓐ

● ☐ + **I63.413** Cerebral infarction due to embolism of bilateral middle cerebral arteries

☐ + **I63.419** Cerebral infarction due to embolism of unspecified middle cerebral artery Ⓐ

Ⓖ + **I63.42** Cerebral infarction due to embolism of anterior cerebral artery

☐ + **I63.421** Cerebral infarction due to embolism of right anterior cerebral artery Ⓐ

☐ + **I63.422** Cerebral infarction due to embolism of left anterior cerebral artery Ⓐ

● ☐ + **I63.423** Cerebral infarction due to embolism of bilateral anterior cerebral arteries

☐ + **I63.429** Cerebral infarction due to embolism of unspecified anterior cerebral artery Ⓐ

Ⓖ + **I63.43** Cerebral infarction due to embolism of posterior cerebral artery

☐ + **I63.431** Cerebral infarction due to embolism of right posterior cerebral artery Ⓐ

☐ + **I63.432** Cerebral infarction due to embolism of left posterior cerebral artery Ⓐ

● ☐ + **I63.433** Cerebral infarction due to embolism of bilateral posterior cerebral arteries

☐ + **I63.439** Cerebral infarction due to embolism of unspecified posterior cerebral artery Ⓐ

Ⓖ + **I63.44** Cerebral infarction due to embolism of cerebellar artery

☐ + **I63.441** Cerebral infarction due to embolism of right cerebellar artery Ⓐ

☐ + **I63.442** Cerebral infarction due to embolism of left cerebellar artery Ⓐ

● ☐ + **I63.443** Cerebral infarction due to embolism of bilateral cerebellar arteries

☐ + **I63.449** Cerebral infarction due to embolism of unspecified cerebellar artery Ⓐ

+ **I63.49** Cerebral infarction due to embolism of other cerebral artery Ⓐ

Ⓢ + **I63.5** Cerebral infarction due to unspecified occlusion or stenosis of cerebral arteries

+ **I63.50** Cerebral infarction due to unspecified occlusion or stenosis of unspecified cerebral artery

Ⓖ + **I63.51** Cerebral infarction due to unspecified occlusion or stenosis of middle cerebral artery

☐ + **I63.511** Cerebral infarction due to unspecified occlusion or stenosis of right middle cerebral artery

☐ + **I63.512** Cerebral infarction due to unspecified occlusion or stenosis of left middle cerebral artery

● ☐ + **I63.513** Cerebral infarction due to unspecified occlusion or stenosis of bilateral middle arteries

☐ + **I63.519** Cerebral infarction due to unspecified occlusion or stenosis of unspecified middle cerebral artery

Ⓖ + **I63.52** Cerebral infarction due to unspecified occlusion or stenosis of anterior cerebral artery

☐ + **I63.521** Cerebral infarction due to unspecified occlusion or stenosis of right anterior cerebral artery

☐ + **I63.522** Cerebral infarction due to unspecified occlusion or stenosis of left anterior cerebral artery

● ☐ + **I63.523** Cerebral infarction due to unspecified occlusion or stenosis of bilateral anterior arteries

☐ + **I63.529** Cerebral infarction due to unspecified occlusion or stenosis of unspecified anterior cerebral artery

Ⓖ + **I63.53** Cerebral infarction due to unspecified occlusion or stenosis of posterior cerebral artery

☐ + **I63.531** Cerebral infarction due to unspecified occlusion or stenosis of right posterior cerebral artery

☐ + **I63.532** Cerebral infarction due to unspecified occlusion or stenosis of left posterior cerebral artery

● ☐ + **I63.533** Cerebral infarction due to unspecified occlusion or stenosis of bilateral posterior arteries

☐ + **I63.539** Cerebral infarction due to unspecified occlusion or stenosis of unspecified posterior cerebral artery

Ⓖ + **I63.54** Cerebral infarction due to unspecified occlusion or stenosis of cerebellar artery

☐ + **I63.541** Cerebral infarction due to unspecified occlusion or stenosis of right cerebellar artery

☐ + **I63.542** Cerebral infarction due to unspecified occlusion or stenosis of left cerebellar artery

● ☐ + **I63.543** Cerebral infarction due to unspecified occlusion or stenosis of bilateral cerebellar arteries

☐ + **I63.549** Cerebral infarction due to unspecified occlusion or stenosis of unspecified cerebellar artery

+ **I63.59** Cerebral infarction due to unspecified occlusion or stenosis of other cerebral artery

+ **I63.6** Cerebral infarction due to cerebral venous thrombosis, nonpyogenic Ⓐ

+ **I63.8** Other cerebral infarction

+ **I63.9** Cerebral infarction, unspecified

Stroke NOS

AHA: 1Q 2015, 26

④ **I65** **Occlusion and stenosis of precerebral arteries, not resulting in cerebral infarction**

INCLUDES embolism of precerebral artery
narrowing of precerebral artery
obstruction (complete) (partial) of precerebral artery
thrombosis of precerebral artery

EXCLUDES 1 *insufficiency, NOS, of precerebral artery (G45.-)*
insufficiency of precerebral arteries causing cerebral infarction (I63.0-I63.2)

CODING TIP ✓ Codes from categories I65.- and I66.- are used to indicate stenosis and occlusion that do not result in infarction. Assign the most specific code as appropriate according to diagnostic statements provided by the physician. If the affected artery is not specified, do not assume a code for an affected location, but rather use an unspecified code. If more than one arterial location is affected and a specific code is available for separate locations, separate codes should be assigned.

AHA: 4Q 2012, 92

⑤ **I65.0** **Occlusion and stenosis of vertebral artery**

⊟ **I65.01** Occlusion and stenosis of right vertebral artery A

⊟ **I65.02** Occlusion and stenosis of left vertebral artery A

⊟ **I65.03** Occlusion and stenosis of bilateral vertebral arteries A

⊟ **I65.09** Occlusion and stenosis of unspecified vertebral artery A

I65.1 Occlusion and stenosis of basilar artery A

⑤ **I65.2** **Occlusion and stenosis of carotid artery**

⊟ **I65.21** Occlusion and stenosis of right carotid artery A

⊟ **I65.22** Occlusion and stenosis of left carotid artery A

⊟ **I65.23** Occlusion and stenosis of bilateral carotid arteries A

⊟ **I65.29** Occlusion and stenosis of unspecified carotid artery A

I65.8 Occlusion and stenosis of other precerebral arteries A

I65.9 Occlusion and stenosis of unspecified precerebral artery A

Occlusion and stenosis of precerebral artery NOS

④ **I66** **Occlusion and stenosis of cerebral arteries, not resulting in cerebral infarction**

INCLUDES embolism of cerebral artery
narrowing of cerebral artery
obstruction (complete) (partial) of cerebral artery
thrombosis of cerebral artery

EXCLUDES 1 *Occlusion and stenosis of cerebral artery causing cerebral infarction (I63.3-I63.5)*

CODING TIP ✓ Codes from categories I65.- and I66.- are used to indicate stenosis and occlusion that do not result in infarction. Assign the most specific code as appropriate according to diagnostic statements provided by the physician. If the affected artery is not specified, do not assume a code for an affected location, but rather use an unspecified code. If more than one arterial location is affected and a specific code is available for separate locations, separate codes should be assigned.

AHA: 4Q 2012, 92

⑤ **I66.0** **Occlusion and stenosis of middle cerebral artery**

⊟ **I66.01** Occlusion and stenosis of right middle cerebral artery A

⊟ **I66.02** Occlusion and stenosis of left middle cerebral artery A

⊟ **I66.03** Occlusion and stenosis of bilateral middle cerebral arteries A

⊟ **I66.09** Occlusion and stenosis of unspecified middle cerebral artery A

⑤ **I66.1** **Occlusion and stenosis of anterior cerebral artery**

⊟ **I66.11** Occlusion and stenosis of right anterior cerebral artery A

⊟ **I66.12** Occlusion and stenosis of left anterior cerebral artery A

⊟ **I66.13** Occlusion and stenosis of bilateral anterior cerebral arteries A

⊟ **I66.19** Occlusion and stenosis of unspecified anterior cerebral artery A

⑤ **I66.2** **Occlusion and stenosis of posterior cerebral artery**

⊟ **I66.21** Occlusion and stenosis of right posterior cerebral artery A

⊟ **I66.22** Occlusion and stenosis of left posterior cerebral artery A

⊟ **I66.23** Occlusion and stenosis of bilateral posterior cerebral arteries A

⊟ **I66.29** Occlusion and stenosis of unspecified posterior cerebral artery A

I66.3 Occlusion and stenosis of cerebellar arteries A

I66.8 Occlusion and stenosis of other cerebral arteries A

Occlusion and stenosis of perforating arteries

I66.9 Occlusion and stenosis of unspecified cerebral artery A

▲④ **I67** **Other cerebrovascular diseases**

EXCLUDES 2 *sequelae of the listed conditions (I69.8)*

AHA: 4Q 2012, 92

I67.0 **Dissection of cerebral arteries, nonruptured**

EXCLUDES 1 *ruptured cerebral arteries (I60.7)*

I67.1 **Cerebral aneurysm, nonruptured**
Cerebral aneurysm NOS
Cerebral arteriovenous fistula, acquired
Internal carotid artery aneurysm, intracranial portion
Internal carotid artery aneurysm, NOS

EXCLUDES 1 *congenital cerebral aneurysm, nonruptured (Q28.-)*
ruptured cerebral aneurysm (I60.7)

I67.2 **Cerebral atherosclerosis** A
Atheroma of cerebral and precerebral arteries

I67.3 **Progressive vascular leukoencephalopathy**
Binswanger's disease

I67.4 **Hypertensive encephalopathy**

I67.5 **Moyamoya disease**

I67.6 **Nonpyogenic thrombosis of intracranial venous system**
Nonpyogenic thrombosis of cerebral vein
Nonpyogenic thrombosis of intracranial venous sinus

EXCLUDES 1 *nonpyogenic thrombosis of intracranial venous system causing infarction (I63.6)*

I67.7 **Cerebral arteritis, not elsewhere classified**
Granulomatous angiitis of the nervous system

EXCLUDES 1 *allergic granulomatous angiitis (M30.1)*

DEFINITION Inflammation of an artery in the head.

⑤ **I67.8** **Other specified cerebrovascular diseases**

I67.81 **Acute cerebrovascular insufficiency**
Acute cerebrovascular insufficiency unspecified as to location or reversibility

I67.82 **Cerebral ischemia**
Chronic cerebral ischemia

I67.83 **Posterior reversible encephalopathy syndrome**
PRES

⑤ **I67.84** **Cerebral vasospasm and vasoconstriction**

I67.841 **Reversible cerebrovascular vasoconstriction syndrome** A
Call-Fleming syndrome
Code first:
underlying condition, if applicable, such as eclampsia (O15.00-O15.9)

I67.848 **Other cerebrovascular vasospasm and vasoconstriction** A

I67.89 **Other cerebrovascular disease**

I67.9 **Cerebrovascular disease, unspecified**

CODING TIP ✓ Do not assign I67.9 for sequelae of cerebral vascular accident. Do not assign I67.9 for cerebral atherosclerosis or any other known type of cerebral vascular disorder. If the type of cerebral vascular disease is not specified in the record, query the physician to attempt to obtain a more specific diagnosis.

④ **I68** **Cerebrovascular disorders in diseases classified elsewhere**

I68.0 *Cerebral amyloid angiopathy*
Code first:
underlying amyloidosis (E85.-)

I68.2 *Cerebral arteritis in other diseases classified elsewhere*
Code first:
underlying disease

EXCLUDES 1 *cerebral arteritis (in) :*
listerosis (A32.89)
systemic lupus erythematosus (M32.19)
syphilis (A52.04)
tuberculosis (A18.89)

I68.8 *Other cerebrovascular disorders in diseases classified elsewhere*
Code first:
underlying disease

EXCLUDES 1 *syphilitic cerebral aneurysm (A52.05)*

● New   ▲ Revised   *Manifestation*   ④-⑦ Digit Indicators   ⊟ Laterality   A Adult (15+ years)   M Maternity (12-55 years)   N Newborn   P Pediatric (0-17 years)   ♂ Male   ♀ Female
✖ Deleted   Unspecified   + Additional code

650   © 2017 DecisionHealth   2017 ICD-10-CM Expert for Physicians

4 I69   Sequelae of cerebrovascular disease

Note: Category I69 is to be used to indicate conditions in I60-I67 as the cause of sequelae. The 'sequelae' include conditions specified as such or as residuals which may occur at any time after the onset of the causal condition

EXCLUDES 1   *personal history of cerebral infarction without residual deficit (Z86.73)*
personal history of prolonged reversible ischemic neurologic deficit (PRIND) (Z86.73)
personal history of reversible ischemic neurol#gical deficit (RIND) (Z86.73)
sequelae of traumatic intracranial injury (S06.-)
transient ischemic attack (TIA) (G45.9)

GUIDELINES   Section I.C.9.d.1)

Category I69 is used to indicate conditions classifiable to categories I60-I67 as the causes of sequela (neurologic deficits), themselves classified elsewhere. These "late effects" include neurologic deficits that persist after initial onset of conditions classifiable to categories I60-I67. The neurologic deficits caused by cerebrovascular disease may be present from the onset or may arise at any time after the onset or may arise at any time after the onset of the condition classifiable to categories I60-I67.

Codes from category I69, Sequelae of cerebrovascular disease, that specify hemiplegia, hemiparesis and monoplegia identify whether the dominant or nondominant side is affected. Should the affected side be documented, but not specified as dominant or nondominant, and the classification system does not indicate a default, code selection is as follows:

• For ambidextrous patients, the default should be dominant.
• If the left side is affected, the default is non-dominant.
• If the right side is affected, the default is dominant.

GUIDELINES   Section I.C.9.d.3)

Codes from category I69 should not be assigned if the patient does not have neurologic deficits.

AHA: 4Q 2012, 92, 107

5 I69.0   Sequelae of nontraumatic subarachnoid hemorrhage

I69.00   Unspecified sequelae of nontraumatic subarachnoid hemorrhage

▲ 6 **I69.01**   Cognitive deficits following nontraumatic subarachnoid hemorrhage

● **I69.010**   Attention and concentration deficit following nontraumatic subarachnoid hemorrhage

● **I69.011**   Memory deficit following nontraumatic subarachnoid hemorrhage

● **I69.012**   Visuospatial deficit and spatial neglect following nontraumatic subarachnoid hemorrhage

● **I69.013**   Psychomotor deficit following nontraumatic subarachnoid hemorrhage

● **I69.014**   Frontal lobe and executive function deficit following nontraumatic subarachnoid hemorrhage

● **I69.015**   Cognitive social or emotional deficit following nontraumatic subarachnoid hemorrhage

● **I69.018**   Other symptoms and signs involving cognitive functions following nontraumatic subarachnoid hemorrhage

● **I69.019**   Unspecified symptoms and signs involving cognitive functions following nontraumatic subarachnoid hemorrhage

6 **I69.02**   Speech and language deficits following nontraumatic subarachnoid hemorrhage

I69.020   Aphasia following nontraumatic subarachnoid hemorrhage

I69.021   Dysphasia following nontraumatic subarachnoid hemorrhage

I69.022   Dysarthria following nontraumatic subarachnoid hemorrhage

I69.023   Fluency disorder following nontraumatic subarachnoid hemorrhage
Stuttering following nontraumatic subarachnoid hemorrhage

I69.028   Other speech and language deficits following nontraumatic subarachnoid hemorrhage

6 **I69.03**   Monoplegia of upper limb following nontraumatic subarachnoid hemorrhage
AHA: 4Q 2012, 105-106

□ **I69.031**   Monoplegia of upper limb following nontraumatic subarachnoid hemorrhage affecting right dominant side

□ **I69.032**   Monoplegia of upper limb following nontraumatic subarachnoid hemorrhage affecting left dominant side

□ **I69.033**   Monoplegia of upper limb following nontraumatic subarachnoid hemorrhage affecting right non-dominant side

□ **I69.034**   Monoplegia of upper limb following nontraumatic subarachnoid hemorrhage affecting left non-dominant side

□ **I69.039**   Monoplegia of upper limb following nontraumatic subarachnoid hemorrhage affecting unspecified side

6 **I69.04**   Monoplegia of lower limb following nontraumatic subarachnoid hemorrhage
AHA: 4Q 2012, 105-106

□ **I69.041**   Monoplegia of lower limb following nontraumatic subarachnoid hemorrhage affecting right dominant side

□ **I69.042**   Monoplegia of lower limb following nontraumatic subarachnoid hemorrhage affecting left dominant side

□ **I69.043**   Monoplegia of lower limb following nontraumatic subarachnoid hemorrhage affecting right non-dominant side

□ **I69.044**   Monoplegia of lower limb following nontraumatic subarachnoid hemorrhage affecting left non-dominant side

□ **I69.049**   Monoplegia of lower limb following nontraumatic subarachnoid hemorrhage affecting unspecified side

6 **I69.05**   Hemiplegia and hemiparesis following nontraumatic subarachnoid hemorrhage

□ **I69.051**   Hemiplegia and hemiparesis following nontraumatic subarachnoid hemorrhage affecting right dominant side

□ **I69.052**   Hemiplegia and hemiparesis following nontraumatic subarachnoid hemorrhage affecting left dominant side

□ **I69.053**   Hemiplegia and hemiparesis following nontraumatic subarachnoid hemorrhage affecting right non-dominant side

□ **I69.054**   Hemiplegia and hemiparesis following nontraumatic subarachnoid hemorrhage affecting left non-dominant side

□ **I69.059**   Hemiplegia and hemiparesis following nontraumatic subarachnoid hemorrhage affecting unspecified side

6 + **I69.06**   Other paralytic syndrome following nontraumatic subarachnoid hemorrhage
Use additional code to identify type of paralytic syndrome, such as:
locked-in state (G83.5)
quadriplegia (G82.5-)

EXCLUDES 1   *hemiplegia/hemiparesis following nontraumatic subarachnoid hemorrhage (I69.05-)*
monoplegia of lower limb following nontraumatic subarachnoid hemorrhage (I69.04-)
monoplegia of upper limb following nontraumatic subarachnoid hemorrhage (I69.03-)

□ + **I69.061**   Other paralytic syndrome following nontraumatic subarachnoid hemorrhage affecting right dominant side

□ + **I69.062**   Other paralytic syndrome following nontraumatic subarachnoid hemorrhage affecting left dominant side

□ + **I69.063**   Other paralytic syndrome following nontraumatic subarachnoid hemorrhage affecting right non-dominant side

□ + **I69.064**   Other paralytic syndrome following nontraumatic subarachnoid hemorrhage affecting left non-dominant side

□ + **I69.065**   Other paralytic syndrome following nontraumatic subarachnoid hemorrhage, bilateral

---

● New   ▲ Revised   *Manifestation*   4-7 Digit Indicators   ⊟ Laterality   A Adult (15+ years)   M Maternity (12-55 years)   N Newborn   P Pediatric (0-17 years)   ♂ Male   ♀ Female
✕ Deleted   Unspecified   + Additional code

□ + **I69.069** **Other paralytic syndrome following nontraumatic subarachnoid hemorrhage affecting unspecified side**

⑥ **I69.09** **Other sequelae of nontraumatic subarachnoid hemorrhage**

I69.090 **Apraxia following nontraumatic subarachnoid hemorrhage**

+ **I69.091** **Dysphagia following nontraumatic subarachnoid hemorrhage**
Use additional code to identify the type of dysphagia, if known (R13.1-)

I69.092 **Facial weakness following nontraumatic subarachnoid hemorrhage**
Facial droop following nontraumatic subarachnoid hemorrhage

I69.093 **Ataxia following nontraumatic subarachnoid hemorrhage**

+ **I69.098** **Other sequelae following nontraumatic subarachnoid hemorrhage**
Alterations of sensation following nontraumatic subarachnoid hemorrhage
Disturbance of vision following nontraumatic subarachnoid hemorrhage
Use additional code to identify the sequelae

⑤ **I69.1** **Sequelae of nontraumatic intracerebral hemorrhage**

I69.10 **Unspecified sequelae of nontraumatic intracerebral hemorrhage**

▲ ⑥ **I69.11** **Cognitive deficits following nontraumatic intracerebral hemorrhage**

● **I69.110** **Attention and concentration deficit following nontraumatic intracerebral hemorrhage**

● **I69.111** **Memory deficit following nontraumatic intracerebral hemorrhage**

● **I69.112** **Visuospatial deficit and spatial neglect following nontraumatic intracerebral hemorrhage**

● **I69.113** **Psychomotor deficit following nontraumatic intracerebral hemorrhage**

● **I69.114** **Frontal lobe and executive function deficit following nontraumatic intracerebral hemorrhage**

● **I69.115** **Cognitive social or emotional deficit following nontraumatic intracerebral hemorrhage**

● **I69.118** **Other symptoms and signs involving cognitive functions following nontraumatic intracerebral hemorrhage**

● **I69.119** **Unspecified symptoms and signs involving cognitive functions following nontraumatic intracerebral hemorrhage**

⑥ **I69.12** **Speech and language deficits following nontraumatic intracerebral hemorrhage**

I69.120 **Aphasia following nontraumatic intracerebral hemorrhage**

I69.121 **Dysphasia following nontraumatic intracerebral hemorrhage**

I69.122 **Dysarthria following nontraumatic intracerebral hemorrhage**

▲ **I69.123** **Fluency disorder following nontraumatic intracerebral hemorrhage**
Stuttering following nontraumatic intracerebral hemorrhage

I69.128 **Other speech and language deficits following nontraumatic intracerebral hemorrhage**

⑥ **I69.13** **Monoplegia of upper limb following nontraumatic intracerebral hemorrhage**
AHA: 4Q 2012, 105-106

□ **I69.131** **Monoplegia of upper limb following nontraumatic intracerebral hemorrhage affecting right dominant side**

□ **I69.132** **Monoplegia of upper limb following nontraumatic intracerebral hemorrhage affecting left dominant side**

□ **I69.133** **Monoplegia of upper limb following nontraumatic intracerebral hemorrhage affecting right non-dominant side**

□ **I69.134** **Monoplegia of upper limb following nontraumatic intracerebral hemorrhage affecting left non-dominant side**

□ **I69.139** **Monoplegia of upper limb following nontraumatic intracerebral hemorrhage affecting unspecified side**

⑥ **I69.14** **Monoplegia of lower limb following nontraumatic intracerebral hemorrhage**
AHA: 4Q 2012, 105-106

□ **I69.141** **Monoplegia of lower limb following nontraumatic intracerebral hemorrhage affecting right dominant side**

□ **I69.142** **Monoplegia of lower limb following nontraumatic intracerebral hemorrhage affecting left dominant side**

□ **I69.143** **Monoplegia of lower limb following nontraumatic intracerebral hemorrhage affecting right non-dominant side**

□ **I69.144** **Monoplegia of lower limb following nontraumatic intracerebral hemorrhage affecting left non-dominant side**

□ **I69.149** **Monoplegia of lower limb following nontraumatic intracerebral hemorrhage affecting unspecified side**

⑥ **I69.15** **Hemiplegia and hemiparesis following nontraumatic intracerebral hemorrhage**

□ **I69.151** **Hemiplegia and hemiparesis following nontraumatic intracerebral hemorrhage affecting right dominant side**

□ **I69.152** **Hemiplegia and hemiparesis following nontraumatic intracerebral hemorrhage affecting left dominant side**

□ **I69.153** **Hemiplegia and hemiparesis following nontraumatic intracerebral hemorrhage affecting right non-dominant side**

□ **I69.154** **Hemiplegia and hemiparesis following nontraumatic intracerebral hemorrhage affecting left non-dominant side**

□ **I69.159** **Hemiplegia and hemiparesis following nontraumatic intracerebral hemorrhage affecting unspecified side**

⑥ + **I69.16** **Other paralytic syndrome following nontraumatic intracerebral hemorrhage**
Use additional code to identify type of paralytic syndrome, such as:
locked-in state (G83.5)
quadriplegia (G82.5-)
EXCLUDES 1 *hemiplegia/hemiparesis following nontraumatic intracerebral hemorrhage (I69.15-)*
monoplegia of lower limb following nontraumatic intracerebral hemorrhage (I69.14-)
monoplegia of upper limb following nontraumatic intracerebral hemorrhage (I69.13-)

□ + **I69.161** **Other paralytic syndrome following nontraumatic intracerebral hemorrhage affecting right dominant side**

□ + **I69.162** **Other paralytic syndrome following nontraumatic intracerebral hemorrhage affecting left dominant side**

□ + **I69.163** **Other paralytic syndrome following nontraumatic intracerebral hemorrhage affecting right non-dominant side**

□ + **I69.164** **Other paralytic syndrome following nontraumatic intracerebral hemorrhage affecting left non-dominant side**

□ + **I69.165** **Other paralytic syndrome following nontraumatic intracerebral hemorrhage, bilateral**

□ + **I69.169** **Other paralytic syndrome following nontraumatic intracerebral hemorrhage affecting unspecified side**

⑥ **I69.19** **Other sequelae of nontraumatic intracerebral hemorrhage**

I69.190 **Apraxia following nontraumatic intracerebral hemorrhage**

+ **I69.191** **Dysphagia following nontraumatic intracerebral hemorrhage**
Use additional code to identify the type of dysphagia, if known (R13.1-)

I69.192 **Facial weakness following nontraumatic intracerebral hemorrhage**
Facial droop following nontraumatic intracerebral hemorrhage

I69.193 **Ataxia following nontraumatic intracerebral hemorrhage**

● New   ▲ Revised   *Manifestation*   ◪-◪ Digit Indicators   □ Laterality   Ⓐ Adult (15+ years)   Ⓜ Maternity (12-55 years)   Ⓝ Newborn   Ⓟ Pediatric (0-17 years)   ♂ Male   ♀ Female
✖ ~~Deleted~~   Unspecified   + Additional code

652   © 2017 DecisionHealth   2017 ICD-10-CM Expert for Physicians

+ I69.198 Other sequelae of nontraumatic intracerebral hemorrhage
Alteration of sensations following nontraumatic intracerebral hemorrhage
Disturbance of vision following nontraumatic intracerebral hemorrhage
Use additional code to identify the sequelae

⑤ I69.2 **Sequelae of other nontraumatic intracranial hemorrhage**

I69.20 **Unspecified sequelae of other nontraumatic intracranial hemorrhage**

▲ ⑥ I69.21 **Cognitive deficits following other nontraumatic intracranial hemorrhage**

● I69.210 Attention and concentration deficit following other nontraumatic intracranial hemorrhage

● I69.211 Memory deficit following other nontraumatic intracranial hemorrhage

● I69.212 Visuospatial deficit and spatial neglect following other nontraumatic intracranial hemorrhage

● I69.213 Psychomotor deficit following other nontraumatic intracranial hemorrhage

● I69.214 Frontal lobe and executive function deficit following other nontraumatic intracranial hemorrhage

● I69.215 Cognitive social or emotional deficit following other nontraumatic intracranial hemorrhage

● I69.218 Other symptoms and signs involving cognitive functions following other nontraumatic intracranial hemorrhage

● I69.219 Unspecified symptoms and signs involving cognitive functions following other nontraumatic intracranial hemorrhage

⑥ I69.22 **Speech and language deficits following other nontraumatic intracranial hemorrhage**

I69.220 Aphasia following other nontraumatic intracranial hemorrhage

I69.221 Dysphasia following other nontraumatic intracranial hemorrhage

I69.222 Dysarthria following other nontraumatic intracranial hemorrhage

▲ I69.223 Fluency disorder following other nontraumatic intracranial hemorrhage
Stuttering following other nontraumatic intracranial hemorrhage

I69.228 Other speech and language deficits following other nontraumatic intracranial hemorrhage

⑥ I69.23 **Monoplegia of upper limb following other nontraumatic intracranial hemorrhage**

⊟ I69.231 Monoplegia of upper limb following other nontraumatic intracranial hemorrhage affecting right dominant side

⊟ I69.232 Monoplegia of upper limb following other nontraumatic intracranial hemorrhage affecting left dominant side

⊟ I69.233 Monoplegia of upper limb following other nontraumatic intracranial hemorrhage affecting right non-dominant side

⊟ I69.234 Monoplegia of upper limb following other nontraumatic intracranial hemorrhage affecting left non-dominant side

⊟ I69.239 Monoplegia of upper limb following other nontraumatic intracranial hemorrhage affecting unspecified side

⑥ I69.24 **Monoplegia of lower limb following other nontraumatic intracranial hemorrhage**

⊟ I69.241 Monoplegia of lower limb following other nontraumatic intracranial hemorrhage affecting right dominant side

⊟ I69.242 Monoplegia of lower limb following other nontraumatic intracranial hemorrhage affecting left dominant side

⊟ I69.243 Monoplegia of lower limb following other nontraumatic intracranial hemorrhage affecting right non-dominant side

⊟ I69.244 Monoplegia of lower limb following other nontraumatic intracranial hemorrhage affecting left non-dominant side

⊟ I69.249 Monoplegia of lower limb following other nontraumatic intracranial hemorrhage affecting unspecified side

⑥ I69.25 **Hemiplegia and hemiparesis following other nontraumatic intracranial hemorrhage**

⊟ I69.251 Hemiplegia and hemiparesis following other nontraumatic intracranial hemorrhage affecting right dominant side

⊟ I69.252 Hemiplegia and hemiparesis following other nontraumatic intracranial hemorrhage affecting left dominant side

⊟ I69.253 Hemiplegia and hemiparesis following other nontraumatic intracranial hemorrhage affecting right non-dominant side

⊟ I69.254 Hemiplegia and hemiparesis following other nontraumatic intracranial hemorrhage affecting left non-dominant side

⊟ I69.259 Hemiplegia and hemiparesis following other nontraumatic intracranial hemorrhage affecting unspecified side

⑥ + I69.26 Other paralytic syndrome following other nontraumatic intracranial hemorrhage
Use additional code to identify type of paralytic syndrome, such as:
locked-in state (G83.5)
quadriplegia (G82.5-)
EXCLUDES 1 *hemiplegia/hemiparesis following other nontraumatic intracranial hemorrhage (I69.25-)*
monoplegia of lower limb following other nontraumatic intracranial hemorrhage (I69.24-)
monoplegia of upper limb following other nontraumatic intracranial hemorrhage (I69.23-)

⊟ + I69.261 Other paralytic syndrome following other nontraumatic intracranial hemorrhage affecting right dominant side

⊟ + I69.262 Other paralytic syndrome following other nontraumatic intracranial hemorrhage affecting left dominant side

⊟ + I69.263 Other paralytic syndrome following other nontraumatic intracranial hemorrhage affecting right non-dominant side

⊟ + I69.264 Other paralytic syndrome following other nontraumatic intracranial hemorrhage affecting left non-dominant side

⊟ + I69.265 Other paralytic syndrome following other nontraumatic intracranial hemorrhage, bilateral

⊟ + I69.269 Other paralytic syndrome following other nontraumatic intracranial hemorrhage affecting unspecified side

⑥ I69.29 **Other sequelae of other nontraumatic intracranial hemorrhage**

I69.290 Apraxia following other nontraumatic intracranial hemorrhage

+ I69.291 Dysphagia following other nontraumatic intracranial hemorrhage
Use additional code to identify the type of dysphagia, if known (R13.1-)

I69.292 Facial weakness following other nontraumatic intracranial hemorrhage
Facial droop following other nontraumatic intracranial hemorrhage

I69.293 Ataxia following other nontraumatic intracranial hemorrhage

+ I69.298 Other sequelae of other nontraumatic intracranial hemorrhage
Alteration of sensation following other nontraumatic intracranial hemorrhage
Disturbance of vision following other nontraumatic intracranial hemorrhage
Use additional code to identify the sequelae

⑤ I69.3 **Sequelae of cerebral infarction**
Sequelae of stroke NOS
AHA: 4Q 2013, 127
AHA: 4Q 2012, 92, 95

I69.30 **Unspecified sequelae of cerebral infarction**

▲ ⑥ I69.31 **Cognitive deficits following cerebral infarction**

● I69.310 Attention and concentration deficit following cerebral infarction

● I69.311 Memory deficit following cerebral infarction

● I69.312 Visuospatial deficit and spatial neglect following cerebral infarction

● I69.313 Psychomotor deficit following cerebral infarction

● New ▲ Revised *Manifestation* ④-⑦ Digit Indicators ⊟ Laterality Ⓐ Adult (15+ years) Ⓜ Maternity (12-55 years) Ⓝ Newborn Ⓟ Pediatric (0-17 years) ♂ Male ♀ Female
✗ ~~Deleted~~ Unspecified + Additional code

2017 ICD-10-CM Expert for Physicians © 2017 DecisionHealth 653

● I69.314   **Frontal lobe and executive function deficit following cerebral infarction**

● I69.315   **Cognitive social or emotional deficit following cerebral infarction**

● I69.318   **Other symptoms and signs involving cognitive functions following cerebral infarction**

● I69.319   **Unspecified symptoms and signs involving cognitive functions following cerebral infarction**

I69.32   **Speech and language deficits following cerebral infarction**

     I69.320   **Aphasia following cerebral infarction**
           AHA: 4Q 2013, 128

     I69.321   **Dysphasia following cerebral infarction**
           AHA: 4Q 2012, 91-92, 95

     I69.322   **Dysarthria following cerebral infarction**

▲ I69.323   **Fluency disorder following cerebral infarction**
           Stuttering following cerebral infarction

     I69.328   **Other speech and language deficits following cerebral infarction**

I69.33   **Monoplegia of upper limb following cerebral infarction**

     I69.331   **Monoplegia of upper limb following cerebral infarction affecting right dominant side**

     I69.332   **Monoplegia of upper limb following cerebral infarction affecting left dominant side**

     I69.333   **Monoplegia of upper limb following cerebral infarction affecting right non-dominant side**

     I69.334   **Monoplegia of upper limb following cerebral infarction affecting left non-dominant side**

     I69.339   **Monoplegia of upper limb following cerebral infarction affecting unspecified side**

I69.34   **Monoplegia of lower limb following cerebral infarction**

     I69.341   **Monoplegia of lower limb following cerebral infarction affecting right dominant side**

     I69.342   **Monoplegia of lower limb following cerebral infarction affecting left dominant side**

     I69.343   **Monoplegia of lower limb following cerebral infarction affecting right non-dominant side**

     I69.344   **Monoplegia of lower limb following cerebral infarction affecting left non-dominant side**

     I69.349   **Monoplegia of lower limb following cerebral infarction affecting unspecified side**

I69.35   **Hemiplegia and hemiparesis following cerebral infarction**

     I69.351   **Hemiplegia and hemiparesis following cerebral infarction affecting right dominant side**
           AHA: 1Q 2015, 25
           AHA: 4Q 2013, 128

     I69.352   **Hemiplegia and hemiparesis following cerebral infarction affecting left dominant side**

     I69.353   **Hemiplegia and hemiparesis following cerebral infarction affecting right non-dominant side**

     I69.354   **Hemiplegia and hemiparesis following cerebral infarction affecting left non-dominant side**
           AHA: 4Q 2012, 91-92, 95

     I69.359   **Hemiplegia and hemiparesis following cerebral infarction affecting unspecified side**

+ I69.36   **Other paralytic syndrome following cerebral infarction**
           Use additional code to identify type of paralytic syndrome, such as:
           locked-in state (G83.5)
           quadriplegia (G82.5-)
           EXCLUDES 1   *hemiplegia/hemiparesis following cerebral infarction (I69.35-)*
                       monoplegia of lower limb following cerebral infarction (I69.34-)
                       monoplegia of upper limb following cerebral infarction (I69.33-)

     + I69.361   **Other paralytic syndrome following cerebral infarction affecting right dominant side**

     + I69.362   **Other paralytic syndrome following cerebral infarction affecting left dominant side**

     + I69.363   **Other paralytic syndrome following cerebral infarction affecting right non-dominant side**

     + I69.364   **Other paralytic syndrome following cerebral infarction affecting left non-dominant side**

     + I69.365   **Other paralytic syndrome following cerebral infarction, bilateral**

     + I69.369   **Other paralytic syndrome following cerebral infarction affecting unspecified side**

I69.39   **Other sequelae of cerebral infarction**

     I69.390   **Apraxia following cerebral infarction**

     + I69.391   **Dysphagia following cerebral infarction**
           Use additional code to identify the type of dysphagia, if known (R13.1-)

     I69.392   **Facial weakness following cerebral infarction**
           Facial droop following cerebral infarction

     I69.393   **Ataxia following cerebral infarction**

     + I69.398   **Other sequelae of cerebral infarction**
           Alteration of sensation following cerebral infarction
           Disturbance of vision following cerebral infarction
           Use additional code to identify the sequelae

I69.8   **Sequelae of other cerebrovascular diseases**
     EXCLUDES 1   *sequelae of traumatic intracranial injury (S06.-)*

I69.80   **Unspecified sequelae of other cerebrovascular disease**

▲ I69.81   **Cognitive deficits following other cerebrovascular disease**

     ● I69.810   **Attention and concentration deficit following other cerebrovascular disease**

     ● I69.811   **Memory deficit following other cerebrovascular disease**

     ● I69.812   **Visuospatial deficit and spatial neglect following other cerebrovascular disease**

     ● I69.813   **Psychomotor deficit following other cerebrovascular disease**

     ● I69.814   **Frontal lobe and executive function deficit following other cerebrovascular disease**

     ● I69.815   **Cognitive social or emotional deficit following other cerebrovascular disease**

     ● I69.818   **Other symptoms and signs involving cognitive functions following other cerebrovascular disease**

     ● I69.819   **Unspecified symptoms and signs involving cognitive functions following other cerebrovascular disease**

I69.82   **Speech and language deficits following other cerebrovascular disease**

     I69.820   **Aphasia following other cerebrovascular disease**

     I69.821   **Dysphasia following other cerebrovascular disease**

     I69.822   **Dysarthria following other cerebrovascular disease**

▲ I69.823   **Fluency disorder following other cerebrovascular disease**
           Stuttering following other cerebrovascular disease

     I69.828   **Other speech and language deficits following other cerebrovascular disease**

I69.83   **Monoplegia of upper limb following other cerebrovascular disease**

     I69.831   **Monoplegia of upper limb following other cerebrovascular disease affecting right dominant side**

     I69.832   **Monoplegia of upper limb following other cerebrovascular disease affecting left dominant side**

     I69.833   **Monoplegia of upper limb following other cerebrovascular disease affecting right non-dominant side**

     I69.834   **Monoplegia of upper limb following other cerebrovascular disease affecting left non-dominant side**

     I69.839   **Monoplegia of upper limb following other cerebrovascular disease affecting unspecified side**

I69.84   **Monoplegia of lower limb following other cerebrovascular disease**

     I69.841   **Monoplegia of lower limb following other cerebrovascular disease affecting right dominant side**

     I69.842   **Monoplegia of lower limb following other cerebrovascular disease affecting left dominant side**

     I69.843   **Monoplegia of lower limb following other cerebrovascular disease affecting right non-dominant side**

● New   ▲ Revised   *Manifestation*   ◪-◪ Digit Indicators   ⊟ Laterality   Ⓐ Adult (15+ years)   Ⓜ Maternity (12-55 years)   Ⓝ Newborn   Ⓟ Pediatric (0-17 years)   ♂ Male   ♀ Female
✖ ~~Deleted~~   Unspecified   + Additional code

654   © 2017 DecisionHealth   2017 ICD-10-CM Expert for Physicians

⊟ **I69.844** **Monoplegia of lower limb following other cerebrovascular disease affecting left non-dominant side**

⊟ **I69.849** **Monoplegia of lower limb following other cerebrovascular disease affecting unspecified side**

◨ **I69.85** **Hemiplegia and hemiparesis following other cerebrovascular disease**

⊟ **I69.851** **Hemiplegia and hemiparesis following other cerebrovascular disease affecting right dominant side**

⊟ **I69.852** **Hemiplegia and hemiparesis following other cerebrovascular disease affecting left dominant side**

⊟ **I69.853** **Hemiplegia and hemiparesis following other cerebrovascular disease affecting right non-dominant side**

⊟ **I69.854** **Hemiplegia and hemiparesis following other cerebrovascular disease affecting left non-dominant side**

⊟ **I69.859** **Hemiplegia and hemiparesis following other cerebrovascular disease affecting unspecified side**

◨ ✚ **I69.86** **Other paralytic syndrome following other cerebrovascular disease**
Use additional code to identify type of paralytic syndrome, such as:
locked-in state (G83.5)
quadriplegia (G82.5-)

EXCLUDES 1 *hemiplegia/hemiparesis following other cerebrovascular disease (I69.85-)*
monoplegia of lower limb following other cerebrovascular disease (I69.84-)
monoplegia of upper limb following other cerebrovascular disease (I69.83-)

⊟ ✚ **I69.861** **Other paralytic syndrome following other cerebrovascular disease affecting right dominant side**

⊟ ✚ **I69.862** **Other paralytic syndrome following other cerebrovascular disease affecting left dominant side**

⊟ ✚ **I69.863** **Other paralytic syndrome following other cerebrovascular disease affecting right non-dominant side**

⊟ ✚ **I69.864** **Other paralytic syndrome following other cerebrovascular disease affecting left non-dominant side**

⊟ ✚ **I69.865** **Other paralytic syndrome following other cerebrovascular disease, bilateral**

⊟ ✚ **I69.869** **Other paralytic syndrome following other cerebrovascular disease affecting unspecified side**

◨ **I69.89** **Other sequelae of other cerebrovascular disease**

I69.890 **Apraxia following other cerebrovascular disease**

✚ **I69.891** **Dysphagia following other cerebrovascular disease**
Use additional code to identify the type of dysphagia, if known (R13.1-)

I69.892 **Facial weakness following other cerebrovascular disease**
Facial droop following other cerebrovascular disease

I69.893 **Ataxia following other cerebrovascular disease**

✚ **I69.898** **Other sequelae of other cerebrovascular disease**
Alteration of sensation following other cerebrovascular disease
Disturbance of vision following other cerebrovascular disease
Use additional code to identify the sequelae

�⊟ **I69.9** **Sequelae of unspecified cerebrovascular diseases**

EXCLUDES 1 *sequelae of stroke (I69.3)*
sequelae of traumatic intracranial injury (S06.-)

I69.90 **Unspecified sequelae of unspecified cerebrovascular disease**

▲ ◨ **I69.91** **Cognitive deficits following unspecified cerebrovascular disease**

● **I69.910** **Attention and concentration deficit following unspecified cerebrovascular disease**

● **I69.911** **Memory deficit following unspecified cerebrovascular disease**

● **I69.912** **Visuospatial deficit and spatial neglect following unspecified cerebrovascular disease**

● **I69.913** **Psychomotor deficit following unspecified cerebrovascular disease**

● **I69.914** **Frontal lobe and executive function deficit following unspecified cerebrovascular disease**

● **I69.915** **Cognitive social or emotional deficit following unspecified cerebrovascular disease**

● **I69.918** **Other symptoms and signs involving cognitive functions following unspecified cerebrovascular disease**

● **I69.919** **Unspecified symptoms and signs involving cognitive functions following unspecified cerebrovascular disease**

◨ **I69.92** **Speech and language deficits following unspecified cerebrovascular disease**

I69.920 **Aphasia following unspecified cerebrovascular disease**

DEFINITION Impaired or complete loss of the ability to communicate with language or symbols resulting from brain damage.

I69.921 **Dysphasia following unspecified cerebrovascular disease**

DEFINITION Impairment in the ability to speak or understand words resulting from brain damage.

I69.922 **Dysarthria following unspecified cerebrovascular disease**

▲ **I69.923** **Fluency disorder following unspecified cerebrovascular disease**
Stuttering following unspecified cerebrovascular disease

I69.928 **Other speech and language deficits following unspecified cerebrovascular disease**

◨ **I69.93** **Monoplegia of upper limb following unspecified cerebrovascular disease**

⊟ **I69.931** **Monoplegia of upper limb following unspecified cerebrovascular disease affecting right dominant side**

⊟ **I69.932** **Monoplegia of upper limb following unspecified cerebrovascular disease affecting left dominant side**

⊟ **I69.933** **Monoplegia of upper limb following unspecified cerebrovascular disease affecting right non-dominant side**

⊟ **I69.934** **Monoplegia of upper limb following unspecified cerebrovascular disease affecting left non-dominant side**

⊟ **I69.939** **Monoplegia of upper limb following unspecified cerebrovascular disease affecting unspecified side**

◨ **I69.94** **Monoplegia of lower limb following unspecified cerebrovascular disease**

⊟ **I69.941** **Monoplegia of lower limb following unspecified cerebrovascular disease affecting right dominant side**

⊟ **I69.942** **Monoplegia of lower limb following unspecified cerebrovascular disease affecting left dominant side**

⊟ **I69.943** **Monoplegia of lower limb following unspecified cerebrovascular disease affecting right non-dominant side**

⊟ **I69.944** **Monoplegia of lower limb following unspecified cerebrovascular disease affecting left non-dominant side**

⊟ **I69.949** **Monoplegia of lower limb following unspecified cerebrovascular disease affecting unspecified side**

◨ **I69.95** **Hemiplegia and hemiparesis following unspecified cerebrovascular disease**

DEFINITION Paralysis affecting one side of the body.

● New ▲ Revised *Manifestation* ◨-◨ Digit Indicators ⊟ Laterality �82 Adult (15+ years) �82 Maternity (12-55 years) �82 Newborn �82 Pediatric (0-17 years) ♂ Male ♀ Female
✖ Deleted Unspecified ✚ Additional code

⊟ **I69.951** **Hemiplegia and hemiparesis following unspecified cerebrovascular disease affecting right dominant side**

⊟ **I69.952** **Hemiplegia and hemiparesis following unspecified cerebrovascular disease affecting left dominant side**

⊟ **I69.953** **Hemiplegia and hemiparesis following unspecified cerebrovascular disease affecting right non-dominant side**

⊟ **I69.954** **Hemiplegia and hemiparesis following unspecified cerebrovascular disease affecting left non-dominant side**

⊟ **I69.959** **Hemiplegia and hemiparesis following unspecified cerebrovascular disease affecting unspecified side**

6 + **I69.96** **Other paralytic syndrome following unspecified cerebrovascular disease**

Use additional code to identify type of paralytic syndrome, such as:
locked-in state (G83.5)
quadriplegia (G82.5-)

EXCLUDES 1 *hemiplegia/hemiparesis following unspecified cerebrovascular disease (I69.95-)*
monoplegia of lower limb following unspecified cerebrovascular disease (I69.94-)
monoplegia of upper limb following unspecified cerebrovascular disease (I69.93-)

⊟ + **I69.961** **Other paralytic syndrome following unspecified cerebrovascular disease affecting right dominant side**

⊟ + **I69.962** **Other paralytic syndrome following unspecified cerebrovascular disease affecting left dominant side**

⊟ + **I69.963** **Other paralytic syndrome following unspecified cerebrovascular disease affecting right non-dominant side**

⊟ + **I69.964** **Other paralytic syndrome following unspecified cerebrovascular disease affecting left non-dominant side**

⊟ + **I69.965** **Other paralytic syndrome following unspecified cerebrovascular disease, bilateral**

⊟ + **I69.969** **Other paralytic syndrome following unspecified cerebrovascular disease affecting unspecified side**

6 **I69.99** **Other sequelae of unspecified cerebrovascular disease**

I69.990 **Apraxia following unspecified cerebrovascular disease**

+ **I69.991** **Dysphagia following unspecified cerebrovascular disease**

Use additional code to identify the type of dysphagia, if known (R13.1-)

I69.992 **Facial weakness following unspecified cerebrovascular disease**

Facial droop following unspecified cerebrovascular disease

I69.993 **Ataxia following unspecified cerebrovascular disease**

DEFINITION Inability to coordinate muscle movement.

+ **I69.998** **Other sequelae following unspecified cerebrovascular disease**

Alteration in sensation following unspecified cerebrovascular disease
Disturbance of vision following unspecified cerebrovascular disease
Use additional code to identify the sequelae

Diseases of arteries, arterioles and capillaries (I70-I79)

▲ 4 + **I70** **Atherosclerosis**

INCLUDES arteriolosclerosis
arterial degeneration
arteriosclerosis
arteriosclerotic vascular disease
arteriovascular degeneration
atheroma
endarteritis deformans or obliterans
senile arteritis
senile endarteritis
vascular degeneration

Use additional code to identify:
exposure to environmental tobacco smoke (Z77.22)
history of tobacco dependence (Z87.891)
occupational exposure to environmental tobacco smoke (Z57.31)
tobacco dependence (F17.-)
tobacco use (Z72.0)

EXCLUDES 2 *arteriosclerotic cardiovascular disease (I25.1-)*
arteriosclerotic heart disease (I25.1-)
atheroembolism (I75.-)
cerebral atherosclerosis (I67.2)
coronary atherosclerosis (I25.1-)
mesenteric atherosclerosis (K55.1)
precerebral atherosclerosis (I67.2)
primary pulmonary atherosclerosis (I27.0)

+ **I70.0** **Atherosclerosis of aorta** A

DEFINITION Fatty plaque deposits in the aorta that reduce its diameter and elasticity.

+ **I70.1** **Atherosclerosis of renal artery** A

Goldblatt's kidney

EXCLUDES 2 *atherosclerosis of renal arterioles (I12.-)*

CODING TIP ✓ Atherosclerosis of renal artery may also be reported as renal artery stenosis. When renal artery stenosis is reported as causative of hypertension, an additional code of I15.0, Renovascular hypertension, should be reported.

5 + **I70.2** **Atherosclerosis of native arteries of the extremities**

Mönckeberg's (medial) sclerosis
Use additional code, if applicable, to identify chronic total occlusion of artery of extremity (I70.92)

EXCLUDES 2 *atherosclerosis of bypass graft of extremities (I70.30-I70.79)*

6 + **I70.20** **Unspecified atherosclerosis of native arteries of extremities**

⊟ + **I70.201** **Unspecified atherosclerosis of native arteries of extremities, right leg** A

⊟ + **I70.202** **Unspecified atherosclerosis of native arteries of extremities, left leg** A

⊟ + **I70.203** **Unspecified atherosclerosis of native arteries of extremities, bilateral legs** A

⊟ + **I70.208** **Unspecified atherosclerosis of native arteries of extremities, other extremity** A

⊟ + **I70.209** **Unspecified atherosclerosis of native arteries of extremities, unspecified extremity** A

6 + **I70.21** **Atherosclerosis of native arteries of extremities with intermittent claudication**

⊟ + **I70.211** **Atherosclerosis of native arteries of extremities with intermittent claudication, right leg** A

⊟ + **I70.212** **Atherosclerosis of native arteries of extremities with intermittent claudication, left leg** A

⊟ + **I70.213** **Atherosclerosis of native arteries of extremities with intermittent claudication, bilateral legs** A

⊟ + **I70.218** **Atherosclerosis of native arteries of extremities with intermittent claudication, other extremity** A

⊟ + **I70.219** **Atherosclerosis of native arteries of extremities with intermittent claudication, unspecified extremity** A

● New ▲ Revised *Manifestation* 4 - 7 Digit Indicators ⊟ Laterality A Adult (15+ years) M Maternity (12-55 years) N Newborn P Pediatric (0-17 years) ♂ Male ♀ Female
✖ Deleted Unspecified + Additional code

⑥ + I70.22 Atherosclerosis of native arteries of extremities with rest pain
> INCLUDES any condition classifiable to I70.21-

⑤ + I70.221 Atherosclerosis of native arteries of extremities with rest pain, right leg Ⓐ

⑤ + I70.222 Atherosclerosis of native arteries of extremities with rest pain, left leg Ⓐ

⑤ + I70.223 Atherosclerosis of native arteries of extremities with rest pain, bilateral legs Ⓐ

⑤ + I70.228 Atherosclerosis of native arteries of extremities with rest pain, other extremity Ⓐ

⑤ + I70.229 Atherosclerosis of native arteries of extremities with rest pain, unspecified extremity Ⓐ

⑥ + I70.23 Atherosclerosis of native arteries of right leg with ulceration
> INCLUDES any condition classifiable to I70.211 and I70.221

Use additional code to identify severity of ulcer (L97.-)

> CODING TIP ✓ When bilateral ulcers are present or ulcers of multiple specified areas classifiable in a patient with atherosclerosis of the extremities, assign a code for each specific site, taking laterality into account. A second code from category L97.- to specify the severity of the ulcer must be used following each reported site of atherosclerosis to the extremity with ulceration.

⑤ + I70.231 Atherosclerosis of native arteries of right leg with ulceration of thigh Ⓐ

⑤ + I70.232 Atherosclerosis of native arteries of right leg with ulceration of calf Ⓐ

⑤ + I70.233 Atherosclerosis of native arteries of right leg with ulceration of ankle Ⓐ

⑤ + I70.234 Atherosclerosis of native arteries of right leg with ulceration of heel and midfoot Ⓐ
> Atherosclerosis of native arteries of right leg with ulceration of plantar surface of midfoot

⑤ + I70.235 Atherosclerosis of native arteries of right leg with ulceration of other part of foot Ⓐ
> Atherosclerosis of native arteries of right leg extremities with ulceration of toe

⑤ + I70.238 Atherosclerosis of native arteries of right leg with ulceration of other part of lower right leg Ⓐ

⑤ + I70.239 Atherosclerosis of native arteries of right leg with ulceration of unspecified site Ⓐ

⑥ + I70.24 Atherosclerosis of native arteries of left leg with ulceration
> INCLUDES any condition classifiable to I70.212 and I70.222

Use additional code to identify severity of ulcer (L97.-)

> CODING TIP ✓ When bilateral ulcers are present or ulcers of multiple specified areas classifiable in a patient with atherosclerosis of the extremities, assign a code for each specific site, taking laterality into account. A second code from category L97.- to specify the severity of the ulcer must be used following each reported site of atherosclerosis to the extremity with ulceration.

⑤ + I70.241 Atherosclerosis of native arteries of left leg with ulceration of thigh Ⓐ

⑤ + I70.242 Atherosclerosis of native arteries of left leg with ulceration of calf Ⓐ

⑤ + I70.243 Atherosclerosis of native arteries of left leg with ulceration of ankle Ⓐ

⑤ + I70.244 Atherosclerosis of native arteries of left leg with ulceration of heel and midfoot Ⓐ
> Atherosclerosis of native arteries of left leg with ulceration of plantar surface of midfoot

⑤ + I70.245 Atherosclerosis of native arteries of left leg with ulceration of other part of foot Ⓐ
> Atherosclerosis of native arteries of left leg extremities with ulceration of toe

⑤ + I70.248 Atherosclerosis of native arteries of left leg with ulceration of other part of lower left leg Ⓐ

⑤ + I70.249 Atherosclerosis of native arteries of left leg with ulceration of unspecified site Ⓐ

⑤ + I70.25 Atherosclerosis of native arteries of other extremities with ulceration Ⓐ
> INCLUDES any condition classifiable to I70.218 and I70.228

Use additional code to identify the severity of the ulcer (L98.49-)

> CODING TIP ✓ When bilateral ulcers are present or ulcers of multiple specified areas classifiable in a patient with atherosclerosis of the extremities, assign a code for each specific site, taking laterality into account. A second code from category L97.- to specify the severity of the ulcer must be used following each reported site of atherosclerosis to the extremity with ulceration.

⑥ + I70.26 Atherosclerosis of native arteries of extremities with gangrene
> INCLUDES any condition classifiable to I70.21-, I70.22-, I70.23-, I70.24-, and I70.25-

Use additional code to identify the severity of any ulcer (L97.-, L98.49-), if applicable

> CODING TIP ✓ When the clinical record reports atherosclerosis of the lower extremities with ulceration and gangrene, assign a code from I70.26-. Do not code the gangrene separately. An additional code from category L97.- should be assigned to report the severity of any ulceration.

⑤ + I70.261 Atherosclerosis of native arteries of extremities with gangrene, right leg Ⓐ

⑤ + I70.262 Atherosclerosis of native arteries of extremities with gangrene, left leg Ⓐ

⑤ + I70.263 Atherosclerosis of native arteries of extremities with gangrene, bilateral legs Ⓐ

⑤ + I70.268 Atherosclerosis of native arteries of extremities with gangrene, other extremity Ⓐ

⑤ + I70.269 Atherosclerosis of native arteries of extremities with gangrene, unspecified extremity Ⓐ

⑥ + I70.29 Other atherosclerosis of native arteries of extremities

⑤ + I70.291 Other atherosclerosis of native arteries of extremities, right leg Ⓐ

⑤ + I70.292 Other atherosclerosis of native arteries of extremities, left leg Ⓐ

⑤ + I70.293 Other atherosclerosis of native arteries of extremities, bilateral legs Ⓐ

⑤ + I70.298 Other atherosclerosis of native arteries of extremities, other extremity Ⓐ

⑤ + I70.299 Other atherosclerosis of native arteries of extremities, unspecified extremity Ⓐ

⑤ + I70.3 Atherosclerosis of unspecified type of bypass graft(s) of the extremities

Use additional code, if applicable, to identify chronic total occlusion of artery of extremity (I70.92)

> EXCLUDES 1 embolism or thrombus of bypass graft (s) of extremities (T82.8-)

⑥ + I70.30 Unspecified atherosclerosis of unspecified type of bypass graft(s) of the extremities

⑤ + I70.301 Unspecified atherosclerosis of unspecified type of bypass graft(s) of the extremities, right leg Ⓐ

⑤ + I70.302 Unspecified atherosclerosis of unspecified type of bypass graft(s) of the extremities, left leg Ⓐ

⑤ + I70.303 Unspecified atherosclerosis of unspecified type of bypass graft(s) of the extremities, bilateral legs Ⓐ

⑤ + I70.308 Unspecified atherosclerosis of unspecified type of bypass graft(s) of the extremities, other extremity Ⓐ

⑤ + I70.309 Unspecified atherosclerosis of unspecified type of bypass graft(s) of the extremities, unspecified extremity Ⓐ

⑥ + I70.31 Atherosclerosis of unspecified type of bypass graft(s) of the extremities with intermittent claudication

⑤ + I70.311 Atherosclerosis of unspecified type of bypass graft(s) of the extremities with intermittent claudication, right leg Ⓐ

● New	▲ Revised	*Manifestation*	④-⑦ Digit Indicators	⊟ Laterality	Ⓐ Adult (15+ years)	Ⓜ Maternity (12-55 years)	Ⓝ Newborn	Ⓟ Pediatric (0-17 years)	♂ Male	♀ Female
✖ ~~Deleted~~		Unspecified	+ Additional code							

☐+ **I70.312** **Atherosclerosis of unspecified type of bypass graft(s) of the extremities with intermittent claudication, left leg** Ⓐ

☐+ **I70.313** **Atherosclerosis of unspecified type of bypass graft(s) of the extremities with intermittent claudication, bilateral legs** Ⓐ

☐+ **I70.318** **Atherosclerosis of unspecified type of bypass graft(s) of the extremities with intermittent claudication, other extremity** Ⓐ

☐+ **I70.319** **Atherosclerosis of unspecified type of bypass graft(s) of the extremities with intermittent claudication, unspecified extremity** Ⓐ

⑥+ **I70.32** **Atherosclerosis of unspecified type of bypass graft(s) of the extremities with rest pain**

> INCLUDES any condition classifiable to I70.31-

☐+ **I70.321** **Atherosclerosis of unspecified type of bypass graft(s) of the extremities with rest pain, right leg** Ⓐ

☐+ **I70.322** **Atherosclerosis of unspecified type of bypass graft(s) of the extremities with rest pain, left leg** Ⓐ

☐+ **I70.323** **Atherosclerosis of unspecified type of bypass graft(s) of the extremities with rest pain, bilateral legs** Ⓐ

☐+ **I70.328** **Atherosclerosis of unspecified type of bypass graft(s) of the extremities with rest pain, other extremity** Ⓐ

☐+ **I70.329** **Atherosclerosis of unspecified type of bypass graft(s) of the extremities with rest pain, unspecified extremity** Ⓐ

⑥+ **I70.33** **Atherosclerosis of unspecified type of bypass graft(s) of the right leg with ulceration**

> INCLUDES any condition classifiable to I70.311 and I70.321

Use additional code to identify severity of ulcer (L97.-)

☐+ **I70.331** **Atherosclerosis of unspecified type of bypass graft(s) of the right leg with ulceration of thigh** Ⓐ

☐+ **I70.332** **Atherosclerosis of unspecified type of bypass graft(s) of the right leg with ulceration of calf** Ⓐ

☐+ **I70.333** **Atherosclerosis of unspecified type of bypass graft(s) of the right leg with ulceration of ankle** Ⓐ

☐+ **I70.334** **Atherosclerosis of unspecified type of bypass graft(s) of the right leg with ulceration of heel and midfoot** Ⓐ

Atherosclerosis of unspecified type of bypass graft(s) of right leg with ulceration of plantar surface of midfoot

☐+ **I70.335** **Atherosclerosis of unspecified type of bypass graft(s) of the right leg with ulceration of other part of foot** Ⓐ

Atherosclerosis of unspecified type of bypass graft(s) of the right leg with ulceration of toe

☐+ **I70.338** **Atherosclerosis of unspecified type of bypass graft(s) of the right leg with ulceration of other part of lower leg** Ⓐ

☐+ **I70.339** **Atherosclerosis of unspecified type of bypass graft(s) of the right leg with ulceration of unspecified site** Ⓐ

⑥+ **I70.34** **Atherosclerosis of unspecified type of bypass graft(s) of the left leg with ulceration**

> INCLUDES any condition classifiable to I70.312 and I70.322

Use additional code to identify severity of ulcer (L97.-)

☐+ **I70.341** **Atherosclerosis of unspecified type of bypass graft(s) of the left leg with ulceration of thigh** Ⓐ

☐+ **I70.342** **Atherosclerosis of unspecified type of bypass graft(s) of the left leg with ulceration of calf** Ⓐ

☐+ **I70.343** **Atherosclerosis of unspecified type of bypass graft(s) of the left leg with ulceration of ankle** Ⓐ

☐+ **I70.344** **Atherosclerosis of unspecified type of bypass graft(s) of the left leg with ulceration of heel and midfoot** Ⓐ

Atherosclerosis of unspecified type of bypass graft(s) of left leg with ulceration of plantar surface of midfoot

☐+ **I70.345** **Atherosclerosis of unspecified type of bypass graft(s) of the left leg with ulceration of other part of foot** Ⓐ

Atherosclerosis of unspecified type of bypass graft(s) of the left leg with ulceration of toe

☐+ **I70.348** **Atherosclerosis of unspecified type of bypass graft(s) of the left leg with ulceration of other part of lower leg** Ⓐ

☐+ **I70.349** **Atherosclerosis of unspecified type of bypass graft(s) of the left leg with ulceration of unspecified site** Ⓐ

☐+ **I70.35** **Atherosclerosis of unspecified type of bypass graft(s) of other extremity with ulceration** Ⓐ

> INCLUDES any condition classifiable to I70.318 and I70.328

Use additional code to identify severity of ulcer (L98.49-)

⑥+ **I70.36** **Atherosclerosis of unspecified type of bypass graft(s) of the extremities with gangrene**

> INCLUDES any condition classifiable to I70.31-, I70.32-, I70.33-, I70.34-, I70.35

Use additional code to identify the severity of any ulcer (L97.-, L98.49-), if applicable

☐+ **I70.361** **Atherosclerosis of unspecified type of bypass graft(s) of the extremities with gangrene, right leg** Ⓐ

☐+ **I70.362** **Atherosclerosis of unspecified type of bypass graft(s) of the extremities with gangrene, left leg** Ⓐ

☐+ **I70.363** **Atherosclerosis of unspecified type of bypass graft(s) of the extremities with gangrene, bilateral legs** Ⓐ

☐+ **I70.368** **Atherosclerosis of unspecified type of bypass graft(s) of the extremities with gangrene, other extremity** Ⓐ

☐+ **I70.369** **Atherosclerosis of unspecified type of bypass graft(s) of the extremities with gangrene, unspecified extremity** Ⓐ

⑥+ **I70.39** **Other atherosclerosis of unspecified type of bypass graft(s) of the extremities**

☐+ **I70.391** **Other atherosclerosis of unspecified type of bypass graft(s) of the extremities, right leg** Ⓐ

☐+ **I70.392** **Other atherosclerosis of unspecified type of bypass graft(s) of the extremities, left leg** Ⓐ

☐+ **I70.393** **Other atherosclerosis of unspecified type of bypass graft(s) of the extremities, bilateral legs** Ⓐ

☐+ **I70.398** **Other atherosclerosis of unspecified type of bypass graft(s) of the extremities, other extremity** Ⓐ

☐+ **I70.399** **Other atherosclerosis of unspecified type of bypass graft(s) of the extremities, unspecified extremity** Ⓐ

⑤+ **I70.4** **Atherosclerosis of autologous vein bypass graft(s) of the extremities**

Use additional code, if applicable, to identify chronic total occlusion of artery of extremity (I70.92)

⑥+ **I70.40** **Unspecified atherosclerosis of autologous vein bypass graft(s) of the extremities**

☐+ **I70.401** **Unspecified atherosclerosis of autologous vein bypass graft(s) of the extremities, right leg** Ⓐ

☐+ **I70.402** **Unspecified atherosclerosis of autologous vein bypass graft(s) of the extremities, left leg** Ⓐ

☐+ **I70.403** **Unspecified atherosclerosis of autologous vein bypass graft(s) of the extremities, bilateral legs** Ⓐ

☐+ **I70.408** **Unspecified atherosclerosis of autologous vein bypass graft(s) of the extremities, other extremity** Ⓐ

● New ▲ Revised *Manifestation* ❹-❼ Digit Indicators ☐ Laterality Ⓐ Adult (15+ years) Ⓜ Maternity (12-55 years) Ⓝ Newborn Ⓟ Pediatric (0-17 years) ♂ Male ♀ Female ✖ Deleted Unspecified + Additional code

658   © 2017 DecisionHealth   2017 ICD-10-CM Expert for Physicians

+ I70.409 Unspecified atherosclerosis of autologous vein bypass graft(s) of the extremities, unspecified extremity [A]

+ I70.41 Atherosclerosis of autologous vein bypass graft(s) of the extremities with intermittent claudication

+ I70.411 Atherosclerosis of autologous vein bypass graft(s) of the extremities with intermittent claudication, right leg [A]

+ I70.412 Atherosclerosis of autologous vein bypass graft(s) of the extremities with intermittent claudication, left leg [A]

+ I70.413 Atherosclerosis of autologous vein bypass graft(s) of the extremities with intermittent claudication, bilateral legs [A]

+ I70.418 Atherosclerosis of autologous vein bypass graft(s) of the extremities with intermittent claudication, other extremity [A]

+ I70.419 Atherosclerosis of autologous vein bypass graft(s) of the extremities with intermittent claudication, unspecified extremity [A]

+ I70.42 Atherosclerosis of autologous vein bypass graft(s) of the extremities with rest pain

> **INCLUDES** any condition classifiable to I70.41-

+ I70.421 Atherosclerosis of autologous vein bypass graft(s) of the extremities with rest pain, right leg [A]

+ I70.422 Atherosclerosis of autologous vein bypass graft(s) of the extremities with rest pain, left leg [A]

+ I70.423 Atherosclerosis of autologous vein bypass graft(s) of the extremities with rest pain, bilateral legs [A]

+ I70.428 Atherosclerosis of autologous vein bypass graft(s) of the extremities with rest pain, other extremity [A]

+ I70.429 Atherosclerosis of autologous vein bypass graft(s) of the extremities with rest pain, unspecified extremity [A]

+ I70.43 Atherosclerosis of autologous vein bypass graft(s) of the right leg with ulceration

> **INCLUDES** any condition classifiable to I70.411 and I70.421

Use additional code to identify severity of ulcer (L97.-)

+ I70.431 Atherosclerosis of autologous vein bypass graft(s) of the right leg with ulceration of thigh [A]

+ I70.432 Atherosclerosis of autologous vein bypass graft(s) of the right leg with ulceration of calf [A]

+ I70.433 Atherosclerosis of autologous vein bypass graft(s) of the right leg with ulceration of ankle [A]

+ I70.434 Atherosclerosis of autologous vein bypass graft(s) of the right leg with ulceration of heel and midfoot [A]
Atherosclerosis of autologous vein bypass graft(s) of right leg with ulceration of plantar surface of midfoot

+ I70.435 Atherosclerosis of autologous vein bypass graft(s) of the right leg with ulceration of other part of foot [A]
Atherosclerosis of autologous vein bypass graft(s) of right leg with ulceration of toe

+ I70.438 Atherosclerosis of autologous vein bypass graft(s) of the right leg with ulceration of other part of lower leg [A]

+ I70.439 Atherosclerosis of autologous vein bypass graft(s) of the right leg with ulceration of unspecified site [A]

+ I70.44 Atherosclerosis of autologous vein bypass graft(s) of the left leg with ulceration

> **INCLUDES** any condition classifiable to I70.412 and I70.422

Use additional code to identify severity of ulcer (L97.-)

+ I70.441 Atherosclerosis of autologous vein bypass graft(s) of the left leg with ulceration of thigh [A]

+ I70.442 Atherosclerosis of autologous vein bypass graft(s) of the left leg with ulceration of calf [A]

+ I70.443 Atherosclerosis of autologous vein bypass graft(s) of the left leg with ulceration of ankle [A]

+ I70.444 Atherosclerosis of autologous vein bypass graft(s) of the left leg with ulceration of heel and midfoot [A]
Atherosclerosis of autologous vein bypass graft(s) of left leg with ulceration of plantar surface of midfoot

+ I70.445 Atherosclerosis of autologous vein bypass graft(s) of the left leg with ulceration of other part of foot [A]
Atherosclerosis of autologous vein bypass graft(s) of left leg with ulceration of toe

+ I70.448 Atherosclerosis of autologous vein bypass graft(s) of the left leg with ulceration of other part of lower leg [A]

+ I70.449 Atherosclerosis of autologous vein bypass graft(s) of the left leg with ulceration of unspecified site [A]

+ I70.45 Atherosclerosis of autologous vein bypass graft(s) of other extremity with ulceration [A]

> **INCLUDES** any condition classifiable to I70.418, I70.428, and I70.438

Use additional code to identify severity of ulcer (L98.49)

+ I70.46 Atherosclerosis of autologous vein bypass graft(s) of the extremities with gangrene

> **INCLUDES** any condition classifiable to I70.41-, I70.42-, and I70.43-, I70.44-, I70.45

Use additional code to identify the severity of any ulcer (L97.-, L98.49-), if applicable

+ I70.461 Atherosclerosis of autologous vein bypass graft(s) of the extremities with gangrene, right leg [A]

+ I70.462 Atherosclerosis of autologous vein bypass graft(s) of the extremities with gangrene, left leg [A]

+ I70.463 Atherosclerosis of autologous vein bypass graft(s) of the extremities with gangrene, bilateral legs [A]

+ I70.468 Atherosclerosis of autologous vein bypass graft(s) of the extremities with gangrene, other extremity [A]

+ I70.469 Atherosclerosis of autologous vein bypass graft(s) of the extremities with gangrene, unspecified extremity [A]

+ I70.49 Other atherosclerosis of autologous vein bypass graft(s) of the extremities

+ I70.491 Other atherosclerosis of autologous vein bypass graft(s) of the extremities, right leg [A]

+ I70.492 Other atherosclerosis of autologous vein bypass graft(s) of the extremities, left leg [A]

+ I70.493 Other atherosclerosis of autologous vein bypass graft(s) of the extremities, bilateral legs [A]

+ I70.498 Other atherosclerosis of autologous vein bypass graft(s) of the extremities, other extremity [A]

+ I70.499 Other atherosclerosis of autologous vein bypass graft(s) of the extremities, unspecified extremity [A]

+ I70.5 Atherosclerosis of nonautologous biological bypass graft(s) of the extremities

Use additional code, if applicable, to identify chronic total occlusion of artery of extremity (I70.92)

+ I70.50 Unspecified atherosclerosis of nonautologous biological bypass graft(s) of the extremities

+ I70.501 Unspecified atherosclerosis of nonautologous biological bypass graft(s) of the extremities, right leg [A]

+ I70.502 Unspecified atherosclerosis of nonautologous biological bypass graft(s) of the extremities, left leg [A]

+ I70.503 Unspecified atherosclerosis of nonautologous biological bypass graft(s) of the extremities, bilateral legs [A]

+ I70.508 Unspecified atherosclerosis of nonautologous biological bypass graft(s) of the extremities, other extremity [A]

● New   ▲ Revised   *Manifestation*   4-7 Digit Indicators   ▤ Laterality   ▣ Adult (15+ years)   M Maternity (12-55 years)   N Newborn   P Pediatric (0-17 years)   ♂ Male   ♀ Female
✖ Deleted   Unspecified   + Additional code

I70.509 Unspecified atherosclerosis of nonautologous biological bypass graft(s) of the extremities, unspecified extremity Ⓐ

I70.51 Atherosclerosis of nonautologous biological bypass graft(s) of the extremities intermittent claudication

I70.511 Atherosclerosis of nonautologous biological bypass graft(s) of the extremities with intermittent claudication, right leg Ⓐ

I70.512 Atherosclerosis of nonautologous biological bypass graft(s) of the extremities with intermittent claudication, left leg Ⓐ

I70.513 Atherosclerosis of nonautologous biological bypass graft(s) of the extremities with intermittent claudication, bilateral legs Ⓐ

I70.518 Atherosclerosis of nonautologous biological bypass graft(s) of the extremities with intermittent claudication, other extremity Ⓐ

I70.519 Atherosclerosis of nonautologous biological bypass graft(s) of the extremities with intermittent claudication, unspecified extremity Ⓐ

I70.52 Atherosclerosis of nonautologous biological bypass graft(s) of the extremities with rest pain

> INCLUDES   any condition classifiable to I70.51-

I70.521 Atherosclerosis of nonautologous biological bypass graft(s) of the extremities with rest pain, right leg Ⓐ

I70.522 Atherosclerosis of nonautologous biological bypass graft(s) of the extremities with rest pain, left leg Ⓐ

I70.523 Atherosclerosis of nonautologous biological bypass graft(s) of the extremities with rest pain, bilateral legs Ⓐ

I70.528 Atherosclerosis of nonautologous biological bypass graft(s) of the extremities with rest pain, other extremity Ⓐ

I70.529 Atherosclerosis of nonautologous biological bypass graft(s) of the extremities with rest pain, unspecified extremity Ⓐ

I70.53 Atherosclerosis of nonautologous biological bypass graft(s) of the right leg with ulceration

> INCLUDES   any condition classifiable to I70.511 and I70.521

Use additional code to identify severity of ulcer (L97.-)

I70.531 Atherosclerosis of nonautologous biological bypass graft(s) of the right leg with ulceration of thigh Ⓐ

I70.532 Atherosclerosis of nonautologous biological bypass graft(s) of the right leg with ulceration of calf Ⓐ

I70.533 Atherosclerosis of nonautologous biological bypass graft(s) of the right leg with ulceration of ankle Ⓐ

I70.534 Atherosclerosis of nonautologous biological bypass graft(s) of the right leg with ulceration of heel and midfoot Ⓐ
Atherosclerosis of nonautologous biological bypass graft(s) of right leg with ulceration of plantar surface of midfoot

I70.535 Atherosclerosis of nonautologous biological bypass graft(s) of the right leg with ulceration of other part of foot Ⓐ
Atherosclerosis of nonautologous biological bypass graft(s) of the right leg with ulceration of toe

I70.538 Atherosclerosis of nonautologous biological bypass graft(s) of the right leg with ulceration of other part of lower leg Ⓐ

I70.539 Atherosclerosis of nonautologous biological bypass graft(s) of the right leg with ulceration of unspecified site Ⓐ

I70.54 Atherosclerosis of nonautologous biological bypass graft(s) of the left leg with ulceration

> INCLUDES   any condition classifiable to I70.512 and I70.522

Use additional code to identify severity of ulcer (L97.-)

I70.541 Atherosclerosis of nonautologous biological bypass graft(s) of the left leg with ulceration of thigh Ⓐ

I70.542 Atherosclerosis of nonautologous biological bypass graft(s) of the left leg with ulceration of calf Ⓐ

I70.543 Atherosclerosis of nonautologous biological bypass graft(s) of the left leg with ulceration of ankle Ⓐ

I70.544 Atherosclerosis of nonautologous biological bypass graft(s) of the left leg with ulceration of heel and midfoot Ⓐ
Atherosclerosis of nonautologous biological bypass graft(s) of left leg with ulceration of plantar surface of midfoot

I70.545 Atherosclerosis of nonautologous biological bypass graft(s) of the left leg with ulceration of other part of foot Ⓐ
Atherosclerosis of nonautologous biological bypass graft(s) of the left leg with ulceration of toe

I70.548 Atherosclerosis of nonautologous biological bypass graft(s) of the left leg with ulceration of other part of lower leg Ⓐ

I70.549 Atherosclerosis of nonautologous biological bypass graft(s) of the left leg with ulceration of unspecified site Ⓐ

I70.55 Atherosclerosis of nonautologous biological bypass graft(s) of other extremity with ulceration Ⓐ

> INCLUDES   any condition classifiable to I70.518, I70.528, and I70.538

Use additional code to identify severity of ulcer (L98.49)

I70.56 Atherosclerosis of nonautologous biological bypass graft(s) of the extremities with gangrene

> INCLUDES   any condition classifiable to I70.51-, I70.52-, and I70.53-, I70.54-, I70.55

Use additional code to identify the severity of any ulcer (L97.-, L98.49-), if applicable

I70.561 Atherosclerosis of nonautologous biological bypass graft(s) of the extremities with gangrene, right leg Ⓐ

I70.562 Atherosclerosis of nonautologous biological bypass graft(s) of the extremities with gangrene, left leg Ⓐ

I70.563 Atherosclerosis of nonautologous biological bypass graft(s) of the extremities with gangrene, bilateral legs Ⓐ

I70.568 Atherosclerosis of nonautologous biological bypass graft(s) of the extremities with gangrene, other extremity Ⓐ

I70.569 Atherosclerosis of nonautologous biological bypass graft(s) of the extremities with gangrene, unspecified extremity Ⓐ

I70.59 Other atherosclerosis of nonautologous biological bypass graft(s) of the extremities

I70.591 Other atherosclerosis of nonautologous biological bypass graft(s) of the extremities, right leg Ⓐ

I70.592 Other atherosclerosis of nonautologous biological bypass graft(s) of the extremities, left leg Ⓐ

I70.593 Other atherosclerosis of nonautologous biological bypass graft(s) of the extremities, bilateral legs Ⓐ

I70.598 Other atherosclerosis of nonautologous biological bypass graft(s) of the extremities, other extremity Ⓐ

I70.599 Other atherosclerosis of nonautologous biological bypass graft(s) of the extremities, unspecified extremity Ⓐ

I70.6 Atherosclerosis of nonbiological bypass graft(s) of the extremities

Use additional code, if applicable, to identify chronic total occlusion of artery of extremity (I70.92)

I70.60 Unspecified atherosclerosis of nonbiological bypass graft(s) of the extremities

I70.601 Unspecified atherosclerosis of nonbiological bypass graft(s) of the extremities, right leg Ⓐ

I70.602 Unspecified atherosclerosis of nonbiological bypass graft(s) of the extremities, left leg Ⓐ

I70.603 Unspecified atherosclerosis of nonbiological bypass graft(s) of the extremities, bilateral legs Ⓐ

● New   ▲ Revised   *Manifestation*   ❹-❼ Digit Indicators   ⊟ Laterality   Ⓐ Adult (15+ years)   Ⓜ Maternity (12-55 years)   Ⓝ Newborn   Ⓟ Pediatric (0-17 years)   ♂ Male   ♀ Female

✖ Deleted   Unspecified   + Additional code

660   © 2017 DecisionHealth   2017 ICD-10-CM Expert for Physicians

I70.509 — I70.603

☐ + **I70.608** **Unspecified atherosclerosis of nonbiological bypass graft(s) of the extremities, other extremity** Ⓐ

☐ + **I70.609** **Unspecified atherosclerosis of nonbiological bypass graft(s) of the extremities, unspecified extremity** Ⓐ

Ⓖ + **I70.61** **Atherosclerosis of nonbiological bypass graft(s) of the extremities with intermittent claudication**

☐ + **I70.611** **Atherosclerosis of nonbiological bypass graft(s) of the extremities with intermittent claudication, right leg** Ⓐ

☐ + **I70.612** **Atherosclerosis of nonbiological bypass graft(s) of the extremities with intermittent claudication, left leg** Ⓐ

☐ + **I70.613** **Atherosclerosis of nonbiological bypass graft(s) of the extremities with intermittent claudication, bilateral legs** Ⓐ

☐ + **I70.618** **Atherosclerosis of nonbiological bypass graft(s) of the extremities with intermittent claudication, other extremity** Ⓐ

☐ + **I70.619** **Atherosclerosis of nonbiological bypass graft(s) of the extremities with intermittent claudication, unspecified extremity** Ⓐ

Ⓖ + **I70.62** **Atherosclerosis of nonbiological bypass graft(s) of the extremities with rest pain**

| INCLUDES | any condition classifiable to I70.61-

☐ + **I70.621** **Atherosclerosis of nonbiological bypass graft(s) of the extremities with rest pain, right leg** Ⓐ

☐ + **I70.622** **Atherosclerosis of nonbiological bypass graft(s) of the extremities with rest pain, left leg** Ⓐ

☐ + **I70.623** **Atherosclerosis of nonbiological bypass graft(s) of the extremities with rest pain, bilateral legs** Ⓐ

☐ + **I70.628** **Atherosclerosis of nonbiological bypass graft(s) of the extremities with rest pain, other extremity** Ⓐ

☐ + **I70.629** **Atherosclerosis of nonbiological bypass graft(s) of the extremities with rest pain, unspecified extremity** Ⓐ

Ⓖ + **I70.63** **Atherosclerosis of nonbiological bypass graft(s) of the right leg with ulceration**

| INCLUDES | any condition classifiable to I70.611 and I70.621

Use additional code to identify severity of ulcer (L97.-)

☐ + **I70.631** **Atherosclerosis of nonbiological bypass graft(s) of the right leg with ulceration of thigh** Ⓐ

☐ + **I70.632** **Atherosclerosis of nonbiological bypass graft(s) of the right leg with ulceration of calf** Ⓐ

☐ + **I70.633** **Atherosclerosis of nonbiological bypass graft(s) of the right leg with ulceration of ankle** Ⓐ

☐ + **I70.634** **Atherosclerosis of nonbiological bypass graft(s) of the right leg with ulceration of heel and midfoot** Ⓐ

Atherosclerosis of nonbiological bypass graft(s) of right leg with ulceration of plantar surface of midfoot

☐ + **I70.635** **Atherosclerosis of nonbiological bypass graft(s) of the right leg with ulceration of other part of foot** Ⓐ

Atherosclerosis of nonbiological bypass graft(s) of the right leg with ulceration of toe

☐ + **I70.638** **Atherosclerosis of nonbiological bypass graft(s) of the right leg with ulceration of other part of lower leg** Ⓐ

☐ + **I70.639** **Atherosclerosis of nonbiological bypass graft(s) of the right leg with ulceration of unspecified site** Ⓐ

Ⓖ + **I70.64** **Atherosclerosis of nonbiological bypass graft(s) of the left leg with ulceration**

| INCLUDES | any condition classifiable to I70.612 and I70.622

Use additional code to identify severity of ulcer (L97.-)

☐ + **I70.641** **Atherosclerosis of nonbiological bypass graft(s) of the left leg with ulceration of thigh** Ⓐ

☐ + **I70.642** **Atherosclerosis of nonbiological bypass graft(s) of the left leg with ulceration of calf** Ⓐ

☐ + **I70.643** **Atherosclerosis of nonbiological bypass graft(s) of the left leg with ulceration of ankle** Ⓐ

☐ + **I70.644** **Atherosclerosis of nonbiological bypass graft(s) of the left leg with ulceration of heel and midfoot** Ⓐ

Atherosclerosis of nonbiological bypass graft(s) of left leg with ulceration of plantar surface of midfoot

☐ + **I70.645** **Atherosclerosis of nonbiological bypass graft(s) of the left leg with ulceration of other part of foot** Ⓐ

Atherosclerosis of nonbiological bypass graft(s) of the left leg with ulceration of toe

☐ + **I70.648** **Atherosclerosis of nonbiological bypass graft(s) of the left leg with ulceration of other part of lower leg** Ⓐ

☐ + **I70.649** **Atherosclerosis of nonbiological bypass graft(s) of the left leg with ulceration of unspecified site** Ⓐ

Ⓖ + **I70.65** **Atherosclerosis of nonbiological bypass graft(s) of other extremity with ulceration** Ⓐ

| INCLUDES | any condition classifiable to I70.618 and I70.628

Use additional code to identify severity of ulcer (L98.49)

Ⓖ + **I70.66** **Atherosclerosis of nonbiological bypass graft(s) of the extremities with gangrene**

| INCLUDES | any condition classifiable to I70.61-, I70.62-, I70.63-, I70.64-, I70.65

Use additional code to identify the severity of any ulcer (L97.-, L98.49-), if applicable

☐ + **I70.661** **Atherosclerosis of nonbiological bypass graft(s) of the extremities with gangrene, right leg** Ⓐ

☐ + **I70.662** **Atherosclerosis of nonbiological bypass graft(s) of the extremities with gangrene, left leg** Ⓐ

☐ + **I70.663** **Atherosclerosis of nonbiological bypass graft(s) of the extremities with gangrene, bilateral legs** Ⓐ

☐ + **I70.668** **Atherosclerosis of nonbiological bypass graft(s) of the extremities with gangrene, other extremity** Ⓐ

☐ + **I70.669** **Atherosclerosis of nonbiological bypass graft(s) of the extremities with gangrene, unspecified extremity** Ⓐ

Ⓖ + **I70.69** **Other atherosclerosis of nonbiological bypass graft(s) of the extremities**

☐ + **I70.691** **Other atherosclerosis of nonbiological bypass graft(s) of the extremities, right leg** Ⓐ

☐ + **I70.692** **Other atherosclerosis of nonbiological bypass graft(s) of the extremities, left leg** Ⓐ

☐ + **I70.693** **Other atherosclerosis of nonbiological bypass graft(s) of the extremities, bilateral legs** Ⓐ

☐ + **I70.698** **Other atherosclerosis of nonbiological bypass graft(s) of the extremities, other extremity** Ⓐ

☐ + **I70.699** **Other atherosclerosis of nonbiological bypass graft(s) of the extremities, unspecified extremity** Ⓐ

Ⓢ + **I70.7** **Atherosclerosis of other type of bypass graft(s) of the extremities**

Use additional code, if applicable, to identify chronic total occlusion of artery of extremity (I70.92)

Ⓖ + **I70.70** **Unspecified atherosclerosis of other type of bypass graft(s) of the extremities**

☐ + **I70.701** **Unspecified atherosclerosis of other type of bypass graft(s) of the extremities, right leg** Ⓐ

☐ + **I70.702** **Unspecified atherosclerosis of other type of bypass graft(s) of the extremities, left leg** Ⓐ

☐ + **I70.703** **Unspecified atherosclerosis of other type of bypass graft(s) of the extremities, bilateral legs** Ⓐ

☐ + **I70.708** **Unspecified atherosclerosis of other type of bypass graft(s) of the extremities, other extremity** Ⓐ

● New   ▲ Revised   *Manifestation*   ④-⑦ Digit Indicators   ☐ Laterality   Ⓐ Adult (15+ years)   Ⓜ Maternity (12-55 years)   Ⓝ Newborn   Ⓟ Pediatric (0-17 years)   ♂ Male   ♀ Female
✖ Deleted   Unspecified   + Additional code

⊟+ I70.709 Unspecified atherosclerosis of other type of bypass graft(s) of the extremities, unspecified extremity Ⓐ

🄶+ I70.71 Atherosclerosis of other type of bypass graft(s) of the extremities with intermittent claudication

⊟+ I70.711 Atherosclerosis of other type of bypass graft(s) of the extremities with intermittent claudication, right leg Ⓐ

⊟+ I70.712 Atherosclerosis of other type of bypass graft(s) of the extremities with intermittent claudication, left leg Ⓐ

⊟+ I70.713 Atherosclerosis of other type of bypass graft(s) of the extremities with intermittent claudication, bilateral legs Ⓐ

⊟+ I70.718 Atherosclerosis of other type of bypass graft(s) of the extremities with intermittent claudication, other extremity Ⓐ

⊟+ I70.719 Atherosclerosis of other type of bypass graft(s) of the extremities with intermittent claudication, unspecified extremity Ⓐ

🄶+ I70.72 Atherosclerosis of other type of bypass graft(s) of the extremities with rest pain

INCLUDES any condition classifiable to I70.71-

⊟+ I70.721 Atherosclerosis of other type of bypass graft(s) of the extremities with rest pain, right leg Ⓐ

⊟+ I70.722 Atherosclerosis of other type of bypass graft(s) of the extremities with rest pain, left leg Ⓐ

⊟+ I70.723 Atherosclerosis of other type of bypass graft(s) of the extremities with rest pain, bilateral legs Ⓐ

⊟+ I70.728 Atherosclerosis of other type of bypass graft(s) of the extremities with rest pain, other extremity Ⓐ

⊟+ I70.729 Atherosclerosis of other type of bypass graft(s) of the extremities with rest pain, unspecified extremity Ⓐ

🄶+ I70.73 Atherosclerosis of other type of bypass graft(s) of the right leg with ulceration

INCLUDES any condition classifiable to I70.711 and I70.721

Use additional code to identify severity of ulcer (L97.-)

⊟+ I70.731 Atherosclerosis of other type of bypass graft(s) of the right leg with ulceration of thigh Ⓐ

⊟+ I70.732 Atherosclerosis of other type of bypass graft(s) of the right leg with ulceration of calf Ⓐ

⊟+ I70.733 Atherosclerosis of other type of bypass graft(s) of the right leg with ulceration of ankle Ⓐ

⊟+ I70.734 Atherosclerosis of other type of bypass graft(s) of the right leg with ulceration of heel and midfoot Ⓐ

Atherosclerosis of other type of bypass graft(s) of right leg with ulceration of plantar surface of midfoot

⊟+ I70.735 Atherosclerosis of other type of bypass graft(s) of the right leg with ulceration of other part of foot Ⓐ

Atherosclerosis of other type of bypass graft(s) of right leg with ulceration of toe

⊟+ I70.738 Atherosclerosis of other type of bypass graft(s) of the right leg with ulceration of other part of lower leg Ⓐ

⊟+ I70.739 Atherosclerosis of other type of bypass graft(s) of the right leg with ulceration of unspecified site Ⓐ

🄶+ I70.74 Atherosclerosis of other type of bypass graft(s) of the left leg with ulceration

INCLUDES any condition classifiable to I70.712 and I70.722

Use additional code to identify severity of ulcer (L97.-)

⊟+ I70.741 Atherosclerosis of other type of bypass graft(s) of the left leg with ulceration of thigh Ⓐ

⊟+ I70.742 Atherosclerosis of other type of bypass graft(s) of the left leg with ulceration of calf Ⓐ

⊟+ I70.743 Atherosclerosis of other type of bypass graft(s) of the left leg with ulceration of ankle Ⓐ

⊟+ I70.744 Atherosclerosis of other type of bypass graft(s) of the left leg with ulceration of heel and midfoot Ⓐ

Atherosclerosis of other type of bypass graft(s) of left leg with ulceration of plantar surface of midfoot

⊟+ I70.745 Atherosclerosis of other type of bypass graft(s) of the left leg with ulceration of other part of foot Ⓐ

Atherosclerosis of other type of bypass graft(s) of left leg with ulceration of toe

⊟+ I70.748 Atherosclerosis of other type of bypass graft(s) of the left leg with ulceration of other part of lower leg Ⓐ

⊟+ I70.749 Atherosclerosis of other type of bypass graft(s) of the left leg with ulceration of unspecified site Ⓐ

🄶+ I70.75 Atherosclerosis of other type of bypass graft(s) of other extremity with ulceration Ⓐ

INCLUDES any condition classifiable to I70.718 and I70.728

Use additional code to identify severity of ulcer (L98.49)

🄶+ I70.76 Atherosclerosis of other type of bypass graft(s) of the extremities with gangrene

INCLUDES any condition classifiable to I70.71-, I70.72-, I70.73-, I70.74-, I70.75

Use additional code to identify the severity of any ulcer (L97.-, L98.49-), if applicable

⊟+ I70.761 Atherosclerosis of other type of bypass graft(s) of the extremities with gangrene, right leg Ⓐ

⊟+ I70.762 Atherosclerosis of other type of bypass graft(s) of the extremities with gangrene, left leg Ⓐ

⊟+ I70.763 Atherosclerosis of other type of bypass graft(s) of the extremities with gangrene, bilateral legs Ⓐ

⊟+ I70.768 Atherosclerosis of other type of bypass graft(s) of the extremities with gangrene, other extremity Ⓐ

⊟+ I70.769 Atherosclerosis of other type of bypass graft(s) of the extremities with gangrene, unspecified extremity Ⓐ

🄶+ I70.79 Other atherosclerosis of other type of bypass graft(s) of the extremities

⊟+ I70.791 Other atherosclerosis of other type of bypass graft(s) of the extremities, right leg Ⓐ

⊟+ I70.792 Other atherosclerosis of other type of bypass graft(s) of the extremities, left leg Ⓐ

⊟+ I70.793 Other atherosclerosis of other type of bypass graft(s) of the extremities, bilateral legs Ⓐ

⊟+ I70.798 Other atherosclerosis of other type of bypass graft(s) of the extremities, other extremity Ⓐ

⊟+ I70.799 Other atherosclerosis of other type of bypass graft(s) of the extremities, unspecified extremity Ⓐ

+ I70.8 Atherosclerosis of other arteries Ⓐ

🄢+ I70.9 Other and unspecified atherosclerosis

+ I70.90 Unspecified atherosclerosis Ⓐ

+ I70.91 Generalized atherosclerosis Ⓐ

+ I70.92 Chronic total occlusion of artery of the extremities Ⓐ

Complete occlusion of artery of the extremities
Total occlusion of artery of the extremities
Code first:
    atherosclerosis of arteries of the extremities (I70.2-, I70.3-, I70.4-, I70.5-, I70.6-, I70.7-)

🄸 I71 **Aortic aneurysm and dissection**

EXCLUDES 1 *aortic ectasia (I77.81-)*
syphilitic aortic aneurysm (A52.01)
traumatic aortic aneurysm (S25.09, S35.09)

🄢 I71.0 Dissection of aorta

I71.00 Dissection of unspecified site of aorta Ⓐ

I71.01 Dissection of thoracic aorta Ⓐ

I71.02 Dissection of abdominal aorta Ⓐ

I71.03 Dissection of thoracoabdominal aorta Ⓐ

● New ▲ Revised *Manifestation* 🄸-🄵 Digit Indicators ⊟ Laterality Ⓐ Adult (15+ years) Ⓜ Maternity (12-55 years) Ⓝ Newborn Ⓟ Pediatric (0-17 years) ♂ Male ♀ Female
✖ Deleted Unspecified + Additional code

I71.1	Thoracic aortic aneurysm, ruptured	A
I71.2	Thoracic aortic aneurysm, without rupture	A
I71.3	Abdominal aortic aneurysm, ruptured	A
I71.4	Abdominal aortic aneurysm, without rupture	A

Abdominal aortic aneurysm, without rupture

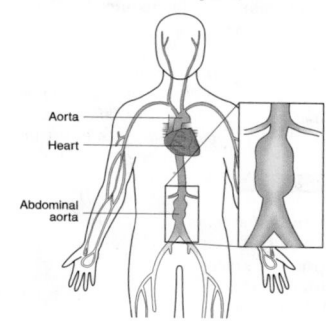

I71.5	Thoracoabdominal aortic aneurysm, ruptured	A
I71.6	Thoracoabdominal aortic aneurysm, without rupture	A
I71.8	Aortic aneurysm of unspecified site, ruptured	A

Rupture of aorta NOS

| I71.9 | Aortic aneurysm of unspecified site, without rupture | A |

Aneurysm of aorta
Dilatation of aorta
Hyaline necrosis of aorta

▲ ④ **I72** **Other aneurysm**

INCLUDES aneurysm (cirsoid) (false) (ruptured)

EXCLUDES 2 *acquired aneurysm (I77.0)*
aneurysm (of) aorta (I71.-)
aneurysm (of) arteriovenous NOS (Q27.3-)
carotid artery dissection (I77.71)
cerebral (nonruptured) aneurysm (I67.1)
coronary aneurysm (I25.4)
coronary artery dissection (I25.42)
dissection of artery NEC (I77.79)
dissection of precerebral artery, congenital (nonruptured) (Q28.1)
heart aneurysm (I25.3)
iliac artery dissection (I77.72)
pulmonary artery aneurysm (I28.1)
renal artery dissection (I77.73)
retinal aneurysm (H35.0)
ruptured cerebral aneurysm (I60.7)
varicose aneurysm (I77.0)
vertebral artery dissection (I77.74)

I72.0 **Aneurysm of carotid artery** A

Aneurysm of common carotid artery
Aneurysm of external carotid artery
Aneurysm of internal carotid artery, extracranial portion

EXCLUDES 1 *aneurysm of internal carotid artery, intracranial portion (I67.1)*
aneurysm of internal carotid artery NOS (I67.1)

I72.1	Aneurysm of artery of upper extremity	A
I72.2	Aneurysm of renal artery	A
I72.3	Aneurysm of iliac artery	A
I72.4	Aneurysm of artery of lower extremity	A

● **I72.5** **Aneurysm of other precerebral arteries**

Aneurysm of basilar artery (trunk)

EXCLUDES 2 *aneurysm of carotid artery (I72.0)*
aneurysm of vertebral artery (I72.6)
dissection of carotid artery (I77.71)
dissection of other precerebral arteries (I77.75)
dissection of vertebral artery (I77.74)

● **I72.6** **Aneurysm of vertebral artery**

EXCLUDES 2 *dissection of vertebral artery (I77.74)*

| I72.8 | Aneurysm of other specified arteries | A |
| I72.9 | Aneurysm of unspecified site | A |

④ **I73** **Other peripheral vascular diseases**

EXCLUDES 2 *chilblains (T69.1)*
frostbite (T33-T34)
immersion hand or foot (T69.0-)
spasm of cerebral artery (G45.9)

⑤ **I73.0** **Raynaud's syndrome**

Raynaud's disease
Raynaud's phenomenon (secondary)

I73.00 **Raynaud's syndrome without gangrene**

I73.01 **Raynaud's syndrome with gangrene**

DEFINITION Medium-sized blood vessels of the hands and feet become inflamed and blocked by blood clots, causing gangrene of the extremities.

I73.1 **Thromboangiitis obliterans [Buerger's disease]**

⑤ **I73.8** **Other specified peripheral vascular diseases**

EXCLUDES 1 *diabetic (peripheral) angiopathy (E08-E13 with .51-.52)*

I73.81 **Erythromelalgia**

DEFINITION Abnormal dilation of extremity blood vessels, especially in the feet, causing a painful, burning sensation, and redness.

I73.89 **Other specified peripheral vascular diseases**

Acrocyanosis
Erythrocyanosis
Simple acroparesthesia [Schultze's type]
Vasomotor acroparesthesia [Nothnagel's type]

I73.9 **Peripheral vascular disease, unspecified**

Intermittent claudication
Peripheral angiopathy NOS
Spasm of artery

EXCLUDES 1 *atherosclerosis of the extremities (I70.2--I70.7-)*

CODING TIP ✓ Do not assign I73.9 when peripheral atherosclerosis is reported in the clinical record. Note, atherosclerosis of the extremities is a more specific diagnosis and should be coded using a code from I70.2- through I70.7-.

Peripheral vascular disease, unspecified

● New ▲ Revised *Manifestation* ④-⑦ Digit Indicators ▭ Laterality A Adult (15+ years) M Maternity (12-55 years) N Newborn P Pediatric (0-17 years) ♂ Male ♀ Female
✖ Deleted Unspecified + Additional code

2017 ICD-10-CM Expert for Physicians

© 2017 DecisionHealth

663

▲ ☐ **I74   Arterial embolism and thrombosis**

INCLUDES	embolic infarction

embolic infarction
embolic occlusion
thrombotic infarction
thrombotic occlusion

Code first:
embolism and thrombosis complicating abortion or ectopic or
molar pregnancy (O00-O07, O08.2)
embolism and thrombosis complicating pregnancy, childbirth
and the puerperium (O88.-)

EXCLUDES 2	*atheroembolism (I75.-)*

atheroembolism (I75.-)
basilar embolism and thrombosis
(I63.0-I63.2, I65.1)
carotid embolism and thrombosis
(I63.0-I63.2, I65.2)
cerebral embolism and thrombosis
(I63.3-I63.5, I66.-)
coronary embolism and thrombosis (I21-I25)
mesenteric embolism and thrombosis (K55.0-)
ophthalmic embolism and thrombosis (H34.-)
precerebral embolism and thrombosis NOS
(I63.0-I63.2, I65.9)
pulmonary embolism and thrombosis (I26.-)
renal embolism and thrombosis (N28.0)
retinal embolism and thrombosis (H34.-)
septic embolism and thrombosis (I76)
vertebral embolism and thrombosis
(I63.0-I63.2, I65.0)

⑤ **I74.0   Embolism and thrombosis of abdominal aorta**

I74.01   Saddle embolus of abdominal aorta

I74.09   Other arterial embolism and thrombosis of
abdominal aorta
Aortic bifurcation syndrome
Aortoiliac obstruction
Leriche's syndrome

⑤ **I74.1   Embolism and thrombosis of other and unspecified parts**
of aorta

I74.10   Embolism and thrombosis of unspecified parts of
aorta

I74.11   Embolism and thrombosis of thoracic aorta

I74.19   Embolism and thrombosis of other parts of aorta

I74.2   Embolism and thrombosis of arteries of the upper
extremities

I74.3   Embolism and thrombosis of arteries of the lower
extremities

I74.4   Embolism and thrombosis of arteries of extremities,
unspecified
Peripheral arterial embolism NOS

I74.5   Embolism and thrombosis of iliac artery

I74.8   Embolism and thrombosis of other arteries

I74.9   Embolism and thrombosis of unspecified artery

☐ **I75   Atheroembolism**

INCLUDES	atherothrombotic microembolism

atherothrombotic microembolism
cholesterol embolism

⑤ **I75.0   Atheroembolism of extremities**

⑥ **I75.01   Atheroembolism of upper extremity**

⊟ **I75.011   Atheroembolism of right upper extremity**

⊟ **I75.012   Atheroembolism of left upper extremity**

⊟ **I75.013   Atheroembolism of bilateral upper extremities**

⊟ **I75.019   Atheroembolism of unspecified upper extremity**

⑥ **I75.02   Atheroembolism of lower extremity**

⊟ **I75.021   Atheroembolism of right lower extremity**

⊟ **I75.022   Atheroembolism of left lower extremity**

⊟ **I75.023   Atheroembolism of bilateral lower extremities**

⊟ **I75.029   Atheroembolism of unspecified lower extremity**

⑤ **I75.8   Atheroembolism of other sites**

✚ **I75.81   Atheroembolism of kidney**
Use additional code for any associated acute kidney
failure and chronic kidney disease (N17.-, N18.-)

I75.89   Atheroembolism of other site

✚ **I76   Septic arterial embolism**
Code first underlying infection, such as:
infective endocarditis (I33.0)
lung abscess (J85.-)
Use additional code to identify the site of the embolism (I74.-)

EXCLUDES 2	*septic pulmonary embolism (I26.01, I26.90)*

DEFINITION	Dislodged material from a centralized

Dislodged material from a centralized
infection lodged in a small arteriole, causing tissue death
due to bacteria and lack of blood supply.

☐ **I77   Other disorders of arteries and arterioles**

EXCLUDES 2	*collagen (vascular) diseases (M30-M36)*

collagen (vascular) diseases (M30-M36)
hypersensitivity angiitis (M31.0)
pulmonary artery (I28.-)

I77.0   Arteriovenous fistula, acquired
Aneurysmal varix
Arteriovenous aneurysm, acquired

EXCLUDES 1	*arteriovenous aneurysm NOS (Q27.3-)*

arteriovenous aneurysm NOS (Q27.3-)
presence of arteriovenous shunt (fistula) for
dialysis (Z99.2)
traumatic - see injury of blood vessel by
body region

EXCLUDES 2	*cerebral (I67.1)*

cerebral (I67.1)
coronary (I25.4)

I77.1   Stricture of artery
Narrowing of artery

I77.2   Rupture of artery
Erosion of artery
Fistula of artery
Ulcer of artery

EXCLUDES 1	*traumatic rupture of artery - see injury of*

traumatic rupture of artery - see injury of
blood vessel by body region

CODING TIP ✓	Do not assign code I77.2 for a traumatic

Do not assign code I77.2 for a traumatic
rupture of the artery. A fistula, ulcer, or arterial erosion
would be coded to I77.2.

I77.3   Arterial fibromuscular dysplasia
Fibromuscular hyperplasia (of) carotid artery
Fibromuscular hyperplasia (of) renal artery

I77.4   Celiac artery compression syndrome

I77.5   Necrosis of artery

I77.6   Arteritis, unspecified
Aortitis NOS
Endarteritis NOS

EXCLUDES 1	*arteritis or endarteritis:*

arteritis or endarteritis:
aortic arch (M31.4)
cerebral NEC (I67.7)
coronary (I25.89)
deformans (I70.-)
giant cell (M31.5., M31.6)
obliterans (I70.-)
senile (I70.-)

⑤ **I77.7   Other arterial dissection**

EXCLUDES 2	*dissection of aorta (I71.0-)*

dissection of aorta (I71.0-)
dissection of coronary artery (I25.42)

● **I77.70   Dissection of unspecified artery**

I77.71   Dissection of carotid artery

I77.72   Dissection of iliac artery

I77.73   Dissection of renal artery

▲ **I77.74   Dissection of vertebral artery**

EXCLUDES 2	*aneurysm of vertebral artery (I72.6)*

● **I77.75   Dissection of other precerebral arteries**
Dissection of basilar artery (trunk)

EXCLUDES 2	*aneurysm of carotid artery (I72.0)*

aneurysm of carotid artery (I72.0)
aneurysm of other precerebral arteries
(I72.5)
aneurysm of vertebral artery (I72.6)
dissection of carotid artery (I77.71)
dissection of vertebral artery (I77.74)

● **I77.76   Dissection of artery of upper extremity**

● **I77.77   Dissection of artery of lower extremity**

▲ **I77.79   Dissection of other specified artery**

⑤ **I77.8   Other specified disorders of arteries and arterioles**

⑥ **I77.81   Aortic ectasia**
Ectasis aorta

EXCLUDES 1	*aortic aneurysm and dissection*

aortic aneurysm and dissection
(I71.0-)

I77.810   Thoracic aortic ectasia

I77.811   Abdominal aortic ectasia

I77.812   Thoracoabdominal aortic ectasia

I77.819   Aortic ectasia, unspecified site

I77.89   Other specified disorders of arteries and arterioles

I77.9   Disorder of arteries and arterioles, unspecified

☐ **I78   Diseases of capillaries**

I78.0   Hereditary hemorrhagic telangiectasia
Rendu-Osler-Weber disease

● New   ▲ Revised   *Manifestation*   ☐-☐ Digit Indicators   ⊟ Laterality   Ⓐ Adult   Ⓜ Maternity   Ⓝ Newborn   Ⓟ Pediatric   ♂ Male   ♀ Female
                                                                                                                                      (15+ years)   (12-55 years)   (0-17 years)
✖ Deleted   Unspecified   ✚ Additional code

I78.1 **Nevus, non-neoplastic**
Araneus nevus
Senile nevus
Spider nevus
Stellar nevus

> **EXCLUDES 1** *nevus NOS (D22.-)*
> *vascular NOS (Q82.5)*
> **EXCLUDES 2** *blue nevus (D22.-)*
> *flammeus nevus (Q82.5)*
> *hairy nevus (D22.-)*
> *melanocytic nevus (D22.-)*
> *pigmented nevus (D22.-)*
> *portwine nevus (Q82.5)*
> *sanguineous nevus (Q82.5)*
> *strawberry nevus (Q82.5)*
> *verrucous nevus (Q82.5)*

I78.8 **Other diseases of capillaries**
I78.9 **Disease of capillaries, unspecified**

I79 **Disorders of arteries, arterioles and capillaries in diseases classified elsewhere**

> **CODING TIP ✓** Codes from category I79.- should be coded only when an the arterial disease/dysfunction is specified as due to another primary disease process. The causative disease process should be coded first.

I79.0 *Aneurysm of aorta in diseases classified elsewhere* 🅰
Code first:
underlying disease

> **EXCLUDES 1** *syphilitic aneurysm (A52.01)*

> **CODING TIP ✓** I79.0 should be coded only when an aortic aneurysm is specified as due to another primary disease process. The causative disease process should be coded first.

I79.1 *Aortitis in diseases classified elsewhere*
Code first:
underlying disease

> **EXCLUDES 1** *syphilitic aortitis (A52.02)*

I79.8 *Other disorders of arteries, arterioles and capillaries in diseases classified elsewhere*
Code first underlying disease, such as:
amyloidosis (E85.-)

> **EXCLUDES 1** *diabetic (peripheral) angiopathy (E08-E13 with .51-.52)*
> *syphilitic endarteritis (A52.09)*
> *tuberculous endarteritis (A18.89)*

Diseases of veins, lymphatic vessels and lymph nodes, not elsewhere classified (I80-I89)

I80 **Phlebitis and thrombophlebitis**

> **INCLUDES** endophlebitis
> inflammation, vein
> periphlebitis
> suppurative phlebitis

Code first:
phlebitis and thrombophlebitis complicating abortion, ectopic or molar pregnancy (O00-O07, O08.7)
phlebitis and thrombophlebitis complicating pregnancy, childbirth and the puerperium (O22.-, O87.-)

> **EXCLUDES 1** *venous embolism and thrombosis of lower extremities (I82.4-, I82.5-, I82.81-)*

I80.0 **Phlebitis and thrombophlebitis of superficial vessels of lower extremities**
Phlebitis and thrombophlebitis of femoropopliteal vein

I80.00 **Phlebitis and thrombophlebitis of superficial vessels of unspecified lower extremity**

I80.01 **Phlebitis and thrombophlebitis of superficial vessels of right lower extremity**

I80.02 **Phlebitis and thrombophlebitis of superficial vessels of left lower extremity**

I80.03 **Phlebitis and thrombophlebitis of superficial vessels of lower extremities, bilateral**

I80.1 **Phlebitis and thrombophlebitis of femoral vein**

I80.10 **Phlebitis and thrombophlebitis of unspecified femoral vein**

I80.11 **Phlebitis and thrombophlebitis of right femoral vein**

I80.12 **Phlebitis and thrombophlebitis of left femoral vein**

I80.13 **Phlebitis and thrombophlebitis of femoral vein, bilateral**

I80.2 **Phlebitis and thrombophlebitis of other and unspecified deep vessels of lower extremities**

I80.20 **Phlebitis and thrombophlebitis of unspecified deep vessels of lower extremities**

I80.201 **Phlebitis and thrombophlebitis of unspecified deep vessels of right lower extremity**

I80.202 **Phlebitis and thrombophlebitis of unspecified deep vessels of left lower extremity**

I80.203 **Phlebitis and thrombophlebitis of unspecified deep vessels of lower extremities, bilateral**

I80.209 **Phlebitis and thrombophlebitis of unspecified deep vessels of unspecified lower extremity**

I80.21 **Phlebitis and thrombophlebitis of iliac vein**

I80.211 **Phlebitis and thrombophlebitis of right iliac vein**

I80.212 **Phlebitis and thrombophlebitis of left iliac vein**

I80.213 **Phlebitis and thrombophlebitis of iliac vein, bilateral**

I80.219 **Phlebitis and thrombophlebitis of unspecified iliac vein**

I80.22 **Phlebitis and thrombophlebitis of popliteal vein**

I80.221 **Phlebitis and thrombophlebitis of right popliteal vein**

I80.222 **Phlebitis and thrombophlebitis of left popliteal vein**

I80.223 **Phlebitis and thrombophlebitis of popliteal vein, bilateral**

I80.229 **Phlebitis and thrombophlebitis of unspecified popliteal vein**

I80.23 **Phlebitis and thrombophlebitis of tibial vein**

I80.231 **Phlebitis and thrombophlebitis of right tibial vein**

I80.232 **Phlebitis and thrombophlebitis of left tibial vein**

I80.233 **Phlebitis and thrombophlebitis of tibial vein, bilateral**

I80.239 **Phlebitis and thrombophlebitis of unspecified tibial vein**

I80.29 **Phlebitis and thrombophlebitis of other deep vessels of lower extremities**

I80.291 **Phlebitis and thrombophlebitis of other deep vessels of right lower extremity**

I80.292 **Phlebitis and thrombophlebitis of other deep vessels of left lower extremity**

I80.293 **Phlebitis and thrombophlebitis of other deep vessels of lower extremity, bilateral**

I80.299 **Phlebitis and thrombophlebitis of other deep vessels of unspecified lower extremity**

I80.3 **Phlebitis and thrombophlebitis of lower extremities, unspecified**

I80.8 **Phlebitis and thrombophlebitis of other sites**

I80.9 **Phlebitis and thrombophlebitis of unspecified site**

I81 **Portal vein thrombosis**
Portal (vein) obstruction

> **EXCLUDES 2** *hepatic vein thrombosis (I82.0)*
> *phlebitis of portal vein (K75.1)*

> **CODING TIP ✓** Portal vein thrombosis is a specific clinical condition caused by the occlusion/obstruction of the portal vein but does not include occlusion of the hepatic vein, and is relatively common in cirrhosis patients. It often leads to portal hypertension. When this condition occurs, any comorbid hepatic vein thrombosis and/or portal hypertension should also be coded.

● New ▲ Revised *Manifestation* 🔢-🔢 Digit Indicators ▱ Laterality 🅰 Adult (15+ years) Ⓜ Maternity (12-55 years) ℕ Newborn 🅿 Pediatric (0-17 years) ♂ Male ♀ Female
✖ Deleted Unspecified + Additional code

▲ ⓓ I82   Other venous embolism and thrombosis

Code first venous embolism and thrombosis complicating:
abortion, ectopic or molar pregnancy (O00-O07, O08.7)
pregnancy, childbirth and the puerperium (O22.-, O87.-)

> **EXCLUDES 2**   *venous embolism and thrombosis (of) :*
> *cerebral (I63.6, I67.6)*
> *coronary (I21-I25)*
> *intracranial and intraspinal, septic or NOS (G08)*
> *intracranial, nonpyogenic (I67.6)*
> *intraspinal, nonpyogenic (G95.1)*
> *mesenteric (K55.0-)*
> *portal (I81)*
> *pulmonary (I26.-)*

I82.0   Budd-Chiari syndrome

Hepatic vein thrombosis

> **DEFINITION**   Obstruction or occlusion of the hepatic veins, causing an enlarged liver, abdominal pain/tenderness, intractable ascites, mild jaundice, portal hypertension, and liver failure.

I82.1   Thrombophlebitis migrans

Ⓢ I82.2   Embolism and thrombosis of vena cava and other thoracic veins

ⓖ I82.21   Embolism and thrombosis of superior vena cava

I82.210   Acute embolism and thrombosis of superior vena cava
Embolism and thrombosis of superior vena cava NOS

I82.211   Chronic embolism and thrombosis of superior vena cava

ⓖ I82.22   Embolism and thrombosis of inferior vena cava

I82.220   Acute embolism and thrombosis of inferior vena cava
Embolism and thrombosis of inferior vena cava NOS

I82.221   Chronic embolism and thrombosis of inferior vena cava

ⓖ I82.29   Embolism and thrombosis of other thoracic veins

Embolism and thrombosis of brachiocephalic (innominate) vein

I82.290   Acute embolism and thrombosis of other thoracic veins

I82.291   Chronic embolism and thrombosis of other thoracic veins

I82.3   Embolism and thrombosis of renal vein

Ⓢ I82.4   Acute embolism and thrombosis of deep veins of lower extremity

ⓖ I82.40   Acute embolism and thrombosis of unspecified deep veins of lower extremity

Deep vein thrombosis NOS
DVT NOS

> **EXCLUDES 1**   *acute embolism and thrombosis of unspecified deep veins of distal lower extremity (I82.4Z-)*
> *acute embolism and thrombosis of unspecified deep veins of proximal lower extremity (I82.4Y-)*

⊟ I82.401   Acute embolism and thrombosis of unspecified deep veins of right lower extremity

⊟ I82.402   Acute embolism and thrombosis of unspecified deep veins of left lower extremity

⊟ I82.403   Acute embolism and thrombosis of unspecified deep veins of lower extremity, bilateral

⊟ I82.409   Acute embolism and thrombosis of unspecified deep veins of unspecified lower extremity

ⓖ I82.41   Acute embolism and thrombosis of femoral vein

⊟ I82.411   Acute embolism and thrombosis of right femoral vein

⊟ I82.412   Acute embolism and thrombosis of left femoral vein

⊟ I82.413   Acute embolism and thrombosis of femoral vein, bilateral

⊟ I82.419   Acute embolism and thrombosis of unspecified femoral vein

ⓖ I82.42   Acute embolism and thrombosis of iliac vein

⊟ I82.421   Acute embolism and thrombosis of right iliac vein

⊟ I82.422   Acute embolism and thrombosis of left iliac vein

⊟ I82.423   Acute embolism and thrombosis of iliac vein, bilateral

⊟ I82.429   Acute embolism and thrombosis of unspecified iliac vein

ⓖ I82.43   Acute embolism and thrombosis of popliteal vein

⊟ I82.431   Acute embolism and thrombosis of right popliteal vein

⊟ I82.432   Acute embolism and thrombosis of left popliteal vein

⊟ I82.433   Acute embolism and thrombosis of popliteal vein, bilateral

⊟ I82.439   Acute embolism and thrombosis of unspecified popliteal vein

ⓖ I82.44   Acute embolism and thrombosis of tibial vein

⊟ I82.441   Acute embolism and thrombosis of right tibial vein

⊟ I82.442   Acute embolism and thrombosis of left tibial vein

⊟ I82.443   Acute embolism and thrombosis of tibial vein, bilateral

⊟ I82.449   Acute embolism and thrombosis of unspecified tibial vein

ⓖ I82.49   Acute embolism and thrombosis of other specified deep vein of lower extremity

⊟ I82.491   Acute embolism and thrombosis of other specified deep vein of right lower extremity

⊟ I82.492   Acute embolism and thrombosis of other specified deep vein of left lower extremity

⊟ I82.493   Acute embolism and thrombosis of other specified deep vein of lower extremity, bilateral

⊟ I82.499   Acute embolism and thrombosis of other specified deep vein of unspecified lower extremity

ⓖ I82.4Y   Acute embolism and thrombosis of unspecified deep veins of proximal lower extremity

Acute embolism and thrombosis of deep vein of thigh NOS
Acute embolism and thrombosis of deep vein of upper leg NOS

⊟ I82.4Y1   Acute embolism and thrombosis of unspecified deep veins of right proximal lower extremity

⊟ I82.4Y2   Acute embolism and thrombosis of unspecified deep veins of left proximal lower extremity

⊟ I82.4Y3   Acute embolism and thrombosis of unspecified deep veins of proximal lower extremity, bilateral

⊟ I82.4Y9   Acute embolism and thrombosis of unspecified deep veins of unspecified proximal lower extremity

ⓖ I82.4Z   Acute embolism and thrombosis of unspecified deep veins of distal lower extremity

Acute embolism and thrombosis of deep vein of calf NOS
Acute embolism and thrombosis of deep vein of lower leg NOS

⊟ I82.4Z1   Acute embolism and thrombosis of unspecified deep veins of right distal lower extremity

⊟ I82.4Z2   Acute embolism and thrombosis of unspecified deep veins of left distal lower extremity

⊟ I82.4Z3   Acute embolism and thrombosis of unspecified deep veins of distal lower extremity, bilateral

⊟ I82.4Z9   Acute embolism and thrombosis of unspecified deep veins of unspecified distal lower extremity

Ⓢ ✚ I82.5   Chronic embolism and thrombosis of deep veins of lower extremity

Use additional code, if applicable, for associated long-term (current) use of anticoagulants (Z79.01)

> **EXCLUDES 1**   *personal history of venous embolism and thrombosis (Z86.718)*

ⓖ ✚ I82.50   Chronic embolism and thrombosis of unspecified deep veins of lower extremity

> **EXCLUDES 1**   *chronic embolism and thrombosis of unspecified deep veins of distal lower extremity (I82.5Z-)*
> *chronic embolism and thrombosis of unspecified deep veins of proximal lower extremity (I82.5Y-)*

⊟ ✚ I82.501   Chronic embolism and thrombosis of unspecified deep veins of right lower extremity

---

● New   ▲ Revised   *Manifestation*   ⓓ-⓻ Digit Indicators   ⊟Laterality   Ⓐ Adult (15+ years)   Ⓜ Maternity (12-55 years)   Ⓝ Newborn   Ⓟ Pediatric (0-17 years)   ♂ Male   ♀Female
✖ ̶D̶e̶l̶e̶t̶e̶d̶   Unspecified   ✚ Additional code

☐ + **I82.502** Chronic embolism and thrombosis of unspecified deep veins of left lower extremity

☐ + **I82.503** Chronic embolism and thrombosis of unspecified deep veins of lower extremity, bilateral

☐ + **I82.509** Chronic embolism and thrombosis of unspecified deep veins of unspecified lower extremity

⑥ + **I82.51** Chronic embolism and thrombosis of femoral vein

☐ + **I82.511** Chronic embolism and thrombosis of right femoral vein

☐ + **I82.512** Chronic embolism and thrombosis of left femoral vein

☐ + **I82.513** Chronic embolism and thrombosis of femoral vein, bilateral

☐ + **I82.519** Chronic embolism and thrombosis of unspecified femoral vein

⑥ + **I82.52** Chronic embolism and thrombosis of iliac vein

☐ + **I82.521** Chronic embolism and thrombosis of right iliac vein

☐ + **I82.522** Chronic embolism and thrombosis of left iliac vein

☐ + **I82.523** Chronic embolism and thrombosis of iliac vein, bilateral

☐ + **I82.529** Chronic embolism and thrombosis of unspecified iliac vein

⑥ + **I82.53** Chronic embolism and thrombosis of popliteal vein

☐ + **I82.531** Chronic embolism and thrombosis of right popliteal vein

☐ + **I82.532** Chronic embolism and thrombosis of left popliteal vein

☐ + **I82.533** Chronic embolism and thrombosis of popliteal vein, bilateral

☐ + **I82.539** Chronic embolism and thrombosis of unspecified popliteal vein

⑥ + **I82.54** Chronic embolism and thrombosis of tibial vein

☐ + **I82.541** Chronic embolism and thrombosis of right tibial vein

☐ + **I82.542** Chronic embolism and thrombosis of left tibial vein

☐ + **I82.543** Chronic embolism and thrombosis of tibial vein, bilateral

☐ + **I82.549** Chronic embolism and thrombosis of unspecified tibial vein

⑥ + **I82.59** Chronic embolism and thrombosis of other specified deep vein of lower extremity

☐ + **I82.591** Chronic embolism and thrombosis of other specified deep vein of right lower extremity

☐ + **I82.592** Chronic embolism and thrombosis of other specified deep vein of left lower extremity

☐ + **I82.593** Chronic embolism and thrombosis of other specified deep vein of lower extremity, bilateral

☐ + **I82.599** Chronic embolism and thrombosis of other specified deep vein of unspecified lower extremity

⑥ + **I82.5Y** Chronic embolism and thrombosis of unspecified deep veins of proximal lower extremity

Chronic embolism and thrombosis of deep veins of thigh NOS

Chronic embolism and thrombosis of deep veins of upper leg NOS

☐ + **I82.5Y1** Chronic embolism and thrombosis of unspecified deep veins of right proximal lower extremity

☐ + **I82.5Y2** Chronic embolism and thrombosis of unspecified deep veins of left proximal lower extremity

☐ + **I82.5Y3** Chronic embolism and thrombosis of unspecified deep veins of proximal lower extremity, bilateral

☐ + **I82.5Y9** Chronic embolism and thrombosis of unspecified deep veins of unspecified proximal lower extremity

⑥ + **I82.5Z** Chronic embolism and thrombosis of unspecified deep veins of distal lower extremity

Chronic embolism and thrombosis of deep veins of calf NOS

Chronic embolism and thrombosis of deep veins of lower leg NOS

☐ + **I82.5Z1** Chronic embolism and thrombosis of unspecified deep veins of right distal lower extremity

☐ + **I82.5Z2** Chronic embolism and thrombosis of unspecified deep veins of left distal lower extremity

☐ + **I82.5Z3** Chronic embolism and thrombosis of unspecified deep veins of distal lower extremity, bilateral

☐ + **I82.5Z9** Chronic embolism and thrombosis of unspecified deep veins of unspecified distal lower extremity

Ⓢ **I82.6** Acute embolism and thrombosis of veins of upper extremity

⑥ **I82.60** Acute embolism and thrombosis of unspecified veins of upper extremity

☐ **I82.601** Acute embolism and thrombosis of unspecified veins of right upper extremity

☐ **I82.602** Acute embolism and thrombosis of unspecified veins of left upper extremity

☐ **I82.603** Acute embolism and thrombosis of unspecified veins of upper extremity, bilateral

☐ **I82.609** Acute embolism and thrombosis of unspecified veins of unspecified upper extremity

⑥ **I82.61** Acute embolism and thrombosis of superficial veins of upper extremity

Acute embolism and thrombosis of antecubital vein
Acute embolism and thrombosis of basilic vein
Acute embolism and thrombosis of cephalic vein

☐ **I82.611** Acute embolism and thrombosis of superficial veins of right upper extremity

☐ **I82.612** Acute embolism and thrombosis of superficial veins of left upper extremity

☐ **I82.613** Acute embolism and thrombosis of superficial veins of upper extremity, bilateral

☐ **I82.619** Acute embolism and thrombosis of superficial veins of unspecified upper extremity

⑥ **I82.62** Acute embolism and thrombosis of deep veins of upper extremity

Acute embolism and thrombosis of brachial vein
Acute embolism and thrombosis of radial vein
Acute embolism and thrombosis of ulnar vein

☐ **I82.621** Acute embolism and thrombosis of deep veins of right upper extremity

☐ **I82.622** Acute embolism and thrombosis of deep veins of left upper extremity

☐ **I82.623** Acute embolism and thrombosis of deep veins of upper extremity, bilateral

☐ **I82.629** Acute embolism and thrombosis of deep veins of unspecified upper extremity

Ⓢ + **I82.7** Chronic embolism and thrombosis of veins of upper extremity

Use additional code, if applicable, for associated long-term (current) use of anticoagulants (Z79.01)

EXCLUDES 1 *personal history of venous embolism and thrombosis (Z86.718)*

⑥ + **I82.70** Chronic embolism and thrombosis of unspecified veins of upper extremity

☐ + **I82.701** Chronic embolism and thrombosis of unspecified veins of right upper extremity

☐ + **I82.702** Chronic embolism and thrombosis of unspecified veins of left upper extremity

☐ + **I82.703** Chronic embolism and thrombosis of unspecified veins of upper extremity, bilateral

☐ + **I82.709** Chronic embolism and thrombosis of unspecified veins of unspecified upper extremity

⑥ + **I82.71** Chronic embolism and thrombosis of superficial veins of upper extremity

Chronic embolism and thrombosis of antecubital vein
Chronic embolism and thrombosis of basilic vein
Chronic embolism and thrombosis of cephalic vein

☐ + **I82.711** Chronic embolism and thrombosis of superficial veins of right upper extremity

☐ + **I82.712** Chronic embolism and thrombosis of superficial veins of left upper extremity

☐ + **I82.713** Chronic embolism and thrombosis of superficial veins of upper extremity, bilateral

● New ▲ Revised *Manifestation* ❹-❼ Digit Indicators ☐ Laterality Ⓐ Adult (15+ years) Ⓜ Maternity (12-55 years) Ⓝ Newborn Ⓟ Pediatric (0-17 years) ♂ Male ♀ Female

✖ ~~Deleted~~ Unspecified + Additional code

2017 ICD-10-CM Expert for Physicians

© 2017 DecisionHealth

667

☐+ **I82.719**   **Chronic embolism and thrombosis of superficial veins of unspecified upper extremity**

⑥+ **I82.72**   **Chronic embolism and thrombosis of deep veins of upper extremity**
Chronic embolism and thrombosis of brachial vein
Chronic embolism and thrombosis of radial vein
Chronic embolism and thrombosis of ulnar vein

☐+ **I82.721**   **Chronic embolism and thrombosis of deep veins of right upper extremity**

☐+ **I82.722**   **Chronic embolism and thrombosis of deep veins of left upper extremity**

☐+ **I82.723**   **Chronic embolism and thrombosis of deep veins of upper extremity, bilateral**

☐+ **I82.729**   **Chronic embolism and thrombosis of deep veins of unspecified upper extremity**

⑤ **I82.A**   **Embolism and thrombosis of axillary vein**

⑥ **I82.A1**   **Acute embolism and thrombosis of axillary vein**

☐ **I82.A11**   **Acute embolism and thrombosis of right axillary vein**

☐ **I82.A12**   **Acute embolism and thrombosis of left axillary vein**

☐ **I82.A13**   **Acute embolism and thrombosis of axillary vein, bilateral**

☐ **I82.A19**   **Acute embolism and thrombosis of unspecified axillary vein**

⑥ **I82.A2**   **Chronic embolism and thrombosis of axillary vein**

☐ **I82.A21**   **Chronic embolism and thrombosis of right axillary vein**

☐ **I82.A22**   **Chronic embolism and thrombosis of left axillary vein**

☐ **I82.A23**   **Chronic embolism and thrombosis of axillary vein, bilateral**

☐ **I82.A29**   **Chronic embolism and thrombosis of unspecified axillary vein**

⑤ **I82.B**   **Embolism and thrombosis of subclavian vein**

⑥ **I82.B1**   **Acute embolism and thrombosis of subclavian vein**

☐ **I82.B11**   **Acute embolism and thrombosis of right subclavian vein**

☐ **I82.B12**   **Acute embolism and thrombosis of left subclavian vein**

☐ **I82.B13**   **Acute embolism and thrombosis of subclavian vein, bilateral**

☐ **I82.B19**   **Acute embolism and thrombosis of unspecified subclavian vein**

⑥ **I82.B2**   **Chronic embolism and thrombosis of subclavian vein**

☐ **I82.B21**   **Chronic embolism and thrombosis of right subclavian vein**

☐ **I82.B22**   **Chronic embolism and thrombosis of left subclavian vein**

☐ **I82.B23**   **Chronic embolism and thrombosis of subclavian vein, bilateral**

☐ **I82.B29**   **Chronic embolism and thrombosis of unspecified subclavian vein**

⑤ **I82.C**   **Embolism and thrombosis of internal jugular vein**

⑥ **I82.C1**   **Acute embolism and thrombosis of internal jugular vein**

☐ **I82.C11**   **Acute embolism and thrombosis of right internal jugular vein**

☐ **I82.C12**   **Acute embolism and thrombosis of left internal jugular vein**

☐ **I82.C13**   **Acute embolism and thrombosis of internal jugular vein, bilateral**

☐ **I82.C19**   **Acute embolism and thrombosis of unspecified internal jugular vein**

⑥ **I82.C2**   **Chronic embolism and thrombosis of internal jugular vein**

☐ **I82.C21**   **Chronic embolism and thrombosis of right internal jugular vein**

☐ **I82.C22**   **Chronic embolism and thrombosis of left internal jugular vein**

☐ **I82.C23**   **Chronic embolism and thrombosis of internal jugular vein, bilateral**

☐ **I82.C29**   **Chronic embolism and thrombosis of unspecified internal jugular vein**

⑤+ **I82.8**   **Embolism and thrombosis of other specified veins**
Use additional code, if applicable, for associated long-term (current) use of anticoagulants (Z79.01)

⑥+ **I82.81**   **Embolism and thrombosis of superficial veins of lower extremities**
Embolism and thrombosis of saphenous vein (greater) (lesser)

☐+ **I82.811**   **Embolism and thrombosis of superficial veins of right lower extremities**

☐+ **I82.812**   **Embolism and thrombosis of superficial veins of left lower extremities**

☐+ **I82.813**   **Embolism and thrombosis of superficial veins of lower extremities, bilateral**

☐+ **I82.819**   **Embolism and thrombosis of superficial veins of unspecified lower extremities**

⑥+ **I82.89**   **Embolism and thrombosis of other specified veins**

+ **I82.890**   **Acute embolism and thrombosis of other specified veins**

+ **I82.891**   **Chronic embolism and thrombosis of other specified veins**

⑤ **I82.9**   **Embolism and thrombosis of unspecified vein**

I82.90   **Acute embolism and thrombosis of unspecified vein**
Embolism of vein NOS
Thrombosis (vein) NOS

I82.91   **Chronic embolism and thrombosis of unspecified vein**

④ **I83**   **Varicose veins of lower extremities**

EXCLUDES 1   *varicose veins complicating pregnancy (O22.0-)*
varicose veins complicating the puerperium (O87.4)

CODING TIP ✓   **Documentation:** When assigning a code from I83.-, coders should assign the most specific code applicable, but cannot assume a specific code. A relationship between a lower extremity wound and varicosity must be stated in the clinical record as a cause and effect relationship by the patient's physician in order to assign a code from I83.2- or I83.0-. Inflammation should not be assumed to be related to varicosities but should be verified by a physician as related before assigning a code from category I83.1-. An additional code from category L97.- should be assigned to report the severity of the ulceration.

⑤+ **I83.0**   **Varicose veins of lower extremities with ulcer**
Use additional code to identify severity of ulcer (L97.-)

⑥+ **I83.00**   **Varicose veins of unspecified lower extremity with ulcer**

+ **I83.001**   **Varicose veins of unspecified lower extremity with ulcer of thigh** Ⓐ

+ **I83.002**   **Varicose veins of unspecified lower extremity with ulcer of calf** Ⓐ

+ **I83.003**   **Varicose veins of unspecified lower extremity with ulcer of ankle** Ⓐ

+ **I83.004**   **Varicose veins of unspecified lower extremity with ulcer of heel and midfoot** Ⓐ
Varicose veins of unspecified lower extremity with ulcer of plantar surface of midfoot

+ **I83.005**   **Varicose veins of unspecified lower extremity with ulcer other part of foot** Ⓐ
Varicose veins of unspecified lower extremity with ulcer of toe

+ **I83.008**   **Varicose veins of unspecified lower extremity with ulcer other part of lower leg** Ⓐ

+ **I83.009**   **Varicose veins of unspecified lower extremity with ulcer of unspecified site** Ⓐ

⑥+ **I83.01**   **Varicose veins of right lower extremity with ulcer**

☐+ **I83.011**   **Varicose veins of right lower extremity with ulcer of thigh** Ⓐ

☐+ **I83.012**   **Varicose veins of right lower extremity with ulcer of calf** Ⓐ

☐+ **I83.013**   **Varicose veins of right lower extremity with ulcer of ankle** Ⓐ

☐+ **I83.014**   **Varicose veins of right lower extremity with ulcer of heel and midfoot** Ⓐ
Varicose veins of right lower extremity with ulcer of plantar surface of midfoot

☐+ **I83.015**   **Varicose veins of right lower extremity with ulcer other part of foot** Ⓐ
Varicose veins of right lower extremity with ulcer of toe

☐+ **I83.018**   **Varicose veins of right lower extremity with ulcer other part of lower leg** Ⓐ

● New   ▲ Revised   *Manifestation*   ④-⑦ Digit Indicators   ☐ Laterality   Ⓐ Adult (15+ years)   Ⓜ Maternity (12-55 years)   Ⓝ Newborn   Ⓟ Pediatric (0-17 years)   ♂ Male   ♀ Female
✖ Deleted   Unspecified   + Additional code

668   © 2017 DecisionHealth   2017 ICD-10-CM Expert for Physicians

I82.719 — I83.018

☐ **+ I83.019** Varicose veins of right lower extremity with ulcer of unspecified site Ⓐ

Ⓖ **+ I83.02** Varicose veins of left lower extremity with ulcer

☐ **+ I83.021** Varicose veins of left lower extremity with ulcer of thigh Ⓐ

☐ **+ I83.022** Varicose veins of left lower extremity with ulcer of calf Ⓐ

☐ **+ I83.023** Varicose veins of left lower extremity with ulcer of ankle Ⓐ

☐ **+ I83.024** Varicose veins of left lower extremity with ulcer of heel and midfoot Ⓐ
Varicose veins of left lower extremity with ulcer of plantar surface of midfoot

☐ **+ I83.025** Varicose veins of left lower extremity with ulcer other part of foot Ⓐ
Varicose veins of left lower extremity with ulcer of toe

☐ **+ I83.028** Varicose veins of left lower extremity with ulcer other part of lower leg Ⓐ

☐ **+ I83.029** Varicose veins of left lower extremity with ulcer of unspecified site Ⓐ

▲ Ⓢ **I83.1** Varicose veins of lower extremities with inflammation

CODING TIP ✓ Documentation: Do not assume inflammation of the lower extremities to be related to varicosities when present. A cause and effect relationship should be confirmed in order to assign a code from category I83.1-.

☐ **I83.10** Varicose veins of unspecified lower extremity with inflammation Ⓐ

☐ **I83.11** Varicose veins of right lower extremity with inflammation Ⓐ

☐ **I83.12** Varicose veins of left lower extremity with inflammation Ⓐ

Ⓢ **+ I83.2** Varicose veins of lower extremities with both ulcer and inflammation
Use additional code to identify severity of ulcer (L97.-)

CODING TIP ✓ If the clinical record reports a confirmed diagnosis of ulcers due to varicosity (condition classifiable to I83.0), as well as inflammation due to varicosity (condition classifiable to I83.1-), then a code from category I83.2- should be reported instead. An additional code is required to indicate the severity of the ulcer.

Ⓖ **+ I83.20** Varicose veins of unspecified lower extremity with both ulcer and inflammation

+ I83.201 Varicose veins of unspecified lower extremity with both ulcer of thigh and inflammation Ⓐ

+ I83.202 Varicose veins of unspecified lower extremity with both ulcer of calf and inflammation Ⓐ

+ I83.203 Varicose veins of unspecified lower extremity with both ulcer of ankle and inflammation Ⓐ

+ I83.204 Varicose veins of unspecified lower extremity with both ulcer of heel and midfoot and inflammation Ⓐ
Varicose veins of unspecified lower extremity with both ulcer of plantar surface of midfoot and inflammation

+ I83.205 Varicose veins of unspecified lower extremity with both ulcer other part of foot and inflammation Ⓐ
Varicose veins of unspecified lower extremity with both ulcer of toe and inflammation

+ I83.208 Varicose veins of unspecified lower extremity with both ulcer of other part of lower extremity and inflammation Ⓐ

+ I83.209 Varicose veins of unspecified lower extremity with both ulcer of unspecified site and inflammation Ⓐ

Ⓖ **+ I83.21** Varicose veins of right lower extremity with both ulcer and inflammation

☐ **+ I83.211** Varicose veins of right lower extremity with both ulcer of thigh and inflammation Ⓐ

☐ **+ I83.212** Varicose veins of right lower extremity with both ulcer of calf and inflammation Ⓐ

☐ **+ I83.213** Varicose veins of right lower extremity with both ulcer of ankle and inflammation Ⓐ

☐ **+ I83.214** Varicose veins of right lower extremity with both ulcer of heel and midfoot and inflammation Ⓐ
Varicose veins of right lower extremity with both ulcer of plantar surface of midfoot and inflammation

☐ **+ I83.215** Varicose veins of right lower extremity with both ulcer other part of foot and inflammation Ⓐ
Varicose veins of right lower extremity with both ulcer of toe and inflammation

☐ **+ I83.218** Varicose veins of right lower extremity with both ulcer of other part of lower extremity and inflammation Ⓐ

☐ **+ I83.219** Varicose veins of right lower extremity with both ulcer of unspecified site and inflammation Ⓐ

Ⓖ **+ I83.22** Varicose veins of left lower extremity with both ulcer and inflammation

☐ **+ I83.221** Varicose veins of left lower extremity with both ulcer of thigh and inflammation Ⓐ

☐ **+ I83.222** Varicose veins of left lower extremity with both ulcer of calf and inflammation Ⓐ

☐ **+ I83.223** Varicose veins of left lower extremity with both ulcer of ankle and inflammation Ⓐ

☐ **+ I83.224** Varicose veins of left lower extremity with both ulcer of heel and midfoot and inflammation Ⓐ
Varicose veins of left lower extremity with both ulcer of plantar surface of midfoot and inflammation

☐ **+ I83.225** Varicose veins of left lower extremity with both ulcer other part of foot and inflammation Ⓐ
Varicose veins of left lower extremity with both ulcer of toe and inflammation

☐ **+ I83.228** Varicose veins of left lower extremity with both ulcer of other part of lower extremity and inflammation Ⓐ

☐ **+ I83.229** Varicose veins of left lower extremity with both ulcer of unspecified site and inflammation Ⓐ

Ⓢ **I83.8** Varicose veins of lower extremities with other complications

Ⓖ **I83.81** Varicose veins of lower extremities with pain

☐ **I83.811** Varicose veins of right lower extremities with pain Ⓐ

☐ **I83.812** Varicose veins of left lower extremities with pain Ⓐ

☐ **I83.813** Varicose veins of bilateral lower extremities with pain Ⓐ

☐ **I83.819** Varicose veins of unspecified lower extremities with pain Ⓐ

Ⓖ **I83.89** Varicose veins of lower extremities with other complications
Varicose veins of lower extremities with edema
Varicose veins of lower extremities with swelling

☐ **I83.891** Varicose veins of right lower extremities with other complications Ⓐ

☐ **I83.892** Varicose veins of left lower extremities with other complications Ⓐ

☐ **I83.893** Varicose veins of bilateral lower extremities with other complications Ⓐ

☐ **I83.899** Varicose veins of unspecified lower extremities with other complications Ⓐ

Ⓢ **I83.9** Asymptomatic varicose veins of lower extremities
Phlebectasia of lower extremities
Varicose veins of lower extremities
Varix of lower extremities

● New ▲ Revised *Manifestation* ▯-▯ Digit Indicators ☐ Laterality Ⓐ Adult (15+ years) Ⓜ Maternity (12-55 years) Ⓝ Newborn Ⓟ Pediatric (0-17 years) ♂ Male ♀ Female
✖ ~~Deleted~~ Unspecified + Additional code

CODING TIP ✓ When assigning a code from I83.9-, coders should consider if this diagnosis is the correct diagnosis, as I83.9- codes indicate asymptomatic varicosities. Also, coders should consider the appropriateness of including I83.9- codes, as these codes indicate a stable and asymptomatic condition, that should require little to no intervention.

Asymptomatic varicose veins of lower extremities

	I83.90	**Asymptomatic varicose veins of unspecified lower extremity**	A
		Varicose veins NOS	
	I83.91	**Asymptomatic varicose veins of right lower extremity**	A
	I83.92	**Asymptomatic varicose veins of left lower extremity**	A
	I83.93	**Asymptomatic varicose veins of bilateral lower extremities**	A

4 + I85   Esophageal varices

Use additional code to identify:
alcohol abuse and dependence (F10.-)

CODING TIP ✓ Esophageal varices are coded to vascular disorders, rather than gastrointestinal disorders, due to the nature of their pathophysiology. Bleeding varices can be life threatening and cause additional complex cardiovascular complications.

5 + I85.0   Esophageal varices
Idiopathic esophageal varices
Primary esophageal varices

+ I85.00   Esophageal varices without bleeding
Esophageal varices NOS

CODING TIP ✓ When the clinical record does not specify bleeding or absence of bleeding in a patient with esophageal varices, assign code I85.00, when the varices are not specified as related to any other cause.

+ I85.01   Esophageal varices with bleeding

5 + I85.1   Secondary esophageal varices
Esophageal varices secondary to alcoholic liver disease
Esophageal varices secondary to cirrhosis of liver
Esophageal varices secondary to schistosomiasis
Esophageal varices secondary to toxic liver disease
Code first:
    underlying disease

+ I85.10   Secondary esophageal varices without bleeding
+ I85.11   Secondary esophageal varices with bleeding

4 I86   Varicose veins of other sites

EXCLUDES 1 *varicose veins of unspecified site (I83.9-)*
EXCLUDES 2 *retinal varices (H35.0-)*

I86.0	**Sublingual varices**	
I86.1	**Scrotal varices**	♂
	Varicocele	
I86.2	**Pelvic varices**	
I86.3	**Vulval varices**	♀A

EXCLUDES 1 *vulval varices complicating childbirth and the puerperium (O87.8)*
vulval varices complicating pregnancy (O22.1-)

I86.4	**Gastric varices**	

I86.8	**Varicose veins of other specified sites**	A
	Varicose ulcer of nasal septum	

4 I87   Other disorders of veins

5 I87.0   Postthrombotic syndrome
Chronic venous hypertension due to deep vein thrombosis
Postphlebitic syndrome

EXCLUDES 1 *chronic venous hypertension without deep vein thrombosis (I87.3-)*

6 I87.00   Postthrombotic syndrome without complications
Asymptomatic Postthrombotic syndrome

	I87.001	**Postthrombotic syndrome without complications of right lower extremity**
	I87.002	**Postthrombotic syndrome without complications of left lower extremity**
	I87.003	**Postthrombotic syndrome without complications of bilateral lower extremity**
	I87.009	**Postthrombotic syndrome without complications of unspecified extremity**
		Postthrombotic syndrome NOS

6 + I87.01   Postthrombotic syndrome with ulcer
Use additional code to specify site and severity of ulcer (L97.-)

	I87.011	**Postthrombotic syndrome with ulcer of right lower extremity**
	I87.012	**Postthrombotic syndrome with ulcer of left lower extremity**
	I87.013	**Postthrombotic syndrome with ulcer of bilateral lower extremity**
	I87.019	**Postthrombotic syndrome with ulcer of unspecified lower extremity**

6 I87.02   Postthrombotic syndrome with inflammation

	I87.021	**Postthrombotic syndrome with inflammation of right lower extremity**
	I87.022	**Postthrombotic syndrome with inflammation of left lower extremity**
	I87.023	**Postthrombotic syndrome with inflammation of bilateral lower extremity**
	I87.029	**Postthrombotic syndrome with inflammation of unspecified lower extremity**

6 + I87.03   Postthrombotic syndrome with ulcer and inflammation
Use additional code to specify site and severity of ulcer (L97.-)

	I87.031	**Postthrombotic syndrome with ulcer and inflammation of right lower extremity**
	I87.032	**Postthrombotic syndrome with ulcer and inflammation of left lower extremity**
	I87.033	**Postthrombotic syndrome with ulcer and inflammation of bilateral lower extremity**
	I87.039	**Postthrombotic syndrome with ulcer and inflammation of unspecified lower extremity**

6 I87.09   Postthrombotic syndrome with other complications

	I87.091	**Postthrombotic syndrome with other complications of right lower extremity**
	I87.092	**Postthrombotic syndrome with other complications of left lower extremity**
	I87.093	**Postthrombotic syndrome with other complications of bilateral lower extremity**
	I87.099	**Postthrombotic syndrome with other complications of unspecified lower extremity**

I87.1   Compression of vein
Stricture of vein
Vena cava syndrome (inferior) (superior)

EXCLUDES 2 *compression of pulmonary vein (I28.8)*

▲ I87.2   Venous insufficiency (chronic) (peripheral)
Stasis dermatitis

EXCLUDES 1 *stasis dermatitis with varicose veins of lower extremities (I83.1-, I83.2-)*

5 I87.3   Chronic venous hypertension (idiopathic)
Stasis edema

EXCLUDES 1 *chronic venous hypertension due to deep vein thrombosis (I87.0-)*
varicose veins of lower extremities (I83.-)

6 I87.30   Chronic venous hypertension (idiopathic) without complications
Asymptomatic chronic venous hypertension (idiopathic)

● New   ▲ Revised   *Manifestation*   4-7 Digit Indicators   ⊟ Laterality   A Adult (15+ years)   M Maternity (12-55 years)   N Newborn   P Pediatric (0-17 years)   ♂ Male   ♀ Female
✖ Deleted   Unspecified   + Additional code

670   © 2017 DecisionHealth   2017 ICD-10-CM Expert for Physicians

☐ I87.301 Chronic venous hypertension (idiopathic) without complications of right lower extremity

☐ I87.302 Chronic venous hypertension (idiopathic) without complications of left lower extremity

☐ I87.303 Chronic venous hypertension (idiopathic) without complications of bilateral lower extremity

☐ I87.309 Chronic venous hypertension (idiopathic) without complications of unspecified lower extremity
Chronic venous hypertension NOS

⑥➕ I87.31 Chronic venous hypertension (idiopathic) with ulcer
Use additional code to specify site and severity of ulcer (L97.-)

☐➕ I87.311 Chronic venous hypertension (idiopathic) with ulcer of right lower extremity

☐➕ I87.312 Chronic venous hypertension (idiopathic) with ulcer of left lower extremity

☐➕ I87.313 Chronic venous hypertension (idiopathic) with ulcer of bilateral lower extremity

☐➕ I87.319 Chronic venous hypertension (idiopathic) with ulcer of unspecified lower extremity

⑥ I87.32 Chronic venous hypertension (idiopathic) with inflammation

☐ I87.321 Chronic venous hypertension (idiopathic) with inflammation of right lower extremity

☐ I87.322 Chronic venous hypertension (idiopathic) with inflammation of left lower extremity

☐ I87.323 Chronic venous hypertension (idiopathic) with inflammation of bilateral lower extremity

☐ I87.329 Chronic venous hypertension (idiopathic) with inflammation of unspecified lower extremity

⑥➕ I87.33 Chronic venous hypertension (idiopathic) with ulcer and inflammation
Use additional code to specify site and severity of ulcer (L97.-)

☐➕ I87.331 Chronic venous hypertension (idiopathic) with ulcer and inflammation of right lower extremity

☐➕ I87.332 Chronic venous hypertension (idiopathic) with ulcer and inflammation of left lower extremity

☐➕ I87.333 Chronic venous hypertension (idiopathic) with ulcer and inflammation of bilateral lower extremity

☐➕ I87.339 Chronic venous hypertension (idiopathic) with ulcer and inflammation of unspecified lower extremity

⑥ I87.39 Chronic venous hypertension (idiopathic) with other complications

☐ I87.391 Chronic venous hypertension (idiopathic) with other complications of right lower extremity

☐ I87.392 Chronic venous hypertension (idiopathic) with other complications of left lower extremity

☐ I87.393 Chronic venous hypertension (idiopathic) with other complications of bilateral lower extremity

☐ I87.399 Chronic venous hypertension (idiopathic) with other complications of unspecified lower extremity

I87.8 **Other specified disorders of veins**
Phlebosclerosis
Venofibrosis

I87.9 **Disorder of vein, unspecified**

④ I88 **Nonspecific lymphadenitis**
EXCLUDES 1 *acute lymphadenitis, except mesenteric (L04.-)*
enlarged lymph nodes NOS (R59.-)
human immunodeficiency virus [HIV] disease resulting in generalized lymphadenopathy (B20)

I88.0 **Nonspecific mesenteric lymphadenitis**
Mesenteric lymphadenitis (acute)(chronic)

I88.1 **Chronic lymphadenitis, except mesenteric**
Adenitis
Lymphadenitis
DEFINITION Chronic enlargement of the lymphatic glands.

I88.8 **Other nonspecific lymphadenitis**

I88.9 **Nonspecific lymphadenitis, unspecified**
Lymphadenitis NOS

Nonspecific lymphadenitis, unspecified
Inflammation of one or more lymph nodes

▲ ④ I89 **Other noninfective disorders of lymphatic vessels and lymph nodes**
EXCLUDES 1 *chylocele, tunica vaginalis (nonfilarial) NOS (N50.89)*
enlarged lymph nodes NOS (R59.-)
filarial chylocele (B74.-)
hereditary lymphedema (Q82.0)

I89.0 **Lymphedema, not elsewhere classified**
Elephantiasis (nonfilarial) NOS
Lymphangiectasis
Obliteration, lymphatic vessel
Praecox lymphedema
Secondary lymphedema
EXCLUDES 1 *postmastectomy lymphedema (I97.2)*

I89.1 **Lymphangitis**
Chronic lymphangitis
Lymphangitis NOS
Subacute lymphangitis
EXCLUDES 1 *acute lymphangitis (L03.-)*

I89.8 **Other specified noninfective disorders of lymphatic vessels and lymph nodes**
Chylocele (nonfilarial)
Chylous ascites
Chylous cyst
Lipomelanotic reticulosis
Lymph node or vessel fistula
Lymph node or vessel infarction
Lymph node or vessel rupture

I89.9 **Noninfective disorder of lymphatic vessels and lymph nodes, unspecified**
Disease of lymphatic vessels NOS

Other and unspecified disorders of the circulatory system (I95-I99)

④ I95 **Hypotension**
EXCLUDES 1 *cardiovascular collapse (R57.9)*
maternal hypotension syndrome (O26.5-)
nonspecific low blood pressure reading NOS (R03.1)
CODING TIP ✓ A low blood pressure reading in the absence of a diagnosis of hypotension should not be coded to I95.-. A singular low blood pressure reading with no diagnosis of hypotension should be coded to R03.1.

I95.0 **Idiopathic hypotension**
CODING TIP ✓ **Documentation:** Idiopathic hypotension requires a confirmed diagnosis by the patient's physician and may not be assumed. Do not assign I95.0 for a patient with hypotension of uncertain cause, with no physician report of idiopathic etiology and do not assign for a singular low blood pressure reading.

● New ▲ Revised *Manifestation* ④-⑦ Digit Indicators ☐ Laterality ▲ Adult (15+ years) Ⓜ Maternity (12-55 years) Ⓝ Newborn Ⓟ Pediatric (0-17 years) ♂ Male ♀ Female
✗ Deleted Unspecified ➕ Additional code

2017 ICD-10-CM Expert for Physicians   © 2017 DecisionHealth   671

I95.1   Orthostatic hypotension
Hypotension, postural

> **EXCLUDES 1** *neurogenic orthostatic hypotension [Shy-Drager] (G90.3)*
> *orthostatic hypotension due to drugs (I95.2)*

> **CODING TIP ✓** Do not assign code I95.1 for orthostasis resulting from medication effects. Hypotension secondary to medication/drug effects is coded to I95.2 and is coded as an adverse effect.

> **DEFINITION** Abnormally low blood pressure that occurs when the patient moves to a standing or upright position.

+ I95.2   Hypotension due to drugs
Orthostatic hypotension due to drugs
Use additional code for adverse effect, if applicable, to identify drug (T36-T50 with fifth or sixth character 5)

> **CODING TIP ✓** When hypotension or orthostasis is confirmed and reported in the medical record as resulting from the effects of medications or other drugs, code I95.2 should be assigned. An additional code from category T36-T50 should be assigned to identify the drug.

I95.3   Hypotension of hemodialysis
Intra-dialytic hypotension

⑤ I95.8   Other hypotension
  I95.81   Postprocedural hypotension
  I95.89   Other hypotension
    Chronic hypotension

I95.9   Hypotension, unspecified

▲ I96   Gangrene, not elsewhere classified
Gangrenous cellulitis

> **EXCLUDES 1** *gangrene in atherosclerosis of native arteries of the extremities (I70.26)*
> *gangrene in diabetes mellitus (E08-E13 with .52)*
> *gangrene in hernia (K40.1, K40.4, K41.1, K41.4, K42.1, K43.1-, K44.1, K45.1, K46.1)*
> *gangrene in other peripheral vascular diseases (I73.-)*
> *gangrene of certain specified sites - see Alphabetical Index*
> *gas gangrene (A48.0)*
> *pyoderma gangrenosum (L88)*

> **CODING TIP ✓** I96 should be assigned to indicate gangrenous cellulitis, such as in the case of gangrene in a pressure ulcer. The L89.- codes for pressure ulcers indicate that coders should "code first" any associated gangrene. In this case, I96 should be assigned. Do not use I96 to indicate gangrene in diabetes, atherosclerosis or other vascular disease, pyoderma gangrenosum, gas gangrene, or gangrene in a hernia.

> **DEFINITION** Complication of cell death (necrosis), characterized by tissue decay, which becomes black and malodorous, caused by infection or ischemia, resulting from insufficient blood supply.

AHA: 2Q 2013, 34-35

④ I97   Intraoperative and postprocedural complications and disorders of circulatory system, not elsewhere classified

> **EXCLUDES 2** *postprocedural shock (T81.1-)*

> **CODING TIP ✓** Documentation: Codes in category I97.- are complication codes and require physician documentation and confirmation of a cause and effect relationship between the procedure and the complicated condition.

I97.0   Postcardiotomy syndrome
⑤ I97.1   Other postprocedural cardiac functional disturbances

> **EXCLUDES 2** *acute pulmonary insufficiency following thoracic surgery (J95.1)*
> *intraoperative cardiac functional disturbances (I97.7-)*

⑥ I97.11   Postprocedural cardiac insufficiency
  I97.110   Postprocedural cardiac insufficiency following cardiac surgery
  I97.111   Postprocedural cardiac insufficiency following other surgery
⑥ I97.12   Postprocedural cardiac arrest

I97.120   Postprocedural cardiac arrest following cardiac surgery
I97.121   Postprocedural cardiac arrest following other surgery
⑥ + I97.13   Postprocedural heart failure
Use additional code to identify the heart failure (I50.-)
+ I97.130   Postprocedural heart failure following cardiac surgery
+ I97.131   Postprocedural heart failure following other surgery
⑥ + I97.19   Other postprocedural cardiac functional disturbances
Use additional code, if applicable, to further specify disorder
+ I97.190   Other postprocedural cardiac functional disturbances following cardiac surgery
+ I97.191   Other postprocedural cardiac functional disturbances following other surgery
I97.2   Postmastectomy lymphedema syndrome Ⓐ
Elephantiasis due to mastectomy
Obliteration of lymphatic vessels

> **CODING TIP ✓** Assign code I97.2 only when lymphedema is specifically reported as related to the effects of a mastectomy.

> **DEFINITION** Localized edema in the arm following breast and lymph node removal due to lack of lymph circulation through the chest area.

I97.3   Postprocedural hypertension
⑤ I97.4   Intraoperative hemorrhage and hematoma of a circulatory system organ or structure complicating a procedure

> **EXCLUDES 1** *intraoperative hemorrhage and hematoma of a circulatory system organ or structure due to accidental puncture and laceration during a procedure (I97.5-)*
> **EXCLUDES 2** *intraoperative cerebrovascular hemorrhage complicating a procedure (G97.3-)*

⑥ I97.41   Intraoperative hemorrhage and hematoma of a circulatory system organ or structure complicating a circulatory system procedure
  I97.410   Intraoperative hemorrhage and hematoma of a circulatory system organ or structure complicating a cardiac catheterization
  I97.411   Intraoperative hemorrhage and hematoma of a circulatory system organ or structure complicating a cardiac bypass
  I97.418   Intraoperative hemorrhage and hematoma of a circulatory system organ or structure complicating other circulatory system procedure
I97.42   Intraoperative hemorrhage and hematoma of a circulatory system organ or structure complicating other procedure
⑤ I97.5   Accidental puncture and laceration of a circulatory system organ or structure during a procedure

> **EXCLUDES 2** *accidental puncture and laceration of brain during a procedure (G97.4-)*

I97.51   Accidental puncture and laceration of a circulatory system organ or structure during a circulatory system procedure
I97.52   Accidental puncture and laceration of a circulatory system organ or structure during other procedure
▲ ⑤ I97.6   Postprocedural hemorrhage, hematoma and seroma of a circulatory system organ or structure following a procedure

> **EXCLUDES 2** *postprocedural cerebrovascular hemorrhage complicating a procedure (G97.5-)*

AHA: 1Q 2014, 7

▲ ⑥ I97.61   Postprocedural hemorrhage of a circulatory system organ or structure following a circulatory system procedure
  ▲ I97.610   Postprocedural hemorrhage of a circulatory system organ or structure following a cardiac catheterization
  ▲ I97.611   Postprocedural hemorrhage of a circulatory system organ or structure following cardiac bypass
  ▲ I97.618   Postprocedural hemorrhage of a circulatory system organ or structure following other circulatory system procedure

▲ ⑥ **I97.62**   **Postprocedural hemorrhage, hematoma and seroma of a circulatory system organ or structure following other procedure**

● **I97.620**   **Postprocedural hemorrhage of a circulatory system organ or structure following other procedure**

● **I97.621**   **Postprocedural hematoma of a circulatory system organ or structure following other procedure**

● **I97.622**   **Postprocedural seroma of a circulatory system organ or structure following other procedure**

● ⑥ **I97.63**   **Postprocedural hematoma of a circulatory system organ or structure following a circulatory system procedure**

● **I97.630**   **Postprocedural hematoma of a circulatory system organ or structure following a cardiac catheterization**

● **I97.631**   **Postprocedural hematoma of a circulatory system organ or structure following cardiac bypass**

● **I97.638**   **Postprocedural hematoma of a circulatory system organ or structure following other circulatory system procedure**

● ⑥ **I97.64**   **Postprocedural seroma of a circulatory system organ or structure following a circulatory system procedure**

● **I97.640**   **Postprocedural seroma of a circulatory system organ or structure following a cardiac catheterization**

● **I97.641**   **Postprocedural seroma of a circulatory system organ or structure following cardiac bypass**

● **I97.648**   **Postprocedural seroma of a circulatory system organ or structure following other circulatory system procedure**

⑤ **I97.7**   **Intraoperative cardiac functional disturbances**

EXCLUDES 2	*acute pulmonary insufficiency following thoracic surgery (J95.1)*
	postprocedural cardiac functional disturbances (I97.1-)

⑥ **I97.71**   **Intraoperative cardiac arrest**

I97.710   **Intraoperative cardiac arrest during cardiac surgery**

I97.711   **Intraoperative cardiac arrest during other surgery**

⑥ + **I97.79**   **Other intraoperative cardiac functional disturbances**

Use additional code, if applicable, to further specify disorder

+ **I97.790**   **Other intraoperative cardiac functional disturbances during cardiac surgery**

+ **I97.791**   **Other intraoperative cardiac functional disturbances during other surgery**

⑤ + **I97.8**   **Other intraoperative and postprocedural complications and disorders of the circulatory system, not elsewhere classified**

Use additional code, if applicable, to further specify disorder

⑥ + **I97.81**   **Intraoperative cerebrovascular infarction**

+ **I97.810**   **Intraoperative cerebrovascular infarction during cardiac surgery**

+ **I97.811**   **Intraoperative cerebrovascular infarction during other surgery**

⑥ + **I97.82**   **Postprocedural cerebrovascular infarction**

▲ + **I97.820**   **Postprocedural cerebrovascular infarction following cardiac surgery**

▲ + **I97.821**   **Postprocedural cerebrovascular infarction following other surgery**

+ **I97.88**   **Other intraoperative complications of the circulatory system, not elsewhere classified**

+ **I97.89**   **Other postprocedural complications and disorders of the circulatory system, not elsewhere classified**

④ **I99**   **Other and unspecified disorders of circulatory system**

I99.8   **Other disorder of circulatory system**

I99.9   **Unspecified disorder of circulatory system**

● New	▲ Revised	*Manifestation*	④-⑦ Digit Indicators	▤ Laterality	▣ Adult (15+ years)	▥ Maternity (12-55 years)	▨ Newborn	▣ Pediatric (0-17 years)	♂ Male	♀ Female
✖ Deleted		Unspecified	+ Additional code							

2017 ICD-10-CM Expert for Physicians   © 2017 DecisionHealth   673

CHAPTER 10: DISEASES OF THE RESPIRATORY SYSTEM (J00-J99)

Note: When a respiratory condition is described as occurring in more than one site and is not specifically indexed, it should be classified to the lower anatomic site (e.g. tracheobronchitis to bronchitis in J40).

Use additional code, where applicable, to identify:
exposure to environmental tobacco smoke (Z77.22)
exposure to tobacco smoke in the perinatal period (P96.81)
history of tobacco dependence (Z87.891)
occupational exposure to environmental tobacco smoke (Z57.31)
tobacco dependence (F17.-)
tobacco use (Z72.0)

EXCLUDES 2 *certain conditions originating in the perinatal period (P04-P96)*
certain infectious and parasitic diseases (A00-B99)
complications of pregnancy, childbirth and the puerperium (O00-O9A)
congenital malformations, deformations and chromosomal abnormalities (Q00-Q99)
endocrine, nutritional and metabolic diseases (E00-E88)
injury, poisoning and certain other consequences of external causes (S00-T88)
neoplasms (C00-D49)
smoke inhalation (T59.81-)
symptoms, signs and abnormal clinical and laboratory findings, not elsewhere classified (R00-R94)

This chapter contains the following blocks:

J00-J06	Acute upper respiratory infections
J09-J18	Influenza and pneumonia
J20-J22	Other acute lower respiratory infections
J30-J39	Other diseases of upper respiratory tract
J40-J47	Chronic lower respiratory diseases
J60-J70	Lung diseases due to external agents
J80-J84	Other respiratory diseases principally affecting the interstitium
J85-J86	Suppurative and necrotic conditions of the lower respiratory tract
J90-J94	Other diseases of the pleura
J95	Intraoperative and postprocedural complications and disorders of respiratory system, not elsewhere classified
J96-J99	Other diseases of the respiratory system

Acute upper respiratory infections (J00-J06)

EXCLUDES 1 *chronic obstructive pulmonary disease with acute lower respiratory infection (J44.0)*
influenza virus with other respiratory manifestations (J09.X2, J10.1, J11.1)

J00 **Acute nasopharyngitis [common cold]**
Acute rhinitis
Coryza (acute)
Infective nasopharyngitis NOS
Infective rhinitis
Nasal catarrh, acute
Nasopharyngitis NOS

EXCLUDES 1 *acute pharyngitis (J02.-)*
acute sore throat NOS (J02.9)
pharyngitis NOS (J02.9)
rhinitis NOS (J31.0)
sore throat NOS (J02.9)

EXCLUDES 2 *allergic rhinitis (J30.1-J30.9)*
chronic pharyngitis (J31.2)
chronic rhinitis (J31.0)
chronic sore throat (J31.2)
nasopharyngitis, chronic (J31.1)
vasomotor rhinitis (J30.0)

Upper respiratory system

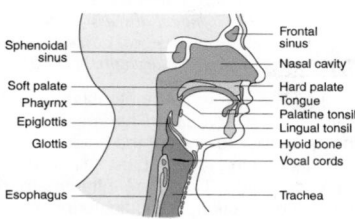

4 + J01 **Acute sinusitis**

INCLUDES acute abscess of sinus
acute empyema of sinus
acute infection of sinus
acute inflammation of sinus
acute suppuration of sinus

Use additional code (B95-B97) to identify infectious agent.

EXCLUDES 1 *sinusitis NOS (J32.9)*

EXCLUDES 2 *chronic sinusitis (J32.0-J32.8)*

5 + J01.0 **Acute maxillary sinusitis**
Acute antritis

Acute maxillary sinusitis

+ J01.00	**Acute maxillary sinusitis, unspecified**	
+ J01.01	**Acute recurrent maxillary sinusitis**	
5 + J01.1	**Acute frontal sinusitis**	
+ J01.10	**Acute frontal sinusitis, unspecified**	
+ J01.11	**Acute recurrent frontal sinusitis**	
5 + J01.2	**Acute ethmoidal sinusitis**	
+ J01.20	**Acute ethmoidal sinusitis, unspecified**	
+ J01.21	**Acute recurrent ethmoidal sinusitis**	
5 + J01.3	**Acute sphenoidal sinusitis**	
+ J01.30	**Acute sphenoidal sinusitis, unspecified**	
+ J01.31	**Acute recurrent sphenoidal sinusitis**	
5 + J01.4	**Acute pansinusitis**	
+ J01.40	**Acute pansinusitis, unspecified**	
+ J01.41	**Acute recurrent pansinusitis**	
5 + J01.8	**Other acute sinusitis**	
+ J01.80	**Other acute sinusitis**	
	Acute sinusitis involving more than one sinus but not pansinusitis	
+ J01.81	**Other acute recurrent sinusitis**	
	Acute recurrent sinusitis involving more than one sinus but not pansinusitis	
5 + J01.9	**Acute sinusitis, unspecified**	
+ J01.90	**Acute sinusitis, unspecified**	
+ J01.91	**Acute recurrent sinusitis, unspecified**	

● New ▲ Revised *Manifestation* 4-7 Digit Indicators ▤ Laterality 🅰 Adult (15+ years) Ⓜ Maternity (12-55 years) Ⓝ Newborn 🅟 Pediatric (0-17 years) ♂ Male ♀ Female
✖ Deleted Unspecified + Additional code

2017 ICD-10-CM Expert for Physicians

© 2017 DecisionHealth

675

J00 — J01.91

◄ **J02** **Acute pharyngitis**

INCLUDES acute sore throat

EXCLUDES 1 *acute laryngopharyngitis (J06.0)*
peritonsillar abscess (J36)
pharyngeal abscess (J39.1)
retropharyngeal abscess (J39.0)

EXCLUDES 2 *chronic pharyngitis (J31.2)*

CODING TIP ✓ Note the anatomical differences between pharyngitis and laryngitis. Pharyngitis involves inflammation of the pharynx, the area of the back of the throat between the tonsils and the larynx. Laryngitis involves inflammation of the vocal cords. These are inflammatory conditions, which may involve infection, but indicate inflammation in different anatomical areas. Do not assume that, because the patient has pharyngitis, that the larynx is also inflamed.

J02.0 **Streptococcal pharyngitis**
Septic pharyngitis
Streptococcal sore throat

EXCLUDES 2 *scarlet fever (A38.-)*

+ **J02.8** **Acute pharyngitis due to other specified organisms**
Use additional code (B95-B97) to identify infectious agent

EXCLUDES 1 *acute pharyngitis due to coxsackie virus (B08.5)*
acute pharyngitis due to gonococcus (A54.5)
acute pharyngitis due to herpes [simplex] virus (B00.2)
acute pharyngitis due to infectious mononucleosis (B27.-)
enteroviral vesicular pharyngitis (B08.5)

J02.9 **Acute pharyngitis, unspecified**
Gangrenous pharyngitis (acute)
Infective pharyngitis (acute) NOS
Pharyngitis (acute) NOS
Sore throat (acute) NOS
Suppurative pharyngitis (acute)
Ulcerative pharyngitis (acute)

◄ **J03** **Acute tonsillitis**

EXCLUDES 1 *acute sore throat (J02.-)*
hypertrophy of tonsils (J35.1)
peritonsillar abscess (J36)
sore throat NOS (J02.9)
streptococcal sore throat (J02.0)

EXCLUDES 2 *chronic tonsillitis (J35.0)*

⑤ **J03.0** **Streptococcal tonsillitis**

J03.00 **Acute streptococcal tonsillitis, unspecified**

J03.01 **Acute recurrent streptococcal tonsillitis**

⑤ + **J03.8** **Acute tonsillitis due to other specified organisms**
Use additional code (B95-B97) to identify infectious agent.

EXCLUDES 1 *diphtheritic tonsillitis (A36.0)*
herpesviral pharyngotonsillitis (B00.2)
streptococcal tonsillitis (J03.0)
tuberculous tonsillitis (A15.8)
Vincent's tonsillitis (A69.1)

+ **J03.80** **Acute tonsillitis due to other specified organisms**

+ **J03.81** **Acute recurrent tonsillitis due to other specified organisms**

⑤ **J03.9** **Acute tonsillitis, unspecified**
Follicular tonsillitis (acute)
Gangrenous tonsillitis (acute)
Infective tonsillitis (acute)
Tonsillitis (acute) NOS
Ulcerative tonsillitis (acute)

J03.90 **Acute tonsillitis, unspecified**

J03.91 **Acute recurrent tonsillitis, unspecified**

◄ + **J04** **Acute laryngitis and tracheitis**
Use additional code (B95-B97) to identify infectious agent.

EXCLUDES 1 *acute obstructive laryngitis [croup] and epiglottitis (J05.-)*

EXCLUDES 2 *laryngismus (stridulus) (J38.5)*

+ **J04.0** **Acute laryngitis**
Edematous laryngitis (acute)
Laryngitis (acute) NOS
Subglottic laryngitis (acute)
Suppurative laryngitis (acute)
Ulcerative laryngitis (acute)

EXCLUDES 1 *acute obstructive laryngitis (J05.0)*

EXCLUDES 2 *chronic laryngitis (J37.0)*

⑤ + **J04.1** **Acute tracheitis**
Acute viral tracheitis
Catarrhal tracheitis (acute)
Tracheitis (acute) NOS

EXCLUDES 2 *chronic tracheitis (J42)*

+ **J04.10** **Acute tracheitis without obstruction**

+ **J04.11** **Acute tracheitis with obstruction**

+ **J04.2** **Acute laryngotracheitis**
Laryngotracheitis NOS
Tracheitis (acute) with laryngitis (acute)

EXCLUDES 1 *acute obstructive laryngotracheitis (J05.0)*

EXCLUDES 2 *chronic laryngotracheitis (J37.1)*

CODING TIP ✓ J04.2 is a specific code and should be assigned when the patient is reported as specifically having laryngotracheitis by the physician. This involves inflammation of both the larynx and trachea.

⑤ + **J04.3** **Supraglottitis, unspecified**

CODING TIP ✓ Supraglottitis is a potentially life threatening inflammation of the supraglottic area of the airway. If airway obstruction is documented, assign J04.31.

+ **J04.30** **Supraglottitis, unspecified, without obstruction**

+ **J04.31** **Supraglottitis, unspecified, with obstruction**

◄ + **J05** **Acute obstructive laryngitis [croup] and epiglottitis**
Use additional code (B95-B97) to identify infectious agent.

+ **J05.0** **Acute obstructive laryngitis [croup]**
Obstructive laryngitis (acute) NOS
Obstructive laryngotracheitis NOS

⑤ + **J05.1** **Acute epiglottitis**

EXCLUDES 2 *epiglottitis, chronic (J37.0)*

+ **J05.10** **Acute epiglottitis without obstruction**
Epiglottitis NOS

+ **J05.11** **Acute epiglottitis with obstruction**

◄ **J06** **Acute upper respiratory infections of multiple and unspecified sites**

EXCLUDES 1 *acute respiratory infection NOS (J22)*
streptococcal pharyngitis (J02.0)

J06.0 **Acute laryngopharyngitis**

J06.9 **Acute upper respiratory infection, unspecified**
Upper respiratory disease, acute
Upper respiratory infection NOS

CODING TIP ✓ Assign J06.9 for upper respiratory infection NOS only when a more specific diagnosis to identify the type of infection cannot be identified.

Influenza and pneumonia (J09-J18)

EXCLUDES 2 *allergic or eosinophilic pneumonia (J82)*
aspiration pneumonia NOS (J69.0)
meconium pneumonia (P24.01)
neonatal aspiration pneumonia (P24.-)
pneumonia due to solids and liquids (J69.-)
congenital pneumonia (P23.9)
lipid pneumonia (J69.1)
rheumatic pneumonia (I00)
ventilator associated pneumonia (J95.851)

CODING TIP ✓ Pneumonia should be coded to the specific causative organism using a combination code when a specific code is available. Evaluate all available clinical documentation and assign the most specific code for pneumonia. When the causative organism of bacterial pneumonia is known but no combination code exists, assign J15.8.

CODING TIP ✓ When pneumonia is diagnosed in a patient who also has COPD, the coder should assign J44.0 (Chronic obstructive pulmonary disease with lower respiratory tract infection) followed by the specific code to indicate the type of pneumonia.

● New   ▲ Revised   *Manifestation*   ◄-⑦ Digit Indicators   ▤ Laterality   Ⓐ Adult (15+ years)   Ⓜ Maternity (12-55 years)   Ⓝ Newborn   Ⓟ Pediatric (0-17 years)   ♂ Male   ♀ Female
✖ Deleted   Unspecified   + Additional code

676   © 2017 DecisionHealth

2017 ICD-10-CM Expert for Physicians

☑ J09 Influenza due to certain identified influenza viruses

EXCLUDES 1 *influenza due to other identified influenza virus (J10.-)*
influenza due to unidentified influenza virus (J11.-)
seasonal influenza due to other identified influenza virus (J10.-)
seasonal influenza due to unidentified influenza virus (J11.-)

GUIDELINES Section I.C.10.c
Code only confirmed cases of influenza due to certain identified influenza viruses (category J09), and due to other identified influenza virus (category J10) ... coding should be based on the provider's diagnostic statement that the patient has avian influenza, or other novel influenza A, for category J09, or has another particular identified strain of influenza, such as H1N1 or H3N2, but not identified as novel or variant, for category J10.

If the provider records "suspected" or "possible" or "probable" avian influenza, or novel influenza, or other identified influenza, then the appropriate influenza code from category J11, Influenza due to unidentified influenza virus, should be assigned.

☑ J09.X Influenza due to identified novel influenza A virus
Avian influenza
Bird influenza
Influenza A/H5N1
Influenza of other animal origin, not bird or swine
Swine influenza virus (viruses that normally cause infections in pigs)

J09.X1 Influenza due to identified novel influenza A virus with pneumonia
Code also, if applicable, associated:
lung abscess (J85.1)
other specified type of pneumonia

+ J09.X2 Influenza due to identified novel influenza A virus with other respiratory manifestations
Influenza due to identified novel influenza A virus NOS
Influenza due to identified novel influenza A virus with laryngitis
Influenza due to identified novel influenza A virus with pharyngitis
Influenza due to identified novel influenza A virus with upper respiratory symptoms
Use additional code, if applicable, for associated:
pleural effusion (J91.8)
sinusitis (J01.-)

J09.X3 Influenza due to identified novel influenza A virus with gastrointestinal manifestations
Influenza due to identified novel influenza A virus gastroenteritis
EXCLUDES 1 *'intestinal flu' [viral gastroenteritis] (A08.-)*

+ J09.X9 Influenza due to identified novel influenza A virus with other manifestations
Influenza due to identified novel influenza A virus with encephalopathy
Influenza due to identified novel influenza A virus with myocarditis
Influenza due to identified novel influenza A virus with otitis media
Use additional code to identify manifestation

☑ J10 Influenza due to other identified influenza virus

EXCLUDES 1 *influenza due to avian influenza virus (J09.X-)*
influenza due to swine flu (J09.X-)
influenza due to unidentifed influenza virus (J11.-)

GUIDELINES Section I.C.10.c
Code only confirmed cases of influenza due to certain identified influenza viruses (category J09), and due to other identified influenza virus (category J10) ... coding should be based on the provider's diagnostic statement that the patient has avian influenza, or other novel influenza A, for category J09, or has another particular identified strain of influenza, such as H1N1 or H3N2, but not identified as novel or variant, for category J10.

If the provider records "suspected" or "possible" or "probable" avian influenza, or novel influenza, or other identified influenza, then the appropriate influenza code from category J11, Influenza due to unidentified influenza virus, should be assigned.

☑ J10.0 Influenza due to other identified influenza virus with pneumonia
Code also:
associated lung abscess, if applicable (J85.1)

J10.00 Influenza due to other identified influenza virus with unspecified type of pneumonia

J10.01 Influenza due to other identified influenza virus with the same other identified influenza virus pneumonia

J10.08 Influenza due to other identified influenza virus with other specified pneumonia
Code also:
other specified type of pneumonia

+ J10.1 Influenza due to other identified influenza virus with other respiratory manifestations
Influenza due to other identified influenza virus NOS
Influenza due to other identified influenza virus with laryngitis
Influenza due to other identified influenza virus with pharyngitis
Influenza due to other identified influenza virus with upper respiratory symptoms
Use additional code for associated pleural effusion, if applicable (J91.8)
Use additional code for associated sinusitis, if applicable (J01.-)

J10.2 Influenza due to other identified influenza virus with gastrointestinal manifestations
Influenza due to other identified influenza virus gastroenteritis
EXCLUDES 1 *'intestinal flu' [viral gastroenteritis] (A08.-)*

☑ J10.8 Influenza due to other identified influenza virus with other manifestations

J10.81 Influenza due to other identified influenza virus with encephalopathy

J10.82 Influenza due to other identified influenza virus with myocarditis

+ J10.83 Influenza due to other identified influenza virus with otitis media
Use additional code for any associated perforated tympanic membrane (H72.-)

+ J10.89 Influenza due to other identified influenza virus with other manifestations
Use additional codes to identify the manifestations

☑ J11 Influenza due to unidentified influenza virus

☑ J11.0 Influenza due to unidentified influenza virus with pneumonia
Code also:
associated lung abscess, if applicable (J85.1)

J11.00 Influenza due to unidentified influenza virus with unspecified type of pneumonia
Influenza with pneumonia NOS

J11.08 Influenza due to unidentified influenza virus with specified pneumonia
Code also:
other specified type of pneumonia

+ J11.1 Influenza due to unidentified influenza virus with other respiratory manifestations
Influenza NOS
Influenzal laryngitis NOS
Influenzal pharyngitis NOS
Influenza with upper respiratory symptoms NOS
Use additional code for associated pleural effusion, if applicable (J91.8)
Use additional code for associated sinusitis, if applicable (J01.-)

● New ▲ Revised *Manifestation* ☑-☑ Digit Indicators ⊟ Laterality Ⓐ Adult (15+ years) Ⓜ Maternity (12-55 years) Ⓝ Newborn Ⓟ Pediatric (0-17 years) ♂ Male ♀ Female
✖ Deleted Unspecified + Additional code

2017 ICD-10-CM Expert for Physicians © 2017 DecisionHealth 677

J09 — J11.1

J11.2   **Influenza due to unidentified influenza virus with gastrointestinal manifestations**
Influenza gastroenteritis NOS
> **EXCLUDES 1**   *'intestinal flu' [viral gastroenteritis] (A08.-)*

⑤ **J11.8**   **Influenza due to unidentified influenza virus with other manifestations**

    J11.81   **Influenza due to unidentified influenza virus with encephalopathy**
Influenzal encephalopathy NOS

    J11.82   **Influenza due to unidentified influenza virus with myocarditis**
Influenzal myocarditis NOS

    ✚ **J11.83**   **Influenza due to unidentified influenza virus with otitis media**
Influenzal otitis media NOS
Use additional code for any associated perforated tympanic membrane (H72.-)

    ✚ **J11.89**   **Influenza due to unidentified influenza virus with other manifestations**
Use additional codes to identify the manifestations

④ **J12**   **Viral pneumonia, not elsewhere classified**
> **INCLUDES**   bronchopneumonia due to viruses other than influenza viruses

Code first:
associated influenza, if applicable (J09.X1, J10.0-, J11.0-)
Code also:
associated abscess, if applicable (J85.1)
> **EXCLUDES 1**   *aspiration pneumonia due to anesthesia during labor and delivery (O74.0)*
> *aspiration pneumonia due to anesthesia during pregnancy (O29)*
> *aspiration pneumonia due to anesthesia during puerperium (O89.0)*
> *aspiration pneumonia due to solids and liquids (J69.-)*
> *aspiration pneumonia NOS (J69.0)*
> *congenital pneumonia (P23.0)*
> *congenital rubella pneumonitis (P35.0)*
> *interstitial pneumonia NOS (J84.9)*
> *lipid pneumonia (J69.1)*
> *neonatal aspiration pneumonia (P24.-)*

J12.0   **Adenoviral pneumonia**

J12.1   **Respiratory syncytial virus pneumonia**

J12.2   **Parainfluenza virus pneumonia**

J12.3   **Human metapneumovirus pneumonia**

⑤ **J12.8**   **Other viral pneumonia**

    J12.81   **Pneumonia due to SARS-associated coronavirus**
Severe acute respiratory syndrome NOS

    J12.89   **Other viral pneumonia**

J12.9   **Viral pneumonia, unspecified**

J13   **Pneumonia due to Streptococcus pneumoniae**
Bronchopneumonia due to S. pneumoniae
Code first:
associated influenza, if applicable (J09.X1, J10.0-, J11.0-)
Code also:
associated abscess, if applicable (J85.1)
> **EXCLUDES 1**   *congenital pneumonia due to S. pneumoniae (P23.6)*
> *lobar pneumonia, unspecified organism (J18.1)*
> *pneumonia due to other streptococci (J15.3-J15.4)*

J14   **Pneumonia due to Hemophilus influenzae**
Bronchopneumonia due to H. influenzae
Code first:
associated influenza, if applicable (J09.X1, J10.0-, J11.0-)
Code also:
associated abscess, if applicable (J85.1)
> **EXCLUDES 1**   *congenital pneumonia due to H. influenzae (P23.6)*

④ **J15**   **Bacterial pneumonia, not elsewhere classified**
> **INCLUDES**   bronchopneumonia due to bacteria other than S. pneumoniae and H. influenzae

Code first:
associated influenza, if applicable (J09.X1, J10.0-, J11.0-)
Code also:
associated abscess, if applicable (J85.1)
> **EXCLUDES 1**   *chlamydial pneumonia (J16.0)*
> *congenital pneumonia (P23.-)*
> *Legionnaires' disease (A48.1)*
> *spirochetal pneumonia (A69.8)*

J15.0   **Pneumonia due to Klebsiella pneumoniae**

J15.1   **Pneumonia due to Pseudomonas**

⑤ **J15.2**   **Pneumonia due to staphylococcus**

    J15.20   **Pneumonia due to staphylococcus, unspecified**

    ⑥ **J15.21**   **Pneumonia due to staphylococcus aureus**

      J15.211   **Pneumonia due to Methicillin susceptible Staphylococcus aureus**
MSSA pneumonia
Pneumonia due to Staphylococcus aureus NOS

      J15.212   **Pneumonia due to Methicillin resistant Staphylococcus aureus**
> **GUIDELINES**   Section I.C.1.e.1)

When a patient is diagnosed with an infection that is due to methicillin resistant Staphylococcus aureus (MRSA), and that infection has a combination code that includes the causal organism (e.g., sepsis, pneumonia) assign the appropriate combination code for the condition (e.g., code A41.02, Sepsis due to Methicillin resistant Staphylococcus aureus or code J15.212, Pneumonia due to Methicillin resistant Staphylococcus aureus). Do not assign code B95.62, Methicillin resistant Staphylococcus aureus infection as the cause of diseases classified elsewhere, as an additional code because the combination code includes the type of infection and the MRSA organism. Do not assign a code from subcategory Z16.11, Resistance to penicillins, as an additional diagnosis.

    J15.29   **Pneumonia due to other staphylococcus**

J15.3   **Pneumonia due to streptococcus, group B**

J15.4   **Pneumonia due to other streptococci**
> **EXCLUDES 1**   *pneumonia due to streptococcus, group B (J15.3)*
> *pneumonia due to Streptococcus pneumoniae (J13)*

Pneumonia due to other streptococci

A culture has determined the pneumonia is caused by *Streptococcus pneumoniae*

Streptococcus bacteria

J15.5   **Pneumonia due to Escherichia coli**

J15.6   **Pneumonia due to other aerobic Gram-negative bacteria**
Pneumonia due to Serratia marcescens

J15.7   **Pneumonia due to Mycoplasma pneumoniae**

J15.8   **Pneumonia due to other specified bacteria**
> **CODING TIP ✓**   Do not assign code J15.8 for unspecified pneumonia. J15.8 indicates pneumonia with a specified organism for which no combination code exists.

J15.9   **Unspecified bacterial pneumonia**
Pneumonia due to gram-positive bacteria

④ **J16**   **Pneumonia due to other infectious organisms, not elsewhere classified**
Code first:
associated influenza, if applicable (J09.X1, J10.0-, J11.0-)
Code also:
associated abscess, if applicable (J85.1)
> **EXCLUDES 1**   *congenital pneumonia (P23.-)*
> *ornithosis (A70)*
> *pneumocystosis (B59)*
> *pneumonia NOS (J18.9)*

J16.0   **Chlamydial pneumonia**

J16.8   **Pneumonia due to other specified infectious organisms**

● New   ▲ Revised   *Manifestation*   ❶-❼ Digit Indicators   ⬛ Laterality   Ⓐ Adult (15+ years)   Ⓜ Maternity (12-55 years)   Ⓝ Newborn   Ⓟ Pediatric (0-17 years)   ♂ Male   ♀ Female
✖ ~~Deleted~~   Unspecified   ✚ Additional code

678   © 2017 DecisionHealth   2017 ICD-10-CM Expert for Physicians

J17   *Pneumonia in diseases classified elsewhere*

Code first underlying disease, such as:
Q fever (A78)
rheumatic fever (I00)
schistosomiasis (B65.0-B65.9)

| EXCLUDES 1 | *candidial pneumonia (B37.1)* |

chlamydial pneumonia (J16.0)
gonorrheal pneumonia (A54.84)
histoplasmosis pneumonia (B39.0-B39.2)
measles pneumonia (B05.2)
nocardiosis pneumonia (A43.0)
pneumocystosis (B59)
pneumonia due to Pneumocystis carinii (B59)
pneumonia due to Pneumocystis jiroveci (B59)
pneumonia in actinomycosis (A42.0)
pneumonia in anthrax (A22.1)
pneumonia in ascariasis (B77.81)
pneumonia in aspergillosis (B44.0-B44.1)
pneumonia in coccidioidomycosis (B38.0-B38.2)
pneumonia in cytomegalovirus disease (B25.0)
pneumonia in toxoplasmosis (B58.3)
rubella pneumonia (B06.81)
salmonella pneumonia (A02.22)
spirochetal infection NEC with pneumonia (A69.8)
tularemia pneumonia (A21.2)
typhoid fever with pneumonia (A01.03)
varicella pneumonia (B01.2)
whooping cough with pneumonia (A37 with fifth-character 1)

J18   **Pneumonia, unspecified organism**

Code first:
associated influenza, if applicable (J09.X1, J10.0-, J11.0-)

| EXCLUDES 1 | *abscess of lung with pneumonia (J85.1)* |

aspiration pneumonia due to anesthesia during labor and delivery (O74.0)
aspiration pneumonia due to anesthesia during pregnancy (O29)
aspiration pneumonia due to anesthesia during puerperium (O89.0)
aspiration pneumonia due to solids and liquids (J69.-)
aspiration pneumonia NOS (J69.0)
congenital pneumonia (P23.0)
drug-induced interstitial lung disorder (J70.2-J70.4)
interstitial pneumonia NOS (J84.9)
lipid pneumonia (J69.1)
neonatal aspiration pneumonia (P24.-)
pneumonitis due to external agents (J67-J70)
pneumonitis due to fumes and vapors (J68.0)
usual interstitial pneumonia (J84.17)

J18.0   **Bronchopneumonia, unspecified organism**

EXCLUDES 1	*hypostatic bronchopneumonia (J18.2)*
	lipid pneumonia (J69.1)
EXCLUDES 2	*acute bronchiolitis (J21.-)*
	chronic bronchiolitis (J44.9)

J18.1   **Lobar pneumonia, unspecified organism**

J18.2   **Hypostatic pneumonia, unspecified organism**

Hypostatic bronchopneumonia
Passive pneumonia

J18.8   **Other pneumonia, unspecified organism**

J18.9   **Pneumonia, unspecified organism**

| CODING TIP ✓ | Do not assign J18.9 when the causative organism or underlying cause of pneumonia is reported in the clinical record. If the organism or cause of pneumonia is known, a combination code should be assigned. When pneumonia is diagnosed in a patient who also has COPD, the coder should assign J44.0 (COPD with lower respiratory tract infection) followed by the specific code to indicate the type of pneumonia.
AHA: 3Q 2014, 4
AHA: 4Q 2012, 94 |

Other acute lower respiratory infections (J20-J22)

| EXCLUDES 2 | *chronic obstructive pulmonary disease with acute lower respiratory infection (J44.0)* |

| CODING TIP ✓ | **Documentation:** Be cautious to differentiate the diagnostic differences between bronchitis and bronchiolitis. These are not interchangeable and are not the same disease process. Bronchitis is inflammation of the mucous membranes of the bronchi, while bronchiolitis involves inflammation of the smaller bronchioles which lead directly to the lungs. Bronchiolitis is more commonly diagnosed in children. |

J20   **Acute bronchitis**

| INCLUDES | acute and subacute bronchitis (with) bronchospasm |

acute and subacute bronchitis (with) tracheitis
acute and subacute bronchitis (with) tracheobronchitis, acute
acute and subacute fibrinous bronchitis
acute and subacute membranous bronchitis
acute and subacute purulent bronchitis
acute and subacute septic bronchitis

EXCLUDES 1	*bronchitis NOS (J40)*
	tracheobronchitis NOS (J40)
EXCLUDES 2	*acute bronchitis with bronchiectasis (J47.0)*

acute bronchitis with chronic obstructive asthma (J44.0)
acute bronchitis with chronic obstructive pulmonary disease (J44.0)
allergic bronchitis NOS (J45.909-)
bronchitis due to chemicals, fumes and vapors (J68.0)
chronic bronchitis NOS (J42)
chronic mucopurulent bronchitis (J41.1)
chronic obstructive bronchitis (J44.-)
chronic obstructive tracheobronchitis (J44.-)
chronic simple bronchitis (J41.0)
chronic tracheobronchitis (J42)

J20.0   **Acute bronchitis due to Mycoplasma pneumoniae**

J20.1   **Acute bronchitis due to Hemophilus influenzae**

J20.2   **Acute bronchitis due to streptococcus**

J20.3   **Acute bronchitis due to coxsackievirus**

J20.4   **Acute bronchitis due to parainfluenza virus**

J20.5   **Acute bronchitis due to respiratory syncytial virus**

J20.6   **Acute bronchitis due to rhinovirus**

J20.7   **Acute bronchitis due to echovirus**

J20.8   **Acute bronchitis due to other specified organisms**

J20.9   **Acute bronchitis, unspecified**

J21   **Acute bronchiolitis**

| INCLUDES | acute bronchiolitis with bronchospasm |
| EXCLUDES 2 | *respiratory bronchiolitis interstitial lung disease (J84.115)* |

J21.0   **Acute bronchiolitis due to respiratory syncytial virus**

J21.1   **Acute bronchiolitis due to human metapneumovirus**

J21.8   **Acute bronchiolitis due to other specified organisms**

J21.9   **Acute bronchiolitis, unspecified**

Bronchiolitis (acute)

| EXCLUDES 1 | *chronic bronchiolitis (J44.-)* |

J22   **Unspecified acute lower respiratory infection**

Acute (lower) respiratory (tract) infection NOS

| EXCLUDES 1 | *upper respiratory infection (acute) (J06.9)* |

Other diseases of upper respiratory tract (J30-J39)

J30   **Vasomotor and allergic rhinitis**

INCLUDES	spasmodic rhinorrhea
EXCLUDES 1	*allergic rhinitis with asthma (bronchial) (J45.909)*
	rhinitis NOS (J31.0)

J30.0   **Vasomotor rhinitis**

J30.1   **Allergic rhinitis due to pollen**

Allergy NOS due to pollen
Hay fever
Pollinosis

J30.2   **Other seasonal allergic rhinitis**

J30.5   **Allergic rhinitis due to food**

J30.8   **Other allergic rhinitis**

J30.81   **Allergic rhinitis due to animal (cat) (dog) hair and dander**

● New   ▲ Revised   *Manifestation*   ◢-◢ Digit Indicators   ⊟ Laterality   Ⓐ Adult (15+ years)   Ⓜ Maternity (12-55 years)   Ⓝ Newborn   Ⓟ Pediatric (0-17 years)   ♂ Male   ♀ Female
✖ Deleted   Unspecified   + Additional code

Diseases of the Respiratory System

J30.89   **Other allergic rhinitis**
Perennial allergic rhinitis

J30.9   **Allergic rhinitis, unspecified**

▲ ◳ + **J31**   **Chronic rhinitis, nasopharyngitis and pharyngitis**
Use additional code to identify:
exposure to environmental tobacco smoke (Z77.22)
exposure to tobacco smoke in the perinatal period (P96.81)
history of tobacco dependence (Z87.891)
occupational exposure to environmental tobacco smoke (Z57.31)
tobacco dependence (F17.-)
tobacco use (Z72.0)

+ **J31.0**   **Chronic rhinitis**
Atrophic rhinitis (chronic)
Granulomatous rhinitis (chronic)
Hypertrophic rhinitis (chronic)
Obstructive rhinitis (chronic)
Ozena
Purulent rhinitis (chronic)
Rhinitis (chronic) NOS
Ulcerative rhinitis (chronic)

> **EXCLUDES 1**   *allergic rhinitis (J30.1-J30.9)*
> *vasomotor rhinitis (J30.0)*

> **DEFINITION**   Long-term inflammation of the nasal mucous membrane, with wasting of the mucous membrane and glands.

+ **J31.1**   **Chronic nasopharyngitis**

> **EXCLUDES 2**   *acute nasopharyngitis (J00)*

> **DEFINITION**   Long-term inflammation of the nasal and pharyngeal (throat) mucous membranes.

+ **J31.2**   **Chronic pharyngitis**
Chronic sore throat
Atrophic pharyngitis (chronic)
Granular pharyngitis (chronic)
Hypertrophic pharyngitis (chronic)

> **EXCLUDES 2**   *acute pharyngitis (J02.9)*

▲ ◳ + **J32**   **Chronic sinusitis**

> **INCLUDES**   sinus abscess
> sinus empyema
> sinus infection
> sinus suppuration

Use additional code to identify:
exposure to environmental tobacco smoke (Z77.22)
exposure to tobacco smoke in the perinatal period (P96.81)
history of tobacco dependence (Z87.891)
infectious agent (B95-B97)
occupational exposure to environmental tobacco smoke (Z57.31)
tobacco dependence (F17.-)
tobacco use (Z72.0)

> **EXCLUDES 2**   *acute sinusitis (J01.-)*

> **CODING TIP** ✓   Do not assign a code from J32.- when sinusitis is reported as acute or infectious, unless the patient is reported to have both the chronic and acute form of sinusitis. If both forms are reported as confirmed in the medical record, assign separate and specific codes for each.

+ **J32.0**   **Chronic maxillary sinusitis**
Antritis (chronic)
Maxillary sinusitis NOS

+ **J32.1**   **Chronic frontal sinusitis**
Frontal sinusitis NOS

+ **J32.2**   **Chronic ethmoidal sinusitis**
Ethmoidal sinusitis NOS

> **EXCLUDES 1**   *Woakes' ethmoiditis (J33.1)*

+ **J32.3**   **Chronic sphenoidal sinusitis**
Sphenoidal sinusitis NOS

+ **J32.4**   **Chronic pansinusitis**
Pansinusitis NOS

+ **J32.8**   **Other chronic sinusitis**
Sinusitis (chronic) involving more than one sinus but not pansinusitis

+ **J32.9**   **Chronic sinusitis, unspecified**
Sinusitis (chronic) NOS

▲ ◳ + **J33**   **Nasal polyp**
Use additional code to identify:
exposure to environmental tobacco smoke (Z77.22)
exposure to tobacco smoke in the perinatal period (P96.81)
history of tobacco dependence (Z87.891)
occupational exposure to environmental tobacco smoke (Z57.31)
tobacco dependence (F17.-)
tobacco use (Z72.0)

> **EXCLUDES 1**   *adenomatous polyps (D14.0)*

+ **J33.0**   **Polyp of nasal cavity**
Choanal polyp
Nasopharyngeal polyp

+ **J33.1**   **Polypoid sinus degeneration**
Woakes' syndrome or ethmoiditis

+ **J33.8**   **Other polyp of sinus**
Accessory polyp of sinus
Ethmoidal polyp of sinus
Maxillary polyp of sinus
Sphenoidal polyp of sinus

+ **J33.9**   **Nasal polyp, unspecified**

◳ **J34**   **Other and unspecified disorders of nose and nasal sinuses**

> **EXCLUDES 2**   *varicose ulcer of nasal septum (I86.8)*

J34.0   **Abscess, furuncle and carbuncle of nose**
Cellulitis of nose
Necrosis of nose
Ulceration of nose

J34.1   **Cyst and mucocele of nose and nasal sinus**

J34.2   **Deviated nasal septum**
Deflection or deviation of septum (nasal) (acquired)

> **EXCLUDES 1**   *congenital deviated nasal septum (Q67.4)*

> **DEFINITION**   Cartilage separating the nostrils is shifted out of position, usually due to an old traumatic injury.

J34.3   **Hypertrophy of nasal turbinates**

◰ **J34.8**   **Other specified disorders of nose and nasal sinuses**

J34.81   **Nasal mucositis (ulcerative)**
Code also type of associated therapy, such as:
antineoplastic and immunosuppressive drugs (T45.1X-)
radiological procedure and radiotherapy (Y84.2)

> **EXCLUDES 2**   *gastrointestinal mucositis (ulcerative) (K92.81)*
> *mucositis (ulcerative) of vagina and vulva (N76.81)*
> *oral mucositis (ulcerative) (K12.3-)*

J34.89   **Other specified disorders of nose and nasal sinuses**
Perforation of nasal septum NOS
Rhinolith

J34.9   **Unspecified disorder of nose and nasal sinuses**

▲ ◳ + **J35**   **Chronic diseases of tonsils and adenoids**
Use additional code to identify:
exposure to environmental tobacco smoke (Z77.22)
exposure to tobacco smoke in the perinatal period (P96.81)
history of tobacco dependence (Z87.891)
occupational exposure to environmental tobacco smoke (Z57.31)
tobacco dependence (F17.-)
tobacco use (Z72.0)

◰ + **J35.0**   **Chronic tonsillitis and adenoiditis**

> **EXCLUDES 2**   *acute tonsillitis (J03.-)*

● New   ▲ Revised   *Manifestation*   ◳-◷ Digit Indicators   ▯ Laterality   Ⓐ Adult (15+ years)   Ⓜ Maternity (12-55 years)   Ⓝ Newborn   Ⓟ Pediatric (0-17 years)   ♂ Male   ♀ Female
✖ Deleted   Unspecified   + Additional code

680   © 2017 DecisionHealth   2017 ICD-10-CM Expert for Physicians

+ J35.01   Chronic tonsillitis

Chronic tonsilitis

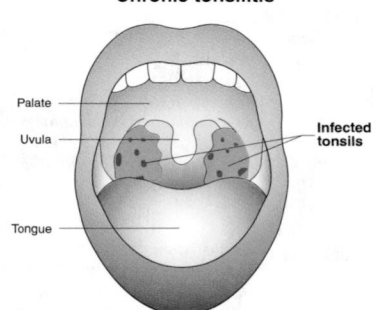

Palate
Uvula
Infected tonsils
Tongue

+ J35.02   Chronic adenoiditis

+ J35.03   Chronic tonsillitis and adenoiditis

+ J35.1   Hypertrophy of tonsils
Enlargement of tonsils
> EXCLUDES 1   *hypertrophy of tonsils with tonsillitis (J35.0-)*

+ J35.2   Hypertrophy of adenoids
Enlargement of adenoids
> EXCLUDES 1   *hypertrophy of adenoids with adenoiditis (J35.0-)*

+ J35.3   Hypertrophy of tonsils with hypertrophy of adenoids
> EXCLUDES 1   *hypertrophy of tonsils and adenoids with tonsillitis and adenoiditis (J35.03)*

+ J35.8   Other chronic diseases of tonsils and adenoids
Adenoid vegetations
Amygdalolith
Calculus, tonsil
Cicatrix of tonsil (and adenoid)
Tonsillar tag
Ulcer of tonsil

+ J35.9   Chronic disease of tonsils and adenoids, unspecified
Disease (chronic) of tonsils and adenoids NOS

+ J36   Peritonsillar abscess
> INCLUDES   abscess of tonsil
> peritonsillar cellulitis
> quinsy

Use additional code (B95-B97) to identify infectious agent.
> EXCLUDES 1   *acute tonsillitis (J03.-)*
> *chronic tonsillitis (J35.0)*
> *retropharyngeal abscess (J39.0)*
> *tonsillitis NOS (J03.9-)*

▲ ◪ + J37   Chronic laryngitis and laryngotracheitis
Use additional code to identify:
exposure to environmental tobacco smoke (Z77.22)
exposure to tobacco smoke in the perinatal period (P96.81)
history of tobacco dependence (Z87.891)
infectious agent (B95-B97)
occupational exposure to environmental tobacco smoke (Z57.31)
tobacco dependence (F17.-)
tobacco use (Z72.0)

> CODING TIP ✓   Assign a code from J37.- only when the physician specifies laryngitis or laryngotracheitis as "chronic."

+ J37.0   Chronic laryngitis
Catarrhal laryngitis
Hypertrophic laryngitis
Sicca laryngitis
> EXCLUDES 2   *acute laryngitis (J04.0)*
> *obstructive (acute) laryngitis (J05.0)*

+ J37.1   Chronic laryngotracheitis
Laryngitis, chronic, with tracheitis (chronic)
Tracheitis, chronic, with laryngitis
> EXCLUDES 1   *chronic tracheitis (J42)*
> EXCLUDES 2   *acute laryngotracheitis (J04.2)*
> *acute tracheitis (J04.1)*

> DEFINITION   Long-term inflammation extending past the vocal cords and into the trachea.

▲ ◪ + J38   Diseases of vocal cords and larynx, not elsewhere classified
Use additional code to identify:
exposure to environmental tobacco smoke (Z77.22)
exposure to tobacco smoke in the perinatal period (P96.81)
history of tobacco dependence (Z87.891)
occupational exposure to environmental tobacco smoke (Z57.31)
tobacco dependence (F17.-)
tobacco use (Z72.0)
> EXCLUDES 1   *congenital laryngeal stridor (P28.89)*
> *obstructive laryngitis (acute) (J05.0)*
> *postprocedural subglottic stenosis (J95.5)*
> *stridor (R06.1)*
> *ulcerative laryngitis (J04.0)*

⑤ + J38.0   Paralysis of vocal cords and larynx
Laryngoplegia
Paralysis of glottis
+ J38.00   Paralysis of vocal cords and larynx, unspecified
+ J38.01   Paralysis of vocal cords and larynx, unilateral
+ J38.02   Paralysis of vocal cords and larynx, bilateral

+ J38.1   Polyp of vocal cord and larynx
> EXCLUDES 1   *adenomatous polyps (D14.1)*

+ J38.2   Nodules of vocal cords
Chorditis (fibrinous)(nodosa)(tuberosa)
Singer's nodes
Teacher's nodes

+ J38.3   Other diseases of vocal cords
Abscess of vocal cords
Cellulitis of vocal cords
Granuloma of vocal cords
Leukokeratosis of vocal cords
Leukoplakia of vocal cords

+ J38.4   Edema of larynx
Edema (of) glottis
Subglottic edema
Supraglottic edema
> EXCLUDES 1   *acute obstructive laryngitis [croup] (J05.0)*
> *edematous laryngitis (J04.0)*

+ J38.5   Laryngeal spasm
Laryngismus (stridulus)

+ J38.6   Stenosis of larynx

Stenosis of larynx
Abnormal narrowing or constriction of larynx

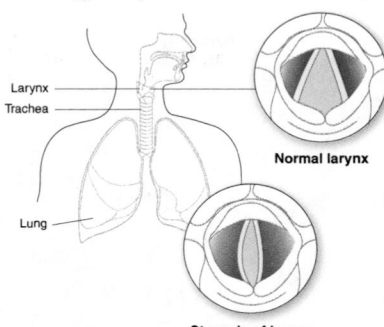

Larynx
Trachea
Normal larynx
Lung
Stenosis of larynx

+ J38.7   Other diseases of larynx
Abscess of larynx
Cellulitis of larynx
Disease of larynx NOS
Necrosis of larynx
Pachyderma of larynx
Perichondritis of larynx
Ulcer of larynx

◪ J39   Other diseases of upper respiratory tract
> EXCLUDES 1   *acute respiratory infection NOS (J22)*
> *acute upper respiratory infection (J06.9)*
> *upper respiratory inflammation due to chemicals, gases, fumes or vapors (J68.2)*

J39.0   Retropharyngeal and parapharyngeal abscess
Peripharyngeal abscess
> EXCLUDES 1   *peritonsillar abscess (J36)*

> DEFINITION   Pus-filled sore at the back of the throat.

● New   ▲ Revised   *Manifestation*   ◪-⑦ Digit Indicators   ☰ Laterality   🅰 Adult (15+ years)   🅼 Maternity (12-55 years)   🅽 Newborn   🅿 Pediatric (0-17 years)   ♂ Male   ♀ Female
✖ ~~Deleted~~   Unspecified   + Additional code

J39.1   **Other abscess of pharynx**
Cellulitis of pharynx
Nasopharyngeal abscess
CODING TIP ✓   Do not assign J39.1 for a diagnosis of pharyngitis. Acute pharyngitis should be coded to J02.-

J39.2   **Other diseases of pharynx**
Cyst of pharynx
Edema of pharynx
EXCLUDES 2   *chronic pharyngitis (J31.2)*
ulcerative pharyngitis (J02.9)

J39.3   **Upper respiratory tract hypersensitivity reaction, site unspecified**
EXCLUDES 1   *hypersensitivity reaction of upper respiratory tract, such as:*
extrinsic allergic alveolitis (J67.9)
pneumoconiosis (J60-J67.9)

J39.8   **Other specified diseases of upper respiratory tract**

J39.9   **Disease of upper respiratory tract, unspecified**

Chronic lower respiratory diseases (J40-J47)

EXCLUDES 1   *bronchitis due to chemicals, gases, fumes and vapors (J68.0)*

EXCLUDES 2   *cystic fibrosis (E84.-)*

▲ + **J40**   **Bronchitis, not specified as acute or chronic**
Bronchitis NOS
Bronchitis with tracheitis NOS
Catarrhal bronchitis
Tracheobronchitis NOS
Use additional code to identify:
exposure to environmental tobacco smoke (Z77.22)
exposure to tobacco smoke in the perinatal period (P96.81)
history of tobacco dependence (Z87.891)
occupational exposure to environmental tobacco smoke (Z57.31)
tobacco dependence (F17.-)
tobacco use (Z72.0)
EXCLUDES 1   *acute bronchitis (J20.-)*
allergic bronchitis NOS (J45.909-)
asthmatic bronchitis NOS (J45.9-)
bronchitis due to chemicals, gases, fumes and vapors (J68.0)
CODING TIP ✓   Do not assign code J40 for chronic, chronic obstructive, or acute bronchitis. J40 should be assigned only when no diagnostic information is available to differentiate the type of bronchitis.

Bronchitis,
not specified as acute or chronic

Trachea

Bronchi

Left lung

Healthy bronchus

Inflamed bronchus

▲ ⬛ + **J41**   **Simple and mucopurulent chronic bronchitis**
Use additional code to identify:
exposure to environmental tobacco smoke (Z77.22)
exposure to tobacco smoke in the perinatal period (P96.81)
history of tobacco dependence (Z87.891)
occupational exposure to environmental tobacco smoke (Z57.31)
tobacco dependence (F17.-)
tobacco use (Z72.0)
EXCLUDES 1   *chronic bronchitis NOS (J42)*
chronic obstructive bronchitis (J44.-)
CODING TIP ✓   Chronic bronchitis not specified as "obstructive" should be coded to J41.0-J42. Chronic bronchitis that is specified as obstructive is coded to category J44.-. Chronic indicates cough with mucous most days of the month for at least 3 months out of the year.

+ **J41.0**   **Simple chronic bronchitis**

+ **J41.1**   **Mucopurulent chronic bronchitis**

+ **J41.8**   **Mixed simple and mucopurulent chronic bronchitis**

▲ + **J42**   **Unspecified chronic bronchitis**
Chronic bronchitis NOS
Chronic tracheitis
Chronic tracheobronchitis
Use additional code to identify:
exposure to environmental tobacco smoke (Z77.22)
exposure to tobacco smoke in the perinatal period (P96.81)
history of tobacco dependence (Z87.891)
occupational exposure to environmental tobacco smoke (Z57.31)
tobacco dependence (F17.-)
tobacco use (Z72.0)
EXCLUDES 1   *chronic asthmatic bronchitis (J44.-)*
chronic bronchitis with airways obstruction (J44.-)
chronic emphysematous bronchitis (J44.-)
chronic obstructive pulmonary disease NOS (J44.9)
simple and mucopurulent chronic bronchitis (J41.-)
CODING TIP ✓   Chronic bronchitis not specified as "obstructive" should be coded to J41.0-J42. Chronic bronchitis that is specified as obstructive is coded to category J44.-. Chronic indicates cough with mucous most days of the month for at least 3 months out of the year.

▲ ⬛ + **J43**   **Emphysema**
Use additional code to identify:
exposure to environmental tobacco smoke (Z77.22)
history of tobacco dependence (Z87.891)
occupational exposure to environmental tobacco smoke (Z57.31)
tobacco dependence (F17.-)
tobacco use (Z72.0)
EXCLUDES 1   *compensatory emphysema (J98.3)*
emphysema due to inhalation of chemicals, gases, fumes or vapors (J68.4)
emphysema with chronic (obstructive) bronchitis (J44.-)
emphysematous (obstructive) bronchitis (J44.-)
interstitial emphysema (J98.2)
mediastinal emphysema (J98.2)
neonatal interstitial emphysema (P25.0)
surgical (subcutaneous) emphysema (T81.82)
traumatic subcutaneous emphysema (T79.7)
CODING TIP ✓   When a diagnosis supports coding a more specific code for emphysema, such as interstitial emphysema (J98.2), compensatory emphysema (J98.3), or subcutaneous emphysema due to trauma (T79.7), then do not assign J43.-, but assign the more specific code.
CODING TIP ✓   Do not assign a code from J43.- when the physician documentation reports emphysema with COPD, chronic obstructive bronchitis or emphysematous bronchitis. Emphysema with COPD, bronchitis and emphysematous bronchitis should be coded to J44.- and cannot be coded on the same claim as J43.-.

+ **J43.0**   **Unilateral pulmonary emphysema [MacLeod's syndrome]**
Swyer-James syndrome
Unilateral emphysema
Unilateral hyperlucent lung
Unilateral pulmonary artery functional hypoplasia
Unilateral transparency of lung

+ **J43.1**   **Panlobular emphysema**
Panacinar emphysema

+ **J43.2**   **Centrilobular emphysema**

+ **J43.8**   **Other emphysema**

+ **J43.9**   **Emphysema, unspecified**
Bullous emphysema (lung)(pulmonary)
Emphysema (lung)(pulmonary) NOS
Emphysematous bleb
Vesicular emphysema (lung)(pulmonary)

● New   ▲ Revised   *Manifestation*   ⬛-⬛ Digit Indicators   ⊟ Laterality   🅰 Adult (15+ years)   Ⓜ Maternity (12-55 years)   Ⓝ Newborn   Ⓟ Pediatric (0-17 years)   ♂ Male   ♀ Female
✖ Deleted   Unspecified   + Additional code

682   © 2017 DecisionHealth   2017 ICD-10-CM Expert for Physicians

DEFINITION Abnormal enlargement of the air sacs in the lungs, which lose their elasticity, making breathing increasingly difficult.

Emphysema, unspecified

Normal alveoli

Emphysemic alveoli

Trachea

Bronchi

Right lung

Damage to air sacs (alveoli)

▲ ⬛ + **J44** **Other chronic obstructive pulmonary disease**

INCLUDES asthma with chronic obstructive pulmonary disease
chronic asthmatic (obstructive) bronchitis
chronic bronchitis with airways obstruction
chronic bronchitis with emphysema
chronic emphysematous bronchitis
chronic obstructive asthma
chronic obstructive bronchitis
chronic obstructive tracheobronchitis

Code also:
type of asthma, if applicable (J45.-)
Use additional code to identify:
exposure to environmental tobacco smoke (Z77.22)
history of tobacco dependence (Z87.891)
occupational exposure to environmental tobacco smoke (Z57.31)
tobacco dependence (F17.-)
tobacco use (Z72.0)

EXCLUDES 1 *bronchiectasis (J47.-)*
chronic bronchitis NOS (J42)
chronic simple and mucopurulent bronchitis (J41.-)
chronic tracheitis (J42)
chronic tracheobronchitis (J42)
emphysema without chronic bronchitis (J43.-)

EXCLUDES 2 *lung diseases due to external agents (J60-J70)*

GUIDELINES Section I.C.10.a
The codes in categories J44 and J45 distinguish between uncomplicated cases and those in acute exacerbation. An acute exacerbation is a worsening or a decompensation of a chronic condition. An acute exacerbation is not equivalent to an infection superimposed on a chronic condition, though an exacerbation may be triggered by an infection.

CODING TIP ✓ When the physician reports chronic obstructive asthma or chronic asthmatic bronchitis, and the type of asthma is specified, an additional code from category J45.- should be reported.

Chronic obstructive pulmonary disease

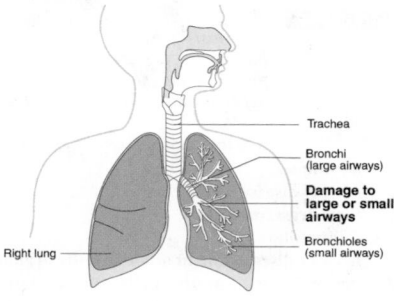

Trachea

Bronchi (large airways)

Damage to large or small airways

Bronchioles (small airways)

Right lung

+ **J44.0** **Chronic obstructive pulmonary disease with acute lower respiratory infection**
Use additional code to identify the infection

CODING TIP ✓ Assign a code from J44.0 when a patient has both COPD and a diagnosis of a lower respiratory tract infection. An additional code should be assigned to report the infection. If the physician confirms both a diagnosis of a lower respiratory tract infection and exacerbation of the chronic obstructive pulmonary disease, both J44.1, Chronic obstructive pulmonary disease with acute exacerbation, and J44.0, Chronic obstructive pulmonary disease with acute lower respiratory infection, should be assigned, followed by a code for the specific lower respiratory infection. Lower respiratory infections include pneumonia, bronchitis and bronchiolitis.

+ **J44.1** **Chronic obstructive pulmonary disease with (acute) exacerbation**
Decompensated COPD
Decompensated COPD with (acute) exacerbation
EXCLUDES 2 *chronic obstructive pulmonary disease [COPD] with acute bronchitis (J44.0)*

CODING TIP ✓ **Documentation:** Do not assign J44.1 unless the physician has confirmed that the condition is exacerbated. An exacerbation may not be assumed without physician confirmation, and changes in treatment and medication regimen do not presume an exacerbation.
AHA: 1Q 2016, 36

+ **J44.9** **Chronic obstructive pulmonary disease, unspecified**
Chronic obstructive airway disease NOS
Chronic obstructive lung disease NOS
AHA: 1Q 2016, 36-37
AHA: 4Q 2014, 21
AHA: 4Q 2013, 109, 129

▲ ⬛ + **J45** **Asthma**

INCLUDES allergic (predominantly) asthma
allergic bronchitis NOS
allergic rhinitis with asthma
atopic asthma
extrinsic allergic asthma
hay fever with asthma
idiosyncratic asthma
intrinsic nonallergic asthma
nonallergic asthma

Use additional code to identify:
exposure to environmental tobacco smoke (Z77.22)
exposure to tobacco smoke in the perinatal period (P96.81)
history of tobacco dependence (Z87.891)
occupational exposure to environmental tobacco smoke (Z57.31)
tobacco dependence (F17.-)
tobacco use (Z72.0)

EXCLUDES 1 *detergent asthma (J69.8)*
eosinophilic asthma (J82)
lung diseases due to external agents (J60-J70)
miner's asthma (J60)
wheezing NOS (R06.2)
wood asthma (J67.8)

EXCLUDES 2 *asthma with chronic obstructive pulmonary disease (J44.9)*
chronic asthmatic (obstructive) bronchitis (J44.9)
chronic obstructive asthma (J44.9)

● New ▲ Revised *Manifestation* ⬛-⬛ Digit Indicators ⊟ Laterality Ⓐ Adult (15+ years) Ⓜ Maternity (12-55 years) Ⓝ Newborn Ⓟ Pediatric (0-17 years) ♂ Male ♀ Female
✖ ~~Deleted~~ Unspecified + Additional code

GUIDELINES   Section I.C.10.a
The codes in categories J44 and J45 distinguish between
uncomplicated cases and those in acute exacerbation. An
acute exacerbation is a worsening or a decompensation of a
chronic condition. An acute exacerbation is not equivalent to
an infection superimposed on a chronic condition, though an
exacerbation may be triggered by an infection.

CODING TIP✓   Documentation: When reporting a code
from category J45.-, do not report the condition as
exacerbated without physician confirmation of the diagnosis.
An exacerbation may not be assumed without physician
confirmation, and changes in treatment and medication
regimen do not presume an exacerbation.

Asthma

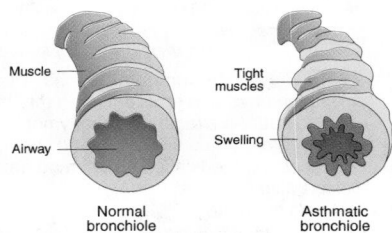

Muscle —

Tight
muscles —

Airway —

Swelling —

Normal
bronchiole

Asthmatic
bronchiole

⑤ + **J45.2**   **Mild intermittent asthma**
  + **J45.20**   **Mild intermittent asthma, uncomplicated**
          Mild intermittent asthma NOS
  + **J45.21**   **Mild intermittent asthma with (acute) exacerbation**
  + **J45.22**   **Mild intermittent asthma with status asthmaticus**
⑤ + **J45.3**   **Mild persistent asthma**
  + **J45.30**   **Mild persistent asthma, uncomplicated**
          Mild persistent asthma NOS
  + **J45.31**   **Mild persistent asthma with (acute) exacerbation**
          AHA: 1Q 2016, 35
  + **J45.32**   **Mild persistent asthma with status asthmaticus**
⑤ + **J45.4**   **Moderate persistent asthma**
  + **J45.40**   **Moderate persistent asthma, uncomplicated**
          Moderate persistent asthma NOS
  + **J45.41**   **Moderate persistent asthma with (acute)
                  exacerbation**
  + **J45.42**   **Moderate persistent asthma with status asthmaticus**
⑤ + **J45.5**   **Severe persistent asthma**
  + **J45.50**   **Severe persistent asthma, uncomplicated**
          Severe persistent asthma NOS
  + **J45.51**   **Severe persistent asthma with (acute) exacerbation**
  + **J45.52**   **Severe persistent asthma with status asthmaticus**
⑤ + **J45.9**   **Other and unspecified asthma**
  ⑥ + **J45.90**   **Unspecified asthma**
          Asthmatic bronchitis NOS
          Childhood asthma NOS
          Late onset asthma
      + **J45.901**   **Unspecified asthma with (acute) exacerbation**
      + **J45.902**   **Unspecified asthma with status asthmaticus**
      + **J45.909**   **Unspecified asthma, uncomplicated**
              Asthma NOS
  ⑥ + **J45.99**   **Other asthma**
      + **J45.990**   **Exercise induced bronchospasm**
      + **J45.991**   **Cough variant asthma**
      + **J45.998**   **Other asthma**
▲ ④ + **J47**   **Bronchiectasis**
      INCLUDES   bronchiolectasis
      Use additional code to identify:
        exposure to environmental tobacco smoke (Z77.22)
        exposure to tobacco smoke in the perinatal period (P96.81)
        history of tobacco dependence (Z87.891)
        *occupational exposure to environmental tobacco smoke
          (Z57.31)*
        tobacco dependence (F17.-)
        tobacco use (Z72.0)
      EXCLUDES 1   *congenital bronchiectasis (Q33.4)*
                *tuberculous bronchiectasis (current disease)
                (A15.0)*

▲ + **J47.0**   **Bronchiectasis with acute lower respiratory infection**
          Bronchiectasis with acute bronchitis
          Use additional code to identify the infection
+ **J47.1**   **Bronchiectasis with (acute) exacerbation**
+ **J47.9**   **Bronchiectasis, uncomplicated**
          Bronchiectasis NOS
      DEFINITION   Destruction and widening of the large
      airways, often due to recurrent, severe infection or
      inflammation, or following foreign body obstruction.

Lung diseases due to external agents (J60-J70)

EXCLUDES 2   *asthma (J45.-)*
          malignant neoplasm of bronchus and lung (C34.-)
J60   **Coalworker's pneumoconiosis**   Ⓐ
          Anthracosilicosis
          Anthracosis
          Black lung disease
          Coalworker's lung
      EXCLUDES 1   *coalworker pneumoconiosis with tuberculosis,
                any type in A15 (J65)*
      DEFINITION   Silicotic nodules and scar-tissue formation
      in the lungs due to prolonged inhalation and collection of
      coal dust particles in the bronchioles.
J61   **Pneumoconiosis due to asbestos and other mineral**   Ⓐ
          fibers
          Asbestosis
      EXCLUDES 1   *pleural plaque with asbestosis (J92.0)*
                *pneumoconiosis with tuberculosis, any type in
                A15 (J65)*
      DEFINITION   Chronic lung disease caused by inhaling
      asbestos particles over a prolonged period.
④ **J62**   **Pneumoconiosis due to dust containing silica**
      INCLUDES   silicotic fibrosis (massive) of lung
      EXCLUDES 1   *pneumoconiosis with tuberculosis, any type in
                A15 (J65)*
  J62.0   **Pneumoconiosis due to talc dust**
  J62.8   **Pneumoconiosis due to other dust containing silica**
          Silicosis NOS
④ **J63**   **Pneumoconiosis due to other inorganic dusts**
      EXCLUDES 1   *pneumoconiosis with tuberculosis, any type in
                A15 (J65)*
  J63.0   **Aluminosis (of lung)**
  J63.1   **Bauxite fibrosis (of lung)**
  J63.2   **Berylliosis**
  J63.3   **Graphite fibrosis (of lung)**
  J63.4   **Siderosis**
  J63.5   **Stannosis**
  J63.6   **Pneumoconiosis due to other specified inorganic dusts**
J64   **Unspecified pneumoconiosis**
      EXCLUDES 1   *pneumonoconiosis with tuberculosis, any type in
                A15 (J65)*
J65   **Pneumoconiosis associated with tuberculosis**
          Any condition in J60-J64 with tuberculosis, any type in A15
          Silicotuberculosis
④ **J66**   **Airway disease due to specific organic dust**
      EXCLUDES 2   *allergic alveolitis (J67.-)*
                asbestosis (J61)
                bagassosis (J67.1)
                farmer's lung (J67.0)
                *hypersensitivity pneumonitis due to organic dust
                (J67.-)*
                reactive airways dysfunction syndrome (J68.3)
  J66.0   **Byssinosis**
          Airway disease due to cotton dust
  J66.1   **Flax-dressers' disease**
  J66.2   **Cannabinosis**
  J66.8   **Airway disease due to other specific organic dusts**
④ **J67**   **Hypersensitivity pneumonitis due to organic dust**
      INCLUDES   allergic alveolitis and pneumonitis due to inhaled
                organic dust and particles of fungal,
                actinomycetic or other origin
      EXCLUDES 1   *pneumonitis due to inhalation of chemicals,
                gases, fumes or vapors (J68.0)*

● New   ▲ Revised   *Manifestation*   ④-⑦ Digit Indicators   ⊟ Laterality   Ⓐ Adult (15+ years)   Ⓜ Maternity (12-55 years)   Ⓝ Newborn   Ⓟ Pediatric (0-17 years)   ♂ Male   ♀ Female
✖ Deleted   Unspecified   + Additional code

684   © 2017 DecisionHealth   2017 ICD-10-CM Expert for Physicians

J67.0 **Farmer's lung**
Harvester's lung
Haymaker's lung
Moldy hay disease

DEFINITION   Inflammation of the small, inner air sacs in the lungs, due to an allergic reaction triggered by inhaled organic substances or microorganisms.

J67.1 **Bagassosis**
Bagasse disease
Bagasse pneumonitis

J67.2 **Bird fancier's lung**
Budgerigar fancier's disease or lung
Pigeon fancier's disease or lung

J67.3 **Suberosis**
Corkhandler's disease or lung
Corkworker's disease or lung

J67.4 **Maltworker's lung**
Alveolitis due to Aspergillus clavatus

J67.5 **Mushroom-worker's lung**

J67.6 **Maple-bark-stripper's lung**
Alveolitis due to Cryptostroma corticale
Cryptostromosis

J67.7 **Air conditioner and humidifier lung**
Allergic alveolitis due to fungal, thermophilic actinomycetes and other organisms growing in ventilation [air conditioning] systems

J67.8 **Hypersensitivity pneumonitis due to other organic dusts**
Cheese-washer's lung
Coffee-worker's lung
Fish-meal worker's lung
Furrier's lung
Sequoiosis

J67.9 **Hypersensitivity pneumonitis due to unspecified organic dust**
Allergic alveolitis (extrinsic) NOS
Hypersensitivity pneumonitis NOS

◢ + **J68** **Respiratory conditions due to inhalation of chemicals, gases, fumes and vapors**
Code first:
(T51-T65) to identify cause
Use additional code to identify associated respiratory conditions, such as:
acute respiratory failure (J96.0-)

+ **J68.0** **Bronchitis and pneumonitis due to chemicals, gases, fumes and vapors**
Chemical bronchitis (acute)

+ **J68.1** **Pulmonary edema due to chemicals, gases, fumes and vapors**
Chemical pulmonary edema (acute) (chronic)
EXCLUDES 1   *pulmonary edema (acute) (chronic) NOS (J81.-)*

+ **J68.2** **Upper respiratory inflammation due to chemicals, gases, fumes and vapors, not elsewhere classified**

+ **J68.3** **Other acute and subacute respiratory conditions due to chemicals, gases, fumes and vapors**
Reactive airways dysfunction syndrome

+ **J68.4** **Chronic respiratory conditions due to chemicals, gases, fumes and vapors**
Emphysema (diffuse) (chronic) due to inhalation of chemicals, gases, fumes and vapors
Obliterative bronchiolitis (chronic) (subacute) due to inhalation of chemicals, gases, fumes and vapors
Pulmonary fibrosis (chronic) due to inhalation of chemicals, gases, fumes and vapors
EXCLUDES 1   *chronic pulmonary edema due to chemicals, gases, fumes and vapors (J68.1)*

+ **J68.8** **Other respiratory conditions due to chemicals, gases, fumes and vapors**

+ **J68.9** **Unspecified respiratory condition due to chemicals, gases, fumes and vapors**

◢ **J69** **Pneumonitis due to solids and liquids**
EXCLUDES 1   *neonatal aspiration syndromes (P24.-)*
postprocedural pneumonitis (J95.4)

J69.0 **Pneumonitis due to inhalation of food and vomit**
Aspiration pneumonia NOS
Aspiration pneumonia (due to) food (regurgitated)
Aspiration pneumonia (due to) gastric secretions
Aspiration pneumonia (due to) milk
Aspiration pneumonia (due to) vomit
Code also:
any associated foreign body in respiratory tract (T17.-)
EXCLUDES 1   *chemical pneumonitis due to anesthesia (J95.4)*
obstetric aspiration pneumonitis (O74.0)

J69.1 **Pneumonitis due to inhalation of oils and essences**
Exogenous lipoid pneumonia
Lipid pneumonia NOS
Code first:
(T51-T65) to identify substance
EXCLUDES 1   *endogenous lipoid pneumonia (J84.89)*

J69.8 **Pneumonitis due to inhalation of other solids and liquids**
Pneumonitis due to aspiration of blood
Pneumonitis due to aspiration of detergent
Code first:
(T51-T65) to identify substance

◢ **J70** **Respiratory conditions due to other external agents**

+ **J70.0** **Acute pulmonary manifestations due to radiation**
Radiation pneumonitis
Use additional code (W88-W90, X39.0-) to identify the external cause

+ **J70.1** **Chronic and other pulmonary manifestations due to radiation**
Fibrosis of lung following radiation
Use additional code (W88-W90, X39.0-) to identify the external cause

+ **J70.2** **Acute drug-induced interstitial lung disorders**
Use additional code for adverse effect, if applicable, to identify drug (T36-T50 with fifth or sixth character 5)
EXCLUDES 1   *interstitial pneumonia NOS (J84.9)*
lymphoid interstitial pneumonia (J84.2)

+ **J70.3** **Chronic drug-induced interstitial lung disorders**
Use additional code for adverse effect, if applicable, to identify drug (T36-T50 with fifth or sixth character 5)
EXCLUDES 1   *interstitial pneumonia NOS (J84.9)*
lymphoid interstitial pneumonia (J84.2)

+ **J70.4** **Drug-induced interstitial lung disorders, unspecified**
Use additional code for adverse effect, if applicable, to identify drug (T36-T50 with fifth or sixth character 5)
EXCLUDES 1   *interstitial pneumonia NOS (J84.9)*
lymphoid interstitial pneumonia (J84.2)

J70.5 **Respiratory conditions due to smoke inhalation**
Smoke inhalation NOS
EXCLUDES 1   *smoke inhalation due to chemicals, gases, fumes and vapors (J68.9)*
AHA: 4Q 2013, 121

J70.8 **Respiratory conditions due to other specified external agents**
Code first:
(T51-T65) to identify the external agent

J70.9 **Respiratory conditions due to unspecified external agent**
Code first:
(T51-T65) to identify the external agent

Other respiratory diseases principally affecting the interstitium (J80-J84)

J80 **Acute respiratory distress syndrome**
Acute respiratory distress syndrome in adult or child
Adult hyaline membrane disease
EXCLUDES 1   *respiratory distress syndrome in newborn (perinatal) (P22.0)*

Diseases of the Respiratory System

▲ 4 + **J81** **Pulmonary edema**
Use additional code to identify:
exposure to environmental tobacco smoke (Z77.22)
history of tobacco dependence (Z87.891)
occupational exposure to environmental tobacco smoke
(Z57.31)
tobacco dependence (F17.-)
tobacco use (Z72.0)
> EXCLUDES 1　*chemical (acute) pulmonary edema (J68.1)*
> *hypostatic pneumonia (J18.2)*
> *passive pneumonia (J18.2)*
> *pulmonary edema due to external agents*
> *(J60-J70)*
> *pulmonary edema with heart disease NOS*
> *(I50.1)*
> *pulmonary edema with heart failure (I50.1)*

+ **J81.0** **Acute pulmonary edema**
Acute edema of lung
> DEFINITION　Sudden, severe accumulation of fluid in the lungs.

+ **J81.1** **Chronic pulmonary edema**
Pulmonary congestion (chronic) (passive)
Pulmonary edema NOS

J82 **Pulmonary eosinophilia, not elsewhere classified**
Allergic pneumonia
Eosinophilic asthma
Eosinophilic pneumonia
Löffler's pneumonia
Tropical (pulmonary) eosinophilia NOS
> EXCLUDES 1　*pulmonary eosinophilia due to aspergillosis*
> *(B44.-)*
> *pulmonary eosinophilia due to drugs*
> *(J70.2-J70.4)*
> *pulmonary eosinophilia due to specified parasitic*
> *infection (B50-B83)*
> *pulmonary eosinophilia due to systemic*
> *connective tissue disorders (M30-M36)*
> *pulmonary infiltrate NOS (R91.8)*

4 **J84** **Other interstitial pulmonary diseases**
> EXCLUDES 1　*drug-induced interstitial lung disorders*
> *(J70.2-J70.4)*
> *interstitial emphysema (J98.2)*
> *lung diseases due to external agents (J60-J70)*

5 **J84.0** **Alveolar and parieto-alveolar conditions**

J84.01 **Alveolar proteinosis**

J84.02 **Pulmonary alveolar microlithiasis**

J84.03 *Idiopathic pulmonary hemosiderosis*
Essential brown induration of lung
Code first underlying disease, such as:
disorders of iron metabolism (E83.1-)
> EXCLUDES 1　*acute idiopathic pulmonary*
> *hemorrhage in infants [AIPHI]*
> *(R04.81)*

J84.09 **Other alveolar and parieto-alveolar conditions**

5 **J84.1** **Other interstitial pulmonary diseases with fibrosis**
> EXCLUDES 1　*pulmonary fibrosis (chronic) due to*
> *inhalation of chemicals, gases, fumes or*
> *vapors (J68.4)*
> *pulmonary fibrosis (chronic) following*
> *radiation (J70.1)*
> DEFINITION　Formation of fibrous tissue and scarring in the lungs after the lungs have been inflamed for a significant period of time.

J84.10 **Pulmonary fibrosis, unspecified**
Capillary fibrosis of lung
Cirrhosis of lung (chronic) NOS
Fibrosis of lung (atrophic) (chronic) (confluent)
(massive) (perialveolar) (peribronchial) NOS
Induration of lung (chronic) NOS
Postinflammatory pulmonary fibrosis

6 **J84.11** **Idiopathic interstitial pneumonia**
> EXCLUDES 1　*lymphoid interstitial pneumonia*
> *(J84.2)*
> *pneumocystis pneumonia (B59)*

J84.111 **Idiopathic interstitial pneumonia, not otherwise specified**

J84.112 **Idiopathic pulmonary fibrosis**
Cryptogenic fibrosing alveolitis
Idiopathic fibrosing alveolitis

J84.113 **Idiopathic non-specific interstitial pneumonitis**
> EXCLUDES 1　*non-specific interstitial*
> *pneumonia NOS, or due to*
> *known underlying cause*
> *(J84.89)*

J84.114 **Acute interstitial pneumonitis**
Hamman-Rich syndrome
> EXCLUDES 1　*pneumocystis pneumonia (B59)*

J84.115 **Respiratory bronchiolitis interstitial lung disease**

J84.116 **Cryptogenic organizing pneumonia**
> EXCLUDES 1　*organizing pneumonia NOS, or*
> *due to known underlying cause*
> *(J84.89)*

J84.117 **Desquamative interstitial pneumonia**

J84.17 **Other interstitial pulmonary diseases with fibrosis in diseases classified elsewhere**
Interstitial pneumonia (nonspecific) (usual) due to
collagen vascular disease
Interstitial pneumonia (nonspecific) (usual) in diseases
classified elsewhere
Organizing pneumonia due to collagen vascular disease
Organizing pneumonia in diseases classified elsewhere
Code first underlying disease, such as:
progressive systemic sclerosis (M34.0)
rheumatoid arthritis (M05.00-M06.9)
systemic lupus erythematosis (M32.0-M32.9)

J84.2 **Lymphoid interstitial pneumonia**
Lymphoid interstitial pneumonitis

5 **J84.8** **Other specified interstitial pulmonary diseases**
> EXCLUDES 1　*exogenous lipoid pneumonia (J69.1)*
> *unspecified lipoid pneumonia (J69.1)*

J84.81 **Lymphangioleiomyomatosis**　　♀
Lymphangiomyomatosis

J84.82 **Adult pulmonary Langerhans cell histiocytosis**　A
Adult PLCH

J84.83 **Surfactant mutations of the lung**

6 **J84.84** **Other interstitial lung diseases of childhood**

J84.841 **Neuroendocrine cell hyperplasia of infancy**

J84.842 **Pulmonary interstitial glycogenosis**

J84.843 **Alveolar capillary dysplasia with vein misalignment**

J84.848 **Other interstitial lung diseases of childhood**　P

▲ + **J84.89** **Other specified interstitial pulmonary diseases**
Endogenous lipoid pneumonia
Interstitial pneumonitis
Non-specific interstitial pneumonitis NOS
Organizing pneumonia NOS
Code first, if applicable:
poisoning due to drug or toxin
(T51-T65 with fifth or sixth character to indicate
intent), for toxic pneumonopathy
underlying cause of pneumonopathy, if known
Use additional code, for adverse effect, to identify drug
(T36-T50 with fifth or sixth character 5), if drug-
induced
> EXCLUDES 1　*cryptogenic organizing pneumonia*
> *(J84.116)*
> *idiopathic non-specific interstitial*
> *pneumonitis (J84.113)*
> *lipoid pneumonia, exogenous or*
> *unspecified (J69.1)*
> *lymphoid interstitial pneumonia*
> *(J84.2)*

J84.9 **Interstitial pulmonary disease, unspecified**
Interstitial pneumonia NOS

Suppurative and necrotic conditions of the lower respiratory tract (J85-J86)

> CODING TIP ✓　When the record specifies the causative organism, use an additional code to report the organism specified, following the instructions to "use an additional code."

4 + **J85** **Abscess of lung and mediastinum**
Use additional code (B95-B97) to identify infectious agent.

+ **J85.0** **Gangrene and necrosis of lung**

+ **J85.1** **Abscess of lung with pneumonia**
Code also:
the type of pneumonia

● New　▲ Revised　*Manifestation*　4-7 Digit Indicators　⊟ Laterality　A Adult (15+ years)　M Maternity (12-55 years)　N Newborn　P Pediatric (0-17 years)　♂ Male　♀ Female
✖ Deleted　Unspecified　+ Additional code

+ **J85.2** **Abscess of lung without pneumonia**
Abscess of lung NOS

+ **J85.3** **Abscess of mediastinum**

◢ + **J86** **Pyothorax**
Use additional code (B95-B97) to identify infectious agent.
> **EXCLUDES 1** *abscess of lung (J85.-)*
> *pyothorax due to tuberculosis (A15.6)*

+ **J86.0** **Pyothorax with fistula**
Bronchocutaneous fistula
Bronchopleural fistula
Hepatopleural fistula
Mediastinal fistula
Pleural fistula
Thoracic fistula
Any condition classifiable to J86.9 with fistula

+ **J86.9** **Pyothorax without fistula**
Abscess of pleura
Abscess of thorax
Empyema (chest) (lung) (pleura)
Fibrinopurulent pleurisy
Purulent pleurisy
Pyopneumothorax
Septic pleurisy
Seropurulent pleurisy
Suppurative pleurisy

Other diseases of the pleura (J90-J94)

J90 **Pleural effusion, not elsewhere classified**
Encysted pleurisy
Pleural effusion NOS
Pleurisy with effusion (exudative) (serous)
> **EXCLUDES 1** *chylous (pleural) effusion (J94.0)*
> *malignant pleural effusion (J91.0))*
> *pleurisy NOS (R09.1)*
> *tuberculous pleural effusion (A15.6)*

> **CODING TIP ✓** Pleural effusion indicates excess pleural fluid built up and accumulated in the pleural lining causing respiratory distress.

◢ **J91** **Pleural effusion in conditions classified elsewhere**
> **EXCLUDES 2** *pleural effusion in heart failure (I50.-)*
> *pleural effusion in systemic lupus erythematosus (M32.13)*

> **CODING TIP ✓** Pleural effusion indicates excess pleural fluid built up and accumulated in the pleural lining causing respiratory distress.

> **CODING TIP ✓** Pleural effusion in systemic lupus erythematosus and in heart failure are to be coded as J91.8. Code first the causative condition. However, if the pleural effusion requires separate treatment, i.e. chest tube for drainage, then add the code for pleural effusion.

J91.0 **Malignant pleural effusion**
Code first:
underlying neoplasm
> **DEFINITION** Dangerous fluid accumulation between the layers of the membrane lining the chest cavity and lungs, most often caused by cancers of the breast, lung, or lymph nodes.

J91.8 *Pleural effusion in other conditions classified elsewhere*
Code first underlying disease, such as:
filariasis (B74.0-B74.9)
influenza (J09.X2, J10.1, J11.1)
AHA: 2Q 2015, 16

◢ **J92** **Pleural plaque**
> **INCLUDES** pleural thickening

J92.0 **Pleural plaque with presence of asbestos**

J92.9 **Pleural plaque without asbestos**
Pleural plaque NOS

◢ **J93** **Pneumothorax and air leak**
> **EXCLUDES 1** *congenital or perinatal pneumothorax (P25.1)*
> *postprocedural air leak (J95.812)*
> *postprocedural pneumothorax (J95.811)*
> *traumatic pneumothorax (S27.0)*
> *tuberculous (current disease) pneumothorax (A15.-)*
> *pyopneumothorax (J86.-)*

J93.0 **Spontaneous tension pneumothorax**

⑤ **J93.1** **Other spontaneous pneumothorax**

J93.11 **Primary spontaneous pneumothorax**

Spontaneous tension pneumothorax

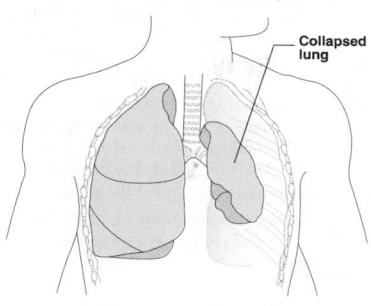

A lung collapses due to an accumulation of air or gas in the chest cavity

Collapsed lung

J93.12 **Secondary spontaneous pneumothorax**
Code first underlying condition, such as:
catamenial pneumothorax due to endometriosis (N80.8)
cystic fibrosis (E84.-)
eosinophilic pneumonia (J82)
lymphangioleiomyomatosis (J84.81)
malignant neoplasm of bronchus and lung (C34.-)
Marfan's syndrome (Q87.4)
pneumonia due to Pneumocystis carinii (B59)
secondary malignant neoplasm of lung (C78.0-)
spontaneous rupture of the esophagus (K22.3)

⑤ **J93.8** **Other pneumothorax and air leak**

J93.81 **Chronic pneumothorax**

J93.82 **Other air leak**
Persistent air leak

J93.83 **Other pneumothorax**
Acute pneumothorax
Spontaneous pneumothorax NOS

J93.9 **Pneumothorax, unspecified**
Pneumothorax NOS

◢ **J94** **Other pleural conditions**
> **EXCLUDES 1** *pleurisy NOS (R09.1)*
> *traumatic hemopneumothorax (S27.2)*
> *traumatic hemothorax (S27.1)*
> *tuberculous pleural conditions (current disease) (A15.-)*

J94.0 **Chylous effusion**
Chyliform effusion

J94.1 **Fibrothorax**

J94.2 **Hemothorax**
Hemopneumothorax

J94.8 **Other specified pleural conditions**
Hydropneumothorax
Hydrothorax

J94.9 **Pleural condition, unspecified**

Intraoperative and postprocedural complications and disorders of respiratory system, not elsewhere classified (J95)

◢ **J95** **Intraoperative and postprocedural complications and disorders of respiratory system, not elsewhere classified**
> **EXCLUDES 2** *aspiration pneumonia (J69.-)*
> *emphysema (subcutaneous) resulting from a procedure (T81.82)*
> *hypostatic pneumonia (J18.2)*
> *pulmonary manifestations due to radiation (J70.0-J70.1)*

> **CODING TIP ✓** Codes in category J95.- are complication codes and require physician documentation and confirmation of a cause and effect relationship between the procedure and the complicated condition.

⑤ **J95.0** **Tracheostomy complications**

J95.00 **Unspecified tracheostomy complication**

J95.01 **Hemorrhage from tracheostomy stoma**

● New ▲ Revised *Manifestation* ◢-⑦ Digit Indicators ▣ Laterality ▲ Adult (15+ years) Ⓜ Maternity (12-55 years) Ⓝ Newborn ▣ Pediatric (0-17 years) ♂ Male ♀ Female
✖ <del>Deleted</del> Unspecified + Additional code

+ J95.02 **Infection of tracheostomy stoma**
Use additional code to identify type of infection, such as:
cellulitis of neck (L03.8)
sepsis (A40, A41.-)
> **CODING TIP ✓** When coding J95.02, always use an additional code to indicate the infection, such as cellulitis, sepsis, or the infectious organism, when the specific information is available.

J95.03 **Malfunction of tracheostomy stoma**
Mechanical complication of tracheostomy stoma
Obstruction of tracheostomy airway
Tracheal stenosis due to tracheostomy

J95.04 **Tracheo-esophageal fistula following tracheostomy**

J95.09 **Other tracheostomy complication**

J95.1 **Acute pulmonary insufficiency following thoracic surgery**
> **EXCLUDES 2** *Functional disturbances following cardiac surgery (I97.0, I97.1-)*

J95.2 **Acute pulmonary insufficiency following nonthoracic surgery**
> **EXCLUDES 2** *Functional disturbances following cardiac surgery (I97.0, I97.1-)*

J95.3 **Chronic pulmonary insufficiency following surgery**
> **EXCLUDES 2** *Functional disturbances following cardiac surgery (I97.0, I97.1-)*

+ J95.4 **Chemical pneumonitis due to anesthesia**
Mendelson's syndrome
Postprocedural aspiration pneumonia
Use additional code for adverse effect, if applicable, to identify drug (T41.- with fifth or sixth character 5)
> **EXCLUDES 1** *aspiration pneumonitis due to anesthesia complicating labor and delivery (O74.0)*
> *aspiration pneumonitis due to anesthesia complicating pregnancy (O29)*
> *aspiration pneumonitis due to anesthesia complicating the puerperium (O89.01)*

J95.5 **Postprocedural subglottic stenosis**

🅢 J95.6 **Intraoperative hemorrhage and hematoma of a respiratory system organ or structure complicating a procedure**
> **EXCLUDES 1** *intraoperative hemorrhage and hematoma of a respiratory system organ or structure due to accidental puncture and laceration during procedure (J95.7-)*

J95.61 **Intraoperative hemorrhage and hematoma of a respiratory system organ or structure complicating a respiratory system procedure**

J95.62 **Intraoperative hemorrhage and hematoma of a respiratory system organ or structure complicating other procedure**

🅢 J95.7 **Accidental puncture and laceration of a respiratory system organ or structure during a procedure**
> **EXCLUDES 2** *postprocedural pneumothorax (J95.811)*

J95.71 **Accidental puncture and laceration of a respiratory system organ or structure during a respiratory system procedure**

J95.72 **Accidental puncture and laceration of a respiratory system organ or structure during other procedure**

🅢 J95.8 **Other intraoperative and postprocedural complications and disorders of respiratory system, not elsewhere classified**

🅖 J95.81 **Postprocedural pneumothorax and air leak**

J95.811 **Postprocedural pneumothorax**

J95.812 **Postprocedural air leak**

🅖 J95.82 **Postprocedural respiratory failure**
> **EXCLUDES 1** *Respiratory failure in other conditions (J96.-)*

J95.821 **Acute postprocedural respiratory failure**
Postprocedural respiratory failure NOS

J95.822 **Acute and chronic postprocedural respiratory failure**

▲ 🅖 J95.83 **Postprocedural hemorrhage of a respiratory system organ or structure following a procedure**

▲ J95.830 **Postprocedural hemorrhage of a respiratory system organ or structure following a respiratory system procedure**

▲ J95.831 **Postprocedural hemorrhage of a respiratory system organ or structure following other procedure**

J95.84 **Transfusion-related acute lung injury (TRALI)**

🅖 J95.85 **Complication of respirator [ventilator]**

J95.850 **Mechanical complication of respirator**
> **EXCLUDES 1** *encounter for respirator [ventilator] dependence during power failure (Z99.12)*

+ J95.851 **Ventilator associated pneumonia**
Ventilator associated pneumonitis
Use additional code to identify the organism, if known (B95.-, B96.-, B97.-)
> **EXCLUDES 1** *ventilator lung in newborn (P27.8)*

J95.859 **Other complication of respirator [ventilator]**

● 🅖 J95.86 **Postprocedural hematoma and seroma of a respiratory system organ or structure following a procedure**

● J95.860 **Postprocedural hematoma of a respiratory system organ or structure following a respiratory system procedure**

● J95.861 **Postprocedural hematoma of a respiratory system organ or structure following other procedure**

● J95.862 **Postprocedural seroma of a respiratory system organ or structure following a respiratory system procedure**

● J95.863 **Postprocedural seroma of a respiratory system organ or structure following other procedure**

J95.88 **Other intraoperative complications of respiratory system, not elsewhere classified**

+ J95.89 **Other postprocedural complications and disorders of respiratory system, not elsewhere classified**
Use additional code to identify disorder, such as:
aspiration pneumonia (J69.-)
bacterial or viral pneumonia (J12-J18)
> **EXCLUDES 2** *acute pulmonary insufficiency following thoracic surgery (J95.1)*
> *postprocedural subglottic stenosis (J95.5)*

Other diseases of the respiratory system (J96-J99)

🄳 J96 **Respiratory failure, not elsewhere classified**
> **EXCLUDES 1** *acute respiratory distress syndrome (J80)*
> *cardiorespiratory failure (R09.2)*
> *newborn respiratory distress syndrome (P22.0)*
> *postprocedural respiratory failure (J95.82-)*
> *respiratory arrest (R09.2)*
> *respiratory arrest of newborn (P28.81)*
> *respiratory failure of newborn (P28.5)*

🅢 J96.0 **Acute respiratory failure**

J96.00 **Acute respiratory failure, unspecified whether with hypoxia or hypercapnia**
AHA: 4Q 2013, 121

J96.01 **Acute respiratory failure with hypoxia**

J96.02 **Acute respiratory failure with hypercapnia**

🅢 J96.1 **Chronic respiratory failure**

J96.10 **Chronic respiratory failure, unspecified whether with hypoxia or hypercapnia**
AHA: 1Q 2016, 38
AHA: 1Q 2015, 21

J96.11 **Chronic respiratory failure with hypoxia**
AHA: 4Q 2013, 129

J96.12 **Chronic respiratory failure with hypercapnia**

🅢 J96.2 **Acute and chronic respiratory failure**
Acute on chronic respiratory failure

J96.20 **Acute and chronic respiratory failure, unspecified whether with hypoxia or hypercapnia**

J96.21 **Acute and chronic respiratory failure with hypoxia**

J96.22 **Acute and chronic respiratory failure with hypercapnia**

🅢 J96.9 **Respiratory failure, unspecified**

J96.90 **Respiratory failure, unspecified, unspecified whether with hypoxia or hypercapnia**

J96.91 **Respiratory failure, unspecified with hypoxia**

J96.92 **Respiratory failure, unspecified with hypercapnia**

● New   ▲ Revised   *Manifestation*   🄳-🆅 Digit Indicators   ▣ Laterality   🄰 Adult (15+ years)   Ⓜ Maternity (12-55 years)   Ⓝ Newborn   🄿 Pediatric (0-17 years)   ♂ Male   ♀ Female
✖ ~~Deleted~~   Unspecified   + Additional code

688   © 2017 DecisionHealth   2017 ICD-10-CM Expert for Physicians

Diseases of the Respiratory System

J95.02 — J96.92

▲ ◢ + **J98**   **Other respiratory disorders**
Use additional code to identify:
exposure to environmental tobacco smoke (Z77.22)
exposure to tobacco smoke in the perinatal period (P96.81)
history of tobacco dependence (Z87.891)
occupational exposure to environmental tobacco smoke
(Z57.31)
tobacco dependence (F17.-)
tobacco use (Z72.0)
EXCLUDES 1   *newborn apnea (P28.4)*
newborn sleep apnea (P28.3)
EXCLUDES 2   *apnea NOS (R06.81)*
sleep apnea (G47.3-)

◢ + **J98.0**   **Diseases of bronchus, not elsewhere classified**
+ **J98.01**   **Acute bronchospasm**
EXCLUDES 1   *acute bronchiolitis with bronchospasm*
(J21.-)
acute bronchitis with bronchospasm
(J20.-)
asthma (J45.-)
exercise induced bronchospasm
(J45.990)
DEFINITION   Constriction or contraction of the
smooth muscle in the large air passages, severely
limiting airflow.

+ **J98.09**   **Other diseases of bronchus, not elsewhere classified**
Broncholithiasis
Calcification of bronchus
Stenosis of bronchus
Tracheobronchial collapse
Tracheobronchial dyskinesia
Ulcer of bronchus

◢ + **J98.1**   **Pulmonary collapse**
EXCLUDES 1   *therapeutic collapse of lung status (Z98.3)*

+ **J98.11**   **Atelectasis**
EXCLUDES 1   *newborn atelectasis*
tuberculous atelectasis
(current disease) (A15)

+ **J98.19**   **Other pulmonary collapse**
+ **J98.2**   **Interstitial emphysema**
Mediastinal emphysema
EXCLUDES 1   *emphysema NOS (J43.9)*
emphysema in newborn (P25.0)
surgical emphysema (subcutaneous)
(T81.82)
traumatic subcutaneous emphysema (T79.7)

+ **J98.3**   **Compensatory emphysema**
+ **J98.4**   **Other disorders of lung**
Calcification of lung
Cystic lung disease (acquired)
Lung disease NOS
Pulmolithiasis
EXCLUDES 1   *acute interstitial pneumonitis (J84.114)*
pulmonary insufficiency following surgery
(J95.1-J95.2)

▲ ◢ + **J98.5**   **Diseases of mediastinum, not elsewhere classified**
EXCLUDES 2   *abscess of mediastinum (J85.3)*

● + **J98.51**   **Mediastinitis**
Code first:
underlying condition, if applicable, such as
postoperative mediastinitis (T81.-)

● + **J98.59**   **Other diseases of mediastinum, not elsewhere classified**
Fibrosis of mediastinum
Hernia of mediastinum
Retraction of mediastinum

+ **J98.6**   **Disorders of diaphragm**
Diaphragmatitis
Paralysis of diaphragm
Relaxation of diaphragm
EXCLUDES 1   *congenital malformation of diaphragm NEC*
(Q79.1)
congenital diaphragmatic hernia (Q79.0)
EXCLUDES 2   *diaphragmatic hernia (K44.-)*

+ **J98.8**   **Other specified respiratory disorders**
+ **J98.9**   **Respiratory disorder, unspecified**
Respiratory disease (chronic) NOS

J99   *Respiratory disorders in diseases classified elsewhere*
Code first underlying disease, such as:
amyloidosis (E85.-)
ankylosing spondylitis (M45)
congenital syphilis (A50.5)
cryoglobulinemia (D89.1)
early congenital syphilis (A50.0)
schistosomiasis (B65.0-B65.9)
EXCLUDES 1   *respiratory disorders in:*
amebiasis (A06.5)
blastomycosis (B40.0-B40.2)
candidiasis (B37.1)
coccidioidomycosis (B38.0-B38.2)
cystic fibrosis with pulmonary manifestations
(E84.0)
dermatomyositis (M33.01, M33.11)
histoplasmosis (B39.0-B39.2)
late syphilis (A52.72, A52.73)
polymyositis (M33.21)
sicca syndrome (M35.02)
systemic lupus erythematosus (M32.13)
systemic sclerosis (M34.81)
Wegener's granulomatosis (M31.30-M31.31)

● New   ▲ Revised   *Manifestation*   ◢-◢ Digit Indicators   ⊟ Laterality   ◮ Adult   Ⓜ Maternity   Ⓝ Newborn   Ⓟ Pediatric   ♂ Male   ♀ Female
✖ Deleted   Unspecified   + Additional code   (15+ years)   (12-55 years)   (0-17 years)

2017 ICD-10-CM Expert for Physicians

© 2017 DecisionHealth   689

Diseases of the Respiratory System

J98 — J99

CHAPTER 11: DISEASES OF THE DIGESTIVE SYSTEM (K00-K95)

EXCLUDES 2   *certain conditions originating in the perinatal period (P04-P96)*
certain infectious and parasitic diseases (A00-B99)
complications of pregnancy, childbirth and the puerperium (O00-O9A)
congenital malformations, deformations and chromosomal abnormalities (Q00-Q99)
endocrine, nutritional and metabolic diseases (E00-E88)
injury, poisoning and certain other consequences of external causes (S00-T88)
neoplasms (C00-D49)
symptoms, signs and abnormal clinical and laboratory findings, not elsewhere classified (R00-R94)

This chapter contains the following blocks:

Diseases of oral cavity and salivary glands (K00-K14)

④ K00   Disorders of tooth development and eruption
> **EXCLUDES 2**   *embedded and impacted teeth (K01.-)*

Oral cavity anatomy

Soft palate
Hard palate
Uvula
Palatine tonsil
Lingual tonsil
Epiglottis
Teeth
Lips
Tongue

K00.0   Anodontia
Hypodontia
Oligodontia
> **EXCLUDES 1**   *acquired absence of teeth (K08.1-)*

> **DEFINITION**   Defect in which many or all of the teeth do not develop and are absent from the mouth.

K00.1   Supernumerary teeth
Distomolar
Fourth molar
Mesiodens
Paramolar
Supplementary teeth
> **EXCLUDES 2**   *supernumerary roots (K00.2)*

K00.2   Abnormalities of size and form of teeth
Concrescence of teeth
Fusion of teeth
Gemination of teeth
Dens evaginatus
Dens in dente
Dens invaginatus
Enamel pearls
Macrodontia
Microdontia
Peg-shaped [conical] teeth
Supernumerary roots
Taurodontism
Tuberculum paramolare
> **EXCLUDES 1**   *abnormalities of teeth due to congenital syphilis (A50.5)*
> *tuberculum Carabelli, which is regarded as a normal variation and should not be coded*

K00.3   Mottled teeth
Dental fluorosis
Mottling of enamel
Nonfluoride enamel opacities
> **EXCLUDES 2**   *deposits [accretions] on teeth (K03.6)*

K00.4   Disturbances in tooth formation
Aplasia and hypoplasia of cementum
Dilaceration of tooth
Enamel hypoplasia (neonatal) (postnatal) (prenatal)
Regional odontodysplasia
Turner's tooth
> **EXCLUDES 1**   *Hutchinson's teeth and mulberry molars in congenital syphilis (A50.5)*
> **EXCLUDES 2**   *mottled teeth (K00.3)*

K00.5   Hereditary disturbances in tooth structure, not elsewhere classified
Amelogenesis imperfecta
Dentinogenesis imperfecta
Odontogenesis imperfecta
Dentinal dysplasia
Shell teeth

K00.6   Disturbances in tooth eruption
Dentia praecox
Natal tooth
Neonatal tooth
Premature eruption of tooth
Premature shedding of primary [deciduous] tooth
Prenatal teeth
Retained [persistent] primary tooth
> **EXCLUDES 2**   *embedded and impacted teeth (K01.-)*

K00.7   Teething syndrome

K00.8   Other disorders of tooth development
Color changes during tooth formation
Intrinsic staining of teeth NOS
> **EXCLUDES 2**   *posteruptive color changes (K03.7)*

K00.9   Disorder of tooth development, unspecified
Disorder of odontogenesis NOS

④ K01   Embedded and impacted teeth
> **EXCLUDES 1**   *abnormal position of fully erupted teeth (M26.3-)*

K01.0   Embedded teeth

K01.1   Impacted teeth

▲ ④ K02   Dental caries
> **INCLUDES**   caries of dentine
> dental cavities
> early childhood caries
> pre-eruptive caries
> recurrent caries (dentino enamel junction) (enamel) (to the pulp)
> tooth decay

K02.3   Arrested dental caries
Arrested coronal and root caries

⑤ K02.5   Dental caries on pit and fissure surface
Dental caries on chewing surface of tooth

K02.51   Dental caries on pit and fissure surface limited to enamel
White spot lesions [initial caries] on pit and fissure surface of tooth

● New   ▲ Revised   *Manifestation*   ④-⑦ Digit Indicators   ⊟ Laterality   Ⓐ Adult (15+ years)   Ⓜ Maternity (12-55 years)   Ⓝ Newborn   Ⓟ Pediatric (0-17 years)   ♂ Male   ♀ Female
✖ Deleted   Unspecified   + Additional code

2017 ICD-10-CM Expert for Physicians

© 2017 DecisionHealth

691

K00 — K02.51

▲ K02.52 **Dental caries on pit and fissure surface penetrating into dentin**
Primary dental caries, cervical origin

K02.53 **Dental caries on pit and fissure surface penetrating into pulp**

⑤ K02.6 **Dental caries on smooth surface**

K02.61 **Dental caries on smooth surface limited to enamel**
White spot lesions [initial caries] on smooth surface of tooth

K02.62 **Dental caries on smooth surface penetrating into dentin**

K02.63 **Dental caries on smooth surface penetrating into pulp**

K02.7 **Dental root caries**

K02.9 **Dental caries, unspecified**

④ **K03** **Other diseases of hard tissues of teeth**
EXCLUDES 2	*bruxism (F45.8)*
	dental caries (K02.-)
	teeth-grinding NOS (F45.8)

K03.0 **Excessive attrition of teeth**
Approximal wear of teeth
Occlusal wear of teeth
DEFINITION Teeth exhibit excessive wear and tear as a result of tooth-to-tooth contact, often due to grinding the teeth.

K03.1 **Abrasion of teeth**
Dentifrice abrasion of teeth
Habitual abrasion of teeth
Occupational abrasion of teeth
Ritual abrasion of teeth
Traditional abrasion of teeth
Wedge defect NOS
DEFINITION Teeth exhibit specific wear and tear as a result of tooth contact with another object.

K03.2 **Erosion of teeth**
Erosion of teeth due to diet
Erosion of teeth due to drugs and medicaments
Erosion of teeth due to persistent vomiting
Erosion of teeth NOS
Idiopathic erosion of teeth
Occupational erosion of teeth

K03.3 **Pathological resorption of teeth**
Internal granuloma of pulp
Resorption of teeth (external)

K03.4 **Hypercementosis**
Cementation hyperplasia

K03.5 **Ankylosis of teeth**
DEFINITION Roots of the teeth grow into and merge with the bone of the jaw; most often occurring during development of baby teeth.

K03.6 **Deposits [accretions] on teeth**
Betel deposits [accretions] on teeth
Black deposits [accretions] on teeth
Extrinsic staining of teeth NOS
Green deposits [accretions] on teeth
Materia alba deposits [accretions] on teeth
Orange deposits [accretions] on teeth
Staining of teeth NOS
Subgingival dental calculus
Supragingival dental calculus
Tobacco deposits [accretions] on teeth
DEFINITION Calculous deposits or tartar build-up that resists removal by normal brushing and requires professional cleaning.

K03.7 **Posteruptive color changes of dental hard tissues**
| EXCLUDES 2 | *deposits [accretions] on teeth (K03.6)* |

⑤ K03.8 **Other specified diseases of hard tissues of teeth**

K03.81 **Cracked tooth**
| EXCLUDES 1 | *asymptomatic craze lines in enamel - omit code* |
| | *broken or fractured tooth due to trauma (S02.5)* |

K03.89 **Other specified diseases of hard tissues of teeth**

K03.9 **Disease of hard tissues of teeth, unspecified**

④ **K04** **Diseases of pulp and periapical tissues**

▲ ⑤ K04.0 **Pulpitis**
Acute pulpitis
Chronic (hyperplastic) (ulcerative) pulpitis
DEFINITION Painful inflammation of the soft living tissue containing nerves within the center of the tooth.

● K04.01 **Reversible pulpitis**

● K04.02 **Irreversible pulpitis**

K04.1 **Necrosis of pulp**
Pulpal gangrene

K04.2 **Pulp degeneration**
Denticles
Pulpal calcifications
Pulpal stones

K04.3 **Abnormal hard tissue formation in pulp**
Secondary or irregular dentine

K04.4 **Acute apical periodontitis of pulpal origin**
Acute apical periodontitis NOS
| EXCLUDES 1 | *acute periodontitis (K05.2-)* |

DEFINITION Severe inflammation of the periodontal ligament connecting the tooth to the jawbone due to infection or necrosis of the soft, living tissue in the center of the tooth.

K04.5 **Chronic apical periodontitis**
Apical or periapical granuloma
Apical periodontitis NOS
| EXCLUDES 1 | *chronic periodontitis (K05.3-)* |

K04.6 **Periapical abscess with sinus**
Dental abscess with sinus
Dentoalveolar abscess with sinus

K04.7 **Periapical abscess without sinus**
Dental abscess without sinus
Dentoalveolar abscess without sinus
Periapical abscess without sinus

K04.8 **Radicular cyst**
Apical (periodontal) cyst
Periapical cyst
Residual radicular cyst
| EXCLUDES 2 | *lateral periodontal cyst (K09.0)* |

⑤ K04.9 **Other and unspecified diseases of pulp and periapical tissues**

K04.90 **Unspecified diseases of pulp and periapical tissues**

K04.99 **Other diseases of pulp and periapical tissues**

▲ ④ + **K05** **Gingivitis and periodontal diseases**
Use additional code to identify:
alcohol abuse and dependence (F10.-)
exposure to environmental tobacco smoke (Z77.22)
exposure to tobacco smoke in the perinatal period (P96.81)
history of tobacco dependence (Z87.891)
occupational exposure to environmental tobacco smoke (Z57.31)
tobacco dependence (F17.-)
tobacco use (Z72.0)

⑤ + K05.0 **Acute gingivitis**
| EXCLUDES 1 | *acute necrotizing ulcerative gingivitis (A69.1)* |
| | *herpesviral [herpes simplex] gingivostomatitis (B00.2)* |

● New   ▲ Revised   *Manifestation*   ④-⑦ Digit Indicators   ▤ Laterality   Ⓐ Adult (15+ years)   Ⓜ Maternity (12-55 years)   Ⓝ Newborn   Ⓟ Pediatric (0-17 years)   ♂ Male   ♀ Female
✖ Deleted   Unspecified   + Additional code

692   © 2017 DecisionHealth   2017 ICD-10-CM Expert for Physicians

▲ + **K05.00** **Acute gingivitis, plaque induced**
Acute gingivitis NOS
Plaque induced gingival disease

Acute gingivitis

An inflammation of the gums
caused by a bacterial infection

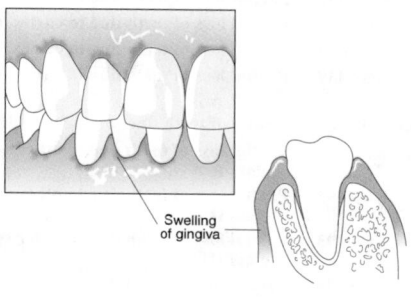

Swelling
of gingiva

+ **K05.01** **Acute gingivitis, non-plaque induced**
▲ ⑤ + **K05.1** **Chronic gingivitis**
Desquamative gingivitis (chronic)
Gingivitis (chronic) NOS
Hyperplastic gingivitis (chronic)
Pregnancy associated gingivitis
Simple marginal gingivitis (chronic)
Ulcerative gingivitis (chronic)
Code first:
, if applicable, diseases of the digestive system
complicating pregnancy (O99.61-)

+ **K05.10** **Chronic gingivitis, plaque induced**
Chronic gingivitis NOS
Gingivitis NOS

+ **K05.11** **Chronic gingivitis, non-plaque induced**
⑤ + **K05.2** **Aggressive periodontitis**
Acute pericoronitis
EXCLUDES 1 *acute apical periodontitis (K04.4)*
periapical abscess (K04.7)
periapical abscess with sinus (K04.6)

+ **K05.20** **Aggressive periodontitis, unspecified**
DEFINITION Serious and destructive
inflammation and infection of the ligaments and
bones supporting the teeth, leading to tooth loss.

▲ ⑥ + **K05.21** **Aggressive periodontitis, localized**
Periodontal abscess

● + **K05.211** **Aggressive periodontitis, localized, slight**
● + **K05.212** **Aggressive periodontitis, localized, moderate**
● + **K05.213** **Aggressive periodontitis, localized, severe**
● + **K05.219** **Aggressive periodontitis, localized, unspecified
severity**

▲ ⑥ + **K05.22** **Aggressive periodontitis, generalized**
● + **K05.221** **Aggressive periodontitis, generalized, slight**
● + **K05.222** **Aggressive periodontitis, generalized, moderate**
● + **K05.223** **Aggressive periodontitis, generalized, severe**
● + **K05.229** **Aggressive periodontitis, generalized,
unspecified severity**

⑤ + **K05.3** **Chronic periodontitis**
Chronic pericoronitis
Complex periodontitis
Periodontitis NOS
Simplex periodontitis
EXCLUDES 1 *chronic apical periodontitis (K04.5)*

+ **K05.30** **Chronic periodontitis, unspecified**
▲ ⑥ + **K05.31** **Chronic periodontitis, localized**
● + **K05.311** **Chronic periodontitis, localized, slight**
● + **K05.312** **Chronic periodontitis, localized, moderate**
● + **K05.313** **Chronic periodontitis, localized, severe**
● + **K05.319** **Chronic periodontitis, localized, unspecified
severity**

▲ ⑥ + **K05.32** **Chronic periodontitis, generalized**
● + **K05.321** **Chronic periodontitis, generalized, slight**
● + **K05.322** **Chronic periodontitis, generalized, moderate**

● + **K05.323** **Chronic periodontitis, generalized, severe**
● + **K05.329** **Chronic periodontitis, generalized, unspecified
severity**

+ **K05.4** **Periodontosis**
Juvenile periodontosis

▲ + **K05.5** **Other periodontal diseases**
Combined periodontic-endodontic lesion
Narrow gingival width (of periodontal soft tissue)
EXCLUDES 2 *leukoplakia of gingiva (K13.21)*

+ **K05.6** **Periodontal disease, unspecified**

④ **K06** **Other disorders of gingiva and edentulous alveolar
ridge**
EXCLUDES 2 *acute gingivitis (K05.0)*
atrophy of edentulous alveolar ridge (K08.2)
chronic gingivitis (K05.1)
gingivitis NOS (K05.1)

K06.0 **Gingival recession**
Gingival recession (generalized) (localized) (postinfective)
(postprocedural)
DEFINITION Gums that have receded, exposing
more tooth.

K06.1 **Gingival enlargement**
Gingival fibromatosis

+ **K06.2** **Gingival and edentulous alveolar ridge lesions associated
with trauma**
Irritative hyperplasia of edentulous ridge [denture
hyperplasia]
*Use additional code (Chapter 20) to identify external cause
or denture status (Z97.2)*

● **K06.3** **Horizontal alveolar bone loss**
▲ **K06.8** **Other specified disorders of gingiva and edentulous
alveolar ridge**
Fibrous epulis
Flabby alveolar ridge
Giant cell epulis
Peripheral giant cell granuloma of gingiva
Pyogenic granuloma of gingiva
Vertical ridge deficiency
EXCLUDES 2 *gingival cyst (K09.0)*

K06.9 **Disorder of gingiva and edentulous alveolar ridge,
unspecified**

④ **K08** **Other disorders of teeth and supporting structures**
EXCLUDES 2 *dentofacial anomalies [including malocclusion]
(M26.-)*
disorders of jaw (M27.-)

K08.0 **Exfoliation of teeth due to systemic causes**
Code also:
underlying systemic condition

⑤ **K08.1** **Complete loss of teeth**
Acquired loss of teeth, complete
EXCLUDES 1 *congenital absence of teeth (K00.0)*
*exfoliation of teeth due to systemic causes
(K08.0)*
partial loss of teeth (K08.4-)

⑥ **K08.10** **Complete loss of teeth, unspecified cause**
K08.101 **Complete loss of teeth, unspecified cause, class I**
K08.102 **Complete loss of teeth, unspecified cause, class
II**
K08.103 **Complete loss of teeth, unspecified cause, class
III**
K08.104 **Complete loss of teeth, unspecified cause, class
IV**
K08.109 **Complete loss of teeth, unspecified cause,
unspecified class**
Edentulism NOS

⑥ **K08.11** **Complete loss of teeth due to trauma**
K08.111 **Complete loss of teeth due to trauma, class I**
K08.112 **Complete loss of teeth due to trauma, class II**
K08.113 **Complete loss of teeth due to trauma, class III**
K08.114 **Complete loss of teeth due to trauma, class IV**
K08.119 **Complete loss of teeth due to trauma,
unspecified class**

⑥ **K08.12** **Complete loss of teeth due to periodontal diseases**
K08.121 **Complete loss of teeth due to periodontal
diseases, class I**

● New ▲ Revised *Manifestation* ④-⑦ Digit Indicators ▭ Laterality ▣ Adult ▣ Maternity ▣ Newborn ▣ Pediatric ♂ Male ♀ Female
✖ Deleted Unspecified + Additional code (15+ years) (12-55 years) (0-17 years)

K08.122   **Complete loss of teeth due to periodontal diseases, class II**

K08.123   **Complete loss of teeth due to periodontal diseases, class III**

K08.124   **Complete loss of teeth due to periodontal diseases, class IV**

K08.129   **Complete loss of teeth due to periodontal diseases, unspecified class**

⑥ K08.13   **Complete loss of teeth due to caries**

K08.131   **Complete loss of teeth due to caries, class I**

K08.132   **Complete loss of teeth due to caries, class II**

K08.133   **Complete loss of teeth due to caries, class III**

K08.134   **Complete loss of teeth due to caries, class IV**

K08.139   **Complete loss of teeth due to caries, unspecified class**

⑥ K08.19   **Complete loss of teeth due to other specified cause**

K08.191   **Complete loss of teeth due to other specified cause, class I**

K08.192   **Complete loss of teeth due to other specified cause, class II**

K08.193   **Complete loss of teeth due to other specified cause, class III**

K08.194   **Complete loss of teeth due to other specified cause, class IV**

K08.199   **Complete loss of teeth due to other specified cause, unspecified class**

⑤ K08.2   **Atrophy of edentulous alveolar ridge**

K08.20   **Unspecified atrophy of edentulous alveolar ridge**
Atrophy of the mandible NOS
Atrophy of the maxilla NOS

K08.21   **Minimal atrophy of the mandible**
Minimal atrophy of the edentulous mandible

K08.22   **Moderate atrophy of the mandible**
Moderate atrophy of the edentulous mandible

K08.23   **Severe atrophy of the mandible**
Severe atrophy of the edentulous mandible

K08.24   **Minimal atrophy of maxilla**
Minimal atrophy of the edentulous maxilla

K08.25   **Moderate atrophy of the maxilla**
Moderate atrophy of the edentulous maxilla

K08.26   **Severe atrophy of the maxilla**
Severe atrophy of the edentulous maxilla

K08.3   **Retained dental root**

DEFINITION   Part or all of the root structure of a tooth remains in the jaw after the tooth is extracted or otherwise lost.

⑤ K08.4   **Partial loss of teeth**
Acquired loss of teeth, partial

EXCLUDES 1   *complete loss of teeth (K08.1-)*
congenital absence of teeth (K00.0)

EXCLUDES 2   *exfoliation of teeth due to systemic causes (K08.0)*

⑥ K08.40   **Partial loss of teeth, unspecified cause**

K08.401   **Partial loss of teeth, unspecified cause, class I**

K08.402   **Partial loss of teeth, unspecified cause, class II**

K08.403   **Partial loss of teeth, unspecified cause, class III**

K08.404   **Partial loss of teeth, unspecified cause, class IV**

K08.409   **Partial loss of teeth, unspecified cause, unspecified class**
Tooth extraction status NOS

⑥ K08.41   **Partial loss of teeth due to trauma**

K08.411   **Partial loss of teeth due to trauma, class I**

K08.412   **Partial loss of teeth due to trauma, class II**

K08.413   **Partial loss of teeth due to trauma, class III**

K08.414   **Partial loss of teeth due to trauma, class IV**

K08.419   **Partial loss of teeth due to trauma, unspecified class**

⑥ K08.42   **Partial loss of teeth due to periodontal diseases**

K08.421   **Partial loss of teeth due to periodontal diseases, class I**

K08.422   **Partial loss of teeth due to periodontal diseases, class II**

K08.423   **Partial loss of teeth due to periodontal diseases, class III**

K08.424   **Partial loss of teeth due to periodontal diseases, class IV**

K08.429   **Partial loss of teeth due to periodontal diseases, unspecified class**

⑥ K08.43   **Partial loss of teeth due to caries**

K08.431   **Partial loss of teeth due to caries, class I**

K08.432   **Partial loss of teeth due to caries, class II**

K08.433   **Partial loss of teeth due to caries, class III**

K08.434   **Partial loss of teeth due to caries, class IV**

K08.439   **Partial loss of teeth due to caries, unspecified class**

⑥ K08.49   **Partial loss of teeth due to other specified cause**

K08.491   **Partial loss of teeth due to other specified cause, class I**

K08.492   **Partial loss of teeth due to other specified cause, class II**

K08.493   **Partial loss of teeth due to other specified cause, class III**

K08.494   **Partial loss of teeth due to other specified cause, class IV**

K08.499   **Partial loss of teeth due to other specified cause, unspecified class**

⑤ K08.5   **Unsatisfactory restoration of tooth**
Defective bridge, crown, filling
Defective dental restoration

EXCLUDES 1   *dental restoration status (Z98.811)*

EXCLUDES 2   *endosseous dental implant failure (M27.6-)*
unsatisfactory endodontic treatment (M27.5-)

K08.50   **Unsatisfactory restoration of tooth, unspecified**
Defective dental restoration NOS

K08.51   **Open restoration margins of tooth**
Dental restoration failure of marginal integrity
Open margin on tooth restoration
Poor gingival margin to tooth restoration

K08.52   **Unrepairable overhanging of dental restorative materials**
Overhanging of tooth restoration

⑥ K08.53   **Fractured dental restorative material**

EXCLUDES 1   *cracked tooth (K03.81)*
traumatic fracture of tooth (S02.5)

K08.530   **Fractured dental restorative material without loss of material**

K08.531   **Fractured dental restorative material with loss of material**

K08.539   **Fractured dental restorative material, unspecified**

K08.54   **Contour of existing restoration of tooth biologically incompatible with oral health**
Dental restoration failure of periodontal anatomical integrity
Unacceptable contours of existing restoration of tooth
Unacceptable morphology of existing restoration of tooth

➕ K08.55   **Allergy to existing dental restorative material**
Use additional code to identify the specific type of allergy

K08.56   **Poor aesthetic of existing restoration of tooth**
Dental restoration aesthetically inadequate or displeasing

K08.59   **Other unsatisfactory restoration of tooth**
Other defective dental restoration

▲ ⑤ K08.8   **Other specified disorders of teeth and supporting structures**

● K08.81   **Primary occlusal trauma**

● K08.82   **Secondary occlusal trauma**

● K08.89   **Other specified disorders of teeth and supporting structures**
Enlargement of alveolar ridge NOS
Insufficient anatomic crown height
Insufficient clinical crown length
Irregular alveolar process
Toothache NOS

K08.9   **Disorder of teeth and supporting structures, unspecified**

● New   ▲ Revised   *Manifestation*   ❹-❼ Digit Indicators   ▤ Laterality   Ⓐ Adult (15+ years)   Ⓜ Maternity (12-55 years)   Ⓝ Newborn   Ⓟ Pediatric (0-17 years)   ♂ Male   ♀ Female

✖ Deleted   Unspecified   ➕ Additional code

◢ **K09** **Cysts of oral region, not elsewhere classified**

INCLUDES lesions showing histological features both of
aneurysmal cyst and of another fibro-osseous
lesion

EXCLUDES 2 *cysts of jaw (M27.0-, M27.4-)*
radicular cyst (K04.8)

K09.0 **Developmental odontogenic cysts**
Dentigerous cyst
Eruption cyst
Follicular cyst
Gingival cyst
Lateral periodontal cyst
Primordial cyst

EXCLUDES 2 *keratocysts (D16.4, D16.5)*
odontogenic keratocystic tumors
(D16.4, D16.5)

K09.1 **Developmental (nonodontogenic) cysts of oral region**
Cyst (of) incisive canal
Cyst (of) palatine of papilla
Globulomaxillary cyst
Median palatal cyst
Nasoalveolar cyst
Nasolabial cyst
Nasopalatine duct cyst

K09.8 **Other cysts of oral region, not elsewhere classified**
Dermoid cyst
Epidermoid cyst
Lymphoepithelial cyst
Epstein's pearl

K09.9 **Cyst of oral region, unspecified**

▲◢ **+ K11** **Diseases of salivary glands**
Use additional code to identify:
alcohol abuse and dependence (F10.-)
exposure to environmental tobacco smoke (Z77.22)
exposure to tobacco smoke in the perinatal period (P96.81)
history of tobacco dependence (Z87.891)
occupational exposure to environmental tobacco smoke
(Z57.31)
tobacco dependence (F17.-)
tobacco use (Z72.0)

+ K11.0 **Atrophy of salivary gland**

DEFINITION Wasting of the saliva glands, resulting
in insufficient saliva production.

+ K11.1 **Hypertrophy of salivary gland**

ⓢ **+ K11.2** **Sialoadenitis**
Parotitis

EXCLUDES 1 *epidemic parotitis (B26.-)*
mumps (B26.-)
uveoparotid fever [Heerfordt] (D86.89)

+ K11.20 **Sialoadenitis, unspecified**

+ K11.21 **Acute sialoadenitis**

EXCLUDES 1 *acute recurrent sialoadenitis (K11.22)*

+ K11.22 **Acute recurrent sialoadenitis**

+ K11.23 **Chronic sialoadenitis**

+ K11.3 **Abscess of salivary gland**

+ K11.4 **Fistula of salivary gland**

EXCLUDES 1 *congenital fistula of salivary gland (Q38.4)*

+ K11.5 **Sialolithiasis**
Calculus of salivary gland or duct
Stone of salivary gland or duct

+ K11.6 **Mucocele of salivary gland**
Mucous extravasation cyst of salivary gland
Mucous retention cyst of salivary gland
Ranula

Mucocele of salivary gland

A type of cyst filled with mucous caused by
the rupturing of a salivary gland duct

Cyst

+ K11.7 **Disturbances of salivary secretion**
Hypoptyalism
Ptyalism
Xerostomia

EXCLUDES 2 *dry mouth NOS (R68.2)*

+ K11.8 **Other diseases of salivary glands**
Benign lymphoepithelial lesion of salivary gland
Mikulicz' disease
Necrotizing sialometaplasia
Sialectasia
Stenosis of salivary duct
Stricture of salivary duct

EXCLUDES 1 *sicca syndrome [Sjögren] (M35.0-)*

+ K11.9 **Disease of salivary gland, unspecified**
Sialoadenopathy NOS

▲◢ **+ K12** **Stomatitis and related lesions**
Use additional code to identify:
alcohol abuse and dependence (F10.-)
exposure to environmental tobacco smoke (Z77.22)
exposure to tobacco smoke in the perinatal period (P96.81)
history of tobacco dependence (Z87.891)
occupational exposure to environmental tobacco smoke
(Z57.31)
tobacco dependence (F17.-)
tobacco use (Z72.0)

EXCLUDES 1 *cancrum oris (A69.0)*
cheilitis (K13.0)
gangrenous stomatitis (A69.0)
herpesviral [herpes simplex] gingivostomatitis
(B00.2)
noma (A69.0)

+ K12.0 **Recurrent oral aphthae**
Aphthous stomatitis (major) (minor)
Bednar's aphthae
Periadenitis mucosa necrotica recurrens
Recurrent aphthous ulcer
Stomatitis herpetiformis

+ K12.1 **Other forms of stomatitis**
Stomatitis NOS
Denture stomatitis
Ulcerative stomatitis
Vesicular stomatitis

EXCLUDES 1 *acute necrotizing ulcerative stomatitis*
(A69.1)
Vincent's stomatitis (A69.1)

DEFINITION Painful inflammation of the mucosal soft
tissues of the mouth, usually from a viral infection that
can lead to ulcers or vesicular lesions.

+ K12.2 **Cellulitis and abscess of mouth**
Cellulitis of mouth (floor)
Submandibular abscess

EXCLUDES 2 *abscess of salivary gland (K11.3)*
abscess of tongue (K14.0)
periapical abscess (K04.6-K04.7)
periodontal abscess (K05.21)
peritonsillar abscess (J36)

● New   ▲ Revised   *Manifestation*   ◢-◪ Digit Indicators   ▤ Laterality   Ⓐ Adult (15+ years)   Ⓜ Maternity (12-55 years)   Ⓝ Newborn   Ⓟ Pediatric (0-17 years)   ♂ Male   ♀ Female
✖ ~~Deleted~~   Unspecified   + Additional code

2017 ICD-10-CM Expert for Physicians

© 2017 DecisionHealth

695

Diseases of the Digestive System

⑤+ K12.3 Oral mucositis (ulcerative)
Mucositis (oral) (oropharyneal)

> EXCLUDES 2   *gastrointestinal mucositis (ulcerative)*
> *(K92.81)*
> *mucositis (ulcerative) of vagina and vulva*
> *(N76.81)*
> *nasal mucositis (ulcerative) (J34.81)*

+ K12.30 Oral mucositis (ulcerative), unspecified

+ K12.31 Oral mucositis (ulcerative) due to antineoplastic therapy
Use additional code for adverse effect, if applicable, to identify antineoplastic and immunosuppressive drugs (T45.1X5)
Use additional code for other antineoplastic therapy, such as:
radiological procedure and radiotherapy (Y84.2)

+ K12.32 Oral mucositis (ulcerative) due to other drugs
Use additional code for adverse effect, if applicable, to identify drug (T36-T50 with fifth or sixth character 5)

+ K12.33 Oral mucositis (ulcerative) due to radiation
Use additional external cause code (W88-W90, X39.0-) to identify cause

+ K12.39 Other oral mucositis (ulcerative)
Viral oral mucositis (ulcerative)

▲ ④+ K13 Other diseases of lip and oral mucosa

> INCLUDES   epithelial disturbances of tongue

Use additional code to identify:
alcohol abuse and dependence (F10.-)
exposure to environmental tobacco smoke (Z77.22)
exposure to tobacco smoke in the perinatal period (P96.81)
history of tobacco dependence (Z87.891)
occupational exposure to environmental tobacco smoke (Z57.31)
tobacco dependence (F17.-)
tobacco use (Z72.0)

> EXCLUDES 2   *certain disorders of gingiva and edentulous*
> *alveolar ridge (K05-K06)*
> *cysts of oral region (K09.-)*
> *diseases of tongue (K14.-)*
> *stomatitis and related lesions (K12.-)*

+ K13.0 Diseases of lips
Abscess of lips
Angular cheilitis
Cellulitis of lips
Cheilitis NOS
Cheilodynia
Cheilosis
Exfoliative cheilitis
Fistula of lips
Glandular cheilitis
Hypertrophy of lips
Perlèche NEC

> EXCLUDES 1   *ariboflavinosis (E53.0)*
> *cheilitis due to radiation-related disorders*
> *(L55-L59)*
> *congenital fistula of lips (Q38.0)*
> *congenital hypertrophy of lips (Q18.6)*
> *Perlèche due to candidiasis (B37.83)*
> *Perlèche due to riboflavin deficiency*
> *(E53.0)*

+ K13.1 Cheek and lip biting

⑤+ K13.2 Leukoplakia and other disturbances of oral epithelium, including tongue

> EXCLUDES 1   *carcinoma in situ of oral epithelium*
> *(D00.0-)*
> *hairy leukoplakia (K13.3)*

+ K13.21 Leukoplakia of oral mucosa, including tongue
Leukokeratosis of oral mucosa
Leukoplakia of gingiva, lips, tongue

> EXCLUDES 1   *hairy leukoplakia (K13.3)*
> *leukokeratosis nicotina palati*
> *(K13.24)*

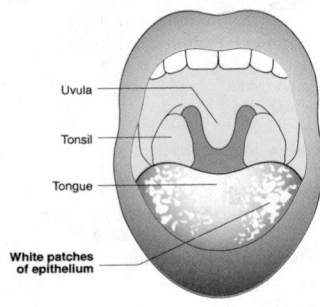

Leukoplakia of oral mucosa, including tongue

Uvula
Tonsil
Tongue
White patches of epithelium

+ K13.22 Minimal keratinized residual ridge mucosa
Minimal keratinization of alveolar ridge mucosa

+ K13.23 Excessive keratinized residual ridge mucosa
Excessive keratinization of alveolar ridge mucosa

+ K13.24 Leukokeratosis nicotina palati
Smoker's palate

+ K13.29 Other disturbances of oral epithelium, including tongue
Erythroplakia of mouth or tongue
Focal epithelial hyperplasia of mouth or tongue
Leukoedema of mouth or tongue
Other oral epithelium disturbances

+ K13.3 Hairy leukoplakia

+ K13.4 Granuloma and granuloma-like lesions of oral mucosa
Eosinophilic granuloma
Granuloma pyogenicum
Verrucous xanthoma

+ K13.5 Oral submucous fibrosis
Submucous fibrosis of tongue

> DEFINITION   Build-up of fibrous (scar-like) tissue within the soft tissues of the mouth, causing rigidity and inability to open the mouth.

+ K13.6 Irritative hyperplasia of oral mucosa

> EXCLUDES 2   *irritative hyperplasia of edentulous ridge [denture hyperplasia] (K06.2)*

⑤+ K13.7 Other and unspecified lesions of oral mucosa

+ K13.70 Unspecified lesions of oral mucosa

+ K13.79 Other lesions of oral mucosa
Focal oral mucinosis

▲ ④+ K14 Diseases of tongue
Use additional code to identify:
alcohol abuse and dependence (F10.-)
exposure to environmental tobacco smoke (Z77.22)
history of tobacco dependence (Z87.891)
occupational exposure to environmental tobacco smoke (Z57.31)
tobacco dependence (F17.-)
tobacco use (Z72.0)

> EXCLUDES 2   *erythroplakia (K13.29)*
> *focal epithelial hyperplasia (K13.29)*
> *leukedema of tongue (K13.29)*
> *leukoplakia of tongue (K13.21)*
> *hairy leukoplakia (K13.3)*
> *macroglossia (congenital) (Q38.2)*
> *submucous fibrosis of tongue (K13.5)*

+ K14.0 Glossitis
Abscess of tongue
Ulceration (traumatic) of tongue

> EXCLUDES 1   *atrophic glossitis (K14.4)*

> DEFINITION   Changes in the appearance of the tongue due to inflammation.

+ K14.1 Geographic tongue
Benign migratory glossitis
Glossitis areata exfoliativa

+ K14.2 Median rhomboid glossitis

● New   ▲ Revised   *Manifestation*   ④-⑦ Digit Indicators   ⊟ Laterality   Ⓐ Adult (15+ years)   Ⓜ Maternity (12-55 years)   Ⓝ Newborn   Ⓟ Pediatric (0-17 years)   ♂ Male   ♀ Female
✖ Deleted   Unspecified   + Additional code

696   © 2017 DecisionHealth   2017 ICD-10-CM Expert for Physicians

K12.3 — K14.2

+ K14.3   **Hypertrophy of tongue papillae**
Black hairy tongue
Coated tongue
Hypertrophy of foliate papillae
Lingua villosa nigra

+ K14.4   **Atrophy of tongue papillae**
Atrophic glossitis

+ K14.5   **Plicated tongue**
Fissured tongue
Furrowed tongue
Scrotal tongue
> **EXCLUDES 1** *fissured tongue, congenital (Q38.3)*

+ K14.6   **Glossodynia**
Glossopyrosis
Painful tongue
> **DEFINITION** Pain and/or a burning sensation in the tongue.

+ K14.8   **Other diseases of tongue**
Atrophy of tongue
Crenated tongue
Enlargement of tongue
Glossocele
Glossoptosis
Hypertrophy of tongue

+ K14.9   **Disease of tongue, unspecified**
Glossopathy NOS

Diseases of esophagus, stomach and duodenum (K20-K31)

> **EXCLUDES 2** *hiatus hernia (K44.-)*

4 + K20   **Esophagitis**
Use additional code to identify:
alcohol abuse and dependence (F10.-)
> **EXCLUDES 1** *erosion of esophagus (K22.1-)*
> *esophagitis with gastro-esophageal reflux disease (K21.0)*
> *reflux esophagitis (K21.0)*
> *ulcerative esophagitis (K22.1-)*
>
> **EXCLUDES 2** *eosinophilic gastritis or gastroenteritis (K52.81)*

> **CODING TIP ✓** Do not assign a code from K20.- if gastroesophageal reflux is also diagnosed. When a patient has confirmed diagnoses of both gastroesophageal reflux and esophagitis, code K21.0 should be assigned.

+ K20.0   **Eosinophilic esophagitis**

+ K20.8   **Other esophagitis**
Abscess of esophagus

+ K20.9   **Esophagitis, unspecified**
Esophagitis NOS

4 K21   **Gastro-esophageal reflux disease**
> **EXCLUDES 1** *newborn esophageal reflux (P78.83)*

K21.0   **Gastro-esophageal reflux disease with esophagitis**
Reflux esophagitis
> **DEFINITION** Esophageal inflammation due to reflux of gastric acid from the stomach back up into the esophagus.

K21.9   **Gastro-esophageal reflux disease without esophagitis**
Esophageal reflux NOS
> **DEFINITION** A burning sensation, usually centered in the middle of the chest near the breast bone, caused by the reflux of acidic stomach fluids that enter the lower end of the esophagus.
AHA: 1Q 2016, 18

4 K22   **Other diseases of esophagus**
> **EXCLUDES 2** *esophageal varices (I85.-)*

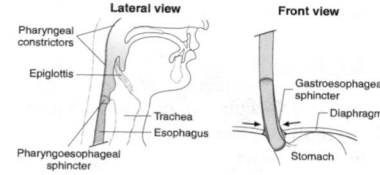

Esophageal anatomy

K22.0   **Achalasia of cardia**
Achalasia NOS
Cardiospasm
> **EXCLUDES 1** *congenital cardiospasm (Q39.5)*

6 + K22.1   **Ulcer of esophagus**
Barrett's ulcer
Erosion of esophagus
Fungal ulcer of esophagus
Peptic ulcer of esophagus
Ulcer of esophagus due to ingestion of chemicals
Ulcer of esophagus due to ingestion of drugs and medicaments
Ulcerative esophagitis
Code first:
poisoning due to drug or toxin, if applicable (T36-T65 with fifth or sixth character 1-4 or 6)
Use additional code for adverse effect, if applicable, to identify drug (T36-T50 with fifth or sixth character 5)
> **EXCLUDES 1** *Barrett's esophagus (K22.7-)*

+ K22.10   **Ulcer of esophagus without bleeding**
Ulcer of esophagus NOS

+ K22.11   **Ulcer of esophagus with bleeding**
> **EXCLUDES 2** *bleeding esophageal varices (I85.01, I85.11)*

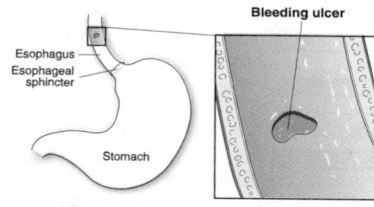

Ulcer of esophagus with bleeding
A lesion that develops on the interior wall of the esophagus

K22.2   **Esophageal obstruction**
Compression of esophagus
Constriction of esophagus
Stenosis of esophagus
Stricture of esophagus
> **EXCLUDES 1** *congenital stenosis or stricture of esophagus (Q39.3)*

K22.3   **Perforation of esophagus**
Rupture of esophagus
> **EXCLUDES 1** *traumatic perforation of (thoracic) esophagus (S27.8-)*

K22.4   **Dyskinesia of esophagus**
Corkscrew esophagus
Diffuse esophageal spasm
Spasm of esophagus
> **EXCLUDES 1** *cardiospasm (K22.0)*
>
> **DEFINITION** Weakened, paralyzed, or uncoordinated movement of esophageal muscles, causing difficulty swallowing.

K22.5   **Diverticulum of esophagus, acquired**
Esophageal pouch, acquired
> **EXCLUDES 1** *diverticulum of esophagus (congenital) (Q39.6)*

K22.6   **Gastro-esophageal laceration-hemorrhage syndrome**
Mallory-Weiss syndrome

● New   ▲ Revised   *Manifestation*   **4-7** Digit Indicators   ▤ Laterality   Ⓐ Adult (15+ years)   Ⓜ Maternity (12-55 years)   Ⓝ Newborn   Ⓟ Pediatric (0-17 years)   ♂ Male   ♀ Female
✖ Deleted   Unspecified   + Additional code

CODING TIP ✓ Code K22.6 should be assigned only for patients diagnosed with Mallory-Weiss syndrome or esophageal laceration and bleeding due to Mallory-Weiss Tears. When esophageal bleeding is documented as due to esophageal varices, assign a code from I85.-.

DEFINITION Esophagus becomes torn and bleeds near its connection to the stomach due to prolonged vomiting, hiccupping, or other spasmodic activity.

Ⓢ K22.7 Barrett's esophagus
Barrett's disease
Barrett's syndrome
EXCLUDES 1 *Barrett's ulcer (K22.1)*
malignant neoplasm of esophagus (C15.-)

K22.70 Barrett's esophagus without dysplasia
Barrett's esophagus NOS
Ⓢ K22.71 Barrett's esophagus with dysplasia
K22.710 Barrett's esophagus with low grade dysplasia
K22.711 Barrett's esophagus with high grade dysplasia
K22.719 Barrett's esophagus with dysplasia, unspecified

K22.8 Other specified diseases of esophagus
Hemorrhage of esophagus NOS
EXCLUDES 2 *esophageal varices (I85.-)*
Paterson-Kelly syndrome (D50.1)

CODING TIP ✓ Do not assign K22.8 when esophageal hemorrhage is documented as due to Mallory-Weiss Syndrome. When Mallory Weiss syndrome causes laceration and esophageal hemorrhage, assign code K22.6. Also do not assign for esophageal bleeding due to varices. When esophageal bleeding is documented as due to esophageal varices, assign a code from I85.-.

K22.9 Disease of esophagus, unspecified

K23 *Disorders of esophagus in diseases classified elsewhere*
Code first underlying disease, such as:
congenital syphilis (A50.5)
EXCLUDES 1 *late syphilis (A52.79)*
megaesophagus due to Chagas' disease (B57.31)
tuberculosis (A18.83)

Ⓓ+ K25 Gastric ulcer
INCLUDES erosion (acute) of stomach
pylorus ulcer (peptic)
stomach ulcer (peptic)
Use additional code to identify:
alcohol abuse and dependence (F10.-)
EXCLUDES 1 *acute gastritis (K29.0-)*
peptic ulcer NOS (K27.-)

CODING TIP ✓ Gastric ulcers are often documented as stomach ulcers. Carefully read all documentation in order to code ulcers to the proper anatomic location.

CODING TIP ✓ When documentation specifies that any gastric, duodenal or peptic ulcer is related to alcohol abuse or dependence, coders should assign an additional code to specify the abuse/dependence as specified.

Gastric ulcer

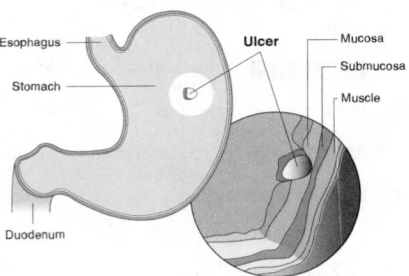

Esophagus — Ulcer — Mucosa
Submucosa
Stomach — Muscle
Duodenum

+ K25.0 Acute gastric ulcer with hemorrhage
+ K25.1 Acute gastric ulcer with perforation
+ K25.2 Acute gastric ulcer with both hemorrhage and perforation
+ K25.3 Acute gastric ulcer without hemorrhage or perforation
+ K25.4 Chronic or unspecified gastric ulcer with hemorrhage

+ K25.5 Chronic or unspecified gastric ulcer with perforation
+ K25.6 Chronic or unspecified gastric ulcer with both hemorrhage and perforation
+ K25.7 Chronic gastric ulcer without hemorrhage or perforation
+ K25.9 Gastric ulcer, unspecified as acute or chronic, without hemorrhage or perforation

Ⓓ+ K26 Duodenal ulcer
INCLUDES erosion (acute) of duodenum
duodenum ulcer (peptic)
postpyloric ulcer (peptic)
Use additional code to identify:
alcohol abuse and dependence (F10.-)
EXCLUDES 1 *peptic ulcer NOS (K27.-)*

CODING TIP ✓ A peptic ulcer should be coded to K26.- only when specified as duodenal or postpyloric. When documentation reports an ulcer as peptic and does not specify to one of these locations, assign a code from K27.-

CODING TIP ✓ When documentation specifies that any gastric, duodenal or peptic ulcer is related to alcohol abuse or dependence, coders should assign an additional code to specify the abuse/dependence as specified.

+ K26.0 Acute duodenal ulcer with hemorrhage
+ K26.1 Acute duodenal ulcer with perforation
+ K26.2 Acute duodenal ulcer with both hemorrhage and perforation
+ K26.3 Acute duodenal ulcer without hemorrhage or perforation
+ K26.4 Chronic or unspecified duodenal ulcer with hemorrhage
AHA: 1Q 2016, 14
+ K26.5 Chronic or unspecified duodenal ulcer with perforation
+ K26.6 Chronic or unspecified duodenal ulcer with both hemorrhage and perforation
+ K26.7 Chronic duodenal ulcer without hemorrhage or perforation
+ K26.9 Duodenal ulcer, unspecified as acute or chronic, without hemorrhage or perforation

Ⓓ+ K27 Peptic ulcer, site unspecified
INCLUDES gastroduodenal ulcer NOS
peptic ulcer NOS
Use additional code to identify:
alcohol abuse and dependence (F10.-)
EXCLUDES 1 *peptic ulcer of newborn (P78.82)*

CODING TIP ✓ When documentation specifies that any gastric, duodenal or peptic ulcer is related to alcohol abuse or dependence, coders should assign an additional code to specify the abuse/dependence as specified.

+ K27.0 Acute peptic ulcer, site unspecified, with hemorrhage
+ K27.1 Acute peptic ulcer, site unspecified, with perforation
+ K27.2 Acute peptic ulcer, site unspecified, with both hemorrhage and perforation
+ K27.3 Acute peptic ulcer, site unspecified, without hemorrhage or perforation
+ K27.4 Chronic or unspecified peptic ulcer, site unspecified, with hemorrhage
+ K27.5 Chronic or unspecified peptic ulcer, site unspecified, with perforation
+ K27.6 Chronic or unspecified peptic ulcer, site unspecified, with both hemorrhage and perforation
+ K27.7 Chronic peptic ulcer, site unspecified, without hemorrhage or perforation
+ K27.9 Peptic ulcer, site unspecified, unspecified as acute or chronic, without hemorrhage or perforation

Ⓓ+ K28 Gastrojejunal ulcer
INCLUDES anastomotic ulcer (peptic) or erosion
gastrocolic ulcer (peptic) or erosion
gastrointestinal ulcer (peptic) or erosion
gastrojejunal ulcer (peptic) or erosion
jejunal ulcer (peptic) or erosion
marginal ulcer (peptic) or erosion
stomal ulcer (peptic) or erosion
Use additional code to identify:
alcohol abuse and dependence (F10.-)
EXCLUDES 1 *primary ulcer of small intestine (K63.3)*

+ K28.0 Acute gastrojejunal ulcer with hemorrhage
+ K28.1 Acute gastrojejunal ulcer with perforation

+ K28.2   Acute gastrojejunal ulcer with both hemorrhage and perforation

+ K28.3   Acute gastrojejunal ulcer without hemorrhage or perforation

+ K28.4   Chronic or unspecified gastrojejunal ulcer with hemorrhage

+ K28.5   Chronic or unspecified gastrojejunal ulcer with perforation

+ K28.6   Chronic or unspecified gastrojejunal ulcer with both hemorrhage and perforation

+ K28.7   Chronic gastrojejunal ulcer without hemorrhage or perforation

+ K28.9   Gastrojejunal ulcer, unspecified as acute or chronic, without hemorrhage or perforation

▣ K29   Gastritis and duodenitis

> **EXCLUDES 1**   *eosinophilic gastritis or gastroenteritis (K52.81)*
> *Zollinger-Ellison syndrome (E16.4)*

⑤+ K29.0   **Acute gastritis**
Use additional code to identify:
alcohol abuse and dependence (F10.-)
> **EXCLUDES 1**   *erosion (acute) of stomach (K25.-)*

  + K29.00   Acute gastritis without bleeding

  + K29.01   Acute gastritis with bleeding

⑤+ K29.2   **Alcoholic gastritis**
Use additional code to identify:
alcohol abuse and dependence (F10.-)

  + K29.20   Alcoholic gastritis without bleeding

  + K29.21   Alcoholic gastritis with bleeding

⑤ K29.3   **Chronic superficial gastritis**

  K29.30   Chronic superficial gastritis without bleeding

  K29.31   Chronic superficial gastritis with bleeding

⑤ K29.4   **Chronic atrophic gastritis**
Gastric atrophy

  K29.40   Chronic atrophic gastritis without bleeding

  K29.41   Chronic atrophic gastritis with bleeding

⑤ K29.5   **Unspecified chronic gastritis**
Chronic antral gastritis
Chronic fundal gastritis

  K29.50   Unspecified chronic gastritis without bleeding

  K29.51   Unspecified chronic gastritis with bleeding

⑤ K29.6   **Other gastritis**
Giant hypertrophic gastritis
Granulomatous gastritis
Ménétrier's disease

  K29.60   Other gastritis without bleeding

  K29.61   Other gastritis with bleeding

⑤ K29.7   **Gastritis, unspecified**

  K29.70   Gastritis, unspecified, without bleeding

  K29.71   Gastritis, unspecified, with bleeding

⑤ K29.8   **Duodenitis**

  K29.80   Duodenitis without bleeding

  K29.81   Duodenitis with bleeding

⑤ K29.9   **Gastroduodenitis, unspecified**

  K29.90   Gastroduodenitis, unspecified, without bleeding

  K29.91   Gastroduodenitis, unspecified, with bleeding

K30   Functional dyspepsia
Indigestion
> **EXCLUDES 1**   *dyspepsia NOS (R10.13)*
> *heartburn (R12)*
> *nervous dyspepsia (F45.8)*
> *neurotic dyspepsia (F45.8)*
> *psychogenic dyspepsia (F45.8)*

▣ K31   Other diseases of stomach and duodenum
> **INCLUDES**   functional disorders of stomach
> **EXCLUDES 2**   *diabetic gastroparesis*
> *(E08.43, E09.43, E10.43, E11.43, E13.43)*
> *diverticulum of duodenum (K57.00-K57.13)*

K31.0   **Acute dilatation of stomach**
Acute distention of stomach
> **DEFINITION**   Distention of the stomach due to excessive gas build-up or bowel obstruction, preventing passage of food.

K31.1   **Adult hypertrophic pyloric stenosis**   ▣
Pyloric stenosis NOS
> **EXCLUDES 1**   *congenital or infantile pyloric stenosis (Q40.0)*

K31.2   **Hourglass stricture and stenosis of stomach**
> **EXCLUDES 1**   *congenital hourglass stomach (Q40.2)*
> *hourglass contraction of stomach (K31.89)*

K31.3   **Pylorospasm, not elsewhere classified**
> **EXCLUDES 1**   *congenital or infantile pylorospasm (Q40.0)*
> *neurotic pylorospasm (F45.8)*
> *psychogenic pylorospasm (F45.8)*

K31.4   **Gastric diverticulum**
> **EXCLUDES 1**   *congenital diverticulum of stomach (Q40.2)*

K31.5   **Obstruction of duodenum**
Constriction of duodenum
Duodenal ileus (chronic)
Stenosis of duodenum
Stricture of duodenum
Volvulus of duodenum
> **EXCLUDES 1**   *congenital stenosis of duodenum (Q41.0)*

K31.6   **Fistula of stomach and duodenum**
Gastrocolic fistula
Gastrojejunocolic fistula

K31.7   **Polyp of stomach and duodenum**
> **EXCLUDES 1**   *adenomatous polyp of stomach (D13.1)*

⑤ K31.8   **Other specified diseases of stomach and duodenum**

  ⑥ K31.81   Angiodysplasia of stomach and duodenum

    K31.811   Angiodysplasia of stomach and duodenum with bleeding

    K31.819   Angiodysplasia of stomach and duodenum without bleeding
Angiodysplasia of stomach and duodenum NOS

  K31.82   Dieulafoy lesion (hemorrhagic) of stomach and duodenum
> **EXCLUDES 2**   *Dieulafoy lesion of intestine (K63.81)*
> **DEFINITION**   Abnormality of arteriole within the digestive tract protruding through a tiny mucosal defect, usually near the gastroesophageal junction, that can cause massive gastrointestinal bleeding.

  K31.83   Achlorhydria
> **DEFINITION**   Absence of hydrochloric acid in the stomach's gastric secretions, most often from antibodies against cells producing gastric acid, or a symptom of H. pylori infection, atrophic gastritis, or cancer.

  K31.84   Gastroparesis
Gastroparalysis
Code first underlying disease, if known, such as:
  anorexia nervosa (F50.0-)
  diabetes mellitus
    (E08.43, E09.43, E10.43, E11.43, E13.43)
  scleroderma (M34.-)
AHA: 4Q 2013, 115

  K31.89   Other diseases of stomach and duodenum

K31.9   **Disease of stomach and duodenum, unspecified**

Diseases of appendix (K35-K38)

▣ K35   Acute appendicitis

K35.2   **Acute appendicitis with generalized peritonitis**
Appendicitis (acute) with generalized (diffuse) peritonitis following rupture or perforation of appendix
Perforated appendix NOS
Ruptured appendix NOS

● New   ▲ Revised   *Manifestation*   ▣-▢ Digit Indicators   ▱ Laterality   ▣ Adult (15+ years)   ▣ Maternity (12-55 years)   ▣ Newborn   ▣ Pediatric (0-17 years)   ♂ Male   ♀ Female
✖ Deleted   Unspecified   + Additional code

▲ **K35.3**   **Acute appendicitis with localized peritonitis**
Acute appendicitis with or without perforation or rupture with peritonitis NOS
Acute appendicitis with or without perforation or rupture with localized peritonitis
Acute appendicitis with peritoneal abscess

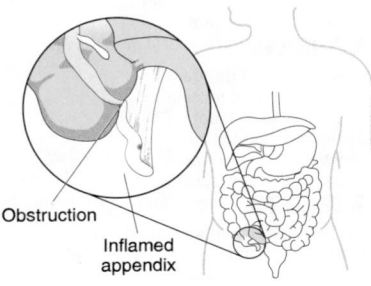

**Acute appendicitis
with localized peritonitis**

Obstruction

Inflamed
appendix

🔲 **K35.8**   **Other and unspecified acute appendicitis**

K35.80   **Unspecified acute appendicitis**
Acute appendicitis NOS
Acute appendicitis without (localized) (generalized) peritonitis

K35.89   **Other acute appendicitis**

K36   **Other appendicitis**
Chronic appendicitis
Recurrent appendicitis

K37   **Unspecified appendicitis**

> **EXCLUDES 1**   *-unspecified appendicitis with peritonitis (K35.2-K35.3)*

🔲 **K38**   **Other diseases of appendix**

K38.0   **Hyperplasia of appendix**

K38.1   **Appendicular concretions**
Fecalith of appendix
Stercolith of appendix

K38.2   **Diverticulum of appendix**

K38.3   **Fistula of appendix**

K38.8   **Other specified diseases of appendix**
Intussusception of appendix

K38.9   **Disease of appendix, unspecified**

Hernia (K40-K46)

Note: Hernia with both gangrene and obstruction is classified to hernia with gangrene.

> **INCLUDES**   acquired hernia
> congenital [except diaphragmatic or hiatus] hernia
> recurrent hernia

🔲 **K40**   **Inguinal hernia**

> **INCLUDES**   bubonocele
> direct inguinal hernia
> double inguinal hernia
> indirect inguinal hernia
> inguinal hernia NOS
> oblique inguinal hernia
> scrotal hernia

> **DEFINITION**   Weakness in the muscles in the groin area between the abdomen and thigh, allowing part of the intestine to bulge through the muscle wall.

Inguinal hernia

Herniated
loop of
intestine

Inguinal canal

Spermatic cord

🔲 **K40.0**   **Bilateral inguinal hernia, with obstruction, without gangrene**
Inguinal hernia (bilateral) causing obstruction without gangrene
Incarcerated inguinal hernia (bilateral) without gangrene
Irreducible inguinal hernia (bilateral) without gangrene
Strangulated inguinal hernia (bilateral) without gangrene

K40.00   **Bilateral inguinal hernia, with obstruction, without gangrene, not specified as recurrent**
Bilateral inguinal hernia, with obstruction, without gangrene NOS

K40.01   **Bilateral inguinal hernia, with obstruction, without gangrene, recurrent**

🔲 **K40.1**   **Bilateral inguinal hernia, with gangrene**

K40.10   **Bilateral inguinal hernia, with gangrene, not specified as recurrent**
Bilateral inguinal hernia, with gangrene NOS

K40.11   **Bilateral inguinal hernia, with gangrene, recurrent**

🔲 **K40.2**   **Bilateral inguinal hernia, without obstruction or gangrene**

K40.20   **Bilateral inguinal hernia, without obstruction or gangrene, not specified as recurrent**
Bilateral inguinal hernia NOS

K40.21   **Bilateral inguinal hernia, without obstruction or gangrene, recurrent**

🔲 **K40.3**   **Unilateral inguinal hernia, with obstruction, without gangrene**
Inguinal hernia (unilateral) causing obstruction without gangrene
Incarcerated inguinal hernia (unilateral) without gangrene
Irreducible inguinal hernia (unilateral) without gangrene
Strangulated inguinal hernia (unilateral) without gangrene

K40.30   **Unilateral inguinal hernia, with obstruction, without gangrene, not specified as recurrent**
Inguinal hernia, with obstruction NOS
Unilateral inguinal hernia, with obstruction, without gangrene NOS

K40.31   **Unilateral inguinal hernia, with obstruction, without gangrene, recurrent**

🔲 **K40.4**   **Unilateral inguinal hernia, with gangrene**

K40.40   **Unilateral inguinal hernia, with gangrene, not specified as recurrent**
Inguinal hernia with gangrene NOS
Unilateral inguinal hernia with gangrene NOS

K40.41   **Unilateral inguinal hernia, with gangrene, recurrent**

🔲 **K40.9**   **Unilateral inguinal hernia, without obstruction or gangrene**

K40.90   **Unilateral inguinal hernia, without obstruction or gangrene, not specified as recurrent**
Inguinal hernia NOS
Unilateral inguinal hernia NOS

K40.91   **Unilateral inguinal hernia, without obstruction or gangrene, recurrent**

🔲 **K41**   **Femoral hernia**

🔲 **K41.0**   **Bilateral femoral hernia, with obstruction, without gangrene**
Femoral hernia (bilateral) causing obstruction, without gangrene
Incarcerated femoral hernia (bilateral), without gangrene
Irreducible femoral hernia (bilateral), without gangrene
Strangulated femoral hernia (bilateral), without gangrene

● New   ▲ Revised   *Manifestation*   🔲-🔢 Digit Indicators   🖫 Laterality   🅰 Adult (15+ years)   🅼 Maternity (12-55 years)   🅽 Newborn   🅿 Pediatric (0-17 years)   ♂ Male   ♀ Female
✱ Deleted   Unspecified   ✚ Additional code

700   © 2017 DecisionHealth

2017 ICD-10-CM Expert for Physicians

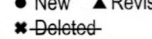

K35.3 — K41.0

K41.00 Bilateral femoral hernia, with obstruction, without gangrene, not specified as recurrent
Bilateral femoral hernia, with obstruction, without gangrene NOS

K41.01 Bilateral femoral hernia, with obstruction, without gangrene, recurrent

⬚ K41.1 Bilateral femoral hernia, with gangrene

K41.10 Bilateral femoral hernia, with gangrene, not specified as recurrent
Bilateral femoral hernia, with gangrene NOS

K41.11 Bilateral femoral hernia, with gangrene, recurrent

⬚ K41.2 Bilateral femoral hernia, without obstruction or gangrene

K41.20 Bilateral femoral hernia, without obstruction or gangrene, not specified as recurrent
Bilateral femoral hernia NOS

K41.21 Bilateral femoral hernia, without obstruction or gangrene, recurrent

⬚ K41.3 Unilateral femoral hernia, with obstruction, without gangrene
Femoral hernia (unilateral) causing obstruction, without gangrene
Incarcerated femoral hernia (unilateral), without gangrene
Irreducible femoral hernia (unilateral), without gangrene
Strangulated femoral hernia (unilateral), without gangrene

K41.30 Unilateral femoral hernia, with obstruction, without gangrene, not specified as recurrent
Femoral hernia, with obstruction NOS
Unilateral femoral hernia, with obstruction NOS

K41.31 Unilateral femoral hernia, with obstruction, without gangrene, recurrent

⬚ K41.4 Unilateral femoral hernia, with gangrene

K41.40 Unilateral femoral hernia, with gangrene, not specified as recurrent
Femoral hernia, with gangrene NOS
Unilateral femoral hernia, with gangrene NOS

K41.41 Unilateral femoral hernia, with gangrene, recurrent

⬚ K41.9 Unilateral femoral hernia, without obstruction or gangrene

K41.90 Unilateral femoral hernia, without obstruction or gangrene, not specified as recurrent
Femoral hernia NOS
Unilateral femoral hernia NOS

K41.91 Unilateral femoral hernia, without obstruction or gangrene, recurrent

⬚ K42 Umbilical hernia

INCLUDES paraumbilical hernia

EXCLUDES 1 omphalocele (Q79.2)

K42.0 Umbilical hernia with obstruction, without gangrene
Umbilical hernia causing obstruction, without gangrene
Incarcerated umbilical hernia, without gangrene
Irreducible umbilical hernia, without gangrene
Strangulated umbilical hernia, without gangrene

K42.1 Umbilical hernia with gangrene
Gangrenous umbilical hernia

K42.9 Umbilical hernia without obstruction or gangrene
Umbilical hernia NOS

⬚ K43 Ventral hernia

Ventral hernia

Hernia appears in the front of the abdomen

K43.0 Incisional hernia with obstruction, without gangrene
Incisional hernia causing obstruction, without gangrene
Incarcerated incisional hernia, without gangrene
Irreducible incisional hernia, without gangrene
Strangulated incisional hernia, without gangrene

K43.1 Incisional hernia with gangrene
Gangrenous incisional hernia

K43.2 Incisional hernia without obstruction or gangrene
Incisional hernia NOS

K43.3 Parastomal hernia with obstruction, without gangrene
Incarcerated parastomal hernia, without gangrene
Irreducible parastomal hernia, without gangrene
Parastomal hernia causing obstruction, without gangrene
Strangulated parastomal hernia, without gangrene

K43.4 Parastomal hernia with gangrene
Gangrenous parastomal hernia

K43.5 Parastomal hernia without obstruction or gangrene
Parastomal hernia NOS

K43.6 Other and unspecified ventral hernia with obstruction, without gangrene
Epigastric hernia causing obstruction, without gangrene
Hypogastric hernia causing obstruction, without gangrene
Incarcerated epigastric hernia without gangrene
Incarcerated hypogastric hernia without gangrene
Incarcerated midline hernia without gangrene
Incarcerated spigelian hernia without gangrene
Incarcerated subxiphoid hernia without gangrene
Irreducible epigastric hernia without gangrene
Irreducible hypogastric hernia without gangrene
Irreducible midline hernia without gangrene
Irreducible spigelian hernia without gangrene
Irreducible subxiphoid hernia without gangrene
Midline hernia causing obstruction, without gangrene
Spigelian hernia causing obstruction, without gangrene
Strangulated epigastric hernia without gangrene
Strangulated hypogastric hernia without gangrene
Strangulated midline hernia without gangrene
Strangulated spigelian hernia without gangrene
Strangulated subxiphoid hernia without gangrene
Subxiphoid hernia causing obstruction, without gangrene

K43.7 Other and unspecified ventral hernia with gangrene
Any condition listed under K43.6 specified as gangrenous

K43.9 Ventral hernia without obstruction or gangrene
Epigastric hernia
Ventral hernia NOS

⬚ K44 Diaphragmatic hernia

INCLUDES hiatus hernia (esophageal) (sliding)
paraesophageal hernia

EXCLUDES 1 congenital diaphragmatic hernia (Q79.0)
congenital hiatus hernia (Q40.1)

K44.0 Diaphragmatic hernia with obstruction, without gangrene
Diaphragmatic hernia causing obstruction
Incarcerated diaphragmatic hernia
Irreducible diaphragmatic hernia
Strangulated diaphragmatic hernia

K44.1 Diaphragmatic hernia with gangrene
Gangrenous diaphragmatic hernia

K44.9 Diaphragmatic hernia without obstruction or gangrene
Diaphragmatic hernia NOS

⬚ K45 Other abdominal hernia

INCLUDES abdominal hernia, specified site NEC
lumbar hernia
obturator hernia
pudendal hernia
retroperitoneal hernia
sciatic hernia

K45.0 Other specified abdominal hernia with obstruction, without gangrene
Other specified abdominal hernia causing obstruction
Other specified incarcerated abdominal hernia
Other specified irreducible abdominal hernia
Other specified strangulated abdominal hernia

K45.1 Other specified abdominal hernia with gangrene
Any condition listed under K45 specified as gangrenous

K45.8 Other specified abdominal hernia without obstruction or gangrene

● New ▲ Revised *Manifestation* ⬚-⬚ Digit Indicators ⬚ Laterality Ⓐ Adult (15+ years) Ⓜ Maternity (12-55 years) Ⓝ Newborn Ⓟ Pediatric (0-17 years) ♂ Male ♀ Female
✖ Deleted Unspecified + Additional code

2017 ICD-10-CM Expert for Physicians

© 2017 DecisionHealth 701

☑ **K46** **Unspecified abdominal hernia**

> INCLUDES enterocele
> epiplocele
> hernia NOS
> interstitial hernia
> intestinal hernia
> intra-abdominal hernia

> EXCLUDES 1 *vaginal enterocele (N81.5)*

K46.0 **Unspecified abdominal hernia with obstruction, without gangrene**

Unspecified abdominal hernia causing obstruction
Unspecified incarcerated abdominal hernia
Unspecified irreducible abdominal hernia
Unspecified strangulated abdominal hernia

K46.1 **Unspecified abdominal hernia with gangrene**

Any condition listed under K46 specified as gangrenous

K46.9 **Unspecified abdominal hernia without obstruction or gangrene**

Abdominal hernia NOS

Noninfective enteritis and colitis (K50-K52)

> INCLUDES noninfective inflammatory bowel disease

> EXCLUDES 1 *irritable bowel syndrome (K58.-)*
> *megacolon (K59.3-)*

> CODING TIP ✓ Do not assign a code from K50-K52 when enteritis/colitis is specified as infectious. Infectious colitis requires assignment of a code from Chapter 1, Certain Infectious and Parasitic Diseases.

☑+ **K50** **Crohn's disease [regional enteritis]**

> INCLUDES granulomatous enteritis

> *Use additional code to identify manifestations, such as:*
> *pyoderma gangrenosum (L88)*

> EXCLUDES 1 *ulcerative colitis (K51.-)*

☑+ **K50.0** **Crohn's disease of small intestine**

Crohn's disease [regional enteritis] of duodenum
Crohn's disease [regional enteritis] of ileum
Crohn's disease [regional enteritis] of jejunum
Regional ileitis
Terminal ileitis

> EXCLUDES 1 *Crohn's disease of both small and large intestine (K50.8-)*

Crohn's disease of small intestine

+ **K50.00** **Crohn's disease of small intestine without complications**

☑+ **K50.01** **Crohn's disease of small intestine with complications**

+ **K50.011** **Crohn's disease of small intestine with rectal bleeding**

+ **K50.012** **Crohn's disease of small intestine with intestinal obstruction**

+ **K50.013** **Crohn's disease of small intestine with fistula**

+ **K50.014** **Crohn's disease of small intestine with abscess**
AHA: 4Q 2012, 104

+ **K50.018** **Crohn's disease of small intestine with other complication**

+ **K50.019** **Crohn's disease of small intestine with unspecified complications**

☑+ **K50.1** **Crohn's disease of large intestine**

Crohn's disease [regional enteritis] of colon
Crohn's disease [regional enteritis] of large bowel
Crohn's disease [regional enteritis] of rectum
Granulomatous colitis
Regional colitis

> EXCLUDES 1 *Crohn's disease of both small and large intestine (K50.8)*

+ **K50.10** **Crohn's disease of large intestine without complications**

☑+ **K50.11** **Crohn's disease of large intestine with complications**

+ **K50.111** **Crohn's disease of large intestine with rectal bleeding**

+ **K50.112** **Crohn's disease of large intestine with intestinal obstruction**

+ **K50.113** **Crohn's disease of large intestine with fistula**

+ **K50.114** **Crohn's disease of large intestine with abscess**
AHA: 4Q 2012, 104

+ **K50.118** **Crohn's disease of large intestine with other complication**

+ **K50.119** **Crohn's disease of large intestine with unspecified complications**

☑+ **K50.8** **Crohn's disease of both small and large intestine**

+ **K50.80** **Crohn's disease of both small and large intestine without complications**

☑+ **K50.81** **Crohn's disease of both small and large intestine with complications**

+ **K50.811** **Crohn's disease of both small and large intestine with rectal bleeding**

+ **K50.812** **Crohn's disease of both small and large intestine with intestinal obstruction**

+ **K50.813** **Crohn's disease of both small and large intestine with fistula**

+ **K50.814** **Crohn's disease of both small and large intestine with abscess**
AHA: 4Q 2012, 104

+ **K50.818** **Crohn's disease of both small and large intestine with other complication**

+ **K50.819** **Crohn's disease of both small and large intestine with unspecified complications**

☑+ **K50.9** **Crohn's disease, unspecified**

+ **K50.90** **Crohn's disease, unspecified, without complications**

Crohn's disease NOS
Regional enteritis NOS

Crohn's disease
Inflammation of the intestinal tract

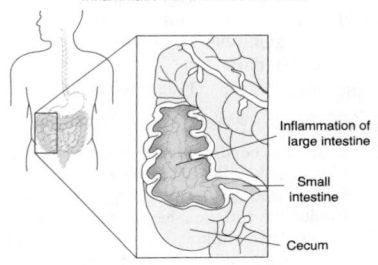

☑+ **K50.91** **Crohn's disease, unspecified, with complications**

+ **K50.911** **Crohn's disease, unspecified, with rectal bleeding**

+ **K50.912** **Crohn's disease, unspecified, with intestinal obstruction**

+ **K50.913** **Crohn's disease, unspecified, with fistula**

+ **K50.914** **Crohn's disease, unspecified, with abscess**
AHA: 4Q 2012, 104

+ **K50.918** **Crohn's disease, unspecified, with other complication**

+ **K50.919** **Crohn's disease, unspecified, with unspecified complications**

☑+ **K51** **Ulcerative colitis**

> *Use additional code to identify manifestations, such as:*
> *pyoderma gangrenosum (L88)*

> EXCLUDES 1 *Crohn's disease [regional enteritis] (K50.-)*

☑+ **K51.0** **Ulcerative (chronic) pancolitis**

Backwash ileitis

+ **K51.00** **Ulcerative (chronic) pancolitis without complications**

Ulcerative (chronic) pancolitis NOS

☑+ **K51.01** **Ulcerative (chronic) pancolitis with complications**

| ● New | ▲ Revised | *Manifestation* | ☑-☑ Digit Indicators | ⊟ Laterality | ⚠ Adult (15+ years) | ⚠ Maternity (12-55 years) | ⚠ Newborn | ⚠ Pediatric (0-17 years) | ♂ Male | ♀ Female |
| ✖ Deleted | | Unspecified | + Additional code | | | | | | | |

702 © 2017 DecisionHealth

2017 ICD-10-CM Expert for Physicians

+ K51.011   **Ulcerative (chronic) pancolitis with rectal bleeding**

+ K51.012   **Ulcerative (chronic) pancolitis with intestinal obstruction**

+ K51.013   **Ulcerative (chronic) pancolitis with fistula**

+ K51.014   **Ulcerative (chronic) pancolitis with abscess**

+ K51.018   **Ulcerative (chronic) pancolitis with other complication**

+ K51.019   **Ulcerative (chronic) pancolitis with unspecified complications**

⑤+ K51.2   **Ulcerative (chronic) proctitis**

+ K51.20   **Ulcerative (chronic) proctitis without complications**
Ulcerative (chronic) proctitis NOS

⑥+ K51.21   **Ulcerative (chronic) proctitis with complications**

+ K51.211   **Ulcerative (chronic) proctitis with rectal bleeding**

+ K51.212   **Ulcerative (chronic) proctitis with intestinal obstruction**

+ K51.213   **Ulcerative (chronic) proctitis with fistula**

+ K51.214   **Ulcerative (chronic) proctitis with abscess**

+ K51.218   **Ulcerative (chronic) proctitis with other complication**

+ K51.219   **Ulcerative (chronic) proctitis with unspecified complications**

⑤+ K51.3   **Ulcerative (chronic) rectosigmoiditis**

+ K51.30   **Ulcerative (chronic) rectosigmoiditis without complications**
Ulcerative (chronic) rectosigmoiditis NOS

⑥+ K51.31   **Ulcerative (chronic) rectosigmoiditis with complications**

+ K51.311   **Ulcerative (chronic) rectosigmoiditis with rectal bleeding**

+ K51.312   **Ulcerative (chronic) rectosigmoiditis with intestinal obstruction**

+ K51.313   **Ulcerative (chronic) rectosigmoiditis with fistula**

+ K51.314   **Ulcerative (chronic) rectosigmoiditis with abscess**

+ K51.318   **Ulcerative (chronic) rectosigmoiditis with other complication**

+ K51.319   **Ulcerative (chronic) rectosigmoiditis with unspecified complications**

⑤+ K51.4   **Inflammatory polyps of colon**
EXCLUDES 1   *adenomatous polyp of colon (D12.6)*
polyposis of colon (D12.6)
polyps of colon NOS (K63.5)

+ K51.40   **Inflammatory polyps of colon without complications**
Inflammatory polyps of colon NOS

⑥+ K51.41   **Inflammatory polyps of colon with complications**

+ K51.411   **Inflammatory polyps of colon with rectal bleeding**

+ K51.412   **Inflammatory polyps of colon with intestinal obstruction**

+ K51.413   **Inflammatory polyps of colon with fistula**

+ K51.414   **Inflammatory polyps of colon with abscess**

+ K51.418   **Inflammatory polyps of colon with other complication**

+ K51.419   **Inflammatory polyps of colon with unspecified complications**

⑤+ K51.5   **Left sided colitis**
Left hemicolitis

+ K51.50   **Left sided colitis without complications**
Left sided colitis NOS

⑥+ K51.51   **Left sided colitis with complications**

+ K51.511   **Left sided colitis with rectal bleeding**

+ K51.512   **Left sided colitis with intestinal obstruction**

+ K51.513   **Left sided colitis with fistula**

+ K51.514   **Left sided colitis with abscess**

+ K51.518   **Left sided colitis with other complication**

+ K51.519   **Left sided colitis with unspecified complications**

⑤+ K51.8   **Other ulcerative colitis**

+ K51.80   **Other ulcerative colitis without complications**
DEFINITION   Inflammation of the intestinal lining with ulcer formation, causing diarrhea as the colon empties frequently.

⑥+ K51.81   **Other ulcerative colitis with complications**

+ K51.811   **Other ulcerative colitis with rectal bleeding**

+ K51.812   **Other ulcerative colitis with intestinal obstruction**

+ K51.813   **Other ulcerative colitis with fistula**

+ K51.814   **Other ulcerative colitis with abscess**

+ K51.818   **Other ulcerative colitis with other complication**

+ K51.819   **Other ulcerative colitis with unspecified complications**

⑤+ K51.9   **Ulcerative colitis, unspecified**

+ K51.90   **Ulcerative colitis, unspecified, without complications**

⑥+ K51.91   **Ulcerative colitis, unspecified, with complications**

+ K51.911   **Ulcerative colitis, unspecified with rectal bleeding**

+ K51.912   **Ulcerative colitis, unspecified with intestinal obstruction**

+ K51.913   **Ulcerative colitis, unspecified with fistula**

+ K51.914   **Ulcerative colitis, unspecified with abscess**

+ K51.918   **Ulcerative colitis, unspecified with other complication**

+ K51.919   **Ulcerative colitis, unspecified with unspecified complications**

④ K52   **Other and unspecified noninfective gastroenteritis and colitis**

K52.0   **Gastroenteritis and colitis due to radiation**

+ K52.1   **Toxic gastroenteritis and colitis**
Drug-induced gastroenteritis and colitis
Code first:
  (T51-T65) to identify toxic agent
Use additional code for adverse effect, if applicable, to identify drug (T36-T50 with fifth or sixth character 5)

▲⑤+ K52.2   **Allergic and dietetic gastroenteritis and colitis**
Food hypersensitivity gastroenteritis or colitis
Use additional code to identify type of food allergy (Z91.01-, Z91.02-)
EXCLUDES 2   *allergic eosinophilic colitis (K52.82)*
allergic eosinophilic esophagitis (K20.0)
allergic eosinophilic gastritis (K52.81)
allergic eosinophilic gastroenteritis (K52.81)
food protein-induced proctocolitis (K52.82)

●+ K52.21   **Food protein-induced enterocolitis syndrome**
Use additional code for hypovolemic shock, if present (R57.1)

●+ K52.22   **Food protein-induced enteropathy**

●+ K52.29   **Other allergic and dietetic gastroenteritis and colitis**
Food hypersensitivity gastroenteritis or colitis
Immediate gastrointestinal hypersensitivity

● K52.3   **Indeterminate colitis**
Colonic inflammatory bowel disease unclassified (IBDU)
EXCLUDES 1   *unspecified colitis (K52.9)*

⑤ K52.8   **Other specified noninfective gastroenteritis and colitis**

▲ K52.81   **Eosinophilic gastritis or gastroenteritis**
Eosinophilic enteritis
EXCLUDES 2   *eosinophilic esophagitis (K20.0)*

▲ K52.82   **Eosinophilic colitis**
Allergic proctocolitis
Food-induced eosinophilic proctocolitis
Food protein-induced proctocolitis
Milk protein-induced proctocolitis

●⑥ K52.83   **Microscopic colitis**

● K52.831   **Collagenous colitis**

● K52.832   **Lymphocytic colitis**

● K52.838   **Other microscopic colitis**

● K52.839   **Microscopic colitis, unspecified**

▲ K52.89   **Other specified noninfective gastroenteritis and colitis**

● New   ▲ Revised   *Manifestation*   ④-❼ Digit Indicators   ⊟ Laterality   Ⓐ Adult (15+ years)   Ⓜ Maternity (12-55 years)   Ⓝ Newborn   Ⓟ Pediatric (0-17 years)   ♂ Male   ♀ Female

✖ Deleted   Unspecified   + Additional code

K52.9   Noninfective gastroenteritis and colitis, unspecified
Colitis NOS
Enteritis NOS
Gastroenteritis NOS
Ileitis NOS
Jejunitis NOS
Sigmoiditis NOS
> **EXCLUDES 1**   *diarrhea NOS (R19.7)*
> *functional diarrhea (K59.1)*
> *infectious gastroenteritis and colitis NOS*
> *(A09)*
> *neonatal diarrhea (noninfective) (P78.3)*
> *psychogenic diarrhea (F45.8)*

Other diseases of intestines (K55-K64)

K55   Vascular disorders of intestine
> **EXCLUDES 1**   *necrotizing enterocolitis of newborn (P77.-)*

▲ K55.0   Acute vascular disorders of intestine
Infarction of appendices epiploicae
Mesenteric (artery) (vein) embolism
Mesenteric (artery) (vein) infarction
Mesenteric (artery) (vein) thrombosis

● K55.01   Acute (reversible) ischemia of small intestine

● K55.011   Focal (segmental) acute (reversible) ischemia of small intestine

● K55.012   Diffuse acute (reversible) ischemia of small intestine

● K55.019   Acute (reversible) ischemia of small intestine, extent unspecified

● K55.02   Acute infarction of small intestine
Gangrene of small intestine
Necrosis of small intestine

● K55.021   Focal (segmental) acute infarction of small intestine

● K55.022   Diffuse acute infarction of small intestine

● K55.029   Acute infarction of small intestine, extent unspecified

● K55.03   Acute (reversible) ischemia of large intestine
Acute fulminant ischemic colitis
Subacute ischemic colitis

● K55.031   Focal (segmental) acute (reversible) ischemia of large intestine

● K55.032   Diffuse acute (reversible) ischemia of large intestine

● K55.039   Acute (reversible) ischemia of large intestine, extent unspecified

● K55.04   Acute infarction of large intestine
Gangrene of large intestine
Necrosis of large intestine

● K55.041   Focal (segmental) acute infarction of large intestine

● K55.042   Diffuse acute infarction of large intestine

● K55.049   Acute infarction of large intestine, extent unspecified

● K55.05   Acute (reversible) ischemia of intestine, part unspecified

● K55.051   Focal (segmental) acute (reversible) ischemia of intestine, part unspecified

● K55.052   Diffuse acute (reversible) ischemia of intestine, part unspecified

● K55.059   Acute (reversible) ischemia of intestine, part and extent unspecified

● K55.06   Acute infarction of intestine, part unspecified
Acute intestinal infarction
Gangrene of intestine
Necrosis of intestine

● K55.061   Focal (segmental) acute infarction of intestine, part unspecified

● K55.062   Diffuse acute infarction of intestine, part unspecified

● K55.069   Acute infarction of intestine, part and extent unspecified

K55.1   Chronic vascular disorders of intestine
Chronic ischemic colitis
Chronic ischemic enteritis
Chronic ischemic enterocolitis
Ischemic stricture of intestine
Mesenteric atherosclerosis
Mesenteric vascular insufficiency

K55.2   Angiodysplasia of colon

K55.20   Angiodysplasia of colon without hemorrhage

K55.21   Angiodysplasia of colon with hemorrhage
> **DEFINITION**   Dilated intestinal blood vessels with corresponding thinning and weakening of vessel walls and bleeding into the intestinal tract.

● K55.3   Necrotizing enterocolitis
> **EXCLUDES 1**   *necrotizing enterocolitis of newborn (P77.-)*
> **EXCLUDES 2**   *necrotizing enterocolitis due to Clostridium difficile (A04.7)*

● K55.30   Necrotizing enterocolitis, unspecified
Necrotizing enterocolitis, NOS

● K55.31   Stage 1 necrotizing enterocolitis
Necrotizing enterocolitis without pneumatosis, without perforation

● K55.32   Stage 2 necrotizing enterocolitis
Necrotizing enterocolitis with pneumatosis, without perforation

● K55.33   Stage 3 necrotizing enterocolitis
Necrotizing enterocolitis with perforation
Necrotizing enterocolitis with pneumatosis and perforation

K55.8   Other vascular disorders of intestine

K55.9   Vascular disorder of intestine, unspecified
Ischemic colitis
Ischemic enteritis
Ischemic enterocolitis

K56   Paralytic ileus and intestinal obstruction without hernia
> **EXCLUDES 1**   *congenital stricture or stenosis of intestine (Q41-Q42)*
> *cystic fibrosis with meconium ileus (E84.11)*
> *ischemic stricture of intestine (K55.1)*
> *meconium ileus NOS (P76.0)*
> *neonatal intestinal obstructions classifiable to P76.-*
> *obstruction of duodenum (K31.5)*
> *postprocedural intestinal obstruction (K91.3)*
> *stenosis of anus or rectum (K62.4)*
> *intestinal obstruction with hernia (K40-K46)*

K56.0   Paralytic ileus
Paralysis of bowel
Paralysis of colon
Paralysis of intestine
> **EXCLUDES 1**   *gallstone ileus (K56.3)*
> *ileus NOS (K56.7)*
> *obstructive ileus NOS (K56.69)*

> **DEFINITION**   Blockage in the small or large intestine due to nonfunctioning muscle wall; may occur due to fluid imbalance, nerve damage, decreased blood supply, or toxins.

K56.1   Intussusception
Intussusception or invagination of bowel
Intussusception or invagination of colon
Intussusception or invagination of intestine
Intussusception or invagination of rectum
> **EXCLUDES 2**   *intussusception of appendix (K38.8)*

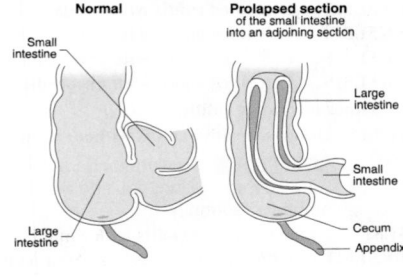
Intussusception

● New   ▲ Revised   *Manifestation*   4-7 Digit Indicators   Laterality   Adult (15+ years)   Maternity (12-55 years)   Newborn   Pediatric (0-17 years)   Male   Female
✖ Deleted   Unspecified   + Additional code

704   © 2017 DecisionHealth   2017 ICD-10-CM Expert for Physicians

K56.2 **Volvulus**
Strangulation of colon or intestine
Torsion of colon or intestine
Twist of colon or intestine
> **EXCLUDES 2** *volvulus of duodenum (K31.5)*

> **DEFINITION** Twisting of the intestine, constricting the passageway and cutting off blood supply to the area; presents with sudden, severe abdominal pain, vomiting, and abdominal distention.

K56.3 **Gallstone ileus**
Obstruction of intestine by gallstone

K56.4 **Other impaction of intestine**
  K56.41 **Fecal impaction**
> **EXCLUDES 1** *constipation (K59.0-)*
> *incomplete defecation (R15.0)*

  K56.49 **Other impaction of intestine**

K56.5 **Intestinal adhesions [bands] with obstruction (postprocedural) (postinfection)**
Abdominal hernia due to adhesions with obstruction
Peritoneal adhesions [bands] with intestinal obstruction (postprocedural) (postinfection)

K56.6 **Other and unspecified intestinal obstruction**
  K56.60 **Unspecified intestinal obstruction**
Intestinal obstruction NOS
> **EXCLUDES 1** *intestinal obstruction due to specified condition-code to condition*

  K56.69 **Other intestinal obstruction**
Enterostenosis NOS
Obstructive ileus NOS
Occlusion of colon or intestine NOS
Stenosis of colon or intestine NOS
Stricture of colon or intestine NOS
> **EXCLUDES 1** *intestinal obstruction due to specified condition-code to condition*

K56.7 **Ileus, unspecified**
> **EXCLUDES 1** *obstructive ileus (K56.69)*

K57 **Diverticular disease of intestine**
> **EXCLUDES 1** *congenital diverticulum of intestine (Q43.8)*
> *Meckel's diverticulum (Q43.0)*
> **EXCLUDES 2** *diverticulum of appendix (K38.2)*

> **CODING TIP ✓** Do not assign a code from K57.- for diverticular conditions reported as congenital. Congenital diverticulum should be coded to the appropriate Q43.- code.

K57.0 **Diverticulitis of small intestine with perforation and abscess**
Diverticulitis of small intestine with peritonitis
> **EXCLUDES 1** *diverticulitis of both small and large intestine with perforation and abscess (K57.4-)*

  K57.00 **Diverticulitis of small intestine with perforation and abscess without bleeding**

  K57.01 **Diverticulitis of small intestine with perforation and abscess with bleeding**

K57.1 **Diverticular disease of small intestine without perforation or abscess**
> **EXCLUDES 1** *diverticular disease of both small and large intestine without perforation or abscess (K57.5-)*

  K57.10 **Diverticulosis of small intestine without perforation or abscess without bleeding**
Diverticular disease of small intestine NOS

  K57.11 **Diverticulosis of small intestine without perforation or abscess with bleeding**

  K57.12 **Diverticulitis of small intestine without perforation or abscess without bleeding**

Diverticulitis of small intestine without perforation or abscess, without bleeding

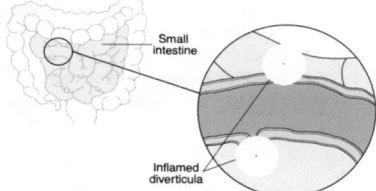
Small intestine
Inflamed diverticula

  K57.13 **Diverticulitis of small intestine without perforation or abscess with bleeding**

K57.2 **Diverticulitis of large intestine with perforation and abscess**
Diverticulitis of colon with peritonitis
> **EXCLUDES 1** *diverticulitis of both small and large intestine with perforation and abscess (K57.4-)*

  K57.20 **Diverticulitis of large intestine with perforation and abscess without bleeding**

  K57.21 **Diverticulitis of large intestine with perforation and abscess with bleeding**

K57.3 **Diverticular disease of large intestine without perforation or abscess**
> **EXCLUDES 1** *diverticular disease of both small and large intestine without perforation or abscess (K57.5-)*

  K57.30 **Diverticulosis of large intestine without perforation or abscess without bleeding**
Diverticular disease of colon NOS

  K57.31 **Diverticulosis of large intestine without perforation or abscess with bleeding**

  K57.32 **Diverticulitis of large intestine without perforation or abscess without bleeding**

  K57.33 **Diverticulitis of large intestine without perforation or abscess with bleeding**

K57.4 **Diverticulitis of both small and large intestine with perforation and abscess**
Diverticulitis of both small and large intestine with peritonitis

  K57.40 **Diverticulitis of both small and large intestine with perforation and abscess without bleeding**

  K57.41 **Diverticulitis of both small and large intestine with perforation and abscess with bleeding**

K57.5 **Diverticular disease of both small and large intestine without perforation or abscess**
  K57.50 **Diverticulosis of both small and large intestine without perforation or abscess without bleeding**
Diverticular disease of both small and large intestine NOS

  K57.51 **Diverticulosis of both small and large intestine without perforation or abscess with bleeding**

  K57.52 **Diverticulitis of both small and large intestine without perforation or abscess without bleeding**

  K57.53 **Diverticulitis of both small and large intestine without perforation or abscess with bleeding**

K57.8 **Diverticulitis of intestine, part unspecified, with perforation and abscess**
Diverticulitis of intestine NOS with peritonitis

  K57.80 **Diverticulitis of intestine, part unspecified, with perforation and abscess without bleeding**

  K57.81 **Diverticulitis of intestine, part unspecified, with perforation and abscess with bleeding**

K57.9 **Diverticular disease of intestine, part unspecified, without perforation or abscess**
  K57.90 **Diverticulosis of intestine, part unspecified, without perforation or abscess without bleeding**
Diverticular disease of intestine NOS

  K57.91 **Diverticulosis of intestine, part unspecified, without perforation or abscess with bleeding**

  K57.92 **Diverticulitis of intestine, part unspecified, without perforation or abscess without bleeding**

  K57.93 **Diverticulitis of intestine, part unspecified, without perforation or abscess with bleeding**

K58 **Irritable bowel syndrome**
> **INCLUDES** irritable colon
> spastic colon

> **DEFINITION** Functional disorder of hypersensitive nerves and muscles in the colon, causing cramping, pain, diarrhea, and/or constipation.

K58.0 **Irritable bowel syndrome with diarrhea**
> **CODING TIP ✓** Do not assign an additional code for the diarrhea. K58.0 is a combination code and does not require additional coding of the included symptom.

● **K58.1** **Irritable bowel syndrome with constipation**
● **K58.2** **Mixed irritable bowel syndrome**
● **K58.8** **Other irritable bowel syndrome**
K58.9 **Irritable bowel syndrome without diarrhea**
Irritable bowel syndrome NOS

● New   ▲ Revised   *Manifestation*   4 - 7 Digit Indicators   ▤ Laterality   Ⓐ Adult (15+ years)   Ⓜ Maternity (12-55 years)   Ⓝ Newborn   Ⓟ Pediatric (0-17 years)   ♂ Male   ♀ Female
✖ Deleted   Unspecified   + Additional code

◩ **K59** **Other functional intestinal disorders**

> **EXCLUDES 1** *change in bowel habit NOS (R19.4)*
> *intestinal malabsorption (K90.-)*
> *psychogenic intestinal disorders (F45.8)*
> **EXCLUDES 2** *functional disorders of stomach (K31.-)*

▲ ⑤ + **K59.0** **Constipation**

> *Use additional code for adverse effect, if applicable, to identify drug (T36-T50 with fifth or sixth character 5)*
> **EXCLUDES 1** *fecal impaction (K56.41)*
> *incomplete defecation (R15.0)*

+ **K59.00** **Constipation, unspecified**

+ **K59.01** **Slow transit constipation**

> **DEFINITION** Dysfunction of intestinal smooth muscles that move fecal matter, causing slow stool movement.

+ **K59.02** **Outlet dysfunction constipation**

● + **K59.03** **Drug induced constipation**

> *Use additional code for adverse effect, if applicable, to identify drug (T36-T50 with fifth or sixth character 5*

● + **K59.04** **Chronic idiopathic constipation**

> Functional constipation

▲ + **K59.09** **Other constipation**

> Chronic constipation

K59.1 **Functional diarrhea**

> **EXCLUDES 1** *diarrhea NOS (R19.7)*
> *irritable bowel syndrome with diarrhea (K58.0)*

K59.2 **Neurogenic bowel, not elsewhere classified**

> **DEFINITION** Intestinal dysfunction due to spinal cord damage.

▲ ⑤ **K59.3** **Megacolon, not elsewhere classified**

> Dilatation of colon
> Code first:
> , if applicable (T51-T65) to identify toxic agent
> **EXCLUDES 1** *congenital megacolon (aganglionic) (Q43.1)*
> *megacolon (due to) (in) Chagas' disease (B57.32)*
> *megacolon (due to) (in) Clostridium difficile (A04.7)*
> *megacolon (due to) (in) Hirschsprung's disease (Q43.1)*

> **CODING TIP ✓** Megacolon is an abnormal dilation of the colon, generally accompanied by reduced peristalsis. Do not assign a code from K59.3- if the cause is known to be due to another condition such as *Clostridium difficile* (A04.7), Hirschsprung's disease (Q43.1), or other congenital or known cause. When the cause is known, code the cause of the megacolon.

> **DEFINITION** Enlargement or dilation of the sigmoid colon.

● **K59.31** **Toxic megacolon**

● **K59.39** **Other megacolon**

> Megacolon NOS

K59.4 **Anal spasm**

> Proctalgia fugax

K59.8 **Other specified functional intestinal disorders**

> Atony of colon
> Pseudo-obstruction (acute) (chronic) of intestine

K59.9 **Functional intestinal disorder, unspecified**

◩ **K60** **Fissure and fistula of anal and rectal regions**

> **EXCLUDES 1** *fissure and fistula of anal and rectal regions with abscess or cellulitis (K61.-)*
> **EXCLUDES 2** *anal sphincter tear (healed) (nontraumatic) (old) (K62.81)*

K60.0 **Acute anal fissure**

K60.1 **Chronic anal fissure**

K60.2 **Anal fissure, unspecified**

K60.3 **Anal fistula**

> **DEFINITION** An abnormal passage from the anus to the skin.

K60.4 **Rectal fistula**

> Fistula of rectum to skin
> **EXCLUDES 1** *rectovaginal fistula (N82.3)*
> *vesicorectal fistual (N32.1)*

K60.5 **Anorectal fistula**

◩ **K61** **Abscess of anal and rectal regions**

> **INCLUDES** abscess of anal and rectal regions
> cellulitis of anal and rectal regions

K61.0 **Anal abscess**

> Perianal abscess
> **EXCLUDES 1** *intrasphincteric abscess (K61.4)*

K61.1 **Rectal abscess**

> Perirectal abscess
> **EXCLUDES 1** *ischiorectal abscess (K61.3)*
> AHA: 4Q 2012, 104

K61.2 **Anorectal abscess**

K61.3 **Ischiorectal abscess**

> Abscess of ischiorectal fossa

K61.4 **Intrasphincteric abscess**

◩ **K62** **Other diseases of anus and rectum**

> **INCLUDES** anal canal
> **EXCLUDES 2** *colostomy and enterostomy malfunction (K94.0-, K94.1-)*
> *fecal incontinence (R15.-)*
> *hemorrhoids (K64.-)*

K62.0 **Anal polyp**

K62.1 **Rectal polyp**

> **EXCLUDES 1** *adenomatous polyp (D12.8)*

K62.2 **Anal prolapse**

> Prolapse of anal canal

K62.3 **Rectal prolapse**

> Prolapse of rectal mucosa
> **DEFINITION** Rectal tissue falls from its usual position, turning itself inside out and protruding from the body in late stages.

Rectal prolapse

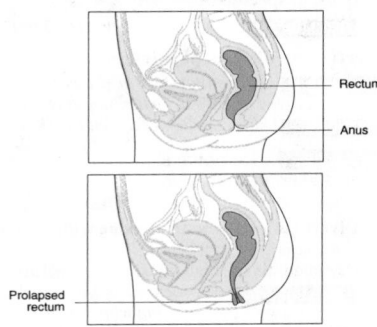

K62.4 **Stenosis of anus and rectum**

> Stricture of anus (sphincter)

K62.5 **Hemorrhage of anus and rectum**

> **EXCLUDES 1** *gastrointestinal bleeding NOS (K92.2)*
> *melena (K92.1)*
> *neonatal rectal hemorrhage (P54.2)*

K62.6 **Ulcer of anus and rectum**

> Solitary ulcer of anus and rectum
> Stercoral ulcer of anus and rectum
> **EXCLUDES 1** *fissure and fistula of anus and rectum (K60.-)*
> *ulcerative colitis (K51.-)*

> **DEFINITION** Open sore in the rectum and/or anus causing pain that worsens during defecation and blood or mucous in the stool.

+ **K62.7** **Radiation proctitis**

> *Use additional code to identify the type of radiation (W90.-)*

> **CODING TIP ✓** Radiation proctitis includes ulceration of the rectal lining due to the adverse effects of radiation. Assign an additional code from W90.- to identify radiation exposure.

⑤ **K62.8** **Other specified diseases of anus and rectum**

> **EXCLUDES 2** *ulcerative proctitis (K51.2)*

● New	▲ Revised	*Manifestation*	◩-◪ Digit Indicators	⊟ Laterality	▲ Adult (15+ years)	Ⓜ Maternity (12-55 years)	Ⓝ Newborn	Ⓟ Pediatric (0-17 years)	♂ Male	♀ Female
✖ Deleted		Unspecified	+ Additional code			

+ K62.81   Anal sphincter tear (healed) (nontraumatic) (old)
Tear of anus, nontraumatic
Use additional code for any associated fecal incontinence (R15.-)
> **EXCLUDES 2**   *anal fissure (K60.-)*
> *anal sphincter tear (healed) (old) complicating delivery (O34.7-)*
> *traumatic tear of anal sphincter (S31.831)*

K62.82   Dysplasia of anus
Anal intraepithelial neoplasia I and II (AIN I and II) (histologically confirmed)
Dysplasia of anus NOS
Mild and moderate dysplasia of anus (histologically confirmed)
> **EXCLUDES 1**   *abnormal results from anal cytologic examination without histologic confirmation (R85.61-)*
> *anal intraepithelial neoplasia III (D01.3)*
> *carcinoma in situ of anus (D01.3)*
> *HGSIL of anus (R85.613)*
> *severe dysplasia of anus (D01.3)*

+ K62.89   Other specified diseases of anus and rectum
Proctitis NOS
Use additional code for any associated fecal incontinence (R15.-)

K62.9   Disease of anus and rectum, unspecified

◁ K63   Other diseases of intestine

K63.0   Abscess of intestine
> **EXCLUDES 1**   *abscess of intestine with Crohn's disease (K50.014, K50.114, K50.814, K50.914,)*
> *abscess of intestine with diverticular disease (K57.0, K57.2, K57.4, K57.8)*
> *abscess of intestine with ulcerative colitis (K51.014, K51.214, K51.314, K51.414, K51.514, K51.814, K51.914)*
> **EXCLUDES 2**   *abscess of anal and rectal regions (K61.-)*
> *abscess of appendix (K35.3)*

K63.1   Perforation of intestine (nontraumatic)
Perforation (nontraumatic) of rectum
> **EXCLUDES 1**   *perforation (nontraumatic) of duodenum (K26.-)*
> *perforation (nontraumatic) of intestine with diverticular disease (K57.0, K57.2, K57.4, K57.8)*
> **EXCLUDES 2**   *perforation (nontraumatic) of appendix (K35.2, K35.3)*
> **DEFINITION**   Hole in the intestinal wall allowing food and/or fecal matter to leak into the abdominal cavity.

Perforation of intestinal (nontraumatic)

Large intestine   Small intestine   Hole in intestinal wall

K63.2   Fistula of intestine
> **EXCLUDES 1**   *fistula of duodenum (K31.6)*
> *fistula of intestine with Crohn's disease (K50.013, K50.113, K50.813, K50.913,)*
> *fistula of intestine with ulcerative colitis (K51.013, K51.213, K51.313, K51.413, K51.513, K51.813, K51.913)*
> **EXCLUDES 2**   *fistula of anal and rectal regions (K60.-)*
> *fistula of appendix (K38.3)*
> *intestinal-genital fistula, female (N82.2-N82.4)*
> *vesicointestinal fistula (N32.1)*

> **DEFINITION**   Abnormal passageway between loops of the intestine or the intestine and another organ or the abdominal wall.

Fistula of intestine

Small intestine   Small intestine   Fistula

K63.3   Ulcer of intestine
Primary ulcer of small intestine
> **EXCLUDES 1**   *duodenal ulcer (K26.-)*
> *gastrointestinal ulcer (K28.-)*
> *gastrojejunal ulcer (K28.-)*
> *jejunal ulcer (K28.-)*
> *peptic ulcer, site unspecified (K27.-)*
> *ulcer of intestine with perforation (K63.1)*
> *ulcer of anus or rectum (K62.6)*
> *ulcerative colitis (K51.-)*

K63.4   Enteroptosis
K63.5   Polyp of colon
> **EXCLUDES 1**   *adenomatous polyp of colon (D12.6)*
> *inflammatory polyp of colon (K51.4-)*
> *polyposis of colon (D12.6)*
AHA: 2Q 2015, 14

⑤ K63.8   Other specified diseases of intestine

K63.81   Dieulafoy lesion of intestine
> **EXCLUDES 2**   *Dieulafoy lesion of stomach and duodenum (K31.82)*

K63.89   Other specified diseases of intestine
AHA: 2Q 2013, 31

K63.9   Disease of intestine, unspecified

◁ K64   Hemorrhoids and perianal venous thrombosis
> **INCLUDES**   piles
> **EXCLUDES 1**   *hemorrhoids complicating childbirth and the puerperium (O87.2)*
> *hemorrhoids complicating pregnancy (O22.4)*

K64.0   First degree hemorrhoids
Grade/stage I hemorrhoids
Hemorrhoids (bleeding) without prolapse outside of anal canal

K64.1   Second degree hemorrhoids
Grade/stage II hemorrhoids
Hemorrhoids (bleeding) that prolapse with straining, but retract spontaneously

K64.2   Third degree hemorrhoids
Grade/stage III hemorrhoids
Hemorrhoids (bleeding) that prolapse with straining and require manual replacement back inside anal canal

K64.3   Fourth degree hemorrhoids
Grade/stage IV hemorrhoids
Hemorrhoids (bleeding) with prolapsed tissue that cannot be manually replaced

K64.4   Residual hemorrhoidal skin tags
External hemorrhoids, NOS
Skin tags of anus

K64.5   Perianal venous thrombosis
External hemorrhoids with thrombosis
Perianal hematoma
Thrombosed hemorrhoids NOS

K64.8   Other hemorrhoids
Internal hemorrhoids, without mention of degree
Prolapsed hemorrhoids, degree not specified

K64.9   Unspecified hemorrhoids
Hemorrhoids (bleeding) NOS
Hemorrhoids (bleeding) without mention of degree

● New   ▲ Revised   *Manifestation*   ◁-⑦ Digit Indicators   ▤ Laterality   Ⓐ Adult (15+ years)   Ⓜ Maternity (12-55 years)   Ⓝ Newborn   Ⓟ Pediatric (0-17 years)   ♂ Male   ♀ Female
✖ Deleted   Unspecified   + Additional code

Diseases of the Digestive System

Diseases of peritoneum and retroperitoneum (K65-K68)

4 + K65   Peritonitis

Use additional code (B95-B97), to identify infectious agent

> **EXCLUDES 1**   *acute appendicitis with generalized peritonitis (K35.2)*
> *aseptic peritonitis (T81.6)*
> *benign paroxysmal peritonitis (E85.0)*
> *chemical peritonitis (T81.6)*
> *diverticulitis of both small and large intestine with peritonitis (K57.4-)*
> *diverticulitis of colon with peritonitis (K57.2-)*
> *diverticulitis of intestine, NOS, with peritonitis (K57.8-)*
> *diverticulitis of small intestine with peritonitis (K57.0-)*
> *gonococcal peritonitis (A54.85)*
> *neonatal peritonitis (P78.0-P78.1)*
> *pelvic peritonitis, female (N73.3-N73.5)*
> *periodic familial peritonitis (E85.0)*
> *peritonitis due to talc or other foreign substance (T81.6)*
> *peritonitis in chlamydia (A74.81)*
> *peritonitis in diphtheria (A36.89)*
> *peritonitis in syphilis (late) (A52.74)*
> *peritonitis in tuberculosis (A18.31)*
> *peritonitis with or following abortion or ectopic or molar pregnancy (O00-O07, O08.0)*
> *peritonitis with or following appendicitis (K35.-)*
> *peritonitis with or following diverticular disease of intestine (K57.-)*
> *puerperal peritonitis (O85)*
> *retroperitoneal infections (K68.-)*

> **CODING TIP ✓**   When the causative infectious organism is known, always assign an additional code from B95-B97 to identify the infectious agent.

+ K65.0   Generalized (acute) peritonitis
Pelvic peritonitis (acute), male
Subphrenic peritonitis (acute)
Suppurative peritonitis (acute)

+ K65.1   Peritoneal abscess
Abdominopelvic abscess
Abscess (of) omentum
Abscess (of) peritoneum
Mesenteric abscess
Retrocecal abscess
Subdiaphragmatic abscess
Subhepatic abscess
Subphrenic abscess

+ K65.2   Spontaneous bacterial peritonitis

> **EXCLUDES 1**   *bacterial peritonitis NOS (K65.9)*

> **CODING TIP ✓**   Do not assign K65.2 unless the physician has specifically provided a diagnosis of "spontaneous" bacterial peritonitis. Bacterial peritonitis not specified as spontaneous is classified to K65.9 (Peritonitis NOS).

+ K65.3   Choleperitonitis
Peritonitis due to bile

+ K65.4   Sclerosing mesenteritis
Fat necrosis of peritoneum
(Idiopathic) sclerosing mesenteric fibrosis
Mesenteric lipodystrophy
Mesenteric panniculitis
Retractile mesenteritis

> **DEFINITION**   Rare, idiopathic lesions of fat necrosis, fibrosis, and chronic inflammation causing single or multiple lesions, with diffuse thickening of the mesentery.

+ K65.8   Other peritonitis
Chronic proliferative peritonitis
Peritonitis due to urine

+ K65.9   Peritonitis, unspecified
Bacterial peritonitis NOS
AHA: 2Q 2013, 31

4 K66   Other disorders of peritoneum

> **EXCLUDES 2**   *ascites (R18.-)*
> *peritoneal effusion (chronic) (R18.8)*

K66.0   Peritoneal adhesions (postprocedural) (postinfection)
Adhesions (of) abdominal (wall)
Adhesions (of) diaphragm
Adhesions (of) intestine
Adhesions (of) male pelvis
Adhesions (of) omentum
Adhesions (of) stomach
Adhesive bands
Mesenteric adhesions

> **EXCLUDES 1**   *female pelvic adhesions [bands] (N73.6)*
> *peritoneal adhesions with intestinal obstruction (K56.5)*

Peritoneal adhesions (postprocedural) (postinfection)

Liver
Pancreas
Stomach
Colon
Small intestine
Colon

Adhesions

Parietal peritoneum (outer lining of the internal organs)

Visceral peritoneum (inner lining of the internal organs)

K66.1   Hemoperitoneum

> **EXCLUDES 1**   *traumatic hemoperitoneum (S36.8-)*

K66.8   Other specified disorders of peritoneum

K66.9   Disorder of peritoneum, unspecified

K67   *Disorders of peritoneum in infectious diseases classified elsewhere*

Code first underlying disease, such as :
congenital syphilis (A50.0)
helminthiasis (B65.0 -B83.9)

> **EXCLUDES 1**   *peritonitis in chlamydia (A74.81)*
> *peritonitis in diphtheria (A36.89)*
> *peritonitis in gonococcal (A54.85)*
> *peritonitis in syphilis (late) (A52.74)*
> *peritonitis in tuberculosis (A18.31)*

4 K68   Disorders of retroperitoneum

5 K68.1   Retroperitoneal abscess

K68.11   Postprocedural retroperitoneal abscess

K68.12   Psoas muscle abscess

K68.19   Other retroperitoneal abscess

K68.9   Other disorders of retroperitoneum

Diseases of liver (K70-K77)

> **EXCLUDES 1**   *jaundice NOS (R17)*

> **EXCLUDES 2**   *hemochromatosis (E83.11-)*
> *Reye's syndrome (G93.7)*
> *viral hepatitis (B15-B19)*
> *Wilson's disease (E83.0)*

4 + K70   Alcoholic liver disease
Use additional code to identify:
alcohol abuse and dependence (F10.-)

● New   ▲ Revised   *Manifestation*   4-7 Digit Indicators   ⊟ Laterality   A Adult (15+ years)   M Maternity (12-55 years)   N Newborn   P Pediatric (0-17 years)   ♂ Male   ♀ Female

✖ Deleted   Unspecified   + Additional code

708   © 2017 DecisionHealth

2017 ICD-10-CM Expert for Physicians

K65 — K70

CODING TIP ✓   Codes from category K70.- indicate liver disease resulting from alcohol use. An additional code should be assigned to identify alcohol abuse or dependence.

Diseases of liver

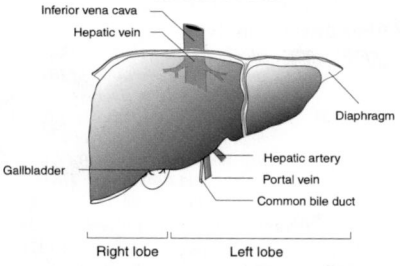

CODING TIP ✓   Codes from category K71.- indicate liver disease resulting from toxicity or toxic damage to the liver due to chemical exposure, including drugs. When a condition from K71.- is caused by poisoning, code first the appropriate T36-T65 code to indicate poisoning. When the condition is diagnosed as an adverse effect, code the appropriate K71.- code followed by the appropriate code from categories T36-T50 to indicate adverse effect.

+ K71.0   Toxic liver disease with cholestasis
Cholestasis with hepatocyte injury
'Pure' cholestasis

Ⓢ + K71.1   Toxic liver disease with hepatic necrosis
Hepatic failure (acute) (chronic) due to drugs

   + K71.10   Toxic liver disease with hepatic necrosis, without coma

   + K71.11   Toxic liver disease with hepatic necrosis, with coma

+ K71.2   Toxic liver disease with acute hepatitis

+ K71.3   Toxic liver disease with chronic persistent hepatitis

+ K71.4   Toxic liver disease with chronic lobular hepatitis

Ⓢ + K71.5   Toxic liver disease with chronic active hepatitis
Toxic liver disease with lupoid hepatitis

   + K71.50   Toxic liver disease with chronic active hepatitis without ascites

   + K71.51   Toxic liver disease with chronic active hepatitis with ascites

+ K71.6   Toxic liver disease with hepatitis, not elsewhere classified

+ K71.7   Toxic liver disease with fibrosis and cirrhosis of liver

+ K71.8   Toxic liver disease with other disorders of liver
Toxic liver disease with focal nodular hyperplasia
Toxic liver disease with hepatic granulomas
Toxic liver disease with peliosis hepatis
Toxic liver disease with veno-occlusive disease of liver

+ K71.9   Toxic liver disease, unspecified

▲ ④ K72   Hepatic failure, not elsewhere classified

  INCLUDES   fulminant hepatitis NEC, with hepatic failure
hepatic encephalopathy NOS
liver (cell) necrosis with hepatic failure
malignant hepatitis NEC, with hepatic failure
yellow liver atrophy or dystrophy

  EXCLUDES 1   *alcoholic hepatic failure (K70.4)*
hepatic failure with toxic liver disease (K71.1-)
icterus of newborn (P55-P59)
postprocedural hepatic failure (K91.82)

  EXCLUDES 2   *hepatic failure complicating abortion or ectopic or molar pregnancy (O00-O07, O08.8)*
hepatic failure complicating pregnancy, childbirth and the puerperium (O26.6-)
viral hepatitis with hepatic coma (B15-B19)

▲ Ⓢ K72.0   Acute and subacute hepatic failure
Acute non-viral hepatitis NOS
AHA: 2Q 2014, 13

   K72.00   Acute and subacute hepatic failure without coma
AHA: 2Q 2015, 17

   K72.01   Acute and subacute hepatic failure with coma

Ⓢ K72.1   Chronic hepatic failure

   K72.10   Chronic hepatic failure without coma

   K72.11   Chronic hepatic failure with coma

Ⓢ K72.9   Hepatic failure, unspecified

   K72.90   Hepatic failure, unspecified without coma
AHA: 2Q 2016, 35

   K72.91   Hepatic failure, unspecified with coma
Hepatic coma NOS

④ K73   Chronic hepatitis, not elsewhere classified

  EXCLUDES 1   *alcoholic hepatitis (chronic) (K70.1-)*
drug-induced hepatitis (chronic) (K71.-)
granulomatous hepatitis (chronic) NEC (K75.3)
reactive, nonspecific hepatitis (chronic) (K75.2)
viral hepatitis (chronic) (B15-B19)

  CODING TIP ✓   Do not assign a code from category K73.- when hepatitis is specified as viral or due to a specific cause, such as alcohol use or toxicity.

  K73.0   Chronic persistent hepatitis, not elsewhere classified

  K73.1   Chronic lobular hepatitis, not elsewhere classified

  K73.2   Chronic active hepatitis, not elsewhere classified

  K73.8   Other chronic hepatitis, not elsewhere classified

  K73.9   Chronic hepatitis, unspecified

+ K70.0   Alcoholic fatty liver   Ⓐ

Ⓢ + K70.1   Alcoholic hepatitis

   + K70.10   Alcoholic hepatitis without ascites   Ⓐ

   + K70.11   Alcoholic hepatitis with ascites   Ⓐ

+ K70.2   Alcoholic fibrosis and sclerosis of liver   Ⓐ

  DEFINITION   Intermediate stage liver disease in which normal, healthy tissue of the liver is replaced by scar tissue due to long-term, excessive alcohol consumption.

Ⓢ + K70.3   Alcoholic cirrhosis of liver
Alcoholic cirrhosis NOS

  DEFINITION   Late stage liver disease characterized by inflammation, debilitating scar tissue, and damaged membranes due to long-term, excessive alcohol consumption.

Alcoholic cirrhosis of liver without ascites

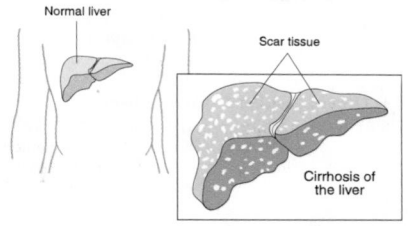

+ K70.30   Alcoholic cirrhosis of liver without ascites   Ⓐ

+ K70.31   Alcoholic cirrhosis of liver with ascites   Ⓐ

Ⓢ + K70.4   Alcoholic hepatic failure
Acute alcoholic hepatic failure
Alcoholic hepatic failure NOS
Chronic alcoholic hepatic failure
Subacute alcoholic hepatic failure

  + K70.40   Alcoholic hepatic failure without coma   Ⓐ

  + K70.41   Alcoholic hepatic failure with coma   Ⓐ

+ K70.9   Alcoholic liver disease, unspecified   Ⓐ

④ + K71   Toxic liver disease

  INCLUDES   drug-induced idiosyncratic (unpredictable) liver disease
drug-induced toxic (predictable) liver disease

  Code first:
  poisoning due to drug or toxin, if applicable (T36-T65 with fifth or sixth character 1-4 or 6)
  Use additional code for adverse effect, if applicable, to identify drug (T36-T50 with fifth or sixth character 5)

  EXCLUDES 2   *alcoholic liver disease (K70.-)*
Budd-Chiari syndrome (I82.0)

● New   ▲ Revised   *Manifestation*   ④-⑦ Digit Indicators   ⊟ Laterality   Ⓐ Adult (15+ years)   Ⓜ Maternity (12-55 years)   Ⓝ Newborn   Ⓟ Pediatric (0-17 years)   ♂ Male   ♀ Female
✖ Deleted   Unspecified   + Additional code

2017 ICD-10-CM Expert for Physicians   © 2017 DecisionHealth   709

K70 — K73.9

▣ **K74** **Fibrosis and cirrhosis of liver**
Code also:
, if applicable, viral hepatitis (acute) (chronic) (B15-B19)

> **EXCLUDES 1** *alcoholic cirrhosis (of liver) (K70.3)*
> *alcoholic fibrosis of liver (K70.2)*
> *cardiac sclerosis of liver (K76.1)*
> *cirrhosis (of liver) with toxic liver disease (K71.7)*
> *congenital cirrhosis (of liver) (P78.81)*
> *pigmentary cirrhosis (of liver) (E83.110)*

> **CODING TIP ✓** When viral hepatitis is also documented as a confirmed diagnosis in a patient with any diagnosis classifiable to K74.-, the appropriate code from B15-B19 should also be assigned.

K74.0 **Hepatic fibrosis**
K74.1 **Hepatic sclerosis**
K74.2 **Hepatic fibrosis with hepatic sclerosis**
K74.3 **Primary biliary cirrhosis**
Chronic nonsuppurative destructive cholangitis

> **DEFINITION** Scar tissue formation of the ducts carrying bile from the liver to the small intestine, resulting in bile build-up and liver damage leading to cirrhosis.

K74.4 **Secondary biliary cirrhosis**
K74.5 **Biliary cirrhosis, unspecified**
▤ **K74.6** **Other and unspecified cirrhosis of liver**
    K74.60 **Unspecified cirrhosis of liver**
        Cirrhosis (of liver) NOS
    K74.69 **Other cirrhosis of liver**
        Cryptogenic cirrhosis (of liver)
        Macronodular cirrhosis (of liver)
        Micronodular cirrhosis (of liver)
        Mixed type cirrhosis (of liver)
        Portal cirrhosis (of liver)
        Postnecrotic cirrhosis (of liver)

▣ **K75** **Other inflammatory liver diseases**
> **EXCLUDES 2** *toxic liver disease (K71.-)*

▲ **K75.0** **Abscess of liver**
Cholangitic hepatic abscess
Hematogenic hepatic abscess
Hepatic abscess NOS
Lymphogenic hepatic abscess
Pylephlebitic hepatic abscess

> **EXCLUDES 1** *amebic liver abscess (A06.4)*
> *cholangitis without liver abscess (K83.0)*
> *pylephlebitis without liver abscess (K75.1)*

> **EXCLUDES 2** *acute or subacute hepatitis NOS (B17.9)*
> *acute or subacute non-viral hepatitis (K72.0)*
> *chronic hepatitis NEC (K73.8)*

K75.1 **Phlebitis of portal vein**
Pylephlebitis

> **EXCLUDES 1** *pylephlebitic liver abscess (K75.0)*

K75.2 **Nonspecific reactive hepatitis**
> **EXCLUDES 1** *acute or subacute hepatitis (K72.0-)*
> *chronic hepatitis NEC (K73.-)*
> *viral hepatitis (B15-B19)*

K75.3 **Granulomatous hepatitis, not elsewhere classified**
> **EXCLUDES 1** *acute or subacute hepatitis (K72.0-)*
> *chronic hepatitis NEC (K73.-)*
> *viral hepatitis (B15-B19)*

K75.4 **Autoimmune hepatitis**
Lupoid hepatitis NEC

> **DEFINITION** Continuous inflammation and necrosis of liver cells that progresses to cirrhosis, in association with autoimmune diseases and not infection, alcohol consumption, or toxic exposure.

▤ **K75.8** **Other specified inflammatory liver diseases**
    K75.81 **Nonalcoholic steatohepatitis (NASH)**
    K75.89 **Other specified inflammatory liver diseases**
K75.9 **Inflammatory liver disease, unspecified**
Hepatitis NOS

> **EXCLUDES 1** *acute or subacute hepatitis (K72.0-)*
> *chronic hepatitis NEC (K73.-)*
> *viral hepatitis (B15-B19)*

> **CODING TIP ✓** **Documentation:** When documentation confirms only that a patient has hepatitis but does not provide any further detail, assign K75.9 to indicate hepatitis NOS. Do not assign this code if specific cause/type of hepatitis is specified in diagnostic information.
> AHA: 2Q 2015, 17

▣ **K76** **Other diseases of liver**
> **EXCLUDES 2** *alcoholic liver disease (K70.-)*
> *amyloid degeneration of liver (E85.-)*
> *cystic disease of liver (congenital) (Q44.6)*
> *hepatic vein thrombosis (I82.0)*
> *hepatomegaly NOS (R16.0)*
> *pigmentary cirrhosis (of liver) (E83.110)*
> *portal vein thrombosis (I81)*
> *toxic liver disease (K71.-)*

K76.0 **Fatty (change of) liver, not elsewhere classified**
Nonalcoholic fatty liver disease (NAFLD)

> **EXCLUDES 1** *nonalcoholic steatohepatitis (NASH) (K75.81)*

K76.1 **Chronic passive congestion of liver**
Cardiac cirrhosis
Cardiac sclerosis
K76.2 **Central hemorrhagic necrosis of liver**
> **EXCLUDES 1** *liver necrosis with hepatic failure (K72.-)*

K76.3 **Infarction of liver**
K76.4 **Peliosis hepatis**
Hepatic angiomatosis
K76.5 **Hepatic veno-occlusive disease**
> **EXCLUDES 1** *Budd-Chiari syndrome (I82.0)*

➕ **K76.6** **Portal hypertension**
Use additional code for any associated complications, such as:
    portal hypertensive gastropathy (K31.89)

> **DEFINITION** Increase in the pressure within the portal vein which carries blood from the digestive organs to the liver, caused by a blockage of blood flow through the liver.

▲ **K76.7** **Hepatorenal syndrome**
> **EXCLUDES 1** *hepatorenal syndrome following labor and delivery (O90.4)*
> *postprocedural hepatorenal syndrome (K91.83)*

▤ **K76.8** **Other specified diseases of liver**
    K76.81 **Hepatopulmonary syndrome**
    Code first underlying liver disease, such as:
        alcoholic cirrhosis of liver (K70.3-)
        cirrhosis of liver without mention of alcohol (K74.6-)
    K76.89 **Other specified diseases of liver**
        Cyst (simple) of liver
        Focal nodular hyperplasia of liver
        Hepatoptosis
    K76.9 **Liver disease, unspecified**

K77 *Liver disorders in diseases classified elsewhere*
Code first underlying disease, such as:
    amyloidosis (E85.-)
    congenital syphilis (A50.0, A50.5)
    congenital toxoplasmosis (P37.1)
    schistosomiasis (B65.0-B65.9)

> **EXCLUDES 1** *alcoholic hepatitis (K70.1-)*
> *alcoholic liver disease (K70.-)*
> *cytomegaloviral hepatitis (B25.1)*
> *herpesviral [herpes simplex] hepatitis (B00.81)*
> *infectious mononucleosis with liver disease (B27.0-B27.9 with .9)*
> *mumps hepatitis (B26.81)*
> *sarcoidosis with liver disease (D86.89)*
> *secondary syphilis with liver disease (A51.45)*
> *syphilis (late) with liver disease (A52.74)*
> *toxoplasmosis (acquired) hepatitis (B58.1)*
> *tuberculosis with liver disease (A18.83)*

Disorders of gallbladder, biliary tract and pancreas (K80-K87)

▣ **K80** **Cholelithiasis**
> **EXCLUDES 1** *retained cholelithiasis following cholecystectomy (K91.86)*

● New ▲ Revised *Manifestation* ▣-▢ Digit Indicators ⊟ Laterality △ Adult (15+ years) Ⓜ Maternity (12-55 years) Ⓝ Newborn Ⓟ Pediatric (0-17 years) ♂ Male ♀ Female
✖ Deleted Unspecified ✚ Additional code

     2017 ICD-10-CM Expert for Physicians

🅢 **K80.0** **Calculus of gallbladder with acute cholecystitis**
Any condition listed in K80.2 with acute cholecystitis

K80.00 Calculus of gallbladder with acute cholecystitis without obstruction

K80.01 Calculus of gallbladder with acute cholecystitis with obstruction

🅢 **K80.1** **Calculus of gallbladder with other cholecystitis**

K80.10 Calculus of gallbladder with chronic cholecystitis without obstruction
Cholelithiasis with cholecystitis NOS

K80.11 Calculus of gallbladder with chronic cholecystitis with obstruction

K80.12 Calculus of gallbladder with acute and chronic cholecystitis without obstruction

K80.13 Calculus of gallbladder with acute and chronic cholecystitis with obstruction

K80.18 Calculus of gallbladder with other cholecystitis without obstruction

K80.19 Calculus of gallbladder with other cholecystitis with obstruction

🅢 **K80.2** **Calculus of gallbladder without cholecystitis**
Cholecystolithiasis without cholecystitis
Cholelithiasis (without cholecystitis)
Colic (recurrent) of gallbladder (without cholecystitis)
Gallstone (impacted) of cystic duct (without cholecystitis)
Gallstone (impacted) of gallbladder (without cholecystitis)

K80.20 Calculus of gallbladder without cholecystitis without obstruction

K80.21 Calculus of gallbladder without cholecystitis with obstruction

Calculus of gallbladder without cholecystities with obstruction

Gallbladder

Gallstones

🅢 **K80.3** **Calculus of bile duct with cholangitis**
Any condition listed in K80.5 with cholangitis

K80.30 Calculus of bile duct with cholangitis, unspecified, without obstruction

K80.31 Calculus of bile duct with cholangitis, unspecified, with obstruction

K80.32 Calculus of bile duct with acute cholangitis without obstruction

K80.33 Calculus of bile duct with acute cholangitis with obstruction

K80.34 Calculus of bile duct with chronic cholangitis without obstruction

K80.35 Calculus of bile duct with chronic cholangitis with obstruction

K80.36 Calculus of bile duct with acute and chronic cholangitis without obstruction

K80.37 Calculus of bile duct with acute and chronic cholangitis with obstruction

🅢 **K80.4** **Calculus of bile duct with cholecystitis**
Any condition listed in K80.5 with cholecystitis (with cholangitis)

K80.40 Calculus of bile duct with cholecystitis, unspecified, without obstruction

K80.41 Calculus of bile duct with cholecystitis, unspecified, with obstruction

K80.42 Calculus of bile duct with acute cholecystitis without obstruction

K80.43 Calculus of bile duct with acute cholecystitis with obstruction

K80.44 Calculus of bile duct with chronic cholecystitis without obstruction

K80.45 Calculus of bile duct with chronic cholecystitis with obstruction

K80.46 Calculus of bile duct with acute and chronic cholecystitis without obstruction

K80.47 Calculus of bile duct with acute and chronic cholecystitis with obstruction

🅢 **K80.5** **Calculus of bile duct without cholangitis or cholecystitis**
Choledocholithiasis (without cholangitis or cholecystitis)
Gallstone (impacted) of bile duct NOS (without cholangitis or cholecystitis)
Gallstone (impacted) of common duct (without cholangitis or cholecystitis)
Gallstone (impacted) of hepatic duct (without cholangitis or cholecystitis)
Hepatic cholelithiasis (without cholangitis or cholecystitis)
Hepatic colic (recurrent) (without cholangitis or cholecystitis)

K80.50 Calculus of bile duct without cholangitis or cholecystitis without obstruction

K80.51 Calculus of bile duct without cholangitis or cholecystitis with obstruction

🅢 **K80.6** **Calculus of gallbladder and bile duct with cholecystitis**

K80.60 Calculus of gallbladder and bile duct with cholecystitis, unspecified, without obstruction

K80.61 Calculus of gallbladder and bile duct with cholecystitis, unspecified, with obstruction

K80.62 Calculus of gallbladder and bile duct with acute cholecystitis without obstruction

K80.63 Calculus of gallbladder and bile duct with acute cholecystitis with obstruction

K80.64 Calculus of gallbladder and bile duct with chronic cholecystitis without obstruction

K80.65 Calculus of gallbladder and bile duct with chronic cholecystitis with obstruction

K80.66 Calculus of gallbladder and bile duct with acute and chronic cholecystitis without obstruction

K80.67 Calculus of gallbladder and bile duct with acute and chronic cholecystitis with obstruction

🅢 **K80.7** **Calculus of gallbladder and bile duct without cholecystitis**

K80.70 Calculus of gallbladder and bile duct without cholecystitis without obstruction

K80.71 Calculus of gallbladder and bile duct without cholecystitis with obstruction

🅢 **K80.8** **Other cholelithiasis**

K80.80 Other cholelithiasis without obstruction

K80.81 Other cholelithiasis with obstruction

K81 **Cholecystitis**
EXCLUDES 1 *cholecystitis with cholelithiasis (K80.-)*

K81.0 **Acute cholecystitis**
Abscess of gallbladder
Angiocholecystitis
Emphysematous (acute) cholecystitis
Empyema of gallbladder
Gangrene of gallbladder
Gangrenous cholecystitis
Suppurative cholecystitis

K81.1 **Chronic cholecystitis**

K81.2 **Acute cholecystitis with chronic cholecystitis**

K81.9 **Cholecystitis, unspecified**

K82 **Other diseases of gallbladder**
EXCLUDES 1 *nonvisualization of gallbladder (R93.2)*
postcholecystectomy syndrome (K91.5)

● New ▲ Revised *Manifestation* 4-7 Digit Indicators ▤ Laterality Ⓐ Adult (15+ years) Ⓜ Maternity (12-55 years) Ⓝ Newborn Ⓟ Pediatric (0-17 years) ♂ Male ♀ Female
✖ Deleted Unspecified + Additional code

2017 ICD-10-CM Expert for Physicians

© 2017 DecisionHealth 711

K80.0 — K82

Diseases of the Digestive System

K82.0   Obstruction of gallbladder
Occlusion of cystic duct or gallbladder without cholelithiasis
Stenosis of cystic duct or gallbladder without cholelithiasis
Stricture of cystic duct or gallbladder without cholelithiasis
EXCLUDES 1   *obstruction of gallbladder with cholelithiasis (K80.-)*

Obstruction of gallbladder

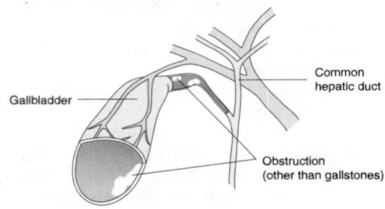

K82.1   Hydrops of gallbladder
Mucocele of gallbladder
DEFINITION   Overly full, distended gallbladder due to accumulation of mucous and watery material rather than stone formation.

K82.2   Perforation of gallbladder
Rupture of cystic duct or gallbladder

K82.3   Fistula of gallbladder
Cholecystocolic fistula
Cholecystoduodenal fistula

K82.4   Cholesterolosis of gallbladder
Strawberry gallbladder
EXCLUDES 1   *cholesterolosis of gallbladder with cholecystitis (K81.-)*
cholesterolosis of gallbladder with cholelithiasis (K80.-)
DEFINITION   Build-up of cholesterol deposits on the surface of the gallbladder, giving it a 'strawberry' appearance.

K82.8   Other specified diseases of gallbladder
Adhesions of cystic duct or gallbladder
Atrophy of cystic duct or gallbladder
Cyst of cystic duct or gallbladder
Dyskinesia of cystic duct or gallbladder
Hypertrophy of cystic duct or gallbladder
Nonfunctioning of cystic duct or gallbladder
Ulcer of cystic duct or gallbladder

K82.9   Disease of gallbladder, unspecified

▲ K83   Other diseases of biliary tract
EXCLUDES 1   *postcholecystectomy syndrome (K91.5)*
EXCLUDES 2   *conditions involving the gallbladder (K81-K82)*
conditions involving the cystic duct (K81-K82)

K83.0   Cholangitis
Ascending cholangitis
Cholangitis NOS
Primary cholangitis
Recurrent cholangitis
Sclerosing cholangitis
Secondary cholangitis
Stenosing cholangitis
Suppurative cholangitis
EXCLUDES 1   *cholangitic liver abscess (K75.0)*
cholangitis with choledocholithiasis (K80.3-, K80.4-)
chronic nonsuppurative destructive cholangitis (K74.3)
DEFINITION   Infection of the biliary tract; presents with pain in the upper-right abdomen which may grow worse after a fatty meal, fever, nausea, vomiting, flatulence, pale-colored stool, and yellowing of the eyes and skin.

K83.1   Obstruction of bile duct
Occlusion of bile duct without cholelithiasis
Stenosis of bile duct without cholelithiasis
Stricture of bile duct without cholelithiasis
EXCLUDES 1   *congenital obstruction of bile duct (Q44.3)*
obstruction of bile duct with cholelithiasis (K80.-)
AHA: 1Q 2016, 18-19

Obstruction of bile duct

K83.2   Perforation of bile duct
Rupture of bile duct

K83.3   Fistula of bile duct
Choledochoduodenal fistula

K83.4   Spasm of sphincter of Oddi

K83.5   Biliary cyst

K83.8   Other specified diseases of biliary tract
Adhesions of biliary tract
Atrophy of biliary tract
Hypertrophy of biliary tract
Ulcer of biliary tract

K83.9   Disease of biliary tract, unspecified

▲ 4 K85   Acute pancreatitis
INCLUDES   acute (recurrent) pancreatitis
subacute pancreatitis

▲ 5 K85.0   Idiopathic acute pancreatitis
● **K85.00   Idiopathic acute pancreatitis without necrosis or infection**
● **K85.01   Idiopathic acute pancreatitis with uninfected necrosis**
● **K85.02   Idiopathic acute pancreatitis with infected necrosis**

▲ 5 K85.1   Biliary acute pancreatitis
Gallstone pancreatitis
● **K85.10   Biliary acute pancreatitis without necrosis or infection**
● **K85.11   Biliary acute pancreatitis with uninfected necrosis**
● **K85.12   Biliary acute pancreatitis with infected necrosis**

▲ 5 K85.2   Alcohol induced acute pancreatitis
EXCLUDES 2   *alcohol induced chronic pancreatitis (K86.0)*
CODING TIP ✓   Assign a code from K85.2- only when physician documentation clearly confirms chronic pancreatitis due to alcohol use. The appropriate F10 code with 5th and 6th digits .88 (F10.188, F10.288, F10.988) should also be added.
● **K85.20   Alcohol induced acute pancreatitis without necrosis or infection**
● **K85.21   Alcohol induced acute pancreatitis with uninfected necrosis**
● **K85.22   Alcohol induced acute pancreatitis with infected necrosis**

▲ 5 + K85.3   Drug induced acute pancreatitis
Use additional code for adverse effect, if applicable, to identify drug (T36-T50 with fifth or sixth character 5)
Use additional code to identify drug abuse and dependence (F11.-F17.-)
● + **K85.30   Drug induced acute pancreatitis without necrosis or infection**
● + **K85.31   Drug induced acute pancreatitis with uninfected necrosis**
● + **K85.32   Drug induced acute pancreatitis with infected necrosis**

▲ 5 K85.8   Other acute pancreatitis
● **K85.80   Other acute pancreatitis without necrosis or infection**
● **K85.81   Other acute pancreatitis with uninfected necrosis**
● **K85.82   Other acute pancreatitis with infected necrosis**

▲ 5 K85.9   Acute pancreatitis, unspecified
Pancreatitis NOS
● **K85.90   Acute pancreatitis without necrosis or infection, unspecified**
● **K85.91   Acute pancreatitis with uninfected necrosis, unspecified**

● New   ▲ Revised   *Manifestation*   4 - 7 Digit Indicators   Laterality   Adult (15+ years)   Maternity (12-55 years)   Newborn   Pediatric (0-17 years)   ♂ Male   ♀ Female
✖ Deleted   Unspecified   + Additional code

712   © 2017 DecisionHealth   2017 ICD-10-CM Expert for Physicians

K82.0 — K85.91

● **K85.92** **Acute pancreatitis with infected necrosis, unspecified**

◢ **K86** **Other diseases of pancreas**

> **EXCLUDES 2** *fibrocystic disease of pancreas (E84.-)*
> *islet cell tumor (of pancreas) (D13.7)*
> *pancreatic steatorrhea (K90.3)*

Other diseases of pancreas

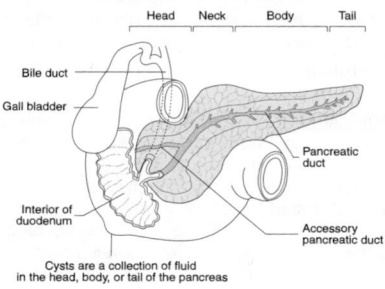

Head | Neck | Body | Tail

Bile duct
Gall bladder
Pancreatic duct
Interior of duodenum
Accessory pancreatic duct

Cysts are a collection of fluid in the head, body, or tail of the pancreas

▲ + **K86.0** **Alcohol-induced chronic pancreatitis**

Code also:
exocrine pancreatic insufficiency (K86.81)
Use additional code to identify:
alcohol abuse and dependence (F10.-)

> **EXCLUDES 2** *alcohol induced acute pancreatitis (K85.2-)*

> **CODING TIP ✓** Assign a code from K86.0- only when physician documentation clearly confirms acute pancreatitis due to alcohol use. The appropriate F10 code with 5th and 6th digits .88 (F10.188, F10.288, F10.988) should also be added.

▲ **K86.1** **Other chronic pancreatitis**

Chronic pancreatitis NOS
Infectious chronic pancreatitis
Recurrent chronic pancreatitis
Relapsing chronic pancreatitis
Code also:
exocrine pancreatic insufficiency (K86.81)

K86.2 **Cyst of pancreas**

K86.3 **Pseudocyst of pancreas**

▲ ⑤ **K86.8** **Other specified diseases of pancreas**

● **K86.81** **Exocrine pancreatic insufficiency**

● **K86.89** **Other specified diseases of pancreas**
Aseptic pancreatic necrosis, unrelated to acute pancreatitis
Atrophy of pancreas
Calculus of pancreas
Cirrhosis of pancreas
Fibrosis of pancreas
Pancreatic fat necrosis, unrelated to acute pancreatitis
Pancreatic infantilism
Pancreatic necrosis NOS, unrelated to acute pancreatitis

K86.9 **Disease of pancreas, unspecified**

K87 **Disorders of gallbladder, biliary tract and pancreas in diseases classified elsewhere**

Code first:
underlying disease

> **EXCLUDES 1** *cytomegaloviral pancreatitis (B25.2)*
> *mumps pancreatitis (B26.3)*
> *syphilitic gallbladder (A52.74)*
> *syphilitic pancreas (A52.74)*
> *tuberculosis of gallbladder (A18.83)*
> *tuberculosis of pancreas (A18.83)*

Other diseases of the digestive system
(K90-K95)

◢ **K90** **Intestinal malabsorption**

> **EXCLUDES 1** *intestinal malabsorption following gastrointestinal surgery (K91.2)*

> **CODING TIP ✓** Do not assign a code from K90.- when malabsorption is reported as post-surgical or post-procedural. Post-procedural / post-surgical complications affecting the gastrointestinal system are coded to category K91.-

▲ + **K90.0** **Celiac disease**

Celiac disease with steatorrhea
Gluten-sensitive enteropathy
Nontropical sprue
Code also:
exocrine pancreatic insufficiency (K86.81)
Use additional code for associated disorders including:
dermatitis herpetiformis (L13.0)
gluten ataxia (G32.81)

> **DEFINITION** Malabsorption syndrome precipitated by ingestion of gluten with loss of villous projections of the intestinal mucosa; manifests with bulky, frothy diarrhea, abdominal distention, flatulence, weight loss, and vitamin and electrolyte depletion.

K90.1 **Tropical sprue**

Sprue NOS
Tropical steatorrhea

> **DEFINITION** A malabsorption syndrome occurring in the tropics and subtropics, marked by inflammation of the mucous tissue of the mouth, diarrhea, and anemia.

K90.2 **Blind loop syndrome, not elsewhere classified**

Blind loop syndrome NOS

> **EXCLUDES 1** *congenital blind loop syndrome (Q43.8)*
> *postsurgical blind loop syndrome (K91.2)*

K90.3 **Pancreatic steatorrhea**

> **DEFINITION** Insufficient pancreatic enzyme excretions causing severe malabsorption and nutrient deficiencies with loose stools containing unabsorbed fat.

▲ ⑤ **K90.4** **Other malabsorption due to intolerance**

> **EXCLUDES 2** *gluten-sensitive enteropathy (K90.0)*
> *lactose intolerance (E73.-)*

● **K90.41** **Non-celiac gluten sensitivity**

Gluten sensitivity NOS
Non-celiac gluten sensitive enteropathy

● **K90.49** **Malabsorption due to intolerance, not elsewhere classified**

Malabsorption due to intolerance to carbohydrate
Malabsorption due to intolerance to fat
Malabsorption due to intolerance to protein
Malabsorption due to intolerance to starch

⑤ **K90.8** **Other intestinal malabsorption**

K90.81 **Whipple's disease**

K90.89 **Other intestinal malabsorption**

K90.9 **Intestinal malabsorption, unspecified**

◢ **K91** **Intraoperative and postprocedural complications and disorders of digestive system, not elsewhere classified**

> **EXCLUDES 2** *complications of artificial opening of digestive system (K94.-)*
> *complications of bariatric procedures (K95.-)*
> *gastrojejunal ulcer (K28.-)*
> *postprocedural (radiation) retroperitoneal abscess (K68.11)*
> *radiation colitis (K52.0)*
> *radiation gastroenteritis (K52.0)*
> *radiation proctitis (K62.7)*

> **CODING TIP ✓** Documentation: Codes in category K91.- are complication codes and require physician documentation and confirmation of a cause and effect relationship between the procedure and the complicated condition. Documentation must also support this relationship.

K91.0 **Vomiting following gastrointestinal surgery**

K91.1 **Postgastric surgery syndromes**

Dumping syndrome
Postgastrectomy syndrome
Postvagotomy syndrome

K91.2 **Postsurgical malabsorption, not elsewhere classified**

Postsurgical blind loop syndrome

> **EXCLUDES 1** *malabsorption osteomalacia in adults (M83.2)*
> *malabsorption osteoporosis, postsurgical (M80.8-, M81.8)*

K91.3 **Postprocedural intestinal obstruction**

K91.5 **Postcholecystectomy syndrome**

● New ▲ Revised *Manifestation* ◢-⑦ Digit Indicators ⊟ Laterality Ⓐ Adult (15+ years) Ⓜ Maternity (12-55 years) Ⓝ Newborn Ⓟ Pediatric (0-17 years) ♂ Male ♀ Female
✖ Deleted Unspecified + Additional code

⑤ **K91.6** **Intraoperative hemorrhage and hematoma of a digestive system organ or structure complicating a procedure**

> EXCLUDES 1 *intraoperative hemorrhage and hematoma of a digestive system organ or structure due to accidental puncture and laceration during a procedure (K91.7-)*

▲ **K91.61** **Intraoperative hemorrhage and hematoma of a digestive system organ or structure complicating a digestive system procedure**

K91.62 **Intraoperative hemorrhage and hematoma of a digestive system organ or structure complicating other procedure**

⑤ **K91.7** **Accidental puncture and laceration of a digestive system organ or structure during a procedure**

K91.71 **Accidental puncture and laceration of a digestive system organ or structure during a digestive system procedure**

K91.72 **Accidental puncture and laceration of a digestive system organ or structure during other procedure**

⑤ **K91.8** **Other intraoperative and postprocedural complications and disorders of digestive system**

K91.81 **Other intraoperative complications of digestive system**

K91.82 **Postprocedural hepatic failure**

K91.83 **Postprocedural hepatorenal syndrome**

▲ ⑥ **K91.84** **Postprocedural hemorrhage of a digestive system organ or structure following a procedure**

▲ **K91.840** **Postprocedural hemorrhage of a digestive system organ or structure following a digestive system procedure**
AHA: 1Q 2016, 15

▲ **K91.841** **Postprocedural hemorrhage of a digestive system organ or structure following other procedure**

⑥ **K91.85** **Complications of intestinal pouch**

K91.850 **Pouchitis**
Inflammation of internal ileoanal pouch

K91.858 **Other complications of intestinal pouch**

K91.86 **Retained cholelithiasis following cholecystectomy**

● ⑥ **K91.87** **Postprocedural hematoma and seroma of a digestive system organ or structure following a procedure**

● **K91.870** **Postprocedural hematoma of a digestive system organ or structure following a digestive system procedure**

● **K91.871** **Postprocedural hematoma of a digestive system organ or structure following other procedure**

● **K91.872** **Postprocedural seroma of a digestive system organ or structure following a digestive system procedure**

● **K91.873** **Postprocedural seroma of a digestive system organ or structure following other procedure**

+ **K91.89** **Other postprocedural complications and disorders of digestive system**
Use additional code, if applicable, to further specify disorder

> EXCLUDES 2 *postprocedural retroperitoneal abscess (K68.11)*

④ **K92** **Other diseases of digestive system**

> EXCLUDES 1 *neonatal gastrointestinal hemorrhage (P54.0-P54.3)*

K92.0 **Hematemesis**

K92.1 **Melena**

> EXCLUDES 1 *occult blood in feces (R19.5)*

K92.2 **Gastrointestinal hemorrhage, unspecified**
Gastric hemorrhage NOS
Intestinal hemorrhage NOS

> EXCLUDES 1 *acute hemorrhagic gastritis (K29.01)*
> *hemorrhage of anus and rectum (K62.5)*
> *angiodysplasia of stomach with hemorrhage (K31.811)*
> *diverticular disease with hemorrhage (K57.-)*
> *gastritis and duodenitis with hemorrhage (K29.-)*
> *peptic ulcer with hemorrhage (K25-K28)*

⑤ **K92.8** **Other specified diseases of the digestive system**

K92.81 **Gastrointestinal mucositis (ulcerative)**
Code also type of associated therapy, such as:
antineoplastic and immunosuppressive drugs (T45.1X-)
radiological procedure and radiotherapy (Y84.2)

> EXCLUDES 2 *mucositis (ulcerative) of vagina and vulva (N76.81)*
> *nasal mucositis (ulcerative) (J34.81)*
> *oral mucositis (ulcerative) (K12.3-)*

K92.89 **Other specified diseases of the digestive system**

K92.9 **Disease of digestive system, unspecified**

④ **K94** **Complications of artificial openings of the digestive system**

> CODING TIP ✓ All colostomy, gastrostomy, enterostomy, and esophagostomy complications are coded to category K94.- . This includes excoriation and denuding of the skin surrounding the ostomy, infection of the ostomy site, hemorrhage of the ostomy site, and other complications. No additional code should be used when coding skin complications unless an infection is present, in which case, an additional code should be used to specify the infection. When an ostomy complication is present, do not assign a Z code for the ostomy. Z codes indicate routine ostomy care, which is not appropriate in the case of a complicated ostomy.

⑤ **K94.0** **Colostomy complications**

K94.00 **Colostomy complication, unspecified**

K94.01 **Colostomy hemorrhage**

+ **K94.02** **Colostomy infection**
Use additional code to specify type of infection, such as:
cellulitis of abdominal wall (L03.311)
sepsis (A40.-, A41.-)

K94.03 **Colostomy malfunction**
Mechanical complication of colostomy

K94.09 **Other complications of colostomy**

⑤ **K94.1** **Enterostomy complications**

K94.10 **Enterostomy complication, unspecified**

K94.11 **Enterostomy hemorrhage**

+ **K94.12** **Enterostomy infection**
Use additional code to specify type of infection, such as:
cellulitis of abdominal wall (L03.311)
sepsis (A40.-, A41.-)

K94.13 **Enterostomy malfunction**
Mechanical complication of enterostomy

K94.19 **Other complications of enterostomy**

⑤ **K94.2** **Gastrostomy complications**

K94.20 **Gastrostomy complication, unspecified**

K94.21 **Gastrostomy hemorrhage**

+ **K94.22** **Gastrostomy infection**
Use additional code to specify type of infection, such as:
cellulitis of abdominal wall (L03.311)
sepsis (A40.-, A41.-)

K94.23 **Gastrostomy malfunction**
Mechanical complication of gastrostomy

K94.29 **Other complications of gastrostomy**

⑤ **K94.3** **Esophagostomy complications**

K94.30 **Esophagostomy complications, unspecified**

K94.31 **Esophagostomy hemorrhage**

+ **K94.32** **Esophagostomy infection**
Use additional code to identify the infection

K94.33 **Esophagostomy malfunction**
Mechanical complication of esophagostomy

K94.39 **Other complications of esophagostomy**

④ **K95** **Complications of bariatric procedures**

> CODING TIP ✓ **Documentation:** Codes in category K95.- are complication codes and require physician documentation and confirmation of a cause and effect relationship between the procedure and the complicated condition. Documentation must also support this relationship.

⑤ **K95.0** **Complications of gastric band procedure**

● New   ▲ Revised   *Manifestation*   ④-⑦ Digit Indicators   ⑤ Laterality   Ⓐ Adult (15+ years)   Ⓜ Maternity (12-55 years)   Ⓝ Newborn   Ⓟ Pediatric (0-17 years)   ♂ Male   ♀ Female

✖ ~~Deleted~~   Unspecified   + Additional code

714   © 2017 DecisionHealth   2017 ICD-10-CM Expert for Physicians

+ K95.01   **Infection due to gastric band procedure**

Use additional code to specify type of infection or organism, such as:
bacterial and viral infectious agents (B95.-, B96.-)
cellulitis of abdominal wall (L03.311)
sepsis (A40.-, A41.-)

+ K95.09   **Other complications of gastric band procedure**

Use additional code, if applicable, to further specify complication

⑤ K95.8   **Complications of other bariatric procedure**

EXCLUDES 1   *complications of gastric band surgery (K95.0-)*

+ K95.81   **Infection due to other bariatric procedure**

Use additional code to specify type of infection or organism, such as:
bacterial and viral infectious agents (B95.-, B96.-)
cellulitis of abdominal wall (L03.311)
sepsis (A40.-, A41.-)

+ K95.89   **Other complications of other bariatric procedure**

Use additional code, if applicable, to further specify complication

---

● New   ▲ Revised   *Manifestation*   ④-⑦ Digit Indicators   ⊟ Laterality   Ⓐ Adult (15+ years)   Ⓜ Maternity (12-55 years)   Ⓝ Newborn   Ⓟ Pediatric (0-17 years)   ♂ Male   ♀ Female

✖ Deleted   Unspecified   + Additional code

2017 ICD-10-CM Expert for Physicians

© 2017 DecisionHealth

715

CHAPTER 12: DISEASES OF THE SKIN AND SUBCUTANEOUS TISSUE (L00 -L99)

EXCLUDES 2 *certain conditions originating in the perinatal period (P04-P96)*
certain infectious and parasitic diseases (A00-B99)
complications of pregnancy, childbirth and the puerperium (O00-O9A)
congenital malformations, deformations, and chromosomal abnormalities (Q00-Q99)
endocrine, nutritional and metabolic diseases (E00-E88)
lipomelanotic reticulosis (I89.8)
neoplasms (C00-D49)
symptoms, signs and abnormal clinical and laboratory findings, not elsewhere classified (R00-R94)
systemic connective tissue disorders (M30-M36)
viral warts (B07.-)

This chapter contains the following blocks:

L00-L08   Infections of the skin and subcutaneous tissue
L10-L14   Bullous disorders
L20-L30   Dermatitis and eczema
L40-L45   Papulosquamous disorders
L49-L54   Urticaria and erythema
L55-L59   Radiation-related disorders of the skin and subcutaneous tissue
L60-L75   Disorders of skin appendages
L76   Intraoperative and postprocedural complications of skin and subcutaneous tissue
L80-L99   Other disorders of the skin and subcutaneous tissue

Infections of the skin and subcutaneous tissue (L00-L08)

Use additional code (B95-B97) to identify infectious agent.

EXCLUDES 2 *hordeolum (H00.0)*
infective dermatitis (L30.3)
local infections of skin classified in Chapter 1
lupus panniculitis (L93.2)
panniculitis NOS (M79.3)
panniculitis of neck and back (M54.0-)
Perlèche NOS (K13.0)
Perlèche due to candidiasis (B37.0)
Perlèche due to riboflavin deficiency (E53.0)
pyogenic granuloma (L98.0)
relapsing panniculitis [Weber-Christian] (M35.6)
viral warts (B07.-)
zoster (B02.-)

+ L00   Staphylococcal scalded skin syndrome
Ritter's disease
Use additional code to identify percentage of skin exfoliation (L49.-)
EXCLUDES 1 *bullous impetigo (L01.03)*
pemphigus neonatorum (L01.03)
toxic epidermal necrolysis [Lyell] (L51.2)
DEFINITION   The breakdown of dermal layer cellular structure by staph bacteria causing large sections of skin to slough off and peel away, leaving raw, exposed areas.

◢ L01   Impetigo
EXCLUDES 1 *impetigo herpetiformis (L40.1)*

⑤ L01.0   Impetigo
Impetigo contagiosa
Impetigo vulgaris
DEFINITION   Bacterial skin infection in children; small pustules form over a reddish rash and burst, leaving an itchy, yellow crust over the affected area.

L01.00   Impetigo, unspecified
Impetigo NOS

L01.01   Non-bullous impetigo
DEFINITION   Most common type of impetigo due to staph or strep bacteria, in which tiny blisters form (particularly on the face), burst quickly, and leave a small, wet, weeping spot that crusts over and disappears, leaving a red mark that later heals.

L01.02   Bockhart's impetigo
Impetigo follicularis
Perifolliculitis NOS
Superficial pustular perifolliculitis
DEFINITION   Superficial, pustular folliculitis caused by *S. aureus*; characterized by small, painful, tense, yellowish-white domed pustules in crops around follicular orifices that heal in a few days.

L01.03   Bullous impetigo
Impetigo neonatorum
Pemphigus neonatorum
DEFINITION   Impetigo of longer duration (generally due to *S. aureus*), in which large, clear, fluid-filled blisters form on red sores, become cloudy, then burst and ooze, leaving a large, yellowish, crusty scab.

L01.09   Other impetigo
Ulcerative impetigo
DEFINITION   Ulcerative impetigo: A deeper dermis form of impetigo with small, shallow, purulent ulcers that form under a thick, brownish-black crusted surface infection, surrounded by erythema.

L01.1   Impetiginization of other dermatoses
DEFINITION   Impetigo occurring in an area already experiencing a dermatosis; the infected blisters burst, leaving a weeping wet patch that crusts over, worsening the existing condition.

◢ + L02   Cutaneous abscess, furuncle and carbuncle
Use additional code to identify organism (B95-B96)
EXCLUDES 2 *abscess of anus and rectal regions (K61.-)*
abscess of female genital organs (external) (N76.4)
abscess of male genital organs (external) (N48.2, N49.-)
CODING TIP ✓   Abscesses, carbuncles and furuncles are coded separately from cellulitis (L03). Furuncles are commonly known as boils. Use an additional code to identify the causative organism.
DEFINITION   Abscess: A pocket of pus that collects within an infected area of skin and is generally red and sore.
DEFINITION   Carbuncle: A group of several infected hair follicles, or furuncles, that join together with more than one opening to drain pus, often extending into deeper tissue.
DEFINITION   Furuncle: A bacterial infection of a hair follicle characterized by a painful, red, swollen bump filled with fluid, pus, and cellular debris; also called a boil.

⑤ + L02.0   Cutaneous abscess, furuncle and carbuncle of face
EXCLUDES 2 *abscess of ear, external (H60.0)*
abscess of eyelid (H00.0)
abscess of head [any part, except face] (L02.8)
abscess of lacrimal gland (H04.0)
abscess of lacrimal passages (H04.3)
abscess of mouth (K12.2)
abscess of nose (J34.0)
abscess of orbit (H05.0)
submandibular abscess (K12.2)

+ L02.01   Cutaneous abscess of face
+ L02.02   Furuncle of face
Boil of face
Folliculitis of face
+ L02.03   Carbuncle of face

⑤ + L02.1   Cutaneous abscess, furuncle and carbuncle of neck
+ L02.11   Cutaneous abscess of neck
+ L02.12   Furuncle of neck
Boil of neck
Folliculitis of neck
+ L02.13   Carbuncle of neck

● New   ▲ Revised   *Manifestation*   ◢-❼ Digit Indicators   ⊟ Laterality   Ⓐ Adult (15+ years)   Ⓜ Maternity (12-55 years)   Ⓝ Newborn   Ⓟ Pediatric (0-17 years)   ♂ Male   ♀ Female
✖ ~~Deleted~~   Unspecified   + Additional code

▲ ▣ ✚ **L02.2**   **Cutaneous abscess, furuncle and carbuncle of trunk**

EXCLUDES 1   *non-newborn omphalitis (L08.82)*
omphalitis of newborn (P38.-)

EXCLUDES 2   *abscess of breast (N61.1)*
abscess of buttocks (L02.3)
abscess of female external genital organs (N76.4)
abscess of male external genital organs (N48.2, N49.-)
abscess of hip (L02.4)

⑥ ✚ **L02.21**   **Cutaneous abscess of trunk**

✚ **L02.211**   **Cutaneous abscess of abdominal wall**

✚ **L02.212**   **Cutaneous abscess of back [any part, except buttock]**

✚ **L02.213**   **Cutaneous abscess of chest wall**

✚ **L02.214**   **Cutaneous abscess of groin**

✚ **L02.215**   **Cutaneous abscess of perineum**

✚ **L02.216**   **Cutaneous abscess of umbilicus**

✚ **L02.219**   **Cutaneous abscess of trunk, unspecified**

⑥ ✚ **L02.22**   **Furuncle of trunk**
Boil of trunk
Folliculitis of trunk

✚ **L02.221**   **Furuncle of abdominal wall**

✚ **L02.222**   **Furuncle of back [any part, except buttock]**

✚ **L02.223**   **Furuncle of chest wall**

✚ **L02.224**   **Furuncle of groin**

✚ **L02.225**   **Furuncle of perineum**

✚ **L02.226**   **Furuncle of umbilicus**

✚ **L02.229**   **Furuncle of trunk, unspecified**

⑥ ✚ **L02.23**   **Carbuncle of trunk**

✚ **L02.231**   **Carbuncle of abdominal wall**

✚ **L02.232**   **Carbuncle of back [any part, except buttock]**

✚ **L02.233**   **Carbuncle of chest wall**

✚ **L02.234**   **Carbuncle of groin**

✚ **L02.235**   **Carbuncle of perineum**

✚ **L02.236**   **Carbuncle of umbilicus**

✚ **L02.239**   **Carbuncle of trunk, unspecified**

▣ ✚ **L02.3**   **Cutaneous abscess, furuncle and carbuncle of buttock**

EXCLUDES 1   *pilonidal cyst with abscess (L05.01)*

✚ **L02.31**   **Cutaneous abscess of buttock**
Cutaneous abscess of gluteal region

✚ **L02.32**   **Furuncle of buttock**
Boil of buttock
Folliculitis of buttock
Furuncle of gluteal region

✚ **L02.33**   **Carbuncle of buttock**
Carbuncle of gluteal region

▣ ✚ **L02.4**   **Cutaneous abscess, furuncle and carbuncle of limb**

EXCLUDES 2   *Cutaneous abscess, furuncle and carbuncle of groin (L02.214, L02.224, L02.234)*
Cutaneous abscess, furuncle and carbuncle of hand (L02.5-)
Cutaneous abscess, furuncle and carbuncle of foot (L02.6-)

⑥ ✚ **L02.41**   **Cutaneous abscess of limb**

▤ ✚ **L02.411**   **Cutaneous abscess of right axilla**

▤ ✚ **L02.412**   **Cutaneous abscess of left axilla**

▤ ✚ **L02.413**   **Cutaneous abscess of right upper limb**

▤ ✚ **L02.414**   **Cutaneous abscess of left upper limb**

▤ ✚ **L02.415**   **Cutaneous abscess of right lower limb**

▤ ✚ **L02.416**   **Cutaneous abscess of left lower limb**

▤ ✚ **L02.419**   **Cutaneous abscess of limb, unspecified**

⑥ ✚ **L02.42**   **Furuncle of limb**
Boil of limb
Folliculitis of limb

▤ ✚ **L02.421**   **Furuncle of right axilla**

▤ ✚ **L02.422**   **Furuncle of left axilla**

▤ ✚ **L02.423**   **Furuncle of right upper limb**

▤ ✚ **L02.424**   **Furuncle of left upper limb**

▤ ✚ **L02.425**   **Furuncle of right lower limb**

▤ ✚ **L02.426**   **Furuncle of left lower limb**

▤ ✚ **L02.429**   **Furuncle of limb, unspecified**

⑥ ✚ **L02.43**   **Carbuncle of limb**

▤ ✚ **L02.431**   **Carbuncle of right axilla**

▤ ✚ **L02.432**   **Carbuncle of left axilla**

▤ ✚ **L02.433**   **Carbuncle of right upper limb**

▤ ✚ **L02.434**   **Carbuncle of left upper limb**

▤ ✚ **L02.435**   **Carbuncle of right lower limb**

▤ ✚ **L02.436**   **Carbuncle of left lower limb**

▤ ✚ **L02.439**   **Carbuncle of limb, unspecified**

▣ ✚ **L02.5**   **Cutaneous abscess, furuncle and carbuncle of hand**

⑥ ✚ **L02.51**   **Cutaneous abscess of hand**

▤ ✚ **L02.511**   **Cutaneous abscess of right hand**

▤ ✚ **L02.512**   **Cutaneous abscess of left hand**

▤ ✚ **L02.519**   **Cutaneous abscess of unspecified hand**

⑥ ✚ **L02.52**   **Furuncle hand**
Boil of hand
Folliculitis of hand

▤ ✚ **L02.521**   **Furuncle right hand**

▤ ✚ **L02.522**   **Furuncle left hand**

▤ ✚ **L02.529**   **Furuncle unspecified hand**

⑥ ✚ **L02.53**   **Carbuncle of hand**

▤ ✚ **L02.531**   **Carbuncle of right hand**

▤ ✚ **L02.532**   **Carbuncle of left hand**

▤ ✚ **L02.539**   **Carbuncle of unspecified hand**

▣ ✚ **L02.6**   **Cutaneous abscess, furuncle and carbuncle of foot**

⑥ ✚ **L02.61**   **Cutaneous abscess of foot**

▤ ✚ **L02.611**   **Cutaneous abscess of right foot**

▤ ✚ **L02.612**   **Cutaneous abscess of left foot**

▤ ✚ **L02.619**   **Cutaneous abscess of unspecified foot**

⑥ ✚ **L02.62**   **Furuncle of foot**
Boil of foot
Folliculitis of foot

▤ ✚ **L02.621**   **Furuncle of right foot**

▤ ✚ **L02.622**   **Furuncle of left foot**

▤ ✚ **L02.629**   **Furuncle of unspecified foot**

⑥ ✚ **L02.63**   **Carbuncle of foot**

▤ ✚ **L02.631**   **Carbuncle of right foot**

▤ ✚ **L02.632**   **Carbuncle of left foot**

▤ ✚ **L02.639**   **Carbuncle of unspecified foot**

▣ ✚ **L02.8**   **Cutaneous abscess, furuncle and carbuncle of other sites**

⑥ ✚ **L02.81**   **Cutaneous abscess of other sites**

✚ **L02.811**   **Cutaneous abscess of head [any part, except face]**

✚ **L02.818**   **Cutaneous abscess of other sites**

⑥ ✚ **L02.82**   **Furuncle of other sites**
Boil of other sites
Folliculitis of other sites

✚ **L02.821**   **Furuncle of head [any part, except face]**

✚ **L02.828**   **Furuncle of other sites**

⑥ ✚ **L02.83**   **Carbuncle of other sites**

✚ **L02.831**   **Carbuncle of head [any part, except face]**

✚ **L02.838**   **Carbuncle of other sites**

▣ ✚ **L02.9**   **Cutaneous abscess, furuncle and carbuncle, unspecified**

✚ **L02.91**   **Cutaneous abscess, unspecified**

✚ **L02.92**   **Furuncle, unspecified**
Boil NOS
Furunculosis NOS

✚ **L02.93**   **Carbuncle, unspecified**

● New   ▲ Revised   *Manifestation*   ❹-❼ Digit Indicators   ▤ Laterality   Ⓐ Adult (15+ years)   Ⓜ Maternity (12-55 years)   Ⓝ Newborn   Ⓟ Pediatric (0-17 years)   ♂ Male   ♀ Female
✖ ̶D̶e̶l̶e̶t̶e̶d̶   Unspecified   ✚ Additional code

718   © 2017 DecisionHealth   2017 ICD-10-CM Expert for Physicians

4 L03   Cellulitis and acute lymphangitis

EXCLUDES 2   *cellulitis of anal and rectal region (K61.-)*
cellulitis of external auditory canal (H60.1)
cellulitis of eyelid (H00.0)
cellulitis of female external genital organs
(N76.4)
cellulitis of lacrimal apparatus (H04.3)
cellulitis of male external genital organs
(N48.2, N49.-)
cellulitis of mouth (K12.2)
cellulitis of nose (J34.0)
eosinophilic cellulitis [Wells] (L98.3)
febrile neutrophilic dermatosis [Sweet] (L98.2)
lymphangitis (chronic) (subacute) (I89.1)

CODING TIP ✓   L03 includes codes for cellulitis. When diagnostic statements indicate abscess, a code from L02 should be coded.

CODING TIP ✓   Cellulitis usually presents as an abrupt onset of redness, swelling, pain, or heat in the affected area. Unless a diagnosis of cellulitis is documented by the physician, a code from category L03 should not be assigned. If cellulitis is associated with a wound or ostomy, code the wound or complicated ostomy first, followed by the appropriate L03 code for cellulitis.

DEFINITION   Acute lymphangitis: A quickly spreading bacterial infection of the lymph vessels appearing as painful, red streaks visible through the skin surface.

DEFINITION   Cellulitis: A spreading bacterial infection of connective soft tissue extending into deep dermal and subcutaneous layers; produces circumscribed swelling, fever, and swollen lymph nodes.

5 L03.0   Cellulitis and acute lymphangitis of finger and toe
Infection of nail
Onychia
Paronychia
Perionychia

6 L03.01   Cellulitis of finger
Felon
Whitlow
EXCLUDES 1   *herpetic whitlow (B00.89)*

- L03.011   **Cellulitis of right finger**
- L03.012   **Cellulitis of left finger**
- L03.019   **Cellulitis of unspecified finger**

6 L03.02   Acute lymphangitis of finger
Hangnail with lymphangitis of finger
- L03.021   **Acute lymphangitis of right finger**
- L03.022   **Acute lymphangitis of left finger**
- L03.029   **Acute lymphangitis of unspecified finger**

6 L03.03   Cellulitis of toe
- L03.031   **Cellulitis of right toe**
- L03.032   **Cellulitis of left toe**
- L03.039   **Cellulitis of unspecified toe**

6 L03.04   Acute lymphangitis of toe
Hangnail with lymphangitis of toe
- L03.041   **Acute lymphangitis of right toe**
- L03.042   **Acute lymphangitis of left toe**
- L03.049   **Acute lymphangitis of unspecified toe**

5 L03.1   Cellulitis and acute lymphangitis of other parts of limb

6 L03.11   Cellulitis of other parts of limb
EXCLUDES 2   *cellulitis of fingers (L03.01-)*
cellulitis of toes (L03.03-)
groin (L03.314)
- L03.111   **Cellulitis of right axilla**
- L03.112   **Cellulitis of left axilla**
- L03.113   **Cellulitis of right upper limb**
- L03.114   **Cellulitis of left upper limb**
- L03.115   **Cellulitis of right lower limb**
- L03.116   **Cellulitis of left lower limb**
- L03.119   **Cellulitis of unspecified part of limb**

6 L03.12   Acute lymphangitis of other parts of limb
EXCLUDES 2   *acute lymphangitis of fingers (L03.2-)*
acute lymphangitis of toes (L03.04-)
acute lymphangitis of groin (L03.324)
- L03.121   **Acute lymphangitis of right axilla**

- L03.122   **Acute lymphangitis of left axilla**
- L03.123   **Acute lymphangitis of right upper limb**
- L03.124   **Acute lymphangitis of left upper limb**
- L03.125   **Acute lymphangitis of right lower limb**
- L03.126   **Acute lymphangitis of left lower limb**
- L03.129   **Acute lymphangitis of unspecified part of limb**

5 L03.2   Cellulitis and acute lymphangitis of face and neck
6 L03.21   Cellulitis and acute lymphangitis of face
▲ L03.211   **Cellulitis of face**
EXCLUDES 2   *abscess of orbit (H05.01-)*
cellulitis of ear (H60.1-)
cellulitis of eyelid (H00.0-)
cellulitis of head (L03.81)
cellulitis of lacrimal apparatus
(H04.3)
cellulitis of lip (K13.0)
cellulitis of mouth (K12.2)
cellulitis of nose (internal)
(J34.0)
cellulitis of orbit (H05.01-)
cellulitis of scalp (L03.81)
L03.212   **Acute lymphangitis of face**
● L03.213   **Periorbital cellulitis**
Preseptal cellulitis

6 L03.22   Cellulitis and acute lymphangitis of neck
L03.221   **Cellulitis of neck**
L03.222   **Acute lymphangitis of neck**

5 L03.3   Cellulitis and acute lymphangitis of trunk
▲ 6 L03.31   **Cellulitis of trunk**
EXCLUDES 2   *cellulitis of anal and rectal regions*
(K61.-)
cellulitis of breast NOS (N61.0)
cellulitis of female external genital
organs (N76.4)
cellulitis of male external genital
organs (N48.2, N49.-)
omphalitis of newborn (P38.-)
puerperal cellulitis of breast (O91.2)
L03.311   **Cellulitis of abdominal wall**
EXCLUDES 2   *cellulitis of umbilicus (L03.316)*
cellulitis of groin (L03.314)
L03.312   **Cellulitis of back [any part except buttock]**
L03.313   **Cellulitis of chest wall**
L03.314   **Cellulitis of groin**
L03.315   **Cellulitis of perineum**
L03.316   **Cellulitis of umbilicus**
L03.317   **Cellulitis of buttock**
L03.319   **Cellulitis of trunk, unspecified**

6 L03.32   Acute lymphangitis of trunk
L03.321   **Acute lymphangitis of abdominal wall**
L03.322   **Acute lymphangitis of back [any part except buttock]**
L03.323   **Acute lymphangitis of chest wall**
L03.324   **Acute lymphangitis of groin**
L03.325   **Acute lymphangitis of perineum**
L03.326   **Acute lymphangitis of umbilicus**
L03.327   **Acute lymphangitis of buttock**
L03.329   **Acute lymphangitis of trunk, unspecified**

5 L03.8   Cellulitis and acute lymphangitis of other sites
6 L03.81   Cellulitis of other sites
L03.811   **Cellulitis of head [any part, except face]**
Cellulitis of scalp
EXCLUDES 2   *cellulitis of face (L03.211)*
L03.818   **Cellulitis of other sites**
6 L03.89   Acute lymphangitis of other sites
L03.891   **Acute lymphangitis of head [any part, except face]**
L03.898   **Acute lymphangitis of other sites**

5 L03.9   Cellulitis and acute lymphangitis, unspecified
L03.90   **Cellulitis, unspecified**
L03.91   **Acute lymphangitis, unspecified**
EXCLUDES 1   *lymphangitis NOS (I89.1)*

● New   ▲ Revised   *Manifestation*   4-7 Digit Indicators   ☐ Laterality   Ⓐ Adult (15+ years)   Ⓜ Maternity (12-55 years)   Ⓝ Newborn   Ⓟ Pediatric (0-17 years)   ♂ Male   ♀ Female
✖ Deleted   Unspecified   + Additional code

Diseases of the Skin and Subcutaneous Tissue

⬚ **L04**   **Acute lymphadenitis**

> **INCLUDES**   abscess (acute) of lymph nodes, except mesenteric
> acute lymphadenitis, except mesenteric
> **EXCLUDES 1**   *chronic or subacute lymphadenitis, except mesenteric (I88.1)*
> *enlarged lymph nodes (R59.-)*
> *human immunodeficiency virus [HIV] disease resulting in generalized lymphadenopathy (B20)*
> *lymphadenitis NOS (I88.9)*
> *nonspecific mesenteric lymphadenitis (I88.0)*

L04.0   **Acute lymphadenitis of face, head and neck**

L04.1   **Acute lymphadenitis of trunk**

Acute lymphadenitis of trunk

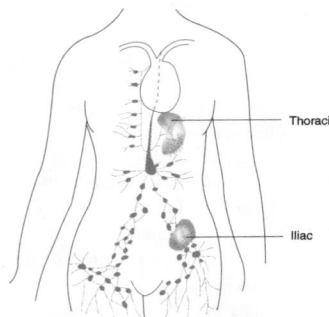

Thoracic

Iliac

L04.2   **Acute lymphadenitis of upper limb**
Acute lymphadenitis of axilla
Acute lymphadenitis of shoulder

L04.3   **Acute lymphadenitis of lower limb**
Acute lymphadenitis of hip
> **EXCLUDES 2**   *acute lymphadenitis of groin (L04.1)*

L04.8   **Acute lymphadenitis of other sites**

L04.9   **Acute lymphadenitis, unspecified**

⬚ **L05**   **Pilonidal cyst and sinus**

⬚ **L05.0**   **Pilonidal cyst and sinus with abscess**
> **DEFINITION**   An abscessed sinus tract draining to the surface and located in the tailbone area, often associated with ingrown hairs.

▲ **L05.01**   **Pilonidal cyst with abscess**
Pilonidal abscess
Pilonidal dimple with abscess
Postanal dimple with abscess
> **EXCLUDES 2**   *congenital sacral dimple (Q82.6)*
> *parasacral dimple (Q82.6)*

L05.02   **Pilonidal sinus with abscess**
Coccygeal fistula with abscess
Coccygeal sinus with abscess
Pilonidal fistula with abscess

⬚ **L05.9**   **Pilonidal cyst and sinus without abscess**

▲ **L05.91**   **Pilonidal cyst without abscess**
Pilonidal dimple
Postanal dimple
Pilonidal cyst NOS
> **EXCLUDES 2**   *congenital sacral dimple (Q82.6)*
> *parasacral dimple (Q82.6)*

L05.92   **Pilonidal sinus without abscess**
Coccygeal fistula
Coccygeal sinus without abscess
Pilonidal fistula

⬚ **L08**   **Other local infections of skin and subcutaneous tissue**

L08.0   **Pyoderma**
Dermatitis gangrenosa
Purulent dermatitis
Septic dermatitis
Suppurative dermatitis
> **EXCLUDES 1**   *pyoderma gangrenosum (L88)*
> *pyoderma vegetans (L08.81)*

> **DEFINITION**   A skin condition producing pus.

L08.1   **Erythrasma**
> **DEFINITION**   Skin infection caused by Corynebacterium minutissimum in which pink-red patches with fine scales and wrinkling appear in perpetually moist skin folds (intergluteal fold, inframammary fold, armpits, groin) and later turn brown and scaly.

⬚ **L08.8**   **Other specified local infections of the skin and subcutaneous tissue**

L08.81   **Pyoderma vegetans**
> **EXCLUDES 1**   *pyoderma gangrenosum (L88)*
> *pyoderma NOS (L08.0)*

L08.82   **Omphalitis not of newborn**
> **EXCLUDES 1**   *omphalitis of newborn (P38.-)*

L08.89   **Other specified local infections of the skin and subcutaneous tissue**

L08.9   **Local infection of the skin and subcutaneous tissue, unspecified**

Bullous disorders (L10-L14)

> **EXCLUDES 1**   *benign familial pemphigus [Hailey-Hailey] (Q82.8)*
> *staphylococcal scalded skin syndrome (L00)*
> *toxic epidermal necrolysis [Lyell] (L51.2)*

⬚ **L10**   **Pemphigus**
> **EXCLUDES 1**   *pemphigus neonatorum (L01.03)*

L10.0   **Pemphigus vulgaris**

L10.1   **Pemphigus vegetans**

L10.2   **Pemphigus foliaceus**

L10.3   **Brazilian pemphigus [fogo selvagem]**

L10.4   **Pemphigus erythematosus**
Senear-Usher syndrome

+ **L10.5**   **Drug-induced pemphigus**
Use additional code for adverse effect, if applicable, to identify drug (T36-T50 with fifth or sixth character 5)
> **CODING TIP** ✓   Code L10.5 should only be assigned when documentation clearly indicates a relationship between pemphigus and a drug or chemical as the underlying cause. Assign a code from T36-T50 following L10.5 to indicate the drug and adverse effect.

⬚ **L10.8**   **Other pemphigus**

L10.81   **Paraneoplastic pemphigus**

L10.89   **Other pemphigus**

L10.9   **Pemphigus, unspecified**

⬚ **L11**   **Other acantholytic disorders**

L11.0   **Acquired keratosis follicularis**
> **EXCLUDES 1**   *keratosis follicularis (congenital) [Darier-White] (Q82.8)*

L11.1   **Transient acantholytic dermatosis [Grover]**

L11.8   **Other specified acantholytic disorders**

L11.9   **Acantholytic disorder, unspecified**

⬚ **L12**   **Pemphigoid**
> **EXCLUDES 1**   *herpes gestationis (O26.4-)*
> *impetigo herpetiformis (L40.1)*

L12.0   **Bullous pemphigoid**

L12.1   **Cicatricial pemphigoid**
Benign mucous membrane pemphigoid

L12.2   **Chronic bullous disease of childhood** ᴾ
Juvenile dermatitis herpetiformis

⬚ **L12.3**   **Acquired epidermolysis bullosa**
> **EXCLUDES 1**   *epidermolysis bullosa (congenital) (Q81.-)*

L12.30   **Acquired epidermolysis bullosa, unspecified**

+ **L12.31**   **Epidermolysis bullosa due to drug**
Use additional code for adverse effect, if applicable, to identify drug (T36-T50 with fifth or sixth character 5)

L12.35   **Other acquired epidermolysis bullosa**

L12.8   **Other pemphigoid**

L12.9   **Pemphigoid, unspecified**

⬚ **L13**   **Other bullous disorders**

● New   ▲ Revised   *Manifestation*   ⬚-❼ Digit Indicators   ⊟ Laterality   🅐 Adult (15+ years)   Ⓜ Maternity (12-55 years)   🅝 Newborn   ᴾ Pediatric (0-17 years)   ♂ Male   ♀ Female
✖ Deleted   Unspecified   + Additional code

720   © 2017 DecisionHealth   2017 ICD-10-CM Expert for Physicians

L04 — L13

L13.0 **Dermatitis herpetiformis**
Duhring's disease
Hydroa herpetiformis
> **EXCLUDES 1** *juvenile dermatitis herpetiformis (L12.2)*
> *senile dermatitis herpetiformis (L12.0)*
>
> **DEFINITION** Chronic skin disease that can persist indefinitely, characterized by intensely itchy, symmetrical excoriations on the elbows, knees, lower back, buttocks, and shoulders, often accompanied by burning and stinging hours before an eruption.

L13.1 **Subcorneal pustular dermatitis**
Sneddon-Wilkinson disease

L13.8 **Other specified bullous disorders**

L13.9 **Bullous disorder, unspecified**

L14 **Bullous disorders in diseases classified elsewhere**
Code first:
underlying disease

Dermatitis and eczema (L20-L30)

Note: In this block the terms dermatitis and eczema are used synonymously and interchangeably.

> **EXCLUDES 2** *chronic (childhood) granulomatous disease (D71)*
> *dermatitis gangrenosa (L08.0)*
> *dermatitis herpetiformis (L13.0)*
> *dry skin dermatitis (L85.3)*
> *factitial dermatitis (L98.1)*
> *perioral dermatitis (L71.0)*
> *radiation-related disorders of the skin and subcutaneous tissue (L55-L59)*
> *stasis dermatitis (I87.2)*

▣ L20 **Atopic dermatitis**

L20.0 **Besnier's prurigo**

▤ L20.8 **Other atopic dermatitis**
> **EXCLUDES 2** *circumscribed neurodermatitis (L28.0)*

L20.81 **Atopic neurodermatitis**
Diffuse neurodermatitis

L20.82 **Flexural eczema**

L20.83 **Infantile (acute) (chronic) eczema** ⓟ

L20.84 **Intrinsic (allergic) eczema**

L20.89 **Other atopic dermatitis**

L20.9 **Atopic dermatitis, unspecified**

▣ L21 **Seborrheic dermatitis**
> **EXCLUDES 2** *infective dermatitis (L30.3)*
> *seborrheic keratosis (L82.-)*

L21.0 **Seborrhea capitis** ⓟ
Cradle cap
> **DEFINITION** Inflammatory skin rash on the scalp of infants, characterized by flaky or scaly skin with redness.

L21.1 **Seborrheic infantile dermatitis** ⓟ

L21.8 **Other seborrheic dermatitis**

L21.9 **Seborrheic dermatitis, unspecified**
Seborrhea NOS
> **DEFINITION** Overactivity of the sebaceous (fat) glands, resulting in an inflammatory skin rash.

L22 **Diaper dermatitis**
Diaper erythema
Diaper rash
Psoriasiform diaper rash

▣ L23 **Allergic contact dermatitis**
> **EXCLUDES 1** *allergy NOS (T78.40)*
> *contact dermatitis NOS (L25.9)*
> *dermatitis NOS (L30.9)*
>
> **EXCLUDES 2** *dermatitis due to substances taken internally (L27.-)*
> *dermatitis of eyelid (H01.1-)*
> *diaper dermatitis (L22)*
> *eczema of external ear (H60.5-)*
> *irritant contact dermatitis (L24.-)*
> *perioral dermatitis (L71.0)*
> *radiation-related disorders of the skin and subcutaneous tissue (L55-L59)*

> **CODING TIP ✓** Do not assign a code from L23 to report a skin reaction or allergy due to drugs or other medications that are ingested (internally). A code from category L27 should be assigned to indicate a skin reaction or allergy due to drugs or other medications ingested internally (with an additional code from T36-T50 assigned to indicate the adverse effect and specific drug).

> **CODING TIP ✓** Contact dermatitis indicates that the inflammation of the skin is related to contact with a substance. The specific causative substance that resulted in the condition should be documented and the plan of care should include appropriate interventions for skin care and instruction on prevention of contact with irritants. If the patient had contact with substances and had a non-allergic type reaction, see L24.

> **DEFINITION** Inflammation of the skin upon contact with an allergen, due to hypersensitization.

L23.0 **Allergic contact dermatitis due to metals**
Allergic contact dermatitis due to chromium
Allergic contact dermatitis due to nickel

L23.1 **Allergic contact dermatitis due to adhesives**

L23.2 **Allergic contact dermatitis due to cosmetics**

+ L23.3 **Allergic contact dermatitis due to drugs in contact with skin**
Use additional code for adverse effect, if applicable, to identify drug (T36-T50 with fifth or sixth character 5)
> **EXCLUDES 2** *dermatitis due to ingested drugs and medicaments (L27.0-L27.1)*

L23.4 **Allergic contact dermatitis due to dyes**

L23.5 **Allergic contact dermatitis due to other chemical products**
Allergic contact dermatitis due to cement
Allergic contact dermatitis due to insecticide
Allergic contact dermatitis due to plastic
Allergic contact dermatitis due to rubber

L23.6 **Allergic contact dermatitis due to food in contact with the skin**
> **EXCLUDES 2** *dermatitis due to ingested food (L27.2)*

L23.7 **Allergic contact dermatitis due to plants, except food**
> **EXCLUDES 2** *allergy NOS due to pollen (J30.1)*

▤ L23.8 **Allergic contact dermatitis due to other agents**

L23.81 **Allergic contact dermatitis due to animal (cat) (dog) dander**
Allergic contact dermatitis due to animal (cat) (dog) hair

L23.89 **Allergic contact dermatitis due to other agents**

L23.9 **Allergic contact dermatitis, unspecified cause**
Allergic contact eczema NOS

▣ L24 **Irritant contact dermatitis**
> **EXCLUDES 1** *allergy NOS (T78.40)*
> *contact dermatitis NOS (L25.9)*
> *dermatitis NOS (L30.9)*
>
> **EXCLUDES 2** *allergic contact dermatitis (L23.-)*
> *dermatitis due to substances taken internally (L27.-)*
> *dermatitis of eyelid (H01.1-)*
> *diaper dermatitis (L22)*
> *eczema of external ear (H60.5-)*
> *perioral dermatitis (L71.0)*
> *radiation-related disorders of the skin and subcutaneous tissue (L55-L59)*

> **CODING TIP ✓** Contact dermatitis indicates that the inflammation of the skin is related to contact with a substance. The specific causative substance that resulted in the condition should be documented and the plan of care should include appropriate interventions for skin care and instruction on prevention of contact with irritants.

L24.0 **Irritant contact dermatitis due to detergents**

L24.1 **Irritant contact dermatitis due to oils and greases**

L24.2 **Irritant contact dermatitis due to solvents**
Irritant contact dermatitis due to chlorocompound
Irritant contact dermatitis due to cyclohexane
Irritant contact dermatitis due to ester
Irritant contact dermatitis due to glycol
Irritant contact dermatitis due to hydrocarbon
Irritant contact dermatitis due to ketone

L24.3 **Irritant contact dermatitis due to cosmetics**

● New ▲ Revised *Manifestation* ▣-▦ Digit Indicators ▤ Laterality Ⓐ Adult (15+ years) Ⓜ Maternity (12-55 years) Ⓝ Newborn Ⓟ Pediatric (0-17 years) ♂ Male ♀ Female
✖ Deleted Unspecified + Additional code

+ L24.4   **Irritant contact dermatitis due to drugs in contact with skin**
Use additional code for adverse effect, if applicable, to identify drug (T36-T50 with fifth or sixth character 5)

L24.5   **Irritant contact dermatitis due to other chemical products**
Irritant contact dermatitis due to cement
Irritant contact dermatitis due to insecticide
Irritant contact dermatitis due to plastic
Irritant contact dermatitis due to rubber

L24.6   **Irritant contact dermatitis due to food in contact with skin**
   `EXCLUDES 2`   *dermatitis due to ingested food (L27.2)*

L24.7   **Irritant contact dermatitis due to plants, except food**
   `EXCLUDES 2`   *allergy NOS to pollen (J30.1)*

⑤ L24.8   **Irritant contact dermatitis due to other agents**

   L24.81   **Irritant contact dermatitis due to metals**
     Irritant contact dermatitis due to chromium
     Irritant contact dermatitis due to nickel

   L24.89   **Irritant contact dermatitis due to other agents**
     Irritant contact dermatitis due to dyes

L24.9   **Irritant contact dermatitis, unspecified cause**
Irritant contact eczema NOS

④ L25   **Unspecified contact dermatitis**
   `EXCLUDES 1`   *allergic contact dermatitis (L23.-)*
          allergy NOS (T78.40)
          dermatitis NOS (L30.9)
          irritant contact dermatitis (L24.-)
   `EXCLUDES 2`   *dermatitis due to ingested substances (L27.-)*
          dermatitis of eyelid (H01.1-)
          eczema of external ear (H60.5-)
          perioral dermatitis (L71.0)
          radiation-related disorders of the skin and
          subcutaneous tissue (L55-L59)

   `CODING TIP ✓`   Contact dermatitis indicates that the inflammation of the skin is related to contact with a substance. The specific causative substance that resulted in the condition should be documented and the plan of care should include appropriate interventions for skin care and instruction on prevention of contact with irritants.

L25.0   **Unspecified contact dermatitis due to cosmetics**

+ L25.1   **Unspecified contact dermatitis due to drugs in contact with skin**
Use additional code for adverse effect, if applicable, to identify drug (T36-T50 with fifth or sixth character 5)
   `EXCLUDES 2`   *dermatitis due to ingested drugs and medicaments (L27.0-L27.1)*

L25.2   **Unspecified contact dermatitis due to dyes**

L25.3   **Unspecified contact dermatitis due to other chemical products**
Unspecified contact dermatitis due to cement
Unspecified contact dermatitis due to insecticide

L25.4   **Unspecified contact dermatitis due to food in contact with skin**
   `EXCLUDES 2`   *dermatitis due to ingested food (L27.2)*

L25.5   **Unspecified contact dermatitis due to plants, except food**
   `EXCLUDES 1`   *nettle rash (L50.9)*
   `EXCLUDES 2`   *allergy NOS due to pollen (J30.1)*

L25.8   **Unspecified contact dermatitis due to other agents**

L25.9   **Unspecified contact dermatitis, unspecified cause**
Contact dermatitis (occupational) NOS
Contact eczema (occupational) NOS

L26   **Exfoliative dermatitis**
Hebra's pityriasis
   `EXCLUDES 1`   *Ritter's disease (L00)*

④ L27   **Dermatitis due to substances taken internally**
   `EXCLUDES 1`   *allergy NOS (T78.40)*
   `EXCLUDES 2`   *adverse food reaction, except dermatitis (T78.0-T78.1)*
          contact dermatitis (L23-L25)
          drug photoallergic response (L56.1)
          drug phototoxic response (L56.0)
          urticaria (L50.-)

+ L27.0   **Generalized skin eruption due to drugs and medicaments taken internally**
Use additional code for adverse effect, if applicable, to identify drug (T36-T50 with fifth or sixth character 5)

+ L27.1   **Localized skin eruption due to drugs and medicaments taken internally**
Use additional code for adverse effect, if applicable, to identify drug (T36-T50 with fifth or sixth character 5)

L27.2   **Dermatitis due to ingested food**
   `EXCLUDES 2`   *dermatitis due to food in contact with skin (L23.6, L24.6, L25.4)*

L27.8   **Dermatitis due to other substances taken internally**

L27.9   **Dermatitis due to unspecified substance taken internally**

④ L28   **Lichen simplex chronicus and prurigo**

   L28.0   **Lichen simplex chronicus**
     Circumscribed neurodermatitis
     Lichen NOS

   L28.1   **Prurigo nodularis**

   L28.2   **Other prurigo**
     Prurigo NOS
     Prurigo Hebra
     Prurigo mitis
     Urticaria papulosa
     `DEFINITION`   Chronic inflammatory skin disease featuring blistering papules and severe itching.

④ L29   **Pruritus**
   `EXCLUDES 1`   *neurotic excoriation (L98.1)*
          psychogenic pruritus (F45.8)
   `CODING TIP ✓`   Do not confuse pruritis with urticaria. Pruritis refers to "itch" or "itching" while urticaria refers to hives. Urticaria should be coded to L50.

   L29.0   **Pruritus ani**
     `DEFINITION`   Severe itching of the perianal region.

   L29.1   **Pruritus scroti**   ♂

   L29.2   **Pruritus vulvae**   ♀

   L29.3   **Anogenital pruritus, unspecified**

   L29.8   **Other pruritus**

   L29.9   **Pruritus, unspecified**
     Itch NOS

▲ ④ L30   **Other and unspecified dermatitis**
   `EXCLUDES 2`   *contact dermatitis (L23-L25)*
          dry skin dermatitis (L85.3)
          small plaque parapsoriasis (L41.3)
          stasis dermatitis (I87.2)

   L30.0   **Nummular dermatitis**

   L30.1   **Dyshidrosis [pompholyx]**

   L30.2   **Cutaneous autosensitization**
     Candidid [levurid]
     Dermatophytid
     Eczematid

   L30.3   **Infective dermatitis**
     Infectious eczematoid dermatitis

   L30.4   **Erythema intertrigo**

   L30.5   **Pityriasis alba**

   L30.8   **Other specified dermatitis**

   L30.9   **Dermatitis, unspecified**
     Eczema NOS

Papulosquamous disorders (L40-L45)

④ L40   **Psoriasis**

   L40.0   **Psoriasis vulgaris**
     Nummular psoriasis
     Plaque psoriasis

   L40.1   **Generalized pustular psoriasis**
     Impetigo herpetiformis
     Von Zumbusch's disease

   L40.2   **Acrodermatitis continua**

   L40.3   **Pustulosis palmaris et plantaris**

   L40.4   **Guttate psoriasis**

   ⑤ L40.5   **Arthropathic psoriasis**

     L40.50   **Arthropathic psoriasis, unspecified**

     L40.51   **Distal interphalangeal psoriatic arthropathy**

     L40.52   **Psoriatic arthritis mutilans**

     L40.53   **Psoriatic spondylitis**

     L40.54   **Psoriatic juvenile arthropathy**

     L40.59   **Other psoriatic arthropathy**

● New   ▲ Revised   *Manifestation* / Unspecified   ④-⑦ Digit Indicators   ▱ Laterality   Ⓐ Adult (15+ years)   Ⓜ Maternity (12-55 years)   Ⓝ Newborn   Ⓟ Pediatric (0-17 years)   ♂ Male   ♀ Female
✖ ̶D̶e̶l̶e̶t̶e̶d̶   + Additional code

L40.8   **Other psoriasis**
Flexural psoriasis

L40.9   **Psoriasis, unspecified**

⁴ **L41**   **Parapsoriasis**

> **EXCLUDES 1**   *poikiloderma vasculare atrophicans (L94.5)*

L41.0   **Pityriasis lichenoides et varioliformis acuta**
Mucha-Habermann disease

L41.1   **Pityriasis lichenoides chronica**

L41.3   **Small plaque parapsoriasis**

L41.4   **Large plaque parapsoriasis**

L41.5   **Retiform parapsoriasis**

L41.8   **Other parapsoriasis**

L41.9   **Parapsoriasis, unspecified**

L42   **Pityriasis rosea**

> **DEFINITION**   Skin that is marked with scaling, pink, oval macules, arranged with the long axes parallel to the cleavage lines of the skin.

⁴ **L43**   **Lichen planus**

> **EXCLUDES 1**   *lichen planopilaris (L66.1)*

L43.0   **Hypertrophic lichen planus**

L43.1   **Bullous lichen planus**

+ **L43.2**   **Lichenoid drug reaction**
Use additional code for adverse effect, if applicable, to identify drug (T36-T50 with fifth or sixth character 5)

L43.3   **Subacute (active) lichen planus**
Lichen planus tropicus

L43.8   **Other lichen planus**

L43.9   **Lichen planus, unspecified**

⁴ **L44**   **Other papulosquamous disorders**

L44.0   **Pityriasis rubra pilaris**

> **DEFINITION**   Rare skin condition of red-orange, scaly patches spreading over the body, thickened palms and soles, and rough, dry plugs within the rash.

L44.1   **Lichen nitidus**

L44.2   **Lichen striatus**

L44.3   **Lichen ruber moniliformis**

L44.4   **Infantile papular acrodermatitis [Gianotti-Crosti]**

L44.8   **Other specified papulosquamous disorders**

L44.9   **Papulosquamous disorder, unspecified**

L45   **Papulosquamous disorders in diseases classified elsewhere**
Code first:
underlying disease.

Urticaria and erythema (L49-L54)

> **EXCLUDES 1**   *Lyme disease (A69.2-)*
> *rosacea (L71.-)*

⁴ **L49**   **Exfoliation due to erythematous conditions according to extent of body surface involved**
Code first erythematous condition causing exfoliation, such as:
Ritter's disease (L00)
(Staphylococcal) scalded skin syndrom (L00)
Stevens-Johnson syndrome (L51.1)
Stevens-Johnson syndrome-toxic epidermal necrolysis overlap syndrome (L51.3)
Toxic epidermal necrolysis (L51.2)

L49.0   **Exfoliation due to erythematous condition involving less than 10 percent of body surface**
Exfoliation due to erythematous condition NOS

L49.1   **Exfoliation due to erythematous condition involving 10-19 percent of body surface**

L49.2   **Exfoliation due to erythematous condition involving 20-29 percent of body surface**

L49.3   **Exfoliation due to erythematous condition involving 30-39 percent of body surface**

L49.4   **Exfoliation due to erythematous condition involving 40-49 percent of body surface**

L49.5   **Exfoliation due to erythematous condition involving 50-59 percent of body surface**

L49.6   **Exfoliation due to erythematous condition involving 60-69 percent of body surface**

L49.7   **Exfoliation due to erythematous condition involving 70-79 percent of body surface**

L49.8   **Exfoliation due to erythematous condition involving 80-89 percent of body surface**

L49.9   **Exfoliation due to erythematous condition involving 90 or more percent of body surface**

⁴ **L50**   **Urticaria**

> **EXCLUDES 1**   *allergic contact dermatitis (L23.-)*
> *angioneurotic edema (T78.3)*
> *giant urticaria (T78.3)*
> *hereditary angio-edema (D84.1)*
> *Quincke's edema (T78.3)*
> *serum urticaria (T80.6-)*
> *solar urticaria (L56.3)*
> *urticaria neonatorum (P83.8)*
> *urticaria papulosa (L28.2)*
> *urticaria pigmentosa (Q82.2)*

> **CODING TIP** ✓   Do not confuse urticaria with pruritis. Pruritis refers to "itch" or "itching" while urticaria refers to hives. Pruritis should be coded to L29.

L50.0   **Allergic urticaria**

> **DEFINITION**   The most common form of hives in which smooth, raised, pink or white, itchy welts appear on or beneath the skin as a hypersensitivity response of the immune system to an allergic trigger.

Allergic urticaria

Characterized by smooth, raised pink or white bumps that appear on or beneath the skin

L50.1   **Idiopathic urticaria**

> **DEFINITION**   The appearance of hives with no known, apparent cause.

▲ **L50.2**   **Urticaria due to cold and heat**

> **EXCLUDES 2**   *familial cold urticaria (M04.2)*

> **DEFINITION**   The appearance of hives in response to external heat or cold that typically fade after moving to a comfortable temperature.

L50.3   **Dermatographic urticaria**

> **DEFINITION**   The appearance of hives in only one particular area of the body.

L50.4   **Vibratory urticaria**

> **DEFINITION**   Hives brought on by intense, prolonged vibration, such as that which occurs with the use of heavy mechanical equipment.

L50.5   **Cholinergic urticaria**

> **DEFINITION**   Hives that occur in response to a rise in body temperature, such as from exercise, stress, or overheating.

L50.6   **Contact urticaria**

L50.8   **Other urticaria**
Chronic urticaria
Recurrent periodic urticaria

L50.9   **Urticaria, unspecified**

● New   ▲ Revised   *Manifestation*   ⁴-⁷ Digit Indicators   ▣ Laterality   Ⓐ Adult (15+ years)   Ⓜ Maternity (12-55 years)   Ⓝ Newborn   Ⓟ Pediatric (0-17 years)   ♂ Male   ♀ Female
✕ Deleted   Unspecified   + Additional code

4 + L51   Erythema multiforme

Use additional code for adverse effect, if applicable, to identify drug (T36-T50 with fifth or sixth character 5)

Use additional code to identify associated manifestations, such as:
arthropathy associated with dermatological disorders (M14.8-)
conjunctival edema (H11.42)
conjunctivitis (H10.22-)
corneal scars and opacities (H17.-)
corneal ulcer (H16.0-)
edema of eyelid (H02.84)
inflammation of eyelid (H01.8)
keratoconjunctivitis sicca (H16.22-)
mechanical lagophthalmos (H02.22-)
stomatitis (K12.-)
symblepharon (H11.23-)
Use additional code to identify percentage of skin exfoliation (L49.-)

> **EXCLUDES 1**   *staphylococcal scalded skin syndrome (L00)*
> *Ritter's disease (L00)*

+ L51.0   Nonbullous erythema multiforme
+ L51.1   Stevens-Johnson syndrome
+ L51.2   Toxic epidermal necrolysis [Lyell]
+ L51.3   Stevens-Johnson syndrome-toxic epidermal necrolysis overlap syndrome
SJS-TEN overlap syndrome
+ L51.8   Other erythema multiforme
+ L51.9   Erythema multiforme, unspecified
Erythema iris
Erythema multiforme major NOS
Erythema multiforme minor NOS
Herpes iris

> **DEFINITION**   Erythema multiforme minor NOS:
> Acute, localized, self-limiting eruption marked by distinctive, classical target lesions of pink-red blotches with a ring around a pale center.

L52   Erythema nodosum

> **EXCLUDES 1**   *tuberculous erythema nodosum (A18.4)*

> **DEFINITION**   An inflammatory skin disorder marked by flat, firm, warm, red, tender, or painful nodules about an inch across under the skin that turn purple and fade to brown after several weeks, commonly found on anterior lower legs.

4 L53   Other erythematous conditions

> **EXCLUDES 1**   *erythema ab igne (L59.0)*
> *erythema due to external agents in contact with skin (L23-L25)*
> *erythema intertrigo (L30.4)*

+ L53.0   Toxic erythema
Code first:
poisoning due to drug or toxin, if applicable (T36-T65 with fifth or sixth character 1-4 or 6)
Use additional code for adverse effect, if applicable, to identify drug (T36-T50 with fifth or sixth character 5)

> **EXCLUDES 1**   *neonatal erythema toxicum (P83.1)*

L53.1   Erythema annulare centrifugum
L53.2   Erythema marginatum
L53.3   Other chronic figurate erythema
L53.8   Other specified erythematous conditions
L53.9   Erythematous condition, unspecified
Erythema NOS
Erythroderma NOS

L54   Erythema in diseases classified elsewhere
Code first:
underlying disease.

Radiation-related disorders of the skin and subcutaneous tissue (L55-L59)

4 L55   Sunburn
L55.0   Sunburn of first degree
L55.1   Sunburn of second degree
L55.2   Sunburn of third degree
L55.9   Sunburn, unspecified

4 + L56   Other acute skin changes due to ultraviolet radiation
Use additional code to identify the source of the ultraviolet radiation (W89, X32)

+ L56.0   Drug phototoxic response
Use additional code for adverse effect, if applicable, to identify drug (T36-T50 with fifth or sixth character 5)
+ L56.1   Drug photoallergic response
Use additional code for adverse effect, if applicable, to identify drug (T36-T50 with fifth or sixth character 5)
+ L56.2   Photocontact dermatitis [berloque dermatitis]
+ L56.3   Solar urticaria
+ L56.4   Polymorphous light eruption
+ L56.5   Disseminated superficial actinic porokeratosis (DSAP)
+ L56.8   Other specified acute skin changes due to ultraviolet radiation
+ L56.9   Acute skin change due to ultraviolet radiation, unspecified

4 + L57   Skin changes due to chronic exposure to nonionizing radiation
Use additional code to identify the source of the ultraviolet radiation (W89, X32)

+ L57.0   Actinic keratosis
Keratosis NOS
Senile keratosis
Solar keratosis

Actinic keratosis
A rough growth on the skin due to chronic exposure to nonionizing radiation

+ L57.1   Actinic reticuloid
+ L57.2   Cutis rhomboidalis nuchae
+ L57.3   Poikiloderma of Civatte
+ L57.4   Cutis laxa senilis
Elastosis senilis
+ L57.5   Actinic granuloma
+ L57.8   Other skin changes due to chronic exposure to nonionizing radiation
Farmer's skin
Sailor's skin
Solar dermatitis

> **DEFINITION**   Solar dermatitis: Premature aging of the skin and degeneration of the elastic tissue of the dermis due to prolonged exposure to sunlight.

+ L57.9   Skin changes due to chronic exposure to nonionizing radiation, unspecified

4 + L58   Radiodermatitis
Use additional code to identify the source of the radiation (W88, W90)

+ L58.0   Acute radiodermatitis
+ L58.1   Chronic radiodermatitis
+ L58.9   Radiodermatitis, unspecified

4 L59   Other disorders of skin and subcutaneous tissue related to radiation

L59.0   Erythema ab igne [dermatitis ab igne]
L59.8   Other specified disorders of the skin and subcutaneous tissue related to radiation
L59.9   Disorder of the skin and subcutaneous tissue related to radiation, unspecified

---

● New   ▲ Revised   *Manifestation*   4-7 Digit Indicators   ⊟ Laterality   Ⓐ Adult (15+ years)   Ⓜ Maternity (12-55 years)   Ⓝ Newborn   Ⓟ Pediatric (0-17 years)   ♂ Male   ♀ Female
✖ Deleted   Unspecified   + Additional code

724   © 2017 DecisionHealth   2017 ICD-10-CM Expert for Physicians

Disorders of skin appendages (L60-L75)

| EXCLUDES 1 | congenital malformations of integument (Q84.-) |

⬚ L60 Nail disorders

| EXCLUDES 2 | clubbing of nails (R68.3) |
| | onychia and paronychia (L03.0-) |

L60.0 Ingrowing nail

Nail disorders, ingrowing nail

Edge of nail growing into nail fold

L60.1 Onycholysis
L60.2 Onychogryphosis
L60.3 Nail dystrophy
L60.4 Beau's lines
L60.5 Yellow nail syndrome
L60.8 Other nail disorders
L60.9 Nail disorder, unspecified

L62 Nail disorders in diseases classified elsewhere

Code first underlying disease, such as:
pachydermoperiostosis (M89.4-)

⬚ L63 Alopecia areata

| DEFINITION | Patchy loss of hair on the head or body. |

L63.0 Alopecia (capitis) totalis
L63.1 Alopecia universalis
L63.2 Ophiasis
L63.8 Other alopecia areata
L63.9 Alopecia areata, unspecified

⬚ L64 Androgenic alopecia

| INCLUDES | male-pattern baldness |

+ L64.0 Drug-induced androgenic alopecia
Use additional code for adverse effect, if applicable, to identify drug (T36-T50 with fifth or sixth character 5)
L64.8 Other androgenic alopecia
L64.9 Androgenic alopecia, unspecified

⬚ + L65 Other nonscarring hair loss

Use additional code for adverse effect, if applicable, to identify drug (T36-T50 with fifth or sixth character 5)

| EXCLUDES 1 | trichotillomania (F63.3) |

+ L65.0 Telogen effluvium
+ L65.1 Anagen effluvium
+ L65.2 Alopecia mucinosa
+ L65.8 Other specified nonscarring hair loss
+ L65.9 Nonscarring hair loss, unspecified
Alopecia NOS

⬚ L66 Cicatricial alopecia [scarring hair loss]

L66.0 Pseudopelade
L66.1 Lichen planopilaris
Follicular lichen planus
L66.2 Folliculitis decalvans
L66.3 Perifolliculitis capitis abscedens
L66.4 Folliculitis ulerythematosa reticulata
L66.8 Other cicatricial alopecia
AHA: 1Q 2015, 19
L66.9 Cicatricial alopecia, unspecified

⬚ L67 Hair color and hair shaft abnormalities

EXCLUDES 1	monilethrix (Q84.1)
	pili annulati (Q84.1)
	telogen effluvium (L65.0)

L67.0 Trichorrhexis nodosa
L67.1 Variations in hair color
Canities
Greyness, hair (premature)
Heterochromia of hair
Poliosis circumscripta, acquired
Poliosis NOS
L67.8 Other hair color and hair shaft abnormalities
Fragilitas crinium
L67.9 Hair color and hair shaft abnormality, unspecified

⬚ L68 Hypertrichosis

INCLUDES	excess hair
EXCLUDES 1	congenital hypertrichosis (Q84.2)
	persistent lanugo (Q84.2)

L68.0 Hirsutism
L68.1 Acquired hypertrichosis lanuginosa
L68.2 Localized hypertrichosis
L68.3 Polytrichia
L68.8 Other hypertrichosis
L68.9 Hypertrichosis, unspecified

⬚ L70 Acne

| EXCLUDES 2 | acne keloid (L73.0) |

L70.0 Acne vulgaris
L70.1 Acne conglobata
L70.2 Acne varioliformis
Acne necrotica miliaris
L70.3 Acne tropica
L70.4 Infantile acne ▣
▲ L70.5 Acné excoriée
Acné excoriée des jeunes filles
Picker's acne
L70.8 Other acne
L70.9 Acne, unspecified

⬚ + L71 Rosacea

Use additional code for adverse effect, if applicable, to identify drug (T36-T50 with fifth or sixth character 5)

+ L71.0 Perioral dermatitis
+ L71.1 Rhinophyma
+ L71.8 Other rosacea

Rosacea

Rosacea

+ L71.9 Rosacea, unspecified

⬚ L72 Follicular cysts of skin and subcutaneous tissue

L72.0 Epidermal cyst
⬚ L72.1 Pilar and trichodermal cyst
L72.11 Pilar cyst
L72.12 Trichodermal cyst
Trichilemmal (proliferating) cyst
L72.2 Steatocystoma multiplex

● New ▲ Revised *Manifestation* ⬚-🗷 Digit Indicators 🖃 Laterality 🅐 Adult (15+ years) 🅜 Maternity (12-55 years) 🅝 Newborn ▣ Pediatric (0-17 years) ♂ Male ♀ Female
✖ Deleted Unspecified + Additional code

L72.3   **Sebaceous cyst**
    EXCLUDES 2 *pilar cyst (L72.11)*
                  trichilemmal (proliferating) cyst (L72.12)

Sebaceous cyst

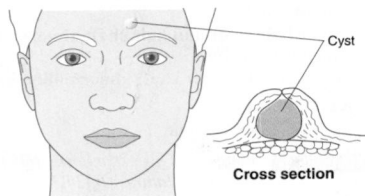

Cross section

L72.8   **Other follicular cysts of the skin and subcutaneous tissue**
L72.9   **Follicular cyst of the skin and subcutaneous tissue, unspecified**

L73   Other follicular disorders

L73.0   **Acne keloid**
L73.1   **Pseudofolliculitis barbae**
L73.2   **Hidradenitis suppurativa**
L73.8   **Other specified follicular disorders**
    Sycosis barbae
L73.9   **Follicular disorder, unspecified**

L74   Eccrine sweat disorders
    EXCLUDES 2 *generalized hyperhidrosis (R61)*

L74.0   **Miliaria rubra**
    DEFINITION Inflammatory heat rash caused by obstruction of the sweat glands with resultant skin rash of small clusters of red pimples on the skin.
L74.1   **Miliaria crystallina**
L74.2   **Miliaria profunda**
    Miliaria tropicalis
L74.3   **Miliaria, unspecified**
L74.4   **Anhidrosis**
    Hypohidrosis
L74.5   **Focal hyperhidrosis**
   L74.51   **Primary focal hyperhidrosis**
      L74.510   **Primary focal hyperhidrosis, axilla**
      L74.511   **Primary focal hyperhidrosis, face**
      L74.512   **Primary focal hyperhidrosis, palms**
      L74.513   **Primary focal hyperhidrosis, soles**
      L74.519   **Primary focal hyperhidrosis, unspecified**
   L74.52   **Secondary focal hyperhidrosis**
      Frey's syndrome
L74.8   **Other eccrine sweat disorders**
L74.9   **Eccrine sweat disorder, unspecified**
    Sweat gland disorder NOS

L75   Apocrine sweat disorders
    EXCLUDES 1 *dyshidrosis (L30.1)*
                  hidradenitis suppurativa (L73.2)

L75.0   **Bromhidrosis**
L75.1   **Chromhidrosis**
L75.2   **Apocrine miliaria**
    Fox-Fordyce disease
L75.8   **Other apocrine sweat disorders**
L75.9   **Apocrine sweat disorder, unspecified**

Intraoperative and postprocedural complications of skin and subcutaneous tissue (L76)

L76   Intraoperative and postprocedural complications of skin and subcutaneous tissue
    CODING TIP ✓ Conditions classifiable to L76 are classifiable as intraoperative and postprocedural complications. These conditions should only be assigned when diagnostic statements clearly indicate that the condition is a complication of a procedure.

L76.0   Intraoperative hemorrhage and hematoma of skin and subcutaneous tissue complicating a procedure
    EXCLUDES 1 *intraoperative hemorrhage and hematoma of skin and subcutaneous tissue due to accidental puncture and laceration during a procedure (L76.1-)*
  L76.01   **Intraoperative hemorrhage and hematoma of skin and subcutaneous tissue complicating a dermatologic procedure**
  L76.02   **Intraoperative hemorrhage and hematoma of skin and subcutaneous tissue complicating other procedure**
L76.1   Accidental puncture and laceration of skin and subcutaneous tissue during a procedure
  L76.11   **Accidental puncture and laceration of skin and subcutaneous tissue during a dermatologic procedure**
  L76.12   **Accidental puncture and laceration of skin and subcutaneous tissue during other procedure**
▲ L76.2   Postprocedural hemorrhage of skin and subcutaneous tissue following a procedure
  ▲ L76.21   Postprocedural hemorrhage of skin and subcutaneous tissue following a dermatologic procedure
  ▲ L76.22   Postprocedural hemorrhage of skin and subcutaneous tissue following other procedure
● L76.3   Postprocedural hematoma and seroma of skin and subcutaneous tissue following a procedure
  ● L76.31   Postprocedural hematoma of skin and subcutaneous tissue following a dermatologic procedure
  ● L76.32   Postprocedural hematoma of skin and subcutaneous tissue following other procedure
  ● L76.33   Postprocedural seroma of skin and subcutaneous tissue following a dermatologic procedure
  ● L76.34   Postprocedural seroma of skin and subcutaneous tissue following other procedure
+ L76.8   Other intraoperative and postprocedural complications of skin and subcutaneous tissue
    Use additional code, if applicable, to further specify disorder
  + L76.81   Other intraoperative complications of skin and subcutaneous tissue
  + L76.82   Other postprocedural complications of skin and subcutaneous tissue

Other disorders of the skin and subcutaneous tissue (L80-L99)

L80   Vitiligo
    EXCLUDES 2 *vitiligo of eyelids (H02.73-)*
                  vitiligo of vulva (N90.89)
    DEFINITION White patches devoid of pigmentation appearing on otherwise normal skin.

L81   Other disorders of pigmentation
    EXCLUDES 1 *birthmark NOS (Q82.5)*
                  Peutz-Jeghers syndrome (Q85.8)
    EXCLUDES 2 *nevus - see Alphabetical Index*

L81.0   **Postinflammatory hyperpigmentation**
L81.1   **Chloasma**
L81.2   **Freckles**
L81.3   **Café au lait spots**
L81.4   **Other melanin hyperpigmentation**
    Lentigo
L81.5   **Leukoderma, not elsewhere classified**
L81.6   **Other disorders of diminished melanin formation**
L81.7   **Pigmented purpuric dermatosis**
    Angioma serpiginosum
L81.8   **Other specified disorders of pigmentation**
    Iron pigmentation
    Tattoo pigmentation
L81.9   **Disorder of pigmentation, unspecified**

▲ L82   Seborrheic keratosis
    INCLUDES basal cell papilloma
              dermatosis papulosa nigra
              Leser-Trélat disease
    EXCLUDES 2 *seborrheic dermatitis (L21.-)*

L82.0   **Inflamed seborrheic keratosis**

● New   ▲ Revised   *Manifestation*   **4 - 7** Digit Indicators   ⊟ Laterality   Ⓐ Adult (15+ years)   Ⓜ Maternity (12-55 years)   Ⓝ Newborn   Ⓟ Pediatric (0-17 years)   ♂ Male   ♀ Female
✖ Deleted   Unspecified   + Additional code

726   © 2017 DecisionHealth   2017 ICD-10-CM Expert for Physicians

DEFINITION Noncancerous, barnacle-like skin lesions appearing in areas of long-term sun exposure in the elderly. Growths are irritated, itchy, inflamed, and may even bleed.

L82.1 Other seborrheic keratosis
Seborrheic keratosis NOS

DEFINITION Noncancerous skin lesion associated with aging and long periods of sun exposure. Growths appear round or oval, slightly elevated, black, brown, or pale in appearance with a crusty or scaly surface.

Other seborrheic keratosis

L83 Acanthosis nigricans
Confluent and reticulated papillomatosis

L84 Corns and callosities
Callus
Clavus

L85 Other epidermal thickening
EXCLUDES 2 hypertrophic disorders of the skin (L91.-)

L85.0 Acquired ichthyosis
EXCLUDES 1 congenital ichthyosis (Q80.-)

L85.1 Acquired keratosis [keratoderma] palmaris et plantaris
EXCLUDES 1 inherited keratosis palmaris et plantaris (Q82.8)

L85.2 Keratosis punctata (palmaris et plantaris)

L85.3 Xerosis cutis
Dry skin dermatitis

L85.8 Other specified epidermal thickening
Cutaneous horn

L85.9 Epidermal thickening, unspecified

L86 Keratoderma in diseases classified elsewhere
Code first underlying disease, such as:
Reiter's disease (M02.3-)
EXCLUDES 1 gonococcal keratoderma (A54.89)
gonococcal keratosis (A54.89)
keratoderma due to vitamin A deficiency (E50.8)
keratosis due to vitamin A deficiency (E50.8)
xeroderma due to vitamin A deficiency (E50.8)

L87 Transepidermal elimination disorders
EXCLUDES 1 granuloma annulare (perforating) (L92.0)

L87.0 Keratosis follicularis et parafollicularis in cutem penetrans
Kyrle disease
Hyperkeratosis follicularis penetrans

L87.1 Reactive perforating collagenosis

L87.2 Elastosis perforans serpiginosa

L87.8 Other transepidermal elimination disorders

L87.9 Transepidermal elimination disorder, unspecified

L88 Pyoderma gangrenosum
Phagedenic pyoderma
EXCLUDES 1 dermatitis gangrenosa (L08.0)

L89 Pressure ulcer
INCLUDES bed sore
decubitus ulcer
plaster ulcer
pressure area
pressure sore

Code first:
any associated gangrene (I96)

EXCLUDES 2 decubitus (trophic) ulcer of cervix (uteri) (N86)
diabetic ulcers
(E08.621, E08.622, E09.621, E09.622, E10.621, E10.622, E11.621, E11.622, E13.621, E13.622)
non-pressure chronic ulcer of skin (L97.-)
skin infections (L00-L08)
varicose ulcer (I83.0, I83.2)

GUIDELINES Section I.B.14
For . . . depth of non-pressure chronic ulcers and pressure ulcer stage codes, code assignment may be based on medical record documentation from clinicians who are not the patient's provider (i.e., physician or other qualified healthcare practitioner legally accountable for establishing the patient's diagnosis), since this information is typically documented by other clinicians involved in the care of the patient (e.g., . . . nurses often documents the pressure ulcer stages). However, the associated diagnosis (such as overweight, obesity, or pressure ulcer) must be documented by the patient's provider. If there is conflicting medical record documentation, either from the same clinician or different clinicians, the patient's attending provider should be queried for clarification.

GUIDELINES Section I.C.12.a.1)
Codes from category L89 are combination codes that identify the site of the pressure ulcer as well as the stage of the ulcer. ... Assign as many codes from category L89 as needed to identify all the pressure ulcers the patient has, if applicable.

GUIDELINES Section I.C.12.a.2)
Assignment of the code for unstageable pressure ulcer (L89.-- 0) should be based on the clinical documentation. These codes are used for pressure ulcers whose stage cannot be clinically determined (e.g., the ulcer is covered by eschar or has been treated with a skin or muscle graft) and pressure ulcers that are documented as deep tissue injury but not documented as due to trauma. This code should not be confused with the codes for unspecified stage (L89.--9). When there is no documentation regarding the stage of the pressure ulcer, assign the appropriate code for unspecified stage (L89.--9).

GUIDELINES Section I.C.12.a.4)
No code is assigned if the documentation states that the pressure ulcer is completely healed.

CODING TIP ✓ When assigning a code for any overweight, obesity, or morbid obesity, physician documentation indicating obesity as a diagnosis is required. If suspected, but not present, the coder may query the provider to obtain confirmation of the condition, but may not code obesity without confirmation from the provider. BMI Z68.- may be calculated and coded based upon documentation from other clinicians and calculated BMI may be coded alone without a diagnosis of obesity. BMI may only be reported as secondary code.

DEFINITION A pressure-induced ulceration or sore of the skin usually occurring when a patient is confined to bed for long periods of time, due to lack of circulation and oxygenation to the affected tissue.

L89.0 Pressure ulcer of elbow

L89.00 Pressure ulcer of unspecified elbow

L89.000 Pressure ulcer of unspecified elbow, unstageable

L89.001 Pressure ulcer of unspecified elbow, stage 1
Healing pressure ulcer of unspecified elbow, stage 1
Pressure pre-ulcer skin changes limited to persistent focal edema, unspecified elbow

● New ▲ Revised *Manifestation* 4-7 Digit Indicators ▤ Laterality ▨ Adult (15+ years) ▥ Maternity (12-55 years) ▨ Newborn ▣ Pediatric (0-17 years) ♂ Male ♀ Female
✖ Deleted Unspecified + Additional code

2017 ICD-10-CM Expert for Physicians

© 2017 decisionhealth

727

L89.002 **Pressure ulcer of unspecified elbow, stage 2**
Healing pressure ulcer of unspecified elbow, stage 2
Pressure ulcer with abrasion, blister, partial thickness skin loss involving epidermis and/or dermis, unspecified elbow

L89.003 **Pressure ulcer of unspecified elbow, stage 3**
Healing pressure ulcer of unspecified elbow, stage 3
Pressure ulcer with full thickness skin loss involving damage or necrosis of subcutaneous tissue, unspecified elbow

L89.004 **Pressure ulcer of unspecified elbow, stage 4**
Healing pressure ulcer of unspecified elbow, stage 4
Pressure ulcer with necrosis of soft tissues through to underlying muscle, tendon, or bone, unspecified elbow

L89.009 **Pressure ulcer of unspecified elbow, unspecified stage**
Healing pressure ulcer of elbow NOS
Healing pressure ulcer of unspecified elbow, unspecified stage

L89.01 **Pressure ulcer of right elbow**

L89.010 **Pressure ulcer of right elbow, unstageable**

L89.011 **Pressure ulcer of right elbow, stage 1**
Healing pressure ulcer of right elbow, stage 1
Pressure pre-ulcer skin changes limited to persistent focal edema, right elbow

L89.012 **Pressure ulcer of right elbow, stage 2**
Healing pressure ulcer of right elbow, stage 2
Pressure ulcer with abrasion, blister, partial thickness skin loss involving epidermis and/or dermis, right elbow

L89.013 **Pressure ulcer of right elbow, stage 3**
Healing pressure ulcer of right elbow, stage 3
Pressure ulcer with full thickness skin loss involving damage or necrosis of subcutaneous tissue, right elbow

L89.014 **Pressure ulcer of right elbow, stage 4**
Healing pressure ulcer of right elbow, stage 4
Pressure ulcer with necrosis of soft tissues through to underlying muscle, tendon, or bone, right elbow

L89.019 **Pressure ulcer of right elbow, unspecified stage**
Healing pressure right of elbow NOS
Healing pressure ulcer of unspecified elbow, unspecified stage

L89.02 **Pressure ulcer of left elbow**

L89.020 **Pressure ulcer of left elbow, unstageable**

L89.021 **Pressure ulcer of left elbow, stage 1**
Healing pressure ulcer of left elbow, stage 1
Pressure pre-ulcer skin changes limited to persistent focal edema, left elbow

L89.022 **Pressure ulcer of left elbow, stage 2**
Healing pressure ulcer of left elbow, stage 2
Pressure ulcer with abrasion, blister, partial thickness skin loss involving epidermis and/or dermis, left elbow

L89.023 **Pressure ulcer of left elbow, stage 3**
Healing pressure ulcer of left elbow, stage 3
Pressure ulcer with full thickness skin loss involving damage or necrosis of subcutaneous tissue, left elbow

L89.024 **Pressure ulcer of left elbow, stage 4**
Healing pressure ulcer of left elbow, stage 4
Pressure ulcer with necrosis of soft tissues through to underlying muscle, tendon, or bone, left elbow

L89.029 **Pressure ulcer of left elbow, unspecified stage**
Healing pressure ulcer of left of elbow NOS
Healing pressure ulcer of unspecified elbow, unspecified stage

L89.1 **Pressure ulcer of back**

L89.10 **Pressure ulcer of unspecified part of back**

L89.100 **Pressure ulcer of unspecified part of back, unstageable**

L89.101 **Pressure ulcer of unspecified part of back, stage 1**
Healing pressure ulcer of unspecified part of back, stage 1
Pressure pre-ulcer skin changes limited to persistent focal edema, unspecified part of back

L89.102 **Pressure ulcer of unspecified part of back, stage 2**
Healing pressure ulcer of unspecified part of back, stage 2
Pressure ulcer with abrasion, blister, partial thickness skin loss involving epidermis and/or dermis, unspecified part of back

L89.103 **Pressure ulcer of unspecified part of back, stage 3**
Healing pressure ulcer of unspecified part of back, stage 3
Pressure ulcer with full thickness skin loss involving damage or necrosis of subcutaneous tissue, unspecified part of back

L89.104 **Pressure ulcer of unspecified part of back, stage 4**
Healing pressure ulcer of unspecified part of back, stage 4
Pressure ulcer with necrosis of soft tissues through to underlying muscle, tendon, or bone, unspecified part of back

L89.109 **Pressure ulcer of unspecified part of back, unspecified stage**
Healing pressure ulcer of unspecified part of back NOS
Healing pressure ulcer of unspecified part of back, unspecified stage

L89.11 **Pressure ulcer of right upper back**
Pressure ulcer of right shoulder blade

L89.110 **Pressure ulcer of right upper back, unstageable**

L89.111 **Pressure ulcer of right upper back, stage 1**
Healing pressure ulcer of right upper back, stage 1
Pressure pre-ulcer skin changes limited to persistent focal edema, right upper back

L89.112 **Pressure ulcer of right upper back, stage 2**
Healing pressure ulcer of right upper back, stage 2
Pressure ulcer with abrasion, blister, partial thickness skin loss involving epidermis and/or dermis, right upper back

L89.113 **Pressure ulcer of right upper back, stage 3**
Healing pressure ulcer of right upper back, stage 3
Pressure ulcer with full thickness skin loss involving damage or necrosis of subcutaneous tissue, right upper back

L89.114 **Pressure ulcer of right upper back, stage 4**
Healing pressure ulcer of right upper back, stage 4
Pressure ulcer with necrosis of soft tissues through to underlying muscle, tendon, or bone, right upper back

L89.119 **Pressure ulcer of right upper back, unspecified stage**
Healing pressure ulcer of right upper back NOS
Healing pressure ulcer of right upper back, unspecified stage

L89.12 **Pressure ulcer of left upper back**
Pressure ulcer of left shoulder blade

L89.120 **Pressure ulcer of left upper back, unstageable**

L89.121 **Pressure ulcer of left upper back, stage 1**
Healing pressure ulcer of left upper back, stage 1
Pressure pre-ulcer skin changes limited to persistent focal edema, left upper back

L89.122 **Pressure ulcer of left upper back, stage 2**
Healing pressure ulcer of left upper back, stage 2
Pressure ulcer with abrasion, blister, partial thickness skin loss involving epidermis and/or dermis, left upper back

L89.123 **Pressure ulcer of left upper back, stage 3**
Healing pressure ulcer of left upper back, stage 3
Pressure ulcer with full thickness skin loss involving damage or necrosis of subcutaneous tissue, left upper back

● New ▲ Revised *Manifestation* Unspecified 🔟-🔢 Digit Indicators + Additional code ▱ Laterality 🅰 Adult (15+ years) Ⓜ Maternity (12-55 years) Ⓝ Newborn 🄿 Pediatric (0-17 years) ♂ Male ♀ Female
✖ Deleted

728   © 2017 DecisionHealth   2017 ICD-10-CM Expert for Physicians

☐ **L89.124** **Pressure ulcer of left upper back, stage 4**
Healing pressure ulcer of left upper back, stage 4
Pressure ulcer with necrosis of soft tissues through to underlying muscle, tendon, or bone, left upper back

☐ **L89.129** **Pressure ulcer of left upper back, unspecified stage**
Healing pressure ulcer of left upper back NOS
Healing pressure ulcer of left upper back, unspecified stage

⑥ **L89.13** **Pressure ulcer of right lower back**

☐ **L89.130** **Pressure ulcer of right lower back, unstageable**

☐ **L89.131** **Pressure ulcer of right lower back, stage 1**
Healing pressure ulcer of right lower back, stage 1
Pressure pre-ulcer skin changes limited to persistent focal edema, right lower back

☐ **L89.132** **Pressure ulcer of right lower back, stage 2**
Healing pressure ulcer of right lower back, stage 2
Pressure ulcer with abrasion, blister, partial thickness skin loss involving epidermis and/or dermis, right lower back

☐ **L89.133** **Pressure ulcer of right lower back, stage 3**
Healing pressure ulcer of right lower back, stage 3
Pressure ulcer with full thickness skin loss involving damage or necrosis of subcutaneous tissue, right lower back

☐ **L89.134** **Pressure ulcer of right lower back, stage 4**
Healing pressure ulcer of right lower back, stage 4
Pressure ulcer with necrosis of soft tissues through to underlying muscle, tendon, or bone, right lower back

☐ **L89.139** **Pressure ulcer of right lower back, unspecified stage**
Healing pressure ulcer of right lower back NOS
Healing pressure ulcer of right lower back, unspecified stage

⑥ **L89.14** **Pressure ulcer of left lower back**

☐ **L89.140** **Pressure ulcer of left lower back, unstageable**

☐ **L89.141** **Pressure ulcer of left lower back, stage 1**
Healing pressure ulcer of left lower back, stage 1
Pressure pre-ulcer skin changes limited to persistent focal edema, left lower back

☐ **L89.142** **Pressure ulcer of left lower back, stage 2**
Healing pressure ulcer of left lower back, stage 2
Pressure ulcer with abrasion, blister, partial thickness skin loss involving epidermis and/or dermis, left lower back

☐ **L89.143** **Pressure ulcer of left lower back, stage 3**
Healing pressure ulcer of left lower back, stage 3
Pressure ulcer with full thickness skin loss involving damage or necrosis of subcutaneous tissue, left lower back

☐ **L89.144** **Pressure ulcer of left lower back, stage 4**
Healing pressure ulcer of left lower back, stage 4
Pressure ulcer with necrosis of soft tissues through to underlying muscle, tendon, or bone, left lower back

☐ **L89.149** **Pressure ulcer of left lower back, unspecified stage**
Healing pressure ulcer of left lower back NOS
Healing pressure ulcer of left lower back, unspecified stage

⑥ **L89.15** **Pressure ulcer of sacral region**
Pressure ulcer of coccyx
Pressure ulcer of tailbone

L89.150 **Pressure ulcer of sacral region, unstageable**

L89.151 **Pressure ulcer of sacral region, stage 1**
Healing pressure ulcer of sacral region, stage 1
Pressure pre-ulcer skin changes limited to persistent focal edema, sacral region

L89.152 **Pressure ulcer of sacral region, stage 2**
Healing pressure ulcer of sacral region, stage 2
Pressure ulcer with abrasion, blister, partial thickness skin loss involving epidermis and/or dermis, sacral region

L89.153 **Pressure ulcer of sacral region, stage 3**
Healing pressure ulcer of sacral region, stage 3
Pressure ulcer with full thickness skin loss involving damage or necrosis of subcutaneous tissue, sacral region

L89.154 **Pressure ulcer of sacral region, stage 4**
Healing pressure ulcer of sacral region, stage 4
Pressure ulcer with necrosis of soft tissues through to underlying muscle, tendon, or bone, sacral region

L89.159 **Pressure ulcer of sacral region, unspecified stage**
Healing pressure ulcer of sacral region NOS
Healing pressure ulcer of sacral region, unspecified stage

⑤ **L89.2** **Pressure ulcer of hip**

⑥ **L89.20** **Pressure ulcer of unspecified hip**

L89.200 **Pressure ulcer of unspecified hip, unstageable**

L89.201 **Pressure ulcer of unspecified hip, stage 1**
Healing pressure ulcer of unspecified hip back, stage 1
Pressure pre-ulcer skin changes limited to persistent focal edema, unspecified hip

L89.202 **Pressure ulcer of unspecified hip, stage 2**
Healing pressure ulcer of unspecified hip, stage 2
Pressure ulcer with abrasion, blister, partial thickness skin loss involving epidermis and/or dermis, unspecified hip

L89.203 **Pressure ulcer of unspecified hip, stage 3**
Healing pressure ulcer of unspecified hip, stage 3
Pressure ulcer with full thickness skin loss involving damage or necrosis of subcutaneous tissue, unspecified hip

L89.204 **Pressure ulcer of unspecified hip, stage 4**
Healing pressure ulcer of unspecified hip, stage 4
Pressure ulcer with necrosis of soft tissues through to underlying muscle, tendon, or bone, unspecified hip

L89.209 **Pressure ulcer of unspecified hip, unspecified stage**
Healing pressure ulcer of unspecified hip NOS
Healing pressure ulcer of unspecified hip, unspecified stage

⑥ **L89.21** **Pressure ulcer of right hip**

☐ **L89.210** **Pressure ulcer of right hip, unstageable**

☐ **L89.211** **Pressure ulcer of right hip, stage 1**
Healing pressure ulcer of right hip back, stage 1
Pressure pre-ulcer skin changes limited to persistent focal edema, right hip

☐ **L89.212** **Pressure ulcer of right hip, stage 2**
Healing pressure ulcer of right hip, stage 2
Pressure ulcer with abrasion, blister, partial thickness skin loss involving epidermis and/or dermis, right hip

☐ **L89.213** **Pressure ulcer of right hip, stage 3**
Healing pressure ulcer of right hip, stage 3
Pressure ulcer with full thickness skin loss involving damage or necrosis of subcutaneous tissue, right hip

☐ **L89.214** **Pressure ulcer of right hip, stage 4**
Healing pressure ulcer of right hip, stage 4
Pressure ulcer with necrosis of soft tissues through to underlying muscle, tendon, or bone, right hip

☐ **L89.219** **Pressure ulcer of right hip, unspecified stage**
Healing pressure ulcer of right hip NOS
Healing pressure ulcer of right hip, unspecified stage

⑥ **L89.22** **Pressure ulcer of left hip**

☐ **L89.220** **Pressure ulcer of left hip, unstageable**

☐ **L89.221** **Pressure ulcer of left hip, stage 1**
Healing pressure ulcer of left hip back, stage 1
Pressure pre-ulcer skin changes limited to persistent focal edema, left hip

☐ **L89.222** **Pressure ulcer of left hip, stage 2**
Healing pressure ulcer of left hip, stage 2
Pressure ulcer with abrasion, blister, partial thickness skin loss involving epidermis and/or dermis, left hip

☐ **L89.223** **Pressure ulcer of left hip, stage 3**
Healing pressure ulcer of left hip, stage 3
Pressure ulcer with full thickness skin loss involving damage or necrosis of subcutaneous tissue, left hip

● New ▲ Revised *Manifestation* ➍-➐ Digit Indicators ☐ Laterality Ⓐ Adult (15+ years) Ⓜ Maternity (12-55 years) Ⓝ Newborn Ⓟ Pediatric (0-17 years) ♂ Male ♀ Female
✖ Deleted Unspecified + Additional code

Diseases of the Skin and Subcutaneous Tissue

L89.224 — L89.504

▣ **L89.224** **Pressure ulcer of left hip, stage 4**
Healing pressure ulcer of left hip, stage 4
Pressure ulcer with necrosis of soft tissues through to underlying muscle, tendon, or bone, left hip

▣ **L89.229** **Pressure ulcer of left hip, unspecified stage**
Healing pressure ulcer of left hip NOS
Healing pressure ulcer of left hip, unspecified stage

⑤ **L89.3** **Pressure ulcer of buttock**

⑥ **L89.30** **Pressure ulcer of unspecified buttock**

L89.300 **Pressure ulcer of unspecified buttock, unstageable**

L89.301 **Pressure ulcer of unspecified buttock, stage 1**
Healing pressure ulcer of unspecified buttock, stage 1
Pressure pre-ulcer skin changes limited to persistent focal edema, unspecified buttock

L89.302 **Pressure ulcer of unspecified buttock, stage 2**
Healing pressure ulcer of unspecified buttock, stage 2
Pressure ulcer with abrasion, blister, partial thickness skin loss involving epidermis and/or dermis, unspecified buttock

L89.303 **Pressure ulcer of unspecified buttock, stage 3**
Healing pressure ulcer of unspecified buttock, stage 3
Pressure ulcer with full thickness skin loss involving damage or necrosis of subcutaneous tissue, unspecified buttock

L89.304 **Pressure ulcer of unspecified buttock, stage 4**
Healing pressure ulcer of unspecified buttock, stage 4
Pressure ulcer with necrosis of soft tissues through to underlying muscle, tendon, or bone, unspecified buttock

L89.309 **Pressure ulcer of unspecified buttock, unspecified stage**
Healing pressure ulcer of unspecified buttock NOS
Healing pressure ulcer of unspecified buttock, unspecified stage

⑥ **L89.31** **Pressure ulcer of right buttock**

▣ **L89.310** **Pressure ulcer of right buttock, unstageable**

▣ **L89.311** **Pressure ulcer of right buttock, stage 1**
Healing pressure ulcer of right buttock, stage 1
Pressure pre-ulcer skin changes limited to persistent focal edema, right buttock

▣ **L89.312** **Pressure ulcer of right buttock, stage 2**
Healing pressure ulcer of right buttock, stage 2
Pressure ulcer with abrasion, blister, partial thickness skin loss involving epidermis and/or dermis, right buttock

▣ **L89.313** **Pressure ulcer of right buttock, stage 3**
Healing pressure ulcer of right buttock, stage 3
Pressure ulcer with full thickness skin loss involving damage or necrosis of subcutaneous tissue, right buttock

▣ **L89.314** **Pressure ulcer of right buttock, stage 4**
Healing pressure ulcer of right buttock, stage 4
Pressure ulcer with necrosis of soft tissues through to underlying muscle, tendon, or bone, right buttock

▣ **L89.319** **Pressure ulcer of right buttock, unspecified stage**
Healing pressure ulcer of right buttock NOS
Healing pressure ulcer of right buttock, unspecified stage

⑥ **L89.32** **Pressure ulcer of left buttock**

▣ **L89.320** **Pressure ulcer of left buttock, unstageable**

▣ **L89.321** **Pressure ulcer of left buttock, stage 1**
Healing pressure ulcer of left buttock, stage 1
Pressure pre-ulcer skin changes limited to persistent focal edema, left buttock

▣ **L89.322** **Pressure ulcer of left buttock, stage 2**
Healing pressure ulcer of left buttock, stage 2
Pressure ulcer with abrasion, blister, partial thickness skin loss involving epidermis and/or dermis, left buttock

▣ **L89.323** **Pressure ulcer of left buttock, stage 3**
Healing pressure ulcer of left buttock, stage 3
Pressure ulcer with full thickness skin loss involving damage or necrosis of subcutaneous tissue, left buttock

▣ **L89.324** **Pressure ulcer of left buttock, stage 4**
Healing pressure ulcer of left buttock, stage 4
Pressure ulcer with necrosis of soft tissues through to underlying muscle, tendon, or bone, left buttock

▣ **L89.329** **Pressure ulcer of left buttock, unspecified stage**
Healing pressure ulcer of left buttock NOS
Healing pressure ulcer of left buttock, unspecified stage

⑤ **L89.4** **Pressure ulcer of contiguous site of back, buttock and hip**

CODING TIP ✓ When a patient presents with a pressure ulcer that is contiguous to the surface area of the back, buttock, and/or hip, a code from L89.4- should be assigned. The stage of the ulcer should be assigned as the worst stage identifiable (the area of the ulcer which has deteriorated to its worst stage).

L89.40 **Pressure ulcer of contiguous site of back, buttock and hip, unspecified stage**
Healing pressure ulcer of contiguous site of back, buttock and hip NOS
Healing pressure ulcer of contiguous site of back, buttock and hip, unspecified stage

L89.41 **Pressure ulcer of contiguous site of back, buttock and hip, stage 1**
Healing pressure ulcer of contiguous site of back, buttock and hip, stage 1
Pressure pre-ulcer skin changes limited to persistent focal edema, contiguous site of back, buttock and hip

L89.42 **Pressure ulcer of contiguous site of back, buttock and hip, stage 2**
Healing pressure ulcer of contiguous site of back, buttock and hip, stage 2
Pressure ulcer with abrasion, blister, partial thickness skin loss involving epidermis and/or dermis, contiguous site of back, buttock and hip

L89.43 **Pressure ulcer of contiguous site of back, buttock and hip, stage 3**
Healing pressure ulcer of contiguous site of back, buttock and hip, stage 3
Pressure ulcer with full thickness skin loss involving damage or necrosis of subcutaneous tissue, contiguous site of back, buttock and hip

L89.44 **Pressure ulcer of contiguous site of back, buttock and hip, stage 4**
Healing pressure ulcer of contiguous site of back, buttock and hip, stage 4
Pressure ulcer with necrosis of soft tissues through to underlying muscle, tendon, or bone, contiguous site of back, buttock and hip

L89.45 **Pressure ulcer of contiguous site of back, buttock and hip, unstageable**

⑤ **L89.5** **Pressure ulcer of ankle**

⑥ **L89.50** **Pressure ulcer of unspecified ankle**

L89.500 **Pressure ulcer of unspecified ankle, unstageable**

L89.501 **Pressure ulcer of unspecified ankle, stage 1**
Healing pressure ulcer of unspecified ankle, stage 1
Pressure pre-ulcer skin changes limited to persistent focal edema, unspecified ankle

L89.502 **Pressure ulcer of unspecified ankle, stage 2**
Healing pressure ulcer of unspecified ankle, stage 2
Pressure ulcer with abrasion, blister, partial thickness skin loss involving epidermis and/or dermis, unspecified ankle

L89.503 **Pressure ulcer of unspecified ankle, stage 3**
Healing pressure ulcer of unspecified ankle, stage 3
Pressure ulcer with full thickness skin loss involving damage or necrosis of subcutaneous tissue, unspecified ankle

L89.504 **Pressure ulcer of unspecified ankle, stage 4**
Healing pressure ulcer of unspecified ankle, stage 4
Pressure ulcer with necrosis of soft tissues through to underlying muscle, tendon, or bone, unspecified ankle

● New ▲ Revised *Manifestation* ◑-◨ Digit Indicators ▤ Laterality ◭ Adult (15+ years) ◫ Maternity (12-55 years) ◩ Newborn ◪ Pediatric (0-17 years) ♂ Male ♀ Female
✖ Deleted Unspecified ✚ Additional code

730   © 2017 DecisionHealth   2017 ICD-10-CM Expert for Physicians

L89.509   **Pressure ulcer of unspecified ankle, unspecified stage**
Healing pressure ulcer of unspecified ankle NOS
Healing pressure ulcer of unspecified ankle, unspecified stage

Ⓖ L89.51   **Pressure ulcer of right ankle**

☐ L89.510   **Pressure ulcer of right ankle, unstageable**

☐ L89.511   **Pressure ulcer of right ankle, stage 1**
Healing pressure ulcer of right ankle, stage 1
Pressure pre-ulcer skin changes limited to persistent focal edema, right ankle

☐ L89.512   **Pressure ulcer of right ankle, stage 2**
Healing pressure ulcer of right ankle, stage 2
Pressure ulcer with abrasion, blister, partial thickness skin loss involving epidermis and/or dermis, right ankle

☐ L89.513   **Pressure ulcer of right ankle, stage 3**
Healing pressure ulcer of right ankle, stage 3
Pressure ulcer with full thickness skin loss involving damage or necrosis of subcutaneous tissue, right ankle

☐ L89.514   **Pressure ulcer of right ankle, stage 4**
Healing pressure ulcer of right ankle, stage 4
Pressure ulcer with necrosis of soft tissues through to underlying muscle, tendon, or bone, right ankle

☐ L89.519   **Pressure ulcer of right ankle, unspecified stage**
Healing pressure ulcer of right ankle NOS
Healing pressure ulcer of right ankle, unspecified stage

Ⓖ L89.52   **Pressure ulcer of left ankle**

☐ L89.520   **Pressure ulcer of left ankle, unstageable**

▲ ☐ L89.521   **Pressure ulcer of left ankle, stage 1**
Healing pressure ulcer of left ankle, stage 1
Pressure pre-ulcer skin changes limited to persistent focal edema, left ankle

☐ L89.522   **Pressure ulcer of left ankle, stage 2**
Healing pressure ulcer of left ankle, stage 2
Pressure ulcer with abrasion, blister, partial thickness skin loss involving epidermis and/or dermis, left ankle

☐ L89.523   **Pressure ulcer of left ankle, stage 3**
Healing pressure ulcer of left ankle, stage 3
Pressure ulcer with full thickness skin loss involving damage or necrosis of subcutaneous tissue, left ankle

☐ L89.524   **Pressure ulcer of left ankle, stage 4**
Healing pressure ulcer of left ankle, stage 4
Pressure ulcer with necrosis of soft tissues through to underlying muscle, tendon, or bone, left ankle

☐ L89.529   **Pressure ulcer of left ankle, unspecified stage**
Healing pressure ulcer of left ankle NOS
Healing pressure ulcer of left ankle, unspecified stage

Ⓢ L89.6   **Pressure ulcer of heel**

Ⓖ L89.60   **Pressure ulcer of unspecified heel**

L89.600   **Pressure ulcer of unspecified heel, unstageable**

L89.601   **Pressure ulcer of unspecified heel, stage 1**
Healing pressure ulcer of unspecified heel, stage 1
Pressure pre-ulcer skin changes limited to persistent focal edema, unspecified heel

L89.602   **Pressure ulcer of unspecified heel, stage 2**
Healing pressure ulcer of unspecified heel, stage 2
Pressure ulcer with abrasion, blister, partial thickness skin loss involving epidermis and/or dermis, unspecified heel

L89.603   **Pressure ulcer of unspecified heel, stage 3**
Healing pressure ulcer of unspecified heel, stage 3
Pressure ulcer with full thickness skin loss involving damage or necrosis of subcutaneous tissue, unspecified heel

L89.604   **Pressure ulcer of unspecified heel, stage 4**
Healing pressure ulcer of unspecified heel, stage 4
Pressure ulcer with necrosis of soft tissues through to underlying muscle, tendon, or bone, unspecified heel

L89.609   **Pressure ulcer of unspecified heel, unspecified stage**
Healing pressure ulcer of unspecified heel NOS
Healing pressure ulcer of unspecified heel, unspecified stage

Ⓖ L89.61   **Pressure ulcer of right heel**

☐ L89.610   **Pressure ulcer of right heel, unstageable**

☐ L89.611   **Pressure ulcer of right heel, stage 1**
Healing pressure ulcer of right heel, stage 1
Pressure pre-ulcer skin changes limited to persistent focal edema, right heel

☐ L89.612   **Pressure ulcer of right heel, stage 2**
Healing pressure ulcer of right heel, stage 2
Pressure ulcer with abrasion, blister, partial thickness skin loss involving epidermis and/or dermis, right heel

☐ L89.613   **Pressure ulcer of right heel, stage 3**
Healing pressure ulcer of right heel, stage 3
Pressure ulcer with full thickness skin loss involving damage or necrosis of subcutaneous tissue, right heel

☐ L89.614   **Pressure ulcer of right heel, stage 4**
Healing pressure ulcer of right heel, stage 4
Pressure ulcer with necrosis of soft tissues through to underlying muscle, tendon, or bone, right heel

☐ L89.619   **Pressure ulcer of right heel, unspecified stage**
Healing pressure ulcer of right heel NOS
Healing pressure ulcer of unspecified heel, right stage

Ⓖ L89.62   **Pressure ulcer of left heel**

☐ L89.620   **Pressure ulcer of left heel, unstageable**

☐ L89.621   **Pressure ulcer of left heel, stage 1**
Healing pressure ulcer of left heel, stage 1
Pressure pre-ulcer skin changes limited to persistent focal edema, left heel

☐ L89.622   **Pressure ulcer of left heel, stage 2**
Healing pressure ulcer of left heel, stage 2
Pressure ulcer with abrasion, blister, partial thickness skin loss involving epidermis and/or dermis, left heel

☐ L89.623   **Pressure ulcer of left heel, stage 3**
Healing pressure ulcer of left heel, stage 3
Pressure ulcer with full thickness skin loss involving damage or necrosis of subcutaneous tissue, left heel

☐ L89.624   **Pressure ulcer of left heel, stage 4**
Healing pressure ulcer of left heel, stage 4
Pressure ulcer with necrosis of soft tissues through to underlying muscle, tendon, or bone, left heel

☐ L89.629   **Pressure ulcer of left heel, unspecified stage**
Healing pressure ulcer of left heel NOS
Healing pressure ulcer of left heel, unspecified stage

Ⓢ L89.8   **Pressure ulcer of other site**

Ⓖ L89.81   **Pressure ulcer of head**
Pressure ulcer of face

L89.810   **Pressure ulcer of head, unstageable**

L89.811   **Pressure ulcer of head, stage 1**
Healing pressure ulcer of head, stage 1
Pressure pre-ulcer skin changes limited to persistent focal edema, head

L89.812   **Pressure ulcer of head, stage 2**
Healing pressure ulcer of head, stage 2
Pressure ulcer with abrasion, blister, partial thickness skin loss involving epidermis and/or dermis, head

L89.813   **Pressure ulcer of head, stage 3**
Healing pressure ulcer of head, stage 3
Pressure ulcer with full thickness skin loss involving damage or necrosis of subcutaneous tissue, head

L89.814   **Pressure ulcer of head, stage 4**
Healing pressure ulcer of head, stage 4
Pressure ulcer with necrosis of soft tissues through to underlying muscle, tendon, or bone, head

L89.819   **Pressure ulcer of head, unspecified stage**
Healing pressure ulcer of head NOS
Healing pressure ulcer of head, unspecified stage

Ⓖ L89.89   **Pressure ulcer of other site**

L89.890   **Pressure ulcer of other site, unstageable**

● New	▲ Revised	*Manifestation*	☐-☐ Digit Indicators	☐ Laterality	Ⓐ Adult (15+ years)	Ⓜ Maternity (12-55 years)	Ⓝ Newborn	Ⓟ Pediatric (0-17 years)	♂ Male	♀ Female
✖ Deleted		Unspecified	+ Additional code					

L89.891 **Pressure ulcer of other site, stage 1**
Healing pressure ulcer of other site, stage 1
Pressure pre-ulcer skin changes limited to
persistent focal edema, other site

L89.892 **Pressure ulcer of other site, stage 2**
Healing pressure ulcer of other site, stage 2
Pressure ulcer with abrasion, blister, partial
thickness skin loss involving epidermis and/or
dermis, other site

L89.893 **Pressure ulcer of other site, stage 3**
Healing pressure ulcer of other site, stage 3
Pressure ulcer with full thickness skin loss
involving damage or necrosis of subcutaneous
tissue, other site

L89.894 **Pressure ulcer of other site, stage 4**
Healing pressure ulcer of other site, stage 4
Pressure ulcer with necrosis of soft tissues through
to underlying muscle, tendon, or bone, other site

L89.899 **Pressure ulcer of other site, unspecified stage**
Healing pressure ulcer of other site NOS
Healing pressure ulcer of other site, unspecified
stage

⑤ L89.9 **Pressure ulcer of unspecified site**

L89.90 **Pressure ulcer of unspecified site, unspecified stage**
Healing pressure ulcer of unspecified site NOS
Healing pressure ulcer of unspecified site, unspecified
stage

L89.91 **Pressure ulcer of unspecified site, stage 1**
Healing pressure ulcer of unspecified site, stage 1
Pressure pre-ulcer skin changes limited to persistent
focal edema, unspecified site

L89.92 **Pressure ulcer of unspecified site, stage 2**
Healing pressure ulcer of unspecified site, stage 2
Pressure ulcer with abrasion, blister, partial thickness
skin loss involving epidermis and/or dermis,
unspecified site

L89.93 **Pressure ulcer of unspecified site, stage 3**
Healing pressure ulcer of unspecified site, stage 3
Pressure ulcer with full thickness skin loss involving
damage or necrosis of subcutaneous tissue,
unspecified site

L89.94 **Pressure ulcer of unspecified site, stage 4**
Healing pressure ulcer of unspecified site, stage 4
Pressure ulcer with necrosis of soft tissues through to
underlying muscle, tendon, or bone, unspecified site

L89.95 **Pressure ulcer of unspecified site, unstageable**

④ L90 **Atrophic disorders of skin**

L90.0 **Lichen sclerosus et atrophicus**
> EXCLUDES 2 *lichen sclerosus of external female genital*
> *organs (N90.4)*
> *lichen sclerosus of external male genital*
> *organs (N48.0)*

L90.1 **Anetoderma of Schweninger-Buzzi**

L90.2 **Anetoderma of Jadassohn-Pellizzari**

L90.3 **Atrophoderma of Pasini and Pierini**

L90.4 **Acrodermatitis chronica atrophicans**

L90.5 **Scar conditions and fibrosis of skin**
Adherent scar (skin)
Cicatrix
Disfigurement of skin due to scar
Fibrosis of skin NOS
Scar NOS
> EXCLUDES 2 *hypertrophic scar (L91.0)*
> *keloid scar (L91.0)*

AHA: 2Q 2016, 5
AHA: 1Q 2015, 19

L90.6 **Striae atrophicae**

L90.8 **Other atrophic disorders of skin**

L90.9 **Atrophic disorder of skin, unspecified**

④ L91 **Hypertrophic disorders of skin**

L91.0 **Hypertrophic scar**
Keloid
Keloid scar
> EXCLUDES 2 *acne keloid (L73.0)*
> *scar NOS (L90.5)*

L91.8 **Other hypertrophic disorders of the skin**

L91.9 **Hypertrophic disorder of the skin, unspecified**

④ L92 **Granulomatous disorders of skin and subcutaneous
tissue**
> EXCLUDES 2 *actinic granuloma (L57.5)*

L92.0 **Granuloma annulare**
Perforating granuloma annulare

L92.1 **Necrobiosis lipoidica, not elsewhere classified**
> EXCLUDES 1 *necrobiosis lipoidica associated with*
> *diabetes mellitus (E08-E13 with .620)*

L92.2 **Granuloma faciale [eosinophilic granuloma of skin]**

+ L92.3 **Foreign body granuloma of the skin and subcutaneous
tissue**
*Use additional code to identify the type of retained foreign
body (Z18.-)*

L92.8 **Other granulomatous disorders of the skin and
subcutaneous tissue**

L92.9 **Granulomatous disorder of the skin and subcutaneous
tissue, unspecified**

④ + L93 **Lupus erythematosus**
*Use additional code for adverse effect, if applicable, to identify
drug (T36-T50 with fifth or sixth character 5)*
> EXCLUDES 1 *lupus exedens (A18.4)*
> *lupus vulgaris (A18.4)*
> *scleroderma (M34.-)*
> *systemic lupus erythematosus (M32.-)*

+ L93.0 **Discoid lupus erythematosus**
Lupus erythematosus NOS

+ L93.1 **Subacute cutaneous lupus erythematosus**

+ L93.2 **Other local lupus erythematosus**
Lupus erythematosus profundus
Lupus panniculitis

④ L94 **Other localized connective tissue disorders**
> EXCLUDES 1 *systemic connective tissue disorders (M30-M36)*

L94.0 **Localized scleroderma [morphea]**
Circumscribed scleroderma

L94.1 **Linear scleroderma**
En coup de sabre lesion

L94.2 **Calcinosis cutis**

L94.3 **Sclerodactyly**

L94.4 **Gottron's papules**

L94.5 **Poikiloderma vasculare atrophicans**

L94.6 **Ainhum**

L94.8 **Other specified localized connective tissue disorders**

L94.9 **Localized connective tissue disorder, unspecified**

④ L95 **Vasculitis limited to skin, not elsewhere classified**
> EXCLUDES 1 *angioma serpiginosum (L81.7)*
> *Henoch (-Schönlein) purpura (D69.0)*
> *hypersensitivity angiitis (M31.0)*
> *lupus panniculitis (L93.2)*
> *panniculitis NOS (M79.3)*
> *panniculitis of neck and back (M54.0-)*
> *polyarteritis nodosa (M30.0)*
> *relapsing panniculitis (M35.6)*
> *rheumatoid vasculitis (M05.2)*
> *serum sickness (T80.6-)*
> *urticaria (L50.-)*
> *Wegener's granulomatosis (M31.3-)*

L95.0 **Livedoid vasculitis**
Atrophie blanche (en plaque)

L95.1 **Erythema elevatum diutinum**

L95.8 **Other vasculitis limited to the skin**

L95.9 **Vasculitis limited to the skin, unspecified**

● New   ▲ Revised   *Manifestation*   ④-⑦ Digit Indicators   ☐ Laterality   Ⓐ Adult (15+ years)   Ⓜ Maternity (12-55 years)   Ⓝ Newborn   Ⓟ Pediatric (0-17 years)   ♂ Male   ♀ Female
✖ Deleted   Unspecified   + Additional code

▣ L97   Non-pressure chronic ulcer of lower limb, not elsewhere classified

> **INCLUDES**   chronic ulcer of skin of lower limb NOS
> non-healing ulcer of skin
> non-infected sinus of skin
> trophic ulcer NOS
> tropical ulcer NOS
> ulcer of skin of lower limb NOS

Code first any associated underlying condition, such as:
any associated gangrene (I96)
atherosclerosis of the lower extremities
(I70.23-, I70.24-, I70.33-, I70.34-, I70.43-, I70.44-, I70.53-, I70.54-, I70.63-, I70.64-, I70.73-, I70.74-)
chronic venous hypertension (I87.31-, I87.33-)
diabetic ulcers
(E08.621, E08.622, E09.621, E09.622, E10.621, E10.622, E11.621, E11.622, E13.621, E13.622)
postphlebitic syndrome (I87.01-, I87.03-)
postthrombotic syndrome (I87.01-, I87.03-)
varicose ulcer (I83.0-, I83.2-)

> **EXCLUDES 2**   *pressure ulcer (pressure area) (L89.-)*
> *skin infections (L00-L08)*
> *specific infections classified to A00-B99*

> **GUIDELINES**   Section I.B.14
> For . . . depth of non-pressure chronic ulcers and pressure ulcer stage codes, code assignment may be based on medical record documentation from clinicians who are not the patient's provider (i.e., physician or other qualified healthcare practitioner legally accountable for establishing the patient's diagnosis), since this information is typically documented by other clinicians involved in the care of the patient (e.g., . . . nurses often documents the pressure ulcer stages). However, the associated diagnosis (such as overweight, obesity, or pressure ulcer) must be documented by the patient's provider. If there is conflicting medical record documentation, either from the same clinician or different clinicians, the patient's attending provider should be queried for clarification.

> **CODING TIP ✓**   When coding any non-pressure chronic ulcer classifiable to L97, first code the underlying cause of the ulcer, followed by the appropriate L97 code to identify the ulcer location, site and severity. Any gangrene associated with the ulcer should also be coded first (prior to sequencing of the L97 code).

> **CODING TIP ✓**   L97 codes are specific for site, laterality, and severity (e.g. skin, fat later exposed, necrosis of muscle, necrosis of bone). The severity of the ulcer may be coded based upon documentation from other clinicians (Official Coding Guidelines I.B.15), but confirmation of necrosis of bone should be obtained by diagnostic testing such as MRI (cannot determine through visualization alone). These codes are for non-pressure chronic ulcers and not for nonhealing surgical wounds.

▣ L97.1   Non-pressure chronic ulcer of thigh

▣ L97.10   Non-pressure chronic ulcer of unspecified thigh

L97.101   Non-pressure chronic ulcer of unspecified thigh limited to breakdown of skin

L97.102   Non-pressure chronic ulcer of unspecified thigh with fat layer exposed

L97.103   Non-pressure chronic ulcer of unspecified thigh with necrosis of muscle

L97.104   Non-pressure chronic ulcer of unspecified thigh with necrosis of bone

L97.109   Non-pressure chronic ulcer of unspecified thigh with unspecified severity

▣ L97.11   Non-pressure chronic ulcer of right thigh

▣ L97.111   Non-pressure chronic ulcer of right thigh limited to breakdown of skin

▣ L97.112   Non-pressure chronic ulcer of right thigh with fat layer exposed

▣ L97.113   Non-pressure chronic ulcer of right thigh with necrosis of muscle

▣ L97.114   Non-pressure chronic ulcer of right thigh with necrosis of bone

▣ L97.119   Non-pressure chronic ulcer of right thigh with unspecified severity

▣ L97.12   Non-pressure chronic ulcer of left thigh

▣ L97.121   Non-pressure chronic ulcer of left thigh limited to breakdown of skin

▣ L97.122   Non-pressure chronic ulcer of left thigh with fat layer exposed

▣ L97.123   Non-pressure chronic ulcer of left thigh with necrosis of muscle

▣ L97.124   Non-pressure chronic ulcer of left thigh with necrosis of bone

▣ L97.129   Non-pressure chronic ulcer of left thigh with unspecified severity

▣ L97.2   Non-pressure chronic ulcer of calf

▣ L97.20   Non-pressure chronic ulcer of unspecified calf

L97.201   Non-pressure chronic ulcer of unspecified calf limited to breakdown of skin

L97.202   Non-pressure chronic ulcer of unspecified calf with fat layer exposed

L97.203   Non-pressure chronic ulcer of unspecified calf with necrosis of muscle

L97.204   Non-pressure chronic ulcer of unspecified calf with necrosis of bone

L97.209   Non-pressure chronic ulcer of unspecified calf with unspecified severity

▣ L97.21   Non-pressure chronic ulcer of right calf

▣ L97.211   Non-pressure chronic ulcer of right calf limited to breakdown of skin

▣ L97.212   Non-pressure chronic ulcer of right calf with fat layer exposed

▣ L97.213   Non-pressure chronic ulcer of right calf with necrosis of muscle

▣ L97.214   Non-pressure chronic ulcer of right calf with necrosis of bone

▣ L97.219   Non-pressure chronic ulcer of right calf with unspecified severity

▣ L97.22   Non-pressure chronic ulcer of left calf

▣ L97.221   Non-pressure chronic ulcer of left calf limited to breakdown of skin

▣ L97.222   Non-pressure chronic ulcer of left calf with fat layer exposed

▣ L97.223   Non-pressure chronic ulcer of left calf with necrosis of muscle

▣ L97.224   Non-pressure chronic ulcer of left calf with necrosis of bone

▣ L97.229   Non-pressure chronic ulcer of left calf with unspecified severity

▣ L97.3   Non-pressure chronic ulcer of ankle

▣ L97.30   Non-pressure chronic ulcer of unspecified ankle

L97.301   Non-pressure chronic ulcer of unspecified ankle limited to breakdown of skin

L97.302   Non-pressure chronic ulcer of unspecified ankle with fat layer exposed

L97.303   Non-pressure chronic ulcer of unspecified ankle with necrosis of muscle

L97.304   Non-pressure chronic ulcer of unspecified ankle with necrosis of bone

L97.309   Non-pressure chronic ulcer of unspecified ankle with unspecified severity

▣ L97.31   Non-pressure chronic ulcer of right ankle

▣ L97.311   Non-pressure chronic ulcer of right ankle limited to breakdown of skin

▣ L97.312   Non-pressure chronic ulcer of right ankle with fat layer exposed

▣ L97.313   Non-pressure chronic ulcer of right ankle with necrosis of muscle

▣ L97.314   Non-pressure chronic ulcer of right ankle with necrosis of bone

▣ L97.319   Non-pressure chronic ulcer of right ankle with unspecified severity

▣ L97.32   Non-pressure chronic ulcer of left ankle

▣ L97.321   Non-pressure chronic ulcer of left ankle limited to breakdown of skin

▣ L97.322   Non-pressure chronic ulcer of left ankle with fat layer exposed

▣ L97.323   Non-pressure chronic ulcer of left ankle with necrosis of muscle

▣ L97.324   Non-pressure chronic ulcer of left ankle with necrosis of bone

▣ L97.329   Non-pressure chronic ulcer of left ankle with unspecified severity

▣ L97.4   Non-pressure chronic ulcer of heel and midfoot
Non-pressure chronic ulcer of plantar surface of midfoot

● New   ▲ Revised   *Manifestation*   ▣-▢ Digit Indicators   ▤ Laterality   Ⓐ Adult (15+ years)   Ⓜ Maternity (12-55 years)   Ⓝ Newborn   Ⓟ Pediatric (0-17 years)   ♂ Male   ♀ Female
✖ Deleted   Unspecified   + Additional code

ⓖ **L97.40** Non-pressure chronic ulcer of unspecified heel and midfoot

　L97.401 Non-pressure chronic ulcer of unspecified heel and midfoot limited to breakdown of skin

　L97.402 Non-pressure chronic ulcer of unspecified heel and midfoot with fat layer exposed

　L97.403 Non-pressure chronic ulcer of unspecified heel and midfoot with necrosis of muscle

　L97.404 Non-pressure chronic ulcer of unspecified heel and midfoot with necrosis of bone

　L97.409 Non-pressure chronic ulcer of unspecified heel and midfoot with unspecified severity

ⓖ **L97.41** Non-pressure chronic ulcer of right heel and midfoot

　▱ L97.411 Non-pressure chronic ulcer of right heel and midfoot limited to breakdown of skin

　▱ L97.412 Non-pressure chronic ulcer of right heel and midfoot with fat layer exposed

　▱ L97.413 Non-pressure chronic ulcer of right heel and midfoot with necrosis of muscle

　▱ L97.414 Non-pressure chronic ulcer of right heel and midfoot with necrosis of bone

　▱ L97.419 Non-pressure chronic ulcer of right heel and midfoot with unspecified severity

ⓖ **L97.42** Non-pressure chronic ulcer of left heel and midfoot

　▱ L97.421 Non-pressure chronic ulcer of left heel and midfoot limited to breakdown of skin
　　AHA: 1Q 2016, 12-13

　▱ L97.422 Non-pressure chronic ulcer of left heel and midfoot with fat layer exposed

　▱ L97.423 Non-pressure chronic ulcer of left heel and midfoot with necrosis of muscle

　▱ L97.424 Non-pressure chronic ulcer of left heel and midfoot with necrosis of bone

　▱ L97.429 Non-pressure chronic ulcer of left heel and midfoot with unspecified severity

ⓢ **L97.5** Non-pressure chronic ulcer of other part of foot
　Non-pressure chronic ulcer of toe

ⓖ **L97.50** Non-pressure chronic ulcer of other part of unspecified foot

　L97.501 Non-pressure chronic ulcer of other part of unspecified foot limited to breakdown of skin

　L97.502 Non-pressure chronic ulcer of other part of unspecified foot with fat layer exposed

　L97.503 Non-pressure chronic ulcer of other part of unspecified foot with necrosis of muscle

　L97.504 Non-pressure chronic ulcer of other part of unspecified foot with necrosis of bone

　L97.509 Non-pressure chronic ulcer of other part of unspecified foot with unspecified severity

ⓖ **L97.51** Non-pressure chronic ulcer of other part of right foot

　▱ L97.511 Non-pressure chronic ulcer of other part of right foot limited to breakdown of skin

　▱ L97.512 Non-pressure chronic ulcer of other part of right foot with fat layer exposed

　▱ L97.513 Non-pressure chronic ulcer of other part of right foot with necrosis of muscle

　▱ L97.514 Non-pressure chronic ulcer of other part of right foot with necrosis of bone

　▱ L97.519 Non-pressure chronic ulcer of other part of right foot with unspecified severity

ⓖ **L97.52** Non-pressure chronic ulcer of other part of left foot

　▱ L97.521 Non-pressure chronic ulcer of other part of left foot limited to breakdown of skin

　▱ L97.522 Non-pressure chronic ulcer of other part of left foot with fat layer exposed

　▱ L97.523 Non-pressure chronic ulcer of other part of left foot with necrosis of muscle

　▱ L97.524 Non-pressure chronic ulcer of other part of left foot with necrosis of bone

　▱ L97.529 Non-pressure chronic ulcer of other part of left foot with unspecified severity

ⓢ **L97.8** Non-pressure chronic ulcer of other part of lower leg

ⓖ **L97.80** Non-pressure chronic ulcer of other part of unspecified lower leg

　L97.801 Non-pressure chronic ulcer of other part of unspecified lower leg limited to breakdown of skin

　L97.802 Non-pressure chronic ulcer of other part of unspecified lower leg with fat layer exposed

　L97.803 Non-pressure chronic ulcer of other part of unspecified lower leg with necrosis of muscle

　L97.804 Non-pressure chronic ulcer of other part of unspecified lower leg with necrosis of bone

　L97.809 Non-pressure chronic ulcer of other part of unspecified lower leg with unspecified severity

ⓖ **L97.81** Non-pressure chronic ulcer of other part of right lower leg

　▱ L97.811 Non-pressure chronic ulcer of other part of right lower leg limited to breakdown of skin

　▱ L97.812 Non-pressure chronic ulcer of other part of right lower leg with fat layer exposed

　▱ L97.813 Non-pressure chronic ulcer of other part of right lower leg with necrosis of muscle

　▱ L97.814 Non-pressure chronic ulcer of other part of right lower leg with necrosis of bone

　▱ L97.819 Non-pressure chronic ulcer of other part of right lower leg with unspecified severity

ⓖ **L97.82** Non-pressure chronic ulcer of other part of left lower leg

　▱ L97.821 Non-pressure chronic ulcer of other part of left lower leg limited to breakdown of skin

　▱ L97.822 Non-pressure chronic ulcer of other part of left lower leg with fat layer exposed

　▱ L97.823 Non-pressure chronic ulcer of other part of left lower leg with necrosis of muscle

　▱ L97.824 Non-pressure chronic ulcer of other part of left lower leg with necrosis of bone

　▱ L97.829 Non-pressure chronic ulcer of other part of left lower leg with unspecified severity

ⓢ **L97.9** Non-pressure chronic ulcer of unspecified part of lower leg

ⓖ **L97.90** Non-pressure chronic ulcer of unspecified part of unspecified lower leg

　L97.901 Non-pressure chronic ulcer of unspecified part of unspecified lower leg limited to breakdown of skin

　L97.902 Non-pressure chronic ulcer of unspecified part of unspecified lower leg with fat layer exposed

　L97.903 Non-pressure chronic ulcer of unspecified part of unspecified lower leg with necrosis of muscle

　L97.904 Non-pressure chronic ulcer of unspecified part of unspecified lower leg with necrosis of bone

　L97.909 Non-pressure chronic ulcer of unspecified part of unspecified lower leg with unspecified severity

ⓖ **L97.91** Non-pressure chronic ulcer of unspecified part of right lower leg

　▱ L97.911 Non-pressure chronic ulcer of unspecified part of right lower leg limited to breakdown of skin

　▱ L97.912 Non-pressure chronic ulcer of unspecified part of right lower leg with fat layer exposed

　▱ L97.913 Non-pressure chronic ulcer of unspecified part of right lower leg with necrosis of muscle

　▱ L97.914 Non-pressure chronic ulcer of unspecified part of right lower leg with necrosis of bone

　▱ L97.919 Non-pressure chronic ulcer of unspecified part of right lower leg with unspecified severity

ⓖ **L97.92** Non-pressure chronic ulcer of unspecified part of left lower leg

　▱ L97.921 Non-pressure chronic ulcer of unspecified part of left lower leg limited to breakdown of skin

　▱ L97.922 Non-pressure chronic ulcer of unspecified part of left lower leg with fat layer exposed

　▱ L97.923 Non-pressure chronic ulcer of unspecified part of left lower leg with necrosis of muscle

　▱ L97.924 Non-pressure chronic ulcer of unspecified part of left lower leg with necrosis of bone

　▱ L97.929 Non-pressure chronic ulcer of unspecified part of left lower leg with unspecified severity

---

● New　▲ Revised　*Manifestation*　④-⑦ Digit Indicators　▱ Laterality　🅰 Adult (15+ years)　Ⓜ Maternity (12-55 years)　ℕ Newborn　🅿 Pediatric (0-17 years)　♂ Male　♀ Female
✖ Deleted　Unspecified　✛ Additional code

L98   Other disorders of skin and subcutaneous tissue, not elsewhere classified

L98.0   Pyogenic granuloma
> EXCLUDES 2   *pyogenic granuloma of gingiva (K06.8)*
> *pyogenic granuloma of maxillary alveolar ridge (K04.5)*
> *pyogenic granuloma of oral mucosa (K13.4)*

▲ L98.1   Factial dermatitis
Neurotic excoriation
> EXCLUDES 1   *Excoriation (skin-picking) disorder (F42.4)*

> CODING TIP ✓   Factial dermatitis, L98.1, may also be referred to as neurotic excoriation or dermatitis artefacta and is characterized by deliberate, self-inflicted skin lesions produced as a result of underlying psychological conditions. When specified, any underlying or additional psychological conditions should also be coded. An example of a psychological condition is obsessive-compulsive disorder (F42).

L98.2   Febrile neutrophilic dermatosis [Sweet]
L98.3   Eosinophilic cellulitis [Wells]
L98.4   Non-pressure chronic ulcer of skin, not elsewhere classified
Chronic ulcer of skin NOS
Tropical ulcer NOS
Ulcer of skin NOS
> EXCLUDES 2   *pressure ulcer (pressure area) (L89.-)*
> *gangrene (I96)*
> *skin infections (L00-L08)*
> *specific infections classified to A00-B99*
> *ulcer of lower limb NEC (L97.-)*
> *varicose ulcer (I83.0-I82.2)*

L98.41   Non-pressure chronic ulcer of buttock
L98.411   Non-pressure chronic ulcer of buttock limited to breakdown of skin
L98.412   Non-pressure chronic ulcer of buttock with fat layer exposed
L98.413   Non-pressure chronic ulcer of buttock with necrosis of muscle
L98.414   Non-pressure chronic ulcer of buttock with necrosis of bone
L98.419   Non-pressure chronic ulcer of buttock with unspecified severity

L98.42   Non-pressure chronic ulcer of back
L98.421   Non-pressure chronic ulcer of back limited to breakdown of skin
L98.422   Non-pressure chronic ulcer of back with fat layer exposed
L98.423   Non-pressure chronic ulcer of back with necrosis of muscle
L98.424   Non-pressure chronic ulcer of back with necrosis of bone
L98.429   Non-pressure chronic ulcer of back with unspecified severity

L98.49   Non-pressure chronic ulcer of skin of other sites
Non-pressure chronic ulcer of skin NOS
L98.491   Non-pressure chronic ulcer of skin of other sites limited to breakdown of skin
L98.492   Non-pressure chronic ulcer of skin of other sites with fat layer exposed
L98.493   Non-pressure chronic ulcer of skin of other sites with necrosis of muscle
L98.494   Non-pressure chronic ulcer of skin of other sites with necrosis of bone
L98.499   Non-pressure chronic ulcer of skin of other sites with unspecified severity

L98.5   Mucinosis of the skin
Focal mucinosis
Lichen myxedematosus
Reticular erythematous mucinosis
> EXCLUDES 1   *focal oral mucinosis (K13.79)*
> *myxedema (E03.9)*

L98.6   Other infiltrative disorders of the skin and subcutaneous tissue
> EXCLUDES 1   *hyalinosis cutis et mucosae (E78.89)*

● L98.7   Excessive and redundant skin and subcutaneous tissue
Loose or sagging skin following bariatric surgery weight loss
Loose or sagging skin following dietary weight loss
Loose or sagging skin, NOS
> EXCLUDES 2   *acquired excess or redundant skin of eyelid (H02.3-)*
> *congenital excess or redundant skin of eyelid (Q10.3)*
> *skin changes due to chronic exposure to nonionizing radiation (L57.-)*

L98.8   Other specified disorders of the skin and subcutaneous tissue
AHA: 2Q 2013, 31-32

L98.9   Disorder of the skin and subcutaneous tissue, unspecified

L99   *Other disorders of skin and subcutaneous tissue in diseases classified elsewhere*
Code first underlying disease, such as:
amyloidosis (E85.-)
> EXCLUDES 1   *skin disorders in diabetes (E08-E13 with .62)*
> *skin disorders in gonorrhea (A54.89)*
> *skin disorders in syphilis (A51.31, A52.79)*

● New   ▲ Revised   *Manifestation*   🔲- 🔢 Digit Indicators   ⊟ Laterality   🅰 Adult (15+ years)   Ⓜ Maternity (12-55 years)   🅽 Newborn   🅿 Pediatric (0-17 years)   ♂ Male   ♀ Female
✖ ~~Deleted~~   Unspecified   + Additional code

CHAPTER 13: DISEASES OF THE MUSCULOSKELETAL SYSTEM AND CONNECTIVE TISSUE (M00-M99)

Note: Use an external cause code following the code for the musculoskeletal condition, if applicable, to identify the cause of the musculoskeletal condition

EXCLUDES 2
arthropathic psoriasis (L40.5-)
certain conditions originating in the perinatal period (P04-P96)
certain infectious and parasitic diseases (A00-B99)
compartment syndrome (traumatic) (T79.A-)
complications of pregnancy, childbirth and the puerperium (O00-O9A)
congenital malformations, deformations, and chromosomal abnormalities (Q00-Q99)
endocrine, nutritional and metabolic diseases (E00-E88)
injury, poisoning and certain other consequences of external causes (S00-T88)
neoplasms (C00-D49)
symptoms, signs and abnormal clinical and laboratory findings, not elsewhere classified (R00-R94)

GUIDELINES Section I.C.13.a
Most of the codes within Chapter 13 have site and laterality designations. The site represents the bone, joint or the muscle involved. For some conditions where more than one bone, joint or muscle is usually involved, such as osteoarthritis, there is a "multiple sites" code available. For categories where no multiple site code is provided and more than one bone, joint or muscle is involved, multiple codes should be used to indicate the different sites involved.

GUIDELINES Section I.C.13.a.1)
For certain conditions, the bone may be affected at the upper or lower end, (e.g., avascular necrosis of bone, M87, Osteoporosis, M80, M81). Though the portion of the bone affected may be at the joint, the site designation will be the bone, not the joint.

GUIDELINES Section I.C.13.b
Many musculoskeletal conditions are a result of previous injury or trauma to a site, or are recurrent conditions. Bone, joint or muscle conditions that are the result of a healed injury are usually found in chapter 13. Recurrent bone, joint or muscle conditions are also usually found in chapter 13. Any current, acute injury should be coded to the appropriate injury code from chapter 19. Chronic or recurrent conditions should generally be coded with a code from chapter 13. If it is difficult to determine from the documentation in the record which code is best to describe a condition, query the provider.

This chapter contains the following blocks:

M00-M02	Infectious arthropathies
M04	Autoinflammatory syndromes
M05-M14	Inflammatory polyarthropathies
M15-M19	Osteoarthritis
M20-M25	Other joint disorders
M26-M27	Dentofacial anomalies [including malocclusion] and other disorders of jaw
M30-M36	Systemic connective tissue disorders
M40-M43	Deforming dorsopathies
M45-M49	Spondylopathies
M50-M54	Other dorsopathies
M60-M63	Disorders of muscles
M65-M67	Disorders of synovium and tendon
M70-M79	Other soft tissue disorders
M80-M85	Disorders of bone density and structure
M86-M90	Other osteopathies
M91-M94	Chondropathies
M95	Other disorders of the musculoskeletal system and connective tissue
M96	Intraoperative and postprocedural complications and disorders of musculoskeletal system, not elsewhere classified
M97	Periprosthetic fracture around internal prosthetic joint
M99	Biomechanical lesions, not elsewhere classified

Arthropathies (M00-M25)

INCLUDES Disorders affecting predominantly peripheral (limb) joints

Infectious arthropathies (M00-M02)

Note: This block comprises arthropathies due to microbiological agents. Distinction is made between the following types of etiological relationship:
a) direct infection of joint, where organisms invade synovial tissue and microbial antigen is present in the joint;
b) indirect infection, which may be of two types: a reactive arthropathy, where microbial infection of the body is established but neither organisms nor antigens can be identified in the joint, and a postinfective arthropathy, where microbial antigen is present but recovery of an organism is inconstant and evidence of local multiplication is lacking.

4 M00 Pyogenic arthritis

  5 + M00.0 Staphylococcal arthritis and polyarthritis
    Use additional code (B95.61-B95.8) to identify bacterial agent

    EXCLUDES 2 *infection and inflammatory reaction due to internal joint prosthesis (T84.5-)*

    + M00.00 Staphylococcal arthritis, unspecified joint
    6 + M00.01 Staphylococcal arthritis, shoulder
      + M00.011 Staphylococcal arthritis, right shoulder
      + M00.012 Staphylococcal arthritis, left shoulder
      + M00.019 Staphylococcal arthritis, unspecified shoulder
    6 + M00.02 Staphylococcal arthritis, elbow
      + M00.021 Staphylococcal arthritis, right elbow
      + M00.022 Staphylococcal arthritis, left elbow
      + M00.029 Staphylococcal arthritis, unspecified elbow
    6 + M00.03 Staphylococcal arthritis, wrist
      Staphylococcal arthritis of carpal bones
      + M00.031 Staphylococcal arthritis, right wrist
      + M00.032 Staphylococcal arthritis, left wrist
      + M00.039 Staphylococcal arthritis, unspecified wrist
    6 + M00.04 Staphylococcal arthritis, hand
      Staphylococcal arthritis of metacarpus and phalanges
      + M00.041 Staphylococcal arthritis, right hand
      + M00.042 Staphylococcal arthritis, left hand
      + M00.049 Staphylococcal arthritis, unspecified hand
    6 + M00.05 Staphylococcal arthritis, hip
      + M00.051 Staphylococcal arthritis, right hip
      + M00.052 Staphylococcal arthritis, left hip
      + M00.059 Staphylococcal arthritis, unspecified hip
    6 + M00.06 Staphylococcal arthritis, knee
      + M00.061 Staphylococcal arthritis, right knee
      + M00.062 Staphylococcal arthritis, left knee
      + M00.069 Staphylococcal arthritis, unspecified knee
    6 + M00.07 Staphylococcal arthritis, ankle and foot
      Staphylococcal arthritis, tarsus, metatarsus and phalanges
      + M00.071 Staphylococcal arthritis, right ankle and foot
      + M00.072 Staphylococcal arthritis, left ankle and foot
      + M00.079 Staphylococcal arthritis, unspecified ankle and foot
    + M00.08 Staphylococcal arthritis, vertebrae
    + M00.09 Staphylococcal polyarthritis
  5 M00.1 Pneumococcal arthritis and polyarthritis
    M00.10 Pneumococcal arthritis, unspecified joint
    6 M00.11 Pneumococcal arthritis, shoulder
      M00.111 Pneumococcal arthritis, right shoulder
      M00.112 Pneumococcal arthritis, left shoulder
      M00.119 Pneumococcal arthritis, unspecified shoulder
    6 M00.12 Pneumococcal arthritis, elbow
      M00.121 Pneumococcal arthritis, right elbow
      M00.122 Pneumococcal arthritis, left elbow
      M00.129 Pneumococcal arthritis, unspecified elbow
    6 M00.13 Pneumococcal arthritis, wrist
      Pneumococcal arthritis of carpal bones
      M00.131 Pneumococcal arthritis, right wrist
      M00.132 Pneumococcal arthritis, left wrist
      M00.139 Pneumococcal arthritis, unspecified wrist
    6 M00.14 Pneumococcal arthritis, hand
      Pneumococcal arthritis of metacarpus and phalanges

● New   ▲ Revised   *Manifestation*   **4 - 7** Digit Indicators   ⊟ Laterality   **A** Adult (15+ years)   **M** Maternity (12-55 years)   **N** Newborn   **P** Pediatric (0-17 years)   ♂ Male   ♀ Female
✖ ~~Deleted~~   Unspecified   + Additional code

⊟ M00.141   Pneumococcal arthritis, right hand
⊟ M00.142   Pneumococcal arthritis, left hand
⊟ M00.149   Pneumococcal arthritis, unspecified hand
⑥ M00.15   Pneumococcal arthritis, hip
⊟ M00.151   Pneumococcal arthritis, right hip
⊟ M00.152   Pneumococcal arthritis, left hip
⊟ M00.159   Pneumococcal arthritis, unspecified hip
⑥ M00.16   Pneumococcal arthritis, knee
⊟ M00.161   Pneumococcal arthritis, right knee
⊟ M00.162   Pneumococcal arthritis, left knee
⊟ M00.169   Pneumococcal arthritis, unspecified knee
⑥ M00.17   Pneumococcal arthritis, ankle and foot
        Pneumococcal arthritis, tarsus, metatarsus and
        phalanges
⊟ M00.171   Pneumococcal arthritis, right ankle and foot
⊟ M00.172   Pneumococcal arthritis, left ankle and foot
⊟ M00.179   Pneumococcal arthritis, unspecified ankle and
        foot
M00.18   Pneumococcal arthritis, vertebrae
M00.19   Pneumococcal polyarthritis
⑤+ M00.2   Other streptococcal arthritis and polyarthritis
        *Use additional code (B95.0-B95.2, B95.4-B95.5) to identify
        bacterial agent*
+ M00.20   Other streptococcal arthritis, unspecified joint
⑥+ M00.21   Other streptococcal arthritis, shoulder
⊟+ M00.211   Other streptococcal arthritis, right shoulder
⊟+ M00.212   Other streptococcal arthritis, left shoulder
⊟+ M00.219   Other streptococcal arthritis, unspecified
        shoulder
⑥+ M00.22   Other streptococcal arthritis, elbow
⊟+ M00.221   Other streptococcal arthritis, right elbow
⊟+ M00.222   Other streptococcal arthritis, left elbow
⊟+ M00.229   Other streptococcal arthritis, unspecified elbow
⑥+ M00.23   Other streptococcal arthritis, wrist
        Other streptococcal arthritis of carpal bones
⊟+ M00.231   Other streptococcal arthritis, right wrist
⊟+ M00.232   Other streptococcal arthritis, left wrist
⊟+ M00.239   Other streptococcal arthritis, unspecified wrist
⑥+ M00.24   Other streptococcal arthritis, hand
        Other streptococcal arthritis metacarpus and phalanges
⊟+ M00.241   Other streptococcal arthritis, right hand
⊟+ M00.242   Other streptococcal arthritis, left hand
⊟+ M00.249   Other streptococcal arthritis, unspecified hand
⑥+ M00.25   Other streptococcal arthritis, hip
⊟+ M00.251   Other streptococcal arthritis, right hip
⊟+ M00.252   Other streptococcal arthritis, left hip
⊟+ M00.259   Other streptococcal arthritis, unspecified hip
⑥+ M00.26   Other streptococcal arthritis, knee
⊟+ M00.261   Other streptococcal arthritis, right knee
⊟+ M00.262   Other streptococcal arthritis, left knee
⊟+ M00.269   Other streptococcal arthritis, unspecified knee
⑥+ M00.27   Other streptococcal arthritis, ankle and foot
        Other streptococcal arthritis, tarsus, metatarsus and
        phalanges
⊟+ M00.271   Other streptococcal arthritis, right ankle and
        foot
⊟+ M00.272   Other streptococcal arthritis, left ankle and foot
⊟+ M00.279   Other streptococcal arthritis, unspecified ankle
        and foot
+ M00.28   Other streptococcal arthritis, vertebrae
+ M00.29   Other streptococcal polyarthritis
⑤+ M00.8   Arthritis and polyarthritis due to other bacteria
        Use additional code (B96) to identify bacteria
+ M00.80   Arthritis due to other bacteria, unspecified joint
⑥+ M00.81   Arthritis due to other bacteria, shoulder
⊟+ M00.811   Arthritis due to other bacteria, right shoulder
⊟+ M00.812   Arthritis due to other bacteria, left shoulder
⊟+ M00.819   Arthritis due to other bacteria, unspecified
        shoulder

⑥+ M00.82   Arthritis due to other bacteria, elbow
⊟+ M00.821   Arthritis due to other bacteria, right elbow
⊟+ M00.822   Arthritis due to other bacteria, left elbow
⊟+ M00.829   Arthritis due to other bacteria, unspecified
        elbow
⑥+ M00.83   Arthritis due to other bacteria, wrist
        Arthritis due to other bacteria, carpal bones
⊟+ M00.831   Arthritis due to other bacteria, right wrist
⊟+ M00.832   Arthritis due to other bacteria, left wrist
⊟+ M00.839   Arthritis due to other bacteria, unspecified
        wrist
⑥+ M00.84   Arthritis due to other bacteria, hand
        Arthritis due to other bacteria, metacarpus and
        phalanges
⊟+ M00.841   Arthritis due to other bacteria, right hand
⊟+ M00.842   Arthritis due to other bacteria, left hand
⊟+ M00.849   Arthritis due to other bacteria, unspecified
        hand
⑥+ M00.85   Arthritis due to other bacteria, hip
⊟+ M00.851   Arthritis due to other bacteria, right hip
⊟+ M00.852   Arthritis due to other bacteria, left hip
⊟+ M00.859   Arthritis due to other bacteria, unspecified hip
⑥+ M00.86   Arthritis due to other bacteria, knee
⊟+ M00.861   Arthritis due to other bacteria, right knee
⊟+ M00.862   Arthritis due to other bacteria, left knee
⊟+ M00.869   Arthritis due to other bacteria, unspecified
        knee
⑥+ M00.87   Arthritis due to other bacteria, ankle and foot
        Arthritis due to other bacteria, tarsus, metatarsus, and
        phalanges
⊟+ M00.871   Arthritis due to other bacteria, right ankle and
        foot
⊟+ M00.872   Arthritis due to other bacteria, left ankle and
        foot
⊟+ M00.879   Arthritis due to other bacteria, unspecified
        ankle and foot
+ M00.88   Arthritis due to other bacteria, vertebrae
+ M00.89   Polyarthritis due to other bacteria
M00.9   Pyogenic arthritis, unspecified
        Infective arthritis NOS
④ M01   **Direct infections of joint in infectious and parasitic
        diseases classified elsewhere**
        Code first underlying disease, such as:
        leprosy [Hansen's disease] (A30.-)
        mycoses (B35-B49)
        O'nyong-nyong fever (A92.1)
        paratyphoid fever (A01.1-A01.4)
        EXCLUDES 1   *arthropathy in Lyme disease (A69.23)
        gonococcal arthritis (A54.42)
        meningococcal arthritis (A39.83)
        mumps arthritis (B26.85)
        postinfective arthropathy (M02.-)
        postmeningococcal arthritis (A39.84)
        reactive arthritis (M02.3)
        rubella arthritis (B06.82)
        sarcoidosis arthritis (D86.86)
        typhoid fever arthritis (A01.04)
        tuberculosis arthritis (A18.01-A18.02)*
⑤ M01.X   **Direct infection of joint in infectious and parasitic
        diseases classified elsewhere**
M01.X0   *Direct infection of unspecified joint in infectious and
        parasitic diseases classified elsewhere*
⑥ M01.X1   **Direct infection of shoulder joint in infectious and
        parasitic diseases classified elsewhere**
⊟ M01.X11   *Direct infection of right shoulder in infectious
        and parasitic diseases classified elsewhere*
⊟ M01.X12   *Direct infection of left shoulder in infectious and
        parasitic diseases classified elsewhere*
⊟ M01.X19   *Direct infection of unspecified shoulder in
        infectious and parasitic diseases classified
        elsewhere*
⑥ M01.X2   **Direct infection of elbow in infectious and parasitic
        diseases classified elsewhere**
⊟ M01.X21   *Direct infection of right elbow in infectious and
        parasitic diseases classified elsewhere*

⊟ **M01.X22** *Direct infection of left elbow in infectious and parasitic diseases classified elsewhere*

⊟ **M01.X29** *Direct infection of unspecified elbow in infectious and parasitic diseases classified elsewhere*

⑥ **M01.X3** Direct infection of wrist in infectious and parasitic diseases classified elsewhere
Direct infection of carpal bones in infectious and parasitic diseases classified elsewhere

⊟ **M01.X31** *Direct infection of right wrist in infectious and parasitic diseases classified elsewhere*

⊟ **M01.X32** *Direct infection of left wrist in infectious and parasitic diseases classified elsewhere*

⊟ **M01.X39** *Direct infection of unspecified wrist in infectious and parasitic diseases classified elsewhere*

⑥ **M01.X4** Direct infection of hand in infectious and parasitic diseases classified elsewhere
Direct infection of metacarpus and phalanges in infectious and parasitic diseases classified elsewhere

⊟ **M01.X41** *Direct infection of right hand in infectious and parasitic diseases classified elsewhere*

⊟ **M01.X42** *Direct infection of left hand in infectious and parasitic diseases classified elsewhere*

⊟ **M01.X49** *Direct infection of unspecified hand in infectious and parasitic diseases classified elsewhere*

⑥ **M01.X5** Direct infection of hip in infectious and parasitic diseases classified elsewhere

⊟ **M01.X51** *Direct infection of right hip in infectious and parasitic diseases classified elsewhere*

⊟ **M01.X52** *Direct infection of left hip in infectious and parasitic diseases classified elsewhere*

⊟ **M01.X59** *Direct infection of unspecified hip in infectious and parasitic diseases classified elsewhere*

⑥ **M01.X6** Direct infection of knee in infectious and parasitic diseases classified elsewhere

⊟ **M01.X61** *Direct infection of right knee in infectious and parasitic diseases classified elsewhere*

⊟ **M01.X62** *Direct infection of left knee in infectious and parasitic diseases classified elsewhere*

⊟ **M01.X69** *Direct infection of unspecified knee in infectious and parasitic diseases classified elsewhere*

⑥ **M01.X7** Direct infection of ankle and foot in infectious and parasitic diseases classified elsewhere
Direct infection of tarsus, metatarsus and phalanges in infectious and parasitic diseases classified elsewhere

⊟ **M01.X71** *Direct infection of right ankle and foot in infectious and parasitic diseases classified elsewhere*

⊟ **M01.X72** *Direct infection of left ankle and foot in infectious and parasitic diseases classified elsewhere*

⊟ **M01.X79** *Direct infection of unspecified ankle and foot in infectious and parasitic diseases classified elsewhere*

M01.X8 *Direct infection of vertebrae in infectious and parasitic diseases classified elsewhere*

M01.X9 *Direct infection of multiple joints in infectious and parasitic diseases classified elsewhere*

④ **M02** **Postinfective and reactive arthropathies**
Code first underlying disease, such as:
congenital syphilis [Clutton's joints] (A50.5)
enteritis due to Yersinia enterocolitica (A04.6)
infective endocarditis (I33.0)
viral hepatitis (B15-B19)

EXCLUDES 1 *Behçet's disease (M35.2)*
direct infections of joint in infectious and parasitic diseases classified elsewhere (M01.-)
postmeningococcal arthritis (A39.84)
mumps arthritis (B26.85)
rubella arthritis (B06.82)
syphilis arthritis (late) (A52.77)
rheumatic fever (I00)
tabetic arthropathy [Charcôt's] (A52.16)

CODING TIP ✓ M02.- codes indicate arthropathy due to another cause. The identified underlying cause should be coded first.

⑤ **M02.0** **Arthropathy following intestinal bypass**

M02.00 Arthropathy following intestinal bypass, unspecified site

⑥ **M02.01** Arthropathy following intestinal bypass, shoulder

⊟ **M02.011** Arthropathy following intestinal bypass, right shoulder

⊟ **M02.012** Arthropathy following intestinal bypass, left shoulder

⊟ **M02.019** Arthropathy following intestinal bypass, unspecified shoulder

⑥ **M02.02** Arthropathy following intestinal bypass, elbow

⊟ **M02.021** Arthropathy following intestinal bypass, right elbow

⊟ **M02.022** Arthropathy following intestinal bypass, left elbow

⊟ **M02.029** Arthropathy following intestinal bypass, unspecified elbow

⑥ **M02.03** Arthropathy following intestinal bypass, wrist
Arthropathy following intestinal bypass, carpal bones

⊟ **M02.031** Arthropathy following intestinal bypass, right wrist

⊟ **M02.032** Arthropathy following intestinal bypass, left wrist

⊟ **M02.039** Arthropathy following intestinal bypass, unspecified wrist

⑥ **M02.04** Arthropathy following intestinal bypass, hand
Arthropathy following intestinal bypass, metacarpals and phalanges

⊟ **M02.041** Arthropathy following intestinal bypass, right hand

⊟ **M02.042** Arthropathy following intestinal bypass, left hand

⊟ **M02.049** Arthropathy following intestinal bypass, unspecified hand

⑥ **M02.05** Arthropathy following intestinal bypass, hip

⊟ **M02.051** Arthropathy following intestinal bypass, right hip

⊟ **M02.052** Arthropathy following intestinal bypass, left hip

⊟ **M02.059** Arthropathy following intestinal bypass, unspecified hip

⑥ **M02.06** Arthropathy following intestinal bypass, knee

⊟ **M02.061** Arthropathy following intestinal bypass, right knee

⊟ **M02.062** Arthropathy following intestinal bypass, left knee

⊟ **M02.069** Arthropathy following intestinal bypass, unspecified knee

⑥ **M02.07** Arthropathy following intestinal bypass, ankle and foot
Arthropathy following intestinal bypass, tarsus, metatarsus and phalanges

⊟ **M02.071** Arthropathy following intestinal bypass, right ankle and foot

⊟ **M02.072** Arthropathy following intestinal bypass, left ankle and foot

⊟ **M02.079** Arthropathy following intestinal bypass, unspecified ankle and foot

M02.08 Arthropathy following intestinal bypass, vertebrae

M02.09 Arthropathy following intestinal bypass, multiple sites

⑤ **M02.1** **Postdysenteric arthropathy**

M02.10 **Postdysenteric arthropathy, unspecified site**

⑥ **M02.11** **Postdysenteric arthropathy, shoulder**

⊟ **M02.111** Postdysenteric arthropathy, right shoulder

⊟ **M02.112** Postdysenteric arthropathy, left shoulder

⊟ **M02.119** Postdysenteric arthropathy, unspecified shoulder

⑥ **M02.12** **Postdysenteric arthropathy, elbow**

⊟ **M02.121** Postdysenteric arthropathy, right elbow

⊟ **M02.122** Postdysenteric arthropathy, left elbow

⊟ **M02.129** Postdysenteric arthropathy, unspecified elbow

⑥ **M02.13** **Postdysenteric arthropathy, wrist**
Postdysenteric arthropathy, carpal bones

⊟ **M02.131** Postdysenteric arthropathy, right wrist

⊟ **M02.132** Postdysenteric arthropathy, left wrist

● New ▲ Revised *Manifestation* ④-⑦ Digit Indicators ⊟ Laterality Ⓐ Adult (15+ years) Ⓜ Maternity (12-55 years) Ⓝ Newborn Ⓟ Pediatric (0-17 years) ♂ Male ♀ Female
✖ ~~Deleted~~ Unspecified + Additional code

⊟ M02.139   Postdysenteric arthropathy, unspecified wrist
⑤ M02.14   Postdysenteric arthropathy, hand
            Postdysenteric arthropathy, metacarpus and phalanges
⊟ M02.141   Postdysenteric arthropathy, right hand
⊟ M02.142   Postdysenteric arthropathy, left hand
⊟ M02.149   Postdysenteric arthropathy, unspecified hand
⑤ M02.15   Postdysenteric arthropathy, hip
⊟ M02.151   Postdysenteric arthropathy, right hip
⊟ M02.152   Postdysenteric arthropathy, left hip
⊟ M02.159   Postdysenteric arthropathy, unspecified hip
⑤ M02.16   Postdysenteric arthropathy, knee
⊟ M02.161   Postdysenteric arthropathy, right knee
⊟ M02.162   Postdysenteric arthropathy, left knee
⊟ M02.169   Postdysenteric arthropathy, unspecified knee
⑤ M02.17   Postdysenteric arthropathy, ankle and foot
            Postdysenteric arthropathy, tarsus, metatarsus and phalanges
⊟ M02.171   Postdysenteric arthropathy, right ankle and foot
⊟ M02.172   Postdysenteric arthropathy, left ankle and foot
⊟ M02.179   Postdysenteric arthropathy, unspecified ankle and foot
   M02.18   Postdysenteric arthropathy, vertebrae
   M02.19   Postdysenteric arthropathy, multiple sites
⑤ M02.2   Postimmunization arthropathy
   M02.20   Postimmunization arthropathy, unspecified site
⑤ M02.21   Postimmunization arthropathy, shoulder
⊟ M02.211   Postimmunization arthropathy, right shoulder
⊟ M02.212   Postimmunization arthropathy, left shoulder
⊟ M02.219   Postimmunization arthropathy, unspecified shoulder
⑤ M02.22   Postimmunization arthropathy, elbow
⊟ M02.221   Postimmunization arthropathy, right elbow
⊟ M02.222   Postimmunization arthropathy, left elbow
⊟ M02.229   Postimmunization arthropathy, unspecified elbow
⑤ M02.23   Postimmunization arthropathy, wrist
            Postimmunization arthropathy, carpal bones
⊟ M02.231   Postimmunization arthropathy, right wrist
⊟ M02.232   Postimmunization arthropathy, left wrist
⊟ M02.239   Postimmunization arthropathy, unspecified wrist
⑤ M02.24   Postimmunization arthropathy, hand
            Postimmunization arthropathy, metacarpus and phalanges
⊟ M02.241   Postimmunization arthropathy, right hand
⊟ M02.242   Postimmunization arthropathy, left hand
⊟ M02.249   Postimmunization arthropathy, unspecified hand
⑤ M02.25   Postimmunization arthropathy, hip
⊟ M02.251   Postimmunization arthropathy, right hip
⊟ M02.252   Postimmunization arthropathy, left hip
⊟ M02.259   Postimmunization arthropathy, unspecified hip
⑤ M02.26   Postimmunization arthropathy, knee
⊟ M02.261   Postimmunization arthropathy, right knee
⊟ M02.262   Postimmunization arthropathy, left knee
⊟ M02.269   Postimmunization arthropathy, unspecified knee
⑤ M02.27   Postimmunization arthropathy, ankle and foot
            Postimmunization arthropathy, tarsus, metatarsus and phalanges
⊟ M02.271   Postimmunization arthropathy, right ankle and foot
⊟ M02.272   Postimmunization arthropathy, left ankle and foot
⊟ M02.279   Postimmunization arthropathy, unspecified ankle and foot
   M02.28   Postimmunization arthropathy, vertebrae
   M02.29   Postimmunization arthropathy, multiple sites
⑤ M02.3   Reiter's disease
           Reactive arthritis

⑤ M02.30   Reiter's disease, unspecified site
⑤ M02.31   Reiter's disease, shoulder
⊟ M02.311   Reiter's disease, right shoulder
⊟ M02.312   Reiter's disease, left shoulder
⊟ M02.319   Reiter's disease, unspecified shoulder
⑤ M02.32   Reiter's disease, elbow
⊟ M02.321   Reiter's disease, right elbow
⊟ M02.322   Reiter's disease, left elbow
⊟ M02.329   Reiter's disease, unspecified elbow
⑤ M02.33   Reiter's disease, wrist
            Reiter's disease, carpal bones
⊟ M02.331   Reiter's disease, right wrist
⊟ M02.332   Reiter's disease, left wrist
⊟ M02.339   Reiter's disease, unspecified wrist
⑤ M02.34   Reiter's disease, hand
            Reiter's disease, metacarpus and phalanges
⊟ M02.341   Reiter's disease, right hand
⊟ M02.342   Reiter's disease, left hand
⊟ M02.349   Reiter's disease, unspecified hand
⑤ M02.35   Reiter's disease, hip
⊟ M02.351   Reiter's disease, right hip
⊟ M02.352   Reiter's disease, left hip
⊟ M02.359   Reiter's disease, unspecified hip
⑤ M02.36   Reiter's disease, knee
⊟ M02.361   Reiter's disease, right knee
⊟ M02.362   Reiter's disease, left knee
⊟ M02.369   Reiter's disease, unspecified knee
⑤ M02.37   Reiter's disease, ankle and foot
            Reiter's disease, tarsus, metatarsus and phalanges
⊟ M02.371   Reiter's disease, right ankle and foot
⊟ M02.372   Reiter's disease, left ankle and foot
⊟ M02.379   Reiter's disease, unspecified ankle and foot
   M02.38   Reiter's disease, vertebrae
   M02.39   Reiter's disease, multiple sites
⑤ M02.8   Other reactive arthropathies
   M02.80   Other reactive arthropathies, unspecified site
⑤ M02.81   Other reactive arthropathies, shoulder
⊟ M02.811   Other reactive arthropathies, right shoulder
⊟ M02.812   Other reactive arthropathies, left shoulder
⊟ M02.819   Other reactive arthropathies, unspecified shoulder
⑤ M02.82   Other reactive arthropathies, elbow
⊟ M02.821   Other reactive arthropathies, right elbow
⊟ M02.822   Other reactive arthropathies, left elbow
⊟ M02.829   Other reactive arthropathies, unspecified elbow
⑤ M02.83   Other reactive arthropathies, wrist
            Other reactive arthropathies, carpal bones
⊟ M02.831   Other reactive arthropathies, right wrist
⊟ M02.832   Other reactive arthropathies, left wrist
⊟ M02.839   Other reactive arthropathies, unspecified wrist
⑤ M02.84   Other reactive arthropathies, hand
            Other reactive arthropathies, metacarpus and phalanges
⊟ M02.841   Other reactive arthropathies, right hand
⊟ M02.842   Other reactive arthropathies, left hand
⊟ M02.849   Other reactive arthropathies, unspecified hand
⑤ M02.85   Other reactive arthropathies, hip
⊟ M02.851   Other reactive arthropathies, right hip
⊟ M02.852   Other reactive arthropathies, left hip
⊟ M02.859   Other reactive arthropathies, unspecified hip
⑤ M02.86   Other reactive arthropathies, knee
⊟ M02.861   Other reactive arthropathies, right knee
⊟ M02.862   Other reactive arthropathies, left knee
⊟ M02.869   Other reactive arthropathies, unspecified knee
⑤ M02.87   Other reactive arthropathies, ankle and foot
            Other reactive arthropathies, tarsus, metatarsus and phalanges
⊟ M02.871   Other reactive arthropathies, right ankle and foot

● New   ▲ Revised   *Manifestation*   ④-⑦ Digit Indicators   ⊟ Laterality   Ⓐ Adult (15+ years)   Ⓜ Maternity (12-55 years)   Ⓝ Newborn   Ⓟ Pediatric (0-17 years)   ♂ Male   ♀ Female
✖ Deleted   Unspecified   + Additional code

740   © 2017 DecisionHealth   2017 ICD-10-CM Expert for Physicians

M02.872　Other reactive arthropathies, left ankle and foot
M02.879　Other reactive arthropathies, unspecified ankle and foot
M02.88　Other reactive arthropathies, vertebrae
M02.89　Other reactive arthropathies, multiple sites
M02.9　Reactive arthropathy, unspecified

Autoinflammatory syndromes (M04)

● ◢ M04　Autoinflammatory syndromes
　　EXCLUDES 2　*Crohn's disease (K50.-)*

● M04.1　Periodic fever syndromes
　Familial Mediterranean fever
　Hyperimmunoglobin D syndrome
　Mevalonate kinase deficiency
　Tumor necrosis factor receptor associated periodic syndrome [TRAPS]

● M04.2　Cryopyrin-associated periodic syndromes
　Chronic infantile neurological, cutaneous and articular syndrome [CINCA]
　Familial cold autoinflammatory syndrome
　Familial cold urticaria
　Muckle-Wells syndrome
　Neonatal onset multisystemic inflammatory disorder [NOMID]

● M04.8　Other autoinflammatory syndromes
　Blau syndrome
　Deficiency of interleukin 1 receptor antagonist [DIRA]
　Majeed syndrome
　Periodic fever, aphthous stomatitis, pharyngitis, and adenopathy syndrome [PFAPA]
　Pyogenic arthritis, pyoderma gangrenosum, and acne syndrome [PAPA]

● M04.9　Autoinflammatory syndrome, unspecified

Inflammatory polyarthropathies (M05-M14)

◢ M05　Rheumatoid arthritis with rheumatoid factor
　　EXCLUDES 1　*rheumatic fever (I00)*
　　juvenile rheumatoid arthritis (M08.-)
　　rheumatoid arthritis of spine (M45.-)

　　CODING TIP ✓　Rheumatoid arthritis classified here includes rheumatoid arthritis and associated conditions (see combination codes) that have an identified rheumatoid factor present. Do not assume the presence of rheumatoid factor when a diagnosis of rheumatoid arthritis is noted in the clinical record. Rheumatoid arthritis that is not specified with rheumatoid factor is coded to M06.-. There are many associated conditions that the classification assumes are related to rheumatoid arthritis. Consult the alphabetic index "arthritis, rheumatoid, with."

⑤ M05.0　Felty's syndrome
　Rheumatoid arthritis with splenoadenomegaly and leukopenia
　　DEFINITION　Atypical form of rheumatoid arthritis presenting with fever, enlarged spleen, recurring infections, and decreased white cell count.

M05.00　Felty's syndrome, unspecified site
⑥ M05.01　Felty's syndrome, shoulder
　M05.011　Felty's syndrome, right shoulder
　M05.012　Felty's syndrome, left shoulder
　M05.019　Felty's syndrome, unspecified shoulder
⑥ M05.02　Felty's syndrome, elbow
　M05.021　Felty's syndrome, right elbow
　M05.022　Felty's syndrome, left elbow
　M05.029　Felty's syndrome, unspecified elbow
⑥ M05.03　Felty's syndrome, wrist
　Felty's syndrome, carpal bones
　M05.031　Felty's syndrome, right wrist
　M05.032　Felty's syndrome, left wrist
　M05.039　Felty's syndrome, unspecified wrist
⑥ M05.04　Felty's syndrome, hand
　Felty's syndrome, metacarpus and phalanges
　M05.041　Felty's syndrome, right hand
　M05.042　Felty's syndrome, left hand

M05.049　Felty's syndrome, unspecified hand
⑥ M05.05　Felty's syndrome, hip
　M05.051　Felty's syndrome, right hip
　M05.052　Felty's syndrome, left hip
　M05.059　Felty's syndrome, unspecified hip
⑥ M05.06　Felty's syndrome, knee
　M05.061　Felty's syndrome, right knee
　M05.062　Felty's syndrome, left knee
　M05.069　Felty's syndrome, unspecified knee
⑥ M05.07　Felty's syndrome, ankle and foot
　Felty's syndrome, tarsus, metatarsus and phalanges
　M05.071　Felty's syndrome, right ankle and foot
　M05.072　Felty's syndrome, left ankle and foot
　M05.079　Felty's syndrome, unspecified ankle and foot
M05.09　Felty's syndrome, multiple sites
⑤ M05.1　Rheumatoid lung disease with rheumatoid arthritis
M05.10　Rheumatoid lung disease with rheumatoid arthritis of unspecified site
⑥ M05.11　Rheumatoid lung disease with rheumatoid arthritis of shoulder
　M05.111　Rheumatoid lung disease with rheumatoid arthritis of right shoulder
　M05.112　Rheumatoid lung disease with rheumatoid arthritis of left shoulder
　M05.119　Rheumatoid lung disease with rheumatoid arthritis of unspecified shoulder
⑥ M05.12　Rheumatoid lung disease with rheumatoid arthritis of elbow
　M05.121　Rheumatoid lung disease with rheumatoid arthritis of right elbow
　M05.122　Rheumatoid lung disease with rheumatoid arthritis of left elbow
　M05.129　Rheumatoid lung disease with rheumatoid arthritis of unspecified elbow
⑥ M05.13　Rheumatoid lung disease with rheumatoid arthritis of wrist
　Rheumatoid lung disease with rheumatoid arthritis, carpal bones
　M05.131　Rheumatoid lung disease with rheumatoid arthritis of right wrist
　M05.132　Rheumatoid lung disease with rheumatoid arthritis of left wrist
　M05.139　Rheumatoid lung disease with rheumatoid arthritis of unspecified wrist
⑥ M05.14　Rheumatoid lung disease with rheumatoid arthritis of hand
　Rheumatoid lung disease with rheumatoid arthritis, metacarpus and phalanges
　M05.141　Rheumatoid lung disease with rheumatoid arthritis of right hand
　M05.142　Rheumatoid lung disease with rheumatoid arthritis of left hand
　M05.149　Rheumatoid lung disease with rheumatoid arthritis of unspecified hand
⑥ M05.15　Rheumatoid lung disease with rheumatoid arthritis of hip
　M05.151　Rheumatoid lung disease with rheumatoid arthritis of right hip
　M05.152　Rheumatoid lung disease with rheumatoid arthritis of left hip
　M05.159　Rheumatoid lung disease with rheumatoid arthritis of unspecified hip
⑥ M05.16　Rheumatoid lung disease with rheumatoid arthritis of knee
　M05.161　Rheumatoid lung disease with rheumatoid arthritis of right knee
　M05.162　Rheumatoid lung disease with rheumatoid arthritis of left knee
　M05.169　Rheumatoid lung disease with rheumatoid arthritis of unspecified knee
⑥ M05.17　Rheumatoid lung disease with rheumatoid arthritis of ankle and foot
　Rheumatoid lung disease with rheumatoid arthritis, tarsus, metatarsus and phalanges
　M05.171　Rheumatoid lung disease with rheumatoid arthritis of right ankle and foot

● New　▲ Revised　*Manifestation*　◢-◿ Digit Indicators　▭ Laterality　Ⓐ Adult (15+ years)　Ⓜ Maternity (12-55 years)　Ⓝ Newborn　Ⓟ Pediatric (0-17 years)　♂ Male　♀ Female
✖ Deleted　Unspecified　+ Additional code

2017 ICD-10-CM Expert for Physicians　　　© 2017 DecisionHealth　　741

⬚ M05.172 **Rheumatoid lung disease with rheumatoid arthritis of left ankle and foot**

⬚ M05.179 **Rheumatoid lung disease with rheumatoid arthritis of unspecified ankle and foot**

M05.19 **Rheumatoid lung disease with rheumatoid arthritis of multiple sites**

⑤ M05.2 **Rheumatoid vasculitis with rheumatoid arthritis**

M05.20 **Rheumatoid vasculitis with rheumatoid arthritis of unspecified site**

⑥ M05.21 **Rheumatoid vasculitis with rheumatoid arthritis of shoulder**

⬚ M05.211 **Rheumatoid vasculitis with rheumatoid arthritis of right shoulder**

⬚ M05.212 **Rheumatoid vasculitis with rheumatoid arthritis of left shoulder**

⬚ M05.219 **Rheumatoid vasculitis with rheumatoid arthritis of unspecified shoulder**

⑥ M05.22 **Rheumatoid vasculitis with rheumatoid arthritis of elbow**

⬚ M05.221 **Rheumatoid vasculitis with rheumatoid arthritis of right elbow**

⬚ M05.222 **Rheumatoid vasculitis with rheumatoid arthritis of left elbow**

⬚ M05.229 **Rheumatoid vasculitis with rheumatoid arthritis of unspecified elbow**

⑥ M05.23 **Rheumatoid vasculitis with rheumatoid arthritis of wrist**
Rheumatoid vasculitis with rheumatoid arthritis, carpal bones

⬚ M05.231 **Rheumatoid vasculitis with rheumatoid arthritis of right wrist**

⬚ M05.232 **Rheumatoid vasculitis with rheumatoid arthritis of left wrist**

⬚ M05.239 **Rheumatoid vasculitis with rheumatoid arthritis of unspecified wrist**

⑥ M05.24 **Rheumatoid vasculitis with rheumatoid arthritis of hand**
Rheumatoid vasculitis with rheumatoid arthritis, metacarpus and phalanges

⬚ M05.241 **Rheumatoid vasculitis with rheumatoid arthritis of right hand**

⬚ M05.242 **Rheumatoid vasculitis with rheumatoid arthritis of left hand**

⬚ M05.249 **Rheumatoid vasculitis with rheumatoid arthritis of unspecified hand**

⑥ M05.25 **Rheumatoid vasculitis with rheumatoid arthritis of hip**

⬚ M05.251 **Rheumatoid vasculitis with rheumatoid arthritis of right hip**

⬚ M05.252 **Rheumatoid vasculitis with rheumatoid arthritis of left hip**

⬚ M05.259 **Rheumatoid vasculitis with rheumatoid arthritis of unspecified hip**

⑥ M05.26 **Rheumatoid vasculitis with rheumatoid arthritis of knee**

⬚ M05.261 **Rheumatoid vasculitis with rheumatoid arthritis of right knee**

⬚ M05.262 **Rheumatoid vasculitis with rheumatoid arthritis of left knee**

⬚ M05.269 **Rheumatoid vasculitis with rheumatoid arthritis of unspecified knee**

⑥ M05.27 **Rheumatoid vasculitis with rheumatoid arthritis of ankle and foot**
Rheumatoid vasculitis with rheumatoid arthritis, tarsus, metatarsus and phalanges

⬚ M05.271 **Rheumatoid vasculitis with rheumatoid arthritis of right ankle and foot**

⬚ M05.272 **Rheumatoid vasculitis with rheumatoid arthritis of left ankle and foot**

⬚ M05.279 **Rheumatoid vasculitis with rheumatoid arthritis of unspecified ankle and foot**

M05.29 **Rheumatoid vasculitis with rheumatoid arthritis of multiple sites**

⑤ M05.3 **Rheumatoid heart disease with rheumatoid arthritis**
Rheumatoid carditis
Rheumatoid endocarditis
Rheumatoid myocarditis
Rheumatoid pericarditis

M05.30 **Rheumatoid heart disease with rheumatoid arthritis of unspecified site**

⑥ M05.31 **Rheumatoid heart disease with rheumatoid arthritis of shoulder**

⬚ M05.311 **Rheumatoid heart disease with rheumatoid arthritis of right shoulder**

⬚ M05.312 **Rheumatoid heart disease with rheumatoid arthritis of left shoulder**

⬚ M05.319 **Rheumatoid heart disease with rheumatoid arthritis of unspecified shoulder**

⑥ M05.32 **Rheumatoid heart disease with rheumatoid arthritis of elbow**

⬚ M05.321 **Rheumatoid heart disease with rheumatoid arthritis of right elbow**

⬚ M05.322 **Rheumatoid heart disease with rheumatoid arthritis of left elbow**

⬚ M05.329 **Rheumatoid heart disease with rheumatoid arthritis of unspecified elbow**

⑥ M05.33 **Rheumatoid heart disease with rheumatoid arthritis of wrist**
Rheumatoid heart disease with rheumatoid arthritis, carpal bones

⬚ M05.331 **Rheumatoid heart disease with rheumatoid arthritis of right wrist**

⬚ M05.332 **Rheumatoid heart disease with rheumatoid arthritis of left wrist**

⬚ M05.339 **Rheumatoid heart disease with rheumatoid arthritis of unspecified wrist**

⑥ M05.34 **Rheumatoid heart disease with rheumatoid arthritis of hand**
Rheumatoid heart disease with rheumatoid arthritis, metacarpus and phalanges

⬚ M05.341 **Rheumatoid heart disease with rheumatoid arthritis of right hand**

⬚ M05.342 **Rheumatoid heart disease with rheumatoid arthritis of left hand**

⬚ M05.349 **Rheumatoid heart disease with rheumatoid arthritis of unspecified hand**

⑥ M05.35 **Rheumatoid heart disease with rheumatoid arthritis of hip**

⬚ M05.351 **Rheumatoid heart disease with rheumatoid arthritis of right hip**

⬚ M05.352 **Rheumatoid heart disease with rheumatoid arthritis of left hip**

⬚ M05.359 **Rheumatoid heart disease with rheumatoid arthritis of unspecified hip**

⑥ M05.36 **Rheumatoid heart disease with rheumatoid arthritis of knee**

⬚ M05.361 **Rheumatoid heart disease with rheumatoid arthritis of right knee**

⬚ M05.362 **Rheumatoid heart disease with rheumatoid arthritis of left knee**

⬚ M05.369 **Rheumatoid heart disease with rheumatoid arthritis of unspecified knee**

⑥ M05.37 **Rheumatoid heart disease with rheumatoid arthritis of ankle and foot**
Rheumatoid heart disease with rheumatoid arthritis, tarsus, metatarsus and phalanges

⬚ M05.371 **Rheumatoid heart disease with rheumatoid arthritis of right ankle and foot**

⬚ M05.372 **Rheumatoid heart disease with rheumatoid arthritis of left ankle and foot**

⬚ M05.379 **Rheumatoid heart disease with rheumatoid arthritis of unspecified ankle and foot**

M05.39 **Rheumatoid heart disease with rheumatoid arthritis of multiple sites**

⑤ M05.4 **Rheumatoid myopathy with rheumatoid arthritis**

M05.40 **Rheumatoid myopathy with rheumatoid arthritis of unspecified site**

⑥ M05.41 **Rheumatoid myopathy with rheumatoid arthritis of shoulder**

⬚ M05.411 **Rheumatoid myopathy with rheumatoid arthritis of right shoulder**

⬚ M05.412 **Rheumatoid myopathy with rheumatoid arthritis of left shoulder**

⬚ M05.419 **Rheumatoid myopathy with rheumatoid arthritis of unspecified shoulder**

● New ▲ Revised *Manifestation* ④-⑦ Digit Indicators ⬚ Laterality Ⓐ Adult (15+ years) Ⓜ Maternity (12-55 years) Ⓝ Newborn Ⓟ Pediatric (0-17 years) ♂ Male ♀ Female
✖ Deleted Unspecified + Additional code

742   © 2017 DecisionHealth   2017 ICD-10-CM Expert for Physicians

🔾 **M05.42** Rheumatoid myopathy with rheumatoid arthritis of elbow

⊟ **M05.421** Rheumatoid myopathy with rheumatoid arthritis of right elbow

⊟ **M05.422** Rheumatoid myopathy with rheumatoid arthritis of left elbow

⊟ **M05.429** Rheumatoid myopathy with rheumatoid arthritis of unspecified elbow

🔾 **M05.43** Rheumatoid myopathy with rheumatoid arthritis of wrist
Rheumatoid myopathy with rheumatoid arthritis, carpal bones

⊟ **M05.431** Rheumatoid myopathy with rheumatoid arthritis of right wrist

⊟ **M05.432** Rheumatoid myopathy with rheumatoid arthritis of left wrist

⊟ **M05.439** Rheumatoid myopathy with rheumatoid arthritis of unspecified wrist

🔾 **M05.44** Rheumatoid myopathy with rheumatoid arthritis of hand
Rheumatoid myopathy with rheumatoid arthritis, metacarpus and phalanges

⊟ **M05.441** Rheumatoid myopathy with rheumatoid arthritis of right hand

⊟ **M05.442** Rheumatoid myopathy with rheumatoid arthritis of left hand

⊟ **M05.449** Rheumatoid myopathy with rheumatoid arthritis of unspecified hand

🔾 **M05.45** Rheumatoid myopathy with rheumatoid arthritis of hip

⊟ **M05.451** Rheumatoid myopathy with rheumatoid arthritis of right hip

⊟ **M05.452** Rheumatoid myopathy with rheumatoid arthritis of left hip

⊟ **M05.459** Rheumatoid myopathy with rheumatoid arthritis of unspecified hip

🔾 **M05.46** Rheumatoid myopathy with rheumatoid arthritis of knee

⊟ **M05.461** Rheumatoid myopathy with rheumatoid arthritis of right knee

⊟ **M05.462** Rheumatoid myopathy with rheumatoid arthritis of left knee

⊟ **M05.469** Rheumatoid myopathy with rheumatoid arthritis of unspecified knee

🔾 **M05.47** Rheumatoid myopathy with rheumatoid arthritis of ankle and foot
Rheumatoid myopathy with rheumatoid arthritis, tarsus, metatarsus and phalanges

⊟ **M05.471** Rheumatoid myopathy with rheumatoid arthritis of right ankle and foot

⊟ **M05.472** Rheumatoid myopathy with rheumatoid arthritis of left ankle and foot

⊟ **M05.479** Rheumatoid myopathy with rheumatoid arthritis of unspecified ankle and foot

M05.49 Rheumatoid myopathy with rheumatoid arthritis of multiple sites

🔾 **M05.5** Rheumatoid polyneuropathy with rheumatoid arthritis

M05.50 Rheumatoid polyneuropathy with rheumatoid arthritis of unspecified site

🔾 **M05.51** Rheumatoid polyneuropathy with rheumatoid arthritis of shoulder

⊟ **M05.511** Rheumatoid polyneuropathy with rheumatoid arthritis of right shoulder

⊟ **M05.512** Rheumatoid polyneuropathy with rheumatoid arthritis of left shoulder

⊟ **M05.519** Rheumatoid polyneuropathy with rheumatoid arthritis of unspecified shoulder

🔾 **M05.52** Rheumatoid polyneuropathy with rheumatoid arthritis of elbow

⊟ **M05.521** Rheumatoid polyneuropathy with rheumatoid arthritis of right elbow

⊟ **M05.522** Rheumatoid polyneuropathy with rheumatoid arthritis of left elbow

⊟ **M05.529** Rheumatoid polyneuropathy with rheumatoid arthritis of unspecified elbow

🔾 **M05.53** Rheumatoid polyneuropathy with rheumatoid arthritis of wrist
Rheumatoid polyneuropathy with rheumatoid arthritis, carpal bones

⊟ **M05.531** Rheumatoid polyneuropathy with rheumatoid arthritis of right wrist

⊟ **M05.532** Rheumatoid polyneuropathy with rheumatoid arthritis of left wrist

⊟ **M05.539** Rheumatoid polyneuropathy with rheumatoid arthritis of unspecified wrist

🔾 **M05.54** Rheumatoid polyneuropathy with rheumatoid arthritis of hand
Rheumatoid polyneuropathy with rheumatoid arthritis, metacarpus and phalanges

⊟ **M05.541** Rheumatoid polyneuropathy with rheumatoid arthritis of right hand

⊟ **M05.542** Rheumatoid polyneuropathy with rheumatoid arthritis of left hand

⊟ **M05.549** Rheumatoid polyneuropathy with rheumatoid arthritis of unspecified hand

🔾 **M05.55** Rheumatoid polyneuropathy with rheumatoid arthritis of hip

⊟ **M05.551** Rheumatoid polyneuropathy with rheumatoid arthritis of right hip

⊟ **M05.552** Rheumatoid polyneuropathy with rheumatoid arthritis of left hip

⊟ **M05.559** Rheumatoid polyneuropathy with rheumatoid arthritis of unspecified hip

🔾 **M05.56** Rheumatoid polyneuropathy with rheumatoid arthritis of knee

⊟ **M05.561** Rheumatoid polyneuropathy with rheumatoid arthritis of right knee

⊟ **M05.562** Rheumatoid polyneuropathy with rheumatoid arthritis of left knee

⊟ **M05.569** Rheumatoid polyneuropathy with rheumatoid arthritis of unspecified knee

🔾 **M05.57** Rheumatoid polyneuropathy with rheumatoid arthritis of ankle and foot
Rheumatoid polyneuropathy with rheumatoid arthritis, tarsus, metatarsus and phalanges

⊟ **M05.571** Rheumatoid polyneuropathy with rheumatoid arthritis of right ankle and foot

⊟ **M05.572** Rheumatoid polyneuropathy with rheumatoid arthritis of left ankle and foot

⊟ **M05.579** Rheumatoid polyneuropathy with rheumatoid arthritis of unspecified ankle and foot

M05.59 Rheumatoid polyneuropathy with rheumatoid arthritis of multiple sites

⑤ **M05.6** Rheumatoid arthritis with involvement of other organs and systems

M05.60 Rheumatoid arthritis of unspecified site with involvement of other organs and systems

🔾 **M05.61** Rheumatoid arthritis of shoulder with involvement of other organs and systems

⊟ **M05.611** Rheumatoid arthritis of right shoulder with involvement of other organs and systems

⊟ **M05.612** Rheumatoid arthritis of left shoulder with involvement of other organs and systems

⊟ **M05.619** Rheumatoid arthritis of unspecified shoulder with involvement of other organs and systems

🔾 **M05.62** Rheumatoid arthritis of elbow with involvement of other organs and systems

⊟ **M05.621** Rheumatoid arthritis of right elbow with involvement of other organs and systems

⊟ **M05.622** Rheumatoid arthritis of left elbow with involvement of other organs and systems

⊟ **M05.629** Rheumatoid arthritis of unspecified elbow with involvement of other organs and systems

🔾 **M05.63** Rheumatoid arthritis of wrist with involvement of other organs and systems
Rheumatoid arthritis of carpal bones with involvement of other organs and systems

⊟ **M05.631** Rheumatoid arthritis of right wrist with involvement of other organs and systems

⊟ **M05.632** Rheumatoid arthritis of left wrist with involvement of other organs and systems

⊟ **M05.639** Rheumatoid arthritis of unspecified wrist with involvement of other organs and systems

🔾 **M05.64** Rheumatoid arthritis of hand with involvement of other organs and systems
Rheumatoid arthritis of metacarpus and phalanges with involvement of other organs and systems

● New ▲ Revised *Manifestation* 🔢-🔢 Digit Indicators ⊟ Laterality Ⓐ Adult (15+ years) Ⓜ Maternity (12-55 years) Ⓝ Newborn Ⓟ Pediatric (0-17 years) ♂ Male ♀ Female
✖ ~~Deleted~~ Unspecified + Additional code

2017 ICD-10-CM Expert for Physicians

© 2017 DecisionHealth

743

⊟ **M05.641**   Rheumatoid arthritis of right hand with involvement of other organs and systems

⊟ **M05.642**   Rheumatoid arthritis of left hand with involvement of other organs and systems

⊟ **M05.649**   Rheumatoid arthritis of unspecified hand with involvement of other organs and systems

⑥ **M05.65**   Rheumatoid arthritis of hip with involvement of other organs and systems

⊟ **M05.651**   Rheumatoid arthritis of right hip with involvement of other organs and systems

⊟ **M05.652**   Rheumatoid arthritis of left hip with involvement of other organs and systems

⊟ **M05.659**   Rheumatoid arthritis of unspecified hip with involvement of other organs and systems

⑥ **M05.66**   Rheumatoid arthritis of knee with involvement of other organs and systems

⊟ **M05.661**   Rheumatoid arthritis of right knee with involvement of other organs and systems

⊟ **M05.662**   Rheumatoid arthritis of left knee with involvement of other organs and systems

⊟ **M05.669**   Rheumatoid arthritis of unspecified knee with involvement of other organs and systems

⑥ **M05.67**   Rheumatoid arthritis of ankle and foot with involvement of other organs and systems
Rheumatoid arthritis of tarsus, metatarsus and phalanges with involvement of other organs and systems

⊟ **M05.671**   Rheumatoid arthritis of right ankle and foot with involvement of other organs and systems

⊟ **M05.672**   Rheumatoid arthritis of left ankle and foot with involvement of other organs and systems

⊟ **M05.679**   Rheumatoid arthritis of unspecified ankle and foot with involvement of other organs and systems

M05.69   Rheumatoid arthritis of multiple sites with involvement of other organs and systems

⑤ **M05.7**   Rheumatoid arthritis with rheumatoid factor without organ or systems involvement

M05.70   Rheumatoid arthritis with rheumatoid factor of unspecified site without organ or systems involvement

⑥ **M05.71**   Rheumatoid arthritis with rheumatoid factor of shoulder without organ or systems involvement

⊟ **M05.711**   Rheumatoid arthritis with rheumatoid factor of right shoulder without organ or systems involvement

⊟ **M05.712**   Rheumatoid arthritis with rheumatoid factor of left shoulder without organ or systems involvement

⊟ **M05.719**   Rheumatoid arthritis with rheumatoid factor of unspecified shoulder without organ or systems involvement

⑥ **M05.72**   Rheumatoid arthritis with rheumatoid factor of elbow without organ or systems involvement

⊟ **M05.721**   Rheumatoid arthritis with rheumatoid factor of right elbow without organ or systems involvement

⊟ **M05.722**   Rheumatoid arthritis with rheumatoid factor of left elbow without organ or systems involvement

⊟ **M05.729**   Rheumatoid arthritis with rheumatoid factor of unspecified elbow without organ or systems involvement

⑥ **M05.73**   Rheumatoid arthritis with rheumatoid factor of wrist without organ or systems involvement

⊟ **M05.731**   Rheumatoid arthritis with rheumatoid factor of right wrist without organ or systems involvement

⊟ **M05.732**   Rheumatoid arthritis with rheumatoid factor of left wrist without organ or systems involvement

⊟ **M05.739**   Rheumatoid arthritis with rheumatoid factor of unspecified wrist without organ or systems involvement

⑥ **M05.74**   Rheumatoid arthritis with rheumatoid factor of hand without organ or systems involvement

⊟ **M05.741**   Rheumatoid arthritis with rheumatoid factor of right hand without organ or systems involvement

⊟ **M05.742**   Rheumatoid arthritis with rheumatoid factor of left hand without organ or systems involvement

⊟ **M05.749**   Rheumatoid arthritis with rheumatoid factor of unspecified hand without organ or systems involvement

⑥ **M05.75**   Rheumatoid arthritis with rheumatoid factor of hip without organ or systems involvement

⊟ **M05.751**   Rheumatoid arthritis with rheumatoid factor of right hip without organ or systems involvement

⊟ **M05.752**   Rheumatoid arthritis with rheumatoid factor of left hip without organ or systems involvement

⊟ **M05.759**   Rheumatoid arthritis with rheumatoid factor of unspecified hip without organ or systems involvement

⑥ **M05.76**   Rheumatoid arthritis with rheumatoid factor of knee without organ or systems involvement

⊟ **M05.761**   Rheumatoid arthritis with rheumatoid factor of right knee without organ or systems involvement

⊟ **M05.762**   Rheumatoid arthritis with rheumatoid factor of left knee without organ or systems involvement

⊟ **M05.769**   Rheumatoid arthritis with rheumatoid factor of unspecified knee without organ or systems involvement

⑥ **M05.77**   Rheumatoid arthritis with rheumatoid factor of ankle and foot without organ or systems involvement

⊟ **M05.771**   Rheumatoid arthritis with rheumatoid factor of right ankle and foot without organ or systems involvement

⊟ **M05.772**   Rheumatoid arthritis with rheumatoid factor of left ankle and foot without organ or systems involvement

⊟ **M05.779**   Rheumatoid arthritis with rheumatoid factor of unspecified ankle and foot without organ or systems involvement

M05.79   Rheumatoid arthritis with rheumatoid factor of multiple sites without organ or systems involvement

⑤ **M05.8**   Other rheumatoid arthritis with rheumatoid factor

M05.80   Other rheumatoid arthritis with rheumatoid factor of unspecified site

⑥ **M05.81**   Other rheumatoid arthritis with rheumatoid factor of shoulder

⊟ **M05.811**   Other rheumatoid arthritis with rheumatoid factor of right shoulder

⊟ **M05.812**   Other rheumatoid arthritis with rheumatoid factor of left shoulder

⊟ **M05.819**   Other rheumatoid arthritis with rheumatoid factor of unspecified shoulder

⑥ **M05.82**   Other rheumatoid arthritis with rheumatoid factor of elbow

⊟ **M05.821**   Other rheumatoid arthritis with rheumatoid factor of right elbow

⊟ **M05.822**   Other rheumatoid arthritis with rheumatoid factor of left elbow

⊟ **M05.829**   Other rheumatoid arthritis with rheumatoid factor of unspecified elbow

⑥ **M05.83**   Other rheumatoid arthritis with rheumatoid factor of wrist

⊟ **M05.831**   Other rheumatoid arthritis with rheumatoid factor of right wrist

⊟ **M05.832**   Other rheumatoid arthritis with rheumatoid factor of left wrist

⊟ **M05.839**   Other rheumatoid arthritis with rheumatoid factor of unspecified wrist

⑥ **M05.84**   Other rheumatoid arthritis with rheumatoid factor of hand

⊟ **M05.841**   Other rheumatoid arthritis with rheumatoid factor of right hand

⊟ **M05.842**   Other rheumatoid arthritis with rheumatoid factor of left hand

⊟ **M05.849**   Other rheumatoid arthritis with rheumatoid factor of unspecified hand

⑥ **M05.85**   Other rheumatoid arthritis with rheumatoid factor of hip

● New   ▲ Revised   *Manifestation*   ④-⑦ Digit Indicators   ⊟ Laterality   Ⓐ Adult (15+ years)   Ⓜ Maternity (12-55 years)   Ⓝ Newborn   Ⓟ Pediatric (0-17 years)   ♂ Male   ♀ Female
✖ Deleted   Unspecified   + Additional code

744   © 2017 DecisionHealth   2017 ICD-10-CM Expert for Physicians

- ⬚ **M05.851** Other rheumatoid arthritis with rheumatoid factor of right hip
- ⬚ **M05.852** Other rheumatoid arthritis with rheumatoid factor of left hip
- ⬚ **M05.859** Other rheumatoid arthritis with rheumatoid factor of unspecified hip
- ⑥ **M05.86** Other rheumatoid arthritis with rheumatoid factor of knee
  - ⬚ **M05.861** Other rheumatoid arthritis with rheumatoid factor of right knee
  - ⬚ **M05.862** Other rheumatoid arthritis with rheumatoid factor of left knee
  - ⬚ **M05.869** Other rheumatoid arthritis with rheumatoid factor of unspecified knee
- ⑥ **M05.87** Other rheumatoid arthritis with rheumatoid factor of ankle and foot
  - ⬚ **M05.871** Other rheumatoid arthritis with rheumatoid factor of right ankle and foot
  - ⬚ **M05.872** Other rheumatoid arthritis with rheumatoid factor of left ankle and foot
  - ⬚ **M05.879** Other rheumatoid arthritis with rheumatoid factor of unspecified ankle and foot
- **M05.89** Other rheumatoid arthritis with rheumatoid factor of multiple sites
- **M05.9** Rheumatoid arthritis with rheumatoid factor, unspecified

④ **M06** Other rheumatoid arthritis
- ⑤ **M06.0** Rheumatoid arthritis without rheumatoid factor
  - **M06.00** Rheumatoid arthritis without rheumatoid factor, unspecified site
  - ⑥ **M06.01** Rheumatoid arthritis without rheumatoid factor, shoulder
    - ⬚ **M06.011** Rheumatoid arthritis without rheumatoid factor, right shoulder
    - ⬚ **M06.012** Rheumatoid arthritis without rheumatoid factor, left shoulder
    - ⬚ **M06.019** Rheumatoid arthritis without rheumatoid factor, unspecified shoulder
  - ⑥ **M06.02** Rheumatoid arthritis without rheumatoid factor, elbow
    - ⬚ **M06.021** Rheumatoid arthritis without rheumatoid factor, right elbow
    - ⬚ **M06.022** Rheumatoid arthritis without rheumatoid factor, left elbow
    - ⬚ **M06.029** Rheumatoid arthritis without rheumatoid factor, unspecified elbow
  - ⑥ **M06.03** Rheumatoid arthritis without rheumatoid factor, wrist
    - ⬚ **M06.031** Rheumatoid arthritis without rheumatoid factor, right wrist
    - ⬚ **M06.032** Rheumatoid arthritis without rheumatoid factor, left wrist
    - ⬚ **M06.039** Rheumatoid arthritis without rheumatoid factor, unspecified wrist
  - ⑥ **M06.04** Rheumatoid arthritis without rheumatoid factor, hand
    - ⬚ **M06.041** Rheumatoid arthritis without rheumatoid factor, right hand
    - ⬚ **M06.042** Rheumatoid arthritis without rheumatoid factor, left hand
    - ⬚ **M06.049** Rheumatoid arthritis without rheumatoid factor, unspecified hand
  - ⑥ **M06.05** Rheumatoid arthritis without rheumatoid factor, hip
    - ⬚ **M06.051** Rheumatoid arthritis without rheumatoid factor, right hip
    - ⬚ **M06.052** Rheumatoid arthritis without rheumatoid factor, left hip
    - ⬚ **M06.059** Rheumatoid arthritis without rheumatoid factor, unspecified hip
  - ⑥ **M06.06** Rheumatoid arthritis without rheumatoid factor, knee
    - ⬚ **M06.061** Rheumatoid arthritis without rheumatoid factor, right knee
    - ⬚ **M06.062** Rheumatoid arthritis without rheumatoid factor, left knee
    - ⬚ **M06.069** Rheumatoid arthritis without rheumatoid factor, unspecified knee

- ⑥ **M06.07** Rheumatoid arthritis without rheumatoid factor, ankle and foot
  - ⬚ **M06.071** Rheumatoid arthritis without rheumatoid factor, right ankle and foot
  - ⬚ **M06.072** Rheumatoid arthritis without rheumatoid factor, left ankle and foot
  - ⬚ **M06.079** Rheumatoid arthritis without rheumatoid factor, unspecified ankle and foot
  - **M06.08** Rheumatoid arthritis without rheumatoid factor, vertebrae
  - **M06.09** Rheumatoid arthritis without rheumatoid factor, multiple sites
- **M06.1** Adult-onset Still's disease Ⓐ
  - **EXCLUDES 1** Still's disease NOS (M08.2-)
- ⑤ **M06.2** Rheumatoid bursitis
  - **M06.20** Rheumatoid bursitis, unspecified site
  - ⑥ **M06.21** Rheumatoid bursitis, shoulder
    - ⬚ **M06.211** Rheumatoid bursitis, right shoulder
    - ⬚ **M06.212** Rheumatoid bursitis, left shoulder
    - ⬚ **M06.219** Rheumatoid bursitis, unspecified shoulder
  - ⑥ **M06.22** Rheumatoid bursitis, elbow
    - ⬚ **M06.221** Rheumatoid bursitis, right elbow
    - ⬚ **M06.222** Rheumatoid bursitis, left elbow
    - ⬚ **M06.229** Rheumatoid bursitis, unspecified elbow
  - ⑥ **M06.23** Rheumatoid bursitis, wrist
    - ⬚ **M06.231** Rheumatoid bursitis, right wrist
    - ⬚ **M06.232** Rheumatoid bursitis, left wrist
    - ⬚ **M06.239** Rheumatoid bursitis, unspecified wrist
  - ⑥ **M06.24** Rheumatoid bursitis, hand
    - ⬚ **M06.241** Rheumatoid bursitis, right hand
    - ⬚ **M06.242** Rheumatoid bursitis, left hand
    - ⬚ **M06.249** Rheumatoid bursitis, unspecified hand
  - ⑥ **M06.25** Rheumatoid bursitis, hip
    - ⬚ **M06.251** Rheumatoid bursitis, right hip
    - ⬚ **M06.252** Rheumatoid bursitis, left hip
    - ⬚ **M06.259** Rheumatoid bursitis, unspecified hip
  - ⑥ **M06.26** Rheumatoid bursitis, knee
    - ⬚ **M06.261** Rheumatoid bursitis, right knee
    - ⬚ **M06.262** Rheumatoid bursitis, left knee
    - ⬚ **M06.269** Rheumatoid bursitis, unspecified knee
  - ⑥ **M06.27** Rheumatoid bursitis, ankle and foot
    - ⬚ **M06.271** Rheumatoid bursitis, right ankle and foot
    - ⬚ **M06.272** Rheumatoid bursitis, left ankle and foot
    - ⬚ **M06.279** Rheumatoid bursitis, unspecified ankle and foot
  - **M06.28** Rheumatoid bursitis, vertebrae
  - **M06.29** Rheumatoid bursitis, multiple sites
- ⑤ **M06.3** Rheumatoid nodule
  - **M06.30** Rheumatoid nodule, unspecified site
  - ⑥ **M06.31** Rheumatoid nodule, shoulder
    - ⬚ **M06.311** Rheumatoid nodule, right shoulder
    - ⬚ **M06.312** Rheumatoid nodule, left shoulder
    - ⬚ **M06.319** Rheumatoid nodule, unspecified shoulder
  - ⑥ **M06.32** Rheumatoid nodule, elbow
    - ⬚ **M06.321** Rheumatoid nodule, right elbow
    - ⬚ **M06.322** Rheumatoid nodule, left elbow
    - ⬚ **M06.329** Rheumatoid nodule, unspecified elbow
  - ⑥ **M06.33** Rheumatoid nodule, wrist
    - ⬚ **M06.331** Rheumatoid nodule, right wrist
    - ⬚ **M06.332** Rheumatoid nodule, left wrist
    - ⬚ **M06.339** Rheumatoid nodule, unspecified wrist
  - ⑥ **M06.34** Rheumatoid nodule, hand
    - ⬚ **M06.341** Rheumatoid nodule, right hand
    - ⬚ **M06.342** Rheumatoid nodule, left hand
    - ⬚ **M06.349** Rheumatoid nodule, unspecified hand
  - ⑥ **M06.35** Rheumatoid nodule, hip
    - ⬚ **M06.351** Rheumatoid nodule, right hip
    - ⬚ **M06.352** Rheumatoid nodule, left hip

● New ▲ Revised *Manifestation* ④-⑦ Digit Indicators ⊟ Laterality Ⓐ Adult (15+ years) Ⓜ Maternity (12-55 years) Ⓝ Newborn Ⓟ Pediatric (0-17 years) ♂ Male ♀ Female
✖ Deleted Unspecified + Additional code

- ⊟ **M06.359** Rheumatoid nodule, unspecified hip
- ⑥ **M06.36** Rheumatoid nodule, knee
  - ⊟ **M06.361** Rheumatoid nodule, right knee
  - ⊟ **M06.362** Rheumatoid nodule, left knee
  - ⊟ **M06.369** Rheumatoid nodule, unspecified knee
- ⑥ **M06.37** Rheumatoid nodule, ankle and foot
  - ⊟ **M06.371** Rheumatoid nodule, right ankle and foot
  - ⊟ **M06.372** Rheumatoid nodule, left ankle and foot
  - ⊟ **M06.379** Rheumatoid nodule, unspecified ankle and foot
  - **M06.38** Rheumatoid nodule, vertebrae
  - **M06.39** Rheumatoid nodule, multiple sites
- **M06.4** Inflammatory polyarthropathy
  - **EXCLUDES 1** *polyarthritis NOS (M13.0)*
- ⑤ **M06.8** Other specified rheumatoid arthritis
  - **M06.80** Other specified rheumatoid arthritis, unspecified site
  - ⑥ **M06.81** Other specified rheumatoid arthritis, shoulder
    - ⊟ **M06.811** Other specified rheumatoid arthritis, right shoulder
    - ⊟ **M06.812** Other specified rheumatoid arthritis, left shoulder
    - ⊟ **M06.819** Other specified rheumatoid arthritis, unspecified shoulder
  - ⑥ **M06.82** Other specified rheumatoid arthritis, elbow
    - ⊟ **M06.821** Other specified rheumatoid arthritis, right elbow
    - ⊟ **M06.822** Other specified rheumatoid arthritis, left elbow
    - ⊟ **M06.829** Other specified rheumatoid arthritis, unspecified elbow
  - ⑥ **M06.83** Other specified rheumatoid arthritis, wrist
    - ⊟ **M06.831** Other specified rheumatoid arthritis, right wrist
    - ⊟ **M06.832** Other specified rheumatoid arthritis, left wrist
    - ⊟ **M06.839** Other specified rheumatoid arthritis, unspecified wrist
  - ⑥ **M06.84** Other specified rheumatoid arthritis, hand
    - ⊟ **M06.841** Other specified rheumatoid arthritis, right hand
    - ⊟ **M06.842** Other specified rheumatoid arthritis, left hand
    - ⊟ **M06.849** Other specified rheumatoid arthritis, unspecified hand
  - ⑥ **M06.85** Other specified rheumatoid arthritis, hip
    - ⊟ **M06.851** Other specified rheumatoid arthritis, right hip
    - ⊟ **M06.852** Other specified rheumatoid arthritis, left hip
    - ⊟ **M06.859** Other specified rheumatoid arthritis, unspecified hip
  - ⑥ **M06.86** Other specified rheumatoid arthritis, knee
    - ⊟ **M06.861** Other specified rheumatoid arthritis, right knee
    - ⊟ **M06.862** Other specified rheumatoid arthritis, left knee
    - ⊟ **M06.869** Other specified rheumatoid arthritis, unspecified knee
  - ⑥ **M06.87** Other specified rheumatoid arthritis, ankle and foot
    - ⊟ **M06.871** Other specified rheumatoid arthritis, right ankle and foot
    - ⊟ **M06.872** Other specified rheumatoid arthritis, left ankle and foot
    - ⊟ **M06.879** Other specified rheumatoid arthritis, unspecified ankle and foot
  - **M06.88** Other specified rheumatoid arthritis, vertebrae
  - **M06.89** Other specified rheumatoid arthritis, multiple sites
- **M06.9** Rheumatoid arthritis, unspecified
- ④ **M07** Enteropathic arthropathies
  - Code also associated enteropathy, such as:
    - regional enteritis [Crohn's disease] (K50.-)
    - ulcerative colitis (K51.-)
  - **EXCLUDES 1** *psoriatic arthropathies (L40.5-)*
- ⑤ **M07.6** Enteropathic arthropathies
  - **M07.60** Enteropathic arthropathies, unspecified site
  - ⑥ **M07.61** Enteropathic arthropathies, shoulder
    - ⊟ **M07.611** Enteropathic arthropathies, right shoulder
    - ⊟ **M07.612** Enteropathic arthropathies, left shoulder

- ⊟ **M07.619** Enteropathic arthropathies, unspecified shoulder
- ⑥ **M07.62** Enteropathic arthropathies, elbow
  - ⊟ **M07.621** Enteropathic arthropathies, right elbow
  - ⊟ **M07.622** Enteropathic arthropathies, left elbow
  - ⊟ **M07.629** Enteropathic arthropathies, unspecified elbow
- ⑥ **M07.63** Enteropathic arthropathies, wrist
  - ⊟ **M07.631** Enteropathic arthropathies, right wrist
  - ⊟ **M07.632** Enteropathic arthropathies, left wrist
  - ⊟ **M07.639** Enteropathic arthropathies, unspecified wrist
- ⑥ **M07.64** Enteropathic arthropathies, hand
  - ⊟ **M07.641** Enteropathic arthropathies, right hand
  - ⊟ **M07.642** Enteropathic arthropathies, left hand
  - ⊟ **M07.649** Enteropathic arthropathies, unspecified hand
- ⑥ **M07.65** Enteropathic arthropathies, hip
  - ⊟ **M07.651** Enteropathic arthropathies, right hip
  - ⊟ **M07.652** Enteropathic arthropathies, left hip
  - ⊟ **M07.659** Enteropathic arthropathies, unspecified hip
- ⑥ **M07.66** Enteropathic arthropathies, knee
  - ⊟ **M07.661** Enteropathic arthropathies, right knee
  - ⊟ **M07.662** Enteropathic arthropathies, left knee
  - ⊟ **M07.669** Enteropathic arthropathies, unspecified knee
- ⑥ **M07.67** Enteropathic arthropathies, ankle and foot
  - ⊟ **M07.671** Enteropathic arthropathies, right ankle and foot
  - ⊟ **M07.672** Enteropathic arthropathies, left ankle and foot
  - ⊟ **M07.679** Enteropathic arthropathies, unspecified ankle and foot
  - **M07.68** Enteropathic arthropathies, vertebrae
  - **M07.69** Enteropathic arthropathies, multiple sites
- ④ **M08** Juvenile arthritis
  - Code also any associated underlying condition, such as:
    - regional enteritis [Crohn's disease] (K50.-)
    - ulcerative colitis (K51.-)
  - **EXCLUDES 1** *arthropathy in Whipple's disease (M14.8)*
    - *Felty's syndrome (M05.0)*
    - *juvenile dermatomyositis (M33.0-)*
    - *psoriatic juvenile arthropathy (L40.54)*
  - **CODING TIP ✓** Juvenile arthritis generally indicates arthritic conditions that have developed in individuals under 16 years of age. Autoimmune disorders are often the cause of these conditions and all available records should be carefully reviewed to assign the most specific diagnosis and identify any underlying conditions.
- ⑤ **M08.0** Unspecified juvenile rheumatoid arthritis
  - Juvenile rheumatoid arthritis with or without rheumatoid factor
  - **M08.00** Unspecified juvenile rheumatoid arthritis of unspecified site
  - ⑥ **M08.01** Unspecified juvenile rheumatoid arthritis, shoulder
    - ⊟ **M08.011** Unspecified juvenile rheumatoid arthritis, right shoulder
    - ⊟ **M08.012** Unspecified juvenile rheumatoid arthritis, left shoulder
    - ⊟ **M08.019** Unspecified juvenile rheumatoid arthritis, unspecified shoulder
  - ⑥ **M08.02** Unspecified juvenile rheumatoid arthritis of elbow
    - ⊟ **M08.021** Unspecified juvenile rheumatoid arthritis, right elbow
    - ⊟ **M08.022** Unspecified juvenile rheumatoid arthritis, left elbow
    - ⊟ **M08.029** Unspecified juvenile rheumatoid arthritis, unspecified elbow
  - ⑥ **M08.03** Unspecified juvenile rheumatoid arthritis, wrist
    - ⊟ **M08.031** Unspecified juvenile rheumatoid arthritis, right wrist
    - ⊟ **M08.032** Unspecified juvenile rheumatoid arthritis, left wrist
    - ⊟ **M08.039** Unspecified juvenile rheumatoid arthritis, unspecified wrist
  - ⑥ **M08.04** Unspecified juvenile rheumatoid arthritis, hand

● New ▲ Revised *Manifestation* ④-⑦ Digit Indicators ⊟ Laterality Ⓐ Adult (15+ years) Ⓜ Maternity (12-55 years) Ⓝ Newborn Ⓟ Pediatric (0-17 years) ♂ Male ♀ Female
✖ Deleted Unspecified + Additional code

746 © 2017 DecisionHealth 2017 ICD-10-CM Expert for Physicians

▣ M08.041   Unspecified juvenile rheumatoid arthritis, right hand

▣ M08.042   Unspecified juvenile rheumatoid arthritis, left hand

▣ M08.049   Unspecified juvenile rheumatoid arthritis, unspecified hand

ⓖ M08.05   Unspecified juvenile rheumatoid arthritis, hip

▣ M08.051   Unspecified juvenile rheumatoid arthritis, right hip

▣ M08.052   Unspecified juvenile rheumatoid arthritis, left hip

▣ M08.059   Unspecified juvenile rheumatoid arthritis, unspecified hip

ⓖ M08.06   Unspecified juvenile rheumatoid arthritis, knee

▣ M08.061   Unspecified juvenile rheumatoid arthritis, right knee

▣ M08.062   Unspecified juvenile rheumatoid arthritis, left knee

▣ M08.069   Unspecified juvenile rheumatoid arthritis, unspecified knee

ⓖ M08.07   Unspecified juvenile rheumatoid arthritis, ankle and foot

▣ M08.071   Unspecified juvenile rheumatoid arthritis, right ankle and foot

▣ M08.072   Unspecified juvenile rheumatoid arthritis, left ankle and foot

▣ M08.079   Unspecified juvenile rheumatoid arthritis, unspecified ankle and foot

M08.08   Unspecified juvenile rheumatoid arthritis, vertebrae

M08.09   Unspecified juvenile rheumatoid arthritis, multiple sites

M08.1   Juvenile ankylosing spondylitis
    EXCLUDES 1   *ankylosing spondylitis in adults (M45.0-)*

Ⓢ M08.2   Juvenile rheumatoid arthritis with systemic onset
    Still's disease NOS
    EXCLUDES 1   *adult-onset Still's disease (M06.1-)*

M08.20   Juvenile rheumatoid arthritis with systemic onset, unspecified site

ⓖ M08.21   Juvenile rheumatoid arthritis with systemic onset, shoulder

▣ M08.211   Juvenile rheumatoid arthritis with systemic onset, right shoulder

▣ M08.212   Juvenile rheumatoid arthritis with systemic onset, left shoulder

▣ M08.219   Juvenile rheumatoid arthritis with systemic onset, unspecified shoulder

ⓖ M08.22   Juvenile rheumatoid arthritis with systemic onset, elbow

▣ M08.221   Juvenile rheumatoid arthritis with systemic onset, right elbow

▣ M08.222   Juvenile rheumatoid arthritis with systemic onset, left elbow

▣ M08.229   Juvenile rheumatoid arthritis with systemic onset, unspecified elbow

ⓖ M08.23   Juvenile rheumatoid arthritis with systemic onset, wrist

▣ M08.231   Juvenile rheumatoid arthritis with systemic onset, right wrist

▣ M08.232   Juvenile rheumatoid arthritis with systemic onset, left wrist

▣ M08.239   Juvenile rheumatoid arthritis with systemic onset, unspecified wrist

ⓖ M08.24   Juvenile rheumatoid arthritis with systemic onset, hand

▣ M08.241   Juvenile rheumatoid arthritis with systemic onset, right hand

▣ M08.242   Juvenile rheumatoid arthritis with systemic onset, left hand

▣ M08.249   Juvenile rheumatoid arthritis with systemic onset, unspecified hand

ⓖ M08.25   Juvenile rheumatoid arthritis with systemic onset, hip

▣ M08.251   Juvenile rheumatoid arthritis with systemic onset, right hip

▣ M08.252   Juvenile rheumatoid arthritis with systemic onset, left hip

▣ M08.259   Juvenile rheumatoid arthritis with systemic onset, unspecified hip

ⓖ M08.26   Juvenile rheumatoid arthritis with systemic onset, knee

▣ M08.261   Juvenile rheumatoid arthritis with systemic onset, right knee

▣ M08.262   Juvenile rheumatoid arthritis with systemic onset, left knee

▣ M08.269   Juvenile rheumatoid arthritis with systemic onset, unspecified knee

ⓖ M08.27   Juvenile rheumatoid arthritis with systemic onset, ankle and foot

▣ M08.271   Juvenile rheumatoid arthritis with systemic onset, right ankle and foot

▣ M08.272   Juvenile rheumatoid arthritis with systemic onset, left ankle and foot

▣ M08.279   Juvenile rheumatoid arthritis with systemic onset, unspecified ankle and foot

M08.28   Juvenile rheumatoid arthritis with systemic onset, vertebrae

M08.29   Juvenile rheumatoid arthritis with systemic onset, multiple sites

M08.3   Juvenile rheumatoid polyarthritis (seronegative)

Ⓢ M08.4   Pauciarticular juvenile rheumatoid arthritis

M08.40   Pauciarticular juvenile rheumatoid arthritis, unspecified site

ⓖ M08.41   Pauciarticular juvenile rheumatoid arthritis, shoulder

▣ M08.411   Pauciarticular juvenile rheumatoid arthritis, right shoulder

▣ M08.412   Pauciarticular juvenile rheumatoid arthritis, left shoulder

▣ M08.419   Pauciarticular juvenile rheumatoid arthritis, unspecified shoulder

ⓖ M08.42   Pauciarticular juvenile rheumatoid arthritis, elbow

▣ M08.421   Pauciarticular juvenile rheumatoid arthritis, right elbow

▣ M08.422   Pauciarticular juvenile rheumatoid arthritis, left elbow

▣ M08.429   Pauciarticular juvenile rheumatoid arthritis, unspecified elbow

ⓖ M08.43   Pauciarticular juvenile rheumatoid arthritis, wrist

▣ M08.431   Pauciarticular juvenile rheumatoid arthritis, right wrist

▣ M08.432   Pauciarticular juvenile rheumatoid arthritis, left wrist

▣ M08.439   Pauciarticular juvenile rheumatoid arthritis, unspecified wrist

ⓖ M08.44   Pauciarticular juvenile rheumatoid arthritis, hand

▣ M08.441   Pauciarticular juvenile rheumatoid arthritis, right hand

▣ M08.442   Pauciarticular juvenile rheumatoid arthritis, left hand

▣ M08.449   Pauciarticular juvenile rheumatoid arthritis, unspecified hand

ⓖ M08.45   Pauciarticular juvenile rheumatoid arthritis, hip

▣ M08.451   Pauciarticular juvenile rheumatoid arthritis, right hip

▣ M08.452   Pauciarticular juvenile rheumatoid arthritis, left hip

▣ M08.459   Pauciarticular juvenile rheumatoid arthritis, unspecified hip

ⓖ M08.46   Pauciarticular juvenile rheumatoid arthritis, knee

▣ M08.461   Pauciarticular juvenile rheumatoid arthritis, right knee

▣ M08.462   Pauciarticular juvenile rheumatoid arthritis, left knee

▣ M08.469   Pauciarticular juvenile rheumatoid arthritis, unspecified knee

ⓖ M08.47   Pauciarticular juvenile rheumatoid arthritis, ankle and foot

▣ M08.471   Pauciarticular juvenile rheumatoid arthritis, right ankle and foot

▣ M08.472   Pauciarticular juvenile rheumatoid arthritis, left ankle and foot

---

● New   ▲ Revised   *Manifestation*   ❹-❼ Digit Indicators   ▣ Laterality   Ⓐ Adult (15+ years)   Ⓜ Maternity (12-55 years)   Ⓝ Newborn   Ⓟ Pediatric (0-17 years)   ♂ Male   ♀ Female
✖ Deleted   Unspecified   + Additional code

⊟ **M08.479** **Pauciarticular juvenile rheumatoid arthritis, unspecified ankle and foot**

M08.48 **Pauciarticular juvenile rheumatoid arthritis, vertebrae**

5 **M08.8** **Other juvenile arthritis**

M08.80 **Other juvenile arthritis, unspecified site**

6 **M08.81** **Other juvenile arthritis, shoulder**

⊟ **M08.811** **Other juvenile arthritis, right shoulder**

⊟ **M08.812** **Other juvenile arthritis, left shoulder**

⊟ **M08.819** **Other juvenile arthritis, unspecified shoulder**

6 **M08.82** **Other juvenile arthritis, elbow**

⊟ **M08.821** **Other juvenile arthritis, right elbow**

⊟ **M08.822** **Other juvenile arthritis, left elbow**

⊟ **M08.829** **Other juvenile arthritis, unspecified elbow**

6 **M08.83** **Other juvenile arthritis, wrist**

⊟ **M08.831** **Other juvenile arthritis, right wrist**

⊟ **M08.832** **Other juvenile arthritis, left wrist**

⊟ **M08.839** **Other juvenile arthritis, unspecified wrist**

6 **M08.84** **Other juvenile arthritis, hand**

⊟ **M08.841** **Other juvenile arthritis, right hand**

⊟ **M08.842** **Other juvenile arthritis, left hand**

⊟ **M08.849** **Other juvenile arthritis, unspecified hand**

6 **M08.85** **Other juvenile arthritis, hip**

⊟ **M08.851** **Other juvenile arthritis, right hip**

⊟ **M08.852** **Other juvenile arthritis, left hip**

⊟ **M08.859** **Other juvenile arthritis, unspecified hip**

6 **M08.86** **Other juvenile arthritis, knee**

⊟ **M08.861** **Other juvenile arthritis, right knee**

⊟ **M08.862** **Other juvenile arthritis, left knee**

⊟ **M08.869** **Other juvenile arthritis, unspecified knee**

6 **M08.87** **Other juvenile arthritis, ankle and foot**

⊟ **M08.871** **Other juvenile arthritis, right ankle and foot**

⊟ **M08.872** **Other juvenile arthritis, left ankle and foot**

⊟ **M08.879** **Other juvenile arthritis, unspecified ankle and foot**

M08.88 **Other juvenile arthritis, other specified site**
Other juvenile arthritis, vertebrae

M08.89 **Other juvenile arthritis, multiple sites**

5 **M08.9** **Juvenile arthritis, unspecified**

> **EXCLUDES 1** *juvenile rheumatoid arthritis, unspecified (M08.0-)*

M08.90 **Juvenile arthritis, unspecified, unspecified site**

6 **M08.91** **Juvenile arthritis, unspecified, shoulder**

⊟ **M08.911** **Juvenile arthritis, unspecified, right shoulder**

⊟ **M08.912** **Juvenile arthritis, unspecified, left shoulder**

⊟ **M08.919** **Juvenile arthritis, unspecified, unspecified shoulder**

6 **M08.92** **Juvenile arthritis, unspecified, elbow**

⊟ **M08.921** **Juvenile arthritis, unspecified, right elbow**

⊟ **M08.922** **Juvenile arthritis, unspecified, left elbow**

⊟ **M08.929** **Juvenile arthritis, unspecified, unspecified elbow**

6 **M08.93** **Juvenile arthritis, unspecified, wrist**

⊟ **M08.931** **Juvenile arthritis, unspecified, right wrist**

⊟ **M08.932** **Juvenile arthritis, unspecified, left wrist**

⊟ **M08.939** **Juvenile arthritis, unspecified, unspecified wrist**

6 **M08.94** **Juvenile arthritis, unspecified, hand**

⊟ **M08.941** **Juvenile arthritis, unspecified, right hand**

⊟ **M08.942** **Juvenile arthritis, unspecified, left hand**

⊟ **M08.949** **Juvenile arthritis, unspecified, unspecified hand**

6 **M08.95** **Juvenile arthritis, unspecified, hip**

⊟ **M08.951** **Juvenile arthritis, unspecified, right hip**

⊟ **M08.952** **Juvenile arthritis, unspecified, left hip**

⊟ **M08.959** **Juvenile arthritis, unspecified, unspecified hip**

6 **M08.96** **Juvenile arthritis, unspecified, knee**

⊟ **M08.961** **Juvenile arthritis, unspecified, right knee**

⊟ **M08.962** **Juvenile arthritis, unspecified, left knee**

⊟ **M08.969** **Juvenile arthritis, unspecified, unspecified knee**

6 **M08.97** **Juvenile arthritis, unspecified, ankle and foot**

⊟ **M08.971** **Juvenile arthritis, unspecified, right ankle and foot**

⊟ **M08.972** **Juvenile arthritis, unspecified, left ankle and foot**

⊟ **M08.979** **Juvenile arthritis, unspecified, unspecified ankle and foot**

M08.98 **Juvenile arthritis, unspecified, vertebrae**

M08.99 **Juvenile arthritis, unspecified, multiple sites**

▲ 4 + **M1A** **Chronic gout**

Use additional code to identify:
Autonomic neuropathy in diseases classified elsewhere (G99.0)
Calculus of urinary tract in diseases classified elsewhere (N22)
Cardiomyopathy in diseases classified elsewhere (I43)
Disorders of external ear in diseases classified elsewhere (H61.1-, H62.8-)
Disorders of iris and ciliary body in diseases classified elsewhere (H22)
Glomerular disorders in diseases classified elsewhere (N08)

> **EXCLUDES 1** *gout NOS (M10.-)*

> **EXCLUDES 2** *acute gout (M10.-)*

The appropriate 7th character is to be added to each code from category M1A
0   without tophus (tophi)
1   with tophus (tophi)

> **CODING TIP ✓** Do not assign a code from category M1A.- unless the physician has specifically provided a diagnosis of "chronic" gout or there is documentation of the presence of tophi.

5 + **M1A.0** **Idiopathic chronic gout**
Chronic gouty bursitis
Primary chronic gout

7 + **M1A.00X-** **Idiopathic chronic gout, unspecified site**

6 + **M1A.01** **Idiopathic chronic gout, shoulder**

7 ⊟ + **M1A.011-** **Idiopathic chronic gout, right shoulder**

7 ⊟ + **M1A.012-** **Idiopathic chronic gout, left shoulder**

7 ⊟ + **M1A.019-** **Idiopathic chronic gout, unspecified shoulder**

6 + **M1A.02** **Idiopathic chronic gout, elbow**

7 ⊟ + **M1A.021-** **Idiopathic chronic gout, right elbow**

7 ⊟ + **M1A.022-** **Idiopathic chronic gout, left elbow**

7 ⊟ + **M1A.029-** **Idiopathic chronic gout, unspecified elbow**

6 + **M1A.03** **Idiopathic chronic gout, wrist**

7 ⊟ + **M1A.031-** **Idiopathic chronic gout, right wrist**

7 ⊟ + **M1A.032-** **Idiopathic chronic gout, left wrist**

7 ⊟ + **M1A.039-** **Idiopathic chronic gout, unspecified wrist**

6 + **M1A.04** **Idiopathic chronic gout, hand**

7 ⊟ + **M1A.041-** **Idiopathic chronic gout, right hand**

7 ⊟ + **M1A.042-** **Idiopathic chronic gout, left hand**

7 ⊟ + **M1A.049-** **Idiopathic chronic gout, unspecified hand**

6 + **M1A.05** **Idiopathic chronic gout, hip**

7 ⊟ + **M1A.051-** **Idiopathic chronic gout, right hip**

7 ⊟ + **M1A.052-** **Idiopathic chronic gout, left hip**

7 ⊟ + **M1A.059-** **Idiopathic chronic gout, unspecified hip**

6 + **M1A.06** **Idiopathic chronic gout, knee**

7 ⊟ + **M1A.061-** **Idiopathic chronic gout, right knee**

7 ⊟ + **M1A.062-** **Idiopathic chronic gout, left knee**

7 ⊟ + **M1A.069-** **Idiopathic chronic gout, unspecified knee**

● New   ▲ Revised   *Manifestation*   4 - 7 Digit Indicators   ⊟ Laterality   A Adult (15+ years)   M Maternity (12-55 years)   N Newborn   P Pediatric (0-17 years)   ♂ Male   ♀ Female
✖ Deleted   Unspecified   + Additional code

6 + M1A.07   Idiopathic chronic gout, ankle and foot

Idiopathic chronic gout, ankle and foot

Inflammation of one or more joints due to gout

Uric acid crystals in big toe joint

Inflammation

7 ⊟ + M1A.071-   Idiopathic chronic gout, right ankle and foot

7 ⊟ + M1A.072-   Idiopathic chronic gout, left ankle and foot

7 ⊟ + M1A.079-   Idiopathic chronic gout, unspecified ankle and foot

7 + M1A.08X-   Idiopathic chronic gout, vertebrae

7 + M1A.09X-   Idiopathic chronic gout, multiple sites

5 + M1A.1   Lead-induced chronic gout
   Code first:
      toxic effects of lead and its compounds (T56.0-)

7 + M1A.10X-   Lead-induced chronic gout, unspecified site

6 + M1A.11   Lead-induced chronic gout, shoulder

7 ⊟ + M1A.111-   Lead-induced chronic gout, right shoulder

7 ⊟ + M1A.112-   Lead-induced chronic gout, left shoulder

7 ⊟ + M1A.119-   Lead-induced chronic gout, unspecified shoulder

6 + M1A.12   Lead-induced chronic gout, elbow

7 ⊟ + M1A.121-   Lead-induced chronic gout, right elbow

7 ⊟ + M1A.122-   Lead-induced chronic gout, left elbow

7 ⊟ + M1A.129-   Lead-induced chronic gout, unspecified elbow

6 + M1A.13   Lead-induced chronic gout, wrist

7 ⊟ + M1A.131-   Lead-induced chronic gout, right wrist

7 ⊟ + M1A.132-   Lead-induced chronic gout, left wrist

7 ⊟ + M1A.139-   Lead-induced chronic gout, unspecified wrist

6 + M1A.14   Lead-induced chronic gout, hand

7 ⊟ + M1A.141-   Lead-induced chronic gout, right hand

7 ⊟ + M1A.142-   Lead-induced chronic gout, left hand

7 ⊟ + M1A.149-   Lead-induced chronic gout, unspecified hand

6 + M1A.15   Lead-induced chronic gout, hip

7 ⊟ + M1A.151-   Lead-induced chronic gout, right hip

7 ⊟ + M1A.152-   Lead-induced chronic gout, left hip

7 ⊟ + M1A.159-   Lead-induced chronic gout, unspecified hip

6 + M1A.16   Lead-induced chronic gout, knee

7 ⊟ + M1A.161-   Lead-induced chronic gout, right knee

7 ⊟ + M1A.162-   Lead-induced chronic gout, left knee

7 ⊟ + M1A.169-   Lead-induced chronic gout, unspecified knee

6 + M1A.17   Lead-induced chronic gout, ankle and foot

7 ⊟ + M1A.171-   Lead-induced chronic gout, right ankle and foot

7 ⊟ + M1A.172-   Lead-induced chronic gout, left ankle and foot

7 ⊟ + M1A.179-   Lead-induced chronic gout, unspecified ankle and foot

7 + M1A.18X-   Lead-induced chronic gout, vertebrae

7 + M1A.19X-   Lead-induced chronic gout, multiple sites

5 + M1A.2   Drug-induced chronic gout
   Use additional code for adverse effect, if applicable, to identify drug (T36-T50 with fifth or sixth character 5)

7 + M1A.20X-   Drug-induced chronic gout, unspecified site

6 + M1A.21   Drug-induced chronic gout, shoulder

7 ⊟ + M1A.211-   Drug-induced chronic gout, right shoulder

7 ⊟ + M1A.212-   Drug-induced chronic gout, left shoulder

7 ⊟ + M1A.219-   Drug-induced chronic gout, unspecified shoulder

6 + M1A.22   Drug-induced chronic gout, elbow

7 ⊟ + M1A.221-   Drug-induced chronic gout, right elbow

7 ⊟ + M1A.222-   Drug-induced chronic gout, left elbow

7 ⊟ + M1A.229-   Drug-induced chronic gout, unspecified elbow

6 + M1A.23   Drug-induced chronic gout, wrist

7 ⊟ + M1A.231-   Drug-induced chronic gout, right wrist

7 ⊟ + M1A.232-   Drug-induced chronic gout, left wrist

7 ⊟ + M1A.239-   Drug-induced chronic gout, unspecified wrist

6 + M1A.24   Drug-induced chronic gout, hand

7 ⊟ + M1A.241-   Drug-induced chronic gout, right hand

7 ⊟ + M1A.242-   Drug-induced chronic gout, left hand

7 ⊟ + M1A.249-   Drug-induced chronic gout, unspecified hand

6 + M1A.25   Drug-induced chronic gout, hip

7 ⊟ + M1A.251-   Drug-induced chronic gout, right hip

7 ⊟ + M1A.252-   Drug-induced chronic gout, left hip

7 ⊟ + M1A.259-   Drug-induced chronic gout, unspecified hip

6 + M1A.26   Drug-induced chronic gout, knee

7 ⊟ + M1A.261-   Drug-induced chronic gout, right knee

7 ⊟ + M1A.262-   Drug-induced chronic gout, left knee

7 ⊟ + M1A.269-   Drug-induced chronic gout, unspecified knee

6 + M1A.27   Drug-induced chronic gout, ankle and foot

7 ⊟ + M1A.271-   Drug-induced chronic gout, right ankle and foot

7 ⊟ + M1A.272-   Drug-induced chronic gout, left ankle and foot

7 ⊟ + M1A.279-   Drug-induced chronic gout, unspecified ankle and foot

7 + M1A.28X-   Drug-induced chronic gout, vertebrae

7 + M1A.29X-   Drug-induced chronic gout, multiple sites

5 + M1A.3   Chronic gout due to renal impairment
   Code first:
      associated renal disease

7 + M1A.30X-   Chronic gout due to renal impairment, unspecified site

6 + M1A.31   Chronic gout due to renal impairment, shoulder

7 ⊟ + M1A.311-   Chronic gout due to renal impairment, right shoulder

7 ⊟ + M1A.312-   Chronic gout due to renal impairment, left shoulder

7 ⊟ + M1A.319-   Chronic gout due to renal impairment, unspecified shoulder

6 + M1A.32   Chronic gout due to renal impairment, elbow

7 ⊟ + M1A.321-   Chronic gout due to renal impairment, right elbow

7 ⊟ + M1A.322-   Chronic gout due to renal impairment, left elbow

7 ⊟ + M1A.329-   Chronic gout due to renal impairment, unspecified elbow

6 + M1A.33   Chronic gout due to renal impairment, wrist

7 ⊟ + M1A.331-   Chronic gout due to renal impairment, right wrist

7 ⊟ + M1A.332-   Chronic gout due to renal impairment, left wrist

7 ⊟ + M1A.339-   Chronic gout due to renal impairment, unspecified wrist

6 + M1A.34   Chronic gout due to renal impairment, hand

7 ⊟ + M1A.341-   Chronic gout due to renal impairment, right hand

7 ⊟ + M1A.342-   Chronic gout due to renal impairment, left hand

7 ⊟ + M1A.349-   Chronic gout due to renal impairment, unspecified hand

6 + M1A.35   Chronic gout due to renal impairment, hip

7 ⊟ + M1A.351-   Chronic gout due to renal impairment, right hip

7 ⊟ + M1A.352-   Chronic gout due to renal impairment, left hip

7 ⊟ + M1A.359-   Chronic gout due to renal impairment, unspecified hip

6 + M1A.36   Chronic gout due to renal impairment, knee

7 ⊟ + M1A.361-   Chronic gout due to renal impairment, right knee

7 ⊟ + M1A.362-   Chronic gout due to renal impairment, left knee

7 ⊟ + M1A.369-   Chronic gout due to renal impairment, unspecified knee

6 + M1A.37   Chronic gout due to renal impairment, ankle and foot

7 ⊟ + M1A.371-   Chronic gout due to renal impairment, right ankle and foot

7 ⊟ + M1A.372-   Chronic gout due to renal impairment, left ankle and foot

---

● New   ▲ Revised   *Manifestation*   4-7 Digit Indicators   ⊟ Laterality   Ⓐ Adult (15+ years)   Ⓜ Maternity (12-55 years)   Ⓝ Newborn   Ⓟ Pediatric (0-17 years)   ♂ Male   ♀ Female

✖ Deleted   Unspecified   + Additional code

7 ⊟ + **M1A.379-** Chronic gout due to renal impairment, unspecified ankle and foot

7 + **M1A.38X-** Chronic gout due to renal impairment, vertebrae

7 + **M1A.39X-** Chronic gout due to renal impairment, multiple sites

5 + **M1A.4** Other secondary chronic gout
Code first:
associated condition

7 + **M1A.40X-** Other secondary chronic gout, unspecified site

6 + **M1A.41** Other secondary chronic gout, shoulder

7 ⊟ + **M1A.411-** Other secondary chronic gout, right shoulder

7 ⊟ + **M1A.412-** Other secondary chronic gout, left shoulder

7 ⊟ + **M1A.419-** Other secondary chronic gout, unspecified shoulder

6 + **M1A.42** Other secondary chronic gout, elbow

7 ⊟ + **M1A.421-** Other secondary chronic gout, right elbow

7 ⊟ + **M1A.422-** Other secondary chronic gout, left elbow

7 ⊟ + **M1A.429-** Other secondary chronic gout, unspecified elbow

6 + **M1A.43** Other secondary chronic gout, wrist

7 ⊟ + **M1A.431-** Other secondary chronic gout, right wrist

7 ⊟ + **M1A.432-** Other secondary chronic gout, left wrist

7 ⊟ + **M1A.439-** Other secondary chronic gout, unspecified wrist

6 + **M1A.44** Other secondary chronic gout, hand

7 ⊟ + **M1A.441-** Other secondary chronic gout, right hand

7 ⊟ + **M1A.442-** Other secondary chronic gout, left hand

7 ⊟ + **M1A.449-** Other secondary chronic gout, unspecified hand

6 + **M1A.45** Other secondary chronic gout, hip

7 ⊟ + **M1A.451-** Other secondary chronic gout, right hip

7 ⊟ + **M1A.452-** Other secondary chronic gout, left hip

7 ⊟ + **M1A.459-** Other secondary chronic gout, unspecified hip

6 + **M1A.46** Other secondary chronic gout, knee

7 ⊟ + **M1A.461-** Other secondary chronic gout, right knee

7 ⊟ + **M1A.462-** Other secondary chronic gout, left knee

7 ⊟ + **M1A.469-** Other secondary chronic gout, unspecified knee

6 + **M1A.47** Other secondary chronic gout, ankle and foot

7 ⊟ + **M1A.471-** Other secondary chronic gout, right ankle and foot

7 ⊟ + **M1A.472-** Other secondary chronic gout, left ankle and foot

7 ⊟ + **M1A.479-** Other secondary chronic gout, unspecified ankle and foot

7 + **M1A.48X-** Other secondary chronic gout, vertebrae

7 + **M1A.49X-** Other secondary chronic gout, multiple sites

7 + **M1A.9XX-** Chronic gout, unspecified

▲ 4 + **M10** **Gout**
Acute gout
Gout attack
Gout flare
Podagra
Use additional code to identify:
Autonomic neuropathy in diseases classified elsewhere (G99.0)
Calculus of urinary tract in diseases classified elsewhere (N22)
Cardiomyopathy in diseases classified elsewhere (I43)
Disorders of external ear in diseases classified elsewhere (H61.1-, H62.8-)
Disorders of iris and ciliary body in diseases classified elsewhere (H22)
Glomerular disorders in diseases classified elsewhere (N08)
EXCLUDES 2 *chronic gout (M1A.-)*

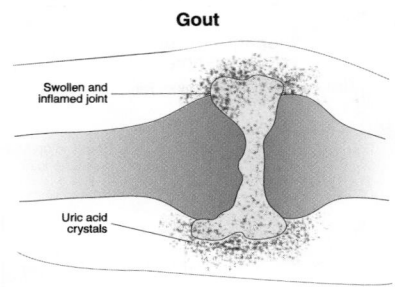

Gout

Swollen and inflamed joint

Uric acid crystals

5 + **M10.0** **Idiopathic gout**
Gouty bursitis
Primary gout

+ **M10.00** Idiopathic gout, unspecified site

6 + **M10.01** Idiopathic gout, shoulder

⊟ + **M10.011** Idiopathic gout, right shoulder

⊟ + **M10.012** Idiopathic gout, left shoulder

⊟ + **M10.019** Idiopathic gout, unspecified shoulder

6 + **M10.02** Idiopathic gout, elbow

⊟ + **M10.021** Idiopathic gout, right elbow

⊟ + **M10.022** Idiopathic gout, left elbow

⊟ + **M10.029** Idiopathic gout, unspecified elbow

6 + **M10.03** Idiopathic gout, wrist

⊟ + **M10.031** Idiopathic gout, right wrist

⊟ + **M10.032** Idiopathic gout, left wrist

⊟ + **M10.039** Idiopathic gout, unspecified wrist

6 + **M10.04** Idiopathic gout, hand

⊟ + **M10.041** Idiopathic gout, right hand

⊟ + **M10.042** Idiopathic gout, left hand

⊟ + **M10.049** Idiopathic gout, unspecified hand

6 + **M10.05** Idiopathic gout, hip

⊟ + **M10.051** Idiopathic gout, right hip

⊟ + **M10.052** Idiopathic gout, left hip

⊟ + **M10.059** Idiopathic gout, unspecified hip

6 + **M10.06** Idiopathic gout, knee

⊟ + **M10.061** Idiopathic gout, right knee

⊟ + **M10.062** Idiopathic gout, left knee

⊟ + **M10.069** Idiopathic gout, unspecified knee

6 + **M10.07** Idiopathic gout, ankle and foot

⊟ + **M10.071** Idiopathic gout, right ankle and foot

⊟ + **M10.072** Idiopathic gout, left ankle and foot

⊟ + **M10.079** Idiopathic gout, unspecified ankle and foot

+ **M10.08** Idiopathic gout, vertebrae

+ **M10.09** Idiopathic gout, multiple sites

5 + **M10.1** **Lead-induced gout**
Code first:
toxic effects of lead and its compounds (T56.0-)

+ **M10.10** Lead-induced gout, unspecified site

6 + **M10.11** Lead-induced gout, shoulder

⊟ + **M10.111** Lead-induced gout, right shoulder

⊟ + **M10.112** Lead-induced gout, left shoulder

⊟ + **M10.119** Lead-induced gout, unspecified shoulder

6 + **M10.12** Lead-induced gout, elbow

⊟ + **M10.121** Lead-induced gout, right elbow

⊟ + **M10.122** Lead-induced gout, left elbow

⊟ + **M10.129** Lead-induced gout, unspecified elbow

6 + **M10.13** Lead-induced gout, wrist

⊟ + **M10.131** Lead-induced gout, right wrist

⊟ + **M10.132** Lead-induced gout, left wrist

⊟ + **M10.139** Lead-induced gout, unspecified wrist

6 + **M10.14** Lead-induced gout, hand

⊟ + **M10.141** Lead-induced gout, right hand

⊟ + **M10.142** Lead-induced gout, left hand

● New　▲ Revised　*Manifestation*　4 - 7 Digit Indicators　⊟ Laterality　Ⓐ Adult (15+ years)　Ⓜ Maternity (12-55 years)　Ⓝ Newborn　Ⓟ Pediatric (0-17 years)　♂ Male　♀ Female
✖ Deleted　Unspecified　+ Additional code

750　© 2017 DecisionHealth　 　2017 ICD-10-CM Expert for Physicians

⑥＋ **M10.149** Lead-induced gout, unspecified hand
⑥＋ **M10.15** Lead-induced gout, hip
　☐＋ **M10.151** Lead-induced gout, right hip
　☐＋ **M10.152** Lead-induced gout, left hip
　☐＋ **M10.159** Lead-induced gout, unspecified hip
⑥＋ **M10.16** Lead-induced gout, knee
　☐＋ **M10.161** Lead-induced gout, right knee
　☐＋ **M10.162** Lead-induced gout, left knee
　☐＋ **M10.169** Lead-induced gout, unspecified knee
⑥＋ **M10.17** Lead-induced gout, ankle and foot
　☐＋ **M10.171** Lead-induced gout, right ankle and foot
　☐＋ **M10.172** Lead-induced gout, left ankle and foot
　☐＋ **M10.179** Lead-induced gout, unspecified ankle and foot
＋ **M10.18** Lead-induced gout, vertebrae
＋ **M10.19** Lead-induced gout, multiple sites
⑤＋ **M10.2** Drug-induced gout
　Use additional code for adverse effect, if applicable, to identify drug (T36-T50 with fifth or sixth character 5)
＋ **M10.20** Drug-induced gout, unspecified site
⑥＋ **M10.21** Drug-induced gout, shoulder
　☐＋ **M10.211** Drug-induced gout, right shoulder
　☐＋ **M10.212** Drug-induced gout, left shoulder
　☐＋ **M10.219** Drug-induced gout, unspecified shoulder
⑥＋ **M10.22** Drug-induced gout, elbow
　☐＋ **M10.221** Drug-induced gout, right elbow
　☐＋ **M10.222** Drug-induced gout, left elbow
　☐＋ **M10.229** Drug-induced gout, unspecified elbow
⑥＋ **M10.23** Drug-induced gout, wrist
　☐＋ **M10.231** Drug-induced gout, right wrist
　☐＋ **M10.232** Drug-induced gout, left wrist
　☐＋ **M10.239** Drug-induced gout, unspecified wrist
⑥＋ **M10.24** Drug-induced gout, hand
　☐＋ **M10.241** Drug-induced gout, right hand
　☐＋ **M10.242** Drug-induced gout, left hand
　☐＋ **M10.249** Drug-induced gout, unspecified hand
⑥＋ **M10.25** Drug-induced gout, hip
　☐＋ **M10.251** Drug-induced gout, right hip
　☐＋ **M10.252** Drug-induced gout, left hip
　☐＋ **M10.259** Drug-induced gout, unspecified hip
⑥＋ **M10.26** Drug-induced gout, knee
　☐＋ **M10.261** Drug-induced gout, right knee
　☐＋ **M10.262** Drug-induced gout, left knee
　☐＋ **M10.269** Drug-induced gout, unspecified knee
⑥＋ **M10.27** Drug-induced gout, ankle and foot
　☐＋ **M10.271** Drug-induced gout, right ankle and foot
　☐＋ **M10.272** Drug-induced gout, left ankle and foot
　☐＋ **M10.279** Drug-induced gout, unspecified ankle and foot
＋ **M10.28** Drug-induced gout, vertebrae
＋ **M10.29** Drug-induced gout, multiple sites
⑤＋ **M10.3** Gout due to renal impairment
　Code first:
　　associated renal disease
＋ **M10.30** Gout due to renal impairment, unspecified site
⑥＋ **M10.31** Gout due to renal impairment, shoulder
　☐＋ **M10.311** Gout due to renal impairment, right shoulder
　☐＋ **M10.312** Gout due to renal impairment, left shoulder
　☐＋ **M10.319** Gout due to renal impairment, unspecified shoulder
⑥＋ **M10.32** Gout due to renal impairment, elbow
　☐＋ **M10.321** Gout due to renal impairment, right elbow
　☐＋ **M10.322** Gout due to renal impairment, left elbow
　☐＋ **M10.329** Gout due to renal impairment, unspecified elbow
⑥＋ **M10.33** Gout due to renal impairment, wrist
　☐＋ **M10.331** Gout due to renal impairment, right wrist
　☐＋ **M10.332** Gout due to renal impairment, left wrist

☐＋ **M10.339** Gout due to renal impairment, unspecified wrist
⑥＋ **M10.34** Gout due to renal impairment, hand
　☐＋ **M10.341** Gout due to renal impairment, right hand
　☐＋ **M10.342** Gout due to renal impairment, left hand
　☐＋ **M10.349** Gout due to renal impairment, unspecified hand
⑥＋ **M10.35** Gout due to renal impairment, hip
　☐＋ **M10.351** Gout due to renal impairment, right hip
　☐＋ **M10.352** Gout due to renal impairment, left hip
　☐＋ **M10.359** Gout due to renal impairment, unspecified hip
⑥＋ **M10.36** Gout due to renal impairment, knee
　☐＋ **M10.361** Gout due to renal impairment, right knee
　☐＋ **M10.362** Gout due to renal impairment, left knee
　☐＋ **M10.369** Gout due to renal impairment, unspecified knee
⑥＋ **M10.37** Gout due to renal impairment, ankle and foot
　☐＋ **M10.371** Gout due to renal impairment, right ankle and foot
　☐＋ **M10.372** Gout due to renal impairment, left ankle and foot
　☐＋ **M10.379** Gout due to renal impairment, unspecified ankle and foot
＋ **M10.38** Gout due to renal impairment, vertebrae
＋ **M10.39** Gout due to renal impairment, multiple sites
⑤＋ **M10.4** Other secondary gout
　Code first:
　　associated condition
＋ **M10.40** Other secondary gout, unspecified site
⑥＋ **M10.41** Other secondary gout, shoulder
　☐＋ **M10.411** Other secondary gout, right shoulder
　☐＋ **M10.412** Other secondary gout, left shoulder
　☐＋ **M10.419** Other secondary gout, unspecified shoulder
⑥＋ **M10.42** Other secondary gout, elbow
　☐＋ **M10.421** Other secondary gout, right elbow
　☐＋ **M10.422** Other secondary gout, left elbow
　☐＋ **M10.429** Other secondary gout, unspecified elbow
⑥＋ **M10.43** Other secondary gout, wrist
　☐＋ **M10.431** Other secondary gout, right wrist
　☐＋ **M10.432** Other secondary gout, left wrist
　☐＋ **M10.439** Other secondary gout, unspecified wrist
⑥＋ **M10.44** Other secondary gout, hand
　☐＋ **M10.441** Other secondary gout, right hand
　☐＋ **M10.442** Other secondary gout, left hand
　☐＋ **M10.449** Other secondary gout, unspecified hand
⑥＋ **M10.45** Other secondary gout, hip
　☐＋ **M10.451** Other secondary gout, right hip
　☐＋ **M10.452** Other secondary gout, left hip
　☐＋ **M10.459** Other secondary gout, unspecified hip
⑥＋ **M10.46** Other secondary gout, knee
　☐＋ **M10.461** Other secondary gout, right knee
　☐＋ **M10.462** Other secondary gout, left knee
　☐＋ **M10.469** Other secondary gout, unspecified knee
⑥＋ **M10.47** Other secondary gout, ankle and foot
　☐＋ **M10.471** Other secondary gout, right ankle and foot
　☐＋ **M10.472** Other secondary gout, left ankle and foot
　☐＋ **M10.479** Other secondary gout, unspecified ankle and foot
＋ **M10.48** Other secondary gout, vertebrae
＋ **M10.49** Other secondary gout, multiple sites
＋ **M10.9** Gout, unspecified
　Gout NOS
④ **M11** Other crystal arthropathies
⑤ **M11.0** Hydroxyapatite deposition disease
　M11.00 Hydroxyapatite deposition disease, unspecified site
⑥ **M11.01** Hydroxyapatite deposition disease, shoulder
　☐ **M11.011** Hydroxyapatite deposition disease, right shoulder
　☐ **M11.012** Hydroxyapatite deposition disease, left shoulder

M11.019 Hydroxyapatite deposition disease, unspecified shoulder
M11.02 Hydroxyapatite deposition disease, elbow
M11.021 Hydroxyapatite deposition disease, right elbow
M11.022 Hydroxyapatite deposition disease, left elbow
M11.029 Hydroxyapatite deposition disease, unspecified elbow
M11.03 Hydroxyapatite deposition disease, wrist
M11.031 Hydroxyapatite deposition disease, right wrist
M11.032 Hydroxyapatite deposition disease, left wrist
M11.039 Hydroxyapatite deposition disease, unspecified wrist
M11.04 Hydroxyapatite deposition disease, hand
M11.041 Hydroxyapatite deposition disease, right hand
M11.042 Hydroxyapatite deposition disease, left hand
M11.049 Hydroxyapatite deposition disease, unspecified hand
M11.05 Hydroxyapatite deposition disease, hip
M11.051 Hydroxyapatite deposition disease, right hip
M11.052 Hydroxyapatite deposition disease, left hip
M11.059 Hydroxyapatite deposition disease, unspecified hip
M11.06 Hydroxyapatite deposition disease, knee
M11.061 Hydroxyapatite deposition disease, right knee
M11.062 Hydroxyapatite deposition disease, left knee
M11.069 Hydroxyapatite deposition disease, unspecified knee
M11.07 Hydroxyapatite deposition disease, ankle and foot
M11.071 Hydroxyapatite deposition disease, right ankle and foot
M11.072 Hydroxyapatite deposition disease, left ankle and foot
M11.079 Hydroxyapatite deposition disease, unspecified ankle and foot
M11.08 Hydroxyapatite deposition disease, vertebrae
M11.09 Hydroxyapatite deposition disease, multiple sites
M11.1 Familial chondrocalcinosis
M11.10 Familial chondrocalcinosis, unspecified site
M11.11 Familial chondrocalcinosis, shoulder
M11.111 Familial chondrocalcinosis, right shoulder
M11.112 Familial chondrocalcinosis, left shoulder
M11.119 Familial chondrocalcinosis, unspecified shoulder
M11.12 Familial chondrocalcinosis, elbow
M11.121 Familial chondrocalcinosis, right elbow
M11.122 Familial chondrocalcinosis, left elbow
M11.129 Familial chondrocalcinosis, unspecified elbow
M11.13 Familial chondrocalcinosis, wrist
M11.131 Familial chondrocalcinosis, right wrist
M11.132 Familial chondrocalcinosis, left wrist
M11.139 Familial chondrocalcinosis, unspecified wrist
M11.14 Familial chondrocalcinosis, hand
M11.141 Familial chondrocalcinosis, right hand
M11.142 Familial chondrocalcinosis, left hand
M11.149 Familial chondrocalcinosis, unspecified hand
M11.15 Familial chondrocalcinosis, hip
M11.151 Familial chondrocalcinosis, right hip
M11.152 Familial chondrocalcinosis, left hip
M11.159 Familial chondrocalcinosis, unspecified hip
M11.16 Familial chondrocalcinosis, knee
M11.161 Familial chondrocalcinosis, right knee
M11.162 Familial chondrocalcinosis, left knee
M11.169 Familial chondrocalcinosis, unspecified knee
M11.17 Familial chondrocalcinosis, ankle and foot
M11.171 Familial chondrocalcinosis, right ankle and foot
M11.172 Familial chondrocalcinosis, left ankle and foot
M11.179 Familial chondrocalcinosis, unspecified ankle and foot
M11.18 Familial chondrocalcinosis, vertebrae
M11.19 Familial chondrocalcinosis, multiple sites
M11.2 Other chondrocalcinosis
Chondrocalcinosis NOS

M11.20 Other chondrocalcinosis, unspecified site
M11.21 Other chondrocalcinosis, shoulder
M11.211 Other chondrocalcinosis, right shoulder
M11.212 Other chondrocalcinosis, left shoulder
M11.219 Other chondrocalcinosis, unspecified shoulder
M11.22 Other chondrocalcinosis, elbow
M11.221 Other chondrocalcinosis, right elbow
M11.222 Other chondrocalcinosis, left elbow
M11.229 Other chondrocalcinosis, unspecified elbow
M11.23 Other chondrocalcinosis, wrist
M11.231 Other chondrocalcinosis, right wrist
M11.232 Other chondrocalcinosis, left wrist
M11.239 Other chondrocalcinosis, unspecified wrist
M11.24 Other chondrocalcinosis, hand
M11.241 Other chondrocalcinosis, right hand
M11.242 Other chondrocalcinosis, left hand
M11.249 Other chondrocalcinosis, unspecified hand
M11.25 Other chondrocalcinosis, hip
M11.251 Other chondrocalcinosis, right hip
M11.252 Other chondrocalcinosis, left hip
M11.259 Other chondrocalcinosis, unspecified hip
M11.26 Other chondrocalcinosis, knee
M11.261 Other chondrocalcinosis, right knee
M11.262 Other chondrocalcinosis, left knee
M11.269 Other chondrocalcinosis, unspecified knee
M11.27 Other chondrocalcinosis, ankle and foot
M11.271 Other chondrocalcinosis, right ankle and foot
M11.272 Other chondrocalcinosis, left ankle and foot
M11.279 Other chondrocalcinosis, unspecified ankle and foot
M11.28 Other chondrocalcinosis, vertebrae
M11.29 Other chondrocalcinosis, multiple sites
M11.8 Other specified crystal arthropathies
M11.80 Other specified crystal arthropathies, unspecified site
M11.81 Other specified crystal arthropathies, shoulder
M11.811 Other specified crystal arthropathies, right shoulder
M11.812 Other specified crystal arthropathies, left shoulder
M11.819 Other specified crystal arthropathies, unspecified shoulder
M11.82 Other specified crystal arthropathies, elbow
M11.821 Other specified crystal arthropathies, right elbow
M11.822 Other specified crystal arthropathies, left elbow
M11.829 Other specified crystal arthropathies, unspecified elbow
M11.83 Other specified crystal arthropathies, wrist
M11.831 Other specified crystal arthropathies, right wrist
M11.832 Other specified crystal arthropathies, left wrist
M11.839 Other specified crystal arthropathies, unspecified wrist
M11.84 Other specified crystal arthropathies, hand
M11.841 Other specified crystal arthropathies, right hand
M11.842 Other specified crystal arthropathies, left hand
M11.849 Other specified crystal arthropathies, unspecified hand
M11.85 Other specified crystal arthropathies, hip
M11.851 Other specified crystal arthropathies, right hip
M11.852 Other specified crystal arthropathies, left hip
M11.859 Other specified crystal arthropathies, unspecified hip
M11.86 Other specified crystal arthropathies, knee
M11.861 Other specified crystal arthropathies, right knee
M11.862 Other specified crystal arthropathies, left knee
M11.869 Other specified crystal arthropathies, unspecified knee
M11.87 Other specified crystal arthropathies, ankle and foot
M11.871 Other specified crystal arthropathies, right ankle and foot
M11.872 Other specified crystal arthropathies, left ankle and foot

☐ M11.879 Other specified crystal arthropathies, unspecified ankle and foot
M11.88 Other specified crystal arthropathies, vertebrae
M11.89 Other specified crystal arthropathies, multiple sites
M11.9 Crystal arthropathy, unspecified

▣ M12 Other and unspecified arthropathy

EXCLUDES 1   *arthrosis (M15-M19)*
              cricoarytenoid arthropathy (J38.7)

⑤ M12.0 Chronic postrheumatic arthropathy [Jaccoud]
M12.00 Chronic postrheumatic arthropathy [Jaccoud], unspecified site
⑥ M12.01 Chronic postrheumatic arthropathy [Jaccoud], shoulder
  ☐ M12.011 Chronic postrheumatic arthropathy [Jaccoud], right shoulder
  ☐ M12.012 Chronic postrheumatic arthropathy [Jaccoud], left shoulder
  ☐ M12.019 Chronic postrheumatic arthropathy [Jaccoud], unspecified shoulder
⑥ M12.02 Chronic postrheumatic arthropathy [Jaccoud], elbow
  ☐ M12.021 Chronic postrheumatic arthropathy [Jaccoud], right elbow
  ☐ M12.022 Chronic postrheumatic arthropathy [Jaccoud], left elbow
  ☐ M12.029 Chronic postrheumatic arthropathy [Jaccoud], unspecified elbow
⑥ M12.03 Chronic postrheumatic arthropathy [Jaccoud], wrist
  ☐ M12.031 Chronic postrheumatic arthropathy [Jaccoud], right wrist
  ☐ M12.032 Chronic postrheumatic arthropathy [Jaccoud], left wrist
  ☐ M12.039 Chronic postrheumatic arthropathy [Jaccoud], unspecified wrist
⑥ M12.04 Chronic postrheumatic arthropathy [Jaccoud], hand
  ☐ M12.041 Chronic postrheumatic arthropathy [Jaccoud], right hand
  ☐ M12.042 Chronic postrheumatic arthropathy [Jaccoud], left hand
  ☐ M12.049 Chronic postrheumatic arthropathy [Jaccoud], unspecified hand
⑥ M12.05 Chronic postrheumatic arthropathy [Jaccoud], hip
  ☐ M12.051 Chronic postrheumatic arthropathy [Jaccoud], right hip
  ☐ M12.052 Chronic postrheumatic arthropathy [Jaccoud], left hip
  ☐ M12.059 Chronic postrheumatic arthropathy [Jaccoud], unspecified hip
⑥ M12.06 Chronic postrheumatic arthropathy [Jaccoud], knee
  ☐ M12.061 Chronic postrheumatic arthropathy [Jaccoud], right knee
  ☐ M12.062 Chronic postrheumatic arthropathy [Jaccoud], left knee
  ☐ M12.069 Chronic postrheumatic arthropathy [Jaccoud], unspecified knee
⑥ M12.07 Chronic postrheumatic arthropathy [Jaccoud], ankle and foot
  ☐ M12.071 Chronic postrheumatic arthropathy [Jaccoud], right ankle and foot
  ☐ M12.072 Chronic postrheumatic arthropathy [Jaccoud], left ankle and foot
  ☐ M12.079 Chronic postrheumatic arthropathy [Jaccoud], unspecified ankle and foot
M12.08 Chronic postrheumatic arthropathy [Jaccoud], other specified site
  Chronic postrheumatic arthropathy [Jaccoud], vertebrae
M12.09 Chronic postrheumatic arthropathy [Jaccoud], multiple sites
⑤ M12.1 Kaschin-Beck disease
  Osteochondroarthrosis deformans endemica
M12.10 Kaschin-Beck disease, unspecified site
⑥ M12.11 Kaschin-Beck disease, shoulder
  ☐ M12.111 Kaschin-Beck disease, right shoulder
  ☐ M12.112 Kaschin-Beck disease, left shoulder
  ☐ M12.119 Kaschin-Beck disease, unspecified shoulder
⑥ M12.12 Kaschin-Beck disease, elbow

  ☐ M12.121 Kaschin-Beck disease, right elbow
  ☐ M12.122 Kaschin-Beck disease, left elbow
  ☐ M12.129 Kaschin-Beck disease, unspecified elbow
⑥ M12.13 Kaschin-Beck disease, wrist
  ☐ M12.131 Kaschin-Beck disease, right wrist
  ☐ M12.132 Kaschin-Beck disease, left wrist
  ☐ M12.139 Kaschin-Beck disease, unspecified wrist
⑥ M12.14 Kaschin-Beck disease, hand
  ☐ M12.141 Kaschin-Beck disease, right hand
  ☐ M12.142 Kaschin-Beck disease, left hand
  ☐ M12.149 Kaschin-Beck disease, unspecified hand
⑥ M12.15 Kaschin-Beck disease, hip
  ☐ M12.151 Kaschin-Beck disease, right hip
  ☐ M12.152 Kaschin-Beck disease, left hip
  ☐ M12.159 Kaschin-Beck disease, unspecified hip
⑥ M12.16 Kaschin-Beck disease, knee
  ☐ M12.161 Kaschin-Beck disease, right knee
  ☐ M12.162 Kaschin-Beck disease, left knee
  ☐ M12.169 Kaschin-Beck disease, unspecified knee
⑥ M12.17 Kaschin-Beck disease, ankle and foot
  ☐ M12.171 Kaschin-Beck disease, right ankle and foot
  ☐ M12.172 Kaschin-Beck disease, left ankle and foot
  ☐ M12.179 Kaschin-Beck disease, unspecified ankle and foot
M12.18 Kaschin-Beck disease, vertebrae
M12.19 Kaschin-Beck disease, multiple sites
⑤ M12.2 Villonodular synovitis (pigmented)
M12.20 Villonodular synovitis (pigmented), unspecified site
⑥ M12.21 Villonodular synovitis (pigmented), shoulder
  ☐ M12.211 Villonodular synovitis (pigmented), right shoulder
  ☐ M12.212 Villonodular synovitis (pigmented), left shoulder
  ☐ M12.219 Villonodular synovitis (pigmented), unspecified shoulder
⑥ M12.22 Villonodular synovitis (pigmented), elbow
  ☐ M12.221 Villonodular synovitis (pigmented), right elbow
  ☐ M12.222 Villonodular synovitis (pigmented), left elbow
  ☐ M12.229 Villonodular synovitis (pigmented), unspecified elbow
⑥ M12.23 Villonodular synovitis (pigmented), wrist
  ☐ M12.231 Villonodular synovitis (pigmented), right wrist
  ☐ M12.232 Villonodular synovitis (pigmented), left wrist
  ☐ M12.239 Villonodular synovitis (pigmented), unspecified wrist
⑥ M12.24 Villonodular synovitis (pigmented), hand
  ☐ M12.241 Villonodular synovitis (pigmented), right hand
  ☐ M12.242 Villonodular synovitis (pigmented), left hand
  ☐ M12.249 Villonodular synovitis (pigmented), unspecified hand
⑥ M12.25 Villonodular synovitis (pigmented), hip
  ☐ M12.251 Villonodular synovitis (pigmented), right hip
  ☐ M12.252 Villonodular synovitis (pigmented), left hip
  ☐ M12.259 Villonodular synovitis (pigmented), unspecified hip
⑥ M12.26 Villonodular synovitis (pigmented), knee
  ☐ M12.261 Villonodular synovitis (pigmented), right knee
  ☐ M12.262 Villonodular synovitis (pigmented), left knee
  ☐ M12.269 Villonodular synovitis (pigmented), unspecified knee
⑥ M12.27 Villonodular synovitis (pigmented), ankle and foot
  ☐ M12.271 Villonodular synovitis (pigmented), right ankle and foot
  ☐ M12.272 Villonodular synovitis (pigmented), left ankle and foot
  ☐ M12.279 Villonodular synovitis (pigmented), unspecified ankle and foot
M12.28 Villonodular synovitis (pigmented), other specified site
  Villonodular synovitis (pigmented), vertebrae
M12.29 Villonodular synovitis (pigmented), multiple sites
⑤ M12.3 Palindromic rheumatism
M12.30 Palindromic rheumatism, unspecified site
⑥ M12.31 Palindromic rheumatism, shoulder
  ☐ M12.311 Palindromic rheumatism, right shoulder

● New   ▲ Revised   *Manifestation*   ④-⑦ Digit Indicators   ☐ Laterality   Ⓐ Adult (15+ years)   Ⓜ Maternity (12-55 years)   Ⓝ Newborn   Ⓟ Pediatric (0-17 years)   ♂ Male   ♀ Female
✖ Deleted   Unspecified   + Additional code

 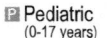

☐ M12.312   **Palindromic rheumatism, left shoulder**
☐ M12.319   **Palindromic rheumatism, unspecified shoulder**
Ⓖ M12.32   **Palindromic rheumatism, elbow**
☐ M12.321   **Palindromic rheumatism, right elbow**
☐ M12.322   **Palindromic rheumatism, left elbow**
☐ M12.329   **Palindromic rheumatism, unspecified elbow**
Ⓖ M12.33   **Palindromic rheumatism, wrist**
☐ M12.331   **Palindromic rheumatism, right wrist**
☐ M12.332   **Palindromic rheumatism, left wrist**
☐ M12.339   **Palindromic rheumatism, unspecified wrist**
Ⓖ M12.34   **Palindromic rheumatism, hand**
☐ M12.341   **Palindromic rheumatism, right hand**
☐ M12.342   **Palindromic rheumatism, left hand**
☐ M12.349   **Palindromic rheumatism, unspecified hand**
Ⓖ M12.35   **Palindromic rheumatism, hip**
☐ M12.351   **Palindromic rheumatism, right hip**
☐ M12.352   **Palindromic rheumatism, left hip**
☐ M12.359   **Palindromic rheumatism, unspecified hip**
Ⓖ M12.36   **Palindromic rheumatism, knee**
☐ M12.361   **Palindromic rheumatism, right knee**
☐ M12.362   **Palindromic rheumatism, left knee**
☐ M12.369   **Palindromic rheumatism, unspecified knee**
Ⓖ M12.37   **Palindromic rheumatism, ankle and foot**
☐ M12.371   **Palindromic rheumatism, right ankle and foot**
☐ M12.372   **Palindromic rheumatism, left ankle and foot**
☐ M12.379   **Palindromic rheumatism, unspecified ankle and foot**
M12.38   **Palindromic rheumatism, other specified site**
          Palindromic rheumatism, vertebrae
M12.39   **Palindromic rheumatism, multiple sites**
Ⓢ M12.4   **Intermittent hydrarthrosis**
M12.40   **Intermittent hydrarthrosis, unspecified site**
Ⓖ M12.41   **Intermittent hydrarthrosis, shoulder**
☐ M12.411   **Intermittent hydrarthrosis, right shoulder**
☐ M12.412   **Intermittent hydrarthrosis, left shoulder**
☐ M12.419   **Intermittent hydrarthrosis, unspecified shoulder**
Ⓖ M12.42   **Intermittent hydrarthrosis, elbow**
☐ M12.421   **Intermittent hydrarthrosis, right elbow**
☐ M12.422   **Intermittent hydrarthrosis, left elbow**
☐ M12.429   **Intermittent hydrarthrosis, unspecified elbow**
Ⓖ M12.43   **Intermittent hydrarthrosis, wrist**
☐ M12.431   **Intermittent hydrarthrosis, right wrist**
☐ M12.432   **Intermittent hydrarthrosis, left wrist**
☐ M12.439   **Intermittent hydrarthrosis, unspecified wrist**
Ⓖ M12.44   **Intermittent hydrarthrosis, hand**
☐ M12.441   **Intermittent hydrarthrosis, right hand**
☐ M12.442   **Intermittent hydrarthrosis, left hand**
☐ M12.449   **Intermittent hydrarthrosis, unspecified hand**
Ⓖ M12.45   **Intermittent hydrarthrosis, hip**
☐ M12.451   **Intermittent hydrarthrosis, right hip**
☐ M12.452   **Intermittent hydrarthrosis, left hip**
☐ M12.459   **Intermittent hydrarthrosis, unspecified hip**
Ⓖ M12.46   **Intermittent hydrarthrosis, knee**
☐ M12.461   **Intermittent hydrarthrosis, right knee**
☐ M12.462   **Intermittent hydrarthrosis, left knee**
☐ M12.469   **Intermittent hydrarthrosis, unspecified knee**
Ⓖ M12.47   **Intermittent hydrarthrosis, ankle and foot**
☐ M12.471   **Intermittent hydrarthrosis, right ankle and foot**
☐ M12.472   **Intermittent hydrarthrosis, left ankle and foot**
☐ M12.479   **Intermittent hydrarthrosis, unspecified ankle and foot**
M12.48   **Intermittent hydrarthrosis, other site**
M12.49   **Intermittent hydrarthrosis, multiple sites**

Ⓢ M12.5   **Traumatic arthropathy**
          EXCLUDES 1   *current injury-see Alphabetic Index*
                          post-traumatic osteoarthritis of first carpometacarpal joint (M18.2-M18.3)
                          post-traumatic osteoarthritis of hip (M16.4-M16.5)
                          post-traumatic osteoarthritis of knee (M17.2-M17.3)
                          post-traumatic osteoarthritis NOS (M19.1-)
                          post-traumatic osteoarthritis of other single joints (M19.1-)
M12.50   **Traumatic arthropathy, unspecified site**
Ⓖ M12.51   **Traumatic arthropathy, shoulder**
☐ M12.511   **Traumatic arthropathy, right shoulder**
☐ M12.512   **Traumatic arthropathy, left shoulder**
☐ M12.519   **Traumatic arthropathy, unspecified shoulder**
Ⓖ M12.52   **Traumatic arthropathy, elbow**
☐ M12.521   **Traumatic arthropathy, right elbow**
☐ M12.522   **Traumatic arthropathy, left elbow**
☐ M12.529   **Traumatic arthropathy, unspecified elbow**
Ⓖ M12.53   **Traumatic arthropathy, wrist**
☐ M12.531   **Traumatic arthropathy, right wrist**
☐ M12.532   **Traumatic arthropathy, left wrist**
☐ M12.539   **Traumatic arthropathy, unspecified wrist**
Ⓖ M12.54   **Traumatic arthropathy, hand**
☐ M12.541   **Traumatic arthropathy, right hand**
☐ M12.542   **Traumatic arthropathy, left hand**
☐ M12.549   **Traumatic arthropathy, unspecified hand**
Ⓖ M12.55   **Traumatic arthropathy, hip**
☐ M12.551   **Traumatic arthropathy, right hip**
☐ M12.552   **Traumatic arthropathy, left hip**
            AHA: 1Q 2015, 17
☐ M12.559   **Traumatic arthropathy, unspecified hip**
Ⓖ M12.56   **Traumatic arthropathy, knee**
☐ M12.561   **Traumatic arthropathy, right knee**
☐ M12.562   **Traumatic arthropathy, left knee**
☐ M12.569   **Traumatic arthropathy, unspecified knee**
Ⓖ M12.57   **Traumatic arthropathy, ankle and foot**
☐ M12.571   **Traumatic arthropathy, right ankle and foot**
☐ M12.572   **Traumatic arthropathy, left ankle and foot**
☐ M12.579   **Traumatic arthropathy, unspecified ankle and foot**
M12.58   **Traumatic arthropathy, other specified site**
          Traumatic arthropathy, vertebrae
M12.59   **Traumatic arthropathy, multiple sites**
Ⓢ M12.8   **Other specific arthropathies, not elsewhere classified**
          Transient arthropathy
M12.80   **Other specific arthropathies, not elsewhere classified, unspecified site**
Ⓖ M12.81   **Other specific arthropathies, not elsewhere classified, shoulder**
☐ M12.811   **Other specific arthropathies, not elsewhere classified, right shoulder**
☐ M12.812   **Other specific arthropathies, not elsewhere classified, left shoulder**
☐ M12.819   **Other specific arthropathies, not elsewhere classified, unspecified shoulder**
Ⓖ M12.82   **Other specific arthropathies, not elsewhere classified, elbow**
☐ M12.821   **Other specific arthropathies, not elsewhere classified, right elbow**
☐ M12.822   **Other specific arthropathies, not elsewhere classified, left elbow**
☐ M12.829   **Other specific arthropathies, not elsewhere classified, unspecified elbow**
Ⓖ M12.83   **Other specific arthropathies, not elsewhere classified, wrist**
☐ M12.831   **Other specific arthropathies, not elsewhere classified, right wrist**
☐ M12.832   **Other specific arthropathies, not elsewhere classified, left wrist**
☐ M12.839   **Other specific arthropathies, not elsewhere classified, unspecified wrist**
Ⓖ M12.84   **Other specific arthropathies, not elsewhere classified, hand**
☐ M12.841   **Other specific arthropathies, not elsewhere classified, right hand**

● New   ▲ Revised   *Manifestation*   4-7 Digit Indicators   ☐ Laterality   Ⓐ Adult (15+ years)   Ⓜ Maternity (12-55 years)   Ⓝ Newborn   Ⓟ Pediatric (0-17 years)   ♂ Male   ♀ Female
✖ Deleted   Unspecified   + Additional code

754   © 2017 DecisionHealth   2017 ICD-10-CM Expert for Physicians

□ **M12.842**   Other specific arthropathies, not elsewhere classified, left hand

□ **M12.849**   Other specific arthropathies, not elsewhere classified, unspecified hand

⑥ **M12.85**   Other specific arthropathies, not elsewhere classified, hip

□ **M12.851**   Other specific arthropathies, not elsewhere classified, right hip

□ **M12.852**   Other specific arthropathies, not elsewhere classified, left hip

□ **M12.859**   Other specific arthropathies, not elsewhere classified, unspecified hip

⑥ **M12.86**   Other specific arthropathies, not elsewhere classified, knee

□ **M12.861**   Other specific arthropathies, not elsewhere classified, right knee

□ **M12.862**   Other specific arthropathies, not elsewhere classified, left knee

□ **M12.869**   Other specific arthropathies, not elsewhere classified, unspecified knee

⑥ **M12.87**   Other specific arthropathies, not elsewhere classified, ankle and foot

□ **M12.871**   Other specific arthropathies, not elsewhere classified, right ankle and foot

□ **M12.872**   Other specific arthropathies, not elsewhere classified, left ankle and foot

□ **M12.879**   Other specific arthropathies, not elsewhere classified, unspecified ankle and foot

M12.88   Other specific arthropathies, not elsewhere classified, other specified site
Other specific arthropathies, not elsewhere classified, vertebrae

M12.89   Other specific arthropathies, not elsewhere classified, multiple sites

M12.9   Arthropathy, unspecified

④ **M13**   **Other arthritis**

> EXCLUDES 1   *arthrosis (M15-M19)*
> *osteoarthritis (M15-M19)*

M13.0   Polyarthritis, unspecified

⑤ **M13.1**   Monoarthritis, not elsewhere classified

M13.10   Monoarthritis, not elsewhere classified, unspecified site

⑥ **M13.11**   Monoarthritis, not elsewhere classified, shoulder

□ **M13.111**   Monoarthritis, not elsewhere classified, right shoulder

□ **M13.112**   Monoarthritis, not elsewhere classified, left shoulder

□ **M13.119**   Monoarthritis, not elsewhere classified, unspecified shoulder

⑥ **M13.12**   Monoarthritis, not elsewhere classified, elbow

□ **M13.121**   Monoarthritis, not elsewhere classified, right elbow

□ **M13.122**   Monoarthritis, not elsewhere classified, left elbow

□ **M13.129**   Monoarthritis, not elsewhere classified, unspecified elbow

⑥ **M13.13**   Monoarthritis, not elsewhere classified, wrist

□ **M13.131**   Monoarthritis, not elsewhere classified, right wrist

□ **M13.132**   Monoarthritis, not elsewhere classified, left wrist

□ **M13.139**   Monoarthritis, not elsewhere classified, unspecified wrist

⑥ **M13.14**   Monoarthritis, not elsewhere classified, hand

□ **M13.141**   Monoarthritis, not elsewhere classified, right hand

□ **M13.142**   Monoarthritis, not elsewhere classified, left hand

□ **M13.149**   Monoarthritis, not elsewhere classified, unspecified hand

⑥ **M13.15**   Monoarthritis, not elsewhere classified, hip

□ **M13.151**   Monoarthritis, not elsewhere classified, right hip

□ **M13.152**   Monoarthritis, not elsewhere classified, left hip

□ **M13.159**   Monoarthritis, not elsewhere classified, unspecified hip

⑥ **M13.16**   Monoarthritis, not elsewhere classified, knee

□ **M13.161**   Monoarthritis, not elsewhere classified, right knee

□ **M13.162**   Monoarthritis, not elsewhere classified, left knee

□ **M13.169**   Monoarthritis, not elsewhere classified, unspecified knee

⑥ **M13.17**   Monoarthritis, not elsewhere classified, ankle and foot

□ **M13.171**   Monoarthritis, not elsewhere classified, right ankle and foot

□ **M13.172**   Monoarthritis, not elsewhere classified, left ankle and foot

□ **M13.179**   Monoarthritis, not elsewhere classified, unspecified ankle and foot

⑤ **M13.8**   Other specified arthritis
Allergic arthritis

> EXCLUDES 1   *osteoarthritis (M15-M19)*

M13.80   Other specified arthritis, unspecified site

⑥ **M13.81**   Other specified arthritis, shoulder

□ **M13.811**   Other specified arthritis, right shoulder

□ **M13.812**   Other specified arthritis, left shoulder

□ **M13.819**   Other specified arthritis, unspecified shoulder

⑥ **M13.82**   Other specified arthritis, elbow

□ **M13.821**   Other specified arthritis, right elbow

□ **M13.822**   Other specified arthritis, left elbow

□ **M13.829**   Other specified arthritis, unspecified elbow

⑥ **M13.83**   Other specified arthritis, wrist

□ **M13.831**   Other specified arthritis, right wrist

□ **M13.832**   Other specified arthritis, left wrist

□ **M13.839**   Other specified arthritis, unspecified wrist

⑥ **M13.84**   Other specified arthritis, hand

□ **M13.841**   Other specified arthritis, right hand

□ **M13.842**   Other specified arthritis, left hand

□ **M13.849**   Other specified arthritis, unspecified hand

⑥ **M13.85**   Other specified arthritis, hip

□ **M13.851**   Other specified arthritis, right hip

□ **M13.852**   Other specified arthritis, left hip

□ **M13.859**   Other specified arthritis, unspecified hip

⑥ **M13.86**   Other specified arthritis, knee

□ **M13.861**   Other specified arthritis, right knee

□ **M13.862**   Other specified arthritis, left knee

□ **M13.869**   Other specified arthritis, unspecified knee

⑥ **M13.87**   Other specified arthritis, ankle and foot

□ **M13.871**   Other specified arthritis, right ankle and foot

□ **M13.872**   Other specified arthritis, left ankle and foot

□ **M13.879**   Other specified arthritis, unspecified ankle and foot

M13.88   Other specified arthritis, other site

M13.89   Other specified arthritis, multiple sites

④ **M14**   **Arthropathies in other diseases classified elsewhere**

> EXCLUDES 1   *arthropathy in:*
> *diabetes mellitus (E08-E13 with .61-)*
> *hematological disorders (M36.2-M36.3)*
> *hypersensitivity reactions (M36.4)*
> *neoplastic disease (M36.1)*
> *neurosyphillis (A52.16)*
> *sarcoidosis (D86.86)*
> *enteropathic arthropathies (M07.-)*
> *juvenile psoriatic arthropathy (L40.54)*
> *lipoid dermatoarthritis (E78.81)*

⑤ **M14.6**   Charcôt's joint
Neuropathic arthropathy

> EXCLUDES 1   *Charcôt's joint in diabetes mellitus (E08-E13 with .610)*
> *Charcôt's joint in tabes dorsalis (A52.16)*

> **CODING TIP** ✓   Do not assign a code from M14.6- to report charcot arthropathy in diabetes. Charcot's joint in diabetes mellitus should be coded to the appropriate combination code from E08-E13 indicating the manifestation.

M14.60   Charcôt's joint, unspecified site

⑥ **M14.61**   Charcôt's joint, shoulder

□ **M14.611**   Charcôt's joint, right shoulder

□ **M14.612**   Charcôt's joint, left shoulder

□ **M14.619**   Charcôt's joint, unspecified shoulder

⑥ **M14.62**   Charcôt's joint, elbow

□ **M14.621**   Charcôt's joint, right elbow

□ **M14.622**   Charcôt's joint, left elbow

● New   ▲ Revised   *Manifestation*   ④-⑦ Digit Indicators   □ Laterality   Ⓐ Adult (15+ years)   Ⓜ Maternity (12-55 years)   Ⓝ Newborn   Ⓟ Pediatric (0-17 years)   ♂ Male   ♀ Female
✖ ~~Deleted~~   Unspecified   + Additional code

2017 ICD-10-CM Expert for Physicians   © 2017 DecisionHealth   755

☐ M14.629   Charcôt's joint, unspecified elbow
🄖 M14.63   Charcôt's joint, wrist
   ☐ M14.631   Charcôt's joint, right wrist
   ☐ M14.632   Charcôt's joint, left wrist
   ☐ M14.639   Charcôt's joint, unspecified wrist
🄖 M14.64   Charcôt's joint, hand
   ☐ M14.641   Charcôt's joint, right hand
   ☐ M14.642   Charcôt's joint, left hand
   ☐ M14.649   Charcôt's joint, unspecified hand
🄖 M14.65   Charcôt's joint, hip
   ☐ M14.651   Charcôt's joint, right hip
   ☐ M14.652   Charcôt's joint, left hip
   ☐ M14.659   Charcôt's joint, unspecified hip
🄖 M14.66   Charcôt's joint, knee
   ☐ M14.661   Charcôt's joint, right knee
   ☐ M14.662   Charcôt's joint, left knee
   ☐ M14.669   Charcôt's joint, unspecified knee
🄖 M14.67   Charcôt's joint, ankle and foot
   ☐ M14.671   Charcôt's joint, right ankle and foot
   ☐ M14.672   Charcôt's joint, left ankle and foot
   ☐ M14.679   Charcôt's joint, unspecified ankle and foot
M14.68   Charcôt's joint, vertebrae
M14.69   Charcôt's joint, multiple sites
🄦 M14.8   Arthropathies in other specified diseases classified elsewhere
   Code first underlying disease, such as:
     amyloidosis (E85.-)
     erythema multiforme (L51.-)
     erythema nodosum (L52)
     hemochromatosis (E83.11-)
     hyperparathyroidism (E21.-)
     hypothyroidism (E00-E03)
     sickle-cell disorders (D57.-)
     thyrotoxicosis [hyperthyroidism] (E05.-)
     Whipple's disease (K90.81)

M14.80   *Arthropathies in other specified diseases classified elsewhere, unspecified site*
🄖 M14.81   Arthropathies in other specified diseases classified elsewhere, shoulder
   ☐ M14.811   *Arthropathies in other specified diseases classified elsewhere, right shoulder*
   ☐ M14.812   *Arthropathies in other specified diseases classified elsewhere, left shoulder*
   ☐ M14.819   *Arthropathies in other specified diseases classified elsewhere, unspecified shoulder*
🄖 M14.82   Arthropathies in other specified diseases classified elsewhere, elbow
   ☐ M14.821   *Arthropathies in other specified diseases classified elsewhere, right elbow*
   ☐ M14.822   *Arthropathies in other specified diseases classified elsewhere, left elbow*
   ☐ M14.829   *Arthropathies in other specified diseases classified elsewhere, unspecified elbow*
🄖 M14.83   Arthropathies in other specified diseases classified elsewhere, wrist
   ☐ M14.831   *Arthropathies in other specified diseases classified elsewhere, right wrist*
   ☐ M14.832   *Arthropathies in other specified diseases classified elsewhere, left wrist*
   ☐ M14.839   *Arthropathies in other specified diseases classified elsewhere, unspecified wrist*
🄖 M14.84   Arthropathies in other specified diseases classified elsewhere, hand
   ☐ M14.841   *Arthropathies in other specified diseases classified elsewhere, right hand*
   ☐ M14.842   *Arthropathies in other specified diseases classified elsewhere, left hand*
   ☐ M14.849   *Arthropathies in other specified diseases classified elsewhere, unspecified hand*
🄖 M14.85   Arthropathies in other specified diseases classified elsewhere, hip
   ☐ M14.851   *Arthropathies in other specified diseases classified elsewhere, right hip*
   ☐ M14.852   *Arthropathies in other specified diseases classified elsewhere, left hip*

☐ M14.859   *Arthropathies in other specified diseases classified elsewhere, unspecified hip*
🄖 M14.86   Arthropathies in other specified diseases classified elsewhere, knee
   ☐ M14.861   *Arthropathies in other specified diseases classified elsewhere, right knee*
   ☐ M14.862   *Arthropathies in other specified diseases classified elsewhere, left knee*
   ☐ M14.869   *Arthropathies in other specified diseases classified elsewhere, unspecified knee*
🄖 M14.87   Arthropathies in other specified diseases classified elsewhere, ankle and foot
   ☐ M14.871   *Arthropathies in other specified diseases classified elsewhere, right ankle and foot*
   ☐ M14.872   *Arthropathies in other specified diseases classified elsewhere, left ankle and foot*
   ☐ M14.879   *Arthropathies in other specified diseases classified elsewhere, unspecified ankle and foot*
M14.88   *Arthropathies in other specified diseases classified elsewhere, vertebrae*
M14.89   *Arthropathies in other specified diseases classified elsewhere, multiple sites*

Osteoarthritis (M15-M19)

EXCLUDES 2   osteoarthritis of spine (M47.-)

CODING TIP ✓   Osteoarthritis/degenerative joint disease (Categories M15-M19) is the most common type of arthritis in the elderly. If the arthritis is in the spine, refer to Category M47. When coding osteoarthrosis, review the medical records to determine whether the OA is localized or generalized; primary or secondary. Bilateral osteoarthrosis of the same site is considered localized. Generalized OA affects multiple joints (M15). Code joints affected separately and avoid the M15 for multiple joints, if multiple joint sites have been identified. Primary osteoarthritis is caused by aging. Secondary OA is caused by other conditions such as obesity.

🄣 M15   **Polyosteoarthritis**
   INCLUDES   arthritis of multiple sites
   EXCLUDES 1   *bilateral involvement of single joint (M16-M19)*

M15.0   **Primary generalized (osteo)arthritis**
M15.1   **Heberden's nodes (with arthropathy)**
   Interphalangeal distal osteoarthritis
M15.2   **Bouchard's nodes (with arthropathy)**
   Juxtaphalangeal distal osteoarthritis
M15.3   **Secondary multiple arthritis**
   Post-traumatic polyosteoarthritis
M15.4   **Erosive (osteo)arthritis**
M15.8   **Other polyosteoarthritis**
M15.9   **Polyosteoarthritis, unspecified**
   Generalized osteoarthritis NOS

🄣 M16   **Osteoarthritis of hip**
M16.0   **Bilateral primary osteoarthritis of hip**
🄦 M16.1   **Unilateral primary osteoarthritis of hip**
   Primary osteoarthritis of hip NOS
   ☐ M16.10   Unilateral primary osteoarthritis, unspecified hip
   ☐ M16.11   Unilateral primary osteoarthritis, right hip
   ☐ M16.12   Unilateral primary osteoarthritis, left hip
M16.2   **Bilateral osteoarthritis resulting from hip dysplasia**
🄦 M16.3   **Unilateral osteoarthritis resulting from hip dysplasia**
   Dysplastic osteoarthritis of hip NOS
   ☐ M16.30   Unilateral osteoarthritis resulting from hip dysplasia, unspecified hip
   ☐ M16.31   Unilateral osteoarthritis resulting from hip dysplasia, right hip
   ☐ M16.32   Unilateral osteoarthritis resulting from hip dysplasia, left hip
M16.4   **Bilateral post-traumatic osteoarthritis of hip**
🄦 M16.5   **Unilateral post-traumatic osteoarthritis of hip**
   Post-traumatic osteoarthritis of hip NOS
   ☐ M16.50   Unilateral post-traumatic osteoarthritis, unspecified hip
   ☐ M16.51   Unilateral post-traumatic osteoarthritis, right hip
   ☐ M16.52   Unilateral post-traumatic osteoarthritis, left hip
M16.6   **Other bilateral secondary osteoarthritis of hip**
M16.7   **Other unilateral secondary osteoarthritis of hip**
   Secondary osteoarthritis of hip NOS

● New   ▲ Revised   *Manifestation*   🄣-🄫 Digit Indicators   ☐ Laterality   🄰 Adult (15+ years)   🄼 Maternity (12-55 years)   🄽 Newborn   🄿 Pediatric (0-17 years)   ♂ Male   ♀ Female
✖ Deleted   Unspecified   + Additional code

M16.9 Osteoarthritis of hip, unspecified

☐ **M17 Osteoarthritis of knee**

M17.0 Bilateral primary osteoarthritis of knee

☐ M17.1 Unilateral primary osteoarthritis of knee
Primary osteoarthritis of knee NOS

☐ M17.10 Unilateral primary osteoarthritis, unspecified knee

☐ M17.11 Unilateral primary osteoarthritis, right knee

☐ M17.12 Unilateral primary osteoarthritis, left knee

M17.2 Bilateral post-traumatic osteoarthritis of knee

☐ M17.3 Unilateral post-traumatic osteoarthritis of knee
Post-traumatic osteoarthritis of knee NOS

☐ M17.30 Unilateral post-traumatic osteoarthritis, unspecified knee

☐ M17.31 Unilateral post-traumatic osteoarthritis, right knee

☐ M17.32 Unilateral post-traumatic osteoarthritis, left knee

M17.4 Other bilateral secondary osteoarthritis of knee

M17.5 Other unilateral secondary osteoarthritis of knee
Secondary osteoarthritis of knee NOS

M17.9 Osteoarthritis of knee, unspecified

☐ **M18 Osteoarthritis of first carpometacarpal joint**

M18.0 Bilateral primary osteoarthritis of first carpometacarpal joints

☐ M18.1 Unilateral primary osteoarthritis of first carpometacarpal joint
Primary osteoarthritis of first carpometacarpal joint NOS

☐ M18.10 Unilateral primary osteoarthritis of first carpometacarpal joint, unspecified hand

☐ M18.11 Unilateral primary osteoarthritis of first carpometacarpal joint, right hand

☐ M18.12 Unilateral primary osteoarthritis of first carpometacarpal joint, left hand

M18.2 Bilateral post-traumatic osteoarthritis of first carpometacarpal joints

☐ M18.3 Unilateral post-traumatic osteoarthritis of first carpometacarpal joint
Post-traumatic osteoarthritis of first carpometacarpal joint NOS

☐ M18.30 Unilateral post-traumatic osteoarthritis of first carpometacarpal joint, unspecified hand

☐ M18.31 Unilateral post-traumatic osteoarthritis of first carpometacarpal joint, right hand

☐ M18.32 Unilateral post-traumatic osteoarthritis of first carpometacarpal joint, left hand

M18.4 Other bilateral secondary osteoarthritis of first carpometacarpal joints

☐ M18.5 Other unilateral secondary osteoarthritis of first carpometacarpal joint
Secondary osteoarthritis of first carpometacarpal joint NOS

☐ M18.50 Other unilateral secondary osteoarthritis of first carpometacarpal joint, unspecified hand

☐ M18.51 Other unilateral secondary osteoarthritis of first carpometacarpal joint, right hand

☐ M18.52 Other unilateral secondary osteoarthritis of first carpometacarpal joint, left hand

M18.9 Osteoarthritis of first carpometacarpal joint, unspecified

☐ **M19 Other and unspecified osteoarthritis**

EXCLUDES 1 *polyarthritis (M15.-)*

EXCLUDES 2 *arthrosis of spine (M47.-)*
hallux rigidus (M20.2)
osteoarthritis of spine (M47.-)

☐ M19.0 Primary osteoarthritis of other joints

☐ M19.01 Primary osteoarthritis, shoulder

☐ M19.011 Primary osteoarthritis, right shoulder

☐ M19.012 Primary osteoarthritis, left shoulder

☐ M19.019 Primary osteoarthritis, unspecified shoulder

☐ M19.02 Primary osteoarthritis, elbow

☐ M19.021 Primary osteoarthritis, right elbow

☐ M19.022 Primary osteoarthritis, left elbow

☐ M19.029 Primary osteoarthritis, unspecified elbow

☐ M19.03 Primary osteoarthritis, wrist

☐ M19.031 Primary osteoarthritis, right wrist

☐ M19.032 Primary osteoarthritis, left wrist

☐ M19.039 Primary osteoarthritis, unspecified wrist

☐ M19.04 Primary osteoarthritis, hand

EXCLUDES 2 *primary osteoarthritis of first carpometacarpal joint (M18.0-, M18.1-)*

☐ M19.041 Primary osteoarthritis, right hand

☐ M19.042 Primary osteoarthritis, left hand

☐ M19.049 Primary osteoarthritis, unspecified hand

☐ M19.07 Primary osteoarthritis ankle and foot

☐ M19.071 Primary osteoarthritis, right ankle and foot

☐ M19.072 Primary osteoarthritis, left ankle and foot

☐ M19.079 Primary osteoarthritis, unspecified ankle and foot

☐ M19.1 Post-traumatic osteoarthritis of other joints

☐ M19.11 Post-traumatic osteoarthritis, shoulder

☐ M19.111 Post-traumatic osteoarthritis, right shoulder

☐ M19.112 Post-traumatic osteoarthritis, left shoulder

☐ M19.119 Post-traumatic osteoarthritis, unspecified shoulder

☐ M19.12 Post-traumatic osteoarthritis, elbow

☐ M19.121 Post-traumatic osteoarthritis, right elbow

☐ M19.122 Post-traumatic osteoarthritis, left elbow

☐ M19.129 Post-traumatic osteoarthritis, unspecified elbow

☐ M19.13 Post-traumatic osteoarthritis, wrist

☐ M19.131 Post-traumatic osteoarthritis, right wrist

☐ M19.132 Post-traumatic osteoarthritis, left wrist

☐ M19.139 Post-traumatic osteoarthritis, unspecified wrist

☐ M19.14 Post-traumatic osteoarthritis, hand

EXCLUDES 2 *post-traumatic osteoarthritis of first carpometacarpal joint (M18.2-, M18.3-)*

☐ M19.141 Post-traumatic osteoarthritis, right hand

☐ M19.142 Post-traumatic osteoarthritis, left hand

☐ M19.149 Post-traumatic osteoarthritis, unspecified hand

☐ M19.17 Post-traumatic osteoarthritis, ankle and foot

☐ M19.171 Post-traumatic osteoarthritis, right ankle and foot

☐ M19.172 Post-traumatic osteoarthritis, left ankle and foot

☐ M19.179 Post-traumatic osteoarthritis, unspecified ankle and foot

☐ M19.2 Secondary osteoarthritis of other joints

☐ M19.21 Secondary osteoarthritis, shoulder

☐ M19.211 Secondary osteoarthritis, right shoulder

☐ M19.212 Secondary osteoarthritis, left shoulder

☐ M19.219 Secondary osteoarthritis, unspecified shoulder

☐ M19.22 Secondary osteoarthritis, elbow

☐ M19.221 Secondary osteoarthritis, right elbow

☐ M19.222 Secondary osteoarthritis, left elbow

☐ M19.229 Secondary osteoarthritis, unspecified elbow

☐ M19.23 Secondary osteoarthritis, wrist

☐ M19.231 Secondary osteoarthritis, right wrist

☐ M19.232 Secondary osteoarthritis, left wrist

☐ M19.239 Secondary osteoarthritis, unspecified wrist

☐ M19.24 Secondary osteoarthritis, hand

☐ M19.241 Secondary osteoarthritis, right hand

☐ M19.242 Secondary osteoarthritis, left hand

☐ M19.249 Secondary osteoarthritis, unspecified hand

☐ M19.27 Secondary osteoarthritis, ankle and foot

☐ M19.271 Secondary osteoarthritis, right ankle and foot

☐ M19.272 Secondary osteoarthritis, left ankle and foot

☐ M19.279 Secondary osteoarthritis, unspecified ankle and foot

☐ M19.9 Osteoarthritis, unspecified site

M19.90 Unspecified osteoarthritis, unspecified site
Arthrosis NOS
Arthritis NOS
Osteoarthritis NOS

M19.91 Primary osteoarthritis, unspecified site
Primary osteoarthritis NOS

M19.92 Post-traumatic osteoarthritis, unspecified site
Post-traumatic osteoarthritis NOS

M19.93 Secondary osteoarthritis, unspecified site
Secondary osteoarthritis NOS

● New ▲ Revised *Manifestation* ☐-☐ Digit Indicators ☐ Laterality Ⓐ Adult (15+ years) Ⓜ Maternity (12-55 years) Ⓝ Newborn Ⓟ Pediatric (0-17 years) ♂ Male ♀ Female
✖ Deleted Unspecified + Additional code

2017 ICD-10-CM Expert for Physicians

© 2017 DecisionHealth 757

Other joint disorders (M20-M25)

EXCLUDES 2   *joints of the spine (M40-M54)*

M20   **Acquired deformities of fingers and toes**

> **EXCLUDES 1**   *acquired absence of fingers and toes (Z89.-)*
> *congenital absence of fingers and toes (Q71.3-, Q72.3-)*
> *congenital deformities and malformations of fingers and toes (Q66.-, Q68-Q70, Q74.-)*

M20.0   **Deformity of finger(s)**

> **EXCLUDES 1**   *clubbing of fingers (R68.3)*
> *palmar fascial fibromatosis [Dupuytren] (M72.0)*
> *trigger finger (M65.3)*

M20.00   **Unspecified deformity of finger(s)**
- **M20.001**   **Unspecified deformity of right finger(s)**
- **M20.002**   **Unspecified deformity of left finger(s)**
- **M20.009**   **Unspecified deformity of unspecified finger(s)**

M20.01   **Mallet finger**
- **M20.011**   **Mallet finger of right finger(s)**
- **M20.012**   **Mallet finger of left finger(s)**
- **M20.019**   **Mallet finger of unspecified finger(s)**

M20.02   **Boutonnière deformity**
- **M20.021**   **Boutonnière deformity of right finger(s)**
- **M20.022**   **Boutonnière deformity of left finger(s)**
- **M20.029**   **Boutonnière deformity of unspecified finger(s)**

M20.03   **Swan-neck deformity**
- **M20.031**   **Swan-neck deformity of right finger(s)**
- **M20.032**   **Swan-neck deformity of left finger(s)**
- **M20.039**   **Swan-neck deformity of unspecified finger(s)**

M20.09   **Other deformity of finger(s)**
- **M20.091**   **Other deformity of right finger(s)**
- **M20.092**   **Other deformity of left finger(s)**
- **M20.099**   **Other deformity of finger(s), unspecified finger(s)**

▲ **M20.1**   **Hallux valgus (acquired)**

> **EXCLUDES 2**   *bunion (M21.6-)*

- **M20.10**   **Hallux valgus (acquired), unspecified foot**

Hallux Valgus
(bunion)

- **M20.11**   **Hallux valgus (acquired), right foot**
- **M20.12**   **Hallux valgus (acquired), left foot**

M20.2   **Hallux rigidus**

> **DEFINITION**   Inflexible, stiff great toe, with limited motion at the metatarsophalangeal joint.

- **M20.20**   **Hallux rigidus, unspecified foot**
- **M20.21**   **Hallux rigidus, right foot**
- **M20.22**   **Hallux rigidus, left foot**

M20.3   **Hallux varus (acquired)**

> **DEFINITION**   Displaced joint of the big toe which is pointed away from the rest of the toes.

- **M20.30**   **Hallux varus (acquired), unspecified foot**
- **M20.31**   **Hallux varus (acquired), right foot**
- **M20.32**   **Hallux varus (acquired), left foot**

M20.4   **Other hammer toe(s) (acquired)**
- **M20.40**   **Other hammer toe(s) (acquired), unspecified foot**
- **M20.41**   **Other hammer toe(s) (acquired), right foot**
- **M20.42**   **Other hammer toe(s) (acquired), left foot**

M20.5   **Other deformities of toe(s) (acquired)**

M20.5X   **Other deformities of toe(s) (acquired)**
- **M20.5X1**   **Other deformities of toe(s) (acquired), right foot**
- **M20.5X2**   **Other deformities of toe(s) (acquired), left foot**
- **M20.5X9**   **Other deformities of toe(s) (acquired), unspecified foot**

M20.6   **Acquired deformities of toe(s), unspecified**
- **M20.60**   **Acquired deformities of toe(s), unspecified, unspecified foot**
- **M20.61**   **Acquired deformities of toe(s), unspecified, right foot**
- **M20.62**   **Acquired deformities of toe(s), unspecified, left foot**

M21   **Other acquired deformities of limbs**

> **EXCLUDES 1**   *acquired absence of limb (Z89.-)*
> *congenital absence of limbs (Q71-Q73)*
> *congenital deformities and malformations of limbs (Q65-Q66, Q68-Q74)*
>
> **EXCLUDES 2**   *acquired deformities of fingers or toes (M20.-)*
> *coxa plana (M91.2)*

M21.0   **Valgus deformity, not elsewhere classified**

> **EXCLUDES 1**   *metatarsus valgus (Q66.6)*
> *talipes calcaneovalgus (Q66.4)*

M21.00   **Valgus deformity, not elsewhere classified, unspecified site**

M21.02   **Valgus deformity, not elsewhere classified, elbow**
Cubitus valgus
- **M21.021**   **Valgus deformity, not elsewhere classified, right elbow**
- **M21.022**   **Valgus deformity, not elsewhere classified, left elbow**
- **M21.029**   **Valgus deformity, not elsewhere classified, unspecified elbow**

M21.05   **Valgus deformity, not elsewhere classified, hip**
- **M21.051**   **Valgus deformity, not elsewhere classified, right hip**
- **M21.052**   **Valgus deformity, not elsewhere classified, left hip**
- **M21.059**   **Valgus deformity, not elsewhere classified, unspecified hip**

M21.06   **Valgus deformity, not elsewhere classified, knee**
Genu valgum
Knock knee

> **DEFINITION**   Deformity in which the knees are angled abnormally close together with the ankles apart when standing erect with the legs straightened.

- **M21.061**   **Valgus deformity, not elsewhere classified, right knee**
- **M21.062**   **Valgus deformity, not elsewhere classified, left knee**
- **M21.069**   **Valgus deformity, not elsewhere classified, unspecified knee**

M21.07   **Valgus deformity, not elsewhere classified, ankle**
- **M21.071**   **Valgus deformity, not elsewhere classified, right ankle**
- **M21.072**   **Valgus deformity, not elsewhere classified, left ankle**
- **M21.079**   **Valgus deformity, not elsewhere classified, unspecified ankle**

▲ **M21.1**   **Varus deformity, not elsewhere classified**

> **EXCLUDES 1**   *metatarsus varus (Q66.22)*
> *tibia vara (M92.5)*

M21.10   **Varus deformity, not elsewhere classified, unspecified site**

● New   ▲ Revised   *Manifestation*   ✚-❼ Digit Indicators   Laterality   Ⓐ Adult (15+ years)   Ⓜ Maternity (12-55 years)   Ⓝ Newborn   Ⓟ Pediatric (0-17 years)   ♂ Male   ♀ Female
✖ Deleted   Unspecified   ✚ Additional code

758   © 2017 DecisionHealth   2017 ICD-10-CM Expert for Physicians

⑥ **M21.12**   **Varus deformity, not elsewhere classified, elbow**
Cubitus varus, elbow

☐ **M21.121**   Varus deformity, not elsewhere classified, right elbow

☐ **M21.122**   Varus deformity, not elsewhere classified, left elbow

☐ **M21.129**   Varus deformity, not elsewhere classified, unspecified elbow

⑥ **M21.15**   **Varus deformity, not elsewhere classified, hip**

☐ **M21.151**   Varus deformity, not elsewhere classified, right hip

☐ **M21.152**   Varus deformity, not elsewhere classified, left hip

☐ **M21.159**   Varus deformity, not elsewhere classified, unspecified

⑥ **M21.16**   **Varus deformity, not elsewhere classified, knee**
Bow leg
Genu varum

☐ **M21.161**   Varus deformity, not elsewhere classified, right knee

☐ **M21.162**   Varus deformity, not elsewhere classified, left knee

☐ **M21.169**   Varus deformity, not elsewhere classified, unspecified knee

⑥ **M21.17**   **Varus deformity, not elsewhere classified, ankle**

DEFINITION   Inward angulation of the tibia and fibula on the talus generally due to trauma or overpull by the tibialis posterior and anterior tendons.

☐ **M21.171**   Varus deformity, not elsewhere classified, right ankle

☐ **M21.172**   Varus deformity, not elsewhere classified, left ankle

☐ **M21.179**   Varus deformity, not elsewhere classified, unspecified ankle

⑤ **M21.2**   **Flexion deformity**

M21.20   **Flexion deformity, unspecified site**

⑥ **M21.21**   **Flexion deformity, shoulder**

☐ **M21.211**   Flexion deformity, right shoulder

☐ **M21.212**   Flexion deformity, left shoulder

☐ **M21.219**   Flexion deformity, unspecified shoulder

⑥ **M21.22**   **Flexion deformity, elbow**

☐ **M21.221**   Flexion deformity, right elbow

☐ **M21.222**   Flexion deformity, left elbow

☐ **M21.229**   Flexion deformity, unspecified elbow

⑥ **M21.23**   **Flexion deformity, wrist**

☐ **M21.231**   Flexion deformity, right wrist

☐ **M21.232**   Flexion deformity, left wrist

☐ **M21.239**   Flexion deformity, unspecified wrist

⑥ **M21.24**   **Flexion deformity, finger joints**

☐ **M21.241**   Flexion deformity, right finger joints

☐ **M21.242**   Flexion deformity, left finger joints

☐ **M21.249**   Flexion deformity, unspecified finger joints

⑥ **M21.25**   **Flexion deformity, hip**

☐ **M21.251**   Flexion deformity, right hip

☐ **M21.252**   Flexion deformity, left hip

☐ **M21.259**   Flexion deformity, unspecified hip

⑥ **M21.26**   **Flexion deformity, knee**

☐ **M21.261**   Flexion deformity, right knee

☐ **M21.262**   Flexion deformity, left knee

☐ **M21.269**   Flexion deformity, unspecified knee

⑥ **M21.27**   **Flexion deformity, ankle and toes**

☐ **M21.271**   Flexion deformity, right ankle and toes

☐ **M21.272**   Flexion deformity, left ankle and toes

☐ **M21.279**   Flexion deformity, unspecified ankle and toes

⑤ **M21.3**   **Wrist or foot drop (acquired)**

⑥ **M21.33**   **Wrist drop (acquired)**

☐ **M21.331**   Wrist drop, right wrist

☐ **M21.332**   Wrist drop, left wrist

☐ **M21.339**   Wrist drop, unspecified wrist

⑥ **M21.37**   **Foot drop (acquired)**

☐ **M21.371**   Foot drop, right foot

☐ **M21.372**   Foot drop, left foot

☐ **M21.379**   Foot drop, unspecified foot

⑤ **M21.4**   **Flat foot [pes planus] (acquired)**

EXCLUDES 1   *congenital pes planus (Q66.5-)*

☐ **M21.40**   **Flat foot [pes planus] (acquired), unspecified foot**

☐ **M21.41**   **Flat foot [pes planus] (acquired), right foot**

☐ **M21.42**   **Flat foot [pes planus] (acquired), left foot**

⑤ **M21.5**   **Acquired clawhand, clubhand, clawfoot and clubfoot**

EXCLUDES 1   *clubfoot, not specified as acquired (Q66.89)*

⑥ **M21.51**   **Acquired clawhand**

☐ **M21.511**   Acquired clawhand, right hand

☐ **M21.512**   Acquired clawhand, left hand

☐ **M21.519**   Acquired clawhand, unspecified hand

⑥ **M21.52**   **Acquired clubhand**

☐ **M21.521**   Acquired clubhand, right hand

☐ **M21.522**   Acquired clubhand, left hand

☐ **M21.529**   Acquired clubhand, unspecified hand

⑥ **M21.53**   **Acquired clawfoot**

☐ **M21.531**   Acquired clawfoot, right foot

☐ **M21.532**   Acquired clawfoot, left foot

☐ **M21.539**   Acquired clawfoot, unspecified foot

⑥ **M21.54**   **Acquired clubfoot**

☐ **M21.541**   Acquired clubfoot, right foot

☐ **M21.542**   Acquired clubfoot, left foot

☐ **M21.549**   Acquired clubfoot, unspecified foot

▲ ⑤ **M21.6**   **Other acquired deformities of foot**

EXCLUDES 2   *deformities of toe (acquired) (M20.1-M20.6-)*

● ⑥ **M21.61**   **Bunion**

● ☐ **M21.611**   **Bunion of right foot**

● ☐ **M21.612**   **Bunion of left foot**

● ☐ **M21.619**   **Bunion of unspecified foot**

● ⑥ **M21.62**   **Bunionette**

● ☐ **M21.621**   **Bunionette of right foot**

● ☐ **M21.622**   **Bunionette of left foot**

● ☐ **M21.629**   **Bunionette of unspecified foot**

⑥ **M21.6X**   **Other acquired deformities of foot**

☐ **M21.6X1**   **Other acquired deformities of right foot**

☐ **M21.6X2**   **Other acquired deformities of left foot**

☐ **M21.6X9**   **Other acquired deformities of unspecified foot**

⑤ **M21.7**   **Unequal limb length (acquired)**
Note: The site used should correspond to the shorter limb

M21.70   **Unequal limb length (acquired), unspecified site**

⑥ **M21.72**   **Unequal limb length (acquired), humerus**

☐ **M21.721**   Unequal limb length (acquired), right humerus

☐ **M21.722**   Unequal limb length (acquired), left humerus

☐ **M21.729**   Unequal limb length (acquired), unspecified humerus

⑥ **M21.73**   **Unequal limb length (acquired), ulna and radius**

☐ **M21.731**   Unequal limb length (acquired), right ulna

☐ **M21.732**   Unequal limb length (acquired), left ulna

☐ **M21.733**   Unequal limb length (acquired), right radius

☐ **M21.734**   Unequal limb length (acquired), left radius

☐ **M21.739**   Unequal limb length (acquired), unspecified ulna and radius

⑥ **M21.75**   **Unequal limb length (acquired), femur**

☐ **M21.751**   Unequal limb length (acquired), right femur

☐ **M21.752**   Unequal limb length (acquired), left femur

☐ **M21.759**   Unequal limb length (acquired), unspecified femur

⑥ **M21.76**   **Unequal limb length (acquired), tibia and fibula**

☐ **M21.761**   Unequal limb length (acquired), right tibia

☐ **M21.762**   Unequal limb length (acquired), left tibia

☐ **M21.763**   Unequal limb length (acquired), right fibula

☐ **M21.764**   Unequal limb length (acquired), left fibula

☐ **M21.769**   Unequal limb length (acquired), unspecified tibia and fibula

⑤ **M21.8**   **Other specified acquired deformities of limbs**

EXCLUDES 2   *coxa plana (M91.2)*

M21.80   **Other specified acquired deformities of unspecified limb**

⑥ **M21.82**   **Other specified acquired deformities of upper arm**

☐ **M21.821**   **Other specified acquired deformities of right upper arm**

● New   ▲ Revised   *Manifestation*   🔲- 🔢 Digit Indicators   ☐ Laterality   Ⓐ Adult (15+ years)   Ⓜ Maternity (12-55 years)   Ⓝ Newborn   Ⓟ Pediatric (0-17 years)   ♂ Male   ♀ Female

✖ Deleted   Unspecified   + Additional code

2017 ICD-10-CM Expert for Physicians   © 2017 DecisionHealth   759

⊟ **M21.822** Other specified acquired deformities of left upper arm

⊟ **M21.829** Other specified acquired deformities of unspecified upper arm

⑥ **M21.83** Other specified acquired deformities of forearm

⊟ **M21.831** Other specified acquired deformities of right forearm

⊟ **M21.832** Other specified acquired deformities of left forearm

⊟ **M21.839** Other specified acquired deformities of unspecified forearm

⑥ **M21.85** Other specified acquired deformities of thigh

⊟ **M21.851** Other specified acquired deformities of right thigh

⊟ **M21.852** Other specified acquired deformities of left thigh

⊟ **M21.859** Other specified acquired deformities of unspecified thigh

⑥ **M21.86** Other specified acquired deformities of lower leg

⊟ **M21.861** Other specified acquired deformities of right lower leg

⊟ **M21.862** Other specified acquired deformities of left lower leg

⊟ **M21.869** Other specified acquired deformities of unspecified lower leg

⑤ **M21.9** Unspecified acquired deformity of limb and hand

M21.90 Unspecified acquired deformity of unspecified limb

⑥ **M21.92** Unspecified acquired deformity of upper arm

⊟ **M21.921** Unspecified acquired deformity of right upper arm

⊟ **M21.922** Unspecified acquired deformity of left upper arm

⊟ **M21.929** Unspecified acquired deformity of unspecified upper arm

⑥ **M21.93** Unspecified acquired deformity of forearm

⊟ **M21.931** Unspecified acquired deformity of right forearm

⊟ **M21.932** Unspecified acquired deformity of left forearm

⊟ **M21.939** Unspecified acquired deformity of unspecified forearm

⑥ **M21.94** Unspecified acquired deformity of hand

⊟ **M21.941** Unspecified acquired deformity of hand, right hand

⊟ **M21.942** Unspecified acquired deformity of hand, left hand

⊟ **M21.949** Unspecified acquired deformity of hand, unspecified hand

⑥ **M21.95** Unspecified acquired deformity of thigh

⊟ **M21.951** Unspecified acquired deformity of right thigh

⊟ **M21.952** Unspecified acquired deformity of left thigh

⊟ **M21.959** Unspecified acquired deformity of unspecified thigh

⑥ **M21.96** Unspecified acquired deformity of lower leg

⊟ **M21.961** Unspecified acquired deformity of right lower leg

⊟ **M21.962** Unspecified acquired deformity of left lower leg

⊟ **M21.969** Unspecified acquired deformity of unspecified lower leg

④ **M22** **Disorder of patella**

> **EXCLUDES 1**   *traumatic dislocation of patella (S83.0-)*

⑤ **M22.0** Recurrent dislocation of patella

⊟ **M22.00** Recurrent dislocation of patella, unspecified knee

⊟ **M22.01** Recurrent dislocation of patella, right knee

⊟ **M22.02** Recurrent dislocation of patella, left knee

⑤ **M22.1** Recurrent subluxation of patella
Incomplete dislocation of patella

⊟ **M22.10** Recurrent subluxation of patella, unspecified knee

⊟ **M22.11** Recurrent subluxation of patella, right knee

⊟ **M22.12** Recurrent subluxation of patella, left knee

⑤ **M22.2** Patellofemoral disorders

⑥ **M22.2X** Patellofemoral disorders

⊟ **M22.2X1** Patellofemoral disorders, right knee

⊟ **M22.2X2** Patellofemoral disorders, left knee

⊟ **M22.2X9** Patellofemoral disorders, unspecified knee

⑤ **M22.3** Other derangements of patella

⑥ **M22.3X** Other derangements of patella

⊟ **M22.3X1** Other derangements of patella, right knee

⊟ **M22.3X2** Other derangements of patella, left knee

⊟ **M22.3X9** Other derangements of patella, unspecified knee

⑤ **M22.4** Chondromalacia patellae

⊟ **M22.40** Chondromalacia patellae, unspecified knee

⊟ **M22.41** Chondromalacia patellae, right knee

⊟ **M22.42** Chondromalacia patellae, left knee

⑤ **M22.8** Other disorders of patella

⑥ **M22.8X** Other disorders of patella

⊟ **M22.8X1** Other disorders of patella, right knee

⊟ **M22.8X2** Other disorders of patella, left knee

⊟ **M22.8X9** Other disorders of patella, unspecified knee

⑤ **M22.9** Unspecified disorder of patella

⊟ **M22.90** Unspecified disorder of patella, unspecified knee

⊟ **M22.91** Unspecified disorder of patella, right knee

⊟ **M22.92** Unspecified disorder of patella, left knee

④ **M23** **Internal derangement of knee**

> **EXCLUDES 1**   *ankylosis (M24.66)*
> *current injury - see injury of knee and lower leg (S80-S89)*
> *deformity of knee (M21.-)*
> *osteochondritis dissecans (M93.2)*
> *recurrent dislocation or subluxation of joints (M24.4)*
> *recurrent dislocation or subluxation of patella (M22.0-M22.1)*

⑤ **M23.0** Cystic meniscus

⑥ **M23.00** Cystic meniscus, unspecified meniscus
Cystic meniscus, unspecified lateral meniscus
Cystic meniscus, unspecified medial meniscus

⊟ **M23.000** Cystic meniscus, unspecified lateral meniscus, right knee

⊟ **M23.001** Cystic meniscus, unspecified lateral meniscus, left knee

⊟ **M23.002** Cystic meniscus, unspecified lateral meniscus, unspecified knee

⊟ **M23.003** Cystic meniscus, unspecified medial meniscus, right knee

⊟ **M23.004** Cystic meniscus, unspecified medial meniscus, left knee

⊟ **M23.005** Cystic meniscus, unspecified medial meniscus, unspecified knee

⊟ **M23.006** Cystic meniscus, unspecified meniscus, right knee

⊟ **M23.007** Cystic meniscus, unspecified meniscus, left knee

⊟ **M23.009** Cystic meniscus, unspecified meniscus, unspecified knee

⑥ **M23.01** Cystic meniscus, anterior horn of medial meniscus

⊟ **M23.011** Cystic meniscus, anterior horn of medial meniscus, right knee

⊟ **M23.012** Cystic meniscus, anterior horn of medial meniscus, left knee

⊟ **M23.019** Cystic meniscus, anterior horn of medial meniscus, unspecified knee

⑥ **M23.02** Cystic meniscus, posterior horn of medial meniscus

⊟ **M23.021** Cystic meniscus, posterior horn of medial meniscus, right knee

⊟ **M23.022** Cystic meniscus, posterior horn of medial meniscus, left knee

⊟ **M23.029** Cystic meniscus, posterior horn of medial meniscus, unspecified knee

⑥ **M23.03** Cystic meniscus, other medial meniscus

⊟ **M23.031** Cystic meniscus, other medial meniscus, right knee

⊟ **M23.032** Cystic meniscus, other medial meniscus, left knee

⊟ **M23.039** Cystic meniscus, other medial meniscus, unspecified knee

⑥ **M23.04** Cystic meniscus, anterior horn of lateral meniscus

⊟ **M23.041** Cystic meniscus, anterior horn of lateral meniscus, right knee

● New   ▲ Revised   *Manifestation*   ④-⑦ Digit Indicators   ⊟ Laterality   Ⓐ Adult (15+ years)   Ⓜ Maternity (12-55 years)   Ⓝ Newborn   Ⓟ Pediatric (0-17 years)   ♂ Male   ♀ Female
✖ ~~Deleted~~   Unspecified   + Additional code

760   © 2017 DecisionHealth   2017 ICD-10-CM Expert for Physicians

⊟ **M23.042** Cystic meniscus, anterior horn of lateral meniscus, left knee

⊟ **M23.049** Cystic meniscus, anterior horn of lateral meniscus, unspecified knee

Ⓖ **M23.05** Cystic meniscus, posterior horn of lateral meniscus

⊟ **M23.051** Cystic meniscus, posterior horn of lateral meniscus, right knee

⊟ **M23.052** Cystic meniscus, posterior horn of lateral meniscus, left knee

⊟ **M23.059** Cystic meniscus, posterior horn of lateral meniscus, unspecified knee

Ⓖ **M23.06** Cystic meniscus, other lateral meniscus

⊟ **M23.061** Cystic meniscus, other lateral meniscus, right knee

⊟ **M23.062** Cystic meniscus, other lateral meniscus, left knee

⊟ **M23.069** Cystic meniscus, other lateral meniscus, unspecified knee

Ⓢ **M23.2** Derangement of meniscus due to old tear or injury
Old bucket-handle tear

Ⓖ **M23.20** Derangement of unspecified meniscus due to old tear or injury
Derangement of unspecified lateral meniscus due to old tear or injury
Derangement of unspecified medial meniscus due to old tear or injury

⊟ **M23.200** Derangement of unspecified lateral meniscus due to old tear or injury, right knee

⊟ **M23.201** Derangement of unspecified lateral meniscus due to old tear or injury, left knee

⊟ **M23.202** Derangement of unspecified lateral meniscus due to old tear or injury, unspecified knee

⊟ **M23.203** Derangement of unspecified medial meniscus due to old tear or injury, right knee

⊟ **M23.204** Derangement of unspecified medial meniscus due to old tear or injury, left knee

⊟ **M23.205** Derangement of unspecified medial meniscus due to old tear or injury, unspecified knee

⊟ **M23.206** Derangement of unspecified meniscus due to old tear or injury, right knee

⊟ **M23.207** Derangement of unspecified meniscus due to old tear or injury, left knee

⊟ **M23.209** Derangement of unspecified meniscus due to old tear or injury, unspecified knee

Ⓖ **M23.21** Derangement of anterior horn of medial meniscus due to old tear or injury

⊟ **M23.211** Derangement of anterior horn of medial meniscus due to old tear or injury, right knee

⊟ **M23.212** Derangement of anterior horn of medial meniscus due to old tear or injury, left knee

⊟ **M23.219** Derangement of anterior horn of medial meniscus due to old tear or injury, unspecified knee

Ⓖ **M23.22** Derangement of posterior horn of medial meniscus due to old tear or injury

⊟ **M23.221** Derangement of posterior horn of medial meniscus due to old tear or injury, right knee

⊟ **M23.222** Derangement of posterior horn of medial meniscus due to old tear or injury, left knee

⊟ **M23.229** Derangement of posterior horn of medial meniscus due to old tear or injury, unspecified knee

Ⓖ **M23.23** Derangement of other medial meniscus due to old tear or injury

⊟ **M23.231** Derangement of other medial meniscus due to old tear or injury, right knee

⊟ **M23.232** Derangement of other medial meniscus due to old tear or injury, left knee

⊟ **M23.239** Derangement of other medial meniscus due to old tear or injury, unspecified knee

Ⓖ **M23.24** Derangement of anterior horn of lateral meniscus due to old tear or injury

⊟ **M23.241** Derangement of anterior horn of lateral meniscus due to old tear or injury, right knee

⊟ **M23.242** Derangement of anterior horn of lateral meniscus due to old tear or injury, left knee

⊟ **M23.249** Derangement of anterior horn of lateral meniscus due to old tear or injury, unspecified knee

Ⓖ **M23.25** Derangement of posterior horn of lateral meniscus due to old tear or injury

⊟ **M23.251** Derangement of posterior horn of lateral meniscus due to old tear or injury, right knee

⊟ **M23.252** Derangement of posterior horn of lateral meniscus due to old tear or injury, left knee

⊟ **M23.259** Derangement of posterior horn of lateral meniscus due to old tear or injury, unspecified knee

Ⓖ **M23.26** Derangement of other lateral meniscus due to old tear or injury

⊟ **M23.261** Derangement of other lateral meniscus due to old tear or injury, right knee

⊟ **M23.262** Derangement of other lateral meniscus due to old tear or injury, left knee

⊟ **M23.269** Derangement of other lateral meniscus due to old tear or injury, unspecified knee

Ⓢ **M23.3** Other meniscus derangements
Degenerate meniscus
Detached meniscus
Retained meniscus

Ⓖ **M23.30** Other meniscus derangements, unspecified meniscus
Other meniscus derangements, unspecified lateral meniscus
Other meniscus derangements, unspecified medial meniscus

⊟ **M23.300** Other meniscus derangements, unspecified lateral meniscus, right knee

⊟ **M23.301** Other meniscus derangements, unspecified lateral meniscus, left knee

⊟ **M23.302** Other meniscus derangements, unspecified lateral meniscus, unspecified knee

⊟ **M23.303** Other meniscus derangements, unspecified medial meniscus, right knee

⊟ **M23.304** Other meniscus derangements, unspecified medial meniscus, left knee

⊟ **M23.305** Other meniscus derangements, unspecified medial meniscus, unspecified knee

⊟ **M23.306** Other meniscus derangements, unspecified meniscus, right knee

⊟ **M23.307** Other meniscus derangements, unspecified meniscus, left knee

⊟ **M23.309** Other meniscus derangements, unspecified meniscus, unspecified knee

Ⓖ **M23.31** Other meniscus derangements, anterior horn of medial meniscus

⊟ **M23.311** Other meniscus derangements, anterior horn of medial meniscus, right knee

⊟ **M23.312** Other meniscus derangements, anterior horn of medial meniscus, left knee

⊟ **M23.319** Other meniscus derangements, anterior horn of medial meniscus, unspecified knee

Ⓖ **M23.32** Other meniscus derangements, posterior horn of medial meniscus

⊟ **M23.321** Other meniscus derangements, posterior horn of medial meniscus, right knee

⊟ **M23.322** Other meniscus derangements, posterior horn of medial meniscus, left knee

⊟ **M23.329** Other meniscus derangements, posterior horn of medial meniscus, unspecified knee

Ⓖ **M23.33** Other meniscus derangements, other medial meniscus

⊟ **M23.331** Other meniscus derangements, other medial meniscus, right knee

⊟ **M23.332** Other meniscus derangements, other medial meniscus, left knee

⊟ **M23.339** Other meniscus derangements, other medial meniscus, unspecified knee

Ⓖ **M23.34** Other meniscus derangements, anterior horn of lateral meniscus

⊟ **M23.341** Other meniscus derangements, anterior horn of lateral meniscus, right knee

⊟ **M23.342** Other meniscus derangements, anterior horn of lateral meniscus, left knee

● New ▲ Revised *Manifestation* ❹-❼ Digit Indicators ⊟ Laterality 🅐 Adult (15+ years) 🅜 Maternity (12-55 years) 🅝 Newborn 🅟 Pediatric (0-17 years) ♂ Male ♀ Female
✖ ̶D̶e̶l̶e̶t̶e̶d̶ Unspecified + Additional code

2017 ICD-10-CM Expert for Physicians

© 2017 DecisionHealth

761

◫ M23.349   **Other meniscus derangements, anterior horn of lateral meniscus, unspecified knee**
⑥ M23.35   **Other meniscus derangements, posterior horn of lateral meniscus**
◫ M23.351   **Other meniscus derangements, posterior horn of lateral meniscus, right knee**
◫ M23.352   **Other meniscus derangements, posterior horn of lateral meniscus, left knee**
◫ M23.359   **Other meniscus derangements, posterior horn of lateral meniscus, unspecified knee**
⑥ M23.36   **Other meniscus derangements, other lateral meniscus**
◫ M23.361   **Other meniscus derangements, other lateral meniscus, right knee**
◫ M23.362   **Other meniscus derangements, other lateral meniscus, left knee**
◫ M23.369   **Other meniscus derangements, other lateral meniscus, unspecified knee**
⑤ M23.4   **Loose body in knee**
◫ M23.40   **Loose body in knee, unspecified knee**
◫ M23.41   **Loose body in knee, right knee**
◫ M23.42   **Loose body in knee, left knee**
⑤ M23.5   **Chronic instability of knee**
◫ M23.50   **Chronic instability of knee, unspecified knee**
◫ M23.51   **Chronic instability of knee, right knee**
◫ M23.52   **Chronic instability of knee, left knee**
⑤ M23.6   **Other spontaneous disruption of ligament(s) of knee**
⑥ M23.60   **Other spontaneous disruption of unspecified ligament of knee**
◫ M23.601   **Other spontaneous disruption of unspecified ligament of right knee**
◫ M23.602   **Other spontaneous disruption of unspecified ligament of left knee**
◫ M23.609   **Other spontaneous disruption of unspecified ligament of unspecified knee**
⑥ M23.61   **Other spontaneous disruption of anterior cruciate ligament of knee**
◫ M23.611   **Other spontaneous disruption of anterior cruciate ligament of right knee**
◫ M23.612   **Other spontaneous disruption of anterior cruciate ligament of left knee**
◫ M23.619   **Other spontaneous disruption of anterior cruciate ligament of unspecified knee**
⑥ M23.62   **Other spontaneous disruption of posterior cruciate ligament of knee**
◫ M23.621   **Other spontaneous disruption of posterior cruciate ligament of right knee**
◫ M23.622   **Other spontaneous disruption of posterior cruciate ligament of left knee**
◫ M23.629   **Other spontaneous disruption of posterior cruciate ligament of unspecified knee**
⑥ M23.63   **Other spontaneous disruption of medial collateral ligament of knee**
◫ M23.631   **Other spontaneous disruption of medial collateral ligament of right knee**
◫ M23.632   **Other spontaneous disruption of medial collateral ligament of left knee**
◫ M23.639   **Other spontaneous disruption of medial collateral ligament of unspecified knee**
⑥ M23.64   **Other spontaneous disruption of lateral collateral ligament of knee**
◫ M23.641   **Other spontaneous disruption of lateral collateral ligament of right knee**
◫ M23.642   **Other spontaneous disruption of lateral collateral ligament of left knee**
◫ M23.649   **Other spontaneous disruption of lateral collateral ligament of unspecified knee**
⑥ M23.67   **Other spontaneous disruption of capsular ligament of knee**
◫ M23.671   **Other spontaneous disruption of capsular ligament of right knee**
◫ M23.672   **Other spontaneous disruption of capsular ligament of left knee**
◫ M23.679   **Other spontaneous disruption of capsular ligament of unspecified knee**
⑤ M23.8   **Other internal derangements of knee**
Laxity of ligament of knee
Snapping knee

⑥ M23.8X   **Other internal derangements of knee**
◫ M23.8X1   **Other internal derangements of right knee**
◫ M23.8X2   **Other internal derangements of left knee**
◫ M23.8X9   **Other internal derangements of unspecified knee**
⑤ M23.9   **Unspecified internal derangement of knee**
◫ M23.90   **Unspecified internal derangement of unspecified knee**
◫ M23.91   **Unspecified internal derangement of right knee**
◫ M23.92   **Unspecified internal derangement of left knee**
④ **M24**   **Other specific joint derangements**
   EXCLUDES 1 *current injury - see injury of joint by body region*
   EXCLUDES 2 *ganglion (M67.4)*
   snapping knee (M23.8-)
   temporomandibular joint disorders (M26.6-)
⑤ M24.0   **Loose body in joint**
   EXCLUDES 2 *loose body in knee (M23.4)*
M24.00   **Loose body in unspecified joint**
⑥ M24.01   **Loose body in shoulder**
◫ M24.011   **Loose body in right shoulder**
◫ M24.012   **Loose body in left shoulder**
◫ M24.019   **Loose body in unspecified shoulder**
⑥ M24.02   **Loose body in elbow**
◫ M24.021   **Loose body in right elbow**
◫ M24.022   **Loose body in left elbow**
◫ M24.029   **Loose body in unspecified elbow**
⑥ M24.03   **Loose body in wrist**
◫ M24.031   **Loose body in right wrist**
◫ M24.032   **Loose body in left wrist**
◫ M24.039   **Loose body in unspecified wrist**
⑥ M24.04   **Loose body in finger joints**
◫ M24.041   **Loose body in right finger joint(s)**
◫ M24.042   **Loose body in left finger joint(s)**
◫ M24.049   **Loose body in unspecified finger joint(s)**
⑥ M24.05   **Loose body in hip**
◫ M24.051   **Loose body in right hip**
◫ M24.052   **Loose body in left hip**
◫ M24.059   **Loose body in unspecified hip**
⑥ M24.07   **Loose body in ankle and toe joints**
◫ M24.071   **Loose body in right ankle**
◫ M24.072   **Loose body in left ankle**
◫ M24.073   **Loose body in unspecified ankle**
◫ M24.074   **Loose body in right toe joint(s)**
◫ M24.075   **Loose body in left toe joint(s)**
◫ M24.076   **Loose body in unspecified toe joints**
M24.08   **Loose body, other site**
⑤ M24.1   **Other articular cartilage disorders**
   EXCLUDES 2 *chondrocalcinosis (M11.1, M11.2-)*
   internal derangement of knee (M23.-)
   metastatic calcification (E83.5)
   ochronosis (E70.2)
M24.10   **Other articular cartilage disorders, unspecified site**
⑥ M24.11   **Other articular cartilage disorders, shoulder**
◫ M24.111   **Other articular cartilage disorders, right shoulder**
◫ M24.112   **Other articular cartilage disorders, left shoulder**
◫ M24.119   **Other articular cartilage disorders, unspecified shoulder**
⑥ M24.12   **Other articular cartilage disorders, elbow**
◫ M24.121   **Other articular cartilage disorders, right elbow**
◫ M24.122   **Other articular cartilage disorders, left elbow**
◫ M24.129   **Other articular cartilage disorders, unspecified elbow**
⑥ M24.13   **Other articular cartilage disorders, wrist**
◫ M24.131   **Other articular cartilage disorders, right wrist**
◫ M24.132   **Other articular cartilage disorders, left wrist**
◫ M24.139   **Other articular cartilage disorders, unspecified wrist**
⑥ M24.14   **Other articular cartilage disorders, hand**
◫ M24.141   **Other articular cartilage disorders, right hand**

M24.142   Other articular cartilage disorders, left hand
M24.149   Other articular cartilage disorders, unspecified hand
M24.15   Other articular cartilage disorders, hip
   M24.151   Other articular cartilage disorders, right hip
   M24.152   Other articular cartilage disorders, left hip
   M24.159   Other articular cartilage disorders, unspecified hip
M24.17   Other articular cartilage disorders, ankle and foot
   M24.171   Other articular cartilage disorders, right ankle
   M24.172   Other articular cartilage disorders, left ankle
   M24.173   Other articular cartilage disorders, unspecified ankle
   M24.174   Other articular cartilage disorders, right foot
   M24.175   Other articular cartilage disorders, left foot
   M24.176   Other articular cartilage disorders, unspecified foot

M24.2   Disorder of ligament
Instability secondary to old ligament injury
Ligamentous laxity NOS
> **EXCLUDES 1**   *familial ligamentous laxity (M35.7)*
> **EXCLUDES 2**   *internal derangement of knee (M23.5-M23.89)*

M24.20   Disorder of ligament, unspecified site
M24.21   Disorder of ligament, shoulder
   M24.211   Disorder of ligament, right shoulder
   M24.212   Disorder of ligament, left shoulder
   M24.219   Disorder of ligament, unspecified shoulder
M24.22   Disorder of ligament, elbow
   M24.221   Disorder of ligament, right elbow
   M24.222   Disorder of ligament, left elbow
   M24.229   Disorder of ligament, unspecified elbow
M24.23   Disorder of ligament, wrist
   M24.231   Disorder of ligament, right wrist
   M24.232   Disorder of ligament, left wrist
   M24.239   Disorder of ligament, unspecified wrist
M24.24   Disorder of ligament, hand
   M24.241   Disorder of ligament, right hand
   M24.242   Disorder of ligament, left hand
   M24.249   Disorder of ligament, unspecified hand
M24.25   Disorder of ligament, hip
   M24.251   Disorder of ligament, right hip
   M24.252   Disorder of ligament, left hip
   M24.259   Disorder of ligament, unspecified hip
M24.27   Disorder of ligament, ankle and foot
   M24.271   Disorder of ligament, right ankle
   M24.272   Disorder of ligament, left ankle
   M24.273   Disorder of ligament, unspecified ankle
   M24.274   Disorder of ligament, right foot
   M24.275   Disorder of ligament, left foot
   M24.276   Disorder of ligament, unspecified foot
M24.28   Disorder of ligament, vertebrae

M24.3   Pathological dislocation of joint, not elsewhere classified
> **EXCLUDES 1**   *congenital dislocation or displacement of joint- see congenital malformations and deformations of the musculoskeletal system (Q65-Q79)*
> *current injury - see injury of joints and ligaments by body region*
> *recurrent dislocation of joint (M24.4-)*

M24.30   Pathological dislocation of unspecified joint, not elsewhere classified
M24.31   Pathological dislocation of shoulder, not elsewhere classified
   M24.311   Pathological dislocation of right shoulder, not elsewhere classified
   M24.312   Pathological dislocation of left shoulder, not elsewhere classified
   M24.319   Pathological dislocation of unspecified shoulder, not elsewhere classified
M24.32   Pathological dislocation of elbow, not elsewhere classified
   M24.321   Pathological dislocation of right elbow, not elsewhere classified

M24.322   Pathological dislocation of left elbow, not elsewhere classified
M24.329   Pathological dislocation of unspecified elbow, not elsewhere classified
M24.33   Pathological dislocation of wrist, not elsewhere classified
   M24.331   Pathological dislocation of right wrist, not elsewhere classified
   M24.332   Pathological dislocation of left wrist, not elsewhere classified
   M24.339   Pathological dislocation of unspecified wrist, not elsewhere classified
M24.34   Pathological dislocation of hand, not elsewhere classified
   M24.341   Pathological dislocation of right hand, not elsewhere classified
   M24.342   Pathological dislocation of left hand, not elsewhere classified
   M24.349   Pathological dislocation of unspecified hand, not elsewhere classified
M24.35   Pathological dislocation of hip, not elsewhere classified
   M24.351   Pathological dislocation of right hip, not elsewhere classified
   M24.352   Pathological dislocation of left hip, not elsewhere classified
   M24.359   Pathological dislocation of unspecified hip, not elsewhere classified
M24.36   Pathological dislocation of knee, not elsewhere classified
   M24.361   Pathological dislocation of right knee, not elsewhere classified
   M24.362   Pathological dislocation of left knee, not elsewhere classified
   M24.369   Pathological dislocation of unspecified knee, not elsewhere classified
M24.37   Pathological dislocation of ankle and foot, not elsewhere classified
   M24.371   Pathological dislocation of right ankle, not elsewhere classified
   M24.372   Pathological dislocation of left ankle, not elsewhere classified
   M24.373   Pathological dislocation of unspecified ankle, not elsewhere classified
   M24.374   Pathological dislocation of right foot, not elsewhere classified
   M24.375   Pathological dislocation of left foot, not elsewhere classified
   M24.376   Pathological dislocation of unspecified foot, not elsewhere classified

M24.4   Recurrent dislocation of joint
Recurrent subluxation of joint
> **EXCLUDES 2**   *recurrent dislocation of patella (M22.0-M22.1)*
> *recurrent vertebral dislocation (M43.3-, M43.4, M43.5-)*

M24.40   Recurrent dislocation, unspecified joint
M24.41   Recurrent dislocation, shoulder
   M24.411   Recurrent dislocation, right shoulder
   M24.412   Recurrent dislocation, left shoulder
   M24.419   Recurrent dislocation, unspecified shoulder
M24.42   Recurrent dislocation, elbow
   M24.421   Recurrent dislocation, right elbow
   M24.422   Recurrent dislocation, left elbow
   M24.429   Recurrent dislocation, unspecified elbow
M24.43   Recurrent dislocation, wrist
   M24.431   Recurrent dislocation, right wrist
   M24.432   Recurrent dislocation, left wrist
   M24.439   Recurrent dislocation, unspecified wrist
M24.44   Recurrent dislocation, hand and finger(s)
   M24.441   Recurrent dislocation, right hand
   M24.442   Recurrent dislocation, left hand
   M24.443   Recurrent dislocation, unspecified hand
   M24.444   Recurrent dislocation, right finger
   M24.445   Recurrent dislocation, left finger
   M24.446   Recurrent dislocation, unspecified finger
M24.45   Recurrent dislocation, hip
   M24.451   Recurrent dislocation, right hip

● New   ▲ Revised   *Manifestation*   **4**-**7** Digit Indicators   ▣ Laterality   **A** Adult (15+ years)   **M** Maternity (12-55 years)   **N** Newborn   **P** Pediatric (0-17 years)   ♂ Male   ♀ Female
✖ Deleted   Unspecified   + Additional code

2017 ICD-10-CM Expert for Physicians

© 2017 DecisionHealth

763

⬡ M24.452   Recurrent dislocation, left hip
⬡ M24.459   Recurrent dislocation, unspecified hip
⑥ M24.46   Recurrent dislocation, knee
⬡ M24.461   Recurrent dislocation, right knee
⬡ M24.462   Recurrent dislocation, left knee
⬡ M24.469   Recurrent dislocation, unspecified knee
⑥ M24.47   Recurrent dislocation, ankle, foot and toes
⬡ M24.471   Recurrent dislocation, right ankle
⬡ M24.472   Recurrent dislocation, left ankle
⬡ M24.473   Recurrent dislocation, unspecified ankle
⬡ M24.474   Recurrent dislocation, right foot
⬡ M24.475   Recurrent dislocation, left foot
⬡ M24.476   Recurrent dislocation, unspecified foot
⬡ M24.477   Recurrent dislocation, right toe(s)
⬡ M24.478   Recurrent dislocation, left toe(s)
⬡ M24.479   Recurrent dislocation, unspecified toe(s)
⑤ M24.5   Contracture of joint

EXCLUDES 1	contracture of muscle without contracture of joint (M62.4-)
	contracture of tendon (sheath) without contracture of joint (M62.4-)
	Dupuytren's contracture (M72.0)
EXCLUDES 2	acquired deformities of limbs (M20-M21)

M24.50   Contracture, unspecified joint
⑥ M24.51   Contracture, shoulder
⬡ M24.511   Contracture, right shoulder
⬡ M24.512   Contracture, left shoulder
⬡ M24.519   Contracture, unspecified shoulder
⑥ M24.52   Contracture, elbow
⬡ M24.521   Contracture, right elbow
⬡ M24.522   Contracture, left elbow
⬡ M24.529   Contracture, unspecified elbow
⑥ M24.53   Contracture, wrist
⬡ M24.531   Contracture, right wrist
⬡ M24.532   Contracture, left wrist
⬡ M24.539   Contracture, unspecified wrist
⑥ M24.54   Contracture, hand
⬡ M24.541   Contracture, right hand
⬡ M24.542   Contracture, left hand
⬡ M24.549   Contracture, unspecified hand
⑥ M24.55   Contracture, hip
⬡ M24.551   Contracture, right hip
           AHA: 2Q 2016, 6
⬡ M24.552   Contracture, left hip
           AHA: 2Q 2016, 6
⬡ M24.559   Contracture, unspecified hip
⑥ M24.56   Contracture, knee
⬡ M24.561   Contracture, right knee
           AHA: 2Q 2016, 6
⬡ M24.562   Contracture, left knee
           AHA: 2Q 2016, 6
⬡ M24.569   Contracture, unspecified knee
⑥ M24.57   Contracture, ankle and foot
⬡ M24.571   Contracture, right ankle
⬡ M24.572   Contracture, left ankle
⬡ M24.573   Contracture, unspecified ankle
⬡ M24.574   Contracture, right foot
⬡ M24.575   Contracture, left foot
⬡ M24.576   Contracture, unspecified foot
⑤ M24.6   Ankylosis of joint

| EXCLUDES 1 | stiffness of joint without ankylosis (M25.6-) |
| EXCLUDES 2 | spine (M43.2-) |

M24.60   Ankylosis, unspecified joint
⑥ M24.61   Ankylosis, shoulder
⬡ M24.611   Ankylosis, right shoulder
⬡ M24.612   Ankylosis, left shoulder
⬡ M24.619   Ankylosis, unspecified shoulder
⑥ M24.62   Ankylosis, elbow
⬡ M24.621   Ankylosis, right elbow
⬡ M24.622   Ankylosis, left elbow
⬡ M24.629   Ankylosis, unspecified elbow

⑥ M24.63   Ankylosis, wrist
⬡ M24.631   Ankylosis, right wrist
⬡ M24.632   Ankylosis, left wrist
⬡ M24.639   Ankylosis, unspecified wrist
⑥ M24.64   Ankylosis, hand
⬡ M24.641   Ankylosis, right hand
⬡ M24.642   Ankylosis, left hand
⬡ M24.649   Ankylosis, unspecified hand
⑥ M24.65   Ankylosis, hip
⬡ M24.651   Ankylosis, right hip
⬡ M24.652   Ankylosis, left hip
⬡ M24.659   Ankylosis, unspecified hip
⑥ M24.66   Ankylosis, knee
⬡ M24.661   Ankylosis, right knee
⬡ M24.662   Ankylosis, left knee
⬡ M24.669   Ankylosis, unspecified knee
⑥ M24.67   Ankylosis, ankle and foot
⬡ M24.671   Ankylosis, right ankle
⬡ M24.672   Ankylosis, left ankle
⬡ M24.673   Ankylosis, unspecified ankle
⬡ M24.674   Ankylosis, right foot
⬡ M24.675   Ankylosis, left foot
⬡ M24.676   Ankylosis, unspecified foot
M24.7   Protrusio acetabuli
⑤ M24.8   Other specific joint derangements, not elsewhere classified

| EXCLUDES 2 | iliotibial band syndrome (M76.3) |

M24.80   Other specific joint derangements of unspecified joint, not elsewhere classified
⑥ M24.81   Other specific joint derangements of shoulder, not elsewhere classified
⬡ M24.811   Other specific joint derangements of right shoulder, not elsewhere classified
⬡ M24.812   Other specific joint derangements of left shoulder, not elsewhere classified
⬡ M24.819   Other specific joint derangements of unspecified shoulder, not elsewhere classified
⑥ M24.82   Other specific joint derangements of elbow, not elsewhere classified
⬡ M24.821   Other specific joint derangements of right elbow, not elsewhere classified
⬡ M24.822   Other specific joint derangements of left elbow, not elsewhere classified
⬡ M24.829   Other specific joint derangements of unspecified elbow, not elsewhere classified
⑥ M24.83   Other specific joint derangements of wrist, not elsewhere classified
⬡ M24.831   Other specific joint derangements of right wrist, not elsewhere classified
⬡ M24.832   Other specific joint derangements of left wrist, not elsewhere classified
⬡ M24.839   Other specific joint derangements of unspecified wrist, not elsewhere classified
⑥ M24.84   Other specific joint derangements of hand, not elsewhere classified
⬡ M24.841   Other specific joint derangements of right hand, not elsewhere classified
⬡ M24.842   Other specific joint derangements of left hand, not elsewhere classified
⬡ M24.849   Other specific joint derangements of unspecified hand, not elsewhere classified
⑥ M24.85   Other specific joint derangements of hip, not elsewhere classified
           Irritable hip
⬡ M24.851   Other specific joint derangements of right hip, not elsewhere classified
⬡ M24.852   Other specific joint derangements of left hip, not elsewhere classified
⬡ M24.859   Other specific joint derangements of unspecified hip, not elsewhere classified
⑥ M24.87   Other specific joint derangements of ankle and foot, not elsewhere classified
⬡ M24.871   Other specific joint derangements of right ankle, not elsewhere classified
⬡ M24.872   Other specific joint derangements of left ankle, not elsewhere classified

● New   ▲ Revised   *Manifestation*   ④-⑦ Digit Indicators   ⊟ Laterality   Ⓐ Adult (15+ years)   Ⓜ Maternity (12-55 years)   Ⓝ Newborn   Ⓟ Pediatric (0-17 years)   ♂ Male   ♀ Female
✖ Deleted   Unspecified   ✚ Additional code

764   © 2017 DecisionHealth   2017 ICD-10-CM Expert for Physicians

⊟ M24.873 Other specific joint derangements of unspecified ankle, not elsewhere classified
⊟ M24.874 Other specific joint derangements of right foot, not elsewhere classified
⊟ M24.875 Other specific joint derangements left foot, not elsewhere classified
⊟ M24.876 Other specific joint derangements of unspecified foot, not elsewhere classified

M24.9 Joint derangement, unspecified

▣ M25 Other joint disorder, not elsewhere classified

> EXCLUDES 2 *abnormality of gait and mobility (R26.-)*
> *acquired deformities of limb (M20-M21)*
> *calcification of bursa (M71.4-)*
> *calcification of shoulder (joint) (M75.3)*
> *calcification of tendon (M65.2-)*
> *difficulty in walking (R26.2)*
> *temporomandibular joint disorder (M26.6-)*

⑤ M25.0 Hemarthrosis

> EXCLUDES 1 *current injury - see injury of joint by body region*
> *hemophilic arthropathy (M36.2)*

M25.00 Hemarthrosis, unspecified joint
⑥ M25.01 Hemarthrosis, shoulder
⊟ M25.011 Hemarthrosis, right shoulder
⊟ M25.012 Hemarthrosis, left shoulder
⊟ M25.019 Hemarthrosis, unspecified shoulder
⑥ M25.02 Hemarthrosis, elbow
⊟ M25.021 Hemarthrosis, right elbow
⊟ M25.022 Hemarthrosis, left elbow
⊟ M25.029 Hemarthrosis, unspecified elbow
⑥ M25.03 Hemarthrosis, wrist
⊟ M25.031 Hemarthrosis, right wrist
⊟ M25.032 Hemarthrosis, left wrist
⊟ M25.039 Hemarthrosis, unspecified wrist
⑥ M25.04 Hemarthrosis, hand
⊟ M25.041 Hemarthrosis, right hand
⊟ M25.042 Hemarthrosis, left hand
⊟ M25.049 Hemarthrosis, unspecified hand
⑥ M25.05 Hemarthrosis, hip
⊟ M25.051 Hemarthrosis, right hip
⊟ M25.052 Hemarthrosis, left hip
⊟ M25.059 Hemarthrosis, unspecified hip
⑥ M25.06 Hemarthrosis, knee
⊟ M25.061 Hemarthrosis, right knee
⊟ M25.062 Hemarthrosis, left knee
⊟ M25.069 Hemarthrosis, unspecified knee
⑥ M25.07 Hemarthrosis, ankle and foot
⊟ M25.071 Hemarthrosis, right ankle
⊟ M25.072 Hemarthrosis, left ankle
⊟ M25.073 Hemarthrosis, unspecified ankle
⊟ M25.074 Hemarthrosis, right foot
⊟ M25.075 Hemarthrosis, left foot
⊟ M25.076 Hemarthrosis, unspecified foot
M25.08 Hemarthrosis, other specified site
Hemarthrosis, vertebrae
⑤ M25.1 Fistula of joint
M25.10 Fistula, unspecified joint
⑥ M25.11 Fistula, shoulder
⊟ M25.111 Fistula, right shoulder
⊟ M25.112 Fistula, left shoulder
⊟ M25.119 Fistula, unspecified shoulder
⑥ M25.12 Fistula, elbow
⊟ M25.121 Fistula, right elbow
⊟ M25.122 Fistula, left elbow
⊟ M25.129 Fistula, unspecified elbow
⑥ M25.13 Fistula, wrist
⊟ M25.131 Fistula, right wrist
⊟ M25.132 Fistula, left wrist
⊟ M25.139 Fistula, unspecified wrist
⑥ M25.14 Fistula, hand
⊟ M25.141 Fistula, right hand

⊟ M25.142 Fistula, left hand
⊟ M25.149 Fistula, unspecified hand
⑥ M25.15 Fistula, hip
⊟ M25.151 Fistula, right hip
⊟ M25.152 Fistula, left hip
⊟ M25.159 Fistula, unspecified hip
⑥ M25.16 Fistula, knee
⊟ M25.161 Fistula, right knee
⊟ M25.162 Fistula, left knee
⊟ M25.169 Fistula, unspecified knee
⑥ M25.17 Fistula, ankle and foot
⊟ M25.171 Fistula, right ankle
⊟ M25.172 Fistula, left ankle
⊟ M25.173 Fistula, unspecified ankle
⊟ M25.174 Fistula, right foot
⊟ M25.175 Fistula, left foot
⊟ M25.176 Fistula, unspecified foot
M25.18 Fistula, other specified site
Fistula, vertebrae
⑤ M25.2 Flail joint
M25.20 Flail joint, unspecified joint
⑥ M25.21 Flail joint, shoulder
⊟ M25.211 Flail joint, right shoulder
⊟ M25.212 Flail joint, left shoulder
⊟ M25.219 Flail joint, unspecified shoulder
⑥ M25.22 Flail joint, elbow
⊟ M25.221 Flail joint, right elbow
⊟ M25.222 Flail joint, left elbow
⊟ M25.229 Flail joint, unspecified elbow
⑥ M25.23 Flail joint, wrist
⊟ M25.231 Flail joint, right wrist
⊟ M25.232 Flail joint, left wrist
⊟ M25.239 Flail joint, unspecified wrist
⑥ M25.24 Flail joint, hand
⊟ M25.241 Flail joint, right hand
⊟ M25.242 Flail joint, left hand
⊟ M25.249 Flail joint, unspecified hand
⑥ M25.25 Flail joint, hip
⊟ M25.251 Flail joint, right hip
⊟ M25.252 Flail joint, left hip
⊟ M25.259 Flail joint, unspecified hip
⑥ M25.26 Flail joint, knee
⊟ M25.261 Flail joint, right knee
⊟ M25.262 Flail joint, left knee
⊟ M25.269 Flail joint, unspecified knee
⑥ M25.27 Flail joint, ankle and foot
⊟ M25.271 Flail joint, right ankle and foot
⊟ M25.272 Flail joint, left ankle and foot
⊟ M25.279 Flail joint, unspecified ankle and foot
M25.28 Flail joint, other site
⑤ M25.3 Other instability of joint

> EXCLUDES 1 *instability of joint secondary to old ligament injury (M24.2-)*
> *instability of joint secondary to removal of joint prosthesis (M96.8-)*
> EXCLUDES 2 *spinal instabilities (M53.2-)*

M25.30 Other instability, unspecified joint
⑥ M25.31 Other instability, shoulder
⊟ M25.311 Other instability, right shoulder
⊟ M25.312 Other instability, left shoulder
⊟ M25.319 Other instability, unspecified shoulder
⑥ M25.32 Other instability, elbow
⊟ M25.321 Other instability, right elbow
⊟ M25.322 Other instability, left elbow
⊟ M25.329 Other instability, unspecified elbow
⑥ M25.33 Other instability, wrist
⊟ M25.331 Other instability, right wrist
⊟ M25.332 Other instability, left wrist
⊟ M25.339 Other instability, unspecified wrist
⑥ M25.34 Other instability, hand
⊟ M25.341 Other instability, right hand
⊟ M25.342 Other instability, left hand

● New ▲ Revised *Manifestation* ▣-▓ Digit Indicators ⊟ Laterality Ⓐ Adult (15+ years) Ⓜ Maternity (12-55 years) Ⓝ Newborn Ⓟ Pediatric (0-17 years) ♂ Male ♀ Female
✖ Deleted Unspecified + Additional code

2017 ICD-10-CM Expert for Physicians

© 2017 DecisionHealth

765

   ⊟ **M25.349**   Other instability, unspecified hand

🄶 **M25.35**   Other instability, hip
   ⊟ **M25.351**   Other instability, right hip
   ⊟ **M25.352**   Other instability, left hip
   ⊟ **M25.359**   Other instability, unspecified hip

🄶 **M25.36**   Other instability, knee
   ⊟ **M25.361**   Other instability, right knee
   ⊟ **M25.362**   Other instability, left knee
   ⊟ **M25.369**   Other instability, unspecified knee

🄶 **M25.37**   Other instability, ankle and foot
   ⊟ **M25.371**   Other instability, right ankle
   ⊟ **M25.372**   Other instability, left ankle
   ⊟ **M25.373**   Other instability, unspecified ankle
   ⊟ **M25.374**   Other instability, right foot
   ⊟ **M25.375**   Other instability, left foot
   ⊟ **M25.376**   Other instability, unspecified foot

🄢 **M25.4**   Effusion of joint
   EXCLUDES 1   *hydrarthrosis in yaws (A66.6)*
      intermittent hydrarthrosis (M12.4-)
      other infective (teno) synovitis (M65.1-)

  M25.40   Effusion, unspecified joint

🄶 **M25.41**   Effusion, shoulder
   ⊟ **M25.411**   Effusion, right shoulder
   ⊟ **M25.412**   Effusion, left shoulder
   ⊟ **M25.419**   Effusion, unspecified shoulder

🄶 **M25.42**   Effusion, elbow
   ⊟ **M25.421**   Effusion, right elbow
   ⊟ **M25.422**   Effusion, left elbow
   ⊟ **M25.429**   Effusion, unspecified elbow

🄶 **M25.43**   Effusion, wrist
   ⊟ **M25.431**   Effusion, right wrist
   ⊟ **M25.432**   Effusion, left wrist
   ⊟ **M25.439**   Effusion, unspecified wrist

🄶 **M25.44**   Effusion, hand
   ⊟ **M25.441**   Effusion, right hand
   ⊟ **M25.442**   Effusion, left hand
   ⊟ **M25.449**   Effusion, unspecified hand

🄶 **M25.45**   Effusion, hip
   ⊟ **M25.451**   Effusion, right hip
   ⊟ **M25.452**   Effusion, left hip
   ⊟ **M25.459**   Effusion, unspecified hip

🄶 **M25.46**   Effusion, knee
   ⊟ **M25.461**   Effusion, right knee
   ⊟ **M25.462**   Effusion, left knee
   ⊟ **M25.469**   Effusion, unspecified knee

🄶 **M25.47**   Effusion, ankle and foot
   ⊟ **M25.471**   Effusion, right ankle
   ⊟ **M25.472**   Effusion, left ankle
   ⊟ **M25.473**   Effusion, unspecified ankle
   ⊟ **M25.474**   Effusion, right foot
   ⊟ **M25.475**   Effusion, left foot
   ⊟ **M25.476**   Effusion, unspecified foot

  M25.48   Effusion, other site

🄢 **M25.5**   Pain in joint
   EXCLUDES 2   *pain in hand (M79.64-)*
      pain in fingers (M79.64-)
      pain in foot (M79.67-)
      pain in limb (M79.6-)
      pain in toes (M79.67-)

  M25.50   Pain in unspecified joint

🄶 **M25.51**   Pain in shoulder
   ⊟ **M25.511**   Pain in right shoulder
   ⊟ **M25.512**   Pain in left shoulder
   ⊟ **M25.519**   Pain in unspecified shoulder

🄶 **M25.52**   Pain in elbow
   ⊟ **M25.521**   Pain in right elbow
   ⊟ **M25.522**   Pain in left elbow
   ⊟ **M25.529**   Pain in unspecified elbow

🄶 **M25.53**   Pain in wrist
   ⊟ **M25.531**   Pain in right wrist
   ⊟ **M25.532**   Pain in left wrist
   ⊟ **M25.539**   Pain in unspecified wrist

● 🄶 **M25.54**   Pain in joints of hand

● ⊟ **M25.541**   Pain in joints of right hand
● ⊟ **M25.542**   Pain in joints of left hand
● ⊟ **M25.549**   Pain in joints of unspecified hand
      Pain in joints of hand NOS

🄶 **M25.55**   Pain in hip
   ⊟ **M25.551**   Pain in right hip
   ⊟ **M25.552**   Pain in left hip
   ⊟ **M25.559**   Pain in unspecified hip

🄶 **M25.56**   Pain in knee
   ⊟ **M25.561**   Pain in right knee
   ⊟ **M25.562**   Pain in left knee
   ⊟ **M25.569**   Pain in unspecified knee

🄶 **M25.57**   Pain in ankle and joints of foot
   ⊟ **M25.571**   Pain in right ankle and joints of right foot
   ⊟ **M25.572**   Pain in left ankle and joints of left foot
   ⊟ **M25.579**   Pain in unspecified ankle and joints of unspecified foot

🄢 **M25.6**   Stiffness of joint, not elsewhere classified
   EXCLUDES 1   *ankylosis of joint (M24.6-)*
      contracture of joint (M24.5-)

  M25.60   Stiffness of unspecified joint, not elsewhere classified

🄶 **M25.61**   Stiffness of shoulder, not elsewhere classified
   ⊟ **M25.611**   Stiffness of right shoulder, not elsewhere classified
   ⊟ **M25.612**   Stiffness of left shoulder, not elsewhere classified
   ⊟ **M25.619**   Stiffness of unspecified shoulder, not elsewhere classified

🄶 **M25.62**   Stiffness of elbow, not elsewhere classified
   ⊟ **M25.621**   Stiffness of right elbow, not elsewhere classified
   ⊟ **M25.622**   Stiffness of left elbow, not elsewhere classified
   ⊟ **M25.629**   Stiffness of unspecified elbow, not elsewhere classified

🄶 **M25.63**   Stiffness of wrist, not elsewhere classified
   ⊟ **M25.631**   Stiffness of right wrist, not elsewhere classified
   ⊟ **M25.632**   Stiffness of left wrist, not elsewhere classified
   ⊟ **M25.639**   Stiffness of unspecified wrist, not elsewhere classified

🄶 **M25.64**   Stiffness of hand, not elsewhere classified
   ⊟ **M25.641**   Stiffness of right hand, not elsewhere classified
   ⊟ **M25.642**   Stiffness of left hand, not elsewhere classified
   ⊟ **M25.649**   Stiffness of unspecified hand, not elsewhere classified

🄶 **M25.65**   Stiffness of hip, not elsewhere classified
   ⊟ **M25.651**   Stiffness of right hip, not elsewhere classified
   ⊟ **M25.652**   Stiffness of left hip, not elsewhere classified
   ⊟ **M25.659**   Stiffness of unspecified hip, not elsewhere classified

🄶 **M25.66**   Stiffness of knee, not elsewhere classified
   ⊟ **M25.661**   Stiffness of right knee, not elsewhere classified
   ⊟ **M25.662**   Stiffness of left knee, not elsewhere classified
   ⊟ **M25.669**   Stiffness of unspecified knee, not elsewhere classified

🄶 **M25.67**   Stiffness of ankle and foot, not elsewhere classified
   ⊟ **M25.671**   Stiffness of right ankle, not elsewhere classified
   ⊟ **M25.672**   Stiffness of left ankle, not elsewhere classified
   ⊟ **M25.673**   Stiffness of unspecified ankle, not elsewhere classified
   ⊟ **M25.674**   Stiffness of right foot, not elsewhere classified
   ⊟ **M25.675**   Stiffness of left foot, not elsewhere classified
   ⊟ **M25.676**   Stiffness of unspecified foot, not elsewhere classified

🄢 **M25.7**   Osteophyte
  M25.70   Osteophyte, unspecified joint

🄶 **M25.71**   Osteophyte, shoulder
   ⊟ **M25.711**   Osteophyte, right shoulder
   ⊟ **M25.712**   Osteophyte, left shoulder
   ⊟ **M25.719**   Osteophyte, unspecified shoulder

🄶 **M25.72**   Osteophyte, elbow
   ⊟ **M25.721**   Osteophyte, right elbow
   ⊟ **M25.722**   Osteophyte, left elbow
   ⊟ **M25.729**   Osteophyte, unspecified elbow

🄶 **M25.73**   Osteophyte, wrist
   ⊟ **M25.731**   Osteophyte, right wrist

● New   ▲ Revised   *Manifestation*   🄸-🄻 Digit Indicators   ⊟ Laterality   Ⓐ Adult (15+ years)   Ⓜ Maternity (12-55 years)   Ⓝ Newborn   Ⓟ Pediatric (0-17 years)   ♂ Male   ♀ Female
✖ Deleted   Unspecified   + Additional code

766   © 2017 DecisionHealth   2017 ICD-10-CM Expert for Physicians

⊟ M25.732   Osteophyte, left wrist
⊟ M25.739   Osteophyte, unspecified wrist
ⓖ M25.74   Osteophyte, hand
⊟ M25.741   Osteophyte, right hand
⊟ M25.742   Osteophyte, left hand
⊟ M25.749   Osteophyte, unspecified hand
ⓖ M25.75   Osteophyte, hip
⊟ M25.751   Osteophyte, right hip
⊟ M25.752   Osteophyte, left hip
⊟ M25.759   Osteophyte, unspecified hip
ⓖ M25.76   Osteophyte, knee
⊟ M25.761   Osteophyte, right knee
⊟ M25.762   Osteophyte, left knee
⊟ M25.769   Osteophyte, unspecified knee
ⓖ M25.77   Osteophyte, ankle and foot
⊟ M25.771   Osteophyte, right ankle
⊟ M25.772   Osteophyte, left ankle
⊟ M25.773   Osteophyte, unspecified ankle
⊟ M25.774   Osteophyte, right foot
⊟ M25.775   Osteophyte, left foot
⊟ M25.776   Osteophyte, unspecified foot
M25.78   Osteophyte, vertebrae
ⓢ M25.8   Other specified joint disorders
M25.80   Other specified joint disorders, unspecified joint
ⓖ M25.81   Other specified joint disorders, shoulder
⊟ M25.811   Other specified joint disorders, right shoulder
⊟ M25.812   Other specified joint disorders, left shoulder
⊟ M25.819   Other specified joint disorders, unspecified shoulder
ⓖ M25.82   Other specified joint disorders, elbow
⊟ M25.821   Other specified joint disorders, right elbow
⊟ M25.822   Other specified joint disorders, left elbow
⊟ M25.829   Other specified joint disorders, unspecified elbow
ⓖ M25.83   Other specified joint disorders, wrist
⊟ M25.831   Other specified joint disorders, right wrist
⊟ M25.832   Other specified joint disorders, left wrist
⊟ M25.839   Other specified joint disorders, unspecified wrist
ⓖ M25.84   Other specified joint disorders, hand
⊟ M25.841   Other specified joint disorders, right hand
⊟ M25.842   Other specified joint disorders, left hand
⊟ M25.849   Other specified joint disorders, unspecified hand
ⓖ M25.85   Other specified joint disorders, hip
⊟ M25.851   Other specified joint disorders, right hip
⊟ M25.852   Other specified joint disorders, left hip
AHA: 4Q 2014, 25
⊟ M25.859   Other specified joint disorders, unspecified hip
ⓖ M25.86   Other specified joint disorders, knee
⊟ M25.861   Other specified joint disorders, right knee
⊟ M25.862   Other specified joint disorders, left knee
⊟ M25.869   Other specified joint disorders, unspecified knee
ⓖ M25.87   Other specified joint disorders, ankle and foot
⊟ M25.871   Other specified joint disorders, right ankle and foot
⊟ M25.872   Other specified joint disorders, left ankle and foot
⊟ M25.879   Other specified joint disorders, unspecified ankle and foot
M25.9   Joint disorder, unspecified

Dentofacial anomalies [including malocclusion] and other disorders of jaw (M26-M27)

⋄ EXCLUDES 1   *hemifacial atrophy or hypertrophy (Q67.4)*
unilateral condylar hyperplasia or hypoplasia (M27.8)
❹ M26   Dentofacial anomalies [including malocclusion]
ⓢ M26.0   Major anomalies of jaw size
EXCLUDES 1   *acromegaly (E22.0)*
Robin's syndrome (Q87.0)
M26.00   Unspecified anomaly of jaw size

M26.01   Maxillary hyperplasia
M26.02   Maxillary hypoplasia
AHA: 3Q 2014, 23
M26.03   Mandibular hyperplasia

Mandibular hyperplasia

Overdevelopment of the lower jaw

M26.04   Mandibular hypoplasia
M26.05   Macrogenia
    DEFINITION   Abnormally large chin.
M26.06   Microgenia
M26.07   Excessive tuberosity of jaw
    Entire maxillary tuberosity
M26.09   Other specified anomalies of jaw size
ⓢ M26.1   Anomalies of jaw-cranial base relationship
M26.10   Unspecified anomaly of jaw-cranial base relationship
M26.11   Maxillary asymmetry
M26.12   Other jaw asymmetry
M26.19   Other specified anomalies of jaw-cranial base relationship
ⓢ M26.2   Anomalies of dental arch relationship
M26.20   Unspecified anomaly of dental arch relationship
ⓖ M26.21   Malocclusion, Angle's class
M26.211   Malocclusion, Angle's class I
    Neutro-occlusion

Malocclusion, Angle's Class 1

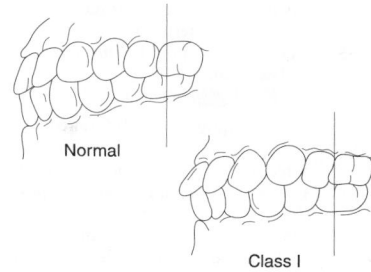

Normal

Class I

M26.212   Malocclusion, Angle's class II
    Disto-occlusion Division I
    Disto-occlusion Division II
M26.213   Malocclusion, Angle's class III
    Mesio-occlusion
M26.219   Malocclusion, Angle's class, unspecified
ⓖ M26.22   Open occlusal relationship
M26.220   Open anterior occlusal relationship
    Anterior openbite
M26.221   Open posterior occlusal relationship
    Posterior openbite
M26.23   Excessive horizontal overlap
    Excessive horizontal overjet
M26.24   Reverse articulation
    Crossbite (anterior) (posterior)
M26.25   Anomalies of interarch distance

● New   ▲ Revised   *Manifestation*   ❹-❼ Digit Indicators   ⊟ Laterality   Ⓐ Adult (15+ years)   Ⓜ Maternity (12-55 years)   Ⓝ Newborn   Ⓟ Pediatric (0-17 years)   ♂ Male   ♀ Female
✖ Deleted   Unspecified   + Additional code

2017 ICD-10-CM Expert for Physicians

© 2017 DecisionHealth

767

M26.29   **Other anomalies of dental arch relationship**
Midline deviation of dental arch
Overbite (excessive) deep
Overbite (excessive) horizontal
Overbite (excessive) vertical
Posterior lingual occlusion of mandibular teeth

☑ **M26.3**   **Anomalies of tooth position of fully erupted tooth or teeth**
> **EXCLUDES 2**   *embedded and impacted teeth (K01.-)*

M26.30   **Unspecified anomaly of tooth position of fully erupted tooth or teeth**
Abnormal spacing of fully erupted tooth or teeth NOS
Displacement of fully erupted tooth or teeth NOS
Transposition of fully erupted tooth or teeth NOS

M26.31   **Crowding of fully erupted teeth**

M26.32   **Excessive spacing of fully erupted teeth**
Diastema of fully erupted tooth or teeth NOS

M26.33   **Horizontal displacement of fully erupted tooth or teeth**
Tipped tooth or teeth
Tipping of fully erupted tooth

M26.34   **Vertical displacement of fully erupted tooth or teeth**
Extruded tooth
Infraeruption of tooth or teeth
Supraeruption of tooth or teeth

M26.35   **Rotation of fully erupted tooth or teeth**

M26.36   **Insufficient interocclusal distance of fully erupted teeth (ridge)**
Lack of adequate intermaxillary vertical dimension of fully erupted teeth

M26.37   **Excessive interocclusal distance of fully erupted teeth**
Excessive intermaxillary vertical dimension of fully erupted teeth
Loss of occlusal vertical dimension of fully erupted teeth

M26.39   **Other anomalies of tooth position of fully erupted tooth or teeth**

M26.4   **Malocclusion, unspecified**

☑ **M26.5**   **Dentofacial functional abnormalities**
> **EXCLUDES 1**   *bruxism (F45.8)*
> *teeth-grinding NOS (F45.8)*

M26.50   **Dentofacial functional abnormalities, unspecified**

M26.51   **Abnormal jaw closure**

M26.52   **Limited mandibular range of motion**

M26.53   **Deviation in opening and closing of the mandible**

M26.54   **Insufficient anterior guidance**
Insufficient anterior occlusal guidance

M26.55   **Centric occlusion maximum intercuspation discrepancy**
> **EXCLUDES 1**   *centric occlusion NOS (M26.59)*

M26.56   **Non-working side interference**
Balancing side interference

M26.57   **Lack of posterior occlusal support**

M26.59   **Other dentofacial functional abnormalities**
Centric occlusion (of teeth) NOS
Malocclusion due to abnormal swallowing
Malocclusion due to mouth breathing
Malocclusion due to tongue, lip or finger habits

☑ **M26.6**   **Temporomandibular joint disorders**
> **EXCLUDES 2**   *current temporomandibular joint dislocation (S03.0)*
> *current temporomandibular joint sprain (S03.4)*

▲ ☑ **M26.60**   **Temporomandibular joint disorder, unspecified**

● ☐ **M26.601**   **Right temporomandibular joint disorder, unspecified**

● ☐ **M26.602**   **Left temporomandibular joint disorder, unspecified**

● ☐ **M26.603**   **Bilateral temporomandibular joint disorder, unspecified**

● ☐ **M26.609**   **Unspecified temporomandibular joint disorder, unspecified side**
Temporomandibular joint disorder NOS

▲ ☑ **M26.61**   **Adhesions and ankylosis of temporomandibular joint**

● ☐ **M26.611**   **Adhesions and ankylosis of right temporomandibular joint**

● ☐ **M26.612**   **Adhesions and ankylosis of left temporomandibular joint**

● ☐ **M26.613**   **Adhesions and ankylosis of bilateral temporomandibular joint**

● ☐ **M26.619**   **Adhesions and ankylosis of temporomandibular joint, unspecified side**

▲ ☑ **M26.62**   **Arthralgia of temporomandibular joint**

Arthralgia of temporomandibular joint

Pain, redness, swelling, and/or stiffness of the joint may accompany temporomandibular arthralgia

● ☐ **M26.621**   **Arthralgia of right temporomandibular joint**

● ☐ **M26.622**   **Arthralgia of left temporomandibular joint**

● ☐ **M26.623**   **Arthralgia of bilateral temporomandibular joint**

● ☐ **M26.629**   **Arthralgia of temporomandibular joint, unspecified side**

▲ ☑ **M26.63**   **Articular disc disorder of temporomandibular joint**

● ☐ **M26.631**   **Articular disc disorder of right temporomandibular joint**

● ☐ **M26.632**   **Articular disc disorder of left temporomandibular joint**

● ☐ **M26.633**   **Articular disc disorder of bilateral temporomandibular joint**

● ☐ **M26.639**   **Articular disc disorder of temporomandibular joint, unspecified side**

M26.69   **Other specified disorders of temporomandibular joint**

☑ **M26.7**   **Dental alveolar anomalies**

M26.70   **Unspecified alveolar anomaly**

M26.71   **Alveolar maxillary hyperplasia**

M26.72   **Alveolar mandibular hyperplasia**

M26.73   **Alveolar maxillary hypoplasia**

M26.74   **Alveolar mandibular hypoplasia**

M26.79   **Other specified alveolar anomalies**

☑ **M26.8**   **Other dentofacial anomalies**

M26.81   **Anterior soft tissue impingement**
Anterior soft tissue impingement on teeth

M26.82   **Posterior soft tissue impingement**
Posterior soft tissue impingement on teeth

M26.89   **Other dentofacial anomalies**

M26.9   **Dentofacial anomaly, unspecified**

☑ **M27**   **Other diseases of jaws**

M27.0   **Developmental disorders of jaws**
Latent bone cyst of jaw
Stafne's cyst
Torus mandibularis
Torus palatinus

M27.1   **Giant cell granuloma, central**
Giant cell granuloma NOS
> **EXCLUDES 1**   *peripheral giant cell granuloma (K06.8)*

✚ **M27.2**   **Inflammatory conditions of jaws**
Osteitis of jaw(s)
Osteomyelitis (neonatal) jaw(s)
Osteoradionecrosis jaw(s)
Periostitis jaw(s)
Sequestrum of jaw bone
Use additional code (W88-W90, X39.0) to identify radiation, if radiation-induced
> **EXCLUDES 2**   *osteonecrosis of jaw due to drug (M87.180)*

M27.3   **Alveolitis of jaws**
Alveolar osteitis
Dry socket
> **DEFINITION**   Inflammation of the tooth sockets.

● New   ▲ Revised   *Manifestation*   ☐-☐ Digit Indicators   ☐ Laterality   Ⓐ Adult (15+ years)   Ⓜ Maternity (12-55 years)   Ⓝ Newborn   Ⓟ Pediatric (0-17 years)   ♂ Male   ♀ Female

✖ Deleted   Unspecified   ✚ Additional code

⑤ **M27.4   Other and unspecified cysts of jaw**

> **EXCLUDES 1** *cysts of oral region (K09.-)*
> *latent bone cyst of jaw (M27.0)*
> *Stafne's cyst (M27.0)*

M27.40   Unspecified cyst of jaw
Cyst of jaw NOS

M27.49   Other cysts of jaw
Aneurysmal cyst of jaw
Hemorrhagic cyst of jaw
Traumatic cyst of jaw

⑤ **M27.5   Periradicular pathology associated with previous endodontic treatment**

M27.51   Perforation of root canal space due to endodontic treatment

M27.52   Endodontic overfill

M27.53   Endodontic underfill

M27.59   Other periradicular pathology associated with previous endodontic treatment

⑤ **M27.6   Endosseous dental implant failure**

M27.61   Osseointegration failure of dental implant
Hemorrhagic complications of dental implant placement
Iatrogenic osseointegration failure of dental implant
Osseointegration failure of dental implant due to complications of systemic disease
Osseointegration failure of dental implant due to poor bone quality
Pre-integration failure of dental implant NOS
Pre-osseointegration failure of dental implant

M27.62   Post-osseointegration biological failure of dental implant
Failure of dental implant due to lack of attached gingiva
Failure of dental implant due to occlusal trauma (caused by poor prosthetic design)
Failure of dental implant due to parafunctional habits
Failure of dental implant due to periodontal infection (peri-implantitis)
Failure of dental implant due to poor oral hygiene
Iatrogenic post-osseointegration failure of dental implant
Post-osseointegration failure of dental implant due to complications of systemic disease

M27.63   Post-osseointegration mechanical failure of dental implant
Failure of dental prosthesis causing loss of dental implant
Fracture of dental implant

> **EXCLUDES 2** *cracked tooth (K03.81)*
> *fractured dental restorative material with loss of material (K08.531)*
> *fractured dental restorative material without loss of material (K08.530)*
> *fractured tooth (S02.5)*

M27.69   Other endosseous dental implant failure
Dental implant failure NOS

M27.8   Other specified diseases of jaws
Cherubism
Exostosis
Fibrous dysplasia
Unilateral condylar hyperplasia
Unilateral condylar hypoplasia

> **EXCLUDES 1** *jaw pain (R68.84)*

M27.9   Disease of jaws, unspecified

Systemic connective tissue disorders (M30-M36)

> **INCLUDES** autoimmune disease NOS
> collagen (vascular) disease NOS
> systemic autoimmune disease
> systemic collagen (vascular) disease

> **EXCLUDES 1** *autoimmune disease, single organ or single cell-type -code to relevant condition category*

④ **M30   Polyarteritis nodosa and related conditions**

> **EXCLUDES 1** *microscopic polyarteritis (M31.7)*

M30.0   Polyarteritis nodosa

> **DEFINITION** The body's immune system mistakenly attacks small and medium-sized blood vessels, resulting in tissue death.

M30.1   Polyarteritis with lung involvement [Churg-Strauss]
Allergic granulomatous angiitis

M30.2   Juvenile polyarteritis

M30.3   Mucocutaneous lymph node syndrome [Kawasaki]

M30.8   Other conditions related to polyarteritis nodosa
Polyangiitis overlap syndrome

④ **M31   Other necrotizing vasculopathies**

M31.0   Hypersensitivity angiitis
Goodpasture's syndrome

M31.1   Thrombotic microangiopathy
Thrombotic thrombocytopenic purpura

M31.2   Lethal midline granuloma

> **DEFINITION** Tumor associated with infection that appears in the nose or sinuses that may be fatal if not diagnosed and treated in time.

⑤ **M31.3   Wegener's granulomatosis**
Necrotizing respiratory granulomatosis

M31.30   Wegener's granulomatosis without renal involvement
Wegener's granulomatosis NOS

M31.31   Wegener's granulomatosis with renal involvement

M31.4   Aortic arch syndrome [Takayasu]

M31.5   Giant cell arteritis with polymyalgia rheumatica

M31.6   Other giant cell arteritis

M31.7   Microscopic polyangiitis
Microscopic polyarteritis

> **EXCLUDES 1** *polyarteritis nodosa (M30.0)*

M31.8   Other specified necrotizing vasculopathies
Hypocomplementemic vasculitis
Septic vasculitis

M31.9   Necrotizing vasculopathy, unspecified

④ **M32   Systemic lupus erythematosus (SLE)**

> **EXCLUDES 1** *lupus erythematosus (discoid) (NOS) (L93.0)*

> **CODING TIP ✓** Do not assign a code from category M32.- unless Lupus is specified as systemic.

✚ **M32.0   Drug-induced systemic lupus erythematosus**
Use additional code for adverse effect, if applicable, to identify drug (T36-T50 with fifth or sixth character 5)

> **CODING TIP ✓** Assign code M32.0 only when documentation clearly confirms that the systemic lupus diagnosis is secondary to the effects of a drug. An additional code from categories T36-T50 should be used to identify the drug.

⑤ **M32.1   Systemic lupus erythematosus with organ or system involvement**

M32.10   Systemic lupus erythematosus, organ or system involvement unspecified

M32.11   Endocarditis in systemic lupus erythematosus
Libman-Sacks disease

M32.12   Pericarditis in systemic lupus erythematosus
Lupus pericarditis

M32.13   Lung involvement in systemic lupus erythematosus
Pleural effusion due to systemic lupus erythematosus

M32.14   Glomerular disease in systemic lupus erythematosus
Lupus renal disease NOS
AHA: 4Q 2013, 125

M32.15   Tubulo-interstitial nephropathy in systemic lupus erythematosus

M32.19   Other organ or system involvement in systemic lupus erythematosus

M32.8   Other forms of systemic lupus erythematosus

M32.9   Systemic lupus erythematosus, unspecified
SLE NOS
Systemic lupus erythematosus NOS
Systemic lupus erythematosus without organ involvement

④ **M33   Dermatopolymyositis**

⑤ **M33.0   Juvenile dermatopolymyositis**

M33.00   Juvenile dermatopolymyositis, organ involvement unspecified

M33.01   Juvenile dermatopolymyositis with respiratory involvement

M33.02   Juvenile dermatopolymyositis with myopathy

M33.09   Juvenile dermatopolymyositis with other organ involvement

⑤ **M33.1   Other dermatopolymyositis**

● New   ▲ Revised   *Manifestation*   ④-⑦ Digit Indicators   ⊟ Laterality   Ⓐ Adult (15+ years)   Ⓜ Maternity (12-55 years)   Ⓝ Newborn   Ⓟ Pediatric (0-17 years)   ♂ Male   ♀ Female
✖ Deleted   Unspecified   ✚ Additional code

M33.10 Other dermatopolymyositis, organ involvement unspecified

M33.11 Other dermatopolymyositis with respiratory involvement

M33.12 Other dermatopolymyositis with myopathy

M33.19 Other dermatopolymyositis with other organ involvement

⑤ **M33.2** Polymyositis

M33.20 Polymyositis, organ involvement unspecified

M33.21 Polymyositis with respiratory involvement

M33.22 Polymyositis with myopathy

M33.29 Polymyositis with other organ involvement

⑤ **M33.9** Dermatopolymyositis, unspecified

M33.90 Dermatopolymyositis, unspecified, organ involvement unspecified

M33.91 Dermatopolymyositis, unspecified with respiratory involvement

M33.92 Dermatopolymyositis, unspecified with myopathy

M33.99 Dermatopolymyositis, unspecified with other organ involvement

④ **M34** Systemic sclerosis [scleroderma]

> **EXCLUDES 1** *circumscribed scleroderma (L94.0)*
> *neonatal scleroderma (P83.8)*

M34.0 Progressive systemic sclerosis

M34.1 CR(E)ST syndrome
Combination of calcinosis, Raynaud's phenomenon, esophageal dysfunction, sclerodactyly, telangiectasia

+ M34.2 Systemic sclerosis induced by drug and chemical
Code first:
poisoning due to drug or toxin, if applicable (T36-T65 with fifth or sixth character 1-4 or 6)
Use additional code for adverse effect, if applicable, to identify drug (T36-T50 with fifth or sixth character 5)

⑤ **M34.8** Other forms of systemic sclerosis

M34.81 Systemic sclerosis with lung involvement

M34.82 Systemic sclerosis with myopathy

M34.83 Systemic sclerosis with polyneuropathy

M34.89 Other systemic sclerosis

M34.9 Systemic sclerosis, unspecified

④ **M35** Other systemic involvement of connective tissue

> **EXCLUDES 1** *reactive perforating collagenosis (L87.1)*

⑤ **M35.0** Sicca syndrome [Sjögren]

M35.00 Sicca syndrome, unspecified

M35.01 Sicca syndrome with keratoconjunctivitis

M35.02 Sicca syndrome with lung involvement

M35.03 Sicca syndrome with myopathy

M35.04 Sicca syndrome with tubulo-interstitial nephropathy
Renal tubular acidosis in sicca syndrome

M35.09 Sicca syndrome with other organ involvement

M35.1 Other overlap syndromes
Mixed connective tissue disease

> **EXCLUDES 1** *polyangiitis overlap syndrome (M30.8)*

M35.2 Behçet's disease

> **DEFINITION** Relapsing inflammatory disorder with recurring painful sores of the mouth, skin, and genitals, swollen joints, severe uveitis, retinal vasculitis, optic atrophy, and digestive system involvement.

M35.3 Polymyalgia rheumatica

> **EXCLUDES 1** *polymyalgia rheumatica with giant cell arteritis (M31.5)*

M35.4 Diffuse (eosinophilic) fasciitis

M35.5 Multifocal fibrosclerosis

M35.6 Relapsing panniculitis [Weber-Christian]

> **EXCLUDES 1** *lupus panniculitis (L93.2)*
> *panniculitis NOS (M79.3-)*

M35.7 Hypermobility syndrome
Familial ligamentous laxity

> **EXCLUDES 1** *Ehlers-Danlos syndrome (Q79.6)*
> *ligamentous laxity, NOS (M24.2-)*

M35.8 Other specified systemic involvement of connective tissue

M35.9 Systemic involvement of connective tissue, unspecified
Autoimmune disease (systemic) NOS
Collagen (vascular) disease NOS

④ **M36** Systemic disorders of connective tissue in diseases classified elsewhere

> **EXCLUDES 2** *arthropathies in diseases classified elsewhere (M14.-)*

M36.0 *Dermato(poly)myositis in neoplastic disease*
Code first:
underlying neoplasm (C00-D49)

M36.1 *Arthropathy in neoplastic disease*
Code first underlying neoplasm, such as:
leukemia (C91-C95)
malignant histiocytosis (C96.A)
multiple myeloma (C90.0)

M36.2 *Hemophilic arthropathy*
Hemarthrosis in hemophilic arthropathy
Code first underlying disease, such as:
factor VIII deficiency (D66)
with vascular defect (D68.0)
factor IX deficiency (D67)
hemophilia (classical) (D66)
hemophilia B (D67)
hemophilia C (D68.1)

M36.3 *Arthropathy in other blood disorders*

M36.4 *Arthropathy in hypersensitivity reactions classified elsewhere*
Code first underlying disease, such as:
Henoch (-Schönlein) purpura (D69.0)
serum sickness (T80.6-)

M36.8 *Systemic disorders of connective tissue in other diseases classified elsewhere*
Code first underlying disease, such as:
alkaptonuria (E70.2)
hypogammaglobulinemia (D80.-)
ochronosis (E70.2)

Dorsopathies (M40-M54)

Deforming dorsopathies (M40-M43)

④ **M40** Kyphosis and lordosis

> **EXCLUDES 1** *congenital kyphosis and lordosis (Q76.4)*
> *kyphoscoliosis (M41.-)*
> *postprocedural kyphosis and lordosis (M96.-)*

⑤ **M40.0** Postural kyphosis

> **EXCLUDES 1** *osteochondrosis of spine (M42.-)*

M40.00 Postural kyphosis, site unspecified

M40.03 Postural kyphosis, cervicothoracic region

M40.04 Postural kyphosis, thoracic region

M40.05 Postural kyphosis, thoracolumbar region

⑤ **M40.1** Other secondary kyphosis

> **CODING TIP ✓** Secondary kyphosis develops as a result of other spinal problems, including other forms of kyphosis. It is often referred to as hyperkyphosis.

M40.10 Other secondary kyphosis, site unspecified

M40.12 Other secondary kyphosis, cervical region

M40.13 Other secondary kyphosis, cervicothoracic region

M40.14 Other secondary kyphosis, thoracic region

M40.15 Other secondary kyphosis, thoracolumbar region

⑤ **M40.2** Other and unspecified kyphosis

⑥ **M40.20** Unspecified kyphosis

M40.202 Unspecified kyphosis, cervical region

M40.203 Unspecified kyphosis, cervicothoracic region

M40.204 Unspecified kyphosis, thoracic region

M40.205 Unspecified kyphosis, thoracolumbar region

M40.209 Unspecified kyphosis, site unspecified

⑥ **M40.29** Other kyphosis

M40.292 Other kyphosis, cervical region

M40.293 Other kyphosis, cervicothoracic region

M40.294 Other kyphosis, thoracic region

M40.295 Other kyphosis, thoracolumbar region

M40.299 Other kyphosis, site unspecified

⑤ **M40.3** Flatback syndrome

M40.30 Flatback syndrome, site unspecified

● New   ▲ Revised   *Manifestation*   ④-❼ Digit Indicators   ⊟ Laterality   Ⓐ Adult (15+ years)   Ⓜ Maternity (12-55 years)   Ⓝ Newborn   Ⓟ Pediatric (0-17 years)   ♂ Male   ♀ Female
✖ Deleted   Unspecified   + Additional code

770   © 2017 DecisionHealth   2017 ICD-10-CM Expert for Physicians

M40.35   Flatback syndrome, thoracolumbar region

M40.36   Flatback syndrome, lumbar region

M40.37   Flatback syndrome, lumbosacral region

⑤ **M40.4 Postural lordosis**
Acquired lordosis

M40.40   **Postural lordosis, site unspecified**

M40.45   **Postural lordosis, thoracolumbar region**

M40.46   **Postural lordosis, lumbar region**

M40.47   **Postural lordosis, lumbosacral region**

⑤ **M40.5 Lordosis, unspecified**

M40.50   **Lordosis, unspecified, site unspecified**

M40.55   **Lordosis, unspecified, thoracolumbar region**

M40.56   **Lordosis, unspecified, lumbar region**

M40.57   **Lordosis, unspecified, lumbosacral region**

④ **M41   Scoliosis**

> **INCLUDES**   kyphoscoliosis
>
> **EXCLUDES 1**   *congenital scoliosis NOS (Q67.5)*
> *congenital scoliosis due to bony malformation*
>   *(Q76.3)*
> *postural congenital scoliosis (Q67.5)*
> *kyphoscoliotic heart disease (I27.1)*
> *postprocedural scoliosis (M96.-)*

⑤ **M41.0 Infantile idiopathic scoliosis**

M41.00   **Infantile idiopathic scoliosis, site unspecified**

M41.02   **Infantile idiopathic scoliosis, cervical region**

M41.03   **Infantile idiopathic scoliosis, cervicothoracic region**

M41.04   **Infantile idiopathic scoliosis, thoracic region**
AHA: 4Q 2014, 27

M41.05   **Infantile idiopathic scoliosis, thoracolumbar region**

M41.06   **Infantile idiopathic scoliosis, lumbar region**

M41.07   **Infantile idiopathic scoliosis, lumbosacral region**

M41.08   **Infantile idiopathic scoliosis, sacral and sacrococcygeal region**

⑤ **M41.1 Juvenile and adolescent idiopathic scoliosis**

⑥ **M41.11 Juvenile idiopathic scoliosis**

M41.112   **Juvenile idiopathic scoliosis, cervical region**

M41.113   **Juvenile idiopathic scoliosis, cervicothoracic region**

M41.114   **Juvenile idiopathic scoliosis, thoracic region**

M41.115   **Juvenile idiopathic scoliosis, thoracolumbar region**

M41.116   **Juvenile idiopathic scoliosis, lumbar region**

M41.117   **Juvenile idiopathic scoliosis, lumbosacral region**

M41.119   **Juvenile idiopathic scoliosis, site unspecified**
AHA: 4Q 2014, 29

⑥ **M41.12 Adolescent scoliosis**

M41.122   **Adolescent idiopathic scoliosis, cervical region**

M41.123   **Adolescent idiopathic scoliosis, cervicothoracic region**

M41.124   **Adolescent idiopathic scoliosis, thoracic region**

M41.125   **Adolescent idiopathic scoliosis, thoracolumbar region**

M41.126   **Adolescent idiopathic scoliosis, lumbar region**

M41.127   **Adolescent idiopathic scoliosis, lumbosacral region**

M41.129   **Adolescent idiopathic scoliosis, site unspecified**

⑤ **M41.2 Other idiopathic scoliosis**

M41.20   **Other idiopathic scoliosis, site unspecified**

M41.22   **Other idiopathic scoliosis, cervical region**

M41.23   **Other idiopathic scoliosis, cervicothoracic region**

M41.24   **Other idiopathic scoliosis, thoracic region**

Idiopathic scoliosis, thoracic region

M41.25   **Other idiopathic scoliosis, thoracolumbar region**

M41.26   **Other idiopathic scoliosis, lumbar region**

M41.27   **Other idiopathic scoliosis, lumbosacral region**

⑤ **M41.3 Thoracogenic scoliosis**

M41.30   **Thoracogenic scoliosis, site unspecified**

M41.34   **Thoracogenic scoliosis, thoracic region**

M41.35   **Thoracogenic scoliosis, thoracolumbar region**

⑤ **M41.4 Neuromuscular scoliosis**
Scoliosis secondary to cerebral palsy, Friedreich's ataxia, poliomyelitis and other neuromuscular disorders
Code also:
   underlying condition

M41.40   **Neuromuscular scoliosis, site unspecified**

M41.41   **Neuromuscular scoliosis, occipito-atlanto-axial region**

M41.42   **Neuromuscular scoliosis, cervical region**

M41.43   **Neuromuscular scoliosis, cervicothoracic region**

M41.44   **Neuromuscular scoliosis, thoracic region**

M41.45   **Neuromuscular scoliosis, thoracolumbar region**
AHA: 4Q 2014, 28

M41.46   **Neuromuscular scoliosis, lumbar region**

M41.47   **Neuromuscular scoliosis, lumbosacral region**

⑤ **M41.5 Other secondary scoliosis**

M41.50   **Other secondary scoliosis, site unspecified**

M41.52   **Other secondary scoliosis, cervical region**

M41.53   **Other secondary scoliosis, cervicothoracic region**

M41.54   **Other secondary scoliosis, thoracic region**

M41.55   **Other secondary scoliosis, thoracolumbar region**

M41.56   **Other secondary scoliosis, lumbar region**

M41.57   **Other secondary scoliosis, lumbosacral region**

⑤ **M41.8 Other forms of scoliosis**

M41.80   **Other forms of scoliosis, site unspecified**

M41.82   **Other forms of scoliosis, cervical region**

M41.83   **Other forms of scoliosis, cervicothoracic region**

M41.84   **Other forms of scoliosis, thoracic region**

M41.85   **Other forms of scoliosis, thoracolumbar region**

M41.86   **Other forms of scoliosis, lumbar region**

M41.87   **Other forms of scoliosis, lumbosacral region**

M41.9   **Scoliosis, unspecified**

④ **M42   Spinal osteochondrosis**

⑤ **M42.0 Juvenile osteochondrosis of spine**
Calvé's disease
Scheuermann's disease

> **EXCLUDES 1**   *postural kyphosis (M40.0)*

M42.00   **Juvenile osteochondrosis of spine, site unspecified**

M42.01   **Juvenile osteochondrosis of spine, occipito-atlanto-axial region**

M42.02   **Juvenile osteochondrosis of spine, cervical region**

M42.03   **Juvenile osteochondrosis of spine, cervicothoracic region**

M42.04   **Juvenile osteochondrosis of spine, thoracic region**

M42.05   **Juvenile osteochondrosis of spine, thoracolumbar region**

M42.06   **Juvenile osteochondrosis of spine, lumbar region**

M42.07   **Juvenile osteochondrosis of spine, lumbosacral region**

M42.08   **Juvenile osteochondrosis of spine, sacral and sacrococcygeal region**

M42.09   **Juvenile osteochondrosis of spine, multiple sites in spine**

● New   ▲ Revised   *Manifestation*   ④-❼ Digit Indicators   ▤ Laterality   🄰 Adult (15+ years)   🄼 Maternity (12-55 years)   🄽 Newborn   🄿 Pediatric (0-17 years)   ♂ Male   ♀ Female

✖ ~~Deleted~~   Unspecified   + Additional code

⑤ **M42.1**   **Adult osteochondrosis of spine**

     M42.10   **Adult osteochondrosis of spine, site unspecified** Ⓐ

     M42.11   **Adult osteochondrosis of spine, occipito-atlanto-axial region**

     M42.12   **Adult osteochondrosis of spine, cervical region** Ⓐ

     M42.13   **Adult osteochondrosis of spine, cervicothoracic region** Ⓐ

     M42.14   **Adult osteochondrosis of spine, thoracic region** Ⓐ

     M42.15   **Adult osteochondrosis of spine, thoracolumbar region** Ⓐ

     M42.16   **Adult osteochondrosis of spine, lumbar region** Ⓐ

     M42.17   **Adult osteochondrosis of spine, lumbosacral region** Ⓐ

     M42.18   **Adult osteochondrosis of spine, sacral and sacrococcygeal region** Ⓐ

     M42.19   **Adult osteochondrosis of spine, multiple sites in spine** Ⓐ

   M42.9   **Spinal osteochondrosis, unspecified**

④ **M43**   **Other deforming dorsopathies**

     EXCLUDES 1   *congenital spondylolysis and spondylolisthesis (Q76.2)*
       hemivertebra (Q76.3-Q76.4)
       Klippel-Feil syndrome (Q76.1)
       lumbarization and sacralization (Q76.4)
       platyspondylisis (Q76.4)
       spina bifida occulta (Q76.0)
       spinal curvature in osteoporosis (M80.-)
       spinal curvature in Paget's disease of bone [osteitis deformans] (M88.-)

⑤ **M43.0**   **Spondylolysis**

     EXCLUDES 1   *congenital spondylolysis (Q76.2)*
       spondylolisthesis (M43.1)

     DEFINITION   A defect of the pars interarticularis segment of vertebral bone that connects the facet joints, causing stress fracture and predisposing to slippage; occurs most commonly in the lumbar region (specifically L5) during adolescence.

     M43.00   **Spondylolysis, site unspecified**

     M43.01   **Spondylolysis, occipito-atlanto-axial region**

     M43.02   **Spondylolysis, cervical region**

     M43.03   **Spondylolysis, cervicothoracic region**

     M43.04   **Spondylolysis, thoracic region**

     M43.05   **Spondylolysis, thoracolumbar region**

     M43.06   **Spondylolysis, lumbar region**

     M43.07   **Spondylolysis, lumbosacral region**

     M43.08   **Spondylolysis, sacral and sacrococcygeal region**

     M43.09   **Spondylolysis, multiple sites in spine**

⑤ **M43.1**   **Spondylolisthesis**

     EXCLUDES 1   *acute traumatic of lumbosacral region (S33.1)*
       acute traumatic of sites other than lumbosacral- code to Fracture, vertebra, by region
       congenital spondylolisthesis (Q76.2)

     DEFINITION   An acquired condition in which one vertebra slips forward over the one below it, often from degenerative aging or a small fracture in the piece of bone (pars interarticularis) connecting the facet joint above to the one below.

     M43.10   **Spondylolisthesis, site unspecified**

     M43.11   **Spondylolisthesis, occipito-atlanto-axial region**

     M43.12   **Spondylolisthesis, cervical region**

     M43.13   **Spondylolisthesis, cervicothoracic region**

     M43.14   **Spondylolisthesis, thoracic region**

     M43.15   **Spondylolisthesis, thoracolumbar region**

     M43.16   **Spondylolisthesis, lumbar region**

     M43.17   **Spondylolisthesis, lumbosacral region**

     M43.18   **Spondylolisthesis, sacral and sacrococcygeal region**

     M43.19   **Spondylolisthesis, multiple sites in spine**

⑤ **M43.2**   **Fusion of spine**

     Ankylosis of spinal joint

     EXCLUDES 1   *ankylosing spondylitis (M45.0-)*
       congenital fusion of spine (Q76.4)

     EXCLUDES 2   *arthrodesis status (Z98.1)*
       pseudoarthrosis after fusion or arthrodesis (M96.0)

     M43.20   **Fusion of spine, site unspecified**

     M43.21   **Fusion of spine, occipito-atlanto-axial region**

     M43.22   **Fusion of spine, cervical region**

     M43.23   **Fusion of spine, cervicothoracic region**

     M43.24   **Fusion of spine, thoracic region**

     M43.25   **Fusion of spine, thoracolumbar region**

     M43.26   **Fusion of spine, lumbar region**

     M43.27   **Fusion of spine, lumbosacral region**

     M43.28   **Fusion of spine, sacral and sacrococcygeal region**

   M43.3   **Recurrent atlantoaxial dislocation with myelopathy**

   M43.4   **Other recurrent atlantoaxial dislocation**

⑤ **M43.5**   **Other recurrent vertebral dislocation**

     EXCLUDES 1   *biomechanical lesions NEC (M99.-)*

⑥ **M43.5X**   **Other recurrent vertebral dislocation**

     M43.5X2   **Other recurrent vertebral dislocation, cervical region**

     M43.5X3   **Other recurrent vertebral dislocation, cervicothoracic region**

     M43.5X4   **Other recurrent vertebral dislocation, thoracic region**

     M43.5X5   **Other recurrent vertebral dislocation, thoracolumbar region**

     M43.5X6   **Other recurrent vertebral dislocation, lumbar region**

     M43.5X7   **Other recurrent vertebral dislocation, lumbosacral region**

     M43.5X8   **Other recurrent vertebral dislocation, sacral and sacrococcygeal region**

     M43.5X9   **Other recurrent vertebral dislocation, site unspecified**

   M43.6   **Torticollis**

     EXCLUDES 1   *congenital (sternomastoid) torticollis (Q68.0)*
       current injury - see Injury, of spine, by body region
       ocular torticollis (R29.891)
       psychogenic torticollis (F45.8)
       spasmodic torticollis (G24.3)
       torticollis due to birth injury (P15.2)

     DEFINITION   Contraction of the neck muscles causing limited neck motion and head positioned to one side.

⑤ **M43.8**   **Other specified deforming dorsopathies**

     EXCLUDES 2   *kyphosis and lordosis (M40.-)*
       scoliosis (M41.-)

⑥ **M43.8X**   **Other specified deforming dorsopathies**

     M43.8X1   **Other specified deforming dorsopathies, occipito-atlanto-axial region**

     M43.8X2   **Other specified deforming dorsopathies, cervical region**

     M43.8X3   **Other specified deforming dorsopathies, cervicothoracic region**

     M43.8X4   **Other specified deforming dorsopathies, thoracic region**

     M43.8X5   **Other specified deforming dorsopathies, thoracolumbar region**

     M43.8X6   **Other specified deforming dorsopathies, lumbar region**

     M43.8X7   **Other specified deforming dorsopathies, lumbosacral region**

     M43.8X8   **Other specified deforming dorsopathies, sacral and sacrococcygeal region**

     M43.8X9   **Other specified deforming dorsopathies, site unspecified**

   M43.9   **Deforming dorsopathy, unspecified**

     Curvature of spine NOS

Spondylopathies (M45-M49)

④ **M45**   **Ankylosing spondylitis**

     Rheumatoid arthritis of spine

     EXCLUDES 1   *arthropathy in Reiter's disease (M02.3-)*
       juvenile (ankylosing) spondylitis (M08.1)

     EXCLUDES 2   *Behçet's disease (M35.2)*

     CODING TIP ✓   Ankylosing spondylosis is a specific inflammatory disease that causes fusion of the vertebrae and reduced mobility/flexion. It may impact more than one area of the vertebrae.

● New   ▲ Revised   *Manifestation*   ④-⑦ Digit Indicators   ⊟ Laterality   Ⓐ Adult (15+ years)   Ⓜ Maternity (12-55 years)   Ⓝ Newborn   Ⓟ Pediatric (0-17 years)   ♂ Male   ♀ Female
✖ Deleted   Unspecified   + Additional code

772   © 2017 DecisionHealth   2017 ICD-10-CM Expert for Physicians

DEFINITION Autoimmune arthritis causing chronic inflammation of the spine and sacroiliac joints, eventually leading to spinal fusion from calcification of ligaments and discs that progresses up the spine, possibly affecting other organs.

M45.0   Ankylosing spondylitis of multiple sites in spine
M45.1   Ankylosing spondylitis of occipito-atlanto-axial region
M45.2   Ankylosing spondylitis of cervical region
M45.3   Ankylosing spondylitis of cervicothoracic region
M45.4   Ankylosing spondylitis of thoracic region
M45.5   Ankylosing spondylitis of thoracolumbar region
M45.6   Ankylosing spondylitis lumbar region
M45.7   Ankylosing spondylitis of lumbosacral region
M45.8   Ankylosing spondylitis sacral and sacrococcygeal region
M45.9   Ankylosing spondylitis of unspecified sites in spine

⬛ **M46   Other inflammatory spondylopathies**

§ **M46.0   Spinal enthesopathy**
     Disorder of ligamentous or muscular attachments of spine

   M46.00   Spinal enthesopathy, site unspecified
   M46.01   Spinal enthesopathy, occipito-atlanto-axial region
   M46.02   Spinal enthesopathy, cervical region
   M46.03   Spinal enthesopathy, cervicothoracic region
   M46.04   Spinal enthesopathy, thoracic region
   M46.05   Spinal enthesopathy, thoracolumbar region
   M46.06   Spinal enthesopathy, lumbar region
   M46.07   Spinal enthesopathy, lumbosacral region
   M46.08   Spinal enthesopathy, sacral and sacrococcygeal region
   M46.09   Spinal enthesopathy, multiple sites in spine

M46.1   Sacroiliitis, not elsewhere classified

§ **M46.2   Osteomyelitis of vertebra**

   M46.20   Osteomyelitis of vertebra, site unspecified
   M46.21   Osteomyelitis of vertebra, occipito-atlanto-axial region
   M46.22   Osteomyelitis of vertebra, cervical region
   M46.23   Osteomyelitis of vertebra, cervicothoracic region
   M46.24   Osteomyelitis of vertebra, thoracic region
   M46.25   Osteomyelitis of vertebra, thoracolumbar region
   M46.26   Osteomyelitis of vertebra, lumbar region
   M46.27   Osteomyelitis of vertebra, lumbosacral region
   M46.28   Osteomyelitis of vertebra, sacral and sacrococcygeal region

§ + **M46.3   Infection of intervertebral disc (pyogenic)**
     Use additional code (B95-B97) to identify infectious agent.

   + M46.30   Infection of intervertebral disc (pyogenic), site unspecified
   + M46.31   Infection of intervertebral disc (pyogenic), occipito-atlanto-axial region
   + M46.32   Infection of intervertebral disc (pyogenic), cervical region
   + M46.33   Infection of intervertebral disc (pyogenic), cervicothoracic region
   + M46.34   Infection of intervertebral disc (pyogenic), thoracic region
   + M46.35   Infection of intervertebral disc (pyogenic), thoracolumbar region
   + M46.36   Infection of intervertebral disc (pyogenic), lumbar region
   + M46.37   Infection of intervertebral disc (pyogenic), lumbosacral region
   + M46.38   Infection of intervertebral disc (pyogenic), sacral and sacrococcygeal region
   + M46.39   Infection of intervertebral disc (pyogenic), multiple sites in spine

§ **M46.4   Discitis, unspecified**

   M46.40   Discitis, unspecified, site unspecified   Ⓐ
   M46.41   Discitis, unspecified, occipito-atlanto-axial region   Ⓐ
   M46.42   Discitis, unspecified, cervical region   Ⓐ
   M46.43   Discitis, unspecified, cervicothoracic region   Ⓐ
   M46.44   Discitis, unspecified, thoracic region   Ⓐ
   M46.45   Discitis, unspecified, thoracolumbar region   Ⓐ
   M46.46   Discitis, unspecified, lumbar region   Ⓐ
   M46.47   Discitis, unspecified, lumbosacral region   Ⓐ
   M46.48   Discitis, unspecified, sacral and sacrococcygeal region   Ⓐ

   M46.49   Discitis, unspecified, multiple sites in spine   Ⓐ

§ **M46.5   Other infective spondylopathies**

   M46.50   Other infective spondylopathies, site unspecified
   M46.51   Other infective spondylopathies, occipito-atlanto-axial region
   M46.52   Other infective spondylopathies, cervical region
   M46.53   Other infective spondylopathies, cervicothoracic region
   M46.54   Other infective spondylopathies, thoracic region
   M46.55   Other infective spondylopathies, thoracolumbar region
   M46.56   Other infective spondylopathies, lumbar region
   M46.57   Other infective spondylopathies, lumbosacral region
   M46.58   Other infective spondylopathies, sacral and sacrococcygeal region
   M46.59   Other infective spondylopathies, multiple sites in spine

§ **M46.8   Other specified inflammatory spondylopathies**

   M46.80   Other specified inflammatory spondylopathies, site unspecified
   M46.81   Other specified inflammatory spondylopathies, occipito-atlanto-axial region
   M46.82   Other specified inflammatory spondylopathies, cervical region
   M46.83   Other specified inflammatory spondylopathies, cervicothoracic region
   M46.84   Other specified inflammatory spondylopathies, thoracic region
   M46.85   Other specified inflammatory spondylopathies, thoracolumbar region
   M46.86   Other specified inflammatory spondylopathies, lumbar region
   M46.87   Other specified inflammatory spondylopathies, lumbosacral region
   M46.88   Other specified inflammatory spondylopathies, sacral and sacrococcygeal region
   M46.89   Other specified inflammatory spondylopathies, multiple sites in spine

§ **M46.9   Unspecified inflammatory spondylopathy**

   M46.90   Unspecified inflammatory spondylopathy, site unspecified
   M46.91   Unspecified inflammatory spondylopathy, occipito-atlanto-axial region
   M46.92   Unspecified inflammatory spondylopathy, cervical region
   M46.93   Unspecified inflammatory spondylopathy, cervicothoracic region
   M46.94   Unspecified inflammatory spondylopathy, thoracic region
   M46.95   Unspecified inflammatory spondylopathy, thoracolumbar region
   M46.96   Unspecified inflammatory spondylopathy, lumbar region
   M46.97   Unspecified inflammatory spondylopathy, lumbosacral region
   M46.98   Unspecified inflammatory spondylopathy, sacral and sacrococcygeal region
   M46.99   Unspecified inflammatory spondylopathy, multiple sites in spine

⬛ **M47   Spondylosis**

   INCLUDES   arthrosis or osteoarthritis of spine
        degeneration of facet joints

§ **M47.0   Anterior spinal and vertebral artery compression syndromes**

⬢ **M47.01   Anterior spinal artery compression syndromes**

   M47.011   Anterior spinal artery compression syndromes, occipito-atlanto-axial region
   M47.012   Anterior spinal artery compression syndromes, cervical region
   M47.013   Anterior spinal artery compression syndromes, cervicothoracic region
   M47.014   Anterior spinal artery compression syndromes, thoracic region
   M47.015   Anterior spinal artery compression syndromes, thoracolumbar region
   M47.016   Anterior spinal artery compression syndromes, lumbar region

● New   ▲ Revised   *Manifestation*   ④-⑦ Digit Indicators   ▤ Laterality   Ⓐ Adult (15+ years)   Ⓜ Maternity (12-55 years)   Ⓝ Newborn   Ⓟ Pediatric (0-17 years)   ♂ Male   ♀ Female
✖ Deleted   Unspecified   + Additional code

2017 ICD-10-CM Expert for Physicians   © 2017 DecisionHealth   773

M47.019   Anterior spinal artery compression syndromes, site unspecified

⑥ M47.02   Vertebral artery compression syndromes

M47.021   Vertebral artery compression syndromes, occipito-atlanto-axial region

M47.022   Vertebral artery compression syndromes, cervical region

M47.029   Vertebral artery compression syndromes, site unspecified

⑤ M47.1   Other spondylosis with myelopathy
Spondylogenic compression of spinal cord
EXCLUDES 1   *vertebral subluxation (M43.3-M43.59)*

M47.10   Other spondylosis with myelopathy, site unspecified

M47.11   Other spondylosis with myelopathy, occipito-atlanto-axial region

M47.12   Other spondylosis with myelopathy, cervical region

M47.13   Other spondylosis with myelopathy, cervicothoracic region

M47.14   Other spondylosis with myelopathy, thoracic region

M47.15   Other spondylosis with myelopathy, thoracolumbar region

M47.16   Other spondylosis with myelopathy, lumbar region

⑤ M47.2   Other spondylosis with radiculopathy

M47.20   Other spondylosis with radiculopathy, site unspecified

M47.21   Other spondylosis with radiculopathy, occipito-atlanto-axial region

M47.22   Other spondylosis with radiculopathy, cervical region

M47.23   Other spondylosis with radiculopathy, cervicothoracic region

M47.24   Other spondylosis with radiculopathy, thoracic region

M47.25   Other spondylosis with radiculopathy, thoracolumbar region

M47.26   Other spondylosis with radiculopathy, lumbar region

M47.27   Other spondylosis with radiculopathy, lumbosacral region

M47.28   Other spondylosis with radiculopathy, sacral and sacrococcygeal region

⑤ M47.8   Other spondylosis

⑥ M47.81   Spondylosis without myelopathy or radiculopathy

M47.811   Spondylosis without myelopathy or radiculopathy, occipito-atlanto-axial region

M47.812   Spondylosis without myelopathy or radiculopathy, cervical region

M47.813   Spondylosis without myelopathy or radiculopathy, cervicothoracic region

M47.814   Spondylosis without myelopathy or radiculopathy, thoracic region

M47.815   Spondylosis without myelopathy or radiculopathy, thoracolumbar region

M47.816   Spondylosis without myelopathy or radiculopathy, lumbar region

M47.817   Spondylosis without myelopathy or radiculopathy, lumbosacral region

M47.818   Spondylosis without myelopathy or radiculopathy, sacral and sacrococcygeal region

M47.819   Spondylosis without myelopathy or radiculopathy, site unspecified

⑥ M47.89   Other spondylosis

M47.891   Other spondylosis, occipito-atlanto-axial region

M47.892   Other spondylosis, cervical region

M47.893   Other spondylosis, cervicothoracic region

M47.894   Other spondylosis, thoracic region

M47.895   Other spondylosis, thoracolumbar region

M47.896   Other spondylosis, lumbar region

M47.897   Other spondylosis, lumbosacral region

M47.898   Other spondylosis, sacral and sacrococcygeal region

M47.899   Other spondylosis, site unspecified

M47.9   Spondylosis, unspecified

④ M48   **Other spondylopathies**

⑤ M48.0   Spinal stenosis
Caudal stenosis

M48.00   Spinal stenosis, site unspecified   Ⓐ

M48.01   Spinal stenosis, occipito-atlanto-axial region

M48.02   Spinal stenosis, cervical region

M48.03   Spinal stenosis, cervicothoracic region

M48.04   Spinal stenosis, thoracic region   Ⓐ

M48.05   Spinal stenosis, thoracolumbar region   Ⓐ

M48.06   Spinal stenosis, lumbar region   Ⓐ

M48.07   Spinal stenosis, lumbosacral region   Ⓐ

M48.08   Spinal stenosis, sacral and sacrococcygeal region   Ⓐ

⑤ M48.1   Ankylosing hyperostosis [Forestier]
Diffuse idiopathic skeletal hyperostosis [DISH]

M48.10   Ankylosing hyperostosis [Forestier], site unspecified

M48.11   Ankylosing hyperostosis [Forestier], occipito-atlanto-axial region

M48.12   Ankylosing hyperostosis [Forestier], cervical region

M48.13   Ankylosing hyperostosis [Forestier], cervicothoracic region

M48.14   Ankylosing hyperostosis [Forestier], thoracic region

M48.15   Ankylosing hyperostosis [Forestier], thoracolumbar region

M48.16   Ankylosing hyperostosis [Forestier], lumbar region

M48.17   Ankylosing hyperostosis [Forestier], lumbosacral region

M48.18   Ankylosing hyperostosis [Forestier], sacral and sacrococcygeal region

M48.19   Ankylosing hyperostosis [Forestier], multiple sites in spine

⑤ M48.2   Kissing spine

M48.20   Kissing spine, site unspecified

M48.21   Kissing spine, occipito-atlanto-axial region

M48.22   Kissing spine, cervical region

M48.23   Kissing spine, cervicothoracic region

M48.24   Kissing spine, thoracic region

M48.25   Kissing spine, thoracolumbar region

M48.26   Kissing spine, lumbar region

M48.27   Kissing spine, lumbosacral region

⑤ M48.3   Traumatic spondylopathy

M48.30   Traumatic spondylopathy, site unspecified

M48.31   Traumatic spondylopathy, occipito-atlanto-axial region

M48.32   Traumatic spondylopathy, cervical region

M48.33   Traumatic spondylopathy, cervicothoracic region

M48.34   Traumatic spondylopathy, thoracic region

M48.35   Traumatic spondylopathy, thoracolumbar region

M48.36   Traumatic spondylopathy, lumbar region

M48.37   Traumatic spondylopathy, lumbosacral region

M48.38   Traumatic spondylopathy, sacral and sacrococcygeal region

⑤ M48.4   Fatigue fracture of vertebra
Stress fracture of vertebra
EXCLUDES 1   *pathological fracture NOS (M84.4-)*
pathological fracture of vertebra due to neoplasm (M84.58)
pathological fracture of vertebra due to other diagnosis (M84.68)
pathological fracture of vertebra due to osteoporosis (M80.-)
traumatic fracture of vertebrae (S12.0-S12.3-, S22.0-, S32.0-)

The appropriate 7th character is to be added to each code from subcategory M48.4:
A   initial encounter for fracture
D   subsequent encounter for fracture with routine healing
G   subsequent encounter for fracture with delayed healing
S   sequela of fracture

⑦ M48.40X-   Fatigue fracture of vertebra, site unspecified

⑦ M48.41X-   Fatigue fracture of vertebra, occipito-atlanto-axial region

⑦ M48.42X-   Fatigue fracture of vertebra, cervical region

⑦ M48.43X-   Fatigue fracture of vertebra, cervicothoracic region

⑦ M48.44X-   Fatigue fracture of vertebra, thoracic region

⑦ M48.45X-   Fatigue fracture of vertebra, thoracolumbar region

⑦ M48.46X-   Fatigue fracture of vertebra, lumbar region

⑦ M48.47X-   Fatigue fracture of vertebra, lumbosacral region

---

● New   ▲ Revised   *Manifestation*   ❹-❼ Digit Indicators   ▤ Laterality   Ⓐ Adult (15+ years)   Ⓜ Maternity (12-55 years)   Ⓝ Newborn   Ⓟ Pediatric (0-17 years)   ♂ Male   ♀ Female
✖ Deleted   Unspecified   + Additional code

774   © 2017 DecisionHealth   2017 ICD-10-CM Expert for Physicians

7 M48.48X- Fatigue fracture of vertebra, sacral and sacrococcygeal region

▲ **5 M48.5** Collapsed vertebra, not elsewhere classified
Collapsed vertebra NOS
Compression fracture of vertebra NOS
Wedging of vertebra NOS

> **EXCLUDES 1** current injury - see Injury of spine, by body region
> fatigue fracture of vertebra (M48.4)
> pathological fracture of vertebra due to neoplasm (M84.58)
> pathological fracture of vertebra due to other diagnosis (M84.68)
> pathological fracture of vertebra due to osteoporosis (M80.-)
> pathological fracture NOS (M84.4-)
> stress fracture of vertebra (M48.4-)
> traumatic fracture of vertebra (S12.-, S22.-, S32.-)

The appropriate 7th character is to be added to each code from subcategory M48.5:

A initial encounter for fracture
D subsequent encounter for fracture with routine healing
G subsequent encounter for fracture with delayed healing
S sequela of fracture

7 M48.50X- Collapsed vertebra, not elsewhere classified, site unspecified

7 M48.51X- Collapsed vertebra, not elsewhere classified, occipito-atlanto-axial region

7 M48.52X- Collapsed vertebra, not elsewhere classified, cervical region

7 M48.53X- Collapsed vertebra, not elsewhere classified, cervicothoracic region

7 M48.54X- Collapsed vertebra, not elsewhere classified, thoracic region

7 M48.55X- Collapsed vertebra, not elsewhere classified, thoracolumbar region

7 M48.56X- Collapsed vertebra, not elsewhere classified, lumbar region

7 M48.57X- Collapsed vertebra, not elsewhere classified, lumbosacral region

7 M48.58X- Collapsed vertebra, not elsewhere classified, sacral and sacrococcygeal region

5 M48.8 Other specified spondylopathies
Ossification of posterior longitudinal ligament

6 M48.8X Other specified spondylopathies

M48.8X1 Other specified spondylopathies, occipito-atlanto-axial region

M48.8X2 Other specified spondylopathies, cervical region

M48.8X3 Other specified spondylopathies, cervicothoracic region

M48.8X4 Other specified spondylopathies, thoracic region

M48.8X5 Other specified spondylopathies, thoracolumbar region

M48.8X6 Other specified spondylopathies, lumbar region

M48.8X7 Other specified spondylopathies, lumbosacral region

M48.8X8 Other specified spondylopathies, sacral and sacrococcygeal region

M48.8X9 Other specified spondylopathies, site unspecified

M48.9 Spondylopathy, unspecified

4 M49 Spondylopathies in diseases classified elsewhere

> **INCLUDES** curvature of spine in diseases classified elsewhere
> deformity of spine in diseases classified elsewhere
> kyphosis in diseases classified elsewhere
> scoliosis in diseases classified elsewhere
> spondylopathy in diseases classified elsewhere

Code first underlying disease, such as:
brucellosis (A23.-)
Charcot-Marie-Tooth disease (G60.0)
enterobacterial infections (A01-A04)
osteitis fibrosa cystica (E21.0)

> **EXCLUDES 1** curvature of spine in tuberculosis [Pott's] (A18.01)
> enteropathic arthropathies (M07.-)
> gonococcal spondylitis (A54.41)
> neuropathic [tabes dorsalis] spondylitis (A52.11)
> neuropathic spondylopathy in syringomyelia (G95.0)
> neuropathic spondylopathy in tabes dorsalis (A52.11)
> nonsyphilitic neuropathic spondylopathy NEC (G98.0)
> spondylitis in syphilis (acquired) (A52.77)
> tuberculous spondylitis (A18.01)
> typhoid fever spondylitis (A01.05)

5 M49.8 Spondylopathy in diseases classified elsewhere

> **CODING TIP ✓** M49.8- codes indicate spondylopathy due to an underlying condition. The underlying condition should be identified and coded first.

M49.80 Spondylopathy in diseases classified elsewhere, site unspecified

M49.81 Spondylopathy in diseases classified elsewhere, occipito-atlanto-axial region

M49.82 Spondylopathy in diseases classified elsewhere, cervical region

M49.83 Spondylopathy in diseases classified elsewhere, cervicothoracic region

M49.84 Spondylopathy in diseases classified elsewhere, thoracic region

M49.85 Spondylopathy in diseases classified elsewhere, thoracolumbar region

M49.86 Spondylopathy in diseases classified elsewhere, lumbar region

M49.87 Spondylopathy in diseases classified elsewhere, lumbosacral region

M49.88 Spondylopathy in diseases classified elsewhere, sacral and sacrococcygeal region

M49.89 Spondylopathy in diseases classified elsewhere, multiple sites in spine

Other dorsopathies (M50-M54)

> **EXCLUDES 1** current injury - see injury of spine by body region
> discitis NOS (M46.4-)

4 M50 Cervical disc disorders
Note: code to the most superior level of disorder

> **INCLUDES** cervicothoracic disc disorders with cervicalgia
> cervicothoracic disc disorders

5 M50.0 Cervical disc disorder with myelopathy
AHA: 1Q 2016, 17

M50.00 Cervical disc disorder with myelopathy, unspecified cervical region 🄰

M50.01 Cervical disc disorder with myelopathy, high cervical region 🄰
C2-C3 disc disorder with myelopathy
C3-C4 disc disorder with myelopathy

▲ **6 M50.02** Cervical disc disorder with myelopathy, mid-cervical region 🄰

● **M50.020** Cervical disc disorder with myelopathy, mid-cervical region, unspecified level

● **M50.021** Cervical disc disorder at C4-C5 level with myelopathy
C4-C5 disc disorder with myelopathy

● **M50.022** Cervical disc disorder at C5-C6 level with myelopathy
C5-C6 disc disorder with myelopathy

● New ▲ Revised *Manifestation* 4-7 Digit Indicators ⊟ Laterality 🄰 Adult (15+ years) 🄼 Maternity (12-55 years) 🄽 Newborn (0-17 years) 🄿 Pediatric ♂ Male ♀ Female
✖ Deleted Unspecified + Additional code

● M50.023   Cervical disc disorder at C6-C7 level with
            myelopathy
            C6-C7 disc disorder with myelopathy

M50.03   Cervical disc disorder with myelopathy,   A
         cervicothoracic region
         C7-T1 disc disorder with myelopathy

⑤ M50.1   Cervical disc disorder with radiculopathy
          EXCLUDES 2   brachial radiculitis NOS (M54.13)

          AHA: 1Q 2016, 17

M50.10   Cervical disc disorder with radiculopathy,
         unspecified cervical region

M50.11   Cervical disc disorder with radiculopathy, high
         cervical region
         C2-C3 disc disorder with radiculopathy
         C3 radiculopathy due to disc disorder
         C3-C4 disc disorder with radiculopathy
         C4 radiculopathy due to disc disorder

▲ ⑥ M50.12   Cervical disc disorder with radiculopathy, mid-
             cervical region
    ● M50.120   Mid-cervical disc disorder, unspecified
    ● M50.121   Cervical disc disorder at C4-C5 level with
                radiculopathy
                C4-C5 disc disorder with radiculopathy
                C5 radiculopathy due to disc disorder
    ● M50.122   Cervical disc disorder at C5-C6 level with
                radiculopathy
                C5-C6 disc disorder with radiculopathy
                C6 radiculopathy due to disc disorder
    ● M50.123   Cervical disc disorder at C6-C7 level with
                radiculopathy
                C6-C7 disc disorder with radiculopathy
                C7 radiculopathy due to disc disorder

M50.13   Cervical disc disorder with radiculopathy,
         cervicothoracic region
         C7-T1 disc disorder with radiculopathy
         C8 radiculopathy due to disc disorder

⑤ M50.2   Other cervical disc displacement
M50.20   Other cervical disc displacement, unspecified   A
         cervical region

M50.21   Other cervical disc displacement, high cervical   A
         region
         Other C2-C3 cervical disc displacement
         Other C3-C4 cervical disc displacement

▲ ⑥ M50.22   Other cervical disc displacement, mid-cervical   A
             region
    ● M50.220   Other cervical disc displacement, mid-cervical
                region, unspecified level
    ● M50.221   Other cervical disc displacement at C4-C5 level
                Other C4-C5 cervical disc displacement
    ● M50.222   Other cervical disc displacement at C5-C6 level
                Other C5-C6 cervical disc displacement
    ● M50.223   Other cervical disc displacement at C6-C7 level
                Other C6-C7 cervical disc displacement

M50.23   Other cervical disc displacement, cervicothoracic   A
         region
         Other C7-T1 cervical disc displacement

⑤ M50.3   Other cervical disc degeneration
M50.30   Other cervical disc degeneration, unspecified   A
         cervical region

M50.31   Other cervical disc degeneration, high cervical   A
         region
         Other C2-C3 cervical disc degeneration
         Other C3-C4 cervical disc degeneration

▲ ⑥ M50.32   Other cervical disc degeneration, mid-cervical   A
             region
    ● M50.320   Other cervical disc degeneration, mid-cervical
                region, unspecified level
    ● M50.321   Other cervical disc degeneration at C4-C5 level
                Other C4-C5 cervical disc degeneration
    ● M50.322   Other cervical disc degeneration at C5-C6 level
                Other C5-C6 cervical disc degeneration
    ● M50.323   Other cervical disc degeneration at C6-C7 level
                Other C6-C7 cervical disc degeneration

M50.33   Other cervical disc degeneration, cervicothoracic   A
         region
         Other C7-T1 cervical disc degeneration

⑤ M50.8   Other cervical disc disorders

M50.80   Other cervical disc disorders, unspecified cervical A
         region

M50.81   Other cervical disc disorders, high cervical region A
         Other C2-C3 cervical disc disorders
         Other C3-C4 cervical disc disorders

▲ ⑥ M50.82   Other cervical disc disorders, mid-cervical region A
    ● M50.820   Other cervical disc disorders, mid-cervical
                region, unspecified level
    ● M50.821   Other cervical disc disorders at C4-C5 level
                Other C4-C5 cervical disc disorders
    ● M50.822   Other cervical disc disorders at C5-C6 level
                Other C5-C6 cervical disc disorders
    ● M50.823   Other cervical disc disorders at C6-C7 level
                Other C6-C7 cervical disc disorders

M50.83   Other cervical disc disorders, cervicothoracic   A
         region
         Other C7-T1 cervical disc disorders

⑤ M50.9   Cervical disc disorder, unspecified
M50.90   Cervical disc disorder, unspecified, unspecified   A
         cervical region

M50.91   Cervical disc disorder, unspecified, high cervical   A
         region
         C2-C3 cervical disc disorder, unspecified
         C3-C4 cervical disc disorder, unspecified

▲ ⑥ M50.92   Cervical disc disorder, unspecified, mid-cervical A
             region
    ● M50.920   Unspecified cervical disc disorder, mid-cervical
                region, unspecified level
    ● M50.921   Unspecified cervical disc disorder at C4-C5
                level
                Unspecified C4-C5 cervical disc disorder
    ● M50.922   Unspecified cervical disc disorder at C5-C6
                level
                Unspecified C5-C6 cervical disc disorder
    ● M50.923   Unspecified cervical disc disorder at C6-C7
                level
                Unspecified C6-C7 cervical disc disorder

M50.93   Cervical disc disorder, unspecified,   A
         cervicothoracic region
         C7-T1 cervical disc disorder, unspecified

④ M51   Thoracic, thoracolumbar, and lumbosacral
        intervertebral disc disorders
        EXCLUDES 2   cervical and cervicothoracic disc disorders
                         (M50.-)
                         sacral and sacrococcygeal disorders (M53.3)

⑤ M51.0   Thoracic, thoracolumbar and lumbosacral intervertebral
          disc disorders with myelopathy
M51.04   Intervertebral disc disorders with myelopathy,   A
         thoracic region
M51.05   Intervertebral disc disorders with myelopathy,   A
         thoracolumbar region
M51.06   Intervertebral disc disorders with myelopathy,   A
         lumbar region

⑤ M51.1   Thoracic, thoracolumbar and lumbosacral intervertebral
          disc disorders with radiculopathy
          Sciatica due to intervertebral disc disorder
          EXCLUDES 1   lumbar radiculitis NOS (M54.16)
                           sciatica NOS (M54.3)
M51.14   Intervertebral disc disorders with radiculopathy,
         thoracic region
M51.15   Intervertebral disc disorders with radiculopathy,
         thoracolumbar region
M51.16   Intervertebral disc disorders with radiculopathy,
         lumbar region
M51.17   Intervertebral disc disorders with radiculopathy,
         lumbosacral region

⑤ M51.2   Other thoracic, thoracolumbar and lumbosacral
          intervertebral disc displacement
          Lumbago due to displacement of intervertebral disc
M51.24   Other intervertebral disc displacement, thoracic   A
         region
M51.25   Other intervertebral disc displacement,   A
         thoracolumbar region
M51.26   Other intervertebral disc displacement, lumbar   A
         region
M51.27   Other intervertebral disc displacement,   A
         lumbosacral region

● New   ▲ Revised   *Manifestation*   ④-⑦ Digit Indicators   ⊟ Laterality   A Adult   M Maternity   N Newborn   P Pediatric   ♂ Male   ♀ Female
✖ ~~Deleted~~   Unspecified   + Additional code   (15+ years)   (12-55 years)   (0-17 years)

⑤ M51.3   Other thoracic, thoracolumbar and lumbosacral intervertebral disc degeneration

M51.34   Other intervertebral disc degeneration, thoracic region   Ⓐ

M51.35   Other intervertebral disc degeneration, thoracolumbar region   Ⓐ

M51.36   Other intervertebral disc degeneration, lumbar region

M51.37   Other intervertebral disc degeneration, lumbosacral region

⑤ M51.4   Schmorl's nodes

M51.44   Schmorl's nodes, thoracic region   Ⓐ

M51.45   Schmorl's nodes, thoracolumbar region   Ⓐ

M51.46   Schmorl's nodes, lumbar region   Ⓐ

M51.47   Schmorl's nodes, lumbosacral region   Ⓐ

⑤ M51.8   Other thoracic, thoracolumbar and lumbosacral intervertebral disc disorders

M51.84   Other intervertebral disc disorders, thoracic region   Ⓐ

M51.85   Other intervertebral disc disorders, thoracolumbar region   Ⓐ

M51.86   Other intervertebral disc disorders, lumbar region   Ⓐ

M51.87   Other intervertebral disc disorders, lumbosacral region   Ⓐ

M51.9   Unspecified thoracic, thoracolumbar and lumbosacral intervertebral disc disorder   Ⓐ

④ M53   Other and unspecified dorsopathies, not elsewhere classified

M53.0   Cervicocranial syndrome
Posterior cervical sympathetic syndrome

M53.1   Cervicobrachial syndrome
> **EXCLUDES 2**   *cervical disc disorder (M50.-)*
> *thoracic outlet syndrome (G54.0)*

⑤ M53.2   Spinal instabilities

⑥ M53.2X   Spinal instabilities

M53.2X1   Spinal instabilities, occipito-atlanto-axial region

M53.2X2   Spinal instabilities, cervical region

M53.2X3   Spinal instabilities, cervicothoracic region

M53.2X4   Spinal instabilities, thoracic region

M53.2X5   Spinal instabilities, thoracolumbar region

M53.2X6   Spinal instabilities, lumbar region

M53.2X7   Spinal instabilities, lumbosacral region

M53.2X8   Spinal instabilities, sacral and sacrococcygeal region

M53.2X9   Spinal instabilities, site unspecified

M53.3   Sacrococcygeal disorders, not elsewhere classified
Coccygodynia

⑤ M53.8   Other specified dorsopathies

M53.80   Other specified dorsopathies, site unspecified

M53.81   Other specified dorsopathies, occipito-atlanto-axial region

M53.82   Other specified dorsopathies, cervical region

M53.83   Other specified dorsopathies, cervicothoracic region

M53.84   Other specified dorsopathies, thoracic region

M53.85   Other specified dorsopathies, thoracolumbar region

M53.86   Other specified dorsopathies, lumbar region

M53.87   Other specified dorsopathies, lumbosacral region

M53.88   Other specified dorsopathies, sacral and sacrococcygeal region

M53.9   Dorsopathy, unspecified

④ M54   Dorsalgia
> **EXCLUDES 1**   *psychogenic dorsalgia (F45.41)*

⑤ M54.0   Panniculitis affecting regions of neck and back
> **EXCLUDES 1**   *lupus panniculitis (L93.2)*
> *panniculitis NOS (M79.3)*
> *relapsing [Weber-Christian] panniculitis (M35.6)*

M54.00   Panniculitis affecting regions of neck and back, site unspecified

M54.01   Panniculitis affecting regions of neck and back, occipito-atlanto-axial region

M54.02   Panniculitis affecting regions of neck and back, cervical region

M54.03   Panniculitis affecting regions of neck and back, cervicothoracic region

M54.04   Panniculitis affecting regions of neck and back, thoracic region

M54.05   Panniculitis affecting regions of neck and back, thoracolumbar region

M54.06   Panniculitis affecting regions of neck and back, lumbar region

M54.07   Panniculitis affecting regions of neck and back, lumbosacral region

M54.08   Panniculitis affecting regions of neck and back, sacral and sacrococcygeal region

M54.09   Panniculitis affecting regions, neck and back, multiple sites in spine

⑤ M54.1   Radiculopathy
Brachial neuritis or radiculitis NOS
Lumbar neuritis or radiculitis NOS
Lumbosacral neuritis or radiculitis NOS
Thoracic neuritis or radiculitis NOS
Radiculitis NOS
> **EXCLUDES 1**   *neuralgia and neuritis NOS (M79.2)*
> *radiculopathy with cervical disc disorder (M50.1)*
> *radiculopathy with lumbar and other intervertebral disc disorder (M51.1-)*
> *radiculopathy with spondylosis (M47.2-)*

M54.10   Radiculopathy, site unspecified

M54.11   Radiculopathy, occipito-atlanto-axial region

M54.12   Radiculopathy, cervical region

M54.13   Radiculopathy, cervicothoracic region

M54.14   Radiculopathy, thoracic region

M54.15   Radiculopathy, thoracolumbar region

M54.16   Radiculopathy, lumbar region

M54.17   Radiculopathy, lumbosacral region

M54.18   Radiculopathy, sacral and sacrococcygeal region

M54.2   Cervicalgia
> **EXCLUDES 1**   *cervicalgia due to intervertebral cervical disc disorder (M50.-)*

⑤ M54.3   Sciatica
> **EXCLUDES 1**   *lesion of sciatic nerve (G57.0)*
> *sciatica due to intervertebral disc disorder (M51.1-)*
> *sciatica with lumbago (M54.4-)*

> **DEFINITION**   Severe pain in the sciatic nerve running down the lower back through the leg; usually resulting from nerve compression or pinching.

⊟ M54.30   Sciatica, unspecified side

⊟ M54.31   Sciatica, right side

⊟ M54.32   Sciatica, left side

⑤ M54.4   Lumbago with sciatica
> **EXCLUDES 1**   *lumbago with sciatica due to intervertebral disc disorder (M51.1-)*

⊟ M54.40   Lumbago with sciatica, unspecified side

⊟ M54.41   Lumbago with sciatica, right side

⊟ M54.42   Lumbago with sciatica, left side
AHA: 2Q 2016, 7

M54.5   Low back pain
Loin pain
Lumbago NOS
> **EXCLUDES 1**   *low back strain (S39.012)*
> *lumbago due to intervertebral disc displacement (M51.2-)*
> *lumbago with sciatica (M54.4-)*

M54.6   Pain in thoracic spine
> **EXCLUDES 1**   *pain in thoracic spine due to intervertebral disc disorder (M51.-)*

⑤ M54.8   Other dorsalgia
> **EXCLUDES 1**   *dorsalgia in thoracic region (M54.6)*
> *low back pain (M54.5)*

M54.81   Occipital neuralgia

M54.89   Other dorsalgia

M54.9   Dorsalgia, unspecified
Backache NOS
Back pain NOS

● New   ▲ Revised   *Manifestation*   ④-⑦ Digit Indicators   ⊟ Laterality   Ⓐ Adult (15+ years)   Ⓜ Maternity (12-55 years)   Ⓝ Newborn   Ⓟ Pediatric (0-17 years)   ♂ Male   ♀ Female
✖ ~~Deleted~~   Unspecified   + Additional code

2017 ICD-10-CM Expert for Physicians   © 2017 DecisionHealth   777

Soft tissue disorders (M60-M79)

Disorders of muscles (M60-M63)

EXCLUDES 1 *dermatopolymyositis (M33.-)*
muscular dystrophies and myopathies (G71-G72)
myopathy in amyloidosis (E85.-)
myopathy in polyarteritis nodosa (M30.0)
myopathy in rheumatoid arthritis (M05.32)
myopathy in scleroderma (M34.-)
myopathy in Sjögren's syndrome (M35.03)
myopathy in systemic lupus erythematosus (M32.-)

◪ **M60   Myositis**

   EXCLUDES 2 *inclusion body myositis [IBM] (G72.41)*

   CODING TIP ✓   Documentation: Myositis indicates inflammation of the muscles. This may be caused by inflammatory disorders/autoimmune conditions, infection, or injury. Review all clinical documentation carefully to identify any cause and assign the most specific code for the condition.

⑤ ✚ **M60.0   Infective myositis**
     Tropical pyomyositis
     Use additional code (B95-B97) to identify infectious agent

  ⑥ ✚ **M60.00   Infective myositis, unspecified site**

    ▤ ✚ **M60.000   Infective myositis, unspecified right arm**
       Infective myositis, right upper limb NOS

    ▤ ✚ **M60.001   Infective myositis, unspecified left arm**
       Infective myositis, left upper limb NOS

    ▤ ✚ **M60.002   Infective myositis, unspecified arm**
       Infective myositis, upper limb NOS

    ▤ ✚ **M60.003   Infective myositis, unspecified right leg**
       Infective myositis, right lower limb NOS

    ▤ ✚ **M60.004   Infective myositis, unspecified left leg**
       Infective myositis, left lower limb NOS

    ▤ ✚ **M60.005   Infective myositis, unspecified leg**
       Infective myositis, lower limb NOS

    ▤ ✚ **M60.009   Infective myositis, unspecified site**

  ⑥ ✚ **M60.01   Infective myositis, shoulder**

    ▤ ✚ **M60.011   Infective myositis, right shoulder**

    ▤ ✚ **M60.012   Infective myositis, left shoulder**

    ▤ ✚ **M60.019   Infective myositis, unspecified shoulder**

  ⑥ ✚ **M60.02   Infective myositis, upper arm**

    ▤ ✚ **M60.021   Infective myositis, right upper arm**

    ▤ ✚ **M60.022   Infective myositis, left upper arm**

    ▤ ✚ **M60.029   Infective myositis, unspecified upper arm**

  ⑥ ✚ **M60.03   Infective myositis, forearm**

    ▤ ✚ **M60.031   Infective myositis, right forearm**

    ▤ ✚ **M60.032   Infective myositis, left forearm**

    ▤ ✚ **M60.039   Infective myositis, unspecified forearm**

  ⑥ ✚ **M60.04   Infective myositis, hand and fingers**

    ▤ ✚ **M60.041   Infective myositis, right hand**

    ▤ ✚ **M60.042   Infective myositis, left hand**

    ▤ ✚ **M60.043   Infective myositis, unspecified hand**

    ▤ ✚ **M60.044   Infective myositis, right finger(s)**

    ▤ ✚ **M60.045   Infective myositis, left finger(s)**

    ▤ ✚ **M60.046   Infective myositis, unspecified finger(s)**

  ⑥ ✚ **M60.05   Infective myositis, thigh**

    ▤ ✚ **M60.051   Infective myositis, right thigh**

    ▤ ✚ **M60.052   Infective myositis, left thigh**

    ▤ ✚ **M60.059   Infective myositis, unspecified thigh**

  ⑥ ✚ **M60.06   Infective myositis, lower leg**

    ▤ ✚ **M60.061   Infective myositis, right lower leg**

    ▤ ✚ **M60.062   Infective myositis, left lower leg**

    ▤ ✚ **M60.069   Infective myositis, unspecified lower leg**

  ⑥ ✚ **M60.07   Infective myositis, ankle, foot and toes**

    ▤ ✚ **M60.070   Infective myositis, right ankle**

    ▤ ✚ **M60.071   Infective myositis, left ankle**

    ▤ ✚ **M60.072   Infective myositis, unspecified ankle**

    ▤ ✚ **M60.073   Infective myositis, right foot**

    ▤ ✚ **M60.074   Infective myositis, left foot**

    ▤ ✚ **M60.075   Infective myositis, unspecified foot**

    ▤ ✚ **M60.076   Infective myositis, right toe(s)**

    ▤ ✚ **M60.077   Infective myositis, left toe(s)**

    ▤ ✚ **M60.078   Infective myositis, unspecified toe(s)**

  ✚ **M60.08   Infective myositis, other site**

  ✚ **M60.09   Infective myositis, multiple sites**

⑤ **M60.1   Interstitial myositis**

  M60.10   Interstitial myositis of unspecified site

  ⑥ **M60.11   Interstitial myositis, shoulder**

    ▤ **M60.111   Interstitial myositis, right shoulder**

    ▤ **M60.112   Interstitial myositis, left shoulder**

    ▤ **M60.119   Interstitial myositis, unspecified shoulder**

  ⑥ **M60.12   Interstitial myositis, upper arm**

    ▤ **M60.121   Interstitial myositis, right upper arm**

    ▤ **M60.122   Interstitial myositis, left upper arm**

    ▤ **M60.129   Interstitial myositis, unspecified upper arm**

  ⑥ **M60.13   Interstitial myositis, forearm**

    ▤ **M60.131   Interstitial myositis, right forearm**

    ▤ **M60.132   Interstitial myositis, left forearm**

    ▤ **M60.139   Interstitial myositis, unspecified forearm**

  ⑥ **M60.14   Interstitial myositis, hand**

    ▤ **M60.141   Interstitial myositis, right hand**

    ▤ **M60.142   Interstitial myositis, left hand**

    ▤ **M60.149   Interstitial myositis, unspecified hand**

  ⑥ **M60.15   Interstitial myositis, thigh**

    ▤ **M60.151   Interstitial myositis, right thigh**

    ▤ **M60.152   Interstitial myositis, left thigh**

    ▤ **M60.159   Interstitial myositis, unspecified thigh**

  ⑥ **M60.16   Interstitial myositis, lower leg**

    ▤ **M60.161   Interstitial myositis, right lower leg**

    ▤ **M60.162   Interstitial myositis, left lower leg**

    ▤ **M60.169   Interstitial myositis, unspecified lower leg**

  ⑥ **M60.17   Interstitial myositis, ankle and foot**

    ▤ **M60.171   Interstitial myositis, right ankle and foot**

    ▤ **M60.172   Interstitial myositis, left ankle and foot**

    ▤ **M60.179   Interstitial myositis, unspecified ankle and foot**

  M60.18   Interstitial myositis, other site

  M60.19   Interstitial myositis, multiple sites

⑤ ✚ **M60.2   Foreign body granuloma of soft tissue, not elsewhere classified**
    Use additional code to identify the type of retained foreign body (Z18.-)

    EXCLUDES 1 *foreign body granuloma of skin and subcutaneous tissue (L92.3)*

  ✚ **M60.20   Foreign body granuloma of soft tissue, not elsewhere classified, unspecified site**

  ⑥ ✚ **M60.21   Foreign body granuloma of soft tissue, not elsewhere classified, shoulder**

    ▤ ✚ **M60.211   Foreign body granuloma of soft tissue, not elsewhere classified, right shoulder**

    ▤ ✚ **M60.212   Foreign body granuloma of soft tissue, not elsewhere classified, left shoulder**

    ▤ ✚ **M60.219   Foreign body granuloma of soft tissue, not elsewhere classified, unspecified shoulder**

  ⑥ ✚ **M60.22   Foreign body granuloma of soft tissue, not elsewhere classified, upper arm**

    ▤ ✚ **M60.221   Foreign body granuloma of soft tissue, not elsewhere classified, right upper arm**

    ▤ ✚ **M60.222   Foreign body granuloma of soft tissue, not elsewhere classified, left upper arm**

    ▤ ✚ **M60.229   Foreign body granuloma of soft tissue, not elsewhere classified, unspecified upper arm**

  ⑥ ✚ **M60.23   Foreign body granuloma of soft tissue, not elsewhere classified, forearm**

    ▤ ✚ **M60.231   Foreign body granuloma of soft tissue, not elsewhere classified, right forearm**

    ▤ ✚ **M60.232   Foreign body granuloma of soft tissue, not elsewhere classified, left forearm**

    ▤ ✚ **M60.239   Foreign body granuloma of soft tissue, not elsewhere classified, unspecified forearm**

● New   ▲ Revised   *Manifestation*   ❹-❼ Digit Indicators   ▤ Laterality   Ⓐ Adult (15+ years)   Ⓜ Maternity (12-55 years)   Ⓝ Newborn   Ⓟ Pediatric (0-17 years)   ♂ Male   ♀ Female
✖ Deleted   Unspecified   ✚ Additional code

Diseases of the Musculoskeletal System and Connective Tissue

⑥+ **M60.24** Foreign body granuloma of soft tissue, not elsewhere classified, hand
  ⊟+ **M60.241** Foreign body granuloma of soft tissue, not elsewhere classified, right hand
  ⊟+ **M60.242** Foreign body granuloma of soft tissue, not elsewhere classified, left hand
  ⊟+ **M60.249** Foreign body granuloma of soft tissue, not elsewhere classified, unspecified hand
⑥+ **M60.25** Foreign body granuloma of soft tissue, not elsewhere classified, thigh
  ⊟+ **M60.251** Foreign body granuloma of soft tissue, not elsewhere classified, right thigh
  ⊟+ **M60.252** Foreign body granuloma of soft tissue, not elsewhere classified, left thigh
  ⊟+ **M60.259** Foreign body granuloma of soft tissue, not elsewhere classified, unspecified thigh
⑥+ **M60.26** Foreign body granuloma of soft tissue, not elsewhere classified, lower leg
  ⊟+ **M60.261** Foreign body granuloma of soft tissue, not elsewhere classified, right lower leg
  ⊟+ **M60.262** Foreign body granuloma of soft tissue, not elsewhere classified, left lower leg
  ⊟+ **M60.269** Foreign body granuloma of soft tissue, not elsewhere classified, unspecified lower leg
⑥+ **M60.27** Foreign body granuloma of soft tissue, not elsewhere classified, ankle and foot
  ⊟+ **M60.271** Foreign body granuloma of soft tissue, not elsewhere classified, right ankle and foot
  ⊟+ **M60.272** Foreign body granuloma of soft tissue, not elsewhere classified, left ankle and foot
  ⊟+ **M60.279** Foreign body granuloma of soft tissue, not elsewhere classified, unspecified ankle and foot
  + **M60.28** Foreign body granuloma of soft tissue, not elsewhere classified, other site
⑤ **M60.8** Other myositis
  M60.80 Other myositis, unspecified site
⑥ **M60.81** Other myositis shoulder
  ⊟ **M60.811** Other myositis, right shoulder
  ⊟ **M60.812** Other myositis, left shoulder
  ⊟ **M60.819** Other myositis, unspecified shoulder
⑥ **M60.82** Other myositis, upper arm
  ⊟ **M60.821** Other myositis, right upper arm
  ⊟ **M60.822** Other myositis, left upper arm
  ⊟ **M60.829** Other myositis, unspecified upper arm
⑥ **M60.83** Other myositis, forearm
  ⊟ **M60.831** Other myositis, right forearm
  ⊟ **M60.832** Other myositis, left forearm
  ⊟ **M60.839** Other myositis, unspecified forearm
⑥ **M60.84** Other myositis, hand
  ⊟ **M60.841** Other myositis, right hand
  ⊟ **M60.842** Other myositis, left hand
  ⊟ **M60.849** Other myositis, unspecified hand
⑥ **M60.85** Other myositis, thigh
  ⊟ **M60.851** Other myositis, right thigh
  ⊟ **M60.852** Other myositis, left thigh
  ⊟ **M60.859** Other myositis, unspecified thigh
⑥ **M60.86** Other myositis, lower leg
  ⊟ **M60.861** Other myositis, right lower leg
  ⊟ **M60.862** Other myositis, left lower leg
  ⊟ **M60.869** Other myositis, unspecified lower leg
⑥ **M60.87** Other myositis, ankle and foot
  ⊟ **M60.871** Other myositis, right ankle and foot
  ⊟ **M60.872** Other myositis, left ankle and foot
  ⊟ **M60.879** Other myositis, unspecified ankle and foot
  M60.88 Other myositis, other site
  M60.89 Other myositis, multiple sites
  M60.9 Myositis, unspecified
④ **M61** Calcification and ossification of muscle
⑤ **M61.0** Myositis ossificans traumatica
  M61.00 Myositis ossificans traumatica, unspecified site

⑥ **M61.01** Myositis ossificans traumatica, shoulder
  ⊟ **M61.011** Myositis ossificans traumatica, right shoulder
  ⊟ **M61.012** Myositis ossificans traumatica, left shoulder
  ⊟ **M61.019** Myositis ossificans traumatica, unspecified shoulder
⑥ **M61.02** Myositis ossificans traumatica, upper arm
  ⊟ **M61.021** Myositis ossificans traumatica, right upper arm
  ⊟ **M61.022** Myositis ossificans traumatica, left upper arm
  ⊟ **M61.029** Myositis ossificans traumatica, unspecified upper arm
⑥ **M61.03** Myositis ossificans traumatica, forearm
  ⊟ **M61.031** Myositis ossificans traumatica, right forearm
  ⊟ **M61.032** Myositis ossificans traumatica, left forearm
  ⊟ **M61.039** Myositis ossificans traumatica, unspecified forearm
⑥ **M61.04** Myositis ossificans traumatica, hand
  ⊟ **M61.041** Myositis ossificans traumatica, right hand
  ⊟ **M61.042** Myositis ossificans traumatica, left hand
  ⊟ **M61.049** Myositis ossificans traumatica, unspecified hand
⑥ **M61.05** Myositis ossificans traumatica, thigh
  ⊟ **M61.051** Myositis ossificans traumatica, right thigh
  ⊟ **M61.052** Myositis ossificans traumatica, left thigh
  ⊟ **M61.059** Myositis ossificans traumatica, unspecified thigh
⑥ **M61.06** Myositis ossificans traumatica, lower leg
  ⊟ **M61.061** Myositis ossificans traumatica, right lower leg
  ⊟ **M61.062** Myositis ossificans traumatica, left lower leg
  ⊟ **M61.069** Myositis ossificans traumatica, unspecified lower leg
⑥ **M61.07** Myositis ossificans traumatica, ankle and foot
  ⊟ **M61.071** Myositis ossificans traumatica, right ankle and foot
  ⊟ **M61.072** Myositis ossificans traumatica, left ankle and foot
  ⊟ **M61.079** Myositis ossificans traumatica, unspecified ankle and foot
  M61.08 Myositis ossificans traumatica, other site
  M61.09 Myositis ossificans traumatica, multiple sites
⑤ **M61.1** Myositis ossificans progressiva
  Fibrodysplasia ossificans progressiva
  M61.10 Myositis ossificans progressiva, unspecified site
⑥ **M61.11** Myositis ossificans progressiva, shoulder
  ⊟ **M61.111** Myositis ossificans progressiva, right shoulder
  ⊟ **M61.112** Myositis ossificans progressiva, left shoulder
  ⊟ **M61.119** Myositis ossificans progressiva, unspecified shoulder
⑥ **M61.12** Myositis ossificans progressiva, upper arm
  ⊟ **M61.121** Myositis ossificans progressiva, right upper arm
  ⊟ **M61.122** Myositis ossificans progressiva, left upper arm
  ⊟ **M61.129** Myositis ossificans progressiva, unspecified arm
⑥ **M61.13** Myositis ossificans progressiva, forearm
  ⊟ **M61.131** Myositis ossificans progressiva, right forearm
  ⊟ **M61.132** Myositis ossificans progressiva, left forearm
  ⊟ **M61.139** Myositis ossificans progressiva, unspecified forearm
⑥ **M61.14** Myositis ossificans progressiva, hand and finger(s)
  ⊟ **M61.141** Myositis ossificans progressiva, right hand
  ⊟ **M61.142** Myositis ossificans progressiva, left hand
  ⊟ **M61.143** Myositis ossificans progressiva, unspecified hand
  ⊟ **M61.144** Myositis ossificans progressiva, right finger(s)
  ⊟ **M61.145** Myositis ossificans progressiva, left finger(s)
  ⊟ **M61.146** Myositis ossificans progressiva, unspecified finger(s)
⑥ **M61.15** Myositis ossificans progressiva, thigh
  ⊟ **M61.151** Myositis ossificans progressiva, right thigh
  ⊟ **M61.152** Myositis ossificans progressiva, left thigh
  ⊟ **M61.159** Myositis ossificans progressiva, unspecified thigh
⑥ **M61.16** Myositis ossificans progressiva, lower leg
  ⊟ **M61.161** Myositis ossificans progressiva, right lower leg

● New ▲ Revised *Manifestation* ④-⑦ Digit Indicators ⊟ Laterality Ⓐ Adult (15+ years) Ⓜ Maternity (12-55 years) Ⓝ Newborn Ⓟ Pediatric (0-17 years) ♂ Male ♀ Female ✖ Deleted Unspecified + Additional code

⊟ **M61.162** Myositis ossificans progressiva, left lower leg
⊟ **M61.169** Myositis ossificans progressiva, unspecified lower leg
Ⓖ **M61.17** Myositis ossificans progressiva, ankle, foot and toe(s)
⊟ **M61.171** Myositis ossificans progressiva, right ankle
⊟ **M61.172** Myositis ossificans progressiva, left ankle
⊟ **M61.173** Myositis ossificans progressiva, unspecified ankle
⊟ **M61.174** Myositis ossificans progressiva, right foot
⊟ **M61.175** Myositis ossificans progressiva, left foot
⊟ **M61.176** Myositis ossificans progressiva, unspecified foot
⊟ **M61.177** Myositis ossificans progressiva, right toe(s)
⊟ **M61.178** Myositis ossificans progressiva, left toe(s)
⊟ **M61.179** Myositis ossificans progressiva, unspecified toe(s)
M61.18 Myositis ossificans progressiva, other site
M61.19 Myositis ossificans progressiva, multiple sites
Ⓢ **M61.2** Paralytic calcification and ossification of muscle
Myositis ossificans associated with quadriplegia or paraplegia
M61.20 Paralytic calcification and ossification of muscle, unspecified site
Ⓖ **M61.21** Paralytic calcification and ossification of muscle, shoulder
⊟ **M61.211** Paralytic calcification and ossification of muscle, right shoulder
⊟ **M61.212** Paralytic calcification and ossification of muscle, left shoulder
⊟ **M61.219** Paralytic calcification and ossification of muscle, unspecified shoulder
Ⓖ **M61.22** Paralytic calcification and ossification of muscle, upper arm
⊟ **M61.221** Paralytic calcification and ossification of muscle, right upper arm
⊟ **M61.222** Paralytic calcification and ossification of muscle, left upper arm
⊟ **M61.229** Paralytic calcification and ossification of muscle, unspecified upper arm
Ⓖ **M61.23** Paralytic calcification and ossification of muscle, forearm
⊟ **M61.231** Paralytic calcification and ossification of muscle, right forearm
⊟ **M61.232** Paralytic calcification and ossification of muscle, left forearm
⊟ **M61.239** Paralytic calcification and ossification of muscle, unspecified forearm
Ⓖ **M61.24** Paralytic calcification and ossification of muscle, hand
⊟ **M61.241** Paralytic calcification and ossification of muscle, right hand
⊟ **M61.242** Paralytic calcification and ossification of muscle, left hand
⊟ **M61.249** Paralytic calcification and ossification of muscle, unspecified hand
Ⓖ **M61.25** Paralytic calcification and ossification of muscle, thigh
⊟ **M61.251** Paralytic calcification and ossification of muscle, right thigh
⊟ **M61.252** Paralytic calcification and ossification of muscle, left thigh
⊟ **M61.259** Paralytic calcification and ossification of muscle, unspecified thigh
Ⓖ **M61.26** Paralytic calcification and ossification of muscle, lower leg
⊟ **M61.261** Paralytic calcification and ossification of muscle, right lower leg
⊟ **M61.262** Paralytic calcification and ossification of muscle, left lower leg
⊟ **M61.269** Paralytic calcification and ossification of muscle, unspecified lower leg
Ⓖ **M61.27** Paralytic calcification and ossification of muscle, ankle and foot
⊟ **M61.271** Paralytic calcification and ossification of muscle, right ankle and foot
⊟ **M61.272** Paralytic calcification and ossification of muscle, left ankle and foot
⊟ **M61.279** Paralytic calcification and ossification of muscle, unspecified ankle and foot
M61.28 Paralytic calcification and ossification of muscle, other site

M61.29 Paralytic calcification and ossification of muscle, multiple sites
Ⓢ **M61.3** Calcification and ossification of muscles associated with burns
Myositis ossificans associated with burns
M61.30 Calcification and ossification of muscles associated with burns, unspecified site
Ⓖ **M61.31** Calcification and ossification of muscles associated with burns, shoulder
⊟ **M61.311** Calcification and ossification of muscles associated with burns, right shoulder
⊟ **M61.312** Calcification and ossification of muscles associated with burns, left shoulder
⊟ **M61.319** Calcification and ossification of muscles associated with burns, unspecified shoulder
Ⓖ **M61.32** Calcification and ossification of muscles associated with burns, upper arm
⊟ **M61.321** Calcification and ossification of muscles associated with burns, right upper arm
⊟ **M61.322** Calcification and ossification of muscles associated with burns, left upper arm
⊟ **M61.329** Calcification and ossification of muscles associated with burns, unspecified upper arm
Ⓖ **M61.33** Calcification and ossification of muscles associated with burns, forearm
⊟ **M61.331** Calcification and ossification of muscles associated with burns, right forearm
⊟ **M61.332** Calcification and ossification of muscles associated with burns, left forearm
⊟ **M61.339** Calcification and ossification of muscles associated with burns, unspecified forearm
Ⓖ **M61.34** Calcification and ossification of muscles associated with burns, hand
⊟ **M61.341** Calcification and ossification of muscles associated with burns, right hand
⊟ **M61.342** Calcification and ossification of muscles associated with burns, left hand
⊟ **M61.349** Calcification and ossification of muscles associated with burns, unspecified hand
Ⓖ **M61.35** Calcification and ossification of muscles associated with burns, thigh
⊟ **M61.351** Calcification and ossification of muscles associated with burns, right thigh
⊟ **M61.352** Calcification and ossification of muscles associated with burns, left thigh
⊟ **M61.359** Calcification and ossification of muscles associated with burns, unspecified thigh
Ⓖ **M61.36** Calcification and ossification of muscles associated with burns, lower leg
⊟ **M61.361** Calcification and ossification of muscles associated with burns, right lower leg
⊟ **M61.362** Calcification and ossification of muscles associated with burns, left lower leg
⊟ **M61.369** Calcification and ossification of muscles associated with burns, unspecified lower leg
Ⓖ **M61.37** Calcification and ossification of muscles associated with burns, ankle and foot
⊟ **M61.371** Calcification and ossification of muscles associated with burns, right ankle and foot
⊟ **M61.372** Calcification and ossification of muscles associated with burns, left ankle and foot
⊟ **M61.379** Calcification and ossification of muscles associated with burns, unspecified ankle and foot
M61.38 Calcification and ossification of muscles associated with burns, other site
M61.39 Calcification and ossification of muscles associated with burns, multiple sites
Ⓢ **M61.4** Other calcification of muscle
EXCLUDES 1 *calcific tendinitis NOS (M65.2-)*
calcific tendinitis of shoulder (M75.3)
M61.40 Other calcification of muscle, unspecified site
Ⓖ **M61.41** Other calcification of muscle, shoulder
⊟ **M61.411** Other calcification of muscle, right shoulder
⊟ **M61.412** Other calcification of muscle, left shoulder
⊟ **M61.419** Other calcification of muscle, unspecified shoulder
Ⓖ **M61.42** Other calcification of muscle, upper arm
⊟ **M61.421** Other calcification of muscle, right upper arm
⊟ **M61.422** Other calcification of muscle, left upper arm

M61.429   Other calcification of muscle, unspecified upper arm
M61.43   Other calcification of muscle, forearm
　M61.431   Other calcification of muscle, right forearm
　M61.432   Other calcification of muscle, left forearm
　M61.439   Other calcification of muscle, unspecified forearm
M61.44   Other calcification of muscle, hand
　M61.441   Other calcification of muscle, right hand
　M61.442   Other calcification of muscle, left hand
　M61.449   Other calcification of muscle, unspecified hand
M61.45   Other calcification of muscle, thigh
　M61.451   Other calcification of muscle, right thigh
　M61.452   Other calcification of muscle, left thigh
　M61.459   Other calcification of muscle, unspecified thigh
M61.46   Other calcification of muscle, lower leg
　M61.461   Other calcification of muscle, right lower leg
　M61.462   Other calcification of muscle, left lower leg
　M61.469   Other calcification of muscle, unspecified lower leg
M61.47   Other calcification of muscle, ankle and foot
　M61.471   Other calcification of muscle, right ankle and foot
　M61.472   Other calcification of muscle, left ankle and foot
　M61.479   Other calcification of muscle, unspecified ankle and foot
M61.48   Other calcification of muscle, other site
M61.49   Other calcification of muscle, multiple sites
M61.5   Other ossification of muscle
M61.50   Other ossification of muscle, unspecified site
M61.51   Other ossification of muscle, shoulder
　M61.511   Other ossification of muscle, right shoulder
　M61.512   Other ossification of muscle, left shoulder
　M61.519   Other ossification of muscle, unspecified shoulder
M61.52   Other ossification of muscle, upper arm
　M61.521   Other ossification of muscle, right upper arm
　M61.522   Other ossification of muscle, left upper arm
　M61.529   Other ossification of muscle, unspecified upper arm
M61.53   Other ossification of muscle, forearm
　M61.531   Other ossification of muscle, right forearm
　M61.532   Other ossification of muscle, left forearm
　M61.539   Other ossification of muscle, unspecified forearm
M61.54   Other ossification of muscle, hand
　M61.541   Other ossification of muscle, right hand
　M61.542   Other ossification of muscle, left hand
　M61.549   Other ossification of muscle, unspecified hand
M61.55   Other ossification of muscle, thigh
　M61.551   Other ossification of muscle, right thigh
　M61.552   Other ossification of muscle, left thigh
　M61.559   Other ossification of muscle, unspecified thigh
M61.56   Other ossification of muscle, lower leg
　M61.561   Other ossification of muscle, right lower leg
　M61.562   Other ossification of muscle, left lower leg
　M61.569   Other ossification of muscle, unspecified lower leg
M61.57   Other ossification of muscle, ankle and foot
　M61.571   Other ossification of muscle, right ankle and foot
　M61.572   Other ossification of muscle, left ankle and foot
　M61.579   Other ossification of muscle, unspecified ankle and foot
M61.58   Other ossification of muscle, other site
M61.59   Other ossification of muscle, multiple sites
M61.9   Calcification and ossification of muscle, unspecified

M62   Other disorders of muscle
　EXCLUDES 1   *alcoholic myopathy (G72.1)*
cramp and spasm (R25.2)
drug-induced myopathy (G72.0)
myalgia (M79.1)
stiff-man syndrome (G25.82)
　EXCLUDES 2   *nontraumatic hematoma of muscle (M79.81)*

M62.0   Separation of muscle (nontraumatic)
Diastasis of muscle
　EXCLUDES 1   *diastasis recti complicating pregnancy, labor and delivery (O71.8)*
traumatic separation of muscle- see strain of muscle by body region
　CODING TIP ✓   Codes classified in M62.0- through M62.28 indicate muscle separation, rupture, and ischemia of a non-traumatic origin. When a traumatic muscle injury is reported do not assign a code from M62.0- through M62.28, but instead assign a code from chapter 19, Injury, poisoning and other certain consequences of external causes.
M62.00   Separation of muscle (nontraumatic), unspecified site
M62.01   Separation of muscle (nontraumatic), shoulder
　M62.011   Separation of muscle (nontraumatic), right shoulder
　M62.012   Separation of muscle (nontraumatic), left shoulder
　M62.019   Separation of muscle (nontraumatic), unspecified shoulder
M62.02   Separation of muscle (nontraumatic), upper arm
　M62.021   Separation of muscle (nontraumatic), right upper arm
　M62.022   Separation of muscle (nontraumatic), left upper arm
　M62.029   Separation of muscle (nontraumatic), unspecified upper arm
M62.03   Separation of muscle (nontraumatic), forearm
　M62.031   Separation of muscle (nontraumatic), right forearm
　M62.032   Separation of muscle (nontraumatic), left forearm
　M62.039   Separation of muscle (nontraumatic), unspecified forearm
M62.04   Separation of muscle (nontraumatic), hand
　M62.041   Separation of muscle (nontraumatic), right hand
　M62.042   Separation of muscle (nontraumatic), left hand
　M62.049   Separation of muscle (nontraumatic), unspecified hand
M62.05   Separation of muscle (nontraumatic), thigh
　M62.051   Separation of muscle (nontraumatic), right thigh
　M62.052   Separation of muscle (nontraumatic), left thigh
　M62.059   Separation of muscle (nontraumatic), unspecified thigh
M62.06   Separation of muscle (nontraumatic), lower leg
　M62.061   Separation of muscle (nontraumatic), right lower leg
　M62.062   Separation of muscle (nontraumatic), left lower leg
　M62.069   Separation of muscle (nontraumatic), unspecified lower leg
M62.07   Separation of muscle (nontraumatic), ankle and foot
　M62.071   Separation of muscle (nontraumatic), right ankle and foot
　M62.072   Separation of muscle (nontraumatic), left ankle and foot
　M62.079   Separation of muscle (nontraumatic), unspecified ankle and foot
M62.08   Separation of muscle (nontraumatic), other site
M62.1   Other rupture of muscle (nontraumatic)
　EXCLUDES 1   *traumatic rupture of muscle - see strain of muscle by body region*
　EXCLUDES 2   *rupture of tendon (M66.-)*
　CODING TIP ✓   Codes classified in M62.0- through M62.28 indicate muscle separation, rupture, and ischemia of a non-traumatic origin. When a traumatic muscle injury is reported do not assign a code from M62.0- through M62.28, but instead assign a code from chapter 19, Injury, poisoning and other certain consequences of external causes.
M62.10   Other rupture of muscle (nontraumatic), unspecified site

● New   ▲ Revised   *Manifestation*   ④-❼ Digit Indicators   ⊟ Laterality   Ⓐ Adult (15+ years)   Ⓜ Maternity (12-55 years)   Ⓝ Newborn   Ⓟ Pediatric (0-17 years)   ♂ Male   ♀ Female
✖ Deleted   Unspecified   + Additional code

2017 ICD-10-CM Expert for Physicians   © 2017 DecisionHealth   781

⑥ **M62.11**   Other rupture of muscle (nontraumatic), shoulder
   ⊟ **M62.111**   Other rupture of muscle (nontraumatic), right shoulder
   ⊟ **M62.112**   Other rupture of muscle (nontraumatic), left shoulder
   ⊟ **M62.119**   Other rupture of muscle (nontraumatic), unspecified shoulder
⑥ **M62.12**   Other rupture of muscle (nontraumatic), upper arm
   ⊟ **M62.121**   Other rupture of muscle (nontraumatic), right upper arm
   ⊟ **M62.122**   Other rupture of muscle (nontraumatic), left upper arm
   ⊟ **M62.129**   Other rupture of muscle (nontraumatic), unspecified upper arm
⑥ **M62.13**   Other rupture of muscle (nontraumatic), forearm
   ⊟ **M62.131**   Other rupture of muscle (nontraumatic), right forearm
   ⊟ **M62.132**   Other rupture of muscle (nontraumatic), left forearm
   ⊟ **M62.139**   Other rupture of muscle (nontraumatic), unspecified forearm
⑥ **M62.14**   Other rupture of muscle (nontraumatic), hand
   ⊟ **M62.141**   Other rupture of muscle (nontraumatic), right hand
   ⊟ **M62.142**   Other rupture of muscle (nontraumatic), left hand
   ⊟ **M62.149**   Other rupture of muscle (nontraumatic), unspecified hand
⑥ **M62.15**   Other rupture of muscle (nontraumatic), thigh
   ⊟ **M62.151**   Other rupture of muscle (nontraumatic), right thigh
   ⊟ **M62.152**   Other rupture of muscle (nontraumatic), left thigh
   ⊟ **M62.159**   Other rupture of muscle (nontraumatic), unspecified thigh
⑥ **M62.16**   Other rupture of muscle (nontraumatic), lower leg
   ⊟ **M62.161**   Other rupture of muscle (nontraumatic), right lower leg
   ⊟ **M62.162**   Other rupture of muscle (nontraumatic), left lower leg
   ⊟ **M62.169**   Other rupture of muscle (nontraumatic), unspecified lower leg
⑥ **M62.17**   Other rupture of muscle (nontraumatic), ankle and foot
   ⊟ **M62.171**   Other rupture of muscle (nontraumatic), right ankle and foot
   ⊟ **M62.172**   Other rupture of muscle (nontraumatic), left ankle and foot
   ⊟ **M62.179**   Other rupture of muscle (nontraumatic), unspecified ankle and foot
   M62.18   Other rupture of muscle (nontraumatic), other site
⑤ **M62.2**   Nontraumatic ischemic infarction of muscle

> **EXCLUDES 1**   *compartment syndrome (traumatic) (T79.A-)*
> *nontraumatic compartment syndrome (M79.A-)*
> *traumatic ischemia of muscle (T79.6)*
> *rhabdomyolysis (M62.82)*
> *Volkmann's ischemic contracture (T79.6)*

> **CODING TIP ✓**   Codes classified in M62.0- through M62.28 indicate muscle separation, rupture, and ischemia of a non-traumatic origin. When a traumatic muscle injury is reported do not assign a code from M62.0- through M62.28, but instead assign a code from chapter 19, Injury, poisoning and other certain consequences of external causes.

   M62.20   Nontraumatic ischemic infarction of muscle, unspecified site
⑥ **M62.21**   Nontraumatic ischemic infarction of muscle, shoulder
   ⊟ **M62.211**   Nontraumatic ischemic infarction of muscle, right shoulder
   ⊟ **M62.212**   Nontraumatic ischemic infarction of muscle, left shoulder
   ⊟ **M62.219**   Nontraumatic ischemic infarction of muscle, unspecified shoulder
⑥ **M62.22**   Nontraumatic ischemic infarction of muscle, upper arm
   ⊟ **M62.221**   Nontraumatic ischemic infarction of muscle, right upper arm
   ⊟ **M62.222**   Nontraumatic ischemic infarction of muscle, left upper arm
   ⊟ **M62.229**   Nontraumatic ischemic infarction of muscle, unspecified upper arm
⑥ **M62.23**   Nontraumatic ischemic infarction of muscle, forearm
   ⊟ **M62.231**   Nontraumatic ischemic infarction of muscle, right forearm
   ⊟ **M62.232**   Nontraumatic ischemic infarction of muscle, left forearm
   ⊟ **M62.239**   Nontraumatic ischemic infarction of muscle, unspecified forearm
⑥ **M62.24**   Nontraumatic ischemic infarction of muscle, hand
   ⊟ **M62.241**   Nontraumatic ischemic infarction of muscle, right hand
   ⊟ **M62.242**   Nontraumatic ischemic infarction of muscle, left hand
   ⊟ **M62.249**   Nontraumatic ischemic infarction of muscle, unspecified hand
⑥ **M62.25**   Nontraumatic ischemic infarction of muscle, thigh
   ⊟ **M62.251**   Nontraumatic ischemic infarction of muscle, right thigh
   ⊟ **M62.252**   Nontraumatic ischemic infarction of muscle, left thigh
   ⊟ **M62.259**   Nontraumatic ischemic infarction of muscle, unspecified thigh
⑥ **M62.26**   Nontraumatic ischemic infarction of muscle, lower leg
   ⊟ **M62.261**   Nontraumatic ischemic infarction of muscle, right lower leg
   ⊟ **M62.262**   Nontraumatic ischemic infarction of muscle, left lower leg
   ⊟ **M62.269**   Nontraumatic ischemic infarction of muscle, unspecified lower leg
⑥ **M62.27**   Nontraumatic ischemic infarction of muscle, ankle and foot
   ⊟ **M62.271**   Nontraumatic ischemic infarction of muscle, right ankle and foot
   ⊟ **M62.272**   Nontraumatic ischemic infarction of muscle, left ankle and foot
   ⊟ **M62.279**   Nontraumatic ischemic infarction of muscle, unspecified ankle and foot
   M62.28   Nontraumatic ischemic infarction of muscle, other site
M62.3   Immobility syndrome (paraplegic)

> **CODING TIP ✓**   Do not assign M62.3 for paraplegia that is due to a neurologic condition or injury. M62.3 indicates paraplegia of a non-neurologic origin due to immobility.

⑤ **M62.4**   Contracture of muscle
   Contracture of tendon (sheath)

> **EXCLUDES 1**   *contracture of joint (M24.5-)*

   M62.40   Contracture of muscle, unspecified site
⑥ **M62.41**   Contracture of muscle, shoulder
   ⊟ **M62.411**   Contracture of muscle, right shoulder
   ⊟ **M62.412**   Contracture of muscle, left shoulder
   ⊟ **M62.419**   Contracture of muscle, unspecified shoulder
⑥ **M62.42**   Contracture of muscle, upper arm
   ⊟ **M62.421**   Contracture of muscle, right upper arm
   ⊟ **M62.422**   Contracture of muscle, left upper arm
   ⊟ **M62.429**   Contracture of muscle, unspecified upper arm
⑥ **M62.43**   Contracture of muscle, forearm
   ⊟ **M62.431**   Contracture of muscle, right forearm
   ⊟ **M62.432**   Contracture of muscle, left forearm
   ⊟ **M62.439**   Contracture of muscle, unspecified forearm
⑥ **M62.44**   Contracture of muscle, hand
   ⊟ **M62.441**   Contracture of muscle, right hand
   ⊟ **M62.442**   Contracture of muscle, left hand
   ⊟ **M62.449**   Contracture of muscle, unspecified hand
⑥ **M62.45**   Contracture of muscle, thigh
   ⊟ **M62.451**   Contracture of muscle, right thigh
   ⊟ **M62.452**   Contracture of muscle, left thigh
   ⊟ **M62.459**   Contracture of muscle, unspecified thigh
⑥ **M62.46**   Contracture of muscle, lower leg

● New   ▲ Revised   *Manifestation*   ❹-❼ Digit Indicators   ⊟ Laterality   Ⓐ Adult (15+ years)   Ⓜ Maternity (12-55 years)   Ⓝ Newborn   Ⓟ Pediatric (0-17 years)   ♂ Male   ♀ Female
✖ ~~Deleted~~   Unspecified   + Additional code

782   © 2017 DecisionHealth   2017 ICD-10-CM Expert for Physicians

M62.461 Contracture of muscle, right lower leg
M62.462 Contracture of muscle, left lower leg
M62.469 Contracture of muscle, unspecified lower leg
🄖 M62.47 Contracture of muscle, ankle and foot
M62.471 Contracture of muscle, right ankle and foot
M62.472 Contracture of muscle, left ankle and foot
M62.479 Contracture of muscle, unspecified ankle and foot
M62.48 Contracture of muscle, other site
M62.49 Contracture of muscle, multiple sites
▲ 🄓 M62.5 Muscle wasting and atrophy, not elsewhere classified
Disuse atrophy NEC

EXCLUDES 1 neuralgic amyotrophy (G54.5)
progressive muscular atrophy (G12.29)
sarcopenia (M62.84)

EXCLUDES 2 pelvic muscle wasting (N81.84)

M62.50 Muscle wasting and atrophy, not elsewhere classified, unspecified site
🄖 M62.51 Muscle wasting and atrophy, not elsewhere classified, shoulder
M62.511 Muscle wasting and atrophy, not elsewhere classified, right shoulder
M62.512 Muscle wasting and atrophy, not elsewhere classified, left shoulder
M62.519 Muscle wasting and atrophy, not elsewhere classified, unspecified shoulder
🄖 M62.52 Muscle wasting and atrophy, not elsewhere classified, upper arm
M62.521 Muscle wasting and atrophy, not elsewhere classified, right upper arm
M62.522 Muscle wasting and atrophy, not elsewhere classified, left upper arm
M62.529 Muscle wasting and atrophy, not elsewhere classified, unspecified upper arm
🄖 M62.53 Muscle wasting and atrophy, not elsewhere classified, forearm
M62.531 Muscle wasting and atrophy, not elsewhere classified, right forearm
M62.532 Muscle wasting and atrophy, not elsewhere classified, left forearm
M62.539 Muscle wasting and atrophy, not elsewhere classified, unspecified forearm
🄖 M62.54 Muscle wasting and atrophy, not elsewhere classified, hand
M62.541 Muscle wasting and atrophy, not elsewhere classified, right hand
M62.542 Muscle wasting and atrophy, not elsewhere classified, left hand
M62.549 Muscle wasting and atrophy, not elsewhere classified, unspecified hand
🄖 M62.55 Muscle wasting and atrophy, not elsewhere classified, thigh
M62.551 Muscle wasting and atrophy, not elsewhere classified, right thigh
M62.552 Muscle wasting and atrophy, not elsewhere classified, left thigh
M62.559 Muscle wasting and atrophy, not elsewhere classified, unspecified thigh
🄖 M62.56 Muscle wasting and atrophy, not elsewhere classified, lower leg
M62.561 Muscle wasting and atrophy, not elsewhere classified, right lower leg
M62.562 Muscle wasting and atrophy, not elsewhere classified, left lower leg
M62.569 Muscle wasting and atrophy, not elsewhere classified, unspecified lower leg
🄖 M62.57 Muscle wasting and atrophy, not elsewhere classified, ankle and foot
M62.571 Muscle wasting and atrophy, not elsewhere classified, right ankle and foot
M62.572 Muscle wasting and atrophy, not elsewhere classified, left ankle and foot
M62.579 Muscle wasting and atrophy, not elsewhere classified, unspecified ankle and foot
M62.58 Muscle wasting and atrophy, not elsewhere classified, other site
M62.59 Muscle wasting and atrophy, not elsewhere classified, multiple sites

🄓 M62.8 Other specified disorders of muscle
EXCLUDES 2 nontraumatic hematoma of muscle (M79.81)
▲ M62.81 Muscle weakness (generalized)
EXCLUDES 1 muscle weakness in sarcopenia (M62.84)
M62.82 Rhabdomyolysis
EXCLUDES 1 traumatic rhabdomyolysis (T79.6)
🄖 M62.83 Muscle spasm
M62.830 Muscle spasm of back
M62.831 Muscle spasm of calf
Charley-horse
M62.838 Other muscle spasm
● M62.84 Sarcopenia
Age-related sarcopenia
Code first underlying disease, if applicable, such as:
disorders of myoneural junction and muscle disease in diseases classified elsewhere (G73.-)
other and unspecified myopathies (G72.-)
primary disorders of muscles (G71.-)
M62.89 Other specified disorders of muscle
Muscle (sheath) hernia
M62.9 Disorder of muscle, unspecified

🄬 M63 Disorders of muscle in diseases classified elsewhere
Code first underlying disease, such as:
leprosy (A30.-)
neoplasm (C49.-, C79.89, D21.-, D48.1)
schistosomiasis (B65.-)
trichinellosis (B75)
EXCLUDES 1 myopathy in cysticercosis (B69.81)
myopathy in endocrine diseases (G73.7)
myopathy in metabolic diseases (G73.7)
myopathy in sarcoidosis (D86.87)
myopathy in secondary syphilis (A51.49)
myopathy in syphilis (late) (A52.78)
myopathy in toxoplasmosis (B58.82)
myopathy in tuberculosis (A18.09)
🄓 M63.8 Disorders of muscle in diseases classified elsewhere
M63.80 Disorders of muscle in diseases classified elsewhere, unspecified site
🄖 M63.81 Disorders of muscle in diseases classified elsewhere, shoulder
M63.811 Disorders of muscle in diseases classified elsewhere, right shoulder
M63.812 Disorders of muscle in diseases classified elsewhere, left shoulder
M63.819 Disorders of muscle in diseases classified elsewhere, unspecified shoulder
🄖 M63.82 Disorders of muscle in diseases classified elsewhere, upper arm
M63.821 Disorders of muscle in diseases classified elsewhere, right upper arm
M63.822 Disorders of muscle in diseases classified elsewhere, left upper arm
M63.829 Disorders of muscle in diseases classified elsewhere, unspecified upper arm
🄖 M63.83 Disorders of muscle in diseases classified elsewhere, forearm
M63.831 Disorders of muscle in diseases classified elsewhere, right forearm
M63.832 Disorders of muscle in diseases classified elsewhere, left forearm
M63.839 Disorders of muscle in diseases classified elsewhere, unspecified forearm
🄖 M63.84 Disorders of muscle in diseases classified elsewhere, hand
M63.841 Disorders of muscle in diseases classified elsewhere, right hand
M63.842 Disorders of muscle in diseases classified elsewhere, left hand
M63.849 Disorders of muscle in diseases classified elsewhere, unspecified hand
🄖 M63.85 Disorders of muscle in diseases classified elsewhere, thigh
M63.851 Disorders of muscle in diseases classified elsewhere, right thigh
M63.852 Disorders of muscle in diseases classified elsewhere, left thigh

● New   ▲ Revised   *Manifestation*   🄓-🄱 Digit Indicators   🖿 Laterality   🅰 Adult (15+ years)   🅼 Maternity (12-55 years)   🅽 Newborn (0-17 years)   🅿 Pediatric   ♂ Male   ♀ Female
✖ Deleted   Unspecified   + Additional code

2017 ICD-10-CM Expert for Physicians

© 2017 DecisionHealth   783

☐ M63.859 *Disorders of muscle in diseases classified elsewhere, unspecified thigh*

Ⓖ M63.86 Disorders of muscle in diseases classified elsewhere, lower leg

☐ M63.861 *Disorders of muscle in diseases classified elsewhere, right lower leg*

☐ M63.862 *Disorders of muscle in diseases classified elsewhere, left lower leg*

☐ M63.869 *Disorders of muscle in diseases classified elsewhere, unspecified lower leg*

Ⓖ M63.87 Disorders of muscle in diseases classified elsewhere, ankle and foot

☐ M63.871 *Disorders of muscle in diseases classified elsewhere, right ankle and foot*

☐ M63.872 *Disorders of muscle in diseases classified elsewhere, left ankle and foot*

☐ M63.879 *Disorders of muscle in diseases classified elsewhere, unspecified ankle and foot*

M63.88 *Disorders of muscle in diseases classified elsewhere, other site*

M63.89 *Disorders of muscle in diseases classified elsewhere, multiple sites*

Disorders of synovium and tendon (M65-M67)

Ⓐ M65 **Synovitis and tenosynovitis**

> **EXCLUDES 1** *chronic crepitant synovitis of hand and wrist (M70.0-)*
> *current injury - see injury of ligament or tendon by body region*
> *soft tissue disorders related to use, overuse and pressure (M70.-)*

Ⓢ➕ M65.0 **Abscess of tendon sheath**
Use additional code (B95-B96) to identify bacterial agent.

➕ M65.00 Abscess of tendon sheath, unspecified site

Ⓖ➕ M65.01 Abscess of tendon sheath, shoulder

☐➕ M65.011 Abscess of tendon sheath, right shoulder

☐➕ M65.012 Abscess of tendon sheath, left shoulder

☐➕ M65.019 Abscess of tendon sheath, unspecified shoulder

Ⓖ➕ M65.02 Abscess of tendon sheath, upper arm

☐➕ M65.021 Abscess of tendon sheath, right upper arm

☐➕ M65.022 Abscess of tendon sheath, left upper arm

☐➕ M65.029 Abscess of tendon sheath, unspecified upper arm

Ⓖ➕ M65.03 Abscess of tendon sheath, forearm

☐➕ M65.031 Abscess of tendon sheath, right forearm

☐➕ M65.032 Abscess of tendon sheath, left forearm

☐➕ M65.039 Abscess of tendon sheath, unspecified forearm

Ⓖ➕ M65.04 Abscess of tendon sheath, hand

☐➕ M65.041 Abscess of tendon sheath, right hand

☐➕ M65.042 Abscess of tendon sheath, left hand

☐➕ M65.049 Abscess of tendon sheath, unspecified hand

Ⓖ➕ M65.05 Abscess of tendon sheath, thigh

☐➕ M65.051 Abscess of tendon sheath, right thigh

☐➕ M65.052 Abscess of tendon sheath, left thigh

☐➕ M65.059 Abscess of tendon sheath, unspecified thigh

Ⓖ➕ M65.06 Abscess of tendon sheath, lower leg

☐➕ M65.061 Abscess of tendon sheath, right lower leg

☐➕ M65.062 Abscess of tendon sheath, left lower leg

☐➕ M65.069 Abscess of tendon sheath, unspecified lower leg

Ⓖ➕ M65.07 Abscess of tendon sheath, ankle and foot

☐➕ M65.071 Abscess of tendon sheath, right ankle and foot

☐➕ M65.072 Abscess of tendon sheath, left ankle and foot

☐➕ M65.079 Abscess of tendon sheath, unspecified ankle and foot

➕ M65.08 Abscess of tendon sheath, other site

Ⓢ M65.1 Other infective (teno)synovitis

M65.10 Other infective (teno)synovitis, unspecified site

Ⓖ M65.11 Other infective (teno)synovitis, shoulder

☐ M65.111 Other infective (teno)synovitis, right shoulder

☐ M65.112 Other infective (teno)synovitis, left shoulder

☐ M65.119 Other infective (teno)synovitis, unspecified shoulder

Ⓖ M65.12 Other infective (teno)synovitis, elbow

☐ M65.121 Other infective (teno)synovitis, right elbow

☐ M65.122 Other infective (teno)synovitis, left elbow

☐ M65.129 Other infective (teno)synovitis, unspecified elbow

Ⓖ M65.13 Other infective (teno)synovitis, wrist

☐ M65.131 Other infective (teno)synovitis, right wrist

☐ M65.132 Other infective (teno)synovitis, left wrist

☐ M65.139 Other infective (teno)synovitis, unspecified wrist

Ⓖ M65.14 Other infective (teno)synovitis, hand

☐ M65.141 Other infective (teno)synovitis, right hand

☐ M65.142 Other infective (teno)synovitis, left hand

☐ M65.149 Other infective (teno)synovitis, unspecified hand

Ⓖ M65.15 Other infective (teno)synovitis, hip

☐ M65.151 Other infective (teno)synovitis, right hip

☐ M65.152 Other infective (teno)synovitis, left hip

☐ M65.159 Other infective (teno)synovitis, unspecified hip

Ⓖ M65.16 Other infective (teno)synovitis, knee

☐ M65.161 Other infective (teno)synovitis, right knee

☐ M65.162 Other infective (teno)synovitis, left knee

☐ M65.169 Other infective (teno)synovitis, unspecified knee

Ⓖ M65.17 Other infective (teno)synovitis, ankle and foot

☐ M65.171 Other infective (teno)synovitis, right ankle and foot

☐ M65.172 Other infective (teno)synovitis, left ankle and foot

☐ M65.179 Other infective (teno)synovitis, unspecified ankle and foot

M65.18 Other infective (teno)synovitis, other site

M65.19 Other infective (teno)synovitis, multiple sites

Ⓢ M65.2 Calcific tendinitis

> **EXCLUDES 1** *tendinitis as classified in M75-M77*
> *calcified tendinitis of shoulder (M75.3)*

M65.20 Calcific tendinitis, unspecified site

Ⓖ M65.22 Calcific tendinitis, upper arm

☐ M65.221 Calcific tendinitis, right upper arm

☐ M65.222 Calcific tendinitis, left upper arm

☐ M65.229 Calcific tendinitis, unspecified upper arm

Ⓖ M65.23 Calcific tendinitis, forearm

☐ M65.231 Calcific tendinitis, right forearm

☐ M65.232 Calcific tendinitis, left forearm

☐ M65.239 Calcific tendinitis, unspecified forearm

Ⓖ M65.24 Calcific tendinitis, hand

☐ M65.241 Calcific tendinitis, right hand

☐ M65.242 Calcific tendinitis, left hand

☐ M65.249 Calcific tendinitis, unspecified hand

Ⓖ M65.25 Calcific tendinitis, thigh

☐ M65.251 Calcific tendinitis, right thigh

☐ M65.252 Calcific tendinitis, left thigh

☐ M65.259 Calcific tendinitis, unspecified thigh

Ⓖ M65.26 Calcific tendinitis, lower leg

☐ M65.261 Calcific tendinitis, right lower leg

☐ M65.262 Calcific tendinitis, left lower leg

☐ M65.269 Calcific tendinitis, unspecified lower leg

Ⓖ M65.27 Calcific tendinitis, ankle and foot

☐ M65.271 Calcific tendinitis, right ankle and foot

☐ M65.272 Calcific tendinitis, left ankle and foot

☐ M65.279 Calcific tendinitis, unspecified ankle and foot

M65.28 Calcific tendinitis, other site

M65.29 Calcific tendinitis, multiple sites

Ⓢ M65.3 Trigger finger
Nodular tendinous disease

M65.30 Trigger finger, unspecified finger

Ⓖ M65.31 Trigger thumb

☐ M65.311 Trigger thumb, right thumb

☐ M65.312 Trigger thumb, left thumb

☐ M65.319 Trigger thumb, unspecified thumb

Ⓖ M65.32 Trigger finger, index finger

☐ M65.321 Trigger finger, right index finger

● New   ▲ Revised   *Manifestation*   Ⓐ-❼ Digit Indicators   ☐ Laterality   Ⓐ Adult (15+ years)   Ⓜ Maternity (12-55 years)   Ⓝ Newborn   Ⓟ Pediatric (0-17 years)   ♂ Male   ♀ Female
✖ Deleted   Unspecified   ➕ Additional code

784   © 2017 DecisionHealth   2017 ICD-10-CM Expert for Physicians

- ⊟ M65.322 Trigger finger, left index finger
- ⊟ M65.329 Trigger finger, unspecified index finger
- ⑤ M65.33 Trigger finger, middle finger
  - ⊟ M65.331 Trigger finger, right middle finger
  - ⊟ M65.332 Trigger finger, left middle finger
  - ⊟ M65.339 Trigger finger, unspecified middle finger
- ⑤ M65.34 Trigger finger, ring finger
  - ⊟ M65.341 Trigger finger, right ring finger
  - ⊟ M65.342 Trigger finger, left ring finger
  - ⊟ M65.349 Trigger finger, unspecified ring finger
- ⑤ M65.35 Trigger finger, little finger
  - ⊟ M65.351 Trigger finger, right little finger
  - ⊟ M65.352 Trigger finger, left little finger
  - ⊟ M65.359 Trigger finger, unspecified little finger
- M65.4 Radial styloid tenosynovitis [de Quervain]
- ⑤ M65.8 Other synovitis and tenosynovitis
  - M65.80 Other synovitis and tenosynovitis, unspecified site
  - ⑤ M65.81 Other synovitis and tenosynovitis, shoulder
    - ⊟ M65.811 Other synovitis and tenosynovitis, right shoulder
    - ⊟ M65.812 Other synovitis and tenosynovitis, left shoulder
    - ⊟ M65.819 Other synovitis and tenosynovitis, unspecified shoulder
  - ⑤ M65.82 Other synovitis and tenosynovitis, upper arm
    - ⊟ M65.821 Other synovitis and tenosynovitis, right upper arm
    - ⊟ M65.822 Other synovitis and tenosynovitis, left upper arm
    - ⊟ M65.829 Other synovitis and tenosynovitis, unspecified upper arm
  - ⑤ M65.83 Other synovitis and tenosynovitis, forearm
    - ⊟ M65.831 Other synovitis and tenosynovitis, right forearm
    - ⊟ M65.832 Other synovitis and tenosynovitis, left forearm
    - ⊟ M65.839 Other synovitis and tenosynovitis, unspecified forearm
  - ⑤ M65.84 Other synovitis and tenosynovitis, hand
    - ⊟ M65.841 Other synovitis and tenosynovitis, right hand
    - ⊟ M65.842 Other synovitis and tenosynovitis, left hand
    - ⊟ M65.849 Other synovitis and tenosynovitis, unspecified hand
  - ⑤ M65.85 Other synovitis and tenosynovitis, thigh
    - ⊟ M65.851 Other synovitis and tenosynovitis, right thigh
    - ⊟ M65.852 Other synovitis and tenosynovitis, left thigh
    - ⊟ M65.859 Other synovitis and tenosynovitis, unspecified thigh
  - ⑤ M65.86 Other synovitis and tenosynovitis, lower leg
    - ⊟ M65.861 Other synovitis and tenosynovitis, right lower leg
    - ⊟ M65.862 Other synovitis and tenosynovitis, left lower leg
    - ⊟ M65.869 Other synovitis and tenosynovitis, unspecified lower leg
  - ⑤ M65.87 Other synovitis and tenosynovitis, ankle and foot
    - ⊟ M65.871 Other synovitis and tenosynovitis, right ankle and foot
    - ⊟ M65.872 Other synovitis and tenosynovitis, left ankle and foot
    - ⊟ M65.879 Other synovitis and tenosynovitis, unspecified ankle and foot
  - M65.88 Other synovitis and tenosynovitis, other site
  - M65.89 Other synovitis and tenosynovitis, multiple sites
- M65.9 Synovitis and tenosynovitis, unspecified
- ④ M66 Spontaneous rupture of synovium and tendon

  INCLUDES rupture that occurs when a normal force is applied to tissues that are inferred to have less than normal strength

  EXCLUDES 2 *rotator cuff syndrome (M75.1-)*
  rupture where an abnormal force is applied to normal tissue - see injury of tendon by body region

  - M66.0 Rupture of popliteal cyst
  - ⑤ M66.1 Rupture of synovium
    Rupture of synovial cyst

    EXCLUDES 2 *rupture of popliteal cyst (M66.0)*

    - M66.10 Rupture of synovium, unspecified joint
    - ⑤ M66.11 Rupture of synovium, shoulder

- ⊟ M66.111 Rupture of synovium, right shoulder
- ⊟ M66.112 Rupture of synovium, left shoulder
- ⊟ M66.119 Rupture of synovium, unspecified shoulder
- ⑤ M66.12 Rupture of synovium, elbow
  - ⊟ M66.121 Rupture of synovium, right elbow
  - ⊟ M66.122 Rupture of synovium, left elbow
  - ⊟ M66.129 Rupture of synovium, unspecified elbow
- ⑤ M66.13 Rupture of synovium, wrist
  - ⊟ M66.131 Rupture of synovium, right wrist
  - ⊟ M66.132 Rupture of synovium, left wrist
  - ⊟ M66.139 Rupture of synovium, unspecified wrist
- ⑤ M66.14 Rupture of synovium, hand and fingers
  - ⊟ M66.141 Rupture of synovium, right hand
  - ⊟ M66.142 Rupture of synovium, left hand
  - ⊟ M66.143 Rupture of synovium, unspecified hand
  - ⊟ M66.144 Rupture of synovium, right finger(s)
  - ⊟ M66.145 Rupture of synovium, left finger(s)
  - ⊟ M66.146 Rupture of synovium, unspecified finger(s)
- ⑤ M66.15 Rupture of synovium, hip
  - ⊟ M66.151 Rupture of synovium, right hip
  - ⊟ M66.152 Rupture of synovium, left hip
  - ⊟ M66.159 Rupture of synovium, unspecified hip
- ⑤ M66.17 Rupture of synovium, ankle, foot and toes
  - ⊟ M66.171 Rupture of synovium, right ankle
  - ⊟ M66.172 Rupture of synovium, left ankle
  - ⊟ M66.173 Rupture of synovium, unspecified ankle
  - ⊟ M66.174 Rupture of synovium, right foot
  - ⊟ M66.175 Rupture of synovium, left foot
  - ⊟ M66.176 Rupture of synovium, unspecified foot
  - ⊟ M66.177 Rupture of synovium, right toe(s)
  - ⊟ M66.178 Rupture of synovium, left toe(s)
  - ⊟ M66.179 Rupture of synovium, unspecified toe(s)
- M66.18 Rupture of synovium, other site
- ⑤ M66.2 Spontaneous rupture of extensor tendons
  - M66.20 Spontaneous rupture of extensor tendons, unspecified site
  - ⑤ M66.21 Spontaneous rupture of extensor tendons, shoulder
    - ⊟ M66.211 Spontaneous rupture of extensor tendons, right shoulder
    - ⊟ M66.212 Spontaneous rupture of extensor tendons, left shoulder
    - ⊟ M66.219 Spontaneous rupture of extensor tendons, unspecified shoulder
  - ⑤ M66.22 Spontaneous rupture of extensor tendons, upper arm
    - ⊟ M66.221 Spontaneous rupture of extensor tendons, right upper arm
    - ⊟ M66.222 Spontaneous rupture of extensor tendons, left upper arm
    - ⊟ M66.229 Spontaneous rupture of extensor tendons, unspecified upper arm
  - ⑤ M66.23 Spontaneous rupture of extensor tendons, forearm
    - ⊟ M66.231 Spontaneous rupture of extensor tendons, right forearm
    - ⊟ M66.232 Spontaneous rupture of extensor tendons, left forearm
    - ⊟ M66.239 Spontaneous rupture of extensor tendons, unspecified forearm
  - ⑤ M66.24 Spontaneous rupture of extensor tendons, hand
    - ⊟ M66.241 Spontaneous rupture of extensor tendons, right hand
    - ⊟ M66.242 Spontaneous rupture of extensor tendons, left hand
    - ⊟ M66.249 Spontaneous rupture of extensor tendons, unspecified hand
  - ⑤ M66.25 Spontaneous rupture of extensor tendons, thigh
    - ⊟ M66.251 Spontaneous rupture of extensor tendons, right thigh
    - ⊟ M66.252 Spontaneous rupture of extensor tendons, left thigh
    - ⊟ M66.259 Spontaneous rupture of extensor tendons, unspecified thigh
  - ⑤ M66.26 Spontaneous rupture of extensor tendons, lower leg
    - ⊟ M66.261 Spontaneous rupture of extensor tendons, right lower leg

---

● New ▲ Revised *Manifestation* ④-⑦ Digit Indicators ⊟ Laterality Ⓐ Adult (15+ years) Ⓜ Maternity (12-55 years) Ⓝ Newborn Ⓟ Pediatric (0-17 years) ♂ Male ♀ Female
✖ Deleted Unspecified + Additional code

☐ **M66.262** Spontaneous rupture of extensor tendons, left lower leg

☐ **M66.269** Spontaneous rupture of extensor tendons, unspecified lower leg

Ⓖ **M66.27** Spontaneous rupture of extensor tendons, ankle and foot

☐ **M66.271** Spontaneous rupture of extensor tendons, right ankle and foot

☐ **M66.272** Spontaneous rupture of extensor tendons, left ankle and foot

☐ **M66.279** Spontaneous rupture of extensor tendons, unspecified ankle and foot

M66.28 Spontaneous rupture of extensor tendons, other site

M66.29 Spontaneous rupture of extensor tendons, multiple sites

Ⓢ **M66.3** Spontaneous rupture of flexor tendons

M66.30 Spontaneous rupture of flexor tendons, unspecified site

Ⓖ **M66.31** Spontaneous rupture of flexor tendons, shoulder

☐ **M66.311** Spontaneous rupture of flexor tendons, right shoulder

☐ **M66.312** Spontaneous rupture of flexor tendons, left shoulder

☐ **M66.319** Spontaneous rupture of flexor tendons, unspecified shoulder

Ⓖ **M66.32** Spontaneous rupture of flexor tendons, upper arm

☐ **M66.321** Spontaneous rupture of flexor tendons, right upper arm

☐ **M66.322** Spontaneous rupture of flexor tendons, left upper arm

☐ **M66.329** Spontaneous rupture of flexor tendons, unspecified upper arm

Ⓖ **M66.33** Spontaneous rupture of flexor tendons, forearm

☐ **M66.331** Spontaneous rupture of flexor tendons, right forearm

☐ **M66.332** Spontaneous rupture of flexor tendons, left forearm

☐ **M66.339** Spontaneous rupture of flexor tendons, unspecified forearm

Ⓖ **M66.34** Spontaneous rupture of flexor tendons, hand

☐ **M66.341** Spontaneous rupture of flexor tendons, right hand

☐ **M66.342** Spontaneous rupture of flexor tendons, left hand

☐ **M66.349** Spontaneous rupture of flexor tendons, unspecified hand

Ⓖ **M66.35** Spontaneous rupture of flexor tendons, thigh

☐ **M66.351** Spontaneous rupture of flexor tendons, right thigh

☐ **M66.352** Spontaneous rupture of flexor tendons, left thigh

☐ **M66.359** Spontaneous rupture of flexor tendons, unspecified thigh

Ⓖ **M66.36** Spontaneous rupture of flexor tendons, lower leg

☐ **M66.361** Spontaneous rupture of flexor tendons, right lower leg

☐ **M66.362** Spontaneous rupture of flexor tendons, left lower leg

☐ **M66.369** Spontaneous rupture of flexor tendons, unspecified lower leg

Ⓖ **M66.37** Spontaneous rupture of flexor tendons, ankle and foot

☐ **M66.371** Spontaneous rupture of flexor tendons, right ankle and foot

☐ **M66.372** Spontaneous rupture of flexor tendons, left ankle and foot

☐ **M66.379** Spontaneous rupture of flexor tendons, unspecified ankle and foot

M66.38 Spontaneous rupture of flexor tendons, other site

M66.39 Spontaneous rupture of flexor tendons, multiple sites

Ⓢ **M66.8** Spontaneous rupture of other tendons

M66.80 Spontaneous rupture of other tendons, unspecified site

Ⓖ **M66.81** Spontaneous rupture of other tendons, shoulder

☐ **M66.811** Spontaneous rupture of other tendons, right shoulder

☐ **M66.812** Spontaneous rupture of other tendons, left shoulder

☐ **M66.819** Spontaneous rupture of other tendons, unspecified shoulder

Ⓖ **M66.82** Spontaneous rupture of other tendons, upper arm

☐ **M66.821** Spontaneous rupture of other tendons, right upper arm

☐ **M66.822** Spontaneous rupture of other tendons, left upper arm

☐ **M66.829** Spontaneous rupture of other tendons, unspecified upper arm

Ⓖ **M66.83** Spontaneous rupture of other tendons, forearm

☐ **M66.831** Spontaneous rupture of other tendons, right forearm

☐ **M66.832** Spontaneous rupture of other tendons, left forearm

☐ **M66.839** Spontaneous rupture of other tendons, unspecified forearm

Ⓖ **M66.84** Spontaneous rupture of other tendons, hand

☐ **M66.841** Spontaneous rupture of other tendons, right hand

☐ **M66.842** Spontaneous rupture of other tendons, left hand

☐ **M66.849** Spontaneous rupture of other tendons, unspecified hand

Ⓖ **M66.85** Spontaneous rupture of other tendons, thigh

☐ **M66.851** Spontaneous rupture of other tendons, right thigh

☐ **M66.852** Spontaneous rupture of other tendons, left thigh

☐ **M66.859** Spontaneous rupture of other tendons, unspecified thigh

Ⓖ **M66.86** Spontaneous rupture of other tendons, lower leg

☐ **M66.861** Spontaneous rupture of other tendons, right lower leg

☐ **M66.862** Spontaneous rupture of other tendons, left lower leg

☐ **M66.869** Spontaneous rupture of other tendons, unspecified lower leg

Ⓖ **M66.87** Spontaneous rupture of other tendons, ankle and foot

☐ **M66.871** Spontaneous rupture of other tendons, right ankle and foot

☐ **M66.872** Spontaneous rupture of other tendons, left ankle and foot

☐ **M66.879** Spontaneous rupture of other tendons, unspecified ankle and foot

M66.88 Spontaneous rupture of other tendons, other

M66.89 Spontaneous rupture of other tendons, multiple sites

M66.9 Spontaneous rupture of unspecified tendon

Rupture at musculotendinous junction, nontraumatic

Ⓐ **M67** **Other disorders of synovium and tendon**

EXCLUDES 1 *palmar fascial fibromatosis [Dupuytren] (M72.0)*
tendinitis NOS (M77.9-)
xanthomatosis localized to tendons (E78.2)

Ⓢ **M67.0** Short Achilles tendon (acquired)

☐ **M67.00** Short Achilles tendon (acquired), unspecified ankle

☐ **M67.01** Short Achilles tendon (acquired), right ankle

☐ **M67.02** Short Achilles tendon (acquired), left ankle

Ⓢ **M67.2** Synovial hypertrophy, not elsewhere classified

EXCLUDES 1 *villonodular synovitis (pigmented) (M12.2-)*

M67.20 Synovial hypertrophy, not elsewhere classified, unspecified site

Ⓖ **M67.21** Synovial hypertrophy, not elsewhere classified, shoulder

☐ **M67.211** Synovial hypertrophy, not elsewhere classified, right shoulder

☐ **M67.212** Synovial hypertrophy, not elsewhere classified, left shoulder

☐ **M67.219** Synovial hypertrophy, not elsewhere classified, unspecified shoulder

Ⓖ **M67.22** Synovial hypertrophy, not elsewhere classified, upper arm

☐ **M67.221** Synovial hypertrophy, not elsewhere classified, right upper arm

☐ **M67.222** Synovial hypertrophy, not elsewhere classified, left upper arm

☐ **M67.229** Synovial hypertrophy, not elsewhere classified, unspecified upper arm

Ⓖ **M67.23** Synovial hypertrophy, not elsewhere classified, forearm

● New   ▲ Revised   *Manifestation*   ❹-❼ Digit Indicators   ☐ Laterality   Ⓐ Adult (15+ years)   Ⓜ Maternity (12-55 years)   Ⓝ Newborn   Ⓟ Pediatric (0-17 years)   ♂ Male   ♀ Female
✖ ~~Deleted~~   Unspecified   + Additional code

786   © 2017 DecisionHealth   2017 ICD-10-CM Expert for Physicians

⬛ M67.231 Synovial hypertrophy, not elsewhere classified, right forearm

⬛ M67.232 Synovial hypertrophy, not elsewhere classified, left forearm

⬛ M67.239 Synovial hypertrophy, not elsewhere classified, unspecified forearm

Ⓖ M67.24 Synovial hypertrophy, not elsewhere classified, hand

⬛ M67.241 Synovial hypertrophy, not elsewhere classified, right hand

⬛ M67.242 Synovial hypertrophy, not elsewhere classified, left hand

⬛ M67.249 Synovial hypertrophy, not elsewhere classified, unspecified hand

Ⓖ M67.25 Synovial hypertrophy, not elsewhere classified, thigh

⬛ M67.251 Synovial hypertrophy, not elsewhere classified, right thigh

⬛ M67.252 Synovial hypertrophy, not elsewhere classified, left thigh

⬛ M67.259 Synovial hypertrophy, not elsewhere classified, unspecified thigh

Ⓖ M67.26 Synovial hypertrophy, not elsewhere classified, lower leg

⬛ M67.261 Synovial hypertrophy, not elsewhere classified, right lower leg

⬛ M67.262 Synovial hypertrophy, not elsewhere classified, left lower leg

⬛ M67.269 Synovial hypertrophy, not elsewhere classified, unspecified lower leg

Ⓖ M67.27 Synovial hypertrophy, not elsewhere classified, ankle and foot

⬛ M67.271 Synovial hypertrophy, not elsewhere classified, right ankle and foot

⬛ M67.272 Synovial hypertrophy, not elsewhere classified, left ankle and foot

⬛ M67.279 Synovial hypertrophy, not elsewhere classified, unspecified ankle and foot

M67.28 Synovial hypertrophy, not elsewhere classified, other site

M67.29 Synovial hypertrophy, not elsewhere classified, multiple sites

Ⓢ M67.3 Transient synovitis
Toxic synovitis

EXCLUDES 1 palindromic rheumatism (M12.3-)

M67.30 Transient synovitis, unspecified site

Ⓖ M67.31 Transient synovitis, shoulder

⬛ M67.311 Transient synovitis, right shoulder

⬛ M67.312 Transient synovitis, left shoulder

⬛ M67.319 Transient synovitis, unspecified shoulder

Ⓖ M67.32 Transient synovitis, elbow

⬛ M67.321 Transient synovitis, right elbow

⬛ M67.322 Transient synovitis, left elbow

⬛ M67.329 Transient synovitis, unspecified elbow

Ⓖ M67.33 Transient synovitis, wrist

⬛ M67.331 Transient synovitis, right wrist

⬛ M67.332 Transient synovitis, left wrist

⬛ M67.339 Transient synovitis, unspecified wrist

Ⓖ M67.34 Transient synovitis, hand

⬛ M67.341 Transient synovitis, right hand

⬛ M67.342 Transient synovitis, left hand

⬛ M67.349 Transient synovitis, unspecified hand

Ⓖ M67.35 Transient synovitis, hip

⬛ M67.351 Transient synovitis, right hip

⬛ M67.352 Transient synovitis, left hip

⬛ M67.359 Transient synovitis, unspecified hip

Ⓖ M67.36 Transient synovitis, knee

⬛ M67.361 Transient synovitis, right knee

⬛ M67.362 Transient synovitis, left knee

⬛ M67.369 Transient synovitis, unspecified knee

Ⓖ M67.37 Transient synovitis, ankle and foot

⬛ M67.371 Transient synovitis, right ankle and foot

⬛ M67.372 Transient synovitis, left ankle and foot

⬛ M67.379 Transient synovitis, unspecified ankle and foot

M67.38 Transient synovitis, other site

M67.39 Transient synovitis, multiple sites

Ⓢ M67.4 Ganglion
Ganglion of joint or tendon (sheath)

EXCLUDES 1 ganglion in yaws (A66.6)

EXCLUDES 2 cyst of bursa (M71.2-M71.3)
cyst of synovium (M71.2-M71.3)

M67.40 Ganglion, unspecified site

Ⓖ M67.41 Ganglion, shoulder

⬛ M67.411 Ganglion, right shoulder

⬛ M67.412 Ganglion, left shoulder

⬛ M67.419 Ganglion, unspecified shoulder

Ⓖ M67.42 Ganglion, elbow

⬛ M67.421 Ganglion, right elbow

⬛ M67.422 Ganglion, left elbow

⬛ M67.429 Ganglion, unspecified elbow

Ⓖ M67.43 Ganglion, wrist

Ganglion, wrist

⬛ M67.431 Ganglion, right wrist

⬛ M67.432 Ganglion, left wrist

⬛ M67.439 Ganglion, unspecified wrist

Ⓖ M67.44 Ganglion, hand

⬛ M67.441 Ganglion, right hand

⬛ M67.442 Ganglion, left hand

⬛ M67.449 Ganglion, unspecified hand

Ⓖ M67.45 Ganglion, hip

⬛ M67.451 Ganglion, right hip

⬛ M67.452 Ganglion, left hip

⬛ M67.459 Ganglion, unspecified hip

Ⓖ M67.46 Ganglion, knee

⬛ M67.461 Ganglion, right knee

⬛ M67.462 Ganglion, left knee

⬛ M67.469 Ganglion, unspecified knee

Ⓖ M67.47 Ganglion, ankle and foot

⬛ M67.471 Ganglion, right ankle and foot

⬛ M67.472 Ganglion, left ankle and foot

⬛ M67.479 Ganglion, unspecified ankle and foot

M67.48 Ganglion, other site

M67.49 Ganglion, multiple sites

Ⓢ M67.5 Plica syndrome
Plica knee

⬛ M67.50 Plica syndrome, unspecified knee

⬛ M67.51 Plica syndrome, right knee

⬛ M67.52 Plica syndrome, left knee

Ⓢ M67.8 Other specified disorders of synovium and tendon

M67.80 Other specified disorders of synovium and tendon, unspecified site

Ⓖ M67.81 Other specified disorders of synovium and tendon, shoulder

⬛ M67.811 Other specified disorders of synovium, right shoulder

⬛ M67.812 Other specified disorders of synovium, left shoulder

⬛ M67.813 Other specified disorders of tendon, right shoulder

⬛ M67.814 Other specified disorders of tendon, left shoulder

⬛ M67.819 Other specified disorders of synovium and tendon, unspecified shoulder

Ⓖ M67.82 Other specified disorders of synovium and tendon, elbow

⬛ M67.821 Other specified disorders of synovium, right elbow

⬛ M67.822 Other specified disorders of synovium, left elbow

⬛ M67.823 Other specified disorders of tendon, right elbow

● New   ▲ Revised   *Manifestation*   ④-⑦ Digit Indicators   ⬛ Laterality   Ⓐ Adult (15+ years)   Ⓜ Maternity (12-55 years)   Ⓝ Newborn   Ⓟ Pediatric (0-17 years)   ♂ Male   ♀ Female
✖ Deleted   Unspecified   + Additional code

2017 ICD-10-CM Expert for Physicians   © 2017 DecisionHealth   787

▤ M67.824   Other specified disorders of tendon, left elbow
▤ M67.829   Other specified disorders of synovium and tendon, unspecified elbow
◪ M67.83   Other specified disorders of synovium and tendon, wrist
▤ M67.831   Other specified disorders of synovium, right wrist
▤ M67.832   Other specified disorders of synovium, left wrist
▤ M67.833   Other specified disorders of tendon, right wrist
▤ M67.834   Other specified disorders of tendon, left wrist
▤ M67.839   Other specified disorders of synovium and tendon, unspecified forearm
◪ M67.84   Other specified disorders of synovium and tendon, hand
▤ M67.841   Other specified disorders of synovium, right hand
▤ M67.842   Other specified disorders of synovium, left hand
▤ M67.843   Other specified disorders of tendon, right hand
▤ M67.844   Other specified disorders of tendon, left hand
▤ M67.849   Other specified disorders of synovium and tendon, unspecified hand
◪ M67.85   Other specified disorders of synovium and tendon, hip
▤ M67.851   Other specified disorders of synovium, right hip
▤ M67.852   Other specified disorders of synovium, left hip
▤ M67.853   Other specified disorders of tendon, right hip
▤ M67.854   Other specified disorders of tendon, left hip
▤ M67.859   Other specified disorders of synovium and tendon, unspecified hip
◪ M67.86   Other specified disorders of synovium and tendon, knee
▤ M67.861   Other specified disorders of synovium, right knee
▤ M67.862   Other specified disorders of synovium, left knee
▤ M67.863   Other specified disorders of tendon, right knee
▤ M67.864   Other specified disorders of tendon, left knee
▤ M67.869   Other specified disorders of synovium and tendon, unspecified knee
◪ M67.87   Other specified disorders of synovium and tendon, ankle and foot
▤ M67.871   Other specified disorders of synovium, right ankle and foot
▤ M67.872   Other specified disorders of synovium, left ankle and foot
▤ M67.873   Other specified disorders of tendon, right ankle and foot
▤ M67.874   Other specified disorders of tendon, left ankle and foot
▤ M67.879   Other specified disorders of synovium and tendon, unspecified ankle and foot
M67.88   Other specified disorders of synovium and tendon, other site
M67.89   Other specified disorders of synovium and tendon, multiple sites
⑤ M67.9   Unspecified disorder of synovium and tendon
M67.90   Unspecified disorder of synovium and tendon, unspecified site
◪ M67.91   Unspecified disorder of synovium and tendon, shoulder
▤ M67.911   Unspecified disorder of synovium and tendon, right shoulder
▤ M67.912   Unspecified disorder of synovium and tendon, left shoulder
▤ M67.919   Unspecified disorder of synovium and tendon, unspecified shoulder
◪ M67.92   Unspecified disorder of synovium and tendon, upper arm
▤ M67.921   Unspecified disorder of synovium and tendon, right upper arm
▤ M67.922   Unspecified disorder of synovium and tendon, left upper arm
▤ M67.929   Unspecified disorder of synovium and tendon, unspecified upper arm
◪ M67.93   Unspecified disorder of synovium and tendon, forearm
▤ M67.931   Unspecified disorder of synovium and tendon, right forearm

▤ M67.932   Unspecified disorder of synovium and tendon, left forearm
▤ M67.939   Unspecified disorder of synovium and tendon, unspecified forearm
◪ M67.94   Unspecified disorder of synovium and tendon, hand
▤ M67.941   Unspecified disorder of synovium and tendon, right hand
▤ M67.942   Unspecified disorder of synovium and tendon, left hand
▤ M67.949   Unspecified disorder of synovium and tendon, unspecified hand
◪ M67.95   Unspecified disorder of synovium and tendon, thigh
▤ M67.951   Unspecified disorder of synovium and tendon, right thigh
▤ M67.952   Unspecified disorder of synovium and tendon, left thigh
▤ M67.959   Unspecified disorder of synovium and tendon, unspecified thigh
◪ M67.96   Unspecified disorder of synovium and tendon, lower leg
▤ M67.961   Unspecified disorder of synovium and tendon, right lower leg
▤ M67.962   Unspecified disorder of synovium and tendon, left lower leg
▤ M67.969   Unspecified disorder of synovium and tendon, unspecified lower leg
◪ M67.97   Unspecified disorder of synovium and tendon, ankle and foot
▤ M67.971   Unspecified disorder of synovium and tendon, right ankle and foot
▤ M67.972   Unspecified disorder of synovium and tendon, left ankle and foot
▤ M67.979   Unspecified disorder of synovium and tendon, unspecified ankle and foot
M67.98   Unspecified disorder of synovium and tendon, other site
M67.99   Unspecified disorder of synovium and tendon, multiple sites

Other soft tissue disorders (M70-M79)

④+ M70   Soft tissue disorders related to use, overuse and pressure

INCLUDES   soft tissue disorders of occupational origin

Use additional external cause code to identify activity causing disorder (Y93.-)

EXCLUDES 1   *bursitis NOS (M71.9-)*

EXCLUDES 2   *bursitis of shoulder (M75.5)*
enthesopathies (M76-M77)
pressure ulcer (pressure area) (L89.-)

⑤+ M70.0   Crepitant synovitis (acute) (chronic) of hand and wrist
◪+ M70.03   Crepitant synovitis (acute) (chronic), wrist
▤+ M70.031   Crepitant synovitis (acute) (chronic), right wrist
▤+ M70.032   Crepitant synovitis (acute) (chronic), left wrist
▤+ M70.039   Crepitant synovitis (acute) (chronic), unspecified wrist
◪+ M70.04   Crepitant synovitis (acute) (chronic), hand
▤+ M70.041   Crepitant synovitis (acute) (chronic), right hand
▤+ M70.042   Crepitant synovitis (acute) (chronic), left hand
▤+ M70.049   Crepitant synovitis (acute) (chronic), unspecified hand
⑤+ M70.1   Bursitis of hand
▤+ M70.10   Bursitis, unspecified hand
▤+ M70.11   Bursitis, right hand
▤+ M70.12   Bursitis, left hand
⑤+ M70.2   Olecranon bursitis
▤+ M70.20   Olecranon bursitis, unspecified elbow
▤+ M70.21   Olecranon bursitis, right elbow
▤+ M70.22   Olecranon bursitis, left elbow
⑤+ M70.3   Other bursitis of elbow
▤+ M70.30   Other bursitis of elbow, unspecified elbow
▤+ M70.31   Other bursitis of elbow, right elbow

● New   ▲ Revised   *Manifestation*   ④-⑦ Digit Indicators   ▤ Laterality   Ⓐ Adult (15+ years)   Ⓜ Maternity (12-55 years)   Ⓝ Newborn   Ⓟ Pediatric (0-17 years)   ♂ Male   ♀ Female
✖ Deleted   Unspecified   + Additional code

788   © 2017 DecisionHealth   2017 ICD-10-CM Expert for Physicians

☐+ M70.32   Other bursitis of elbow, left elbow

⑤+ M70.4   Prepatellar bursitis
   ☐+ M70.40   Prepatellar bursitis, unspecified knee
   ☐+ M70.41   Prepatellar bursitis, right knee
   ☐+ M70.42   Prepatellar bursitis, left knee

⑤+ M70.5   Other bursitis of knee
   ☐+ M70.50   Other bursitis of knee, unspecified knee
   ☐+ M70.51   Other bursitis of knee, right knee
   ☐+ M70.52   Other bursitis of knee, left knee

⑤+ M70.6   Trochanteric bursitis
   Trochanteric tendinitis
   ☐+ M70.60   Trochanteric bursitis, unspecified hip
   ☐+ M70.61   Trochanteric bursitis, right hip
   ☐+ M70.62   Trochanteric bursitis, left hip

⑤+ M70.7   Other bursitis of hip
   Ischial bursitis
   ☐+ M70.70   Other bursitis of hip, unspecified hip
   ☐+ M70.71   Other bursitis of hip, right hip
   ☐+ M70.72   Other bursitis of hip, left hip

⑤+ M70.8   Other soft tissue disorders related to use, overuse and pressure
   + M70.80   Other soft tissue disorders related to use, overuse and pressure of unspecified site
   ⑥+ M70.81   Other soft tissue disorders related to use, overuse and pressure of shoulder
      ☐+ M70.811   Other soft tissue disorders related to use, overuse and pressure, right shoulder
      ☐+ M70.812   Other soft tissue disorders related to use, overuse and pressure, left shoulder
      ☐+ M70.819   Other soft tissue disorders related to use, overuse and pressure, unspecified shoulder
   ⑥+ M70.82   Other soft tissue disorders related to use, overuse and pressure of upper arm
      ☐+ M70.821   Other soft tissue disorders related to use, overuse and pressure, right upper arm
      ☐+ M70.822   Other soft tissue disorders related to use, overuse and pressure, left upper arm
      ☐+ M70.829   Other soft tissue disorders related to use, overuse and pressure, unspecified upper arms
   ⑥+ M70.83   Other soft tissue disorders related to use, overuse and pressure of forearm
      ☐+ M70.831   Other soft tissue disorders related to use, overuse and pressure, right forearm
      ☐+ M70.832   Other soft tissue disorders related to use, overuse and pressure, left forearm
      ☐+ M70.839   Other soft tissue disorders related to use, overuse and pressure, unspecified forearm
   ⑥+ M70.84   Other soft tissue disorders related to use, overuse and pressure of hand
      ☐+ M70.841   Other soft tissue disorders related to use, overuse and pressure, right hand
      ☐+ M70.842   Other soft tissue disorders related to use, overuse and pressure, left hand
      ☐+ M70.849   Other soft tissue disorders related to use, overuse and pressure, unspecified hand
   ⑥+ M70.85   Other soft tissue disorders related to use, overuse and pressure of thigh
      ☐+ M70.851   Other soft tissue disorders related to use, overuse and pressure, right thigh
      ☐+ M70.852   Other soft tissue disorders related to use, overuse and pressure, left thigh
      ☐+ M70.859   Other soft tissue disorders related to use, overuse and pressure, unspecified thigh
   ⑥+ M70.86   Other soft tissue disorders related to use, overuse and pressure lower leg
      ☐+ M70.861   Other soft tissue disorders related to use, overuse and pressure, right lower leg
      ☐+ M70.862   Other soft tissue disorders related to use, overuse and pressure, left lower leg
      ☐+ M70.869   Other soft tissue disorders related to use, overuse and pressure, unspecified leg
   ⑥+ M70.87   Other soft tissue disorders related to use, overuse and pressure of ankle and foot

      ☐+ M70.871   Other soft tissue disorders related to use, overuse and pressure, right ankle and foot
      ☐+ M70.872   Other soft tissue disorders related to use, overuse and pressure, left ankle and foot
      ☐+ M70.879   Other soft tissue disorders related to use, overuse and pressure, unspecified ankle and foot
   + M70.88   Other soft tissue disorders related to use, overuse and pressure other site
   + M70.89   Other soft tissue disorders related to use, overuse and pressure multiple sites

⑤+ M70.9   Unspecified soft tissue disorder related to use, overuse and pressure
   + M70.90   Unspecified soft tissue disorder related to use, overuse and pressure of unspecified site
   ⑥+ M70.91   Unspecified soft tissue disorder related to use, overuse and pressure of shoulder
      ☐+ M70.911   Unspecified soft tissue disorder related to use, overuse and pressure, right shoulder
      ☐+ M70.912   Unspecified soft tissue disorder related to use, overuse and pressure, left shoulder
      ☐+ M70.919   Unspecified soft tissue disorder related to use, overuse and pressure, unspecified shoulder
   ⑥+ M70.92   Unspecified soft tissue disorder related to use, overuse and pressure of upper arm
      ☐+ M70.921   Unspecified soft tissue disorder related to use, overuse and pressure, right upper arm
      ☐+ M70.922   Unspecified soft tissue disorder related to use, overuse and pressure, left upper arm
      ☐+ M70.929   Unspecified soft tissue disorder related to use, overuse and pressure, unspecified upper arm
   ⑥+ M70.93   Unspecified soft tissue disorder related to use, overuse and pressure of forearm
      ☐+ M70.931   Unspecified soft tissue disorder related to use, overuse and pressure, right forearm
      ☐+ M70.932   Unspecified soft tissue disorder related to use, overuse and pressure, left forearm
      ☐+ M70.939   Unspecified soft tissue disorder related to use, overuse and pressure, unspecified forearm
   ⑥+ M70.94   Unspecified soft tissue disorder related to use, overuse and pressure of hand
      ☐+ M70.941   Unspecified soft tissue disorder related to use, overuse and pressure, right hand
      ☐+ M70.942   Unspecified soft tissue disorder related to use, overuse and pressure, left hand
      ☐+ M70.949   Unspecified soft tissue disorder related to use, overuse and pressure, unspecified hand
   ⑥+ M70.95   Unspecified soft tissue disorder related to use, overuse and pressure of thigh
      ☐+ M70.951   Unspecified soft tissue disorder related to use, overuse and pressure, right thigh
      ☐+ M70.952   Unspecified soft tissue disorder related to use, overuse and pressure, left thigh
      ☐+ M70.959   Unspecified soft tissue disorder related to use, overuse and pressure, unspecified thigh
   ⑥+ M70.96   Unspecified soft tissue disorder related to use, overuse and pressure lower leg
      ☐+ M70.961   Unspecified soft tissue disorder related to use, overuse and pressure, right lower leg
      ☐+ M70.962   Unspecified soft tissue disorder related to use, overuse and pressure, left lower leg
      ☐+ M70.969   Unspecified soft tissue disorder related to use, overuse and pressure, unspecified lower leg
   ⑥+ M70.97   Unspecified soft tissue disorder related to use, overuse and pressure of ankle and foot
      ☐+ M70.971   Unspecified soft tissue disorder related to use, overuse and pressure, right ankle and foot
      ☐+ M70.972   Unspecified soft tissue disorder related to use, overuse and pressure, left ankle and foot
      ☐+ M70.979   Unspecified soft tissue disorder related to use, overuse and pressure, unspecified ankle and foot
   + M70.98   Unspecified soft tissue disorder related to use, overuse and pressure other

---

● New   ▲ Revised   *Manifestation*   ❹-❼ Digit Indicators   ☐ Laterality   Ⓐ Adult (15+ years)   Ⓜ Maternity (12-55 years)   Ⓝ Newborn   Ⓟ Pediatric (0-17 years)   ♂ Male   ♀ Female
✖ Deleted   Unspecified   + Additional code

+ M70.99　Unspecified soft tissue disorder related to use, overuse and pressure multiple sites

M71　Other bursopathies
　EXCLUDES 1　bunion (M20.1)
　　bursitis related to use, overuse or pressure (M70.-)
　　enthesopathies (M76-M77)

+ M71.0　Abscess of bursa
　Use additional code (B95.-, B96.-) to identify causative organism

+ M71.00　Abscess of bursa, unspecified site
+ M71.01　Abscess of bursa, shoulder
　+ M71.011　Abscess of bursa, right shoulder
　+ M71.012　Abscess of bursa, left shoulder
　+ M71.019　Abscess of bursa, unspecified shoulder
+ M71.02　Abscess of bursa, elbow
　+ M71.021　Abscess of bursa, right elbow
　+ M71.022　Abscess of bursa, left elbow
　+ M71.029　Abscess of bursa, unspecified elbow
+ M71.03　Abscess of bursa, wrist
　+ M71.031　Abscess of bursa, right wrist
　+ M71.032　Abscess of bursa, left wrist
　+ M71.039　Abscess of bursa, unspecified wrist
+ M71.04　Abscess of bursa, hand
　+ M71.041　Abscess of bursa, right hand
　+ M71.042　Abscess of bursa, left hand
　+ M71.049　Abscess of bursa, unspecified hand
+ M71.05　Abscess of bursa, hip
　+ M71.051　Abscess of bursa, right hip
　+ M71.052　Abscess of bursa, left hip
　+ M71.059　Abscess of bursa, unspecified hip
+ M71.06　Abscess of bursa, knee
　+ M71.061　Abscess of bursa, right knee
　+ M71.062　Abscess of bursa, left knee
　+ M71.069　Abscess of bursa, unspecified knee
+ M71.07　Abscess of bursa, ankle and foot
　+ M71.071　Abscess of bursa, right ankle and foot
　+ M71.072　Abscess of bursa, left ankle and foot
　+ M71.079　Abscess of bursa, unspecified ankle and foot
+ M71.08　Abscess of bursa, other site
+ M71.09　Abscess of bursa, multiple sites

+ M71.1　Other infective bursitis
　Use additional code (B95.-, B96.-) to identify causative organism

+ M71.10　Other infective bursitis, unspecified site
+ M71.11　Other infective bursitis, shoulder
　+ M71.111　Other infective bursitis, right shoulder
　+ M71.112　Other infective bursitis, left shoulder
　+ M71.119　Other infective bursitis, unspecified shoulder
+ M71.12　Other infective bursitis, elbow
　+ M71.121　Other infective bursitis, right elbow
　+ M71.122　Other infective bursitis, left elbow
　+ M71.129　Other infective bursitis, unspecified elbow
+ M71.13　Other infective bursitis, wrist
　+ M71.131　Other infective bursitis, right wrist
　+ M71.132　Other infective bursitis, left wrist
　+ M71.139　Other infective bursitis, unspecified wrist
+ M71.14　Other infective bursitis, hand
　+ M71.141　Other infective bursitis, right hand
　+ M71.142　Other infective bursitis, left hand
　+ M71.149　Other infective bursitis, unspecified hand
+ M71.15　Other infective bursitis, hip
　+ M71.151　Other infective bursitis, right hip
　+ M71.152　Other infective bursitis, left hip
　+ M71.159　Other infective bursitis, unspecified hip
+ M71.16　Other infective bursitis, knee
　+ M71.161　Other infective bursitis, right knee
　+ M71.162　Other infective bursitis, left knee
　+ M71.169　Other infective bursitis, unspecified knee
+ M71.17　Other infective bursitis, ankle and foot

+ M71.171　Other infective bursitis, right ankle and foot
+ M71.172　Other infective bursitis, left ankle and foot
+ M71.179　Other infective bursitis, unspecified ankle and foot
+ M71.18　Other infective bursitis, other site
+ M71.19　Other infective bursitis, multiple sites

M71.2　Synovial cyst of popliteal space [Baker]
　EXCLUDES 1　synovial cyst of popliteal space with rupture (M66.0)
　DEFINITION　Collection of synovial fluid that has escaped from the knee joint or bursa and has formed a synovial-lined sac behind the knee.

M71.20　Synovial cyst of popliteal space [Baker], unspecified knee
M71.21　Synovial cyst of popliteal space [Baker], right knee
M71.22　Synovial cyst of popliteal space [Baker], left knee

M71.3　Other bursal cyst
　Synovial cyst NOS
　EXCLUDES 1　synovial cyst with rupture (M66.1-)

M71.30　Other bursal cyst, unspecified site
M71.31　Other bursal cyst, shoulder
　M71.311　Other bursal cyst, right shoulder
　M71.312　Other bursal cyst, left shoulder
　M71.319　Other bursal cyst, unspecified shoulder
M71.32　Other bursal cyst, elbow
　M71.321　Other bursal cyst, right elbow
　M71.322　Other bursal cyst, left elbow
　M71.329　Other bursal cyst, unspecified elbow
M71.33　Other bursal cyst, wrist
　M71.331　Other bursal cyst, right wrist
　M71.332　Other bursal cyst, left wrist
　M71.339　Other bursal cyst, unspecified wrist
M71.34　Other bursal cyst, hand
　M71.341　Other bursal cyst, right hand
　M71.342　Other bursal cyst, left hand
　M71.349　Other bursal cyst, unspecified hand
M71.35　Other bursal cyst, hip
　M71.351　Other bursal cyst, right hip
　M71.352　Other bursal cyst, left hip
　M71.359　Other bursal cyst, unspecified hip
M71.37　Other bursal cyst, ankle and foot
　M71.371　Other bursal cyst, right ankle and foot
　M71.372　Other bursal cyst, left ankle and foot
　M71.379　Other bursal cyst, unspecified ankle and foot
M71.38　Other bursal cyst, other site
M71.39　Other bursal cyst, multiple sites

M71.4　Calcium deposit in bursa
　EXCLUDES 2　calcium deposit in bursa of shoulder (M75.3)

M71.40　Calcium deposit in bursa, unspecified site
M71.42　Calcium deposit in bursa, elbow
　M71.421　Calcium deposit in bursa, right elbow
　M71.422　Calcium deposit in bursa, left elbow
　M71.429　Calcium deposit in bursa, unspecified elbow
M71.43　Calcium deposit in bursa, wrist
　M71.431　Calcium deposit in bursa, right wrist
　M71.432　Calcium deposit in bursa, left wrist
　M71.439　Calcium deposit in bursa, unspecified wrist
M71.44　Calcium deposit in bursa, hand
　M71.441　Calcium deposit in bursa, right hand
　M71.442　Calcium deposit in bursa, left hand
　M71.449　Calcium deposit in bursa, unspecified hand
M71.45　Calcium deposit in bursa, hip
　M71.451　Calcium deposit in bursa, right hip
　M71.452　Calcium deposit in bursa, left hip
　M71.459　Calcium deposit in bursa, unspecified hip
M71.46　Calcium deposit in bursa, knee
　M71.461　Calcium deposit in bursa, right knee
　M71.462　Calcium deposit in bursa, left knee
　M71.469　Calcium deposit in bursa, unspecified knee
M71.47　Calcium deposit in bursa, ankle and foot
　M71.471　Calcium deposit in bursa, right ankle and foot

M71.472   Calcium deposit in bursa, left ankle and foot
M71.479   Calcium deposit in bursa, unspecified ankle and foot
M71.48   Calcium deposit in bursa, other site
M71.49   Calcium deposit in bursa, multiple sites
▲ ⑤ M71.5   Other bursitis, not elsewhere classified
    EXCLUDES 1   bursitis NOS (M71.9-)
    EXCLUDES 2   bursitis of shoulder (M75.5)
                  bursitis of tibial collateral [Pellegrini-Stieda] (M76.4-)
M71.50   Other bursitis, not elsewhere classified, unspecified site
⑥ M71.52   Other bursitis, not elsewhere classified, elbow
    M71.521   Other bursitis, not elsewhere classified, right elbow
    M71.522   Other bursitis, not elsewhere classified, left elbow
    M71.529   Other bursitis, not elsewhere classified, unspecified elbow
⑥ M71.53   Other bursitis, not elsewhere classified, wrist
    M71.531   Other bursitis, not elsewhere classified, right wrist
    M71.532   Other bursitis, not elsewhere classified, left wrist
    M71.539   Other bursitis, not elsewhere classified, unspecified wrist
⑥ M71.54   Other bursitis, not elsewhere classified, hand
    M71.541   Other bursitis, not elsewhere classified, right hand
    M71.542   Other bursitis, not elsewhere classified, left hand
    M71.549   Other bursitis, not elsewhere classified, unspecified hand
⑥ M71.55   Other bursitis, not elsewhere classified, hip
    M71.551   Other bursitis, not elsewhere classified, right hip
    M71.552   Other bursitis, not elsewhere classified, left hip
    M71.559   Other bursitis, not elsewhere classified, unspecified hip
⑥ M71.56   Other bursitis, not elsewhere classified, knee
    M71.561   Other bursitis, not elsewhere classified, right knee
    M71.562   Other bursitis, not elsewhere classified, left knee
    M71.569   Other bursitis, not elsewhere classified, unspecified knee
⑥ M71.57   Other bursitis, not elsewhere classified, ankle and foot
    M71.571   Other bursitis, not elsewhere classified, right ankle and foot
    M71.572   Other bursitis, not elsewhere classified, left ankle and foot
    M71.579   Other bursitis, not elsewhere classified, unspecified ankle and foot
M71.58   Other bursitis, not elsewhere classified, other site
⑤ M71.8   Other specified bursopathies
M71.80   Other specified bursopathies, unspecified site
⑥ M71.81   Other specified bursopathies, shoulder
    M71.811   Other specified bursopathies, right shoulder
    M71.812   Other specified bursopathies, left shoulder
    M71.819   Other specified bursopathies, unspecified shoulder
⑥ M71.82   Other specified bursopathies, elbow
    M71.821   Other specified bursopathies, right elbow
    M71.822   Other specified bursopathies, left elbow
    M71.829   Other specified bursopathies, unspecified elbow
⑥ M71.83   Other specified bursopathies, wrist
    M71.831   Other specified bursopathies, right wrist
    M71.832   Other specified bursopathies, left wrist
    M71.839   Other specified bursopathies, unspecified wrist
⑥ M71.84   Other specified bursopathies, hand
    M71.841   Other specified bursopathies, right hand
    M71.842   Other specified bursopathies, left hand
    M71.849   Other specified bursopathies, unspecified hand
⑥ M71.85   Other specified bursopathies, hip
    M71.851   Other specified bursopathies, right hip
    M71.852   Other specified bursopathies, left hip

M71.859   Other specified bursopathies, unspecified hip
⑥ M71.86   Other specified bursopathies, knee
    M71.861   Other specified bursopathies, right knee
    M71.862   Other specified bursopathies, left knee
    M71.869   Other specified bursopathies, unspecified knee
⑥ M71.87   Other specified bursopathies, ankle and foot
    M71.871   Other specified bursopathies, right ankle and foot
    M71.872   Other specified bursopathies, left ankle and foot
    M71.879   Other specified bursopathies, unspecified ankle and foot
M71.88   Other specified bursopathies, other site
M71.89   Other specified bursopathies, multiple sites
M71.9   Bursopathy, unspecified
    Bursitis NOS
④ M72   Fibroblastic disorders
    EXCLUDES 2   retroperitoneal fibromatosis (D48.3)
M72.0   Palmar fascial fibromatosis [Dupuytren]   Ⓐ
M72.1   Knuckle pads
M72.2   Plantar fascial fibromatosis
    Plantar fasciitis

Plantar fascial fibromatosis

Achilles tendon
Inflammation
Plantar fascia

M72.4   Pseudosarcomatous fibromatosis
    Nodular fasciitis
➕ M72.6   Necrotizing fasciitis
    Use additional code (B95.-, B96.-) to identify causative organism
➕ M72.8   Other fibroblastic disorders
    Abscess of fascia
    Fasciitis NEC
    Other infective fasciitis
    Use additional code to (B95.-, B96.-) identify causative organism
    EXCLUDES 1   diffuse (eosinophilic) fasciitis (M35.4)
                  necrotizing fasciitis (M72.6)
                  nodular fasciitis (M72.4)
                  perirenal fasciitis NOS (N13.5)
                  perirenal fasciitis with infection (N13.6)
                  plantar fasciitis (M72.2)
M72.9   Fibroblastic disorder, unspecified
    Fasciitis NOS
    Fibromatosis NOS
④ M75   Shoulder lesions
    EXCLUDES 2   shoulder-hand syndrome (M89.0-)
⑤ M75.0   Adhesive capsulitis of shoulder
    Frozen shoulder
    Periarthritis of shoulder
    M75.00   Adhesive capsulitis of unspecified shoulder
    M75.01   Adhesive capsulitis of right shoulder
    M75.02   Adhesive capsulitis of left shoulder
        AHA: 2Q 2015, 23
⑤ M75.1   Rotator cuff tear or rupture, not specified as traumatic
    Rotator cuff syndrome
    Supraspinatus tear or rupture, not specified as traumatic
    Supraspinatus syndrome
    EXCLUDES 1   tear of rotator cuff, traumatic (S46.01-)

● New   ▲ Revised   *Manifestation*   ④-⑦ Digit Indicators   ▤ Laterality   Ⓐ Adult (15+ years)   Ⓜ Maternity (12-55 years)   Ⓝ Newborn (0-17 years)   Ⓟ Pediatric (0-17 years)   ♂ Male   ♀ Female
✖ Deleted   Unspecified   ➕ Additional code

2017 ICD-10-CM Expert for Physicians   © 2017 DecisionHealth   791

Ⓖ **M75.10**   Unspecified rotator cuff tear or rupture, not specified as traumatic

Unspecified rotator cuff tear or rupture, not specified as traumatic

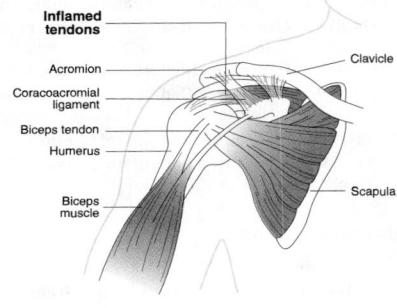

⊟ **M75.100**   Unspecified rotator cuff tear or rupture of unspecified shoulder, not specified as traumatic

⊟ **M75.101**   Unspecified rotator cuff tear or rupture of right shoulder, not specified as traumatic

⊟ **M75.102**   Unspecified rotator cuff tear or rupture of left shoulder, not specified as traumatic

Ⓖ **M75.11**   Incomplete rotator cuff tear or rupture not specified as traumatic

⊟ **M75.110**   Incomplete rotator cuff tear or rupture of unspecified shoulder, not specified as traumatic

⊟ **M75.111**   Incomplete rotator cuff tear or rupture of right shoulder, not specified as traumatic

⊟ **M75.112**   Incomplete rotator cuff tear or rupture of left shoulder, not specified as traumatic

Ⓖ **M75.12**   Complete rotator cuff tear or rupture not specified as traumatic

Complete rotator cuff tear or rupture

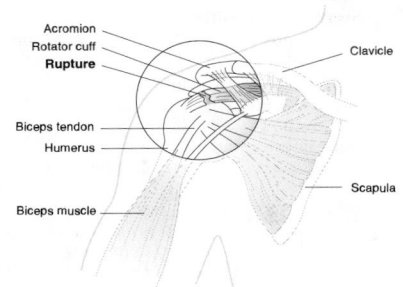

⊟ **M75.120**   Complete rotator cuff tear or rupture of unspecified shoulder, not specified as traumatic

⊟ **M75.121**   Complete rotator cuff tear or rupture of right shoulder, not specified as traumatic

⊟ **M75.122**   Complete rotator cuff tear or rupture of left shoulder, not specified as traumatic

Ⓢ **M75.2**   Bicipital tendinitis

⊟ **M75.20**   Bicipital tendinitis, unspecified shoulder

⊟ **M75.21**   Bicipital tendinitis, right shoulder

⊟ **M75.22**   Bicipital tendinitis, left shoulder

Ⓢ **M75.3**   Calcific tendinitis of shoulder
Calcified bursa of shoulder

⊟ **M75.30**   Calcific tendinitis of unspecified shoulder

⊟ **M75.31**   Calcific tendinitis of right shoulder

⊟ **M75.32**   Calcific tendinitis of left shoulder

Ⓢ **M75.4**   Impingement syndrome of shoulder

⊟ **M75.40**   Impingement syndrome of unspecified shoulder

⊟ **M75.41**   Impingement syndrome of right shoulder

⊟ **M75.42**   Impingement syndrome of left shoulder

Ⓢ **M75.5**   Bursitis of shoulder

⊟ **M75.50**   Bursitis of unspecified shoulder

⊟ **M75.51**   Bursitis of right shoulder

⊟ **M75.52**   Bursitis of left shoulder

Ⓢ **M75.8**   Other shoulder lesions

⊟ **M75.80**   Other shoulder lesions, unspecified shoulder

⊟ **M75.81**   Other shoulder lesions, right shoulder

⊟ **M75.82**   Other shoulder lesions, left shoulder

Ⓢ **M75.9**   Shoulder lesion, unspecified

⊟ **M75.90**   Shoulder lesion, unspecified, unspecified shoulder

⊟ **M75.91**   Shoulder lesion, unspecified, right shoulder

⊟ **M75.92**   Shoulder lesion, unspecified, left shoulder

Ⓐ **M76**   Enthesopathies, lower limb, excluding foot

EXCLUDES 2   *bursitis due to use, overuse and pressure (M70.-)*
enthesopathies of ankle and foot (M77.5-)

Ⓢ **M76.0**   Gluteal tendinitis

⊟ **M76.00**   Gluteal tendinitis, unspecified hip

⊟ **M76.01**   Gluteal tendinitis, right hip

⊟ **M76.02**   Gluteal tendinitis, left hip

Ⓢ **M76.1**   Psoas tendinitis

⊟ **M76.10**   Psoas tendinitis, unspecified hip

⊟ **M76.11**   Psoas tendinitis, right hip

⊟ **M76.12**   Psoas tendinitis, left hip

Ⓢ **M76.2**   Iliac crest spur

⊟ **M76.20**   Iliac crest spur, unspecified hip

⊟ **M76.21**   Iliac crest spur, right hip

⊟ **M76.22**   Iliac crest spur, left hip

Ⓢ **M76.3**   Iliotibial band syndrome

⊟ **M76.30**   Iliotibial band syndrome, unspecified leg

⊟ **M76.31**   Iliotibial band syndrome, right leg

⊟ **M76.32**   Iliotibial band syndrome, left leg

Ⓢ **M76.4**   Tibial collateral bursitis [Pellegrini-Stieda]

⊟ **M76.40**   Tibial collateral bursitis [Pellegrini-Stieda], unspecified leg

⊟ **M76.41**   Tibial collateral bursitis [Pellegrini-Stieda], right leg

⊟ **M76.42**   Tibial collateral bursitis [Pellegrini-Stieda], left leg

Ⓢ **M76.5**   Patellar tendinitis

⊟ **M76.50**   Patellar tendinitis, unspecified knee

⊟ **M76.51**   Patellar tendinitis, right knee

⊟ **M76.52**   Patellar tendinitis, left knee

Ⓢ **M76.6**   Achilles tendinitis
Achilles bursitis

⊟ **M76.60**   Achilles tendinitis, unspecified leg

⊟ **M76.61**   Achilles tendinitis, right leg

⊟ **M76.62**   Achilles tendinitis, left leg

Ⓢ **M76.7**   Peroneal tendinitis

⊟ **M76.70**   Peroneal tendinitis, unspecified leg

⊟ **M76.71**   Peroneal tendinitis, right leg

⊟ **M76.72**   Peroneal tendinitis, left leg

Ⓢ **M76.8**   Other specified enthesopathies of lower limb, excluding foot

Ⓖ **M76.81**   Anterior tibial syndrome

⊟ **M76.811**   Anterior tibial syndrome, right leg

⊟ **M76.812**   Anterior tibial syndrome, left leg

⊟ **M76.819**   Anterior tibial syndrome, unspecified leg

Ⓖ **M76.82**   Posterior tibial tendinitis

⊟ **M76.821**   Posterior tibial tendinitis, right leg

⊟ **M76.822**   Posterior tibial tendinitis, left leg

⊟ **M76.829**   Posterior tibial tendinitis, unspecified leg

Ⓖ **M76.89**   Other specified enthesopathies of lower limb, excluding foot

⊟ **M76.891**   Other specified enthesopathies of right lower limb, excluding foot

⊟ **M76.892**   Other specified enthesopathies of left lower limb, excluding foot

⊟ **M76.899**   Other specified enthesopathies of unspecified lower limb, excluding foot

M76.9   Unspecified enthesopathy, lower limb, excluding foot

⁴ **M77   Other enthesopathies**

| EXCLUDES 1 | *bursitis NOS (M71.9-)* |

EXCLUDES 2	*bursitis due to use, overuse and pressure (M70.-)*
	osteophyte (M25.7)
	spinal enthesopathy (M46.0-)

⁵ **M77.0   Medial epicondylitis**

◻ **M77.00   Medial epicondylitis, unspecified elbow**

◻ **M77.01   Medial epicondylitis, right elbow**

◻ **M77.02   Medial epicondylitis, left elbow**

⁵ **M77.1   Lateral epicondylitis**

Tennis elbow

| DEFINITION | A painful inflammation of the tendons that anchor the extensor carpi radialis brevis muscle to the outer aspect of the humerus at the elbow. |

◻ **M77.10   Lateral epicondylitis, unspecified elbow**

◻ **M77.11   Lateral epicondylitis, right elbow**

◻ **M77.12   Lateral epicondylitis, left elbow**

⁵ **M77.2   Periarthritis of wrist**

◻ **M77.20   Periarthritis, unspecified wrist**

◻ **M77.21   Periarthritis, right wrist**

◻ **M77.22   Periarthritis, left wrist**

⁵ **M77.3   Calcaneal spur**

Calcaneal spur

Talus

Overgrowth of calcaneus bone

◻ **M77.30   Calcaneal spur, unspecified foot**

◻ **M77.31   Calcaneal spur, right foot**

◻ **M77.32   Calcaneal spur, left foot**

⁵ **M77.4   Metatarsalgia**

| EXCLUDES 1 | *Morton's metatarsalgia (G57.6)* |

◻ **M77.40   Metatarsalgia, unspecified foot**

◻ **M77.41   Metatarsalgia, right foot**

◻ **M77.42   Metatarsalgia, left foot**

⁵ **M77.5   Other enthesopathy of foot**

◻ **M77.50   Other enthesopathy of unspecified foot**

◻ **M77.51   Other enthesopathy of right foot**

◻ **M77.52   Other enthesopathy of left foot**

M77.8   Other enthesopathies, not elsewhere classified

M77.9   Enthesopathy, unspecified

Bone spur NOS
Capsulitis NOS
Periarthritis NOS
Tendinitis NOS

⁴ **M79   Other and unspecified soft tissue disorders, not elsewhere classified**

| EXCLUDES 1 | *psychogenic rheumatism (F45.8)* |
| | *soft tissue pain, psychogenic (F45.41)* |

M79.0   Rheumatism, unspecified

| EXCLUDES 1 | *fibromyalgia (M79.7)* |
| | *palindromic rheumatism (M12.3-)* |

M79.1   Myalgia

Myofascial pain syndrome

| EXCLUDES 1 | *fibromyalgia (M79.7)* |
| | *myositis (M60.-)* |

M79.2   Neuralgia and neuritis, unspecified

EXCLUDES 1	*brachial radiculitis NOS (M54.1)*
	lumbosacral radiculitis NOS (M54.1)
	mononeuropathies (G56-G58)
	radiculitis NOS (M54.1)
	sciatica (M54.3-M54.4)

M79.3   Panniculitis, unspecified

EXCLUDES 1	*lupus panniculitis (L93.2)*
	neck and back panniculitis (M54.0-)
	relapsing [Weber-Christian] panniculitis (M35.6)

M79.4   Hypertrophy of (infrapatellar) fat pad

M79.5   Residual foreign body in soft tissue

| EXCLUDES 1 | *foreign body granuloma of skin and subcutaneous tissue (L92.3)* |
| | *foreign body granuloma of soft tissue (M60.2-)* |

⁵ **M79.6   Pain in limb, hand, foot, fingers and toes**

| EXCLUDES 2 | *pain in joint (M25.5-)* |

⁶ **M79.60   Pain in limb, unspecified**

◻ **M79.601   Pain in right arm**
Pain in right upper limb NOS

◻ **M79.602   Pain in left arm**
Pain in left upper limb NOS

◻ **M79.603   Pain in arm, unspecified**
Pain in upper limb NOS

◻ **M79.604   Pain in right leg**
Pain in right lower limb NOS

◻ **M79.605   Pain in left leg**
Pain in left lower limb NOS

◻ **M79.606   Pain in leg, unspecified**
Pain in lower limb NOS

◻ **M79.609   Pain in unspecified limb**
Pain in limb NOS

⁶ **M79.62   Pain in upper arm**
Pain in axillary region

◻ **M79.621   Pain in right upper arm**

◻ **M79.622   Pain in left upper arm**

◻ **M79.629   Pain in unspecified upper arm**

⁶ **M79.63   Pain in forearm**

◻ **M79.631   Pain in right forearm**

◻ **M79.632   Pain in left forearm**

◻ **M79.639   Pain in unspecified forearm**

⁶ **M79.64   Pain in hand and fingers**

◻ **M79.641   Pain in right hand**

◻ **M79.642   Pain in left hand**

◻ **M79.643   Pain in unspecified hand**

◻ **M79.644   Pain in right finger(s)**

◻ **M79.645   Pain in left finger(s)**

◻ **M79.646   Pain in unspecified finger(s)**

⁶ **M79.65   Pain in thigh**

◻ **M79.651   Pain in right thigh**

◻ **M79.652   Pain in left thigh**

◻ **M79.659   Pain in unspecified thigh**

⁶ **M79.66   Pain in lower leg**

◻ **M79.661   Pain in right lower leg**

◻ **M79.662   Pain in left lower leg**

◻ **M79.669   Pain in unspecified lower leg**

⁶ **M79.67   Pain in foot and toes**

◻ **M79.671   Pain in right foot**

◻ **M79.672   Pain in left foot**

◻ **M79.673   Pain in unspecified foot**

◻ **M79.674   Pain in right toe(s)**

◻ **M79.675   Pain in left toe(s)**

◻ **M79.676   Pain in unspecified toe(s)**

M79.7   Fibromyalgia
Fibromyositis
Fibrositis
Myofibrositis

⁵ **M79.A   Nontraumatic compartment syndrome**
Code first:
, if applicable, associated postprocedural complication

EXCLUDES 1	*compartment syndrome NOS (T79.A-)*
	fibromyalgia (M79.7)
	nontraumatic ischemic infarction of muscle (M62.2-)
	traumatic compartment syndrome (T79.A-)

⁶ **M79.A1   Nontraumatic compartment syndrome of upper extremity**
Nontraumatic compartment syndrome of shoulder, arm, forearm, wrist, hand, and fingers

□ **M79.A11** **Nontraumatic compartment syndrome of right upper extremity**

□ **M79.A12** **Nontraumatic compartment syndrome of left upper extremity**

□ **M79.A19** **Nontraumatic compartment syndrome of unspecified upper extremity**

⑥ **M79.A2** **Nontraumatic compartment syndrome of lower extremity**
Nontraumatic compartment syndrome of hip, buttock, thigh, leg, foot, and toes

□ **M79.A21** **Nontraumatic compartment syndrome of right lower extremity**

□ **M79.A22** **Nontraumatic compartment syndrome of left lower extremity**

□ **M79.A29** **Nontraumatic compartment syndrome of unspecified lower extremity**

M79.A3 **Nontraumatic compartment syndrome of abdomen**

M79.A9 **Nontraumatic compartment syndrome of other sites**

⑤ **M79.8** **Other specified soft tissue disorders**

M79.81 **Nontraumatic hematoma of soft tissue**
Nontraumatic hematoma of muscle
Nontraumatic seroma of muscle and soft tissue

DEFINITION   A spontaneous, nontraumatic localized collection of partially clotted blood within a soft tissue such as muscle.

M79.89 **Other specified soft tissue disorders**
Polyalgia

M79.9 **Soft tissue disorder, unspecified**

Osteopathies and chondropathies (M80-M94)

Disorders of bone density and structure (M80-M85)

④+ **M80** **Osteoporosis with current pathological fracture**

INCLUDES   osteoporosis with current fragility fracture

Use additional code to identify major osseous defect, if applicable (M89.7-)

EXCLUDES 1   *collapsed vertebra NOS (M48.5)*
pathological fracture NOS (M84.4)
wedging of vertebra NOS (M48.5)

EXCLUDES 2   *personal history of (healed) osteoporosis fracture (Z87.310)*

The appropriate 7th character is to be added to each code from category M80:
A   initial encounter for fracture
D   subsequent encounter for fracture with routine healing
G   subsequent encounter for fracture with delayed healing
K   subsequent encounter for fracture with nonunion
P   subsequent encounter for fracture with malunion
S   sequela

GUIDELINES   **Section I.C.13.c**
Coding of Pathologic Fractures: 7th character D is to be used for encounters after the patient has completed active treatment. The other 7th characters, listed under each subcategory in the Tabular List, are to be used for subsequent encounters for treatment of problems associated with the healing, such as malunions, nonunions, and sequelae. Care for complications of surgical treatment for fracture repairs during the healing or recovery phase should be coded with the appropriate complication codes.

GUIDELINES   **Section I.C.13.d.2)**
Category M80, Osteoporosis with current pathological fracture, is for patients who have a current pathologic fracture at the time of an encounter. The codes under M80 identify the site of the fracture. A code from category M80, not a traumatic fracture code, should be used for any patient with known osteoporosis who suffers a fracture, even if the patient had a minor fall or trauma, if that fall or trauma would not usually break a normal, healthy bone.

CODING TIP ✓   When a patient with osteoporosis is noted to have an active fracture, use the osteoporosis fracture codes, even if the patient had a minor fall or trauma (fall from standing height or less), unless the physician has identified the fracture as a traumatic fracture. Age-related osteoporosis includes post-menopausal and senile osteoporosis, as well as unspecified. Age-related osteoporosis is the default if the type of osteoporosis is not identified. Code Z87.310 is assigned only for an osteoporosis fracture that has healed.

⑤+ **M80.0** **Age-related osteoporosis with current pathological fracture**
Involutional osteoporosis with current pathological fracture
Osteoporosis NOS with current pathological fracture
Postmenopausal osteoporosis with current pathological fracture
Senile osteoporosis with current pathological fracture

⑦+ **M80.00X-** **Age-related osteoporosis with current pathological fracture, unspecified site**   Ⓐ

⑥+ **M80.01** **Age-related osteoporosis with current pathological fracture, shoulder**   Ⓐ

⑦□+ **M80.011-** **Age-related osteoporosis with current pathological fracture, right shoulder**   Ⓐ

⑦□+ **M80.012-** **Age-related osteoporosis with current pathological fracture, left shoulder**   Ⓐ

⑦□+ **M80.019-** **Age-related osteoporosis with current pathological fracture, unspecified shoulder**   Ⓐ

⑥+ **M80.02** **Age-related osteoporosis with current pathological fracture, humerus**

⑦□+ **M80.021-** **Age-related osteoporosis with current pathological fracture, right humerus**   Ⓐ

⑦□+ **M80.022-** **Age-related osteoporosis with current pathological fracture, left humerus**   Ⓐ

⑦□+ **M80.029-** **Age-related osteoporosis with current pathological fracture, unspecified humerus**   Ⓐ

⑥+ **M80.03** **Age-related osteoporosis with current pathological fracture, forearm**
Age-related osteoporosis with current pathological fracture of wrist

⑦□+ **M80.031-** **Age-related osteoporosis with current pathological fracture, right forearm**   Ⓐ

⑦□+ **M80.032-** **Age-related osteoporosis with current pathological fracture, left forearm**   Ⓐ

⑦□+ **M80.039-** **Age-related osteoporosis with current pathological fracture, unspecified forearm**   Ⓐ

⑥+ **M80.04** **Age-related osteoporosis with current pathological fracture, hand**

⑦□+ **M80.041-** **Age-related osteoporosis with current pathological fracture, right hand**   Ⓐ

⑦□+ **M80.042-** **Age-related osteoporosis with current pathological fracture, left hand**   Ⓐ

⑦□+ **M80.049-** **Age-related osteoporosis with current pathological fracture, unspecified hand**   Ⓐ

⑥+ **M80.05** **Age-related osteoporosis with current pathological fracture, femur**
Age-related osteoporosis with current pathological fracture of hip

⑦□+ **M80.051-** **Age-related osteoporosis with current pathological fracture, right femur**   Ⓐ

⑦□+ **M80.052-** **Age-related osteoporosis with current pathological fracture, left femur**   Ⓐ

⑦□+ **M80.059-** **Age-related osteoporosis with current pathological fracture, unspecified femur**   Ⓐ

⑥+ **M80.06** **Age-related osteoporosis with current pathological fracture, lower leg**   Ⓐ

⑦□+ **M80.061-** **Age-related osteoporosis with current pathological fracture, right lower leg**   Ⓐ

⑦□+ **M80.062-** **Age-related osteoporosis with current pathological fracture, left lower leg**   Ⓐ

⑦□+ **M80.069-** **Age-related osteoporosis with current pathological fracture, unspecified lower leg**   Ⓐ

⑥+ **M80.07** **Age-related osteoporosis with current pathological fracture, ankle and foot**

⑦□+ **M80.071-** **Age-related osteoporosis with current pathological fracture, right ankle and foot**   Ⓐ

● New   ▲ Revised   *Manifestation*   ④-⑦ Digit Indicators   □ Laterality   Ⓐ Adult (15+ years)   Ⓜ Maternity (12-55 years)   Ⓝ Newborn   Ⓟ Pediatric (0-17 years)   ♂ Male   ♀ Female
�excludes Deleted   Unspecified   + Additional code

794   © 2017 DecisionHealth   2017 ICD-10-CM Expert for Physicians

M79.A11 — M80.071-

7 🔲 ✚ **M80.072-** Age-related osteoporosis with current pathological fracture, left ankle and foot 🅰

7 🔲 ✚ **M80.079-** Age-related osteoporosis with current pathological fracture, unspecified ankle and foot 🅰

7 ✚ **M80.08X-** Age-related osteoporosis with current pathological fracture, vertebra(e) 🅰

Age related osteoporosis
with current pathological fracture, vertebra(e)

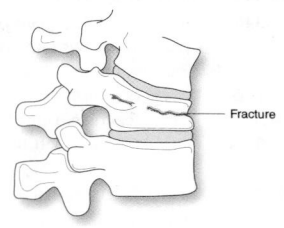

Fracture

6 ✚ **M80.8** Other osteoporosis with current pathological fracture
Drug-induced osteoporosis with current pathological fracture
Idiopathic osteoporosis with current pathological fracture
Osteoporosis of disuse with current pathological fracture
Postoophorectomy osteoporosis with current pathological fracture
Postsurgical malabsorption osteoporosis with current pathological fracture
Post-traumatic osteoporosis with current pathological fracture
Use additional code for adverse effect, if applicable, to identify drug (T36-T50 with fifth or sixth character 5)

7 ✚ **M80.80X-** Other osteoporosis with current pathological fracture, unspecified site

6 ✚ **M80.81** Other osteoporosis with pathological fracture, shoulder

7 🔲 ✚ **M80.811-** Other osteoporosis with current pathological fracture, right shoulder

7 🔲 ✚ **M80.812-** Other osteoporosis with current pathological fracture, left shoulder

7 🔲 ✚ **M80.819-** Other osteoporosis with current pathological fracture, unspecified shoulder

6 ✚ **M80.82** Other osteoporosis with current pathological fracture, humerus

7 🔲 ✚ **M80.821-** Other osteoporosis with current pathological fracture, right humerus

7 🔲 ✚ **M80.822-** Other osteoporosis with current pathological fracture, left humerus

7 🔲 ✚ **M80.829-** Other osteoporosis with current pathological fracture, unspecified humerus

6 ✚ **M80.83** Other osteoporosis with current pathological fracture, forearm
Other osteoporosis with current pathological fracture of wrist

7 🔲 ✚ **M80.831-** Other osteoporosis with current pathological fracture, right forearm

7 🔲 ✚ **M80.832-** Other osteoporosis with current pathological fracture, left forearm

7 🔲 ✚ **M80.839-** Other osteoporosis with current pathological fracture, unspecified forearm

6 ✚ **M80.84** Other osteoporosis with current pathological fracture, hand

7 🔲 ✚ **M80.841-** Other osteoporosis with current pathological fracture, right hand

7 🔲 ✚ **M80.842-** Other osteoporosis with current pathological fracture, left hand

7 🔲 ✚ **M80.849-** Other osteoporosis with current pathological fracture, unspecified hand

6 ✚ **M80.85** Other osteoporosis with current pathological fracture, femur
Other osteoporosis with current pathological fracture of hip

7 🔲 ✚ **M80.851-** Other osteoporosis with current pathological fracture, right femur

7 🔲 ✚ **M80.852-** Other osteoporosis with current pathological fracture, left femur

7 🔲 ✚ **M80.859-** Other osteoporosis with current pathological fracture, unspecified femur

6 ✚ **M80.86** Other osteoporosis with current pathological fracture, lower leg

7 🔲 ✚ **M80.861-** Other osteoporosis with current pathological fracture, right lower leg

7 🔲 ✚ **M80.862-** Other osteoporosis with current pathological fracture, left lower leg

7 🔲 ✚ **M80.869-** Other osteoporosis with current pathological fracture, unspecified lower leg

6 ✚ **M80.87** Other osteoporosis with current pathological fracture, ankle and foot

7 🔲 ✚ **M80.871-** Other osteoporosis with current pathological fracture, right ankle and foot

7 🔲 ✚ **M80.872-** Other osteoporosis with current pathological fracture, left ankle and foot

7 🔲 ✚ **M80.879-** Other osteoporosis with current pathological fracture, unspecified ankle and foot

7 ✚ **M80.88X-** Other osteoporosis with current pathological fracture, vertebra(e)

4 ✚ **M81** Osteoporosis without current pathological fracture
Use additional code to identify:
major osseous defect, if applicable (M89.7-)
personal history of (healed) osteoporosis fracture, if applicable (Z87.310)
EXCLUDES 1 *osteoporosis with current pathological fracture (M80.-)*
Sudeck's atrophy (M89.0)
GUIDELINES Section I.C.13.d.1)
Category M81, Osteoporosis without current pathological fracture, is for use for patients with osteoporosis who do not currently have a pathologic fracture due to the osteoporosis, even if they have had a fracture in the past. For patients with a history of osteoporosis fractures, status code Z87.310, Personal history of (healed) osteoporosis fracture, should follow the code from M81.

Osteoporosis
without current pathological fracture

Healthy bone

Low bone density

Osteoporotic bone

✚ **M81.0** Age-related osteoporosis without current pathological fracture 🅰
Involutional osteoporosis without current pathological fracture
Osteoporosis NOS
Postmenopausal osteoporosis without current pathological fracture
Senile osteoporosis without current pathological fracture

✚ **M81.6** Localized osteoporosis [Lequesne]
EXCLUDES 1 *Sudeck's atrophy (M89.0)*

✚ **M81.8** Other osteoporosis without current pathological fracture
Drug-induced osteoporosis without current pathological fracture
Idiopathic osteoporosis without current pathological fracture
Osteoporosis of disuse without current pathological fracture
Postoophorectomy osteoporosis without current pathological fracture
Postsurgical malabsorption osteoporosis without current pathological fracture
Post-traumatic osteoporosis without current pathological fracture
Use additional code for adverse effect, if applicable, to identify drug (T36-T50 with fifth or sixth character 5)

● New ▲ Revised *Manifestation* 4-7 Digit Indicators 🔲 Laterality 🅰 Adult (15+ years) Ⓜ Maternity (12-55 years) Ⓝ Newborn Ⓟ Pediatric (0-17 years) ♂ Male ♀ Female
✖ Deleted Unspecified ✚ Additional code

4 **M83   Adult osteomalacia**

EXCLUDES 1   *infantile and juvenile osteomalacia (E55.0)*
renal osteodystrophy (N25.0)
rickets (active) (E55.0)
rickets (active) sequelae (E64.3)
vitamin D-resistant osteomalacia (E83.3)
vitamin D-resistant rickets (active) (E83.3)

CODING TIP ✓   Osteomalacia differs from osteoporosis in that osteomalacia implies softening of the bone due to demineralization. Osteoporosis indicates a clear reduction in bone density/mass with porousness of the bones.

DEFINITION   Deficient levels of calcium in the bone, resulting in bone softening.

M83.0   **Puerperal osteomalacia**   ♀ Ⓜ
M83.1   **Senile osteomalacia**   Ⓐ
M83.2   **Adult osteomalacia due to malabsorption**   Ⓐ
         Postsurgical malabsorption osteomalacia in adults
M83.3   **Adult osteomalacia due to malnutrition**   Ⓐ
M83.4   **Aluminum bone disease**
+ M83.5   **Other drug-induced osteomalacia in adults**   Ⓐ
         Use additional code for adverse effect, if applicable, to identify drug (T36-T50 with fifth or sixth character 5)
M83.8   **Other adult osteomalacia**   Ⓐ
M83.9   **Adult osteomalacia, unspecified**   Ⓐ

4 **M84   Disorder of continuity of bone**

EXCLUDES 2   *traumatic fracture of bone-see fracture, by site*

GUIDELINES   Section I.C.13.c
Coding of Pathologic Fractures: 7th character D is to be used for encounters after the patient has completed active treatment. The other 7th characters, listed under each subcategory in the Tabular List, are to be used for subsequent encounters for treatment of problems associated with the healing, such as malunions, nonunions, and sequelae. Care for complications of surgical treatment for fracture repairs during the healing or recovery phase should be coded with the appropriate complication codes.

5 + **M84.3   Stress fracture**
         Fatigue fracture
         March fracture
         Stress fracture NOS
         Stress reaction
         Use additional external cause code(s) to identify the cause of the stress fracture

EXCLUDES 1   *pathological fracture NOS (M84.4.-)*
pathological fracture due to osteoporosis (M80.-)
traumatic fracture
(S12.-, S22.-, S32.-, S42.-, S52.-, S62.-, S72.-, S82.-, S92.-)

EXCLUDES 2   *personal history of (healed) stress (fatigue) fracture (Z87.312)*
stress fracture of vertebra (M48.4-)

The appropriate 7th character is to be added to each code from subcategory M84.3:
A   initial encounter for fracture
D   subsequent encounter for fracture with routine healing
G   subsequent encounter for fracture with delayed healing
K   subsequent encounter for fracture with nonunion
P   subsequent encounter for fracture with malunion
S   sequela

DEFINITION   Small, hairline crack(s) in the surface of a bone due to overuse or activity that applies a repetitive force to a particular area, most commonly occurring in the lower legs and feet.

7 + **M84.30X-   Stress fracture, unspecified site**
6 + **M84.31   Stress fracture, shoulder**
   7 🖛 + **M84.311-   Stress fracture, right shoulder**
   7 🖛 + **M84.312-   Stress fracture, left shoulder**
   7 🖛 + **M84.319-   Stress fracture, unspecified shoulder**
6 + **M84.32   Stress fracture, humerus**
   7 🖛 + **M84.321-   Stress fracture, right humerus**
   7 🖛 + **M84.322-   Stress fracture, left humerus**
   7 🖛 + **M84.329-   Stress fracture, unspecified humerus**
6 + **M84.33   Stress fracture, ulna and radius**

   7 🖛 + **M84.331-   Stress fracture, right ulna**
   7 🖛 + **M84.332-   Stress fracture, left ulna**
   7 🖛 + **M84.333-   Stress fracture, right radius**
   7 🖛 + **M84.334-   Stress fracture, left radius**
   7 🖛 + **M84.339-   Stress fracture, unspecified ulna and radius**
6 + **M84.34   Stress fracture, hand and fingers**
   7 🖛 + **M84.341-   Stress fracture, right hand**
   7 🖛 + **M84.342-   Stress fracture, left hand**
   7 🖛 + **M84.343-   Stress fracture, unspecified hand**
   7 🖛 + **M84.344-   Stress fracture, right finger(s)**
   7 🖛 + **M84.345-   Stress fracture, left finger(s)**
   7 🖛 + **M84.346-   Stress fracture, unspecified finger(s)**
6 + **M84.35   Stress fracture, pelvis and femur**
         Stress fracture, hip
   7 🖛 + **M84.350-   Stress fracture, pelvis**
   7 🖛 + **M84.351-   Stress fracture, right femur**
   7 🖛 + **M84.352-   Stress fracture, left femur**
   7 🖛 + **M84.353-   Stress fracture, unspecified femur**
   7 🖛 + **M84.359-   Stress fracture, hip, unspecified**
6 + **M84.36   Stress fracture, tibia and fibula**
   7 🖛 + **M84.361-   Stress fracture, right tibia**
   7 🖛 + **M84.362-   Stress fracture, left tibia**
   7 🖛 + **M84.363-   Stress fracture, right fibula**
   7 🖛 + **M84.364-   Stress fracture, left fibula**
   7 🖛 + **M84.369-   Stress fracture, unspecified tibia and fibula**
6 + **M84.37   Stress fracture, ankle, foot and toes**
   7 🖛 + **M84.371-   Stress fracture, right ankle**
   7 🖛 + **M84.372-   Stress fracture, left ankle**
   7 🖛 + **M84.373-   Stress fracture, unspecified ankle**
   7 🖛 + **M84.374-   Stress fracture, right foot**
   7 🖛 + **M84.375-   Stress fracture, left foot**
   7 🖛 + **M84.376-   Stress fracture, unspecified foot**
   7 🖛 + **M84.377-   Stress fracture, right toe(s)**
   7 🖛 + **M84.378-   Stress fracture, left toe(s)**
   7 🖛 + **M84.379-   Stress fracture, unspecified toe(s)**
7 + **M84.38X-   Stress fracture, other site**

EXCLUDES 2   *stress fracture of vertebra (M48.4-)*

5 **M84.4   Pathological fracture, not elsewhere classified**
         Chronic fracture
         Pathological fracture NOS

EXCLUDES 1   *collapsed vertebra NEC (M48.5)*
pathological fracture in neoplastic disease (M84.5-)
pathological fracture in osteoporosis (M80.-)
pathological fracture in other disease (M84.6-)
stress fracture (M84.3-)
traumatic fracture
(S12.-, S22.-, S32.-, S42.-, S52.-, S62.-, S72.-, S82.-, S92.-)

EXCLUDES 2   *personal history of (healed) pathological fracture (Z87.311)*

The appropriate 7th character is to be added to each code from subcategory M84.4:
A   initial encounter for fracture
D   subsequent encounter for fracture with routine healing
G   subsequent encounter for fracture with delayed healing
K   subsequent encounter for fracture with nonunion
P   subsequent encounter for fracture with malunion
S   sequela

DEFINITION   A break resulting from widespread lesions or disease process that destroys normal bone mass, causing the weakened bone to break spontaneously without obvious external force.

7 **M84.40X-   Pathological fracture, unspecified site**
6 **M84.41   Pathological fracture, shoulder**
   7 🖛 **M84.411-   Pathological fracture, right shoulder**
   7 🖛 **M84.412-   Pathological fracture, left shoulder**
   7 🖛 **M84.419-   Pathological fracture, unspecified shoulder**
6 **M84.42   Pathological fracture, humerus**
   7 🖛 **M84.421-   Pathological fracture, right humerus**

● New   ▲ Revised   *Manifestation*   4-7 Digit Indicators   🖛 Laterality   Ⓐ Adult (15+ years)   Ⓜ Maternity (12-55 years)   Ⓝ Newborn   Ⓟ Pediatric (0-17 years)   ♂ Male   ♀ Female
✖ Deleted   Unspecified   + Additional code

796   © 2017 DecisionHealth   2017 ICD-10-CM Expert for Physicians

7 ⊟ M84.422-　Pathological fracture, left humerus
7 ⊟ M84.429-　Pathological fracture, unspecified humerus
6 M84.43　Pathological fracture, ulna and radius
7 ⊟ M84.431-　Pathological fracture, right ulna
7 ⊟ M84.432-　Pathological fracture, left ulna
7 ⊟ M84.433-　Pathological fracture, right radius
7 ⊟ M84.434-　Pathological fracture, left radius
7 ⊟ M84.439-　Pathological fracture, unspecified ulna and radius
6 M84.44　Pathological fracture, hand and fingers
7 ⊟ M84.441-　Pathological fracture, right hand
7 ⊟ M84.442-　Pathological fracture, left hand
7 ⊟ M84.443-　Pathological fracture, unspecified hand
7 ⊟ M84.444-　Pathological fracture, right finger(s)
7 ⊟ M84.445-　Pathological fracture, left finger(s)
7 ⊟ M84.446-　Pathological fracture, unspecified finger(s)
6 M84.45　Pathological fracture, femur and pelvis
7 ⊟ M84.451-　Pathological fracture, right femur
7 ⊟ M84.452-　Pathological fracture, left femur
7 ⊟ M84.453-　Pathological fracture, unspecified femur
7 ⊟ M84.454-　Pathological fracture, pelvis
7 ⊟ M84.459-　Pathological fracture, hip, unspecified
6 M84.46　Pathological fracture, tibia and fibula
7 ⊟ M84.461-　Pathological fracture, right tibia
7 ⊟ M84.462-　Pathological fracture, left tibia
7 ⊟ M84.463-　Pathological fracture, right fibula
7 ⊟ M84.464-　Pathological fracture, left fibula
7 ⊟ M84.469-　Pathological fracture, unspecified tibia and fibula
6 M84.47　Pathological fracture, ankle, foot and toes
7 ⊟ M84.471-　Pathological fracture, right ankle
7 ⊟ M84.472-　Pathological fracture, left ankle
7 ⊟ M84.473-　Pathological fracture, unspecified ankle
7 ⊟ M84.474-　Pathological fracture, right foot
7 ⊟ M84.475-　Pathological fracture, left foot
7 ⊟ M84.476-　Pathological fracture, unspecified foot
7 ⊟ M84.477-　Pathological fracture, right toe(s)
7 ⊟ M84.478-　Pathological fracture, left toe(s)
7 ⊟ M84.479-　Pathological fracture, unspecified toe(s)
7 M84.48X-　Pathological fracture, other site
5 M84.5　Pathological fracture in neoplastic disease
Code also:
underlying neoplasm

The appropriate 7th character is to be added to each code from subcategory M84.5:
A　initial encounter for fracture
D　subsequent encounter for fracture with routine healing
G　subsequent encounter for fracture with delayed healing
K　subsequent encounter for fracture with nonunion
P　subsequent encounter for fracture with malunion
S　sequela

GUIDELINES　Section I.C.2.I.6)
When an encounter is for a pathological fracture due to a neoplasm, and the focus of treatment is the fracture, a code from subcategory M84.5, Pathological fracture in neoplastic disease, should be sequenced first, followed by the code for the neoplasm. If the focus of treatment is the neoplasm with an associated pathological fracture, the neoplasm code should be sequenced first, followed by a code from M84.5 for the pathological fracture.

DEFINITION　A break resulting from metastatic invasion or tumor growth that destroys normal bone mass, resulting in fracture without obvious trauma to the bone.

7 M84.50X-　Pathological fracture in neoplastic disease, unspecified site
6 M84.51　Pathological fracture in neoplastic disease, shoulder
7 ⊟ M84.511-　Pathological fracture in neoplastic disease, right shoulder
7 ⊟ M84.512-　Pathological fracture in neoplastic disease, left shoulder

7 ⊟ M84.519-　Pathological fracture in neoplastic disease, unspecified shoulder
6 M84.52　Pathological fracture in neoplastic disease, humerus
7 ⊟ M84.521-　Pathological fracture in neoplastic disease, right humerus
7 ⊟ M84.522-　Pathological fracture in neoplastic disease, left humerus
7 ⊟ M84.529-　Pathological fracture in neoplastic disease, unspecified humerus
6 M84.53　Pathological fracture in neoplastic disease, ulna and radius
7 ⊟ M84.531-　Pathological fracture in neoplastic disease, right ulna
7 ⊟ M84.532-　Pathological fracture in neoplastic disease, left ulna
7 ⊟ M84.533-　Pathological fracture in neoplastic disease, right radius
7 ⊟ M84.534-　Pathological fracture in neoplastic disease, left radius
7 ⊟ M84.539-　Pathological fracture in neoplastic disease, unspecified ulna and radius
6 M84.54　Pathological fracture in neoplastic disease, hand
7 ⊟ M84.541-　Pathological fracture in neoplastic disease, right hand
7 ⊟ M84.542-　Pathological fracture in neoplastic disease, left hand
7 ⊟ M84.549-　Pathological fracture in neoplastic disease, unspecified hand
6 M84.55　Pathological fracture in neoplastic disease, pelvis and femur
7 ⊟ M84.550-　Pathological fracture in neoplastic disease, pelvis
7 ⊟ M84.551-　Pathological fracture in neoplastic disease, right femur
7 ⊟ M84.552-　Pathological fracture in neoplastic disease, left femur
7 ⊟ M84.553-　Pathological fracture in neoplastic disease, unspecified femur
7 ⊟ M84.559-　Pathological fracture in neoplastic disease, hip, unspecified
6 M84.56　Pathological fracture in neoplastic disease, tibia and fibula
7 ⊟ M84.561-　Pathological fracture in neoplastic disease, right tibia
7 ⊟ M84.562-　Pathological fracture in neoplastic disease, left tibia
7 ⊟ M84.563-　Pathological fracture in neoplastic disease, right fibula
7 ⊟ M84.564-　Pathological fracture in neoplastic disease, left fibula
7 ⊟ M84.569-　Pathological fracture in neoplastic disease, unspecified tibia and fibula
6 M84.57　Pathological fracture in neoplastic disease, ankle and foot
7 ⊟ M84.571-　Pathological fracture in neoplastic disease, right ankle
7 ⊟ M84.572-　Pathological fracture in neoplastic disease, left ankle
7 ⊟ M84.573-　Pathological fracture in neoplastic disease, unspecified ankle
7 ⊟ M84.574-　Pathological fracture in neoplastic disease, right foot
7 ⊟ M84.575-　Pathological fracture in neoplastic disease, left foot
7 ⊟ M84.576-　Pathological fracture in neoplastic disease, unspecified foot
7 M84.58X-　Pathological fracture in neoplastic disease, other specified site
Pathological fracture in neoplastic disease, vertebrae

⑤ **M84.6**   **Pathological fracture in other disease**
Code also:
    underlying condition
EXCLUDES 1   *pathological fracture in osteoporosis (M80.-)*

The appropriate 7th character is to be added to each code from subcategory M84.6:
A   initial encounter for fracture
D   subsequent encounter for fracture with routine healing
G   subsequent encounter for fracture with delayed healing
K   subsequent encounter for fracture with nonunion
P   subsequent encounter for fracture with malunion
S   sequela

⑦ **M84.60X-**   **Pathological fracture in other disease, unspecified site**

⑥ **M84.61**   **Pathological fracture in other disease, shoulder**
⑦⊟ **M84.611-**   Pathological fracture in other disease, right shoulder
⑦⊟ **M84.612-**   Pathological fracture in other disease, left shoulder
⑦⊟ **M84.619-**   **Pathological fracture in other disease, unspecified shoulder**

⑥ **M84.62**   **Pathological fracture in other disease, humerus**
⑦⊟ **M84.621-**   Pathological fracture in other disease, right humerus
⑦⊟ **M84.622-**   Pathological fracture in other disease, left humerus
⑦⊟ **M84.629-**   **Pathological fracture in other disease, unspecified humerus**

⑥ **M84.63**   **Pathological fracture in other disease, ulna and radius**
⑦⊟ **M84.631-**   Pathological fracture in other disease, right ulna
⑦⊟ **M84.632-**   Pathological fracture in other disease, left ulna
⑦⊟ **M84.633-**   Pathological fracture in other disease, right radius
⑦⊟ **M84.634-**   Pathological fracture in other disease, left radius
⑦⊟ **M84.639-**   **Pathological fracture in other disease, unspecified ulna and radius**

⑥ **M84.64**   **Pathological fracture in other disease, hand**
⑦⊟ **M84.641-**   Pathological fracture in other disease, right hand
⑦⊟ **M84.642-**   Pathological fracture in other disease, left hand
⑦⊟ **M84.649-**   **Pathological fracture in other disease, unspecified hand**

⑥ **M84.65**   **Pathological fracture in other disease, pelvis and femur**
⑦⊟ **M84.650-**   Pathological fracture in other disease, pelvis
⑦⊟ **M84.651-**   Pathological fracture in other disease, right femur
⑦⊟ **M84.652-**   Pathological fracture in other disease, left femur
⑦⊟ **M84.653-**   **Pathological fracture in other disease, unspecified femur**
⑦⊟ **M84.659-**   **Pathological fracture in other disease, hip, unspecified**

⑥ **M84.66**   **Pathological fracture in other disease, tibia and fibula**
⑦⊟ **M84.661-**   Pathological fracture in other disease, right tibia
⑦⊟ **M84.662-**   Pathological fracture in other disease, left tibia
⑦⊟ **M84.663-**   Pathological fracture in other disease, right fibula
⑦⊟ **M84.664-**   Pathological fracture in other disease, left fibula
⑦⊟ **M84.669-**   **Pathological fracture in other disease, unspecified tibia and fibula**

⑥ **M84.67**   **Pathological fracture in other disease, ankle and foot**
⑦⊟ **M84.671-**   Pathological fracture in other disease, right ankle
⑦⊟ **M84.672-**   Pathological fracture in other disease, left ankle
⑦⊟ **M84.673-**   **Pathological fracture in other disease, unspecified ankle**

⑦⊟ **M84.674-**   Pathological fracture in other disease, right foot
⑦⊟ **M84.675-**   Pathological fracture in other disease, left foot
⑦⊟ **M84.676-**   **Pathological fracture in other disease, unspecified foot**
⑦ **M84.68X-**   Pathological fracture in other disease, other site

● ⑤ **M84.7**   **Nontraumatic fracture, not elsewhere classified**
● ⑥ **M84.75**   **Atypical femoral fracture**

The appropriate 7th character is to be added to each code from M84.75:
A   initial encounter for fracture
D   subsequent encounter for fracture with routine healing
G   subsequent encounter for fracture with delayed healing
K   subsequent encounter for fracture with nonunion
P   subsequent encounter for fracture with malunion
S   sequela

● ⑦ **M84.750-**   Atypical femoral fracture, unspecified
● ⑦⊟ **M84.751-**   Incomplete atypical femoral fracture, right leg
● ⑦⊟ **M84.752-**   Incomplete atypical femoral fracture, left leg
● ⑦⊟ **M84.753-**   **Incomplete atypical femoral fracture, unspecified leg**
● ⑦⊟ **M84.754-**   Complete transverse atypical femoral fracture, right leg
● ⑦⊟ **M84.755-**   Complete transverse atypical femoral fracture, left leg
● ⑦⊟ **M84.756-**   **Complete transverse atypical femoral fracture, unspecified leg**
● ⑦⊟ **M84.757-**   Complete oblique atypical femoral fracture, right leg
● ⑦⊟ **M84.758-**   Complete oblique atypical femoral fracture, left leg
● ⑦⊟ **M84.759-**   **Complete oblique atypical femoral fracture, unspecified leg**

⑤ **M84.8**   **Other disorders of continuity of bone**
M84.80   Other disorders of continuity of bone, unspecified site

⑥ **M84.81**   Other disorders of continuity of bone, shoulder
⊟ **M84.811**   Other disorders of continuity of bone, right shoulder
⊟ **M84.812**   Other disorders of continuity of bone, left shoulder
⊟ **M84.819**   **Other disorders of continuity of bone, unspecified shoulder**

⑥ **M84.82**   Other disorders of continuity of bone, humerus
⊟ **M84.821**   Other disorders of continuity of bone, right humerus
⊟ **M84.822**   Other disorders of continuity of bone, left humerus
⊟ **M84.829**   **Other disorders of continuity of bone, unspecified humerus**

⑥ **M84.83**   Other disorders of continuity of bone, ulna and radius
⊟ **M84.831**   Other disorders of continuity of bone, right ulna
⊟ **M84.832**   Other disorders of continuity of bone, left ulna
⊟ **M84.833**   Other disorders of continuity of bone, right radius
⊟ **M84.834**   Other disorders of continuity of bone, left radius
⊟ **M84.839**   **Other disorders of continuity of bone, unspecified ulna and radius**

⑥ **M84.84**   Other disorders of continuity of bone, hand
⊟ **M84.841**   Other disorders of continuity of bone, right hand
⊟ **M84.842**   Other disorders of continuity of bone, left hand
⊟ **M84.849**   **Other disorders of continuity of bone, unspecified hand**

⑥ **M84.85**   Other disorders of continuity of bone, pelvic region and thigh
⊟ **M84.851**   Other disorders of continuity of bone, right pelvic region and thigh
⊟ **M84.852**   Other disorders of continuity of bone, left pelvic region and thigh

● New   ▲ Revised   *Manifestation*   ④-⑦ Digit Indicators   ⊟ Laterality   Ⓐ Adult (15+ years)   Ⓜ Maternity (12-55 years)   Ⓝ Newborn   Ⓟ Pediatric (0-17 years)   ♂ Male   ♀ Female
✖ Deleted   Unspecified   + Additional code

798   © 2017 DecisionHealth   2017 ICD-10-CM Expert for Physicians

⬡ M84.859   Other disorders of continuity of bone, unspecified pelvic region and thigh
◻ M84.86   Other disorders of continuity of bone, tibia and fibula
⬡ M84.861   Other disorders of continuity of bone, right tibia
⬡ M84.862   Other disorders of continuity of bone, left tibia
⬡ M84.863   Other disorders of continuity of bone, right fibula
⬡ M84.864   Other disorders of continuity of bone, left fibula
⬡ M84.869   Other disorders of continuity of bone, unspecified tibia and fibula
◻ M84.87   Other disorders of continuity of bone, ankle and foot
⬡ M84.871   Other disorders of continuity of bone, right ankle and foot
⬡ M84.872   Other disorders of continuity of bone, left ankle and foot
⬡ M84.879   Other disorders of continuity of bone, unspecified ankle and foot
M84.88   Other disorders of continuity of bone, other site
M84.9   Disorder of continuity of bone, unspecified
◪ M85   Other disorders of bone density and structure

EXCLUDES 1	osteogenesis imperfecta (Q78.0)
	osteopetrosis (Q78.2)
	osteopoikilosis (Q78.8)
	polyostotic fibrous dysplasia (Q78.1)

⑤ M85.0   Fibrous dysplasia (monostotic)

| EXCLUDES 2 | fibrous dysplasia of jaw (M27.8) |

M85.00   Fibrous dysplasia (monostotic), unspecified site
◻ M85.01   Fibrous dysplasia (monostotic), shoulder
⬡ M85.011   Fibrous dysplasia (monostotic), right shoulder
⬡ M85.012   Fibrous dysplasia (monostotic), left shoulder
⬡ M85.019   Fibrous dysplasia (monostotic), unspecified shoulder
◻ M85.02   Fibrous dysplasia (monostotic), upper arm
⬡ M85.021   Fibrous dysplasia (monostotic), right upper arm
⬡ M85.022   Fibrous dysplasia (monostotic), left upper arm
⬡ M85.029   Fibrous dysplasia (monostotic), unspecified upper arm
◻ M85.03   Fibrous dysplasia (monostotic), forearm
⬡ M85.031   Fibrous dysplasia (monostotic), right forearm
⬡ M85.032   Fibrous dysplasia (monostotic), left forearm
⬡ M85.039   Fibrous dysplasia (monostotic), unspecified forearm
◻ M85.04   Fibrous dysplasia (monostotic), hand
⬡ M85.041   Fibrous dysplasia (monostotic), right hand
⬡ M85.042   Fibrous dysplasia (monostotic), left hand
⬡ M85.049   Fibrous dysplasia (monostotic), unspecified hand
◻ M85.05   Fibrous dysplasia (monostotic), thigh
⬡ M85.051   Fibrous dysplasia (monostotic), right thigh
⬡ M85.052   Fibrous dysplasia (monostotic), left thigh
⬡ M85.059   Fibrous dysplasia (monostotic), unspecified thigh
◻ M85.06   Fibrous dysplasia (monostotic), lower leg
⬡ M85.061   Fibrous dysplasia (monostotic), right lower leg
⬡ M85.062   Fibrous dysplasia (monostotic), left lower leg
⬡ M85.069   Fibrous dysplasia (monostotic), unspecified lower leg
◻ M85.07   Fibrous dysplasia (monostotic), ankle and foot
⬡ M85.071   Fibrous dysplasia (monostotic), right ankle and foot
⬡ M85.072   Fibrous dysplasia (monostotic), left ankle and foot
⬡ M85.079   Fibrous dysplasia (monostotic), unspecified ankle and foot
M85.08   Fibrous dysplasia (monostotic), other site
M85.09   Fibrous dysplasia (monostotic), multiple sites
⑤ M85.1   Skeletal fluorosis
M85.10   Skeletal fluorosis, unspecified site
◻ M85.11   Skeletal fluorosis, shoulder
⬡ M85.111   Skeletal fluorosis, right shoulder
⬡ M85.112   Skeletal fluorosis, left shoulder

⬡ M85.119   Skeletal fluorosis, unspecified shoulder
◻ M85.12   Skeletal fluorosis, upper arm
⬡ M85.121   Skeletal fluorosis, right upper arm
⬡ M85.122   Skeletal fluorosis, left upper arm
⬡ M85.129   Skeletal fluorosis, unspecified upper arm
◻ M85.13   Skeletal fluorosis, forearm
⬡ M85.131   Skeletal fluorosis, right forearm
⬡ M85.132   Skeletal fluorosis, left forearm
⬡ M85.139   Skeletal fluorosis, unspecified forearm
◻ M85.14   Skeletal fluorosis, hand
⬡ M85.141   Skeletal fluorosis, right hand
⬡ M85.142   Skeletal fluorosis, left hand
⬡ M85.149   Skeletal fluorosis, unspecified hand
◻ M85.15   Skeletal fluorosis, thigh
⬡ M85.151   Skeletal fluorosis, right thigh
⬡ M85.152   Skeletal fluorosis, left thigh
⬡ M85.159   Skeletal fluorosis, unspecified thigh
◻ M85.16   Skeletal fluorosis, lower leg
⬡ M85.161   Skeletal fluorosis, right lower leg
⬡ M85.162   Skeletal fluorosis, left lower leg
⬡ M85.169   Skeletal fluorosis, unspecified lower leg
◻ M85.17   Skeletal fluorosis, ankle and foot
⬡ M85.171   Skeletal fluorosis, right ankle and foot
⬡ M85.172   Skeletal fluorosis, left ankle and foot
⬡ M85.179   Skeletal fluorosis, unspecified ankle and foot
M85.18   Skeletal fluorosis, other site
M85.19   Skeletal fluorosis, multiple sites
M85.2   Hyperostosis of skull
⑤ M85.3   Osteitis condensans
M85.30   Osteitis condensans, unspecified site
◻ M85.31   Osteitis condensans, shoulder
⬡ M85.311   Osteitis condensans, right shoulder
⬡ M85.312   Osteitis condensans, left shoulder
⬡ M85.319   Osteitis condensans, unspecified shoulder
◻ M85.32   Osteitis condensans, upper arm
⬡ M85.321   Osteitis condensans, right upper arm
⬡ M85.322   Osteitis condensans, left upper arm
⬡ M85.329   Osteitis condensans, unspecified upper arm
◻ M85.33   Osteitis condensans, forearm
⬡ M85.331   Osteitis condensans, right forearm
⬡ M85.332   Osteitis condensans, left forearm
⬡ M85.339   Osteitis condensans, unspecified forearm
◻ M85.34   Osteitis condensans, hand
⬡ M85.341   Osteitis condensans, right hand
⬡ M85.342   Osteitis condensans, left hand
⬡ M85.349   Osteitis condensans, unspecified hand
◻ M85.35   Osteitis condensans, thigh
⬡ M85.351   Osteitis condensans, right thigh
⬡ M85.352   Osteitis condensans, left thigh
⬡ M85.359   Osteitis condensans, unspecified thigh
◻ M85.36   Osteitis condensans, lower leg
⬡ M85.361   Osteitis condensans, right lower leg
⬡ M85.362   Osteitis condensans, left lower leg
⬡ M85.369   Osteitis condensans, unspecified lower leg
◻ M85.37   Osteitis condensans, ankle and foot
⬡ M85.371   Osteitis condensans, right ankle and foot
⬡ M85.372   Osteitis condensans, left ankle and foot
⬡ M85.379   Osteitis condensans, unspecified ankle and foot
M85.38   Osteitis condensans, other site
M85.39   Osteitis condensans, multiple sites
⑤ M85.4   Solitary bone cyst

| EXCLUDES 2 | solitary cyst of jaw (M27.4) |

M85.40   Solitary bone cyst, unspecified site
◻ M85.41   Solitary bone cyst, shoulder
⬡ M85.411   Solitary bone cyst, right shoulder
⬡ M85.412   Solitary bone cyst, left shoulder
⬡ M85.419   Solitary bone cyst, unspecified shoulder
◻ M85.42   Solitary bone cyst, humerus
⬡ M85.421   Solitary bone cyst, right humerus
⬡ M85.422   Solitary bone cyst, left humerus
⬡ M85.429   Solitary bone cyst, unspecified humerus
◻ M85.43   Solitary bone cyst, ulna and radius

● New   ▲ Revised   *Manifestation*   ◪-⬢ Digit Indicators   ▣ Laterality   Ⓐ Adult (15+ years)   Ⓜ Maternity (12-55 years)   Ⓝ Newborn   Ⓟ Pediatric (0-17 years)   ♂ Male   ♀ Female
✖ Deleted   Unspecified   + Additional code

2017 ICD-10-CM Expert for Physicians   © 2017 DecisionHealth   799

- ⊟ M85.431   Solitary bone cyst, right ulna and radius
- ⊟ M85.432   Solitary bone cyst, left ulna and radius
- ⊟ M85.439   Solitary bone cyst, unspecified ulna and radius
- ⑤ M85.44   Solitary bone cyst, hand
  - ⊟ M85.441   Solitary bone cyst, right hand
  - ⊟ M85.442   Solitary bone cyst, left hand
  - ⊟ M85.449   Solitary bone cyst, unspecified hand
- ⑤ M85.45   Solitary bone cyst, pelvis
  - ⊟ M85.451   Solitary bone cyst, right pelvis
  - ⊟ M85.452   Solitary bone cyst, left pelvis
  - ⊟ M85.459   Solitary bone cyst, unspecified pelvis
- ⑤ M85.46   Solitary bone cyst, tibia and fibula
  - ⊟ M85.461   Solitary bone cyst, right tibia and fibula
  - ⊟ M85.462   Solitary bone cyst, left tibia and fibula
  - ⊟ M85.469   Solitary bone cyst, unspecified tibia and fibula
- ⑤ M85.47   Solitary bone cyst, ankle and foot
  - ⊟ M85.471   Solitary bone cyst, right ankle and foot
  - ⊟ M85.472   Solitary bone cyst, left ankle and foot
  - ⊟ M85.479   Solitary bone cyst, unspecified ankle and foot
  - M85.48   Solitary bone cyst, other site
- ⑤ M85.5   Aneurysmal bone cyst
  - **EXCLUDES 2**   aneurysmal cyst of jaw (M27.4)
  - M85.50   Aneurysmal bone cyst, unspecified site
- ⑤ M85.51   Aneurysmal bone cyst, shoulder
  - ⊟ M85.511   Aneurysmal bone cyst, right shoulder
  - ⊟ M85.512   Aneurysmal bone cyst, left shoulder
  - ⊟ M85.519   Aneurysmal bone cyst, unspecified shoulder
- ⑤ M85.52   Aneurysmal bone cyst, upper arm
  - ⊟ M85.521   Aneurysmal bone cyst, right upper arm
  - ⊟ M85.522   Aneurysmal bone cyst, left upper arm
  - ⊟ M85.529   Aneurysmal bone cyst, unspecified upper arm
- ⑤ M85.53   Aneurysmal bone cyst, forearm
  - ⊟ M85.531   Aneurysmal bone cyst, right forearm
  - ⊟ M85.532   Aneurysmal bone cyst, left forearm
  - ⊟ M85.539   Aneurysmal bone cyst, unspecified forearm
- ⑤ M85.54   Aneurysmal bone cyst, hand
  - ⊟ M85.541   Aneurysmal bone cyst, right hand
  - ⊟ M85.542   Aneurysmal bone cyst, left hand
  - ⊟ M85.549   Aneurysmal bone cyst, unspecified hand
- ⑤ M85.55   Aneurysmal bone cyst, thigh
  - ⊟ M85.551   Aneurysmal bone cyst, right thigh
  - ⊟ M85.552   Aneurysmal bone cyst, left thigh
  - ⊟ M85.559   Aneurysmal bone cyst, unspecified thigh
- ⑤ M85.56   Aneurysmal bone cyst, lower leg
  - ⊟ M85.561   Aneurysmal bone cyst, right lower leg
  - ⊟ M85.562   Aneurysmal bone cyst, left lower leg
  - ⊟ M85.569   Aneurysmal bone cyst, unspecified lower leg
- ⑤ M85.57   Aneurysmal bone cyst, ankle and foot
  - ⊟ M85.571   Aneurysmal bone cyst, right ankle and foot
  - ⊟ M85.572   Aneurysmal bone cyst, left ankle and foot
  - ⊟ M85.579   Aneurysmal bone cyst, unspecified ankle and foot
  - M85.58   Aneurysmal bone cyst, other site
  - M85.59   Aneurysmal bone cyst, multiple sites
- ⑤ M85.6   Other cyst of bone
  - **EXCLUDES 1**   cyst of jaw NEC (M27.4)
  - osteitis fibrosa cystica generalisata [von Recklinghausen's disease of bone] (E21.0)
  - M85.60   Other cyst of bone, unspecified site
- ⑤ M85.61   Other cyst of bone, shoulder
  - ⊟ M85.611   Other cyst of bone, right shoulder
  - ⊟ M85.612   Other cyst of bone, left shoulder
  - ⊟ M85.619   Other cyst of bone, unspecified shoulder
- ⑤ M85.62   Other cyst of bone, upper arm
  - ⊟ M85.621   Other cyst of bone, right upper arm
  - ⊟ M85.622   Other cyst of bone, left upper arm
  - ⊟ M85.629   Other cyst of bone, unspecified upper arm
- ⑤ M85.63   Other cyst of bone, forearm
  - ⊟ M85.631   Other cyst of bone, right forearm
  - ⊟ M85.632   Other cyst of bone, left forearm
  - ⊟ M85.639   Other cyst of bone, unspecified forearm

- ⑤ M85.64   Other cyst of bone, hand
  - ⊟ M85.641   Other cyst of bone, right hand
  - ⊟ M85.642   Other cyst of bone, left hand
  - ⊟ M85.649   Other cyst of bone, unspecified hand
- ⑤ M85.65   Other cyst of bone, thigh
  - ⊟ M85.651   Other cyst of bone, right thigh
  - ⊟ M85.652   Other cyst of bone, left thigh
  - ⊟ M85.659   Other cyst of bone, unspecified thigh
- ⑤ M85.66   Other cyst of bone, lower leg
  - ⊟ M85.661   Other cyst of bone, right lower leg
  - ⊟ M85.662   Other cyst of bone, left lower leg
  - ⊟ M85.669   Other cyst of bone, unspecified lower leg
- ⑤ M85.67   Other cyst of bone, ankle and foot
  - ⊟ M85.671   Other cyst of bone, right ankle and foot
  - ⊟ M85.672   Other cyst of bone, left ankle and foot
  - ⊟ M85.679   Other cyst of bone, unspecified ankle and foot
  - M85.68   Other cyst of bone, other site
  - M85.69   Other cyst of bone, multiple sites
- ⑤ M85.8   Other specified disorders of bone density and structure
  - Hyperostosis of bones, except skull
  - Osteosclerosis, acquired
  - **EXCLUDES 1**   diffuse idiopathic skeletal hyperostosis [DISH] (M48.1)
  - osteosclerosis congenita (Q77.4)
  - osteosclerosis fragilitas (generalista) (Q78.2)
  - osteosclerosis myelofibrosis (D75.81)
  - M85.80   Other specified disorders of bone density and structure, unspecified site
- ⑤ M85.81   Other specified disorders of bone density and structure, shoulder
  - ⊟ M85.811   Other specified disorders of bone density and structure, right shoulder
  - ⊟ M85.812   Other specified disorders of bone density and structure, left shoulder
  - ⊟ M85.819   Other specified disorders of bone density and structure, unspecified shoulder
- ⑤ M85.82   Other specified disorders of bone density and structure, upper arm
  - ⊟ M85.821   Other specified disorders of bone density and structure, right upper arm
  - ⊟ M85.822   Other specified disorders of bone density and structure, left upper arm
  - ⊟ M85.829   Other specified disorders of bone density and structure, unspecified upper arm
- ⑤ M85.83   Other specified disorders of bone density and structure, forearm
  - ⊟ M85.831   Other specified disorders of bone density and structure, right forearm
  - ⊟ M85.832   Other specified disorders of bone density and structure, left forearm
  - ⊟ M85.839   Other specified disorders of bone density and structure, unspecified forearm
- ⑤ M85.84   Other specified disorders of bone density and structure, hand
  - ⊟ M85.841   Other specified disorders of bone density and structure, right hand
  - ⊟ M85.842   Other specified disorders of bone density and structure, left hand
  - ⊟ M85.849   Other specified disorders of bone density and structure, unspecified hand
- ⑤ M85.85   Other specified disorders of bone density and structure, thigh
  - ⊟ M85.851   Other specified disorders of bone density and structure, right thigh
  - ⊟ M85.852   Other specified disorders of bone density and structure, left thigh
  - ⊟ M85.859   Other specified disorders of bone density and structure, unspecified thigh
- ⑤ M85.86   Other specified disorders of bone density and structure, lower leg
  - ⊟ M85.861   Other specified disorders of bone density and structure, right lower leg
  - ⊟ M85.862   Other specified disorders of bone density and structure, left lower leg
  - ⊟ M85.869   Other specified disorders of bone density and structure, unspecified lower leg
- ⑤ M85.87   Other specified disorders of bone density and structure, ankle and foot

---

● New   ▲ Revised   *Manifestation*   ④-❼ Digit Indicators   ⊟ Laterality   Ⓐ Adult (15+ years)   Ⓜ Maternity (12-55 years)   Ⓝ Newborn   Ⓟ Pediatric (0-17 years)   ♂ Male   ♀ Female
✖ Deleted   Unspecified   + Additional code

M85.871 Other specified disorders of bone density and structure, right ankle and foot

M85.872 Other specified disorders of bone density and structure, left ankle and foot

M85.879 Other specified disorders of bone density and structure, unspecified ankle and foot

M85.88 Other specified disorders of bone density and structure, other site

M85.89 Other specified disorders of bone density and structure, multiple sites

M85.9 Disorder of bone density and structure, unspecified

Other osteopathies (M86-M90)

EXCLUDES 1   *postprocedural osteopathies (M96.-)*

4 + M86   Osteomyelitis

Use additional code (B95-B97) to identify infectious agent
Use additional code to identify major osseous defect, if applicable (M89.7-)

EXCLUDES 1   *osteomyelitis due to:*
echinococcus (B67.2)
gonococcus (A54.43)
salmonella (A02.24)

EXCLUDES 2   *ostemyelitis of:*
orbit (H05.0-)
petrous bone (H70.2-)
vertebra (M46.2-)

CODING TIP ✓   Codes classified to M86.- do not include osteomyelitis of the orbit, petrous bone, or vertebrae.

CODING TIP ✓   Osteomyelitis commonly occurs in diabetic patients. However, no manifestation combination code pairing for diabetic osteomyelitis exists. When osteomyelitis occurs in a diabetic patient and is confirmed as due to diabetes, the appropriate code from E08-E13 should be assigned with 4th & 5th characters -.69 followed by the appropriate code for osteomyelitis. Documentation must include the type (acute or chronic) and site.

5 + M86.0   Acute hematogenous osteomyelitis

+ M86.00   Acute hematogenous osteomyelitis, unspecified site

6 + M86.01   Acute hematogenous osteomyelitis, shoulder

M86.011   Acute hematogenous osteomyelitis, right shoulder

M86.012   Acute hematogenous osteomyelitis, left shoulder

M86.019   Acute hematogenous osteomyelitis, unspecified shoulder

6 + M86.02   Acute hematogenous osteomyelitis, humerus

M86.021   Acute hematogenous osteomyelitis, right humerus

M86.022   Acute hematogenous osteomyelitis, left humerus

M86.029   Acute hematogenous osteomyelitis, unspecified humerus

6 + M86.03   Acute hematogenous osteomyelitis, radius and ulna

M86.031   Acute hematogenous osteomyelitis, right radius and ulna

M86.032   Acute hematogenous osteomyelitis, left radius and ulna

M86.039   Acute hematogenous osteomyelitis, unspecified radius and ulna

6 + M86.04   Acute hematogenous osteomyelitis, hand

M86.041   Acute hematogenous osteomyelitis, right hand

M86.042   Acute hematogenous osteomyelitis, left hand

M86.049   Acute hematogenous osteomyelitis, unspecified hand

6 + M86.05   Acute hematogenous osteomyelitis, femur

M86.051   Acute hematogenous osteomyelitis, right femur

M86.052   Acute hematogenous osteomyelitis, left femur

M86.059   Acute hematogenous osteomyelitis, unspecified femur

6 + M86.06   Acute hematogenous osteomyelitis, tibia and fibula

M86.061   Acute hematogenous osteomyelitis, right tibia and fibula

M86.062   Acute hematogenous osteomyelitis, left tibia and fibula

M86.069   Acute hematogenous osteomyelitis, unspecified tibia and fibula

6 + M86.07   Acute hematogenous osteomyelitis, ankle and foot

M86.071   Acute hematogenous osteomyelitis, right ankle and foot

M86.072   Acute hematogenous osteomyelitis, left ankle and foot

M86.079   Acute hematogenous osteomyelitis, unspecified ankle and foot

+ M86.08   Acute hematogenous osteomyelitis, other sites

+ M86.09   Acute hematogenous osteomyelitis, multiple sites

5 + M86.1   Other acute osteomyelitis

+ M86.10   Other acute osteomyelitis, unspecified site

6 + M86.11   Other acute osteomyelitis, shoulder

M86.111   Other acute osteomyelitis, right shoulder

M86.112   Other acute osteomyelitis, left shoulder

M86.119   Other acute osteomyelitis, unspecified shoulder

6 + M86.12   Other acute osteomyelitis, humerus

M86.121   Other acute osteomyelitis, right humerus

M86.122   Other acute osteomyelitis, left humerus

M86.129   Other acute osteomyelitis, unspecified humerus

6 + M86.13   Other acute osteomyelitis, radius and ulna

M86.131   Other acute osteomyelitis, right radius and ulna

M86.132   Other acute osteomyelitis, left radius and ulna

M86.139   Other acute osteomyelitis, unspecified radius and ulna

6 + M86.14   Other acute osteomyelitis, hand

M86.141   Other acute osteomyelitis, right hand

M86.142   Other acute osteomyelitis, left hand

M86.149   Other acute osteomyelitis, unspecified hand

6 + M86.15   Other acute osteomyelitis, femur

M86.151   Other acute osteomyelitis, right femur

M86.152   Other acute osteomyelitis, left femur

M86.159   Other acute osteomyelitis, unspecified femur

6 + M86.16   Other acute osteomyelitis, tibia and fibula

M86.161   Other acute osteomyelitis, right tibia and fibula

M86.162   Other acute osteomyelitis, left tibia and fibula

M86.169   Other acute osteomyelitis, unspecified tibia and fibula

6 + M86.17   Other acute osteomyelitis, ankle and foot

M86.171   Other acute osteomyelitis, right ankle and foot

M86.172   Other acute osteomyelitis, left ankle and foot

M86.179   Other acute osteomyelitis, unspecified ankle and foot

+ M86.18   Other acute osteomyelitis, other site

+ M86.19   Other acute osteomyelitis, multiple sites

5 + M86.2   Subacute osteomyelitis

+ M86.20   Subacute osteomyelitis, unspecified site

6 + M86.21   Subacute osteomyelitis, shoulder

M86.211   Subacute osteomyelitis, right shoulder

M86.212   Subacute osteomyelitis, left shoulder

M86.219   Subacute osteomyelitis, unspecified shoulder

6 + M86.22   Subacute osteomyelitis, humerus

M86.221   Subacute osteomyelitis, right humerus

M86.222   Subacute osteomyelitis, left humerus

M86.229   Subacute osteomyelitis, unspecified humerus

6 + M86.23   Subacute osteomyelitis, radius and ulna

M86.231   Subacute osteomyelitis, right radius and ulna

M86.232   Subacute osteomyelitis, left radius and ulna

M86.239   Subacute osteomyelitis, unspecified radius and ulna

6 + M86.24   Subacute osteomyelitis, hand

M86.241   Subacute osteomyelitis, right hand

M86.242   Subacute osteomyelitis, left hand

M86.249   Subacute osteomyelitis, unspecified hand

6 + M86.25   Subacute osteomyelitis, femur

M86.251   Subacute osteomyelitis, right femur

M86.252   Subacute osteomyelitis, left femur

M86.259   Subacute osteomyelitis, unspecified femur

6 + M86.26   Subacute osteomyelitis, tibia and fibula

M86.261   Subacute osteomyelitis, right tibia and fibula

M86.262   Subacute osteomyelitis, left tibia and fibula

M86.269   Subacute osteomyelitis, unspecified tibia and fibula

● New   ▲ Revised   *Manifestation*   4 - 7 Digit Indicators   ▤ Laterality   A Adult (15+ years)   M Maternity (12-55 years)   N Newborn   P Pediatric (0-17 years)   ♂ Male   ♀ Female
✖ Deleted   Unspecified   + Additional code

2017 ICD-10-CM Expert for Physicians   © 2017 DecisionHealth   801

6 + **M86.27**   Subacute osteomyelitis, ankle and foot
  ▤+ **M86.271**   Subacute osteomyelitis, right ankle and foot
  ▤+ **M86.272**   Subacute osteomyelitis, left ankle and foot
  ▤+ **M86.279**   Subacute osteomyelitis, unspecified ankle and foot
    + **M86.28**   Subacute osteomyelitis, other site
    + **M86.29**   Subacute osteomyelitis, multiple sites
5 + **M86.3**   Chronic multifocal osteomyelitis
    + **M86.30**   Chronic multifocal osteomyelitis, unspecified site
6 + **M86.31**   Chronic multifocal osteomyelitis, shoulder
  ▤+ **M86.311**   Chronic multifocal osteomyelitis, right shoulder
  ▤+ **M86.312**   Chronic multifocal osteomyelitis, left shoulder
  ▤+ **M86.319**   Chronic multifocal osteomyelitis, unspecified shoulder
6 + **M86.32**   Chronic multifocal osteomyelitis, humerus
  ▤+ **M86.321**   Chronic multifocal osteomyelitis, right humerus
  ▤+ **M86.322**   Chronic multifocal osteomyelitis, left humerus
  ▤+ **M86.329**   Chronic multifocal osteomyelitis, unspecified humerus
6 + **M86.33**   Chronic multifocal osteomyelitis, radius and ulna
  ▤+ **M86.331**   Chronic multifocal osteomyelitis, right radius and ulna
  ▤+ **M86.332**   Chronic multifocal osteomyelitis, left radius and ulna
  ▤+ **M86.339**   Chronic multifocal osteomyelitis, unspecified radius and ulna
6 + **M86.34**   Chronic multifocal osteomyelitis, hand
  ▤+ **M86.341**   Chronic multifocal osteomyelitis, right hand
  ▤+ **M86.342**   Chronic multifocal osteomyelitis, left hand
  ▤+ **M86.349**   Chronic multifocal osteomyelitis, unspecified hand
6 + **M86.35**   Chronic multifocal osteomyelitis, femur
  ▤+ **M86.351**   Chronic multifocal osteomyelitis, right femur
  ▤+ **M86.352**   Chronic multifocal osteomyelitis, left femur
  ▤+ **M86.359**   Chronic multifocal osteomyelitis, unspecified femur
6 + **M86.36**   Chronic multifocal osteomyelitis, tibia and fibula
  ▤+ **M86.361**   Chronic multifocal osteomyelitis, right tibia and fibula
  ▤+ **M86.362**   Chronic multifocal osteomyelitis, left tibia and fibula
  ▤+ **M86.369**   Chronic multifocal osteomyelitis, unspecified tibia and fibula
6 + **M86.37**   Chronic multifocal osteomyelitis, ankle and foot
  ▤+ **M86.371**   Chronic multifocal osteomyelitis, right ankle and foot
  ▤+ **M86.372**   Chronic multifocal osteomyelitis, left ankle and foot
  ▤+ **M86.379**   Chronic multifocal osteomyelitis, unspecified ankle and foot
    + **M86.38**   Chronic multifocal osteomyelitis, other site
    + **M86.39**   Chronic multifocal osteomyelitis, multiple sites
5 + **M86.4**   Chronic osteomyelitis with draining sinus
    + **M86.40**   Chronic osteomyelitis with draining sinus, unspecified site
6 + **M86.41**   Chronic osteomyelitis with draining sinus, shoulder
  ▤+ **M86.411**   Chronic osteomyelitis with draining sinus, right shoulder
  ▤+ **M86.412**   Chronic osteomyelitis with draining sinus, left shoulder
  ▤+ **M86.419**   Chronic osteomyelitis with draining sinus, unspecified shoulder
6 + **M86.42**   Chronic osteomyelitis with draining sinus, humerus
  ▤+ **M86.421**   Chronic osteomyelitis with draining sinus, right humerus
  ▤+ **M86.422**   Chronic osteomyelitis with draining sinus, left humerus
  ▤+ **M86.429**   Chronic osteomyelitis with draining sinus, unspecified humerus
6 + **M86.43**   Chronic osteomyelitis with draining sinus, radius and ulna
  ▤+ **M86.431**   Chronic osteomyelitis with draining sinus, right radius and ulna
  ▤+ **M86.432**   Chronic osteomyelitis with draining sinus, left radius and ulna
  ▤+ **M86.439**   Chronic osteomyelitis with draining sinus, unspecified radius and ulna

6 + **M86.44**   Chronic osteomyelitis with draining sinus, hand
  ▤+ **M86.441**   Chronic osteomyelitis with draining sinus, right hand
  ▤+ **M86.442**   Chronic osteomyelitis with draining sinus, left hand
  ▤+ **M86.449**   Chronic osteomyelitis with draining sinus, unspecified hand
6 + **M86.45**   Chronic osteomyelitis with draining sinus, femur
  ▤+ **M86.451**   Chronic osteomyelitis with draining sinus, right femur
  ▤+ **M86.452**   Chronic osteomyelitis with draining sinus, left femur
  ▤+ **M86.459**   Chronic osteomyelitis with draining sinus, unspecified femur
6 + **M86.46**   Chronic osteomyelitis with draining sinus, tibia and fibula
  ▤+ **M86.461**   Chronic osteomyelitis with draining sinus, right tibia and fibula
  ▤+ **M86.462**   Chronic osteomyelitis with draining sinus, left tibia and fibula
  ▤+ **M86.469**   Chronic osteomyelitis with draining sinus, unspecified tibia and fibula
6 + **M86.47**   Chronic osteomyelitis with draining sinus, ankle and foot
  ▤+ **M86.471**   Chronic osteomyelitis with draining sinus, right ankle and foot
  ▤+ **M86.472**   Chronic osteomyelitis with draining sinus, left ankle and foot
  ▤+ **M86.479**   Chronic osteomyelitis with draining sinus, unspecified ankle and foot
    + **M86.48**   Chronic osteomyelitis with draining sinus, other site
    + **M86.49**   Chronic osteomyelitis with draining sinus, multiple sites
5 + **M86.5**   Other chronic hematogenous osteomyelitis
    + **M86.50**   Other chronic hematogenous osteomyelitis, unspecified site
6 + **M86.51**   Other chronic hematogenous osteomyelitis, shoulder
  ▤+ **M86.511**   Other chronic hematogenous osteomyelitis, right shoulder
  ▤+ **M86.512**   Other chronic hematogenous osteomyelitis, left shoulder
  ▤+ **M86.519**   Other chronic hematogenous osteomyelitis, unspecified shoulder
6 + **M86.52**   Other chronic hematogenous osteomyelitis, humerus
  ▤+ **M86.521**   Other chronic hematogenous osteomyelitis, right humerus
  ▤+ **M86.522**   Other chronic hematogenous osteomyelitis, left humerus
  ▤+ **M86.529**   Other chronic hematogenous osteomyelitis, unspecified humerus
6 + **M86.53**   Other chronic hematogenous osteomyelitis, radius and ulna
  ▤+ **M86.531**   Other chronic hematogenous osteomyelitis, right radius and ulna
  ▤+ **M86.532**   Other chronic hematogenous osteomyelitis, left radius and ulna
  ▤+ **M86.539**   Other chronic hematogenous osteomyelitis, unspecified radius and ulna
6 + **M86.54**   Other chronic hematogenous osteomyelitis, hand
  ▤+ **M86.541**   Other chronic hematogenous osteomyelitis, right hand
  ▤+ **M86.542**   Other chronic hematogenous osteomyelitis, left hand
  ▤+ **M86.549**   Other chronic hematogenous osteomyelitis, unspecified hand
6 + **M86.55**   Other chronic hematogenous osteomyelitis, femur
  ▤+ **M86.551**   Other chronic hematogenous osteomyelitis, right femur
  ▤+ **M86.552**   Other chronic hematogenous osteomyelitis, left femur
  ▤+ **M86.559**   Other chronic hematogenous osteomyelitis, unspecified femur
6 + **M86.56**   Other chronic hematogenous osteomyelitis, tibia and fibula
  ▤+ **M86.561**   Other chronic hematogenous osteomyelitis, right tibia and fibula
  ▤+ **M86.562**   Other chronic hematogenous osteomyelitis, left tibia and fibula

● New   ▲ Revised   *Manifestation*   4 - 7 Digit Indicators   ▤ Laterality   Ⓐ Adult (15+ years)   Ⓜ Maternity (12-55 years)   Ⓝ Newborn   Ⓟ Pediatric (0-17 years)   ♂ Male   ♀ Female
✖ Deleted   Unspecified   + Additional code

☐ + M86.569   Other chronic hematogenous osteomyelitis, unspecified tibia and fibula

⑥ + M86.57   Other chronic hematogenous osteomyelitis, ankle and foot

☐ + M86.571   Other chronic hematogenous osteomyelitis, right ankle and foot

☐ + M86.572   Other chronic hematogenous osteomyelitis, left ankle and foot

☐ + M86.579   Other chronic hematogenous osteomyelitis, unspecified ankle and foot

+ M86.58   Other chronic hematogenous osteomyelitis, other site

+ M86.59   Other chronic hematogenous osteomyelitis, multiple sites

⑥ + M86.6   Other chronic osteomyelitis

+ M86.60   Other chronic osteomyelitis, unspecified site

⑥ + M86.61   Other chronic osteomyelitis, shoulder

☐ + M86.611   Other chronic osteomyelitis, right shoulder

☐ + M86.612   Other chronic osteomyelitis, left shoulder

☐ + M86.619   Other chronic osteomyelitis, unspecified shoulder

⑥ + M86.62   Other chronic osteomyelitis, humerus

☐ + M86.621   Other chronic osteomyelitis, right humerus

☐ + M86.622   Other chronic osteomyelitis, left humerus

☐ + M86.629   Other chronic osteomyelitis, unspecified humerus

⑥ + M86.63   Other chronic osteomyelitis, radius and ulna

☐ + M86.631   Other chronic osteomyelitis, right radius and ulna

☐ + M86.632   Other chronic osteomyelitis, left radius and ulna

☐ + M86.639   Other chronic osteomyelitis, unspecified radius and ulna

⑥ + M86.64   Other chronic osteomyelitis, hand

☐ + M86.641   Other chronic osteomyelitis, right hand

☐ + M86.642   Other chronic osteomyelitis, left hand

☐ + M86.649   Other chronic osteomyelitis, unspecified hand

⑥ + M86.65   Other chronic osteomyelitis, thigh

☐ + M86.651   Other chronic osteomyelitis, right thigh

☐ + M86.652   Other chronic osteomyelitis, left thigh

☐ + M86.659   Other chronic osteomyelitis, unspecified thigh

⑥ + M86.66   Other chronic osteomyelitis, tibia and fibula

☐ + M86.661   Other chronic osteomyelitis, right tibia and fibula

☐ + M86.662   Other chronic osteomyelitis, left tibia and fibula

☐ + M86.669   Other chronic osteomyelitis, unspecified tibia and fibula

⑥ + M86.67   Other chronic osteomyelitis, ankle and foot

☐ + M86.671   Other chronic osteomyelitis, right ankle and foot
          AHA: 1Q 2016, 13

☐ + M86.672   Other chronic osteomyelitis, left ankle and foot

☐ + M86.679   Other chronic osteomyelitis, unspecified ankle and foot

+ M86.68   Other chronic osteomyelitis, other site

+ M86.69   Other chronic osteomyelitis, multiple sites

☐ + M86.8   Other osteomyelitis
     Brodie's abscess

⑥ + M86.8X   Other osteomyelitis

+ M86.8X0   Other osteomyelitis, multiple sites

+ M86.8X1   Other osteomyelitis, shoulder

+ M86.8X2   Other osteomyelitis, upper arm

+ M86.8X3   Other osteomyelitis, forearm

+ M86.8X4   Other osteomyelitis, hand

+ M86.8X5   Other osteomyelitis, thigh

+ M86.8X6   Other osteomyelitis, lower leg

+ M86.8X7   Other osteomyelitis, ankle and foot

+ M86.8X8   Other osteomyelitis, other site

+ M86.8X9   Other osteomyelitis, unspecified sites

+ M86.9   Osteomyelitis, unspecified
     Infection of bone NOS
     Periostitis without osteomyelitis

④ + M87   **Osteonecrosis**

     INCLUDES   avascular necrosis of bone

     Use additional code to identify major osseous defect, if applicable (M89.7-)

     EXCLUDES 1   *juvenile osteonecrosis (M91-M92)*
                        osteochondropathies (M90-M93)

     GUIDELINES   Section I.C.13.a.1)
For certain conditions, the bone may be affected at the upper or lower end, (e.g., avascular necrosis of bone, M87, Osteoporosis, M80, M81). Though the portion of the bone affected may be at the joint, the site designation will be the bone, not the joint.

     CODING TIP ✓   Documentation: Osteonecrosis also may be termed avascular necrosis or aseptic necrosis of the bone. The condition indicates a necrosis of bone due to impaired blood supply and may be related to trauma, use of drugs or another cause. Review documentation carefully to determine if a causative condition is known.

     DEFINITION   The death of bone tissue from an interruption of its blood supply.

☐ + M87.0   Idiopathic aseptic necrosis of bone

     DEFINITION   The death of bone tissue from ischemia of unknown cause.

+ M87.00   Idiopathic aseptic necrosis of unspecified bone

⑥ + M87.01   Idiopathic aseptic necrosis of shoulder
     Idiopathic aseptic necrosis of clavicle and scapula

☐ + M87.011   Idiopathic aseptic necrosis of right shoulder

☐ + M87.012   Idiopathic aseptic necrosis of left shoulder

☐ + M87.019   Idiopathic aseptic necrosis of unspecified shoulder

⑥ + M87.02   Idiopathic aseptic necrosis of humerus

☐ + M87.021   Idiopathic aseptic necrosis of right humerus

☐ + M87.022   Idiopathic aseptic necrosis of left humerus

☐ + M87.029   Idiopathic aseptic necrosis of unspecified humerus

⑥ + M87.03   Idiopathic aseptic necrosis of radius, ulna and carpus

☐ + M87.031   Idiopathic aseptic necrosis of right radius

☐ + M87.032   Idiopathic aseptic necrosis of left radius

☐ + M87.033   Idiopathic aseptic necrosis of unspecified radius

☐ + M87.034   Idiopathic aseptic necrosis of right ulna

☐ + M87.035   Idiopathic aseptic necrosis of left ulna

☐ + M87.036   Idiopathic aseptic necrosis of unspecified ulna

☐ + M87.037   Idiopathic aseptic necrosis of right carpus

☐ + M87.038   Idiopathic aseptic necrosis of left carpus

☐ + M87.039   Idiopathic aseptic necrosis of unspecified carpus

⑥ + M87.04   Idiopathic aseptic necrosis of hand and fingers
     Idiopathic aseptic necrosis of metacarpals and phalanges of hands

☐ + M87.041   Idiopathic aseptic necrosis of right hand

☐ + M87.042   Idiopathic aseptic necrosis of left hand

☐ + M87.043   Idiopathic aseptic necrosis of unspecified hand

☐ + M87.044   Idiopathic aseptic necrosis of right finger(s)

☐ + M87.045   Idiopathic aseptic necrosis of left finger(s)

☐ + M87.046   Idiopathic aseptic necrosis of unspecified finger(s)

⑥ + M87.05   Idiopathic aseptic necrosis of pelvis and femur

☐ + M87.050   Idiopathic aseptic necrosis of pelvis

☐ + M87.051   Idiopathic aseptic necrosis of right femur

☐ + M87.052   Idiopathic aseptic necrosis of left femur

☐ + M87.059   Idiopathic aseptic necrosis of unspecified femur
     Idiopathic aseptic necrosis of hip NOS

⑥ + M87.06   Idiopathic aseptic necrosis of tibia and fibula

☐ + M87.061   Idiopathic aseptic necrosis of right tibia

☐ + M87.062   Idiopathic aseptic necrosis of left tibia

☐ + M87.063   Idiopathic aseptic necrosis of unspecified tibia

☐ + M87.064   Idiopathic aseptic necrosis of right fibula

☐ + M87.065   Idiopathic aseptic necrosis of left fibula

☐ + M87.066   Idiopathic aseptic necrosis of unspecified fibula

---

● New   ▲ Revised   *Manifestation*   ④-⑦ Digit Indicators   ☐ Laterality   Ⓐ Adult (15+ years)   Ⓜ Maternity (12-55 years)   Ⓝ Newborn   Ⓟ Pediatric (0-17 years)   ♂ Male   ♀ Female
✖ Deleted   Unspecified   + Additional code

2017 ICD-10-CM Expert for Physicians   © 2017 DecisionHealth   803

6 + M87.07   Idiopathic aseptic necrosis of ankle, foot and toes
Idiopathic aseptic necrosis of metatarsus, tarsus, and phalanges of toes
6 + M87.071   Idiopathic aseptic necrosis of right ankle
6 + M87.072   Idiopathic aseptic necrosis of left ankle
6 + M87.073   Idiopathic aseptic necrosis of unspecified ankle
6 + M87.074   Idiopathic aseptic necrosis of right foot
6 + M87.075   Idiopathic aseptic necrosis of left foot
6 + M87.076   Idiopathic aseptic necrosis of unspecified foot
6 + M87.077   Idiopathic aseptic necrosis of right toe(s)
6 + M87.078   Idiopathic aseptic necrosis of left toe(s)
6 + M87.079   Idiopathic aseptic necrosis of unspecified toe(s)
+ M87.08   Idiopathic aseptic necrosis of bone, other site
+ M87.09   Idiopathic aseptic necrosis of bone, multiple sites
5 + M87.1   Osteonecrosis due to drugs
Use additional code for adverse effect, if applicable, to identify drug (T36-T50 with fifth or sixth character 5)
+ M87.10   Osteonecrosis due to drugs, unspecified bone
6 + M87.11   Osteonecrosis due to drugs, shoulder
6 + M87.111   Osteonecrosis due to drugs, right shoulder
6 + M87.112   Osteonecrosis due to drugs, left shoulder
6 + M87.119   Osteonecrosis due to drugs, unspecified shoulder
6 + M87.12   Osteonecrosis due to drugs, humerus
6 + M87.121   Osteonecrosis due to drugs, right humerus
6 + M87.122   Osteonecrosis due to drugs, left humerus
6 + M87.129   Osteonecrosis due to drugs, unspecified humerus
6 + M87.13   Osteonecrosis due to drugs of radius, ulna and carpus
6 + M87.131   Osteonecrosis due to drugs of right radius
6 + M87.132   Osteonecrosis due to drugs of left radius
6 + M87.133   Osteonecrosis due to drugs of unspecified radius
6 + M87.134   Osteonecrosis due to drugs of right ulna
6 + M87.135   Osteonecrosis due to drugs of left ulna
6 + M87.136   Osteonecrosis due to drugs of unspecified ulna
6 + M87.137   Osteonecrosis due to drugs of right carpus
6 + M87.138   Osteonecrosis due to drugs of left carpus
6 + M87.139   Osteonecrosis due to drugs of unspecified carpus
6 + M87.14   Osteonecrosis due to drugs, hand and fingers
6 + M87.141   Osteonecrosis due to drugs, right hand
6 + M87.142   Osteonecrosis due to drugs, left hand
6 + M87.143   Osteonecrosis due to drugs, unspecified hand
6 + M87.144   Osteonecrosis due to drugs, right finger(s)
6 + M87.145   Osteonecrosis due to drugs, left finger(s)
6 + M87.146   Osteonecrosis due to drugs, unspecified finger(s)
6 + M87.15   Osteonecrosis due to drugs, pelvis and femur
6 + M87.150   Osteonecrosis due to drugs, pelvis
6 + M87.151   Osteonecrosis due to drugs, right femur
6 + M87.152   Osteonecrosis due to drugs, left femur
6 + M87.159   Osteonecrosis due to drugs, unspecified femur
6 + M87.16   Osteonecrosis due to drugs, tibia and fibula
6 + M87.161   Osteonecrosis due to drugs, right tibia
6 + M87.162   Osteonecrosis due to drugs, left tibia
6 + M87.163   Osteonecrosis due to drugs, unspecified tibia
6 + M87.164   Osteonecrosis due to drugs, right fibula
6 + M87.165   Osteonecrosis due to drugs, left fibula
6 + M87.166   Osteonecrosis due to drugs, unspecified fibula
6 + M87.17   Osteonecrosis due to drugs, ankle, foot and toes
6 + M87.171   Osteonecrosis due to drugs, right ankle
6 + M87.172   Osteonecrosis due to drugs, left ankle
6 + M87.173   Osteonecrosis due to drugs, unspecified ankle
6 + M87.174   Osteonecrosis due to drugs, right foot
6 + M87.175   Osteonecrosis due to drugs, left foot
6 + M87.176   Osteonecrosis due to drugs, unspecified foot
6 + M87.177   Osteonecrosis due to drugs, right toe(s)
6 + M87.178   Osteonecrosis due to drugs, left toe(s)
6 + M87.179   Osteonecrosis due to drugs, unspecified toe(s)
6 + M87.18   Osteonecrosis due to drugs, other site

+ M87.180   Osteonecrosis due to drugs, jaw
+ M87.188   Osteonecrosis due to drugs, other site
+ M87.19   Osteonecrosis due to drugs, multiple sites
5 + M87.2   Osteonecrosis due to previous trauma
+ M87.20   Osteonecrosis due to previous trauma, unspecified bone
6 + M87.21   Osteonecrosis due to previous trauma, shoulder
6 + M87.211   Osteonecrosis due to previous trauma, right shoulder
6 + M87.212   Osteonecrosis due to previous trauma, left shoulder
6 + M87.219   Osteonecrosis due to previous trauma, unspecified shoulder
6 + M87.22   Osteonecrosis due to previous trauma, humerus
6 + M87.221   Osteonecrosis due to previous trauma, right humerus
6 + M87.222   Osteonecrosis due to previous trauma, left humerus
6 + M87.229   Osteonecrosis due to previous trauma, unspecified humerus
6 + M87.23   Osteonecrosis due to previous trauma of radius, ulna and carpus
6 + M87.231   Osteonecrosis due to previous trauma of right radius
6 + M87.232   Osteonecrosis due to previous trauma of left radius
6 + M87.233   Osteonecrosis due to previous trauma of unspecified radius
6 + M87.234   Osteonecrosis due to previous trauma of right ulna
6 + M87.235   Osteonecrosis due to previous trauma of left ulna
6 + M87.236   Osteonecrosis due to previous trauma of unspecified ulna
6 + M87.237   Osteonecrosis due to previous trauma of right carpus
6 + M87.238   Osteonecrosis due to previous trauma of left carpus
6 + M87.239   Osteonecrosis due to previous trauma of unspecified carpus
6 + M87.24   Osteonecrosis due to previous trauma, hand and fingers
6 + M87.241   Osteonecrosis due to previous trauma, right hand
6 + M87.242   Osteonecrosis due to previous trauma, left hand
6 + M87.243   Osteonecrosis due to previous trauma, unspecified hand
6 + M87.244   Osteonecrosis due to previous trauma, right finger(s)
6 + M87.245   Osteonecrosis due to previous trauma, left finger(s)
6 + M87.246   Osteonecrosis due to previous trauma, unspecified finger(s)
6 + M87.25   Osteonecrosis due to previous trauma, pelvis and femur
6 + M87.250   Osteonecrosis due to previous trauma, pelvis
6 + M87.251   Osteonecrosis due to previous trauma, right femur
6 + M87.252   Osteonecrosis due to previous trauma, left femur
6 + M87.256   Osteonecrosis due to previous trauma, unspecified femur
6 + M87.26   Osteonecrosis due to previous trauma, tibia and fibula
6 + M87.261   Osteonecrosis due to previous trauma, right tibia
6 + M87.262   Osteonecrosis due to previous trauma, left tibia
6 + M87.263   Osteonecrosis due to previous trauma, unspecified tibia
6 + M87.264   Osteonecrosis due to previous trauma, right fibula
6 + M87.265   Osteonecrosis due to previous trauma, left fibula
6 + M87.266   Osteonecrosis due to previous trauma, unspecified fibula
6 + M87.27   Osteonecrosis due to previous trauma, ankle, foot and toes
6 + M87.271   Osteonecrosis due to previous trauma, right ankle

☐ + M87.272   Osteonecrosis due to previous trauma, left ankle
☐ + M87.273   Osteonecrosis due to previous trauma, unspecified ankle
☐ + M87.274   Osteonecrosis due to previous trauma, right foot
☐ + M87.275   Osteonecrosis due to previous trauma, left foot
☐ + M87.276   Osteonecrosis due to previous trauma, unspecified foot
☐ + M87.277   Osteonecrosis due to previous trauma, right toe(s)
☐ + M87.278   Osteonecrosis due to previous trauma, left toe(s)
☐ + M87.279   Osteonecrosis due to previous trauma, unspecified toe(s)
   + M87.28   Osteonecrosis due to previous trauma, other site
   + M87.29   Osteonecrosis due to previous trauma, multiple sites
Ⓢ + M87.3   Other secondary osteonecrosis
   + M87.30   Other secondary osteonecrosis, unspecified bone
Ⓖ + M87.31   Other secondary osteonecrosis, shoulder
☐ + M87.311   Other secondary osteonecrosis, right shoulder
☐ + M87.312   Other secondary osteonecrosis, left shoulder
☐ + M87.319   Other secondary osteonecrosis, unspecified shoulder
Ⓖ + M87.32   Other secondary osteonecrosis, humerus
☐ + M87.321   Other secondary osteonecrosis, right humerus
☐ + M87.322   Other secondary osteonecrosis, left humerus
☐ + M87.329   Other secondary osteonecrosis, unspecified humerus
Ⓖ + M87.33   Other secondary osteonecrosis of radius, ulna and carpus
☐ + M87.331   Other secondary osteonecrosis of right radius
☐ + M87.332   Other secondary osteonecrosis of left radius
☐ + M87.333   Other secondary osteonecrosis of unspecified radius
☐ + M87.334   Other secondary osteonecrosis of right ulna
☐ + M87.335   Other secondary osteonecrosis of left ulna
☐ + M87.336   Other secondary osteonecrosis of unspecified ulna
☐ + M87.337   Other secondary osteonecrosis of right carpus
☐ + M87.338   Other secondary osteonecrosis of left carpus
☐ + M87.339   Other secondary osteonecrosis of unspecified carpus
Ⓖ + M87.34   Other secondary osteonecrosis, hand and fingers
☐ + M87.341   Other secondary osteonecrosis, right hand
☐ + M87.342   Other secondary osteonecrosis, left hand
☐ + M87.343   Other secondary osteonecrosis, unspecified hand
☐ + M87.344   Other secondary osteonecrosis, right finger(s)
☐ + M87.345   Other secondary osteonecrosis, left finger(s)
☐ + M87.346   Other secondary osteonecrosis, unspecified finger(s)
Ⓖ + M87.35   Other secondary osteonecrosis, pelvis and femur
☐ + M87.350   Other secondary osteonecrosis, pelvis
☐ + M87.351   Other secondary osteonecrosis, right femur
☐ + M87.352   Other secondary osteonecrosis, left femur
☐ + M87.353   Other secondary osteonecrosis, unspecified femur
Ⓖ + M87.36   Other secondary osteonecrosis, tibia and fibula
☐ + M87.361   Other secondary osteonecrosis, right tibia
☐ + M87.362   Other secondary osteonecrosis, left tibia
☐ + M87.363   Other secondary osteonecrosis, unspecified tibia
☐ + M87.364   Other secondary osteonecrosis, right fibula
☐ + M87.365   Other secondary osteonecrosis, left fibula
☐ + M87.366   Other secondary osteonecrosis, unspecified fibula
Ⓖ + M87.37   Other secondary osteonecrosis, ankle and foot
☐ + M87.371   Other secondary osteonecrosis, right ankle
☐ + M87.372   Other secondary osteonecrosis, left ankle
☐ + M87.373   Other secondary osteonecrosis, unspecified ankle
☐ + M87.374   Other secondary osteonecrosis, right foot
☐ + M87.375   Other secondary osteonecrosis, left foot
☐ + M87.376   Other secondary osteonecrosis, unspecified foot
☐ + M87.377   Other secondary osteonecrosis, right toe(s)
☐ + M87.378   Other secondary osteonecrosis, left toe(s)

☐ + M87.379   Other secondary osteonecrosis, unspecified toe(s)
   + M87.38   Other secondary osteonecrosis, other site
   + M87.39   Other secondary osteonecrosis, multiple sites
Ⓢ + M87.8   Other osteonecrosis
   + M87.80   Other osteonecrosis, unspecified bone
Ⓖ + M87.81   Other osteonecrosis, shoulder
☐ + M87.811   Other osteonecrosis, right shoulder
☐ + M87.812   Other osteonecrosis, left shoulder
☐ + M87.819   Other osteonecrosis, unspecified shoulder
Ⓖ + M87.82   Other osteonecrosis, humerus
☐ + M87.821   Other osteonecrosis, right humerus
☐ + M87.822   Other osteonecrosis, left humerus
☐ + M87.829   Other osteonecrosis, unspecified humerus
Ⓖ + M87.83   Other osteonecrosis of radius, ulna and carpus
☐ + M87.831   Other osteonecrosis of right radius
☐ + M87.832   Other osteonecrosis of left radius
☐ + M87.833   Other osteonecrosis of unspecified radius
☐ + M87.834   Other osteonecrosis of right ulna
☐ + M87.835   Other osteonecrosis of left ulna
☐ + M87.836   Other osteonecrosis of unspecified ulna
☐ + M87.837   Other osteonecrosis of right carpus
☐ + M87.838   Other osteonecrosis of left carpus
☐ + M87.839   Other osteonecrosis of unspecified carpus
Ⓖ + M87.84   Other osteonecrosis, hand and fingers
☐ + M87.841   Other osteonecrosis, right hand
☐ + M87.842   Other osteonecrosis, left hand
☐ + M87.843   Other osteonecrosis, unspecified hand
☐ + M87.844   Other osteonecrosis, right finger(s)
☐ + M87.845   Other osteonecrosis, left finger(s)
☐ + M87.849   Other osteonecrosis, unspecified finger(s)
Ⓖ + M87.85   Other osteonecrosis, pelvis and femur
☐ + M87.850   Other osteonecrosis, pelvis
☐ + M87.851   Other osteonecrosis, right femur
☐ + M87.852   Other osteonecrosis, left femur
☐ + M87.859   Other osteonecrosis, unspecified femur
Ⓖ + M87.86   Other osteonecrosis, tibia and fibula
☐ + M87.861   Other osteonecrosis, right tibia
☐ + M87.862   Other osteonecrosis, left tibia
☐ + M87.863   Other osteonecrosis, unspecified tibia
☐ + M87.864   Other osteonecrosis, right fibula
☐ + M87.865   Other osteonecrosis, left fibula
☐ + M87.869   Other osteonecrosis, unspecified fibula
Ⓖ + M87.87   Other osteonecrosis, ankle, foot and toes
☐ + M87.871   Other osteonecrosis, right ankle
☐ + M87.872   Other osteonecrosis, left ankle
☐ + M87.873   Other osteonecrosis, unspecified ankle
☐ + M87.874   Other osteonecrosis, right foot
☐ + M87.875   Other osteonecrosis, left foot
☐ + M87.876   Other osteonecrosis, unspecified foot
☐ + M87.877   Other osteonecrosis, right toe(s)
☐ + M87.878   Other osteonecrosis, left toe(s)
☐ + M87.879   Other osteonecrosis, unspecified toe(s)
   + M87.88   Other osteonecrosis, other site
   + M87.89   Other osteonecrosis, multiple sites
   + M87.9   Osteonecrosis, unspecified
             Necrosis of bone NOS
◭ M88   Osteitis deformans [Paget's disease of bone]
        EXCLUDES 1   osteitis deformans in neoplastic disease (M90.6)
        DEFINITION   A bone disorder characterized by cycles of bone loss followed by excessive attempts at repair; results in painful, deformed, enlarged bones of porous tissue prone to fractures and arthritic affected joints.
   M88.0   Osteitis deformans of skull
           DEFINITION   Excessive breakdown and rebuilding of bone tissue in the skull, resulting in an enlarged head with abnormally remodeled skull bones that may press on nerves causing headache, vertigo, tinnitus, or hearing loss.
   M88.1   Osteitis deformans of vertebrae

● New   ▲ Revised   *Manifestation*   4-7 Digit Indicators   ☐ Laterality   Ⓐ Adult (15+ years)   Ⓜ Maternity (12-55 years)   Ⓝ Newborn   Ⓟ Pediatric (0-17 years)   ♂ Male   ♀ Female
✖ Deleted   Unspecified   + Additional code

2017 ICD-10-CM Expert for Physicians   © 2017 DecisionHealth   805

DEFINITION Excessive breakdown and rebuilding of the vertebrae with bone material that is less dense, resulting in an abnormally remodeled, thickened spine prone to fracture that may compress nerve roots causing pain, numbness, and tingling in arms or legs.

⑤ **M88.8 Osteitis deformans of other bones**
　⑥ **M88.81 Osteitis deformans of shoulder**
　　⊟ M88.811 Osteitis deformans of right shoulder
　　⊟ M88.812 Osteitis deformans of left shoulder
　　⊟ M88.819 Osteitis deformans of unspecified shoulder
　⑥ **M88.82 Osteitis deformans of upper arm**
　　⊟ M88.821 Osteitis deformans of right upper arm
　　⊟ M88.822 Osteitis deformans of left upper arm
　　⊟ M88.829 Osteitis deformans of unspecified upper arm
　⑥ **M88.83 Osteitis deformans of forearm**
　　⊟ M88.831 Osteitis deformans of right forearm
　　⊟ M88.832 Osteitis deformans of left forearm
　　⊟ M88.839 Osteitis deformans of unspecified forearm
　⑥ **M88.84 Osteitis deformans of hand**
　　⊟ M88.841 Osteitis deformans of right hand
　　⊟ M88.842 Osteitis deformans of left hand
　　⊟ M88.849 Osteitis deformans of unspecified hand
　⑥ **M88.85 Osteitis deformans of thigh**
　　⊟ M88.851 Osteitis deformans of right thigh
　　⊟ M88.852 Osteitis deformans of left thigh
　　⊟ M88.859 Osteitis deformans of unspecified thigh
　⑥ **M88.86 Osteitis deformans of lower leg**
　　⊟ M88.861 Osteitis deformans of right lower leg
　　⊟ M88.862 Osteitis deformans of left lower leg
　　⊟ M88.869 Osteitis deformans of unspecified lower leg
　⑥ **M88.87 Osteitis deformans of ankle and foot**
　　⊟ M88.871 Osteitis deformans of right ankle and foot
　　⊟ M88.872 Osteitis deformans of left ankle and foot
　　⊟ M88.879 Osteitis deformans of unspecified ankle and foot
　　M88.88 Osteitis deformans of other bones
　　　EXCLUDES 2 *osteitis deformans of skull (M88.0)*
　　　osteitis deformans of vertebrae (M88.1)
　　M88.89 Osteitis deformans of multiple sites
　M88.9 Osteitis deformans of unspecified bone
④ **M89 Other disorders of bone**
　⑤ **M89.0 Algoneurodystrophy**
　　Shoulder-hand syndrome
　　Sudeck's atrophy
　　　EXCLUDES 1 *causalgia, lower limb (G57.7-)*
　　　causalgia, upper limb (G56.4-)
　　　complex regional pain syndrome II, lower limb (G57.7-)
　　　complex regional pain syndrome II, upper limb (G56.4-)
　　　reflex sympathetic dystrophy (G90.5-)
　　　DEFINITION Acute wasting away of bone(s) following relatively minor injury; presents with severe burning pain in the affected extremity, trophic changes in bone, and vasomotor disturbances without specific nerve injury.
　　M89.00 Algoneurodystrophy, unspecified site
　　⑥ **M89.01 Algoneurodystrophy, shoulder**
　　　⊟ M89.011 Algoneurodystrophy, right shoulder
　　　⊟ M89.012 Algoneurodystrophy, left shoulder
　　　⊟ M89.019 Algoneurodystrophy, unspecified shoulder
　　⑥ **M89.02 Algoneurodystrophy, upper arm**
　　　⊟ M89.021 Algoneurodystrophy, right upper arm
　　　⊟ M89.022 Algoneurodystrophy, left upper arm
　　　⊟ M89.029 Algoneurodystrophy, unspecified upper arm
　　⑥ **M89.03 Algoneurodystrophy, forearm**
　　　⊟ M89.031 Algoneurodystrophy, right forearm
　　　⊟ M89.032 Algoneurodystrophy, left forearm
　　　⊟ M89.039 Algoneurodystrophy, unspecified forearm
　　⑥ **M89.04 Algoneurodystrophy, hand**
　　　⊟ M89.041 Algoneurodystrophy, right hand
　　　⊟ M89.042 Algoneurodystrophy, left hand

　　　⊟ M89.049 Algoneurodystrophy, unspecified hand
　　⑥ **M89.05 Algoneurodystrophy, thigh**
　　　⊟ M89.051 Algoneurodystrophy, right thigh
　　　⊟ M89.052 Algoneurodystrophy, left thigh
　　　⊟ M89.059 Algoneurodystrophy, unspecified thigh
　　⑥ **M89.06 Algoneurodystrophy, lower leg**
　　　⊟ M89.061 Algoneurodystrophy, right lower leg
　　　⊟ M89.062 Algoneurodystrophy, left lower leg
　　　⊟ M89.069 Algoneurodystrophy, unspecified lower leg
　　⑥ **M89.07 Algoneurodystrophy, ankle and foot**
　　　⊟ M89.071 Algoneurodystrophy, right ankle and foot
　　　⊟ M89.072 Algoneurodystrophy, left ankle and foot
　　　⊟ M89.079 Algoneurodystrophy, unspecified ankle and foot
　　M89.08 Algoneurodystrophy, other site
　　M89.09 Algoneurodystrophy, multiple sites
　⑤ **M89.1 Physeal arrest**
　　Arrest of growth plate
　　Epiphyseal arrest
　　Growth plate arrest
　　⑥ **M89.12 Physeal arrest, humerus**
　　　⊟ M89.121 Complete physeal arrest, right proximal humerus
　　　⊟ M89.122 Complete physeal arrest, left proximal humerus
　　　⊟ M89.123 Partial physeal arrest, right proximal humerus
　　　⊟ M89.124 Partial physeal arrest, left proximal humerus
　　　⊟ M89.125 Complete physeal arrest, right distal humerus
　　　⊟ M89.126 Complete physeal arrest, left distal humerus
　　　⊟ M89.127 Partial physeal arrest, right distal humerus
　　　⊟ M89.128 Partial physeal arrest, left distal humerus
　　　⊟ M89.129 Physeal arrest, humerus, unspecified
　　⑥ **M89.13 Physeal arrest, forearm**
　　　⊟ M89.131 Complete physeal arrest, right distal radius
　　　⊟ M89.132 Complete physeal arrest, left distal radius
　　　⊟ M89.133 Partial physeal arrest, right distal radius
　　　⊟ M89.134 Partial physeal arrest, left distal radius
　　　⊟ M89.138 Other physeal arrest of forearm
　　　⊟ M89.139 Physeal arrest, forearm, unspecified
　　⑥ **M89.15 Physeal arrest, femur**
　　　⊟ M89.151 Complete physeal arrest, right proximal femur
　　　⊟ M89.152 Complete physeal arrest, left proximal femur
　　　⊟ M89.153 Partial physeal arrest, right proximal femur
　　　⊟ M89.154 Partial physeal arrest, left proximal femur
　　　⊟ M89.155 Complete physeal arrest, right distal femur
　　　⊟ M89.156 Complete physeal arrest, left distal femur
　　　⊟ M89.157 Partial physeal arrest, right distal femur
　　　⊟ M89.158 Partial physeal arrest, left distal femur
　　　⊟ M89.159 Physeal arrest, femur, unspecified
　　⑥ **M89.16 Physeal arrest, lower leg**
　　　⊟ M89.160 Complete physeal arrest, right proximal tibia
　　　⊟ M89.161 Complete physeal arrest, left proximal tibia
　　　⊟ M89.162 Partial physeal arrest, right proximal tibia
　　　⊟ M89.163 Partial physeal arrest, left proximal tibia
　　　⊟ M89.164 Complete physeal arrest, right distal tibia
　　　⊟ M89.165 Complete physeal arrest, left distal tibia
　　　⊟ M89.166 Partial physeal arrest, right distal tibia
　　　⊟ M89.167 Partial physeal arrest, left distal tibia
　　　⊟ M89.168 Other physeal arrest of lower leg
　　　⊟ M89.169 Physeal arrest, lower leg, unspecified
　　M89.18 Physeal arrest, other site
　⑤ **M89.2 Other disorders of bone development and growth**
　　M89.20 Other disorders of bone development and growth, unspecified site
　　⑥ **M89.21 Other disorders of bone development and growth, shoulder**
　　　⊟ M89.211 Other disorders of bone development and growth, right shoulder
　　　⊟ M89.212 Other disorders of bone development and growth, left shoulder
　　　⊟ M89.219 Other disorders of bone development and growth, unspecified shoulder
　　⑥ **M89.22 Other disorders of bone development and growth, humerus**

● New　▲ Revised　*Manifestation*　❹-❼ Digit Indicators　⊟ Laterality　Ⓐ Adult (15+ years)　Ⓜ Maternity (12-55 years)　Ⓝ Newborn　Ⓟ Pediatric (0-17 years)　♂ Male　♀ Female
✖ Deleted　Unspecified　+ Additional code

Diseases of the Musculoskeletal System and Connective Tissue

- ▫ M89.221 Other disorders of bone development and growth, right humerus
- ▫ M89.222 Other disorders of bone development and growth, left humerus
- ▫ M89.229 Other disorders of bone development and growth, unspecified humerus
- ◚ M89.23 Other disorders of bone development and growth, ulna and radius
  - ▫ M89.231 Other disorders of bone development and growth, right ulna
  - ▫ M89.232 Other disorders of bone development and growth, left ulna
  - ▫ M89.233 Other disorders of bone development and growth, right radius
  - ▫ M89.234 Other disorders of bone development and growth, left radius
  - ▫ M89.239 Other disorders of bone development and growth, unspecified ulna and radius
- ◚ M89.24 Other disorders of bone development and growth, hand
  - ▫ M89.241 Other disorders of bone development and growth, right hand
  - ▫ M89.242 Other disorders of bone development and growth, left hand
  - ▫ M89.249 Other disorders of bone development and growth, unspecified hand
- ◚ M89.25 Other disorders of bone development and growth, femur
  - ▫ M89.251 Other disorders of bone development and growth, right femur
  - ▫ M89.252 Other disorders of bone development and growth, left femur
  - ▫ M89.259 Other disorders of bone development and growth, unspecified femur
- ◚ M89.26 Other disorders of bone development and growth, tibia and fibula
  - ▫ M89.261 Other disorders of bone development and growth, right tibia
  - ▫ M89.262 Other disorders of bone development and growth, left tibia
  - ▫ M89.263 Other disorders of bone development and growth, right fibula
  - ▫ M89.264 Other disorders of bone development and growth, left fibula
  - ▫ M89.269 Other disorders of bone development and growth, unspecified lower leg
- ◚ M89.27 Other disorders of bone development and growth, ankle and foot
  - ▫ M89.271 Other disorders of bone development and growth, right ankle and foot
  - ▫ M89.272 Other disorders of bone development and growth, left ankle and foot
  - ▫ M89.279 Other disorders of bone development and growth, unspecified ankle and foot
- M89.28 Other disorders of bone development and growth, other site
- M89.29 Other disorders of bone development and growth, multiple sites
- ⑤ M89.3 Hypertrophy of bone
  - M89.30 Hypertrophy of bone, unspecified site
  - ◚ M89.31 Hypertrophy of bone, shoulder
    - ▫ M89.311 Hypertrophy of bone, right shoulder
    - ▫ M89.312 Hypertrophy of bone, left shoulder
    - ▫ M89.319 Hypertrophy of bone, unspecified shoulder
  - ◚ M89.32 Hypertrophy of bone, humerus
    - ▫ M89.321 Hypertrophy of bone, right humerus
    - ▫ M89.322 Hypertrophy of bone, left humerus
    - ▫ M89.329 Hypertrophy of bone, unspecified humerus
  - ◚ M89.33 Hypertrophy of bone, ulna and radius
    - ▫ M89.331 Hypertrophy of bone, right ulna
    - ▫ M89.332 Hypertrophy of bone, left ulna
    - ▫ M89.333 Hypertrophy of bone, right radius
    - ▫ M89.334 Hypertrophy of bone, left radius
    - ▫ M89.339 Hypertrophy of bone, unspecified ulna and radius
  - ◚ M89.34 Hypertrophy of bone, hand
    - ▫ M89.341 Hypertrophy of bone, right hand
    - ▫ M89.342 Hypertrophy of bone, left hand

- ▫ M89.349 Hypertrophy of bone, unspecified hand
- ◚ M89.35 Hypertrophy of bone, femur
  - ▫ M89.351 Hypertrophy of bone, right femur
  - ▫ M89.352 Hypertrophy of bone, left femur
  - ▫ M89.359 Hypertrophy of bone, unspecified femur
- ◚ M89.36 Hypertrophy of bone, tibia and fibula
  - ▫ M89.361 Hypertrophy of bone, right tibia
  - ▫ M89.362 Hypertrophy of bone, left tibia
  - ▫ M89.363 Hypertrophy of bone, right fibula
  - ▫ M89.364 Hypertrophy of bone, left fibula
  - ▫ M89.369 Hypertrophy of bone, unspecified tibia and fibula
- ◚ M89.37 Hypertrophy of bone, ankle and foot
  - ▫ M89.371 Hypertrophy of bone, right ankle and foot
  - ▫ M89.372 Hypertrophy of bone, left ankle and foot
  - ▫ M89.379 Hypertrophy of bone, unspecified ankle and foot
- M89.38 Hypertrophy of bone, other site
- M89.39 Hypertrophy of bone, multiple sites
- ⑤ M89.4 Other hypertrophic osteoarthropathy
  - Marie-Bamberger disease
  - Pachydermoperiostosis
  - M89.40 Other hypertrophic osteoarthropathy, unspecified site
  - ◚ M89.41 Other hypertrophic osteoarthropathy, shoulder
    - ▫ M89.411 Other hypertrophic osteoarthropathy, right shoulder
    - ▫ M89.412 Other hypertrophic osteoarthropathy, left shoulder
    - ▫ M89.419 Other hypertrophic osteoarthropathy, unspecified shoulder
  - ◚ M89.42 Other hypertrophic osteoarthropathy, upper arm
    - ▫ M89.421 Other hypertrophic osteoarthropathy, right upper arm
    - ▫ M89.422 Other hypertrophic osteoarthropathy, left upper arm
    - ▫ M89.429 Other hypertrophic osteoarthropathy, unspecified upper arm
  - ◚ M89.43 Other hypertrophic osteoarthropathy, forearm
    - ▫ M89.431 Other hypertrophic osteoarthropathy, right forearm
    - ▫ M89.432 Other hypertrophic osteoarthropathy, left forearm
    - ▫ M89.439 Other hypertrophic osteoarthropathy, unspecified forearm
  - ◚ M89.44 Other hypertrophic osteoarthropathy, hand
    - ▫ M89.441 Other hypertrophic osteoarthropathy, right hand
    - ▫ M89.442 Other hypertrophic osteoarthropathy, left hand
    - ▫ M89.449 Other hypertrophic osteoarthropathy, unspecified hand
  - ◚ M89.45 Other hypertrophic osteoarthropathy, thigh
    - ▫ M89.451 Other hypertrophic osteoarthropathy, right thigh
    - ▫ M89.452 Other hypertrophic osteoarthropathy, left thigh
    - ▫ M89.459 Other hypertrophic osteoarthropathy, unspecified thigh
  - ◚ M89.46 Other hypertrophic osteoarthropathy, lower leg
    - ▫ M89.461 Other hypertrophic osteoarthropathy, right lower leg
    - ▫ M89.462 Other hypertrophic osteoarthropathy, left lower leg
    - ▫ M89.469 Other hypertrophic osteoarthropathy, unspecified lower leg
  - ◚ M89.47 Other hypertrophic osteoarthropathy, ankle and foot
    - ▫ M89.471 Other hypertrophic osteoarthropathy, right ankle and foot
    - ▫ M89.472 Other hypertrophic osteoarthropathy, left ankle and foot
    - ▫ M89.479 Other hypertrophic osteoarthropathy, unspecified ankle and foot
  - M89.48 Other hypertrophic osteoarthropathy, other site
  - M89.49 Other hypertrophic osteoarthropathy, multiple sites

● New ▲ Revised *Manifestation* ❹-❼ Digit Indicators ▯ Laterality ☒ Adult (15+ years) ⓜ Maternity (12-55 years) ⓝ Newborn ⓟ Pediatric (0-17 years) ♂ Male ♀ Female
✖ Deleted Unspecified + Additional code

2017 ICD-10-CM Expert for Physicians
© 2017 DecisionHealth
807

M89.221 — M89.49

⑤＋ **M89.5** **Osteolysis**

Use additional code to identify major osseous defect, if applicable (M89.7-)

EXCLUDES 2 *periprosthetic osteolysis of internal prosthetic joint (T84.05-)*

  ＋ **M89.50** Osteolysis, unspecified site

⑥＋ **M89.51** Osteolysis, shoulder
- ＋ **M89.511** Osteolysis, right shoulder
- ＋ **M89.512** Osteolysis, left shoulder
- ＋ **M89.519** Osteolysis, unspecified shoulder

⑥＋ **M89.52** Osteolysis, upper arm
- ＋ **M89.521** Osteolysis, right upper arm
- ＋ **M89.522** Osteolysis, left upper arm
- ＋ **M89.529** Osteolysis, unspecified upper arm

⑥＋ **M89.53** Osteolysis, forearm
- ＋ **M89.531** Osteolysis, right forearm
- ＋ **M89.532** Osteolysis, left forearm
- ＋ **M89.539** Osteolysis, unspecified forearm

⑥＋ **M89.54** Osteolysis, hand
- ＋ **M89.541** Osteolysis, right hand
- ＋ **M89.542** Osteolysis, left hand
- ＋ **M89.549** Osteolysis, unspecified hand

⑥＋ **M89.55** Osteolysis, thigh
- ＋ **M89.551** Osteolysis, right thigh
- ＋ **M89.552** Osteolysis, left thigh
- ＋ **M89.559** Osteolysis, unspecified thigh

⑥＋ **M89.56** Osteolysis, lower leg
- ＋ **M89.561** Osteolysis, right lower leg
- ＋ **M89.562** Osteolysis, left lower leg
- ＋ **M89.569** Osteolysis, unspecified lower leg

⑥＋ **M89.57** Osteolysis, ankle and foot
- ＋ **M89.571** Osteolysis, right ankle and foot
- ＋ **M89.572** Osteolysis, left ankle and foot
- ＋ **M89.579** Osteolysis, unspecified ankle and foot

  ＋ **M89.58** Osteolysis, other site
  ＋ **M89.59** Osteolysis, multiple sites

⑤＋ **M89.6** **Osteopathy after poliomyelitis**

Use additional code (B91) to identify previous poliomyelitis

EXCLUDES 1 *postpolio syndrome (G14)*

  ＋ **M89.60** Osteopathy after poliomyelitis, unspecified site

⑥＋ **M89.61** Osteopathy after poliomyelitis, shoulder
- ＋ **M89.611** Osteopathy after poliomyelitis, right shoulder
- ＋ **M89.612** Osteopathy after poliomyelitis, left shoulder
- ＋ **M89.619** Osteopathy after poliomyelitis, unspecified shoulder

⑥＋ **M89.62** Osteopathy after poliomyelitis, upper arm
- ＋ **M89.621** Osteopathy after poliomyelitis, right upper arm
- ＋ **M89.622** Osteopathy after poliomyelitis, left upper arm
- ＋ **M89.629** Osteopathy after poliomyelitis, unspecified upper arm

⑥＋ **M89.63** Osteopathy after poliomyelitis, forearm
- ＋ **M89.631** Osteopathy after poliomyelitis, right forearm
- ＋ **M89.632** Osteopathy after poliomyelitis, left forearm
- ＋ **M89.639** Osteopathy after poliomyelitis, unspecified forearm

⑥＋ **M89.64** Osteopathy after poliomyelitis, hand
- ＋ **M89.641** Osteopathy after poliomyelitis, right hand
- ＋ **M89.642** Osteopathy after poliomyelitis, left hand
- ＋ **M89.649** Osteopathy after poliomyelitis, unspecified hand

⑥＋ **M89.65** Osteopathy after poliomyelitis, thigh
- ＋ **M89.651** Osteopathy after poliomyelitis, right thigh
- ＋ **M89.652** Osteopathy after poliomyelitis, left thigh
- ＋ **M89.659** Osteopathy after poliomyelitis, unspecified thigh

⑥＋ **M89.66** Osteopathy after poliomyelitis, lower leg
- ＋ **M89.661** Osteopathy after poliomyelitis, right lower leg
- ＋ **M89.662** Osteopathy after poliomyelitis, left lower leg
- ＋ **M89.669** Osteopathy after poliomyelitis, unspecified lower leg

⑥＋ **M89.67** Osteopathy after poliomyelitis, ankle and foot
- ＋ **M89.671** Osteopathy after poliomyelitis, right ankle and foot

- ＋ **M89.672** Osteopathy after poliomyelitis, left ankle and foot
- ＋ **M89.679** Osteopathy after poliomyelitis, unspecified ankle and foot

  ＋ **M89.68** Osteopathy after poliomyelitis, other site
  ＋ **M89.69** Osteopathy after poliomyelitis, multiple sites

⑤ **M89.7** **Major osseous defect**

Code first underlying disease, if known, such as:
aseptic necrosis of bone (M87.-)
malignant neoplasm of bone (C40.-)
osteolysis (M89.5)
osteomyelitis (M86.-)
osteonecrosis (M87.-)
osteoporosis (M80.-, M81.-)
periprosthetic osteolysis (T84.05-)

  M89.70 Major osseous defect, unspecified site

⑥ **M89.71** Major osseous defect, shoulder region
    Major osseous defect clavicle or scapula
- **M89.711** Major osseous defect, right shoulder region
- **M89.712** Major osseous defect, left shoulder region
- **M89.719** Major osseous defect, unspecified shoulder region

⑥ **M89.72** Major osseous defect, humerus
- **M89.721** Major osseous defect, right humerus
- **M89.722** Major osseous defect, left humerus
- **M89.729** Major osseous defect, unspecified humerus

⑥ **M89.73** Major osseous defect, forearm
    Major osseous defect of radius and ulna
- **M89.731** Major osseous defect, right forearm
- **M89.732** Major osseous defect, left forearm
- **M89.739** Major osseous defect, unspecified forearm

⑥ **M89.74** Major osseous defect, hand
    Major osseous defect of carpus, fingers, metacarpus
- **M89.741** Major osseous defect, right hand
- **M89.742** Major osseous defect, left hand
- **M89.749** Major osseous defect, unspecified hand

⑥ **M89.75** Major osseous defect, pelvic region and thigh
    Major osseous defect of femur and pelvis
- **M89.751** Major osseous defect, right pelvic region and thigh
- **M89.752** Major osseous defect, left pelvic region and thigh
- **M89.759** Major osseous defect, unspecified pelvic region and thigh

⑥ **M89.76** Major osseous defect, lower leg
    Major osseous defect of fibula and tibia
- **M89.761** Major osseous defect, right lower leg
- **M89.762** Major osseous defect, left lower leg
- **M89.769** Major osseous defect, unspecified lower leg

⑥ **M89.77** Major osseous defect, ankle and foot
    Major osseous defect of metatarsus, tarsus, toes
- **M89.771** Major osseous defect, right ankle and foot
- **M89.772** Major osseous defect, left ankle and foot
- **M89.779** Major osseous defect, unspecified ankle and foot

  M89.78 Major osseous defect, other site
  M89.79 Major osseous defect, multiple sites

⑤ **M89.8** **Other specified disorders of bone**
    Infantile cortical hyperostoses
    Post-traumatic subperiosteal ossification

⑥ **M89.8X** Other specified disorders of bone
  M89.8X0 Other specified disorders of bone, multiple sites
  M89.8X1 Other specified disorders of bone, shoulder
  M89.8X2 Other specified disorders of bone, upper arm
  M89.8X3 Other specified disorders of bone, forearm
  M89.8X4 Other specified disorders of bone, hand
  M89.8X5 Other specified disorders of bone, thigh
  M89.8X6 Other specified disorders of bone, lower leg
  M89.8X7 Other specified disorders of bone, ankle and foot
  M89.8X8 Other specified disorders of bone, other site
  M89.8X9 Other specified disorders of bone, unspecified site

  M89.9 **Disorder of bone, unspecified**

● New ▲ Revised *Manifestation* **4-7** Digit Indicators ▤ Laterality Ⓐ Adult (15+ years) Ⓜ Maternity (12-55 years) Ⓝ Newborn Ⓟ Pediatric (0-17 years) ♂ Male ♀ Female
✖ Deleted Unspecified ＋ Additional code

▲ ◪ **M90   Osteopathies in diseases classified elsewhere**

　　EXCLUDES 1　*osteochondritis, osteomyelitis, and osteopathy*
(in) :
cryptococcosis (B45.3)
diabetes mellitus (E08-E13 with .69-)
gonococcal (A54.43)
neurogenic syphilis (A52.11)
renal osteodystrophy (N25.0)
salmonellosis (A02.24)
secondary syphilis (A51.46)
syphilis (late) (A52.77)

◪ **M90.5   Osteonecrosis in diseases classified elsewhere**

　　Code first underlying disease, such as:
　　caisson disease (T70.3)
　　hemoglobinopathy (D50-D64)

　　M90.50　*Osteonecrosis in diseases classified elsewhere,*
unspecified site

　◪ **M90.51**　Osteonecrosis in diseases classified elsewhere,
shoulder

　　　▤ **M90.511**　*Osteonecrosis in diseases classified elsewhere,*
right shoulder

　　　▤ **M90.512**　*Osteonecrosis in diseases classified elsewhere,*
left shoulder

　　　▤ **M90.519**　*Osteonecrosis in diseases classified elsewhere,*
unspecified shoulder

　◪ **M90.52**　Osteonecrosis in diseases classified elsewhere, upper
arm

　　　▤ **M90.521**　*Osteonecrosis in diseases classified elsewhere,*
right upper arm

　　　▤ **M90.522**　*Osteonecrosis in diseases classified elsewhere,*
left upper arm

　　　▤ **M90.529**　*Osteonecrosis in diseases classified elsewhere,*
unspecified upper arm

　◪ **M90.53**　Osteonecrosis in diseases classified elsewhere,
forearm

　　　▤ **M90.531**　*Osteonecrosis in diseases classified elsewhere,*
right forearm

　　　▤ **M90.532**　*Osteonecrosis in diseases classified elsewhere,*
left forearm

　　　▤ **M90.539**　*Osteonecrosis in diseases classified elsewhere,*
unspecified forearm

　◪ **M90.54**　Osteonecrosis in diseases classified elsewhere, hand

　　　▤ **M90.541**　*Osteonecrosis in diseases classified elsewhere,*
right hand

　　　▤ **M90.542**　*Osteonecrosis in diseases classified elsewhere,*
left hand

　　　▤ **M90.549**　*Osteonecrosis in diseases classified elsewhere,*
unspecified hand

　◪ **M90.55**　Osteonecrosis in diseases classified elsewhere, thigh

　　　▤ **M90.551**　*Osteonecrosis in diseases classified elsewhere,*
right thigh

　　　▤ **M90.552**　*Osteonecrosis in diseases classified elsewhere,*
left thigh

　　　▤ **M90.559**　*Osteonecrosis in diseases classified elsewhere,*
unspecified thigh

　◪ **M90.56**　Osteonecrosis in diseases classified elsewhere, lower
leg

　　　▤ **M90.561**　*Osteonecrosis in diseases classified elsewhere,*
right lower leg

　　　▤ **M90.562**　*Osteonecrosis in diseases classified elsewhere,*
left lower leg

　　　▤ **M90.569**　*Osteonecrosis in diseases classified elsewhere,*
unspecified lower leg

　◪ **M90.57**　Osteonecrosis in diseases classified elsewhere, ankle
and foot

　　　▤ **M90.571**　*Osteonecrosis in diseases classified elsewhere,*
right ankle and foot

　　　▤ **M90.572**　*Osteonecrosis in diseases classified elsewhere,*
left ankle and foot

　　　▤ **M90.579**　*Osteonecrosis in diseases classified elsewhere,*
unspecified ankle and foot

　　M90.58　*Osteonecrosis in diseases classified elsewhere, other*
site

　　M90.59　*Osteonecrosis in diseases classified elsewhere,*
multiple sites

◪ **M90.6   Osteitis deformans in neoplastic diseases**

Osteitis deformans in malignant neoplasm of bone
Code first:
　the neoplasm (C40.-, C41.-)
　　EXCLUDES 1　*osteitis deformans [Paget's disease of bone]*
(M88.-)
　　DEFINITION　Excessive breakdown with abnormal
reformation of bone tissue in the presence of a
malignant neoplasm of the bone; results in painful,
deformed bones prone to pathological fractures.

　　M90.60　*Osteitis deformans in neoplastic diseases, unspecified*
site

　◪ **M90.61**　Osteitis deformans in neoplastic diseases, shoulder

　　　▤ **M90.611**　*Osteitis deformans in neoplastic diseases, right*
shoulder

　　　▤ **M90.612**　*Osteitis deformans in neoplastic diseases, left*
shoulder

　　　▤ **M90.619**　*Osteitis deformans in neoplastic diseases,*
unspecified shoulder

　◪ **M90.62**　Osteitis deformans in neoplastic diseases, upper arm

　　　▤ **M90.621**　*Osteitis deformans in neoplastic diseases, right*
upper arm

　　　▤ **M90.622**　*Osteitis deformans in neoplastic diseases, left*
upper arm

　　　▤ **M90.629**　*Osteitis deformans in neoplastic diseases,*
unspecified upper arm

　◪ **M90.63**　Osteitis deformans in neoplastic diseases, forearm

　　　▤ **M90.631**　*Osteitis deformans in neoplastic diseases, right*
forearm

　　　▤ **M90.632**　*Osteitis deformans in neoplastic diseases, left*
forearm

　　　▤ **M90.639**　*Osteitis deformans in neoplastic diseases,*
unspecified forearm

　◪ **M90.64**　Osteitis deformans in neoplastic diseases, hand

　　　▤ **M90.641**　*Osteitis deformans in neoplastic diseases, right*
hand

　　　▤ **M90.642**　*Osteitis deformans in neoplastic diseases, left*
hand

　　　▤ **M90.649**　*Osteitis deformans in neoplastic diseases,*
unspecified hand

　◪ **M90.65**　Osteitis deformans in neoplastic diseases, thigh

　　　▤ **M90.651**　*Osteitis deformans in neoplastic diseases, right*
thigh

　　　▤ **M90.652**　*Osteitis deformans in neoplastic diseases, left*
thigh

　　　▤ **M90.659**　*Osteitis deformans in neoplastic diseases,*
unspecified thigh

　◪ **M90.66**　Osteitis deformans in neoplastic diseases, lower leg

　　　▤ **M90.661**　*Osteitis deformans in neoplastic diseases, right*
lower leg

　　　▤ **M90.662**　*Osteitis deformans in neoplastic diseases, left*
lower leg

　　　▤ **M90.669**　*Osteitis deformans in neoplastic diseases,*
unspecified lower leg

　◪ **M90.67**　Osteitis deformans in neoplastic diseases, ankle and
foot

　　　▤ **M90.671**　*Osteitis deformans in neoplastic diseases, right*
ankle and foot

　　　▤ **M90.672**　*Osteitis deformans in neoplastic diseases, left*
ankle and foot

　　　▤ **M90.679**　*Osteitis deformans in neoplastic diseases,*
unspecified ankle and foot

　　M90.68　*Osteitis deformans in neoplastic diseases, other site*

　　M90.69　*Osteitis deformans in neoplastic diseases, multiple*
sites

◪ **M90.8   Osteopathy in diseases classified elsewhere**

Code first underlying disease, such as:
　rickets (E55.0)
　vitamin-D-resistant rickets (E83.3)

　　M90.80　*Osteopathy in diseases classified elsewhere,*
unspecified site

　◪ **M90.81**　Osteopathy in diseases classified elsewhere, shoulder

　　　▤ **M90.811**　*Osteopathy in diseases classified elsewhere, right*
shoulder

● New	▲ Revised	*Manifestation*	◪-▨ Digit Indicators	▤ Laterality	Ⓐ Adult (15+ years)	Ⓜ Maternity (12-55 years)	Ⓝ Newborn	Ⓟ Pediatric (0-17 years)	♂ Male	♀ Female
✖ Deleted		Unspecified	+ Additional code							

Diseases of the Musculoskeletal System and Connective Tissue

- **M90.812** *Osteopathy in diseases classified elsewhere, left shoulder*
- **M90.819** *Osteopathy in diseases classified elsewhere, unspecified shoulder*
- **M90.82** Osteopathy in diseases classified elsewhere, upper arm
  - **M90.821** *Osteopathy in diseases classified elsewhere, right upper arm*
  - **M90.822** *Osteopathy in diseases classified elsewhere, left upper arm*
  - **M90.829** *Osteopathy in diseases classified elsewhere, unspecified upper arm*
- **M90.83** Osteopathy in diseases classified elsewhere, forearm
  - **M90.831** *Osteopathy in diseases classified elsewhere, right forearm*
  - **M90.832** *Osteopathy in diseases classified elsewhere, left forearm*
  - **M90.839** *Osteopathy in diseases classified elsewhere, unspecified forearm*
- **M90.84** Osteopathy in diseases classified elsewhere, hand
  - **M90.841** *Osteopathy in diseases classified elsewhere, right hand*
  - **M90.842** *Osteopathy in diseases classified elsewhere, left hand*
  - **M90.849** *Osteopathy in diseases classified elsewhere, unspecified hand*
- **M90.85** Osteopathy in diseases classified elsewhere, thigh
  - **M90.851** *Osteopathy in diseases classified elsewhere, right thigh*
  - **M90.852** *Osteopathy in diseases classified elsewhere, left thigh*
  - **M90.859** *Osteopathy in diseases classified elsewhere, unspecified thigh*
- **M90.86** Osteopathy in diseases classified elsewhere, lower leg
  - **M90.861** *Osteopathy in diseases classified elsewhere, right lower leg*
  - **M90.862** *Osteopathy in diseases classified elsewhere, left lower leg*
  - **M90.869** *Osteopathy in diseases classified elsewhere, unspecified lower leg*
- **M90.87** Osteopathy in diseases classified elsewhere, ankle and foot
  - **M90.871** *Osteopathy in diseases classified elsewhere, right ankle and foot*
  - **M90.872** *Osteopathy in diseases classified elsewhere, left ankle and foot*
  - **M90.879** *Osteopathy in diseases classified elsewhere, unspecified ankle and foot*
- **M90.88** *Osteopathy in diseases classified elsewhere, other site*
- **M90.89** *Osteopathy in diseases classified elsewhere, multiple sites*

Chondropathies (M91-M94)

EXCLUDES 1 *postprocedural chondropathies (M96.-)*

- **M91 Juvenile osteochondrosis of hip and pelvis**
  - **EXCLUDES 1** *slipped upper femoral epiphysis (nontraumatic) (M93.0)*
  - **M91.0 Juvenile osteochondrosis of pelvis**
    Osteochondrosis (juvenile) of acetabulum
    Osteochondrosis (juvenile) of iliac crest [Buchanan]
    Osteochondrosis (juvenile) of ischiopubic synchondrosis [van Neck]
    Osteochondrosis (juvenile) of symphysis pubis [Pierson]
  - **M91.1 Juvenile osteochondrosis of head of femur [Legg-Calvé-Perthes]**
    DEFINITION Disruption of blood supply to the femoral head epiphysis in children, resulting in death of bone; occurs most commonly in boys age 4-8.
    - **M91.10 Juvenile osteochondrosis of head of femur [Legg-Calvé-Perthes], unspecified leg**
    - **M91.11 Juvenile osteochondrosis of head of femur [Legg-Calvé-Perthes], right leg**
    - **M91.12 Juvenile osteochondrosis of head of femur [Legg-Calvé-Perthes], left leg**

- **M91.2 Coxa plana**
  Hip deformity due to previous juvenile osteochondrosis
  DEFINITION Residual effect of Legg-Calve-Perthes in which the necrotic bone of the normally rounded femoral head is flattened due to gradual bone replacement; secondary deformity of the acetabulum occurs with growth.
  - **M91.20 Coxa plana, unspecified hip**
  - **M91.21 Coxa plana, right hip**
  - **M91.22 Coxa plana, left hip**
- **M91.3 Pseudocoxalgia**
  - **M91.30 Pseudocoxalgia, unspecified hip**
  - **M91.31 Pseudocoxalgia, right hip**
  - **M91.32 Pseudocoxalgia, left hip**
- **M91.4 Coxa magna**
  DEFINITION Residual effect of Legg-Calve-Perthes in which the femoral head is enlarged, becoming broad and overgrown due to the gradual bone replacement process.
  - **M91.40 Coxa magna, unspecified hip**
  - **M91.41 Coxa magna, right hip**
  - **M91.42 Coxa magna, left hip**
- **M91.8 Other juvenile osteochondrosis of hip and pelvis**
  Juvenile osteochondrosis after reduction of congenital dislocation of hip
  - **M91.80 Other juvenile osteochondrosis of hip and pelvis, unspecified leg**
  - **M91.81 Other juvenile osteochondrosis of hip and pelvis, right leg**
  - **M91.82 Other juvenile osteochondrosis of hip and pelvis, left leg**
- **M91.9 Juvenile osteochondrosis of hip and pelvis, unspecified**
  - **M91.90 Juvenile osteochondrosis of hip and pelvis, unspecified, unspecified leg**
  - **M91.91 Juvenile osteochondrosis of hip and pelvis, unspecified, right leg**
  - **M91.92 Juvenile osteochondrosis of hip and pelvis, unspecified, left leg**

- **M92 Other juvenile osteochondrosis**
  DEFINITION Condition of unknown etiology affecting the developing growth plate and ossification centers in children where increased stress occurs; genetics, repeated trauma, mechanical factors, hormone imbalances, and vascular abnormalities may be a factor.
  - **M92.0 Juvenile osteochondrosis of humerus**
    Osteochondrosis (juvenile) of capitulum of humerus [Panner]
    Osteochondrosis (juvenile) of head of humerus [Haas]
    - **M92.00 Juvenile osteochondrosis of humerus, unspecified arm**
    - **M92.01 Juvenile osteochondrosis of humerus, right arm**
    - **M92.02 Juvenile osteochondrosis of humerus, left arm**
  - **M92.1 Juvenile osteochondrosis of radius and ulna**
    Osteochondrosis (juvenile) of lower ulna [Burns]
    Osteochondrosis (juvenile) of radial head [Brailsford]
    - **M92.10 Juvenile osteochondrosis of radius and ulna, unspecified arm**
    - **M92.11 Juvenile osteochondrosis of radius and ulna, right arm**
    - **M92.12 Juvenile osteochondrosis of radius and ulna, left arm**
  - **M92.2 Juvenile osteochondrosis, hand**
    - **M92.20 Unspecified juvenile osteochondrosis, hand**
      - **M92.201 Unspecified juvenile osteochondrosis, right hand**
      - **M92.202 Unspecified juvenile osteochondrosis, left hand**
      - **M92.209 Unspecified juvenile osteochondrosis, unspecified hand**
    - **M92.21 Osteochondrosis (juvenile) of carpal lunate [Kienböck]**
      - **M92.211 Osteochondrosis (juvenile) of carpal lunate [Kienböck], right hand**
      - **M92.212 Osteochondrosis (juvenile) of carpal lunate [Kienböck], left hand**
      - **M92.219 Osteochondrosis (juvenile) of carpal lunate [Kienböck], unspecified hand**

● New ▲ Revised *Manifestation* 4-7 Digit Indicators Laterality Adult (15+ years) Maternity (12-55 years) Newborn Pediatric (0-17 years) ♂ Male ♀ Female
✖ Deleted Unspecified + Additional code

810   © 2017 DecisionHealth   2017 ICD-10-CM Expert for Physicians

⑥ **M92.22** Osteochondrosis (juvenile) of metacarpal heads [Mauclaire]
   ☐ **M92.221** Osteochondrosis (juvenile) of metacarpal heads [Mauclaire], right hand
   ☐ **M92.222** Osteochondrosis (juvenile) of metacarpal heads [Mauclaire], left hand
   ☐ **M92.229** Osteochondrosis (juvenile) of metacarpal heads [Mauclaire], unspecified hand

⑥ **M92.29** Other juvenile osteochondrosis, hand
   ☐ **M92.291** Other juvenile osteochondrosis, right hand
   ☐ **M92.292** Other juvenile osteochondrosis, left hand
   ☐ **M92.299** Other juvenile osteochondrosis, unspecified hand

⑤ **M92.3** Other juvenile osteochondrosis, upper limb
   ☐ **M92.30** Other juvenile osteochondrosis, unspecified upper limb
   ☐ **M92.31** Other juvenile osteochondrosis, right upper limb
   ☐ **M92.32** Other juvenile osteochondrosis, left upper limb

⑤ **M92.4** Juvenile osteochondrosis of patella
   Osteochondrosis (juvenile) of primary patellar center [Köhler]
   Osteochondrosis (juvenile) of secondary patellar centre [Sinding Larsen]
   ☐ **M92.40** Juvenile osteochondrosis of patella, unspecified knee
   ☐ **M92.41** Juvenile osteochondrosis of patella, right knee
   ☐ **M92.42** Juvenile osteochondrosis of patella, left knee

⑤ **M92.5** Juvenile osteochondrosis of tibia and fibula
   Osteochondrosis (juvenile) of proximal tibia [Blount]
   Osteochondrosis (juvenile) of tibial tubercle [Osgood-Schlatter]
   Tibia vara
   ☐ **M92.50** Juvenile osteochondrosis of tibia and fibula, unspecified leg
   ☐ **M92.51** Juvenile osteochondrosis of tibia and fibula, right leg
   ☐ **M92.52** Juvenile osteochondrosis of tibia and fibula, left leg

⑤ **M92.6** Juvenile osteochondrosis of tarsus
   Osteochondrosis (juvenile) of calcaneum [Sever]
   Osteochondrosis (juvenile) of os tibiale externum [Haglund]
   Osteochondrosis (juvenile) of talus [Diaz]
   Osteochondrosis (juvenile) of tarsal navicular [Köhler]
   ☐ **M92.60** Juvenile osteochondrosis of tarsus, unspecified ankle
   ☐ **M92.61** Juvenile osteochondrosis of tarsus, right ankle
   ☐ **M92.62** Juvenile osteochondrosis of tarsus, left ankle

⑤ **M92.7** Juvenile osteochondrosis of metatarsus
   Osteochondrosis (juvenile) of fifth metatarsus [Iselin]
   Osteochondrosis (juvenile) of second metatarsus [Freiberg]
   ☐ **M92.70** Juvenile osteochondrosis of metatarsus, unspecified foot
   ☐ **M92.71** Juvenile osteochondrosis of metatarsus, right foot
   ☐ **M92.72** Juvenile osteochondrosis of metatarsus, left foot

M92.8 Other specified juvenile osteochondrosis
   Calcaneal apophysitis

M92.9 Juvenile osteochondrosis, unspecified
   Juvenile apophysitis NOS
   Juvenile epiphysitis NOS
   Juvenile osteochondritis NOS
   Juvenile osteochondrosis NOS

④ **M93** Other osteochondropathies
   EXCLUDES 2 *osteochondrosis of spine (M42.-)*

⑤ ✚ **M93.0** Slipped upper femoral epiphysis (nontraumatic)
   Use additional code for associated chondrolysis (M94.3)
   DEFINITION Nontraumatic slippage of the femoral head of the epiphysis occurring in adolescence.

   ⑥ ✚ **M93.00** Unspecified slipped upper femoral epiphysis (nontraumatic)
     ☐ ✚ **M93.001** Unspecified slipped upper femoral epiphysis (nontraumatic), right hip
     ☐ ✚ **M93.002** Unspecified slipped upper femoral epiphysis (nontraumatic), left hip
     ☐ ✚ **M93.003** Unspecified slipped upper femoral epiphysis (nontraumatic), unspecified hip

   ⑥ ✚ **M93.01** Acute slipped upper femoral epiphysis (nontraumatic)
     ☐ ✚ **M93.011** Acute slipped upper femoral epiphysis (nontraumatic), right hip
     ☐ ✚ **M93.012** Acute slipped upper femoral epiphysis (nontraumatic), left hip
     ☐ ✚ **M93.013** Acute slipped upper femoral epiphysis (nontraumatic), unspecified hip

   ⑥ ✚ **M93.02** Chronic slipped upper femoral epiphysis (nontraumatic)
     ☐ ✚ **M93.021** Chronic slipped upper femoral epiphysis (nontraumatic), right hip
     ☐ ✚ **M93.022** Chronic slipped upper femoral epiphysis (nontraumatic), left hip
     ☐ ✚ **M93.023** Chronic slipped upper femoral epiphysis (nontraumatic), unspecified hip

   ⑥ ✚ **M93.03** Acute on chronic slipped upper femoral epiphysis (nontraumatic)
     ☐ ✚ **M93.031** Acute on chronic slipped upper femoral epiphysis (nontraumatic), right hip
     ☐ ✚ **M93.032** Acute on chronic slipped upper femoral epiphysis (nontraumatic), left hip
     ☐ ✚ **M93.033** Acute on chronic slipped upper femoral epiphysis (nontraumatic), unspecified hip

M93.1 Kienböck's disease of adults   Ⓐ
   Adult osteochondrosis of carpal lunates
   DEFINITION Idiopathic disruption of blood supply to the carpal lunate bone in adults, resulting in death of the bone tissue.

⑤ **M93.2** Osteochondritis dissecans
   DEFINITION Joint condition in which a piece of cartilage and thin, underlying bone detaches from the bone's end; occurs most often in boys age 10-20 after a joint injury, and commonly affecting the knee.

   M93.20 Osteochondritis dissecans of unspecified site
   ⑥ **M93.21** Osteochondritis dissecans of shoulder
     ☐ **M93.211** Osteochondritis dissecans, right shoulder
     ☐ **M93.212** Osteochondritis dissecans, left shoulder
     ☐ **M93.219** Osteochondritis dissecans, unspecified shoulder
   ⑥ **M93.22** Osteochondritis dissecans of elbow
     ☐ **M93.221** Osteochondritis dissecans, right elbow
     ☐ **M93.222** Osteochondritis dissecans, left elbow
     ☐ **M93.229** Osteochondritis dissecans, unspecified elbow
   ⑥ **M93.23** Osteochondritis dissecans of wrist
     ☐ **M93.231** Osteochondritis dissecans, right wrist
     ☐ **M93.232** Osteochondritis dissecans, left wrist
     ☐ **M93.239** Osteochondritis dissecans, unspecified wrist
   ⑥ **M93.24** Osteochondritis dissecans of joints of hand
     ☐ **M93.241** Osteochondritis dissecans, joints of right hand
     ☐ **M93.242** Osteochondritis dissecans, joints of left hand
     ☐ **M93.249** Osteochondritis dissecans, joints of unspecified hand
   ⑥ **M93.25** Osteochondritis dissecans of hip
     ☐ **M93.251** Osteochondritis dissecans, right hip
     ☐ **M93.252** Osteochondritis dissecans, left hip
     ☐ **M93.259** Osteochondritis dissecans, unspecified hip
   ⑥ **M93.26** Osteochondritis dissecans knee
     ☐ **M93.261** Osteochondritis dissecans, right knee
     ☐ **M93.262** Osteochondritis dissecans, left knee
     ☐ **M93.269** Osteochondritis dissecans, unspecified knee
   ⑥ **M93.27** Osteochondritis dissecans of ankle and joints of foot
     ☐ **M93.271** Osteochondritis dissecans, right ankle and joints of right foot
     ☐ **M93.272** Osteochondritis dissecans, left ankle and joints of left foot
     ☐ **M93.279** Osteochondritis dissecans, unspecified ankle and joints of foot
   M93.28 Osteochondritis dissecans other site
   M93.29 Osteochondritis dissecans multiple sites

⑤ **M93.8** Other specified osteochondropathies
   DEFINITION Other conditions affecting bone and cartilage at any age, noted by abnormal endochondral ossification.
   M93.80 Other specified osteochondropathies of unspecified site
   ⑥ **M93.81** Other specified osteochondropathies of shoulder
     ☐ **M93.811** Other specified osteochondropathies, right shoulder

---

● New   ▲ Revised   *Manifestation*   ④-⑦ Digit Indicators   ☐ Laterality   Ⓐ Adult (15+ years)   Ⓜ Maternity (12-55 years)   Ⓝ Newborn   Ⓟ Pediatric (0-17 years)   ♂ Male   ♀ Female
✕ Deleted   Unspecified   ✚ Additional code

⊟ M93.812   Other specified osteochondropathies, left shoulder

⊟ M93.819   Other specified osteochondropathies, unspecified shoulder

Ⓖ M93.82   Other specified osteochondropathies of upper arm

⊟ M93.821   Other specified osteochondropathies, right upper arm

⊟ M93.822   Other specified osteochondropathies, left upper arm

⊟ M93.829   Other specified osteochondropathies, unspecified upper arm

Ⓖ M93.83   Other specified osteochondropathies of forearm

⊟ M93.831   Other specified osteochondropathies, right forearm

⊟ M93.832   Other specified osteochondropathies, left forearm

⊟ M93.839   Other specified osteochondropathies, unspecified forearm

Ⓖ M93.84   Other specified osteochondropathies of hand

⊟ M93.841   Other specified osteochondropathies, right hand

⊟ M93.842   Other specified osteochondropathies, left hand

⊟ M93.849   Other specified osteochondropathies, unspecified hand

Ⓖ M93.85   Other specified osteochondropathies of thigh

⊟ M93.851   Other specified osteochondropathies, right thigh

⊟ M93.852   Other specified osteochondropathies, left thigh

⊟ M93.859   Other specified osteochondropathies, unspecified thigh

Ⓖ M93.86   Other specified osteochondropathies lower leg

⊟ M93.861   Other specified osteochondropathies, right lower leg

⊟ M93.862   Other specified osteochondropathies, left lower leg

⊟ M93.869   Other specified osteochondropathies, unspecified lower leg

Ⓖ M93.87   Other specified osteochondropathies of ankle and foot

⊟ M93.871   Other specified osteochondropathies, right ankle and foot

⊟ M93.872   Other specified osteochondropathies, left ankle and foot

⊟ M93.879   Other specified osteochondropathies, unspecified ankle and foot

M93.88   Other specified osteochondropathies other

M93.89   Other specified osteochondropathies multiple sites

Ⓢ M93.9   Osteochondropathy, unspecified

Apophysitis NOS
Epiphysitis NOS
Osteochondritis NOS
Osteochondrosis NOS

M93.90   Osteochondropathy, unspecified of unspecified site

Ⓖ M93.91   Osteochondropathy, unspecified of shoulder

⊟ M93.911   Osteochondropathy, unspecified, right shoulder

⊟ M93.912   Osteochondropathy, unspecified, left shoulder

⊟ M93.919   Osteochondropathy, unspecified, unspecified shoulder

Ⓖ M93.92   Osteochondropathy, unspecified of upper arm

⊟ M93.921   Osteochondropathy, unspecified, right upper arm

⊟ M93.922   Osteochondropathy, unspecified, left upper arm

⊟ M93.929   Osteochondropathy, unspecified, unspecified upper arm

Ⓖ M93.93   Osteochondropathy, unspecified of forearm

⊟ M93.931   Osteochondropathy, unspecified, right forearm

⊟ M93.932   Osteochondropathy, unspecified, left forearm

⊟ M93.939   Osteochondropathy, unspecified, unspecified forearm

Ⓖ M93.94   Osteochondropathy, unspecified of hand

⊟ M93.941   Osteochondropathy, unspecified, right hand

⊟ M93.942   Osteochondropathy, unspecified, left hand

⊟ M93.949   Osteochondropathy, unspecified, unspecified hand

Ⓖ M93.95   Osteochondropathy, unspecified of thigh

⊟ M93.951   Osteochondropathy, unspecified, right thigh

⊟ M93.952   Osteochondropathy, unspecified, left thigh

⊟ M93.959   Osteochondropathy, unspecified, unspecified thigh

Ⓖ M93.96   Osteochondropathy, unspecified lower leg

⊟ M93.961   Osteochondropathy, unspecified, right lower leg

⊟ M93.962   Osteochondropathy, unspecified, left lower leg

⊟ M93.969   Osteochondropathy, unspecified, unspecified lower leg

Ⓖ M93.97   Osteochondropathy, unspecified of ankle and foot

⊟ M93.971   Osteochondropathy, unspecified, right ankle and foot

⊟ M93.972   Osteochondropathy, unspecified, left ankle and foot

⊟ M93.979   Osteochondropathy, unspecified, unspecified ankle and foot

M93.98   Osteochondropathy, unspecified other

M93.99   Osteochondropathy, unspecified multiple sites

④ M94   **Other disorders of cartilage**

M94.0   Chondrocostal junction syndrome [Tietze]
Costochondritis

M94.1   Relapsing polychondritis

Ⓢ M94.2   Chondromalacia

> **EXCLUDES 1**   *chondromalacia patellae (M22.4)*

> **DEFINITION**   Joint cartilage softens and degenerates, causing tenderness, pain, and a grinding sensation.

M94.20   Chondromalacia, unspecified site

Ⓖ M94.21   Chondromalacia, shoulder

⊟ M94.211   Chondromalacia, right shoulder

⊟ M94.212   Chondromalacia, left shoulder

⊟ M94.219   Chondromalacia, unspecified shoulder

Ⓖ M94.22   Chondromalacia, elbow

⊟ M94.221   Chondromalacia, right elbow

⊟ M94.222   Chondromalacia, left elbow

⊟ M94.229   Chondromalacia, unspecified elbow

Ⓖ M94.23   Chondromalacia, wrist

⊟ M94.231   Chondromalacia, right wrist

⊟ M94.232   Chondromalacia, left wrist

⊟ M94.239   Chondromalacia, unspecified wrist

Ⓖ M94.24   Chondromalacia, joints of hand

⊟ M94.241   Chondromalacia, joints of right hand

⊟ M94.242   Chondromalacia, joints of left hand

⊟ M94.249   Chondromalacia, joints of unspecified hand

Ⓖ M94.25   Chondromalacia, hip

⊟ M94.251   Chondromalacia, right hip

⊟ M94.252   Chondromalacia, left hip

⊟ M94.259   Chondromalacia, unspecified hip

Ⓖ M94.26   Chondromalacia, knee

> **CODING TIP ✓**   Do not assign M94.26 for chondromalacia patellae (also called 'runner's knee' or CMP). Chondromalacia patellae is an inflammation of the underside of the patella and is coded to M22.4.

⊟ M94.261   Chondromalacia, right knee

⊟ M94.262   Chondromalacia, left knee

⊟ M94.269   Chondromalacia, unspecified knee

Ⓖ M94.27   Chondromalacia, ankle and joints of foot

⊟ M94.271   Chondromalacia, right ankle and joints of right foot

⊟ M94.272   Chondromalacia, left ankle and joints of left foot

⊟ M94.279   Chondromalacia, unspecified ankle and joints of foot

M94.28   Chondromalacia, other site

M94.29   Chondromalacia, multiple sites

Ⓢ M94.3   Chondrolysis

Code first:
any associated slipped upper femoral epiphysis (nontraumatic) (M93.0-)

> **DEFINITION**   Sudden, severe damage to joint cartilage causing rapid death of normal cartilage cells and abrupt loss of the joint's cartilage layer.

Ⓖ M94.35   Chondrolysis, hip

⊟ M94.351   Chondrolysis, right hip

● New   ▲ Revised   *Manifestation*   ④-❼ Digit Indicators   ⊟ Laterality   Ⓐ Adult (15+ years)   Ⓜ Maternity (12-55 years)   Ⓝ Newborn   Ⓟ Pediatric (0-17 years)   ♂ Male   ♀ Female

✖ Deleted   Unspecified   + Additional code

   ☐ **M94.352**   Chondrolysis, left hip
   ☐ **M94.359**   Chondrolysis, unspecified hip
 ⑤ **M94.8**   Other specified disorders of cartilage
  ⑥ **M94.8X**   Other specified disorders of cartilage

    M94.8X0   Other specified disorders of cartilage, multiple sites
    M94.8X1   Other specified disorders of cartilage, shoulder
    M94.8X2   Other specified disorders of cartilage, upper arm
    M94.8X3   Other specified disorders of cartilage, forearm
    M94.8X4   Other specified disorders of cartilage, hand
    M94.8X5   Other specified disorders of cartilage, thigh
    M94.8X6   Other specified disorders of cartilage, lower leg
    M94.8X7   Other specified disorders of cartilage, ankle and foot
    M94.8X8   Other specified disorders of cartilage, other site
    M94.8X9   Other specified disorders of cartilage, unspecified sites

 M94.9   Disorder of cartilage, unspecified

Other disorders of the musculoskeletal system and connective tissue (M95)

④ **M95**   Other acquired deformities of musculoskeletal system and connective tissue

   EXCLUDES 2   *acquired absence of limbs and organs (Z89-Z90)*
     acquired deformities of limbs (M20-M21)
     congenital malformations and deformations of the musculoskeletal system (Q65-Q79)
     deforming dorsopathies (M40-M43)
     dentofacial anomalies [including malocclusion] (M26.-)
     postprocedural musculoskeletal disorders (M96.-)

 M95.0   Acquired deformity of nose
   EXCLUDES 2   *deviated nasal septum (J34.2)*

⑤ **M95.1**   Cauliflower ear
   EXCLUDES 2   *other acquired deformities of ear (H61.1)*

Cauliflower ear

Normal ear   Cauliflower ear

Abnormal external ear as a result of injury

   ☐ **M95.10**   Cauliflower ear, unspecified ear
   ☐ **M95.11**   Cauliflower ear, right ear
   ☐ **M95.12**   Cauliflower ear, left ear
 M95.2   Other acquired deformity of head
 M95.3   Acquired deformity of neck
 M95.4   Acquired deformity of chest and rib
    AHA: 4Q 2014, 26, 27
 M95.5   Acquired deformity of pelvis
   EXCLUDES 1   *maternal care for known or suspected disproportion (O33.-)*
 M95.8   Other specified acquired deformities of musculoskeletal system
 M95.9   Acquired deformity of musculoskeletal system, unspecified

Intraoperative and postprocedural complications and disorders of musculoskeletal system, not elsewhere classified (M96)

▲ ④ **M96**   Intraoperative and postprocedural complications and disorders of musculoskeletal system, not elsewhere classified

   EXCLUDES 2   *arthropathy following intestinal bypass (M02.0-)*
     complications of internal orthopedic prosthetic devices, implants and grafts (T84.-)
     disorders associated with osteoporosis (M80)
     periprosthetic fracture around internal prosthetic joint (M97.-)
     presence of functional implants and other devices (Z96-Z97)

   CODING TIP ✓   **Documentation:** Codes in category M96.- are complication codes and require physician documentation and confirmation of a cause and effect relationship between the procedure and the complicated condition.

 M96.0   Pseudarthrosis after fusion or arthrodesis
 M96.1   Postlaminectomy syndrome, not elsewhere classified   Ⓐ
 M96.2   Postradiation kyphosis
 M96.3   Postlaminectomy kyphosis
 M96.4   Postsurgical lordosis
 M96.5   Postradiation scoliosis
⑤ **M96.6**   Fracture of bone following insertion of orthopedic implant, joint prosthesis, or bone plate

    Intraoperative fracture of bone during insertion of orthopedic implant, joint prosthesis, or bone plate

   EXCLUDES 2   *complication of internal orthopedic devices, implants or grafts (T84.-)*

 ⑥ **M96.62**   Fracture of humerus following insertion of orthopedic implant, joint prosthesis, or bone plate
   ☐ **M96.621**   Fracture of humerus following insertion of orthopedic implant, joint prosthesis, or bone plate, right arm
   ☐ **M96.622**   Fracture of humerus following insertion of orthopedic implant, joint prosthesis, or bone plate, left arm
   ☐ **M96.629**   Fracture of humerus following insertion of orthopedic implant, joint prosthesis, or bone plate, unspecified arm

 ⑥ **M96.63**   Fracture of radius or ulna following insertion of orthopedic implant, joint prosthesis, or bone plate
   ☐ **M96.631**   Fracture of radius or ulna following insertion of orthopedic implant, joint prosthesis, or bone plate, right arm
   ☐ **M96.632**   Fracture of radius or ulna following insertion of orthopedic implant, joint prosthesis, or bone plate, left arm
   ☐ **M96.639**   Fracture of radius or ulna following insertion of orthopedic implant, joint prosthesis, or bone plate, unspecified arm

 M96.65   Fracture of pelvis following insertion of orthopedic implant, joint prosthesis, or bone plate
 ⑥ **M96.66**   Fracture of femur following insertion of orthopedic implant, joint prosthesis, or bone plate
   ☐ **M96.661**   Fracture of femur following insertion of orthopedic implant, joint prosthesis, or bone plate, right leg
   ☐ **M96.662**   Fracture of femur following insertion of orthopedic implant, joint prosthesis, or bone plate, left leg
   ☐ **M96.669**   Fracture of femur following insertion of orthopedic implant, joint prosthesis, or bone plate, unspecified leg

 ⑥ **M96.67**   Fracture of tibia or fibula following insertion of orthopedic implant, joint prosthesis, or bone plate
   ☐ **M96.671**   Fracture of tibia or fibula following insertion of orthopedic implant, joint prosthesis, or bone plate, right leg
   ☐ **M96.672**   Fracture of tibia or fibula following insertion of orthopedic implant, joint prosthesis, or bone plate, left leg
   ☐ **M96.679**   Fracture of tibia or fibula following insertion of orthopedic implant, joint prosthesis, or bone plate, unspecified leg

---

● New   ▲ Revised   *Manifestation*   ④-⑦ Digit Indicators   ☐ Laterality   Ⓐ Adult (15+ years)   Ⓜ Maternity (12-55 years)   Ⓝ Newborn   Ⓟ Pediatric (0-17 years)   ♂ Male   ♀ Female
✖ Deleted   Unspecified   + Additional code

M96.69   Fracture of other bone following insertion of orthopedic implant, joint prosthesis, or bone plate

⑤ **M96.8**   Other intraoperative and postprocedural complications and disorders of musculoskeletal system, not elsewhere classified

⑥ **M96.81**   Intraoperative hemorrhage and hematoma of a musculoskeletal structure complicating a procedure

> **EXCLUDES 1**   *intraoperative hemorrhage and hematoma of a musculoskeletal structure due to accidental puncture and laceration during a procedure (M96.82-)*

    M96.810   Intraoperative hemorrhage and hematoma of a musculoskeletal structure complicating a musculoskeletal system procedure

    M96.811   Intraoperative hemorrhage and hematoma of a musculoskeletal structure complicating other procedure

⑥ **M96.82**   Accidental puncture and laceration of a musculoskeletal structure during a procedure

    M96.820   Accidental puncture and laceration of a musculoskeletal structure during a musculoskeletal system procedure

    M96.821   Accidental puncture and laceration of a musculoskeletal structure during other procedure

▲ ⑥ **M96.83**   Postprocedural hemorrhage of a musculoskeletal structure following a procedure

▲ **M96.830**   Postprocedural hemorrhage of a musculoskeletal structure following a musculoskeletal system procedure

▲ **M96.831**   Postprocedural hemorrhage of a musculoskeletal structure following other procedure

● ⑥ **M96.84**   Postprocedural hematoma and seroma of a musculoskeletal structure following a procedure

● **M96.840**   Postprocedural hematoma of a musculoskeletal structure following a musculoskeletal system procedure

● **M96.841**   Postprocedural hematoma of a musculoskeletal structure following other procedure

● **M96.842**   Postprocedural seroma of a musculoskeletal structure following a musculoskeletal system procedure

● **M96.843**   Postprocedural seroma of a musculoskeletal structure following other procedure

＋ **M96.89**   Other intraoperative and postprocedural complications and disorders of the musculoskeletal system

    Instability of joint secondary to removal of joint prosthesis

    Use additional code, if applicable, to further specify disorder

Periprosthetic fracture around internal prosthetic joint (M97)

● ④ **M97**   Periprosthetic fracture around internal prosthetic joint

> **EXCLUDES 2**   *fracture of bone following insertion of orthopedic implant, joint prosthesis or bone plate (M96.6-)*
> *breakage (fracture) of prosthetic joint (T84.01-)*

The appropriate 7th character is to be added to each code from category M97
A   initial encounter
D   subsequent encounter
S   sequela

● ⑤ **M97.0**   Periprosthetic fracture around internal prosthetic hip joint

● ⑦ ☐ **M97.01X-**   Periprosthetic fracture around internal prosthetic right hip joint

● ⑦ ☐ **M97.02X-**   Periprosthetic fracture around internal prosthetic left hip joint

● ⑤ **M97.1**   Periprosthetic fracture around internal prosthetic knee joint

● ⑦ ☐ **M97.11X-**   Periprosthetic fracture around internal prosthetic right knee joint

● ⑦ ☐ **M97.12X-**   Periprosthetic fracture around internal prosthetic left knee joint

● ⑤ **M97.2**   Periprosthetic fracture around internal prosthetic ankle joint

● ⑦ ☐ **M97.21X-**   Periprosthetic fracture around internal prosthetic right ankle joint

● ⑦ ☐ **M97.22X-**   Periprosthetic fracture around internal prosthetic left ankle joint

● ⑤ **M97.3**   Periprosthetic fracture around internal prosthetic shoulder joint

● ⑦ ☐ **M97.31X-**   Periprosthetic fracture around internal prosthetic right shoulder joint

● ⑦ ☐ **M97.32X-**   Periprosthetic fracture around internal prosthetic left shoulder joint

● ⑤ **M97.4**   Periprosthetic fracture around internal prosthetic elbow joint

● ⑦ ☐ **M97.41X-**   Periprosthetic fracture around internal prosthetic right elbow joint

● ⑦ ☐ **M97.42X-**   Periprosthetic fracture around internal prosthetic left elbow joint

● ⑦ ＋ **M97.8XX-**   Periprosthetic fracture around other internal prosthetic joint

    Periprosthetic fracture around internal prosthetic finger joint
    Periprosthetic fracture around internal prosthetic spinal joint
    Periprosthetic fracture around internal prosthetic toe joint
    Periprosthetic fracture around internal prosthetic wrist joint
    Use additional code to identify the joint (Z96.6-)

● ⑦ **M97.9XX-**   Periprosthetic fracture around unspecified internal prosthetic joint

Biomechanical lesions, not elsewhere classified (M99)

④ **M99**   Biomechanical lesions, not elsewhere classified

    Note: This category should not be used if the condition can be classified elsewhere.

⑤ **M99.0**   Segmental and somatic dysfunction

    M99.00   Segmental and somatic dysfunction of head region

    M99.01   Segmental and somatic dysfunction of cervical region

    M99.02   Segmental and somatic dysfunction of thoracic region

    M99.03   Segmental and somatic dysfunction of lumbar region

    M99.04   Segmental and somatic dysfunction of sacral region

    M99.05   Segmental and somatic dysfunction of pelvic region

    M99.06   Segmental and somatic dysfunction of lower extremity

    M99.07   Segmental and somatic dysfunction of upper extremity

    M99.08   Segmental and somatic dysfunction of rib cage

    M99.09   Segmental and somatic dysfunction of abdomen and other regions

⑤ **M99.1**   Subluxation complex (vertebral)

    M99.10   Subluxation complex (vertebral) of head region

    M99.11   Subluxation complex (vertebral) of cervical region

    M99.12   Subluxation complex (vertebral) of thoracic region

    M99.13   Subluxation complex (vertebral) of lumbar region

    M99.14   Subluxation complex (vertebral) of sacral region

    M99.15   Subluxation complex (vertebral) of pelvic region

    M99.16   Subluxation complex (vertebral) of lower extremity

    M99.17   Subluxation complex (vertebral) of upper extremity

    M99.18   Subluxation complex (vertebral) of rib cage

    M99.19   Subluxation complex (vertebral) of abdomen and other regions

⑤ **M99.2**   Subluxation stenosis of neural canal

    M99.20   Subluxation stenosis of neural canal of head region

    M99.21   Subluxation stenosis of neural canal of cervical region

    M99.22   Subluxation stenosis of neural canal of thoracic region   Ⓐ

    M99.23   Subluxation stenosis of neural canal of lumbar region   Ⓐ

    M99.24   Subluxation stenosis of neural canal of sacral region   Ⓐ

    M99.25   Subluxation stenosis of neural canal of pelvic region   Ⓐ

● New   ▲ Revised   *Manifestation*   ④-⑦ Digit Indicators   ☐ Laterality   Adult (15+ years)   Maternity (12-55 years)   Newborn   Pediatric (0-17 years)   ♂ Male   ♀ Female
✖ Deleted   Unspecified   ＋ Additional code

M99.26   Subluxation stenosis of neural canal of lower extremity Ⓐ

M99.27   Subluxation stenosis of neural canal of upper extremity Ⓐ

M99.28   Subluxation stenosis of neural canal of rib cage Ⓐ

M99.29   Subluxation stenosis of neural canal of abdomen and other regions Ⓐ

Ⓢ M99.3   Osseous stenosis of neural canal

M99.30   Osseous stenosis of neural canal of head region

M99.31   Osseous stenosis of neural canal of cervical region

M99.32   Osseous stenosis of neural canal of thoracic region Ⓐ

M99.33   Osseous stenosis of neural canal of lumbar region Ⓐ

M99.34   Osseous stenosis of neural canal of sacral region Ⓐ

M99.35   Osseous stenosis of neural canal of pelvic region Ⓐ

M99.36   Osseous stenosis of neural canal of lower extremity Ⓐ

M99.37   Osseous stenosis of neural canal of upper extremity Ⓐ

M99.38   Osseous stenosis of neural canal of rib cage Ⓐ

M99.39   Osseous stenosis of neural canal of abdomen and other regions Ⓐ

Ⓢ M99.4   Connective tissue stenosis of neural canal

M99.40   Connective tissue stenosis of neural canal of head region

M99.41   Connective tissue stenosis of neural canal of cervical region

M99.42   Connective tissue stenosis of neural canal of thoracic region Ⓐ

M99.43   Connective tissue stenosis of neural canal of lumbar region Ⓐ

M99.44   Connective tissue stenosis of neural canal of sacral region Ⓐ

M99.45   Connective tissue stenosis of neural canal of pelvic region Ⓐ

M99.46   Connective tissue stenosis of neural canal of lower extremity Ⓐ

M99.47   Connective tissue stenosis of neural canal of upper extremity Ⓐ

M99.48   Connective tissue stenosis of neural canal of rib cage Ⓐ

M99.49   Connective tissue stenosis of neural canal of abdomen and other regions Ⓐ

Ⓢ M99.5   Intervertebral disc stenosis of neural canal

M99.50   Intervertebral disc stenosis of neural canal of head region

M99.51   Intervertebral disc stenosis of neural canal of cervical region

M99.52   Intervertebral disc stenosis of neural canal of thoracic region Ⓐ

M99.53   Intervertebral disc stenosis of neural canal of lumbar region Ⓐ

M99.54   Intervertebral disc stenosis of neural canal of sacral region Ⓐ

M99.55   Intervertebral disc stenosis of neural canal of pelvic region Ⓐ

M99.56   Intervertebral disc stenosis of neural canal of lower extremity Ⓐ

M99.57   Intervertebral disc stenosis of neural canal of upper extremity Ⓐ

M99.58   Intervertebral disc stenosis of neural canal of rib cage Ⓐ

M99.59   Intervertebral disc stenosis of neural canal of abdomen and other regions Ⓐ

Ⓢ M99.6   Osseous and subluxation stenosis of intervertebral foramina

M99.60   Osseous and subluxation stenosis of intervertebral foramina of head region

M99.61   Osseous and subluxation stenosis of intervertebral foramina of cervical region

M99.62   Osseous and subluxation stenosis of intervertebral foramina of thoracic region Ⓐ

M99.63   Osseous and subluxation stenosis of intervertebral foramina of lumbar region Ⓐ

M99.64   Osseous and subluxation stenosis of intervertebral foramina of sacral region Ⓐ

M99.65   Osseous and subluxation stenosis of intervertebral foramina of pelvic region Ⓐ

M99.66   Osseous and subluxation stenosis of intervertebral foramina of lower extremity Ⓐ

M99.67   Osseous and subluxation stenosis of intervertebral foramina of upper extremity Ⓐ

M99.68   Osseous and subluxation stenosis of intervertebral foramina of rib cage Ⓐ

M99.69   Osseous and subluxation stenosis of intervertebral foramina of abdomen and other regions Ⓐ

Ⓢ M99.7   Connective tissue and disc stenosis of intervertebral foramina

M99.70   Connective tissue and disc stenosis of intervertebral foramina of head region

M99.71   Connective tissue and disc stenosis of intervertebral foramina of cervical region

M99.72   Connective tissue and disc stenosis of intervertebral foramina of thoracic region Ⓐ

M99.73   Connective tissue and disc stenosis of intervertebral foramina of lumbar region Ⓐ

M99.74   Connective tissue and disc stenosis of intervertebral foramina of sacral region Ⓐ

M99.75   Connective tissue and disc stenosis of intervertebral foramina of pelvic region Ⓐ

M99.76   Connective tissue and disc stenosis of intervertebral foramina of lower extremity Ⓐ

M99.77   Connective tissue and disc stenosis of intervertebral foramina of upper extremity Ⓐ

M99.78   Connective tissue and disc stenosis of intervertebral foramina of rib cage Ⓐ

M99.79   Connective tissue and disc stenosis of intervertebral foramina of abdomen and other regions Ⓐ

Ⓢ M99.8   Other biomechanical lesions

M99.80   Other biomechanical lesions of head region

M99.81   Other biomechanical lesions of cervical region

M99.82   Other biomechanical lesions of thoracic region

M99.83   Other biomechanical lesions of lumbar region

M99.84   Other biomechanical lesions of sacral region

M99.85   Other biomechanical lesions of pelvic region

M99.86   Other biomechanical lesions of lower extremity

M99.87   Other biomechanical lesions of upper extremity

M99.88   Other biomechanical lesions of rib cage

M99.89   Other biomechanical lesions of abdomen and other regions

M99.9   Biomechanical lesion, unspecified

| ● New | ▲ Revised | *Manifestation* | 🔢-🔢 Digit Indicators | ▤ Laterality | Ⓐ Adult (15+ years) | Ⓜ Maternity (12-55 years) | Ⓝ Newborn | Ⓟ Pediatric (0-17 years) | ♂ Male | ♀ Female |
| ✖ Deleted | | Unspecified | + Additional code | | | | | | | |

CHAPTER 14: DISEASES OF THE GENITOURINARY SYSTEM (N00-N99)

EXCLUDES 2 *certain conditions originating in the perinatal period (P04-P96)*
certain infectious and parasitic diseases (A00-B99)
complications of pregnancy, childbirth and the puerperium (O00-O9A)
congenital malformations, deformations and chromosomal abnormalities (Q00-Q99)
endocrine, nutritional and metabolic diseases (E00-E88)
injury, poisoning and certain other consequences of external causes (S00-T88)
neoplasms (C00-D49)
symptoms, signs and abnormal clinical and laboratory findings, not elsewhere classified (R00-R94)

This chapter contains the following blocks:
N00-N08   Glomerular diseases
N10-N16   Renal tubulo-interstitial diseases
N17-N19   Acute kidney failure and chronic kidney disease
N20-N23   Urolithiasis
N25-N29   Other disorders of kidney and ureter
N30-N39   Other diseases of the urinary system
N40-N53   Diseases of male genital organs
N60-N65   Disorders of breast
N70-N77   Inflammatory diseases of female pelvic organs
N80-N98   Noninflammatory disorders of female genital tract
N99   Intraoperative and postprocedural complications and disorders of genitourinary system, not elsewhere classified

Glomerular diseases (N00-N08)

Code also:
  any associated kidney failure (N17-N19) .
EXCLUDES 1 *hypertensive chronic kidney disease (I12.-)*

◢ N00   Acute nephritic syndrome

INCLUDES   acute glomerular disease
acute glomerulonephritis
acute nephritis

EXCLUDES 1   *acute tubulo-interstitial nephritis (N10)*
nephritic syndrome NOS (N05.-)

N00.0   Acute nephritic syndrome with minor glomerular abnormality
Acute nephritic syndrome with minimal change lesion

N00.1   Acute nephritic syndrome with focal and segmental glomerular lesions
Acute nephritic syndrome with focal and segmental hyalinosis
Acute nephritic syndrome with focal and segmental sclerosis
Acute nephritic syndrome with focal glomerulonephritis

N00.2   Acute nephritic syndrome with diffuse membranous glomerulonephritis

N00.3   Acute nephritic syndrome with diffuse mesangial proliferative glomerulonephritis

N00.4   Acute nephritic syndrome with diffuse endocapillary proliferative glomerulonephritis

N00.5   Acute nephritic syndrome with diffuse mesangiocapillary glomerulonephritis
Acute nephritic syndrome with membranoproliferative glomerulonephritis, types 1 and 3, or NOS

N00.6   Acute nephritic syndrome with dense deposit disease
Acute nephritic syndrome with membranoproliferative glomerulonephritis, type 2

N00.7   Acute nephritic syndrome with diffuse crescentic glomerulonephritis
Acute nephritic syndrome with extracapillary glomerulonephritis

N00.8   Acute nephritic syndrome with other morphologic changes
Acute nephritic syndrome with proliferative glomerulonephritis NOS

N00.9   Acute nephritic syndrome with unspecified morphologic changes

◢ N01   Rapidly progressive nephritic syndrome

INCLUDES   rapidly progressive glomerular disease
rapidly progressive glomerulonephritis
rapidly progressive nephritis

EXCLUDES 1   *nephritic syndrome NOS (N05.-)*

N01.0   Rapidly progressive nephritic syndrome with minor glomerular abnormality
Rapidly progressive nephritic syndrome with minimal change lesion

N01.1   Rapidly progressive nephritic syndrome with focal and segmental glomerular lesions
Rapidly progressive nephritic syndrome with focal and segmental hyalinosis
Rapidly progressive nephritic syndrome with focal and segmental sclerosis
Rapidly progressive nephritic syndrome with focal glomerulonephritis

N01.2   Rapidly progressive nephritic syndrome with diffuse membranous glomerulonephritis

N01.3   Rapidly progressive nephritic syndrome with diffuse mesangial proliferative glomerulonephritis

N01.4   Rapidly progressive nephritic syndrome with diffuse endocapillary proliferative glomerulonephritis

N01.5   Rapidly progressive nephritic syndrome with diffuse mesangiocapillary glomerulonephritis
Rapidly progressive nephritic syndrome with membranoproliferative glomerulonephritis, types 1 and 3, or NOS

N01.6   Rapidly progressive nephritic syndrome with dense deposit disease
Rapidly progressive nephritic syndrome with membranoproliferative glomerulonephritis, type 2

N01.7   Rapidly progressive nephritic syndrome with diffuse crescentic glomerulonephritis
Rapidly progressive nephritic syndrome with extracapillary glomerulonephritis

N01.8   Rapidly progressive nephritic syndrome with other morphologic changes
Rapidly progressive nephritic syndrome with proliferative glomerulonephritis NOS

N01.9   Rapidly progressive nephritic syndrome with unspecified morphologic changes

◢ N02   Recurrent and persistent hematuria

EXCLUDES 1   *acute cystitis with hematuria (N30.01)*
hematuria NOS (R31.9)
hematuria not associated with specified morphologic lesions (R31.-)

N02.0   Recurrent and persistent hematuria with minor glomerular abnormality
Recurrent and persistent hematuria with minimal change lesion

N02.1   Recurrent and persistent hematuria with focal and segmental glomerular lesions
Recurrent and persistent hematuria with focal and segmental hyalinosis
Recurrent and persistent hematuria with focal and segmental sclerosis
Recurrent and persistent hematuria with focal glomerulonephritis

N02.2   Recurrent and persistent hematuria with diffuse membranous glomerulonephritis

N02.3   Recurrent and persistent hematuria with diffuse mesangial proliferative glomerulonephritis

N02.4   Recurrent and persistent hematuria with diffuse endocapillary proliferative glomerulonephritis

N02.5   Recurrent and persistent hematuria with diffuse mesangiocapillary glomerulonephritis
Recurrent and persistent hematuria with membranoproliferative glomerulonephritis, types 1 and 3, or NOS

N02.6   Recurrent and persistent hematuria with dense deposit disease
Recurrent and persistent hematuria with membranoproliferative glomerulonephritis, type 2

N02.7   Recurrent and persistent hematuria with diffuse crescentic glomerulonephritis
Recurrent and persistent hematuria with extracapillary glomerulonephritis

N02.8   Recurrent and persistent hematuria with other morphologic changes
Recurrent and persistent hematuria with proliferative glomerulonephritis NOS

N02.9   Recurrent and persistent hematuria with unspecified morphologic changes

---

● New   ▲ Revised   *Manifestation*   �४-�7 Digit Indicators   ⊟ Laterality   🅰 Adult (15+ years)   Ⓜ Maternity (12-55 years)   Ⓝ Newborn   🅿 Pediatric (0-17 years)   ♂ Male   ♀ Female
✖ Deleted   Unspecified   + Additional code

2017 ICD-10-CM Expert for Physicians

© 2017 DecisionHealth   817

N00 — N02.9

Diseases of the Genitourinary System

⁴ **N03**   **Chronic nephritic syndrome**

INCLUDES   chronic glomerular disease
chronic glomerulonephritis
chronic nephritis

EXCLUDES 1   *chronic tubulo-interstitial nephritis (N11.-)*
diffuse sclerosing glomerulonephritis (N05.8-)
nephritic syndrome NOS (N05.-)

N03.0   **Chronic nephritic syndrome with minor glomerular abnormality**
Chronic nephritic syndrome with minimal change lesion

N03.1   **Chronic nephritic syndrome with focal and segmental glomerular lesions**
Chronic nephritic syndrome with focal and segmental hyalinosis
Chronic nephritic syndrome with focal and segmental sclerosis
Chronic nephritic syndrome with focal glomerulonephritis

N03.2   **Chronic nephritic syndrome with diffuse membranous glomerulonephritis**

N03.3   **Chronic nephritic syndrome with diffuse mesangial proliferative glomerulonephritis**

N03.4   **Chronic nephritic syndrome with diffuse endocapillary proliferative glomerulonephritis**

N03.5   **Chronic nephritic syndrome with diffuse mesangiocapillary glomerulonephritis**
Chronic nephritic syndrome with membranoproliferative glomerulonephritis, types 1 and 3, or NOS

N03.6   **Chronic nephritic syndrome with dense deposit disease**
Chronic nephritic syndrome with membranoproliferative glomerulonephritis, type 2

N03.7   **Chronic nephritic syndrome with diffuse crescentic glomerulonephritis**
Chronic nephritic syndrome with extracapillary glomerulonephritis

N03.8   **Chronic nephritic syndrome with other morphologic changes**
Chronic nephritic syndrome with proliferative glomerulonephritis NOS

N03.9   **Chronic nephritic syndrome with unspecified morphologic changes**

⁴ **N04**   **Nephrotic syndrome**

INCLUDES   congenital nephrotic syndrome
lipoid nephrosis

N04.0   **Nephrotic syndrome with minor glomerular abnormality**
Nephrotic syndrome with minimal change lesion

N04.1   **Nephrotic syndrome with focal and segmental glomerular lesions**
Nephrotic syndrome with focal and segmental hyalinosis
Nephrotic syndrome with focal and segmental sclerosis
Nephrotic syndrome with focal glomerulonephritis

N04.2   **Nephrotic syndrome with diffuse membranous glomerulonephritis**

N04.3   **Nephrotic syndrome with diffuse mesangial proliferative glomerulonephritis**

N04.4   **Nephrotic syndrome with diffuse endocapillary proliferative glomerulonephritis**

N04.5   **Nephrotic syndrome with diffuse mesangiocapillary glomerulonephritis**
Nephrotic syndrome with membranoproliferative glomerulonephritis, types 1 and 3, or NOS

N04.6   **Nephrotic syndrome with dense deposit disease**
Nephrotic syndrome with membranoproliferative glomerulonephritis, type 2

N04.7   **Nephrotic syndrome with diffuse crescentic glomerulonephritis**
Nephrotic syndrome with extracapillary glomerulonephritis

N04.8   **Nephrotic syndrome with other morphologic changes**
Nephrotic syndrome with proliferative glomerulonephritis NOS

N04.9   **Nephrotic syndrome with unspecified morphologic changes**

Nephrotic syndrome with unspecified morphologic changes

Damage to kidneys

Protein from blood leaks into urine, leaving blood deficient

Ureter

Bladder

⁴ **N05**   **Unspecified nephritic syndrome**

INCLUDES   glomerular disease NOS
glomerulonephritis NOS
nephritis NOS
nephropathy NOS and renal disease NOS with morphological lesion specified in .0-.8

EXCLUDES 1   *nephropathy NOS with no stated morphological lesion (N28.9)*
renal disease NOS with no stated morphological lesion (N28.9)
tubulo-interstitial nephritis NOS (N12)

N05.0   **Unspecified nephritic syndrome with minor glomerular abnormality**
Unspecified nephritic syndrome with minimal change lesion

N05.1   **Unspecified nephritic syndrome with focal and segmental glomerular lesions**
Unspecified nephritic syndrome with focal and segmental hyalinosis
Unspecified nephritic syndrome with focal and segmental sclerosis
Unspecified nephritic syndrome with focal glomerulonephritis

N05.2   **Unspecified nephritic syndrome with diffuse membranous glomerulonephritis**

N05.3   **Unspecified nephritic syndrome with diffuse mesangial proliferative glomerulonephritis**

N05.4   **Unspecified nephritic syndrome with diffuse endocapillary proliferative glomerulonephritis**

N05.5   **Unspecified nephritic syndrome with diffuse mesangiocapillary glomerulonephritis**
Unspecified nephritic syndrome with membranoproliferative glomerulonephritis, types 1 and 3, or NOS

N05.6   **Unspecified nephritic syndrome with dense deposit disease**
Unspecified nephritic syndrome with membranoproliferative glomerulonephritis, type 2

N05.7   **Unspecified nephritic syndrome with diffuse crescentic glomerulonephritis**
Unspecified nephritic syndrome with extracapillary glomerulonephritis

N05.8   **Unspecified nephritic syndrome with other morphologic changes**
Unspecified nephritic syndrome with proliferative glomerulonephritis NOS

N05.9   **Unspecified nephritic syndrome with unspecified morphologic changes**

⁴ **N06**   **Isolated proteinuria with specified morphological lesion**

EXCLUDES 1   *Proteinuria not associated with specific morphologic lesions (R80.0)*

N06.0   **Isolated proteinuria with minor glomerular abnormality**
Isolated proteinuria with minimal change lesion

N06.1   **Isolated proteinuria with focal and segmental glomerular lesions**
Isolated proteinuria with focal and segmental hyalinosis
Isolated proteinuria with focal and segmental sclerosis
Isolated proteinuria with focal glomerulonephritis

N06.2   **Isolated proteinuria with diffuse membranous glomerulonephritis**

N06.3   **Isolated proteinuria with diffuse mesangial proliferative glomerulonephritis**

● New   ▲ Revised   *Manifestation*   ⁴-⁷ Digit Indicators   ▱ Laterality   Ⓐ Adult (15+ years)   Ⓜ Maternity (12-55 years)   Ⓝ Newborn   Ⓟ Pediatric (0-17 years)   ♂ Male   ♀ Female
✖ Deleted   Unspecified   + Additional code

818   © 2017 DecisionHealth   2017 ICD-10-CM Expert for Physicians

N06.4 Isolated proteinuria with diffuse endocapillary proliferative glomerulonephritis

N06.5 Isolated proteinuria with diffuse mesangiocapillary glomerulonephritis
Isolated proteinuria with membranoproliferative glomerulonephritis, types 1 and 3, or NOS

N06.6 Isolated proteinuria with dense deposit disease
Isolated proteinuria with membranoproliferative glomerulonephritis, type 2

N06.7 Isolated proteinuria with diffuse crescentic glomerulonephritis
Isolated proteinuria with extracapillary glomerulonephritis

N06.8 Isolated proteinuria with other morphologic lesion
Isolated proteinuria with proliferative glomerulonephritis NOS

N06.9 Isolated proteinuria with unspecified morphologic lesion

▣ **N07** Hereditary nephropathy, not elsewhere classified

EXCLUDES 2   *Alport's syndrome (Q87.81-)*
hereditary amyloid nephropathy (E85.-)
nail patella syndrome (Q87.2)
non-neuropathic heredofamilial amyloidosis (E85.-)

N07.0 Hereditary nephropathy, not elsewhere classified with minor glomerular abnormality
Hereditary nephropathy, not elsewhere classified with minimal change lesion

N07.1 Hereditary nephropathy, not elsewhere classified with focal and segmental glomerular lesions
Hereditary nephropathy, not elsewhere classified with focal and segmental hyalinosis
Hereditary nephropathy, not elsewhere classified with focal and segmental sclerosis
Hereditary nephropathy, not elsewhere classified with focal glomerulonephritis

N07.2 Hereditary nephropathy, not elsewhere classified with diffuse membranous glomerulonephritis

N07.3 Hereditary nephropathy, not elsewhere classified with diffuse mesangial proliferative glomerulonephritis

N07.4 Hereditary nephropathy, not elsewhere classified with diffuse endocapillary proliferative glomerulonephritis

N07.5 Hereditary nephropathy, not elsewhere classified with diffuse mesangiocapillary glomerulonephritis
Hereditary nephropathy, not elsewhere classified with membranoproliferative glomerulonephritis, types 1 and 3, or NOS

N07.6 Hereditary nephropathy, not elsewhere classified with dense deposit disease
Hereditary nephropathy, not elsewhere classified with membranoproliferative glomerulonephritis, type 2

N07.7 Hereditary nephropathy, not elsewhere classified with diffuse crescentic glomerulonephritis
Hereditary nephropathy, not elsewhere classified with extracapillary glomerulonephritis

N07.8 Hereditary nephropathy, not elsewhere classified with other morphologic lesions
Hereditary nephropathy, not elsewhere classified with proliferative glomerulonephritis NOS

N07.9 Hereditary nephropathy, not elsewhere classified with unspecified morphologic lesions

N08   *Glomerular disorders in diseases classified elsewhere*
Glomerulonephritis
Nephritis
Nephropathy
Code first underlying disease, such as:
amyloidosis (E85.-)
congenital syphilis (A50.5)
cryoglobulinemia (D89.1)
disseminated intravascular coagulation (D65)
gout (M1A.-, M10.-)
microscopic polyangiitis (M31.7)
multiple myeloma (C90.0-)
sepsis (A40.0-A41.9)
sickle-cell disease (D57.0-D57.8)

EXCLUDES 1   *glomerulonephritis, nephritis and nephropathy (in):*
antiglomerular basement membrane disease (M31.0)
diabetes (E08-E13 with .21)
gonococcal (A54.21)
Goodpasture's syndrome (M31.0)
hemolytic-uremic syndrome (D59.3)
lupus (M32.14)
mumps (B26.83)
syphilis (A52.75)
systemic lupus erythematosus (M32.14)
Wegener's granulomatosis (M31.31)
pyelonephritis in diseases classified elsewhere (N16)
renal tubulo-interstitial disorders classified elsewhere (N16)

CODING TIP ✓   Do not assign code N08 for a patient diagnosed with diabetic nephropathy. For a patient diagnosed with diabetic nephropathy, choose and assign the appropriate combination code to specify the manifestation from categories E08-E13 with 4th and 5th characters .21.

Renal tubulo-interstitial diseases (N10-N16)

INCLUDES   pyelonephritis

EXCLUDES 1   *pyeloureteritis cystica (N28.85)*

▲ ✚ **N10** Acute pyelonephritis
Acute infectious interstitial nephritis
Acute pyelitis
Acute tubulo-interstitial nephritis
Hemoglobin nephrosis
Myoglobin nephrosis
Use additional code (B95-B97), to identify infectious agent.

▣ ✚ **N11** Chronic tubulo-interstitial nephritis
INCLUDES   chronic infectious interstitial nephritis
chronic pyelitis
chronic pyelonephritis
Use additional code (B95-B97), to identify infectious agent.

✚ **N11.0** Nonobstructive reflux-associated chronic pyelonephritis
Pyelonephritis (chronic) associated with (vesicoureteral) reflux

EXCLUDES 1   *vesicoureteral reflux NOS (N13.70)*

✚ **N11.1** Chronic obstructive pyelonephritis
Pyelonephritis (chronic) associated with anomaly of pelviureteric junction
Pyelonephritis (chronic) associated with anomaly of pyeloureteric junction
Pyelonephritis (chronic) associated with crossing of vessel
Pyelonephritis (chronic) associated with kinking of ureter
Pyelonephritis (chronic) associated with obstruction of ureter
Pyelonephritis (chronic) associated with stricture of pelviureteric junction
Pyelonephritis (chronic) associated with stricture of ureter

EXCLUDES 1   *calculous pyelonephritis (N20.9)*
obstructive uropathy (N13.-)

✚ **N11.8** Other chronic tubulo-interstitial nephritis
Nonobstructive chronic pyelonephritis NOS

✚ **N11.9** Chronic tubulo-interstitial nephritis, unspecified
Chronic interstitial nephritis NOS
Chronic pyelitis NOS
Chronic pyelonephritis NOS

● New ▲ Revised *Manifestation* ▣-▭ Digit Indicators ▤ Laterality Ⓐ Adult (15+ years) Ⓜ Maternity (12-55 years) Ⓝ Newborn Ⓟ Pediatric (0-17 years) ♂ Male ♀ Female
✖ Deleted Unspecified ✚ Additional code

2017 ICD-10-CM Expert for Physicians   © 2017 DecisionHealth   819

N12 **Tubulo-interstitial nephritis, not specified as acute or chronic**
Interstitial nephritis NOS
Pyelitis NOS
Pyelonephritis NOS
EXCLUDES 1 *calculous pyelonephritis (N20.9)*

⬛ N13 **Obstructive and reflux uropathy**
EXCLUDES 2 *calculus of kidney and ureter without hydronephrosis (N20.-)*
congenital obstructive defects of renal pelvis and ureter (Q62.0-Q62.3)
hydronephrosis with ureteropelvic junction obstruction (Q62.1)
obstructive pyelonephritis (N11.1)

● **N13.0** **Hydronephrosis with ureteropelvic junction obstruction**
Hydronephrosis due to acquired occlusion of ureteropelvic junction
EXCLUDES 2 *Hydronephrosis with ureteropelvic junction obstruction due to calculus (N13.2)*

N13.1 **Hydronephrosis with ureteral stricture, not elsewhere classified**
EXCLUDES 1 *Hydronephrosis with ureteral stricture with infection (N13.6)*

N13.2 **Hydronephrosis with renal and ureteral calculous obstruction**
EXCLUDES 1 *Hydronephrosis with renal and ureteral calculous obstruction with infection (N13.6)*

⬛ N13.3 **Other and unspecified hydronephrosis**
EXCLUDES 1 *hydronephrosis with infection (N13.6)*

N13.30 **Unspecified hydronephrosis**
N13.39 **Other hydronephrosis**

N13.4 **Hydroureter**
EXCLUDES 1 *congenital hydroureter (Q62.3-)*
hydroureter with infection (N13.6)
vesicoureteral-reflux with hydroureter (N13.73-)

N13.5 **Crossing vessel and stricture of ureter without hydronephrosis**
Kinking and stricture of ureter without hydronephrosis
EXCLUDES 1 *Crossing vessel and stricture of ureter without hydronephrosis with infection (N13.6)*

Crossing vessel and stricture of ureter without hydronephrosis

▲ + **N13.6** **Pyonephrosis**
Conditions in N13.0-N13.5 with infection
Obstructive uropathy with infection
Use additional code (B95-B97), to identify infectious agent.

⬛ N13.7 **Vesicoureteral-reflux**
EXCLUDES 1 *reflux-associated pyelonephritis (N11.0)*

N13.70 **Vesicoureteral-reflux, unspecified**
Vesicoureteral-reflux NOS
DEFINITION Abnormal retrograde flow of urine from bladder back into the ureter and kidney; may cause progressive, long-term damage.

N13.71 **Vesicoureteral-reflux without reflux nephropathy**
⬛ N13.72 **Vesicoureteral-reflux with reflux nephropathy without hydroureter**
N13.721 **Vesicoureteral-reflux with reflux nephropathy without hydroureter, unilateral**
N13.722 **Vesicoureteral-reflux with reflux nephropathy without hydroureter, bilateral**

N13.729 **Vesicoureteral-reflux with reflux nephropathy without hydroureter, unspecified**
⬛ N13.73 **Vesicoureteral-reflux with reflux nephropathy with hydroureter**
N13.731 **Vesicoureteral-reflux with reflux nephropathy with hydroureter, unilateral**
N13.732 **Vesicoureteral-reflux with reflux nephropathy with hydroureter, bilateral**
N13.739 **Vesicoureteral-reflux with reflux nephropathy with hydroureter, unspecified**

N13.8 **Other obstructive and reflux uropathy**
Urinary tract obstruction due to specified cause
Code first, if applicable, any causal condition, such as:
enlarged prostate (N40.1)

N13.9 **Obstructive and reflux uropathy, unspecified**
Urinary tract obstruction NOS

Obstructive and reflux uropathy, unspecified

Kidney
Ureter
Bladder
Prostate
Urethra
Obstruction anywhere in urinary tract

⬛ + N14 **Drug- and heavy-metal-induced tubulo-interstitial and tubular conditions**
Code first:
poisoning due to drug or toxin, if applicable
(T36-T65 with fifth or sixth character 1-4 or 6)
Use additional code for adverse effect, if applicable, to identify drug (T36-T50 with fifth or sixth character 5)
CODING TIP ✓ Conditions classified to N14.- indicate nephropathy due to drugs, metals, or other toxic exposure. When one of these conditions has been specifically reported, first assign the appropriate code from T36-T65 when the condition is due to a poisoning. Or, to indicate adverse effect, assign a second code from T36-T50 following the appropriate N14.- code.

+ **N14.0** **Analgesic nephropathy**
+ **N14.1** **Nephropathy induced by other drugs, medicaments and biological substances**
+ **N14.2** **Nephropathy induced by unspecified drug, medicament or biological substance**
+ **N14.3** **Nephropathy induced by heavy metals**
+ **N14.4** **Toxic nephropathy, not elsewhere classified**

⬛ N15 **Other renal tubulo-interstitial diseases**
N15.0 **Balkan nephropathy**
Balkan endemic nephropathy
N15.1 **Renal and perinephric abscess**
N15.8 **Other specified renal tubulo-interstitial diseases**
N15.9 **Renal tubulo-interstitial disease, unspecified**
Infection of kidney NOS
EXCLUDES 1 *urinary tract infection NOS (N39.0)*

N16   *Renal tubulo-interstitial disorders in diseases classified elsewhere*

Pyelonephritis
Tubulo-interstitial nephritis
Code first underlying disease, such as:
  brucellosis (A23.0-A23.9)
  cryoglobulinemia (D89.1)
  glycogen storage disease (E74.0)
  leukemia (C91-C95)
  lymphoma (C81.0-C85.9, C96.0-C96.9)
  multiple myeloma (C90.0-)
  sepsis (A40.0-A41.9)
  Wilson's disease (E83.0)

> **EXCLUDES 1**   *diphtheritic pyelonephritis and tubulo-interstitial nephritis (A36.84)*
> *pyelonephritis and tubulo-interstitial nephritis in candidiasis (B37.49)*
> *pyelonephritis and tubulo-interstitial nephritis in cystinosis (E72.04)*
> *pyelonephritis and tubulo-interstitial nephritis in salmonella infection (A02.25)*
> *pyelonephritis and tubulo-interstitial nephritis in sarcoidosis (D86.84)*
> *pyelonephritis and tubulo-interstitial nephritis in sicca syndrome [Sjogren's] (M35.04)*
> *pyelonephritis and tubulo-interstitial nephritis in systemic lupus erythematosus (M32.15)*
> *pyelonephritis and tubulo-interstitial nephritis in toxoplasmosis (B58.83)*
> *renal tubular degeneration in diabetes (E08-E13 with .29)*
> *syphilitic pyelonephritis and tubulo-interstitial nephritis (A52.75)*

Acute kidney failure and chronic kidney disease (N17-N19)

> **EXCLUDES 2**   *congenital renal failure (P96.0)*
> *drug- and heavy-metal-induced tubulo-interstitial and tubular conditions (N14.-)*
> *extrarenal uremia (R39.2)*
> *hemolytic-uremic syndrome (D59.3)*
> *hepatorenal syndrome (K76.7)*
> *postpartum hepatorenal syndrome (O90.4)*
> *posttraumatic renal failure (T79.5)*
> *prerenal uremia (R39.2)*
> *renal failure complicating abortion or ectopic or molar pregnancy (O00-O07, O08.4)*
> *renal failure following labor and delivery (O90.4)*
> *renal failure postprocedural (N99.0)*

N17   **Acute kidney failure**

Code also:
  associated underlying condition

> **EXCLUDES 1**   *posttraumatic renal failure (T79.5)*

> **GUIDELINES**   **Section I.C.9.a.2)**
> If a patient has hypertensive chronic kidney disease and acute renal failure, an additional code for the acute renal failure [category N17] is required.

> **CODING TIP ✓**   When both acute kidney failure and chronic kidney disease (CKD) are present, both conditions should be coded.

N17.0   **Acute kidney failure with tubular necrosis**
Acute tubular necrosis
Renal tubular necrosis
Tubular necrosis NOS

Acute kidney failure
with tubular necrosis

Kidney
Renal artery
Renal vein
Ureter
Destruction
of tubules

N17.1   **Acute kidney failure with acute cortical necrosis**
Acute cortical necrosis
Cortical necrosis NOS
Renal cortical necrosis

N17.2   **Acute kidney failure with medullary necrosis**
Medullary [papillary] necrosis NOS
Acute medullary [papillary] necrosis
Renal medullary [papillary] necrosis

N17.8   **Other acute kidney failure**

N17.9   **Acute kidney failure, unspecified**
Acute kidney injury (nontraumatic)

> **EXCLUDES 2**   *traumatic kidney injury (S37.0-)*

N18   **Chronic kidney disease (CKD)**

Code first any associated:
  diabetic chronic kidney disease (E08.22, E09.22, E10.22, E11.22, E13.22)
  hypertensive chronic kidney disease (I12.-, I13.-)
Use additional code to identify kidney transplant status, if applicable, (Z94.0)

> **GUIDELINES**   **Section I.C.14.a.1)**
> The ICD-10-CM classifies CKD based on severity. The severity of CKD is designated by stages 1-5. Stage 2, code N18.2, equates to mild CKD; stage 3, code N18.3, equates to moderate CKD; and stage 4, code N18.4, equates to severe CKD. Code N18.6, End stage renal disease (ESRD), is assigned when the provider has documented end-stage-renal disease (ESRD). If both a stage of CKD and ESRD are documented, assign code N18.6 only.

> **GUIDELINES**   **Section I.C.14.a.2)**
> Patients who have undergone kidney transplant may still have some form of chronic kidney disease (CKD) because the kidney transplant may not fully restore kidney function. Therefore, the presence of CKD alone does not constitute a transplant complication. Assign the appropriate N18 code for the patient's stage of CKD and code Z94.0, Kidney transplant status. If a transplant complication such as failure or rejection or other transplant complication is documented, see section I.C.19.g for information on coding complications of a kidney transplant. If the documentation is unclear as to whether the patient has a complication of the transplant, query the provider.

> **GUIDELINES**   **Section I.C.14.a.3)**
> Patients with CKD may also suffer from other serious conditions, most commonly diabetes mellitus and hypertension. The sequencing of the CKD code in relationship to codes for other contributing conditions is based on the conventions in the Tabular List.

> **CODING TIP ✓**   Note that when assigning a code from N18.- as a confirmed manifestation of Diabetes Mellitus, that the code N18.9 is not an allowed pairing. Only N18.1-N18.6 may be assigned as additional diagnoses to identify the stage of chronic kidney disease when this is a confirmed manifestation of Diabetes Mellitus.

> **CODING TIP ✓**   **Documentation:** The stage of chronic kidney disease may be identified and determined by referencing any available current lab work in the clinical record and configuring the stage according to the Glomerular Filtration Rate (GFR).

+ **N18.1**   **Chronic kidney disease, stage 1**
+ **N18.2**   **Chronic kidney disease, stage 2 (mild)**
+ **N18.3**   **Chronic kidney disease, stage 3 (moderate)**

● New   ▲ Revised   *Manifestation*   ❹-❼ Digit Indicators   ⊟ Laterality   🄰 Adult (15+ years)   🄼 Maternity (12-55 years)   🄽 Newborn   🄿 Pediatric (0-17 years)   ♂ Male   ♀ Female
✖ Deleted   Unspecified   + Additional code

+ N18.4   **Chronic kidney disease, stage 4 (severe)**
AHA: 1Q 2013, 24

+ N18.5   **Chronic kidney disease, stage 5**
EXCLUDES 1   *chronic kidney disease, stage 5 requiring chronic dialysis (N18.6)*

+ N18.6   **End stage renal disease**
Chronic kidney disease requiring chronic dialysis
Use additional code to identify dialysis status (Z99.2)
AHA: 1Q 2016, 12-13
AHA: 4Q 2013, 124, 125

+ N18.9   **Chronic kidney disease, unspecified**
Chronic renal disease
Chronic renal failure NOS
Chronic renal insufficiency
Chronic uremia

N19   **Unspecified kidney failure**
Uremia NOS
EXCLUDES 1   *acute kidney failure (N17.-)*
chronic kidney disease (N18.-)
chronic uremia (N18.9)
extrarenal uremia (R39.2)
prerenal uremia (R39.2)
renal insufficiency (acute) (N28.9)
uremia of newborn (P96.0)

Urolithiasis (N20-N23)

◰ N20   **Calculus of kidney and ureter**
Calculous pyelonephritis
EXCLUDES 1   *nephrocalcinosis (E83.5)*
that with hydronephrosis (N13.2)

N20.0   **Calculus of kidney**
Nephrolithiasis NOS
Renal calculus
Renal stone
Staghorn calculus
Stone in kidney

N20.1   **Calculus of ureter**
Ureteric stone

Calculus of ureter

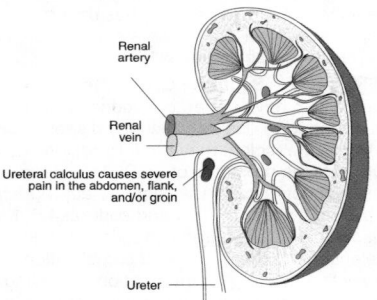

Renal artery
Renal vein
Ureteral calculus causes severe pain in the abdomen, flank, and/or groin
Ureter

N20.2   **Calculus of kidney with calculus of ureter**
N20.9   **Urinary calculus, unspecified**

◰ N21   **Calculus of lower urinary tract**
INCLUDES   calculus of lower urinary tract with cystitis and urethritis

N21.0   **Calculus in bladder**
Calculus in diverticulum of bladder
Urinary bladder stone
EXCLUDES 2   *staghorn calculus (N20.0)*

DEFINITION   An abnormal concretion of mineral salts, occurring in the bladder.

N21.1   **Calculus in urethra**
EXCLUDES 2   *calculus of prostate (N42.0)*

Calculus in urethra

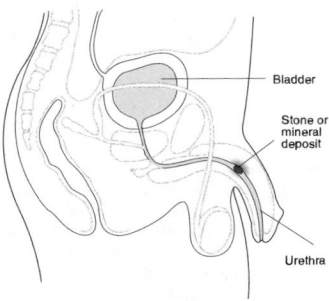

Bladder
Stone or mineral deposit
Urethra

N21.8   **Other lower urinary tract calculus**
N21.9   **Calculus of lower urinary tract, unspecified**
EXCLUDES 1   *calculus of urinary tract NOS (N20.9)*

N22   *Calculus of urinary tract in diseases classified elsewhere*
Code first underlying disease, such as:
gout (M1A.-, M10.-)
schistosomiasis (B65.0-B65.9)

N23   **Unspecified renal colic**

Other disorders of kidney and ureter (N25-N29)

EXCLUDES 2   *disorders of kidney and ureter with urolithiasis (N20-N23)*

◰ N25   **Disorders resulting from impaired renal tubular function**
EXCLUDES 1   *metabolic disorders classifiable to E70-E88*

N25.0   **Renal osteodystrophy**
Azotemic osteodystrophy
Phosphate-losing tubular disorders
Renal rickets
Renal short stature

N25.1   **Nephrogenic diabetes insipidus**
EXCLUDES 1   *diabetes insipidus NOS (E23.2)*

◳ N25.8   **Other disorders resulting from impaired renal tubular function**

N25.81   **Secondary hyperparathyroidism of renal origin**
EXCLUDES 1   *secondary hyperparathyroidism, non-renal (E21.1)*

N25.89   **Other disorders resulting from impaired renal tubular function**
Hypokalemic nephropathy
Lightwood-Albright syndrome
Renal tubular acidosis NOS

N25.9   **Disorder resulting from impaired renal tubular function, unspecified**

◰ N26   **Unspecified contracted kidney**
EXCLUDES 1   *contracted kidney due to hypertension (I12.-)*
diffuse sclerosing glomerulonephritis (N05.8.-)
hypertensive nephrosclerosis (arteriolar) (arteriosclerotic) (I12.-)
small kidney of unknown cause (N27.-)

CODING TIP ✓   When a condition classifiable to N26.- is present in combination with a diagnosis of hypertension, I12.9 should be assigned followed by the appropriate N26.- code.

N26.1   **Atrophy of kidney (terminal)**
N26.2   **Page kidney**

● New   ▲ Revised   *Manifestation*   ◰-◷ Digit Indicators   ⊟ Laterality   Ⓐ Adult (15+ years)   Ⓜ Maternity (12-55 years)   Ⓝ Newborn   Ⓟ Pediatric (0-17 years)   ♂ Male   ♀ Female
✖ Deleted   Unspecified   + Additional code

822   © 2017 DecisionHealth   2017 ICD-10-CM Expert for Physicians

N26.9   Renal sclerosis, unspecified

Renal sclerosis

Renal artery — Renal vein — Ureter — Kidney hardens — Fibrous tissue deposits develop

N27   Small kidney of unknown cause

INCLUDES   oligonephronia

N27.0   **Small kidney, unilateral**
N27.1   **Small kidney, bilateral**
N27.9   **Small kidney, unspecified**

N28   Other disorders of kidney and ureter, not elsewhere classified

N28.0   **Ischemia and infarction of kidney**
Renal artery embolism
Renal artery obstruction
Renal artery occlusion
Renal artery thrombosis
Renal infarct

EXCLUDES 1   *atherosclerosis of renal artery (extrarenal part) (I70.1)*
congenital stenosis of renal artery (Q27.1)
Goldblatt's kidney (I70.1)

N28.1   **Cyst of kidney, acquired**
Cyst (multiple)(solitary) of kidney, acquired

EXCLUDES 1   *cystic kidney disease (congenital) (Q61.-)*

CODING TIP ✓   N28.1 is coded only for acquired renal cysts. Note that cysts documented as single or solitary are considered congenital while those documented as simple are considered acquired. If the medical record is not clear as to whether the cyst is acquired or congenital the provider should be queried. Carefully review documentation provided to assure that the location of cyst is in the kidney. Cysts noted to be present in the ureters are not classified here.

N28.8   **Other specified disorders of kidney and ureter**

EXCLUDES 1   *hydroureter (N13.4)*
ureteric stricture with hydronephrosis (N13.1)
ureteric stricture without hydronephrosis (N13.5)

N28.81   **Hypertrophy of kidney**
N28.82   **Megaloureter**
N28.83   **Nephroptosis**
N28.84   **Pyelitis cystica**
N28.85   **Pyeloureteritis cystica**

DEFINITION   Infection of the renal pelvis and ureter with development of small cysts in the kidney and ureter.

N28.86   **Ureteritis cystica**
N28.89   **Other specified disorders of kidney and ureter**
N28.9   **Disorder of kidney and ureter, unspecified**
Nephropathy NOS
Renal disease (acute) NOS
Renal insufficiency (acute)

EXCLUDES 1   *chronic renal insufficiency (N18.9)*
unspecified nephritic syndrome (N05.-)

AHA: 1Q 2016, 13

N29   *Other disorders of kidney and ureter in diseases classified elsewhere*
Code first underlying disease, such as:
amyloidosis (E85.-)
nephrocalcinosis (E83.5)
schistosomiasis (B65.0-B65.9)

EXCLUDES 1   *disorders of kidney and ureter in:*
cystinosis (E72.0)
gonorrhea (A54.21)
syphilis (A52.75)
tuberculosis (A18.11)

Other diseases of the urinary system (N30-N39)

EXCLUDES 1   *urinary infection (complicating) :*
abortion or ectopic or molar pregnancy (O00-O07, O08.8)
pregnancy, childbirth and the puerperium (O23.-, O75.3, O86.2-)

N30   Cystitis
Use additional code to identify infectious agent (B95-B97)

EXCLUDES 1   *prostatocystitis (N41.3)*

CODING TIP ✓   Cystitis indicates inflammation and/or infection localized to the bladder. When a urinary tract infection is specified as cystitis, assign the appropriate N30.- code. Also assign a code for the causative organism, when known. An unspecified urinary tract infection should be coded to N39.0.

N30.0   Acute cystitis

EXCLUDES 1   *irradiation cystitis (N30.4-)*
trigonitis (N30.3-)

N30.00   **Acute cystitis without hematuria**
N30.01   **Acute cystitis with hematuria**

N30.1   Interstitial cystitis (chronic)
N30.10   **Interstitial cystitis (chronic) without hematuria**
N30.11   **Interstitial cystitis (chronic) with hematuria**

N30.2   Other chronic cystitis
N30.20   **Other chronic cystitis without hematuria**
N30.21   **Other chronic cystitis with hematuria**

N30.3   Trigonitis
Urethrotrigonitis

DEFINITION   Inflammation of the mouth of the bladder where it drains into the urethra.

N30.30   **Trigonitis without hematuria**
N30.31   **Trigonitis with hematuria**

N30.4   Irradiation cystitis
N30.40   **Irradiation cystitis without hematuria**
N30.41   **Irradiation cystitis with hematuria**

N30.8   Other cystitis
Abscess of bladder
N30.80   **Other cystitis without hematuria**
N30.81   **Other cystitis with hematuria**

DEFINITION   Bullous (cystic) cystitis: Inflammation of the bladder with formation of cysts on the interior bladder wall.

N30.9   Cystitis, unspecified
N30.90   **Cystitis, unspecified without hematuria**
N30.91   **Cystitis, unspecified with hematuria**

N31   Neuromuscular dysfunction of bladder, not elsewhere classified
Use additional code to identify any associated urinary incontinence (N39.3-N39.4-)

EXCLUDES 1   *cord bladder NOS (G95.89)*
neurogenic bladder due to cauda equina syndrome (G83.4)
neuromuscular dysfunction due to spinal cord lesion (G95.89)

N31.0   **Uninhibited neuropathic bladder, not elsewhere classified**
N31.1   **Reflex neuropathic bladder, not elsewhere classified**

● New   ▲ Revised   *Manifestation*   ◆-❼ Digit Indicators   ⊟ Laterality   Ⓐ Adult (15+ years)   Ⓜ Maternity (12-55 years)   Ⓝ Newborn   Ⓟ Pediatric (0-17 years)   ♂ Male   ♀ Female
✖ Deleted   Unspecified   ✚ Additional code

2017 ICD-10-CM Expert for Physicians

© 2017 DecisionHealth   823

N26.9 — N31.1

+ N31.2   Flaccid neuropathic bladder, not elsewhere classified
Atonic (motor) (sensory) neuropathic bladder
Autonomous neuropathic bladder
Nonreflex neuropathic bladder

Flaccid neuropthic bladder, not elsewhere classified

+ N31.8   Other neuromuscular dysfunction of bladder
+ N31.9   Neuromuscular dysfunction of bladder, unspecified
Neurogenic bladder dysfunction NOS

▣ N32   Other disorders of bladder

> EXCLUDES 2   *calculus of bladder (N21.0)*
> *cystocele (N81.1-)*
> *hernia or prolapse of bladder, female (N81.1-)*

N32.0   Bladder-neck obstruction
Bladder-neck stenosis (acquired)

> EXCLUDES 1   *congenital bladder-neck obstruction*
> *(Q64.3-)*

> DEFINITION   Blockage in the opening between the bladder and the urethra, causing bladder distention and decreased urine output.

N32.1   Vesicointestinal fistula
Vesicorectal fistula

> DEFINITION   Abnormal passage between the bladder and the intestines.

N32.2   Vesical fistula, not elsewhere classified

> EXCLUDES 1   *fistula between bladder and female genital tract (N82.0-N82.1)*

N32.3   Diverticulum of bladder

> EXCLUDES 1   *congenital diverticulum of bladder (Q64.6)*
> *diverticulitis of bladder (N30.8-)*

▣ N32.8   Other specified disorders of bladder

N32.81   Overactive bladder
Detrusor muscle hyperactivity

> EXCLUDES 1   *frequent urination due to specified bladder condition- code to condition*

N32.89   Other specified disorders of bladder
Bladder hemorrhage
Bladder hypertrophy
Calcified bladder
Contracted bladder

N32.9   Bladder disorder, unspecified

N33   *Bladder disorders in diseases classified elsewhere*

Code first underlying disease, such as:
schistosomiasis (B65.0-B65.9)

> EXCLUDES 1   *bladder disorder in syphilis (A52.76)*
> *bladder disorder in tuberculosis (A18.12)*
> *candidal cystitis (B37.41)*
> *chlamydial cystitis (A56.01)*
> *cystitis in gonorrhea (A54.01)*
> *cystitis in neurogenic bladder (N31.-)*
> *diphtheritic cystitis (A36.85)*
> *syphilitic cystitis (A52.76)*
> *trichomonal cystitis (A59.03)*

▣+ N34   Urethritis and urethral syndrome
Use additional code (B95-B97), to identify infectious agent.

> EXCLUDES 2   *Reiter's disease (M02.3-)*
> *urethritis in diseases with a predominantly sexual mode of transmission (A50-A64)*
> *urethrotrigonitis (N30.3-)*

+ N34.0   Urethral abscess
Abscess (of) Cowper's gland
Abscess (of) Littré's gland
Abscess (of) urethral (gland)
Periurethral abscess

> EXCLUDES 1   *urethral caruncle (N36.2)*

Urethral abscess

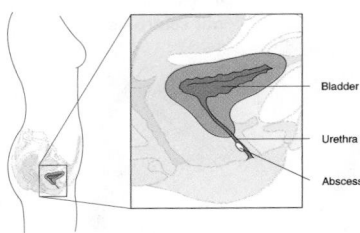

- Bladder
- Urethra
- Abscess

+ N34.1   Nonspecific urethritis
Nongonococcal urethritis
Nonvenereal urethritis

+ N34.2   Other urethritis
Meatitis, urethral
Postmenopausal urethritis
Ulcer of urethra (meatus)
Urethritis NOS

+ N34.3   Urethral syndrome, unspecified

▣ N35   Urethral stricture

> EXCLUDES 1   *congenital urethral stricture (Q64.3-)*
> *postprocedural urethral stricture (N99.1-)*

⑤ N35.0   Post-traumatic urethral stricture
Urethral stricture due to injury

> EXCLUDES 1   *postprocedural urethral stricture (N99.1-)*

⑥ N35.01   Post-traumatic urethral stricture, male

N35.010   Post-traumatic urethral stricture, male, meatal   ♂

N35.011   Post-traumatic bulbous urethral stricture

N35.012   Post-traumatic membranous urethral stricture

N35.013   Post-traumatic anterior urethral stricture

N35.014   Post-traumatic urethral stricture, male, unspecified   ♂

⑥ N35.02   Post-traumatic urethral stricture, female

N35.021   Urethral stricture due to childbirth   ♀

N35.028   Other post-traumatic urethral stricture, female   ♀

⑤ N35.1   Postinfective urethral stricture, not elsewhere classified

> EXCLUDES 1   *urethral stricture associated with schistosomiasis (B65.-, N29)*
> *gonococcal urethral stricture (A54.01)*
> *syphilitic urethral stricture (A52.76)*

⑥ N35.11   Postinfective urethral stricture, not elsewhere classified, male

N35.111   Postinfective urethral stricture, not elsewhere classified, male, meatal   ♂

N35.112   Postinfective bulbous urethral stricture, not elsewhere classified

N35.113   Postinfective membranous urethral stricture, not elsewhere classified

N35.114   Postinfective anterior urethral stricture, not elsewhere classified

N35.119   Postinfective urethral stricture, not elsewhere classified, male, unspecified   ♂

N35.12   Postinfective urethral stricture, not elsewhere classified, female   ♀

N35.8   Other urethral stricture

> EXCLUDES 1   *postprocedural urethral stricture (N99.1-)*

N35.9   Urethral stricture, unspecified

▣ N36   Other disorders of urethra

▲ N36.0   Urethral fistula
Urethroperineal fistula
Urethrorectal fistula
Urinary fistula NOS

> EXCLUDES 1   *urethroscrotal fistula (N50.89)*
> *urethrovaginal fistula (N82.1)*
> *urethrovesicovaginal fistula (N82.1)*

> DEFINITION   An abnormal passage communicating with the urethra.

N36.1   Urethral diverticulum

> DEFINITION   Sac-like out-pouching of the urethral wall.

● New   ▲ Revised   *Manifestation*   ▣-❼ Digit Indicators   ▤ Laterality   Ⓐ Adult (15+ years)   Ⓜ Maternity (12-55 years)   Ⓝ Newborn   Ⓟ Pediatric (0-17 years)   ♂ Male   ♀ Female
✖ Deleted   Unspecified   + Additional code

824   © 2017 DecisionHealth   2017 ICD-10-CM Expert for Physicians

Diseases of the Genitourinary System

N36.2 **Urethral caruncle**

DEFINITION A fleshy outgrowth in the urethra that may be normal or abnormal, often growing from mucous membranes.

⑤➕ N36.4 **Urethral functional and muscular disorders**
Use additional code to identify associated urinary stress incontinence (N39.3)

➕ N36.41 **Hypermobility of urethra**
➕ N36.42 **Intrinsic sphincter deficiency (ISD)**
➕ N36.43 **Combined hypermobility of urethra and intrinsic sphincter deficiency**
➕ N36.44 **Muscular disorders of urethra**
Bladder sphincter dyssynergy

N36.5 **Urethral false passage**
▲ N36.8 **Other specified disorders of urethra**
EXCLUDES 1 *congenital urethrocele (Q64.7)*
female urethrocele (N81.0)

N36.9 **Urethral disorder, unspecified**

N37 *Urethral disorders in diseases classified elsewhere*
Code first:
underlying disease
EXCLUDES 1 *urethritis (in) :*
candidal infection (B37.41)
chlamydial (A56.01)
gonorrhea (A54.01)
syphilis (A52.76)
trichomonal infection (A59.03)
tuberculosis (A18.13)

④ N39 **Other disorders of urinary system**
EXCLUDES 2 *hematuria NOS (R31.-)*
recurrent or persistent hematuria (N02.-)
recurrent or persistent hematuria with specified morphological lesion (N02.-)
proteinuria NOS (R80.-)

➕ N39.0 **Urinary tract infection, site not specified**
Use additional code (B95-B97), to identify infectious agent.
EXCLUDES 1 *candidiasis of urinary tract (B37.4-)*
neonatal urinary tract infection (P39.3)
urinary tract infection of specified site, such as:
cystitis (N30.-)
urethritis (N34.-)
AHA: 4Q 2012, 94

N39.3 **Stress incontinence (female) (male)**
Code also:
any associated overactive bladder (N32.81)
EXCLUDES 1 *mixed incontinence (N39.46)*
DEFINITION Involuntary loss of bladder control during physical movements, such as coughing, sneezing, or other strenuous activity.

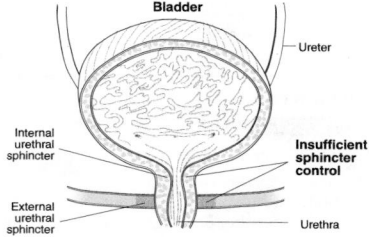

Stress incontinence, (female) (male)

Bladder
Ureter
Internal urethral sphincter
Insufficient sphincter control
External urethral sphincter
Urethra

⑤ N39.4 **Other specified urinary incontinence**
Code also:
any associated overactive bladder (N32.81)
EXCLUDES 1 *enuresis NOS (R32)*
functional urinary incontinence (R39.81)
urinary incontinence associated with cognitive impairment (R39.81)
urinary incontinence NOS (R32)
urinary incontinence of nonorganic origin (F98.0)

N39.41 **Urge incontinence**
EXCLUDES 1 *mixed incontinence (N39.46)*

DEFINITION Inability to control urination after the urge to urinate.

▲ N39.42 **Incontinence without sensory awareness**
Insensible (urinary) incontinence
N39.43 **Post-void dribbling**
N39.44 **Nocturnal enuresis**
N39.45 **Continuous leakage**
N39.46 **Mixed incontinence**
Urge and stress incontinence
⑥ N39.49 **Other specified urinary incontinence**
N39.490 **Overflow incontinence**
DEFINITION Urinary incontinence due to pressure of retained urine in the bladder, after the bladder has contracted to its limits, with dribbling urine.
● N39.491 **Coital incontinence**
● N39.492 **Postural (urinary) incontinence**
N39.498 **Other specified urinary incontinence**
Reflex incontinence
Total incontinence

N39.8 **Other specified disorders of urinary system**
N39.9 **Disorder of urinary system, unspecified**

Diseases of male genital organs (N40-N53)

▲ ④ N40 **Benign prostatic hyperplasia**
INCLUDES adenofibromatous hypertrophy of prostate
benign hypertrophy of the prostate
benign prostatic hypertrophy
BPH
enlarged prostate
nodular prostate
polyp of prostate
EXCLUDES 1 *benign neoplasms of prostate (adenoma, benign) (fibroadenoma) (fibroma) (myoma) (D29.1)*
EXCLUDES 2 *malignant neoplasm of prostate (C61)*

CODING TIP✓ Although hyperplasia (increase in number of cells) and hypertrophy (increase in size of cells) are not synonymous, Benign Prostatic Hyperplasia and Benign Prostatic Hypertrophy are classified to the same code. When a patient diagnosed with a condition classifiable to N40.- also has lower urinary tract symptoms present – such as obstruction, incontinence, hesitancy, frequency, urgency, or other included conditions – assign code N40.1. and the associated symptoms.

▲ N40.0 **Benign prostatic hyperplasia without lower urinary tract symptoms** ♂ 🅰
Enlarged prostate without LUTS
Enlarged prostate NOS

Enlarged prostate without lower urinary tract symptoms

Normal prostate   Enlarged prostate

Bladder
Prostate
Urethra
Sphincter

▲ ➕ N40.1 **Benign prostatic hyperplasia with lower urinary tract symptoms** ♂ 🅰
Enlarged prostate with LUTS
Use additional code for associated symptoms, when specified:
incomplete bladder emptying (R39.14)
nocturia (R35.1)
straining on urination (R39.16)
urinary frequency (R35.0)
urinary hesitancy (R39.11)
urinary incontinence (N39.4-)
urinary obstruction (N13.8)
urinary retention (R33.8)
urinary urgency (R39.15)
weak urinary stream (R39.12)

● New ▲ Revised *Manifestation* ④-⑦ Digit Indicators ⊟ Laterality 🅰 Adult (15+ years) Ⓜ Maternity (12-55 years) Ⓝ Newborn Ⓟ Pediatric (0-17 years) ♂ Male ♀ Female
✖ Deleted Unspecified ➕ Additional code

N40.2 **Nodular prostate without lower urinary tract symptoms** ♂ 🅰
Nodular prostate without LUTS

+ N40.3 **Nodular prostate with lower urinary tract symptoms** ♂ 🅰
Use additional code for associated symptoms, when
specified:
incomplete bladder emptying (R39.14)
nocturia (R35.1)
straining on urination (R39.16)
urinary frequency (R35.0)
urinary hesitancy (R39.11)
urinary incontinence (N39.4-)
urinary obstruction (N13.8)
urinary retention (R33.8)
urinary urgency (R39.15)
weak urinary stream (R39.12)

4️ + N41 **Inflammatory diseases of prostate**
Use additional code (B95-B97), to identify infectious agent.

+ N41.0 **Acute prostatitis** ♂ 🅰
+ N41.1 **Chronic prostatitis** ♂ 🅰
+ N41.2 **Abscess of prostate** ♂ 🅰
+ N41.3 **Prostatocystitis** ♂ 🅰
+ N41.4 **Granulomatous prostatitis** ♂ 🅰
+ N41.8 **Other inflammatory diseases of prostate** ♂ 🅰
+ N41.9 **Inflammatory disease of prostate, unspecified** ♂ 🅰
Prostatitis NOS

4️ N42 **Other and unspecified disorders of prostate**

N42.0 **Calculus of prostate** ♂ 🅰
Prostatic stone

N42.1 **Congestion and hemorrhage of prostate** ♂ 🅰

> **EXCLUDES 1** *enlarged prostate (N40.-)*
> *hematuria (R31.-)*
> *hyperplasia of prostate (N40.-)*
> *inflammatory diseases of prostate (N41.-)*

▲ 5️ N42.3 **Dysplasia of prostate**
● N42.30 **Unspecified dysplasia of prostate** ♂
● N42.31 **Prostatic intraepithelial neoplasia** ♂
PIN
Prostatic intraepithelial neoplasia I (PIN I)
Prostatic intraepithelial neoplasia II (PIN II)

> **EXCLUDES 1** *prostatic intraepithelial neoplasia III*
> *(PIN III) (D07.5)*

● N42.32 **Atypical small acinar proliferation of prostate** ♂
● N42.39 **Other dysplasia of prostate** ♂
5️ N42.8 **Other specified disorders of prostate**
N42.81 **Prostatodynia syndrome** ♂ 🅰
Painful prostate syndrome
N42.82 **Prostatosis syndrome** ♂ 🅰
N42.83 **Cyst of prostate** ♂ 🅰
N42.89 **Other specified disorders of prostate** ♂ 🅰
N42.9 **Disorder of prostate, unspecified** ♂ 🅰

4️ N43 **Hydrocele and spermatocele**

> **INCLUDES** hydrocele of spermatic cord, testis or tunica
> vaginalis

> **EXCLUDES 1** *congenital hydrocele (P83.5)*

> **CODING TIP ✓** Conditions classifiable to N43.- indicate
cysts of fluid that develop near the head of the epididymis
(spermatocele), or surrounding the testicle (hydrocele). They
are often painless but may cause discomfort due to pressure
on surrounding areas. When a hydrocele is reported as
infected, assign N43.1 with an additional code for the
causative organism, if known.

Hydrocele

Spermatic cord
Penis
Testicle
Fluid buildup
Scrotum

Normal   Hydrocele

N43.0 **Encysted hydrocele** ♂
+ N43.1 **Infected hydrocele** ♂
Use additional code (B95-B97), to identify infectious agent.
N43.2 **Other hydrocele** ♂
N43.3 **Hydrocele, unspecified** ♂

> **DEFINITION** Collection of serous fluid on the tunica
> vaginalis, spermatic cord, or testicle from acute local
> injury, infection, radiotherapy, or gradual fluid
> accumulation.

5️ N43.4 **Spermatocele of epididymis**
Spermatic cyst

> **DEFINITION** Cyst on the epididymis containing
> sperm.

N43.40 **Spermatocele of epididymis, unspecified** ♂
N43.41 **Spermatocele of epididymis, single** ♂
N43.42 **Spermatocele of epididymis, multiple** ♂

4️ N44 **Noninflammatory disorders of testis**

5️ N44.0 **Torsion of testis**
N44.00 **Torsion of testis, unspecified** ♂

> **DEFINITION** Testicle becomes twisted inside
> the scrotum, cutting off the blood supply.

N44.01 **Extravaginal torsion of spermatic cord** ♂
N44.02 **Intravaginal torsion of spermatic cord** ♂
Torsion of spermatic cord NOS
N44.03 **Torsion of appendix testis** ♂
N44.04 **Torsion of appendix epididymis** ♂
N44.1 **Cyst of tunica albuginea testis** ♂
N44.2 **Benign cyst of testis** ♂
N44.8 **Other noninflammatory disorders of the testis** ♂

4️ + N45 **Orchitis and epididymitis**
Use additional code (B95-B97), to identify infectious agent.

> **CODING TIP ✓** When coding conditions classifiable to N45.-
> , review documentation to identify the causative organism(s)
> if known, and assign an additional code.

+ N45.1 **Epididymitis** ♂
+ N45.2 **Orchitis** ♂
+ N45.3 **Epididymo-orchitis** ♂
+ N45.4 **Abscess of epididymis or testis** ♂

Abscess of epididymis or testis

Inflammation
Abscess
Testes
Penis
Epididymis

4️ N46 **Male infertility**

> **EXCLUDES 1** *vasectomy status (Z98.52)*

5️ N46.0 **Azoospermia**
Absolute male infertility
Male infertility due to germinal (cell) aplasia
Male infertility due to spermatogenic arrest (complete)
N46.01 **Organic azoospermia** ♂ 🅰
Azoospermia NOS
6️ N46.02 **Azoospermia due to extratesticular causes**
Code also:
associated cause
N46.021 **Azoospermia due to drug therapy** ♂ 🅰
N46.022 **Azoospermia due to infection** ♂ 🅰
N46.023 **Azoospermia due to obstruction of efferent** ♂ 🅰
ducts
N46.024 **Azoospermia due to radiation** ♂ 🅰
N46.025 **Azoospermia due to systemic disease** ♂ 🅰
N46.029 **Azoospermia due to other extratesticular** ♂ 🅰
causes

● New ▲ Revised *Manifestation* 4️-7️ Digit Indicators ▤ Laterality 🅰 Adult (15+ years) Ⓜ Maternity (12-55 years) Ⓝ Newborn Ⓟ Pediatric (0-17 years) ♂ Male ♀ Female

✖ Deleted Unspecified + Additional code

826   © 2017 DecisionHealth   2017 ICD-10-CM Expert for Physicians

⑤ **N46.1** **Oligospermia**
Male infertility due to germinal cell desquamation
Male infertility due to hypospermatogenesis
Male infertility due to incomplete spermatogenic arrest

DEFINITION Insufficient spermatozoa in the semen.

N46.11 **Organic oligospermia** ♂ Ⓐ
Oligospermia NOS

⑥ **N46.12** **Oligospermia due to extratesticular causes**
Code also:
associated cause

N46.121 **Oligospermia due to drug therapy** ♂ Ⓐ
N46.122 **Oligospermia due to infection** ♂ Ⓐ
N46.123 **Oligospermia due to obstruction of efferent** ♂ Ⓐ
ducts
N46.124 **Oligospermia due to radiation** ♂ Ⓐ
N46.125 **Oligospermia due to systemic disease** ♂ Ⓐ
N46.129 **Oligospermia due to other extratesticular** ♂ Ⓐ
causes

N46.8 **Other male infertility** ♂ Ⓐ
N46.9 **Male infertility, unspecified** ♂ Ⓐ

④ **N47** **Disorders of prepuce**
N47.0 **Adherent prepuce, newborn** ♂ Ⓝ
N47.1 **Phimosis** ♂
N47.2 **Paraphimosis** ♂
N47.3 **Deficient foreskin** ♂
N47.4 **Benign cyst of prepuce** ♂
N47.5 **Adhesions of prepuce and glans penis** ♂
+ **N47.6** **Balanoposthitis** ♂
Use additional code (B95-B97), to identify infectious agent.

EXCLUDES 1 balanitis (N48.1)

DEFINITION Inflammation of the head of the penis
and foreskin.

+ **N47.7** **Other inflammatory diseases of prepuce** ♂
Use additional code (B95-B97), to identify infectious agent.
N47.8 **Other disorders of prepuce** ♂

④ **N48** **Other disorders of penis**
N48.0 **Leukoplakia of penis** ♂
Balanitis xerotica obliterans
Kraurosis of penis
Lichen sclerosus of external male genital organs

EXCLUDES 1 carcinoma in situ of penis (D07.4)

DEFINITION Chronic skin condition of the penis
causing atrophic, white, patches on the foreskin and
glans with hardened, indurated tissue near the meatus.

+ **N48.1** **Balanitis** ♂
Use additional code (B95-B97), to identify infectious agent

EXCLUDES 1 amebic balanitis (A06.8)
balanitis xerotica obliterans (N48.0)
candidal balanitis (B37.42)
gonococcal balanitis (A54.23)
herpesviral [herpes simplex] balanitis
(A60.01)

DEFINITION Inflammation of the glans penis (the
head of the penis).

⑤+ **N48.2** **Other inflammatory disorders of penis**
Use additional code (B95-B97), to identify infectious agent.

EXCLUDES 1 balanitis (N48.1)
balanitis xerotica obliterans (N48.0)
balanoposthitis (N47.6)

+ **N48.21** **Abscess of corpus cavernosum and penis** ♂
+ **N48.22** **Cellulitis of corpus cavernosum and penis** ♂
+ **N48.29** **Other inflammatory disorders of penis** ♂
⑤ **N48.3** **Priapism**
Painful erection
Code first:
underlying cause

N48.30 **Priapism, unspecified** ♂
N48.31 **Priapism due to trauma** ♂
N48.32 **Priapism due to disease classified elsewhere** ♂
N48.33 **Priapism, drug-induced** ♂
N48.39 **Other priapism** ♂
N48.5 **Ulcer of penis** ♂
N48.6 **Induration penis plastica** ♂ Ⓐ
Peyronie's disease
Plastic induration of penis

⑤ **N48.8** **Other specified disorders of penis**
N48.81 **Thrombosis of superficial vein of penis** ♂
N48.82 **Acquired torsion of penis** ♂
Acquired torsion of penis NOS

EXCLUDES 1 congenital torsion of penis (Q55.63)

N48.83 **Acquired buried penis** ♂

EXCLUDES 1 congenital hidden penis (Q55.64)

N48.89 **Other specified disorders of penis** ♂
N48.9 **Disorder of penis, unspecified** ♂

④+ **N49** **Inflammatory disorders of male genital organs, not
elsewhere classified**
Use additional code (B95-B97), to identify infectious agent

EXCLUDES 1 inflammation of penis (N48.1, N48.2-)
orchitis and epididymitis (N45.-)

+ **N49.0** **Inflammatory disorders of seminal vesicle** ♂
Vesiculitis NOS

Inflammatory disorders of seminal vesicle

Bladder
Ureter
Seminal
vesicle is
inflamed
Prostate
gland
Ejaculatory
duct
Bulbourethral
gland
Penis
Ductus
deferens
Urethra
Epididymis
Testis
Glans penis

+ **N49.1** **Inflammatory disorders of spermatic cord, tunica** ♂
vaginalis and vas deferens
Vasitis
+ **N49.2** **Inflammatory disorders of scrotum** ♂
+ **N49.3** **Fournier gangrene** ♂

CODING TIP ✓ Fournier gangrene is a specific
condition occurring in males, which includes a
necrotizing or gangrenous infection of the perineal
region often including a mix of aerobic and anaerobic
bacteria. An additional code should be assigned to
identify causative organism(s).

DEFINITION Necrosis affecting the perineal, genital,
or perianal regions, characterized by black and
malodorous tissue decay caused by infection or
ischemia.

+ **N49.8** **Inflammatory disorders of other specified male genital** ♂
organs
Inflammation of multiple sites in male genital organs
+ **N49.9** **Inflammatory disorder of unspecified male genital** ♂
organ
Abscess of unspecified male genital organ
Boil of unspecified male genital organ
Carbuncle of unspecified male genital organ
Cellulitis of unspecified male genital organ

④ **N50** **Other and unspecified disorders of male genital organs**

EXCLUDES 2 torsion of testis (N44.0-)

N50.0 **Atrophy of testis** ♂
N50.1 **Vascular disorders of male genital organs** ♂
Hematocele, NOS, of male genital organs
Hemorrhage of male genital organs
Thrombosis of male genital organs
N50.3 **Cyst of epididymis** ♂
▲⑤ **N50.8** **Other specified disorders of male genital organs**

DEFINITION Chylocele: A cyst-like lesion resulting
from the escape of chyle (milky fluid consisting of lymph
and emulsified fat) into the tunica vaginalis of the
testes.

● ⑥ **N50.81** **Testicular pain** ♂
● ▣ **N50.811** **Right testicular pain** ♂
● ▣ **N50.812** **Left testicular pain** ♂
● ▣ **N50.819** **Testicular pain, unspecified** ♂
● **N50.82** **Scrotal pain** ♂

● New ▲ Revised *Manifestation* ④-⑦ Digit Indicators ▣ Laterality Ⓐ Adult Ⓜ Maternity Ⓝ Newborn Ⓟ Pediatric ♂ Male ♀ Female
✖ Deleted Unspecified + Additional code (15+ years) (12-55 years) (0-17 years)

Diseases of the Genitourinary System

● **N50.89** **Other specified disorders of the male genital organs** ♂

Atrophy of scrotum, seminal vesicle, spermatic cord, tunica vaginalis and vas deferens

Chylocele, tunica vaginalis (nonfilarial) NOS

Edema of scrotum, seminal vesicle, spermatic cord, tunica vaginalis and vas deferens

Hypertrophy of scrotum, seminal vesicle, spermatic cord, tunica vaginalis and vas deferens

Stricture of spermatic cord, tunica vaginalis, and vas deferens

Ulcer of scrotum, seminal vesicle, spermatic cord, testis, tunica vaginalis and vas deferens

Urethroscrotal fistula

N50.9 **Disorder of male genital organs, unspecified** ♂

N51 *Disorders of male genital organs in diseases classified elsewhere* ♂

Code first underlying disease, such as:
filariasis (B74.0-B74.9)

EXCLUDES 1   *amebic balanitis (A06.8)*
candidal balanitis (B37.42)
gonococcal balanitis (A54.23)
gonococcal prostatitis (A54.22)
herpesviral [herpes simplex] balanitis (A60.01)
trichomonal prostatitis (A59.02)
tuberculous prostatitis (A18.14)

▣ **N52** **Male erectile dysfunction**

EXCLUDES 1   *psychogenic impotence (F52.21)*

▣ **N52.0** **Vasculogenic erectile dysfunction**

N52.01 **Erectile dysfunction due to arterial insufficiency** ♂ Ⓐ

N52.02 **Corporo-venous occlusive erectile dysfunction** ♂ Ⓐ

N52.03 **Combined arterial insufficiency and corporo-venous occlusive erectile dysfunction** ♂ Ⓐ

N52.1 **Erectile dysfunction due to diseases classified elsewhere** ♂ Ⓐ

Code first:
underlying disease

N52.2 **Drug-induced erectile dysfunction** ♂ Ⓐ

▲ ▣ **N52.3** **Postprocedural erectile dysfunction**

N52.31 **Erectile dysfunction following radical prostatectomy** ♂ Ⓐ

N52.32 **Erectile dysfunction following radical cystectomy** ♂ Ⓐ

N52.33 **Erectile dysfunction following urethral surgery** ♂ Ⓐ

N52.34 **Erectile dysfunction following simple prostatectomy** ♂ Ⓐ

● **N52.35** **Erectile dysfunction following radiation therapy** ♂

● **N52.36** **Erectile dysfunction following interstitial seed therapy** ♂

● **N52.37** **Erectile dysfunction following prostate ablative therapy** ♂

Erectile dysfunction following cryotherapy

Erectile dysfunction following other prostate ablative therapies

Erectile dysfunction following ultrasound ablative therapies

▲ **N52.39** **Other and unspecified postprocedural erectile dysfunction** ♂ Ⓐ

N52.8 **Other male erectile dysfunction** ♂ Ⓐ

N52.9 **Male erectile dysfunction, unspecified** ♂ Ⓐ

Impotence NOS

▣ **N53** **Other male sexual dysfunction**

EXCLUDES 1   *psychogenic sexual dysfunction (F52.-)*

▣ **N53.1** **Ejaculatory dysfunction**

EXCLUDES 1   *premature ejaculation (F52.4)*

N53.11 **Retarded ejaculation** ♂ Ⓐ

N53.12 **Painful ejaculation** ♂

N53.13 **Anejaculatory orgasm** ♂ Ⓐ

N53.14 **Retrograde ejaculation** ♂ Ⓐ

N53.19 **Other ejaculatory dysfunction** ♂ Ⓐ

Ejaculatory dysfunction NOS

N53.8 **Other male sexual dysfunction** ♂

N53.9 **Unspecified male sexual dysfunction** ♂

Disorders of breast (N60-N65)

EXCLUDES 1   *disorders of breast associated with childbirth (O91-O92)*

▣ **N60** **Benign mammary dysplasia**

INCLUDES   fibrocystic mastopathy

▣ **N60.0** **Solitary cyst of breast**

Cyst of breast

Solitary cyst of breast

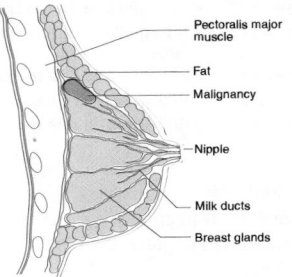

Pectoralis major muscle
Fat
Malignancy
Nipple
Milk ducts
Breast glands

▣ **N60.01** **Solitary cyst of right breast**

▣ **N60.02** **Solitary cyst of left breast**

▣ **N60.09** **Solitary cyst of unspecified breast**

▣ **N60.1** **Diffuse cystic mastopathy**

Cystic breast

Fibrocystic disease of breast

EXCLUDES 1   *diffuse cystic mastopathy with epithelial proliferation (N60.3-)*

▣ **N60.11** **Diffuse cystic mastopathy of right breast** Ⓐ

▣ **N60.12** **Diffuse cystic mastopathy of left breast** Ⓐ

▣ **N60.19** **Diffuse cystic mastopathy of unspecified breast** Ⓐ

▣ **N60.2** **Fibroadenosis of breast**

Adenofibrosis of breast

EXCLUDES 2   *fibroadenoma of breast (D24.-)*

▣ **N60.21** **Fibroadenosis of right breast**

▣ **N60.22** **Fibroadenosis of left breast**

▣ **N60.29** **Fibroadenosis of unspecified breast**

▣ **N60.3** **Fibrosclerosis of breast**

Cystic mastopathy with epithelial proliferation

▣ **N60.31** **Fibrosclerosis of right breast**

▣ **N60.32** **Fibrosclerosis of left breast**

▣ **N60.39** **Fibrosclerosis of unspecified breast**

▣ **N60.4** **Mammary duct ectasia**

DEFINITION   Dilated milk duct filled with fluid; becomes inflamed and clogged with a thick, sticky substance, causing discharge and tenderness.

▣ **N60.41** **Mammary duct ectasia of right breast**

▣ **N60.42** **Mammary duct ectasia of left breast**

▣ **N60.49** **Mammary duct ectasia of unspecified breast**

▣ **N60.8** **Other benign mammary dysplasias**

▣ **N60.81** **Other benign mammary dysplasias of right breast**

▣ **N60.82** **Other benign mammary dysplasias of left breast**

▣ **N60.89** **Other benign mammary dysplasias of unspecified breast**

▣ **N60.9** **Unspecified benign mammary dysplasia**

▣ **N60.91** **Unspecified benign mammary dysplasia of right breast**

▣ **N60.92** **Unspecified benign mammary dysplasia of left breast**

▣ **N60.99** **Unspecified benign mammary dysplasia of unspecified breast**

▲ ▣ **N61** **Inflammatory disorders of breast**

EXCLUDES 1   *inflammatory carcinoma of breast (C50.9)*
inflammatory disorder of breast associated with childbirth (O91.-)
neonatal infective mastitis (P39.0)
thrombophlebitis of breast [Mondor's disease] (I80.8)

● New   ▲ Revised   *Manifestation*   ▣-▣ Digit Indicators   ▣ Laterality   Ⓐ Adult (15+ years)   Ⓜ Maternity (12-55 years)   Ⓝ Newborn   Ⓟ Pediatric (0-17 years)   ♂ Male   ♀ Female

✖ Deleted   Unspecified   ✚ Additional code

828   © 2017 DecisionHealth   2017 ICD-10-CM Expert for Physicians

N50.89 — N61

CODING TIP ✓ Do not assign a code from N61.- for patients who also have breast cancer.

● **N61.0 Mastitis without abscess**
Infective mastitis (acute) (nonpuerperal) (subacute)
Mastitis (acute) (nonpuerperal) (subacute) NOS
Cellulitis (acute) (nonpuerperal) (subacute) of breast NOS
Cellulitis (acute) (nonpuerperal) (subacute) of nipple NOS

● **N61.1 Abscess of the breast and nipple**
Abscess (acute) (chronic) (nonpuerperal) of areola
Abscess (acute) (chronic) (nonpuerperal) of breast
Carbuncle of breast
Mastitis with abscess

N62 Hypertrophy of breast
Gynecomastia
Hypertrophy of breast NOS
Massive pubertal hypertrophy of breast
EXCLUDES 1 *breast engorgement of newborn (P83.4)*
disproportion of reconstructed breast (N65.1)
DEFINITION Abnormal largeness of the breast.

N63 Unspecified lump in breast
Nodule(s) NOS in breast

④ **N64 Other disorders of breast**
EXCLUDES 2 *mechanical complication of breast prosthesis and implant (T85.4-)*

N64.0 **Fissure and fistula of nipple**
▲ N64.1 **Fat necrosis of breast**
Fat necrosis (segmental) of breast
Code first:
breast necrosis due to breast graft (T85.898)

N64.2 **Atrophy of breast**
N64.3 **Galactorrhea not associated with childbirth**
DEFINITION Inappropriate discharge of milk from the breast.

N64.4 **Mastodynia**
⑤ N64.5 **Other signs and symptoms in breast**
EXCLUDES 2 *abnormal findings on diagnostic imaging of breast (R92.-)*

N64.51 **Induration of breast**
N64.52 **Nipple discharge**
EXCLUDES 1 *abnormal findings in nipple discharge (R89.-)*
N64.53 **Retraction of nipple**
N64.59 **Other signs and symptoms in breast**
⑤ N64.8 **Other specified disorders of breast**
N64.81 **Ptosis of breast** Ⓐ
EXCLUDES 1 *ptosis of native breast in relation to reconstructed breast (N65.1)*
DEFINITION Falling, drooping, or sagging of the breast tissue which can occur naturally, or following pregnancy or weight gain and loss.
N64.82 **Hypoplasia of breast** Ⓐ
Micromastia
EXCLUDES 1 *congenital absence of breast (Q83.0)*
hypoplasia of native breast in relation to reconstructed breast (N65.1)
N64.89 **Other specified disorders of breast**
Galactocele
Subinvolution of breast (postlactational)
N64.9 **Disorder of breast, unspecified**

④ **N65 Deformity and disproportion of reconstructed breast**
N65.0 **Deformity of reconstructed breast** Ⓐ
Contour irregularity in reconstructed breast
Excess tissue in reconstructed breast
Misshapen reconstructed breast
N65.1 **Disproportion of reconstructed breast** Ⓐ
Breast asymmetry between native breast and reconstructed breast
Disproportion between native breast and reconstructed breast

Inflammatory diseases of female pelvic organs (N70-N77)

EXCLUDES 1 *inflammatory diseases of female pelvic organs complicating: abortion or ectopic or molar pregnancy (O00-O07, O08.0) pregnancy, childbirth and the puerperium (O23.-, O75.3, O85, O86.-)*

④ ➕ **N70 Salpingitis and oophoritis**
INCLUDES abscess (of) fallopian tube
abscess (of) ovary
pyosalpinx
salpingo-oophoritis
tubo-ovarian abscess
tubo-ovarian inflammatory disease
Use additional code (B95-B97), to identify infectious agent
EXCLUDES 1 *gonococcal infection (A54.24)*
tuberculous infection (A18.17)
CODING TIP ✓ Conditions classifiable to N70.- should have an additional code assigned to identify the causative organism of infection, when this is known.
⑤ ➕ N70.0 **Acute salpingitis and oophoritis**
➕ N70.01 **Acute salpingitis** ♀
➕ N70.02 **Acute oophoritis** ♀
➕ N70.03 **Acute salpingitis and oophoritis** ♀
⑤ ➕ N70.1 **Chronic salpingitis and oophoritis**
Hydrosalpinx
➕ N70.11 **Chronic salpingitis** ♀
➕ N70.12 **Chronic oophoritis** ♀
➕ N70.13 **Chronic salpingitis and oophoritis** ♀
⑤ ➕ N70.9 **Salpingitis and oophoritis, unspecified**
DEFINITION Inflammation of appendages of the uterus (adnexa uteri).
➕ N70.91 **Salpingitis, unspecified** ♀
➕ N70.92 **Oophoritis, unspecified** ♀
➕ N70.93 **Salpingitis and oophoritis, unspecified** ♀
④ ➕ **N71 Inflammatory disease of uterus, except cervix**
INCLUDES endo (myo) metritis
metritis
myometritis
pyometra
uterine abscess
Use additional code (B95-B97), to identify infectious agent
EXCLUDES 1 *hyperplastic endometritis (N85.0-)*
infection of uterus following delivery (O85, O86.-)
➕ N71.0 **Acute inflammatory disease of uterus** ♀
➕ N71.1 **Chronic inflammatory disease of uterus** ♀
➕ N71.9 **Inflammatory disease of uterus, unspecified** ♀
➕ **N72 Inflammatory disease of cervix uteri** ♀
INCLUDES cervicitis (with or without erosion or ectropion)
endocervicitis (with or without erosion or ectropion)
exocervicitis (with or without erosion or ectropion)
Use additional code (B95-B97), to identify infectious agent
EXCLUDES 1 *erosion and ectropion of cervix without cervicitis (N86)*
④ ➕ **N73 Other female pelvic inflammatory diseases**
Use additional code (B95-B97), to identify infectious agent.
➕ N73.0 **Acute parametritis and pelvic cellulitis** ♀
Abscess of broad ligament
Abscess of parametrium
Pelvic cellulitis, female

Acute parametritis and pelvic cellulitis

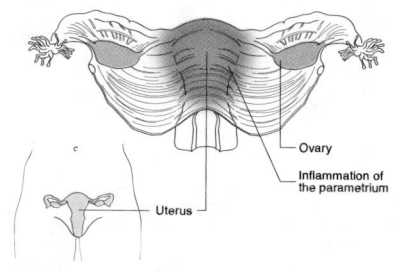
Ovary
Inflammation of the parametrium
Uterus

➕ N73.1 **Chronic parametritis and pelvic cellulitis** ♀
Any condition in N73.0 specified as chronic
EXCLUDES 1 *tuberculous parametritis and pelvic cellultis (A18.17)*

● New ▲ Revised *Manifestation* ④-⑦ Digit Indicators ▤ Laterality Ⓐ Adult (15+ years) Ⓜ Maternity (12-55 years) Ⓝ Newborn Ⓟ Pediatric (0-17 years) ♂ Male ♀ Female
✖ Deleted Unspecified ➕ Additional code
2017 ICD-10-CM Expert for Physicians
© 2017 DecisionHealth
829
N61 — N73.1

Diseases of the Genitourinary System

+ N73.2 **Unspecified parametritis and pelvic cellulitis** ♀
Any condition in N73.0 unspecified whether acute or chronic

+ N73.3 **Female acute pelvic peritonitis** ♀

+ N73.4 **Female chronic pelvic peritonitis** ♀
EXCLUDES 1 *tuberculous pelvic (female) peritonitis (A18.17)*

+ N73.5 **Female pelvic peritonitis, unspecified** ♀

+ N73.6 **Female pelvic peritoneal adhesions (postinfective)** ♀
EXCLUDES 2 *postprocedural pelvic peritoneal adhesions (N99.4)*
AHA: 1Q 2014, 6

+ N73.8 **Other specified female pelvic inflammatory diseases** ♀

+ N73.9 **Female pelvic inflammatory disease, unspecified** ♀
Female pelvic infection or inflammation NOS

N74 **Female pelvic inflammatory disorders in diseases classified elsewhere** ♀
Code first:
underlying disease
EXCLUDES 1 *chlamydial cervicitis (A56.02)*
chlamydial pelvic inflammatory disease (A56.11)
gonococcal cervicitis (A54.03)
gonococcal pelvic inflammatory disease (A54.24)
herpesviral [herpes simplex] cervicitis (A60.03)
herpesviral [herpes simplex] pelvic inflammatory disease (A60.09)
syphilitic cervicitis (A52.76)
syphilitic pelvic inflammatory disease (A52.76)
trichomonal cervicitis (A59.09)
tuberculous cervicitis (A18.16)
tuberculous pelvic inflammatory disease (A18.17)

4 N75 **Diseases of Bartholin's gland**
N75.0 Cyst of Bartholin's gland ♀

Cyst of Bartholin's gland

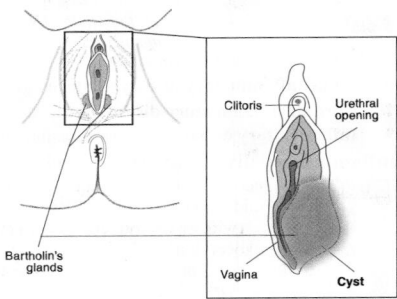

Clitoris · Urethral opening · Bartholin's glands · Vagina · Cyst

N75.1 **Abscess of Bartholin's gland** ♀

Abscess of Bartholin's gland

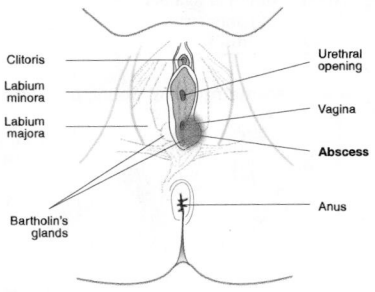

Clitoris · Labium minora · Labium majora · Bartholin's glands · Urethral opening · Vagina · Abscess · Anus

N75.8 **Other diseases of Bartholin's gland** ♀
Bartholinitis

N75.9 **Disease of Bartholin's gland, unspecified** ♀

4 + N76 **Other inflammation of vagina and vulva**
Use additional code (B95-B97), to identify infectious agent
EXCLUDES 2 *senile (atrophic) vaginitis (N95.2)*
vulvar vestibulitis (N94.810)

+ N76.0 **Acute vaginitis** ♀
Acute vulvovaginitis
Vaginitis NOS
Vulvovaginitis NOS

+ N76.1 **Subacute and chronic vaginitis** ♀
Chronic vulvovaginitis
Subacute vulvovaginitis

+ N76.2 **Acute vulvitis** ♀
Vulvitis NOS

+ N76.3 **Subacute and chronic vulvitis** ♀

+ N76.4 **Abscess of vulva** ♀
Furuncle of vulva

+ N76.5 **Ulceration of vagina** ♀

+ N76.6 **Ulceration of vulva** ♀

5 + N76.8 **Other specified inflammation of vagina and vulva**
+ N76.81 **Mucositis (ulcerative) of vagina and vulva** ♀
Code also type of associated therapy, such as:
antineoplastic and immunosuppressive drugs (T45.1X-)
radiological procedure and radiotherapy (Y84.2)
EXCLUDES 2 *gastrointestinal mucositis (ulcerative) (K92.81)*
nasal mucositis (ulcerative) (J34.81)
oral mucositis (ulcerative) (K12.3-)

+ N76.89 **Other specified inflammation of vagina and vulva** ♀

4 N77 **Vulvovaginal ulceration and inflammation in diseases classified elsewhere**
N77.0 *Ulceration of vulva in diseases classified elsewhere* ♀
Code first underlying disease, such as:
Behçet's disease (M35.2)
EXCLUDES 1 *ulceration of vulva in gonococcal infection (A54.02)*
ulceration of vulva in herpesviral [herpes simplex] infection (A60.04)
ulceration of vulva in syphilis (A51.0)
ulceration of vulva in tuberculosis (A18.18)

N77.1 *Vaginitis, vulvitis and vulvovaginitis in diseases classified elsewhere* ♀
Code first underlying disease, such as:
pinworm (B80)
EXCLUDES 1 *candidal vulvovaginitis (B37.3)*
chlamydial vulvovaginitis (A56.02)
gonococcal vulvovaginitts (A54.02)
herpesviral [herpes simplex] vulvovaginitis (A60.04)
trichomonal vulvovaginitis (A59.01)
tuberculous vulvovaginitis (A18.18)
vulvovaginitis in early syphilis (A51.0)
vulvovaginitis in late syphilis (A52.76)

Noninflammatory disorders of female genital tract (N80-N98)

4 N80 **Endometriosis**
DEFINITION Tissue that lines the uterus growing outside the uterus in the pelvis, abdomen, and on other organs; causes pain and infertility.

N80.0 **Endometriosis of uterus** ♀
Adenomyosis
EXCLUDES 1 *stromal endometriosis (D39.0)*

N80.1 **Endometriosis of ovary** ♀

Endometriosis of ovary

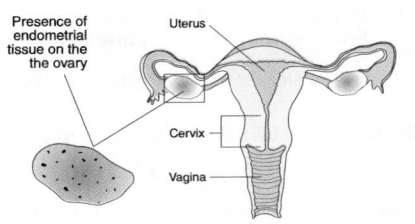

Presence of endometrial tissue on the the ovary · Uterus · Cervix · Vagina

N80.2 **Endometriosis of fallopian tube** ♀

N80.3 **Endometriosis of pelvic peritoneum** ♀

● New ▲ Revised *Manifestation* 4-7 Digit Indicators ⊟ Laterality A Adult (15+ years) M Maternity (12-55 years) N Newborn P Pediatric (0-17 years) ♂ Male ♀ Female
✖ Deleted Unspecified + Additional code

830 © 2017 DecisionHealth
2017 ICD-10-CM Expert for Physicians

N73.2 — N80.3

N80.4   **Endometriosis of rectovaginal septum and vagina** ♀

N80.5   **Endometriosis of intestine** ♀

N80.6   **Endometriosis in cutaneous scar** ♀

N80.8   **Other endometriosis** ♀

N80.9   **Endometriosis, unspecified** ♀

▲ ▣ **N81**   **Female genital prolapse**

> **EXCLUDES 1**   *genital prolapse complicating pregnancy, labor or delivery (O34.5-)*
> *prolapse and hernia of ovary and fallopian tube (N83.4-)*
> *prolapse of vaginal vault after hysterectomy (N99.3)*

N81.0   **Urethrocele** ♀

> **EXCLUDES 1**   *urethrocele with cystocele (N81.1-)*
> *urethrocele with prolapse of uterus (N81.2-N81.4)*

> **CODING TIP ✓**   Urethrocele is identified by prolapse of the urethra into the vaginal canal and may result in urinary disorders, including incontinence.

Ⓢ N81.1   **Cystocele**
Cystocele with urethrocele
Cystourethrocele

> **EXCLUDES 1**   *cystocele with prolapse of uterus (N81.2-N81.4)*

> **CODING TIP ✓**   Cystocele is identified by the prolapse of the bladder into the vaginal canal, due to muscle weakening in the pelvic floor, and may result in discomfort and urinary dysfunction, including incontinence.

    N81.10   **Cystocele, unspecified** ♀
      Prolapse of (anterior) vaginal wall NOS

    N81.11   **Cystocele, midline** ♀

    N81.12   **Cystocele, lateral** ♀
      Paravaginal cystocele

> **DEFINITION**   Bladder bulges through the side wall of the vagina.

N81.2   **Incomplete uterovaginal prolapse** ♀
First degree uterine prolapse
Prolapse of cervix NOS
Second degree uterine prolapse

> **EXCLUDES 1**   *cervical stump prolaspe (N81.85)*

N81.3   **Complete uterovaginal prolapse** ♀
Procidentia (uteri) NOS
Third degree uterine prolapse

N81.4   **Uterovaginal prolapse, unspecified** ♀
Prolapse of uterus NOS

N81.5   **Vaginal enterocele** ♀

> **EXCLUDES 1**   *enterocele with prolapse of uterus (N81.2-N81.4)*

✚ N81.6   **Rectocele**
Prolapse of posterior vaginal wall
Use additional code for any associated fecal incontinence, if applicable (R15.-)

> **EXCLUDES 2**   *perineocele (N81.81)*
> *rectal prolapse (K62.3)*
> *rectocele with prolapse of uterus (N81.2-N81.4)*

Ⓢ N81.8   **Other female genital prolapse**

    N81.81   **Perineocele** ♀

    N81.82   **Incompetence or weakening of pubocervical tissue** ♀

    N81.83   **Incompetence or weakening of rectovaginal tissue** ♀

    N81.84   **Pelvic muscle wasting** ♀
      Disuse atrophy of pelvic muscles and anal sphincter

    N81.85   **Cervical stump prolapse** ♀

    N81.89   **Other female genital prolapse** ♀
      Deficient perineum
      Old laceration of muscles of pelvic floor

N81.9   **Female genital prolapse, unspecified** ♀

▣ **N82**   **Fistulae involving female genital tract**

> **EXCLUDES 1**   *vesicointestinal fistulae (N32.1)*

N82.0   **Vesicovaginal fistula** ♀

N82.1   **Other female urinary-genital tract fistulae** ♀
Cervicovesical fistula
Ureterovaginal fistula
Urethrovaginal fistula
Uteroureteric fistula
Uterovesical fistula

N82.2   **Fistula of vagina to small intestine** ♀

N82.3   **Fistula of vagina to large intestine** ♀
Rectovaginal fistula

N82.4   **Other female intestinal-genital tract fistulae** ♀
Intestinouterine fistula

N82.5   **Female genital tract-skin fistulae** ♀
Uterus to abdominal wall fistula
Vaginoperineal fistula

Female genital tract-skin fistula
An abnormal tube-like passage connecting the genital tract to the skin surface

N82.8   **Other female genital tract fistulae** ♀

N82.9   **Female genital tract fistula, unspecified** ♀

▣ **N83**   **Noninflammatory disorders of ovary, fallopian tube and broad ligament**

> **EXCLUDES 2**   *hydrosalpinx (N70.1-)*

▲ Ⓢ N83.0   **Follicular cyst of ovary**
Cyst of graafian follicle
Hemorrhagic follicular cyst (of ovary)

> **DEFINITION**   Fluid-filled sac on the ovary caused by larger than normal growth of a follicle that does not rupture to release the egg.

   ● ▣ N83.00   **Follicular cyst of ovary, unspecified side** ♀

   ● ▣ N83.01   **Follicular cyst of right ovary** ♀

   ● ▣ N83.02   **Follicular cyst of left ovary** ♀

▲ Ⓢ N83.1   **Corpus luteum cyst**
Hemorrhagic corpus luteum cyst

   ● ▣ N83.10   **Corpus luteum cyst of ovary, unspecified side** ♀

   ● ▣ N83.11   **Corpus luteum cyst of right ovary** ♀

   ● ▣ N83.12   **Corpus luteum cyst of left ovary** ♀

Ⓢ N83.2   **Other and unspecified ovarian cysts**

> **EXCLUDES 1**   *developmental ovarian cyst (Q50.1)*
> *neoplastic ovarian cyst (D27.-)*
> *polycystic ovarian syndrome (E28.2)*
> *Stein-Leventhal syndrome (E28.2)*

▲ Ⓖ N83.20   **Unspecified ovarian cysts**

   ● ▣ N83.201   **Unspecified ovarian cyst, right side** ♀

   ● ▣ N83.202   **Unspecified ovarian cyst, left side** ♀

   ● ▣ N83.209   **Unspecified ovarian cyst, unspecified side** ♀
      Ovarian cyst, NOS

▲ Ⓖ N83.29   **Other ovarian cysts**
      Retention cyst of ovary
      Simple cyst of ovary

   ● ▣ N83.291   **Other ovarian cyst, right side** ♀

   ● ▣ N83.292   **Other ovarian cyst, left side** ♀

   ● ▣ N83.299   **Other ovarian cyst, unspecified side** ♀

Ⓢ N83.3   **Acquired atrophy of ovary and fallopian tube**

▲ Ⓖ N83.31   **Acquired atrophy of ovary**

   ● ▣ N83.311   **Acquired atrophy of right ovary** ♀

   ● ▣ N83.312   **Acquired atrophy of left ovary** ♀

● New   ▲ Revised   *Manifestation*   ▣-▣ Digit Indicators   ▣ Laterality   Ⓐ Adult (15+ years)   Ⓜ Maternity (12-55 years)   Ⓝ Newborn   Ⓟ Pediatric (0-17 years)   ♂ Male   ♀ Female
✖ Deleted   Unspecified   ✚ Additional code

● ⊟ N83.319   **Acquired atrophy of ovary, unspecified side** ♀
               Acquired atrophy of ovary, NOS
▲ ⑥ N83.32   **Acquired atrophy of fallopian tube**
● ⊟ N83.321   **Acquired atrophy of right fallopian tube** ♀
● ⊟ N83.322   **Acquired atrophy of left fallopian tube** ♀
● ⊟ N83.329   **Acquired atrophy of fallopian tube,** ♀
               unspecified side
               Acquired atrophy of fallopian tube, NOS
▲ ⑥ N83.33   **Acquired atrophy of ovary and fallopian tube**
● ⊟ N83.331   **Acquired atrophy of right ovary and fallopian** ♀
               tube
● ⊟ N83.332   **Acquired atrophy of left ovary and fallopian** ♀
               tube
● ⊟ N83.339   **Acquired atrophy of ovary and fallopian** ♀
               tube, unspecified side
               Acquired atrophy of ovary and fallopian tube, NOS
▲ ⑤ N83.4   **Prolapse and hernia of ovary and fallopian tube**
● ⊟ N83.40   **Prolapse and hernia of ovary and fallopian tube,** ♀
               unspecified side
               Prolapse and hernia of ovary and fallopian tube, NOS
● ⊟ N83.41   **Prolapse and hernia of right ovary and fallopian** ♀
               tube
● ⊟ N83.42   **Prolapse and hernia of left ovary and fallopian** ♀
               tube
⑤ N83.5   **Torsion of ovary, ovarian pedicle and fallopian tube**
               Torsion of accessory tube
▲ ⑥ N83.51   **Torsion of ovary and ovarian pedicle**
● ⊟ N83.511   **Torsion of right ovary and ovarian pedicle** ♀
● ⊟ N83.512   **Torsion of left ovary and ovarian pedicle** ♀
● ⊟ N83.519   **Torsion of ovary and ovarian pedicle,** ♀
               unspecified side
               Torsion of ovary and ovarian pedicle, NOS
▲ ⑥ N83.52   **Torsion of fallopian tube**
               Torsion of hydatid of Morgagni
● ⊟ N83.521   **Torsion of right fallopian tube** ♀
● ⊟ N83.522   **Torsion of left fallopian tube** ♀
● ⊟ N83.529   **Torsion of fallopian tube, unspecified side** ♀
               Torsion of fallopian tube, NOS
   N83.53   **Torsion of ovary, ovarian pedicle and fallopian** ♀
               tube
▲ N83.6   **Hematosalpinx** ♀
               | EXCLUDES 1 | hematosalpinx (with) (in):
                              hematocolpos (N89.7)
                              hematometra (N85.7)
                              tubal pregnancy (O00.1-)
   N83.7   **Hematoma of broad ligament** ♀
   N83.8   **Other noninflammatory disorders of ovary, fallopian** ♀
               tube and broad ligament
               Broad ligament laceration syndrome [Allen-Masters]
   N83.9   **Noninflammatory disorder of ovary, fallopian tube and** ♀
               broad ligament, unspecified

④ N84   **Polyp of female genital tract**
         | EXCLUDES 1 | adenomatous polyp (D28.-)
                        placental polyp (O90.89)
   N84.0   **Polyp of corpus uteri** ♀
            Polyp of endometrium
            Polyp of uterus NOS
            | EXCLUDES 1 | polypoid endometrial hyperplasia (N85.0-)
   N84.1   **Polyp of cervix uteri** ♀
            Mucous polyp of cervix
   N84.2   **Polyp of vagina** ♀
   N84.3   **Polyp of vulva** ♀
            Polyp of labia
   N84.8   **Polyp of other parts of female genital tract** ♀
   N84.9   **Polyp of female genital tract, unspecified** ♀

④ N85   **Other noninflammatory disorders of uterus, except**
         cervix
         | EXCLUDES 1 | endometriosis (N80.-)
                        inflammatory diseases of uterus (N71.-)
                        noninflammatory disorders of cervix, except
                           malposition (N86-N88)
                        polyp of corpus uteri (N84.0)
                        uterine prolapse (N81.-)
   ⑤ N85.0   **Endometrial hyperplasia**
             | DEFINITION | Overgrowth of cells lining the uterus.

Endometrial hyperplasia

Normal endometrium

Endometrial hyperplasia

Uterus   Endometrium

   N85.00   **Endometrial hyperplasia, unspecified** ♀
            Hyperplasia (adenomatous) (cystic) (glandular) of
               endometrium
            Hyperplastic endometritis
   N85.01   **Benign endometrial hyperplasia** ♀
            Endometrial hyperplasia (complex) (simple) without
               atypia
   N85.02   **Endometrial intraepithelial neoplasia [EIN]** ♀
            Endometrial hyperplasia with atypia
            | EXCLUDES 1 | malignant neoplasm of endometrium
                           (with endometrial intraepithelial
                           neoplasia [EIN]) (C54.1)
   N85.2   **Hypertrophy of uterus** ♀
            Bulky or enlarged uterus
            | EXCLUDES 1 | puerperal hypertrophy of uterus (O90.89)
   N85.3   **Subinvolution of uterus** ♀
            | EXCLUDES 1 | puerperal subinvolution of uterus (O90.89)
   N85.4   **Malposition of uterus** ♀
            Anteversion of uterus
            Retroflexion of uterus
            Retroversion of uterus
            | EXCLUDES 1 | malposition of uterus complicating
                           pregnancy, labor or delivery
                           (O34.5-, O65.5)
   N85.5   **Inversion of uterus** ♀
            | EXCLUDES 1 | current obstetric trauma (O71.2)
                           postpartum inversion of uterus (O71.2)
   N85.6   **Intrauterine synechiae** ♀
   N85.7   **Hematometra** ♀
            Hematosalpinx with hematometra
            | EXCLUDES 1 | hematometra with hematocolpos (N89.7)
            | DEFINITION | Blood accumulated in the uterus.
   N85.8   **Other specified noninflammatory disorders of uterus** ♀
            Atrophy of uterus, acquired
            Fibrosis of uterus NOS
   N85.9   **Noninflammatory disorder of uterus, unspecified** ♀
            Disorder of uterus NOS

N86   **Erosion and ectropion of cervix uteri** ♀
      Decubitus (trophic) ulcer of cervix
      Eversion of cervix
      | EXCLUDES 1 | erosion and ectropion of cervix with cervicitis
                     (N72)

④ N87   **Dysplasia of cervix uteri**
         | EXCLUDES 1 | abnormal results from cervical cytologic
                        examination without histologic confirmation
                        (R87.61-)
                        carcinoma in situ of cervix uteri (D06.-)
                        cervical intraepithelial neoplasia III [CIN III]
                           (D06.-)
                        HGSIL of cervix (R87.613)
                        severe dysplasia of cervix uteri (D06.-)
   N87.0   **Mild cervical dysplasia** ♀
            Cervical intraepithelial neoplasia I [CIN I]
   N87.1   **Moderate cervical dysplasia** ♀
            Cervical intraepithelial neoplasia II [CIN II]
   N87.9   **Dysplasia of cervix uteri, unspecified** ♀
            Anaplasia of cervix
            Cervical atypism
            Cervical dysplasia NOS

④ N88   **Other noninflammatory disorders of cervix uteri**
         | EXCLUDES 2 | inflammatory disease of cervix (N72)
                        polyp of cervix (N84.1)
   N88.0   **Leukoplakia of cervix uteri** ♀

| ● New | ▲ Revised | *Manifestation* | ④-⑦ Digit Indicators | ⊟ Laterality | Ⓐ Adult (15+ years) | Ⓜ Maternity (12-55 years) | Ⓝ Newborn | Ⓟ Pediatric (0-17 years) | ♂ Male | ♀ Female |
| ✖ Deleted | | Unspecified | + Additional code | | | | | | | |

N88.1 **Old laceration of cervix uteri** ♀
Adhesions of cervix
EXCLUDES 1 *current obstetric trauma (O71.3)*

N88.2 **Stricture and stenosis of cervix uteri** ♀
EXCLUDES 1 *stricture and stenosis of cervix uteri complicating labor (O65.5)*

Stricture and stenosis of cervix uteri

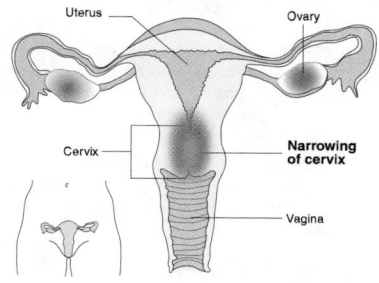

N88.3 **Incompetence of cervix uteri** ♀
Investigation and management of (suspected) cervical incompetence in a nonpregnant woman
EXCLUDES 1 *cervical incompetence complicating pregnancy (O34.3-)*

N88.4 **Hypertrophic elongation of cervix uteri** ♀

N88.8 **Other specified noninflammatory disorders of cervix uteri** ♀
EXCLUDES 1 *current obstetric trauma (O71.3)*

N88.9 **Noninflammatory disorder of cervix uteri, unspecified** ♀

④ N89 **Other noninflammatory disorders of vagina**
EXCLUDES 1 *abnormal results from vaginal cytologic examination without histologic confirmation (R87.62-)*
carcinoma in situ of vagina (D07.2)
HGSIL of vagina (R87.623)
inflammation of vagina (N76.-)
senile (atrophic) vaginitis (N95.2)
severe dysplasia of vagina (D07.2)
trichomonal leukorrhea (A59.00)
vaginal intraepithelial neoplasia [VAIN], grade III (D07.2)

N89.0 **Mild vaginal dysplasia** ♀
Vaginal intraepithelial neoplasia [VAIN], grade I

N89.1 **Moderate vaginal dysplasia** ♀
Vaginal intraepithelial neoplasia [VAIN], grade II

N89.3 **Dysplasia of vagina, unspecified** ♀

N89.4 **Leukoplakia of vagina** ♀
DEFINITION White plaque on the mucosal surface of the vagina that develops into thickened, rough-textured grayish white lesions.

N89.5 **Stricture and atresia of vagina** ♀
Vaginal adhesions
Vaginal stenosis
EXCLUDES 1 *congenital atresia or stricture (Q52.4)*
postprocedural adhesions of vagina (N99.2)

N89.6 **Tight hymenal ring** ♀
Rigid hymen
Tight introitus
EXCLUDES 1 *imperforate hymen (Q52.3)*

N89.7 **Hematocolpos** ♀
Hematocolpos with hematometra or hematosalpinx

N89.8 **Other specified noninflammatory disorders of vagina** ♀
Leukorrhea NOS
Old vaginal laceration
Pessary ulcer of vagina
EXCLUDES 1 *current obstetric trauma (O70.-, O71.4, O71.7-O71.8)*
old laceration involving muscles of pelvic floor (N81.8)

N89.9 **Noninflammatory disorder of vagina, unspecified** ♀

④ N90 **Other noninflammatory disorders of vulva and perineum**
EXCLUDES 1 *anogenital (venereal) warts (A63.0)*
carcinoma in situ of vulva (D07.1)
condyloma acuminatum (A63.0)
current obstetric trauma (O70.-, O71.7-O71.8)
inflammation of vulva (N76.-)
severe dysplasia of vulva (D07.1)
vulvar intraepithelial neoplasm III [VIN III] (D07.1)

N90.0 **Mild vulvar dysplasia** ♀
Vulvar intraepithelial neoplasia [VIN], grade I

N90.1 **Moderate vulvar dysplasia** ♀
Vulvar intraepithelial neoplasia [VIN], grade II

N90.3 **Dysplasia of vulva, unspecified** ♀

N90.4 **Leukoplakia of vulva** ♀
Dystrophy of vulva
Kraurosis of vulva
Lichen sclerosus of external female genital organs

N90.5 **Atrophy of vulva** ♀
Stenosis of vulva

▲ ⑤ N90.6 **Hypertrophy of vulva**
● N90.60 **Unspecified hypertrophy of vulva** ♀
Unspecified hypertrophy of labia

● N90.61 **Childhood asymmetric labium majus enlargement** ♀ ℙ
CALME

● N90.69 **Other specified hypertrophy of vulva** ♀
Other specified hypertrophy of labia

N90.7 **Vulvar cyst** ♀

⑤ N90.8 **Other specified noninflammatory disorders of vulva and perineum**
⑥ N90.81 **Female genital mutilation status**
Female genital cutting status

N90.810 **Female genital mutilation status, unspecified** ♀
Female genital cutting status, unspecified
Female genital mutilation status NOS

N90.811 **Female genital mutilation Type I status** ♀
Clitorectomy status
Female genital cutting Type I status

N90.812 **Female genital mutilation Type II status** ♀
Clitorectomy with excision of labia minora status
Female genital cutting Type II status

N90.813 **Female genital mutilation Type III status** ♀
Female genital cutting Type III status
Infibulation status

N90.818 **Other female genital mutilation status** ♀
Female genital cutting Type IV status
Female genital mutilation Type IV status
Other female genital cutting status

N90.89 **Other specified noninflammatory disorders of vulva and perineum** ♀
Adhesions of vulva
Hypertrophy of clitoris

N90.9 **Noninflammatory disorder of vulva and perineum, unspecified** ♀

④ N91 **Absent, scanty and rare menstruation**
EXCLUDES 1 *ovarian dysfunction (E28.-)*

N91.0 **Primary amenorrhea** ♀
N91.1 **Secondary amenorrhea** ♀
N91.2 **Amenorrhea, unspecified** ♀
N91.3 **Primary oligomenorrhea** ♀
N91.4 **Secondary oligomenorrhea** ♀
N91.5 **Oligomenorrhea, unspecified** ♀
Hypomenorrhea NOS

④ N92 **Excessive, frequent and irregular menstruation**
EXCLUDES 1 *postmenopausal bleeding (N95.0)*
precocious puberty (menstruation) (E30.1)

N92.0 **Excessive and frequent menstruation with regular cycle** ♀
Heavy periods NOS
Menorrhagia NOS
Polymenorrhea

● New ▲ Revised *Manifestation* ④-⑦ Digit Indicators ▤ Laterality Ⓐ Adult (15+ years) Ⓜ Maternity (12-55 years) Ⓝ Newborn ℙ Pediatric (0-17 years) ♂ Male ♀ Female
✖ ~~Deleted~~ Unspecified + Additional code

2017 ICD-10-CM Expert for Physicians

© 2017 DecisionHealth

833

N92.1   **Excessive and frequent menstruation with irregular cycle**   ♀
Irregular intermenstrual bleeding
Irregular, shortened intervals between menstrual bleeding
Menometrorrhagia
Metrorrhagia

N92.2   **Excessive menstruation at puberty**   ♀ ⓟ
Excessive bleeding associated with onset of menstrual periods
Pubertal menorrhagia
Puberty bleeding

N92.3   **Ovulation bleeding**   ♀
Regular intermenstrual bleeding

N92.4   **Excessive bleeding in the premenopausal period**   ♀
Climacteric menorrhagia or metrorrhagia
Menopausal menorrhagia or metrorrhagia
Preclimacteric menorrhagia or metrorrhagia
Premenopausal menorrhagia or metrorrhagia

N92.5   **Other specified irregular menstruation**   ♀

N92.6   **Irregular menstruation, unspecified**   ♀
Irregular bleeding NOS
Irregular periods NOS
> **EXCLUDES 1**   *irregular menstruation with:*
> *lengthened intervals or scanty bleeding (N91.3-N91.5)*
> *shortened intervals or excessive bleeding (N92.1)*

④ **N93**   **Other abnormal uterine and vaginal bleeding**
> **EXCLUDES 1**   *neonatal vaginal hemorrhage (P54.6)*
> *precocious puberty (menstruation) (E30.1)*
> *pseudomenses (P54.6)*

N93.0   **Postcoital and contact bleeding**   ♀
> **DEFINITION**   Bleeding after sexual intercourse.

● **N93.1**   **Pre-pubertal vaginal bleeding**   ♀ ⓟ

N93.8   **Other specified abnormal uterine and vaginal bleeding**   ♀
Dysfunctional or functional uterine or vaginal bleeding NOS

N93.9   **Abnormal uterine and vaginal bleeding, unspecified**   ♀

④ **N94**   **Pain and other conditions associated with female genital organs and menstrual cycle**

N94.0   **Mittelschmerz**   ♀
> **DEFINITION**   Pain accompanying ovulation, usually occurring midway between menstruation periods.

▲ ⑤ **N94.1**   **Dyspareunia**
> **EXCLUDES 1**   *psychogenic dyspareunia (F52.6)*
> **DEFINITION**   Pain during sexual intercourse.

● **N94.10**   **Unspecified dyspareunia**   ♀
● **N94.11**   **Superficial (introital) dyspareunia**   ♀
● **N94.12**   **Deep dyspareunia**   ♀
● **N94.19**   **Other specified dyspareunia**   ♀

N94.2   **Vaginismus**   ♀
> **EXCLUDES 1**   *psychogenic vaginismus (F52.5)*
> **DEFINITION**   Severe, painful spasms of the vaginal muscles that prevent sexual intercourse.

▲ **N94.3**   **Premenstrual tension syndrome**   ♀
Premenstrual dysphoric disorder
Code also:
   associated menstrual migraine (G43.82-, G43.83-)
> **EXCLUDES 1**   *Premenstrual dysphoric disorder (F32.81)*

N94.4   **Primary dysmenorrhea**   ♀
N94.5   **Secondary dysmenorrhea**   ♀
N94.6   **Dysmenorrhea, unspecified**   ♀
> **EXCLUDES 1**   *psychogenic dysmenorrhea (F45.8)*

⑤ **N94.8**   **Other specified conditions associated with female genital organs and menstrual cycle**

⑥ **N94.81**   **Vulvodynia**

N94.810   **Vulvar vestibulitis**   ♀
> **DEFINITION**   Pain, tenderness, and redness in the vestibule area of the female external genitalia of unknown cause.

N94.818   **Other vulvodynia**   ♀
N94.819   **Vulvodynia, unspecified**   ♀
Vulvodynia NOS

N94.89   **Other specified conditions associated with female genital organs and menstrual cycle**   ♀

N94.9   **Unspecified condition associated with female genital organs and menstrual cycle**   ♀

④ **N95**   **Menopausal and other perimenopausal disorders**
Menopausal and other perimenopausal disorders due to naturally occurring (age-related) menopause and perimenopause
> **EXCLUDES 1**   *excessive bleeding in the premenopausal period (N92.4)*
> *menopausal and perimenopausal disorders due to artificial or premature menopause (E89.4-, E28.31-)*
> *premature menopause (E28.31-)*
> **EXCLUDES 2**   *postmenopausal osteoporosis (M81.0-)*
> *postmenopausal osteoporosis with current pathological fracture (M80.0-)*
> *postmenopausal urethritis (N34.2)*

N95.0   **Postmenopausal bleeding**   ♀

+ **N95.1**   **Menopausal and female climacteric states**   ♀
Symptoms such as flushing, sleeplessness, headache, lack of concentration, associated with natural (age-related) menopause
Use additional code for associated symptoms
> **EXCLUDES 1**   *asymptomatic menopausal state (Z78.0)*
> *symptoms associated with artificial menopause (E89.41)*
> *symptoms associated with premature menopause (E28.310)*

N95.2   **Postmenopausal atrophic vaginitis**   ♀
Senile (atrophic) vaginitis
> **DEFINITION**   Thinning of vaginal epithelium due to decreased estrogen levels.

Postmenopausal atrophic vaginitis

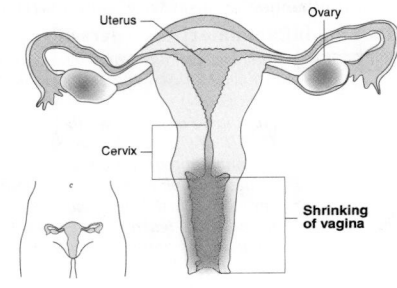

N95.8   **Other specified menopausal and perimenopausal disorders**   ♀
N95.9   **Unspecified menopausal and perimenopausal disorder**   ♀

N96   **Recurrent pregnancy loss**   ♀
Investigation or care in a nonpregnant woman with history of recurrent pregnancy loss
> **EXCLUDES 1**   *recurrent pregancy loss with current pregnancy (O26.2-)*

④ **N97**   **Female infertility**
> **INCLUDES**   inability to achieve a pregnancy
> sterility, female NOS
> **EXCLUDES 1**   *female infertility associated with:*
> *hypopituitarism (E23.0)*
> *Stein-Leventhal syndrome (E28.2)*
> **EXCLUDES 2**   *incompetence of cervix uteri (N88.3)*

N97.0   **Female infertility associated with anovulation**   ♀

● New   ▲ Revised   *Manifestation*   ④-⑦ Digit Indicators   ⊟ Laterality   Ⓐ Adult (15+ years)   Ⓜ Maternity (12-55 years)   Ⓝ Newborn   Ⓟ Pediatric (0-17 years)   ♂ Male   ♀ Female
✖ Deleted   Unspecified   + Additional code

834   © 2017 DecisionHealth   2017 ICD-10-CM Expert for Physicians

N97.1 **Female infertility of tubal origin** ♀
Female infertility associated with congenital anomaly of tube
Female infertility due to tubal block
Female infertility due to tubal occlusion
Female infertility due to tubal stenosis

Female Infertility of tubal origin

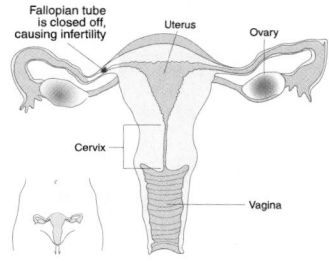

N97.2 **Female infertility of uterine origin** ♀
Female infertility associated with congenital anomaly of uterus
Female infertility due to nonimplantation of ovum
N97.8 **Female infertility of other origin** ♀
N97.9 **Female infertility, unspecified** ♀

◪ N98 **Complications associated with artificial fertilization**
N98.0 **Infection associated with artificial insemination** ♀
N98.1 **Hyperstimulation of ovaries** ♀
Hyperstimulation of ovaries NOS
Hyperstimulation of ovaries associated with induced ovulation
N98.2 **Complications of attempted introduction of fertilized ovum following in vitro fertilization** ♀
N98.3 **Complications of attempted introduction of embryo in embryo transfer** ♀
N98.8 **Other complications associated with artificial fertilization** ♀
N98.9 **Complication associated with artificial fertilization, unspecified** ♀

Intraoperative and postprocedural complications and disorders of genitourinary system, not elsewhere classified (N99)

◪ N99 **Intraoperative and postprocedural complications and disorders of genitourinary system, not elsewhere classified**

EXCLUDES 2   *irradiation cystitis (N30.4-)*
postoophorectomy osteoporosis with current pathological fracture (M80.8-)
postoophorectomy osteoporosis without current pathological fracture (M81.8)

CODING TIP ✓   **Documentation:** Codes in category N99.- are complication codes and require physician documentation and confirmation of a cause and effect relationship between any specified procedure and the complicated condition.

+ N99.0 **Postprocedural (acute) (chronic) kidney failure**
Use additional code to type of kidney disease
⑤ N99.1 **Postprocedural urethral stricture**
Postcatheterization urethral stricture
⑥ N99.11 **Postprocedural urethral stricture, male**
N99.110 **Postprocedural urethral stricture, male, meatal** ♂
N99.111 **Postprocedural bulbous urethral stricture**
N99.112 **Postprocedural membranous urethral stricture**
▲ N99.113 **Postprocedural anterior bulbous urethral stricture**

N99.114 **Postprocedural urethral stricture, male, unspecified** ♂
● N99.115 **Postprocedural fossa navicularis urethral stricture** ♂
N99.12 **Postprocedural urethral stricture, female** ♀
N99.2 **Postprocedural adhesions of vagina** ♀
N99.3 **Prolapse of vaginal vault after hysterectomy** ♀
N99.4 **Postprocedural pelvic peritoneal adhesions**
EXCLUDES 2   *pelvic peritoneal adhesions NOS (N73.6)*
postinfective pelvic peritoneal adhesions (N73.6)
▲ ⑤ N99.5 **Complications of stoma of urinary tract**
EXCLUDES 2   *mechanical complication of urinary catheter (T83.0-)*

CODING TIP ✓   All cystostomy and other urinary stoma complications (including ileocondiut, urostomy, and nephrostomy) are coded to N99.51-N99.53 This includes excoriation and denuding of the skin surrounding the ostomy, infection of the ostomy site, hemorrhage of the ostomy site, and other complications. No additional code should be used when coding skin complications unless an infection is present, in which case, an additional code should be used to specify the infection. When an ostomy complication is present, do not assign a Z code for the ostomy. Z codes indicate routine ostomy care, which is not appropriate in the case of a complicated ostomy.

⑥ N99.51 **Complication of cystostomy**
N99.510 **Cystostomy hemorrhage**
N99.511 **Cystostomy infection**
N99.512 **Cystostomy malfunction**
N99.518 **Other cystostomy complication**
▲ ⑥ N99.52 **Complication of incontinent external stoma of urinary tract**
▲ N99.520 **Hemorrhage of incontinent external stoma of urinary tract**
▲ N99.521 **Infection of incontinent external stoma of urinary tract**
▲ N99.522 **Malfunction of incontinent external stoma of urinary tract**
● N99.523 **Herniation of incontinent stoma of urinary tract**
● N99.524 **Stenosis of incontinent stoma of urinary tract**
▲ N99.528 **Other complication of incontinent external stoma of urinary tract**
▲ ⑥ N99.53 **Complication of continent stoma of urinary tract**
▲ N99.530 **Hemorrhage of continent stoma of urinary tract**
▲ N99.531 **Infection of continent stoma of urinary tract**
▲ N99.532 **Malfunction of continent stoma of urinary tract**
● N99.533 **Herniation of continent stoma of urinary tract**
● N99.534 **Stenosis of continent stoma of urinary tract**
▲ N99.538 **Other complication of continent stoma of urinary tract**
⑤ N99.6 **Intraoperative hemorrhage and hematoma of a genitourinary system organ or structure complicating a procedure**
EXCLUDES 1   *intraoperative hemorrhage and hematoma of a genitourinary system organ or structure due to accidental puncture or laceration during a procedure (N99.7-)*
N99.61 **Intraoperative hemorrhage and hematoma of a genitourinary system organ or structure complicating a genitourinary system procedure**
N99.62 **Intraoperative hemorrhage and hematoma of a genitourinary system organ or structure complicating other procedure**
⑤ N99.7 **Accidental puncture and laceration of a genitourinary system organ or structure during a procedure**
N99.71 **Accidental puncture and laceration of a genitourinary system organ or structure during a genitourinary system procedure**
N99.72 **Accidental puncture and laceration of a genitourinary system organ or structure during other procedure**
⑤ N99.8 **Other intraoperative and postprocedural complications and disorders of genitourinary system**
N99.81 **Other intraoperative complications of genitourinary system**
▲ ⑥ N99.82 **Postprocedural hemorrhage of a genitourinary system organ or structure following a procedure**

● New ▲ Revised *Manifestation* ◪-◪ Digit Indicators ▤ Laterality Ⓐ Adult (15+ years) Ⓜ Maternity (12-55 years) Ⓝ Newborn Ⓟ Pediatric (0-17 years) ♂ Male ♀ Female
✖ Deleted Unspecified + Additional code

2017 ICD-10-CM Expert for Physicians   © 2017 DecisionHealth   835

   ▲ N99.820   Postprocedural hemorrhage of a genitourinary system organ or structure following a genitourinary system procedure

   ▲ N99.821   Postprocedural hemorrhage of a genitourinary system organ or structure following other procedure

   N99.83   Residual ovary syndrome   ♀

● ⑤ N99.84   Postprocedural hematoma and seroma of a genitourinary system organ or structure following a procedure

   ● N99.840   Postprocedural hematoma of a genitourinary system organ or structure following a genitourinary system procedure

   ● N99.841   Postprocedural hematoma of a genitourinary system organ or structure following other procedure

   ● N99.842   Postprocedural seroma of a genitourinary system organ or structure following a genitourinary system procedure

   ● N99.843   Postprocedural seroma of a genitourinary system organ or structure following other procedure

   N99.89   Other postprocedural complications and disorders of genitourinary system

CHAPTER 15: PREGNANCY, CHILDBIRTH AND THE PUERPERIUM (O00-O9A)

Note: CODES FROM THIS CHAPTER ARE FOR USE ONLY ON MATERNAL RECORDS, NEVER ON NEWBORN RECORDS

Codes from this chapter are for use for conditions related to or aggravated by the pregnancy, childbirth, or by the puerperium (maternal causes or obstetric causes)

Trimesters are counted from the first day of the last menstrual period. They are defined as follows:

1st trimester- less than 14 weeks 0 days
2nd trimester- 14 weeks 0 days to less than 28 weeks 0 days
3rd trimester- 28 weeks 0 days until delivery

Use additional code from category Z3A, Weeks of gestation, to identify the specific week of the pregnancy, if known.

EXCLUDES 1 *supervision of normal pregnancy (Z34.-)*

EXCLUDES 2 *mental and behavioral disorders associated with the puerperium (F53)*
obstetrical tetanus (A34)
postpartum necrosis of pituitary gland (E23.0)
puerperal osteomalacia (M83.0)

GUIDELINES **Section I.C.15.a.1)**
Obstetric cases require codes from chapter 15, codes in the range O00-O9A, Pregnancy, Childbirth, and the Puerperium. Chapter 15 codes have sequencing priority over codes from other chapters. Additional codes from other chapters may be used in conjunction with chapter 15 codes to further specify conditions. Should the provider document that the pregnancy is incidental to the encounter, then code Z33.1, Pregnant state, incidental, should be used in place of any chapter 15 codes. It is the provider's responsibility to state that the condition being treated is not affecting the pregnancy.

GUIDELINES **Section I.C.15.a.2)**
Chapter 15 codes are to be used only on the maternal record, never on the record of the newborn.

GUIDELINES **Section I.C.15.c**
When assigning codes from Chapter 15, it is important to assess if a condition was pre-existing prior to pregnancy or developed during or due to the pregnancy in order to assign the correct code. Categories that do not distinguish between pre-existing and pregnancy related conditions may be used for either. It is acceptable to use codes specifically for the puerperium with codes complicating pregnancy and childbirth if a condition arises postpartum during the delivery encounter.

This chapter contains the following blocks:

O00-O08   Pregnancy with abortive outcome
O09   Supervision of high risk pregnancy
O10-O16   Edema, proteinuria and hypertensive disorders in pregnancy, childbirth and the puerperium
O20-O29   Other maternal disorders predominantly related to pregnancy
O30-O48   Maternal care related to the fetus and amniotic cavity and possible delivery problems
O60-O77   Complications of labor and delivery
O80-O82   Encounter for delivery
O85-O92   Complications predominantly related to the puerperium
O94-O9A   Other obstetric conditions, not elsewhere classified

Pregnancy with abortive outcome (O00-O08)

EXCLUDES 1 *continuing pregnancy in multiple gestation after abortion of one fetus or more (O31.1-, O31.3-)*

4️⃣+ O00 **Ectopic pregnancy**

    INCLUDES ruptured ectopic pregnancy

    Use additional code from category O08 to identify any associated complication

▲⑤+ O00.0 **Abdominal pregnancy**
    EXCLUDES 1 *maternal care for viable fetus in abdominal pregnancy (O36.7-)*

●+ O00.00 **Abdominal pregnancy without intrauterine pregnancy** ♀Ⓜ
    Abdominal pregnancy NOS

●+ O00.01 **Abdominal pregnancy with intrauterine pregnancy** ♀Ⓜ

▲⑤+ O00.1 **Tubal pregnancy**
    Fallopian pregnancy
    Rupture of (fallopian) tube due to pregnancy
    Tubal abortion

DEFINITION Fertilized egg implants itself within the fallopian tube where the embryo grows and may rupture the tube.

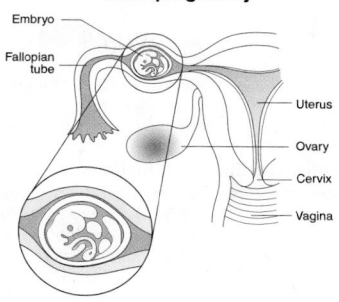

Tubal pregnancy

●+ O00.10 **Tubal pregnancy without intrauterine pregnancy** ♀Ⓜ
    Tubal pregnancy NOS

●+ O00.11 **Tubal pregnancy with intrauterine pregnancy** ♀Ⓜ

▲⑤+ O00.2 **Ovarian pregnancy**

●+ O00.20 **Ovarian pregnancy without intrauterine pregnancy** ♀Ⓜ
    Ovarian pregnancy NOS

●+ O00.21 **Ovarian pregnancy with intrauterine pregnancy** ♀Ⓜ

▲⑤+ O00.8 **Other ectopic pregnancy**
    Cervical pregnancy
    Cornual pregnancy
    Intraligamentous pregnancy
    Mural pregnancy

●+ O00.80 **Other ectopic pregnancy without intrauterine pregnancy** ♀Ⓜ
    Other ectopic pregnancy NOS

●+ O00.81 **Other ectopic pregnancy with intrauterine pregnancy** ♀Ⓜ

▲⑤+ O00.9 **Ectopic pregnancy, unspecified**

●+ O00.90 **Unspecified ectopic pregnancy without intrauterine pregnancy** ♀Ⓜ
    Ectopic pregnancy NOS

●+ O00.91 **Unspecified ectopic pregnancy with intrauterine pregnancy** ♀Ⓜ

4️⃣+ O01 **Hydatidiform mole**
    Use additional code from category O08 to identify any associated complication.
    EXCLUDES 1 *chorioadenoma (destruens) (D39.2)*
    malignant hydatidiform mole (D39.2)

+ O01.0 **Classical hydatidiform mole** ♀Ⓜ
    Complete hydatidiform mole

+ O01.1 **Incomplete and partial hydatidiform mole** ♀Ⓜ

+ O01.9 **Hydatidiform mole, unspecified** ♀Ⓜ
    Trophoblastic disease NOS
    Vesicular mole NOS

4️⃣+ O02 **Other abnormal products of conception**
    Use additional code from category O08 to identify any associated complication.
    EXCLUDES 1 *papyraceous fetus (O31.0-)*

+ O02.0 **Blighted ovum and nonhydatidiform mole** ♀Ⓜ
    Carneous mole
    Fleshy mole
    Intrauterine mole NOS
    Molar pregnancy NEC
    Pathological ovum

● New ▲ Revised *Manifestation* 4️⃣-7️⃣ Digit Indicators ⊟ Laterality 🅰 Adult (15+ years) Ⓜ Maternity (12-55 years) 🅽 Newborn 🅟 Pediatric (0-17 years) ♂ Male ♀ Female
✖ ~~Deleted~~ Unspecified + Additional code

+ O02.1   Missed abortion ♀ⓜ
Early fetal death, before completion of 20 weeks of gestation, with retention of dead fetus
EXCLUDES 1	*failed induced abortion (O07.-)*
	fetal death (intrauterine) (late) (O36.4)
	missed abortion with blighted ovum (O02.0)
	missed abortion with hydatidiform mole (O01.-)
	missed abortion with nonhydatidiform (O02.0)
	missed abortion with other abnormal products of conception (O02.8-)
	missed delivery (O36.4)
	stillbirth (P95)

⑤+ O02.8   Other specified abnormal products of conception ♀ⓜ
EXCLUDES 1	*abnormal products of conception with blighted ovum (O02.0)*
	abnormal products of conception with hydatidiform mole (O01.-)
	abnormal products of conception with nonhydatidiform mole (O02.0)

+ O02.81   Inappropriate change in quantitative human chorionic gonadotropin (hCG) in early pregnancy ♀ⓜ
Biochemical pregnancy
Chemical pregnancy
Inappropriate level of quantitative human chorionic gonadotropin (hCG) for gestational age in early pregnancy

+ O02.89   Other abnormal products of conception ♀ⓜ

+ O02.9   Abnormal product of conception, unspecified ♀ⓜ

④ O03   Spontaneous abortion
Note: Incomplete abortion includes retained products of conception following spontaneous abortion
| **INCLUDES** | miscarriage |

O03.0   Genital tract and pelvic infection following incomplete spontaneous abortion ♀ⓜ
Endometritis following incomplete spontaneous abortion
Oophoritis following incomplete spontaneous abortion
Parametritis following incomplete spontaneous abortion
Pelvic peritonitis following incomplete spontaneous abortion
Salpingitis following incomplete spontaneous abortion
Salpingo-oophoritis following incomplete spontaneous abortion
| **EXCLUDES 1** | *sepsis following incomplete spontaneous abortion (O03.37)* |
| | *urinary tract infection following incomplete spontaneous abortion (O03.38)* |

O03.1   Delayed or excessive hemorrhage following incomplete spontaneous abortion ♀ⓜ
Afibrinogenemia following incomplete spontaneous abortion
Defibrination syndrome following incomplete spontaneous abortion
Hemolysis following incomplete spontaneous abortion
Intravascular coagulation following incomplete spontaneous abortion

O03.2   Embolism following incomplete spontaneous abortion ♀ⓜ
Air embolism following incomplete spontaneous abortion
Amniotic fluid embolism following incomplete spontaneous abortion
Blood-clot embolism following incomplete spontaneous abortion
Embolism NOS following incomplete spontaneous abortion
Fat embolism following incomplete spontaneous abortion
Pulmonary embolism following incomplete spontaneous abortion
Pyemic embolism following incomplete spontaneous abortion
Septic or septicopyemic embolism following incomplete spontaneous abortion
Soap embolism following incomplete spontaneous abortion

⑤ O03.3   Other and unspecified complications following incomplete spontaneous abortion ♀ⓜ

O03.30   Unspecified complication following incomplete spontaneous abortion ♀ⓜ

O03.31   Shock following incomplete spontaneous abortion ♀ⓜ
Circulatory collapse following incomplete spontaneous abortion
Shock (postprocedural) following incomplete spontaneous abortion
| **EXCLUDES 1** | *shock due to infection following incomplete spontaneous abortion (O03.37)* |

O03.32   Renal failure following incomplete spontaneous abortion ♀ⓜ
Kidney failure (acute) following incomplete spontaneous abortion
Oliguria following incomplete spontaneous abortion
Renal shutdown following incomplete spontaneous abortion
Renal tubular necrosis following incomplete spontaneous abortion
Uremia following incomplete spontaneous abortion

O03.33   Metabolic disorder following incomplete spontaneous abortion ♀ⓜ

O03.34   Damage to pelvic organs following incomplete spontaneous abortion ♀ⓜ
Laceration, perforation, tear or chemical damage of bladder following incomplete spontaneous abortion
Laceration, perforation, tear or chemical damage of bowel following incomplete spontaneous abortion
Laceration, perforation, tear or chemical damage of broad ligament following incomplete spontaneous abortion
Laceration, perforation, tear or chemical damage of cervix following incomplete spontaneous abortion
Laceration, perforation, tear or chemical damage of periurethral tissue following incomplete spontaneous abortion
Laceration, perforation, tear or chemical damage of uterus following incomplete spontaneous abortion
Laceration, perforation, tear or chemical damage of vagina following incomplete spontaneous abortion

O03.35   Other venous complications following incomplete spontaneous abortion ♀ⓜ

O03.36   Cardiac arrest following incomplete spontaneous abortion ♀ⓜ

+ O03.37   Sepsis following incomplete spontaneous abortion ♀ⓜ
Use additional code to identify infectious agent (B95-B97)
Use additional code to identify severe sepsis, if applicable (R65.2-)
| **EXCLUDES 1** | *septic or septicopyemic embolism following incomplete spontaneous abortion (O03.2)* |

O03.38   Urinary tract infection following incomplete spontaneous abortion ♀ⓜ
Cystitis following incomplete spontaneous abortion

O03.39   Incomplete spontaneous abortion with other complications ♀ⓜ

O03.4   Incomplete spontaneous abortion without complication ♀ⓜ

O03.5   Genital tract and pelvic infection following complete or unspecified spontaneous abortion ♀ⓜ
Endometritis following complete or unspecified spontaneous abortion
Oophoritis following complete or unspecified spontaneous abortion
Parametritis following complete or unspecified spontaneous abortion
Pelvic peritonitis following complete or unspecified spontaneous abortion
Salpingitis following complete or unspecified spontaneous abortion
Salpingo-oophoritis following complete or unspecified spontaneous abortion
| **EXCLUDES 1** | *sepsis following complete or unspecified spontaneous abortion (O03.87)* |
| | *urinary tract infection following complete or unspecified spontaneous abortion (O03.88)* |

● New   ▲ Revised   *Manifestation*   ④-⑦ Digit Indicators   ⊟ Laterality   Ⓐ Adult (15+ years)   Ⓜ Maternity (12-55 years)   Ⓝ Newborn   Ⓟ Pediatric (0-17 years)   ♂ Male   ♀ Female
✖ Deleted   Unspecified   + Additional code

838   © 2017 DecisionHealth   2017 ICD-10-CM Expert for Physicians

O03.6   **Delayed or excessive hemorrhage following complete or unspecified spontaneous abortion**   ♀ⓜ

Afibrinogenemia following complete or unspecified spontaneous abortion

Defibrination syndrome following complete or unspecified spontaneous abortion

Hemolysis following complete or unspecified spontaneous abortion

Intravascular coagulation following complete or unspecified spontaneous abortion

O03.7   **Embolism following complete or unspecified spontaneous abortion**   ♀ⓜ

Air embolism following complete or unspecified spontaneous abortion

Amniotic fluid embolism following complete or unspecified spontaneous abortion

Blood-clot embolism following complete or unspecified spontaneous abortion

Embolism NOS following complete or unspecified spontaneous abortion

Fat embolism following complete or unspecified spontaneous abortion

Pulmonary embolism following complete or unspecified spontaneous abortion

Pyemic embolism following complete or unspecified spontaneous abortion

Septic or septicopyemic embolism following complete or unspecified spontaneous abortion

Soap embolism following complete or unspecified spontaneous abortion

⑤ O03.8   **Other and unspecified complications following complete or unspecified spontaneous abortion**   ♀ⓜ

   O03.80   **Unspecified complication following complete or unspecified spontaneous abortion**   ♀ⓜ

   O03.81   **Shock following complete or unspecified spontaneous abortion**   ♀ⓜ

Circulatory collapse following complete or unspecified spontaneous abortion

Shock (postprocedural) following complete or unspecified spontaneous abortion

     EXCLUDES 1   *shock due to infection following complete or unspecified spontaneous abortion (O03.87)*

   O03.82   **Renal failure following complete or unspecified spontaneous abortion**   ♀ⓜ

Kidney failure (acute) following complete or unspecified spontaneous abortion

Oliguria following complete or unspecified spontaneous abortion

Renal shutdown following complete or unspecified spontaneous abortion

Renal tubular necrosis following complete or unspecified spontaneous abortion

Uremia following complete or unspecified spontaneous abortion

   O03.83   **Metabolic disorder following complete or unspecified spontaneous abortion**   ♀ⓜ

   O03.84   **Damage to pelvic organs following complete or unspecified spontaneous abortion**   ♀ⓜ

Laceration, perforation, tear or chemical damage of bladder following complete or unspecified spontaneous abortion

Laceration, perforation, tear or chemical damage of bowel following complete or unspecified spontaneous abortion

Laceration, perforation, tear or chemical damage of broad ligament following complete or unspecified spontaneous abortion

Laceration, perforation, tear or chemical damage of cervix following complete or unspecified spontaneous abortion

Laceration, perforation, tear or chemical damage of periurethral tissue following complete or unspecified spontaneous abortion

Laceration, perforation, tear or chemical damage of uterus following complete or unspecified spontaneous abortion

Laceration, perforation, tear or chemical damage of vagina following complete or unspecified spontaneous abortion

   O03.85   **Other venous complications following complete or unspecified spontaneous abortion**   ♀ⓜ

   O03.86   **Cardiac arrest following complete or unspecified spontaneous abortion**   ♀ⓜ

   + O03.87   **Sepsis following complete or unspecified spontaneous abortion**   ♀ⓜ

Use additional code to identify infectious agent (B95-B97)

Use additional code to identify severe sepsis, if applicable (R65.2-)

     EXCLUDES 1   *septic or septicopyemic embolism following complete or unspecified spontaneous abortion (O03.7)*

   O03.88   **Urinary tract infection following complete or unspecified spontaneous abortion**   ♀ⓜ

Cystitis following complete or unspecified spontaneous abortion

   O03.89   **Complete or unspecified spontaneous abortion with other complications**   ♀ⓜ

O03.9   **Complete or unspecified spontaneous abortion without complication**   ♀ⓜ

Miscarriage NOS

Spontaneous abortion NOS

④ O04   **Complications following (induced) termination of pregnancy**

     INCLUDES   complications following (induced) termination of pregnancy

     EXCLUDES 1   *encounter for elective termination of pregnancy, uncomplicated (Z33.2)*

failed attempted termination of pregnancy (O07.-)

O04.5   **Genital tract and pelvic infection following (induced) termination of pregnancy**   ♀ⓜ

Endometritis following (induced) termination of pregnancy

Oophoritis following (induced) termination of pregnancy

Parametritis following (induced) termination of pregnancy

Pelvic peritonitis following (induced) termination of pregnancy

Salpingitis following (induced) termination of pregnancy

Salpingo-oophoritis following (induced) termination of pregnancy

     EXCLUDES 1   *sepsis following (induced) termination of pregnancy (O04.87)*

urinary tract infection following (induced) termination of pregnancy (O04.88)

O04.6   **Delayed or excessive hemorrhage following (induced) termination of pregnancy**   ♀ⓜ

Afibrinogenemia following (induced) termination of pregnancy

Defibrination syndrome following (induced) termination of pregnancy

Hemolysis following (induced) termination of pregnancy

Intravascular coagulation following (induced) termination of pregnancy

O04.7   **Embolism following (induced) termination of pregnancy**   ♀ⓜ

Air embolism following (induced) termination of pregnancy

Amniotic fluid embolism following (induced) termination of pregnancy

Blood-clot embolism following (induced) termination of pregnancy

Embolism NOS following (induced) termination of pregnancy

Fat embolism following (induced) termination of pregnancy

Pulmonary embolism following (induced) termination of pregnancy

Pyemic embolism following (induced) termination of pregnancy

Septic or septicopyemic embolism following (induced) termination of pregnancy

Soap embolism following (induced) termination of pregnancy

⑤ O04.8   **(Induced) termination of pregnancy with other and unspecified complications**   ♀ⓜ

   O04.80   **(Induced) termination of pregnancy with unspecified complications**   ♀ⓜ

O04.81 Shock following (induced) termination of ♀Ⓜ
pregnancy
Circulatory collapse following (induced) termination of
pregnancy
Shock (postprocedural) following (induced) termination
of pregnancy
> **EXCLUDES 1**   *shock due to infection following
(induced) termination of pregnancy
(O04.87)*

O04.82 Renal failure following (induced) termination of ♀Ⓜ
pregnancy
Kidney failure (acute) following (induced) termination
of pregnancy
Oliguria following (induced) termination of pregnancy
Renal shutdown following (induced) termination of
pregnancy
Renal tubular necrosis following (induced) termination
of pregnancy
Uremia following (induced) termination of pregnancy

O04.83 Metabolic disorder following (induced) ♀Ⓜ
termination of pregnancy

O04.84 Damage to pelvic organs following (induced) ♀Ⓜ
termination of pregnancy
Laceration, perforation, tear or chemical damage of
bladder following (induced) termination of pregnancy
Laceration, perforation, tear or chemical damage of
bowel following (induced) termination of pregnancy
Laceration, perforation, tear or chemical damage of
broad ligament following (induced) termination of
pregnancy
Laceration, perforation, tear or chemical damage of
cervix following (induced) termination of pregnancy
Laceration, perforation, tear or chemical damage of
periurethral tissue following (induced) termination of
pregnancy
Laceration, perforation, tear or chemical damage of
uterus following (induced) termination of pregnancy
Laceration, perforation, tear or chemical damage of
vagina following (induced) termination of pregnancy

O04.85 Other venous complications following (induced) ♀Ⓜ
termination of pregnancy

O04.86 Cardiac arrest following (induced) termination ♀Ⓜ
of pregnancy

+ O04.87 Sepsis following (induced) termination of ♀Ⓜ
pregnancy
*Use additional code to identify infectious agent (B95-
B97)*
*Use additional code to identify severe sepsis, if
applicable (R65.2-)*
> **EXCLUDES 1**   *septic or septicopyemic embolism
following (induced) termination of
pregnancy (O04.7)*

O04.88 Urinary tract infection following (induced) ♀Ⓜ
termination of pregnancy
Cystitis following (induced) termination of pregnancy

O04.89 (Induced) termination of pregnancy with other ♀Ⓜ
complications

Ⓐ **O07   Failed attempted termination of pregnancy**
> **INCLUDES**   failure of attempted induction of termination of
pregnancy
incomplete elective abortion
> **EXCLUDES 1**   *incomplete spontaneous abortion (O03.0-)*

O07.0 Genital tract and pelvic infection following failed ♀Ⓜ
attempted termination of pregnancy
Endometritis following failed attempted termination of
pregnancy
Oophoritis following failed attempted termination of
pregnancy
Parametritis following failed attempted termination of
pregnancy
Pelvic peritonitis following failed attempted termination of
pregnancy
Salpingitis following failed attempted termination of
pregnancy
Salpingo-oophoritis following failed attempted termination of
pregnancy
> **EXCLUDES 1**   *sepsis following failed attempted termination
of pregnancy (O07.37)*
> *urinary tract infection following failed
attempted termination of pregnancy
(O07.38)*

O07.1 Delayed or excessive hemorrhage following failed ♀Ⓜ
attempted termination of pregnancy
Afibrinogenemia following failed attempted termination of
pregnancy
Defibrination syndrome following failed attempted
termination of pregnancy
Hemolysis following failed attempted termination of
pregnancy
Intravascular coagulation following failed attempted
termination of pregnancy

O07.2 Embolism following failed attempted termination of ♀Ⓜ
pregnancy
Air embolism following failed attempted termination of
pregnancy
Amniotic fluid embolism following failed attempted
termination of pregnancy
Blood-clot embolism following failed attempted termination
of pregnancy
Embolism NOS following failed attempted termination of
pregnancy
Fat embolism following failed attempted termination of
pregnancy
Pulmonary embolism following failed attempted termination
of pregnancy
Pyemic embolism following failed attempted termination of
pregnancy
Septic or septicopyemic embolism following failed attempted
termination of pregnancy
Soap embolism following failed attempted termination of
pregnancy

Ⓢ **O07.3   Failed attempted termination of pregnancy with** ♀Ⓜ
other and unspecified complications

O07.30 Failed attempted termination of pregnancy with ♀Ⓜ
unspecified complications

O07.31 Shock following failed attempted termination of ♀Ⓜ
pregnancy
Circulatory collapse following failed attempted
termination of pregnancy
Shock (postprocedural) following failed attempted
termination of pregnancy
> **EXCLUDES 1**   *shock due to infection following failed
attempted termination of pregnancy
(O07.37)*

O07.32 Renal failure following failed attempted ♀Ⓜ
termination of pregnancy
Kidney failure (acute) following failed attempted
termination of pregnancy
Oliguria following failed attempted termination of
pregnancy
Renal shutdown following failed attempted termination
of pregnancy
Renal tubular necrosis following failed attempted
termination of pregnancy
Uremia following failed attempted termination of
pregnancy

O07.33 Metabolic disorder following failed attempted ♀Ⓜ
termination of pregnancy

O07.34 Damage to pelvic organs following failed ♀Ⓜ
attempted termination of pregnancy
Laceration, perforation, tear or chemical damage of
bladder following failed attempted termination of
pregnancy
Laceration, perforation, tear or chemical damage of
bowel following failed attempted termination of
pregnancy
Laceration, perforation, tear or chemical damage of
broad ligament following failed attempted
termination of pregnancy
Laceration, perforation, tear or chemical damage of
cervix following failed attempted termination of
pregnancy
Laceration, perforation, tear or chemical damage of
periurethral tissue following failed attempted
termination of pregnancy
Laceration, perforation, tear or chemical damage of
uterus following failed attempted termination of
pregnancy
Laceration, perforation, tear or chemical damage of
vagina following failed attempted termination of
pregnancy

O07.35 Other venous complications following failed ♀Ⓜ
attempted termination of pregnancy

● New ▲ Revised *Manifestation* Ⓐ-Ⓩ Digit Indicators ▤ Laterality Ⓐ Adult Ⓜ Maternity Ⓝ Newborn Ⓟ Pediatric ♂ Male ♀ Female
✖ D̶e̶l̶e̶t̶e̶d̶ Unspecified + Additional code (15+ years) (12-55 years) (0-17 years)

840   © 2017 DecisionHealth   2017 ICD-10-CM Expert for Physicians

O04.81 — O07.35

- **O07.36** Cardiac arrest following failed attempted termination of pregnancy ♀Ⓜ
+ **O07.37** Sepsis following failed attempted termination of pregnancy ♀Ⓜ

    Use additional code (B95-B97), to identify infectious agent

    Use additional code (R65.2-) to identify severe sepsis, if applicable

    EXCLUDES 1 *septic or septicopyemic embolism following failed attempted termination of pregnancy (O07.2)*

- **O07.38** Urinary tract infection following failed attempted termination of pregnancy ♀Ⓜ

    Cystitis following failed attempted termination of pregnancy

- **O07.39** Failed attempted termination of pregnancy with other complications ♀Ⓜ
- **O07.4** Failed attempted termination of pregnancy without complication ♀Ⓜ

④ **O08** Complications following ectopic and molar pregnancy

This category is for use with categories O00-O02 to identify any associated complications

- **O08.0** Genital tract and pelvic infection following ectopic and molar pregnancy ♀Ⓜ

    Endometritis following ectopic and molar pregnancy
    Oophoritis following ectopic and molar pregnancy
    Parametritis following ectopic and molar pregnancy
    Pelvic peritonitis following ectopic and molar pregnancy
    Salpingitis following ectopic and molar pregnancy
    Salpingo-oophoritis following ectopic and molar pregnancy

    EXCLUDES 1 *sepsis following ectopic and molar pregnancy (O08.82)*
    urinary tract infection (O08.83)

- **O08.1** Delayed or excessive hemorrhage following ectopic and molar pregnancy ♀Ⓜ

    Afibrinogenemia following ectopic and molar pregnancy
    Defibrination syndrome following ectopic and molar pregnancy
    Hemolysis following ectopic and molar pregnancy
    Intravascular coagulation following ectopic and molar pregnancy

    EXCLUDES 1 *delayed or excessive hemorrhage due to incomplete abortion (O03.1)*

- **O08.2** Embolism following ectopic and molar pregnancy ♀Ⓜ

    Air embolism following ectopic and molar pregnancy
    Amniotic fluid embolism following ectopic and molar pregnancy
    Blood-clot embolism following ectopic and molar pregnancy
    Embolism NOS following ectopic and molar pregnancy
    Fat embolism following ectopic and molar pregnancy
    Pulmonary embolism following ectopic and molar pregnancy
    Pyemic embolism following ectopic and molar pregnancy
    Septic or septicopyemic embolism following ectopic and molar pregnancy
    Soap embolism following ectopic and molar pregnancy

- **O08.3** Shock following ectopic and molar pregnancy ♀Ⓜ

    Circulatory collapse following ectopic and molar pregnancy
    Shock (postprocedural) following ectopic and molar pregnancy

    EXCLUDES 1 *shock due to infection following ectopic and molar pregnancy (O08.82)*

- **O08.4** Renal failure following ectopic and molar pregnancy ♀Ⓜ

    Kidney failure (acute) following ectopic and molar pregnancy
    Oliguria following ectopic and molar pregnancy
    Renal shutdown following ectopic and molar pregnancy
    Renal tubular necrosis following ectopic and molar pregnancy
    Uremia following ectopic and molar pregnancy

- **O08.5** Metabolic disorders following an ectopic and molar pregnancy ♀Ⓜ

- **O08.6** Damage to pelvic organs and tissues following an ectopic and molar pregnancy ♀Ⓜ

    Laceration, perforation, tear or chemical damage of bladder following an ectopic and molar pregnancy
    Laceration, perforation, tear or chemical damage of bowel following an ectopic and molar pregnancy
    Laceration, perforation, tear or chemical damage of broad ligament following an ectopic and molar pregnancy
    Laceration, perforation, tear or chemical damage of cervix following an ectopic and molar pregnancy
    Laceration, perforation, tear or chemical damage of periurethral tissue following an ectopic and molar pregnancy
    Laceration, perforation, tear or chemical damage of uterus following an ectopic and molar pregnancy
    Laceration, perforation, tear or chemical damage of vagina following an ectopic and molar pregnancy

- **O08.7** Other venous complications following an ectopic and molar pregnancy ♀Ⓜ

⑤ **O08.8** Other complications following an ectopic and molar pregnancy ♀Ⓜ

- **O08.81** Cardiac arrest following an ectopic and molar pregnancy ♀Ⓜ
+ **O08.82** Sepsis following ectopic and molar pregnancy ♀Ⓜ

    Use additional code (B95-B97), to identify infectious agent

    Use additional code (R65.2-) to identify severe sepsis, if applicable

    EXCLUDES 1 *septic or septicopyemic embolism following ectopic and molar pregnancy (O08.2)*

- **O08.83** Urinary tract infection following an ectopic and molar pregnancy ♀Ⓜ

    Cystitis following an ectopic and molar pregnancy

- **O08.89** Other complications following an ectopic and molar pregnancy ♀Ⓜ

- **O08.9** Unspecified complication following an ectopic and molar pregnancy ♀Ⓜ

Supervision of high risk pregnancy (O09)

④ **O09** Supervision of high risk pregnancy

⑤ **O09.0** Supervision of pregnancy with history of infertility ♀Ⓜ

- **O09.00** Supervision of pregnancy with history of infertility, unspecified trimester ♀Ⓜ
- **O09.01** Supervision of pregnancy with history of infertility, first trimester ♀Ⓜ
- **O09.02** Supervision of pregnancy with history of infertility, second trimester ♀Ⓜ
- **O09.03** Supervision of pregnancy with history of infertility, third trimester ♀Ⓜ

▲⑤ **O09.1** Supervision of pregnancy with history of ectopic pregnancy ♀Ⓜ

- ▲ **O09.10** Supervision of pregnancy with history of ectopic pregnancy, unspecified trimester ♀Ⓜ
- ▲ **O09.11** Supervision of pregnancy with history of ectopic pregnancy, first trimester ♀Ⓜ
- ▲ **O09.12** Supervision of pregnancy with history of ectopic pregnancy, second trimester ♀Ⓜ
- ▲ **O09.13** Supervision of pregnancy with history of ectopic pregnancy, third trimester ♀Ⓜ

●⑤ **O09.A** Supervision of pregnancy with history of molar pregnancy ♀Ⓜ

- ● **O09.A0** Supervision of pregnancy with history of molar pregnancy, unspecified trimester ♀Ⓜ
- ● **O09.A1** Supervision of pregnancy with history of molar pregnancy, first trimester ♀Ⓜ
- ● **O09.A2** Supervision of pregnancy with history of molar pregnancy, second trimester ♀Ⓜ
- ● **O09.A3** Supervision of pregnancy with history of molar pregnancy, third trimester ♀Ⓜ

⑤ **O09.2** Supervision of pregnancy with other poor reproductive or obstetric history ♀Ⓜ

    EXCLUDES 2 *pregnancy care for patient with history of recurrent pregnancy loss (O26.2-)*

⑥ **O09.21** Supervision of pregnancy with history of pre-term labor

- **O09.211** Supervision of pregnancy with history of pre-term labor, first trimester ♀Ⓜ

● New ▲ Revised *Manifestation* ④-⑦ Digit Indicators ▤ Laterality Ⓐ Adult (15+ years) Ⓜ Maternity (12-55 years) Ⓝ Newborn Ⓟ Pediatric (0-17 years) ♂ Male ♀ Female
✖ ~~Deleted~~ Unspecified + Additional code

Pregnancy, Childbirth and the Puerperium

O07.36 — O09.211

O09.212 Supervision of pregnancy with history of
pre-term labor, second trimester ♀Ⓜ

O09.213 Supervision of pregnancy with history of
pre-term labor, third trimester ♀Ⓜ

O09.219 Supervision of pregnancy with history of
pre-term labor, unspecified trimester ♀Ⓜ

Ⓢ O09.29 Supervision of pregnancy with other poor
reproductive or obstetric history
Supervision of pregnancy with history of neonatal death
Supervision of pregnancy with history of stillbirth

O09.291 Supervision of pregnancy with other poor
reproductive or obstetric history, first
trimester ♀Ⓜ

O09.292 Supervision of pregnancy with other poor
reproductive or obstetric history, second
trimester ♀Ⓜ

O09.293 Supervision of pregnancy with other poor
reproductive or obstetric history, third
trimester ♀Ⓜ

O09.299 Supervision of pregnancy with other poor
reproductive or obstetric history,
unspecified trimester ♀Ⓜ

Ⓢ O09.3 Supervision of pregnancy with insufficient antenatal
care ♀Ⓜ
Supervision of concealed pregnancy
Supervision of hidden pregnancy

O09.30 Supervision of pregnancy with insufficient
antenatal care, unspecified trimester ♀Ⓜ

O09.31 Supervision of pregnancy with insufficient
antenatal care, first trimester ♀Ⓜ

O09.32 Supervision of pregnancy with insufficient
antenatal care, second trimester ♀Ⓜ

O09.33 Supervision of pregnancy with insufficient
antenatal care, third trimester ♀Ⓜ

Ⓢ O09.4 Supervision of pregnancy with grand multiparity ♀Ⓜ

O09.40 Supervision of pregnancy with grand
multiparity, unspecified trimester ♀Ⓜ

O09.41 Supervision of pregnancy with grand
multiparity, first trimester ♀Ⓜ

O09.42 Supervision of pregnancy with grand
multiparity, second trimester ♀Ⓜ

O09.43 Supervision of pregnancy with grand
multiparity, third trimester ♀Ⓜ

Ⓢ O09.5 Supervision of elderly primigravida and multigravida ♀Ⓜ
Pregnancy for a female 35 years and older at expected date of
delivery

Ⓢ O09.51 Supervision of elderly primigravida

O09.511 Supervision of elderly primigravida, first
trimester ♀Ⓜ

O09.512 Supervision of elderly primigravida, second
trimester ♀Ⓜ

O09.513 Supervision of elderly primigravida, third
trimester ♀Ⓜ

O09.519 Supervision of elderly primigravida,
unspecified trimester ♀Ⓜ

Ⓢ O09.52 Supervision of elderly multigravida

O09.521 Supervision of elderly multigravida, first
trimester ♀Ⓜ

O09.522 Supervision of elderly multigravida, second
trimester ♀Ⓜ

O09.523 Supervision of elderly multigravida, third
trimester ♀Ⓜ

O09.529 Supervision of elderly multigravida,
unspecified trimester ♀Ⓜ

Ⓢ O09.6 Supervision of young primigravida and multigravida ♀Ⓜ
Supervision of pregnancy for a female less than 16 years old
at expected date of delivery

Ⓢ O09.61 Supervision of young primigravida

O09.611 Supervision of young primigravida, first
trimester ♀Ⓜ

O09.612 Supervision of young primigravida, second
trimester ♀Ⓜ

O09.613 Supervision of young primigravida, third
trimester ♀Ⓜ

O09.619 Supervision of young primigravida,
unspecified trimester ♀Ⓜ

Ⓢ O09.62 Supervision of young multigravida

O09.621 Supervision of young multigravida, first
trimester ♀Ⓜ

O09.622 Supervision of young multigravida, second
trimester ♀Ⓜ

O09.623 Supervision of young multigravida, third
trimester ♀Ⓜ

O09.629 Supervision of young multigravida,
unspecified trimester ♀Ⓜ

Ⓢ O09.7 Supervision of high risk pregnancy due to social
problems ♀Ⓜ

O09.70 Supervision of high risk pregnancy due to social
problems, unspecified trimester ♀Ⓜ

O09.71 Supervision of high risk pregnancy due to social
problems, first trimester ♀Ⓜ

O09.72 Supervision of high risk pregnancy due to social
problems, second trimester ♀Ⓜ

O09.73 Supervision of high risk pregnancy due to social
problems, third trimester ♀Ⓜ

Ⓢ O09.8 Supervision of other high risk pregnancies ♀Ⓜ

▲ Ⓢ O09.81 Supervision of pregnancy resulting from assisted
reproductive technology
Supervision of pregnancy resulting from in-vitro
fertilization
EXCLUDES 2 gestational carrier status (Z33.3)

O09.811 Supervision of pregnancy resulting from
assisted reproductive technology, first
trimester ♀Ⓜ

O09.812 Supervision of pregnancy resulting from
assisted reproductive technology, second
trimester ♀Ⓜ

O09.813 Supervision of pregnancy resulting from
assisted reproductive technology, third
trimester ♀Ⓜ

O09.819 Supervision of pregnancy resulting from
assisted reproductive technology,
unspecified trimester ♀Ⓜ

Ⓢ O09.82 Supervision of pregnancy with history of in utero
procedure during previous pregnancy

O09.821 Supervision of pregnancy with history of in
utero procedure during previous
pregnancy, first trimester ♀Ⓜ

O09.822 Supervision of pregnancy with history of in
utero procedure during previous
pregnancy, second trimester ♀Ⓜ

O09.823 Supervision of pregnancy with history of in
utero procedure during previous
pregnancy, third trimester ♀Ⓜ

O09.829 Supervision of pregnancy with history of in
utero procedure during previous
pregnancy, unspecified trimester ♀Ⓜ

EXCLUDES 1 supervision of pregnancy affected
by in utero procedure during
current pregnancy (O35.7)

Ⓢ O09.89 Supervision of other high risk pregnancies ♀Ⓜ

O09.891 Supervision of other high risk pregnancies,
first trimester ♀Ⓜ

O09.892 Supervision of other high risk pregnancies,
second trimester ♀Ⓜ

O09.893 Supervision of other high risk pregnancies,
third trimester ♀Ⓜ

O09.899 Supervision of other high risk pregnancies,
unspecified trimester ♀Ⓜ

Ⓢ O09.9 Supervision of high risk pregnancy, unspecified ♀Ⓜ

O09.90 Supervision of high risk pregnancy, unspecified,
unspecified trimester ♀Ⓜ

O09.91 Supervision of high risk pregnancy, unspecified,
first trimester ♀Ⓜ

O09.92 Supervision of high risk pregnancy, unspecified,
second trimester ♀Ⓜ

O09.93 Supervision of high risk pregnancy, unspecified,
third trimester ♀Ⓜ

Edema, proteinuria and hypertensive disorders in pregnancy, childbirth and the puerperium (O10-O16)

◢ **O10** **Pre-existing hypertension complicating pregnancy, childbirth and the puerperium**

> **INCLUDES** pre-existing hypertension with pre-existing proteinuria complicating pregnancy, childbirth and the puerperium

> **EXCLUDES 2** *pre-existing hypertension with superimposed pre-eclampsia complicating pregnancy, childbirth and the puerperium (O11.-)*

> **GUIDELINES** Section I.C.15.d
> Category O10 includes codes for hypertensive heart and hypertensive chronic kidney disease. When assigning one of the O10 codes that includes hypertensive heart disease or hypertensive chronic kidney disease, it is necessary to add a secondary code from the appropriate hypertension category to specify the type of heart failure or chronic kidney disease.

⑤ **O10.0** **Pre-existing essential hypertension complicating pregnancy, childbirth and the puerperium**
> Any condition in I10 specified as a reason for obstetric care during pregnancy, childbirth or the puerperium

⑥ **O10.01** **Pre-existing essential hypertension complicating pregnancy,**

O10.011 Pre-existing essential hypertension complicating pregnancy, first trimester ♀M

O10.012 Pre-existing essential hypertension complicating pregnancy, second trimester ♀M

O10.013 Pre-existing essential hypertension complicating pregnancy, third trimester ♀M

O10.019 Pre-existing essential hypertension complicating pregnancy, unspecified trimester ♀M

O10.02 Pre-existing essential hypertension complicating childbirth ♀M

O10.03 Pre-existing essential hypertension complicating the puerperium ♀M

⑤＋ **O10.1** **Pre-existing hypertensive heart disease complicating pregnancy, childbirth and the puerperium**
> Any condition in I11 specified as a reason for obstetric care during pregnancy, childbirth or the puerperium
> *Use additional code from I11 to identify the type of hypertensive heart disease*

⑥＋ **O10.11** **Pre-existing hypertensive heart disease complicating pregnancy**

＋ **O10.111** Pre-existing hypertensive heart disease complicating pregnancy, first trimester ♀M

＋ **O10.112** Pre-existing hypertensive heart disease complicating pregnancy, second trimester ♀M

＋ **O10.113** Pre-existing hypertensive heart disease complicating pregnancy, third trimester ♀M

＋ **O10.119** Pre-existing hypertensive heart disease complicating pregnancy, unspecified trimester ♀M

＋ **O10.12** Pre-existing hypertensive heart disease complicating childbirth ♀M

＋ **O10.13** Pre-existing hypertensive heart disease complicating the puerperium ♀M

⑤＋ **O10.2** **Pre-existing hypertensive chronic kidney disease complicating pregnancy, childbirth and the puerperium**
> Any condition in I12 specified as a reason for obstetric care during pregnancy, childbirth or the puerperium
> *Use additional code from I12 to identify the type of hypertensive chronic kidney disease*

⑥＋ **O10.21** **Pre-existing hypertensive chronic kidney disease complicating pregnancy**

＋ **O10.211** Pre-existing hypertensive chronic kidney disease complicating pregnancy, first trimester ♀M

＋ **O10.212** Pre-existing hypertensive chronic kidney disease complicating pregnancy, second trimester ♀M

＋ **O10.213** Pre-existing hypertensive chronic kidney disease complicating pregnancy, third trimester ♀M

＋ **O10.219** Pre-existing hypertensive chronic kidney disease complicating pregnancy, unspecified trimester ♀M

＋ **O10.22** Pre-existing hypertensive chronic kidney disease complicating childbirth ♀M

＋ **O10.23** Pre-existing hypertensive chronic kidney disease complicating the puerperium ♀M

⑤＋ **O10.3** **Pre-existing hypertensive heart and chronic kidney disease complicating pregnancy, childbirth and the puerperium**
> Any condition in I13 specified as a reason for obstetric care during pregnancy, childbirth or the puerperium
> *Use additional code from I13 to identify the type of hypertensive heart and chronic kidney disease*

⑥＋ **O10.31** **Pre-existing hypertensive heart and chronic kidney disease complicating pregnancy**

＋ **O10.311** Pre-existing hypertensive heart and chronic kidney disease complicating pregnancy, first trimester ♀M

＋ **O10.312** Pre-existing hypertensive heart and chronic kidney disease complicating pregnancy, second trimester ♀M

＋ **O10.313** Pre-existing hypertensive heart and chronic kidney disease complicating pregnancy, third trimester ♀M

＋ **O10.319** Pre-existing hypertensive heart and chronic kidney disease complicating pregnancy, unspecified trimester ♀M

＋ **O10.32** Pre-existing hypertensive heart and chronic kidney disease complicating childbirth ♀M

＋ **O10.33** Pre-existing hypertensive heart and chronic kidney disease complicating the puerperium ♀M

⑤＋ **O10.4** **Pre-existing secondary hypertension complicating pregnancy, childbirth and the puerperium**
> Any condition in I15 specified as a reason for obstetric care during pregnancy, childbirth or the puerperium
> *Use additional code from I15 to identify the type of secondary hypertension*

⑥＋ **O10.41** **Pre-existing secondary hypertension complicating pregnancy**

＋ **O10.411** Pre-existing secondary hypertension complicating pregnancy, first trimester ♀M

＋ **O10.412** Pre-existing secondary hypertension complicating pregnancy, second trimester ♀M

＋ **O10.413** Pre-existing secondary hypertension complicating pregnancy, third trimester ♀M

＋ **O10.419** Pre-existing secondary hypertension complicating pregnancy, unspecified trimester ♀M

＋ **O10.42** Pre-existing secondary hypertension complicating childbirth ♀M

＋ **O10.43** Pre-existing secondary hypertension complicating the puerperium ♀M

⑤ **O10.9** **Unspecified pre-existing hypertension complicating pregnancy, childbirth and the puerperium**

⑥ **O10.91** **Unspecified pre-existing hypertension complicating pregnancy**

O10.911 Unspecified pre-existing hypertension complicating pregnancy, first trimester ♀M

O10.912 Unspecified pre-existing hypertension complicating pregnancy, second trimester ♀M

O10.913 Unspecified pre-existing hypertension complicating pregnancy, third trimester ♀M

O10.919 Unspecified pre-existing hypertension complicating pregnancy, unspecified trimester ♀M

O10.92 Unspecified pre-existing hypertension complicating childbirth ♀M

O10.93 Unspecified pre-existing hypertension complicating the puerperium ♀M

● New ▲ Revised *Manifestation* ④-❼ Digit Indicators ▤ Laterality ▲ Adult (15+ years) ▨ Maternity (12-55 years) ▧ Newborn ▣ Pediatric (0-17 years) ♂ Male ♀ Female
✖ Deleted Unspecified ＋ Additional code

Pregnancy, Childbirth and the Puerperium

④+ **O11** **Pre-existing hypertension with pre-eclampsia**

INCLUDES conditions in O10 complicated by pre-eclampsia
pre-eclampsia superimposed pre-existing
hypertension

Use additional code from O10 to identify the type of hypertension

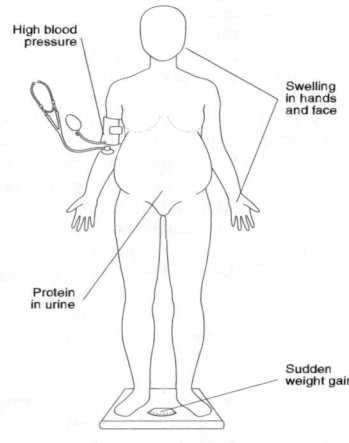

Pre-existing hypertension with pre-eclampsia

High blood pressure

Swelling in hands and face

Protein in urine

Sudden weight gain

+ **O11.1** Pre-existing hypertension with pre-eclampsia, first trimester ♀Ⓜ

+ **O11.2** Pre-existing hypertension with pre-eclampsia, second trimester ♀Ⓜ

+ **O11.3** Pre-existing hypertension with pre-eclampsia, third trimester ♀Ⓜ

●+ **O11.4** Pre-existing hypertension with pre-eclampsia, complicating childbirth ♀Ⓜ

●+ **O11.5** Pre-existing hypertension with pre-eclampsia, complicating the puerperium ♀Ⓜ

+ **O11.9** Pre-existing hypertension with pre-eclampsia, unspecified trimester ♀Ⓜ

④ **O12** **Gestational [pregnancy-induced] edema and proteinuria without hypertension**

⑤ **O12.0** **Gestational edema**

O12.00 Gestational edema, unspecified trimester ♀Ⓜ

O12.01 Gestational edema, first trimester ♀Ⓜ

O12.02 Gestational edema, second trimester ♀Ⓜ

O12.03 Gestational edema, third trimester ♀Ⓜ

● **O12.04** Gestational edema, complicating childbirth ♀Ⓜ

● **O12.05** Gestational edema, complicating the puerperium ♀Ⓜ

⑤ **O12.1** **Gestational proteinuria**

O12.10 Gestational proteinuria, unspecified trimester ♀Ⓜ

O12.11 Gestational proteinuria, first trimester ♀Ⓜ

O12.12 Gestational proteinuria, second trimester ♀Ⓜ

O12.13 Gestational proteinuria, third trimester ♀Ⓜ

● **O12.14** Gestational proteinuria, complicating childbirth ♀Ⓜ

● **O12.15** Gestational proteinuria, complicating the puerperium ♀Ⓜ

⑤ **O12.2** **Gestational edema with proteinuria**

O12.20 Gestational edema with proteinuria, unspecified trimester ♀Ⓜ

O12.21 Gestational edema with proteinuria, first trimester ♀Ⓜ

O12.22 Gestational edema with proteinuria, second trimester ♀Ⓜ

O12.23 Gestational edema with proteinuria, third trimester ♀Ⓜ

● **O12.24** Gestational edema with proteinuria, complicating childbirth ♀Ⓜ

● **O12.25** Gestational edema with proteinuria, complicating the puerperium ♀Ⓜ

▲④ **O13** **Gestational [pregnancy-induced] hypertension without significant proteinuria**

INCLUDES gestational hypertension NOS
transient hypertension of pregnancy

GUIDELINES Section I.9.a.7)
Unless patient has an established diagnosis of hypertension, assign code O13.-, Gestational [pregnancy-induced] hypertension without significant proteinuria, or O14.-, Pre-eclampsia, for transient hypertension of pregnancy.

O13.1 Gestational [pregnancy-induced] hypertension without significant proteinuria, first trimester ♀Ⓜ

O13.2 Gestational [pregnancy-induced] hypertension without significant proteinuria, second trimester ♀Ⓜ

O13.3 Gestational [pregnancy-induced] hypertension without significant proteinuria, third trimester ♀Ⓜ

● **O13.4** Gestational [pregnancy-induced] hypertension without significant proteinuria, complicating childbirth ♀Ⓜ

● **O13.5** Gestational [pregnancy-induced] hypertension without significant proteinuria, complicating the puerperium ♀Ⓜ

O13.9 Gestational [pregnancy-induced] hypertension without significant proteinuria, unspecified trimester ♀Ⓜ

④ **O14** **Pre-eclampsia**

EXCLUDES 1 *pre-existing hypertension with pre-eclampsia (O11)*

GUIDELINES Section I.9.a.7)
Unless patient has an established diagnosis of hypertension, assign code O13.-, Gestational [pregnancy-induced] hypertension without significant proteinuria, or O14.-, Pre-eclampsia, for transient hypertension of pregnancy.

⑤ **O14.0** **Mild to moderate pre-eclampsia**

DEFINITION Hypertension (BP >140/90 mmHg) after the 20th week of gestation and up to 6 weeks postpartum, with proteinuria.

O14.00 Mild to moderate pre-eclampsia, unspecified trimester ♀Ⓜ

O14.02 Mild to moderate pre-eclampsia, second trimester ♀Ⓜ

O14.03 Mild to moderate pre-eclampsia, third trimester ♀Ⓜ

● **O14.04** Mild to moderate pre-eclampsia, complicating childbirth ♀Ⓜ

● **O14.05** Mild to moderate pre-eclampsia, complicating the puerperium ♀

⑤ **O14.1** **Severe pre-eclampsia**

EXCLUDES 1 *HELLP syndrome (O14.2-)*

DEFINITION Severe hypertension (BP >160/110 mmHg) after the 20th week of gestation and up to 6 weeks postpartum, with proteinuria, and additional symptoms such as pulmonary edema, upper abdominal pain, severe headaches, and blurred vision.

O14.10 Severe pre-eclampsia, unspecified trimester ♀Ⓜ

O14.12 Severe pre-eclampsia, second trimester ♀Ⓜ

O14.13 Severe pre-eclampsia, third trimester ♀Ⓜ

● **O14.14** Severe pre-eclampsia complicating childbirth ♀Ⓜ

● **O14.15** Severe pre-eclampsia, complicating the puerperium ♀Ⓜ

⑤ **O14.2** **HELLP syndrome**

Severe pre-eclampsia with hemolysis, elevated liver enzymes and low platelet count (HELLP)

DEFINITION Severe pre-eclampsia with hemolysis, elevated liver enzymes and low platelet count (HELLP).

O14.20 HELLP syndrome (HELLP), unspecified trimester ♀Ⓜ

O14.22 HELLP syndrome (HELLP), second trimester ♀Ⓜ

O14.23 HELLP syndrome (HELLP), third trimester ♀Ⓜ

● **O14.24** HELLP syndrome, complicating childbirth ♀Ⓜ

● **O14.25** HELLP syndrome, complicating the puerperium ♀Ⓜ

⑤ **O14.9** **Unspecified pre-eclampsia**

O14.90 Unspecified pre-eclampsia, unspecified trimester ♀Ⓜ

O14.92 Unspecified pre-eclampsia, second trimester ♀Ⓜ

O14.93 Unspecified pre-eclampsia, third trimester ♀Ⓜ

● **O14.94** Unspecified pre-eclampsia, complicating childbirth ♀Ⓜ

● **O14.95** Unspecified pre-eclampsia, complicating the puerperium ♀Ⓜ

● New ▲ Revised *Manifestation* ④-⑦ Digit Indicators ▭ Laterality Ⓐ Adult (15+ years) Ⓜ Maternity (12-55 years) Ⓝ Newborn Ⓟ Pediatric (0-17 years) ♂ Male ♀ Female

✖ ~~Deleted~~ Unspecified + Additional code

844   © 2017 DecisionHealth   2017 ICD-10-CM Expert for Physicians

⊿ **O15   Eclampsia**

⬛ INCLUDES   convulsions following conditions in O10-O14 and O16

▲ ⑤ **O15.0   Eclampsia complicating pregnancy**

▲ **O15.00   Eclampsia complicating pregnancy, unspecified trimester**   ♀Ⓜ

▲ **O15.02   Eclampsia complicating pregnancy, second trimester**   ♀Ⓜ

▲ **O15.03   Eclampsia complicating pregnancy, third trimester**   ♀Ⓜ

▲ **O15.1   Eclampsia complicating labor**   ♀Ⓜ

▲ **O15.2   Eclampsia complicating the puerperium**   ♀Ⓜ

O15.9   Eclampsia, unspecified as to time period   ♀Ⓜ
Eclampsia NOS

⊿ **O16   Unspecified maternal hypertension**

O16.1   Unspecified maternal hypertension, first trimester   ♀Ⓜ

O16.2   Unspecified maternal hypertension, second trimester   ♀Ⓜ

O16.3   Unspecified maternal hypertension, third trimester   ♀Ⓜ

● **O16.4   Unspecified maternal hypertension, complicating childbirth**   ♀Ⓜ

● **O16.5   Unspecified maternal hypertension, complicating the puerperium**   ♀Ⓜ

O16.9   Unspecified maternal hypertension, unspecified trimester   ♀Ⓜ

Other maternal disorders predominantly related to pregnancy (O20-O29)

⬛ EXCLUDES 2   *maternal care related to the fetus and amniotic cavity and possible delivery problems (O30-O48)*
maternal diseases classifiable elsewhere but complicating pregnancy, labor and delivery, and the puerperium (O98-O99)

⊿ **O20   Hemorrhage in early pregnancy**

⬛ INCLUDES   hemorrhage before completion of 20 weeks gestation

⬛ EXCLUDES 1   *pregnancy with abortive outcome (O00-O08)*

O20.0   Threatened abortion   ♀Ⓜ
Hemorrhage specified as due to threatened abortion

O20.8   Other hemorrhage in early pregnancy   ♀Ⓜ

O20.9   Hemorrhage in early pregnancy, unspecified   ♀Ⓜ

⊿ **O21   Excessive vomiting in pregnancy**

O21.0   Mild hyperemesis gravidarum   ♀Ⓜ
Hyperemesis gravidarum, mild or unspecified, starting before the end of the 20th week of gestation

O21.1   Hyperemesis gravidarum with metabolic disturbance   ♀Ⓜ
Hyperemesis gravidarum, starting before the end of the 20th week of gestation, with metabolic disturbance such as carbohydrate depletion
Hyperemesis gravidarum, starting before the end of the 20th week of gestation, with metabolic disturbance such as dehydration
Hyperemesis gravidarum, starting before the end of the 20th week of gestation, with metabolic disturbance such as electrolyte imbalance

O21.2   Late vomiting of pregnancy   ♀Ⓜ
Excessive vomiting starting after 20 completed weeks of gestation

➕ **O21.8   Other vomiting complicating pregnancy**   ♀Ⓜ
Vomiting due to diseases classified elsewhere, complicating pregnancy
Use additional code, to identify cause.

O21.9   Vomiting of pregnancy, unspecified   ♀Ⓜ

⊿ **O22   Venous complications and hemorrhoids in pregnancy**

⬛ EXCLUDES 1   *venous complications of:*
abortion NOS (O03.9)
ectopic or molar pregnancy (O08.7)
failed attempted abortion (O07.35)
induced abortion (O04.85)
spontaneous abortion (O03.89)

⬛ EXCLUDES 2   *obstetric pulmonary embolism (O88.-)*
venous complications and hemorrhoids of childbirth and the puerperium (O87.-)

⑤ **O22.0   Varicose veins of lower extremity in pregnancy**
Varicose veins NOS in pregnancy

O22.00   Varicose veins of lower extremity in pregnancy, unspecified trimester   ♀Ⓜ

O22.01   Varicose veins of lower extremity in pregnancy, first trimester   ♀Ⓜ

O22.02   Varicose veins of lower extremity in pregnancy, second trimester   ♀Ⓜ

O22.03   Varicose veins of lower extremity in pregnancy, third trimester   ♀Ⓜ

⑤ **O22.1   Genital varices in pregnancy**
Perineal varices in pregnancy
Vaginal varices in pregnancy
Vulval varices in pregnancy

O22.10   Genital varices in pregnancy, unspecified trimester   ♀Ⓜ

O22.11   Genital varices in pregnancy, first trimester   ♀Ⓜ

O22.12   Genital varices in pregnancy, second trimester   ♀Ⓜ

O22.13   Genital varices in pregnancy, third trimester   ♀Ⓜ

⑤➕ **O22.2   Superficial thrombophlebitis in pregnancy**
Phlebitis in pregnancy NOS
Thrombophlebitis of legs in pregnancy
Thrombosis in pregnancy NOS
Use additional code to identify the superficial thrombophlebitis (I80.0-)

➕ **O22.20   Superficial thrombophlebitis in pregnancy, unspecified trimester**   ♀Ⓜ

➕ **O22.21   Superficial thrombophlebitis in pregnancy, first trimester**   ♀Ⓜ

➕ **O22.22   Superficial thrombophlebitis in pregnancy, second trimester**   ♀Ⓜ

➕ **O22.23   Superficial thrombophlebitis in pregnancy, third trimester**   ♀Ⓜ

⑤➕ **O22.3   Deep phlebothrombosis in pregnancy**
Deep vein thrombosis, antepartum
Use additional code to identify the deep vein thrombosis (I82.4-, I82.5-, I82.62-. I82.72-)
Use additional code, if applicable, for associated long-term (current) use of anticoagulants (Z79.01)

➕ **O22.30   Deep phlebothrombosis in pregnancy, unspecified trimester**   ♀Ⓜ

➕ **O22.31   Deep phlebothrombosis in pregnancy, first trimester**   ♀Ⓜ

➕ **O22.32   Deep phlebothrombosis in pregnancy, second trimester**   ♀Ⓜ

➕ **O22.33   Deep phlebothrombosis in pregnancy, third trimester**   ♀Ⓜ

⑤ **O22.4   Hemorrhoids in pregnancy**

O22.40   Hemorrhoids in pregnancy, unspecified trimester   ♀Ⓜ

O22.41   Hemorrhoids in pregnancy, first trimester   ♀Ⓜ

O22.42   Hemorrhoids in pregnancy, second trimester   ♀Ⓜ

O22.43   Hemorrhoids in pregnancy, third trimester   ♀Ⓜ

⑤ **O22.5   Cerebral venous thrombosis in pregnancy**
Cerebrovenous sinus thrombosis in pregnancy

O22.50   Cerebral venous thrombosis in pregnancy, unspecified trimester   ♀Ⓜ

O22.51   Cerebral venous thrombosis in pregnancy, first trimester   ♀Ⓜ

O22.52   Cerebral venous thrombosis in pregnancy, second trimester   ♀Ⓜ

O22.53   Cerebral venous thrombosis in pregnancy, third trimester   ♀Ⓜ

⑤ **O22.8   Other venous complications in pregnancy**

⑥ **O22.8X   Other venous complications in pregnancy**

O22.8X1   Other venous complications in pregnancy, first trimester   ♀Ⓜ

O22.8X2   Other venous complications in pregnancy, second trimester   ♀Ⓜ

O22.8X3   Other venous complications in pregnancy, third trimester   ♀Ⓜ

O22.8X9   Other venous complications in pregnancy, unspecified trimester   ♀Ⓜ

⑤ **O22.9   Venous complication in pregnancy, unspecified**
Gestational phlebitis NOS
Gestational phlebopathy NOS
Gestational thrombosis NOS

O22.90   Venous complication in pregnancy, unspecified, unspecified trimester   ♀Ⓜ

O22.91   Venous complication in pregnancy, unspecified, first trimester   ♀Ⓜ

O22.92   Venous complication in pregnancy, unspecified, second trimester   ♀Ⓜ

● New   ▲ Revised   *Manifestation*   ⊿-❼ Digit Indicators   ⬛ Laterality   Ⓐ Adult (15+ years)   Ⓜ Maternity (12-55 years)   Ⓝ Newborn   Ⓟ Pediatric (0-17 years)   ♂ Male   ♀ Female
✖ Deleted   Unspecified   ➕ Additional code

O22.93   Venous complication in pregnancy, unspecified, third trimester ♀Ⓜ

⁴+ O23   **Infections of genitourinary tract in pregnancy**
Use additional code to identify organism (B95.-, B96.-)

> EXCLUDES 2   *gonococcal infections complicating pregnancy, childbirth and the puerperium (O98.2)*
> *infections with a predominantly sexual mode of transmission NOS complicating pregnancy, childbirth and the puerperium (O98.3)*
> *syphilis complicating pregnancy, childbirth and the puerperium (O98.1)*
> *tuberculosis of genitourinary system complicating pregnancy, childbirth and the puerperium (O98.0)*
> *venereal disease NOS complicating pregnancy, childbirth and the puerperium (O98.3)*

⑤+ O23.0   **Infections of kidney in pregnancy**
Pyelonephritis in pregnancy

   + O23.00   Infections of kidney in pregnancy, unspecified trimester ♀Ⓜ

   + O23.01   Infections of kidney in pregnancy, first trimester ♀Ⓜ

   + O23.02   Infections of kidney in pregnancy, second trimester ♀Ⓜ

   + O23.03   Infections of kidney in pregnancy, third trimester ♀Ⓜ

⑤+ O23.1   **Infections of bladder in pregnancy**

   + O23.10   Infections of bladder in pregnancy, unspecified trimester ♀Ⓜ

   + O23.11   Infections of bladder in pregnancy, first trimester ♀Ⓜ

   + O23.12   Infections of bladder in pregnancy, second trimester ♀Ⓜ

   + O23.13   Infections of bladder in pregnancy, third trimester ♀Ⓜ

⑤+ O23.2   **Infections of urethra in pregnancy**

   + O23.20   Infections of urethra in pregnancy, unspecified trimester ♀Ⓜ

   + O23.21   Infections of urethra in pregnancy, first trimester ♀Ⓜ

   + O23.22   Infections of urethra in pregnancy, second trimester ♀Ⓜ

   + O23.23   Infections of urethra in pregnancy, third trimester ♀Ⓜ

⑤+ O23.3   **Infections of other parts of urinary tract in pregnancy**

   + O23.30   Infections of other parts of urinary tract in pregnancy, unspecified trimester ♀Ⓜ

   + O23.31   Infections of other parts of urinary tract in pregnancy, first trimester ♀Ⓜ

   + O23.32   Infections of other parts of urinary tract in pregnancy, second trimester ♀Ⓜ

   + O23.33   Infections of other parts of urinary tract in pregnancy, third trimester ♀Ⓜ

⑤+ O23.4   **Unspecified infection of urinary tract in pregnancy**

   + O23.40   Unspecified infection of urinary tract in pregnancy, unspecified trimester ♀Ⓜ

   + O23.41   Unspecified infection of urinary tract in pregnancy, first trimester ♀Ⓜ

   + O23.42   Unspecified infection of urinary tract in pregnancy, second trimester ♀Ⓜ

   + O23.43   Unspecified infection of urinary tract in pregnancy, third trimester ♀Ⓜ

⑤+ O23.5   **Infections of the genital tract in pregnancy**

   ⑥+ O23.51   **Infection of cervix in pregnancy**

     + O23.511   Infections of cervix in pregnancy, first trimester ♀Ⓜ

     + O23.512   Infections of cervix in pregnancy, second trimester ♀Ⓜ

     + O23.513   Infections of cervix in pregnancy, third trimester ♀Ⓜ

     + O23.519   Infections of cervix in pregnancy, unspecified trimester ♀Ⓜ

   ⑥+ O23.52   **Salpingo-oophoritis in pregnancy**
Oophoritis in pregnancy
Salpingitis in pregnancy

     + O23.521   Salpingo-oophoritis in pregnancy, first trimester ♀Ⓜ

     + O23.522   Salpingo-oophoritis in pregnancy, second trimester ♀Ⓜ

     + O23.523   Salpingo-oophoritis in pregnancy, third trimester ♀Ⓜ

     + O23.529   Salpingo-oophoritis in pregnancy, unspecified trimester ♀Ⓜ

   ⑥+ O23.59   **Infection of other part of genital tract in pregnancy**

     + O23.591   Infection of other part of genital tract in pregnancy, first trimester ♀Ⓜ

     + O23.592   Infection of other part of genital tract in pregnancy, second trimester ♀Ⓜ

     + O23.593   Infection of other part of genital tract in pregnancy, third trimester ♀Ⓜ

     + O23.599   Infection of other part of genital tract in pregnancy, unspecified trimester ♀Ⓜ

⑤+ O23.9   **Unspecified genitourinary tract infection in pregnancy**
Genitourinary tract infection in pregnancy NOS

   + O23.90   Unspecified genitourinary tract infection in pregnancy, unspecified trimester ♀Ⓜ

   + O23.91   Unspecified genitourinary tract infection in pregnancy, first trimester ♀Ⓜ

   + O23.92   Unspecified genitourinary tract infection in pregnancy, second trimester ♀Ⓜ

   + O23.93   Unspecified genitourinary tract infection in pregnancy, third trimester ♀Ⓜ

⁴ O24   **Diabetes mellitus in pregnancy, childbirth, and the puerperium**

> GUIDELINES   **Section I.C.15.g-h**
> Diabetes mellitus is a significant complicating factor in pregnancy. Pregnant women who are diabetic should be assigned a code from category O24 first, followed by the appropriate diabetes code(s) (E08-E13) from Chapter 4. Code Z79.4, Long-term (current) use of insulin, should also be assigned if the diabetes mellitus is being treated with insulin.

▲⑤+ O24.0   **Pre-existing type 1 diabetes mellitus, in pregnancy, childbirth and the puerperium** ♀Ⓜ
Juvenile onset diabetes mellitus, in pregnancy, childbirth and the puerperium
Ketosis-prone diabetes mellitus in pregnancy, childbirth and the puerperium
Use additional code from category E10 to further identify any manifestations

> CODING TIP✓   Use the appropriate code from category O24.0, O24.1, O24.3 or O24.8 for the obstetric patient who had pre-existing diabetes before pregnancy. Use an additional code for the type of diabetes E08-E13.

   ▲⑥+ O24.01   **Pre-existing type 1 diabetes mellitus, in pregnancy**

     ▲+ O24.011   Pre-existing type 1 diabetes mellitus, in pregnancy, first trimester ♀Ⓜ

     ▲+ O24.012   Pre-existing type 1 diabetes mellitus, in pregnancy, second trimester ♀Ⓜ

     ▲+ O24.013   Pre-existing type 1 diabetes mellitus, in pregnancy, third trimester ♀Ⓜ

     ▲+ O24.019   Pre-existing type 1 diabetes mellitus, in pregnancy, unspecified trimester ♀Ⓜ

   ▲+ O24.02   Pre-existing type 1 diabetes mellitus, in childbirth ♀Ⓜ

   ▲+ O24.03   Pre-existing type 1 diabetes mellitus, in the puerperium ♀Ⓜ

▲⑤+ O24.1   **Pre-existing type 2 diabetes mellitus, in pregnancy, childbirth and the puerperium** ♀Ⓜ
Insulin-resistant diabetes mellitus in pregnancy, childbirth and the puerperium
Use additional code (for):
from category E11 to further identify any manifestations
long-term (current) use of insulin (Z79.4)

> CODING TIP✓   Use the appropriate code from category O24.0, O24.1, O24.3 or O24.8 for the obstetric patient who had pre-existing diabetes before pregnancy. Use an additional code for the type of diabetes E08-E13.

   ▲⑥+ O24.11   **Pre-existing type 2 diabetes mellitus, in pregnancy**

     ▲+ O24.111   Pre-existing type 2 diabetes mellitus, in pregnancy, first trimester ♀Ⓜ

     ▲+ O24.112   Pre-existing type 2 diabetes mellitus, in pregnancy, second trimester ♀Ⓜ

     ▲+ O24.113   Pre-existing type 2 diabetes mellitus, in pregnancy, third trimester ♀Ⓜ

     ▲+ O24.119   Pre-existing type 2 diabetes mellitus, in pregnancy, unspecified trimester ♀Ⓜ

● New   ▲ Revised   *Manifestation*   ④-⑦ Digit Indicators   ▤ Laterality   ▣ Adult (15+ years)   Ⓜ Maternity (12-55 years)   Ⓝ Newborn   ▣ Pediatric (0-17 years)   ♂ Male   ♀ Female

✖ Deleted   Unspecified   + Additional code

846   © 2017 DecisionHealth   2017 ICD-10-CM Expert for Physicians

▲ + **O24.12** **Pre-existing type 2 diabetes mellitus, in** ♀Ⓜ
childbirth

▲ + **O24.13** **Pre-existing type 2 diabetes mellitus, in the** ♀Ⓜ
puerperium

⑤ + **O24.3** **Unspecified pre-existing diabetes mellitus in** ♀Ⓜ
pregnancy, childbirth and the puerperium
Use additional code (for):
from category E11 to further identify any manifestation
long-term (current) use of insulin (Z79.4)

CODING TIP ✓ Use the appropriate code from category O24.0, O24.1, O24.3 or O24.8 for the obstetric patient who had pre-existing diabetes before pregnancy. Use an additional code for the type of diabetes E08-E13.

⑥ + **O24.31** **Unspecified pre-existing diabetes mellitus in** ♀Ⓜ
pregnancy

+ **O24.311** **Unspecified pre-existing diabetes mellitus in** ♀Ⓜ
pregnancy, first trimester

+ **O24.312** **Unspecified pre-existing diabetes mellitus in** ♀Ⓜ
pregnancy, second trimester

+ **O24.313** **Unspecified pre-existing diabetes mellitus in** ♀Ⓜ
pregnancy, third trimester

+ **O24.319** **Unspecified pre-existing diabetes mellitus in** ♀Ⓜ
pregnancy, unspecified trimester

+ **O24.32** **Unspecified pre-existing diabetes mellitus in** ♀Ⓜ
childbirth

+ **O24.33** **Unspecified pre-existing diabetes mellitus in the** ♀Ⓜ
puerperium

⑤ **O24.4** **Gestational diabetes mellitus** ♀Ⓜ
Diabetes mellitus arising in pregnancy
Gestational diabetes mellitus NOS

GUIDELINES Section I.C.15.i
Codes for gestational diabetes are in subcategory O24.4. No other code from category O24 should be used with a code from O24.4. The codes under subcategory O24.4 include diet controlled and insulin controlled. If a patient with gestational diabetes is treated with both diet and insulin, only the code for insulin-controlled is required. Code Z79.4, Long-term (current) use of insulin, should not be assigned with codes from subcategory O24.4.

An abnormal glucose tolerance in pregnancy is assigned a code from subcategory O99.81, Abnormal glucose complicating pregnancy, childbirth, and the puerperium.

CODING TIP ✓ Do not use O24.4 if diabetes persists after pregnancy. Use E08 -E13 code.

⑥ **O24.41** **Gestational diabetes mellitus in pregnancy**

O24.410 **Gestational diabetes mellitus in pregnancy,** ♀Ⓜ
diet controlled

O24.414 **Gestational diabetes mellitus in pregnancy,** ♀Ⓜ
insulin controlled

● **O24.415** **Gestational diabetes mellitus in pregnancy,** ♀Ⓜ
controlled by oral hypoglycemic drugs
Gestational diabetes mellitus in pregnancy, controlled by oral antidiabetic drugs

O24.419 **Gestational diabetes mellitus in pregnancy,** ♀Ⓜ
unspecified control
AHA: 4Q 2015, 34

⑥ **O24.42** **Gestational diabetes mellitus in childbirth**

O24.420 **Gestational diabetes mellitus in childbirth,** ♀Ⓜ
diet controlled

O24.424 **Gestational diabetes mellitus in childbirth,** ♀Ⓜ
insulin controlled

● **O24.425** **Gestational diabetes mellitus in childbirth,** ♀Ⓜ
controlled by oral hypoglycemic drugs
Gestational diabetes mellitus in childbirth, controlled by oral antidiabetic drugs

O24.429 **Gestational diabetes mellitus in childbirth,** ♀Ⓜ
unspecified control

⑥ **O24.43** **Gestational diabetes mellitus in the puerperium**

O24.430 **Gestational diabetes mellitus in the** ♀Ⓜ
puerperium, diet controlled

O24.434 **Gestational diabetes mellitus in the** ♀Ⓜ
puerperium, insulin controlled

● **O24.435** **Gestational diabetes mellitus in puerperium,** ♀Ⓜ
controlled by oral hypoglycemic drugs
Gestational diabetes mellitus in puerperium, controlled by oral antidiabetic drugs

O24.439 **Gestational diabetes mellitus in the** ♀Ⓜ
puerperium, unspecified control

⑤ + **O24.8** **Other pre-existing diabetes mellitus in pregnancy,** ♀Ⓜ
childbirth, and the puerperium
Use additional code (for):
from categories E08, E09 and E13 to further identify any manifestation
long-term (current) use of insulin (Z79.4)

CODING TIP ✓ Use the appropriate code from category O24.0, O24.1, O24.3 or O24.8 for the obstetric patient who had pre-existing diabetes before pregnancy. Use an additional code for the type of diabetes E08-E13.

⑥ + **O24.81** **Other pre-existing diabetes mellitus in pregnancy**

+ **O24.811** **Other pre-existing diabetes mellitus in** ♀Ⓜ
pregnancy, first trimester

+ **O24.812** **Other pre-existing diabetes mellitus in** ♀Ⓜ
pregnancy, second trimester

+ **O24.813** **Other pre-existing diabetes mellitus in** ♀Ⓜ
pregnancy, third trimester

+ **O24.819** **Other pre-existing diabetes mellitus in** ♀Ⓜ
pregnancy, unspecified trimester

+ **O24.82** **Other pre-existing diabetes mellitus in childbirth** ♀Ⓜ

+ **O24.83** **Other pre-existing diabetes mellitus in the** ♀Ⓜ
puerperium

⑤ + **O24.9** **Unspecified diabetes mellitus in pregnancy, childbirth** ♀Ⓜ
and the puerperium
Use additional code for long-term (current) use of insulin (Z79.4)

⑥ + **O24.91** **Unspecified diabetes mellitus in pregnancy**

+ **O24.911** **Unspecified diabetes mellitus in pregnancy,** ♀Ⓜ
first trimester

+ **O24.912** **Unspecified diabetes mellitus in pregnancy,** ♀Ⓜ
second trimester

+ **O24.913** **Unspecified diabetes mellitus in pregnancy,** ♀Ⓜ
third trimester

+ **O24.919** **Unspecified diabetes mellitus in pregnancy,** ♀Ⓜ
unspecified trimester

+ **O24.92** **Unspecified diabetes mellitus in childbirth** ♀Ⓜ

+ **O24.93** **Unspecified diabetes mellitus in the puerperium** ♀Ⓜ

④ **O25** **Malnutrition in pregnancy, childbirth and the**
puerperium

⑤ **O25.1** **Malnutrition in pregnancy**

O25.10 **Malnutrition in pregnancy, unspecified** ♀Ⓜ
trimester

O25.11 **Malnutrition in pregnancy, first trimester** ♀Ⓜ

O25.12 **Malnutrition in pregnancy, second trimester** ♀Ⓜ

O25.13 **Malnutrition in pregnancy, third trimester** ♀Ⓜ

O25.2 **Malnutrition in childbirth** ♀Ⓜ

O25.3 **Malnutrition in the puerperium** ♀Ⓜ

④ **O26** **Maternal care for other conditions predominantly**
related to pregnancy

⑤ **O26.0** **Excessive weight gain in pregnancy**

EXCLUDES 2 *gestational edema (O12.0, O12.2)*

O26.00 **Excessive weight gain in pregnancy, unspecified** ♀Ⓜ
trimester

O26.01 **Excessive weight gain in pregnancy, first** ♀Ⓜ
trimester

O26.02 **Excessive weight gain in pregnancy, second** ♀Ⓜ
trimester

O26.03 **Excessive weight gain in pregnancy, third** ♀Ⓜ
trimester

⑤ **O26.1** **Low weight gain in pregnancy**

O26.10 **Low weight gain in pregnancy, unspecified** ♀Ⓜ
trimester

O26.11 **Low weight gain in pregnancy, first trimester** ♀Ⓜ

O26.12 **Low weight gain in pregnancy, second trimester** ♀Ⓜ

O26.13 **Low weight gain in pregnancy, third trimester** ♀Ⓜ

⑤ **O26.2** **Pregnancy care for patient with recurrent pregnancy loss**

O26.20 **Pregnancy care for patient with recurrent** ♀Ⓜ
pregnancy loss, unspecified trimester

O26.21 **Pregnancy care for patient with recurrent** ♀Ⓜ
pregnancy loss, first trimester

O26.22 **Pregnancy care for patient with recurrent** ♀Ⓜ
pregnancy loss, second trimester

O26.23 **Pregnancy care for patient with recurrent** ♀Ⓜ
pregnancy loss, third trimester

⑤ **O26.3**   Retained intrauterine contraceptive device in pregnancy

   O26.30   Retained intrauterine contraceptive device in pregnancy, unspecified trimester ♀Ⓜ

   O26.31   Retained intrauterine contraceptive device in pregnancy, first trimester ♀Ⓜ

   O26.32   Retained intrauterine contraceptive device in pregnancy, second trimester ♀Ⓜ

   O26.33   Retained intrauterine contraceptive device in pregnancy, third trimester ♀Ⓜ

⑤ **O26.4**   Herpes gestationis

   O26.40   Herpes gestationis, unspecified trimester ♀Ⓜ

   O26.41   Herpes gestationis, first trimester ♀Ⓜ

   O26.42   Herpes gestationis, second trimester ♀Ⓜ

   O26.43   Herpes gestationis, third trimester ♀Ⓜ

⑤ **O26.5**   Maternal hypotension syndrome

   Supine hypotensive syndrome

   O26.50   Maternal hypotension syndrome, unspecified trimester ♀Ⓜ

   O26.51   Maternal hypotension syndrome, first trimester ♀Ⓜ

   O26.52   Maternal hypotension syndrome, second trimester ♀Ⓜ

   O26.53   Maternal hypotension syndrome, third trimester ♀Ⓜ

⑤➕ **O26.6**   Liver and biliary tract disorders in pregnancy, childbirth and the puerperium

   Use additional code to identify the specific disorder

   EXCLUDES 2   *hepatorenal syndrome following labor and delivery (O90.4)*

  ⑥➕ **O26.61**   Liver and biliary tract disorders in pregnancy

   ➕ **O26.611**   Liver and biliary tract disorders in pregnancy, first trimester ♀Ⓜ

   ➕ **O26.612**   Liver and biliary tract disorders in pregnancy, second trimester ♀Ⓜ

   ➕ **O26.613**   Liver and biliary tract disorders in pregnancy, third trimester ♀Ⓜ

   ➕ **O26.619**   Liver and biliary tract disorders in pregnancy, unspecified trimester ♀Ⓜ

  ➕ **O26.62**   Liver and biliary tract disorders in childbirth ♀Ⓜ

  ➕ **O26.63**   Liver and biliary tract disorders in the puerperium ♀Ⓜ

⑤ **O26.7**   Subluxation of symphysis (pubis) in pregnancy, childbirth and the puerperium

   EXCLUDES 1   *traumatic separation of symphysis (pubis) during childbirth (O71.6)*

  ⑥ **O26.71**   Subluxation of symphysis (pubis) in pregnancy

   O26.711   Subluxation of symphysis (pubis) in pregnancy, first trimester ♀Ⓜ

   O26.712   Subluxation of symphysis (pubis) in pregnancy, second trimester ♀Ⓜ

   O26.713   Subluxation of symphysis (pubis) in pregnancy, third trimester ♀Ⓜ

   O26.719   Subluxation of symphysis (pubis) in pregnancy, unspecified trimester ♀Ⓜ

  O26.72   Subluxation of symphysis (pubis) in childbirth ♀Ⓜ

  O26.73   Subluxation of symphysis (pubis) in the puerperium ♀Ⓜ

⑤ **O26.8**   Other specified pregnancy related conditions

  ⑥ **O26.81**   Pregnancy related exhaustion and fatigue

   O26.811   Pregnancy related exhaustion and fatigue, first trimester ♀Ⓜ

   O26.812   Pregnancy related exhaustion and fatigue, second trimester ♀Ⓜ

   O26.813   Pregnancy related exhaustion and fatigue, third trimester ♀Ⓜ

   O26.819   Pregnancy related exhaustion and fatigue, unspecified trimester ♀Ⓜ

  ⑥ **O26.82**   Pregnancy related peripheral neuritis

   O26.821   Pregnancy related peripheral neuritis, first trimester ♀Ⓜ

   O26.822   Pregnancy related peripheral neuritis, second trimester ♀Ⓜ

   O26.823   Pregnancy related peripheral neuritis, third trimester ♀Ⓜ

   O26.829   Pregnancy related peripheral neuritis, unspecified trimester ♀Ⓜ

  ⑥ **O26.83**   Pregnancy related renal disease

   Use additional code to identify the specific disorder

   O26.831   Pregnancy related renal disease, first trimester ♀Ⓜ

   O26.832   Pregnancy related renal disease, second trimester ♀Ⓜ

   O26.833   Pregnancy related renal disease, third trimester ♀Ⓜ

   O26.839   Pregnancy related renal disease, unspecified trimester ♀Ⓜ

  ⑥ **O26.84**   Uterine size-date discrepancy complicating pregnancy

   EXCLUDES 1   *encounter for suspected problem with fetal growth ruled out (Z03.74)*

   O26.841   Uterine size-date discrepancy, first trimester ♀Ⓜ

   O26.842   Uterine size-date discrepancy, second trimester ♀Ⓜ

   O26.843   Uterine size-date discrepancy, third trimester ♀Ⓜ

   O26.849   Uterine size-date discrepancy, unspecified trimester ♀Ⓜ

  ⑥ **O26.85**   Spotting complicating pregnancy

   O26.851   Spotting complicating pregnancy, first trimester ♀Ⓜ

   O26.852   Spotting complicating pregnancy, second trimester ♀Ⓜ

   O26.853   Spotting complicating pregnancy, third trimester ♀Ⓜ

   O26.859   Spotting complicating pregnancy, unspecified trimester ♀Ⓜ

  O26.86   Pruritic urticarial papules and plaques of pregnancy (PUPPP) ♀Ⓜ

   Polymorphic eruption of pregnancy

  ⑥ **O26.87**   Cervical shortening

   EXCLUDES 1   *encounter for suspected cervical shortening ruled out (Z03.75)*

   O26.872   Cervical shortening, second trimester ♀Ⓜ

   DEFINITION   Sonographic evidence of a cervix shortened to 2.5 cm or less in the second trimester; a warning of impending premature birth in women with a prior history of early delivery.

   O26.873   Cervical shortening, third trimester ♀Ⓜ

   O26.879   Cervical shortening, unspecified trimester ♀Ⓜ

  ⑥ **O26.89**   Other specified pregnancy related conditions

   O26.891   Other specified pregnancy related conditions, first trimester ♀Ⓜ

   O26.892   Other specified pregnancy related conditions, second trimester ♀Ⓜ

   O26.893   Other specified pregnancy related conditions, third trimester ♀Ⓜ

   AHA: 3Q 2015, 40

   O26.899   Other specified pregnancy related conditions, unspecified trimester ♀Ⓜ

⑤ **O26.9**   Pregnancy related conditions, unspecified

   O26.90   Pregnancy related conditions, unspecified, unspecified trimester ♀Ⓜ

   O26.91   Pregnancy related conditions, unspecified, first trimester ♀Ⓜ

   O26.92   Pregnancy related conditions, unspecified, second trimester ♀Ⓜ

   O26.93   Pregnancy related conditions, unspecified, third trimester ♀Ⓜ

④ **O28**   **Abnormal findings on antenatal screening of mother**

   EXCLUDES 1   *diagnostic findings classified elsewhere - see Alphabetical Index*

  O28.0   Abnormal hematological finding on antenatal screening of mother ♀Ⓜ

  O28.1   Abnormal biochemical finding on antenatal screening of mother ♀Ⓜ

  O28.2   Abnormal cytological finding on antenatal screening of mother ♀Ⓜ

  O28.3   Abnormal ultrasonic finding on antenatal screening of mother ♀Ⓜ

  O28.4   Abnormal radiological finding on antenatal screening of mother ♀Ⓜ

  O28.5   Abnormal chromosomal and genetic finding on antenatal screening of mother ♀Ⓜ

  O28.8   Other abnormal findings on antenatal screening of mother ♀Ⓜ

  O28.9   Unspecified abnormal findings on antenatal screening of mother ♀Ⓜ

● New   ▲ Revised   *Manifestation*   ④-⑦ Digit Indicators   ⊟ Laterality   Ⓐ Adult (15+ years)   Ⓜ Maternity (12-55 years)   Ⓝ Newborn   Ⓟ Pediatric (0-17 years)   ♂ Male   ♀ Female
✖ Deleted   Unspecified   ➕ Additional code

848   © 2017 DecisionHealth   2017 ICD-10-CM Expert for Physicians

4+ O29   Complications of anesthesia during pregnancy

> INCLUDES   maternal complications arising from the administration of a general, regional or local anesthetic, analgesic or other sedation during pregnancy

Use additional code, if necessary, to identify the complication

> EXCLUDES 2   *complications of anesthesia during labor and delivery (O74.-)*
> *complications of anesthesia during the puerperium (O89.-)*

5+ O29.0   Pulmonary complications of anesthesia during pregnancy   ♀Ⓜ

6+ O29.01   Aspiration pneumonitis due to anesthesia during pregnancy

Inhalation of stomach contents or secretions NOS due to anesthesia during pregnancy

Mendelson's syndrome due to anesthesia during pregnancy

+ **O29.011   Aspiration pneumonitis due to anesthesia during pregnancy, first trimester**   ♀Ⓜ

+ **O29.012   Aspiration pneumonitis due to anesthesia during pregnancy, second trimester**   ♀Ⓜ

+ **O29.013   Aspiration pneumonitis due to anesthesia during pregnancy, third trimester**   ♀Ⓜ

+ **O29.019   Aspiration pneumonitis due to anesthesia during pregnancy, unspecified trimester**   ♀Ⓜ

6+ O29.02   Pressure collapse of lung due to anesthesia during pregnancy

+ **O29.021   Pressure collapse of lung due to anesthesia during pregnancy, first trimester**   ♀Ⓜ

+ **O29.022   Pressure collapse of lung due to anesthesia during pregnancy, second trimester**   ♀Ⓜ

+ **O29.023   Pressure collapse of lung due to anesthesia during pregnancy, third trimester**   ♀Ⓜ

+ **O29.029   Pressure collapse of lung due to anesthesia during pregnancy, unspecified trimester**   ♀Ⓜ

6+ O29.09   Other pulmonary complications of anesthesia during pregnancy

+ **O29.091   Other pulmonary complications of anesthesia during pregnancy, first trimester**   ♀Ⓜ

+ **O29.092   Other pulmonary complications of anesthesia during pregnancy, second trimester**   ♀Ⓜ

+ **O29.093   Other pulmonary complications of anesthesia during pregnancy, third trimester**   ♀Ⓜ

+ **O29.099   Other pulmonary complications of anesthesia during pregnancy, unspecified trimester**   ♀Ⓜ

5+ O29.1   Cardiac complications of anesthesia during pregnancy   ♀Ⓜ

6+ O29.11   Cardiac arrest due to anesthesia during pregnancy

+ **O29.111   Cardiac arrest due to anesthesia during pregnancy, first trimester**   ♀Ⓜ

+ **O29.112   Cardiac arrest due to anesthesia during pregnancy, second trimester**   ♀Ⓜ

+ **O29.113   Cardiac arrest due to anesthesia during pregnancy, third trimester**   ♀Ⓜ

+ **O29.119   Cardiac arrest due to anesthesia during pregnancy, unspecified trimester**   ♀Ⓜ

6+ O29.12   Cardiac failure due to anesthesia during pregnancy

+ **O29.121   Cardiac failure due to anesthesia during pregnancy, first trimester**   ♀Ⓜ

+ **O29.122   Cardiac failure due to anesthesia during pregnancy, second trimester**   ♀Ⓜ

+ **O29.123   Cardiac failure due to anesthesia during pregnancy, third trimester**   ♀Ⓜ

+ **O29.129   Cardiac failure due to anesthesia during pregnancy, unspecified trimester**   ♀Ⓜ

6+ O29.19   Other cardiac complications of anesthesia during pregnancy

+ **O29.191   Other cardiac complications of anesthesia during pregnancy, first trimester**   ♀Ⓜ

+ **O29.192   Other cardiac complications of anesthesia during pregnancy, second trimester**   ♀Ⓜ

+ **O29.193   Other cardiac complications of anesthesia during pregnancy, third trimester**   ♀Ⓜ

+ **O29.199   Other cardiac complications of anesthesia during pregnancy, unspecified trimester**   ♀Ⓜ

5+ O29.2   Central nervous system complications of anesthesia during pregnancy   ♀Ⓜ

6+ O29.21   Cerebral anoxia due to anesthesia during pregnancy

+ **O29.211   Cerebral anoxia due to anesthesia during pregnancy, first trimester**   ♀Ⓜ

+ **O29.212   Cerebral anoxia due to anesthesia during pregnancy, second trimester**   ♀Ⓜ

+ **O29.213   Cerebral anoxia due to anesthesia during pregnancy, third trimester**   ♀Ⓜ

+ **O29.219   Cerebral anoxia due to anesthesia during pregnancy, unspecified trimester**   ♀Ⓜ

6+ O29.29   Other central nervous system complications of anesthesia during pregnancy

+ **O29.291   Other central nervous system complications of anesthesia during pregnancy, first trimester**   ♀Ⓜ

+ **O29.292   Other central nervous system complications of anesthesia during pregnancy, second trimester**   ♀Ⓜ

+ **O29.293   Other central nervous system complications of anesthesia during pregnancy, third trimester**   ♀Ⓜ

+ **O29.299   Other central nervous system complications of anesthesia during pregnancy, unspecified trimester**   ♀Ⓜ

5+ O29.3   Toxic reaction to local anesthesia during pregnancy   ♀Ⓜ

6+ O29.3X   Toxic reaction to local anesthesia during pregnancy

+ **O29.3X1   Toxic reaction to local anesthesia during pregnancy, first trimester**   ♀Ⓜ

+ **O29.3X2   Toxic reaction to local anesthesia during pregnancy, second trimester**   ♀Ⓜ

+ **O29.3X3   Toxic reaction to local anesthesia during pregnancy, third trimester**   ♀Ⓜ

+ **O29.3X9   Toxic reaction to local anesthesia during pregnancy, unspecified trimester**   ♀Ⓜ

5+ O29.4   Spinal and epidural anesthesia induced headache during pregnancy   ♀Ⓜ

+ **O29.40   Spinal and epidural anesthesia induced headache during pregnancy, unspecified trimester**   ♀Ⓜ

+ **O29.41   Spinal and epidural anesthesia induced headache during pregnancy, first trimester**   ♀Ⓜ

+ **O29.42   Spinal and epidural anesthesia induced headache during pregnancy, second trimester**   ♀Ⓜ

+ **O29.43   Spinal and epidural anesthesia induced headache during pregnancy, third trimester**   ♀Ⓜ

5+ O29.5   Other complications of spinal and epidural anesthesia during pregnancy   ♀Ⓜ

6+ O29.5X   Other complications of spinal and epidural anesthesia during pregnancy

+ **O29.5X1   Other complications of spinal and epidural anesthesia during pregnancy, first trimester**   ♀Ⓜ

+ **O29.5X2   Other complications of spinal and epidural anesthesia during pregnancy, second trimester**   ♀Ⓜ

+ **O29.5X3   Other complications of spinal and epidural anesthesia during pregnancy, third trimester**   ♀Ⓜ

+ **O29.5X9   Other complications of spinal and epidural anesthesia during pregnancy, unspecified trimester**   ♀Ⓜ

5+ O29.6   Failed or difficult intubation for anesthesia during pregnancy   ♀Ⓜ

+ **O29.60   Failed or difficult intubation for anesthesia during pregnancy, unspecified trimester**   ♀Ⓜ

+ **O29.61   Failed or difficult intubation for anesthesia during pregnancy, first trimester**   ♀Ⓜ

+ **O29.62   Failed or difficult intubation for anesthesia during pregnancy, second trimester**   ♀Ⓜ

+ **O29.63   Failed or difficult intubation for anesthesia during pregnancy, third trimester**   ♀Ⓜ

5+ O29.8   Other complications of anesthesia during pregnancy   ♀Ⓜ

6+ O29.8X   Other complications of anesthesia during pregnancy

+ **O29.8X1   Other complications of anesthesia during pregnancy, first trimester**   ♀Ⓜ

+ **O29.8X2   Other complications of anesthesia during pregnancy, second trimester**   ♀Ⓜ

+ **O29.8X3   Other complications of anesthesia during pregnancy, third trimester**   ♀Ⓜ

● New   ▲ Revised   *Manifestation*   4-7 Digit Indicators   ▱ Laterality   Ⓐ Adult (15+ years)   Ⓜ Maternity (12-55 years)   Ⓝ Newborn   Ⓟ Pediatric (0-17 years)   ♂ Male   ♀ Female
✖ Deleted   Unspecified   + Additional code

+ O29.8X9 Other complications of anesthesia during pregnancy, unspecified trimester ♀Ⓜ

⑤+ O29.9 Unspecified complication of anesthesia during pregnancy ♀Ⓜ

+ O29.90 Unspecified complication of anesthesia during pregnancy, unspecified trimester ♀Ⓜ

+ O29.91 Unspecified complication of anesthesia during pregnancy, first trimester ♀Ⓜ

+ O29.92 Unspecified complication of anesthesia during pregnancy, second trimester ♀Ⓜ

+ O29.93 Unspecified complication of anesthesia during pregnancy, third trimester ♀Ⓜ

Maternal care related to the fetus and amniotic cavity and possible delivery problems (O30-O48)

④ O30 **Multiple gestation**
Code also:
any complications specific to multiple gestation

⑤ O30.0 **Twin pregnancy**

⑥ O30.00 Twin pregnancy, unspecified number of placenta and unspecified number of amniotic sacs

O30.001 Twin pregnancy, unspecified number of placenta and unspecified number of amniotic sacs, first trimester ♀Ⓜ

O30.002 Twin pregnancy, unspecified number of placenta and unspecified number of amniotic sacs, second trimester ♀Ⓜ

O30.003 Twin pregnancy, unspecified number of placenta and unspecified number of amniotic sacs, third trimester ♀Ⓜ

O30.009 Twin pregnancy, unspecified number of placenta and unspecified number of amniotic sacs, unspecified trimester ♀Ⓜ

⑥ O30.01 Twin pregnancy, monochorionic/monoamniotic
Twin pregnancy, one placenta, one amniotic sac
EXCLUDES 1 *conjoined twins (O30.02-)*

O30.011 Twin pregnancy, monochorionic/monoamniotic, first trimester ♀Ⓜ

O30.012 Twin pregnancy, monochorionic/monoamniotic, second trimester ♀Ⓜ

O30.013 Twin pregnancy, monochorionic/monoamniotic, third trimester ♀Ⓜ

O30.019 Twin pregnancy, monochorionic/monoamniotic, unspecified trimester ♀Ⓜ

⑥ O30.02 Conjoined twin pregnancy

O30.021 Conjoined twin pregnancy, first trimester ♀Ⓜ

O30.022 Conjoined twin pregnancy, second trimester ♀Ⓜ

O30.023 Conjoined twin pregnancy, third trimester ♀Ⓜ

O30.029 Conjoined twin pregnancy, unspecified trimester ♀Ⓜ

⑥ O30.03 Twin pregnancy, monochorionic/diamniotic
Twin pregnancy, one placenta, two amniotic sacs

O30.031 Twin pregnancy, monochorionic/diamniotic, first trimester ♀Ⓜ

O30.032 Twin pregnancy, monochorionic/diamniotic, second trimester ♀Ⓜ

O30.033 Twin pregnancy, monochorionic/diamniotic, third trimester ♀Ⓜ

O30.039 Twin pregnancy, monochorionic/diamniotic, unspecified trimester ♀Ⓜ

⑥ O30.04 Twin pregnancy, dichorionic/diamniotic
Twin pregnancy, two placentae, two amniotic sacs

O30.041 Twin pregnancy, dichorionic/diamniotic, first trimester ♀Ⓜ

O30.042 Twin pregnancy, dichorionic/diamniotic, second trimester ♀Ⓜ

O30.043 Twin pregnancy, dichorionic/diamniotic, third trimester ♀Ⓜ

O30.049 Twin pregnancy, dichorionic/diamniotic, unspecified trimester ♀Ⓜ

⑥ O30.09 Twin pregnancy, unable to determine number of placenta and number of amniotic sacs

O30.091 Twin pregnancy, unable to determine number of placenta and number of amniotic sacs, first trimester ♀Ⓜ

O30.092 Twin pregnancy, unable to determine number of placenta and number of amniotic sacs, second trimester ♀Ⓜ

O30.093 Twin pregnancy, unable to determine number of placenta and number of amniotic sacs, third trimester ♀Ⓜ

O30.099 Twin pregnancy, unable to determine number of placenta and number of amniotic sacs, unspecified trimester ♀Ⓜ

⑤ O30.1 **Triplet pregnancy**

⑥ O30.10 Triplet pregnancy, unspecified number of placenta and unspecified number of amniotic sacs

O30.101 Triplet pregnancy, unspecified number of placenta and unspecified number of amniotic sacs, first trimester ♀Ⓜ

O30.102 Triplet pregnancy, unspecified number of placenta and unspecified number of amniotic sacs, second trimester ♀Ⓜ

O30.103 Triplet pregnancy, unspecified number of placenta and unspecified number of amniotic sacs, third trimester ♀Ⓜ
AHA: 2Q 2016, 8

O30.109 Triplet pregnancy, unspecified number of placenta and unspecified number of amniotic sacs, unspecified trimester ♀Ⓜ

⑥ O30.11 Triplet pregnancy with two or more monochorionic fetuses

O30.111 Triplet pregnancy with two or more monochorionic fetuses, first trimester ♀Ⓜ

O30.112 Triplet pregnancy with two or more monochorionic fetuses, second trimester ♀Ⓜ

O30.113 Triplet pregnancy with two or more monochorionic fetuses, third trimester ♀Ⓜ

O30.119 Triplet pregnancy with two or more monochorionic fetuses, unspecified trimester ♀Ⓜ

⑥ O30.12 Triplet pregnancy with two or more monoamniotic fetuses

O30.121 Triplet pregnancy with two or more monoamniotic fetuses, first trimester ♀Ⓜ

O30.122 Triplet pregnancy with two or more monoamniotic fetuses, second trimester ♀Ⓜ

O30.123 Triplet pregnancy with two or more monoamniotic fetuses, third trimester ♀Ⓜ

O30.129 Triplet pregnancy with two or more monoamniotic fetuses, unspecified trimester ♀Ⓜ

⑥ O30.19 Triplet pregnancy, unable to determine number of placenta and number of amniotic sacs

O30.191 Triplet pregnancy, unable to determine number of placenta and number of amniotic sacs, first trimester ♀Ⓜ

O30.192 Triplet pregnancy, unable to determine number of placenta and number of amniotic sacs, second trimester ♀Ⓜ

O30.193 Triplet pregnancy, unable to determine number of placenta and number of amniotic sacs, third trimester ♀Ⓜ

O30.199 Triplet pregnancy, unable to determine number of placenta and number of amniotic sacs, unspecified trimester ♀Ⓜ

⑤ O30.2 **Quadruplet pregnancy** ♀Ⓜ

⑥ O30.20 Quadruplet pregnancy, unspecified number of placenta and unspecified number of amniotic sacs

O30.201 Quadruplet pregnancy, unspecified number of placenta and unspecified number of amniotic sacs, first trimester ♀Ⓜ

O30.202 Quadruplet pregnancy, unspecified number of placenta and unspecified number of amniotic sacs, second trimester ♀Ⓜ

● New ▲ Revised *Manifestation* ④-⑦ Digit Indicators ▤ Laterality ⒶAdult (15+ years) Ⓜ Maternity (12-55 years) Ⓝ Newborn �Ⓟ Pediatric (0-17 years) ♂ Male ♀ Female
✖ Deleted Unspecified + Additional code

850　© 2017 DecisionHealth

2017 ICD-10-CM Expert for Physicians

O29.8X9 — O30.202

O30.203 Quadruplet pregnancy, unspecified number ♀Ⓜ
of placenta and unspecified number of
amniotic sacs, third trimester

O30.209 Quadruplet pregnancy, unspecified number ♀Ⓜ
of placenta and unspecified number of
amniotic sacs, unspecified trimester

Ⓖ O30.21 Quadruplet pregnancy with two or more
monochorionic fetuses

O30.211 Quadruplet pregnancy with two or more ♀Ⓜ
monochorionic fetuses, first trimester

O30.212 Quadruplet pregnancy with two or more ♀Ⓜ
monochorionic fetuses, second trimester

O30.213 Quadruplet pregnancy with two or more ♀Ⓜ
monochorionic fetuses, third trimester

O30.219 Quadruplet pregnancy with two or more ♀Ⓜ
monochorionic fetuses, unspecified
trimester

Ⓖ O30.22 Quadruplet pregnancy with two or more
monoamniotic fetuses

O30.221 Quadruplet pregnancy with two or more ♀Ⓜ
monoamniotic fetuses, first trimester

O30.222 Quadruplet pregnancy with two or more ♀Ⓜ
monoamniotic fetuses, second trimester

O30.223 Quadruplet pregnancy with two or more ♀Ⓜ
monoamniotic fetuses, third trimester

O30.229 Quadruplet pregnancy with two or more ♀Ⓜ
monoamniotic fetuses, unspecified
trimester

Ⓖ O30.29 Quadruplet pregnancy, unable to determine ♀Ⓜ
number of placenta and number of amniotic
sacs

O30.291 Quadruplet pregnancy, unable to determine ♀Ⓜ
number of placenta and number of
amniotic sacs, first trimester

O30.292 Quadruplet pregnancy, unable to determine ♀Ⓜ
number of placenta and number of
amniotic sacs, second trimester

O30.293 Quadruplet pregnancy, unable to determine ♀Ⓜ
number of placenta and number of
amniotic sacs, third trimester

O30.299 Quadruplet pregnancy, unable to determine ♀Ⓜ
number of placenta and number of
amniotic sacs, unspecified trimester

Ⓢ O30.8 Other specified multiple gestation ♀Ⓜ
Multiple gestation pregnancy greater then quadruplets

Ⓖ O30.80 Other specified multiple gestation, unspecified
number of placenta and unspecified number of
amniotic sacs

O30.801 Other specified multiple gestation, ♀Ⓜ
unspecified number of placenta and
unspecified number of amniotic sacs, first
trimester

O30.802 Other specified multiple gestation, ♀Ⓜ
unspecified number of placenta and
unspecified number of amniotic sacs,
second trimester

O30.803 Other specified multiple gestation, ♀Ⓜ
unspecified number of placenta and
unspecified number of amniotic sacs,
third trimester

O30.809 Other specified multiple gestation, ♀Ⓜ
unspecified number of placenta and
unspecified number of amniotic sacs,
unspecified trimester

Ⓖ O30.81 Other specified multiple gestation with two or more
monochorionic fetuses

O30.811 Other specified multiple gestation with two ♀Ⓜ
or more monochorionic fetuses, first
trimester

O30.812 Other specified multiple gestation with two ♀Ⓜ
or more monochorionic fetuses, second
trimester

O30.813 Other specified multiple gestation with two ♀Ⓜ
or more monochorionic fetuses, third
trimester

O30.819 Other specified multiple gestation with two ♀Ⓜ
or more monochorionic fetuses,
unspecified trimester

Ⓖ O30.82 Other specified multiple gestation with two or more
monoamniotic fetuses

O30.821 Other specified multiple gestation with two ♀Ⓜ
or more monoamniotic fetuses, first
trimester

O30.822 Other specified multiple gestation with two ♀Ⓜ
or more monoamniotic fetuses, second
trimester

O30.823 Other specified multiple gestation with two ♀Ⓜ
or more monoamniotic fetuses, third
trimester

O30.829 Other specified multiple gestation with two ♀Ⓜ
or more monoamniotic fetuses,
unspecified trimester

Ⓖ O30.89 Other specified multiple gestation, unable to
determine number of placenta and number of
amniotic sacs

O30.891 Other specified multiple gestation, unable to ♀Ⓜ
determine number of placenta and
number of amniotic sacs, first trimester

O30.892 Other specified multiple gestation, unable to ♀Ⓜ
determine number of placenta and
number of amniotic sacs, second trimester

O30.893 Other specified multiple gestation, unable to ♀Ⓜ
determine number of placenta and
number of amniotic sacs, third trimester

O30.899 Other specified multiple gestation, unable ♀Ⓜ
to determine number of placenta and
number of amniotic sacs, unspecified
trimester

Ⓢ O30.9 Multiple gestation, unspecified ♀Ⓜ
Multiple pregnancy NOS

O30.90 Multiple gestation, unspecified, unspecified ♀Ⓜ
trimester

O30.91 Multiple gestation, unspecified, first trimester ♀Ⓜ

O30.92 Multiple gestation, unspecified, second trimester ♀Ⓜ

O30.93 Multiple gestation, unspecified, third trimester ♀Ⓜ

Ⓐ O31 **Complications specific to multiple gestation**

EXCLUDES 2	*delayed delivery of second twin, triplet, etc. (O63.2)*
	malpresentation of one fetus or more (O32.9)
	placental transfusion syndromes (O43.0-)

One of the following 7th characters is to be assigned to each code
under category O31. 7th character 0 is for single gestations and
multiple gestations where the fetus is unspecified. 7th characters 1
through 9 are for cases of multiple gestations to identify the fetus
for which the code applies. The appropriate code from category
O30, Multiple gestation, must also be assigned when assigning a
code from category O31 that has a 7th character of 1 through 9.

0	not applicable or unspecified
1	fetus 1
2	fetus 2
3	fetus 3
4	fetus 4
5	fetus 5
9	other fetus

AHA: 4Q 2012, 107-108

Ⓢ O31.0 **Papyraceous fetus**
Fetus compressus

Ⓩ O31.00X- **Papyraceous fetus, unspecified trimester** ♀Ⓜ

Ⓩ O31.01X- **Papyraceous fetus, first trimester** Ⓜ

Ⓩ O31.02X- **Papyraceous fetus, second trimester** Ⓜ

Ⓩ O31.03X- **Papyraceous fetus, third trimester** Ⓜ

Ⓢ O31.1 **Continuing pregnancy after spontaneous abortion of one
fetus or more**

Ⓩ O31.10X- **Continuing pregnancy after spontaneous** Ⓜ
**abortion of one fetus or more, unspecified
trimester**

Ⓩ O31.11X- **Continuing pregnancy after spontaneous** Ⓜ
abortion of one fetus or more, first trimester

Ⓩ O31.12X- **Continuing pregnancy after spontaneous** Ⓜ
**abortion of one fetus or more, second
trimester**

Ⓩ O31.13X- **Continuing pregnancy after spontaneous** Ⓜ
abortion of one fetus or more, third trimester

Ⓢ O31.2 **Continuing pregnancy after intrauterine death of one
fetus or more**

● New ▲ Revised *Manifestation* Ⓐ-Ⓩ Digit Indicators ▤ Laterality Ⓐ Adult (15+ years) Ⓜ Maternity (12-55 years) Ⓝ Newborn Ⓟ Pediatric (0-17 years) ♂ Male ♀ Female
✖ Deleted Unspecified + Additional code

2017 ICD-10-CM Expert for Physicians   © 2017 DecisionHealth   851

7 O31.20X- Continuing pregnancy after intrauterine death of one fetus or more, unspecified trimester M

7 O31.21X- Continuing pregnancy after intrauterine death of one fetus or more, first trimester M

7 O31.22X- Continuing pregnancy after intrauterine death of one fetus or more, second trimester M

7 O31.23X- Continuing pregnancy after intrauterine death of one fetus or more, third trimester M

S O31.3 Continuing pregnancy after elective fetal reduction of one fetus or more

Continuing pregnancy after selective termination of one fetus or more

7 O31.30X- Continuing pregnancy after elective fetal reduction of one fetus or more, unspecified trimester M

7 O31.31X- Continuing pregnancy after elective fetal reduction of one fetus or more, first trimester M

7 O31.32X- Continuing pregnancy after elective fetal reduction of one fetus or more, second trimester M

7 O31.33X- Continuing pregnancy after elective fetal reduction of one fetus or more, third trimester M

S O31.8 Other complications specific to multiple gestation

6 O31.8X Other complications specific to multiple gestation

7 O31.8X1- Other complications specific to multiple gestation, first trimester ♀M

7 O31.8X2- Other complications specific to multiple gestation, second trimester ♀M

7 O31.8X3- Other complications specific to multiple gestation, third trimester

7 O31.8X9- Other complications specific to multiple gestation, unspecified trimester

4 O32 Maternal care for malpresentation of fetus

> | INCLUDES | the listed conditions as a reason for observation, hospitalization or other obstetric care of the mother, or for cesarean delivery before onset of labor |

> | EXCLUDES 1 | *malpresentation of fetus with obstructed labor (O64.-)* |

One of the following 7th characters is to be assigned to each code under category O32. 7th character 0 is for single gestations and multiple gestations where the fetus is unspecified. 7th characters 1 through 9 are for cases of multiple gestations to identify the fetus for which the code applies. The appropriate code from category O30, Multiple gestation, must also be assigned when assigning a code from category O32 that has a 7th character of 1 through 9.

0	not applicable or unspecified
1	fetus 1
2	fetus 2
3	fetus 3
4	fetus 4
5	fetus 5
9	other fetus

AHA: 4Q 2012, 107-108

7 O32.0XX- Maternal care for unstable lie

7 O32.1XX- Maternal care for breech presentation
Maternal care for buttocks presentation
Maternal care for complete breech
Maternal care for frank breech

> | EXCLUDES 1 | *footling presentation (O32.8)* |
> | | *incomplete breech (O32.8)* |

7 O32.2XX- Maternal care for transverse and oblique lie
Maternal care for oblique presentation
Maternal care for transverse presentation

7 O32.3XX- Maternal care for face, brow and chin presentation

7 O32.4XX- Maternal care for high head at term
Maternal care for failure of head to enter pelvic brim

7 O32.6XX- Maternal care for compound presentation

7 O32.8XX- Maternal care for other malpresentation of fetus
Maternal care for footling presentation
Maternal care for incomplete breech

7 O32.9XX- Maternal care for malpresentation of fetus, unspecified

4 O33 Maternal care for disproportion

> | INCLUDES | the listed conditions as a reason for observation, hospitalization or other obstetric care of the mother, or for cesarean delivery before onset of labor |

> | EXCLUDES 1 | *disproportion with obstructed labor (O65-O66)* |

O33.0 Maternal care for disproportion due to deformity of maternal pelvic bones ♀M
Maternal care for disproportion due to pelvic deformity causing disproportion NOS

O33.1 Maternal care for disproportion due to generally contracted pelvis ♀M
Maternal care for disproportion due to contracted pelvis NOS causing disproportion

O33.2 Maternal care for disproportion due to inlet contraction of pelvis ♀M
Maternal care for disproportion due to inlet contraction (pelvis) causing disproportion

7 O33.3XX- Maternal care for disproportion due to outlet contraction of pelvis
Maternal care for disproportion due to mid-cavity contraction (pelvis)
Maternal care for disproportion due to outlet contraction (pelvis)

One of the following 7th characters is to be assigned to code O33.3. 7th character 0 is for single gestations and multiple gestations where the fetus is unspecified. 7th characters 1 through 9 are for cases of multiple gestations to identify the fetus for which the code applies. The appropriate code from category O30, Multiple gestation, must also be assigned when assigning code O33.3 with a 7th character of 1 through 9.

0	not applicable or unspecified
1	fetus 1
2	fetus 2
3	fetus 3
4	fetus 4
5	fetus 5
9	other fetus

7 O33.4XX- Maternal care for disproportion of mixed maternal and fetal origin

One of the following 7th characters is to be assigned to code O33.4. 7th character 0 is for single gestations and multiple gestations where the fetus is unspecified. 7th characters 1 through 9 are for cases of multiple gestations to identify the fetus for which the code applies. The appropriate code from category O30, Multiple gestation, must also be assigned when assigning code O33.4 with a 7th character of 1 through 9.

0	not applicable or unspecified
1	fetus 1
2	fetus 2
3	fetus 3
4	fetus 4
5	fetus 5
9	other fetus

● New ▲ Revised *Manifestation* 4-7 Digit Indicators ⊟ Laterality A Adult (15+ years) M Maternity (12-55 years) N Newborn P Pediatric (0-17 years) ♂ Male ♀ Female
✖ Deleted Unspecified + Additional code

7 O33.5XX- Maternal care for disproportion due to unusually large fetus
Maternal care for disproportion due to disproportion of fetal origin with normally formed fetus
Maternal care for disproportion due to fetal disproportion NOS

One of the following 7th characters is to be assigned to code O33.5. 7th character 0 is for single gestations and multiple gestations where the fetus is unspecified. 7th characters 1 through 9 are for cases of multiple gestations to identify the fetus for which the code applies. The appropriate code from category O30, Multiple gestation, must also be assigned when assigning code O33.5 with a 7th character of 1 through 9.
0   not applicable or unspecified
1   fetus 1
2   fetus 2
3   fetus 3
4   fetus 4
5   fetus 5
9   other fetus

7 O33.6XX- Maternal care for disproportion due to hydrocephalic fetus

One of the following 7th characters is to be assigned to code O33.6. 7th character 0 is for single gestations and multiple gestations where the fetus is unspecified. 7th characters 1 through 9 are for cases of multiple gestations to identify the fetus for which the code applies. The appropriate code from category O30, Multiple gestation, must also be assigned when assigning code O33.6 with a 7th character of 1 through 9.
0   not applicable or unspecified
1   fetus 1
2   fetus 2
3   fetus 3
4   fetus 4
5   fetus 5
9   other fetus

▲ 7 O33.7XX- Maternal care for disproportion due to other fetal deformities ♀Ⓜ
Maternal care for disproportion due to fetal ascites
Maternal care for disproportion due to fetal hydrops
Maternal care for disproportion due to fetal meningomyelocele
Maternal care for disproportion due to fetal sacral teratoma
Maternal care for disproportion due to fetal tumor

EXCLUDES 1   obstructed labor due to other fetal deformities (O66.3)

One of the following 7th characters is to be assigned to code O33.7. 7th character 0 is for single gestations and multiple gestations where the fetus is unspecified. 7th characters 1 through 9 are for cases of multiple gestations to identify the fetus for which the code applies. The appropriate code from category O30, Multiple gestation, must also be assigned when assigning code O33.7 with a 7th character of 1 through 9.
0   not applicable or unspecified
1   fetus 1
2   fetus 2
3   fetus 3
4   fetus 4
5   fetus 5
9   other fetus

O33.8   Maternal care for disproportion of other origin ♀Ⓜ
O33.9   Maternal care for disproportion, unspecified ♀Ⓜ
Maternal care for disproportion due to cephalopelvic disproportion NOS
Maternal care for disproportion due to fetopelvic disproportion NOS

4 + O34 Maternal care for abnormality of pelvic organs

INCLUDES   the listed conditions as a reason for hospitalization or other obstetric care of the mother, or for cesarean delivery before onset of labor

Code first:
any associated obstructed labor (O65.5)
Use additional code for specific condition

Maternal care for cervical incompetence

Uterus
Fetus
Rectum
Bladder
Vagina
Cervix dilates early in pregnancy

▲ 5 + O34.0 Maternal care for congenital malformation of uterus
Maternal care for double uterus
Maternal care for uterus bicornis

+ O34.00 Maternal care for unspecified congenital malformation of uterus, unspecified trimester ♀Ⓜ
+ O34.01 Maternal care for unspecified congenital malformation of uterus, first trimester ♀Ⓜ
+ O34.02 Maternal care for unspecified congenital malformation of uterus, second trimester ♀Ⓜ
+ O34.03 Maternal care for unspecified congenital malformation of uterus, third trimester ♀Ⓜ

5 + O34.1 Maternal care for benign tumor of corpus uteri
EXCLUDES 2   *maternal care for benign tumor of cervix (O34.4-)*
maternal care for malignant neoplasm of uterus (O9A.1-)
+ O34.10 Maternal care for benign tumor of corpus uteri, unspecified trimester ♀Ⓜ
+ O34.11 Maternal care for benign tumor of corpus uteri, first trimester ♀Ⓜ
+ O34.12 Maternal care for benign tumor of corpus uteri, second trimester ♀Ⓜ
+ O34.13 Maternal care for benign tumor of corpus uteri, third trimester ♀Ⓜ

5 + O34.2 Maternal care due to uterine scar from previous surgery
▲ 6 + O34.21 Maternal care for scar from previous cesarean delivery
● + O34.211 Maternal care for low transverse scar from previous cesarean delivery ♀Ⓜ
● + O34.212 Maternal care for vertical scar from previous cesarean delivery ♀Ⓜ
Maternal care for classical scar from previous cesarean delivery
● + O34.219 Maternal care for unspecified type scar from previous cesarean delivery ♀Ⓜ
▲ + O34.29 Maternal care due to uterine scar from other previous surgery ♀Ⓜ
Maternal care due to uterine scar from other transmural uterine incision

5 + O34.3 Maternal care for cervical incompetence
Maternal care for cerclage with or without cervical incompetence
Maternal care for Shirodkar suture with or without cervical incompetence
+ O34.30 Maternal care for cervical incompetence, unspecified trimester ♀Ⓜ
+ O34.31 Maternal care for cervical incompetence, first trimester ♀Ⓜ
+ O34.32 Maternal care for cervical incompetence, second trimester ♀Ⓜ
+ O34.33 Maternal care for cervical incompetence, third trimester ♀Ⓜ

5 + O34.4 Maternal care for other abnormalities of cervix ♀Ⓜ
+ O34.40 Maternal care for other abnormalities of cervix, unspecified trimester ♀Ⓜ

● New   ▲ Revised   *Manifestation*   4-7 Digit Indicators   ⊟ Laterality   Ⓐ Adult (15+ years)   Ⓜ Maternity (12-55 years)   Ⓝ Newborn   Ⓟ Pediatric (0-17 years)   ♂ Male   ♀ Female
✖ Deleted   Unspecified   + Additional code

2017 ICD-10-CM Expert for Physicians

© 2017 DecisionHealth   853

+ O34.41 Maternal care for other abnormalities of cervix, ♀Ⓜ
first trimester

+ O34.42 Maternal care for other abnormalities of cervix, ♀Ⓜ
second trimester

+ O34.43 Maternal care for other abnormalities of cervix, ♀Ⓜ
third trimester

Ⓢ+ O34.5 Maternal care for other abnormalities of gravid ♀Ⓜ
uterus

Ⓖ+ O34.51 Maternal care for incarceration of gravid uterus

+ O34.511 Maternal care for incarceration of gravid ♀Ⓜ
uterus, first trimester

+ O34.512 Maternal care for incarceration of gravid ♀Ⓜ
uterus, second trimester

+ O34.513 Maternal care for incarceration of gravid ♀Ⓜ
uterus, third trimester

+ O34.519 Maternal care for incarceration of gravid ♀Ⓜ
uterus, unspecified trimester

Ⓖ+ O34.52 Maternal care for prolapse of gravid uterus

+ O34.521 Maternal care for prolapse of gravid uterus, ♀Ⓜ
first trimester

+ O34.522 Maternal care for prolapse of gravid uterus, ♀Ⓜ
second trimester

+ O34.523 Maternal care for prolapse of gravid uterus, ♀Ⓜ
third trimester

+ O34.529 Maternal care for prolapse of gravid ♀Ⓜ
uterus, unspecified trimester

Ⓖ+ O34.53 Maternal care for retroversion of gravid uterus

+ O34.531 Maternal care for retroversion of gravid ♀Ⓜ
uterus, first trimester

+ O34.532 Maternal care for retroversion of gravid ♀Ⓜ
uterus, second trimester

+ O34.533 Maternal care for retroversion of gravid ♀Ⓜ
uterus, third trimester

+ O34.539 Maternal care for retroversion of gravid ♀Ⓜ
uterus, unspecified trimester

Ⓖ+ O34.59 Maternal care for other abnormalities of gravid
uterus

+ O34.591 Maternal care for other abnormalities of ♀Ⓜ
gravid uterus, first trimester

+ O34.592 Maternal care for other abnormalities of ♀Ⓜ
gravid uterus, second trimester

+ O34.593 Maternal care for other abnormalities of ♀Ⓜ
gravid uterus, third trimester

+ O34.599 Maternal care for other abnormalities of ♀Ⓜ
gravid uterus, unspecified trimester

Ⓢ+ O34.6 Maternal care for abnormality of vagina ♀Ⓜ

EXCLUDES 2 *maternal care for vaginal varices in pregnancy (O22.1-)*

+ O34.60 Maternal care for abnormality of vagina, ♀Ⓜ
unspecified trimester

+ O34.61 Maternal care for abnormality of vagina, first ♀Ⓜ
trimester

+ O34.62 Maternal care for abnormality of vagina, second ♀Ⓜ
trimester

+ O34.63 Maternal care for abnormality of vagina, third ♀Ⓜ
trimester

Ⓢ+ O34.7 Maternal care for abnormality of vulva and perineum ♀Ⓜ

EXCLUDES 2 *maternal care for perineal and vulval varices in pregnancy (O22.1-)*

+ O34.70 Maternal care for abnormality of vulva and ♀Ⓜ
perineum, unspecified trimester

+ O34.71 Maternal care for abnormality of vulva and ♀Ⓜ
perineum, first trimester

+ O34.72 Maternal care for abnormality of vulva and ♀Ⓜ
perineum, second trimester

+ O34.73 Maternal care for abnormality of vulva and ♀Ⓜ
perineum, third trimester

Ⓢ+ O34.8 Maternal care for other abnormalities of pelvic ♀Ⓜ
organs

+ O34.80 Maternal care for other abnormalities of pelvic ♀Ⓜ
organs, unspecified trimester

+ O34.81 Maternal care for other abnormalities of pelvic ♀Ⓜ
organs, first trimester

+ O34.82 Maternal care for other abnormalities of pelvic ♀Ⓜ
organs, second trimester

+ O34.83 Maternal care for other abnormalities of pelvic ♀Ⓜ
organs, third trimester

Ⓢ+ O34.9 Maternal care for abnormality of pelvic organ, ♀Ⓜ
unspecified

+ O34.90 Maternal care for abnormality of pelvic organ, ♀Ⓜ
unspecified, unspecified trimester

+ O34.91 Maternal care for abnormality of pelvic organ, ♀Ⓜ
unspecified, first trimester

+ O34.92 Maternal care for abnormality of pelvic organ, ♀Ⓜ
unspecified, second trimester

+ O34.93 Maternal care for abnormality of pelvic organ, ♀Ⓜ
unspecified, third trimester

④ O35 **Maternal care for known or suspected fetal abnormality and damage**

INCLUDES the listed conditions in the fetus as a reason for hospitalization or other obstetric care to the mother, or for termination of pregnancy

Code also:
any associated maternal condition
EXCLUDES 1 *encounter for suspected maternal and fetal conditions ruled out (Z03.7-)*

One of the following 7th characters is to be assigned to each code under category O35. 7th character 0 is for single gestations and multiple gestations where the fetus is unspecified. 7th characters 1 through 9 are for cases of multiple gestations to identify the fetus for which the code applies. The appropriate code from category O30, Multiple gestation, must also be assigned when assigning a code from category O35 that has a 7th character of 1 through 9.
0   not applicable or unspecified
1   fetus 1
2   fetus 2
3   fetus 3
4   fetus 4
5   fetus 5
9   other fetus

⑦ O35.0XX- **Maternal care for (suspected) central nervous system malformation in fetus**
Maternal care for fetal anencephaly
Maternal care for fetal hydrocephalus
Maternal care for fetal spina bifida
EXCLUDES 2 *chromosomal abnormality in fetus (O35.1)*

⑦ O35.1XX- **Maternal care for (suspected) chromosomal abnormality in fetus**

⑦ O35.2XX- **Maternal care for (suspected) hereditary disease in fetus**
EXCLUDES 2 *chromosomal abnormality in fetus (O35.1)*

⑦ O35.3XX- **Maternal care for (suspected) damage to fetus from viral disease in mother**
Maternal care for damage to fetus from maternal cytomegalovirus infection
Maternal care for damage to fetus from maternal rubella

⑦ O35.4XX- **Maternal care for (suspected) damage to fetus from alcohol**

⑦ O35.5XX- **Maternal care for (suspected) damage to fetus by drugs**
Maternal care for damage to fetus from drug addiction

⑦ O35.6XX- **Maternal care for (suspected) damage to fetus by radiation**

⑦ O35.7XX- **Maternal care for (suspected) damage to fetus by other medical procedures**
Maternal care for damage to fetus by amniocentesis
Maternal care for damage to fetus by biopsy procedures
Maternal care for damage to fetus by hematological investigation
Maternal care for damage to fetus by intrauterine contraceptive device
Maternal care for damage to fetus by intrauterine surgery

⑦ O35.8XX- **Maternal care for other (suspected) fetal abnormality and damage**
Maternal care for damage to fetus from maternal listeriosis
Maternal care for damage to fetus from maternal toxoplasmosis

⑦ O35.9XX- **Maternal care for (suspected) fetal abnormality and damage, unspecified**

◢ O36   Maternal care for other fetal problems

> **INCLUDES**   the listed conditions in the fetus as a reason for hospitalization or other obstetric care of the mother, or for termination of pregnancy
> **EXCLUDES 1**   encounter for suspected maternal and fetal conditions ruled out (Z03.7-)
> placental transfusion syndromes (O43.0-)
> **EXCLUDES 2**   labor and delivery complicated by fetal stress (O77.-)

> One of the following 7th characters is to be assigned to each code under category O36. 7th character 0 is for single gestations and multiple gestations where the fetus is unspecified. 7th characters 1 through 9 are for cases of multiple gestations to identify the fetus for which the code applies. The appropriate code from category O30, Multiple gestation, must also be assigned when assigning a code from category O36 that has a 7th character of 1 through 9.
> 0   not applicable or unspecified
> 1   fetus 1
> 2   fetus 2
> 3   fetus 3
> 4   fetus 4
> 5   fetus 5
> 9   other fetus

⑤ O36.0   Maternal care for rhesus isoimmunization
Maternal care for Rh incompatibility (with hydrops fetalis)

⑥ O36.01   Maternal care for anti-D [Rh] antibodies
AHA: 4Q 2014, 17

⑦ O36.011-   Maternal care for anti-D [Rh] antibodies, first trimester

⑦ O36.012-   Maternal care for anti-D [Rh] antibodies, second trimester

⑦ O36.013-   Maternal care for anti-D [Rh] antibodies, third trimester
AHA: 4Q 2014, 17

⑦ O36.019-   Maternal care for anti-D [Rh] antibodies, unspecified trimester

⑥ O36.09   Maternal care for other rhesus isoimmunization

⑦ O36.091-   Maternal care for other rhesus isoimmunization, first trimester

⑦ O36.092-   Maternal care for other rhesus isoimmunization, second trimester

⑦ O36.093-   Maternal care for other rhesus isoimmunization, third trimester
AHA: 3Q 2015, 40

⑦ O36.099-   Maternal care for other rhesus isoimmunization, unspecified trimester

⑤ O36.1   Maternal care for other isoimmunization
Maternal care for ABO isoimmunization

⑥ O36.11   Maternal care for Anti-A sensitization
Maternal care for isoimmunization NOS (with hydrops fetalis)

⑦ O36.111-   Maternal care for Anti-A sensitization, first trimester

⑦ O36.112-   Maternal care for Anti-A sensitization, second trimester

⑦ O36.113-   Maternal care for Anti-A sensitization, third trimester

⑦ O36.119-   Maternal care for Anti-A sensitization, unspecified trimester

⑥ O36.19   Maternal care for other isoimmunization
Maternal care for Anti-B sensitization

⑦ O36.191-   Maternal care for other isoimmunization, first trimester

⑦ O36.192-   Maternal care for other isoimmunization, second trimester

⑦ O36.193-   Maternal care for other isoimmunization, third trimester

⑦ O36.199-   Maternal care for other isoimmunization, unspecified trimester

⑤ O36.2   Maternal care for hydrops fetalis
Maternal care for hydrops fetalis NOS
Maternal care for hydrops fetalis not associated with isoimmunization

> **EXCLUDES 1**   hydrops fetalis associated with ABO isoimmunization (O36.1-)
> hydrops fetalis associated with rhesus isoimmunization (O36.0-)

⑦ O36.20X-   Maternal care for hydrops fetalis, unspecified trimester

⑦ O36.21X-   Maternal care for hydrops fetalis, first trimester

⑦ O36.22X-   Maternal care for hydrops fetalis, second trimester

⑦ O36.23X-   Maternal care for hydrops fetalis, third trimester

⑦ O36.4XX-   Maternal care for intrauterine death
Maternal care for intrauterine fetal death NOS
Maternal care for intrauterine fetal death after completion of 20 weeks of gestation
Maternal care for late fetal death
Maternal care for missed delivery

> **EXCLUDES 1**   missed abortion (O02.1)
> stillbirth (P95)

⑤ O36.5   Maternal care for known or suspected poor fetal growth

⑥ O36.51   Maternal care for known or suspected placental insufficiency

⑦ O36.511-   Maternal care for known or suspected placental insufficiency, first trimester

⑦ O36.512-   Maternal care for known or suspected placental insufficiency, second trimester

⑦ O36.513-   Maternal care for known or suspected placental insufficiency, third trimester

⑦ O36.519-   Maternal care for known or suspected placental insufficiency, unspecified trimester

⑥ O36.59   Maternal care for other known or suspected poor fetal growth
Maternal care for known or suspected light-for-dates NOS
Maternal care for known or suspected small-for-dates NOS

⑦ O36.591-   Maternal care for other known or suspected poor fetal growth, first trimester

⑦ O36.592-   Maternal care for other known or suspected poor fetal growth, second trimester

⑦ O36.593-   Maternal care for other known or suspected poor fetal growth, third trimester

⑦ O36.599-   Maternal care for other known or suspected poor fetal growth, unspecified trimester

⑤ O36.6   Maternal care for excessive fetal growth
Maternal care for known or suspected large-for-dates

⑦ O36.60X-   Maternal care for excessive fetal growth, unspecified trimester

⑦ O36.61X-   Maternal care for excessive fetal growth, first trimester

⑦ O36.62X-   Maternal care for excessive fetal growth, second trimester

⑦ O36.63X-   Maternal care for excessive fetal growth, third trimester

⑤ O36.7   Maternal care for viable fetus in abdominal pregnancy

⑦ O36.70X-   Maternal care for viable fetus in abdominal pregnancy, unspecified trimester

⑦ O36.71X-   Maternal care for viable fetus in abdominal pregnancy, first trimester

⑦ O36.72X-   Maternal care for viable fetus in abdominal pregnancy, second trimester

⑦ O36.73X-   Maternal care for viable fetus in abdominal pregnancy, third trimester

⑤ O36.8   Maternal care for other specified fetal problems

⑦ O36.80X-   Pregnancy with inconclusive fetal viability
Encounter to determine fetal viability of pregnancy

⑥ O36.81   Decreased fetal movements

⑦ O36.812-   Decreased fetal movements, second trimester

⑦ O36.813-   Decreased fetal movements, third trimester   ♀Ⓜ

⑦ O36.819-   Decreased fetal movements, unspecified trimester   ♀Ⓜ

⑥ O36.82   Fetal anemia and thrombocytopenia   ♀Ⓜ

⑦ O36.821-   Fetal anemia and thrombocytopenia, first trimester   ♀Ⓜ

⑦ O36.822-   Fetal anemia and thrombocytopenia, second trimester   ♀Ⓜ

⑦ O36.823-   Fetal anemia and thrombocytopenia, third trimester   ♀Ⓜ

⑦ O36.829-   Fetal anemia and thrombocytopenia, unspecified trimester   ♀Ⓜ

⑥ O36.89   Maternal care for other specified fetal problems   ♀Ⓜ

⑦ O36.891-   Maternal care for other specified fetal problems, first trimester   ♀Ⓜ

● New   ▲ Revised   *Manifestation*   ④-⑦ Digit Indicators   ⊟ Laterality   Ⓐ Adult (15+ years)   Ⓜ Maternity (12-55 years)   Ⓝ Newborn   Ⓟ Pediatric (0-17 years)   ♂ Male   ♀ Female
✖ ~~Deleted~~   Unspecified   + Additional code

O36.892- Maternal care for other specified fetal problems, second trimester ♀Ⓜ

O36.893- Maternal care for other specified fetal problems, third trimester ♀Ⓜ

O36.899- Maternal care for other specified fetal problems, unspecified trimester ♀Ⓜ

§ O36.9 Maternal care for fetal problem, unspecified

O36.90X- Maternal care for fetal problem, unspecified, unspecified trimester

O36.91X- Maternal care for fetal problem, unspecified, first trimester ♀Ⓜ

O36.92X- Maternal care for fetal problem, unspecified, second trimester ♀Ⓜ

O36.93X- Maternal care for fetal problem, unspecified, third trimester ♀Ⓜ

O40 Polyhydramnios

INCLUDES hydramnios

EXCLUDES 1 encounter for suspected maternal and fetal conditions ruled out (Z03.7-)

One of the following 7th characters is to be assigned to each code under category O40. 7th character 0 is for single gestations and multiple gestations where the fetus is unspecified. 7th characters 1 through 9 are for cases of multiple gestations to identify the fetus for which the code applies. The appropriate code from category O30, Multiple gestation, must also be assigned when assigning a code from category O40 that has a 7th character of 1 through 9.
0 not applicable or unspecified
1 fetus 1
2 fetus 2
3 fetus 3
4 fetus 4
5 fetus 5
9 other fetus

O40.1XX- Polyhydramnios, first trimester ♀Ⓜ

O40.2XX- Polyhydramnios, second trimester ♀Ⓜ

O40.3XX- Polyhydramnios, third trimester ♀Ⓜ

O40.9XX- Polyhydramnios, unspecified trimester ♀Ⓜ

O41 Other disorders of amniotic fluid and membranes

EXCLUDES 1 encounter for suspected maternal and fetal conditions ruled out (Z03.7-)

One of the following 7th characters is to be assigned to each code under category O41. 7th character 0 is for single gestations and multiple gestations where the fetus is unspecified. 7th characters 1 through 9 are for cases of multiple gestations to identify the fetus for which the code applies. The appropriate code from category O30, Multiple gestation, must also be assigned when assigning a code from category O41 that has a 7th character of 1 through 9.
0 not applicable or unspecified
1 fetus 1
2 fetus 2
3 fetus 3
4 fetus 4
5 fetus 5
9 other fetus

§ O41.0 Oligohydramnios
Oligohydramnios without rupture of membranes

O41.00X- Oligohydramnios, unspecified trimester ♀Ⓜ

O41.01X- Oligohydramnios, first trimester ♀Ⓜ

O41.02X- Oligohydramnios, second trimester ♀Ⓜ

O41.03X- Oligohydramnios, third trimester ♀Ⓜ

§ O41.1 Infection of amniotic sac and membranes

Ⓖ O41.10 Infection of amniotic sac and membranes, unspecified

O41.101- Infection of amniotic sac and membranes, unspecified, first trimester ♀Ⓜ

O41.102- Infection of amniotic sac and membranes, unspecified, second trimester ♀Ⓜ

O41.103- Infection of amniotic sac and membranes, unspecified, third trimester ♀Ⓜ

O41.109- Infection of amniotic sac and membranes, unspecified, unspecified trimester ♀Ⓜ

Ⓖ O41.12 Chorioamnionitis

O41.121- Chorioamnionitis, first trimester ♀Ⓜ

O41.122- Chorioamnionitis, second trimester ♀Ⓜ

O41.123- Chorioamnionitis, third trimester ♀Ⓜ

O41.129- Chorioamnionitis, unspecified trimester ♀Ⓜ

Ⓖ O41.14 Placentitis

O41.141- Placentitis, first trimester ♀Ⓜ

O41.142- Placentitis, second trimester ♀Ⓜ

O41.143- Placentitis, third trimester ♀Ⓜ

O41.149- Placentitis, unspecified trimester ♀Ⓜ

§ O41.8 Other specified disorders of amniotic fluid and membranes

Ⓖ O41.8X Other specified disorders of amniotic fluid and membranes

O41.8X1- Other specified disorders of amniotic fluid and membranes, first trimester ♀Ⓜ

O41.8X2- Other specified disorders of amniotic fluid and membranes, second trimester ♀Ⓜ

O41.8X3- Other specified disorders of amniotic fluid and membranes, third trimester ♀Ⓜ

O41.8X9- Other specified disorders of amniotic fluid and membranes, unspecified trimester ♀Ⓜ

§ O41.9 Disorder of amniotic fluid and membranes, unspecified

O41.90X- Disorder of amniotic fluid and membranes, unspecified, unspecified trimester ♀Ⓜ

O41.91X- Disorder of amniotic fluid and membranes, unspecified, first trimester ♀Ⓜ

O41.92X- Disorder of amniotic fluid and membranes, unspecified, second trimester ♀Ⓜ

O41.93X- Disorder of amniotic fluid and membranes, unspecified, third trimester ♀Ⓜ

O42 Premature rupture of membranes

§ O42.0 Premature rupture of membranes, onset of labor within 24 hours of rupture ♀Ⓜ

O42.00 Premature rupture of membranes, onset of labor within 24 hours of rupture, unspecified weeks of gestation ♀Ⓜ

Ⓖ O42.01 Preterm premature rupture of membranes, onset of labor within 24 hours of rupture
Premature rupture of membranes before 37 completed weeks of gestation

O42.011 Preterm premature rupture of membranes, onset of labor within 24 hours of rupture, first trimester ♀Ⓜ

O42.012 Preterm premature rupture of membranes, onset of labor within 24 hours of rupture, second trimester ♀Ⓜ

O42.013 Preterm premature rupture of membranes, onset of labor within 24 hours of rupture, third trimester ♀Ⓜ

O42.019 Preterm premature rupture of membranes, onset of labor within 24 hours of rupture, unspecified trimester ♀Ⓜ

▲ O42.02 Full-term premature rupture of membranes, onset of labor within 24 hours of rupture ♀Ⓜ
Premature rupture of membranes at or after 37 completed weeks of gestation, onset of labor within 24 hours of rupture

§ O42.1 Premature rupture of membranes, onset of labor more than 24 hours following rupture ♀Ⓜ

O42.10 Premature rupture of membranes, onset of labor more than 24 hours following rupture, unspecified weeks of gestation ♀Ⓜ

Ⓖ O42.11 Preterm premature rupture of membranes, onset of labor more than 24 hours following rupture
Premature rupture of membranes before 37 completed weeks of gestation

O42.111 Preterm premature rupture of membranes, onset of labor more than 24 hours following rupture, first trimester ♀Ⓜ

O42.112 Preterm premature rupture of membranes, onset of labor more than 24 hours following rupture, second trimester ♀Ⓜ

O42.113 Preterm premature rupture of membranes, onset of labor more than 24 hours following rupture, third trimester ♀Ⓜ

O42.119 Preterm premature rupture of membranes, onset of labor more than 24 hours following rupture, unspecified trimester ♀Ⓜ

● New ▲ Revised Manifestation ◆-🟥 Digit Indicators ⬒ Laterality 🅰 Adult (15+ years) Ⓜ Maternity (12-55 years) 🅽 Newborn 🅿 Pediatric (0-17 years) ♂ Male ♀ Female
✖ Deleted Unspecified ✚ Additional code

856 © 2017 DecisionHealth 2017 ICD-10-CM Expert for Physicians

▲ **O42.12** **Full-term premature rupture of membranes, onset of labor more than 24 hours following rupture** ♀Ⓜ
Premature rupture of membranes at or after 37 completed weeks of gestation, onset of labor more than 24 hours following rupture

⑤ **O42.9** **Premature rupture of membranes, unspecified as to length of time between rupture and onset of labor** ♀Ⓜ

O42.90 **Premature rupture of membranes, unspecified as to length of time between rupture and onset of labor, unspecified weeks of gestation** ♀Ⓜ

⑥ **O42.91** **Preterm premature rupture of membranes, unspecified as to length of time between rupture and onset of labor**
Premature rupture of membranes before 37 completed weeks of gestation

O42.911 **Preterm premature rupture of membranes, unspecified as to length of time between rupture and onset of labor, first trimester** ♀Ⓜ

O42.912 **Preterm premature rupture of membranes, unspecified as to length of time between rupture and onset of labor, second trimester** ♀Ⓜ

O42.913 **Preterm premature rupture of membranes, unspecified as to length of time between rupture and onset of labor, third trimester** ♀Ⓜ

O42.919 **Preterm premature rupture of membranes, unspecified as to length of time between rupture and onset of labor, unspecified trimester** ♀Ⓜ

▲ **O42.92** **Full-term premature rupture of membranes, unspecified as to length of time between rupture and onset of labor** ♀Ⓜ
Premature rupture of membranes at or after 37 completed weeks of gestation, unspecified as to length of time between rupture and onset of labor

④ **O43** **Placental disorders**
EXCLUDES 2 *maternal care for poor fetal growth due to placental insufficiency (O36.5-)*
placenta previa (O44.-)
placental polyp (O90.89)
placentitis (O41.14-)
premature separation of placenta [abruptio placentae] (O45.-)

⑤ **O43.0** **Placental transfusion syndromes** ♀Ⓜ

⑥ **O43.01** **Fetomaternal placental transfusion syndrome**
Maternofetal placental transfusion syndrome

O43.011 **Fetomaternal placental transfusion syndrome, first trimester** ♀Ⓜ

O43.012 **Fetomaternal placental transfusion syndrome, second trimester** ♀Ⓜ

O43.013 **Fetomaternal placental transfusion syndrome, third trimester** ♀Ⓜ

O43.019 **Fetomaternal placental transfusion syndrome, unspecified trimester** ♀Ⓜ

⑥ **O43.02** **Fetus-to-fetus placental transfusion syndrome**

O43.021 **Fetus-to-fetus placental transfusion syndrome, first trimester** ♀Ⓜ

O43.022 **Fetus-to-fetus placental transfusion syndrome, second trimester** ♀Ⓜ

O43.023 **Fetus-to-fetus placental transfusion syndrome, third trimester** ♀Ⓜ

O43.029 **Fetus-to-fetus placental transfusion syndrome, unspecified trimester** ♀Ⓜ

⑤ **O43.1** **Malformation of placenta** ♀Ⓜ

⑥ **O43.10** **Malformation of placenta, unspecified**
Abnormal placenta NOS

O43.101 **Malformation of placenta, unspecified, first trimester** ♀Ⓜ

O43.102 **Malformation of placenta, unspecified, second trimester** ♀Ⓜ

O43.103 **Malformation of placenta, unspecified, third trimester** ♀Ⓜ

O43.109 **Malformation of placenta, unspecified, unspecified trimester** ♀Ⓜ

⑥ **O43.11** **Circumvallate placenta**

O43.111 **Circumvallate placenta, first trimester** ♀Ⓜ

O43.112 **Circumvallate placenta, second trimester** ♀Ⓜ

O43.113 **Circumvallate placenta, third trimester** ♀Ⓜ

O43.119 **Circumvallate placenta, unspecified trimester** ♀Ⓜ

⑥ **O43.12** **Velamentous insertion of umbilical cord**

O43.121 **Velamentous insertion of umbilical cord, first trimester** ♀Ⓜ

O43.122 **Velamentous insertion of umbilical cord, second trimester** ♀Ⓜ

O43.123 **Velamentous insertion of umbilical cord, third trimester** ♀Ⓜ

O43.129 **Velamentous insertion of umbilical cord, unspecified trimester** ♀Ⓜ

⑥ **O43.19** **Other malformation of placenta**

O43.191 **Other malformation of placenta, first trimester** ♀Ⓜ

O43.192 **Other malformation of placenta, second trimester** ♀Ⓜ

O43.193 **Other malformation of placenta, third trimester** ♀Ⓜ

O43.199 **Other malformation of placenta, unspecified trimester** ♀Ⓜ

⑤ **O43.2** **Morbidly adherent placenta** ♀Ⓜ
Code also:
associated third stage postpartum hemorrhage, if applicable (O72.0)
EXCLUDES 1 *retained placenta (O73.-)*

⑥ **O43.21** **Placenta accreta**

O43.211 **Placenta accreta, first trimester** ♀Ⓜ

O43.212 **Placenta accreta, second trimester** ♀Ⓜ

O43.213 **Placenta accreta, third trimester** ♀Ⓜ

O43.219 **Placenta accreta, unspecified trimester** ♀Ⓜ

⑥ **O43.22** **Placenta increta**

O43.221 **Placenta increta, first trimester** ♀Ⓜ

O43.222 **Placenta increta, second trimester** ♀Ⓜ

O43.223 **Placenta increta, third trimester** ♀Ⓜ

O43.229 **Placenta increta, unspecified trimester** ♀Ⓜ

⑥ **O43.23** **Placenta percreta**

O43.231 **Placenta percreta, first trimester** ♀Ⓜ

O43.232 **Placenta percreta, second trimester** ♀Ⓜ

O43.233 **Placenta percreta, third trimester** ♀Ⓜ

O43.239 **Placenta percreta, unspecified trimester** ♀Ⓜ

⑤ **O43.8** **Other placental disorders** ♀Ⓜ

⑥ **O43.81** **Placental infarction**

O43.811 **Placental infarction, first trimester** ♀Ⓜ

O43.812 **Placental infarction, second trimester** ♀Ⓜ

O43.813 **Placental infarction, third trimester** ♀Ⓜ

O43.819 **Placental infarction, unspecified trimester** ♀Ⓜ

⑥ **O43.89** **Other placental disorders**
Placental dysfunction

O43.891 **Other placental disorders, first trimester** ♀Ⓜ

O43.892 **Other placental disorders, second trimester** ♀Ⓜ

O43.893 **Other placental disorders, third trimester** ♀Ⓜ

O43.899 **Other placental disorders, unspecified trimester** ♀Ⓜ

⑤ **O43.9** **Unspecified placental disorder** ♀Ⓜ

O43.90 **Unspecified placental disorder, unspecified trimester** ♀Ⓜ

O43.91 **Unspecified placental disorder, first trimester** ♀Ⓜ

O43.92 **Unspecified placental disorder, second trimester** ♀Ⓜ

O43.93 **Unspecified placental disorder, third trimester** ♀Ⓜ

④ **O44** **Placenta previa**

▲⑤ **O44.0** **Complete placenta previa NOS or without hemorrhage** ♀Ⓜ
Placenta previa NOS

▲ **O44.00** **Complete placenta previa NOS or without hemorrhage, unspecified trimester** ♀Ⓜ

▲ **O44.01** **Complete placenta previa NOS or without hemorrhage, first trimester** ♀Ⓜ

▲ **O44.02** **Complete placenta previa NOS or without hemorrhage, second trimester** ♀Ⓜ

▲ **O44.03** **Complete placenta previa NOS or without hemorrhage, third trimester** ♀Ⓜ

▲ ⑤ O44.1   Complete placenta previa with hemorrhage   ♀Ⓜ
              EXCLUDES 1   *labor and delivery complicated by*
                              hemorrhage from vasa previa (O69.4)

Placenta previa hemorrhage

Marginal   Total   Partial

▲ O44.10   Complete placenta previa with hemorrhage,   ♀Ⓜ
            unspecified trimester
▲ O44.11   Complete placenta previa with hemorrhage, first   ♀Ⓜ
            trimester
▲ O44.12   Complete placenta previa with hemorrhage,   ♀Ⓜ
            second trimester
▲ O44.13   Complete placenta previa with hemorrhage,   ♀Ⓜ
            third trimester
● ⑤ O44.2   Partial placenta previa without hemorrhage
            Marginal placenta previa, NOS or without hemorrhage
● O44.20   Partial placenta previa NOS or without   ♀Ⓜ
            hemorrhage, unspecified trimester
● O44.21   Partial placenta previa NOS or without   ♀Ⓜ
            hemorrhage, first trimester
● O44.22   Partial placenta previa NOS or without   ♀Ⓜ
            hemorrhage, second trimester
● O44.23   Partial placenta previa NOS or without   ♀Ⓜ
            hemorrhage, third trimester
● ⑤ O44.3   Partial placenta previa with hemorrhage
            Marginal placenta previa with hemorrhage
● O44.30   Partial placenta previa with hemorrhage,   ♀Ⓜ
            unspecified trimester
● O44.31   Partial placenta previa with hemorrhage, first   ♀Ⓜ
            trimester
● O44.32   Partial placenta previa with hemorrhage, second   ♀Ⓜ
            trimester
● O44.33   Partial placenta previa with hemorrhage, third   ♀Ⓜ
            trimester
● ⑤ O44.4   Low lying placenta NOS or without hemorrhage
            Low implantation of placenta NOS or without hemorrhage
● O44.40   Low lying placenta NOS or without   ♀Ⓜ
            hemorrhage, unspecified trimester
● O44.41   Low lying placenta NOS or without hemorrhage,   ♀Ⓜ
            first trimester
● O44.42   Low lying placenta NOS or without hemorrhage,   ♀Ⓜ
            second trimester
● O44.43   Low lying placenta NOS or without hemorrhage,   ♀Ⓜ
            third trimester
● ⑤ O44.5   Low lying placenta with hemorrhage
            Low implantation of placenta with hemorrhage
● O44.50   Low lying placenta with hemorrhage,   ♀Ⓜ
            unspecified trimester
● O44.51   Low lying placenta with hemorrhage, first   ♀Ⓜ
            trimester
● O44.52   Low lying placenta with hemorrhage, second   ♀Ⓜ
            trimester
● O44.53   Low lying placenta with hemorrhage, third   ♀Ⓜ
            trimester
④ O45   Premature separation of placenta [abruptio placentae]
⑤ O45.0   Premature separation of placenta with coagulation   ♀Ⓜ
            defect
⑥ O45.00   Premature separation of placenta with coagulation
            defect, unspecified
O45.001   Premature separation of placenta with   ♀Ⓜ
            coagulation defect, unspecified, first
            trimester
O45.002   Premature separation of placenta with   ♀Ⓜ
            coagulation defect, unspecified, second
            trimester

O45.003   Premature separation of placenta with   ♀Ⓜ
            coagulation defect, unspecified, third
            trimester
O45.009   Premature separation of placenta with   ♀Ⓜ
            coagulation defect, unspecified,
            unspecified trimester
⑥ O45.01   Premature separation of placenta with
            afibrinogenemia
            Premature separation of placenta with
            hypofibrinogenemia
O45.011   Premature separation of placenta with   ♀Ⓜ
            afibrinogenemia, first trimester
O45.012   Premature separation of placenta with   ♀Ⓜ
            afibrinogenemia, second trimester
O45.013   Premature separation of placenta with   ♀Ⓜ
            afibrinogenemia, third trimester
O45.019   Premature separation of placenta with   ♀Ⓜ
            afibrinogenemia, unspecified trimester
⑥ O45.02   Premature separation of placenta with disseminated
            intravascular coagulation
O45.021   Premature separation of placenta with   ♀Ⓜ
            disseminated intravascular coagulation,
            first trimester
O45.022   Premature separation of placenta with   ♀Ⓜ
            disseminated intravascular coagulation,
            second trimester
O45.023   Premature separation of placenta with   ♀Ⓜ
            disseminated intravascular coagulation,
            third trimester
O45.029   Premature separation of placenta with   ♀Ⓜ
            disseminated intravascular coagulation,
            unspecified trimester
⑥ O45.09   Premature separation of placenta with other
            coagulation defect
O45.091   Premature separation of placenta with other ♀Ⓜ
            coagulation defect, first trimester
O45.092   Premature separation of placenta with other ♀Ⓜ
            coagulation defect, second trimester
O45.093   Premature separation of placenta with other ♀Ⓜ
            coagulation defect, third trimester
O45.099   Premature separation of placenta with   ♀Ⓜ
            other coagulation defect, unspecified
            trimester
⑤ O45.8   Other premature separation of placenta   ♀Ⓜ
⑥ O45.8X   Other premature separation of placenta
O45.8X1   Other premature separation of placenta,   ♀Ⓜ
            first trimester
O45.8X2   Other premature separation of placenta,   ♀Ⓜ
            second trimester
O45.8X3   Other premature separation of placenta,   ♀Ⓜ
            third trimester
O45.8X9   Other premature separation of placenta,   ♀Ⓜ
            unspecified trimester
⑤ O45.9   Premature separation of placenta, unspecified   ♀Ⓜ
            Abruptio placentae NOS
O45.90   Premature separation of placenta, unspecified,   ♀Ⓜ
            unspecified trimester
O45.91   Premature separation of placenta, unspecified,   ♀Ⓜ
            first trimester
O45.92   Premature separation of placenta, unspecified,   ♀Ⓜ
            second trimester
O45.93   Premature separation of placenta, unspecified,   ♀Ⓜ
            third trimester
④ O46   Antepartum hemorrhage, not elsewhere classified
            EXCLUDES 1   *hemorrhage in early pregnancy (O20.-)*
                            intrapartum hemorrhage NEC (O67.-)
                            placenta previa (O44.-)
                            premature separation of placenta [abruptio
                            placentae] (O45.-)
⑤ O46.0   Antepartum hemorrhage with coagulation defect   ♀Ⓜ
⑥ O46.00   Antepartum hemorrhage with coagulation defect,
            unspecified
O46.001   Antepartum hemorrhage with coagulation   ♀Ⓜ
            defect, unspecified, first trimester
O46.002   Antepartum hemorrhage with coagulation   ♀Ⓜ
            defect, unspecified, second trimester
O46.003   Antepartum hemorrhage with coagulation   ♀Ⓜ
            defect, unspecified, third trimester

● New   ▲ Revised   *Manifestation*   ④-⑦ Digit Indicators   ⊟ Laterality   Ⓐ Adult   Ⓜ Maternity   Ⓝ Newborn   Ⓟ Pediatric   ♂ Male   ♀ Female
✖ Deleted   Unspecified   + Additional code   (15+ years)   (12-55 years)   (0-17 years)

858   © 2017 DecisionHealth   2017 ICD-10-CM Expert for Physicians

O46.009	Antepartum hemorrhage with coagulation defect, unspecified, unspecified trimester	♀▩

⑥ **O46.01** Antepartum hemorrhage with afibrinogenemia
Antepartum hemorrhage with hypofibrinogenemia

O46.011	Antepartum hemorrhage with afibrinogenemia, first trimester	♀▩
O46.012	Antepartum hemorrhage with afibrinogenemia, second trimester	
O46.013	Antepartum hemorrhage with afibrinogenemia, third trimester	♀▩
O46.019	Antepartum hemorrhage with afibrinogenemia, unspecified trimester	

⑥ **O46.02** Antepartum hemorrhage with disseminated intravascular coagulation

O46.021	Antepartum hemorrhage with disseminated intravascular coagulation, first trimester	♀▩
O46.022	Antepartum hemorrhage with disseminated intravascular coagulation, second trimester	♀▩
O46.023	Antepartum hemorrhage with disseminated intravascular coagulation, third trimester	♀▩
O46.029	Antepartum hemorrhage with disseminated intravascular coagulation, unspecified trimester	♀▩

⑥ **O46.09** Antepartum hemorrhage with other coagulation defect

O46.091	Antepartum hemorrhage with other coagulation defect, first trimester	♀▩
O46.092	Antepartum hemorrhage with other coagulation defect, second trimester	♀▩
O46.093	Antepartum hemorrhage with other coagulation defect, third trimester	♀▩
O46.099	Antepartum hemorrhage with other coagulation defect, unspecified trimester	♀▩

⑤ **O46.8** Other antepartum hemorrhage ♀▩
⑥ **O46.8X** Other antepartum hemorrhage

O46.8X1	Other antepartum hemorrhage, first trimester	♀▩
O46.8X2	Other antepartum hemorrhage, second trimester	♀▩
O46.8X3	Other antepartum hemorrhage, third trimester	♀▩
O46.8X9	Other antepartum hemorrhage, unspecified trimester	♀▩

⑤ **O46.9** Antepartum hemorrhage, unspecified ♀▩

O46.90	Antepartum hemorrhage, unspecified, unspecified trimester	♀▩
O46.91	Antepartum hemorrhage, unspecified, first trimester	♀▩
O46.92	Antepartum hemorrhage, unspecified, second trimester	♀▩
O46.93	Antepartum hemorrhage, unspecified, third trimester	♀▩

④ **O47** False labor
INCLUDES Braxton Hicks contractions
threatened labor
EXCLUDES 1 *preterm labor (O60.-)*

⑤ **O47.0** False labor before 37 completed weeks of gestation

O47.00	False labor before 37 completed weeks of gestation, unspecified trimester	♀▩
O47.02	False labor before 37 completed weeks of gestation, second trimester	♀▩
O47.03	False labor before 37 completed weeks of gestation, third trimester	♀▩
O47.1	False labor at or after 37 completed weeks of gestation	♀▩
O47.9	False labor, unspecified	♀▩

④ **O48** Late pregnancy

| O48.0 | Post-term pregnancy | ♀▩ |

Pregnancy over 40 completed weeks to 42 completed weeks gestation

| O48.1 | Prolonged pregnancy | ♀▩ |

Pregnancy which has advanced beyond 42 completed weeks gestation

Complications of labor and delivery (O60-O77)

④ **O60** Preterm labor
INCLUDES onset (spontaneous) of labor before 37 completed weeks of gestation
EXCLUDES 1 *false labor (O47.0-)*
threatened labor NOS (O47.0-)

⑤ **O60.0** Preterm labor without delivery

O60.00	Preterm labor without delivery, unspecified trimester	♀▩
O60.02	Preterm labor without delivery, second trimester	♀▩
O60.03	Preterm labor without delivery, third trimester	♀▩

⑤ **O60.1** Preterm labor with preterm delivery

One of the following 7th characters is to be assigned to each code under subcategory O60.1. 7th character 0 is for single gestations and multiple gestations where the fetus is unspecified. 7th characters 1 through 9 are for cases of multiple gestations to identify the fetus for which the code applies. The appropriate code from category O30, Multiple gestation, must also be assigned when assigning a code from subcategory O60.1 that has a 7th character of 1 through 9.
0 not applicable or unspecified
1 fetus 1
2 fetus 2
3 fetus 3
4 fetus 4
5 fetus 5
9 other fetus

| ⑦ O60.10X- | Preterm labor with preterm delivery, unspecified trimester | ♀▩ |

Preterm labor with delivery NOS

⑦ O60.12X-	Preterm labor second trimester with preterm delivery second trimester	♀▩
⑦ O60.13X-	Preterm labor second trimester with preterm delivery third trimester	♀▩
⑦ O60.14X-	Preterm labor third trimester with preterm delivery third trimester	♀▩

AHA: (O60.14X0) 2Q 2016, 10
AHA: (O60.14X1) 2Q 2016, 10
AHA: (O60.14X2) 2Q 2016, 10

⑤ **O60.2** Term delivery with preterm labor

One of the following 7th characters is to be assigned to each code under subcategory O60.2. 7th character 0 is for single gestations and multiple gestations where the fetus is unspecified. 7th characters 1 through 9 are for cases of multiple gestations to identify the fetus for which the code applies. The appropriate code from category O30, Multiple gestation, must also be assigned when assigning a code from subcategory O60.2 that has a 7th character of 1 through 9.
0 not applicable or unspecified
1 fetus 1
2 fetus 2
3 fetus 3
4 fetus 4
5 fetus 5
9 other fetus

⑦ O60.20X-	Term delivery with preterm labor, unspecified trimester	♀▩
⑦ O60.22X-	Term delivery with preterm labor, second trimester	♀▩
⑦ O60.23X-	Term delivery with preterm labor, third trimester	♀▩

④ **O61** Failed induction of labor

| O61.0 | Failed medical induction of labor | ♀▩ |

Failed induction (of labor) by oxytocin
Failed induction (of labor) by prostaglandins

| O61.1 | Failed instrumental induction of labor | ♀▩ |

Failed mechanical induction (of labor)
Failed surgical induction (of labor)

| O61.8 | Other failed induction of labor | ♀▩ |
| O61.9 | Failed induction of labor, unspecified | ♀▩ |

④ **O62** Abnormalities of forces of labor

O62.0   **Primary inadequate contractions** ♀Ⓜ
Failure of cervical dilatation
Primary hypotonic uterine dysfunction
Uterine inertia during latent phase of labor

O62.1   **Secondary uterine inertia** ♀Ⓜ
Arrested active phase of labor
Secondary hypotonic uterine dysfunction

O62.2   **Other uterine inertia** ♀Ⓜ
Atony of uterus without hemorrhage
Atony of uterus NOS
Desultory labor
Hypotonic uterine dysfunction NOS
Irregular labor
Poor contractions
Slow slope active phase of labor
Uterine inertia NOS

> **EXCLUDES 1**   *atony of uterus with hemorrhage (postpartum) (O72.1)*
> *postpartum atony of uterus without hemorrhage (O75.89)*

O62.3   **Precipitate labor** ♀Ⓜ
> **DEFINITION**   Labor occurring quickly, with rapid expulsion of the fetus.

O62.4   **Hypertonic, incoordinate, and prolonged uterine contractions** ♀Ⓜ
Cervical spasm
Contraction ring dystocia
Dyscoordinate labor
Hour-glass contraction of uterus
Hypertonic uterine dysfunction
Incoordinate uterine action
Tetanic contractions
Uterine dystocia NOS
Uterine spasm

> **EXCLUDES 1**   *dystocia (fetal) (maternal) NOS (O66.9)*

O62.8   **Other abnormalities of forces of labor** ♀Ⓜ
O62.9   **Abnormality of forces of labor, unspecified** ♀Ⓜ

④ O63   **Long labor**
O63.0   **Prolonged first stage (of labor)** ♀Ⓜ
O63.1   **Prolonged second stage (of labor)** ♀Ⓜ
O63.2   **Delayed delivery of second twin, triplet, etc.** ♀Ⓜ
O63.9   **Long labor, unspecified** ♀Ⓜ
Prolonged labor NOS

④ O64   **Obstructed labor due to malposition and malpresentation of fetus**

> One of the following 7th characters is to be assigned to each code under category O64. 7th character 0 is for single gestations and multiple gestations where the fetus is unspecified. 7th characters 1 through 9 are for cases of multiple gestations to identify the fetus for which the code applies. The appropriate code from category O30, Multiple gestation, must also be assigned when assigning a code from category O64 that has a 7th character of 1 through 9.
>
> 0   not applicable or unspecified
> 1   fetus 1
> 2   fetus 2
> 3   fetus 3
> 4   fetus 4
> 5   fetus 5
> 9   other fetus

⑦ O64.0XX-   **Obstructed labor due to incomplete rotation of fetal head** ♀Ⓜ
Deep transverse arrest
Obstructed labor due to persistent occipitoiliac (position)
Obstructed labor due to persistent occipitoposterior (position)
Obstructed labor due to persistent occipitosacral (position)
Obstructed labor due to persistent occipitotransverse (position)

⑦ O64.1XX-   **Obstructed labor due to breech presentation** ♀Ⓜ
Obstructed labor due to buttocks presentation
Obstructed labor due to complete breech presentation
Obstructed labor due to frank breech presentation

⑦ O64.2XX-   **Obstructed labor due to face presentation** ♀Ⓜ
Obstructed labor due to chin presentation

⑦ O64.3XX-   **Obstructed labor due to brow presentation** ♀Ⓜ

⑦ O64.4XX-   **Obstructed labor due to shoulder presentation** ♀Ⓜ
Prolapsed arm
> **EXCLUDES 1**   *impacted shoulders (O66.0)*
> *shoulder dystocia (O66.0)*

⑦ O64.5XX-   **Obstructed labor due to compound presentation** ♀Ⓜ
⑦ O64.8XX-   **Obstructed labor due to other malposition and malpresentation** ♀Ⓜ
Obstructed labor due to footling presentation
Obstructed labor due to incomplete breech presentation

⑦ O64.9XX-   **Obstructed labor due to malposition and malpresentation, unspecified** ♀Ⓜ

④ O65   **Obstructed labor due to maternal pelvic abnormality**
O65.0   **Obstructed labor due to deformed pelvis** ♀Ⓜ
O65.1   **Obstructed labor due to generally contracted pelvis** ♀Ⓜ
O65.2   **Obstructed labor due to pelvic inlet contraction** ♀Ⓜ
O65.3   **Obstructed labor due to pelvic outlet and mid-cavity contraction** ♀Ⓜ
O65.4   **Obstructed labor due to fetopelvic disproportion, unspecified** ♀Ⓜ

> **EXCLUDES 1**   *dystocia due to abnormality of fetus (O66.2-O66.3)*

➕ O65.5   **Obstructed labor due to abnormality of maternal pelvic organs** ♀Ⓜ
Obstructed labor due to conditions listed in O34.-
Use additional code to identify abnormality of pelvic organs O34.-

O65.8   **Obstructed labor due to other maternal pelvic abnormalities** ♀Ⓜ
O65.9   **Obstructed labor due to maternal pelvic abnormality, unspecified** ♀Ⓜ

④ O66   **Other obstructed labor**
O66.0   **Obstructed labor due to shoulder dystocia** ♀Ⓜ
Impacted shoulders
> **DEFINITION**   Shoulders of the fetus become caught in the pelvis during delivery.

O66.1   **Obstructed labor due to locked twins** ♀Ⓜ
O66.2   **Obstructed labor due to unusually large fetus** ♀Ⓜ
➕ O66.3   **Obstructed labor due to other abnormalities of fetus** ♀Ⓜ
Dystocia due to fetal ascites
Dystocia due to fetal hydrops
Dystocia due to fetal meningomyelocele
Dystocia due to fetal sacral teratoma
Dystocia due to fetal tumor
Dystocia due to hydrocephalic fetus
Use additional code to identify cause of obstruction

⑤ O66.4   **Failed trial of labor**
O66.40   **Failed trial of labor, unspecified** ♀Ⓜ
O66.41   **Failed attempted vaginal birth after previous cesarean delivery** ♀Ⓜ
Code first:
rupture of uterus, if applicable (O71.0-, O71.1)

O66.5   **Attempted application of vacuum extractor and forceps** ♀Ⓜ
Attempted application of vacuum or forceps, with subsequent delivery by forceps or cesarean delivery

O66.6   **Obstructed labor due to other multiple fetuses** ♀Ⓜ
➕ O66.8   **Other specified obstructed labor** ♀Ⓜ
Use additional code to identify cause of obstruction

O66.9   **Obstructed labor, unspecified** ♀Ⓜ
Dystocia NOS
Fetal dystocia NOS
Maternal dystocia NOS

④ O67   **Labor and delivery complicated by intrapartum hemorrhage, not elsewhere classified**
> **EXCLUDES 1**   *antepartum hemorrhage NEC (O46.-)*
> *placenta previa (O44.-)*
> *premature separation of placenta [abruptio placentae] (O45.-)*
> **EXCLUDES 2**   *postpartum hemorrhage (O72.-)*

O67.0   **Intrapartum hemorrhage with coagulation defect** ♀Ⓜ
Intrapartum hemorrhage (excessive) associated with afibrinogenemia
Intrapartum hemorrhage (excessive) associated with disseminated intravascular coagulation
Intrapartum hemorrhage (excessive) associated with hyperfibrinolysis
Intrapartum hemorrhage (excessive) associated with hypofibrinogenemia

● New   ▲ Revised   *Manifestation*   ④-⑦ Digit Indicators   ▤ Laterality   ▲ Adult (15+ years)   Ⓜ Maternity (12-55 years)   Ⓝ Newborn   Ⓟ Pediatric (0-17 years)   ♂ Male   ♀ Female
✖ Deleted   Unspecified   ➕ Additional code

860   © 2017 DecisionHealth   2017 ICD-10-CM Expert for Physicians

O67.8   **Other intrapartum hemorrhage**   ♀Ⓜ
Excessive intrapartum hemorrhage
O67.9   **Intrapartum hemorrhage, unspecified**   ♀Ⓜ

O68   Labor and delivery complicated by abnormality of   ♀Ⓜ
fetal acid-base balance
Fetal acidemia complicating labor and delivery
Fetal acidosis complicating labor and delivery
Fetal alkalosis complicating labor and delivery
Fetal metabolic acidemia complicating labor and delivery
> **EXCLUDES 1**   *fetal stress NOS (O77.9)*
> *labor and delivery complicated by*
> *electrocardiographic evidence of fetal stress*
> *(O77.8)*
> *labor and delivery complicated by ultrasonic*
> *evidence of fetal stress (O77.8)*
> **EXCLUDES 2**   *abnormality in fetal heart rate or rhythm (O76)*
> *labor and delivery complicated by meconium in*
> *amniotic fluid (O77.0)*

④ **O69   Labor and delivery complicated by umbilical cord**
complications

> One of the following 7th characters is to be assigned to each code
> under category O69. 7th character 0 is for single gestations and
> multiple gestations where the fetus is unspecified. 7th characters 1
> through 9 are for cases of multiple gestations to identify the fetus
> for which the code applies. The appropriate code from category
> O30, Multiple gestation, must also be assigned when assigning a
> code from category O69 that has a 7th character of 1 through 9.
>
> 0   not applicable or unspecified
> 1   fetus 1
> 2   fetus 2
> 3   fetus 3
> 4   fetus 4
> 5   fetus 5
> 9   other fetus

⑦ O69.0XX-   **Labor and delivery complicated by prolapse of**   ♀Ⓜ
cord
⑦ O69.1XX-   **Labor and delivery complicated by cord around**   ♀Ⓜ
neck, with compression
> **EXCLUDES 1**   *labor and delivery complicated by*
> *cord around neck, without*
> *compression (O69.81)*
⑦ O69.2XX-   **Labor and delivery complicated by other cord**   ♀Ⓜ
entanglement, with compression
Labor and delivery complicated by compression of cord
NOS
Labor and delivery complicated by entanglement of
cords of twins in monoamniotic sac
Labor and delivery complicated by knot in cord
> **EXCLUDES 1**   *labor and delivery complicated by*
> *other cord entanglement, without*
> *compression (O69.82)*
⑦ O69.3XX-   **Labor and delivery complicated by short cord**   ♀Ⓜ
⑦ O69.4XX-   **Labor and delivery complicated by vasa previa**   ♀Ⓜ
Labor and delivery complicated by hemorrhage from
vasa previa
⑦ O69.5XX-   **Labor and delivery complicated by vascular**   ♀Ⓜ
lesion of cord
Labor and delivery complicated by cord bruising
Labor and delivery complicated by cord hematoma
Labor and delivery complicated by thrombosis of
umbilical vessels
⑤ O69.8   **Labor and delivery complicated by other cord**
complications
⑦ O69.81X-   **Labor and delivery complicated by cord**   ♀Ⓜ
around neck, without compression
⑦ O69.82X-   **Labor and delivery complicated by other cord**   ♀Ⓜ
entanglement, without compression
⑦ O69.89X-   **Labor and delivery complicated by other cord**   ♀Ⓜ
complications
⑦ O69.9XX-   **Labor and delivery complicated by cord**   ♀Ⓜ
complication, unspecified

④ **O70   Perineal laceration during delivery**
> **INCLUDES**   episiotomy extended by laceration
> **EXCLUDES 1**   *obstetric high vaginal laceration alone (O71.4)*

O70.0   **First degree perineal laceration during delivery**   ♀Ⓜ
Perineal laceration, rupture or tear involving fourchette
during delivery
Perineal laceration, rupture or tear involving labia during
delivery
Perineal laceration, rupture or tear involving skin during
delivery
Perineal laceration, rupture or tear involving vagina during
delivery
Perineal laceration, rupture or tear involving vulva during
delivery
Slight perineal laceration, rupture or tear during delivery
O70.1   **Second degree perineal laceration during delivery**   ♀Ⓜ
Perineal laceration, rupture or tear during delivery as in
O70.0, also involving pelvic floor
Perineal laceration, rupture or tear during delivery as in
O70.0, also involving perineal muscles
Perineal laceration, rupture or tear during delivery as in
O70.0, also involving vaginal muscles
> **EXCLUDES 1**   *perineal laceration involving anal sphincter*
> *(O70.2)*
> AHA: 2Q 2016, 34
▲ ⑤ O70.2   **Third degree perineal laceration during delivery**
Perineal laceration, rupture or tear during delivery as in
O70.1, also involving anal sphincter
Perineal laceration, rupture or tear during delivery as in
O70.1, also involving rectovaginal septum
Perineal laceration, rupture or tear during delivery as in
O70.1, also involving sphincter NOS
> **EXCLUDES 1**   *anal sphincter tear during delivery without*
> *third degree perineal laceration (O70.4)*
> *perineal laceration involving anal or rectal*
> *mucosa (O70.3)*
● O70.20   **Third degree perineal laceration during**   ♀Ⓜ
delivery, unspecified
● O70.21   **Third degree perineal laceration during**   ♀Ⓜ
delivery, IIIa
Third degree perineal laceration during delivery with
less than 50% of external anal sphincter (EAS)
thickness torn
● O70.22   **Third degree perineal laceration during**   ♀Ⓜ
delivery, IIIb
Third degree perineal laceration during delivery with
more than 50% external anal sphincter (EAS)
thickness torn
● O70.23   **Third degree perineal laceration during**   ♀Ⓜ
delivery, IIIc
Third degree perineal laceration during delivery with
both external anal sphincter (EAS) and internal anal
sphincter (IAS) torn
O70.3   **Fourth degree perineal laceration during delivery**   ♀Ⓜ
Perineal laceration, rupture or tear during delivery as in
O70.2, also involving anal mucosa
Perineal laceration, rupture or tear during delivery as in
O70.2, also involving rectal mucosa
O70.4   **Anal sphincter tear complicating delivery, not**   ♀Ⓜ
associated with third degree laceration
> **EXCLUDES 1**   *anal sphincter tear with third degree*
> *perineal laceration (O70.2)*
O70.9   **Perineal laceration during delivery, unspecified**   ♀Ⓜ
④ **O71   Other obstetric trauma**
> **INCLUDES**   obstetric damage from instruments
⑤ O71.0   **Rupture of uterus (spontaneous) before onset of labor**   ♀Ⓜ
> **EXCLUDES 1**   *disruption of (current) cesarean delivery*
> *wound (O90.0)*
> *laceration of uterus, NEC (O71.81)*
O71.00   **Rupture of uterus before onset of labor,**   ♀Ⓜ
unspecified trimester
O71.02   **Rupture of uterus before onset of labor, second**   ♀Ⓜ
trimester
O71.03   **Rupture of uterus before onset of labor, third**   ♀Ⓜ
trimester
O71.1   **Rupture of uterus during labor**   ♀Ⓜ
Rupture of uterus not stated as occurring before onset of labor
> **EXCLUDES 1**   *disruption of cesarean delivery wound*
> *(O90.0)*
> *laceration of uterus, NEC (O71.81)*
O71.2   **Postpartum inversion of uterus**   ♀Ⓜ
O71.3   **Obstetric laceration of cervix**   ♀Ⓜ
Annular detachment of cervix

● New   ▲ Revised   *Manifestation*   ④-⑦ Digit Indicators   ▤ Laterality   ▲ Adult   Ⓜ Maternity   Ⓝ Newborn   ▣ Pediatric   ♂ Male   ♀ Female
✖ ~~Deleted~~   Unspecified   + Additional code   (15+ years)   (12-55 years)   (0-17 years)

O71.4   Obstetric high vaginal laceration alone ♀▣
Laceration of vaginal wall without perineal laceration
EXCLUDES 1   *obstetric high vaginal laceration with perineal laceration (O70.-)*

O71.5   Other obstetric injury to pelvic organs ♀▣
Obstetric injury to bladder
Obstetric injury to urethra
EXCLUDES 2   *obstetric periurethral trauma (O71.82)*
AHA: 4Q 2014, 18

O71.6   Obstetric damage to pelvic joints and ligaments ♀▣
Obstetric avulsion of inner symphyseal cartilage
Obstetric damage to coccyx
Obstetric traumatic separation of symphysis (pubis)

O71.7   Obstetric hematoma of pelvis ♀▣
Obstetric hematoma of perineum
Obstetric hematoma of vagina
Obstetric hematoma of vulva

Ⓢ **O71.8   Other specified obstetric trauma** ♀▣
  O71.81   Laceration of uterus, not elsewhere classified ♀▣
  O71.82   Other specified trauma to perineum and vulva ♀▣
Obstetric periurethral trauma
AHA: 4Q 2014, 18
  O71.89   Other specified obstetric trauma ♀▣
O71.9   Obstetric trauma, unspecified ♀▣

Ⓐ **O72   Postpartum hemorrhage**
INCLUDES   hemorrhage after delivery of fetus or infant

O72.0   Third-stage hemorrhage ♀▣
Hemorrhage associated with retained, trapped or adherent placenta
Retained placenta NOS
Code also:
  type of adherent placenta (O43.2-)

O72.1   Other immediate postpartum hemorrhage ♀▣
Hemorrhage following delivery of placenta
Postpartum hemorrhage (atonic) NOS
Uterine atony with hemorrhage
EXCLUDES 1   *uterine atony NOS (O62.2)*
  uterine atony without hemorrhage (O62.2)
  postpartum atony of uterus without hemorrhage (O75.89)

O72.2   Delayed and secondary postpartum hemorrhage ♀▣
Hemorrhage associated with retained portions of placenta or membranes after the first 24 hours following delivery of placenta
Retained products of conception NOS, following delivery

O72.3   Postpartum coagulation defects ♀▣
Postpartum afibrinogenemia
Postpartum fibrinolysis

Ⓐ **O73   Retained placenta and membranes, without hemorrhage**
EXCLUDES 1   *placenta accreta (O43.21-)*
  placenta increta (O43.22-)
  placenta percreta (O43.23-)

O73.0   Retained placenta without hemorrhage ♀▣
Adherent placenta, without hemorrhage
Trapped placenta without hemorrhage

O73.1   Retained portions of placenta and membranes, without hemorrhage ♀▣
Retained products of conception following delivery, without hemorrhage

Ⓐ✛ **O74   Complications of anesthesia during labor and delivery**
INCLUDES   maternal complications arising from the administration of a general, regional or local anesthetic, analgesic or other sedation during labor and delivery
Use additional code, if applicable, to identify specific complication

✛ **O74.0   Aspiration pneumonitis due to anesthesia during labor and delivery** ♀▣
Inhalation of stomach contents or secretions NOS due to anesthesia during labor and delivery
Mendelson's syndrome due to anesthesia during labor and delivery

✛ **O74.1   Other pulmonary complications of anesthesia during labor and delivery** ♀▣

✛ **O74.2   Cardiac complications of anesthesia during labor and delivery** ♀▣

✛ **O74.3   Central nervous system complications of anesthesia during labor and delivery** ♀▣

✛ **O74.4   Toxic reaction to local anesthesia during labor and delivery** ♀▣

✛ **O74.5   Spinal and epidural anesthesia-induced headache during labor and delivery** ♀▣

✛ **O74.6   Other complications of spinal and epidural anesthesia during labor and delivery** ♀▣

✛ **O74.7   Failed or difficult intubation for anesthesia during labor and delivery** ♀▣

✛ **O74.8   Other complications of anesthesia during labor and delivery** ♀▣

✛ **O74.9   Complication of anesthesia during labor and delivery, unspecified** ♀▣

Ⓐ **O75   Other complications of labor and delivery, not elsewhere classified**
EXCLUDES 2   *puerperal (postpartum) infection (O86.-)*
  puerperal (postpartum) sepsis (O85)

O75.0   Maternal distress during labor and delivery ♀▣

O75.1   Shock during or following labor and delivery ♀▣
Obstetric shock following labor and delivery

O75.2   Pyrexia during labor, not elsewhere classified ♀▣

✛ **O75.3   Other infection during labor** ♀▣
Sepsis during labor
Use additional code (B95-B97), to identify infectious agent

✛ **O75.4   Other complications of obstetric surgery and procedures** ♀▣
Cardiac arrest following obstetric surgery or procedures
Cardiac failure following obstetric surgery or procedures
Cerebral anoxia following obstetric surgery or procedures
Pulmonary edema following obstetric surgery or procedures
Use additional code to identify specific complication
EXCLUDES 2   *complications of anesthesia during labor and delivery (O74.-)*
  disruption of obstetrical (surgical) wound (O90.0-O90.1)
  hematoma of obstetrical (surgical) wound (O90.2)
  infection of obstetrical (surgical) wound (O86.0)

O75.5   Delayed delivery after artificial rupture of membranes ♀▣

Ⓢ **O75.8   Other specified complications of labor and delivery** ♀▣
  O75.81   Maternal exhaustion complicating labor and delivery ♀▣
  O75.82   Onset (spontaneous) of labor after 37 completed weeks of gestation but before 39 completed weeks gestation, with delivery by (planned) cesarean section ♀▣
Delivery by (planned) cesarean section occurring after 37 completed weeks of gestation but before 39 completed weeks gestation due to (spontaneous) onset of labor
Code first to specify reason for planned cesarean section such as:
  cephalopelvic disproportion (normally formed fetus) (O33.9)
  previous cesarean delivery (O34.21)
  O75.89   Other specified complications of labor and delivery ♀▣

O75.9   Complication of labor and delivery, unspecified ♀▣

O76   Abnormality in fetal heart rate and rhythm complicating labor and delivery ♀▣
Depressed fetal heart rate tones complicating labor and delivery
Fetal bradycardia complicating labor and delivery
Fetal heart rate decelerations complicating labor and delivery
Fetal heart rate irregularity complicating labor and delivery
Fetal heart rate abnormal variability complicating labor and delivery
Fetal tachycardia complicating labor and delivery
Non-reassuring fetal heart rate or rhythm complicating labor and delivery
EXCLUDES 1   *fetal stress NOS (O77.9)*
  labor and delivery complicated by electrocardiographic evidence of fetal stress (O77.8)
  labor and delivery complicated by ultrasonic evidence of fetal stress (O77.8)
EXCLUDES 2   *fetal metabolic acidemia (O68)*
  other fetal stress (O77.0-O77.1)
AHA: 4Q 2013, 118

Ⓐ **O77   Other fetal stress complicating labor and delivery**

O77.0   **Labor and delivery complicated by meconium in amniotic fluid**   ♀ⓂI
AHA: 4Q 2013, 118

O77.1   **Fetal stress in labor or delivery due to drug administration**   ♀Ⓜ

O77.8   **Labor and delivery complicated by other evidence of fetal stress**   ♀Ⓜ
Labor and delivery complicated by electrocardiographic evidence of fetal stress
Labor and delivery complicated by ultrasonic evidence of fetal stress
> EXCLUDES 1   *abnormality of fetal acid-base balance (O68)*
> *abnormality in fetal heart rate or rhythm (O76)*
> *fetal metabolic acidemia (O68)*

O77.9   **Labor and delivery complicated by fetal stress, unspecified**   ♀Ⓜ
> EXCLUDES 1   *abnormality of fetal acid-base balance (O68)*
> *abnormality in fetal heart rate or rhythm (O76)*
> *fetal metabolic acidemia (O68)*

Encounter for delivery (O80-O82)

+ O80   **Encounter for full-term uncomplicated delivery**   ♀Ⓜ
Delivery requiring minimal or no assistance, with or without episiotomy, without fetal manipulation [e.g., rotation version] or instrumentation [forceps] of a spontaneous, cephalic, vaginal, full-term, single, live-born infant. This code is for use as a single diagnosis code and is not to be used with any other code from chapter 15.
Use additional code to indicate outcome of delivery (Z37.0)
AHA: 2Q 2014, 9

+ O82   **Encounter for cesarean delivery without indication**   ♀Ⓜ
Use additional code to indicate outcome of delivery (Z37.0)

Complications predominantly related to the puerperium (O85-O92)

> EXCLUDES 2   *mental and behavioral disorders associated with the puerperium (F53)*
> *obstetrical tetanus (A34)*
> *puerperal osteomalacia (M83.0)*

> GUIDELINES   Section I.C.15.a.2)
Chapter 15 codes are to be used only on the maternal record, never on the record of the newborn.

+ O85   **Puerperal sepsis**   ♀Ⓜ
Postpartum sepsis
Puerperal peritonitis
Puerperal pyemia
Use additional code (B95-B97), to identify infectious agent
Use additional code (R65.2-) to identify severe sepsis, if applicable
> EXCLUDES 1   *fever of unknown origin following delivery (O86.4)*
> *genital tract infection following delivery (O86.1-)*
> *obstetric pyemic and septic embolism (O88.3-)*
> *puerperal septic thrombophlebitis (O86.81)*
> *urinary tract infection following delivery (O86.2-)*
> EXCLUDES 2   *sepsis during labor (O75.3)*

> GUIDELINES   Section I.C.15.k
Code O85, Puerperal sepsis, should be assigned with a secondary code to identify the causal organism (e.g., for a bacterial infection, assign a code from category B95-B96, Bacterial infections in conditions classified elsewhere). A code from category A40, Streptococcal sepsis, or A41, Other sepsis, should not be used for puerperal sepsis. If applicable, use additional codes to identify severe sepsis (R65.2-) and any associated acute organ dysfunction.

◢ + O86   **Other puerperal infections**
Use additional code (B95-B97), to identify infectious agent
> EXCLUDES 2   *infection during labor (O75.3)*
> *obstetrical tetanus (A34)*

> GUIDELINES   Section I.C.1.d.5)(c)
In cases where a postprocedural infection has occurred and has resulted in severe sepsis, the code for the precipitating complication such as code T81.4, Infection following a procedure, or O86.0, Infection of obstetrical surgical wound, should be coded first followed by code R65.20, Severe sepsis without septic shock. A code for the systemic infection should also be assigned.

If the postprocedural infection has resulted in postprocedural septic shock, the code for the precipitating complication such as code T81.4 or O86.0 should be coded first followed by code T81.12-, Postprocedural septic shock. A code for the systemic infection should also be assigned.

+ O86.0   **Infection of obstetric surgical wound**   ♀Ⓜ
Infected cesarean delivery wound following delivery
Infected perineal repair following delivery

ⓢ + O86.1   **Other infection of genital tract following delivery**   ♀Ⓜ
   + O86.11   **Cervicitis following delivery**   ♀Ⓜ
   + O86.12   **Endometritis following delivery**   ♀Ⓜ
   + O86.13   **Vaginitis following delivery**   ♀Ⓜ
   + O86.19   **Other infection of genital tract following delivery**   ♀Ⓜ

ⓢ + O86.2   **Urinary tract infection following delivery**   ♀Ⓜ
   + O86.20   **Urinary tract infection following delivery, unspecified**   ♀Ⓜ
     Puerperal urinary tract infection NOS
   + O86.21   **Infection of kidney following delivery**   ♀Ⓜ
   + O86.22   **Infection of bladder following delivery**   ♀Ⓜ
     Infection of urethra following delivery
   + O86.29   **Other urinary tract infection following delivery**   ♀Ⓜ

+ O86.4   **Pyrexia of unknown origin following delivery**   ♀Ⓜ
Puerperal infection NOS following delivery
Puerperal pyrexia NOS following delivery
> EXCLUDES 2   *pyrexia during labor (O75.2)*

ⓢ + O86.8   **Other specified puerperal infections**   ♀Ⓜ
   + O86.81   **Puerperal septic thrombophlebitis**   ♀Ⓜ
   + O86.89   **Other specified puerperal infections**   ♀Ⓜ

◢ O87   **Venous complications and hemorrhoids in the puerperium**
> INCLUDES   venous complications in labor, delivery and the puerperium
> EXCLUDES 2   *obstetric embolism (O88.-)*
> *puerperal septic thrombophlebitis (O86.81)*
> *venous complications in pregnancy (O22.-)*

O87.0   **Superficial thrombophlebitis in the puerperium**   ♀Ⓜ
Puerperal phlebitis NOS
Puerperal thrombosis NOS

+ O87.1   **Deep phlebothrombosis in the puerperium**   ♀Ⓜ
Deep vein thrombosis, postpartum
Pelvic thrombophlebitis, postpartum
Use additional code to identify the deep vein thrombosis (I82.4-, I82.5-, I82.62-. I82.72-)
Use additional code, if applicable, for associated long-term (current) use of anticoagulants (Z79.01)

O87.2   **Hemorrhoids in the puerperium**   ♀Ⓜ

O87.3   **Cerebral venous thrombosis in the puerperium**   ♀Ⓜ
Cerebrovenous sinus thrombosis in the puerperium

O87.4   **Varicose veins of lower extremity in the puerperium**   ♀Ⓜ

O87.8   **Other venous complications in the puerperium**   ♀Ⓜ
Genital varices in the puerperium

O87.9   **Venous complication in the puerperium, unspecified**   ♀Ⓜ
Puerperal phlebopathy NOS

◢ O88   **Obstetric embolism**
> EXCLUDES 1   *embolism complicating abortion NOS (O03.2)*
> *embolism complicating ectopic or molar pregnancy (O08.2)*
> *embolism complicating failed attempted abortion (O07.2)*
> *embolism complicating induced abortion (O04.7)*
> *embolism complicating spontaneous abortion (O03.2, O03.7)*

ⓢ O88.0   **Obstetric air embolism**   ♀Ⓜ
   ⓖ O88.01   **Obstetric air embolism in pregnancy**
     O88.011   **Air embolism in pregnancy, first trimester**   ♀Ⓜ
     O88.012   **Air embolism in pregnancy, second trimester**   ♀Ⓜ

● New   ▲ Revised   *Manifestation*   ◢-◿ Digit Indicators   ▤ Laterality   ▣ Adult (15+ years)   Ⓜ Maternity (12-55 years)   Ⓝ Newborn   Ⓟ Pediatric (0-17 years)   ♂ Male   ♀ Female
✖ Deleted   Unspecified   + Additional code

2017 ICD-10-CM Expert for Physicians   © 2017 DecisionHealth   863

O88.013   Air embolism in pregnancy, third trimester ♀Ⓜ

O88.019   Air embolism in pregnancy, unspecified trimester ♀Ⓜ

O88.02   Air embolism in childbirth ♀Ⓜ

O88.03   Air embolism in the puerperium ♀Ⓜ

⑤ **O88.1**   Amniotic fluid embolism ♀Ⓜ
Anaphylactoid syndrome in pregnancy

⑥ **O88.11**   Amniotic fluid embolism in pregnancy

O88.111   Amniotic fluid embolism in pregnancy, first trimester ♀Ⓜ

O88.112   Amniotic fluid embolism in pregnancy, second trimester ♀Ⓜ

O88.113   Amniotic fluid embolism in pregnancy, third trimester ♀Ⓜ

O88.119   Amniotic fluid embolism in pregnancy, unspecified trimester ♀Ⓜ

O88.12   Amniotic fluid embolism in childbirth ♀Ⓜ

O88.13   Amniotic fluid embolism in the puerperium ♀Ⓜ

⑤ **O88.2**   Obstetric thromboembolism ♀Ⓜ

⑥ **O88.21**   Thromboembolism in pregnancy
Obstetric (pulmonary) embolism NOS

O88.211   Thromboembolism in pregnancy, first trimester ♀Ⓜ

O88.212   Thromboembolism in pregnancy, second trimester ♀Ⓜ

O88.213   Thromboembolism in pregnancy, third trimester ♀Ⓜ

O88.219   Thromboembolism in pregnancy, unspecified trimester ♀Ⓜ

O88.22   Thromboembolism in childbirth ♀Ⓜ

O88.23   Thromboembolism in the puerperium ♀Ⓜ
Puerperal (pulmonary) embolism NOS

⑤ **O88.3**   Obstetric pyemic and septic embolism ♀Ⓜ

⑥ **O88.31**   Pyemic and septic embolism in pregnancy

O88.311   Pyemic and septic embolism in pregnancy, first trimester ♀Ⓜ

O88.312   Pyemic and septic embolism in pregnancy, second trimester ♀Ⓜ

O88.313   Pyemic and septic embolism in pregnancy, third trimester ♀Ⓜ

O88.319   Pyemic and septic embolism in pregnancy, unspecified trimester ♀Ⓜ

O88.32   Pyemic and septic embolism in childbirth ♀Ⓜ

O88.33   Pyemic and septic embolism in the puerperium ♀Ⓜ

⑤ **O88.8**   Other obstetric embolism ♀Ⓜ
Obstetric fat embolism

⑥ **O88.81**   Other embolism in pregnancy

O88.811   Other embolism in pregnancy, first trimester ♀Ⓜ

O88.812   Other embolism in pregnancy, second trimester ♀Ⓜ

O88.813   Other embolism in pregnancy, third trimester ♀Ⓜ

O88.819   Other embolism in pregnancy, unspecified trimester ♀Ⓜ

O88.82   Other embolism in childbirth ♀Ⓜ

O88.83   Other embolism in the puerperium ♀Ⓜ

④ + **O89**   **Complications of anesthesia during the puerperium**

INCLUDES   maternal complications arising from the administration of a general, regional or local anesthetic, analgesic or other sedation during the puerperium

Use additional code, if applicable, to identify specific complication

⑤ + **O89.0**   Pulmonary complications of anesthesia during the puerperium ♀Ⓜ

+ **O89.01**   Aspiration pneumonitis due to anesthesia during the puerperium ♀Ⓜ
Inhalation of stomach contents or secretions NOS due to anesthesia during the puerperium
Mendelson's syndrome due to anesthesia during the puerperium

+ **O89.09**   Other pulmonary complications of anesthesia during the puerperium ♀Ⓜ

+ **O89.1**   Cardiac complications of anesthesia during the puerperium ♀Ⓜ

+ **O89.2**   Central nervous system complications of anesthesia during the puerperium ♀Ⓜ

+ **O89.3**   Toxic reaction to local anesthesia during the puerperium ♀Ⓜ

+ **O89.4**   Spinal and epidural anesthesia-induced headache during the puerperium ♀Ⓜ

+ **O89.5**   Other complications of spinal and epidural anesthesia during the puerperium ♀Ⓜ

+ **O89.6**   Failed or difficult intubation for anesthesia during the puerperium ♀Ⓜ

+ **O89.8**   Other complications of anesthesia during the puerperium ♀Ⓜ

+ **O89.9**   Complication of anesthesia during the puerperium, unspecified ♀Ⓜ

④ **O90**   **Complications of the puerperium, not elsewhere classified**

O90.0   Disruption of cesarean delivery wound ♀Ⓜ
Dehiscence of cesarean delivery wound
EXCLUDES 1   *rupture of uterus (spontaneous) before onset of labor (O71.0-)*
rupture of uterus during labor (O71.1)

O90.1   Disruption of perineal obstetric wound ♀Ⓜ
Disruption of wound of episiotomy
Disruption of wound of perineal laceration
Secondary perineal tear

Disruption of perineal obstetric wound

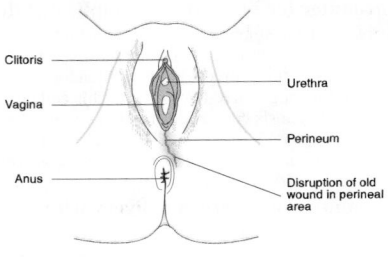

Clitoris   Urethra   Vagina   Perineum   Anus   Disruption of old wound in perineal area

O90.2   Hematoma of obstetric wound ♀Ⓜ

O90.3   Peripartum cardiomyopathy ♀Ⓜ
Conditions in I42.- arising during pregnancy and the puerperium
EXCLUDES 1   *pre-existing heart disease complicating pregnancy and the puerperium (O99.4-)*
GUIDELINES   Section I.C.15.o.5)
Pregnancy associated cardiomyopathy, code O90.3, is unique in that it may be diagnosed in the third trimester of pregnancy but may continue to progress months after delivery. For this reason, it is referred to as peripartum cardiomyopathy. Code O90.3 is only for use when the cardiomyopathy develops as a result of pregnancy in a woman who did not have pre-existing heart disease.

O90.4   Postpartum acute kidney failure ♀Ⓜ
Hepatorenal syndrome following labor and delivery

O90.5   Postpartum thyroiditis ♀Ⓜ

O90.6   Postpartum mood disturbance ♀Ⓜ
Postpartum blues
Postpartum dysphoria
Postpartum sadness
EXCLUDES 1   *postpartum depression (F53)*
puerperal psychosis (F53)

⑤ **O90.8**   Other complications of the puerperium, not elsewhere classified ♀Ⓜ

O90.81   Anemia of the puerperium ♀Ⓜ
Postpartum anemia NOS
EXCLUDES 1   *pre-existing anemia complicating the puerperium (O99.03)*
CODING TIP ✓   Use O90.81 for diagnosed anemia complicating the postpartum period. Use O99.01 for anemia complicating pregnancy. Use O99.03 for pre-existing anemia complicating the puerperium.

O90.89   Other complications of the puerperium, not elsewhere classified ♀Ⓜ
Placental polyp

O90.9   Complication of the puerperium, unspecified ♀Ⓜ

● New   ▲ Revised   *Manifestation*   ④-⑦ Digit Indicators   ⊟ Laterality   Ⓐ Adult (15+ years)   Ⓜ Maternity (12-55 years)   Ⓝ Newborn   Ⓟ Pediatric (0-17 years)   ♂ Male   ♀ Female

✖ Deleted   Unspecified   + Additional code

864   © 2017 DecisionHealth   2017 ICD-10-CM Expert for Physicians

⁴+ **O91**   **Infections of breast associated with pregnancy, the puerperium and lactation**
Use additional code to identify infection

⁵+ **O91.0**   **Infection of nipple associated with pregnancy, the puerperium and lactation**   ♀Ⓜ

⁶+ **O91.01**   **Infection of nipple associated with pregnancy**   ♀Ⓜ
Gestational abscess of nipple

+ **O91.011**   **Infection of nipple associated with pregnancy, first trimester**   ♀Ⓜ

+ **O91.012**   **Infection of nipple associated with pregnancy, second trimester**   ♀Ⓜ

+ **O91.013**   **Infection of nipple associated with pregnancy, third trimester**   ♀Ⓜ

+ **O91.019**   **Infection of nipple associated with pregnancy, unspecified trimester**   ♀Ⓜ

+ **O91.02**   **Infection of nipple associated with the puerperium**   ♀Ⓜ
Puerperal abscess of nipple

+ **O91.03**   **Infection of nipple associated with lactation**   ♀Ⓜ
Abscess of nipple associated with lactation

⁵+ **O91.1**   **Abscess of breast associated with pregnancy, the puerperium and lactation**   ♀Ⓜ

⁶+ **O91.11**   **Abscess of breast associated with pregnancy**   ♀Ⓜ
Gestational mammary abscess
Gestational purulent mastitis
Gestational subareolar abscess

+ **O91.111**   **Abscess of breast associated with pregnancy, first trimester**   ♀Ⓜ

+ **O91.112**   **Abscess of breast associated with pregnancy, second trimester**   ♀Ⓜ

+ **O91.113**   **Abscess of breast associated with pregnancy, third trimester**   ♀Ⓜ

+ **O91.119**   **Abscess of breast associated with pregnancy, unspecified trimester**   ♀Ⓜ

+ **O91.12**   **Abscess of breast associated with the puerperium**   ♀Ⓜ
Puerperal mammary abscess
Puerperal purulent mastitis
Puerperal subareolar abscess

+ **O91.13**   **Abscess of breast associated with lactation**   ♀Ⓜ
Mammary abscess associated with lactation
Purulent mastitis associated with lactation
Subareolar abscess associated with lactation

⁵+ **O91.2**   **Nonpurulent mastitis associated with pregnancy, the puerperium and lactation**   ♀Ⓜ

⁶+ **O91.21**   **Nonpurulent mastitis associated with pregnancy**   ♀Ⓜ
Gestational interstitial mastitis
Gestational lymphangitis of breast
Gestational mastitis NOS
Gestational parenchymatous mastitis

+ **O91.211**   **Nonpurulent mastitis associated with pregnancy, first trimester**   ♀Ⓜ

+ **O91.212**   **Nonpurulent mastitis associated with pregnancy, second trimester**   ♀Ⓜ

+ **O91.213**   **Nonpurulent mastitis associated with pregnancy, third trimester**   ♀Ⓜ

+ **O91.219**   **Nonpurulent mastitis associated with pregnancy, unspecified trimester**   ♀Ⓜ

+ **O91.22**   **Nonpurulent mastitis associated with the puerperium**   ♀Ⓜ
Puerperal interstitial mastitis
Puerperal lymphangitis of breast
Puerperal mastitis NOS
Puerperal parenchymatous mastitis

+ **O91.23**   **Nonpurulent mastitis associated with lactation**   ♀Ⓜ
Interstitial mastitis associated with lactation
Lymphangitis of breast associated with lactation
Mastitis NOS associated with lactation
Parenchymatous mastitis associated with lactation

⁴ **O92**   **Other disorders of breast and disorders of lactation associated with pregnancy and the puerperium**

⁵ **O92.0**   **Retracted nipple associated with pregnancy, the puerperium, and lactation**   ♀Ⓜ

⁶ **O92.01**   **Retracted nipple associated with pregnancy**

O92.011   **Retracted nipple associated with pregnancy, first trimester**   ♀Ⓜ

O92.012   **Retracted nipple associated with pregnancy, second trimester**   ♀Ⓜ

O92.013   **Retracted nipple associated with pregnancy, third trimester**   ♀Ⓜ

O92.019   **Retracted nipple associated with pregnancy, unspecified trimester**   ♀Ⓜ

O92.02   **Retracted nipple associated with the puerperium**   ♀Ⓜ

O92.03   **Retracted nipple associated with lactation**   ♀Ⓜ

⁵ **O92.1**   **Cracked nipple associated with pregnancy, the puerperium, and lactation**   ♀Ⓜ
Fissure of nipple, gestational or puerperal

⁶ **O92.11**   **Cracked nipple associated with pregnancy**

O92.111   **Cracked nipple associated with pregnancy, first trimester**   ♀Ⓜ

O92.112   **Cracked nipple associated with pregnancy, second trimester**   ♀Ⓜ

O92.113   **Cracked nipple associated with pregnancy, third trimester**   ♀Ⓜ

O92.119   **Cracked nipple associated with pregnancy, unspecified trimester**   ♀Ⓜ

O92.12   **Cracked nipple associated with the puerperium**   ♀Ⓜ

O92.13   **Cracked nipple associated with lactation**   ♀Ⓜ

⁵ **O92.2**   **Other and unspecified disorders of breast associated with pregnancy and the puerperium**   ♀Ⓜ

O92.20   **Unspecified disorder of breast associated with pregnancy and the puerperium**   ♀Ⓜ

O92.29   **Other disorders of breast associated with pregnancy and the puerperium**   ♀Ⓜ

O92.3   **Agalactia**   ♀Ⓜ
Primary agalactia
EXCLUDES 1	*Elective agalactia (O92.5)*
	Secondary agalactia (O92.5)
	Therapeutic agalactia (O92.5)

O92.4   **Hypogalactia**   ♀Ⓜ

O92.5   **Suppressed lactation**   ♀Ⓜ
Elective agalactia
Secondary agalactia
Therapeutic agalactia
| **EXCLUDES 1** | *primary agalactia (O92.3)* |

O92.6   **Galactorrhea**   ♀Ⓜ

⁵ **O92.7**   **Other and unspecified disorders of lactation**   ♀Ⓜ

O92.70   **Unspecified disorders of lactation**   ♀Ⓜ

O92.79   **Other disorders of lactation**   ♀Ⓜ
Puerperal galactocele

Other obstetric conditions, not elsewhere classified (O94-O9A)

O94   **Sequelae of complication of pregnancy, childbirth, and the puerperium**   ♀Ⓜ
Note: This category is to be used to indicate conditions in O00-O77.-, O85-O94 and O98-O9A.- as the cause of late effects. The sequelae include conditions specified as such, or as late effects, which may occur at any time after the puerperium
Code first:
   condition resulting from (sequela) of complication of pregnancy, childbirth, and the puerperium
| **GUIDELINES**   Section I.C.15.p.1)-3) |

Code O94 is for use in those cases when an initial complication of a pregnancy develops a sequelae requiring care or treatment at a future date. This code may be used at any time after the initial postpartum period. This code, like all sequela codes, is to be sequenced following the code describing the sequelae of the complication.

⁴+ **O98**   **Maternal infectious and parasitic diseases classifiable elsewhere but complicating pregnancy, childbirth and the puerperium**
| **INCLUDES**   the listed conditions when complicating the pregnant state, when aggravated by the pregnancy, or as a reason for obstetric care |

Use additional code (Chapter 1), to identify specific infectious or parasitic disease
EXCLUDES 2	*herpes gestationis (O26.4-)*
	infectious carrier state (O99.82-, O99.83-)
	obstetrical tetanus (A34)
	puerperal infection (O86.-)
	puerperal sepsis (O85)
	when the reason for maternal care is that the disease is known or suspected to have affected the fetus (O35-O36)

● New   ▲ Revised   *Manifestation*   ④-⑦ Digit Indicators   ⊟ Laterality   Ⓐ Adult (15+ years)   Ⓜ Maternity (12-55 years)   Ⓝ Newborn   Ⓟ Pediatric (0-17 years)   ♂ Male   ♀ Female
✖ Deleted   Unspecified   + Additional code

2017 ICD-10-CM Expert for Physicians   © 2017 DecisionHealth   865

Pregnancy, Childbirth and the Puerperium

O91 — O98

5 + O98.0 Tuberculosis complicating pregnancy, childbirth and ♀ M
the puerperium
Conditions in A15-A19
  6 + O98.01 Tuberculosis complicating pregnancy
    + O98.011 Tuberculosis complicating pregnancy, first ♀ M
trimester
    + O98.012 Tuberculosis complicating pregnancy, ♀ M
second trimester
    + O98.013 Tuberculosis complicating pregnancy, third ♀ M
trimester
    + O98.019 Tuberculosis complicating pregnancy, ♀ M
unspecified trimester
  + O98.02 Tuberculosis complicating childbirth ♀ M
  + O98.03 Tuberculosis complicating the puerperium ♀ M

5 + O98.1 Syphilis complicating pregnancy, childbirth and the ♀ M
puerperium
Conditions in A50-A53
  6 + O98.11 Syphilis complicating pregnancy
    + O98.111 Syphilis complicating pregnancy, first ♀ M
trimester
    + O98.112 Syphilis complicating pregnancy, second ♀ M
trimester
    + O98.113 Syphilis complicating pregnancy, third ♀ M
trimester
    + O98.119 Syphilis complicating pregnancy, ♀ M
unspecified trimester
  + O98.12 Syphilis complicating childbirth ♀ M
  + O98.13 Syphilis complicating the puerperium ♀ M

5 + O98.2 Gonorrhea complicating pregnancy, childbirth and ♀ M
the puerperium
Conditions in A54.-
  6 + O98.21 Gonorrhea complicating pregnancy
    + O98.211 Gonorrhea complicating pregnancy, first ♀ M
trimester
    + O98.212 Gonorrhea complicating pregnancy, second ♀ M
trimester
    + O98.213 Gonorrhea complicating pregnancy, third ♀ M
trimester
    + O98.219 Gonorrhea complicating pregnancy, ♀ M
unspecified trimester
  + O98.22 Gonorrhea complicating childbirth ♀ M
  + O98.23 Gonorrhea complicating the puerperium ♀ M

5 + O98.3 Other infections with a predominantly sexual mode of ♀ M
transmission complicating pregnancy, childbirth
and the puerperium
Conditions in A55-A64
  6 + O98.31 Other infections with a predominantly sexual mode
of transmission complicating pregnancy
    + O98.311 Other infections with a predominantly ♀ M
sexual mode of transmission complicating
pregnancy, first trimester
    + O98.312 Other infections with a predominantly ♀ M
sexual mode of transmission complicating
pregnancy, second trimester
    + O98.313 Other infections with a predominantly ♀ M
sexual mode of transmission complicating
pregnancy, third trimester
    + O98.319 Other infections with a predominantly ♀ M
sexual mode of transmission complicating
pregnancy, unspecified trimester
  + O98.32 Other infections with a predominantly sexual ♀ M
mode of transmission complicating childbirth
  + O98.33 Other infections with a predominantly sexual ♀ M
mode of transmission complicating the
puerperium

5 + O98.4 Viral hepatitis complicating pregnancy, childbirth ♀ M
and the puerperium
Conditions in B15-B19
  6 + O98.41 Viral hepatitis complicating pregnancy
    + O98.411 Viral hepatitis complicating pregnancy, first ♀ M
trimester
    + O98.412 Viral hepatitis complicating pregnancy, ♀ M
second trimester
    + O98.413 Viral hepatitis complicating pregnancy, ♀ M
third trimester
    + O98.419 Viral hepatitis complicating pregnancy, ♀ M
unspecified trimester
  + O98.42 Viral hepatitis complicating childbirth ♀ M
  + O98.43 Viral hepatitis complicating the puerperium ♀ M

5 + O98.5 Other viral diseases complicating pregnancy, ♀ M
childbirth and the puerperium
Conditions in A80-B09, B25-B34, R87.81-, R87.82-
  EXCLUDES 1 *human immunodeficiency virus [HIV]
disease complicating pregnancy,
childbirth and the puerperium (O98.7-)*
  6 + O98.51 Other viral diseases complicating pregnancy
    + O98.511 Other viral diseases complicating ♀ M
pregnancy, first trimester
    + O98.512 Other viral diseases complicating ♀ M
pregnancy, second trimester
    + O98.513 Other viral diseases complicating ♀ M
pregnancy, third trimester
    + O98.519 Other viral diseases complicating ♀ M
pregnancy, unspecified trimester
  + O98.52 Other viral diseases complicating childbirth ♀ M
  + O98.53 Other viral diseases complicating the ♀ M
puerperium

5 + O98.6 Protozoal diseases complicating pregnancy, childbirth ♀ M
and the puerperium
Conditions in B50-B64
  6 + O98.61 Protozoal diseases complicating pregnancy
    + O98.611 Protozoal diseases complicating pregnancy, ♀ M
first trimester
    + O98.612 Protozoal diseases complicating pregnancy, ♀ M
second trimester
    + O98.613 Protozoal diseases complicating pregnancy, ♀ M
third trimester
    + O98.619 Protozoal diseases complicating pregnancy, ♀ M
unspecified trimester
  + O98.62 Protozoal diseases complicating childbirth ♀ M
  + O98.63 Protozoal diseases complicating the puerperium ♀ M

5 + O98.7 Human immunodeficiency virus [HIV] disease ♀ M
complicating pregnancy, childbirth and the
puerperium
*Use additional code to identify the type of HIV disease:
Acquired immune deficiency syndrome (AIDS) (B20)
Asymptomatic HIV status (Z21)
HIV positive NOS (Z21)
Symptomatic HIV disease (B20)*
  GUIDELINES Section I.C.1.a.2)(g)
During pregnancy, childbirth or the puerperium, a
patient admitted (or presenting for a health care
encounter) because of an HIV-related illness should
receive a principal diagnosis code of O98.7-, followed
by B20 and the code(s) for the HIV-related illness(es).
Codes from Chapter 15 always take sequencing priority.

Patients with asymptomatic HIV infection status
admitted (or presenting for a health care encounter)
during pregnancy, childbirth, or the puerperium should
receive codes of O98.7- and Z21.
  6 + O98.71 Human immunodeficiency virus [HIV] disease
complicating pregnancy
    + O98.711 Human immunodeficiency virus [HIV] ♀ M
disease complicating pregnancy, first
trimester
    + O98.712 Human immunodeficiency virus [HIV] ♀ M
disease complicating pregnancy, second
trimester
    + O98.713 Human immunodeficiency virus [HIV] ♀ M
disease complicating pregnancy, third
trimester
    + O98.719 Human immunodeficiency virus [HIV] ♀ M
disease complicating pregnancy,
unspecified trimester
  + O98.72 Human immunodeficiency virus [HIV] disease ♀ M
complicating childbirth
  + O98.73 Human immunodeficiency virus [HIV] disease ♀ M
complicating the puerperium

5 + O98.8 Other maternal infectious and parasitic diseases ♀ M
complicating pregnancy, childbirth and the
puerperium
  6 + O98.81 Other maternal infectious and parasitic diseases
complicating pregnancy
    + O98.811 Other maternal infectious and parasitic ♀ M
diseases complicating pregnancy, first
trimester
    + O98.812 Other maternal infectious and parasitic ♀ M
diseases complicating pregnancy, second
trimester

● New   ▲ Revised   *Manifestation*   4-7 Digit Indicators   ⊟ Laterality   A Adult (15+ years)   M Maternity (12-55 years)   N Newborn   P Pediatric (0-17 years)   ♂ Male   ♀ Female
✖ Deleted   Unspecified   + Additional code

+ O98.813 Other maternal infectious and parasitic diseases complicating pregnancy, third trimester ♀Ⓜ

+ O98.819 Other maternal infectious and parasitic diseases complicating pregnancy, unspecified trimester ♀Ⓜ

+ O98.82 Other maternal infectious and parasitic diseases complicating childbirth ♀Ⓜ

+ O98.83 Other maternal infectious and parasitic diseases complicating the puerperium ♀Ⓜ

⑤+ O98.9 Unspecified maternal infectious and parasitic disease complicating pregnancy, childbirth and the puerperium ♀Ⓜ

⑥+ O98.91 Unspecified maternal infectious and parasitic disease complicating pregnancy

+ O98.911 Unspecified maternal infectious and parasitic disease complicating pregnancy, first trimester ♀Ⓜ

+ O98.912 Unspecified maternal infectious and parasitic disease complicating pregnancy, second trimester ♀Ⓜ

+ O98.913 Unspecified maternal infectious and parasitic disease complicating pregnancy, third trimester ♀Ⓜ

+ O98.919 Unspecified maternal infectious and parasitic disease complicating pregnancy, unspecified trimester ♀Ⓜ

+ O98.92 Unspecified maternal infectious and parasitic disease complicating childbirth ♀Ⓜ

+ O98.93 Unspecified maternal infectious and parasitic disease complicating the puerperium ♀Ⓜ

④+ O99 Other maternal diseases classifiable elsewhere but complicating pregnancy, childbirth and the puerperium

> INCLUDES conditions which complicate the pregnant state, are aggravated by the pregnancy or are a main reason for obstetric care

Use additional code to identify specific condition

> EXCLUDES 2 *when the reason for maternal care is that the condition is known or suspected to have affected the fetus (O35-O36)*

⑤+ O99.0 Anemia complicating pregnancy, childbirth and the puerperium
Conditions in D50-D64

> EXCLUDES 1 *anemia arising in the puerperium (O90.81)*
> *postpartum anemia NOS (O90.81)*

⑥+ O99.01 Anemia complicating pregnancy

> CODING TIP ✓ Use O90.81 for diagnosed anemia complicating the postpartum period. Use O99.01 for anemia complicating pregnancy. Use O99.03 for pre-existing anemia complicating the puerperium.

+ O99.011 Anemia complicating pregnancy, first trimester ♀Ⓜ

+ O99.012 Anemia complicating pregnancy, second trimester ♀Ⓜ

+ O99.013 Anemia complicating pregnancy, third trimester ♀Ⓜ

+ O99.019 Anemia complicating pregnancy, unspecified trimester ♀Ⓜ

+ O99.02 Anemia complicating childbirth ♀Ⓜ

+ O99.03 Anemia complicating the puerperium ♀Ⓜ

> EXCLUDES 1 *postpartum anemia not pre-existing prior to delivery (O90.81)*

> CODING TIP ✓ Use O90.81 for diagnosed anemia complicating the postpartum period. Use O99.01 for anemia complicating pregnancy. Use O99.03 for pre-existing anemia complicating the puerperium.

⑤+ O99.1 Other diseases of the blood and blood-forming organs and certain disorders involving the immune mechanism complicating pregnancy, childbirth and the puerperium ♀Ⓜ
Conditions in D65-D89

> EXCLUDES 2 *hemorrhage with coagulation defects (O45.-, O46.0-, O67.0, O72.3)*

⑥+ O99.11 Other diseases of the blood and blood-forming organs and certain disorders involving the immune mechanism complicating pregnancy

+ O99.111 Other diseases of the blood and blood-forming organs and certain disorders involving the immune mechanism complicating pregnancy, first trimester ♀Ⓜ

+ O99.112 Other diseases of the blood and blood-forming organs and certain disorders involving the immune mechanism complicating pregnancy, second trimester ♀Ⓜ

+ O99.113 Other diseases of the blood and blood-forming organs and certain disorders involving the immune mechanism complicating pregnancy, third trimester ♀Ⓜ

+ O99.119 Other diseases of the blood and blood-forming organs and certain disorders involving the immune mechanism complicating pregnancy, unspecified trimester ♀Ⓜ

+ O99.12 Other diseases of the blood and blood-forming organs and certain disorders involving the immune mechanism complicating childbirth ♀Ⓜ

+ O99.13 Other diseases of the blood and blood-forming organs and certain disorders involving the immune mechanism complicating the puerperium ♀Ⓜ

⑤+ O99.2 Endocrine, nutritional and metabolic diseases complicating pregnancy, childbirth and the puerperium ♀Ⓜ
Conditions in E00-E88

> EXCLUDES 2 *diabetes mellitus (O24.-)*
> *malnutrition (O25.-)*
> *postpartum thyroiditis (O90.5)*

⑥+ O99.21 Obesity complicating pregnancy, childbirth, and the puerperium

Use additional code to identify the type of obesity (E66.-)

+ O99.210 Obesity complicating pregnancy, unspecified trimester ♀Ⓜ

+ O99.211 Obesity complicating pregnancy, first trimester ♀Ⓜ

+ O99.212 Obesity complicating pregnancy, second trimester ♀Ⓜ

+ O99.213 Obesity complicating pregnancy, third trimester ♀Ⓜ

+ O99.214 Obesity complicating childbirth ♀Ⓜ

+ O99.215 Obesity complicating the puerperium ♀Ⓜ

⑥+ O99.28 Other endocrine, nutritional and metabolic diseases complicating pregnancy, childbirth and the puerperium

+ O99.280 Endocrine, nutritional and metabolic diseases complicating pregnancy, unspecified trimester ♀Ⓜ

+ O99.281 Endocrine, nutritional and metabolic diseases complicating pregnancy, first trimester ♀Ⓜ

+ O99.282 Endocrine, nutritional and metabolic diseases complicating pregnancy, second trimester ♀Ⓜ

+ O99.283 Endocrine, nutritional and metabolic diseases complicating pregnancy, third trimester ♀Ⓜ

+ O99.284 Endocrine, nutritional and metabolic diseases complicating childbirth ♀Ⓜ

+ O99.285 Endocrine, nutritional and metabolic diseases complicating the puerperium ♀Ⓜ

⑤+ O99.3 Mental disorders and diseases of the nervous system complicating pregnancy, childbirth and the puerperium ♀Ⓜ

⑥+ O99.31 Alcohol use complicating pregnancy, childbirth, and the puerperium

Use additional code(s) from F10 to identify manifestations of the alcohol use

+ O99.310 Alcohol use complicating pregnancy, unspecified trimester ♀Ⓜ

+ O99.311 Alcohol use complicating pregnancy, first trimester ♀Ⓜ

+ O99.312 Alcohol use complicating pregnancy, second trimester ♀Ⓜ

+ O99.313 Alcohol use complicating pregnancy, third trimester ♀Ⓜ

+ O99.314 Alcohol use complicating childbirth ♀Ⓜ

+ O99.315 Alcohol use complicating the puerperium ♀Ⓜ

● New ▲ Revised *Manifestation* ④-⑦ Digit Indicators ⊟ Laterality Ⓐ Adult (15+ years) Ⓜ Maternity (12-55 years) Ⓝ Newborn Ⓟ Pediatric (0-17 years) ♂ Male ♀ Female
✖ Deleted Unspecified + Additional code

2017 ICD-10-CM Expert for Physicians

© 2017 DecisionHealth

867

Pregnancy, Childbirth and the Puerperium

O98.813 — O99.315

⑥+ **O99.32**   **Drug use complicating pregnancy, childbirth, and the puerperium**
Use additional code(s) from F11-F16 and F18-F19 to identify manifestations of the drug use

+ **O99.320**   **Drug use complicating pregnancy, unspecified trimester**   ♀Ⓜ

+ **O99.321**   **Drug use complicating pregnancy, first trimester**   ♀Ⓜ

+ **O99.322**   **Drug use complicating pregnancy, second trimester**   ♀Ⓜ

+ **O99.323**   **Drug use complicating pregnancy, third trimester**   ♀Ⓜ

+ **O99.324**   **Drug use complicating childbirth**   ♀Ⓜ

+ **O99.325**   **Drug use complicating the puerperium**   ♀Ⓜ

▲⑥+ **O99.33**   **Tobacco use disorder complicating pregnancy, childbirth, and the puerperium**
Smoking complicating pregnancy, childbirth, and the puerperium
Use additional code from category F17 to identify type of tobacco nicotine dependence

+ **O99.330**   **Smoking (tobacco) complicating pregnancy, unspecified trimester**   ♀Ⓜ

+ **O99.331**   **Smoking (tobacco) complicating pregnancy, first trimester**   ♀Ⓜ

+ **O99.332**   **Smoking (tobacco) complicating pregnancy, second trimester**   ♀Ⓜ

+ **O99.333**   **Smoking (tobacco) complicating pregnancy, third trimester**   ♀Ⓜ

+ **O99.334**   **Smoking (tobacco) complicating childbirth**   ♀Ⓜ

+ **O99.335**   **Smoking (tobacco) complicating the puerperium**   ♀Ⓜ

⑥+ **O99.34**   **Other mental disorders complicating pregnancy, childbirth, and the puerperium**
Conditions in F01-F09 and F20-F99

EXCLUDES 2   *postpartum mood disturbance (O90.6)*
postnatal psychosis (F53)
puerperal psychosis (F53)

+ **O99.340**   **Other mental disorders complicating pregnancy, unspecified trimester**   ♀Ⓜ

+ **O99.341**   **Other mental disorders complicating pregnancy, first trimester**   ♀Ⓜ

+ **O99.342**   **Other mental disorders complicating pregnancy, second trimester**   ♀Ⓜ

+ **O99.343**   **Other mental disorders complicating pregnancy, third trimester**   ♀Ⓜ

+ **O99.344**   **Other mental disorders complicating childbirth**   ♀Ⓜ

+ **O99.345**   **Other mental disorders complicating the puerperium**   ♀Ⓜ

⑥+ **O99.35**   **Diseases of the nervous system complicating pregnancy, childbirth, and the puerperium**
Conditions in G00-G99

EXCLUDES 2   *pregnancy related peripheral neuritis (O26.8-)*

+ **O99.350**   **Diseases of the nervous system complicating pregnancy, unspecified trimester**   ♀Ⓜ

+ **O99.351**   **Diseases of the nervous system complicating pregnancy, first trimester**   ♀Ⓜ

+ **O99.352**   **Diseases of the nervous system complicating pregnancy, second trimester**   ♀Ⓜ

+ **O99.353**   **Diseases of the nervous system complicating pregnancy, third trimester**   ♀Ⓜ

+ **O99.354**   **Diseases of the nervous system complicating childbirth**   ♀Ⓜ

+ **O99.355**   **Diseases of the nervous system complicating the puerperium**   ♀Ⓜ

⑥+ **O99.4**   **Diseases of the circulatory system complicating pregnancy, childbirth and the puerperium**   ♀Ⓜ
Conditions in I00-I99

EXCLUDES 1   *peripartum cardiomyopathy (O90.3)*

EXCLUDES 2   *hypertensive disorders (O10-O16)*
obstetric embolism (O88.-)
venous complications and cerebrovenous sinus thrombosis in labor, childbirth and the puerperium (O87.-)
venous complications and cerebrovenous sinus thrombosis in pregnancy (O22.-)

⑥+ **O99.41**   **Diseases of the circulatory system complicating pregnancy**
AHA: 2Q 2016, 8

+ **O99.411**   **Diseases of the circulatory system complicating pregnancy, first trimester**   ♀Ⓜ

+ **O99.412**   **Diseases of the circulatory system complicating pregnancy, second trimester**   ♀Ⓜ

+ **O99.413**   **Diseases of the circulatory system complicating pregnancy, third trimester**   ♀Ⓜ

+ **O99.419**   **Diseases of the circulatory system complicating pregnancy, unspecified trimester**   ♀Ⓜ

+ **O99.42**   **Diseases of the circulatory system complicating childbirth**   ♀Ⓜ

+ **O99.43**   **Diseases of the circulatory system complicating the puerperium**   ♀Ⓜ

⑥+ **O99.5**   **Diseases of the respiratory system complicating pregnancy, childbirth and the puerperium**   ♀Ⓜ
Conditions in J00-J99

⑥+ **O99.51**   **Diseases of the respiratory system complicating pregnancy**

+ **O99.511**   **Diseases of the respiratory system complicating pregnancy, first trimester**   ♀Ⓜ

+ **O99.512**   **Diseases of the respiratory system complicating pregnancy, second trimester**   ♀Ⓜ

+ **O99.513**   **Diseases of the respiratory system complicating pregnancy, third trimester**   ♀Ⓜ

+ **O99.519**   **Diseases of the respiratory system complicating pregnancy, unspecified trimester**   ♀Ⓜ

+ **O99.52**   **Diseases of the respiratory system complicating childbirth**   ♀Ⓜ

+ **O99.53**   **Diseases of the respiratory system complicating the puerperium**   ♀Ⓜ

▲⑥+ **O99.6**   **Diseases of the digestive system complicating pregnancy, childbirth and the puerperium**   ♀Ⓜ
Conditions in K00-K93

EXCLUDES 2   *hemorrhoids in pregnancy (O22.4-)*
liver and biliary tract disorders in pregnancy, childbirth and the puerperium (O26.6-)

⑥+ **O99.61**   **Diseases of the digestive system complicating pregnancy**

+ **O99.611**   **Diseases of the digestive system complicating pregnancy, first trimester**   ♀Ⓜ

+ **O99.612**   **Diseases of the digestive system complicating pregnancy, second trimester**   ♀Ⓜ

+ **O99.613**   **Diseases of the digestive system complicating pregnancy, third trimester**   ♀Ⓜ

+ **O99.619**   **Diseases of the digestive system complicating pregnancy, unspecified trimester**   ♀Ⓜ

+ **O99.62**   **Diseases of the digestive system complicating childbirth**   ♀Ⓜ

+ **O99.63**   **Diseases of the digestive system complicating the puerperium**   ♀Ⓜ

⑥+ **O99.7**   **Diseases of the skin and subcutaneous tissue complicating pregnancy, childbirth and the puerperium**   ♀Ⓜ
Conditions in L00-L99

EXCLUDES 2   *herpes gestationis (O26.4)*
pruritic urticarial papules and plaques of pregnancy (PUPPP) (O26.86)

⑥+ **O99.71**   **Diseases of the skin and subcutaneous tissue complicating pregnancy**

+ **O99.711**   **Diseases of the skin and subcutaneous tissue complicating pregnancy, first trimester**   ♀Ⓜ

+ **O99.712**   **Diseases of the skin and subcutaneous tissue complicating pregnancy, second trimester**   ♀Ⓜ

+ **O99.713**   **Diseases of the skin and subcutaneous tissue complicating pregnancy, third trimester**   ♀Ⓜ

+ **O99.719**   **Diseases of the skin and subcutaneous tissue complicating pregnancy, unspecified trimester**   ♀Ⓜ

+ **O99.72**   **Diseases of the skin and subcutaneous tissue complicating childbirth**   ♀Ⓜ

+ **O99.73**   **Diseases of the skin and subcutaneous tissue complicating the puerperium**   ♀Ⓜ

● New   ▲ Revised   *Manifestation*   ❹-❼ Digit Indicators   ⊟ Laterality   Ⓐ Adult (15+ years)   Ⓜ Maternity (12-55 years)   Ⓝ Newborn   Ⓟ Pediatric (0-17 years)   ♂ Male   ♀ Female
✖ ~~Deleted~~   Unspecified   + Additional code

⑤＋ O99.8 Other specified diseases and conditions complicating ♀Ⓜ
pregnancy, childbirth and the puerperium
Conditions in D00-D48, H00-H95, M00-N99, and Q00-Q99
Use additional code to identify condition
> **EXCLUDES 2** *genitourinary infections in pregnancy*
> *(O23.-)*
> *infection of genitourinary tract following*
> *delivery (O86.1-O86.3)*
> *malignant neoplasm complicating*
> *pregnancy, childbirth and the puerperium*
> *(O9A.1-)*
> *maternal care for known or suspected*
> *abnormality of maternal pelvic organs*
> *(O34.-)*
> *postpartum acute kidney failure (O90.4)*
> *traumatic injuries in pregnancy (O9A.2-)*

⑥＋ O99.81 Abnormal glucose complicating pregnancy,
childbirth and the puerperium
> **EXCLUDES 1** *gestational diabetes (O24.4-)*

＋ O99.810 Abnormal glucose complicating pregnancy ♀Ⓜ
＋ O99.814 Abnormal glucose complicating childbirth ♀Ⓜ
＋ O99.815 Abnormal glucose complicating the ♀Ⓜ
puerperium

▲⑥＋ O99.82 Streptococcus B carrier state complicating
pregnancy, childbirth and the puerperium
> **EXCLUDES 1** *Carrier of streptococcus group B*
> *(GBS) in a nonpregnant woman*
> *(Z22.330)*

＋ O99.820 Streptococcus B carrier state complicating ♀Ⓜ
pregnancy
＋ O99.824 Streptococcus B carrier state complicating ♀Ⓜ
childbirth
＋ O99.825 Streptococcus B carrier state complicating ♀Ⓜ
the puerperium

⑥＋ O99.83 Other infection carrier state complicating
pregnancy, childbirth and the puerperium
> *Use additional code to identify the carrier state (Z22.-)*

＋ O99.830 Other infection carrier state complicating ♀Ⓜ
pregnancy
＋ O99.834 Other infection carrier state complicating ♀Ⓜ
childbirth
＋ O99.835 Other infection carrier state complicating ♀Ⓜ
the puerperium

⑥＋ O99.84 Bariatric surgery status complicating pregnancy,
childbirth and the puerperium
Gastric banding status complicating pregnancy,
childbirth and the puerperium
Gastric bypass status for obesity complicating
pregnancy, childbirth and the puerperium
Obesity surgery status complicating pregnancy,
childbirth and the puerperium

＋ O99.840 Bariatric surgery status complicating ♀Ⓜ
pregnancy, unspecified trimester
＋ O99.841 Bariatric surgery status complicating ♀Ⓜ
pregnancy, first trimester
＋ O99.842 Bariatric surgery status complicating ♀Ⓜ
pregnancy, second trimester
＋ O99.843 Bariatric surgery status complicating ♀Ⓜ
pregnancy, third trimester
＋ O99.844 Bariatric surgery status complicating ♀Ⓜ
childbirth
＋ O99.845 Bariatric surgery status complicating the ♀Ⓜ
puerperium

＋ O99.89 Other specified diseases and conditions ♀Ⓜ
complicating pregnancy, childbirth and the
puerperium

④ O9A Maternal malignant neoplasms, traumatic injuries and
abuse classifiable elsewhere but complicating
pregnancy, childbirth and the puerperium

⑤＋ O9A.1 Malignant neoplasm complicating pregnancy, ♀Ⓜ
childbirth and the puerperium
Conditions in C00-C96
Use additional code to identify neoplasm
> **EXCLUDES 2** *maternal care for benign tumor of corpus*
> *uteri (O34.1-)*
> *maternal care for benign tumor of cervix*
> *(O34.4-)*

⑥＋ O9A.11 Malignant neoplasm complicating pregnancy
＋ O9A.111 Malignant neoplasm complicating ♀Ⓜ
pregnancy, first trimester

＋ O9A.112 Malignant neoplasm complicating ♀Ⓜ
pregnancy, second trimester
＋ O9A.113 Malignant neoplasm complicating ♀Ⓜ
pregnancy, third trimester
＋ O9A.119 Malignant neoplasm complicating ♀Ⓜ
pregnancy, unspecified trimester
＋ O9A.12 Malignant neoplasm complicating childbirth ♀Ⓜ
＋ O9A.13 Malignant neoplasm complicating the ♀Ⓜ
puerperium
AHA: 3Q 2015, 19-20

⑤＋ O9A.2 Injury, poisoning and certain other consequences of ♀Ⓜ
external causes complicating pregnancy, childbirth
and the puerperium
Conditions in S00-T88, except T74 and T76
Use additional code(s) to identify the injury or poisoning
> **EXCLUDES 2** *physical, sexual and psychological abuse*
> *complicating pregnancy, childbirth and*
> *the puerperium (O9A.3-, O9A.4-, O9A.5-)*

⑥＋ O9A.21 Injury, poisoning and certain other consequences of
external causes complicating pregnancy
＋ O9A.211 Injury, poisoning and certain other ♀Ⓜ
consequences of external causes
complicating pregnancy, first trimester
＋ O9A.212 Injury, poisoning and certain other ♀Ⓜ
consequences of external causes
complicating pregnancy, second trimester
＋ O9A.213 Injury, poisoning and certain other ♀Ⓜ
consequences of external causes
complicating pregnancy, third trimester
＋ O9A.219 Injury, poisoning and certain other ♀Ⓜ
consequences of external causes
complicating pregnancy, unspecified
trimester
＋ O9A.22 Injury, poisoning and certain other ♀Ⓜ
consequences of external causes complicating
childbirth
＋ O9A.23 Injury, poisoning and certain other ♀Ⓜ
consequences of external causes complicating
the puerperium

⑤＋ O9A.3 Physical abuse complicating pregnancy, childbirth ♀Ⓜ
and the puerperium
Conditions in T74.11 or T76.11
Use additional code (if applicable):
> *to identify any associated current injury due to physical*
> *abuse*
> *to identify the perpetrator of abuse (Y07.-)*
> **EXCLUDES 2** *sexual abuse complicating pregnancy,*
> *childbirth and the puerperium (O9A.4)*

> **GUIDELINES** Section I.C.15.r
> For suspected or confirmed cases of abuse of a
> pregnant patient, a code(s) from subcategories O9A.3,
> O9A.4, and O9A.5, should be sequenced first, followed
> by the appropriate codes (if applicable) to identify any
> associated current injury due to physical abuse, sexual
> abuse, and the perpetrator of abuse.

⑥＋ O9A.31 Physical abuse complicating pregnancy
＋ O9A.311 Physical abuse complicating pregnancy, first ♀Ⓜ
trimester
＋ O9A.312 Physical abuse complicating pregnancy, ♀Ⓜ
second trimester
＋ O9A.313 Physical abuse complicating pregnancy, ♀Ⓜ
third trimester
＋ O9A.319 Physical abuse complicating pregnancy, ♀Ⓜ
unspecified trimester
＋ O9A.32 Physical abuse complicating childbirth ♀Ⓜ
＋ O9A.33 Physical abuse complicating the puerperium ♀Ⓜ

⑤＋ O9A.4 Sexual abuse complicating pregnancy, childbirth and ♀Ⓜ
the puerperium
Conditions in T74.21 or T76.21
Use additional code (if applicable):
> *to identify any associated current injury due to sexual*
> *abuse*
> *to identify the perpetrator of abuse (Y07.-)*

⑥＋ O9A.41 Sexual abuse complicating pregnancy
＋ O9A.411 Sexual abuse complicating pregnancy, first ♀Ⓜ
trimester
＋ O9A.412 Sexual abuse complicating pregnancy, ♀Ⓜ
second trimester
＋ O9A.413 Sexual abuse complicating pregnancy, third ♀Ⓜ
trimester

● New ▲ Revised *Manifestation* ④-⑦ Digit Indicators ⊟ Laterality Ⓐ Adult (15+ years) Ⓜ Maternity (12-55 years) Ⓝ Newborn Ⓟ Pediatric (0-17 years) ♂ Male ♀ Female
✖ Deleted Unspecified ＋ Additional code

2017 ICD-10-CM Expert for Physicians

© 2017 DecisionHealth

869

+ **O9A.419**   Sexual abuse complicating pregnancy, unspecified trimester   ♀ⓜ

+ **O9A.42**   Sexual abuse complicating childbirth   ♀ⓜ

+ **O9A.43**   Sexual abuse complicating the puerperium   ♀ⓜ

🖬 + **O9A.5**   Psychological abuse complicating pregnancy, childbirth and the puerperium   ♀ⓜ
    Conditions in T74.31 or T76.31
    Use additional code to identify the perpetrator of abuse (Y07.-)

⑥ + **O9A.51**   Psychological abuse complicating pregnancy

+ **O9A.511**   Psychological abuse complicating pregnancy, first trimester   ♀ⓜ

+ **O9A.512**   Psychological abuse complicating pregnancy, second trimester   ♀ⓜ

+ **O9A.513**   Psychological abuse complicating pregnancy, third trimester   ♀ⓜ

+ **O9A.519**   Psychological abuse complicating pregnancy, unspecified trimester   ♀ⓜ

+ **O9A.52**   Psychological abuse complicating childbirth   ♀ⓜ

+ **O9A.53**   Psychological abuse complicating the puerperium   ♀ⓜ

● New   ▲ Revised   *Manifestation*   ❹-❼ Digit Indicators   ⊟ Laterality   🅰 Adult (15+ years)   ⓜ Maternity (12-55 years)   ⓝ Newborn   🅿 Pediatric (0-17 years)   ♂ Male   ♀ Female

✖ Deleted   Unspecified   + Additional code

870   © 2017 DecisionHealth   2017 ICD-10-CM Expert for Physicians

CHAPTER 16: CERTAIN CONDITIONS ORIGINATING IN THE PERINATAL PERIOD (P00-P96)

Note: Codes from this chapter are for use on newborn records only, never on maternal records

INCLUDES   conditions that have their origin in the fetal or perinatal period (before birth through the first 28 days after birth) even if morbidity occurs later

EXCLUDES 2   *congenital malformations, deformations and chromosomal abnormalities (Q00-Q99)*
endocrine, nutritional and metabolic diseases (E00-E88)
injury, poisoning and certain other consequences of external causes (S00-T88)
neoplasms (C00-D49)
tetanus neonatorum (A33)

This chapter contains the following blocks:

P00-P04	Newborn affected by maternal factors and by complications of pregnancy, labor, and delivery
P05-P08	Disorders of newborn related to length of gestation and fetal growth
P09	Abnormal findings on neonatal screening
P10-P15	Birth trauma
P19-P29	Respiratory and cardiovascular disorders specific to the perinatal period
P35-P39	Infections specific to the perinatal period
P50-P61	Hemorrhagic and hematological disorders of newborn
P70-P74	Transitory endocrine and metabolic disorders specific to newborn
P76-P78	Digestive system disorders of newborn
P80-P83	Conditions involving the integument and temperature regulation of newborn
P84	Other problems with newborn
P90-P96	Other disorders originating in the perinatal period

Newborn affected by maternal factors and by complications of pregnancy, labor, and delivery (P00-P04)

Note: These codes are for use when the listed maternal conditions are specified as the cause of confirmed morbidity or potential morbidity which have their origin in the perinatal period (before birth through the first 28 days after birth).

▲ 🔲 **P00**   **Newborn affected by maternal conditions that may be unrelated to present pregnancy**
Code first:
any current condition in newborn
EXCLUDES 2   *encounter for observation of newborn for suspected diseases and conditions ruled out (Z05.-)*
newborn affected by maternal complications of pregnancy (P01.-)
newborn affected by maternal endocrine and metabolic disorders (P70-P74)
newborn affected by noxious substances transmitted via placenta or breast milk (P04.-)

▲ **P00.0**   **Newborn affected by maternal hypertensive disorders** 🔳
Newborn affected by maternal conditions classifiable to O10-O11, O13-O16

▲ **P00.1**   **Newborn affected by maternal renal and urinary tract diseases** 🔳
Newborn affected by maternal conditions classifiable to N00-N39

▲ **P00.2**   **Newborn affected by maternal infectious and parasitic diseases** 🔳
Newborn affected by maternal infectious disease classifiable to A00-B99, J09 and J10
EXCLUDES 1   *infections specific to the perinatal period (P35-P39)*
maternal genital tract or other localized infections (P00.8)
AHA: 3Q 2015, 20-21

▲ **P00.3**   **Newborn affected by other maternal circulatory and respiratory diseases** 🔳
Newborn affected by maternal conditions classifiable to I00-I99, J00-J99, Q20-Q34 and not included in P00.0, P00.2

▲ **P00.4**   **Newborn affected by maternal nutritional disorders** 🔳
Newborn affected by maternal disorders classifiable to E40-E64
Maternal malnutrition NOS

▲ **P00.5**   **Newborn affected by maternal injury** 🔳
Newborn affected by maternal conditions classifiable to O9A.2-

▲ **P00.6**   **Newborn affected by surgical procedure on mother** 🔳
Newborn affected by amniocentesis
EXCLUDES 1   *Cesarean delivery for present delivery (P03.4)*
damage to placenta from amniocentesis, Cesarean delivery or surgical induction (P02.1)
previous surgery to uterus or pelvic organs (P03.89)
EXCLUDES 2   *newborn affected by complication of (fetal) intrauterine procedure (P96.5)*

▲ **P00.7**   **Newborn affected by other medical procedures on mother, not elsewhere classified** 🔳
Newborn affected by radiation to mother
EXCLUDES 1   *damage to placenta from amniocentesis, cesarean delivery or surgical induction (P02.1)*
newborn affected by other complications of labor and delivery (P03.-)

▲ 🔢 **P00.8**   **Newborn affected by other maternal conditions**

     ▲ **P00.81**   **Newborn affected by periodontal disease in mother** 🔳

     ▲ **P00.89**   **Newborn affected by other maternal conditions** 🔳
Newborn affected by conditions classifiable to T80-T88
Newborn affected by maternal genital tract or other localized infections
Newborn affected by maternal systemic lupus erythematosus

▲ **P00.9**   **Newborn affected by unspecified maternal condition** 🔳

▲ 🔲 **P01**   **Newborn affected by maternal complications of pregnancy**
Code first:
any current condition in newborn
EXCLUDES 2   *encounter for observation of newborn for suspected diseases and conditions ruled out (Z05.-)*

▲ **P01.0**   **Newborn affected by incompetent cervix** 🔳

▲ **P01.1**   **Newborn affected by premature rupture of membranes** 🔳

▲ **P01.2**   **Newborn affected by oligohydramnios** 🔳
EXCLUDES 1   *oligohydramnios due to premature rupture of membranes (P01.1)*
DEFINITION   Inadequate amount of amniotic fluid in the womb affecting the fetus.

▲ **P01.3**   **Newborn affected by polyhydramnios** 🔳
Newborn affected by hydramnios
DEFINITION   Excessive amount of amniotic fluid in the womb affecting the fetus.

▲ **P01.4**   **Newborn affected by ectopic pregnancy** 🔳
Newborn affected by abdominal pregnancy

▲ **P01.5**   **Newborn affected by multiple pregnancy** 🔳
Newborn affected by triplet (pregnancy)
Newborn affected by twin (pregnancy)

▲ **P01.6**   **Newborn affected by maternal death** 🔳

▲ **P01.7**   **Newborn affected by malpresentation before labor** 🔳
Newborn affected by breech presentation before labor
Newborn affected by external version before labor
Newborn affected by face presentation before labor
Newborn affected by transverse lie before labor
Newborn affected by unstable lie before labor

▲ **P01.8**   **Newborn affected by other maternal complications of pregnancy** 🔳

▲ **P01.9**   **Newborn affected by maternal complication of pregnancy, unspecified** 🔳

▲ 🔲 **P02**   **Newborn affected by complications of placenta, cord and membranes**
Code first:
any current condition in newborn
EXCLUDES 2   *encounter for observation of newborn for suspected diseases and conditions ruled out (Z05.-)*

▲ **P02.0**   **Newborn affected by placenta previa** 🔳

● New   ▲ Revised   *Manifestation*   🔲 **4**-**7** Digit Indicators   🖪 Laterality   🅐 Adult (15+ years)   🅜 Maternity (12-55 years)   🔳 Newborn   🅟 Pediatric (0-17 years)   ♂ Male   ♀ Female
✖ Deleted   Unspecified   + Additional code

▲ **P02.1** **Newborn affected by other forms of placental separation and hemorrhage** N
Newborn affected by abruptio placenta
Newborn affected by accidental hemorrhage
Newborn affected by antepartum hemorrhage
Newborn affected by damage to placenta from amniocentesis, cesarean delivery or surgical induction
Newborn affected by maternal blood loss
Newborn affected by premature separation of placenta

▲ 5 **P02.2** **Newborn affected by other and unspecified morphological and functional abnormalities of placenta**

▲ **P02.20** **Newborn affected by unspecified morphological and functional abnormalities of placenta** N

▲ **P02.29** **Newborn affected by other morphological and functional abnormalities of placenta** N
Newborn affected by placental dysfunction
Newborn affected by placental infarction
Newborn affected by placental insufficiency

▲ **P02.3** **Newborn affected by placental transfusion syndromes** N
Newborn affected by placental and cord abnormalities resulting in twin-to-twin or other transplacental transfusion

▲ **P02.4** **Newborn affected by prolapsed cord** N

Prolapsed umbilical cord

Fetus

Uterus

Prolapsed umbilical cord

Cervix

▲ **P02.5** **Newborn affected by other compression of umbilical cord** N
Newborn affected by umbilical cord (tightly) around neck
Newborn affected by entanglement of umbilical cord
Newborn affected by knot in umbilical cord

▲ 5 **P02.6** **Newborn affected by other and unspecified conditions of umbilical cord**

▲ **P02.60** **Newborn affected by unspecified conditions of umbilical cord** N

▲ **P02.69** **Newborn affected by other conditions of umbilical cord** N
Newborn affected by short umbilical cord
Newborn affected by vasa previa
EXCLUDES 1 *newborn affected by single umbilical artery (Q27.0)*

▲ **P02.7** **Newborn affected by chorioamnionitis** N
Newborn affected by amnionitis
Newborn affected by membranitis
Newborn affected by placentitis

▲ **P02.8** **Newborn affected by other abnormalities of membranes** N

▲ **P02.9** **Newborn affected by abnormality of membranes, unspecified** N

▲ 4 **P03** **Newborn affected by other complications of labor and delivery**
Code first:
any current condition in newborn
EXCLUDES 2 *encounter for observation of newborn for suspected diseases and conditions ruled out (Z05.-)*

▲ **P03.0** **Newborn affected by breech delivery and extraction** N

▲ **P03.1** **Newborn affected by other malpresentation, malposition and disproportion during labor and delivery** N
Newborn affected by contracted pelvis
Newborn affected by conditions classifiable to O64-O66
Newborn affected by persistent occipitoposterior
Newborn affected by transverse lie

▲ **P03.2** **Newborn affected by forceps delivery** N

▲ **P03.3** **Newborn affected by delivery by vacuum extractor [ventouse]** N

▲ **P03.4** **Newborn affected by Cesarean delivery** N

▲ **P03.5** **Newborn affected by precipitate delivery** N
Newborn affected by rapid second stage
DEFINITION Fetus affected by labor occurring quickly, with rapid expulsion.

▲ **P03.6** **Newborn affected by abnormal uterine contractions** N
Newborn affected by conditions classifiable to O62.-, except O62.3
Newborn affected by hypertonic labor
Newborn affected by uterine inertia

▲ 5 **P03.8** **Newborn affected by other specified complications of labor and delivery**

▲ 6 **P03.81** **Newborn affected by abnormality in fetal (intrauterine) heart rate or rhythm**
EXCLUDES 1 *neonatal cardiac dysrhythmia (P29.1-)*

▲ **P03.810** **Newborn affected by abnormality in fetal (intrauterine) heart rate or rhythm before the onset of labor** N

▲ **P03.811** **Newborn affected by abnormality in fetal (intrauterine) heart rate or rhythm during labor** N

▲ **P03.819** **Newborn affected by abnormality in fetal (intrauterine) heart rate or rhythm, unspecified as to time of onset** N

P03.82 **Meconium passage during delivery** N
EXCLUDES 1 *meconium aspiration (P24.00, P24.01)*
meconium staining (P96.83)

▲ **P03.89** **Newborn affected by other specified complications of labor and delivery** N
Newborn affected by abnormality of maternal soft tissues
Newborn affected by conditions classifiable to O60-O75 and by procedures used in labor and delivery not included in P02.- and P03.0-P03.6
Newborn affected by induction of labor

▲ **P03.9** **Newborn affected by complication of labor and delivery, unspecified** N

▲ 4 **P04** **Newborn affected by noxious substances transmitted via placenta or breast milk**
INCLUDES nonteratogenic effects of substances transmitted via placenta
EXCLUDES 2 *congenital malformations (Q00-Q99)*
encounter for observation of newborn for suspected diseases and conditions ruled out (Z05.-)
neonatal jaundice from excessive hemolysis due to drugs or toxins transmitted from mother (P58.4)
newborn in contact with and (suspected) exposures hazardous to health not transmitted via placenta or breast milk (Z77.-)

▲ **P04.0** **Newborn affected by maternal anesthesia and analgesia in pregnancy, labor and delivery** N
Newborn affected by reactions and intoxications from maternal opiates and tranquilizers administered during labor and delivery

▲ **P04.1** **Newborn affected by other maternal medication** N
Newborn affected by cancer chemotherapy
Newborn affected by cytotoxic drugs
EXCLUDES 1 *dysmorphism due to warfarin (Q86.2)*
fetal hydantoin syndrome (Q86.1)
maternal use of drugs of addiction (P04.4-)

▲ **P04.2** **Newborn affected by maternal use of tobacco** N
Newborn affected by exposure in utero to tobacco smoke
EXCLUDES 2 *newborn exposure to environmental tobacco smoke (P96.81)*

▲ **P04.3** **Newborn affected by maternal use of alcohol** N
EXCLUDES 1 *fetal alcohol syndrome (Q86.0)*

● New   ▲ Revised   *Manifestation*   4-7 Digit Indicators   ▤ Laterality   A Adult (15+ years)   M Maternity (12-55 years)   N Newborn   P Pediatric (0-17 years)   ♂ Male   ♀ Female
✖ Deleted   Unspecified   + Additional code

872   © 2017 DecisionHealth   2017 ICD-10-CM Expert for Physicians

▲ ⑤ **P04.4** **Newborn affected by maternal use of drugs of addiction** N

  ▲ **P04.41** **Newborn affected by maternal use of cocaine** N
    'Crack baby'

  ▲ **P04.49** **Newborn affected by maternal use of other drugs of addiction** N

    EXCLUDES 2 *newborn affected by maternal anesthesia and analgesia (P04.0) withdrawal symptoms from maternal use of drugs of addiction (P96.1)*

▲ **P04.5** **Newborn affected by maternal use of nutritional chemical substances** N

▲ **P04.6** **Newborn affected by maternal exposure to environmental chemical substances** N

▲ **P04.8** **Newborn affected by other maternal noxious substances** N

▲ **P04.9** **Newborn affected by maternal noxious substance, unspecified** N

Disorders of newborn related to length of gestation and fetal growth (P05-P08)

④ **P05** **Disorders of newborn related to slow fetal growth and fetal malnutrition**

▲ ⑤ **P05.0** **Newborn light for gestational age**
Newborn light-for-dates
Weight below but length above 10th percentile for gestational age

  P05.00 **Newborn light for gestational age, unspecified weight** N

  P05.01 **Newborn light for gestational age, less than 500 grams** N

  P05.02 **Newborn light for gestational age, 500-749 grams** N

  P05.03 **Newborn light for gestational age, 750-999 grams** N

  P05.04 **Newborn light for gestational age, 1000-1249 grams** N

  P05.05 **Newborn light for gestational age, 1250-1499 grams** N

  P05.06 **Newborn light for gestational age, 1500-1749 grams** N

  P05.07 **Newborn light for gestational age, 1750-1999 grams** N

  P05.08 **Newborn light for gestational age, 2000-2499 grams** N

  ● **P05.09** **Newborn light for gestational age, 2500 grams and over** N
    Newborn light for gestational age, other

▲ ⑤ **P05.1** **Newborn small for gestational age**
Newborn small-and-light-for-dates
Newborn small-for-dates
Weight and length below 10th percentile for gestational age

  P05.10 **Newborn small for gestational age, unspecified weight** N

  P05.11 **Newborn small for gestational age, less than 500 grams** N

  P05.12 **Newborn small for gestational age, 500-749 grams** N

  P05.13 **Newborn small for gestational age, 750-999 grams** N

  P05.14 **Newborn small for gestational age, 1000-1249 grams** N

  P05.15 **Newborn small for gestational age, 1250-1499 grams** N

  P05.16 **Newborn small for gestational age, 1500-1749 grams** N

  P05.17 **Newborn small for gestational age, 1750-1999 grams** N

  P05.18 **Newborn small for gestational age, 2000-2499 grams** N

  ● **P05.19** **Newborn small for gestational age, other** N
    Newborn small for gestational age, 2500 grams and over

P05.2 **Newborn affected by fetal (intrauterine) malnutrition not light or small for gestational age** N
Infant, not light or small for gestational age, showing signs of fetal malnutrition, such as dry, peeling skin and loss of subcutaneous tissue

  EXCLUDES 1 *newborn affected by fetal malnutrition with light for gestational age (P05.0-) newborn affected by fetal malnutrition with small for gestational age (P05.1-)*

P05.9 **Newborn affected by slow intrauterine growth, unspecified** N
Newborn affected by fetal growth retardation NOS

▲ ④ **P07** **Disorders of newborn related to short gestation and low birth weight, not elsewhere classified**
Note: When both birth weight and gestational age of the newborn are available, both should be coded with birth weight sequenced before gestational age

  INCLUDES the listed conditions, without further specification, as the cause of morbidity or additional care, in newborn

▲ ⑤ **P07.0** **Extremely low birth weight newborn**
Newborn birth weight 999 g. or less

  EXCLUDES 1 *low birth weight due to slow fetal growth and fetal malnutrition (P05.-)*

  P07.00 **Extremely low birth weight newborn, unspecified weight** N

  P07.01 **Extremely low birth weight newborn, less than 500 grams** N

  P07.02 **Extremely low birth weight newborn, 500-749 grams** N

  P07.03 **Extremely low birth weight newborn, 750-999 grams** N

▲ ⑤ **P07.1** **Other low birth weight newborn**
Newborn birth weight 1000-2499 g.

  EXCLUDES 1 *low birth weight due to slow fetal growth and fetal malnutrition (P05.-)*

  P07.10 **Other low birth weight newborn, unspecified weight** N

  P07.14 **Other low birth weight newborn, 1000-1249 grams** N

  P07.15 **Other low birth weight newborn, 1250-1499 grams** N

  P07.16 **Other low birth weight newborn, 1500-1749 grams** N

  P07.17 **Other low birth weight newborn, 1750-1999 grams** N

  P07.18 **Other low birth weight newborn, 2000-2499 grams** N

⑤ **P07.2** **Extreme immaturity of newborn**
Less than 28 completed weeks (less than 196 completed days) of gestation.

  P07.20 **Extreme immaturity of newborn, unspecified weeks of gestation** N
    Gestational age less than 28 completed weeks NOS

  P07.21 **Extreme immaturity of newborn, gestational age less than 23 completed weeks** N
    Extreme immaturity of newborn, gestational age less than 23 weeks, 0 days

  P07.22 **Extreme immaturity of newborn, gestational age 23 completed weeks** N
    Extreme immaturity of newborn, gestational age 23 weeks, 0 days through 23 weeks, 6 days

  P07.23 **Extreme immaturity of newborn, gestational age 24 completed weeks** N
    Extreme immaturity of newborn, gestational age 24 weeks, 0 days through 24 weeks, 6 days

  P07.24 **Extreme immaturity of newborn, gestational age 25 completed weeks** N
    Extreme immaturity of newborn, gestational age 25 weeks, 0 days through 25 weeks, 6 days

  P07.25 **Extreme immaturity of newborn, gestational age 26 completed weeks** N
    Extreme immaturity of newborn, gestational age 26 weeks, 0 days through 26 weeks, 6 days

  P07.26 **Extreme immaturity of newborn, gestational age 27 completed weeks** N
    Extreme immaturity of newborn, gestational age 27 weeks, 0 days through 27 weeks, 6 days

⑤ **P07.3** **Preterm [premature] newborn [other]**
28 completed weeks or more but less than 37 completed weeks (196 completed days but less than 259 completed days) of gestation.
Prematurity NOS

  P07.30 **Preterm newborn, unspecified weeks of gestation** N

  P07.31 **Preterm newborn, gestational age 28 completed weeks** N
    Preterm newborn, gestational age 28 weeks, 0 days through 28 weeks, 6 days

● New ▲ Revised *Manifestation* ④-⑦ Digit Indicators ⊟ Laterality 🅐 Adult (15+ years) Ⓜ Maternity (12-55 years) N Newborn 🅟 Pediatric (0-17 years) ♂ Male ♀ Female
✖ Deleted Unspecified + Additional code

2017 ICD-10-CM Expert for Physicians

© 2017 DecisionHealth   873

P07.32 Preterm newborn, gestational age 29 completed weeks ◨
Preterm newborn, gestational age 29 weeks, 0 days through 29 weeks, 6 days

P07.33 Preterm newborn, gestational age 30 completed weeks ◨
Preterm newborn, gestational age 30 weeks, 0 days through 30 weeks, 6 days

P07.34 Preterm newborn, gestational age 31 completed weeks ◨
Preterm newborn, gestational age 31 weeks, 0 days through 31 weeks, 6 days

P07.35 Preterm newborn, gestational age 32 completed weeks ◨
Preterm newborn, gestational age 32 weeks, 0 days through 32 weeks, 6 days

P07.36 Preterm newborn, gestational age 33 completed weeks ◨
Preterm newborn, gestational age 33 weeks, 0 days through 33 weeks, 6 days

P07.37 Preterm newborn, gestational age 34 completed weeks ◨
Preterm newborn, gestational age 34 weeks, 0 days through 34 weeks, 6 days

P07.38 Preterm newborn, gestational age 35 completed weeks ◨
Preterm newborn, gestational age 35 weeks, 0 days through 35 weeks, 6 days

P07.39 Preterm newborn, gestational age 36 completed weeks ◨
Preterm newborn, gestational age 36 weeks, 0 days through 36 weeks, 6 days

◩ **P08** **Disorders of newborn related to long gestation and high birth weight**
Note: When both birth weight and gestational age of the newborn are available, priority of assignment should be given to birth weight
INCLUDES the listed conditions, without further specification, as causes of morbidity or additional care, in newborn

P08.0 **Exceptionally large newborn baby** ◨
Usually implies a birth weight of 4500 g. or more
EXCLUDES 1 *syndrome of infant of diabetic mother (P70.1)*
syndrome of infant of mother with gestational diabetes (P70.0)

P08.1 **Other heavy for gestational age newborn** ◨
Other newborn heavy- or large-for-dates regardless of period of gestation
Usually implies a birth weight of 4000 g. to 4499 g.
EXCLUDES 1 *newborn with a birth weight of 4500 or more (P08.0)*
syndrome of infant of diabetic mother (P70.1)
syndrome of infant of mother with gestational diabetes (P70.0) .

◫ **P08.2** **Late newborn, not heavy for gestational age**

P08.21 **Post-term newborn** ◨
Newborn with gestation period over 40 completed weeks to 42 completed weeks
AHA: 1Q 2014, 14

P08.22 **Prolonged gestation of newborn** ◨
Newborn with gestation period over 42 completed weeks (294 days or more), not heavy- or large-for-dates.
Postmaturity NOS
AHA: 1Q 2014, 14

Abnormal findings on neonatal screening (P09)

+ **P09** **Abnormal findings on neonatal screening** ◨
Use additional code to identify signs, symptoms and conditions associated with the screening
EXCLUDES 2 *nonspecific serologic evidence of human immunodeficiency virus [HIV] (R75)*

Birth trauma (P10-P15)

◩ **P10** **Intracranial laceration and hemorrhage due to birth injury**
EXCLUDES 1 *intracranial hemorrhage of newborn NOS (P52.9)*
intracranial hemorrhage of newborn due to anoxia or hypoxia (P52.-)
nontraumatic intracranial hemorrhage of newborn (P52.-)

P10.0 **Subdural hemorrhage due to birth injury** ◨
Subdural hematoma (localized) due to birth injury
EXCLUDES 1 *subdural hemorrhage accompanying tentorial tear (P10.4)*

P10.1 **Cerebral hemorrhage due to birth injury** ◨

P10.2 **Intraventricular hemorrhage due to birth injury** ◨

P10.3 **Subarachnoid hemorrhage due to birth injury** ◨

P10.4 **Tentorial tear due to birth injury** ◨

P10.8 **Other intracranial lacerations and hemorrhages due to birth injury** ◨

P10.9 **Unspecified intracranial laceration and hemorrhage due to birth injury** ◨

◩ **P11** **Other birth injuries to central nervous system**

P11.0 **Cerebral edema due to birth injury** ◨

P11.1 **Other specified brain damage due to birth injury** ◨

P11.2 **Unspecified brain damage due to birth injury** ◨

P11.3 **Birth injury to facial nerve** ◨
Facial palsy due to birth injury
DEFINITION Facial muscle weakness or paralysis resulting from damage or trauma to one of the paired facial nerves.

P11.4 **Birth injury to other cranial nerves** ◨

P11.5 **Birth injury to spine and spinal cord** ◨
Fracture of spine due to birth injury

P11.9 **Birth injury to central nervous system, unspecified** ◨

◩ **P12** **Birth injury to scalp**

P12.0 **Cephalhematoma due to birth injury** ◨

P12.1 **Chignon (from vacuum extraction) due to birth injury** ◨

P12.2 **Epicranial subaponeurotic hemorrhage due to birth injury** ◨
Subgaleal hemorrhage

P12.3 **Bruising of scalp due to birth injury** ◨

P12.4 **Injury of scalp of newborn due to monitoring equipment** ◨
Sampling incision of scalp of newborn
Scalp clip (electrode) injury of newborn

◫ **P12.8** **Other birth injuries to scalp**

P12.81 **Caput succedaneum** ◨

P12.89 **Other birth injuries to scalp** ◨

P12.9 **Birth injury to scalp, unspecified** ◨

◩ **P13** **Birth injury to skeleton**
EXCLUDES 2 *birth injury to spine (P11.5)*

P13.0 **Fracture of skull due to birth injury** ◨

P13.1 **Other birth injuries to skull** ◨
EXCLUDES 1 *cephalhematoma (P12.0)*

P13.2 **Birth injury to femur** ◨

P13.3 **Birth injury to other long bones** ◨

P13.4 **Fracture of clavicle due to birth injury** ◨

P13.8 **Birth injuries to other parts of skeleton** ◨

P13.9 **Birth injury to skeleton, unspecified** ◨

◩ **P14** **Birth injury to peripheral nervous system**

P14.0 **Erb's paralysis due to birth injury** ◨

P14.1 **Klumpke's paralysis due to birth injury** ◨

P14.2 **Phrenic nerve paralysis due to birth injury** ◨

P14.3 **Other brachial plexus birth injuries** ◨

P14.8 **Birth injuries to other parts of peripheral nervous system** ◨

P14.9 **Birth injury to peripheral nervous system, unspecified** ◨

◩ **P15** **Other birth injuries**

P15.0 **Birth injury to liver** ◨
Rupture of liver due to birth injury

P15.1 **Birth injury to spleen** ◨
Rupture of spleen due to birth injury

● New   ▲ Revised   *Manifestation*   ◪-◨ Digit Indicators   ⊟ Laterality   ⬟ Adult (15+ years)   ◩ Maternity (12-55 years)   ◲ Newborn   ⊡ Pediatric (0-17 years)   ♂ Male   ♀ Female
✖ Deleted   Unspecified   + Additional code

874   © 2017 DecisionHealth   2017 ICD-10-CM Expert for Physicians

P15.2 **Sternomastoid injury due to birth injury**

P15.3 **Birth injury to eye**
Subconjunctival hemorrhage due to birth injury
Traumatic glaucoma due to birth injury

P15.4 **Birth injury to face**
Facial congestion due to birth injury

P15.5 **Birth injury to external genitalia**

P15.6 **Subcutaneous fat necrosis due to birth injury**

P15.8 **Other specified birth injuries**

P15.9 **Birth injury, unspecified**

Respiratory and cardiovascular disorders specific to the perinatal period (P19-P29)

⬛ **P19** **Metabolic acidemia in newborn**
INCLUDES   metabolic acidemia in newborn

P19.0 **Metabolic acidemia in newborn first noted before onset of labor**

P19.1 **Metabolic acidemia in newborn first noted during labor**

P19.2 **Metabolic acidemia noted at birth**

P19.9 **Metabolic acidemia, unspecified**

⬛ **P22** **Respiratory distress of newborn**
EXCLUDES 1   *respiratory arrest of newborn (P28.81)*
respiratory failure of newborn NOS (P28.5)

P22.0 **Respiratory distress syndrome of newborn**
Cardiorespiratory distress syndrome of newborn
Hyaline membrane disease
Idiopathic respiratory distress syndrome [IRDS or RDS] of newborn
Pulmonary hypoperfusion syndrome
Respiratory distress syndrome, type I

P22.1 **Transient tachypnea of newborn**
Idiopathic tachypnea of newborn
Respiratory distress syndrome, type II
Wet lung syndrome
DEFINITION   Rapid breathing of a newborn.

P22.8 **Other respiratory distress of newborn**

P22.9 **Respiratory distress of newborn, unspecified**

⬛ **P23** **Congenital pneumonia**
INCLUDES   infective pneumonia acquired in utero or during birth
EXCLUDES 1   *neonatal pneumonia resulting from aspiration (P24.-)*

➕ P23.0 **Congenital pneumonia due to viral agent**
Use additional code (B97) to identify organism
EXCLUDES 1   *congenital rubella pneumonitis (P35.0)*

P23.1 **Congenital pneumonia due to Chlamydia**

P23.2 **Congenital pneumonia due to staphylococcus**

P23.3 **Congenital pneumonia due to streptococcus, group B**

P23.4 **Congenital pneumonia due to Escherichia coli**

P23.5 **Congenital pneumonia due to Pseudomonas**

➕ P23.6 **Congenital pneumonia due to other bacterial agents**
Congenital pneumonia due to Hemophilus influenzae
Congenital pneumonia due to Klebsiella pneumoniae
Congenital pneumonia due to Mycoplasma
Congenital pneumonia due to Streptococcus, except group B
Use additional code (B95-B96) to identify organism

P23.8 **Congenital pneumonia due to other organisms**

P23.9 **Congenital pneumonia, unspecified**

⬛ **P24** **Neonatal aspiration**
INCLUDES   aspiration in utero and during delivery

⬛ P24.0 **Meconium aspiration**
EXCLUDES 1   *meconium passage (without aspiration) during delivery (P03.82)*
meconium staining (P96.83)

P24.00 **Meconium aspiration without respiratory symptoms**
Meconium aspiration NOS

➕ P24.01 **Meconium aspiration with respiratory symptoms**
Meconium aspiration pneumonia
Meconium aspiration pneumonitis
Meconium aspiration syndrome NOS
Use additional code to identify any secondary pulmonary hypertension, if applicable (I27.2)

⬛ P24.1 **Neonatal aspiration of (clear) amniotic fluid and mucus**
Neonatal aspiration of liquor (amnii)

P24.10 **Neonatal aspiration of (clear) amniotic fluid and mucus without respiratory symptoms**
Neonatal aspiration of amniotic fluid and mucus NOS

➕ P24.11 **Neonatal aspiration of (clear) amniotic fluid and mucus with respiratory symptoms**
Neonatal aspiration of amniotic fluid and mucus with pneumonia
Neonatal aspiration of amniotic fluid and mucus with pneumonitis
Use additional code to identify any secondary pulmonary hypertension, if applicable (I27.2)

⬛ P24.2 **Neonatal aspiration of blood**

P24.20 **Neonatal aspiration of blood without respiratory symptoms**
Neonatal aspiration of blood NOS

➕ P24.21 **Neonatal aspiration of blood with respiratory symptoms**
Neonatal aspiration of blood with pneumonia
Neonatal aspiration of blood with pneumonitis
Use additional code to identify any secondary pulmonary hypertension, if applicable (I27.2)

⬛ P24.3 **Neonatal aspiration of milk and regurgitated food**
Neonatal aspiration of stomach contents

P24.30 **Neonatal aspiration of milk and regurgitated food without respiratory symptoms**
Neonatal aspiration of milk and regurgitated food NOS

➕ P24.31 **Neonatal aspiration of milk and regurgitated food with respiratory symptoms**
Neonatal aspiration of milk and regurgitated food with pneumonia
Neonatal aspiration of milk and regurgitated food with pneumonitis
Use additional code to identify any secondary pulmonary hypertension, if applicable (I27.2)

⬛ P24.8 **Other neonatal aspiration**

P24.80 **Other neonatal aspiration without respiratory symptoms**
Neonatal aspiration NEC

➕ P24.81 **Other neonatal aspiration with respiratory symptoms**
Neonatal aspiration pneumonia NEC
Neonatal aspiration with pneumonitis NEC
Neonatal aspiration with pneumonia NOS
Neonatal aspiration with pneumonitis NOS
Use additional code to identify any secondary pulmonary hypertension, if applicable (I27.2)

P24.9 **Neonatal aspiration, unspecified**

⬛ **P25** **Interstitial emphysema and related conditions originating in the perinatal period**

P25.0 **Interstitial emphysema originating in the perinatal period**

P25.1 **Pneumothorax originating in the perinatal period**

P25.2 **Pneumomediastinum originating in the perinatal period**

P25.3 **Pneumopericardium originating in the perinatal period**

P25.8 **Other conditions related to interstitial emphysema originating in the perinatal period**

⬛ **P26** **Pulmonary hemorrhage originating in the perinatal period**
EXCLUDES 1   *acute idiopathic hemorrhage in infants over 28 days old (R04.81)*

P26.0 **Tracheobronchial hemorrhage originating in the perinatal period**

P26.1 **Massive pulmonary hemorrhage originating in the perinatal period**

P26.8 **Other pulmonary hemorrhages originating in the perinatal period**

P26.9 **Unspecified pulmonary hemorrhage originating in the perinatal period**

⬛ **P27** **Chronic respiratory disease originating in the perinatal period**
EXCLUDES 1   *respiratory distress of newborn (P22.0-P22.9)*

P27.0 **Wilson-Mikity syndrome**
Pulmonary dysmaturity

P27.1 **Bronchopulmonary dysplasia originating in the perinatal period**

● New   ▲ Revised   *Manifestation*   ⬛-⬛ Digit Indicators   ⊟ Laterality   🅐 Adult (15+ years)   Ⓜ Maternity (12-55 years)   🅝 Newborn   🅟 Pediatric (0-17 years)   ♂ Male   ♀ Female
✖ ~~Deleted~~   Unspecified   + Additional code

Certain Conditions Originating in the Perinatal Period

P27.8 **Other chronic respiratory diseases originating in the perinatal period**
Congenital pulmonary fibrosis
Ventilator lung in newborn

P27.9 **Unspecified chronic respiratory disease originating in the perinatal period**

4️⃣ **P28** **Other respiratory conditions originating in the perinatal period**

> EXCLUDES 1   *congenital malformations of the respiratory system (Q30-Q34)*

P28.0 **Primary atelectasis of newborn** Ⓝ
Primary failure to expand terminal respiratory units
Pulmonary hypoplasia associated with short gestation
Pulmonary immaturity NOS

5️⃣ **P28.1** **Other and unspecified atelectasis of newborn**

P28.10 **Unspecified atelectasis of newborn** Ⓝ
Atelectasis of newborn NOS

P28.11 **Resorption atelectasis without respiratory distress syndrome** Ⓝ

> EXCLUDES 1   *resorption atelectasis with respiratory distress syndrome (P22.0)*

P28.19 **Other atelectasis of newborn** Ⓝ
Partial atelectasis of newborn
Secondary atelectasis of newborn

P28.2 **Cyanotic attacks of newborn** Ⓝ

> EXCLUDES 1   *apnea of newborn (P28.3-P28.4)*

> DEFINITION   A newborn with normal skin tone suddenly turns blue due to a lack of oxygen for a certain period of time before returning to normal color.

P28.3 **Primary sleep apnea of newborn** Ⓝ
Central sleep apnea of newborn
Obstructive sleep apnea of newborn
Sleep apnea of newborn NOS

P28.4 **Other apnea of newborn** Ⓝ
Apnea of prematurity
Obstructive apnea of newborn

> EXCLUDES 1   *obstructive sleep apnea of newborn (P28.3)*

P28.5 **Respiratory failure of newborn** Ⓝ

> EXCLUDES 1   *respiratory arrest of newborn (P28.81)*
> *respiratory distress of newborn (P22.0-)*

5️⃣ **P28.8** **Other specified respiratory conditions of newborn**

P28.81 **Respiratory arrest of newborn** Ⓝ

P28.89 **Other specified respiratory conditions of newborn** Ⓝ
Congenital laryngeal stridor
Sniffles in newborn
Snuffles in newborn

> EXCLUDES 1   *early congenital syphilitic rhinitis (A50.05)*

P28.9 **Respiratory condition of newborn, unspecified** Ⓝ
Respiratory depression in newborn

4️⃣ **P29** **Cardiovascular disorders originating in the perinatal period**

> EXCLUDES 1   *congenital malformations of the circulatory system (Q20-Q28)*

P29.0 **Neonatal cardiac failure** Ⓝ

5️⃣ **P29.1** **Neonatal cardiac dysrhythmia**

P29.11 **Neonatal tachycardia** Ⓝ

P29.12 **Neonatal bradycardia** Ⓝ

> DEFINITION   Abnormally slow newborn heartbeat.

P29.2 **Neonatal hypertension** Ⓝ

P29.3 **Persistent fetal circulation** Ⓝ
Delayed closure of ductus arteriosus
(Persistent) pulmonary hypertension of newborn

P29.4 **Transient myocardial ischemia in newborn** Ⓝ

5️⃣ **P29.8** **Other cardiovascular disorders originating in the perinatal period**

P29.81 **Cardiac arrest of newborn** Ⓝ

P29.89 **Other cardiovascular disorders originating in the perinatal period** Ⓝ
AHA: 4Q 2014, 23

P29.9 **Cardiovascular disorder originating in the perinatal period, unspecified** Ⓝ

Infections specific to the perinatal period (P35-P39)

Infections acquired in utero, during birth via the umbilicus, or during the first 28 days after birth

> EXCLUDES 2   *asymptomatic human immunodeficiency virus [HIV] infection status (Z21)*
> *congenital gonococcal infection (A54.-)*
> *congenital pneumonia (P23.-)*
> *congenital syphilis (A50.-)*
> *human immunodeficiency virus [HIV] disease (B20)*
> *infant botulism (A48.51)*
> *infectious diseases not specific to the perinatal period (A00-B99, J09, J10.-)*
> *intestinal infectious disease (A00-A09)*
> *laboratory evidence of human immunodeficiency virus [HIV] (R75)*
> *tetanus neonatorum (A33)*

4️⃣ **P35** **Congenital viral diseases**

> INCLUDES   infections acquired in utero or during birth

P35.0 **Congenital rubella syndrome** Ⓝ
Congenital rubella pneumonitis

P35.1 **Congenital cytomegalovirus infection** Ⓝ

P35.2 **Congenital herpesviral [herpes simplex] infection** Ⓝ

P35.3 **Congenital viral hepatitis** Ⓝ

P35.8 **Other congenital viral diseases** Ⓝ
Congenital varicella [chickenpox]

P35.9 **Congenital viral disease, unspecified** Ⓝ

4️⃣➕ **P36** **Bacterial sepsis of newborn**

> INCLUDES   congenital sepsis

Use additional code(s), if applicable, to identify severe sepsis (R65.2-) and associated acute organ dysfunction(s)

➕ **P36.0** **Sepsis of newborn due to streptococcus, group B** Ⓝ

5️⃣➕ **P36.1** **Sepsis of newborn due to other and unspecified streptococci**

➕ **P36.10** **Sepsis of newborn due to unspecified streptococci** Ⓝ

➕ **P36.19** **Sepsis of newborn due to other streptococci** Ⓝ

➕ **P36.2** **Sepsis of newborn due to Staphylococcus aureus** Ⓝ

5️⃣➕ **P36.3** **Sepsis of newborn due to other and unspecified staphylococci**

➕ **P36.30** **Sepsis of newborn due to unspecified staphylococci** Ⓝ

➕ **P36.39** **Sepsis of newborn due to other staphylococci** Ⓝ

➕ **P36.4** **Sepsis of newborn due to Escherichia coli** Ⓝ

➕ **P36.5** **Sepsis of newborn due to anaerobes** Ⓝ

➕ **P36.8** **Other bacterial sepsis of newborn** Ⓝ
Use additional code from category B96 to identify organism

➕ **P36.9** **Bacterial sepsis of newborn, unspecified** Ⓝ

4️⃣ **P37** **Other congenital infectious and parasitic diseases**

> EXCLUDES 2   *congenital syphilis (A50.-)*
> *infectious neonatal diarrhea (A00-A09)*
> *necrotizing enterocolitis in newborn (P77.-)*
> *noninfectious neonatal diarrhea (P78.3)*
> *ophthalmia neonatorum due to gonococcus (A54.31)*
> *tetanus neonatorum (A33)*

P37.0 **Congenital tuberculosis** Ⓝ

P37.1 **Congenital toxoplasmosis** Ⓝ
Hydrocephalus due to congenital toxoplasmosis

P37.2 **Neonatal (disseminated) listeriosis** Ⓝ

P37.3 **Congenital falciparum malaria** Ⓝ

P37.4 **Other congenital malaria** Ⓝ

P37.5 **Neonatal candidiasis** Ⓝ

P37.8 **Other specified congenital infectious and parasitic diseases** Ⓝ

P37.9 **Congenital infectious or parasitic disease, unspecified** Ⓝ

4️⃣ **P38** **Omphalitis of newborn**

> EXCLUDES 1   *omphalitis not of newborn (L08.82)*
> *tetanus omphalitis (A33)*
> *umbilical hemorrhage of newborn (P51.-)*

P38.1 **Omphalitis with mild hemorrhage** Ⓝ

P38.9 **Omphalitis without hemorrhage** Ⓝ
Omphalitis of newborn NOS

4️⃣➕ **P39** **Other infections specific to the perinatal period**
Use additional code to identify organism or specific infection

---

● New   ▲ Revised   *Manifestation*   4️⃣-7️⃣ Digit Indicators   ▤ Laterality   Ⓐ Adult (15+ years)   Ⓜ Maternity (12-55 years)   Ⓝ Newborn   Ⓟ Pediatric (0-17 years)   ♂ Male   ♀ Female
✖ D̶e̶l̶e̶t̶e̶d̶   Unspecified   ➕ Additional code

+ **P39.0**   **Neonatal infective mastitis**   N

  EXCLUDES 1   *breast engorgement of newborn (P83.4)*
  noninfective mastitis of newborn (P83.4)

  DEFINITION   Inflammation of the breast in a newborn.

+ **P39.1**   **Neonatal conjunctivitis and dacryocystitis**   N
  Neonatal chlamydial conjunctivitis
  Ophthalmia neonatorum NOS

  EXCLUDES 1   *gonococcal conjunctivitis (A54.31)*

+ **P39.2**   **Intra-amniotic infection affecting newborn, not elsewhere classified**   N

+ **P39.3**   **Neonatal urinary tract infection**   N

+ **P39.4**   **Neonatal skin infection**   N
  Neonatal pyoderma

  EXCLUDES 1   *pemphigus neonatorum (L00)*
  staphylococcal scalded skin syndrome (L00)

+ **P39.8**   **Other specified infections specific to the perinatal period**   N

+ **P39.9**   **Infection specific to the perinatal period, unspecified**   N

Hemorrhagic and hematological disorders of newborn (P50-P61)

EXCLUDES 1   *congenital stenosis and stricture of bile ducts (Q44.3)*
Crigler-Najjar syndrome (E80.5)
Dubin-Johnson syndrome (E80.6)
Gilbert syndrome (E80.4)
hereditary hemolytic anemias (D55-D58)

⊿ **P50**   **Newborn affected by intrauterine (fetal) blood loss**

  EXCLUDES 1   *congenital anemia from intrauterine (fetal) blood loss (P61.3)*

  P50.0   **Newborn affected by intrauterine (fetal) blood loss from vasa previa**   N

  P50.1   **Newborn affected by intrauterine (fetal) blood loss from ruptured cord**   N

  P50.2   **Newborn affected by intrauterine (fetal) blood loss from placenta**   N

  P50.3   **Newborn affected by hemorrhage into co-twin**   N

  P50.4   **Newborn affected by hemorrhage into maternal circulation**   N

  P50.5   **Newborn affected by intrauterine (fetal) blood loss from cut end of co-twin's cord**   N

  P50.8   **Newborn affected by other intrauterine (fetal) blood loss**   N

  P50.9   **Newborn affected by intrauterine (fetal) blood loss, unspecified**   N
  Newborn affected by fetal hemorrhage NOS

⊿ **P51**   **Umbilical hemorrhage of newborn**

  EXCLUDES 1   *omphalitis with mild hemorrhage (P38.1)*
  umbilical hemorrhage from cut end of co-twins cord (P50.5)

  P51.0   **Massive umbilical hemorrhage of newborn**   N

  P51.8   **Other umbilical hemorrhages of newborn**   N
  Slipped umbilical ligature NOS

  P51.9   **Umbilical hemorrhage of newborn, unspecified**   N

⊿ **P52**   **Intracranial nontraumatic hemorrhage of newborn**

  INCLUDES   intracranial hemorrhage due to anoxia or hypoxia

  EXCLUDES 1   *intracranial hemorrhage due to birth injury (P10.-)*
  intracranial hemorrhage due to other injury (S06.-)

  P52.0   **Intraventricular (nontraumatic) hemorrhage, grade 1, of newborn**   N
  Subependymal hemorrhage (without intraventricular extension)
  Bleeding into germinal matrix

  P52.1   **Intraventricular (nontraumatic) hemorrhage, grade 2, of newborn**   N
  Subependymal hemorrhage with intraventricular extension
  Bleeding into ventricle

  ⑤ **P52.2**   **Intraventricular (nontraumatic) hemorrhage, grade 3 and grade 4, of newborn**

    P52.21   **Intraventricular (nontraumatic) hemorrhage, grade 3, of newborn**   N
    Subependymal hemorrhage with intraventricular extension with enlargement of ventricle

    P52.22   **Intraventricular (nontraumatic) hemorrhage, grade 4, of newborn**   N
    Bleeding into cerebral cortex
    Subependymal hemorrhage with intracerebral extension

  P52.3   **Unspecified intraventricular (nontraumatic) hemorrhage of newborn**   N

  P52.4   **Intracerebral (nontraumatic) hemorrhage of newborn**   N

  P52.5   **Subarachnoid (nontraumatic) hemorrhage of newborn**   N

  P52.6   **Cerebellar (nontraumatic) and posterior fossa hemorrhage of newborn**   N

  P52.8   **Other intracranial (nontraumatic) hemorrhages of newborn**   N

  P52.9   **Intracranial (nontraumatic) hemorrhage of newborn, unspecified**   N

P53   **Hemorrhagic disease of newborn**   N
  Vitamin K deficiency of newborn

⊿ **P54**   **Other neonatal hemorrhages**

  EXCLUDES 1   *newborn affected by (intrauterine) blood loss (P50.-)*
  pulmonary hemorrhage originating in the perinatal period (P26.-)

  P54.0   **Neonatal hematemesis**   N

  EXCLUDES 1   *neonatal hematemesis due to swallowed maternal blood (P78.2)*

  P54.1   **Neonatal melena**   N

  EXCLUDES 1   *neonatal melena due to swallowed maternal blood (P78.2)*

  P54.2   **Neonatal rectal hemorrhage**   N

  P54.3   **Other neonatal gastrointestinal hemorrhage**   N

  P54.4   **Neonatal adrenal hemorrhage**   N

  P54.5   **Neonatal cutaneous hemorrhage**   N
  Neonatal bruising
  Neonatal ecchymoses
  Neonatal petechiae
  Neonatal superficial hematomata

  EXCLUDES 2   *bruising of scalp due to birth injury (P12.3)*
  cephalhematoma due to birth injury (P12.0)

  DEFINITION   Minute red spots on the surface of the skin, due to escape of a small amount of blood from the vessels.

  P54.6   **Neonatal vaginal hemorrhage**   ♀N
  Neonatal pseudomenses

  P54.8   **Other specified neonatal hemorrhages**   N

  P54.9   **Neonatal hemorrhage, unspecified**   N

⊿ **P55**   **Hemolytic disease of newborn**

  P55.0   **Rh isoimmunization of newborn**   N

  P55.1   **ABO isoimmunization of newborn**   N
  AHA: 3Q 2015, 20

  P55.8   **Other hemolytic diseases of newborn**   N

  P55.9   **Hemolytic disease of newborn, unspecified**   N

⊿ **P56**   **Hydrops fetalis due to hemolytic disease**

  EXCLUDES 1   *hydrops fetalis NOS (P83.2)*

  P56.0   **Hydrops fetalis due to isoimmunization**   N

  ⑤ **P56.9**   **Hydrops fetalis due to other and unspecified hemolytic disease**

    P56.90   **Hydrops fetalis due to unspecified hemolytic disease**   N

    P56.99   **Hydrops fetalis due to other hemolytic disease**   N

⊿ **P57**   **Kernicterus**

  P57.0   **Kernicterus due to isoimmunization**   N

  DEFINITION   Encephalopathy due to severe jaundice caused by destruction of the infant's red blood cells by the mother's immune system. Excess bilirubin crosses the blood-brain barrier and accumulates toxically in the brain.

  P57.8   **Other specified kernicterus**   N

  EXCLUDES 1   *Crigler-Najjar syndrome (E80.5)*

  P57.9   **Kernicterus, unspecified**   N

⊿ **P58**   **Neonatal jaundice due to other excessive hemolysis**

  EXCLUDES 1   *jaundice due to isoimmunization (P55-P57)*

  P58.0   **Neonatal jaundice due to bruising**   N

  P58.1   **Neonatal jaundice due to bleeding**   N

  P58.2   **Neonatal jaundice due to infection**   N

  P58.3   **Neonatal jaundice due to polycythemia**   N

● New   ▲ Revised   *Manifestation*   ⊿-☑ Digit Indicators   ⊟ Laterality   A Adult (15+ years)   M Maternity (12-55 years)   N Newborn   P Pediatric (0-17 years)   ♂ Male   ♀ Female
✖ Deleted   Unspecified   + Additional code

⑤✚ P58.4   Neonatal jaundice due to drugs or toxins transmitted from mother or given to newborn
Code first:
   poisoning due to drug or toxin, if applicable
      (T36-T65 with fifth or sixth character 1-4 or 6)
   Use additional code for adverse effect, if applicable, to identify drug (T36-T50 with fifth or sixth character 5)

✚ P58.41   Neonatal jaundice due to drugs or toxins transmitted from mother

✚ P58.42   Neonatal jaundice due to drugs or toxins given to newborn

P58.5   Neonatal jaundice due to swallowed maternal blood

P58.8   Neonatal jaundice due to other specified excessive hemolysis

P58.9   Neonatal jaundice due to excessive hemolysis, unspecified

④ P59   Neonatal jaundice from other and unspecified causes
   EXCLUDES 1   *jaundice due to inborn errors of metabolism (E70-E88)*
               kernicterus (P57.-)

P59.0   Neonatal jaundice associated with preterm delivery
   Hyperbilirubinemia of prematurity
   Jaundice due to delayed conjugation associated with preterm delivery

P59.1   Inspissated bile syndrome

⑤ P59.2   Neonatal jaundice from other and unspecified hepatocellular damage
   EXCLUDES 1   *congenital viral hepatitis (P35.3)*

P59.20   Neonatal jaundice from unspecified hepatocellular damage

P59.29   Neonatal jaundice from other hepatocellular damage
   Neonatal giant cell hepatitis
   Neonatal (idiopathic) hepatitis

P59.3   Neonatal jaundice from breast milk inhibitor

P59.8   Neonatal jaundice from other specified causes

P59.9   Neonatal jaundice, unspecified
   Neonatal physiological jaundice (intense)(prolonged) NOS
   AHA: 3Q 2015, 20

P60   Disseminated intravascular coagulation of newborn
   Defibrination syndrome of newborn

④ P61   Other perinatal hematological disorders
   EXCLUDES 1   *transient hypogammaglobulinemia of infancy (D80.7)*

P61.0   Transient neonatal thrombocytopenia
   Neonatal thrombocytopenia due to exchange transfusion
   Neonatal thrombocytopenia due to idiopathic maternal thrombocytopenia
   Neonatal thrombocytopenia due to isoimmunization

P61.1   Polycythemia neonatorum
   DEFINITION   Abnormally increased number of red blood cells in the neonate's bloodstream.

P61.2   Anemia of prematurity

P61.3   Congenital anemia from fetal blood loss

P61.4   Other congenital anemias, not elsewhere classified
   Congenital anemia NOS

P61.5   Transient neonatal neutropenia
   EXCLUDES 1   *congenital neutropenia (nontransient) (D70.0)*

P61.6   Other transient neonatal disorders of coagulation

P61.8   Other specified perinatal hematological disorders

P61.9   Perinatal hematological disorder, unspecified

Transitory endocrine and metabolic disorders specific to newborn (P70-P74)

INCLUDES   transitory endocrine and metabolic disturbances caused by the infant's response to maternal endocrine and metabolic factors, or its adjustment to extrauterine environment

④ P70   Transitory disorders of carbohydrate metabolism specific to newborn

P70.0   Syndrome of infant of mother with gestational diabetes
   Newborn (with hypoglycemia) affected by maternal gestational diabetes
   EXCLUDES 1   *newborn (with hypoglycemia) affected by maternal (pre-existing) diabetes mellitus (P70.1)*
               syndrome of infant of a diabetic mother (P70.1)

P70.1   Syndrome of infant of a diabetic mother
   Newborn (with hypoglycemia) affected by maternal (pre-existing) diabetes mellitus
   EXCLUDES 1   *newborn (with hypoglycemia) affected by maternal gestational diabetes (P70.0)*
               syndrome of infant of mother with gestational diabetes (P70.0)

P70.2   Neonatal diabetes mellitus

P70.3   Iatrogenic neonatal hypoglycemia

P70.4   Other neonatal hypoglycemia
   Transitory neonatal hypoglycemia

P70.8   Other transitory disorders of carbohydrate metabolism of newborn

P70.9   Transitory disorder of carbohydrate metabolism of newborn, unspecified

④ P71   Transitory neonatal disorders of calcium and magnesium metabolism

P71.0   Cow's milk hypocalcemia in newborn

P71.1   Other neonatal hypocalcemia
   EXCLUDES 1   *neonatal hypoparathyroidism (P71.4)*

P71.2   Neonatal hypomagnesemia

P71.3   Neonatal tetany without calcium or magnesium deficiency
   Neonatal tetany NOS

P71.4   Transitory neonatal hypoparathyroidism

P71.8   Other transitory neonatal disorders of calcium and magnesium metabolism

P71.9   Transitory neonatal disorder of calcium and magnesium metabolism, unspecified

④ P72   Other transitory neonatal endocrine disorders
   EXCLUDES 1   *congenital hypothyroidism with or without goiter (E03.0-E03.1)*
               dyshormogenetic goiter (E07.1)
               Pendred's syndrome (E07.1)

P72.0   Neonatal goiter, not elsewhere classified
   Transitory congenital goiter with normal functioning

P72.1   Transitory neonatal hyperthyroidism
   Neonatal thyrotoxicosis
   DEFINITION   Abnormally high levels of thyroid hormone in the neonate.

P72.2   Other transitory neonatal disorders of thyroid function, not elsewhere classified
   Transitory neonatal hypothyroidism

P72.8   Other specified transitory neonatal endocrine disorders

P72.9   Transitory neonatal endocrine disorder, unspecified

④ P74   Other transitory neonatal electrolyte and metabolic disturbances

P74.0   Late metabolic acidosis of newborn
   EXCLUDES 1   *(fetal) metabolic acidosis of newborn (P19)*
   DEFINITION   Imbalance in the acid to alkaline ratio in the blood, most often affecting premature infants in the 2nd and 3rd week of life.

P74.1   Dehydration of newborn

P74.2   Disturbances of sodium balance of newborn

P74.3   Disturbances of potassium balance of newborn

P74.4   Other transitory electrolyte disturbances of newborn

P74.5   Transitory tyrosinemia of newborn

P74.6   Transitory hyperammonemia of newborn

P74.8   Other transitory metabolic disturbances of newborn
   Amino-acid metabolic disorders described as transitory

P74.9   Transitory metabolic disturbance of newborn, unspecified

● New   ▲ Revised   *Manifestation*   ④-❼ Digit Indicators   ⊟ Laterality   Ⓐ Adult (15+ years)   Ⓜ Maternity (12-55 years)   Ⓝ Newborn   Ⓟ Pediatric (0-17 years)   ♂ Male   ♀ Female
✖ Deleted   Unspecified   ✚ Additional code

878   © 2017 DecisionHealth   2017 ICD-10-CM Expert for Physicians

Digestive system disorders of newborn (P76-P78)

⚃ **P76** **Other intestinal obstruction of newborn**

P76.0 **Meconium plug syndrome**
Meconium ileus NOS

> **EXCLUDES 1** *meconium ileus in cystic fibrosis (E84.11)*

> **DEFINITION** Dark green feces that normally comprises a newborn's first bowel movement does not pass through the bowel, causing blockage of the intestine.

P76.1 **Transitory ileus of newborn**
> **EXCLUDES 1** *Hirschsprung's disease (Q43.1)*

P76.2 **Intestinal obstruction due to inspissated milk**

P76.8 **Other specified intestinal obstruction of newborn**
> **EXCLUDES 1** *intestinal obstruction classifiable to K56.-*

P76.9 **Intestinal obstruction of newborn, unspecified**

⚃ **P77** **Necrotizing enterocolitis of newborn**

P77.1 **Stage 1 necrotizing enterocolitis in newborn**
Necrotizing enterocolitis without pneumatosis, without perforation

P77.2 **Stage 2 necrotizing enterocolitis in newborn**
Necrotizing enterocolitis with pneumatosis, without perforation

P77.3 **Stage 3 necrotizing enterocolitis in newborn**
Necrotizing enterocolitis with perforation
Necrotizing enterocolitis with pneumatosis and perforation

P77.9 **Necrotizing enterocolitis in newborn, unspecified**
Necrotizing enterocolitis in newborn, NOS

⚃ **P78** **Other perinatal digestive system disorders**
> **EXCLUDES 1** *cystic fibrosis (E84.0-E84.9)*
> *neonatal gastrointestinal hemorrhages (P54.0-P54.3)*

P78.0 **Perinatal intestinal perforation**
Meconium peritonitis

Perinatal intestinal perforation

Large intestines
Small intestines
Rectum
Holes/tears in intestines

P78.1 **Other neonatal peritonitis**
Neonatal peritonitis NOS

P78.2 **Neonatal hematemesis and melena due to swallowed maternal blood**

P78.3 **Noninfective neonatal diarrhea**
Neonatal diarrhea NOS

⑤ **P78.8** **Other specified perinatal digestive system disorders**

P78.81 **Congenital cirrhosis (of liver)**

P78.82 **Peptic ulcer of newborn**

P78.83 **Newborn esophageal reflux**
Neonatal esophageal reflux

P78.89 **Other specified perinatal digestive system disorders**

P78.9 **Perinatal digestive system disorder, unspecified**

Conditions involving the integument and temperature regulation of newborn (P80-P83)

⚃ **P80** **Hypothermia of newborn**

P80.0 **Cold injury syndrome**
Severe and usually chronic hypothermia associated with a pink flushed appearance, edema and neurological and biochemical abnormalities.
> **EXCLUDES 1** *mild hypothermia of newborn (P80.8)*

P80.8 **Other hypothermia of newborn**
Mild hypothermia of newborn

P80.9 **Hypothermia of newborn, unspecified**

⚃ **P81** **Other disturbances of temperature regulation of newborn**

P81.0 **Environmental hyperthermia of newborn**

P81.8 **Other specified disturbances of temperature regulation of newborn**

P81.9 **Disturbance of temperature regulation of newborn, unspecified**
Fever of newborn NOS

⚃ **P83** **Other conditions of integument specific to newborn**
> **EXCLUDES 1** *congenital malformations of skin and integument (Q80-Q84)*
> *hydrops fetalis due to hemolytic disease (P56.-)*
> *neonatal skin infection (P39.4)*
> *staphylococcal scalded skin syndrome (L00)*
> **EXCLUDES 2** *cradle cap (L21.0)*
> *diaper [napkin] dermatitis (L22)*

P83.0 **Sclerema neonatorum**

P83.1 **Neonatal erythema toxicum**

P83.2 **Hydrops fetalis not due to hemolytic disease**
Hydrops fetalis NOS

⑤ **P83.3** **Other and unspecified edema specific to newborn**

P83.30 **Unspecified edema specific to newborn**

P83.39 **Other edema specific to newborn**

P83.4 **Breast engorgement of newborn**
Noninfective mastitis of newborn

P83.5 **Congenital hydrocele** ♂

P83.6 **Umbilical polyp of newborn**

P83.8 **Other specified conditions of integument specific to newborn**
Bronze baby syndrome
Neonatal scleroderma
Urticaria neonatorum

P83.9 **Condition of the integument specific to newborn, unspecified**

Other problems with newborn (P84)

P84 **Other problems with newborn**
Acidemia of newborn
Acidosis of newborn
Anoxia of newborn NOS
Asphyxia of newborn NOS
Hypercapnia of newborn
Hypoxemia of newborn
Hypoxia of newborn NOS
Mixed metabolic and respiratory acidosis of newborn
> **EXCLUDES 1** *intracranial hemorrhage due to anoxia or hypoxia (P52.-)*
> *hypoxic ischemic encephalopathy [HIE] (P91.6-)*
> *late metabolic acidosis of newborn (P74.0)*

Other disorders originating in the perinatal period (P90-P96)

P90 **Convulsions of newborn**
> **EXCLUDES 1** *benign myoclonic epilepsy in infancy (G40.3-)*
> *benign neonatal convulsions (familial) (G40.3-)*

⚃ **P91** **Other disturbances of cerebral status of newborn**

P91.0 **Neonatal cerebral ischemia**

P91.1 **Acquired periventricular cysts of newborn**

P91.2 **Neonatal cerebral leukomalacia**
Periventricular leukomalacia

P91.3 **Neonatal cerebral irritability**

P91.4 **Neonatal cerebral depression**

P91.5 **Neonatal coma**

⑤ **P91.6** **Hypoxic ischemic encephalopathy [HIE]**

P91.60 **Hypoxic ischemic encephalopathy [HIE], unspecified**

P91.61 **Mild hypoxic ischemic encephalopathy [HIE]**

P91.62 **Moderate hypoxic ischemic encephalopathy [HIE]**

P91.63 **Severe hypoxic ischemic encephalopathy [HIE]**

● New ▲ Revised *Manifestation* ⚃-⚇ Digit Indicators ▤ Laterality Ⓐ Adult (15+ years) Ⓜ Maternity (12-55 years) Ⓝ Newborn Ⓟ Pediatric (0-17 years) ♂ Male ♀ Female
✖ Deleted Unspecified + Additional code

Certain Conditions Originating in the Perinatal Period

P91.8   **Other specified disturbances of cerebral status of newborn**   N

P91.9   **Disturbance of cerebral status of newborn, unspecified**   N

4 **P92**   **Feeding problems of newborn**

> EXCLUDES 1   *feeding problems in child over 28 days old (R63.3)*

5 **P92.0**   **Vomiting of newborn**

> EXCLUDES 1   *vomiting of child over 28 days old (R11.-)*

     P92.01   **Bilious vomiting of newborn**   N

> EXCLUDES 1   *bilious vomiting in child over 28 days old (R11.14)*

     P92.09   **Other vomiting of newborn**   N

> EXCLUDES 1   *regurgitation of food in newborn (P92.1)*

P92.1   **Regurgitation and rumination of newborn**   N

P92.2   **Slow feeding of newborn**   N

P92.3   **Underfeeding of newborn**   N

P92.4   **Overfeeding of newborn**   N

P92.5   **Neonatal difficulty in feeding at breast**   N

P92.6   **Failure to thrive in newborn**   N

> EXCLUDES 1   *failure to thrive in child over 28 days old (R62.51)*

P92.8   **Other feeding problems of newborn**   N

P92.9   **Feeding problem of newborn, unspecified**   N

4 **P93**   **Reactions and intoxications due to drugs administered to newborn**

> INCLUDES   reactions and intoxications due to drugs administered to fetus affecting newborn
>
> EXCLUDES 1   *jaundice due to drugs or toxins transmitted from mother or given to newborn (P58.4-)*
> *reactions and intoxications from maternal opiates, tranquilizers and other medication (P04.0-P04.1, P04.4)*
> *withdrawal symptoms from maternal use of drugs of addiction (P96.1)*
> *withdrawal symptoms from therapeutic use of drugs in newborn (P96.2)*

P93.0   **Grey baby syndrome**   N
Grey syndrome from chloramphenicol administration in newborn

+ **P93.8**   **Other reactions and intoxications due to drugs administered to newborn**   N
Use additional code for adverse effect, if applicable, to identify drug (T36-T50 with fifth or sixth character 5)

4 **P94**   **Disorders of muscle tone of newborn**

P94.0   **Transient neonatal myasthenia gravis**   N

> EXCLUDES 1   *myasthenia gravis (G70.0)*

P94.1   **Congenital hypertonia**   N

P94.2   **Congenital hypotonia**   N
Floppy baby syndrome, unspecified

P94.8   **Other disorders of muscle tone of newborn**   N

P94.9   **Disorder of muscle tone of newborn, unspecified**   N

P95   **Stillbirth**   N
Deadborn fetus NOS
Fetal death of unspecified cause
Stillbirth NOS

> EXCLUDES 1   *maternal care for intrauterine death (O36.4)*
> *missed abortion (O02.1)*
> *outcome of delivery, stillbirth (Z37.1, Z37.3, Z37.4, Z37.7)*

4 **P96**   **Other conditions originating in the perinatal period**

P96.0   **Congenital renal failure**   N
Uremia of newborn

P96.1   **Neonatal withdrawal symptoms from maternal use of drugs of addiction**   N
Drug withdrawal syndrome in infant of dependent mother
Neonatal abstinence syndrome

> EXCLUDES 1   *reactions and intoxications from maternal opiates and tranquilizers administered during labor and delivery (P04.0)*

P96.2   **Withdrawal symptoms from therapeutic use of drugs in newborn**   N

P96.3   **Wide cranial sutures of newborn**   N
Neonatal craniotabes

▲ **P96.5**   **Complication to newborn due to (fetal) intrauterine procedure**   N

> EXCLUDES 2   *newborn affected by amniocentesis (P00.6)*

5 **P96.8**   **Other specified conditions originating in the perinatal period**

P96.81   **Exposure to (parental) (environmental) tobacco smoke in the perinatal period**

> EXCLUDES 2   *newborn affected by in utero exposure to tobacco (P04.2)*
> *exposure to environmental tobacco smoke after the perinatal period (Z77.22)*

P96.82   **Delayed separation of umbilical cord**   N

P96.83   **Meconium staining**   N

> EXCLUDES 1   *meconium aspiration (P24.00, P24.01)*
> *meconium passage during delivery (P03.82)*

+ **P96.89**   **Other specified conditions originating in the perinatal period**   N
Use additional code to specify condition

P96.9   **Condition originating in the perinatal period, unspecified**   N
Congenital debility NOS

● New   ▲ Revised   *Manifestation*   4 - 7 Digit Indicators   ⊟ Laterality   A Adult (15+ years)   M Maternity (12-55 years)   N Newborn   P Pediatric (0-17 years)   ♂ Male   ♀ Female
✖ Deleted   Unspecified   + Additional code

CHAPTER 17: CONGENITAL MALFORMATIONS, DEFORMATIONS AND CHROMOSOMAL ABNORMALITIES (Q00-Q99)

Note: Codes from this chapter are not for use on maternal or fetal records

EXCLUDES 2 *inborn errors of metabolism (E70-E88)*

GUIDELINES Section I.C.17

Codes from Chapter 17 may be used throughout the life of the patient. If a congenital malformation or deformity has been corrected, a personal history code should be used to identify the history of the malformation or deformity. Although present at birth, malformation/deformation/or chromosomal abnormality may not be identified until later in life. Whenever the condition is diagnosed by the physician, it is appropriate to assign a code from codes Q00-Q99. For the birth admission, the appropriate code from category Z38, Liveborn infants, according to place of birth and type of delivery, should be sequenced as the principal diagnosis, followed by any congenital anomaly codes, Q00- Q99.

This chapter contains the following blocks:
Q00-Q07   Congenital malformations of the nervous system
Q10-Q18   Congenital malformations of eye, ear, face and neck
Q20-Q28   Congenital malformations of the circulatory system
Q30-Q34   Congenital malformations of the respiratory system
Q35-Q37   Cleft lip and cleft palate
Q38-Q45   Other congenital malformations of the digestive system
Q50-Q56   Congenital malformations of genital organs
Q60-Q64   Congenital malformations of the urinary system
Q65-Q79   Congenital malformations and deformations of the musculoskeletal system
Q80-Q89   Other congenital malformations
Q90-Q99   Chromosomal abnormalities, not elsewhere classified

Congenital malformations of the nervous system (Q00-Q07)

⬔ Q00   Anencephaly and similar malformations

Q00.0   Anencephaly
Acephaly
Acrania
Amyelencephaly
Hemianencephaly
Hemicephaly

Q00.1   Craniorachischisis

Q00.2   Iniencephaly

DEFINITION   Neural tube birth defect in which the fetal head is severely bent backwards, the neck is usually absent, and other severe birth defects are present.

⬔ Q01   Encephalocele

INCLUDES   Arnold-Chiari syndrome, type III
encephalocystocele
encephalomyelocele
hydroencephalocele
hydromeningocele, cranial
meningocele, cerebral
meningoencephalocele

EXCLUDES 1   *Meckel-Gruber syndrome (Q61.9)*

Q01.0   Frontal encephalocele

Q01.1   Nasofrontal encephalocele

Q01.2   Occipital encephalocele

Q01.8   Encephalocele of other sites

Q01.9   Encephalocele, unspecified

Q02   Microcephaly

INCLUDES   hydromicrocephaly
micrencephalon

EXCLUDES 1   *Meckel-Gruber syndrome (Q61.9)*

DEFINITION   Abnormal smallness of the head.

⬔ Q03   Congenital hydrocephalus

INCLUDES   hydrocephalus in newborn

EXCLUDES 1   *Arnold-Chiari syndrome, type II (Q07.0-)*
acquired hydrocephalus (G91.-)
hydrocephalus due to congenital toxoplasmosis (P37.1)
hydrocephalus with spina bifida (Q05.0-Q05.4)

Q03.0   Malformations of aqueduct of Sylvius
Anomaly of aqueduct of Sylvius
Obstruction of aqueduct of Sylvius, congenital
Stenosis of aqueduct of Sylvius

Q03.1   Atresia of foramina of Magendie and Luschka
Dandy-Walker syndrome

Q03.8   Other congenital hydrocephalus

Other congenital hydrocephalus

Ventricles fill with fluid, pushing the brain outward

Q03.9   Congenital hydrocephalus, unspecified

⬔ Q04   Other congenital malformations of brain

EXCLUDES 1   *cyclopia (Q87.0)*
macrocephaly (Q75.3)

Q04.0   Congenital malformations of corpus callosum
Agenesis of corpus callosum

Q04.1   Arhinencephaly

Q04.2   Holoprosencephaly

Q04.3   Other reduction deformities of brain
Absence of part of brain
Agenesis of part of brain
Agyria
Aplasia of part of brain
Hydranencephaly
Hypoplasia of part of brain
Lissencephaly
Microgyria
Pachygyria

EXCLUDES 1   *congenital malformations of corpus callosum (Q04.0)*

Q04.4   Septo-optic dysplasia of brain

Q04.5   Megalencephaly

Q04.6   Congenital cerebral cysts
Porencephaly
Schizencephaly

EXCLUDES 1   *acquired porencephalic cyst (G93.0)*

Q04.8   Other specified congenital malformations of brain
Arnold-Chiari syndrome, type IV
Macrogyria

CODING TIP ✓   Chiari malformation, also referred to as Arnold Chiari malformation, is an anomaly where cerebellar tissue extends into the spinal canal. The rarest form, type IV, the back of the brain fails to develop normally. Type IV is an anomaly where cerebellar hypoplasia is present.

Q04.9   Congenital malformation of brain, unspecified
Congenital anomaly NOS of brain
Congenital deformity NOS of brain
Congenital disease or lesion NOS of brain
Multiple anomalies NOS of brain, congenital

● New ▲ Revised *Manifestation* ⬔-⬕ Digit Indicators ⊟ Laterality Ⓐ Adult (15+ years) Ⓜ Maternity (12-55 years) Ⓝ Newborn Ⓟ Pediatric (0-17 years) ♂ Male ♀ Female
✖ Deleted Unspecified + Additional code

2017 ICD-10-CM Expert for Physicians   © 2017 DecisionHealth   881

▣+ Q05   Spina bifida

> **INCLUDES**   hydromeningocele (spinal)
> meningocele (spinal)
> meningomyelocele
> myelocele
> myelomeningocele
> rachischisis
> spina bifida (aperta) (cystica)
> syringomyelocele

Use additional code for any associated paraplegia (paraparesis) (G82.2-)

> **EXCLUDES 1**   *Arnold-Chiari syndrome, type II (Q07.0-)*
> *spina bifida occulta (Q76.0)*

+ Q05.0   Cervical spina bifida with hydrocephalus

+ Q05.1   Thoracic spina bifida with hydrocephalus
> Dorsal spina bifida with hydrocephalus
> Thoracolumbar spina bifida with hydrocephalus

+ Q05.2   Lumbar spina bifida with hydrocephalus
> Lumbosacral spina bifida with hydrocephalus

+ Q05.3   Sacral spina bifida with hydrocephalus

+ Q05.4   Unspecified spina bifida with hydrocephalus

+ Q05.5   Cervical spina bifida without hydrocephalus

+ Q05.6   Thoracic spina bifida without hydrocephalus
> Dorsal spina bifida NOS
> Thoracolumbar spina bifida NOS

+ Q05.7   Lumbar spina bifida without hydrocephalus
> Lumbosacral spina bifida NOS

+ Q05.8   Sacral spina bifida without hydrocephalus

+ Q05.9   Spina bifida, unspecified

▣ Q06   Other congenital malformations of spinal cord

Q06.0   Amyelia

Q06.1   Hypoplasia and dysplasia of spinal cord
> Atelomyelia
> Myelatelia
> Myelodysplasia of spinal cord

Q06.2   Diastematomyelia

Q06.3   Other congenital cauda equina malformations

Q06.4   Hydromyelia
> Hydrorachis

Q06.8   Other specified congenital malformations of spinal cord

Q06.9   Congenital malformation of spinal cord, unspecified
> Congenital anomaly NOS of spinal cord
> Congenital deformity NOS of spinal cord
> Congenital disease or lesion NOS of spinal cord

▣ Q07   Other congenital malformations of nervous system

> **EXCLUDES 2**   *congenital central alveolar hypoventilation syndrome (G47.35)*
> *familial dysautonomia [Riley-Day] (G90.1)*
> *neurofibromatosis (nonmalignant) (Q85.0-)*

▤ Q07.0   Arnold-Chiari syndrome
> Arnold-Chiari syndrome, type II
> **EXCLUDES 1**   *Arnold-Chiari syndrome, type III (Q01.-)*
> *Arnold-Chiari syndrome, type IV (Q04.8)*

Q07.00   Arnold-Chiari syndrome without spina bifida or hydrocephalus

Q07.01   Arnold-Chiari syndrome with spina bifida

Q07.02   Arnold-Chiari syndrome with hydrocephalus

Q07.03   Arnold-Chiari syndrome with spina bifida and hydrocephalus

Q07.8   Other specified congenital malformations of nervous system
> Agenesis of nerve
> Displacement of brachial plexus
> Jaw-winking syndrome
> Marcus Gunn's syndrome

Q07.9   Congenital malformation of nervous system, unspecified
> Congenital anomaly NOS of nervous system
> Congenital deformity NOS of nervous system
> Congenital disease or lesion NOS of nervous system

Congenital malformations of eye, ear, face and neck (Q10-Q18)

> **EXCLUDES 2**   *cleft lip and cleft palate (Q35-Q37)*
> *congenital malformation of cervical spine (Q05.0, Q05.5, Q67.5, Q76.0-Q76.4)*
> *congenital malformation of larynx (Q31.-)*
> *congenital malformation of lip NEC (Q38.0)*
> *congenital malformation of nose (Q30.-)*
> *congenital malformation of parathyroid gland (Q89.2)*
> *congenital malformation of thyroid gland (Q89.2)*

▣ Q10   Congenital malformations of eyelid, lacrimal apparatus and orbit
> **EXCLUDES 1**   *cryptophthalmos NOS (Q11.2)*
> *cryptophthalmos syndrome (Q87.0)*

Q10.0   Congenital ptosis
> **DEFINITION**   Congenital drooping of the upper eyelid.

Q10.1   Congenital ectropion

Q10.2   Congenital entropion

Q10.3   Other congenital malformations of eyelid
> Ablepharon
> Blepharophimosis, congenital
> Coloboma of eyelid
> Congenital absence or agenesis of cilia
> Congenital absence or agenesis of eyelid
> Congenital accessory eyelid
> Congenital accessory eye muscle
> Congenital malformation of eyelid NOS

Q10.4   Absence and agenesis of lacrimal apparatus
> Congenital absence of punctum lacrimale

Q10.5   Congenital stenosis and stricture of lacrimal duct

Q10.6   Other congenital malformations of lacrimal apparatus
> Congenital malformation of lacrimal apparatus NOS

Q10.7   Congenital malformation of orbit

▣ Q11   Anophthalmos, microphthalmos and macrophthalmos

Q11.0   Cystic eyeball

Q11.1   Other anophthalmos
> Anophthalmos NOS
> Agenesis of eye
> Aplasia of eye

Q11.2   Microphthalmos
> Cryptophthalmos NOS
> Dysplasia of eye
> Hypoplasia of eye
> Rudimentary eye
> **EXCLUDES 1**   *cryptophthalmos syndrome (Q87.0)*
> **DEFINITION**   Abnormal smallness in all dimensions of one or both eyes.

Q11.3   Macrophthalmos
> **EXCLUDES 1**   *macrophthalmos in congenital glaucoma (Q15.0)*

▣ Q12   Congenital lens malformations

Q12.0   Congenital cataract

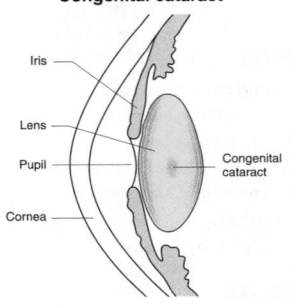

Congenital cataract

Iris
Lens
Pupil
Cornea
Congenital cataract

Q12.1   Congenital displaced lens

Q12.2   Coloboma of lens

Q12.3   Congenital aphakia

Q12.4   Spherophakia

● New   ▲ Revised   *Manifestation*   ▣-▰ Digit Indicators   ▱ Laterality   ▲ Adult (15+ years)   ▤ Maternity (12-55 years)   ▯ Newborn   ▣ Pediatric (0-17 years)   ♂ Male   ♀ Female
✖ ~~Deleted~~   Unspecified   + Additional code

882   © 2017 DecisionHealth   2017 ICD-10-CM Expert for Physicians

Q12.8 Other congenital lens malformations
Microphakia

Q12.9 Congenital lens malformation, unspecified

⊿ **Q13 Congenital malformations of anterior segment of eye**

Q13.0 Coloboma of iris
Coloboma NOS

➕ **Q13.1 Absence of iris**
Aniridia
Use additional code for associated glaucoma (H42)

Q13.2 Other congenital malformations of iris
Anisocoria, congenital
Atresia of pupil
Congenital malformation of iris NOS
Corectopia

Q13.3 Congenital corneal opacity

Q13.4 Other congenital corneal malformations
Congenital malformation of cornea NOS
Microcornea
Peter's anomaly

Q13.5 Blue sclera

⑤ **Q13.8 Other congenital malformations of anterior segment of eye**

➕ **Q13.81 Rieger's anomaly**
Use additional code for associated glaucoma (H42)

Q13.89 Other congenital malformations of anterior segment of eye

Q13.9 Congenital malformation of anterior segment of eye, unspecified

⊿ **Q14 Congenital malformations of posterior segment of eye**
EXCLUDES 2 *optic nerve hypoplasia (H47.03-)*

Q14.0 Congenital malformation of vitreous humor
Congenital vitreous opacity

Q14.1 Congenital malformation of retina
Congenital retinal aneurysm

Q14.2 Congenital malformation of optic disc
Coloboma of optic disc

Q14.3 Congenital malformation of choroid

Q14.8 Other congenital malformations of posterior segment of eye
Coloboma of the fundus

Q14.9 Congenital malformation of posterior segment of eye, unspecified

⊿ **Q15 Other congenital malformations of eye**
EXCLUDES 1 *congenital nystagmus (H55.01)*
ocular albinism (E70.31-)
optic nerve hypoplasia (H47.03-)
retinitis pigmentosa (H35.52)

Q15.0 Congenital glaucoma
Axenfeld's anomaly
Buphthalmos
Glaucoma of childhood
Glaucoma of newborn
Hydrophthalmos
Keratoglobus, congenital, with glaucoma
Macrocornea with glaucoma
Macrophthalmos in congenital glaucoma
Megalocornea with glaucoma
DEFINITION Disease of infancy, marked by an increase of intraocular fluid, elevated eye pressure, and enlargement of the eyeball.

Q15.8 Other specified congenital malformations of eye

Q15.9 Congenital malformation of eye, unspecified
Congenital anomaly of eye
Congenital deformity of eye

⊿ **Q16 Congenital malformations of ear causing impairment of hearing**
EXCLUDES 1 *congenital deafness (H90.-)*

Q16.0 Congenital absence of (ear) auricle

Q16.1 Congenital absence, atresia and stricture of auditory canal (external)
Congenital atresia or stricture of osseous meatus

Q16.2 Absence of eustachian tube

Q16.3 Congenital malformation of ear ossicles
Congenital fusion of ear ossicles

Q16.4 Other congenital malformations of middle ear
Congenital malformation of middle ear NOS

Q16.5 Congenital malformation of inner ear
Congenital anomaly of membranous labyrinth
Congenital anomaly of organ of Corti

Q16.9 Congenital malformation of ear causing impairment of hearing, unspecified
Congenital absence of ear NOS

⊿ **Q17 Other congenital malformations of ear**
EXCLUDES 1 *congenital malformations of ear with impairment of hearing (Q16.0-Q16.9)*
preauricular sinus (Q18.1)

Q17.0 Accessory auricle
Accessory tragus
Polyotia
Preauricular appendage or tag
Supernumerary ear
Supernumerary lobule

Q17.1 Macrotia
DEFINITION Excessive enlargement of the auricle (outer portion of ear).

Q17.2 Microtia

Q17.3 Other misshapen ear
Pointed ear

Q17.4 Misplaced ear
Low-set ears
EXCLUDES 1 *cervical auricle (Q18.2)*

Q17.5 Prominent ear
Bat ear

Q17.8 Other specified congenital malformations of ear
Congenital absence of lobe of ear

Q17.9 Congenital malformation of ear, unspecified
Congenital anomaly of ear NOS

⊿ **Q18 Other congenital malformations of face and neck**
EXCLUDES 1 *cleft lip and cleft palate (Q35-Q37)*
conditions classified to Q67.0-Q67.4
congenital malformations of skull and face bones (Q75.-)
cyclopia (Q87.0)
dentofacial anomalies [including malocclusion] (M26.-)
malformation syndromes affecting facial appearance (Q87.0)
persistent thyroglossal duct (Q89.2)

Q18.0 Sinus, fistula and cyst of branchial cleft
Branchial vestige

Q18.1 Preauricular sinus and cyst
Fistula of auricle, congenital
Cervicoaural fistula

Q18.2 Other branchial cleft malformations
Branchial cleft malformation NOS
Cervical auricle
Otocephaly

Q18.3 Webbing of neck
Pterygium colli
DEFINITION A thick flap of skin extending from the side of the neck to the shoulder, often in concert with other birth defects.

Q18.4 Macrostomia
DEFINITION Abnormally large mouth.

Q18.5 Microstomia
DEFINITION Abnormally small mouth.

Q18.6 Macrocheilia
Hypertrophy of lip, congenital
DEFINITION Abnormally large lips.

Q18.7 Microcheilia

Q18.8 Other specified congenital malformations of face and neck
Medial cyst of face and neck
Medial fistula of face and neck
Medial sinus of face and neck

Q18.9 Congenital malformation of face and neck, unspecified
Congenital anomaly NOS of face and neck

Congenital malformations of the circulatory system (Q20-Q28)

⊿ **Q20 Congenital malformations of cardiac chambers and connections**
EXCLUDES 1 *dextrocardia with situs inversus (Q89.3)*
mirror-image atrial arrangement with situs inversus (Q89.3)

● New ▲ Revised *Manifestation* ⊿-❼ Digit Indicators ⊟ Laterality Ⓐ Adult (15+ years) Ⓜ Maternity (12-55 years) Ⓝ Newborn Ⓟ Pediatric (0-17 years) ♂ Male ♀ Female
✖ ~~Deleted~~ Unspecified ➕ Additional code

Q20.0   Common arterial trunk
Persistent truncus arteriosus
EXCLUDES 1   *aortic septal defect (Q21.4)*

DEFINITION   Congenital anomaly in which there is abnormal communication between the ascending aorta and pulmonary artery, near the semilunar valve.

Q20.1   Double outlet right ventricle
Taussig-Bing syndrome

Q20.2   Double outlet left ventricle

Q20.3   Discordant ventriculoarterial connection
Dextrotransposition of aorta
Transposition of great vessels (complete)

Q20.4   Double inlet ventricle
Common ventricle
Cor triloculare biatriatum
Single ventricle
DEFINITION   No septum or membrane is present dividing the right ventricle from the left ventricle.

Q20.5   Discordant atrioventricular connection
Corrected transposition
Levotransposition
Ventricular inversion

Q20.6   Isomerism of atrial appendages
Isomerism of atrial appendages with asplenia or polysplenia

Q20.8   Other congenital malformations of cardiac chambers and connections
Cor binoculare

Q20.9   Congenital malformation of cardiac chambers and connections, unspecified

4 Q21   Congenital malformations of cardiac septa
EXCLUDES 1   *acquired cardiac septal defect (I51.0)*

Q21.0   Ventricular septal defect
Roger's disease

Ventricular septal defect

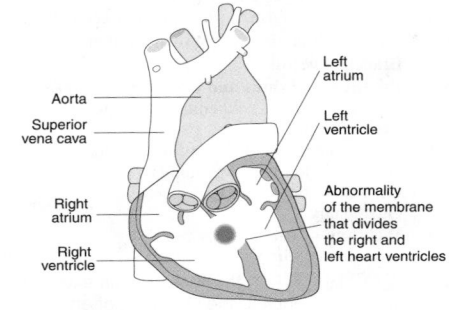

Aorta
Superior vena cava
Right atrium
Right ventricle
Left atrium
Left ventricle
Abnormality of the membrane that divides the right and left heart ventricles

Q21.1   Atrial septal defect
Coronary sinus defect
Patent or persistent foramen ovale
Patent or persistent ostium secundum defect (type II)
Patent or persistent sinus venosus defect

Q21.2   Atrioventricular septal defect
Common atrioventricular canal
Endocardial cushion defect
Ostium primum atrial septal defect (type I)

Q21.3   Tetralogy of Fallot
Ventricular septal defect with pulmonary stenosis or atresia, dextroposition of aorta and hypertrophy of right ventricle.
AHA: 3Q 2014, 17

Tetralogy of Fallot

Displacement of aorta over ventricular septal defect
Narrowing of the pulmonary valve
Ventricular septal defect—opening between the left and right ventricles
Thickening of wall of right ventricle

Q21.4   Aortopulmonary septal defect
Aortic septal defect
Aortopulmonary window

Q21.8   Other congenital malformations of cardiac septa
Eisenmenger's defect
Pentalogy of Fallot
EXCLUDES 1   *Eisenmenger's complex (I27.8)*
                   Eisenmenger's syndrome (I27.8)

Q21.9   Congenital malformation of cardiac septum, unspecified
Septal (heart) defect NOS

4 Q22   Congenital malformations of pulmonary and tricuspid valves

Q22.0   Pulmonary valve atresia
DEFINITION   Congenital absence of a normal valvular opening into the pulmonary artery.

Q22.1   Congenital pulmonary valve stenosis

Q22.2   Congenital pulmonary valve insufficiency
Congenital pulmonary valve regurgitation

Q22.3   Other congenital malformations of pulmonary valve
Congenital malformation of pulmonary valve NOS
Supernumerary cusps of pulmonary valve

Q22.4   Congenital tricuspid stenosis
Congenital tricuspid atresia
DEFINITION   Abnormal narrowing of the valve that prevents blood from flowing back into the right atrium from the right ventricle.

Q22.5   Ebstein's anomaly

Q22.6   Hypoplastic right heart syndrome

Q22.8   Other congenital malformations of tricuspid valve

Q22.9   Congenital malformation of tricuspid valve, unspecified

4 Q23   Congenital malformations of aortic and mitral valves

Q23.0   Congenital stenosis of aortic valve
Congenital aortic atresia
Congenital aortic stenosis NOS
EXCLUDES 1   *congenital stenosis of aortic valve in hypoplastic left heart syndrome (Q23.4)*
                   congenital subaortic stenosis (Q24.4)
                   supravalvular aortic stenosis (congenital) (Q25.3)

Q23.1   Congenital insufficiency of aortic valve
Bicuspid aortic valve
Congenital aortic insufficiency

Q23.2   Congenital mitral stenosis
Congenital mitral atresia

Congenital mitral stenosis

Aorta
Superior vena cava
Left atrium
Narrowed mitral valve
Left ventricle

● New   ▲ Revised   *Manifestation*   4 - 7 Digit Indicators   ▣ Laterality   Ⓐ Adult (15+ years)   Ⓜ Maternity (12-55 years)   Ⓝ Newborn   Ⓟ Pediatric (0-17 years)   ♂ Male   ♀ Female
✖ Deleted   Unspecified   + Additional code

884   © 2017 DecisionHealth   2017 ICD-10-CM Expert for Physicians

Q23.3 **Congenital mitral insufficiency**

Q23.4 **Hypoplastic left heart syndrome**

Q23.8 **Other congenital malformations of aortic and mitral valves**

Q23.9 **Congenital malformation of aortic and mitral valves, unspecified**

④ Q24 **Other congenital malformations of heart**

> **EXCLUDES 1** *endocardial fibroelastosis (I42.4)*

Q24.0 **Dextrocardia**

> **EXCLUDES 1** *dextrocardia with situs inversus (Q89.3)*
> *isomerism of atrial appendages (with asplenia or polysplenia) (Q20.6)*
> *mirror-image atrial arrangement with situs inversus (Q89.3)*

Q24.1 **Levocardia**

Q24.2 **Cor triatriatum**

> **DEFINITION** The heart has three atrial chambers with the left atrium divided into two segments.

Q24.3 **Pulmonary infundibular stenosis**
Subvalvular pulmonic stenosis

Q24.4 **Congenital subaortic stenosis**

Q24.5 **Malformation of coronary vessels**
Congenital coronary (artery) aneurysm

Q24.6 **Congenital heart block**

Q24.8 **Other specified congenital malformations of heart**
Congenital diverticulum of left ventricle
Congenital malformation of myocardium
Congenital malformation of pericardium
Malposition of heart
Uhl's disease

Q24.9 **Congenital malformation of heart, unspecified**
Congenital anomaly of heart
Congenital disease of heart

④ Q25 **Congenital malformations of great arteries**

> **CODING TIP ✓** If the condition has been corrected or is no longer a problem, then code Z87.74, personal history of (corrected) congenital malformations of heart and circulatory system.

Q25.0 **Patent ductus arteriosus**
Patent ductus Botallo
Persistent ductus arteriosus

▲ Q25.1 **Coarctation of aorta**
Coarctation of aorta (preductal) (postductal)
Stenosis of aorta

▲ ⑤ Q25.2 **Atresia of aorta**

● Q25.21 **Interruption of aortic arch**
Atresia of aortic arch

● Q25.29 **Other atresia of aorta**
Atresia of aorta

Q25.3 **Supravalvular aortic stenosis**

> **EXCLUDES 1** *congenital aortic stenosis NOS (Q23.0)*
> *congenital stenosis of aortic valve (Q23.0)*

▲ ⑤ Q25.4 **Other congenital malformations of aorta**

> **EXCLUDES 1** *hypoplasia of aorta in hypoplastic left heart syndrome (Q23.4)*

● Q25.40 **Congenital malformation of aorta unspecified**

● Q25.41 **Absence and aplasia of aorta**

● Q25.42 **Hypoplasia of aorta**

● Q25.43 **Congenital aneurysm of aorta**
Congenital aneurysm of aortic root
Congenital aneurysm of aortic sinus

● Q25.44 **Congenital dilation of aorta**

● Q25.45 **Double aortic arch**
Vascular ring of aorta

● Q25.46 **Tortuous aortic arch**
Persistent convolutions of aortic arch

● Q25.47 **Right aortic arch**
Persistent right aortic arch

● Q25.48 **Anomalous origin of subclavian artery**

● Q25.49 **Other congenital malformations of aorta**

Q25.5 **Atresia of pulmonary artery**

Q25.6 **Stenosis of pulmonary artery**
Supravalvular pulmonary stenosis

⑤ Q25.7 **Other congenital malformations of pulmonary artery**

Q25.71 **Coarctation of pulmonary artery**

Q25.72 **Congenital pulmonary arteriovenous malformation**
Congenital pulmonary arteriovenous aneurysm

Q25.79 **Other congenital malformations of pulmonary artery**
Aberrant pulmonary artery
Agenesis of pulmonary artery
Congenital aneurysm of pulmonary artery
Congenital anomaly of pulmonary artery
Hypoplasia of pulmonary artery

Q25.8 **Other congenital malformations of other great arteries**

Q25.9 **Congenital malformation of great arteries, unspecified**

④ Q26 **Congenital malformations of great veins**

Q26.0 **Congenital stenosis of vena cava**
Congenital stenosis of vena cava (inferior)(superior)

Q26.1 **Persistent left superior vena cava**

Q26.2 **Total anomalous pulmonary venous connection**
Total anomalous pulmonary venous return [TAPVR], subdiaphragmatic
Total anomalous pulmonary venous return [TAPVR], supradiaphragmatic

Q26.3 **Partial anomalous pulmonary venous connection**
Partial anomalous pulmonary venous return

Q26.4 **Anomalous pulmonary venous connection, unspecified**

Q26.5 **Anomalous portal venous connection**

Q26.6 **Portal vein-hepatic artery fistula**

Q26.8 **Other congenital malformations of great veins**
Absence of vena cava (inferior) (superior)
Azygos continuation of inferior vena cava
Persistent left posterior cardinal vein
Scimitar syndrome

Q26.9 **Congenital malformation of great vein, unspecified**
Congenital anomaly of vena cava (inferior) (superior) NOS

④ Q27 **Other congenital malformations of peripheral vascular system**

> **EXCLUDES 2** *anomalies of cerebral and precerebral vessels (Q28.0-Q28.3)*
> *anomalies of coronary vessels (Q24.5)*
> *anomalies of pulmonary artery (Q25.5-Q25.7)*
> *congenital retinal aneurysm (Q14.1)*
> *hemangioma and lymphangioma (D18.-)*

Q27.0 **Congenital absence and hypoplasia of umbilical artery**
Single umbilical artery

Q27.1 **Congenital renal artery stenosis**

Q27.2 **Other congenital malformations of renal artery**
Congenital malformation of renal artery NOS
Multiple renal arteries

⑤ Q27.3 **Arteriovenous malformation (peripheral)**
Arteriovenous aneurysm

> **EXCLUDES 1** *acquired arteriovenous aneurysm (I77.0)*

> **EXCLUDES 2** *arteriovenous malformation of cerebral vessels (Q28.2)*
> *arteriovenous malformation of precerebral vessels (Q28.0)*

Q27.30 **Arteriovenous malformation, site unspecified**

Q27.31 **Arteriovenous malformation of vessel of upper limb**

Q27.32 **Arteriovenous malformation of vessel of lower limb**

Q27.33 **Arteriovenous malformation of digestive system vessel**

Q27.34 **Arteriovenous malformation of renal vessel**

Q27.39 **Arteriovenous malformation, other site**

Q27.4 **Congenital phlebectasia**

Q27.8 **Other specified congenital malformations of peripheral vascular system**
Absence of peripheral vascular system
Atresia of peripheral vascular system
Congenital aneurysm (peripheral)
Congenital stricture, artery
Congenital varix

> **EXCLUDES 1** *arteriovenous malformation (Q27.3-)*

Q27.9 **Congenital malformation of peripheral vascular system, unspecified**
Anomaly of artery or vein NOS

● New ▲ Revised *Manifestation* ④-⑦ Digit Indicators ⊟ Laterality ⒶAdult (15+ years) ⓂMaternity (12-55 years) ⓃNewborn ⓅPediatric (0-17 years) ♂ Male ♀ Female
✖ Deleted Unspecified + Additional code

Q28   Other congenital malformations of circulatory system
> EXCLUDES 1   congenital aneurysm NOS (Q27.8)
> congenital coronary aneurysm (Q24.5)
> ruptured cerebral arteriovenous malformation (I60.8)
> ruptured malformation of precerebral vessels (I72.0)
> EXCLUDES 2   congenital peripheral aneurysm (Q27.8)
> congenital pulmonary aneurysm (Q25.79)
> congenital retinal aneurysm (Q14.1)

Q28.0   **Arteriovenous malformation of precerebral vessels**
Congenital arteriovenous precerebral aneurysm (nonruptured)

Q28.1   **Other malformations of precerebral vessels**
Congenital malformation of precerebral vessels NOS
Congenital precerebral aneurysm (nonruptured)

Q28.2   **Arteriovenous malformation of cerebral vessels**
Arteriovenous malformation of brain NOS
Congenital arteriovenous cerebral aneurysm (nonruptured)

Q28.3   **Other malformations of cerebral vessels**
Congenital cerebral aneurysm (nonruptured)
Congenital malformation of cerebral vessels NOS
Developmental venous anomaly

Q28.8   **Other specified congenital malformations of circulatory system**
Congenital aneurysm, specified site NEC
Spinal vessel anomaly

Q28.9   **Congenital malformation of circulatory system, unspecified**

Congenital malformations of the respiratory system (Q30-Q34)

Q30   Congenital malformations of nose
> EXCLUDES 1   congenital deviation of nasal septum (Q67.4)

Q30.0   **Choanal atresia**
Atresia of nares (anterior) (posterior)
Congenital stenosis of nares (anterior) (posterior)
> DEFINITION   Fetal nasal airways are obstructed by membranous or bony tissue; infant is unable to breathe and nurse simultaneously.

Q30.1   **Agenesis and underdevelopment of nose**
Congenital absent of nose

Q30.2   **Fissured, notched and cleft nose**

Q30.3   **Congenital perforated nasal septum**

Q30.8   **Other congenital malformations of nose**
Accessory nose
Congenital anomaly of nasal sinus wall

Q30.9   **Congenital malformation of nose, unspecified**

Q31   Congenital malformations of larynx
> EXCLUDES 1   congenital laryngeal stridor NOS (P28.89)

Q31.0   **Web of larynx**
Glottic web of larynx
Subglottic web of larynx
Web of larynx NOS

Q31.1   **Congenital subglottic stenosis**

Q31.2   **Laryngeal hypoplasia**

Q31.3   **Laryngocele**

Q31.5   **Congenital laryngomalacia**

Q31.8   **Other congenital malformations of larynx**
Absence of larynx
Agenesis of larynx
Atresia of larynx
Congenital cleft thyroid cartilage
Congenital fissure of epiglottis
Congenital stenosis of larynx NEC
Posterior cleft of cricoid cartilage

Q31.9   **Congenital malformation of larynx, unspecified**

Q32   Congenital malformations of trachea and bronchus
> EXCLUDES 1   congenital bronchiectasis (Q33.4)

Q32.0   **Congenital tracheomalacia**

Q32.1   **Other congenital malformations of trachea**
Atresia of trachea
Congenital anomaly of tracheal cartilage
Congenital dilatation of trachea
Congenital malformation of trachea
Congenital stenosis of trachea
Congenital tracheocele

Q32.2   **Congenital bronchomalacia**

Q32.3   **Congenital stenosis of bronchus**

Q32.4   **Other congenital malformations of bronchus**
Absence of bronchus
Agenesis of bronchus
Atresia of bronchus
Congenital diverticulum of bronchus
Congenital malformation of bronchus NOS

Q33   Congenital malformations of lung

Q33.0   **Congenital cystic lung**
Congenital cystic lung disease
Congenital honeycomb lung
Congenital polycystic lung disease
> EXCLUDES 1   cystic fibrosis (E84.0)
> cystic lung disease, acquired or unspecified (J98.4)

Q33.1   **Accessory lobe of lung**
Azygos lobe (fissured), lung

Q33.2   **Sequestration of lung**

Q33.3   **Agenesis of lung**
Congenital absence of lung (lobe)

Q33.4   **Congenital bronchiectasis**

Q33.5   **Ectopic tissue in lung**

Q33.6   **Congenital hypoplasia and dysplasia of lung**
> EXCLUDES 1   pulmonary hypoplasia associated with short gestation (P28.0)

Q33.8   **Other congenital malformations of lung**

Q33.9   **Congenital malformation of lung, unspecified**

Q34   Other congenital malformations of respiratory system
> EXCLUDES 2   congenital central alveolar hypoventilation syndrome (G47.35)

Q34.0   **Anomaly of pleura**

Q34.1   **Congenital cyst of mediastinum**

Q34.8   **Other specified congenital malformations of respiratory system**
Atresia of nasopharynx

Q34.9   **Congenital malformation of respiratory system, unspecified**
Congenital absence of respiratory system
Congenital anomaly of respiratory system NOS

Cleft lip and cleft palate (Q35-Q37)

Use additional code to identify associated malformation of the nose (Q30.2)
> EXCLUDES 1   Robin's syndrome (Q87.0)

Q35   Cleft palate
> INCLUDES   fissure of palate
> palatoschisis
> EXCLUDES 1   cleft palate with cleft lip (Q37.-)

Q35.1   **Cleft hard palate**

Q35.3   **Cleft soft palate**

Q35.5   **Cleft hard palate with cleft soft palate**

Q35.7   **Cleft uvula**

Q35.9   **Cleft palate, unspecified**
Cleft palate NOS
> DEFINITION   A congenital fissure in the roof of the mouth, resulting from incomplete fusion of the palate during embryonic development.

Q36   Cleft lip
> INCLUDES   cheiloschisis
> congenital fissure of lip
> harelip
> labium leporinum
> EXCLUDES 1   cleft lip with cleft palate (Q37.-)
> CODING TIP ✓   If the cleft palate/cleft lip has been corrected, use Z87.730, personal history of (corrected) congenital malformations of cleft lip and palate.

Q36.0   **Cleft lip, bilateral**

Q36.1   **Cleft lip, median**

Q36.9   **Cleft lip, unilateral**
Cleft lip NOS

Q37   Cleft palate with cleft lip
> INCLUDES   cheilopalatoschisis
> CODING TIP ✓   If the cleft palate/cleft lip has been corrected, use Z87.730, personal history of (corrected) congenital malformations of cleft lip and palate.

Q37.0   **Cleft hard palate with bilateral cleft lip**

● New   ▲ Revised   *Manifestation*   ◀-▶ Digit Indicators   ⊟ Laterality   ⓐ Adult (15+ years)   Ⓜ Maternity (12-55 years)   Ⓝ Newborn   Ⓟ Pediatric (0-17 years)   ♂ Male   ♀ Female
✖ Deleted   Unspecified   + Additional code

886   © 2017 DecisionHealth   2017 ICD-10-CM Expert for Physicians

Q28 — Q37.0

Q37.1   **Cleft hard palate with unilateral cleft lip**
          Cleft hard palate with cleft lip NOS
Q37.2   **Cleft soft palate with bilateral cleft lip**
Q37.3   **Cleft soft palate with unilateral cleft lip**
          Cleft soft palate with cleft lip NOS
Q37.4   **Cleft hard and soft palate with bilateral cleft lip**
Q37.5   **Cleft hard and soft palate with unilateral cleft lip**
          Cleft hard and soft palate with cleft lip NOS
Q37.8   **Unspecified cleft palate with bilateral cleft lip**
Q37.9   **Unspecified cleft palate with unilateral cleft lip**
          Cleft palate with cleft lip NOS

Cleft palate with unilateral cleft lip

Cleft lip   Cleft palate

Other congenital malformations of the digestive system (Q38-Q45)

Q38   Other congenital malformations of tongue, mouth and pharynx

> **EXCLUDES 1**   *dentofacial anomalies (M26.-)*
> *macrostomia (Q18.4)*
> *microstomia (Q18.5)*

Q38.0   **Congenital malformations of lips, not elsewhere classified**
          Congenital fistula of lip
          Congenital malformation of lip NOS
          Van der Woude's syndrome

> **EXCLUDES 1**   *cleft lip (Q36.-)*
> *cleft lip with cleft palate (Q37.-)*
> *macrocheilia (Q18.6)*
> *microcheilia (Q18.7)*

Q38.1   **Ankyloglossia**
          Tongue tie
Q38.2   **Macroglossia**
          Congenital hypertrophy of tongue

> **DEFINITION**   Congenital enlargement of the tongue.

Q38.3   **Other congenital malformations of tongue**
          Aglossia
          Bifid tongue
          Congenital adhesion of tongue
          Congenital fissure of tongue
          Congenital malformation of tongue NOS
          Double tongue
          Hypoglossia
          Hypoplasia of tongue
          Microglossia
Q38.4   **Congenital malformations of salivary glands and ducts**
          Atresia of salivary glands and ducts
          Congenital absence of salivary glands and ducts
          Congenital accessory salivary glands and ducts
          Congenital fistula of salivary gland

> **DEFINITION**   Congenital salivary gland fistula:
> Abnormal passage communicating with a salivary gland
> and present at birth.

Q38.5   **Congenital malformations of palate, not elsewhere classified**
          Congenital absence of uvula
          Congenital malformation of palate NOS
          Congenital high arched palate

> **EXCLUDES 1**   *cleft palate (Q35.-)*
> *cleft palate with cleft lip (Q37.-)*

Q38.6   **Other congenital malformations of mouth**
          Congenital malformation of mouth NOS
Q38.7   **Congenital pharyngeal pouch**
          Congenital diverticulum of pharynx

> **EXCLUDES 1**   *pharyngeal pouch syndrome (D82.1)*

Q38.8   **Other congenital malformations of pharynx**
          Congenital malformation of pharynx NOS
          Imperforate pharynx
Q39   Congenital malformations of esophagus
Q39.0   **Atresia of esophagus without fistula**
          Atresia of esophagus NOS
Q39.1   **Atresia of esophagus with tracheo-esophageal fistula**
          Atresia of esophagus with broncho-esophageal fistula

> **CODING TIP ✓**   Code Q39.1 is used for a congenital
> tracheoesophageal fistula [TE fistula]. A fistula as a
> complication of a tracheostomy is coded J95.04.

Q39.2   **Congenital tracheo-esophageal fistula without atresia**
          Congenital tracheo-esophageal fistula NOS
Q39.3   **Congenital stenosis and stricture of esophagus**
Q39.4   **Esophageal web**
Q39.5   **Congenital dilatation of esophagus**
          Congenital cardiospasm
Q39.6   **Congenital diverticulum of esophagus**
          Congenital esophageal pouch
Q39.8   **Other congenital malformations of esophagus**
          Congenital absence of esophagus
          Congenital displacement of esophagus
          Congenital duplication of esophagus
Q39.9   **Congenital malformation of esophagus, unspecified**
Q40   Other congenital malformations of upper alimentary tract
Q40.0   **Congenital hypertrophic pyloric stenosis**
          Congenital or infantile constriction
          Congenital or infantile hypertrophy
          Congenital or infantile spasm
          Congenital or infantile stenosis
          Congenital or infantile stricture

> **DEFINITION**   Congenital narrowing and partial
> obstruction of the gastric outlet due to muscular
> hypertrophy and mucosal edema of the ring-like muscle
> at the lower end of the stomach (pyloric orifice) in
> newborns.

Q40.1   **Congenital hiatus hernia**
          Congenital displacement of cardia through esophageal hiatus

> **EXCLUDES 1**   *congenital diaphragmatic hernia (Q79.0)*

Q40.2   **Other specified congenital malformations of stomach**
          Congenital displacement of stomach
          Congenital diverticulum of stomach
          Congenital hourglass stomach
          Congenital duplication of stomach
          Megalogastria
          Microgastria
Q40.3   **Congenital malformation of stomach, unspecified**
Q40.8   **Other specified congenital malformations of upper alimentary tract**
Q40.9   **Congenital malformation of upper alimentary tract, unspecified**

          Congenital anomaly of upper alimentary tract
          Congenital deformity of upper alimentary tract
Q41   Congenital absence, atresia and stenosis of small intestine

> **INCLUDES**   congenital obstruction, occlusion or stricture of
> small intestine or intestine NOS
> **EXCLUDES 1**   *cystic fibrosis with intestinal manifestation*
> *(E84.11)*
> *meconium ileus NOS (without cystic fibrosis)*
> *(P76.0)*

Q41.0   **Congenital absence, atresia and stenosis of duodenum**
Q41.1   **Congenital absence, atresia and stenosis of jejunum**
          Apple peel syndrome
          Imperforate jejunum
Q41.2   **Congenital absence, atresia and stenosis of ileum**
Q41.8   **Congenital absence, atresia and stenosis of other specified parts of small intestine**
Q41.9   **Congenital absence, atresia and stenosis of small intestine, part unspecified**

          Congenital absence, atresia and stenosis of intestine NOS
Q42   Congenital absence, atresia and stenosis of large intestine

> **INCLUDES**   congenital obstruction, occlusion and stricture of
> large intestine

Q42.0   **Congenital absence, atresia and stenosis of rectum with fistula**

● New   ▲ Revised   *Manifestation*   **◨-◮** Digit Indicators   ▤ Laterality   ▣ Adult   ▥ Maternity   ▨ Newborn   ▦ Pediatric   ♂ Male   ♀Female
✖ Deleted   Unspecified   ✚ Additional code   (15+ years)   (12-55 years)   (0-17 years)

Q42.1   **Congenital absence, atresia and stenosis of rectum without fistula**
Imperforate rectum

Q42.2   **Congenital absence, atresia and stenosis of anus with fistula**

Q42.3   **Congenital absence, atresia and stenosis of anus without fistula**
Imperforate anus

Q42.8   **Congenital absence, atresia and stenosis of other parts of large intestine**

Q42.9   **Congenital absence, atresia and stenosis of large intestine, part unspecified**

4 Q43   **Other congenital malformations of intestine**

Q43.0   **Meckel's diverticulum (displaced) (hypertrophic)**
Persistent omphalomesenteric duct
Persistent vitelline duct

Q43.1   **Hirschsprung's disease**
Aganglionosis
Congenital (aganglionic) megacolon

Q43.2   **Other congenital functional disorders of colon**
Congenital dilatation of colon

Q43.3   **Congenital malformations of intestinal fixation**
Congenital omental, anomalous adhesions [bands]
Congenital peritoneal adhesions [bands]
Incomplete rotation of cecum and colon
Insufficient rotation of cecum and colon
Jackson's membrane
Malrotation of colon
Rotation failure of cecum and colon
Universal mesentery

Q43.4   **Duplication of intestine**

Q43.5   **Ectopic anus**

Q43.6   **Congenital fistula of rectum and anus**
> **EXCLUDES 1**   *congenital fistula of anus with absence, atresia and stenosis (Q42.2)*
> *congenital fistula of rectum with absence, atresia and stenosis (Q42.0)*
> *congenital rectovaginal fistula (Q52.2)*
> *congenital urethrorectal fistula (Q64.73)*
> *pilonidal fistula or sinus (L05.-)*

Q43.7   **Persistent cloaca**
Cloaca NOS

Q43.8   **Other specified congenital malformations of intestine**
Congenital blind loop syndrome
Congenital diverticulitis, colon
Congenital diverticulum, intestine
Dolichocolon
Megaloappendix
Megaloduodenum
Microcolon
Transposition of appendix
Transposition of colon
Transposition of intestine
AHA: 2Q 2013, 31

Q43.9   **Congenital malformation of intestine, unspecified**

4 Q44   **Congenital malformations of gallbladder, bile ducts and liver**

Q44.0   **Agenesis, aplasia and hypoplasia of gallbladder**
Congenital absence of gallbladder

Q44.1   **Other congenital malformations of gallbladder**
Congenital malformation of gallbladder NOS
Intrahepatic gallbladder

Q44.2   **Atresia of bile ducts**

Q44.3   **Congenital stenosis and stricture of bile ducts**

Q44.4   **Choledochal cyst**

Q44.5   **Other congenital malformations of bile ducts**
Accessory hepatic duct
Biliary duct duplication
Congenital malformation of bile duct NOS
Cystic duct duplication

Q44.6   **Cystic disease of liver**
Fibrocystic disease of liver

Q44.7   **Other congenital malformations of liver**
Accessory liver
Alagille's syndrome
Congenital absence of liver
Congenital hepatomegaly
Congenital malformation of liver NOS

4 Q45   **Other congenital malformations of digestive system**
> **EXCLUDES 2**   *congenital diaphragmatic hernia (Q79.0)*
> *congenital hiatus hernia (Q40.1)*

Q45.0   **Agenesis, aplasia and hypoplasia of pancreas**
Congenital absence of pancreas

Q45.1   **Annular pancreas**

Q45.2   **Congenital pancreatic cyst**

Q45.3   **Other congenital malformations of pancreas and pancreatic duct**
Accessory pancreas
Congenital malformation of pancreas or pancreatic duct NOS
> **EXCLUDES 1**   *congenital diabetes mellitus (E10.-)*
> *cystic fibrosis (E84.0-E84.9)*
> *fibrocystic disease of pancreas (E84.-)*
> *neonatal diabetes mellitus (P70.2)*

Q45.8   **Other specified congenital malformations of digestive system**
Absence (complete) (partial) of alimentary tract NOS
Duplication of digestive system
Malposition, congenital of digestive system

Q45.9   **Congenital malformation of digestive system, unspecified**
Congenital anomaly of digestive system
Congenital deformity of digestive system

Congenital malformations of genital organs (Q50-Q56)

> **EXCLUDES 1**   *androgen insensitivity syndrome (E34.5-)*
> *syndromes associated with anomalies in the number and form of chromosomes (Q90-Q99)*

4 Q50   **Congenital malformations of ovaries, fallopian tubes and broad ligaments**

5 Q50.0   **Congenital absence of ovary**
> **EXCLUDES 1**   *Turner's syndrome (Q96.-)*

     Q50.01   **Congenital absence of ovary, unilateral** ♀

     Q50.02   **Congenital absence of ovary, bilateral** ♀

   Q50.1   **Developmental ovarian cyst** ♀

   Q50.2   **Congenital torsion of ovary** ♀

5 Q50.3   **Other congenital malformations of ovary**

     Q50.31   **Accessory ovary** ♀

     Q50.32   **Ovarian streak** ♀
46, XX with streak gonads

     Q50.39   **Other congenital malformation of ovary** ♀
Congenital malformation of ovary NOS

   Q50.4   **Embryonic cyst of fallopian tube** ♀
Fimbrial cyst

   Q50.5   **Embryonic cyst of broad ligament** ♀
Epoophoron cyst
Parovarian cyst

   Q50.6   **Other congenital malformations of fallopian tube and broad ligament** ♀
Absence of fallopian tube and broad ligament
Accessory fallopian tube and broad ligament
Atresia of fallopian tube and broad ligament
Congenital malformation of fallopian tube or broad ligament NOS

4 Q51   **Congenital malformations of uterus and cervix**

   Q51.0   **Agenesis and aplasia of uterus** ♀
Congenital absence of uterus

5 Q51.1   **Doubling of uterus with doubling of cervix and vagina**

● New   ▲ Revised   *Manifestation*   **4 - 7** Digit Indicators   ☰ Laterality   Ⓐ Adult (15+ years)   Ⓜ Maternity (12-55 years)   Ⓝ Newborn   Ⓟ Pediatric (0-17 years)   ♂ Male   ♀ Female
✖ Deleted   Unspecified   + Additional code

888   © 2017 DecisionHealth   2017 ICD-10-CM Expert for Physicians

Q51.10 **Doubling of uterus with doubling of cervix and vagina without obstruction** ♀
Doubling of uterus with doubling of cervix and vagina NOS

Bicornate uterus

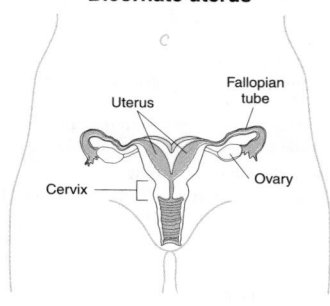

Q51.11 **Doubling of uterus with doubling of cervix and vagina with obstruction** ♀

Q51.2 **Other doubling of uterus** ♀
Doubling of uterus NOS
Septate uterus, complete or partial

Q51.3 **Bicornate uterus** ♀
Bicornate uterus, complete or partial

Q51.4 **Unicornate uterus** ♀
Unicornate uterus with or without a separate uterine horn
Uterus with only one functioning horn

Q51.5 **Agenesis and aplasia of cervix** ♀
Congenital absence of cervix

Q51.6 **Embryonic cyst of cervix** ♀

Q51.7 **Congenital fistulae between uterus and digestive and urinary tracts** ♀

⑤ Q51.8 **Other congenital malformations of uterus and cervix**

⑥ Q51.81 **Other congenital malformations of uterus**

Q51.810 **Arcuate uterus** ♀
Arcuatus uterus

Q51.811 **Hypoplasia of uterus** ♀

Q51.818 **Other congenital malformations of uterus** ♀
Müllerian anomaly of uterus NEC

⑥ Q51.82 **Other congenital malformations of cervix**

Q51.820 **Cervical duplication** ♀

Q51.821 **Hypoplasia of cervix** ♀

Q51.828 **Other congenital malformations of cervix** ♀

Q51.9 **Congenital malformation of uterus and cervix, unspecified** ♀

④ Q52 **Other congenital malformations of female genitalia**

Q52.0 **Congenital absence of vagina** ♀
Vaginal agenesis, total or partial

⑤ Q52.1 **Doubling of vagina**

> **EXCLUDES 1** *doubling of vagina with doubling of uterus and cervix (Q51.1-)*

Q52.10 **Doubling of vagina, unspecified** ♀
Septate vagina NOS

Q52.11 **Transverse vaginal septum** ♀

▲⑥ Q52.12 **Longitudinal vaginal septum**

● Q52.120 **Longitudinal vaginal septum, nonobstructing** ♀

●⊟ Q52.121 **Longitudinal vaginal septum, obstructing, right side** ♀

●⊟ Q52.122 **Longitudinal vaginal septum, obstructing, left side** ♀

●⊟ Q52.123 **Longitudinal vaginal septum, microperforate, right side** ♀

●⊟ Q52.124 **Longitudinal vaginal septum, microperforate, left side** ♀

● Q52.129 **Other and unspecified longitudinal vaginal septum** ♀

Q52.2 **Congenital rectovaginal fistula** ♀

> **EXCLUDES 1** *cloaca (Q43.7)*

Q52.3 **Imperforate hymen** ♀

Q52.4 **Other congenital malformations of vagina** ♀
Canal of Nuck cyst, congenital
Congenital malformation of vagina NOS
Embryonic vaginal cyst
Gartner's duct cyst

Q52.5 **Fusion of labia** ♀

Q52.6 **Congenital malformation of clitoris** ♀

⑤ Q52.7 **Other and unspecified congenital malformations of vulva**

Q52.70 **Unspecified congenital malformations of vulva** ♀
Congenital malformation of vulva NOS

Q52.71 **Congenital absence of vulva** ♀

Q52.79 **Other congenital malformations of vulva** ♀
Congenital cyst of vulva

Q52.8 **Other specified congenital malformations of female genitalia** ♀

Q52.9 **Congenital malformation of female genitalia, unspecified** ♀

④ Q53 **Undescended and ectopic testicle**

⑤ Q53.0 **Ectopic testis**

Q53.00 **Ectopic testis, unspecified** ♂

Q53.01 **Ectopic testis, unilateral** ♂

Q53.02 **Ectopic testes, bilateral** ♂

⑤ Q53.1 **Undescended testicle, unilateral**

Q53.10 **Unspecified undescended testicle, unilateral** ♂

Q53.11 **Abdominal testis, unilateral** ♂

Q53.12 **Ectopic perineal testis, unilateral** ♂

⑤ Q53.2 **Undescended testicle, bilateral**

Q53.20 **Undescended testicle, unspecified, bilateral** ♂

Q53.21 **Abdominal testis, bilateral** ♂

Q53.22 **Ectopic perineal testis, bilateral** ♂

Q53.9 **Undescended testicle, unspecified** ♂
Cryptorchism NOS

④ Q54 **Hypospadias**

> **EXCLUDES 1** *epispadias (Q64.0)*

> **CODING TIP ✓** Use category Q54 when hypospadias is still present. If the condition has been corrected, then code Z87.710, personal history of hypospadias.

Q54.0 **Hypospadias, balanic** ♂
Hypospadias, coronal
Hypospadias, glandular

Q54.1 **Hypospadias, penile** ♂

Q54.2 **Hypospadias, penoscrotal** ♂

Q54.3 **Hypospadias, perineal** ♂

Q54.4 **Congenital chordee** ♂
Chordee without hypospadias

> **DEFINITION** Abnormal downward or upward bowing of the penis, due to a congenital anomaly.

Q54.8 **Other hypospadias** ♂
Hypospadias with intersex state

Q54.9 **Hypospadias, unspecified** ♂

④ Q55 **Other congenital malformations of male genital organs**

> **EXCLUDES 1** *congenital hydrocele (P83.5)*
> *hypospadias (Q54.-)*

Q55.0 **Absence and aplasia of testis** ♂
Monorchism

Q55.1 **Hypoplasia of testis and scrotum** ♂
Fusion of testes

⑤ Q55.2 **Other and unspecified congenital malformations of testis and scrotum**

Q55.20 **Unspecified congenital malformations of testis and scrotum** ♂
Congenital malformation of testis or scrotum NOS

Q55.21 **Polyorchism** ♂

Q55.22 **Retractile testis** ♂

Q55.23 **Scrotal transposition** ♂

Q55.29 **Other congenital malformations of testis and scrotum** ♂

Q55.3 **Atresia of vas deferens** ♂
Code first:
any associated cystic fibrosis (E84.-)

● New ▲ Revised *Manifestation* ④-⑦ Digit Indicators ⊟ Laterality Ⓐ Adult (15+ years) Ⓜ Maternity (12-55 years) Ⓝ Newborn Ⓟ Pediatric (0-17 years) ♂ Male ♀ Female
✖ Deleted Unspecified ✚ Additional code

2017 ICD-10-CM Expert for Physicians

© 2017 DecisionHealth

889

Q55.4   **Other congenital malformations of vas deferens, epididymis, seminal vesicles and prostate**   ♂
Absence or aplasia of prostate
Absence or aplasia of spermatic cord
Congenital malformation of vas deferens, epididymis, seminal vesicles or prostate NOS

Q55.5   **Congenital absence and aplasia of penis**   ♂

Ⓢ **Q55.6**   **Other congenital malformations of penis**

   Q55.61   **Curvature of penis (lateral)**   ♂

   Q55.62   **Hypoplasia of penis**   ♂
   Micropenis

   Q55.63   **Congenital torsion of penis**   ♂
       EXCLUDES 1   *acquired torsion of penis (N48.82)*

   Q55.64   **Hidden penis**   ♂
   Buried penis
   Concealed penis
       EXCLUDES 1   *acquired buried penis (N48.83)*

   Q55.69   **Other congenital malformation of penis**   ♂
   Congenital malformation of penis NOS

Q55.7   **Congenital vasocutaneous fistula**   ♂

Q55.8   **Other specified congenital malformations of male genital organs**   ♂

Q55.9   **Congenital malformation of male genital organ, unspecified**   ♂
Congenital anomaly of male genital organ
Congenital deformity of male genital organ

④ **Q56**   **Indeterminate sex and pseudohermaphroditism**
     EXCLUDES 1   *46,XX true hermaphrodite (Q99.1)*
         androgen insensitivity syndrome (E34.5-)
         chimera 46,XX/46,XY true hermaphrodite (Q99.0)
         female pseudohermaphroditism with adrenocortical disorder (E25.-)
         pseudohermaphroditism with specified chromosomal anomaly (Q96-Q99)
         pure gonadal dysgenesis (Q99.1)

Q56.0   **Hermaphroditism, not elsewhere classified**
Ovotestis

Q56.1   **Male pseudohermaphroditism, not elsewhere classified**   ♂
46, XY with streak gonads
Male pseudohermaphroditism NOS

Q56.2   **Female pseudohermaphroditism, not elsewhere classified**   ♀
Female pseudohermaphroditism NOS

Q56.3   **Pseudohermaphroditism, unspecified**

Q56.4   **Indeterminate sex, unspecified**
Ambiguous genitalia

Congenital malformations of the urinary system (Q60-Q64)

④ **Q60**   **Renal agenesis and other reduction defects of kidney**
     INCLUDES   congenital absence of kidney
         congenital atrophy of kidney
         infantile atrophy of kidney

Q60.0   **Renal agenesis, unilateral**

Q60.1   **Renal agenesis, bilateral**

Q60.2   **Renal agenesis, unspecified**

Q60.3   **Renal hypoplasia, unilateral**

Q60.4   **Renal hypoplasia, bilateral**

Q60.5   **Renal hypoplasia, unspecified**

Q60.6   **Potter's syndrome**

④ **Q61**   **Cystic kidney disease**
     EXCLUDES 1   *acquired cyst of kidney (N28.1)*
         Potter's syndrome (Q60.6)

Ⓢ **Q61.0**   **Congenital renal cyst**

   Q61.00   **Congenital renal cyst, unspecified**
   Cyst of kidney NOS (congenital)

   Q61.01   **Congenital single renal cyst**

   Q61.02   **Congenital multiple renal cysts**

Ⓢ **Q61.1**   **Polycystic kidney, infantile type**
Polycystic kidney, autosomal recessive

   Q61.11   **Cystic dilatation of collecting ducts**

   Q61.19   **Other polycystic kidney, infantile type**

Q61.2   **Polycystic kidney, adult type**
Polycystic kidney, autosomal dominant

Q61.3   **Polycystic kidney, unspecified**

Q61.4   **Renal dysplasia**
Multicystic dysplastic kidney
Multicystic kidney (development)
Multicystic kidney disease
Multicystic renal dysplasia
     EXCLUDES 1   *polycystic kidney disease (Q61.11-Q61.3)*

Q61.5   **Medullary cystic kidney**
Nephronopthisis
Sponge kidney NOS

Q61.8   **Other cystic kidney diseases**
Fibrocystic kidney
Fibrocystic renal degeneration or disease

Q61.9   **Cystic kidney disease, unspecified**
Meckel-Gruber syndrome

④ **Q62**   **Congenital obstructive defects of renal pelvis and congenital malformations of ureter**

Q62.0   **Congenital hydronephrosis**

Ⓢ **Q62.1**   **Congenital occlusion of ureter**
Atresia and stenosis of ureter

   Q62.10   **Congenital occlusion of ureter, unspecified**

   Q62.11   **Congenital occlusion of ureteropelvic junction**

   Q62.12   **Congenital occlusion of ureterovesical orifice**

Q62.2   **Congenital megaureter**
Congenital dilatation of ureter

Ⓢ **Q62.3**   **Other obstructive defects of renal pelvis and ureter**

   Q62.31   **Congenital ureterocele, orthotopic**

   Q62.32   **Cecoureterocele**
   Ectopic ureterocele

   Q62.39   **Other obstructive defects of renal pelvis and ureter**
   Ureteropelvic junction obstruction NOS

Q62.4   **Agenesis of ureter**
Congenital absence ureter

Q62.5   **Duplication of ureter**
Accessory ureter
Double ureter

Ⓢ **Q62.6**   **Malposition of ureter**

   Q62.60   **Malposition of ureter, unspecified**

   Q62.61   **Deviation of ureter**

   Q62.62   **Displacement of ureter**

   Q62.63   **Anomalous implantation of ureter**
   Ectopia of ureter
   Ectopic ureter

   Q62.69   **Other malposition of ureter**

Q62.7   **Congenital vesico-uretero-renal reflux**

Q62.8   **Other congenital malformations of ureter**
Anomaly of ureter NOS

④ **Q63**   **Other congenital malformations of kidney**
     EXCLUDES 1   *congenital nephrotic syndrome (N04.-)*

Q63.0   **Accessory kidney**

Q63.1   **Lobulated, fused and horseshoe kidney**

Q63.2   **Ectopic kidney**
Congenital displaced kidney
Malrotation of kidney

Q63.3   **Hyperplastic and giant kidney**
Compensatory hypertrophy of kidney

Q63.8   **Other specified congenital malformations of kidney**
Congenital renal calculi

Q63.9   **Congenital malformation of kidney, unspecified**

④ **Q64**   **Other congenital malformations of urinary system**

Q64.0   **Epispadias**   ♂
     EXCLUDES 1   *hypospadias (Q54.-)*
     DEFINITION   A rare, congenital defect in which the urethra typically opens on the upper penile surface in boys, although, the urethral opening may also be positioned in the abdomen.

Ⓢ **Q64.1**   **Exstrophy of urinary bladder**

   Q64.10   **Exstrophy of urinary bladder, unspecified**
   Ectopia vesicae

   Q64.11   **Supravesical fissure of urinary bladder**

   Q64.12   **Cloacal extrophy of urinary bladder**

   Q64.19   **Other exstrophy of urinary bladder**
   Extroversion of bladder

Q64.2   **Congenital posterior urethral valves**

Ⓢ **Q64.3**   **Other atresia and stenosis of urethra and bladder neck**

   Q64.31   **Congenital bladder neck obstruction**
   Congenital obstruction of vesicourethral orifice

● New   ▲ Revised   *Manifestation*   ④-⑦ Digit Indicators   ▣ Laterality   Ⓐ Adult (15+ years)   Ⓜ Maternity (12-55 years)   Ⓝ Newborn   Ⓟ Pediatric (0-17 years)   ♂ Male   ♀ Female
✖ Deleted   Unspecified   ✦ Additional code

Q64.32   **Congenital stricture of urethra**

Q64.33   **Congenital stricture of urinary meatus**

Q64.39   **Other atresia and stenosis of urethra and bladder neck**

Atresia and stenosis of urethra and bladder neck NOS

Q64.4   **Malformation of urachus**

Cyst of urachus

Patent urachus

Prolapse of urachus

Q64.5   **Congenital absence of bladder and urethra**

Q64.6   **Congenital diverticulum of bladder**

5 Q64.7   **Other and unspecified congenital malformations of bladder and urethra**

> **EXCLUDES 1**   *congenital prolapse of bladder (mucosa) (Q79.4)*

Q64.70   **Unspecified congenital malformation of bladder and urethra**

Malformation of bladder or urethra NOS

Q64.71   **Congenital prolapse of urethra**

Q64.72   **Congenital prolapse of urinary meatus**

Q64.73   **Congenital urethrorectal fistula**

Q64.74   **Double urethra**

Q64.75   **Double urinary meatus**

Q64.79   **Other congenital malformations of bladder and urethra**

Q64.8   **Other specified congenital malformations of urinary system**

Q64.9   **Congenital malformation of urinary system, unspecified**

Congenital anomaly NOS of urinary system

Congenital deformity NOS of urinary system

Congenital malformations and deformations of the musculoskeletal system (Q65-Q79)

4 Q65   **Congenital deformities of hip**

> **EXCLUDES 1**   *clicking hip (R29.4)*

5 Q65.0   **Congenital dislocation of hip, unilateral**

Q65.00   **Congenital dislocation of unspecified hip, unilateral**

Q65.01   **Congenital dislocation of right hip, unilateral**

Q65.02   **Congenital dislocation of left hip, unilateral**

Q65.1   **Congenital dislocation of hip, bilateral**

Q65.2   **Congenital dislocation of hip, unspecified**

5 Q65.3   **Congenital partial dislocation of hip, unilateral**

Q65.30   **Congenital partial dislocation of unspecified hip, unilateral**

Q65.31   **Congenital partial dislocation of right hip, unilateral**

Q65.32   **Congenital partial dislocation of left hip, unilateral**

Q65.4   **Congenital partial dislocation of hip, bilateral**

Q65.5   **Congenital partial dislocation of hip, unspecified**

Q65.6   **Congenital unstable hip**

Congenital dislocatable hip

5 Q65.8   **Other congenital deformities of hip**

Q65.81   **Congenital coxa valga**

Q65.82   **Congenital coxa vara**

Q65.89   **Other specified congenital deformities of hip**

Anteversion of femoral neck

Congenital acetabular dysplasia

Q65.9   **Congenital deformity of hip, unspecified**

4 Q66   **Congenital deformities of feet**

> **EXCLUDES 1**   *reduction defects of feet (Q72.-)*
> *valgus deformities (acquired) (M21.0-)*
> *varus deformities (acquired) (M21.1-)*

Q66.0   **Congenital talipes equinovarus**

Congenital talipes equinovarus

Normal   Clubfoot

Q66.1   **Congenital talipes calcaneovarus**

▲ 5 Q66.2   **Congenital metatarsus (primus) varus**

● Q66.21   **Congenital metatarsus primus varus**

● Q66.22   **Congenital metatarsus adductus**

Congenital metatarsus varus

Q66.3   **Other congenital varus deformities of feet**

Hallux varus, congenital

Q66.4   **Congenital talipes calcaneovalgus**

5 Q66.5   **Congenital pes planus**

Congenital flat foot

Congenital rigid flat foot

Congenital spastic (everted) flat foot

> **EXCLUDES 1**   *pes planus, acquired (M21.4)*

Q66.50   **Congenital pes planus, unspecified foot**

Q66.51   **Congenital pes planus, right foot**

Q66.52   **Congenital pes planus, left foot**

Q66.6   **Other congenital valgus deformities of feet**

Congenital metatarsus valgus

Q66.7   **Congenital pes cavus**

5 Q66.8   **Other congenital deformities of feet**

Q66.80   **Congenital vertical talus deformity, unspecified foot**

Q66.81   **Congenital vertical talus deformity, right foot**

Q66.82   **Congenital vertical talus deformity, left foot**

Q66.89   **Other specified congenital deformities of feet**

Congenital asymmetric talipes

Congenital clubfoot NOS

Congenital talipes NOS

Congenital tarsal coalition

Hammer toe, congenital

Q66.9   **Congenital deformity of feet, unspecified**

4 Q67   **Congenital musculoskeletal deformities of head, face, spine and chest**

> **EXCLUDES 1**   *congenital malformation syndromes classified to Q87.-*
> *Potter's syndrome (Q60.6)*

Q67.0   **Congenital facial asymmetry**

Q67.1   **Congenital compression facies**

Q67.2   **Dolichocephaly**

Q67.3   **Plagiocephaly**

Q67.4   **Other congenital deformities of skull, face and jaw**

Congenital depressions in skull

Congenital hemifacial atrophy or hypertrophy

Deviation of nasal septum, congenital

Squashed or bent nose, congenital

> **EXCLUDES 1**   *dentofacial anomalies [including malocclusion] (M26.-)*
> *syphilitic saddle nose (A50.5)*

Q67.5   **Congenital deformity of spine**

Congenital postural scoliosis

Congenital scoliosis NOS

> **EXCLUDES 1**   *infantile idiopathic scoliosis (M41.0)*
> *scoliosis due to congenital bony malformation (Q76.3)*

AHA: 4Q 2014, 26

Q67.6   **Pectus excavatum**

Congenital funnel chest

Q67.7   **Pectus carinatum**

Congenital pigeon chest

> **DEFINITION**   A protrusion deformity of the chest wall in which the sternum and ribs are prominent, due to obstruction of infantile respiration or to rickets.

● New   ▲ Revised   *Manifestation*   4-7 Digit Indicators   ☐ Laterality   A Adult (15+ years)   M Maternity (12-55 years)   N Newborn   P Pediatric (0-17 years)   ♂ Male   ♀ Female

✖ Deleted   Unspecified   + Additional code

2017 ICD-10-CM Expert for Physicians   © 2017 DecisionHealth   891

Q67.8   **Other congenital deformities of chest**
Congenital deformity of chest wall NOS

⬛ Q68   **Other congenital musculoskeletal deformities**

> **EXCLUDES 1** *reduction defects of limb (s) (Q71-Q73)*
>
> **EXCLUDES 2** *congenital myotonic chondrodystrophy (G71.13)*

Q68.0   **Congenital deformity of sternocleidomastoid muscle**
Congenital contracture of sternocleidomastoid (muscle)
Congenital (sternomastoid) torticollis
Sternomastoid tumor (congenital)

Q68.1   **Congenital deformity of finger(s) and hand**
Congenital clubfinger
Spade-like hand (congenital)

Q68.2   **Congenital deformity of knee**
Congenital dislocation of knee
Congenital genu recurvatum

Q68.3   **Congenital bowing of femur**

> **EXCLUDES 1** *anteversion of femur (neck) (Q65.89)*

Q68.4   **Congenital bowing of tibia and fibula**

Q68.5   **Congenital bowing of long bones of leg, unspecified**

Q68.6   **Discoid meniscus**

Q68.8   **Other specified congenital musculoskeletal deformities**
Congenital deformity of clavicle
Congenital deformity of elbow
Congenital deformity of forearm
Congenital deformity of scapula
Congenital deformity of wrist
Congenital dislocation of elbow
Congenital dislocation of shoulder
Congenital dislocation of wrist

⬛ Q69   **Polydactyly**

Q69.0   **Accessory finger(s)**

Q69.1   **Accessory thumb(s)**

Q69.2   **Accessory toe(s)**
Accessory hallux

Q69.9   **Polydactyly, unspecified**
Supernumerary digit(s) NOS

> **DEFINITION** An extra number of digits on a hand or foot.

⬛ Q70   **Syndactyly**

Q70.0   **Fused fingers**
Complex syndactyly of fingers with synostosis
- **Q70.00**   **Fused fingers, unspecified hand**
- **Q70.01**   **Fused fingers, right hand**
- **Q70.02**   **Fused fingers, left hand**
- **Q70.03**   **Fused fingers, bilateral**

Q70.1   **Webbed fingers**
Simple syndactyly of fingers without synostosis
- **Q70.10**   **Webbed fingers, unspecified hand**
- **Q70.11**   **Webbed fingers, right hand**
- **Q70.12**   **Webbed fingers, left hand**
- **Q70.13**   **Webbed fingers, bilateral**

Q70.2   **Fused toes**
Complex syndactyly of toes with synostosis
- **Q70.20**   **Fused toes, unspecified foot**
- **Q70.21**   **Fused toes, right foot**
- **Q70.22**   **Fused toes, left foot**
- **Q70.23**   **Fused toes, bilateral**

Q70.3   **Webbed toes**
Simple syndactyly of toes without synostosis
- **Q70.30**   **Webbed toes, unspecified foot**
- **Q70.31**   **Webbed toes, right foot**
- **Q70.32**   **Webbed toes, left foot**
- **Q70.33**   **Webbed toes, bilateral**

Q70.4   **Polysyndactyly, unspecified**

> **EXCLUDES 1** *specified syndactyly of hand and feet - code to specified conditions (Q70.0- -Q70.3-)*

Q70.9   **Syndactyly, unspecified**
Symphalangy NOS

> **DEFINITION** Partial or total webbing connecting two or more fingers or toes; may involve skin/soft tissue only or include fusion of bone.

⬛ Q71   **Reduction defects of upper limb**

Q71.0   **Congenital complete absence of upper limb**
- **Q71.00**   **Congenital complete absence of unspecified upper limb**
- **Q71.01**   **Congenital complete absence of right upper limb**
- **Q71.02**   **Congenital complete absence of left upper limb**
- **Q71.03**   **Congenital complete absence of upper limb, bilateral**

Q71.1   **Congenital absence of upper arm and forearm with hand present**
- **Q71.10**   **Congenital absence of unspecified upper arm and forearm with hand present**
- **Q71.11**   **Congenital absence of right upper arm and forearm with hand present**
- **Q71.12**   **Congenital absence of left upper arm and forearm with hand present**
- **Q71.13**   **Congenital absence of upper arm and forearm with hand present, bilateral**

Q71.2   **Congenital absence of both forearm and hand**
- **Q71.20**   **Congenital absence of both forearm and hand, unspecified upper limb**
- **Q71.21**   **Congenital absence of both forearm and hand, right upper limb**
- **Q71.22**   **Congenital absence of both forearm and hand, left upper limb**
- **Q71.23**   **Congenital absence of both forearm and hand, bilateral**

Q71.3   **Congenital absence of hand and finger**
- **Q71.30**   **Congenital absence of unspecified hand and finger**
- **Q71.31**   **Congenital absence of right hand and finger**
- **Q71.32**   **Congenital absence of left hand and finger**
- **Q71.33**   **Congenital absence of hand and finger, bilateral**

Q71.4   **Longitudinal reduction defect of radius**
Clubhand (congenital)
Radial clubhand
- **Q71.40**   **Longitudinal reduction defect of unspecified radius**
- **Q71.41**   **Longitudinal reduction defect of right radius**
- **Q71.42**   **Longitudinal reduction defect of left radius**
- **Q71.43**   **Longitudinal reduction defect of radius, bilateral**

Q71.5   **Longitudinal reduction defect of ulna**
- **Q71.50**   **Longitudinal reduction defect of unspecified ulna**
- **Q71.51**   **Longitudinal reduction defect of right ulna**
- **Q71.52**   **Longitudinal reduction defect of left ulna**
- **Q71.53**   **Longitudinal reduction defect of ulna, bilateral**

Q71.6   **Lobster-claw hand**
- **Q71.60**   **Lobster-claw hand, unspecified hand**
- **Q71.61**   **Lobster-claw right hand**
- **Q71.62**   **Lobster-claw left hand**
- **Q71.63**   **Lobster-claw hand, bilateral**

Q71.8   **Other reduction defects of upper limb**
- **Q71.81**   **Congenital shortening of upper limb**
  - **Q71.811**   **Congenital shortening of right upper limb**
  - **Q71.812**   **Congenital shortening of left upper limb**
  - **Q71.813**   **Congenital shortening of upper limb, bilateral**
  - **Q71.819**   **Congenital shortening of unspecified upper limb**
- **Q71.89**   **Other reduction defects of upper limb**
  - **Q71.891**   **Other reduction defects of right upper limb**
  - **Q71.892**   **Other reduction defects of left upper limb**
  - **Q71.893**   **Other reduction defects of upper limb, bilateral**
  - **Q71.899**   **Other reduction defects of unspecified upper limb**

Q71.9   **Unspecified reduction defect of upper limb**
- **Q71.90**   **Unspecified reduction defect of unspecified upper limb**
- **Q71.91**   **Unspecified reduction defect of right upper limb**
- **Q71.92**   **Unspecified reduction defect of left upper limb**
- **Q71.93**   **Unspecified reduction defect of upper limb, bilateral**

⬛ Q72   **Reduction defects of lower limb**

Q72.0   **Congenital complete absence of lower limb**
- **Q72.00**   **Congenital complete absence of unspecified lower limb**
- **Q72.01**   **Congenital complete absence of right lower limb**
- **Q72.02**   **Congenital complete absence of left lower limb**
- **Q72.03**   **Congenital complete absence of lower limb, bilateral**

Q72.1   **Congenital absence of thigh and lower leg with foot present**

● New   ▲ Revised   *Manifestation*   ⬛-⬛ Digit Indicators   Laterality   A Adult (15+ years)   M Maternity (12-55 years)   N Newborn   P Pediatric (0-17 years)   ♂ Male   ♀ Female
✖ Deleted   Unspecified   ✚ Additional code

⊟ Q72.10   **Congenital absence of unspecified thigh and lower leg with foot present**

⊟ Q72.11   **Congenital absence of right thigh and lower leg with foot present**

⊟ Q72.12   **Congenital absence of left thigh and lower leg with foot present**

⊟ Q72.13   **Congenital absence of thigh and lower leg with foot present, bilateral**

⑤ Q72.2   **Congenital absence of both lower leg and foot**

⊟ Q72.20   **Congenital absence of both lower leg and foot, unspecified lower limb**

⊟ Q72.21   **Congenital absence of both lower leg and foot, right lower limb**

⊟ Q72.22   **Congenital absence of both lower leg and foot, left lower limb**

⊟ Q72.23   **Congenital absence of both lower leg and foot, bilateral**

⑤ Q72.3   **Congenital absence of foot and toe(s)**

⊟ Q72.30   **Congenital absence of unspecified foot and toe(s)**

⊟ Q72.31   **Congenital absence of right foot and toe(s)**

⊟ Q72.32   **Congenital absence of left foot and toe(s)**

⊟ Q72.33   **Congenital absence of foot and toe(s), bilateral**

⑤ Q72.4   **Longitudinal reduction defect of femur**
Proximal femoral focal deficiency

⊟ Q72.40   **Longitudinal reduction defect of unspecified femur**

⊟ Q72.41   **Longitudinal reduction defect of right femur**

⊟ Q72.42   **Longitudinal reduction defect of left femur**

⊟ Q72.43   **Longitudinal reduction defect of femur, bilateral**

⑤ Q72.5   **Longitudinal reduction defect of tibia**

⊟ Q72.50   **Longitudinal reduction defect of unspecified tibia**

⊟ Q72.51   **Longitudinal reduction defect of right tibia**

⊟ Q72.52   **Longitudinal reduction defect of left tibia**

⊟ Q72.53   **Longitudinal reduction defect of tibia, bilateral**

⑤ Q72.6   **Longitudinal reduction defect of fibula**

⊟ Q72.60   **Longitudinal reduction defect of unspecified fibula**

⊟ Q72.61   **Longitudinal reduction defect of right fibula**

⊟ Q72.62   **Longitudinal reduction defect of left fibula**

⊟ Q72.63   **Longitudinal reduction defect of fibula, bilateral**

⑤ Q72.7   **Split foot**

⊟ Q72.70   **Split foot, unspecified lower limb**

⊟ Q72.71   **Split foot, right lower limb**

⊟ Q72.72   **Split foot, left lower limb**

⊟ Q72.73   **Split foot, bilateral**

⑤ Q72.8   **Other reduction defects of lower limb**

⑥ Q72.81   **Congenital shortening of lower limb**

⊟ Q72.811   **Congenital shortening of right lower limb**

⊟ Q72.812   **Congenital shortening of left lower limb**

⊟ Q72.813   **Congenital shortening of lower limb, bilateral**

⊟ Q72.819   **Congenital shortening of unspecified lower limb**

⑥ Q72.89   **Other reduction defects of lower limb**

⊟ Q72.891   **Other reduction defects of right lower limb**

⊟ Q72.892   **Other reduction defects of left lower limb**

⊟ Q72.893   **Other reduction defects of lower limb, bilateral**

⊟ Q72.899   **Other reduction defects of unspecified lower limb**

⑤ Q72.9   **Unspecified reduction defect of lower limb**

⊟ Q72.90   **Unspecified reduction defect of unspecified lower limb**

⊟ Q72.91   **Unspecified reduction defect of right lower limb**

⊟ Q72.92   **Unspecified reduction defect of left lower limb**

⊟ Q72.93   **Unspecified reduction defect of lower limb, bilateral**

④ **Q73**   **Reduction defects of unspecified limb**

Q73.0   **Congenital absence of unspecified limb(s)**
Amelia NOS

Q73.1   **Phocomelia, unspecified limb(s)**
Phocomelia NOS

Q73.8   **Other reduction defects of unspecified limb(s)**
Longitudinal reduction deformity of unspecified limb(s)
Ectromelia of limb NOS
Hemimelia of limb NOS
Reduction defect of limb NOS

④ **Q74**   **Other congenital malformations of limb(s)**

EXCLUDES 1   *polydactyly (Q69.-)*
reduction defect of limb (Q71-Q73)
syndactyly (Q70.-)

Q74.0   **Other congenital malformations of upper limb(s), including shoulder girdle**
Accessory carpal bones
Cleidocranial dysostosis
Congenital pseudarthrosis of clavicle
Macrodactylia (fingers)
Madelung's deformity
Radioulnar synostosis
Sprengel's deformity
Triphalangeal thumb

Q74.1   **Congenital malformation of knee**
Congenital absence of patella
Congenital dislocation of patella
Congenital genu valgum
Congenital genu varum
Rudimentary patella

EXCLUDES 1   *congenital dislocation of knee (Q68.2)*
congenital genu recurvatum (Q68.2)
nail patella syndrome (Q87.2)

Q74.2   **Other congenital malformations of lower limb(s), including pelvic girdle**
Congenital fusion of sacroiliac joint
Congenital malformation of ankle joint
Congenital malformation of sacroiliac joint

EXCLUDES 1   *anteversion of femur (neck) (Q65.89)*

Q74.3   **Arthrogryposis multiplex congenita**

Q74.8   **Other specified congenital malformations of limb(s)**

Q74.9   **Unspecified congenital malformation of limb(s)**
Congenital anomaly of limb(s) NOS

④ **Q75**   **Other congenital malformations of skull and face bones**

EXCLUDES 1   *congenital malformation of face NOS (Q18.-)*
congenital malformation syndromes classified to Q87.-
dentofacial anomalies [including malocclusion] (M26.-)
musculoskeletal deformities of head and face (Q67.0-Q67.4)
skull defects associated with congenital anomalies of brain such as:
anencephaly (Q00.0)
encephalocele (Q01.-)
hydrocephalus (Q03.-)
microcephaly (Q02)

Q75.0   **Craniosynostosis**
Acrocephaly
Imperfect fusion of skull
Oxycephaly
Trigonocephaly

Q75.1   **Craniofacial dysostosis**
Crouzon's disease

Q75.2   **Hypertelorism**

Q75.3   **Macrocephaly**

Q75.4   **Mandibulofacial dysostosis**
Franceschetti syndrome
Treacher Collins syndrome

Q75.5   **Oculomandibular dysostosis**

Q75.8   **Other specified congenital malformations of skull and face bones**
Absence of skull bone, congenital
Congenital deformity of forehead
Platybasia

Q75.9   **Congenital malformation of skull and face bones, unspecified**
Congenital anomaly of face bones NOS
Congenital anomaly of skull NOS

④ **Q76**   **Congenital malformations of spine and bony thorax**

EXCLUDES 1   *congenital musculoskeletal deformities of spine and chest (Q67.5-Q67.8)*

Q76.0   **Spina bifida occulta**

EXCLUDES 1   *meningocele (spinal) (Q05.-)*
spina bifida (aperta) (cystica) (Q05.-)

Q76.1   **Klippel-Feil syndrome**
Cervical fusion syndrome

● New   ▲ Revised   *Manifestation*   ④-⑦ Digit Indicators   ⊟ Laterality   Ⓐ Adult (15+ years)   Ⓜ Maternity (12-55 years)   Ⓝ Newborn   Ⓟ Pediatric (0-17 years)   ♂ Male   ♀ Female
✖ Deleted   Unspecified   + Additional code

Q76.2   Congenital spondylolisthesis
Congenital spondylolysis
EXCLUDES 1 *spondylolisthesis (acquired) (M43.1-)*
spondylolysis (acquired) (M43.0-)

Congenital spondylolisthesis

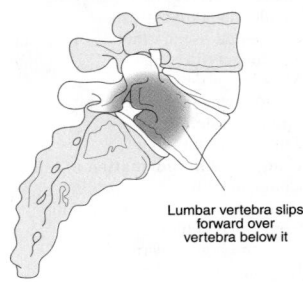

Lumbar vertebra slips
forward over
vertebra below it

Q76.3   Congenital scoliosis due to congenital bony malformation
Hemivertebra fusion or failure of segmentation with scoliosis
**Q76.4   Other congenital malformations of spine, not associated
with scoliosis**
Q76.41   Congenital kyphosis
**Q76.411   Congenital kyphosis, occipito-atlanto-axial
region**
Q76.412   Congenital kyphosis, cervical region
Q76.413   Congenital kyphosis, cervicothoracic region
Q76.414   Congenital kyphosis, thoracic region
Q76.415   Congenital kyphosis, thoracolumbar region
Q76.419   Congenital kyphosis, unspecified region
Q76.42   Congenital lordosis
Q76.425   Congenital lordosis, thoracolumbar region
Q76.426   Congenital lordosis, lumbar region
Q76.427   Congenital lordosis, lumbosacral region
**Q76.428   Congenital lordosis, sacral and sacrococcygeal
region**
Q76.429   Congenital lordosis, unspecified region
**Q76.49   Other congenital malformations of spine, not
associated with scoliosis**
Congenital absence of vertebra NOS
Congenital fusion of spine NOS
Congenital malformation of lumbosacral (joint) (region)
NOS
Congenital malformation of spine NOS
Hemivertebra NOS
Malformation of spine NOS
Platyspondylisis NOS
Supernumerary vertebra NOS
Q76.5   Cervical rib
Supernumerary rib in cervical region
Q76.6   Other congenital malformations of ribs
Accessory rib
Congenital absence of rib
Congenital fusion of ribs
Congenital malformation of ribs NOS
EXCLUDES 1 *short rib syndrome (Q77.2)*
Q76.7   Congenital malformation of sternum
Congenital absence of sternum
Sternum bifidum
Q76.8   Other congenital malformations of bony thorax
Q76.9   Congenital malformation of bony thorax, unspecified
**Q77   Osteochondrodysplasia with defects of growth of
tubular bones and spine**
EXCLUDES 1 *mucopolysaccharidosis (E76.0-E76.3)*
EXCLUDES 2 *congenital myotonic chondrodystrophy (G71.13)*
Q77.0   Achondrogenesis
Hypochondrogenesis
Q77.1   Thanatophoric short stature
Q77.2   Short rib syndrome
Asphyxiating thoracic dysplasia [Jeune]
Q77.3   Chondrodysplasia punctata
EXCLUDES 1 *Rhizomelic chondrodysplasia punctata
(E71.43)*

Q77.4   Achondroplasia
Hypochondroplasia
Osteosclerosis congenita
Q77.5   Diastrophic dysplasia
Q77.6   Chondroectodermal dysplasia
Ellis-van Creveld syndrome
Q77.7   Spondyloepiphyseal dysplasia
**Q77.8   Other osteochondrodysplasia with defects of growth of
tubular bones and spine**
**Q77.9   Osteochondrodysplasia with defects of growth of tubular
bones and spine, unspecified**
Q78   Other osteochondrodysplasias
EXCLUDES 2 *congenital myotonic chondrodystrophy (G71.13)*
Q78.0   Osteogenesis imperfecta
Fragilitas ossium
Osteopsathyrosis
Q78.1   Polyostotic fibrous dysplasia
Albright(-McCune)(-Sternberg) syndrome
DEFINITION   Genetic bone disorder causing multiple
areas of normal bone to be replaced by bands of
abnormal fibrous tissue, causing pain, fractures, and
deformity.
Q78.2   Osteopetrosis
Albers-Schönberg syndrome
Osteosclerosis NOS
Q78.3   Progressive diaphyseal dysplasia
Camurati-Engelmann syndrome
Q78.4   Enchondromatosis
Maffucci's syndrome
Ollier's disease
Q78.5   Metaphyseal dysplasia
Pyle's syndrome
Q78.6   Multiple congenital exostoses
Diaphyseal aclasis
Q78.8   Other specified osteochondrodysplasias
Osteopoikilosis
Q78.9   Osteochondrodysplasia, unspecified
Chondrodystrophy NOS
Osteodystrophy NOS
**Q79   Congenital malformations of musculoskeletal system,
not elsewhere classified**
EXCLUDES 2 *congenital (sternomastoid) torticollis (Q68.0)*
Q79.0   Congenital diaphragmatic hernia
EXCLUDES 1 *congenital hiatus hernia (Q40.1)*
Q79.1   Other congenital malformations of diaphragm
Absence of diaphragm
Congenital malformation of diaphragm NOS
Eventration of diaphragm
Q79.2   Exomphalos
Omphalocele
EXCLUDES 1 *umbilical hernia (K42.-)*
Q79.3   Gastroschisis
Q79.4   Prune belly syndrome
Congenital prolapse of bladder mucosa
Eagle-Barrett syndrome
Q79.5   Other congenital malformations of abdominal wall
EXCLUDES 1 *umbilical hernia (K42.-)*
Q79.51   Congenital hernia of bladder
Q79.59   Other congenital malformations of abdominal wall
Q79.6   Ehlers-Danlos syndrome
**Q79.8   Other congenital malformations of musculoskeletal
system**
Absence of muscle
Absence of tendon
Accessory muscle
Amyotrophia congenita
Congenital constricting bands
Congenital shortening of tendon
Poland syndrome
**Q79.9   Congenital malformation of musculoskeletal system,
unspecified**
Congenital anomaly of musculoskeletal system NOS
Congenital deformity of musculoskeletal system NOS

● New   ▲ Revised   *Manifestation*   4- 7 Digit Indicators   ▤ Laterality   ▨ Adult (15+ years)   ▧ Maternity (12-55 years)   ▨ Newborn   ▣ Pediatric (0-17 years)   ♂ Male   ♀ Female

✕ Deleted   Unspecified   + Additional code

894   © 2017 DecisionHealth   2017 ICD-10-CM Expert for Physicians

Other congenital malformations (Q80-Q89)

▣ Q80   Congenital ichthyosis
EXCLUDES 1   *Refsum's disease (G60.1)*

Q80.0   Ichthyosis vulgaris
Q80.1   X-linked ichthyosis
Q80.2   Lamellar ichthyosis
Collodion baby
Q80.3   Congenital bullous ichthyosiform erythroderma
Q80.4   Harlequin fetus
Q80.8   Other congenital ichthyosis
Q80.9   Congenital ichthyosis, unspecified

▣ Q81   Epidermolysis bullosa
Q81.0   Epidermolysis bullosa simplex
EXCLUDES 1   *Cockayne's syndrome (Q87.1)*

Q81.1   Epidermolysis bullosa letalis
Herlitz' syndrome
Q81.2   Epidermolysis bullosa dystrophica
Q81.8   Other epidermolysis bullosa
Q81.9   Epidermolysis bullosa, unspecified

▣ Q82   Other congenital malformations of skin
EXCLUDES 1   *acrodermatitis enteropathica (E83.2)*
congenital erythropoietic porphyria (E80.0)
pilonidal cyst or sinus (L05.-)
Sturge-Weber (-Dimitri) syndrome (Q85.8)

Q82.0   Hereditary lymphedema
Q82.1   Xeroderma pigmentosum
Q82.2   Mastocytosis
Urticaria pigmentosa
EXCLUDES 1   *malignant mastocytosis (C96.2)*

Q82.3   Incontinentia pigmenti
Q82.4   Ectodermal dysplasia (anhidrotic)
EXCLUDES 1   *Ellis-van Creveld syndrome (Q77.6)*

Q82.5   Congenital non-neoplastic nevus
Birthmark NOS
Flammeus Nevus
Portwine Nevus
Sanguineous Nevus
Strawberry Nevus
Vascular Nevus NOS
Verrucous Nevus
EXCLUDES 2   *Café au lait spots (L81.3)*
lentigo (L81.4)
nevus NOS (D22.-)
araneus nevus (I78.1)
melanocytic nevus (D22.-)
pigmented nevus (D22.-)
spider nevus (I78.1)
stellar nevus (I78.1)

● Q82.6   Congenital sacral dimple
Parasacral dimple
EXCLUDES 2   *pilonidal cyst with abscess (L05.01)*
pilonidal cyst without abscess (L05.91)

Q82.8   Other specified congenital malformations of skin
Abnormal palmar creases
Accessory skin tags
Benign familial pemphigus [Hailey-Hailey]
Congenital poikiloderma
Cutis laxa (hyperelastica)
Dermatoglyphic anomalies
Inherited keratosis palmaris et plantaris
Keratosis follicularis [Darier-White]
EXCLUDES 1   *Ehlers-Danlos syndrome (Q79.6)*
AHA: 1Q 2016, 17
Q82.9   Congenital malformation of skin, unspecified

▣ Q83   Congenital malformations of breast
EXCLUDES 2   *absence of pectoral muscle (Q79.8)*
hypoplasia of breast (N64.82)
micromastia (N64.82)

Q83.0   Congenital absence of breast with absent nipple
Q83.1   Accessory breast
Supernumerary breast
Q83.2   Absent nipple
Q83.3   Accessory nipple
Supernumerary nipple
Q83.8   Other congenital malformations of breast

Q83.9   Congenital malformation of breast, unspecified

▣ Q84   Other congenital malformations of integument
Q84.0   Congenital alopecia
Congenital atrichosis
Q84.1   Congenital morphological disturbances of hair, not elsewhere classified
Beaded hair
Monilethrix
Pili annulati
EXCLUDES 1   *Menkes' kinky hair syndrome (E83.0)*

Q84.2   Other congenital malformations of hair
Congenital hypertrichosis
Congenital malformation of hair NOS
Persistent lanugo
Q84.3   Anonychia
EXCLUDES 1   *nail patella syndrome (Q87.2)*

Q84.4   Congenital leukonychia
Q84.5   Enlarged and hypertrophic nails
Congenital onychauxis
Pachyonychia
Q84.6   Other congenital malformations of nails
Congenital clubnail
Congenital koilonychia
Congenital malformation of nail NOS
Q84.8   Other specified congenital malformations of integument
Aplasia cutis congenita
Q84.9   Congenital malformation of integument, unspecified
Congenital anomaly of integument NOS
Congenital deformity of integument NOS

▣ Q85   Phakomatoses, not elsewhere classified
EXCLUDES 1   *ataxia telangiectasia [Louis-Bar] (G11.3)*
familial dysautonomia [Riley-Day] (G90.1)

▤ Q85.0   Neurofibromatosis (nonmalignant)
Q85.00   Neurofibromatosis, unspecified
Q85.01   Neurofibromatosis, type 1
Von Recklinghausen disease
Q85.02   Neurofibromatosis, type 2
Acoustic neurofibromatosis
Q85.03   Schwannomatosis
DEFINITION   A rare type of neurofibromatosis causing tumors on nerve sheaths of spinal, peripheral, and cranial nerves - except the eighth (vestibular) cranial nerve.

Q85.09   Other neurofibromatosis
Q85.1   Tuberous sclerosis
Bourneville's disease
Epiloia
Q85.8   Other phakomatoses, not elsewhere classified
Peutz-Jeghers Syndrome
Sturge-Weber(-Dimitri) syndrome
von Hippel-Lindau syndrome
EXCLUDES 1   *Meckel-Gruber syndrome (Q61.9)*

Q85.9   Phakomatosis, unspecified
Hamartosis NOS

▣ Q86   Congenital malformation syndromes due to known exogenous causes, not elsewhere classified
EXCLUDES 2   *iodine-deficiency-related hypothyroidism (E00-E02)*
nonteratogenic effects of substances transmitted via placenta or breast milk (P04.-)

Q86.0   Fetal alcohol syndrome (dysmorphic)
Q86.1   Fetal hydantoin syndrome   ℕ
Meadow's syndrome
Q86.2   Dysmorphism due to warfarin
Q86.8   Other congenital malformation syndromes due to known exogenous causes

▣ + Q87   Other specified congenital malformation syndromes affecting multiple systems
Use additional code(s) to identify all associated manifestations

---

● New   ▲ Revised   *Manifestation*   ▣-▦ Digit Indicators   ▤ Laterality   ⒶAdult (15+ years)   ⓂMaternity (12-55 years)   ℕ Newborn   ⓅPediatric (0-17 years)   ♂ Male   ♀Female
✖ Deleted   Unspecified   + Additional code

+ Q87.0   Congenital malformation syndromes predominantly affecting facial appearance
Acrocephalopolysyndactyly
Acrocephalosyndactyly [Apert]
Cryptophthalmos syndrome
Cyclopia
Goldenhar syndrome
Moebius syndrome
Oro-facial-digital syndrome
Robin syndrome
Whistling face

+ Q87.1   Congenital malformation syndromes predominantly associated with short stature
Aarskog syndrome
Cockayne syndrome
De Lange syndrome
Dubowitz syndrome
Noonan syndrome
Prader-Willi syndrome
Robinow-Silverman-Smith syndrome
Russell-Silver syndrome
Seckel syndrome
> **EXCLUDES 1**   *Ellis-van Creveld syndrome (Q77.6)*
> *Smith-Lemli-Opitz syndrome (E78.72)*

+ Q87.2   Congenital malformation syndromes predominantly involving limbs
Holt-Oram syndrome
Klippel-Trenaunay-Weber syndrome
Nail patella syndrome
Rubinstein-Taybi syndrome
Sirenomelia
Thrombocytopenia with absent radius [TAR] syndrome
VATER syndrome

+ Q87.3   Congenital malformation syndromes involving early overgrowth
Beckwith-Wiedemann syndrome
Sotos syndrome
Weaver syndrome

⑤+ Q87.4   Marfan's syndrome

+ Q87.40   Marfan's syndrome, unspecified

⑥+ Q87.41   Marfan's syndrome with cardiovascular manifestations

+ Q87.410   Marfan's syndrome with aortic dilation

+ Q87.418   Marfan's syndrome with other cardiovascular manifestations

+ Q87.42   Marfan's syndrome with ocular manifestations

+ Q87.43   Marfan's syndrome with skeletal manifestation

+ Q87.5   Other congenital malformation syndromes with other skeletal changes

⑤+ Q87.8   Other specified congenital malformation syndromes, not elsewhere classified
> **EXCLUDES 1**   *Zellweger syndrome (E71.510)*

+ Q87.81   Alport syndrome
Use additional code to identify stage of chronic kidney disease (N18.1-N18.6)

●+ Q87.82   Arterial tortuosity syndrome

+ Q87.89   Other specified congenital malformation syndromes, not elsewhere classified
Laurence-Moon (-Bardet)-Biedl syndrome

④ Q89   Other congenital malformations, not elsewhere classified

⑤ Q89.0   Congenital absence and malformations of spleen
> **EXCLUDES 1**   *isomerism of atrial appendages (with asplenia or polysplenia) (Q20.6)*

Q89.01   Asplenia (congenital)

Q89.09   Congenital malformations of spleen
Congenital splenomegaly

Q89.1   Congenital malformations of adrenal gland
> **EXCLUDES 1**   *adrenogenital disorders (E25.-)*
> *congenital adrenal hyperplasia (E25.0)*

Q89.2   Congenital malformations of other endocrine glands
Congenital malformation of parathyroid or thyroid gland
Persistent thyroglossal duct
Thyroglossal cyst
> **EXCLUDES 1**   *congenital goiter (E03.0)*
> *congenital hypothyroidism (E03.1)*

Q89.3   Situs inversus
Dextrocardia with situs inversus
Mirror-image atrial arrangement with situs inversus
Situs inversus or transversus abdominalis
Situs inversus or transversus thoracis
Transposition of abdominal viscera
Transposition of thoracic viscera
> **EXCLUDES 1**   *dextrocardia NOS (Q24.0)*

> **DEFINITION**   Congenital disorder in which the position of all major organs in the chest and abdomen are reversed horizontally.

Q89.4   Conjoined twins
Craniopagus
Dicephaly
Pygopagus
Thoracopagus

Q89.7   Multiple congenital malformations, not elsewhere classified
Multiple congenital anomalies NOS
Multiple congenital deformities NOS
> **EXCLUDES 1**   *congenital malformation syndromes affecting multiple systems (Q87.-)*

+ Q89.8   Other specified congenital malformations
Use additional code(s) to identify all associated manifestations

Q89.9   Congenital malformation, unspecified
Congenital anomaly NOS
Congenital deformity NOS

Chromosomal abnormalities, not elsewhere classified (Q90-Q99)

> **EXCLUDES 2**   *mitochondrial metabolic disorders (E88.4-)*

④+ Q90   Down syndrome
Use additional code(s) to identify any associated physical conditions and degree of intellectual disabilities (F70-F79)

+ Q90.0   Trisomy 21, nonmosaicism (meiotic nondisjunction)

+ Q90.1   Trisomy 21, mosaicism (mitotic nondisjunction)

+ Q90.2   Trisomy 21, translocation

+ Q90.9   Down syndrome, unspecified
Trisomy 21 NOS

④ Q91   Trisomy 18 and Trisomy 13

Q91.0   Trisomy 18, nonmosaicism (meiotic nondisjunction)

Q91.1   Trisomy 18, mosaicism (mitotic nondisjunction)

Q91.2   Trisomy 18, translocation

Q91.3   Trisomy 18, unspecified

Q91.4   Trisomy 13, nonmosaicism (meiotic nondisjunction)

Q91.5   Trisomy 13, mosaicism (mitotic nondisjunction)

Q91.6   Trisomy 13, translocation

Q91.7   Trisomy 13, unspecified

④ Q92   Other trisomies and partial trisomies of the autosomes, not elsewhere classified
> **INCLUDES**   unbalanced translocations and insertions
> **EXCLUDES 1**   *trisomies of chromosomes 13, 18, 21 (Q90-Q91)*

Q92.0   Whole chromosome trisomy, nonmosaicism (meiotic nondisjunction)

Q92.1   Whole chromosome trisomy, mosaicism (mitotic nondisjunction)

Q92.2   Partial trisomy
Less than whole arm duplicated
Whole arm or more duplicated
> **EXCLUDES 1**   *partial trisomy due to unbalanced translocation (Q92.5)*

Q92.5   Duplications with other complex rearrangements
Partial trisomy due to unbalanced translocations
Code also:
> any associated deletions due to unbalanced translocations, inversions and insertions (Q93.7)

⑤ Q92.6   Marker chromosomes
Trisomies due to dicentrics
Trisomies due to extra rings
Trisomies due to isochromosomes
Individual with marker heterochromatin

Q92.61   Marker chromosomes in normal individual

Q92.62   Marker chromosomes in abnormal individual

Q92.7   Triploidy and polyploidy

● New   ▲ Revised   *Manifestation*   ④-⑦ Digit Indicators   ⊟ Laterality   🅰 Adult (15+ years)   🅼 Maternity (12-55 years)   🅽 Newborn   🅿 Pediatric (0-17 years)   ♂ Male   ♀ Female
✖ Deleted   Unspecified   + Additional code

Q92.8 Other specified trisomies and partial trisomies of autosomes
Duplications identified by fluorescence in situ hybridization (FISH)
Duplications identified by in situ hybridization (ISH)
Duplications seen only at prometaphase

Q92.9 Trisomy and partial trisomy of autosomes, unspecified

⬛ Q93 Monosomies and deletions from the autosomes, not elsewhere classified

Q93.0 Whole chromosome monosomy, nonmosaicism (meiotic nondisjunction)

Q93.1 Whole chromosome monosomy, mosaicism (mitotic nondisjunction)

Q93.2 Chromosome replaced with ring, dicentric or isochromosome

Q93.3 Deletion of short arm of chromosome 4
Wolff-Hirschorn syndrome

Q93.4 Deletion of short arm of chromosome 5
Cri-du-chat syndrome

Q93.5 Other deletions of part of a chromosome
Angelman syndrome

Q93.7 Deletions with other complex rearrangements
Deletions due to unbalanced translocations, inversions and insertions
Code also:
any associated duplications due to unbalanced translocations, inversions and insertions (Q92.5)

⬛ Q93.8 Other deletions from the autosomes

Q93.81 Velo-cardio-facial syndrome
Deletion 22q11.2

Q93.88 Other microdeletions
Miller-Dieker syndrome
Smith-Magenis syndrome

Q93.89 Other deletions from the autosomes
Deletions identified by fluorescence in situ hybridization (FISH)
Deletions identified by in situ hybridization (ISH)
Deletions seen only at prometaphase

Q93.9 Deletion from autosomes, unspecified

⬛ Q95 Balanced rearrangements and structural markers, not elsewhere classified
| INCLUDES | Robertsonian and balanced reciprocal translocations and insertions

Q95.0 Balanced translocation and insertion in normal individual

Q95.1 Chromosome inversion in normal individual

Q95.2 Balanced autosomal rearrangement in abnormal individual

Q95.3 Balanced sex/autosomal rearrangement in abnormal individual

Q95.5 Individual with autosomal fragile site

Q95.8 Other balanced rearrangements and structural markers

Q95.9 Balanced rearrangement and structural marker, unspecified

⬛ Q96 Turner's syndrome
EXCLUDES 1 Noonan syndrome (Q87.1)

Q96.0 Karyotype 45, X ♀

Q96.1 Karyotype 46, X iso (Xq) ♀
Karyotype 46, isochromosome Xq

Q96.2 Karyotype 46, X with abnormal sex chromosome, except iso (Xq) ♀
Karyotype 46, X with abnormal sex chromosome, except isochromosome Xq

Q96.3 Mosaicism, 45, X/46, XX or XY ♀

Q96.4 Mosaicism, 45, X/other cell line(s) with abnormal sex chromosome ♀

Q96.8 Other variants of Turner's syndrome ♀

Q96.9 Turner's syndrome, unspecified ♀

⬛ Q97 Other sex chromosome abnormalities, female phenotype, not elsewhere classified
EXCLUDES 1 Turner's syndrome (Q96.-)

Q97.0 Karyotype 47, XXX ♀

Q97.1 Female with more than three X chromosomes ♀

Q97.2 Mosaicism, lines with various numbers of X chromosomes ♀

Q97.3 Female with 46, XY karyotype ♀

Q97.8 Other specified sex chromosome abnormalities, female phenotype ♀

Q97.9 Sex chromosome abnormality, female phenotype, unspecified ♀

⬛ Q98 Other sex chromosome abnormalities, male phenotype, not elsewhere classified

Q98.0 Klinefelter syndrome karyotype 47, XXY ♂

Q98.1 Klinefelter syndrome, male with more than two X chromosomes ♂

Q98.3 Other male with 46, XX karyotype ♂

Q98.4 Klinefelter syndrome, unspecified ♂

Q98.5 Karyotype 47, XYY ♂

Q98.6 Male with structurally abnormal sex chromosome ♂

Q98.7 Male with sex chromosome mosaicism ♂

Q98.8 Other specified sex chromosome abnormalities, male phenotype ♂

Q98.9 Sex chromosome abnormality, male phenotype, unspecified ♂

⬛ Q99 Other chromosome abnormalities, not elsewhere classified

Q99.0 Chimera 46, XX/46, XY
Chimera 46, XX/46, XY true hermaphrodite

Q99.1 46, XX true hermaphrodite
46, XX with streak gonads
46, XY with streak gonads
Pure gonadal dysgenesis

Q99.2 Fragile X chromosome
Fragile X syndrome

Q99.8 Other specified chromosome abnormalities

Q99.9 Chromosomal abnormality, unspecified

Congenital Malformations, Deformations and Chromosomal Abnormalities   Q92.8 — Q99.9

CHAPTER 18: SYMPTOMS, SIGNS AND ABNORMAL CLINICAL AND LABORATORY FINDINGS, NOT ELSEWHERE CLASSIFIED (R00-R99)

Note: This chapter includes symptoms, signs, abnormal results of clinical or other investigative procedures, and ill-defined conditions regarding which no diagnosis classifiable elsewhere is recorded.

Signs and symptoms that point rather definitely to a given diagnosis have been assigned to a category in other chapters of the classification. In general, categories in this chapter include the less well-defined conditions and symptoms that, without the necessary study of the case to establish a final diagnosis, point perhaps equally to two or more diseases or to two or more systems of the body. Practically all categories in the chapter could be designated 'not otherwise specified', 'unknown etiology' or 'transient'. The Alphabetical Index should be consulted to determine which symptoms and signs are to be allocated here and which to other chapters. The residual subcategories, numbered .8, are generally provided for other relevant symptoms that cannot be allocated elsewhere in the classification.

The conditions and signs or symptoms included in categories R00-R94 consist of:

(a) cases for which no more specific diagnosis can be made even after all the facts bearing on the case have been investigated;

(b) signs or symptoms existing at the time of initial encounter that proved to be transient and whose causes could not be determined;

(c) provisional diagnosis in a patient who failed to return for further investigation or care;

(d) cases referred elsewhere for investigation or treatment before the diagnosis was made;

(e) cases in which a more precise diagnosis was not available for any other reason;

(f) certain symptoms, for which supplementary information is provided, that represent important problems in medical care in their own right.

> **EXCLUDES 2** *abnormal findings on antenatal screening of mother (O28.-)*
> *certain conditions originating in the perinatal period (P04-P96)*
> *signs and symptoms classified in the body system chapters*
> *signs and symptoms of breast (N63, N64.5)*

GUIDELINES Section I.C.18.a-c

Codes that describe symptoms and signs are acceptable for reporting purposes when a related definitive diagnosis has not been established (confirmed) by the provider.

Codes for signs and symptoms may be reported in addition to a related definitive diagnosis when the sign or symptom is not routinely associated with that diagnosis, such as the various signs and symptoms associated with complex syndromes. The definitive diagnosis code should be sequenced before the symptom code. Signs or symptoms that are associated routinely with a disease process should not be assigned as additional codes, unless otherwise instructed by the classification.

ICD-10-CM contains a number of combination codes that identify both the definitive diagnosis and common symptoms of that diagnosis. When using one of these combination codes, an additional code should not be assigned for the symptom.

This chapter contains the following blocks:

R00-R09	Symptoms and signs involving the circulatory and respiratory systems
R10-R19	Symptoms and signs involving the digestive system and abdomen
R20-R23	Symptoms and signs involving the skin and subcutaneous tissue
R25-R29	Symptoms and signs involving the nervous and musculoskeletal systems
R30-R39	Symptoms and signs involving the genitourinary system
R40-R46	Symptoms and signs involving cognition, perception, emotional state and behavior
R47-R49	Symptoms and signs involving speech and voice
R50-R69	General symptoms and signs
R70-R79	Abnormal findings on examination of blood, without diagnosis
R80-R82	Abnormal findings on examination of urine, without diagnosis
R83-R89	Abnormal findings on examination of other body fluids, substances and tissues, without diagnosis
R90-R94	Abnormal findings on diagnostic imaging and in function studies, without diagnosis
R97	Abnormal tumor markers
R99	Ill-defined and unknown cause of mortality

Symptoms and signs involving the circulatory and respiratory systems (R00-R09)

▲ ⁴ R00   Abnormalities of heart beat

> **EXCLUDES 1** *abnormalities originating in the perinatal period (P29.1-)*
> **EXCLUDES 2** *specified arrhythmias (I47-I49)*

R00.0   Tachycardia, unspecified
Rapid heart beat
Sinoauricular tachycardia NOS
Sinus [sinusal] tachycardia NOS

> **EXCLUDES 1** *neonatal tachycardia (P29.11)*
> *paroxysmal tachycardia (I47.-)*

CODING TIP ✓ Tachycardia that is not specified as due to a specific arrhythmia or any particular cause is coded here. When the record reports "sinus tachycardia", assign code R00.0. Sinus tachycardia indicates a high heart rate with an impulse that continues to originate from the SA node.

Tachycardia, unspecified

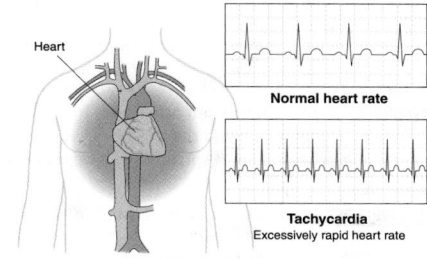

Heart

Normal heart rate

Tachycardia
Excessively rapid heart rate

+ R00.1   Bradycardia, unspecified
Sinoatrial bradycardia
Sinus bradycardia
Slow heart beat
Vagal bradycardia
Use additional code for adverse effect, if applicable, to identify drug (T36-T50 with fifth or sixth character 5)

> **EXCLUDES 1** *neonatal bradycardia (P29.12)*

R00.2   Palpitations
Awareness of heart beat

> **DEFINITION** Sensation of feeling the heart beat.

R00.8   Other abnormalities of heart beat

R00.9   Unspecified abnormalities of heart beat

⁴ R01   Cardiac murmurs and other cardiac sounds

> **EXCLUDES 1** *cardiac murmurs and sounds originating in the perinatal period (P29.8)*

R01.0   Benign and innocent cardiac murmurs
Functional cardiac murmur

▲ R01.1   Cardiac murmur, unspecified
Cardiac bruit NOS
Heart murmur NOS
Systolic murmur NOS

R01.2   Other cardiac sounds
Cardiac dullness, increased or decreased
Precordial friction

⁴ R03   Abnormal blood-pressure reading, without diagnosis

R03.0   Elevated blood-pressure reading, without diagnosis of hypertension
Note: This category is to be used to record an episode of elevated blood pressure in a patient in whom no formal diagnosis of hypertension has been made, or as an isolated incidental finding.

GUIDELINES Section I.C.9.a.7)

Assign code R03.0, Elevated blood pressure reading without diagnosis of hypertension, unless patient has an established diagnosis of hypertension. Assign code O13.-, Gestational [pregnancy-induced] hypertension without significant proteinuria, or O14.-, Pre-eclampsia, for transient hypertension of pregnancy.

CODING TIP ✓ Do not assign this code for a patient with a diagnosis of hypertension (I10-I13).

R03.1 Nonspecific low blood-pressure reading
> **EXCLUDES 1** *hypotension (I95.-)*
> *maternal hypotension syndrome (O26.5-)*
> *neurogenic orthostatic hypotension (G90.3)*

> **CODING TIP ✓** Assign code R03.1 when a patient has a low blood pressure reading but has not been diagnosed with hypotension or orthostasis.

R04 Hemorrhage from respiratory passages

R04.0 Epistaxis
Hemorrhage from nose
Nosebleed

R04.1 Hemorrhage from throat
> **EXCLUDES 2** *hemoptysis (R04.2)*

R04.2 Hemoptysis
Blood-stained sputum
Cough with hemorrhage
> **DEFINITION** Coughing up blood or bloody mucous.
AHA: 4Q 2013, 118

R04.8 Hemorrhage from other sites in respiratory passages

R04.81 Acute idiopathic pulmonary hemorrhage in infants
AIPHI
Acute idiopathic hemorrhage in infants over 28 days old
> **EXCLUDES 1** *perinatal pulmonary hemorrhage (P26.-)*
> *von Willebrand's disease (D68.0)*

R04.89 Hemorrhage from other sites in respiratory passages
Pulmonary hemorrhage NOS

R04.9 Hemorrhage from respiratory passages, unspecified

R05 Cough
> **EXCLUDES 1** *cough with hemorrhage (R04.2)*
> *smoker's cough (J41.0)*

> **CODING TIP ✓** Do not assign R05 as an additional code when the cough is an integral symptom of another disease process also coded, such as COPD, bronchitis, asthma, or another pulmonary condition known to be the cause of the cough.
AHA: 2Q 2016, 34

R06 Abnormalities of breathing
> **EXCLUDES 1** *acute respiratory distress syndrome (J80)*
> *respiratory arrest (R09.2)*
> *respiratory arrest of newborn (P28.81)*
> *respiratory distress syndrome of newborn (P22.-)*
> *respiratory failure (J96.-)*
> *respiratory failure of newborn (P28.5)*

> **CODING TIP ✓** Do not assign a code from R06.- as an additional code when the respiratory symptom is an integral symptom of another disease process also coded, such as COPD, bronchitis, asthma, or another condition known to be the cause of the presenting symptom. The more specific condition should be coded.

R06.0 Dyspnea
> **EXCLUDES 1** *tachypnea NOS (R06.82)*
> *transient tachypnea of newborn (P22.1)*

R06.00 Dyspnea, unspecified
R06.01 Orthopnea
> **DEFINITION** Difficulty breathing while lying down, necessitating sleeping propped up or in a chair.

R06.02 Shortness of breath
R06.09 Other forms of dyspnea
R06.1 Stridor
> **EXCLUDES 1** *congenital laryngeal stridor (P28.89)*
> *laryngismus (stridulus) (J38.5)*

> **DEFINITION** A whistling sound when breathing, usually heard on inspiration, indicating obstruction of the trachea or larynx.

R06.2 Wheezing
> **EXCLUDES 1** *Asthma (J45.-)*
AHA: 2Q 2016, 34

R06.3 Periodic breathing
Cheyne-Stokes breathing

R06.4 Hyperventilation
> **EXCLUDES 1** *psychogenic hyperventilation (F45.8)*

R06.5 Mouth breathing
> **EXCLUDES 2** *dry mouth NOS (R68.2)*

R06.6 Hiccough
> **EXCLUDES 1** *psychogenic hiccough (F45.8)*
> **DEFINITION** Sharp sound of inhalation, with spasm of the glottis and diaphragm.

R06.7 Sneezing
R06.8 Other abnormalities of breathing

R06.81 Apnea, not elsewhere classified
Apnea NOS
> **EXCLUDES 1** *apnea (of) newborn (P28.4)*
> *sleep apnea (G47.3-)*
> *sleep apnea of newborn (primary) (P28.3)*
> **DEFINITION** Temporary cessation of breathing.

R06.82 Tachypnea, not elsewhere classified
Tachypnea NOS
> **EXCLUDES 1** *transitory tachypnea of newborn (P22.1)*
> **DEFINITION** Rapid breathing.

R06.83 Snoring
R06.89 Other abnormalities of breathing
Breath-holding (spells)
Sighing

R06.9 Unspecified abnormalities of breathing

R07 Pain in throat and chest
> **EXCLUDES 1** *epidemic myalgia (B33.0)*
> **EXCLUDES 2** *jaw pain R68.84*
> *pain in breast (N64.4)*

> **CODING TIP ✓** Do not assign a code from R07.- for a patient with angina. Chest pain due to angina should be coded to the appropriate I20.- or I25.- code

R07.0 Pain in throat
> **EXCLUDES 1** *chronic sore throat (J31.2)*
> *sore throat (acute) NOS (J02.9)*
> **EXCLUDES 2** *dysphagia (R13.1-)*
> *pain in neck (M54.2)*

R07.1 Chest pain on breathing
Painful respiration
R07.2 Precordial pain
R07.8 Other chest pain

R07.81 Pleurodynia
Pleurodynia NOS
> **EXCLUDES 1** *epidemic pleurodynia (B33.0)*

R07.82 Intercostal pain
R07.89 Other chest pain
Anterior chest-wall pain NOS

R07.9 Chest pain, unspecified

R09 Other symptoms and signs involving the circulatory and respiratory system
> **EXCLUDES 1** *acute respiratory distress syndrome (J80)*
> *respiratory arrest of newborn (P28.81)*
> *respiratory distress syndrome of newborn (P22.0)*
> *respiratory failure (J96.-)*
> *respiratory failure of newborn (P28.5)*

R09.0 Asphyxia and hypoxemia
> **EXCLUDES 1** *asphyxia due to carbon monoxide (T58.-)*
> *asphyxia due to foreign body in respiratory tract (T17.-)*
> *birth (intrauterine) asphyxia (P84)*
> *hypercapnia (R06.4)*
> *hyperventilation (R06.4)*
> *traumatic asphyxia (T71.-)*

R09.01 Asphyxia
> **DEFINITION** Extreme decrease in the amount of oxygen in the body, accompanied by an increase of carbon dioxide, leading to loss of consciousness or death.

R09.02 Hypoxemia
> **DEFINITION** Abnormally low levels of oxygen in arterial blood.

R09.1 Pleurisy
> **EXCLUDES 1** *pleurisy with effusion (J90)*

R09.2 **Respiratory arrest**
Cardiorespiratory failure
> **EXCLUDES 1** *cardiac arrest (I46.-)*
> *respiratory arrest of newborn (P28.81)*
> *respiratory distress of newborn (P22.0)*
> *respiratory failure (J96.-)*
> *respiratory failure of newborn (P28.5)*
> *respiratory insufficiency (R06.89)*
> *respiratory insufficiency of newborn (P28.5)*

R09.3 **Abnormal sputum**
Abnormal amount of sputum
Abnormal color of sputum
Abnormal odor of sputum
Excessive sputum
> **EXCLUDES 1** *blood-stained sputum (R04.2)*

R09.8 **Other specified symptoms and signs involving the circulatory and respiratory systems**

R09.81 **Nasal congestion**

R09.82 **Postnasal drip**

R09.89 **Other specified symptoms and signs involving the circulatory and respiratory systems**
Bruit (arterial)
Abnormal chest percussion
Feeling of foreign body in throat
Friction sounds in chest
Chest tympany
Choking sensation
Rales
Weak pulse
> **EXCLUDES 2** *foreign body in throat (T17.2-)*
> *wheezing (R06.2)*

Symptoms and signs involving the digestive system and abdomen (R10-R19)

> **EXCLUDES 2** *congenital or infantile pylorospasm (Q40.0)*
> *gastrointestinal hemorrhage (K92.0-K92.2)*
> *intestinal obstruction (K56.-)*
> *newborn gastrointestinal hemorrhage (P54.0-P54.3)*
> *newborn intestinal obstruction (P76.-)*
> *pylorospasm (K31.3)*
> *signs and symptoms involving the urinary system (R30-R39)*
> *symptoms referable to female genital organs (N94.-)*
> *symptoms referable to male genital organs (N48-N50)*

R10 **Abdominal and pelvic pain**
> **EXCLUDES 1** *renal colic (N23)*
> **EXCLUDES 2** *dorsalgia (M54.-)*
> *flatulence and related conditions (R14.-)*

R10.0 **Acute abdomen**
Severe abdominal pain (generalized) (with abdominal rigidity)
> **EXCLUDES 1** *abdominal rigidity NOS (R19.3)*
> *generalized abdominal pain NOS (R10.84)*
> *localized abdominal pain (R10.1-R10.3-)*

R10.1 **Pain localized to upper abdomen**

R10.10 **Upper abdominal pain, unspecified**

R10.11 **Right upper quadrant pain**

R10.12 **Left upper quadrant pain**

R10.13 **Epigastric pain**
Dyspepsia
> **EXCLUDES 1** *functional dyspepsia (K30)*

R10.2 **Pelvic and perineal pain**
> **EXCLUDES 1** *vulvodynia (N94.81)*

R10.3 **Pain localized to other parts of lower abdomen**

R10.30 **Lower abdominal pain, unspecified**

R10.31 **Right lower quadrant pain**

R10.32 **Left lower quadrant pain**

R10.33 **Periumbilical pain**

R10.8 **Other abdominal pain**

R10.81 **Abdominal tenderness**
Abdominal tenderness NOS

R10.811 **Right upper quadrant abdominal tenderness**

R10.812 **Left upper quadrant abdominal tenderness**

R10.813 **Right lower quadrant abdominal tenderness**

R10.814 **Left lower quadrant abdominal tenderness**

R10.815 **Periumbilic abdominal tenderness**

R10.816 **Epigastric abdominal tenderness**

R10.817 **Generalized abdominal tenderness**

R10.819 **Abdominal tenderness, unspecified site**

R10.82 **Rebound abdominal tenderness**

R10.821 **Right upper quadrant rebound abdominal tenderness**

R10.822 **Left upper quadrant rebound abdominal tenderness**

R10.823 **Right lower quadrant rebound abdominal tenderness**

R10.824 **Left lower quadrant rebound abdominal tenderness**

R10.825 **Periumbilic rebound abdominal tenderness**

R10.826 **Epigastric rebound abdominal tenderness**

R10.827 **Generalized rebound abdominal tenderness**

R10.829 **Rebound abdominal tenderness, unspecified site**

R10.83 **Colic**   P
Colic NOS
Infantile colic
> **EXCLUDES 1** *colic in adult and child over 12 months old (R10.84)*

R10.84 **Generalized abdominal pain**
> **EXCLUDES 1** *generalized abdominal pain associated with acute abdomen (R10.0)*

R10.9 **Unspecified abdominal pain**

▲ R11 **Nausea and vomiting**
> **EXCLUDES 1** *cyclical vomiting associated with migraine (G43.A-)*
> *excessive vomiting in pregnancy (O21.-)*
> *hematemesis (K92.0)*
> *neonatal hematemesis (P54.0)*
> *newborn vomiting (P92.0-)*
> *psychogenic vomiting (F50.89)*
> *vomiting associated with bulimia nervosa (F50.2)*
> *vomiting following gastrointestinal surgery (K91.0)*

R11.0 **Nausea**
Nausea NOS
Nausea without vomiting

R11.1 **Vomiting**

R11.10 **Vomiting, unspecified**
Vomiting NOS

R11.11 **Vomiting without nausea**

R11.12 **Projectile vomiting**

R11.13 **Vomiting of fecal matter**

R11.14 **Bilious vomiting**
Bilious emesis

R11.2 **Nausea with vomiting, unspecified**
Persistent nausea with vomiting NOS

R12 **Heartburn**
> **EXCLUDES 1** *dyspepsia NOS (R10.13)*
> *functional dyspepsia (K30)*

R13 **Aphagia and dysphagia**

R13.0 **Aphagia**
Inability to swallow
> **EXCLUDES 1** *psychogenic aphagia (F50.9)*

R13.1 **Dysphagia**
Code first:
, if applicable, dysphagia following cerebrovascular disease (I69. with final characters -91)
> **EXCLUDES 1** *psychogenic dysphagia (F45.8)*

> **CODING TIP ✓** Assign a code from R13.1- following a code from I69.- when dysphagia is reported as a sequela of cerebral vascular disease to report the specified level of dysphagia.

> **DEFINITION** Difficulty in swallowing.

● New	▲ Revised	*Manifestation*	◢-ⁿ Digit Indicators	▤ Laterality	Ⓐ Adult (15+ years)	Ⓜ Maternity (12-55 years)	Ⓝ Newborn	Ⓟ Pediatric (0-17 years)	♂ Male	♀ Female
✖ Deleted		Unspecified	+ Additional code					

R13.10   **Dysphagia, unspecified**
Difficulty in swallowing NOS

Dysphagia, unspecified
Lateral view

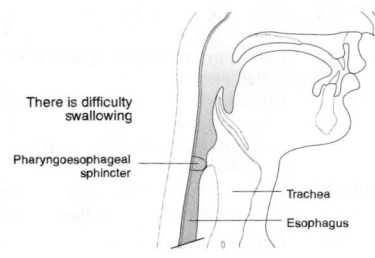

There is difficulty swallowing

Pharyngoesophageal sphincter

Trachea

Esophagus

R13.11   **Dysphagia, oral phase**
R13.12   **Dysphagia, oropharyngeal phase**
R13.13   **Dysphagia, pharyngeal phase**
R13.14   **Dysphagia, pharyngoesophageal phase**
R13.19   **Other dysphagia**
Cervical dysphagia
Neurogenic dysphagia

R14   **Flatulence and related conditions**
> **EXCLUDES 1**   *psychogenic aerophagy (F45.8)*

R14.0   **Abdominal distension (gaseous)**
Bloating
Tympanites (abdominal) (intestinal)
R14.1   **Gas pain**
R14.2   **Eructation**
R14.3   **Flatulence**

R15   **Fecal incontinence**
> **INCLUDES**   encopresis NOS
> **EXCLUDES 1**   *fecal incontinence of nonorganic origin (F98.1)*

R15.0   **Incomplete defecation**
> **EXCLUDES 1**   *constipation (K59.0-)*
> *fecal impaction (K56.41)*
R15.1   **Fecal smearing**
Fecal soiling
R15.2   **Fecal urgency**
R15.9   **Full incontinence of feces**
Fecal incontinence NOS

R16   **Hepatomegaly and splenomegaly, not elsewhere classified**
R16.0   **Hepatomegaly, not elsewhere classified**
Hepatomegaly NOS
R16.1   **Splenomegaly, not elsewhere classified**
Splenomegaly NOS
R16.2   **Hepatomegaly with splenomegaly, not elsewhere classified**
Hepatosplenomegaly NOS

R17   **Unspecified jaundice**
> **EXCLUDES 1**   *neonatal jaundice (P55, P57-P59)*

R18   **Ascites**
> **INCLUDES**   fluid in peritoneal cavity
> **EXCLUDES 1**   *ascites in alcoholic cirrhosis (K70.31)*
> *ascites in alcoholic hepatitis (K70.11)*
> *ascites in toxic liver disease with chronic active hepatitis (K71.51)*

R18.0   **Malignant ascites**
Code first malignancy, such as:
malignant neoplasm of ovary (C56.-)
secondary malignant neoplasm of retroperitoneum and peritoneum (C78.6)
> **DEFINITION**   Abnormal accumulation of fluid containing cancer cells in the peritoneal cavity, usually from metastatic spread of a malignancy.
R18.8   **Other ascites**
Ascites NOS
Peritoneal effusion (chronic)

R19   **Other symptoms and signs involving the digestive system and abdomen**
> **EXCLUDES 1**   *acute abdomen (R10.0)*

R19.0   **Intra-abdominal and pelvic swelling, mass and lump**
> **EXCLUDES 1**   *abdominal distension (gaseous) (R14.-)*
> *ascites (R18.-)*

> **CODING TIP ✓**   A mass should not be coded for an area that has been clearly identified as a neoplasm. If a mass has been biopsied and reported as a neoplasm, code the appropriate neoplasm code.

R19.00   **Intra-abdominal and pelvic swelling, mass and lump, unspecified site**
R19.01   **Right upper quadrant abdominal swelling, mass and lump**
R19.02   **Left upper quadrant abdominal swelling, mass and lump**
R19.03   **Right lower quadrant abdominal swelling, mass and lump**
R19.04   **Left lower quadrant abdominal swelling, mass and lump**
R19.05   **Periumbilic swelling, mass or lump**
Diffuse or generalized umbilical swelling or mass
R19.06   **Epigastric swelling, mass or lump**
R19.07   **Generalized intra-abdominal and pelvic swelling, mass and lump**
Diffuse or generalized intra-abdominal swelling or mass NOS
Diffuse or generalized pelvic swelling or mass NOS
R19.09   **Other intra-abdominal and pelvic swelling, mass and lump**

R19.1   **Abnormal bowel sounds**
R19.11   **Absent bowel sounds**
R19.12   **Hyperactive bowel sounds**
R19.15   **Other abnormal bowel sounds**
Abnormal bowel sounds NOS
R19.2   **Visible peristalsis**
Hyperperistalsis
R19.3   **Abdominal rigidity**
> **EXCLUDES 1**   *abdominal rigidity with severe abdominal pain (R10.0)*
R19.30   **Abdominal rigidity, unspecified site**
R19.31   **Right upper quadrant abdominal rigidity**
R19.32   **Left upper quadrant abdominal rigidity**
R19.33   **Right lower quadrant abdominal rigidity**
R19.34   **Left lower quadrant abdominal rigidity**
R19.35   **Periumbilic abdominal rigidity**
R19.36   **Epigastric abdominal rigidity**
R19.37   **Generalized abdominal rigidity**
R19.4   **Change in bowel habit**
> **EXCLUDES 1**   *constipation (K59.0-)*
> *functional diarrhea (K59.1)*
R19.5   **Other fecal abnormalities**
Abnormal stool color
Bulky stools
Mucus in stools
Occult blood in feces
Occult blood in stools
> **EXCLUDES 1**   *melena (K92.1)*
> *neonatal melena (P54.1)*
R19.6   **Halitosis**
R19.7   **Diarrhea, unspecified**
Diarrhea NOS
> **EXCLUDES 1**   *functional diarrhea (K59.1)*
> *neonatal diarrhea (P78.3)*
> *psychogenic diarrhea (F45.8)*
R19.8   **Other specified symptoms and signs involving the digestive system and abdomen**

Symptoms and signs involving the skin and subcutaneous tissue (R20-R23)

> **EXCLUDES 2**   *symptoms relating to breast (N64.4-N64.5)*

R20   **Disturbances of skin sensation**
> **EXCLUDES 1**   *dissociative anesthesia and sensory loss (F44.6)*
> *psychogenic disturbances (F45.8)*
R20.0   **Anesthesia of skin**
R20.1   **Hypoesthesia of skin**

● New   ▲ Revised   *Manifestation*   **4-7** Digit Indicators   ⊟ Laterality   Ⓐ Adult (15+ years)   Ⓜ Maternity (12-55 years)   Ⓝ Newborn   Ⓟ Pediatric (0-17 years)   ♂ Male   ♀ Female
✖ Deleted   Unspecified   + Additional code

902   © 2017 DecisionHealth   2017 ICD-10-CM Expert for Physicians

R13.10 — R20.1   Symptoms, Signs and Abnormal Clinical and Laboratory Findings, Not Elsewhere Classified

R20.2   **Paresthesia of skin**
Formication
Pins and needles
Tingling skin
> **EXCLUDES 1**   *acroparesthesia (I73.8)*

R20.3   **Hyperesthesia**

R20.8   **Other disturbances of skin sensation**

R20.9   **Unspecified disturbances of skin sensation**

R21   **Rash and other nonspecific skin eruption**
> **INCLUDES**   rash NOS
> **EXCLUDES 1**   *specified type of rash- code to condition*
> *vesicular eruption (R23.8)*

R22   **Localized swelling, mass and lump of skin and subcutaneous tissue**
> **INCLUDES**   subcutaneous nodules (localized) (superficial)
> **EXCLUDES 1**   *abnormal findings on diagnostic imaging (R90-R93)*
> *edema (R60.-)*
> *enlarged lymph nodes (R59.-)*
> *localized adiposity (E65)*
> *swelling of joint (M25.4-)*

R22.0   **Localized swelling, mass and lump, head**

R22.1   **Localized swelling, mass and lump, neck**

R22.2   **Localized swelling, mass and lump, trunk**
> **EXCLUDES 1**   *intra-abdominal or pelvic mass and lump (R19.0-)*
> *intra-abdominal or pelvic swelling (R19.0-)*
> **EXCLUDES 2**   *breast mass and lump (N63)*

R22.3   **Localized swelling, mass and lump, upper limb**

R22.30   **Localized swelling, mass and lump, unspecified upper limb**

R22.31   **Localized swelling, mass and lump, right upper limb**

R22.32   **Localized swelling, mass and lump, left upper limb**

R22.33   **Localized swelling, mass and lump, upper limb, bilateral**

R22.4   **Localized swelling, mass and lump, lower limb**

R22.40   **Localized swelling, mass and lump, unspecified lower limb**

R22.41   **Localized swelling, mass and lump, right lower limb**

R22.42   **Localized swelling, mass and lump, left lower limb**

R22.43   **Localized swelling, mass and lump, lower limb, bilateral**

R22.9   **Localized swelling, mass and lump, unspecified**

R23   **Other skin changes**

R23.0   **Cyanosis**
> **EXCLUDES 1**   *acrocyanosis (I73.8)*
> *cyanotic attacks of newborn (P28.2)*
> **DEFINITION**   Bluish tint of the skin from lack of oxygen.

R23.1   **Pallor**
Clammy skin
> **DEFINITION**   Excessive paleness of the skin, especially the face.

R23.2   **Flushing**
Excessive blushing
Code first:
, if applicable, menopausal and female climacteric states (N95.1)

R23.3   **Spontaneous ecchymoses**
Petechiae
> **EXCLUDES 1**   *ecchymoses of newborn (P54.5)*
> *purpura (D69.-)*
> **DEFINITION**   Minute red spots on the skin, due to escape of a small amount of blood from the vessels.

R23.4   **Changes in skin texture**
Desquamation of skin
Induration of skin
Scaling of skin
> **EXCLUDES 1**   *epidermal thickening NOS (L85.9)*

R23.8   **Other skin changes**

> **CODING TIP ✓**   When vesicular ulcerations (weeping ulcers) occur to the lower extremities as a result of edema (such as due to CHF or other edema producing conditions), assign R23.8 to indicate the resulting open vesicular (blister) ulceration. Do not assign this code to indicate other ulcerations such as due to friction or unspecified ulcers.

R23.9   **Unspecified skin changes**

Symptoms and signs involving the nervous and musculoskeletal systems (R25-R29)

R25   **Abnormal involuntary movements**
> **EXCLUDES 1**   *specific movement disorders (G20-G26)*
> *stereotyped movement disorders (F98.4)*
> *tic disorders (F95.-)*

R25.0   **Abnormal head movements**

R25.1   **Tremor, unspecified**
> **EXCLUDES 1**   *chorea NOS (G25.5)*
> *essential tremor (G25.0)*
> *hysterical tremor (F44.4)*
> *intention tremor (G25.2)*

R25.2   **Cramp and spasm**
> **EXCLUDES 2**   *carpopedal spasm (R29.0)*
> *charley-horse (M62.831)*
> *infantile spasms (G40.4-)*
> *muscle spasm of back (M62.830)*
> *muscle spasm of calf (M62.831)*

R25.3   **Fasciculation**
Twitching NOS

R25.8   **Other abnormal involuntary movements**

R25.9   **Unspecified abnormal involuntary movements**

R26   **Abnormalities of gait and mobility**
> **EXCLUDES 1**   *ataxia NOS (R27.0)*
> *hereditary ataxia (G11.-)*
> *locomotor (syphilitic) ataxia (A52.11)*
> *immobility syndrome (paraplegic) (M62.3)*

R26.0   **Ataxic gait**
Staggering gait
> **CODING TIP ✓**   Note the definition of ataxia, which indicates a lack of muscle coordination. This term is not interchangeable with the term gait abnormality, which indicates an abnormal gait pattern.

R26.1   **Paralytic gait**
Spastic gait

R26.2   **Difficulty in walking, not elsewhere classified**
> **EXCLUDES 1**   *falling (R29.6)*
> *unsteadiness on feet (R26.81)*
AHA: 2Q 2016, 7

R26.8   **Other abnormalities of gait and mobility**

R26.81   **Unsteadiness on feet**

R26.89   **Other abnormalities of gait and mobility**

R26.9   **Unspecified abnormalities of gait and mobility**
> **CODING TIP ✓**   Keep in mind when assigning R26.9 that if the cause of the gait abnormality is known, the code for the underlying cause of the gait abnormality should be assigned. It is not appropriate to assign the code for a symptom when a more specific code is identified.

R27   **Other lack of coordination**
> **EXCLUDES 1**   *ataxic gait (R26.0)*
> *hereditary ataxia (G11.-)*
> *vertigo NOS (R42)*

R27.0   **Ataxia, unspecified**
> **EXCLUDES 1**   *ataxia following cerebrovascular disease (I69. with final characters -93)*
> **DEFINITION**   Distortion or impairment of voluntary movement.

R27.8   **Other lack of coordination**

R27.9   **Unspecified lack of coordination**

R29   **Other symptoms and signs involving the nervous and musculoskeletal systems**

● New   ▲ Revised   *Manifestation*   ◀-▶ Digit Indicators   ▤ Laterality   Ⓐ Adult (15+ years)   Ⓜ Maternity (12-55 years)   Ⓝ Newborn   Ⓟ Pediatric (0-17 years)   ♂ Male   ♀ Female
✖ Deleted   Unspecified   + Additional code

2017 ICD-10-CM Expert for Physicians   © 2017 DecisionHealth   903

R29.0   Tetany
Carpopedal spasm
> **EXCLUDES 1**   *hysterical tetany (F44.5)*
> *neonatal tetany (P71.3)*
> *parathyroid tetany (E20.9)*
> *post-thyroidectomy tetany (E89.2)*

R29.1   Meningismus

R29.2   Abnormal reflex
> **EXCLUDES 2**   *abnormal pupillary reflex (H57.0)*
> *hyperactive gag reflex (J39.2)*
> *vasovagal reaction or syncope (R55)*

R29.3   Abnormal posture

R29.4   Clicking hip
> **EXCLUDES 1**   *congenital deformities of hip (Q65.-)*

R29.5   Transient paralysis
Code first:
any associated spinal cord injury
(S14.0, S14.1-, S24.0, S24.1-, S34.0-, S34.1-)
> **EXCLUDES 1**   *transient ischemic attack (G45.9)*

R29.6   Repeated falls
Falling
Tendency to fall
> **EXCLUDES 2**   *at risk for falling (Z91.81)*
> *history of falling (Z91.81)*

> **GUIDELINES**   **Section I.C.18.d**
> Code R29.6, Repeated falls, is for use for encounters when a patient has recently fallen and the reason for the fall is being investigated. Code Z91.81, History of falling, is for use when a patient has fallen in the past and is at risk for future falls. When appropriate, both codes R29.6 and Z91.81 may be assigned together.
> AHA: 2Q 2016, 7

● ⑤ **R29.7   National Institutes of Health Stroke Scale (NIHSS) score**
Code first:
the type of cerebral infarction (I63-)

● ⑥ **R29.70   NIHSS score 0-9**
● **R29.700   NIHSS score 0**
● **R29.701   NIHSS score 1**
● **R29.702   NIHSS score 2**
● **R29.703   NIHSS score 3**
● **R29.704   NIHSS score 4**
● **R29.705   NIHSS score 5**
● **R29.706   NIHSS score 6**
● **R29.707   NIHSS score 7**
● **R29.708   NIHSS score 8**
● **R29.709   NIHSS score 9**
● ⑥ **R29.71   NIHSS score 10-19**
● **R29.710   NIHSS score 10**
● **R29.711   NIHSS score 11**
● **R29.712   NIHSS score 12**
● **R29.713   NIHSS score 13**
● **R29.714   NIHSS score 14**
● **R29.715   NIHSS score 15**
● **R29.716   NIHSS score 16**
● **R29.717   NIHSS score 17**
● **R29.718   NIHSS score 18**
● **R29.719   NIHSS score 19**
● ⑥ **R29.72   NIHSS score 20-29**
● **R29.720   NIHSS score 20**
● **R29.721   NIHSS score 21**
● **R29.722   NIHSS score 22**
● **R29.723   NIHSS score 23**
● **R29.724   NIHSS score 24**
● **R29.725   NIHSS score 25**
● **R29.726   NIHSS score 26**
● **R29.727   NIHSS score 27**
● **R29.728   NIHSS score 28**
● **R29.729   NIHSS score 29**
● ⑥ **R29.73   NIHSS score 30-39**
● **R29.730   NIHSS score 30**
● **R29.731   NIHSS score 31**
● **R29.732   NIHSS score 32**
● **R29.733   NIHSS score 33**
● **R29.734   NIHSS score 34**

● **R29.735   NIHSS score 35**
● **R29.736   NIHSS score 36**
● **R29.737   NIHSS score 37**
● **R29.738   NIHSS score 38**
● **R29.739   NIHSS score 39**
● ⑥ **R29.74   NIHSS score 40-42**
● **R29.740   NIHSS score 40**
● **R29.741   NIHSS score 41**
● **R29.742   NIHSS score 42**

⑤ **R29.8   Other symptoms and signs involving the nervous and musculoskeletal systems**
⑥ **R29.81   Other symptoms and signs involving the nervous system**
R29.810   Facial weakness
Facial droop
> **EXCLUDES 1**   *Bell's palsy (G51.0)*
> *facial weakness following cerebrovascular disease (I69. with final characters -92)*

R29.818   Other symptoms and signs involving the nervous system

⑥ **R29.89   Other symptoms and signs involving the musculoskeletal system**
> **EXCLUDES 2**   *pain in limb (M79.6-)*

R29.890   Loss of height
> **EXCLUDES 1**   *osteoporosis (M80-M81)*

R29.891   Ocular torticollis
> **EXCLUDES 1**   *congenital (sternomastoid) torticollis Q68.0*
> *psychogenic torticollis (F45.8)*
> *spasmodic torticollis (G24.3)*
> *torticollis due to birth injury (P15.8)*
> *torticollis NOS M43.6*

R29.898   Other symptoms and signs involving the musculoskeletal system

⑤ **R29.9   Unspecified symptoms and signs involving the nervous and musculoskeletal systems**
R29.90   Unspecified symptoms and signs involving the nervous system
R29.91   Unspecified symptoms and signs involving the musculoskeletal system

Symptoms and signs involving the genitourinary system (R30-R39)

④ **R30   Pain associated with micturition**
> **EXCLUDES 1**   *psychogenic pain associated with micturition (F45.8)*

R30.0   Dysuria
Strangury

R30.1   Vesical tenesmus

R30.9   Painful micturition, unspecified
Painful urination NOS

④ **R31   Hematuria**
> **EXCLUDES 1**   *hematuria included with underlying conditions, such as:*
> *acute cystitis with hematuria (N30.01)*
> *recurrent and persistent hematuria in glomerular diseases (N02.-)*

R31.0   Gross hematuria

R31.1   Benign essential microscopic hematuria

▲ ⑤ **R31.2   Other microscopic hematuria**
● **R31.21   Asymptomatic microscopic hematuria**
AMH
● **R31.29   Other microscopic hematuria**

R31.9   Hematuria, unspecified
> **DEFINITION**   Presence of blood in the urine.

R32   Unspecified urinary incontinence
Enuresis NOS
| EXCLUDES 1 | *functional urinary incontinence (R39.81)*
nonorganic enuresis (F98.0)
stress incontinence and other specified urinary
incontinence (N39.3-N39.4-)
urinary incontinence associated with cognitive
impairment (R39.81) |

Unspecified urinary incontinence

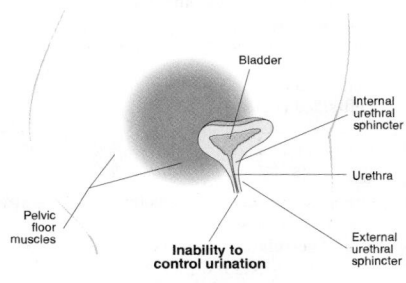

Bladder
Internal urethral sphincter
Urethra
Pelvic floor muscles
External urethral sphincter
Inability to control urination

4 R33   Retention of urine
| EXCLUDES 1 | *psychogenic retention of urine (F45.8)* |

+ R33.0   Drug induced retention of urine
Use additional code for adverse effect, if applicable, to
identify drug (T36-T50 with fifth or sixth character 5)

R33.8   Other retention of urine
Code first, if applicable, any causal condition, such as:
enlarged prostate (N40.1)

R33.9   Retention of urine, unspecified

R34   Anuria and oliguria
| EXCLUDES 1 | *anuria and oliguria complicating abortion or*
ectopic or molar pregnancy (O00-O07, O08.4)
anuria and oliguria complicating pregnancy
(O26.83-)
anuria and oliguria complicating the puerperium
(O90.4) |

4 R35   Polyuria
Code first, if applicable, any causal condition, such as:
enlarged prostate (N40.1)
| EXCLUDES 1 | *psychogenic polyuria (F45.8)* |

R35.0   Frequency of micturition
R35.1   Nocturia
R35.8   Other polyuria
Polyuria NOS

4 R36   Urethral discharge
R36.0   Urethral discharge without blood
R36.1   Hematospermia   ♂
R36.9   Urethral discharge, unspecified
Penile discharge NOS
Urethrorrhea

R37   Sexual dysfunction, unspecified

4 R39   Other and unspecified symptoms and signs involving the genitourinary system
R39.0   Extravasation of urine
5 R39.1   Other difficulties with micturition
Code first, if applicable, any causal condition, such as:
enlarged prostate (N40.1)
R39.11   Hesitancy of micturition
| DEFINITION | Difficulty starting urination. |
R39.12   Poor urinary stream
Weak urinary steam
R39.13   Splitting of urinary stream
R39.14   Feeling of incomplete bladder emptying
R39.15   Urgency of urination
| EXCLUDES 1 | *urge incontinence (N39.41, N39.46)* |
R39.16   Straining to void
▲ 6 R39.19   Other difficulties with micturition
● **R39.191   Need to immediately re-void**
● **R39.192   Position dependent micturition**
● **R39.198   Other difficulties with micturition**

R39.2   Extrarenal uremia
Prerenal uremia
| EXCLUDES 1 | *uremia NOS (N19)* |

5 R39.8   Other symptoms and signs involving the genitourinary system
R39.81   Functional urinary incontinence
Urinary incontinence due to cognitive impairment, or
severe physical disability or immobility
| EXCLUDES 1 | *stress incontinence and other specified*
urinary incontinence
(N39.3-N39.4-)
urinary incontinence NOS (R32) |
| DEFINITION | Leaking urine due to cognitive
impairment or physical disability leading to the
inability for volitional control over bladder function. |
● **R39.82   Chronic bladder pain**
R39.89   Other symptoms and signs involving the genitourinary system
R39.9   Unspecified symptoms and signs involving the genitourinary system

Symptoms and signs involving cognition, perception, emotional state and behavior (R40-R46)

| EXCLUDES 2 | *symptoms and signs constituting part of a pattern of mental*
disorder (F01-F99) |

4 R40   Somnolence, stupor and coma
| EXCLUDES 1 | *neonatal coma (P91.5)*
somnolence, stupor and coma in diabetes
(E08-E13)
somnolence, stupor and coma in hepatic failure
(K72.-)
somnolence, stupor and coma in hypoglycemia
(nondiabetic) (E15) |

R40.0   Somnolence
Drowsiness
| EXCLUDES 1 | *coma (R40.2-)* |

R40.1   Stupor
Catatonic stupor
Semicoma
| EXCLUDES 1 | *catatonic schizophrenia (F20.2)*
coma (R40.2-)
depressive stupor (F31-F33)
dissociative stupor (F44.2)
manic stupor (F30.2) |

▲ 5 R40.2   Coma
Note: One code from each subcategory, R40.21-R40.23, is
required to complete the coma scale
Code first any associated:
fracture of skull (S02.-)
intracranial injury (S06.-)
R40.20   Unspecified coma
Coma NOS
Unconsciousness NOS
6 R40.21   Coma scale, eyes open

The following appropriate 7th character is to be added
to subcategory R40.21-:
0	unspecified time
1	in the field [EMT or ambulance]
2	at arrival to emergency department
3	at hospital admission
4	24 hours or more after hospital admission

AHA: 2Q 2015, 18
7 R40.211-   Coma scale, eyes open, never
7 R40.212-   Coma scale, eyes open, to pain
7 R40.213-   Coma scale, eyes open, to sound
7 R40.214-   Coma scale, eyes open, spontaneous

● New   ▲ Revised   *Manifestation*   **4**-**7** Digit Indicators   ⊟ Laterality   **A** Adult (15+ years)   **M** Maternity (12-55 years)   **N** Newborn   **P** Pediatric (0-17 years)   ♂ Male   ♀ Female
✖ ~~Deleted~~   Unspecified   + Additional code

2017 ICD-10-CM Expert for Physicians   © 2017 DecisionHealth   905

⑥ **R40.22**   **Coma scale, best verbal response**

The following appropriate 7th character is to be added to subcategory R40.22-:
0   unspecified time
1   in the field [EMT or ambulance]
2   at arrival to emergency department
3   at hospital admission
4   24 hours or more after hospital admission

AHA: 2Q 2015, 18

⑦ **R40.221-**   **Coma scale, best verbal response, none**
⑦ **R40.222-**   **Coma scale, best verbal response, incomprehensible words**
⑦ **R40.223-**   **Coma scale, best verbal response, inappropriate words**
⑦ **R40.224-**   **Coma scale, best verbal response, confused conversation**
⑦ **R40.225-**   **Coma scale, best verbal response, oriented**

⑥ **R40.23**   **Coma scale, best motor response**

The following appropriate 7th character is to be added to subcategory R40.23-:
0   unspecified time
1   in the field [EMT or ambulance]
2   at arrival to emergency department
3   at hospital admission
4   24 hours or more after hospital admission

AHA: 2Q 2015, 18

⑦ **R40.231-**   **Coma scale, best motor response, none**
⑦ **R40.232-**   **Coma scale, best motor response, extension**
⑦ **R40.233-**   **Coma scale, best motor response, abnormal**
⑦ **R40.234-**   **Coma scale, best motor response, flexion withdrawal**
⑦ **R40.235-**   **Coma scale, best motor response, localizes pain**
⑦ **R40.236-**   **Coma scale, best motor response, obeys commands**

▲ ⑥ **R40.24**   **Glasgow coma scale, total score**

Note: Assign a code from subcategory R40.24, when only the total coma score is documented

The following appropriate 7th character is to be added to subcategory R40.24-:
0   unspecified time
1   in the field [EMT or ambulance]
2   at arrival to emergency department
3   at hospital admission
4   24 hours or more after hospital admission

AHA: 2Q 2015, 18

⑦ **R40.241-**   **Glasgow coma scale score 13-15**
⑦ **R40.242-**   **Glasgow coma scale score 9-12**
⑦ **R40.243-**   **Glasgow coma scale score 3-8**
⑦ **R40.244-**   **Other coma, without documented Glasgow coma scale score, or with partial score reported**

R40.3   **Persistent vegetative state**

CODING TIP ✓   Assign code R40.3 only when the physician has specifically confirmed persistent vegetative state (PVS). Also note that PVS differs from coma.

R40.4   **Transient alteration of awareness**

④ **R41**   **Other symptoms and signs involving cognitive functions and awareness**
EXCLUDES 1   *dissociative [conversion] disorders (F44.-)*
mild cognitive impairment, so stated (G31.84)

R41.0   **Disorientation, unspecified**
Confusion NOS
Delirium NOS

R41.1   **Anterograde amnesia**
R41.2   **Retrograde amnesia**

R41.3   **Other amnesia**
Amnesia NOS
Memory loss NOS
EXCLUDES 1   *amnestic disorder due to known physiologic condition (F04)*
amnestic syndrome due to psychoactive substance use (F10-F19 with 5th character .6)
mild memory disturbance due to known physiological condition (F06.8)
transient global amnesia (G45.4)

R41.4   **Neurologic neglect syndrome**
Asomatognosia
Hemi-akinesia
Hemi-inattention
Hemispatial neglect
Left-sided neglect
Sensory neglect
Visuospatial neglect
EXCLUDES 1   *visuospatial deficit (R41.842)*

⑤ **R41.8**   **Other symptoms and signs involving cognitive functions and awareness**
R41.81   **Age-related cognitive decline**   Ⓐ
Senility NOS
R41.82   **Altered mental status, unspecified**
Change in mental status NOS
EXCLUDES 1   *altered level of consciousness (R40.-)*
altered mental status due to known condition - code to condition
delirium NOS (R41.0)
AHA: 4Q 2012, 98
R41.83   **Borderline intellectual functioning**
IQ level 71 to 84
EXCLUDES 1   *intellectual disabilities (F70-F79)*
▲ ⑥ **R41.84**   **Other specified cognitive deficit**
EXCLUDES 1   *cognitive deficits as sequelae of cerebrovascular disease (I69.01-, I69.11-, I69.21-, I69.31-, I69.81-, I69.91-)*
R41.840   **Attention and concentration deficit**
EXCLUDES 1   *attention-deficit hyperactivity disorders (F90.-)*
R41.841   **Cognitive communication deficit**
R41.842   **Visuospatial deficit**
R41.843   **Psychomotor deficit**
R41.844   **Frontal lobe and executive function deficit**
R41.89   **Other symptoms and signs involving cognitive functions and awareness**
Anosognosia
R41.9   **Unspecified symptoms and signs involving cognitive functions and awareness**

R42   **Dizziness and giddiness**
Light-headedness
Vertigo NOS
EXCLUDES 1   *vertiginous syndromes (H81.-)*
vertigo from infrasound (T75.23)

④ **R43**   **Disturbances of smell and taste**
R43.0   **Anosmia**
R43.1   **Parosmia**
R43.2   **Parageusia**
R43.8   **Other disturbances of smell and taste**
Mixed disturbance of smell and taste
R43.9   **Unspecified disturbances of smell and taste**

④ **R44**   **Other symptoms and signs involving general sensations and perceptions**
EXCLUDES 1   *alcoholic hallucinations (F1.5)*
hallucinations in drug psychosis (F11-F19 with .5)
hallucinations in mood disorders with psychotic symptoms (F30.2, F31.5, F32.3, F33.3)
hallucinations in schizophrenia, schizotypal and delusional disorders (F20-F29)
EXCLUDES 2   *disturbances of skin sensation (R20.-)*

R44.0   **Auditory hallucinations**
R44.1   **Visual hallucinations**
R44.2   **Other hallucinations**
R44.3   **Hallucinations, unspecified**
R44.8   **Other symptoms and signs involving general sensations and perceptions**

● New   ▲ Revised   *Manifestation*   ④-⑦ Digit Indicators   ▤ Laterality   Ⓐ Adult (15+ years)   Ⓜ Maternity (12-55 years)   Ⓝ Newborn   Ⓟ Pediatric (0-17 years)   ♂ Male   ♀ Female
✖ Deleted   Unspecified   + Additional code

906   © 2017 DecisionHealth   2017 ICD-10-CM Expert for Physicians

R44.9   Unspecified symptoms and signs involving general sensations and perceptions

4 R45   Symptoms and signs involving emotional state

R45.0   Nervousness
Nervous tension

R45.1   Restlessness and agitation

R45.2   Unhappiness

R45.3   Demoralization and apathy
EXCLUDES 1   *anhedonia (R45.84)*

R45.4   Irritability and anger

R45.5   Hostility

R45.6   Violent behavior

R45.7   State of emotional shock and stress, unspecified

5 R45.8   Other symptoms and signs involving emotional state

R45.81   Low self-esteem

R45.82   Worries

R45.83   Excessive crying of child, adolescent or adult
EXCLUDES 1   *excessive crying of infant (baby) R68.11*

R45.84   Anhedonia

6 R45.85   Homicidal and suicidal ideations
EXCLUDES 1   *suicide attempt (T14.91)*

R45.850   Homicidal ideations

R45.851   Suicidal ideations

R45.86   Emotional lability

R45.87   Impulsiveness

R45.89   Other symptoms and signs involving emotional state

4 R46   Symptoms and signs involving appearance and behavior
EXCLUDES 1   *appearance and behavior in schizophrenia, schizotypal and delusional disorders (F20-F29)*
mental and behavioral disorders (F01-F99)

R46.0   Very low level of personal hygiene

R46.1   Bizarre personal appearance

R46.2   Strange and inexplicable behavior

R46.3   Overactivity

R46.4   Slowness and poor responsiveness
EXCLUDES 1   *stupor (R40.1)*

R46.5   Suspiciousness and marked evasiveness

R46.6   Undue concern and preoccupation with stressful events

R46.7   Verbosity and circumstantial detail obscuring reason for contact

5 R46.8   Other symptoms and signs involving appearance and behavior

▲ R46.81   Obsessive-compulsive behavior
EXCLUDES 1   *obsessive-compulsive disorder (F42-)*

CODING TIP ✓   Do not assign R46.81 for obsessive compulsive disorder, which is a specific syndrome coded to F42. R46.81 indicates the presence of behaviors in the absence of a specific diagnosis.

R46.89   Other symptoms and signs involving appearance and behavior

Symptoms and signs involving speech and voice (R47-R49)

4 R47   Speech disturbances, not elsewhere classified
EXCLUDES 1   *autism (F84.0)*
cluttering (F80.81)
specific developmental disorders of speech and language (F80.-)
stuttering (F80.81)

5 R47.0   Dysphasia and aphasia

R47.01   Aphasia
EXCLUDES 1   *aphasia following cerebrovascular disease (I69. with final characters -20)*
progressive isolated aphasia (G31.01)

DEFINITION   The inability to speak, write, or understand spoken or written language.

R47.02   Dysphasia
EXCLUDES 1   *dysphasia following cerebrovascular disease (I69. with final characters -21)*

R47.1   Dysarthria and anarthria
EXCLUDES 1   *dysarthria following cerebrovascular disease (I69. with final characters -22)*

5 R47.8   Other speech disturbances
EXCLUDES 1   *dysarthria following cerebrovascular disease (I69. with final characters -28)*

R47.81   Slurred speech

R47.82   Fluency disorder in conditions classified elsewhere
Stuttering in conditions classified elsewhere
Code first underlying disease or condition, such as:
Parkinson's disease (G20)
EXCLUDES 1   *adult onset fluency disorder (F98.5)*
childhood onset fluency disorder (F80.81)
fluency disorder (stuttering) following cerebrovascular disease (I69. with final characters -23)

R47.89   Other speech disturbances

R47.9   Unspecified speech disturbances

4 R48   Dyslexia and other symbolic dysfunctions, not elsewhere classified
EXCLUDES 1   *specific developmental disorders of scholastic skills (F81.-)*

R48.0   Dyslexia and alexia

R48.1   Agnosia
Astereognosia (astereognosis)
Autotopagnosia
EXCLUDES 1   *visual object agnosia (R48.3)*

R48.2   Apraxia
EXCLUDES 1   *apraxia following cerebrovascular disease (I69. with final characters -90)*

R48.3   Visual agnosia
Prosopagnosia
Simultanagnosia (asimultagnosia)

R48.8   Other symbolic dysfunctions
Acalculia
Agraphia

R48.9   Unspecified symbolic dysfunctions

4 R49   Voice and resonance disorders
EXCLUDES 1   *psychogenic voice and resonance disorders (F44.4)*

R49.0   Dysphonia
Hoarseness

R49.1   Aphonia
Loss of voice
DEFINITION   Inability to produce vocal sounds.

5 R49.2   Hypernasality and hyponasality

R49.21   Hypernasality

R49.22   Hyponasality

R49.8   Other voice and resonance disorders

R49.9   Unspecified voice and resonance disorder
Change in voice NOS
Resonance disorder NOS

General symptoms and signs (R50-R69)

4 R50   Fever of other and unknown origin
EXCLUDES 1   *chills without fever (R68.83)*
febrile convulsions (R56.0-)
fever of unknown origin during labor (O75.2)
fever of unknown origin in newborn (P81.9)
hypothermia due to illness (R68.0)
malignant hyperthermia due to anesthesia (T88.3)
puerperal pyrexia NOS (O86.4)

+ R50.2   Drug induced fever
Use additional code for adverse effect, if applicable, to identify drug (T36-T50 with fifth or sixth character 5)
EXCLUDES 1   *postvaccination (postimmunization) fever (R50.83)*

5 R50.8   Other specified fever

R50.81   Fever presenting with conditions classified elsewhere
Code first underlying condition when associated fever is present, such as with:
leukemia (C91-C95)
neutropenia (D70.-)
sickle-cell disease (D57.-)
AHA: 4Q 2014, 22

● New   ▲ Revised   *Manifestation*   4-7 Digit Indicators   ⊟ Laterality   Ⓐ Adult (15+ years)   Ⓜ Maternity (12-55 years)   Ⓝ Newborn   Ⓟ Pediatric (0-17 years)   ♂ Male   ♀ Female
✖ Deleted   Unspecified   + Additional code

▲ R50.82   **Postprocedural fever**
> EXCLUDES 1   *postprocedural infection (T81.4-)*
> *posttransfusion fever (R50.84)*
> *postvaccination (postimmunization)*
> *fever (R50.83)*

R50.83   **Postvaccination fever**
Postimmunization fever

R50.84   **Febrile nonhemolytic transfusion reaction**
FNHTR
Posttransfusion fever

R50.9   **Fever, unspecified**
Fever NOS
Fever of unknown origin [FUO]
Fever with chills
Fever with rigors
Hyperpyrexia NOS
Persistent fever
Pyrexia NOS

> CODING TIP ✓   When an infection causing a fever has been diagnosed, do not assign R50.9, but instead code the causative infectious disease specifically.

R51   **Headache**
Facial pain NOS
> EXCLUDES 1   *atypical face pain (G50.1)*
> *migraine and other headache syndromes (G43-G44)*
> *trigeminal neuralgia (G50.0)*

R52   **Pain, unspecified**
Acute pain NOS
Generalized pain NOS
Pain NOS
> EXCLUDES 1   *acute and chronic pain, not elsewhere classified (G89.-)*
> *localized pain, unspecified type - code to pain by site, such as:*
> *abdomen pain (R10.-)*
> *back pain (M54.9)*
> *breast pain (N64.4)*
> *chest pain (R07.1-R07.9)*
> *ear pain (H92.0-)*
> *eye pain (H57.1)*
> *headache (R51)*
> *joint pain (M25.5-)*
> *limb pain (M79.6-)*
> *lumbar region pain (M54.5)*
> *pelvic and perineal pain (R10.2)*
> *shoulder pain (M25.51-)*
> *spine pain (M54.-)*
> *throat pain (R07.0)*
> *tongue pain (K14.6)*
> *tooth pain (K08.8)*
> *renal colic (N23)*
> *pain disorders exclusively related to psychological factors (F45.41)*

> CODING TIP ✓   R52 should not be coded to identify pain when the underlying cause of pain is known. Code the specific cause of the pain when a diagnosis is present for the cause, such as osteoarthritis. Pay special attention to the Excludes 1 note.

④ R53   **Malaise and fatigue**

R53.0   **Neoplastic (malignant) related fatigue**
Code first:
associated neoplasm

▲ R53.1   **Weakness**
Asthenia NOS
> EXCLUDES 1   *age-related weakness (R54)*
> *muscle weakness (M62.8-)*
> *sarcopenia (M62.84)*
> *senile asthenia (R54)*

> CODING TIP ✓   Do not assign R53.1 to indicate muscle weakness or weakness resulting as a sequela of a cerebral vascular accident. Muscle weakness is coded to M62.8-

> CODING TIP ✓   Also known as general weakness. If code R53.1 is used to support therapy, documentation should establish medical necessity. The condition may include excessive tiredness, lacking energy, listlessness, and/or sleepiness. Excludes generalized muscle weakness.
> Generally used for patients with cardiorespiratory diseases. May be part of many different illnesses, including the flu, pneumonia, congestive heart failure (CHF) and arteriosclerotic heart disease (ASHD).

R53.2   **Functional quadriplegia**
Complete immobility due to severe physical disability or frailty
> EXCLUDES 1   *frailty NOS (R54)*
> *hysterical paralysis (F44.4)*
> *immobility syndrome (M62.3)*
> *neurologic quadriplegia (G82.5-)*
> *quadriplegia (G82.50)*

> GUIDELINES   **Section I.C.18.f**
> Functional quadriplegia is the lack of ability to use one's limbs or to ambulate due to extreme debility. It is not associated with neurologic deficit or injury, and code R53.2 should not be used for cases of neurologic quadriplegia. It should only be assigned if functional quadriplegia is specifically documented in the medical record.

> DEFINITION   Inability to move due to non-neurological condition, such as severe spasticity, arthritis, or severe muscle contracture.
> AHA: 2Q 2016, 6

⑤ R53.8   **Other malaise and fatigue**
> EXCLUDES 1   *combat exhaustion and fatigue (F43.0)*
> *congenital debility (P96.9)*
> *exhaustion and fatigue due to depressive episode (F32.-)*
> *exhaustion and fatigue due to excessive exertion (T73.3)*
> *exhaustion and fatigue due to exposure (T73.2)*
> *exhaustion and fatigue due to heat (T67.-)*
> *exhaustion and fatigue due to pregnancy (O26.8-)*
> *exhaustion and fatigue due to recurrent depressive episode (F33)*
> *exhaustion and fatigue due to senile debility (R54)*

R53.81   **Other malaise**
Chronic debility
Debility NOS
General physical deterioration
Malaise NOS
Nervous debility
> EXCLUDES 1   *age-related physical debility (R54)*

> CODING TIP ✓   Note that debility is a non-specific condition characterized by weight loss, functional decline, malnutrition, and multiple chronic conditions. Coding non-specific diagnosis such as this should be avoided if possible. If the diagnosis causing the debility is known, code that condition.

R53.82   **Chronic fatigue, unspecified**
Chronic fatigue syndrome NOS
> EXCLUDES 1   *postviral fatigue syndrome (G93.3)*

R53.83   **Other fatigue**
Fatigue NOS
Lack of energy
Lethargy
Tiredness

▲ R54   **Age-related physical debility**   Ⓐ
Frailty
Old age
Senescence
Senile asthenia
Senile debility
> EXCLUDES 1   *age-related cognitive decline (R41.81)*
> *sarcopenia (M62.84)*
> *senile psychosis (F03)*
> *senility NOS (R41.81)*

● New   ▲ Revised   *Manifestation*   ④-⑦ Digit Indicators   ⊟ Laterality   Ⓐ Adult (15+ years)   Ⓜ Maternity (12-55 years)   Ⓝ Newborn   Ⓟ Pediatric (0-17 years)   ♂ Male   ♀ Female
✖ ~~Deleted~~   Unspecified   + Additional code

908   © 2017 DecisionHealth   2017 ICD-10-CM Expert for Physicians

CODING TIP ✓   Note that debility is a non-specific condition characterized by weight loss, functional decline, malnutrition, and multiple chronic conditions. Coding non-specific diagnosis such as this should be avoided if possible. If the diagnosis causing the debility is known, code that condition.

R55   Syncope and collapse
Blackout
Fainting
Vasovagal attack

EXCLUDES 1   cardiogenic shock (R57.0)
carotid sinus syncope (G90.01)
heat syncope (T67.1)
neurocirculatory asthenia (F45.8)
neurogenic orthostatic hypotension (G90.3)
orthostatic hypotension (I95.1)
postprocedural shock (T81.1-)
psychogenic syncope (F48.8)
shock NOS (R57.9)
shock complicating or following abortion or ectopic or molar pregnancy (O00-O07, O08.3)
shock complicating or following labor and delivery (O75.1)
Stokes-Adams attack (I45.9)
unconsciousness NOS (R40.2-)

DEFINITION   Fainting and collapse due to a lack of blood flow to the brain.

R56   Convulsions, not elsewhere classified
EXCLUDES 1   dissociative convulsions and seizures (F44.5)
epileptic convulsions and seizures (G40.-)
newborn convulsions and seizures (P90)

R56.0   Febrile convulsions

DEFINITION   A convulsion accompanying high fever, characterized by loss of consciousness with stiffness and jerking of the limbs. The skin may become pale or turn blue. Once the jerking subsides, the child goes limp and then normal color and consciousness return.

R56.00   Simple febrile convulsions
Febrile convulsion NOS
Febrile seizure NOS

R56.01   Complex febrile convulsions
Atypical febrile seizure
Complex febrile seizure
Complicated febrile seizure
EXCLUDES 1   status epilepticus (G40.901)

R56.1   Post traumatic seizures
EXCLUDES 1   post traumatic epilepsy (G40.-)

R56.9   Unspecified convulsions
Convulsion disorder
Fit NOS
Recurrent convulsions
Seizure(s) (convulsive) NOS

CODING TIP ✓   Do not assign R56.9 when a patient has had recurrent seizures or a seizure disorder. When recurrent seizures or seizure disorder are present, report the appropriate code from category G40.-.

R57   Shock, not elsewhere classified
EXCLUDES 1   anaphylactic shock NOS (T78.2)
anaphylactic reaction or shock due to adverse food reaction (T78.0-)
anaphylactic shock due to adverse effect of correct drug or medicament properly administered (T88.6)
anaphylactic shock due to serum (T80.5-)
anesthetic shock (T88.3)
electric shock (T75.4)
obstetric shock (O75.1)
postprocedural shock (T81.1-)
psychic shock (F43.0)
septic shock (R65.21)
shock complicating or following ectopic or molar pregnancy (O00-O07, O08.3)
shock due to lightning (T75.01)
traumatic shock (T79.4)
toxic shock syndrome (A48.3)

R57.0   Cardiogenic shock
R57.1   Hypovolemic shock
R57.8   Other shock

R57.9   Shock, unspecified
Failure of peripheral circulation NOS

R58   Hemorrhage, not elsewhere classified
Hemorrhage NOS
EXCLUDES 1   hemorrhage included with underlying conditions, such as:
acute duodenal ulcer with hemorrhage (K26.0)
acute gastritis with bleeding (K29.01)
ulcerative enterocolitis with rectal bleeding (K51.01)

R59   Enlarged lymph nodes
INCLUDES   swollen glands
EXCLUDES 1   lymphadenitis NOS (I88.9)
acute lymphadenitis (L04.-)
chronic lymphadenitis (I88.1)
mesenteric (acute) (chronic) lymphadenitis (I88.0)

R59.0   Localized enlarged lymph nodes
R59.1   Generalized enlarged lymph nodes
Lymphadenopathy NOS
R59.9   Enlarged lymph nodes, unspecified

R60   Edema, not elsewhere classified
EXCLUDES 1   angioneurotic edema (T78.3)
ascites (R18.-)
cerebral edema (G93.6)
cerebral edema due to birth injury (P11.0)
edema of larynx (J38.4)
edema of nasopharynx (J39.2)
edema of pharynx (J39.2)
gestational edema (O12.0-)
hereditary edema (Q82.0)
hydrops fetalis NOS (P83.2)
hydrothorax (J94.8)
nutritional edema (E40-E46)
hydrops fetalis NOS (P83.2)
newborn edema (P83.3)
pulmonary edema (J81.-)

R60.0   Localized edema
CODING TIP ✓   Do not report R60.0 in a patient with heart failure or any other known cause for the edema.

R60.1   Generalized edema

Generalized edema

Edema—the swelling of tissues or organs with fluid

R60.9   Edema, unspecified
Fluid retention NOS

R61   Generalized hyperhidrosis
Excessive sweating
Night sweats
Secondary hyperhidrosis
Code first:
, if applicable, menopausal and female climacteric states (N95.1)
EXCLUDES 1   focal (primary) (secondary) hyperhidrosis (L74.5-)
Frey's syndrome (L74.52)
localized (primary) (secondary) hyperhidrosis (L74.5-)

R62   Lack of expected normal physiological development in childhood and adults
EXCLUDES 1   delayed puberty (E30.0)
gonadal dysgenesis (Q99.1)
hypopituitarism (E23.0)

● New   ▲ Revised   *Manifestation*   ④-❼ Digit Indicators   ⊟ Laterality   Ⓐ Adult (15+ years)   Ⓜ Maternity (12-55 years)   Ⓝ Newborn (0-17 years)   ♂ Male   ♀ Female
✖ Deleted   Unspecified   + Additional code

2017 ICD-10-CM Expert for Physicians   © 2017 DecisionHealth   909

R62.0 **Delayed milestone in childhood** 🅿
Delayed attainment of expected physiological developmental stage
Late talker
Late walker

⑤ R62.5 **Other and unspecified lack of expected normal physiological development in childhood**
> **EXCLUDES 1** *HIV disease resulting in failure to thrive (B20)*
> *physical retardation due to malnutrition (E45)*

R62.50 **Unspecified lack of expected normal physiological development in childhood** 🅿
Infantilism NOS

R62.51 **Failure to thrive (child)** 🅿
Failure to gain weight
> **EXCLUDES 1** *failure to thrive in child under 28 days old (P92.6)*

R62.52 **Short stature (child)** 🅿
Lack of growth
Physical retardation
Short stature NOS
> **EXCLUDES 1** *short stature due to endocrine disorder (E34.3)*

R62.59 **Other lack of expected normal physiological development in childhood** 🅿

R62.7 **Adult failure to thrive** 🅰
> **CODING TIP ✓** When coding failure to thrive, identify the conditions leading to the patient's failure to thrive and code these underlying conditions first.

④ R63 **Symptoms and signs concerning food and fluid intake**
> **EXCLUDES 1** *bulimia NOS (F50.2)*
> *eating disorders of nonorganic origin (F50.-)*
> *malnutrition (E40-E46)*

▲ R63.0 **Anorexia**
Loss of appetite
> **EXCLUDES 1** *anorexia nervosa (F50.0-)*
> *loss of appetite of nonorganic origin (F50.89)*

> **CODING TIP ✓** Anorexia indicates a loss of appetite or intake resulting from appetite loss. Note that anorexia nervosa, which is coded to F50.0-, differs from anorexia coded to R53.0 in that anorexia nervosa includes a psychological component of body image disturbance.

R63.1 **Polydipsia**
Excessive thirst

R63.2 **Polyphagia**
Excessive eating
Hyperalimentation NOS

R63.3 **Feeding difficulties**
Feeding problem (elderly) (infant) NOS
> **EXCLUDES 1** *feeding problems of newborn (P92.-)*
> *infant feeding disorder of nonorganic origin (F98.2-)*

R63.4 **Abnormal weight loss**
R63.5 **Abnormal weight gain**
> **EXCLUDES 1** *excessive weight gain in pregnancy (O26.0-)*
> *obesity (E66.-)*

✚ R63.6 **Underweight**
Use additional code to identify body mass index (BMI), if known (Z68.-)
> **EXCLUDES 1** *abnormal weight loss (R63.4)*
> *anorexia nervosa (F50.0-)*
> *malnutrition (E40-E46)*

R63.8 **Other symptoms and signs concerning food and fluid intake**

R64 **Cachexia**
Wasting syndrome
Code first:
underlying condition, if known
> **EXCLUDES 1** *abnormal weight loss (R63.4)*
> *nutritional marasmus (E41)*

④ R65 **Symptoms and signs specifically associated with systemic inflammation and infection**

> **GUIDELINES** **Section I.C.1.d.6)**
> Only one code from category R65, Symptoms and signs specifically associated with systemic inflammation and infection, should be assigned. Therefore, when a non-infectious condition leads to an infection resulting in severe sepsis, assign the appropriate code from subcategory R65.2, Severe sepsis. Do not additionally assign a code from subcategory R65.1, Systemic inflammatory response syndrome (SIRS) of noninfectious origin.

⑤ R65.1 **Systemic inflammatory response syndrome (SIRS) of non-infectious origin**
Code first underlying condition, such as:
heatstroke (T67.0)
injury and trauma (S00-T88)
> **EXCLUDES 1** *sepsis- code to infection*
> *severe sepsis (R65.2)*

> **CODING TIP ✓** R65.1 codes are used for systemic inflammatory response syndrome (SIRS) of non-infectious origin. Some physicians will document 'sepsis', but not indicate an infectious process, for example, 'due to a Pulmonary Embolism'. Sepsis implies an infection so the physician should be queried. SIRS is defined as 2 or more of the following: fever <38° C or >36°C, heart rate >90 beats/min, respirations >30/min or PaCO2 < 32mmHg and/or abnormal WBC count.

R65.10 **Systemic inflammatory response syndrome (SIRS) of non-infectious origin without acute organ dysfunction**
Systemic inflammatory response syndrome (SIRS) NOS

✚ R65.11 **Systemic inflammatory response syndrome (SIRS) of non-infectious origin with acute organ dysfunction**
Use additional code to identify specific acute organ dysfunction, such as:
acute kidney failure (N17.-)
acute respiratory failure (J96.0-)
critical illness myopathy (G72.81)
critical illness polyneuropathy (G62.81)
disseminated intravascular coagulopathy [DIC] (D65)
encephalopathy (metabolic) (septic) (G93.41)
hepatic failure (K72.0-)

> **GUIDELINES** **Section I.C.18.g**
> The systemic inflammatory response syndrome (SIRS) can develop as a result of certain non-infectious disease processes, such as trauma, malignant neoplasm, or pancreatitis. When SIRS is documented with a noninfectious condition, and no subsequent infection is documented, the code for the underlying condition, such as an injury, should be assigned, followed by code R65.10, Systemic inflammatory response syndrome (SIRS) of non-infectious origin without acute organ dysfunction, or code R65.11, Systemic inflammatory response syndrome (SIRS) of non-infectious origin with acute organ dysfunction. If an associated acute organ dysfunction is documented, the appropriate code(s) for the specific type of organ dysfunction(s) should be assigned in addition to code R65.11. If acute organ dysfunction is documented, but it cannot be determined if the acute organ dysfunction is associated with SIRS or due to another condition (e.g., directly due to the trauma), the provider should be queried.

● New ▲ Revised *Manifestation* ④-❼ Digit Indicators ⊟ Laterality 🅰 Adult (15+ years) Ⓜ Maternity (12-55 years) Ⓝ Newborn 🅿 Pediatric (0-17 years) ♂ Male ♀ Female
✖ ~~Deleted~~ Unspecified ✚ Additional code

910   © 2017 DecisionHealth   2017 ICD-10-CM Expert for Physicians

▲ ⑤ ✚ **R65.2**   **Severe sepsis**
Infection with associated acute organ dysfunction
Sepsis with acute organ dysfunction
Sepsis with multiple organ dysfunction
Systemic inflammatory response syndrome due to infectious process with acute organ dysfunction
Code first underlying infection, such as:
  infection following a procedure (T81.4-)
  infections following infusion, transfusion and therapeutic injection (T80.2-)
  puerperal sepsis (O85)
  sepsis following complete or unspecified spontaneous abortion (O03.87)
  sepsis following ectopic and molar pregnancy (O08.82)
  sepsis following incomplete spontaneous abortion (O03.37)
  sepsis following (induced) termination of pregnancy (O04.87)
  sepsis NOS (A41.9)
Use additional code to identify specific acute organ dysfunction, such as:
  acute kidney failure (N17.-)
  acute respiratory failure (J96.0-)
  critical illness myopathy (G72.81)
  critical illness polyneuropathy (G62.81)
  disseminated intravascular coagulopathy [DIC] (D65)
  encephalopathy (metabolic) (septic) (G93.41)
  hepatic failure (K72.0-)

GUIDELINES   Section I.C.1.d.1)(b)
The coding of severe sepsis requires a minimum of two codes: first a code for the underlying systemic infection, followed by a code from subcategory R65.2, Severe sepsis. If the causal organism is not documented, assign code A41.9, Sepsis, unspecified organism, for the infection. Additional code(s) for the associated acute organ dysfunction are also required. Due to the complex nature of severe sepsis, some cases may require querying the provider prior to assignment of the codes.

GUIDELINES   Section I.C.1.d.1)(a)(iv)
If a patient has sepsis and an acute organ dysfunction, but the medical record documentation indicates that the acute organ dysfunction is related to a medical condition other than the sepsis, do not assign a code from subcategory R65.2, Severe sepsis. An acute organ dysfunction must be associated with the sepsis in order to assign the severe sepsis code. If the documentation is not clear as to whether an acute organ dysfunction is related to the sepsis or another medical condition, query the provider.

GUIDELINES   Section I.C.1.d.4)
If the reason for admission is both sepsis or severe sepsis and a localized infection, such as pneumonia or cellulitis, a code(s) for the underlying systemic infection should be assigned first and the code for the localized infection should be assigned as a secondary diagnosis. If the patient has severe sepsis, a code from subcategory R65.2 should also be assigned as a secondary diagnosis. If the patient is admitted with a localized infection, such as pneumonia, and sepsis/severe sepsis doesn't develop until after admission, the localized infection should be assigned first, followed by the appropriate sepsis/severe sepsis codes.

CODING TIP ✓   When severe sepsis is present in a patient (sepsis with the additional presence of organ dysfunction, hypotension, or hypoperfusion), a code from R65.2- must be assigned in addition to the code identifying the underlying infection. An additional code(s) also should be assigned to identify all organ dysfunction present.

✚ **R65.20**   **Severe sepsis without septic shock**
Severe sepsis NOS

GUIDELINES   Section I.C.1.d.5)(c)
In cases where a postprocedural infection has occurred and has resulted in severe sepsis, the code for the precipitating complication such as code T81.4, Infection following a procedure, or O86.0, Infection of obstetrical surgical wound, should be coded first followed by code R65.20, Severe sepsis without septic shock. A code for the systemic infection should also be assigned.

If the postprocedural infection has resulted in postprocedural septic shock, the code for the precipitating complication such as code T81.4 or O86.0 should be coded first followed by code T81.12-, Postprocedural septic shock. A code for the systemic infection should also be assigned.

✚ **R65.21**   **Severe sepsis with septic shock**
GUIDELINES   Section I.C.1.d.2)(a)
Septic shock generally refers to circulatory failure associated with severe sepsis, and therefore, it represents a type of acute organ dysfunction. For cases of septic shock, the code for the systemic infection should be sequenced first, followed by code R65.21, Severe sepsis with septic shock or code T81.12, Postprocedural septic shock. Any additional codes for the other acute organ dysfunctions should also be assigned. As noted in the sequencing instructions in the Tabular List, the code for septic shock cannot be assigned as a principal diagnosis.

④ **R68**   **Other general symptoms and signs**

R68.0   **Hypothermia, not associated with low environmental temperature**
  EXCLUDES 1   *hypothermia NOS (accidental) (T68)*
      hypothermia due to anesthesia (T88.51)
      hypothermia due to low environmental temperature (T68)
      newborn hypothermia (P80.-)

⑤ **R68.1**   **Nonspecific symptoms peculiar to infancy**
  EXCLUDES 1   *colic, infantile (R10.83)*
      neonatal cerebral irritability (P91.3)
      teething syndrome (K00.7)
  R68.11   **Excessive crying of infant (baby)**   ℙ
    EXCLUDES 1   *excessive crying of child, adolescent, or adult (R45.83)*
  R68.12   **Fussy infant (baby)**   ℙ
    Irritable infant
  ✚ **R68.13**   **Apparent life threatening event in infant (ALTE)**   ℙ
    Apparent life threatening event in newborn
    Code first:
      confirmed diagnosis, if known
    Use additional code(s) for associated signs and symptoms if no confirmed diagnosis established, or if signs and symptoms are not associated routinely with confirmed diagnosis, or provide additional information for cause of ALTE
  R68.19   **Other nonspecific symptoms peculiar to infancy**   ℙ

R68.2   **Dry mouth, unspecified**
  EXCLUDES 1   *dry mouth due to dehydration (E86.0)*
      dry mouth due to sicca syndrome [Sjögren] (M35.0-)
      salivary gland hyposecretion (K11.7)

R68.3   **Clubbing of fingers**
  Clubbing of nails
  EXCLUDES 1   *congenital clubfinger (Q68.1)*

⑤ **R68.8**   **Other general symptoms and signs**
  R68.81   **Early satiety**
  R68.82   **Decreased libido**   Ⓐ
    Decreased sexual desire
  R68.83   **Chills (without fever)**
    Chills NOS
    EXCLUDES 1   *chills with fever (R50.9)*
  ▲ **R68.84**   **Jaw pain**
    Mandibular pain
    Maxilla pain
    EXCLUDES 1   *temporomandibular joint arthralgia (M26.62-)*
  R68.89   **Other general symptoms and signs**

● New   ▲ Revised   *Manifestation*   ④-⑦ Digit Indicators   ⊟ Laterality   Ⓐ Adult (15+ years)   Ⓜ Maternity (12-55 years)   Ⓝ Newborn   ℙ Pediatric (0-17 years)   ♂ Male   ♀ Female
✖ ~~Deleted~~   Unspecified   ✚ Additional code

R69   Illness, unspecified
Unknown and unspecified cases of morbidity

Abnormal findings on examination of blood, without diagnosis (R70-R79)

EXCLUDES 2   *abnormal findings on antenatal screening of mother (O28.-)*
abnormalities of lipids (E78.-)
abnormalities of platelets and thrombocytes (D69.-)
abnormalities of white blood cells classified elsewhere (D70-D72)
coagulation hemorrhagic disorders (D65-D68)
diagnostic abnormal findings classified elsewhere - see Alphabetical Index
hemorrhagic and hematological disorders of newborn (P50-P61)

4 R70   Elevated erythrocyte sedimentation rate and abnormality of plasma viscosity

 R70.0   Elevated erythrocyte sedimentation rate

 R70.1   Abnormal plasma viscosity

4 R71   Abnormality of red blood cells

 EXCLUDES 1   *anemias (D50-D64)*
anemia of premature infant (P61.2)
benign (familial) polycythemia (D75.0)
congenital anemias (P61.2-P61.4)
newborn anemia due to isoimmunization (P55.-)
polycythemia neonatorum (P61.1)
polycythemia NOS (D75.1)
polycythemia vera (D45)
secondary polycythemia (D75.1)

 R71.0   Precipitous drop in hematocrit
Drop (precipitous) in hemoglobin
Drop in hematocrit

 R71.8   Other abnormality of red blood cells
Abnormal red-cell morphology NOS
Abnormal red-cell volume NOS
Anisocytosis
Poikilocytosis

4 R73   Elevated blood glucose level

 EXCLUDES 1   *diabetes mellitus (E08-E13)*
diabetes mellitus in pregnancy, childbirth and the puerperium (O24.-)
neonatal disorders (P70.0-P70.2)
postsurgical hypoinsulinemia (E89.1)

 5 R73.0   Abnormal glucose

  EXCLUDES 1   *abnormal glucose in pregnancy (O99.81-)*
diabetes mellitus (E08-E13)
dysmetabolic syndrome X (E88.81)
gestational diabetes (O24.4-)
glycosuria (R81)
hypoglycemia (E16.2)

  R73.01   Impaired fasting glucose
Elevated fasting glucose

  R73.02   Impaired glucose tolerance (oral)
Elevated glucose tolerance

  ● **R73.03   Prediabetes**
Latent diabetes

  R73.09   Other abnormal glucose
Abnormal glucose NOS
Abnormal non-fasting glucose tolerance

 R73.9   Hyperglycemia, unspecified

 CODING TIP ✓   Hyperglycemia should be coded to R73.9 only when not associated with diabetes mellitus or any form of post-procedural hyperinsulinemia. R73.9 indicates hyperglycemia that is of an unspecified origin.

4 R74   Abnormal serum enzyme levels

 R74.0   Nonspecific elevation of levels of transaminase and lactic acid dehydrogenase [LDH]

 R74.8   Abnormal levels of other serum enzymes
Abnormal level of acid phosphatase
Abnormal level of alkaline phosphatase
Abnormal level of amylase
Abnormal level of lipase [triacylglycerol lipase]

 R74.9   Abnormal serum enzyme level, unspecified

R75   Inconclusive laboratory evidence of human immunodeficiency virus [HIV]
Nonconclusive HIV-test finding in infants

 EXCLUDES 1   *asymptomatic human immunodeficiency virus [HIV] infection status (Z21)*
human immunodeficiency virus [HIV] disease (B20)

 GUIDELINES   **Section I.C.1.a.2)(e)**
Patients with inconclusive HIV serology, but no definitive diagnosis or manifestations of the illness, may be assigned code R75, Inconclusive laboratory evidence of human immunodeficiency virus [HIV].

 GUIDELINES   **Section I.C.1.a.2)(f)**
Patients previously diagnosed with any HIV illness (B20) should never be assigned to R75 or Z21, Asymptomatic human immunodeficiency virus [HIV] infection status.

4 R76   Other abnormal immunological findings in serum

 R76.0   Raised antibody titer

  EXCLUDES 1   *isoimmunization in pregnancy (O36.0-O36.1)*
isoimmunization affecting newborn (P55.-)

 5 R76.1   Nonspecific reaction to test for tuberculosis

  R76.11   Nonspecific reaction to tuberculin skin test without active tuberculosis
Abnormal result of Mantoux test
PPD positive
Tuberculin (skin test) positive
Tuberculin (skin test) reactor

   EXCLUDES 1   *nonspecific reaction to cell mediated immunity measurement of gamma interferon antigen response without active tuberculosis (R76.12)*

  R76.12   Nonspecific reaction to cell mediated immunity measurement of gamma interferon antigen response without active tuberculosis
Nonspecific reaction to QuantiFERON-TB test (QFT) without active tuberculosis

   EXCLUDES 1   *nonspecific reaction to tuberculin skin test without active tuberculosis (R76.11)*
positive tuberculin skin test (R76.11)

 R76.8   Other specified abnormal immunological findings in serum
Raised level of immunoglobulins NOS

 R76.9   Abnormal immunological finding in serum, unspecified

4 R77   Other abnormalities of plasma proteins

 EXCLUDES 1   *disorders of plasma-protein metabolism (E88.0)*

 R77.0   Abnormality of albumin

 R77.1   Abnormality of globulin
Hyperglobulinemia NOS

 R77.2   Abnormality of alphafetoprotein

 R77.8   Other specified abnormalities of plasma proteins

 R77.9   Abnormality of plasma protein, unspecified

4 + R78   Findings of drugs and other substances, not normally found in blood
Use additional code to identify the any retained foreign body, if applicable (Z18.-)

 EXCLUDES 1   *mental or behavioral disorders due to psychoactive substance use (F10-F19)*

 + R78.0   Finding of alcohol in blood
Use additional external cause code (Y90.-), for detail regarding alcohol level.

 + R78.1   Finding of opiate drug in blood

 + R78.2   Finding of cocaine in blood

 + R78.3   Finding of hallucinogen in blood

 + R78.4   Finding of other drugs of addictive potential in blood

 + R78.5   Finding of other psychotropic drug in blood

 + R78.6   Finding of steroid agent in blood

 5 + R78.7   Finding of abnormal level of heavy metals in blood

  + R78.71   Abnormal lead level in blood

   EXCLUDES 1   *lead poisoning (T56.0-)*

  + R78.79   Finding of abnormal level of heavy metals in blood

 5 + R78.8   Finding of other specified substances, not normally found in blood

  ▲ **+ R78.81   Bacteremia**

   EXCLUDES 1   *sepsis-code to specified infection*

● New   ▲ Revised   *Manifestation*   **4 - 7** Digit Indicators   ⊟ Laterality   Ⓐ Adult (15+ years)   Ⓜ Maternity (12-55 years)   Ⓝ Newborn (0-17 years)   Ⓟ Pediatric (0-17 years)   ♂ Male   ♀ Female

✖ ~~Deleted~~   Unspecified   + Additional code

912   © 2017 DecisionHealth   2017 ICD-10-CM Expert for Physicians

CODING TIP ✓ Do not assign code R78.81 to indicate the presence of sepsis. Bacteremia only indicates the presence of bacteria identified in the bloodstream, not the infectious process. Do not assign R78.81 with any code identifying sepsis. Sepsis should be coded to the appropriate code identifying the specific type of sepsis present.

DEFINITION The presence of small numbers of bacteria in the bloodstream, usually as a temporary condition, and without causing symptoms.

+ **R78.89** **Finding of other specified substances, not normally found in blood**
Finding of abnormal level of lithium in blood

+ **R78.9** **Finding of unspecified substance, not normally found in blood**

▣ + **R79** **Other abnormal findings of blood chemistry**
Use additional code to identify any retained foreign body, if applicable (Z18.-)

EXCLUDES 1 *abnormality of fluid, electrolyte or acid-base balance (E86-E87)*
asymptomatic hyperuricemia (E79.0)
hyperglycemia NOS (R73.9)
hypoglycemia NOS (E16.2)
neonatal hypoglycemia (P70.3-P70.4)
specific findings indicating disorder of amino-acid metabolism (E70-E72)
specific findings indicating disorder of carbohydrate metabolism (E73-E74)
specific findings indicating disorder of lipid metabolism (E75.-)

+ **R79.0** **Abnormal level of blood mineral**
Abnormal blood level of cobalt
Abnormal blood level of copper
Abnormal blood level of iron
Abnormal blood level of magnesium
Abnormal blood level of mineral NEC
Abnormal blood level of zinc

EXCLUDES 1 *abnormal level of lithium (R78.89)*
disorders of mineral metabolism (E83.-)
neonatal hypomagnesemia (P71.2)
nutritional mineral deficiency (E58-E61)

+ **R79.1** **Abnormal coagulation profile**
Abnormal or prolonged bleeding time
Abnormal or prolonged coagulation time
Abnormal or prolonged partial thromboplastin time [PTT]
Abnormal or prolonged prothrombin time [PT]

EXCLUDES 1 *coagulation defects (D68.-)*

▣ + **R79.8** **Other specified abnormal findings of blood chemistry**

+ **R79.81** **Abnormal blood-gas level**

DEFINITION Abnormal oxygen or carbon dioxide level in the blood.

+ **R79.82** **Elevated C-reactive protein (CRP)**

+ **R79.89** **Other specified abnormal findings of blood chemistry**

+ **R79.9** **Abnormal finding of blood chemistry, unspecified**

Abnormal findings on examination of urine, without diagnosis (R80-R82)

EXCLUDES 1 *abnormal findings on antenatal screening of mother (O28.-)*
diagnostic abnormal findings classified elsewhere - see Alphabetical Index
specific findings indicating disorder of amino-acid metabolism (E70-E72)
specific findings indicating disorder of carbohydrate metabolism (E73-E74)

▣ **R80** **Proteinuria**

EXCLUDES 1 *gestational proteinuria (O12.1-)*

R80.0 **Isolated proteinuria**
Idiopathic proteinuria

EXCLUDES 1 *isolated proteinuria with specific morphological lesion (N06.-)*

R80.1 **Persistent proteinuria, unspecified**

R80.2 **Orthostatic proteinuria, unspecified**
Postural proteinuria

R80.3 **Bence Jones proteinuria**

R80.8 **Other proteinuria**

R80.9 **Proteinuria, unspecified**
Albuminuria NOS

R81 **Glycosuria**

EXCLUDES 1 *renal glycosuria (E74.8)*

▣ + **R82** **Other and unspecified abnormal findings in urine**

INCLUDES chromoabnormalities in urine

Use additional code to identify any retained foreign body, if applicable (Z18.-)

EXCLUDES 2 *hematuria (R31.-)*

+ **R82.0** **Chyluria**

EXCLUDES 1 *filarial chyluria (B74.-)*

+ **R82.1** **Myoglobinuria**

+ **R82.2** **Biliuria**

+ **R82.3** **Hemoglobinuria**

EXCLUDES 1 *hemoglobinuria due to hemolysis from external causes NEC (D59.6)*
hemoglobinuria due to paroxysmal nocturnal [Marchiafava-Micheli] (D59.5)

+ **R82.4** **Acetonuria**
Ketonuria

+ **R82.5** **Elevated urine levels of drugs, medicaments and biological substances**
Elevated urine levels of catecholamines
Elevated urine levels of indoleacetic acid
Elevated urine levels of 17-ketosteroids
Elevated urine levels of steroids

+ **R82.6** **Abnormal urine levels of substances chiefly nonmedicinal as to source**
Abnormal urine level of heavy metals

▲ ▣ + **R82.7** **Abnormal findings on microbiological examination of urine**

EXCLUDES 1 *colonization status (Z22.-)*

● + **R82.71** **Bacteriuria**

● + **R82.79** **Other abnormal findings on microbiological examination of urine**
Positive culture findings of urine

+ **R82.8** **Abnormal findings on cytological and histological examination of urine**

▣ + **R82.9** **Other and unspecified abnormal findings in urine**

+ **R82.90** **Unspecified abnormal findings in urine**

+ **R82.91** **Other chromoabnormalities of urine**
Chromoconversion (dipstick)
Idiopathic dipstick converts positive for blood with no cellular forms in sediment

EXCLUDES 1 *hemoglobinuria (R82.3)*
myoglobinuria (R82.1)

+ **R82.99** **Other abnormal findings in urine**
Cells and casts in urine
Crystalluria
Melanuria

Abnormal findings on examination of other body fluids, substances and tissues, without diagnosis (R83-R89)

EXCLUDES 1 *abnormal findings on antenatal screening of mother (O28.-)*
diagnostic abnormal findings classified elsewhere - see Alphabetical Index

EXCLUDES 2 *abnormal findings on examination of blood, without diagnosis (R70-R79)*
abnormal findings on examination of urine, without diagnosis (R80-R82)
abnormal tumor markers (R97.-)

▣ **R83** **Abnormal findings in cerebrospinal fluid**

R83.0 **Abnormal level of enzymes in cerebrospinal fluid**

R83.1 **Abnormal level of hormones in cerebrospinal fluid**

R83.2 **Abnormal level of other drugs, medicaments and biological substances in cerebrospinal fluid**

R83.3 **Abnormal level of substances chiefly nonmedicinal as to source in cerebrospinal fluid**

R83.4 **Abnormal immunological findings in cerebrospinal fluid**

R83.5 **Abnormal microbiological findings in cerebrospinal fluid**
Positive culture findings in cerebrospinal fluid

EXCLUDES 1 *colonization status (Z22.-)*

R83.6 **Abnormal cytological findings in cerebrospinal fluid**

● New ▲ Revised *Manifestation* ▣-▣ Digit Indicators ▤ Laterality ▣ Adult (15+ years) ▣ Maternity (12-55 years) ▣ Newborn ▣ Pediatric (0-17 years) ♂ Male ♀ Female
✖ Deleted Unspecified + Additional code

R83.8   **Other abnormal findings in cerebrospinal fluid**
Abnormal chromosomal findings in cerebrospinal fluid

R83.9   **Unspecified abnormal finding in cerebrospinal fluid**

◢ R84   **Abnormal findings in specimens from respiratory organs and thorax**

INCLUDES   abnormal findings in bronchial washings
abnormal findings in nasal secretions
abnormal findings in pleural fluid
abnormal findings in sputum
abnormal findings in throat scrapings

EXCLUDES 1   *blood-stained sputum (R04.2)*

R84.0   **Abnormal level of enzymes in specimens from respiratory organs and thorax**

R84.1   **Abnormal level of hormones in specimens from respiratory organs and thorax**

R84.2   **Abnormal level of other drugs, medicaments and biological substances in specimens from respiratory organs and thorax**

R84.3   **Abnormal level of substances chiefly nonmedicinal as to source in specimens from respiratory organs and thorax**

R84.4   **Abnormal immunological findings in specimens from respiratory organs and thorax**

R84.5   **Abnormal microbiological findings in specimens from respiratory organs and thorax**
Positive culture findings in specimens from respiratory organs and thorax

EXCLUDES 1   *colonization status (Z22.-)*

R84.6   **Abnormal cytological findings in specimens from respiratory organs and thorax**

R84.7   **Abnormal histological findings in specimens from respiratory organs and thorax**

R84.8   **Other abnormal findings in specimens from respiratory organs and thorax**
Abnormal chromosomal findings in specimens from respiratory organs and thorax

R84.9   **Unspecified abnormal finding in specimens from respiratory organs and thorax**

◢ R85   **Abnormal findings in specimens from digestive organs and abdominal cavity**

INCLUDES   abnormal findings in peritoneal fluid
abnormal findings in saliva

EXCLUDES 1   *cloudy peritoneal dialysis effluent (R88.0)*
fecal abnormalities (R19.5)

R85.0   **Abnormal level of enzymes in specimens from digestive organs and abdominal cavity**

R85.1   **Abnormal level of hormones in specimens from digestive organs and abdominal cavity**

R85.2   **Abnormal level of other drugs, medicaments and biological substances in specimens from digestive organs and abdominal cavity**

R85.3   **Abnormal level of substances chiefly nonmedicinal as to source in specimens from digestive organs and abdominal cavity**

R85.4   **Abnormal immunological findings in specimens from digestive organs and abdominal cavity**

R85.5   **Abnormal microbiological findings in specimens from digestive organs and abdominal cavity**
Positive culture findings in specimens from digestive organs and abdominal cavity

EXCLUDES 1   *colonization status (Z22.-)*

⑤ R85.6   **Abnormal cytological findings in specimens from digestive organs and abdominal cavity**

⑥ R85.61   **Abnormal cytologic smear of anus**

EXCLUDES 1   *abnormal cytological findings in specimens from other digestive organs and abdominal cavity (R85.69)*
carcinoma in situ of anus (histologically confirmed) (D01.3)
anal intraepithelial neoplasia I [AIN I] (K62.82)
anal intraepithelial neoplasia II [AIN II] (K62.82)
anal intraepithelial neoplasia III [AIN III] (D01.3)
dysplasia (mild) (moderate) of anus (histologically confirmed) (K62.82)
severe dysplasia of anus (histologically confirmed) (D01.3)

EXCLUDES 2   *anal high risk human papillomavirus (HPV) DNA test positive (R85.81)*
anal low risk human papillomavirus (HPV) DNA test positive (R85.82)

R85.610   **Atypical squamous cells of undetermined significance on cytologic smear of anus (ASC-US)**

R85.611   **Atypical squamous cells cannot exclude high grade squamous intraepithelial lesion on cytologic smear of anus (ASC-H)**

R85.612   **Low grade squamous intraepithelial lesion on cytologic smear of anus (LGSIL)**

R85.613   **High grade squamous intraepithelial lesion on cytologic smear of anus (HGSIL)**

R85.614   **Cytologic evidence of malignancy on smear of anus**

R85.615   **Unsatisfactory cytologic smear of anus**
Inadequate sample of cytologic smear of anus

R85.616   **Satisfactory anal smear but lacking transformation zone**

R85.618   **Other abnormal cytological findings on specimens from anus**

R85.619   **Unspecified abnormal cytological findings in specimens from anus**
Abnormal anal cytology NOS
Atypical glandular cells of anus NOS

R85.69   **Abnormal cytological findings in specimens from other digestive organs and abdominal cavity**

R85.7   **Abnormal histological findings in specimens from digestive organs and abdominal cavity**

⑤ R85.8   **Other abnormal findings in specimens from digestive organs and abdominal cavity**

R85.81   **Anal high risk human papillomavirus (HPV) DNA test positive**

EXCLUDES 1   *anogenital warts due to human papillomavirus (HPV) (A63.0)*
condyloma acuminatum (A63.0)

✚ R85.82   **Anal low risk human papillomavirus (HPV) DNA test positive**
Use additional code for associated human papillomavirus (B97.7)

R85.89   **Other abnormal findings in specimens from digestive organs and abdominal cavity**
Abnormal chromosomal findings in specimens from digestive organs and abdominal cavity

R85.9   **Unspecified abnormal finding in specimens from digestive organs and abdominal cavity**

◢ R86   **Abnormal findings in specimens from male genital organs**

INCLUDES   abnormal findings in prostatic secretions
abnormal findings in semen, seminal fluid
abnormal spermatozoa

EXCLUDES 1   *azoospermia (N46.0-)*
oligospermia (N46.1-)

R86.0   **Abnormal level of enzymes in specimens from male genital organs**   ♂

R86.1   **Abnormal level of hormones in specimens from male genital organs**   ♂

R86.2   **Abnormal level of other drugs, medicaments and biological substances in specimens from male genital organs**   ♂

R86.3   **Abnormal level of substances chiefly nonmedicinal as to source in specimens from male genital organs**   ♂

R86.4   **Abnormal immunological findings in specimens from male genital organs**   ♂

● New   ▲ Revised   *Manifestation*   ◢-◪ Digit Indicators   ▤ Laterality   Ⓐ Adult (15+ years)   Ⓜ Maternity (12-55 years)   Ⓝ Newborn   Ⓟ Pediatric (0-17 years)   ♂ Male   ♀ Female
✖ Deleted   Unspecified   ✚ Additional code

914   © 2017 DecisionHealth   2017 ICD-10-CM Expert for Physicians

R86.5   **Abnormal microbiological findings in specimens from**   ♂
     male genital organs
     Positive culture findings in specimens from male genital
     organs
     EXCLUDES 1   *colonization status (Z22.-)*

R86.6   **Abnormal cytological findings in specimens from male**   ♂
     genital organs

R86.7   **Abnormal histological findings in specimens from male**   ♂
     genital organs

R86.8   **Other abnormal findings in specimens from male**   ♂
     genital organs
     Abnormal chromosomal findings in specimens from male
     genital organs

R86.9   **Unspecified abnormal finding in specimens from male**   ♂
     genital organs

⁴ R87   **Abnormal findings in specimens from female genital**
     organs
     INCLUDES   abnormal findings in secretion and smears from
           cervix uteri
           abnormal findings in secretion and smears from
           vagina
           abnormal findings in secretion and smears from
           vulva

R87.0   **Abnormal level of enzymes in specimens from female**   ♀
     genital organs

R87.1   **Abnormal level of hormones in specimens from female**   ♀
     genital organs

R87.2   **Abnormal level of other drugs, medicaments and**   ♀
     biological substances in specimens from female
     genital organs

R87.3   **Abnormal level of substances chiefly nonmedicinal as to**   ♀
     source in specimens from female genital organs

R87.4   **Abnormal immunological findings in specimens from**   ♀
     female genital organs

R87.5   **Abnormal microbiological findings in specimens from**   ♀
     female genital organs
     Positive culture findings in specimens from female genital
     organs
     EXCLUDES 1   *colonization status (Z22.-)*

⁵ R87.6   **Abnormal cytological findings in specimens from female**
     genital organs

     ⁶ R87.61   **Abnormal cytological findings in specimens from**
           cervix uteri
           EXCLUDES 1   *abnormal cytological findings in*
                specimens from other female genital
                organs (R87.69)
                abnormal cytological findings in
                specimens from vagina (R87.62-)
                carcinoma in situ of cervix uteri
                (histologically confirmed) (D06.-)
                cervical intraepithelial neoplasia I
                [CIN I] (N87.0)
                cervical intraepithelial neoplasia II
                [CIN II] (N87.1)
                cervical intraepithelial neoplasia III
                [CIN III] (D06.-)
                dysplasia (mild) (moderate) of cervix
                uteri (histologically confirmed)
                (N87.-)
                severe dysplasia of cervix uteri
                (histologically confirmed) (D06.-)
           EXCLUDES 2   *cervical high risk human*
                papillomavirus (HPV) DNA test
                positive (R87.810)
                cervical low risk human
                papillomavirus (HPV) DNA test
                positive (R87.820)

           R87.610   **Atypical squamous cells of undetermined**   ♀
                significance on cytologic smear of cervix
                (ASC-US)

           R87.611   **Atypical squamous cells cannot exclude high**   ♀
                grade squamous intraepithelial lesion on
                cytologic smear of cervix (ASC-H)

           R87.612   **Low grade squamous intraepithelial lesion on**   ♀
                cytologic smear of cervix (LGSIL)

           R87.613   **High grade squamous intraepithelial lesion on**   ♀
                cytologic smear of cervix (HGSIL)

           R87.614   **Cytologic evidence of malignancy on smear of**   ♀
                cervix

           R87.615   **Unsatisfactory cytologic smear of cervix**   ♀
                Inadequate sample of cytologic smear of cervix

R87.616   **Satisfactory cervical smear but lacking**   ♀
           transformation zone

R87.618   **Other abnormal cytological findings on**   ♀
           specimens from cervix uteri

R87.619   **Unspecified abnormal cytological findings in**   ♀
           specimens from cervix uteri
           Abnormal cervical cytology NOS
           Abnormal Papanicolaou smear of cervix NOS
           Abnormal thin preparation smear of cervix NOS
           Atypical endocervical cells of cervix NOS
           Atypical endometrial cells of cervix NOS
           Atypical glandular cells of cervix NOS

⁶ ➕ R87.62   **Abnormal cytological findings in specimens from**
           vagina
           Use additional code to identify acquired absence of
           uterus and cervix, if applicable (Z90.71-)
           EXCLUDES 1   *abnormal cytological findings in*
                specimens from cervix uteri
                (R87.61-)
                abnormal cytological findings in
                specimens from other female genital
                organs (R87.69)
                carcinoma in situ of vagina
                (histologically confirmed) (D07.2)
                vaginal intraepithelial neoplasia I
                [VAIN I] (N89.0)
                vaginal intraepithelial neoplasia II
                [VAIN II] (N89.1)
                vaginal intraepithelial neoplasia III
                [VAIN III] (D07.2)
                dysplasia (mild) (moderate) of vagina
                (histologically confirmed) (N89.-)
                severe dysplasia of vagina
                (histologically confirmed) (D07.2)
           EXCLUDES 2   *vaginal high risk human*
                papillomavirus (HPV) DNA test
                positive (R87.811)
                vaginal low risk human papillomavirus
                (HPV) DNA test positive (R87.821)

   ➕ **R87.620**   **Atypical squamous cells of undetermined**   ♀
                significance on cytologic smear of vagina
                (ASC-US)

   ➕ **R87.621**   **Atypical squamous cells cannot exclude high**   ♀
                grade squamous intraepithelial lesion on
                cytologic smear of vagina (ASC-H)

   ➕ **R87.622**   **Low grade squamous intraepithelial lesion on**   ♀
                cytologic smear of vagina (LGSIL)

   ➕ **R87.623**   **High grade squamous intraepithelial lesion on**   ♀
                cytologic smear of vagina (HGSIL)

   ➕ **R87.624**   **Cytologic evidence of malignancy on smear of**   ♀
                vagina

   ➕ **R87.625**   **Unsatisfactory cytologic smear of vagina**   ♀
                Inadequate sample of cytologic smear of vagina

   ➕ **R87.628**   **Other abnormal cytological findings on**   ♀
                specimens from vagina

   ➕ **R87.629**   **Unspecified abnormal cytological findings in**   ♀
                specimens from vagina
                Abnormal Papanicolaou smear of vagina NOS
                Abnormal thin preparation smear of vagina NOS
                Abnormal vaginal cytology NOS
                Atypical endocervical cells of vagina NOS
                Atypical endometrial cells of vagina NOS
                Atypical glandular cells of vagina NOS

R87.69   **Abnormal cytological findings in specimens from**   ♀
           other female genital organs
           Abnormal cytological findings in specimens from
           female genital organs NOS
           EXCLUDES 1   *dysplasia of vulva*
                (histologically confirmed) (N90.0-
                N90.3)

● New   ▲ Revised   *Manifestation*   **4 - 7** Digit Indicators   ▣ Laterality   Ⓐ Adult   Ⓜ Maternity   Ⓝ Newborn   Ⓟ Pediatric   ♂ Male   ♀ Female
✖ Deleted   Unspecified   ➕ Additional code   (15+ years)   (12-55 years)   (0-17 years)

R87.7   **Abnormal histological findings in specimens from female genital organs**   ♀

> EXCLUDES 1   *carcinoma in situ (histologically confirmed) of female genital organs (D06-D07.3)*
> *cervical intraepithelial neoplasia I [CIN I] (N87.0)*
> *cervical intraepithelial neoplasia II [CIN II] (N87.1)*
> *cervical intraepithelial neoplasia III [CIN III] (D06.-)*
> *dysplasia (mild) (moderate) of cervix uteri (histologically confirmed) (N87.-)*
> *dysplasia (mild) (moderate) of vagina (histologically confirmed) (N89.-)*
> *vaginal intraepithelial neoplasia I [VAIN I] (N89.0)*
> *vaginal intraepithelial neoplasia II [VAIN II] (N89.1)*
> *vaginal intraepithelial neoplasia III [VAIN III] (D07.2)*
> *severe dysplasia of cervix uteri (histologically confirmed) (D06.-)*
> *severe dysplasia of vagina (histologically confirmed) (D07.2)*

⑤ R87.8   **Other abnormal findings in specimens from female genital organs**

   ⑥ R87.81   **High risk human papillomavirus (HPV) DNA test positive from female genital organs**

> EXCLUDES 1   *anogenital warts due to human papillomavirus (HPV) (A63.0)*
> *condyloma acuminatum (A63.0)*

     R87.810   **Cervical high risk human papillomavirus (HPV) DNA test positive**   ♀

     R87.811   **Vaginal high risk human papillomavirus (HPV) DNA test positive**   ♀

   ⑥ ✛ R87.82   **Low risk human papillomavirus (HPV) DNA test positive from female genital organs**

     Use additional code for associated human papillomavirus (B97.7)

     ✛ R87.820   **Cervical low risk human papillomavirus (HPV) DNA test positive**   ♀

     ✛ R87.821   **Vaginal low risk human papillomavirus (HPV) DNA test positive**   ♀

   R87.89   **Other abnormal findings in specimens from female genital organs**   ♀

     Abnormal chromosomal findings in specimens from female genital organs

R87.9   **Unspecified abnormal finding in specimens from female genital organs**   ♀

④ R88   **Abnormal findings in other body fluids and substances**

   R88.0   **Cloudy (hemodialysis) (peritoneal) dialysis effluent**

   R88.8   **Abnormal findings in other body fluids and substances**

④ R89   **Abnormal findings in specimens from other organs, systems and tissues**

> INCLUDES   abnormal findings in nipple discharge
> abnormal findings in synovial fluid
> abnormal findings in wound secretions

   R89.0   **Abnormal level of enzymes in specimens from other organs, systems and tissues**

   R89.1   **Abnormal level of hormones in specimens from other organs, systems and tissues**

   R89.2   **Abnormal level of other drugs, medicaments and biological substances in specimens from other organs, systems and tissues**

   R89.3   **Abnormal level of substances chiefly nonmedicinal as to source in specimens from other organs, systems and tissues**

   R89.4   **Abnormal immunological findings in specimens from other organs, systems and tissues**

   R89.5   **Abnormal microbiological findings in specimens from other organs, systems and tissues**

     Positive culture findings in specimens from other organs, systems and tissues

> EXCLUDES 1   *colonization status (Z22.-)*

   R89.6   **Abnormal cytological findings in specimens from other organs, systems and tissues**

   R89.7   **Abnormal histological findings in specimens from other organs, systems and tissues**

   R89.8   **Other abnormal findings in specimens from other organs, systems and tissues**

     Abnormal chromosomal findings in specimens from other organs, systems and tissues

   R89.9   **Unspecified abnormal finding in specimens from other organs, systems and tissues**

Abnormal findings on diagnostic imaging and in function studies, without diagnosis (R90-R94)

> INCLUDES   nonspecific abnormal findings on diagnostic imaging by computerized axial tomography [CAT scan]
> nonspecific abnormal findings on diagnostic imaging by magnetic resonance imaging [MRI][NMR]
> nonspecific abnormal findings on diagnostic imaging by positron emission tomography [PET scan]
> nonspecific abnormal findings on diagnostic imaging by thermography
> nonspecific abnormal findings on diagnostic imaging by ultrasound [echogram]
> nonspecific abnormal findings on diagnostic imaging by X-ray examination

> EXCLUDES 1   *abnormal findings on antenatal screening of mother (O28.-)*
> *diagnostic abnormal findings classified elsewhere - see Alphabetical Index*

④ R90   **Abnormal findings on diagnostic imaging of central nervous system**

   R90.0   **Intracranial space-occupying lesion found on diagnostic imaging of central nervous system**

   ⑤ R90.8   **Other abnormal findings on diagnostic imaging of central nervous system**

     R90.81   **Abnormal echoencephalogram**

     R90.82   **White matter disease, unspecified**

     R90.89   **Other abnormal findings on diagnostic imaging of central nervous system**

       Other cerebrovascular abnormality found on diagnostic imaging of central nervous system

④ R91   **Abnormal findings on diagnostic imaging of lung**

   R91.1   **Solitary pulmonary nodule**

     Coin lesion lung
     Solitary pulmonary nodule, subsegmental branch of the bronchial tree

   R91.8   **Other nonspecific abnormal finding of lung field**

     Lung mass NOS found on diagnostic imaging of lung
     Pulmonary infiltrate NOS
     Shadow, lung

④ R92   **Abnormal and inconclusive findings on diagnostic imaging of breast**

   R92.0   **Mammographic microcalcification found on diagnostic imaging of breast**

> EXCLUDES 2   *mammographic calcification (calculus) found on diagnostic imaging of breast (R92.1)*

   R92.1   **Mammographic calcification found on diagnostic imaging of breast**

     Mammographic calculus found on diagnostic imaging of breast

   R92.2   **Inconclusive mammogram**

     Dense breasts NOS
     Inconclusive mammogram NEC
     Inconclusive mammography due to dense breasts
     Inconclusive mammography NEC
     AHA: 1Q 2015, 24

   R92.8   **Other abnormal and inconclusive findings on diagnostic imaging of breast**

④ R93   **Abnormal findings on diagnostic imaging of other body structures**

   R93.0   **Abnormal findings on diagnostic imaging of skull and head, not elsewhere classified**

> EXCLUDES 1   *intracranial space-occupying lesion found on diagnostic imaging (R90.0)*

   R93.1   **Abnormal findings on diagnostic imaging of heart and coronary circulation**

     Abnormal echocardiogram NOS
     Abnormal heart shadow

   R93.2   **Abnormal findings on diagnostic imaging of liver and biliary tract**

     Nonvisualization of gallbladder

   R93.3   **Abnormal findings on diagnostic imaging of other parts of digestive tract**

● New   ▲ Revised   *Manifestation*   ④-❼ Digit Indicators   ▤ Laterality   Ⓐ Adult (15+ years)   Ⓜ Maternity (12-55 years)   Ⓝ Newborn   Ⓟ Pediatric (0-17 years)   ♂ Male   ♀ Female
✖ Deleted   Unspecified   ✛ Additional code

916   © 2017 DecisionHealth   2017 ICD-10-CM Expert for Physicians

▲ 🅂 **R93.4** **Abnormal findings on diagnostic imaging of urinary organs**
> **EXCLUDES 2** *hypertrophy of kidney (N28.81)*

● **R93.41** **Abnormal radiologic findings on diagnostic imaging of renal pelvis, ureter, or bladder**
Filling defect of bladder found on diagnostic imaging
Filling defect of renal pelvis found on diagnostic imaging
Filling defect of ureter found on diagnostic imaging

● 🄶 **R93.42** **Abnormal radiologic findings on diagnostic imaging of kidney**

● 🄴 **R93.421** **Abnormal radiologic findings on diagnostic imaging of right kidney**

● 🄴 **R93.422** **Abnormal radiologic findings on diagnostic imaging of left kidney**

● 🄴 **R93.429** **Abnormal radiologic findings on diagnostic imaging of unspecified kidney**

● **R93.49** **Abnormal radiologic findings on diagnostic imaging of other urinary organs**

R93.5 **Abnormal findings on diagnostic imaging of other abdominal regions, including retroperitoneum**

R93.6 **Abnormal findings on diagnostic imaging of limbs**
> **EXCLUDES 2** *abnormal finding in skin and subcutaneous tissue (R93.8)*

R93.7 **Abnormal findings on diagnostic imaging of other parts of musculoskeletal system**
> **EXCLUDES 2** *abnormal findings on diagnostic imaging of skull (R93.0)*

R93.8 **Abnormal findings on diagnostic imaging of other specified body structures**
Abnormal finding by radioisotope localization of placenta
Abnormal radiological finding in skin and subcutaneous tissue
Mediastinal shift

R93.9 **Diagnostic imaging inconclusive due to excess body fat of patient**

🄴 **R94** **Abnormal results of function studies**
> **INCLUDES** abnormal results of radionuclide [radioisotope] uptake studies
> abnormal results of scintigraphy

🅂 **R94.0** **Abnormal results of function studies of central nervous system**

R94.01 **Abnormal electroencephalogram [EEG]**
R94.02 **Abnormal brain scan**
R94.09 **Abnormal results of other function studies of central nervous system**

🅂 **R94.1** **Abnormal results of function studies of peripheral nervous system and special senses**

🄶 **R94.11** **Abnormal results of function studies of eye**
R94.110 **Abnormal electro-oculogram [EOG]**
R94.111 **Abnormal electroretinogram [ERG]**
Abnormal retinal function study
R94.112 **Abnormal visually evoked potential [VEP]**
R94.113 **Abnormal oculomotor study**
R94.118 **Abnormal results of other function studies of eye**

🄶 **R94.12** **Abnormal results of function studies of ear and other special senses**
R94.120 **Abnormal auditory function study**
R94.121 **Abnormal vestibular function study**
R94.128 **Abnormal results of other function studies of ear and other special senses**

🄶 **R94.13** **Abnormal results of function studies of peripheral nervous system**
R94.130 **Abnormal response to nerve stimulation, unspecified**
R94.131 **Abnormal electromyogram [EMG]**
> **EXCLUDES 1** *electromyogram of eye (R94.113)*

R94.138 **Abnormal results of other function studies of peripheral nervous system**

R94.2 **Abnormal results of pulmonary function studies**
Reduced ventilatory capacity
Reduced vital capacity

🅂 **R94.3** **Abnormal results of cardiovascular function studies**
R94.30 **Abnormal result of cardiovascular function study, unspecified**
R94.31 **Abnormal electrocardiogram [ECG] [EKG]**
> **EXCLUDES 1** *long QT syndrome (I45.81)*

R94.39 **Abnormal result of other cardiovascular function study**
Abnormal electrophysiological intracardiac studies
Abnormal phonocardiogram
Abnormal vectorcardiogram

R94.4 **Abnormal results of kidney function studies**
Abnormal renal function test

R94.5 **Abnormal results of liver function studies**
R94.6 **Abnormal results of thyroid function studies**
R94.7 **Abnormal results of other endocrine function studies**
> **EXCLUDES 2** *abnormal glucose (R73.0-)*

R94.8 **Abnormal results of function studies of other organs and systems**
Abnormal basal metabolic rate [BMR]
Abnormal bladder function test
Abnormal splenic function test

Abnormal tumor markers (R97)

🄴 **R97** **Abnormal tumor markers**
Elevated tumor associated antigens [TAA]
Elevated tumor specific antigens [TSA]
R97.0 **Elevated carcinoembryonic antigen [CEA]**
R97.1 **Elevated cancer antigen 125 [CA 125]** ♀
▲ 🅂 **R97.2** **Elevated prostate specific antigen [PSA]** ♂🄰
● **R97.20** **Elevated prostate specific antigen [PSA]** ♂🄰
● **R97.21** **Rising PSA following treatment for malignant neoplasm of prostate** ♂🄰
R97.8 **Other abnormal tumor markers**

Ill-defined and unknown cause of mortality (R99)

R99 **Ill-defined and unknown cause of mortality**
Death (unexplained) NOS
Unspecified cause of mortality

CHAPTER 19: INJURY, POISONING AND CERTAIN OTHER CONSEQUENCES OF EXTERNAL CAUSES (S00-T88)

Note: Use secondary code(s) from Chapter 20, External causes of morbidity, to indicate cause of injury. Codes within the T section that include the external cause do not require an additional external cause code

The chapter uses the S-section for coding different types of injuries related to single body regions and the T-section to cover injuries to unspecified body regions as well as poisoning and certain other consequences of external causes.

Use additional code to identify any retained foreign body, if applicable (Z18.-)

EXCLUDES 1   birth trauma (P10-P15)
         obstetric trauma (O70-O71)

GUIDELINES   **Section I.C.19.a**

Most categories in chapter 19 have a 7th character requirement for each applicable code ... While the patient may be seen by a new or different provider over the course of treatment for an injury, assignment of the 7th character is based on whether the patient is undergoing active treatment and not whether the provider is seeing the patient for the first time ... 7th character "D" subsequent encounter is used for encounters after the patient has received active treatment of the condition and is receiving routine care for the condition during the healing or recovery phase.

The aftercare Z codes should not be used for aftercare for conditions such as injuries or poisonings, where 7th characters are provided to identify subsequent care. For example, for aftercare of an injury, assign the acute injury code with the 7th character "D" (subsequent encounter).

7th character "S", sequela, is for use for complications or conditions that arise as a direct result of a condition, such as scar formation after a burn. The scars are sequelae of the burn. When using 7th character "S", it is necessary to use both the injury code that precipitated the sequela and the code for the sequela itself. The "S" is added only to the injury code, not the sequela code. The 7th character "S" identifies the injury responsible for the sequela. The specific type of sequela (e.g. scar) is sequenced first, followed by the injury code.

This chapter contains the following blocks:

S00-S09	Injuries to the head
S10-S19	Injuries to the neck
S20-S29	Injuries to the thorax
S30-S39	Injuries to the abdomen, lower back, lumbar spine, pelvis and external genitals
S40-S49	Injuries to the shoulder and upper arm
S50-S59	Injuries to the elbow and forearm
S60-S69	Injuries to the wrist, hand and fingers
S70-S79	Injuries to the hip and thigh
S80-S89	Injuries to the knee and lower leg
S90-S99	Injuries to the ankle and foot
T07	Injuries involving multiple body regions
T14	Injury of unspecified body region
T15-T19	Effects of foreign body entering through natural orifice
T20-T32	Burns and corrosions
T20-T25	Burns and corrosions of external body surface, specified by site
T26-T28	Burns and corrosions confined to eye and internal organs
T30-T32	Burns and corrosions of multiple and unspecified body regions
T33-T34	Frostbite
T36-T50	Poisoning by, adverse effect of and underdosing of drugs, medicaments and biological substances
T51-T65	Toxic effects of substances chiefly nonmedicinal as to source
T66-T78	Other and unspecified effects of external causes
T79	Certain early complications of trauma
T80-T88	Complications of surgical and medical care, not elsewhere classified

Injuries to the head (S00-S09)

INCLUDES   injuries of ear
         injuries of eye
         injuries of face [any part]
         injuries of gum
         injuries of jaw
         injuries of oral cavity
         injuries of palate
         injuries of periocular area
         injuries of scalp
         injuries of temporomandibular joint area
         injuries of tongue
         injuries of tooth

Code also:
   for any associated infection

EXCLUDES 2   burns and corrosions (T20-T32)
         effects of foreign body in ear (T16)
         effects of foreign body in larynx (T17.3)
         effects of foreign body in mouth NOS (T18.0)
         effects of foreign body in nose (T17.0-T17.1)
         effects of foreign body in pharynx (T17.2)
         effects of foreign body on external eye (T15.-)
         frostbite (T33-T34)
         insect bite or sting, venomous (T63.4)

GUIDELINES   **Section I.C.19.c.2)**
Multiple fractures are sequenced in accordance with the severity of the fracture.

GUIDELINES   **Section I.C.19.b.1)-2)**
When coding injuries, assign separate codes for each injury unless a combination code is provided, in which case the combination code is assigned ... Traumatic injury codes (S00-T14.9) are not to be used for normal, healing surgical wounds or to identify complications of surgical wounds. The code for the most serious injury, as determined by the provider and the focus of treatment, is sequenced first.

1) Superficial injuries such as abrasions or contusions are not coded when associated with more severe injuries of the same site.

2) When a primary injury results in minor damage to peripheral nerves or blood vessels, the primary injury is sequenced first with additional code(s) for injuries to nerves and spinal cord (such as category S04), and/or injury to blood vessels (such as category S15). When the primary injury is to the blood vessels or nerves, that injury should be sequenced first.

GUIDELINES   **Section I.C.19.c**
Coding of Traumatic Fractures: The principles of multiple coding of injuries should be followed in coding fractures. Fractures of specified sites are coded individually by site in accordance with both the provisions within categories S02, S12, S22, S32, S42, S49, S52, S59, S62, S72, S79, S82, S89, S92 and the level of detail furnished by medical record content. A fracture not indicated as open or closed should be coded to closed. A fracture not indicated whether displaced or not displaced should be coded to displaced.

4 S00   **Superficial injury of head**
     EXCLUDES 1   diffuse cerebral contusion (S06.2-)
                    focal cerebral contusion (S06.3-)
                    injury of eye and orbit (S05.-)
                    open wound of head (S01.-)

The appropriate 7th character is to be added to each code from category S00
A   initial encounter
D   subsequent encounter
S   sequela

   5 S00.0   **Superficial injury of scalp**
     7 S00.00X-   **Unspecified superficial injury of scalp**
     7 S00.01X-   **Abrasion of scalp**
     7 S00.02X-   **Blister (nonthermal) of scalp**
     7 S00.03X-   **Contusion of scalp**
                        Bruise of scalp
                        Hematoma of scalp
     7 S00.04X-   **External constriction of part of scalp**
     7 S00.05X-   **Superficial foreign body of scalp**
                        Splinter in the scalp
     7 S00.06X-   **Insect bite (nonvenomous) of scalp**

● New   ▲ Revised   *Manifestation*   4-7 Digit Indicators   ▤ Laterality   ▣ Adult (15+ years)   ▣ Maternity (12-55 years)   ▣ Newborn   ▣ Pediatric (0-17 years)   ♂ Male   ♀ Female
✖ Deleted   Unspecified   + Additional code

2017 ICD-10-CM Expert for Physicians   © 2017 DecisionHealth   919

7 S00.07X-   **Other superficial bite of scalp**
> EXCLUDES 1   *open bite of scalp (S01.05)*

5 S00.1   **Contusion of eyelid and periocular area**
Black eye
> EXCLUDES 2   *contusion of eyeball and orbital tissues (S05.1)*

7 6 S00.10X-   **Contusion of unspecified eyelid and periocular area**

7 6 S00.11X-   **Contusion of right eyelid and periocular area**

7 6 S00.12X-   **Contusion of left eyelid and periocular area**

5 S00.2   **Other and unspecified superficial injuries of eyelid and periocular area**
> EXCLUDES 2   *superficial injury of conjunctiva and cornea (S05.0-)*

6 S00.20   **Unspecified superficial injury of eyelid and periocular area**

7 6 S00.201-   **Unspecified superficial injury of right eyelid and periocular area**

7 6 S00.202-   **Unspecified superficial injury of left eyelid and periocular area**

7 6 S00.209-   **Unspecified superficial injury of unspecified eyelid and periocular area**

6 S00.21   **Abrasion of eyelid and periocular area**

7 6 S00.211-   **Abrasion of right eyelid and periocular area**

7 6 S00.212-   **Abrasion of left eyelid and periocular area**

7 6 S00.219-   **Abrasion of unspecified eyelid and periocular area**

6 S00.22   **Blister (nonthermal) of eyelid and periocular area**

7 6 S00.221-   **Blister (nonthermal) of right eyelid and periocular area**

7 6 S00.222-   **Blister (nonthermal) of left eyelid and periocular area**

7 6 S00.229-   **Blister (nonthermal) of unspecified eyelid and periocular area**

6 S00.24   **External constriction of eyelid and periocular area**

7 6 S00.241-   **External constriction of right eyelid and periocular area**

7 6 S00.242-   **External constriction of left eyelid and periocular area**

7 6 S00.249-   **External constriction of unspecified eyelid and periocular area**

6 S00.25   **Superficial foreign body of eyelid and periocular area**
Splinter of eyelid and periocular area
> EXCLUDES 2   *retained foreign body in eyelid (H02.81-)*

7 6 S00.251-   **Superficial foreign body of right eyelid and periocular area**

7 6 S00.252-   **Superficial foreign body of left eyelid and periocular area**

7 6 S00.259-   **Superficial foreign body of unspecified eyelid and periocular area**

6 S00.26   **Insect bite (nonvenomous) of eyelid and periocular area**

7 6 S00.261-   **Insect bite (nonvenomous) of right eyelid and periocular area**

7 6 S00.262-   **Insect bite (nonvenomous) of left eyelid and periocular area**

7 6 S00.269-   **Insect bite (nonvenomous) of unspecified eyelid and periocular area**

6 S00.27   **Other superficial bite of eyelid and periocular area**
> EXCLUDES 1   *open bite of eyelid and periocular area (S01.15)*

7 6 S00.271-   **Other superficial bite of right eyelid and periocular area**

7 6 S00.272-   **Other superficial bite of left eyelid and periocular area**

7 6 S00.279-   **Other superficial bite of unspecified eyelid and periocular area**

5 S00.3   **Superficial injury of nose**

7 S00.30X-   **Unspecified superficial injury of nose**

7 S00.31X-   **Abrasion of nose**

7 S00.32X-   **Blister (nonthermal) of nose**

7 S00.33X-   **Contusion of nose**
Bruise of nose
Hematoma of nose

7 S00.34X-   **External constriction of nose**

7 S00.35X-   **Superficial foreign body of nose**
Splinter in the nose

7 S00.36X-   **Insect bite (nonvenomous) of nose**

7 S00.37X-   **Other superficial bite of nose**
> EXCLUDES 1   *open bite of nose (S01.25)*

5 S00.4   **Superficial injury of ear**

6 S00.40   **Unspecified superficial injury of ear**

7 6 S00.401-   **Unspecified superficial injury of right ear**

7 6 S00.402-   **Unspecified superficial injury of left ear**

7 6 S00.409-   **Unspecified superficial injury of unspecified ear**

6 S00.41   **Abrasion of ear**

7 6 S00.411-   **Abrasion of right ear**

7 6 S00.412-   **Abrasion of left ear**

7 6 S00.419-   **Abrasion of unspecified ear**

6 S00.42   **Blister (nonthermal) of ear**

7 6 S00.421-   **Blister (nonthermal) of right ear**

7 6 S00.422-   **Blister (nonthermal) of left ear**

7 6 S00.429-   **Blister (nonthermal) of unspecified ear**

6 S00.43   **Contusion of ear**
Bruise of ear
Hematoma of ear

7 6 S00.431-   **Contusion of right ear**

7 6 S00.432-   **Contusion of left ear**

7 6 S00.439-   **Contusion of unspecified ear**

6 S00.44   **External constriction of ear**

7 6 S00.441-   **External constriction of right ear**

7 6 S00.442-   **External constriction of left ear**

7 6 S00.449-   **External constriction of unspecified ear**

6 S00.45   **Superficial foreign body of ear**
Splinter in the ear

7 6 S00.451-   **Superficial foreign body of right ear**

7 6 S00.452-   **Superficial foreign body of left ear**

7 6 S00.459-   **Superficial foreign body of unspecified ear**

6 S00.46   **Insect bite (nonvenomous) of ear**

7 6 S00.461-   **Insect bite (nonvenomous) of right ear**

7 6 S00.462-   **Insect bite (nonvenomous) of left ear**

7 6 S00.469-   **Insect bite (nonvenomous) of unspecified ear**

6 S00.47   **Other superficial bite of ear**
> EXCLUDES 1   *open bite of ear (S01.35)*

7 6 S00.471-   **Other superficial bite of right ear**

7 6 S00.472-   **Other superficial bite of left ear**

7 6 S00.479-   **Other superficial bite of unspecified ear**

5 S00.5   **Superficial injury of lip and oral cavity**

6 S00.50   **Unspecified superficial injury of lip and oral cavity**

7 S00.501-   **Unspecified superficial injury of lip**

7 S00.502-   **Unspecified superficial injury of oral cavity**

6 S00.51   **Abrasion of lip and oral cavity**

7 S00.511-   **Abrasion of lip**

7 S00.512-   **Abrasion of oral cavity**

6 S00.52   **Blister (nonthermal) of lip and oral cavity**

7 S00.521-   **Blister (nonthermal) of lip**

7 S00.522-   **Blister (nonthermal) of oral cavity**

6 S00.53   **Contusion of lip and oral cavity**

7 S00.531-   **Contusion of lip**
Bruise of lip
Hematoma of oral cavity

7 S00.532-   **Contusion of oral cavity**
Bruise of lip
Hematoma of oral cavity

6 S00.54   **External constriction of lip and oral cavity**

7 S00.541-   **External constriction of lip**

7 S00.542-   **External constriction of oral cavity**

6 S00.55   **Superficial foreign body of lip and oral cavity**

● New   ▲ Revised   *Manifestation*   **4 - 7** Digit Indicators   ⊟ Laterality   Ⓐ Adult (15+ years)   Ⓜ Maternity (12-55 years)   Ⓝ Newborn   Ⓟ Pediatric (0-17 years)   ♂ Male   ♀ Female

✖ Deleted   Unspecified   ✚ Additional code

920   © 2017 DecisionHealth   2017 ICD-10-CM Expert for Physicians

☑ S00.551- **Superficial foreign body of lip**
Splinter of lip and oral cavity

☑ S00.552- **Superficial foreign body of oral cavity**
Splinter of lip and oral cavity

⑥ S00.56 **Insect bite (nonvenomous) of lip and oral cavity**

☑ S00.561- **Insect bite (nonvenomous) of lip**

☑ S00.562- **Insect bite (nonvenomous) of oral cavity**

⑥ S00.57 **Other superficial bite of lip and oral cavity**

☑ S00.571- **Other superficial bite of lip**
EXCLUDES 1 *open bite of lip (S01.551)*

☑ S00.572- **Other superficial bite of oral cavity**
EXCLUDES 1 *open bite of oral cavity (S01.552)*

▲ ⑤ S00.8 **Superficial injury of other parts of head**
Superficial injuries of face [any part]

☑ S00.80X- **Unspecified superficial injury of other part of head**

☑ S00.81X- **Abrasion of other part of head**

☑ S00.82X- **Blister (nonthermal) of other part of head**

☑ S00.83X- **Contusion of other part of head**
Bruise of other part of head
Hematoma of other part of head

☑ S00.84X- **External constriction of other part of head**

☑ S00.85X- **Superficial foreign body of other part of head**
Splinter in other part of head

☑ S00.86X- **Insect bite (nonvenomous) of other part of head**

☑ S00.87X- **Other superficial bite of other part of head**
EXCLUDES 1 *open bite of other part of head (S01.85)*

⑤ S00.9 **Superficial injury of unspecified part of head**

☑ S00.90X- **Unspecified superficial injury of unspecified part of head**

☑ S00.91X- **Abrasion of unspecified part of head**

☑ S00.92X- **Blister (nonthermal) of unspecified part of head**

☑ S00.93X- **Contusion of unspecified part of head**
Bruise of head
Hematoma of head

☑ S00.94X- **External constriction of unspecified part of head**

☑ S00.95X- **Superficial foreign body of unspecified part of head**
Splinter of head

☑ S00.96X- **Insect bite (nonvenomous) of unspecified part of head**

☑ S00.97X- **Other superficial bite of unspecified part of head**
EXCLUDES 1 *open bite of head (S01.95)*

④ S01 **Open wound of head**
Code also any associated:
injury of cranial nerve (S04.-)
injury of muscle and tendon of head (S09.1-)
intracranial injury (S06.-)
wound infection
EXCLUDES 1 *open skull fracture (S02.- with 7th character B)*
EXCLUDES 2 *injury of eye and orbit (S05.-)*
traumatic amputation of part of head (S08.-)

The appropriate 7th character is to be added to each code from category S01
A   initial encounter
D   subsequent encounter
S   sequela

CODING TIP✓ Open wound codes are used for wounds caused by trauma. Do not assign a code for "open wound" unless the etiology of the wound is related to trauma.

⑤ S01.0 **Open wound of scalp**
EXCLUDES 1 *avulsion of scalp (S08.0)*

☑ S01.00X- **Unspecified open wound of scalp**

☑ S01.01X- **Laceration without foreign body of scalp**

☑ S01.02X- **Laceration with foreign body of scalp**
AHA: (S01.02XA) 1Q 2015, 5
AHA: (S01.02XD) 1Q 2015, 6, 7

☑ S01.03X- **Puncture wound without foreign body of scalp**

☑ S01.04X- **Puncture wound with foreign body of scalp**

☑ S01.05X- **Open bite of scalp**
Bite of scalp NOS
EXCLUDES 1 *superficial bite of scalp (S00.06, S00.07-)*

⑤ S01.1 **Open wound of eyelid and periocular area**
Open wound of eyelid and periocular area with or without involvement of lacrimal passages

⑥ S01.10 **Unspecified open wound of eyelid and periocular area**

☑ ⊟ S01.101- **Unspecified open wound of right eyelid and periocular area**

☑ ⊟ S01.102- **Unspecified open wound of left eyelid and periocular area**

☑ ⊟ S01.109- **Unspecified open wound of unspecified eyelid and periocular area**

⑥ S01.11 **Laceration without foreign body of eyelid and periocular area**

☑ ⊟ S01.111- **Laceration without foreign body of right eyelid and periocular area**

☑ ⊟ S01.112- **Laceration without foreign body of left eyelid and periocular area**

☑ ⊟ S01.119- **Laceration without foreign body of unspecified eyelid and periocular area**

⑥ S01.12 **Laceration with foreign body of eyelid and periocular area**

☑ ⊟ S01.121- **Laceration with foreign body of right eyelid and periocular area**

☑ ⊟ S01.122- **Laceration with foreign body of left eyelid and periocular area**

☑ ⊟ S01.129- **Laceration with foreign body of unspecified eyelid and periocular area**

⑥ S01.13 **Puncture wound without foreign body of eyelid and periocular area**

☑ ⊟ S01.131- **Puncture wound without foreign body of right eyelid and periocular area**

☑ ⊟ S01.132- **Puncture wound without foreign body of left eyelid and periocular area**

☑ ⊟ S01.139- **Puncture wound without foreign body of unspecified eyelid and periocular area**

⑥ S01.14 **Puncture wound with foreign body of eyelid and periocular area**

☑ ⊟ S01.141- **Puncture wound with foreign body of right eyelid and periocular area**

☑ ⊟ S01.142- **Puncture wound with foreign body of left eyelid and periocular area**

☑ ⊟ S01.149- **Puncture wound with foreign body of unspecified eyelid and periocular area**

⑥ S01.15 **Open bite of eyelid and periocular area**
Bite of eyelid and periocular area NOS
EXCLUDES 1 *superficial bite of eyelid and periocular area (S00.26, S00.27)*

☑ ⊟ S01.151- **Open bite of right eyelid and periocular area**

☑ ⊟ S01.152- **Open bite of left eyelid and periocular area**

☑ ⊟ S01.159- **Open bite of unspecified eyelid and periocular area**

⑤ S01.2 **Open wound of nose**

☑ S01.20X- **Unspecified open wound of nose**

☑ S01.21X- **Laceration without foreign body of nose**
AHA: (S01.21XA) 1Q 2015, 5
AHA: (S01.21XD) 1Q 2015, 6

☑ S01.22X- **Laceration with foreign body of nose**

☑ S01.23X- **Puncture wound without foreign body of nose**

☑ S01.24X- **Puncture wound with foreign body of nose**

☑ S01.25X- **Open bite of nose**
Bite of nose NOS
EXCLUDES 1 *superficial bite of nose (S00.36, S00.37)*

⑤ S01.3 **Open wound of ear**

⑥ S01.30 **Unspecified open wound of ear**

☑ ⊟ S01.301- **Unspecified open wound of right ear**

☑ ⊟ S01.302- **Unspecified open wound of left ear**

☑ ⊟ S01.309- **Unspecified open wound of unspecified ear**

⑥ S01.31 **Laceration without foreign body of ear**

☑ ⊟ S01.311- **Laceration without foreign body of right ear**

● New ▲ Revised *Manifestation* ④-☑ Digit Indicators ⊟ Laterality Ⓐ Adult (15+ years) Ⓜ Maternity (12-55 years) Ⓝ Newborn Ⓟ Pediatric (0-17 years) ♂ Male ♀ Female
✖ Deleted Unspecified + Additional code

2017 ICD-10-CM Expert for Physicians

© 2017 DecisionHealth

921

7 ⊟ **S01.312-**   Laceration without foreign body of left ear

7 ⊟ **S01.319-**   Laceration without foreign body of unspecified ear

6 **S01.32**   Laceration with foreign body of ear

7 ⊟ **S01.321-**   Laceration with foreign body of right ear

7 ⊟ **S01.322-**   Laceration with foreign body of left ear

7 ⊟ **S01.329-**   Laceration with foreign body of unspecified ear

6 **S01.33**   Puncture wound without foreign body of ear

7 ⊟ **S01.331-**   Puncture wound without foreign body of right ear

7 ⊟ **S01.332-**   Puncture wound without foreign body of left ear

7 ⊟ **S01.339-**   Puncture wound without foreign body of unspecified ear

6 **S01.34**   Puncture wound with foreign body of ear

7 ⊟ **S01.341-**   Puncture wound with foreign body of right ear

7 ⊟ **S01.342-**   Puncture wound with foreign body of left ear

7 ⊟ **S01.349-**   Puncture wound with foreign body of unspecified ear

6 **S01.35**   Open bite of ear
Bite of ear NOS
EXCLUDES 1   *superficial bite of ear (S00.46, S00.47)*

7 ⊟ **S01.351-**   Open bite of right ear

7 ⊟ **S01.352-**   Open bite of left ear

7 ⊟ **S01.359-**   Open bite of unspecified ear

5 **S01.4**   Open wound of cheek and temporomandibular area

6 **S01.40**   Unspecified open wound of cheek and temporomandibular area

7 ⊟ **S01.401-**   Unspecified open wound of right cheek and temporomandibular area

7 ⊟ **S01.402-**   Unspecified open wound of left cheek and temporomandibular area

7 ⊟ **S01.409-**   Unspecified open wound of unspecified cheek and temporomandibular area

6 **S01.41**   Laceration without foreign body of cheek and temporomandibular area

7 ⊟ **S01.411-**   Laceration without foreign body of right cheek and temporomandibular area
AHA: (S01.411A) 1Q 2015, 5
AHA: (S01.411D) 1Q 2015, 6, 7

7 ⊟ **S01.412-**   Laceration without foreign body of left cheek and temporomandibular area

7 ⊟ **S01.419-**   Laceration without foreign body of unspecified cheek and temporomandibular area

6 **S01.42**   Laceration with foreign body of cheek and temporomandibular area

7 ⊟ **S01.421-**   Laceration with foreign body of right cheek and temporomandibular area

7 ⊟ **S01.422-**   Laceration with foreign body of left cheek and temporomandibular area

7 ⊟ **S01.429-**   Laceration with foreign body of unspecified cheek and temporomandibular area

6 **S01.43**   Puncture wound without foreign body of cheek and temporomandibular area

7 ⊟ **S01.431-**   Puncture wound without foreign body of right cheek and temporomandibular area

7 ⊟ **S01.432-**   Puncture wound without foreign body of left cheek and temporomandibular area

7 ⊟ **S01.439-**   Puncture wound without foreign body of unspecified cheek and temporomandibular area

6 **S01.44**   Puncture wound with foreign body of cheek and temporomandibular area

7 ⊟ **S01.441-**   Puncture wound with foreign body of right cheek and temporomandibular area

7 ⊟ **S01.442-**   Puncture wound with foreign body of left cheek and temporomandibular area

7 ⊟ **S01.449-**   Puncture wound with foreign body of unspecified cheek and temporomandibular area

6 **S01.45**   Open bite of cheek and temporomandibular area
Bite of cheek and temporomandibular area NOS
EXCLUDES 2   *superficial bite of cheek and temporomandibular area (S00.86, S00.87)*

7 ⊟ **S01.451-**   Open bite of right cheek and temporomandibular area

7 ⊟ **S01.452-**   Open bite of left cheek and temporomandibular area

7 ⊟ **S01.459-**   Open bite of unspecified cheek and temporomandibular area

5 **S01.5**   Open wound of lip and oral cavity
EXCLUDES 2   *tooth dislocation (S03.2)*
tooth fracture (S02.5)

6 **S01.50**   Unspecified open wound of lip and oral cavity

7 **S01.501-**   Unspecified open wound of lip

7 **S01.502-**   Unspecified open wound of oral cavity

6 **S01.51**   Laceration of lip and oral cavity without foreign body

7 **S01.511-**   Laceration without foreign body of lip

7 **S01.512-**   Laceration without foreign body of oral cavity

6 **S01.52**   Laceration of lip and oral cavity with foreign body

7 **S01.521-**   Laceration with foreign body of lip

7 **S01.522-**   Laceration with foreign body of oral cavity

6 **S01.53**   Puncture wound of lip and oral cavity without foreign body

7 **S01.531-**   Puncture wound without foreign body of lip

7 **S01.532-**   Puncture wound without foreign body of oral cavity

6 **S01.54**   Puncture wound of lip and oral cavity with foreign body

7 **S01.541-**   Puncture wound with foreign body of lip

7 **S01.542-**   Puncture wound with foreign body of oral cavity

6 **S01.55**   Open bite of lip and oral cavity

7 **S01.551-**   Open bite of lip
Bite of lip NOS
EXCLUDES 1   *superficial bite of lip (S00.571)*

7 **S01.552-**   Open bite of oral cavity
Bite of oral cavity NOS
EXCLUDES 1   *superficial bite of oral cavity (S00.572)*

5 **S01.8**   Open wound of other parts of head

7 **S01.80X-**   Unspecified open wound of other part of head

7 **S01.81X-**   Laceration without foreign body of other part of head

7 **S01.82X-**   Laceration with foreign body of other part of head

7 **S01.83X-**   Puncture wound without foreign body of other part of head

7 **S01.84X-**   Puncture wound with foreign body of other part of head

7 **S01.85X-**   Open bite of other part of head
Bite of other part of head NOS
EXCLUDES 1   *superficial bite of other part of head (S00.85)*

5 **S01.9**   Open wound of unspecified part of head

7 **S01.90X-**   Unspecified open wound of unspecified part of head

7 **S01.91X-**   Laceration without foreign body of unspecified part of head

7 **S01.92X-**   Laceration with foreign body of unspecified part of head

7 **S01.93X-**   Puncture wound without foreign body of unspecified part of head

7 **S01.94X-**   Puncture wound with foreign body of unspecified part of head

7 **S01.95X-**   Open bite of unspecified part of head
Bite of head NOS
EXCLUDES 1   *superficial bite of head NOS (S00.97)*

● New   ▲ Revised   *Manifestation*   4-7 Digit Indicators   ⊟ Laterality   ▲ Adult (15+ years)   Ⓜ Maternity (12-55 years)   Ⓝ Newborn   Ⓟ Pediatric (0-17 years)   ♂ Male   ♀ Female
✖ ~~Deleted~~   Unspecified   ✚ Additional code

4 **S02**   **Fracture of skull and facial bones**
Note: A fracture not indicated as open or closed should be coded to closed
Code also:
  any associated intracranial injury (S06.-)

The appropriate 7th character is to be added to each code from category S02
A   initial encounter for closed fracture
B   initial encounter for open fracture
D   subsequent encounter for fracture with routine healing
G   subsequent encounter for fracture with delayed healing
K   subsequent encounter for fracture with nonunion
S   sequela

CODING TIP ✓   A fracture not indicated as open or closed should be coded to closed.

7 **S02.0XX-**   **Fracture of vault of skull**
Fracture of frontal bone
Fracture of parietal bone

5 **S02.1**   **Fracture of base of skull**
EXCLUDES 1   orbit NOS (S02.8)
EXCLUDES 2   orbital floor (S02.3-)

▲ 6 **S02.10**   **Unspecified fracture of base of skull**

Unspecified fracture of base of skull

Exterior view

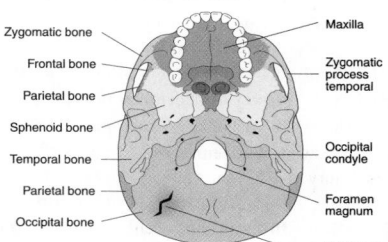

Zygomatic bone
Frontal bone
Parietal bone
Sphenoid bone
Temporal bone
Parietal bone
Occipital bone
Maxilla
Zygomatic process temporal
Occipital condyle
Foramen magnum
Fracture

● 7 ⊟ **S02.101-**   **Fracture of base of skull, right side**
● 7 ⊟ **S02.102-**   **Fracture of base of skull, left side**
● 7 ⊟ **S02.109-**   **Fracture of base of skull, unspecified side**
6 **S02.11**   **Fracture of occiput**
▲ 7 ⊟ **S02.110-**   **Type I occipital condyle fracture, unspecified side**
▲ 7 ⊟ **S02.111-**   **Type II occipital condyle fracture, unspecified side**
▲ 7 ⊟ **S02.112-**   **Type III occipital condyle fracture, unspecified side**
7 **S02.113-**   **Unspecified occipital condyle fracture**
▲ 7 ⊟ **S02.118-**   **Other fracture of occiput, unspecified side**
7 **S02.119-**   **Unspecified fracture of occiput**
● 7 ⊟ **S02.11A-**   **Type I occipital condyle fracture, right side**
● 7 ⊟ **S02.11B-**   **Type I occipital condyle fracture, left side**
● 7 ⊟ **S02.11C-**   **Type II occipital condyle fracture, right side**
● 7 ⊟ **S02.11D-**   **Type II occipital condyle fracture, left side**
● 7 ⊟ **S02.11E-**   **Type III occipital condyle fracture, right side**
● 7 ⊟ **S02.11F-**   **Type III occipital condyle fracture, left side**
● 7 ⊟ **S02.11G-**   **Other fracture of occiput, right side**
● 7 ⊟ **S02.11H-**   **Other fracture of occiput, left side**
7 **S02.19X-**   **Other fracture of base of skull**
Fracture of anterior fossa of base of skull
Fracture of ethmoid sinus
Fracture of frontal sinus
Fracture of middle fossa of base of skull
Fracture of orbital roof
Fracture of posterior fossa of base of skull
Fracture of sphenoid
Fracture of temporal bone
7 **S02.2XX-**   **Fracture of nasal bones**
▲ 5 **S02.3**   **Fracture of orbital floor**
EXCLUDES 1   orbit NOS (S02.8)
EXCLUDES 2   orbital roof (S02.1-)

● 7 ⊟ **S02.30X-**   **Fracture of orbital floor, unspecified side**
● 7 ⊟ **S02.31X-**   **Fracture of orbital floor, right side**
● 7 ⊟ **S02.32X-**   **Fracture of orbital floor, left side**
5 **S02.4**   **Fracture of malar, maxillary and zygoma bones**
Fracture of superior maxilla
Fracture of upper jaw (bone)
Fracture of zygomatic process of temporal bone
6 **S02.40**   **Fracture of malar, maxillary and zygoma bones, unspecified**
▲ 7 ⊟ **S02.400-**   **Malar fracture, unspecified side**
▲ 7 ⊟ **S02.401-**   **Maxillary fracture, unspecified side**
▲ 7 ⊟ **S02.402-**   **Zygomatic fracture, unspecified side**
● 7 ⊟ **S02.40A-**   **Malar fracture, right side**
● 7 ⊟ **S02.40B-**   **Malar fracture, left side**
● 7 ⊟ **S02.40C-**   **Maxillary fracture, right side**
● 7 ⊟ **S02.40D-**   **Maxillary fracture, left side**
● 7 ⊟ **S02.40E-**   **Zygomatic fracture, right side**
● 7 ⊟ **S02.40F-**   **Zygomatic fracture, left side**
6 **S02.41**   **LeFort fracture**
7 **S02.411-**   **LeFort I fracture**
7 **S02.412-**   **LeFort II fracture**
7 **S02.413-**   **LeFort III fracture**
7 **S02.42X-**   **Fracture of alveolus of maxilla**
7 **S02.5XX-**   **Fracture of tooth (traumatic)**
Broken tooth
EXCLUDES 1   cracked tooth (nontraumatic) (K03.81)
5 **S02.6**   **Fracture of mandible**
Fracture of lower jaw (bone)
6 **S02.60**   **Fracture of mandible, unspecified**
▲ 7 ⊟ **S02.600-**   **Fracture of unspecified part of body of mandible, unspecified side**
● 7 ⊟ **S02.601-**   **Fracture of unspecified part of body of right mandible**
● 7 ⊟ **S02.602-**   **Fracture of unspecified part of body of left mandible**
7 **S02.609-**   **Fracture of mandible, unspecified**
▲ 6 **S02.61**   **Fracture of condylar process of mandible**
● 7 ⊟ **S02.610-**   **Fracture of condylar process of mandible, unspecified side**
● 7 ⊟ **S02.611-**   **Fracture of condylar process of right mandible**
● 7 ⊟ **S02.612-**   **Fracture of condylar process of left mandible**
▲ 6 **S02.62**   **Fracture of subcondylar process of mandible**
● 7 ⊟ **S02.620-**   **Fracture of subcondylar process of mandible, unspecified side**
● 7 ⊟ **S02.621-**   **Fracture of subcondylar process of right mandible**
● 7 ⊟ **S02.622-**   **Fracture of subcondylar process of left mandible**
▲ 6 **S02.63**   **Fracture of coronoid process of mandible**
● 7 ⊟ **S02.630-**   **Fracture of coronoid process of mandible, unspecified side**
● 7 ⊟ **S02.631-**   **Fracture of coronoid process of right mandible**
● 7 ⊟ **S02.632-**   **Fracture of coronoid process of left mandible**
▲ 6 **S02.64**   **Fracture of ramus of mandible**
● 7 ⊟ **S02.640-**   **Fracture of ramus of mandible, unspecified side**
● 7 ⊟ **S02.641-**   **Fracture of ramus of right mandible**
● 7 ⊟ **S02.642-**   **Fracture of ramus of left mandible**
▲ 6 **S02.65**   **Fracture of angle of mandible**
● 7 ⊟ **S02.650-**   **Fracture of angle of mandible, unspecified side**
● 7 ⊟ **S02.651-**   **Fracture of angle of right mandible**
● 7 ⊟ **S02.652-**   **Fracture of angle of left mandible**
7 **S02.66X-**   **Fracture of symphysis of mandible**
▲ 6 **S02.67**   **Fracture of alveolus of mandible**
● 7 ⊟ **S02.670-**   **Fracture of alveolus of mandible, unspecified side**
● 7 ⊟ **S02.671-**   **Fracture of alveolus of right mandible**
● 7 ⊟ **S02.672-**   **Fracture of alveolus of left mandible**

● New   ▲ Revised   *Manifestation*   4-7 Digit Indicators   ⊟ Laterality   🅐 Adult (15+ years)   🅜 Maternity (12-55 years)   🅝 Newborn   🅟 Pediatric (0-17 years)   ♂ Male   ♀ Female
✖ ~~Deleted~~   Unspecified   + Additional code

2017 ICD-10-CM Expert for Physicians
© 2017 DecisionHealth   923

⑦ **S02.69X-**   **Fracture of mandible of other specified site**

▲⑤ **S02.8**   **Fractures of other specified skull and facial bones**
Fracture of orbit NOS
Fracture of palate

> **EXCLUDES 1**   *fracture of orbital floor (S02.3-)*
> *fracture of orbital roof (S02.1-)*

●⑦⊟ **S02.80X-**   **Fracture of other specified skull and facial bones, unspecified side**

●⑦⊟ **S02.81X-**   **Fracture of other specified skull and facial bones, right side**

●⑦⊟ **S02.82X-**   **Fracture of other specified skull and facial bones, left side**

⑤ **S02.9**   **Fracture of unspecified skull and facial bones**

⑦ **S02.91X-**   **Unspecified fracture of skull**

⑦ **S02.92X-**   **Unspecified fracture of facial bones**

④ **S03**   **Dislocation and sprain of joints and ligaments of head**

> **INCLUDES**   avulsion of joint (capsule) or ligament of head
> laceration of cartilage, joint (capsule) or ligament of head
> sprain of cartilage, joint (capsule) or ligament of head
> traumatic hemarthrosis of joint or ligament of head
> traumatic rupture of joint or ligament of head
> traumatic subluxation of joint or ligament of head
> traumatic tear of joint or ligament of head

Code also:
any associated open wound

> **EXCLUDES 2**   *Strain of muscle or tendon of head (S09.1)*

The appropriate 7th character is to be added to each code from category S03
A   initial encounter
D   subsequent encounter
S   sequela

▲⑤ **S03.0**   **Dislocation of jaw**
Dislocation of jaw (cartilage) (meniscus)
Dislocation of mandible
Dislocation of temporomandibular (joint)

●⑦⊟ **S03.00X-**   **Dislocation of jaw, unspecified side**
●⑦⊟ **S03.01X-**   **Dislocation of jaw, right side**
●⑦⊟ **S03.02X-**   **Dislocation of jaw, left side**
●⑦⊟ **S03.03X-**   **Dislocation of jaw, bilateral**
⑦ **S03.1XX-**   **Dislocation of septal cartilage of nose**
⑦ **S03.2XX-**   **Dislocation of tooth**

▲⑤ **S03.4**   **Sprain of jaw**
Sprain of temporomandibular (joint) (ligament)

●⑦⊟ **S03.40X-**   **Sprain of jaw, unspecified side**
●⑦⊟ **S03.41X-**   **Sprain of jaw, right side**
●⑦⊟ **S03.42X-**   **Sprain of jaw, left side**
●⑦⊟ **S03.43X-**   **Sprain of jaw, bilateral**
⑦ **S03.8XX-**   **Sprain of joints and ligaments of other parts of head**
⑦ **S03.9XX-**   **Sprain of joints and ligaments of unspecified parts of head**

④ **S04**   **Injury of cranial nerve**
The selection of side should be based on the side of the body being affected
Code first:
any associated intracranial injury (S06.-)
Code also any associated:
open wound of head (S01.-)
skull fracture (S02.-)

The appropriate 7th character is to be added to each code from category S04
A   initial encounter
D   subsequent encounter
S   sequela

⑤✚ **S04.0**   **Injury of optic nerve and pathways**
Use additional code to identify any visual field defect or blindness (H53.4-, H54)

⑥✚ **S04.01**   **Injury of optic nerve**
Injury of 2nd cranial nerve

⑦⊟✚ **S04.011-**   **Injury of optic nerve, right eye**
⑦⊟✚ **S04.012-**   **Injury of optic nerve, left eye**

⑦⊟✚ **S04.019-**   **Injury of optic nerve, unspecified eye**
Injury of optic nerve NOS

⑦✚ **S04.02X-**   **Injury of optic chiasm**

⑥✚ **S04.03**   **Injury of optic tract and pathways**
Injury of optic radiation

⑦⊟✚ **S04.031-**   **Injury of optic tract and pathways, right eye**
⑦⊟✚ **S04.032-**   **Injury of optic tract and pathways, left eye**
⑦⊟✚ **S04.039-**   **Injury of optic tract and pathways, unspecified eye**
Injury of optic tract and pathways NOS

⑥✚ **S04.04**   **Injury of visual cortex**
⑦⊟✚ **S04.041-**   **Injury of visual cortex, right eye**
⑦⊟✚ **S04.042-**   **Injury of visual cortex, left eye**
⑦⊟✚ **S04.049-**   **Injury of visual cortex, unspecified eye**
Injury of visual cortex NOS

⑤ **S04.1**   **Injury of oculomotor nerve**
Injury of 3rd cranial nerve

⑦⊟ **S04.10X-**   **Injury of oculomotor nerve, unspecified side**
⑦⊟ **S04.11X-**   **Injury of oculomotor nerve, right side**
⑦⊟ **S04.12X-**   **Injury of oculomotor nerve, left side**

⑤ **S04.2**   **Injury of trochlear nerve**
Injury of 4th cranial nerve

⑦⊟ **S04.20X-**   **Injury of trochlear nerve, unspecified side**
⑦⊟ **S04.21X-**   **Injury of trochlear nerve, right side**
⑦⊟ **S04.22X-**   **Injury of trochlear nerve, left side**

⑤ **S04.3**   **Injury of trigeminal nerve**
Injury of 5th cranial nerve

⑦⊟ **S04.30X-**   **Injury of trigeminal nerve, unspecified side**
⑦⊟ **S04.31X-**   **Injury of trigeminal nerve, right side**
⑦⊟ **S04.32X-**   **Injury of trigeminal nerve, left side**

⑤ **S04.4**   **Injury of abducent nerve**
Injury of 6th cranial nerve

⑦⊟ **S04.40X-**   **Injury of abducent nerve, unspecified side**
⑦⊟ **S04.41X-**   **Injury of abducent nerve, right side**
⑦⊟ **S04.42X-**   **Injury of abducent nerve, left side**

⑤ **S04.5**   **Injury of facial nerve**
Injury of 7th cranial nerve

⑦⊟ **S04.50X-**   **Injury of facial nerve, unspecified side**
⑦⊟ **S04.51X-**   **Injury of facial nerve, right side**
⑦⊟ **S04.52X-**   **Injury of facial nerve, left side**

⑤ **S04.6**   **Injury of acoustic nerve**
Injury of auditory nerve
Injury of 8th cranial nerve

⑦⊟ **S04.60X-**   **Injury of acoustic nerve, unspecified side**
⑦⊟ **S04.61X-**   **Injury of acoustic nerve, right side**
⑦⊟ **S04.62X-**   **Injury of acoustic nerve, left side**

⑤ **S04.7**   **Injury of accessory nerve**
Injury of 11th cranial nerve

⑦⊟ **S04.70X-**   **Injury of accessory nerve, unspecified side**
⑦⊟ **S04.71X-**   **Injury of accessory nerve, right side**
⑦⊟ **S04.72X-**   **Injury of accessory nerve, left side**

⑤ **S04.8**   **Injury of other cranial nerves**
⑥ **S04.81**   **Injury of olfactory [1st] nerve**
⑦⊟ **S04.811-**   **Injury of olfactory [1st] nerve, right side**
⑦⊟ **S04.812-**   **Injury of olfactory [1st] nerve, left side**
⑦⊟ **S04.819-**   **Injury of olfactory [1st] nerve, unspecified side**

⑥ **S04.89**   **Injury of other cranial nerves**
Injury of vagus [10th] nerve
⑦⊟ **S04.891-**   **Injury of other cranial nerves, right side**
⑦⊟ **S04.892-**   **Injury of other cranial nerves, left side**
⑦⊟ **S04.899-**   **Injury of other cranial nerves, unspecified side**

⑦ **S04.9XX-**   **Injury of unspecified cranial nerve**

● New   ▲ Revised   *Manifestation*   ④-⑦ Digit Indicators   ⊟ Laterality   Ⓐ Adult (15+ years)   Ⓜ Maternity (12-55 years)   Ⓝ Newborn   Ⓟ Pediatric (0-17 years)   ♂ Male   ♀ Female
✖ Deleted   Unspecified   ✚ Additional code

924   © 2017 DecisionHealth   2017 ICD-10-CM Expert for Physicians

S05   Injury of eye and orbit

> INCLUDES   open wound of eye and orbit
>
> EXCLUDES 2   2nd cranial [optic] nerve injury (S04.0-)
> 3rd cranial [oculomotor] nerve injury (S04.1-)
> open wound of eyelid and periocular area (S01.1-)
> orbital bone fracture (S02.1-, S02.3-, S02.8-)
> superficial injury of eyelid (S00.1-S00.2)

> The appropriate 7th character is to be added to each code from category S05
> A   initial encounter
> D   subsequent encounter
> S   sequela

S05.0   Injury of conjunctiva and corneal abrasion without foreign body

> EXCLUDES 1   foreign body in conjunctival sac (T15.1)
> foreign body in cornea (T15.0)

S05.00X-   Injury of conjunctiva and corneal abrasion without foreign body, unspecified eye

S05.01X-   Injury of conjunctiva and corneal abrasion without foreign body, right eye

S05.02X-   Injury of conjunctiva and corneal abrasion without foreign body, left eye

S05.1   Contusion of eyeball and orbital tissues
Traumatic hyphema

> EXCLUDES 2   black eye NOS (S00.1)
> contusion of eyelid and periocular area (S00.1)

S05.10X-   Contusion of eyeball and orbital tissues, unspecified eye

S05.11X-   Contusion of eyeball and orbital tissues, right eye

S05.12X-   Contusion of eyeball and orbital tissues, left eye

S05.2   Ocular laceration and rupture with prolapse or loss of intraocular tissue

S05.20X-   Ocular laceration and rupture with prolapse or loss of intraocular tissue, unspecified eye

S05.21X-   Ocular laceration and rupture with prolapse or loss of intraocular tissue, right eye

S05.22X-   Ocular laceration and rupture with prolapse or loss of intraocular tissue, left eye

S05.3   Ocular laceration without prolapse or loss of intraocular tissue
Laceration of eye NOS

S05.30X-   Ocular laceration without prolapse or loss of intraocular tissue, unspecified eye

S05.31X-   Ocular laceration without prolapse or loss of intraocular tissue, right eye

S05.32X-   Ocular laceration without prolapse or loss of intraocular tissue, left eye

S05.4   Penetrating wound of orbit with or without foreign body

> EXCLUDES 2   retained (old) foreign body following penetrating wound in orbit (H05.5-)

S05.40X-   Penetrating wound of orbit with or without foreign body, unspecified eye

S05.41X-   Penetrating wound of orbit with or without foreign body, right eye

S05.42X-   Penetrating wound of orbit with or without foreign body, left eye

S05.5   Penetrating wound with foreign body of eyeball

> EXCLUDES 2   retained (old) intraocular foreign body (H44.6-, H44.7)

S05.50X-   Penetrating wound with foreign body of unspecified eyeball

S05.51X-   Penetrating wound with foreign body of right eyeball

S05.52X-   Penetrating wound with foreign body of left eyeball

S05.6   Penetrating wound without foreign body of eyeball
Ocular penetration NOS

S05.60X-   Penetrating wound without foreign body of unspecified eyeball

S05.61X-   Penetrating wound without foreign body of right eyeball

S05.62X-   Penetrating wound without foreign body of left eyeball

S05.7   Avulsion of eye
Traumatic enucleation

S05.70X-   Avulsion of unspecified eye

S05.71X-   Avulsion of right eye

S05.72X-   Avulsion of left eye

S05.8   Other injuries of eye and orbit
Lacrimal duct injury

S05.8X   Other injuries of eye and orbit

S05.8X1-   Other injuries of right eye and orbit

S05.8X2-   Other injuries of left eye and orbit

S05.8X9-   Other injuries of unspecified eye and orbit

S05.9   Unspecified injury of eye and orbit
Injury of eye NOS

S05.90X-   Unspecified injury of unspecified eye and orbit

S05.91X-   Unspecified injury of right eye and orbit

S05.92X-   Unspecified injury of left eye and orbit

S06   Intracranial injury

> INCLUDES   traumatic brain injury
>
> Code also any associated:
> open wound of head (S01.-)
> skull fracture (S02.-)
>
> EXCLUDES 1   head injury NOS (S09.90)

> The appropriate 7th character is to be added to each code from category S06
> A   initial encounter
> D   subsequent encounter
> S   sequela

> CODING TIP ✓   When coding sequelae of a traumatic brain injury, the guideline indicates to first list the residual condition(s), followed by the specific traumatic brain injury diagnosed, using the appropriate code from category S06 with the seventh character 'S' to indicate sequelae. In some cases with traumatic brain injury, there is a tabular convention that indicates to code the intracranial injury first and then the residual, e.g. R40.2-. A convention always overrules a conflicting guideline.

▲ S06.0   Concussion
Commotio cerebri

> EXCLUDES 1   concussion with other intracranial injuries classified in subcategories S06.1- to S06.6- , S06.81- and S06.82- code to specified intracranial injury

S06.0X   Concussion

S06.0X0-   Concussion without loss of consciousness

S06.0X1-   Concussion with loss of consciousness of 30 minutes or less

✖ S06.0X2-   ~~Concussion with loss of consciousness of 31 minutes to 59 minutes~~

✖ S06.0X3-   ~~Concussion with loss of consciousness of 1 hour to 5 hours 59 minutes~~

✖ S06.0X4-   ~~Concussion with loss of consciousness of 6 hours to 24 hours~~

✖ S06.0X5-   ~~Concussion with loss of consciousness greater than 24 hours with return to pre-existing conscious level~~

✖ S06.0X6-   ~~Concussion with loss of consciousness greater than 24 hours without return to pre-existing conscious level with patient surviving~~

✖ S06.0X7-   ~~Concussion with loss of consciousness of any duration with death due to brain injury prior to regaining consciousness~~

✖ S06.0X8-   ~~Concussion with loss of consciousness of any duration with death due to other cause prior to regaining consciousness~~

S06.0X9-   Concussion with loss of consciousness of unspecified duration
Concussion NOS

S06.1   Traumatic cerebral edema
Diffuse traumatic cerebral edema
Focal traumatic cerebral edema
AHA: (S06.1X0A) 1Q 2015, 12

S06.1X   Traumatic cerebral edema

S06.1X0-   Traumatic cerebral edema without loss of consciousness

S06.1X1-   Traumatic cerebral edema with loss of consciousness of 30 minutes or less

● New   ▲ Revised   *Manifestation*   🄳-🄷 Digit Indicators   ▤ Laterality   🄰 Adult (15+ years)   🄼 Maternity (12-55 years)   🄽 Newborn   🄿 Pediatric (0-17 years)   ♂ Male   ♀ Female
✖ ~~Deleted~~   Unspecified   + Additional code

2017 ICD-10-CM Expert for Physicians   © 2017 DecisionHealth   925

7 S06.1X2- Traumatic cerebral edema with loss of consciousness of 31 minutes to 59 minutes

7 S06.1X3- Traumatic cerebral edema with loss of consciousness of 1 hour to 5 hours 59 minutes

7 S06.1X4- Traumatic cerebral edema with loss of consciousness of 6 hours to 24 hours

7 S06.1X5- Traumatic cerebral edema with loss of consciousness greater than 24 hours with return to pre-existing conscious level

7 S06.1X6- Traumatic cerebral edema with loss of consciousness greater than 24 hours without return to pre-existing conscious level with patient surviving

7 S06.1X7- Traumatic cerebral edema with loss of consciousness of any duration with death due to brain injury prior to regaining consciousness

7 S06.1X8- Traumatic cerebral edema with loss of consciousness of any duration with death due to other cause prior to regaining consciousness

7 S06.1X9- Traumatic cerebral edema with loss of consciousness of unspecified duration
Traumatic cerebral edema NOS

5 S06.2 Diffuse traumatic brain injury
Diffuse axonal brain injury
    EXCLUDES 1   *traumatic diffuse cerebral edema (S06.1X-)*

6 S06.2X Diffuse traumatic brain injury

7 S06.2X0- Diffuse traumatic brain injury without loss of consciousness

7 S06.2X1- Diffuse traumatic brain injury with loss of consciousness of 30 minutes or less

7 S06.2X2- Diffuse traumatic brain injury with loss of consciousness of 31 minutes to 59 minutes

7 S06.2X3- Diffuse traumatic brain injury with loss of consciousness of 1 hour to 5 hours 59 minutes

7 S06.2X4- Diffuse traumatic brain injury with loss of consciousness of 6 hours to 24 hours

7 S06.2X5- Diffuse traumatic brain injury with loss of consciousness greater than 24 hours with return to pre-existing conscious levels

7 S06.2X6- Diffuse traumatic brain injury with loss of consciousness greater than 24 hours without return to pre-existing conscious level with patient surviving

7 S06.2X7- Diffuse traumatic brain injury with loss of consciousness of any duration with death due to brain injury prior to regaining consciousness

7 S06.2X8- Diffuse traumatic brain injury with loss of consciousness of any duration with death due to other cause prior to regaining consciousness

7 S06.2X9- Diffuse traumatic brain injury with loss of consciousness of unspecified duration
Diffuse traumatic brain injury NOS

5 S06.3 Focal traumatic brain injury
    EXCLUDES 1   *any condition classifiable to S06.4-S06.6 focal cerebral edema (S06.1)*

6 S06.30 Unspecified focal traumatic brain injury

7 S06.300- Unspecified focal traumatic brain injury without loss of consciousness

7 S06.301- Unspecified focal traumatic brain injury with loss of consciousness of 30 minutes or less

7 S06.302- Unspecified focal traumatic brain injury with loss of consciousness of 31 minutes to 59 minutes

7 S06.303- Unspecified focal traumatic brain injury with loss of consciousness of 1 hour to 5 hours 59 minutes

7 S06.304- Unspecified focal traumatic brain injury with loss of consciousness of 6 hours to 24 hours

7 S06.305- Unspecified focal traumatic brain injury with loss of consciousness greater than 24 hours with return to pre-existing conscious level

7 S06.306- Unspecified focal traumatic brain injury with loss of consciousness greater than 24 hours without return to pre-existing conscious level with patient surviving

7 S06.307- Unspecified focal traumatic brain injury with loss of consciousness of any duration with death due to brain injury prior to regaining consciousness

7 S06.308- Unspecified focal traumatic brain injury with loss of consciousness of any duration with death due to other cause prior to regaining consciousness

7 S06.309- Unspecified focal traumatic brain injury with loss of consciousness of unspecified duration
Unspecified focal traumatic brain injury NOS

6 S06.31 Contusion and laceration of right cerebrum

7 □ S06.310- Contusion and laceration of right cerebrum without loss of consciousness

7 □ S06.311- Contusion and laceration of right cerebrum with loss of consciousness of 30 minutes or less

7 □ S06.312- Contusion and laceration of right cerebrum with loss of consciousness of 31 minutes to 59 minutes

7 □ S06.313- Contusion and laceration of right cerebrum with loss of consciousness of 1 hour to 5 hours 59 minutes

7 □ S06.314- Contusion and laceration of right cerebrum with loss of consciousness of 6 hours to 24 hours

7 □ S06.315- Contusion and laceration of right cerebrum with loss of consciousness greater than 24 hours with return to pre-existing conscious level

7 □ S06.316- Contusion and laceration of right cerebrum with loss of consciousness greater than 24 hours without return to pre-existing conscious level with patient surviving

7 □ S06.317- Contusion and laceration of right cerebrum with loss of consciousness of any duration with death due to brain injury prior to regaining consciousness

7 □ S06.318- Contusion and laceration of right cerebrum with loss of consciousness of any duration with death due to other cause prior to regaining consciousness

7 □ S06.319- Contusion and laceration of right cerebrum with loss of consciousness of unspecified duration
Contusion and laceration of right cerebrum NOS

6 S06.32 Contusion and laceration of left cerebrum

7 □ S06.320- Contusion and laceration of left cerebrum without loss of consciousness

7 □ S06.321- Contusion and laceration of left cerebrum with loss of consciousness of 30 minutes or less

7 □ S06.322- Contusion and laceration of left cerebrum with loss of consciousness of 31 minutes to 59 minutes

7 □ S06.323- Contusion and laceration of left cerebrum with loss of consciousness of 1 hour to 5 hours 59 minutes

7 □ S06.324- Contusion and laceration of left cerebrum with loss of consciousness of 6 hours to 24 hours

7 □ S06.325- Contusion and laceration of left cerebrum with loss of consciousness greater than 24 hours with return to pre-existing conscious level

7 □ S06.326- Contusion and laceration of left cerebrum with loss of consciousness greater than 24 hours without return to pre-existing conscious level with patient surviving

7 □ S06.327- Contusion and laceration of left cerebrum with loss of consciousness of any duration with death due to brain injury prior to regaining consciousness

7 □ S06.328- Contusion and laceration of left cerebrum with loss of consciousness of any duration with death due to other cause prior to regaining consciousness

● New   ▲ Revised   *Manifestation*   4-7 Digit Indicators   □ Laterality   A Adult (15+ years)   M Maternity (12-55 years)   N Newborn   P Pediatric (0-17 years)   ♂ Male   ♀ Female
✖ Deleted   Unspecified   + Additional code

926   © 2017 DecisionHealth   2017 ICD-10-CM Expert for Physicians

7️⃣🔲 **S06.329-** **Contusion and laceration of left cerebrum with loss of consciousness of unspecified duration**
Contusion and laceration of left cerebrum NOS

6️⃣ **S06.33** **Contusion and laceration of cerebrum, unspecified**

7️⃣ **S06.330-** **Contusion and laceration of cerebrum, unspecified, without loss of consciousness**

7️⃣ **S06.331-** **Contusion and laceration of cerebrum, unspecified, with loss of consciousness of 30 minutes or less**

7️⃣ **S06.332-** **Contusion and laceration of cerebrum, unspecified, with loss of consciousness of 31 minutes to 59 minutes**

7️⃣ **S06.333-** **Contusion and laceration of cerebrum, unspecified, with loss of consciousness of 1 hour to 5 hours 59 minutes**

7️⃣ **S06.334-** **Contusion and laceration of cerebrum, unspecified, with loss of consciousness of 6 hours to 24 hours**

7️⃣ **S06.335-** **Contusion and laceration of cerebrum, unspecified, with loss of consciousness greater than 24 hours with return to pre-existing conscious level**

7️⃣ **S06.336-** **Contusion and laceration of cerebrum, unspecified, with loss of consciousness greater than 24 hours without return to pre-existing conscious level with patient surviving**

7️⃣ **S06.337-** **Contusion and laceration of cerebrum, unspecified, with loss of consciousness of any duration with death due to brain injury prior to regaining consciousness**

7️⃣ **S06.338-** **Contusion and laceration of cerebrum, unspecified, with loss of consciousness of any duration with death due to other cause prior to regaining consciousness**

7️⃣ **S06.339-** **Contusion and laceration of cerebrum, unspecified, with loss of consciousness of unspecified duration**
Contusion and laceration of cerebrum NOS

6️⃣ **S06.34** **Traumatic hemorrhage of right cerebrum**
Traumatic intracerebral hemorrhage and hematoma of right cerebrum

7️⃣🔲 **S06.340-** **Traumatic hemorrhage of right cerebrum without loss of consciousness**
AHA: (S06.340A) 1Q 2015, 12

7️⃣🔲 **S06.341-** **Traumatic hemorrhage of right cerebrum with loss of consciousness of 30 minutes or less**

7️⃣🔲 **S06.342-** **Traumatic hemorrhage of right cerebrum with loss of consciousness of 31 minutes to 59 minutes**

7️⃣🔲 **S06.343-** **Traumatic hemorrhage of right cerebrum with loss of consciousness of 1 hours to 5 hours 59 minutes**

7️⃣🔲 **S06.344-** **Traumatic hemorrhage of right cerebrum with loss of consciousness of 6 hours to 24 hours**

7️⃣🔲 **S06.345-** **Traumatic hemorrhage of right cerebrum with loss of consciousness greater than 24 hours with return to pre-existing conscious level**

7️⃣🔲 **S06.346-** **Traumatic hemorrhage of right cerebrum with loss of consciousness greater than 24 hours without return to pre-existing conscious level with patient surviving**

7️⃣🔲 **S06.347-** **Traumatic hemorrhage of right cerebrum with loss of consciousness of any duration with death due to brain injury prior to regaining consciousness**

7️⃣🔲 **S06.348-** **Traumatic hemorrhage of right cerebrum with loss of consciousness of any duration with death due to other cause prior to regaining consciousness**

7️⃣🔲 **S06.349-** **Traumatic hemorrhage of right cerebrum with loss of consciousness of unspecified duration**
Traumatic hemorrhage of right cerebrum NOS

6️⃣ **S06.35** **Traumatic hemorrhage of left cerebrum**
Traumatic intracerebral hemorrhage and hematoma of left cerebrum

7️⃣🔲 **S06.350-** **Traumatic hemorrhage of left cerebrum without loss of consciousness**

7️⃣🔲 **S06.351-** **Traumatic hemorrhage of left cerebrum with loss of consciousness of 30 minutes or less**

7️⃣🔲 **S06.352-** **Traumatic hemorrhage of left cerebrum with loss of consciousness of 31 minutes to 59 minutes**

7️⃣🔲 **S06.353-** **Traumatic hemorrhage of left cerebrum with loss of consciousness of 1 hours to 5 hours 59 minutes**

7️⃣🔲 **S06.354-** **Traumatic hemorrhage of left cerebrum with loss of consciousness of 6 hours to 24 hours**

7️⃣🔲 **S06.355-** **Traumatic hemorrhage of left cerebrum with loss of consciousness greater than 24 hours with return to pre-existing conscious level**

7️⃣🔲 **S06.356-** **Traumatic hemorrhage of left cerebrum with loss of consciousness greater than 24 hours without return to pre-existing conscious level with patient surviving**

7️⃣🔲 **S06.357-** **Traumatic hemorrhage of left cerebrum with loss of consciousness of any duration with death due to brain injury prior to regaining consciousness**

7️⃣🔲 **S06.358-** **Traumatic hemorrhage of left cerebrum with loss of consciousness of any duration with death due to other cause prior to regaining consciousness**

7️⃣🔲 **S06.359-** **Traumatic hemorrhage of left cerebrum with loss of consciousness of unspecified duration**
Traumatic hemorrhage of left cerebrum NOS

6️⃣ **S06.36** **Traumatic hemorrhage of cerebrum, unspecified**
Traumatic intracerebral hemorrhage and hematoma, unspecified

7️⃣ **S06.360-** **Traumatic hemorrhage of cerebrum, unspecified, without loss of consciousness**

7️⃣ **S06.361-** **Traumatic hemorrhage of cerebrum, unspecified, with loss of consciousness of 30 minutes or less**

7️⃣ **S06.362-** **Traumatic hemorrhage of cerebrum, unspecified, with loss of consciousness of 31 minutes to 59 minutes**

7️⃣ **S06.363-** **Traumatic hemorrhage of cerebrum, unspecified, with loss of consciousness of 1 hours to 5 hours 59 minutes**

7️⃣ **S06.364-** **Traumatic hemorrhage of cerebrum, unspecified, with loss of consciousness of 6 hours to 24 hours**

7️⃣ **S06.365-** **Traumatic hemorrhage of cerebrum, unspecified, with loss of consciousness greater than 24 hours with return to pre-existing conscious level**

7️⃣ **S06.366-** **Traumatic hemorrhage of cerebrum, unspecified, with loss of consciousness greater than 24 hours without return to pre-existing conscious level with patient surviving**

7️⃣ **S06.367-** **Traumatic hemorrhage of cerebrum, unspecified, with loss of consciousness of any duration with death due to brain injury prior to regaining consciousness**

7️⃣ **S06.368-** **Traumatic hemorrhage of cerebrum, unspecified, with loss of consciousness of any duration with death due to other cause prior to regaining consciousness**

7️⃣ **S06.369-** **Traumatic hemorrhage of cerebrum, unspecified, with loss of consciousness of unspecified duration**
Traumatic hemorrhage of cerebrum NOS

6️⃣ **S06.37** **Contusion, laceration, and hemorrhage of cerebellum**

7️⃣ **S06.370-** **Contusion, laceration, and hemorrhage of cerebellum without loss of consciousness**

7️⃣ **S06.371-** **Contusion, laceration, and hemorrhage of cerebellum with loss of consciousness of 30 minutes or less**

7️⃣ **S06.372-** **Contusion, laceration, and hemorrhage of cerebellum with loss of consciousness of 31 minutes to 59 minutes**

● New ▲ Revised *Manifestation* 4️⃣-7️⃣ Digit Indicators 🔲 Laterality 🅰 Adult (15+ years) Ⓜ Maternity (12-55 years) Ⓝ Newborn 🅿 Pediatric (0-17 years) ♂ Male ♀ Female
✖ Deleted Unspecified + Additional code

7 S06.373-   Contusion, laceration, and hemorrhage of cerebellum with loss of consciousness of 1 hour to 5 hours 59 minutes

7 S06.374-   Contusion, laceration, and hemorrhage of cerebellum with loss of consciousness of 6 hours to 24 hours

7 S06.375-   Contusion, laceration, and hemorrhage of cerebellum with loss of consciousness greater than 24 hours with return to pre-existing conscious level

7 S06.376-   Contusion, laceration, and hemorrhage of cerebellum with loss of consciousness greater than 24 hours without return to pre-existing conscious level with patient surviving

7 S06.377-   Contusion, laceration, and hemorrhage of cerebellum with loss of consciousness of any duration with death due to brain injury prior to regaining consciousness

7 S06.378-   Contusion, laceration, and hemorrhage of cerebellum with loss of consciousness of any duration with death due to other cause prior to regaining consciousness

7 S06.379-   Contusion, laceration, and hemorrhage of cerebellum with loss of consciousness of unspecified duration
            Contusion, laceration, and hemorrhage of cerebellum NOS

6 S06.38   Contusion, laceration, and hemorrhage of brainstem

7 S06.380-   Contusion, laceration, and hemorrhage of brainstem without loss of consciousness

7 S06.381-   Contusion, laceration, and hemorrhage of brainstem with loss of consciousness of 30 minutes or less

7 S06.382-   Contusion, laceration, and hemorrhage of brainstem with loss of consciousness of 31 minutes to 59 minutes

7 S06.383-   Contusion, laceration, and hemorrhage of brainstem with loss of consciousness of 1 hour to 5 hours 59 minutes

7 S06.384-   Contusion, laceration, and hemorrhage of brainstem with loss of consciousness of 6 hours to 24 hours

7 S06.385-   Contusion, laceration, and hemorrhage of brainstem with loss of consciousness greater than 24 hours with return to pre-existing conscious level

7 S06.386-   Contusion, laceration, and hemorrhage of brainstem with loss of consciousness greater than 24 hours without return to pre-existing conscious level with patient surviving

7 S06.387-   Contusion, laceration, and hemorrhage of brainstem with loss of consciousness of any duration with death due to brain injury prior to regaining consciousness

7 S06.388-   Contusion, laceration, and hemorrhage of brainstem with loss of consciousness of any duration with death due to other cause prior to regaining consciousness

7 S06.389-   Contusion, laceration, and hemorrhage of brainstem with loss of consciousness of unspecified duration
            Contusion, laceration, and hemorrhage of brainstem NOS

5 S06.4   Epidural hemorrhage
            Extradural hemorrhage NOS
            Extradural hemorrhage (traumatic)

6 S06.4X   Epidural hemorrhage

7 S06.4X0-   Epidural hemorrhage without loss of consciousness

7 S06.4X1-   Epidural hemorrhage with loss of consciousness of 30 minutes or less

7 S06.4X2-   Epidural hemorrhage with loss of consciousness of 31 minutes to 59 minutes

7 S06.4X3-   Epidural hemorrhage with loss of consciousness of 1 hour to 5 hours 59 minutes

7 S06.4X4-   Epidural hemorrhage with loss of consciousness of 6 hours to 24 hours

7 S06.4X5-   Epidural hemorrhage with loss of consciousness greater than 24 hours with return to pre-existing conscious level

7 S06.4X6-   Epidural hemorrhage with loss of consciousness greater than 24 hours without return to pre-existing conscious level with patient surviving

7 S06.4X7-   Epidural hemorrhage with loss of consciousness of any duration with death due to brain injury prior to regaining consciousness

7 S06.4X8-   Epidural hemorrhage with loss of consciousness of any duration with death due to other causes prior to regaining consciousness

7 S06.4X9-   Epidural hemorrhage with loss of consciousness of unspecified duration
            Epidural hemorrhage NOS

5 S06.5   Traumatic subdural hemorrhage
            AHA: (S06.5X0A) 3Q 2015, 37

6 S06.5X   Traumatic subdural hemorrhage

7 S06.5X0-   Traumatic subdural hemorrhage without loss of consciousness

7 S06.5X1-   Traumatic subdural hemorrhage with loss of consciousness of 30 minutes or less

7 S06.5X2-   Traumatic subdural hemorrhage with loss of consciousness of 31 minutes to 59 minutes

7 S06.5X3-   Traumatic subdural hemorrhage with loss of consciousness of 1 hour to 5 hours 59 minutes

7 S06.5X4-   Traumatic subdural hemorrhage with loss of consciousness of 6 hours to 24 hours

7 S06.5X5-   Traumatic subdural hemorrhage with loss of consciousness greater than 24 hours with return to pre-existing conscious level

7 S06.5X6-   Traumatic subdural hemorrhage with loss of consciousness greater than 24 hours without return to pre-existing conscious level with patient surviving

7 S06.5X7-   Traumatic subdural hemorrhage with loss of consciousness of any duration with death due to brain injury before regaining consciousness

7 S06.5X8-   Traumatic subdural hemorrhage with loss of consciousness of any duration with death due to other cause before regaining consciousness

7 S06.5X9-   Traumatic subdural hemorrhage with loss of consciousness of unspecified duration
            Traumatic subdural hemorrhage NOS

5 S06.6   Traumatic subarachnoid hemorrhage
            AHA: (S06.6X0A) 3Q 2015, 37

6 S06.6X   Traumatic subarachnoid hemorrhage

7 S06.6X0-   Traumatic subarachnoid hemorrhage without loss of consciousness

7 S06.6X1-   Traumatic subarachnoid hemorrhage with loss of consciousness of 30 minutes or less

7 S06.6X2-   Traumatic subarachnoid hemorrhage with loss of consciousness of 31 minutes to 59 minutes

7 S06.6X3-   Traumatic subarachnoid hemorrhage with loss of consciousness of 1 hour to 5 hours 59 minutes

7 S06.6X4-   Traumatic subarachnoid hemorrhage with loss of consciousness of 6 hours to 24 hours

7 S06.6X5-   Traumatic subarachnoid hemorrhage with loss of consciousness greater than 24 hours with return to pre-existing conscious level

7 S06.6X6-   Traumatic subarachnoid hemorrhage with loss of consciousness greater than 24 hours without return to pre-existing conscious level with patient surviving

7 S06.6X7-   Traumatic subarachnoid hemorrhage with loss of consciousness of any duration with death due to brain injury prior to regaining consciousness

7 S06.6X8-   Traumatic subarachnoid hemorrhage with loss of consciousness of any duration with death due to other cause prior to regaining consciousness

● New   ▲ Revised   *Manifestation*   4-7 Digit Indicators   ⊟ Laterality   A Adult (15+ years)   M Maternity (12-55 years)   N Newborn   P Pediatric (0-17 years)   ♂ Male   ♀ Female
✖ Deleted   Unspecified   + Additional code

928   © 2017 DecisionHealth   2017 ICD-10-CM Expert for Physicians

[7] S06.6X9-   **Traumatic subarachnoid hemorrhage with loss of consciousness of unspecified duration**
Traumatic subarachnoid hemorrhage NOS

[S] **S06.8   Other specified intracranial injuries**

[6] **S06.81   Injury of right internal carotid artery, intracranial portion, not elsewhere classified**

[7] S06.810-   Injury of right internal carotid artery, intracranial portion, not elsewhere classified without loss of consciousness

[7] S06.811-   Injury of right internal carotid artery, intracranial portion, not elsewhere classified with loss of consciousness of 30 minutes or less

[7] S06.812-   Injury of right internal carotid artery, intracranial portion, not elsewhere classified with loss of consciousness of 31 minutes to 59 minutes

[7] S06.813-   Injury of right internal carotid artery, intracranial portion, not elsewhere classified with loss of consciousness of 1 hour to 5 hours 59 minutes

[7] S06.814-   Injury of right internal carotid artery, intracranial portion, not elsewhere classified with loss of consciousness of 6 hours to 24 hours

[7] S06.815-   Injury of right internal carotid artery, intracranial portion, not elsewhere classified with loss of consciousness greater than 24 hours with return to pre-existing conscious level

[7] S06.816-   Injury of right internal carotid artery, intracranial portion, not elsewhere classified with loss of consciousness greater than 24 hours without return to pre-existing conscious level with patient surviving

[7] S06.817-   Injury of right internal carotid artery, intracranial portion, not elsewhere classified with loss of consciousness of any duration with death due to brain injury prior to regaining consciousness

[7] S06.818-   Injury of right internal carotid artery, intracranial portion, not elsewhere classified with loss of consciousness of any duration with death due to other cause prior to regaining consciousness

[7] S06.819-   **Injury of right internal carotid artery, intracranial portion, not elsewhere classified with loss of consciousness of unspecified duration**
Injury of right internal carotid artery, intracranial portion, not elsewhere classified NOS

[6] **S06.82   Injury of left internal carotid artery, intracranial portion, not elsewhere classified**

[7] S06.820-   Injury of left internal carotid artery, intracranial portion, not elsewhere classified without loss of consciousness

[7] S06.821-   Injury of left internal carotid artery, intracranial portion, not elsewhere classified with loss of consciousness of 30 minutes or less

[7] S06.822-   Injury of left internal carotid artery, intracranial portion, not elsewhere classified with loss of consciousness of 31 minutes to 59 minutes

[7] S06.823-   Injury of left internal carotid artery, intracranial portion, not elsewhere classified with loss of consciousness of 1 hour to 5 hours 59 minutes

[7] S06.824-   Injury of left internal carotid artery, intracranial portion, not elsewhere classified with loss of consciousness of 6 hours to 24 hours

[7] S06.825-   Injury of left internal carotid artery, intracranial portion, not elsewhere classified with loss of consciousness greater than 24 hours with return to pre-existing conscious level

[7] S06.826-   Injury of left internal carotid artery, intracranial portion, not elsewhere classified with loss of consciousness greater than 24 hours without return to pre-existing conscious level with patient surviving

[7] S06.827-   Injury of left internal carotid artery, intracranial portion, not elsewhere classified with loss of consciousness of any duration with death due to brain injury prior to regaining consciousness

[7] S06.828-   Injury of left internal carotid artery, intracranial portion, not elsewhere classified with loss of consciousness of any duration with death due to other cause prior to regaining consciousness

[7] S06.829-   **Injury of left internal carotid artery, intracranial portion, not elsewhere classified with loss of consciousness of unspecified duration**
Injury of left internal carotid artery, intracranial portion, not elsewhere classified NOS

▲ [6] **S06.89   Other specified intracranial injury**
EXCLUDES 1   *concussion (S06.0X-)*

[7] S06.890-   Other specified intracranial injury without loss of consciousness

[7] S06.891-   Other specified intracranial injury with loss of consciousness of 30 minutes or less

[7] S06.892-   Other specified intracranial injury with loss of consciousness of 31 minutes to 59 minutes

[7] S06.893-   Other specified intracranial injury with loss of consciousness of 1 hour to 5 hours 59 minutes

[7] S06.894-   Other specified intracranial injury with loss of consciousness of 6 hours to 24 hours

[7] S06.895-   Other specified intracranial injury with loss of consciousness greater than 24 hours with return to pre-existing conscious level

[7] S06.896-   Other specified intracranial injury with loss of consciousness greater than 24 hours without return to pre-existing conscious level with patient surviving

[7] S06.897-   Other specified intracranial injury with loss of consciousness of any duration with death due to brain injury prior to regaining consciousness

[7] S06.898-   Other specified intracranial injury with loss of consciousness of any duration with death due to other cause prior to regaining consciousness

[7] S06.899-   Other specified intracranial injury with loss of consciousness of unspecified duration

▲ [S] **S06.9   Unspecified intracranial injury**
Brain injury NOS
Head injury NOS with loss of consciousness
Traumatic brain injury NOS
EXCLUDES 1   *conditions classifiable to S06.0- to S06.8-
code to specified intracranial injury
head injury NOS (S09.90)*

[6] **S06.9X   Unspecified intracranial injury**

[7] S06.9X0-   Unspecified intracranial injury without loss of consciousness

[7] S06.9X1-   Unspecified intracranial injury with loss of consciousness of 30 minutes or less

[7] S06.9X2-   Unspecified intracranial injury with loss of consciousness of 31 minutes to 59 minutes

[7] S06.9X3-   Unspecified intracranial injury with loss of consciousness of 1 hour to 5 hours 59 minutes

[7] S06.9X4-   Unspecified intracranial injury with loss of consciousness of 6 hours to 24 hours

[7] S06.9X5-   Unspecified intracranial injury with loss of consciousness greater than 24 hours with return to pre-existing conscious level

[7] S06.9X6-   Unspecified intracranial injury with loss of consciousness greater than 24 hours without return to pre-existing conscious level with patient surviving

[7] S06.9X7-   Unspecified intracranial injury with loss of consciousness of any duration with death due to brain injury prior to regaining consciousness

☷ **S06.9X8-**   Unspecified intracranial injury with loss of consciousness of any duration with death due to other cause prior to regaining consciousness

☷ **S06.9X9-**   Unspecified intracranial injury with loss of consciousness of unspecified duration

❹+ **S07**   **Crushing injury of head**

Use additional code for all associated injuries, such as:
intracranial injuries (S06.-)
skull fractures (S02.-)

The appropriate 7th character is to be added to each code from category S07
A   initial encounter
D   subsequent encounter
S   sequela

☷+ **S07.0XX-**   **Crushing injury of face**
☷+ **S07.1XX-**   **Crushing injury of skull**
☷+ **S07.8XX-**   **Crushing injury of other parts of head**
☷+ **S07.9XX-**   **Crushing injury of head, part unspecified**

❹ **S08**   **Avulsion and traumatic amputation of part of head**

An amputation not identified as partial or complete should be coded to complete

The appropriate 7th character is to be added to each code from category S08
A   initial encounter
D   subsequent encounter
S   sequela

☷ **S08.0XX-**   **Avulsion of scalp**
❺ **S08.1**   **Traumatic amputation of ear**
❻ **S08.11**   **Complete traumatic amputation of ear**
☷⊟ **S08.111-**   **Complete traumatic amputation of right ear**
☷⊟ **S08.112-**   **Complete traumatic amputation of left ear**
☷⊟ **S08.119-**   **Complete traumatic amputation of unspecified ear**
❻ **S08.12**   **Partial traumatic amputation of ear**
☷⊟ **S08.121-**   **Partial traumatic amputation of right ear**
☷⊟ **S08.122-**   **Partial traumatic amputation of left ear**
☷⊟ **S08.129-**   **Partial traumatic amputation of unspecified ear**
❺ **S08.8**   **Traumatic amputation of other parts of head**
❻ **S08.81**   **Traumatic amputation of nose**
☷ **S08.811-**   **Complete traumatic amputation of nose**
☷ **S08.812-**   **Partial traumatic amputation of nose**
☷ **S08.89X-**   **Traumatic amputation of other parts of head**

❹ **S09**   **Other and unspecified injuries of head**

The appropriate 7th character is to be added to each code from category S09
A   initial encounter
D   subsequent encounter
S   sequela

☷ **S09.0XX-**   **Injury of blood vessels of head, not elsewhere classified**

EXCLUDES 1   *injury of cerebral blood vessels (S06.-)*
injury of precerebral blood vessels (S15.-)

❺ **S09.1**   **Injury of muscle and tendon of head**
Code also:
any associated open wound (S01.-)

EXCLUDES 2   *sprain to joints and ligament of head (S03.9)*

☷ **S09.10X-**   **Unspecified injury of muscle and tendon of head**
Injury of muscle and tendon of head NOS
☷ **S09.11X-**   **Strain of muscle and tendon of head**
☷ **S09.12X-**   **Laceration of muscle and tendon of head**
☷ **S09.19X-**   **Other specified injury of muscle and tendon of head**
❺ **S09.2**   **Traumatic rupture of ear drum**

EXCLUDES 1   *traumatic rupture of ear drum due to blast injury (S09.31-)*

☷⊟ **S09.20X-**   **Traumatic rupture of unspecified ear drum**
☷⊟ **S09.21X-**   **Traumatic rupture of right ear drum**

☷⊟ **S09.22X-**   **Traumatic rupture of left ear drum**
❺ **S09.3**   **Other specified and unspecified injury of middle and inner ear**

EXCLUDES 1   *injury to ear NOS (S09.91-)*
EXCLUDES 2   *injury to external ear (S00.4-, S01.3-, S08.1-)*

❻ **S09.30**   **Unspecified injury of middle and inner ear**
☷⊟ **S09.301-**   **Unspecified injury of right middle and inner ear**
☷⊟ **S09.302-**   **Unspecified injury of left middle and inner ear**
☷⊟ **S09.309-**   **Unspecified injury of unspecified middle and inner ear**
❻ **S09.31**   **Primary blast injury of ear**
Blast injury of ear NOS
☷⊟ **S09.311-**   **Primary blast injury of right ear**
☷⊟ **S09.312-**   **Primary blast injury of left ear**
☷⊟ **S09.313-**   **Primary blast injury of ear, bilateral**
☷⊟ **S09.319-**   **Primary blast injury of unspecified ear**
❻ **S09.39**   **Other specified injury of middle and inner ear**
Secondary blast injury to ear
☷⊟ **S09.391-**   **Other specified injury of right middle and inner ear**
☷⊟ **S09.392-**   **Other specified injury of left middle and inner ear**
☷⊟ **S09.399-**   **Other specified injury of unspecified middle and inner ear**
☷ **S09.8XX-**   **Other specified injuries of head**
❺ **S09.9**   **Unspecified injury of face and head**
☷ **S09.90X-**   **Unspecified injury of head**
Head injury NOS

EXCLUDES 1   *brain injury NOS (S06.9-)*
head injury NOS with loss of consciousness (S06.9-)
intracranial injury NOS (S06.9-)

☷ **S09.91X-**   **Unspecified injury of ear**
Injury of ear NOS
☷ **S09.92X-**   **Unspecified injury of nose**
Injury of nose NOS
☷ **S09.93X-**   **Unspecified injury of face**
Injury of face NOS

Injuries to the neck (S10-S19)

INCLUDES   injuries of nape
injuries of supraclavicular region
injuries of throat
EXCLUDES 2   *burns and corrosions (T20-T32)*
effects of foreign body in esophagus (T18.1)
effects of foreign body in larynx (T17.3)
effects of foreign body in pharynx (T17.2)
effects of foreign body in trachea (T17.4)
frostbite (T33-T34)
insect bite or sting, venomous (T63.4)

GUIDELINES   Section I.C.19.c.2)
Multiple fractures are sequenced in accordance with the severity of the fracture.

GUIDELINES   Section I.C.19.b.1)-2)
When coding injuries, assign separate codes for each injury unless a combination code is provided, in which case the combination code is assigned ... Traumatic injury codes (S00-T14.9) are not to be used for normal, healing surgical wounds or to identify complications of surgical wounds. The code for the most serious injury, as determined by the provider and the focus of treatment, is sequenced first.

1) Superficial injuries such as abrasions or contusions are not coded when associated with more severe injuries of the same site.

2) When a primary injury results in minor damage to peripheral nerves or blood vessels, the primary injury is sequenced first with additional code(s) for injuries to nerves and spinal cord (such as category S04), and/or injury to blood vessels (such as category S15). When the primary injury is to the blood vessels or nerves, that injury should be sequenced first.

GUIDELINES Section I.C.19.c

Coding of Traumatic Fractures: The principles of multiple coding of injuries should be followed in coding fractures. Fractures of specified sites are coded individually by site in accordance with both the provisions within categories S02, S12, S22, S32, S42, S49, S52, S59, S62, S72, S79, S82, S89, S92 and the level of detail furnished by medical record content. A fracture not indicated as open or closed should be coded to closed. A fracture not indicated whether displaced or not displaced should be coded to displaced.

▲ **S10** **Superficial injury of neck**

The appropriate 7th character is to be added to each code from category S10
A initial encounter
D subsequent encounter
S sequela

7 **S10.0XX-** **Contusion of throat**
Contusion of cervical esophagus
Contusion of larynx
Contusion of pharynx
Contusion of trachea

5 **S10.1** **Other and unspecified superficial injuries of throat**

7 **S10.10X-** **Unspecified superficial injuries of throat**

7 **S10.11X-** **Abrasion of throat**

7 **S10.12X-** **Blister (nonthermal) of throat**

7 **S10.14X-** **External constriction of part of throat**

7 **S10.15X-** **Superficial foreign body of throat**
Splinter in the throat

7 **S10.16X-** **Insect bite (nonvenomous) of throat**

7 **S10.17X-** **Other superficial bite of throat**
EXCLUDES 1 *open bite of throat (S11.85)*

5 **S10.8** **Superficial injury of other specified parts of neck**

7 **S10.80X-** **Unspecified superficial injury of other specified part of neck**

7 **S10.81X-** **Abrasion of other specified part of neck**

7 **S10.82X-** **Blister (nonthermal) of other specified part of neck**

7 **S10.83X-** **Contusion of other specified part of neck**

7 **S10.84X-** **External constriction of other specified part of neck**

7 **S10.85X-** **Superficial foreign body of other specified part of neck**
Splinter in other specified part of neck

7 **S10.86X-** **Insect bite of other specified part of neck**

7 **S10.87X-** **Other superficial bite of other specified part of neck**
EXCLUDES 1 *open bite of other specified parts of neck (S11.85)*

5 **S10.9** **Superficial injury of unspecified part of neck**

7 **S10.90X-** **Unspecified superficial injury of unspecified part of neck**

7 **S10.91X-** **Abrasion of unspecified part of neck**

7 **S10.92X-** **Blister (nonthermal) of unspecified part of neck**

7 **S10.93X-** **Contusion of unspecified part of neck**

7 **S10.94X-** **External constriction of unspecified part of neck**

7 **S10.95X-** **Superficial foreign body of unspecified part of neck**

7 **S10.96X-** **Insect bite of unspecified part of neck**

7 **S10.97X-** **Other superficial bite of unspecified part of neck**

▲ **S11** **Open wound of neck**
Code also any associated:
spinal cord injury (S14.0, S14.1-)
wound infection
EXCLUDES 2 *open fracture of vertebra (S12.- with 7th character B)*

The appropriate 7th character is to be added to each code from category S11
A initial encounter
D subsequent encounter
S sequela

CODING TIP ✓ Open wound codes are used for wounds caused by trauma. Do not assign a code for "open wound" unless the etiology of the wound is related to trauma.

5 **S11.0** **Open wound of larynx and trachea**

6 **S11.01** **Open wound of larynx**
EXCLUDES 2 *open wound of vocal cord (S11.03)*

7 **S11.011-** **Laceration without foreign body of larynx**

7 **S11.012-** **Laceration with foreign body of larynx**

7 **S11.013-** **Puncture wound without foreign body of larynx**

7 **S11.014-** **Puncture wound with foreign body of larynx**

7 **S11.015-** **Open bite of larynx**
Bite of larynx NOS

7 **S11.019-** **Unspecified open wound of larynx**

6 **S11.02** **Open wound of trachea**
Open wound of cervical trachea
Open wound of trachea NOS
EXCLUDES 2 *open wound of thoracic trachea (S27.5-)*

7 **S11.021-** **Laceration without foreign body of trachea**

7 **S11.022-** **Laceration with foreign body of trachea**

7 **S11.023-** **Puncture wound without foreign body of trachea**

7 **S11.024-** **Puncture wound with foreign body of trachea**

7 **S11.025-** **Open bite of trachea**
Bite of trachea NOS

7 **S11.029-** **Unspecified open wound of trachea**

6 **S11.03** **Open wound of vocal cord**

7 **S11.031-** **Laceration without foreign body of vocal cord**

7 **S11.032-** **Laceration with foreign body of vocal cord**

7 **S11.033-** **Puncture wound without foreign body of vocal cord**

7 **S11.034-** **Puncture wound with foreign body of vocal cord**

7 **S11.035-** **Open bite of vocal cord**
Bite of vocal cord NOS

7 **S11.039-** **Unspecified open wound of vocal cord**

5 **S11.1** **Open wound of thyroid gland**

7 **S11.10X-** **Unspecified open wound of thyroid gland**

7 **S11.11X-** **Laceration without foreign body of thyroid gland**

7 **S11.12X-** **Laceration with foreign body of thyroid gland**

7 **S11.13X-** **Puncture wound without foreign body of thyroid gland**

7 **S11.14X-** **Puncture wound with foreign body of thyroid gland**

7 **S11.15X-** **Open bite of thyroid gland**
Bite of thyroid gland NOS

5 **S11.2** **Open wound of pharynx and cervical esophagus**
EXCLUDES 1 *open wound of esophagus NOS (S27.8-)*

7 **S11.20X-** **Unspecified open wound of pharynx and cervical esophagus**

7 **S11.21X-** **Laceration without foreign body of pharynx and cervical esophagus**

7 **S11.22X-** **Laceration with foreign body of pharynx and cervical esophagus**

7 **S11.23X-** **Puncture wound without foreign body of pharynx and cervical esophagus**

7 **S11.24X-** **Puncture wound with foreign body of pharynx and cervical esophagus**

7 **S11.25X-** **Open bite of pharynx and cervical esophagus**
Bite of pharynx and cervical esophagus NOS

5 **S11.8** **Open wound of other specified parts of neck**

7 **S11.80X-** **Unspecified open wound of other specified part of neck**

7 **S11.81X-** **Laceration without foreign body of other specified part of neck**

7 **S11.82X-** **Laceration with foreign body of other specified part of neck**

7 **S11.83X-** **Puncture wound without foreign body of other specified part of neck**

7 **S11.84X-** **Puncture wound with foreign body of other specified part of neck**

7 **S11.85X-** **Open bite of other specified part of neck**
Bite of other specified part of neck NOS
EXCLUDES 1 *superficial bite of other specified part of neck (S10.87)*

7 **S11.89X-** **Other open wound of other specified part of neck**

5 **S11.9** **Open wound of unspecified part of neck**

● New ▲ Revised *Manifestation* 4-7 Digit Indicators ▤ Laterality ▢A Adult (15+ years) ▢M Maternity (12-55 years) ▢N Newborn ▢P Pediatric (0-17 years) ♂ Male ♀ Female
✖ ~~Deleted~~ Unspecified + Additional code

7 S11.90X-   Unspecified open wound of unspecified part of neck

7 S11.91X-   Laceration without foreign body of unspecified part of neck

7 S11.92X-   Laceration with foreign body of unspecified part of neck

7 S11.93X-   Puncture wound without foreign body of unspecified part of neck

7 S11.94X-   Puncture wound with foreign body of unspecified part of neck

7 S11.95X-   Open bite of unspecified part of neck
Bite of neck NOS

EXCLUDES 1   *superficial bite of neck (S10.97)*

4 **S12**   **Fracture of cervical vertebra and other parts of neck**
Note: A fracture not indicated as displaced or nondisplaced should be coded to displaced
A fracture not indicated as open or closed should be coded to closed

INCLUDES   fracture of cervical neural arch
fracture of cervical spine
fracture of cervical spinous process
fracture of cervical transverse process
fracture of cervical vertebral arch
fracture of neck

Code first:
any associated cervical spinal cord injury (S14.0, S14.1-)

The appropriate 7th character is to be added to all codes from subcategories S12.0-S12.6
A   initial encounter for closed fracture
B   initial encounter for open fracture
D   subsequent encounter for fracture with routine healing
G   subsequent encounter for fracture with delayed healing
K   subsequent encounter for fracture with nonunion
S   sequela

CODING TIP ✓   A fracture not indicated as displaced or nondisplaced should be coded to displaced. A fracture not indicated as open or closed should be coded to closed. Query providers on fractures not documented as displaced/nondisplaced otherwise displaced fracture diagnosis could be assigned without reduction being performed potentially resulting in claim denials.

5 **S12.0**   **Fracture of first cervical vertebra**
Atlas

6 **S12.00**   **Unspecified fracture of first cervical vertebra**

7 S12.000-   Unspecified displaced fracture of first cervical vertebra

7 S12.001-   Unspecified nondisplaced fracture of first cervical vertebra

7 S12.01X-   Stable burst fracture of first cervical vertebra

7 S12.02X-   Unstable burst fracture of first cervical vertebra

6 **S12.03**   **Posterior arch fracture of first cervical vertebra**

7 S12.030-   Displaced posterior arch fracture of first cervical vertebra

7 S12.031-   Nondisplaced posterior arch fracture of first cervical vertebra

6 **S12.04**   **Lateral mass fracture of first cervical vertebra**

7 S12.040-   Displaced lateral mass fracture of first cervical vertebra

7 S12.041-   Nondisplaced lateral mass fracture of first cervical vertebra

6 **S12.09**   **Other fracture of first cervical vertebra**

7 S12.090-   Other displaced fracture of first cervical vertebra

7 S12.091-   Other nondisplaced fracture of first cervical vertebra

5 **S12.1**   **Fracture of second cervical vertebra**
Axis

6 **S12.10**   **Unspecified fracture of second cervical vertebra**

7 S12.100-   Unspecified displaced fracture of second cervical vertebra

7 S12.101-   Unspecified nondisplaced fracture of second cervical vertebra

6 **S12.11**   **Type II dens fracture**

7 S12.110-   Anterior displaced Type II dens fracture

7 S12.111-   Posterior displaced Type II dens fracture

7 S12.112-   Nondisplaced Type II dens fracture

6 **S12.12**   **Other dens fracture**

7 S12.120-   Other displaced dens fracture

7 S12.121-   Other nondisplaced dens fracture

6 **S12.13**   **Unspecified traumatic spondylolisthesis of second cervical vertebra**

7 S12.130-   Unspecified traumatic displaced spondylolisthesis of second cervical vertebra

7 S12.131-   Unspecified traumatic nondisplaced spondylolisthesis of second cervical vertebra

7 S12.14X-   Type III traumatic spondylolisthesis of second cervical vertebra

6 **S12.15**   **Other traumatic spondylolisthesis of second cervical vertebra**

7 S12.150-   Other traumatic displaced spondylolisthesis of second cervical vertebra

7 S12.151-   Other traumatic nondisplaced spondylolisthesis of second cervical vertebra

6 **S12.19**   **Other fracture of second cervical vertebra**

7 S12.190-   Other displaced fracture of second cervical vertebra

7 S12.191-   Other nondisplaced fracture of second cervical vertebra

5 **S12.2**   **Fracture of third cervical vertebra**

6 **S12.20**   **Unspecified fracture of third cervical vertebra**

7 S12.200-   Unspecified displaced fracture of third cervical vertebra

7 S12.201-   Unspecified nondisplaced fracture of third cervical vertebra

6 **S12.23**   **Unspecified traumatic spondylolisthesis of third cervical vertebra**

7 S12.230-   Unspecified traumatic displaced spondylolisthesis of third cervical vertebra

7 S12.231-   Unspecified traumatic nondisplaced spondylolisthesis of third cervical vertebra

7 S12.24X-   Type III traumatic spondylolisthesis of third cervical vertebra

6 **S12.25**   **Other traumatic spondylolisthesis of third cervical vertebra**

7 S12.250-   Other traumatic displaced spondylolisthesis of third cervical vertebra

7 S12.251-   Other traumatic nondisplaced spondylolisthesis of third cervical vertebra

6 **S12.29**   **Other fracture of third cervical vertebra**

7 S12.290-   Other displaced fracture of third cervical vertebra

7 S12.291-   Other nondisplaced fracture of third cervical vertebra

5 **S12.3**   **Fracture of fourth cervical vertebra**

6 **S12.30**   **Unspecified fracture of fourth cervical vertebra**

7 S12.300-   Unspecified displaced fracture of fourth cervical vertebra

7 S12.301-   Unspecified nondisplaced fracture of fourth cervical vertebra

6 **S12.33**   **Unspecified traumatic spondylolisthesis of fourth cervical vertebra**

7 S12.330-   Unspecified traumatic displaced spondylolisthesis of fourth cervical vertebra

7 S12.331-   Unspecified traumatic nondisplaced spondylolisthesis of fourth cervical vertebra

7 S12.34X-   Type III traumatic spondylolisthesis of fourth cervical vertebra

6 **S12.35**   **Other traumatic spondylolisthesis of fourth cervical vertebra**

7 S12.350-   Other traumatic displaced spondylolisthesis of fourth cervical vertebra

7 S12.351-   Other traumatic nondisplaced spondylolisthesis of fourth cervical vertebra

6 **S12.39**   **Other fracture of fourth cervical vertebra**

7 S12.390-   Other displaced fracture of fourth cervical vertebra

7 S12.391-   Other nondisplaced fracture of fourth cervical vertebra

5 **S12.4**   **Fracture of fifth cervical vertebra**

6 **S12.40**   **Unspecified fracture of fifth cervical vertebra**

7 S12.400-   Unspecified displaced fracture of fifth cervical vertebra

● New   ▲ Revised   *Manifestation*   4-7 Digit Indicators   ▤ Laterality   A Adult (15+ years)   M Maternity (12-55 years)   N Newborn   P Pediatric (0-17 years)   ♂ Male   ♀ Female
✖ Deleted   Unspecified   + Additional code

932   © 2017 DecisionHealth   2017 ICD-10-CM Expert for Physicians

7 **S12.401-** Unspecified nondisplaced fracture of fifth cervical vertebra

6 **S12.43** Unspecified traumatic spondylolisthesis of fifth cervical vertebra

  7 **S12.430-** Unspecified traumatic displaced spondylolisthesis of fifth cervical vertebra

  7 **S12.431-** Unspecified traumatic nondisplaced spondylolisthesis of fifth cervical vertebra

7 **S12.44X-** Type III traumatic spondylolisthesis of fifth cervical vertebra

6 **S12.45** Other traumatic spondylolisthesis of fifth cervical vertebra

  7 **S12.450-** Other traumatic displaced spondylolisthesis of fifth cervical vertebra

  7 **S12.451-** Other traumatic nondisplaced spondylolisthesis of fifth cervical vertebra

6 **S12.49** Other fracture of fifth cervical vertebra

  7 **S12.490-** Other displaced fracture of fifth cervical vertebra

  7 **S12.491-** Other nondisplaced fracture of fifth cervical vertebra

5 **S12.5** Fracture of sixth cervical vertebra

6 **S12.50** Unspecified fracture of sixth cervical vertebra

  7 **S12.500-** Unspecified displaced fracture of sixth cervical vertebra

  7 **S12.501-** Unspecified nondisplaced fracture of sixth cervical vertebra

6 **S12.53** Unspecified traumatic spondylolisthesis of sixth cervical vertebra

  7 **S12.530-** Unspecified traumatic displaced spondylolisthesis of sixth cervical vertebra

  7 **S12.531-** Unspecified traumatic nondisplaced spondylolisthesis of sixth cervical vertebra

7 **S12.54X-** Type III traumatic spondylolisthesis of sixth cervical vertebra

6 **S12.55** Other traumatic spondylolisthesis of sixth cervical vertebra

  7 **S12.550-** Other traumatic displaced spondylolisthesis of sixth cervical vertebra

  7 **S12.551-** Other traumatic nondisplaced spondylolisthesis of sixth cervical vertebra

6 **S12.59** Other fracture of sixth cervical vertebra

  7 **S12.590-** Other displaced fracture of sixth cervical vertebra

  7 **S12.591-** Other nondisplaced fracture of sixth cervical vertebra

5 **S12.6** Fracture of seventh cervical vertebra

6 **S12.60** Unspecified fracture of seventh cervical vertebra

  7 **S12.600-** Unspecified displaced fracture of seventh cervical vertebra

  7 **S12.601-** Unspecified nondisplaced fracture of seventh cervical vertebra

6 **S12.63** Unspecified traumatic spondylolisthesis of seventh cervical vertebra

  7 **S12.630-** Unspecified traumatic displaced spondylolisthesis of seventh cervical vertebra

  7 **S12.631-** Unspecified traumatic nondisplaced spondylolisthesis of seventh cervical vertebra

7 **S12.64X-** Type III traumatic spondylolisthesis of seventh cervical vertebra

6 **S12.65** Other traumatic spondylolisthesis of seventh cervical vertebra

  7 **S12.650-** Other traumatic displaced spondylolisthesis of seventh cervical vertebra

  7 **S12.651-** Other traumatic nondisplaced spondylolisthesis of seventh cervical vertebra

6 **S12.69** Other fracture of seventh cervical vertebra

  7 **S12.690-** Other displaced fracture of seventh cervical vertebra

  7 **S12.691-** Other nondisplaced fracture of seventh cervical vertebra

7 **S12.8XX-** **Fracture of other parts of neck**
Hyoid bone
Larynx
Thyroid cartilage
Trachea

The appropriate 7th character is to be added to code S12.8
A   initial encounter
D   subsequent encounter
S   sequela

7 **S12.9XX-** **Fracture of neck, unspecified**
Fracture of neck NOS
Fracture of cervical spine NOS
Fracture of cervical vertebra NOS

The appropriate 7th character is to be added to code S12.9
A   initial encounter
D   subsequent encounter
S   sequela

4 **S13** **Dislocation and sprain of joints and ligaments at neck level**

  INCLUDES   avulsion of joint or ligament at neck level
laceration of cartilage, joint or ligament at neck level
sprain of cartilage, joint or ligament at neck level
traumatic hemarthrosis of joint or ligament at neck level
traumatic rupture of joint or ligament at neck level
traumatic subluxation of joint or ligament at neck level
traumatic tear of joint or ligament at neck level

Code also:
any associated open wound

  EXCLUDES 2   *strain of muscle or tendon at neck level (S16.1)*

The appropriate 7th character is to be added to each code from category S13
A   initial encounter
D   subsequent encounter
S   sequela

  CODING TIP ✓   Unlike ICD-9 there is no code for open dislocations. When documented as open an additional code for the open wound must be applied.

7 **S13.0XX-** **Traumatic rupture of cervical intervertebral disc**
  EXCLUDES 1   *rupture or displacement (nontraumatic) of cervical intervertebral disc NOS (M50.-)*

5 **S13.1** Subluxation and dislocation of cervical vertebrae
Code also any associated:
open wound of neck (S11.-)
spinal cord injury (S14.1-)
  EXCLUDES 2   *fracture of cervical vertebrae (S12.0-S12.3-)*

6 **S13.10** **Subluxation and dislocation of unspecified cervical vertebrae**

  7 **S13.100-** **Subluxation of unspecified cervical vertebrae**

  7 **S13.101-** **Dislocation of unspecified cervical vertebrae**

6 **S13.11** **Subluxation and dislocation of C0/C1 cervical vertebrae**
Subluxation and dislocation of atlantooccipital joint
Subluxation and dislocation of atloidooccipital joint
Subluxation and dislocation of occipitoatloid joint

  7 **S13.110-** **Subluxation of C0/C1 cervical vertebrae**
  7 **S13.111-** **Dislocation of C0/C1 cervical vertebrae**

6 **S13.12** **Subluxation and dislocation of C1/C2 cervical vertebrae**
Subluxation and dislocation of atlantoaxial joint

  7 **S13.120-** **Subluxation of C1/C2 cervical vertebrae**
  7 **S13.121-** **Dislocation of C1/C2 cervical vertebrae**

6 **S13.13** **Subluxation and dislocation of C2/C3 cervical vertebrae**

  7 **S13.130-** **Subluxation of C2/C3 cervical vertebrae**
  7 **S13.131-** **Dislocation of C2/C3 cervical vertebrae**

6 **S13.14** **Subluxation and dislocation of C3/C4 cervical vertebrae**

  7 **S13.140-** **Subluxation of C3/C4 cervical vertebrae**
  7 **S13.141-** **Dislocation of C3/C4 cervical vertebrae**

● New   ▲ Revised   *Manifestation*   4-7 Digit Indicators   ▤ Laterality   Ⓐ Adult (15+ years)   Ⓜ Maternity (12-55 years)   Ⓝ Newborn   Ⓟ Pediatric (0-17 years)   ♂ Male   ♀ Female
✖ Deleted   Unspecified   + Additional code

◨ **S13.15** **Subluxation and dislocation of C4/C5 cervical vertebrae**
　　☷ S13.150- **Subluxation of C4/C5 cervical vertebrae**
　　☷ S13.151- **Dislocation of C4/C5 cervical vertebrae**
◨ **S13.16** **Subluxation and dislocation of C5/C6 cervical vertebrae**
　　☷ S13.160- **Subluxation of C5/C6 cervical vertebrae**
　　☷ S13.161- **Dislocation of C5/C6 cervical vertebrae**
◨ **S13.17** **Subluxation and dislocation of C6/C7 cervical vertebrae**
　　☷ S13.170- **Subluxation of C6/C7 cervical vertebrae**
　　☷ S13.171- **Dislocation of C6/C7 cervical vertebrae**
◨ **S13.18** **Subluxation and dislocation of C7/T1 cervical vertebrae**
　　☷ S13.180- **Subluxation of C7/T1 cervical vertebrae**
　　☷ S13.181- **Dislocation of C7/T1 cervical vertebrae**
▤ **S13.2** **Dislocation of other and unspecified parts of neck**
　☷ **S13.20X-** **Dislocation of unspecified parts of neck**
　☷ **S13.29X-** **Dislocation of other parts of neck**
☷ **S13.4XX-** **Sprain of ligaments of cervical spine**
　　Sprain of anterior longitudinal (ligament), cervical
　　Sprain of atlanto-axial (joints)
　　Sprain of atlanto-occipital (joints)
　　Whiplash injury of cervical spine
☷ **S13.5XX-** **Sprain of thyroid region**
　　Sprain of cricoarytenoid (joint) (ligament)
　　Sprain of cricothyroid (joint) (ligament)
　　Sprain of thyroid cartilage
☷ **S13.8XX-** **Sprain of joints and ligaments of other parts of neck**
☷ **S13.9XX-** **Sprain of joints and ligaments of unspecified parts of neck**

▦ **S14** **Injury of nerves and spinal cord at neck level**
　　Note: Code to highest level of cervical cord injury
　　Code also any associated:
　　　fracture of cervical vertebra (S12.0--S12.6.-)
　　　open wound of neck (S11.-)
　　　transient paralysis (R29.5)

> The appropriate 7th character is to be added to each code from category S14
> A initial encounter
> D subsequent encounter
> S sequela

CODING TIP ✓ When coding sequelae of a spinal cord injury, first list the residual condition(s), followed by the specific spinal cord injury diagnosed using the appropriate code from this category with the seventh character "S" to indicate sequelae. If there are multiple levels of injury, code only the highest injury.

☷ **S14.0XX-** **Concussion and edema of cervical spinal cord**
▤ **S14.1** **Other and unspecified injuries of cervical spinal cord**
　◨ **S14.10** **Unspecified injury of cervical spinal cord**
　　☷ S14.101- **Unspecified injury at C1 level of cervical spinal cord**
　　☷ S14.102- **Unspecified injury at C2 level of cervical spinal cord**
　　☷ S14.103- **Unspecified injury at C3 level of cervical spinal cord**
　　☷ S14.104- **Unspecified injury at C4 level of cervical spinal cord**
　　☷ S14.105- **Unspecified injury at C5 level of cervical spinal cord**
　　☷ S14.106- **Unspecified injury at C6 level of cervical spinal cord**
　　☷ S14.107- **Unspecified injury at C7 level of cervical spinal cord**
　　☷ S14.108- **Unspecified injury at C8 level of cervical spinal cord**
　　☷ S14.109- **Unspecified injury at unspecified level of cervical spinal cord**
　　　　Injury of cervical spinal cord NOS
　◨ **S14.11** **Complete lesion of cervical spinal cord**
　　☷ S14.111- **Complete lesion at C1 level of cervical spinal cord**
　　☷ S14.112- **Complete lesion at C2 level of cervical spinal cord**

　　☷ S14.113- **Complete lesion at C3 level of cervical spinal cord**
　　☷ S14.114- **Complete lesion at C4 level of cervical spinal cord**
　　☷ S14.115- **Complete lesion at C5 level of cervical spinal cord**
　　☷ S14.116- **Complete lesion at C6 level of cervical spinal cord**
　　☷ S14.117- **Complete lesion at C7 level of cervical spinal cord**
　　☷ S14.118- **Complete lesion at C8 level of cervical spinal cord**
　　☷ S14.119- **Complete lesion at unspecified level of cervical spinal cord**
　◨ **S14.12** **Central cord syndrome of cervical spinal cord**
　　☷ S14.121- **Central cord syndrome at C1 level of cervical spinal cord**
　　☷ S14.122- **Central cord syndrome at C2 level of cervical spinal cord**
　　☷ S14.123- **Central cord syndrome at C3 level of cervical spinal cord**
　　☷ S14.124- **Central cord syndrome at C4 level of cervical spinal cord**
　　☷ S14.125- **Central cord syndrome at C5 level of cervical spinal cord**
　　☷ S14.126- **Central cord syndrome at C6 level of cervical spinal cord**
　　☷ S14.127- **Central cord syndrome at C7 level of cervical spinal cord**
　　☷ S14.128- **Central cord syndrome at C8 level of cervical spinal cord**
　　☷ S14.129- **Central cord syndrome at unspecified level of cervical spinal cord**
　◨ **S14.13** **Anterior cord syndrome of cervical spinal cord**
　　☷ S14.131- **Anterior cord syndrome at C1 level of cervical spinal cord**
　　☷ S14.132- **Anterior cord syndrome at C2 level of cervical spinal cord**
　　☷ S14.133- **Anterior cord syndrome at C3 level of cervical spinal cord**
　　☷ S14.134- **Anterior cord syndrome at C4 level of cervical spinal cord**
　　☷ S14.135- **Anterior cord syndrome at C5 level of cervical spinal cord**
　　☷ S14.136- **Anterior cord syndrome at C6 level of cervical spinal cord**
　　☷ S14.137- **Anterior cord syndrome at C7 level of cervical spinal cord**
　　☷ S14.138- **Anterior cord syndrome at C8 level of cervical spinal cord**
　　☷ S14.139- **Anterior cord syndrome at unspecified level of cervical spinal cord**
　◨ **S14.14** **Brown-Séquard syndrome of cervical spinal cord**
　　☷ S14.141- **Brown-Séquard syndrome at C1 level of cervical spinal cord**
　　☷ S14.142- **Brown-Séquard syndrome at C2 level of cervical spinal cord**
　　☷ S14.143- **Brown-Séquard syndrome at C3 level of cervical spinal cord**
　　☷ S14.144- **Brown-Séquard syndrome at C4 level of cervical spinal cord**
　　☷ S14.145- **Brown-Séquard syndrome at C5 level of cervical spinal cord**
　　☷ S14.146- **Brown-Séquard syndrome at C6 level of cervical spinal cord**
　　☷ S14.147- **Brown-Séquard syndrome at C7 level of cervical spinal cord**
　　☷ S14.148- **Brown-Séquard syndrome at C8 level of cervical spinal cord**
　　☷ S14.149- **Brown-Séquard syndrome at unspecified level of cervical spinal cord**
　◨ **S14.15** **Other incomplete lesions of cervical spinal cord**
　　　Incomplete lesion of cervical spinal cord NOS
　　　Posterior cord syndrome of cervical spinal cord
　　☷ S14.151- **Other incomplete lesion at C1 level of cervical spinal cord**
　　☷ S14.152- **Other incomplete lesion at C2 level of cervical spinal cord**
　　☷ S14.153- **Other incomplete lesion at C3 level of cervical spinal cord**

7 ⊟ **S14.154-**   Other incomplete lesion at C4 level of cervical spinal cord

7 ⊟ **S14.155-**   Other incomplete lesion at C5 level of cervical spinal cord

7 ⊟ **S14.156-**   Other incomplete lesion at C6 level of cervical spinal cord

7 ⊟ **S14.157-**   Other incomplete lesion at C7 level of cervical spinal cord

7 ⊟ **S14.158-**   Other incomplete lesion at C8 level of cervical spinal cord

7 ⊟ **S14.159-**   Other incomplete lesion at unspecified level of cervical spinal cord

7 **S14.2XX-**   **Injury of nerve root of cervical spine**

7 **S14.3XX-**   **Injury of brachial plexus**

7 **S14.4XX-**   **Injury of peripheral nerves of neck**

7 **S14.5XX-**   **Injury of cervical sympathetic nerves**

7 **S14.8XX-**   **Injury of other specified nerves of neck**

7 **S14.9XX-**   **Injury of unspecified nerves of neck**

4 **S15**   **Injury of blood vessels at neck level**

Code also:
　any associated open wound (S11.-)

The appropriate 7th character is to be added to each code from category S15
A   initial encounter
D   subsequent encounter
S   sequela

5 **S15.0**   **Injury of carotid artery of neck**

Injury of carotid artery (common) (external) (internal, extracranial portion)
Injury of carotid artery NOS

> **EXCLUDES 1**   *injury of internal carotid artery, intracranial portion (S06.8)*

6 **S15.00**   **Unspecified injury of carotid artery**

7 ⊟ **S15.001-**   Unspecified injury of right carotid artery

7 ⊟ **S15.002-**   Unspecified injury of left carotid artery

7 ⊟ **S15.009-**   Unspecified injury of unspecified carotid artery

6 **S15.01**   **Minor laceration of carotid artery**

Incomplete transection of carotid artery
Laceration of carotid artery NOS
Superficial laceration of carotid artery

7 ⊟ **S15.011-**   Minor laceration of right carotid artery

7 ⊟ **S15.012-**   Minor laceration of left carotid artery

7 ⊟ **S15.019-**   Minor laceration of unspecified carotid artery

6 **S15.02**   **Major laceration of carotid artery**

Complete transection of carotid artery
Traumatic rupture of carotid artery

7 ⊟ **S15.021-**   Major laceration of right carotid artery

7 ⊟ **S15.022-**   Major laceration of left carotid artery

7 ⊟ **S15.029-**   Major laceration of unspecified carotid artery

6 **S15.09**   **Other specified injury of carotid artery**

7 ⊟ **S15.091-**   Other specified injury of right carotid artery

7 ⊟ **S15.092-**   Other specified injury of left carotid artery

7 ⊟ **S15.099-**   Other specified injury of unspecified carotid artery

5 **S15.1**   **Injury of vertebral artery**

6 **S15.10**   **Unspecified injury of vertebral artery**

7 ⊟ **S15.101-**   Unspecified injury of right vertebral artery

7 ⊟ **S15.102-**   Unspecified injury of left vertebral artery

7 ⊟ **S15.109-**   Unspecified injury of unspecified vertebral artery

6 **S15.11**   **Minor laceration of vertebral artery**

Incomplete transection of vertebral artery
Laceration of vertebral artery NOS
Superficial laceration of vertebral artery

7 ⊟ **S15.111-**   Minor laceration of right vertebral artery

7 ⊟ **S15.112-**   Minor laceration of left vertebral artery

7 ⊟ **S15.119-**   Minor laceration of unspecified vertebral artery

6 **S15.12**   **Major laceration of vertebral artery**

Complete transection of vertebral artery
Traumatic rupture of vertebral artery

7 ⊟ **S15.121-**   Major laceration of right vertebral artery

7 ⊟ **S15.122-**   Major laceration of left vertebral artery

7 ⊟ **S15.129-**   Major laceration of unspecified vertebral artery

6 **S15.19**   **Other specified injury of vertebral artery**

7 ⊟ **S15.191-**   Other specified injury of right vertebral artery

7 ⊟ **S15.192-**   Other specified injury of left vertebral artery

7 ⊟ **S15.199-**   Other specified injury of unspecified vertebral artery

5 **S15.2**   **Injury of external jugular vein**

6 **S15.20**   **Unspecified injury of external jugular vein**

7 ⊟ **S15.201-**   Unspecified injury of right external jugular vein

7 ⊟ **S15.202-**   Unspecified injury of left external jugular vein

7 ⊟ **S15.209-**   Unspecified injury of unspecified external jugular vein

6 **S15.21**   **Minor laceration of external jugular vein**

Incomplete transection of external jugular vein
Laceration of external jugular vein NOS
Superficial laceration of external jugular vein

7 ⊟ **S15.211-**   Minor laceration of right external jugular vein

7 ⊟ **S15.212-**   Minor laceration of left external jugular vein

7 ⊟ **S15.219-**   Minor laceration of unspecified external jugular vein

6 **S15.22**   **Major laceration of external jugular vein**

Complete transection of external jugular vein
Traumatic rupture of external jugular vein

7 ⊟ **S15.221-**   Major laceration of right external jugular vein

7 ⊟ **S15.222-**   Major laceration of left external jugular vein

7 ⊟ **S15.229-**   Major laceration of unspecified external jugular vein

6 **S15.29**   **Other specified injury of external jugular vein**

7 ⊟ **S15.291-**   Other specified injury of right external jugular vein

7 ⊟ **S15.292-**   Other specified injury of left external jugular vein

7 ⊟ **S15.299-**   Other specified injury of unspecified external jugular vein

5 **S15.3**   **Injury of internal jugular vein**

6 **S15.30**   **Unspecified injury of internal jugular vein**

7 ⊟ **S15.301-**   Unspecified injury of right internal jugular vein

7 ⊟ **S15.302-**   Unspecified injury of left internal jugular vein

7 ⊟ **S15.309-**   Unspecified injury of unspecified internal jugular vein

6 **S15.31**   **Minor laceration of internal jugular vein**

Incomplete transection of internal jugular vein
Laceration of internal jugular vein NOS
Superficial laceration of internal jugular vein

7 ⊟ **S15.311-**   Minor laceration of right internal jugular vein

7 ⊟ **S15.312-**   Minor laceration of left internal jugular vein

7 ⊟ **S15.319-**   Minor laceration of unspecified internal jugular vein

6 **S15.32**   **Major laceration of internal jugular vein**

Complete transection of internal jugular vein
Traumatic rupture of internal jugular vein

7 ⊟ **S15.321-**   Major laceration of right internal jugular vein

7 ⊟ **S15.322-**   Major laceration of left internal jugular vein

7 ⊟ **S15.329-**   Major laceration of unspecified internal jugular vein

6 **S15.39**   **Other specified injury of internal jugular vein**

7 ⊟ **S15.391-**   Other specified injury of right internal jugular vein

7 ⊟ **S15.392-**   Other specified injury of left internal jugular vein

7 ⊟ **S15.399-**   Other specified injury of unspecified internal jugular vein

7 **S15.8XX-**   **Injury of other specified blood vessels at neck level**

7 **S15.9XX-**   **Injury of unspecified blood vessel at neck level**

● New   ▲ Revised   *Manifestation*   4-7 Digit Indicators   ⊟ Laterality   A Adult (15+ years)   M Maternity (12-55 years)   N Newborn   P Pediatric (0-17 years)   ♂ Male   ♀ Female
✖ Deleted   Unspecified   + Additional code

4 S16   Injury of muscle, fascia and tendon at neck level

Code also:
any associated open wound (S11.-)

EXCLUDES 2   *sprain of joint or ligament at neck level (S13.9)*

The appropriate 7th character is to be added to each code from category S16
A   initial encounter
D   subsequent encounter
S   sequela

7 S16.1XX-   **Strain of muscle, fascia and tendon at neck level**
7 S16.2XX-   **Laceration of muscle, fascia and tendon at neck level**
7 S16.8XX-   **Other specified injury of muscle, fascia and tendon at neck level**
7 S16.9XX-   **Unspecified injury of muscle, fascia and tendon at neck level**

4 + S17   Crushing injury of neck

Use additional code for all associated injuries, such as:
injury of blood vessels (S15.-)
open wound of neck (S11.-)
spinal cord injury (S14.0, S14.1-)
vertebral fracture (S12.0--S12.3-)

The appropriate 7th character is to be added to each code from category S17
A   initial encounter
D   subsequent encounter
S   sequela

7 + S17.0XX-   **Crushing injury of larynx and trachea**
7 + S17.8XX-   **Crushing injury of other specified parts of neck**
7 + S17.9XX-   **Crushing injury of neck, part unspecified**

4 S19   Other specified and unspecified injuries of neck

The appropriate 7th character is to be added to each code from category S19
A   initial encounter
D   subsequent encounter
S   sequela

5 S19.8   Other specified injuries of neck
7 S19.80X-   **Other specified injuries of unspecified part of neck**
7 S19.81X-   **Other specified injuries of larynx**
7 S19.82X-   **Other specified injuries of cervical trachea**

EXCLUDES 2   *other specified injury of thoracic trachea (S27.5-)*

7 S19.83X-   **Other specified injuries of vocal cord**
7 S19.84X-   **Other specified injuries of thyroid gland**
7 S19.85X-   **Other specified injuries of pharynx and cervical esophagus**
7 S19.89X-   **Other specified injuries of other specified part of neck**
7 S19.9XX-   **Unspecified injury of neck**

Injuries to the thorax (S20-S29)

INCLUDES   injuries of breast
injuries of chest (wall)
injuries of interscapular area

EXCLUDES 2   *burns and corrosions (T20-T32)*
effects of foreign body in bronchus (T17.5)
effects of foreign body in esophagus (T18.1)
effects of foreign body in lung (T17.8)
effects of foreign body in trachea (T17.4)
frostbite (T33-T34)
injuries of axilla
injuries of clavicle
injuries of scapular region
injuries of shoulder
insect bite or sting, venomous (T63.4)

GUIDELINES   **Section I.C.19.c.2)**
Multiple fractures are sequenced in accordance with the severity of the fracture.

GUIDELINES   **Section I.C.19.b.1)-2)**
When coding injuries, assign separate codes for each injury unless a combination code is provided, in which case the combination code is assigned ... Traumatic injury codes (S00-T14.9) are not to be used for normal, healing surgical wounds or to identify complications of surgical wounds. The code for the most serious injury, as determined by the provider and the focus of treatment, is sequenced first.

1) Superficial injuries such as abrasions or contusions are not coded when associated with more severe injuries of the same site.

2) When a primary injury results in minor damage to peripheral nerves or blood vessels, the primary injury is sequenced first with additional code(s) for injuries to nerves and spinal cord (such as category S04), and/or injury to blood vessels (such as category S15). When the primary injury is to the blood vessels or nerves, that injury should be sequenced first.

GUIDELINES   **Section I.C.19.c**
Coding of Traumatic Fractures: The principles of multiple coding of injuries should be followed in coding fractures. Fractures of specified sites are coded individually by site in accordance with both the provisions within categories S02, S12, S22, S32, S42, S49, S52, S59, S62, S72, S79, S82, S89, S92 and the level of detail furnished by medical record content. A fracture not indicated as open or closed should be coded to closed. A fracture not indicated whether displaced or not displaced should be coded to displaced.

4 S20   Superficial injury of thorax

The appropriate 7th character is to be added to each code from category S20
A   initial encounter
D   subsequent encounter
S   sequela

5 S20.0   Contusion of breast
7 S20.00X-   **Contusion of breast, unspecified breast**
7 S20.01X-   **Contusion of right breast**
7 S20.02X-   **Contusion of left breast**
5 S20.1   Other and unspecified superficial injuries of breast
6 S20.10   Unspecified superficial injuries of breast
7 S20.101-   **Unspecified superficial injuries of breast, right breast**
7 S20.102-   **Unspecified superficial injuries of breast, left breast**
7 S20.109-   **Unspecified superficial injuries of breast, unspecified breast**
6 S20.11   Abrasion of breast
7 S20.111-   **Abrasion of breast, right breast**
7 S20.112-   **Abrasion of breast, left breast**
7 S20.119-   **Abrasion of breast, unspecified breast**
6 S20.12   Blister (nonthermal) of breast
7 S20.121-   **Blister (nonthermal) of breast, right breast**
7 S20.122-   **Blister (nonthermal) of breast, left breast**
7 S20.129-   **Blister (nonthermal) of breast, unspecified breast**
6 S20.14   External constriction of part of breast
7 S20.141-   **External constriction of part of breast, right breast**
7 S20.142-   **External constriction of part of breast, left breast**
7 S20.149-   **External constriction of part of breast, unspecified breast**
6 S20.15   Superficial foreign body of breast
Splinter in the breast
7 S20.151-   **Superficial foreign body of breast, right breast**
7 S20.152-   **Superficial foreign body of breast, left breast**
7 S20.159-   **Superficial foreign body of breast, unspecified breast**
6 S20.16   Insect bite (nonvenomous) of breast
7 S20.161-   **Insect bite (nonvenomous) of breast, right breast**
7 S20.162-   **Insect bite (nonvenomous) of breast, left breast**
7 S20.169-   **Insect bite (nonvenomous) of breast, unspecified breast**

● New   ▲ Revised   *Manifestation*   **4 - 7** Digit Indicators   ⊟ Laterality   🅰 Adult (15+ years)   🅼 Maternity (12-55 years)   🅽 Newborn   🅿 Pediatric (0-17 years)   ♂ Male   ♀ Female
✖ Deleted   Unspecified   + Additional code

6 S20.17   Other superficial bite of breast

    EXCLUDES 1   *open bite of breast (S21.05-)*

7 S20.171-   Other superficial bite of breast, right breast

7 S20.172-   Other superficial bite of breast, left breast

7 S20.179-   Other superficial bite of breast, unspecified breast

5 S20.2   Contusion of thorax

7 S20.20X-   Contusion of thorax, unspecified

6 S20.21   Contusion of front wall of thorax

7 S20.211-   Contusion of right front wall of thorax

7 S20.212-   Contusion of left front wall of thorax

7 S20.219-   Contusion of unspecified front wall of thorax

6 S20.22   Contusion of back wall of thorax

7 S20.221-   Contusion of right back wall of thorax

7 S20.222-   Contusion of left back wall of thorax

7 S20.229-   Contusion of unspecified back wall of thorax

5 S20.3   Other and unspecified superficial injuries of front wall of thorax

6 S20.30   Unspecified superficial injuries of front wall of thorax

7 S20.301-   Unspecified superficial injuries of right front wall of thorax

7 S20.302-   Unspecified superficial injuries of left front wall of thorax

7 S20.309-   Unspecified superficial injuries of unspecified front wall of thorax

6 S20.31   Abrasion of front wall of thorax

7 S20.311-   Abrasion of right front wall of thorax

7 S20.312-   Abrasion of left front wall of thorax

7 S20.319-   Abrasion of unspecified front wall of thorax

6 S20.32   Blister (nonthermal) of front wall of thorax

7 S20.321-   Blister (nonthermal) of right front wall of thorax

7 S20.322-   Blister (nonthermal) of left front wall of thorax

7 S20.329-   Blister (nonthermal) of unspecified front wall of thorax

6 S20.34   External constriction of front wall of thorax

7 S20.341-   External constriction of right front wall of thorax

7 S20.342-   External constriction of left front wall of thorax

7 S20.349-   External constriction of unspecified front wall of thorax

6 S20.35   Superficial foreign body of front wall of thorax

    Splinter in front wall of thorax

7 S20.351-   Superficial foreign body of right front wall of thorax

7 S20.352-   Superficial foreign body of left front wall of thorax

7 S20.359-   Superficial foreign body of unspecified front wall of thorax

6 S20.36   Insect bite (nonvenomous) of front wall of thorax

7 S20.361-   Insect bite (nonvenomous) of right front wall of thorax

7 S20.362-   Insect bite (nonvenomous) of left front wall of thorax

7 S20.369-   Insect bite (nonvenomous) of unspecified front wall of thorax

6 S20.37   Other superficial bite of front wall of thorax

    EXCLUDES 1   *open bite of front wall of thorax (S21.14)*

7 S20.371-   Other superficial bite of right front wall of thorax

7 S20.372-   Other superficial bite of left front wall of thorax

7 S20.379-   Other superficial bite of unspecified front wall of thorax

5 S20.4   Other and unspecified superficial injuries of back wall of thorax

6 S20.40   Unspecified superficial injuries of back wall of thorax

7 S20.401-   Unspecified superficial injuries of right back wall of thorax

7 S20.402-   Unspecified superficial injuries of left back wall of thorax

7 S20.409-   Unspecified superficial injuries of unspecified back wall of thorax

6 S20.41   Abrasion of back wall of thorax

7 S20.411-   Abrasion of right back wall of thorax

7 S20.412-   Abrasion of left back wall of thorax

7 S20.419-   Abrasion of unspecified back wall of thorax

6 S20.42   Blister (nonthermal) of back wall of thorax

7 S20.421-   Blister (nonthermal) of right back wall of thorax

7 S20.422-   Blister (nonthermal) of left back wall of thorax

7 S20.429-   Blister (nonthermal) of unspecified back wall of thorax

6 S20.44   External constriction of back wall of thorax

7 S20.441-   External constriction of right back wall of thorax

7 S20.442-   External constriction of left back wall of thorax

7 S20.449-   External constriction of unspecified back wall of thorax

6 S20.45   Superficial foreign body of back wall of thorax

    Splinter of back wall of thorax

7 S20.451-   Superficial foreign body of right back wall of thorax

7 S20.452-   Superficial foreign body of left back wall of thorax

7 S20.459-   Superficial foreign body of unspecified back wall of thorax

6 S20.46   Insect bite (nonvenomous) of back wall of thorax

7 S20.461-   Insect bite (nonvenomous) of right back wall of thorax

7 S20.462-   Insect bite (nonvenomous) of left back wall of thorax

7 S20.469-   Insect bite (nonvenomous) of unspecified back wall of thorax

6 S20.47   Other superficial bite of back wall of thorax

    EXCLUDES 1   *open bite of back wall of thorax (S21.24)*

7 S20.471-   Other superficial bite of right back wall of thorax

7 S20.472-   Other superficial bite of left back wall of thorax

7 S20.479-   Other superficial bite of unspecified back wall of thorax

5 S20.9   Superficial injury of unspecified parts of thorax

    EXCLUDES 1   *contusion of thorax NOS (S20.20)*

7 S20.90X-   Unspecified superficial injury of unspecified parts of thorax

    Superficial injury of thoracic wall NOS

7 S20.91X-   Abrasion of unspecified parts of thorax

7 S20.92X-   Blister (nonthermal) of unspecified parts of thorax

7 S20.94X-   External constriction of unspecified parts of thorax

7 S20.95X-   Superficial foreign body of unspecified parts of thorax

    Splinter in thorax NOS

7 S20.96X-   Insect bite (nonvenomous) of unspecified parts of thorax

7 S20.97X-   Other superficial bite of unspecified parts of thorax

    EXCLUDES 1   *open bite of thorax NOS (S21.95)*

● New   ▲ Revised   *Manifestation*   4-7 Digit Indicators   ⊟ Laterality   A Adult (15+ years)   M Maternity (12-55 years)   N Newborn   P Pediatric (0-17 years)   ♂ Male   ♀ Female

✖ Deleted   Unspecified   + Additional code

2017 ICD-10-CM Expert for Physicians   © 2017 DecisionHealth   937

⑤ S21   Open wound of thorax

Code also any associated injury, such as:
  injury of heart (S26.-)
  injury of intrathoracic organs (S27.-)
  rib fracture (S22.3-, S22.4-)
  spinal cord injury (S24.0-, S24.1-)
  traumatic hemopneumothorax (S27.3)
  traumatic hemothorax (S27.1)
  traumatic pneumothorax (S27.0)
  wound infection

EXCLUDES 1   *traumatic amputation (partial) of thorax (S28.1)*

The appropriate 7th character is to be added to each code from category S21
A   initial encounter
D   subsequent encounter
S   sequela

CODING TIP ✓   Open wound codes are used for wounds caused by trauma. Do not assign a code for "open wound" unless the etiology of the wound is related to trauma.

⑤ S21.0   Open wound of breast

⑥ S21.00   Unspecified open wound of breast

⑦ ⊟ S21.001-   Unspecified open wound of right breast

⑦ ⊟ S21.002-   Unspecified open wound of left breast

⑦ ⊟ S21.009-   Unspecified open wound of unspecified breast

⑥ S21.01   Laceration without foreign body of breast

⑦ ⊟ S21.011-   Laceration without foreign body of right breast

⑦ ⊟ S21.012-   Laceration without foreign body of left breast

⑦ ⊟ S21.019-   Laceration without foreign body of unspecified breast

⑥ S21.02   Laceration with foreign body of breast

⑦ ⊟ S21.021-   Laceration with foreign body of right breast

⑦ ⊟ S21.022-   Laceration with foreign body of left breast

⑦ ⊟ S21.029-   Laceration with foreign body of unspecified breast

⑥ S21.03   Puncture wound without foreign body of breast

⑦ ⊟ S21.031-   Puncture wound without foreign body of right breast

⑦ ⊟ S21.032-   Puncture wound without foreign body of left breast

⑦ ⊟ S21.039-   Puncture wound without foreign body of unspecified breast

⑥ S21.04   Puncture wound with foreign body of breast

⑦ ⊟ S21.041-   Puncture wound with foreign body of right breast

⑦ ⊟ S21.042-   Puncture wound with foreign body of left breast

⑦ ⊟ S21.049-   Puncture wound with foreign body of unspecified breast

⑥ S21.05   Open bite of breast
Bite of breast NOS

EXCLUDES 1   *superficial bite of breast (S20.17)*

⑦ ⊟ S21.051-   Open bite of right breast

⑦ ⊟ S21.052-   Open bite of left breast

⑦ ⊟ S21.059-   Open bite of unspecified breast

⑤ S21.1   Open wound of front wall of thorax without penetration into thoracic cavity
Open wound of chest without penetration into thoracic cavity

⑥ S21.10   Unspecified open wound of front wall of thorax without penetration into thoracic cavity

⑦ ⊟ S21.101-   Unspecified open wound of right front wall of thorax without penetration into thoracic cavity

⑦ ⊟ S21.102-   Unspecified open wound of left front wall of thorax without penetration into thoracic cavity

⑦ ⊟ S21.109-   Unspecified open wound of unspecified front wall of thorax without penetration into thoracic cavity

⑥ S21.11   Laceration without foreign body of front wall of thorax without penetration into thoracic cavity

⑦ ⊟ S21.111-   Laceration without foreign body of right front wall of thorax without penetration into thoracic cavity

⑦ ⊟ S21.112-   Laceration without foreign body of left front wall of thorax without penetration into thoracic cavity

⑦ ⊟ S21.119-   Laceration without foreign body of unspecified front wall of thorax without penetration into thoracic cavity

⑥ S21.12   Laceration with foreign body of front wall of thorax without penetration into thoracic cavity

⑦ ⊟ S21.121-   Laceration with foreign body of right front wall of thorax without penetration into thoracic cavity

⑦ ⊟ S21.122-   Laceration with foreign body of left front wall of thorax without penetration into thoracic cavity

⑦ ⊟ S21.129-   Laceration with foreign body of unspecified front wall of thorax without penetration into thoracic cavity

⑥ S21.13   Puncture wound without foreign body of front wall of thorax without penetration into thoracic cavity

⑦ ⊟ S21.131-   Puncture wound without foreign body of right front wall of thorax without penetration into thoracic cavity

⑦ ⊟ S21.132-   Puncture wound without foreign body of left front wall of thorax without penetration into thoracic cavity

⑦ ⊟ S21.139-   Puncture wound without foreign body of unspecified front wall of thorax without penetration into thoracic cavity

⑥ S21.14   Puncture wound with foreign body of front wall of thorax without penetration into thoracic cavity

⑦ ⊟ S21.141-   Puncture wound with foreign body of right front wall of thorax without penetration into thoracic cavity

⑦ ⊟ S21.142-   Puncture wound with foreign body of left front wall of thorax without penetration into thoracic cavity

⑦ ⊟ S21.149-   Puncture wound with foreign body of unspecified front wall of thorax without penetration into thoracic cavity

⑥ S21.15   Open bite of front wall of thorax without penetration into thoracic cavity
Bite of front wall of thorax NOS

EXCLUDES 1   *superficial bite of front wall of thorax (S20.37)*

⑦ ⊟ S21.151-   Open bite of right front wall of thorax without penetration into thoracic cavity

⑦ ⊟ S21.152-   Open bite of left front wall of thorax without penetration into thoracic cavity

⑦ ⊟ S21.159-   Open bite of unspecified front wall of thorax without penetration into thoracic cavity

⑤ S21.2   Open wound of back wall of thorax without penetration into thoracic cavity

⑥ S21.20   Unspecified open wound of back wall of thorax without penetration into thoracic cavity

⑦ ⊟ S21.201-   Unspecified open wound of right back wall of thorax without penetration into thoracic cavity

⑦ ⊟ S21.202-   Unspecified open wound of left back wall of thorax without penetration into thoracic cavity

⑦ ⊟ S21.209-   Unspecified open wound of unspecified back wall of thorax without penetration into thoracic cavity

⑥ S21.21   Laceration without foreign body of back wall of thorax without penetration into thoracic cavity

⑦ ⊟ S21.211-   Laceration without foreign body of right back wall of thorax without penetration into thoracic cavity

⑦ ⊟ S21.212-   Laceration without foreign body of left back wall of thorax without penetration into thoracic cavity

⑦ ⊟ S21.219-   Laceration without foreign body of unspecified back wall of thorax without penetration into thoracic cavity

⑥ S21.22   Laceration with foreign body of back wall of thorax without penetration into thoracic cavity

⑦ ⊟ S21.221-   Laceration with foreign body of right back wall of thorax without penetration into thoracic cavity

● New ▲ Revised *Manifestation* ❹-❼ Digit Indicators ⊟ Laterality 🄰 Adult (15+ years) 🄼 Maternity (12-55 years) 🄽 Newborn 🄿 Pediatric (0-17 years) ♂ Male ♀ Female
✖ Deleted Unspecified + Additional code

938   © 2017 DecisionHealth   2017 ICD-10-CM Expert for Physicians

7 ⊟ **S21.222-** Laceration with foreign body of left back wall of thorax without penetration into thoracic cavity

7 ⊟ **S21.229-** Laceration with foreign body of unspecified back wall of thorax without penetration into thoracic cavity

6 **S21.23** Puncture wound without foreign body of back wall of thorax without penetration into thoracic cavity

7 ⊟ **S21.231-** Puncture wound without foreign body of right back wall of thorax without penetration into thoracic cavity

7 ⊟ **S21.232-** Puncture wound without foreign body of left back wall of thorax without penetration into thoracic cavity

7 ⊟ **S21.239-** Puncture wound without foreign body of unspecified back wall of thorax without penetration into thoracic cavity

6 **S21.24** Puncture wound with foreign body of back wall of thorax without penetration into thoracic cavity

7 ⊟ **S21.241-** Puncture wound with foreign body of right back wall of thorax without penetration into thoracic cavity

7 ⊟ **S21.242-** Puncture wound with foreign body of left back wall of thorax without penetration into thoracic cavity

7 ⊟ **S21.249-** Puncture wound with foreign body of unspecified back wall of thorax without penetration into thoracic cavity

6 **S21.25** Open bite of back wall of thorax without penetration into thoracic cavity
Bite of back wall of thorax NOS

EXCLUDES 1 *superficial bite of back wall of thorax (S20.47)*

7 ⊟ **S21.251-** Open bite of right back wall of thorax without penetration into thoracic cavity

7 ⊟ **S21.252-** Open bite of left back wall of thorax without penetration into thoracic cavity

7 ⊟ **S21.259-** Open bite of unspecified back wall of thorax without penetration into thoracic cavity

5 **S21.3** Open wound of front wall of thorax with penetration into thoracic cavity
Open wound of chest with penetration into thoracic cavity

6 **S21.30** Unspecified open wound of front wall of thorax with penetration into thoracic cavity

7 ⊟ **S21.301-** Unspecified open wound of right front wall of thorax with penetration into thoracic cavity

7 ⊟ **S21.302-** Unspecified open wound of left front wall of thorax with penetration into thoracic cavity

7 ⊟ **S21.309-** Unspecified open wound of unspecified front wall of thorax with penetration into thoracic cavity

6 **S21.31** Laceration without foreign body of front wall of thorax with penetration into thoracic cavity

7 ⊟ **S21.311-** Laceration without foreign body of right front wall of thorax with penetration into thoracic cavity

7 ⊟ **S21.312-** Laceration without foreign body of left front wall of thorax with penetration into thoracic cavity

7 ⊟ **S21.319-** Laceration without foreign body of unspecified front wall of thorax with penetration into thoracic cavity

6 **S21.32** Laceration with foreign body of front wall of thorax with penetration into thoracic cavity

7 ⊟ **S21.321-** Laceration with foreign body of right front wall of thorax with penetration into thoracic cavity

7 ⊟ **S21.322-** Laceration with foreign body of left front wall of thorax with penetration into thoracic cavity

7 ⊟ **S21.329-** Laceration with foreign body of unspecified front wall of thorax with penetration into thoracic cavity

6 **S21.33** Puncture wound without foreign body of front wall of thorax with penetration into thoracic cavity

7 ⊟ **S21.331-** Puncture wound without foreign body of right front wall of thorax with penetration into thoracic cavity

7 ⊟ **S21.332-** Puncture wound without foreign body of left front wall of thorax with penetration into thoracic cavity

7 ⊟ **S21.339-** Puncture wound without foreign body of unspecified front wall of thorax with penetration into thoracic cavity

6 **S21.34** Puncture wound with foreign body of front wall of thorax with penetration into thoracic cavity

7 ⊟ **S21.341-** Puncture wound with foreign body of right front wall of thorax with penetration into thoracic cavity

7 ⊟ **S21.342-** Puncture wound with foreign body of left front wall of thorax with penetration into thoracic cavity

7 ⊟ **S21.349-** Puncture wound with foreign body of unspecified front wall of thorax with penetration into thoracic cavity

6 **S21.35** Open bite of front wall of thorax with penetration into thoracic cavity

EXCLUDES 1 *superficial bite of front wall of thorax (S20.37)*

7 ⊟ **S21.351-** Open bite of right front wall of thorax with penetration into thoracic cavity

7 ⊟ **S21.352-** Open bite of left front wall of thorax with penetration into thoracic cavity

7 ⊟ **S21.359-** Open bite of unspecified front wall of thorax with penetration into thoracic cavity

5 **S21.4** Open wound of back wall of thorax with penetration into thoracic cavity

6 **S21.40** Unspecified open wound of back wall of thorax with penetration into thoracic cavity

7 ⊟ **S21.401-** Unspecified open wound of right back wall of thorax with penetration into thoracic cavity

7 ⊟ **S21.402-** Unspecified open wound of left back wall of thorax with penetration into thoracic cavity

7 ⊟ **S21.409-** Unspecified open wound of unspecified back wall of thorax with penetration into thoracic cavity

6 **S21.41** Laceration without foreign body of back wall of thorax with penetration into thoracic cavity

7 ⊟ **S21.411-** Laceration without foreign body of right back wall of thorax with penetration into thoracic cavity

7 ⊟ **S21.412-** Laceration without foreign body of left back wall of thorax with penetration into thoracic cavity

7 ⊟ **S21.419-** Laceration without foreign body of unspecified back wall of thorax with penetration into thoracic cavity

6 **S21.42** Laceration with foreign body of back wall of thorax with penetration into thoracic cavity

7 ⊟ **S21.421-** Laceration with foreign body of right back wall of thorax with penetration into thoracic cavity

7 ⊟ **S21.422-** Laceration with foreign body of left back wall of thorax with penetration into thoracic cavity

7 ⊟ **S21.429-** Laceration with foreign body of unspecified back wall of thorax with penetration into thoracic cavity

6 **S21.43** Puncture wound without foreign body of back wall of thorax with penetration into thoracic cavity

7 ⊟ **S21.431-** Puncture wound without foreign body of right back wall of thorax with penetration into thoracic cavity

7 ⊟ **S21.432-** Puncture wound without foreign body of left back wall of thorax with penetration into thoracic cavity

7 ⊟ **S21.439-** Puncture wound without foreign body of unspecified back wall of thorax with penetration into thoracic cavity

6 **S21.44** Puncture wound with foreign body of back wall of thorax with penetration into thoracic cavity

7 ⊟ **S21.441-** Puncture wound with foreign body of right back wall of thorax with penetration into thoracic cavity

7 ⊟ **S21.442-** Puncture wound with foreign body of left back wall of thorax with penetration into thoracic cavity

7 ⊟ **S21.449-** Puncture wound with foreign body of unspecified back wall of thorax with penetration into thoracic cavity

● New ▲ Revised *Manifestation* 4-7 Digit Indicators ⊟ Laterality Ⓐ Adult (15+ years) Ⓜ Maternity (12-55 years) Ⓝ Newborn (0-17 years) Ⓟ Pediatric ♂ Male ♀ Female
✖ Deleted Unspecified + Additional code

2017 ICD-10-CM Expert for Physicians

© 2017 DecisionHealth

939

6 **S21.45**   **Open bite of back wall of thorax with penetration into thoracic cavity**
Bite of back wall of thorax NOS
EXCLUDES 1   *superficial bite of back wall of thorax (S20.47)*

7 ⊟ **S21.451-**   **Open bite of right back wall of thorax with penetration into thoracic cavity**

7 ⊟ **S21.452-**   **Open bite of left back wall of thorax with penetration into thoracic cavity**

7 **S21.459-**   **Open bite of unspecified back wall of thorax with penetration into thoracic cavity**

5 **S21.9**   **Open wound of unspecified part of thorax**
Open wound of thoracic wall NOS

7 **S21.90X-**   **Unspecified open wound of unspecified part of thorax**

7 **S21.91X-**   **Laceration without foreign body of unspecified part of thorax**

7 **S21.92X-**   **Laceration with foreign body of unspecified part of thorax**

7 **S21.93X-**   **Puncture wound without foreign body of unspecified part of thorax**

7 **S21.94X-**   **Puncture wound with foreign body of unspecified part of thorax**

7 **S21.95X-**   **Open bite of unspecified part of thorax**
EXCLUDES 1   *superficial bite of thorax (S20.97)*

4 **S22**   **Fracture of rib(s), sternum and thoracic spine**
Note: A fracture not indicated as displaced or nondisplaced should be coded to displaced
A fracture not indicated as open or closed should be coded to closed
INCLUDES   fracture of thoracic neural arch
fracture of thoracic spinous process
fracture of thoracic transverse process
fracture of thoracic vertebra
fracture of thoracic vertebral arch
Code first any associated:
injury of intrathoracic organ (S27.-)
spinal cord injury (S24.0-, S24.1-)
EXCLUDES 1   *transection of thorax (S28.1)*
EXCLUDES 2   *fracture of clavicle (S42.0-)*
fracture of scapula (S42.1-)

The appropriate 7th character is to be added to each code from category S22
A   initial encounter for closed fracture
B   initial encounter for open fracture
D   subsequent encounter for fracture with routine healing
G   subsequent encounter for fracture with delayed healing
K   subsequent encounter for fracture with nonunion
S   sequela

CODING TIP ✓   A fracture not indicated as displaced or nondisplaced should be coded to displaced. A fracture not indicated as open or closed should be coded to closed. Query providers on fractures not documented as displaced/nondisplaced otherwise displaced fracture diagnosis could be assigned without reduction being performed potentially resulting in claim denials.

5 **S22.0**   **Fracture of thoracic vertebra**

6 **S22.00**   **Fracture of unspecified thoracic vertebra**

7 **S22.000-**   **Wedge compression fracture of unspecified thoracic vertebra**

7 **S22.001-**   **Stable burst fracture of unspecified thoracic vertebra**

7 **S22.002-**   **Unstable burst fracture of unspecified thoracic vertebra**

7 **S22.008-**   **Other fracture of unspecified thoracic vertebra**

7 **S22.009-**   **Unspecified fracture of unspecified thoracic vertebra**

6 **S22.01**   **Fracture of first thoracic vertebra**

7 **S22.010-**   **Wedge compression fracture of first thoracic vertebra**

7 **S22.011-**   **Stable burst fracture of first thoracic vertebra**

7 **S22.012-**   **Unstable burst fracture of first thoracic vertebra**

7 **S22.018-**   **Other fracture of first thoracic vertebra**

7 **S22.019-**   **Unspecified fracture of first thoracic vertebra**

6 **S22.02**   **Fracture of second thoracic vertebra**

7 **S22.020-**   **Wedge compression fracture of second thoracic vertebra**

7 **S22.021-**   **Stable burst fracture of second thoracic vertebra**

7 **S22.022-**   **Unstable burst fracture of second thoracic vertebra**

7 **S22.028-**   **Other fracture of second thoracic vertebra**

7 **S22.029-**   **Unspecified fracture of second thoracic vertebra**

6 **S22.03**   **Fracture of third thoracic vertebra**

7 **S22.030-**   **Wedge compression fracture of third thoracic vertebra**

7 **S22.031-**   **Stable burst fracture of third thoracic vertebra**

7 **S22.032-**   **Unstable burst fracture of third thoracic vertebra**

7 **S22.038-**   **Other fracture of third thoracic vertebra**

7 **S22.039-**   **Unspecified fracture of third thoracic vertebra**

6 **S22.04**   **Fracture of fourth thoracic vertebra**

7 **S22.040-**   **Wedge compression fracture of fourth thoracic vertebra**

7 **S22.041-**   **Stable burst fracture of fourth thoracic vertebra**

7 **S22.042-**   **Unstable burst fracture of fourth thoracic vertebra**

7 **S22.048-**   **Other fracture of fourth thoracic vertebra**

7 **S22.049-**   **Unspecified fracture of fourth thoracic vertebra**

6 **S22.05**   **Fracture of T5-T6 vertebra**

7 **S22.050-**   **Wedge compression fracture of T5-T6 vertebra**

7 **S22.051-**   **Stable burst fracture of T5-T6 vertebra**

7 **S22.052-**   **Unstable burst fracture of T5-T6 vertebra**

7 **S22.058-**   **Other fracture of T5-T6 vertebra**

7 **S22.059-**   **Unspecified fracture of T5-T6 vertebra**

6 **S22.06**   **Fracture of T7-T8 vertebra**

7 **S22.060-**   **Wedge compression fracture of T7-T8 vertebra**

7 **S22.061-**   **Stable burst fracture of T7-T8 vertebra**

7 **S22.062-**   **Unstable burst fracture of T7-T8 vertebra**

7 **S22.068-**   **Other fracture of T7-T8 thoracic vertebra**

7 **S22.069-**   **Unspecified fracture of T7-T8 vertebra**

6 **S22.07**   **Fracture of T9-T10 vertebra**

7 **S22.070-**   **Wedge compression fracture of T9-T10 vertebra**

7 **S22.071-**   **Stable burst fracture of T9-T10 vertebra**

7 **S22.072-**   **Unstable burst fracture of T9-T10 vertebra**

7 **S22.078-**   **Other fracture of T9-T10 vertebra**

7 **S22.079-**   **Unspecified fracture of T9-T10 vertebra**

6 **S22.08**   **Fracture of T11-T12 vertebra**

7 **S22.080-**   **Wedge compression fracture of T11-T12 vertebra**

7 **S22.081-**   **Stable burst fracture of T11-T12 vertebra**

7 **S22.082-**   **Unstable burst fracture of T11-T12 vertebra**

7 **S22.088-**   **Other fracture of T11-T12 vertebra**

7 **S22.089-**   **Unspecified fracture of T11-T12 vertebra**

5 **S22.2**   **Fracture of sternum**

7 **S22.20X-**   **Unspecified fracture of sternum**

7 **S22.21X-**   **Fracture of manubrium**

7 **S22.22X-**   **Fracture of body of sternum**

7 **S22.23X-**   **Sternal manubrial dissociation**

7 **S22.24X-**   **Fracture of xiphoid process**

5 **S22.3**   **Fracture of one rib**

7 ⊟ **S22.31X-**   **Fracture of one rib, right side**

7 ⊟ **S22.32X-**   **Fracture of one rib, left side**

7 ⊟ **S22.39X-**   **Fracture of one rib, unspecified side**

5 **S22.4**   **Multiple fractures of ribs**
Fractures of two or more ribs
EXCLUDES 1   *flail chest (S22.5-)*

7 ⊟ **S22.41X-**   **Multiple fractures of ribs, right side**

7 ⊟ **S22.42X-**   **Multiple fractures of ribs, left side**

7 ⊟ **S22.43X-**   **Multiple fractures of ribs, bilateral**

7 ⊟ **S22.49X-**   **Multiple fractures of ribs, unspecified side**

● New   ▲ Revised   *Manifestation*   4-7 Digit Indicators   ⊟ Laterality   A Adult (15+ years)   M Maternity (12-55 years)   N Newborn (0-17 years)   ♂ Male   ♀ Female
✖ Deleted   Unspecified   + Additional code

7️⃣ **S22.5XX-**   Flail chest

7️⃣ **S22.9XX-**   Fracture of bony thorax, part unspecified

4️⃣ **S23**   **Dislocation and sprain of joints and ligaments of thorax**

INCLUDES   avulsion of joint or ligament of thorax
laceration of cartilage, joint or ligament of thorax
sprain of cartilage, joint or ligament of thorax
traumatic hemarthrosis of joint or ligament of thorax
traumatic rupture of joint or ligament of thorax
traumatic subluxation of joint or ligament of thorax
traumatic tear of joint or ligament of thorax

Code also:
  any associated open wound

EXCLUDES 2   *dislocation, sprain of sternoclavicular joint (S43.2, S43.6)*
strain of muscle or tendon of thorax (S29.01-)

The appropriate 7th character is to be added to each code from category S23
A   initial encounter
D   subsequent encounter
S   sequela

CODING TIP✓   Unlike ICD-9 there is no code for open dislocations. When documented as open an additional code for the open wound must be applied.

7️⃣ **S23.0XX-**   **Traumatic rupture of thoracic intervertebral disc**

EXCLUDES 1   *rupture or displacement (nontraumatic) of thoracic intervertebral disc NOS (M51.- with fifth character 4)*

5️⃣ **S23.1**   **Subluxation and dislocation of thoracic vertebra**
Code also:
  any associated
  open wound of thorax (S21.-)
  spinal cord injury (S24.0-, S24.1-)

EXCLUDES 2   *fracture of thoracic vertebrae (S22.0-)*

6️⃣ **S23.10**   **Subluxation and dislocation of unspecified thoracic vertebra**
7️⃣ **S23.100-**   Subluxation of unspecified thoracic vertebra
7️⃣ **S23.101-**   Dislocation of unspecified thoracic vertebra
6️⃣ **S23.11**   **Subluxation and dislocation of T1/T2 thoracic vertebra**
7️⃣ **S23.110-**   Subluxation of T1/T2 thoracic vertebra
7️⃣ **S23.111-**   Dislocation of T1/T2 thoracic vertebra
6️⃣ **S23.12**   **Subluxation and dislocation of T2/T3-T3/T4 thoracic vertebra**
7️⃣ **S23.120-**   Subluxation of T2/T3 thoracic vertebra
7️⃣ **S23.121-**   Dislocation of T2/T3 thoracic vertebra
7️⃣ **S23.122-**   Subluxation of T3/T4 thoracic vertebra
7️⃣ **S23.123-**   Dislocation of T3/T4 thoracic vertebra
6️⃣ **S23.13**   **Subluxation and dislocation of T4/T5-T5/T6 thoracic vertebra**
7️⃣ **S23.130-**   Subluxation of T4/T5 thoracic vertebra
7️⃣ **S23.131-**   Dislocation of T4/T5 thoracic vertebra
7️⃣ **S23.132-**   Subluxation of T5/T6 thoracic vertebra
7️⃣ **S23.133-**   Dislocation of T5/T6 thoracic vertebra
6️⃣ **S23.14**   **Subluxation and dislocation of T6/T7-T7/T8 thoracic vertebra**
7️⃣ **S23.140-**   Subluxation of T6/T7 thoracic vertebra
7️⃣ **S23.141-**   Dislocation of T6/T7 thoracic vertebra
7️⃣ **S23.142-**   Subluxation of T7/T8 thoracic vertebra
7️⃣ **S23.143-**   Dislocation of T7/T8 thoracic vertebra
6️⃣ **S23.15**   **Subluxation and dislocation of T8/T9-T9/T10 thoracic vertebra**
7️⃣ **S23.150-**   Subluxation of T8/T9 thoracic vertebra
7️⃣ **S23.151-**   Dislocation of T8/T9 thoracic vertebra
7️⃣ **S23.152-**   Subluxation of T9/T10 thoracic vertebra
7️⃣ **S23.153-**   Dislocation of T9/T10 thoracic vertebra
6️⃣ **S23.16**   **Subluxation and dislocation of T10/T11-T11/T12 thoracic vertebra**
7️⃣ **S23.160-**   Subluxation of T10/T11 thoracic vertebra
7️⃣ **S23.161-**   Dislocation of T10/T11 thoracic vertebra
7️⃣ **S23.162-**   Subluxation of T11/T12 thoracic vertebra
7️⃣ **S23.163-**   Dislocation of T11/T12 thoracic vertebra

6️⃣ **S23.17**   **Subluxation and dislocation of T12/L1 thoracic vertebra**
7️⃣ **S23.170-**   Subluxation of T12/L1 thoracic vertebra
7️⃣ **S23.171-**   Dislocation of T12/L1 thoracic vertebra
5️⃣ **S23.2**   **Dislocation of other and unspecified parts of thorax**
7️⃣ **S23.20X-**   Dislocation of unspecified part of thorax
7️⃣ **S23.29X-**   Dislocation of other parts of thorax
7️⃣ **S23.3XX-**   Sprain of ligaments of thoracic spine
5️⃣ **S23.4**   Sprain of ribs and sternum
7️⃣ **S23.41X-**   Sprain of ribs
6️⃣ **S23.42**   Sprain of sternum
7️⃣ **S23.420-**   Sprain of sternoclavicular (joint) (ligament)
7️⃣ **S23.421-**   Sprain of chondrosternal joint
7️⃣ **S23.428-**   Other sprain of sternum
7️⃣ **S23.429-**   Unspecified sprain of sternum
7️⃣ **S23.8XX-**   Sprain of other specified parts of thorax
7️⃣ **S23.9XX-**   Sprain of unspecified parts of thorax

4️⃣ **S24**   **Injury of nerves and spinal cord at thorax level**
Note: Code to highest level of thoracic spinal cord injury
Injuries to the spinal cord (S24.0 and S24.1) refer to the cord level and not bone level injury, and can affect nerve roots at and below the level given.
Code also any associated:
  fracture of thoracic vertebra (S22.0-)
  open wound of thorax (S21.-)
  transient paralysis (R29.5)

EXCLUDES 2   *injury of brachial plexus (S14.3)*

The appropriate 7th character is to be added to each code from category S24
A   initial encounter
D   subsequent encounter
S   sequela

CODING TIP✓   When coding sequelae of a thoracic spinal cord injury, first list the residual condition(s), followed by the specific spinal cord injury diagnosed using the appropriate code from category S24 with the seventh character "S" to indicate sequelae.

CODING TIP✓   When coding sequelae of a spinal cord injury, first list the residual condition(s), followed by the specific spinal cord injury diagnosed using the appropriate code from this category with the seventh character "S" to indicate sequelae. If there are multiple levels of injury, code only the highest injury.

7️⃣ **S24.0XX-**   Concussion and edema of thoracic spinal cord
5️⃣ **S24.1**   Other and unspecified injuries of thoracic spinal cord
6️⃣ **S24.10**   Unspecified injury of thoracic spinal cord
7️⃣ **S24.101-**   Unspecified injury at T1 level of thoracic spinal cord
7️⃣ **S24.102-**   Unspecified injury at T2-T6 level of thoracic spinal cord
7️⃣ **S24.103-**   Unspecified injury at T7-T10 level of thoracic spinal cord
7️⃣ **S24.104-**   Unspecified injury at T11-T12 level of thoracic spinal cord
7️⃣ **S24.109-**   Unspecified injury at unspecified level of thoracic spinal cord
  Injury of thoracic spinal cord NOS
6️⃣ **S24.11**   Complete lesion of thoracic spinal cord
7️⃣ **S24.111-**   Complete lesion at T1 level of thoracic spinal cord
7️⃣ **S24.112-**   Complete lesion at T2-T6 level of thoracic spinal cord
7️⃣ **S24.113-**   Complete lesion at T7-T10 level of thoracic spinal cord
7️⃣ **S24.114-**   Complete lesion at T11-T12 level of thoracic spinal cord
7️⃣ **S24.119-**   Complete lesion at unspecified level of thoracic spinal cord
6️⃣ **S24.13**   Anterior cord syndrome of thoracic spinal cord
7️⃣ **S24.131-**   Anterior cord syndrome at T1 level of thoracic spinal cord
7️⃣ **S24.132-**   Anterior cord syndrome at T2-T6 level of thoracic spinal cord
7️⃣ **S24.133-**   Anterior cord syndrome at T7-T10 level of thoracic spinal cord

● New ▲ Revised *Manifestation* 4️⃣-7️⃣ Digit Indicators ⊟ Laterality 🅰 Adult (15+ years) 🅼 Maternity (12-55 years) 🅽 Newborn 🅿 Pediatric (0-17 years) ♂ Male ♀ Female ✖ Deleted Unspecified + Additional code

2017 ICD-10-CM Expert for Physicians   © 2017 DecisionHealth   941

7 S24.134-   **Anterior cord syndrome at T11-T12 level of thoracic spinal cord**

7 S24.139-   **Anterior cord syndrome at unspecified level of thoracic spinal cord**

6 S24.14   **Brown-Séquard syndrome of thoracic spinal cord**

7 S24.141-   **Brown-Séquard syndrome at T1 level of thoracic spinal cord**

7 S24.142-   **Brown-Séquard syndrome at T2-T6 level of thoracic spinal cord**

7 S24.143-   **Brown-Séquard syndrome at T7-T10 level of thoracic spinal cord**

7 S24.144-   **Brown-Séquard syndrome at T11-T12 level of thoracic spinal cord**

7 S24.149-   **Brown-Séquard syndrome at unspecified level of thoracic spinal cord**

6 S24.15   **Other incomplete lesions of thoracic spinal cord**
Incomplete lesion of thoracic spinal cord NOS
Posterior cord syndrome of thoracic spinal cord

7 S24.151-   **Other incomplete lesion at T1 level of thoracic spinal cord**

7 S24.152-   **Other incomplete lesion at T2-T6 level of thoracic spinal cord**

7 S24.153-   **Other incomplete lesion at T7-T10 level of thoracic spinal cord**

7 S24.154-   **Other incomplete lesion at T11-T12 level of thoracic spinal cord**

7 S24.159-   **Other incomplete lesion at unspecified level of thoracic spinal cord**

7 S24.2XX-   **Injury of nerve root of thoracic spine**

7 S24.3XX-   **Injury of peripheral nerves of thorax**

7 S24.4XX-   **Injury of thoracic sympathetic nervous system**
Injury of cardiac plexus
Injury of esophageal plexus
Injury of pulmonary plexus
Injury of stellate ganglion
Injury of thoracic sympathetic ganglion

7 S24.8XX-   **Injury of other specified nerves of thorax**

7 S24.9XX-   **Injury of unspecified nerve of thorax**

4 S25   **Injury of blood vessels of thorax**
Code also:
  any associated open wound (S21.-)

The appropriate 7th character is to be added to each code from category S25
A   initial encounter
D   subsequent encounter
S   sequela

5 S25.0   **Injury of thoracic aorta**
Injury of aorta NOS

7 S25.00X-   **Unspecified injury of thoracic aorta**

7 S25.01X-   **Minor laceration of thoracic aorta**
Incomplete transection of thoracic aorta
Laceration of thoracic aorta NOS
Superficial laceration of thoracic aorta

7 S25.02X-   **Major laceration of thoracic aorta**
Complete transection of thoracic aorta
Traumatic rupture of thoracic aorta

7 S25.09X-   **Other specified injury of thoracic aorta**

5 S25.1   **Injury of innominate or subclavian artery**

6 S25.10   **Unspecified injury of innominate or subclavian artery**

7 S25.101-   **Unspecified injury of right innominate or subclavian artery**

7 S25.102-   **Unspecified injury of left innominate or subclavian artery**

7 S25.109-   **Unspecified injury of unspecified innominate or subclavian artery**

6 S25.11   **Minor laceration of innominate or subclavian artery**
Incomplete transection of innominate or subclavian artery
Laceration of innominate or subclavian artery NOS
Superficial laceration of innominate or subclavian artery

7 S25.111-   **Minor laceration of right innominate or subclavian artery**

7 S25.112-   **Minor laceration of left innominate or subclavian artery**

7 S25.119-   **Minor laceration of unspecified innominate or subclavian artery**

6 S25.12   **Major laceration of innominate or subclavian artery**
Complete transection of innominate or subclavian artery
Traumatic rupture of innominate or subclavian artery

7 S25.121-   **Major laceration of right innominate or subclavian artery**

7 S25.122-   **Major laceration of left innominate or subclavian artery**

7 S25.129-   **Major laceration of unspecified innominate or subclavian artery**

6 S25.19   **Other specified injury of innominate or subclavian artery**

7 S25.191-   **Other specified injury of right innominate or subclavian artery**

7 S25.192-   **Other specified injury of left innominate or subclavian artery**

7 S25.199-   **Other specified injury of unspecified innominate or subclavian artery**

5 S25.2   **Injury of superior vena cava**
Injury of vena cava NOS

7 S25.20X-   **Unspecified injury of superior vena cava**

7 S25.21X-   **Minor laceration of superior vena cava**
Incomplete transection of superior vena cava
Laceration of superior vena cava NOS
Superficial laceration of superior vena cava

7 S25.22X-   **Major laceration of superior vena cava**
Complete transection of superior vena cava
Traumatic rupture of superior vena cava

7 S25.29X-   **Other specified injury of superior vena cava**

5 S25.3   **Injury of innominate or subclavian vein**

6 S25.30   **Unspecified injury of innominate or subclavian vein**

7 S25.301-   **Unspecified injury of right innominate or subclavian vein**

7 S25.302-   **Unspecified injury of left innominate or subclavian vein**

7 S25.309-   **Unspecified injury of unspecified innominate or subclavian vein**

6 S25.31   **Minor laceration of innominate or subclavian vein**
Incomplete transection of innominate or subclavian vein
Laceration of innominate or subclavian vein NOS
Superficial laceration of innominate or subclavian vein

7 S25.311-   **Minor laceration of right innominate or subclavian vein**

7 S25.312-   **Minor laceration of left innominate or subclavian vein**

7 S25.319-   **Minor laceration of unspecified innominate or subclavian vein**

6 S25.32   **Major laceration of innominate or subclavian vein**
Complete transection of innominate or subclavian vein
Traumatic rupture of innominate or subclavian vein

7 S25.321-   **Major laceration of right innominate or subclavian vein**

7 S25.322-   **Major laceration of left innominate or subclavian vein**

7 S25.329-   **Major laceration of unspecified innominate or subclavian vein**

6 S25.39   **Other specified injury of innominate or subclavian vein**

7 S25.391-   **Other specified injury of right innominate or subclavian vein**

7 S25.392-   **Other specified injury of left innominate or subclavian vein**

7 S25.399-   **Other specified injury of unspecified innominate or subclavian vein**

5 S25.4   **Injury of pulmonary blood vessels**

6 S25.40   **Unspecified injury of pulmonary blood vessels**

7 S25.401-   **Unspecified injury of right pulmonary blood vessels**

7 S25.402-   **Unspecified injury of left pulmonary blood vessels**

7 S25.409-   **Unspecified injury of unspecified pulmonary blood vessels**

6 S25.41   **Minor laceration of pulmonary blood vessels**
Incomplete transection of pulmonary blood vessels
Laceration of pulmonary blood vessels NOS
Superficial laceration of pulmonary blood vessels

● New   ▲ Revised   *Manifestation*   4-7 Digit Indicators   ☐ Laterality   A Adult (15+ years)   M Maternity (12-55 years)   N Newborn   P Pediatric (0-17 years)   ♂ Male   ♀ Female
✖ Deleted   Unspecified   + Additional code

942   © 2017 DecisionHealth   2017 ICD-10-CM Expert for Physicians

7 ▤ **S25.411-**   **Minor laceration of right pulmonary blood vessels**

7 ▤ **S25.412-**   **Minor laceration of left pulmonary blood vessels**

7 ▤ **S25.419-**   **Minor laceration of unspecified pulmonary blood vessels**

6 **S25.42**   **Major laceration of pulmonary blood vessels**
Complete transection of pulmonary blood vessels
Traumatic rupture of pulmonary blood vessels

7 ▤ **S25.421-**   **Major laceration of right pulmonary blood vessels**

7 ▤ **S25.422-**   **Major laceration of left pulmonary blood vessels**

7 ▤ **S25.429-**   **Major laceration of unspecified pulmonary blood vessels**

6 **S25.49**   **Other specified injury of pulmonary blood vessels**

7 ▤ **S25.491-**   **Other specified injury of right pulmonary blood vessels**

7 ▤ **S25.492-**   **Other specified injury of left pulmonary blood vessels**

7 ▤ **S25.499-**   **Other specified injury of unspecified pulmonary blood vessels**

5 **S25.5**   **Injury of intercostal blood vessels**

6 **S25.50**   **Unspecified injury of intercostal blood vessels**

7 ▤ **S25.501-**   **Unspecified injury of intercostal blood vessels, right side**

7 ▤ **S25.502-**   **Unspecified injury of intercostal blood vessels, left side**

7 ▤ **S25.509-**   **Unspecified injury of intercostal blood vessels, unspecified side**

6 **S25.51**   **Laceration of intercostal blood vessels**

7 ▤ **S25.511-**   **Laceration of intercostal blood vessels, right side**

7 ▤ **S25.512-**   **Laceration of intercostal blood vessels, left side**

7 ▤ **S25.519-**   **Laceration of intercostal blood vessels, unspecified side**

6 **S25.59**   **Other specified injury of intercostal blood vessels**

7 ▤ **S25.591-**   **Other specified injury of intercostal blood vessels, right side**

7 ▤ **S25.592-**   **Other specified injury of intercostal blood vessels, left side**

7 ▤ **S25.599-**   **Other specified injury of intercostal blood vessels, unspecified side**

5 **S25.8**   **Injury of other blood vessels of thorax**
Injury of azygos vein
Injury of mammary artery or vein

6 **S25.80**   **Unspecified injury of other blood vessels of thorax**

7 ▤ **S25.801-**   **Unspecified injury of other blood vessels of thorax, right side**

7 ▤ **S25.802-**   **Unspecified injury of other blood vessels of thorax, left side**

7 ▤ **S25.809-**   **Unspecified injury of other blood vessels of thorax, unspecified side**

6 **S25.81**   **Laceration of other blood vessels of thorax**

7 ▤ **S25.811-**   **Laceration of other blood vessels of thorax, right side**

7 ▤ **S25.812-**   **Laceration of other blood vessels of thorax, left side**

7 ▤ **S25.819-**   **Laceration of other blood vessels of thorax, unspecified side**

6 **S25.89**   **Other specified injury of other blood vessels of thorax**

7 ▤ **S25.891-**   **Other specified injury of other blood vessels of thorax, right side**

7 ▤ **S25.892-**   **Other specified injury of other blood vessels of thorax, left side**

7 ▤ **S25.899-**   **Other specified injury of other blood vessels of thorax, unspecified side**

5 **S25.9**   **Injury of unspecified blood vessel of thorax**

7 **S25.90X-**   **Unspecified injury of unspecified blood vessel of thorax**

7 **S25.91X-**   **Laceration of unspecified blood vessel of thorax**

7 **S25.99X-**   **Other specified injury of unspecified blood vessel of thorax**

---

4 **S26**   **Injury of heart**
Code also any associated:
   open wound of thorax (S21.-)
   traumatic hemopneumothorax (S27.2)
   traumatic hemothorax (S27.1)
   traumatic pneumothorax (S27.0)

The appropriate 7th character is to be added to each code from category S26
A   initial encounter
D   subsequent encounter
S   sequela

5 **S26.0**   **Injury of heart with hemopericardium**

7 **S26.00X-**   **Unspecified injury of heart with hemopericardium**

7 **S26.01X-**   **Contusion of heart with hemopericardium**

6 **S26.02**   **Laceration of heart with hemopericardium**

7 **S26.020-**   **Mild laceration of heart with hemopericardium**
Laceration of heart without penetration of heart chamber

7 **S26.021-**   **Moderate laceration of heart with hemopericardium**
Laceration of heart with penetration of heart chamber

7 **S26.022-**   **Major laceration of heart with hemopericardium**
Laceration of heart with penetration of multiple heart chambers

7 **S26.09X-**   **Other injury of heart with hemopericardium**

5 **S26.1**   **Injury of heart without hemopericardium**

7 **S26.10X-**   **Unspecified injury of heart without hemopericardium**

7 **S26.11X-**   **Contusion of heart without hemopericardium**

7 **S26.12X-**   **Laceration of heart without hemopericardium**

7 **S26.19X-**   **Other injury of heart without hemopericardium**

5 **S26.9**   **Injury of heart, unspecified with or without hemopericardium**

7 **S26.90X-**   **Unspecified injury of heart, unspecified with or without hemopericardium**

7 **S26.91X-**   **Contusion of heart, unspecified with or without hemopericardium**

7 **S26.92X-**   **Laceration of heart, unspecified with or without hemopericardium**
Laceration of heart NOS

7 **S26.99X-**   **Other injury of heart, unspecified with or without hemopericardium**

4 **S27**   **Injury of other and unspecified intrathoracic organs**
Code also:
   any associated open wound of thorax (S21.-)
   EXCLUDES 2   *injury of cervical esophagus (S10-S19)*
               injury of trachea (cervical) (S10-S19)

The appropriate 7th character is to be added to each code from category S27
A   initial encounter
D   subsequent encounter
S   sequela

7 **S27.0XX-**   **Traumatic pneumothorax**

   EXCLUDES 1   *spontaneous pneumothorax (J93.-)*

   CODING TIP ✓   Do not assign S27.0- to indicate a pneumothorax that is not specifically identified as due to trauma. Chapter 19 codes are for those diagnoses due to injury and trauma. S27.0- indicates pneumothorax resulting from traumatic origin. Nontraumatic (spontaneous or unspecified pneumothorax) should be coded to J93.-.

7 **S27.1XX-**   **Traumatic hemothorax**

7 **S27.2XX-**   **Traumatic hemopneumothorax**

5 **S27.3**   **Other and unspecified injuries of lung**

6 **S27.30**   **Unspecified injury of lung**

7 **S27.301-**   **Unspecified injury of lung, unilateral**

7 **S27.302-**   **Unspecified injury of lung, bilateral**

7 **S27.309-**   **Unspecified injury of lung, unspecified**

6 **S27.31**   **Primary blast injury of lung**
Blast injury of lung NOS

● New   ▲ Revised   *Manifestation*   4-7 Digit Indicators   ▤ Laterality   Ⓐ Adult (15+ years)   Ⓜ Maternity (12-55 years)   Ⓝ Newborn   Ⓟ Pediatric (0-17 years)   ♂ Male   ♀ Female
✖ ~~Deleted~~   Unspecified   + Additional code

2017 ICD-10-CM Expert for Physicians   © 2017 DecisionHealth   943

☑ S27.311- Primary blast injury of lung, unilateral
☑ S27.312- Primary blast injury of lung, bilateral
☑ S27.319- Primary blast injury of lung, unspecified
◩ S27.32 Contusion of lung
　☑ S27.321- Contusion of lung, unilateral
　☑ S27.322- Contusion of lung, bilateral
　☑ S27.329- Contusion of lung, unspecified
◩ S27.33 Laceration of lung
　☑ S27.331- Laceration of lung, unilateral
　☑ S27.332- Laceration of lung, bilateral
　☑ S27.339- Laceration of lung, unspecified
◩ S27.39 Other injuries of lung
　Secondary blast injury of lung
　☑ S27.391- Other injuries of lung, unilateral
　☑ S27.392- Other injuries of lung, bilateral
　☑ S27.399- Other injuries of lung, unspecified
⑤ S27.4 Injury of bronchus
　◩ S27.40 Unspecified injury of bronchus
　　☑ S27.401- Unspecified injury of bronchus, unilateral
　　☑ S27.402- Unspecified injury of bronchus, bilateral
　　☑ S27.409- Unspecified injury of bronchus, unspecified
　◩ S27.41 Primary blast injury of bronchus
　　Blast injury of bronchus NOS
　　☑ S27.411- Primary blast injury of bronchus, unilateral
　　☑ S27.412- Primary blast injury of bronchus, bilateral
　　☑ S27.419- Primary blast injury of bronchus, unspecified
　◩ S27.42 Contusion of bronchus
　　☑ S27.421- Contusion of bronchus, unilateral
　　☑ S27.422- Contusion of bronchus, bilateral
　　☑ S27.429- Contusion of bronchus, unspecified
　◩ S27.43 Laceration of bronchus
　　☑ S27.431- Laceration of bronchus, unilateral
　　☑ S27.432- Laceration of bronchus, bilateral
　　☑ S27.439- Laceration of bronchus, unspecified
　◩ S27.49 Other injury of bronchus
　　Secondary blast injury of bronchus
　　☑ S27.491- Other injury of bronchus, unilateral
　　☑ S27.492- Other injury of bronchus, bilateral
　　☑ S27.499- Other injury of bronchus, unspecified
⑤ S27.5 Injury of thoracic trachea
　☑ S27.50X- Unspecified injury of thoracic trachea
　☑ S27.51X- Primary blast injury of thoracic trachea
　　Blast injury of thoracic trachea NOS
　☑ S27.52X- Contusion of thoracic trachea
　☑ S27.53X- Laceration of thoracic trachea
　☑ S27.59X- Other injury of thoracic trachea
　　Secondary blast injury of thoracic trachea
⑤ S27.6 Injury of pleura
　☑ S27.60X- Unspecified injury of pleura
　☑ S27.63X- Laceration of pleura
　☑ S27.69X- Other injury of pleura
⑤ S27.8 Injury of other specified intrathoracic organs
　◩ S27.80 Injury of diaphragm
　　☑ S27.802- Contusion of diaphragm
　　☑ S27.803- Laceration of diaphragm
　　☑ S27.808- Other injury of diaphragm
　　☑ S27.809- Unspecified injury of diaphragm
　◩ S27.81 Injury of esophagus (thoracic part)
　　☑ S27.812- Contusion of esophagus (thoracic part)
　　☑ S27.813- Laceration of esophagus (thoracic part)
　　☑ S27.818- Other injury of esophagus (thoracic part)
　　☑ S27.819- Unspecified injury of esophagus (thoracic part)
　◩ S27.89 Injury of other specified intrathoracic organs
　　Injury of lymphatic thoracic duct
　　Injury of thymus gland
　　☑ S27.892- Contusion of other specified intrathoracic organs
　　☑ S27.893- Laceration of other specified intrathoracic organs
　　☑ S27.898- Other injury of other specified intrathoracic organs

☑ S27.899- Unspecified injury of other specified intrathoracic organs
☑ S27.9XX- Injury of unspecified intrathoracic organ
④ S28 **Crushing injury of thorax, and traumatic amputation of part of thorax**

> The appropriate 7th character is to be added to each code from category S28
> A　initial encounter
> D　subsequent encounter
> S　sequela

☑ ✛ S28.0XX- Crushed chest
　Use additional code for all associated injuries
　EXCLUDES 1　*flail chest (S22.5)*
☑ S28.1XX- Traumatic amputation (partial) of part of thorax, except breast
⑤ S28.2 Traumatic amputation of breast
　◩ S28.21 Complete traumatic amputation of breast
　　Traumatic amputation of breast NOS
　　☑ ⊟ S28.211- Complete traumatic amputation of right breast
　　☑ ⊟ S28.212- Complete traumatic amputation of left breast
　　☑ ⊟ S28.219- Complete traumatic amputation of unspecified breast
　◩ S28.22 Partial traumatic amputation of breast
　　☑ ⊟ S28.221- Partial traumatic amputation of right breast
　　☑ ⊟ S28.222- Partial traumatic amputation of left breast
　　☑ ⊟ S28.229- Partial traumatic amputation of unspecified breast

④ S29 **Other and unspecified injuries of thorax**

> Code also:
> 　any associated open wound (S21.-)

> The appropriate 7th character is to be added to each code from category S29
> A　initial encounter
> D　subsequent encounter
> S　sequela

⑤ S29.0 Injury of muscle and tendon at thorax level
　◩ S29.00 Unspecified injury of muscle and tendon of thorax
　　☑ S29.001- Unspecified injury of muscle and tendon of front wall of thorax
　　☑ S29.002- Unspecified injury of muscle and tendon of back wall of thorax
　　☑ S29.009- Unspecified injury of muscle and tendon of unspecified wall of thorax
　◩ S29.01 Strain of muscle and tendon of thorax
　　☑ S29.011- Strain of muscle and tendon of front wall of thorax
　　☑ S29.012- Strain of muscle and tendon of back wall of thorax
　　☑ S29.019- Strain of muscle and tendon of unspecified wall of thorax
　◩ S29.02 Laceration of muscle and tendon of thorax
　　☑ S29.021- Laceration of muscle and tendon of front wall of thorax
　　☑ S29.022- Laceration of muscle and tendon of back wall of thorax
　　☑ S29.029- Laceration of muscle and tendon of unspecified wall of thorax
　◩ S29.09 Other injury of muscle and tendon of thorax
　　☑ S29.091- Other injury of muscle and tendon of front wall of thorax
　　☑ S29.092- Other injury of muscle and tendon of back wall of thorax
　　☑ S29.099- Other injury of muscle and tendon of unspecified wall of thorax
☑ S29.8XX- Other specified injuries of thorax
☑ S29.9XX- Unspecified injury of thorax

● New　▲ Revised　*Manifestation*　④-☑ Digit Indicators　⊟ Laterality　Ⓐ Adult (15+ years)　Ⓜ Maternity (12-55 years)　Ⓝ Newborn　Ⓟ Pediatric (0-17 years)　♂ Male　♀ Female
✖ Deleted　Unspecified　✛ Additional code

944　© 2017 DecisionHealth　　　　2017 ICD-10-CM Expert for Physicians

Injuries to the abdomen, lower back, lumbar spine, pelvis and external genitals (S30-S39)

INCLUDES
injuries to the abdominal wall
injuries to the anus
injuries to the buttock
injuries to the external genitalia
injuries to the flank
injuries to the groin

EXCLUDES 2
burns and corrosions (T20-T32)
effects of foreign body in anus and rectum (T18.5)
effects of foreign body in genitourinary tract (T19.-)
effects of foreign body in stomach, small intestine and colon (T18.2-T18.4)
frostbite (T33-T34)
insect bite or sting, venomous (T63.4)

GUIDELINES Section I.C.19.c.2)
Multiple fractures are sequenced in accordance with the severity of the fracture.

GUIDELINES Section I.C.19.b.1)-2)
When coding injuries, assign separate codes for each injury unless a combination code is provided, in which case the combination code is assigned ... Traumatic injury codes (S00-T14.9) are not to be used for normal, healing surgical wounds or to identify complications of surgical wounds. The code for the most serious injury, as determined by the provider and the focus of treatment, is sequenced first.

1) Superficial injuries such as abrasions or contusions are not coded when associated with more severe injuries of the same site.

2) When a primary injury results in minor damage to peripheral nerves or blood vessels, the primary injury is sequenced first with additional code(s) for injuries to nerves and spinal cord (such as category S04), and/or injury to blood vessels (such as category S15). When the primary injury is to the blood vessels or nerves, that injury should be sequenced first.

GUIDELINES Section I.C.19.c
Coding of Traumatic Fractures: The principles of multiple coding of injuries should be followed in coding fractures. Fractures of specified sites are coded individually by site in accordance with both the provisions within categories S02, S12, S22, S32, S42, S49, S52, S59, S62, S72, S79, S82, S89, S92 and the level of detail furnished by medical record content. A fracture not indicated as open or closed should be coded to closed. A fracture not indicated whether displaced or not displaced should be coded to displaced.

4 S30   Superficial injury of abdomen, lower back, pelvis and external genitals

EXCLUDES 2 *superficial injury of hip (S70.-)*

The appropriate 7th character is to be added to each code from category S30
A   initial encounter
D   subsequent encounter
S   sequela

7 S30.0XX-   Contusion of lower back and pelvis
Contusion of buttock

7 S30.1XX-   Contusion of abdominal wall
Contusion of flank
Contusion of groin

5 S30.2   Contusion of external genital organs

6 S30.20   Contusion of unspecified external genital organ

7 S30.201-   Contusion of unspecified external genital organ, male

7 S30.202-   Contusion of unspecified external genital organ, female

7 S30.21X-   Contusion of penis

7 S30.22X-   Contusion of scrotum and testes

7 S30.23X-   Contusion of vagina and vulva

7 S30.3XX-   Contusion of anus

5 S30.8   Other superficial injuries of abdomen, lower back, pelvis and external genitals

6 S30.81   Abrasion of abdomen, lower back, pelvis and external genitals

7 S30.810-   Abrasion of lower back and pelvis

7 S30.811-   Abrasion of abdominal wall

7 S30.812-   Abrasion of penis

7 S30.813-   Abrasion of scrotum and testes

7 S30.814-   Abrasion of vagina and vulva

7 S30.815-   Abrasion of unspecified external genital organs, male

7 S30.816-   Abrasion of unspecified external genital organs, female

7 S30.817-   Abrasion of anus

6 S30.82   Blister (nonthermal) of abdomen, lower back, pelvis and external genitals

7 S30.820-   Blister (nonthermal) of lower back and pelvis

7 S30.821-   Blister (nonthermal) of abdominal wall

7 S30.822-   Blister (nonthermal) of penis

7 S30.823-   Blister (nonthermal) of scrotum and testes

7 S30.824-   Blister (nonthermal) of vagina and vulva

7 S30.825-   Blister (nonthermal) of unspecified external genital organs, male

7 S30.826-   Blister (nonthermal) of unspecified external genital organs, female

7 S30.827-   Blister (nonthermal) of anus

6 S30.84   External constriction of abdomen, lower back, pelvis and external genitals

7 S30.840-   External constriction of lower back and pelvis

7 S30.841-   External constriction of abdominal wall

7 + S30.842-   External constriction of penis
Hair tourniquet syndrome of penis
Use additional cause code to identify the constricting item (W49.0-)

7 S30.843-   External constriction of scrotum and testes

7 S30.844-   External constriction of vagina and vulva

7 S30.845-   External constriction of unspecified external genital organs, male

7 S30.846-   External constriction of unspecified external genital organs, female

6 S30.85   Superficial foreign body of abdomen, lower back, pelvis and external genitals
Splinter in the abdomen, lower back, pelvis and external genitals

7 S30.850-   Superficial foreign body of lower back and pelvis

7 S30.851-   Superficial foreign body of abdominal wall

7 S30.852-   Superficial foreign body of penis

7 S30.853-   Superficial foreign body of scrotum and testes

7 S30.854-   Superficial foreign body of vagina and vulva

7 S30.855-   Superficial foreign body of unspecified external genital organs, male

7 S30.856-   Superficial foreign body of unspecified external genital organs, female

7 S30.857-   Superficial foreign body of anus

6 S30.86   Insect bite (nonvenomous) of abdomen, lower back, pelvis and external genitals

7 S30.860-   Insect bite (nonvenomous) of lower back and pelvis

7 S30.861-   Insect bite (nonvenomous) of abdominal wall

7 S30.862-   Insect bite (nonvenomous) of penis

7 S30.863-   Insect bite (nonvenomous) of scrotum and testes

7 S30.864-   Insect bite (nonvenomous) of vagina and vulva

7 S30.865-   Insect bite (nonvenomous) of unspecified external genital organs, male

7 S30.866-   Insect bite (nonvenomous) of unspecified external genital organs, female

7 S30.867-   Insect bite (nonvenomous) of anus

6 S30.87   Other superficial bite of abdomen, lower back, pelvis and external genitals

EXCLUDES 1 *open bite of abdomen, lower back, pelvis and external genitals (S31.05, S31.15, S31.25, S31.35, S31.45, S31.55)*

7 S30.870-   Other superficial bite of lower back and pelvis

7 S30.871-   Other superficial bite of abdominal wall

7 S30.872-   Other superficial bite of penis

● New   ▲ Revised   *Manifestation*   4-7 Digit Indicators   ▤ Laterality   ▣ Adult (15+ years)   ▣ Maternity (12-55 years)   ▣ Newborn   ▣ Pediatric (0-17 years)   ♂ Male   ♀ Female
✖ Deleted   Unspecified   + Additional code

Injury, Poisoning and Certain Other Consequences of External Causes

S30 — S30.872-

7 **S30.873-** Other superficial bite of scrotum and testes

7 **S30.874-** Other superficial bite of vagina and vulva

7 **S30.875-** Other superficial bite of unspecified external genital organs, male

7 **S30.876-** Other superficial bite of unspecified external genital organs, female

7 **S30.877-** Other superficial bite of anus

5 **S30.9** Unspecified superficial injury of abdomen, lower back, pelvis and external genitals

7 **S30.91X-** Unspecified superficial injury of lower back and pelvis

7 **S30.92X-** Unspecified superficial injury of abdominal wall

7 **S30.93X-** Unspecified superficial injury of penis

7 **S30.94X-** Unspecified superficial injury of scrotum and testes

7 **S30.95X-** Unspecified superficial injury of vagina and vulva

7 **S30.96X-** Unspecified superficial injury of unspecified external genital organs, male

7 **S30.97X-** Unspecified superficial injury of unspecified external genital organs, female

7 **S30.98X-** Unspecified superficial injury of anus

4 **S31** **Open wound of abdomen, lower back, pelvis and external genitals**

Code also any associated:
spinal cord injury (S24.0, S24.1-, S34.0-, S34.1-)
wound infection

> **EXCLUDES 1** *traumatic amputation of part of abdomen, lower back and pelvis (S38.2-, S38.3)*

> **EXCLUDES 2** *open wound of hip (S71.00-S71.02)*
> *open fracture of pelvis*
> *(S32.1--S32.9 with 7th character B)*

The appropriate 7th character is to be added to each code from category S31
A   initial encounter
D   subsequent encounter
S   sequela

> **CODING TIP ✓** Open wound codes are used for wounds caused by trauma. Do not assign a code for "open wound" unless the etiology of the wound is related to trauma.

5 **S31.0** Open wound of lower back and pelvis

6 **S31.00** Unspecified open wound of lower back and pelvis

7 **S31.000-** Unspecified open wound of lower back and pelvis without penetration into retroperitoneum
Unspecified open wound of lower back and pelvis NOS

7 **S31.001-** Unspecified open wound of lower back and pelvis with penetration into retroperitoneum

6 **S31.01** Laceration without foreign body of lower back and pelvis

7 **S31.010-** Laceration without foreign body of lower back and pelvis without penetration into retroperitoneum
Laceration without foreign body of lower back and pelvis NOS

7 **S31.011-** Laceration without foreign body of lower back and pelvis with penetration into retroperitoneum

6 **S31.02** Laceration with foreign body of lower back and pelvis

7 **S31.020-** Laceration with foreign body of lower back and pelvis without penetration into retroperitoneum
Laceration with foreign body of lower back and pelvis NOS

7 **S31.021-** Laceration with foreign body of lower back and pelvis with penetration into retroperitoneum

6 **S31.03** Puncture wound without foreign body of lower back and pelvis

7 **S31.030-** Puncture wound without foreign body of lower back and pelvis without penetration into retroperitoneum
Puncture wound without foreign body of lower back and pelvis NOS

7 **S31.031-** Puncture wound without foreign body of lower back and pelvis with penetration into retroperitoneum

6 **S31.04** Puncture wound with foreign body of lower back and pelvis

7 **S31.040-** Puncture wound with foreign body of lower back and pelvis without penetration into retroperitoneum
Puncture wound with foreign body of lower back and pelvis NOS

7 **S31.041-** Puncture wound with foreign body of lower back and pelvis with penetration into retroperitoneum

6 **S31.05** Open bite of lower back and pelvis
Bite of lower back and pelvis NOS

> **EXCLUDES 1** *superficial bite of lower back and pelvis (S30.860, S30.870)*

7 **S31.050-** Open bite of lower back and pelvis without penetration into retroperitoneum
Open bite of lower back and pelvis NOS

7 **S31.051-** Open bite of lower back and pelvis with penetration into retroperitoneum

5 **S31.1** Open wound of abdominal wall without penetration into peritoneal cavity
Open wound of abdominal wall NOS

> **EXCLUDES 2** *open wound of abdominal wall with penetration into peritoneal cavity (S31.6-)*

6 **S31.10** Unspecified open wound of abdominal wall without penetration into peritoneal cavity

7 ⊟ **S31.100-** Unspecified open wound of abdominal wall, right upper quadrant without penetration into peritoneal cavity

7 ⊟ **S31.101-** Unspecified open wound of abdominal wall, left upper quadrant without penetration into peritoneal cavity

7 ⊟ **S31.102-** Unspecified open wound of abdominal wall, epigastric region without penetration into peritoneal cavity

7 ⊟ **S31.103-** Unspecified open wound of abdominal wall, right lower quadrant without penetration into peritoneal cavity

7 ⊟ **S31.104-** Unspecified open wound of abdominal wall, left lower quadrant without penetration into peritoneal cavity

7 ⊟ **S31.105-** Unspecified open wound of abdominal wall, periumbilic region without penetration into peritoneal cavity

7 ⊟ **S31.109-** Unspecified open wound of abdominal wall, unspecified quadrant without penetration into peritoneal cavity
Unspecified open wound of abdominal wall NOS

6 **S31.11** Laceration without foreign body of abdominal wall without penetration into peritoneal cavity

7 ⊟ **S31.110-** Laceration without foreign body of abdominal wall, right upper quadrant without penetration into peritoneal cavity

7 ⊟ **S31.111-** Laceration without foreign body of abdominal wall, left upper quadrant without penetration into peritoneal cavity

7 ⊟ **S31.112-** Laceration without foreign body of abdominal wall, epigastric region without penetration into peritoneal cavity

7 ⊟ **S31.113-** Laceration without foreign body of abdominal wall, right lower quadrant without penetration into peritoneal cavity

7 ⊟ **S31.114-** Laceration without foreign body of abdominal wall, left lower quadrant without penetration into peritoneal cavity

7 ⊟ **S31.115-** Laceration without foreign body of abdominal wall, periumbilic region without penetration into peritoneal cavity

7 ⊟ **S31.119-** Laceration without foreign body of abdominal wall, unspecified quadrant without penetration into peritoneal cavity

---

● New   ▲ Revised   *Manifestation*   **4**-**7** Digit Indicators   ⊟ Laterality   Ⓐ Adult (15+ years)   Ⓜ Maternity (12-55 years)   Ⓝ Newborn   Ⓟ Pediatric (0-17 years)   ♂ Male   ♀ Female

✖ Deleted   Unspecified   + Additional code

⑥ S31.12   Laceration with foreign body of abdominal wall
            without penetration into peritoneal cavity
⑦ ▤ S31.120-   Laceration of abdominal wall with foreign
                body, right upper quadrant without
                penetration into peritoneal cavity
⑦ ▤ S31.121-   Laceration of abdominal wall with foreign
                body, left upper quadrant without
                penetration into peritoneal cavity
⑦ ▤ S31.122-   Laceration of abdominal wall with foreign
                body, epigastric region without penetration
                into peritoneal cavity
⑦ ▤ S31.123-   Laceration of abdominal wall with foreign
                body, right lower quadrant without
                penetration into peritoneal cavity
⑦ ▤ S31.124-   Laceration of abdominal wall with foreign
                body, left lower quadrant without
                penetration into peritoneal cavity
⑦ ▤ S31.125-   Laceration of abdominal wall with foreign
                body, periumbilic region without
                penetration into peritoneal cavity
⑦ ▤ S31.129-   Laceration of abdominal wall with foreign
                body, unspecified quadrant without
                penetration into peritoneal cavity

⑥ S31.13   Puncture wound of abdominal wall without foreign
            body without penetration into peritoneal cavity
⑦ ▤ S31.130-   Puncture wound of abdominal wall without
                foreign body, right upper quadrant without
                penetration into peritoneal cavity
⑦ ▤ S31.131-   Puncture wound of abdominal wall without
                foreign body, left upper quadrant without
                penetration into peritoneal cavity
⑦ ▤ S31.132-   Puncture wound of abdominal wall without
                foreign body, epigastric region without
                penetration into peritoneal cavity
⑦ ▤ S31.133-   Puncture wound of abdominal wall without
                foreign body, right lower quadrant without
                penetration into peritoneal cavity
⑦ ▤ S31.134-   Puncture wound of abdominal wall without
                foreign body, left lower quadrant without
                penetration into peritoneal cavity
⑦ ▤ S31.135-   Puncture wound of abdominal wall without
                foreign body, periumbilic region without
                penetration into peritoneal cavity
⑦ ▤ S31.139-   Puncture wound of abdominal wall without
                foreign body, unspecified quadrant without
                penetration into peritoneal cavity

⑥ S31.14   Puncture wound of abdominal wall with foreign
            body without penetration into peritoneal cavity
⑦ ▤ S31.140-   Puncture wound of abdominal wall with
                foreign body, right upper quadrant without
                penetration into peritoneal cavity
⑦ ▤ S31.141-   Puncture wound of abdominal wall with
                foreign body, left upper quadrant without
                penetration into peritoneal cavity
⑦ ▤ S31.142-   Puncture wound of abdominal wall with
                foreign body, epigastric region without
                penetration into peritoneal cavity
⑦ ▤ S31.143-   Puncture wound of abdominal wall with
                foreign body, right lower quadrant without
                penetration into peritoneal cavity
⑦ ▤ S31.144-   Puncture wound of abdominal wall with
                foreign body, left lower quadrant without
                penetration into peritoneal cavity
⑦ ▤ S31.145-   Puncture wound of abdominal wall with
                foreign body, periumbilic region without
                penetration into peritoneal cavity
⑦ ▤ S31.149-   Puncture wound of abdominal wall with
                foreign body, unspecified quadrant without
                penetration into peritoneal cavity

⑥ S31.15   Open bite of abdominal wall without penetration
            into peritoneal cavity
            Bite of abdominal wall NOS
            EXCLUDES 1   superficial bite of abdominal wall
                              (S30.871)
⑦ ▤ S31.150-   Open bite of abdominal wall, right upper
                quadrant without penetration into
                peritoneal cavity
⑦ ▤ S31.151-   Open bite of abdominal wall, left upper
                quadrant without penetration into
                peritoneal cavity
⑦ ▤ S31.152-   Open bite of abdominal wall, epigastric region
                without penetration into peritoneal cavity

⑦ ▤ S31.153-   Open bite of abdominal wall, right lower
                quadrant without penetration into
                peritoneal cavity
⑦ ▤ S31.154-   Open bite of abdominal wall, left lower
                quadrant without penetration into
                peritoneal cavity
⑦ ▤ S31.155-   Open bite of abdominal wall, periumbilic
                region without penetration into peritoneal
                cavity
⑦ ▤ S31.159-   Open bite of abdominal wall, unspecified
                quadrant without penetration into
                peritoneal cavity

⑤ S31.2   Open wound of penis
⑦ S31.20X-   Unspecified open wound of penis
⑦ S31.21X-   Laceration without foreign body of penis
⑦ S31.22X-   Laceration with foreign body of penis
⑦ S31.23X-   Puncture wound without foreign body of penis
⑦ S31.24X-   Puncture wound with foreign body of penis
⑦ S31.25X-   Open bite of penis
              Bite of penis NOS
              EXCLUDES 1   superficial bite of penis
                                (S30.862, S30.872)

⑤ S31.3   Open wound of scrotum and testes
⑦ S31.30X-   Unspecified open wound of scrotum and testes
⑦ S31.31X-   Laceration without foreign body of scrotum and
              testes
⑦ S31.32X-   Laceration with foreign body of scrotum and
              testes
⑦ S31.33X-   Puncture wound without foreign body of scrotum
              and testes
⑦ S31.34X-   Puncture wound with foreign body of scrotum
              and testes
⑦ S31.35X-   Open bite of scrotum and testes
              Bite of scrotum and testes NOS
              EXCLUDES 1   superficial bite of scrotum and
                                testes (S30.863, S30.873)

⑤ S31.4   Open wound of vagina and vulva
            EXCLUDES 1   injury to vagina and vulva during delivery
                              (O70.-, O71.4)
⑦ S31.40X-   Unspecified open wound of vagina and vulva
⑦ S31.41X-   Laceration without foreign body of vagina and
              vulva
⑦ S31.42X-   Laceration with foreign body of vagina and vulva
⑦ S31.43X-   Puncture wound without foreign body of vagina
              and vulva
⑦ S31.44X-   Puncture wound with foreign body of vagina and
              vulva
⑦ S31.45X-   Open bite of vagina and vulva
              Bite of vagina and vulva NOS
              EXCLUDES 1   superficial bite of vagina and vulva
                                (S30.864, S30.874)

⑤ S31.5   Open wound of unspecified external genital organs
            EXCLUDES 1   traumatic amputation of external genital
                              organs (S38.21, S38.22)
⑥ S31.50   Unspecified open wound of unspecified external
            genital organs
⑦ S31.501-   Unspecified open wound of unspecified
              external genital organs, male
⑦ S31.502-   Unspecified open wound of unspecified
              external genital organs, female
⑥ S31.51   Laceration without foreign body of unspecified
            external genital organs
⑦ S31.511-   Laceration without foreign body of
              unspecified external genital organs, male
⑦ S31.512-   Laceration without foreign body of
              unspecified external genital organs, female
⑥ S31.52   Laceration with foreign body of unspecified external
            genital organs
⑦ S31.521-   Laceration with foreign body of unspecified
              external genital organs, male
⑦ S31.522-   Laceration with foreign body of unspecified
              external genital organs, female
⑥ S31.53   Puncture wound without foreign body of
            unspecified external genital organs
⑦ S31.531-   Puncture wound without foreign body of
              unspecified external genital organs, male
⑦ S31.532-   Puncture wound without foreign body of
              unspecified external genital organs, female

● New   ▲ Revised   *Manifestation*   ④-⑦ Digit Indicators   ▤ Laterality   Ⓐ Adult   Ⓜ Maternity   Ⓝ Newborn   Ⓟ Pediatric   ♂ Male   ♀ Female
✖ Deleted   Unspecified   + Additional code   (15+ years)   (12-55 years)   (0-17 years)

⑥ S31.54   Puncture wound with foreign body of unspecified external genital organs

⑦ S31.541-   Puncture wound with foreign body of unspecified external genital organs, male

⑦ S31.542-   Puncture wound with foreign body of unspecified external genital organs, female

⑥ S31.55   Open bite of unspecified external genital organs

Bite of unspecified external genital organs NOS

EXCLUDES 1   *superficial bite of unspecified external genital organs (S30.865, S30.866, S30.875, S30.876)*

⑦ S31.551-   Open bite of unspecified external genital organs, male

⑦ S31.552-   Open bite of unspecified external genital organs, female

⑤ S31.6   Open wound of abdominal wall with penetration into peritoneal cavity

⑥ S31.60   Unspecified open wound of abdominal wall with penetration into peritoneal cavity

⑦ ⊟ S31.600-   Unspecified open wound of abdominal wall, right upper quadrant with penetration into peritoneal cavity

⑦ ⊟ S31.601-   Unspecified open wound of abdominal wall, left upper quadrant with penetration into peritoneal cavity

⑦ ⊟ S31.602-   Unspecified open wound of abdominal wall, epigastric region with penetration into peritoneal cavity

⑦ ⊟ S31.603-   Unspecified open wound of abdominal wall, right lower quadrant with penetration into peritoneal cavity

⑦ ⊟ S31.604-   Unspecified open wound of abdominal wall, left lower quadrant with penetration into peritoneal cavity

⑦ ⊟ S31.605-   Unspecified open wound of abdominal wall, periumbilic region with penetration into peritoneal cavity

⑦ ⊟ S31.609-   Unspecified open wound of abdominal wall, unspecified quadrant with penetration into peritoneal cavity

⑥ S31.61   Laceration without foreign body of abdominal wall with penetration into peritoneal cavity

⑦ ⊟ S31.610-   Laceration without foreign body of abdominal wall, right upper quadrant with penetration into peritoneal cavity

⑦ ⊟ S31.611-   Laceration without foreign body of abdominal wall, left upper quadrant with penetration into peritoneal cavity

⑦ ⊟ S31.612-   Laceration without foreign body of abdominal wall, epigastric region with penetration into peritoneal cavity

⑦ ⊟ S31.613-   Laceration without foreign body of abdominal wall, right lower quadrant with penetration into peritoneal cavity

AHA: (S31.613A) 4Q 2015, 37-38

⑦ ⊟ S31.614-   Laceration without foreign body of abdominal wall, left lower quadrant with penetration into peritoneal cavity

⑦ ⊟ S31.615-   Laceration without foreign body of abdominal wall, periumbilic region with penetration into peritoneal cavity

⑦ ⊟ S31.619-   Laceration without foreign body of abdominal wall, unspecified quadrant with penetration into peritoneal cavity

⑥ S31.62   Laceration with foreign body of abdominal wall with penetration into peritoneal cavity

⑦ ⊟ S31.620-   Laceration with foreign body of abdominal wall, right upper quadrant with penetration into peritoneal cavity

⑦ ⊟ S31.621-   Laceration with foreign body of abdominal wall, left upper quadrant with penetration into peritoneal cavity

⑦ ⊟ S31.622-   Laceration with foreign body of abdominal wall, epigastric region with penetration into peritoneal cavity

⑦ ⊟ S31.623-   Laceration with foreign body of abdominal wall, right lower quadrant with penetration into peritoneal cavity

⑦ ⊟ S31.624-   Laceration with foreign body of abdominal wall, left lower quadrant with penetration into peritoneal cavity

⑦ ⊟ S31.625-   Laceration with foreign body of abdominal wall, periumbilic region with penetration into peritoneal cavity

⑦ ⊟ S31.629-   Laceration with foreign body of abdominal wall, unspecified quadrant with penetration into peritoneal cavity

⑥ S31.63   Puncture wound without foreign body of abdominal wall with penetration into peritoneal cavity

⑦ ⊟ S31.630-   Puncture wound without foreign body of abdominal wall, right upper quadrant with penetration into peritoneal cavity

⑦ ⊟ S31.631-   Puncture wound without foreign body of abdominal wall, left upper quadrant with penetration into peritoneal cavity

⑦ ⊟ S31.632-   Puncture wound without foreign body of abdominal wall, epigastric region with penetration into peritoneal cavity

⑦ ⊟ S31.633-   Puncture wound without foreign body of abdominal wall, right lower quadrant with penetration into peritoneal cavity

⑦ ⊟ S31.634-   Puncture wound without foreign body of abdominal wall, left lower quadrant with penetration into peritoneal cavity

⑦ ⊟ S31.635-   Puncture wound without foreign body of abdominal wall, periumbilic region with penetration into peritoneal cavity

⑦ ⊟ S31.639-   Puncture wound without foreign body of abdominal wall, unspecified quadrant with penetration into peritoneal cavity

⑥ S31.64   Puncture wound with foreign body of abdominal wall with penetration into peritoneal cavity

⑦ ⊟ S31.640-   Puncture wound with foreign body of abdominal wall, right upper quadrant with penetration into peritoneal cavity

⑦ ⊟ S31.641-   Puncture wound with foreign body of abdominal wall, left upper quadrant with penetration into peritoneal cavity

⑦ ⊟ S31.642-   Puncture wound with foreign body of abdominal wall, epigastric region with penetration into peritoneal cavity

⑦ ⊟ S31.643-   Puncture wound with foreign body of abdominal wall, right lower quadrant with penetration into peritoneal cavity

⑦ ⊟ S31.644-   Puncture wound with foreign body of abdominal wall, left lower quadrant with penetration into peritoneal cavity

⑦ ⊟ S31.645-   Puncture wound with foreign body of abdominal wall, periumbilic region with penetration into peritoneal cavity

⑦ ⊟ S31.649-   Puncture wound with foreign body of abdominal wall, unspecified quadrant with penetration into peritoneal cavity

⑥ S31.65   Open bite of abdominal wall with penetration into peritoneal cavity

EXCLUDES 1   *superficial bite of abdominal wall (S30.861, S30.871)*

⑦ ⊟ S31.650-   Open bite of abdominal wall, right upper quadrant with penetration into peritoneal cavity

⑦ ⊟ S31.651-   Open bite of abdominal wall, left upper quadrant with penetration into peritoneal cavity

⑦ ⊟ S31.652-   Open bite of abdominal wall, epigastric region with penetration into peritoneal cavity

⑦ ⊟ S31.653-   Open bite of abdominal wall, right lower quadrant with penetration into peritoneal cavity

⑦ ⊟ S31.654-   Open bite of abdominal wall, left lower quadrant with penetration into peritoneal cavity

⑦ ⊟ S31.655-   Open bite of abdominal wall, periumbilic region with penetration into peritoneal cavity

⑦ ⊟ S31.659-   Open bite of abdominal wall, unspecified quadrant with penetration into peritoneal cavity

⑤ S31.8   Open wound of other parts of abdomen, lower back and pelvis

⑥ S31.80   Open wound of unspecified buttock

● New	▲ Revised	*Manifestation*	④-⑦ Digit Indicators	⊟ Laterality	Ⓐ Adult (15+ years)	Ⓜ Maternity (12-55 years)	Ⓝ Newborn	Ⓟ Pediatric (0-17 years)	♂ Male	♀ Female
✖ Deleted		Unspecified	+ Additional code							

948   © 2017 DecisionHealth   2017 ICD-10-CM Expert for Physicians

☑ S31.801-   Laceration without foreign body of unspecified buttock

☑ S31.802-   Laceration with foreign body of unspecified buttock

☑ S31.803-   Puncture wound without foreign body of unspecified buttock

☑ S31.804-   Puncture wound with foreign body of unspecified buttock

☑ S31.805-   Open bite of unspecified buttock
Bite of buttock NOS
> **EXCLUDES 1**   *superficial bite of buttock (S30.870)*

☑ S31.809-   Unspecified open wound of unspecified buttock

⑥ S31.81   Open wound of right buttock

☑⊟ S31.811-   Laceration without foreign body of right buttock

☑⊟ S31.812-   Laceration with foreign body of right buttock

☑⊟ S31.813-   Puncture wound without foreign body of right buttock

☑⊟ S31.814-   Puncture wound with foreign body of right buttock

☑⊟ S31.815-   Open bite of right buttock
Bite of right buttock NOS
> **EXCLUDES 1**   *superficial bite of buttock (S30.870)*

☑⊟ S31.819-   Unspecified open wound of right buttock

⑥ S31.82   Open wound of left buttock

☑⊟ S31.821-   Laceration without foreign body of left buttock

☑⊟ S31.822-   Laceration with foreign body of left buttock

☑⊟ S31.823-   Puncture wound without foreign body of left buttock

☑⊟ S31.824-   Puncture wound with foreign body of left buttock

☑⊟ S31.825-   Open bite of left buttock
Bite of left buttock NOS
> **EXCLUDES 1**   *superficial bite of buttock (S30.870)*

☑⊟ S31.829-   Unspecified open wound of left buttock

⑥ S31.83   Open wound of anus

☑ S31.831-   Laceration without foreign body of anus

☑ S31.832-   Laceration with foreign body of anus

☑ S31.833-   Puncture wound without foreign body of anus

☑ S31.834-   Puncture wound with foreign body of anus

☑ S31.835-   Open bite of anus
Bite of anus NOS
> **EXCLUDES 1**   *superficial bite of anus (S30.877)*

☑ S31.839-   Unspecified open wound of anus

◢ S32   **Fracture of lumbar spine and pelvis**
Note: A fracture not indicated as displaced or nondisplaced should be coded to displaced
A fracture not indicated as opened or closed should be coded to closed

> **INCLUDES**   fracture of lumbosacral neural arch
> fracture of lumbosacral spinous process
> fracture of lumbosacral transverse process
> fracture of lumbosacral vertebra
> fracture of lumbosacral vertebral arch

Code first:
any associated spinal cord and spinal nerve injury (S34.-)

> **EXCLUDES 1**   *transection of abdomen (S38.3)*

> **EXCLUDES 2**   *fracture of hip NOS (S72.0-)*

The appropriate 7th character is to be added to each code from category S32
A   initial encounter for closed fracture
B   initial encounter for open fracture
D   subsequent encounter for fracture with routine healing
G   subsequent encounter for fracture with delayed healing
K   subsequent encounter for fracture with nonunion
S   sequela

> **CODING TIP ✓**   A fracture not indicated as displaced or nondisplaced should be coded to displaced. A fracture not indicated as open or closed should be coded to closed. Query providers on fractures not documented as displaced/nondisplaced otherwise displaced fracture diagnosis could be assigned without reduction being performed potentially resulting in claim denials.

⑤ S32.0   **Fracture of lumbar vertebra**
Fracture of lumbar spine NOS

⑥ S32.00   Fracture of unspecified lumbar vertebra

☑ S32.000-   Wedge compression fracture of unspecified lumbar vertebra

☑ S32.001-   Stable burst fracture of unspecified lumbar vertebra

☑ S32.002-   Unstable burst fracture of unspecified lumbar vertebra

☑ S32.008-   Other fracture of unspecified lumbar vertebra

☑ S32.009-   Unspecified fracture of unspecified lumbar vertebra

⑥ S32.01   Fracture of first lumbar vertebra

☑ S32.010-   Wedge compression fracture of first lumbar vertebra

☑ S32.011-   Stable burst fracture of first lumbar vertebra

☑ S32.012-   Unstable burst fracture of first lumbar vertebra

☑ S32.018-   Other fracture of first lumbar vertebra

☑ S32.019-   Unspecified fracture of first lumbar vertebra

⑥ S32.02   Fracture of second lumbar vertebra

☑ S32.020-   Wedge compression fracture of second lumbar vertebra

☑ S32.021-   Stable burst fracture of second lumbar vertebra

☑ S32.022-   Unstable burst fracture of second lumbar vertebra

☑ S32.028-   Other fracture of second lumbar vertebra

☑ S32.029-   Unspecified fracture of second lumbar vertebra

⑥ S32.03   Fracture of third lumbar vertebra

☑ S32.030-   Wedge compression fracture of third lumbar vertebra

☑ S32.031-   Stable burst fracture of third lumbar vertebra

☑ S32.032-   Unstable burst fracture of third lumbar vertebra

☑ S32.038-   Other fracture of third lumbar vertebra

☑ S32.039-   Unspecified fracture of third lumbar vertebra

⑥ S32.04   Fracture of fourth lumbar vertebra

☑ S32.040-   Wedge compression fracture of fourth lumbar vertebra

☑ S32.041-   Stable burst fracture of fourth lumbar vertebra

☑ S32.042-   Unstable burst fracture of fourth lumbar vertebra

☑ S32.048-   Other fracture of fourth lumbar vertebra

☑ S32.049-   Unspecified fracture of fourth lumbar vertebra

⑥ S32.05   Fracture of fifth lumbar vertebra

☑ S32.050-   Wedge compression fracture of fifth lumbar vertebra

☑ S32.051-   Stable burst fracture of fifth lumbar vertebra

☑ S32.052-   Unstable burst fracture of fifth lumbar vertebra

☑ S32.058-   Other fracture of fifth lumbar vertebra

☑ S32.059-   Unspecified fracture of fifth lumbar vertebra

⑤ S32.1   **Fracture of sacrum**
For vertical fractures, code to most medial fracture extension
Use two codes if both a vertical and transverse fracture are present
Code also:
any associated fracture of pelvic ring (S32.8-)

☑ S32.10X-   Unspecified fracture of sacrum

⑥ S32.11   Zone I fracture of sacrum
Vertical sacral ala fracture of sacrum

☑ S32.110-   Nondisplaced Zone I fracture of sacrum

☑ S32.111-   Minimally displaced Zone I fracture of sacrum

● New ▲ Revised *Manifestation* ④-☑ Digit Indicators ⊟ Laterality Ⓐ Adult (15+ years) Ⓜ Maternity (12-55 years) Ⓝ Newborn Ⓟ Pediatric (0-17 years) ♂ Male ♀ Female
✖ Deleted Unspecified ✚ Additional code

2017 ICD-10-CM Expert for Physicians   © 2017 DecisionHealth   949

⑦ S32.112-   Severely displaced Zone I fracture of sacrum
⑦ S32.119-   Unspecified Zone I fracture of sacrum
⑥ S32.12   Zone II fracture of sacrum
              Vertical foraminal region fracture of sacrum
⑦ S32.120-   Nondisplaced Zone II fracture of sacrum
⑦ S32.121-   Minimally displaced Zone II fracture of sacrum
⑦ S32.122-   Severely displaced Zone II fracture of sacrum
⑦ S32.129-   Unspecified Zone II fracture of sacrum
⑥ S32.13   Zone III fracture of sacrum
              Vertical fracture into spinal canal region of sacrum
⑦ S32.130-   Nondisplaced Zone III fracture of sacrum
⑦ S32.131-   Minimally displaced Zone III fracture of sacrum
⑦ S32.132-   Severely displaced Zone III fracture of sacrum
⑦ S32.139-   Unspecified Zone III fracture of sacrum
⑦ S32.14X-   Type 1 fracture of sacrum
              Transverse flexion fracture of sacrum without displacement
⑦ S32.15X-   Type 2 fracture of sacrum
              Transverse flexion fracture of sacrum with posterior displacement
⑦ S32.16X-   Type 3 fracture of sacrum
              Transverse extension fracture of sacrum with anterior displacement
⑦ S32.17X-   Type 4 fracture of sacrum
              Transverse segmental comminution of upper sacrum
⑦ S32.19X-   Other fracture of sacrum
⑦ S32.2XX-   Fracture of coccyx
⑧ S32.3   Fracture of ilium
              EXCLUDES 1 *fracture of ilium with associated disruption of pelvic ring (S32.8-)*
⑥ S32.30   Unspecified fracture of ilium
⑦⊟ S32.301-   Unspecified fracture of right ilium
⑦⊟ S32.302-   Unspecified fracture of left ilium
⑦⊟ S32.309-   Unspecified fracture of unspecified ilium
⑥ S32.31   Avulsion fracture of ilium
⑦⊟ S32.311-   Displaced avulsion fracture of right ilium
⑦⊟ S32.312-   Displaced avulsion fracture of left ilium
⑦⊟ S32.313-   Displaced avulsion fracture of unspecified ilium
⑦⊟ S32.314-   Nondisplaced avulsion fracture of right ilium
⑦⊟ S32.315-   Nondisplaced avulsion fracture of left ilium
⑦⊟ S32.316-   Nondisplaced avulsion fracture of unspecified ilium
⑥ S32.39   Other fracture of ilium
⑦⊟ S32.391-   Other fracture of right ilium
⑦⊟ S32.392-   Other fracture of left ilium
⑦⊟ S32.399-   Other fracture of unspecified ilium
⑧ S32.4   Fracture of acetabulum
              Code also:
                any associated fracture of pelvic ring (S32.8-)
⑥ S32.40   Unspecified fracture of acetabulum
⑦⊟ S32.401-   Unspecified fracture of right acetabulum
⑦⊟ S32.402-   Unspecified fracture of left acetabulum
⑦⊟ S32.409-   Unspecified fracture of unspecified acetabulum
⑥ S32.41   Fracture of anterior wall of acetabulum
⑦⊟ S32.411-   Displaced fracture of anterior wall of right acetabulum
⑦⊟ S32.412-   Displaced fracture of anterior wall of left acetabulum
⑦⊟ S32.413-   Displaced fracture of anterior wall of unspecified acetabulum
⑦⊟ S32.414-   Nondisplaced fracture of anterior wall of right acetabulum
⑦⊟ S32.415-   Nondisplaced fracture of anterior wall of left acetabulum
⑦⊟ S32.416-   Nondisplaced fracture of anterior wall of unspecified acetabulum
⑥ S32.42   Fracture of posterior wall of acetabulum
⑦⊟ S32.421-   Displaced fracture of posterior wall of right acetabulum
⑦⊟ S32.422-   Displaced fracture of posterior wall of left acetabulum

⑦⊟ S32.423-   Displaced fracture of posterior wall of unspecified acetabulum
⑦⊟ S32.424-   Nondisplaced fracture of posterior wall of right acetabulum
⑦⊟ S32.425-   Nondisplaced fracture of posterior wall of left acetabulum
⑦⊟ S32.426-   Nondisplaced fracture of posterior wall of unspecified acetabulum
⑥ S32.43   Fracture of anterior column [iliopubic] of acetabulum
⑦⊟ S32.431-   Displaced fracture of anterior column [iliopubic] of right acetabulum
⑦⊟ S32.432-   Displaced fracture of anterior column [iliopubic] of left acetabulum
⑦⊟ S32.433-   Displaced fracture of anterior column [iliopubic] of unspecified acetabulum
⑦⊟ S32.434-   Nondisplaced fracture of anterior column [iliopubic] of right acetabulum
⑦⊟ S32.435-   Nondisplaced fracture of anterior column [iliopubic] of left acetabulum
⑦⊟ S32.436-   Nondisplaced fracture of anterior column [iliopubic] of unspecified acetabulum
⑥ S32.44   Fracture of posterior column [ilioischial] of acetabulum
⑦⊟ S32.441-   Displaced fracture of posterior column [ilioischial] of right acetabulum
⑦⊟ S32.442-   Displaced fracture of posterior column [ilioischial] of left acetabulum
⑦⊟ S32.443-   Displaced fracture of posterior column [ilioischial] of unspecified acetabulum
⑦⊟ S32.444-   Nondisplaced fracture of posterior column [ilioischial] of right acetabulum
⑦⊟ S32.445-   Nondisplaced fracture of posterior column [ilioischial] of left acetabulum
⑦⊟ S32.446-   Nondisplaced fracture of posterior column [ilioischial] of unspecified acetabulum
⑥ S32.45   Transverse fracture of acetabulum
⑦⊟ S32.451-   Displaced transverse fracture of right acetabulum
⑦⊟ S32.452-   Displaced transverse fracture of left acetabulum
⑦⊟ S32.453-   Displaced transverse fracture of unspecified acetabulum
⑦⊟ S32.454-   Nondisplaced transverse fracture of right acetabulum
⑦⊟ S32.455-   Nondisplaced transverse fracture of left acetabulum
⑦⊟ S32.456-   Nondisplaced transverse fracture of unspecified acetabulum
⑥ S32.46   Associated transverse-posterior fracture of acetabulum
⑦⊟ S32.461-   Displaced associated transverse-posterior fracture of right acetabulum
⑦⊟ S32.462-   Displaced associated transverse-posterior fracture of left acetabulum
⑦⊟ S32.463-   Displaced associated transverse-posterior fracture of unspecified acetabulum
⑦⊟ S32.464-   Nondisplaced associated transverse-posterior fracture of right acetabulum
⑦⊟ S32.465-   Nondisplaced associated transverse-posterior fracture of left acetabulum
⑦⊟ S32.466-   Nondisplaced associated transverse-posterior fracture of unspecified acetabulum
⑥ S32.47   Fracture of medial wall of acetabulum
⑦⊟ S32.471-   Displaced fracture of medial wall of right acetabulum
⑦⊟ S32.472-   Displaced fracture of medial wall of left acetabulum
⑦⊟ S32.473-   Displaced fracture of medial wall of unspecified acetabulum
⑦⊟ S32.474-   Nondisplaced fracture of medial wall of right acetabulum
⑦⊟ S32.475-   Nondisplaced fracture of medial wall of left acetabulum
⑦⊟ S32.476-   Nondisplaced fracture of medial wall of unspecified acetabulum
⑥ S32.48   Dome fracture of acetabulum
⑦⊟ S32.481-   Displaced dome fracture of right acetabulum
⑦⊟ S32.482-   Displaced dome fracture of left acetabulum

● New   ▲ Revised   *Manifestation*   ④-⑦ Digit Indicators   ⊟ Laterality   🅐 Adult (15+ years)   🅜 Maternity (12-55 years)   🅝 Newborn   🅟 Pediatric (0-17 years)   ♂ Male   ♀ Female
✖ Deleted   Unspecified   + Additional code

7 ▢ **S32.483-** Displaced dome fracture of unspecified acetabulum

7 ▢ **S32.484-** Nondisplaced dome fracture of right acetabulum

7 ▢ **S32.485-** Nondisplaced dome fracture of left acetabulum

7 ▢ **S32.486-** Nondisplaced dome fracture of unspecified acetabulum

6 **S32.49** Other specified fracture of acetabulum

7 ▢ **S32.491-** Other specified fracture of right acetabulum

7 ▢ **S32.492-** Other specified fracture of left acetabulum

7 ▢ **S32.499-** Other specified fracture of unspecified acetabulum

5 **S32.5** Fracture of pubis

> **EXCLUDES 1** *fracture of pubis with associated disruption of pelvic ring (S32.8-)*

6 **S32.50** Unspecified fracture of pubis

7 ▢ **S32.501-** Unspecified fracture of right pubis

7 ▢ **S32.502-** Unspecified fracture of left pubis

7 ▢ **S32.509-** Unspecified fracture of unspecified pubis

6 **S32.51** Fracture of superior rim of pubis

7 ▢ **S32.511-** Fracture of superior rim of right pubis

7 ▢ **S32.512-** Fracture of superior rim of left pubis

7 ▢ **S32.519-** Fracture of superior rim of unspecified pubis

6 **S32.59** Other specified fracture of pubis

7 ▢ **S32.591-** Other specified fracture of right pubis

7 ▢ **S32.592-** Other specified fracture of left pubis

7 ▢ **S32.599-** Other specified fracture of unspecified pubis

5 **S32.6** Fracture of ischium

> **EXCLUDES 1** *fracture of ischium with associated disruption of pelvic ring (S32.8-)*

6 **S32.60** Unspecified fracture of ischium

7 ▢ **S32.601-** Unspecified fracture of right ischium

7 ▢ **S32.602-** Unspecified fracture of left ischium

7 ▢ **S32.609-** Unspecified fracture of unspecified ischium

6 **S32.61** Avulsion fracture of ischium

7 ▢ **S32.611-** Displaced avulsion fracture of right ischium

7 ▢ **S32.612-** Displaced avulsion fracture of left ischium

7 ▢ **S32.613-** Displaced avulsion fracture of unspecified ischium

7 ▢ **S32.614-** Nondisplaced avulsion fracture of right ischium

7 ▢ **S32.615-** Nondisplaced avulsion fracture of left ischium

7 ▢ **S32.616-** Nondisplaced avulsion fracture of unspecified ischium

6 **S32.69** Other specified fracture of ischium

7 ▢ **S32.691-** Other specified fracture of right ischium

7 ▢ **S32.692-** Other specified fracture of left ischium

7 ▢ **S32.699-** Other specified fracture of unspecified ischium

5 **S32.8** Fracture of other parts of pelvis

Code also any associated:
fracture of acetabulum (S32.4-)
sacral fracture (S32.1-)

6 **S32.81** Multiple fractures of pelvis with disruption of pelvic ring

Multiple pelvic fractures with disruption of pelvic circle

7 **S32.810-** Multiple fractures of pelvis with stable disruption of pelvic ring

7 **S32.811-** Multiple fractures of pelvis with unstable disruption of pelvic ring

7 **S32.82X-** Multiple fractures of pelvis without disruption of pelvic ring

Multiple pelvic fractures without disruption of pelvic circle

7 **S32.89X-** Fracture of other parts of pelvis

7 **S32.9XX-** Fracture of unspecified parts of lumbosacral spine and pelvis

Fracture of lumbosacral spine NOS
Fracture of pelvis NOS
AHA: (S32.9XXD) 4Q 2012, 93

---

4 **S33** Dislocation and sprain of joints and ligaments of lumbar spine and pelvis

> **INCLUDES** avulsion of joint or ligament of lumbar spine and pelvis
> laceration of cartilage, joint or ligament of lumbar spine and pelvis
> sprain of cartilage, joint or ligament of lumbar spine and pelvis
> traumatic hemarthrosis of joint or ligament of lumbar spine and pelvis
> traumatic rupture of joint or ligament of lumbar spine and pelvis
> traumatic subluxation of joint or ligament of lumbar spine and pelvis
> traumatic tear of joint or ligament of lumbar spine and pelvis

Code also:
any associated open wound

> **EXCLUDES 1** *nontraumatic rupture or displacement of lumbar intervertebral disc NOS (M51.-)*
> *obstetric damage to pelvic joints and ligaments (O71.6)*

> **EXCLUDES 2** *dislocation and sprain of joints and ligaments of hip (S73.-)*
> *strain of muscle of lower back and pelvis (S39.01-)*

The appropriate 7th character is to be added to each code from category S33
A initial encounter
D subsequent encounter
S sequela

> **CODING TIP ✓** Unlike ICD-9 there is no code for open dislocations. When documented as open an additional code for the open wound must be applied.

7 **S33.0XX-** Traumatic rupture of lumbar intervertebral disc

> **EXCLUDES 1** *rupture or displacement (nontraumatic) of lumbar intervertebral disc NOS (M51.- with fifth character 6)*

5 **S33.1** Subluxation and dislocation of lumbar vertebra

Code also any associated:
open wound of abdomen, lower back and pelvis (S31)
spinal cord injury (S24.0, S24.1-, S34.0-, S34.1-)

> **EXCLUDES 2** *fracture of lumbar vertebrae (S32.0-)*

6 **S33.10** Subluxation and dislocation of unspecified lumbar vertebra

7 **S33.100-** Subluxation of unspecified lumbar vertebra

7 **S33.101-** Dislocation of unspecified lumbar vertebra

6 **S33.11** Subluxation and dislocation of L1/L2 lumbar vertebra

7 **S33.110-** Subluxation of L1/L2 lumbar vertebra

7 **S33.111-** Dislocation of L1/L2 lumbar vertebra

6 **S33.12** Subluxation and dislocation of L2/L3 lumbar vertebra

7 **S33.120-** Subluxation of L2/L3 lumbar vertebra

7 **S33.121-** Dislocation of L2/L3 lumbar vertebra

6 **S33.13** Subluxation and dislocation of L3/L4 lumbar vertebra

7 **S33.130-** Subluxation of L3/L4 lumbar vertebra

7 **S33.131-** Dislocation of L3/L4 lumbar vertebra

6 **S33.14** Subluxation and dislocation of L4/L5 lumbar vertebra

7 **S33.140-** Subluxation of L4/L5 lumbar vertebra

7 **S33.141-** Dislocation of L4/L5 lumbar vertebra

7 **S33.2XX-** Dislocation of sacroiliac and sacrococcygeal joint

5 **S33.3** Dislocation of other and unspecified parts of lumbar spine and pelvis

7 **S33.30X-** Dislocation of unspecified parts of lumbar spine and pelvis

7 **S33.39X-** Dislocation of other parts of lumbar spine and pelvis

7 **S33.4XX-** Traumatic rupture of symphysis pubis

7 **S33.5XX-** Sprain of ligaments of lumbar spine

7 **S33.6XX-** Sprain of sacroiliac joint

7 **S33.8XX-** Sprain of other parts of lumbar spine and pelvis

7 **S33.9XX-** Sprain of unspecified parts of lumbar spine and pelvis

---

● New ▲ Revised *Manifestation* 4-7 Digit Indicators ▢ Laterality Ⓐ Adult (15+ years) Ⓜ Maternity (12-55 years) Ⓝ Newborn Ⓟ Pediatric (0-17 years) ♂ Male ♀ Female
✖ ~~Deleted~~ Unspecified + Additional code

⬛ S34   Injury of lumbar and sacral spinal cord and nerves at abdomen, lower back and pelvis level

Note: Code to highest level of lumbar cord injury
Injuries to the spinal cord (S34.0 and S34.1) refer to the cord level and not bone level injury, and can affect nerve roots at and below the level given.
Code also any associated:
   fracture of vertebra (S22.0-, S32.0-)
   open wound of abdomen, lower back and pelvis (S31.-)
   transient paralysis (R29.5)

The appropriate 7th character is to be added to each code from category S34
A   initial encounter
D   subsequent encounter
S   sequela

> **CODING TIP ✓** When coding sequelae of a lumbar and/or sacral spinal cord injury, first list the residual condition(s), followed by the specific spinal cord injury diagnosed using the appropriate code from category S34 with the seventh character "S" to indicate sequelae.

> **CODING TIP ✓** When coding sequelae of a spinal cord injury, first list the residual condition(s), followed by the specific spinal cord injury diagnosed using the appropriate code from this category with the seventh character "S" to indicate sequelae. If there are multiple levels of injury, code only the highest injury.

⑤ S34.0   Concussion and edema of lumbar and sacral spinal cord
  ⑦ S34.01X-   Concussion and edema of lumbar spinal cord
  ⑦ S34.02X-   Concussion and edema of sacral spinal cord
     Concussion and edema of conus medullaris

⑤ S34.1   Other and unspecified injury of lumbar and sacral spinal cord
  Ⓖ S34.10   Unspecified injury to lumbar spinal cord
    ▲ ⑦ S34.101-   Unspecified injury to L1 level of lumbar spinal cord
      Unspecified injury to lumbar spinal cord level 1
    ▲ ⑦ S34.102-   Unspecified injury to L2 level of lumbar spinal cord
      Unspecified injury to lumbar spinal cord level 2
    ▲ ⑦ S34.103-   Unspecified injury to L3 level of lumbar spinal cord
      Unspecified injury to lumbar spinal cord level 3
    ▲ ⑦ S34.104-   Unspecified injury to L4 level of lumbar spinal cord
      Unspecified injury to lumbar spinal cord level 4
    ▲ ⑦ S34.105-   Unspecified injury to L5 level of lumbar spinal cord
      Unspecified injury to lumbar spinal cord level 5
    ⑦ S34.109-   Unspecified injury to unspecified level of lumbar spinal cord

  Ⓖ S34.11   Complete lesion of lumbar spinal cord
    ▲ ⑦ S34.111-   Complete lesion of L1 level of lumbar spinal cord
      Complete lesion of lumbar spinal cord level 1
    ▲ ⑦ S34.112-   Complete lesion of L2 level of lumbar spinal cord
      Complete lesion of lumbar spinal cord level 2
    ▲ ⑦ S34.113-   Complete lesion of L3 level of lumbar spinal cord
      Complete lesion of lumbar spinal cord level 3
    ▲ ⑦ S34.114-   Complete lesion of L4 level of lumbar spinal cord
      Complete lesion of lumbar spinal cord level 4
    ▲ ⑦ S34.115-   Complete lesion of L5 level of lumbar spinal cord
      Complete lesion of lumbar spinal cord level 5
    ⑦ S34.119-   Complete lesion of unspecified level of lumbar spinal cord

  Ⓖ S34.12   Incomplete lesion of lumbar spinal cord
    ▲ ⑦ S34.121-   Incomplete lesion of L1 level of lumbar spinal cord
      Incomplete lesion of lumbar spinal cord level 1
    ▲ ⑦ S34.122-   Incomplete lesion of L2 level of lumbar spinal cord
      Incomplete lesion of lumbar spinal cord level 2
    ▲ ⑦ S34.123-   Incomplete lesion of L3 level of lumbar spinal cord
      Incomplete lesion of lumbar spinal cord level 3

    ▲ ⑦ S34.124-   Incomplete lesion of L4 level of lumbar spinal cord
      Incomplete lesion of lumbar spinal cord level 4
    ▲ ⑦ S34.125-   Incomplete lesion of L5 level of lumbar spinal cord
      Incomplete lesion of lumbar spinal cord level 5
    ⑦ S34.129-   Incomplete lesion of unspecified level of lumbar spinal cord

  Ⓖ S34.13   Other and unspecified injury to sacral spinal cord
    Other injury to conus medullaris
    ⑦ S34.131-   Complete lesion of sacral spinal cord
      Complete lesion of conus medullaris
    ⑦ S34.132-   Incomplete lesion of sacral spinal cord
      Incomplete lesion of conus medullaris
    ⑦ S34.139-   Unspecified injury to sacral spinal cord
      Unspecified injury of conus medullaris

⑤ S34.2   Injury of nerve root of lumbar and sacral spine
  ⑦ S34.21X-   Injury of nerve root of lumbar spine
  ⑦ S34.22X-   Injury of nerve root of sacral spine
⑦ S34.3XX-   Injury of cauda equina
⑦ S34.4XX-   Injury of lumbosacral plexus
⑦ S34.5XX-   Injury of lumbar, sacral and pelvic sympathetic nerves
  Injury of celiac ganglion or plexus
  Injury of hypogastric plexus
  Injury of mesenteric plexus (inferior) (superior)
  Injury of splanchnic nerve
⑦ S34.6XX-   Injury of peripheral nerve(s) at abdomen, lower back and pelvis level
⑦ S34.8XX-   Injury of other nerves at abdomen, lower back and pelvis level
⑦ S34.9XX-   Injury of unspecified nerves at abdomen, lower back and pelvis level

⬛ S35   Injury of blood vessels at abdomen, lower back and pelvis level

Code also:
   any associated open wound (S31.-)

The appropriate 7th character is to be added to each code from category S35
A   initial encounter
D   subsequent encounter
S   sequela

⑤ S35.0   Injury of abdominal aorta
   EXCLUDES 1 *injury of aorta NOS (S25.0)*
  ⑦ S35.00X-   Unspecified injury of abdominal aorta
  ⑦ S35.01X-   Minor laceration of abdominal aorta
    Incomplete transection of abdominal aorta
    Laceration of abdominal aorta NOS
    Superficial laceration of abdominal aorta
  ⑦ S35.02X-   Major laceration of abdominal aorta
    Complete transection of abdominal aorta
    Traumatic rupture of abdominal aorta
  ⑦ S35.09X-   Other injury of abdominal aorta

⑤ S35.1   Injury of inferior vena cava
   Injury of hepatic vein
   EXCLUDES 1 *injury of vena cava NOS (S25.2)*
  ⑦ S35.10X-   Unspecified injury of inferior vena cava
  ⑦ S35.11X-   Minor laceration of inferior vena cava
    Incomplete transection of inferior vena cava
    Laceration of inferior vena cava NOS
    Superficial laceration of inferior vena cava
  ⑦ S35.12X-   Major laceration of inferior vena cava
    Complete transection of inferior vena cava
    Traumatic rupture of inferior vena cava
  ⑦ S35.19X-   Other injury of inferior vena cava

⑤ S35.2   Injury of celiac or mesenteric artery and branches
  Ⓖ S35.21   Injury of celiac artery
    ⑦ S35.211-   Minor laceration of celiac artery
      Incomplete transection of celiac artery
      Laceration of celiac artery NOS
      Superficial laceration of celiac artery
    ⑦ S35.212-   Major laceration of celiac artery
      Complete transection of celiac artery
      Traumatic rupture of celiac artery
    ⑦ S35.218-   Other injury of celiac artery
    ⑦ S35.219-   Unspecified injury of celiac artery

● New   ▲ Revised   *Manifestation*   ⬛-⑦ Digit Indicators   ▤ Laterality   Ⓐ Adult (15+ years)   Ⓜ Maternity (12-55 years)   Ⓝ Newborn   Ⓟ Pediatric (0-17 years)   ♂ Male   ♀ Female
✖ Deleted   Unspecified   ✚ Additional code

952   © 2017 DecisionHealth   2017 ICD-10-CM Expert for Physicians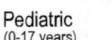

6 S35.22 Injury of superior mesenteric artery
- **7 S35.221- Minor laceration of superior mesenteric artery**
  Incomplete transection of superior mesenteric artery
  Laceration of superior mesenteric artery NOS
  Superficial laceration of superior mesenteric artery
- **7 S35.222- Major laceration of superior mesenteric artery**
  Complete transection of superior mesenteric artery
  Traumatic rupture of superior mesenteric artery
- **7 S35.228- Other injury of superior mesenteric artery**
- **7 S35.229- Unspecified injury of superior mesenteric artery**

6 S35.23 Injury of inferior mesenteric artery
- **7 S35.231- Minor laceration of inferior mesenteric artery**
  Incomplete transection of inferior mesenteric artery
  Laceration of inferior mesenteric artery NOS
  Superficial laceration of inferior mesenteric artery
- **7 S35.232- Major laceration of inferior mesenteric artery**
  Complete transection of inferior mesenteric artery
  Traumatic rupture of inferior mesenteric artery
- **7 S35.238- Other injury of inferior mesenteric artery**
- **7 S35.239- Unspecified injury of inferior mesenteric artery**

6 S35.29 Injury of branches of celiac and mesenteric artery
  Injury of gastric artery
  Injury of gastroduodenal artery
  Injury of hepatic artery
  Injury of splenic artery
- **7 S35.291- Minor laceration of branches of celiac and mesenteric artery**
  Incomplete transection of branches of celiac and mesenteric artery
  Laceration of branches of celiac and mesenteric artery NOS
  Superficial laceration of branches of celiac and mesenteric artery
- **7 S35.292- Major laceration of branches of celiac and mesenteric artery**
  Complete transection of branches of celiac and mesenteric artery
  Traumatic rupture of branches of celiac and mesenteric artery
- **7 S35.298- Other injury of branches of celiac and mesenteric artery**
- **7 S35.299- Unspecified injury of branches of celiac and mesenteric artery**

5 S35.3 Injury of portal or splenic vein and branches
6 S35.31 Injury of portal vein
- **7 S35.311- Laceration of portal vein**
- **7 S35.318- Other specified injury of portal vein**
- **7 S35.319- Unspecified injury of portal vein**
6 S35.32 Injury of splenic vein
- **7 S35.321- Laceration of splenic vein**
- **7 S35.328- Other specified injury of splenic vein**
- **7 S35.329- Unspecified injury of splenic vein**
6 S35.33 Injury of superior mesenteric vein
- **7 S35.331- Laceration of superior mesenteric vein**
- **7 S35.338- Other specified injury of superior mesenteric vein**
- **7 S35.339- Unspecified injury of superior mesenteric vein**
6 S35.34 Injury of inferior mesenteric vein
- **7 S35.341- Laceration of inferior mesenteric vein**
- **7 S35.348- Other specified injury of inferior mesenteric vein**
- **7 S35.349- Unspecified injury of inferior mesenteric vein**

5 S35.4 Injury of renal blood vessels
6 S35.40 Unspecified injury of renal blood vessel
- **7 S35.401- Unspecified injury of right renal artery**
- **7 S35.402- Unspecified injury of left renal artery**
- **7 S35.403- Unspecified injury of unspecified renal artery**
- **7 S35.404- Unspecified injury of right renal vein**
- **7 S35.405- Unspecified injury of left renal vein**
- **7 S35.406- Unspecified injury of unspecified renal vein**
6 S35.41 Laceration of renal blood vessel
- **7 S35.411- Laceration of right renal artery**
- **7 S35.412- Laceration of left renal artery**
- **7 S35.413- Laceration of unspecified renal artery**
- **7 S35.414- Laceration of right renal vein**
- **7 S35.415- Laceration of left renal vein**
- **7 S35.416- Laceration of unspecified renal vein**
6 S35.49 Other specified injury of renal blood vessel
- **7 S35.491- Other specified injury of right renal artery**
- **7 S35.492- Other specified injury of left renal artery**
- **7 S35.493- Other specified injury of unspecified renal artery**
- **7 S35.494- Other specified injury of right renal vein**
- **7 S35.495- Other specified injury of left renal vein**
- **7 S35.496- Other specified injury of unspecified renal vein**

5 S35.5 Injury of iliac blood vessels
- **7 S35.50X- Injury of unspecified iliac blood vessel(s)**
6 S35.51 Injury of iliac artery or vein
  Injury of hypogastric artery or vein
- **7 S35.511- Injury of right iliac artery**
- **7 S35.512- Injury of left iliac artery**
- **7 S35.513- Injury of unspecified iliac artery**
- **7 S35.514- Injury of right iliac vein**
- **7 S35.515- Injury of left iliac vein**
- **7 S35.516- Injury of unspecified iliac vein**
6 S35.53 Injury of uterine artery or vein
- **7 S35.531- Injury of right uterine artery**
- **7 S35.532- Injury of left uterine artery**
- **7 S35.533- Injury of unspecified uterine artery**
- **7 S35.534- Injury of right uterine vein**
- **7 S35.535- Injury of left uterine vein**
- **7 S35.536- Injury of unspecified uterine vein**
- **7 S35.59X- Injury of other iliac blood vessels**
5 S35.8 Injury of other blood vessels at abdomen, lower back and pelvis level
  Injury of ovarian artery or vein
6 S35.8X Injury of other blood vessels at abdomen, lower back and pelvis level
- **7 S35.8X1- Laceration of other blood vessels at abdomen, lower back and pelvis level**
- **7 S35.8X8- Other specified injury of other blood vessels at abdomen, lower back and pelvis level**
- **7 S35.8X9- Unspecified injury of other blood vessels at abdomen, lower back and pelvis level**
5 S35.9 Injury of unspecified blood vessel at abdomen, lower back and pelvis level
- **7 S35.90X- Unspecified injury of unspecified blood vessel at abdomen, lower back and pelvis level**
- **7 S35.91X- Laceration of unspecified blood vessel at abdomen, lower back and pelvis level**
- **7 S35.99X- Other specified injury of unspecified blood vessel at abdomen, lower back and pelvis level**

4 S36 Injury of intra-abdominal organs
Code also:
  any associated open wound (S31.-)

The appropriate 7th character is to be added to each code from category S36
A   initial encounter
D   subsequent encounter
S   sequela

CODING TIP ✓ Codes from category S36 do not include injury to intra-abdominal organs resulting from intra-operative complications. When Intra-operative complications occur, the appropriate complication code from the disease-specific chapter should be assigned (Intraoperative and postprocedural complications), as well as any T codes indicating further information on the complication.

5 S36.0 Injury of spleen
- **7 S36.00X- Unspecified injury of spleen**
6 S36.02 Contusion of spleen
- **7 S36.020- Minor contusion of spleen**
  Contusion of spleen less than 2 cm
- **7 S36.021- Major contusion of spleen**
  Contusion of spleen greater than 2 cm

7 **S36.029-** **Unspecified contusion of spleen**
AHA: (S36.029A) 1Q 2015, 11

6 **S36.03** **Laceration of spleen**

7 **S36.030-** **Superficial (capsular) laceration of spleen**
Laceration of spleen less than 1 cm
Minor laceration of spleen

7 **S36.031-** **Moderate laceration of spleen**
Laceration of spleen 1 to 3 cm
AHA: (S36.031A) 1Q 2015, 11

7 **S36.032-** **Major laceration of spleen**
Avulsion of spleen
Laceration of spleen greater than 3 cm
Massive laceration of spleen
Multiple moderate lacerations of spleen
Stellate laceration of spleen

7 **S36.039-** **Unspecified laceration of spleen**

7 **S36.09X-** **Other injury of spleen**

5 **S36.1** **Injury of liver and gallbladder and bile duct**

6 **S36.11** **Injury of liver**

7 **S36.112-** **Contusion of liver**

7 **S36.113-** **Laceration of liver, unspecified degree**

7 **S36.114-** **Minor laceration of liver**
Laceration involving capsule only, or, without
significant involvement of hepatic parenchyma
[i.e., less than 1 cm deep]

7 **S36.115-** **Moderate laceration of liver**
Laceration involving parenchyma but without
major disruption of parenchyma [i.e., less than
10 cm long and less than 3 cm deep]

7 **S36.116-** **Major laceration of liver**
Laceration with significant disruption of hepatic
parenchyma [i.e., greater than 10 cm long and 3
cm deep]
Multiple moderate lacerations, with or without
hematoma
Stellate laceration of liver

7 **S36.118-** **Other injury of liver**

7 **S36.119-** **Unspecified injury of liver**
AHA: 2Q 2015, 17

6 **S36.12** **Injury of gallbladder**

7 **S36.122-** **Contusion of gallbladder**

7 **S36.123-** **Laceration of gallbladder**

7 **S36.128-** **Other injury of gallbladder**

7 **S36.129-** **Unspecified injury of gallbladder**

7 **S36.13X-** **Injury of bile duct**

5 **S36.2** **Injury of pancreas**

6 **S36.20** **Unspecified injury of pancreas**

7 **S36.200-** **Unspecified injury of head of pancreas**

7 **S36.201-** **Unspecified injury of body of pancreas**

7 **S36.202-** **Unspecified injury of tail of pancreas**

7 **S36.209-** **Unspecified injury of unspecified part of
pancreas**

6 **S36.22** **Contusion of pancreas**

7 **S36.220-** **Contusion of head of pancreas**

7 **S36.221-** **Contusion of body of pancreas**

7 **S36.222-** **Contusion of tail of pancreas**

7 **S36.229-** **Contusion of unspecified part of pancreas**

6 **S36.23** **Laceration of pancreas, unspecified degree**

7 **S36.230-** **Laceration of head of pancreas, unspecified
degree**

7 **S36.231-** **Laceration of body of pancreas, unspecified
degree**

7 **S36.232-** **Laceration of tail of pancreas, unspecified
degree**

7 **S36.239-** **Laceration of unspecified part of pancreas,
unspecified degree**

6 **S36.24** **Minor laceration of pancreas**

7 **S36.240-** **Minor laceration of head of pancreas**

7 **S36.241-** **Minor laceration of body of pancreas**

7 **S36.242-** **Minor laceration of tail of pancreas**

7 **S36.249-** **Minor laceration of unspecified part of
pancreas**

6 **S36.25** **Moderate laceration of pancreas**

7 **S36.250-** **Moderate laceration of head of pancreas**

7 **S36.251-** **Moderate laceration of body of pancreas**

7 **S36.252-** **Moderate laceration of tail of pancreas**

7 **S36.259-** **Moderate laceration of unspecified part of
pancreas**

6 **S36.26** **Major laceration of pancreas**

7 **S36.260-** **Major laceration of head of pancreas**

7 **S36.261-** **Major laceration of body of pancreas**

7 **S36.262-** **Major laceration of tail of pancreas**

7 **S36.269-** **Major laceration of unspecified part of
pancreas**

6 **S36.29** **Other injury of pancreas**

7 **S36.290-** **Other injury of head of pancreas**

7 **S36.291-** **Other injury of body of pancreas**

7 **S36.292-** **Other injury of tail of pancreas**

7 **S36.299-** **Other injury of unspecified part of pancreas**

5 **S36.3** **Injury of stomach**

7 **S36.30X-** **Unspecified injury of stomach**

7 **S36.32X-** **Contusion of stomach**

7 **S36.33X-** **Laceration of stomach**

7 **S36.39X-** **Other injury of stomach**

5 **S36.4** **Injury of small intestine**

6 **S36.40** **Unspecified injury of small intestine**

7 **S36.400-** **Unspecified injury of duodenum**

7 **S36.408-** **Unspecified injury of other part of small
intestine**

7 **S36.409-** **Unspecified injury of unspecified part of small
intestine**

6 **S36.41** **Primary blast injury of small intestine**
Blast injury of small intestine NOS

7 **S36.410-** **Primary blast injury of duodenum**

7 **S36.418-** **Primary blast injury of other part of small
intestine**

7 **S36.419-** **Primary blast injury of unspecified part of
small intestine**

6 **S36.42** **Contusion of small intestine**

7 **S36.420-** **Contusion of duodenum**

7 **S36.428-** **Contusion of other part of small intestine**

7 **S36.429-** **Contusion of unspecified part of small
intestine**

6 **S36.43** **Laceration of small intestine**

7 **S36.430-** **Laceration of duodenum**

7 **S36.438-** **Laceration of other part of small intestine**

7 **S36.439-** **Laceration of unspecified part of small
intestine**

6 **S36.49** **Other injury of small intestine**

7 **S36.490-** **Other injury of duodenum**

7 **S36.498-** **Other injury of other part of small intestine**

7 **S36.499-** **Other injury of unspecified part of small
intestine**

5 **S36.5** **Injury of colon**
EXCLUDES 2 *injury of rectum (S36.6-)*

6 **S36.50** **Unspecified injury of colon**

7 **S36.500-** **Unspecified injury of ascending [right] colon**

7 **S36.501-** **Unspecified injury of transverse colon**

7 **S36.502-** **Unspecified injury of descending [left] colon**

7 **S36.503-** **Unspecified injury of sigmoid colon**

7 **S36.508-** **Unspecified injury of other part of colon**

7 **S36.509-** **Unspecified injury of unspecified part of colon**

6 **S36.51** **Primary blast injury of colon**
Blast injury of colon NOS

7 **S36.510-** **Primary blast injury of ascending [right] colon**

7 **S36.511-** **Primary blast injury of transverse colon**

7 **S36.512-** **Primary blast injury of descending [left] colon**

7 **S36.513-** **Primary blast injury of sigmoid colon**

7 **S36.518-** **Primary blast injury of other part of colon**

7 **S36.519-** **Primary blast injury of unspecified part of
colon**

6 **S36.52** **Contusion of colon**

7 **S36.520-** **Contusion of ascending [right] colon**

7 **S36.521-** **Contusion of transverse colon**

7 **S36.522-** **Contusion of descending [left] colon**

● New   ▲ Revised   *Manifestation*   4-7 Digit Indicators   ▱ Laterality   A Adult (15+ years)   M Maternity (12-55 years)   N Newborn   P Pediatric (0-17 years)   ♂ Male   ♀ Female
✖ Deleted   Unspecified   + Additional code

954   © 2017 DecisionHealth   2017 ICD-10-CM Expert for Physicians

7	S36.523-	Contusion of sigmoid colon
7	S36.528-	Contusion of other part of colon
7	S36.529-	Contusion of unspecified part of colon
6	S36.53	Laceration of colon
7	S36.530-	Laceration of ascending [right] colon
7	S36.531-	Laceration of transverse colon
7	S36.532-	Laceration of descending [left] colon
7	S36.533-	Laceration of sigmoid colon
7	S36.538-	Laceration of other part of colon
7	S36.539-	Laceration of unspecified part of colon

6 S36.59   **Other injury of colon**
Secondary blast injury of colon

7	S36.590-	Other injury of ascending [right] colon
7	S36.591-	Other injury of transverse colon
7	S36.592-	Other injury of descending [left] colon
7	S36.593-	Other injury of sigmoid colon
7	S36.598-	Other injury of other part of colon
7	S36.599-	Other injury of unspecified part of colon

5 S36.6   **Injury of rectum**

7	S36.60X-	Unspecified injury of rectum
7	S36.61X-	Primary blast injury of rectum

Blast injury of rectum NOS

7	S36.62X-	Contusion of rectum
7	S36.63X-	Laceration of rectum
7	S36.69X-	Other injury of rectum

Secondary blast injury of rectum

5 S36.8   **Injury of other intra-abdominal organs**

7	S36.81X-	Injury of peritoneum
6	S36.89	Injury of other intra-abdominal organs

Injury of retroperitoneum

7	S36.892-	Contusion of other intra-abdominal organs
7	S36.893-	Laceration of other intra-abdominal organs
7	S36.898-	Other injury of other intra-abdominal organs
7	S36.899-	Unspecified injury of other intra-abdominal organs

5 S36.9   **Injury of unspecified intra-abdominal organ**

7	S36.90X-	Unspecified injury of unspecified intra-abdominal organ
7	S36.92X-	Contusion of unspecified intra-abdominal organ
7	S36.93X-	Laceration of unspecified intra-abdominal organ
7	S36.99X-	Other injury of unspecified intra-abdominal organ

4 **S37   Injury of urinary and pelvic organs**

Code also:
any associated open wound (S31.-)

EXCLUDES 1   *obstetric trauma to pelvic organs (O71.-)*

EXCLUDES 2   *injury of peritoneum (S36.81)*
injury of retroperitoneum (S36.89-)

The appropriate 7th character is to be added to each code from category S37
A   initial encounter
D   subsequent encounter
S   sequela

CODING TIP ✓   Codes from category S37 do not include injury to urinary and pelvic organs resulting from intra-operative complications. When Intra-operative complications occur, the appropriate complication code from the disease-specific chapter should be assigned (Intraoperative and postprocedural complications), as well as any T codes indicating further information on the complication.

5 S37.0   **Injury of kidney**

EXCLUDES 2   *acute kidney injury (nontraumatic) (N17.9)*

6 S37.00   **Unspecified injury of kidney**

7 ⊟	S37.001-	Unspecified injury of right kidney
7 ⊟	S37.002-	Unspecified injury of left kidney
7 ⊟	S37.009-	Unspecified injury of unspecified kidney

6 S37.01   **Minor contusion of kidney**
Contusion of kidney less than 2 cm
Contusion of kidney NOS

7 ⊟	S37.011-	Minor contusion of right kidney
7 ⊟	S37.012-	Minor contusion of left kidney
7 ⊟	S37.019-	Minor contusion of unspecified kidney

6 S37.02   **Major contusion of kidney**
Contusion of kidney greater than 2 cm

7 ⊟	S37.021-	Major contusion of right kidney
7 ⊟	S37.022-	Major contusion of left kidney
7 ⊟	S37.029-	Major contusion of unspecified kidney

6 S37.03   **Laceration of kidney, unspecified degree**

7 ⊟	S37.031-	Laceration of right kidney, unspecified degree
7 ⊟	S37.032-	Laceration of left kidney, unspecified degree
7 ⊟	S37.039-	Laceration of unspecified kidney, unspecified degree

6 S37.04   **Minor laceration of kidney**
Laceration of kidney less than 1 cm

7 ⊟	S37.041-	Minor laceration of right kidney
7 ⊟	S37.042-	Minor laceration of left kidney
7 ⊟	S37.049-	Minor laceration of unspecified kidney

6 S37.05   **Moderate laceration of kidney**
Laceration of kidney 1 to 3 cm

7 ⊟	S37.051-	Moderate laceration of right kidney
7 ⊟	S37.052-	Moderate laceration of left kidney
7 ⊟	S37.059-	Moderate laceration of unspecified kidney

6 S37.06   **Major laceration of kidney**
Avulsion of kidney
Laceration of kidney greater than 3 cm
Massive laceration of kidney
Multiple moderate lacerations of kidney
Stellate laceration of kidney

7 ⊟	S37.061-	Major laceration of right kidney
7 ⊟	S37.062-	Major laceration of left kidney
7 ⊟	S37.069-	Major laceration of unspecified kidney

6 S37.09   **Other injury of kidney**

7 ⊟	S37.091-	Other injury of right kidney
7 ⊟	S37.092-	Other injury of left kidney
7 ⊟	S37.099-	Other injury of unspecified kidney

5 S37.1   **Injury of ureter**

7	S37.10X-	Unspecified injury of ureter
7	S37.12X-	Contusion of ureter
7	S37.13X-	Laceration of ureter
7	S37.19X-	Other injury of ureter

5 S37.2   **Injury of bladder**

7	S37.20X-	Unspecified injury of bladder
7	S37.22X-	Contusion of bladder
7	S37.23X-	Laceration of bladder
7	S37.29X-	Other injury of bladder

5 S37.3   **Injury of urethra**

7	S37.30X-	Unspecified injury of urethra
7	S37.32X-	Contusion of urethra
7	S37.33X-	Laceration of urethra
7	S37.39X-	Other injury of urethra

5 S37.4   **Injury of ovary**

6 S37.40   **Unspecified injury of ovary**

7	S37.401-	Unspecified injury of ovary, unilateral
7	S37.402-	Unspecified injury of ovary, bilateral
7	S37.409-	Unspecified injury of ovary, unspecified

6 S37.42   **Contusion of ovary**

7	S37.421-	Contusion of ovary, unilateral
7	S37.422-	Contusion of ovary, bilateral
7	S37.429-	Contusion of ovary, unspecified

6 S37.43   **Laceration of ovary**

7	S37.431-	Laceration of ovary, unilateral
7	S37.432-	Laceration of ovary, bilateral
7	S37.439-	Laceration of ovary, unspecified

6 S37.49   **Other injury of ovary**

7	S37.491-	Other injury of ovary, unilateral
7	S37.492-	Other injury of ovary, bilateral
7	S37.499-	Other injury of ovary, unspecified

5 S37.5   **Injury of fallopian tube**

6 S37.50   **Unspecified injury of fallopian tube**

7	S37.501-	Unspecified injury of fallopian tube, unilateral
7	S37.502-	Unspecified injury of fallopian tube, bilateral

● New   ▲ Revised   *Manifestation*   4-7 Digit Indicators   ⊟ Laterality   Ⓐ Adult (15+ years)   Ⓜ Maternity (12-55 years)   Ⓝ Newborn   Ⓟ Pediatric (0-17 years)   ♂ Male   ♀ Female
✖ Deleted   Unspecified   + Additional code

7 S37.509- Unspecified injury of fallopian tube, unspecified

6 S37.51 Primary blast injury of fallopian tube
Blast injury of fallopian tube NOS

7 S37.511- Primary blast injury of fallopian tube, unilateral

7 S37.512- Primary blast injury of fallopian tube, bilateral

7 S37.519- Primary blast injury of fallopian tube, unspecified

6 S37.52 Contusion of fallopian tube

7 S37.521- Contusion of fallopian tube, unilateral

7 S37.522- Contusion of fallopian tube, bilateral

7 S37.529- Contusion of fallopian tube, unspecified

6 S37.53 Laceration of fallopian tube

7 S37.531- Laceration of fallopian tube, unilateral

7 S37.532- Laceration of fallopian tube, bilateral

7 S37.539- Laceration of fallopian tube, unspecified

6 S37.59 Other injury of fallopian tube
Secondary blast injury of fallopian tube

7 S37.591- Other injury of fallopian tube, unilateral

7 S37.592- Other injury of fallopian tube, bilateral

7 S37.599- Other injury of fallopian tube, unspecified

5 S37.6 Injury of uterus

> **EXCLUDES 1** *injury to gravid uterus (O9A.2-)*
> *injury to uterus during delivery (O71.-)*

7 S37.60X- Unspecified injury of uterus

7 S37.62X- Contusion of uterus

7 S37.63X- Laceration of uterus

7 S37.69X- Other injury of uterus

5 S37.8 Injury of other urinary and pelvic organs

6 S37.81 Injury of adrenal gland

7 S37.812- Contusion of adrenal gland

7 S37.813- Laceration of adrenal gland

7 S37.818- Other injury of adrenal gland

7 S37.819- Unspecified injury of adrenal gland

6 S37.82 Injury of prostate

7 S37.822- Contusion of prostate

7 S37.823- Laceration of prostate

7 S37.828- Other injury of prostate

7 S37.829- Unspecified injury of prostate

6 S37.89 Injury of other urinary and pelvic organ

7 S37.892- Contusion of other urinary and pelvic organ

7 S37.893- Laceration of other urinary and pelvic organ

7 S37.898- Other injury of other urinary and pelvic organ

7 S37.899- Unspecified injury of other urinary and pelvic organ

5 S37.9 Injury of unspecified urinary and pelvic organ

7 S37.90X- Unspecified injury of unspecified urinary and pelvic organ

7 S37.92X- Contusion of unspecified urinary and pelvic organ

7 S37.93X- Laceration of unspecified urinary and pelvic organ

7 S37.99X- Other injury of unspecified urinary and pelvic organ

4 S38 **Crushing injury and traumatic amputation of abdomen, lower back, pelvis and external genitals**
An amputation not identified as partial or complete should be coded to complete

The appropriate 7th character is to be added to each code from category S38
A   initial encounter
D   subsequent encounter
S   sequela

5 + S38.0 Crushing injury of external genital organs
Use additional code for any associated injuries

6 + S38.00 Crushing injury of unspecified external genital organs

7 + S38.001- Crushing injury of unspecified external genital organs, male

7 + S38.002- Crushing injury of unspecified external genital organs, female

7 + S38.01X- Crushing injury of penis

7 + S38.02X- Crushing injury of scrotum and testis

7 + S38.03X- Crushing injury of vulva

7 + S38.1XX- Crushing injury of abdomen, lower back, and pelvis
Use additional code for all associated injuries, such as:
fracture of thoracic or lumbar spine and pelvis
(S22.0-, S32.-)
injury to intra-abdominal organs (S36.-)
injury to urinary and pelvic organs (S37.-)
open wound of abdominal wall (S31.-)
spinal cord injury (S34.0, S34.1-)

> **EXCLUDES 2** *crushing injury of external genital organs (S38.0-)*

5 S38.2 Traumatic amputation of external genital organs

6 S38.21 Traumatic amputation of female external genital organs
Traumatic amputation of clitoris
Traumatic amputation of labium (majus) (minus)
Traumatic amputation of vulva

7 S38.211- Complete traumatic amputation of female external genital organs

7 S38.212- Partial traumatic amputation of female external genital organs

6 S38.22 Traumatic amputation of penis

7 S38.221- Complete traumatic amputation of penis

7 S38.222- Partial traumatic amputation of penis

6 S38.23 Traumatic amputation of scrotum and testis

7 S38.231- Complete traumatic amputation of scrotum and testis

7 S38.232- Partial traumatic amputation of scrotum and testis

7 S38.3XX- Transection (partial) of abdomen

4 S39 **Other and unspecified injuries of abdomen, lower back, pelvis and external genitals**
Code also:
any associated open wound (S31.-)

> **EXCLUDES 2** *sprain of joints and ligaments of lumbar spine and pelvis (S33.-)*

The appropriate 7th character is to be added to each code from category S39
A   initial encounter
D   subsequent encounter
S   sequela

5 S39.0 Injury of muscle, fascia and tendon of abdomen, lower back and pelvis

6 S39.00 Unspecified injury of muscle, fascia and tendon of abdomen, lower back and pelvis

7 S39.001- Unspecified injury of muscle, fascia and tendon of abdomen

7 S39.002- Unspecified injury of muscle, fascia and tendon of lower back

7 S39.003- Unspecified injury of muscle, fascia and tendon of pelvis

6 S39.01 Strain of muscle, fascia and tendon of abdomen, lower back and pelvis

7 S39.011- Strain of muscle, fascia and tendon of abdomen

7 S39.012- Strain of muscle, fascia and tendon of lower back

7 S39.013- Strain of muscle, fascia and tendon of pelvis

6 S39.02 Laceration of muscle, fascia and tendon of abdomen, lower back and pelvis

7 S39.021- Laceration of muscle, fascia and tendon of abdomen

7 S39.022- Laceration of muscle, fascia and tendon of lower back

7 S39.023- Laceration of muscle, fascia and tendon of pelvis

6 S39.09 Other injury of muscle, fascia and tendon of abdomen, lower back and pelvis

7 S39.091- Other injury of muscle, fascia and tendon of abdomen

7 S39.092- Other injury of muscle, fascia and tendon of lower back

7 S39.093- Other injury of muscle, fascia and tendon of pelvis

5 S39.8 Other specified injuries of abdomen, lower back, pelvis and external genitals

7 S39.81X- Other specified injuries of abdomen

● New   ▲ Revised   *Manifestation*   4 - 7 Digit Indicators   ⊟ Laterality   A Adult (15+ years)   M Maternity (12-55 years)   N Newborn   P Pediatric (0-17 years)   ♂ Male   ♀ Female
✖ Deleted   Unspecified   + Additional code

956   © 2017 DecisionHealth   2017 ICD-10-CM Expert for Physicians

7 S39.82X-   Other specified injuries of lower back
7 S39.83X-   Other specified injuries of pelvis
6 S39.84   Other specified injuries of external genitals
   7 S39.840-   Fracture of corpus cavernosum penis
   7 S39.848-   Other specified injuries of external genitals
5 S39.9   Unspecified injury of abdomen, lower back, pelvis and external genitals
7 S39.91X-   Unspecified injury of abdomen
7 S39.92X-   Unspecified injury of lower back
7 S39.93X-   Unspecified injury of pelvis
7 S39.94X-   Unspecified injury of external genitals

Injuries to the shoulder and upper arm (S40-S49)

INCLUDES injuries of axilla
           injuries of scapular region
EXCLUDES 2 *burns and corrosions (T20-T32)*
           frostbite (T33-T34)
           injuries of elbow (S50-S59)
           insect bite or sting, venomous (T63.4)

GUIDELINES Section I.C.19.c.2)
Multiple fractures are sequenced in accordance with the severity of the fracture.

GUIDELINES Section I.C.19.b.1)-2)
When coding injuries, assign separate codes for each injury unless a combination code is provided, in which case the combination code is assigned ... Traumatic injury codes (S00-T14.9) are not to be used for normal, healing surgical wounds or to identify complications of surgical wounds. The code for the most serious injury, as determined by the provider and the focus of treatment, is sequenced first.

1) Superficial injuries such as abrasions or contusions are not coded when associated with more severe injuries of the same site.

2) When a primary injury results in minor damage to peripheral nerves or blood vessels, the primary injury is sequenced first with additional code(s) for injuries to nerves and spinal cord (such as category S04), and/or injury to blood vessels (such as category S15). When the primary injury is to the blood vessels or nerves, that injury should be sequenced first.

GUIDELINES Section I.C.19.c
Coding of Traumatic Fractures: The principles of multiple coding of injuries should be followed in coding fractures. Fractures of specified sites are coded individually by site in accordance with both the provisions within categories S02, S12, S22, S32, S42, S49, S52, S59, S62, S72, S79, S82, S89, S92 and the level of detail furnished by medical record content. A fracture not indicated as open or closed should be coded to closed. A fracture not indicated whether displaced or not displaced should be coded to displaced.

4 S40   **Superficial injury of shoulder and upper arm**

The appropriate 7th character is to be added to each code from category S40
  A   initial encounter
  D   subsequent encounter
  S   sequela

5 S40.0   Contusion of shoulder and upper arm
6 S40.01   Contusion of shoulder
7 S40.011-   Contusion of right shoulder
7 S40.012-   Contusion of left shoulder
7 S40.019-   Contusion of unspecified shoulder
6 S40.02   Contusion of upper arm
7 S40.021-   Contusion of right upper arm
7 S40.022-   Contusion of left upper arm
7 S40.029-   Contusion of unspecified upper arm
5 S40.2   Other superficial injuries of shoulder
6 S40.21   Abrasion of shoulder
7 S40.211-   Abrasion of right shoulder
7 S40.212-   Abrasion of left shoulder
7 S40.219-   Abrasion of unspecified shoulder
6 S40.22   Blister (nonthermal) of shoulder

7 S40.221-   Blister (nonthermal) of right shoulder
7 S40.222-   Blister (nonthermal) of left shoulder
7 S40.229-   Blister (nonthermal) of unspecified shoulder
6 S40.24   External constriction of shoulder
7 S40.241-   External constriction of right shoulder
7 S40.242-   External constriction of left shoulder
7 S40.249-   External constriction of unspecified shoulder
6 S40.25   Superficial foreign body of shoulder
    Splinter in the shoulder
7 S40.251-   Superficial foreign body of right shoulder
7 S40.252-   Superficial foreign body of left shoulder
7 S40.259-   Superficial foreign body of unspecified shoulder
6 S40.26   Insect bite (nonvenomous) of shoulder
7 S40.261-   Insect bite (nonvenomous) of right shoulder
7 S40.262-   Insect bite (nonvenomous) of left shoulder
7 S40.269-   Insect bite (nonvenomous) of unspecified shoulder
6 S40.27   Other superficial bite of shoulder
    EXCLUDES 1 *open bite of shoulder (S41.05)*
7 S40.271-   Other superficial bite of right shoulder
7 S40.272-   Other superficial bite of left shoulder
7 S40.279-   Other superficial bite of unspecified shoulder
5 S40.8   Other superficial injuries of upper arm
6 S40.81   Abrasion of upper arm
7 S40.811-   Abrasion of right upper arm
7 S40.812-   Abrasion of left upper arm
7 S40.819-   Abrasion of unspecified upper arm
6 S40.82   Blister (nonthermal) of upper arm
7 S40.821-   Blister (nonthermal) of right upper arm
7 S40.822-   Blister (nonthermal) of left upper arm
7 S40.829-   Blister (nonthermal) of unspecified upper arm
6 S40.84   External constriction of upper arm
7 S40.841-   External constriction of right upper arm
7 S40.842-   External constriction of left upper arm
7 S40.849-   External constriction of unspecified upper arm
6 S40.85   Superficial foreign body of upper arm
    Splinter in the upper arm
7 S40.851-   Superficial foreign body of right upper arm
7 S40.852-   Superficial foreign body of left upper arm
7 S40.859-   Superficial foreign body of unspecified upper arm
6 S40.86   Insect bite (nonvenomous) of upper arm
7 S40.861-   Insect bite (nonvenomous) of right upper arm
7 S40.862-   Insect bite (nonvenomous) of left upper arm
7 S40.869-   Insect bite (nonvenomous) of unspecified upper arm
6 S40.87   Other superficial bite of upper arm
    EXCLUDES 1 *open bite of upper arm (S41.14)*
    EXCLUDES 2 *other superficial bite of shoulder (S40.27-)*
7 S40.871-   Other superficial bite of right upper arm
7 S40.872-   Other superficial bite of left upper arm
7 S40.879-   Other superficial bite of unspecified upper arm
5 S40.9   Unspecified superficial injury of shoulder and upper arm
6 S40.91   Unspecified superficial injury of shoulder
7 S40.911-   Unspecified superficial injury of right shoulder
7 S40.912-   Unspecified superficial injury of left shoulder
7 S40.919-   Unspecified superficial injury of unspecified shoulder
6 S40.92   Unspecified superficial injury of upper arm
7 S40.921-   Unspecified superficial injury of right upper arm
7 S40.922-   Unspecified superficial injury of left upper arm

● New ▲ Revised *Manifestation* 4-7 Digit Indicators ⊟ Laterality A Adult (15+ years) M Maternity (12-55 years) N Newborn P Pediatric (0-17 years) ♂ Male ♀ Female
✖ Deleted Unspecified + Additional code

2017 ICD-10-CM Expert for Physicians   © 2017 DecisionHealth   957

7 ⊟ **S40.929-**   Unspecified superficial injury of unspecified upper arm

4 **S41**   **Open wound of shoulder and upper arm**

Code also:
any associated wound infection

> **EXCLUDES 1**   *traumatic amputation of shoulder and upper arm (S48.-)*

> **EXCLUDES 2**   *open fracture of shoulder and upper arm (S42.- with 7th character B or C)*

The appropriate 7th character is to be added to each code from category S41
A   initial encounter
D   subsequent encounter
S   sequela

> **CODING TIP ✓**   Open wound codes indicate a wound resulting from a traumatic origin. Do not assign a code for "open wound" unless the etiology of the wound is related to trauma.

5 **S41.0**   **Open wound of shoulder**

6 **S41.00**   **Unspecified open wound of shoulder**

7 ⊟ **S41.001-**   Unspecified open wound of right shoulder

7 ⊟ **S41.002-**   Unspecified open wound of left shoulder

7 ⊟ **S41.009-**   Unspecified open wound of unspecified shoulder

6 **S41.01**   **Laceration without foreign body of shoulder**

7 ⊟ **S41.011-**   Laceration without foreign body of right shoulder

7 ⊟ **S41.012-**   Laceration without foreign body of left shoulder

7 ⊟ **S41.019-**   Laceration without foreign body of unspecified shoulder

6 **S41.02**   **Laceration with foreign body of shoulder**

7 ⊟ **S41.021-**   Laceration with foreign body of right shoulder

7 ⊟ **S41.022-**   Laceration with foreign body of left shoulder

7 ⊟ **S41.029-**   Laceration with foreign body of unspecified shoulder

6 **S41.03**   **Puncture wound without foreign body of shoulder**

7 ⊟ **S41.031-**   Puncture wound without foreign body of right shoulder

7 ⊟ **S41.032-**   Puncture wound without foreign body of left shoulder

7 ⊟ **S41.039-**   Puncture wound without foreign body of unspecified shoulder

6 **S41.04**   **Puncture wound with foreign body of shoulder**

7 ⊟ **S41.041-**   Puncture wound with foreign body of right shoulder

7 ⊟ **S41.042-**   Puncture wound with foreign body of left shoulder

7 ⊟ **S41.049-**   Puncture wound with foreign body of unspecified shoulder

6 **S41.05**   **Open bite of shoulder**
Bite of shoulder NOS

> **EXCLUDES 1**   *superficial bite of shoulder (S40.27)*

7 ⊟ **S41.051-**   Open bite of right shoulder

7 ⊟ **S41.052-**   Open bite of left shoulder

7 ⊟ **S41.059-**   Open bite of unspecified shoulder

5 **S41.1**   **Open wound of upper arm**

6 **S41.10**   **Unspecified open wound of upper arm**

7 ⊟ **S41.101-**   Unspecified open wound of right upper arm

7 ⊟ **S41.102-**   Unspecified open wound of left upper arm

7 ⊟ **S41.109-**   Unspecified open wound of unspecified upper arm

6 **S41.11**   **Laceration without foreign body of upper arm**

7 ⊟ **S41.111-**   Laceration without foreign body of right upper arm

7 ⊟ **S41.112-**   Laceration without foreign body of left upper arm

7 ⊟ **S41.119-**   Laceration without foreign body of unspecified upper arm

6 **S41.12**   **Laceration with foreign body of upper arm**

7 ⊟ **S41.121-**   Laceration with foreign body of right upper arm

7 ⊟ **S41.122-**   Laceration with foreign body of left upper arm

7 ⊟ **S41.129-**   Laceration with foreign body of unspecified upper arm

6 **S41.13**   **Puncture wound without foreign body of upper arm**

7 ⊟ **S41.131-**   Puncture wound without foreign body of right upper arm

7 ⊟ **S41.132-**   Puncture wound without foreign body of left upper arm

7 ⊟ **S41.139-**   Puncture wound without foreign body of unspecified upper arm

6 **S41.14**   **Puncture wound with foreign body of upper arm**

7 ⊟ **S41.141-**   Puncture wound with foreign body of right upper arm

7 ⊟ **S41.142-**   Puncture wound with foreign body of left upper arm

7 ⊟ **S41.149-**   Puncture wound with foreign body of unspecified upper arm

6 **S41.15**   **Open bite of upper arm**
Bite of upper arm NOS

> **EXCLUDES 1**   *superficial bite of upper arm (S40.87)*

7 ⊟ **S41.151-**   Open bite of right upper arm

7 ⊟ **S41.152-**   Open bite of left upper arm

7 ⊟ **S41.159-**   Open bite of unspecified upper arm

4 **S42**   **Fracture of shoulder and upper arm**

Note: A fracture not indicated as displaced or nondisplaced should be coded to displaced
A fracture not indicated as open or closed should be coded to closed

> **EXCLUDES 1**   *traumatic amputation of shoulder and upper arm (S48.-)*

The appropriate 7th character is to be added to all codes from category S42
A   initial encounter for closed fracture
B   initial encounter for open fracture
D   subsequent encounter for fracture with routine healing
G   subsequent encounter for fracture with delayed healing
K   subsequent encounter for fracture with nonunion
P   subsequent encounter for fracture with malunion
S   sequela

> **CODING TIP ✓**   A fracture not indicated as displaced or nondisplaced should be coded to displaced. A fracture not indicated as open or closed should be coded to closed. Query providers on fractures not documented as displaced/nondisplaced otherwise displaced fracture diagnosis could be assigned without reduction being performed potentially resulting in claim denials.

5 **S42.0**   **Fracture of clavicle**

6 **S42.00**   **Fracture of unspecified part of clavicle**

7 ⊟ **S42.001-**   Fracture of unspecified part of right clavicle

7 ⊟ **S42.002-**   Fracture of unspecified part of left clavicle

7 ⊟ **S42.009-**   Fracture of unspecified part of unspecified clavicle
AHA: (S42.009D) 4Q 2012, 93

6 **S42.01**   **Fracture of sternal end of clavicle**

7 ⊟ **S42.011-**   Anterior displaced fracture of sternal end of right clavicle

7 ⊟ **S42.012-**   Anterior displaced fracture of sternal end of left clavicle

7 ⊟ **S42.013-**   Anterior displaced fracture of sternal end of unspecified clavicle
Displaced fracture of sternal end of clavicle NOS

7 ⊟ **S42.014-**   Posterior displaced fracture of sternal end of right clavicle

7 ⊟ **S42.015-**   Posterior displaced fracture of sternal end of left clavicle

7 ⊟ **S42.016-**   Posterior displaced fracture of sternal end of unspecified clavicle

7 ⊟ **S42.017-**   Nondisplaced fracture of sternal end of right clavicle

7 ⊟ **S42.018-**   Nondisplaced fracture of sternal end of left clavicle

7 ⊟ **S42.019-**   Nondisplaced fracture of sternal end of unspecified clavicle

6 **S42.02**   **Fracture of shaft of clavicle**

7 ⊟ **S42.021-**   Displaced fracture of shaft of right clavicle

7 ⊟ **S42.022-**   Displaced fracture of shaft of left clavicle

● New   ▲ Revised   *Manifestation*   4-7 Digit Indicators   ⊟ Laterality   ▲ Adult (15+ years)   Ⓜ Maternity (12-55 years)   Ⓝ Newborn   Ⓟ Pediatric (0-17 years)   ♂ Male   ♀ Female

✖ Deleted   Unspecified   ✚ Additional code

958   © 2017 DecisionHealth   2017 ICD-10-CM Expert for Physicians

7 ⊟ **S42.023-** Displaced fracture of shaft of unspecified clavicle
7 ⊟ **S42.024-** Nondisplaced fracture of shaft of right clavicle
7 ⊟ **S42.025-** Nondisplaced fracture of shaft of left clavicle
7 ⊟ **S42.026-** Nondisplaced fracture of shaft of unspecified clavicle

6 **S42.03** Fracture of lateral end of clavicle
Fracture of acromial end of clavicle
7 ⊟ **S42.031-** Displaced fracture of lateral end of right clavicle
7 ⊟ **S42.032-** Displaced fracture of lateral end of left clavicle
7 ⊟ **S42.033-** Displaced fracture of lateral end of unspecified clavicle
7 ⊟ **S42.034-** Nondisplaced fracture of lateral end of right clavicle
7 ⊟ **S42.035-** Nondisplaced fracture of lateral end of left clavicle
7 ⊟ **S42.036-** Nondisplaced fracture of lateral end of unspecified clavicle

5 **S42.1** Fracture of scapula
6 **S42.10** Fracture of unspecified part of scapula
7 ⊟ **S42.101-** Fracture of unspecified part of scapula, right shoulder
7 ⊟ **S42.102-** Fracture of unspecified part of scapula, left shoulder
7 ⊟ **S42.109-** Fracture of unspecified part of scapula, unspecified shoulder

6 **S42.11** Fracture of body of scapula
7 ⊟ **S42.111-** Displaced fracture of body of scapula, right shoulder
7 ⊟ **S42.112-** Displaced fracture of body of scapula, left shoulder
7 ⊟ **S42.113-** Displaced fracture of body of scapula, unspecified shoulder
7 ⊟ **S42.114-** Nondisplaced fracture of body of scapula, right shoulder
7 ⊟ **S42.115-** Nondisplaced fracture of body of scapula, left shoulder
7 ⊟ **S42.116-** Nondisplaced fracture of body of scapula, unspecified shoulder

6 **S42.12** Fracture of acromial process
7 ⊟ **S42.121-** Displaced fracture of acromial process, right shoulder
7 ⊟ **S42.122-** Displaced fracture of acromial process, left shoulder
7 ⊟ **S42.123-** Displaced fracture of acromial process, unspecified shoulder
7 ⊟ **S42.124-** Nondisplaced fracture of acromial process, right shoulder
7 ⊟ **S42.125-** Nondisplaced fracture of acromial process, left shoulder
7 ⊟ **S42.126-** Nondisplaced fracture of acromial process, unspecified shoulder

6 **S42.13** Fracture of coracoid process
7 ⊟ **S42.131-** Displaced fracture of coracoid process, right shoulder
7 ⊟ **S42.132-** Displaced fracture of coracoid process, left shoulder
7 ⊟ **S42.133-** Displaced fracture of coracoid process, unspecified shoulder
7 ⊟ **S42.134-** Nondisplaced fracture of coracoid process, right shoulder
7 ⊟ **S42.135-** Nondisplaced fracture of coracoid process, left shoulder
7 ⊟ **S42.136-** Nondisplaced fracture of coracoid process, unspecified shoulder

6 **S42.14** Fracture of glenoid cavity of scapula
7 ⊟ **S42.141-** Displaced fracture of glenoid cavity of scapula, right shoulder
7 ⊟ **S42.142-** Displaced fracture of glenoid cavity of scapula, left shoulder
7 ⊟ **S42.143-** Displaced fracture of glenoid cavity of scapula, unspecified shoulder
7 ⊟ **S42.144-** Nondisplaced fracture of glenoid cavity of scapula, right shoulder
7 ⊟ **S42.145-** Nondisplaced fracture of glenoid cavity of scapula, left shoulder
7 ⊟ **S42.146-** Nondisplaced fracture of glenoid cavity of scapula, unspecified shoulder

6 **S42.15** Fracture of neck of scapula
7 ⊟ **S42.151-** Displaced fracture of neck of scapula, right shoulder
7 ⊟ **S42.152-** Displaced fracture of neck of scapula, left shoulder
7 ⊟ **S42.153-** Displaced fracture of neck of scapula, unspecified shoulder
7 ⊟ **S42.154-** Nondisplaced fracture of neck of scapula, right shoulder
7 ⊟ **S42.155-** Nondisplaced fracture of neck of scapula, left shoulder
7 ⊟ **S42.156-** Nondisplaced fracture of neck of scapula, unspecified shoulder

6 **S42.19** Fracture of other part of scapula
7 ⊟ **S42.191-** Fracture of other part of scapula, right shoulder
7 ⊟ **S42.192-** Fracture of other part of scapula, left shoulder
7 ⊟ **S42.199-** Fracture of other part of scapula, unspecified shoulder

5 **S42.2** Fracture of upper end of humerus
Fracture of proximal end of humerus
EXCLUDES 2 *fracture of shaft of humerus (S42.3-)*
physeal fracture of upper end of humerus (S49.0-)

6 **S42.20** Unspecified fracture of upper end of humerus
7 ⊟ **S42.201-** Unspecified fracture of upper end of right humerus
7 ⊟ **S42.202-** Unspecified fracture of upper end of left humerus
7 ⊟ **S42.209-** Unspecified fracture of upper end of unspecified humerus

6 **S42.21** Unspecified fracture of surgical neck of humerus
Fracture of neck of humerus NOS
7 ⊟ **S42.211-** Unspecified displaced fracture of surgical neck of right humerus
7 ⊟ **S42.212-** Unspecified displaced fracture of surgical neck of left humerus
7 ⊟ **S42.213-** Unspecified displaced fracture of surgical neck of unspecified humerus
7 ⊟ **S42.214-** Unspecified nondisplaced fracture of surgical neck of right humerus
7 ⊟ **S42.215-** Unspecified nondisplaced fracture of surgical neck of left humerus
7 ⊟ **S42.216-** Unspecified nondisplaced fracture of surgical neck of unspecified humerus

6 **S42.22** 2-part fracture of surgical neck of humerus
7 ⊟ **S42.221-** 2-part displaced fracture of surgical neck of right humerus
7 ⊟ **S42.222-** 2-part displaced fracture of surgical neck of left humerus
7 ⊟ **S42.223-** 2-part displaced fracture of surgical neck of unspecified humerus
7 ⊟ **S42.224-** 2-part nondisplaced fracture of surgical neck of right humerus
7 ⊟ **S42.225-** 2-part nondisplaced fracture of surgical neck of left humerus
7 ⊟ **S42.226-** 2-part nondisplaced fracture of surgical neck of unspecified humerus

6 **S42.23** 3-part fracture of surgical neck of humerus

7 ⊟ S42.231-   3-part fracture of surgical neck of right humerus

3-part fracture of surgical neck of humerus

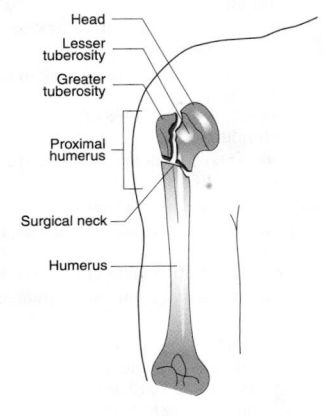

Head
Lesser tuberosity
Greater tuberosity
Proximal humerus
Surgical neck
Humerus

7 ⊟ S42.232-   3-part fracture of surgical neck of left humerus

7 ⊟ S42.239-   3-part fracture of surgical neck of unspecified humerus

6 S42.24   4-part fracture of surgical neck of humerus

7 ⊟ S42.241-   4-part fracture of surgical neck of right humerus

4-part fracture of surgical neck of humerus

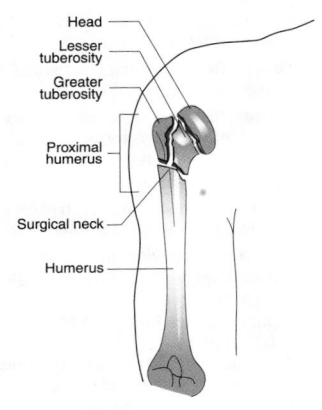

Head
Lesser tuberosity
Greater tuberosity
Proximal humerus
Surgical neck
Humerus

7 ⊟ S42.242-   4-part fracture of surgical neck of left humerus

7 ⊟ S42.249-   4-part fracture of surgical neck of unspecified humerus

6 S42.25   Fracture of greater tuberosity of humerus

7 ⊟ S42.251-   Displaced fracture of greater tuberosity of right humerus

7 ⊟ S42.252-   Displaced fracture of greater tuberosity of left humerus

7 ⊟ S42.253-   Displaced fracture of greater tuberosity of unspecified humerus

7 ⊟ S42.254-   Nondisplaced fracture of greater tuberosity of right humerus

7 ⊟ S42.255-   Nondisplaced fracture of greater tuberosity of left humerus

7 ⊟ S42.256-   Nondisplaced fracture of greater tuberosity of unspecified humerus

6 S42.26   Fracture of lesser tuberosity of humerus

7 ⊟ S42.261-   Displaced fracture of lesser tuberosity of right humerus

7 ⊟ S42.262-   Displaced fracture of lesser tuberosity of left humerus

7 ⊟ S42.263-   Displaced fracture of lesser tuberosity of unspecified humerus

7 ⊟ S42.264-   Nondisplaced fracture of lesser tuberosity of right humerus

7 ⊟ S42.265-   Nondisplaced fracture of lesser tuberosity of left humerus

7 ⊟ S42.266-   Nondisplaced fracture of lesser tuberosity of unspecified humerus

6 S42.27   Torus fracture of upper end of humerus

The appropriate 7th character is to be added to all codes in subcategory S42.27
A   initial encounter for closed fracture
D   subsequent encounter for fracture with routine healing
G   subsequent encounter for fracture with delayed healing
K   subsequent encounter for fracture with nonunion
P   subsequent encounter for fracture with malunion
S   sequela

7 ⊟ S42.271-   Torus fracture of upper end of right humerus

7 ⊟ S42.272-   Torus fracture of upper end of left humerus

7 ⊟ S42.279-   Torus fracture of upper end of unspecified humerus

6 S42.29   Other fracture of upper end of humerus
Fracture of anatomical neck of humerus
Fracture of articular head of humerus

7 ⊟ S42.291-   Other displaced fracture of upper end of right humerus

7 ⊟ S42.292-   Other displaced fracture of upper end of left humerus

7 ⊟ S42.293-   Other displaced fracture of upper end of unspecified humerus

7 ⊟ S42.294-   Other nondisplaced fracture of upper end of right humerus

7 ⊟ S42.295-   Other nondisplaced fracture of upper end of left humerus

7 ⊟ S42.296-   Other nondisplaced fracture of upper end of unspecified humerus

5 S42.3   Fracture of shaft of humerus
Fracture of humerus NOS
Fracture of upper arm NOS
EXCLUDES 2   *physeal fractures of upper end of humerus (S49.0-)*
physeal fractures of lower end of humerus (S49.1-)

6 S42.30   Unspecified fracture of shaft of humerus

7 ⊟ S42.301-   Unspecified fracture of shaft of humerus, right arm

7 ⊟ S42.302-   Unspecified fracture of shaft of humerus, left arm

7 ⊟ S42.309-   Unspecified fracture of shaft of humerus, unspecified arm

Humerus fracture

Scapula
Humerus
Ulna
Radius

● New   ▲ Revised   *Manifestation*   ◄-7 Digit Indicators   ⊟ Laterality   Ⓐ Adult (15+ years)   Ⓜ Maternity (12-55 years)   Ⓝ Newborn   Ⓟ Pediatric (0-17 years)   ♂ Male   ♀ Female
✖ Deleted   Unspecified   + Additional code

960   © 2017 DecisionHealth   2017 ICD-10-CM Expert for Physicians

⑥ S42.31   Greenstick fracture of shaft of humerus

The appropriate 7th character is to be added to all codes in subcategory S42.31
A   initial encounter for closed fracture
D   subsequent encounter for fracture with routine healing
G   subsequent encounter for fracture with delayed healing
K   subsequent encounter for fracture with nonunion
P   subsequent encounter for fracture with malunion
S   sequela

7 ⊟ S42.311-   **Greenstick fracture of shaft of humerus, right arm**

7 ⊟ S42.312-   **Greenstick fracture of shaft of humerus, left arm**

7 ⊟ S42.319-   **Greenstick fracture of shaft of humerus, unspecified arm**

⑥ S42.32   Transverse fracture of shaft of humerus

7 ⊟ S42.321-   **Displaced transverse fracture of shaft of humerus, right arm**

7 ⊟ S42.322-   **Displaced transverse fracture of shaft of humerus, left arm**

7 ⊟ S42.323-   **Displaced transverse fracture of shaft of humerus, unspecified arm**

7 ⊟ S42.324-   **Nondisplaced transverse fracture of shaft of humerus, right arm**

7 ⊟ S42.325-   **Nondisplaced transverse fracture of shaft of humerus, left arm**

7 ⊟ S42.326-   **Nondisplaced transverse fracture of shaft of humerus, unspecified arm**

⑥ S42.33   Oblique fracture of shaft of humerus

7 ⊟ S42.331-   **Displaced oblique fracture of shaft of humerus, right arm**

7 ⊟ S42.332-   **Displaced oblique fracture of shaft of humerus, left arm**

7 ⊟ S42.333-   **Displaced oblique fracture of shaft of humerus, unspecified arm**

7 ⊟ S42.334-   **Nondisplaced oblique fracture of shaft of humerus, right arm**

7 ⊟ S42.335-   **Nondisplaced oblique fracture of shaft of humerus, left arm**

7 ⊟ S42.336-   **Nondisplaced oblique fracture of shaft of humerus, unspecified arm**

⑥ S42.34   Spiral fracture of shaft of humerus

7 ⊟ S42.341-   **Displaced spiral fracture of shaft of humerus, right arm**

7 ⊟ S42.342-   **Displaced spiral fracture of shaft of humerus, left arm**

7 ⊟ S42.343-   **Displaced spiral fracture of shaft of humerus, unspecified arm**

7 ⊟ S42.344-   **Nondisplaced spiral fracture of shaft of humerus, right arm**

7 ⊟ S42.345-   **Nondisplaced spiral fracture of shaft of humerus, left arm**

7 ⊟ S42.346-   **Nondisplaced spiral fracture of shaft of humerus, unspecified arm**

⑥ S42.35   Comminuted fracture of shaft of humerus

7 ⊟ S42.351-   **Displaced comminuted fracture of shaft of humerus, right arm**

7 ⊟ S42.352-   **Displaced comminuted fracture of shaft of humerus, left arm**

7 ⊟ S42.353-   **Displaced comminuted fracture of shaft of humerus, unspecified arm**

7 ⊟ S42.354-   **Nondisplaced comminuted fracture of shaft of humerus, right arm**

7 ⊟ S42.355-   **Nondisplaced comminuted fracture of shaft of humerus, left arm**

7 ⊟ S42.356-   **Nondisplaced comminuted fracture of shaft of humerus, unspecified arm**

⑥ S42.36   Segmental fracture of shaft of humerus

7 ⊟ S42.361-   **Displaced segmental fracture of shaft of humerus, right arm**

7 ⊟ S42.362-   **Displaced segmental fracture of shaft of humerus, left arm**

7 ⊟ S42.363-   **Displaced segmental fracture of shaft of humerus, unspecified arm**

7 ⊟ S42.364-   **Nondisplaced segmental fracture of shaft of humerus, right arm**

7 ⊟ S42.365-   **Nondisplaced segmental fracture of shaft of humerus, left arm**

7 ⊟ S42.366-   **Nondisplaced segmental fracture of shaft of humerus, unspecified arm**

⑥ S42.39   Other fracture of shaft of humerus

7 ⊟ S42.391-   **Other fracture of shaft of right humerus**

7 ⊟ S42.392-   **Other fracture of shaft of left humerus**

7 ⊟ S42.399-   **Other fracture of shaft of unspecified humerus**

⑤ S42.4   Fracture of lower end of humerus

Fracture of distal end of humerus

EXCLUDES 2   *fracture of shaft of humerus (S42.3-)*
physeal fracture of lower end of humerus (S49.1-)

⑥ S42.40   **Unspecified fracture of lower end of humerus**

Fracture of elbow NOS

7 ⊟ S42.401-   **Unspecified fracture of lower end of right humerus**

7 ⊟ S42.402-   **Unspecified fracture of lower end of left humerus**

7 ⊟ S42.409-   **Unspecified fracture of lower end of unspecified humerus**

⑥ S42.41   **Simple supracondylar fracture without intercondylar fracture of humerus**

7 ⊟ S42.411-   **Displaced simple supracondylar fracture without intercondylar fracture of right humerus**

7 ⊟ S42.412-   **Displaced simple supracondylar fracture without intercondylar fracture of left humerus**

7 ⊟ S42.413-   **Displaced simple supracondylar fracture without intercondylar fracture of unspecified humerus**

7 ⊟ S42.414-   **Nondisplaced simple supracondylar fracture without intercondylar fracture of right humerus**

7 ⊟ S42.415-   **Nondisplaced simple supracondylar fracture without intercondylar fracture of left humerus**

7 ⊟ S42.416-   **Nondisplaced simple supracondylar fracture without intercondylar fracture of unspecified humerus**

⑥ S42.42   **Comminuted supracondylar fracture without intercondylar fracture of humerus**

7 ⊟ S42.421-   **Displaced comminuted supracondylar fracture without intercondylar fracture of right humerus**

7 ⊟ S42.422-   **Displaced comminuted supracondylar fracture without intercondylar fracture of left humerus**

7 ⊟ S42.423-   **Displaced comminuted supracondylar fracture without intercondylar fracture of unspecified humerus**

7 ⊟ S42.424-   **Nondisplaced comminuted supracondylar fracture without intercondylar fracture of right humerus**

7 ⊟ S42.425-   **Nondisplaced comminuted supracondylar fracture without intercondylar fracture of left humerus**

7 ⊟ S42.426-   **Nondisplaced comminuted supracondylar fracture without intercondylar fracture of unspecified humerus**

⑥ S42.43   **Fracture (avulsion) of lateral epicondyle of humerus**

7 ⊟ S42.431-   **Displaced fracture (avulsion) of lateral epicondyle of right humerus**

7 ⊟ S42.432-   **Displaced fracture (avulsion) of lateral epicondyle of left humerus**

7 ⊟ S42.433-   **Displaced fracture (avulsion) of lateral epicondyle of unspecified humerus**

7 ⊟ S42.434-   **Nondisplaced fracture (avulsion) of lateral epicondyle of right humerus**

7 ⊟ S42.435-   **Nondisplaced fracture (avulsion) of lateral epicondyle of left humerus**

7 ⊟ S42.436-   **Nondisplaced fracture (avulsion) of lateral epicondyle of unspecified humerus**

⑥ S42.44   **Fracture (avulsion) of medial epicondyle of humerus**

7 ⊟ S42.441-   **Displaced fracture (avulsion) of medial epicondyle of right humerus**

● New   ▲ Revised   *Manifestation*   4-7 Digit Indicators   ⊟ Laterality   Ⓐ Adult (15+ years)   Ⓜ Maternity (12-55 years)   Ⓝ Newborn   Ⓟ Pediatric (0-17 years)   ♂ Male   ♀ Female
✖ Deleted   Unspecified   + Additional code

2017 ICD-10-CM Expert for Physicians   © 2017 DecisionHealth   961

7 ⊟ **S42.442-**   Displaced fracture (avulsion) of medial epicondyle of left humerus

7 ⊟ **S42.443-**   Displaced fracture (avulsion) of medial epicondyle of unspecified humerus

7 ⊟ **S42.444-**   Nondisplaced fracture (avulsion) of medial epicondyle of right humerus

7 ⊟ **S42.445-**   Nondisplaced fracture (avulsion) of medial epicondyle of left humerus

7 ⊟ **S42.446-**   Nondisplaced fracture (avulsion) of medial epicondyle of unspecified humerus

7 ⊟ **S42.447-**   Incarcerated fracture (avulsion) of medial epicondyle of right humerus

7 ⊟ **S42.448-**   Incarcerated fracture (avulsion) of medial epicondyle of left humerus

7 ⊟ **S42.449-**   Incarcerated fracture (avulsion) of medial epicondyle of unspecified humerus

6 **S42.45**   **Fracture of lateral condyle of humerus**
Fracture of capitellum of humerus

7 ⊟ **S42.451-**   Displaced fracture of lateral condyle of right humerus

7 ⊟ **S42.452-**   Displaced fracture of lateral condyle of left humerus

7 ⊟ **S42.453-**   Displaced fracture of lateral condyle of unspecified humerus

7 ⊟ **S42.454-**   Nondisplaced fracture of lateral condyle of right humerus

7 ⊟ **S42.455-**   Nondisplaced fracture of lateral condyle of left humerus

7 ⊟ **S42.456-**   Nondisplaced fracture of lateral condyle of unspecified humerus

6 **S42.46**   **Fracture of medial condyle of humerus**
Trochlea fracture of humerus

7 ⊟ **S42.461-**   Displaced fracture of medial condyle of right humerus

7 ⊟ **S42.462-**   Displaced fracture of medial condyle of left humerus

7 ⊟ **S42.463-**   Displaced fracture of medial condyle of unspecified humerus

7 ⊟ **S42.464-**   Nondisplaced fracture of medial condyle of right humerus

7 ⊟ **S42.465-**   Nondisplaced fracture of medial condyle of left humerus

7 ⊟ **S42.466-**   Nondisplaced fracture of medial condyle of unspecified humerus

6 **S42.47**   **Transcondylar fracture of humerus**

7 ⊟ **S42.471-**   Displaced transcondylar fracture of right humerus

7 ⊟ **S42.472-**   Displaced transcondylar fracture of left humerus

7 ⊟ **S42.473-**   Displaced transcondylar fracture of unspecified humerus

7 ⊟ **S42.474-**   Nondisplaced transcondylar fracture of right humerus

7 ⊟ **S42.475-**   Nondisplaced transcondylar fracture of left humerus

7 ⊟ **S42.476-**   Nondisplaced transcondylar fracture of unspecified humerus

6 **S42.48**   **Torus fracture of lower end of humerus**

The appropriate 7th character is to be added to all codes in subcategory S42.48
A   initial encounter for closed fracture
D   subsequent encounter for fracture with routine healing
G   subsequent encounter for fracture with delayed healing
K   subsequent encounter for fracture with nonunion
P   subsequent encounter for fracture with malunion
S   sequela

7 ⊟ **S42.481-**   Torus fracture of lower end of right humerus

7 ⊟ **S42.482-**   Torus fracture of lower end of left humerus

7 ⊟ **S42.489-**   Torus fracture of lower end of unspecified humerus

6 **S42.49**   **Other fracture of lower end of humerus**

7 ⊟ **S42.491-**   Other displaced fracture of lower end of right humerus

7 ⊟ **S42.492-**   Other displaced fracture of lower end of left humerus

7 ⊟ **S42.493-**   Other displaced fracture of lower end of unspecified humerus

7 ⊟ **S42.494-**   Other nondisplaced fracture of lower end of right humerus

7 ⊟ **S42.495-**   Other nondisplaced fracture of lower end of left humerus

7 ⊟ **S42.496-**   Other nondisplaced fracture of lower end of unspecified humerus

5 **S42.9**   **Fracture of shoulder girdle, part unspecified**
Fracture of shoulder NOS

7 ⊟ **S42.90X-**   Fracture of unspecified shoulder girdle, part unspecified

7 ⊟ **S42.91X-**   Fracture of right shoulder girdle, part unspecified

7 ⊟ **S42.92X-**   Fracture of left shoulder girdle, part unspecified

4 **S43**   **Dislocation and sprain of joints and ligaments of shoulder girdle**

INCLUDES	avulsion of joint or ligament of shoulder girdle
	laceration of cartilage, joint or ligament of shoulder girdle
	sprain of cartilage, joint or ligament of shoulder girdle
	traumatic hemarthrosis of joint or ligament of shoulder girdle
	traumatic rupture of joint or ligament of shoulder girdle
	traumatic subluxation of joint or ligament of shoulder girdle
	traumatic tear of joint or ligament of shoulder girdle

Code also:
any associated open wound

EXCLUDES 2	*strain of muscle, fascia and tendon of shoulder and upper arm (S46.-)*

The appropriate 7th character is to be added to each code from category S43
A   initial encounter
D   subsequent encounter
S   sequela

CODING TIP ✓   Unlike ICD-9 there is no code for open dislocations. When documented as open an additional code for the open wound must be applied.

5 **S43.0**   **Subluxation and dislocation of shoulder joint**
Dislocation of glenohumeral joint
Subluxation of glenohumeral joint

6 **S43.00**   **Unspecified subluxation and dislocation of shoulder joint**
Dislocation of humerus NOS
Subluxation of humerus NOS

7 ⊟ **S43.001-**   Unspecified subluxation of right shoulder joint

7 ⊟ **S43.002-**   Unspecified subluxation of left shoulder joint

7 ⊟ **S43.003-**   Unspecified subluxation of unspecified shoulder joint

7 ⊟ **S43.004-**   Unspecified dislocation of right shoulder joint

7 ⊟ **S43.005-**   Unspecified dislocation of left shoulder joint

7 ⊟ **S43.006-**   Unspecified dislocation of unspecified shoulder joint

6 **S43.01**   **Anterior subluxation and dislocation of humerus**

7 ⊟ **S43.011-**   Anterior subluxation of right humerus

7 ⊟ **S43.012-**   Anterior subluxation of left humerus

7 ⊟ **S43.013-**   Anterior subluxation of unspecified humerus

7 ⊟ **S43.014-**   Anterior dislocation of right humerus

7 ⊟ **S43.015-**   Anterior dislocation of left humerus

7 ⊟ **S43.016-**   Anterior dislocation of unspecified humerus

6 **S43.02**   **Posterior subluxation and dislocation of humerus**

7 ⊟ **S43.021-**   Posterior subluxation of right humerus

7 ⊟ **S43.022-**   Posterior subluxation of left humerus

7 ⊟ **S43.023-**   Posterior subluxation of unspecified humerus

7 ⊟ **S43.024-**   Posterior dislocation of right humerus

7 ⊟ **S43.025-**   Posterior dislocation of left humerus

7 ⊟ **S43.026-**   Posterior dislocation of unspecified humerus

6 **S43.03**   **Inferior subluxation and dislocation of humerus**

7 ⊟ **S43.031-**   Inferior subluxation of right humerus

● New   ▲ Revised   *Manifestation*   �4-7 Digit Indicators   ⊟ Laterality   Ⓐ Adult (15+ years)   Ⓜ Maternity (12-55 years)   Ⓝ Newborn   Ⓟ Pediatric (0-17 years)   ♂ Male   ♀ Female
✖ Deleted   Unspecified   + Additional code

7 ⊟ S43.032-	Inferior subluxation of left humerus
7 ⊟ S43.033-	**Inferior subluxation of unspecified humerus**
7 ⊟ S43.034-	Inferior dislocation of right humerus
7 ⊟ S43.035-	Inferior dislocation of left humerus
7 ⊟ S43.036-	**Inferior dislocation of unspecified humerus**

6 **S43.08** Other subluxation and dislocation of shoulder joint

7 ⊟ S43.081-	Other subluxation of right shoulder joint
7 ⊟ S43.082-	Other subluxation of left shoulder joint
7 ⊟ S43.083-	Other subluxation of unspecified shoulder joint
7 ⊟ S43.084-	Other dislocation of right shoulder joint
7 ⊟ S43.085-	Other dislocation of left shoulder joint
7 ⊟ S43.086-	Other dislocation of unspecified shoulder joint

5 **S43.1** Subluxation and dislocation of acromioclavicular joint

6 **S43.10** Unspecified dislocation of acromioclavicular joint

7 ⊟ S43.101-	Unspecified dislocation of right acromioclavicular joint
7 ⊟ S43.102-	Unspecified dislocation of left acromioclavicular joint
7 ⊟ S43.109-	Unspecified dislocation of unspecified acromioclavicular joint

6 **S43.11** Subluxation of acromioclavicular joint

7 ⊟ S43.111-	Subluxation of right acromioclavicular joint
7 ⊟ S43.112-	Subluxation of left acromioclavicular joint
7 ⊟ S43.119-	Subluxation of unspecified acromioclavicular joint

6 **S43.12** Dislocation of acromioclavicular joint, 100%-200% displacement

7 ⊟ S43.121-	Dislocation of right acromioclavicular joint, 100%-200% displacement
7 ⊟ S43.122-	Dislocation of left acromioclavicular joint, 100%-200% displacement
7 ⊟ S43.129-	Dislocation of unspecified acromioclavicular joint, 100%-200% displacement

6 **S43.13** Dislocation of acromioclavicular joint, greater than 200% displacement

7 ⊟ S43.131-	Dislocation of right acromioclavicular joint, greater than 200% displacement
7 ⊟ S43.132-	Dislocation of left acromioclavicular joint, greater than 200% displacement
7 ⊟ S43.139-	Dislocation of unspecified acromioclavicular joint, greater than 200% displacement

6 **S43.14** Inferior dislocation of acromioclavicular joint

7 ⊟ S43.141-	Inferior dislocation of right acromioclavicular joint
7 ⊟ S43.142-	Inferior dislocation of left acromioclavicular joint
7 ⊟ S43.149-	Inferior dislocation of unspecified acromioclavicular joint

6 **S43.15** Posterior dislocation of acromioclavicular joint

7 ⊟ S43.151-	Posterior dislocation of right acromioclavicular joint
7 ⊟ S43.152-	Posterior dislocation of left acromioclavicular joint
7 ⊟ S43.159-	Posterior dislocation of unspecified acromioclavicular joint

5 **S43.2** Subluxation and dislocation of sternoclavicular joint

6 **S43.20** Unspecified subluxation and dislocation of sternoclavicular joint

7 ⊟ S43.201-	Unspecified subluxation of right sternoclavicular joint
7 ⊟ S43.202-	Unspecified subluxation of left sternoclavicular joint
7 ⊟ S43.203-	Unspecified subluxation of unspecified sternoclavicular joint
7 ⊟ S43.204-	Unspecified dislocation of right sternoclavicular joint
7 ⊟ S43.205-	Unspecified dislocation of left sternoclavicular joint
7 ⊟ S43.206-	Unspecified dislocation of unspecified sternoclavicular joint

6 **S43.21** Anterior subluxation and dislocation of sternoclavicular joint

7 ⊟ S43.211-	Anterior subluxation of right sternoclavicular joint
7 ⊟ S43.212-	Anterior subluxation of left sternoclavicular joint
7 ⊟ S43.213-	Anterior subluxation of unspecified sternoclavicular joint
7 ⊟ S43.214-	Anterior dislocation of right sternoclavicular joint
7 ⊟ S43.215-	Anterior dislocation of left sternoclavicular joint
7 ⊟ S43.216-	Anterior dislocation of unspecified sternoclavicular joint

6 **S43.22** Posterior subluxation and dislocation of sternoclavicular joint

7 ⊟ S43.221-	Posterior subluxation of right sternoclavicular joint
7 ⊟ S43.222-	Posterior subluxation of left sternoclavicular joint
7 ⊟ S43.223-	Posterior subluxation of unspecified sternoclavicular joint
7 ⊟ S43.224-	Posterior dislocation of right sternoclavicular joint
7 ⊟ S43.225-	Posterior dislocation of left sternoclavicular joint
7 ⊟ S43.226-	Posterior dislocation of unspecified sternoclavicular joint

5 **S43.3** Subluxation and dislocation of other and unspecified parts of shoulder girdle

6 **S43.30** Subluxation and dislocation of unspecified parts of shoulder girdle

Dislocation of shoulder girdle NOS
Subluxation of shoulder girdle NOS

7 ⊟ S43.301-	Subluxation of unspecified parts of right shoulder girdle
7 ⊟ S43.302-	Subluxation of unspecified parts of left shoulder girdle
7 ⊟ S43.303-	Subluxation of unspecified parts of unspecified shoulder girdle
7 ⊟ S43.304-	Dislocation of unspecified parts of right shoulder girdle
7 ⊟ S43.305-	Dislocation of unspecified parts of left shoulder girdle
7 ⊟ S43.306-	Dislocation of unspecified parts of unspecified shoulder girdle

6 **S43.31** Subluxation and dislocation of scapula

7 ⊟ S43.311-	Subluxation of right scapula
7 ⊟ S43.312-	Subluxation of left scapula
7 ⊟ S43.313-	Subluxation of unspecified scapula
7 ⊟ S43.314-	Dislocation of right scapula
7 ⊟ S43.315-	Dislocation of left scapula
7 ⊟ S43.316-	Dislocation of unspecified scapula

6 **S43.39** Subluxation and dislocation of other parts of shoulder girdle

7 ⊟ S43.391-	Subluxation of other parts of right shoulder girdle
7 ⊟ S43.392-	Subluxation of other parts of left shoulder girdle
7 ⊟ S43.393-	Subluxation of other parts of unspecified shoulder girdle
7 ⊟ S43.394-	Dislocation of other parts of right shoulder girdle
7 ⊟ S43.395-	Dislocation of other parts of left shoulder girdle
7 ⊟ S43.396-	Dislocation of other parts of unspecified shoulder girdle

5 **S43.4** Sprain of shoulder joint

6 **S43.40** Unspecified sprain of shoulder joint

7 ⊟ S43.401-	Unspecified sprain of right shoulder joint
7 ⊟ S43.402-	Unspecified sprain of left shoulder joint
7 ⊟ S43.409-	Unspecified sprain of unspecified shoulder joint

6 **S43.41** Sprain of coracohumeral (ligament)

7 ⊟ S43.411-	Sprain of right coracohumeral (ligament)
7 ⊟ S43.412-	Sprain of left coracohumeral (ligament)
7 ⊟ S43.419-	Sprain of unspecified coracohumeral (ligament)

● New ▲ Revised *Manifestation* 4-7 Digit Indicators ⊟ Laterality A Adult (15+ years) M Maternity (12-55 years) N Newborn P Pediatric (0-17 years) ♂ Male ♀ Female
✖ Deleted Unspecified + Additional code

2017 ICD-10-CM Expert for Physicians © 2017 DecisionHealth 963

⑥ **S43.42**   **Sprain of rotator cuff capsule**
   EXCLUDES 1 *rotator cuff syndrome (complete) (incomplete), not specified as traumatic (M75.1-)*
   EXCLUDES 2 *injury of tendon of rotator cuff (S46.0-)*
   ⑦⊟ **S43.421-**   **Sprain of right rotator cuff capsule**
   ⑦⊟ **S43.422-**   **Sprain of left rotator cuff capsule**
   ⑦⊟ **S43.429-**   **Sprain of unspecified rotator cuff capsule**
⑥ **S43.43**   **Superior glenoid labrum lesion**
   SLAP lesion
   ⑦⊟ **S43.431-**   **Superior glenoid labrum lesion of right shoulder**
   ⑦⊟ **S43.432-**   **Superior glenoid labrum lesion of left shoulder**
   ⑦⊟ **S43.439-**   **Superior glenoid labrum lesion of unspecified shoulder**
⑥ **S43.49**   **Other sprain of shoulder joint**
   ⑦⊟ **S43.491-**   **Other sprain of right shoulder joint**
   ⑦⊟ **S43.492-**   **Other sprain of left shoulder joint**
   ⑦⊟ **S43.499-**   **Other sprain of unspecified shoulder joint**
⑤ **S43.5**   **Sprain of acromioclavicular joint**
   Sprain of acromioclavicular ligament
   ⑦⊟ **S43.50X-**   **Sprain of unspecified acromioclavicular joint**
   ⑦⊟ **S43.51X-**   **Sprain of right acromioclavicular joint**
   ⑦⊟ **S43.52X-**   **Sprain of left acromioclavicular joint**
⑤ **S43.6**   **Sprain of sternoclavicular joint**
   ⑦⊟ **S43.60X-**   **Sprain of unspecified sternoclavicular joint**
   ⑦⊟ **S43.61X-**   **Sprain of right sternoclavicular joint**
   ⑦⊟ **S43.62X-**   **Sprain of left sternoclavicular joint**
⑤ **S43.8**   **Sprain of other specified parts of shoulder girdle**
   ⑦⊟ **S43.80X-**   **Sprain of other specified parts of unspecified shoulder girdle**
   ⑦⊟ **S43.81X-**   **Sprain of other specified parts of right shoulder girdle**
   ⑦⊟ **S43.82X-**   **Sprain of other specified parts of left shoulder girdle**
⑤ **S43.9**   **Sprain of unspecified parts of shoulder girdle**
   ⑦⊟ **S43.90X-**   **Sprain of unspecified parts of unspecified shoulder girdle**
   Sprain of shoulder girdle NOS
   ⑦⊟ **S43.91X-**   **Sprain of unspecified parts of right shoulder girdle**
   ⑦⊟ **S43.92X-**   **Sprain of unspecified parts of left shoulder girdle**
④ **S44**   **Injury of nerves at shoulder and upper arm level**
   Code also:
   any associated open wound (S41.-)
   EXCLUDES 2 *injury of brachial plexus (S14.3-)*

   The appropriate 7th character is to be added to each code from category S44
   A   initial encounter
   D   subsequent encounter
   S   sequela

⑤ **S44.0**   **Injury of ulnar nerve at upper arm level**
   EXCLUDES 1 *ulnar nerve NOS (S54.0)*
   ⑦⊟ **S44.00X-**   **Injury of ulnar nerve at upper arm level, unspecified arm**
   ⑦⊟ **S44.01X-**   **Injury of ulnar nerve at upper arm level, right arm**
   ⑦⊟ **S44.02X-**   **Injury of ulnar nerve at upper arm level, left arm**
⑤ **S44.1**   **Injury of median nerve at upper arm level**
   EXCLUDES 1 *median nerve NOS (S54.1)*
   ⑦⊟ **S44.10X-**   **Injury of median nerve at upper arm level, unspecified arm**
   ⑦⊟ **S44.11X-**   **Injury of median nerve at upper arm level, right arm**
   ⑦⊟ **S44.12X-**   **Injury of median nerve at upper arm level, left arm**
⑤ **S44.2**   **Injury of radial nerve at upper arm level**
   EXCLUDES 1 *radial nerve NOS (S54.2)*
   ⑦⊟ **S44.20X-**   **Injury of radial nerve at upper arm level, unspecified arm**
   ⑦⊟ **S44.21X-**   **Injury of radial nerve at upper arm level, right arm**
   ⑦⊟ **S44.22X-**   **Injury of radial nerve at upper arm level, left arm**

⑤ **S44.3**   **Injury of axillary nerve**
   ⑦⊟ **S44.30X-**   **Injury of axillary nerve, unspecified arm**
   ⑦⊟ **S44.31X-**   **Injury of axillary nerve, right arm**
   ⑦⊟ **S44.32X-**   **Injury of axillary nerve, left arm**
⑤ **S44.4**   **Injury of musculocutaneous nerve**
   ⑦⊟ **S44.40X-**   **Injury of musculocutaneous nerve, unspecified arm**
   ⑦⊟ **S44.41X-**   **Injury of musculocutaneous nerve, right arm**
   ⑦⊟ **S44.42X-**   **Injury of musculocutaneous nerve, left arm**
⑤ **S44.5**   **Injury of cutaneous sensory nerve at shoulder and upper arm level**
   ⑦⊟ **S44.50X-**   **Injury of cutaneous sensory nerve at shoulder and upper arm level, unspecified arm**
   ⑦⊟ **S44.51X-**   **Injury of cutaneous sensory nerve at shoulder and upper arm level, right arm**
   ⑦⊟ **S44.52X-**   **Injury of cutaneous sensory nerve at shoulder and upper arm level, left arm**
⑤ **S44.8**   **Injury of other nerves at shoulder and upper arm level**
   ⑥ **S44.8X**   **Injury of other nerves at shoulder and upper arm level**
   ⑦⊟ **S44.8X1-**   **Injury of other nerves at shoulder and upper arm level, right arm**
   ⑦⊟ **S44.8X2-**   **Injury of other nerves at shoulder and upper arm level, left arm**
   ⑦⊟ **S44.8X9-**   **Injury of other nerves at shoulder and upper arm level, unspecified arm**
⑤ **S44.9**   **Injury of unspecified nerve at shoulder and upper arm level**
   ⑦⊟ **S44.90X-**   **Injury of unspecified nerve at shoulder and upper arm level, unspecified arm**
   ⑦⊟ **S44.91X-**   **Injury of unspecified nerve at shoulder and upper arm level, right arm**
   ⑦⊟ **S44.92X-**   **Injury of unspecified nerve at shoulder and upper arm level, left arm**
④ **S45**   **Injury of blood vessels at shoulder and upper arm level**
   Code also:
   any associated open wound (S41.-)
   EXCLUDES 2 *injury of subclavian artery (S25.1)*
   injury of subclavian vein (S25.3)

   The appropriate 7th character is to be added to each code from category S45
   A   initial encounter
   D   subsequent encounter
   S   sequela

⑤ **S45.0**   **Injury of axillary artery**
   ⑥ **S45.00**   **Unspecified injury of axillary artery**
   ⑦⊟ **S45.001-**   **Unspecified injury of axillary artery, right side**
   ⑦⊟ **S45.002-**   **Unspecified injury of axillary artery, left side**
   ⑦⊟ **S45.009-**   **Unspecified injury of axillary artery, unspecified side**
   ⑥ **S45.01**   **Laceration of axillary artery**
   CODING TIP ✓ Code also any associated open wound S41.-
   ⑦⊟ **S45.011-**   **Laceration of axillary artery, right side**
   ⑦⊟ **S45.012-**   **Laceration of axillary artery, left side**
   ⑦⊟ **S45.019-**   **Laceration of axillary artery, unspecified side**
   ⑥ **S45.09**   **Other specified injury of axillary artery**
   ⑦⊟ **S45.091-**   **Other specified injury of axillary artery, right side**
   ⑦⊟ **S45.092-**   **Other specified injury of axillary artery, left side**
   ⑦⊟ **S45.099-**   **Other specified injury of axillary artery, unspecified side**
⑤ **S45.1**   **Injury of brachial artery**
   ⑥ **S45.10**   **Unspecified injury of brachial artery**
   ⑦⊟ **S45.101-**   **Unspecified injury of brachial artery, right side**
   ⑦⊟ **S45.102-**   **Unspecified injury of brachial artery, left side**
   ⑦⊟ **S45.109-**   **Unspecified injury of brachial artery, unspecified side**
   ⑥ **S45.11**   **Laceration of brachial artery**
   CODING TIP ✓ Code also any associated open wound S41.-
   ⑦⊟ **S45.111-**   **Laceration of brachial artery, right side**

7 ⊟ S45.112- Laceration of brachial artery, left side
7 ⊟ S45.119- Laceration of brachial artery, unspecified side
6 S45.19 Other specified injury of brachial artery
7 ⊟ S45.191- Other specified injury of brachial artery, right side
7 ⊟ S45.192- Other specified injury of brachial artery, left side
7 ⊟ S45.199- Other specified injury of brachial artery, unspecified side

5 S45.2 Injury of axillary or brachial vein
6 S45.20 Unspecified injury of axillary or brachial vein
7 ⊟ S45.201- Unspecified injury of axillary or brachial vein, right side
7 ⊟ S45.202- Unspecified injury of axillary or brachial vein, left side
7 ⊟ S45.209- Unspecified injury of axillary or brachial vein, unspecified side

6 S45.21 Laceration of axillary or brachial vein
CODING TIP ✓ Code also any associated open wound S41.-
7 ⊟ S45.211- Laceration of axillary or brachial vein, right side
7 ⊟ S45.212- Laceration of axillary or brachial vein, left side
7 ⊟ S45.219- Laceration of axillary or brachial vein, unspecified side

6 S45.29 Other specified injury of axillary or brachial vein
7 ⊟ S45.291- Other specified injury of axillary or brachial vein, right side
7 ⊟ S45.292- Other specified injury of axillary or brachial vein, left side
7 ⊟ S45.299- Other specified injury of axillary or brachial vein, unspecified side

5 S45.3 Injury of superficial vein at shoulder and upper arm level
6 S45.30 Unspecified injury of superficial vein at shoulder and upper arm level
7 ⊟ S45.301- Unspecified injury of superficial vein at shoulder and upper arm level, right arm
7 ⊟ S45.302- Unspecified injury of superficial vein at shoulder and upper arm level, left arm
7 ⊟ S45.309- Unspecified injury of superficial vein at shoulder and upper arm level, unspecified arm

6 S45.31 Laceration of superficial vein at shoulder and upper arm level
CODING TIP ✓ Code also any associated open wound S41.-
7 ⊟ S45.311- Laceration of superficial vein at shoulder and upper arm level, right arm
7 ⊟ S45.312- Laceration of superficial vein at shoulder and upper arm level, left arm
7 ⊟ S45.319- Laceration of superficial vein at shoulder and upper arm level, unspecified arm

6 S45.39 Other specified injury of superficial vein at shoulder and upper arm level
7 ⊟ S45.391- Other specified injury of superficial vein at shoulder and upper arm level, right arm
7 ⊟ S45.392- Other specified injury of superficial vein at shoulder and upper arm level, left arm
7 ⊟ S45.399- Other specified injury of superficial vein at shoulder and upper arm level, unspecified arm

5 S45.8 Injury of other specified blood vessels at shoulder and upper arm level
6 S45.80 Unspecified injury of other specified blood vessels at shoulder and upper arm level
7 ⊟ S45.801- Unspecified injury of other specified blood vessels at shoulder and upper arm level, right arm
7 ⊟ S45.802- Unspecified injury of other specified blood vessels at shoulder and upper arm level, left arm
7 ⊟ S45.809- Unspecified injury of other specified blood vessels at shoulder and upper arm level, unspecified arm

6 S45.81 Laceration of other specified blood vessels at shoulder and upper arm level
CODING TIP ✓ Code also any associated open wound S41.-
7 ⊟ S45.811- Laceration of other specified blood vessels at shoulder and upper arm level, right arm
7 ⊟ S45.812- Laceration of other specified blood vessels at shoulder and upper arm level, left arm
7 ⊟ S45.819- Laceration of other specified blood vessels at shoulder and upper arm level, unspecified arm

6 S45.89 Other specified injury of other specified blood vessels at shoulder and upper arm level
7 ⊟ S45.891- Other specified injury of other specified blood vessels at shoulder and upper arm level, right arm
7 ⊟ S45.892- Other specified injury of other specified blood vessels at shoulder and upper arm level, left arm
7 ⊟ S45.899- Other specified injury of other specified blood vessels at shoulder and upper arm level, unspecified arm

5 S45.9 Injury of unspecified blood vessel at shoulder and upper arm level
6 S45.90 Unspecified injury of unspecified blood vessel at shoulder and upper arm level
7 ⊟ S45.901- Unspecified injury of unspecified blood vessel at shoulder and upper arm level, right arm
7 ⊟ S45.902- Unspecified injury of unspecified blood vessel at shoulder and upper arm level, left arm
7 ⊟ S45.909- Unspecified injury of unspecified blood vessel at shoulder and upper arm level, unspecified arm

6 S45.91 Laceration of unspecified blood vessel at shoulder and upper arm level
CODING TIP ✓ Code also any associated open wound S41.-
7 ⊟ S45.911- Laceration of unspecified blood vessel at shoulder and upper arm level, right arm
7 ⊟ S45.912- Laceration of unspecified blood vessel at shoulder and upper arm level, left arm
7 ⊟ S45.919- Laceration of unspecified blood vessel at shoulder and upper arm level, unspecified arm

6 S45.99 Other specified injury of unspecified blood vessel at shoulder and upper arm level
7 ⊟ S45.991- Other specified injury of unspecified blood vessel at shoulder and upper arm level, right arm
7 ⊟ S45.992- Other specified injury of unspecified blood vessel at shoulder and upper arm level, left arm
7 ⊟ S45.999- Other specified injury of unspecified blood vessel at shoulder and upper arm level, unspecified arm

4 S46 Injury of muscle, fascia and tendon at shoulder and upper arm level
Code also:
  any associated open wound (S41.-)
  EXCLUDES 2 injury of muscle, fascia and tendon at elbow (S56.-)
  sprain of joints and ligaments of shoulder girdle (S43.9)

The appropriate 7th character is to be added to each code from category S46
A   initial encounter
D   subsequent encounter
S   sequela

5 S46.0 Injury of muscle(s) and tendon(s) of the rotator cuff of shoulder
6 S46.00 Unspecified injury of muscle(s) and tendon(s) of the rotator cuff of shoulder
7 ⊟ S46.001- Unspecified injury of muscle(s) and tendon(s) of the rotator cuff of right shoulder
7 ⊟ S46.002- Unspecified injury of muscle(s) and tendon(s) of the rotator cuff of left shoulder
7 ⊟ S46.009- Unspecified injury of muscle(s) and tendon(s) of the rotator cuff of unspecified shoulder

● New ▲ Revised *Manifestation* 4-7 Digit Indicators ⊟ Laterality Ⓐ Adult (15+ years) Ⓜ Maternity (12-55 years) Ⓝ Newborn (0-17 years) Ⓟ Pediatric (0-17 years) ♂ Male ♀ Female
✖ Deleted Unspecified + Additional code

2017 ICD-10-CM Expert for Physicians

© 2017 DecisionHealth

965

⑥ S46.01   Strain of muscle(s) and tendon(s) of the rotator cuff of shoulder

⑦ ⊟ S46.011-   Strain of muscle(s) and tendon(s) of the rotator cuff of right shoulder

⑦ ⊟ S46.012-   Strain of muscle(s) and tendon(s) of the rotator cuff of left shoulder

⑦ ⊟ S46.019-   Strain of muscle(s) and tendon(s) of the rotator cuff of unspecified shoulder

⑥ S46.02   Laceration of muscle(s) and tendon(s) of the rotator cuff of shoulder

> **CODING TIP ✓**   Code also any associated open wound S41.-

⑦ ⊟ S46.021-   Laceration of muscle(s) and tendon(s) of the rotator cuff of right shoulder

⑦ ⊟ S46.022-   Laceration of muscle(s) and tendon(s) of the rotator cuff of left shoulder

⑦ ⊟ S46.029-   Laceration of muscle(s) and tendon(s) of the rotator cuff of unspecified shoulder

⑥ S46.09   Other injury of muscle(s) and tendon(s) of the rotator cuff of shoulder

⑦ ⊟ S46.091-   Other injury of muscle(s) and tendon(s) of the rotator cuff of right shoulder

⑦ ⊟ S46.092-   Other injury of muscle(s) and tendon(s) of the rotator cuff of left shoulder

⑦ ⊟ S46.099-   Other injury of muscle(s) and tendon(s) of the rotator cuff of unspecified shoulder

⑤ S46.1   Injury of muscle, fascia and tendon of long head of biceps

⑥ S46.10   Unspecified injury of muscle, fascia and tendon of long head of biceps

⑦ ⊟ S46.101-   Unspecified injury of muscle, fascia and tendon of long head of biceps, right arm

⑦ ⊟ S46.102-   Unspecified injury of muscle, fascia and tendon of long head of biceps, left arm

⑦ ⊟ S46.109-   Unspecified injury of muscle, fascia and tendon of long head of biceps, unspecified arm

⑥ S46.11   Strain of muscle, fascia and tendon of long head of biceps

⑦ ⊟ S46.111-   Strain of muscle, fascia and tendon of long head of biceps, right arm

⑦ ⊟ S46.112-   Strain of muscle, fascia and tendon of long head of biceps, left arm

⑦ ⊟ S46.119-   Strain of muscle, fascia and tendon of long head of biceps, unspecified arm

⑥ S46.12   Laceration of muscle, fascia and tendon of long head of biceps

> **CODING TIP ✓**   Code also any associated open wound S41.-

⑦ ⊟ S46.121-   Laceration of muscle, fascia and tendon of long head of biceps, right arm

⑦ ⊟ S46.122-   Laceration of muscle, fascia and tendon of long head of biceps, left arm

⑦ ⊟ S46.129-   Laceration of muscle, fascia and tendon of long head of biceps, unspecified arm

⑥ S46.19   Other injury of muscle, fascia and tendon of long head of biceps

⑦ ⊟ S46.191-   Other injury of muscle, fascia and tendon of long head of biceps, right arm

⑦ ⊟ S46.192-   Other injury of muscle, fascia and tendon of long head of biceps, left arm

⑦ ⊟ S46.199-   Other injury of muscle, fascia and tendon of long head of biceps, unspecified arm

⑤ S46.2   Injury of muscle, fascia and tendon of other parts of biceps

⑥ S46.20   Unspecified injury of muscle, fascia and tendon of other parts of biceps

⑦ ⊟ S46.201-   Unspecified injury of muscle, fascia and tendon of other parts of biceps, right arm

⑦ ⊟ S46.202-   Unspecified injury of muscle, fascia and tendon of other parts of biceps, left arm

⑦ ⊟ S46.209-   Unspecified injury of muscle, fascia and tendon of other parts of biceps, unspecified arm

⑥ S46.21   Strain of muscle, fascia and tendon of other parts of biceps

⑦ ⊟ S46.211-   Strain of muscle, fascia and tendon of other parts of biceps, right arm

⑦ ⊟ S46.212-   Strain of muscle, fascia and tendon of other parts of biceps, left arm

⑦ ⊟ S46.219-   Strain of muscle, fascia and tendon of other parts of biceps, unspecified arm

⑥ S46.22   Laceration of muscle, fascia and tendon of other parts of biceps

> **CODING TIP ✓**   Code also any associated open wound S41.-

⑦ ⊟ S46.221-   Laceration of muscle, fascia and tendon of other parts of biceps, right arm

⑦ ⊟ S46.222-   Laceration of muscle, fascia and tendon of other parts of biceps, left arm

⑦ ⊟ S46.229-   Laceration of muscle, fascia and tendon of other parts of biceps, unspecified arm

⑥ S46.29   Other injury of muscle, fascia and tendon of other parts of biceps

⑦ ⊟ S46.291-   Other injury of muscle, fascia and tendon of other parts of biceps, right arm

⑦ ⊟ S46.292-   Other injury of muscle, fascia and tendon of other parts of biceps, left arm

⑦ ⊟ S46.299-   Other injury of muscle, fascia and tendon of other parts of biceps, unspecified arm

⑤ S46.3   Injury of muscle, fascia and tendon of triceps

⑥ S46.30   Unspecified injury of muscle, fascia and tendon of triceps

⑦ ⊟ S46.301-   Unspecified injury of muscle, fascia and tendon of triceps, right arm

⑦ ⊟ S46.302-   Unspecified injury of muscle, fascia and tendon of triceps, left arm

⑦ ⊟ S46.309-   Unspecified injury of muscle, fascia and tendon of triceps, unspecified arm

⑥ S46.31   Strain of muscle, fascia and tendon of triceps

⑦ ⊟ S46.311-   Strain of muscle, fascia and tendon of triceps, right arm

⑦ ⊟ S46.312-   Strain of muscle, fascia and tendon of triceps, left arm

⑦ ⊟ S46.319-   Strain of muscle, fascia and tendon of triceps, unspecified arm

⑥ S46.32   Laceration of muscle, fascia and tendon of triceps

> **CODING TIP ✓**   Code also any associated open wound S41.-

⑦ ⊟ S46.321-   Laceration of muscle, fascia and tendon of triceps, right arm

⑦ ⊟ S46.322-   Laceration of muscle, fascia and tendon of triceps, left arm

⑦ ⊟ S46.329-   Laceration of muscle, fascia and tendon of triceps, unspecified arm

⑥ S46.39   Other injury of muscle, fascia and tendon of triceps

⑦ ⊟ S46.391-   Other injury of muscle, fascia and tendon of triceps, right arm

⑦ ⊟ S46.392-   Other injury of muscle, fascia and tendon of triceps, left arm

⑦ ⊟ S46.399-   Other injury of muscle, fascia and tendon of triceps, unspecified arm

⑤ S46.8   Injury of other muscles, fascia and tendons at shoulder and upper arm level

⑥ S46.80   Unspecified injury of other muscles, fascia and tendons at shoulder and upper arm level

⑦ ⊟ S46.801-   Unspecified injury of other muscles, fascia and tendons at shoulder and upper arm level, right arm

⑦ ⊟ S46.802-   Unspecified injury of other muscles, fascia and tendons at shoulder and upper arm level, left arm

⑦ ⊟ S46.809-   Unspecified injury of other muscles, fascia and tendons at shoulder and upper arm level, unspecified arm

⑥ S46.81   Strain of other muscles, fascia and tendons at shoulder and upper arm level

⑦ ⊟ S46.811-   Strain of other muscles, fascia and tendons at shoulder and upper arm level, right arm

⑦ ⊟ S46.812-   Strain of other muscles, fascia and tendons at shoulder and upper arm level, left arm

⑦ ⊟ S46.819-   Strain of other muscles, fascia and tendons at shoulder and upper arm level, unspecified arm

⑥ S46.82   Laceration of other muscles, fascia and tendons at shoulder and upper arm level

● New   ▲ Revised   *Manifestation*   ④-⑦ Digit Indicators   ⊟ Laterality   Ⓐ Adult (15+ years)   Ⓜ Maternity (12-55 years)   Ⓝ Newborn   Ⓟ Pediatric (0-17 years)   ♂ Male   ♀ Female
✖ Deleted   Unspecified   + Additional code

966   © 2017 DecisionHealth   2017 ICD-10-CM Expert for Physicians

CODING TIP ✓ Code also any associated open wound S41.-

7 ⊟ S46.821- Laceration of other muscles, fascia and tendons at shoulder and upper arm level, right arm

7 ⊟ S46.822- Laceration of other muscles, fascia and tendons at shoulder and upper arm level, left arm

7 ⊟ S46.829- Laceration of other muscles, fascia and tendons at shoulder and upper arm level, unspecified arm

6 S46.89 Other injury of other muscles, fascia and tendons at shoulder and upper arm level

7 ⊟ S46.891- Other injury of other muscles, fascia and tendons at shoulder and upper arm level, right arm

7 ⊟ S46.892- Other injury of other muscles, fascia and tendons at shoulder and upper arm level, left arm

7 ⊟ S46.899- Other injury of other muscles, fascia and tendons at shoulder and upper arm level, unspecified arm

5 S46.9 Injury of unspecified muscle, fascia and tendon at shoulder and upper arm level

6 S46.90 Unspecified injury of unspecified muscle, fascia and tendon at shoulder and upper arm level

7 ⊟ S46.901- Unspecified injury of unspecified muscle, fascia and tendon at shoulder and upper arm level, right arm

7 ⊟ S46.902- Unspecified injury of unspecified muscle, fascia and tendon at shoulder and upper arm level, left arm

7 ⊟ S46.909- Unspecified injury of unspecified muscle, fascia and tendon at shoulder and upper arm level, unspecified arm

6 S46.91 Strain of unspecified muscle, fascia and tendon at shoulder and upper arm level

7 ⊟ S46.911- Strain of unspecified muscle, fascia and tendon at shoulder and upper arm level, right arm

7 ⊟ S46.912- Strain of unspecified muscle, fascia and tendon at shoulder and upper arm level, left arm

7 ⊟ S46.919- Strain of unspecified muscle, fascia and tendon at shoulder and upper arm level, unspecified arm

6 S46.92 Laceration of unspecified muscle, fascia and tendon at shoulder and upper arm level

CODING TIP ✓ Code also any associated open wound S41.-

7 ⊟ S46.921- Laceration of unspecified muscle, fascia and tendon at shoulder and upper arm level, right arm

7 ⊟ S46.922- Laceration of unspecified muscle, fascia and tendon at shoulder and upper arm level, left arm

7 ⊟ S46.929- Laceration of unspecified muscle, fascia and tendon at shoulder and upper arm level, unspecified arm

6 S46.99 Other injury of unspecified muscle, fascia and tendon at shoulder and upper arm level

7 ⊟ S46.991- Other injury of unspecified muscle, fascia and tendon at shoulder and upper arm level, right arm

7 ⊟ S46.992- Other injury of unspecified muscle, fascia and tendon at shoulder and upper arm level, left arm

7 ⊟ S46.999- Other injury of unspecified muscle, fascia and tendon at shoulder and upper arm level, unspecified arm

4 + S47 Crushing injury of shoulder and upper arm

Use additional code for all associated injuries

EXCLUDES 2 *crushing injury of elbow (S57.0-)*

The appropriate 7th character is to be added to each code from category S47
A   initial encounter
D   subsequent encounter
S   sequela

7 ⊟ + S47.1XX- Crushing injury of right shoulder and upper arm
7 ⊟ + S47.2XX- Crushing injury of left shoulder and upper arm
7 ⊟ + S47.9XX- Crushing injury of shoulder and upper arm, unspecified arm

4 S48 Traumatic amputation of shoulder and upper arm

An amputation not identified as partial or complete should be coded to complete

EXCLUDES 1 *traumatic amputation at elbow level (S58.0)*

The appropriate 7th character is to be added to each code from category S48
A   initial encounter
D   subsequent encounter
S   sequela

5 S48.0 Traumatic amputation at shoulder joint

6 S48.01 Complete traumatic amputation at shoulder joint

7 ⊟ S48.011- Complete traumatic amputation at right shoulder joint

7 ⊟ S48.012- Complete traumatic amputation at left shoulder joint

7 ⊟ S48.019- Complete traumatic amputation at unspecified shoulder joint

6 S48.02 Partial traumatic amputation at shoulder joint

7 ⊟ S48.021- Partial traumatic amputation at right shoulder joint

7 ⊟ S48.022- Partial traumatic amputation at left shoulder joint

7 ⊟ S48.029- Partial traumatic amputation at unspecified shoulder joint

5 S48.1 Traumatic amputation at level between shoulder and elbow

6 S48.11 Complete traumatic amputation at level between shoulder and elbow

7 ⊟ S48.111- Complete traumatic amputation at level between right shoulder and elbow

7 ⊟ S48.112- Complete traumatic amputation at level between left shoulder and elbow

7 ⊟ S48.119- Complete traumatic amputation at level between unspecified shoulder and elbow

6 S48.12 Partial traumatic amputation at level between shoulder and elbow

7 ⊟ S48.121- Partial traumatic amputation at level between right shoulder and elbow

7 ⊟ S48.122- Partial traumatic amputation at level between left shoulder and elbow

7 ⊟ S48.129- Partial traumatic amputation at level between unspecified shoulder and elbow

5 S48.9 Traumatic amputation of shoulder and upper arm, level unspecified

6 S48.91 Complete traumatic amputation of shoulder and upper arm, level unspecified

7 ⊟ S48.911- Complete traumatic amputation of right shoulder and upper arm, level unspecified

7 ⊟ S48.912- Complete traumatic amputation of left shoulder and upper arm, level unspecified

7 ⊟ S48.919- Complete traumatic amputation of unspecified shoulder and upper arm, level unspecified

6 S48.92 Partial traumatic amputation of shoulder and upper arm, level unspecified

7 ⊟ S48.921- Partial traumatic amputation of right shoulder and upper arm, level unspecified

7 ⊟ S48.922- Partial traumatic amputation of left shoulder and upper arm, level unspecified

7 ⊟ S48.929- Partial traumatic amputation of unspecified shoulder and upper arm, level unspecified

---

● New   ▲ Revised   *Manifestation*   4-7 Digit Indicators   ⊟ Laterality   A Adult (15+ years)   M Maternity (12-55 years)   N Newborn   P Pediatric (0-17 years)   ♂ Male   ♀ Female
✖ Deleted   Unspecified   + Additional code

◪ **S49   Other and unspecified injuries of shoulder and upper arm**

The appropriate 7th character is to be added to each code from subcategories S49.0 and S49.1
A   initial encounter for closed fracture
D   subsequent encounter for fracture with routine healing
G   subsequent encounter for fracture with delayed healing
K   subsequent encounter for fracture with nonunion
P   subsequent encounter for fracture with malunion
S   sequela

Ⓢ **S49.0   Physeal fracture of upper end of humerus**

Ⓖ **S49.00   Unspecified physeal fracture of upper end of humerus**

🗗 **S49.001-   Unspecified physeal fracture of upper end of humerus, right arm**

🗗 **S49.002-   Unspecified physeal fracture of upper end of humerus, left arm**

🗗 **S49.009-   Unspecified physeal fracture of upper end of humerus, unspecified arm**

Ⓖ **S49.01   Salter-Harris Type I physeal fracture of upper end of humerus**

🗗 **S49.011-   Salter-Harris Type I physeal fracture of upper end of humerus, right arm**

🗗 **S49.012-   Salter-Harris Type I physeal fracture of upper end of humerus, left arm**

🗗 **S49.019-   Salter-Harris Type I physeal fracture of upper end of humerus, unspecified arm**

Ⓖ **S49.02   Salter-Harris Type II physeal fracture of upper end of humerus**

🗗 **S49.021-   Salter-Harris Type II physeal fracture of upper end of humerus, right arm**

🗗 **S49.022-   Salter-Harris Type II physeal fracture of upper end of humerus, left arm**

🗗 **S49.029-   Salter-Harris Type II physeal fracture of upper end of humerus, unspecified arm**

Ⓖ **S49.03   Salter-Harris Type III physeal fracture of upper end of humerus**

▲ 🗗 **S49.031-   Salter-Harris Type III physeal fracture of upper end of humerus, right arm**

▲ 🗗 **S49.032-   Salter-Harris Type III physeal fracture of upper end of humerus, left arm**

▲ 🗗 **S49.039-   Salter-Harris Type III physeal fracture of upper end of humerus, unspecified arm**

Ⓖ **S49.04   Salter-Harris Type IV physeal fracture of upper end of humerus**

🗗 **S49.041-   Salter-Harris Type IV physeal fracture of upper end of humerus, right arm**

🗗 **S49.042-   Salter-Harris Type IV physeal fracture of upper end of humerus, left arm**

🗗 **S49.049-   Salter-Harris Type IV physeal fracture of upper end of humerus, unspecified arm**

Ⓖ **S49.09   Other physeal fracture of upper end of humerus**

🗗 **S49.091-   Other physeal fracture of upper end of humerus, right arm**

🗗 **S49.092-   Other physeal fracture of upper end of humerus, left arm**

🗗 **S49.099-   Other physeal fracture of upper end of humerus, unspecified arm**

Ⓢ **S49.1   Physeal fracture of lower end of humerus**

Ⓖ **S49.10   Unspecified physeal fracture of lower end of humerus**

🗗 **S49.101-   Unspecified physeal fracture of lower end of humerus, right arm**

🗗 **S49.102-   Unspecified physeal fracture of lower end of humerus, left arm**

🗗 **S49.109-   Unspecified physeal fracture of lower end of humerus, unspecified arm**

Ⓖ **S49.11   Salter-Harris Type I physeal fracture of lower end of humerus**

🗗 **S49.111-   Salter-Harris Type I physeal fracture of lower end of humerus, right arm**

🗗 **S49.112-   Salter-Harris Type I physeal fracture of lower end of humerus, left arm**

🗗 **S49.119-   Salter-Harris Type I physeal fracture of lower end of humerus, unspecified arm**

Ⓖ **S49.12   Salter-Harris Type II physeal fracture of lower end of humerus**

🗗 **S49.121-   Salter-Harris Type II physeal fracture of lower end of humerus, right arm**

🗗 **S49.122-   Salter-Harris Type II physeal fracture of lower end of humerus, left arm**

🗗 **S49.129-   Salter-Harris Type II physeal fracture of lower end of humerus, unspecified arm**

Ⓖ **S49.13   Salter-Harris Type III physeal fracture of lower end of humerus**

▲ 🗗 **S49.131-   Salter-Harris Type III physeal fracture of lower end of humerus, right arm**

▲ 🗗 **S49.132-   Salter-Harris Type III physeal fracture of lower end of humerus, left arm**

▲ 🗗 **S49.139-   Salter-Harris Type III physeal fracture of lower end of humerus, unspecified arm**

Ⓖ **S49.14   Salter-Harris Type IV physeal fracture of lower end of humerus**

🗗 **S49.141-   Salter-Harris Type IV physeal fracture of lower end of humerus, right arm**

🗗 **S49.142-   Salter-Harris Type IV physeal fracture of lower end of humerus, left arm**

🗗 **S49.149-   Salter-Harris Type IV physeal fracture of lower end of humerus, unspecified arm**

Ⓖ **S49.19   Other physeal fracture of lower end of humerus**

🗗 **S49.191-   Other physeal fracture of lower end of humerus, right arm**

🗗 **S49.192-   Other physeal fracture of lower end of humerus, left arm**

🗗 **S49.199-   Other physeal fracture of lower end of humerus, unspecified arm**

Ⓢ **S49.8   Other specified injuries of shoulder and upper arm**

The appropriate 7th character is to be added to each code in subcategory S49.8
A   initial encounter
D   subsequent encounter
S   sequela

🗗 **S49.80X-   Other specified injuries of shoulder and upper arm, unspecified arm**

🗗 **S49.81X-   Other specified injuries of right shoulder and upper arm**

🗗 **S49.82X-   Other specified injuries of left shoulder and upper arm**

Ⓢ **S49.9   Unspecified injury of shoulder and upper arm**

The appropriate 7th character is to be added to each code in subcategory S49.9
A   initial encounter
D   subsequent encounter
S   sequela

🗗 **S49.90X-   Unspecified injury of shoulder and upper arm, unspecified arm**

🗗 **S49.91X-   Unspecified injury of right shoulder and upper arm**

🗗 **S49.92X-   Unspecified injury of left shoulder and upper arm**

Injuries to the elbow and forearm (S50-S59)

EXCLUDES 2   *burns and corrosions (T20-T32)*
frostbite (T33-T34)
injuries of wrist and hand (S60-S69)
insect bite or sting, venomous (T63.4)

GUIDELINES   Section I.C.19.c.2)
Multiple fractures are sequenced in accordance with the severity of the fracture.

● New   ▲ Revised   *Manifestation*   ◪-🗗 Digit Indicators   ⊟ Laterality   Ⓐ Adult (15+ years)   Ⓜ Maternity (12-55 years)   Ⓝ Newborn (0-17 years)   Ⓟ Pediatric (0-17 years)   ♂ Male   ♀ Female
✖ Deleted   Unspecified   + Additional code

968   © 2017 DecisionHealth   2017 ICD-10-CM Expert for Physicians

GUIDELINES   Section I.C.19.b.1)-2)

When coding injuries, assign separate codes for each injury unless a combination code is provided, in which case the combination code is assigned ... Traumatic injury codes (S00-T14.9) are not to be used for normal, healing surgical wounds or to identify complications of surgical wounds. The code for the most serious injury, as determined by the provider and the focus of treatment, is sequenced first.

1) Superficial injuries such as abrasions or contusions are not coded when associated with more severe injuries of the same site.

2) When a primary injury results in minor damage to peripheral nerves or blood vessels, the primary injury is sequenced first with additional code(s) for injuries to nerves and spinal cord (such as category S04), and/or injury to blood vessels (such as category S15). When the primary injury is to the blood vessels or nerves, that injury should be sequenced first.

GUIDELINES   Section I.C.19.c

Coding of Traumatic Fractures: The principles of multiple coding of injuries should be followed in coding fractures. Fractures of specified sites are coded individually by site in accordance with both the provisions within categories S02, S12, S22, S32, S42, S49, S52, S59, S62, S72, S79, S82, S89, S92 and the level of detail furnished by medical record content. A fracture not indicated as open or closed should be coded to closed. A fracture not indicated whether displaced or not displaced should be coded to displaced.

⁴ **S50**   **Superficial injury of elbow and forearm**

    EXCLUDES 2   *superficial injury of wrist and hand (S60.-)*

> The appropriate 7th character is to be added to each code from category S50
> A   initial encounter
> D   subsequent encounter
> S   sequela

⁵ **S50.0**   **Contusion of elbow**
  7 ⊟ **S50.00X-**   **Contusion of unspecified elbow**
  7 ⊟ **S50.01X-**   **Contusion of right elbow**
  7 ⊟ **S50.02X-**   **Contusion of left elbow**

⁵ **S50.1**   **Contusion of forearm**
  7 ⊟ **S50.10X-**   **Contusion of unspecified forearm**
  7 ⊟ **S50.11X-**   **Contusion of right forearm**
  7 ⊟ **S50.12X-**   **Contusion of left forearm**

⁵ **S50.3**   **Other superficial injuries of elbow**
  ⁶ **S50.31**   **Abrasion of elbow**
    7 ⊟ **S50.311-**   **Abrasion of right elbow**
    7 ⊟ **S50.312-**   **Abrasion of left elbow**
    7 ⊟ **S50.319-**   **Abrasion of unspecified elbow**
  ⁶ **S50.32**   **Blister (nonthermal) of elbow**
    7 ⊟ **S50.321-**   **Blister (nonthermal) of right elbow**
    7 ⊟ **S50.322-**   **Blister (nonthermal) of left elbow**
    7 ⊟ **S50.329-**   **Blister (nonthermal) of unspecified elbow**
  ⁶ **S50.34**   **External constriction of elbow**
    7 ⊟ **S50.341-**   **External constriction of right elbow**
    7 ⊟ **S50.342-**   **External constriction of left elbow**
    7 ⊟ **S50.349-**   **External constriction of unspecified elbow**
  ⁶ **S50.35**   **Superficial foreign body of elbow**
    Splinter in the elbow
    7 ⊟ **S50.351-**   **Superficial foreign body of right elbow**
    7 ⊟ **S50.352-**   **Superficial foreign body of left elbow**
    7 ⊟ **S50.359-**   **Superficial foreign body of unspecified elbow**
  ⁶ **S50.36**   **Insect bite (nonvenomous) of elbow**
    7 ⊟ **S50.361-**   **Insect bite (nonvenomous) of right elbow**
    7 ⊟ **S50.362-**   **Insect bite (nonvenomous) of left elbow**
    7 ⊟ **S50.369-**   **Insect bite (nonvenomous) of unspecified elbow**
  ⁶ **S50.37**   **Other superficial bite of elbow**
    EXCLUDES 1   *open bite of elbow (S51.04)*
    7 ⊟ **S50.371-**   **Other superficial bite of right elbow**
    7 ⊟ **S50.372-**   **Other superficial bite of left elbow**
    7 ⊟ **S50.379-**   **Other superficial bite of unspecified elbow**

⁵ **S50.8**   **Other superficial injuries of forearm**

  ⁶ **S50.81**   **Abrasion of forearm**
    7 ⊟ **S50.811-**   **Abrasion of right forearm**
    7 ⊟ **S50.812-**   **Abrasion of left forearm**
    7 ⊟ **S50.819-**   **Abrasion of unspecified forearm**
  ⁶ **S50.82**   **Blister (nonthermal) of forearm**
    7 ⊟ **S50.821-**   **Blister (nonthermal) of right forearm**
    7 ⊟ **S50.822-**   **Blister (nonthermal) of left forearm**
    7 ⊟ **S50.829-**   **Blister (nonthermal) of unspecified forearm**
  ⁶ **S50.84**   **External constriction of forearm**
    7 ⊟ **S50.841-**   **External constriction of right forearm**
    7 ⊟ **S50.842-**   **External constriction of left forearm**
    7 ⊟ **S50.849-**   **External constriction of unspecified forearm**
  ⁶ **S50.85**   **Superficial foreign body of forearm**
    Splinter in the forearm
    7 ⊟ **S50.851-**   **Superficial foreign body of right forearm**
    7 ⊟ **S50.852-**   **Superficial foreign body of left forearm**
    7 ⊟ **S50.859-**   **Superficial foreign body of unspecified forearm**
  ⁶ **S50.86**   **Insect bite (nonvenomous) of forearm**
    7 ⊟ **S50.861-**   **Insect bite (nonvenomous) of right forearm**
    7 ⊟ **S50.862-**   **Insect bite (nonvenomous) of left forearm**
    7 ⊟ **S50.869-**   **Insect bite (nonvenomous) of unspecified forearm**
  ⁶ **S50.87**   **Other superficial bite of forearm**
    EXCLUDES 1   *open bite of forearm (S51.84)*
    7 ⊟ **S50.871-**   **Other superficial bite of right forearm**
    7 ⊟ **S50.872-**   **Other superficial bite of left forearm**
    7 ⊟ **S50.879-**   **Other superficial bite of unspecified forearm**

⁵ **S50.9**   **Unspecified superficial injury of elbow and forearm**
  ⁶ **S50.90**   **Unspecified superficial injury of elbow**
    7 ⊟ **S50.901-**   **Unspecified superficial injury of right elbow**
    7 ⊟ **S50.902-**   **Unspecified superficial injury of left elbow**
    7 ⊟ **S50.909-**   **Unspecified superficial injury of unspecified elbow**
  ⁶ **S50.91**   **Unspecified superficial injury of forearm**
    7 ⊟ **S50.911-**   **Unspecified superficial injury of right forearm**
    7 ⊟ **S50.912-**   **Unspecified superficial injury of left forearm**
    7 ⊟ **S50.919-**   **Unspecified superficial injury of unspecified forearm**

⁴ **S51**   **Open wound of elbow and forearm**
    Code also:
      any associated wound infection
    EXCLUDES 1   *open fracture of elbow and forearm*
        (S52.- with open fracture 7th character)
        traumatic amputation of elbow and forearm
        (S58.-)
    EXCLUDES 2   *open wound of wrist and hand (S61.-)*

> The appropriate 7th character is to be added to each code from category S51
> A   initial encounter
> D   subsequent encounter
> S   sequela

CODING TIP ✓   Open wound codes indicate a wound resulting from a traumatic origin. Do not assign a code for "open wound" unless the etiology of the wound is related to trauma.

⁵ **S51.0**   **Open wound of elbow**
  ⁶ **S51.00**   **Unspecified open wound of elbow**
    7 ⊟ **S51.001-**   **Unspecified open wound of right elbow**
      AHA: (S51.001A) 4Q 2012, 108
    7 ⊟ **S51.002-**   **Unspecified open wound of left elbow**
    7 ⊟ **S51.009-**   **Unspecified open wound of unspecified elbow**
      Open wound of elbow NOS
  ⁶ **S51.01**   **Laceration without foreign body of elbow**
    7 ⊟ **S51.011-**   **Laceration without foreign body of right elbow**
    7 ⊟ **S51.012-**   **Laceration without foreign body of left elbow**
    7 ⊟ **S51.019-**   **Laceration without foreign body of unspecified elbow**
  ⁶ **S51.02**   **Laceration with foreign body of elbow**

● New ▲ Revised *Manifestation* ④-⑦ Digit Indicators ⊟ Laterality Ⓐ Adult (15+ years) Ⓜ Maternity (12-55 years) Ⓝ Newborn Ⓟ Pediatric (0-17 years) ♂ Male ♀ Female
✖ ~~Deleted~~ Unspecified + Additional code

7 ⊟ **S51.021-**   Laceration with foreign body of right elbow

7 ⊟ **S51.022-**   Laceration with foreign body of left elbow

7 ⊟ **S51.029-**   Laceration with foreign body of unspecified elbow

6 **S51.03**   Puncture wound without foreign body of elbow

7 ⊟ **S51.031-**   Puncture wound without foreign body of right elbow

7 ⊟ **S51.032-**   Puncture wound without foreign body of left elbow

7 ⊟ **S51.039-**   Puncture wound without foreign body of unspecified elbow

6 **S51.04**   Puncture wound with foreign body of elbow

7 ⊟ **S51.041-**   Puncture wound with foreign body of right elbow

7 ⊟ **S51.042-**   Puncture wound with foreign body of left elbow

7 ⊟ **S51.049-**   Puncture wound with foreign body of unspecified elbow

6 **S51.05**   Open bite of elbow
Bite of elbow NOS
EXCLUDES 1   *superficial bite of elbow (S50.36, S50.37)*

7 ⊟ **S51.051-**   Open bite, right elbow

7 ⊟ **S51.052-**   Open bite, left elbow

7 ⊟ **S51.059-**   Open bite, unspecified elbow

5 **S51.8**   Open wound of forearm
EXCLUDES 2   *open wound of elbow (S51.0-)*

6 **S51.80**   Unspecified open wound of forearm

7 ⊟ **S51.801-**   Unspecified open wound of right forearm

7 ⊟ **S51.802-**   Unspecified open wound of left forearm

7 ⊟ **S51.809-**   Unspecified open wound of unspecified forearm
Open wound of forearm NOS

6 **S51.81**   Laceration without foreign body of forearm

7 ⊟ **S51.811-**   Laceration without foreign body of right forearm

7 ⊟ **S51.812-**   Laceration without foreign body of left forearm

7 ⊟ **S51.819-**   Laceration without foreign body of unspecified forearm

6 **S51.82**   Laceration with foreign body of forearm

7 ⊟ **S51.821-**   Laceration with foreign body of right forearm

7 ⊟ **S51.822-**   Laceration with foreign body of left forearm

7 ⊟ **S51.829-**   Laceration with foreign body of unspecified forearm

6 **S51.83**   Puncture wound without foreign body of forearm

7 ⊟ **S51.831-**   Puncture wound without foreign body of right forearm

7 ⊟ **S51.832-**   Puncture wound without foreign body of left forearm

7 ⊟ **S51.839-**   Puncture wound without foreign body of unspecified forearm

6 **S51.84**   Puncture wound with foreign body of forearm

7 ⊟ **S51.841-**   Puncture wound with foreign body of right forearm

7 ⊟ **S51.842-**   Puncture wound with foreign body of left forearm

7 ⊟ **S51.849-**   Puncture wound with foreign body of unspecified forearm

6 **S51.85**   Open bite of forearm
Bite of forearm NOS
EXCLUDES 1   *superficial bite of forearm (S50.86, S50.87)*

7 ⊟ **S51.851-**   Open bite of right forearm

7 ⊟ **S51.852-**   Open bite of left forearm

7 ⊟ **S51.859-**   Open bite of unspecified forearm

4 **S52**   **Fracture of forearm**
Note: A fracture not indicated as displaced or nondisplaced should be coded to displaced
A fracture not indicated as open or closed should be coded to closed
The open fracture designations are based on the Gustilo open fracture classification
EXCLUDES 1   *traumatic amputation of forearm (S58.-)*
EXCLUDES 2   *fracture at wrist and hand level (S62.-)*

The appropriate 7th character is to be added to all codes from category S52

A	initial encounter for closed fracture
B	initial encounter for open fracture type I or II
C	initial encounter for open fracture type IIIA, IIIB, or IIIC
D	subsequent encounter for closed fracture with routine healing
E	subsequent encounter for open fracture type I or II with routine healing
F	subsequent encounter for open fracture type IIIA, IIIB, or IIIC with routine healing
G	subsequent encounter for closed fracture with delayed healing
H	subsequent encounter for open fracture type I or II with delayed healing
J	subsequent encounter for open fracture type IIIA, IIIB, or IIIC with delayed healing
K	subsequent encounter for closed fracture with nonunion
M	subsequent encounter for open fracture type I or II with nonunion
N	subsequent encounter for open fracture type IIIA, IIIB, or IIIC with nonunion
P	subsequent encounter for closed fracture with malunion
Q	subsequent encounter for open fracture type I or II with malunion
R	subsequent encounter for open fracture type IIIA, IIIB, or IIIC with malunion
S	sequela

CODING TIP ✓   A fracture not indicated as displaced or nondisplaced should be coded to displaced. A fracture not indicated as open or closed should be coded to closed. Query providers on fractures not documented as displaced/nondisplaced otherwise displaced fracture diagnosis could be assigned without reduction being performed potentially resulting in claim denials.

5 **S52.0**   **Fracture of upper end of ulna**
Fracture of proximal end of ulna
EXCLUDES 2   *fracture of elbow NOS (S42.40-)*
fractures of shaft of ulna (S52.2-)

6 **S52.00**   Unspecified fracture of upper end of ulna

7 ⊟ **S52.001-**   Unspecified fracture of upper end of right ulna

7 ⊟ **S52.002-**   Unspecified fracture of upper end of left ulna

7 ⊟ **S52.009-**   Unspecified fracture of upper end of unspecified ulna

6 **S52.01**   Torus fracture of upper end of ulna

The appropriate 7th character is to be added to all codes in subcategory S52.01

A	initial encounter for closed fracture
D	subsequent encounter for fracture with routine healing
G	subsequent encounter for fracture with delayed healing
K	subsequent encounter for fracture with nonunion
P	subsequent encounter for fracture with malunion
S	sequela

7 ⊟ **S52.011-**   Torus fracture of upper end of right ulna

7 ⊟ **S52.012-**   Torus fracture of upper end of left ulna

7 ⊟ **S52.019-**   Torus fracture of upper end of unspecified ulna

6 **S52.02**   Fracture of olecranon process without intraarticular extension of ulna

7 ⊟ **S52.021-**   Displaced fracture of olecranon process without intraarticular extension of right ulna

● New   ▲ Revised   *Manifestation*   **4**-**7** Digit Indicators   ⊟ Laterality   **A** Adult (15+ years)   **M** Maternity (12-55 years)   **N** Newborn   **P** Pediatric (0-17 years)   ♂ Male   ♀ Female
✖ Deleted   Unspecified   + Additional code

970   © 2017 DecisionHealth   2017 ICD-10-CM Expert for Physicians

☑ ⊟ **S52.022-** Displaced fracture of olecranon process without intraarticular extension of left ulna

☑ ⊟ **S52.023-** **Displaced fracture of olecranon process without intraarticular extension of unspecified ulna**

☑ ⊟ **S52.024-** Nondisplaced fracture of olecranon process without intraarticular extension of right ulna

☑ ⊟ **S52.025-** **Nondisplaced fracture of olecranon process without intraarticular extension of left ulna**

☑ ⊟ **S52.026-** **Nondisplaced fracture of olecranon process without intraarticular extension of unspecified ulna**

⑥ **S52.03** Fracture of olecranon process with intraarticular extension of ulna

☑ ⊟ **S52.031-** Displaced fracture of olecranon process with intraarticular extension of right ulna

☑ ⊟ **S52.032-** Displaced fracture of olecranon process with intraarticular extension of left ulna

☑ ⊟ **S52.033-** **Displaced fracture of olecranon process with intraarticular extension of unspecified ulna**

☑ ⊟ **S52.034-** Nondisplaced fracture of olecranon process with intraarticular extension of right ulna

☑ ⊟ **S52.035-** **Nondisplaced fracture of olecranon process with intraarticular extension of left ulna**

☑ ⊟ **S52.036-** **Nondisplaced fracture of olecranon process with intraarticular extension of unspecified ulna**

⑥ **S52.04** Fracture of coronoid process of ulna

☑ ⊟ **S52.041-** Displaced fracture of coronoid process of right ulna

☑ ⊟ **S52.042-** Displaced fracture of coronoid process of left ulna

☑ ⊟ **S52.043-** **Displaced fracture of coronoid process of unspecified ulna**

☑ ⊟ **S52.044-** Nondisplaced fracture of coronoid process of right ulna

☑ ⊟ **S52.045-** Nondisplaced fracture of coronoid process of left ulna

☑ ⊟ **S52.046-** **Nondisplaced fracture of coronoid process of unspecified ulna**

⑥ **S52.09** Other fracture of upper end of ulna

☑ ⊟ **S52.091-** Other fracture of upper end of right ulna

☑ ⊟ **S52.092-** Other fracture of upper end of left ulna

☑ ⊟ **S52.099-** **Other fracture of upper end of unspecified ulna**

Ⓢ **S52.1** **Fracture of upper end of radius**
Fracture of proximal end of radius
EXCLUDES 2 *physeal fractures of upper end of radius (S59.2-)*
fracture of shaft of radius (S52.3-)

⑥ **S52.10** Unspecified fracture of upper end of radius

☑ ⊟ **S52.101-** **Unspecified fracture of upper end of right radius**

☑ ⊟ **S52.102-** **Unspecified fracture of upper end of left radius**

☑ ⊟ **S52.109-** **Unspecified fracture of upper end of unspecified radius**

⑥ **S52.11** Torus fracture of upper end of radius

The appropriate 7th character is to be added to all codes in subcategory S52.11
A   initial encounter for closed fracture
D   subsequent encounter for fracture with routine healing
G   subsequent encounter for fracture with delayed healing
K   subsequent encounter for fracture with nonunion
P   subsequent encounter for fracture with malunion
S   sequela

☑ ⊟ **S52.111-** Torus fracture of upper end of right radius
☑ ⊟ **S52.112-** Torus fracture of upper end of left radius
☑ ⊟ **S52.119-** **Torus fracture of upper end of unspecified radius**

⑥ **S52.12** **Fracture of head of radius**

☑ ⊟ **S52.121-** Displaced fracture of head of right radius
☑ ⊟ **S52.122-** Displaced fracture of head of left radius
☑ ⊟ **S52.123-** **Displaced fracture of head of unspecified radius**

☑ ⊟ **S52.124-** Nondisplaced fracture of head of right radius
☑ ⊟ **S52.125-** Nondisplaced fracture of head of left radius
☑ ⊟ **S52.126-** **Nondisplaced fracture of head of unspecified radius**

⑥ **S52.13** Fracture of neck of radius

☑ ⊟ **S52.131-** Displaced fracture of neck of right radius
☑ ⊟ **S52.132-** Displaced fracture of neck of left radius
☑ ⊟ **S52.133-** **Displaced fracture of neck of unspecified radius**

☑ ⊟ **S52.134-** Nondisplaced fracture of neck of right radius
☑ ⊟ **S52.135-** Nondisplaced fracture of neck of left radius
☑ ⊟ **S52.136-** **Nondisplaced fracture of neck of unspecified radius**

⑥ **S52.18** Other fracture of upper end of radius

☑ ⊟ **S52.181-** Other fracture of upper end of right radius
☑ ⊟ **S52.182-** Other fracture of upper end of left radius
☑ ⊟ **S52.189-** **Other fracture of upper end of unspecified radius**

Ⓢ **S52.2** **Fracture of shaft of ulna**

⑥ **S52.20** **Unspecified fracture of shaft of ulna**
Fracture of ulna NOS

☑ ⊟ **S52.201-** **Unspecified fracture of shaft of right ulna**
☑ ⊟ **S52.202-** **Unspecified fracture of shaft of left ulna**
☑ ⊟ **S52.209-** **Unspecified fracture of shaft of unspecified ulna**

Displaced transverse fracture, shafts and radius of ulna

Ulna
Radius

Two codes are required to report fractures of the radius and ulna

⑥ **S52.21** **Greenstick fracture of shaft of ulna**

The appropriate 7th character is to be added to all codes in subcategory S52.21
A   initial encounter for closed fracture
D   subsequent encounter for fracture with routine healing
G   subsequent encounter for fracture with delayed healing
K   subsequent encounter for fracture with nonunion
P   subsequent encounter for fracture with malunion
S   sequela

☑ ⊟ **S52.211-** Greenstick fracture of shaft of right ulna
☑ ⊟ **S52.212-** Greenstick fracture of shaft of left ulna
☑ ⊟ **S52.219-** **Greenstick fracture of shaft of unspecified ulna**

⑥ **S52.22** Transverse fracture of shaft of ulna

☑ ⊟ **S52.221-** Displaced transverse fracture of shaft of right ulna
☑ ⊟ **S52.222-** Displaced transverse fracture of shaft of left ulna
☑ ⊟ **S52.223-** **Displaced transverse fracture of shaft of unspecified ulna**
☑ ⊟ **S52.224-** Nondisplaced transverse fracture of shaft of right ulna

---

● New   ▲ Revised   *Manifestation*   ④-☑ Digit Indicators   ⊟ Laterality   Ⓐ Adult (15+ years)   Ⓜ Maternity (12-55 years)   Ⓝ Newborn   Ⓟ Pediatric (0-17 years)   ♂ Male   ♀ Female
✖ Deleted   Unspecified   + Additional code

7 ⊟ S52.225-   Nondisplaced transverse fracture of shaft of left ulna

7 ⊟ S52.226-   Nondisplaced transverse fracture of shaft of unspecified ulna

6 S52.23   Oblique fracture of shaft of ulna

7 ⊟ S52.231-   Displaced oblique fracture of shaft of right ulna

7 ⊟ S52.232-   Displaced oblique fracture of shaft of left ulna

7 ⊟ S52.233-   Displaced oblique fracture of shaft of unspecified ulna

7 ⊟ S52.234-   Nondisplaced oblique fracture of shaft of right ulna

7 ⊟ S52.235-   Nondisplaced oblique fracture of shaft of left ulna

7 ⊟ S52.236-   Nondisplaced oblique fracture of shaft of unspecified ulna

6 S52.24   Spiral fracture of shaft of ulna

7 ⊟ S52.241-   Displaced spiral fracture of shaft of ulna, right arm

7 ⊟ S52.242-   Displaced spiral fracture of shaft of ulna, left arm

7 ⊟ S52.243-   Displaced spiral fracture of shaft of ulna, unspecified arm

7 ⊟ S52.244-   Nondisplaced spiral fracture of shaft of ulna, right arm

7 ⊟ S52.245-   Nondisplaced spiral fracture of shaft of ulna, left arm

7 ⊟ S52.246-   Nondisplaced spiral fracture of shaft of ulna, unspecified arm

6 S52.25   Comminuted fracture of shaft of ulna

7 ⊟ S52.251-   Displaced comminuted fracture of shaft of ulna, right arm

7 ⊟ S52.252-   Displaced comminuted fracture of shaft of ulna, left arm

7 ⊟ S52.253-   Displaced comminuted fracture of shaft of ulna, unspecified arm

7 ⊟ S52.254-   Nondisplaced comminuted fracture of shaft of ulna, right arm

7 ⊟ S52.255-   Nondisplaced comminuted fracture of shaft of ulna, left arm

7 ⊟ S52.256-   Nondisplaced comminuted fracture of shaft of ulna, unspecified arm

6 S52.26   Segmental fracture of shaft of ulna

7 ⊟ S52.261-   Displaced segmental fracture of shaft of ulna, right arm

7 ⊟ S52.262-   Displaced segmental fracture of shaft of ulna, left arm

7 ⊟ S52.263-   Displaced segmental fracture of shaft of ulna, unspecified arm

7 ⊟ S52.264-   Nondisplaced segmental fracture of shaft of ulna, right arm

7 ⊟ S52.265-   Nondisplaced segmental fracture of shaft of ulna, left arm

7 ⊟ S52.266-   Nondisplaced segmental fracture of shaft of ulna, unspecified arm

6 S52.27   Monteggia's fracture of ulna

Fracture of upper shaft of ulna with dislocation of radial head

7 ⊟ S52.271-   Monteggia's fracture of right ulna

7 ⊟ S52.272-   Monteggia's fracture of left ulna

7 ⊟ S52.279-   Monteggia's fracture of unspecified ulna

6 S52.28   Bent bone of ulna

7 ⊟ S52.281-   Bent bone of right ulna

7 ⊟ S52.282-   Bent bone of left ulna

7 ⊟ S52.283-   Bent bone of unspecified ulna

6 S52.29   Other fracture of shaft of ulna

7 ⊟ S52.291-   Other fracture of shaft of right ulna

7 ⊟ S52.292-   Other fracture of shaft of left ulna

7 ⊟ S52.299-   Other fracture of shaft of unspecified ulna

5 S52.3   Fracture of shaft of radius

6 S52.30   Unspecified fracture of shaft of radius

7 ⊟ S52.301-   Unspecified fracture of shaft of right radius

7 ⊟ S52.302-   Unspecified fracture of shaft of left radius

7 ⊟ S52.309-   Unspecified fracture of shaft of unspecified radius

6 S52.31   Greenstick fracture of shaft of radius

The appropriate 7th character is to be added to all codes in subcategory S52.31

A   initial encounter for closed fracture

D   subsequent encounter for fracture with routine healing

G   subsequent encounter for fracture with delayed healing

K   subsequent encounter for fracture with nonunion

P   subsequent encounter for fracture with malunion

S   sequela

7 ⊟ S52.311-   Greenstick fracture of shaft of radius, right arm

7 ⊟ S52.312-   Greenstick fracture of shaft of radius, left arm

7 ⊟ S52.319-   Greenstick fracture of shaft of radius, unspecified arm

6 S52.32   Transverse fracture of shaft of radius

7 ⊟ S52.321-   Displaced transverse fracture of shaft of right radius

7 ⊟ S52.322-   Displaced transverse fracture of shaft of left radius

7 ⊟ S52.323-   Displaced transverse fracture of shaft of unspecified radius

7 ⊟ S52.324-   Nondisplaced transverse fracture of shaft of right radius

7 ⊟ S52.325-   Nondisplaced transverse fracture of shaft of left radius

7 ⊟ S52.326-   Nondisplaced transverse fracture of shaft of unspecified radius

6 S52.33   Oblique fracture of shaft of radius

7 ⊟ S52.331-   Displaced oblique fracture of shaft of right radius

7 ⊟ S52.332-   Displaced oblique fracture of shaft of left radius

7 ⊟ S52.333-   Displaced oblique fracture of shaft of unspecified radius

7 ⊟ S52.334-   Nondisplaced oblique fracture of shaft of right radius

7 ⊟ S52.335-   Nondisplaced oblique fracture of shaft of left radius

7 ⊟ S52.336-   Nondisplaced oblique fracture of shaft of unspecified radius

6 S52.34   Spiral fracture of shaft of radius

7 ⊟ S52.341-   Displaced spiral fracture of shaft of radius, right arm

7 ⊟ S52.342-   Displaced spiral fracture of shaft of radius, left arm

7 ⊟ S52.343-   Displaced spiral fracture of shaft of radius, unspecified arm

7 ⊟ S52.344-   Nondisplaced spiral fracture of shaft of radius, right arm

7 ⊟ S52.345-   Nondisplaced spiral fracture of shaft of radius, left arm

7 ⊟ S52.346-   Nondisplaced spiral fracture of shaft of radius, unspecified arm

6 S52.35   Comminuted fracture of shaft of radius

7 ⊟ S52.351-   Displaced comminuted fracture of shaft of radius, right arm

7 ⊟ S52.352-   Displaced comminuted fracture of shaft of radius, left arm

7 ⊟ S52.353-   Displaced comminuted fracture of shaft of radius, unspecified arm

7 ⊟ S52.354-   Nondisplaced comminuted fracture of shaft of radius, right arm

7 ⊟ S52.355-   Nondisplaced comminuted fracture of shaft of radius, left arm

7 ⊟ S52.356-   Nondisplaced comminuted fracture of shaft of radius, unspecified arm

6 S52.36   Segmental fracture of shaft of radius

7 ⊟ S52.361-   Displaced segmental fracture of shaft of radius, right arm

7 ⊟ S52.362-   Displaced segmental fracture of shaft of radius, left arm

7 ⊟ S52.363-   Displaced segmental fracture of shaft of radius, unspecified arm

7 ⊟ S52.364-   Nondisplaced segmental fracture of shaft of radius, right arm

● New   ▲ Revised   *Manifestation*   **4**-**7** Digit Indicators   ⊟ Laterality   Ⓐ Adult (15+ years)   Ⓜ Maternity (12-55 years)   Ⓝ Newborn   Ⓟ Pediatric (0-17 years)   ♂ Male   ♀ Female

✖ Deleted   Unspecified   + Additional code

972   © 2017 DecisionHealth   2017 ICD-10-CM Expert for Physicians

7 ⊟ S52.365- **Nondisplaced segmental fracture of shaft of radius, left arm**

7 ⊟ S52.366- **Nondisplaced segmental fracture of shaft of radius, unspecified arm**

6 S52.37 Galeazzi's fracture
Fracture of lower shaft of radius with radioulnar joint dislocation

7 ⊟ S52.371- **Galeazzi's fracture of right radius**

7 ⊟ S52.372- **Galeazzi's fracture of left radius**

7 ⊟ S52.379- **Galeazzi's fracture of unspecified radius**

6 S52.38 Bent bone of radius

7 ⊟ S52.381- **Bent bone of right radius**

7 ⊟ S52.382- **Bent bone of left radius**

7 ⊟ S52.389- **Bent bone of unspecified radius**

6 S52.39 Other fracture of shaft of radius

7 ⊟ S52.391- **Other fracture of shaft of radius, right arm**

7 ⊟ S52.392- **Other fracture of shaft of radius, left arm**

7 ⊟ S52.399- **Other fracture of shaft of radius, unspecified arm**

5 S52.5 Fracture of lower end of radius
Fracture of distal end of radius

EXCLUDES 2 *physeal fractures of lower end of radius (S59.2-)*

6 S52.50 Unspecified fracture of the lower end of radius

7 ⊟ S52.501- **Unspecified fracture of the lower end of right radius**

7 ⊟ S52.502- **Unspecified fracture of the lower end of left radius**

7 ⊟ S52.509- **Unspecified fracture of the lower end of unspecified radius**

6 S52.51 Fracture of radial styloid process

7 ⊟ S52.511- **Displaced fracture of right radial styloid process**

7 ⊟ S52.512- **Displaced fracture of left radial styloid process**

7 ⊟ S52.513- **Displaced fracture of unspecified radial styloid process**

7 ⊟ S52.514- **Nondisplaced fracture of right radial styloid process**

7 ⊟ S52.515- **Nondisplaced fracture of left radial styloid process**

7 ⊟ S52.516- **Nondisplaced fracture of unspecified radial styloid process**

6 S52.52 Torus fracture of lower end of radius

The appropriate 7th character is to be added to all codes in subcategory S52.52
A   initial encounter for closed fracture
D   subsequent encounter for fracture with routine healing
G   subsequent encounter for fracture with delayed healing
K   subsequent encounter for fracture with nonunion
P   subsequent encounter for fracture with malunion
S   sequela

7 ⊟ S52.521- **Torus fracture of lower end of right radius**

7 ⊟ S52.522- **Torus fracture of lower end of left radius**

7 ⊟ S52.529- **Torus fracture of lower end of unspecified radius**

6 S52.53 Colles' fracture

DEFINITION Break in the lower end of the radius with posterior displacement of the wrist, often caused by breaking a fall with an extended, outstretched hand.

7 ⊟ S52.531- **Colles' fracture of right radius**

7 ⊟ S52.532- **Colles' fracture of left radius**
AHA: (S52.532D) 2Q 2016, 5

7 ⊟ S52.539- **Colles' fracture of unspecified radius**

6 S52.54 Smith's fracture

DEFINITION Break in the lower end of the radius with palmar displacement of the wrist; a reverse Colles' fracture.

7 ⊟ S52.541- **Smith's fracture of right radius**

7 ⊟ S52.542- **Smith's fracture of left radius**

7 ⊟ S52.549- **Smith's fracture of unspecified radius**

6 S52.55 Other extraarticular fracture of lower end of radius

7 ⊟ S52.551- **Other extraarticular fracture of lower end of right radius**

7 ⊟ S52.552- **Other extraarticular fracture of lower end of left radius**

7 ⊟ S52.559- **Other extraarticular fracture of lower end of unspecified radius**

6 S52.56 Barton's fracture

7 ⊟ S52.561- **Barton's fracture of right radius**

7 ⊟ S52.562- **Barton's fracture of left radius**

7 ⊟ S52.569- **Barton's fracture of unspecified radius**

6 S52.57 Other intraarticular fracture of lower end of radius

7 ⊟ S52.571- **Other intraarticular fracture of lower end of right radius**

7 ⊟ S52.572- **Other intraarticular fracture of lower end of left radius**

7 ⊟ S52.579- **Other intraarticular fracture of lower end of unspecified radius**

6 S52.59 Other fractures of lower end of radius

7 ⊟ S52.591- **Other fractures of lower end of right radius**

7 ⊟ S52.592- **Other fractures of lower end of left radius**

7 ⊟ S52.599- **Other fractures of lower end of unspecified radius**

5 S52.6 Fracture of lower end of ulna

6 S52.60 Unspecified fracture of lower end of ulna

7 ⊟ S52.601- **Unspecified fracture of lower end of right ulna**

7 ⊟ S52.602- **Unspecified fracture of lower end of left ulna**

7 ⊟ S52.609- **Unspecified fracture of lower end of unspecified ulna**

6 S52.61 Fracture of ulna styloid process

7 ⊟ S52.611- **Displaced fracture of right ulna styloid process**

7 ⊟ S52.612- **Displaced fracture of left ulna styloid process**

7 ⊟ S52.613- **Displaced fracture of unspecified ulna styloid process**

7 ⊟ S52.614- **Nondisplaced fracture of right ulna styloid process**

7 ⊟ S52.615- **Nondisplaced fracture of left ulna styloid process**

7 ⊟ S52.616- **Nondisplaced fracture of unspecified ulna styloid process**

6 S52.62 Torus fracture of lower end of ulna

The appropriate 7th character is to be added to all codes in subcategory S52.62
A   initial encounter for closed fracture
D   subsequent encounter for fracture with routine healing
G   subsequent encounter for fracture with delayed healing
K   subsequent encounter for fracture with nonunion
P   subsequent encounter for fracture with malunion
S   sequela

7 ⊟ S52.621- **Torus fracture of lower end of right ulna**

7 ⊟ S52.622- **Torus fracture of lower end of left ulna**

7 ⊟ S52.629- **Torus fracture of lower end of unspecified ulna**

6 S52.69 Other fracture of lower end of ulna

7 ⊟ S52.691- **Other fracture of lower end of right ulna**

7 ⊟ S52.692- **Other fracture of lower end of left ulna**

7 ⊟ S52.699- **Other fracture of lower end of unspecified ulna**

5 S52.9 Unspecified fracture of forearm

7 ⊟ S52.90X- **Unspecified fracture of unspecified forearm**

7 ⊟ S52.91X- **Unspecified fracture of right forearm**

7 ⊟ S52.92X- **Unspecified fracture of left forearm**

● New   ▲ Revised   *Manifestation*   4-7 Digit Indicators   ⊟ Laterality   A Adult (15+ years)   M Maternity (12-55 years)   N Newborn (0-17 years)   P Pediatric (0-17 years)   ♂ Male   ♀ Female
✖ Deleted   Unspecified   + Additional code

2017 ICD-10-CM Expert for Physicians

© 2017 DecisionHealth   973

◢ **S53**   **Dislocation and sprain of joints and ligaments of elbow**

INCLUDES   avulsion of joint or ligament of elbow
laceration of cartilage, joint or ligament of elbow
sprain of cartilage, joint or ligament of elbow
traumatic hemarthrosis of joint or ligament of elbow
traumatic rupture of joint or ligament of elbow
traumatic subluxation of joint or ligament of elbow
traumatic tear of joint or ligament of elbow

Code also:
any associated open wound

EXCLUDES 2   *strain of muscle, fascia and tendon at forearm level (S56.-)*

The appropriate 7th character is to be added to each code from category S53
A   initial encounter
D   subsequent encounter
S   sequela

CODING TIP ✓   Unlike ICD-9 there is no code for open dislocations. When documented as open an additional code for the open wound must be applied.

⑤ **S53.0**   **Subluxation and dislocation of radial head**
Dislocation of radiohumeral joint
Subluxation of radiohumeral joint

EXCLUDES 1   *Monteggia's fracture-dislocation (S52.27-)*

⑥ **S53.00**   **Unspecified subluxation and dislocation of radial head**

⑦ ▤ S53.001-   Unspecified subluxation of right radial head

⑦ ▤ S53.002-   Unspecified subluxation of left radial head

⑦ ▤ S53.003-   Unspecified subluxation of unspecified radial head

⑦ ▤ S53.004-   Unspecified dislocation of right radial head

⑦ ▤ S53.005-   Unspecified dislocation of left radial head

⑦ ▤ S53.006-   Unspecified dislocation of unspecified radial head

⑥ **S53.01**   **Anterior subluxation and dislocation of radial head**
Anteriomedial subluxation and dislocation of radial head

⑦ ▤ S53.011-   Anterior subluxation of right radial head

⑦ ▤ S53.012-   Anterior subluxation of left radial head

⑦ ▤ S53.013-   Anterior subluxation of unspecified radial head

⑦ ▤ S53.014-   Anterior dislocation of right radial head

⑦ ▤ S53.015-   Anterior dislocation of left radial head

⑦ ▤ S53.016-   Anterior dislocation of unspecified radial head

⑥ **S53.02**   **Posterior subluxation and dislocation of radial head**
Posteriolateral subluxation and dislocation of radial head

⑦ ▤ S53.021-   Posterior subluxation of right radial head

⑦ ▤ S53.022-   Posterior subluxation of left radial head

⑦ ▤ S53.023-   Posterior subluxation of unspecified radial head

⑦ ▤ S53.024-   Posterior dislocation of right radial head

⑦ ▤ S53.025-   Posterior dislocation of left radial head

⑦ ▤ S53.026-   Posterior dislocation of unspecified radial head

⑥ **S53.03**   **Nursemaid's elbow**

⑦ ▤ S53.031-   Nursemaid's elbow, right elbow
AHA: (S53.031A) 1Q 2015, 7
AHA: (S53.031D) 1Q 2015, 8

⑦ ▤ S53.032-   Nursemaid's elbow, left elbow

⑦ ▤ S53.033-   Nursemaid's elbow, unspecified elbow

⑥ **S53.09**   **Other subluxation and dislocation of radial head**

⑦ ▤ S53.091-   Other subluxation of right radial head

⑦ ▤ S53.092-   Other subluxation of left radial head

⑦ ▤ S53.093-   Other subluxation of unspecified radial head

⑦ ▤ S53.094-   Other dislocation of right radial head

⑦ ▤ S53.095-   Other dislocation of left radial head

⑦ ▤ S53.096-   Other dislocation of unspecified radial head

⑤ **S53.1**   **Subluxation and dislocation of ulnohumeral joint**
Subluxation and dislocation of elbow NOS

EXCLUDES 1   *dislocation of radial head alone (S53.0-)*

⑥ **S53.10**   **Unspecified subluxation and dislocation of ulnohumeral joint**

⑦ ▤ S53.101-   Unspecified subluxation of right ulnohumeral joint

⑦ ▤ S53.102-   Unspecified subluxation of left ulnohumeral joint

⑦ ▤ S53.103-   Unspecified subluxation of unspecified ulnohumeral joint

⑦ ▤ S53.104-   Unspecified dislocation of right ulnohumeral joint

⑦ ▤ S53.105-   Unspecified dislocation of left ulnohumeral joint

⑦ ▤ S53.106-   Unspecified dislocation of unspecified ulnohumeral joint

⑥ **S53.11**   **Anterior subluxation and dislocation of ulnohumeral joint**

⑦ ▤ S53.111-   Anterior subluxation of right ulnohumeral joint

⑦ ▤ S53.112-   Anterior subluxation of left ulnohumeral joint

⑦ ▤ S53.113-   Anterior subluxation of unspecified ulnohumeral joint

⑦ ▤ S53.114-   Anterior dislocation of right ulnohumeral joint
AHA: (S53.114A) 4Q 2012, 108

⑦ ▤ S53.115-   Anterior dislocation of left ulnohumeral joint

⑦ ▤ S53.116-   Anterior dislocation of unspecified ulnohumeral joint

⑥ **S53.12**   **Posterior subluxation and dislocation of ulnohumeral joint**

⑦ ▤ S53.121-   Posterior subluxation of right ulnohumeral joint

⑦ ▤ S53.122-   Posterior subluxation of left ulnohumeral joint

⑦ ▤ S53.123-   Posterior subluxation of unspecified ulnohumeral joint

⑦ ▤ S53.124-   Posterior dislocation of right ulnohumeral joint

⑦ ▤ S53.125-   Posterior dislocation of left ulnohumeral joint

⑦ ▤ S53.126-   Posterior dislocation of unspecified ulnohumeral joint

⑥ **S53.13**   **Medial subluxation and dislocation of ulnohumeral joint**

⑦ ▤ S53.131-   Medial subluxation of right ulnohumeral joint

⑦ ▤ S53.132-   Medial subluxation of left ulnohumeral joint

⑦ ▤ S53.133-   Medial subluxation of unspecified ulnohumeral joint

⑦ ▤ S53.134-   Medial dislocation of right ulnohumeral joint

⑦ ▤ S53.135-   Medial dislocation of left ulnohumeral joint

⑦ ▤ S53.136-   Medial dislocation of unspecified ulnohumeral joint

⑥ **S53.14**   **Lateral subluxation and dislocation of ulnohumeral joint**

⑦ ▤ S53.141-   Lateral subluxation of right ulnohumeral joint

⑦ ▤ S53.142-   Lateral subluxation of left ulnohumeral joint

⑦ ▤ S53.143-   Lateral subluxation of unspecified ulnohumeral joint

⑦ ▤ S53.144-   Lateral dislocation of right ulnohumeral joint

⑦ ▤ S53.145-   Lateral dislocation of left ulnohumeral joint

⑦ ▤ S53.146-   Lateral dislocation of unspecified ulnohumeral joint

⑥ **S53.19**   **Other subluxation and dislocation of ulnohumeral joint**

⑦ ▤ S53.191-   Other subluxation of right ulnohumeral joint

⑦ ▤ S53.192-   Other subluxation of left ulnohumeral joint

⑦ ▤ S53.193-   Other subluxation of unspecified ulnohumeral joint

⑦ ▤ S53.194-   Other dislocation of right ulnohumeral joint

⑦ ▤ S53.195-   Other dislocation of left ulnohumeral joint

⑦ ▤ S53.196-   Other dislocation of unspecified ulnohumeral joint

⑤ **S53.2**   **Traumatic rupture of radial collateral ligament**

EXCLUDES 1   *sprain of radial collateral ligament NOS (S53.43-)*

⑦ ▤ S53.20X-   **Traumatic rupture of unspecified radial collateral ligament**

● New   ▲ Revised   *Manifestation*   ◀-⑦ Digit Indicators   ▤ Laterality   🄰 Adult (15+ years)   🄼 Maternity (12-55 years)   🄽 Newborn   🄿 Pediatric (0-17 years)   ♂ Male   ♀ Female
✖ Deleted   Unspecified   + Additional code

974   © 2017 DecisionHealth   2017 ICD-10-CM Expert for Physicians

7 ⊟ **S53.21X-** **Traumatic rupture of right radial collateral ligament**

7 ⊟ **S53.22X-** **Traumatic rupture of left radial collateral ligament**

5 **S53.3** **Traumatic rupture of ulnar collateral ligament**

EXCLUDES 1 *sprain of ulnar collateral ligament (S53.44-)*

7 ⊟ **S53.30X-** **Traumatic rupture of unspecified ulnar collateral ligament**

7 ⊟ **S53.31X-** **Traumatic rupture of right ulnar collateral ligament**

7 ⊟ **S53.32X-** **Traumatic rupture of left ulnar collateral ligament**

5 **S53.4** **Sprain of elbow**

EXCLUDES 2 *traumatic rupture of radial collateral ligament (S53.2-)*
traumatic rupture of ulnar collateral ligament (S53.3-)

6 **S53.40** **Unspecified sprain of elbow**

7 ⊟ **S53.401-** **Unspecified sprain of right elbow**

7 ⊟ **S53.402-** **Unspecified sprain of left elbow**

7 ⊟ **S53.409-** **Unspecified sprain of unspecified elbow**
Sprain of elbow NOS

6 **S53.41** **Radiohumeral (joint) sprain**

7 ⊟ **S53.411-** **Radiohumeral (joint) sprain of right elbow**

7 ⊟ **S53.412-** **Radiohumeral (joint) sprain of left elbow**

7 ⊟ **S53.419-** **Radiohumeral (joint) sprain of unspecified elbow**

6 **S53.42** **Ulnohumeral (joint) sprain**

7 ⊟ **S53.421-** **Ulnohumeral (joint) sprain of right elbow**

7 ⊟ **S53.422-** **Ulnohumeral (joint) sprain of left elbow**

7 ⊟ **S53.429-** **Ulnohumeral (joint) sprain of unspecified elbow**

6 **S53.43** **Radial collateral ligament sprain**

7 ⊟ **S53.431-** **Radial collateral ligament sprain of right elbow**

7 ⊟ **S53.432-** **Radial collateral ligament sprain of left elbow**

7 ⊟ **S53.439-** **Radial collateral ligament sprain of unspecified elbow**

6 **S53.44** **Ulnar collateral ligament sprain**

7 ⊟ **S53.441-** **Ulnar collateral ligament sprain of right elbow**

7 ⊟ **S53.442-** **Ulnar collateral ligament sprain of left elbow**

7 ⊟ **S53.449-** **Ulnar collateral ligament sprain of unspecified elbow**

6 **S53.49** **Other sprain of elbow**

7 ⊟ **S53.491-** **Other sprain of right elbow**

7 ⊟ **S53.492-** **Other sprain of left elbow**

7 ⊟ **S53.499-** **Other sprain of unspecified elbow**

4 **S54** **Injury of nerves at forearm level**
Code also:
any associated open wound (S51.-)

EXCLUDES 2 *injury of nerves at wrist and hand level (S64.-)*

The appropriate 7th character is to be added to each code from category S54
A   initial encounter
D   subsequent encounter
S   sequela

5 **S54.0** **Injury of ulnar nerve at forearm level**
Injury of ulnar nerve NOS

7 ⊟ **S54.00X-** **Injury of ulnar nerve at forearm level, unspecified arm**

7 ⊟ **S54.01X-** **Injury of ulnar nerve at forearm level, right arm**

7 ⊟ **S54.02X-** **Injury of ulnar nerve at forearm level, left arm**

5 **S54.1** **Injury of median nerve at forearm level**
Injury of median nerve NOS

7 ⊟ **S54.10X-** **Injury of median nerve at forearm level, unspecified arm**

7 ⊟ **S54.11X-** **Injury of median nerve at forearm level, right arm**

7 ⊟ **S54.12X-** **Injury of median nerve at forearm level, left arm**

5 **S54.2** **Injury of radial nerve at forearm level**
Injury of radial nerve NOS

7 ⊟ **S54.20X-** **Injury of radial nerve at forearm level, unspecified arm**

7 ⊟ **S54.21X-** **Injury of radial nerve at forearm level, right arm**

7 ⊟ **S54.22X-** **Injury of radial nerve at forearm level, left arm**

5 **S54.3** **Injury of cutaneous sensory nerve at forearm level**

7 ⊟ **S54.30X-** **Injury of cutaneous sensory nerve at forearm level, unspecified arm**

7 ⊟ **S54.31X-** **Injury of cutaneous sensory nerve at forearm level, right arm**

7 ⊟ **S54.32X-** **Injury of cutaneous sensory nerve at forearm level, left arm**

5 **S54.8** **Injury of other nerves at forearm level**

▲ 6 **S54.8X** **Injury of other nerves at forearm level**

▲ 7 ⊟ **S54.8X1-** **Injury of other nerves at forearm level, right arm**

▲ 7 ⊟ **S54.8X2-** **Injury of other nerves at forearm level, left arm**

▲ 7 ⊟ **S54.8X9-** **Injury of other nerves at forearm level, unspecified arm**

5 **S54.9** **Injury of unspecified nerve at forearm level**

7 ⊟ **S54.90X-** **Injury of unspecified nerve at forearm level, unspecified arm**

7 ⊟ **S54.91X-** **Injury of unspecified nerve at forearm level, right arm**

7 ⊟ **S54.92X-** **Injury of unspecified nerve at forearm level, left arm**

4 **S55** **Injury of blood vessels at forearm level**
Code also:
any associated open wound (S51.-)

EXCLUDES 2 *injury of blood vessels at wrist and hand level (S65.-)*
injury of brachial vessels (S45.1-S45.2)

The appropriate 7th character is to be added to each code from category S55
A   initial encounter
D   subsequent encounter
S   sequela

5 **S55.0** **Injury of ulnar artery at forearm level**

6 **S55.00** **Unspecified injury of ulnar artery at forearm level**

7 ⊟ **S55.001-** **Unspecified injury of ulnar artery at forearm level, right arm**

7 ⊟ **S55.002-** **Unspecified injury of ulnar artery at forearm level, left arm**

7 ⊟ **S55.009-** **Unspecified injury of ulnar artery at forearm level, unspecified arm**

6 **S55.01** **Laceration of ulnar artery at forearm level**

CODING TIP ✓ Code also any associated open wound S51.-

7 ⊟ **S55.011-** **Laceration of ulnar artery at forearm level, right arm**

7 ⊟ **S55.012-** **Laceration of ulnar artery at forearm level, left arm**

7 ⊟ **S55.019-** **Laceration of ulnar artery at forearm level, unspecified arm**

6 **S55.09** **Other specified injury of ulnar artery at forearm level**

7 ⊟ **S55.091-** **Other specified injury of ulnar artery at forearm level, right arm**

7 ⊟ **S55.092-** **Other specified injury of ulnar artery at forearm level, left arm**

7 ⊟ **S55.099-** **Other specified injury of ulnar artery at forearm level, unspecified arm**

5 **S55.1** **Injury of radial artery at forearm level**

6 **S55.10** **Unspecified injury of radial artery at forearm level**

7 ⊟ **S55.101-** **Unspecified injury of radial artery at forearm level, right arm**

7 ⊟ **S55.102-** **Unspecified injury of radial artery at forearm level, left arm**

7 ⊟ **S55.109-** **Unspecified injury of radial artery at forearm level, unspecified arm**

6 **S55.11** **Laceration of radial artery at forearm level**

CODING TIP ✓ Code also any associated open wound S51.-

7 ⊟ **S55.111-** **Laceration of radial artery at forearm level, right arm**

7 ⊟ **S55.112-** **Laceration of radial artery at forearm level, left arm**

● New ▲ Revised *Manifestation* 4-7 Digit Indicators ⊟ Laterality Ⓐ Adult (15+ years) Ⓜ Maternity (12-55 years) Ⓝ Newborn (0-17 years) Ⓟ Pediatric (0-17 years) ♂ Male ♀ Female
✖ Deleted Unspecified + Additional code

2017 ICD-10-CM Expert for Physicians

© 2017 DecisionHealth

975

7 ⊟ **S55.119-**   Laceration of radial artery at forearm level, unspecified arm

6 **S55.19**   Other specified injury of radial artery at forearm level

7 ⊟ **S55.191-**   Other specified injury of radial artery at forearm level, right arm

7 ⊟ **S55.192-**   Other specified injury of radial artery at forearm level, left arm

7 ⊟ **S55.199-**   Other specified injury of radial artery at forearm level, unspecified arm

5 **S55.2**   Injury of vein at forearm level

6 **S55.20**   Unspecified injury of vein at forearm level

7 ⊟ **S55.201-**   Unspecified injury of vein at forearm level, right arm

7 ⊟ **S55.202-**   Unspecified injury of vein at forearm level, left arm

7 ⊟ **S55.209-**   Unspecified injury of vein at forearm level, unspecified arm

6 **S55.21**   Laceration of vein at forearm level

> **CODING TIP ✓**   Code also any associated open wound S51.-

7 ⊟ **S55.211-**   Laceration of vein at forearm level, right arm

7 ⊟ **S55.212-**   Laceration of vein at forearm level, left arm

7 ⊟ **S55.219-**   Laceration of vein at forearm level, unspecified arm

6 **S55.29**   Other specified injury of vein at forearm level

7 ⊟ **S55.291-**   Other specified injury of vein at forearm level, right arm

7 ⊟ **S55.292-**   Other specified injury of vein at forearm level, left arm

7 ⊟ **S55.299-**   Other specified injury of vein at forearm level, unspecified arm

5 **S55.8**   Injury of other blood vessels at forearm level

6 **S55.80**   Unspecified injury of other blood vessels at forearm level

7 ⊟ **S55.801-**   Unspecified injury of other blood vessels at forearm level, right arm

7 ⊟ **S55.802-**   Unspecified injury of other blood vessels at forearm level, left arm

7 ⊟ **S55.809-**   Unspecified injury of other blood vessels at forearm level, unspecified arm

6 **S55.81**   Laceration of other blood vessels at forearm level

> **CODING TIP ✓**   Code also any associated open wound S51.-

7 ⊟ **S55.811-**   Laceration of other blood vessels at forearm level, right arm

7 ⊟ **S55.812-**   Laceration of other blood vessels at forearm level, left arm

7 ⊟ **S55.819-**   Laceration of other blood vessels at forearm level, unspecified arm

6 **S55.89**   Other specified injury of other blood vessels at forearm level

7 ⊟ **S55.891-**   Other specified injury of other blood vessels at forearm level, right arm

7 ⊟ **S55.892-**   Other specified injury of other blood vessels at forearm level, left arm

7 ⊟ **S55.899-**   Other specified injury of other blood vessels at forearm level, unspecified arm

5 **S55.9**   Injury of unspecified blood vessel at forearm level

6 **S55.90**   Unspecified injury of unspecified blood vessel at forearm level

7 ⊟ **S55.901-**   Unspecified injury of unspecified blood vessel at forearm level, right arm

7 ⊟ **S55.902-**   Unspecified injury of unspecified blood vessel at forearm level, left arm

7 ⊟ **S55.909-**   Unspecified injury of unspecified blood vessel at forearm level, unspecified arm

6 **S55.91**   Laceration of unspecified blood vessel at forearm level

> **CODING TIP ✓**   Code also any associated open wound S51.-

7 ⊟ **S55.911-**   Laceration of unspecified blood vessel at forearm level, right arm

7 ⊟ **S55.912-**   Laceration of unspecified blood vessel at forearm level, left arm

7 ⊟ **S55.919-**   Laceration of unspecified blood vessel at forearm level, unspecified arm

6 **S55.99**   Other specified injury of unspecified blood vessel at forearm level

7 ⊟ **S55.991-**   Other specified injury of unspecified blood vessel at forearm level, right arm

7 ⊟ **S55.992-**   Other specified injury of unspecified blood vessel at forearm level, left arm

7 ⊟ **S55.999-**   Other specified injury of unspecified blood vessel at forearm level, unspecified arm

4 **S56**   Injury of muscle, fascia and tendon at forearm level

Code also:
  any associated open wound (S51.-)

EXCLUDES 2   *injury of muscle, fascia and tendon at or below wrist (S66.-)*
  sprain of joints and ligaments of elbow (S53.4-)

The appropriate 7th character is to be added to each code from category S56.
A   initial encounter
D   subsequent encounter
S   sequela

5 **S56.0**   Injury of flexor muscle, fascia and tendon of thumb at forearm level

6 **S56.00**   Unspecified injury of flexor muscle, fascia and tendon of thumb at forearm level

7 ⊟ **S56.001-**   Unspecified injury of flexor muscle, fascia and tendon of right thumb at forearm level

7 ⊟ **S56.002-**   Unspecified injury of flexor muscle, fascia and tendon of left thumb at forearm level

7 ⊟ **S56.009-**   Unspecified injury of flexor muscle, fascia and tendon of unspecified thumb at forearm level

6 **S56.01**   Strain of flexor muscle, fascia and tendon of thumb at forearm level

7 ⊟ **S56.011-**   Strain of flexor muscle, fascia and tendon of right thumb at forearm level

7 ⊟ **S56.012-**   Strain of flexor muscle, fascia and tendon of left thumb at forearm level

7 ⊟ **S56.019-**   Strain of flexor muscle, fascia and tendon of unspecified thumb at forearm level

6 **S56.02**   Laceration of flexor muscle, fascia and tendon of thumb at forearm level

> **CODING TIP ✓**   Code also any associated open wound S51.-

7 ⊟ **S56.021-**   Laceration of flexor muscle, fascia and tendon of right thumb at forearm level

7 ⊟ **S56.022-**   Laceration of flexor muscle, fascia and tendon of left thumb at forearm level

7 ⊟ **S56.029-**   Laceration of flexor muscle, fascia and tendon of unspecified thumb at forearm level

6 **S56.09**   Other injury of flexor muscle, fascia and tendon of thumb at forearm level

7 ⊟ **S56.091-**   Other injury of flexor muscle, fascia and tendon of right thumb at forearm level

7 ⊟ **S56.092-**   Other injury of flexor muscle, fascia and tendon of left thumb at forearm level

7 ⊟ **S56.099-**   Other injury of flexor muscle, fascia and tendon of unspecified thumb at forearm level

5 **S56.1**   Injury of flexor muscle, fascia and tendon of other and unspecified finger at forearm level

6 **S56.10**   Unspecified injury of flexor muscle, fascia and tendon of other and unspecified finger at forearm level

7 ⊟ **S56.101-**   Unspecified injury of flexor muscle, fascia and tendon of right index finger at forearm level

7 ⊟ **S56.102-**   Unspecified injury of flexor muscle, fascia and tendon of left index finger at forearm level

7 ⊟ **S56.103-**   Unspecified injury of flexor muscle, fascia and tendon of right middle finger at forearm level

7 ⊟ **S56.104-**   Unspecified injury of flexor muscle, fascia and tendon of left middle finger at forearm level

7 ⊟ **S56.105-**   Unspecified injury of flexor muscle, fascia and tendon of right ring finger at forearm level

---

● New   ▲ Revised   *Manifestation*   4-7 Digit Indicators   ⊟ Laterality   A Adult (15+ years)   M Maternity (12-55 years)   N Newborn   P Pediatric (0-17 years)   ♂ Male   ♀ Female
✖ Deleted   Unspecified   ✚ Additional code

7 ⊟ S56.106- Unspecified injury of flexor muscle, fascia and tendon of left ring finger at forearm level

7 ⊟ S56.107- Unspecified injury of flexor muscle, fascia and tendon of right little finger at forearm level

7 ⊟ S56.108- Unspecified injury of flexor muscle, fascia and tendon of left little finger at forearm level

7 ⊟ S56.109- Unspecified injury of flexor muscle, fascia and tendon of unspecified finger at forearm level

6 S56.11 Strain of flexor muscle, fascia and tendon of other and unspecified finger at forearm level

7 ⊟ S56.111- Strain of flexor muscle, fascia and tendon of right index finger at forearm level

7 ⊟ S56.112- Strain of flexor muscle, fascia and tendon of left index finger at forearm level

7 ⊟ S56.113- Strain of flexor muscle, fascia and tendon of right middle finger at forearm level

7 ⊟ S56.114- Strain of flexor muscle, fascia and tendon of left middle finger at forearm level

7 ⊟ S56.115- Strain of flexor muscle, fascia and tendon of right ring finger at forearm level

7 ⊟ S56.116- Strain of flexor muscle, fascia and tendon of left ring finger at forearm level

7 ⊟ S56.117- Strain of flexor muscle, fascia and tendon of right little finger at forearm level

7 ⊟ S56.118- Strain of flexor muscle, fascia and tendon of left little finger at forearm level

7 ⊟ S56.119- Strain of flexor muscle, fascia and tendon of finger of unspecified finger at forearm level

6 S56.12 Laceration of flexor muscle, fascia and tendon of other and unspecified finger at forearm level

CODING TIP ✓ Code also any associated open wound S51.-

7 ⊟ S56.121- Laceration of flexor muscle, fascia and tendon of right index finger at forearm level

7 ⊟ S56.122- Laceration of flexor muscle, fascia and tendon of left index finger at forearm level

7 ⊟ S56.123- Laceration of flexor muscle, fascia and tendon of right middle finger at forearm level

7 ⊟ S56.124- Laceration of flexor muscle, fascia and tendon of left middle finger at forearm level

7 ⊟ S56.125- Laceration of flexor muscle, fascia and tendon of right ring finger at forearm level

7 ⊟ S56.126- Laceration of flexor muscle, fascia and tendon of left ring finger at forearm level

7 ⊟ S56.127- Laceration of flexor muscle, fascia and tendon of right little finger at forearm level

7 ⊟ S56.128- Laceration of flexor muscle, fascia and tendon of left little finger at forearm level

7 ⊟ S56.129- Laceration of flexor muscle, fascia and tendon of unspecified finger at forearm level

6 S56.19 Other injury of flexor muscle, fascia and tendon of other and unspecified finger at forearm level

7 ⊟ S56.191- Other injury of flexor muscle, fascia and tendon of right index finger at forearm level

7 ⊟ S56.192- Other injury of flexor muscle, fascia and tendon of left index finger at forearm level

7 ⊟ S56.193- Other injury of flexor muscle, fascia and tendon of right middle finger at forearm level

7 ⊟ S56.194- Other injury of flexor muscle, fascia and tendon of left middle finger at forearm level

7 ⊟ S56.195- Other injury of flexor muscle, fascia and tendon of right ring finger at forearm level

7 ⊟ S56.196- Other injury of flexor muscle, fascia and tendon of left ring finger at forearm level

7 ⊟ S56.197- Other injury of flexor muscle, fascia and tendon of right little finger at forearm level

7 ⊟ S56.198- Other injury of flexor muscle, fascia and tendon of left little finger at forearm level

7 ⊟ S56.199- Other injury of flexor muscle, fascia and tendon of unspecified finger at forearm level

5 S56.2 Injury of other flexor muscle, fascia and tendon at forearm level

6 S56.20 Unspecified injury of other flexor muscle, fascia and tendon at forearm level

7 ⊟ S56.201- Unspecified injury of other flexor muscle, fascia and tendon at forearm level, right arm

7 ⊟ S56.202- Unspecified injury of other flexor muscle, fascia and tendon at forearm level, left arm

7 ⊟ S56.209- Unspecified injury of other flexor muscle, fascia and tendon at forearm level, unspecified arm

6 S56.21 Strain of other flexor muscle, fascia and tendon at forearm level

7 ⊟ S56.211- Strain of other flexor muscle, fascia and tendon at forearm level, right arm

7 ⊟ S56.212- Strain of other flexor muscle, fascia and tendon at forearm level, left arm

7 ⊟ S56.219- Strain of other flexor muscle, fascia and tendon at forearm level, unspecified arm

6 S56.22 Laceration of other flexor muscle, fascia and tendon at forearm level

CODING TIP ✓ Code also any associated open wound S51.-

7 ⊟ S56.221- Laceration of other flexor muscle, fascia and tendon at forearm level, right arm

7 ⊟ S56.222- Laceration of other flexor muscle, fascia and tendon at forearm level, left arm

7 ⊟ S56.229- Laceration of other flexor muscle, fascia and tendon at forearm level, unspecified arm

6 S56.29 Other injury of other flexor muscle, fascia and tendon at forearm level

7 ⊟ S56.291- Other injury of other flexor muscle, fascia and tendon at forearm level, right arm

7 ⊟ S56.292- Other injury of other flexor muscle, fascia and tendon at forearm level, left arm

7 ⊟ S56.299- Other injury of other flexor muscle, fascia and tendon at forearm level, unspecified arm

5 S56.3 Injury of extensor or abductor muscles, fascia and tendons of thumb at forearm level

6 S56.30 Unspecified injury of extensor or abductor muscles, fascia and tendons of thumb at forearm level

7 ⊟ S56.301- Unspecified injury of extensor or abductor muscles, fascia and tendons of right thumb at forearm level

7 ⊟ S56.302- Unspecified injury of extensor or abductor muscles, fascia and tendons of left thumb at forearm level

7 ⊟ S56.309- Unspecified injury of extensor or abductor muscles, fascia and tendons of unspecified thumb at forearm level

6 S56.31 Strain of extensor or abductor muscles, fascia and tendons of thumb at forearm level

7 ⊟ S56.311- Strain of extensor or abductor muscles, fascia and tendons of right thumb at forearm level

7 ⊟ S56.312- Strain of extensor or abductor muscles, fascia and tendons of left thumb at forearm level

7 ⊟ S56.319- Strain of extensor or abductor muscles, fascia and tendons of unspecified thumb at forearm level

6 S56.32 Laceration of extensor or abductor muscles, fascia and tendons of thumb at forearm level

CODING TIP ✓ Code also any associated open wound S51.-

7 ⊟ S56.321- Laceration of extensor or abductor muscles, fascia and tendons of right thumb at forearm level

7 ⊟ S56.322- Laceration of extensor or abductor muscles, fascia and tendons of left thumb at forearm level

7 ⊟ S56.329- Laceration of extensor or abductor muscles, fascia and tendons of unspecified thumb at forearm level

6 S56.39 Other injury of extensor or abductor muscles, fascia and tendons of thumb at forearm level

7 ⊟ S56.391- Other injury of extensor or abductor muscles, fascia and tendons of right thumb at forearm level

7 ⊟ S56.392- Other injury of extensor or abductor muscles, fascia and tendons of left thumb at forearm level

7 ⊟ S56.399- Other injury of extensor or abductor muscles, fascia and tendons of unspecified thumb at forearm level

5 S56.4 Injury of extensor muscle, fascia and tendon of other and unspecified finger at forearm level

---

● New ▲ Revised *Manifestation* 4-7 Digit Indicators ⊟ Laterality Ⓐ Adult (15+ years) Ⓜ Maternity (12-55 years) Ⓝ Newborn (0-17 years) Ⓟ Pediatric (0-17 years) ♂ Male ♀ Female
✖ Deleted Unspecified + Additional code

6 S56.40 Unspecified injury of extensor muscle, fascia and tendon of other and unspecified finger at forearm level

7 ⊟ S56.401- Unspecified injury of extensor muscle, fascia and tendon of right index finger at forearm level

7 ⊟ S56.402- Unspecified injury of extensor muscle, fascia and tendon of left index finger at forearm level

7 ⊟ S56.403- Unspecified injury of extensor muscle, fascia and tendon of right middle finger at forearm level

7 ⊟ S56.404- Unspecified injury of extensor muscle, fascia and tendon of left middle finger at forearm level

7 ⊟ S56.405- Unspecified injury of extensor muscle, fascia and tendon of right ring finger at forearm level

7 ⊟ S56.406- Unspecified injury of extensor muscle, fascia and tendon of left ring finger at forearm level

7 ⊟ S56.407- Unspecified injury of extensor muscle, fascia and tendon of right little finger at forearm level

7 ⊟ S56.408- Unspecified injury of extensor muscle, fascia and tendon of left little finger at forearm level

7 ⊟ S56.409- Unspecified injury of extensor muscle, fascia and tendon of unspecified finger at forearm level

6 S56.41 Strain of extensor muscle, fascia and tendon of other and unspecified finger at forearm level

7 ⊟ S56.411- Strain of extensor muscle, fascia and tendon of right index finger at forearm level

7 ⊟ S56.412- Strain of extensor muscle, fascia and tendon of left index finger at forearm level

7 ⊟ S56.413- Strain of extensor muscle, fascia and tendon of right middle finger at forearm level

7 ⊟ S56.414- Strain of extensor muscle, fascia and tendon of left middle finger at forearm level

7 ⊟ S56.415- Strain of extensor muscle, fascia and tendon of right ring finger at forearm level

7 ⊟ S56.416- Strain of extensor muscle, fascia and tendon of left ring finger at forearm level

7 ⊟ S56.417- Strain of extensor muscle, fascia and tendon of right little finger at forearm level

7 ⊟ S56.418- Strain of extensor muscle, fascia and tendon of left little finger at forearm level

7 ⊟ S56.419- Strain of extensor muscle, fascia and tendon of finger, unspecified finger at forearm level

6 S56.42 Laceration of extensor muscle, fascia and tendon of other and unspecified finger at forearm level

CODING TIP ✓ Code also any associated open wound S51.-

7 ⊟ S56.421- Laceration of extensor muscle, fascia and tendon of right index finger at forearm level

7 ⊟ S56.422- Laceration of extensor muscle, fascia and tendon of left index finger at forearm level

7 ⊟ S56.423- Laceration of extensor muscle, fascia and tendon of right middle finger at forearm level

7 ⊟ S56.424- Laceration of extensor muscle, fascia and tendon of left middle finger at forearm level

7 ⊟ S56.425- Laceration of extensor muscle, fascia and tendon of right ring finger at forearm level

7 ⊟ S56.426- Laceration of extensor muscle, fascia and tendon of left ring finger at forearm level

7 ⊟ S56.427- Laceration of extensor muscle, fascia and tendon of right little finger at forearm level

7 ⊟ S56.428- Laceration of extensor muscle, fascia and tendon of left little finger at forearm level

7 ⊟ S56.429- Laceration of extensor muscle, fascia and tendon of unspecified finger at forearm level

6 S56.49 Other injury of extensor muscle, fascia and tendon of other and unspecified finger at forearm level

7 ⊟ S56.491- Other injury of extensor muscle, fascia and tendon of right index finger at forearm level

7 ⊟ S56.492- Other injury of extensor muscle, fascia and tendon of left index finger at forearm level

7 ⊟ S56.493- Other injury of extensor muscle, fascia and tendon of right middle finger at forearm level

7 ⊟ S56.494- Other injury of extensor muscle, fascia and tendon of left middle finger at forearm level

7 ⊟ S56.495- Other injury of extensor muscle, fascia and tendon of right ring finger at forearm level

7 ⊟ S56.496- Other injury of extensor muscle, fascia and tendon of left ring finger at forearm level

7 ⊟ S56.497- Other injury of extensor muscle, fascia and tendon of right little finger at forearm level

7 ⊟ S56.498- Other injury of extensor muscle, fascia and tendon of left little finger at forearm level

7 ⊟ S56.499- Other injury of extensor muscle, fascia and tendon of unspecified finger at forearm level

5 S56.5 Injury of other extensor muscle, fascia and tendon at forearm level

6 S56.50 Unspecified injury of other extensor muscle, fascia and tendon at forearm level

7 ⊟ S56.501- Unspecified injury of other extensor muscle, fascia and tendon at forearm level, right arm

7 ⊟ S56.502- Unspecified injury of other extensor muscle, fascia and tendon at forearm level, left arm

7 ⊟ S56.509- Unspecified injury of other extensor muscle, fascia and tendon at forearm level, unspecified arm

6 S56.51 Strain of other extensor muscle, fascia and tendon at forearm level

7 ⊟ S56.511- Strain of other extensor muscle, fascia and tendon at forearm level, right arm

7 ⊟ S56.512- Strain of other extensor muscle, fascia and tendon at forearm level, left arm

7 ⊟ S56.519- Strain of other extensor muscle, fascia and tendon at forearm level, unspecified arm

6 S56.52 Laceration of other extensor muscle, fascia and tendon at forearm level

CODING TIP ✓ Code also any associated open wound S51.-

7 ⊟ S56.521- Laceration of other extensor muscle, fascia and tendon at forearm level, right arm

7 ⊟ S56.522- Laceration of other extensor muscle, fascia and tendon at forearm level, left arm

7 ⊟ S56.529- Laceration of other extensor muscle, fascia and tendon at forearm level, unspecified arm

6 S56.59 Other injury of other extensor muscle, fascia and tendon at forearm level

7 ⊟ S56.591- Other injury of other extensor muscle, fascia and tendon at forearm level, right arm

7 ⊟ S56.592- Other injury of other extensor muscle, fascia and tendon at forearm level, left arm

7 ⊟ S56.599- Other injury of other extensor muscle, fascia and tendon at forearm level, unspecified arm

5 S56.8 Injury of other muscles, fascia and tendons at forearm level

6 S56.80 Unspecified injury of other muscles, fascia and tendons at forearm level

7 ⊟ S56.801- Unspecified injury of other muscles, fascia and tendons at forearm level, right arm

7 ⊟ S56.802- Unspecified injury of other muscles, fascia and tendons at forearm level, left arm

7 ⊟ S56.809- Unspecified injury of other muscles, fascia and tendons at forearm level, unspecified arm

6 S56.81 Strain of other muscles, fascia and tendons at forearm level

7 ⊟ S56.811- Strain of other muscles, fascia and tendons at forearm level, right arm

7 ⊟ S56.812- Strain of other muscles, fascia and tendons at forearm level, left arm

7 ⊟ S56.819- Strain of other muscles, fascia and tendons at forearm level, unspecified arm

6 S56.82 Laceration of other muscles, fascia and tendons at forearm level

CODING TIP ✓ Code also any associated open wound S51.-

7 ⊟ S56.821- Laceration of other muscles, fascia and tendons at forearm level, right arm

---

● New   ▲ Revised   *Manifestation*   **4 - 7** Digit Indicators   ⊟ Laterality   Ⓐ Adult (15+ years)   Ⓜ Maternity (12-55 years)   Ⓝ Newborn   Ⓟ Pediatric (0-17 years)   ♂ Male   ♀ Female

✖ Deleted   Unspecified   + Additional code

978   © 2017 DecisionHealth   2017 ICD-10-CM Expert for Physicians

7 ▣ S56.822-   Laceration of other muscles, fascia and tendons at forearm level, left arm
7 ▣ S56.829-   Laceration of other muscles, fascia and tendons at forearm level, unspecified arm
6 S56.89   Other injury of other muscles, fascia and tendons at forearm level
7 ▣ S56.891-   Other injury of other muscles, fascia and tendons at forearm level, right arm
7 ▣ S56.892-   Other injury of other muscles, fascia and tendons at forearm level, left arm
7 ▣ S56.899-   Other injury of other muscles, fascia and tendons at forearm level, unspecified arm
5 S56.9   Injury of unspecified muscles, fascia and tendons at forearm level
6 S56.90   Unspecified injury of unspecified muscles, fascia and tendons at forearm level
7 ▣ S56.901-   Unspecified injury of unspecified muscles, fascia and tendons at forearm level, right arm
7 ▣ S56.902-   Unspecified injury of unspecified muscles, fascia and tendons at forearm level, left arm
7 ▣ S56.909-   Unspecified injury of unspecified muscles, fascia and tendons at forearm level, unspecified arm
6 S56.91   Strain of unspecified muscles, fascia and tendons at forearm level
7 ▣ S56.911-   Strain of unspecified muscles, fascia and tendons at forearm level, right arm
7 ▣ S56.912-   Strain of unspecified muscles, fascia and tendons at forearm level, left arm
7 ▣ S56.919-   Strain of unspecified muscles, fascia and tendons at forearm level, unspecified arm
6 S56.92   Laceration of unspecified muscles, fascia and tendons at forearm level

CODING TIP ✓   Code also any associated open wound S51.-

7 ▣ S56.921-   Laceration of unspecified muscles, fascia and tendons at forearm level, right arm
7 ▣ S56.922-   Laceration of unspecified muscles, fascia and tendons at forearm level, left arm
7 ▣ S56.929-   Laceration of unspecified muscles, fascia and tendons at forearm level, unspecified arm
6 S56.99   Other injury of unspecified muscles, fascia and tendons at forearm level
7 ▣ S56.991-   Other injury of unspecified muscles, fascia and tendons at forearm level, right arm
7 ▣ S56.992-   Other injury of unspecified muscles, fascia and tendons at forearm level, left arm
7 ▣ S56.999-   Other injury of unspecified muscles, fascia and tendons at forearm level, unspecified arm

4 + S57   **Crushing injury of elbow and forearm**
Use additional code(s) for all associated injuries
EXCLUDES 2   *crushing injury of wrist and hand (S67.-)*

The appropriate 7th character is to be added to each code from category S57
A   initial encounter
D   subsequent encounter
S   sequela

5 + S57.0   Crushing injury of elbow
7 ▣ + S57.00X-   Crushing injury of unspecified elbow
7 ▣ + S57.01X-   Crushing injury of right elbow
7 ▣ + S57.02X-   Crushing injury of left elbow
5 + S57.8   Crushing injury of forearm
7 ▣ + S57.80X-   Crushing injury of unspecified forearm
7 ▣ + S57.81X-   Crushing injury of right forearm
7 ▣ + S57.82X-   Crushing injury of left forearm

4 S58   **Traumatic amputation of elbow and forearm**
An amputation not identified as partial or complete should be coded to complete
EXCLUDES 1   *traumatic amputation of wrist and hand (S68.-)*

The appropriate 7th character is to be added to each code from category S58
A   initial encounter
D   subsequent encounter
S   sequela

5 S58.0   Traumatic amputation at elbow level
6 S58.01   Complete traumatic amputation at elbow level
7 ▣ S58.011-   Complete traumatic amputation at elbow level, right arm
7 ▣ S58.012-   Complete traumatic amputation at elbow level, left arm
7 ▣ S58.019-   Complete traumatic amputation at elbow level, unspecified arm
6 S58.02   Partial traumatic amputation at elbow level
7 ▣ S58.021-   Partial traumatic amputation at elbow level, right arm
7 ▣ S58.022-   Partial traumatic amputation at elbow level, left arm
7 ▣ S58.029-   Partial traumatic amputation at elbow level, unspecified arm
5 S58.1   Traumatic amputation at level between elbow and wrist
6 S58.11   Complete traumatic amputation at level between elbow and wrist
7 ▣ S58.111-   Complete traumatic amputation at level between elbow and wrist, right arm
7 ▣ S58.112-   Complete traumatic amputation at level between elbow and wrist, left arm
7 ▣ S58.119-   Complete traumatic amputation at level between elbow and wrist, unspecified arm
6 S58.12   Partial traumatic amputation at level between elbow and wrist
7 ▣ S58.121-   Partial traumatic amputation at level between elbow and wrist, right arm
7 ▣ S58.122-   Partial traumatic amputation at level between elbow and wrist, left arm
7 ▣ S58.129-   Partial traumatic amputation at level between elbow and wrist, unspecified arm
5 S58.9   Traumatic amputation of forearm, level unspecified
EXCLUDES 1   *traumatic amputation of wrist (S68.-)*
6 S58.91   Complete traumatic amputation of forearm, level unspecified
7 ▣ S58.911-   Complete traumatic amputation of right forearm, level unspecified
7 ▣ S58.912-   Complete traumatic amputation of left forearm, level unspecified
7 ▣ S58.919-   Complete traumatic amputation of unspecified forearm, level unspecified
6 S58.92   Partial traumatic amputation of forearm, level unspecified
7 ▣ S58.921-   Partial traumatic amputation of right forearm, level unspecified
7 ▣ S58.922-   Partial traumatic amputation of left forearm, level unspecified
7 ▣ S58.929-   Partial traumatic amputation of unspecified forearm, level unspecified

4 S59   **Other and unspecified injuries of elbow and forearm**
EXCLUDES 2   *other and unspecified injuries of wrist and hand (S69.-)*

The appropriate 7th character is to be added to each code from subcategories S59.0, S59.1, and S59.2
A   initial encounter for closed fracture
D   subsequent encounter for fracture with routine healing
G   subsequent encounter for fracture with delayed healing
K   subsequent encounter for fracture with nonunion
P   subsequent encounter for fracture with malunion
S   sequela

5 S59.0   Physeal fracture of lower end of ulna
6 S59.00   Unspecified physeal fracture of lower end of ulna
7 ▣ S59.001-   Unspecified physeal fracture of lower end of ulna, right arm

● New   ▲ Revised   *Manifestation*   4-7 Digit Indicators   ▣ Laterality   A Adult (15+ years)   M Maternity (12-55 years)   N Newborn   P Pediatric (0-17 years)   ♂ Male   ♀ Female
✖ Deleted   Unspecified   + Additional code

2017 ICD-10-CM Expert for Physicians   © 2017 DecisionHealth   979

7 ⊟ **S59.002-** Unspecified physeal fracture of lower end of ulna, left arm

7 ⊟ **S59.009-** Unspecified physeal fracture of lower end of ulna, unspecified arm

6 **S59.01** Salter-Harris Type I physeal fracture of lower end of ulna

7 ⊟ **S59.011-** Salter-Harris Type I physeal fracture of lower end of ulna, right arm

7 ⊟ **S59.012-** Salter-Harris Type I physeal fracture of lower end of ulna, left arm

7 ⊟ **S59.019-** Salter-Harris Type I physeal fracture of lower end of ulna, unspecified arm

6 **S59.02** Salter-Harris Type II physeal fracture of lower end of ulna

7 ⊟ **S59.021-** Salter-Harris Type II physeal fracture of lower end of ulna, right arm

7 ⊟ **S59.022-** Salter-Harris Type II physeal fracture of lower end of ulna, left arm

7 ⊟ **S59.029-** Salter-Harris Type II physeal fracture of lower end of ulna, unspecified arm

6 **S59.03** Salter-Harris Type III physeal fracture of lower end of ulna

7 ⊟ **S59.031-** Salter-Harris Type III physeal fracture of lower end of ulna, right arm

7 ⊟ **S59.032-** Salter-Harris Type III physeal fracture of lower end of ulna, left arm

7 ⊟ **S59.039-** Salter-Harris Type III physeal fracture of lower end of ulna, unspecified arm

6 **S59.04** Salter-Harris Type IV physeal fracture of lower end of ulna

7 ⊟ **S59.041-** Salter-Harris Type IV physeal fracture of lower end of ulna, right arm

7 ⊟ **S59.042-** Salter-Harris Type IV physeal fracture of lower end of ulna, left arm

7 ⊟ **S59.049-** Salter-Harris Type IV physeal fracture of lower end of ulna, unspecified arm

6 **S59.09** Other physeal fracture of lower end of ulna

7 ⊟ **S59.091-** Other physeal fracture of lower end of ulna, right arm

7 ⊟ **S59.092-** Other physeal fracture of lower end of ulna, left arm

7 ⊟ **S59.099-** Other physeal fracture of lower end of ulna, unspecified arm

5 **S59.1** Physeal fracture of upper end of radius

6 **S59.10** Unspecified physeal fracture of upper end of radius

7 ⊟ **S59.101-** Unspecified physeal fracture of upper end of radius, right arm

7 ⊟ **S59.102-** Unspecified physeal fracture of upper end of radius, left arm

7 ⊟ **S59.109-** Unspecified physeal fracture of upper end of radius, unspecified arm

6 **S59.11** Salter-Harris Type I physeal fracture of upper end of radius

7 ⊟ **S59.111-** Salter-Harris Type I physeal fracture of upper end of radius, right arm

7 ⊟ **S59.112-** Salter-Harris Type I physeal fracture of upper end of radius, left arm

7 ⊟ **S59.119-** Salter-Harris Type I physeal fracture of upper end of radius, unspecified arm

6 **S59.12** Salter-Harris Type II physeal fracture of upper end of radius

7 ⊟ **S59.121-** Salter-Harris Type II physeal fracture of upper end of radius, right arm

7 ⊟ **S59.122-** Salter-Harris Type II physeal fracture of upper end of radius, left arm

7 ⊟ **S59.129-** Salter-Harris Type II physeal fracture of upper end of radius, unspecified arm

6 **S59.13** Salter-Harris Type III physeal fracture of upper end of radius

7 ⊟ **S59.131-** Salter-Harris Type III physeal fracture of upper end of radius, right arm

7 ⊟ **S59.132-** Salter-Harris Type III physeal fracture of upper end of radius, left arm

7 ⊟ **S59.139-** Salter-Harris Type III physeal fracture of upper end of radius, unspecified arm

6 **S59.14** Salter-Harris Type IV physeal fracture of upper end of radius

7 ⊟ **S59.141-** Salter-Harris Type IV physeal fracture of upper end of radius, right arm

7 ⊟ **S59.142-** Salter-Harris Type IV physeal fracture of upper end of radius, left arm

7 ⊟ **S59.149-** Salter-Harris Type IV physeal fracture of upper end of radius, unspecified arm

6 **S59.19** Other physeal fracture of upper end of radius

7 ⊟ **S59.191-** Other physeal fracture of upper end of radius, right arm

7 ⊟ **S59.192-** Other physeal fracture of upper end of radius, left arm

7 ⊟ **S59.199-** Other physeal fracture of upper end of radius, unspecified arm

5 **S59.2** Physeal fracture of lower end of radius

6 **S59.20** Unspecified physeal fracture of lower end of radius

7 ⊟ **S59.201-** Unspecified physeal fracture of lower end of radius, right arm

7 ⊟ **S59.202-** Unspecified physeal fracture of lower end of radius, left arm

7 ⊟ **S59.209-** Unspecified physeal fracture of lower end of radius, unspecified arm

6 **S59.21** Salter-Harris Type I physeal fracture of lower end of radius

7 ⊟ **S59.211-** Salter-Harris Type I physeal fracture of lower end of radius, right arm

7 ⊟ **S59.212-** Salter-Harris Type I physeal fracture of lower end of radius, left arm

7 ⊟ **S59.219-** Salter-Harris Type I physeal fracture of lower end of radius, unspecified arm

6 **S59.22** Salter-Harris Type II physeal fracture of lower end of radius

7 ⊟ **S59.221-** Salter-Harris Type II physeal fracture of lower end of radius, right arm

7 ⊟ **S59.222-** Salter-Harris Type II physeal fracture of lower end of radius, left arm

7 ⊟ **S59.229-** Salter-Harris Type II physeal fracture of lower end of radius, unspecified arm

6 **S59.23** Salter-Harris Type III physeal fracture of lower end of radius

7 ⊟ **S59.231-** Salter-Harris Type III physeal fracture of lower end of radius, right arm

7 ⊟ **S59.232-** Salter-Harris Type III physeal fracture of lower end of radius, left arm

7 ⊟ **S59.239-** Salter-Harris Type III physeal fracture of lower end of radius, unspecified arm

6 **S59.24** Salter-Harris Type IV physeal fracture of lower end of radius

7 ⊟ **S59.241-** Salter-Harris Type IV physeal fracture of lower end of radius, right arm

7 ⊟ **S59.242-** Salter-Harris Type IV physeal fracture of lower end of radius, left arm

7 ⊟ **S59.249-** Salter-Harris Type IV physeal fracture of lower end of radius, unspecified arm

6 **S59.29** Other physeal fracture of lower end of radius

7 ⊟ **S59.291-** Other physeal fracture of lower end of radius, right arm

7 ⊟ **S59.292-** Other physeal fracture of lower end of radius, left arm

7 ⊟ **S59.299-** Other physeal fracture of lower end of radius, unspecified arm

5 **S59.8** Other specified injuries of elbow and forearm

> The appropriate 7th character is to be added to each code in subcategory S59.8
> A   initial encounter
> D   subsequent encounter
> S   sequela

6 **S59.80** Other specified injuries of elbow

7 ⊟ **S59.801-** Other specified injuries of right elbow

7 ⊟ **S59.802-** Other specified injuries of left elbow

7 ⊟ **S59.809-** Other specified injuries of unspecified elbow

6 **S59.81** Other specified injuries of forearm

7 ⊟ **S59.811-** Other specified injuries right forearm

7 ⊟ **S59.812-** Other specified injuries left forearm

7 ⊟ **S59.819-** Other specified injuries unspecified forearm

Ⓖ **S59.9**   **Unspecified injury of elbow and forearm**

The appropriate 7th character is to be added to each code in subcategory S59.9
A   initial encounter
D   subsequent encounter
S   sequela

Ⓖ **S59.90**   **Unspecified injury of elbow**

7️⃣🔲 **S59.901-**   **Unspecified injury of right elbow**

7️⃣🔲 **S59.902-**   **Unspecified injury of left elbow**

7️⃣🔲 **S59.909-**   **Unspecified injury of unspecified elbow**

Ⓖ **S59.91**   **Unspecified injury of forearm**

7️⃣🔲 **S59.911-**   **Unspecified injury of right forearm**

7️⃣🔲 **S59.912-**   **Unspecified injury of left forearm**

7️⃣🔲 **S59.919-**   **Unspecified injury of unspecified forearm**

Injuries to the wrist, hand and fingers (S60-S69)

EXCLUDES 2   *burns and corrosions (T20-T32)*
frostbite (T33-T34)
insect bite or sting, venomous (T63.4)

GUIDELINES   **Section I.C.19.c.2)**
Multiple fractures are sequenced in accordance with the severity of the fracture.

GUIDELINES   **Section I.C.19.b.1)-2)**
When coding injuries, assign separate codes for each injury unless a combination code is provided, in which case the combination code is assigned ... Traumatic injury codes (S00-T14.9) are not to be used for normal, healing surgical wounds or to identify complications of surgical wounds. The code for the most serious injury, as determined by the provider and the focus of treatment, is sequenced first.

1) Superficial injuries such as abrasions or contusions are not coded when associated with more severe injuries of the same site.

2) When a primary injury results in minor damage to peripheral nerves or blood vessels, the primary injury is sequenced first with additional code(s) for injuries to nerves and spinal cord (such as category S04), and/or injury to blood vessels (such as category S15). When the primary injury is to the blood vessels or nerves, that injury should be sequenced first.

GUIDELINES   **Section I.C.19.c**
Coding of Traumatic Fractures: The principles of multiple coding of injuries should be followed in coding fractures. Fractures of specified sites are coded individually by site in accordance with both the provisions within categories S02, S12, S22, S32, S42, S49, S52, S59, S62, S72, S79, S82, S89, S92 and the level of detail furnished by medical record content. A fracture not indicated as open or closed should be coded to closed. A fracture not indicated whether displaced or not displaced should be coded to displaced.

4️⃣ **S60**   **Superficial injury of wrist, hand and fingers**

The appropriate 7th character is to be added to each code from category S60
A   initial encounter
D   subsequent encounter
S   sequela

Ⓢ **S60.0**   **Contusion of finger without damage to nail**

EXCLUDES 1   *contusion involving nail (matrix) (S60.1)*

7️⃣ **S60.00X-**   **Contusion of unspecified finger without damage to nail**
Contusion of finger(s) NOS

Ⓖ **S60.01**   **Contusion of thumb without damage to nail**

7️⃣🔲 **S60.011-**   **Contusion of right thumb without damage to nail**

7️⃣🔲 **S60.012-**   **Contusion of left thumb without damage to nail**

7️⃣🔲 **S60.019-**   **Contusion of unspecified thumb without damage to nail**

Ⓖ **S60.02**   **Contusion of index finger without damage to nail**

7️⃣🔲 **S60.021-**   **Contusion of right index finger without damage to nail**

7️⃣🔲 **S60.022-**   **Contusion of left index finger without damage to nail**

7️⃣🔲 **S60.029-**   **Contusion of unspecified index finger without damage to nail**

Ⓖ **S60.03**   **Contusion of middle finger without damage to nail**

7️⃣🔲 **S60.031-**   **Contusion of right middle finger without damage to nail**

7️⃣🔲 **S60.032-**   **Contusion of left middle finger without damage to nail**

7️⃣🔲 **S60.039-**   **Contusion of unspecified middle finger without damage to nail**

Ⓖ **S60.04**   **Contusion of ring finger without damage to nail**

7️⃣🔲 **S60.041-**   **Contusion of right ring finger without damage to nail**

7️⃣🔲 **S60.042-**   **Contusion of left ring finger without damage to nail**

7️⃣🔲 **S60.049-**   **Contusion of unspecified ring finger without damage to nail**

Ⓖ **S60.05**   **Contusion of little finger without damage to nail**

7️⃣🔲 **S60.051-**   **Contusion of right little finger without damage to nail**

7️⃣🔲 **S60.052-**   **Contusion of left little finger without damage to nail**

7️⃣🔲 **S60.059-**   **Contusion of unspecified little finger without damage to nail**

Ⓢ **S60.1**   **Contusion of finger with damage to nail**

7️⃣ **S60.10X-**   **Contusion of unspecified finger with damage to nail**

Ⓖ **S60.11**   **Contusion of thumb with damage to nail**

7️⃣🔲 **S60.111-**   **Contusion of right thumb with damage to nail**

7️⃣🔲 **S60.112-**   **Contusion of left thumb with damage to nail**

7️⃣🔲 **S60.119-**   **Contusion of unspecified thumb with damage to nail**

Ⓖ **S60.12**   **Contusion of index finger with damage to nail**

7️⃣🔲 **S60.121-**   **Contusion of right index finger with damage to nail**

7️⃣🔲 **S60.122-**   **Contusion of left index finger with damage to nail**

7️⃣🔲 **S60.129-**   **Contusion of unspecified index finger with damage to nail**

Ⓖ **S60.13**   **Contusion of middle finger with damage to nail**

7️⃣🔲 **S60.131-**   **Contusion of right middle finger with damage to nail**

7️⃣🔲 **S60.132-**   **Contusion of left middle finger with damage to nail**

7️⃣🔲 **S60.139-**   **Contusion of unspecified middle finger with damage to nail**

Ⓖ **S60.14**   **Contusion of ring finger with damage to nail**

7️⃣🔲 **S60.141-**   **Contusion of right ring finger with damage to nail**

7️⃣🔲 **S60.142-**   **Contusion of left ring finger with damage to nail**

7️⃣🔲 **S60.149-**   **Contusion of unspecified ring finger with damage to nail**

Ⓖ **S60.15**   **Contusion of little finger with damage to nail**

7️⃣🔲 **S60.151-**   **Contusion of right little finger with damage to nail**

7️⃣🔲 **S60.152-**   **Contusion of left little finger with damage to nail**

7️⃣🔲 **S60.159-**   **Contusion of unspecified little finger with damage to nail**

Ⓢ **S60.2**   **Contusion of wrist and hand**

EXCLUDES 2   *contusion of fingers (S60.0-, S60.1-)*

Ⓖ **S60.21**   **Contusion of wrist**

7️⃣🔲 **S60.211-**   **Contusion of right wrist**

7️⃣🔲 **S60.212-**   **Contusion of left wrist**

7️⃣🔲 **S60.219-**   **Contusion of unspecified wrist**

Ⓖ **S60.22**   **Contusion of hand**

7️⃣🔲 **S60.221-**   **Contusion of right hand**

7️⃣🔲 **S60.222-**   **Contusion of left hand**

7️⃣🔲 **S60.229-**   **Contusion of unspecified hand**

Ⓢ **S60.3**   **Other superficial injuries of thumb**

Ⓖ **S60.31**   **Abrasion of thumb**

● New   ▲ Revised   *Manifestation*   4️⃣-7️⃣ Digit Indicators   🔲 Laterality   🅰 Adult (15+ years)   🅼 Maternity (12-55 years)   🅽 Newborn   🅿 Pediatric (0-17 years)   ♂ Male   ♀ Female
✖ Deleted   Unspecified   ✚ Additional code

7 ⊟ S60.311-　Abrasion of right thumb
7 ⊟ S60.312-　Abrasion of left thumb
7 ⊟ S60.319-　Abrasion of unspecified thumb
6 S60.32　Blister (nonthermal) of thumb
7 ⊟ S60.321-　Blister (nonthermal) of right thumb
7 ⊟ S60.322-　Blister (nonthermal) of left thumb
7 ⊟ S60.329-　Blister (nonthermal) of unspecified thumb
6 + S60.34　External constriction of thumb
　　Hair tourniquet syndrome of thumb
　　Use additional cause code to identify the constricting item (W49.0-)
7 ⊟ + S60.341-　External constriction of right thumb
7 ⊟ + S60.342-　External constriction of left thumb
7 ⊟ + S60.349-　External constriction of unspecified thumb
6 S60.35　Superficial foreign body of thumb
　　Splinter in the thumb
7 ⊟ S60.351-　Superficial foreign body of right thumb
7 ⊟ S60.352-　Superficial foreign body of left thumb
7 ⊟ S60.359-　Superficial foreign body of unspecified thumb
6 S60.36　Insect bite (nonvenomous) of thumb
7 ⊟ S60.361-　Insect bite (nonvenomous) of right thumb
7 ⊟ S60.362-　Insect bite (nonvenomous) of left thumb
7 ⊟ S60.369-　Insect bite (nonvenomous) of unspecified thumb
6 S60.37　Other superficial bite of thumb
　　EXCLUDES 1　*open bite of thumb (S61.05-, S61.15-)*
7 ⊟ S60.371-　Other superficial bite of right thumb
7 ⊟ S60.372-　Other superficial bite of left thumb
7 ⊟ S60.379-　Other superficial bite of unspecified thumb
6 S60.39　Other superficial injuries of thumb
7 ⊟ S60.391-　Other superficial injuries of right thumb
7 ⊟ S60.392-　Other superficial injuries of left thumb
7 ⊟ S60.399-　Other superficial injuries of unspecified thumb
5 S60.4　Other superficial injuries of other fingers
6 S60.41　Abrasion of fingers
7 ⊟ S60.410-　Abrasion of right index finger
7 ⊟ S60.411-　Abrasion of left index finger
7 ⊟ S60.412-　Abrasion of right middle finger
7 ⊟ S60.413-　Abrasion of left middle finger
7 ⊟ S60.414-　Abrasion of right ring finger
7 ⊟ S60.415-　Abrasion of left ring finger
7 ⊟ S60.416-　Abrasion of right little finger
7 ⊟ S60.417-　Abrasion of left little finger
7 ⊟ S60.418-　Abrasion of other finger
　　Abrasion of specified finger with unspecified laterality
7 ⊟ S60.419-　Abrasion of unspecified finger
6 S60.42　Blister (nonthermal) of fingers
7 ⊟ S60.420-　Blister (nonthermal) of right index finger
7 ⊟ S60.421-　Blister (nonthermal) of left index finger
7 ⊟ S60.422-　Blister (nonthermal) of right middle finger
7 ⊟ S60.423-　Blister (nonthermal) of left middle finger
7 ⊟ S60.424-　Blister (nonthermal) of right ring finger
7 ⊟ S60.425-　Blister (nonthermal) of left ring finger
7 ⊟ S60.426-　Blister (nonthermal) of right little finger
7 ⊟ S60.427-　Blister (nonthermal) of left little finger
7 ⊟ S60.428-　Blister (nonthermal) of other finger
　　Blister (nonthermal) of specified finger with unspecified laterality
7 ⊟ S60.429-　Blister (nonthermal) of unspecified finger
6 + S60.44　External constriction of fingers
　　Hair tourniquet syndrome of finger
　　Use additional cause code to identify the constricting item (W49.0-)
7 ⊟ + S60.440-　External constriction of right index finger
7 ⊟ + S60.441-　External constriction of left index finger
7 ⊟ + S60.442-　External constriction of right middle finger
7 ⊟ + S60.443-　External constriction of left middle finger
7 ⊟ + S60.444-　External constriction of right ring finger
7 ⊟ + S60.445-　External constriction of left ring finger
7 ⊟ + S60.446-　External constriction of right little finger
7 ⊟ + S60.447-　External constriction of left little finger
7 ⊟ + S60.448-　External constriction of other finger
　　External constriction of specified finger with unspecified laterality
7 ⊟ + S60.449-　External constriction of unspecified finger
6 S60.45　Superficial foreign body of fingers
　　Splinter in the finger(s)
7 ⊟ S60.450-　Superficial foreign body of right index finger
7 ⊟ S60.451-　Superficial foreign body of left index finger
7 ⊟ S60.452-　Superficial foreign body of right middle finger
7 ⊟ S60.453-　Superficial foreign body of left middle finger
7 ⊟ S60.454-　Superficial foreign body of right ring finger
7 ⊟ S60.455-　Superficial foreign body of left ring finger
7 ⊟ S60.456-　Superficial foreign body of right little finger
7 ⊟ S60.457-　Superficial foreign body of left little finger
7 ⊟ S60.458-　Superficial foreign body of other finger
　　Superficial foreign body of specified finger with unspecified laterality
7 ⊟ S60.459-　Superficial foreign body of unspecified finger
6 S60.46　Insect bite (nonvenomous) of fingers
7 ⊟ S60.460-　Insect bite (nonvenomous) of right index finger
7 ⊟ S60.461-　Insect bite (nonvenomous) of left index finger
7 ⊟ S60.462-　Insect bite (nonvenomous) of right middle finger
7 ⊟ S60.463-　Insect bite (nonvenomous) of left middle finger
7 ⊟ S60.464-　Insect bite (nonvenomous) of right ring finger
7 ⊟ S60.465-　Insect bite (nonvenomous) of left ring finger
7 ⊟ S60.466-　Insect bite (nonvenomous) of right little finger
7 ⊟ S60.467-　Insect bite (nonvenomous) of left little finger
7 ⊟ S60.468-　Insect bite (nonvenomous) of other finger
　　Insect bite (nonvenomous) of specified finger with unspecified laterality
7 ⊟ S60.469-　Insect bite (nonvenomous) of unspecified finger
6 S60.47　Other superficial bite of fingers
　　EXCLUDES 1　*open bite of fingers (S61.25-, S61.35-)*
7 ⊟ S60.470-　Other superficial bite of right index finger
7 ⊟ S60.471-　Other superficial bite of left index finger
7 ⊟ S60.472-　Other superficial bite of right middle finger
7 ⊟ S60.473-　Other superficial bite of left middle finger
7 ⊟ S60.474-　Other superficial bite of right ring finger
7 ⊟ S60.475-　Other superficial bite of left ring finger
7 ⊟ S60.476-　Other superficial bite of right little finger
7 ⊟ S60.477-　Other superficial bite of left little finger
7 ⊟ S60.478-　Other superficial bite of other finger
　　Other superficial bite of specified finger with unspecified laterality
7 ⊟ S60.479-　Other superficial bite of unspecified finger
5 S60.5　Other superficial injuries of hand
　　EXCLUDES 2　*superficial injuries of fingers (S60.3-, S60.4-)*
6 S60.51　Abrasion of hand
7 ⊟ S60.511-　Abrasion of right hand
7 ⊟ S60.512-　Abrasion of left hand
7 ⊟ S60.519-　Abrasion of unspecified hand
6 S60.52　Blister (nonthermal) of hand
7 ⊟ S60.521-　Blister (nonthermal) of right hand
7 ⊟ S60.522-　Blister (nonthermal) of left hand
7 ⊟ S60.529-　Blister (nonthermal) of unspecified hand
6 S60.54　External constriction of hand
7 ⊟ S60.541-　External constriction of right hand
7 ⊟ S60.542-　External constriction of left hand
7 ⊟ S60.549-　External constriction of unspecified hand
6 S60.55　Superficial foreign body of hand
　　Splinter in the hand

7 ⊟ **S60.551-** Superficial foreign body of right hand

7 ⊟ **S60.552-** Superficial foreign body of left hand

7 ⊟ **S60.559-** Superficial foreign body of unspecified hand

6 **S60.56** Insect bite (nonvenomous) of hand

7 ⊟ **S60.561-** Insect bite (nonvenomous) of right hand

7 ⊟ **S60.562-** Insect bite (nonvenomous) of left hand

7 ⊟ **S60.569-** Insect bite (nonvenomous) of unspecified hand

6 **S60.57** Other superficial bite of hand

> **EXCLUDES 1** *open bite of hand (S61.45-)*

7 ⊟ **S60.571-** Other superficial bite of hand of right hand

7 ⊟ **S60.572-** Other superficial bite of hand of left hand

7 ⊟ **S60.579-** Other superficial bite of hand of unspecified hand

5 **S60.8** Other superficial injuries of wrist

6 **S60.81** Abrasion of wrist

7 ⊟ **S60.811-** Abrasion of right wrist

7 ⊟ **S60.812-** Abrasion of left wrist

7 ⊟ **S60.819-** Abrasion of unspecified wrist

6 **S60.82** Blister (nonthermal) of wrist

7 ⊟ **S60.821-** Blister (nonthermal) of right wrist

7 ⊟ **S60.822-** Blister (nonthermal) of left wrist

7 ⊟ **S60.829-** Blister (nonthermal) of unspecified wrist

6 **S60.84** External constriction of wrist

7 ⊟ **S60.841-** External constriction of right wrist

7 ⊟ **S60.842-** External constriction of left wrist

7 ⊟ **S60.849-** External constriction of unspecified wrist

6 **S60.85** Superficial foreign body of wrist
Splinter in the wrist

7 ⊟ **S60.851-** Superficial foreign body of right wrist

7 ⊟ **S60.852-** Superficial foreign body of left wrist

7 ⊟ **S60.859-** Superficial foreign body of unspecified wrist

6 **S60.86** Insect bite (nonvenomous) of wrist

7 ⊟ **S60.861-** Insect bite (nonvenomous) of right wrist

7 ⊟ **S60.862-** Insect bite (nonvenomous) of left wrist

7 ⊟ **S60.869-** Insect bite (nonvenomous) of unspecified wrist

6 **S60.87** Other superficial bite of wrist

> **EXCLUDES 1** *open bite of wrist (S61.55)*

7 ⊟ **S60.871-** Other superficial bite of right wrist

7 ⊟ **S60.872-** Other superficial bite of left wrist

7 ⊟ **S60.879-** Other superficial bite of unspecified wrist

5 **S60.9** Unspecified superficial injury of wrist, hand and fingers

6 **S60.91** Unspecified superficial injury of wrist

7 ⊟ **S60.911-** Unspecified superficial injury of right wrist

7 ⊟ **S60.912-** Unspecified superficial injury of left wrist

7 ⊟ **S60.919-** Unspecified superficial injury of unspecified wrist

6 **S60.92** Unspecified superficial injury of hand

7 ⊟ **S60.921-** Unspecified superficial injury of right hand

7 ⊟ **S60.922-** Unspecified superficial injury of left hand

7 ⊟ **S60.929-** Unspecified superficial injury of unspecified hand

6 **S60.93** Unspecified superficial injury of thumb

7 ⊟ **S60.931-** Unspecified superficial injury of right thumb

7 ⊟ **S60.932-** Unspecified superficial injury of left thumb

7 ⊟ **S60.939-** Unspecified superficial injury of unspecified thumb

6 **S60.94** Unspecified superficial injury of other fingers

7 ⊟ **S60.940-** Unspecified superficial injury of right index finger

7 ⊟ **S60.941-** Unspecified superficial injury of left index finger

7 ⊟ **S60.942-** Unspecified superficial injury of right middle finger

7 ⊟ **S60.943-** Unspecified superficial injury of left middle finger

7 ⊟ **S60.944-** Unspecified superficial injury of right ring finger

7 ⊟ **S60.945-** Unspecified superficial injury of left ring finger

7 ⊟ **S60.946-** Unspecified superficial injury of right little finger

7 ⊟ **S60.947-** Unspecified superficial injury of left little finger

7 ⊟ **S60.948-** Unspecified superficial injury of other finger
Unspecified superficial injury of specified finger with unspecified laterality

7 ⊟ **S60.949-** Unspecified superficial injury of unspecified finger

4 **S61** **Open wound of wrist, hand and fingers**
Code also:
any associated wound infection

> **EXCLUDES 1** *open fracture of wrist, hand and finger (S62.- with 7th character B)*
> *traumatic amputation of wrist and hand (S68.-)*

The appropriate 7th character is to be added to each code from category S61
A   initial encounter
D   subsequent encounter
S   sequela

> **CODING TIP ✓** Open wound codes indicate a wound resulting from a traumatic origin. Do not assign a code for "open wound" unless the etiology of the wound is related to trauma.

5 **S61.0** Open wound of thumb without damage to nail

> **EXCLUDES 1** *open wound of thumb with damage to nail (S61.1-)*

6 **S61.00** Unspecified open wound of thumb without damage to nail

7 ⊟ **S61.001-** Unspecified open wound of right thumb without damage to nail

7 ⊟ **S61.002-** Unspecified open wound of left thumb without damage to nail

7 ⊟ **S61.009-** Unspecified open wound of unspecified thumb without damage to nail

6 **S61.01** Laceration without foreign body of thumb without damage to nail

7 ⊟ **S61.011-** Laceration without foreign body of right thumb without damage to nail

7 ⊟ **S61.012-** Laceration without foreign body of left thumb without damage to nail

7 ⊟ **S61.019-** Laceration without foreign body of unspecified thumb without damage to nail

6 **S61.02** Laceration with foreign body of thumb without damage to nail

7 ⊟ **S61.021-** Laceration with foreign body of right thumb without damage to nail

7 ⊟ **S61.022-** Laceration with foreign body of left thumb without damage to nail

7 ⊟ **S61.029-** Laceration with foreign body of unspecified thumb without damage to nail

6 **S61.03** Puncture wound without foreign body of thumb without damage to nail

7 ⊟ **S61.031-** Puncture wound without foreign body of right thumb without damage to nail

7 ⊟ **S61.032-** Puncture wound without foreign body of left thumb without damage to nail

7 ⊟ **S61.039-** Puncture wound without foreign body of unspecified thumb without damage to nail

6 **S61.04** Puncture wound with foreign body of thumb without damage to nail

7 ⊟ **S61.041-** Puncture wound with foreign body of right thumb without damage to nail

7 ⊟ **S61.042-** Puncture wound with foreign body of left thumb without damage to nail

7 ⊟ **S61.049-** Puncture wound with foreign body of unspecified thumb without damage to nail

6 **S61.05** Open bite of thumb without damage to nail
Bite of thumb NOS

> **EXCLUDES 1** *superficial bite of thumb (S60.36-, S60.37-)*

7 ⊟ **S61.051-** Open bite of right thumb without damage to nail

7 ⊟ **S61.052-** Open bite of left thumb without damage to nail

---

● New   ▲ Revised   *Manifestation*   ✖ ~~Deleted~~   Unspecified   4 - 7 Digit Indicators   + Additional code   ⊟ Laterality   🅰 Adult (15+ years)   🅼 Maternity (12-55 years)   🅽 Newborn   🅿 Pediatric (0-17 years)   ♂ Male   ♀ Female

7 ⊟ **S61.059-**   Open bite of unspecified thumb without damage to nail

5 **S61.1**   Open wound of thumb with damage to nail

6 **S61.10**   Unspecified open wound of thumb with damage to nail

7 ⊟ **S61.101-**   Unspecified open wound of right thumb with damage to nail

7 ⊟ **S61.102-**   Unspecified open wound of left thumb with damage to nail

7 ⊟ **S61.109-**   Unspecified open wound of unspecified thumb with damage to nail

6 **S61.11**   Laceration without foreign body of thumb with damage to nail

7 ⊟ **S61.111-**   Laceration without foreign body of right thumb with damage to nail

7 ⊟ **S61.112-**   Laceration without foreign body of left thumb with damage to nail

7 ⊟ **S61.119-**   Laceration without foreign body of unspecified thumb with damage to nail

6 **S61.12**   Laceration with foreign body of thumb with damage to nail

7 ⊟ **S61.121-**   Laceration with foreign body of right thumb with damage to nail

7 ⊟ **S61.122-**   Laceration with foreign body of left thumb with damage to nail

7 ⊟ **S61.129-**   Laceration with foreign body of unspecified thumb with damage to nail

6 **S61.13**   Puncture wound without foreign body of thumb with damage to nail

7 ⊟ **S61.131-**   Puncture wound without foreign body of right thumb with damage to nail

7 ⊟ **S61.132-**   Puncture wound without foreign body of left thumb with damage to nail

7 ⊟ **S61.139-**   Puncture wound without foreign body of unspecified thumb with damage to nail

6 **S61.14**   Puncture wound with foreign body of thumb with damage to nail

7 ⊟ **S61.141-**   Puncture wound with foreign body of right thumb with damage to nail

7 ⊟ **S61.142-**   Puncture wound with foreign body of left thumb with damage to nail

7 ⊟ **S61.149-**   Puncture wound with foreign body of unspecified thumb with damage to nail

6 **S61.15**   Open bite of thumb with damage to nail
Bite of thumb with damage to nail NOS

> **EXCLUDES 1**   *superficial bite of thumb (S60.36-, S60.37-)*

7 ⊟ **S61.151-**   Open bite of right thumb with damage to nail

7 ⊟ **S61.152-**   Open bite of left thumb with damage to nail

7 ⊟ **S61.159-**   Open bite of unspecified thumb with damage to nail

5 **S61.2**   Open wound of other finger without damage to nail

> **EXCLUDES 1**   *open wound of finger involving nail (matrix) (S61.3-)*

> **EXCLUDES 2**   *open wound of thumb without damage to nail (S61.0-)*

6 **S61.20**   Unspecified open wound of other finger without damage to nail

7 ⊟ **S61.200-**   Unspecified open wound of right index finger without damage to nail

7 ⊟ **S61.201-**   Unspecified open wound of left index finger without damage to nail

7 ⊟ **S61.202-**   Unspecified open wound of right middle finger without damage to nail

7 ⊟ **S61.203-**   Unspecified open wound of left middle finger without damage to nail

7 ⊟ **S61.204-**   Unspecified open wound of right ring finger without damage to nail

7 ⊟ **S61.205-**   Unspecified open wound of left ring finger without damage to nail

7 ⊟ **S61.206-**   Unspecified open wound of right little finger without damage to nail

7 ⊟ **S61.207-**   Unspecified open wound of left little finger without damage to nail

7 ⊟ **S61.208-**   Unspecified open wound of other finger without damage to nail
Unspecified open wound of specified finger with unspecified laterality without damage to nail

7 ⊟ **S61.209-**   Unspecified open wound of unspecified finger without damage to nail

6 **S61.21**   Laceration without foreign body of finger without damage to nail

7 ⊟ **S61.210-**   Laceration without foreign body of right index finger without damage to nail

7 ⊟ **S61.211-**   Laceration without foreign body of left index finger without damage to nail

7 ⊟ **S61.212-**   Laceration without foreign body of right middle finger without damage to nail

7 ⊟ **S61.213-**   Laceration without foreign body of left middle finger without damage to nail

7 ⊟ **S61.214-**   Laceration without foreign body of right ring finger without damage to nail

7 ⊟ **S61.215-**   Laceration without foreign body of left ring finger without damage to nail

7 ⊟ **S61.216-**   Laceration without foreign body of right little finger without damage to nail

7 ⊟ **S61.217-**   Laceration without foreign body of left little finger without damage to nail

7 ⊟ **S61.218-**   Laceration without foreign body of other finger without damage to nail
Laceration without foreign body of specified finger with unspecified laterality without damage to nail

7 ⊟ **S61.219-**   Laceration without foreign body of unspecified finger without damage to nail

6 **S61.22**   Laceration with foreign body of finger without damage to nail

7 ⊟ **S61.220-**   Laceration with foreign body of right index finger without damage to nail

7 ⊟ **S61.221-**   Laceration with foreign body of left index finger without damage to nail

7 ⊟ **S61.222-**   Laceration with foreign body of right middle finger without damage to nail

7 ⊟ **S61.223-**   Laceration with foreign body of left middle finger without damage to nail

7 ⊟ **S61.224-**   Laceration with foreign body of right ring finger without damage to nail

7 ⊟ **S61.225-**   Laceration with foreign body of left ring finger without damage to nail

7 ⊟ **S61.226-**   Laceration with foreign body of right little finger without damage to nail

7 ⊟ **S61.227-**   Laceration with foreign body of left little finger without damage to nail

7 ⊟ **S61.228-**   Laceration with foreign body of other finger without damage to nail
Laceration with foreign body of specified finger with unspecified laterality without damage to nail

7 ⊟ **S61.229-**   Laceration with foreign body of unspecified finger without damage to nail

6 **S61.23**   Puncture wound without foreign body of finger without damage to nail

7 ⊟ **S61.230-**   Puncture wound without foreign body of right index finger without damage to nail

7 ⊟ **S61.231-**   Puncture wound without foreign body of left index finger without damage to nail

7 ⊟ **S61.232-**   Puncture wound without foreign body of right middle finger without damage to nail

7 ⊟ **S61.233-**   Puncture wound without foreign body of left middle finger without damage to nail

7 ⊟ **S61.234-**   Puncture wound without foreign body of right ring finger without damage to nail

7 ⊟ **S61.235-**   Puncture wound without foreign body of left ring finger without damage to nail

7 ⊟ **S61.236-**   Puncture wound without foreign body of right little finger without damage to nail

7 ⊟ **S61.237-**   Puncture wound without foreign body of left little finger without damage to nail

7 ⊟ **S61.238-**   Puncture wound without foreign body of other finger without damage to nail
Puncture wound without foreign body of specified finger with unspecified laterality without damage to nail

7 ⊟ **S61.239-**   Puncture wound without foreign body of unspecified finger without damage to nail

---

● New   ▲ Revised   *Manifestation*   4-7 Digit Indicators   ⊟ Laterality   Ⓐ Adult (15+ years)   Ⓜ Maternity (12-55 years)   Ⓝ Newborn   Ⓟ Pediatric (0-17 years)   ♂ Male   ♀ Female
✖ Deleted   Unspecified   + Additional code

984   © 2017 DecisionHealth   2017 ICD-10-CM Expert for Physicians

6 S61.24   Puncture wound with foreign body of finger without damage to nail

7 ⊟ **S61.240-**   Puncture wound with foreign body of right index finger without damage to nail

7 ⊟ **S61.241-**   Puncture wound with foreign body of left index finger without damage to nail

7 ⊟ **S61.242-**   Puncture wound with foreign body of right middle finger without damage to nail

7 ⊟ **S61.243-**   Puncture wound with foreign body of left middle finger without damage to nail

7 ⊟ **S61.244-**   Puncture wound with foreign body of right ring finger without damage to nail

7 ⊟ **S61.245-**   Puncture wound with foreign body of left ring finger without damage to nail

7 ⊟ **S61.246-**   Puncture wound with foreign body of right little finger without damage to nail

7 ⊟ **S61.247-**   Puncture wound with foreign body of left little finger without damage to nail

7 ⊟ **S61.248-**   Puncture wound with foreign body of other finger without damage to nail

     Puncture wound with foreign body of specified finger with unspecified laterality without damage to nail

7 ⊟ **S61.249-**   **Puncture wound with foreign body of unspecified finger without damage to nail**

6 S61.25   Open bite of finger without damage to nail

     Bite of finger without damage to nail NOS

     EXCLUDES 1   *superficial bite of finger (S60.46-, S60.47-)*

7 ⊟ **S61.250-**   Open bite of right index finger without damage to nail

7 ⊟ **S61.251-**   Open bite of left index finger without damage to nail

7 ⊟ **S61.252-**   Open bite of right middle finger without damage to nail

7 ⊟ **S61.253-**   Open bite of left middle finger without damage to nail

7 ⊟ **S61.254-**   Open bite of right ring finger without damage to nail

7 ⊟ **S61.255-**   Open bite of left ring finger without damage to nail

7 ⊟ **S61.256-**   Open bite of right little finger without damage to nail

7 ⊟ **S61.257-**   Open bite of left little finger without damage to nail

7 ⊟ **S61.258-**   Open bite of other finger without damage to nail

     Open bite of specified finger with unspecified laterality without damage to nail

7 ⊟ **S61.259-**   **Open bite of unspecified finger without damage to nail**

5 S61.3   Open wound of other finger with damage to nail

6 S61.30   **Unspecified open wound of finger with damage to nail**

7 ⊟ **S61.300-**   **Unspecified open wound of right index finger with damage to nail**

7 ⊟ **S61.301-**   **Unspecified open wound of left index finger with damage to nail**

7 ⊟ **S61.302-**   **Unspecified open wound of right middle finger with damage to nail**

7 ⊟ **S61.303-**   **Unspecified open wound of left middle finger with damage to nail**

7 ⊟ **S61.304-**   **Unspecified open wound of right ring finger with damage to nail**

7 ⊟ **S61.305-**   **Unspecified open wound of left ring finger with damage to nail**

7 ⊟ **S61.306-**   **Unspecified open wound of right little finger with damage to nail**

7 ⊟ **S61.307-**   **Unspecified open wound of left little finger with damage to nail**

7 ⊟ **S61.308-**   **Unspecified open wound of other finger with damage to nail**

     Unspecified open wound of specified finger with unspecified laterality with damage to nail

7 ⊟ **S61.309-**   **Unspecified open wound of unspecified finger with damage to nail**

6 S61.31   Laceration without foreign body of finger with damage to nail

---

7 ⊟ **S61.310-**   Laceration without foreign body of right index finger with damage to nail

7 ⊟ **S61.311-**   Laceration without foreign body of left index finger with damage to nail

7 ⊟ **S61.312-**   Laceration without foreign body of right middle finger with damage to nail

7 ⊟ **S61.313-**   Laceration without foreign body of left middle finger with damage to nail

7 ⊟ **S61.314-**   Laceration without foreign body of right ring finger with damage to nail

7 ⊟ **S61.315-**   Laceration without foreign body of left ring finger with damage to nail

7 ⊟ **S61.316-**   Laceration without foreign body of right little finger with damage to nail

7 ⊟ **S61.317-**   Laceration without foreign body of left little finger with damage to nail

7 ⊟ **S61.318-**   Laceration without foreign body of other finger with damage to nail

     Laceration without foreign body of specified finger with unspecified laterality with damage to nail

7 ⊟ **S61.319-**   **Laceration without foreign body of unspecified finger with damage to nail**

6 S61.32   Laceration with foreign body of finger with damage to nail

7 ⊟ **S61.320-**   Laceration with foreign body of right index finger with damage to nail

7 ⊟ **S61.321-**   Laceration with foreign body of left index finger with damage to nail

7 ⊟ **S61.322-**   Laceration with foreign body of right middle finger with damage to nail

7 ⊟ **S61.323-**   Laceration with foreign body of left middle finger with damage to nail

7 ⊟ **S61.324-**   Laceration with foreign body of right ring finger with damage to nail

7 ⊟ **S61.325-**   Laceration with foreign body of left ring finger with damage to nail

7 ⊟ **S61.326-**   Laceration with foreign body of right little finger with damage to nail

7 ⊟ **S61.327-**   Laceration with foreign body of left little finger with damage to nail

7 ⊟ **S61.328-**   Laceration with foreign body of other finger with damage to nail

     Laceration with foreign body of specified finger with unspecified laterality with damage to nail

7 ⊟ **S61.329-**   **Laceration with foreign body of unspecified finger with damage to nail**

6 S61.33   Puncture wound without foreign body of finger with damage to nail

7 ⊟ **S61.330-**   Puncture wound without foreign body of right index finger with damage to nail

7 ⊟ **S61.331-**   Puncture wound without foreign body of left index finger with damage to nail

7 ⊟ **S61.332-**   Puncture wound without foreign body of right middle finger with damage to nail

7 ⊟ **S61.333-**   Puncture wound without foreign body of left middle finger with damage to nail

7 ⊟ **S61.334-**   Puncture wound without foreign body of right ring finger with damage to nail

7 ⊟ **S61.335-**   Puncture wound without foreign body of left ring finger with damage to nail

7 ⊟ **S61.336-**   Puncture wound without foreign body of right little finger with damage to nail

7 ⊟ **S61.337-**   Puncture wound without foreign body of left little finger with damage to nail

7 ⊟ **S61.338-**   Puncture wound without foreign body of other finger with damage to nail

     Puncture wound without foreign body of specified finger with unspecified laterality with damage to nail

7 ⊟ **S61.339-**   **Puncture wound without foreign body of unspecified finger with damage to nail**

6 S61.34   Puncture wound with foreign body of finger with damage to nail

7 ⊟ **S61.340-**   Puncture wound with foreign body of right index finger with damage to nail

7 ⊟ **S61.341-**   Puncture wound with foreign body of left index finger with damage to nail

7 ⊟ **S61.342-**   Puncture wound with foreign body of right middle finger with damage to nail

7 ⊟ **S61.343-**   Puncture wound with foreign body of left middle finger with damage to nail

---

● New   ▲ Revised   *Manifestation*   4-7 Digit Indicators   ⊟ Laterality   A Adult (15+ years)   M Maternity (12-55 years)   N Newborn   P Pediatric (0-17 years)   ♂ Male   ♀ Female

✖ Deleted   Unspecified   + Additional code

7⃞ S61.344-	Puncture wound with foreign body of right ring finger with damage to nail
7⃞ S61.345-	Puncture wound with foreign body of left ring finger with damage to nail
7⃞ S61.346-	Puncture wound with foreign body of right little finger with damage to nail
7⃞ S61.347-	Puncture wound with foreign body of left little finger with damage to nail
7⃞ S61.348-	Puncture wound with foreign body of other finger with damage to nail
	Puncture wound with foreign body of specified finger with unspecified laterality with damage to nail
7⃞ S61.349-	Puncture wound with foreign body of unspecified finger with damage to nail
6⃞ S61.35	Open bite of finger with damage to nail

Bite of finger with damage to nail NOS

EXCLUDES 1 *superficial bite of finger (S60.46-, S60.47-)*

7⃞ S61.350-	Open bite of right index finger with damage to nail
7⃞ S61.351-	Open bite of left index finger with damage to nail
7⃞ S61.352-	Open bite of right middle finger with damage to nail
7⃞ S61.353-	Open bite of left middle finger with damage to nail
7⃞ S61.354-	Open bite of right ring finger with damage to nail
7⃞ S61.355-	Open bite of left ring finger with damage to nail
7⃞ S61.356-	Open bite of right little finger with damage to nail
7⃞ S61.357-	Open bite of left little finger with damage to nail
7⃞ S61.358-	Open bite of other finger with damage to nail
	Open bite of specified finger with unspecified laterality with damage to nail
7⃞ S61.359-	Open bite of unspecified finger with damage to nail
5⃞ S61.4	Open wound of hand
6⃞ S61.40	Unspecified open wound of hand
7⃞ S61.401-	Unspecified open wound of right hand
7⃞ S61.402-	Unspecified open wound of left hand
7⃞ S61.409-	Unspecified open wound of unspecified hand
6⃞ S61.41	Laceration without foreign body of hand
7⃞ S61.411-	Laceration without foreign body of right hand
7⃞ S61.412-	Laceration without foreign body of left hand
7⃞ S61.419-	Laceration without foreign body of unspecified hand
6⃞ S61.42	Laceration with foreign body of hand
7⃞ S61.421-	Laceration with foreign body of right hand
7⃞ S61.422-	Laceration with foreign body of left hand
7⃞ S61.429-	Laceration with foreign body of unspecified hand
6⃞ S61.43	Puncture wound without foreign body of hand
7⃞ S61.431-	Puncture wound without foreign body of right hand
7⃞ S61.432-	Puncture wound without foreign body of left hand
7⃞ S61.439-	Puncture wound without foreign body of unspecified hand
6⃞ S61.44	Puncture wound with foreign body of hand
7⃞ S61.441-	Puncture wound with foreign body of right hand
7⃞ S61.442-	Puncture wound with foreign body of left hand
7⃞ S61.449-	Puncture wound with foreign body of unspecified hand
6⃞ S61.45	Open bite of hand

Bite of hand NOS

EXCLUDES 1 *superficial bite of hand (S60.56-, S60.57-)*

7⃞ S61.451-	Open bite of right hand
7⃞ S61.452-	Open bite of left hand
7⃞ S61.459-	Open bite of unspecified hand
5⃞ S61.5	Open wound of wrist
6⃞ S61.50	Unspecified open wound of wrist
7⃞ S61.501-	Unspecified open wound of right wrist
7⃞ S61.502-	Unspecified open wound of left wrist
7⃞ S61.509-	Unspecified open wound of unspecified wrist
6⃞ S61.51	Laceration without foreign body of wrist
7⃞ S61.511-	Laceration without foreign body of right wrist
7⃞ S61.512-	Laceration without foreign body of left wrist
7⃞ S61.519-	Laceration without foreign body of unspecified wrist
6⃞ S61.52	Laceration with foreign body of wrist
7⃞ S61.521-	Laceration with foreign body of right wrist
7⃞ S61.522-	Laceration with foreign body of left wrist
7⃞ S61.529-	Laceration with foreign body of unspecified wrist
6⃞ S61.53	Puncture wound without foreign body of wrist
7⃞ S61.531-	Puncture wound without foreign body of right wrist
7⃞ S61.532-	Puncture wound without foreign body of left wrist
7⃞ S61.539-	Puncture wound without foreign body of unspecified wrist
6⃞ S61.54	Puncture wound with foreign body of wrist
7⃞ S61.541-	Puncture wound with foreign body of right wrist
7⃞ S61.542-	Puncture wound with foreign body of left wrist
7⃞ S61.549-	Puncture wound with foreign body of unspecified wrist
6⃞ S61.55	Open bite of wrist

Bite of wrist NOS

EXCLUDES 1 *superficial bite of wrist (S60.86-, S60.87-)*

7⃞ S61.551-	Open bite of right wrist
7⃞ S61.552-	Open bite of left wrist
7⃞ S61.559-	Open bite of unspecified wrist
4⃞ S62	**Fracture at wrist and hand level**

Note: A fracture not indicated as displaced or nondisplaced should be coded to displaced
A fracture not indicated as open or closed should be coded to closed

EXCLUDES 1 *traumatic amputation of wrist and hand (S68.-)*

EXCLUDES 2 *fracture of distal parts of ulna and radius (S52.-)*

The appropriate 7th character is to be added to each code from category S62
A	initial encounter for closed fracture
B	initial encounter for open fracture
D	subsequent encounter for fracture with routine healing
G	subsequent encounter for fracture with delayed healing
K	subsequent encounter for fracture with nonunion
P	subsequent encounter for fracture with malunion
S	sequela

CODING TIP ✓ A fracture not indicated as displaced or nondisplaced should be coded to displaced. A fracture not indicated as open or closed should be coded to closed. Query providers on fractures not documented as displaced/nondisplaced otherwise displaced fracture diagnosis could be assigned without reduction being performed potentially resulting in claim denials.

5⃞ S62.0	Fracture of navicular [scaphoid] bone of wrist
6⃞ S62.00	Unspecified fracture of navicular [scaphoid] bone of wrist
7⃞ S62.001-	Unspecified fracture of navicular [scaphoid] bone of right wrist
7⃞ S62.002-	Unspecified fracture of navicular [scaphoid] bone of left wrist
	AHA: (S62.002A) 4Q 2012, 106
7⃞ S62.009-	Unspecified fracture of navicular [scaphoid] bone of unspecified wrist
6⃞ S62.01	Fracture of distal pole of navicular [scaphoid] bone of wrist
	Fracture of volar tuberosity of navicular [scaphoid] bone of wrist
7⃞ S62.011-	Displaced fracture of distal pole of navicular [scaphoid] bone of right wrist
7⃞ S62.012-	Displaced fracture of distal pole of navicular [scaphoid] bone of left wrist
7⃞ S62.013-	Displaced fracture of distal pole of navicular [scaphoid] bone of unspecified wrist

7️⃣ 🔲 **S62.014-**   Nondisplaced fracture of distal pole of navicular [scaphoid] bone of right wrist

7️⃣ 🔲 **S62.015-**   Nondisplaced fracture of distal pole of navicular [scaphoid] bone of left wrist

7️⃣ 🔲 **S62.016-**   Nondisplaced fracture of distal pole of navicular [scaphoid] bone of unspecified wrist

🅖 **S62.02**   **Fracture of middle third of navicular [scaphoid] bone of wrist**

7️⃣ 🔲 **S62.021-**   Displaced fracture of middle third of navicular [scaphoid] bone of right wrist

7️⃣ 🔲 **S62.022-**   Displaced fracture of middle third of navicular [scaphoid] bone of left wrist

7️⃣ 🔲 **S62.023-**   Displaced fracture of middle third of navicular [scaphoid] bone of unspecified wrist

7️⃣ 🔲 **S62.024-**   Nondisplaced fracture of middle third of navicular [scaphoid] bone of right wrist

7️⃣ 🔲 **S62.025-**   Nondisplaced fracture of middle third of navicular [scaphoid] bone of left wrist

7️⃣ 🔲 **S62.026-**   Nondisplaced fracture of middle third of navicular [scaphoid] bone of unspecified wrist

🅖 **S62.03**   **Fracture of proximal third of navicular [scaphoid] bone of wrist**

7️⃣ 🔲 **S62.031-**   Displaced fracture of proximal third of navicular [scaphoid] bone of right wrist

7️⃣ 🔲 **S62.032-**   Displaced fracture of proximal third of navicular [scaphoid] bone of left wrist

7️⃣ 🔲 **S62.033-**   Displaced fracture of proximal third of navicular [scaphoid] bone of unspecified wrist

7️⃣ 🔲 **S62.034-**   Nondisplaced fracture of proximal third of navicular [scaphoid] bone of right wrist

7️⃣ 🔲 **S62.035-**   Nondisplaced fracture of proximal third of navicular [scaphoid] bone of left wrist

7️⃣ 🔲 **S62.036-**   Nondisplaced fracture of proximal third of navicular [scaphoid] bone of unspecified wrist

🅢 **S62.1**   **Fracture of other and unspecified carpal bone(s)**

    EXCLUDES 2   *fracture of scaphoid of wrist (S62.0-)*

🅖 **S62.10**   **Fracture of unspecified carpal bone**
    Fracture of wrist NOS

7️⃣ 🔲 **S62.101-**   Fracture of unspecified carpal bone, right wrist

7️⃣ 🔲 **S62.102-**   Fracture of unspecified carpal bone, left wrist
    AHA: (S62.102D) 4Q 2012, 95

7️⃣ 🔲 **S62.109-**   Fracture of unspecified carpal bone, unspecified wrist

🅖 **S62.11**   **Fracture of triquetrum [cuneiform] bone of wrist**

7️⃣ 🔲 **S62.111-**   Displaced fracture of triquetrum [cuneiform] bone, right wrist

7️⃣ 🔲 **S62.112-**   Displaced fracture of triquetrum [cuneiform] bone, left wrist

7️⃣ 🔲 **S62.113-**   Displaced fracture of triquetrum [cuneiform] bone, unspecified wrist

7️⃣ 🔲 **S62.114-**   Nondisplaced fracture of triquetrum [cuneiform] bone, right wrist

7️⃣ 🔲 **S62.115-**   Nondisplaced fracture of triquetrum [cuneiform] bone, left wrist

7️⃣ 🔲 **S62.116-**   Nondisplaced fracture of triquetrum [cuneiform] bone, unspecified wrist

🅖 **S62.12**   **Fracture of lunate [semilunar]**

7️⃣ 🔲 **S62.121-**   Displaced fracture of lunate [semilunar], right wrist

7️⃣ 🔲 **S62.122-**   Displaced fracture of lunate [semilunar], left wrist

7️⃣ 🔲 **S62.123-**   Displaced fracture of lunate [semilunar], unspecified wrist

7️⃣ 🔲 **S62.124-**   Nondisplaced fracture of lunate [semilunar], right wrist

7️⃣ 🔲 **S62.125-**   Nondisplaced fracture of lunate [semilunar], left wrist

7️⃣ 🔲 **S62.126-**   Nondisplaced fracture of lunate [semilunar], unspecified wrist

🅖 **S62.13**   **Fracture of capitate [os magnum] bone**

7️⃣ 🔲 **S62.131-**   Displaced fracture of capitate [os magnum] bone, right wrist

7️⃣ 🔲 **S62.132-**   Displaced fracture of capitate [os magnum] bone, left wrist

7️⃣ 🔲 **S62.133-**   Displaced fracture of capitate [os magnum] bone, unspecified wrist

7️⃣ 🔲 **S62.134-**   Nondisplaced fracture of capitate [os magnum] bone, right wrist

7️⃣ 🔲 **S62.135-**   Nondisplaced fracture of capitate [os magnum] bone, left wrist

7️⃣ 🔲 **S62.136-**   Nondisplaced fracture of capitate [os magnum] bone, unspecified wrist

🅖 **S62.14**   **Fracture of body of hamate [unciform] bone**
    Fracture of hamate [unciform] bone NOS

7️⃣ 🔲 **S62.141-**   Displaced fracture of body of hamate [unciform] bone, right wrist

7️⃣ 🔲 **S62.142-**   Displaced fracture of body of hamate [unciform] bone, left wrist

7️⃣ 🔲 **S62.143-**   Displaced fracture of body of hamate [unciform] bone, unspecified wrist

7️⃣ 🔲 **S62.144-**   Nondisplaced fracture of body of hamate [unciform] bone, right wrist

7️⃣ 🔲 **S62.145-**   Nondisplaced fracture of body of hamate [unciform] bone, left wrist

7️⃣ 🔲 **S62.146-**   Nondisplaced fracture of body of hamate [unciform] bone, unspecified wrist

🅖 **S62.15**   **Fracture of hook process of hamate [unciform] bone**
    Fracture of unciform process of hamate [unciform] bone

7️⃣ 🔲 **S62.151-**   Displaced fracture of hook process of hamate [unciform] bone, right wrist

7️⃣ 🔲 **S62.152-**   Displaced fracture of hook process of hamate [unciform] bone, left wrist

7️⃣ 🔲 **S62.153-**   Displaced fracture of hook process of hamate [unciform] bone, unspecified wrist

7️⃣ 🔲 **S62.154-**   Nondisplaced fracture of hook process of hamate [unciform] bone, right wrist

7️⃣ 🔲 **S62.155-**   Nondisplaced fracture of hook process of hamate [unciform] bone, left wrist

7️⃣ 🔲 **S62.156-**   Nondisplaced fracture of hook process of hamate [unciform] bone, unspecified wrist

🅖 **S62.16**   **Fracture of pisiform**

7️⃣ 🔲 **S62.161-**   Displaced fracture of pisiform, right wrist

7️⃣ 🔲 **S62.162-**   Displaced fracture of pisiform, left wrist

7️⃣ 🔲 **S62.163-**   Displaced fracture of pisiform, unspecified wrist

7️⃣ 🔲 **S62.164-**   Nondisplaced fracture of pisiform, right wrist

7️⃣ 🔲 **S62.165-**   Nondisplaced fracture of pisiform, left wrist

7️⃣ 🔲 **S62.166-**   Nondisplaced fracture of pisiform, unspecified wrist

🅖 **S62.17**   **Fracture of trapezium [larger multangular]**

7️⃣ 🔲 **S62.171-**   Displaced fracture of trapezium [larger multangular], right wrist

7️⃣ 🔲 **S62.172-**   Displaced fracture of trapezium [larger multangular], left wrist

7️⃣ 🔲 **S62.173-**   Displaced fracture of trapezium [larger multangular], unspecified wrist

7️⃣ 🔲 **S62.174-**   Nondisplaced fracture of trapezium [larger multangular], right wrist

7️⃣ 🔲 **S62.175-**   Nondisplaced fracture of trapezium [larger multangular], left wrist

7️⃣ 🔲 **S62.176-**   Nondisplaced fracture of trapezium [larger multangular], unspecified wrist

🅖 **S62.18**   **Fracture of trapezoid [smaller multangular]**

7️⃣ 🔲 **S62.181-**   Displaced fracture of trapezoid [smaller multangular], right wrist

7️⃣ 🔲 **S62.182-**   Displaced fracture of trapezoid [smaller multangular], left wrist

7️⃣ 🔲 **S62.183-**   Displaced fracture of trapezoid [smaller multangular], unspecified wrist

7️⃣ 🔲 **S62.184-**   Nondisplaced fracture of trapezoid [smaller multangular], right wrist

7️⃣ 🔲 **S62.185-**   Nondisplaced fracture of trapezoid [smaller multangular], left wrist

7️⃣ 🔲 **S62.186-**   Nondisplaced fracture of trapezoid [smaller multangular], unspecified wrist

🅢 **S62.2**   **Fracture of first metacarpal bone**

🅖 **S62.20**   **Unspecified fracture of first metacarpal bone**

7️⃣ 🔲 **S62.201-**   Unspecified fracture of first metacarpal bone, right hand

● New   ▲ Revised   *Manifestation*   4️⃣-7️⃣ Digit Indicators   🔲 Laterality   🅰 Adult (15+ years)   🅼 Maternity (12-55 years)   🅽 Newborn   🅿 Pediatric (0-17 years)   ♂ Male   ♀ Female
✖ ~~Deleted~~   Unspecified   + Additional code

2017 ICD-10-CM Expert for Physicians   © 2017 DecisionHealth   987

7 ⊟ **S62.202-** Unspecified fracture of first metacarpal bone, left hand

7 ⊟ **S62.209-** Unspecified fracture of first metacarpal bone, unspecified hand

6 **S62.21** Bennett's fracture

> **DEFINITION** An intra-articular fracture dislocation of the base of the first metacarpal bone (thumb) extending into the carpometacarpal joint.

7 ⊟ **S62.211-** Bennett's fracture, right hand

7 ⊟ **S62.212-** Bennett's fracture, left hand

7 ⊟ **S62.213-** Bennett's fracture, unspecified hand

6 **S62.22** Rolando's fracture

7 ⊟ **S62.221-** Displaced Rolando's fracture, right hand

7 ⊟ **S62.222-** Displaced Rolando's fracture, left hand

7 ⊟ **S62.223-** Displaced Rolando's fracture, unspecified hand

7 ⊟ **S62.224-** Nondisplaced Rolando's fracture, right hand

7 ⊟ **S62.225-** Nondisplaced Rolando's fracture, left hand

7 ⊟ **S62.226-** Nondisplaced Rolando's fracture, unspecified hand

6 **S62.23** Other fracture of base of first metacarpal bone

7 ⊟ **S62.231-** Other displaced fracture of base of first metacarpal bone, right hand

7 ⊟ **S62.232-** Other displaced fracture of base of first metacarpal bone, left hand

7 ⊟ **S62.233-** Other displaced fracture of base of first metacarpal bone, unspecified hand

7 ⊟ **S62.234-** Other nondisplaced fracture of base of first metacarpal bone, right hand

7 ⊟ **S62.235-** Other nondisplaced fracture of base of first metacarpal bone, left hand

7 ⊟ **S62.236-** Other nondisplaced fracture of base of first metacarpal bone, unspecified hand

6 **S62.24** Fracture of shaft of first metacarpal bone

7 ⊟ **S62.241-** Displaced fracture of shaft of first metacarpal bone, right hand

7 ⊟ **S62.242-** Displaced fracture of shaft of first metacarpal bone, left hand

7 ⊟ **S62.243-** Displaced fracture of shaft of first metacarpal bone, unspecified hand

7 ⊟ **S62.244-** Nondisplaced fracture of shaft of first metacarpal bone, right hand

7 ⊟ **S62.245-** Nondisplaced fracture of shaft of first metacarpal bone, left hand

7 ⊟ **S62.246-** Nondisplaced fracture of shaft of first metacarpal bone, unspecified hand

6 **S62.25** Fracture of neck of first metacarpal bone

7 ⊟ **S62.251-** Displaced fracture of neck of first metacarpal bone, right hand

7 ⊟ **S62.252-** Displaced fracture of neck of first metacarpal bone, left hand

7 ⊟ **S62.253-** Displaced fracture of neck of first metacarpal bone, unspecified hand

7 ⊟ **S62.254-** Nondisplaced fracture of neck of first metacarpal bone, right hand

7 ⊟ **S62.255-** Nondisplaced fracture of neck of first metacarpal bone, left hand

7 ⊟ **S62.256-** Nondisplaced fracture of neck of first metacarpal bone, unspecified hand

6 **S62.29** Other fracture of first metacarpal bone

7 ⊟ **S62.291-** Other fracture of first metacarpal bone, right hand

7 ⊟ **S62.292-** Other fracture of first metacarpal bone, left hand

7 ⊟ **S62.299-** Other fracture of first metacarpal bone, unspecified hand

5 **S62.3** Fracture of other and unspecified metacarpal bone

> **EXCLUDES 2** *fracture of first metacarpal bone (S62.2-)*

6 **S62.30** Unspecified fracture of other metacarpal bone

7 ⊟ **S62.300-** Unspecified fracture of second metacarpal bone, right hand

7 ⊟ **S62.301-** Unspecified fracture of second metacarpal bone, left hand

7 ⊟ **S62.302-** Unspecified fracture of third metacarpal bone, right hand

7 ⊟ **S62.303-** Unspecified fracture of third metacarpal bone, left hand

7 ⊟ **S62.304-** Unspecified fracture of fourth metacarpal bone, right hand

7 ⊟ **S62.305-** Unspecified fracture of fourth metacarpal bone, left hand

7 ⊟ **S62.306-** Unspecified fracture of fifth metacarpal bone, right hand

7 ⊟ **S62.307-** Unspecified fracture of fifth metacarpal bone, left hand

7 ⊟ **S62.308-** Unspecified fracture of other metacarpal bone

Unspecified fracture of specified metacarpal bone with unspecified laterality

7 ⊟ **S62.309-** Unspecified fracture of unspecified metacarpal bone

6 **S62.31** Displaced fracture of base of other metacarpal bone

7 ⊟ **S62.310-** Displaced fracture of base of second metacarpal bone, right hand

7 ⊟ **S62.311-** Displaced fracture of base of second metacarpal bone. left hand

7 ⊟ **S62.312-** Displaced fracture of base of third metacarpal bone, right hand

7 ⊟ **S62.313-** Displaced fracture of base of third metacarpal bone, left hand

7 ⊟ **S62.314-** Displaced fracture of base of fourth metacarpal bone, right hand

7 ⊟ **S62.315-** Displaced fracture of base of fourth metacarpal bone, left hand

7 ⊟ **S62.316-** Displaced fracture of base of fifth metacarpal bone, right hand

7 ⊟ **S62.317-** Displaced fracture of base of fifth metacarpal bone. left hand

7 ⊟ **S62.318-** Displaced fracture of base of other metacarpal bone

Displaced fracture of base of specified metacarpal bone with unspecified laterality

7 ⊟ **S62.319-** Displaced fracture of base of unspecified metacarpal bone

6 **S62.32** Displaced fracture of shaft of other metacarpal bone

7 ⊟ **S62.320-** Displaced fracture of shaft of second metacarpal bone, right hand

7 ⊟ **S62.321-** Displaced fracture of shaft of second metacarpal bone, left hand

7 ⊟ **S62.322-** Displaced fracture of shaft of third metacarpal bone, right hand

7 ⊟ **S62.323-** Displaced fracture of shaft of third metacarpal bone, left hand

7 ⊟ **S62.324-** Displaced fracture of shaft of fourth metacarpal bone, right hand

7 ⊟ **S62.325-** Displaced fracture of shaft of fourth metacarpal bone, left hand

7 ⊟ **S62.326-** Displaced fracture of shaft of fifth metacarpal bone, right hand

7 ⊟ **S62.327-** Displaced fracture of shaft of fifth metacarpal bone, left hand

7 ⊟ **S62.328-** Displaced fracture of shaft of other metacarpal bone

Displaced fracture of shaft of specified metacarpal bone with unspecified laterality

7 ⊟ **S62.329-** Displaced fracture of shaft of unspecified metacarpal bone

6 **S62.33** Displaced fracture of neck of other metacarpal bone

7 ⊟ **S62.330-** Displaced fracture of neck of second metacarpal bone, right hand

7 ⊟ **S62.331-** Displaced fracture of neck of second metacarpal bone, left hand

7 ⊟ **S62.332-** Displaced fracture of neck of third metacarpal bone, right hand

7 ⊟ **S62.333-** Displaced fracture of neck of third metacarpal bone, left hand

7 ⊟ **S62.334-** Displaced fracture of neck of fourth metacarpal bone, right hand

7 ⊟ **S62.335-** Displaced fracture of neck of fourth metacarpal bone, left hand

7 ⊟ **S62.336-** Displaced fracture of neck of fifth metacarpal bone, right hand

7 ⊟ **S62.337-** Displaced fracture of neck of fifth metacarpal bone, left hand

---

● New	▲ Revised	*Manifestation*	4 - 7 Digit Indicators	⊟ Laterality	Ⓐ Adult (15+ years)	Ⓜ Maternity (12-55 years)	Ⓝ Newborn	Ⓟ Pediatric (0-17 years)	♂ Male	♀ Female
✖ Deleted		Unspecified	+ Additional code							

7 ▤ **S62.338-** Displaced fracture of neck of other metacarpal bone
Displaced fracture of neck of specified metacarpal bone with unspecified laterality

7 ▤ **S62.339-** Displaced fracture of neck of unspecified metacarpal bone

6 **S62.34** Nondisplaced fracture of base of other metacarpal bone

7 ▤ **S62.340-** Nondisplaced fracture of base of second metacarpal bone, right hand

7 ▤ **S62.341-** Nondisplaced fracture of base of second metacarpal bone. left hand

7 ▤ **S62.342-** Nondisplaced fracture of base of third metacarpal bone, right hand

7 ▤ **S62.343-** Nondisplaced fracture of base of third metacarpal bone, left hand

7 ▤ **S62.344-** Nondisplaced fracture of base of fourth metacarpal bone, right hand

7 ▤ **S62.345-** Nondisplaced fracture of base of fourth metacarpal bone, left hand

7 ▤ **S62.346-** Nondisplaced fracture of base of fifth metacarpal bone, right hand

7 ▤ **S62.347-** Nondisplaced fracture of base of fifth metacarpal bone. left hand

7 ▤ **S62.348-** Nondisplaced fracture of base of other metacarpal bone
Nondisplaced fracture of base of specified metacarpal bone with unspecified laterality

7 ▤ **S62.349-** Nondisplaced fracture of base of unspecified metacarpal bone

6 **S62.35** Nondisplaced fracture of shaft of other metacarpal bone

7 ▤ **S62.350-** Nondisplaced fracture of shaft of second metacarpal bone, right hand

7 ▤ **S62.351-** Nondisplaced fracture of shaft of second metacarpal bone, left hand

7 ▤ **S62.352-** Nondisplaced fracture of shaft of third metacarpal bone, right hand

7 ▤ **S62.353-** Nondisplaced fracture of shaft of third metacarpal bone, left hand

7 ▤ **S62.354-** Nondisplaced fracture of shaft of fourth metacarpal bone, right hand

7 ▤ **S62.355-** Nondisplaced fracture of shaft of fourth metacarpal bone, left hand

7 ▤ **S62.356-** Nondisplaced fracture of shaft of fifth metacarpal bone, right hand

7 ▤ **S62.357-** Nondisplaced fracture of shaft of fifth metacarpal bone, left hand

7 ▤ **S62.358-** Nondisplaced fracture of shaft of other metacarpal bone
Nondisplaced fracture of shaft of specified metacarpal bone with unspecified laterality

7 ▤ **S62.359-** Nondisplaced fracture of shaft of unspecified metacarpal bone

6 **S62.36** Nondisplaced fracture of neck of other metacarpal bone

7 ▤ **S62.360-** Nondisplaced fracture of neck of second metacarpal bone, right hand

7 ▤ **S62.361-** Nondisplaced fracture of neck of second metacarpal bone, left hand

7 ▤ **S62.362-** Nondisplaced fracture of neck of third metacarpal bone, right hand

7 ▤ **S62.363-** Nondisplaced fracture of neck of third metacarpal bone, left hand

7 ▤ **S62.364-** Nondisplaced fracture of neck of fourth metacarpal bone, right hand

7 ▤ **S62.365-** Nondisplaced fracture of neck of fourth metacarpal bone, left hand

7 ▤ **S62.366-** Nondisplaced fracture of neck of fifth metacarpal bone, right hand

7 ▤ **S62.367-** Nondisplaced fracture of neck of fifth metacarpal bone, left hand

7 ▤ **S62.368-** Nondisplaced fracture of neck of other metacarpal bone
Nondisplaced fracture of neck of specified metacarpal bone with unspecified laterality

7 ▤ **S62.369-** Nondisplaced fracture of neck of unspecified metacarpal bone

6 **S62.39** Other fracture of other metacarpal bone

7 ▤ **S62.390-** Other fracture of second metacarpal bone, right hand

7 ▤ **S62.391-** Other fracture of second metacarpal bone, left hand

7 ▤ **S62.392-** Other fracture of third metacarpal bone, right hand

7 ▤ **S62.393-** Other fracture of third metacarpal bone, left hand

7 ▤ **S62.394-** Other fracture of fourth metacarpal bone, right hand

7 ▤ **S62.395-** Other fracture of fourth metacarpal bone, left hand

7 ▤ **S62.396-** Other fracture of fifth metacarpal bone, right hand

7 ▤ **S62.397-** Other fracture of fifth metacarpal bone, left hand

7 ▤ **S62.398-** Other fracture of other metacarpal bone
Other fracture of specified metacarpal bone with unspecified laterality

7 ▤ **S62.399-** Other fracture of unspecified metacarpal bone

5 **S62.5** Fracture of thumb

6 **S62.50** Fracture of unspecified phalanx of thumb

7 ▤ **S62.501-** Fracture of unspecified phalanx of right thumb

7 ▤ **S62.502-** Fracture of unspecified phalanx of left thumb

7 ▤ **S62.509-** Fracture of unspecified phalanx of unspecified thumb

6 **S62.51** Fracture of proximal phalanx of thumb

7 ▤ **S62.511-** Displaced fracture of proximal phalanx of right thumb

7 ▤ **S62.512-** Displaced fracture of proximal phalanx of left thumb

7 ▤ **S62.513-** Displaced fracture of proximal phalanx of unspecified thumb

7 ▤ **S62.514-** Nondisplaced fracture of proximal phalanx of right thumb

7 ▤ **S62.515-** Nondisplaced fracture of proximal phalanx of left thumb

7 ▤ **S62.516-** Nondisplaced fracture of proximal phalanx of unspecified thumb

6 **S62.52** Fracture of distal phalanx of thumb

7 ▤ **S62.521-** Displaced fracture of distal phalanx of right thumb

7 ▤ **S62.522-** Displaced fracture of distal phalanx of left thumb

7 ▤ **S62.523-** Displaced fracture of distal phalanx of unspecified thumb

7 ▤ **S62.524-** Nondisplaced fracture of distal phalanx of right thumb

7 ▤ **S62.525-** Nondisplaced fracture of distal phalanx of left thumb

7 ▤ **S62.526-** Nondisplaced fracture of distal phalanx of unspecified thumb

5 **S62.6** Fracture of other and unspecified finger(s)

EXCLUDES 2 *fracture of thumb (S62.5-)*

6 **S62.60** Fracture of unspecified phalanx of finger

7 ▤ **S62.600-** Fracture of unspecified phalanx of right index finger

7 ▤ **S62.601-** Fracture of unspecified phalanx of left index finger

7 ▤ **S62.602-** Fracture of unspecified phalanx of right middle finger

7 ▤ **S62.603-** Fracture of unspecified phalanx of left middle finger

7 ▤ **S62.604-** Fracture of unspecified phalanx of right ring finger

7 ▤ **S62.605-** Fracture of unspecified phalanx of left ring finger

7 ▤ **S62.606-** Fracture of unspecified phalanx of right little finger

7 ▤ **S62.607-** Fracture of unspecified phalanx of left little finger

7 ▤ **S62.608-** Fracture of unspecified phalanx of other finger
Fracture of unspecified phalanx of specified finger with unspecified laterality

7 ▤ **S62.609-** Fracture of unspecified phalanx of unspecified finger

6 **S62.61** Displaced fracture of proximal phalanx of finger

---

● New ▲ Revised *Manifestation* ◣-7 Digit Indicators ▤ Laterality ▲ Adult (15+ years) Ⓜ Maternity (12-55 years) Ⓝ Newborn Ⓟ Pediatric (0-17 years) ♂ Male ♀ Female
✖ Deleted Unspecified + Additional code

7 ⊟ **S62.610-** Displaced fracture of proximal phalanx of right index finger

7 ⊟ **S62.611-** Displaced fracture of proximal phalanx of left index finger

7 ⊟ **S62.612-** Displaced fracture of proximal phalanx of right middle finger

7 ⊟ **S62.613-** Displaced fracture of proximal phalanx of left middle finger

7 ⊟ **S62.614-** Displaced fracture of proximal phalanx of right ring finger

7 ⊟ **S62.615-** Displaced fracture of proximal phalanx of left ring finger

7 ⊟ **S62.616-** Displaced fracture of proximal phalanx of right little finger

7 ⊟ **S62.617-** Displaced fracture of proximal phalanx of left little finger

7 ⊟ **S62.618-** Displaced fracture of proximal phalanx of other finger

Displaced fracture of proximal phalanx of specified finger with unspecified laterality

7 ⊟ **S62.619-** **Displaced fracture of proximal phalanx of unspecified finger**

6 **S62.62** Displaced fracture of medial phalanx of finger

7 ⊟ **S62.620-** Displaced fracture of medial phalanx of right index finger

7 ⊟ **S62.621-** Displaced fracture of medial phalanx of left index finger

7 ⊟ **S62.622-** Displaced fracture of medial phalanx of right middle finger

7 ⊟ **S62.623-** Displaced fracture of medial phalanx of left middle finger

7 ⊟ **S62.624-** Displaced fracture of medial phalanx of right ring finger

7 ⊟ **S62.625-** Displaced fracture of medial phalanx of left ring finger

7 ⊟ **S62.626-** Displaced fracture of medial phalanx of right little finger

7 ⊟ **S62.627-** Displaced fracture of medial phalanx of left little finger

7 ⊟ **S62.628-** Displaced fracture of medial phalanx of other finger

Displaced fracture of medial phalanx of specified finger with unspecified laterality

7 ⊟ **S62.629-** **Displaced fracture of medial phalanx of unspecified finger**

6 **S62.63** Displaced fracture of distal phalanx of finger

7 ⊟ **S62.630-** Displaced fracture of distal phalanx of right index finger

7 ⊟ **S62.631-** Displaced fracture of distal phalanx of left index finger

7 ⊟ **S62.632-** Displaced fracture of distal phalanx of right middle finger

7 ⊟ **S62.633-** Displaced fracture of distal phalanx of left middle finger

7 ⊟ **S62.634-** Displaced fracture of distal phalanx of right ring finger

7 ⊟ **S62.635-** Displaced fracture of distal phalanx of left ring finger

7 ⊟ **S62.636-** Displaced fracture of distal phalanx of right little finger

7 ⊟ **S62.637-** Displaced fracture of distal phalanx of left little finger

7 ⊟ **S62.638-** Displaced fracture of distal phalanx of other finger

Displaced fracture of distal phalanx of specified finger with unspecified laterality

7 ⊟ **S62.639-** **Displaced fracture of distal phalanx of unspecified finger**

6 **S62.64** Nondisplaced fracture of proximal phalanx of finger

7 ⊟ **S62.640-** Nondisplaced fracture of proximal phalanx of right index finger

7 ⊟ **S62.641-** Nondisplaced fracture of proximal phalanx of left index finger

7 ⊟ **S62.642-** Nondisplaced fracture of proximal phalanx of right middle finger

7 ⊟ **S62.643-** Nondisplaced fracture of proximal phalanx of left middle finger

7 ⊟ **S62.644-** Nondisplaced fracture of proximal phalanx of right ring finger

7 ⊟ **S62.645-** Nondisplaced fracture of proximal phalanx of left ring finger

7 ⊟ **S62.646-** Nondisplaced fracture of proximal phalanx of right little finger

7 ⊟ **S62.647-** Nondisplaced fracture of proximal phalanx of left little finger

7 ⊟ **S62.648-** Nondisplaced fracture of proximal phalanx of other finger

Nondisplaced fracture of proximal phalanx of specified finger with unspecified laterality

7 ⊟ **S62.649-** **Nondisplaced fracture of proximal phalanx of unspecified finger**

6 **S62.65** Nondisplaced fracture of medial phalanx of finger

7 ⊟ **S62.650-** Nondisplaced fracture of medial phalanx of right index finger

7 ⊟ **S62.651-** Nondisplaced fracture of medial phalanx of left index finger

7 ⊟ **S62.652-** Nondisplaced fracture of medial phalanx of right middle finger

7 ⊟ **S62.653-** Nondisplaced fracture of medial phalanx of left middle finger

7 ⊟ **S62.654-** Nondisplaced fracture of medial phalanx of right ring finger

7 ⊟ **S62.655-** Nondisplaced fracture of medial phalanx of left ring finger

7 ⊟ **S62.656-** Nondisplaced fracture of medial phalanx of right little finger

7 ⊟ **S62.657-** Nondisplaced fracture of medial phalanx of left little finger

7 ⊟ **S62.658-** Nondisplaced fracture of medial phalanx of other finger

Nondisplaced fracture of medial phalanx of specified finger with unspecified laterality

7 ⊟ **S62.659-** **Nondisplaced fracture of medial phalanx of unspecified finger**

6 **S62.66** Nondisplaced fracture of distal phalanx of finger

7 ⊟ **S62.660-** Nondisplaced fracture of distal phalanx of right index finger

7 ⊟ **S62.661-** Nondisplaced fracture of distal phalanx of left index finger

7 ⊟ **S62.662-** Nondisplaced fracture of distal phalanx of right middle finger

7 ⊟ **S62.663-** Nondisplaced fracture of distal phalanx of left middle finger

7 ⊟ **S62.664-** Nondisplaced fracture of distal phalanx of right ring finger

7 ⊟ **S62.665-** Nondisplaced fracture of distal phalanx of left ring finger

7 ⊟ **S62.666-** Nondisplaced fracture of distal phalanx of right little finger

7 ⊟ **S62.667-** Nondisplaced fracture of distal phalanx of left little finger

7 ⊟ **S62.668-** Nondisplaced fracture of distal phalanx of other finger

Nondisplaced fracture of distal phalanx of specified finger with unspecified laterality

7 ⊟ **S62.669-** **Nondisplaced fracture of distal phalanx of unspecified finger**

5 **S62.9** Unspecified fracture of wrist and hand

7 ⊟ **S62.90X-** **Unspecified fracture of unspecified wrist and hand**

7 ⊟ **S62.91X-** **Unspecified fracture of right wrist and hand**

7 ⊟ **S62.92X-** **Unspecified fracture of left wrist and hand**

● New   ▲ Revised   *Manifestation*   4-7 Digit Indicators   ⊟ Laterality   🅰 Adult (15+ years)   🅼 Maternity (12-55 years)   🅽 Newborn   🅿 Pediatric (0-17 years)   ♂ Male   ♀ Female
✖ Deleted   Unspecified   + Additional code

990   © 2017 DecisionHealth   2017 ICD-10-CM Expert for Physicians

S62.610- — S62.92X-   Injury, Poisoning and Certain Other Consequences of External Causes

4 **S63**   **Dislocation and sprain of joints and ligaments at wrist and hand level**

INCLUDES   avulsion of joint or ligament at wrist and hand level

laceration of cartilage, joint or ligament at wrist and hand level

sprain of cartilage, joint or ligament at wrist and hand level

traumatic hemarthrosis of joint or ligament at wrist and hand level

traumatic rupture of joint or ligament at wrist and hand level

traumatic subluxation of joint or ligament at wrist and hand level

traumatic tear of joint or ligament at wrist and hand level

Code also:

any associated open wound

EXCLUDES 2   *strain of muscle, fascia and tendon of wrist and hand (S66.-)*

The appropriate 7th character is to be added to each code from category S63
A   initial encounter
D   subsequent encounter
S   sequela

CODING TIP ✓   Unlike ICD-9 there is no code for open dislocations. When documented as open an additional code for the open wound must be applied.

5 **S63.0**   **Subluxation and dislocation of wrist and hand joints**

6 **S63.00**   **Unspecified subluxation and dislocation of wrist and hand**

Dislocation of carpal bone NOS
Dislocation of distal end of radius NOS
Subluxation of carpal bone NOS
Subluxation of distal end of radius NOS

7 ⊟ **S63.001-**   **Unspecified subluxation of right wrist and hand**

7 ⊟ **S63.002-**   **Unspecified subluxation of left wrist and hand**

7 ⊟ **S63.003-**   **Unspecified subluxation of unspecified wrist and hand**

7 ⊟ **S63.004-**   **Unspecified dislocation of right wrist and hand**

7 ⊟ **S63.005-**   **Unspecified dislocation of left wrist and hand**

7 ⊟ **S63.006-**   **Unspecified dislocation of unspecified wrist and hand**

6 **S63.01**   **Subluxation and dislocation of distal radioulnar joint**

7 ⊟ **S63.011-**   **Subluxation of distal radioulnar joint of right wrist**

7 ⊟ **S63.012-**   **Subluxation of distal radioulnar joint of left wrist**

7 ⊟ **S63.013-**   **Subluxation of distal radioulnar joint of unspecified wrist**

7 ⊟ **S63.014-**   **Dislocation of distal radioulnar joint of right wrist**

7 ⊟ **S63.015-**   **Dislocation of distal radioulnar joint of left wrist**

7 ⊟ **S63.016-**   **Dislocation of distal radioulnar joint of unspecified wrist**

6 **S63.02**   **Subluxation and dislocation of radiocarpal joint**

7 ⊟ **S63.021-**   **Subluxation of radiocarpal joint of right wrist**

7 ⊟ **S63.022-**   **Subluxation of radiocarpal joint of left wrist**

7 ⊟ **S63.023-**   **Subluxation of radiocarpal joint of unspecified wrist**

7 ⊟ **S63.024-**   **Dislocation of radiocarpal joint of right wrist**

7 ⊟ **S63.025-**   **Dislocation of radiocarpal joint of left wrist**

7 ⊟ **S63.026-**   **Dislocation of radiocarpal joint of unspecified wrist**

6 **S63.03**   **Subluxation and dislocation of midcarpal joint**

7 ⊟ **S63.031-**   **Subluxation of midcarpal joint of right wrist**

7 ⊟ **S63.032-**   **Subluxation of midcarpal joint of left wrist**

7 ⊟ **S63.033-**   **Subluxation of midcarpal joint of unspecified wrist**

7 ⊟ **S63.034-**   **Dislocation of midcarpal joint of right wrist**

7 ⊟ **S63.035-**   **Dislocation of midcarpal joint of left wrist**

7 ⊟ **S63.036-**   **Dislocation of midcarpal joint of unspecified wrist**

6 **S63.04**   **Subluxation and dislocation of carpometacarpal joint of thumb**

EXCLUDES 2   *interphalangeal subluxation and dislocation of thumb (S63.1-)*

7 ⊟ **S63.041-**   **Subluxation of carpometacarpal joint of right thumb**

7 ⊟ **S63.042-**   **Subluxation of carpometacarpal joint of left thumb**

7 ⊟ **S63.043-**   **Subluxation of carpometacarpal joint of unspecified thumb**

7 ⊟ **S63.044-**   **Dislocation of carpometacarpal joint of right thumb**

7 ⊟ **S63.045-**   **Dislocation of carpometacarpal joint of left thumb**

7 ⊟ **S63.046-**   **Dislocation of carpometacarpal joint of unspecified thumb**

6 **S63.05**   **Subluxation and dislocation of other carpometacarpal joint**

EXCLUDES 2   *subluxation and dislocation of carpometacarpal joint of thumb (S63.04-)*

7 ⊟ **S63.051-**   **Subluxation of other carpometacarpal joint of right hand**

7 ⊟ **S63.052-**   **Subluxation of other carpometacarpal joint of left hand**

7 ⊟ **S63.053-**   **Subluxation of other carpometacarpal joint of unspecified hand**

7 ⊟ **S63.054-**   **Dislocation of other carpometacarpal joint of right hand**

7 ⊟ **S63.055-**   **Dislocation of other carpometacarpal joint of left hand**

7 ⊟ **S63.056-**   **Dislocation of other carpometacarpal joint of unspecified hand**

6 **S63.06**   **Subluxation and dislocation of metacarpal (bone), proximal end**

7 ⊟ **S63.061-**   **Subluxation of metacarpal (bone), proximal end of right hand**

7 ⊟ **S63.062-**   **Subluxation of metacarpal (bone), proximal end of left hand**

7 ⊟ **S63.063-**   **Subluxation of metacarpal (bone), proximal end of unspecified hand**

7 ⊟ **S63.064-**   **Dislocation of metacarpal (bone), proximal end of right hand**

7 ⊟ **S63.065-**   **Dislocation of metacarpal (bone), proximal end of left hand**

7 ⊟ **S63.066-**   **Dislocation of metacarpal (bone), proximal end of unspecified hand**

6 **S63.07**   **Subluxation and dislocation of distal end of ulna**

7 ⊟ **S63.071-**   **Subluxation of distal end of right ulna**

7 ⊟ **S63.072-**   **Subluxation of distal end of left ulna**

7 ⊟ **S63.073-**   **Subluxation of distal end of unspecified ulna**

7 ⊟ **S63.074-**   **Dislocation of distal end of right ulna**

7 ⊟ **S63.075-**   **Dislocation of distal end of left ulna**

7 ⊟ **S63.076-**   **Dislocation of distal end of unspecified ulna**

6 **S63.09**   **Other subluxation and dislocation of wrist and hand**

7 ⊟ **S63.091-**   **Other subluxation of right wrist and hand**

7 ⊟ **S63.092-**   **Other subluxation of left wrist and hand**

7 ⊟ **S63.093-**   **Other subluxation of unspecified wrist and hand**

7 ⊟ **S63.094-**   **Other dislocation of right wrist and hand**

7 ⊟ **S63.095-**   **Other dislocation of left wrist and hand**

7 ⊟ **S63.096-**   **Other dislocation of unspecified wrist and hand**

5 **S63.1**   **Subluxation and dislocation of thumb**

6 **S63.10**   **Unspecified subluxation and dislocation of thumb**

7 ⊟ **S63.101-**   **Unspecified subluxation of right thumb**

7 ⊟ **S63.102-**   **Unspecified subluxation of left thumb**

7 ⊟ **S63.103-**   **Unspecified subluxation of unspecified thumb**

7 ⊟ **S63.104-**   **Unspecified dislocation of right thumb**

7 ⊟ **S63.105-**   **Unspecified dislocation of left thumb**

7 ⊟ **S63.106-**   **Unspecified dislocation of unspecified thumb**

● New   ▲ Revised   *Manifestation*   4-7 Digit Indicators   ⊟ Laterality   A Adult (15+ years)   M Maternity (12-55 years)   N Newborn   P Pediatric (0-17 years)   ♂ Male   ♀ Female
✖ Deleted   Unspecified   + Additional code

⑥ S63.11 Subluxation and dislocation of metacarpophalangeal joint of thumb
- ⑦ ⊟ S63.111- Subluxation of metacarpophalangeal joint of right thumb
- ⑦ ⊟ S63.112- Subluxation of metacarpophalangeal joint of left thumb
- ⑦ ⊟ S63.113- Subluxation of metacarpophalangeal joint of unspecified thumb
- ⑦ ⊟ S63.114- Dislocation of metacarpophalangeal joint of right thumb
- ⑦ ⊟ S63.115- Dislocation of metacarpophalangeal joint of left thumb
- ⑦ ⊟ S63.116- Dislocation of metacarpophalangeal joint of unspecified thumb

⑥ S63.12 Subluxation and dislocation of unspecified interphalangeal joint of thumb
- ⑦ ⊟ S63.121- Subluxation of unspecified interphalangeal joint of right thumb
- ⑦ ⊟ S63.122- Subluxation of unspecified interphalangeal joint of left thumb
- ⑦ ⊟ S63.123- Subluxation of unspecified interphalangeal joint of unspecified thumb
- ⑦ ⊟ S63.124- Dislocation of unspecified interphalangeal joint of right thumb
- ⑦ ⊟ S63.125- Dislocation of unspecified interphalangeal joint of left thumb
- ⑦ ⊟ S63.126- Dislocation of unspecified interphalangeal joint of unspecified thumb

⑥ S63.13 Subluxation and dislocation of proximal interphalangeal joint of thumb
- ⑦ ⊟ S63.131- Subluxation of proximal interphalangeal joint of right thumb
- ⑦ ⊟ S63.132- Subluxation of proximal interphalangeal joint of left thumb
- ⑦ ⊟ S63.133- Subluxation of proximal interphalangeal joint of unspecified thumb
- ⑦ ⊟ S63.134- Dislocation of proximal interphalangeal joint of right thumb
- ⑦ ⊟ S63.135- Dislocation of proximal interphalangeal joint of left thumb
- ⑦ ⊟ S63.136- Dislocation of proximal interphalangeal joint of unspecified thumb

⑥ S63.14 Subluxation and dislocation of distal interphalangeal joint of thumb
- ⑦ ⊟ S63.141- Subluxation of distal interphalangeal joint of right thumb
- ⑦ ⊟ S63.142- Subluxation of distal interphalangeal joint of left thumb
- ⑦ ⊟ S63.143- Subluxation of distal interphalangeal joint of unspecified thumb
- ⑦ ⊟ S63.144- Dislocation of distal interphalangeal joint of right thumb
- ⑦ ⊟ S63.145- Dislocation of distal interphalangeal joint of left thumb
- ⑦ ⊟ S63.146- Dislocation of distal interphalangeal joint of unspecified thumb

⑥ S63.2 Subluxation and dislocation of other finger(s)
> **EXCLUDES 2** *subluxation and dislocation of thumb (S63.1-)*

⑥ S63.20 Unspecified subluxation of other finger
- ⑦ ⊟ S63.200- Unspecified subluxation of right index finger
- ⑦ ⊟ S63.201- Unspecified subluxation of left index finger
- ⑦ ⊟ S63.202- Unspecified subluxation of right middle finger
- ⑦ ⊟ S63.203- Unspecified subluxation of left middle finger
- ⑦ ⊟ S63.204- Unspecified subluxation of right ring finger
- ⑦ ⊟ S63.205- Unspecified subluxation of left ring finger
- ⑦ ⊟ S63.206- Unspecified subluxation of right little finger
- ⑦ ⊟ S63.207- Unspecified subluxation of left little finger
- ⑦ ⊟ S63.208- Unspecified subluxation of other finger
  Unspecified subluxation of specified finger with unspecified laterality
- ⑦ ⊟ S63.209- Unspecified subluxation of unspecified finger

⑥ S63.21 Subluxation of metacarpophalangeal joint of finger
- ⑦ ⊟ S63.210- Subluxation of metacarpophalangeal joint of right index finger
- ⑦ ⊟ S63.211- Subluxation of metacarpophalangeal joint of left index finger
- ⑦ ⊟ S63.212- Subluxation of metacarpophalangeal joint of right middle finger
- ⑦ ⊟ S63.213- Subluxation of metacarpophalangeal joint of left middle finger
- ⑦ ⊟ S63.214- Subluxation of metacarpophalangeal joint of right ring finger
- ⑦ ⊟ S63.215- Subluxation of metacarpophalangeal joint of left ring finger
- ⑦ ⊟ S63.216- Subluxation of metacarpophalangeal joint of right little finger
- ⑦ ⊟ S63.217- Subluxation of metacarpophalangeal joint of left little finger
- ⑦ ⊟ S63.218- Subluxation of metacarpophalangeal joint of other finger
  Subluxation of metacarpophalangeal joint of specified finger with unspecified laterality
- ⑦ ⊟ S63.219- Subluxation of metacarpophalangeal joint of unspecified finger

⑥ S63.22 Subluxation of unspecified interphalangeal joint of finger
- ⑦ ⊟ S63.220- Subluxation of unspecified interphalangeal joint of right index finger
- ⑦ ⊟ S63.221- Subluxation of unspecified interphalangeal joint of left index finger
- ⑦ ⊟ S63.222- Subluxation of unspecified interphalangeal joint of right middle finger
- ⑦ ⊟ S63.223- Subluxation of unspecified interphalangeal joint of left middle finger
- ⑦ ⊟ S63.224- Subluxation of unspecified interphalangeal joint of right ring finger
- ⑦ ⊟ S63.225- Subluxation of unspecified interphalangeal joint of left ring finger
- ⑦ ⊟ S63.226- Subluxation of unspecified interphalangeal joint of right little finger
- ⑦ ⊟ S63.227- Subluxation of unspecified interphalangeal joint of left little finger
- ⑦ ⊟ S63.228- Subluxation of unspecified interphalangeal joint of other finger
  Subluxation of unspecified interphalangeal joint of specified finger with unspecified laterality
- ⑦ ⊟ S63.229- Subluxation of unspecified interphalangeal joint of unspecified finger

⑥ S63.23 Subluxation of proximal interphalangeal joint of finger
- ⑦ ⊟ S63.230- Subluxation of proximal interphalangeal joint of right index finger
- ⑦ ⊟ S63.231- Subluxation of proximal interphalangeal joint of left index finger
- ⑦ ⊟ S63.232- Subluxation of proximal interphalangeal joint of right middle finger
- ⑦ ⊟ S63.233- Subluxation of proximal interphalangeal joint of left middle finger
- ⑦ ⊟ S63.234- Subluxation of proximal interphalangeal joint of right ring finger
- ⑦ ⊟ S63.235- Subluxation of proximal interphalangeal joint of left ring finger
- ⑦ ⊟ S63.236- Subluxation of proximal interphalangeal joint of right little finger
- ⑦ ⊟ S63.237- Subluxation of proximal interphalangeal joint of left little finger
- ⑦ ⊟ S63.238- Subluxation of proximal interphalangeal joint of other finger
  Subluxation of proximal interphalangeal joint of specified finger with unspecified laterality
- ⑦ ⊟ S63.239- Subluxation of proximal interphalangeal joint of unspecified finger

⑥ S63.24 Subluxation of distal interphalangeal joint of finger
- ⑦ ⊟ S63.240- Subluxation of distal interphalangeal joint of right index finger
- ⑦ ⊟ S63.241- Subluxation of distal interphalangeal joint of left index finger
- ⑦ ⊟ S63.242- Subluxation of distal interphalangeal joint of right middle finger
- ⑦ ⊟ S63.243- Subluxation of distal interphalangeal joint of left middle finger
- ⑦ ⊟ S63.244- Subluxation of distal interphalangeal joint of right ring finger
- ⑦ ⊟ S63.245- Subluxation of distal interphalangeal joint of left ring finger

● New ▲ Revised *Manifestation* ④-⑦ Digit Indicators ⊟ Laterality Ⓐ Adult (15+ years) Ⓜ Maternity (12-55 years) Ⓝ Newborn Ⓟ Pediatric (0-17 years) ♂ Male ♀ Female
✖ Deleted Unspecified + Additional code

992 © 2017 DecisionHealth   2017 ICD-10-CM Expert for Physicians

7 ⊟ S63.246-   **Subluxation of distal interphalangeal joint of right little finger**

7 ⊟ S63.247-   **Subluxation of distal interphalangeal joint of left little finger**

7 ⊟ S63.248-   **Subluxation of distal interphalangeal joint of other finger**
   Subluxation of distal interphalangeal joint of specified finger with unspecified laterality

7 ⊟ S63.249-   **Subluxation of distal interphalangeal joint of unspecified finger**

6 S63.25   **Unspecified dislocation of other finger**

7 ⊟ S63.250-   **Unspecified dislocation of right index finger**

7 ⊟ S63.251-   **Unspecified dislocation of left index finger**

7 ⊟ S63.252-   **Unspecified dislocation of right middle finger**

7 ⊟ S63.253-   **Unspecified dislocation of left middle finger**

7 ⊟ S63.254-   **Unspecified dislocation of right ring finger**

7 ⊟ S63.255-   **Unspecified dislocation of left ring finger**

7 ⊟ S63.256-   **Unspecified dislocation of right little finger**

7 ⊟ S63.257-   **Unspecified dislocation of left little finger**

7 ⊟ S63.258-   **Unspecified dislocation of other finger**
   Unspecified dislocation of specified finger with unspecified laterality

7 ⊟ S63.259-   **Unspecified dislocation of unspecified finger**
   Unspecified dislocation of specified finger with unspecified laterality

6 S63.26   **Dislocation of metacarpophalangeal joint of finger**

7 ⊟ S63.260-   **Dislocation of metacarpophalangeal joint of right index finger**

7 ⊟ S63.261-   **Dislocation of metacarpophalangeal joint of left index finger**

7 ⊟ S63.262-   **Dislocation of metacarpophalangeal joint of right middle finger**

7 ⊟ S63.263-   **Dislocation of metacarpophalangeal joint of left middle finger**

7 ⊟ S63.264-   **Dislocation of metacarpophalangeal joint of right ring finger**

7 ⊟ S63.265-   **Dislocation of metacarpophalangeal joint of left ring finger**

7 ⊟ S63.266-   **Dislocation of metacarpophalangeal joint of right little finger**

7 ⊟ S63.267-   **Dislocation of metacarpophalangeal joint of left little finger**

7 ⊟ S63.268-   **Dislocation of metacarpophalangeal joint of other finger**
   Dislocation of metacarpophalangeal joint of specified finger with unspecified laterality

7 ⊟ S63.269-   **Dislocation of metacarpophalangeal joint of unspecified finger**

6 S63.27   **Dislocation of unspecified interphalangeal joint of finger**

7 ⊟ S63.270-   **Dislocation of unspecified interphalangeal joint of right index finger**

7 ⊟ S63.271-   **Dislocation of unspecified interphalangeal joint of left index finger**

7 ⊟ S63.272-   **Dislocation of unspecified interphalangeal joint of right middle finger**

7 ⊟ S63.273-   **Dislocation of unspecified interphalangeal joint of left middle finger**

7 ⊟ S63.274-   **Dislocation of unspecified interphalangeal joint of right ring finger**

7 ⊟ S63.275-   **Dislocation of unspecified interphalangeal joint of left ring finger**

7 ⊟ S63.276-   **Dislocation of unspecified interphalangeal joint of right little finger**

7 ⊟ S63.277-   **Dislocation of unspecified interphalangeal joint of left little finger**

7 ⊟ S63.278-   **Dislocation of unspecified interphalangeal joint of other finger**
   Dislocation of unspecified interphalangeal joint of specified finger with unspecified laterality

7 ⊟ S63.279-   **Dislocation of unspecified interphalangeal joint of unspecified finger**
   Dislocation of unspecified interphalangeal joint of specified finger without specified laterality

6 S63.28   **Dislocation of proximal interphalangeal joint of finger**

7 ⊟ S63.280-   **Dislocation of proximal interphalangeal joint of right index finger**

7 ⊟ S63.281-   **Dislocation of proximal interphalangeal joint of left index finger**

7 ⊟ S63.282-   **Dislocation of proximal interphalangeal joint of right middle finger**

7 ⊟ S63.283-   **Dislocation of proximal interphalangeal joint of left middle finger**

7 ⊟ S63.284-   **Dislocation of proximal interphalangeal joint of right ring finger**

7 ⊟ S63.285-   **Dislocation of proximal interphalangeal joint of left ring finger**

7 ⊟ S63.286-   **Dislocation of proximal interphalangeal joint of right little finger**

7 ⊟ S63.287-   **Dislocation of proximal interphalangeal joint of left little finger**

7 ⊟ S63.288-   **Dislocation of proximal interphalangeal joint of other finger**
   Dislocation of proximal interphalangeal joint of specified finger with unspecified laterality

7 ⊟ S63.289-   **Dislocation of proximal interphalangeal joint of unspecified finger**

6 S63.29   **Dislocation of distal interphalangeal joint of finger**

7 ⊟ S63.290-   **Dislocation of distal interphalangeal joint of right index finger**

7 ⊟ S63.291-   **Dislocation of distal interphalangeal joint of left index finger**

7 ⊟ S63.292-   **Dislocation of distal interphalangeal joint of right middle finger**

7 ⊟ S63.293-   **Dislocation of distal interphalangeal joint of left middle finger**

7 ⊟ S63.294-   **Dislocation of distal interphalangeal joint of right ring finger**

7 ⊟ S63.295-   **Dislocation of distal interphalangeal joint of left ring finger**

7 ⊟ S63.296-   **Dislocation of distal interphalangeal joint of right little finger**

7 ⊟ S63.297-   **Dislocation of distal interphalangeal joint of left little finger**

7 ⊟ S63.298-   **Dislocation of distal interphalangeal joint of other finger**
   Dislocation of distal interphalangeal joint of specified finger with unspecified laterality

7 ⊟ S63.299-   **Dislocation of distal interphalangeal joint of unspecified finger**

⊟ S63.3   **Traumatic rupture of ligament of wrist**

6 S63.30   **Traumatic rupture of unspecified ligament of wrist**

7 ⊟ S63.301-   **Traumatic rupture of unspecified ligament of right wrist**

7 ⊟ S63.302-   **Traumatic rupture of unspecified ligament of left wrist**

7 ⊟ S63.309-   **Traumatic rupture of unspecified ligament of unspecified wrist**

6 S63.31   **Traumatic rupture of collateral ligament of wrist**

7 ⊟ S63.311-   **Traumatic rupture of collateral ligament of right wrist**

7 ⊟ S63.312-   **Traumatic rupture of collateral ligament of left wrist**

7 ⊟ S63.319-   **Traumatic rupture of collateral ligament of unspecified wrist**

6 S63.32   **Traumatic rupture of radiocarpal ligament**

7 ⊟ S63.321-   **Traumatic rupture of right radiocarpal ligament**

7 ⊟ S63.322-   **Traumatic rupture of left radiocarpal ligament**

7 ⊟ S63.329-   **Traumatic rupture of unspecified radiocarpal ligament**

6 S63.33   **Traumatic rupture of ulnocarpal (palmar) ligament**

7 ⊟ S63.331-   **Traumatic rupture of right ulnocarpal (palmar) ligament**

7 ⊟ S63.332-   **Traumatic rupture of left ulnocarpal (palmar) ligament**

7 ⊟ S63.339-   **Traumatic rupture of unspecified ulnocarpal (palmar) ligament**

6 S63.39   **Traumatic rupture of other ligament of wrist**

7 ⊟ S63.391-   **Traumatic rupture of other ligament of right wrist**

7 ⊟ S63.392-   **Traumatic rupture of other ligament of left wrist**

7 ⊟ S63.399-   **Traumatic rupture of other ligament of unspecified wrist**

● New   ▲ Revised   *Manifestation*   4-7 Digit Indicators   ⊟ Laterality   Ⓐ Adult (15+ years)   Ⓜ Maternity (12-55 years)   Ⓝ Newborn   Ⓟ Pediatric (0-17 years)   ♂ Male   ♀ Female
✖ Deleted   Unspecified   + Additional code

⑤ **S63.4**   **Traumatic rupture of ligament of finger at metacarpophalangeal and interphalangeal joint(s)**

⑥ **S63.40**   **Traumatic rupture of unspecified ligament of finger at metacarpophalangeal and interphalangeal joint**

☷⊟ **S63.400-**   **Traumatic rupture of unspecified ligament of right index finger at metacarpophalangeal and interphalangeal joint**

☷⊟ **S63.401-**   **Traumatic rupture of unspecified ligament of left index finger at metacarpophalangeal and interphalangeal joint**

☷⊟ **S63.402-**   **Traumatic rupture of unspecified ligament of right middle finger at metacarpophalangeal and interphalangeal joint**

☷⊟ **S63.403-**   **Traumatic rupture of unspecified ligament of left middle finger at metacarpophalangeal and interphalangeal joint**

☷⊟ **S63.404-**   **Traumatic rupture of unspecified ligament of right ring finger at metacarpophalangeal and interphalangeal joint**

☷⊟ **S63.405-**   **Traumatic rupture of unspecified ligament of left ring finger at metacarpophalangeal and interphalangeal joint**

☷⊟ **S63.406-**   **Traumatic rupture of unspecified ligament of right little finger at metacarpophalangeal and interphalangeal joint**

☷⊟ **S63.407-**   **Traumatic rupture of unspecified ligament of left little finger at metacarpophalangeal and interphalangeal joint**

☷⊟ **S63.408-**   **Traumatic rupture of unspecified ligament of other finger at metacarpophalangeal and interphalangeal joint**

Traumatic rupture of unspecified ligament of specified finger with unspecified laterality at metacarpophalangeal and interphalangeal joint

☷⊟ **S63.409-**   **Traumatic rupture of unspecified ligament of unspecified finger at metacarpophalangeal and interphalangeal joint**

⑥ **S63.41**   **Traumatic rupture of collateral ligament of finger at metacarpophalangeal and interphalangeal joint**

☷⊟ **S63.410-**   **Traumatic rupture of collateral ligament of right index finger at metacarpophalangeal and interphalangeal joint**

☷⊟ **S63.411-**   **Traumatic rupture of collateral ligament of left index finger at metacarpophalangeal and interphalangeal joint**

☷⊟ **S63.412-**   **Traumatic rupture of collateral ligament of right middle finger at metacarpophalangeal and interphalangeal joint**

☷⊟ **S63.413-**   **Traumatic rupture of collateral ligament of left middle finger at metacarpophalangeal and interphalangeal joint**

☷⊟ **S63.414-**   **Traumatic rupture of collateral ligament of right ring finger at metacarpophalangeal and interphalangeal joint**

☷⊟ **S63.415-**   **Traumatic rupture of collateral ligament of left ring finger at metacarpophalangeal and interphalangeal joint**

☷⊟ **S63.416-**   **Traumatic rupture of collateral ligament of right little finger at metacarpophalangeal and interphalangeal joint**

☷⊟ **S63.417-**   **Traumatic rupture of collateral ligament of left little finger at metacarpophalangeal and interphalangeal joint**

☷⊟ **S63.418-**   **Traumatic rupture of collateral ligament of other finger at metacarpophalangeal and interphalangeal joint**

Traumatic rupture of collateral ligament of specified finger with unspecified laterality at metacarpophalangeal and interphalangeal joint

☷⊟ **S63.419-**   **Traumatic rupture of collateral ligament of unspecified finger at metacarpophalangeal and interphalangeal joint**

⑥ **S63.42**   **Traumatic rupture of palmar ligament of finger at metacarpophalangeal and interphalangeal joint**

☷⊟ **S63.420-**   **Traumatic rupture of palmar ligament of right index finger at metacarpophalangeal and interphalangeal joint**

☷⊟ **S63.421-**   **Traumatic rupture of palmar ligament of left index finger at metacarpophalangeal and interphalangeal joint**

☷⊟ **S63.422-**   **Traumatic rupture of palmar ligament of right middle finger at metacarpophalangeal and interphalangeal joint**

☷⊟ **S63.423-**   **Traumatic rupture of palmar ligament of left middle finger at metacarpophalangeal and interphalangeal joint**

☷⊟ **S63.424-**   **Traumatic rupture of palmar ligament of right ring finger at metacarpophalangeal and interphalangeal joint**

☷⊟ **S63.425-**   **Traumatic rupture of palmar ligament of left ring finger at metacarpophalangeal and interphalangeal joint**

☷⊟ **S63.426-**   **Traumatic rupture of palmar ligament of right little finger at metacarpophalangeal and interphalangeal joint**

☷⊟ **S63.427-**   **Traumatic rupture of palmar ligament of left little finger at metacarpophalangeal and interphalangeal joint**

☷⊟ **S63.428-**   **Traumatic rupture of palmar ligament of other finger at metacarpophalangeal and interphalangeal joint**

Traumatic rupture of palmar ligament of specified finger with unspecified laterality at metacarpophalangeal and interphalangeal joint

☷⊟ **S63.429-**   **Traumatic rupture of palmar ligament of unspecified finger at metacarpophalangeal and interphalangeal joint**

⑥ **S63.43**   **Traumatic rupture of volar plate of finger at metacarpophalangeal and interphalangeal joint**

☷⊟ **S63.430-**   **Traumatic rupture of volar plate of right index finger at metacarpophalangeal and interphalangeal joint**

☷⊟ **S63.431-**   **Traumatic rupture of volar plate of left index finger at metacarpophalangeal and interphalangeal joint**

☷⊟ **S63.432-**   **Traumatic rupture of volar plate of right middle finger at metacarpophalangeal and interphalangeal joint**

☷⊟ **S63.433-**   **Traumatic rupture of volar plate of left middle finger at metacarpophalangeal and interphalangeal joint**

☷⊟ **S63.434-**   **Traumatic rupture of volar plate of right ring finger at metacarpophalangeal and interphalangeal joint**

☷⊟ **S63.435-**   **Traumatic rupture of volar plate of left ring finger at metacarpophalangeal and interphalangeal joint**

☷⊟ **S63.436-**   **Traumatic rupture of volar plate of right little finger at metacarpophalangeal and interphalangeal joint**

☷⊟ **S63.437-**   **Traumatic rupture of volar plate of left little finger at metacarpophalangeal and interphalangeal joint**

☷⊟ **S63.438-**   **Traumatic rupture of volar plate of other finger at metacarpophalangeal and interphalangeal joint**

Traumatic rupture of volar plate of specified finger with unspecified laterality at metacarpophalangeal and interphalangeal joint

☷⊟ **S63.439-**   **Traumatic rupture of volar plate of unspecified finger at metacarpophalangeal and interphalangeal joint**

⑥ **S63.49**   **Traumatic rupture of other ligament of finger at metacarpophalangeal and interphalangeal joint**

☷⊟ **S63.490-**   **Traumatic rupture of other ligament of right index finger at metacarpophalangeal and interphalangeal joint**

☷⊟ **S63.491-**   **Traumatic rupture of other ligament of left index finger at metacarpophalangeal and interphalangeal joint**

☷⊟ **S63.492-**   **Traumatic rupture of other ligament of right middle finger at metacarpophalangeal and interphalangeal joint**

☷⊟ **S63.493-**   **Traumatic rupture of other ligament of left middle finger at metacarpophalangeal and interphalangeal joint**

☷⊟ **S63.494-**   **Traumatic rupture of other ligament of right ring finger at metacarpophalangeal and interphalangeal joint**

☷⊟ **S63.495-**   **Traumatic rupture of other ligament of left ring finger at metacarpophalangeal and interphalangeal joint**

● New   ▲ Revised   *Manifestation*   ④-☷ Digit Indicators   ⊟ Laterality   Ⓐ Adult (15+ years)   Ⓜ Maternity (12-55 years)   Ⓝ Newborn   Ⓟ Pediatric (0-17 years)   ♂ Male   ♀ Female

✖ Deleted   Unspecified   + Additional code

994   © 2017 DecisionHealth   2017 ICD-10-CM Expert for Physicians

7 ⊟ S63.496- Traumatic rupture of other ligament of right little finger at metacarpophalangeal and interphalangeal joint

7 ⊟ S63.497- Traumatic rupture of other ligament of left little finger at metacarpophalangeal and interphalangeal joint

7 ⊟ S63.498- Traumatic rupture of other ligament of other finger at metacarpophalangeal and interphalangeal joint
Traumatic rupture of ligament of specified finger with unspecified laterality at metacarpophalangeal and interphalangeal joint

7 ⊟ S63.499- Traumatic rupture of other ligament of unspecified finger at metacarpophalangeal and interphalangeal joint

5 S63.5 Other and unspecified sprain of wrist

6 S63.50 Unspecified sprain of wrist

7 ⊟ S63.501- Unspecified sprain of right wrist

7 ⊟ S63.502- Unspecified sprain of left wrist

7 ⊟ S63.509- Unspecified sprain of unspecified wrist

6 S63.51 Sprain of carpal (joint)

7 ⊟ S63.511- Sprain of carpal joint of right wrist

7 ⊟ S63.512- Sprain of carpal joint of left wrist

7 ⊟ S63.519- Sprain of carpal joint of unspecified wrist

6 S63.52 Sprain of radiocarpal joint

EXCLUDES 1 *traumatic rupture of radiocarpal ligament (S63.32-)*

7 ⊟ S63.521- Sprain of radiocarpal joint of right wrist

7 ⊟ S63.522- Sprain of radiocarpal joint of left wrist

7 ⊟ S63.529- Sprain of radiocarpal joint of unspecified wrist

6 S63.59 Other specified sprain of wrist

7 ⊟ S63.591- Other specified sprain of right wrist

7 ⊟ S63.592- Other specified sprain of left wrist

7 ⊟ S63.599- Other specified sprain of unspecified wrist

5 S63.6 Other and unspecified sprain of finger(s)

EXCLUDES 1 *traumatic rupture of ligament of finger at metacarpophalangeal and interphalangeal joint (s) (S63.4-)*

6 S63.60 Unspecified sprain of thumb

7 ⊟ S63.601- Unspecified sprain of right thumb

7 ⊟ S63.602- Unspecified sprain of left thumb

7 ⊟ S63.609- Unspecified sprain of unspecified thumb

6 S63.61 Unspecified sprain of other and unspecified finger(s)

7 ⊟ S63.610- Unspecified sprain of right index finger

7 ⊟ S63.611- Unspecified sprain of left index finger

7 ⊟ S63.612- Unspecified sprain of right middle finger

7 ⊟ S63.613- Unspecified sprain of left middle finger

7 ⊟ S63.614- Unspecified sprain of right ring finger

7 ⊟ S63.615- Unspecified sprain of left ring finger

7 ⊟ S63.616- Unspecified sprain of right little finger

7 ⊟ S63.617- Unspecified sprain of left little finger

7 ⊟ S63.618- Unspecified sprain of other finger
Unspecified sprain of specified finger with unspecified laterality

7 ⊟ S63.619- Unspecified sprain of unspecified finger

6 S63.62 Sprain of interphalangeal joint of thumb

7 ⊟ S63.621- Sprain of interphalangeal joint of right thumb

7 ⊟ S63.622- Sprain of interphalangeal joint of left thumb

7 ⊟ S63.629- Sprain of interphalangeal joint of unspecified thumb

6 S63.63 Sprain of interphalangeal joint of other and unspecified finger(s)

7 ⊟ S63.630- Sprain of interphalangeal joint of right index finger

7 ⊟ S63.631- Sprain of interphalangeal joint of left index finger

7 ⊟ S63.632- Sprain of interphalangeal joint of right middle finger

7 ⊟ S63.633- Sprain of interphalangeal joint of left middle finger

7 ⊟ S63.634- Sprain of interphalangeal joint of right ring finger

7 ⊟ S63.635- Sprain of interphalangeal joint of left ring finger

7 ⊟ S63.636- Sprain of interphalangeal joint of right little finger

7 ⊟ S63.637- Sprain of interphalangeal joint of left little finger

7 ⊟ S63.638- Sprain of interphalangeal joint of other finger

7 ⊟ S63.639- Sprain of interphalangeal joint of unspecified finger

6 S63.64 Sprain of metacarpophalangeal joint of thumb

7 ⊟ S63.641- Sprain of metacarpophalangeal joint of right thumb

7 ⊟ S63.642- Sprain of metacarpophalangeal joint of left thumb

7 ⊟ S63.649- Sprain of metacarpophalangeal joint of unspecified thumb

6 S63.65 Sprain of metacarpophalangeal joint of other and unspecified finger(s)

7 ⊟ S63.650- Sprain of metacarpophalangeal joint of right index finger

7 ⊟ S63.651- Sprain of metacarpophalangeal joint of left index finger

7 ⊟ S63.652- Sprain of metacarpophalangeal joint of right middle finger

7 ⊟ S63.653- Sprain of metacarpophalangeal joint of left middle finger

7 ⊟ S63.654- Sprain of metacarpophalangeal joint of right ring finger

7 ⊟ S63.655- Sprain of metacarpophalangeal joint of left ring finger

7 ⊟ S63.656- Sprain of metacarpophalangeal joint of right little finger

7 ⊟ S63.657- Sprain of metacarpophalangeal joint of left little finger

7 ⊟ S63.658- Sprain of metacarpophalangeal joint of other finger
Sprain of metacarpophalangeal joint of specified finger with unspecified laterality

7 ⊟ S63.659- Sprain of metacarpophalangeal joint of unspecified finger

6 S63.68 Other sprain of thumb

7 ⊟ S63.681- Other sprain of right thumb

7 ⊟ S63.682- Other sprain of left thumb

7 ⊟ S63.689- Other sprain of unspecified thumb

6 S63.69 Other sprain of other and unspecified finger(s)

7 ⊟ S63.690- Other sprain of right index finger

7 ⊟ S63.691- Other sprain of left index finger

7 ⊟ S63.692- Other sprain of right middle finger

7 ⊟ S63.693- Other sprain of left middle finger

7 ⊟ S63.694- Other sprain of right ring finger

7 ⊟ S63.695- Other sprain of left ring finger

7 ⊟ S63.696- Other sprain of right little finger

7 ⊟ S63.697- Other sprain of left little finger

7 ⊟ S63.698- Other sprain of other finger
Other sprain of specified finger with unspecified laterality

7 ⊟ S63.699- Other sprain of unspecified finger

5 S63.8 Sprain of other part of wrist and hand

6 S63.8X Sprain of other part of wrist and hand

7 ⊟ S63.8X1- Sprain of other part of right wrist and hand

7 ⊟ S63.8X2- Sprain of other part of left wrist and hand

7 ⊟ S63.8X9- Sprain of other part of unspecified wrist and hand

5 S63.9 Sprain of unspecified part of wrist and hand

7 ⊟ S63.90X- Sprain of unspecified part of unspecified wrist and hand

7 ⊟ S63.91X- Sprain of unspecified part of right wrist and hand

7 ⊟ S63.92X- Sprain of unspecified part of left wrist and hand

● New ▲ Revised *Manifestation* 4-7 Digit Indicators ⊟ Laterality ▲ Adult (15+ years) Ⓜ Maternity (12-55 years) Ⓝ Newborn Ⓟ Pediatric (0-17 years) ♂ Male ♀ Female
✖ Deleted Unspecified + Additional code

2017 ICD-10-CM Expert for Physicians

© 2017 DecisionHealth

995

④ **S64**   **Injury of nerves at wrist and hand level**

Code also:
    any associated open wound (S61.-)

The appropriate 7th character is to be added to each code from category S64
A   initial encounter
D   subsequent encounter
S   sequela

⑤ **S64.0**   **Injury of ulnar nerve at wrist and hand level**

7 ⊟ **S64.00X-**   **Injury of ulnar nerve at wrist and hand level of unspecified arm**

7 ⊟ **S64.01X-**   **Injury of ulnar nerve at wrist and hand level of right arm**

7 ⊟ **S64.02X-**   **Injury of ulnar nerve at wrist and hand level of left arm**

⑤ **S64.1**   **Injury of median nerve at wrist and hand level**

7 ⊟ **S64.10X-**   **Injury of median nerve at wrist and hand level of unspecified arm**

7 ⊟ **S64.11X-**   **Injury of median nerve at wrist and hand level of right arm**

7 ⊟ **S64.12X-**   **Injury of median nerve at wrist and hand level of left arm**

⑤ **S64.2**   **Injury of radial nerve at wrist and hand level**

7 ⊟ **S64.20X-**   **Injury of radial nerve at wrist and hand level of unspecified arm**

7 ⊟ **S64.21X-**   **Injury of radial nerve at wrist and hand level of right arm**

7 ⊟ **S64.22X-**   **Injury of radial nerve at wrist and hand level of left arm**

⑤ **S64.3**   **Injury of digital nerve of thumb**

7 ⊟ **S64.30X-**   **Injury of digital nerve of unspecified thumb**

7 ⊟ **S64.31X-**   **Injury of digital nerve of right thumb**

7 ⊟ **S64.32X-**   **Injury of digital nerve of left thumb**

⑤ **S64.4**   **Injury of digital nerve of other and unspecified finger**

7 **S64.40X-**   **Injury of digital nerve of unspecified finger**

⑥ **S64.49**   **Injury of digital nerve of other finger**

7 ⊟ **S64.490-**   **Injury of digital nerve of right index finger**

7 ⊟ **S64.491-**   **Injury of digital nerve of left index finger**

7 ⊟ **S64.492-**   **Injury of digital nerve of right middle finger**

7 ⊟ **S64.493-**   **Injury of digital nerve of left middle finger**

7 ⊟ **S64.494-**   **Injury of digital nerve of right ring finger**

7 ⊟ **S64.495-**   **Injury of digital nerve of left ring finger**

7 ⊟ **S64.496-**   **Injury of digital nerve of right little finger**

7 ⊟ **S64.497-**   **Injury of digital nerve of left little finger**

7 ⊟ **S64.498-**   **Injury of digital nerve of other finger**
    Injury of digital nerve of specified finger with unspecified laterality

⑤ **S64.8**   **Injury of other nerves at wrist and hand level**

⑥ **S64.8X**   **Injury of other nerves at wrist and hand level**

7 ⊟ **S64.8X1-**   **Injury of other nerves at wrist and hand level of right arm**

7 ⊟ **S64.8X2-**   **Injury of other nerves at wrist and hand level of left arm**

7 ⊟ **S64.8X9-**   **Injury of other nerves at wrist and hand level of unspecified arm**

⑤ **S64.9**   **Injury of unspecified nerve at wrist and hand level**

7 ⊟ **S64.90X-**   **Injury of unspecified nerve at wrist and hand level of unspecified arm**

7 ⊟ **S64.91X-**   **Injury of unspecified nerve at wrist and hand level of right arm**

7 ⊟ **S64.92X-**   **Injury of unspecified nerve at wrist and hand level of left arm**

④ **S65**   **Injury of blood vessels at wrist and hand level**

Code also:
    any associated open wound (S61.-)

The appropriate 7th character is to be added to each code from category S65
A   initial encounter
D   subsequent encounter
S   sequela

⑤ **S65.0**   **Injury of ulnar artery at wrist and hand level**

⑥ **S65.00**   **Unspecified injury of ulnar artery at wrist and hand level**

7 ⊟ **S65.001-**   **Unspecified injury of ulnar artery at wrist and hand level of right arm**

7 ⊟ **S65.002-**   **Unspecified injury of ulnar artery at wrist and hand level of left arm**

7 ⊟ **S65.009-**   **Unspecified injury of ulnar artery at wrist and hand level of unspecified arm**

⑥ **S65.01**   **Laceration of ulnar artery at wrist and hand level**

CODING TIP ✓ Code also any associated open wound S61.-

7 ⊟ **S65.011-**   **Laceration of ulnar artery at wrist and hand level of right arm**

7 ⊟ **S65.012-**   **Laceration of ulnar artery at wrist and hand level of left arm**

7 ⊟ **S65.019-**   **Laceration of ulnar artery at wrist and hand level of unspecified arm**

⑥ **S65.09**   **Other specified injury of ulnar artery at wrist and hand level**

7 ⊟ **S65.091-**   **Other specified injury of ulnar artery at wrist and hand level of right arm**

7 ⊟ **S65.092-**   **Other specified injury of ulnar artery at wrist and hand level of left arm**

7 ⊟ **S65.099-**   **Other specified injury of ulnar artery at wrist and hand level of unspecified arm**

⑤ **S65.1**   **Injury of radial artery at wrist and hand level**

⑥ **S65.10**   **Unspecified injury of radial artery at wrist and hand level**

7 ⊟ **S65.101-**   **Unspecified injury of radial artery at wrist and hand level of right arm**

7 ⊟ **S65.102-**   **Unspecified injury of radial artery at wrist and hand level of left arm**

7 ⊟ **S65.109-**   **Unspecified injury of radial artery at wrist and hand level of unspecified arm**

⑥ **S65.11**   **Laceration of radial artery at wrist and hand level**

CODING TIP ✓ Code also any associated open wound S61.-

7 ⊟ **S65.111-**   **Laceration of radial artery at wrist and hand level of right arm**

7 ⊟ **S65.112-**   **Laceration of radial artery at wrist and hand level of left arm**

7 ⊟ **S65.119-**   **Laceration of radial artery at wrist and hand level of unspecified arm**

⑥ **S65.19**   **Other specified injury of radial artery at wrist and hand level**

7 ⊟ **S65.191-**   **Other specified injury of radial artery at wrist and hand level of right arm**

7 ⊟ **S65.192-**   **Other specified injury of radial artery at wrist and hand level of left arm**

7 ⊟ **S65.199-**   **Other specified injury of radial artery at wrist and hand level of unspecified arm**

⑤ **S65.2**   **Injury of superficial palmar arch**

⑥ **S65.20**   **Unspecified injury of superficial palmar arch**

7 ⊟ **S65.201-**   **Unspecified injury of superficial palmar arch of right hand**

7 ⊟ **S65.202-**   **Unspecified injury of superficial palmar arch of left hand**

7 ⊟ **S65.209-**   **Unspecified injury of superficial palmar arch of unspecified hand**

⑥ **S65.21**   **Laceration of superficial palmar arch**

CODING TIP ✓ Code also any associated open wound S61.-

7 ⊟ **S65.211-**   **Laceration of superficial palmar arch of right hand**

7 ⊟ **S65.212-**   **Laceration of superficial palmar arch of left hand**

7 ⊟ **S65.219-**   **Laceration of superficial palmar arch of unspecified hand**

⑥ **S65.29**   **Other specified injury of superficial palmar arch**

7 ⊟ **S65.291-**   **Other specified injury of superficial palmar arch of right hand**

7 ⊟ **S65.292-**   **Other specified injury of superficial palmar arch of left hand**

7 ⊟ **S65.299-**   **Other specified injury of superficial palmar arch of unspecified hand**

⑤ **S65.3**   **Injury of deep palmar arch**

⑥ **S65.30**   **Unspecified injury of deep palmar arch**

● New   ▲ Revised   *Manifestation*   ④-7 Digit Indicators   ⊟ Laterality   Ⓐ Adult (15+ years)   Ⓜ Maternity (12-55 years)   Ⓝ Newborn   Ⓟ Pediatric (0-17 years)   ♂ Male   ♀ Female

✖ Deleted   Unspecified   + Additional code

996   © 2017 DecisionHealth   2017 ICD-10-CM Expert for Physicians

7 ⊟ S65.301-	Unspecified injury of deep palmar arch of right hand	
7 ⊟ S65.302-	Unspecified injury of deep palmar arch of left hand	
7 ⊟ S65.309-	Unspecified injury of deep palmar arch of unspecified hand	

⑥ S65.31   Laceration of deep palmar arch

> CODING TIP ✓   Code also any associated open wound S61.-

7 ⊟ S65.311-	Laceration of deep palmar arch of right hand
7 ⊟ S65.312-	Laceration of deep palmar arch of left hand
7 ⊟ S65.319-	Laceration of deep palmar arch of unspecified hand

⑥ S65.39   Other specified injury of deep palmar arch

7 ⊟ S65.391-	Other specified injury of deep palmar arch of right hand
7 ⊟ S65.392-	Other specified injury of deep palmar arch of left hand
7 ⊟ S65.399-	Other specified injury of deep palmar arch of unspecified hand

⑤ S65.4   Injury of blood vessel of thumb

⑥ S65.40   Unspecified injury of blood vessel of thumb

7 ⊟ S65.401-	Unspecified injury of blood vessel of right thumb
7 ⊟ S65.402-	Unspecified injury of blood vessel of left thumb
7 ⊟ S65.409-	Unspecified injury of blood vessel of unspecified thumb

⑥ S65.41   Laceration of blood vessel of thumb

> CODING TIP ✓   Code also any associated open wound S61.-

7 ⊟ S65.411-	Laceration of blood vessel of right thumb
7 ⊟ S65.412-	Laceration of blood vessel of left thumb
7 ⊟ S65.419-	Laceration of blood vessel of unspecified thumb

⑥ S65.49   Other specified injury of blood vessel of thumb

7 ⊟ S65.491-	Other specified injury of blood vessel of right thumb
7 ⊟ S65.492-	Other specified injury of blood vessel of left thumb
7 ⊟ S65.499-	Other specified injury of blood vessel of unspecified thumb

⑤ S65.5   Injury of blood vessel of other and unspecified finger

⑥ S65.50   Unspecified injury of blood vessel of other and unspecified finger

7 ⊟ S65.500-	Unspecified injury of blood vessel of right index finger
7 ⊟ S65.501-	Unspecified injury of blood vessel of left index finger
7 ⊟ S65.502-	Unspecified injury of blood vessel of right middle finger
7 ⊟ S65.503-	Unspecified injury of blood vessel of left middle finger
7 ⊟ S65.504-	Unspecified injury of blood vessel of right ring finger
7 ⊟ S65.505-	Unspecified injury of blood vessel of left ring finger
7 ⊟ S65.506-	Unspecified injury of blood vessel of right little finger
7 ⊟ S65.507-	Unspecified injury of blood vessel of left little finger
7 ⊟ S65.508-	Unspecified injury of blood vessel of other finger
	Unspecified injury of blood vessel of specified finger with unspecified laterality
7 ⊟ S65.509-	Unspecified injury of blood vessel of unspecified finger

⑥ S65.51   Laceration of blood vessel of other and unspecified finger

> CODING TIP ✓   Code also any associated open wound S61.-

7 ⊟ S65.510-	Laceration of blood vessel of right index finger
7 ⊟ S65.511-	Laceration of blood vessel of left index finger
7 ⊟ S65.512-	Laceration of blood vessel of right middle finger
7 ⊟ S65.513-	Laceration of blood vessel of left middle finger
7 ⊟ S65.514-	Laceration of blood vessel of right ring finger
7 ⊟ S65.515-	Laceration of blood vessel of left ring finger
7 ⊟ S65.516-	Laceration of blood vessel of right little finger
7 ⊟ S65.517-	Laceration of blood vessel of left little finger
7 ⊟ S65.518-	Laceration of blood vessel of other finger
	Laceration of blood vessel of specified finger with unspecified laterality
7 ⊟ S65.519-	Laceration of blood vessel of unspecified finger

⑥ S65.59   Other specified injury of blood vessel of other and unspecified finger

7 ⊟ S65.590-	Other specified injury of blood vessel of right index finger
7 ⊟ S65.591-	Other specified injury of blood vessel of left index finger
7 ⊟ S65.592-	Other specified injury of blood vessel of right middle finger
7 ⊟ S65.593-	Other specified injury of blood vessel of left middle finger
7 ⊟ S65.594-	Other specified injury of blood vessel of right ring finger
7 ⊟ S65.595-	Other specified injury of blood vessel of left ring finger
7 ⊟ S65.596-	Other specified injury of blood vessel of right little finger
7 ⊟ S65.597-	Other specified injury of blood vessel of left little finger
7 ⊟ S65.598-	Other specified injury of blood vessel of other finger
	Other specified injury of blood vessel of specified finger with unspecified laterality
7 ⊟ S65.599-	Other specified injury of blood vessel of unspecified finger

⑤ S65.8   Injury of other blood vessels at wrist and hand level

⑥ S65.80   Unspecified injury of other blood vessels at wrist and hand level

7 ⊟ S65.801-	Unspecified injury of other blood vessels at wrist and hand level of right arm
7 ⊟ S65.802-	Unspecified injury of other blood vessels at wrist and hand level of left arm
7 ⊟ S65.809-	Unspecified injury of other blood vessels at wrist and hand level of unspecified arm

⑥ S65.81   Laceration of other blood vessels at wrist and hand level

> CODING TIP ✓   Code also any associated open wound S61.-

7 ⊟ S65.811-	Laceration of other blood vessels at wrist and hand level of right arm
7 ⊟ S65.812-	Laceration of other blood vessels at wrist and hand level of left arm
7 ⊟ S65.819-	Laceration of other blood vessels at wrist and hand level of unspecified arm

⑥ S65.89   Other specified injury of other blood vessels at wrist and hand level

7 ⊟ S65.891-	Other specified injury of other blood vessels at wrist and hand level of right arm
7 ⊟ S65.892-	Other specified injury of other blood vessels at wrist and hand level of left arm
7 ⊟ S65.899-	Other specified injury of other blood vessels at wrist and hand level of unspecified arm

⑤ S65.9   Injury of unspecified blood vessel at wrist and hand level

⑥ S65.90   Unspecified injury of unspecified blood vessel at wrist and hand level

7 ⊟ S65.901-	Unspecified injury of unspecified blood vessel at wrist and hand level of right arm
7 ⊟ S65.902-	Unspecified injury of unspecified blood vessel at wrist and hand level of left arm
7 ⊟ S65.909-	Unspecified injury of unspecified blood vessel at wrist and hand level of unspecified arm

⑥ S65.91   Laceration of unspecified blood vessel at wrist and hand level

> CODING TIP ✓   Code also any associated open wound S61.-

● New   ▲ Revised   *Manifestation*   ❹-❼ Digit Indicators   ⊟ Laterality   Ⓐ Adult (15+ years)   Ⓜ Maternity (12-55 years)   Ⓝ Newborn   Ⓟ Pediatric (0-17 years)   ♂ Male   ♀ Female
✖ Deleted   Unspecified   + Additional code

2017 ICD-10-CM Expert for Physicians   © 2017 DecisionHealth   997

Injury, Poisoning and Certain Other Consequences of External Causes

7 ⊟ **S65.911-** Laceration of unspecified blood vessel at wrist and hand level of right arm

7 ⊟ **S65.912-** Laceration of unspecified blood vessel at wrist and hand level of left arm

7 ⊟ **S65.919-** Laceration of unspecified blood vessel at wrist and hand level of unspecified arm

6 **S65.99** Other specified injury of unspecified blood vessel at wrist and hand level

7 ⊟ **S65.991-** Other specified injury of unspecified blood vessel at wrist and hand of right arm

7 ⊟ **S65.992-** Other specified injury of unspecified blood vessel at wrist and hand of left arm

7 ⊟ **S65.999-** Other specified injury of unspecified blood vessel at wrist and hand of unspecified arm

4 **S66** **Injury of muscle, fascia and tendon at wrist and hand level**

Code also:
any associated open wound (S61.-)

EXCLUDES 2 *sprain of joints and ligaments of wrist and hand (S63.-)*

The appropriate 7th character is to be added to each code from category S66

A initial encounter
D subsequent encounter
S sequela

5 **S66.0** **Injury of long flexor muscle, fascia and tendon of thumb at wrist and hand level**

6 **S66.00** Unspecified injury of long flexor muscle, fascia and tendon of thumb at wrist and hand level

7 ⊟ **S66.001-** Unspecified injury of long flexor muscle, fascia and tendon of right thumb at wrist and hand level

7 ⊟ **S66.002-** Unspecified injury of long flexor muscle, fascia and tendon of left thumb at wrist and hand level

7 ⊟ **S66.009-** Unspecified injury of long flexor muscle, fascia and tendon of unspecified thumb at wrist and hand level

6 **S66.01** Strain of long flexor muscle, fascia and tendon of thumb at wrist and hand level

7 ⊟ **S66.011-** Strain of long flexor muscle, fascia and tendon of right thumb at wrist and hand level

7 ⊟ **S66.012-** Strain of long flexor muscle, fascia and tendon of left thumb at wrist and hand level

7 ⊟ **S66.019-** Strain of long flexor muscle, fascia and tendon of unspecified thumb at wrist and hand level

6 **S66.02** Laceration of long flexor muscle, fascia and tendon of thumb at wrist and hand level

CODING TIP ✓ Code also any associated open wound S61.-

7 ⊟ **S66.021-** Laceration of long flexor muscle, fascia and tendon of right thumb at wrist and hand level

7 ⊟ **S66.022-** Laceration of long flexor muscle, fascia and tendon of left thumb at wrist and hand level

7 ⊟ **S66.029-** Laceration of long flexor muscle, fascia and tendon of unspecified thumb at wrist and hand level

6 **S66.09** Other specified injury of long flexor muscle, fascia and tendon of thumb at wrist and hand level

7 ⊟ **S66.091-** Other specified injury of long flexor muscle, fascia and tendon of right thumb at wrist and hand level

7 ⊟ **S66.092-** Other specified injury of long flexor muscle, fascia and tendon of left thumb at wrist and hand level

7 ⊟ **S66.099-** Other specified injury of long flexor muscle, fascia and tendon of unspecified thumb at wrist and hand level

5 **S66.1** **Injury of flexor muscle, fascia and tendon of other and unspecified finger at wrist and hand level**

EXCLUDES 2 *Injury of long flexor muscle, fascia and tendon of thumb at wrist and hand level (S66.0-)*

6 **S66.10** Unspecified injury of flexor muscle, fascia and tendon of other and unspecified finger at wrist and hand level

7 ⊟ **S66.100-** Unspecified injury of flexor muscle, fascia and tendon of right index finger at wrist and hand level

7 ⊟ **S66.101-** Unspecified injury of flexor muscle, fascia and tendon of left index finger at wrist and hand level

7 ⊟ **S66.102-** Unspecified injury of flexor muscle, fascia and tendon of right middle finger at wrist and hand level

7 ⊟ **S66.103-** Unspecified injury of flexor muscle, fascia and tendon of left middle finger at wrist and hand level

7 ⊟ **S66.104-** Unspecified injury of flexor muscle, fascia and tendon of right ring finger at wrist and hand level

7 ⊟ **S66.105-** Unspecified injury of flexor muscle, fascia and tendon of left ring finger at wrist and hand level

7 ⊟ **S66.106-** Unspecified injury of flexor muscle, fascia and tendon of right little finger at wrist and hand level

7 ⊟ **S66.107-** Unspecified injury of flexor muscle, fascia and tendon of left little finger at wrist and hand level

7 ⊟ **S66.108-** Unspecified injury of flexor muscle, fascia and tendon of other finger at wrist and hand level

Unspecified injury of flexor muscle, fascia and tendon of specified finger with unspecified laterality at wrist and hand level

7 ⊟ **S66.109-** Unspecified injury of flexor muscle, fascia and tendon of unspecified finger at wrist and hand level

6 **S66.11** Strain of flexor muscle, fascia and tendon of other and unspecified finger at wrist and hand level

7 ⊟ **S66.110-** Strain of flexor muscle, fascia and tendon of right index finger at wrist and hand level

7 ⊟ **S66.111-** Strain of flexor muscle, fascia and tendon of left index finger at wrist and hand level

7 ⊟ **S66.112-** Strain of flexor muscle, fascia and tendon of right middle finger at wrist and hand level

7 ⊟ **S66.113-** Strain of flexor muscle, fascia and tendon of left middle finger at wrist and hand level

7 ⊟ **S66.114-** Strain of flexor muscle, fascia and tendon of right ring finger at wrist and hand level

7 ⊟ **S66.115-** Strain of flexor muscle, fascia and tendon of left ring finger at wrist and hand level

7 ⊟ **S66.116-** Strain of flexor muscle, fascia and tendon of right little finger at wrist and hand level

7 ⊟ **S66.117-** Strain of flexor muscle, fascia and tendon of left little finger at wrist and hand level

7 ⊟ **S66.118-** Strain of flexor muscle, fascia and tendon of other finger at wrist and hand level

Strain of flexor muscle, fascia and tendon of specified finger with unspecified laterality at wrist and hand level

7 ⊟ **S66.119-** Strain of flexor muscle, fascia and tendon of unspecified finger at wrist and hand level

6 **S66.12** Laceration of flexor muscle, fascia and tendon of other and unspecified finger at wrist and hand level

CODING TIP ✓ Code also any associated open wound S61.-

7 ⊟ **S66.120-** Laceration of flexor muscle, fascia and tendon of right index finger at wrist and hand level

7 ⊟ **S66.121-** Laceration of flexor muscle, fascia and tendon of left index finger at wrist and hand level

7 ⊟ **S66.122-** Laceration of flexor muscle, fascia and tendon of right middle finger at wrist and hand level

7 ⊟ **S66.123-** Laceration of flexor muscle, fascia and tendon of left middle finger at wrist and hand level

7 ⊟ **S66.124-** Laceration of flexor muscle, fascia and tendon of right ring finger at wrist and hand level

7 ⊟ **S66.125-** Laceration of flexor muscle, fascia and tendon of left ring finger at wrist and hand level

● New ▲ Revised *Manifestation* 4-7 Digit Indicators ⊟ Laterality Ⓐ Adult (15+ years) Ⓜ Maternity (12-55 years) Ⓝ Newborn Ⓟ Pediatric (0-17 years) ♂ Male ♀ Female
✖ Deleted Unspecified + Additional code

998   © 2017 DecisionHealth   2017 ICD-10-CM Expert for Physicians

S65.911- — S66.125-

7️⃣⊟ **S66.126-** Laceration of flexor muscle, fascia and tendon of right little finger at wrist and hand level

7️⃣⊟ **S66.127-** Laceration of flexor muscle, fascia and tendon of left little finger at wrist and hand level

7️⃣⊟ **S66.128-** Laceration of flexor muscle, fascia and tendon of other finger at wrist and hand level
Laceration of flexor muscle, fascia and tendon of specified finger with unspecified laterality at wrist and hand level

7️⃣⊟ **S66.129-** Laceration of flexor muscle, fascia and tendon of unspecified finger at wrist and hand level

6️⃣ **S66.19** Other injury of flexor muscle, fascia and tendon of other and unspecified finger at wrist and hand level

7️⃣⊟ **S66.190-** Other injury of flexor muscle, fascia and tendon of right index finger at wrist and hand level

7️⃣⊟ **S66.191-** Other injury of flexor muscle, fascia and tendon of left index finger at wrist and hand level

7️⃣⊟ **S66.192-** Other injury of flexor muscle, fascia and tendon of right middle finger at wrist and hand level

7️⃣⊟ **S66.193-** Other injury of flexor muscle, fascia and tendon of left middle finger at wrist and hand level

7️⃣⊟ **S66.194-** Other injury of flexor muscle, fascia and tendon of right ring finger at wrist and hand level

7️⃣⊟ **S66.195-** Other injury of flexor muscle, fascia and tendon of left ring finger at wrist and hand level

7️⃣⊟ **S66.196-** Other injury of flexor muscle, fascia and tendon of right little finger at wrist and hand level

7️⃣⊟ **S66.197-** Other injury of flexor muscle, fascia and tendon of left little finger at wrist and hand level

7️⃣⊟ **S66.198-** Other injury of flexor muscle, fascia and tendon of other finger at wrist and hand level
Other injury of flexor muscle, fascia and tendon of specified finger with unspecified laterality at wrist and hand level

7️⃣⊟ **S66.199-** Other injury of flexor muscle, fascia and tendon of unspecified finger at wrist and hand level

5️⃣ **S66.2** Injury of extensor muscle, fascia and tendon of thumb at wrist and hand level

6️⃣ **S66.20** Unspecified injury of extensor muscle, fascia and tendon of thumb at wrist and hand level

7️⃣⊟ **S66.201-** Unspecified injury of extensor muscle, fascia and tendon of right thumb at wrist and hand level

7️⃣⊟ **S66.202-** Unspecified injury of extensor muscle, fascia and tendon of left thumb at wrist and hand level

7️⃣⊟ **S66.209-** Unspecified injury of extensor muscle, fascia and tendon of unspecified thumb at wrist and hand level

6️⃣ **S66.21** Strain of extensor muscle, fascia and tendon of thumb at wrist and hand level

7️⃣⊟ **S66.211-** Strain of extensor muscle, fascia and tendon of right thumb at wrist and hand level

7️⃣⊟ **S66.212-** Strain of extensor muscle, fascia and tendon of left thumb at wrist and hand level

7️⃣⊟ **S66.219-** Strain of extensor muscle, fascia and tendon of unspecified thumb at wrist and hand level

6️⃣ **S66.22** Laceration of extensor muscle, fascia and tendon of thumb at wrist and hand level

CODING TIP ✓ Code also any associated open wound S61.-

7️⃣⊟ **S66.221-** Laceration of extensor muscle, fascia and tendon of right thumb at wrist and hand level

7️⃣⊟ **S66.222-** Laceration of extensor muscle, fascia and tendon of left thumb at wrist and hand level

7️⃣⊟ **S66.229-** Laceration of extensor muscle, fascia and tendon of unspecified thumb at wrist and hand level

6️⃣ **S66.29** Other specified injury of extensor muscle, fascia and tendon of thumb at wrist and hand level

7️⃣⊟ **S66.291-** Other specified injury of extensor muscle, fascia and tendon of right thumb at wrist and hand level

7️⃣⊟ **S66.292-** Other specified injury of extensor muscle, fascia and tendon of left thumb at wrist and hand level

7️⃣⊟ **S66.299-** Other specified injury of extensor muscle, fascia and tendon of unspecified thumb at wrist and hand level

5️⃣ **S66.3** Injury of extensor muscle, fascia and tendon of other and unspecified finger at wrist and hand level

EXCLUDES 2 *Injury of extensor muscle, fascia and tendon of thumb at wrist and hand level (S66.2-)*

6️⃣ **S66.30** Unspecified injury of extensor muscle, fascia and tendon of other and unspecified finger at wrist and hand level

7️⃣⊟ **S66.300-** Unspecified injury of extensor muscle, fascia and tendon of right index finger at wrist and hand level

7️⃣⊟ **S66.301-** Unspecified injury of extensor muscle, fascia and tendon of left index finger at wrist and hand level

7️⃣⊟ **S66.302-** Unspecified injury of extensor muscle, fascia and tendon of right middle finger at wrist and hand level

7️⃣⊟ **S66.303-** Unspecified injury of extensor muscle, fascia and tendon of left middle finger at wrist and hand level

7️⃣⊟ **S66.304-** Unspecified injury of extensor muscle, fascia and tendon of right ring finger at wrist and hand level

7️⃣⊟ **S66.305-** Unspecified injury of extensor muscle, fascia and tendon of left ring finger at wrist and hand level

7️⃣⊟ **S66.306-** Unspecified injury of extensor muscle, fascia and tendon of right little finger at wrist and hand level

7️⃣⊟ **S66.307-** Unspecified injury of extensor muscle, fascia and tendon of left little finger at wrist and hand level

7️⃣⊟ **S66.308-** Unspecified injury of extensor muscle, fascia and tendon of other finger at wrist and hand level
Unspecified injury of extensor muscle, fascia and tendon of specified finger with unspecified laterality at wrist and hand level

7️⃣⊟ **S66.309-** Unspecified injury of extensor muscle, fascia and tendon of unspecified finger at wrist and hand level

6️⃣ **S66.31** Strain of extensor muscle, fascia and tendon of other and unspecified finger at wrist and hand level

7️⃣⊟ **S66.310-** Strain of extensor muscle, fascia and tendon of right index finger at wrist and hand level

7️⃣⊟ **S66.311-** Strain of extensor muscle, fascia and tendon of left index finger at wrist and hand level

7️⃣⊟ **S66.312-** Strain of extensor muscle, fascia and tendon of right middle finger at wrist and hand level

7️⃣⊟ **S66.313-** Strain of extensor muscle, fascia and tendon of left middle finger at wrist and hand level

7️⃣⊟ **S66.314-** Strain of extensor muscle, fascia and tendon of right ring finger at wrist and hand level

7️⃣⊟ **S66.315-** Strain of extensor muscle, fascia and tendon of left ring finger at wrist and hand level

7️⃣⊟ **S66.316-** Strain of extensor muscle, fascia and tendon of right little finger at wrist and hand level

7️⃣⊟ **S66.317-** Strain of extensor muscle, fascia and tendon of left little finger at wrist and hand level

7️⃣⊟ **S66.318-** Strain of extensor muscle, fascia and tendon of other finger at wrist and hand level
Strain of extensor muscle, fascia and tendon of specified finger with unspecified laterality at wrist and hand level

7️⃣⊟ **S66.319-** Strain of extensor muscle, fascia and tendon of unspecified finger at wrist and hand level

6️⃣ **S66.32** Laceration of extensor muscle, fascia and tendon of other and unspecified finger at wrist and hand level

---

● New   ▲ Revised   *Manifestation*   4️⃣-7️⃣ Digit Indicators   ⊟ Laterality   🅰 Adult (15+ years)   Ⓜ Maternity (12-55 years)   Ⓝ Newborn   🅿 Pediatric (0-17 years)   ♂ Male   ♀ Female
✖ Deleted   Unspecified   + Additional code

CODING TIP ✓ Code also any associated open wound S61.-

☑ ⊟ **S66.320-** **Laceration of extensor muscle, fascia and tendon of right index finger at wrist and hand level**

☑ ⊟ **S66.321-** **Laceration of extensor muscle, fascia and tendon of left index finger at wrist and hand level**

☑ ⊟ **S66.322-** **Laceration of extensor muscle, fascia and tendon of right middle finger at wrist and hand level**

☑ ⊟ **S66.323-** **Laceration of extensor muscle, fascia and tendon of left middle finger at wrist and hand level**

☑ ⊟ **S66.324-** **Laceration of extensor muscle, fascia and tendon of right ring finger at wrist and hand level**

☑ ⊟ **S66.325-** **Laceration of extensor muscle, fascia and tendon of left ring finger at wrist and hand level**

☑ ⊟ **S66.326-** **Laceration of extensor muscle, fascia and tendon of right little finger at wrist and hand level**

☑ ⊟ **S66.327-** **Laceration of extensor muscle, fascia and tendon of left little finger at wrist and hand level**

☑ ⊟ **S66.328-** **Laceration of extensor muscle, fascia and tendon of other finger at wrist and hand level**

Laceration of extensor muscle, fascia and tendon of specified finger with unspecified laterality at wrist and hand level

☑ ⊟ **S66.329-** **Laceration of extensor muscle, fascia and tendon of unspecified finger at wrist and hand level**

⑥ **S66.39** **Other injury of extensor muscle, fascia and tendon of other and unspecified finger at wrist and hand level**

☑ ⊟ **S66.390-** **Other injury of extensor muscle, fascia and tendon of right index finger at wrist and hand level**

☑ ⊟ **S66.391-** **Other injury of extensor muscle, fascia and tendon of left index finger at wrist and hand level**

☑ ⊟ **S66.392-** **Other injury of extensor muscle, fascia and tendon of right middle finger at wrist and hand level**

☑ ⊟ **S66.393-** **Other injury of extensor muscle, fascia and tendon of left middle finger at wrist and hand level**

☑ ⊟ **S66.394-** **Other injury of extensor muscle, fascia and tendon of right ring finger at wrist and hand level**

☑ ⊟ **S66.395-** **Other injury of extensor muscle, fascia and tendon of left ring finger at wrist and hand level**

☑ ⊟ **S66.396-** **Other injury of extensor muscle, fascia and tendon of right little finger at wrist and hand level**

☑ ⊟ **S66.397-** **Other injury of extensor muscle, fascia and tendon of left little finger at wrist and hand level**

☑ ⊟ **S66.398-** **Other injury of extensor muscle, fascia and tendon of other finger at wrist and hand level**

Other injury of extensor muscle, fascia and tendon of specified finger with unspecified laterality at wrist and hand level

☑ ⊟ **S66.399-** **Other injury of extensor muscle, fascia and tendon of unspecified finger at wrist and hand level**

⑤ **S66.4** **Injury of intrinsic muscle, fascia and tendon of thumb at wrist and hand level**

⑥ **S66.40** **Unspecified injury of intrinsic muscle, fascia and tendon of thumb at wrist and hand level**

☑ ⊟ **S66.401-** **Unspecified injury of intrinsic muscle, fascia and tendon of right thumb at wrist and hand level**

☑ ⊟ **S66.402-** **Unspecified injury of intrinsic muscle, fascia and tendon of left thumb at wrist and hand level**

☑ ⊟ **S66.409-** Unspecified injury of intrinsic muscle, fascia and tendon of unspecified thumb at wrist and hand level

⑥ **S66.41** Strain of intrinsic muscle, fascia and tendon of thumb at wrist and hand level

☑ ⊟ **S66.411-** Strain of intrinsic muscle, fascia and tendon of right thumb at wrist and hand level

☑ ⊟ **S66.412-** Strain of intrinsic muscle, fascia and tendon of left thumb at wrist and hand level

☑ ⊟ **S66.419-** Strain of intrinsic muscle, fascia and tendon of unspecified thumb at wrist and hand level

⑥ **S66.42** Laceration of intrinsic muscle, fascia and tendon of thumb at wrist and hand level

CODING TIP ✓ Code also any associated open wound S61.-

☑ ⊟ **S66.421-** Laceration of intrinsic muscle, fascia and tendon of right thumb at wrist and hand level

☑ ⊟ **S66.422-** Laceration of intrinsic muscle, fascia and tendon of left thumb at wrist and hand level

☑ ⊟ **S66.429-** Laceration of intrinsic muscle, fascia and tendon of unspecified thumb at wrist and hand level

⑥ **S66.49** Other specified injury of intrinsic muscle, fascia and tendon of thumb at wrist and hand level

☑ ⊟ **S66.491-** Other specified injury of intrinsic muscle, fascia and tendon of right thumb at wrist and hand level

☑ ⊟ **S66.492-** Other specified injury of intrinsic muscle, fascia and tendon of left thumb at wrist and hand level

☑ ⊟ **S66.499-** Other specified injury of intrinsic muscle, fascia and tendon of unspecified thumb at wrist and hand level

⑤ **S66.5** Injury of intrinsic muscle, fascia and tendon of other and unspecified finger at wrist and hand level

EXCLUDES 2 *injury of intrinsic muscle, fascia and tendon of thumb at wrist and hand level (S66.4-)*

⑥ **S66.50** Unspecified injury of intrinsic muscle, fascia and tendon of other and unspecified finger at wrist and hand level

☑ ⊟ **S66.500-** **Unspecified injury of intrinsic muscle, fascia and tendon of right index finger at wrist and hand level**

☑ ⊟ **S66.501-** **Unspecified injury of intrinsic muscle, fascia and tendon of left index finger at wrist and hand level**

☑ ⊟ **S66.502-** **Unspecified injury of intrinsic muscle, fascia and tendon of right middle finger at wrist and hand level**

☑ ⊟ **S66.503-** **Unspecified injury of intrinsic muscle, fascia and tendon of left middle finger at wrist and hand level**

☑ ⊟ **S66.504-** **Unspecified injury of intrinsic muscle, fascia and tendon of right ring finger at wrist and hand level**

☑ ⊟ **S66.505-** **Unspecified injury of intrinsic muscle, fascia and tendon of left ring finger at wrist and hand level**

☑ ⊟ **S66.506-** **Unspecified injury of intrinsic muscle, fascia and tendon of right little finger at wrist and hand level**

☑ ⊟ **S66.507-** **Unspecified injury of intrinsic muscle, fascia and tendon of left little finger at wrist and hand level**

☑ ⊟ **S66.508-** **Unspecified injury of intrinsic muscle, fascia and tendon of other finger at wrist and hand level**

Unspecified injury of intrinsic muscle, fascia and tendon of specified finger with unspecified laterality at wrist and hand level

☑ ⊟ **S66.509-** **Unspecified injury of intrinsic muscle, fascia and tendon of unspecified finger at wrist and hand level**

⑥ **S66.51** Strain of intrinsic muscle, fascia and tendon of other and unspecified finger at wrist and hand level

☑ ⊟ **S66.510-** **Strain of intrinsic muscle, fascia and tendon of right index finger at wrist and hand level**

● New ▲ Revised *Manifestation* ④-☑ Digit Indicators ⊟ Laterality Ⓐ Adult (15+ years) Ⓜ Maternity (12-55 years) Ⓝ Newborn Ⓟ Pediatric (0-17 years) ♂ Male ♀ Female
✖ ~~Deleted~~ Unspecified ＋ Additional code

1000   © 2017 DecisionHealth   2017 ICD-10-CM Expert for Physicians

7 ⊟ S66.511- Strain of intrinsic muscle, fascia and tendon of left index finger at wrist and hand level

7 ⊟ S66.512- Strain of intrinsic muscle, fascia and tendon of right middle finger at wrist and hand level

7 ⊟ S66.513- Strain of intrinsic muscle, fascia and tendon of left middle finger at wrist and hand level

7 ⊟ S66.514- Strain of intrinsic muscle, fascia and tendon of right ring finger at wrist and hand level

7 ⊟ S66.515- Strain of intrinsic muscle, fascia and tendon of left ring finger at wrist and hand level

7 ⊟ S66.516- Strain of intrinsic muscle, fascia and tendon of right little finger at wrist and hand level

7 ⊟ S66.517- Strain of intrinsic muscle, fascia and tendon of left little finger at wrist and hand level

7 ⊟ S66.518- Strain of intrinsic muscle, fascia and tendon of other finger at wrist and hand level

Strain of intrinsic muscle, fascia and tendon of specified finger with unspecified laterality at wrist and hand level

7 ⊟ S66.519- Strain of intrinsic muscle, fascia and tendon of unspecified finger at wrist and hand level

6 S66.52 Laceration of intrinsic muscle, fascia and tendon of other and unspecified finger at wrist and hand level

CODING TIP ✓ Code also any associated open wound S61.-

7 ⊟ S66.520- Laceration of intrinsic muscle, fascia and tendon of right index finger at wrist and hand level

7 ⊟ S66.521- Laceration of intrinsic muscle, fascia and tendon of left index finger at wrist and hand level

7 ⊟ S66.522- Laceration of intrinsic muscle, fascia and tendon of right middle finger at wrist and hand level

7 ⊟ S66.523- Laceration of intrinsic muscle, fascia and tendon of left middle finger at wrist and hand level

7 ⊟ S66.524- Laceration of intrinsic muscle, fascia and tendon of right ring finger at wrist and hand level

7 ⊟ S66.525- Laceration of intrinsic muscle, fascia and tendon of left ring finger at wrist and hand level

7 ⊟ S66.526- Laceration of intrinsic muscle, fascia and tendon of right little finger at wrist and hand level

7 ⊟ S66.527- Laceration of intrinsic muscle, fascia and tendon of left little finger at wrist and hand level

7 ⊟ S66.528- Laceration of intrinsic muscle, fascia and tendon of other finger at wrist and hand level

Laceration of intrinsic muscle, fascia and tendon of specified finger with unspecified laterality at wrist and hand level

7 ⊟ S66.529- Laceration of intrinsic muscle, fascia and tendon of unspecified finger at wrist and hand level

6 S66.59 Other injury of intrinsic muscle, fascia and tendon of other and unspecified finger at wrist and hand level

7 ⊟ S66.590- Other injury of intrinsic muscle, fascia and tendon of right index finger at wrist and hand level

7 ⊟ S66.591- Other injury of intrinsic muscle, fascia and tendon of left index finger at wrist and hand level

7 ⊟ S66.592- Other injury of intrinsic muscle, fascia and tendon of right middle finger at wrist and hand level

7 ⊟ S66.593- Other injury of intrinsic muscle, fascia and tendon of left middle finger at wrist and hand level

7 ⊟ S66.594- Other injury of intrinsic muscle, fascia and tendon of right ring finger at wrist and hand level

7 ⊟ S66.595- Other injury of intrinsic muscle, fascia and tendon of left ring finger at wrist and hand level

7 ⊟ S66.596- Other injury of intrinsic muscle, fascia and tendon of right little finger at wrist and hand level

7 ⊟ S66.597- Other injury of intrinsic muscle, fascia and tendon of left little finger at wrist and hand level

7 ⊟ S66.598- Other injury of intrinsic muscle, fascia and tendon of other finger at wrist and hand level

Other injury of intrinsic muscle, fascia and tendon of specified finger with unspecified laterality at wrist and hand level

7 ⊟ S66.599- Other injury of intrinsic muscle, fascia and tendon of unspecified finger at wrist and hand level

5 S66.8 Injury of other specified muscles, fascia and tendons at wrist and hand level

6 S66.80 Unspecified injury of other specified muscles, fascia and tendons at wrist and hand level

7 ⊟ S66.801- Unspecified injury of other specified muscles, fascia and tendons at wrist and hand level, right hand

7 ⊟ S66.802- Unspecified injury of other specified muscles, fascia and tendons at wrist and hand level, left hand

7 ⊟ S66.809- Unspecified injury of other specified muscles, fascia and tendons at wrist and hand level, unspecified hand

6 S66.81 Strain of other specified muscles, fascia and tendons at wrist and hand level

7 ⊟ S66.811- Strain of other specified muscles, fascia and tendons at wrist and hand level, right hand

7 ⊟ S66.812- Strain of other specified muscles, fascia and tendons at wrist and hand level, left hand

7 ⊟ S66.819- Strain of other specified muscles, fascia and tendons at wrist and hand level, unspecified hand

6 S66.82 Laceration of other specified muscles, fascia and tendons at wrist and hand level

CODING TIP ✓ Code also any associated open wound S61.-

7 ⊟ S66.821- Laceration of other specified muscles, fascia and tendons at wrist and hand level, right hand

7 ⊟ S66.822- Laceration of other specified muscles, fascia and tendons at wrist and hand level, left hand

7 ⊟ S66.829- Laceration of other specified muscles, fascia and tendons at wrist and hand level, unspecified hand

6 S66.89 Other injury of other specified muscles, fascia and tendons at wrist and hand level

7 ⊟ S66.891- Other injury of other specified muscles, fascia and tendons at wrist and hand level, right hand

7 ⊟ S66.892- Other injury of other specified muscles, fascia and tendons at wrist and hand level, left hand

7 ⊟ S66.899- Other injury of other specified muscles, fascia and tendons at wrist and hand level, unspecified hand

5 S66.9 Injury of unspecified muscle, fascia and tendon at wrist and hand level

6 S66.90 Unspecified injury of unspecified muscle, fascia and tendon at wrist and hand level

7 ⊟ S66.901- Unspecified injury of unspecified muscle, fascia and tendon at wrist and hand level, right hand

7 ⊟ S66.902- Unspecified injury of unspecified muscle, fascia and tendon at wrist and hand level, left hand

7 ⊟ S66.909- Unspecified injury of unspecified muscle, fascia and tendon at wrist and hand level, unspecified hand

6 S66.91 Strain of unspecified muscle, fascia and tendon at wrist and hand level

7 ⊟ S66.911- Strain of unspecified muscle, fascia and tendon at wrist and hand level, right hand

---

● New ▲ Revised | *Manifestation* | 4-7 Digit Indicators ⊟ Laterality | 🅐 Adult (15+ years) | 🅜 Maternity (12-55 years) | 🅝 Newborn | 🅟 Pediatric (0-17 years) | ♂ Male | ♀ Female
✖ Deleted | Unspecified | + Additional code

7 ⊟ S66.912-   Strain of unspecified muscle, fascia and tendon at wrist and hand level, left hand

7 ⊟ S66.919-   Strain of unspecified muscle, fascia and tendon at wrist and hand level, unspecified hand

6 S66.92   Laceration of unspecified muscle, fascia and tendon at wrist and hand level

> **CODING TIP ✓**   Code also any associated open wound S61.-

7 ⊟ S66.921-   Laceration of unspecified muscle, fascia and tendon at wrist and hand level, right hand

7 ⊟ S66.922-   Laceration of unspecified muscle, fascia and tendon at wrist and hand level, left hand

7 ⊟ S66.929-   Laceration of unspecified muscle, fascia and tendon at wrist and hand level, unspecified hand

6 S66.99   Other injury of unspecified muscle, fascia and tendon at wrist and hand level

7 ⊟ S66.991-   Other injury of unspecified muscle, fascia and tendon at wrist and hand level, right hand

7 ⊟ S66.992-   Other injury of unspecified muscle, fascia and tendon at wrist and hand level, left hand

7 ⊟ S66.999-   Other injury of unspecified muscle, fascia and tendon at wrist and hand level, unspecified hand

4 + S67   Crushing injury of wrist, hand and fingers

> *Use additional code for all associated injuries, such as:*
> *fracture of wrist and hand (S62.-)*
> *open wound of wrist and hand (S61.-)*

> The appropriate 7th character is to be added to each code from category S67
> A   initial encounter
> D   subsequent encounter
> S   sequela

5 + S67.0   Crushing injury of thumb

7 ⊟ + S67.00X-   Crushing injury of unspecified thumb
7 ⊟ + S67.01X-   Crushing injury of right thumb
7 ⊟ + S67.02X-   Crushing injury of left thumb

5 + S67.1   Crushing injury of other and unspecified finger(s)

> **EXCLUDES 2**   *crushing injury of thumb (S67.0-)*

7 + S67.10X-   Crushing injury of unspecified finger(s)

6 + S67.19   Crushing injury of other finger(s)

7 ⊟ + S67.190-   Crushing injury of right index finger
7 ⊟ + S67.191-   Crushing injury of left index finger
7 ⊟ + S67.192-   Crushing injury of right middle finger
7 ⊟ + S67.193-   Crushing injury of left middle finger
7 ⊟ + S67.194-   Crushing injury of right ring finger
7 ⊟ + S67.195-   Crushing injury of left ring finger
7 ⊟ + S67.196-   Crushing injury of right little finger
7 ⊟ + S67.197-   Crushing injury of left little finger
7 ⊟ + S67.198-   Crushing injury of other finger
Crushing injury of specified finger with unspecified laterality

5 + S67.2   Crushing injury of hand

> **EXCLUDES 2**   *crushing injury of fingers (S67.1-)*
> *crushing injury of thumb (S67.0-)*

7 ⊟ + S67.20X-   Crushing injury of unspecified hand
7 ⊟ + S67.21X-   Crushing injury of right hand
7 ⊟ + S67.22X-   Crushing injury of left hand

5 + S67.3   Crushing injury of wrist

7 ⊟ + S67.30X-   Crushing injury of unspecified wrist
7 ⊟ + S67.31X-   Crushing injury of right wrist
7 ⊟ + S67.32X-   Crushing injury of left wrist

5 + S67.4   Crushing injury of wrist and hand

> **EXCLUDES 1**   *crushing injury of hand alone (S67.2-)*
> *crushing injury of wrist alone (S67.3-)*

> **EXCLUDES 2**   *crushing injury of fingers (S67.1-)*
> *crushing injury of thumb (S67.0-)*

7 ⊟ + S67.40X-   Crushing injury of unspecified wrist and hand
7 ⊟ + S67.41X-   Crushing injury of right wrist and hand
7 ⊟ + S67.42X-   Crushing injury of left wrist and hand

5 + S67.9   Crushing injury of unspecified part(s) of wrist, hand and fingers

7 ⊟ + S67.90X-   Crushing injury of unspecified part(s) of unspecified wrist, hand and fingers

7 ⊟ + S67.91X-   Crushing injury of unspecified part(s) of right wrist, hand and fingers

7 ⊟ + S67.92X-   Crushing injury of unspecified part(s) of left wrist, hand and fingers

4 S68   Traumatic amputation of wrist, hand and fingers

> An amputation not identified as partial or complete should be coded to complete

> The appropriate 7th character is to be added to each code from category S68
> A   initial encounter
> D   subsequent encounter
> S   sequela

5 S68.0   Traumatic metacarpophalangeal amputation of thumb

Traumatic amputation of thumb NOS

6 S68.01   Complete traumatic metacarpophalangeal amputation of thumb

7 ⊟ S68.011-   Complete traumatic metacarpophalangeal amputation of right thumb
7 ⊟ S68.012-   Complete traumatic metacarpophalangeal amputation of left thumb
7 ⊟ S68.019-   Complete traumatic metacarpophalangeal amputation of unspecified thumb

6 S68.02   Partial traumatic metacarpophalangeal amputation of thumb

7 ⊟ S68.021-   Partial traumatic metacarpophalangeal amputation of right thumb
7 ⊟ S68.022-   Partial traumatic metacarpophalangeal amputation of left thumb
7 ⊟ S68.029-   Partial traumatic metacarpophalangeal amputation of unspecified thumb

5 S68.1   Traumatic metacarpophalangeal amputation of other and unspecified finger

Traumatic amputation of finger NOS

> **EXCLUDES 2**   *traumatic metacarpophalangeal amputation of thumb (S68.0-)*

6 S68.11   Complete traumatic metacarpophalangeal amputation of other and unspecified finger

7 ⊟ S68.110-   Complete traumatic metacarpophalangeal amputation of right index finger
7 ⊟ S68.111-   Complete traumatic metacarpophalangeal amputation of left index finger
7 ⊟ S68.112-   Complete traumatic metacarpophalangeal amputation of right middle finger
7 ⊟ S68.113-   Complete traumatic metacarpophalangeal amputation of left middle finger
7 ⊟ S68.114-   Complete traumatic metacarpophalangeal amputation of right ring finger
7 ⊟ S68.115-   Complete traumatic metacarpophalangeal amputation of left ring finger
7 ⊟ S68.116-   Complete traumatic metacarpophalangeal amputation of right little finger
7 ⊟ S68.117-   Complete traumatic metacarpophalangeal amputation of left little finger
7 ⊟ S68.118-   Complete traumatic metacarpophalangeal amputation of other finger
Complete traumatic metacarpophalangeal amputation of specified finger with unspecified laterality
7 ⊟ S68.119-   Complete traumatic metacarpophalangeal amputation of unspecified finger

6 S68.12   Partial traumatic metacarpophalangeal amputation of other and unspecified finger

7 ⊟ S68.120-   Partial traumatic metacarpophalangeal amputation of right index finger
7 ⊟ S68.121-   Partial traumatic metacarpophalangeal amputation of left index finger
7 ⊟ S68.122-   Partial traumatic metacarpophalangeal amputation of right middle finger
7 ⊟ S68.123-   Partial traumatic metacarpophalangeal amputation of left middle finger
7 ⊟ S68.124-   Partial traumatic metacarpophalangeal amputation of right ring finger
7 ⊟ S68.125-   Partial traumatic metacarpophalangeal amputation of left ring finger
7 ⊟ S68.126-   Partial traumatic metacarpophalangeal amputation of right little finger

---

● New   ▲ Revised   *Manifestation*   **4 - 7** Digit Indicators   ⊟ Laterality   🅰 Adult (15+ years)   🅼 Maternity (12-55 years)   🅽 Newborn   🅿 Pediatric (0-17 years)   ♂ Male   ♀ Female
✖ Deleted   Unspecified   + Additional code

1002   © 2017 DecisionHealth   2017 ICD-10-CM Expert for Physicians

7 ⊟ S68.127- **Partial traumatic metacarpophalangeal amputation of left little finger**

7 ⊟ S68.128- **Partial traumatic metacarpophalangeal amputation of other finger**
Partial traumatic metacarpophalangeal amputation of specified finger with unspecified laterality

7 ⊟ S68.129- **Partial traumatic metacarpophalangeal amputation of unspecified finger**

5 S68.4 **Traumatic amputation of hand at wrist level**
Traumatic amputation of hand NOS
Traumatic amputation of wrist

6 S68.41 **Complete traumatic amputation of hand at wrist level**

7 ⊟ S68.411- **Complete traumatic amputation of right hand at wrist level**

7 ⊟ S68.412- **Complete traumatic amputation of left hand at wrist level**

7 ⊟ S68.419- **Complete traumatic amputation of unspecified hand at wrist level**

6 S68.42 **Partial traumatic amputation of hand at wrist level**

7 ⊟ S68.421- **Partial traumatic amputation of right hand at wrist level**

7 ⊟ S68.422- **Partial traumatic amputation of left hand at wrist level**

7 ⊟ S68.429- **Partial traumatic amputation of unspecified hand at wrist level**

5 S68.5 **Traumatic transphalangeal amputation of thumb**
Traumatic interphalangeal joint amputation of thumb

6 S68.51 **Complete traumatic transphalangeal amputation of thumb**

7 ⊟ S68.511- **Complete traumatic transphalangeal amputation of right thumb**

7 ⊟ S68.512- **Complete traumatic transphalangeal amputation of left thumb**

7 ⊟ S68.519- **Complete traumatic transphalangeal amputation of unspecified thumb**

6 S68.52 **Partial traumatic transphalangeal amputation of thumb**

7 ⊟ S68.521- **Partial traumatic transphalangeal amputation of right thumb**

7 ⊟ S68.522- **Partial traumatic transphalangeal amputation of left thumb**

7 ⊟ S68.529- **Partial traumatic transphalangeal amputation of unspecified thumb**

5 S68.6 **Traumatic transphalangeal amputation of other and unspecified finger**

6 S68.61 **Complete traumatic transphalangeal amputation of other and unspecified finger(s)**

7 ⊟ S68.610- **Complete traumatic transphalangeal amputation of right index finger**

7 ⊟ S68.611- **Complete traumatic transphalangeal amputation of left index finger**

7 ⊟ S68.612- **Complete traumatic transphalangeal amputation of right middle finger**

7 ⊟ S68.613- **Complete traumatic transphalangeal amputation of left middle finger**

7 ⊟ S68.614- **Complete traumatic transphalangeal amputation of right ring finger**

7 ⊟ S68.615- **Complete traumatic transphalangeal amputation of left ring finger**

7 ⊟ S68.616- **Complete traumatic transphalangeal amputation of right little finger**

7 ⊟ S68.617- **Complete traumatic transphalangeal amputation of left little finger**

7 ⊟ S68.618- **Complete traumatic transphalangeal amputation of other finger**
Complete traumatic transphalangeal amputation of specified finger with unspecified laterality

7 ⊟ S68.619- **Complete traumatic transphalangeal amputation of unspecified finger**

6 S68.62 **Partial traumatic transphalangeal amputation of other and unspecified finger**

7 ⊟ S68.620- **Partial traumatic transphalangeal amputation of right index finger**

7 ⊟ S68.621- **Partial traumatic transphalangeal amputation of left index finger**

7 ⊟ S68.622- **Partial traumatic transphalangeal amputation of right middle finger**

7 ⊟ S68.623- **Partial traumatic transphalangeal amputation of left middle finger**

7 ⊟ S68.624- **Partial traumatic transphalangeal amputation of right ring finger**

7 ⊟ S68.625- **Partial traumatic transphalangeal amputation of left ring finger**

7 ⊟ S68.626- **Partial traumatic transphalangeal amputation of right little finger**

7 ⊟ S68.627- **Partial traumatic transphalangeal amputation of left little finger**

7 ⊟ S68.628- **Partial traumatic transphalangeal amputation of other finger**
Partial traumatic transphalangeal amputation of specified finger with unspecified laterality

7 ⊟ S68.629- **Partial traumatic transphalangeal amputation of unspecified finger**

5 S68.7 **Traumatic transmetacarpal amputation of hand**

6 S68.71 **Complete traumatic transmetacarpal amputation of hand**

7 ⊟ S68.711- **Complete traumatic transmetacarpal amputation of right hand**

7 ⊟ S68.712- **Complete traumatic transmetacarpal amputation of left hand**

7 ⊟ S68.719- **Complete traumatic transmetacarpal amputation of unspecified hand**

6 S68.72 **Partial traumatic transmetacarpal amputation of hand**

7 ⊟ S68.721- **Partial traumatic transmetacarpal amputation of right hand**

7 ⊟ S68.722- **Partial traumatic transmetacarpal amputation of left hand**

7 ⊟ S68.729- **Partial traumatic transmetacarpal amputation of unspecified hand**

4 S69 **Other and unspecified injuries of wrist, hand and finger(s)**

The appropriate 7th character is to be added to each code from category S69
A   initial encounter
D   subsequent encounter
S   sequela

5 S69.8 **Other specified injuries of wrist, hand and finger(s)**

7 ⊟ S69.80X- **Other specified injuries of unspecified wrist, hand and finger(s)**

7 ⊟ S69.81X- **Other specified injuries of right wrist, hand and finger(s)**

7 ⊟ S69.82X- **Other specified injuries of left wrist, hand and finger(s)**

5 S69.9 **Unspecified injury of wrist, hand and finger(s)**

7 ⊟ S69.90X- **Unspecified injury of unspecified wrist, hand and finger(s)**

7 ⊟ S69.91X- **Unspecified injury of right wrist, hand and finger(s)**

7 ⊟ S69.92X- **Unspecified injury of left wrist, hand and finger(s)**

Injuries to the hip and thigh (S70-S79)

EXCLUDES 2   *burns and corrosions (T20-T32)*
frostbite (T33-T34)
snake bite (T63.0-)
venomous insect bite or sting (T63.4-)

GUIDELINES   Section I.C.19.c.2)
Multiple fractures are sequenced in accordance with the severity of the fracture.

GUIDELINES Section I.C.19.b.1)-2)

When coding injuries, assign separate codes for each injury unless a combination code is provided, in which case the combination code is assigned ... Traumatic injury codes (S00-T14.9) are not to be used for normal, healing surgical wounds or to identify complications of surgical wounds. The code for the most serious injury, as determined by the provider and the focus of treatment, is sequenced first.

1) Superficial injuries such as abrasions or contusions are not coded when associated with more severe injuries of the same site.

2) When a primary injury results in minor damage to peripheral nerves or blood vessels, the primary injury is sequenced first with additional code(s) for injuries to nerves and spinal cord (such as category S04), and/or injury to blood vessels (such as category S15). When the primary injury is to the blood vessels or nerves, that injury should be sequenced first.

GUIDELINES Section I.C.19.c

Coding of Traumatic Fractures: The principles of multiple coding of injuries should be followed in coding fractures. Fractures of specified sites are coded individually by site in accordance with both the provisions within categories S02, S12, S22, S32, S42, S49, S52, S59, S62, S72, S79, S82, S89, S92 and the level of detail furnished by medical record content. A fracture not indicated as open or closed should be coded to closed. A fracture not indicated whether displaced or not displaced should be coded to displaced.

4 S70   Superficial injury of hip and thigh

> The appropriate 7th character is to be added to each code from category S70
> A   initial encounter
> D   subsequent encounter
> S   sequela

5 S70.0   Contusion of hip
- **7 S70.00X-   Contusion of unspecified hip**
- **7 S70.01X-   Contusion of right hip**
- **7 S70.02X-   Contusion of left hip**

5 S70.1   Contusion of thigh
- **7 S70.10X-   Contusion of unspecified thigh**
- **7 S70.11X-   Contusion of right thigh**
- **7 S70.12X-   Contusion of left thigh**

5 S70.2   Other superficial injuries of hip
- **6 S70.21   Abrasion of hip**
  - **7 S70.211-   Abrasion, right hip**
  - **7 S70.212-   Abrasion, left hip**
  - **7 S70.219-   Abrasion, unspecified hip**
- **6 S70.22   Blister (nonthermal) of hip**
  - **7 S70.221-   Blister (nonthermal), right hip**
  - **7 S70.222-   Blister (nonthermal), left hip**
  - **7 S70.229-   Blister (nonthermal), unspecified hip**
- **6 S70.24   External constriction of hip**
  - **7 S70.241-   External constriction, right hip**
  - **7 S70.242-   External constriction, left hip**
  - **7 S70.249-   External constriction, unspecified hip**
- **6 S70.25   Superficial foreign body of hip**
  > Splinter in the hip
  - **7 S70.251-   Superficial foreign body, right hip**
  - **7 S70.252-   Superficial foreign body, left hip**
  - **7 S70.259-   Superficial foreign body, unspecified hip**
- **6 S70.26   Insect bite (nonvenomous) of hip**
  - **7 S70.261-   Insect bite (nonvenomous), right hip**
  - **7 S70.262-   Insect bite (nonvenomous), left hip**
  - **7 S70.269-   Insect bite (nonvenomous), unspecified hip**
- **6 S70.27   Other superficial bite of hip**
  > **EXCLUDES 1**   *open bite of hip (S71.05-)*
  - **7 S70.271-   Other superficial bite of hip, right hip**
  - **7 S70.272-   Other superficial bite of hip, left hip**
  - **7 S70.279-   Other superficial bite of hip, unspecified hip**

5 S70.3   Other superficial injuries of thigh
- **6 S70.31   Abrasion of thigh**

- **7 S70.311-   Abrasion, right thigh**
- **7 S70.312-   Abrasion, left thigh**
- **7 S70.319-   Abrasion, unspecified thigh**
- **6 S70.32   Blister (nonthermal) of thigh**
  - **7 S70.321-   Blister (nonthermal), right thigh**
  - **7 S70.322-   Blister (nonthermal), left thigh**
  - **7 S70.329-   Blister (nonthermal), unspecified thigh**
- **6 S70.34   External constriction of thigh**
  - **7 S70.341-   External constriction, right thigh**
  - **7 S70.342-   External constriction, left thigh**
  - **7 S70.349-   External constriction, unspecified thigh**
- **6 S70.35   Superficial foreign body of thigh**
  > Splinter in the thigh
  - **7 S70.351-   Superficial foreign body, right thigh**
  - **7 S70.352-   Superficial foreign body, left thigh**
  - **7 S70.359-   Superficial foreign body, unspecified thigh**
- **6 S70.36   Insect bite (nonvenomous) of thigh**
  - **7 S70.361-   Insect bite (nonvenomous), right thigh**
  - **7 S70.362-   Insect bite (nonvenomous), left thigh**
  - **7 S70.369-   Insect bite (nonvenomous), unspecified thigh**
- **6 S70.37   Other superficial bite of thigh**
  > **EXCLUDES 1**   *open bite of thigh (S71.15)*
  - **7 S70.371-   Other superficial bite of right thigh**
  - **7 S70.372-   Other superficial bite of left thigh**
  - **7 S70.379-   Other superficial bite of unspecified thigh**

5 S70.9   Unspecified superficial injury of hip and thigh
- **6 S70.91   Unspecified superficial injury of hip**
  - **7 S70.911-   Unspecified superficial injury of right hip**
  - **7 S70.912-   Unspecified superficial injury of left hip**
  - **7 S70.919-   Unspecified superficial injury of unspecified hip**
- **6 S70.92   Unspecified superficial injury of thigh**
  - **7 S70.921-   Unspecified superficial injury of right thigh**
  - **7 S70.922-   Unspecified superficial injury of left thigh**
  - **7 S70.929-   Unspecified superficial injury of unspecified thigh**

4 S71   Open wound of hip and thigh

> Code also:
> any associated wound infection
> **EXCLUDES 1**   *open fracture of hip and thigh (S72.-)*
> *traumatic amputation of hip and thigh (S78.-)*
> **EXCLUDES 2**   *bite of venomous animal (T63.-)*
> *open wound of ankle, foot and toes (S91.-)*
> *open wound of knee and lower leg (S81.-)*

> The appropriate 7th character is to be added to each code from category S71
> A   initial encounter
> D   subsequent encounter
> S   sequela

CODING TIP ✓ Open wound codes indicate a wound resulting from a traumatic origin. Do not assign a code for "open wound" unless the etiology of the wound is related to trauma.

5 S71.0   Open wound of hip
- **6 S71.00   Unspecified open wound of hip**
  - **7 S71.001-   Unspecified open wound, right hip**
  - **7 S71.002-   Unspecified open wound, left hip**
  - **7 S71.009-   Unspecified open wound, unspecified hip**
- **6 S71.01   Laceration without foreign body of hip**
  - **7 S71.011-   Laceration without foreign body, right hip**
  - **7 S71.012-   Laceration without foreign body, left hip**
  - **7 S71.019-   Laceration without foreign body, unspecified hip**
- **6 S71.02   Laceration with foreign body of hip**
  - **7 S71.021-   Laceration with foreign body, right hip**
  - **7 S71.022-   Laceration with foreign body, left hip**
  - **7 S71.029-   Laceration with foreign body, unspecified hip**
- **6 S71.03   Puncture wound without foreign body of hip**

● New   ▲ Revised   *Manifestation*   4-7 Digit Indicators   ⊟ Laterality   Ⓐ Adult (15+ years)   Ⓜ Maternity (12-55 years)   Ⓝ Newborn   Ⓟ Pediatric (0-17 years)   ♂ Male   ♀ Female

✖ ~~Deleted~~   Unspecified   + Additional code

1004   © 2017 DecisionHealth   2017 ICD-10-CM Expert for Physicians

7 ⊟	**S71.031-**	**Puncture wound without foreign body, right hip**
7 ⊟	**S71.032-**	**Puncture wound without foreign body, left hip**
7 ⊟	**S71.039-**	**Puncture wound without foreign body, unspecified hip**
6	**S71.04**	**Puncture wound with foreign body of hip**
7 ⊟	**S71.041-**	**Puncture wound with foreign body, right hip**
7 ⊟	**S71.042-**	**Puncture wound with foreign body, left hip**
7 ⊟	**S71.049-**	**Puncture wound with foreign body, unspecified hip**
6	**S71.05**	**Open bite of hip**

Bite of hip NOS

EXCLUDES 1 *superficial bite of hip (S70.26, S70.27)*

7 ⊟	**S71.051-**	**Open bite, right hip**
7 ⊟	**S71.052-**	**Open bite, left hip**
7 ⊟	**S71.059-**	**Open bite, unspecified hip**
5	**S71.1**	**Open wound of thigh**
6	**S71.10**	**Unspecified open wound of thigh**
7 ⊟	**S71.101-**	**Unspecified open wound, right thigh**
7 ⊟	**S71.102-**	**Unspecified open wound, left thigh**
7 ⊟	**S71.109-**	**Unspecified open wound, unspecified thigh**
6	**S71.11**	**Laceration without foreign body of thigh**
7 ⊟	**S71.111-**	**Laceration without foreign body, right thigh**
7 ⊟	**S71.112-**	**Laceration without foreign body, left thigh**
7 ⊟	**S71.119-**	**Laceration without foreign body, unspecified thigh**
6	**S71.12**	**Laceration with foreign body of thigh**
7 ⊟	**S71.121-**	**Laceration with foreign body, right thigh**
7 ⊟	**S71.122-**	**Laceration with foreign body, left thigh**
7 ⊟	**S71.129-**	**Laceration with foreign body, unspecified thigh**
6	**S71.13**	**Puncture wound without foreign body of thigh**
7 ⊟	**S71.131-**	**Puncture wound without foreign body, right thigh**
7 ⊟	**S71.132-**	**Puncture wound without foreign body, left thigh**
7 ⊟	**S71.139-**	**Puncture wound without foreign body, unspecified thigh**
6	**S71.14**	**Puncture wound with foreign body of thigh**
7 ⊟	**S71.141-**	**Puncture wound with foreign body, right thigh**
7 ⊟	**S71.142-**	**Puncture wound with foreign body, left thigh**
7 ⊟	**S71.149-**	**Puncture wound with foreign body, unspecified thigh**
6	**S71.15**	**Open bite of thigh**

Bite of thigh NOS

EXCLUDES 1 *superficial bite of thigh (S70.37-)*

7 ⊟	**S71.151-**	**Open bite, right thigh**
7 ⊟	**S71.152-**	**Open bite, left thigh**
7 ⊟	**S71.159-**	**Open bite, unspecified thigh**

4 **S72   Fracture of femur**

Note: A fracture not indicated as displaced or nondisplaced should be coded to displaced

A fracture not indicated as open or closed should be coded to closed

The open fracture designations are based on the Gustilo open fracture classification

EXCLUDES 1 *traumatic amputation of hip and thigh (S78.-)*

EXCLUDES 2 *fracture of lower leg and ankle (S82.-)*
fracture of foot (S92.-)
periprosthetic fracture of prosthetic implant of hip (T84.040, T84.041)

The appropriate 7th character is to be added to all codes from category S72

A	initial encounter for closed fracture
B	initial encounter for open fracture type I or II
C	initial encounter for open fracture type IIIA, IIIB, or IIIC
D	subsequent encounter for closed fracture with routine healing
E	subsequent encounter for open fracture type I or II with routine healing
F	subsequent encounter for open fracture type IIIA, IIIB, or IIIC with routine healing
G	subsequent encounter for closed fracture with delayed healing
H	subsequent encounter for open fracture type I or II with delayed healing
J	subsequent encounter for open fracture type IIIA, IIIB, or IIIC with delayed healing
K	subsequent encounter for closed fracture with nonunion
M	subsequent encounter for open fracture type I or II with nonunion
N	subsequent encounter for open fracture type IIIA, IIIB, or IIIC with nonunion
P	subsequent encounter for closed fracture with malunion
Q	subsequent encounter for open fracture type I or II with malunion
R	subsequent encounter for open fracture type IIIA, IIIB, or IIIC with malunion
S	sequela

CODING TIP ✓   A fracture not indicated as displaced or nondisplaced should be coded to displaced. A fracture not indicated as open or closed should be coded to closed. Query providers on fractures not documented as displaced/nondisplaced otherwise displaced fracture diagnosis could be assigned without reduction being performed potentially resulting in claim denials.

5 **S72.0   Fracture of head and neck of femur**

EXCLUDES 2 *physeal fracture of upper end of femur (S79.0-)*

6 **S72.00   Fracture of unspecified part of neck of femur**

Fracture of hip NOS
Fracture of neck of femur NOS

CODING TIP ✓   A fracture that is only reported as a "hip fracture" should be coded to S72.00- with the appropriate 6th character to indicate laterality, and a 7th character to indicate healing status and episode of care.

7 ⊟	**S72.001-**	**Fracture of unspecified part of neck of right femur**
7 ⊟	**S72.002-**	**Fracture of unspecified part of neck of left femur**

AHA: (S72.002D) 4Q 2015, 36-37
AHA: (S72.002S) 1Q 2015, 17

7 ⊟	**S72.009-**	**Fracture of unspecified part of neck of unspecified femur**
6	**S72.01**	**Unspecified intracapsular fracture of femur**

Subcapital fracture of femur

7 ⊟	**S72.011-**	**Unspecified intracapsular fracture of right femur**
7 ⊟	**S72.012-**	**Unspecified intracapsular fracture of left femur**
7 ⊟	**S72.019-**	**Unspecified intracapsular fracture of unspecified femur**

⑥ S72.02   Fracture of epiphysis (separation) (upper) of femur
Transepiphyseal fracture of femur
> **EXCLUDES 1** *capital femoral epiphyseal fracture (pediatric) of femur (S79.01-)*
> *Salter-Harris Type I physeal fracture of upper end of femur (S79.01-)*

7 ⊟ S72.021-   Displaced fracture of epiphysis (separation) (upper) of right femur

7 ⊟ S72.022-   Displaced fracture of epiphysis (separation) (upper) of left femur

7 ⊟ S72.023-   Displaced fracture of epiphysis (separation) (upper) of unspecified femur

7 ⊟ S72.024-   Nondisplaced fracture of epiphysis (separation) (upper) of right femur

7 ⊟ S72.025-   Nondisplaced fracture of epiphysis (separation) (upper) of left femur

7 ⊟ S72.026-   Nondisplaced fracture of epiphysis (separation) (upper) of unspecified femur

⑥ S72.03   Midcervical fracture of femur
Transcervical fracture of femur NOS

7 ⊟ S72.031-   Displaced midcervical fracture of right femur

7 ⊟ S72.032-   Displaced midcervical fracture of left femur

7 ⊟ S72.033-   Displaced midcervical fracture of unspecified femur

7 ⊟ S72.034-   Nondisplaced midcervical fracture of right femur

7 ⊟ S72.035-   Nondisplaced midcervical fracture of left femur

7 ⊟ S72.036-   Nondisplaced midcervical fracture of unspecified femur

⑥ S72.04   Fracture of base of neck of femur
Cervicotrochanteric fracture of femur

7 ⊟ S72.041-   Displaced fracture of base of neck of right femur

7 ⊟ S72.042-   Displaced fracture of base of neck of left femur

7 ⊟ S72.043-   Displaced fracture of base of neck of unspecified femur

7 ⊟ S72.044-   Nondisplaced fracture of base of neck of right femur

7 ⊟ S72.045-   Nondisplaced fracture of base of neck of left femur

7 ⊟ S72.046-   Nondisplaced fracture of base of neck of unspecified femur

⑥ S72.05   Unspecified fracture of head of femur
Fracture of head of femur NOS

7 ⊟ S72.051-   Unspecified fracture of head of right femur

7 ⊟ S72.052-   Unspecified fracture of head of left femur

7 ⊟ S72.059-   Unspecified fracture of head of unspecified femur

⑥ S72.06   Articular fracture of head of femur

7 ⊟ S72.061-   Displaced articular fracture of head of right femur

7 ⊟ S72.062-   Displaced articular fracture of head of left femur

7 ⊟ S72.063-   Displaced articular fracture of head of unspecified femur

7 ⊟ S72.064-   Nondisplaced articular fracture of head of right femur

7 ⊟ S72.065-   Nondisplaced articular fracture of head of left femur

7 ⊟ S72.066-   Nondisplaced articular fracture of head of unspecified femur

⑥ S72.09   Other fracture of head and neck of femur

7 ⊟ S72.091-   Other fracture of head and neck of right femur

7 ⊟ S72.092-   Other fracture of head and neck of left femur

7 ⊟ S72.099-   Other fracture of head and neck of unspecified femur

⑤ S72.1   Pertrochanteric fracture

⑥ S72.10   Unspecified trochanteric fracture of femur
Fracture of trochanter NOS

7 ⊟ S72.101-   Unspecified trochanteric fracture of right femur

7 ⊟ S72.102-   Unspecified trochanteric fracture of left femur

7 ⊟ S72.109-   Unspecified trochanteric fracture of unspecified femur

⑥ S72.11   Fracture of greater trochanter of femur

7 ⊟ S72.111-   Displaced fracture of greater trochanter of right femur

7 ⊟ S72.112-   Displaced fracture of greater trochanter of left femur

7 ⊟ S72.113-   Displaced fracture of greater trochanter of unspecified femur

7 ⊟ S72.114-   Nondisplaced fracture of greater trochanter of right femur

7 ⊟ S72.115-   Nondisplaced fracture of greater trochanter of left femur

7 ⊟ S72.116-   Nondisplaced fracture of greater trochanter of unspecified femur

⑥ S72.12   Fracture of lesser trochanter of femur

7 ⊟ S72.121-   Displaced fracture of lesser trochanter of right femur

7 ⊟ S72.122-   Displaced fracture of lesser trochanter of left femur

7 ⊟ S72.123-   Displaced fracture of lesser trochanter of unspecified femur

7 ⊟ S72.124-   Nondisplaced fracture of lesser trochanter of right femur

7 ⊟ S72.125-   Nondisplaced fracture of lesser trochanter of left femur

7 ⊟ S72.126-   Nondisplaced fracture of lesser trochanter of unspecified femur

⑥ S72.13   Apophyseal fracture of femur
> **EXCLUDES 1** *chronic (nontraumatic) slipped upper femoral epiphysis (M93.0-)*

7 ⊟ S72.131-   Displaced apophyseal fracture of right femur

7 ⊟ S72.132-   Displaced apophyseal fracture of left femur

7 ⊟ S72.133-   Displaced apophyseal fracture of unspecified femur

7 ⊟ S72.134-   Nondisplaced apophyseal fracture of right femur

7 ⊟ S72.135-   Nondisplaced apophyseal fracture of left femur

7 ⊟ S72.136-   Nondisplaced apophyseal fracture of unspecified femur

⑥ S72.14   Intertrochanteric fracture of femur

7 ⊟ S72.141-   Displaced intertrochanteric fracture of right femur
AHA: 4Q 2013, 129

7 ⊟ S72.142-   Displaced intertrochanteric fracture of left femur

7 ⊟ S72.143-   Displaced intertrochanteric fracture of unspecified femur

7 ⊟ S72.144-   Nondisplaced intertrochanteric fracture of right femur

7 ⊟ S72.145-   Nondisplaced intertrochanteric fracture of left femur

7 ⊟ S72.146-   Nondisplaced intertrochanteric fracture of unspecified femur

⑤ S72.2   Subtrochanteric fracture of femur

7 ⊟ S72.21X-   Displaced subtrochanteric fracture of right femur

7 ⊟ S72.22X-   Displaced subtrochanteric fracture of left femur

7 ⊟ S72.23X-   Displaced subtrochanteric fracture of unspecified femur

7 ⊟ S72.24X-   Nondisplaced subtrochanteric fracture of right femur

7 ⊟ S72.25X-   Nondisplaced subtrochanteric fracture of left femur

7 ⊟ S72.26X-   Nondisplaced subtrochanteric fracture of unspecified femur

⑤ S72.3   Fracture of shaft of femur

⑥ S72.30   Unspecified fracture of shaft of femur

7 ⊟ S72.301-   Unspecified fracture of shaft of right femur

7 ⊟ S72.302-   Unspecified fracture of shaft of left femur

7 ⊟ S72.309-   Unspecified fracture of shaft of unspecified femur

⑥ S72.32   Transverse fracture of shaft of femur

7 ⊟ S72.321-   Displaced transverse fracture of shaft of right femur

7 ⊟ S72.322-   Displaced transverse fracture of shaft of left femur

7 ⊟ S72.323-   Displaced transverse fracture of shaft of unspecified femur

---

● New   ▲ Revised   *Manifestation*   ◀-7 Digit Indicators   ⊟ Laterality   Ⓐ Adult (15+ years)   Ⓜ Maternity (12-55 years)   Ⓝ Newborn   Ⓟ Pediatric (0-17 years)   ♂ Male   ♀ Female
✖ Deleted   Unspecified   ＋ Additional code

1006   © 2017 DecisionHealth   2017 ICD-10-CM Expert for Physicians

7 ⊟ **S72.324-**   **Nondisplaced transverse fracture of shaft of right femur**

7 ⊟ **S72.325-**   **Nondisplaced transverse fracture of shaft of left femur**

7 ⊟ **S72.326-**   **Nondisplaced transverse fracture of shaft of unspecified femur**

6 **S72.33**   **Oblique fracture of shaft of femur**

7 ⊟ **S72.331-**   **Displaced oblique fracture of shaft of right femur**

7 ⊟ **S72.332-**   **Displaced oblique fracture of shaft of left femur**

7 ⊟ **S72.333-**   **Displaced oblique fracture of shaft of unspecified femur**

7 ⊟ **S72.334-**   **Nondisplaced oblique fracture of shaft of right femur**

7 ⊟ **S72.335-**   **Nondisplaced oblique fracture of shaft of left femur**

7 ⊟ **S72.336-**   **Nondisplaced oblique fracture of shaft of unspecified femur**

6 **S72.34**   **Spiral fracture of shaft of femur**

7 ⊟ **S72.341-**   **Displaced spiral fracture of shaft of right femur**

7 ⊟ **S72.342-**   **Displaced spiral fracture of shaft of left femur**

7 ⊟ **S72.343-**   **Displaced spiral fracture of shaft of unspecified femur**

7 ⊟ **S72.344-**   **Nondisplaced spiral fracture of shaft of right femur**

7 ⊟ **S72.345-**   **Nondisplaced spiral fracture of shaft of left femur**

7 ⊟ **S72.346-**   **Nondisplaced spiral fracture of shaft of unspecified femur**

6 **S72.35**   **Comminuted fracture of shaft of femur**

7 ⊟ **S72.351-**   **Displaced comminuted fracture of shaft of right femur**

7 ⊟ **S72.352-**   **Displaced comminuted fracture of shaft of left femur**

7 ⊟ **S72.353-**   **Displaced comminuted fracture of shaft of unspecified femur**

7 ⊟ **S72.354-**   **Nondisplaced comminuted fracture of shaft of right femur**

7 ⊟ **S72.355-**   **Nondisplaced comminuted fracture of shaft of left femur**

7 ⊟ **S72.356-**   **Nondisplaced comminuted fracture of shaft of unspecified femur**

6 **S72.36**   **Segmental fracture of shaft of femur**

7 ⊟ **S72.361-**   **Displaced segmental fracture of shaft of right femur**

7 ⊟ **S72.362-**   **Displaced segmental fracture of shaft of left femur**

7 ⊟ **S72.363-**   **Displaced segmental fracture of shaft of unspecified femur**

7 ⊟ **S72.364-**   **Nondisplaced segmental fracture of shaft of right femur**

7 ⊟ **S72.365-**   **Nondisplaced segmental fracture of shaft of left femur**

7 ⊟ **S72.366-**   **Nondisplaced segmental fracture of shaft of unspecified femur**

6 **S72.39**   **Other fracture of shaft of femur**

7 ⊟ **S72.391-**   **Other fracture of shaft of right femur**

7 ⊟ **S72.392-**   **Other fracture of shaft of left femur**

7 ⊟ **S72.399-**   **Other fracture of shaft of unspecified femur**

5 **S72.4**   **Fracture of lower end of femur**
Fracture of distal end of femur
EXCLUDES 2   *fracture of shaft of femur (S72.3-)*
physeal fracture of lower end of femur (S79.1-)

6 **S72.40**   **Unspecified fracture of lower end of femur**

7 ⊟ **S72.401-**   **Unspecified fracture of lower end of right femur**

7 ⊟ **S72.402-**   **Unspecified fracture of lower end of left femur**

7 ⊟ **S72.409-**   **Unspecified fracture of lower end of unspecified femur**

6 **S72.41**   **Unspecified condyle fracture of lower end of femur**
Condyle fracture of femur NOS

7 ⊟ **S72.411-**   **Displaced unspecified condyle fracture of lower end of right femur**

7 ⊟ **S72.412-**   **Displaced unspecified condyle fracture of lower end of left femur**

7 ⊟ **S72.413-**   **Displaced unspecified condyle fracture of lower end of unspecified femur**

7 ⊟ **S72.414-**   **Nondisplaced unspecified condyle fracture of lower end of right femur**

7 ⊟ **S72.415-**   **Nondisplaced unspecified condyle fracture of lower end of left femur**

7 ⊟ **S72.416-**   **Nondisplaced unspecified condyle fracture of lower end of unspecified femur**

6 **S72.42**   **Fracture of lateral condyle of femur**

7 ⊟ **S72.421-**   **Displaced fracture of lateral condyle of right femur**

7 ⊟ **S72.422-**   **Displaced fracture of lateral condyle of left femur**

7 ⊟ **S72.423-**   **Displaced fracture of lateral condyle of unspecified femur**

7 ⊟ **S72.424-**   **Nondisplaced fracture of lateral condyle of right femur**

7 ⊟ **S72.425-**   **Nondisplaced fracture of lateral condyle of left femur**

7 ⊟ **S72.426-**   **Nondisplaced fracture of lateral condyle of unspecified femur**

6 **S72.43**   **Fracture of medial condyle of femur**

7 ⊟ **S72.431-**   **Displaced fracture of medial condyle of right femur**

7 ⊟ **S72.432-**   **Displaced fracture of medial condyle of left femur**

7 ⊟ **S72.433-**   **Displaced fracture of medial condyle of unspecified femur**

7 ⊟ **S72.434-**   **Nondisplaced fracture of medial condyle of right femur**

7 ⊟ **S72.435-**   **Nondisplaced fracture of medial condyle of left femur**

7 ⊟ **S72.436-**   **Nondisplaced fracture of medial condyle of unspecified femur**

6 **S72.44**   **Fracture of lower epiphysis (separation) of femur**
EXCLUDES 1   *Salter-Harris Type I physeal fracture of lower end of femur (S79.11-)*

7 ⊟ **S72.441-**   **Displaced fracture of lower epiphysis (separation) of right femur**

7 ⊟ **S72.442-**   **Displaced fracture of lower epiphysis (separation) of left femur**

7 ⊟ **S72.443-**   **Displaced fracture of lower epiphysis (separation) of unspecified femur**

7 ⊟ **S72.444-**   **Nondisplaced fracture of lower epiphysis (separation) of right femur**

7 ⊟ **S72.445-**   **Nondisplaced fracture of lower epiphysis (separation) of left femur**

7 ⊟ **S72.446-**   **Nondisplaced fracture of lower epiphysis (separation) of unspecified femur**

6 **S72.45**   **Supracondylar fracture without intracondylar extension of lower end of femur**
Supracondylar fracture of lower end of femur NOS
EXCLUDES 1   *supracondylar fracture with intracondylar extension of lower end of femur (S72.46-)*

7 ⊟ **S72.451-**   **Displaced supracondylar fracture without intracondylar extension of lower end of right femur**

7 ⊟ **S72.452-**   **Displaced supracondylar fracture without intracondylar extension of lower end of left femur**

7 ⊟ **S72.453-**   **Displaced supracondylar fracture without intracondylar extension of lower end of unspecified femur**

7 ⊟ **S72.454-**   **Nondisplaced supracondylar fracture without intracondylar extension of lower end of right femur**

7 ⊟ **S72.455-**   **Nondisplaced supracondylar fracture without intracondylar extension of lower end of left femur**

7 ⊟ **S72.456-**   **Nondisplaced supracondylar fracture without intracondylar extension of lower end of unspecified femur**

6 **S72.46**   **Supracondylar fracture with intracondylar extension of lower end of femur**
EXCLUDES 1   *supracondylar fracture without intracondylar extension of lower end of femur (S72.45-)*

● New   ▲ Revised   *Manifestation*   4-7 Digit Indicators   ⊟ Laterality   A Adult (15+ years)   M Maternity (12-55 years)   N Newborn   P Pediatric (0-17 years)   ♂ Male   ♀ Female
✖ Deleted   Unspecified   + Additional code

7 🖃 **S72.461-**	**Displaced supracondylar fracture with intracondylar extension of lower end of right femur**
7 🖃 **S72.462-**	**Displaced supracondylar fracture with intracondylar extension of lower end of left femur**
7 🖃 **S72.463-**	**Displaced supracondylar fracture with intracondylar extension of lower end of unspecified femur**
7 🖃 **S72.464-**	**Nondisplaced supracondylar fracture with intracondylar extension of lower end of right femur**
7 🖃 **S72.465-**	**Nondisplaced supracondylar fracture with intracondylar extension of lower end of left femur**
7 🖃 **S72.466-**	**Nondisplaced supracondylar fracture with intracondylar extension of lower end of unspecified femur**
6 **S72.47**	**Torus fracture of lower end of femur**

The appropriate 7th character is to be added to all codes in subcategory S72.47

A	initial encounter for closed fracture
D	subsequent encounter for fracture with routine healing
G	subsequent encounter for fracture with delayed healing
K	subsequent encounter for fracture with nonunion
P	subsequent encounter for fracture with malunion
S	sequela

7 🖃 **S72.471-**	**Torus fracture of lower end of right femur**
7 🖃 **S72.472-**	**Torus fracture of lower end of left femur**
7 🖃 **S72.479-**	**Torus fracture of lower end of unspecified femur**
6 **S72.49**	**Other fracture of lower end of femur**
7 🖃 **S72.491-**	**Other fracture of lower end of right femur**
7 🖃 **S72.492-**	**Other fracture of lower end of left femur**
7 🖃 **S72.499-**	**Other fracture of lower end of unspecified femur**
5 **S72.8**	**Other fracture of femur**
6 **S72.8X**	**Other fracture of femur**
7 🖃 **S72.8X1-**	**Other fracture of right femur**
7 🖃 **S72.8X2-**	**Other fracture of left femur**
7 🖃 **S72.8X9-**	**Other fracture of unspecified femur**
5 **S72.9**	**Unspecified fracture of femur**

Fracture of thigh NOS
Fracture of upper leg NOS

EXCLUDES 1 *fracture of hip NOS (S72.00-, S72.01-)*

7 🖃 **S72.90X-**	**Unspecified fracture of unspecified femur**
	AHA: (S72.90XD) 4Q 2012, 93-94
7 🖃 **S72.91X-**	**Unspecified fracture of right femur**
7 🖃 **S72.92X-**	**Unspecified fracture of left femur**
4 **S73**	**Dislocation and sprain of joint and ligaments of hip**

INCLUDES
avulsion of joint or ligament of hip
laceration of cartilage, joint or ligament of hip
sprain of cartilage, joint or ligament of hip
traumatic hemarthrosis of joint or ligament of hip
traumatic rupture of joint or ligament of hip
traumatic subluxation of joint or ligament of hip
traumatic tear of joint or ligament of hip

Code also:
any associated open wound

EXCLUDES 2 *strain of muscle, fascia and tendon of hip and thigh (S76.-)*

The appropriate 7th character is to be added to each code from category S73

A	initial encounter
D	subsequent encounter
S	sequela

CODING TIP ✓   Unlike ICD-9 there is no code for open dislocations. When documented as open an additional code for the open wound must be applied.

5 **S73.0**	**Subluxation and dislocation of hip**
	EXCLUDES 2 *dislocation and subluxation of hip prosthesis (T84.020, T84.021)*
6 **S73.00**	**Unspecified subluxation and dislocation of hip**

Dislocation of hip NOS
Subluxation of hip NOS

7 🖃 **S73.001-**	**Unspecified subluxation of right hip**
7 🖃 **S73.002-**	**Unspecified subluxation of left hip**
7 🖃 **S73.003-**	**Unspecified subluxation of unspecified hip**
7 🖃 **S73.004-**	**Unspecified dislocation of right hip**
7 🖃 **S73.005-**	**Unspecified dislocation of left hip**
7 🖃 **S73.006-**	**Unspecified dislocation of unspecified hip**
6 **S73.01**	**Posterior subluxation and dislocation of hip**
7 🖃 **S73.011-**	**Posterior subluxation of right hip**
7 🖃 **S73.012-**	**Posterior subluxation of left hip**
7 🖃 **S73.013-**	**Posterior subluxation of unspecified hip**
7 🖃 **S73.014-**	**Posterior dislocation of right hip**
7 🖃 **S73.015-**	**Posterior dislocation of left hip**
7 🖃 **S73.016-**	**Posterior dislocation of unspecified hip**
6 **S73.02**	**Obturator subluxation and dislocation of hip**
7 🖃 **S73.021-**	**Obturator subluxation of right hip**
7 🖃 **S73.022-**	**Obturator subluxation of left hip**
7 🖃 **S73.023-**	**Obturator subluxation of unspecified hip**
7 🖃 **S73.024-**	**Obturator dislocation of right hip**
7 🖃 **S73.025-**	**Obturator dislocation of left hip**
7 🖃 **S73.026-**	**Obturator dislocation of unspecified hip**
6 **S73.03**	**Other anterior dislocation of hip**
7 🖃 **S73.031-**	**Other anterior subluxation of right hip**
7 🖃 **S73.032-**	**Other anterior subluxation of left hip**
7 🖃 **S73.033-**	**Other anterior subluxation of unspecified hip**
7 🖃 **S73.034-**	**Other anterior dislocation of right hip**
7 🖃 **S73.035-**	**Other anterior dislocation of left hip**
7 🖃 **S73.036-**	**Other anterior dislocation of unspecified hip**
6 **S73.04**	**Central dislocation of hip**
7 🖃 **S73.041-**	**Central subluxation of right hip**
7 🖃 **S73.042-**	**Central subluxation of left hip**
7 🖃 **S73.043-**	**Central subluxation of unspecified hip**
7 🖃 **S73.044-**	**Central dislocation of right hip**
7 🖃 **S73.045-**	**Central dislocation of left hip**
7 🖃 **S73.046-**	**Central dislocation of unspecified hip**
5 **S73.1**	**Sprain of hip**
	AHA: 4Q 2014, 25
6 **S73.10**	**Unspecified sprain of hip**
7 🖃 **S73.101-**	**Unspecified sprain of right hip**
7 🖃 **S73.102-**	**Unspecified sprain of left hip**
7 🖃 **S73.109-**	**Unspecified sprain of unspecified hip**
6 **S73.11**	**Iliofemoral ligament sprain of hip**
7 🖃 **S73.111-**	**Iliofemoral ligament sprain of right hip**
7 🖃 **S73.112-**	**Iliofemoral ligament sprain of left hip**
7 🖃 **S73.119-**	**Iliofemoral ligament sprain of unspecified hip**
6 **S73.12**	**Ischiocapsular (ligament) sprain of hip**
7 🖃 **S73.121-**	**Ischiocapsular ligament sprain of right hip**
7 🖃 **S73.122-**	**Ischiocapsular ligament sprain of left hip**
7 🖃 **S73.129-**	**Ischiocapsular ligament sprain of unspecified hip**
6 **S73.19**	**Other sprain of hip**
7 🖃 **S73.191-**	**Other sprain of right hip**
7 🖃 **S73.192-**	**Other sprain of left hip**
	AHA: (S73.192A) 4Q 2014, 25
7 🖃 **S73.199-**	**Other sprain of unspecified hip**
4 **S74**	**Injury of nerves at hip and thigh level**

Code also:
any associated open wound (S71.-)

EXCLUDES 2 *injury of nerves at ankle and foot level (S94.-)*
injury of nerves at lower leg level (S84.-)

The appropriate 7th character is to be added to each code from category S74

A	initial encounter
D	subsequent encounter
S	sequela

5 **S74.0**	**Injury of sciatic nerve at hip and thigh level**

● New   ▲ Revised   *Manifestation*   4-7 Digit Indicators   🖃 Laterality   A Adult (15+ years)   M Maternity (12-55 years)   N Newborn   P Pediatric (0-17 years)   ♂ Male   ♀ Female

✖ Deleted   Unspecified   ✦ Additional code

1008   © 2017 DecisionHealth   2017 ICD-10-CM Expert for Physicians

7 ⊟ **S74.00X-** Injury of sciatic nerve at hip and thigh level, unspecified leg

7 ⊟ **S74.01X-** Injury of sciatic nerve at hip and thigh level, right leg

7 ⊟ **S74.02X-** Injury of sciatic nerve at hip and thigh level, left leg

S **S74.1** Injury of femoral nerve at hip and thigh level

7 ⊟ **S74.10X-** Injury of femoral nerve at hip and thigh level, unspecified leg

7 ⊟ **S74.11X-** Injury of femoral nerve at hip and thigh level, right leg

7 ⊟ **S74.12X-** Injury of femoral nerve at hip and thigh level, left leg

S **S74.2** Injury of cutaneous sensory nerve at hip and thigh level

7 ⊟ **S74.20X-** Injury of cutaneous sensory nerve at hip and thigh level, unspecified leg

7 ⊟ **S74.21X-** Injury of cutaneous sensory nerve at hip and high level, right leg

7 ⊟ **S74.22X-** Injury of cutaneous sensory nerve at hip and thigh level, left leg

S **S74.8** Injury of other nerves at hip and thigh level

6 **S74.8X** Injury of other nerves at hip and thigh level

7 ⊟ **S74.8X1-** Injury of other nerves at hip and thigh level, right leg

7 ⊟ **S74.8X2-** Injury of other nerves at hip and thigh level, left leg

7 ⊟ **S74.8X9-** Injury of other nerves at hip and thigh level, unspecified leg

S **S74.9** Injury of unspecified nerve at hip and thigh level

7 ⊟ **S74.90X-** Injury of unspecified nerve at hip and thigh level, unspecified leg

7 ⊟ **S74.91X-** Injury of unspecified nerve at hip and thigh level, right leg

7 ⊟ **S74.92X-** Injury of unspecified nerve at hip and thigh level, left leg

4 **S75** **Injury of blood vessels at hip and thigh level**

Code also:

any associated open wound (S71.-)

EXCLUDES 2 *injury of blood vessels at lower leg level (S85.-)*
injury of popliteal artery (S85.0)

The appropriate 7th character is to be added to each code from category S75
A   initial encounter
D   subsequent encounter
S   sequela

S **S75.0** Injury of femoral artery

6 **S75.00** Unspecified injury of femoral artery

7 ⊟ **S75.001-** Unspecified injury of femoral artery, right leg

7 ⊟ **S75.002-** Unspecified injury of femoral artery, left leg

7 ⊟ **S75.009-** Unspecified injury of femoral artery, unspecified leg

6 **S75.01** Minor laceration of femoral artery
Incomplete transection of femoral artery
Laceration of femoral artery NOS
Superficial laceration of femoral artery
CODING TIP ✓ Code also any associated open wound S71.-

7 ⊟ **S75.011-** Minor laceration of femoral artery, right leg

7 ⊟ **S75.012-** Minor laceration of femoral artery, left leg

7 ⊟ **S75.019-** Minor laceration of femoral artery, unspecified leg

6 **S75.02** Major laceration of femoral artery
Complete transection of femoral artery
Traumatic rupture of femoral artery
CODING TIP ✓ Code also any associated open wound S71.-

7 ⊟ **S75.021-** Major laceration of femoral artery, right leg

7 ⊟ **S75.022-** Major laceration of femoral artery, left leg

7 ⊟ **S75.029-** Major laceration of femoral artery, unspecified leg

6 **S75.09** Other specified injury of femoral artery

7 ⊟ **S75.091-** Other specified injury of femoral artery, right leg

7 ⊟ **S75.092-** Other specified injury of femoral artery, left leg

7 ⊟ **S75.099-** Other specified injury of femoral artery, unspecified leg

S **S75.1** Injury of femoral vein at hip and thigh level

6 **S75.10** Unspecified injury of femoral vein at hip and thigh level

7 ⊟ **S75.101-** Unspecified injury of femoral vein at hip and thigh level, right leg

7 ⊟ **S75.102-** Unspecified injury of femoral vein at hip and thigh level, left leg

7 ⊟ **S75.109-** Unspecified injury of femoral vein at hip and thigh level, unspecified leg

6 **S75.11** Minor laceration of femoral vein at hip and thigh level
Incomplete transection of femoral vein at hip and thigh level
Laceration of femoral vein at hip and thigh level NOS
Superficial laceration of femoral vein at hip and thigh level
CODING TIP ✓ Code also any associated open wound S71.-

7 ⊟ **S75.111-** Minor laceration of femoral vein at hip and thigh level, right leg

7 ⊟ **S75.112-** Minor laceration of femoral vein at hip and thigh level, left leg

7 ⊟ **S75.119-** Minor laceration of femoral vein at hip and thigh level, unspecified leg

6 **S75.12** Major laceration of femoral vein at hip and thigh level
Complete transection of femoral vein at hip and thigh level
Traumatic rupture of femoral vein at hip and thigh level
CODING TIP ✓ Code also any associated open wound S71.-

7 ⊟ **S75.121-** Major laceration of femoral vein at hip and thigh level, right leg

7 ⊟ **S75.122-** Major laceration of femoral vein at hip and thigh level, left leg

7 ⊟ **S75.129-** Major laceration of femoral vein at hip and thigh level, unspecified leg

6 **S75.19** Other specified injury of femoral vein at hip and thigh level

7 ⊟ **S75.191-** Other specified injury of femoral vein at hip and thigh level, right leg

7 ⊟ **S75.192-** Other specified injury of femoral vein at hip and thigh level, left leg

7 ⊟ **S75.199-** Other specified injury of femoral vein at hip and thigh level, unspecified leg

S **S75.2** Injury of greater saphenous vein at hip and thigh level
EXCLUDES 1 *greater saphenous vein NOS (S85.3)*

6 **S75.20** Unspecified injury of greater saphenous vein at hip and thigh level

7 ⊟ **S75.201-** Unspecified injury of greater saphenous vein at hip and thigh level, right leg

7 ⊟ **S75.202-** Unspecified injury of greater saphenous vein at hip and thigh level, left leg

7 ⊟ **S75.209-** Unspecified injury of greater saphenous vein at hip and thigh level, unspecified leg

6 **S75.21** Minor laceration of greater saphenous vein at hip and thigh level
Incomplete transection of greater saphenous vein at hip and thigh level
Laceration of greater saphenous vein at hip and thigh level NOS
Superficial laceration of greater saphenous vein at hip and thigh level
CODING TIP ✓ Code also any associated open wound S71.-

7 ⊟ **S75.211-** Minor laceration of greater saphenous vein at hip and thigh level, right leg

7 ⊟ **S75.212-** Minor laceration of greater saphenous vein at hip and thigh level, left leg

7 ⊟ **S75.219-** Minor laceration of greater saphenous vein at hip and thigh level, unspecified leg

---

● New   ▲ Revised   *Manifestation*   4-7 Digit Indicators   ⊟ Laterality   Ⓐ Adult (15+ years)   Ⓜ Maternity (12-55 years)   Ⓝ Newborn   Ⓟ Pediatric (0-17 years)   ♂ Male   ♀ Female
✖ Deleted   Unspecified   + Additional code

2017 ICD-10-CM Expert for Physicians

© 2017 DecisionHealth

1009

ⓖ **S75.22**　**Major laceration of greater saphenous vein at hip and thigh level**
Complete transection of greater saphenous vein at hip and thigh level
Traumatic rupture of greater saphenous vein at hip and thigh level

CODING TIP ✓　Code also any associated open wound S71.-

⑦⊟ **S75.221-**　**Major laceration of greater saphenous vein at hip and thigh level, right leg**

⑦⊟ **S75.222-**　**Major laceration of greater saphenous vein at hip and thigh level, left leg**

⑦⊟ **S75.229-**　**Major laceration of greater saphenous vein at hip and thigh level, unspecified leg**

ⓖ **S75.29**　**Other specified injury of greater saphenous vein at hip and thigh level**

⑦⊟ **S75.291-**　**Other specified injury of greater saphenous vein at hip and thigh level, right leg**

⑦⊟ **S75.292-**　**Other specified injury of greater saphenous vein at hip and thigh level, left leg**

⑦⊟ **S75.299-**　**Other specified injury of greater saphenous vein at hip and thigh level, unspecified leg**

ⓢ **S75.8**　**Injury of other blood vessels at hip and thigh level**

ⓖ **S75.80**　**Unspecified injury of other blood vessels at hip and thigh level**

⑦⊟ **S75.801-**　**Unspecified injury of other blood vessels at hip and thigh level, right leg**

⑦⊟ **S75.802-**　**Unspecified injury of other blood vessels at hip and thigh level, left leg**

⑦⊟ **S75.809-**　**Unspecified injury of other blood vessels at hip and thigh level, unspecified leg**

ⓖ **S75.81**　**Laceration of other blood vessels at hip and thigh level**

CODING TIP ✓　Code also any associated open wound S71.-

⑦⊟ **S75.811-**　**Laceration of other blood vessels at hip and thigh level, right leg**

⑦⊟ **S75.812-**　**Laceration of other blood vessels at hip and thigh level, left leg**

⑦⊟ **S75.819-**　**Laceration of other blood vessels at hip and thigh level, unspecified leg**

ⓖ **S75.89**　**Other specified injury of other blood vessels at hip and thigh level**

⑦⊟ **S75.891-**　**Other specified injury of other blood vessels at hip and thigh level, right leg**

⑦⊟ **S75.892-**　**Other specified injury of other blood vessels at hip and thigh level, left leg**

⑦⊟ **S75.899-**　**Other specified injury of other blood vessels at hip and thigh level, unspecified leg**

ⓢ **S75.9**　**Injury of unspecified blood vessel at hip and thigh level**

ⓖ **S75.90**　**Unspecified injury of unspecified blood vessel at hip and thigh level**

⑦⊟ **S75.901-**　**Unspecified injury of unspecified blood vessel at hip and thigh level, right leg**

⑦⊟ **S75.902-**　**Unspecified injury of unspecified blood vessel at hip and thigh level, left leg**

⑦⊟ **S75.909-**　**Unspecified injury of unspecified blood vessel at hip and thigh level, unspecified leg**

ⓖ **S75.91**　**Laceration of unspecified blood vessel at hip and thigh level**

CODING TIP ✓　Code also any associated open wound S71.-

⑦⊟ **S75.911-**　**Laceration of unspecified blood vessel at hip and thigh level, right leg**

⑦⊟ **S75.912-**　**Laceration of unspecified blood vessel at hip and thigh level, left leg**

⑦⊟ **S75.919-**　**Laceration of unspecified blood vessel at hip and thigh level, unspecified leg**

ⓖ **S75.99**　**Other specified injury of unspecified blood vessel at hip and thigh level**

⑦⊟ **S75.991-**　**Other specified injury of unspecified blood vessel at hip and thigh level, right leg**

⑦⊟ **S75.992-**　**Other specified injury of unspecified blood vessel at hip and thigh level, left leg**

⑦⊟ **S75.999-**　**Other specified injury of unspecified blood vessel at hip and thigh level, unspecified leg**

④ **S76**　**Injury of muscle, fascia and tendon at hip and thigh level**
Code also:
any associated open wound (S71.-)

EXCLUDES 2　*injury of muscle, fascia and tendon at lower leg level (S86)*
sprain of joint and ligament of hip (S73.1)

The appropriate 7th character is to be added to each code from category S76
A　　initial encounter
D　　subsequent encounter
S　　sequela

ⓢ **S76.0**　**Injury of muscle, fascia and tendon of hip**

ⓖ **S76.00**　**Unspecified injury of muscle, fascia and tendon of hip**

⑦⊟ **S76.001-**　**Unspecified injury of muscle, fascia and tendon of right hip**

⑦⊟ **S76.002-**　**Unspecified injury of muscle, fascia and tendon of left hip**

⑦⊟ **S76.009-**　**Unspecified injury of muscle, fascia and tendon of unspecified hip**

ⓖ **S76.01**　**Strain of muscle, fascia and tendon of hip**

⑦⊟ **S76.011-**　**Strain of muscle, fascia and tendon of right hip**

⑦⊟ **S76.012-**　**Strain of muscle, fascia and tendon of left hip**

⑦⊟ **S76.019-**　**Strain of muscle, fascia and tendon of unspecified hip**

ⓖ **S76.02**　**Laceration of muscle, fascia and tendon of hip**

CODING TIP ✓　Code also any associated open wound S71.-

⑦⊟ **S76.021-**　**Laceration of muscle, fascia and tendon of right hip**

⑦⊟ **S76.022-**　**Laceration of muscle, fascia and tendon of left hip**

⑦⊟ **S76.029-**　**Laceration of muscle, fascia and tendon of unspecified hip**

ⓖ **S76.09**　**Other specified injury of muscle, fascia and tendon of hip**

⑦⊟ **S76.091-**　**Other specified injury of muscle, fascia and tendon of right hip**

⑦⊟ **S76.092-**　**Other specified injury of muscle, fascia and tendon of left hip**

⑦⊟ **S76.099-**　**Other specified injury of muscle, fascia and tendon of unspecified hip**

ⓢ **S76.1**　**Injury of quadriceps muscle, fascia and tendon**
Injury of patellar ligament (tendon)

ⓖ **S76.10**　**Unspecified injury of quadriceps muscle, fascia and tendon**

⑦⊟ **S76.101-**　**Unspecified injury of right quadriceps muscle, fascia and tendon**

⑦⊟ **S76.102-**　**Unspecified injury of left quadriceps muscle, fascia and tendon**

⑦⊟ **S76.109-**　**Unspecified injury of unspecified quadriceps muscle, fascia and tendon**

ⓖ **S76.11**　**Strain of quadriceps muscle, fascia and tendon**

⑦⊟ **S76.111-**　**Strain of right quadriceps muscle, fascia and tendon**

⑦⊟ **S76.112-**　**Strain of left quadriceps muscle, fascia and tendon**

⑦⊟ **S76.119-**　**Strain of unspecified quadriceps muscle, fascia and tendon**

ⓖ **S76.12**　**Laceration of quadriceps muscle, fascia and tendon**

CODING TIP ✓　Code also any associated open wound S71.-

⑦⊟ **S76.121-**　**Laceration of right quadriceps muscle, fascia and tendon**

⑦⊟ **S76.122-**　**Laceration of left quadriceps muscle, fascia and tendon**

⑦⊟ **S76.129-**　**Laceration of unspecified quadriceps muscle, fascia and tendon**

ⓖ **S76.19**　**Other specified injury of quadriceps muscle, fascia and tendon**

⑦⊟ **S76.191-**　**Other specified injury of right quadriceps muscle, fascia and tendon**

⑦⊟ **S76.192-**　**Other specified injury of left quadriceps muscle, fascia and tendon**

● New　▲ Revised　*Manifestation*　④-⑦ Digit Indicators　⊟ Laterality　🅰 Adult (15+ years)　🅼 Maternity (12-55 years)　🅽 Newborn　🅿 Pediatric (0-17 years)　♂ Male　♀ Female
✖ Deleted　Unspecified　+ Additional code

1010　　© 2017 DecisionHealth　　　　2017 ICD-10-CM Expert for Physicians

7 🗐 **S76.199-** Other specified injury of unspecified quadriceps muscle, fascia and tendon

5 **S76.2** Injury of adductor muscle, fascia and tendon of thigh

6 **S76.20** Unspecified injury of adductor muscle, fascia and tendon of thigh

7 🗐 **S76.201-** Unspecified injury of adductor muscle, fascia and tendon of right thigh

7 🗐 **S76.202-** Unspecified injury of adductor muscle, fascia and tendon of left thigh

7 🗐 **S76.209-** Unspecified injury of adductor muscle, fascia and tendon of unspecified thigh

6 **S76.21** Strain of adductor muscle, fascia and tendon of thigh

7 🗐 **S76.211-** Strain of adductor muscle, fascia and tendon of right thigh

7 🗐 **S76.212-** Strain of adductor muscle, fascia and tendon of left thigh

7 🗐 **S76.219-** Strain of adductor muscle, fascia and tendon of unspecified thigh

6 **S76.22** Laceration of adductor muscle, fascia and tendon of thigh

CODING TIP ✓ Code also any associated open wound S71.-

7 🗐 **S76.221-** Laceration of adductor muscle, fascia and tendon of right thigh

7 🗐 **S76.222-** Laceration of adductor muscle, fascia and tendon of left thigh

7 🗐 **S76.229-** Laceration of adductor muscle, fascia and tendon of unspecified thigh

6 **S76.29** Other injury of adductor muscle, fascia and tendon of thigh

7 🗐 **S76.291-** Other injury of adductor muscle, fascia and tendon of right thigh

7 🗐 **S76.292-** Other injury of adductor muscle, fascia and tendon of left thigh

7 🗐 **S76.299-** Other injury of adductor muscle, fascia and tendon of unspecified thigh

5 **S76.3** Injury of muscle, fascia and tendon of the posterior muscle group at thigh level

6 **S76.30** Unspecified injury of muscle, fascia and tendon of the posterior muscle group at thigh level

7 🗐 **S76.301-** Unspecified injury of muscle, fascia and tendon of the posterior muscle group at thigh level, right thigh

7 🗐 **S76.302-** Unspecified injury of muscle, fascia and tendon of the posterior muscle group at thigh level, left thigh

7 🗐 **S76.309-** Unspecified injury of muscle, fascia and tendon of the posterior muscle group at thigh level, unspecified thigh

6 **S76.31** Strain of muscle, fascia and tendon of the posterior muscle group at thigh level

7 🗐 **S76.311-** Strain of muscle, fascia and tendon of the posterior muscle group at thigh level, right thigh

7 🗐 **S76.312-** Strain of muscle, fascia and tendon of the posterior muscle group at thigh level, left thigh

7 🗐 **S76.319-** Strain of muscle, fascia and tendon of the posterior muscle group at thigh level, unspecified thigh

6 **S76.32** Laceration of muscle, fascia and tendon of the posterior muscle group at thigh level

CODING TIP ✓ Code also any associated open wound S71.-

7 🗐 **S76.321-** Laceration of muscle, fascia and tendon of the posterior muscle group at thigh level, right thigh

7 🗐 **S76.322-** Laceration of muscle, fascia and tendon of the posterior muscle group at thigh level, left thigh

7 🗐 **S76.329-** Laceration of muscle, fascia and tendon of the posterior muscle group at thigh level, unspecified thigh

6 **S76.39** Other specified injury of muscle, fascia and tendon of the posterior muscle group at thigh level

7 🗐 **S76.391-** Other specified injury of muscle, fascia and tendon of the posterior muscle group at thigh level, right thigh

7 🗐 **S76.392-** Other specified injury of muscle, fascia and tendon of the posterior muscle group at thigh level, left thigh

7 🗐 **S76.399-** Other specified injury of muscle, fascia and tendon of the posterior muscle group at thigh level, unspecified thigh

5 **S76.8** Injury of other specified muscles, fascia and tendons at thigh level

6 **S76.80** Unspecified injury of other specified muscles, fascia and tendons at thigh level

7 🗐 **S76.801-** Unspecified injury of other specified muscles, fascia and tendons at thigh level, right thigh

7 🗐 **S76.802-** Unspecified injury of other specified muscles, fascia and tendons at thigh level, left thigh

7 🗐 **S76.809-** Unspecified injury of other specified muscles, fascia and tendons at thigh level, unspecified thigh

6 **S76.81** Strain of other specified muscles, fascia and tendons at thigh level

7 🗐 **S76.811-** Strain of other specified muscles, fascia and tendons at thigh level, right thigh

7 🗐 **S76.812-** Strain of other specified muscles, fascia and tendons at thigh level, left thigh

7 🗐 **S76.819-** Strain of other specified muscles, fascia and tendons at thigh level, unspecified thigh

6 **S76.82** Laceration of other specified muscles, fascia and tendons at thigh level

CODING TIP ✓ Code also any associated open wound S71.-

7 🗐 **S76.821-** Laceration of other specified muscles, fascia and tendons at thigh level, right thigh

7 🗐 **S76.822-** Laceration of other specified muscles, fascia and tendons at thigh level, left thigh

7 🗐 **S76.829-** Laceration of other specified muscles, fascia and tendons at thigh level, unspecified thigh

6 **S76.89** Other injury of other specified muscles, fascia and tendons at thigh level

7 🗐 **S76.891-** Other injury of other specified muscles, fascia and tendons at thigh level, right thigh

7 🗐 **S76.892-** Other injury of other specified muscles, fascia and tendons at thigh level, left thigh

7 🗐 **S76.899-** Other injury of other specified muscles, fascia and tendons at thigh level, unspecified thigh

5 **S76.9** Injury of unspecified muscles, fascia and tendons at thigh level

6 **S76.90** Unspecified injury of unspecified muscles, fascia and tendons at thigh level

7 🗐 **S76.901-** Unspecified injury of unspecified muscles, fascia and tendons at thigh level, right thigh

7 🗐 **S76.902-** Unspecified injury of unspecified muscles, fascia and tendons at thigh level, left thigh

7 🗐 **S76.909-** Unspecified injury of unspecified muscles, fascia and tendons at thigh level, unspecified thigh

6 **S76.91** Strain of unspecified muscles, fascia and tendons at thigh level

7 🗐 **S76.911-** Strain of unspecified muscles, fascia and tendons at thigh level, right thigh

7 🗐 **S76.912-** Strain of unspecified muscles, fascia and tendons at thigh level, left thigh

7 🗐 **S76.919-** Strain of unspecified muscles, fascia and tendons at thigh level, unspecified thigh

6 **S76.92** Laceration of unspecified muscles, fascia and tendons at thigh level

CODING TIP ✓ Code also any associated open wound S71.-

7 🗐 **S76.921-** Laceration of unspecified muscles, fascia and tendons at thigh level, right thigh

7 🗐 **S76.922-** Laceration of unspecified muscles, fascia and tendons at thigh level, left thigh

7 🗐 **S76.929-** Laceration of unspecified muscles, fascia and tendons at thigh level, unspecified thigh

6 **S76.99** Other specified injury of unspecified muscles, fascia and tendons at thigh level

7 🗐 **S76.991-** Other specified injury of unspecified muscles, fascia and tendons at thigh level, right thigh

---

● New ▲ Revised *Manifestation* 4-7 Digit Indicators 🗐 Laterality A Adult (15+ years) M Maternity (12-55 years) N Newborn P Pediatric (0-17 years) ♂ Male ♀ Female
✖ ~~Deleted~~ Unspecified + Additional code

7 ⊟ **S76.992-**   Other specified injury of unspecified muscles, fascia and tendons at thigh level, left thigh

7 ⊟ **S76.999-**   Other specified injury of unspecified muscles, fascia and tendons at thigh level, unspecified thigh

4 + **S77**   **Crushing injury of hip and thigh**
Use additional code(s) for all associated injuries
EXCLUDES 2   *crushing injury of ankle and foot (S97.-)*
crushing injury of lower leg (S87.-)

The appropriate 7th character is to be added to each code from category S77
A   initial encounter
D   subsequent encounter
S   sequela

5 + **S77.0**   **Crushing injury of hip**
7 ⊟ + **S77.00X-**   **Crushing injury of unspecified hip**
7 ⊟ + **S77.01X-**   **Crushing injury of right hip**
7 ⊟ + **S77.02X-**   **Crushing injury of left hip**
5 + **S77.1**   **Crushing injury of thigh**
7 ⊟ + **S77.10X-**   **Crushing injury of unspecified thigh**
7 ⊟ + **S77.11X-**   **Crushing injury of right thigh**
7 ⊟ + **S77.12X-**   **Crushing injury of left thigh**
5 + **S77.2**   **Crushing injury of hip with thigh**
7 ⊟ + **S77.20X-**   **Crushing injury of unspecified hip with thigh**
7 ⊟ + **S77.21X-**   **Crushing injury of right hip with thigh**
7 ⊟ + **S77.22X-**   **Crushing injury of left hip with thigh**

4 **S78**   **Traumatic amputation of hip and thigh**
An amputation not identified as partial or complete should be coded to complete
EXCLUDES 1   *traumatic amputation of knee (S88.0-)*

The appropriate 7th character is to be added to each code from category S78
A   initial encounter
D   subsequent encounter
S   sequela

5 **S78.0**   **Traumatic amputation at hip joint**
6 **S78.01**   **Complete traumatic amputation at hip joint**
7 ⊟ **S78.011-**   Complete traumatic amputation at right hip joint
7 ⊟ **S78.012-**   Complete traumatic amputation at left hip joint
7 ⊟ **S78.019-**   Complete traumatic amputation at unspecified hip joint
6 **S78.02**   **Partial traumatic amputation at hip joint**
7 ⊟ **S78.021-**   Partial traumatic amputation at right hip joint
7 ⊟ **S78.022-**   Partial traumatic amputation at left hip joint
7 ⊟ **S78.029-**   Partial traumatic amputation at unspecified hip joint
5 **S78.1**   **Traumatic amputation at level between hip and knee**
EXCLUDES 1   *traumatic amputation of knee (S88.0-)*
6 **S78.11**   **Complete traumatic amputation at level between hip and knee**
7 ⊟ **S78.111-**   Complete traumatic amputation at level between right hip and knee
7 ⊟ **S78.112-**   Complete traumatic amputation at level between left hip and knee
7 ⊟ **S78.119-**   Complete traumatic amputation at level between unspecified hip and knee
6 **S78.12**   **Partial traumatic amputation at level between hip and knee**
7 ⊟ **S78.121-**   Partial traumatic amputation at level between right hip and knee
7 ⊟ **S78.122-**   Partial traumatic amputation at level between left hip and knee
7 ⊟ **S78.129-**   Partial traumatic amputation at level between unspecified hip and knee
5 **S78.9**   **Traumatic amputation of hip and thigh, level unspecified**
6 **S78.91**   **Complete traumatic amputation of hip and thigh, level unspecified**
7 ⊟ **S78.911-**   Complete traumatic amputation of right hip and thigh, level unspecified
7 ⊟ **S78.912-**   Complete traumatic amputation of left hip and thigh, level unspecified

7 ⊟ **S78.919-**   Complete traumatic amputation of unspecified hip and thigh, level unspecified
6 **S78.92**   **Partial traumatic amputation of hip and thigh, level unspecified**
7 ⊟ **S78.921-**   Partial traumatic amputation of right hip and thigh, level unspecified
7 ⊟ **S78.922-**   Partial traumatic amputation of left hip and thigh, level unspecified
7 ⊟ **S78.929-**   Partial traumatic amputation of unspecified hip and thigh, level unspecified

4 **S79**   **Other and unspecified injuries of hip and thigh**
Note: A fracture not indicated as open or closed should be coded to closed

The appropriate 7th character is to be added to each code from subcategories S79.0 and S79.1
A   initial encounter for closed fracture
D   subsequent encounter for fracture with routine healing
G   subsequent encounter for fracture with delayed healing
K   subsequent encounter for fracture with nonunion
P   subsequent encounter for fracture with malunion
S   sequela

5 **S79.0**   **Physeal fracture of upper end of femur**
EXCLUDES 1   *apophyseal fracture of upper end of femur (S72.13-)*
nontraumatic slipped upper femoral epiphysis (M93.0-)
6 **S79.00**   **Unspecified physeal fracture of upper end of femur**
7 ⊟ **S79.001-**   Unspecified physeal fracture of upper end of right femur
7 ⊟ **S79.002-**   Unspecified physeal fracture of upper end of left femur
7 ⊟ **S79.009-**   Unspecified physeal fracture of upper end of unspecified femur
6 **S79.01**   **Salter-Harris Type I physeal fracture of upper end of femur**
Acute on chronic slipped capital femoral epiphysis (traumatic)
Acute slipped capital femoral epiphysis (traumatic)
Capital femoral epiphyseal fracture
EXCLUDES 1   *chronic slipped upper femoral epiphysis (nontraumatic) (M93.02-)*
7 ⊟ **S79.011-**   Salter-Harris Type I physeal fracture of upper end of right femur

**Physeal fracture (Salter-Harris) Type 1
upper end of right femur**

Type 1 physeal fracture
Upper end of femur
Epiphysys
Growth (epiphyseal) disks
Metaphysys

7 ⊟ **S79.012-**   Salter-Harris Type I physeal fracture of upper end of left femur
7 ⊟ **S79.019-**   Salter-Harris Type I physeal fracture of upper end of unspecified femur
6 **S79.09**   **Other physeal fracture of upper end of femur**
7 ⊟ **S79.091-**   Other physeal fracture of upper end of right femur
7 ⊟ **S79.092-**   Other physeal fracture of upper end of left femur
7 ⊟ **S79.099-**   Other physeal fracture of upper end of unspecified femur
5 **S79.1**   **Physeal fracture of lower end of femur**

● New   ▲ Revised   *Manifestation*   4-7 Digit Indicators   ⊟ Laterality   A Adult (15+ years)   M Maternity (12-55 years)   N Newborn   P Pediatric (0-17 years)   ♂ Male   ♀ Female
✖ Deleted   Unspecified   + Additional code

⑥ **S79.10** Unspecified physeal fracture of lower end of femur

⑦⊟ **S79.101-** Unspecified physeal fracture of lower end of right femur

⑦⊟ **S79.102-** Unspecified physeal fracture of lower end of left femur

⑦⊟ **S79.109-** Unspecified physeal fracture of lower end of unspecified femur

⑥ **S79.11** Salter-Harris Type I physeal fracture of lower end of femur

⑦⊟ **S79.111-** Salter-Harris Type I physeal fracture of lower end of right femur

⑦⊟ **S79.112-** Salter-Harris Type I physeal fracture of lower end of left femur

⑦⊟ **S79.119-** Salter-Harris Type I physeal fracture of lower end of unspecified femur

⑥ **S79.12** Salter-Harris Type II physeal fracture of lower end of femur

⑦⊟ **S79.121-** Salter-Harris Type II physeal fracture of lower end of right femur

⑦⊟ **S79.122-** Salter-Harris Type II physeal fracture of lower end of left femur

⑦⊟ **S79.129-** Salter-Harris Type II physeal fracture of lower end of unspecified femur

⑥ **S79.13** Salter-Harris Type III physeal fracture of lower end of femur

⑦⊟ **S79.131-** Salter-Harris Type III physeal fracture of lower end of right femur

⑦⊟ **S79.132-** Salter-Harris Type III physeal fracture of lower end of left femur

⑦⊟ **S79.139-** Salter-Harris Type III physeal fracture of lower end of unspecified femur

⑥ **S79.14** Salter-Harris Type IV physeal fracture of lower end of femur

⑦⊟ **S79.141-** Salter-Harris Type IV physeal fracture of lower end of right femur

⑦⊟ **S79.142-** Salter-Harris Type IV physeal fracture of lower end of left femur

⑦⊟ **S79.149-** Salter-Harris Type IV physeal fracture of lower end of unspecified femur

⑥ **S79.19** Other physeal fracture of lower end of femur

⑦⊟ **S79.191-** Other physeal fracture of lower end of right femur

⑦⊟ **S79.192-** Other physeal fracture of lower end of left femur

⑦⊟ **S79.199-** Other physeal fracture of lower end of unspecified femur

⑤ **S79.8** Other specified injuries of hip and thigh

The appropriate 7th character is to be added to each code in subcategory S79.8
A   initial encounter
D   subsequent encounter
S   sequela

⑥ **S79.81** Other specified injuries of hip

⑦⊟ **S79.811-** Other specified injuries of right hip

⑦⊟ **S79.812-** Other specified injuries of left hip

⑦⊟ **S79.819-** Other specified injuries of unspecified hip

⑥ **S79.82** Other specified injuries of thigh

⑦⊟ **S79.821-** Other specified injuries of right thigh

⑦⊟ **S79.822-** Other specified injuries of left thigh

⑦⊟ **S79.829-** Other specified injuries of unspecified thigh

⑤ **S79.9** Unspecified injury of hip and thigh

The appropriate 7th character is to be added to each code in subcategory S79.9
A   initial encounter
D   subsequent encounter
S   sequela

⑥ **S79.91** Unspecified injury of hip

⑦⊟ **S79.911-** Unspecified injury of right hip

⑦⊟ **S79.912-** Unspecified injury of left hip

⑦⊟ **S79.919-** Unspecified injury of unspecified hip

⑥ **S79.92** Unspecified injury of thigh

⑦⊟ **S79.921-** Unspecified injury of right thigh

⑦⊟ **S79.922-** Unspecified injury of left thigh

⑦⊟ **S79.929-** Unspecified injury of unspecified thigh

Injuries to the knee and lower leg (S80-S89)

EXCLUDES 2   *burns and corrosions (T20-T32)*
frostbite (T33-T34)
injuries of ankle and foot, except fracture of ankle and malleolus (S90-S99)
insect bite or sting, venomous (T63.4)

GUIDELINES   **Section I.C.19.c.2)**
Multiple fractures are sequenced in accordance with the severity of the fracture.

GUIDELINES   **Section I.C.19.b.1)-2)**
When coding injuries, assign separate codes for each injury unless a combination code is provided, in which case the combination code is assigned ... Traumatic injury codes (S00-T14.9) are not to be used for normal, healing surgical wounds or to identify complications of surgical wounds. The code for the most serious injury, as determined by the provider and the focus of treatment, is sequenced first.

1) Superficial injuries such as abrasions or contusions are not coded when associated with more severe injuries of the same site.

2) When a primary injury results in minor damage to peripheral nerves or blood vessels, the primary injury is sequenced first with additional code(s) for injuries to nerves and spinal cord (such as category S04), and/or injury to blood vessels (such as category S15). When the primary injury is to the blood vessels or nerves, that injury should be sequenced first.

GUIDELINES   **Section I.C.19.c**
Coding of Traumatic Fractures: The principles of multiple coding of injuries should be followed in coding fractures. Fractures of specified sites are coded individually by site in accordance with both the provisions within categories S02, S12, S22, S32, S42, S49, S52, S59, S62, S72, S79, S82, S89, S92 and the level of detail furnished by medical record content. A fracture not indicated as open or closed should be coded to closed. A fracture not indicated whether displaced or not displaced should be coded to displaced.

④ **S80**   **Superficial injury of knee and lower leg**

EXCLUDES 2   *superficial injury of ankle and foot (S90.-)*

The appropriate 7th character is to be added to each code from category S80
A   initial encounter
D   subsequent encounter
S   sequela

⑤ **S80.0**   Contusion of knee

⑦⊟ **S80.00X-**   Contusion of unspecified knee

⑦⊟ **S80.01X-**   Contusion of right knee

⑦⊟ **S80.02X-**   Contusion of left knee

⑤ **S80.1**   Contusion of lower leg

⑦⊟ **S80.10X-**   Contusion of unspecified lower leg

⑦⊟ **S80.11X-**   Contusion of right lower leg

⑦⊟ **S80.12X-**   Contusion of left lower leg

⑤ **S80.2**   Other superficial injuries of knee

⑥ **S80.21**   Abrasion of knee

⑦⊟ **S80.211-**   Abrasion, right knee

⑦⊟ **S80.212-**   Abrasion, left knee

⑦⊟ **S80.219-**   Abrasion, unspecified knee

⑥ **S80.22**   Blister (nonthermal) of knee

⑦⊟ **S80.221-**   Blister (nonthermal), right knee

⑦⊟ **S80.222-**   Blister (nonthermal), left knee

⑦⊟ **S80.229-**   Blister (nonthermal), unspecified knee

⑥ **S80.24**   External constriction of knee

⑦⊟ **S80.241-**   External constriction, right knee

⑦⊟ **S80.242-**   External constriction, left knee

⑦⊟ **S80.249-**   External constriction, unspecified knee

⑥ **S80.25**   Superficial foreign body of knee
Splinter in the knee

⑦⊟ **S80.251-**   Superficial foreign body, right knee

⑦⊟ **S80.252-**   Superficial foreign body, left knee

⑦⊟ **S80.259-**   Superficial foreign body, unspecified knee

⑥ **S80.26**   Insect bite (nonvenomous) of knee

● New   ▲ Revised   *Manifestation*   ④-⑦ Digit Indicators   ⊟ Laterality   Ⓐ Adult (15+ years)   Ⓜ Maternity (12-55 years)   Ⓝ Newborn   Ⓟ Pediatric (0-17 years)   ♂ Male   ♀ Female
✖ Deleted   Unspecified   + Additional code

7️⃣⊟ S80.261-   Insect bite (nonvenomous), right knee
7️⃣⊟ S80.262-   Insect bite (nonvenomous), left knee
7️⃣⊟ S80.269-   Insect bite (nonvenomous), unspecified knee
6️⃣ S80.27   Other superficial bite of knee
      EXCLUDES 1   *open bite of knee (S81.05-)*
7️⃣⊟ S80.271-   Other superficial bite of right knee
7️⃣⊟ S80.272-   Other superficial bite of left knee
7️⃣⊟ S80.279-   Other superficial bite of unspecified knee
5️⃣ S80.8   Other superficial injuries of lower leg
   6️⃣ S80.81   Abrasion of lower leg
7️⃣⊟ S80.811-   Abrasion, right lower leg
7️⃣⊟ S80.812-   Abrasion, left lower leg
7️⃣⊟ S80.819-   Abrasion, unspecified lower leg
   6️⃣ S80.82   Blister (nonthermal) of lower leg
7️⃣⊟ S80.821-   Blister (nonthermal), right lower leg
7️⃣⊟ S80.822-   Blister (nonthermal), left lower leg
7️⃣⊟ S80.829-   Blister (nonthermal), unspecified lower leg
   6️⃣ S80.84   External constriction of lower leg
7️⃣⊟ S80.841-   External constriction, right lower leg
7️⃣⊟ S80.842-   External constriction, left lower leg
7️⃣⊟ S80.849-   External constriction, unspecified lower leg
   6️⃣ S80.85   Superficial foreign body of lower leg
      Splinter in the lower leg
7️⃣⊟ S80.851-   Superficial foreign body, right lower leg
7️⃣⊟ S80.852-   Superficial foreign body, left lower leg
7️⃣⊟ S80.859-   Superficial foreign body, unspecified lower leg
   6️⃣ S80.86   Insect bite (nonvenomous) of lower leg
7️⃣⊟ S80.861-   Insect bite (nonvenomous), right lower leg
7️⃣⊟ S80.862-   Insect bite (nonvenomous), left lower leg
7️⃣⊟ S80.869-   Insect bite (nonvenomous), unspecified lower leg
   6️⃣ S80.87   Other superficial bite of lower leg
      EXCLUDES 1   *open bite of lower leg (S81.85-)*
7️⃣⊟ S80.871-   Other superficial bite, right lower leg
7️⃣⊟ S80.872-   Other superficial bite, left lower leg
7️⃣⊟ S80.879-   Other superficial bite, unspecified lower leg
5️⃣ S80.9   Unspecified superficial injury of knee and lower leg
   6️⃣ S80.91   Unspecified superficial injury of knee
7️⃣⊟ S80.911-   Unspecified superficial injury of right knee
7️⃣⊟ S80.912-   Unspecified superficial injury of left knee
7️⃣⊟ S80.919-   Unspecified superficial injury of unspecified knee
   6️⃣ S80.92   Unspecified superficial injury of lower leg
7️⃣⊟ S80.921-   Unspecified superficial injury of right lower leg
7️⃣⊟ S80.922-   Unspecified superficial injury of left lower leg
7️⃣⊟ S80.929-   Unspecified superficial injury of unspecified lower leg

4️⃣ S81   Open wound of knee and lower leg
      Code also:
         any associated wound infection
      EXCLUDES 1   *open fracture of knee and lower leg (S82.-)*
                    traumatic amputation of lower leg (S88.-)
      EXCLUDES 2   *open wound of ankle and foot (S91.-)*

The appropriate 7th character is to be added to each code from category S81.
A   initial encounter
D   subsequent encounter
S   sequela

CODING TIP ✓   Open wound codes indicate a wound resulting from a traumatic origin. Do not assign a code for "open wound" unless the etiology of the wound is related to trauma.

5️⃣ S81.0   Open wound of knee
   6️⃣ S81.00   Unspecified open wound of knee
7️⃣⊟ S81.001-   Unspecified open wound, right knee
7️⃣⊟ S81.002-   Unspecified open wound, left knee
7️⃣⊟ S81.009-   Unspecified open wound, unspecified knee

   6️⃣ S81.01   Laceration without foreign body of knee
7️⃣⊟ S81.011-   Laceration without foreign body, right knee
7️⃣⊟ S81.012-   Laceration without foreign body, left knee
7️⃣⊟ S81.019-   Laceration without foreign body, unspecified knee
   6️⃣ S81.02   Laceration with foreign body of knee
7️⃣⊟ S81.021-   Laceration with foreign body, right knee
7️⃣⊟ S81.022-   Laceration with foreign body, left knee
7️⃣⊟ S81.029-   Laceration with foreign body, unspecified knee
   6️⃣ S81.03   Puncture wound without foreign body of knee
7️⃣⊟ S81.031-   Puncture wound without foreign body, right knee
7️⃣⊟ S81.032-   Puncture wound without foreign body, left knee
7️⃣⊟ S81.039-   Puncture wound without foreign body, unspecified knee
   6️⃣ S81.04   Puncture wound with foreign body of knee
7️⃣⊟ S81.041-   Puncture wound with foreign body, right knee
7️⃣⊟ S81.042-   Puncture wound with foreign body, left knee
7️⃣⊟ S81.049-   Puncture wound with foreign body, unspecified knee
   6️⃣ S81.05   Open bite of knee
      Bite of knee NOS
      EXCLUDES 1   *superficial bite of knee (S80.27-)*
7️⃣⊟ S81.051-   Open bite, right knee
7️⃣⊟ S81.052-   Open bite, left knee
7️⃣⊟ S81.059-   Open bite, unspecified knee
5️⃣ S81.8   Open wound of lower leg
   6️⃣ S81.80   Unspecified open wound of lower leg
7️⃣⊟ S81.801-   Unspecified open wound, right lower leg
7️⃣⊟ S81.802-   Unspecified open wound, left lower leg
7️⃣⊟ S81.809-   Unspecified open wound, unspecified lower leg
   6️⃣ S81.81   Laceration without foreign body of lower leg
7️⃣⊟ S81.811-   Laceration without foreign body, right lower leg
7️⃣⊟ S81.812-   Laceration without foreign body, left lower leg
7️⃣⊟ S81.819-   Laceration without foreign body, unspecified lower leg
   6️⃣ S81.82   Laceration with foreign body of lower leg
7️⃣⊟ S81.821-   Laceration with foreign body, right lower leg
7️⃣⊟ S81.822-   Laceration with foreign body, left lower leg
7️⃣⊟ S81.829-   Laceration with foreign body, unspecified lower leg
   6️⃣ S81.83   Puncture wound without foreign body of lower leg
7️⃣⊟ S81.831-   Puncture wound without foreign body, right lower leg
7️⃣⊟ S81.832-   Puncture wound without foreign body, left lower leg
7️⃣⊟ S81.839-   Puncture wound without foreign body, unspecified lower leg
   6️⃣ S81.84   Puncture wound with foreign body of lower leg
7️⃣⊟ S81.841-   Puncture wound with foreign body, right lower leg
7️⃣⊟ S81.842-   Puncture wound with foreign body, left lower leg
7️⃣⊟ S81.849-   Puncture wound with foreign body, unspecified lower leg
   6️⃣ S81.85   Open bite of lower leg
      Bite of lower leg NOS
      EXCLUDES 1   *superficial bite of lower leg (S80.86-, S80.87-)*
7️⃣⊟ S81.851-   Open bite, right lower leg
7️⃣⊟ S81.852-   Open bite, left lower leg
7️⃣⊟ S81.859-   Open bite, unspecified lower leg

◢ S82   **Fracture of lower leg, including ankle**

Note: A fracture not indicated as displaced or nondisplaced should be coded to displaced

A fracture not indicated as open or closed should be coded to closed

The open fracture designations are based on the Gustilo open fracture classification

| INCLUDES | fracture of malleolus |

| EXCLUDES 1 | *traumatic amputation of lower leg (S88.-)* |

| EXCLUDES 2 | *fracture of foot, except ankle (S92.-)* |
| | *periprosthetic fracture of prosthetic implant of knee (T84.042, T84.043)* |

The appropriate 7th character is to be added to all codes from category S82

A   initial encounter for closed fracture

B   initial encounter for open fracture type I or II

C   initial encounter for open fracture type IIIA, IIIB, or IIIC

D   subsequent encounter for closed fracture with routine healing

E   subsequent encounter for open fracture type I or II with routine healing

F   subsequent encounter for open fracture type IIIA, IIIB, or IIIC with routine healing

G   subsequent encounter for closed fracture with delayed healing

H   subsequent encounter for open fracture type I or II with delayed healing

J   subsequent encounter for open fracture type IIIA, IIIB, or IIIC with delayed healing

K   subsequent encounter for closed fracture with nonunion

M   subsequent encounter for open fracture type I or II with nonunion

N   subsequent encounter for open fracture type IIIA, IIIB, or IIIC with nonunion

P   subsequent encounter for closed fracture with malunion

Q   subsequent encounter for open fracture type I or II with malunion

R   subsequent encounter for open fracture type IIIA, IIIB, or IIIC with malunion

S   sequela

| CODING TIP ✓ | A fracture not indicated as displaced or nondisplaced should be coded to displaced. A fracture not indicated as open or closed should be coded to closed. Query providers on fractures not documented as displaced/nondisplaced otherwise displaced fracture diagnosis could be assigned without reduction being performed potentially resulting in claim denials. |

⑤ S82.0   **Fracture of patella**

　　Knee cap

⑥ S82.00   **Unspecified fracture of patella**

　⑦ S82.001-   Unspecified fracture of right patella

　⑦ S82.002-   Unspecified fracture of left patella

　⑦ S82.009-   Unspecified fracture of unspecified patella

⑥ S82.01   **Osteochondral fracture of patella**

　⑦ S82.011-   Displaced osteochondral fracture of right patella

　⑦ S82.012-   Displaced osteochondral fracture of left patella

　⑦ S82.013-   Displaced osteochondral fracture of unspecified patella

　⑦ S82.014-   Nondisplaced osteochondral fracture of right patella

　⑦ S82.015-   Nondisplaced osteochondral fracture of left patella

　⑦ S82.016-   Nondisplaced osteochondral fracture of unspecified patella

⑥ S82.02   **Longitudinal fracture of patella**

　⑦ S82.021-   Displaced longitudinal fracture of right patella

　⑦ S82.022-   Displaced longitudinal fracture of left patella

　⑦ S82.023-   Displaced longitudinal fracture of unspecified patella

　⑦ S82.024-   Nondisplaced longitudinal fracture of right patella

　⑦ S82.025-   Nondisplaced longitudinal fracture of left patella

　⑦ S82.026-   Nondisplaced longitudinal fracture of unspecified patella

⑥ S82.03   **Transverse fracture of patella**

　⑦ S82.031-   Displaced transverse fracture of right patella

　⑦ S82.032-   Displaced transverse fracture of left patella

　⑦ S82.033-   Displaced transverse fracture of unspecified patella

　⑦ S82.034-   Nondisplaced transverse fracture of right patella

　⑦ S82.035-   Nondisplaced transverse fracture of left patella

　⑦ S82.036-   Nondisplaced transverse fracture of unspecified patella

⑥ S82.04   **Comminuted fracture of patella**

　⑦ S82.041-   Displaced comminuted fracture of right patella

　⑦ S82.042-   Displaced comminuted fracture of left patella

　⑦ S82.043-   Displaced comminuted fracture of unspecified patella

　⑦ S82.044-   Nondisplaced comminuted fracture of right patella

　⑦ S82.045-   Nondisplaced comminuted fracture of left patella

　⑦ S82.046-   Nondisplaced comminuted fracture of unspecified patella

⑥ S82.09   **Other fracture of patella**

　⑦ S82.091-   Other fracture of right patella

　⑦ S82.092-   Other fracture of left patella

　⑦ S82.099-   Other fracture of unspecified patella

⑤ S82.1   **Fracture of upper end of tibia**

　　Fracture of proximal end of tibia

| EXCLUDES 2 | *fracture of shaft of tibia (S82.2-)* |
| | *physeal fracture of upper end of tibia (S89.0-)* |

⑥ S82.10   **Unspecified fracture of upper end of tibia**

　⑦ S82.101-   Unspecified fracture of upper end of right tibia

　⑦ S82.102-   Unspecified fracture of upper end of left tibia

　⑦ S82.109-   Unspecified fracture of upper end of unspecified tibia

⑥ S82.11   **Fracture of tibial spine**

　⑦ S82.111-   Displaced fracture of right tibial spine

　⑦ S82.112-   Displaced fracture of left tibial spine

　⑦ S82.113-   Displaced fracture of unspecified tibial spine

　⑦ S82.114-   Nondisplaced fracture of right tibial spine

　⑦ S82.115-   Nondisplaced fracture of left tibial spine

　⑦ S82.116-   Nondisplaced fracture of unspecified tibial spine

⑥ S82.12   **Fracture of lateral condyle of tibia**

　⑦ S82.121-   Displaced fracture of lateral condyle of right tibia

　⑦ S82.122-   Displaced fracture of lateral condyle of left tibia

　⑦ S82.123-   Displaced fracture of lateral condyle of unspecified tibia

　⑦ S82.124-   Nondisplaced fracture of lateral condyle of right tibia

　⑦ S82.125-   Nondisplaced fracture of lateral condyle of left tibia

　⑦ S82.126-   Nondisplaced fracture of lateral condyle of unspecified tibia

⑥ S82.13   **Fracture of medial condyle of tibia**

　⑦ S82.131-   Displaced fracture of medial condyle of right tibia

　⑦ S82.132-   Displaced fracture of medial condyle of left tibia

　⑦ S82.133-   Displaced fracture of medial condyle of unspecified tibia

　⑦ S82.134-   Nondisplaced fracture of medial condyle of right tibia

　⑦ S82.135-   Nondisplaced fracture of medial condyle of left tibia

　⑦ S82.136-   Nondisplaced fracture of medial condyle of unspecified tibia

⑥ S82.14   **Bicondylar fracture of tibia**

　　Fracture of tibial plateau NOS

　⑦ S82.141-   Displaced bicondylar fracture of right tibia

　⑦ S82.142-   Displaced bicondylar fracture of left tibia

● New   ▲ Revised   *Manifestation*   ◢-⑦ Digit Indicators   ⊟ Laterality   🅐 Adult (15+ years)   🅜 Maternity (12-55 years)   🅝 Newborn   🅟 Pediatric (0-17 years)   ♂ Male   ♀ Female

✖ ̶D̶e̶l̶e̶t̶e̶d̶   Unspecified   ＋ Additional code

2017 ICD-10-CM Expert for Physicians

© 2017 DecisionHealth

1015

7️⃣🔲 **S82.143-**   **Displaced bicondylar fracture of unspecified tibia**

7️⃣🔲 **S82.144-**   **Nondisplaced bicondylar fracture of right tibia**

7️⃣🔲 **S82.145-**   **Nondisplaced bicondylar fracture of left tibia**

7️⃣🔲 **S82.146-**   **Nondisplaced bicondylar fracture of unspecified tibia**

6️⃣ **S82.15**   **Fracture of tibial tuberosity**

7️⃣🔲 **S82.151-**   **Displaced fracture of right tibial tuberosity**

7️⃣🔲 **S82.152-**   **Displaced fracture of left tibial tuberosity**

7️⃣🔲 **S82.153-**   **Displaced fracture of unspecified tibial tuberosity**

7️⃣🔲 **S82.154-**   **Nondisplaced fracture of right tibial tuberosity**

7️⃣🔲 **S82.155-**   **Nondisplaced fracture of left tibial tuberosity**

7️⃣🔲 **S82.156-**   **Nondisplaced fracture of unspecified tibial tuberosity**

6️⃣ **S82.16**   **Torus fracture of upper end of tibia**

> The appropriate 7th character is to be added to all codes in subcategory S82.16
>
> A   initial encounter for closed fracture
> D   subsequent encounter for fracture with routine healing
> G   subsequent encounter for fracture with delayed healing
> K   subsequent encounter for fracture with nonunion
> P   subsequent encounter for fracture with malunion
> S   sequela

7️⃣🔲 **S82.161-**   **Torus fracture of upper end of right tibia**

7️⃣🔲 **S82.162-**   **Torus fracture of upper end of left tibia**

7️⃣🔲 **S82.169-**   **Torus fracture of upper end of unspecified tibia**

6️⃣ **S82.19**   **Other fracture of upper end of tibia**

7️⃣🔲 **S82.191-**   **Other fracture of upper end of right tibia**

7️⃣🔲 **S82.192-**   **Other fracture of upper end of left tibia**

7️⃣🔲 **S82.199-**   **Other fracture of upper end of unspecified tibia**

5️⃣ **S82.2**   **Fracture of shaft of tibia**

6️⃣ **S82.20**   **Unspecified fracture of shaft of tibia**
Fracture of tibia NOS

7️⃣🔲 **S82.201-**   **Unspecified fracture of shaft of right tibia**

7️⃣🔲 **S82.202-**   **Unspecified fracture of shaft of left tibia**

7️⃣🔲 **S82.209-**   **Unspecified fracture of shaft of unspecified tibia**

6️⃣ **S82.22**   **Transverse fracture of shaft of tibia**

7️⃣🔲 **S82.221-**   **Displaced transverse fracture of shaft of right tibia**

7️⃣🔲 **S82.222-**   **Displaced transverse fracture of shaft of left tibia**

7️⃣🔲 **S82.223-**   **Displaced transverse fracture of shaft of unspecified tibia**

7️⃣🔲 **S82.224-**   **Nondisplaced transverse fracture of shaft of right tibia**

7️⃣🔲 **S82.225-**   **Nondisplaced transverse fracture of shaft of left tibia**

7️⃣🔲 **S82.226-**   **Nondisplaced transverse fracture of shaft of unspecified tibia**

6️⃣ **S82.23**   **Oblique fracture of shaft of tibia**

7️⃣🔲 **S82.231-**   **Displaced oblique fracture of shaft of right tibia**

7️⃣🔲 **S82.232-**   **Displaced oblique fracture of shaft of left tibia**

7️⃣🔲 **S82.233-**   **Displaced oblique fracture of shaft of unspecified tibia**

7️⃣🔲 **S82.234-**   **Nondisplaced oblique fracture of shaft of right tibia**
AHA: (S82.234A) 1Q 2015, 9
AHA: (S82.234D) 1Q 2015, 10

7️⃣🔲 **S82.235-**   **Nondisplaced oblique fracture of shaft of left tibia**

7️⃣🔲 **S82.236-**   **Nondisplaced oblique fracture of shaft of unspecified tibia**

6️⃣ **S82.24**   **Spiral fracture of shaft of tibia**
Toddler fracture

7️⃣🔲 **S82.241-**   **Displaced spiral fracture of shaft of right tibia**

7️⃣🔲 **S82.242-**   **Displaced spiral fracture of shaft of left tibia**

7️⃣🔲 **S82.243-**   **Displaced spiral fracture of shaft of unspecified tibia**

7️⃣🔲 **S82.244-**   **Nondisplaced spiral fracture of shaft of right tibia**

7️⃣🔲 **S82.245-**   **Nondisplaced spiral fracture of shaft of left tibia**

7️⃣🔲 **S82.246-**   **Nondisplaced spiral fracture of shaft of unspecified tibia**

6️⃣ **S82.25**   **Comminuted fracture of shaft of tibia**

7️⃣🔲 **S82.251-**   **Displaced comminuted fracture of shaft of right tibia**
AHA: (S82.251D) 2Q 2015, 6

7️⃣🔲 **S82.252-**   **Displaced comminuted fracture of shaft of left tibia**

7️⃣🔲 **S82.253-**   **Displaced comminuted fracture of shaft of unspecified tibia**

7️⃣🔲 **S82.254-**   **Nondisplaced comminuted fracture of shaft of right tibia**

7️⃣🔲 **S82.255-**   **Nondisplaced comminuted fracture of shaft of left tibia**

7️⃣🔲 **S82.256-**   **Nondisplaced comminuted fracture of shaft of unspecified tibia**

6️⃣ **S82.26**   **Segmental fracture of shaft of tibia**

7️⃣🔲 **S82.261-**   **Displaced segmental fracture of shaft of right tibia**

7️⃣🔲 **S82.262-**   **Displaced segmental fracture of shaft of left tibia**

7️⃣🔲 **S82.263-**   **Displaced segmental fracture of shaft of unspecified tibia**

7️⃣🔲 **S82.264-**   **Nondisplaced segmental fracture of shaft of right tibia**

7️⃣🔲 **S82.265-**   **Nondisplaced segmental fracture of shaft of left tibia**

7️⃣🔲 **S82.266-**   **Nondisplaced segmental fracture of shaft of unspecified tibia**

6️⃣ **S82.29**   **Other fracture of shaft of tibia**

7️⃣🔲 **S82.291-**   **Other fracture of shaft of right tibia**

7️⃣🔲 **S82.292-**   **Other fracture of shaft of left tibia**

7️⃣🔲 **S82.299-**   **Other fracture of shaft of unspecified tibia**

5️⃣ **S82.3**   **Fracture of lower end of tibia**

> **EXCLUDES 1**   *bimalleolar fracture of lower leg (S82.84-)*
> *fracture of medial malleolus alone (S82.5-)*
> *Maisonneuve's fracture (S82.86-)*
> *pilon fracture of distal tibia (S82.87-)*
> *trimalleolar fractures of lower leg (S82.85-)*

6️⃣ **S82.30**   **Unspecified fracture of lower end of tibia**

7️⃣🔲 **S82.301-**   **Unspecified fracture of lower end of right tibia**

7️⃣🔲 **S82.302-**   **Unspecified fracture of lower end of left tibia**

7️⃣🔲 **S82.309-**   **Unspecified fracture of lower end of unspecified tibia**

6️⃣ **S82.31**   **Torus fracture of lower end of tibia**

> The appropriate 7th character is to be added to all codes in subcategory S82.31
>
> A   initial encounter for closed fracture
> D   subsequent encounter for fracture with routine healing
> G   subsequent encounter for fracture with delayed healing
> K   subsequent encounter for fracture with nonunion
> P   subsequent encounter for fracture with malunion
> S   sequela

7️⃣🔲 **S82.311-**   **Torus fracture of lower end of right tibia**

7️⃣🔲 **S82.312-**   **Torus fracture of lower end of left tibia**

7️⃣🔲 **S82.319-**   **Torus fracture of lower end of unspecified tibia**

6️⃣ **S82.39**   **Other fracture of lower end of tibia**

7️⃣🔲 **S82.391-**   **Other fracture of lower end of right tibia**

7️⃣🔲 **S82.392-**   **Other fracture of lower end of left tibia**
AHA: 1Q 2015, 25

7️⃣🔲 **S82.399-**   **Other fracture of lower end of unspecified tibia**

5️⃣ **S82.4**   **Fracture of shaft of fibula**

> **EXCLUDES 2**   *fracture of lateral malleolus alone (S82.6-)*

6️⃣ **S82.40**   **Unspecified fracture of shaft of fibula**

● New   ▲ Revised   *Manifestation*   4️⃣-7️⃣ Digit Indicators   🔲 Laterality   🅰 Adult (15+ years)   Ⓜ Maternity (12-55 years)   Ⓝ Newborn   🅿 Pediatric (0-17 years)   ♂ Male   ♀ Female

✖ ~~Deleted~~   Unspecified   + Additional code

7 ⊟	**S82.401-**	Unspecified fracture of shaft of right fibula
7 ⊟	**S82.402-**	Unspecified fracture of shaft of left fibula
7 ⊟	**S82.409-**	Unspecified fracture of shaft of unspecified fibula

6 **S82.42** Transverse fracture of shaft of fibula

7 ⊟	**S82.421-**	Displaced transverse fracture of shaft of right fibula
7 ⊟	**S82.422-**	Displaced transverse fracture of shaft of left fibula
7 ⊟	**S82.423-**	Displaced transverse fracture of shaft of unspecified fibula
7 ⊟	**S82.424-**	Nondisplaced transverse fracture of shaft of right fibula
7 ⊟	**S82.425-**	Nondisplaced transverse fracture of shaft of left fibula
7 ⊟	**S82.426-**	Nondisplaced transverse fracture of shaft of unspecified fibula

6 **S82.43** Oblique fracture of shaft of fibula

7 ⊟	**S82.431-**	Displaced oblique fracture of shaft of right fibula
7 ⊟	**S82.432-**	Displaced oblique fracture of shaft of left fibula
7 ⊟	**S82.433-**	Displaced oblique fracture of shaft of unspecified fibula
7 ⊟	**S82.434-**	Nondisplaced oblique fracture of shaft of right fibula
7 ⊟	**S82.435-**	Nondisplaced oblique fracture of shaft of left fibula
7 ⊟	**S82.436-**	Nondisplaced oblique fracture of shaft of unspecified fibula

6 **S82.44** Spiral fracture of shaft of fibula

7 ⊟	**S82.441-**	Displaced spiral fracture of shaft of right fibula
7 ⊟	**S82.442-**	Displaced spiral fracture of shaft of left fibula
7 ⊟	**S82.443-**	Displaced spiral fracture of shaft of unspecified fibula
7 ⊟	**S82.444-**	Nondisplaced spiral fracture of shaft of right fibula
7 ⊟	**S82.445-**	Nondisplaced spiral fracture of shaft of left fibula
7 ⊟	**S82.446-**	Nondisplaced spiral fracture of shaft of unspecified fibula

6 **S82.45** Comminuted fracture of shaft of fibula

7 ⊟	**S82.451-**	Displaced comminuted fracture of shaft of right fibula
7 ⊟	**S82.452-**	Displaced comminuted fracture of shaft of left fibula
7 ⊟	**S82.453-**	Displaced comminuted fracture of shaft of unspecified fibula
7 ⊟	**S82.454-**	Nondisplaced comminuted fracture of shaft of right fibula
7 ⊟	**S82.455-**	Nondisplaced comminuted fracture of shaft of left fibula
7 ⊟	**S82.456-**	Nondisplaced comminuted fracture of shaft of unspecified fibula

6 **S82.46** Segmental fracture of shaft of fibula

7 ⊟	**S82.461-**	Displaced segmental fracture of shaft of right fibula
7 ⊟	**S82.462-**	Displaced segmental fracture of shaft of left fibula
7 ⊟	**S82.463-**	Displaced segmental fracture of shaft of unspecified fibula
7 ⊟	**S82.464-**	Nondisplaced segmental fracture of shaft of right fibula
7 ⊟	**S82.465-**	Nondisplaced segmental fracture of shaft of left fibula
7 ⊟	**S82.466-**	Nondisplaced segmental fracture of shaft of unspecified fibula

6 **S82.49** Other fracture of shaft of fibula

7 ⊟	**S82.491-**	Other fracture of shaft of right fibula
7 ⊟	**S82.492-**	Other fracture of shaft of left fibula
7 ⊟	**S82.499-**	Other fracture of shaft of unspecified fibula

5 **S82.5** Fracture of medial malleolus

> **EXCLUDES 1** *pilon fracture of distal tibia (S82.87-)*
> *Salter-Harris type III of lower end of tibia (S89.13-)*
> *Salter-Harris type IV of lower end of tibia (S89.14-)*

7 ⊟	**S82.51X-**	Displaced fracture of medial malleolus of right tibia
7 ⊟	**S82.52X-**	Displaced fracture of medial malleolus of left tibia
7 ⊟	**S82.53X-**	Displaced fracture of medial malleolus of unspecified tibia
7 ⊟	**S82.54X-**	Nondisplaced fracture of medial malleolus of right tibia
7 ⊟	**S82.55X-**	Nondisplaced fracture of medial malleolus of left tibia
7 ⊟	**S82.56X-**	Nondisplaced fracture of medial malleolus of unspecified tibia

5 **S82.6** Fracture of lateral malleolus

> **EXCLUDES 1** *pilon fracture of distal tibia (S82.87-)*

7 ⊟	**S82.61X-**	Displaced fracture of lateral malleolus of right fibula
7 ⊟	**S82.62X-**	Displaced fracture of lateral malleolus of left fibula
7 ⊟	**S82.63X-**	Displaced fracture of lateral malleolus of unspecified fibula
7 ⊟	**S82.64X-**	Nondisplaced fracture of lateral malleolus of right fibula
7 ⊟	**S82.65X-**	Nondisplaced fracture of lateral malleolus of left fibula
7 ⊟	**S82.66X-**	Nondisplaced fracture of lateral malleolus of unspecified fibula

5 **S82.8** Other fractures of lower leg

6 **S82.81** Torus fracture of upper end of fibula

> The appropriate 7th character is to be added to all codes in subcategory S82.81
> A   initial encounter for closed fracture
> D   subsequent encounter for fracture with routine healing
> G   subsequent encounter for fracture with delayed healing
> K   subsequent encounter for fracture with nonunion
> P   subsequent encounter for fracture with malunion
> S   sequela

7 ⊟	**S82.811-**	Torus fracture of upper end of right fibula
7 ⊟	**S82.812-**	Torus fracture of upper end of left fibula
7 ⊟	**S82.819-**	Torus fracture of upper end of unspecified fibula

6 **S82.82** Torus fracture of lower end of fibula

> The appropriate 7th character is to be added to all codes in subcategory S82.82
> A   initial encounter for closed fracture
> D   subsequent encounter for fracture with routine healing
> G   subsequent encounter for fracture with delayed healing
> K   subsequent encounter for fracture with nonunion
> P   subsequent encounter for fracture with malunion
> S   sequela

7 ⊟	**S82.821-**	Torus fracture of lower end of right fibula
7 ⊟	**S82.822-**	Torus fracture of lower end of left fibula
7 ⊟	**S82.829-**	Torus fracture of lower end of unspecified fibula

6 **S82.83** Other fracture of upper and lower end of fibula

7 ⊟	**S82.831-**	Other fracture of upper and lower end of right fibula
7 ⊟	**S82.832-**	Other fracture of upper and lower end of left fibula AHA: 1Q 2015, 25
7 ⊟	**S82.839-**	Other fracture of upper and lower end of unspecified fibula

6 **S82.84** Bimalleolar fracture of lower leg

7 ⊟	**S82.841-**	Displaced bimalleolar fracture of right lower leg
7 ⊟	**S82.842-**	Displaced bimalleolar fracture of left lower leg
7 ⊟	**S82.843-**	Displaced bimalleolar fracture of unspecified lower leg
7 ⊟	**S82.844-**	Nondisplaced bimalleolar fracture of right lower leg

● New   ▲ Revised   *Manifestation*   4-7 Digit Indicators   ⊟ Laterality   A Adult (15+ years)   M Maternity (12-55 years)   N Newborn   P Pediatric (0-17 years)   ♂ Male   ♀ Female
✖ Deleted   Unspecified   ✚ Additional code

2017 ICD-10-CM Expert for Physicians

© 2017 DecisionHealth

1017

Injury, Poisoning and Certain Other Consequences of External Causes

S82.401- — S82.844-

7 S82.845- Nondisplaced bimalleolar fracture of left lower leg

7 S82.846- Nondisplaced bimalleolar fracture of unspecified lower leg

G S82.85 Trimalleolar fracture of lower leg

7 S82.851- Displaced trimalleolar fracture of right lower leg

7 S82.852- Displaced trimalleolar fracture of left lower leg

7 S82.853- Displaced trimalleolar fracture of unspecified lower leg

7 S82.854- Nondisplaced trimalleolar fracture of right lower leg

7 S82.855- Nondisplaced trimalleolar fracture of left lower leg

7 S82.856- Nondisplaced trimalleolar fracture of unspecified lower leg

G S82.86 Maisonneuve's fracture

7 S82.861- Displaced Maisonneuve's fracture of right leg

7 S82.862- Displaced Maisonneuve's fracture of left leg

7 S82.863- Displaced Maisonneuve's fracture of unspecified leg

7 S82.864- Nondisplaced Maisonneuve's fracture of right leg

7 S82.865- Nondisplaced Maisonneuve's fracture of left leg

7 S82.866- Nondisplaced Maisonneuve's fracture of unspecified leg

G S82.87 Pilon fracture of tibia

7 S82.871- Displaced pilon fracture of right tibia

7 S82.872- Displaced pilon fracture of left tibia

7 S82.873- Displaced pilon fracture of unspecified tibia

7 S82.874- Nondisplaced pilon fracture of right tibia

7 S82.875- Nondisplaced pilon fracture of left tibia

7 S82.876- Nondisplaced pilon fracture of unspecified tibia

G S82.89 Other fractures of lower leg
Fracture of ankle NOS

7 S82.891- Other fracture of right lower leg

7 S82.892- Other fracture of left lower leg

7 S82.899- Other fracture of unspecified lower leg

5 S82.9 Unspecified fracture of lower leg

7 S82.90X- Unspecified fracture of unspecified lower leg

7 S82.91X- Unspecified fracture of right lower leg

7 S82.92X- Unspecified fracture of left lower leg

4 S83 Dislocation and sprain of joints and ligaments of knee

INCLUDES avulsion of joint or ligament of knee
laceration of cartilage, joint or ligament of knee
sprain of cartilage, joint or ligament of knee
traumatic hemarthrosis of joint or ligament of knee
traumatic rupture of joint or ligament of knee
traumatic subluxation of joint or ligament of knee
traumatic tear of joint or ligament of knee

Code also:
any associated open wound

EXCLUDES 1 *derangement of patella (M22.0-M22.3)*
injury of patellar ligament (tendon) (S76.1-)
internal derangement of knee (M23.-)
old dislocation of knee (M24.36)
pathological dislocation of knee (M24.36)
recurrent dislocation of knee (M22.0)

EXCLUDES 2 *strain of muscle, fascia and tendon of lower leg (S86.-)*

The appropriate 7th character is to be added to each code from category S83
A initial encounter
D subsequent encounter
S sequela

CODING TIP ✓ Unlike ICD-9 there is no code for open dislocations. When documented as open an additional code for the open wound must be applied.

5 S83.0 Subluxation and dislocation of patella

G S83.00 Unspecified subluxation and dislocation of patella

7 S83.001- Unspecified subluxation of right patella

7 S83.002- Unspecified subluxation of left patella

7 S83.003- Unspecified subluxation of unspecified patella

7 S83.004- Unspecified dislocation of right patella

7 S83.005- Unspecified dislocation of left patella

7 S83.006- Unspecified dislocation of unspecified patella

G S83.01 Lateral subluxation and dislocation of patella

7 S83.011- Lateral subluxation of right patella

7 S83.012- Lateral subluxation of left patella

7 S83.013- Lateral subluxation of unspecified patella

7 S83.014- Lateral dislocation of right patella

7 S83.015- Lateral dislocation of left patella

7 S83.016- Lateral dislocation of unspecified patella

G S83.09 Other subluxation and dislocation of patella

7 S83.091- Other subluxation of right patella

7 S83.092- Other subluxation of left patella

7 S83.093- Other subluxation of unspecified patella

7 S83.094- Other dislocation of right patella

7 S83.095- Other dislocation of left patella

7 S83.096- Other dislocation of unspecified patella

5 S83.1 Subluxation and dislocation of knee

EXCLUDES 2 *instability of knee prosthesis (T84.022, T84.023)*

G S83.10 Unspecified subluxation and dislocation of knee

7 S83.101- Unspecified subluxation of right knee

7 S83.102- Unspecified subluxation of left knee

7 S83.103- Unspecified subluxation of unspecified knee

7 S83.104- Unspecified dislocation of right knee

7 S83.105- Unspecified dislocation of left knee

7 S83.106- Unspecified dislocation of unspecified knee

Unspecified dislocation of unspecified knee

Front view / Side view. Femur, Dislocation of patella, Tibia, Fibula, Patella, Dislocation of tibia, Fibula

G S83.11 Anterior subluxation and dislocation of proximal end of tibia
Posterior subluxation and dislocation of distal end of femur

7 S83.111- Anterior subluxation of proximal end of tibia, right knee

7 S83.112- Anterior subluxation of proximal end of tibia, left knee

7 S83.113- Anterior subluxation of proximal end of tibia, unspecified knee

7 S83.114- Anterior dislocation of proximal end of tibia, right knee

7 S83.115- Anterior dislocation of proximal end of tibia, left knee

7 S83.116- Anterior dislocation of proximal end of tibia, unspecified knee

G S83.12 Posterior subluxation and dislocation of proximal end of tibia
Anterior dislocation of distal end of femur

7 S83.121- Posterior subluxation of proximal end of tibia, right knee

7 S83.122- Posterior subluxation of proximal end of tibia, left knee

7 S83.123- Posterior subluxation of proximal end of tibia, unspecified knee

7 S83.124- Posterior dislocation of proximal end of tibia, right knee

7 S83.125- Posterior dislocation of proximal end of tibia, left knee

● New ▲ Revised *Manifestation* 4-7 Digit Indicators ▭ Laterality Ⓐ Adult (15+ years) Ⓜ Maternity (12-55 years) Ⓝ Newborn Ⓟ Pediatric (0-17 years) ♂ Male ♀ Female
✖ Deleted Unspecified + Additional code

1018 © 2017 DecisionHealth 2017 ICD-10-CM Expert for Physicians

7 ☐ S83.126-   Posterior dislocation of proximal end of tibia, unspecified knee

6 S83.13   Medial subluxation and dislocation of proximal end of tibia

7 ☐ S83.131-   Medial subluxation of proximal end of tibia, right knee

7 ☐ S83.132-   Medial subluxation of proximal end of tibia, left knee

7 ☐ S83.133-   Medial subluxation of proximal end of tibia, unspecified knee

7 ☐ S83.134-   Medial dislocation of proximal end of tibia, right knee

7 ☐ S83.135-   Medial dislocation of proximal end of tibia, left knee

7 ☐ S83.136-   Medial dislocation of proximal end of tibia, unspecified knee

6 S83.14   Lateral subluxation and dislocation of proximal end of tibia

7 ☐ S83.141-   Lateral subluxation of proximal end of tibia, right knee

7 ☐ S83.142-   Lateral subluxation of proximal end of tibia, left knee

7 ☐ S83.143-   Lateral subluxation of proximal end of tibia, unspecified knee

7 ☐ S83.144-   Lateral dislocation of proximal end of tibia, right knee

7 ☐ S83.145-   Lateral dislocation of proximal end of tibia, left knee

7 ☐ S83.146-   Lateral dislocation of proximal end of tibia, unspecified knee

6 S83.19   Other subluxation and dislocation of knee

7 ☐ S83.191-   Other subluxation of right knee

7 ☐ S83.192-   Other subluxation of left knee

7 ☐ S83.193-   Other subluxation of unspecified knee

7 ☐ S83.194-   Other dislocation of right knee

7 ☐ S83.195-   Other dislocation of left knee

7 ☐ S83.196-   Other dislocation of unspecified knee

5 S83.2   Tear of meniscus, current injury

> **EXCLUDES 1**   *old bucket-handle tear (M23.2)*

6 S83.20   Tear of unspecified meniscus, current injury
Tear of meniscus of knee NOS

7 ☐ S83.200-   Bucket-handle tear of unspecified meniscus, current injury, right knee

7 ☐ S83.201-   Bucket-handle tear of unspecified meniscus, current injury, left knee

7 ☐ S83.202-   Bucket-handle tear of unspecified meniscus, current injury, unspecified knee

7 ☐ S83.203-   Other tear of unspecified meniscus, current injury, right knee

7 ☐ S83.204-   Other tear of unspecified meniscus, current injury, left knee

7 ☐ S83.205-   Other tear of unspecified meniscus, current injury, unspecified knee

7 ☐ S83.206-   Unspecified tear of unspecified meniscus, current injury, right knee

7 ☐ S83.207-   Unspecified tear of unspecified meniscus, current injury, left knee

7 ☐ S83.209-   Unspecified tear of unspecified meniscus, current injury, unspecified knee

6 S83.21   Bucket-handle tear of medial meniscus, current injury

7 ☐ S83.211-   Bucket-handle tear of medial meniscus, current injury, right knee

7 ☐ S83.212-   Bucket-handle tear of medial meniscus, current injury, left knee

7 ☐ S83.219-   Bucket-handle tear of medial meniscus, current injury, unspecified knee

6 S83.22   Peripheral tear of medial meniscus, current injury

7 ☐ S83.221-   Peripheral tear of medial meniscus, current injury, right knee

7 ☐ S83.222-   Peripheral tear of medial meniscus, current injury, left knee

7 ☐ S83.229-   Peripheral tear of medial meniscus, current injury, unspecified knee

6 S83.23   Complex tear of medial meniscus, current injury

7 ☐ S83.231-   Complex tear of medial meniscus, current injury, right knee

7 ☐ S83.232-   Complex tear of medial meniscus, current injury, left knee

7 ☐ S83.239-   Complex tear of medial meniscus, current injury, unspecified knee

6 S83.24   Other tear of medial meniscus, current injury

7 ☐ S83.241-   Other tear of medial meniscus, current injury, right knee

7 ☐ S83.242-   Other tear of medial meniscus, current injury, left knee

7 ☐ S83.249-   Other tear of medial meniscus, current injury, unspecified knee

6 S83.25   Bucket-handle tear of lateral meniscus, current injury

7 ☐ S83.251-   Bucket-handle tear of lateral meniscus, current injury, right knee

7 ☐ S83.252-   Bucket-handle tear of lateral meniscus, current injury, left knee

7 ☐ S83.259-   Bucket-handle tear of lateral meniscus, current injury, unspecified knee

6 S83.26   Peripheral tear of lateral meniscus, current injury

7 ☐ S83.261-   Peripheral tear of lateral meniscus, current injury, right knee

7 ☐ S83.262-   Peripheral tear of lateral meniscus, current injury, left knee

7 ☐ S83.269-   Peripheral tear of lateral meniscus, current injury, unspecified knee

6 S83.27   Complex tear of lateral meniscus, current injury

7 ☐ S83.271-   Complex tear of lateral meniscus, current injury, right knee

7 ☐ S83.272-   Complex tear of lateral meniscus, current injury, left knee

7 ☐ S83.279-   Complex tear of lateral meniscus, current injury, unspecified knee

6 S83.28   Other tear of lateral meniscus, current injury

7 ☐ S83.281-   Other tear of lateral meniscus, current injury, right knee

7 ☐ S83.282-   Other tear of lateral meniscus, current injury, left knee

7 ☐ S83.289-   Other tear of lateral meniscus, current injury, unspecified knee

5 S83.3   Tear of articular cartilage of knee, current

7 ☐ S83.30X-   Tear of articular cartilage of unspecified knee, current

7 ☐ S83.31X-   Tear of articular cartilage of right knee, current

7 ☐ S83.32X-   Tear of articular cartilage of left knee, current

5 S83.4   Sprain of collateral ligament of knee

6 S83.40   Sprain of unspecified collateral ligament of knee

7 ☐ S83.401-   Sprain of unspecified collateral ligament of right knee

7 ☐ S83.402-   Sprain of unspecified collateral ligament of left knee

7 ☐ S83.409-   Sprain of unspecified collateral ligament of unspecified knee

6 S83.41   Sprain of medial collateral ligament of knee
Sprain of tibial collateral ligament

7 ☐ S83.411-   Sprain of medial collateral ligament of right knee

7 ☐ S83.412-   Sprain of medial collateral ligament of left knee

7 ☐ S83.419-   Sprain of medial collateral ligament of unspecified knee

6 S83.42   Sprain of lateral collateral ligament of knee
Sprain of fibular collateral ligament

7 ☐ S83.421-   Sprain of lateral collateral ligament of right knee

7 ☐ S83.422-   Sprain of lateral collateral ligament of left knee

7 ☐ S83.429-   Sprain of lateral collateral ligament of unspecified knee

5 S83.5   Sprain of cruciate ligament of knee

6 S83.50   Sprain of unspecified cruciate ligament of knee

7 ☐ S83.501-   Sprain of unspecified cruciate ligament of right knee

7 ☐ S83.502-   Sprain of unspecified cruciate ligament of left knee

7 ☐ S83.509-   Sprain of unspecified cruciate ligament of unspecified knee

---

● New   ▲ Revised   *Manifestation*   4-7 Digit Indicators   ☐ Laterality   A Adult (15+ years)   M Maternity (12-55 years)   N Newborn   P Pediatric (0-17 years)   ♂ Male   ♀ Female

✖ Deleted   Unspecified   + Additional code

⑥ **S83.51**   Sprain of anterior cruciate ligament of knee
   ⑦ ▤ **S83.511-**   Sprain of anterior cruciate ligament of right knee
          AHA: (S83.511D) 2Q 2016, 3
   ⑦ ▤ **S83.512-**   Sprain of anterior cruciate ligament of left knee
   ⑦ ▤ **S83.519-**   Sprain of anterior cruciate ligament of unspecified knee

⑥ **S83.52**   Sprain of posterior cruciate ligament of knee
   ⑦ ▤ **S83.521-**   Sprain of posterior cruciate ligament of right knee
   ⑦ ▤ **S83.522-**   Sprain of posterior cruciate ligament of left knee
   ⑦ ▤ **S83.529-**   Sprain of posterior cruciate ligament of unspecified knee

⑤ **S83.6**   Sprain of the superior tibiofibular joint and ligament
   ⑦ ▤ **S83.60X-**   Sprain of the superior tibiofibular joint and ligament, unspecified knee
   ⑦ ▤ **S83.61X-**   Sprain of the superior tibiofibular joint and ligament, right knee
   ⑦ ▤ **S83.62X-**   Sprain of the superior tibiofibular joint and ligament, left knee

⑤ **S83.8**   Sprain of other specified parts of knee
   ⑥ **S83.8X**   Sprain of other specified parts of knee
      ⑦ ▤ **S83.8X1-**   Sprain of other specified parts of right knee
      ⑦ ▤ **S83.8X2-**   Sprain of other specified parts of left knee
      ⑦ ▤ **S83.8X9-**   Sprain of other specified parts of unspecified knee

⑤ **S83.9**   Sprain of unspecified site of knee
   ⑦ ▤ **S83.90X-**   Sprain of unspecified site of unspecified knee
   ⑦ ▤ **S83.91X-**   Sprain of unspecified site of right knee
   ⑦ ▤ **S83.92X-**   Sprain of unspecified site of left knee

④ **S84**   **Injury of nerves at lower leg level**
   Code also:
     any associated open wound (S81.-)
   EXCLUDES 2   *injury of nerves at ankle and foot level (S94.-)*

   The appropriate 7th character is to be added to each code from category S84
   A   initial encounter
   D   subsequent encounter
   S   sequela

⑤ **S84.0**   Injury of tibial nerve at lower leg level
   ⑦ ▤ **S84.00X-**   Injury of tibial nerve at lower leg level, unspecified leg
   ⑦ ▤ **S84.01X-**   Injury of tibial nerve at lower leg level, right leg
   ⑦ ▤ **S84.02X-**   Injury of tibial nerve at lower leg level, left leg

⑤ **S84.1**   Injury of peroneal nerve at lower leg level
   ⑦ ▤ **S84.10X-**   Injury of peroneal nerve at lower leg level, unspecified leg
   ⑦ ▤ **S84.11X-**   Injury of peroneal nerve at lower leg level, right leg
   ⑦ ▤ **S84.12X-**   Injury of peroneal nerve at lower leg level, left leg

⑤ **S84.2**   Injury of cutaneous sensory nerve at lower leg level
   ⑦ ▤ **S84.20X-**   Injury of cutaneous sensory nerve at lower leg level, unspecified leg
   ⑦ ▤ **S84.21X-**   Injury of cutaneous sensory nerve at lower leg level, right leg
   ⑦ ▤ **S84.22X-**   Injury of cutaneous sensory nerve at lower leg level, left leg

⑤ **S84.8**   Injury of other nerves at lower leg level
   ⑥ **S84.80**   Injury of other nerves at lower leg level
      ⑦ ▤ **S84.801-**   Injury of other nerves at lower leg level, right leg
      ⑦ ▤ **S84.802-**   Injury of other nerves at lower leg level, left leg
      ⑦ ▤ **S84.809-**   Injury of other nerves at lower leg level, unspecified leg

⑤ **S84.9**   Injury of unspecified nerve at lower leg level
   ⑦ ▤ **S84.90X-**   Injury of unspecified nerve at lower leg level, unspecified leg
   ⑦ ▤ **S84.91X-**   Injury of unspecified nerve at lower leg level, right leg
   ⑦ ▤ **S84.92X-**   Injury of unspecified nerve at lower leg level, left leg

④ **S85**   **Injury of blood vessels at lower leg level**
   Code also:
     any associated open wound (S81.-)
   EXCLUDES 2   *injury of blood vessels at ankle and foot level (S95.-)*

   The appropriate 7th character is to be added to each code from category S85
   A   initial encounter
   D   subsequent encounter
   S   sequela

⑤ **S85.0**   Injury of popliteal artery
   ⑥ **S85.00**   Unspecified injury of popliteal artery
      ⑦ ▤ **S85.001-**   Unspecified injury of popliteal artery, right leg
      ⑦ ▤ **S85.002-**   Unspecified injury of popliteal artery, left leg
      ⑦ ▤ **S85.009-**   Unspecified injury of popliteal artery, unspecified leg
   ⑥ **S85.01**   Laceration of popliteal artery
      CODING TIP ✓   Code also any associated open wound S81.-
      ⑦ ▤ **S85.011-**   Laceration of popliteal artery, right leg
      ⑦ ▤ **S85.012-**   Laceration of popliteal artery, left leg
      ⑦ ▤ **S85.019-**   Laceration of popliteal artery, unspecified leg
   ⑥ **S85.09**   Other specified injury of popliteal artery
      ⑦ ▤ **S85.091-**   Other specified injury of popliteal artery, right leg
      ⑦ ▤ **S85.092-**   Other specified injury of popliteal artery, left leg
      ⑦ ▤ **S85.099-**   Other specified injury of popliteal artery, unspecified leg

⑤ **S85.1**   Injury of tibial artery
   ⑥ **S85.10**   Unspecified injury of unspecified tibial artery
      Injury of tibial artery NOS
      ⑦ ▤ **S85.101-**   Unspecified injury of unspecified tibial artery, right leg
      ⑦ ▤ **S85.102-**   Unspecified injury of unspecified tibial artery, left leg
      ⑦ ▤ **S85.109-**   Unspecified injury of unspecified tibial artery, unspecified leg
   ⑥ **S85.11**   Laceration of unspecified tibial artery
      CODING TIP ✓   Code also any associated open wound S81.-
      ⑦ ▤ **S85.111-**   Laceration of unspecified tibial artery, right leg
      ⑦ ▤ **S85.112-**   Laceration of unspecified tibial artery, left leg
      ⑦ ▤ **S85.119-**   Laceration of unspecified tibial artery, unspecified leg
   ⑥ **S85.12**   Other specified injury of unspecified tibial artery
      ⑦ ▤ **S85.121-**   Other specified injury of unspecified tibial artery, right leg
      ⑦ ▤ **S85.122-**   Other specified injury of unspecified tibial artery, left leg
      ⑦ ▤ **S85.129-**   Other specified injury of unspecified tibial artery, unspecified leg
   ⑥ **S85.13**   Unspecified injury of anterior tibial artery
      ⑦ ▤ **S85.131-**   Unspecified injury of anterior tibial artery, right leg
      ⑦ ▤ **S85.132-**   Unspecified injury of anterior tibial artery, left leg
      ⑦ ▤ **S85.139-**   Unspecified injury of anterior tibial artery, unspecified leg
   ⑥ **S85.14**   Laceration of anterior tibial artery
      CODING TIP ✓   Code also any associated open wound S81.-
      ⑦ ▤ **S85.141-**   Laceration of anterior tibial artery, right leg
      ⑦ ▤ **S85.142-**   Laceration of anterior tibial artery, left leg
      ⑦ ▤ **S85.149-**   Laceration of anterior tibial artery, unspecified leg
   ⑥ **S85.15**   Other specified injury of anterior tibial artery
      ⑦ ▤ **S85.151-**   Other specified injury of anterior tibial artery, right leg
      ⑦ ▤ **S85.152-**   Other specified injury of anterior tibial artery, left leg

---

● New   ▲ Revised   *Manifestation*   ④-⑦ Digit Indicators   ▤ Laterality   Ⓐ Adult (15+ years)   Ⓜ Maternity (12-55 years)   Ⓝ Newborn   Ⓟ Pediatric (0-17 years)   ♂ Male   ♀ Female
✖ Deleted   Unspecified   + Additional code

1020   © 2017 DecisionHealth   2017 ICD-10-CM Expert for Physicians

7 ⊟ **S85.159-** Other specified injury of anterior tibial artery, unspecified leg

6 **S85.16** Unspecified injury of posterior tibial artery

7 ⊟ **S85.161-** Unspecified injury of posterior tibial artery, right leg

7 ⊟ **S85.162-** Unspecified injury of posterior tibial artery, left leg

7 ⊟ **S85.169-** Unspecified injury of posterior tibial artery, unspecified leg

6 **S85.17** Laceration of posterior tibial artery

> **CODING TIP ✓** Code also any associated open wound S81.-

7 ⊟ **S85.171-** Laceration of posterior tibial artery, right leg

7 ⊟ **S85.172-** Laceration of posterior tibial artery, left leg

7 ⊟ **S85.179-** Laceration of posterior tibial artery, unspecified leg

6 **S85.18** Other specified injury of posterior tibial artery

7 ⊟ **S85.181-** Other specified injury of posterior tibial artery, right leg

7 ⊟ **S85.182-** Other specified injury of posterior tibial artery, left leg

7 ⊟ **S85.189-** Other specified injury of posterior tibial artery, unspecified leg

5 **S85.2** Injury of peroneal artery

6 **S85.20** Unspecified injury of peroneal artery

7 ⊟ **S85.201-** Unspecified injury of peroneal artery, right leg

7 ⊟ **S85.202-** Unspecified injury of peroneal artery, left leg

7 ⊟ **S85.209-** Unspecified injury of peroneal artery, unspecified leg

6 **S85.21** Laceration of peroneal artery

> **CODING TIP ✓** Code also any associated open wound S81.-

7 ⊟ **S85.211-** Laceration of peroneal artery, right leg

7 ⊟ **S85.212-** Laceration of peroneal artery, left leg

7 ⊟ **S85.219-** Laceration of peroneal artery, unspecified leg

6 **S85.29** Other specified injury of peroneal artery

7 ⊟ **S85.291-** Other specified injury of peroneal artery, right leg

7 ⊟ **S85.292-** Other specified injury of peroneal artery, left leg

7 ⊟ **S85.299-** Other specified injury of peroneal artery, unspecified leg

5 **S85.3** Injury of greater saphenous vein at lower leg level
Injury of greater saphenous vein NOS
Injury of saphenous vein NOS

6 **S85.30** Unspecified injury of greater saphenous vein at lower leg level

7 ⊟ **S85.301-** Unspecified injury of greater saphenous vein at lower leg level, right leg

7 ⊟ **S85.302-** Unspecified injury of greater saphenous vein at lower leg level, left leg

7 ⊟ **S85.309-** Unspecified injury of greater saphenous vein at lower leg level, unspecified leg

6 **S85.31** Laceration of greater saphenous vein at lower leg level

> **CODING TIP ✓** Code also any associated open wound S81.-

7 ⊟ **S85.311-** Laceration of greater saphenous vein at lower leg level, right leg

7 ⊟ **S85.312-** Laceration of greater saphenous vein at lower leg level, left leg

7 ⊟ **S85.319-** Laceration of greater saphenous vein at lower leg level, unspecified leg

6 **S85.39** Other specified injury of greater saphenous vein at lower leg level

7 ⊟ **S85.391-** Other specified injury of greater saphenous vein at lower leg level, right leg

7 ⊟ **S85.392-** Other specified injury of greater saphenous vein at lower leg level, left leg

7 ⊟ **S85.399-** Other specified injury of greater saphenous vein at lower leg level, unspecified leg

5 **S85.4** Injury of lesser saphenous vein at lower leg level

6 **S85.40** Unspecified injury of lesser saphenous vein at lower leg level

7 ⊟ **S85.401-** Unspecified injury of lesser saphenous vein at lower leg level, right leg

7 ⊟ **S85.402-** Unspecified injury of lesser saphenous vein at lower leg level, left leg

7 ⊟ **S85.409-** Unspecified injury of lesser saphenous vein at lower leg level, unspecified leg

6 **S85.41** Laceration of lesser saphenous vein at lower leg level

> **CODING TIP ✓** Code also any associated open wound S81.-

7 ⊟ **S85.411-** Laceration of lesser saphenous vein at lower leg level, right leg

7 ⊟ **S85.412-** Laceration of lesser saphenous vein at lower leg level, left leg

7 ⊟ **S85.419-** Laceration of lesser saphenous vein at lower leg level, unspecified leg

6 **S85.49** Other specified injury of lesser saphenous vein at lower leg level

7 ⊟ **S85.491-** Other specified injury of lesser saphenous vein at lower leg level, right leg

7 ⊟ **S85.492-** Other specified injury of lesser saphenous vein at lower leg level, left leg

7 ⊟ **S85.499-** Other specified injury of lesser saphenous vein at lower leg level, unspecified leg

5 **S85.5** Injury of popliteal vein

6 **S85.50** Unspecified injury of popliteal vein

7 ⊟ **S85.501-** Unspecified injury of popliteal vein, right leg

7 ⊟ **S85.502-** Unspecified injury of popliteal vein, left leg

7 ⊟ **S85.509-** Unspecified injury of popliteal vein, unspecified leg

6 **S85.51** Laceration of popliteal vein

> **CODING TIP ✓** Code also any associated open wound S81.-

7 ⊟ **S85.511-** Laceration of popliteal vein, right leg

7 ⊟ **S85.512-** Laceration of popliteal vein, left leg

7 ⊟ **S85.519-** Laceration of popliteal vein, unspecified leg

6 **S85.59** Other specified injury of popliteal vein

7 ⊟ **S85.591-** Other specified injury of popliteal vein, right leg

7 ⊟ **S85.592-** Other specified injury of popliteal vein, left leg

7 ⊟ **S85.599-** Other specified injury of popliteal vein, unspecified leg

5 **S85.8** Injury of other blood vessels at lower leg level

6 **S85.80** Unspecified injury of other blood vessels at lower leg level

7 ⊟ **S85.801-** Unspecified injury of other blood vessels at lower leg level, right leg

7 ⊟ **S85.802-** Unspecified injury of other blood vessels at lower leg level, left leg

7 ⊟ **S85.809-** Unspecified injury of other blood vessels at lower leg level, unspecified leg

6 **S85.81** Laceration of other blood vessels at lower leg level

> **CODING TIP ✓** Code also any associated open wound S81.-

7 ⊟ **S85.811-** Laceration of other blood vessels at lower leg level, right leg

7 ⊟ **S85.812-** Laceration of other blood vessels at lower leg level, left leg

7 ⊟ **S85.819-** Laceration of other blood vessels at lower leg level, unspecified leg

6 **S85.89** Other specified injury of other blood vessels at lower leg level

7 ⊟ **S85.891-** Other specified injury of other blood vessels at lower leg level, right leg

7 ⊟ **S85.892-** Other specified injury of other blood vessels at lower leg level, left leg

7 ⊟ **S85.899-** Other specified injury of other blood vessels at lower leg level, unspecified leg

5 **S85.9** Injury of unspecified blood vessel at lower leg level

6 **S85.90** Unspecified injury of unspecified blood vessel at lower leg level

7 ⊟ **S85.901-** Unspecified injury of unspecified blood vessel at lower leg level, right leg

7 ⊟ **S85.902-** Unspecified injury of unspecified blood vessel at lower leg level, left leg

---

● New ▲ Revised *Manifestation* 4-7 Digit Indicators ⊟ Laterality Ⓐ Adult (15+ years) Ⓜ Maternity (12-55 years) Ⓝ Newborn Ⓟ Pediatric (0-17 years) ♂ Male ♀ Female
✖ Deleted Unspecified + Additional code

7 ⊟ **S85.909-** Unspecified injury of unspecified blood vessel at lower leg level, unspecified leg

6 **S85.91** Laceration of unspecified blood vessel at lower leg level

> **CODING TIP ✓** Code also any associated open wound S81.-

7 ⊟ **S85.911-** Laceration of unspecified blood vessel at lower leg level, right leg

7 ⊟ **S85.912-** Laceration of unspecified blood vessel at lower leg level, left leg

7 ⊟ **S85.919-** Laceration of unspecified blood vessel at lower leg level, unspecified leg

6 **S85.99** Other specified injury of unspecified blood vessel at lower leg level

7 ⊟ **S85.991-** Other specified injury of unspecified blood vessel at lower leg level, right leg

7 ⊟ **S85.992-** Other specified injury of unspecified blood vessel at lower leg level, left leg

7 ⊟ **S85.999-** Other specified injury of unspecified blood vessel at lower leg level, unspecified leg

4 **S86** **Injury of muscle, fascia and tendon at lower leg level**

Code also:
  any associated open wound (S81.-)

> **EXCLUDES 2** injury of muscle, fascia and tendon at ankle (S96.-)
> injury of patellar ligament (tendon) (S76.1-)
> sprain of joints and ligaments of knee (S83.-)

The appropriate 7th character is to be added to each code from category S86
A   initial encounter
D   subsequent encounter
S   sequela

5 **S86.0** **Injury of Achilles tendon**

6 **S86.00** Unspecified injury of Achilles tendon

7 ⊟ **S86.001-** Unspecified injury of right Achilles tendon

7 ⊟ **S86.002-** Unspecified injury of left Achilles tendon

7 ⊟ **S86.009-** Unspecified injury of unspecified Achilles tendon

6 **S86.01** Strain of Achilles tendon

7 ⊟ **S86.011-** Strain of right Achilles tendon

7 ⊟ **S86.012-** Strain of left Achilles tendon

7 ⊟ **S86.019-** Strain of unspecified Achilles tendon

6 **S86.02** Laceration of Achilles tendon

> **CODING TIP ✓** Code also any associated open wound S81.-

7 ⊟ **S86.021-** Laceration of right Achilles tendon

7 ⊟ **S86.022-** Laceration of left Achilles tendon

7 ⊟ **S86.029-** Laceration of unspecified Achilles tendon

6 **S86.09** Other specified injury of Achilles tendon

7 ⊟ **S86.091-** Other specified injury of right Achilles tendon

7 ⊟ **S86.092-** Other specified injury of left Achilles tendon

7 ⊟ **S86.099-** Other specified injury of unspecified Achilles tendon

5 **S86.1** **Injury of other muscle(s) and tendon(s) of posterior muscle group at lower leg level**

6 **S86.10** Unspecified injury of other muscle(s) and tendon(s) of posterior muscle group at lower leg level

7 ⊟ **S86.101-** Unspecified injury of other muscle(s) and tendon(s) of posterior muscle group at lower leg level, right leg

7 ⊟ **S86.102-** Unspecified injury of other muscle(s) and tendon(s) of posterior muscle group at lower leg level, left leg

7 ⊟ **S86.109-** Unspecified injury of other muscle(s) and tendon(s) of posterior muscle group at lower leg level, unspecified leg

6 **S86.11** Strain of other muscle(s) and tendon(s) of posterior muscle group at lower leg level

7 ⊟ **S86.111-** Strain of other muscle(s) and tendon(s) of posterior muscle group at lower leg level, right leg

7 ⊟ **S86.112-** Strain of other muscle(s) and tendon(s) of posterior muscle group at lower leg level, left leg

7 ⊟ **S86.119-** Strain of other muscle(s) and tendon(s) of posterior muscle group at lower leg level, unspecified leg

6 **S86.12** Laceration of other muscle(s) and tendon(s) of posterior muscle group at lower leg level

> **CODING TIP ✓** Code also any associated open wound S81.-

7 ⊟ **S86.121-** Laceration of other muscle(s) and tendon(s) of posterior muscle group at lower leg level, right leg

7 ⊟ **S86.122-** Laceration of other muscle(s) and tendon(s) of posterior muscle group at lower leg level, left leg

7 ⊟ **S86.129-** Laceration of other muscle(s) and tendon(s) of posterior muscle group at lower leg level, unspecified leg

6 **S86.19** Other injury of other muscle(s) and tendon(s) of posterior muscle group at lower leg level

7 ⊟ **S86.191-** Other injury of other muscle(s) of posterior muscle group at lower leg level, right leg

7 ⊟ **S86.192-** Other injury of other muscle(s) of posterior muscle group at lower leg level, left leg

7 ⊟ **S86.199-** Other injury of other muscle(s) of posterior muscle group at lower leg level, unspecified leg

5 **S86.2** **Injury of muscle(s) and tendon(s) of anterior muscle group at lower leg level**

6 **S86.20** Unspecified injury of muscle(s) and tendon(s) of anterior muscle group at lower leg level

7 ⊟ **S86.201-** Unspecified injury of muscle(s) and tendon(s) of anterior muscle group at lower leg level, right leg

7 ⊟ **S86.202-** Unspecified injury of muscle(s) and tendon(s) of anterior muscle group at lower leg level, left leg

7 ⊟ **S86.209-** Unspecified injury of muscle(s) and tendon(s) of anterior muscle group at lower leg level, unspecified leg

6 **S86.21** Strain of muscle(s) and tendon(s) of anterior muscle group at lower leg level

7 ⊟ **S86.211-** Strain of muscle(s) and tendon(s) of anterior muscle group at lower leg level, right leg

7 ⊟ **S86.212-** Strain of muscle(s) and tendon(s) of anterior muscle group at lower leg level, left leg

7 ⊟ **S86.219-** Strain of muscle(s) and tendon(s) of anterior muscle group at lower leg level, unspecified leg

6 **S86.22** Laceration of muscle(s) and tendon(s) of anterior muscle group at lower leg level

> **CODING TIP ✓** Code also any associated open wound S81.-

7 ⊟ **S86.221-** Laceration of muscle(s) and tendon(s) of anterior muscle group at lower leg level, right leg

7 ⊟ **S86.222-** Laceration of muscle(s) and tendon(s) of anterior muscle group at lower leg level, left leg

7 ⊟ **S86.229-** Laceration of muscle(s) and tendon(s) of anterior muscle group at lower leg level, unspecified leg

6 **S86.29** Other injury of muscle(s) and tendon(s) of anterior muscle group at lower leg level

7 ⊟ **S86.291-** Other injury of muscle(s) and tendon(s) of anterior muscle group at lower leg level, right leg

7 ⊟ **S86.292-** Other injury of muscle(s) and tendon(s) of anterior muscle group at lower leg level, left leg

7 ⊟ **S86.299-** Other injury of muscle(s) and tendon(s) of anterior muscle group at lower leg level, unspecified leg

5 **S86.3** **Injury of muscle(s) and tendon(s) of peroneal muscle group at lower leg level**

6 **S86.30** Unspecified injury of muscle(s) and tendon(s) of peroneal muscle group at lower leg level

7 ⊟ **S86.301-** Unspecified injury of muscle(s) and tendon(s) of peroneal muscle group at lower leg level, right leg

---

● New ▲ Revised *Manifestation* 4-7 Digit Indicators ⊟ Laterality Ⓐ Adult (15+ years) Ⓜ Maternity (12-55 years) Ⓝ Newborn Ⓟ Pediatric (0-17 years) ♂ Male ♀ Female
✖ Deleted Unspecified + Additional code

1022   © 2017 DecisionHealth   2017 ICD-10-CM Expert for Physicians

7 ⊟ S86.302- Unspecified injury of muscle(s) and tendon(s) of peroneal muscle group at lower leg level, left leg

7 ⊟ S86.309- Unspecified injury of muscle(s) and tendon(s) of peroneal muscle group at lower leg level, unspecified leg

6 S86.31 Strain of muscle(s) and tendon(s) of peroneal muscle group at lower leg level

7 ⊟ S86.311- Strain of muscle(s) and tendon(s) of peroneal muscle group at lower leg level, right leg

7 ⊟ S86.312- Strain of muscle(s) and tendon(s) of peroneal muscle group at lower leg level, left leg

7 ⊟ S86.319- Strain of muscle(s) and tendon(s) of peroneal muscle group at lower leg level, unspecified leg

6 S86.32 Laceration of muscle(s) and tendon(s) of peroneal muscle group at lower leg level

CODING TIP ✓ Code also any associated open wound S81.-

7 ⊟ S86.321- Laceration of muscle(s) and tendon(s) of peroneal muscle group at lower leg level, right leg

7 ⊟ S86.322- Laceration of muscle(s) and tendon(s) of peroneal muscle group at lower leg level, left leg

7 ⊟ S86.329- Laceration of muscle(s) and tendon(s) of peroneal muscle group at lower leg level, unspecified leg

6 S86.39 Other injury of muscle(s) and tendon(s) of peroneal muscle group at lower leg level

7 ⊟ S86.391- Other injury of muscle(s) and tendon(s) of peroneal muscle group at lower leg level, right leg

7 ⊟ S86.392- Other injury of muscle(s) and tendon(s) of peroneal muscle group at lower leg level, left leg

7 ⊟ S86.399- Other injury of muscle(s) and tendon(s) of peroneal muscle group at lower leg level, unspecified leg

5 S86.8 Injury of other muscles and tendons at lower leg level

6 S86.80 Unspecified injury of other muscles and tendons at lower leg level

7 ⊟ S86.801- Unspecified injury of other muscle(s) and tendon(s) at lower leg level, right leg

7 ⊟ S86.802- Unspecified injury of other muscle(s) and tendon(s) at lower leg level, left leg

7 ⊟ S86.809- Unspecified injury of other muscle(s) and tendon(s) at lower leg level, unspecified leg

6 S86.81 Strain of other muscles and tendons at lower leg level

7 ⊟ S86.811- Strain of other muscle(s) and tendon(s) at lower leg level, right leg

7 ⊟ S86.812- Strain of other muscle(s) and tendon(s) at lower leg level, left leg

7 ⊟ S86.819- Strain of other muscle(s) and tendon(s) at lower leg level, unspecified leg

6 S86.82 Laceration of other muscles and tendons at lower leg level

CODING TIP ✓ Code also any associated open wound S81.-

7 ⊟ S86.821- Laceration of other muscle(s) and tendon(s) at lower leg level, right leg

7 ⊟ S86.822- Laceration of other muscle(s) and tendon(s) at lower leg level, left leg

7 ⊟ S86.829- Laceration of other muscle(s) and tendon(s) at lower leg level, unspecified leg

6 S86.89 Other injury of other muscles and tendons at lower leg level

7 ⊟ S86.891- Other injury of other muscle(s) and tendon(s) at lower leg level, right leg

7 ⊟ S86.892- Other injury of other muscle(s) and tendon(s) at lower leg level, left leg

7 ⊟ S86.899- Other injury of other muscle(s) and tendon(s) at lower leg level, unspecified leg

5 S86.9 Injury of unspecified muscle and tendon at lower leg level

6 S86.90 Unspecified injury of unspecified muscle and tendon at lower leg level

7 ⊟ S86.901- Unspecified injury of unspecified muscle(s) and tendon(s) at lower leg level, right leg

7 ⊟ S86.902- Unspecified injury of unspecified muscle(s) and tendon(s) at lower leg level, left leg

7 ⊟ S86.909- Unspecified injury of unspecified muscle(s) and tendon(s) at lower leg level, unspecified leg

6 S86.91 Strain of unspecified muscle and tendon at lower leg level

7 ⊟ S86.911- Strain of unspecified muscle(s) and tendon(s) at lower leg level, right leg

7 ⊟ S86.912- Strain of unspecified muscle(s) and tendon(s) at lower leg level, left leg

7 ⊟ S86.919- Strain of unspecified muscle(s) and tendon(s) at lower leg level, unspecified leg

6 S86.92 Laceration of unspecified muscle and tendon at lower leg level

CODING TIP ✓ Code also any associated open wound S81.-

7 ⊟ S86.921- Laceration of unspecified muscle(s) and tendon(s) at lower leg level, right leg

7 ⊟ S86.922- Laceration of unspecified muscle(s) and tendon(s) at lower leg level, left leg

7 ⊟ S86.929- Laceration of unspecified muscle(s) and tendon(s) at lower leg level, unspecified leg

6 S86.99 Other injury of unspecified muscle and tendon at lower leg level

7 ⊟ S86.991- Other injury of unspecified muscle(s) and tendon(s) at lower leg level, right leg

7 ⊟ S86.992- Other injury of unspecified muscle(s) and tendon(s) at lower leg level, left leg

7 ⊟ S86.999- Other injury of unspecified muscle(s) and tendon(s) at lower leg level, unspecified leg

4 + S87 **Crushing injury of lower leg**

Use additional code(s) for all associated injuries

EXCLUDES 2 *crushing injury of ankle and foot (S97.-)*

The appropriate 7th character is to be added to each code from category S87
A initial encounter
D subsequent encounter
S sequela

5 + S87.0 Crushing injury of knee

7 ⊟ + S87.00X- Crushing injury of unspecified knee

7 ⊟ + S87.01X- Crushing injury of right knee

7 ⊟ + S87.02X- Crushing injury of left knee

5 + S87.8 Crushing injury of lower leg

7 ⊟ + S87.80X- Crushing injury of unspecified lower leg

7 ⊟ + S87.81X- Crushing injury of right lower leg

7 ⊟ + S87.82X- Crushing injury of left lower leg

4 S88 **Traumatic amputation of lower leg**

An amputation not identified as partial or complete should be coded to complete

EXCLUDES 1 *traumatic amputation of ankle and foot (S98.-)*

The appropriate 7th character is to be added to each code from category S88
A initial encounter
D subsequent encounter
S sequela

5 S88.0 Traumatic amputation at knee level

6 S88.01 Complete traumatic amputation at knee level

7 ⊟ S88.011- Complete traumatic amputation at knee level, right lower leg

7 ⊟ S88.012- Complete traumatic amputation at knee level, left lower leg

7 ⊟ S88.019- Complete traumatic amputation at knee level, unspecified lower leg

6 S88.02 Partial traumatic amputation at knee level

7 ⊟ S88.021- Partial traumatic amputation at knee level, right lower leg

7 ⊟ S88.022- Partial traumatic amputation at knee level, left lower leg

7 ⊟ S88.029- Partial traumatic amputation at knee level, unspecified lower leg

5 S88.1 Traumatic amputation at level between knee and ankle

● New ▲ Revised *Manifestation* 4-7 Digit Indicators ⊟ Laterality A Adult (15+ years) M Maternity (12-55 years) N Newborn P Pediatric (0-17 years) ♂ Male ♀ Female
✖ Deleted Unspecified + Additional code

2017 ICD-10-CM Expert for Physicians

© 2017 DecisionHealth

1023

⑥ S88.11   Complete traumatic amputation at level between knee and ankle

⑦ ⊟ S88.111-   Complete traumatic amputation at level between knee and ankle, right lower leg

⑦ ⊟ S88.112-   Complete traumatic amputation at level between knee and ankle, left lower leg

⑦ ⊟ S88.119-   Complete traumatic amputation at level between knee and ankle, unspecified lower leg

⑥ S88.12   Partial traumatic amputation at level between knee and ankle

⑦ ⊟ S88.121-   Partial traumatic amputation at level between knee and ankle, right lower leg

⑦ ⊟ S88.122-   Partial traumatic amputation at level between knee and ankle, left lower leg

⑦ ⊟ S88.129-   Partial traumatic amputation at level between knee and ankle, unspecified lower leg

⑤ S88.9   Traumatic amputation of lower leg, level unspecified

⑥ S88.91   Complete traumatic amputation of lower leg, level unspecified

⑦ ⊟ S88.911-   Complete traumatic amputation of right lower leg, level unspecified

⑦ ⊟ S88.912-   Complete traumatic amputation of left lower leg, level unspecified

⑦ ⊟ S88.919-   Complete traumatic amputation of unspecified lower leg, level unspecified

⑥ S88.92   Partial traumatic amputation of lower leg, level unspecified

⑦ ⊟ S88.921-   Partial traumatic amputation of right lower leg, level unspecified

⑦ ⊟ S88.922-   Partial traumatic amputation of left lower leg, level unspecified

⑦ ⊟ S88.929-   Partial traumatic amputation of unspecified lower leg, level unspecified

④ S89   **Other and unspecified injuries of lower leg**

Note: A fracture not indicated as open or closed should be coded to closed

EXCLUDES 2   *other and unspecified injuries of ankle and foot (S99.-)*

The appropriate 7th character is to be added to each code from subcategories S89.0, S89.1, S89.2, and S89.3
A   initial encounter for closed fracture
D   subsequent encounter for fracture with routine healing
G   subsequent encounter for fracture with delayed healing
K   subsequent encounter for fracture with nonunion
P   subsequent encounter for fracture with malunion
S   sequela

CODING TIP ✓   A fracture not indicated as open or closed should be coded to closed.

⑤ S89.0   Physeal fracture of upper end of tibia

⑥ S89.00   Unspecified physeal fracture of upper end of tibia

⑦ ⊟ S89.001-   Unspecified physeal fracture of upper end of right tibia

⑦ ⊟ S89.002-   Unspecified physeal fracture of upper end of left tibia

⑦ ⊟ S89.009-   Unspecified physeal fracture of upper end of unspecified tibia

⑥ S89.01   Salter-Harris Type I physeal fracture of upper end of tibia

⑦ ⊟ S89.011-   Salter-Harris Type I physeal fracture of upper end of right tibia

Physeal fracture (Salter-Harris) Type 1
upper end of right tibia

Upper end of tibia

Type 1 physeal fracture

⑦ ⊟ S89.012-   Salter-Harris Type I physeal fracture of upper end of left tibia

⑦ ⊟ S89.019-   Salter-Harris Type I physeal fracture of upper end of unspecified tibia

⑥ S89.02   Salter-Harris Type II physeal fracture of upper end of tibia

⑦ ⊟ S89.021-   Salter-Harris Type II physeal fracture of upper end of right tibia

⑦ ⊟ S89.022-   Salter-Harris Type II physeal fracture of upper end of left tibia

⑦ ⊟ S89.029-   Salter-Harris Type II physeal fracture of upper end of unspecified tibia

⑥ S89.03   Salter-Harris Type III physeal fracture of upper end of tibia

⑦ ⊟ S89.031-   Salter-Harris Type III physeal fracture of upper end of right tibia

Salter-Harris Type III physeal
fracture of upper end of right tibia

Upper end of tibia
Epiphysis
Growth plate (epiphyseal disk)
Metaphysis

Type III physeal fracture

⑦ ⊟ S89.032-   Salter-Harris Type III physeal fracture of upper end of left tibia

⑦ ⊟ S89.039-   Salter-Harris Type III physeal fracture of upper end of unspecified tibia

⑥ S89.04   Salter-Harris Type IV physeal fracture of upper end of tibia

⑦ ⊟ S89.041-   Salter-Harris Type IV physeal fracture of upper end of right tibia

⑦ ⊟ S89.042-   Salter-Harris Type IV physeal fracture of upper end of left tibia

⑦ ⊟ S89.049-   Salter-Harris Type IV physeal fracture of upper end of unspecified tibia

⑥ S89.09   Other physeal fracture of upper end of tibia

⑦ ⊟ S89.091-   Other physeal fracture of upper end of right tibia

⑦ ⊟ S89.092-   Other physeal fracture of upper end of left tibia

⑦ ⊟ S89.099-   Other physeal fracture of upper end of unspecified tibia

⑤ S89.1   Physeal fracture of lower end of tibia

● New   ▲ Revised   *Manifestation*   ④-⑦ Digit Indicators   ⊟ Laterality   Ⓐ Adult (15+ years)   Ⓜ Maternity (12-55 years)   Ⓝ Newborn   Ⓟ Pediatric (0-17 years)   ♂ Male   ♀ Female
✖ Deleted   Unspecified   + Additional code

1024   © 2017 DecisionHealth   2017 ICD-10-CM Expert for Physicians

⑥ S89.10 Unspecified physeal fracture of lower end of tibia

⑦ ⊟ S89.101- Unspecified physeal fracture of lower end of right tibia

⑦ ⊟ S89.102- Unspecified physeal fracture of lower end of left tibia

⑦ ⊟ S89.109- Unspecified physeal fracture of lower end of unspecified tibia

⑥ S89.11 Salter-Harris Type I physeal fracture of lower end of tibia

⑦ ⊟ S89.111- Salter-Harris Type I physeal fracture of lower end of right tibia

⑦ ⊟ S89.112- Salter-Harris Type I physeal fracture of lower end of left tibia

⑦ ⊟ S89.119- Salter-Harris Type I physeal fracture of lower end of unspecified tibia

⑥ S89.12 Salter-Harris Type II physeal fracture of lower end of tibia

⑦ ⊟ S89.121- Salter-Harris Type II physeal fracture of lower end of right tibia

⑦ ⊟ S89.122- Salter-Harris Type II physeal fracture of lower end of left tibia

⑦ ⊟ S89.129- Salter-Harris Type II physeal fracture of lower end of unspecified tibia

⑥ S89.13 Salter-Harris Type III physeal fracture of lower end of tibia

> **EXCLUDES 1** *fracture of medial malleolus (adult) (S82.5-)*

⑦ ⊟ S89.131- Salter-Harris Type III physeal fracture of lower end of right tibia

⑦ ⊟ S89.132- Salter-Harris Type III physeal fracture of lower end of left tibia

⑦ ⊟ S89.139- Salter-Harris Type III physeal fracture of lower end of unspecified tibia

⑥ S89.14 Salter-Harris Type IV physeal fracture of lower end of tibia

> **EXCLUDES 1** *fracture of medial malleolus (adult) (S82.5-)*

⑦ ⊟ S89.141- Salter-Harris Type IV physeal fracture of lower end of right tibia

⑦ ⊟ S89.142- Salter-Harris Type IV physeal fracture of lower end of left tibia

⑦ ⊟ S89.149- Salter-Harris Type IV physeal fracture of lower end of unspecified tibia

⑥ S89.19 Other physeal fracture of lower end of tibia

⑦ ⊟ S89.191- Other physeal fracture of lower end of right tibia

⑦ ⊟ S89.192- Other physeal fracture of lower end of left tibia

⑦ ⊟ S89.199- Other physeal fracture of lower end of unspecified tibia

⑤ S89.2 Physeal fracture of upper end of fibula

⑥ S89.20 Unspecified physeal fracture of upper end of fibula

⑦ ⊟ S89.201- Unspecified physeal fracture of upper end of right fibula

⑦ ⊟ S89.202- Unspecified physeal fracture of upper end of left fibula

⑦ ⊟ S89.209- Unspecified physeal fracture of upper end of unspecified fibula

⑥ S89.21 Salter-Harris Type I physeal fracture of upper end of fibula

⑦ ⊟ S89.211- Salter-Harris Type I physeal fracture of upper end of right fibula

⑦ ⊟ S89.212- Salter-Harris Type I physeal fracture of upper end of left fibula

⑦ ⊟ S89.219- Salter-Harris Type I physeal fracture of upper end of unspecified fibula

⑥ S89.22 Salter-Harris Type II physeal fracture of upper end of fibula

⑦ ⊟ S89.221- Salter-Harris Type II physeal fracture of upper end of right fibula

⑦ ⊟ S89.222- Salter-Harris Type II physeal fracture of upper end of left fibula

⑦ ⊟ S89.229- Salter-Harris Type II physeal fracture of upper end of unspecified fibula

⑥ S89.29 Other physeal fracture of upper end of fibula

⑦ ⊟ S89.291- Other physeal fracture of upper end of right fibula

⑦ ⊟ S89.292- Other physeal fracture of upper end of left fibula

⑦ ⊟ S89.299- Other physeal fracture of upper end of unspecified fibula

⑤ S89.3 Physeal fracture of lower end of fibula

⑥ S89.30 Unspecified physeal fracture of lower end of fibula

⑦ ⊟ S89.301- Unspecified physeal fracture of lower end of right fibula

⑦ ⊟ S89.302- Unspecified physeal fracture of lower end of left fibula

⑦ ⊟ S89.309- Unspecified physeal fracture of lower end of unspecified fibula

⑥ S89.31 Salter-Harris Type I physeal fracture of lower end of fibula

⑦ ⊟ S89.311- Salter-Harris Type I physeal fracture of lower end of right fibula

⑦ ⊟ S89.312- Salter-Harris Type I physeal fracture of lower end of left fibula

⑦ ⊟ S89.319- Salter-Harris Type I physeal fracture of lower end of unspecified fibula

⑥ S89.32 Salter-Harris Type II physeal fracture of lower end of fibula

⑦ ⊟ S89.321- Salter-Harris Type II physeal fracture of lower end of right fibula

⑦ ⊟ S89.322- Salter-Harris Type II physeal fracture of lower end of left fibula

⑦ ⊟ S89.329- Salter-Harris Type II physeal fracture of lower end of unspecified fibula

⑥ S89.39 Other physeal fracture of lower end of fibula

⑦ ⊟ S89.391- Other physeal fracture of lower end of right fibula

⑦ ⊟ S89.392- Other physeal fracture of lower end of left fibula

⑦ ⊟ S89.399- Other physeal fracture of lower end of unspecified fibula

⑤ S89.8 Other specified injuries of lower leg

> The appropriate 7th character is to be added to each code in subcategory S89.8
> A initial encounter
> D subsequent encounter
> S sequela

⑦ ⊟ S89.80X- Other specified injuries of unspecified lower leg

⑦ ⊟ S89.81X- Other specified injuries of right lower leg

⑦ ⊟ S89.82X- Other specified injuries of left lower leg

⑤ S89.9 Unspecified injury of lower leg

> The appropriate 7th character is to be added to each code in subcategory S89.9
> A initial encounter
> D subsequent encounter
> S sequela

⑦ ⊟ S89.90X- Unspecified injury of unspecified lower leg

⑦ ⊟ S89.91X- Unspecified injury of right lower leg

⑦ ⊟ S89.92X- Unspecified injury of left lower leg

Injuries to the ankle and foot (S90-S99)

> **EXCLUDES 2** *burns and corrosions (T20-T32)*
> *fracture of ankle and malleolus (S82.-)*
> *frostbite (T33-T34)*
> *insect bite or sting, venomous (T63.4)*

> **GUIDELINES** **Section I.C.19.c.2)**
> Multiple fractures are sequenced in accordance with the severity of the fracture.

● New ▲ Revised *Manifestation* ④-⑦ Digit Indicators ⊟ Laterality Ⓐ Adult (15+ years) Ⓜ Maternity (12-55 years) Ⓝ Newborn Ⓟ Pediatric (0-17 years) ♂ Male ♀ Female

✖ ̶D̶e̶l̶e̶t̶e̶d̶ Unspecified + Additional code

GUIDELINES Section I.C.19.b.1)-2)

When coding injuries, assign separate codes for each injury unless a combination code is provided, in which case the combination code is assigned ... Traumatic injury codes (S00-T14.9) are not to be used for normal, healing surgical wounds or to identify complications of surgical wounds. The code for the most serious injury, as determined by the provider and the focus of treatment, is sequenced first.

1) Superficial injuries such as abrasions or contusions are not coded when associated with more severe injuries of the same site.

2) When a primary injury results in minor damage to peripheral nerves or blood vessels, the primary injury is sequenced first with additional code(s) for injuries to nerves and spinal cord (such as category S04), and/or injury to blood vessels (such as category S15). When the primary injury is to the blood vessels or nerves, that injury should be sequenced first.

GUIDELINES Section I.C.19.c

Coding of Traumatic Fractures: The principles of multiple coding of injuries should be followed in coding fractures. Fractures of specified sites are coded individually by site in accordance with both the provisions within categories S02, S12, S22, S32, S42, S49, S52, S59, S62, S72, S79, S82, S89, S92 and the level of detail furnished by medical record content. A fracture not indicated as open or closed should be coded to closed. A fracture not indicated whether displaced or not displaced should be coded to displaced.

4 **S90** **Superficial injury of ankle, foot and toes**

> The appropriate 7th character is to be added to each code from category S90
> A   initial encounter
> D   subsequent encounter
> S   sequela

5 **S90.0** **Contusion of ankle**

7 **S90.00X-** **Contusion of unspecified ankle**

7 **S90.01X-** **Contusion of right ankle**

7 **S90.02X-** **Contusion of left ankle**

5 **S90.1** **Contusion of toe without damage to nail**

6 **S90.11** **Contusion of great toe without damage to nail**

7 **S90.111-** **Contusion of right great toe without damage to nail**

7 **S90.112-** **Contusion of left great toe without damage to nail**

7 **S90.119-** **Contusion of unspecified great toe without damage to nail**

6 **S90.12** **Contusion of lesser toe without damage to nail**

7 **S90.121-** **Contusion of right lesser toe(s) without damage to nail**

7 **S90.122-** **Contusion of left lesser toe(s) without damage to nail**

7 **S90.129-** **Contusion of unspecified lesser toe(s) without damage to nail**
> Contusion of toe NOS

5 **S90.2** **Contusion of toe with damage to nail**

6 **S90.21** **Contusion of great toe with damage to nail**

7 **S90.211-** **Contusion of right great toe with damage to nail**

7 **S90.212-** **Contusion of left great toe with damage to nail**

7 **S90.219-** **Contusion of unspecified great toe with damage to nail**

6 **S90.22** **Contusion of lesser toe with damage to nail**

7 **S90.221-** **Contusion of right lesser toe(s) with damage to nail**

7 **S90.222-** **Contusion of left lesser toe(s) with damage to nail**

7 **S90.229-** **Contusion of unspecified lesser toe(s) with damage to nail**

5 **S90.3** **Contusion of foot**

> **EXCLUDES 2** *contusion of toes (S90.1-, S90.2-)*

7 **S90.30X-** **Contusion of unspecified foot**
> Contusion of foot NOS

7 **S90.31X-** **Contusion of right foot**

7 **S90.32X-** **Contusion of left foot**

5 **S90.4** **Other superficial injuries of toe**

6 **S90.41** **Abrasion of toe**

7 **S90.411-** **Abrasion, right great toe**

7 **S90.412-** **Abrasion, left great toe**

7 **S90.413-** **Abrasion, unspecified great toe**

7 **S90.414-** **Abrasion, right lesser toe(s)**

7 **S90.415-** **Abrasion, left lesser toe(s)**

7 **S90.416-** **Abrasion, unspecified lesser toe(s)**

6 **S90.42** **Blister (nonthermal) of toe**

7 **S90.421-** **Blister (nonthermal), right great toe**

7 **S90.422-** **Blister (nonthermal), left great toe**

7 **S90.423-** **Blister (nonthermal), unspecified great toe**

7 **S90.424-** **Blister (nonthermal), right lesser toe(s)**

7 **S90.425-** **Blister (nonthermal), left lesser toe(s)**

7 **S90.426-** **Blister (nonthermal), unspecified lesser toe(s)**

6 **S90.44** **External constriction of toe**
> Hair tourniquet syndrome of toe

7 **S90.441-** **External constriction, right great toe**

7 **S90.442-** **External constriction, left great toe**

7 **S90.443-** **External constriction, unspecified great toe**

7 **S90.444-** **External constriction, right lesser toe(s)**

7 **S90.445-** **External constriction, left lesser toe(s)**

7 **S90.446-** **External constriction, unspecified lesser toe(s)**

6 **S90.45** **Superficial foreign body of toe**
> Splinter in the toe

7 **S90.451-** **Superficial foreign body, right great toe**

7 **S90.452-** **Superficial foreign body, left great toe**

7 **S90.453-** **Superficial foreign body, unspecified great toe**

7 **S90.454-** **Superficial foreign body, right lesser toe(s)**

7 **S90.455-** **Superficial foreign body, left lesser toe(s)**

7 **S90.456-** **Superficial foreign body, unspecified lesser toe(s)**

6 **S90.46** **Insect bite (nonvenomous) of toe**

7 **S90.461-** **Insect bite (nonvenomous), right great toe**

7 **S90.462-** **Insect bite (nonvenomous), left great toe**

7 **S90.463-** **Insect bite (nonvenomous), unspecified great toe**

7 **S90.464-** **Insect bite (nonvenomous), right lesser toe(s)**

7 **S90.465-** **Insect bite (nonvenomous), left lesser toe(s)**

7 **S90.466-** **Insect bite (nonvenomous), unspecified lesser toe(s)**

6 **S90.47** **Other superficial bite of toe**
> **EXCLUDES 1** *open bite of toe (S91.15-, S91.25-)*

7 **S90.471-** **Other superficial bite of right great toe**

7 **S90.472-** **Other superficial bite of left great toe**

7 **S90.473-** **Other superficial bite of unspecified great toe**

7 **S90.474-** **Other superficial bite of right lesser toe(s)**

7 **S90.475-** **Other superficial bite of left lesser toe(s)**

7 **S90.476-** **Other superficial bite of unspecified lesser toe(s)**

5 **S90.5** **Other superficial injuries of ankle**

6 **S90.51** **Abrasion of ankle**

7 **S90.511-** **Abrasion, right ankle**

7 **S90.512-** **Abrasion, left ankle**

7 **S90.519-** **Abrasion, unspecified ankle**

6 **S90.52** **Blister (nonthermal) of ankle**

7 **S90.521-** **Blister (nonthermal), right ankle**

7 **S90.522-** **Blister (nonthermal), left ankle**

7 **S90.529-** **Blister (nonthermal), unspecified ankle**

6 **S90.54** **External constriction of ankle**

7 **S90.541-** **External constriction, right ankle**

7 **S90.542-** **External constriction, left ankle**

7 **S90.549-** **External constriction, unspecified ankle**

6 **S90.55** **Superficial foreign body of ankle**
> Splinter in the ankle

7 **S90.551-** **Superficial foreign body, right ankle**

7 **S90.552-** **Superficial foreign body, left ankle**

7 **S90.559-** **Superficial foreign body, unspecified ankle**

● New ▲ Revised *Manifestation* 4-7 Digit Indicators ▣ Laterality ⒶAdult (15+ years) ⓂMaternity (12-55 years) ⓃNewborn ⓅPediatric (0-17 years) ♂Male ♀Female
✖ Deleted Unspecified + Additional code

⑥ **S90.56**   **Insect bite (nonvenomous) of ankle**
   7️⃣ ⊟ **S90.561-**   Insect bite (nonvenomous), right ankle
   7️⃣ ⊟ **S90.562-**   Insect bite (nonvenomous), left ankle
   7️⃣ ⊟ **S90.569-**   **Insect bite (nonvenomous), unspecified ankle**

⑥ **S90.57**   **Other superficial bite of ankle**
        EXCLUDES 1   *open bite of ankle (S91.05-)*
   7️⃣ ⊟ **S90.571-**   Other superficial bite of ankle, right ankle
   7️⃣ ⊟ **S90.572-**   Other superficial bite of ankle, left ankle
   7️⃣ ⊟ **S90.579-**   **Other superficial bite of ankle, unspecified ankle**

⑤ **S90.8**   **Other superficial injuries of foot**

⑥ **S90.81**   **Abrasion of foot**
   7️⃣ ⊟ **S90.811-**   **Abrasion, right foot**
   7️⃣ ⊟ **S90.812-**   **Abrasion, left foot**
   7️⃣ ⊟ **S90.819-**   **Abrasion, unspecified foot**

⑥ **S90.82**   **Blister (nonthermal) of foot**
   7️⃣ ⊟ **S90.821-**   **Blister (nonthermal), right foot**
   7️⃣ ⊟ **S90.822-**   **Blister (nonthermal), left foot**
   7️⃣ ⊟ **S90.829-**   **Blister (nonthermal), unspecified foot**

⑥ **S90.84**   **External constriction of foot**
   7️⃣ ⊟ **S90.841-**   **External constriction, right foot**
   7️⃣ ⊟ **S90.842-**   **External constriction, left foot**
   7️⃣ ⊟ **S90.849-**   **External constriction, unspecified foot**

⑥ **S90.85**   **Superficial foreign body of foot**
        Splinter in the foot
   7️⃣ ⊟ **S90.851-**   **Superficial foreign body, right foot**
   7️⃣ ⊟ **S90.852-**   **Superficial foreign body, left foot**
   7️⃣ ⊟ **S90.859-**   **Superficial foreign body, unspecified foot**

⑥ **S90.86**   **Insect bite (nonvenomous) of foot**
   7️⃣ ⊟ **S90.861-**   **Insect bite (nonvenomous), right foot**
   7️⃣ ⊟ **S90.862-**   **Insect bite (nonvenomous), left foot**
   7️⃣ ⊟ **S90.869-**   **Insect bite (nonvenomous), unspecified foot**

⑥ **S90.87**   **Other superficial bite of foot**
        EXCLUDES 1   *open bite of foot (S91.35-)*
   7️⃣ ⊟ **S90.871-**   **Other superficial bite of right foot**
   7️⃣ ⊟ **S90.872-**   **Other superficial bite of left foot**
   7️⃣ ⊟ **S90.879-**   **Other superficial bite of unspecified foot**

⑤ **S90.9**   **Unspecified superficial injury of ankle, foot and toe**

⑥ **S90.91**   **Unspecified superficial injury of ankle**
   7️⃣ ⊟ **S90.911-**   **Unspecified superficial injury of right ankle**
   7️⃣ ⊟ **S90.912-**   **Unspecified superficial injury of left ankle**
   7️⃣ ⊟ **S90.919-**   **Unspecified superficial injury of unspecified ankle**

⑥ **S90.92**   **Unspecified superficial injury of foot**
   7️⃣ ⊟ **S90.921-**   **Unspecified superficial injury of right foot**
   7️⃣ ⊟ **S90.922-**   **Unspecified superficial injury of left foot**
   7️⃣ ⊟ **S90.929-**   **Unspecified superficial injury of unspecified foot**

⑥ **S90.93**   **Unspecified superficial injury of toes**
   7️⃣ ⊟ **S90.931-**   **Unspecified superficial injury of right great toe**
   7️⃣ ⊟ **S90.932-**   **Unspecified superficial injury of left great toe**
   7️⃣ ⊟ **S90.933-**   **Unspecified superficial injury of unspecified great toe**
   7️⃣ ⊟ **S90.934-**   **Unspecified superficial injury of right lesser toe(s)**
   7️⃣ ⊟ **S90.935-**   **Unspecified superficial injury of left lesser toe(s)**
   7️⃣ ⊟ **S90.936-**   **Unspecified superficial injury of unspecified lesser toe(s)**

④ **S91**   **Open wound of ankle, foot and toes**
     Code also:
       any associated wound infection
       EXCLUDES 1   *open fracture of ankle, foot and toes (S92.-with 7th character B)*
                  traumatic amputation of ankle and foot (S98.-)

The appropriate 7th character is to be added to each code from category S91
A   initial encounter
D   subsequent encounter
S   sequela

CODING TIP ✓   Open wound codes indicate a wound resulting from a traumatic origin. Do not assign a code for "open wound" unless the etiology of the wound is related to trauma.

⑤ **S91.0**   **Open wound of ankle**

⑥ **S91.00**   **Unspecified open wound of ankle**
   7️⃣ ⊟ **S91.001-**   **Unspecified open wound, right ankle**
   7️⃣ ⊟ **S91.002-**   **Unspecified open wound, left ankle**
   7️⃣ ⊟ **S91.009-**   **Unspecified open wound, unspecified ankle**

⑥ **S91.01**   **Laceration without foreign body of ankle**
   7️⃣ ⊟ **S91.011-**   **Laceration without foreign body, right ankle**
   7️⃣ ⊟ **S91.012-**   **Laceration without foreign body, left ankle**
   7️⃣ ⊟ **S91.019-**   **Laceration without foreign body, unspecified ankle**

⑥ **S91.02**   **Laceration with foreign body of ankle**
   7️⃣ ⊟ **S91.021-**   **Laceration with foreign body, right ankle**
   7️⃣ ⊟ **S91.022-**   **Laceration with foreign body, left ankle**
   7️⃣ ⊟ **S91.029-**   **Laceration with foreign body, unspecified ankle**

⑥ **S91.03**   **Puncture wound without foreign body of ankle**
   7️⃣ ⊟ **S91.031-**   **Puncture wound without foreign body, right ankle**
   7️⃣ ⊟ **S91.032-**   **Puncture wound without foreign body, left ankle**
   7️⃣ ⊟ **S91.039-**   **Puncture wound without foreign body, unspecified ankle**

⑥ **S91.04**   **Puncture wound with foreign body of ankle**
   7️⃣ ⊟ **S91.041-**   **Puncture wound with foreign body, right ankle**
   7️⃣ ⊟ **S91.042-**   **Puncture wound with foreign body, left ankle**
   7️⃣ ⊟ **S91.049-**   **Puncture wound with foreign body, unspecified ankle**

⑥ **S91.05**   **Open bite of ankle**
        EXCLUDES 1   *superficial bite of ankle (S90.56-, S90.57-)*
   7️⃣ ⊟ **S91.051-**   **Open bite, right ankle**
   7️⃣ ⊟ **S91.052-**   **Open bite, left ankle**
   7️⃣ ⊟ **S91.059-**   **Open bite, unspecified ankle**

⑤ **S91.1**   **Open wound of toe without damage to nail**

⑥ **S91.10**   **Unspecified open wound of toe without damage to nail**
   7️⃣ ⊟ **S91.101-**   **Unspecified open wound of right great toe without damage to nail**
   7️⃣ ⊟ **S91.102-**   **Unspecified open wound of left great toe without damage to nail**
   7️⃣ ⊟ **S91.103-**   **Unspecified open wound of unspecified great toe without damage to nail**
   7️⃣ ⊟ **S91.104-**   **Unspecified open wound of right lesser toe(s) without damage to nail**
   7️⃣ ⊟ **S91.105-**   **Unspecified open wound of left lesser toe(s) without damage to nail**
   7️⃣ ⊟ **S91.106-**   **Unspecified open wound of unspecified lesser toe(s) without damage to nail**
   7️⃣ ⊟ **S91.109-**   **Unspecified open wound of unspecified toe(s) without damage to nail**

⑥ **S91.11**   **Laceration without foreign body of toe without damage to nail**
   7️⃣ ⊟ **S91.111-**   **Laceration without foreign body of right great toe without damage to nail**
   7️⃣ ⊟ **S91.112-**   **Laceration without foreign body of left great toe without damage to nail**
   7️⃣ ⊟ **S91.113-**   **Laceration without foreign body of unspecified great toe without damage to nail**

● New   ▲ Revised   *Manifestation*   ④-⑦ Digit Indicators   ⊟ Laterality   Ⓐ Adult (15+ years)   Ⓜ Maternity (12-55 years)   Ⓝ Newborn   Ⓟ Pediatric (0-17 years)   ♂ Male   ♀ Female
✖ ~~Deleted~~   Unspecified   ✚ Additional code

7 🔲 S91.114-   Laceration without foreign body of right lesser toe(s) without damage to nail

7 🔲 S91.115-   Laceration without foreign body of left lesser toe(s) without damage to nail

7 🔲 S91.116-   Laceration without foreign body of unspecified lesser toe(s) without damage to nail

7 🔲 S91.119-   Laceration without foreign body of unspecified toe without damage to nail

6 S91.12   Laceration with foreign body of toe without damage to nail

7 🔲 S91.121-   Laceration with foreign body of right great toe without damage to nail

7 🔲 S91.122-   Laceration with foreign body of left great toe without damage to nail

7 🔲 S91.123-   Laceration with foreign body of unspecified great toe without damage to nail

7 🔲 S91.124-   Laceration with foreign body of right lesser toe(s) without damage to nail

7 🔲 S91.125-   Laceration with foreign body of left lesser toe(s) without damage to nail

7 🔲 S91.126-   Laceration with foreign body of unspecified lesser toe(s) without damage to nail

7 🔲 S91.129-   Laceration with foreign body of unspecified toe(s) without damage to nail

6 S91.13   Puncture wound without foreign body of toe without damage to nail

7 🔲 S91.131-   Puncture wound without foreign body of right great toe without damage to nail

7 🔲 S91.132-   Puncture wound without foreign body of left great toe without damage to nail

7 🔲 S91.133-   Puncture wound without foreign body of unspecified great toe without damage to nail

7 🔲 S91.134-   Puncture wound without foreign body of right lesser toe(s) without damage to nail

7 🔲 S91.135-   Puncture wound without foreign body of left lesser toe(s) without damage to nail

7 🔲 S91.136-   Puncture wound without foreign body of unspecified lesser toe(s) without damage to nail

7 🔲 S91.139-   Puncture wound without foreign body of unspecified toe(s) without damage to nail

6 S91.14   Puncture wound with foreign body of toe without damage to nail

7 🔲 S91.141-   Puncture wound with foreign body of right great toe without damage to nail

7 🔲 S91.142-   Puncture wound with foreign body of left great toe without damage to nail

7 🔲 S91.143-   Puncture wound with foreign body of unspecified great toe without damage to nail

7 🔲 S91.144-   Puncture wound with foreign body of right lesser toe(s) without damage to nail

7 🔲 S91.145-   Puncture wound with foreign body of left lesser toe(s) without damage to nail

7 🔲 S91.146-   Puncture wound with foreign body of unspecified lesser toe(s) without damage to nail

7 🔲 S91.149-   Puncture wound with foreign body of unspecified toe(s) without damage to nail

6 S91.15   Open bite of toe without damage to nail

     Bite of toe NOS

     EXCLUDES 1   *superficial bite of toe (S90.46-, S90.47-)*

7 🔲 S91.151-   Open bite of right great toe without damage to nail

7 🔲 S91.152-   Open bite of left great toe without damage to nail

7 🔲 S91.153-   Open bite of unspecified great toe without damage to nail

7 🔲 S91.154-   Open bite of right lesser toe(s) without damage to nail

7 🔲 S91.155-   Open bite of left lesser toe(s) without damage to nail

7 🔲 S91.156-   Open bite of unspecified lesser toe(s) without damage to nail

7 🔲 S91.159-   Open bite of unspecified toe(s) without damage to nail

5 S91.2   Open wound of toe with damage to nail

6 S91.20   Unspecified open wound of toe with damage to nail

7 🔲 S91.201-   Unspecified open wound of right great toe with damage to nail

7 🔲 S91.202-   Unspecified open wound of left great toe with damage to nail

7 🔲 S91.203-   Unspecified open wound of unspecified great toe with damage to nail

7 🔲 S91.204-   Unspecified open wound of right lesser toe(s) with damage to nail

7 🔲 S91.205-   Unspecified open wound of left lesser toe(s) with damage to nail

7 🔲 S91.206-   Unspecified open wound of unspecified lesser toe(s) with damage to nail

7 🔲 S91.209-   Unspecified open wound of unspecified toe(s) with damage to nail

6 S91.21   Laceration without foreign body of toe with damage to nail

7 🔲 S91.211-   Laceration without foreign body of right great toe with damage to nail

7 🔲 S91.212-   Laceration without foreign body of left great toe with damage to nail

7 🔲 S91.213-   Laceration without foreign body of unspecified great toe with damage to nail

7 🔲 S91.214-   Laceration without foreign body of right lesser toe(s) with damage to nail

7 🔲 S91.215-   Laceration without foreign body of left lesser toe(s) with damage to nail

7 🔲 S91.216-   Laceration without foreign body of unspecified lesser toe(s) with damage to nail

7 🔲 S91.219-   Laceration without foreign body of unspecified toe(s) with damage to nail

6 S91.22   Laceration with foreign body of toe with damage to nail

7 🔲 S91.221-   Laceration with foreign body of right great toe with damage to nail

7 🔲 S91.222-   Laceration with foreign body of left great toe with damage to nail

7 🔲 S91.223-   Laceration with foreign body of unspecified great toe with damage to nail

7 🔲 S91.224-   Laceration with foreign body of right lesser toe(s) with damage to nail

7 🔲 S91.225-   Laceration with foreign body of left lesser toe(s) with damage to nail

7 🔲 S91.226-   Laceration with foreign body of unspecified lesser toe(s) with damage to nail

7 🔲 S91.229-   Laceration with foreign body of unspecified toe(s) with damage to nail

6 S91.23   Puncture wound without foreign body of toe with damage to nail

7 🔲 S91.231-   Puncture wound without foreign body of right great toe with damage to nail

7 🔲 S91.232-   Puncture wound without foreign body of left great toe with damage to nail

7 🔲 S91.233-   Puncture wound without foreign body of unspecified great toe with damage to nail

7 🔲 S91.234-   Puncture wound without foreign body of right lesser toe(s) with damage to nail

7 🔲 S91.235-   Puncture wound without foreign body of left lesser toe(s) with damage to nail

7 🔲 S91.236-   Puncture wound without foreign body of unspecified lesser toe(s) with damage to nail

7 🔲 S91.239-   Puncture wound without foreign body of unspecified toe(s) with damage to nail

6 S91.24   Puncture wound with foreign body of toe with damage to nail

7 🔲 S91.241-   Puncture wound with foreign body of right great toe with damage to nail

7 🔲 S91.242-   Puncture wound with foreign body of left great toe with damage to nail

7 🔲 S91.243-   Puncture wound with foreign body of unspecified great toe with damage to nail

7 🔲 S91.244-   Puncture wound with foreign body of right lesser toe(s) with damage to nail

7 🔲 S91.245-   Puncture wound with foreign body of left lesser toe(s) with damage to nail

7 🔲 S91.246-   Puncture wound with foreign body of unspecified lesser toe(s) with damage to nail

7 🔲 S91.249-   Puncture wound with foreign body of unspecified toe(s) with damage to nail

---

● New   ▲ Revised   *Manifestation*   4 - 7 Digit Indicators   🔲 Laterality   Ⓐ Adult (15+ years)   Ⓜ Maternity (12-55 years)   Ⓝ Newborn   Ⓟ Pediatric (0-17 years)   ♂ Male   ♀ Female

✖ Deleted   Unspecified   + Additional code

S91.25 Open bite of toe with damage to nail
Bite of toe with damage to nail NOS
EXCLUDES 1 *superficial bite of toe (S90.46-, S90.47-)*

7☐ **S91.251-** Open bite of right great toe with damage to nail

7☐ **S91.252-** Open bite of left great toe with damage to nail

7☐ **S91.253-** Open bite of unspecified great toe with damage to nail

7☐ **S91.254-** Open bite of right lesser toe(s) with damage to nail

7☐ **S91.255-** Open bite of left lesser toe(s) with damage to nail

7☐ **S91.256-** Open bite of unspecified lesser toe(s) with damage to nail

7☐ **S91.259-** Open bite of unspecified toe(s) with damage to nail

S91.3 Open wound of foot

6 **S91.30** Unspecified open wound of foot

7☐ **S91.301-** Unspecified open wound, right foot

7☐ **S91.302-** Unspecified open wound, left foot

7☐ **S91.309-** Unspecified open wound, unspecified foot

6 **S91.31** Laceration without foreign body of foot

7☐ **S91.311-** Laceration without foreign body, right foot

7☐ **S91.312-** Laceration without foreign body, left foot

7☐ **S91.319-** Laceration without foreign body, unspecified foot

6 **S91.32** Laceration with foreign body of foot

7☐ **S91.321-** Laceration with foreign body, right foot

7☐ **S91.322-** Laceration with foreign body, left foot

7☐ **S91.329-** Laceration with foreign body, unspecified foot

6 **S91.33** Puncture wound without foreign body of foot

7☐ **S91.331-** Puncture wound without foreign body, right foot

7☐ **S91.332-** Puncture wound without foreign body, left foot

7☐ **S91.339-** Puncture wound without foreign body, unspecified foot

6 **S91.34** Puncture wound with foreign body of foot

7☐ **S91.341-** Puncture wound with foreign body, right foot

7☐ **S91.342-** Puncture wound with foreign body, left foot

7☐ **S91.349-** Puncture wound with foreign body, unspecified foot

6 **S91.35** Open bite of foot
EXCLUDES 1 *superficial bite of foot (S90.86-, S90.87-)*

7☐ **S91.351-** Open bite, right foot

7☐ **S91.352-** Open bite, left foot

7☐ **S91.359-** Open bite, unspecified foot

4 **S92** **Fracture of foot and toe, except ankle**
Note: A fracture not indicated as displaced or nondisplaced should be coded to displaced
A fracture not indicated as open or closed should be coded to closed
EXCLUDES 1 *traumatic amputation of ankle and foot (S98.-)*
EXCLUDES 2 *fracture of ankle (S82.-)*
fracture of malleolus (S82.-)

The appropriate 7th character is to be added to each code from category S92
A initial encounter for closed fracture
B initial encounter for open fracture
D subsequent encounter for fracture with routine healing
G subsequent encounter for fracture with delayed healing
K subsequent encounter for fracture with nonunion
P subsequent encounter for fracture with malunion
S sequela

CODING TIP ✓ A fracture not indicated as displaced or nondisplaced should be coded to displaced. A fracture not indicated as open or closed should be coded to closed. Query providers on fractures not documented as displaced/nondisplaced otherwise displaced fracture diagnosis could be assigned without reduction being performed potentially resulting in claim denials.

▲ 5 **S92.0** **Fracture of calcaneus**
Heel bone
Os calcis
EXCLUDES 2 *Physeal fracture of calcaneus (S99.0-)*

6 **S92.00** Unspecified fracture of calcaneus

7☐ **S92.001-** Unspecified fracture of right calcaneus

7☐ **S92.002-** Unspecified fracture of left calcaneus

7☐ **S92.009-** Unspecified fracture of unspecified calcaneus

6 **S92.01** Fracture of body of calcaneus

7☐ **S92.011-** Displaced fracture of body of right calcaneus

7☐ **S92.012-** Displaced fracture of body of left calcaneus

7☐ **S92.013-** Displaced fracture of body of unspecified calcaneus

7☐ **S92.014-** Nondisplaced fracture of body of right calcaneus

7☐ **S92.015-** Nondisplaced fracture of body of left calcaneus

7☐ **S92.016-** Nondisplaced fracture of body of unspecified calcaneus

6 **S92.02** Fracture of anterior process of calcaneus

7☐ **S92.021-** Displaced fracture of anterior process of right calcaneus

7☐ **S92.022-** Displaced fracture of anterior process of left calcaneus

7☐ **S92.023-** Displaced fracture of anterior process of unspecified calcaneus

7☐ **S92.024-** Nondisplaced fracture of anterior process of right calcaneus

7☐ **S92.025-** Nondisplaced fracture of anterior process of left calcaneus

7☐ **S92.026-** Nondisplaced fracture of anterior process of unspecified calcaneus

6 **S92.03** Avulsion fracture of tuberosity of calcaneus

7☐ **S92.031-** Displaced avulsion fracture of tuberosity of right calcaneus

7☐ **S92.032-** Displaced avulsion fracture of tuberosity of left calcaneus

7☐ **S92.033-** Displaced avulsion fracture of tuberosity of unspecified calcaneus

7☐ **S92.034-** Nondisplaced avulsion fracture of tuberosity of right calcaneus

7☐ **S92.035-** Nondisplaced avulsion fracture of tuberosity of left calcaneus

7☐ **S92.036-** Nondisplaced avulsion fracture of tuberosity of unspecified calcaneus

6 **S92.04** Other fracture of tuberosity of calcaneus

7☐ **S92.041-** Displaced other fracture of tuberosity of right calcaneus

7☐ **S92.042-** Displaced other fracture of tuberosity of left calcaneus

7☐ **S92.043-** Displaced other fracture of tuberosity of unspecified calcaneus

7☐ **S92.044-** Nondisplaced other fracture of tuberosity of right calcaneus

7☐ **S92.045-** Nondisplaced other fracture of tuberosity of left calcaneus

7☐ **S92.046-** Nondisplaced other fracture of tuberosity of unspecified calcaneus

6 **S92.05** Other extraarticular fracture of calcaneus

7☐ **S92.051-** Displaced other extraarticular fracture of right calcaneus

7☐ **S92.052-** Displaced other extraarticular fracture of left calcaneus

7☐ **S92.053-** Displaced other extraarticular fracture of unspecified calcaneus

7☐ **S92.054-** Nondisplaced other extraarticular fracture of right calcaneus

7☐ **S92.055-** Nondisplaced other extraarticular fracture of left calcaneus

7☐ **S92.056-** Nondisplaced other extraarticular fracture of unspecified calcaneus

6 **S92.06** Intraarticular fracture of calcaneus

7☐ **S92.061-** Displaced intraarticular fracture of right calcaneus

7☐ **S92.062-** Displaced intraarticular fracture of left calcaneus

7 ☰ **S92.063-**   **Displaced intraarticular fracture of unspecified calcaneus**

7 ☰ **S92.064-**   **Nondisplaced intraarticular fracture of right calcaneus**

7 ☰ **S92.065-**   **Nondisplaced intraarticular fracture of left calcaneus**

7 ☰ **S92.066-**   **Nondisplaced intraarticular fracture of unspecified calcaneus**

Ⓢ **S92.1**   **Fracture of talus**
    Astragalus

Ⓖ **S92.10**   **Unspecified fracture of talus**

7 ☰ **S92.101-**   **Unspecified fracture of right talus**

7 ☰ **S92.102-**   **Unspecified fracture of left talus**

7 ☰ **S92.109-**   **Unspecified fracture of unspecified talus**

Ⓖ **S92.11**   **Fracture of neck of talus**

7 ☰ **S92.111-**   **Displaced fracture of neck of right talus**

7 ☰ **S92.112-**   **Displaced fracture of neck of left talus**

7 ☰ **S92.113-**   **Displaced fracture of neck of unspecified talus**

7 ☰ **S92.114-**   **Nondisplaced fracture of neck of right talus**

7 ☰ **S92.115-**   **Nondisplaced fracture of neck of left talus**

7 ☰ **S92.116-**   **Nondisplaced fracture of neck of unspecified talus**

Ⓖ **S92.12**   **Fracture of body of talus**

7 ☰ **S92.121-**   **Displaced fracture of body of right talus**

7 ☰ **S92.122-**   **Displaced fracture of body of left talus**

7 ☰ **S92.123-**   **Displaced fracture of body of unspecified talus**

7 ☰ **S92.124-**   **Nondisplaced fracture of body of right talus**

7 ☰ **S92.125-**   **Nondisplaced fracture of body of left talus**

7 ☰ **S92.126-**   **Nondisplaced fracture of body of unspecified talus**

Ⓖ **S92.13**   **Fracture of posterior process of talus**

7 ☰ **S92.131-**   **Displaced fracture of posterior process of right talus**

7 ☰ **S92.132-**   **Displaced fracture of posterior process of left talus**

7 ☰ **S92.133-**   **Displaced fracture of posterior process of unspecified talus**

7 ☰ **S92.134-**   **Nondisplaced fracture of posterior process of right talus**

7 ☰ **S92.135-**   **Nondisplaced fracture of posterior process of left talus**

7 ☰ **S92.136-**   **Nondisplaced fracture of posterior process of unspecified talus**

Ⓖ **S92.14**   **Dome fracture of talus**

    EXCLUDES 1   *osteochondritis dissecans (M93.2)*

7 ☰ **S92.141-**   **Displaced dome fracture of right talus**

7 ☰ **S92.142-**   **Displaced dome fracture of left talus**

7 ☰ **S92.143-**   **Displaced dome fracture of unspecified talus**

7 ☰ **S92.144-**   **Nondisplaced dome fracture of right talus**

7 ☰ **S92.145-**   **Nondisplaced dome fracture of left talus**

7 ☰ **S92.146-**   **Nondisplaced dome fracture of unspecified talus**

Ⓖ **S92.15**   **Avulsion fracture (chip fracture) of talus**

7 ☰ **S92.151-**   **Displaced avulsion fracture (chip fracture) of right talus**

7 ☰ **S92.152-**   **Displaced avulsion fracture (chip fracture) of left talus**

7 ☰ **S92.153-**   **Displaced avulsion fracture (chip fracture) of unspecified talus**

7 ☰ **S92.154-**   **Nondisplaced avulsion fracture (chip fracture) of right talus**

7 ☰ **S92.155-**   **Nondisplaced avulsion fracture (chip fracture) of left talus**

7 ☰ **S92.156-**   **Nondisplaced avulsion fracture (chip fracture) of unspecified talus**

Ⓖ **S92.19**   **Other fracture of talus**

7 ☰ **S92.191-**   **Other fracture of right talus**

7 ☰ **S92.192-**   **Other fracture of left talus**

7 ☰ **S92.199-**   **Other fracture of unspecified talus**

Ⓢ **S92.2**   **Fracture of other and unspecified tarsal bone(s)**

Ⓖ **S92.20**   **Fracture of unspecified tarsal bone(s)**

7 ☰ **S92.201-**   **Fracture of unspecified tarsal bone(s) of right foot**

7 ☰ **S92.202-**   **Fracture of unspecified tarsal bone(s) of left foot**

7 ☰ **S92.209-**   **Fracture of unspecified tarsal bone(s) of unspecified foot**

Ⓖ **S92.21**   **Fracture of cuboid bone**

7 ☰ **S92.211-**   **Displaced fracture of cuboid bone of right foot**

7 ☰ **S92.212-**   **Displaced fracture of cuboid bone of left foot**

7 ☰ **S92.213-**   **Displaced fracture of cuboid bone of unspecified foot**

7 ☰ **S92.214-**   **Nondisplaced fracture of cuboid bone of right foot**

7 ☰ **S92.215-**   **Nondisplaced fracture of cuboid bone of left foot**

7 ☰ **S92.216-**   **Nondisplaced fracture of cuboid bone of unspecified foot**

Ⓖ **S92.22**   **Fracture of lateral cuneiform**

7 ☰ **S92.221-**   **Displaced fracture of lateral cuneiform of right foot**

7 ☰ **S92.222-**   **Displaced fracture of lateral cuneiform of left foot**

7 ☰ **S92.223-**   **Displaced fracture of lateral cuneiform of unspecified foot**

7 ☰ **S92.224-**   **Nondisplaced fracture of lateral cuneiform of right foot**

7 ☰ **S92.225-**   **Nondisplaced fracture of lateral cuneiform of left foot**

7 ☰ **S92.226-**   **Nondisplaced fracture of lateral cuneiform of unspecified foot**

Ⓖ **S92.23**   **Fracture of intermediate cuneiform**

7 ☰ **S92.231-**   **Displaced fracture of intermediate cuneiform of right foot**

7 ☰ **S92.232-**   **Displaced fracture of intermediate cuneiform of left foot**

7 ☰ **S92.233-**   **Displaced fracture of intermediate cuneiform of unspecified foot**

7 ☰ **S92.234-**   **Nondisplaced fracture of intermediate cuneiform of right foot**

7 ☰ **S92.235-**   **Nondisplaced fracture of intermediate cuneiform of left foot**

7 ☰ **S92.236-**   **Nondisplaced fracture of intermediate cuneiform of unspecified foot**

Ⓖ **S92.24**   **Fracture of medial cuneiform**

7 ☰ **S92.241-**   **Displaced fracture of medial cuneiform of right foot**

7 ☰ **S92.242-**   **Displaced fracture of medial cuneiform of left foot**

7 ☰ **S92.243-**   **Displaced fracture of medial cuneiform of unspecified foot**

7 ☰ **S92.244-**   **Nondisplaced fracture of medial cuneiform of right foot**

7 ☰ **S92.245-**   **Nondisplaced fracture of medial cuneiform of left foot**

7 ☰ **S92.246-**   **Nondisplaced fracture of medial cuneiform of unspecified foot**

Ⓖ **S92.25**   **Fracture of navicular [scaphoid] of foot**

7 ☰ **S92.251-**   **Displaced fracture of navicular [scaphoid] of right foot**

7 ☰ **S92.252-**   **Displaced fracture of navicular [scaphoid] of left foot**

7 ☰ **S92.253-**   **Displaced fracture of navicular [scaphoid] of unspecified foot**

7 ☰ **S92.254-**   **Nondisplaced fracture of navicular [scaphoid] of right foot**

7 ☰ **S92.255-**   **Nondisplaced fracture of navicular [scaphoid] of left foot**

7 ☰ **S92.256-**   **Nondisplaced fracture of navicular [scaphoid] of unspecified foot**

▲ Ⓢ **S92.3**   **Fracture of metatarsal bone(s)**

    EXCLUDES 2   *Physeal fracture of metatarsal (S99.1-)*

Ⓖ **S92.30**   **Fracture of unspecified metatarsal bone(s)**

7 ☰ **S92.301-**   **Fracture of unspecified metatarsal bone(s), right foot**

7 ☰ **S92.302-**   **Fracture of unspecified metatarsal bone(s), left foot**

7 ☰ **S92.309-**   **Fracture of unspecified metatarsal bone(s), unspecified foot**

Ⓖ **S92.31**   **Fracture of first metatarsal bone**

● New   ▲ Revised   *Manifestation*   4 - 7 Digit Indicators   ☰ Laterality   Ⓐ Adult (15+ years)   Ⓜ Maternity (12-55 years)   Ⓝ Newborn   Ⓟ Pediatric (0-17 years)   ♂ Male   ♀ Female

✖ Deleted   Unspecified   + Additional code

1030   © 2017 DecisionHealth   2017 ICD-10-CM Expert for Physicians

7 ☐ S92.311-   Displaced fracture of first metatarsal bone, right foot
7 ☐ S92.312-   Displaced fracture of first metatarsal bone, left foot
7 ☐ S92.313-   Displaced fracture of first metatarsal bone, unspecified foot
7 ☐ S92.314-   Nondisplaced fracture of first metatarsal bone, right foot
7 ☐ S92.315-   Nondisplaced fracture of first metatarsal bone, left foot
7 ☐ S92.316-   Nondisplaced fracture of first metatarsal bone, unspecified foot

6 S92.32   Fracture of second metatarsal bone
7 ☐ S92.321-   Displaced fracture of second metatarsal bone, right foot
7 ☐ S92.322-   Displaced fracture of second metatarsal bone, left foot
7 ☐ S92.323-   Displaced fracture of second metatarsal bone, unspecified foot
7 ☐ S92.324-   Nondisplaced fracture of second metatarsal bone, right foot
7 ☐ S92.325-   Nondisplaced fracture of second metatarsal bone, left foot
7 ☐ S92.326-   Nondisplaced fracture of second metatarsal bone, unspecified foot

6 S92.33   Fracture of third metatarsal bone
7 ☐ S92.331-   Displaced fracture of third metatarsal bone, right foot
7 ☐ S92.332-   Displaced fracture of third metatarsal bone, left foot
7 ☐ S92.333-   Displaced fracture of third metatarsal bone, unspecified foot
7 ☐ S92.334-   Nondisplaced fracture of third metatarsal bone, right foot
7 ☐ S92.335-   Nondisplaced fracture of third metatarsal bone, left foot
7 ☐ S92.336-   Nondisplaced fracture of third metatarsal bone, unspecified foot

6 S92.34   Fracture of fourth metatarsal bone
7 ☐ S92.341-   Displaced fracture of fourth metatarsal bone, right foot
7 ☐ S92.342-   Displaced fracture of fourth metatarsal bone, left foot
7 ☐ S92.343-   Displaced fracture of fourth metatarsal bone, unspecified foot
7 ☐ S92.344-   Nondisplaced fracture of fourth metatarsal bone, right foot
7 ☐ S92.345-   Nondisplaced fracture of fourth metatarsal bone, left foot
7 ☐ S92.346-   Nondisplaced fracture of fourth metatarsal bone, unspecified foot

6 S92.35   Fracture of fifth metatarsal bone
7 ☐ S92.351-   Displaced fracture of fifth metatarsal bone, right foot
7 ☐ S92.352-   Displaced fracture of fifth metatarsal bone, left foot
7 ☐ S92.353-   Displaced fracture of fifth metatarsal bone, unspecified foot
7 ☐ S92.354-   Nondisplaced fracture of fifth metatarsal bone, right foot
7 ☐ S92.355-   Nondisplaced fracture of fifth metatarsal bone, left foot
7 ☐ S92.356-   Nondisplaced fracture of fifth metatarsal bone, unspecified foot

▲ ☐ S92.4   Fracture of great toe
EXCLUDES 2   *Physeal fracture of phalanx of toe (S99.2-)*

6 S92.40   Unspecified fracture of great toe
7 ☐ S92.401-   Displaced unspecified fracture of right great toe
7 ☐ S92.402-   Displaced unspecified fracture of left great toe
7 ☐ S92.403-   Displaced unspecified fracture of unspecified great toe
7 ☐ S92.404-   Nondisplaced unspecified fracture of right great toe
7 ☐ S92.405-   Nondisplaced unspecified fracture of left great toe
7 ☐ S92.406-   Nondisplaced unspecified fracture of unspecified great toe

6 S92.41   Fracture of proximal phalanx of great toe
7 ☐ S92.411-   Displaced fracture of proximal phalanx of right great toe
7 ☐ S92.412-   Displaced fracture of proximal phalanx of left great toe
7 ☐ S92.413-   Displaced fracture of proximal phalanx of unspecified great toe
7 ☐ S92.414-   Nondisplaced fracture of proximal phalanx of right great toe
7 ☐ S92.415-   Nondisplaced fracture of proximal phalanx of left great toe
7 ☐ S92.416-   Nondisplaced fracture of proximal phalanx of unspecified great toe

6 S92.42   Fracture of distal phalanx of great toe
7 ☐ S92.421-   Displaced fracture of distal phalanx of right great toe
7 ☐ S92.422-   Displaced fracture of distal phalanx of left great toe
7 ☐ S92.423-   Displaced fracture of distal phalanx of unspecified great toe
7 ☐ S92.424-   Nondisplaced fracture of distal phalanx of right great toe
7 ☐ S92.425-   Nondisplaced fracture of distal phalanx of left great toe
7 ☐ S92.426-   Nondisplaced fracture of distal phalanx of unspecified great toe

6 S92.49   Other fracture of great toe
7 ☐ S92.491-   Other fracture of right great toe
7 ☐ S92.492-   Other fracture of left great toe
7 ☐ S92.499-   Other fracture of unspecified great toe

▲ ☐ S92.5   Fracture of lesser toe(s)
EXCLUDES 2   *Physeal fracture of phalanx of toe (S99.2-)*

6 S92.50   Unspecified fracture of lesser toe(s)
7 ☐ S92.501-   Displaced unspecified fracture of right lesser toe(s)
7 ☐ S92.502-   Displaced unspecified fracture of left lesser toe(s)
7 ☐ S92.503-   Displaced unspecified fracture of unspecified lesser toe(s)
7 ☐ S92.504-   Nondisplaced unspecified fracture of right lesser toe(s)
7 ☐ S92.505-   Nondisplaced unspecified fracture of left lesser toe(s)
7 ☐ S92.506-   Nondisplaced unspecified fracture of unspecified lesser toe(s)

6 S92.51   Fracture of proximal phalanx of lesser toe(s)
7 ☐ S92.511-   Displaced fracture of proximal phalanx of right lesser toe(s)
7 ☐ S92.512-   Displaced fracture of proximal phalanx of left lesser toe(s)
7 ☐ S92.513-   Displaced fracture of proximal phalanx of unspecified lesser toe(s)
7 ☐ S92.514-   Nondisplaced fracture of proximal phalanx of right lesser toe(s)
7 ☐ S92.515-   Nondisplaced fracture of proximal phalanx of left lesser toe(s)
7 ☐ S92.516-   Nondisplaced fracture of proximal phalanx of unspecified lesser toe(s)

6 S92.52   Fracture of medial phalanx of lesser toe(s)
7 ☐ S92.521-   Displaced fracture of medial phalanx of right lesser toe(s)
7 ☐ S92.522-   Displaced fracture of medial phalanx of left lesser toe(s)
7 ☐ S92.523-   Displaced fracture of medial phalanx of unspecified lesser toe(s)
7 ☐ S92.524-   Nondisplaced fracture of medial phalanx of right lesser toe(s)
7 ☐ S92.525-   Nondisplaced fracture of medial phalanx of left lesser toe(s)
7 ☐ S92.526-   Nondisplaced fracture of medial phalanx of unspecified lesser toe(s)

6 S92.53   Fracture of distal phalanx of lesser toe(s)
7 ☐ S92.531-   Displaced fracture of distal phalanx of right lesser toe(s)
7 ☐ S92.532-   Displaced fracture of distal phalanx of left lesser toe(s)

7 ⊟ S92.533- Displaced fracture of distal phalanx of unspecified lesser toe(s)

7 ⊟ S92.534- Nondisplaced fracture of distal phalanx of right lesser toe(s)

7 ⊟ S92.535- Nondisplaced fracture of distal phalanx of left lesser toe(s)

7 ⊟ S92.536- Nondisplaced fracture of distal phalanx of unspecified lesser toe(s)

6 S92.59 Other fracture of lesser toe(s)

7 ⊟ S92.591- Other fracture of right lesser toe(s)

7 ⊟ S92.592- Other fracture of left lesser toe(s)

7 ⊟ S92.599- Other fracture of unspecified lesser toe(s)

● 5 S92.8 Other fracture of foot, except ankle

● 6 S92.81 Other fracture of foot
Sesamoid fracture of foot

● 7 ⊟ S92.811- Other fracture of right foot

● 7 ⊟ S92.812- Other fracture of left foot

● 7 ⊟ S92.819- Other fracture of unspecified foot

5 S92.9 Unspecified fracture of foot and toe

6 S92.90 Unspecified fracture of foot

7 ⊟ S92.901- Unspecified fracture of right foot

7 ⊟ S92.902- Unspecified fracture of left foot

7 ⊟ S92.909- Unspecified fracture of unspecified foot

6 S92.91 Unspecified fracture of toe

7 ⊟ S92.911- Unspecified fracture of right toe(s)

7 ⊟ S92.912- Unspecified fracture of left toe(s)

7 ⊟ S92.919- Unspecified fracture of unspecified toe(s)

4 S93 Dislocation and sprain of joints and ligaments at ankle, foot and toe level

| INCLUDES | avulsion of joint or ligament of ankle, foot and toe |

laceration of cartilage, joint or ligament of ankle, foot and toe

sprain of cartilage, joint or ligament of ankle, foot and toe

traumatic hemarthrosis of joint or ligament of ankle, foot and toe

traumatic rupture of joint or ligament of ankle, foot and toe

traumatic subluxation of joint or ligament of ankle, foot and toe

traumatic tear of joint or ligament of ankle, foot and toe

Code also:
any associated open wound

| EXCLUDES 2 | *strain of muscle and tendon of ankle and foot (S96.-)* |

The appropriate 7th character is to be added to each code from category S93
A   initial encounter
D   subsequent encounter
S   sequela

| CODING TIP ✓ | Unlike ICD-9 there is no code for open dislocations. When documented as open an additional code for the open wound must be applied. |

5 S93.0 Subluxation and dislocation of ankle joint
Subluxation and dislocation of astragalus
Subluxation and dislocation of fibula, lower end
Subluxation and dislocation of talus
Subluxation and dislocation of tibia, lower end

7 ⊟ S93.01X- Subluxation of right ankle joint

7 ⊟ S93.02X- Subluxation of left ankle joint

7 ⊟ S93.03X- Subluxation of unspecified ankle joint

7 ⊟ S93.04X- Dislocation of right ankle joint

7 ⊟ S93.05X- Dislocation of left ankle joint

7 ⊟ S93.06X- Dislocation of unspecified ankle joint

5 S93.1 Subluxation and dislocation of toe

6 S93.10 Unspecified subluxation and dislocation of toe
Dislocation of toe NOS
Subluxation of toe NOS

7 ⊟ S93.101- Unspecified subluxation of right toe(s)

7 ⊟ S93.102- Unspecified subluxation of left toe(s)

7 ⊟ S93.103- Unspecified subluxation of unspecified toe(s)

7 ⊟ S93.104- Unspecified dislocation of right toe(s)

7 ⊟ S93.105- Unspecified dislocation of left toe(s)

7 ⊟ S93.106- Unspecified dislocation of unspecified toe(s)

6 S93.11 Dislocation of interphalangeal joint

7 ⊟ S93.111- Dislocation of interphalangeal joint of right great toe

7 ⊟ S93.112- Dislocation of interphalangeal joint of left great toe

7 ⊟ S93.113- Dislocation of interphalangeal joint of unspecified great toe

7 ⊟ S93.114- Dislocation of interphalangeal joint of right lesser toe(s)

7 ⊟ S93.115- Dislocation of interphalangeal joint of left lesser toe(s)

7 ⊟ S93.116- Dislocation of interphalangeal joint of unspecified lesser toe(s)

7 ⊟ S93.119- Dislocation of interphalangeal joint of unspecified toe(s)

6 S93.12 Dislocation of metatarsophalangeal joint

7 ⊟ S93.121- Dislocation of metatarsophalangeal joint of right great toe

7 ⊟ S93.122- Dislocation of metatarsophalangeal joint of left great toe

7 ⊟ S93.123- Dislocation of metatarsophalangeal joint of unspecified great toe

7 ⊟ S93.124- Dislocation of metatarsophalangeal joint of right lesser toe(s)

7 ⊟ S93.125- Dislocation of metatarsophalangeal joint of left lesser toe(s)

7 ⊟ S93.126- Dislocation of metatarsophalangeal joint of unspecified lesser toe(s)

7 ⊟ S93.129- Dislocation of metatarsophalangeal joint of unspecified toe(s)

6 S93.13 Subluxation of interphalangeal joint

7 ⊟ S93.131- Subluxation of interphalangeal joint of right great toe

7 ⊟ S93.132- Subluxation of interphalangeal joint of left great toe

7 ⊟ S93.133- Subluxation of interphalangeal joint of unspecified great toe

7 ⊟ S93.134- Subluxation of interphalangeal joint of right lesser toe(s)

7 ⊟ S93.135- Subluxation of interphalangeal joint of left lesser toe(s)

7 ⊟ S93.136- Subluxation of interphalangeal joint of unspecified lesser toe(s)

7 ⊟ S93.139- Subluxation of interphalangeal joint of unspecified toe(s)

6 S93.14 Subluxation of metatarsophalangeal joint

7 ⊟ S93.141- Subluxation of metatarsophalangeal joint of right great toe

7 ⊟ S93.142- Subluxation of metatarsophalangeal joint of left great toe

7 ⊟ S93.143- Subluxation of metatarsophalangeal joint of unspecified great toe

7 ⊟ S93.144- Subluxation of metatarsophalangeal joint of right lesser toe(s)

7 ⊟ S93.145- Subluxation of metatarsophalangeal joint of left lesser toe(s)

7 ⊟ S93.146- Subluxation of metatarsophalangeal joint of unspecified lesser toe(s)

7 ⊟ S93.149- Subluxation of metatarsophalangeal joint of unspecified toe(s)

5 S93.3 Subluxation and dislocation of foot

| EXCLUDES 2 | *dislocation of toe (S93.1-)* |

6 S93.30 Unspecified subluxation and dislocation of foot
Dislocation of foot NOS
Subluxation of foot NOS

7 ⊟ S93.301- Unspecified subluxation of right foot

7 ⊟ S93.302- Unspecified subluxation of left foot

7 ⊟ S93.303- Unspecified subluxation of unspecified foot

7 ⊟ S93.304- Unspecified dislocation of right foot

7 ⊟ S93.305- Unspecified dislocation of left foot

7 ⊟ S93.306- Unspecified dislocation of unspecified foot

6 S93.31 Subluxation and dislocation of tarsal joint

7 ⊟ S93.311- Subluxation of tarsal joint of right foot

7 ⊟ S93.312- Subluxation of tarsal joint of left foot

● New   ▲ Revised   *Manifestation*   4-7 Digit Indicators   ⊟ Laterality   A Adult (15+ years)   M Maternity (12-55 years)   N Newborn   P Pediatric (0-17 years)   ♂ Male   ♀ Female
✖ Deleted   Unspecified   + Additional code

1032   © 2017 DecisionHealth   2017 ICD-10-CM Expert for Physicians

7 ⊟	S93.313-	Subluxation of tarsal joint of unspecified foot
7 ⊟	S93.314-	Dislocation of tarsal joint of right foot
7 ⊟	S93.315-	Dislocation of tarsal joint of left foot
7 ⊟	S93.316-	Dislocation of tarsal joint of unspecified foot
6	S93.32	Subluxation and dislocation of tarsometatarsal joint
7 ⊟	S93.321-	Subluxation of tarsometatarsal joint of right foot
7 ⊟	S93.322-	Subluxation of tarsometatarsal joint of left foot
7 ⊟	S93.323-	Subluxation of tarsometatarsal joint of unspecified foot
7 ⊟	S93.324-	Dislocation of tarsometatarsal joint of right foot
7 ⊟	S93.325-	Dislocation of tarsometatarsal joint of left foot
7 ⊟	S93.326-	Dislocation of tarsometatarsal joint of unspecified foot
6	S93.33	Other subluxation and dislocation of foot
7 ⊟	S93.331-	Other subluxation of right foot
7 ⊟	S93.332-	Other subluxation of left foot
7 ⊟	S93.333-	Other subluxation of unspecified foot
7 ⊟	S93.334-	Other dislocation of right foot
7 ⊟	S93.335-	Other dislocation of left foot
7 ⊟	S93.336-	Other dislocation of unspecified foot

S S93.4   Sprain of ankle

EXCLUDES 2   *injury of Achilles tendon (S86.0-)*

6	S93.40	Sprain of unspecified ligament of ankle
		Sprain of ankle NOS
		Sprained ankle NOS
7 ⊟	S93.401-	Sprain of unspecified ligament of right ankle
7 ⊟	S93.402-	Sprain of unspecified ligament of left ankle
7 ⊟	S93.409-	Sprain of unspecified ligament of unspecified ankle
6	S93.41	Sprain of calcaneofibular ligament
7 ⊟	S93.411-	Sprain of calcaneofibular ligament of right ankle
7 ⊟	S93.412-	Sprain of calcaneofibular ligament of left ankle
7 ⊟	S93.419-	Sprain of calcaneofibular ligament of unspecified ankle
6	S93.42	Sprain of deltoid ligament
7 ⊟	S93.421-	Sprain of deltoid ligament of right ankle
7 ⊟	S93.422-	Sprain of deltoid ligament of left ankle
7 ⊟	S93.429-	Sprain of deltoid ligament of unspecified ankle
6	S93.43	Sprain of tibiofibular ligament
7 ⊟	S93.431-	Sprain of tibiofibular ligament of right ankle
7 ⊟	S93.432-	Sprain of tibiofibular ligament of left ankle
7 ⊟	S93.439-	Sprain of tibiofibular ligament of unspecified ankle
6	S93.49	Sprain of other ligament of ankle
		Sprain of internal collateral ligament
		Sprain of talofibular ligament
7 ⊟	S93.491-	Sprain of other ligament of right ankle
7 ⊟	S93.492-	Sprain of other ligament of left ankle
7 ⊟	S93.499-	Sprain of other ligament of unspecified ankle

S S93.5   Sprain of toe

6	S93.50	Unspecified sprain of toe
7 ⊟	S93.501-	Unspecified sprain of right great toe
7 ⊟	S93.502-	Unspecified sprain of left great toe
7 ⊟	S93.503-	Unspecified sprain of unspecified great toe
7 ⊟	S93.504-	Unspecified sprain of right lesser toe(s)
7 ⊟	S93.505-	Unspecified sprain of left lesser toe(s)
7 ⊟	S93.506-	Unspecified sprain of unspecified lesser toe(s)
7 ⊟	S93.509-	Unspecified sprain of unspecified toe(s)
6	S93.51	Sprain of interphalangeal joint of toe
7 ⊟	S93.511-	Sprain of interphalangeal joint of right great toe
7 ⊟	S93.512-	Sprain of interphalangeal joint of left great toe
7 ⊟	S93.513-	Sprain of interphalangeal joint of unspecified great toe
7 ⊟	S93.514-	Sprain of interphalangeal joint of right lesser toe(s)
7 ⊟	S93.515-	Sprain of interphalangeal joint of left lesser toe(s)
7 ⊟	S93.516-	Sprain of interphalangeal joint of unspecified lesser toe(s)
7 ⊟	S93.519-	Sprain of interphalangeal joint of unspecified toe(s)
6	S93.52	Sprain of metatarsophalangeal joint of toe
7 ⊟	S93.521-	Sprain of metatarsophalangeal joint of right great toe
7 ⊟	S93.522-	Sprain of metatarsophalangeal joint of left great toe
7 ⊟	S93.523-	Sprain of metatarsophalangeal joint of unspecified great toe
7 ⊟	S93.524-	Sprain of metatarsophalangeal joint of right lesser toe(s)
7 ⊟	S93.525-	Sprain of metatarsophalangeal joint of left lesser toe(s)
7 ⊟	S93.526-	Sprain of metatarsophalangeal joint of unspecified lesser toe(s)
7 ⊟	S93.529-	Sprain of metatarsophalangeal joint of unspecified toe(s)

S S93.6   Sprain of foot

EXCLUDES 2   *sprain of metatarsophalangeal joint of toe (S93.52-)*
sprain of toe (S93.5-)

6	S93.60	Unspecified sprain of foot
7 ⊟	S93.601-	Unspecified sprain of right foot
7 ⊟	S93.602-	Unspecified sprain of left foot
7 ⊟	S93.609-	Unspecified sprain of unspecified foot
6	S93.61	Sprain of tarsal ligament of foot
7 ⊟	S93.611-	Sprain of tarsal ligament of right foot
7 ⊟	S93.612-	Sprain of tarsal ligament of left foot
7 ⊟	S93.619-	Sprain of tarsal ligament of unspecified foot
6	S93.62	Sprain of tarsometatarsal ligament of foot
7 ⊟	S93.621-	Sprain of tarsometatarsal ligament of right foot
7 ⊟	S93.622-	Sprain of tarsometatarsal ligament of left foot
7 ⊟	S93.629-	Sprain of tarsometatarsal ligament of unspecified foot
6	S93.69	Other sprain of foot
7 ⊟	S93.691-	Other sprain of right foot
7 ⊟	S93.692-	Other sprain of left foot
7 ⊟	S93.699-	Other sprain of unspecified foot

4 S94   Injury of nerves at ankle and foot level

Code also:
   any associated open wound (S91.-)

The appropriate 7th character is to be added to each code from category S94
A   initial encounter
D   subsequent encounter
S   sequela

S S94.0   Injury of lateral plantar nerve

7 ⊟	S94.00X-	Injury of lateral plantar nerve, unspecified leg
7 ⊟	S94.01X-	Injury of lateral plantar nerve, right leg
7 ⊟	S94.02X-	Injury of lateral plantar nerve, left leg

S S94.1   Injury of medial plantar nerve

7 ⊟	S94.10X-	Injury of medial plantar nerve, unspecified leg
7 ⊟	S94.11X-	Injury of medial plantar nerve, right leg
7 ⊟	S94.12X-	Injury of medial plantar nerve, left leg

S S94.2   Injury of deep peroneal nerve at ankle and foot level

Injury of terminal, lateral branch of deep peroneal nerve

7 ⊟	S94.20X-	Injury of deep peroneal nerve at ankle and foot level, unspecified leg
7 ⊟	S94.21X-	Injury of deep peroneal nerve at ankle and foot level, right leg
7 ⊟	S94.22X-	Injury of deep peroneal nerve at ankle and foot level, left leg

S S94.3   Injury of cutaneous sensory nerve at ankle and foot level

7 ⊟	S94.30X-	Injury of cutaneous sensory nerve at ankle and foot level, unspecified leg
7 ⊟	S94.31X-	Injury of cutaneous sensory nerve at ankle and foot level, right leg
7 ⊟	S94.32X-	Injury of cutaneous sensory nerve at ankle and foot level, left leg

S S94.8   Injury of other nerves at ankle and foot level

6	S94.8X	Injury of other nerves at ankle and foot level

● New   ▲ Revised   *Manifestation*   4-7 Digit Indicators   ⊟ Laterality   A Adult (15+ years)   M Maternity (12-55 years)   N Newborn   P Pediatric (0-17 years)   ♂ Male   ♀ Female
✖ Deleted   Unspecified   + Additional code

2017 ICD-10-CM Expert for Physicians   © 2017 DecisionHealth   1033

7 ⊟ **S94.8X1-** Injury of other nerves at ankle and foot level, right leg

7 ⊟ **S94.8X2-** Injury of other nerves at ankle and foot level, left leg

7 ⊟ **S94.8X9-** Injury of other nerves at ankle and foot level, unspecified leg

5 **S94.9** **Injury of unspecified nerve at ankle and foot level**

7 ⊟ **S94.90X-** Injury of unspecified nerve at ankle and foot level, unspecified leg

7 ⊟ **S94.91X-** Injury of unspecified nerve at ankle and foot level, right leg

7 ⊟ **S94.92X-** Injury of unspecified nerve at ankle and foot level, left leg

4 **S95** **Injury of blood vessels at ankle and foot level**

Code also:
any associated open wound (S91.-)

EXCLUDES 2 *injury of posterior tibial artery and vein (S85.1-, S85.8-)*

The appropriate 7th character is to be added to each code from category S95
A   initial encounter
D   subsequent encounter
S   sequela

5 **S95.0** **Injury of dorsal artery of foot**

6 **S95.00** **Unspecified injury of dorsal artery of foot**

7 ⊟ **S95.001-** Unspecified injury of dorsal artery of right foot

7 ⊟ **S95.002-** Unspecified injury of dorsal artery of left foot

7 ⊟ **S95.009-** Unspecified injury of dorsal artery of unspecified foot

6 **S95.01** **Laceration of dorsal artery of foot**

CODING TIP ✓ Code also any associated open wound S91.-

7 ⊟ **S95.011-** Laceration of dorsal artery of right foot

7 ⊟ **S95.012-** Laceration of dorsal artery of left foot

7 ⊟ **S95.019-** Laceration of dorsal artery of unspecified foot

6 **S95.09** **Other specified injury of dorsal artery of foot**

7 ⊟ **S95.091-** Other specified injury of dorsal artery of right foot

7 ⊟ **S95.092-** Other specified injury of dorsal artery of left foot

7 ⊟ **S95.099-** Other specified injury of dorsal artery of unspecified foot

5 **S95.1** **Injury of plantar artery of foot**

6 **S95.10** **Unspecified injury of plantar artery of foot**

7 ⊟ **S95.101-** Unspecified injury of plantar artery of right foot

7 ⊟ **S95.102-** Unspecified injury of plantar artery of left foot

7 ⊟ **S95.109-** Unspecified injury of plantar artery of unspecified foot

6 **S95.11** **Laceration of plantar artery of foot**

CODING TIP ✓ Code also any associated open wound S91.-

7 ⊟ **S95.111-** Laceration of plantar artery of right foot

7 ⊟ **S95.112-** Laceration of plantar artery of left foot

7 ⊟ **S95.119-** Laceration of plantar artery of unspecified foot

6 **S95.19** **Other specified injury of plantar artery of foot**

7 ⊟ **S95.191-** Other specified injury of plantar artery of right foot

7 ⊟ **S95.192-** Other specified injury of plantar artery of left foot

7 ⊟ **S95.199-** Other specified injury of plantar artery of unspecified foot

5 **S95.2** **Injury of dorsal vein of foot**

6 **S95.20** **Unspecified injury of dorsal vein of foot**

7 ⊟ **S95.201-** Unspecified injury of dorsal vein of right foot

7 ⊟ **S95.202-** Unspecified injury of dorsal vein of left foot

7 ⊟ **S95.209-** Unspecified injury of dorsal vein of unspecified foot

6 **S95.21** **Laceration of dorsal vein of foot**

CODING TIP ✓ Code also any associated open wound S91.-

7 ⊟ **S95.211-** Laceration of dorsal vein of right foot

7 ⊟ **S95.212-** Laceration of dorsal vein of left foot

7 ⊟ **S95.219-** Laceration of dorsal vein of unspecified foot

6 **S95.29** **Other specified injury of dorsal vein of foot**

7 ⊟ **S95.291-** Other specified injury of dorsal vein of right foot

7 ⊟ **S95.292-** Other specified injury of dorsal vein of left foot

7 ⊟ **S95.299-** Other specified injury of dorsal vein of unspecified foot

5 **S95.8** **Injury of other blood vessels at ankle and foot level**

6 **S95.80** **Unspecified injury of other blood vessels at ankle and foot level**

7 ⊟ **S95.801-** Unspecified injury of other blood vessels at ankle and foot level, right leg

7 ⊟ **S95.802-** Unspecified injury of other blood vessels at ankle and foot level, left leg

7 ⊟ **S95.809-** Unspecified injury of other blood vessels at ankle and foot level, unspecified leg

6 **S95.81** **Laceration of other blood vessels at ankle and foot level**

CODING TIP ✓ Code also any associated open wound S91.-

7 ⊟ **S95.811-** Laceration of other blood vessels at ankle and foot level, right leg

7 ⊟ **S95.812-** Laceration of other blood vessels at ankle and foot level, left leg

7 ⊟ **S95.819-** Laceration of other blood vessels at ankle and foot level, unspecified leg

6 **S95.89** **Other specified injury of other blood vessels at ankle and foot level**

7 ⊟ **S95.891-** Other specified injury of other blood vessels at ankle and foot level, right leg

7 ⊟ **S95.892-** Other specified injury of other blood vessels at ankle and foot level, left leg

7 ⊟ **S95.899-** Other specified injury of other blood vessels at ankle and foot level, unspecified leg

5 **S95.9** **Injury of unspecified blood vessel at ankle and foot level**

6 **S95.90** **Unspecified injury of unspecified blood vessel at ankle and foot level**

7 ⊟ **S95.901-** Unspecified injury of unspecified blood vessel at ankle and foot level, right leg

7 ⊟ **S95.902-** Unspecified injury of unspecified blood vessel at ankle and foot level, left leg

7 ⊟ **S95.909-** Unspecified injury of unspecified blood vessel at ankle and foot level, unspecified leg

6 **S95.91** **Laceration of unspecified blood vessel at ankle and foot level**

CODING TIP ✓ Code also any associated open wound S91.-

7 ⊟ **S95.911-** Laceration of unspecified blood vessel at ankle and foot level, right leg

7 ⊟ **S95.912-** Laceration of unspecified blood vessel at ankle and foot level, left leg

7 ⊟ **S95.919-** Laceration of unspecified blood vessel at ankle and foot level, unspecified leg

6 **S95.99** **Other specified injury of unspecified blood vessel at ankle and foot level**

7 ⊟ **S95.991-** Other specified injury of unspecified blood vessel at ankle and foot level, right leg

7 ⊟ **S95.992-** Other specified injury of unspecified blood vessel at ankle and foot level, left leg

7 ⊟ **S95.999-** Other specified injury of unspecified blood vessel at ankle and foot level, unspecified leg

---

④ **S96** **Injury of muscle and tendon at ankle and foot level**
    Code also:
        any associated open wound (S91.-)
    EXCLUDES 2   *injury of Achilles tendon (S86.0-)*
                     sprain of joints and ligaments of ankle and foot
                     (S93.-)

    The appropriate 7th character is to be added to each code from
    category S96
    A   initial encounter
    D   subsequent encounter
    S   sequela

⑤ **S96.0**   **Injury of muscle and tendon of long flexor muscle of toe**
              at ankle and foot level

   ⑥ **S96.00**   **Unspecified injury of muscle and tendon of long**
                  flexor muscle of toe at ankle and foot level

   ⑦ **S96.001-**   **Unspecified injury of muscle and tendon of**
                    long flexor muscle of toe at ankle and foot
                    level, right foot

   ⑦ **S96.002-**   **Unspecified injury of muscle and tendon of**
                    long flexor muscle of toe at ankle and foot
                    level, left foot

   ⑦ **S96.009-**   **Unspecified injury of muscle and tendon of**
                    long flexor muscle of toe at ankle and foot
                    level, unspecified foot

   ⑥ **S96.01**   **Strain of muscle and tendon of long flexor muscle of**
                  toe at ankle and foot level

   ⑦ **S96.011-**   **Strain of muscle and tendon of long flexor**
                    muscle of toe at ankle and foot level, right
                    foot

   ⑦ **S96.012-**   **Strain of muscle and tendon of long flexor**
                    muscle of toe at ankle and foot level, left foot

   ⑦ **S96.019-**   **Strain of muscle and tendon of long flexor**
                    muscle of toe at ankle and foot level,
                    unspecified foot

   ⑥ **S96.02**   **Laceration of muscle and tendon of long flexor**
                  muscle of toe at ankle and foot level
                  CODING TIP ✓   Code also any associated open
                  wound S91.-

   ⑦ **S96.021-**   **Laceration of muscle and tendon of long flexor**
                    muscle of toe at ankle and foot level, right
                    foot

   ⑦ **S96.022-**   **Laceration of muscle and tendon of long flexor**
                    muscle of toe at ankle and foot level, left foot

   ⑦ **S96.029-**   **Laceration of muscle and tendon of long flexor**
                    muscle of toe at ankle and foot level,
                    unspecified foot

   ⑥ **S96.09**   **Other injury of muscle and tendon of long flexor**
                  muscle of toe at ankle and foot level

   ⑦ **S96.091-**   **Other injury of muscle and tendon of long**
                    flexor muscle of toe at ankle and foot level,
                    right foot

   ⑦ **S96.092-**   **Other injury of muscle and tendon of long**
                    flexor muscle of toe at ankle and foot level,
                    left foot

   ⑦ **S96.099-**   **Other injury of muscle and tendon of long**
                    flexor muscle of toe at ankle and foot level,
                    unspecified foot

⑤ **S96.1**   **Injury of muscle and tendon of long extensor muscle of**
              toe at ankle and foot level

   ⑥ **S96.10**   **Unspecified injury of muscle and tendon of long**
                  extensor muscle of toe at ankle and foot level

   ⑦ **S96.101-**   **Unspecified injury of muscle and tendon of**
                    long extensor muscle of toe at ankle and foot
                    level, right foot

   ⑦ **S96.102-**   **Unspecified injury of muscle and tendon of**
                    long extensor muscle of toe at ankle and foot
                    level, left foot

   ⑦ **S96.109-**   **Unspecified injury of muscle and tendon of**
                    long extensor muscle of toe at ankle and foot
                    level, unspecified foot

   ⑥ **S96.11**   **Strain of muscle and tendon of long extensor muscle**
                  of toe at ankle and foot level

   ⑦ **S96.111-**   **Strain of muscle and tendon of long extensor**
                    muscle of toe at ankle and foot level, right
                    foot

   ⑦ **S96.112-**   **Strain of muscle and tendon of long extensor**
                    muscle of toe at ankle and foot level, left foot

   ⑦ **S96.119-**   **Strain of muscle and tendon of long extensor**
                    muscle of toe at ankle and foot level,
                    unspecified foot

   ⑥ **S96.12**   **Laceration of muscle and tendon of long extensor**
                  muscle of toe at ankle and foot level
                  CODING TIP ✓   Code also any associated open
                  wound S91.-

   ⑦ **S96.121-**   **Laceration of muscle and tendon of long**
                    extensor muscle of toe at ankle and foot
                    level, right foot

   ⑦ **S96.122-**   **Laceration of muscle and tendon of long**
                    extensor muscle of toe at ankle and foot
                    level, left foot

   ⑦ **S96.129-**   **Laceration of muscle and tendon of long**
                    extensor muscle of toe at ankle and foot
                    level, unspecified foot

   ⑥ **S96.19**   **Other specified injury of muscle and tendon of long**
                  extensor muscle of toe at ankle and foot level

   ⑦ **S96.191-**   **Other specified injury of muscle and tendon of**
                    long extensor muscle of toe at ankle and foot
                    level, right foot

   ⑦ **S96.192-**   **Other specified injury of muscle and tendon of**
                    long extensor muscle of toe at ankle and foot
                    level, left foot

   ⑦ **S96.199-**   **Other specified injury of muscle and tendon of**
                    long extensor muscle of toe at ankle and foot
                    level, unspecified foot

⑤ **S96.2**   **Injury of intrinsic muscle and tendon at ankle and foot**
              level

   ⑥ **S96.20**   **Unspecified injury of intrinsic muscle and tendon at**
                  ankle and foot level

   ⑦ **S96.201-**   **Unspecified injury of intrinsic muscle and**
                    tendon at ankle and foot level, right foot

   ⑦ **S96.202-**   **Unspecified injury of intrinsic muscle and**
                    tendon at ankle and foot level, left foot

   ⑦ **S96.209-**   **Unspecified injury of intrinsic muscle and**
                    tendon at ankle and foot level, unspecified
                    foot

   ⑥ **S96.21**   **Strain of intrinsic muscle and tendon at ankle and**
                  foot level

   ⑦ **S96.211-**   **Strain of intrinsic muscle and tendon at ankle**
                    and foot level, right foot

   ⑦ **S96.212-**   **Strain of intrinsic muscle and tendon at ankle**
                    and foot level, left foot

   ⑦ **S96.219-**   **Strain of intrinsic muscle and tendon at ankle**
                    and foot level, unspecified foot

   ⑥ **S96.22**   **Laceration of intrinsic muscle and tendon at ankle**
                  and foot level
                  CODING TIP ✓   Code also any associated open
                  wound S91.-

   ⑦ **S96.221-**   **Laceration of intrinsic muscle and tendon at**
                    ankle and foot level, right foot

   ⑦ **S96.222-**   **Laceration of intrinsic muscle and tendon at**
                    ankle and foot level, left foot

   ⑦ **S96.229-**   **Laceration of intrinsic muscle and tendon at**
                    ankle and foot level, unspecified foot

   ⑥ **S96.29**   **Other specified injury of intrinsic muscle and**
                  tendon at ankle and foot level

   ⑦ **S96.291-**   **Other specified injury of intrinsic muscle and**
                    tendon at ankle and foot level, right foot

   ⑦ **S96.292-**   **Other specified injury of intrinsic muscle and**
                    tendon at ankle and foot level, left foot

   ⑦ **S96.299-**   **Other specified injury of intrinsic muscle and**
                    tendon at ankle and foot level, unspecified
                    foot

⑤ **S96.8**   **Injury of other specified muscles and tendons at ankle**
              and foot level

   ⑥ **S96.80**   **Unspecified injury of other specified muscles and**
                  tendons at ankle and foot level

   ⑦ **S96.801-**   **Unspecified injury of other specified muscles**
                    and tendons at ankle and foot level, right
                    foot

   ⑦ **S96.802-**   **Unspecified injury of other specified muscles**
                    and tendons at ankle and foot level, left foot

   ⑦ **S96.809-**   **Unspecified injury of other specified muscles**
                    and tendons at ankle and foot level,
                    unspecified foot

   ⑥ **S96.81**   **Strain of other specified muscles and tendons at**
                  ankle and foot level

● New   ▲ Revised   *Manifestation*   ④-⑦ Digit Indicators   ⊟ Laterality   Ⓐ Adult   Ⓜ Maternity   Ⓝ Newborn   Ⓟ Pediatric   ♂ Male   ♀ Female
✖ Deleted   Unspecified   ✚ Additional code   (15+ years)   (12-55 years)   (0-17 years)

2017 ICD-10-CM Expert for Physicians

© 2017 DecisionHealth   1035

7 S96.811- **Strain of other specified muscles and tendons at ankle and foot level, right foot**

7 S96.812- **Strain of other specified muscles and tendons at ankle and foot level, left foot**

7 S96.819- **Strain of other specified muscles and tendons at ankle and foot level, unspecified foot**

6 S96.82 **Laceration of other specified muscles and tendons at ankle and foot level**

> **CODING TIP ✓** Code also any associated open wound S91.-

7 S96.821- **Laceration of other specified muscles and tendons at ankle and foot level, right foot**

7 S96.822- **Laceration of other specified muscles and tendons at ankle and foot level, left foot**

7 S96.829- **Laceration of other specified muscles and tendons at ankle and foot level, unspecified foot**

6 S96.89 **Other specified injury of other specified muscles and tendons at ankle and foot level**

7 S96.891- **Other specified injury of other specified muscles and tendons at ankle and foot level, right foot**

7 S96.892- **Other specified injury of other specified muscles and tendons at ankle and foot level, left foot**

7 S96.899- **Other specified injury of other specified muscles and tendons at ankle and foot level, unspecified foot**

5 S96.9 **Injury of unspecified muscle and tendon at ankle and foot level**

6 S96.90 **Unspecified injury of unspecified muscle and tendon at ankle and foot level**

7 S96.901- **Unspecified injury of unspecified muscle and tendon at ankle and foot level, right foot**

7 S96.902- **Unspecified injury of unspecified muscle and tendon at ankle and foot level, left foot**

7 S96.909- **Unspecified injury of unspecified muscle and tendon at ankle and foot level, unspecified foot**

6 S96.91 **Strain of unspecified muscle and tendon at ankle and foot level**

7 S96.911- **Strain of unspecified muscle and tendon at ankle and foot level, right foot**

7 S96.912- **Strain of unspecified muscle and tendon at ankle and foot level, left foot**

7 S96.919- **Strain of unspecified muscle and tendon at ankle and foot level, unspecified foot**

6 S96.92 **Laceration of unspecified muscle and tendon at ankle and foot level**

> **CODING TIP ✓** Code also any associated open wound S91.-

7 S96.921- **Laceration of unspecified muscle and tendon at ankle and foot level, right foot**

7 S96.922- **Laceration of unspecified muscle and tendon at ankle and foot level, left foot**

7 S96.929- **Laceration of unspecified muscle and tendon at ankle and foot level, unspecified foot**

6 S96.99 **Other specified injury of unspecified muscle and tendon at ankle and foot level**

7 S96.991- **Other specified injury of unspecified muscle and tendon at ankle and foot level, right foot**

7 S96.992- **Other specified injury of unspecified muscle and tendon at ankle and foot level, left foot**

7 S96.999- **Other specified injury of unspecified muscle and tendon at ankle and foot level, unspecified foot**

4 + S97 **Crushing injury of ankle and foot**

Use additional code(s) for all associated injuries

The appropriate 7th character is to be added to each code from category S97
A   initial encounter
D   subsequent encounter
S   sequela

5 + S97.0 **Crushing injury of ankle**

7 + S97.00X- **Crushing injury of unspecified ankle**

7 + S97.01X- **Crushing injury of right ankle**

7 + S97.02X- **Crushing injury of left ankle**

5 + S97.1 **Crushing injury of toe**

6 + S97.10 **Crushing injury of unspecified toe(s)**

7 + S97.101- **Crushing injury of unspecified right toe(s)**

7 + S97.102- **Crushing injury of unspecified left toe(s)**

7 + S97.109- **Crushing injury of unspecified toe(s)**
Crushing injury of toe NOS

6 + S97.11 **Crushing injury of great toe**

7 + S97.111- **Crushing injury of right great toe**

7 + S97.112- **Crushing injury of left great toe**

7 + S97.119- **Crushing injury of unspecified great toe**

6 + S97.12 **Crushing injury of lesser toe(s)**

7 + S97.121- **Crushing injury of right lesser toe(s)**

7 + S97.122- **Crushing injury of left lesser toe(s)**

7 + S97.129- **Crushing injury of unspecified lesser toe(s)**

5 + S97.8 **Crushing injury of foot**

7 + S97.80X- **Crushing injury of unspecified foot**
Crushing injury of foot NOS

7 + S97.81X- **Crushing injury of right foot**

7 + S97.82X- **Crushing injury of left foot**

4 S98 **Traumatic amputation of ankle and foot**
An amputation not identified as partial or complete should be coded to complete

The appropriate 7th character is to be added to each code from category S98
A   initial encounter
D   subsequent encounter
S   sequela

5 S98.0 **Traumatic amputation of foot at ankle level**

6 S98.01 **Complete traumatic amputation of foot at ankle level**

7 S98.011- **Complete traumatic amputation of right foot at ankle level**

7 S98.012- **Complete traumatic amputation of left foot at ankle level**

7 S98.019- **Complete traumatic amputation of unspecified foot at ankle level**

6 S98.02 **Partial traumatic amputation of foot at ankle level**

7 S98.021- **Partial traumatic amputation of right foot at ankle level**

7 S98.022- **Partial traumatic amputation of left foot at ankle level**

7 S98.029- **Partial traumatic amputation of unspecified foot at ankle level**

5 S98.1 **Traumatic amputation of one toe**

6 S98.11 **Complete traumatic amputation of great toe**

7 S98.111- **Complete traumatic amputation of right great toe**

7 S98.112- **Complete traumatic amputation of left great toe**

7 S98.119- **Complete traumatic amputation of unspecified great toe**

6 S98.12 **Partial traumatic amputation of great toe**

7 S98.121- **Partial traumatic amputation of right great toe**

7 S98.122- **Partial traumatic amputation of left great toe**

7 S98.129- **Partial traumatic amputation of unspecified great toe**

6 S98.13 **Complete traumatic amputation of one lesser toe**
Traumatic amputation of toe NOS

7 S98.131- **Complete traumatic amputation of one right lesser toe**

7 S98.132- **Complete traumatic amputation of one left lesser toe**

7 S98.139- **Complete traumatic amputation of one unspecified lesser toe**

6 S98.14 **Partial traumatic amputation of one lesser toe**

7 S98.141- **Partial traumatic amputation of one right lesser toe**

7 S98.142- **Partial traumatic amputation of one left lesser toe**

7 S98.149- **Partial traumatic amputation of one unspecified lesser toe**

5 S98.2 **Traumatic amputation of two or more lesser toes**

● New   ▲ Revised   *Manifestation*   4-7 Digit Indicators   ⊟ Laterality   Ⓐ Adult (15+ years)   Ⓜ Maternity (12-55 years)   Ⓝ Newborn (0-17 years)   ♂ Male   ♀ Female
✖ Deleted   Unspecified   + Additional code   Ⓟ Pediatric (0-17 years)

⑥ S98.21   Complete traumatic amputation of two or more lesser toes
- ⑦ ⊟ S98.211-   Complete traumatic amputation of two or more right lesser toes
- ⑦ ⊟ S98.212-   Complete traumatic amputation of two or more left lesser toes
- ⑦ ⊟ S98.219-   Complete traumatic amputation of two or more unspecified lesser toes

⑥ S98.22   Partial traumatic amputation of two or more lesser toes
- ⑦ ⊟ S98.221-   Partial traumatic amputation of two or more right lesser toes
- ⑦ ⊟ S98.222-   Partial traumatic amputation of two or more left lesser toes
- ⑦ ⊟ S98.229-   Partial traumatic amputation of two or more unspecified lesser toes

⑤ S98.3   Traumatic amputation of midfoot
   ⑥ S98.31   Complete traumatic amputation of midfoot
- ⑦ ⊟ S98.311-   Complete traumatic amputation of right midfoot
- ⑦ ⊟ S98.312-   Complete traumatic amputation of left midfoot
- ⑦ ⊟ S98.319-   Complete traumatic amputation of unspecified midfoot
   ⑥ S98.32   Partial traumatic amputation of midfoot
- ⑦ ⊟ S98.321-   Partial traumatic amputation of right midfoot
- ⑦ ⊟ S98.322-   Partial traumatic amputation of left midfoot
- ⑦ ⊟ S98.329-   Partial traumatic amputation of unspecified midfoot

⑤ S98.9   Traumatic amputation of foot, level unspecified
   ⑥ S98.91   Complete traumatic amputation of foot, level unspecified
- ⑦ ⊟ S98.911-   Complete traumatic amputation of right foot, level unspecified
- ⑦ ⊟ S98.912-   Complete traumatic amputation of left foot, level unspecified
- ⑦ ⊟ S98.919-   Complete traumatic amputation of unspecified foot, level unspecified
   ⑥ S98.92   Partial traumatic amputation of foot, level unspecified
- ⑦ ⊟ S98.921-   Partial traumatic amputation of right foot, level unspecified
- ⑦ ⊟ S98.922-   Partial traumatic amputation of left foot, level unspecified
- ⑦ ⊟ S98.929-   Partial traumatic amputation of unspecified foot, level unspecified

▲ ④ S99   **Other and unspecified injuries of ankle and foot**
● ⑤ S99.0   Physeal fracture of calcaneus

> The appropriate 7th character is to be added to each code from subcategories S99.0
> A   initial encounter for closed fracture
> B   initial encounter for open fracture
> D   subsequent encounter for fracture with routine healing
> G   subsequent encounter for fracture with delayed healing
> K   subsequent encounter for fracture with nonunion
> P   subsequent encounter for fracture with malunion
> S   sequela

● ⑥ S99.00   Unspecified physeal fracture of calcaneus
- ● ⑦ ⊟ S99.001-   Unspecified physeal fracture of right calcaneus
- ● ⑦ ⊟ S99.002-   Unspecified physeal fracture of left calcaneus
- ● ⑦ ⊟ S99.009-   Unspecified physeal fracture of unspecified calcaneus

● ⑥ S99.01   Salter-Harris Type I physeal fracture of calcaneus
- ● ⑦ ⊟ S99.011-   Salter-Harris Type I physeal fracture of right calcaneus
- ● ⑦ ⊟ S99.012-   Salter-Harris Type I physeal fracture of left calcaneus
- ● ⑦ ⊟ S99.019-   Salter-Harris Type I physeal fracture of unspecified calcaneus

● ⑥ S99.02   Salter-Harris Type II physeal fracture of calcaneus
- ● ⑦ ⊟ S99.021-   Salter-Harris Type II physeal fracture of right calcaneus
- ● ⑦ ⊟ S99.022-   Salter-Harris Type II physeal fracture of left calcaneus
- ● ⑦ ⊟ S99.029-   Salter-Harris Type II physeal fracture of unspecified calcaneus

● ⑥ S99.03   Salter-Harris Type III physeal fracture of calcaneus
- ● ⑦ ⊟ S99.031-   Salter-Harris Type III physeal fracture of right calcaneus
- ● ⑦ ⊟ S99.032-   Salter-Harris Type III physeal fracture of left calcaneus
- ● ⑦ ⊟ S99.039-   Salter-Harris Type III physeal fracture of unspecified calcaneus

● ⑥ S99.04   Salter-Harris Type IV physeal fracture of calcaneus
- ● ⑦ ⊟ S99.041-   Salter-Harris Type IV physeal fracture of right calcaneus
- ● ⑦ ⊟ S99.042-   Salter-Harris Type IV physeal fracture of left calcaneus
- ● ⑦ ⊟ S99.049-   Salter-Harris Type IV physeal fracture of unspecified calcaneus

● ⑥ S99.09   Other physeal fracture of calcaneus
- ● ⑦ ⊟ S99.091-   Other physeal fracture of right calcaneus
- ● ⑦ ⊟ S99.092-   Other physeal fracture of left calcaneus
- ● ⑦ ⊟ S99.099-   Other physeal fracture of unspecified calcaneus

● ⑤ S99.1   Physeal fracture of metatarsal

> The appropriate 7th character is to be added to each code from subcategories S99.1
> A   initial encounter for closed fracture
> B   initial encounter for open fracture
> D   subsequent encounter for fracture with routine healing
> G   subsequent encounter for fracture with delayed healing
> K   subsequent encounter for fracture with nonunion
> P   subsequent encounter for fracture with malunion
> S   sequela

● ⑥ S99.10   Unspecified physeal fracture of metatarsal
- ● ⑦ ⊟ S99.101-   Unspecified physeal fracture of right metatarsal
- ● ⑦ ⊟ S99.102-   Unspecified physeal fracture of left metatarsal
- ● ⑦ ⊟ S99.109-   Unspecified physeal fracture of unspecified metatarsal

● ⑥ S99.11   Salter-Harris Type I physeal fracture of metatarsal
- ● ⑦ ⊟ S99.111-   Salter-Harris Type I physeal fracture of right metatarsal
- ● ⑦ ⊟ S99.112-   Salter-Harris Type I physeal fracture of left metatarsal
- ● ⑦ ⊟ S99.119-   Salter-Harris Type I physeal fracture of unspecified metatarsal

● ⑥ S99.12   Salter-Harris Type II physeal fracture of metatarsal
- ● ⑦ ⊟ S99.121-   Salter-Harris Type II physeal fracture of right metatarsal
- ● ⑦ ⊟ S99.122-   Salter-Harris Type II physeal fracture of left metatarsal
- ● ⑦ ⊟ S99.129-   Salter-Harris Type II physeal fracture of unspecified metatarsal

● ⑥ S99.13   Salter-Harris Type III physeal fracture of metatarsal
- ● ⑦ ⊟ S99.131-   Salter-Harris Type III physeal fracture of right metatarsal
- ● ⑦ ⊟ S99.132-   Salter-Harris Type III physeal fracture of left metatarsal
- ● ⑦ ⊟ S99.139-   Salter-Harris Type III physeal fracture of unspecified metatarsal

● ⑥ S99.14   Salter-Harris Type IV physeal fracture of metatarsal
- ● ⑦ ⊟ S99.141-   Salter-Harris Type IV physeal fracture of right metatarsal
- ● ⑦ ⊟ S99.142-   Salter-Harris Type IV physeal fracture of left metatarsal
- ● ⑦ ⊟ S99.149-   Salter-Harris Type IV physeal fracture of unspecified metatarsal

● ⑥ S99.19   Other physeal fracture of metatarsal
- ● ⑦ ⊟ S99.191-   Other physeal fracture of right metatarsal
- ● ⑦ ⊟ S99.192-   Other physeal fracture of left metatarsal
- ● ⑦ ⊟ S99.199-   Other physeal fracture of unspecified metatarsal

---

● New   ▲ Revised   *Manifestation*   ④-⑦ Digit Indicators   ⊟ Laterality   Ⓐ Adult (15+ years)   Ⓜ Maternity (12-55 years)   Ⓝ Newborn   Ⓟ Pediatric (0-17 years)   ♂ Male   ♀ Female
✖ Deleted   Unspecified   + Additional code

● Ⓢ **S99.2** **Physeal fracture of phalanx of toe**

The appropriate 7th character is to be added to each code from subcategories S99.2
A   initial encounter for closed fracture
B   initial encounter for open fracture
D   subsequent encounter for fracture with routine healing
G   subsequent encounter for fracture with delayed healing
K   subsequent encounter for fracture with nonunion
P   subsequent encounter for fracture with malunion
S   sequela

● Ⓖ **S99.20** **Unspecified physeal fracture of phalanx of toe**

● ⑦ ▭ **S99.201-** **Unspecified physeal fracture of right toe**

● ⑦ ▭ **S99.202-** **Unspecified physeal fracture of left toe**

● ⑦ ▭ **S99.209-** **Unspecified physeal fracture of unspecified toe**

● Ⓖ **S99.21** **Salter-Harris Type I physeal fracture of phalanx of toe**

● ⑦ ▭ **S99.211-** **Salter-Harris Type I physeal fracture of phalanx of right toe**

● ⑦ ▭ **S99.212-** **Salter-Harris Type I physeal fracture of phalanx of left toe**

● ⑦ ▭ **S99.219-** **Salter-Harris Type I physeal fracture of phalanx of unspecified toe**

● Ⓖ **S99.22** **Salter-Harris Type II physeal fracture of phalanx of toe**

● ⑦ ▭ **S99.221-** **Salter-Harris Type II physeal fracture of phalanx of right toe**

● ⑦ ▭ **S99.222-** **Salter-Harris Type II physeal fracture of phalanx of left toe**

● ⑦ ▭ **S99.229-** **Salter-Harris Type II physeal fracture of phalanx of unspecified toe**

● Ⓖ **S99.23** **Salter-Harris Type III physeal fracture of phalanx of toe**

● ⑦ ▭ **S99.231-** **Salter-Harris Type III physeal fracture of phalanx of right toe**

● ⑦ ▭ **S99.232-** **Salter-Harris Type III physeal fracture of phalanx of left toe**

● ⑦ ▭ **S99.239-** **Salter-Harris Type III physeal fracture of phalanx of unspecified toe**

● Ⓖ **S99.24** **Salter-Harris Type IV physeal fracture of phalanx of toe**

● ⑦ ▭ **S99.241-** **Salter-Harris Type IV physeal fracture of phalanx of right toe**

● ⑦ ▭ **S99.242-** **Salter-Harris Type IV physeal fracture of phalanx of left toe**

● ⑦ ▭ **S99.249-** **Salter-Harris Type IV physeal fracture of phalanx of unspecified toe**

● Ⓖ **S99.29** **Other physeal fracture of phalanx of toe**

● ⑦ ▭ **S99.291-** **Other physeal fracture of phalanx of right toe**

● ⑦ ▭ **S99.292-** **Other physeal fracture of phalanx of left toe**

● ⑦ ▭ **S99.299-** **Other physeal fracture of phalanx of unspecified toe**

▲ Ⓢ **S99.8** **Other specified injuries of ankle and foot**

The appropriate 7th character is to be added to each code from subcategory S99.8
A   initial encounter
D   subsequent encounter
S   sequela

Ⓖ **S99.81** **Other specified injuries of ankle**
⑦ ▭ **S99.811-** **Other specified injuries of right ankle**
⑦ ▭ **S99.812-** **Other specified injuries of left ankle**
⑦ ▭ **S99.819-** **Other specified injuries of unspecified ankle**
Ⓖ **S99.82** **Other specified injuries of foot**
⑦ ▭ **S99.821-** **Other specified injuries of right foot**
⑦ ▭ **S99.822-** **Other specified injuries of left foot**
⑦ ▭ **S99.829-** **Other specified injuries of unspecified foot**

▲ Ⓢ **S99.9** **Unspecified injury of ankle and foot**

The appropriate 7th character is to be added to each code from subcategory S99.9
A   initial encounter
D   subsequent encounter
S   sequela

Ⓖ **S99.91** **Unspecified injury of ankle**
⑦ ▭ **S99.911-** **Unspecified injury of right ankle**
⑦ ▭ **S99.912-** **Unspecified injury of left ankle**
⑦ ▭ **S99.919-** **Unspecified injury of unspecified ankle**
Ⓖ **S99.92** **Unspecified injury of foot**
⑦ ▭ **S99.921-** **Unspecified injury of right foot**
⑦ ▭ **S99.922-** **Unspecified injury of left foot**
⑦ ▭ **S99.929-** **Unspecified injury of unspecified foot**

Injury, poisoning and certain other consequences of external causes (T07-T88)

Injuries involving multiple body regions (T07)

EXCLUDES 1 *burns and corrosions (T20-T32)*
frostbite (T33-T34)
insect bite or sting, venomous (T63.4)
sunburn (L55.-)

T07 **Unspecified multiple injuries**
EXCLUDES 1 *injury NOS (T14)*

Injury of unspecified body region (T14)

◪ **T14** **Injury of unspecified body region**
EXCLUDES 1 *multiple unspecified injuries (T07)*

T14.8 **Other injury of unspecified body region**
Abrasion NOS
Contusion NOS
Crush injury NOS
Fracture NOS
Skin injury NOS
Vascular injury NOS
Ⓢ **T14.9** **Unspecified injury**
T14.90 **Injury, unspecified**
Injury NOS
T14.91 **Suicide attempt**
Attempted suicide NOS

Effects of foreign body entering through natural orifice (T15-T19)

EXCLUDES 2 *foreign body accidentally left in operation wound (T81.5-)*
foreign body in penetrating wound - See open wound by body region
residual foreign body in soft tissue (M79.5)
splinter, without open wound - See superficial injury by body region

◪ **T15** **Foreign body on external eye**
EXCLUDES 2 *foreign body in penetrating wound of orbit and eye ball (S05.4-, S05.5-)*
open wound of eyelid and periocular area (S01.1-)
retained foreign body in eyelid (H02.8-)
retained (old) foreign body in penetrating wound of orbit and eye ball (H05.5-, H44.6-, H44.7-)
superficial foreign body of eyelid and periocular area (S00.25-)

The appropriate 7th character is to be added to each code from category T15
A   initial encounter
D   subsequent encounter
S   sequela

Ⓢ **T15.0** **Foreign body in cornea**
⑦ ▭ **T15.00X-** **Foreign body in cornea, unspecified eye**
⑦ ▭ **T15.01X-** **Foreign body in cornea, right eye**
⑦ ▭ **T15.02X-** **Foreign body in cornea, left eye**

● New   ▲ Revised   *Manifestation*   ◪- ⑦ Digit Indicators   ▭ Laterality   Ⓐ Adult (15+ years)   Ⓜ Maternity (12-55 years)   Ⓝ Newborn   Ⓟ Pediatric (0-17 years)   ♂ Male   ♀ Female
✖ Deleted   Unspecified   + Additional code

1038   © 2017 DecisionHealth   2017 ICD-10-CM Expert for Physicians

⑤ T15.1   Foreign body in conjunctival sac
  ⑦⊟ T15.10X-   Foreign body in conjunctival sac, unspecified eye
  ⑦⊟ T15.11X-   Foreign body in conjunctival sac, right eye
  ⑦⊟ T15.12X-   Foreign body in conjunctival sac, left eye
⑤ T15.8   Foreign body in other and multiple parts of external eye
            Foreign body in lacrimal punctum
  ⑦⊟ T15.80X-   Foreign body in other and multiple parts of
                 external eye, unspecified eye
  ⑦⊟ T15.81X-   Foreign body in other and multiple parts of
                 external eye, right eye
  ⑦⊟ T15.82X-   Foreign body in other and multiple parts of
                 external eye, left eye
⑤ T15.9   Foreign body on external eye, part unspecified
  ⑦⊟ T15.90X-   Foreign body on external eye, part unspecified,
                 unspecified eye
  ⑦⊟ T15.91X-   Foreign body on external eye, part unspecified,
                 right eye
  ⑦⊟ T15.92X-   Foreign body on external eye, part unspecified,
                 left eye

④ T16   Foreign body in ear

  [INCLUDES]   foreign body in auditory canal

  The appropriate 7th character is to be added to each code from
  category T16
  A   initial encounter
  D   subsequent encounter
  S   sequela

  ⑦⊟ T16.1XX-   Foreign body in right ear
  ⑦⊟ T16.2XX-   Foreign body in left ear
  ⑦⊟ T16.9XX-   Foreign body in ear, unspecified ear

④ T17   Foreign body in respiratory tract

  The appropriate 7th character is to be added to each code from
  category T17
  A   initial encounter
  D   subsequent encounter
  S   sequela

  ⑦ T17.0XX-   Foreign body in nasal sinus
  ⑦ T17.1XX-   Foreign body in nostril
               Foreign body in nose NOS
⑤ T17.2   Foreign body in pharynx
            Foreign body in nasopharynx
            Foreign body in throat NOS
  ⑥ T17.20   Unspecified foreign body in pharynx
    ⑦ T17.200-   Unspecified foreign body in pharynx causing
                  asphyxiation
    ⑦ T17.208-   Unspecified foreign body in pharynx causing
                  other injury
  ⑥ T17.21   Gastric contents in pharynx
              Aspiration of gastric contents into pharynx
              Vomitus in pharynx
    ⑦ T17.210-   Gastric contents in pharynx causing
                  asphyxiation
    ⑦ T17.218-   Gastric contents in pharynx causing other
                  injury
  ⑥ T17.22   Food in pharynx
              Bones in pharynx
              Seeds in pharynx
    ⑦ T17.220-   Food in pharynx causing asphyxiation
    ⑦ T17.228-   Food in pharynx causing other injury
  ⑥ T17.29   Other foreign object in pharynx
    ⑦ T17.290-   Other foreign object in pharynx causing
                  asphyxiation
    ⑦ T17.298-   Other foreign object in pharynx causing other
                  injury
⑤ T17.3   Foreign body in larynx
  ⑥ T17.30   Unspecified foreign body in larynx
    ⑦ T17.300-   Unspecified foreign body in larynx causing
                  asphyxiation
    ⑦ T17.308-   Unspecified foreign body in larynx causing
                  other injury
  ⑥ T17.31   Gastric contents in larynx
              Aspiration of gastric contents into larynx
              Vomitus in larynx
    ⑦ T17.310-   Gastric contents in larynx causing
                  asphyxiation

  ⑦ T17.318-   Gastric contents in larynx causing other injury
  ▲ ⑥ T17.32   Food in larynx
              Bones in larynx
              Seeds in larynx
    ⑦ T17.320-   Food in larynx causing asphyxiation
    ⑦ T17.328-   Food in larynx causing other injury
  ⑥ T17.39   Other foreign object in larynx
    ⑦ T17.390-   Other foreign object in larynx causing
                  asphyxiation
    ⑦ T17.398-   Other foreign object in larynx causing other
                  injury
⑤ T17.4   Foreign body in trachea
  ⑥ T17.40   Unspecified foreign body in trachea
    ⑦ T17.400-   Unspecified foreign body in trachea causing
                  asphyxiation
    ⑦ T17.408-   Unspecified foreign body in trachea causing
                  other injury
  ⑥ T17.41   Gastric contents in trachea
              Aspiration of gastric contents into trachea
              Vomitus in trachea
    ⑦ T17.410-   Gastric contents in trachea causing
                  asphyxiation
    ⑦ T17.418-   Gastric contents in trachea causing other
                  injury
  ⑥ T17.42   Food in trachea
              Bones in trachea
              Seeds in trachea
    ⑦ T17.420-   Food in trachea causing asphyxiation
    ⑦ T17.428-   Food in trachea causing other injury
  ⑥ T17.49   Other foreign object in trachea
    ⑦ T17.490-   Other foreign object in trachea causing
                  asphyxiation
    ⑦ T17.498-   Other foreign object in trachea causing other
                  injury
⑤ T17.5   Foreign body in bronchus
  ⑥ T17.50   Unspecified foreign body in bronchus
    ⑦ T17.500-   Unspecified foreign body in bronchus causing
                  asphyxiation
    ⑦ T17.508-   Unspecified foreign body in bronchus causing
                  other injury
  ⑥ T17.51   Gastric contents in bronchus
              Aspiration of gastric contents into bronchus
              Vomitus in bronchus
    ⑦ T17.510-   Gastric contents in bronchus causing
                  asphyxiation
    ⑦ T17.518-   Gastric contents in bronchus causing other
                  injury
  ⑥ T17.52   Food in bronchus
              Bones in bronchus
              Seeds in bronchus
    ⑦ T17.520-   Food in bronchus causing asphyxiation
    ⑦ T17.528-   Food in bronchus causing other injury
  ⑥ T17.59   Other foreign object in bronchus
    ⑦ T17.590-   Other foreign object in bronchus causing
                  asphyxiation
    ⑦ T17.598-   Other foreign object in bronchus causing other
                  injury
⑤ T17.8   Foreign body in other parts of respiratory tract
            Foreign body in bronchioles
            Foreign body in lung
  ⑥ T17.80   Unspecified foreign body in other parts of
              respiratory tract
    ⑦ T17.800-   Unspecified foreign body in other parts of
                  respiratory tract causing asphyxiation
    ⑦ T17.808-   Unspecified foreign body in other parts of
                  respiratory tract causing other injury
  ⑥ T17.81   Gastric contents in other parts of respiratory tract
              Aspiration of gastric contents into other parts of
                  respiratory tract
              Vomitus in other parts of respiratory tract
    ⑦ T17.810-   Gastric contents in other parts of respiratory
                  tract causing asphyxiation
    ⑦ T17.818-   Gastric contents in other parts of respiratory
                  tract causing other injury
  ⑥ T17.82   Food in other parts of respiratory tract
              Bones in other parts of respiratory tract
              Seeds in other parts of respiratory tract

● New   ▲ Revised   *Manifestation*   ④-⑦ Digit Indicators   ⊟ Laterality   🅐 Adult   🅜 Maternity   🅝 Newborn   🅟 Pediatric   ♂ Male   ♀ Female
✖ Deleted   Unspecified   + Additional code   (15+ years)   (12-55 years)   (0-17 years)

☑ **T17.820-**   **Food in other parts of respiratory tract causing asphyxiation**

☑ **T17.828-**   **Food in other parts of respiratory tract causing other injury**

⑥ **T17.89**   **Other foreign object in other parts of respiratory tract**

☑ **T17.890-**   **Other foreign object in other parts of respiratory tract causing asphyxiation**

☑ **T17.898-**   **Other foreign object in other parts of respiratory tract causing other injury**

⑤ **T17.9**   **Foreign body in respiratory tract, part unspecified**

⑥ **T17.90**   **Unspecified foreign body in respiratory tract, part unspecified**

☑ **T17.900-**   **Unspecified foreign body in respiratory tract, part unspecified causing asphyxiation**

☑ **T17.908-**   **Unspecified foreign body in respiratory tract, part unspecified causing other injury**

⑥ **T17.91**   **Gastric contents in respiratory tract, part unspecified**

Aspiration of gastric contents into respiratory tract, part unspecified
Vomitus in trachea respiratory tract, part unspecified

☑ **T17.910-**   **Gastric contents in respiratory tract, part unspecified causing asphyxiation**

☑ **T17.918-**   **Gastric contents in respiratory tract, part unspecified causing other injury**

⑥ **T17.92**   **Food in respiratory tract, part unspecified**

Bones in respiratory tract, part unspecified
Seeds in respiratory tract, part unspecified

☑ **T17.920-**   **Food in respiratory tract, part unspecified causing asphyxiation**

☑ **T17.928-**   **Food in respiratory tract, part unspecified causing other injury**

⑥ **T17.99**   **Other foreign object in respiratory tract, part unspecified**

☑ **T17.990-**   **Other foreign object in respiratory tract, part unspecified in causing asphyxiation**

☑ **T17.998-**   **Other foreign object in respiratory tract, part unspecified causing other injury**

④ **T18**   **Foreign body in alimentary tract**

| EXCLUDES 2 | *foreign body in pharynx (T17.2-)* |

The appropriate 7th character is to be added to each code from category T18
A   initial encounter
D   subsequent encounter
S   sequela

☑ **T18.0XX-**   **Foreign body in mouth**

⑤ **T18.1**   **Foreign body in esophagus**

| EXCLUDES 2 | *foreign body in respiratory tract (T17.-)* |

⑥ **T18.10**   **Unspecified foreign body in esophagus**

☑ **T18.100-**   **Unspecified foreign body in esophagus causing compression of trachea**

Unspecified foreign body in esophagus causing obstruction of respiration

☑ **T18.108-**   **Unspecified foreign body in esophagus causing other injury**

⑥ **T18.11**   **Gastric contents in esophagus**

Vomitus in esophagus

☑ **T18.110-**   **Gastric contents in esophagus causing compression of trachea**

Gastric contents in esophagus causing obstruction of respiration

☑ **T18.118-**   **Gastric contents in esophagus causing other injury**

⑥ **T18.12**   **Food in esophagus**

Bones in esophagus
Seeds in esophagus

☑ **T18.120-**   **Food in esophagus causing compression of trachea**

Food in esophagus causing obstruction of respiration

☑ **T18.128-**   **Food in esophagus causing other injury**

⑥ **T18.19**   **Other foreign object in esophagus**

☑ **T18.190-**   **Other foreign object in esophagus causing compression of trachea**

Other foreign body in esophagus causing obstruction of respiration
AHA: 1Q 2015, 24

☑ **T18.198-**   **Other foreign object in esophagus causing other injury**

AHA: 1Q 2015, 24

☑ **T18.2XX-**   **Foreign body in stomach**

☑ **T18.3XX-**   **Foreign body in small intestine**

☑ **T18.4XX-**   **Foreign body in colon**

☑ **T18.5XX-**   **Foreign body in anus and rectum**

Foreign body in rectosigmoid (junction)

☑ **T18.8XX-**   **Foreign body in other parts of alimentary tract**

☑ **T18.9XX-**   **Foreign body of alimentary tract, part unspecified**

Foreign body in digestive system NOS
Swallowed foreign body NOS

④ **T19**   **Foreign body in genitourinary tract**

EXCLUDES 2	*complications due to implanted mesh (T83.7-)*
	mechanical complications of contraceptive device (intrauterine) (vaginal) (T83.3-)
	presence of contraceptive device (intrauterine) (vaginal) (Z97.5)

The appropriate 7th character is to be added to each code from category T19
A   initial encounter
D   subsequent encounter
S   sequela

☑ **T19.0XX-**   **Foreign body in urethra**

☑ **T19.1XX-**   **Foreign body in bladder**

☑ **T19.2XX-**   **Foreign body in vulva and vagina**

☑ **T19.3XX-**   **Foreign body in uterus**

☑ **T19.4XX-**   **Foreign body in penis**

☑ **T19.8XX-**   **Foreign body in other parts of genitourinary tract**

☑ **T19.9XX-**   **Foreign body in genitourinary tract, part unspecified**

Burns and corrosions (T20-T32)

INCLUDES	burns (thermal) from electrical heating appliances
	burns (thermal) from electricity
	burns (thermal) from flame
	burns (thermal) from friction
	burns (thermal) from hot air and hot gases
	burns (thermal) from hot objects
	burns (thermal) from lightning
	burns (thermal) from radiation
	chemical burn [corrosion] (external) (internal)
	scalds
EXCLUDES 2	*erythema [dermatitis] ab igne (L59.0)*
	radiation-related disorders of the skin and subcutaneous tissue (L55-L59)
	sunburn (L55.-)

| GUIDELINES | Section I.C.19.d |

The ICD-10-CM makes a distinction between burns and corrosions. The burn codes are for thermal burns, except sunburns, that come from a heat source, such as a fire or hot appliance. The burn codes are also for burns resulting from electricity and radiation. Corrosions are burns due to chemicals. The guidelines are the same for burns and corrosions.

● New   ▲ Revised   *Manifestation*   ④-☑ Digit Indicators   ⊟ Laterality   Ⓐ Adult (15+ years)   Ⓜ Maternity (12-55 years)   Ⓝ Newborn   Ⓟ Pediatric (0-17 years)   ♂ Male   ♀ Female
✖ Deleted   Unspecified   + Additional code

1040   © 2017 DecisionHealth   2017 ICD-10-CM Expert for Physicians

GUIDELINES   Section I.C.19.d.1)-5)
Sequence first the code that reflects the highest degree of burn when more than one burn is present.
a. When the reason for the admission or encounter is for treatment of external multiple burns, sequence first the code that reflects the burn of the highest degree.
b. When a patient has both internal and external burns, the circumstances of admission govern the selection of the principal diagnosis or first-listed diagnosis.
c. When a patient is admitted for burn injuries and other related conditions such as smoke inhalation and/or respiratory failure, the circumstances of admission govern the selection of the principal or first-listed diagnosis.

Classify burns of the same local site (three-character category level, T20-T28) but of different degrees to the subcategory identifying the highest degree recorded in the diagnosis.

Non-healing burns are coded as acute burns. Necrosis of burned skin should be coded as a non-healed burn.

For any documented infected burn site, use an additional code for the infection.

When coding burns, assign separate codes for each burn site.

CODING TIP ✓   When a patient presents with a burn (other than sunburn), an additional code from Chapter 20 (External causes) should be added to indicate the cause (intent) of the burn.

CODING TIP ✓   A burn that is referred to as "not healing" should be coded as an acute burn using 7th character "A" or "D" depending upon treatment stage. Sequelae of a burn, such as contracture or keloid scarring, should be coded by first assigning the code for the residual condition, followed by the appropriate code to identify the burn with the 7th character "S" to indicate sequelae.

Burns and corrosions of external body surface, specified by site (T20-T25)

INCLUDES   burns and corrosions of first degree [erythema]
burns and corrosions of second degree [blisters][epidermal loss]
burns and corrosions of third degree [deep necrosis of underlying tissue] [full- thickness skin loss]

Use additional code from category T31 or T32 to identify extent of body surface involved

GUIDELINES   Section I.C.19.d
Current burns (T20-T25) are classified by depth, extent and by agent (X code). Burns are classified by depth as first degree (erythema), second degree (blistering), and third degree (full-thickness involvement). Burns of the eye and internal organs (T26-T28) are classified by site, but not by degree.

4 **T20**   **Burn and corrosion of head, face, and neck**

   EXCLUDES 2   *burn and corrosion of ear drum (T28.41, T28.91)*
   burn and corrosion of eye and adnexa (T26.-)
   burn and corrosion of mouth and pharynx (T28.0)

   The appropriate 7th character is to be added to each code from category T20
   A   initial encounter
   D   subsequent encounter
   S   sequela

5 + **T20.0**   **Burn of unspecified degree of head, face, and neck**
   Use additional external cause code to identify the source, place and intent of the burn (X00-X19, X75-X77, X96-X98, Y92)

   7 + **T20.00X-**   Burn of unspecified degree of head, face, and neck, unspecified site

   6 + **T20.01**   Burn of unspecified degree of ear [any part, except ear drum]
      EXCLUDES 2   *burn of ear drum (T28.41-)*

      7 ▣ + **T20.011-**   Burn of unspecified degree of right ear [any part, except ear drum]

      7 ▣ + **T20.012-**   Burn of unspecified degree of left ear [any part, except ear drum]

      7 ▣ + **T20.019-**   Burn of unspecified degree of unspecified ear [any part, except ear drum]

   7 + **T20.02X-**   Burn of unspecified degree of lip(s)
   7 + **T20.03X-**   Burn of unspecified degree of chin

   7 + **T20.04X-**   Burn of unspecified degree of nose (septum)
   7 + **T20.05X-**   Burn of unspecified degree of scalp [any part]
   7 + **T20.06X-**   Burn of unspecified degree of forehead and cheek
   7 + **T20.07X-**   Burn of unspecified degree of neck
   7 + **T20.09X-**   Burn of unspecified degree of multiple sites of head, face, and neck

5 + **T20.1**   **Burn of first degree of head, face, and neck**
   Use additional external cause code to identify the source, place and intent of the burn (X00-X19, X75-X77, X96-X98, Y92)

   7 + **T20.10X-**   Burn of first degree of head, face, and neck, unspecified site

   6 + **T20.11**   Burn of first degree of ear [any part, except ear drum]
      EXCLUDES 2   *burn of ear drum (T28.41-)*

      7 ▣ + **T20.111-**   Burn of first degree of right ear [any part, except ear drum]

      7 ▣ + **T20.112-**   Burn of first degree of left ear [any part, except ear drum]

      7 ▣ + **T20.119-**   Burn of first degree of unspecified ear [any part, except ear drum]

   7 + **T20.12X-**   Burn of first degree of lip(s)
   7 + **T20.13X-**   Burn of first degree of chin
   7 + **T20.14X-**   Burn of first degree of nose (septum)
   7 + **T20.15X-**   Burn of first degree of scalp [any part]
   7 + **T20.16X-**   Burn of first degree of forehead and cheek
   7 + **T20.17X-**   Burn of first degree of neck
   7 + **T20.19X-**   Burn of first degree of multiple sites of head, face, and neck

5 + **T20.2**   **Burn of second degree of head, face, and neck**
   Use additional external cause code to identify the source, place and intent of the burn (X00-X19, X75-X77, X96-X98, Y92)

   7 + **T20.20X-**   Burn of second degree of head, face, and neck, unspecified site

   6 + **T20.21**   Burn of second degree of ear [any part, except ear drum]
      EXCLUDES 2   *burn of ear drum (T28.41-)*

      7 ▣ + **T20.211-**   Burn of second degree of right ear [any part, except ear drum]

      7 ▣ + **T20.212-**   Burn of second degree of left ear [any part, except ear drum]

      7 ▣ + **T20.219-**   Burn of second degree of unspecified ear [any part, except ear drum]

   7 + **T20.22X-**   Burn of second degree of lip(s)
   7 + **T20.23X-**   Burn of second degree of chin
   7 + **T20.24X-**   Burn of second degree of nose (septum)
   7 + **T20.25X-**   Burn of second degree of scalp [any part]
      AHA: (T20.25XS) 1Q 2015, 19
   7 + **T20.26X-**   Burn of second degree of forehead and cheek
   7 + **T20.27X-**   Burn of second degree of neck
   7 + **T20.29X-**   Burn of second degree of multiple sites of head, face, and neck

5 + **T20.3**   **Burn of third degree of head, face, and neck**
   Use additional external cause code to identify the source, place and intent of the burn (X00-X19, X75-X77, X96-X98, Y92)

   7 + **T20.30X-**   Burn of third degree of head, face, and neck, unspecified site

   6 + **T20.31**   Burn of third degree of ear [any part, except ear drum]
      EXCLUDES 2   *burn of ear drum (T28.41-)*

      7 ▣ + **T20.311-**   Burn of third degree of right ear [any part, except ear drum]

      7 ▣ + **T20.312-**   Burn of third degree of left ear [any part, except ear drum]
         AHA: (T20.312S) 1Q 2015, 18

      7 ▣ + **T20.319-**   Burn of third degree of unspecified ear [any part, except ear drum]

   7 + **T20.32X-**   Burn of third degree of lip(s)
   7 + **T20.33X-**   Burn of third degree of chin
   7 + **T20.34X-**   Burn of third degree of nose (septum)
   7 + **T20.35X-**   Burn of third degree of scalp [any part]

● New   ▲ Revised   *Manifestation*   4-7 Digit Indicators   ▣ Laterality   Ⓐ Adult (15+ years)   Ⓜ Maternity (12-55 years)   Ⓝ Newborn (0-17 years)   Ⓟ Pediatric (0-17 years)   ♂ Male   ♀ Female
✖ Deleted   Unspecified   + Additional code

7 + T20.36X-   Burn of third degree of forehead and cheek

7 + T20.37X-   Burn of third degree of neck

7 + T20.39X-   Burn of third degree of multiple sites of head, face, and neck

5 + T20.4   Corrosion of unspecified degree of head, face, and neck
    Code first:
      (T51-T65) to identify chemical and intent
    Use additional external cause code to identify place (Y92)

7 + T20.40X-   Corrosion of unspecified degree of head, face, and neck, unspecified site

6 + T20.41   Corrosion of unspecified degree of ear [any part, except ear drum]
    EXCLUDES 2   *corrosion of ear drum (T28.91-)*

7 ⊟ + T20.411-   Corrosion of unspecified degree of right ear [any part, except ear drum]

7 ⊟ + T20.412-   Corrosion of unspecified degree of left ear [any part, except ear drum]

7 ⊟ + T20.419-   Corrosion of unspecified degree of unspecified ear [any part, except ear drum]

7 + T20.42X-   Corrosion of unspecified degree of lip(s)

7 + T20.43X-   Corrosion of unspecified degree of chin

7 + T20.44X-   Corrosion of unspecified degree of nose (septum)

7 + T20.45X-   Corrosion of unspecified degree of scalp [any part]

7 + T20.46X-   Corrosion of unspecified degree of forehead and cheek

7 + T20.47X-   Corrosion of unspecified degree of neck

7 + T20.49X-   Corrosion of unspecified degree of multiple sites of head, face, and neck

5 + T20.5   Corrosion of first degree of head, face, and neck
    Code first:
      (T51-T65) to identify chemical and intent
    Use additional external cause code to identify place (Y92)

7 + T20.50X-   Corrosion of first degree of head, face, and neck, unspecified site

6 + T20.51   Corrosion of first degree of ear [any part, except ear drum]
    EXCLUDES 2   *corrosion of ear drum (T28.91-)*

7 ⊟ + T20.511-   Corrosion of first degree of right ear [any part, except ear drum]

7 ⊟ + T20.512-   Corrosion of first degree of left ear [any part, except ear drum]

7 ⊟ + T20.519-   Corrosion of first degree of unspecified ear [any part, except ear drum]

7 + T20.52X-   Corrosion of first degree of lip(s)

7 + T20.53X-   Corrosion of first degree of chin

7 + T20.54X-   Corrosion of first degree of nose (septum)

7 + T20.55X-   Corrosion of first degree of scalp [any part]

7 + T20.56X-   Corrosion of first degree of forehead and cheek

7 + T20.57X-   Corrosion of first degree of neck

7 + T20.59X-   Corrosion of first degree of multiple sites of head, face, and neck

5 + T20.6   Corrosion of second degree of head, face, and neck
    Code first:
      (T51-T65) to identify chemical and intent
    Use additional external cause code to identify place (Y92)

7 + T20.60X-   Corrosion of second degree of head, face, and neck, unspecified site

6 + T20.61   Corrosion of second degree of ear [any part, except ear drum]
    EXCLUDES 2   *corrosion of ear drum (T28.91-)*

7 ⊟ + T20.611-   Corrosion of second degree of right ear [any part, except ear drum]

7 ⊟ + T20.612-   Corrosion of second degree of left ear [any part, except ear drum]

7 ⊟ + T20.619-   Corrosion of second degree of unspecified ear [any part, except ear drum]

7 + T20.62X-   Corrosion of second degree of lip(s)

7 + T20.63X-   Corrosion of second degree of chin

7 + T20.64X-   Corrosion of second degree of nose (septum)

7 + T20.65X-   Corrosion of second degree of scalp [any part]

7 + T20.66X-   Corrosion of second degree of forehead and cheek

7 + T20.67X-   Corrosion of second degree of neck

7 + T20.69X-   Corrosion of second degree of multiple sites of head, face, and neck

5 + T20.7   Corrosion of third degree of head, face, and neck
    Code first:
      (T51-T65) to identify chemical and intent
    Use additional external cause code to identify place (Y92)

7 + T20.70X-   Corrosion of third degree of head, face, and neck, unspecified site

6 + T20.71   Corrosion of third degree of ear [any part, except ear drum]
    EXCLUDES 2   *corrosion of ear drum (T28.91-)*

7 ⊟ + T20.711-   Corrosion of third degree of right ear [any part, except ear drum]

7 ⊟ + T20.712-   Corrosion of third degree of left ear [any part, except ear drum]

7 ⊟ + T20.719-   Corrosion of third degree of unspecified ear [any part, except ear drum]

7 + T20.72X-   Corrosion of third degree of lip(s)

7 + T20.73X-   Corrosion of third degree of chin

7 + T20.74X-   Corrosion of third degree of nose (septum)

7 + T20.75X-   Corrosion of third degree of scalp [any part]

7 + T20.76X-   Corrosion of third degree of forehead and cheek

7 + T20.77X-   Corrosion of third degree of neck

7 + T20.79X-   Corrosion of third degree of multiple sites of head, face, and neck

4 T21   **Burn and corrosion of trunk**
    INCLUDES   burns and corrosion of hip region
    EXCLUDES 2   *burns and corrosion of axilla*
        (T22.- with fifth character 4)
        burns and corrosion of scapular region
        (T22.- with fifth character 6)
        burns and corrosion of shoulder
        (T22.- with fifth character 5)

The appropriate 7th character is to be added to each code from category T21

A   initial encounter
D   subsequent encounter
S   sequela

5 + T21.0   **Burn of unspecified degree of trunk**
    Use additional external cause code to identify the source, place and intent of the burn (X00-X19, X75-X77, X96-X98, Y92)

7 + T21.00X-   Burn of unspecified degree of trunk, unspecified site

7 + T21.01X-   Burn of unspecified degree of chest wall
    Burn of of unspecified degree of breast

7 + T21.02X-   Burn of unspecified degree of abdominal wall
    Burn of unspecified degree of flank
    Burn of unspecified degree of groin

7 + T21.03X-   Burn of unspecified degree of upper back
    Burn of unspecified degree of interscapular region

7 + T21.04X-   Burn of unspecified degree of lower back

7 + T21.05X-   Burn of unspecified degree of buttock
    Burn of unspecified degree of anus

7 + T21.06X-   Burn of unspecified degree of male genital region
    Burn of unspecified degree of penis
    Burn of unspecified degree of scrotum
    Burn of unspecified degree of testis

7 + T21.07X-   Burn of unspecified degree of female genital region
    Burn of unspecified degree of labium (majus) (minus)
    Burn of unspecified degree of perineum
    Burn of unspecified degree of vulva
    EXCLUDES 2   *burn of vagina (T28.3)*

7 + T21.09X-   Burn of unspecified degree of other site of trunk

5 + T21.1   **Burn of first degree of trunk**
    Use additional external cause code to identify the source, place and intent of the burn (X00-X19, X75-X77, X96-X98, Y92)

7 + T21.10X-   Burn of first degree of trunk, unspecified site

7 + T21.11X-   Burn of first degree of chest wall
    Burn of first degree of breast

● New   ▲ Revised   *Manifestation*   **4-7** Digit Indicators   ⊟ Laterality   Ⓐ Adult (15+ years)   Ⓜ Maternity (12-55 years)   Ⓝ Newborn   Ⓟ Pediatric (0-17 years)   ♂ Male   ♀ Female
✖ Deleted   Unspecified   + Additional code

1042   © 2017 DecisionHealth   2017 ICD-10-CM Expert for Physicians

7 + T21.12X- **Burn of first degree of abdominal wall**
Burn of first degree of flank
Burn of first degree of groin

7 + T21.13X- **Burn of first degree of upper back**
Burn of first degree of interscapular region

7 + T21.14X- **Burn of first degree of lower back**

7 + T21.15X- **Burn of first degree of buttock**
Burn of first degree of anus

7 + T21.16X- **Burn of first degree of male genital region**
Burn of first degree of penis
Burn of first degree of scrotum
Burn of first degree of testis

7 + T21.17X- **Burn of first degree of female genital region**
Burn of first degree of labium (majus) (minus)
Burn of first degree of perineum
Burn of first degree of vulva
EXCLUDES 2 *burn of vagina (T28.3)*

7 + T21.19X- **Burn of first degree of other site of trunk**

5 + T21.2 **Burn of second degree of trunk**
Use additional external cause code to identify the source, place and intent of the burn (X00-X19, X75-X77, X96-X98, Y92)

7 + T21.20X- **Burn of second degree of trunk, unspecified site**

7 + T21.21X- **Burn of second degree of chest wall**
Burn of second degree of breast

7 + T21.22X- **Burn of second degree of abdominal wall**
Burn of second degree of flank
Burn of second degree of groin

7 + T21.23X- **Burn of second degree of upper back**
Burn of second degree of interscapular region

7 + T21.24X- **Burn of second degree of lower back**

7 + T21.25X- **Burn of second degree of buttock**
Burn of second degree of anus

7 + T21.26X- **Burn of second degree of male genital region**
Burn of second degree of penis
Burn of second degree of scrotum
Burn of second degree of testis

7 + T21.27X- **Burn of second degree of female genital region**
Burn of second degree of labium (majus) (minus)
Burn of second degree of perineum
Burn of second degree of vulva
EXCLUDES 2 *burn of vagina (T28.3)*

7 + T21.29X- **Burn of second degree of other site of trunk**

5 + T21.3 **Burn of third degree of trunk**
Use additional external cause code to identify the source, place and intent of the burn (X00-X19, X75-X77, X96-X98, Y92)

7 + T21.30X- **Burn of third degree of trunk, unspecified site**

7 + T21.31X- **Burn of third degree of chest wall**
Burn of third degree of breast
AHA: (T21.31XD) 2Q 2016, 6

7 + T21.32X- **Burn of third degree of abdominal wall**
Burn of third degree of flank
Burn of third degree of groin

7 + T21.33X- **Burn of third degree of upper back**
Burn of third degree of interscapular region

7 + T21.34X- **Burn of third degree of lower back**

7 + T21.35X- **Burn of third degree of buttock**
Burn of third degree of anus

7 + T21.36X- **Burn of third degree of male genital region**
Burn of third degree of penis
Burn of third degree of scrotum
Burn of third degree of testis

7 + T21.37X- **Burn of third degree of female genital region**
Burn of third degree of labium (majus) (minus)
Burn of third degree of perineum
Burn of third degree of vulva
EXCLUDES 2 *burn of vagina (T28.3)*

7 + T21.39X- **Burn of third degree of other site of trunk**

5 + T21.4 **Corrosion of unspecified degree of trunk**
Code first:
(T51-T65) to identify chemical and intent
Use additional external cause code to identify place (Y92)

7 + T21.40X- **Corrosion of unspecified degree of trunk, unspecified site**

7 + T21.41X- **Corrosion of unspecified degree of chest wall**
Corrosion of unspecified degree of breast

7 + T21.42X- **Corrosion of unspecified degree of abdominal wall**
Corrosion of unspecified degree of flank
Corrosion of unspecified degree of groin

7 + T21.43X- **Corrosion of unspecified degree of upper back**
Corrosion of unspecified degree of interscapular region

7 + T21.44X- **Corrosion of unspecified degree of lower back**

7 + T21.45X- **Corrosion of unspecified degree of buttock**
Corrosion of unspecified degree of anus

7 + T21.46X- **Corrosion of unspecified degree of male genital region**
Corrosion of unspecified degree of penis
Corrosion of unspecified degree of scrotum
Corrosion of unspecified degree of testis

7 + T21.47X- **Corrosion of unspecified degree of female genital region**
Corrosion of unspecified degree of labium (majus) (minus)
Corrosion of unspecified degree of perineum
Corrosion of unspecified degree of vulva
EXCLUDES 2 *corrosion of vagina (T28.8)*

7 + T21.49X- **Corrosion of unspecified degree of other site of trunk**

5 + T21.5 **Corrosion of first degree of trunk**
Code first:
(T51-T65) to identify chemical and intent
Use additional external cause code to identify place (Y92)

7 + T21.50X- **Corrosion of first degree of trunk, unspecified site**

7 + T21.51X- **Corrosion of first degree of chest wall**
Corrosion of first degree of breast

7 + T21.52X- **Corrosion of first degree of abdominal wall**
Corrosion of first degree of flank
Corrosion of first degree of groin

7 + T21.53X- **Corrosion of first degree of upper back**
Corrosion of first degree of interscapular region

7 + T21.54X- **Corrosion of first degree of lower back**

7 + T21.55X- **Corrosion of first degree of buttock**
Corrosion of first degree of anus

7 + T21.56X- **Corrosion of first degree of male genital region**
Corrosion of first degree of penis
Corrosion of first degree of scrotum
Corrosion of first degree of testis

7 + T21.57X- **Corrosion of first degree of female genital region**
Corrosion of first degree of labium (majus) (minus)
Corrosion of first degree of perineum
Corrosion of first degree of vulva
EXCLUDES 2 *corrosion of vagina (T28.8)*

7 + T21.59X- **Corrosion of first degree of other site of trunk**

5 + T21.6 **Corrosion of second degree of trunk**
Code first:
(T51-T65) to identify chemical and intent
Use additional external cause code to identify place (Y92)

7 + T21.60X- **Corrosion of second degree of trunk, unspecified site**

7 + T21.61X- **Corrosion of second degree of chest wall**
Corrosion of second degree of breast

7 + T21.62X- **Corrosion of second degree of abdominal wall**
Corrosion of second degree of flank
Corrosion of second degree of groin

7 + T21.63X- **Corrosion of second degree of upper back**
Corrosion of second degree of interscapular region

7 + T21.64X- **Corrosion of second degree of lower back**

7 + T21.65X- **Corrosion of second degree of buttock**
Corrosion of second degree of anus

7 + T21.66X- **Corrosion of second degree of male genital region**
Corrosion of second degree of penis
Corrosion of second degree of scrotum
Corrosion of second degree of testis

7 + T21.67X- **Corrosion of second degree of female genital region**
Corrosion of second degree of labium (majus) (minus)
Corrosion of second degree of perineum
Corrosion of second degree of vulva
EXCLUDES 2 *corrosion of vagina (T28.8)*

7 + T21.69X- **Corrosion of second degree of other site of trunk**

● New ▲ Revised *Manifestation* 4-7 Digit Indicators ▤ Laterality Ⓐ Adult (15+ years) Ⓜ Maternity (12-55 years) Ⓝ Newborn Ⓟ Pediatric (0-17 years) ♂ Male ♀ Female
✖ Deleted Unspecified + Additional code

2017 ICD-10-CM Expert for Physicians

© 2017 DecisionHealth 1043

⑤+ T21.7   Corrosion of third degree of trunk
Code first:
(T51-T65) to identify chemical and intent
Use additional external cause code to identify place (Y92)

⑦+ T21.70X-   Corrosion of third degree of trunk, unspecified site

⑦+ T21.71X-   Corrosion of third degree of chest wall
Corrosion of third degree of breast

⑦+ T21.72X-   Corrosion of third degree of abdominal wall
Corrosion of third degree of flank
Corrosion of third degree of groin

⑦+ T21.73X-   Corrosion of third degree of upper back
Corrosion of third degree of interscapular region

⑦+ T21.74X-   Corrosion of third degree of lower back

⑦+ T21.75X-   Corrosion of third degree of buttock
Corrosion of third degree of anus

⑦+ T21.76X-   Corrosion of third degree of male genital region
Corrosion of third degree of penis
Corrosion of third degree of scrotum
Corrosion of third degree of testis

⑦+ T21.77X-   Corrosion of third degree of female genital region
Corrosion of third degree of labium (majus) (minus)
Corrosion of third degree of perineum
Corrosion of third degree of vulva
EXCLUDES 2   *corrosion of vagina (T28.8)*

⑦+ T21.79X-   Corrosion of third degree of other site of trunk

④ T22   Burn and corrosion of shoulder and upper limb, except wrist and hand
EXCLUDES 2   *burn and corrosion of interscapular region (T21.-)*
burn and corrosion of wrist and hand (T23.-)

The appropriate 7th character is to be added to each code from category T22
A   initial encounter
D   subsequent encounter
S   sequela

⑤+ T22.0   Burn of unspecified degree of shoulder and upper limb, except wrist and hand
Use additional external cause code to identify the source, place and intent of the burn (X00-X19, X75-X77, X96-X98, Y92)

⑦+ T22.00X-   Burn of unspecified degree of shoulder and upper limb, except wrist and hand, unspecified site

⑥+ T22.01   Burn of unspecified degree of forearm
⑦☐+ T22.011-   Burn of unspecified degree of right forearm
⑦☐+ T22.012-   Burn of unspecified degree of left forearm
⑦☐+ T22.019-   Burn of unspecified degree of unspecified forearm

⑥+ T22.02   Burn of unspecified degree of elbow
⑦☐+ T22.021-   Burn of unspecified degree of right elbow
⑦☐+ T22.022-   Burn of unspecified degree of left elbow
⑦☐+ T22.029-   Burn of unspecified degree of unspecified elbow

⑥+ T22.03   Burn of unspecified degree of upper arm
⑦☐+ T22.031-   Burn of unspecified degree of right upper arm
⑦☐+ T22.032-   Burn of unspecified degree of left upper arm
⑦☐+ T22.039-   Burn of unspecified degree of unspecified upper arm

⑥+ T22.04   Burn of unspecified degree of axilla
⑦☐+ T22.041-   Burn of unspecified degree of right axilla
⑦☐+ T22.042-   Burn of unspecified degree of left axilla
⑦☐+ T22.049-   Burn of unspecified degree of unspecified axilla

⑥+ T22.05   Burn of unspecified degree of shoulder
⑦☐+ T22.051-   Burn of unspecified degree of right shoulder
⑦☐+ T22.052-   Burn of unspecified degree of left shoulder
⑦☐+ T22.059-   Burn of unspecified degree of unspecified shoulder

⑥+ T22.06   Burn of unspecified degree of scapular region
⑦☐+ T22.061-   Burn of unspecified degree of right scapular region
⑦☐+ T22.062-   Burn of unspecified degree of left scapular region

⑦☐+ T22.069-   Burn of unspecified degree of unspecified scapular region

⑥+ T22.09   Burn of unspecified degree of multiple sites of shoulder and upper limb, except wrist and hand
⑦☐+ T22.091-   Burn of unspecified degree of multiple sites of right shoulder and upper limb, except wrist and hand
⑦☐+ T22.092-   Burn of unspecified degree of multiple sites of left shoulder and upper limb, except wrist and hand
⑦☐+ T22.099-   Burn of unspecified degree of multiple sites of unspecified shoulder and upper limb, except wrist and hand

⑤+ T22.1   Burn of first degree of shoulder and upper limb, except wrist and hand
Use additional external cause code to identify the source, place and intent of the burn (X00-X19, X75-X77, X96-X98, Y92)

⑦+ T22.10X-   Burn of first degree of shoulder and upper limb, except wrist and hand, unspecified site

⑥+ T22.11   Burn of first degree of forearm
⑦☐+ T22.111-   Burn of first degree of right forearm
⑦☐+ T22.112-   Burn of first degree of left forearm
⑦☐+ T22.119-   Burn of first degree of unspecified forearm

⑥+ T22.12   Burn of first degree of elbow
⑦☐+ T22.121-   Burn of first degree of right elbow
⑦☐+ T22.122-   Burn of first degree of left elbow
⑦☐+ T22.129-   Burn of first degree of unspecified elbow

⑥+ T22.13   Burn of first degree of upper arm
⑦☐+ T22.131-   Burn of first degree of right upper arm
⑦☐+ T22.132-   Burn of first degree of left upper arm
⑦☐+ T22.139-   Burn of first degree of unspecified upper arm

⑥+ T22.14   Burn of first degree of axilla
⑦☐+ T22.141-   Burn of first degree of right axilla
⑦☐+ T22.142-   Burn of first degree of left axilla
⑦☐+ T22.149-   Burn of first degree of unspecified axilla

⑥+ T22.15   Burn of first degree of shoulder
⑦☐+ T22.151-   Burn of first degree of right shoulder
⑦☐+ T22.152-   Burn of first degree of left shoulder
⑦☐+ T22.159-   Burn of first degree of unspecified shoulder

⑥+ T22.16   Burn of first degree of scapular region
⑦☐+ T22.161-   Burn of first degree of right scapular region
⑦☐+ T22.162-   Burn of first degree of left scapular region
⑦☐+ T22.169-   Burn of first degree of unspecified scapular region

⑥+ T22.19   Burn of first degree of multiple sites of shoulder and upper limb, except wrist and hand
⑦☐+ T22.191-   Burn of first degree of multiple sites of right shoulder and upper limb, except wrist and hand
⑦☐+ T22.192-   Burn of first degree of multiple sites of left shoulder and upper limb, except wrist and hand
⑦☐+ T22.199-   Burn of first degree of multiple sites of unspecified shoulder and upper limb, except wrist and hand

⑤+ T22.2   Burn of second degree of shoulder and upper limb, except wrist and hand
Use additional external cause code to identify the source, place and intent of the burn (X00-X19, X75-X77, X96-X98, Y92)

⑦+ T22.20X-   Burn of second degree of shoulder and upper limb, except wrist and hand, unspecified site

⑥+ T22.21   Burn of second degree of forearm
⑦☐+ T22.211-   Burn of second degree of right forearm
⑦☐+ T22.212-   Burn of second degree of left forearm
⑦☐+ T22.219-   Burn of second degree of unspecified forearm

⑥+ T22.22   Burn of second degree of elbow
⑦☐+ T22.221-   Burn of second degree of right elbow
⑦☐+ T22.222-   Burn of second degree of left elbow
⑦☐+ T22.229-   Burn of second degree of unspecified elbow

⑥+ T22.23   Burn of second degree of upper arm
⑦☐+ T22.231-   Burn of second degree of right upper arm
⑦☐+ T22.232-   Burn of second degree of left upper arm
⑦☐+ T22.239-   Burn of second degree of unspecified upper arm

6 + **T22.24** Burn of second degree of axilla
  7 + **T22.241-** Burn of second degree of right axilla
  7 + **T22.242-** Burn of second degree of left axilla
  7 + **T22.249-** Burn of second degree of unspecified axilla
6 + **T22.25** Burn of second degree of shoulder
  7 + **T22.251-** Burn of second degree of right shoulder
  7 + **T22.252-** Burn of second degree of left shoulder
  7 + **T22.259-** Burn of second degree of unspecified shoulder
6 + **T22.26** Burn of second degree of scapular region
  7 + **T22.261-** Burn of second degree of right scapular region
  7 + **T22.262-** Burn of second degree of left scapular region
  7 + **T22.269-** Burn of second degree of unspecified scapular region
6 + **T22.29** Burn of second degree of multiple sites of shoulder and upper limb, except wrist and hand
  7 + **T22.291-** Burn of second degree of multiple sites of right shoulder and upper limb, except wrist and hand
  7 + **T22.292-** Burn of second degree of multiple sites of left shoulder and upper limb, except wrist and hand
  7 + **T22.299-** Burn of second degree of multiple sites of unspecified shoulder and upper limb, except wrist and hand
5 + **T22.3** Burn of third degree of shoulder and upper limb, except wrist and hand
Use additional external cause code to identify the source, place and intent of the burn (X00-X19, X75-X77, X96-X98, Y92)
  7 + **T22.30X-** Burn of third degree of shoulder and upper limb, except wrist and hand, unspecified site
6 + **T22.31** Burn of third degree of forearm
  7 + **T22.311-** Burn of third degree of right forearm
  7 + **T22.312-** Burn of third degree of left forearm
  7 + **T22.319-** Burn of third degree of unspecified forearm
6 + **T22.32** Burn of third degree of elbow
  7 + **T22.321-** Burn of third degree of right elbow
  7 + **T22.322-** Burn of third degree of left elbow
  7 + **T22.329-** Burn of third degree of unspecified elbow
6 + **T22.33** Burn of third degree of upper arm
  7 + **T22.331-** Burn of third degree of right upper arm
  7 + **T22.332-** Burn of third degree of left upper arm
  7 + **T22.339-** Burn of third degree of unspecified upper arm
6 + **T22.34** Burn of third degree of axilla
  7 + **T22.341-** Burn of third degree of right axilla
  7 + **T22.342-** Burn of third degree of left axilla
  7 + **T22.349-** Burn of third degree of unspecified axilla
6 + **T22.35** Burn of third degree of shoulder
  7 + **T22.351-** Burn of third degree of right shoulder
  7 + **T22.352-** Burn of third degree of left shoulder
  7 + **T22.359-** Burn of third degree of unspecified shoulder
6 + **T22.36** Burn of third degree of scapular region
  7 + **T22.361-** Burn of third degree of right scapular region
  7 + **T22.362-** Burn of third degree of left scapular region
  7 + **T22.369-** Burn of third degree of unspecified scapular region
6 + **T22.39** Burn of third degree of multiple sites of shoulder and upper limb, except wrist and hand
  7 + **T22.391-** Burn of third degree of multiple sites of right shoulder and upper limb, except wrist and hand
  7 + **T22.392-** Burn of third degree of multiple sites of left shoulder and upper limb, except wrist and hand
  7 + **T22.399-** Burn of third degree of multiple sites of unspecified shoulder and upper limb, except wrist and hand
5 + **T22.4** Corrosion of unspecified degree of shoulder and upper limb, except wrist and hand
Code first:
(T51-T65) to identify chemical and intent
Use additional external cause code to identify place (Y92)
  7 + **T22.40X-** Corrosion of unspecified degree of shoulder and upper limb, except wrist and hand, unspecified site
6 + **T22.41** Corrosion of unspecified degree of forearm

  7 + **T22.411-** Corrosion of unspecified degree of right forearm
  7 + **T22.412-** Corrosion of unspecified degree of left forearm
  7 + **T22.419-** Corrosion of unspecified degree of unspecified forearm
6 + **T22.42** Corrosion of unspecified degree of elbow
  7 + **T22.421-** Corrosion of unspecified degree of right elbow
  7 + **T22.422-** Corrosion of unspecified degree of left elbow
  7 + **T22.429-** Corrosion of unspecified degree of unspecified elbow
6 + **T22.43** Corrosion of unspecified degree of upper arm
  7 + **T22.431-** Corrosion of unspecified degree of right upper arm
  7 + **T22.432-** Corrosion of unspecified degree of left upper arm
  7 + **T22.439-** Corrosion of unspecified degree of unspecified upper arm
6 + **T22.44** Corrosion of unspecified degree of axilla
  7 + **T22.441-** Corrosion of unspecified degree of right axilla
  7 + **T22.442-** Corrosion of unspecified degree of left axilla
  7 + **T22.449-** Corrosion of unspecified degree of unspecified axilla
6 + **T22.45** Corrosion of unspecified degree of shoulder
  7 + **T22.451-** Corrosion of unspecified degree of right shoulder
  7 + **T22.452-** Corrosion of unspecified degree of left shoulder
  7 + **T22.459-** Corrosion of unspecified degree of unspecified shoulder
6 + **T22.46** Corrosion of unspecified degree of scapular region
  7 + **T22.461-** Corrosion of unspecified degree of right scapular region
  7 + **T22.462-** Corrosion of unspecified degree of left scapular region
  7 + **T22.469-** Corrosion of unspecified degree of unspecified scapular region
6 + **T22.49** Corrosion of unspecified degree of multiple sites of shoulder and upper limb, except wrist and hand
  7 + **T22.491-** Corrosion of unspecified degree of multiple sites of right shoulder and upper limb, except wrist and hand
  7 + **T22.492-** Corrosion of unspecified degree of multiple sites of left shoulder and upper limb, except wrist and hand
  7 + **T22.499-** Corrosion of unspecified degree of multiple sites of unspecified shoulder and upper limb, except wrist and hand
5 + **T22.5** Corrosion of first degree of shoulder and upper limb, except wrist and hand
Code first:
(T51-T65) to identify chemical and intent
Use additional external cause code to identify place (Y92)
  7 + **T22.50X-** Corrosion of first degree of shoulder and upper limb, except wrist and hand unspecified site
6 + **T22.51** Corrosion of first degree of forearm
  7 + **T22.511-** Corrosion of first degree of right forearm
  7 + **T22.512-** Corrosion of first degree of left forearm
  7 + **T22.519-** Corrosion of first degree of unspecified forearm
6 + **T22.52** Corrosion of first degree of elbow
  7 + **T22.521-** Corrosion of first degree of right elbow
  7 + **T22.522-** Corrosion of first degree of left elbow
  7 + **T22.529-** Corrosion of first degree of unspecified elbow
6 + **T22.53** Corrosion of first degree of upper arm
  7 + **T22.531-** Corrosion of first degree of right upper arm
  7 + **T22.532-** Corrosion of first degree of left upper arm
  7 + **T22.539-** Corrosion of first degree of unspecified upper arm
6 + **T22.54** Corrosion of first degree of axilla
  7 + **T22.541-** Corrosion of first degree of right axilla
  7 + **T22.542-** Corrosion of first degree of left axilla
  7 + **T22.549-** Corrosion of first degree of unspecified axilla
6 + **T22.55** Corrosion of first degree of shoulder
  7 + **T22.551-** Corrosion of first degree of right shoulder

---

● New ▲ Revised *Manifestation* 4-7 Digit Indicators ⊟ Laterality Ⓐ Adult (15+ years) Ⓜ Maternity (12-55 years) Ⓝ Newborn Ⓟ Pediatric (0-17 years) ♂ Male ♀ Female
✖ Deleted   Unspecified + Additional code

7 ⬚ + T22.552-   Corrosion of first degree of left shoulder

7 ⬚ + T22.559-   Corrosion of first degree of unspecified shoulder

6 + T22.56   Corrosion of first degree of scapular region

7 ⬚ + T22.561-   Corrosion of first degree of right scapular region

7 ⬚ + T22.562-   Corrosion of first degree of left scapular region

7 ⬚ + T22.569-   Corrosion of first degree of unspecified scapular region

6 + T22.59   Corrosion of first degree of multiple sites of shoulder and upper limb, except wrist and hand

7 ⬚ + T22.591-   Corrosion of first degree of multiple sites of right shoulder and upper limb, except wrist and hand

7 ⬚ + T22.592-   Corrosion of first degree of multiple sites of left shoulder and upper limb, except wrist and hand

7 ⬚ + T22.599-   Corrosion of first degree of multiple sites of unspecified shoulder and upper limb, except wrist and hand

5 + T22.6   Corrosion of second degree of shoulder and upper limb, except wrist and hand

Code first:
(T51-T65) to identify chemical and intent
Use additional external cause code to identify place (Y92)

7 + T22.60X-   Corrosion of second degree of shoulder and upper limb, except wrist and hand, unspecified site

6 + T22.61   Corrosion of second degree of forearm

7 ⬚ + T22.611-   Corrosion of second degree of right forearm

7 ⬚ + T22.612-   Corrosion of second degree of left forearm

7 ⬚ + T22.619-   Corrosion of second degree of unspecified forearm

6 + T22.62   Corrosion of second degree of elbow

7 ⬚ + T22.621-   Corrosion of second degree of right elbow

7 ⬚ + T22.622-   Corrosion of second degree of left elbow

7 ⬚ + T22.629-   Corrosion of second degree of unspecified elbow

6 + T22.63   Corrosion of second degree of upper arm

7 ⬚ + T22.631-   Corrosion of second degree of right upper arm

7 ⬚ + T22.632-   Corrosion of second degree of left upper arm

7 ⬚ + T22.639-   Corrosion of second degree of unspecified upper arm

6 + T22.64   Corrosion of second degree of axilla

7 ⬚ + T22.641-   Corrosion of second degree of right axilla

7 ⬚ + T22.642-   Corrosion of second degree of left axilla

7 ⬚ + T22.649-   Corrosion of second degree of unspecified axilla

6 + T22.65   Corrosion of second degree of shoulder

7 ⬚ + T22.651-   Corrosion of second degree of right shoulder

7 ⬚ + T22.652-   Corrosion of second degree of left shoulder

7 ⬚ + T22.659-   Corrosion of second degree of unspecified shoulder

6 + T22.66   Corrosion of second degree of scapular region

7 ⬚ + T22.661-   Corrosion of second degree of right scapular region

7 ⬚ + T22.662-   Corrosion of second degree of left scapular region

7 ⬚ + T22.669-   Corrosion of second degree of unspecified scapular region

6 + T22.69   Corrosion of second degree of multiple sites of shoulder and upper limb, except wrist and hand

7 ⬚ + T22.691-   Corrosion of second degree of multiple sites of right shoulder and upper limb, except wrist and hand

7 ⬚ + T22.692-   Corrosion of second degree of multiple sites of left shoulder and upper limb, except wrist and hand

7 ⬚ + T22.699-   Corrosion of second degree of multiple sites of unspecified shoulder and upper limb, except wrist and hand

5 + T22.7   Corrosion of third degree of shoulder and upper limb, except wrist and hand

Code first:
(T51-T65) to identify chemical and intent
Use additional external cause code to identify place (Y92)

7 + T22.70X-   Corrosion of third degree of shoulder and upper limb, except wrist and hand, unspecified site

6 + T22.71   Corrosion of third degree of forearm

7 ⬚ + T22.711-   Corrosion of third degree of right forearm

7 ⬚ + T22.712-   Corrosion of third degree of left forearm

7 ⬚ + T22.719-   Corrosion of third degree of unspecified forearm

6 + T22.72   Corrosion of third degree of elbow

7 ⬚ + T22.721-   Corrosion of third degree of right elbow

7 ⬚ + T22.722-   Corrosion of third degree of left elbow

7 ⬚ + T22.729-   Corrosion of third degree of unspecified elbow

6 + T22.73   Corrosion of third degree of upper arm

7 ⬚ + T22.731-   Corrosion of third degree of right upper arm

7 ⬚ + T22.732-   Corrosion of third degree of left upper arm

7 ⬚ + T22.739-   Corrosion of third degree of unspecified upper arm

6 + T22.74   Corrosion of third degree of axilla

7 ⬚ + T22.741-   Corrosion of third degree of right axilla

7 ⬚ + T22.742-   Corrosion of third degree of left axilla

7 ⬚ + T22.749-   Corrosion of third degree of unspecified axilla

6 + T22.75   Corrosion of third degree of shoulder

7 ⬚ + T22.751-   Corrosion of third degree of right shoulder

7 ⬚ + T22.752-   Corrosion of third degree of left shoulder

7 ⬚ + T22.759-   Corrosion of third degree of unspecified shoulder

6 + T22.76   Corrosion of third degree of scapular region

7 ⬚ + T22.761-   Corrosion of third degree of right scapular region

7 ⬚ + T22.762-   Corrosion of third degree of left scapular region

7 ⬚ + T22.769-   Corrosion of third degree of unspecified scapular region

6 + T22.79   Corrosion of third degree of multiple sites of shoulder and upper limb, except wrist and hand

7 ⬚ + T22.791-   Corrosion of third degree of multiple sites of right shoulder and upper limb, except wrist and hand

7 ⬚ + T22.792-   Corrosion of third degree of multiple sites of left shoulder and upper limb, except wrist and hand

7 ⬚ + T22.799-   Corrosion of third degree of multiple sites of unspecified shoulder and upper limb, except wrist and hand

4 T23   **Burn and corrosion of wrist and hand**

The appropriate 7th character is to be added to each code from category T23
A   initial encounter
D   subsequent encounter
S   sequela

5 + T23.0   **Burn of unspecified degree of wrist and hand**

Use additional external cause code to identify the source, place and intent of the burn (X00-X19, X75-X77, X96-X98, Y92)

6 + T23.00   Burn of unspecified degree of hand, unspecified site

7 ⬚ + T23.001-   Burn of unspecified degree of right hand, unspecified site

7 ⬚ + T23.002-   Burn of unspecified degree of left hand, unspecified site

7 ⬚ + T23.009-   Burn of unspecified degree of unspecified hand, unspecified site

6 + T23.01   Burn of unspecified degree of thumb (nail)

7 ⬚ + T23.011-   Burn of unspecified degree of right thumb (nail)

7 ⬚ + T23.012-   Burn of unspecified degree of left thumb (nail)

7 ⬚ + T23.019-   Burn of unspecified degree of unspecified thumb (nail)

6 + T23.02   Burn of unspecified degree of single finger (nail) except thumb

7 ⬚ + T23.021-   Burn of unspecified degree of single right finger (nail) except thumb

7 ⬚ + T23.022-   Burn of unspecified degree of single left finger (nail) except thumb

7 ⬚ + T23.029-   Burn of unspecified degree of unspecified single finger (nail) except thumb

6 + T23.03   Burn of unspecified degree of multiple fingers (nail), not including thumb

---

● New   ▲ Revised   *Manifestation*   4-7 Digit Indicators   ⬚ Laterality   Ⓐ Adult (15+ years)   Ⓜ Maternity (12-55 years)   Ⓝ Newborn   Ⓟ Pediatric (0-17 years)   ♂ Male   ♀ Female

✖ Deleted   Unspecified   + Additional code

1046   © 2017 DecisionHealth   2017 ICD-10-CM Expert for Physicians

7 ⊟ + T23.031- Burn of unspecified degree of multiple right fingers (nail), not including thumb

7 ⊟ + T23.032- Burn of unspecified degree of multiple left fingers (nail), not including thumb

7 ⊟ + T23.039- Burn of unspecified degree of unspecified multiple fingers (nail), not including thumb

6 + T23.04 Burn of unspecified degree of multiple fingers (nail), including thumb

7 ⊟ + T23.041- Burn of unspecified degree of multiple right fingers (nail), including thumb

7 ⊟ + T23.042- Burn of unspecified degree of multiple left fingers (nail), including thumb

7 ⊟ + T23.049- Burn of unspecified degree of unspecified multiple fingers (nail), including thumb

6 + T23.05 Burn of unspecified degree of palm

7 ⊟ + T23.051- Burn of unspecified degree of right palm

7 ⊟ + T23.052- Burn of unspecified degree of left palm

7 ⊟ + T23.059- Burn of unspecified degree of unspecified palm

6 + T23.06 Burn of unspecified degree of back of hand

7 ⊟ + T23.061- Burn of unspecified degree of back of right hand

7 ⊟ + T23.062- Burn of unspecified degree of back of left hand

7 ⊟ + T23.069- Burn of unspecified degree of back of unspecified hand

6 + T23.07 Burn of unspecified degree of wrist

7 ⊟ + T23.071- Burn of unspecified degree of right wrist

7 ⊟ + T23.072- Burn of unspecified degree of left wrist

7 ⊟ + T23.079- Burn of unspecified degree of unspecified wrist

6 + T23.09 Burn of unspecified degree of multiple sites of wrist and hand

7 ⊟ + T23.091- Burn of unspecified degree of multiple sites of right wrist and hand

7 ⊟ + T23.092- Burn of unspecified degree of multiple sites of left wrist and hand

7 ⊟ + T23.099- Burn of unspecified degree of multiple sites of unspecified wrist and hand

5 + T23.1 Burn of first degree of wrist and hand
Use additional external cause code to identify the source, place and intent of the burn (X00-X19, X75-X77, X96-X98, Y92)

6 + T23.10 Burn of first degree of hand, unspecified site

7 ⊟ + T23.101- Burn of first degree of right hand, unspecified site

7 ⊟ + T23.102- Burn of first degree of left hand, unspecified site

7 ⊟ + T23.109- Burn of first degree of unspecified hand, unspecified site

6 + T23.11 Burn of first degree of thumb (nail)

7 ⊟ + T23.111- Burn of first degree of right thumb (nail)

7 ⊟ + T23.112- Burn of first degree of left thumb (nail)

7 ⊟ + T23.119- Burn of first degree of unspecified thumb (nail)

6 + T23.12 Burn of first degree of single finger (nail) except thumb

7 ⊟ + T23.121- Burn of first degree of single right finger (nail) except thumb

7 ⊟ + T23.122- Burn of first degree of single left finger (nail) except thumb

7 ⊟ + T23.129- Burn of first degree of unspecified single finger (nail) except thumb

6 + T23.13 Burn of first degree of multiple fingers (nail), not including thumb

7 ⊟ + T23.131- Burn of first degree of multiple right fingers (nail), not including thumb

7 ⊟ + T23.132- Burn of first degree of multiple left fingers (nail), not including thumb

7 ⊟ + T23.139- Burn of first degree of unspecified multiple fingers (nail), not including thumb

6 + T23.14 Burn of first degree of multiple fingers (nail), including thumb

7 ⊟ + T23.141- Burn of first degree of multiple right fingers (nail), including thumb

7 ⊟ + T23.142- Burn of first degree of multiple left fingers (nail), including thumb

7 ⊟ + T23.149- Burn of first degree of unspecified multiple fingers (nail), including thumb

6 + T23.15 Burn of first degree of palm

7 ⊟ + T23.151- Burn of first degree of right palm

7 ⊟ + T23.152- Burn of first degree of left palm

7 ⊟ + T23.159- Burn of first degree of unspecified palm

6 + T23.16 Burn of first degree of back of hand

7 ⊟ + T23.161- Burn of first degree of back of right hand

7 ⊟ + T23.162- Burn of first degree of back of left hand

7 ⊟ + T23.169- Burn of first degree of back of unspecified hand

6 + T23.17 Burn of first degree of wrist

7 ⊟ + T23.171- Burn of first degree of right wrist

7 ⊟ + T23.172- Burn of first degree of left wrist

7 ⊟ + T23.179- Burn of first degree of unspecified wrist

6 + T23.19 Burn of first degree of multiple sites of wrist and hand

7 ⊟ + T23.191- Burn of first degree of multiple sites of right wrist and hand

7 ⊟ + T23.192- Burn of first degree of multiple sites of left wrist and hand

7 ⊟ + T23.199- Burn of first degree of multiple sites of unspecified wrist and hand

5 + T23.2 Burn of second degree of wrist and hand
Use additional external cause code to identify the source, place and intent of the burn (X00-X19, X75-X77, X96-X98, Y92)

6 + T23.20 Burn of second degree of hand, unspecified site

7 ⊟ + T23.201- Burn of second degree of right hand, unspecified site

7 ⊟ + T23.202- Burn of second degree of left hand, unspecified site

7 ⊟ + T23.209- Burn of second degree of unspecified hand, unspecified site

6 + T23.21 Burn of second degree of thumb (nail)

7 ⊟ + T23.211- Burn of second degree of right thumb (nail)

7 ⊟ + T23.212- Burn of second degree of left thumb (nail)

7 ⊟ + T23.219- Burn of second degree of unspecified thumb (nail)

6 + T23.22 Burn of second degree of single finger (nail) except thumb

7 ⊟ + T23.221- Burn of second degree of single right finger (nail) except thumb

7 ⊟ + T23.222- Burn of second degree of single left finger (nail) except thumb

7 ⊟ + T23.229- Burn of second degree of unspecified single finger (nail) except thumb

6 + T23.23 Burn of second degree of multiple fingers (nail), not including thumb

7 ⊟ + T23.231- Burn of second degree of multiple right fingers (nail), not including thumb

7 ⊟ + T23.232- Burn of second degree of multiple left fingers (nail), not including thumb

7 ⊟ + T23.239- Burn of second degree of unspecified multiple fingers (nail), not including thumb

6 + T23.24 Burn of second degree of multiple fingers (nail), including thumb

7 ⊟ + T23.241- Burn of second degree of multiple right fingers (nail), including thumb

7 ⊟ + T23.242- Burn of second degree of multiple left fingers (nail), including thumb

7 ⊟ + T23.249- Burn of second degree of unspecified multiple fingers (nail), including thumb

6 + T23.25 Burn of second degree of palm

7 ⊟ + T23.251- Burn of second degree of right palm

7 ⊟ + T23.252- Burn of second degree of left palm

7 ⊟ + T23.259- Burn of second degree of unspecified palm

6 + T23.26 Burn of second degree of back of hand

7 ⊟ + T23.261- Burn of second degree of back of right hand

7 ⊟ + T23.262- Burn of second degree of back of left hand

7 ⊟ + T23.269- Burn of second degree of back of unspecified hand

6 + T23.27 Burn of second degree of wrist

7 ⊟ + T23.271- Burn of second degree of right wrist

7 ⊟ + T23.272- Burn of second degree of left wrist

● New ▲ Revised *Manifestation* 4-7 Digit Indicators ⊟ Laterality A Adult (15+ years) M Maternity (12-55 years) N Newborn P Pediatric (0-17 years) ♂ Male ♀ Female
✖ Deleted Unspecified + Additional code

2017 ICD-10-CM Expert for Physicians

© 2017 DecisionHealth 1047

7 ⊟ **+** T23.279-   Burn of second degree of unspecified wrist

6 **+** T23.29   Burn of second degree of multiple sites of wrist and hand

7 ⊟ **+** T23.291-   Burn of second degree of multiple sites of right wrist and hand

7 ⊟ **+** T23.292-   Burn of second degree of multiple sites of left wrist and hand

7 ⊟ **+** T23.299-   Burn of second degree of multiple sites of unspecified wrist and hand

5 **+** T23.3   Burn of third degree of wrist and hand
Use additional external cause code to identify the source, place and intent of the burn (X00-X19, X75-X77, X96-X98, Y92)

6 **+** T23.30   Burn of third degree of hand, unspecified site

7 ⊟ **+** T23.301-   Burn of third degree of right hand, unspecified site
AHA: (T23.301S) 1Q 2015, 19

7 ⊟ **+** T23.302-   Burn of third degree of left hand, unspecified site
AHA: (T23.302S) 2Q 2016, 5

7 ⊟ **+** T23.309-   Burn of third degree of unspecified hand, unspecified site

6 **+** T23.31   Burn of third degree of thumb (nail)

7 ⊟ **+** T23.311-   Burn of third degree of right thumb (nail)

7 ⊟ **+** T23.312-   Burn of third degree of left thumb (nail)

7 ⊟ **+** T23.319-   Burn of third degree of unspecified thumb (nail)

6 **+** T23.32   Burn of third degree of single finger (nail) except thumb

7 ⊟ **+** T23.321-   Burn of third degree of single right finger (nail) except thumb

7 ⊟ **+** T23.322-   Burn of third degree of single left finger (nail) except thumb

7 ⊟ **+** T23.329-   Burn of third degree of unspecified single finger (nail) except thumb

6 **+** T23.33   Burn of third degree of multiple fingers (nail), not including thumb

7 ⊟ **+** T23.331-   Burn of third degree of multiple right fingers (nail), not including thumb

7 ⊟ **+** T23.332-   Burn of third degree of multiple left fingers (nail), not including thumb

7 ⊟ **+** T23.339-   Burn of third degree of unspecified multiple fingers (nail), not including thumb

6 **+** T23.34   Burn of third degree of multiple fingers (nail), including thumb

7 ⊟ **+** T23.341-   Burn of third degree of multiple right fingers (nail), including thumb

7 ⊟ **+** T23.342-   Burn of third degree of multiple left fingers (nail), including thumb

7 ⊟ **+** T23.349-   Burn of third degree of unspecified multiple fingers (nail), including thumb

6 **+** T23.35   Burn of third degree of palm

7 ⊟ **+** T23.351-   Burn of third degree of right palm

7 ⊟ **+** T23.352-   Burn of third degree of left palm

7 ⊟ **+** T23.359-   Burn of third degree of unspecified palm

6 **+** T23.36   Burn of third degree of back of hand

7 ⊟ **+** T23.361-   Burn of third degree of back of right hand

7 ⊟ **+** T23.362-   Burn of third degree of back of left hand

7 ⊟ **+** T23.369-   Burn of third degree of back of unspecified hand

6 **+** T23.37   Burn of third degree of wrist

7 ⊟ **+** T23.371-   Burn of third degree of right wrist

7 ⊟ **+** T23.372-   Burn of third degree of left wrist

7 ⊟ **+** T23.379-   Burn of third degree of unspecified wrist

6 **+** T23.39   Burn of third degree of multiple sites of wrist and hand

7 ⊟ **+** T23.391-   Burn of third degree of multiple sites of right wrist and hand

7 ⊟ **+** T23.392-   Burn of third degree of multiple sites of left wrist and hand

7 ⊟ **+** T23.399-   Burn of third degree of multiple sites of unspecified wrist and hand

5 **+** T23.4   Corrosion of unspecified degree of wrist and hand
Code first:
(T51-T65) to identify chemical and intent
Use additional external cause code to identify place (Y92)

6 **+** T23.40   Corrosion of unspecified degree of hand, unspecified site

7 ⊟ **+** T23.401-   Corrosion of unspecified degree of right hand, unspecified site

7 ⊟ **+** T23.402-   Corrosion of unspecified degree of left hand, unspecified site

7 ⊟ **+** T23.409-   Corrosion of unspecified degree of unspecified hand, unspecified site

6 **+** T23.41   Corrosion of unspecified degree of thumb (nail)

7 ⊟ **+** T23.411-   Corrosion of unspecified degree of right thumb (nail)

7 ⊟ **+** T23.412-   Corrosion of unspecified degree of left thumb (nail)

7 ⊟ **+** T23.419-   Corrosion of unspecified degree of unspecified thumb (nail)

6 **+** T23.42   Corrosion of unspecified degree of single finger (nail) except thumb

7 ⊟ **+** T23.421-   Corrosion of unspecified degree of single right finger (nail) except thumb

7 ⊟ **+** T23.422-   Corrosion of unspecified degree of single left finger (nail) except thumb

7 ⊟ **+** T23.429-   Corrosion of unspecified degree of unspecified single finger (nail) except thumb

6 **+** T23.43   Corrosion of unspecified degree of multiple fingers (nail), not including thumb

7 ⊟ **+** T23.431-   Corrosion of unspecified degree of multiple right fingers (nail), not including thumb

7 ⊟ **+** T23.432-   Corrosion of unspecified degree of multiple left fingers (nail), not including thumb

7 ⊟ **+** T23.439-   Corrosion of unspecified degree of unspecified multiple fingers (nail), not including thumb

6 **+** T23.44   Corrosion of unspecified degree of multiple fingers (nail), including thumb

7 ⊟ **+** T23.441-   Corrosion of unspecified degree of multiple right fingers (nail), including thumb

7 ⊟ **+** T23.442-   Corrosion of unspecified degree of multiple left fingers (nail), including thumb

7 ⊟ **+** T23.449-   Corrosion of unspecified degree of unspecified multiple fingers (nail), including thumb

6 **+** T23.45   Corrosion of unspecified degree of palm

7 ⊟ **+** T23.451-   Corrosion of unspecified degree of right palm

7 ⊟ **+** T23.452-   Corrosion of unspecified degree of left palm

7 ⊟ **+** T23.459-   Corrosion of unspecified degree of unspecified palm

6 **+** T23.46   Corrosion of unspecified degree of back of hand

7 ⊟ **+** T23.461-   Corrosion of unspecified degree of back of right hand

7 ⊟ **+** T23.462-   Corrosion of unspecified degree of back of left hand

7 ⊟ **+** T23.469-   Corrosion of unspecified degree of back of unspecified hand

6 **+** T23.47   Corrosion of unspecified degree of wrist

7 ⊟ **+** T23.471-   Corrosion of unspecified degree of right wrist

7 ⊟ **+** T23.472-   Corrosion of unspecified degree of left wrist

7 ⊟ **+** T23.479-   Corrosion of unspecified degree of unspecified wrist

6 **+** T23.49   Corrosion of unspecified degree of multiple sites of wrist and hand

7 ⊟ **+** T23.491-   Corrosion of unspecified degree of multiple sites of right wrist and hand

7 ⊟ **+** T23.492-   Corrosion of unspecified degree of multiple sites of left wrist and hand

7 ⊟ **+** T23.499-   Corrosion of unspecified degree of multiple sites of unspecified wrist and hand

5 **+** T23.5   Corrosion of first degree of wrist and hand
Code first:
(T51-T65) to identify chemical and intent
Use additional external cause code to identify place (Y92)

6 **+** T23.50   Corrosion of first degree of hand, unspecified site

7 ⊟ **+** T23.501-   Corrosion of first degree of right hand, unspecified site

7 ⊟ **+** T23.502-   Corrosion of first degree of left hand, unspecified site

---

● New   ▲ Revised   *Manifestation*   4 - 7 Digit Indicators   ⊟ Laterality   Ⓐ Adult (15+ years)   Ⓜ Maternity (12-55 years)   Ⓝ Newborn   Ⓟ Pediatric (0-17 years)   ♂ Male   ♀ Female

✖ Deleted   Unspecified   **+** Additional code

1048   © 2017 DecisionHealth   2017 ICD-10-CM Expert for Physicians

7 ⊟ + T23.509- Corrosion of first degree of unspecified hand, unspecified site

6 + T23.51 Corrosion of first degree of thumb (nail)
7 ⊟ + T23.511- Corrosion of first degree of right thumb (nail)
7 ⊟ + T23.512- Corrosion of first degree of left thumb (nail)
7 ⊟ + T23.519- Corrosion of first degree of unspecified thumb (nail)

6 + T23.52 Corrosion of first degree of single finger (nail) except thumb
7 ⊟ + T23.521- Corrosion of first degree of single right finger (nail) except thumb
7 ⊟ + T23.522- Corrosion of first degree of single left finger (nail) except thumb
7 ⊟ + T23.529- Corrosion of first degree of unspecified single finger (nail) except thumb

6 + T23.53 Corrosion of first degree of multiple fingers (nail), not including thumb
7 ⊟ + T23.531- Corrosion of first degree of multiple right fingers (nail), not including thumb
7 ⊟ + T23.532- Corrosion of first degree of multiple left fingers (nail), not including thumb
7 ⊟ + T23.539- Corrosion of first degree of unspecified multiple fingers (nail), not including thumb

6 + T23.54 Corrosion of first degree of multiple fingers (nail), including thumb
7 ⊟ + T23.541- Corrosion of first degree of multiple right fingers (nail), including thumb
7 ⊟ + T23.542- Corrosion of first degree of multiple left fingers (nail), including thumb
7 ⊟ + T23.549- Corrosion of first degree of unspecified multiple fingers (nail), including thumb

6 + T23.55 Corrosion of first degree of palm
7 ⊟ + T23.551- Corrosion of first degree of right palm
7 ⊟ + T23.552- Corrosion of first degree of left palm
7 ⊟ + T23.559- Corrosion of first degree of unspecified palm

6 + T23.56 Corrosion of first degree of back of hand
7 ⊟ + T23.561- Corrosion of first degree of back of right hand
7 ⊟ + T23.562- Corrosion of first degree of back of left hand
7 ⊟ + T23.569- Corrosion of first degree of back of unspecified hand

6 + T23.57 Corrosion of first degree of wrist
7 ⊟ + T23.571- Corrosion of first degree of right wrist
7 ⊟ + T23.572- Corrosion of first degree of left wrist
7 ⊟ + T23.579- Corrosion of first degree of unspecified wrist

6 + T23.59 Corrosion of first degree of multiple sites of wrist and hand
7 ⊟ + T23.591- Corrosion of first degree of multiple sites of right wrist and hand
7 ⊟ + T23.592- Corrosion of first degree of multiple sites of left wrist and hand
7 ⊟ + T23.599- Corrosion of first degree of multiple sites of unspecified wrist and hand

5 + T23.6 Corrosion of second degree of wrist and hand
Code first:
(T51-T65) to identify chemical and intent
Use additional external cause code to identify place (Y92)

6 + T23.60 Corrosion of second degree of hand, unspecified site
7 ⊟ + T23.601- Corrosion of second degree of right hand, unspecified site
7 ⊟ + T23.602- Corrosion of second degree of left hand, unspecified site
7 ⊟ + T23.609- Corrosion of second degree of unspecified hand, unspecified site

6 + T23.61 Corrosion of second degree of thumb (nail)
7 ⊟ + T23.611- Corrosion of second degree of right thumb (nail)
7 ⊟ + T23.612- Corrosion of second degree of left thumb (nail)
7 ⊟ + T23.619- Corrosion of second degree of unspecified thumb (nail)

6 + T23.62 Corrosion of second degree of single finger (nail) except thumb
7 ⊟ + T23.621- Corrosion of second degree of single right finger (nail) except thumb
7 ⊟ + T23.622- Corrosion of second degree of single left finger (nail) except thumb
7 ⊟ + T23.629- Corrosion of second degree of unspecified single finger (nail) except thumb

6 + T23.63 Corrosion of second degree of multiple fingers (nail), not including thumb
7 ⊟ + T23.631- Corrosion of second degree of multiple right fingers (nail), not including thumb
7 ⊟ + T23.632- Corrosion of second degree of multiple left fingers (nail), not including thumb
7 ⊟ + T23.639- Corrosion of second degree of unspecified multiple fingers (nail), not including thumb

6 + T23.64 Corrosion of second degree of multiple fingers (nail), including thumb
7 ⊟ + T23.641- Corrosion of second degree of multiple right fingers (nail), including thumb
7 ⊟ + T23.642- Corrosion of second degree of multiple left fingers (nail), including thumb
7 ⊟ + T23.649- Corrosion of second degree of unspecified multiple fingers (nail), including thumb

6 + T23.65 Corrosion of second degree of palm
7 ⊟ + T23.651- Corrosion of second degree of right palm
7 ⊟ + T23.652- Corrosion of second degree of left palm
7 ⊟ + T23.659- Corrosion of second degree of unspecified palm

6 + T23.66 Corrosion of second degree of back of hand
7 ⊟ + T23.661- Corrosion of second degree back of right hand
7 ⊟ + T23.662- Corrosion of second degree back of left hand
7 ⊟ + T23.669- Corrosion of second degree back of unspecified hand

6 + T23.67 Corrosion of second degree of wrist
7 ⊟ + T23.671- Corrosion of second degree of right wrist
7 ⊟ + T23.672- Corrosion of second degree of left wrist
7 ⊟ + T23.679- Corrosion of second degree of unspecified wrist

6 + T23.69 Corrosion of second degree of multiple sites of wrist and hand
7 ⊟ + T23.691- Corrosion of second degree of multiple sites of right wrist and hand
7 ⊟ + T23.692- Corrosion of second degree of multiple sites of left wrist and hand
7 ⊟ + T23.699- Corrosion of second degree of multiple sites of unspecified wrist and hand

5 + T23.7 Corrosion of third degree of wrist and hand
Code first:
(T51-T65) to identify chemical and intent
Use additional external cause code to identify place (Y92)

6 + T23.70 Corrosion of third degree of hand, unspecified site
7 ⊟ + T23.701- Corrosion of third degree of right hand, unspecified site
7 ⊟ + T23.702- Corrosion of third degree of left hand, unspecified site
7 ⊟ + T23.709- Corrosion of third degree of unspecified hand, unspecified site

6 + T23.71 Corrosion of third degree of thumb (nail)
7 ⊟ + T23.711- Corrosion of third degree of right thumb (nail)
7 ⊟ + T23.712- Corrosion of third degree of left thumb (nail)
7 ⊟ + T23.719- Corrosion of third degree of unspecified thumb (nail)

6 + T23.72 Corrosion of third degree of single finger (nail) except thumb
7 ⊟ + T23.721- Corrosion of third degree of single right finger (nail) except thumb
7 ⊟ + T23.722- Corrosion of third degree of single left finger (nail) except thumb
7 ⊟ + T23.729- Corrosion of third degree of unspecified single finger (nail) except thumb

6 + T23.73 Corrosion of third degree of multiple fingers (nail), not including thumb
7 ⊟ + T23.731- Corrosion of third degree of multiple right fingers (nail), not including thumb
7 ⊟ + T23.732- Corrosion of third degree of multiple left fingers (nail), not including thumb
7 ⊟ + T23.739- Corrosion of third degree of unspecified multiple fingers (nail), not including thumb

6 + T23.74 Corrosion of third degree of multiple fingers (nail), including thumb
7 ⊟ + T23.741- Corrosion of third degree of multiple right fingers (nail), including thumb
7 ⊟ + T23.742- Corrosion of third degree of multiple left fingers (nail), including thumb

● New ▲ Revised *Manifestation* 4 - 7 Digit Indicators ⊟ Laterality A Adult (15+ years) M Maternity (12-55 years) N Newborn P Pediatric (0-17 years) ♂ Male ♀ Female
✖ Deleted Unspecified + Additional code

2017 ICD-10-CM Expert for Physicians © 2017 DecisionHealth 1049

[6] [≡] **+ T23.749-** Corrosion of third degree of unspecified multiple fingers (nail), including thumb

[6] **+ T23.75** Corrosion of third degree of palm
  [7] [≡] **+ T23.751-** Corrosion of third degree of right palm
  [7] [≡] **+ T23.752-** Corrosion of third degree of left palm
  [7] [≡] **+ T23.759-** Corrosion of third degree of unspecified palm

[6] **+ T23.76** Corrosion of third degree of back of hand
  [7] [≡] **+ T23.761-** Corrosion of third degree of back of right hand
  [7] [≡] **+ T23.762-** Corrosion of third degree of back of left hand
  [7] [≡] **+ T23.769-** Corrosion of third degree back of unspecified hand

[6] **+ T23.77** Corrosion of third degree of wrist
  [7] [≡] **+ T23.771-** Corrosion of third degree of right wrist
  [7] [≡] **+ T23.772-** Corrosion of third degree of left wrist
  [7] [≡] **+ T23.779-** Corrosion of third degree of unspecified wrist

[6] **+ T23.79** Corrosion of third degree of multiple sites of wrist and hand
  [7] [≡] **+ T23.791-** Corrosion of third degree of multiple sites of right wrist and hand
  [7] [≡] **+ T23.792-** Corrosion of third degree of multiple sites of left wrist and hand
  [7] [≡] **+ T23.799-** Corrosion of third degree of multiple sites of unspecified wrist and hand

[4] **T24** **Burn and corrosion of lower limb, except ankle and foot**

> **EXCLUDES 2** *burn and corrosion of ankle and foot (T25.-)*
> *burn and corrosion of hip region (T21.-)*

The appropriate 7th character is to be added to each code from category T24
A   initial encounter
D   subsequent encounter
S   sequela

[5] **+ T24.0** **Burn of unspecified degree of lower limb, except ankle and foot**
Use additional external cause code to identify the source, place and intent of the burn (X00-X19, X75-X77, X96-X98, Y92)

  [6] **+ T24.00** Burn of unspecified degree of unspecified site of lower limb, except ankle and foot
    [7] [≡] **+ T24.001-** Burn of unspecified degree of unspecified site of right lower limb, except ankle and foot
    [7] [≡] **+ T24.002-** Burn of unspecified degree of unspecified site of left lower limb, except ankle and foot
    [7] [≡] **+ T24.009-** Burn of unspecified degree of unspecified site of unspecified lower limb, except ankle and foot

  [6] **+ T24.01** Burn of unspecified degree of thigh
    [7] [≡] **+ T24.011-** Burn of unspecified degree of right thigh
    [7] [≡] **+ T24.012-** Burn of unspecified degree of left thigh
    [7] [≡] **+ T24.019-** Burn of unspecified degree of unspecified thigh

  [6] **+ T24.02** Burn of unspecified degree of knee
    [7] [≡] **+ T24.021-** Burn of unspecified degree of right knee
    [7] [≡] **+ T24.022-** Burn of unspecified degree of left knee
    [7] [≡] **+ T24.029-** Burn of unspecified degree of unspecified knee

  [6] **+ T24.03** Burn of unspecified degree of lower leg
    [7] [≡] **+ T24.031-** Burn of unspecified degree of right lower leg
    [7] [≡] **+ T24.032-** Burn of unspecified degree of left lower leg
    [7] [≡] **+ T24.039-** Burn of unspecified degree of unspecified lower leg

  [6] **+ T24.09** Burn of unspecified degree of multiple sites of lower limb, except ankle and foot
    [7] [≡] **+ T24.091-** Burn of unspecified degree of multiple sites of right lower limb, except ankle and foot
    [7] [≡] **+ T24.092-** Burn of unspecified degree of multiple sites of left lower limb, except ankle and foot
    [7] [≡] **+ T24.099-** Burn of unspecified degree of multiple sites of unspecified lower limb, except ankle and foot

[5] **+ T24.1** **Burn of first degree of lower limb, except ankle and foot**
Use additional external cause code to identify the source, place and intent of the burn (X00-X19, X75-X77, X96-X98, Y92)

  [6] **+ T24.10** Burn of first degree of unspecified site of lower limb, except ankle and foot
    [7] [≡] **+ T24.101-** Burn of first degree of unspecified site of right lower limb, except ankle and foot
    [7] [≡] **+ T24.102-** Burn of first degree of unspecified site of left lower limb, except ankle and foot
    [7] [≡] **+ T24.109-** Burn of first degree of unspecified site of unspecified lower limb, except ankle and foot

  [6] **+ T24.11** Burn of first degree of thigh
    [7] [≡] **+ T24.111-** Burn of first degree of right thigh
    [7] [≡] **+ T24.112-** Burn of first degree of left thigh
    [7] [≡] **+ T24.119-** Burn of first degree of unspecified thigh

  [6] **+ T24.12** Burn of first degree of knee
    [7] [≡] **+ T24.121-** Burn of first degree of right knee
    [7] [≡] **+ T24.122-** Burn of first degree of left knee
    [7] [≡] **+ T24.129-** Burn of first degree of unspecified knee

  [6] **+ T24.13** Burn of first degree of lower leg
    [7] [≡] **+ T24.131-** Burn of first degree of right lower leg
    [7] [≡] **+ T24.132-** Burn of first degree of left lower leg
    [7] [≡] **+ T24.139-** Burn of first degree of unspecified lower leg

  [6] **+ T24.19** Burn of first degree of multiple sites of lower limb, except ankle and foot
    [7] [≡] **+ T24.191-** Burn of first degree of multiple sites of right lower limb, except ankle and foot
    [7] [≡] **+ T24.192-** Burn of first degree of multiple sites of left lower limb, except ankle and foot
    [7] [≡] **+ T24.199-** Burn of first degree of multiple sites of unspecified lower limb, except ankle and foot

[5] **+ T24.2** **Burn of second degree of lower limb, except ankle and foot**
Use additional external cause code to identify the source, place and intent of the burn (X00-X19, X75-X77, X96-X98, Y92)

  [6] **+ T24.20** Burn of second degree of unspecified site of lower limb, except ankle and foot
    [7] [≡] **+ T24.201-** Burn of second degree of unspecified site of right lower limb, except ankle and foot
    [7] [≡] **+ T24.202-** Burn of second degree of unspecified site of left lower limb, except ankle and foot
    [7] [≡] **+ T24.209-** Burn of second degree of unspecified site of unspecified lower limb, except ankle and foot

  [6] **+ T24.21** Burn of second degree of thigh
    [7] [≡] **+ T24.211-** Burn of second degree of right thigh
    [7] [≡] **+ T24.212-** Burn of second degree of left thigh
    [7] [≡] **+ T24.219-** Burn of second degree of unspecified thigh

  [6] **+ T24.22** Burn of second degree of knee
    [7] [≡] **+ T24.221-** Burn of second degree of right knee
    [7] [≡] **+ T24.222-** Burn of second degree of left knee
    [7] [≡] **+ T24.229-** Burn of second degree of unspecified knee

  [6] **+ T24.23** Burn of second degree of lower leg
    [7] [≡] **+ T24.231-** Burn of second degree of right lower leg
    [7] [≡] **+ T24.232-** Burn of second degree of left lower leg
    [7] [≡] **+ T24.239-** Burn of second degree of unspecified lower leg

  [6] **+ T24.29** Burn of second degree of multiple sites of lower limb, except ankle and foot
    [7] [≡] **+ T24.291-** Burn of second degree of multiple sites of right lower limb, except ankle and foot
    [7] [≡] **+ T24.292-** Burn of second degree of multiple sites of left lower limb, except ankle and foot
    [7] [≡] **+ T24.299-** Burn of second degree of multiple sites of unspecified lower limb, except ankle and foot

[5] **+ T24.3** **Burn of third degree of lower limb, except ankle and foot**
Use additional external cause code to identify the source, place and intent of the burn (X00-X19, X75-X77, X96-X98, Y92)

  [6] **+ T24.30** Burn of third degree of unspecified site of lower limb, except ankle and foot
    [7] [≡] **+ T24.301-** Burn of third degree of unspecified site of right lower limb, except ankle and foot
    [7] [≡] **+ T24.302-** Burn of third degree of unspecified site of left lower limb, except ankle and foot

7 ⊟ + T24.309-   Burn of third degree of unspecified site of unspecified lower limb, except ankle and foot

6 + T24.31   Burn of third degree of thigh

7 ⊟ + T24.311-   Burn of third degree of right thigh

7 ⊟ + T24.312-   Burn of third degree of left thigh

7 ⊟ + T24.319-   Burn of third degree of unspecified thigh

6 + T24.32   Burn of third degree of knee

7 ⊟ + T24.321-   Burn of third degree of right knee

7 ⊟ + T24.322-   Burn of third degree of left knee

7 ⊟ + T24.329-   Burn of third degree of unspecified knee

6 + T24.33   Burn of third degree of lower leg

7 ⊟ + T24.331-   Burn of third degree of right lower leg

7 ⊟ + T24.332-   Burn of third degree of left lower leg

7 ⊟ + T24.339-   Burn of third degree of unspecified lower leg

6 + T24.39   Burn of third degree of multiple sites of lower limb, except ankle and foot

7 ⊟ + T24.391-   Burn of third degree of multiple sites of right lower limb, except ankle and foot
     AHA: (T24.391A) 2Q 2016, 4

7 ⊟ + T24.392-   Burn of third degree of multiple sites of left lower limb, except ankle and foot
     AHA: (T24.392A) 2Q 2016, 4

7 ⊟ + T24.399-   Burn of third degree of multiple sites of unspecified lower limb, except ankle and foot

5 + T24.4   Corrosion of unspecified degree of lower limb, except ankle and foot
     Code first:
       (T51-T65) to identify chemical and intent
     Use additional external cause code to identify place (Y92)

6 + T24.40   Corrosion of unspecified degree of unspecified site of lower limb, except ankle and foot

7 ⊟ + T24.401-   Corrosion of unspecified degree of unspecified site of right lower limb, except ankle and foot

7 ⊟ + T24.402-   Corrosion of unspecified degree of unspecified site of left lower limb, except ankle and foot

7 ⊟ + T24.409-   Corrosion of unspecified degree of unspecified site of unspecified lower limb, except ankle and foot

6 + T24.41   Corrosion of unspecified degree of thigh

7 ⊟ + T24.411-   Corrosion of unspecified degree of right thigh

7 ⊟ + T24.412-   Corrosion of unspecified degree of left thigh

7 ⊟ + T24.419-   Corrosion of unspecified degree of unspecified thigh

6 + T24.42   Corrosion of unspecified degree of knee

7 ⊟ + T24.421-   Corrosion of unspecified degree of right knee

7 ⊟ + T24.422-   Corrosion of unspecified degree of left knee

7 ⊟ + T24.429-   Corrosion of unspecified degree of unspecified knee

6 + T24.43   Corrosion of unspecified degree of lower leg

7 ⊟ + T24.431-   Corrosion of unspecified degree of right lower leg

7 ⊟ + T24.432-   Corrosion of unspecified degree of left lower leg

7 ⊟ + T24.439-   Corrosion of unspecified degree of unspecified lower leg

6 + T24.49   Corrosion of unspecified degree of multiple sites of lower limb, except ankle and foot

7 ⊟ + T24.491-   Corrosion of unspecified degree of multiple sites of right lower limb, except ankle and foot

7 ⊟ + T24.492-   Corrosion of unspecified degree of multiple sites of left lower limb, except ankle and foot

7 ⊟ + T24.499-   Corrosion of unspecified degree of multiple sites of unspecified lower limb, except ankle and foot

5 + T24.5   Corrosion of first degree of lower limb, except ankle and foot
     Code first:
       (T51-T65) to identify chemical and intent
     Use additional external cause code to identify place (Y92)

6 + T24.50   Corrosion of first degree of unspecified site of lower limb, except ankle and foot

7 ⊟ + T24.501-   Corrosion of first degree of unspecified site of right lower limb, except ankle and foot

7 ⊟ + T24.502-   Corrosion of first degree of unspecified site of left lower limb, except ankle and foot

7 ⊟ + T24.509-   Corrosion of first degree of unspecified site of unspecified lower limb, except ankle and foot

6 + T24.51   Corrosion of first degree of thigh

7 ⊟ + T24.511-   Corrosion of first degree of right thigh

7 ⊟ + T24.512-   Corrosion of first degree of left thigh

7 ⊟ + T24.519-   Corrosion of first degree of unspecified thigh

6 + T24.52   Corrosion of first degree of knee

7 ⊟ + T24.521-   Corrosion of first degree of right knee

7 ⊟ + T24.522-   Corrosion of first degree of left knee

7 ⊟ + T24.529-   Corrosion of first degree of unspecified knee

6 + T24.53   Corrosion of first degree of lower leg

7 ⊟ + T24.531-   Corrosion of first degree of right lower leg

7 ⊟ + T24.532-   Corrosion of first degree of left lower leg

7 ⊟ + T24.539-   Corrosion of first degree of unspecified lower leg

6 + T24.59   Corrosion of first degree of multiple sites of lower limb, except ankle and foot

7 ⊟ + T24.591-   Corrosion of first degree of multiple sites of right lower limb, except ankle and foot

7 ⊟ + T24.592-   Corrosion of first degree of multiple sites of left lower limb, except ankle and foot

7 ⊟ + T24.599-   Corrosion of first degree of multiple sites of unspecified lower limb, except ankle and foot

5 + T24.6   Corrosion of second degree of lower limb, except ankle and foot
     Code first:
       (T51-T65) to identify chemical and intent
     Use additional external cause code to identify place (Y92)

6 + T24.60   Corrosion of second degree of unspecified site of lower limb, except ankle and foot

7 ⊟ + T24.601-   Corrosion of second degree of unspecified site of right lower limb, except ankle and foot

7 ⊟ + T24.602-   Corrosion of second degree of unspecified site of left lower limb, except ankle and foot

7 ⊟ + T24.609-   Corrosion of second degree of unspecified site of unspecified lower limb, except ankle and foot

6 + T24.61   Corrosion of second degree of thigh

7 ⊟ + T24.611-   Corrosion of second degree of right thigh

7 ⊟ + T24.612-   Corrosion of second degree of left thigh

7 ⊟ + T24.619-   Corrosion of second degree of unspecified thigh

6 + T24.62   Corrosion of second degree of knee

7 ⊟ + T24.621-   Corrosion of second degree of right knee

7 ⊟ + T24.622-   Corrosion of second degree of left knee

7 ⊟ + T24.629-   Corrosion of second degree of unspecified knee

6 + T24.63   Corrosion of second degree of lower leg

7 ⊟ + T24.631-   Corrosion of second degree of right lower leg

7 ⊟ + T24.632-   Corrosion of second degree of left lower leg

7 ⊟ + T24.639-   Corrosion of second degree of unspecified lower leg

6 + T24.69   Corrosion of second degree of multiple sites of lower limb, except ankle and foot

7 ⊟ + T24.691-   Corrosion of second degree of multiple sites of right lower limb, except ankle and foot

7 ⊟ + T24.692-   Corrosion of second degree of multiple sites of left lower limb, except ankle and foot

7 ⊟ + T24.699-   Corrosion of second degree of multiple sites of unspecified lower limb, except ankle and foot

5 + T24.7   Corrosion of third degree of lower limb, except ankle and foot
     Code first:
       (T51-T65) to identify chemical and intent
     Use additional external cause code to identify place (Y92)

6 + T24.70   Corrosion of third degree of unspecified site of lower limb, except ankle and foot

7 ⊟ + T24.701-   Corrosion of third degree of unspecified site of right lower limb, except ankle and foot

● New   ▲ Revised   *Manifestation*   4-7 Digit Indicators   ⊟ Laterality   A Adult (15+ years)   M Maternity (12-55 years)   N Newborn   P Pediatric (0-17 years)   ♂ Male   ♀ Female
✖ Deleted   Unspecified   + Additional code

2017 ICD-10-CM Expert for Physicians   © 2017 DecisionHealth   1051

7 ⊟ + T24.702- Corrosion of third degree of unspecified site of left lower limb, except ankle and foot

7 ⊟ + T24.709- Corrosion of third degree of unspecified site of unspecified lower limb, except ankle and foot

6 + T24.71 Corrosion of third degree of thigh

7 ⊟ + T24.711- Corrosion of third degree of right thigh

7 ⊟ + T24.712- Corrosion of third degree of left thigh

7 ⊟ + T24.719- Corrosion of third degree of unspecified thigh

6 + T24.72 Corrosion of third degree of knee

7 ⊟ + T24.721- Corrosion of third degree of right knee

7 ⊟ + T24.722- Corrosion of third degree of left knee

7 ⊟ + T24.729- Corrosion of third degree of unspecified knee

6 + T24.73 Corrosion of third degree of lower leg

7 ⊟ + T24.731- Corrosion of third degree of right lower leg

7 ⊟ + T24.732- Corrosion of third degree of left lower leg

7 ⊟ + T24.739- Corrosion of third degree of unspecified lower leg

6 + T24.79 Corrosion of third degree of multiple sites of lower limb, except ankle and foot

7 ⊟ + T24.791- Corrosion of third degree of multiple sites of right lower limb, except ankle and foot

7 ⊟ + T24.792- Corrosion of third degree of multiple sites of left lower limb, except ankle and foot

7 ⊟ + T24.799- Corrosion of third degree of multiple sites of unspecified lower limb, except ankle and foot

4 ▢ T25 **Burn and corrosion of ankle and foot**

The appropriate 7th character is to be added to each code from category T25
A   initial encounter
D   subsequent encounter
S   sequela

5 + T25.0 **Burn of unspecified degree of ankle and foot**
Use additional external cause code to identify the source, place and intent of the burn (X00-X19, X75-X77, X96-X98, Y92)

6 + T25.01 Burn of unspecified degree of ankle

7 ⊟ + T25.011- Burn of unspecified degree of right ankle

7 ⊟ + T25.012- Burn of unspecified degree of left ankle

7 ⊟ + T25.019- Burn of unspecified degree of unspecified ankle

6 + T25.02 Burn of unspecified degree of foot
EXCLUDES 2 *burn of unspecified degree of toe (s) (nail) (T25.03-)*

7 ⊟ + T25.021- Burn of unspecified degree of right foot

7 ⊟ + T25.022- Burn of unspecified degree of left foot

7 ⊟ + T25.029- Burn of unspecified degree of unspecified foot

6 + T25.03 Burn of unspecified degree of toe(s) (nail)

7 ⊟ + T25.031- Burn of unspecified degree of right toe(s) (nail)

7 ⊟ + T25.032- Burn of unspecified degree of left toe(s) (nail)

7 ⊟ + T25.039- Burn of unspecified degree of unspecified toe(s) (nail)

6 + T25.09 Burn of unspecified degree of multiple sites of ankle and foot

7 ⊟ + T25.091- Burn of unspecified degree of multiple sites of right ankle and foot

7 ⊟ + T25.092- Burn of unspecified degree of multiple sites of left ankle and foot

7 ⊟ + T25.099- Burn of unspecified degree of multiple sites of unspecified ankle and foot

5 + T25.1 **Burn of first degree of ankle and foot**
Use additional external cause code to identify the source, place and intent of the burn (X00-X19, X75-X77, X96-X98, Y92)

6 + T25.11 Burn of first degree of ankle

7 ⊟ + T25.111- Burn of first degree of right ankle

7 ⊟ + T25.112- Burn of first degree of left ankle

7 ⊟ + T25.119- Burn of first degree of unspecified ankle

6 + T25.12 Burn of first degree of foot
EXCLUDES 2 *burn of first degree of toe (s) (nail) (T25.13-)*

7 ⊟ + T25.121- Burn of first degree of right foot

7 ⊟ + T25.122- Burn of first degree of left foot

7 ⊟ + T25.129- Burn of first degree of unspecified foot

6 + T25.13 Burn of first degree of toe(s) (nail)

7 ⊟ + T25.131- Burn of first degree of right toe(s) (nail)

7 ⊟ + T25.132- Burn of first degree of left toe(s) (nail)

7 ⊟ + T25.139- Burn of first degree of unspecified toe(s) (nail)

6 + T25.19 Burn of first degree of multiple sites of ankle and foot

7 ⊟ + T25.191- Burn of first degree of multiple sites of right ankle and foot

7 ⊟ + T25.192- Burn of first degree of multiple sites of left ankle and foot

7 ⊟ + T25.199- Burn of first degree of multiple sites of unspecified ankle and foot

5 + T25.2 **Burn of second degree of ankle and foot**
Use additional external cause code to identify the source, place and intent of the burn (X00-X19, X75-X77, X96-X98, Y92)

6 + T25.21 Burn of second degree of ankle

7 ⊟ + T25.211- Burn of second degree of right ankle

7 ⊟ + T25.212- Burn of second degree of left ankle

7 ⊟ + T25.219- Burn of second degree of unspecified ankle

6 + T25.22 Burn of second degree of foot
EXCLUDES 2 *burn of second degree of toe (s) (nail) (T25.23-)*

7 ⊟ + T25.221- Burn of second degree of right foot

7 ⊟ + T25.222- Burn of second degree of left foot

7 ⊟ + T25.229- Burn of second degree of unspecified foot

6 + T25.23 Burn of second degree of toe(s) (nail)

7 ⊟ + T25.231- Burn of second degree of right toe(s) (nail)

7 ⊟ + T25.232- Burn of second degree of left toe(s) (nail)

7 ⊟ + T25.239- Burn of second degree of unspecified toe(s) (nail)

6 + T25.29 Burn of second degree of multiple sites of ankle and foot

7 ⊟ + T25.291- Burn of second degree of multiple sites of right ankle and foot

7 ⊟ + T25.292- Burn of second degree of multiple sites of left ankle and foot

7 ⊟ + T25.299- Burn of second degree of multiple sites of unspecified ankle and foot

5 + T25.3 **Burn of third degree of ankle and foot**
Use additional external cause code to identify the source, place and intent of the burn (X00-X19, X75-X77, X96-X98, Y92)

6 + T25.31 Burn of third degree of ankle

7 ⊟ + T25.311- Burn of third degree of right ankle

7 ⊟ + T25.312- Burn of third degree of left ankle

7 ⊟ + T25.319- Burn of third degree of unspecified ankle

6 + T25.32 Burn of third degree of foot
EXCLUDES 2 *burn of third degree of toe (s) (nail) (T25.33-)*

7 ⊟ + T25.321- Burn of third degree of right foot

7 ⊟ + T25.322- Burn of third degree of left foot

7 ⊟ + T25.329- Burn of third degree of unspecified foot

6 + T25.33 Burn of third degree of toe(s) (nail)

7 ⊟ + T25.331- Burn of third degree of right toe(s) (nail)

7 ⊟ + T25.332- Burn of third degree of left toe(s) (nail)

7 ⊟ + T25.339- Burn of third degree of unspecified toe(s) (nail)

6 + T25.39 Burn of third degree of multiple sites of ankle and foot

7 ⊟ + T25.391- Burn of third degree of multiple sites of right ankle and foot

7 ⊟ + T25.392- Burn of third degree of multiple sites of left ankle and foot

7 ⊟ + T25.399- Burn of third degree of multiple sites of unspecified ankle and foot

5 + T25.4 **Corrosion of unspecified degree of ankle and foot**
Code first:
(T51-T65) to identify chemical and intent
Use additional external cause code to identify place (Y92)

6 + T25.41 Corrosion of unspecified degree of ankle

7 ⊟ + T25.411- Corrosion of unspecified degree of right ankle

7 ⊟ + T25.412- Corrosion of unspecified degree of left ankle

● New   ▲ Revised   *Manifestation*   ◩-**7** Digit Indicators   ⊟ Laterality   Ⓐ Adult (15+ years)   Ⓜ Maternity (12-55 years)   Ⓝ Newborn   Ⓟ Pediatric (0-17 years)   ♂ Male   ♀ Female
✖ Deleted   Unspecified   + Additional code

1052   © 2017 DecisionHealth   2017 ICD-10-CM Expert for Physicians

7 ⊟ + **T25.419-** Corrosion of unspecified degree of unspecified ankle

6 + **T25.42** Corrosion of unspecified degree of foot

> **EXCLUDES 2** *corrosion of unspecified degree of toe(s) (nail) (T25.43-)*

7 ⊟ + **T25.421-** Corrosion of unspecified degree of right foot

7 ⊟ + **T25.422-** Corrosion of unspecified degree of left foot

7 ⊟ + **T25.429-** Corrosion of unspecified degree of unspecified foot

6 + **T25.43** Corrosion of unspecified degree of toe(s) (nail)

7 ⊟ + **T25.431-** Corrosion of unspecified degree of right toe(s) (nail)

7 ⊟ + **T25.432-** Corrosion of unspecified degree of left toe(s) (nail)

7 ⊟ + **T25.439-** Corrosion of unspecified degree of unspecified toe(s) (nail)

6 + **T25.49** Corrosion of unspecified degree of multiple sites of ankle and foot

7 ⊟ + **T25.491-** Corrosion of unspecified degree of multiple sites of right ankle and foot

7 ⊟ + **T25.492-** Corrosion of unspecified degree of multiple sites of left ankle and foot

7 ⊟ + **T25.499-** Corrosion of unspecified degree of multiple sites of unspecified ankle and foot

5 + **T25.5** Corrosion of first degree of ankle and foot

> Code first:
>   (T51-T65) to identify chemical and intent
> *Use additional external cause code to identify place (Y92)*

6 + **T25.51** Corrosion of first degree of ankle

7 ⊟ + **T25.511-** Corrosion of first degree of right ankle

7 ⊟ + **T25.512-** Corrosion of first degree of left ankle

7 ⊟ + **T25.519-** Corrosion of first degree of unspecified ankle

6 + **T25.52** Corrosion of first degree of foot

> **EXCLUDES 2** *corrosion of first degree of toe(s) (nail) (T25.53-)*

7 ⊟ + **T25.521-** Corrosion of first degree of right foot

7 ⊟ + **T25.522-** Corrosion of first degree of left foot

7 ⊟ + **T25.529-** Corrosion of first degree of unspecified foot

6 + **T25.53** Corrosion of first degree of toe(s) (nail)

7 ⊟ + **T25.531-** Corrosion of first degree of right toe(s) (nail)

7 ⊟ + **T25.532-** Corrosion of first degree of left toe(s) (nail)

7 ⊟ + **T25.539-** Corrosion of first degree of unspecified toe(s) (nail)

6 + **T25.59** Corrosion of first degree of multiple sites of ankle and foot

7 ⊟ + **T25.591-** Corrosion of first degree of multiple sites of right ankle and foot

7 ⊟ + **T25.592-** Corrosion of first degree of multiple sites of left ankle and foot

7 ⊟ + **T25.599-** Corrosion of first degree of multiple sites of unspecified ankle and foot

5 + **T25.6** Corrosion of second degree of ankle and foot

> Code first:
>   (T51-T65) to identify chemical and intent
> *Use additional external cause code to identify place (Y92)*

6 + **T25.61** Corrosion of second degree of ankle

7 ⊟ + **T25.611-** Corrosion of second degree of right ankle

7 ⊟ + **T25.612-** Corrosion of second degree of left ankle

7 ⊟ + **T25.619-** Corrosion of second degree of unspecified ankle

6 + **T25.62** Corrosion of second degree of foot

> **EXCLUDES 2** *corrosion of second degree of toe(s) (nail) (T25.63-)*

7 ⊟ + **T25.621-** Corrosion of second degree of right foot

7 ⊟ + **T25.622-** Corrosion of second degree of left foot

7 ⊟ + **T25.629-** Corrosion of second degree of unspecified foot

6 + **T25.63** Corrosion of second degree of toe(s) (nail)

7 ⊟ + **T25.631-** Corrosion of second degree of right toe(s) (nail)

7 ⊟ + **T25.632-** Corrosion of second degree of left toe(s) (nail)

7 ⊟ + **T25.639-** Corrosion of second degree of unspecified toe(s) (nail)

6 + **T25.69** Corrosion of second degree of multiple sites of ankle and foot

7 ⊟ + **T25.691-** Corrosion of second degree of right ankle and foot

7 ⊟ + **T25.692-** Corrosion of second degree of left ankle and foot

7 ⊟ + **T25.699-** Corrosion of second degree of unspecified ankle and foot

5 + **T25.7** Corrosion of third degree of ankle and foot

> Code first:
>   (T51-T65) to identify chemical and intent
> *Use additional external cause code to identify place (Y92)*

6 + **T25.71** Corrosion of third degree of ankle

7 ⊟ + **T25.711-** Corrosion of third degree of right ankle

7 ⊟ + **T25.712-** Corrosion of third degree of left ankle

7 ⊟ + **T25.719-** Corrosion of third degree of unspecified ankle

6 + **T25.72** Corrosion of third degree of foot

> **EXCLUDES 2** *corrosion of third degree of toe(s) (nail) (T25.73-)*

7 ⊟ + **T25.721-** Corrosion of third degree of right foot

7 ⊟ + **T25.722-** Corrosion of third degree of left foot

7 ⊟ + **T25.729-** Corrosion of third degree of unspecified foot

6 + **T25.73** Corrosion of third degree of toe(s) (nail)

7 ⊟ + **T25.731-** Corrosion of third degree of right toe(s) (nail)

7 ⊟ + **T25.732-** Corrosion of third degree of left toe(s) (nail)

7 ⊟ + **T25.739-** Corrosion of third degree of unspecified toe(s) (nail)

6 + **T25.79** Corrosion of third degree of multiple sites of ankle and foot

7 ⊟ + **T25.791-** Corrosion of third degree of multiple sites of right ankle and foot

7 ⊟ + **T25.792-** Corrosion of third degree of multiple sites of left ankle and foot

7 ⊟ + **T25.799-** Corrosion of third degree of multiple sites of unspecified ankle and foot

Burns and corrosions confined to eye and internal organs (T26-T28)

4 **T26** **Burn and corrosion confined to eye and adnexa**

> The appropriate 7th character is to be added to each code from category T26
> A   initial encounter
> D   subsequent encounter
> S   sequela

5 + **T26.0** **Burn of eyelid and periocular area**

> *Use additional external cause code to identify the source, place and intent of the burn (X00-X19, X75-X77, X96-X98, Y92)*

7 ⊟ + **T26.00X-** Burn of unspecified eyelid and periocular area

7 ⊟ + **T26.01X-** Burn of right eyelid and periocular area

7 ⊟ + **T26.02X-** Burn of left eyelid and periocular area

5 + **T26.1** **Burn of cornea and conjunctival sac**

> *Use additional external cause code to identify the source, place and intent of the burn (X00-X19, X75-X77, X96-X98, Y92)*

7 ⊟ + **T26.10X-** Burn of cornea and conjunctival sac, unspecified eye

7 ⊟ + **T26.11X-** Burn of cornea and conjunctival sac, right eye

7 ⊟ + **T26.12X-** Burn of cornea and conjunctival sac, left eye

5 + **T26.2** **Burn with resulting rupture and destruction of eyeball**

> *Use additional external cause code to identify the source, place and intent of the burn (X00-X19, X75-X77, X96-X98, Y92)*

7 ⊟ + **T26.20X-** Burn with resulting rupture and destruction of unspecified eyeball

7 ⊟ + **T26.21X-** Burn with resulting rupture and destruction of right eyeball

7 ⊟ + **T26.22X-** Burn with resulting rupture and destruction of left eyeball

5 + **T26.3** **Burns of other specified parts of eye and adnexa**

> *Use additional external cause code to identify the source, place and intent of the burn (X00-X19, X75-X77, X96-X98, Y92)*

7 ⊟ + **T26.30X-** Burns of other specified parts of unspecified eye and adnexa

7 ⊟ + **T26.31X-** Burns of other specified parts of right eye and adnexa

7 ⊟ + **T26.32X-** Burns of other specified parts of left eye and adnexa

---

● New ▲ Revised *Manifestation* 4-7 Digit Indicators ⊟ Laterality 🅰 Adult (15+ years) 🅼 Maternity (12-55 years) 🅽 Newborn 🅿 Pediatric (0-17 years) ♂ Male ♀ Female

✖ Deleted Unspecified + Additional code

2017 ICD-10-CM Expert for Physicians   © 2017 DecisionHealth   1053

⑤+ **T26.4**   **Burn of eye and adnexa, part unspecified**
Use additional external cause code to identify the source, place and intent of the burn (X00-X19, X75-X77, X96-X98, Y92)

⑦◨+ **T26.40X-**   **Burn of unspecified eye and adnexa, part unspecified**

⑦◨+ **T26.41X-**   **Burn of right eye and adnexa, part unspecified**

⑦◨+ **T26.42X-**   **Burn of left eye and adnexa, part unspecified**

⑤+ **T26.5**   **Corrosion of eyelid and periocular area**
Code first:
    (T51-T65) to identify chemical and intent
Use additional external cause code to identify place (Y92)

⑦◨+ **T26.50X-**   **Corrosion of unspecified eyelid and periocular area**

⑦◨+ **T26.51X-**   **Corrosion of right eyelid and periocular area**

⑦◨+ **T26.52X-**   **Corrosion of left eyelid and periocular area**

⑤+ **T26.6**   **Corrosion of cornea and conjunctival sac**
Code first:
    (T51-T65) to identify chemical and intent
Use additional external cause code to identify place (Y92)

⑦◨+ **T26.60X-**   **Corrosion of cornea and conjunctival sac, unspecified eye**

⑦◨+ **T26.61X-**   **Corrosion of cornea and conjunctival sac, right eye**

⑦◨+ **T26.62X-**   **Corrosion of cornea and conjunctival sac, left eye**

⑤+ **T26.7**   **Corrosion with resulting rupture and destruction of eyeball**
Code first:
    (T51-T65) to identify chemical and intent
Use additional external cause code to identify place (Y92)

⑦◨+ **T26.70X-**   **Corrosion with resulting rupture and destruction of unspecified eyeball**

⑦◨+ **T26.71X-**   **Corrosion with resulting rupture and destruction of right eyeball**

⑦◨+ **T26.72X-**   **Corrosion with resulting rupture and destruction of left eyeball**

⑤+ **T26.8**   **Corrosions of other specified parts of eye and adnexa**
Code first:
    (T51-T65) to identify chemical and intent
Use additional external cause code to identify place (Y92)

⑦◨+ **T26.80X-**   **Corrosions of other specified parts of unspecified eye and adnexa**

⑦◨+ **T26.81X-**   **Corrosions of other specified parts of right eye and adnexa**

⑦◨+ **T26.82X-**   **Corrosions of other specified parts of left eye and adnexa**

⑤+ **T26.9**   **Corrosion of eye and adnexa, part unspecified**
Code first:
    (T51-T65) to identify chemical and intent
Use additional external cause code to identify place (Y92)

⑦◨+ **T26.90X-**   **Corrosion of unspecified eye and adnexa, part unspecified**

⑦◨+ **T26.91X-**   **Corrosion of right eye and adnexa, part unspecified**

⑦◨+ **T26.92X-**   **Corrosion of left eye and adnexa, part unspecified**

④+ **T27**   **Burn and corrosion of respiratory tract**
Use additional external cause code to identify the source and intent of the burn (X00-X19, X75-X77, X96-X98)
Use additional external cause code to identify place (Y92)

The appropriate 7th character is to be added to each code from category T27
A   initial encounter
D   subsequent encounter
S   sequela

⑦+ **T27.0XX-**   **Burn of larynx and trachea**

⑦+ **T27.1XX-**   **Burn involving larynx and trachea with lung**

⑦+ **T27.2XX-**   **Burn of other parts of respiratory tract**
Burn of thoracic cavity

⑦+ **T27.3XX-**   **Burn of respiratory tract, part unspecified**
Code first:
    (T51-T65) to identify chemical and intent for codes T27.4-T27.7

⑦+ **T27.4XX-**   **Corrosion of larynx and trachea**

⑦+ **T27.5XX-**   **Corrosion involving larynx and trachea with lung**

⑦+ **T27.6XX-**   **Corrosion of other parts of respiratory tract**

⑦+ **T27.7XX-**   **Corrosion of respiratory tract, part unspecified**

④+ **T28**   **Burn and corrosion of other internal organs**
Use additional external cause code to identify the source and intent of the burn (X00-X19, X75-X77, X96-X98)
Use additional external cause code to identify place (Y92)

The appropriate 7th character is to be added to each code from category T28
A   initial encounter
D   subsequent encounter
S   sequela

⑦+ **T28.0XX-**   **Burn of mouth and pharynx**

⑦+ **T28.1XX-**   **Burn of esophagus**

⑦+ **T28.2XX-**   **Burn of other parts of alimentary tract**

⑦+ **T28.3XX-**   **Burn of internal genitourinary organs**

⑤+ **T28.4**   **Burns of other and unspecified internal organs**

⑦+ **T28.40X-**   **Burn of unspecified internal organ**

⑥+ **T28.41**   **Burn of ear drum**

⑦◨+ **T28.411-**   **Burn of right ear drum**

⑦◨+ **T28.412-**   **Burn of left ear drum**

⑦◨+ **T28.419-**   **Burn of unspecified ear drum**

⑦+ **T28.49X-**   **Burn of other internal organ**
Code first:
    (T51-T65) to identify chemical and intent for T28.5-T28.9-

⑦+ **T28.5XX-**   **Corrosion of mouth and pharynx**

⑦+ **T28.6XX-**   **Corrosion of esophagus**

⑦+ **T28.7XX-**   **Corrosion of other parts of alimentary tract**

⑦+ **T28.8XX-**   **Corrosion of internal genitourinary organs**

⑤+ **T28.9**   **Corrosions of other and unspecified internal organs**

⑦+ **T28.90X-**   **Corrosions of unspecified internal organs**

⑥+ **T28.91**   **Corrosions of ear drum**

⑦◨+ **T28.911-**   **Corrosions of right ear drum**

⑦◨+ **T28.912-**   **Corrosions of left ear drum**

⑦◨+ **T28.919-**   **Corrosions of unspecified ear drum**

⑦+ **T28.99X-**   **Corrosions of other internal organs**

Burns and corrosions of multiple and unspecified body regions (T30-T32)

GUIDELINES   Section I.C.19.d.6)-9)
Categories T31 and T32 are based on the classic "rule of nines" in estimating body surface involved: head and neck are assigned nine percent, each arm nine percent, each leg 18 percent, the anterior trunk 18 percent, posterior trunk 18 percent, and genitalia one percent. Providers may change these percentage assignments where necessary to accommodate infants and children who have proportionately larger heads than adults, and patients who have large buttocks, thighs, or abdomen that involve burns.

Encounters for the treatment of the late effects of burns or corrosions (i.e., scars or joint contractures) should be coded with a burn or corrosion code with the 7th character "S" for sequela.

When appropriate, both a code for a current burn or corrosion with 7th character "A" or "D" and a burn or corrosion code with 7th character "S" may be assigned on the same record (when both a current burn and sequelae of an old burn exist). Burns and corrosions do not heal at the same rate and a current healing wound may still exist with sequela of a healed burn or corrosion.

An external cause code should be used with burns and corrosions to identify the source and intent of the burn, as well as the place where it occurred.

④ **T30**   **Burn and corrosion, body region unspecified**

GUIDELINES   Section I.C.19.d.5)
Category T30, Burn and corrosion, body region unspecified is extremely vague and should rarely be used.

T30.0   **Burn of unspecified body region, unspecified degree**
This code is not for inpatient use. Code to specified site and degree of burns
Burn NOS
Multiple burns NOS

● New   ▲ Revised   *Manifestation*   ④-⑦ Digit Indicators   ◨ Laterality   Ⓐ Adult (15+ years)   Ⓜ Maternity (12-55 years)   Ⓝ Newborn   Ⓟ Pediatric (0-17 years)   ♂ Male   ♀ Female
✖ Deleted   Unspecified   + Additional code

T30.4   **Corrosion of unspecified body region, unspecified degree**
This code is not for inpatient use. Code to specified site and degree of corrosion
Corrosion NOS
Multiple corrosion NOS

▣ **T31**   **Burns classified according to extent of body surface involved**
Note: This category is to be used as the primary code only when the site of the burn is unspecified. It should be used as a supplementary code with categories T20-T25 when the site is specified.

Burns classified according to extent of body surface involved

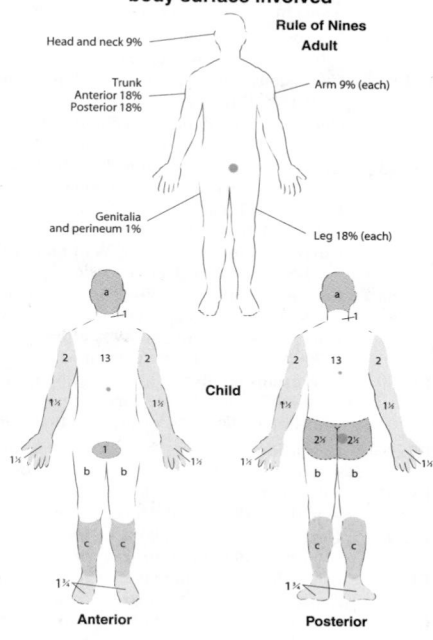

T31.0   **Burns involving less than 10% of body surface**

⑤ T31.1   **Burns involving 10-19% of body surface**

  T31.10   **Burns involving 10-19% of body surface with 0% to 9% third degree burns**
Burns involving 10-19% of body surface NOS

  T31.11   **Burns involving 10-19% of body surface with 10-19% third degree burns**

⑤ T31.2   **Burns involving 20-29% of body surface**

  T31.20   **Burns involving 20-29% of body surface with 0% to 9% third degree burns**
Burns involving 20-29% of body surface NOS

  T31.21   **Burns involving 20-29% of body surface with 10-19% third degree burns**

  T31.22   **Burns involving 20-29% of body surface with 20-29% third degree burns**

⑤ T31.3   **Burns involving 30-39% of body surface**

  T31.30   **Burns involving 30-39% of body surface with 0% to 9% third degree burns**
Burns involving 30-39% of body surface NOS

  T31.31   **Burns involving 30-39% of body surface with 10-19% third degree burns**

  T31.32   **Burns involving 30-39% of body surface with 20-29% third degree burns**

  T31.33   **Burns involving 30-39% of body surface with 30-39% third degree burns**

⑤ T31.4   **Burns involving 40-49% of body surface**

  T31.40   **Burns involving 40-49% of body surface with 0% to 9% third degree burns**
Burns involving 40-49% of body surface NOS

  T31.41   **Burns involving 40-49% of body surface with 10-19% third degree burns**

  T31.42   **Burns involving 40-49% of body surface with 20-29% third degree burns**

  T31.43   **Burns involving 40-49% of body surface with 30-39% third degree burns**

  T31.44   **Burns involving 40-49% of body surface with 40-49% third degree burns**

⑤ T31.5   **Burns involving 50-59% of body surface**

  T31.50   **Burns involving 50-59% of body surface with 0% to 9% third degree burns**
Burns involving 50-59% of body surface NOS

  T31.51   **Burns involving 50-59% of body surface with 10-19% third degree burns**

  T31.52   **Burns involving 50-59% of body surface with 20-29% third degree burns**

  T31.53   **Burns involving 50-59% of body surface with 30-39% third degree burns**

  T31.54   **Burns involving 50-59% of body surface with 40-49% third degree burns**

  T31.55   **Burns involving 50-59% of body surface with 50-59% third degree burns**

⑤ T31.6   **Burns involving 60-69% of body surface**

  T31.60   **Burns involving 60-69% of body surface with 0% to 9% third degree burns**
Burns involving 60-69% of body surface NOS

  T31.61   **Burns involving 60-69% of body surface with 10-19% third degree burns**

  T31.62   **Burns involving 60-69% of body surface with 20-29% third degree burns**

  T31.63   **Burns involving 60-69% of body surface with 30-39% third degree burns**

  T31.64   **Burns involving 60-69% of body surface with 40-49% third degree burns**

  T31.65   **Burns involving 60-69% of body surface with 50-59% third degree burns**

  T31.66   **Burns involving 60-69% of body surface with 60-69% third degree burns**

⑤ T31.7   **Burns involving 70-79% of body surface**

  T31.70   **Burns involving 70-79% of body surface with 0% to 9% third degree burns**
Burns involving 70-79% of body surface NOS

  T31.71   **Burns involving 70-79% of body surface with 10-19% third degree burns**

  T31.72   **Burns involving 70-79% of body surface with 20-29% third degree burns**

  T31.73   **Burns involving 70-79% of body surface with 30-39% third degree burns**

  T31.74   **Burns involving 70-79% of body surface with 40-49% third degree burns**

  T31.75   **Burns involving 70-79% of body surface with 50-59% third degree burns**

  T31.76   **Burns involving 70-79% of body surface with 60-69% third degree burns**

  T31.77   **Burns involving 70-79% of body surface with 70-79% third degree burns**

⑤ T31.8   **Burns involving 80-89% of body surface**

  T31.80   **Burns involving 80-89% of body surface with 0% to 9% third degree burns**
Burns involving 80-89% of body surface NOS

  T31.81   **Burns involving 80-89% of body surface with 10-19% third degree burns**

  T31.82   **Burns involving 80-89% of body surface with 20-29% third degree burns**

  T31.83   **Burns involving 80-89% of body surface with 30-39% third degree burns**

  T31.84   **Burns involving 80-89% of body surface with 40-49% third degree burns**

  T31.85   **Burns involving 80-89% of body surface with 50-59% third degree burns**

  T31.86   **Burns involving 80-89% of body surface with 60-69% third degree burns**

  T31.87   **Burns involving 80-89% of body surface with 70-79% third degree burns**

  T31.88   **Burns involving 80-89% of body surface with 80-89% third degree burns**

⑤ T31.9   **Burns involving 90% or more of body surface**

  T31.90   **Burns involving 90% or more of body surface with 0% to 9% third degree burns**
Burns involving 90% or more of body surface NOS

  T31.91   **Burns involving 90% or more of body surface with 10-19% third degree burns**

  T31.92   **Burns involving 90% or more of body surface with 20-29% third degree burns**

  T31.93   **Burns involving 90% or more of body surface with 30-39% third degree burns**

  T31.94   **Burns involving 90% or more of body surface with 40-49% third degree burns**

● New   ▲ Revised   *Manifestation*   ▣-▸ Digit Indicators   ▤ Laterality   ▣ Adult (15+ years)   ▣ Maternity (12-55 years)   ▣ Newborn   ▣ Pediatric (0-17 years)   ♂ Male   ♀ Female
✕ Deleted   Unspecified   + Additional code

2017 ICD-10-CM Expert for Physicians   © 2017 DecisionHealth   1055

T31.95 Burns involving 90% or more of body surface with 50-59% third degree burns

T31.96 Burns involving 90% or more of body surface with 60-69% third degree burns

T31.97 Burns involving 90% or more of body surface with 70-79% third degree burns

T31.98 Burns involving 90% or more of body surface with 80-89% third degree burns

T31.99 Burns involving 90% or more of body surface with 90% or more third degree burns

☑ T32 **Corrosions classified according to extent of body surface involved**

Note: This category is to be used as the primary code only when the site of the corrosion is unspecified. It may be used as a supplementary code with categories T20-T25 when the site is specified.

T32.0 Corrosions involving less than 10% of body surface

☑ T32.1 Corrosions involving 10-19% of body surface

T32.10 Corrosions involving 10-19% of body surface with 0% to 9% third degree corrosion
Corrosions involving 10-19% of body surface NOS

T32.11 Corrosions involving 10-19% of body surface with 10-19% third degree corrosion

☑ T32.2 Corrosions involving 20-29% of body surface

T32.20 Corrosions involving 20-29% of body surface with 0% to 9% third degree corrosion

T32.21 Corrosions involving 20-29% of body surface with 10-19% third degree corrosion

T32.22 Corrosions involving 20-29% of body surface with 20-29% third degree corrosion

☑ T32.3 Corrosions involving 30-39% of body surface

T32.30 Corrosions involving 30-39% of body surface with 0% to 9% third degree corrosion

T32.31 Corrosions involving 30-39% of body surface with 10-19% third degree corrosion

T32.32 Corrosions involving 30-39% of body surface with 20-29% third degree corrosion

T32.33 Corrosions involving 30-39% of body surface with 30-39% third degree corrosion

☑ T32.4 Corrosions involving 40-49% of body surface

T32.40 Corrosions involving 40-49% of body surface with 0% to 9% third degree corrosion

T32.41 Corrosions involving 40-49% of body surface with 10-19% third degree corrosion

T32.42 Corrosions involving 40-49% of body surface with 20-29% third degree corrosion

T32.43 Corrosions involving 40-49% of body surface with 30-39% third degree corrosion

T32.44 Corrosions involving 40-49% of body surface with 40-49% third degree corrosion

☑ T32.5 Corrosions involving 50-59% of body surface

T32.50 Corrosions involving 50-59% of body surface with 0% to 9% third degree corrosion

T32.51 Corrosions involving 50-59% of body surface with 10-19% third degree corrosion

T32.52 Corrosions involving 50-59% of body surface with 20-29% third degree corrosion

T32.53 Corrosions involving 50-59% of body surface with 30-39% third degree corrosion

T32.54 Corrosions involving 50-59% of body surface with 40-49% third degree corrosion

T32.55 Corrosions involving 50-59% of body surface with 50-59% third degree corrosion

☑ T32.6 Corrosions involving 60-69% of body surface

T32.60 Corrosions involving 60-69% of body surface with 0% to 9% third degree corrosion

T32.61 Corrosions involving 60-69% of body surface with 10-19% third degree corrosion

T32.62 Corrosions involving 60-69% of body surface with 20-29% third degree corrosion

T32.63 Corrosions involving 60-69% of body surface with 30-39% third degree corrosion

T32.64 Corrosions involving 60-69% of body surface with 40-49% third degree corrosion

T32.65 Corrosions involving 60-69% of body surface with 50-59% third degree corrosion

T32.66 Corrosions involving 60-69% of body surface with 60-69% third degree corrosion

☑ T32.7 Corrosions involving 70-79% of body surface

T32.70 Corrosions involving 70-79% of body surface with 0% to 9% third degree corrosion

T32.71 Corrosions involving 70-79% of body surface with 10-19% third degree corrosion

T32.72 Corrosions involving 70-79% of body surface with 20-29% third degree corrosion

T32.73 Corrosions involving 70-79% of body surface with 30-39% third degree corrosion

T32.74 Corrosions involving 70-79% of body surface with 40-49% third degree corrosion

T32.75 Corrosions involving 70-79% of body surface with 50-59% third degree corrosion

T32.76 Corrosions involving 70-79% of body surface with 60-69% third degree corrosion

T32.77 Corrosions involving 70-79% of body surface with 70-79% third degree corrosion

☑ T32.8 Corrosions involving 80-89% of body surface

T32.80 Corrosions involving 80-89% of body surface with 0% to 9% third degree corrosion

T32.81 Corrosions involving 80-89% of body surface with 10-19% third degree corrosion

T32.82 Corrosions involving 80-89% of body surface with 20-29% third degree corrosion

T32.83 Corrosions involving 80-89% of body surface with 30-39% third degree corrosion

T32.84 Corrosions involving 80-89% of body surface with 40-49% third degree corrosion

T32.85 Corrosions involving 80-89% of body surface with 50-59% third degree corrosion

T32.86 Corrosions involving 80-89% of body surface with 60-69% third degree corrosion

T32.87 Corrosions involving 80-89% of body surface with 70-79% third degree corrosion

T32.88 Corrosions involving 80-89% of body surface with 80-89% third degree corrosion

☑ T32.9 Corrosions involving 90% or more of body surface

T32.90 Corrosions involving 90% or more of body surface with 0% to 9% third degree corrosion

T32.91 Corrosions involving 90% or more of body surface with 10-19% third degree corrosion

T32.92 Corrosions involving 90% or more of body surface with 20-29% third degree corrosion

T32.93 Corrosions involving 90% or more of body surface with 30-39% third degree corrosion

T32.94 Corrosions involving 90% or more of body surface with 40-49% third degree corrosion

T32.95 Corrosions involving 90% or more of body surface with 50-59% third degree corrosion

T32.96 Corrosions involving 90% or more of body surface with 60-69% third degree corrosion

T32.97 Corrosions involving 90% or more of body surface with 70-79% third degree corrosion

T32.98 Corrosions involving 90% or more of body surface with 80-89% third degree corrosion

T32.99 Corrosions involving 90% or more of body surface with 90% or more third degree corrosion

Frostbite (T33-T34)

EXCLUDES 2 *hypothermia and other effects of reduced temperature (T68, T69.-)*

☑ T33 **Superficial frostbite**

INCLUDES frostbite with partial thickness skin loss

The appropriate 7th character is to be added to each code from category T33
A   initial encounter
D   subsequent encounter
S   sequela

☑ T33.0 Superficial frostbite of head

☑ T33.01 Superficial frostbite of ear

☑ T33.011- Superficial frostbite of right ear

☑ T33.012- Superficial frostbite of left ear

☑ T33.019- Superficial frostbite of unspecified ear

☑ T33.02X- Superficial frostbite of nose

☑ T33.09X- Superficial frostbite of other part of head

☑ T33.1XX- Superficial frostbite of neck

☑ T33.2XX- Superficial frostbite of thorax

☑ T33.3XX- Superficial frostbite of abdominal wall, lower back and pelvis

● New ▲ Revised *Manifestation* ☑-☑ Digit Indicators ⊟ Laterality 🅰 Adult (15+ years) 🅼 Maternity (12-55 years) 🅽 Newborn 🅿 Pediatric (0-17 years) ♂ Male ♀ Female
✖ Deleted Unspecified + Additional code

1056   © 2017 DecisionHealth   2017 ICD-10-CM Expert for Physicians

⑤ T33.4 Superficial frostbite of arm

> **EXCLUDES 2** *superficial frostbite of wrist and hand (T33.5-)*

⑦ ⊟ T33.40X- Superficial frostbite of unspecified arm
⑦ ⊟ T33.41X- Superficial frostbite of right arm
⑦ ⊟ T33.42X- Superficial frostbite of left arm

⑤ T33.5 Superficial frostbite of wrist, hand, and fingers

⑥ T33.51 Superficial frostbite of wrist
⑦ ⊟ T33.511- Superficial frostbite of right wrist
⑦ ⊟ T33.512- Superficial frostbite of left wrist
⑦ ⊟ T33.519- Superficial frostbite of unspecified wrist

⑥ T33.52 Superficial frostbite of hand

> **EXCLUDES 2** *superficial frostbite of fingers (T33.53-)*

⑦ ⊟ T33.521- Superficial frostbite of right hand
⑦ ⊟ T33.522- Superficial frostbite of left hand
⑦ ⊟ T33.529- Superficial frostbite of unspecified hand

⑥ T33.53 Superficial frostbite of finger(s)
⑦ ⊟ T33.531- Superficial frostbite of right finger(s)
⑦ ⊟ T33.532- Superficial frostbite of left finger(s)
⑦ ⊟ T33.539- Superficial frostbite of unspecified finger(s)

⑤ T33.6 Superficial frostbite of hip and thigh

⑦ ⊟ T33.60X- Superficial frostbite of unspecified hip and thigh
⑦ ⊟ T33.61X- Superficial frostbite of right hip and thigh
⑦ ⊟ T33.62X- Superficial frostbite of left hip and thigh

⑤ T33.7 Superficial frostbite of knee and lower leg

> **EXCLUDES 2** *superficial frostbite of ankle and foot (T33.8-)*

⑦ ⊟ T33.70X- Superficial frostbite of unspecified knee and lower leg
⑦ ⊟ T33.71X- Superficial frostbite of right knee and lower leg
⑦ ⊟ T33.72X- Superficial frostbite of left knee and lower leg

⑤ T33.8 Superficial frostbite of ankle, foot, and toe(s)

⑥ T33.81 Superficial frostbite of ankle
⑦ ⊟ T33.811- Superficial frostbite of right ankle
⑦ ⊟ T33.812- Superficial frostbite of left ankle
⑦ ⊟ T33.819- Superficial frostbite of unspecified ankle

⑥ T33.82 Superficial frostbite of foot
⑦ ⊟ T33.821- Superficial frostbite of right foot
⑦ ⊟ T33.822- Superficial frostbite of left foot
⑦ ⊟ T33.829- Superficial frostbite of unspecified foot

⑥ T33.83 Superficial frostbite of toe(s)
⑦ ⊟ T33.831- Superficial frostbite of right toe(s)
⑦ ⊟ T33.832- Superficial frostbite of left toe(s)
⑦ ⊟ T33.839- Superficial frostbite of unspecified toe(s)

⑤ T33.9 Superficial frostbite of other and unspecified sites

⑦ T33.90X- Superficial frostbite of unspecified sites
Superficial frostbite NOS

⑦ T33.99X- Superficial frostbite of other sites
Superficial frostbite of leg NOS
Superficial frostbite of trunk NOS

④ T34 Frostbite with tissue necrosis

> The appropriate 7th character is to be added to each code from category T34
> A   initial encounter
> D   subsequent encounter
> S   sequela

⑤ T34.0 Frostbite with tissue necrosis of head

⑥ T34.01 Frostbite with tissue necrosis of ear
⑦ ⊟ T34.011- Frostbite with tissue necrosis of right ear
⑦ ⊟ T34.012- Frostbite with tissue necrosis of left ear
⑦ ⊟ T34.019- Frostbite with tissue necrosis of unspecified ear

⑦ T34.02X- Frostbite with tissue necrosis of nose
⑦ T34.09X- Frostbite with tissue necrosis of other part of head
⑦ T34.1XX- Frostbite with tissue necrosis of neck
⑦ T34.2XX- Frostbite with tissue necrosis of thorax
⑦ T34.3XX- Frostbite with tissue necrosis of abdominal wall, lower back and pelvis

⑤ T34.4 Frostbite with tissue necrosis of arm

> **EXCLUDES 2** *frostbite with tissue necrosis of wrist and hand (T34.5-)*

⑦ ⊟ T34.40X- Frostbite with tissue necrosis of unspecified arm

⑦ ⊟ T34.41X- Frostbite with tissue necrosis of right arm
⑦ ⊟ T34.42X- Frostbite with tissue necrosis of left arm

⑤ T34.5 Frostbite with tissue necrosis of wrist, hand, and finger(s)

⑥ T34.51 Frostbite with tissue necrosis of wrist
⑦ ⊟ T34.511- Frostbite with tissue necrosis of right wrist
⑦ ⊟ T34.512- Frostbite with tissue necrosis of left wrist
⑦ ⊟ T34.519- Frostbite with tissue necrosis of unspecified wrist

⑥ T34.52 Frostbite with tissue necrosis of hand

> **EXCLUDES 2** *frostbite with tissue necrosis of finger(s) (T34.53-)*

⑦ ⊟ T34.521- Frostbite with tissue necrosis of right hand
⑦ ⊟ T34.522- Frostbite with tissue necrosis of left hand
⑦ ⊟ T34.529- Frostbite with tissue necrosis of unspecified hand

⑥ T34.53 Frostbite with tissue necrosis of finger(s)
⑦ ⊟ T34.531- Frostbite with tissue necrosis of right finger(s)
⑦ ⊟ T34.532- Frostbite with tissue necrosis of left finger(s)
⑦ ⊟ T34.539- Frostbite with tissue necrosis of unspecified finger(s)

⑤ T34.6 Frostbite with tissue necrosis of hip and thigh

⑦ ⊟ T34.60X- Frostbite with tissue necrosis of unspecified hip and thigh
⑦ ⊟ T34.61X- Frostbite with tissue necrosis of right hip and thigh
⑦ ⊟ T34.62X- Frostbite with tissue necrosis of left hip and thigh

⑤ T34.7 Frostbite with tissue necrosis of knee and lower leg

> **EXCLUDES 2** *frostbite with tissue necrosis of ankle and foot (T34.8-)*

⑦ ⊟ T34.70X- Frostbite with tissue necrosis of unspecified knee and lower leg
⑦ ⊟ T34.71X- Frostbite with tissue necrosis of right knee and lower leg
⑦ ⊟ T34.72X- Frostbite with tissue necrosis of left knee and lower leg

⑤ T34.8 Frostbite with tissue necrosis of ankle, foot, and toe(s)

⑥ T34.81 Frostbite with tissue necrosis of ankle
⑦ ⊟ T34.811- Frostbite with tissue necrosis of right ankle
⑦ ⊟ T34.812- Frostbite with tissue necrosis of left ankle
⑦ ⊟ T34.819- Frostbite with tissue necrosis of unspecified ankle

⑥ T34.82 Frostbite with tissue necrosis of foot
⑦ ⊟ T34.821- Frostbite with tissue necrosis of right foot
⑦ ⊟ T34.822- Frostbite with tissue necrosis of left foot
⑦ ⊟ T34.829- Frostbite with tissue necrosis of unspecified foot

⑥ T34.83 Frostbite with tissue necrosis of toe(s)
⑦ ⊟ T34.831- Frostbite with tissue necrosis of right toe(s)
⑦ ⊟ T34.832- Frostbite with tissue necrosis of left toe(s)
⑦ ⊟ T34.839- Frostbite with tissue necrosis of unspecified toe(s)

⑤ T34.9 Frostbite with tissue necrosis of other and unspecified sites

⑦ T34.90X- Frostbite with tissue necrosis of unspecified sites
Frostbite with tissue necrosis NOS

⑦ T34.99X- Frostbite with tissue necrosis of other sites
Frostbite with tissue necrosis of leg NOS
Frostbite with tissue necrosis of trunk NOS

● New   ▲ Revised   *Manifestation*   ④-⑦ Digit Indicators   ⊟ Laterality   Ⓐ Adult (15+ years)   Ⓜ Maternity (12-55 years)   Ⓝ Newborn   Ⓟ Pediatric (0-17 years)   ♂ Male   ♀ Female
✖ Deleted   Unspecified   + Additional code

2017 ICD-10-CM Expert for Physicians   © 2017 DecisionHealth   1057

Poisoning by, adverse effects of and underdosing of drugs, medicaments and biological substances (T36-T50)

Note: The drug giving rise to the adverse effect should be identified by use of codes from categories T36-T50 with fifth or sixth character 5.

INCLUDES adverse effect of correct substance properly administered
poisoning by overdose of substance
poisoning by wrong substance given or taken in error
underdosing by (inadvertently) (deliberately) taking less substance than prescribed or instructed

Code first, for adverse effects, the nature of the adverse effect, such as:
adverse effect NOS (T88.7)
aspirin gastritis (K29.-)
blood disorders (D56-D76)
contact dermatitis (L23-L25)
dermatitis due to substances taken internally (L27.-)
nephropathy (N14.0-N14.2)
Use additional code(s) to specify:
manifestations of poisoning
underdosing or failure in dosage during medical and surgical care (Y63.6, Y63.8-Y63.9)
underdosing of medication regimen (Z91.12-, Z91.13-)

EXCLUDES 1 *toxic reaction to local anesthesia in pregnancy (O29.3-)*

EXCLUDES 2 *abuse and dependence of psychoactive substances (F10-F19)*
abuse of non-dependence-producing substances (F55.-)
drug reaction and poisoning affecting newborn (P00-P96)
pathological drug intoxication (inebriation) (F10-F19)

GUIDELINES Section I.C.19.e.1)-4)
Codes in categories T36-T65 are combination codes that include the substance that was taken as well as the intent. No additional external cause code is required for poisonings, toxic effects, adverse effects and underdosing codes.

Do not code directly from the Table of Drugs and Chemicals. Always refer back to the Tabular List. Use as many codes as necessary to describe completely all drugs, medicinal or biological substances. If the same code would describe the causative agent for more than one adverse reaction, poisoning, toxic effect or underdosing, assign the code only once. If two or more drugs, medicinal or biological substances are reported, code each individually unless a combination code is listed in the Table of Drugs and Chemicals.

GUIDELINES Section I.C.19.e.5)(a)
When coding an adverse effect of a drug that has been correctly prescribed and properly administered, assign the appropriate code for the nature of the adverse effect followed by the appropriate code for the adverse effect of the drug (T36-T50). The code for the drug should have a 5th or 6th character "5" (for example T36.0X5-). Examples of the nature of an adverse effect are tachycardia, delirium, gastrointestinal hemorrhaging, vomiting, hypokalemia, hepatitis, renal failure, or respiratory failure.

CODING TIP ✓ When coding any adverse effect of a drug that has been correctly prescribed and administered, assign the appropriate code for the drug giving rise to the nature of the adverse effect, using the fifth or sixth character "5."

CODING TIP ✓ Poisonings are coded as accidental unless there is physician documentation to indicate otherwise. 7th character 'A' means the effect of the drug/chemical requires active treatment. 'D' should be the 7th character if the effect is healing/resolving. 'S' should be used as the 7th character if the condition resulting is still a factor after the medication has long cleared from the body, i.e., glucocorticoids were taken last year resulting in diabetes.

④ **T36** **Poisoning by, adverse effect of and underdosing of systemic antibiotics**

EXCLUDES 1 *antineoplastic antibiotics (T45.1-)*
locally applied antibiotic NEC (T49.0)
topically used antibiotic for ear, nose and throat (T49.6)
topically used antibiotic for eye (T49.5)

The appropriate 7th character is to be added to each code from category T36
A   initial encounter
D   subsequent encounter
S   sequela

GUIDELINES Section I.C.19.e.5)(b)
When coding a poisoning or reaction to the improper use of a medication (e.g., overdose, wrong substance given or taken in error, wrong route of administration), first assign the appropriate code from categories T36-T50. The poisoning codes have an associated intent as their 5th or 6th character (accidental, intentional self harm, assault and undetermined). Use additional code(s) for all manifestations of poisonings. If there is also a diagnosis of abuse or dependence of the substance, the abuse or dependence is assigned as an additional code.
See Section I.C.4. if poisoning is the result of insulin pump malfunctions.

GUIDELINES Section I.C.19.e.5)(c)
Underdosing refers to taking less of a medication than is prescribed by a provider or a manufacturer's instruction. For underdosing, assign the code from categories T36-T50 (fifth or sixth character "6"). Codes for underdosing should never be assigned as principal or first-listed codes. If a patient has a relapse or exacerbation of the medical condition for which the drug is prescribed because of the reduction in dose, then the medical condition itself should be coded. Noncompliance (Z91.12-, Z91.13-) or complication of care (Y63.6-Y63.9) codes are to be used with an underdosing code to indicate intent, if known.

⑤ **T36.0** Poisoning by, adverse effect of and underdosing of penicillins

⑥ **T36.0X** Poisoning by, adverse effect of and underdosing of penicillins

⑦ **T36.0X1-** Poisoning by penicillins, accidental (unintentional)
Poisoning by penicillins NOS

⑦ **T36.0X2-** Poisoning by penicillins, intentional self-harm

⑦ **T36.0X3-** Poisoning by penicillins, assault

⑦ **T36.0X4-** Poisoning by penicillins, undetermined

⑦ **T36.0X5-** Adverse effect of penicillins

⑦ **T36.0X6-** Underdosing of penicillins

⑤ **T36.1** Poisoning by, adverse effect of and underdosing of cephalosporins and other beta-lactam antibiotics

⑥ **T36.1X** Poisoning by, adverse effect of and underdosing of cephalosporins and other beta-lactam antibiotics

⑦ **T36.1X1-** Poisoning by cephalosporins and other beta-lactam antibiotics, accidental (unintentional)
Poisoning by cephalosporins and other beta-lactam antibiotics NOS

⑦ **T36.1X2-** Poisoning by cephalosporins and other beta-lactam antibiotics, intentional self-harm

⑦ **T36.1X3-** Poisoning by cephalosporins and other beta-lactam antibiotics, assault

⑦ **T36.1X4-** Poisoning by cephalosporins and other beta-lactam antibiotics, undetermined

⑦ **T36.1X5-** Adverse effect of cephalosporins and other beta-lactam antibiotics

⑦ **T36.1X6-** Underdosing of cephalosporins and other beta-lactam antibiotics

⑤ **T36.2** Poisoning by, adverse effect of and underdosing of chloramphenicol group

⑥ **T36.2X** Poisoning by, adverse effect of and underdosing of chloramphenicol group

⑦ **T36.2X1-** Poisoning by chloramphenicol group, accidental (unintentional)
Poisoning by chloramphenicol group NOS

⑦ **T36.2X2-** Poisoning by chloramphenicol group, intentional self-harm

⑦ **T36.2X3-** Poisoning by chloramphenicol group, assault

⑦ **T36.2X4-** Poisoning by chloramphenicol group, undetermined

⑦ **T36.2X5-** Adverse effect of chloramphenicol group

⑦ **T36.2X6-** Underdosing of chloramphenicol group

⑤ **T36.3** Poisoning by, adverse effect of and underdosing of macrolides

⑥ **T36.3X** Poisoning by, adverse effect of and underdosing of macrolides

⑦ **T36.3X1-** Poisoning by macrolides, accidental (unintentional)
Poisoning by macrolides NOS

⑦ **T36.3X2-** Poisoning by macrolides, intentional self-harm

⑦ **T36.3X3-** Poisoning by macrolides, assault

⑦ **T36.3X4-** Poisoning by macrolides, undetermined

☑ **T36.3X5-**   **Adverse effect of macrolides**

☑ **T36.3X6-**   **Underdosing of macrolides**

⑤ **T36.4**   **Poisoning by, adverse effect of and underdosing of tetracyclines**

   ⑥ **T36.4X**   **Poisoning by, adverse effect of and underdosing of tetracyclines**

     ☑ **T36.4X1-**   **Poisoning by tetracyclines, accidental (unintentional)**
Poisoning by tetracyclines NOS

     ☑ **T36.4X2-**   **Poisoning by tetracyclines, intentional self-harm**

     ☑ **T36.4X3-**   **Poisoning by tetracyclines, assault**

     ☑ **T36.4X4-**   **Poisoning by tetracyclines, undetermined**

     ☑ **T36.4X5-**   **Adverse effect of tetracyclines**

     ☑ **T36.4X6-**   **Underdosing of tetracyclines**

⑤ **T36.5**   **Poisoning by, adverse effect of and underdosing of aminoglycosides**
Poisoning by, adverse effect of and underdosing of streptomycin

   ⑥ **T36.5X**   **Poisoning by, adverse effect of and underdosing of aminoglycosides**

     ☑ **T36.5X1-**   **Poisoning by aminoglycosides, accidental (unintentional)**
Poisoning by aminoglycosides NOS

     ☑ **T36.5X2-**   **Poisoning by aminoglycosides, intentional self-harm**

     ☑ **T36.5X3-**   **Poisoning by aminoglycosides, assault**

     ☑ **T36.5X4-**   **Poisoning by aminoglycosides, undetermined**

     ☑ **T36.5X5-**   **Adverse effect of aminoglycosides**

     ☑ **T36.5X6-**   **Underdosing of aminoglycosides**

⑤ **T36.6**   **Poisoning by, adverse effect of and underdosing of rifampicins**

   ⑥ **T36.6X**   **Poisoning by, adverse effect of and underdosing of rifampicins**

     ☑ **T36.6X1-**   **Poisoning by rifampicins, accidental (unintentional)**
Poisoning by rifampicins NOS

     ☑ **T36.6X2-**   **Poisoning by rifampicins, intentional self-harm**

     ☑ **T36.6X3-**   **Poisoning by rifampicins, assault**

     ☑ **T36.6X4-**   **Poisoning by rifampicins, undetermined**

     ☑ **T36.6X5-**   **Adverse effect of rifampicins**

     ☑ **T36.6X6-**   **Underdosing of rifampicins**

⑤ **T36.7**   **Poisoning by, adverse effect of and underdosing of antifungal antibiotics, systemically used**

   ⑥ **T36.7X**   **Poisoning by, adverse effect of and underdosing of antifungal antibiotics, systemically used**

     ☑ **T36.7X1-**   **Poisoning by antifungal antibiotics, systemically used, accidental (unintentional)**
Poisoning by antifungal antibiotics, systemically used NOS

     ☑ **T36.7X2-**   **Poisoning by antifungal antibiotics, systemically used, intentional self-harm**

     ☑ **T36.7X3-**   **Poisoning by antifungal antibiotics, systemically used, assault**

     ☑ **T36.7X4-**   **Poisoning by antifungal antibiotics, systemically used, undetermined**

     ☑ **T36.7X5-**   **Adverse effect of antifungal antibiotics, systemically used**

     ☑ **T36.7X6-**   **Underdosing of antifungal antibiotics, systemically used**

⑤ **T36.8**   **Poisoning by, adverse effect of and underdosing of other systemic antibiotics**

   ⑥ **T36.8X**   **Poisoning by, adverse effect of and underdosing of other systemic antibiotics**

     ☑ **T36.8X1-**   **Poisoning by other systemic antibiotics, accidental (unintentional)**
Poisoning by other systemic antibiotics NOS

     ☑ **T36.8X2-**   **Poisoning by other systemic antibiotics, intentional self-harm**

     ☑ **T36.8X3-**   **Poisoning by other systemic antibiotics, assault**

     ☑ **T36.8X4-**   **Poisoning by other systemic antibiotics, undetermined**

     ☑ **T36.8X5-**   **Adverse effect of other systemic antibiotics**

     ☑ **T36.8X6-**   **Underdosing of other systemic antibiotics**

⑤ **T36.9**   **Poisoning by, adverse effect of and underdosing of unspecified systemic antibiotic**

     ☑ **T36.91X-**   **Poisoning by unspecified systemic antibiotic, accidental (unintentional)**
Poisoning by systemic antibiotic NOS

☑ **T36.92X-**   **Poisoning by unspecified systemic antibiotic, intentional self-harm**

☑ **T36.93X-**   **Poisoning by unspecified systemic antibiotic, assault**

☑ **T36.94X-**   **Poisoning by unspecified systemic antibiotic, undetermined**

☑ **T36.95X-**   **Adverse effect of unspecified systemic antibiotic**

☑ **T36.96X-**   **Underdosing of unspecified systemic antibiotic**

④ **T37**   **Poisoning by, adverse effect of and underdosing of other systemic anti- infectives and antiparasitics**

   EXCLUDES 1   *anti-infectives topically used for ear, nose and throat (T49.6-)*
anti-infectives topically used for eye (T49.5-)
locally applied anti-infectives NEC (T49.0-)

   The appropriate 7th character is to be added to each code from category T37
   A   initial encounter
   D   subsequent encounter
   S   sequela

⑤ **T37.0**   **Poisoning by, adverse effect of and underdosing of sulfonamides**

   ⑥ **T37.0X**   **Poisoning by, adverse effect of and underdosing of sulfonamides**

     ☑ **T37.0X1-**   **Poisoning by sulfonamides, accidental (unintentional)**
Poisoning by sulfonamides NOS

     ☑ **T37.0X2-**   **Poisoning by sulfonamides, intentional self-harm**

     ☑ **T37.0X3-**   **Poisoning by sulfonamides, assault**

     ☑ **T37.0X4-**   **Poisoning by sulfonamides, undetermined**

     ☑ **T37.0X5-**   **Adverse effect of sulfonamides**

     ☑ **T37.0X6-**   **Underdosing of sulfonamides**

⑤ **T37.1**   **Poisoning by, adverse effect of and underdosing of antimycobacterial drugs**

   EXCLUDES 1   *rifampicins (T36.6-)*
streptomycin (T36.5-)

   ⑥ **T37.1X**   **Poisoning by, adverse effect of and underdosing of antimycobacterial drugs**

     ☑ **T37.1X1-**   **Poisoning by antimycobacterial drugs, accidental (unintentional)**
Poisoning by antimycobacterial drugs NOS

     ☑ **T37.1X2-**   **Poisoning by antimycobacterial drugs, intentional self-harm**

     ☑ **T37.1X3-**   **Poisoning by antimycobacterial drugs, assault**

     ☑ **T37.1X4-**   **Poisoning by antimycobacterial drugs, undetermined**

     ☑ **T37.1X5-**   **Adverse effect of antimycobacterial drugs**

     ☑ **T37.1X6-**   **Underdosing of antimycobacterial drugs**

⑤ **T37.2**   **Poisoning by, adverse effect of and underdosing of antimalarials and drugs acting on other blood protozoa**

   EXCLUDES 1   *hydroxyquinoline derivatives (T37.8-)*

   ⑥ **T37.2X**   **Poisoning by, adverse effect of and underdosing of antimalarials and drugs acting on other blood protozoa**

     ☑ **T37.2X1-**   **Poisoning by antimalarials and drugs acting on other blood protozoa, accidental (unintentional)**
Poisoning by antimalarials and drugs acting on other blood protozoa NOS

     ☑ **T37.2X2-**   **Poisoning by antimalarials and drugs acting on other blood protozoa, intentional self-harm**

     ☑ **T37.2X3-**   **Poisoning by antimalarials and drugs acting on other blood protozoa, assault**

     ☑ **T37.2X4-**   **Poisoning by antimalarials and drugs acting on other blood protozoa, undetermined**

     ☑ **T37.2X5-**   **Adverse effect of antimalarials and drugs acting on other blood protozoa**

     ☑ **T37.2X6-**   **Underdosing of antimalarials and drugs acting on other blood protozoa**

⑤ **T37.3**   **Poisoning by, adverse effect of and underdosing of other antiprotozoal drugs**

   ⑥ **T37.3X**   **Poisoning by, adverse effect of and underdosing of other antiprotozoal drugs**

     ☑ **T37.3X1-**   **Poisoning by other antiprotozoal drugs, accidental (unintentional)**
Poisoning by other antiprotozoal drugs NOS

● New   ▲ Revised   *Manifestation*   ④-☑ Digit Indicators   ⊟ Laterality   Ⓐ Adult (15+ years)   Ⓜ Maternity (12-55 years)   Ⓝ Newborn (0-17 years)   ♂ Male   ♀ Female
✖ ~~Deleted~~   Unspecified   + Additional code

7 T37.3X2- Poisoning by other antiprotozoal drugs, intentional self-harm
7 T37.3X3- Poisoning by other antiprotozoal drugs, assault
7 T37.3X4- Poisoning by other antiprotozoal drugs, undetermined
7 T37.3X5- Adverse effect of other antiprotozoal drugs
7 T37.3X6- Underdosing of other antiprotozoal drugs
5 T37.4 Poisoning by, adverse effect of and underdosing of anthelminthics
6 T37.4X Poisoning by, adverse effect of and underdosing of anthelminthics
7 T37.4X1- Poisoning by anthelminthics, accidental (unintentional)
Poisoning by anthelminthics NOS
7 T37.4X2- Poisoning by anthelminthics, intentional self-harm
7 T37.4X3- Poisoning by anthelminthics, assault
7 T37.4X4- Poisoning by anthelminthics, undetermined
7 T37.4X5- Adverse effect of anthelminthics
7 T37.4X6- Underdosing of anthelminthics
5 T37.5 Poisoning by, adverse effect of and underdosing of antiviral drugs
EXCLUDES 1 *amantadine (T42.8-)*
cytarabine (T45.1-)
6 T37.5X Poisoning by, adverse effect of and underdosing of antiviral drugs
7 T37.5X1- Poisoning by antiviral drugs, accidental (unintentional)
Poisoning by antiviral drugs NOS
7 T37.5X2- Poisoning by antiviral drugs, intentional self-harm
7 T37.5X3- Poisoning by antiviral drugs, assault
7 T37.5X4- Poisoning by antiviral drugs, undetermined
7 T37.5X5- Adverse effect of antiviral drugs
7 T37.5X6- Underdosing of antiviral drugs
5 T37.8 Poisoning by, adverse effect of and underdosing of other specified systemic anti-infectives and antiparasitics
Poisoning by, adverse effect of and underdosing of hydroxyquinoline derivatives
EXCLUDES 1 *antimalarial drugs (T37.2-)*
6 T37.8X Poisoning by, adverse effect of and underdosing of other specified systemic anti-infectives and antiparasitics
7 T37.8X1- Poisoning by other specified systemic anti-infectives and antiparasitics, accidental (unintentional)
Poisoning by other specified systemic anti-infectives and antiparasitics NOS
7 T37.8X2- Poisoning by other specified systemic anti-infectives and antiparasitics, intentional self-harm
7 T37.8X3- Poisoning by other specified systemic anti-infectives and antiparasitics, assault
7 T37.8X4- Poisoning by other specified systemic anti-infectives and antiparasitics, undetermined
7 T37.8X5- Adverse effect of other specified systemic anti-infectives and antiparasitics
7 T37.8X6- Underdosing of other specified systemic anti-infectives and antiparasitics
5 T37.9 Poisoning by, adverse effect of and underdosing of unspecified systemic anti-infective and antiparasitics
7 T37.91X- Poisoning by unspecified systemic anti-infective and antiparasitics, accidental (unintentional)
Poisoning by, adverse effect of and underdosing of systemic anti-infective and antiparasitics NOS
7 T37.92X- Poisoning by unspecified systemic anti-infective and antiparasitics, intentional self-harm
7 T37.93X- Poisoning by unspecified systemic anti-infective and antiparasitics, assault
7 T37.94X- Poisoning by unspecified systemic anti-infective and antiparasitics, undetermined
7 T37.95X- Adverse effect of unspecified systemic anti-infective and antiparasitic
7 T37.96X- Underdosing of unspecified systemic anti-infectives and antiparasitics

4 T38 Poisoning by, adverse effect of and underdosing of hormones and their synthetic substitutes and antagonists, not elsewhere classified
EXCLUDES 1 *mineralocorticoids and their antagonists (T50.0-)*
oxytocic hormones (T48.0-)
parathyroid hormones and derivatives (T50.9-)

The appropriate 7th character is to be added to each code from category T38
A   initial encounter
D   subsequent encounter
S   sequela

5 T38.0 Poisoning by, adverse effect of and underdosing of glucocorticoids and synthetic analogues
EXCLUDES 1 *glucocorticoids, topically used (T49.-)*
6 T38.0X Poisoning by, adverse effect of and underdosing of glucocorticoids and synthetic analogues
7 T38.0X1- Poisoning by glucocorticoids and synthetic analogues, accidental (unintentional)
Poisoning by glucocorticoids and synthetic analogues NOS
7 T38.0X2- Poisoning by glucocorticoids and synthetic analogues, intentional self-harm
7 T38.0X3- Poisoning by glucocorticoids and synthetic analogues, assault
7 T38.0X4- Poisoning by glucocorticoids and synthetic analogues, undetermined
7 T38.0X5- Adverse effect of glucocorticoids and synthetic analogues
7 T38.0X6- Underdosing of glucocorticoids and synthetic analogues
5 T38.1 Poisoning by, adverse effect of and underdosing of thyroid hormones and substitutes
6 T38.1X Poisoning by, adverse effect of and underdosing of thyroid hormones and substitutes
7 T38.1X1- Poisoning by thyroid hormones and substitutes, accidental (unintentional)
Poisoning by thyroid hormones and substitutes NOS
7 T38.1X2- Poisoning by thyroid hormones and substitutes, intentional self-harm
7 T38.1X3- Poisoning by thyroid hormones and substitutes, assault
7 T38.1X4- Poisoning by thyroid hormones and substitutes, undetermined
7 T38.1X5- Adverse effect of thyroid hormones and substitutes
7 T38.1X6- Underdosing of thyroid hormones and substitutes
5 T38.2 Poisoning by, adverse effect of and underdosing of antithyroid drugs
6 T38.2X Poisoning by, adverse effect of and underdosing of antithyroid drugs
7 T38.2X1- Poisoning by antithyroid drugs, accidental (unintentional)
Poisoning by antithyroid drugs NOS
7 T38.2X2- Poisoning by antithyroid drugs, intentional self-harm
7 T38.2X3- Poisoning by antithyroid drugs, assault
7 T38.2X4- Poisoning by antithyroid drugs, undetermined
7 T38.2X5- Adverse effect of antithyroid drugs
7 T38.2X6- Underdosing of antithyroid drugs
5 T38.3 Poisoning by, adverse effect of and underdosing of insulin and oral hypoglycemic [antidiabetic] drugs
6 T38.3X Poisoning by, adverse effect of and underdosing of insulin and oral hypoglycemic [antidiabetic] drugs
7 T38.3X1- Poisoning by insulin and oral hypoglycemic [antidiabetic] drugs, accidental (unintentional)
Poisoning by insulin and oral hypoglycemic [antidiabetic] drugs NOS
GUIDELINES Section I.C.4.a.5)(b)
The principal or first-listed code for an encounter due to an insulin pump malfunction resulting in an overdose of insulin, should also be T85.6-, Mechanical complication of other specified internal and external prosthetic devices, implants and grafts, followed by code T38.3x1-.

7️⃣ T38.3X2- **Poisoning by insulin and oral hypoglycemic [antidiabetic] drugs, intentional self-harm**

7️⃣ T38.3X3- **Poisoning by insulin and oral hypoglycemic [antidiabetic] drugs, assault**

7️⃣ T38.3X4- **Poisoning by insulin and oral hypoglycemic [antidiabetic] drugs, undetermined**

7️⃣ T38.3X5- **Adverse effect of insulin and oral hypoglycemic [antidiabetic] drugs**

7️⃣ T38.3X6- **Underdosing of insulin and oral hypoglycemic [antidiabetic] drugs**

GUIDELINES Section I.C.4.a.5)(a)
An underdose of insulin due to an insulin pump failure should be assigned to a code from subcategory T85.6, Mechanical complication of other specified internal and external prosthetic devices, implants and grafts, followed by code T38.3x6-. Additional codes for the type of diabetes mellitus and any associated complications due to the underdosing should also be assigned.

5️⃣ T38.4 **Poisoning by, adverse effect of and underdosing of oral contraceptives**
Poisoning by, adverse effect of and underdosing of multiple- and single-ingredient oral contraceptive preparations

6️⃣ T38.4X **Poisoning by, adverse effect of and underdosing of oral contraceptives**

7️⃣ T38.4X1- **Poisoning by oral contraceptives, accidental (unintentional)**
Poisoning by oral contraceptives NOS

7️⃣ T38.4X2- **Poisoning by oral contraceptives, intentional self-harm**

7️⃣ T38.4X3- **Poisoning by oral contraceptives, assault**

7️⃣ T38.4X4- **Poisoning by oral contraceptives, undetermined**

7️⃣ T38.4X5- **Adverse effect of oral contraceptives**

7️⃣ T38.4X6- **Underdosing of oral contraceptives**

5️⃣ T38.5 **Poisoning by, adverse effect of and underdosing of other estrogens and progestogens**
Poisoning by, adverse effect of and underdosing of estrogens and progestogens mixtures and substitutes

6️⃣ T38.5X **Poisoning by, adverse effect of and underdosing of other estrogens and progestogens**

7️⃣ T38.5X1- **Poisoning by other estrogens and progestogens, accidental (unintentional)**
Poisoning by other estrogens and progestogens NOS

7️⃣ T38.5X2- **Poisoning by other estrogens and progestogens, intentional self-harm**

7️⃣ T38.5X3- **Poisoning by other estrogens and progestogens, assault**

7️⃣ T38.5X4- **Poisoning by other estrogens and progestogens, undetermined**

7️⃣ T38.5X5- **Adverse effect of other estrogens and progestogens**

7️⃣ T38.5X6- **Underdosing of other estrogens and progestogens**

5️⃣ T38.6 **Poisoning by, adverse effect of and underdosing of antigonadotrophins, antiestrogens, antiandrogens, not elsewhere classified**
Poisoning by, adverse effect of and underdosing of tamoxifen

6️⃣ T38.6X **Poisoning by, adverse effect of and underdosing of antigonadotrophins, antiestrogens, antiandrogens, not elsewhere classified**

7️⃣ T38.6X1- **Poisoning by antigonadotrophins, antiestrogens, antiandrogens, not elsewhere classified, accidental (unintentional)**
Poisoning by antigonadotrophins, antiestrogens, antiandrogens, not elsewhere classified NOS

7️⃣ T38.6X2- **Poisoning by antigonadotrophins, antiestrogens, antiandrogens, not elsewhere classified, intentional self-harm**

7️⃣ T38.6X3- **Poisoning by antigonadotrophins, antiestrogens, antiandrogens, not elsewhere classified, assault**

7️⃣ T38.6X4- **Poisoning by antigonadotrophins, antiestrogens, antiandrogens, not elsewhere classified, undetermined**

7️⃣ T38.6X5- **Adverse effect of antigonadotrophins, antiestrogens, antiandrogens, not elsewhere classified**

7️⃣ T38.6X6- **Underdosing of antigonadotrophins, antiestrogens, antiandrogens, not elsewhere classified**

5️⃣ T38.7 **Poisoning by, adverse effect of and underdosing of androgens and anabolic congeners**

6️⃣ T38.7X **Poisoning by, adverse effect of and underdosing of androgens and anabolic congeners**

7️⃣ T38.7X1- **Poisoning by androgens and anabolic congeners, accidental (unintentional)**
Poisoning by androgens and anabolic congeners NOS

7️⃣ T38.7X2- **Poisoning by androgens and anabolic congeners, intentional self-harm**

7️⃣ T38.7X3- **Poisoning by androgens and anabolic congeners, assault**

7️⃣ T38.7X4- **Poisoning by androgens and anabolic congeners, undetermined**

7️⃣ T38.7X5- **Adverse effect of androgens and anabolic congeners**

7️⃣ T38.7X6- **Underdosing of androgens and anabolic congeners**

5️⃣ T38.8 **Poisoning by, adverse effect of and underdosing of other and unspecified hormones and synthetic substitutes**

6️⃣ T38.80 **Poisoning by, adverse effect of and underdosing of unspecified hormones and synthetic substitutes**

7️⃣ T38.801- **Poisoning by unspecified hormones and synthetic substitutes, accidental (unintentional)**
Poisoning by unspecified hormones and synthetic substitutes NOS

7️⃣ T38.802- **Poisoning by unspecified hormones and synthetic substitutes, intentional self-harm**

7️⃣ T38.803- **Poisoning by unspecified hormones and synthetic substitutes, assault**

7️⃣ T38.804- **Poisoning by unspecified hormones and synthetic substitutes, undetermined**

7️⃣ T38.805- **Adverse effect of unspecified hormones and synthetic substitutes**

7️⃣ T38.806- **Underdosing of unspecified hormones and synthetic substitutes**

6️⃣ T38.81 **Poisoning by, adverse effect of and underdosing of anterior pituitary [adenohypophyseal] hormones**

7️⃣ T38.811- **Poisoning by anterior pituitary [adenohypophyseal] hormones, accidental (unintentional)**
Poisoning by anterior pituitary [adenohypophyseal] hormones NOS

7️⃣ T38.812- **Poisoning by anterior pituitary [adenohypophyseal] hormones, intentional self-harm**

7️⃣ T38.813- **Poisoning by anterior pituitary [adenohypophyseal] hormones, assault**

7️⃣ T38.814- **Poisoning by anterior pituitary [adenohypophyseal] hormones, undetermined**

7️⃣ T38.815- **Adverse effect of anterior pituitary [adenohypophyseal] hormones**

7️⃣ T38.816- **Underdosing of anterior pituitary [adenohypophyseal] hormones**

6️⃣ T38.89 **Poisoning by, adverse effect of and underdosing of other hormones and synthetic substitutes**

7️⃣ T38.891- **Poisoning by other hormones and synthetic substitutes, accidental (unintentional)**
Poisoning by other hormones and synthetic substitutes NOS

7️⃣ T38.892- **Poisoning by other hormones and synthetic substitutes, intentional self-harm**

7️⃣ T38.893- **Poisoning by other hormones and synthetic substitutes, assault**

7️⃣ T38.894- **Poisoning by other hormones and synthetic substitutes, undetermined**

7️⃣ T38.895- **Adverse effect of other hormones and synthetic substitutes**

7️⃣ T38.896- **Underdosing of other hormones and synthetic substitutes**

5️⃣ T38.9 **Poisoning by, adverse effect of and underdosing of other and unspecified hormone antagonists**

6️⃣ T38.90 **Poisoning by, adverse effect of and underdosing of unspecified hormone antagonists**

● New ▲ Revised *Manifestation* 4️⃣-7️⃣ Digit Indicators ⊟ Laterality 🅰 Adult (15+ years) 🅼 Maternity (12-55 years) 🅽 Newborn 🅿 Pediatric (0-17 years) ♂ Male ♀ Female
✖ Deleted Unspecified ✛ Additional code

2017 ICD-10-CM Expert for Physicians

© 2017 decisionHealth

1061

7 **T38.901-** **Poisoning by unspecified hormone antagonists, accidental (unintentional)**
Poisoning by unspecified hormone antagonists NOS

7 **T38.902-** **Poisoning by unspecified hormone antagonists, intentional self-harm**

7 **T38.903-** **Poisoning by unspecified hormone antagonists, assault**

7 **T38.904-** **Poisoning by unspecified hormone antagonists, undetermined**

7 **T38.905-** **Adverse effect of unspecified hormone antagonists**

7 **T38.906-** **Underdosing of unspecified hormone antagonists**

6 **T38.99** **Poisoning by, adverse effect of and underdosing of other hormone antagonists**

7 **T38.991-** **Poisoning by other hormone antagonists, accidental (unintentional)**
Poisoning by other hormone antagonists NOS

7 **T38.992-** **Poisoning by other hormone antagonists, intentional self-harm**

7 **T38.993-** **Poisoning by other hormone antagonists, assault**

7 **T38.994-** **Poisoning by other hormone antagonists, undetermined**

7 **T38.995-** **Adverse effect of other hormone antagonists**

7 **T38.996-** **Underdosing of other hormone antagonists**

4 **T39** **Poisoning by, adverse effect of and underdosing of nonopioid analgesics, antipyretics and antirheumatics**

The appropriate 7th character is to be added to each code from category T39
A   initial encounter
D   subsequent encounter
S   sequela

5 **T39.0** **Poisoning by, adverse effect of and underdosing of salicylates**

6 **T39.01** **Poisoning by, adverse effect of and underdosing of aspirin**
Poisoning by, adverse effect of and underdosing of acetylsalicylic acid

7 **T39.011-** **Poisoning by aspirin, accidental (unintentional)**

7 **T39.012-** **Poisoning by aspirin, intentional self-harm**

7 **T39.013-** **Poisoning by aspirin, assault**

7 **T39.014-** **Poisoning by aspirin, undetermined**

7 **T39.015-** **Adverse effect of aspirin**
AHA: (T39.015A) 1Q 2016, 15

7 **T39.016-** **Underdosing of aspirin**

6 **T39.09** **Poisoning by, adverse effect of and underdosing of other salicylates**

7 **T39.091-** **Poisoning by salicylates, accidental (unintentional)**
Poisoning by salicylates NOS

7 **T39.092-** **Poisoning by salicylates, intentional self-harm**

7 **T39.093-** **Poisoning by salicylates, assault**

7 **T39.094-** **Poisoning by salicylates, undetermined**

7 **T39.095-** **Adverse effect of salicylates**

7 **T39.096-** **Underdosing of salicylates**

5 **T39.1** **Poisoning by, adverse effect of and underdosing of 4-Aminophenol derivatives**

6 **T39.1X** **Poisoning by, adverse effect of and underdosing of 4-Aminophenol derivatives**

7 **T39.1X1-** **Poisoning by 4-Aminophenol derivatives, accidental (unintentional)**
Poisoning by 4-Aminophenol derivatives NOS

7 **T39.1X2-** **Poisoning by 4-Aminophenol derivatives, intentional self-harm**

7 **T39.1X3-** **Poisoning by 4-Aminophenol derivatives, assault**

7 **T39.1X4-** **Poisoning by 4-Aminophenol derivatives, undetermined**

7 **T39.1X5-** **Adverse effect of 4-Aminophenol derivatives**

7 **T39.1X6-** **Underdosing of 4-Aminophenol derivatives**

5 **T39.2** **Poisoning by, adverse effect of and underdosing of pyrazolone derivatives**

6 **T39.2X** **Poisoning by, adverse effect of and underdosing of pyrazolone derivatives**

7 **T39.2X1-** **Poisoning by pyrazolone derivatives, accidental (unintentional)**
Poisoning by pyrazolone derivatives NOS

7 **T39.2X2-** **Poisoning by pyrazolone derivatives, intentional self-harm**

7 **T39.2X3-** **Poisoning by pyrazolone derivatives, assault**

7 **T39.2X4-** **Poisoning by pyrazolone derivatives, undetermined**

7 **T39.2X5-** **Adverse effect of pyrazolone derivatives**

7 **T39.2X6-** **Underdosing of pyrazolone derivatives**

5 **T39.3** **Poisoning by, adverse effect of and underdosing of other nonsteroidal anti-inflammatory drugs [NSAID]**

6 **T39.31** **Poisoning by, adverse effect of and underdosing of propionic acid derivatives**
Poisoning by, adverse effect of and underdosing of fenoprofen
Poisoning by, adverse effect of and underdosing of flurbiprofen
Poisoning by, adverse effect of and underdosing of ibuprofen
Poisoning by, adverse effect of and underdosing of ketoprofen
Poisoning by, adverse effect of and underdosing of naproxen
Poisoning by, adverse effect of and underdosing of oxaprozin

7 **T39.311-** **Poisoning by propionic acid derivatives, accidental (unintentional)**

7 **T39.312-** **Poisoning by propionic acid derivatives, intentional self-harm**

7 **T39.313-** **Poisoning by propionic acid derivatives, assault**

7 **T39.314-** **Poisoning by propionic acid derivatives, undetermined**

7 **T39.315-** **Adverse effect of propionic acid derivatives**

7 **T39.316-** **Underdosing of propionic acid derivatives**

6 **T39.39** **Poisoning by, adverse effect of and underdosing of other nonsteroidal anti-inflammatory drugs [NSAID]**

7 **T39.391-** **Poisoning by other nonsteroidal anti-inflammatory drugs [NSAID], accidental (unintentional)**
Poisoning by other nonsteroidal anti-inflammatory drugs NOS

7 **T39.392-** **Poisoning by other nonsteroidal anti-inflammatory drugs [NSAID], intentional self-harm**

7 **T39.393-** **Poisoning by other nonsteroidal anti-inflammatory drugs [NSAID], assault**

7 **T39.394-** **Poisoning by other nonsteroidal anti-inflammatory drugs [NSAID], undetermined**

7 **T39.395-** **Adverse effect of other nonsteroidal anti-inflammatory drugs [NSAID]**

7 **T39.396-** **Underdosing of other nonsteroidal anti-inflammatory drugs [NSAID]**

5 **T39.4** **Poisoning by, adverse effect of and underdosing of antirheumatics, not elsewhere classified**

EXCLUDES 1 *poisoning by, adverse effect of and underdosing of glucocorticoids (T38.0-)*
poisoning by, adverse effect of and underdosing of salicylates (T39.0-)

6 **T39.4X** **Poisoning by, adverse effect of and underdosing of antirheumatics, not elsewhere classified**

7 **T39.4X1-** **Poisoning by antirheumatics, not elsewhere classified, accidental (unintentional)**
Poisoning by antirheumatics, not elsewhere classified NOS

7 **T39.4X2-** **Poisoning by antirheumatics, not elsewhere classified, intentional self-harm**

7 **T39.4X3-** **Poisoning by antirheumatics, not elsewhere classified, assault**

7 **T39.4X4-** **Poisoning by antirheumatics, not elsewhere classified, undetermined**

7 **T39.4X5-** **Adverse effect of antirheumatics, not elsewhere classified**

7 **T39.4X6-** **Underdosing of antirheumatics, not elsewhere classified**

5 **T39.8** **Poisoning by, adverse effect of and underdosing of other nonopioid analgesics and antipyretics, not elsewhere classified**

● New   ▲ Revised   *Manifestation*   4 - 7 Digit Indicators   ⊟ Laterality   Ⓐ Adult (15+ years)   Ⓜ Maternity (12-55 years)   Ⓝ Newborn   Ⓟ Pediatric (0-17 years)   ♂ Male   ♀ Female
✖ Deleted   Unspecified   + Additional code

1062   © 2017 DecisionHealth   2017 ICD-10-CM Expert for Physicians

6 **T39.8X**   **Poisoning by, adverse effect of and underdosing of other nonopioid analgesics and antipyretics, not elsewhere classified**

   7 **T39.8X1-**   **Poisoning by other nonopioid analgesics and antipyretics, not elsewhere classified, accidental (unintentional)**
      Poisoning by other nonopioid analgesics and antipyretics, not elsewhere classified NOS

   7 **T39.8X2-**   **Poisoning by other nonopioid analgesics and antipyretics, not elsewhere classified, intentional self-harm**

   7 **T39.8X3-**   **Poisoning by other nonopioid analgesics and antipyretics, not elsewhere classified, assault**

   7 **T39.8X4-**   **Poisoning by other nonopioid analgesics and antipyretics, not elsewhere classified, undetermined**

   7 **T39.8X5-**   **Adverse effect of other nonopioid analgesics and antipyretics, not elsewhere classified**

   7 **T39.8X6-**   **Underdosing of other nonopioid analgesics and antipyretics, not elsewhere classified**

5 **T39.9**   **Poisoning by, adverse effect of and underdosing of unspecified nonopioid analgesic, antipyretic and antirheumatic**

   7 **T39.91X-**   **Poisoning by unspecified nonopioid analgesic, antipyretic and antirheumatic, accidental (unintentional)**
      Poisoning by nonopioid analgesic, antipyretic and antirheumatic NOS

   7 **T39.92X-**   **Poisoning by unspecified nonopioid analgesic, antipyretic and antirheumatic, intentional self-harm**

   7 **T39.93X-**   **Poisoning by unspecified nonopioid analgesic, antipyretic and antirheumatic, assault**

   7 **T39.94X-**   **Poisoning by unspecified nonopioid analgesic, antipyretic and antirheumatic, undetermined**

   7 **T39.95X-**   **Adverse effect of unspecified nonopioid analgesic, antipyretic and antirheumatic**

   7 **T39.96X-**   **Underdosing of unspecified nonopioid analgesic, antipyretic and antirheumatic**

4 **T40**   **Poisoning by, adverse effect of and underdosing of narcotics and psychodysleptics [hallucinogens]**

   EXCLUDES 2   *drug dependence and related mental and behavioral disorders due to psychoactive substance use (F10.-F19.-)*

The appropriate 7th character is to be added to each code from category T40
A   initial encounter
D   subsequent encounter
S   sequela

5 **T40.0**   **Poisoning by, adverse effect of and underdosing of opium**

  6 **T40.0X**   **Poisoning by, adverse effect of and underdosing of opium**

   7 **T40.0X1-**   **Poisoning by opium, accidental (unintentional)**
      Poisoning by opium NOS

   7 **T40.0X2-**   **Poisoning by opium, intentional self-harm**

   7 **T40.0X3-**   **Poisoning by opium, assault**

   7 **T40.0X4-**   **Poisoning by opium, undetermined**

   7 **T40.0X5-**   **Adverse effect of opium**

   7 **T40.0X6-**   **Underdosing of opium**

5 **T40.1**   **Poisoning by and adverse effect of heroin**

  6 **T40.1X**   **Poisoning by and adverse effect of heroin**

   7 **T40.1X1-**   **Poisoning by heroin, accidental (unintentional)**
      Poisoning by heroin NOS

   7 **T40.1X2-**   **Poisoning by heroin, intentional self-harm**

   7 **T40.1X3-**   **Poisoning by heroin, assault**

   7 **T40.1X4-**   **Poisoning by heroin, undetermined**

5 **T40.2**   **Poisoning by, adverse effect of and underdosing of other opioids**

  6 **T40.2X**   **Poisoning by, adverse effect of and underdosing of other opioids**

   7 **T40.2X1-**   **Poisoning by other opioids, accidental (unintentional)**
      Poisoning by other opioids NOS

   7 **T40.2X2-**   **Poisoning by other opioids, intentional self-harm**

   7 **T40.2X3-**   **Poisoning by other opioids, assault**

   7 **T40.2X4-**   **Poisoning by other opioids, undetermined**

   7 **T40.2X5-**   **Adverse effect of other opioids**

   7 **T40.2X6-**   **Underdosing of other opioids**

5 **T40.3**   **Poisoning by, adverse effect of and underdosing of methadone**

  6 **T40.3X**   **Poisoning by, adverse effect of and underdosing of methadone**

   7 **T40.3X1-**   **Poisoning by methadone, accidental (unintentional)**
      Poisoning by methadone NOS

   7 **T40.3X2-**   **Poisoning by methadone, intentional self-harm**

   7 **T40.3X3-**   **Poisoning by methadone, assault**

   7 **T40.3X4-**   **Poisoning by methadone, undetermined**

   7 **T40.3X5-**   **Adverse effect of methadone**

   7 **T40.3X6-**   **Underdosing of methadone**

5 **T40.4**   **Poisoning by, adverse effect of and underdosing of other synthetic narcotics**

  6 **T40.4X**   **Poisoning by, adverse effect of and underdosing of other synthetic narcotics**

   7 **T40.4X1-**   **Poisoning by other synthetic narcotics, accidental (unintentional)**
      Poisoning by other synthetic narcotics NOS

   7 **T40.4X2-**   **Poisoning by other synthetic narcotics, intentional self-harm**

   7 **T40.4X3-**   **Poisoning by other synthetic narcotics, assault**

   7 **T40.4X4-**   **Poisoning by other synthetic narcotics, undetermined**

   7 **T40.4X5-**   **Adverse effect of other synthetic narcotics**

   7 **T40.4X6-**   **Underdosing of other synthetic narcotics**

5 **T40.5**   **Poisoning by, adverse effect of and underdosing of cocaine**
    AHA: (T40.5X1A) 2Q 2016, 9

  6 **T40.5X**   **Poisoning by, adverse effect of and underdosing of cocaine**

   7 **T40.5X1-**   **Poisoning by cocaine, accidental (unintentional)**
      Poisoning by cocaine NOS

   7 **T40.5X2-**   **Poisoning by cocaine, intentional self-harm**

   7 **T40.5X3-**   **Poisoning by cocaine, assault**

   7 **T40.5X4-**   **Poisoning by cocaine, undetermined**

   7 **T40.5X5-**   **Adverse effect of cocaine**

   7 **T40.5X6-**   **Underdosing of cocaine**

5 **T40.6**   **Poisoning by, adverse effect of and underdosing of other and unspecified narcotics**

  6 **T40.60**   **Poisoning by, adverse effect of and underdosing of unspecified narcotics**

   7 **T40.601-**   **Poisoning by unspecified narcotics, accidental (unintentional)**
      Poisoning by narcotics NOS

   7 **T40.602-**   **Poisoning by unspecified narcotics, intentional self-harm**

   7 **T40.603-**   **Poisoning by unspecified narcotics, assault**

   7 **T40.604-**   **Poisoning by unspecified narcotics, undetermined**

   7 **T40.605-**   **Adverse effect of unspecified narcotics**

   7 **T40.606-**   **Underdosing of unspecified narcotics**

  6 **T40.69**   **Poisoning by, adverse effect of and underdosing of other narcotics**

   7 **T40.691-**   **Poisoning by other narcotics, accidental (unintentional)**
      Poisoning by other narcotics NOS

   7 **T40.692-**   **Poisoning by other narcotics, intentional self-harm**

   7 **T40.693-**   **Poisoning by other narcotics, assault**

   7 **T40.694-**   **Poisoning by other narcotics, undetermined**

   7 **T40.695-**   **Adverse effect of other narcotics**

   7 **T40.696-**   **Underdosing of other narcotics**

5 **T40.7**   **Poisoning by, adverse effect of and underdosing of cannabis (derivatives)**

  6 **T40.7X**   **Poisoning by, adverse effect of and underdosing of cannabis (derivatives)**

   7 **T40.7X1-**   **Poisoning by cannabis (derivatives), accidental (unintentional)**
      Poisoning by cannabis NOS

● New   ▲ Revised   *Manifestation*   4 - 7 Digit Indicators   ⊟ Laterality   A Adult (15+ years)   M Maternity (12-55 years)   N Newborn   P Pediatric (0-17 years)   ♂ Male   ♀ Female
✖ Deleted   Unspecified   + Additional code

7️⃣ T40.7X2- Poisoning by cannabis (derivatives), intentional self-harm

7️⃣ T40.7X3- Poisoning by cannabis (derivatives), assault

7️⃣ T40.7X4- Poisoning by cannabis (derivatives), undetermined

7️⃣ T40.7X5- Adverse effect of cannabis (derivatives)

7️⃣ T40.7X6- Underdosing of cannabis (derivatives)

5️⃣ T40.8 Poisoning by and adverse effect of lysergide [LSD]

6️⃣ T40.8X Poisoning by and adverse effect of lysergide [LSD]

7️⃣ T40.8X1- Poisoning by lysergide [LSD], accidental (unintentional)
Poisoning by lysergide [LSD]NOS

7️⃣ T40.8X2- Poisoning by lysergide [LSD], intentional self-harm

7️⃣ T40.8X3- Poisoning by lysergide [LSD], assault

7️⃣ T40.8X4- Poisoning by lysergide [LSD], undetermined

5️⃣ T40.9 Poisoning by, adverse effect of and underdosing of other and unspecified psychodysleptics [hallucinogens]

6️⃣ T40.90 Poisoning by, adverse effect of and underdosing of unspecified psychodysleptics [hallucinogens]

7️⃣ T40.901- Poisoning by unspecified psychodysleptics [hallucinogens], accidental (unintentional)

7️⃣ T40.902- Poisoning by unspecified psychodysleptics [hallucinogens], intentional self-harm

7️⃣ T40.903- Poisoning by unspecified psychodysleptics [hallucinogens], assault

7️⃣ T40.904- Poisoning by unspecified psychodysleptics [hallucinogens], undetermined

7️⃣ T40.905- Adverse effect of unspecified psychodysleptics [hallucinogens]

7️⃣ T40.906- Underdosing of unspecified psychodysleptics

6️⃣ T40.99 Poisoning by, adverse effect of and underdosing of other psychodysleptics [hallucinogens]

7️⃣ T40.991- Poisoning by other psychodysleptics [hallucinogens], accidental (unintentional)
Poisoning by other psychodysleptics [hallucinogens] NOS

7️⃣ T40.992- Poisoning by other psychodysleptics [hallucinogens], intentional self-harm

7️⃣ T40.993- Poisoning by other psychodysleptics [hallucinogens], assault

7️⃣ T40.994- Poisoning by other psychodysleptics [hallucinogens], undetermined

7️⃣ T40.995- Adverse effect of other psychodysleptics [hallucinogens]

7️⃣ T40.996- Underdosing of other psychodysleptics

4️⃣ T41 Poisoning by, adverse effect of and underdosing of anesthetics and therapeutic gases

EXCLUDES 1
benzodiazepines (T42.4-)
cocaine (T40.5-)
complications of anesthesia during pregnancy (O29.-)
complications of anesthesia during labor and delivery (O74.-)
complications of anesthesia during the puerperium (O89.-)
opioids (T40.0-T40.2-)

The appropriate 7th character is to be added to each code from category T41
A   initial encounter
D   subsequent encounter
S   sequela

5️⃣ T41.0 Poisoning by, adverse effect of and underdosing of inhaled anesthetics

EXCLUDES 1 oxygen (T41.5-)

6️⃣ T41.0X Poisoning by, adverse effect of and underdosing of inhaled anesthetics

7️⃣ T41.0X1- Poisoning by inhaled anesthetics, accidental (unintentional)
Poisoning by inhaled anesthetics NOS

7️⃣ T41.0X2- Poisoning by inhaled anesthetics, intentional self-harm

7️⃣ T41.0X3- Poisoning by inhaled anesthetics, assault

7️⃣ T41.0X4- Poisoning by inhaled anesthetics, undetermined

7️⃣ T41.0X5- Adverse effect of inhaled anesthetics

7️⃣ T41.0X6- Underdosing of inhaled anesthetics

5️⃣ T41.1 Poisoning by, adverse effect of and underdosing of intravenous anesthetics
Poisoning by, adverse effect of and underdosing of thiobarbiturates

6️⃣ T41.1X Poisoning by, adverse effect of and underdosing of intravenous anesthetics

7️⃣ T41.1X1- Poisoning by intravenous anesthetics, accidental (unintentional)
Poisoning by intravenous anesthetics NOS

7️⃣ T41.1X2- Poisoning by intravenous anesthetics, intentional self-harm

7️⃣ T41.1X3- Poisoning by intravenous anesthetics, assault

7️⃣ T41.1X4- Poisoning by intravenous anesthetics, undetermined

7️⃣ T41.1X5- Adverse effect of intravenous anesthetics

7️⃣ T41.1X6- Underdosing of intravenous anesthetics

5️⃣ T41.2 Poisoning by, adverse effect of and underdosing of other and unspecified general anesthetics

6️⃣ T41.20 Poisoning by, adverse effect of and underdosing of unspecified general anesthetics

7️⃣ T41.201- Poisoning by unspecified general anesthetics, accidental (unintentional)
Poisoning by general anesthetics NOS

7️⃣ T41.202- Poisoning by unspecified general anesthetics, intentional self-harm

7️⃣ T41.203- Poisoning by unspecified general anesthetics, assault

7️⃣ T41.204- Poisoning by unspecified general anesthetics, undetermined

7️⃣ T41.205- Adverse effect of unspecified general anesthetics

7️⃣ T41.206- Underdosing of unspecified general anesthetics

6️⃣ T41.29 Poisoning by, adverse effect of and underdosing of other general anesthetics

7️⃣ T41.291- Poisoning by other general anesthetics, accidental (unintentional)
Poisoning by other general anesthetics NOS

7️⃣ T41.292- Poisoning by other general anesthetics, intentional self-harm

7️⃣ T41.293- Poisoning by other general anesthetics, assault

7️⃣ T41.294- Poisoning by other general anesthetics, undetermined

7️⃣ T41.295- Adverse effect of other general anesthetics

7️⃣ T41.296- Underdosing of other general anesthetics

5️⃣ T41.3 Poisoning by, adverse effect of and underdosing of local anesthetics
Cocaine (topical)

EXCLUDES 2 poisoning by cocaine used as a central nervous system stimulant (T40.5X1-T40.5X4)

6️⃣ T41.3X Poisoning by, adverse effect of and underdosing of local anesthetics

7️⃣ T41.3X1- Poisoning by local anesthetics, accidental (unintentional)
Poisoning by local anesthetics NOS

7️⃣ T41.3X2- Poisoning by local anesthetics, intentional self-harm

7️⃣ T41.3X3- Poisoning by local anesthetics, assault

7️⃣ T41.3X4- Poisoning by local anesthetics, undetermined

7️⃣ T41.3X5- Adverse effect of local anesthetics

7️⃣ T41.3X6- Underdosing of local anesthetics

5️⃣ T41.4 Poisoning by, adverse effect of and underdosing of unspecified anesthetic

7️⃣ T41.41X- Poisoning by unspecified anesthetic, accidental (unintentional)
Poisoning by anesthetic NOS

7️⃣ T41.42X- Poisoning by unspecified anesthetic, intentional self-harm

7️⃣ T41.43X- Poisoning by unspecified anesthetic, assault

7️⃣ T41.44X- Poisoning by unspecified anesthetic, undetermined

7️⃣ T41.45X- Adverse effect of unspecified anesthetic

7️⃣ T41.46X- Underdosing of unspecified anesthetics

5️⃣ T41.5 Poisoning by, adverse effect of and underdosing of therapeutic gases

---

● New ▲ Revised *Manifestation* 4️⃣-7️⃣ Digit Indicators ▣ Laterality 🅰 Adult (15+ years) Ⓜ Maternity (12-55 years) Ⓝ Newborn Ⓟ Pediatric (0-17 years) ♂ Male ♀ Female
✖ Deleted Unspecified + Additional code

1064   © 2017 DecisionHealth   2017 ICD-10-CM Expert for Physicians

☑ **T41.5X** Poisoning by, adverse effect of and underdosing of therapeutic gases

  ☑ **T41.5X1-** Poisoning by therapeutic gases, accidental (unintentional)
      Poisoning by therapeutic gases NOS

  ☑ **T41.5X2-** Poisoning by therapeutic gases, intentional self-harm

  ☑ **T41.5X3-** Poisoning by therapeutic gases, assault

  ☑ **T41.5X4-** Poisoning by therapeutic gases, undetermined

  ☑ **T41.5X5-** Adverse effect of therapeutic gases

  ☑ **T41.5X6-** Underdosing of therapeutic gases

☑ **T42** **Poisoning by, adverse effect of and underdosing of antiepileptic, sedative- hypnotic and antiparkinsonism drugs**

  EXCLUDES 2 *drug dependence and related mental and behavioral disorders due to psychoactive substance use (F10.--F19.-)*

  The appropriate 7th character is to be added to each code from category T42
  A   initial encounter
  D   subsequent encounter
  S   sequela

☑ **T42.0** Poisoning by, adverse effect of and underdosing of hydantoin derivatives

  ☑ **T42.0X** Poisoning by, adverse effect of and underdosing of hydantoin derivatives

    ☑ **T42.0X1-** Poisoning by hydantoin derivatives, accidental (unintentional)
       Poisoning by hydantoin derivatives NOS

    ☑ **T42.0X2-** Poisoning by hydantoin derivatives, intentional self-harm

    ☑ **T42.0X3-** Poisoning by hydantoin derivatives, assault

    ☑ **T42.0X4-** Poisoning by hydantoin derivatives, undetermined

    ☑ **T42.0X5-** Adverse effect of hydantoin derivatives

    ☑ **T42.0X6-** Underdosing of hydantoin derivatives

☑ **T42.1** Poisoning by, adverse effect of and underdosing of iminostilbenes
  Poisoning by, adverse effect of and underdosing of carbamazepine

  ☑ **T42.1X** Poisoning by, adverse effect of and underdosing of iminostilbenes

    ☑ **T42.1X1-** Poisoning by iminostilbenes, accidental (unintentional)
       Poisoning by iminostilbenes NOS

    ☑ **T42.1X2-** Poisoning by iminostilbenes, intentional self-harm

    ☑ **T42.1X3-** Poisoning by iminostilbenes, assault

    ☑ **T42.1X4-** Poisoning by iminostilbenes, undetermined

    ☑ **T42.1X5-** Adverse effect of iminostilbenes

    ☑ **T42.1X6-** Underdosing of iminostilbenes

☑ **T42.2** Poisoning by, adverse effect of and underdosing of succinimides and oxazolidinediones

  ☑ **T42.2X** Poisoning by, adverse effect of and underdosing of succinimides and oxazolidinediones

    ☑ **T42.2X1-** Poisoning by succinimides and oxazolidinediones, accidental (unintentional)
       Poisoning by succinimides and oxazolidinediones NOS

    ☑ **T42.2X2-** Poisoning by succinimides and oxazolidinediones, intentional self-harm

    ☑ **T42.2X3-** Poisoning by succinimides and oxazolidinediones, assault

    ☑ **T42.2X4-** Poisoning by succinimides and oxazolidinediones, undetermined

    ☑ **T42.2X5-** Adverse effect of succinimides and oxazolidinediones

    ☑ **T42.2X6-** Underdosing of succinimides and oxazolidinediones

☑ **T42.3** Poisoning by, adverse effect of and underdosing of barbiturates

  EXCLUDES 1 *poisoning by, adverse effect of and underdosing of thiobarbiturates (T41.1-)*

  ☑ **T42.3X** Poisoning by, adverse effect of and underdosing of barbiturates

    ☑ **T42.3X1-** Poisoning by barbiturates, accidental (unintentional)
       Poisoning by barbiturates NOS

    ☑ **T42.3X2-** Poisoning by barbiturates, intentional self-harm

    ☑ **T42.3X3-** Poisoning by barbiturates, assault

    ☑ **T42.3X4-** Poisoning by barbiturates, undetermined

    ☑ **T42.3X5-** Adverse effect of barbiturates

    ☑ **T42.3X6-** Underdosing of barbiturates

☑ **T42.4** Poisoning by, adverse effect of and underdosing of benzodiazepines

  ☑ **T42.4X** Poisoning by, adverse effect of and underdosing of benzodiazepines

    ☑ **T42.4X1-** Poisoning by benzodiazepines, accidental (unintentional)
       Poisoning by benzodiazepines NOS

    ☑ **T42.4X2-** Poisoning by benzodiazepines, intentional self-harm

    ☑ **T42.4X3-** Poisoning by benzodiazepines, assault

    ☑ **T42.4X4-** Poisoning by benzodiazepines, undetermined

    ☑ **T42.4X5-** Adverse effect of benzodiazepines

    ☑ **T42.4X6-** Underdosing of benzodiazepines

☑ **T42.5** Poisoning by, adverse effect of and underdosing of mixed antiepileptics

  ☑ **T42.5X** Poisoning by, adverse effect of and underdosing of antiepileptics

    ☑ **T42.5X1-** Poisoning by mixed antiepileptics, accidental (unintentional)
       Poisoning by mixed antiepileptics NOS

    ☑ **T42.5X2-** Poisoning by mixed antiepileptics, intentional self-harm

    ☑ **T42.5X3-** Poisoning by mixed antiepileptics, assault

    ☑ **T42.5X4-** Poisoning by mixed antiepileptics, undetermined

    ☑ **T42.5X5-** Adverse effect of mixed antiepileptics

    ☑ **T42.5X6-** Underdosing of mixed antiepileptics

☑ **T42.6** Poisoning by, adverse effect of and underdosing of other antiepileptic and sedative-hypnotic drugs
  Poisoning by, adverse effect of and underdosing of methaqualone
  Poisoning by, adverse effect of and underdosing of valproic acid

  EXCLUDES 1 *poisoning by, adverse effect of and underdosing of carbamazepine (T42.1-)*

  ☑ **T42.6X** Poisoning by, adverse effect of and underdosing of other antiepileptic and sedative-hypnotic drugs

    ☑ **T42.6X1-** Poisoning by other antiepileptic and sedative-hypnotic drugs, accidental (unintentional)
       Poisoning by other antiepileptic and sedative-hypnotic drugs NOS

    ☑ **T42.6X2-** Poisoning by other antiepileptic and sedative-hypnotic drugs, intentional self-harm

    ☑ **T42.6X3-** Poisoning by other antiepileptic and sedative-hypnotic drugs, assault

    ☑ **T42.6X4-** Poisoning by other antiepileptic and sedative-hypnotic drugs, undetermined

    ☑ **T42.6X5-** Adverse effect of other antiepileptic and sedative-hypnotic drugs

    ☑ **T42.6X6-** Underdosing of other antiepileptic and sedative-hypnotic drugs

☑ **T42.7** Poisoning by, adverse effect of and underdosing of unspecified antiepileptic and sedative-hypnotic drugs

  ☑ **T42.71X-** Poisoning by unspecified antiepileptic and sedative-hypnotic drugs, accidental (unintentional)
    Poisoning by antiepileptic and sedative-hypnotic drugs NOS

  ☑ **T42.72X-** Poisoning by unspecified antiepileptic and sedative-hypnotic drugs, intentional self-harm

  ☑ **T42.73X-** Poisoning by unspecified antiepileptic and sedative-hypnotic drugs, assault

  ☑ **T42.74X-** Poisoning by unspecified antiepileptic and sedative-hypnotic drugs, undetermined

  ☑ **T42.75X-** Adverse effect of unspecified antiepileptic and sedative-hypnotic drugs

  ☑ **T42.76X-** Underdosing of unspecified antiepileptic and sedative-hypnotic drugs

☑ **T42.8** Poisoning by, adverse effect of and underdosing of antiparkinsonism drugs and other central muscle-tone depressants
  Poisoning by, adverse effect of and underdosing of amantadine

---

● New ▲ Revised *Manifestation* **4-7** Digit Indicators ▤ Laterality Ⓐ Adult (15+ years) Ⓜ Maternity (12-55 years) Ⓝ Newborn Ⓟ Pediatric (0-17 years) ♂ Male ♀ Female
✖ Deleted Unspecified + Additional code

⑥ T42.8X Poisoning by, adverse effect of and underdosing of antiparkinsonism drugs and other central muscle-tone depressants

⑦ T42.8X1- Poisoning by antiparkinsonism drugs and other central muscle-tone depressants, accidental (unintentional)
Poisoning by antiparkinsonism drugs and other central muscle-tone depressants NOS

⑦ T42.8X2- Poisoning by antiparkinsonism drugs and other central muscle-tone depressants, intentional self-harm

⑦ T42.8X3- Poisoning by antiparkinsonism drugs and other central muscle-tone depressants, assault

⑦ T42.8X4- Poisoning by antiparkinsonism drugs and other central muscle-tone depressants, undetermined

⑦ T42.8X5- Adverse effect of antiparkinsonism drugs and other central muscle-tone depressants

⑦ T42.8X6- Underdosing of antiparkinsonism drugs and other central muscle-tone depressants

④ T43 Poisoning by, adverse effect of and underdosing of psychotropic drugs, not elsewhere classified

EXCLUDES 1 *appetite depressants (T50.5-)*
barbiturates (T42.3-)
benzodiazepines (T42.4-)
methaqualone (T42.6-)
psychodysleptics [hallucinogens] (T40.7-T40.9-)

EXCLUDES 2 *drug dependence and related mental and behavioral disorders due to psychoactive substance use (F10.- -F19.-)*

The appropriate 7th character is to be added to each code from category T43
A   initial encounter
D   subsequent encounter
S   sequela

⑤ T43.0 Poisoning by, adverse effect of and underdosing of tricyclic and tetracyclic antidepressants

⑥ T43.01 Poisoning by, adverse effect of and underdosing of tricyclic antidepressants

⑦ T43.011- Poisoning by tricyclic antidepressants, accidental (unintentional)
Poisoning by tricyclic antidepressants NOS

⑦ T43.012- Poisoning by tricyclic antidepressants, intentional self-harm

⑦ T43.013- Poisoning by tricyclic antidepressants, assault

⑦ T43.014- Poisoning by tricyclic antidepressants, undetermined

⑦ T43.015- Adverse effect of tricyclic antidepressants

⑦ T43.016- Underdosing of tricyclic antidepressants

⑥ T43.02 Poisoning by, adverse effect of and underdosing of tetracyclic antidepressants

⑦ T43.021- Poisoning by tetracyclic antidepressants, accidental (unintentional)
Poisoning by tetracyclic antidepressants NOS

⑦ T43.022- Poisoning by tetracyclic antidepressants, intentional self-harm

⑦ T43.023- Poisoning by tetracyclic antidepressants, assault

⑦ T43.024- Poisoning by tetracyclic antidepressants, undetermined

⑦ T43.025- Adverse effect of tetracyclic antidepressants

⑦ T43.026- Underdosing of tetracyclic antidepressants

⑤ T43.1 Poisoning by, adverse effect of and underdosing of monoamine-oxidase-inhibitor antidepressants

⑥ T43.1X Poisoning by, adverse effect of and underdosing of monoamine-oxidase-inhibitor antidepressants

⑦ T43.1X1- Poisoning by monoamine-oxidase-inhibitor antidepressants, accidental (unintentional)
Poisoning by monoamine-oxidase-inhibitor antidepressants NOS

⑦ T43.1X2- Poisoning by monoamine-oxidase-inhibitor antidepressants, intentional self-harm

⑦ T43.1X3- Poisoning by monoamine-oxidase-inhibitor antidepressants, assault

⑦ T43.1X4- Poisoning by monoamine-oxidase-inhibitor antidepressants, undetermined

⑦ T43.1X5- Adverse effect of monoamine-oxidase-inhibitor antidepressants

⑦ T43.1X6- Underdosing of monoamine-oxidase-inhibitor antidepressants

⑤ T43.2 Poisoning by, adverse effect of and underdosing of other and unspecified antidepressants

⑥ T43.20 Poisoning by, adverse effect of and underdosing of unspecified antidepressants

⑦ T43.201- Poisoning by unspecified antidepressants, accidental (unintentional)
Poisoning by antidepressants NOS

⑦ T43.202- Poisoning by unspecified antidepressants, intentional self-harm

⑦ T43.203- Poisoning by unspecified antidepressants, assault

⑦ T43.204- Poisoning by unspecified antidepressants, undetermined

⑦ T43.205- Adverse effect of unspecified antidepressants

⑦ T43.206- Underdosing of unspecified antidepressants

⑥ T43.21 Poisoning by, adverse effect of and underdosing of selective serotonin and norepinephrine reuptake inhibitors
Poisoning by, adverse effect of and underdosing of SSNRI antidepressants

⑦ T43.211- Poisoning by selective serotonin and norepinephrine reuptake inhibitors, accidental (unintentional)

⑦ T43.212- Poisoning by selective serotonin and norepinephrine reuptake inhibitors, intentional self-harm

⑦ T43.213- Poisoning by selective serotonin and norepinephrine reuptake inhibitors, assault

⑦ T43.214- Poisoning by selective serotonin and norepinephrine reuptake inhibitors, undetermined

⑦ T43.215- Adverse effect of selective serotonin and norepinephrine reuptake inhibitors

⑦ T43.216- Underdosing of selective serotonin and norepinephrine reuptake inhibitors

⑥ T43.22 Poisoning by, adverse effect of and underdosing of selective serotonin reuptake inhibitors
Poisoning by, adverse effect of and underdosing of SSRI antidepressants

⑦ T43.221- Poisoning by selective serotonin reuptake inhibitors, accidental (unintentional)

⑦ T43.222- Poisoning by selective serotonin reuptake inhibitors, intentional self-harm

⑦ T43.223- Poisoning by selective serotonin reuptake inhibitors, assault

⑦ T43.224- Poisoning by selective serotonin reuptake inhibitors, undetermined

⑦ T43.225- Adverse effect of selective serotonin reuptake inhibitors

⑦ T43.226- Underdosing of selective serotonin reuptake inhibitors

⑥ T43.29 Poisoning by, adverse effect of and underdosing of other antidepressants

⑦ T43.291- Poisoning by other antidepressants, accidental (unintentional)
Poisoning by other antidepressants NOS

⑦ T43.292- Poisoning by other antidepressants, intentional self-harm

⑦ T43.293- Poisoning by other antidepressants, assault

⑦ T43.294- Poisoning by other antidepressants, undetermined

⑦ T43.295- Adverse effect of other antidepressants

⑦ T43.296- Underdosing of other antidepressants

⑤ T43.3 Poisoning by, adverse effect of and underdosing of phenothiazine antipsychotics and neuroleptics

⑥ T43.3X Poisoning by, adverse effect of and underdosing of phenothiazine antipsychotics and neuroleptics

⑦ T43.3X1- Poisoning by phenothiazine antipsychotics and neuroleptics, accidental (unintentional)
Poisoning by phenothiazine antipsychotics and neuroleptics NOS

⑦ T43.3X2- Poisoning by phenothiazine antipsychotics and neuroleptics, intentional self-harm

⑦ T43.3X3- Poisoning by phenothiazine antipsychotics and neuroleptics, assault

⑦ T43.3X4- Poisoning by phenothiazine antipsychotics and neuroleptics, undetermined

● New ▲ Revised *Manifestation* ④-⑦ Digit Indicators ▣ Laterality Ⓐ Adult (15+ years) Ⓜ Maternity (12-55 years) Ⓝ Newborn Ⓟ Pediatric (0-17 years) ♂ Male ♀ Female
✖ Deleted Unspecified + Additional code

�7 **T43.3X5-** Adverse effect of phenothiazine antipsychotics and neuroleptics

�7 **T43.3X6-** Underdosing of phenothiazine antipsychotics and neuroleptics

⑤ **T43.4** Poisoning by, adverse effect of and underdosing of butyrophenone and thiothixene neuroleptics

⑥ **T43.4X** Poisoning by, adverse effect of and underdosing of butyrophenone and thiothixene neuroleptics

☐ **T43.4X1-** Poisoning by butyrophenone and thiothixene neuroleptics, accidental (unintentional)
Poisoning by butyrophenone and thiothixene neuroleptics NOS

☐ **T43.4X2-** Poisoning by butyrophenone and thiothixene neuroleptics, intentional self-harm

☐ **T43.4X3-** Poisoning by butyrophenone and thiothixene neuroleptics, assault

☐ **T43.4X4-** Poisoning by butyrophenone and thiothixene neuroleptics, undetermined

☐ **T43.4X5-** Adverse effect of butyrophenone and thiothixene neuroleptics

☐ **T43.4X6-** Underdosing of butyrophenone and thiothixene neuroleptics

⑤ **T43.5** Poisoning by, adverse effect of and underdosing of other and unspecified antipsychotics and neuroleptics

EXCLUDES 1 *poisoning by, adverse effect of and underdosing of rauwolfia (T46.5-)*

⑥ **T43.50** Poisoning by, adverse effect of and underdosing of unspecified antipsychotics and neuroleptics

☐ **T43.501-** Poisoning by unspecified antipsychotics and neuroleptics, accidental (unintentional)
Poisoning by antipsychotics and neuroleptics NOS

☐ **T43.502-** Poisoning by unspecified antipsychotics and neuroleptics, intentional self-harm

☐ **T43.503-** Poisoning by unspecified antipsychotics and neuroleptics, assault

☐ **T43.504-** Poisoning by unspecified antipsychotics and neuroleptics, undetermined

☐ **T43.505-** Adverse effect of unspecified antipsychotics and neuroleptics

☐ **T43.506-** Underdosing of unspecified antipsychotics and neuroleptics

⑥ **T43.59** Poisoning by, adverse effect of and underdosing of other antipsychotics and neuroleptics

☐ **T43.591-** Poisoning by other antipsychotics and neuroleptics, accidental (unintentional)
Poisoning by other antipsychotics and neuroleptics NOS

☐ **T43.592-** Poisoning by other antipsychotics and neuroleptics, intentional self-harm

☐ **T43.593-** Poisoning by other antipsychotics and neuroleptics, assault

☐ **T43.594-** Poisoning by other antipsychotics and neuroleptics, undetermined

☐ **T43.595-** Adverse effect of other antipsychotics and neuroleptics

☐ **T43.596-** Underdosing of other antipsychotics and neuroleptics

⑤ **T43.6** Poisoning by, adverse effect of and underdosing of psychostimulants

EXCLUDES 1 *poisoning by, adverse effect of and underdosing of cocaine (T40.5-)*

⑥ **T43.60** Poisoning by, adverse effect of and underdosing of unspecified psychostimulant

☐ **T43.601-** Poisoning by unspecified psychostimulants, accidental (unintentional)
Poisoning by psychostimulants NOS

☐ **T43.602-** Poisoning by unspecified psychostimulants, intentional self-harm

☐ **T43.603-** Poisoning by unspecified psychostimulants, assault

☐ **T43.604-** Poisoning by unspecified psychostimulants, undetermined

☐ **T43.605-** Adverse effect of unspecified psychostimulants

☐ **T43.606-** Underdosing of unspecified psychostimulants

⑥ **T43.61** Poisoning by, adverse effect of and underdosing of caffeine

☐ **T43.611-** Poisoning by caffeine, accidental (unintentional)
Poisoning by caffeine NOS

☐ **T43.612-** Poisoning by caffeine, intentional self-harm

☐ **T43.613-** Poisoning by caffeine, assault

☐ **T43.614-** Poisoning by caffeine, undetermined

☐ **T43.615-** Adverse effect of caffeine

☐ **T43.616-** Underdosing of caffeine

⑥ **T43.62** Poisoning by, adverse effect of and underdosing of amphetamines
Poisoning by, adverse effect of and underdosing of methamphetamines

☐ **T43.621-** Poisoning by amphetamines, accidental (unintentional)
Poisoning by amphetamines NOS

☐ **T43.622-** Poisoning by amphetamines, intentional self-harm

☐ **T43.623-** Poisoning by amphetamines, assault

☐ **T43.624-** Poisoning by amphetamines, undetermined

☐ **T43.625-** Adverse effect of amphetamines

☐ **T43.626-** Underdosing of amphetamines

⑥ **T43.63** Poisoning by, adverse effect of and underdosing of methylphenidate

☐ **T43.631-** Poisoning by methylphenidate, accidental (unintentional)
Poisoning by methylphenidate NOS

☐ **T43.632-** Poisoning by methylphenidate, intentional self-harm

☐ **T43.633-** Poisoning by methylphenidate, assault

☐ **T43.634-** Poisoning by methylphenidate, undetermined

☐ **T43.635-** Adverse effect of methylphenidate

☐ **T43.636-** Underdosing of methylphenidate

⑥ **T43.69** Poisoning by, adverse effect of and underdosing of other psychostimulants

☐ **T43.691-** Poisoning by other psychostimulants, accidental (unintentional)
Poisoning by other psychostimulants NOS

☐ **T43.692-** Poisoning by other psychostimulants, intentional self-harm

☐ **T43.693-** Poisoning by other psychostimulants, assault

☐ **T43.694-** Poisoning by other psychostimulants, undetermined

☐ **T43.695-** Adverse effect of other psychostimulants

☐ **T43.696-** Underdosing of other psychostimulants

⑤ **T43.8** Poisoning by, adverse effect of and underdosing of other psychotropic drugs

⑥ **T43.8X** Poisoning by, adverse effect of and underdosing of other psychotropic drugs

☐ **T43.8X1-** Poisoning by other psychotropic drugs, accidental (unintentional)
Poisoning by other psychotropic drugs NOS

☐ **T43.8X2-** Poisoning by other psychotropic drugs, intentional self-harm

☐ **T43.8X3-** Poisoning by other psychotropic drugs, assault

☐ **T43.8X4-** Poisoning by other psychotropic drugs, undetermined

☐ **T43.8X5-** Adverse effect of other psychotropic drugs

☐ **T43.8X6-** Underdosing of other psychotropic drugs

⑤ **T43.9** Poisoning by, adverse effect of and underdosing of unspecified psychotropic drug

☐ **T43.91X-** Poisoning by unspecified psychotropic drug, accidental (unintentional)
Poisoning by psychotropic drug NOS

☐ **T43.92X-** Poisoning by unspecified psychotropic drug, intentional self-harm

☐ **T43.93X-** Poisoning by unspecified psychotropic drug, assault

☐ **T43.94X-** Poisoning by unspecified psychotropic drug, undetermined

☐ **T43.95X-** Adverse effect of unspecified psychotropic drug

☐ **T43.96X-** Underdosing of unspecified psychotropic drug

● New ▲ Revised *Manifestation* ☐-☐ Digit Indicators ⊟ Laterality Ⓐ Adult (15+ years) Ⓜ Maternity (12-55 years) Ⓝ Newborn Ⓟ Pediatric (0-17 years) ♂ Male ♀ Female
✖ ~~Deleted~~ Unspecified + Additional code

2017 ICD-10-CM Expert for Physicians

© 2017 DecisionHealth

1067

④ **T44** **Poisoning by, adverse effect of and underdosing of drugs primarily affecting the autonomic nervous system**

The appropriate 7th character is to be added to each code from category T44
A   initial encounter
D   subsequent encounter
S   sequela

⑤ **T44.0** **Poisoning by, adverse effect of and underdosing of anticholinesterase agents**

⑥ **T44.0X** **Poisoning by, adverse effect of and underdosing of anticholinesterase agents**

⑦ **T44.0X1-** **Poisoning by anticholinesterase agents, accidental (unintentional)**
Poisoning by anticholinesterase agents NOS

⑦ **T44.0X2-** **Poisoning by anticholinesterase agents, intentional self-harm**

⑦ **T44.0X3-** **Poisoning by anticholinesterase agents, assault**

⑦ **T44.0X4-** **Poisoning by anticholinesterase agents, undetermined**

⑦ **T44.0X5-** **Adverse effect of anticholinesterase agents**

⑦ **T44.0X6-** **Underdosing of anticholinesterase agents**

⑤ **T44.1** **Poisoning by, adverse effect of and underdosing of other parasympathomimetics [cholinergics]**

⑥ **T44.1X** **Poisoning by, adverse effect of and underdosing of other parasympathomimetics [cholinergics]**

⑦ **T44.1X1-** **Poisoning by other parasympathomimetics [cholinergics], accidental (unintentional)**
Poisoning by other parasympathomimetics [cholinergics] NOS

⑦ **T44.1X2-** **Poisoning by other parasympathomimetics [cholinergics], intentional self-harm**

⑦ **T44.1X3-** **Poisoning by other parasympathomimetics [cholinergics], assault**

⑦ **T44.1X4-** **Poisoning by other parasympathomimetics [cholinergics], undetermined**

⑦ **T44.1X5-** **Adverse effect of other parasympathomimetics [cholinergics]**

⑦ **T44.1X6-** **Underdosing of other parasympathomimetics**

⑤ **T44.2** **Poisoning by, adverse effect of and underdosing of ganglionic blocking drugs**

⑥ **T44.2X** **Poisoning by, adverse effect of and underdosing of ganglionic blocking drugs**

⑦ **T44.2X1-** **Poisoning by ganglionic blocking drugs, accidental (unintentional)**
Poisoning by ganglionic blocking drugs NOS

⑦ **T44.2X2-** **Poisoning by ganglionic blocking drugs, intentional self-harm**

⑦ **T44.2X3-** **Poisoning by ganglionic blocking drugs, assault**

⑦ **T44.2X4-** **Poisoning by ganglionic blocking drugs, undetermined**

⑦ **T44.2X5-** **Adverse effect of ganglionic blocking drugs**

⑦ **T44.2X6-** **Underdosing of ganglionic blocking drugs**

⑤ **T44.3** **Poisoning by, adverse effect of and underdosing of other parasympatholytics [anticholinergics and antimuscarinics] and spasmolytics**
Poisoning by, adverse effect of and underdosing of papaverine

⑥ **T44.3X** **Poisoning by, adverse effect of and underdosing of other parasympatholytics [anticholinergics and antimuscarinics] and spasmolytics**

⑦ **T44.3X1-** **Poisoning by other parasympatholytics [anticholinergics and antimuscarinics] and spasmolytics, accidental (unintentional)**
Poisoning by other parasympatholytics [anticholinergics and antimuscarinics] and spasmolytics NOS

⑦ **T44.3X2-** **Poisoning by other parasympatholytics [anticholinergics and antimuscarinics] and spasmolytics, intentional self-harm**

⑦ **T44.3X3-** **Poisoning by other parasympatholytics [anticholinergics and antimuscarinics] and spasmolytics, assault**

⑦ **T44.3X4-** **Poisoning by other parasympatholytics [anticholinergics and antimuscarinics] and spasmolytics, undetermined**

⑦ **T44.3X5-** **Adverse effect of other parasympatholytics [anticholinergics and antimuscarinics] and spasmolytics**

⑦ **T44.3X6-** **Underdosing of other parasympatholytics [anticholinergics and antimuscarinics] and spasmolytics**

⑤ **T44.4** **Poisoning by, adverse effect of and underdosing of predominantly alpha-adrenoreceptor agonists**
Poisoning by, adverse effect of and underdosing of metaraminol

⑥ **T44.4X** **Poisoning by, adverse effect of and underdosing of predominantly alpha-adrenoreceptor agonists**

⑦ **T44.4X1-** **Poisoning by predominantly alpha-adrenoreceptor agonists, accidental (unintentional)**
Poisoning by predominantly alpha-adrenoreceptor agonists NOS

⑦ **T44.4X2-** **Poisoning by predominantly alpha-adrenoreceptor agonists, intentional self-harm**

⑦ **T44.4X3-** **Poisoning by predominantly alpha-adrenoreceptor agonists, assault**

⑦ **T44.4X4-** **Poisoning by predominantly alpha-adrenoreceptor agonists, undetermined**

⑦ **T44.4X5-** **Adverse effect of predominantly alpha-adrenoreceptor agonists**

⑦ **T44.4X6-** **Underdosing of predominantly alpha-adrenoreceptor agonists**

⑤ **T44.5** **Poisoning by, adverse effect of and underdosing of predominantly beta-adrenoreceptor agonists**

EXCLUDES 1 *poisoning by, adverse effect of and underdosing of beta-adrenoreceptor agonists used in asthma therapy (T48.6-)*

⑥ **T44.5X** **Poisoning by, adverse effect of and underdosing of predominantly beta-adrenoreceptor agonists**

⑦ **T44.5X1-** **Poisoning by predominantly beta-adrenoreceptor agonists, accidental (unintentional)**
Poisoning by predominantly beta-adrenoreceptor agonists NOS

⑦ **T44.5X2-** **Poisoning by predominantly beta-adrenoreceptor agonists, intentional self-harm**

⑦ **T44.5X3-** **Poisoning by predominantly beta-adrenoreceptor agonists, assault**

⑦ **T44.5X4-** **Poisoning by predominantly beta-adrenoreceptor agonists, undetermined**

⑦ **T44.5X5-** **Adverse effect of predominantly beta-adrenoreceptor agonists**

⑦ **T44.5X6-** **Underdosing of predominantly beta-adrenoreceptor agonists**

⑤ **T44.6** **Poisoning by, adverse effect of and underdosing of alpha-adrenoreceptor antagonists**

EXCLUDES 1 *poisoning by, adverse effect of and underdosing of ergot alkaloids (T48.0)*

⑥ **T44.6X** **Poisoning by, adverse effect of and underdosing of alpha-adrenoreceptor antagonists**

⑦ **T44.6X1-** **Poisoning by alpha-adrenoreceptor antagonists, accidental (unintentional)**
Poisoning by alpha-adrenoreceptor antagonists NOS

⑦ **T44.6X2-** **Poisoning by alpha-adrenoreceptor antagonists, intentional self-harm**

⑦ **T44.6X3-** **Poisoning by alpha-adrenoreceptor antagonists, assault**

⑦ **T44.6X4-** **Poisoning by alpha-adrenoreceptor antagonists, undetermined**

⑦ **T44.6X5-** **Adverse effect of alpha-adrenoreceptor antagonists**

⑦ **T44.6X6-** **Underdosing of alpha-adrenoreceptor antagonists**

⑤ **T44.7** **Poisoning by, adverse effect of and underdosing of beta-adrenoreceptor antagonists**

⑥ **T44.7X** **Poisoning by, adverse effect of and underdosing of beta-adrenoreceptor antagonists**

⑦ **T44.7X1-** **Poisoning by beta-adrenoreceptor antagonists, accidental (unintentional)**
Poisoning by beta-adrenoreceptor antagonists NOS

⑦ **T44.7X2-** **Poisoning by beta-adrenoreceptor antagonists, intentional self-harm**

⑦ **T44.7X3-** **Poisoning by beta-adrenoreceptor antagonists, assault**

⑦ **T44.7X4-** **Poisoning by beta-adrenoreceptor antagonists, undetermined**

● New   ▲ Revised   *Manifestation*   ④-⑦ Digit Indicators   ⊟ Laterality   Ⓐ Adult (15+ years)   Ⓜ Maternity (12-55 years)   Ⓝ Newborn   Ⓟ Pediatric (0-17 years)   ♂ Male   ♀ Female
✖ Deleted   Unspecified   + Additional code

T44.7X5- Adverse effect of beta-adrenoreceptor antagonists

T44.7X6- Underdosing of beta-adrenoreceptor antagonists

T44.8 Poisoning by, adverse effect of and underdosing of centrally-acting and adrenergic-neuron- blocking agents

> **EXCLUDES 1** *poisoning by, adverse effect of and underdosing of clonidine (T46.5)*
> *poisoning by, adverse effect of and underdosing of guanethidine (T46.5)*

T44.8X Poisoning by, adverse effect of and underdosing of centrally-acting and adrenergic- neuron-blocking agents

T44.8X1- Poisoning by centrally-acting and adrenergic-neuron-blocking agents, accidental (unintentional)

Poisoning by centrally-acting and adrenergic-neuron-blocking agents NOS

T44.8X2- Poisoning by centrally-acting and adrenergic-neuron-blocking agents, intentional self-harm

T44.8X3- Poisoning by centrally-acting and adrenergic-neuron-blocking agents, assault

T44.8X4- Poisoning by centrally-acting and adrenergic-neuron-blocking agents, undetermined

T44.8X5- Adverse effect of centrally-acting and adrenergic-neuron-blocking agents

T44.8X6- Underdosing of centrally-acting and adrenergic-neuron-blocking agents

T44.9 Poisoning by, adverse effect of and underdosing of other and unspecified drugs primarily affecting the autonomic nervous system

Poisoning by, adverse effect of and underdosing of drug stimulating both alpha and beta-adrenoreceptors

T44.90 Poisoning by, adverse effect of and underdosing of unspecified drugs primarily affecting the autonomic nervous system

T44.901- Poisoning by unspecified drugs primarily affecting the autonomic nervous system, accidental (unintentional)

Poisoning by unspecified drugs primarily affecting the autonomic nervous system NOS

T44.902- Poisoning by unspecified drugs primarily affecting the autonomic nervous system, intentional self-harm

T44.903- Poisoning by unspecified drugs primarily affecting the autonomic nervous system, assault

T44.904- Poisoning by unspecified drugs primarily affecting the autonomic nervous system, undetermined

T44.905- Adverse effect of unspecified drugs primarily affecting the autonomic nervous system

T44.906- Underdosing of unspecified drugs primarily affecting the autonomic nervous system

T44.99 Poisoning by, adverse effect of and underdosing of other drugs primarily affecting the autonomic nervous system

T44.991- Poisoning by other drug primarily affecting the autonomic nervous system, accidental (unintentional)

Poisoning by other drugs primarily affecting the autonomic nervous system NOS

T44.992- Poisoning by other drug primarily affecting the autonomic nervous system, intentional self-harm

T44.993- Poisoning by other drug primarily affecting the autonomic nervous system, assault

T44.994- Poisoning by other drug primarily affecting the autonomic nervous system, undetermined

T44.995- Adverse effect of other drug primarily affecting the autonomic nervous system

T44.996- Underdosing of other drug primarily affecting the autonomic nervous system

T45 Poisoning by, adverse effect of and underdosing of primarily systemic and hematological agents, not elsewhere classified

> The appropriate 7th character is to be added to each code from category T45.
> A initial encounter
> D subsequent encounter
> S sequela

T45.0 Poisoning by, adverse effect of and underdosing of antiallergic and antiemetic drugs

> **EXCLUDES 1** *poisoning by, adverse effect of and underdosing of phenothiazine-based neuroleptics (T43.3)*

T45.0X Poisoning by, adverse effect of and underdosing of antiallergic and antiemetic drugs

T45.0X1- Poisoning by antiallergic and antiemetic drugs, accidental (unintentional)

Poisoning by antiallergic and antiemetic drugs NOS

T45.0X2- Poisoning by antiallergic and antiemetic drugs, intentional self-harm

T45.0X3- Poisoning by antiallergic and antiemetic drugs, assault

T45.0X4- Poisoning by antiallergic and antiemetic drugs, undetermined

T45.0X5- Adverse effect of antiallergic and antiemetic drugs

T45.0X6- Underdosing of antiallergic and antiemetic drugs

T45.1 Poisoning by, adverse effect of and underdosing of antineoplastic and immunosuppressive drugs

> **EXCLUDES 1** *poisoning by, adverse effect of and underdosing of tamoxifen (T38.6)*

T45.1X Poisoning by, adverse effect of and underdosing of antineoplastic and immunosuppressive drugs

T45.1X1- Poisoning by antineoplastic and immunosuppressive drugs, accidental (unintentional)

Poisoning by antineoplastic and immunosuppressive drugs NOS

T45.1X2- Poisoning by antineoplastic and immunosuppressive drugs, intentional self-harm

T45.1X3- Poisoning by antineoplastic and immunosuppressive drugs, assault

T45.1X4- Poisoning by antineoplastic and immunosuppressive drugs, undetermined

T45.1X5- Adverse effect of antineoplastic and immunosuppressive drugs

AHA: (T45.1X5A) 4Q 2014, 22

T45.1X6- Underdosing of antineoplastic and immunosuppressive drugs

T45.2 Poisoning by, adverse effect of and underdosing of vitamins

> **EXCLUDES 2** *poisoning by, adverse effect of and underdosing of nicotinic acid (derivatives) (T46.7)*
> *poisoning by, adverse effect of and underdosing of iron (T45.4)*
> *poisoning by, adverse effect of and underdosing of vitamin K (T45.7)*

T45.2X Poisoning by, adverse effect of and underdosing of vitamins

T45.2X1- Poisoning by vitamins, accidental (unintentional)

Poisoning by vitamins NOS

T45.2X2- Poisoning by vitamins, intentional self-harm

T45.2X3- Poisoning by vitamins, assault

T45.2X4- Poisoning by vitamins, undetermined

T45.2X5- Adverse effect of vitamins

T45.2X6- Underdosing of vitamins

> **EXCLUDES 1** *vitamin deficiencies (E50-E56)*

T45.3 Poisoning by, adverse effect of and underdosing of enzymes

T45.3X Poisoning by, adverse effect of and underdosing of enzymes

T45.3X1- Poisoning by enzymes, accidental (unintentional)

Poisoning by enzymes NOS

T45.3X2- Poisoning by enzymes, intentional self-harm

● New ▲ Revised *Manifestation* ◢-�%0 Digit Indicators ▣ Laterality Ⓐ Adult (15+ years) Ⓜ Maternity (12-55 years) Ⓝ Newborn Ⓟ Pediatric (0-17 years) ♂ Male ♀ Female
✖ Deleted Unspecified ✚ Additional code

2017 ICD-10-CM Expert for Physicians © 2017 DecisionHealth 1069

7 T45.3X3- **Poisoning by enzymes, assault**
7 T45.3X4- **Poisoning by enzymes, undetermined**
7 T45.3X5- **Adverse effect of enzymes**
7 T45.3X6- **Underdosing of enzymes**
5 T45.4 **Poisoning by, adverse effect of and underdosing of iron and its compounds**
6 T45.4X **Poisoning by, adverse effect of and underdosing of iron and its compounds**
7 T45.4X1- **Poisoning by iron and its compounds, accidental (unintentional)**
Poisoning by iron and its compounds NOS
7 T45.4X2- **Poisoning by iron and its compounds, intentional self-harm**
7 T45.4X3- **Poisoning by iron and its compounds, assault**
7 T45.4X4- **Poisoning by iron and its compounds, undetermined**
7 T45.4X5- **Adverse effect of iron and its compounds**
7 T45.4X6- **Underdosing of iron and its compounds**
EXCLUDES 1 *iron deficiency (E61.1)*
5 T45.5 **Poisoning by, adverse effect of and underdosing of anticoagulants and antithrombotic drugs**
6 T45.51 **Poisoning by, adverse effect of and underdosing of anticoagulants**
7 T45.511- **Poisoning by anticoagulants, accidental (unintentional)**
Poisoning by anticoagulants NOS
7 T45.512- **Poisoning by anticoagulants, intentional self-harm**
7 T45.513- **Poisoning by anticoagulants, assault**
7 T45.514- **Poisoning by anticoagulants, undetermined**
7 T45.515- **Adverse effect of anticoagulants**
AHA: 1Q 2016, 14
AHA: 2Q 2013, 35
7 T45.516- **Underdosing of anticoagulants**
6 T45.52 **Poisoning by, adverse effect of and underdosing of antithrombotic drugs**
Poisoning by, adverse effect of and underdosing of antiplatelet drugs
EXCLUDES 2 *poisoning by, adverse effect of and underdosing of aspirin (T39.01-)*
poisoning by, adverse effect of and underdosing of acetylsalicylic acid (T39.01-)
7 T45.521- **Poisoning by antithrombotic drugs, accidental (unintentional)**
Poisoning by antithrombotic drug NOS
7 T45.522- **Poisoning by antithrombotic drugs, intentional self-harm**
7 T45.523- **Poisoning by antithrombotic drugs, assault**
7 T45.524- **Poisoning by antithrombotic drugs, undetermined**
7 T45.525- **Adverse effect of antithrombotic drugs**
AHA: (T45.525A) 1Q 2016, 15
7 T45.526- **Underdosing of antithrombotic drugs**
5 T45.6 **Poisoning by, adverse effect of and underdosing of fibrinolysis-affecting drugs**
6 T45.60 **Poisoning by, adverse effect of and underdosing of unspecified fibrinolysis-affecting drugs**
7 T45.601- **Poisoning by unspecified fibrinolysis-affecting drugs, accidental (unintentional)**
Poisoning by fibrinolysis-affecting drug NOS
7 T45.602- **Poisoning by unspecified fibrinolysis-affecting drugs, intentional self-harm**
7 T45.603- **Poisoning by unspecified fibrinolysis-affecting drugs, assault**
7 T45.604- **Poisoning by unspecified fibrinolysis-affecting drugs, undetermined**
7 T45.605- **Adverse effect of unspecified fibrinolysis-affecting drugs**
7 T45.606- **Underdosing of unspecified fibrinolysis-affecting drugs**
6 T45.61 **Poisoning by, adverse effect of and underdosing of thrombolytic drugs**
7 T45.611- **Poisoning by thrombolytic drug, accidental (unintentional)**
Poisoning by thrombolytic drug NOS
7 T45.612- **Poisoning by thrombolytic drug, intentional self-harm**

7 T45.613- **Poisoning by thrombolytic drug, assault**
7 T45.614- **Poisoning by thrombolytic drug, undetermined**
7 T45.615- **Adverse effect of thrombolytic drugs**
7 T45.616- **Underdosing of thrombolytic drugs**
6 T45.62 **Poisoning by, adverse effect of and underdosing of hemostatic drugs**
7 T45.621- **Poisoning by hemostatic drug, accidental (unintentional)**
Poisoning by hemostatic drug NOS
7 T45.622- **Poisoning by hemostatic drug, intentional self-harm**
7 T45.623- **Poisoning by hemostatic drug, assault**
7 T45.624- **Poisoning by hemostatic drug, undetermined**
7 T45.625- **Adverse effect of hemostatic drug**
7 T45.626- **Underdosing of hemostatic drugs**
6 T45.69 **Poisoning by, adverse effect of and underdosing of other fibrinolysis-affecting drugs**
7 T45.691- **Poisoning by other fibrinolysis-affecting drugs, accidental (unintentional)**
Poisoning by other fibrinolysis-affecting drug NOS
7 T45.692- **Poisoning by other fibrinolysis-affecting drugs, intentional self-harm**
7 T45.693- **Poisoning by other fibrinolysis-affecting drugs, assault**
7 T45.694- **Poisoning by other fibrinolysis-affecting drugs, undetermined**
7 T45.695- **Adverse effect of other fibrinolysis-affecting drugs**
7 T45.696- **Underdosing of other fibrinolysis-affecting drugs**
5 T45.7 **Poisoning by, adverse effect of and underdosing of anticoagulant antagonists, vitamin K and other coagulants**
6 T45.7X **Poisoning by, adverse effect of and underdosing of anticoagulant antagonists, vitamin K and other coagulants**
7 T45.7X1- **Poisoning by anticoagulant antagonists, vitamin K and other coagulants, accidental (unintentional)**
Poisoning by anticoagulant antagonists, vitamin K and other coagulants NOS
7 T45.7X2- **Poisoning by anticoagulant antagonists, vitamin K and other coagulants, intentional self-harm**
7 T45.7X3- **Poisoning by anticoagulant antagonists, vitamin K and other coagulants, assault**
7 T45.7X4- **Poisoning by anticoagulant antagonists, vitamin K and other coagulants, undetermined**
7 T45.7X5- **Adverse effect of anticoagulant antagonists, vitamin K and other coagulants**
7 T45.7X6- **Underdosing of anticoagulant antagonist, vitamin K and other coagulants**
EXCLUDES 1 *vitamin K deficiency (E56.1)*
5 T45.8 **Poisoning by, adverse effect of and underdosing of other primarily systemic and hematological agents**
Poisoning by, adverse effect of and underdosing of liver preparations and other antianemic agents
Poisoning by, adverse effect of and underdosing of natural blood and blood products
Poisoning by, adverse effect of and underdosing of plasma substitute
EXCLUDES 2 *poisoning by, adverse effect of and underdosing of immunoglobulin (T50.Z1)*
poisoning by, adverse effect of and underdosing of iron (T45.4)
transfusion reactions (T80.-)
6 T45.8X **Poisoning by, adverse effect of and underdosing of other primarily systemic and hematological agents**
7 T45.8X1- **Poisoning by other primarily systemic and hematological agents, accidental (unintentional)**
Poisoning by other primarily systemic and hematological agents NOS
7 T45.8X2- **Poisoning by other primarily systemic and hematological agents, intentional self-harm**
7 T45.8X3- **Poisoning by other primarily systemic and hematological agents, assault**
7 T45.8X4- **Poisoning by other primarily systemic and hematological agents, undetermined**

● New ▲ Revised *Manifestation* 4-7 Digit Indicators ⊟ Laterality Ⓐ Adult (15+ years) Ⓜ Maternity (12-55 years) Ⓝ Newborn Ⓟ Pediatric (0-17 years) ♂ Male ♀ Female
✖ Deleted Unspecified + Additional code

☑ **T45.8X5-** Adverse effect of other primarily systemic and hematological agents

☑ **T45.8X6-** Underdosing of other primarily systemic and hematological agents

⑤ **T45.9** Poisoning by, adverse effect of and underdosing of unspecified primarily systemic and hematological agent

☑ **T45.91X-** Poisoning by unspecified primarily systemic and hematological agent, accidental (unintentional)
Poisoning by primarily systemic and hematological agent NOS

☑ **T45.92X-** Poisoning by unspecified primarily systemic and hematological agent, intentional self-harm

☑ **T45.93X-** Poisoning by unspecified primarily systemic and hematological agent, assault

☑ **T45.94X-** Poisoning by unspecified primarily systemic and hematological agent, undetermined

☑ **T45.95X-** Adverse effect of unspecified primarily systemic and hematological agent

☑ **T45.96X-** Underdosing of unspecified primarily systemic and hematological agent

④ **T46** **Poisoning by, adverse effect of and underdosing of agents primarily affecting the cardiovascular system**
EXCLUDES 1 *poisoning by, adverse effect of and underdosing of metaraminol (T44.4)*

The appropriate 7th character is to be added to each code from category T46
A   initial encounter
D   subsequent encounter
S   sequela

⑤ **T46.0** Poisoning by, adverse effect of and underdosing of cardiac-stimulant glycosides and drugs of similar action

⑥ **T46.0X** Poisoning by, adverse effect of and underdosing of cardiac-stimulant glycosides and drugs of similar action

☑ **T46.0X1-** Poisoning by cardiac-stimulant glycosides and drugs of similar action, accidental (unintentional)
Poisoning by cardiac-stimulant glycosides and drugs of similar action NOS

☑ **T46.0X2-** Poisoning by cardiac-stimulant glycosides and drugs of similar action, intentional self-harm

☑ **T46.0X3-** Poisoning by cardiac-stimulant glycosides and drugs of similar action, assault

☑ **T46.0X4-** Poisoning by cardiac-stimulant glycosides and drugs of similar action, undetermined

☑ **T46.0X5-** Adverse effect of cardiac-stimulant glycosides and drugs of similar action

☑ **T46.0X6-** Underdosing of cardiac-stimulant glycosides and drugs of similar action

⑤ **T46.1** Poisoning by, adverse effect of and underdosing of calcium-channel blockers

⑥ **T46.1X** Poisoning by, adverse effect of and underdosing of calcium-channel blockers

☑ **T46.1X1-** Poisoning by calcium-channel blockers, accidental (unintentional)
Poisoning by calcium-channel blockers NOS

☑ **T46.1X2-** Poisoning by calcium-channel blockers, intentional self-harm

☑ **T46.1X3-** Poisoning by calcium-channel blockers, assault

☑ **T46.1X4-** Poisoning by calcium-channel blockers, undetermined

☑ **T46.1X5-** Adverse effect of calcium-channel blockers

☑ **T46.1X6-** Underdosing of calcium-channel blockers

⑤ **T46.2** Poisoning by, adverse effect of and underdosing of other antidysrhythmic drugs, not elsewhere classified
EXCLUDES 1 *poisoning by, adverse effect of and underdosing of beta-adrenoreceptor antagonists (T44.7-)*

⑥ **T46.2X** Poisoning by, adverse effect of and underdosing of other antidysrhythmic drugs

☑ **T46.2X1-** Poisoning by other antidysrhythmic drugs, accidental (unintentional)
Poisoning by other antidysrhythmic drugs NOS

☑ **T46.2X2-** Poisoning by other antidysrhythmic drugs, intentional self-harm

☑ **T46.2X3-** Poisoning by other antidysrhythmic drugs, assault

☑ **T46.2X4-** Poisoning by other antidysrhythmic drugs, undetermined

☑ **T46.2X5-** Adverse effect of other antidysrhythmic drugs

☑ **T46.2X6-** Underdosing of other antidysrhythmic drugs

⑤ **T46.3** Poisoning by, adverse effect of and underdosing of coronary vasodilators
Poisoning by, adverse effect of and underdosing of dipyridamole
EXCLUDES 1 *poisoning by, adverse effect of and underdosing of calcium-channel blockers (T46.1)*

⑥ **T46.3X** Poisoning by, adverse effect of and underdosing of coronary vasodilators

☑ **T46.3X1-** Poisoning by coronary vasodilators, accidental (unintentional)
Poisoning by coronary vasodilators NOS

☑ **T46.3X2-** Poisoning by coronary vasodilators, intentional self-harm

☑ **T46.3X3-** Poisoning by coronary vasodilators, assault

☑ **T46.3X4-** Poisoning by coronary vasodilators, undetermined

☑ **T46.3X5-** Adverse effect of coronary vasodilators

☑ **T46.3X6-** Underdosing of coronary vasodilators

⑤ **T46.4** Poisoning by, adverse effect of and underdosing of angiotensin-converting-enzyme inhibitors

⑥ **T46.4X** Poisoning by, adverse effect of and underdosing of angiotensin-converting-enzyme inhibitors

☑ **T46.4X1-** Poisoning by angiotensin-converting-enzyme inhibitors, accidental (unintentional)
Poisoning by angiotensin-converting-enzyme inhibitors NOS

☑ **T46.4X2-** Poisoning by angiotensin-converting-enzyme inhibitors, intentional self-harm

☑ **T46.4X3-** Poisoning by angiotensin-converting-enzyme inhibitors, assault

☑ **T46.4X4-** Poisoning by angiotensin-converting-enzyme inhibitors, undetermined

☑ **T46.4X5-** Adverse effect of angiotensin-converting-enzyme inhibitors

☑ **T46.4X6-** Underdosing of angiotensin-converting-enzyme inhibitors

⑤ **T46.5** Poisoning by, adverse effect of and underdosing of other antihypertensive drugs
EXCLUDES 2 *poisoning by, adverse effect of and underdosing of beta-adrenoreceptor antagonists (T44.7)*
poisoning by, adverse effect of and underdosing of calcium-channel blockers (T46.1)
poisoning by, adverse effect of and underdosing of diuretics (T50.0-T50.2)

⑥ **T46.5X** Poisoning by, adverse effect of and underdosing of other antihypertensive drugs

☑ **T46.5X1-** Poisoning by other antihypertensive drugs, accidental (unintentional)
Poisoning by other antihypertensive drugs NOS

☑ **T46.5X2-** Poisoning by other antihypertensive drugs, intentional self-harm

☑ **T46.5X3-** Poisoning by other antihypertensive drugs, assault

☑ **T46.5X4-** Poisoning by other antihypertensive drugs, undetermined

☑ **T46.5X5-** Adverse effect of other antihypertensive drugs

☑ **T46.5X6-** Underdosing of other antihypertensive drugs

⑤ **T46.6** Poisoning by, adverse effect of and underdosing of antihyperlipidemic and antiarteriosclerotic drugs

⑥ **T46.6X** Poisoning by, adverse effect of and underdosing of antihyperlipidemic and antiarteriosclerotic drugs

☑ **T46.6X1-** Poisoning by antihyperlipidemic and antiarteriosclerotic drugs, accidental (unintentional)
Poisoning by antihyperlipidemic and antiarteriosclerotic drugs NOS

☑ **T46.6X2-** Poisoning by antihyperlipidemic and antiarteriosclerotic drugs, intentional self-harm

☑ **T46.6X3-** Poisoning by antihyperlipidemic and antiarteriosclerotic drugs, assault

☑ **T46.6X4-** Poisoning by antihyperlipidemic and antiarteriosclerotic drugs, undetermined

☑ **T46.6X5-** Adverse effect of antihyperlipidemic and antiarteriosclerotic drugs

---

● New   ▲ Revised   *Manifestation*   ④-☑ Digit Indicators   ⊟ Laterality   Ⓐ Adult (15+ years)   Ⓜ Maternity (12-55 years)   Ⓝ Newborn   Ⓟ Pediatric (0-17 years)   ♂ Male   ♀ Female
✖ Deleted   Unspecified   + Additional code

T46.6X6- Underdosing of antihyperlipidemic and antiarteriosclerotic drugs

T46.7 Poisoning by, adverse effect of and underdosing of peripheral vasodilators

Poisoning by, adverse effect of and underdosing of nicotinic acid (derivatives)

> **EXCLUDES 1** *poisoning by, adverse effect of and underdosing of papaverine (T44.3)*

T46.7X Poisoning by, adverse effect of and underdosing of peripheral vasodilators

T46.7X1- Poisoning by peripheral vasodilators, accidental (unintentional)

Poisoning by peripheral vasodilators NOS

T46.7X2- Poisoning by peripheral vasodilators, intentional self-harm

T46.7X3- Poisoning by peripheral vasodilators, assault

T46.7X4- Poisoning by peripheral vasodilators, undetermined

T46.7X5- Adverse effect of peripheral vasodilators

T46.7X6- Underdosing of peripheral vasodilators

T46.8 Poisoning by, adverse effect of and underdosing of antivaricose drugs, including sclerosing agents

T46.8X Poisoning by, adverse effect of and underdosing of antivaricose drugs, including sclerosing agents

T46.8X1- Poisoning by antivaricose drugs, including sclerosing agents, accidental (unintentional)

Poisoning by antivaricose drugs, including sclerosing agents NOS

T46.8X2- Poisoning by antivaricose drugs, including sclerosing agents, intentional self-harm

T46.8X3- Poisoning by antivaricose drugs, including sclerosing agents, assault

T46.8X4- Poisoning by antivaricose drugs, including sclerosing agents, undetermined

T46.8X5- Adverse effect of antivaricose drugs, including sclerosing agents

T46.8X6- Underdosing of antivaricose drugs, including sclerosing agents

T46.9 Poisoning by, adverse effect of and underdosing of other and unspecified agents primarily affecting the cardiovascular system

T46.90 Poisoning by, adverse effect of and underdosing of unspecified agents primarily affecting the cardiovascular system

T46.901- Poisoning by unspecified agents primarily affecting the cardiovascular system, accidental (unintentional)

T46.902- Poisoning by unspecified agents primarily affecting the cardiovascular system, intentional self-harm

T46.903- Poisoning by unspecified agents primarily affecting the cardiovascular system, assault

T46.904- Poisoning by unspecified agents primarily affecting the cardiovascular system, undetermined

T46.905- Adverse effect of unspecified agents primarily affecting the cardiovascular system

T46.906- Underdosing of unspecified agents primarily affecting the cardiovascular system

T46.99 Poisoning by, adverse effect of and underdosing of other agents primarily affecting the cardiovascular system

T46.991- Poisoning by other agents primarily affecting the cardiovascular system, accidental (unintentional)

T46.992- Poisoning by other agents primarily affecting the cardiovascular system, intentional self-harm

T46.993- Poisoning by other agents primarily affecting the cardiovascular system, assault

T46.994- Poisoning by other agents primarily affecting the cardiovascular system, undetermined

T46.995- Adverse effect of other agents primarily affecting the cardiovascular system

T46.996- Underdosing of other agents primarily affecting the cardiovascular system

T47 Poisoning by, adverse effect of and underdosing of agents primarily affecting the gastrointestinal system

The appropriate 7th character is to be added to each code from category T47
A   initial encounter
D   subsequent encounter
S   sequela

T47.0 Poisoning by, adverse effect of and underdosing of histamine H2-receptor blockers

T47.0X Poisoning by, adverse effect of and underdosing of histamine H2-receptor blockers

T47.0X1- Poisoning by histamine H2-receptor blockers, accidental (unintentional)

Poisoning by histamine H2-receptor blockers NOS

T47.0X2- Poisoning by histamine H2-receptor blockers, intentional self-harm

T47.0X3- Poisoning by histamine H2-receptor blockers, assault

T47.0X4- Poisoning by histamine H2-receptor blockers, undetermined

T47.0X5- Adverse effect of histamine H2-receptor blockers

T47.0X6- Underdosing of histamine H2-receptor blockers

T47.1 Poisoning by, adverse effect of and underdosing of other antacids and anti-gastric-secretion drugs

T47.1X Poisoning by, adverse effect of and underdosing of other antacids and anti-gastric-secretion drugs

T47.1X1- Poisoning by other antacids and anti-gastric-secretion drugs, accidental (unintentional)

Poisoning by other antacids and anti-gastric-secretion drugs NOS

T47.1X2- Poisoning by other antacids and anti-gastric-secretion drugs, intentional self-harm

T47.1X3- Poisoning by other antacids and anti-gastric-secretion drugs, assault

T47.1X4- Poisoning by other antacids and anti-gastric-secretion drugs, undetermined

T47.1X5- Adverse effect of other antacids and anti-gastric-secretion drugs

T47.1X6- Underdosing of other antacids and anti-gastric-secretion drugs

T47.2 Poisoning by, adverse effect of and underdosing of stimulant laxatives

T47.2X Poisoning by, adverse effect of and underdosing of stimulant laxatives

T47.2X1- Poisoning by stimulant laxatives, accidental (unintentional)

Poisoning by stimulant laxatives NOS

T47.2X2- Poisoning by stimulant laxatives, intentional self-harm

T47.2X3- Poisoning by stimulant laxatives, assault

T47.2X4- Poisoning by stimulant laxatives, undetermined

T47.2X5- Adverse effect of stimulant laxatives

T47.2X6- Underdosing of stimulant laxatives

T47.3 Poisoning by, adverse effect of and underdosing of saline and osmotic laxatives

T47.3X Poisoning by and adverse effect of saline and osmotic laxatives

T47.3X1- Poisoning by saline and osmotic laxatives, accidental (unintentional)

Poisoning by saline and osmotic laxatives NOS

T47.3X2- Poisoning by saline and osmotic laxatives, intentional self-harm

T47.3X3- Poisoning by saline and osmotic laxatives, assault

T47.3X4- Poisoning by saline and osmotic laxatives, undetermined

T47.3X5- Adverse effect of saline and osmotic laxatives

T47.3X6- Underdosing of saline and osmotic laxatives

T47.4 Poisoning by, adverse effect of and underdosing of other laxatives

T47.4X Poisoning by, adverse effect of and underdosing of other laxatives

T47.4X1- Poisoning by other laxatives, accidental (unintentional)

Poisoning by other laxatives NOS

● New   ▲ Revised   *Manifestation*   4-7 Digit Indicators   ▤ Laterality   Ⓐ Adult (15+ years)   Ⓜ Maternity (12-55 years)   Ⓝ Newborn   Ⓟ Pediatric (0-17 years)   ♂ Male   ♀ Female
✖ Deleted   Unspecified   + Additional code

7 T47.4X2- **Poisoning by other laxatives, intentional self-harm**

7 T47.4X3- **Poisoning by other laxatives, assault**

7 T47.4X4- **Poisoning by other laxatives, undetermined**

7 T47.4X5- **Adverse effect of other laxatives**

7 T47.4X6- **Underdosing of other laxatives**

5 T47.5 **Poisoning by, adverse effect of and underdosing of digestants**

6 T47.5X **Poisoning by, adverse effect of and underdosing of digestants**

7 T47.5X1- **Poisoning by digestants, accidental (unintentional)**
Poisoning by digestants NOS

7 T47.5X2- **Poisoning by digestants, intentional self-harm**

7 T47.5X3- **Poisoning by digestants, assault**

7 T47.5X4- **Poisoning by digestants, undetermined**

7 T47.5X5- **Adverse effect of digestants**

7 T47.5X6- **Underdosing of digestants**

5 T47.6 **Poisoning by, adverse effect of and underdosing of antidiarrheal drugs**

EXCLUDES 2 *poisoning by, adverse effect of and underdosing of systemic antibiotics and other anti-infectives (T36-T37)*

6 T47.6X **Poisoning by, adverse effect of and underdosing of antidiarrheal drugs**

7 T47.6X1- **Poisoning by antidiarrheal drugs, accidental (unintentional)**
Poisoning by antidiarrheal drugs NOS

7 T47.6X2- **Poisoning by antidiarrheal drugs, intentional self-harm**

7 T47.6X3- **Poisoning by antidiarrheal drugs, assault**

7 T47.6X4- **Poisoning by antidiarrheal drugs, undetermined**

7 T47.6X5- **Adverse effect of antidiarrheal drugs**

7 T47.6X6- **Underdosing of antidiarrheal drugs**

5 T47.7 **Poisoning by, adverse effect of and underdosing of emetics**

6 T47.7X **Poisoning by, adverse effect of and underdosing of emetics**

7 T47.7X1- **Poisoning by emetics, accidental (unintentional)**
Poisoning by emetics NOS

7 T47.7X2- **Poisoning by emetics, intentional self-harm**

7 T47.7X3- **Poisoning by emetics, assault**

7 T47.7X4- **Poisoning by emetics, undetermined**

7 T47.7X5- **Adverse effect of emetics**

7 T47.7X6- **Underdosing of emetics**

5 T47.8 **Poisoning by, adverse effect of and underdosing of other agents primarily affecting gastrointestinal system**

6 T47.8X **Poisoning by, adverse effect of and underdosing of other agents primarily affecting gastrointestinal system**

7 T47.8X1- **Poisoning by other agents primarily affecting gastrointestinal system, accidental (unintentional)**
Poisoning by other agents primarily affecting gastrointestinal system NOS

7 T47.8X2- **Poisoning by other agents primarily affecting gastrointestinal system, intentional self-harm**

7 T47.8X3- **Poisoning by other agents primarily affecting gastrointestinal system, assault**

7 T47.8X4- **Poisoning by other agents primarily affecting gastrointestinal system, undetermined**

7 T47.8X5- **Adverse effect of other agents primarily affecting gastrointestinal system**

7 T47.8X6- **Underdosing of other agents primarily affecting gastrointestinal system**

5 T47.9 **Poisoning by, adverse effect of and underdosing of unspecified agents primarily affecting the gastrointestinal system**

7 T47.91X- **Poisoning by unspecified agents primarily affecting the gastrointestinal system, accidental (unintentional)**
Poisoning by agents primarily affecting the gastrointestinal system NOS

7 T47.92X- **Poisoning by unspecified agents primarily affecting the gastrointestinal system, intentional self-harm**

7 T47.93X- **Poisoning by unspecified agents primarily affecting the gastrointestinal system, assault**

7 T47.94X- **Poisoning by unspecified agents primarily affecting the gastrointestinal system, undetermined**

7 T47.95X- **Adverse effect of unspecified agents primarily affecting the gastrointestinal system**

7 T47.96X- **Underdosing of unspecified agents primarily affecting the gastrointestinal system**

4 T48 **Poisoning by, adverse effect of and underdosing of agents primarily acting on smooth and skeletal muscles and the respiratory system**

The appropriate 7th character is to be added to each code from category T48
A   initial encounter
D   subsequent encounter
S   sequela

5 T48.0 **Poisoning by, adverse effect of and underdosing of oxytocic drugs**

EXCLUDES 1 *poisoning by, adverse effect of and underdosing of estrogens, progestogens and antagonists (T38.4-T38.6)*

6 T48.0X **Poisoning by, adverse effect of and underdosing of oxytocic drugs**

7 T48.0X1- **Poisoning by oxytocic drugs, accidental (unintentional)**
Poisoning by oxytocic drugs NOS

7 T48.0X2- **Poisoning by oxytocic drugs, intentional self-harm**

7 T48.0X3- **Poisoning by oxytocic drugs, assault**

7 T48.0X4- **Poisoning by oxytocic drugs, undetermined**

7 T48.0X5- **Adverse effect of oxytocic drugs**

7 T48.0X6- **Underdosing of oxytocic drugs**

5 T48.1 **Poisoning by, adverse effect of and underdosing of skeletal muscle relaxants [neuromuscular blocking agents]**

6 T48.1X **Poisoning by, adverse effect of and underdosing of skeletal muscle relaxants [neuromuscular blocking agents]**

7 T48.1X1- **Poisoning by skeletal muscle relaxants [neuromuscular blocking agents], accidental (unintentional)**
Poisoning by skeletal muscle relaxants [neuromuscular blocking agents] NOS

7 T48.1X2- **Poisoning by skeletal muscle relaxants [neuromuscular blocking agents], intentional self-harm**

7 T48.1X3- **Poisoning by skeletal muscle relaxants [neuromuscular blocking agents], assault**

7 T48.1X4- **Poisoning by skeletal muscle relaxants [neuromuscular blocking agents], undetermined**

7 T48.1X5- **Adverse effect of skeletal muscle relaxants [neuromuscular blocking agents]**

7 T48.1X6- **Underdosing of skeletal muscle relaxants [neuromuscular blocking agents]**

5 T48.2 **Poisoning by, adverse effect of and underdosing of other and unspecified drugs acting on muscles**

6 T48.20 **Poisoning by, adverse effect of and underdosing of unspecified drugs acting on muscles**

7 T48.201- **Poisoning by unspecified drugs acting on muscles, accidental (unintentional)**
Poisoning by unspecified drugs acting on muscles NOS

7 T48.202- **Poisoning by unspecified drugs acting on muscles, intentional self-harm**

7 T48.203- **Poisoning by unspecified drugs acting on muscles, assault**

7 T48.204- **Poisoning by unspecified drugs acting on muscles, undetermined**

7 T48.205- **Adverse effect of unspecified drugs acting on muscles**

7 T48.206- **Underdosing of unspecified drugs acting on muscles**

6 T48.29 **Poisoning by, adverse effect of and underdosing of other drugs acting on muscles**

7 T48.291- **Poisoning by other drugs acting on muscles, accidental (unintentional)**
Poisoning by other drugs acting on muscles NOS

● New   ▲ Revised   *Manifestation*   4-7 Digit Indicators   ⊟ Laterality   Ａ Adult (15+ years)   Ｍ Maternity (12-55 years)   Ｎ Newborn   Ｐ Pediatric (0-17 years)   ♂ Male   ♀ Female
✖ Deleted   Unspecified   + Additional code

☑ T48.292-   Poisoning by other drugs acting on muscles, intentional self-harm

☑ T48.293-   Poisoning by other drugs acting on muscles, assault

☑ T48.294-   Poisoning by other drugs acting on muscles, undetermined

☑ T48.295-   Adverse effect of other drugs acting on muscles

☑ T48.296-   Underdosing of other drugs acting on muscles

⑤ T48.3   Poisoning by, adverse effect of and underdosing of antitussives

⑥ T48.3X   Poisoning by, adverse effect of and underdosing of antitussives

☑ T48.3X1-   Poisoning by antitussives, accidental (unintentional)
Poisoning by antitussives NOS

☑ T48.3X2-   Poisoning by antitussives, intentional self-harm

☑ T48.3X3-   Poisoning by antitussives, assault

☑ T48.3X4-   Poisoning by antitussives, undetermined

☑ T48.3X5-   Adverse effect of antitussives

☑ T48.3X6-   Underdosing of antitussives

⑤ T48.4   Poisoning by, adverse effect of and underdosing of expectorants

⑥ T48.4X   Poisoning by, adverse effect of and underdosing of expectorants

☑ T48.4X1-   Poisoning by expectorants, accidental (unintentional)
Poisoning by expectorants NOS

☑ T48.4X2-   Poisoning by expectorants, intentional self-harm

☑ T48.4X3-   Poisoning by expectorants, assault

☑ T48.4X4-   Poisoning by expectorants, undetermined

☑ T48.4X5-   Adverse effect of expectorants

☑ T48.4X6-   Underdosing of expectorants

⑤ T48.5   Poisoning by, adverse effect of and underdosing of other anti-common-cold drugs
Poisoning by, adverse effect of and underdosing of decongestants

EXCLUDES 2   *poisoning by, adverse effect of and underdosing of antipyretics, NEC (T39.9-)*
poisoning by, adverse effect of and underdosing of non-steroidal antiinflammatory drugs (T39.3-)
poisoning by, adverse effect of and underdosing of salicylates (T39.0-)

⑥ T48.5X   Poisoning by, adverse effect of and underdosing of other anti-common-cold drugs

☑ T48.5X1-   Poisoning by other anti-common-cold drugs, accidental (unintentional)
Poisoning by other anti-common-cold drugs NOS

☑ T48.5X2-   Poisoning by other anti-common-cold drugs, intentional self-harm

☑ T48.5X3-   Poisoning by other anti-common-cold drugs, assault

☑ T48.5X4-   Poisoning by other anti-common-cold drugs, undetermined

☑ T48.5X5-   Adverse effect of other anti-common-cold drugs

☑ T48.5X6-   Underdosing of other anti-common-cold drugs

⑤ T48.6   Poisoning by, adverse effect of and underdosing of antiasthmatics, not elsewhere classified
Poisoning by, adverse effect of and underdosing of beta-adrenoreceptor agonists used in asthma therapy

EXCLUDES 1   *poisoning by, adverse effect of and underdosing of beta-adrenoreceptor agonists not used in asthma therapy (T44.5)*
poisoning by, adverse effect of and underdosing of anterior pituitary [adenohypophyseal] hormones (T38.8)

⑥ T48.6X   Poisoning by, adverse effect of and underdosing of antiasthmatics

☑ T48.6X1-   Poisoning by antiasthmatics, accidental (unintentional)
Poisoning by antiasthmatics NOS

☑ T48.6X2-   Poisoning by antiasthmatics, intentional self-harm

☑ T48.6X3-   Poisoning by antiasthmatics, assault

☑ T48.6X4-   Poisoning by antiasthmatics, undetermined

☑ T48.6X5-   Adverse effect of antiasthmatics

☑ T48.6X6-   Underdosing of antiasthmatics

⑤ T48.9   Poisoning by, adverse effect of and underdosing of other and unspecified agents primarily acting on the respiratory system

⑥ T48.90   Poisoning by, adverse effect of and underdosing of unspecified agents primarily acting on the respiratory system

☑ T48.901-   Poisoning by unspecified agents primarily acting on the respiratory system, accidental (unintentional)

☑ T48.902-   Poisoning by unspecified agents primarily acting on the respiratory system, intentional self-harm

☑ T48.903-   Poisoning by unspecified agents primarily acting on the respiratory system, assault

☑ T48.904-   Poisoning by unspecified agents primarily acting on the respiratory system, undetermined

☑ T48.905-   Adverse effect of unspecified agents primarily acting on the respiratory system

☑ T48.906-   Underdosing of unspecified agents primarily acting on the respiratory system

⑥ T48.99   Poisoning by, adverse effect of and underdosing of other agents primarily acting on the respiratory system

☑ T48.991-   Poisoning by other agents primarily acting on the respiratory system, accidental (unintentional)

☑ T48.992-   Poisoning by other agents primarily acting on the respiratory system, intentional self-harm

☑ T48.993-   Poisoning by other agents primarily acting on the respiratory system, assault

☑ T48.994-   Poisoning by other agents primarily acting on the respiratory system, undetermined

☑ T48.995-   Adverse effect of other agents primarily acting on the respiratory system

☑ T48.996-   Underdosing of other agents primarily acting on the respiratory system

④ T49   Poisoning by, adverse effect of and underdosing of topical agents primarily affecting skin and mucous membrane and by ophthalmological, otorhinolaryngological and dental drugs

INCLUDES   poisoning by, adverse effect of and underdosing of glucocorticoids, topically used

The appropriate 7th character is to be added to each code from category T49
A   initial encounter
D   subsequent encounter
S   sequela

⑤ T49.0   Poisoning by, adverse effect of and underdosing of local antifungal, anti-infective and anti-inflammatory drugs

⑥ T49.0X   Poisoning by, adverse effect of and underdosing of local antifungal, anti-infective and anti-inflammatory drugs

☑ T49.0X1-   Poisoning by local antifungal, anti-infective and anti-inflammatory drugs, accidental (unintentional)
Poisoning by local antifungal, anti-infective and anti-inflammatory drugs NOS

☑ T49.0X2-   Poisoning by local antifungal, anti-infective and anti-inflammatory drugs, intentional self-harm

☑ T49.0X3-   Poisoning by local antifungal, anti-infective and anti-inflammatory drugs, assault

☑ T49.0X4-   Poisoning by local antifungal, anti-infective and anti-inflammatory drugs, undetermined

☑ T49.0X5-   Adverse effect of local antifungal, anti-infective and anti-inflammatory drugs

☑ T49.0X6-   Underdosing of local antifungal, anti-infective and anti-inflammatory drugs

⑤ T49.1   Poisoning by, adverse effect of and underdosing of antipruritics

⑥ T49.1X   Poisoning by, adverse effect of and underdosing of antipruritics

☑ T49.1X1-   Poisoning by antipruritics, accidental (unintentional)
Poisoning by antipruritics NOS

● New   ▲ Revised   *Manifestation*   ④-☑ Digit Indicators   ▣ Laterality   Ⓐ Adult (15+ years)   Ⓜ Maternity (12-55 years)   Ⓝ Newborn   Ⓟ Pediatric (0-17 years)   ♂ Male   ♀ Female
Unspecified
✖ Deleted   + Additional code

1074   © 2017 DecisionHealth   2017 ICD-10-CM Expert for Physicians

7 T49.1X2- Poisoning by antipruritics, intentional self-harm

7 T49.1X3- Poisoning by antipruritics, assault

7 T49.1X4- Poisoning by antipruritics, undetermined

7 T49.1X5- Adverse effect of antipruritics

7 T49.1X6- Underdosing of antipruritics

5 T49.2 Poisoning by, adverse effect of and underdosing of local astringents and local detergents

6 T49.2X Poisoning by, adverse effect of and underdosing of local astringents and local detergents

7 T49.2X1- Poisoning by local astringents and local detergents, accidental (unintentional)
Poisoning by local astringents and local detergents NOS

7 T49.2X2- Poisoning by local astringents and local detergents, intentional self-harm

7 T49.2X3- Poisoning by local astringents and local detergents, assault

7 T49.2X4- Poisoning by local astringents and local detergents, undetermined

7 T49.2X5- Adverse effect of local astringents and local detergents

7 T49.2X6- Underdosing of local astringents and local detergents

5 T49.3 Poisoning by, adverse effect of and underdosing of emollients, demulcents and protectants

6 T49.3X Poisoning by, adverse effect of and underdosing of emollients, demulcents and protectants

7 T49.3X1- Poisoning by emollients, demulcents and protectants, accidental (unintentional)
Poisoning by emollients, demulcents and protectants NOS

7 T49.3X2- Poisoning by emollients, demulcents and protectants, intentional self-harm

7 T49.3X3- Poisoning by emollients, demulcents and protectants, assault

7 T49.3X4- Poisoning by emollients, demulcents and protectants, undetermined

7 T49.3X5- Adverse effect of emollients, demulcents and protectants

7 T49.3X6- Underdosing of emollients, demulcents and protectants

5 T49.4 Poisoning by, adverse effect of and underdosing of keratolytics, keratoplastics, and other hair treatment drugs and preparations

6 T49.4X Poisoning by, adverse effect of and underdosing of keratolytics, keratoplastics, and other hair treatment drugs and preparations

7 T49.4X1- Poisoning by keratolytics, keratoplastics, and other hair treatment drugs and preparations, accidental (unintentional)
Poisoning by keratolytics, keratoplastics, and other hair treatment drugs and preparations NOS

7 T49.4X2- Poisoning by keratolytics, keratoplastics, and other hair treatment drugs and preparations, intentional self-harm

7 T49.4X3- Poisoning by keratolytics, keratoplastics, and other hair treatment drugs and preparations, assault

7 T49.4X4- Poisoning by keratolytics, keratoplastics, and other hair treatment drugs and preparations, undetermined

7 T49.4X5- Adverse effect of keratolytics, keratoplastics, and other hair treatment drugs and preparations

7 T49.4X6- Underdosing of keratolytics, keratoplastics, and other hair treatment drugs and preparations

5 T49.5 Poisoning by, adverse effect of and underdosing of ophthalmological drugs and preparations

6 T49.5X Poisoning by, adverse effect of and underdosing of ophthalmological drugs and preparations

7 T49.5X1- Poisoning by ophthalmological drugs and preparations, accidental (unintentional)
Poisoning by ophthalmological drugs and preparations NOS

7 T49.5X2- Poisoning by ophthalmological drugs and preparations, intentional self-harm

7 T49.5X3- Poisoning by ophthalmological drugs and preparations, assault

7 T49.5X4- Poisoning by ophthalmological drugs and preparations, undetermined

7 T49.5X5- Adverse effect of ophthalmological drugs and preparations

7 T49.5X6- Underdosing of ophthalmological drugs and preparations

5 T49.6 Poisoning by, adverse effect of and underdosing of otorhinolaryngological drugs and preparations

6 T49.6X Poisoning by, adverse effect of and underdosing of otorhinolaryngological drugs and preparations

7 T49.6X1- Poisoning by otorhinolaryngological drugs and preparations, accidental (unintentional)
Poisoning by otorhinolaryngological drugs and preparations NOS

7 T49.6X2- Poisoning by otorhinolaryngological drugs and preparations, intentional self-harm

7 T49.6X3- Poisoning by otorhinolaryngological drugs and preparations, assault

7 T49.6X4- Poisoning by otorhinolaryngological drugs and preparations, undetermined

7 T49.6X5- Adverse effect of otorhinolaryngological drugs and preparations

7 T49.6X6- Underdosing of otorhinolaryngological drugs and preparations

5 T49.7 Poisoning by, adverse effect of and underdosing of dental drugs, topically applied

6 T49.7X Poisoning by, adverse effect of and underdosing of dental drugs, topically applied

7 T49.7X1- Poisoning by dental drugs, topically applied, accidental (unintentional)
Poisoning by dental drugs, topically applied NOS

7 T49.7X2- Poisoning by dental drugs, topically applied, intentional self-harm

7 T49.7X3- Poisoning by dental drugs, topically applied, assault

7 T49.7X4- Poisoning by dental drugs, topically applied, undetermined

7 T49.7X5- Adverse effect of dental drugs, topically applied

7 T49.7X6- Underdosing of dental drugs, topically applied

5 T49.8 Poisoning by, adverse effect of and underdosing of other topical agents
Poisoning by, adverse effect of and underdosing of spermicides

6 T49.8X Poisoning by, adverse effect of and underdosing of other topical agents

7 T49.8X1- Poisoning by other topical agents, accidental (unintentional)
Poisoning by other topical agents NOS

7 T49.8X2- Poisoning by other topical agents, intentional self-harm

7 T49.8X3- Poisoning by other topical agents, assault

7 T49.8X4- Poisoning by other topical agents, undetermined

7 T49.8X5- Adverse effect of other topical agents

7 T49.8X6- Underdosing of other topical agents

5 T49.9 Poisoning by, adverse effect of and underdosing of unspecified topical agent

7 T49.91X- Poisoning by unspecified topical agent, accidental (unintentional)

7 T49.92X- Poisoning by unspecified topical agent, intentional self-harm

7 T49.93X- Poisoning by unspecified topical agent, assault

7 T49.94X- Poisoning by unspecified topical agent, undetermined

7 T49.95X- Adverse effect of unspecified topical agent

7 T49.96X- Underdosing of unspecified topical agent

4 T50 **Poisoning by, adverse effect of and underdosing of diuretics and other and unspecified drugs, medicaments and biological substances**

The appropriate 7th character is to be added to each code from category T50
A   initial encounter
D   subsequent encounter
S   sequela

5 T50.0 Poisoning by, adverse effect of and underdosing of mineralocorticoids and their antagonists

6 T50.0X Poisoning by, adverse effect of and underdosing of mineralocorticoids and their antagonists

● New ▲ Revised *Manifestation* **4**-**7** Digit Indicators ▭ Laterality Ⓐ Adult (15+ years) Ⓜ Maternity (12-55 years) Ⓝ Newborn (0-17 years) Ⓟ Pediatric (0-17 years) ♂ Male ♀ Female
✖ Deleted Unspecified + Additional code

2017 ICD-10-CM Expert for Physicians

© 2017 DecisionHealth   1075

7 T50.0X1- Poisoning by mineralocorticoids and their antagonists, accidental (unintentional)
Poisoning by mineralocorticoids and their antagonists NOS

7 T50.0X2- Poisoning by mineralocorticoids and their antagonists, intentional self-harm

7 T50.0X3- Poisoning by mineralocorticoids and their antagonists, assault

7 T50.0X4- Poisoning by mineralocorticoids and their antagonists, undetermined

7 T50.0X5- Adverse effect of mineralocorticoids and their antagonists

7 T50.0X6- Underdosing of mineralocorticoids and their antagonists

5 T50.1 Poisoning by, adverse effect of and underdosing of loop [high-ceiling] diuretics

6 T50.1X Poisoning by, adverse effect of and underdosing of loop [high-ceiling] diuretics

7 T50.1X1- Poisoning by loop [high-ceiling] diuretics, accidental (unintentional)
Poisoning by loop [high-ceiling] diuretics NOS

7 T50.1X2- Poisoning by loop [high-ceiling] diuretics, intentional self-harm

7 T50.1X3- Poisoning by loop [high-ceiling] diuretics, assault

7 T50.1X4- Poisoning by loop [high-ceiling] diuretics, undetermined

7 T50.1X5- Adverse effect of loop [high-ceiling] diuretics

7 T50.1X6- Underdosing of loop [high-ceiling] diuretics

5 T50.2 Poisoning by, adverse effect of and underdosing of carbonic-anhydrase inhibitors, benzothiadiazides and other diuretics
Poisoning by, adverse effect of and underdosing of acetazolamide

6 T50.2X Poisoning by, adverse effect of and underdosing of carbonic-anhydrase inhibitors, benzothiadiazides and other diuretics

7 T50.2X1- Poisoning by carbonic-anhydrase inhibitors, benzothiadiazides and other diuretics, accidental (unintentional)
Poisoning by carbonic-anhydrase inhibitors, benzothiadiazides and other diuretics NOS

7 T50.2X2- Poisoning by carbonic-anhydrase inhibitors, benzothiadiazides and other diuretics, intentional self-harm

7 T50.2X3- Poisoning by carbonic-anhydrase inhibitors, benzothiadiazides and other diuretics, assault

7 T50.2X4- Poisoning by carbonic-anhydrase inhibitors, benzothiadiazides and other diuretics, undetermined

7 T50.2X5- Adverse effect of carbonic-anhydrase inhibitors, benzothiadiazides and other diuretics

7 T50.2X6- Underdosing of carbonic-anhydrase inhibitors, benzothiadiazides and other diuretics

5 T50.3 Poisoning by, adverse effect of and underdosing of electrolytic, caloric and water-balance agents
Poisoning by, adverse effect of and underdosing of oral rehydration salts

6 T50.3X Poisoning by, adverse effect of and underdosing of electrolytic, caloric and water-balance agents

7 T50.3X1- Poisoning by electrolytic, caloric and water-balance agents, accidental (unintentional)
Poisoning by electrolytic, caloric and water-balance agents NOS

7 T50.3X2- Poisoning by electrolytic, caloric and water-balance agents, intentional self-harm

7 T50.3X3- Poisoning by electrolytic, caloric and water-balance agents, assault

7 T50.3X4- Poisoning by electrolytic, caloric and water-balance agents, undetermined

7 T50.3X5- Adverse effect of electrolytic, caloric and water-balance agents

7 T50.3X6- Underdosing of electrolytic, caloric and water-balance agents

5 T50.4 Poisoning by, adverse effect of and underdosing of drugs affecting uric acid metabolism

6 T50.4X Poisoning by, adverse effect of and underdosing of drugs affecting uric acid metabolism

7 T50.4X1- Poisoning by drugs affecting uric acid metabolism, accidental (unintentional)
Poisoning by drugs affecting uric acid metabolism NOS

7 T50.4X2- Poisoning by drugs affecting uric acid metabolism, intentional self-harm

7 T50.4X3- Poisoning by drugs affecting uric acid metabolism, assault

7 T50.4X4- Poisoning by drugs affecting uric acid metabolism, undetermined

7 T50.4X5- Adverse effect of drugs affecting uric acid metabolism

7 T50.4X6- Underdosing of drugs affecting uric acid metabolism

5 T50.5 Poisoning by, adverse effect of and underdosing of appetite depressants

6 T50.5X Poisoning by, adverse effect of and underdosing of appetite depressants

7 T50.5X1- Poisoning by appetite depressants, accidental (unintentional)
Poisoning by appetite depressants NOS

7 T50.5X2- Poisoning by appetite depressants, intentional self-harm

7 T50.5X3- Poisoning by appetite depressants, assault

7 T50.5X4- Poisoning by appetite depressants, undetermined

7 T50.5X5- Adverse effect of appetite depressants

7 T50.5X6- Underdosing of appetite depressants

5 T50.6 Poisoning by, adverse effect of and underdosing of antidotes and chelating agents
Poisoning by, adverse effect of and underdosing of alcohol deterrents

6 T50.6X Poisoning by, adverse effect of and underdosing of antidotes and chelating agents

7 T50.6X1- Poisoning by antidotes and chelating agents, accidental (unintentional)
Poisoning by antidotes and chelating agents NOS

7 T50.6X2- Poisoning by antidotes and chelating agents, intentional self-harm

7 T50.6X3- Poisoning by antidotes and chelating agents, assault

7 T50.6X4- Poisoning by antidotes and chelating agents, undetermined

7 T50.6X5- Adverse effect of antidotes and chelating agents

7 T50.6X6- Underdosing of antidotes and chelating agents

5 T50.7 Poisoning by, adverse effect of and underdosing of analeptics and opioid receptor antagonists

6 T50.7X Poisoning by, adverse effect of and underdosing of analeptics and opioid receptor antagonists

7 T50.7X1- Poisoning by analeptics and opioid receptor antagonists, accidental (unintentional)
Poisoning by analeptics and opioid receptor antagonists NOS

7 T50.7X2- Poisoning by analeptics and opioid receptor antagonists, intentional self-harm

7 T50.7X3- Poisoning by analeptics and opioid receptor antagonists, assault

7 T50.7X4- Poisoning by analeptics and opioid receptor antagonists, undetermined

7 T50.7X5- Adverse effect of analeptics and opioid receptor antagonists

7 T50.7X6- Underdosing of analeptics and opioid receptor antagonists

5 T50.8 Poisoning by, adverse effect of and underdosing of diagnostic agents

6 T50.8X Poisoning by, adverse effect of and underdosing of diagnostic agents

7 T50.8X1- Poisoning by diagnostic agents, accidental (unintentional)
Poisoning by diagnostic agents NOS

7 T50.8X2- Poisoning by diagnostic agents, intentional self-harm

7 T50.8X3- Poisoning by diagnostic agents, assault

7 T50.8X4- Poisoning by diagnostic agents, undetermined

7 T50.8X5- Adverse effect of diagnostic agents

7 T50.8X6- Underdosing of diagnostic agents

5 T50.A Poisoning by, adverse effect of and underdosing of bacterial vaccines

---

● New   ▲ Revised   *Manifestation*   **4 - 7** Digit Indicators   ▤ Laterality   Ⓐ Adult (15+ years)   Ⓜ Maternity (12-55 years)   Ⓝ Newborn   Ⓟ Pediatric (0-17 years)   ♂ Male   ♀ Female
✖ Deleted   Unspecified   + Additional code

Injury, Poisoning and Certain Other Consequences of External Causes (side tab)

6 **T50.A1** Poisoning by, adverse effect of and underdosing of pertussis vaccine, including combinations with a pertussis component

7 **T50.A11-** Poisoning by pertussis vaccine, including combinations with a pertussis component, accidental (unintentional)

7 **T50.A12-** Poisoning by pertussis vaccine, including combinations with a pertussis component, intentional self-harm

7 **T50.A13-** Poisoning by pertussis vaccine, including combinations with a pertussis component, assault

7 **T50.A14-** Poisoning by pertussis vaccine, including combinations with a pertussis component, undetermined

7 **T50.A15-** Adverse effect of pertussis vaccine, including combinations with a pertussis component

7 **T50.A16-** Underdosing of pertussis vaccine, including combinations with a pertussis component

6 **T50.A2** Poisoning by, adverse effect of and underdosing of mixed bacterial vaccines without a pertussis component

7 **T50.A21-** Poisoning by mixed bacterial vaccines without a pertussis component, accidental (unintentional)

7 **T50.A22-** Poisoning by mixed bacterial vaccines without a pertussis component, intentional self-harm

7 **T50.A23-** Poisoning by mixed bacterial vaccines without a pertussis component, assault

7 **T50.A24-** Poisoning by mixed bacterial vaccines without a pertussis component, undetermined

7 **T50.A25-** Adverse effect of mixed bacterial vaccines without a pertussis component

7 **T50.A26-** Underdosing of mixed bacterial vaccines without a pertussis component

6 **T50.A9** Poisoning by, adverse effect of and underdosing of other bacterial vaccines

7 **T50.A91-** Poisoning by other bacterial vaccines, accidental (unintentional)

7 **T50.A92-** Poisoning by other bacterial vaccines, intentional self-harm

7 **T50.A93-** Poisoning by other bacterial vaccines, assault

7 **T50.A94-** Poisoning by other bacterial vaccines, undetermined

7 **T50.A95-** Adverse effect of other bacterial vaccines

7 **T50.A96-** Underdosing of other bacterial vaccines

5 **T50.B** Poisoning by, adverse effect of and underdosing of viral vaccines

6 **T50.B1** Poisoning by, adverse effect of and underdosing of smallpox vaccines

7 **T50.B11-** Poisoning by smallpox vaccines, accidental (unintentional)

7 **T50.B12-** Poisoning by smallpox vaccines, intentional self-harm

7 **T50.B13-** Poisoning by smallpox vaccines, assault

7 **T50.B14-** Poisoning by smallpox vaccines, undetermined

7 **T50.B15-** Adverse effect of smallpox vaccines

7 **T50.B16-** Underdosing of smallpox vaccines

6 **T50.B9** Poisoning by, adverse effect of and underdosing of other viral vaccines

7 **T50.B91-** Poisoning by other viral vaccines, accidental (unintentional)

7 **T50.B92-** Poisoning by other viral vaccines, intentional self-harm

7 **T50.B93-** Poisoning by other viral vaccines, assault

7 **T50.B94-** Poisoning by other viral vaccines, undetermined

7 **T50.B95-** Adverse effect of other viral vaccines

7 **T50.B96-** Underdosing of other viral vaccines

5 **T50.Z** Poisoning by, adverse effect of and underdosing of other vaccines and biological substances

6 **T50.Z1** Poisoning by, adverse effect of and underdosing of immunoglobulin

7 **T50.Z11-** Poisoning by immunoglobulin, accidental (unintentional)

7 **T50.Z12-** Poisoning by immunoglobulin, intentional self-harm

7 **T50.Z13-** Poisoning by immunoglobulin, assault

7 **T50.Z14-** Poisoning by immunoglobulin, undetermined

7 **T50.Z15-** Adverse effect of immunoglobulin

7 **T50.Z16-** Underdosing of immunoglobulin

6 **T50.Z9** Poisoning by, adverse effect of and underdosing of other vaccines and biological substances

7 **T50.Z91-** Poisoning by other vaccines and biological substances, accidental (unintentional)

7 **T50.Z92-** Poisoning by other vaccines and biological substances, intentional self-harm

7 **T50.Z93-** Poisoning by other vaccines and biological substances, assault

7 **T50.Z94-** Poisoning by other vaccines and biological substances, undetermined

7 **T50.Z95-** Adverse effect of other vaccines and biological substances

7 **T50.Z96-** Underdosing of other vaccines and biological substances

5 **T50.9** Poisoning by, adverse effect of and underdosing of other and unspecified drugs, medicaments and biological substances

6 **T50.90** Poisoning by, adverse effect of and underdosing of unspecified drugs, medicaments and biological substances

7 **T50.901-** Poisoning by unspecified drugs, medicaments and biological substances, accidental (unintentional)
AHA: (T50.901S) 1Q 2015, 21

7 **T50.902-** Poisoning by unspecified drugs, medicaments and biological substances, intentional self-harm

7 **T50.903-** Poisoning by unspecified drugs, medicaments and biological substances, assault

7 **T50.904-** Poisoning by unspecified drugs, medicaments and biological substances, undetermined

7 **T50.905-** Adverse effect of unspecified drugs, medicaments and biological substances

7 **T50.906-** Underdosing of unspecified drugs, medicaments and biological substances

6 **T50.99** Poisoning by, adverse effect of and underdosing of other drugs, medicaments and biological substances

7 **T50.991-** Poisoning by other drugs, medicaments and biological substances, accidental (unintentional)

7 **T50.992-** Poisoning by other drugs, medicaments and biological substances, intentional self-harm

7 **T50.993-** Poisoning by other drugs, medicaments and biological substances, assault

7 **T50.994-** Poisoning by other drugs, medicaments and biological substances, undetermined

7 **T50.995-** Adverse effect of other drugs, medicaments and biological substances

7 **T50.996-** Underdosing of other drugs, medicaments and biological substances

Toxic effects of substances chiefly nonmedicinal as to source (T51-T65)

Note: When no intent is indicated code to accidental. Undetermined intent is only for use when there is specific documentation in the record that the intent of the toxic effect cannot be determined.

Use additional code(s):
  for all associated manifestations of toxic effect, such as: respiratory conditions due to external agents (J60-J70)
  personal history of foreign body fully removed (Z87.821)
  to identify any retained foreign body, if applicable (Z18.-)

EXCLUDES 1   contact with and (suspected) exposure to toxic substances (Z77.-)

● New ▲ Revised *Manifestation* 4-7 Digit Indicators ⊟ Laterality A Adult (15+ years) M Maternity (12-55 years) N Newborn P Pediatric (0-17 years) ♂ Male ♀ Female
✖ Deleted Unspecified + Additional code

2017 ICD-10-CM Expert for Physicians

© 2017 DecisionHealth

1077

GUIDELINES   Section I.C.19.e.1)-4)
Codes in categories T36-T65 are combination codes that include the substance that was taken as well as the intent. No additional external cause code is required for poisonings, toxic effects, adverse effects and underdosing codes.

Do not code directly from the Table of Drugs and Chemicals. Always refer back to the Tabular List. Use as many codes as necessary to describe completely all drugs, medicinal or biological substances. If the same code would describe the causative agent for more than one adverse reaction, poisoning, toxic effect or underdosing, assign the code only once. If two or more drugs, medicinal or biological substances are reported, code each individually unless a combination code is listed in the Table of Drugs and Chemicals.

GUIDELINES   Section I.C.19.e.5)(d)
When a harmful substance is ingested or comes in contact with a person, this is classified as a toxic effect. The toxic effect codes are in categories T51-T65. Toxic effect codes have an associated intent: accidental, intentional self-harm, assault and undetermined.

CODING TIP ✓   When coding toxic effects, first assign the code from T51-T65 to identify the substance and intent, followed by an additional code to identify the manifestations of the toxic substance that resulted in the effect(s). If the intent is not documented, accidental intent should be coded. Undetermined intent should only be coded when documentation specifically indicates that the intent cannot be determined.

CODING TIP ✓   Note there are only codes for poisonings or toxic effects. There are no therapeutic uses for the following substances, therefore there are no codes for adverse effects or underdosing.

◢ **T51   Toxic effect of alcohol**

> The appropriate 7th character is to be added to each code from category T51
> A   initial encounter
> D   subsequent encounter
> S   sequela

⑤ **T51.0   Toxic effect of ethanol**
Toxic effect of ethyl alcohol
> EXCLUDES 2   *acute alcohol intoxication or 'hangover' effects (F10.129, F10.229, F10.929)*
> *drunkenness (F10.129, F10.229, F10.929)*
> *pathological alcohol intoxication (F10.129, F10.229, F10.929)*

⑥ **T51.0X   Toxic effect of ethanol**
⑦ **T51.0X1-   Toxic effect of ethanol, accidental (unintentional)**
Toxic effect of ethanol NOS
⑦ **T51.0X2-   Toxic effect of ethanol, intentional self-harm**
⑦ **T51.0X3-   Toxic effect of ethanol, assault**
⑦ **T51.0X4-   Toxic effect of ethanol, undetermined**

⑤ **T51.1   Toxic effect of methanol**
Toxic effect of methyl alcohol
⑥ **T51.1X   Toxic effect of methanol**
⑦ **T51.1X1-   Toxic effect of methanol, accidental (unintentional)**
Toxic effect of methanol NOS
⑦ **T51.1X2-   Toxic effect of methanol, intentional self-harm**
⑦ **T51.1X3-   Toxic effect of methanol, assault**
⑦ **T51.1X4-   Toxic effect of methanol, undetermined**

⑤ **T51.2   Toxic effect of 2-Propanol**
Toxic effect of isopropyl alcohol
⑥ **T51.2X   Toxic effect of 2-Propanol**
⑦ **T51.2X1-   Toxic effect of 2-Propanol, accidental (unintentional)**
Toxic effect of 2-Propanol NOS
⑦ **T51.2X2-   Toxic effect of 2-Propanol, intentional self-harm**
⑦ **T51.2X3-   Toxic effect of 2-Propanol, assault**
⑦ **T51.2X4-   Toxic effect of 2-Propanol, undetermined**

⑤ **T51.3   Toxic effect of fusel oil**
Toxic effect of amyl alcohol
Toxic effect of butyl [1-butanol] alcohol
Toxic effect of propyl [1-propanol] alcohol
⑥ **T51.3X   Toxic effect of fusel oil**
⑦ **T51.3X1-   Toxic effect of fusel oil, accidental (unintentional)**
Toxic effect of fusel oil NOS
⑦ **T51.3X2-   Toxic effect of fusel oil, intentional self-harm**
⑦ **T51.3X3-   Toxic effect of fusel oil, assault**

⑦ **T51.3X4-   Toxic effect of fusel oil, undetermined**
⑤ **T51.8   Toxic effect of other alcohols**
⑥ **T51.8X   Toxic effect of other alcohols**
⑦ **T51.8X1-   Toxic effect of other alcohols, accidental (unintentional)**
Toxic effect of other alcohols NOS
⑦ **T51.8X2-   Toxic effect of other alcohols, intentional self-harm**
⑦ **T51.8X3-   Toxic effect of other alcohols, assault**
⑦ **T51.8X4-   Toxic effect of other alcohols, undetermined**

⑤ **T51.9   Toxic effect of unspecified alcohol**
⑦ **T51.91X-   Toxic effect of unspecified alcohol, accidental (unintentional)**
⑦ **T51.92X-   Toxic effect of unspecified alcohol, intentional self-harm**
⑦ **T51.93X-   Toxic effect of unspecified alcohol, assault**
⑦ **T51.94X-   Toxic effect of unspecified alcohol, undetermined**

◢ **T52   Toxic effect of organic solvents**
> EXCLUDES 1   *halogen derivatives of aliphatic and aromatic hydrocarbons (T53.-)*

> The appropriate 7th character is to be added to each code from category T52
> A   initial encounter
> D   subsequent encounter
> S   sequela

⑤ **T52.0   Toxic effects of petroleum products**
Toxic effects of gasoline [petrol]
Toxic effects of kerosene [paraffin oil]
Toxic effects of paraffin wax
Toxic effects of ether petroleum
Toxic effects of naphtha petroleum
Toxic effects of spirit petroleum
⑥ **T52.0X   Toxic effects of petroleum products**
⑦ **T52.0X1-   Toxic effect of petroleum products, accidental (unintentional)**
Toxic effects of petroleum products NOS
⑦ **T52.0X2-   Toxic effect of petroleum products, intentional self-harm**
⑦ **T52.0X3-   Toxic effect of petroleum products, assault**
⑦ **T52.0X4-   Toxic effect of petroleum products, undetermined**

⑤ **T52.1   Toxic effects of benzene**
> EXCLUDES 1   *homologues of benzene (T52.2)*
> *nitroderivatives and aminoderivatives of benzene and its homologues (T65.3)*
⑥ **T52.1X   Toxic effects of benzene**
⑦ **T52.1X1-   Toxic effect of benzene, accidental (unintentional)**
Toxic effects of benzene NOS
⑦ **T52.1X2-   Toxic effect of benzene, intentional self-harm**
⑦ **T52.1X3-   Toxic effect of benzene, assault**
⑦ **T52.1X4-   Toxic effect of benzene, undetermined**

⑤ **T52.2   Toxic effects of homologues of benzene**
Toxic effects of toluene [methylbenzene]
Toxic effects of xylene [dimethylbenzene]
⑥ **T52.2X   Toxic effects of homologues of benzene**
⑦ **T52.2X1-   Toxic effect of homologues of benzene, accidental (unintentional)**
Toxic effects of homologues of benzene NOS
⑦ **T52.2X2-   Toxic effect of homologues of benzene, intentional self-harm**
⑦ **T52.2X3-   Toxic effect of homologues of benzene, assault**
⑦ **T52.2X4-   Toxic effect of homologues of benzene, undetermined**

⑤ **T52.3   Toxic effects of glycols**
⑥ **T52.3X   Toxic effects of glycols**
⑦ **T52.3X1-   Toxic effect of glycols, accidental (unintentional)**
Toxic effects of glycols NOS
⑦ **T52.3X2-   Toxic effect of glycols, intentional self-harm**
⑦ **T52.3X3-   Toxic effect of glycols, assault**
⑦ **T52.3X4-   Toxic effect of glycols, undetermined**

⑤ **T52.4   Toxic effects of ketones**
⑥ **T52.4X   Toxic effects of ketones**
⑦ **T52.4X1-   Toxic effect of ketones, accidental (unintentional)**
Toxic effects of ketones NOS

● New   ▲ Revised   *Manifestation*   ④-⑦ Digit Indicators   ⊟ Laterality   Ⓐ Adult (15+ years)   Ⓜ Maternity (12-55 years)   Ⓝ Newborn   Ⓟ Pediatric (0-17 years)   ♂ Male   ♀ Female
✖ Deleted   Unspecified   + Additional code

1078   © 2017 DecisionHealth   2017 ICD-10-CM Expert for Physicians

[7] **T52.4X2-** Toxic effect of ketones, intentional self-harm
[7] **T52.4X3-** Toxic effect of ketones, assault
[7] **T52.4X4-** Toxic effect of ketones, undetermined
[5] **T52.8** Toxic effects of other organic solvents
[6] **T52.8X** Toxic effects of other organic solvents
[7] **T52.8X1-** Toxic effect of other organic solvents, accidental (unintentional)
Toxic effects of other organic solvents NOS
[7] **T52.8X2-** Toxic effect of other organic solvents, intentional self-harm
[7] **T52.8X3-** Toxic effect of other organic solvents, assault
[7] **T52.8X4-** Toxic effect of other organic solvents, undetermined
[5] **T52.9** Toxic effects of unspecified organic solvent
[7] **T52.91X-** Toxic effect of unspecified organic solvent, accidental (unintentional)
[7] **T52.92X-** Toxic effect of unspecified organic solvent, intentional self-harm
[7] **T52.93X-** Toxic effect of unspecified organic solvent, assault
[7] **T52.94X-** Toxic effect of unspecified organic solvent, undetermined

[4] **T53** Toxic effect of halogen derivatives of aliphatic and aromatic hydrocarbons

The appropriate 7th character is to be added to each code from category T53
A   initial encounter
D   subsequent encounter
S   sequela

[5] **T53.0** Toxic effects of carbon tetrachloride
Toxic effects of tetrachloromethane
[6] **T53.0X** Toxic effects of carbon tetrachloride
[7] **T53.0X1-** Toxic effect of carbon tetrachloride, accidental (unintentional)
Toxic effects of carbon tetrachloride NOS
[7] **T53.0X2-** Toxic effect of carbon tetrachloride, intentional self-harm
[7] **T53.0X3-** Toxic effect of carbon tetrachloride, assault
[7] **T53.0X4-** Toxic effect of carbon tetrachloride, undetermined
[5] **T53.1** Toxic effects of chloroform
Toxic effects of trichloromethane
[6] **T53.1X** Toxic effects of chloroform
[7] **T53.1X1-** Toxic effect of chloroform, accidental (unintentional)
Toxic effects of chloroform NOS
[7] **T53.1X2-** Toxic effect of chloroform, intentional self-harm
[7] **T53.1X3-** Toxic effect of chloroform, assault
[7] **T53.1X4-** Toxic effect of chloroform, undetermined
[5] **T53.2** Toxic effects of trichloroethylene
Toxic effects of trichloroethene
[6] **T53.2X** Toxic effects of trichloroethylene
[7] **T53.2X1-** Toxic effect of trichloroethylene, accidental (unintentional)
Toxic effects of trichloroethylene NOS
[7] **T53.2X2-** Toxic effect of trichloroethylene, intentional self-harm
[7] **T53.2X3-** Toxic effect of trichloroethylene, assault
[7] **T53.2X4-** Toxic effect of trichloroethylene, undetermined
[5] **T53.3** Toxic effects of tetrachloroethylene
Toxic effects of perchloroethylene
Toxic effect of tetrachloroethene
[6] **T53.3X** Toxic effects of tetrachloroethylene
[7] **T53.3X1-** Toxic effect of tetrachloroethylene, accidental (unintentional)
Toxic effects of tetrachloroethylene NOS
[7] **T53.3X2-** Toxic effect of tetrachloroethylene, intentional self-harm
[7] **T53.3X3-** Toxic effect of tetrachloroethylene, assault
[7] **T53.3X4-** Toxic effect of tetrachloroethylene, undetermined
[5] **T53.4** Toxic effects of dichloromethane
Toxic effects of methylene chloride
[6] **T53.4X** Toxic effects of dichloromethane
[7] **T53.4X1-** Toxic effect of dichloromethane, accidental (unintentional)
Toxic effects of dichloromethane NOS

[7] **T53.4X2-** Toxic effect of dichloromethane, intentional self-harm
[7] **T53.4X3-** Toxic effect of dichloromethane, assault
[7] **T53.4X4-** Toxic effect of dichloromethane, undetermined
[5] **T53.5** Toxic effects of chlorofluorocarbons
[6] **T53.5X** Toxic effects of chlorofluorocarbons
[7] **T53.5X1-** Toxic effect of chlorofluorocarbons, accidental (unintentional)
Toxic effects of chlorofluorocarbons NOS
[7] **T53.5X2-** Toxic effect of chlorofluorocarbons, intentional self-harm
[7] **T53.5X3-** Toxic effect of chlorofluorocarbons, assault
[7] **T53.5X4-** Toxic effect of chlorofluorocarbons, undetermined
[5] **T53.6** Toxic effects of other halogen derivatives of aliphatic hydrocarbons
[6] **T53.6X** Toxic effects of other halogen derivatives of aliphatic hydrocarbons
[7] **T53.6X1-** Toxic effect of other halogen derivatives of aliphatic hydrocarbons, accidental (unintentional)
Toxic effects of other halogen derivatives of aliphatic hydrocarbons NOS
[7] **T53.6X2-** Toxic effect of other halogen derivatives of aliphatic hydrocarbons, intentional self-harm
[7] **T53.6X3-** Toxic effect of other halogen derivatives of aliphatic hydrocarbons, assault
[7] **T53.6X4-** Toxic effect of other halogen derivatives of aliphatic hydrocarbons, undetermined
[5] **T53.7** Toxic effects of other halogen derivatives of aromatic hydrocarbons
[6] **T53.7X** Toxic effects of other halogen derivatives of aromatic hydrocarbons
[7] **T53.7X1-** Toxic effect of other halogen derivatives of aromatic hydrocarbons, accidental (unintentional)
Toxic effects of other halogen derivatives of aromatic hydrocarbons NOS
[7] **T53.7X2-** Toxic effect of other halogen derivatives of aromatic hydrocarbons, intentional self-harm
[7] **T53.7X3-** Toxic effect of other halogen derivatives of aromatic hydrocarbons, assault
[7] **T53.7X4-** Toxic effect of other halogen derivatives of aromatic hydrocarbons, undetermined
[5] **T53.9** Toxic effects of unspecified halogen derivatives of aliphatic and aromatic hydrocarbons
[7] **T53.91X-** Toxic effect of unspecified halogen derivatives of aliphatic and aromatic hydrocarbons, accidental (unintentional)
[7] **T53.92X-** Toxic effect of unspecified halogen derivatives of aliphatic and aromatic hydrocarbons, intentional self-harm
[7] **T53.93X-** Toxic effect of unspecified halogen derivatives of aliphatic and aromatic hydrocarbons, assault
[7] **T53.94X-** Toxic effect of unspecified halogen derivatives of aliphatic and aromatic hydrocarbons, undetermined

[4] **T54** Toxic effect of corrosive substances

The appropriate 7th character is to be added to each code from category T54
A   initial encounter
D   subsequent encounter
S   sequela

[5] **T54.0** Toxic effects of phenol and phenol homologues
[6] **T54.0X** Toxic effects of phenol and phenol homologues
[7] **T54.0X1-** Toxic effect of phenol and phenol homologues, accidental (unintentional)
Toxic effects of phenol and phenol homologues NOS
[7] **T54.0X2-** Toxic effect of phenol and phenol homologues, intentional self-harm
[7] **T54.0X3-** Toxic effect of phenol and phenol homologues, assault
[7] **T54.0X4-** Toxic effect of phenol and phenol homologues, undetermined
[5] **T54.1** Toxic effects of other corrosive organic compounds
[6] **T54.1X** Toxic effects of other corrosive organic compounds

---

● New   ▲ Revised   *Manifestation*   [4]-[7] Digit Indicators   ▭ Laterality   Ⓐ Adult (15+ years)   Ⓜ Maternity (12-55 years)   Ⓝ Newborn   Ⓟ Pediatric (0-17 years)   ♂ Male   ♀ Female
✖ Deleted   Unspecified   + Additional code

7 T54.1X1-   Toxic effect of other corrosive organic compounds, accidental (unintentional)
Toxic effects of other corrosive organic compounds NOS

7 T54.1X2-   Toxic effect of other corrosive organic compounds, intentional self-harm

7 T54.1X3-   Toxic effect of other corrosive organic compounds, assault

7 T54.1X4-   Toxic effect of other corrosive organic compounds, undetermined

5 T54.2   Toxic effects of corrosive acids and acid-like substances
Toxic effects of hydrochloric acid
Toxic effects of sulfuric acid

6 T54.2X   Toxic effects of corrosive acids and acid-like substances

7 T54.2X1-   Toxic effect of corrosive acids and acid-like substances, accidental (unintentional)
Toxic effects of corrosive acids and acid-like substances NOS

7 T54.2X2-   Toxic effect of corrosive acids and acid-like substances, intentional self-harm

7 T54.2X3-   Toxic effect of corrosive acids and acid-like substances, assault

7 T54.2X4-   Toxic effect of corrosive acids and acid-like substances, undetermined

5 T54.3   Toxic effects of corrosive alkalis and alkali-like substances
Toxic effects of potassium hydroxide
Toxic effects of sodium hydroxide

6 T54.3X   Toxic effects of corrosive alkalis and alkali-like substances

7 T54.3X1-   Toxic effect of corrosive alkalis and alkali-like substances, accidental (unintentional)
Toxic effects of corrosive alkalis and alkali-like substances NOS

7 T54.3X2-   Toxic effect of corrosive alkalis and alkali-like substances, intentional self-harm

7 T54.3X3-   Toxic effect of corrosive alkalis and alkali-like substances, assault

7 T54.3X4-   Toxic effect of corrosive alkalis and alkali-like substances, undetermined

5 T54.9   Toxic effects of unspecified corrosive substance

7 T54.91X-   Toxic effect of unspecified corrosive substance, accidental (unintentional)

7 T54.92X-   Toxic effect of unspecified corrosive substance, intentional self-harm

7 T54.93X-   Toxic effect of unspecified corrosive substance, assault

7 T54.94X-   Toxic effect of unspecified corrosive substance, undetermined

4 T55   Toxic effect of soaps and detergents

The appropriate 7th character is to be added to each code from category T55
A   initial encounter
D   subsequent encounter
S   sequela

5 T55.0   Toxic effect of soaps

6 T55.0X   Toxic effect of soaps

7 T55.0X1-   Toxic effect of soaps, accidental (unintentional)
Toxic effect of soaps NOS

7 T55.0X2-   Toxic effect of soaps, intentional self-harm

7 T55.0X3-   Toxic effect of soaps, assault

7 T55.0X4-   Toxic effect of soaps, undetermined

5 T55.1   Toxic effect of detergents

6 T55.1X   Toxic effect of detergents

7 T55.1X1-   Toxic effect of detergents, accidental (unintentional)
Toxic effect of detergents NOS

7 T55.1X2-   Toxic effect of detergents, intentional self-harm

7 T55.1X3-   Toxic effect of detergents, assault

7 T55.1X4-   Toxic effect of detergents, undetermined

4 + T56   Toxic effect of metals

| INCLUDES | toxic effects of fumes and vapors of metals
toxic effects of metals from all sources, except medicinal substances |

Use additional code to identify any retained metal foreign body, if applicable (Z18.0-, T18.1-)

| EXCLUDES 1 | arsenic and its compounds (T57.0)
manganese and its compounds (T57.2) |

The appropriate 7th character is to be added to each code from category T56
A   initial encounter
D   subsequent encounter
S   sequela

5 + T56.0   Toxic effects of lead and its compounds

6 + T56.0X   Toxic effects of lead and its compounds

7 + T56.0X1-   Toxic effect of lead and its compounds, accidental (unintentional)
Toxic effects of lead and its compounds NOS

7 + T56.0X2-   Toxic effect of lead and its compounds, intentional self-harm

7 + T56.0X3-   Toxic effect of lead and its compounds, assault

7 + T56.0X4-   Toxic effect of lead and its compounds, undetermined

5 + T56.1   Toxic effects of mercury and its compounds

6 + T56.1X   Toxic effects of mercury and its compounds

7 + T56.1X1-   Toxic effect of mercury and its compounds, accidental (unintentional)
Toxic effects of mercury and its compounds NOS

7 + T56.1X2-   Toxic effect of mercury and its compounds, intentional self-harm

7 + T56.1X3-   Toxic effect of mercury and its compounds, assault

7 + T56.1X4-   Toxic effect of mercury and its compounds, undetermined

5 + T56.2   Toxic effects of chromium and its compounds

6 + T56.2X   Toxic effects of chromium and its compounds

7 + T56.2X1-   Toxic effect of chromium and its compounds, accidental (unintentional)
Toxic effects of chromium and its compounds NOS

7 + T56.2X2-   Toxic effect of chromium and its compounds, intentional self-harm

7 + T56.2X3-   Toxic effect of chromium and its compounds, assault

7 + T56.2X4-   Toxic effect of chromium and its compounds, undetermined

5 + T56.3   Toxic effects of cadmium and its compounds

6 + T56.3X   Toxic effects of cadmium and its compounds

7 + T56.3X1-   Toxic effect of cadmium and its compounds, accidental (unintentional)
Toxic effects of cadmium and its compounds NOS

7 + T56.3X2-   Toxic effect of cadmium and its compounds, intentional self-harm

7 + T56.3X3-   Toxic effect of cadmium and its compounds, assault

7 + T56.3X4-   Toxic effect of cadmium and its compounds, undetermined

5 + T56.4   Toxic effects of copper and its compounds

6 + T56.4X   Toxic effects of copper and its compounds

7 + T56.4X1-   Toxic effect of copper and its compounds, accidental (unintentional)
Toxic effects of copper and its compounds NOS

7 + T56.4X2-   Toxic effect of copper and its compounds, intentional self-harm

7 + T56.4X3-   Toxic effect of copper and its compounds, assault

7 + T56.4X4-   Toxic effect of copper and its compounds, undetermined

5 + T56.5   Toxic effects of zinc and its compounds

6 + T56.5X   Toxic effects of zinc and its compounds

7 + T56.5X1-   Toxic effect of zinc and its compounds, accidental (unintentional)
Toxic effects of zinc and its compounds NOS

7 + T56.5X2-   Toxic effect of zinc and its compounds, intentional self-harm

7 + T56.5X3-   Toxic effect of zinc and its compounds, assault

7 + T56.5X4-   Toxic effect of zinc and its compounds, undetermined

5 + **T56.6** Toxic effects of tin and its compounds
  6 + **T56.6X** Toxic effects of tin and its compounds
    7 + **T56.6X1-** Toxic effect of tin and its compounds, accidental (unintentional)
      Toxic effects of tin and its compounds NOS
    7 + **T56.6X2-** Toxic effect of tin and its compounds, intentional self-harm
    7 + **T56.6X3-** Toxic effect of tin and its compounds, assault
    7 + **T56.6X4-** Toxic effect of tin and its compounds, undetermined
5 + **T56.7** Toxic effects of beryllium and its compounds
  6 + **T56.7X** Toxic effect of beryllium and its compounds
    7 + **T56.7X1-** Toxic effect of beryllium and its compounds, accidental (unintentional)
      Toxic effects of beryllium and its compounds NOS
    7 + **T56.7X2-** Toxic effect of beryllium and its compounds, intentional self-harm
    7 + **T56.7X3-** Toxic effect of beryllium and its compounds, assault
    7 + **T56.7X4-** Toxic effect of beryllium and its compounds, undetermined
5 + **T56.8** Toxic effects of other metals
  6 + **T56.81** Toxic effect of thallium
    7 + **T56.811-** Toxic effect of thallium, accidental (unintentional)
      Toxic effect of thallium NOS
    7 + **T56.812-** Toxic effect of thallium, intentional self-harm
    7 + **T56.813-** Toxic effect of thallium, assault
    7 + **T56.814-** Toxic effect of thallium, undetermined
  6 + **T56.89** Toxic effects of other metals
    7 + **T56.891-** Toxic effect of other metals, accidental (unintentional)
      Toxic effects of other metals NOS
    7 + **T56.892-** Toxic effect of other metals, intentional self-harm
    7 + **T56.893-** Toxic effect of other metals, assault
    7 + **T56.894-** Toxic effect of other metals, undetermined
5 + **T56.9** Toxic effects of unspecified metal
    7 + **T56.91X-** Toxic effect of unspecified metal, accidental (unintentional)
    7 + **T56.92X-** Toxic effect of unspecified metal, intentional self-harm
    7 + **T56.93X-** Toxic effect of unspecified metal, assault
    7 + **T56.94X-** Toxic effect of unspecified metal, undetermined

4 **T57** Toxic effect of other inorganic substances

The appropriate 7th character is to be added to each code from category T57
A   initial encounter
D   subsequent encounter
S   sequela

5 **T57.0** Toxic effect of arsenic and its compounds
  6 **T57.0X** Toxic effect of arsenic and its compounds
    7 **T57.0X1-** Toxic effect of arsenic and its compounds, accidental (unintentional)
      Toxic effect of arsenic and its compounds NOS
    7 **T57.0X2-** Toxic effect of arsenic and its compounds, intentional self-harm
    7 **T57.0X3-** Toxic effect of arsenic and its compounds, assault
    7 **T57.0X4-** Toxic effect of arsenic and its compounds, undetermined
5 **T57.1** Toxic effect of phosphorus and its compounds
    EXCLUDES 1 *organophosphate insecticides (T60.0)*
  6 **T57.1X** Toxic effect of phosphorus and its compounds
    7 **T57.1X1-** Toxic effect of phosphorus and its compounds, accidental (unintentional)
      Toxic effect of phosphorus and its compounds NOS
    7 **T57.1X2-** Toxic effect of phosphorus and its compounds, intentional self-harm
    7 **T57.1X3-** Toxic effect of phosphorus and its compounds, assault
    7 **T57.1X4-** Toxic effect of phosphorus and its compounds, undetermined
5 **T57.2** Toxic effect of manganese and its compounds
  6 **T57.2X** Toxic effect of manganese and its compounds

    7 **T57.2X1-** Toxic effect of manganese and its compounds, accidental (unintentional)
      Toxic effect of manganese and its compounds NOS
    7 **T57.2X2-** Toxic effect of manganese and its compounds, intentional self-harm
    7 **T57.2X3-** Toxic effect of manganese and its compounds, assault
    7 **T57.2X4-** Toxic effect of manganese and its compounds, undetermined
5 **T57.3** Toxic effect of hydrogen cyanide
  6 **T57.3X** Toxic effect of hydrogen cyanide
    7 **T57.3X1-** Toxic effect of hydrogen cyanide, accidental (unintentional)
      Toxic effect of hydrogen cyanide NOS
    7 **T57.3X2-** Toxic effect of hydrogen cyanide, intentional self-harm
    7 **T57.3X3-** Toxic effect of hydrogen cyanide, assault
    7 **T57.3X4-** Toxic effect of hydrogen cyanide, undetermined
5 **T57.8** Toxic effect of other specified inorganic substances
  6 **T57.8X** Toxic effect of other specified inorganic substances
    7 **T57.8X1-** Toxic effect of other specified inorganic substances, accidental (unintentional)
      Toxic effect of other specified inorganic substances NOS
    7 **T57.8X2-** Toxic effect of other specified inorganic substances, intentional self-harm
    7 **T57.8X3-** Toxic effect of other specified inorganic substances, assault
    7 **T57.8X4-** Toxic effect of other specified inorganic substances, undetermined
5 **T57.9** Toxic effect of unspecified inorganic substance
    7 **T57.91X-** Toxic effect of unspecified inorganic substance, accidental (unintentional)
    7 **T57.92X-** Toxic effect of unspecified inorganic substance, intentional self-harm
    7 **T57.93X-** Toxic effect of unspecified inorganic substance, assault
    7 **T57.94X-** Toxic effect of unspecified inorganic substance, undetermined

4 **T58** Toxic effect of carbon monoxide
    INCLUDES asphyxiation from carbon monoxide
      toxic effect of carbon monoxide from all sources

The appropriate 7th character is to be added to each code from category T58
A   initial encounter
D   subsequent encounter
S   sequela

5 **T58.0** Toxic effect of carbon monoxide from motor vehicle exhaust
    Toxic effect of exhaust gas from gas engine
    Toxic effect of exhaust gas from motor pump
    7 **T58.01X-** Toxic effect of carbon monoxide from motor vehicle exhaust, accidental (unintentional)
    7 **T58.02X-** Toxic effect of carbon monoxide from motor vehicle exhaust, intentional self-harm
    7 **T58.03X-** Toxic effect of carbon monoxide from motor vehicle exhaust, assault
    7 **T58.04X-** Toxic effect of carbon monoxide from motor vehicle exhaust, undetermined
5 **T58.1** Toxic effect of carbon monoxide from utility gas
    Toxic effect of acetylene
    Toxic effect of gas NOS used for lighting, heating, cooking
    Toxic effect of water gas
    7 **T58.11X-** Toxic effect of carbon monoxide from utility gas, accidental (unintentional)
    7 **T58.12X-** Toxic effect of carbon monoxide from utility gas, intentional self-harm
    7 **T58.13X-** Toxic effect of carbon monoxide from utility gas, assault
    7 **T58.14X-** Toxic effect of carbon monoxide from utility gas, undetermined
5 **T58.2** Toxic effect of carbon monoxide from incomplete combustion of other domestic fuels
    Toxic effect of carbon monoxide from incomplete combustion of coal, coke, kerosene, wood
  6 **T58.2X** Toxic effect of carbon monoxide from incomplete combustion of other domestic fuels

● New   ▲ Revised   *Manifestation*   4-7 Digit Indicators   ⊟ Laterality   Ⓐ Adult (15+ years)   Ⓜ Maternity (12-55 years)   Ⓝ Newborn   Ⓟ Pediatric (0-17 years)   ♂ Male   ♀ Female
✖ Deleted   Unspecified   + Additional code

2017 ICD-10-CM Expert for Physicians

© 2017 DecisionHealth   1081

7 **T58.2X1-** Toxic effect of carbon monoxide from incomplete combustion of other domestic fuels, accidental (unintentional)

7 **T58.2X2-** Toxic effect of carbon monoxide from incomplete combustion of other domestic fuels, intentional self-harm

7 **T58.2X3-** Toxic effect of carbon monoxide from incomplete combustion of other domestic fuels, assault

7 **T58.2X4-** Toxic effect of carbon monoxide from incomplete combustion of other domestic fuels, undetermined

5 **T58.8** Toxic effect of carbon monoxide from other source
Toxic effect of carbon monoxide from blast furnace gas
Toxic effect of carbon monoxide from fuels in industrial use
Toxic effect of carbon monoxide from kiln vapor

6 **T58.8X** Toxic effect of carbon monoxide from other source

7 **T58.8X1-** Toxic effect of carbon monoxide from other source, accidental (unintentional)

7 **T58.8X2-** Toxic effect of carbon monoxide from other source, intentional self-harm

7 **T58.8X3-** Toxic effect of carbon monoxide from other source, assault

7 **T58.8X4-** Toxic effect of carbon monoxide from other source, undetermined

5 **T58.9** Toxic effect of carbon monoxide from unspecified source

7 **T58.91X-** Toxic effect of carbon monoxide from unspecified source, accidental (unintentional)

7 **T58.92X-** Toxic effect of carbon monoxide from unspecified source, intentional self-harm

7 **T58.93X-** Toxic effect of carbon monoxide from unspecified source, assault

7 **T58.94X-** Toxic effect of carbon monoxide from unspecified source, undetermined

4 **T59** **Toxic effect of other gases, fumes and vapors**

INCLUDES	aerosol propellants

EXCLUDES 1	*chlorofluorocarbons (T53.5)*

The appropriate 7th character is to be added to each code from category T59
A   initial encounter
D   subsequent encounter
S   sequela

5 **T59.0** Toxic effect of nitrogen oxides

6 **T59.0X** Toxic effect of nitrogen oxides

7 **T59.0X1-** Toxic effect of nitrogen oxides, accidental (unintentional)
Toxic effect of nitrogen oxides NOS

7 **T59.0X2-** Toxic effect of nitrogen oxides, intentional self-harm

7 **T59.0X3-** Toxic effect of nitrogen oxides, assault

7 **T59.0X4-** Toxic effect of nitrogen oxides, undetermined

5 **T59.1** Toxic effect of sulfur dioxide

6 **T59.1X** Toxic effect of sulfur dioxide

7 **T59.1X1-** Toxic effect of sulfur dioxide, accidental (unintentional)
Toxic effect of sulfur dioxide NOS

7 **T59.1X2-** Toxic effect of sulfur dioxide, intentional self-harm

7 **T59.1X3-** Toxic effect of sulfur dioxide, assault

7 **T59.1X4-** Toxic effect of sulfur dioxide, undetermined

5 **T59.2** Toxic effect of formaldehyde

6 **T59.2X** Toxic effect of formaldehyde

7 **T59.2X1-** Toxic effect of formaldehyde, accidental (unintentional)
Toxic effect of formaldehyde NOS

7 **T59.2X2-** Toxic effect of formaldehyde, intentional self-harm

7 **T59.2X3-** Toxic effect of formaldehyde, assault

7 **T59.2X4-** Toxic effect of formaldehyde, undetermined

5 **T59.3** Toxic effect of lacrimogenic gas
Toxic effect of tear gas

6 **T59.3X** Toxic effect of lacrimogenic gas

7 **T59.3X1-** Toxic effect of lacrimogenic gas, accidental (unintentional)
Toxic effect of lacrimogenic gas NOS

7 **T59.3X2-** Toxic effect of lacrimogenic gas, intentional self-harm

7 **T59.3X3-** Toxic effect of lacrimogenic gas, assault

7 **T59.3X4-** Toxic effect of lacrimogenic gas, undetermined

5 **T59.4** Toxic effect of chlorine gas

6 **T59.4X** Toxic effect of chlorine gas

7 **T59.4X1-** Toxic effect of chlorine gas, accidental (unintentional)
Toxic effect of chlorine gas NOS

7 **T59.4X2-** Toxic effect of chlorine gas, intentional self-harm

7 **T59.4X3-** Toxic effect of chlorine gas, assault

7 **T59.4X4-** Toxic effect of chlorine gas, undetermined

5 **T59.5** Toxic effect of fluorine gas and hydrogen fluoride

6 **T59.5X** Toxic effect of fluorine gas and hydrogen fluoride

7 **T59.5X1-** Toxic effect of fluorine gas and hydrogen fluoride, accidental (unintentional)
Toxic effect of fluorine gas and hydrogen fluoride NOS

7 **T59.5X2-** Toxic effect of fluorine gas and hydrogen fluoride, intentional self-harm

7 **T59.5X3-** Toxic effect of fluorine gas and hydrogen fluoride, assault

7 **T59.5X4-** Toxic effect of fluorine gas and hydrogen fluoride, undetermined

5 **T59.6** Toxic effect of hydrogen sulfide

6 **T59.6X** Toxic effect of hydrogen sulfide

7 **T59.6X1-** Toxic effect of hydrogen sulfide, accidental (unintentional)
Toxic effect of hydrogen sulfide NOS

7 **T59.6X2-** Toxic effect of hydrogen sulfide, intentional self-harm

7 **T59.6X3-** Toxic effect of hydrogen sulfide, assault

7 **T59.6X4-** Toxic effect of hydrogen sulfide, undetermined

5 **T59.7** Toxic effect of carbon dioxide

6 **T59.7X** Toxic effect of carbon dioxide

7 **T59.7X1-** Toxic effect of carbon dioxide, accidental (unintentional)
Toxic effect of carbon dioxide NOS

7 **T59.7X2-** Toxic effect of carbon dioxide, intentional self-harm

7 **T59.7X3-** Toxic effect of carbon dioxide, assault

7 **T59.7X4-** Toxic effect of carbon dioxide, undetermined

5 **T59.8** Toxic effect of other specified gases, fumes and vapors

6 **T59.81** Toxic effect of smoke
Smoke inhalation

EXCLUDES 2	*toxic effect of cigarette (tobacco) smoke (T65.22-)*

7 **T59.811-** Toxic effect of smoke, accidental (unintentional)
Toxic effect of smoke NOS
AHA: 4Q 2013, 121

7 **T59.812-** Toxic effect of smoke, intentional self-harm

7 **T59.813-** Toxic effect of smoke, assault

7 **T59.814-** Toxic effect of smoke, undetermined

6 **T59.89** Toxic effect of other specified gases, fumes and vapors

7 **T59.891-** Toxic effect of other specified gases, fumes and vapors, accidental (unintentional)

7 **T59.892-** Toxic effect of other specified gases, fumes and vapors, intentional self-harm

7 **T59.893-** Toxic effect of other specified gases, fumes and vapors, assault

7 **T59.894-** Toxic effect of other specified gases, fumes and vapors, undetermined

5 **T59.9** Toxic effect of unspecified gases, fumes and vapors

7 **T59.91X-** Toxic effect of unspecified gases, fumes and vapors, accidental (unintentional)

7 **T59.92X-** Toxic effect of unspecified gases, fumes and vapors, intentional self-harm

7 **T59.93X-** Toxic effect of unspecified gases, fumes and vapors, assault

7 **T59.94X-** Toxic effect of unspecified gases, fumes and vapors, undetermined

● New   ▲ Revised   *Manifestation*   4-7 Digit Indicators   ▣ Laterality   Ⓐ Adult (15+ years)   Ⓜ Maternity (12-55 years)   Ⓝ Newborn   Ⓟ Pediatric (0-17 years)   ♂ Male   ♀ Female
✖ Deleted   Unspecified   ✚ Additional code

1082   © 2017 DecisionHealth   2017 ICD-10-CM Expert for Physicians

4 **T60 Toxic effect of pesticides**

INCLUDES   toxic effect of wood preservatives

The appropriate 7th character is to be added to each code from category T60
A   initial encounter
D   subsequent encounter
S   sequela

5 **T60.0 Toxic effect of organophosphate and carbamate insecticides**

6 **T60.0X Toxic effect of organophosphate and carbamate insecticides**

7 **T60.0X1- Toxic effect of organophosphate and carbamate insecticides, accidental (unintentional)**
Toxic effect of organophosphate and carbamate insecticides NOS

7 **T60.0X2- Toxic effect of organophosphate and carbamate insecticides, intentional self-harm**

7 **T60.0X3- Toxic effect of organophosphate and carbamate insecticides, assault**

7 **T60.0X4- Toxic effect of organophosphate and carbamate insecticides, undetermined**

5 **T60.1 Toxic effect of halogenated insecticides**

EXCLUDES 1   chlorinated hydrocarbon (T53.-)

6 **T60.1X Toxic effect of halogenated insecticides**

7 **T60.1X1- Toxic effect of halogenated insecticides, accidental (unintentional)**
Toxic effect of halogenated insecticides NOS

7 **T60.1X2- Toxic effect of halogenated insecticides, intentional self-harm**

7 **T60.1X3- Toxic effect of halogenated insecticides, assault**

7 **T60.1X4- Toxic effect of halogenated insecticides, undetermined**

5 **T60.2 Toxic effect of other insecticides**

6 **T60.2X Toxic effect of other insecticides**

7 **T60.2X1- Toxic effect of other insecticides, accidental (unintentional)**
Toxic effect of other insecticides NOS

7 **T60.2X2- Toxic effect of other insecticides, intentional self-harm**

7 **T60.2X3- Toxic effect of other insecticides, assault**

7 **T60.2X4- Toxic effect of other insecticides, undetermined**

5 **T60.3 Toxic effect of herbicides and fungicides**

6 **T60.3X Toxic effect of herbicides and fungicides**

7 **T60.3X1- Toxic effect of herbicides and fungicides, accidental (unintentional)**
Toxic effect of herbicides and fungicides NOS

7 **T60.3X2- Toxic effect of herbicides and fungicides, intentional self-harm**

7 **T60.3X3- Toxic effect of herbicides and fungicides, assault**

7 **T60.3X4- Toxic effect of herbicides and fungicides, undetermined**

5 **T60.4 Toxic effect of rodenticides**

EXCLUDES 1   strychnine and its salts (T65.1)
thallium (T56.81-)

6 **T60.4X Toxic effect of rodenticides**

7 **T60.4X1- Toxic effect of rodenticides, accidental (unintentional)**
Toxic effect of rodenticides NOS

7 **T60.4X2- Toxic effect of rodenticides, intentional self-harm**

7 **T60.4X3- Toxic effect of rodenticides, assault**

7 **T60.4X4- Toxic effect of rodenticides, undetermined**

5 **T60.8 Toxic effect of other pesticides**

6 **T60.8X Toxic effect of other pesticides**

7 **T60.8X1- Toxic effect of other pesticides, accidental (unintentional)**
Toxic effect of other pesticides NOS

7 **T60.8X2- Toxic effect of other pesticides, intentional self-harm**

7 **T60.8X3- Toxic effect of other pesticides, assault**

7 **T60.8X4- Toxic effect of other pesticides, undetermined**

5 **T60.9 Toxic effect of unspecified pesticide**

7 **T60.91X- Toxic effect of unspecified pesticide, accidental (unintentional)**

7 **T60.92X- Toxic effect of unspecified pesticide, intentional self-harm**

7 **T60.93X- Toxic effect of unspecified pesticide, assault**

7 **T60.94X- Toxic effect of unspecified pesticide, undetermined**

▲ 4 **T61 Toxic effect of noxious substances eaten as seafood**

EXCLUDES 1   *allergic reaction to food, such as:*
anaphylactic reaction or shock due to adverse food reaction (T78.0-)
bacterial foodborne intoxications (A05.-)
dermatitis (L23.6, L25.4, L27.2)
food protein-induced enterocolitis syndrome (K52.21)
food protein-induced enteropathy (K52.22)
gastroenteritis (noninfective) (K52.29)
toxic effect of aflatoxin and other mycotoxins (T64)
toxic effect of cyanides (T65.0-)
toxic effect of harmful algae bloom (T65.82-)
toxic effect of hydrogen cyanide (T57.3-)
toxic effect of mercury (T56.1-)
toxic effect of red tide (T65.82-)

The appropriate 7th character is to be added to each code from category T61
A   initial encounter
D   subsequent encounter
S   sequela

5 **T61.0 Ciguatera fish poisoning**

7 **T61.01X- Ciguatera fish poisoning, accidental (unintentional)**

7 **T61.02X- Ciguatera fish poisoning, intentional self-harm**

7 **T61.03X- Ciguatera fish poisoning, assault**

7 **T61.04X- Ciguatera fish poisoning, undetermined**

5 **T61.1 Scombroid fish poisoning**
Histamine-like syndrome

7 **T61.11X- Scombroid fish poisoning, accidental (unintentional)**

7 **T61.12X- Scombroid fish poisoning, intentional self-harm**

7 **T61.13X- Scombroid fish poisoning, assault**

7 **T61.14X- Scombroid fish poisoning, undetermined**

5 **T61.7 Other fish and shellfish poisoning**

6 **T61.77 Other fish poisoning**

7 **T61.771- Other fish poisoning, accidental (unintentional)**

7 **T61.772- Other fish poisoning, intentional self-harm**

7 **T61.773- Other fish poisoning, assault**

7 **T61.774- Other fish poisoning, undetermined**

6 **T61.78 Other shellfish poisoning**

7 **T61.781- Other shellfish poisoning, accidental (unintentional)**

7 **T61.782- Other shellfish poisoning, intentional self-harm**

7 **T61.783- Other shellfish poisoning, assault**

7 **T61.784- Other shellfish poisoning, undetermined**

5 **T61.8 Toxic effect of other seafood**

6 **T61.8X Toxic effect of other seafood**

7 **T61.8X1- Toxic effect of other seafood, accidental (unintentional)**

7 **T61.8X2- Toxic effect of other seafood, intentional self-harm**

7 **T61.8X3- Toxic effect of other seafood, assault**

7 **T61.8X4- Toxic effect of other seafood, undetermined**

5 **T61.9 Toxic effect of unspecified seafood**

7 **T61.91X- Toxic effect of unspecified seafood, accidental (unintentional)**

7 **T61.92X- Toxic effect of unspecified seafood, intentional self-harm**

7 **T61.93X- Toxic effect of unspecified seafood, assault**

7 **T61.94X- Toxic effect of unspecified seafood, undetermined**

● New   ▲ Revised   *Manifestation*   4- 7 Digit Indicators   ▭ Laterality   ▲ Adult (15+ years)   Ⓜ Maternity (12-55 years)   Ⓝ Newborn   Ⓟ Pediatric (0-17 years)   ♂ Male   ♀ Female
✖ Deleted   Unspecified   + Additional code

2017 ICD-10-CM Expert for Physicians

© 2017 DecisionHealth

1083

▲ 4️⃣ **T62**   **Toxic effect of other noxious substances eaten as food**

|EXCLUDES 1| *allergic reaction to food, such as:*
anaphylactic shock (reaction) due to adverse food reaction (T78.0-)
bacterial food borne intoxications (A05.-)
dermatitis (L23.6, L25.4, L27.2)
food protein-induced enterocolitis syndrome (K52.21)
food protein-induced enteropathy (K52.22)
gastroenteritis (noninfective) (K52.29)
toxic effect of aflatoxin and other mycotoxins (T64)
toxic effect of cyanides (T65.0-)
toxic effect of hydrogen cyanide (T57.3-)
toxic effect of mercury (T56.1-)

The appropriate 7th character is to be added to each code from category T62
A   initial encounter
D   subsequent encounter
S   sequela

5️⃣ **T62.0**   **Toxic effect of ingested mushrooms**
  6️⃣ **T62.0X**   **Toxic effect of ingested mushrooms**
    7️⃣ **T62.0X1-**   **Toxic effect of ingested mushrooms, accidental (unintentional)**
    Toxic effect of ingested mushrooms NOS
    7️⃣ **T62.0X2-**   **Toxic effect of ingested mushrooms, intentional self-harm**
    7️⃣ **T62.0X3-**   **Toxic effect of ingested mushrooms, assault**
    7️⃣ **T62.0X4-**   **Toxic effect of ingested mushrooms, undetermined**

5️⃣ **T62.1**   **Toxic effect of ingested berries**
  6️⃣ **T62.1X**   **Toxic effect of ingested berries**
    7️⃣ **T62.1X1-**   **Toxic effect of ingested berries, accidental (unintentional)**
    Toxic effect of ingested berries NOS
    7️⃣ **T62.1X2-**   **Toxic effect of ingested berries, intentional self-harm**
    7️⃣ **T62.1X3-**   **Toxic effect of ingested berries, assault**
    7️⃣ **T62.1X4-**   **Toxic effect of ingested berries, undetermined**

5️⃣ **T62.2**   **Toxic effect of other ingested (parts of) plant(s)**
  6️⃣ **T62.2X**   **Toxic effect of other ingested (parts of) plant(s)**
    7️⃣ **T62.2X1-**   **Toxic effect of other ingested (parts of) plant(s), accidental (unintentional)**
    Toxic effect of other ingested (parts of) plant(s) NOS
    7️⃣ **T62.2X2-**   **Toxic effect of other ingested (parts of) plant(s), intentional self-harm**
    7️⃣ **T62.2X3-**   **Toxic effect of other ingested (parts of) plant(s), assault**
    7️⃣ **T62.2X4-**   **Toxic effect of other ingested (parts of) plant(s), undetermined**

5️⃣ **T62.8**   **Toxic effect of other specified noxious substances eaten as food**
  6️⃣ **T62.8X**   **Toxic effect of other specified noxious substances eaten as food**
    7️⃣ **T62.8X1-**   **Toxic effect of other specified noxious substances eaten as food, accidental (unintentional)**
    Toxic effect of other specified noxious substances eaten as food NOS
    7️⃣ **T62.8X2-**   **Toxic effect of other specified noxious substances eaten as food, intentional self-harm**
    7️⃣ **T62.8X3-**   **Toxic effect of other specified noxious substances eaten as food, assault**
    7️⃣ **T62.8X4-**   **Toxic effect of other specified noxious substances eaten as food, undetermined**

5️⃣ **T62.9**   **Toxic effect of unspecified noxious substance eaten as food**
    7️⃣ **T62.91X-**   **Toxic effect of unspecified noxious substance eaten as food, accidental (unintentional)**
    Toxic effect of unspecified noxious substance eaten as food NOS
    7️⃣ **T62.92X-**   **Toxic effect of unspecified noxious substance eaten as food, intentional self-harm**
    7️⃣ **T62.93X-**   **Toxic effect of unspecified noxious substance eaten as food, assault**
    7️⃣ **T62.94X-**   **Toxic effect of unspecified noxious substance eaten as food, undetermined**

4️⃣ **T63**   **Toxic effect of contact with venomous animals and plants**

|INCLUDES| bite or touch of venomous animal
pricked or stuck by thorn or leaf
|EXCLUDES 2| *ingestion of toxic animal or plant (T61.-, T62.-)*

The appropriate 7th character is to be added to each code from category T63
A   initial encounter
D   subsequent encounter
S   sequela

5️⃣ **T63.0**   **Toxic effect of snake venom**
  6️⃣ **T63.00**   **Toxic effect of unspecified snake venom**
    7️⃣ **T63.001-**   **Toxic effect of unspecified snake venom, accidental (unintentional)**
    Toxic effect of unspecified snake venom NOS
    7️⃣ **T63.002-**   **Toxic effect of unspecified snake venom, intentional self-harm**
    7️⃣ **T63.003-**   **Toxic effect of unspecified snake venom, assault**
    7️⃣ **T63.004-**   **Toxic effect of unspecified snake venom, undetermined**

  6️⃣ **T63.01**   **Toxic effect of rattlesnake venom**
    7️⃣ **T63.011-**   **Toxic effect of rattlesnake venom, accidental (unintentional)**
    Toxic effect of rattlesnake venom NOS
    7️⃣ **T63.012-**   **Toxic effect of rattlesnake venom, intentional self-harm**
    7️⃣ **T63.013-**   **Toxic effect of rattlesnake venom, assault**
    7️⃣ **T63.014-**   **Toxic effect of rattlesnake venom, undetermined**

  6️⃣ **T63.02**   **Toxic effect of coral snake venom**
    7️⃣ **T63.021-**   **Toxic effect of coral snake venom, accidental (unintentional)**
    Toxic effect of coral snake venom NOS
    7️⃣ **T63.022-**   **Toxic effect of coral snake venom, intentional self-harm**
    7️⃣ **T63.023-**   **Toxic effect of coral snake venom, assault**
    7️⃣ **T63.024-**   **Toxic effect of coral snake venom, undetermined**

  6️⃣ **T63.03**   **Toxic effect of taipan venom**
    7️⃣ **T63.031-**   **Toxic effect of taipan venom, accidental (unintentional)**
    Toxic effect of taipan venom NOS
    7️⃣ **T63.032-**   **Toxic effect of taipan venom, intentional self-harm**
    7️⃣ **T63.033-**   **Toxic effect of taipan venom, assault**
    7️⃣ **T63.034-**   **Toxic effect of taipan venom, undetermined**

  6️⃣ **T63.04**   **Toxic effect of cobra venom**
    7️⃣ **T63.041-**   **Toxic effect of cobra venom, accidental (unintentional)**
    Toxic effect of cobra venom NOS
    7️⃣ **T63.042-**   **Toxic effect of cobra venom, intentional self-harm**
    7️⃣ **T63.043-**   **Toxic effect of cobra venom, assault**
    7️⃣ **T63.044-**   **Toxic effect of cobra venom, undetermined**

  6️⃣ **T63.06**   **Toxic effect of venom of other North and South American snake**
    7️⃣ **T63.061-**   **Toxic effect of venom of other North and South American snake, accidental (unintentional)**
    Toxic effect of venom of other North and South American snake NOS
    7️⃣ **T63.062-**   **Toxic effect of venom of other North and South American snake, intentional self-harm**
    7️⃣ **T63.063-**   **Toxic effect of venom of other North and South American snake, assault**
    7️⃣ **T63.064-**   **Toxic effect of venom of other North and South American snake, undetermined**

  6️⃣ **T63.07**   **Toxic effect of venom of other Australian snake**
    7️⃣ **T63.071-**   **Toxic effect of venom of other Australian snake, accidental (unintentional)**
    Toxic effect of venom of other Australian snake NOS
    7️⃣ **T63.072-**   **Toxic effect of venom of other Australian snake, intentional self-harm**
    7️⃣ **T63.073-**   **Toxic effect of venom of other Australian snake, assault**

● New   ▲ Revised   *Manifestation*   4️⃣-7️⃣ Digit Indicators   ▭ Laterality   🅰 Adult (15+ years)   Ⓜ Maternity (12-55 years)   Ⓝ Newborn   🅿 Pediatric (0-17 years)   ♂ Male   ♀ Female
✖ ~~Deleted~~   Unspecified   ✚ Additional code

1084   © 2017 DecisionHealth   2017 ICD-10-CM Expert for Physicians

☑ T63.074-   Toxic effect of venom of other Australian snake, undetermined

◯ T63.08   Toxic effect of venom of other African and Asian snake

☑ T63.081-   Toxic effect of venom of other African and Asian snake, accidental (unintentional)
Toxic effect of venom of other African and Asian snake NOS

☑ T63.082-   Toxic effect of venom of other African and Asian snake, intentional self-harm

☑ T63.083-   Toxic effect of venom of other African and Asian snake, assault

☑ T63.084-   Toxic effect of venom of other African and Asian snake, undetermined

◯ T63.09   Toxic effect of venom of other snake

☑ T63.091-   Toxic effect of venom of other snake, accidental (unintentional)
Toxic effect of venom of other snake NOS

☑ T63.092-   Toxic effect of venom of other snake, intentional self-harm

☑ T63.093-   Toxic effect of venom of other snake, assault

☑ T63.094-   Toxic effect of venom of other snake, undetermined

▣ T63.1   Toxic effect of venom of other reptiles

◯ T63.11   Toxic effect of venom of gila monster

☑ T63.111-   Toxic effect of venom of gila monster, accidental (unintentional)
Toxic effect of venom of gila monster NOS

☑ T63.112-   Toxic effect of venom of gila monster, intentional self-harm

☑ T63.113-   Toxic effect of venom of gila monster, assault

☑ T63.114-   Toxic effect of venom of gila monster, undetermined

◯ T63.12   Toxic effect of venom of other venomous lizard

☑ T63.121-   Toxic effect of venom of other venomous lizard, accidental (unintentional)
Toxic effect of venom of other venomous lizard NOS

☑ T63.122-   Toxic effect of venom of other venomous lizard, intentional self-harm

☑ T63.123-   Toxic effect of venom of other venomous lizard, assault

☑ T63.124-   Toxic effect of venom of other venomous lizard, undetermined

◯ T63.19   Toxic effect of venom of other reptiles

☑ T63.191-   Toxic effect of venom of other reptiles, accidental (unintentional)
Toxic effect of venom of other reptiles NOS

☑ T63.192-   Toxic effect of venom of other reptiles, intentional self-harm

☑ T63.193-   Toxic effect of venom of other reptiles, assault

☑ T63.194-   Toxic effect of venom of other reptiles, undetermined

▣ T63.2   Toxic effect of venom of scorpion

◯ T63.2X   Toxic effect of venom of scorpion

☑ T63.2X1-   Toxic effect of venom of scorpion, accidental (unintentional)
Toxic effect of venom of scorpion NOS

☑ T63.2X2-   Toxic effect of venom of scorpion, intentional self-harm

☑ T63.2X3-   Toxic effect of venom of scorpion, assault

☑ T63.2X4-   Toxic effect of venom of scorpion, undetermined

▣ T63.3   Toxic effect of venom of spider

◯ T63.30   Toxic effect of unspecified spider venom

☑ T63.301-   Toxic effect of unspecified spider venom, accidental (unintentional)

☑ T63.302-   Toxic effect of unspecified spider venom, intentional self-harm

☑ T63.303-   Toxic effect of unspecified spider venom, assault

☑ T63.304-   Toxic effect of unspecified spider venom, undetermined

◯ T63.31   Toxic effect of venom of black widow spider

☑ T63.311-   Toxic effect of venom of black widow spider, accidental (unintentional)

☑ T63.312-   Toxic effect of venom of black widow spider, intentional self-harm

☑ T63.313-   Toxic effect of venom of black widow spider, assault

☑ T63.314-   Toxic effect of venom of black widow spider, undetermined

◯ T63.32   Toxic effect of venom of tarantula

☑ T63.321-   Toxic effect of venom of tarantula, accidental (unintentional)

☑ T63.322-   Toxic effect of venom of tarantula, intentional self-harm

☑ T63.323-   Toxic effect of venom of tarantula, assault

☑ T63.324-   Toxic effect of venom of tarantula, undetermined

◯ T63.33   Toxic effect of venom of brown recluse spider

☑ T63.331-   Toxic effect of venom of brown recluse spider, accidental (unintentional)

☑ T63.332-   Toxic effect of venom of brown recluse spider, intentional self-harm

☑ T63.333-   Toxic effect of venom of brown recluse spider, assault

☑ T63.334-   Toxic effect of venom of brown recluse spider, undetermined

◯ T63.39   Toxic effect of venom of other spider

☑ T63.391-   Toxic effect of venom of other spider, accidental (unintentional)

☑ T63.392-   Toxic effect of venom of other spider, intentional self-harm

☑ T63.393-   Toxic effect of venom of other spider, assault

☑ T63.394-   Toxic effect of venom of other spider, undetermined

▣ T63.4   Toxic effect of venom of other arthropods

◯ T63.41   Toxic effect of venom of centipedes and venomous millipedes

☑ T63.411-   Toxic effect of venom of centipedes and venomous millipedes, accidental (unintentional)

☑ T63.412-   Toxic effect of venom of centipedes and venomous millipedes, intentional self-harm

☑ T63.413-   Toxic effect of venom of centipedes and venomous millipedes, assault

☑ T63.414-   Toxic effect of venom of centipedes and venomous millipedes, undetermined

◯ T63.42   Toxic effect of venom of ants

☑ T63.421-   Toxic effect of venom of ants, accidental (unintentional)

☑ T63.422-   Toxic effect of venom of ants, intentional self-harm

☑ T63.423-   Toxic effect of venom of ants, assault

☑ T63.424-   Toxic effect of venom of ants, undetermined

◯ T63.43   Toxic effect of venom of caterpillars

☑ T63.431-   Toxic effect of venom of caterpillars, accidental (unintentional)

☑ T63.432-   Toxic effect of venom of caterpillars, intentional self-harm

☑ T63.433-   Toxic effect of venom of caterpillars, assault

☑ T63.434-   Toxic effect of venom of caterpillars, undetermined

◯ T63.44   Toxic effect of venom of bees

☑ T63.441-   Toxic effect of venom of bees, accidental (unintentional)

☑ T63.442-   Toxic effect of venom of bees, intentional self-harm

☑ T63.443-   Toxic effect of venom of bees, assault

☑ T63.444-   Toxic effect of venom of bees, undetermined

◯ T63.45   Toxic effect of venom of hornets

☑ T63.451-   Toxic effect of venom of hornets, accidental (unintentional)

☑ T63.452-   Toxic effect of venom of hornets, intentional self-harm

☑ T63.453-   Toxic effect of venom of hornets, assault

☑ T63.454-   Toxic effect of venom of hornets, undetermined

◯ T63.46   Toxic effect of venom of wasps
Toxic effect of yellow jacket

☑ T63.461-   Toxic effect of venom of wasps, accidental (unintentional)

☑ T63.462-   Toxic effect of venom of wasps, intentional self-harm

☑ T63.463-   Toxic effect of venom of wasps, assault

☑ T63.464-   Toxic effect of venom of wasps, undetermined

◯ T63.48   Toxic effect of venom of other arthropod

New	▲ Revised	*Manifestation*	◪-☑ Digit Indicators	▭ Laterality	Ⓐ Adult (15+ years)	Ⓜ Maternity (12-55 years)	Ⓝ Newborn	Ⓟ Pediatric (0-17 years)	♂ Male	♀ Female
~~Deleted~~		Unspecified	+ Additional code							

7 T63.481-　Toxic effect of venom of other arthropod, accidental (unintentional)

7 T63.482-　Toxic effect of venom of other arthropod, intentional self-harm

7 T63.483-　Toxic effect of venom of other arthropod, assault

7 T63.484-　Toxic effect of venom of other arthropod, undetermined

5 T63.5　Toxic effect of contact with venomous fish
　　EXCLUDES 2　*poisoning by ingestion of fish (T61.-)*

6 T63.51　Toxic effect of contact with stingray

7 T63.511-　Toxic effect of contact with stingray, accidental (unintentional)

7 T63.512-　Toxic effect of contact with stingray, intentional self-harm

7 T63.513-　Toxic effect of contact with stingray, assault

7 T63.514-　Toxic effect of contact with stingray, undetermined

6 T63.59　Toxic effect of contact with other venomous fish

7 T63.591-　Toxic effect of contact with other venomous fish, accidental (unintentional)

7 T63.592-　Toxic effect of contact with other venomous fish, intentional self-harm

7 T63.593-　Toxic effect of contact with other venomous fish, assault

7 T63.594-　Toxic effect of contact with other venomous fish, undetermined

5 T63.6　Toxic effect of contact with other venomous marine animals
　　EXCLUDES 1　*sea-snake venom (T63.09)*
　　EXCLUDES 2　*poisoning by ingestion of shellfish (T61.78-)*

6 T63.61　Toxic effect of contact with Portugese Man-o-war
　　Toxic effect of contact with bluebottle

7 T63.611-　Toxic effect of contact with Portugese Man-o-war, accidental (unintentional)

7 T63.612-　Toxic effect of contact with Portugese Man-o-war, intentional self-harm

7 T63.613-　Toxic effect of contact with Portugese Man-o-war, assault

7 T63.614-　Toxic effect of contact with Portugese Man-o-war, undetermined

6 T63.62　Toxic effect of contact with other jellyfish

7 T63.621-　Toxic effect of contact with other jellyfish, accidental (unintentional)

7 T63.622-　Toxic effect of contact with other jellyfish, intentional self-harm

7 T63.623-　Toxic effect of contact with other jellyfish, assault

7 T63.624-　Toxic effect of contact with other jellyfish, undetermined

6 T63.63　Toxic effect of contact with sea anemone

7 T63.631-　Toxic effect of contact with sea anemone, accidental (unintentional)

7 T63.632-　Toxic effect of contact with sea anemone, intentional self-harm

7 T63.633-　Toxic effect of contact with sea anemone, assault

7 T63.634-　Toxic effect of contact with sea anemone, undetermined

6 T63.69　Toxic effect of contact with other venomous marine animals

7 T63.691-　Toxic effect of contact with other venomous marine animals, accidental (unintentional)

7 T63.692-　Toxic effect of contact with other venomous marine animals, intentional self-harm

7 T63.693-　Toxic effect of contact with other venomous marine animals, assault

7 T63.694-　Toxic effect of contact with other venomous marine animals, undetermined

5 T63.7　Toxic effect of contact with venomous plant

6 T63.71　Toxic effect of contact with venomous marine plant

7 T63.711-　Toxic effect of contact with venomous marine plant, accidental (unintentional)

7 T63.712-　Toxic effect of contact with venomous marine plant, intentional self-harm

7 T63.713-　Toxic effect of contact with venomous marine plant, assault

7 T63.714-　Toxic effect of contact with venomous marine plant, undetermined

6 T63.79　Toxic effect of contact with other venomous plant

7 T63.791-　Toxic effect of contact with other venomous plant, accidental (unintentional)

7 T63.792-　Toxic effect of contact with other venomous plant, intentional self-harm

7 T63.793-　Toxic effect of contact with other venomous plant, assault

7 T63.794-　Toxic effect of contact with other venomous plant, undetermined

5 T63.8　Toxic effect of contact with other venomous animals

6 T63.81　Toxic effect of contact with venomous frog
　　EXCLUDES 1　*contact with nonvenomous frog (W62.0)*

7 T63.811-　Toxic effect of contact with venomous frog, accidental (unintentional)

7 T63.812-　Toxic effect of contact with venomous frog, intentional self-harm

7 T63.813-　Toxic effect of contact with venomous frog, assault

7 T63.814-　Toxic effect of contact with venomous frog, undetermined

6 T63.82　Toxic effect of contact with venomous toad
　　EXCLUDES 1　*contact with nonvenomous toad (W62.1)*

7 T63.821-　Toxic effect of contact with venomous toad, accidental (unintentional)

7 T63.822-　Toxic effect of contact with venomous toad, intentional self-harm

7 T63.823-　Toxic effect of contact with venomous toad, assault

7 T63.824-　Toxic effect of contact with venomous toad, undetermined

6 T63.83　Toxic effect of contact with other venomous amphibian
　　EXCLUDES 1　*contact with nonvenomous amphibian (W62.9)*

7 T63.831-　Toxic effect of contact with other venomous amphibian, accidental (unintentional)

7 T63.832-　Toxic effect of contact with other venomous amphibian, intentional self-harm

7 T63.833-　Toxic effect of contact with other venomous amphibian, assault

7 T63.834-　Toxic effect of contact with other venomous amphibian, undetermined

6 T63.89　Toxic effect of contact with other venomous animals

7 T63.891-　Toxic effect of contact with other venomous animals, accidental (unintentional)

7 T63.892-　Toxic effect of contact with other venomous animals, intentional self-harm

7 T63.893-　Toxic effect of contact with other venomous animals, assault

7 T63.894-　Toxic effect of contact with other venomous animals, undetermined

5 T63.9　Toxic effect of contact with unspecified venomous animal

7 T63.91X-　Toxic effect of contact with unspecified venomous animal, accidental (unintentional)

7 T63.92X-　Toxic effect of contact with unspecified venomous animal, intentional self-harm

7 T63.93X-　Toxic effect of contact with unspecified venomous animal, assault

7 T63.94X-　Toxic effect of contact with unspecified venomous animal, undetermined

4 T64　Toxic effect of aflatoxin and other mycotoxin food contaminants

The appropriate 7th character is to be added to each code from category T64
A　initial encounter
D　subsequent encounter
S　sequela

5 T64.0　Toxic effect of aflatoxin

7 T64.01X-　Toxic effect of aflatoxin, accidental (unintentional)

7 T64.02X-　Toxic effect of aflatoxin, intentional self-harm

7 T64.03X-　Toxic effect of aflatoxin, assault

7 T64.04X-　Toxic effect of aflatoxin, undetermined

5 T64.8　Toxic effect of other mycotoxin food contaminants

7 T64.81X-　Toxic effect of other mycotoxin food contaminants, accidental (unintentional)

7 T64.82X-　Toxic effect of other mycotoxin food contaminants, intentional self-harm

---

● New　▲ Revised　*Manifestation*　4- 7 Digit Indicators　⊟ Laterality　A Adult (15+ years)　M Maternity (12-55 years)　N Newborn　P Pediatric (0-17 years)　♂ Male　♀ Female
✖ Deleted　Unspecified　+ Additional code

1086　© 2017 DecisionHealth　　2017 ICD-10-CM Expert for Physicians

☑ **T64.83X-** Toxic effect of other mycotoxin food contaminants, assault

☑ **T64.84X-** Toxic effect of other mycotoxin food contaminants, undetermined

◢ **T65** **Toxic effect of other and unspecified substances**

The appropriate 7th character is to be added to each code from category T65
A   initial encounter
D   subsequent encounter
S   sequela

◳ **T65.0** **Toxic effect of cyanides**
    EXCLUDES 1 *hydrogen cyanide (T57.3-)*

  ◳ **T65.0X** Toxic effect of cyanides

    ☑ **T65.0X1-** Toxic effect of cyanides, accidental (unintentional)
        Toxic effect of cyanides NOS

    ☑ **T65.0X2-** Toxic effect of cyanides, intentional self-harm

    ☑ **T65.0X3-** Toxic effect of cyanides, assault

    ☑ **T65.0X4-** Toxic effect of cyanides, undetermined

◳ **T65.1** **Toxic effect of strychnine and its salts**

  ◳ **T65.1X** Toxic effect of strychnine and its salts

    ☑ **T65.1X1-** Toxic effect of strychnine and its salts, accidental (unintentional)
        Toxic effect of strychnine and its salts NOS

    ☑ **T65.1X2-** Toxic effect of strychnine and its salts, intentional self-harm

    ☑ **T65.1X3-** Toxic effect of strychnine and its salts, assault

    ☑ **T65.1X4-** Toxic effect of strychnine and its salts, undetermined

◳ **T65.2** **Toxic effect of tobacco and nicotine**
    EXCLUDES 2 *nicotine dependence (F17.-)*

  ◳ **T65.21** Toxic effect of chewing tobacco

    ☑ **T65.211-** Toxic effect of chewing tobacco, accidental (unintentional)
        Toxic effect of chewing tobacco NOS

    ☑ **T65.212-** Toxic effect of chewing tobacco, intentional self-harm

    ☑ **T65.213-** Toxic effect of chewing tobacco, assault

    ☑ **T65.214-** Toxic effect of chewing tobacco, undetermined

  ◳ **+ T65.22** Toxic effect of tobacco cigarettes
    Toxic effect of tobacco smoke
    Use additional code for exposure to second hand tobacco smoke (Z57.31, Z77.22)

    ☑ **+ T65.221-** Toxic effect of tobacco cigarettes, accidental (unintentional)
        Toxic effect of tobacco cigarettes NOS

    ☑ **+ T65.222-** Toxic effect of tobacco cigarettes, intentional self-harm

    ☑ **+ T65.223-** Toxic effect of tobacco cigarettes, assault

    ☑ **+ T65.224-** Toxic effect of tobacco cigarettes, undetermined

  ◳ **T65.29** Toxic effect of other tobacco and nicotine

    ☑ **T65.291-** Toxic effect of other tobacco and nicotine, accidental (unintentional)
        Toxic effect of other tobacco and nicotine NOS

    ☑ **T65.292-** Toxic effect of other tobacco and nicotine, intentional self-harm

    ☑ **T65.293-** Toxic effect of other tobacco and nicotine, assault

    ☑ **T65.294-** Toxic effect of other tobacco and nicotine, undetermined

◳ **T65.3** **Toxic effect of nitroderivatives and aminoderivatives of benzene and its homologues**
    Toxic effect of anilin [benzenamine]
    Toxic effect of nitrobenzene
    Toxic effect of trinitrotoluene

  ◳ **T65.3X** Toxic effect of nitroderivatives and aminoderivatives of benzene and its homologues

    ☑ **T65.3X1-** Toxic effect of nitroderivatives and aminoderivatives of benzene and its homologues, accidental (unintentional)
        Toxic effect of nitroderivatives and aminoderivatives of benzene and its homologues NOS

    ☑ **T65.3X2-** Toxic effect of nitroderivatives and aminoderivatives of benzene and its homologues, intentional self-harm

    ☑ **T65.3X3-** Toxic effect of nitroderivatives and aminoderivatives of benzene and its homologues, assault

    ☑ **T65.3X4-** Toxic effect of nitroderivatives and aminoderivatives of benzene and its homologues, undetermined

◳ **T65.4** **Toxic effect of carbon disulfide**

  ◳ **T65.4X** Toxic effect of carbon disulfide

    ☑ **T65.4X1-** Toxic effect of carbon disulfide, accidental (unintentional)
        Toxic effect of carbon disulfide NOS

    ☑ **T65.4X2-** Toxic effect of carbon disulfide, intentional self-harm

    ☑ **T65.4X3-** Toxic effect of carbon disulfide, assault

    ☑ **T65.4X4-** Toxic effect of carbon disulfide, undetermined

◳ **T65.5** **Toxic effect of nitroglycerin and other nitric acids and esters**
    Toxic effect of 1,2,3-Propanetriol trinitrate

  ◳ **T65.5X** Toxic effect of nitroglycerin and other nitric acids and esters

    ☑ **T65.5X1-** Toxic effect of nitroglycerin and other nitric acids and esters, accidental (unintentional)
        Toxic effect of nitroglycerin and other nitric acids and esters NOS

    ☑ **T65.5X2-** Toxic effect of nitroglycerin and other nitric acids and esters, intentional self-harm

    ☑ **T65.5X3-** Toxic effect of nitroglycerin and other nitric acids and esters, assault

    ☑ **T65.5X4-** Toxic effect of nitroglycerin and other nitric acids and esters, undetermined

◳ **T65.6** **Toxic effect of paints and dyes, not elsewhere classified**

  ◳ **T65.6X** Toxic effect of paints and dyes, not elsewhere classified

    ☑ **T65.6X1-** Toxic effect of paints and dyes, not elsewhere classified, accidental (unintentional)
        Toxic effect of paints and dyes NOS

    ☑ **T65.6X2-** Toxic effect of paints and dyes, not elsewhere classified, intentional self-harm

    ☑ **T65.6X3-** Toxic effect of paints and dyes, not elsewhere classified, assault

    ☑ **T65.6X4-** Toxic effect of paints and dyes, not elsewhere classified, undetermined

◳ **T65.8** **Toxic effect of other specified substances**

  ◳ **T65.81** Toxic effect of latex

    ☑ **T65.811-** Toxic effect of latex, accidental (unintentional)
        Toxic effect of latex NOS

    ☑ **T65.812-** Toxic effect of latex, intentional self-harm

    ☑ **T65.813-** Toxic effect of latex, assault

    ☑ **T65.814-** Toxic effect of latex, undetermined

  ◳ **T65.82** Toxic effect of harmful algae and algae toxins
    Toxic effect of (harmful) algae bloom NOS
    Toxic effect of blue-green algae bloom
    Toxic effect of brown tide
    Toxic effect of cyanobacteria bloom
    Toxic effect of Florida red tide
    Toxic effect of pfiesteria piscicida
    Toxic effect of red tide

    ☑ **T65.821-** Toxic effect of harmful algae and algae toxins, accidental (unintentional)
        Toxic effect of harmful algae and algae toxins NOS

    ☑ **T65.822-** Toxic effect of harmful algae and algae toxins, intentional self-harm

    ☑ **T65.823-** Toxic effect of harmful algae and algae toxins, assault

    ☑ **T65.824-** Toxic effect of harmful algae and algae toxins, undetermined

  ◳ **T65.83** Toxic effect of fiberglass

    ☑ **T65.831-** Toxic effect of fiberglass, accidental (unintentional)
        Toxic effect of fiberglass NOS

    ☑ **T65.832-** Toxic effect of fiberglass, intentional self-harm

    ☑ **T65.833-** Toxic effect of fiberglass, assault

    ☑ **T65.834-** Toxic effect of fiberglass, undetermined

  ◳ **T65.89** Toxic effect of other specified substances

    ☑ **T65.891-** Toxic effect of other specified substances, accidental (unintentional)
        Toxic effect of other specified substances NOS

    ☑ **T65.892-** Toxic effect of other specified substances, intentional self-harm

---

● New   ▲ Revised   *Manifestation*   ◳-☑ Digit Indicators   ▤ Laterality   Ⓐ Adult (15+ years)   Ⓜ Maternity (12-55 years)   Ⓝ Newborn   Ⓟ Pediatric (0-17 years)   ♂ Male   ♀ Female
✖ Deleted   Unspecified   + Additional code

7 T65.893-   Toxic effect of other specified substances, assault

7 T65.894-   Toxic effect of other specified substances, undetermined

5 T65.9   **Toxic effect of unspecified substance**

7 T65.91X-   Toxic effect of unspecified substance, accidental (unintentional)

Poisoning NOS

7 T65.92X-   Toxic effect of unspecified substance, intentional self-harm

7 T65.93X-   Toxic effect of unspecified substance, assault

7 T65.94X-   Toxic effect of unspecified substance, undetermined

Other and unspecified effects of external causes (T66-T78)

7 T66.XXX-   **Radiation sickness, unspecified**

> **EXCLUDES 1**   specified adverse effects of radiation, such as:
> burns (T20-T31)
> leukemia (C91-C95)
> radiation gastroenteritis and colitis (K52.0)
> radiation pneumonitis (J70.0)
> radiation related disorders of the skin and subcutaneous tissue (L55-L59)
> sunburn (L55.-)

The appropriate 7th character is to be added to code T66
A   initial encounter
D   subsequent encounter
S   sequela

4 T67   **Effects of heat and light**

> **EXCLUDES 1**   erythema [dermatitis] ab igne (L59.0)
> malignant hyperpyrexia due to anesthesia (T88.3)
> radiation-related disorders of the skin and subcutaneous tissue (L55-L59)
>
> **EXCLUDES 2**   burns (T20-T31)
> sunburn (L55.-)
> sweat disorder due to heat (L74-L75)

The appropriate 7th character is to be added to each code from category T67
A   initial encounter
D   subsequent encounter
S   sequela

7 + T67.0XX-   **Heatstroke and sunstroke**

Heat apoplexy
Heat pyrexia
Siriasis
Thermoplegia
Use additional code(s) to identify any associated complications of heatstroke, such as:
coma and stupor (R40.-)
systemic inflammatory response syndrome (R65.1-)

7 T67.1XX-   **Heat syncope**

Heat collapse

7 T67.2XX-   **Heat cramp**

7 T67.3XX-   **Heat exhaustion, anhydrotic**

Heat prostration due to water depletion
> **EXCLUDES 1**   heat exhaustion due to salt depletion (T67.4)

7 T67.4XX-   **Heat exhaustion due to salt depletion**

Heat prostration due to salt (and water) depletion

7 T67.5XX-   **Heat exhaustion, unspecified**

Heat prostration NOS

7 T67.6XX-   **Heat fatigue, transient**

7 T67.7XX-   **Heat edema**

7 T67.8XX-   **Other effects of heat and light**

7 T67.9XX-   **Effect of heat and light, unspecified**

7 + T68.XXX-   **Hypothermia**

Accidental hypothermia
Hypothermia NOS
Use additional code to identify source of exposure:
Exposure to excessive cold of man-made origin (W93)
Exposure to excessive cold of natural origin (X31)
> **EXCLUDES 1**   hypothermia following anesthesia (T88.51)
> hypothermia not associated with low environmental temperature (R68.0)
> hypothermia of newborn (P80.-)
>
> **EXCLUDES 2**   frostbite (T33-T34)

The appropriate 7th character is to be added to code T68
A   initial encounter
D   subsequent encounter
S   sequela

4 + T69   **Other effects of reduced temperature**

Use additional code to identify source of exposure:
Exposure to excessive cold of man-made origin (W93)
Exposure to excessive cold of natural origin (X31)
> **EXCLUDES 2**   frostbite (T33-T34)

The appropriate 7th character is to be added to each code from category T69
A   initial encounter
D   subsequent encounter
S   sequela

5 + T69.0   **Immersion hand and foot**

6 + T69.01   **Immersion hand**

7 6 + T69.011-   **Immersion hand, right hand**

7 6 + T69.012-   **Immersion hand, left hand**

7 6 + T69.019-   **Immersion hand, unspecified hand**

6 + T69.02   **Immersion foot**

Trench foot

7 6 + T69.021-   **Immersion foot, right foot**

7 6 + T69.022-   **Immersion foot, left foot**

7 6 + T69.029-   **Immersion foot, unspecified foot**

7 + T69.1XX-   **Chilblains**

7 + T69.8XX-   **Other specified effects of reduced temperature**

7 + T69.9XX-   **Effect of reduced temperature, unspecified**

4 T70   **Effects of air pressure and water pressure**

The appropriate 7th character is to be added to each code from category T70
A   initial encounter
D   subsequent encounter
S   sequela

7 T70.0XX-   **Otitic barotrauma**

Aero-otitis media
Effects of change in ambient atmospheric pressure or water pressure on ears

7 T70.1XX-   **Sinus barotrauma**

Aerosinusitis
Effects of change in ambient atmospheric pressure on sinuses

5 T70.2   **Other and unspecified effects of high altitude**

> **EXCLUDES 2**   polycythemia due to high altitude (D75.1)

7 T70.20X-   **Unspecified effects of high altitude**

7 T70.29X-   **Other effects of high altitude**

Alpine sickness
Anoxia due to high altitude
Barotrauma NOS
Hypobaropathy
Mountain sickness

7 T70.3XX-   **Caisson disease [decompression sickness]**

Compressed-air disease
Diver's palsy or paralysis

7 T70.4XX-   **Effects of high-pressure fluids**

Hydraulic jet injection (industrial)
Pneumatic jet injection (industrial)
Traumatic jet injection (industrial)

7 T70.8XX-   **Other effects of air pressure and water pressure**

7 T70.9XX-   **Effect of air pressure and water pressure, unspecified**

● New   ▲ Revised   *Manifestation*   4-7 Digit Indicators   ⊟ Laterality   A Adult (15+ years)   M Maternity (12-55 years)   N Newborn   P Pediatric (0-17 years)   ♂ Male   ♀ Female

✖ Deleted   Unspecified   + Additional code

1088   © 2017 DecisionHealth   2017 ICD-10-CM Expert for Physicians

T71   **Asphyxiation**

Mechanical suffocation

Traumatic suffocation

> **EXCLUDES 1**   *acute respiratory distress (syndrome) (J80)*
> *anoxia due to high altitude (T70.2)*
> *asphyxia NOS (R09.01)*
> *asphyxia from carbon monoxide (T58.-)*
> *asphyxia from inhalation of food or foreign body (T17.-)*
> *asphyxia from other gases, fumes and vapors (T59.-)*
> *respiratory distress (syndrome) in newborn (P22.-)*

> The appropriate 7th character is to be added to each code from category T71
> A   initial encounter
> D   subsequent encounter
> S   sequela

T71.1   **Asphyxiation due to mechanical threat to breathing**

Suffocation due to mechanical threat to breathing

T71.11   **Asphyxiation due to smothering under pillow**

T71.111-   **Asphyxiation due to smothering under pillow, accidental**

Asphyxiation due to smothering under pillow NOS

T71.112-   **Asphyxiation due to smothering under pillow, intentional self-harm**

T71.113-   **Asphyxiation due to smothering under pillow, assault**

T71.114-   **Asphyxiation due to smothering under pillow, undetermined**

T71.12   **Asphyxiation due to plastic bag**

T71.121-   **Asphyxiation due to plastic bag, accidental**

Asphyxiation due to plastic bag NOS

T71.122-   **Asphyxiation due to plastic bag, intentional self-harm**

T71.123-   **Asphyxiation due to plastic bag, assault**

T71.124-   **Asphyxiation due to plastic bag, undetermined**

T71.13   **Asphyxiation due to being trapped in bed linens**

T71.131-   **Asphyxiation due to being trapped in bed linens, accidental**

Asphyxiation due to being trapped in bed linens NOS

T71.132-   **Asphyxiation due to being trapped in bed linens, intentional self-harm**

T71.133-   **Asphyxiation due to being trapped in bed linens, assault**

T71.134-   **Asphyxiation due to being trapped in bed linens, undetermined**

T71.14   **Asphyxiation due to smothering under another person's body (in bed)**

T71.141-   **Asphyxiation due to smothering under another person's body (in bed), accidental**

Asphyxiation due to smothering under another person's body (in bed) NOS

T71.143-   **Asphyxiation due to smothering under another person's body (in bed), assault**

T71.144-   **Asphyxiation due to smothering under another person's body (in bed), undetermined**

T71.15   **Asphyxiation due to smothering in furniture**

T71.151-   **Asphyxiation due to smothering in furniture, accidental**

Asphyxiation due to smothering in furniture NOS

T71.152-   **Asphyxiation due to smothering in furniture, intentional self-harm**

T71.153-   **Asphyxiation due to smothering in furniture, assault**

T71.154-   **Asphyxiation due to smothering in furniture, undetermined**

+ T71.16   **Asphyxiation due to hanging**

Hanging by window shade cord

Use additional code for any associated injuries, such as:
crushing injury of neck (S17.-)
fracture of cervical vertebrae (S12.0-S12.2-)
open wound of neck (S11.-)

+ T71.161-   **Asphyxiation due to hanging, accidental**

Asphyxiation due to hanging NOS
Hanging NOS

+ T71.162-   **Asphyxiation due to hanging, intentional self-harm**

+ T71.163-   **Asphyxiation due to hanging, assault**

+ T71.164-   **Asphyxiation due to hanging, undetermined**

T71.19   **Asphyxiation due to mechanical threat to breathing due to other causes**

T71.191-   **Asphyxiation due to mechanical threat to breathing due to other causes, accidental**

Asphyxiation due to other causes NOS

T71.192-   **Asphyxiation due to mechanical threat to breathing due to other causes, intentional self-harm**

T71.193-   **Asphyxiation due to mechanical threat to breathing due to other causes, assault**

T71.194-   **Asphyxiation due to mechanical threat to breathing due to other causes, undetermined**

T71.2   **Asphyxiation due to systemic oxygen deficiency due to low oxygen content in ambient air**

Suffocation due to systemic oxygen deficiency due to low oxygen content in ambient air

T71.20X-   **Asphyxiation due to systemic oxygen deficiency due to low oxygen content in ambient air due to unspecified cause**

+ T71.21X-   **Asphyxiation due to cave-in or falling earth**

Use additional code for any associated cataclysm (X34-X38)

T71.22   **Asphyxiation due to being trapped in a car trunk**

T71.221-   **Asphyxiation due to being trapped in a car trunk, accidental**

T71.222-   **Asphyxiation due to being trapped in a car trunk, intentional self-harm**

T71.223-   **Asphyxiation due to being trapped in a car trunk, assault**

T71.224-   **Asphyxiation due to being trapped in a car trunk, undetermined**

T71.23   **Asphyxiation due to being trapped in a (discarded) refrigerator**

T71.231-   **Asphyxiation due to being trapped in a (discarded) refrigerator, accidental**

T71.232-   **Asphyxiation due to being trapped in a (discarded) refrigerator, intentional self-harm**

T71.233-   **Asphyxiation due to being trapped in a (discarded) refrigerator, assault**

T71.234-   **Asphyxiation due to being trapped in a (discarded) refrigerator, undetermined**

T71.29X-   **Asphyxiation due to being trapped in other low oxygen environment**

T71.9XX-   **Asphyxiation due to unspecified cause**

Suffocation (by strangulation) due to unspecified cause
Suffocation NOS
Systemic oxygen deficiency due to low oxygen content in ambient air due to unspecified cause
Systemic oxygen deficiency due to mechanical threat to breathing due to unspecified cause
Traumatic asphyxia NOS

T73   **Effects of other deprivation**

> The appropriate 7th character is to be added to each code from category T73
> A   initial encounter
> D   subsequent encounter
> S   sequela

T73.0XX-   **Starvation**

Deprivation of food

T73.1XX-   **Deprivation of water**

T73.2XX-   **Exhaustion due to exposure**

T73.3XX-   **Exhaustion due to excessive exertion**

Exhaustion due to overexertion

T73.8XX-   **Other effects of deprivation**

T73.9XX-   **Effect of deprivation, unspecified**

● New   ▲ Revised   *Manifestation*   4-7 Digit Indicators   ▣ Laterality   Ⓐ Adult (15+ years)   Ⓜ Maternity (12-55 years)   Ⓝ Newborn   Ⓟ Pediatric (0-17 years)   ♂ Male   ♀ Female

Deleted   Unspecified   + Additional code

2017 ICD-10-CM Expert for Physicians   © 2017 DecisionHealth   1089

4 + T74   Adult and child abuse, neglect and other maltreatment, confirmed

Use additional code, if applicable, to identify any associated current injury
Use additional external cause code to identify perpetrator, if known (Y07.-)

> **EXCLUDES 1**   *abuse and maltreatment in pregnancy (O9A.3-, O9A.4-, O9A.5-)*
> *adult and child maltreatment, suspected (T76.-)*

The appropriate 7th character is to be added to each code from category T74
A   initial encounter
D   subsequent encounter
S   sequela

GUIDELINES   Section I.C.19.f
Sequence first the appropriate code from categories T74.- (Adult and child abuse, neglect and other maltreatment, confirmed) or T76.- (Adult and child abuse, neglect and other maltreatment, suspected) for abuse, neglect and other maltreatment, followed by any accompanying mental health or injury code(s). If the documentation in the medical record states abuse or neglect it is coded as confirmed (T74.-). It is coded as suspected if it is documented as suspected (T76.-).

For cases of confirmed abuse or neglect an external cause code from the assault section (X92-Y08) should be added to identify the cause of any physical injuries. A perpetrator code (Y07) should be added when the perpetrator of the abuse is known. For suspected cases of abuse or neglect, do not report external cause or perpetrator code. If a suspected case of abuse, neglect or mistreatment is ruled out during an encounter code Z04.71, Encounter for examination and observation following alleged physical adult abuse, ruled out, or code Z04.72, Encounter for examination and observation following alleged child physical abuse, ruled out, should be used, not a code from T76.

5 + T74.0   Neglect or abandonment, confirmed
   7 + T74.01X-   Adult neglect or abandonment, confirmed
   7 + T74.02X-   Child neglect or abandonment, confirmed
5 + T74.1   Physical abuse, confirmed
> **EXCLUDES 2**   *sexual abuse (T74.2-)*
   7 + T74.11X-   Adult physical abuse, confirmed
   7 + T74.12X-   Child physical abuse, confirmed
> **EXCLUDES 2**   *shaken infant syndrome (T74.4)*
5 + T74.2   Sexual abuse, confirmed
   Rape, confirmed
   Sexual assault, confirmed
   7 + T74.21X-   Adult sexual abuse, confirmed
   7 + T74.22X-   Child sexual abuse, confirmed
5 + T74.3   Psychological abuse, confirmed
   7 + T74.31X-   Adult psychological abuse, confirmed
   7 + T74.32X-   Child psychological abuse, confirmed
7 + T74.4XX-   Shaken infant syndrome
5 + T74.9   Unspecified maltreatment, confirmed
   7 + T74.91X-   Unspecified adult maltreatment, confirmed
   7 + T74.92X-   Unspecified child maltreatment, confirmed

4 T75   Other and unspecified effects of other external causes

> **EXCLUDES 1**   *adverse effects NEC (T78.-)*
> **EXCLUDES 2**   *burns (electric) (T20-T31)*

The appropriate 7th character is to be added to each code from category T75
A   initial encounter
D   subsequent encounter
S   sequela

5 T75.0   Effects of lightning
   Struck by lightning
   7 T75.00X-   Unspecified effects of lightning
     Struck by lightning NOS
   7 T75.01X-   Shock due to being struck by lightning
   7 + T75.09X-   Other effects of lightning
     Use additional code for other effects of lightning

7 T75.1XX-   Unspecified effects of drowning and nonfatal submersion
   Immersion
> **EXCLUDES 1**   *specified effects of drowning- code to effects*

5 T75.2   Effects of vibration
   7 T75.20X-   Unspecified effects of vibration
   7 T75.21X-   Pneumatic hammer syndrome
   7 T75.22X-   Traumatic vasospastic syndrome
   7 T75.23X-   Vertigo from infrasound
> **EXCLUDES 1**   *vertigo NOS (R42)*
   7 T75.29X-   Other effects of vibration

7 + T75.3XX-   Motion sickness
   Airsickness
   Seasickness
   Travel sickness
   Use additional external cause code to identify vehicle or type of motion (Y92.81-, Y93.5-)

7 T75.4XX-   Electrocution
   Shock from electric current
   Shock from electroshock gun (taser)

5 T75.8   Other specified effects of external causes
   7 T75.81X-   Effects of abnormal gravitation [G] forces
   7 T75.82X-   Effects of weightlessness
   7 T75.89X-   Other specified effects of external causes

4 + T76   Adult and child abuse, neglect and other maltreatment, suspected

Use additional code, if applicable, to identify any associated current injury

> **EXCLUDES 1**   *adult and child maltreatment, confirmed (T74.-)*
> *suspected abuse and maltreatment in pregnancy (O9A.3-, O9A.4-, O9A.5-)*
> *suspected adult physical abuse, ruled out (Z04.71)*
> *suspected adult sexual abuse, ruled out (Z04.41)*
> *suspected child physical abuse, ruled out (Z04.72)*
> *suspected child sexual abuse, ruled out (Z04.42)*

The appropriate 7th character is to be added to each code from category T76
A   initial encounter
D   subsequent encounter
S   sequela

GUIDELINES   Section I.C.19.f
Sequence first the appropriate code from categories T74.- (Adult and child abuse, neglect and other maltreatment, confirmed) or T76.- (Adult and child abuse, neglect and other maltreatment, suspected) for abuse, neglect and other maltreatment, followed by any accompanying mental health or injury code(s). If the documentation in the medical record states abuse or neglect it is coded as confirmed (T74.-). It is coded as suspected if it is documented as suspected (T76.-).

For cases of confirmed abuse or neglect an external cause code from the assault section (X92-Y08) should be added to identify the cause of any physical injuries. A perpetrator code (Y07) should be added when the perpetrator of the abuse is known. For suspected cases of abuse or neglect, do not report external cause or perpetrator code. If a suspected case of abuse, neglect or mistreatment is ruled out during an encounter code Z04.71, Encounter for examination and observation following alleged physical adult abuse, ruled out, or code Z04.72, Encounter for examination and observation following alleged child physical abuse, ruled out, should be used, not a code from T76.

5 + T76.0   Neglect or abandonment, suspected
   7 + T76.01X-   Adult neglect or abandonment, suspected
   7 + T76.02X-   Child neglect or abandonment, suspected
5 + T76.1   Physical abuse, suspected
   7 + T76.11X-   Adult physical abuse, suspected
   7 + T76.12X-   Child physical abuse, suspected
5 + T76.2   Sexual abuse, suspected
   Rape, suspected
   Sexual abuse, suspected
> **EXCLUDES 1**   *alleged abuse, ruled out (Z04.7)*
   7 + T76.21X-   Adult sexual abuse, suspected

7 + T76.22X-   **Child sexual abuse, suspected**

6 + T76.3   **Psychological abuse, suspected**

    7 + T76.31X-   **Adult psychological abuse, suspected**

    7 + T76.32X-   **Child psychological abuse, suspected**

6 + T76.9   **Unspecified maltreatment, suspected**

    7 + T76.91X-   **Unspecified adult maltreatment, suspected**

    7 + T76.92X-   **Unspecified child maltreatment, suspected**

4 T78   **Adverse effects, not elsewhere classified**

> **EXCLUDES 2**   *complications of surgical and medical care NEC (T80-T88)*

> The appropriate 7th character is to be added to each code from category T78
> A   initial encounter
> D   subsequent encounter
> S   sequela

6 T78.0   **Anaphylactic reaction due to food**

Anaphylactic reaction due to adverse food reaction
Anaphylactic shock or reaction due to nonpoisonous foods
Anaphylactoid reaction due to food

    7 T78.00X-   **Anaphylactic reaction due to unspecified food**

    7 T78.01X-   **Anaphylactic reaction due to peanuts**

    7 T78.02X-   **Anaphylactic reaction due to shellfish (crustaceans)**

    7 T78.03X-   **Anaphylactic reaction due to other fish**

    7 T78.04X-   **Anaphylactic reaction due to fruits and vegetables**

    ▲ 7 T78.05X-   **Anaphylactic reaction due to tree nuts and seeds**

> **EXCLUDES 2**   *anaphylactic reaction due to peanuts (T78.01)*

    7 T78.06X-   **Anaphylactic reaction due to food additives**

    7 T78.07X-   **Anaphylactic reaction due to milk and dairy products**

    7 T78.08X-   **Anaphylactic reaction due to eggs**

    7 T78.09X-   **Anaphylactic reaction due to other food products**

▲ 7 + T78.1XX-   **Other adverse food reactions, not elsewhere classified**

Use additional code to identify the type of reaction, if applicable

> **EXCLUDES 1**   *anaphylactic reaction or shock due to adverse food reaction (T78.0-)*
> *anaphylactic reaction due to food (T78.0-)*
> *bacterial food borne intoxications (A05.-)*

> **EXCLUDES 2**   *allergic and dietetic gastroenteritis and colitis (K52.29)*
> *allergic rhinitis due to food (J30.5)*
> *dermatitis due to food in contact with skin (L23.6, L24.6, L25.4)*
> *dermatitis due to ingested food (L27.2)*
> *food protein-induced enterocolitis syndrome (K52.21)*
> *food protein-induced enteropathy (K52.22)*

7 T78.2XX-   **Anaphylactic shock, unspecified**

Allergic shock
Anaphylactic reaction
Anaphylaxis

> **EXCLUDES 1**   *anaphylactic reaction or shock due to adverse effect of correct medicinal substance properly administered (T88.6)*
> *anaphylactic reaction or shock due to adverse food reaction (T78.0-)*
> *anaphylactic reaction or shock due to serum (T80.5-)*

7 T78.3XX-   **Angioneurotic edema**

Allergic angioedema
Giant urticaria
Quincke's edema

> **EXCLUDES 1**   *serum urticaria (T80.6-)*
> *urticaria (L50.-)*

▲ 5 T78.4   **Other and unspecified allergy**

> **EXCLUDES 1**   *specified types of allergic reaction such as: allergic diarrhea (K52.29)*
> *allergic gastroenteritis and colitis (K52.29)*
> *dermatitis (L23-L25, L27.-)*
> *food protein-induced enterocolitis syndrome (K52.21)*
> *food protein-induced enteropathy (K52.22)*
> *hay fever (J30.1)*

    7 T78.40X-   **Allergy, unspecified**

Allergic reaction NOS
Hypersensitivity NOS

    7 T78.41X-   **Arthus phenomenon**

Arthus reaction

    7 T78.49X-   **Other allergy**

7 T78.8XX-   **Other adverse effects, not elsewhere classified**

Certain early complications of trauma (T79)

4 T79   **Certain early complications of trauma, not elsewhere classified**

> **EXCLUDES 2**   *acute respiratory distress syndrome (J80)*
> *complications occurring during or following medical procedures (T80-T88)*
> *complications of surgical and medical care NEC (T80-T88)*
> *newborn respiratory distress syndrome (P22.0)*

> The appropriate 7th character is to be added to each code from category T79
> A   initial encounter
> D   subsequent encounter
> S   sequela

7 T79.0XX-   **Air embolism (traumatic)**

> **EXCLUDES 1**   *air embolism complicating abortion or ectopic or molar pregnancy (O00-O07, O08.2)*
> *air embolism complicating pregnancy, childbirth and the puerperium (O88.0)*
> *air embolism following infusion, transfusion, and therapeutic injection (T80.0)*
> *air embolism following procedure NEC (T81.7-)*

> **CODING TIP ✓**   Code T79.0- should not be assigned for an air embolus that is not specified as due to a traumatic cause.

7 T79.1XX-   **Fat embolism (traumatic)**

> **EXCLUDES 1**   *fat embolism complicating: abortion or ectopic or molar pregnancy (O00-O07, O08.2)*
> *pregnancy, childbirth and the puerperium (O88.8)*

7 T79.2XX-   **Traumatic secondary and recurrent hemorrhage and seroma**

7 T79.4XX-   **Traumatic shock**

Shock (immediate) (delayed) following injury

> **EXCLUDES 1**   *anaphylactic shock due to adverse food reaction (T78.0-)*
> *anaphylactic shock due to correct medicinal substance properly administered (T88.6)*
> *anaphylactic shock due to serum (T80.5-)*
> *anaphylactic shock NOS (T78.2)*
> *anesthetic shock (T88.2)*
> *electric shock (T75.4)*
> *nontraumatic shock NEC (R57.-)*
> *obstetric shock (O75.1)*
> *postprocedural shock (T81.1-)*
> *septic shock (R65.21)*
> *shock complicating abortion or ectopic or molar pregnancy (O00-O07, O08.3)*
> *shock due to lightning (T75.01)*
> *shock NOS (R57.9)*

7 T79.5XX-   **Traumatic anuria**

Crush syndrome
Renal failure following crushing

▣ T79.6XX-   **Traumatic ischemia of muscle**
Traumatic rhabdomyolysis
Volkmann's ischemic contracture

> **EXCLUDES 2**   *anterior tibial syndrome (M76.8)*
> *compartment syndrome (traumatic)*
> *(T79.A-)*
> *nontraumatic ischemia of muscle*
> *(M62.2-)*

▣ T79.7XX-   **Traumatic subcutaneous emphysema**

> **EXCLUDES 1**   *emphysema NOS (J43)*
> *emphysema (subcutaneous) resulting*
> *from a procedure (T81.82)*

⑤ T79.A   **Traumatic compartment syndrome**

> **EXCLUDES 1**   *fibromyalgia (M79.7)*
> *nontraumatic compartment syndrome*
> *(M79.A-)*
> *traumatic ischemic infarction of muscle*
> *(T79.6)*

> **CODING TIP ✓**   Do not assign any code from subcategory T79.A- to indicate compartment syndrome that is not specifically stated as due to a traumatic cause. Non-traumatic compartment syndrome is coded to M79.A-

▣ T79.A0X-   **Compartment syndrome, unspecified**
Compartment syndrome NOS

⑥ T79.A1   **Traumatic compartment syndrome of upper extremity**
Traumatic compartment syndrome of shoulder, arm, forearm, wrist, hand, and fingers

▣ ▤ T79.A11-   **Traumatic compartment syndrome of right upper extremity**

▣ ▤ T79.A12-   **Traumatic compartment syndrome of left upper extremity**

▣ ▤ T79.A19-   **Traumatic compartment syndrome of unspecified upper extremity**

⑥ T79.A2   **Traumatic compartment syndrome of lower extremity**
Traumatic compartment syndrome of hip, buttock, thigh, leg, foot, and toes

▣ ▤ T79.A21-   **Traumatic compartment syndrome of right lower extremity**

▣ ▤ T79.A22-   **Traumatic compartment syndrome of left lower extremity**

▣ ▤ T79.A29-   **Traumatic compartment syndrome of unspecified lower extremity**

▣ T79.A3X-   **Traumatic compartment syndrome of abdomen**

▣ T79.A9X-   **Traumatic compartment syndrome of other sites**

▣ T79.8XX-   **Other early complications of trauma**

▣ T79.9XX-   **Unspecified early complication of trauma**

Complications of surgical and medical care, not elsewhere classified (T80-T88)

Use additional code for adverse effect, if applicable, to identify drug (T36-T50 with fifth or sixth character 5)
Use additional code(s) to identify the specified condition resulting from the complication
Use additional code to identify devices involved and details of circumstances (Y62-Y82)

> **EXCLUDES 2**   *any encounters with medical care for postprocedural conditions in which no complications are present, such as:*
> *artificial opening status (Z93.-)*
> *closure of external stoma (Z43.-)*
> *fitting and adjustment of external prosthetic device (Z44.-)*
> *burns and corrosions from local applications and irradiation (T20-T32)*
> *complications of surgical procedures during pregnancy, childbirth and the puerperium (O00-O9A)*
> *mechanical complication of respirator [ventilator] (J95.850)*
> *poisoning and toxic effects of drugs and chemicals (T36-T65 with fifth or sixth character 1-4 or 6)*
> *postprocedural fever (R50.82)*
> *specified complications classified elsewhere, such as:*
> *cerebrospinal fluid leak from spinal puncture (G97.0)*
> *colostomy malfunction (K94.0-)*
> *disorders of fluid and electrolyte imbalance (E86-E87)*
> *functional disturbances following cardiac surgery (I97.0-I97.1)*
> *intraoperative and postprocedural complications of specified body systems*
> *(D78.-, E36.-, E89.-, G97.3-, G97.4, H59.3-, H59.-, H95.2-, H95.3, I97.4-, I97.5, J95.6-, J95.7, K91.6-, L76.-, M96.-, N99.-)*
> *ostomy complications (J95.0-, K94.-, N99.5-)*
> *postgastric surgery syndromes (K91.1)*
> *postlaminectomy syndrome NEC (M96.1)*
> *postmastectomy lymphedema syndrome (I97.2)*
> *postsurgical blind-loop syndrome (K91.2)*
> *ventilator associated pneumonia (J95.851)*

> **GUIDELINES**   **Section I.B.16**
> Documentation of Complication of Care: Code assignment is based on the provider's documentation of the relationship between the condition and the care or procedure. The guideline extends to any complications of care, regardless of the chapter the code is located in. It is important to note that not all conditions that occur during or following medical care or surgery are classified as complications. There must be a cause-and-effect relationship between the care provided and the condition, and an indication in the documentation that it is a complication. Query the provider for clarification, if the complication is not clearly documented.

> **GUIDELINES**   **Section I.C.19.g.5)**
> Intraoperative and postprocedural complication codes are found within the body system chapters with codes specific to the organs and structures of that body system. These codes should be sequenced first, followed by a code(s) for the specific complication, if applicable.

> **CODING TIP ✓**   Conditions classifiable to T80-T88 are classifiable as complications of surgical and medical care. These conditions should only be assigned when diagnostic statements clearly indicate that the condition is a complication.

④ T80   **Complications following infusion, transfusion and therapeutic injection**

> **INCLUDES**   complications following perfusion

> **EXCLUDES 2**   *bone marrow transplant rejection (T86.01)*
> *febrile nonhemolytic transfusion reaction (R50.84)*
> *fluid overload due to transfusion (E87.71)*
> *posttransfusion purpura (D69.51)*
> *transfusion associated circulatory overload (TACO) (E87.71)*
> *transfusion (red blood cell) associated hemochromatosis (E83.111)*
> *transfusion related acute lung injury (TRALI) (J95.84)*

> The appropriate 7th character is to be added to each code from category T80
> A   initial encounter
> D   subsequent encounter
> S   sequela

▣ T80.0XX-   **Air embolism following infusion, transfusion and therapeutic injection**

● New   ▲ Revised   *Manifestation*   ④-▣ Digit Indicators   ▤ Laterality   🅰 Adult (15+ years)   🅼 Maternity (12-55 years)   🅽 Newborn   🅿 Pediatric (0-17 years)   ♂ Male   ♀ Female
✘ Deleted   Unspecified   + Additional code

1092   © 2017 DecisionHealth   2017 ICD-10-CM Expert for Physicians

▲ 🗷 + **T80.1XX-** **Vascular complications following infusion, transfusion and therapeutic injection**
Use additional code to identify the vascular complication
EXCLUDES 2 *extravasation of vesicant agent (T80.81-)*
infiltration of vesicant agent (T80.81-)
vascular complications specified as due to prosthetic devices, implants and grafts (T82.8-, T83.8-, T84.8-, T85.8-)
postprocedural vascular complications (T81.7-)

▲ 🗟 + **T80.2** **Infections following infusion, transfusion and therapeutic injection**
Use additional code to identify the specific infection, such as: sepsis (A41.9)
Use additional code (R65.2-) to identify severe sepsis, if applicable
EXCLUDES 2 *infections specified as due to prosthetic devices, implants and grafts (T82.6-T82.7, T83.5-T83.6, T84.5-T84.7, T85.7)*
postprocedural infections (T81.4-)

▲ 🗟 + **T80.21** **Infection due to central venous catheter**
Infection due to pulmonary artery catheter (Swan-Ganz catheter)

▲ 🗷 + **T80.211-** **Bloodstream infection due to central venous catheter**
Catheter-related bloodstream infection (CRBSI) NOS
Central line-associated bloodstream infection (CLABSI)
Bloodstream infection due Hickman catheter
Bloodstream infection due to peripherally inserted central catheter (PICC)
Bloodstream infection due to portacath (port-a-cath)
Bloodstream infection due to pulmonary artery catheter
Bloodstream infection due to triple lumen catheter
Bloodstream infection due to umbilical venous catheter

▲ 🗷 + **T80.212-** **Local infection due to central venous catheter**
Exit or insertion site infection
Local infection due to Hickman catheter
Local infection due to peripherally inserted central catheter (PICC)
Local infection due to portacath (port-a-cath)
Local infection due to pulmonary artery catheter
Local infection due to triple lumen catheter
Local infection due to umbilical venous catheter
Port or reservoir infection
Tunnel infection

▲ 🗷 + **T80.218-** **Other infection due to central venous catheter**
Other central line-associated infection
Other infection due to Hickman catheter
Other infection due to peripherally inserted central catheter (PICC)
Other infection due to portacath (port-a-cath)
Other infection due to pulmonary artery catheter
Other infection due to triple lumen catheter
Other infection due to umbilical venous catheter

▲ 🗷 + **T80.219-** **Unspecified infection due to central venous catheter**
Central line-associated infection NOS
Unspecified infection due to Hickman catheter
Unspecified infection due to peripherally inserted central catheter (PICC)
Unspecified infection due to portacath (port-a-cath)
Unspecified infection due to pulmonary artery catheter
Unspecified infection due to triple lumen catheter
Unspecified infection due to umbilical venous catheter

🗷 + **T80.22X-** **Acute infection following transfusion, infusion, or injection of blood and blood products**

🗷 + **T80.29X-** **Infection following other infusion, transfusion and therapeutic injection**

🗟 **T80.3** **ABO incompatibility reaction due to transfusion of blood or blood products**
EXCLUDES 1 *minor blood group antigens reactions (Duffy) (E) (K(ell)) (Kidd) (Lewis) (M) (N) (P) (S) (T80.A)*

🗷 **T80.30X-** **ABO incompatibility reaction due to transfusion of blood or blood products, unspecified**
ABO incompatibility blood transfusion NOS
Reaction to ABO incompatibility from transfusion NOS

🗟 **T80.31** **ABO incompatibility with hemolytic transfusion reaction**

🗷 **T80.310-** **ABO incompatibility with acute hemolytic transfusion reaction**
ABO incompatibility with hemolytic transfusion reaction less than 24 hours after transfusion
Acute hemolytic transfusion reaction (AHTR) due to ABO incompatibility

🗷 **T80.311-** **ABO incompatibility with delayed hemolytic transfusion reaction**
ABO incompatibility with hemolytic transfusion reaction 24 hours or more after transfusion
Delayed hemolytic transfusion reaction (DHTR) due to ABO incompatibility

🗷 **T80.319-** **ABO incompatibility with hemolytic transfusion reaction, unspecified**
ABO incompatibility with hemolytic transfusion reaction at unspecified time after transfusion
Hemolytic transfusion reaction (HTR) due to ABO incompatibility NOS

🗷 **T80.39X-** **Other ABO incompatibility reaction due to transfusion of blood or blood products**
Delayed serologic transfusion reaction (DSTR) from ABO incompatibility
Other ABO incompatible blood transfusion
Other reaction to ABO incompatible blood transfusion

🗟 **T80.4** **Rh incompatibility reaction due to transfusion of blood or blood products**
Reaction due to incompatibility of Rh antigens (C) (c) (D) (E) (e)

🗷 **T80.40X-** **Rh incompatibility reaction due to transfusion of blood or blood products, unspecified**
Reaction due to Rh factor in transfusion NOS
Rh incompatible blood transfusion NOS

🗟 **T80.41** **Rh incompatibility with hemolytic transfusion reaction**

🗷 **T80.410-** **Rh incompatibility with acute hemolytic transfusion reaction**
Acute hemolytic transfusion reaction (AHTR) due to Rh incompatibility
Rh incompatibility with hemolytic transfusion reaction less than 24 hours after transfusion

🗷 **T80.411-** **Rh incompatibility with delayed hemolytic transfusion reaction**
Delayed hemolytic transfusion reaction (DHTR) due to Rh incompatibility
Rh incompatibility with hemolytic transfusion reaction 24 hours or more after transfusion

🗷 **T80.419-** **Rh incompatibility with hemolytic transfusion reaction, unspecified**
Rh incompatibility with hemolytic transfusion reaction at unspecified time after transfusion
Hemolytic transfusion reaction (HTR) due to Rh incompatibility NOS

🗷 **T80.49X-** **Other Rh incompatibility reaction due to transfusion of blood or blood products**
Delayed serologic transfusion reaction (DSTR) from Rh incompatibility
Other reaction to Rh incompatible blood transfusion

🗟 **T80.A** **Non-ABO incompatibility reaction due to transfusion of blood or blood products**
Reaction due to incompatibility of minor antigens (Duffy) (Kell) (Kidd) (Lewis) (M) (N) (P) (S)

🗷 **T80.A0X-** **Non-ABO incompatibility reaction due to transfusion of blood or blood products, unspecified**
Non-ABO antigen incompatibility reaction from transfusion NOS

🗟 **T80.A1** **Non-ABO incompatibility with hemolytic transfusion reaction**

● New ▲ Revised *Manifestation* 🗗-🗷 Digit Indicators 🗐 Laterality 🗛 Adult (15+ years) 🗏 Maternity (12-55 years) 🗑 Newborn 🄿 Pediatric (0-17 years) ♂ Male ♀ Female
✖ Deleted Unspecified + Additional code
2017 ICD-10-CM Expert for Physicians

© 2017 decisionHealth 1093

7 T80.A10- **Non-ABO incompatibility with acute hemolytic transfusion reaction**

Acute hemolytic transfusion reaction (AHTR) due to non-ABO incompatibility

Non-ABO incompatibility with hemolytic transfusion reaction less than 24 hours after transfusion

7 T80.A11- **Non-ABO incompatibility with delayed hemolytic transfusion reaction**

Delayed hemolytic transfusion reaction (DHTR) due to non-ABO incompatibility

Non-ABO incompatibility with hemolytic transfusion reaction 24 or more hours after transfusion

7 T80.A19- **Non-ABO incompatibility with hemolytic transfusion reaction, unspecified**

Hemolytic transfusion reaction (HTR) due to non-ABO incompatibility NOS

Non-ABO incompatibility with hemolytic transfusion reaction at unspecified time after transfusion

7 T80.A9X- **Other non-ABO incompatibility reaction due to transfusion of blood or blood products**

Delayed serologic transfusion reaction (DSTR) from non-ABO incompatibility

Other reaction to non-ABO incompatible blood transfusion

5 T80.5 **Anaphylactic reaction due to serum**

Allergic shock due to serum
Anaphylactic shock due to serum
Anaphylactoid reaction due to serum
Anaphylaxis due to serum

EXCLUDES 1 *ABO incompatibility reaction due to transfusion of blood or blood products (T80.3-)*
allergic reaction or shock NOS (T78.2)
anaphylactic reaction or shock NOS (T78.2)
anaphylactic reaction or shock due to adverse effect of correct medicinal substance properly administered (T88.6)
other serum reaction (T80.6-)

7 T80.51X- **Anaphylactic reaction due to administration of blood and blood products**

7 T80.52X- **Anaphylactic reaction due to vaccination**

7 T80.59X- **Anaphylactic reaction due to other serum**

▲ 5 T80.6 **Other serum reactions**

Intoxication by serum
Protein sickness
Serum rash
Serum sickness
Serum urticaria

EXCLUDES 2 *serum hepatitis (B16-B19)*

7 T80.61X- **Other serum reaction due to administration of blood and blood products**

7 T80.62X- **Other serum reaction due to vaccination**

7 T80.69X- **Other serum reaction due to other serum**

5 T80.8 **Other complications following infusion, transfusion and therapeutic injection**

6 T80.81 **Extravasation of vesicant agent**

Infiltration of vesicant agent

7 T80.810- **Extravasation of vesicant antineoplastic chemotherapy**

Infiltration of vesicant antineoplastic chemotherapy

7 T80.818- **Extravasation of other vesicant agent**

Infiltration of other vesicant agent

7 + T80.89X- **Other complications following infusion, transfusion and therapeutic injection**

Delayed serologic transfusion reaction (DSTR), unspecified incompatibility

Use additional code to identify graft-versus-host reaction, if applicable, (D89.81-)

5 T80.9 **Unspecified complication following infusion, transfusion and therapeutic injection**

7 T80.90X- **Unspecified complication following infusion and therapeutic injection**

6 T80.91 **Hemolytic transfusion reaction, unspecified incompatibility**

EXCLUDES 1 *ABO incompatibility with hemolytic transfusion reaction (T80.31-)*
Non-ABO incompatibility with hemolytic transfusion reaction (T80.A1-)
Rh incompatibility with hemolytic transfusion reaction (T80.41-)

7 T80.910- **Acute hemolytic transfusion reaction, unspecified incompatibility**

7 T80.911- **Delayed hemolytic transfusion reaction, unspecified incompatibility**

7 T80.919- **Hemolytic transfusion reaction, unspecified incompatibility, unspecified as acute or delayed**

Hemolytic transfusion reaction NOS

7 T80.92X- **Unspecified transfusion reaction**

Transfusion reaction NOS

4 + T81 **Complications of procedures, not elsewhere classified**

Use additional code for adverse effect, if applicable, to identify drug (T36-T50 with fifth or sixth character 5)

EXCLUDES 2 *complications following immunization (T88.0-T88.1)*
complications following infusion, transfusion and therapeutic injection (T80.-)
complications of transplanted organs and tissue (T86.-)
specified complications classified elsewhere, such as:
complication of prosthetic devices, implants and grafts (T82-T85)
dermatitis due to drugs and medicaments (L23.3, L24.4, L25.1, L27.0-L27.1)
endosseous dental implant failure (M27.6-)
floppy iris syndrome (IFIS) (intraoperative) H21.81
intraoperative and postprocedural complications of specific body system (D78.-, E36.-, E89.-, G97.3-, G97.4, H59.3-, H59.-, H95.2-, H95.3, I97.4-, I97.5, J95, K91.-, L76.-, M96.-, N99.-)
ostomy complications (J95.0-, K94.-, N99.5-)
plateau iris syndrome (post-iridectomy) (postprocedural) H21.82
poisoning and toxic effects of drugs and chemicals (T36-T65 with fifth or sixth character 1-4 or 6)

The appropriate 7th character is to be added to each code from category T81
A   initial encounter
D   subsequent encounter
S   sequela

5 + T81.1 **Postprocedural shock**

Shock during or resulting from a procedure, not elsewhere classified

EXCLUDES 1 *anaphylactic shock NOS (T78.2)*
anaphylactic shock due to correct substance properly administered (T88.6)
anaphylactic shock due to serum (T80.5-)
anesthetic shock (T88.2)
electric shock (T75.4)
obstetric shock (O75.1)
septic shock (R65.21)
shock following abortion or ectopic or molar pregnancy (O00-O07, O08.3)
traumatic shock (T79.4)

7 + T81.10X- **Postprocedural shock unspecified**

Collapse NOS during or resulting from a procedure, not elsewhere classified
Postprocedural failure of peripheral circulation
Postprocedural shock NOS

7 + T81.11X- **Postprocedural cardiogenic shock**

● New   ▲ Revised   *Manifestation*   4-7 Digit Indicators   ▱ Laterality   Ⓐ Adult (15+ years)   Ⓜ Maternity (12-55 years)   Ⓝ Newborn   Ⓟ Pediatric (0-17 years)   ♂ Male   ♀ Female
✖ Deleted   Unspecified   + Additional code

1094   © 2017 DecisionHealth   2017 ICD-10-CM Expert for Physicians

▲ 7 + **T81.12X-**   **Postprocedural septic shock**
Postprocedural endotoxic shock resulting from a procedure, not elsewhere classified
Postprocedural gram-negative shock resulting from a procedure, not elsewhere classified
Code first:
underlying infection
Use additional code, to identify any associated acute organ dysfunction, if applicable

> **GUIDELINES**   Section I.C.1.d.5)(c)
> In cases where a postprocedural infection has occurred and has resulted in severe sepsis, the code for the precipitating complication such as code T81.4, Infection following a procedure, or O86.0, Infection of obstetrical surgical wound, should be coded first followed by code R65.20, Severe sepsis without septic shock. A code for the systemic infection should also be assigned.
>
> If the postprocedural infection has resulted in postprocedural septic shock, the code for the precipitating complication such as code T81.4 or O86.0 should be coded first followed by code T81.12-, Postprocedural septic shock. A code for the systemic infection should also be assigned.

> **CODING TIP ✓**   **Documentation:** Only assign T81.12- when the provider diagnostic statements clearly indicate septic shock as a postprocedural complication.

7 + **T81.19X-**   **Other postprocedural shock**
Postprocedural hypovolemic shock

5 + **T81.3**   **Disruption of wound, not elsewhere classified**
Disruption of any suture materials or other closure methods

> **EXCLUDES 1**   *breakdown (mechanical) of permanent sutures (T85.612)*
> *displacement of permanent sutures (T85.622)*
> *disruption of cesarean delivery wound (O90.0)*
> *disruption of perineal obstetric wound (O90.1)*
> *mechanical complication of permanent sutures NEC (T85.692)*

AHA: 1Q 2014, 23

7 + **T81.30X-**   **Disruption of wound, unspecified**
Disruption of wound NOS

7 + **T81.31X-**   **Disruption of external operation (surgical) wound, not elsewhere classified**
Dehiscence of operation wound NOS
Disruption of operation wound NOS
Disruption or dehiscence of closure of cornea
Disruption or dehiscence of closure of mucosa
Disruption or dehiscence of closure of skin and subcutaneous tissue
Full-thickness skin disruption or dehiscence
Superficial disruption or dehiscence of operation wound

> **EXCLUDES 1**   *dehiscence of amputation stump (T87.81)*

> **CODING TIP ✓**   Assign T81.31- for an unspecified dehiscence of a surgical wound.
AHA: (T81.31XA) 1Q 2015, 20

7 + **T81.32X-**   **Disruption of internal operation (surgical) wound, not elsewhere classified**
Deep disruption or dehiscence of operation wound NOS
Disruption or dehiscence of closure of internal organ or other internal tissue
Disruption or dehiscence of closure of muscle or muscle flap
Disruption or dehiscence of closure of ribs or rib cage
Disruption or dehiscence of closure of skull or craniotomy
Disruption or dehiscence of closure of sternum or sternotomy
Disruption or dehiscence of closure of tendon or ligament
Disruption or dehiscence of closure of superficial or muscular fascia

7 + **T81.33X-**   **Disruption of traumatic injury wound repair**
Disruption or dehiscence of closure of traumatic laceration (external) (internal)

> **CODING TIP ✓**   Assign code T81.33- for a repaired (sutured) traumatic laceration, which has dehisced. This code should not be used for surgically created wounds.

7 + **T81.4XX-**   **Infection following a procedure**
Intra-abdominal abscess following a procedure
Postprocedural infection, not elsewhere classified
Sepsis following a procedure
Stitch abscess following a procedure
Subphrenic abscess following a procedure
Wound abscess following a procedure
Use additional code to identify infection
Use additional code (R65.2-) to identify severe sepsis, if applicable

> **EXCLUDES 1**   *obstetric surgical wound infection (O86.0)*
> *postprocedural fever NOS (R50.82)*
> *postprocedural retroperitoneal abscess (K68.11)*

> **EXCLUDES 2**   *bleb associated endophthalmitis (H59.4-)*
> *infection due to infusion, transfusion and therapeutic injection (T80.2-)*
> *infection due to prosthetic devices, implants and grafts (T82.6-T82.7, T83.5-T83.6, T84.5-T84.7, T85.7)*

> **CODING TIP ✓**   Assign code T81.4- to indicate post operative infections such as postprocedural sepsis, postoperative wound infections, and intra-abdominal abscess following a procedure. If severe sepsis also code R65.2-. Use additional code to identify type of infection.
AHA: 1Q 2014, 23
AHA: (T81.4XXD) 4Q 2015, 37

5 + **T81.5**   **Complications of foreign body accidentally left in body following procedure**

6 + **T81.50**   **Unspecified complication of foreign body accidentally left in body following procedure**

7 + **T81.500-**   **Unspecified complication of foreign body accidentally left in body following surgical operation**

7 + **T81.501-**   **Unspecified complication of foreign body accidentally left in body following infusion or transfusion**

7 + **T81.502-**   **Unspecified complication of foreign body accidentally left in body following kidney dialysis**

7 + **T81.503-**   **Unspecified complication of foreign body accidentally left in body following injection or immunization**

7 + **T81.504-**   **Unspecified complication of foreign body accidentally left in body following endoscopic examination**

7 + **T81.505-**   **Unspecified complication of foreign body accidentally left in body following heart catheterization**

7 + **T81.506-**   **Unspecified complication of foreign body accidentally left in body following aspiration, puncture or other catheterization**

7 + **T81.507-**   **Unspecified complication of foreign body accidentally left in body following removal of catheter or packing**

7 + **T81.508-**   **Unspecified complication of foreign body accidentally left in body following other procedure**

7 + **T81.509-**   **Unspecified complication of foreign body accidentally left in body following unspecified procedure**

6 + **T81.51**   **Adhesions due to foreign body accidentally left in body following procedure**

7 + **T81.510-**   **Adhesions due to foreign body accidentally left in body following surgical operation**

7 + **T81.511-**   **Adhesions due to foreign body accidentally left in body following infusion or transfusion**

● New   ▲ Revised   *Manifestation*   4-7 Digit Indicators   ⊟ Laterality   A Adult (15+ years)   M Maternity (12-55 years)   N Newborn   P Pediatric (0-17 years)   ♂ Male   ♀ Female
✖ Deleted   Unspecified   + Additional code

7 + T81.512- Adhesions due to foreign body accidentally left in body following kidney dialysis

7 + T81.513- Adhesions due to foreign body accidentally left in body following injection or immunization

7 + T81.514- Adhesions due to foreign body accidentally left in body following endoscopic examination

7 + T81.515- Adhesions due to foreign body accidentally left in body following heart catheterization

7 + T81.516- Adhesions due to foreign body accidentally left in body following aspiration, puncture or other catheterization

7 + T81.517- Adhesions due to foreign body accidentally left in body following removal of catheter or packing

7 + T81.518- Adhesions due to foreign body accidentally left in body following other procedure

7 + T81.519- Adhesions due to foreign body accidentally left in body following unspecified procedure

6 + T81.52 Obstruction due to foreign body accidentally left in body following procedure

7 + T81.520- Obstruction due to foreign body accidentally left in body following surgical operation

7 + T81.521- Obstruction due to foreign body accidentally left in body following infusion or transfusion

7 + T81.522- Obstruction due to foreign body accidentally left in body following kidney dialysis

7 + T81.523- Obstruction due to foreign body accidentally left in body following injection or immunization

7 + T81.524- Obstruction due to foreign body accidentally left in body following endoscopic examination

7 + T81.525- Obstruction due to foreign body accidentally left in body following heart catheterization

7 + T81.526- Obstruction due to foreign body accidentally left in body following aspiration, puncture or other catheterization

7 + T81.527- Obstruction due to foreign body accidentally left in body following removal of catheter or packing

7 + T81.528- Obstruction due to foreign body accidentally left in body following other procedure

7 + T81.529- Obstruction due to foreign body accidentally left in body following unspecified procedure

6 + T81.53 Perforation due to foreign body accidentally left in body following procedure

7 + T81.530- Perforation due to foreign body accidentally left in body following surgical operation

7 + T81.531- Perforation due to foreign body accidentally left in body following infusion or transfusion

7 + T81.532- Perforation due to foreign body accidentally left in body following kidney dialysis

7 + T81.533- Perforation due to foreign body accidentally left in body following injection or immunization

7 + T81.534- Perforation due to foreign body accidentally left in body following endoscopic examination

7 + T81.535- Perforation due to foreign body accidentally left in body following heart catheterization

7 + T81.536- Perforation due to foreign body accidentally left in body following aspiration, puncture or other catheterization

7 + T81.537- Perforation due to foreign body accidentally left in body following removal of catheter or packing

7 + T81.538- Perforation due to foreign body accidentally left in body following other procedure

7 + T81.539- Perforation due to foreign body accidentally left in body following unspecified procedure

6 + T81.59 Other complications of foreign body accidentally left in body following procedure

> **EXCLUDES 2** *obstruction or perforation due to prosthetic devices and implants intentionally left in body (T82.0-T82.5, T83.0-T83.4, T83.7, T84.0-T84.4, T85.0-T85.6)*

7 + T81.590- Other complications of foreign body accidentally left in body following surgical operation
AHA: (T81.590A) 4Q 2014, 24

7 + T81.591- Other complications of foreign body accidentally left in body following infusion or transfusion

7 + T81.592- Other complications of foreign body accidentally left in body following kidney dialysis

7 + T81.593- Other complications of foreign body accidentally left in body following injection or immunization

7 + T81.594- Other complications of foreign body accidentally left in body following endoscopic examination

7 + T81.595- Other complications of foreign body accidentally left in body following heart catheterization

7 + T81.596- Other complications of foreign body accidentally left in body following aspiration, puncture or other catheterization

7 + T81.597- Other complications of foreign body accidentally left in body following removal of catheter or packing

7 + T81.598- Other complications of foreign body accidentally left in body following other procedure

7 + T81.599- Other complications of foreign body accidentally left in body following unspecified procedure

5 + T81.6 Acute reaction to foreign substance accidentally left during a procedure

> **EXCLUDES 2** *complications of foreign body accidentally left in body cavity or operation wound following procedure (T81.5-)*

7 + T81.60X- Unspecified acute reaction to foreign substance accidentally left during a procedure

7 + T81.61X- Aseptic peritonitis due to foreign substance accidentally left during a procedure
Chemical peritonitis

7 + T81.69X- Other acute reaction to foreign substance accidentally left during a procedure

▲ 5 + T81.7 Vascular complications following a procedure, not elsewhere classified
Air embolism following procedure NEC
Phlebitis or thrombophlebitis resulting from a procedure

> **EXCLUDES 1** *embolism complicating abortion or ectopic or molar pregnancy (O00-O07, O08.2)*
> *embolism complicating pregnancy, childbirth and the puerperium (O88.-)*
> *traumatic embolism (T79.0)*

> **EXCLUDES 2** *embolism due to prosthetic devices, implants and grafts (T82.8-, T83.81, T84.8-, T85.81-)*
> *embolism following infusion, transfusion and therapeutic injection (T80.0)*

6 + T81.71 Complication of artery following a procedure, not elsewhere classified

7 + T81.710- Complication of mesenteric artery following a procedure, not elsewhere classified

7 + T81.711- Complication of renal artery following a procedure, not elsewhere classified

7 + T81.718- Complication of other artery following a procedure, not elsewhere classified

7 + T81.719- Complication of unspecified artery following a procedure, not elsewhere classified

7 + T81.72X- Complication of vein following a procedure, not elsewhere classified

5 + T81.8 Other complications of procedures, not elsewhere classified

> **EXCLUDES 2** *hypothermia following anesthesia (T88.51)*
> *malignant hyperpyrexia due to anesthesia (T88.3)*

7 + T81.81X- Complication of inhalation therapy

7 + T81.82X- Emphysema (subcutaneous) resulting from a procedure

7 + T81.83X- Persistent postprocedural fistula

7 + T81.89X- Other complications of procedures, not elsewhere classified
Use additional code to specify complication, such as:
postprocedural delirium (F05)
AHA: (T81.89X) 1Q 2014, 23

7 + T81.9XX- Unspecified complication of procedure

● New   ▲ Revised   *Manifestation*   **4-7** Digit Indicators   ⊟ Laterality   Ⓐ Adult (15+ years)   Ⓜ Maternity (12-55 years)   Ⓝ Newborn   Ⓟ Pediatric (0-17 years)   ♂ Male   ♀ Female
✖ Deleted   Unspecified   + Additional code

1096   © 2017 DecisionHealth   2017 ICD-10-CM Expert for Physicians

4 **T82** **Complications of cardiac and vascular prosthetic devices, implants and grafts**

> **EXCLUDES 2** *failure and rejection of transplanted organs and tissue (T86.-)*

> The appropriate 7th character is to be added to each code from category T82
> A   initial encounter
> D   subsequent encounter
> S   sequela

5 **T82.0** **Mechanical complication of heart valve prosthesis**
Mechanical complication of artificial heart valve

> **EXCLUDES 1** *mechanical complication of biological heart valve graft (T82.22-)*

7 **T82.01X-** **Breakdown (mechanical) of heart valve prosthesis**

7 **T82.02X-** **Displacement of heart valve prosthesis**
Malposition of heart valve prosthesis

7 **T82.03X-** **Leakage of heart valve prosthesis**

7 **T82.09X-** **Other mechanical complication of heart valve prosthesis**
Obstruction (mechanical) of heart valve prosthesis
Perforation of heart valve prosthesis
Protrusion of heart valve prosthesis

5 **T82.1** **Mechanical complication of cardiac electronic device**
6 **T82.11** **Breakdown (mechanical) of cardiac electronic device**

7 **T82.110-** **Breakdown (mechanical) of cardiac electrode**

7 **T82.111-** **Breakdown (mechanical) of cardiac pulse generator (battery)**

7 **T82.118-** **Breakdown (mechanical) of other cardiac electronic device**

7 **T82.119-** **Breakdown (mechanical) of unspecified cardiac electronic device**

6 **T82.12** **Displacement of cardiac electronic device**
Malposition of cardiac electronic device

7 **T82.120-** **Displacement of cardiac electrode**

7 **T82.121-** **Displacement of cardiac pulse generator (battery)**

7 **T82.128-** **Displacement of other cardiac electronic device**

7 **T82.129-** **Displacement of unspecified cardiac electronic device**

6 **T82.19** **Other mechanical complication of cardiac electronic device**
Leakage of cardiac electronic device
Obstruction of cardiac electronic device
Perforation of cardiac electronic device
Protrusion of cardiac electronic device

7 **T82.190-** **Other mechanical complication of cardiac electrode**

7 **T82.191-** **Other mechanical complication of cardiac pulse generator (battery)**

7 **T82.198-** **Other mechanical complication of other cardiac electronic device**

7 **T82.199-** **Other mechanical complication of unspecified cardiac device**

5 **T82.2** **Mechanical complication of coronary artery bypass graft and biological heart valve graft**

> **EXCLUDES 1** *mechanical complication of artificial heart valve prosthesis (T82.0-)*

6 **T82.21** **Mechanical complication of coronary artery bypass graft**

7 **T82.211-** **Breakdown (mechanical) of coronary artery bypass graft**

7 **T82.212-** **Displacement of coronary artery bypass graft**
Malposition of coronary artery bypass graft

7 **T82.213-** **Leakage of coronary artery bypass graft**

7 **T82.218-** **Other mechanical complication of coronary artery bypass graft**
Obstruction, mechanical of coronary artery bypass graft
Perforation of coronary artery bypass graft
Protrusion of coronary artery bypass graft

6 **T82.22** **Mechanical complication of biological heart valve graft**

7 **T82.221-** **Breakdown (mechanical) of biological heart valve graft**

7 **T82.222-** **Displacement of biological heart valve graft**
Malposition of biological heart valve graft

7 **T82.223-** **Leakage of biological heart valve graft**

7 **T82.228-** **Other mechanical complication of biological heart valve graft**
Obstruction of biological heart valve graft
Perforation of biological heart valve graft
Protrusion of biological heart valve graft

5 **T82.3** **Mechanical complication of other vascular grafts**
6 **T82.31** **Breakdown (mechanical) of other vascular grafts**

7 **T82.310-** **Breakdown (mechanical) of aortic (bifurcation) graft (replacement)**

7 **T82.311-** **Breakdown (mechanical) of carotid arterial graft (bypass)**

7 **T82.312-** **Breakdown (mechanical) of femoral arterial graft (bypass)**

7 **T82.318-** **Breakdown (mechanical) of other vascular grafts**

7 **T82.319-** **Breakdown (mechanical) of unspecified vascular grafts**

6 **T82.32** **Displacement of other vascular grafts**
Malposition of other vascular grafts

7 **T82.320-** **Displacement of aortic (bifurcation) graft (replacement)**

7 **T82.321-** **Displacement of carotid arterial graft (bypass)**

7 **T82.322-** **Displacement of femoral arterial graft (bypass)**

7 **T82.328-** **Displacement of other vascular grafts**

7 **T82.329-** **Displacement of unspecified vascular grafts**

6 **T82.33** **Leakage of other vascular grafts**

7 **T82.330-** **Leakage of aortic (bifurcation) graft (replacement)**

7 **T82.331-** **Leakage of carotid arterial graft (bypass)**

7 **T82.332-** **Leakage of femoral arterial graft (bypass)**

7 **T82.338-** **Leakage of other vascular grafts**

7 **T82.339-** **Leakage of unspecified vascular graft**

6 **T82.39** **Other mechanical complication of other vascular grafts**
Obstruction (mechanical) of other vascular grafts
Perforation of other vascular grafts
Protrusion of other vascular grafts

7 **T82.390-** **Other mechanical complication of aortic (bifurcation) graft (replacement)**

7 **T82.391-** **Other mechanical complication of carotid arterial graft (bypass)**

7 **T82.392-** **Other mechanical complication of femoral arterial graft (bypass)**

7 **T82.398-** **Other mechanical complication of other vascular grafts**

7 **T82.399-** **Other mechanical complication of unspecified vascular grafts**

5 **T82.4** **Mechanical complication of vascular dialysis catheter**
Mechanical complication of hemodialysis catheter

> **EXCLUDES 1** *mechanical complication of intraperitoneal dialysis catheter (T85.62)*

7 **T82.41X-** **Breakdown (mechanical) of vascular dialysis catheter**

7 **T82.42X-** **Displacement of vascular dialysis catheter**
Malposition of vascular dialysis catheter

7 **T82.43X-** **Leakage of vascular dialysis catheter**

7 **T82.49X-** **Other complication of vascular dialysis catheter**
Obstruction (mechanical) of vascular dialysis catheter
Perforation of vascular dialysis catheter
Protrusion of vascular dialysis catheter

5 **T82.5** **Mechanical complication of other cardiac and vascular devices and implants**

> **EXCLUDES 2** *mechanical complication of epidural and subdural infusion catheter (T85.61)*

6 **T82.51** **Breakdown (mechanical) of other cardiac and vascular devices and implants**

7 **T82.510-** **Breakdown (mechanical) of surgically created arteriovenous fistula**

7 **T82.511-** **Breakdown (mechanical) of surgically created arteriovenous shunt**

7 **T82.512-** **Breakdown (mechanical) of artificial heart**

7 **T82.513-** **Breakdown (mechanical) of balloon (counterpulsation) device**

7 **T82.514-** **Breakdown (mechanical) of infusion catheter**

7 **T82.515-** **Breakdown (mechanical) of umbrella device**

7 **T82.518-** **Breakdown (mechanical) of other cardiac and vascular devices and implants**

● New   ▲ Revised   *Manifestation*   4 - 7 Digit Indicators   ▤ Laterality   Ⓐ Adult (15+ years)   Ⓜ Maternity (12-55 years)   Ⓝ Newborn (0-17 years)   Ⓟ Pediatric (0-17 years)   ♂ Male   ♀ Female
✖ Deleted   Unspecified   + Additional code

7 T82.519-   **Breakdown (mechanical) of unspecified cardiac and vascular devices and implants**

6 T82.52   **Displacement of other cardiac and vascular devices and implants**
Malposition of other cardiac and vascular devices and implants

7 T82.520-   **Displacement of surgically created arteriovenous fistula**

7 T82.521-   **Displacement of surgically created arteriovenous shunt**

7 T82.522-   **Displacement of artificial heart**

7 T82.523-   **Displacement of balloon (counterpulsation) device**

7 T82.524-   **Displacement of infusion catheter**

7 T82.525-   **Displacement of umbrella device**

7 T82.528-   **Displacement of other cardiac and vascular devices and implants**

7 T82.529-   **Displacement of unspecified cardiac and vascular devices and implants**

6 T82.53   **Leakage of other cardiac and vascular devices and implants**

7 T82.530-   **Leakage of surgically created arteriovenous fistula**

7 T82.531-   **Leakage of surgically created arteriovenous shunt**

7 T82.532-   **Leakage of artificial heart**

7 T82.533-   **Leakage of balloon (counterpulsation) device**

7 T82.534-   **Leakage of infusion catheter**

7 T82.535-   **Leakage of umbrella device**

7 T82.538-   **Leakage of other cardiac and vascular devices and implants**

7 T82.539-   **Leakage of unspecified cardiac and vascular devices and implants**

6 T82.59   **Other mechanical complication of other cardiac and vascular devices and implants**
Obstruction (mechanical) of other cardiac and vascular devices and implants
Perforation of other cardiac and vascular devices and implants
Protrusion of other cardiac and vascular devices and implants

7 T82.590-   **Other mechanical complication of surgically created arteriovenous fistula**

7 T82.591-   **Other mechanical complication of surgically created arteriovenous shunt**

7 T82.592-   **Other mechanical complication of artificial heart**

7 T82.593-   **Other mechanical complication of balloon (counterpulsation) device**

7 T82.594-   **Other mechanical complication of infusion catheter**

7 T82.595-   **Other mechanical complication of umbrella device**

7 T82.598-   **Other mechanical complication of other cardiac and vascular devices and implants**

7 T82.599-   **Other mechanical complication of unspecified cardiac and vascular devices and implants**

7 + T82.6XX-   **Infection and inflammatory reaction due to cardiac valve prosthesis**
Use additional code to identify infection

7 + T82.7XX-   **Infection and inflammatory reaction due to other cardiac and vascular devices, implants and grafts**
Use additional code to identify infection
AHA: (T82.7XXA) 1Q 2015, 20

5 T82.8   **Other specified complications of cardiac and vascular prosthetic devices, implants and grafts**

▲ 6 T82.81   **Embolism due to cardiac and vascular prosthetic devices, implants and grafts**

▲ 7 T82.817-   **Embolism due to cardiac prosthetic devices, implants and grafts**

▲ 7 T82.818-   **Embolism due to vascular prosthetic devices, implants and grafts**

▲ 6 T82.82   **Fibrosis due to cardiac and vascular prosthetic devices, implants and grafts**

▲ 7 T82.827-   **Fibrosis due to cardiac prosthetic devices, implants and grafts**

▲ 7 T82.828-   **Fibrosis due to vascular prosthetic devices, implants and grafts**

▲ 6 T82.83   **Hemorrhage due to cardiac and vascular prosthetic devices, implants and grafts**

▲ 7 T82.837-   **Hemorrhage due to cardiac prosthetic devices, implants and grafts**

▲ 7 T82.838-   **Hemorrhage due to vascular prosthetic devices, implants and grafts**

▲ 6 T82.84   **Pain due to cardiac and vascular prosthetic devices, implants and grafts**

▲ 7 T82.847-   **Pain due to cardiac prosthetic devices, implants and grafts**

▲ 7 T82.848-   **Pain due to vascular prosthetic devices, implants and grafts**

▲ 6 T82.85   **Stenosis due to cardiac and vascular prosthetic devices, implants and grafts**

● 7 T82.855-   **Stenosis of coronary artery stent**
In-stent stenosis (restenosis) of coronary artery stent
Restenosis of coronary artery stent

● 7 T82.856-   **Stenosis of peripheral vascular stent**
In-stent stenosis (restenosis) of peripheral vascular stent
Restenosis of peripheral vascular stent

▲ 7 T82.857-   **Stenosis of other cardiac prosthetic devices, implants and grafts**

▲ 7 T82.858-   **Stenosis of other vascular prosthetic devices, implants and grafts**

6 T82.86   **Thrombosis of cardiac and vascular prosthetic devices, implants and grafts**

▲ 7 T82.867-   **Thrombosis due to cardiac prosthetic devices, implants and grafts**

▲ 7 T82.868-   **Thrombosis due to vascular prosthetic devices, implants and grafts**

6 T82.89   **Other specified complication of cardiac and vascular prosthetic devices, implants and grafts**

7 T82.897-   **Other specified complication of cardiac prosthetic devices, implants and grafts**

7 T82.898-   **Other specified complication of vascular prosthetic devices, implants and grafts**

7 T82.9XX-   **Unspecified complication of cardiac and vascular prosthetic device, implant and graft**

4 **T83   Complications of genitourinary prosthetic devices, implants and grafts**
EXCLUDES 2   *failure and rejection of transplanted organs and tissue (T86.-)*

The appropriate 7th character is to be added to each code from category T83
A   initial encounter
D   subsequent encounter
S   sequela

▲ 5 T83.0   **Mechanical complication of urinary catheter**
EXCLUDES 2   *complications of stoma of urinary tract (N99.5-)*

▲ 6 T83.01   **Breakdown (mechanical) of urinary catheter**

7 T83.010-   **Breakdown (mechanical) of cystostomy catheter**

● 7 T83.011-   **Breakdown (mechanical) of indwelling urethral catheter**

● 7 T83.012-   **Breakdown (mechanical) of nephrostomy catheter**

▲ 7 T83.018-   **Breakdown (mechanical) of other urinary catheter**
Breakdown (mechanical) of Hopkins catheter
Breakdown (mechanical) of ileostomy catheter
Breakdown (mechanical) urostomy catheter

▲ 6 T83.02   **Displacement of urinary catheter**
Malposition of urinary catheter

7 T83.020-   **Displacement of cystostomy catheter**

● 7 T83.021-   **Displacement of indwelling urethral catheter**

● 7 T83.022-   **Displacement of nephrostomy catheter**

▲ 7 T83.028-   **Displacement of other urinary catheter**
Displacement of Hopkins catheter
Displacement of ileostomy catheter
Displacement of urostomy catheter

▲ 6 T83.03   **Leakage of urinary catheter**

7 T83.030-   **Leakage of cystostomy catheter**

● 7 T83.031-   **Leakage of indwelling urethral catheter**

● 7 T83.032-   **Leakage of nephrostomy catheter**

● New   ▲ Revised   *Manifestation*   4 - 7 Digit Indicators   ⊟ Laterality   A Adult (15+ years)   M Maternity (12-55 years)   N Newborn (0-17 years)   P Pediatric (0-17 years)   ♂ Male   ♀ Female
✖ Deleted   Unspecified   + Additional code

1098   © 2017 DecisionHealth   2017 ICD-10-CM Expert for Physicians

▲ 7 **T83.038-** Leakage of other urinary catheter
Leakage of Hopkins catheter
Leakage of ileostomy catheter
Leakage of urostomy catheter

▲ 6 **T83.09** Other mechanical complication of urinary catheter
Obstruction (mechanical) of urinary catheter
Perforation of urinary catheter
Protrusion of urinary catheter

7 **T83.090-** Other mechanical complication of cystostomy catheter

● 7 **T83.091-** Other mechanical complication of indwelling urethral catheter

● 7 **T83.092-** Other mechanical complication of nephrostomy catheter

▲ 7 **T83.098-** Other mechanical complication of other urinary catheter
Other mechanical complication of Hopkins catheter
Other mechanical complication of ileostomy catheter
Other mechanical complication of urostomy catheter

5 **T83.1** Mechanical complication of other urinary devices and implants

6 **T83.11** Breakdown (mechanical) of other urinary devices and implants

▲ 7 **T83.110-** Breakdown (mechanical) of urinary electronic stimulator device

> **EXCLUDES 2** *Breakdown (mechanical) of electrode (lead) for sacral nerve neurostimulator (T85.111)*
> *Breakdown (mechanical) of implanted electronic sacral neurostimulator, pulse generator or receiver (T85.113)*

▲ 7 **T83.111-** Breakdown (mechanical) of implanted urinary sphincter

▲ 7 **T83.112-** Breakdown (mechanical) of indwelling ureteral stent

● 7 **T83.113-** Breakdown (mechanical) of other urinary stents
Breakdown (mechanical) of ileal conduit stent
Breakdown (mechanical) of nephroureteral stent

7 **T83.118-** Breakdown (mechanical) of other urinary devices and implants

6 **T83.12** Displacement of other urinary devices and implants
Malposition of other urinary devices and implants

▲ 7 **T83.120-** Displacement of urinary electronic stimulator device

> **EXCLUDES 2** *Displacement of electrode (lead) for sacral nerve neurostimulator (T85.121)*
> *Displacement of implanted electronic sacral neurostimulator, pulse generator or receiver (T85.123)*

▲ 7 **T83.121-** Displacement of implanted urinary sphincter

▲ 7 **T83.122-** Displacement of indwelling ureteral stent

● 7 **T83.123-** Displacement of other urinary stents
Displacement of ileal conduit stent
Displacement of nephroureteral stent

7 **T83.128-** Displacement of other urinary devices and implants

6 **T83.19** Other mechanical complication of other urinary devices and implants
Leakage of other urinary devices and implants
Obstruction (mechanical) of other urinary devices and implants
Perforation of other urinary devices and implants
Protrusion of other urinary devices and implants

▲ 7 **T83.190-** Other mechanical complication of urinary electronic stimulator device

> **EXCLUDES 2** *Other mechanical complication of electrode (lead) for sacral nerve neurostimulator (T85.191)*
> *Other mechanical complication of implanted electronic sacral neurostimulator, pulse generator or receiver (T85.193)*

▲ 7 **T83.191-** Other mechanical complication of implanted urinary sphincter

▲ 7 **T83.192-** Other mechanical complication of indwelling ureteral stent

● 7 **T83.193-** Other mechanical complication of other urinary stent
Other mechanical complication of ileal conduit stent
Other mechanical complication of nephroureteral stent

7 **T83.198-** Other mechanical complication of other urinary devices and implants

5 **T83.2** Mechanical complication of graft of urinary organ

7 **T83.21X-** Breakdown (mechanical) of graft of urinary organ

7 **T83.22X-** Displacement of graft of urinary organ
Malposition of graft of urinary organ

7 **T83.23X-** Leakage of graft of urinary organ

● 7 **T83.24X-** Erosion of graft of urinary organ

● 7 **T83.25X-** Exposure of graft of urinary organ

7 **T83.29X-** Other mechanical complication of graft of urinary organ
Obstruction (mechanical) of graft of urinary organ
Perforation of graft of urinary organ
Protrusion of graft of urinary organ

5 **T83.3** Mechanical complication of intrauterine contraceptive device

7 **T83.31X-** Breakdown (mechanical) of intrauterine contraceptive device

▲ 7 **T83.32X-** Displacement of intrauterine contraceptive device
Malposition of intrauterine contraceptive device
Missing string of intrauterine contraceptive device

7 **T83.39X-** Other mechanical complication of intrauterine contraceptive device
Leakage of intrauterine contraceptive device
Obstruction (mechanical) of intrauterine contraceptive device
Perforation of intrauterine contraceptive device
Protrusion of intrauterine contraceptive device

5 **T83.4** Mechanical complication of other prosthetic devices, implants and grafts of genital tract

6 **T83.41** Breakdown (mechanical) of other prosthetic devices, implants and grafts of genital tract

▲ 7 **T83.410-** Breakdown (mechanical) of implanted penile prosthesis
Breakdown (mechanical) of penile prosthesis cylinder
Breakdown (mechanical) of penile prosthesis pump
Breakdown (mechanical) of penile prosthesis reservoir

● 7 **T83.411-** Breakdown (mechanical) of implanted testicular prosthesis

7 **T83.418-** Breakdown (mechanical) of other prosthetic devices, implants and grafts of genital tract

6 **T83.42** Displacement of other prosthetic devices, implants and grafts of genital tract
Malposition of other prosthetic devices, implants and grafts of genital tract

▲ 7 **T83.420-** Displacement of implanted penile prosthesis
Displacement of penile prosthesis cylinder
Displacement of penile prosthesis pump
Displacement of penile prosthesis reservoir

● 7 **T83.421-** Displacement of implanted testicular prosthesis

7 **T83.428-** Displacement of other prosthetic devices, implants and grafts of genital tract

🆖 **T83.49** **Other mechanical complication of other prosthetic devices, implants and grafts of genital tract**
Leakage of other prosthetic devices, implants and grafts of genital tract
Obstruction, mechanical of other prosthetic devices, implants and grafts of genital tract
Perforation of other prosthetic devices, implants and grafts of genital tract
Protrusion of other prosthetic devices, implants and grafts of genital tract

▲ 7 **T83.490-** **Other mechanical complication of implanted penile prosthesis**
Other mechanical complication of penile prosthesis cylinder
Other mechanical complication of penile prosthesis pump
Other mechanical complication of penile prosthesis reservoir

● 7 **T83.491-** **Other mechanical complication of implanted testicular prosthesis**

7 **T83.498-** **Other mechanical complication of other prosthetic devices, implants and grafts of genital tract**

🆕+ **T83.5** **Infection and inflammatory reaction due to prosthetic device, implant and graft in urinary system**
Use additional code to identify infection

▲ 🆖+ **T83.51** **Infection and inflammatory reaction due to urinary catheter**
EXCLUDES 2 *complications of stoma of urinary tract (N99.5-)*

● 7+ **T83.510-** **Infection and inflammatory reaction due to cystostomy catheter**

● 7+ **T83.511-** **Infection and inflammatory reaction due to indwelling urethral catheter**

● 7+ **T83.512-** **Infection and inflammatory reaction due to nephrostomy catheter**

● 7+ **T83.518-** **Infection and inflammatory reaction due to other urinary catheter**
Infection and inflammatory reaction due to Hopkins catheter
Infection and inflammatory reaction due to ileostomy catheter
Infection and inflammatory reaction due to urostomy catheter

▲ 🆖+ **T83.59** **Infection and inflammatory reaction due to prosthetic device, implant and graft in urinary system**

● 7+ **T83.590-** **Infection and inflammatory reaction due to implanted urinary neurostimulation device**
EXCLUDES 2 *Infection and inflammatory reaction due to electrode lead of sacral nerve neurostimulator (T85.732) Infection and inflammatory reaction due to pulse generator or receiver of sacral nerve neurostimulator (T85.734)*

● 7+ **T83.591-** **Infection and inflammatory reaction due to implanted urinary sphincter**

● 7+ **T83.592-** **Infection and inflammatory reaction due to indwelling ureteral stent**

● 7+ **T83.593-** **Infection and inflammatory reaction due to other urinary stents**
Infection and inflammatory reaction due to ileal conduit stents
Infection and inflammatory reaction due to nephroureteral stent

● 7+ **T83.598-** **Infection and inflammatory reaction due to other prosthetic device, implant and graft in urinary system**

▲ 🆕+ **T83.6** **Infection and inflammatory reaction due to prosthetic device, implant and graft in genital tract**
Use additional code to identify infection

● 7+ **T83.61X-** **Infection and inflammatory reaction due to implanted penile prosthesis**
Infection and inflammatory reaction due to penile prosthesis cylinder
Infection and inflammatory reaction due to penile prosthesis pump
Infection and inflammatory reaction due to penile prosthesis reservoir

● 7+ **T83.62X-** **Infection and inflammatory reaction due to implanted testicular prosthesis**

● 7+ **T83.69X-** **Infection and inflammatory reaction due to other prosthetic device, implant and graft in genital tract**

🆕 **T83.7** **Complications due to implanted mesh and other prosthetic materials**

🆖 **T83.71** **Erosion of implanted mesh and other prosthetic materials to surrounding organ or tissue**

▲ 7 **T83.711-** **Erosion of implanted vaginal mesh to surrounding organ or tissue**
Erosion of implanted vaginal mesh into pelvic floor muscles

● 7 **T83.712-** **Erosion of implanted urethral mesh to surrounding organ or tissue**
Erosion of implanted female urethral sling
Erosion of implanted male urethral sling
Erosion of implanted urethral mesh into pelvic floor muscles

● 7 **T83.713-** **Erosion of implanted urethral bulking agent to surrounding organ or tissue**

● 7 **T83.714-** **Erosion of implanted ureteral bulking agent to surrounding organ or tissue**

▲ 7 **T83.718-** **Erosion of other implanted mesh to organ or tissue**

● 7 **T83.719-** **Erosion of other prosthetic materials to surrounding organ or tissue**

▲ 🆖 **T83.72** **Exposure of implanted mesh and other prosthetic materials into surrounding organ or tissue**
Extrusion of implanted mesh

▲ 7 **T83.721-** **Exposure of implanted vaginal mesh into vagina**
Exposure of implanted vaginal mesh through vaginal wall

● 7 **T83.722-** **Exposure of implanted urethral mesh into urethra**
Exposure of implanted female urethral sling
Exposure of implanted male urethral sling
Exposure of implanted urethral mesh through urethral wall

● 7 **T83.723-** **Exposure of implanted urethral bulking agent into urethra**

● 7 **T83.724-** **Exposure of implanted ureteral bulking agent into ureter**

▲ 7 **T83.728-** **Exposure of other implanted mesh into organ or tissue**

● 7 **T83.729-** **Exposure of other prosthetic materials into organ or tissue**

● 7 **T83.79X-** **Other specified complications due to other genitourinary prosthetic materials**

🆕 **T83.8** **Other specified complications of genitourinary prosthetic devices, implants and grafts**

▲ 7 **T83.81X-** **Embolism due to genitourinary prosthetic devices, implants and grafts**

▲ 7 **T83.82X-** **Fibrosis due to genitourinary prosthetic devices, implants and grafts**

▲ 7 **T83.83X-** **Hemorrhage due to genitourinary prosthetic devices, implants and grafts**

▲ 7 **T83.84X-** **Pain due to genitourinary prosthetic devices, implants and grafts**

▲ 7 **T83.85X-** **Stenosis due to genitourinary prosthetic devices, implants and grafts**

▲ 7 **T83.86X-** **Thrombosis due to genitourinary prosthetic devices, implants and grafts**

7 **T83.89X-** **Other specified complication of genitourinary prosthetic devices, implants and grafts**

7 **T83.9XX-** **Unspecified complication of genitourinary prosthetic device, implant and graft**

4 **T84** **Complications of internal orthopedic prosthetic devices, implants and grafts**
EXCLUDES 2 *failure and rejection of transplanted organs and tissues (T86.-) fracture of bone following insertion of orthopedic implant, joint prosthesis or bone plate (M96.6)*

The appropriate 7th character is to be added to each code from category T84
A   initial encounter
D   subsequent encounter
S   sequela

🆕 **T84.0** **Mechanical complication of internal joint prosthesis**

6 **T84.01** **Broken internal joint prosthesis**
Breakage (fracture) of prosthetic joint
Broken prosthetic joint implant
> **EXCLUDES 1** *periprosthetic joint implant fracture (T84.04)*

7 ⊟ **T84.010-** **Broken internal right hip prosthesis**

7 ⊟ **T84.011-** **Broken internal left hip prosthesis**

7 ⊟ **T84.012-** **Broken internal right knee prosthesis**

7 ⊟ **T84.013-** **Broken internal left knee prosthesis**

7 + **T84.018-** **Broken internal joint prosthesis, other site**
> *Use additional code to identify the joint (Z96.6-)*

7 ⊟ **T84.019-** **Broken internal joint prosthesis, unspecified site**

6 **T84.02** **Dislocation of internal joint prosthesis**
Instability of internal joint prosthesis
Subluxation of internal joint prosthesis

7 ⊟ **T84.020-** **Dislocation of internal right hip prosthesis**

7 ⊟ **T84.021-** **Dislocation of internal left hip prosthesis**

7 ⊟ **T84.022-** **Instability of internal right knee prosthesis**

7 ⊟ **T84.023-** **Instability of internal left knee prosthesis**

7 ⊟ + **T84.028-** **Dislocation of other internal joint prosthesis**
> *Use additional code to identify the joint (Z96.6-)*

7 ⊟ **T84.029-** **Dislocation of unspecified internal joint prosthesis**

6 **T84.03** **Mechanical loosening of internal prosthetic joint**
Aseptic loosening of prosthetic joint

7 ⊟ **T84.030-** **Mechanical loosening of internal right hip prosthetic joint**

7 ⊟ **T84.031-** **Mechanical loosening of internal left hip prosthetic joint**

7 ⊟ **T84.032-** **Mechanical loosening of internal right knee prosthetic joint**

7 ⊟ **T84.033-** **Mechanical loosening of internal left knee prosthetic joint**

7 ⊟ + **T84.038-** **Mechanical loosening of other internal prosthetic joint**
> *Use additional code to identify the joint (Z96.6-)*

7 ⊟ **T84.039-** **Mechanical loosening of unspecified internal prosthetic joint**

✖ ~~T84.04~~ ~~Periprosthetic fracture around internal prosthetic joint~~

✖ ~~T84.040-~~ ~~Periprosthetic fracture around internal prosthetic right hip joint~~

✖ ~~T84.041-~~ ~~Periprosthetic fracture around internal prosthetic left hip joint~~

✖ ~~T84.042-~~ ~~Periprosthetic fracture around internal prosthetic right knee joint~~

✖ ~~T84.043-~~ ~~Periprosthetic fracture around internal prosthetic left knee joint~~

✖ ~~T84.048-~~ ~~Periprosthetic fracture around other internal prosthetic joint~~

✖ ~~T84.049-~~ ~~Periprosthetic fracture around unspecified internal prosthetic joint~~

6 + **T84.05** **Periprosthetic osteolysis of internal prosthetic joint**
> *Use additional code to identify major osseous defect, if applicable (M89.7-)*

7 ⊟ + **T84.050-** **Periprosthetic osteolysis of internal prosthetic right hip joint**

7 ⊟ + **T84.051-** **Periprosthetic osteolysis of internal prosthetic left hip joint**

7 ⊟ + **T84.052-** **Periprosthetic osteolysis of internal prosthetic right knee joint**

7 ⊟ + **T84.053-** **Periprosthetic osteolysis of internal prosthetic left knee joint**

7 ⊟ + **T84.058-** **Periprosthetic osteolysis of other internal prosthetic joint**
> *Use additional code to identify the joint (Z96.6-)*

7 ⊟ + **T84.059-** **Periprosthetic osteolysis of unspecified internal prosthetic joint**

6 **T84.06** **Wear of articular bearing surface of internal prosthetic joint**

7 ⊟ **T84.060-** **Wear of articular bearing surface of internal prosthetic right hip joint**

7 ⊟ **T84.061-** **Wear of articular bearing surface of internal prosthetic left hip joint**

7 ⊟ **T84.062-** **Wear of articular bearing surface of internal prosthetic right knee joint**

7 ⊟ **T84.063-** **Wear of articular bearing surface of internal prosthetic left knee joint**

7 ⊟ + **T84.068-** **Wear of articular bearing surface of other internal prosthetic joint**
> *Use additional code to identify the joint (Z96.6-)*

7 ⊟ **T84.069-** **Wear of articular bearing surface of unspecified internal prosthetic joint**

6 **T84.09** **Other mechanical complication of internal joint prosthesis**
Prosthetic joint implant failure NOS

7 ⊟ **T84.090-** **Other mechanical complication of internal right hip prosthesis**

7 ⊟ **T84.091-** **Other mechanical complication of internal left hip prosthesis**

7 ⊟ **T84.092-** **Other mechanical complication of internal right knee prosthesis**

7 ⊟ **T84.093-** **Other mechanical complication of internal left knee prosthesis**

7 ⊟ + **T84.098-** **Other mechanical complication of other internal joint prosthesis**
> *Use additional code to identify the joint (Z96.6-)*

7 ⊟ **T84.099-** **Other mechanical complication of unspecified internal joint prosthesis**

5 **T84.1** **Mechanical complication of internal fixation device of bones of limb**
> **EXCLUDES 2** *mechanical complication of internal fixation device of bones of feet (T84.2-)*
> *mechanical complication of internal fixation device of bones of fingers (T84.2-)*
> *mechanical complication of internal fixation device of bones of hands (T84.2-)*
> *mechanical complication of internal fixation device of bones of toes (T84.2-)*

6 **T84.11** **Breakdown (mechanical) of internal fixation device of bones of limb**

7 ⊟ **T84.110-** **Breakdown (mechanical) of internal fixation device of right humerus**

7 ⊟ **T84.111-** **Breakdown (mechanical) of internal fixation device of left humerus**

7 ⊟ **T84.112-** **Breakdown (mechanical) of internal fixation device of bone of right forearm**

7 ⊟ **T84.113-** **Breakdown (mechanical) of internal fixation device of bone of left forearm**

7 ⊟ **T84.114-** **Breakdown (mechanical) of internal fixation device of right femur**

7 ⊟ **T84.115-** **Breakdown (mechanical) of internal fixation device of left femur**

7 ⊟ **T84.116-** **Breakdown (mechanical) of internal fixation device of bone of right lower leg**

7 ⊟ **T84.117-** **Breakdown (mechanical) of internal fixation device of bone of left lower leg**

7 ⊟ **T84.119-** **Breakdown (mechanical) of internal fixation device of unspecified bone of limb**

6 **T84.12** **Displacement of internal fixation device of bones of limb**
Malposition of internal fixation device of bones of limb

7 ⊟ **T84.120-** **Displacement of internal fixation device of right humerus**

7 ⊟ **T84.121-** **Displacement of internal fixation device of left humerus**

7 ⊟ **T84.122-** **Displacement of internal fixation device of bone of right forearm**

7 ⊟ **T84.123-** **Displacement of internal fixation device of bone of left forearm**

7 ⊟ **T84.124-** **Displacement of internal fixation device of right femur**

7 ⊟ **T84.125-** **Displacement of internal fixation device of left femur**

7 ⊟ **T84.126-** **Displacement of internal fixation device of bone of right lower leg**

7 ⊟ **T84.127-** **Displacement of internal fixation device of bone of left lower leg**

7 ⊟ **T84.129-** **Displacement of internal fixation device of unspecified bone of limb**

6 **T84.19** **Other mechanical complication of internal fixation device of bones of limb**
Obstruction (mechanical) of internal fixation device of bones of limb
Perforation of internal fixation device of bones of limb
Protrusion of internal fixation device of bones of limb

● New ▲ Revised *Manifestation* | 4-7 Digit Indicators ⊟ Laterality | A Adult (15+ years) | M Maternity (12-55 years) | N Newborn | P Pediatric (0-17 years) | ♂ Male | ♀ Female
✖ ~~Deleted~~ | Unspecified + Additional code

7️⃣⊟ **T84.190-** Other mechanical complication of internal fixation device of right humerus

7️⃣⊟ **T84.191-** Other mechanical complication of internal fixation device of left humerus

7️⃣⊟ **T84.192-** Other mechanical complication of internal fixation device of bone of right forearm

7️⃣⊟ **T84.193-** Other mechanical complication of internal fixation device of bone of left forearm

7️⃣⊟ **T84.194-** Other mechanical complication of internal fixation device of right femur

7️⃣⊟ **T84.195-** Other mechanical complication of internal fixation device of left femur

7️⃣⊟ **T84.196-** Other mechanical complication of internal fixation device of bone of right lower leg

7️⃣⊟ **T84.197-** Other mechanical complication of internal fixation device of bone of left lower leg

7️⃣⊟ **T84.199-** Other mechanical complication of internal fixation device of unspecified bone of limb

5️⃣ **T84.2** Mechanical complication of internal fixation device of other bones

6️⃣ **T84.21** Breakdown (mechanical) of internal fixation device of other bones

7️⃣ **T84.210-** Breakdown (mechanical) of internal fixation device of bones of hand and fingers

7️⃣ **T84.213-** Breakdown (mechanical) of internal fixation device of bones of foot and toes

7️⃣ **T84.216-** Breakdown (mechanical) of internal fixation device of vertebrae

7️⃣ **T84.218-** Breakdown (mechanical) of internal fixation device of other bones

6️⃣ **T84.22** Displacement of internal fixation device of other bones

Malposition of internal fixation device of other bones

7️⃣ **T84.220-** Displacement of internal fixation device of bones of hand and fingers

7️⃣ **T84.223-** Displacement of internal fixation device of bones of foot and toes

7️⃣ **T84.226-** Displacement of internal fixation device of vertebrae

7️⃣ **T84.228-** Displacement of internal fixation device of other bones

6️⃣ **T84.29** Other mechanical complication of internal fixation device of other bones

Obstruction (mechanical) of internal fixation device of other bones

Perforation of internal fixation device of other bones

Protrusion of internal fixation device of other bones

7️⃣ **T84.290-** Other mechanical complication of internal fixation device of bones of hand and fingers

7️⃣ **T84.293-** Other mechanical complication of internal fixation device of bones of foot and toes

7️⃣ **T84.296-** Other mechanical complication of internal fixation device of vertebrae

7️⃣ **T84.298-** Other mechanical complication of internal fixation device of other bones

5️⃣ **T84.3** Mechanical complication of other bone devices, implants and grafts

EXCLUDES 2 *other complications of bone graft (T86.83-)*

6️⃣ **T84.31** Breakdown (mechanical) of other bone devices, implants and grafts

7️⃣ **T84.310-** Breakdown (mechanical) of electronic bone stimulator

7️⃣ **T84.318-** Breakdown (mechanical) of other bone devices, implants and grafts

6️⃣ **T84.32** Displacement of other bone devices, implants and grafts

Malposition of other bone devices, implants and grafts

7️⃣ **T84.320-** Displacement of electronic bone stimulator

7️⃣ **T84.328-** Displacement of other bone devices, implants and grafts

AHA: (T84.328A) 4Q 2014, 29

6️⃣ **T84.39** Other mechanical complication of other bone devices, implants and grafts

Obstruction (mechanical) of other bone devices, implants and grafts

Perforation of other bone devices, implants and grafts

Protrusion of other bone devices, implants and grafts

7️⃣ **T84.390-** Other mechanical complication of electronic bone stimulator

7️⃣ **T84.398-** Other mechanical complication of other bone devices, implants and grafts

5️⃣ **T84.4** Mechanical complication of other internal orthopedic devices, implants and grafts

6️⃣ **T84.41** Breakdown (mechanical) of other internal orthopedic devices, implants and grafts

7️⃣ **T84.410-** Breakdown (mechanical) of muscle and tendon graft

7️⃣ **T84.418-** Breakdown (mechanical) of other internal orthopedic devices, implants and grafts

6️⃣ **T84.42** Displacement of other internal orthopedic devices, implants and grafts

Malposition of other internal orthopedic devices, implants and grafts

7️⃣ **T84.420-** Displacement of muscle and tendon graft

7️⃣ **T84.428-** Displacement of other internal orthopedic devices, implants and grafts

6️⃣ **T84.49** Other mechanical complication of other internal orthopedic devices, implants and grafts

Mechanical complication of other internal orthopedic devices, implants and grafts NOS

Obstruction (mechanical) of other internal orthopedic devices, implants and grafts

Perforation of other internal orthopedic devices, implants and grafts

Protrusion of other internal orthopedic devices, implants and grafts

7️⃣ **T84.490-** Other mechanical complication of muscle and tendon graft

7️⃣ **T84.498-** Other mechanical complication of other internal orthopedic devices, implants and grafts

5️⃣＋ **T84.5** Infection and inflammatory reaction due to internal joint prosthesis

Use additional code to identify infection

AHA: 1Q 2015, 16

7️⃣⊟＋ **T84.50X-** Infection and inflammatory reaction due to unspecified internal joint prosthesis

7️⃣⊟＋ **T84.51X-** Infection and inflammatory reaction due to internal right hip prosthesis

AHA: (T84.51XA) 4Q 2015, 36

7️⃣⊟＋ **T84.52X-** Infection and inflammatory reaction due to internal left hip prosthesis

AHA: (T84.52X-) 1Q 2015, 17

AHA: (T84.52XA) 1Q 2015, 16

7️⃣⊟＋ **T84.53X-** Infection and inflammatory reaction due to internal right knee prosthesis

7️⃣⊟＋ **T84.54X-** Infection and inflammatory reaction due to internal left knee prosthesis

7️⃣＋ **T84.59X-** Infection and inflammatory reaction due to other internal joint prosthesis

5️⃣＋ **T84.6** Infection and inflammatory reaction due to internal fixation device

Use additional code to identify infection

7️⃣＋ **T84.60X-** Infection and inflammatory reaction due to internal fixation device of unspecified site

6️⃣＋ **T84.61** Infection and inflammatory reaction due to internal fixation device of arm

7️⃣⊟＋ **T84.610-** Infection and inflammatory reaction due to internal fixation device of right humerus

7️⃣⊟＋ **T84.611-** Infection and inflammatory reaction due to internal fixation device of left humerus

7️⃣⊟＋ **T84.612-** Infection and inflammatory reaction due to internal fixation device of right radius

7️⃣⊟＋ **T84.613-** Infection and inflammatory reaction due to internal fixation device of left radius

7️⃣⊟＋ **T84.614-** Infection and inflammatory reaction due to internal fixation device of right ulna

7️⃣⊟＋ **T84.615-** Infection and inflammatory reaction due to internal fixation device of left ulna

7️⃣⊟＋ **T84.619-** Infection and inflammatory reaction due to internal fixation device of unspecified bone of arm

6️⃣＋ **T84.62** Infection and inflammatory reaction due to internal fixation device of leg

7️⃣⊟＋ **T84.620-** Infection and inflammatory reaction due to internal fixation device of right femur

7️⃣⊟＋ **T84.621-** Infection and inflammatory reaction due to internal fixation device of left femur

7️⃣⊟＋ **T84.622-** Infection and inflammatory reaction due to internal fixation device of right tibia

7️⃣⊟＋ **T84.623-** Infection and inflammatory reaction due to internal fixation device of left tibia

● New ▲ Revised *Manifestation* 4️⃣-7️⃣ Digit Indicators ⊟ Laterality 🅐 Adult (15+ years) 🅜 Maternity (12-55 years) 🅝 Newborn 🅟 Pediatric (0-17 years) ♂ Male ♀ Female

✖ Deleted Unspecified ＋ Additional code

1102   © 2017 DecisionHealth   2017 ICD-10-CM Expert for Physicians

7 ⊟ + **T84.624-** Infection and inflammatory reaction due to internal fixation device of right fibula

7 ⊟ + **T84.625-** Infection and inflammatory reaction due to internal fixation device of left fibula

7 ⊟ + **T84.629-** Infection and inflammatory reaction due to internal fixation device of unspecified bone of leg

7 + **T84.63X-** Infection and inflammatory reaction due to internal fixation device of spine

7 + **T84.69X-** Infection and inflammatory reaction due to internal fixation device of other site

7 + **T84.7XX-** Infection and inflammatory reaction due to other internal orthopedic prosthetic devices, implants and grafts

Use additional code to identify infection

5 **T84.8** Other specified complications of internal orthopedic prosthetic devices, implants and grafts

7 **T84.81X-** Embolism due to internal orthopedic prosthetic devices, implants and grafts

7 **T84.82X-** Fibrosis due to internal orthopedic prosthetic devices, implants and grafts

7 **T84.83X-** Hemorrhage due to internal orthopedic prosthetic devices, implants and grafts

7 **T84.84X-** Pain due to internal orthopedic prosthetic devices, implants and grafts

7 **T84.85X-** Stenosis due to internal orthopedic prosthetic devices, implants and grafts

7 **T84.86X-** Thrombosis due to internal orthopedic prosthetic devices, implants and grafts

7 **T84.89X-** Other specified complication of internal orthopedic prosthetic devices, implants and grafts

7 **T84.9XX-** Unspecified complication of internal orthopedic prosthetic device, implant and graft

4 **T85** **Complications of other internal prosthetic devices, implants and grafts**

EXCLUDES 2 *failure and rejection of transplanted organs and tissue (T86.-)*

The appropriate 7th character is to be added to each code from category T85
A   initial encounter
D   subsequent encounter
S   sequela

5 **T85.0** Mechanical complication of ventricular intracranial (communicating) shunt

7 **T85.01X-** Breakdown (mechanical) of ventricular intracranial (communicating) shunt

7 **T85.02X-** Displacement of ventricular intracranial (communicating) shunt
Malposition of ventricular intracranial (communicating) shunt

7 **T85.03X-** Leakage of ventricular intracranial (communicating) shunt

7 **T85.09X-** Other mechanical complication of ventricular intracranial (communicating) shunt
Obstruction (mechanical) of ventricular intracranial (communicating) shunt
Perforation of ventricular intracranial (communicating) shunt
Protrusion of ventricular intracranial (communicating) shunt

5 **T85.1** Mechanical complication of implanted electronic stimulator of nervous system

6 **T85.11** Breakdown (mechanical) of implanted electronic stimulator of nervous system

▲ 7 **T85.110-** Breakdown (mechanical) of implanted electronic neurostimulator of brain electrode (lead)

▲ 7 **T85.111-** Breakdown (mechanical) of implanted electronic neurostimulator of peripheral nerve electrode (lead)
Breakdown of electrode (lead) for cranial nerve neurostimulators
Breakdown of electrode (lead) for gastric neurostimulator
Breakdown of electrode (lead) for sacral nerve neurostimulator
Breakdown of electrode (lead) for vagal nerve neurostimulators

▲ 7 **T85.112-** Breakdown (mechanical) of implanted electronic neurostimulator of spinal cord electrode (lead)

● 7 **T85.113-** Breakdown (mechanical) of implanted electronic neurostimulator, generator
Breakdown (mechanical) of implanted electronic neurostimuator generator, brain, peripheral, gastric, spinal
Breakdown (mechanical) of implanted electronic sacral neurostimulator, pulse generator or receiver

7 **T85.118-** Breakdown (mechanical) of other implanted electronic stimulator of nervous system

6 **T85.12** Displacement of implanted electronic stimulator of nervous system
Malposition of implanted electronic stimulator of nervous system

▲ 7 **T85.120-** Displacement of implanted electronic neurostimulator of brain electrode (lead)

▲ 7 **T85.121-** Displacement of implanted electronic neurostimulator of peripheral nerve electrode (lead)
Displacement of electrode (lead) for cranial nerve neurostimulators
Displacement of electrode (lead) for gastric neurostimulator
Displacement of electrode (lead) for sacral nerve neurostimulator
Displacement of electrode (lead) for vagal nerve neurostimulators

▲ 7 **T85.122-** Displacement of implanted electronic neurostimulator of spinal cord electrode (lead)

● 7 **T85.123-** Displacement of implanted electronic neurostimulator, generator
Displacement of implanted electronic neurostimulator generator, brain, peripheral, gastric, spinal
Displacement of implanted electronic sacral neurostimulator, pulse generator or receiver

7 **T85.128-** Displacement of other implanted electronic stimulator of nervous system

6 **T85.19** Other mechanical complication of implanted electronic stimulator of nervous system
Leakage of implanted electronic stimulator of nervous system
Obstruction (mechanical) of implanted electronic stimulator of nervous system
Perforation of implanted electronic stimulator of nervous system
Protrusion of implanted electronic stimulator of nervous system

▲ 7 **T85.190-** Other mechanical complication of implanted electronic neurostimulator of brain electrode (lead)

▲ 7 **T85.191-** Other mechanical complication of implanted electronic neurostimulator of peripheral nerve electrode (lead)
Other mechanical complication of electrode (lead) for cranial nerve neurostimulators
Other mechanical complication of electrode (lead) for gastric neurostimulator
Other mechanical complication of electrode (lead) for sacral nerve neurostimulator
Other mechanical complication of electrode (lead) for vagal nerve neurostimulators

▲ 7 **T85.192-** Other mechanical complication of implanted electronic neurostimulator of spinal cord electrode (lead)

● 7 **T85.193-** Other mechanical complication of implanted electronic neurostimulator, generator
Other mechanical complication of implanted electronic neurostimulator generator, brain, peripheral, gastric, spinal
Other mechanical complication of implanted electronic sacral neurostimulator, pulse generator or receiver

7 **T85.199-** Other mechanical complication of other implanted electronic stimulator of nervous system

5 **T85.2** Mechanical complication of intraocular lens

7 **T85.21X-** Breakdown (mechanical) of intraocular lens

● New   ▲ Revised   *Manifestation*   4 - 7 Digit Indicators   ⊟ Laterality   A Adult (15+ years)   M Maternity (12-55 years)   N Newborn   P Pediatric (0-17 years)   ♂ Male   ♀ Female
✖ Deleted   Unspecified   + Additional code

2017 ICD-10-CM Expert for Physicians

© 2017 DecisionHealth   1103

Injury, Poisoning and Certain Other Consequences of External Causes

☑ **T85.22X-** **Displacement of intraocular lens**
Malposition of intraocular lens

☑ **T85.29X-** **Other mechanical complication of intraocular lens**
Obstruction (mechanical) of intraocular lens
Perforation of intraocular lens
Protrusion of intraocular lens

⑤ **T85.3** **Mechanical complication of other ocular prosthetic devices, implants and grafts**
EXCLUDES 2 other complications of corneal graft (T86.84-)

⑥ **T85.31** **Breakdown (mechanical) of other ocular prosthetic devices, implants and grafts**

☑⊟ **T85.310-** **Breakdown (mechanical) of prosthetic orbit of right eye**

☑⊟ **T85.311-** **Breakdown (mechanical) of prosthetic orbit of left eye**

☑⊟ **T85.318-** **Breakdown (mechanical) of other ocular prosthetic devices, implants and grafts**

⑥ **T85.32** **Displacement of other ocular prosthetic devices, implants and grafts**
Malposition of other ocular prosthetic devices, implants and grafts

☑⊟ **T85.320-** **Displacement of prosthetic orbit of right eye**

☑⊟ **T85.321-** **Displacement of prosthetic orbit of left eye**

☑⊟ **T85.328-** **Displacement of other ocular prosthetic devices, implants and grafts**

⑥ **T85.39** **Other mechanical complication of other ocular prosthetic devices, implants and grafts**
Obstruction (mechanical) of other ocular prosthetic devices, implants and grafts
Perforation of other ocular prosthetic devices, implants and grafts
Protrusion of other ocular prosthetic devices, implants and grafts

☑⊟ **T85.390-** **Other mechanical complication of prosthetic orbit of right eye**

☑⊟ **T85.391-** **Other mechanical complication of prosthetic orbit of left eye**

☑⊟ **T85.398-** **Other mechanical complication of other ocular prosthetic devices, implants and grafts**

⑤ **T85.4** **Mechanical complication of breast prosthesis and implant**

☑ **T85.41X-** **Breakdown (mechanical) of breast prosthesis and implant**

☑ **T85.42X-** **Displacement of breast prosthesis and implant**
Malposition of breast prosthesis and implant

☑ **T85.43X-** **Leakage of breast prosthesis and implant**

☑ **T85.44X-** **Capsular contracture of breast implant**

☑ **T85.49X-** **Other mechanical complication of breast prosthesis and implant**
Obstruction (mechanical) of breast prosthesis and implant
Perforation of breast prosthesis and implant
Protrusion of breast prosthesis and implant

⑤ **T85.5** **Mechanical complication of gastrointestinal prosthetic devices, implants and grafts**

⑥ **T85.51** **Breakdown (mechanical) of gastrointestinal prosthetic devices, implants and grafts**

☑ **T85.510-** **Breakdown (mechanical) of bile duct prosthesis**

☑ **T85.511-** **Breakdown (mechanical) of esophageal anti-reflux device**

☑ **T85.518-** **Breakdown (mechanical) of other gastrointestinal prosthetic devices, implants and grafts**

⑥ **T85.52** **Displacement of gastrointestinal prosthetic devices, implants and grafts**
Malposition of gastrointestinal prosthetic devices, implants and grafts

☑ **T85.520-** **Displacement of bile duct prosthesis**

☑ **T85.521-** **Displacement of esophageal anti-reflux device**

☑ **T85.528-** **Displacement of other gastrointestinal prosthetic devices, implants and grafts**

⑥ **T85.59** **Other mechanical complication of gastrointestinal prosthetic devices, implants and**
Obstruction, mechanical of gastrointestinal prosthetic devices, implants and grafts
Perforation of gastrointestinal prosthetic devices, implants and grafts
Protrusion of gastrointestinal prosthetic devices, implants and grafts

☑ **T85.590-** **Other mechanical complication of bile duct prosthesis**

☑ **T85.591-** **Other mechanical complication of esophageal anti-reflux device**

☑ **T85.598-** **Other mechanical complication of other gastrointestinal prosthetic devices, implants and grafts**

⑤ **T85.6** **Mechanical complication of other specified internal and external prosthetic devices, implants and grafts**
GUIDELINES Section I.C.4.a.5)(a)-(b)
An underdose of insulin due to an insulin pump failure should be assigned to a code from subcategory T85.6 followed by code T38.3x6-, Underdosing of insulin and oral hypoglycemic [antidiabetic] drugs. Additional codes for the type of diabetes mellitus and any associated complications due to the underdosing should also be assigned.

The principal or first-listed code for an encounter due to an insulin pump malfunction resulting in an overdose of insulin, should also be T85.6- followed by code T38.3x1-, Poisoning by insulin and oral hypoglycemic [antidiabetic] drugs, accidental (unintentional).

⑥ **T85.61** **Breakdown (mechanical) of other specified internal prosthetic devices, implants and grafts**

▲☑ **T85.610-** **Breakdown (mechanical) of cranial or spinal infusion catheter**
Breakdown (mechanical) of epidural infusion catheter
Breakdown (mechanical) of intrathecal infusion catheter
Breakdown (mechanical) of subarachnoid infusion catheter
Breakdown (mechanical) of subdural infusion catheter

☑ **T85.611-** **Breakdown (mechanical) of intraperitoneal dialysis catheter**
EXCLUDES 1 mechanical complication of vascular dialysis catheter (T82.4-)

☑ **T85.612-** **Breakdown (mechanical) of permanent sutures**
EXCLUDES 1 mechanical complication of permanent (wire) suture used in bone repair (T84.1-T84.2)

☑ **T85.613-** **Breakdown (mechanical) of artificial skin graft and decellularized allodermis**
Failure of artificial skin graft and decellularized allodermis
Non-adherence of artificial skin graft and decellularized allodermis
Poor incorporation of artificial skin graft and decellularized allodermis
Shearing of artificial skin graft and decellularized allodermis

☑ **T85.614-** **Breakdown (mechanical) of insulin pump**

●☑ **T85.615-** **Breakdown (mechanical) of other nervous system device, implant or graft**
Breakdown (mechanical) of intrathecal infusion pump

☑ **T85.618-** **Breakdown (mechanical) of other specified internal prosthetic devices, implants and grafts**

⑥ **T85.62** **Displacement of other specified internal prosthetic devices, implants and grafts**
Malposition of other specified internal prosthetic devices, implants and grafts

▲☑ **T85.620-** **Displacement of cranial or spinal infusion catheter**
Displacement of epidural infusion catheter
Displacement of intrathecal infusion catheter
Displacement of subarachnoid infusion catheter
Displacement of subdural infusion catheter

☑ **T85.621-** **Displacement of intraperitoneal dialysis catheter**
EXCLUDES 1 mechanical complication of vascular dialysis catheter (T82.4-)

☑ **T85.622-** **Displacement of permanent sutures**
EXCLUDES 1 mechanical complication of permanent (wire) suture used in bone repair (T84.1-T84.2)

● New   ▲ Revised   *Manifestation*   ❹-❼ Digit Indicators   ⊟ Laterality   Ⓐ Adult (15+ years)   Ⓜ Maternity (12-55 years)   Ⓝ Newborn   Ⓟ Pediatric (0-17 years)   ♂ Male   ♀ Female
✖ Deleted   Unspecified   + Additional code

▢ T85.623- **Displacement of artificial skin graft and decellularized allodermis**
Dislodgement of artificial skin graft and decellularized allodermis
Displacement of artificial skin graft and decellularized allodermis

▢ T85.624- **Displacement of insulin pump**

● ▢ T85.625- **Displacement of other nervous system device, implant or graft**
Displacement of intrathecal infusion pump

▢ T85.628- **Displacement of other specified internal prosthetic devices, implants and grafts**
AHA: (T85.628A) 1Q 2015, 15

⑥ T85.63 **Leakage of other specified internal prosthetic devices, implants and grafts**

▲ ▢ T85.630- **Leakage of cranial or spinal infusion catheter**
Leakage of epidural infusion catheter
Leakage of intrathecal infusion catheter infusion catheter
Leakage of subdural infusion catheter
Leakage of subarachnoid infusion catheter

▢ T85.631- **Leakage of intraperitoneal dialysis catheter**
> EXCLUDES 1 *mechanical complication of vascular dialysis catheter (T82.4)*

▢ T85.633- **Leakage of insulin pump**

● ▢ T85.635- **Leakage of other nervous system device, implant or graft**
Leakage of intrathecal infusion pump

▢ T85.638- **Leakage of other specified internal prosthetic devices, implants and grafts**

⑥ T85.69 **Other mechanical complication of other specified internal prosthetic devices, implants and grafts**
Obstruction, mechanical of other specified internal prosthetic devices, implants and grafts
Perforation of other specified internal prosthetic devices, implants and grafts
Protrusion of other specified internal prosthetic devices, implants and grafts

▲ ▢ T85.690- **Other mechanical complication of cranial or spinal infusion catheter**
Other mechanical complication of epidural infusion catheter
Other mechanical complication of intrathecal infusion catheter
Other mechanical complication of subarachnoid infusion catheter
Other mechanical complication of subdural infusion catheter

▢ T85.691- **Other mechanical complication of intraperitoneal dialysis catheter**
> EXCLUDES 1 *mechanical complication of vascular dialysis catheter (T82.4)*

▢ T85.692- **Other mechanical complication of permanent sutures**
> EXCLUDES 1 *mechanical complication of permanent (wire) suture used in bone repair (T84.1-T84.2)*

▢ T85.693- **Other mechanical complication of artificial skin graft and decellularized allodermis**

▢ T85.694- **Other mechanical complication of insulin pump**

● ▢ T85.695- **Other mechanical complication of other nervous system device, implant or graft**
Other mechanical complication of intrathecal infusion pump

▢ T85.698- **Other mechanical complication of other specified internal prosthetic devices, implants and grafts**
Mechanical complication of nonabsorbable surgical material NOS

⑤ + T85.7 **Infection and inflammatory reaction due to other internal prosthetic devices, implants and grafts**
Use additional code to identify infection

▢ + T85.71X- **Infection and inflammatory reaction due to peritoneal dialysis catheter**

▢ + T85.72X- **Infection and inflammatory reaction due to insulin pump**

● ⑥ + T85.73 **Infection and inflammatory reaction due to nervous system devices, implants and graft**

● ▢ + T85.730- **Infection and inflammatory reaction due to ventricular intracranial (communicating) shunt**

● ▢ + T85.731- **Infection and inflammatory reaction due to implanted electronic neurostimulator of brain, electrode (lead)**

● ▢ + T85.732- **Infection and inflammatory reaction due to implanted electronic neurostimulator of peripheral nerve, electrode (lead)**
Infection and inflammatory reaction due to electrode (lead) for cranial nerve neurostimulators
Infection and inflammatory reaction due to electrode (lead) for gastric neurostimulator
Infection and inflammatory reaction due to electrode (lead) for sacral nerve neurostimulator
Infection and inflammatory reaction due to electrode (lead) for vagal nerve neurostimulators

● ▢ + T85.733- **Infection and inflammatory reaction due to implanted electronic neurostimulator of spinal cord, electrode (lead)**

● ▢ + T85.734- **Infection and inflammatory reaction due to implanted electronic neurostimulator, generator**
Generator pocket infection

● ▢ + T85.735- **Infection and inflammatory reaction due to cranial or spinal infusion catheter**
Infection and inflammatory reaction due to epidural catheter
Infection and inflammatory reaction due to intrathecal infusion catheter
Infection and inflammatory reaction due to subarachnoid catheter
Infection and inflammatory reaction due to subdural catheter

● ▢ + T85.738- **Infection and inflammatory reaction due to other nervous system device, implant or graft**
Infection and inflammatory reaction due to intrathecal infusion pump

▢ + T85.79X- **Infection and inflammatory reaction due to other internal prosthetic devices, implants and grafts**

⑤ T85.8 **Other specified complications of internal prosthetic devices, implants and grafts, not elsewhere classified**

▲ ⑥ T85.81 **Embolism due to internal prosthetic devices, implants and grafts, not elsewhere classified**

● ▢ T85.810- **Embolism due to nervous system prosthetic devices, implants and grafts**

● ▢ T85.818- **Embolism due to other internal prosthetic devices, implants and grafts**

▲ ⑥ T85.82 **Fibrosis due to internal prosthetic devices, implants and grafts, not elsewhere classified**

● ▢ T85.820- **Fibrosis due to nervous system prosthetic devices, implants and grafts**

● ▢ T85.828- **Fibrosis due to other internal prosthetic devices, implants and grafts**

▲ ⑥ T85.83 **Hemorrhage due to internal prosthetic devices, implants and grafts, not elsewhere classified**

● ▢ T85.830- **Hemorrhage due to nervous system prosthetic devices, implants and grafts**

● ▢ T85.838- **Hemorrhage due to other internal prosthetic devices, implants and grafts**

▲ ⑥ T85.84 **Pain due to internal prosthetic devices, implants and grafts, not elsewhere classified**

● ▢ T85.840- **Pain due to nervous system prosthetic devices, implants and grafts**

● ▢ T85.848- **Pain due to other internal prosthetic devices, implants and grafts**

▲ ⑥ T85.85 **Stenosis due to internal prosthetic devices, implants and grafts, not elsewhere classified**

● ▢ T85.850- **Stenosis due to nervous system prosthetic devices, implants and grafts**

● ▢ T85.858- **Stenosis due to other internal prosthetic devices, implants and grafts**

▲ ⑥ T85.86 **Thrombosis due to internal prosthetic devices, implants and grafts, not elsewhere classified**

● ▢ T85.860- **Thrombosis due to nervous system prosthetic devices, implants and grafts**

● ▢ T85.868- **Thrombosis due to other internal prosthetic devices, implants and grafts**

▲ ⑤ **T85.89**   **Other specified complication of internal prosthetic devices, implants and grafts, not elsewhere classified**
Erosion or breakdown of subcutaneous device pocket

● ⑦ **T85.890-**   **Other specified complication of nervous system prosthetic devices, implants and grafts**

● ⑦ **T85.898-**   **Other specified complication of other internal prosthetic devices, implants and grafts**

⑦ **T85.9XX-**   **Unspecified complication of internal prosthetic device, implant and graft**
Complication of internal prosthetic device, implant and graft NOS

④+ **T86**   **Complications of transplanted organs and tissue**
Use additional code to identify other transplant complications, such as:
graft-versus-host disease (D89.81-)
malignancy associated with organ transplant (C80.2)
post-transplant lymphoproliferative disorders (PTLD) (D47.Z1)

GUIDELINES   **Section I.C.2.r**
A malignant neoplasm of a transplanted organ should be coded as a transplant complication. Assign first the appropriate code from category T86.-, Complications of transplanted organs and tissue, followed by code C80.2. Use an additional code for the specific malignancy.

GUIDELINES   **Section I.C.19.g.3)(a)**
Codes under category T86, Complications of transplanted organs and tissues, are for use for both complications and rejection of transplanted organs. A transplant complication code is only assigned if the complication affects the function of the transplanted organ. Two codes are required to fully describe a transplant complication: the appropriate code from category T86 and a secondary code that identifies the complication.

Pre-existing conditions or conditions that develop after the transplant are not coded as complications unless they affect the function of the transplanted organs.

CODING TIP ✓   Do not assume dysfunction in a transplanted organ to be a complication of a transplanted organ unless specifically stated by a provider diagnostic statement. The only exception to this is a malignant neoplasm of a transplanted organ. A neoplasm associated with a transplant is coded as an "other complication of transplant" unless specified by the physician as a failure or rejection.

⑤+ **T86.0**   **Complications of bone marrow transplant**

+ **T86.00**   **Unspecified complication of bone marrow transplant**

+ **T86.01**   **Bone marrow transplant rejection**

+ **T86.02**   **Bone marrow transplant failure**

+ **T86.03**   **Bone marrow transplant infection**

+ **T86.09**   **Other complications of bone marrow transplant**

⑤+ **T86.1**   **Complications of kidney transplant**

GUIDELINES   **Section I.C.19.g.3)(b)**
Patients who have undergone kidney transplant may still have some form of chronic kidney disease (CKD) because the kidney transplant may not fully restore kidney function ... Code T86.1- should not be assigned for post kidney transplant patients who have CKD unless a transplant complication such as transplant failure or rejection is documented. If the documentation is unclear as to whether the patient has a complication of the transplant, query the provider.

Conditions that affect the function of the transplanted kidney, other than CKD, should be assigned a code from subcategory T86.1 and a secondary code that identifies the complication. For patients with CKD following a kidney transplant, but who do not have a complication such as failure or rejection
, see section I.C.14. Chronic kidney disease and kidney transplant status.

+ **T86.10**   **Unspecified complication of kidney transplant**

+ **T86.11**   **Kidney transplant rejection**

+ **T86.12**   **Kidney transplant failure**
AHA: 1Q 2013, 24

+ **T86.13**   **Kidney transplant infection**
Use additional code to specify infection

+ **T86.19**   **Other complication of kidney transplant**

⑤+ **T86.2**   **Complications of heart transplant**
EXCLUDES 1   *complication of:*
artificial heart device (T82.5)
heart-lung transplant (T86.3)

+ **T86.20**   **Unspecified complication of heart transplant**

+ **T86.21**   **Heart transplant rejection**

+ **T86.22**   **Heart transplant failure**

+ **T86.23**   **Heart transplant infection**
Use additional code to specify infection

⑤+ **T86.29**   **Other complications of heart transplant**

+ **T86.290**   **Cardiac allograft vasculopathy**
EXCLUDES 1   *atherosclerosis of coronary arteries (I25.75-, I25.76-, I25.81-)*

+ **T86.298**   **Other complications of heart transplant**

⑤+ **T86.3**   **Complications of heart-lung transplant**

+ **T86.30**   **Unspecified complication of heart-lung transplant**

+ **T86.31**   **Heart-lung transplant rejection**

+ **T86.32**   **Heart-lung transplant failure**

+ **T86.33**   **Heart-lung transplant infection**
Use additional code to specify infection

+ **T86.39**   **Other complications of heart-lung transplant**

⑤+ **T86.4**   **Complications of liver transplant**

+ **T86.40**   **Unspecified complication of liver transplant**

+ **T86.41**   **Liver transplant rejection**

+ **T86.42**   **Liver transplant failure**

+ **T86.43**   **Liver transplant infection**
Use additional code to identify infection, such as:
Cytomegalovirus (CMV) infection (B25.-)

+ **T86.49**   **Other complications of liver transplant**

+ **T86.5**   **Complications of stem cell transplant**
Complications from stem cells from peripheral blood
Complications from stem cells from umbilical cord

⑤+ **T86.8**   **Complications of other transplanted organs and tissues**

⑤+ **T86.81**   **Complications of lung transplant**
EXCLUDES 1   *complication of heart-lung transplant (T86.3-)*

+ **T86.810**   **Lung transplant rejection**

+ **T86.811**   **Lung transplant failure**

+ **T86.812**   **Lung transplant infection**
Use additional code to specify infection

+ **T86.818**   **Other complications of lung transplant**

+ **T86.819**   **Unspecified complication of lung transplant**

⑤+ **T86.82**   **Complications of skin graft (allograft) (autograft)**
EXCLUDES 2   *complication of artificial skin graft (T85.693)*

+ **T86.820**   **Skin graft (allograft) rejection**

+ **T86.821**   **Skin graft (allograft) (autograft) failure**

+ **T86.822**   **Skin graft (allograft) (autograft) infection**
Use additional code to specify infection

+ **T86.828**   **Other complications of skin graft (allograft) (autograft)**

+ **T86.829**   **Unspecified complication of skin graft (allograft) (autograft)**

⑤+ **T86.83**   **Complications of bone graft**
EXCLUDES 2   *mechanical complications of bone graft (T84.3-)*

+ **T86.830**   **Bone graft rejection**

+ **T86.831**   **Bone graft failure**

+ **T86.832**   **Bone graft infection**
Use additional code to specify infection

+ **T86.838**   **Other complications of bone graft**

+ **T86.839**   **Unspecified complication of bone graft**

⑤+ **T86.84**   **Complications of corneal transplant**
EXCLUDES 2   *mechanical complications of corneal graft (T85.3-)*

+ **T86.840**   **Corneal transplant rejection**

+ **T86.841**   **Corneal transplant failure**

+ **T86.842**   **Corneal transplant infection**
Use additional code to specify infection

+ **T86.848**   **Other complications of corneal transplant**

+ **T86.849**   **Unspecified complication of corneal transplant**

● New   ▲ Revised   *Manifestation*   ④-⑦ Digit Indicators   ⊟ Laterality   🅰 Adult (15+ years)   Ⓜ Maternity (12-55 years)   🅝 Newborn   🅟 Pediatric (0-17 years)   ♂ Male   ♀ Female
✖ Deleted   Unspecified   + Additional code

⑥ + **T86.85**   **Complication of intestine transplant**

   + **T86.850**   **Intestine transplant rejection**

   + **T86.851**   **Intestine transplant failure**

   + **T86.852**   **Intestine transplant infection**

     Use additional code to specify infection

   + **T86.858**   **Other complications of intestine transplant**

   + **T86.859**   **Unspecified complication of intestine transplant**

⑥ + **T86.89**   **Complications of other transplanted tissue**

     Transplant failure or rejection of pancreas

   + **T86.890**   **Other transplanted tissue rejection**

   + **T86.891**   **Other transplanted tissue failure**

   + **T86.892**   **Other transplanted tissue infection**

     Use additional code to specify infection

   + **T86.898**   **Other complications of other transplanted tissue**

   + **T86.899**   **Unspecified complication of other transplanted tissue**

⑤ + **T86.9**   **Complication of unspecified transplanted organ and tissue**

   + **T86.90**   **Unspecified complication of unspecified transplanted organ and tissue**

   + **T86.91**   **Unspecified transplanted organ and tissue rejection**

   + **T86.92**   **Unspecified transplanted organ and tissue failure**

   + **T86.93**   **Unspecified transplanted organ and tissue infection**

     Use additional code to specify infection

   + **T86.99**   **Other complications of unspecified transplanted organ and tissue**

④ **T87**   **Complications peculiar to reattachment and amputation**

⑤ **T87.0**   **Complications of reattached (part of) upper extremity**

   ⑥ **T87.0X**   **Complications of reattached (part of) upper extremity**

     ⑦ **T87.0X1**   **Complications of reattached (part of) right upper extremity**

     ⑦ **T87.0X2**   **Complications of reattached (part of) left upper extremity**

     ⑦ **T87.0X9**   **Complications of reattached (part of) unspecified upper extremity**

⑤ **T87.1**   **Complications of reattached (part of) lower extremity**

   ⑥ **T87.1X**   **Complications of reattached (part of) lower extremity**

     ⑦ **T87.1X1**   **Complications of reattached (part of) right lower extremity**

     ⑦ **T87.1X2**   **Complications of reattached (part of) left lower extremity**

     ⑦ **T87.1X9**   **Complications of reattached (part of) unspecified lower extremity**

T87.2   **Complications of other reattached body part**

⑤ **T87.3**   **Neuroma of amputation stump**

   ⑦ **T87.30**   **Neuroma of amputation stump, unspecified extremity**

   ⑦ **T87.31**   **Neuroma of amputation stump, right upper extremity**

   ⑦ **T87.32**   **Neuroma of amputation stump, left upper extremity**

   ⑦ **T87.33**   **Neuroma of amputation stump, right lower extremity**

   ⑦ **T87.34**   **Neuroma of amputation stump, left lower extremity**

⑤ **T87.4**   **Infection of amputation stump**

   ⑦ **T87.40**   **Infection of amputation stump, unspecified extremity**

   ⑦ **T87.41**   **Infection of amputation stump, right upper extremity**

   ⑦ **T87.42**   **Infection of amputation stump, left upper extremity**

   ⑦ **T87.43**   **Infection of amputation stump, right lower extremity**

   ⑦ **T87.44**   **Infection of amputation stump, left lower extremity**

⑤ **T87.5**   **Necrosis of amputation stump**

   ⑦ **T87.50**   **Necrosis of amputation stump, unspecified extremity**

   ⑦ **T87.51**   **Necrosis of amputation stump, right upper extremity**

   ⑦ **T87.52**   **Necrosis of amputation stump, left upper extremity**

   ⑦ **T87.53**   **Necrosis of amputation stump, right lower extremity**

   ⑦ **T87.54**   **Necrosis of amputation stump, left lower extremity**

⑤ **T87.8**   **Other complications of amputation stump**

   T87.81   **Dehiscence of amputation stump**

CODING TIP ✓   When a patient presents with a dehiscence of an amputation stump wound, assign code T87.81. When both dehiscence and infection are present, code the dehiscence first (T87.81), followed by infection. Use an additional code to specify the infection.

T87.89   **Other complications of amputation stump**

   Amputation stump contracture

   Amputation stump contracture of next proximal joint

   Amputation stump flexion

   Amputation stump edema

   Amputation stump hematoma

   EXCLUDES 2   *phantom limb syndrome (G54.6-G54.7)*

CODING TIP ✓   Do not assign a code for complication of an amputation stump for an ulcer (due to pressure, diabetic ulcer, arterial, trauma, stasis, or other) of the amputation stump. Ulcers of the amputation stump are not considered amputation stump complications. Use the L89 codes for pressure ulcer/injury and the staging system to stage.

T87.9   **Unspecified complications of amputation stump**

④ **T88**   **Other complications of surgical and medical care, not elsewhere classified**

   EXCLUDES 2   *complication following infusion, transfusion and therapeutic injection (T80.-)*

     complication following procedure NEC (T81.-)

     complications of anesthesia in labor and delivery (O74.-)

     complications of anesthesia in pregnancy (O29.-)

     complications of anesthesia in puerperium (O89.-)

     complications of devices, implants and grafts (T82-T85)

     complications of obstetric surgery and procedure (O75.4)

     dermatitis due to drugs and medicaments (L23.3, L24.4, L25.1, L27.0-L27.1)

     poisoning and toxic effects of drugs and chemicals (T36-T65 with fifth or sixth character 1-4 or 6)

     specified complications classified elsewhere

The appropriate 7th character is to be added to each code from category T88

   A   initial encounter

   D   subsequent encounter

   S   sequela

⑦ **T88.0XX-**   **Infection following immunization**

   Sepsis following immunization

⑦ **T88.1XX-**   **Other complications following immunization, not elsewhere classified**

   Generalized vaccinia

   Rash following immunization

   EXCLUDES 1   *vaccinia not from vaccine (B08.011)*

   EXCLUDES 2   *anaphylactic shock due to serum (T80.5-)*

     other serum reactions (T80.6-)

     postimmunization arthropathy (M02.2)

     postimmunization encephalitis (G04.02)

     postimmunization fever (R50.83)

⑦ + **T88.2XX-**   **Shock due to anesthesia**

   Use additional code for adverse effect, if applicable, to identify drug (T41.- with fifth or sixth character 5)

   EXCLUDES 1   *complications of anesthesia (in):*

     labor and delivery (O74.-)

     pregnancy (O29.-)

     puerperium (O89.-)

     postprocedural shock NOS (T81.1-)

⑦ + **T88.3XX-**   **Malignant hyperthermia due to anesthesia**

   Use additional code for adverse effect, if applicable, to identify drug (T41.- with fifth or sixth character 5)

⑦ **T88.4XX-**   **Failed or difficult intubation**

⑤ + **T88.5**   **Other complications of anesthesia**

   Use additional code for adverse effect, if applicable, to identify drug (T41.- with fifth or sixth character 5)

⑦ + **T88.51X-**   **Hypothermia following anesthesia**

● New   ▲ Revised   *Manifestation*   ④-⑦ Digit Indicators   ▱ Laterality   Ⓐ Adult (15+ years)   Ⓜ Maternity (12-55 years)   Ⓝ Newborn   Ⓟ Pediatric (0-17 years)   ♂ Male   ♀ Female

✖ Deleted   Unspecified   + Additional code

2017 ICD-10-CM Expert for Physicians   © 2017 DecisionHealth   1107

7 + T88.52X-   **Failed moderate sedation during procedure**
Failed conscious sedation during procedure
> **EXCLUDES 2**   *personal history of failed moderate sedation (Z92.83)*

● **7 + T88.53X-**   **Unintended awareness under general anesthesia during procedure**
> **EXCLUDES 2**   *personal history of unintended awareness under general anesthesia (Z92.84)*

7 + T88.59X-   **Other complications of anesthesia**

7 + T88.6XX-   **Anaphylactic reaction due to adverse effect of correct drug or medicament properly administered**
Anaphylactic shock due to adverse effect of correct drug or medicament properly administered
Anaphylactoid reaction NOS
Use additional code for adverse effect, if applicable, to identify drug (T36-T50 with fifth or sixth character 5)
> **EXCLUDES 1**   *anaphylactic reaction due to serum (T80.5-)*
> *anaphylactic shock or reaction due to adverse food reaction (T78.0-)*

7 + T88.7XX-   **Unspecified adverse effect of drug or medicament**
Drug hypersensitivity NOS
Drug reaction NOS
Use additional code for adverse effect, if applicable, to identify drug (T36-T50 with fifth or sixth character 5)
> **EXCLUDES 1**   *specified adverse effects of drugs and medicaments (A00-R94 and T80-T88.6, T88.8)*

7 + T88.8XX-   **Other specified complications of surgical and medical care, not elsewhere classified**
Use additional code to identify the complication

7 T88.9XX-   **Complication of surgical and medical care, unspecified**

● New   ▲ Revised   *Manifestation*   4-7 Digit Indicators   ▤ Laterality   Ⓐ Adult (15+ years)   Ⓜ Maternity (12-55 years)   Ⓝ Newborn   Ⓟ Pediatric (0-17 years)   ♂ Male   ♀ Female
✖ Deleted   Unspecified   + Additional code

1108   © 2017 DecisionHealth   2017 ICD-10-CM Expert for Physicians

CHAPTER 20: EXTERNAL CAUSES OF MORBIDITY (V00-Y99)

Note: This chapter permits the classification of environmental events and circumstances as the cause of injury, and other adverse effects. Where a code from this section is applicable, it is intended that it shall be used secondary to a code from another chapter of the Classification indicating the nature of the condition. Most often, the condition will be classifiable to Chapter 19, Injury, poisoning and certain other consequences of external causes (S00-T88). Other conditions that may be stated to be due to external causes are classified in Chapters I to XVIII. For these conditions, codes from Chapter 20 should be used to provide additional information as to the cause of the condition.

GUIDELINES Section I.C.20

The external causes of morbidity codes should never be sequenced as the first-listed or principal diagnosis. External cause codes are intended to provide data for injury research and evaluation of injury prevention strategies. These codes capture how the injury or health condition happened (cause), the intent (unintentional or accidental; or intentional, such as suicide or assault), the place where the event occurred the activity of the patient at the time of the event, and the person's status (e.g., civilian, military).

There is no national requirement for mandatory ICD-10-CM external cause code reporting. Unless a provider is subject to a state-based external cause code reporting mandate or these codes are required by a particular payer, reporting of ICD-10-CM codes in Chapter 20, External Causes of Morbidity, is not required. In the absence of a mandatory reporting requirement, providers are encouraged to voluntarily report external cause codes, as they provide valuable data for injury research and evaluation of injury prevention strategies.

GUIDELINES Section I.C.20.a.2)

Most categories in chapter 20 have a 7th character requirement for each applicable code. ... While the patient may be seen by a new or different provider over the course of treatment for an injury or condition, assignment of the 7th character for external cause should match the 7th character of the code assigned for the associated injury or condition for the encounter.

This chapter contains the following blocks:

V00-X58	Accidents
V00-V99	Transport accidents
V00-V09	Pedestrian injured in transport accident
V10-V19	Pedal cycle rider injured in transport accident
V20-V29	Motorcycle rider injured in transport accident
V30-V39	Occupant of three-wheeled motor vehicle injured in transport accident
V40-V49	Car occupant injured in transport accident
V50-V59	Occupant of pick-up truck or van injured in transport accident
V60-V69	Occupant of heavy transport vehicle injured in transport accident
V70-V79	Bus occupant injured in transport accident
V80-V89	Other land transport accidents
V90-V94	Water transport accidents
V95-V97	Air and space transport accidents
V98-V99	Other and unspecified transport accidents
W00-X58	Other external causes of accidental injury
W00-W19	Slipping, tripping, stumbling and falls
W20-W49	Exposure to inanimate mechanical forces
W50-W64	Exposure to animate mechanical forces
W65-W74	Accidental non-transport drowning and submersion
W85-W99	Exposure to electric current, radiation and extreme ambient air temperature and pressure
X00-X08	Exposure to smoke, fire and flames
X10-X19	Contact with heat and hot substances
X30-X39	Exposure to forces of nature
X50	Overexertion and strenuous or repetitive movements
X52-X58	Accidental exposure to other specified factors
X71-X83	Intentional self-harm
X92-Y09	Assault
Y21-Y33	Event of undetermined intent
Y35-Y38	Legal intervention, operations of war, military operations, and terrorism
Y62-Y84	Complications of medical and surgical care
Y62-Y69	Misadventures to patients during surgical and medical care
Y70-Y82	Medical devices associated with adverse incidents in diagnostic and therapeutic use
Y83-Y84	Surgical and other medical procedures as the cause of abnormal reaction of the patient, or of later complication, without mention of misadventure at the time of the procedure
Y90-Y99	Supplementary factors related to causes of morbidity classified elsewhere

Accidents (V00-X58)

Transport accidents (V00-V99)

Note: This section is structured in 12 groups. Those relating to land transport accidents (V00-V89) reflect the victim's mode of transport and are subdivided to identify the victim's 'counterpart' or the type of event. The vehicle of which the injured person is an occupant is identified in the first two characters since it is seen as the most important factor to identify for prevention purposes. A transport accident is one in which the vehicle involved must be moving or running or in use for transport purposes at the time of the accident.

Definitions related to transport accidents:

(a) A transport accident (V00-V99) is any accident involving a device designed primarily for, or used at the time primarily for, conveying persons or good from one place to another.

(b) A public highway [trafficway] or street is the entire width between property lines (or other boundary lines) of land open to the public as a matter of right or custom for purposes of moving persons or property from one place to another. A roadway is that part of the public highway designed, improved and customarily used for vehicular traffic.

(c) A traffic accident is any vehicle accident occurring on the public highway [i.e. originating on, terminating on, or involving a vehicle partially on the highway]. A vehicle accident is assumed to have occurred on the public highway unless another place is specified, except in the case of accidents involving only off-road motor vehicles, which are classified as nontraffic accidents unless the contrary is stated.

(d) A nontraffic accident is any vehicle accident that occurs entirely in any place other than a public highway.

(e) A pedestrian is any person involved in an accident who was not at the time of the accident riding in or on a motor vehicle, railway train, streetcar or animal-drawn or other vehicle, or on a pedal cycle or animal. This includes, a person changing a tire, working on a parked car, or a person on foot. It also includes the user of a pedestrian conveyance such as a babystroller, ice-skates, skis, sled, roller skates, a skateboard, nonmotorized or motorized wheelchair, motorized mobility scooter, or nonmotorized scooter.

(f) A driver is an occupant of a transport vehicle who is operating or intending to operate it.

(g) A passenger is any occupant of a transport vehicle other than the driver, except a person traveling on the outside of the vehicle.

(h) A person on the outside of a vehicle is any person being transported by a vehicle but not occupying the space normally reserved for the driver or passengers, or the space intended for the transport of property. This includes a person travelling on the bodywork, bumper, fender, roof, running board or step of a vehicle, as well as, hanging on the outside of the vehicle.

(i) A pedal cycle is any land transport vehicle operated solely by nonmotorized pedals including a bicycle or tricycle.

(j) A pedal cyclist is any person riding a pedal cycle or in a sidecar or trailer attached to a pedal cycle.

(k) A motorcycle is a two-wheeled motor vehicle with one or two riding saddles and sometimes with a third wheel for the support of a sidecar. The sidecar is considered part of the motorcycle. This includes a moped, motor scooter, or motorized bicycle.

(l) A motorcycle rider is any person riding a motorcycle or in a sidecar or trailer attached to the motorcycle.

(m) A three-wheeled motor vehicle is a motorized tricycle designed primarily for on-road use. This includes a motor-driven tricycle, a motorized rickshaw, or a three-wheeled motor car.

(n) A car [automobile] is a four-wheeled motor vehicle designed primarily for carrying up to 7 persons. A trailer being towed by the car is considered part of the car. It does not include a van or minivan - see definition (o)

(o) A pick-up truck or van is a four or six-wheeled motor vehicle designed for carrying passengers as well as property or cargo weighing less than the local limit for classification as a heavy goods vehicle, and not requiring a special driver's license. This includes a minivan and a sport-utility vehicle (SUV).

(p) A heavy transport vehicle is a motor vehicle designed primarily for carrying property, meeting local criteria for classification as a heavy goods vehicle in terms of weight and requiring a special driver's license.

(q) A bus (coach) is a motor vehicle designed or adapted primarily for carrying more than 10 passengers, and requiring a special driver's license.

(r) A railway train or railway vehicle is any device, with or without freight or passenger cars couple to it, designed for traffic on a railway track. This includes subterranean (subways) or elevated trains.

(s) A streetcar, is a device designed and used primarily for transporting passengers within a municipality, running on rails, usually subject to normal traffic control signals, and operated principally on a right-of-way that forms part of the roadway. This includes a tram or trolley that runs on rails. A trailer being towed by a streetcar is considered part of the streetcar.

(t) A special vehicle mainly used on industrial premises is a motor vehicle designed primarily for use within the buildings and premises of industrial or commercial establishments. This includes battery-powered airport passenger vehicles or baggage/mail trucks, forklifts, coal-cars in a coal mine, logging cars and trucks used in mines or quarries.

● New ▲ Revised *Manifestation* 🔟-🔢 Digit Indicators ▤ Laterality 🅰 Adult (15+ years) Ⓜ Maternity (12-55 years) Ⓝ Newborn ℙ Pediatric (0-17 years) ♂ Male ♀ Female
✖ ~~Deleted~~ Unspecified + Additional code

External Causes of Morbidity *(left margin)*

(u) A special vehicle mainly used in agriculture is a motor vehicle designed specifically for use in farming and agriculture (horticulture), to work the land, tend and harvest crops and transport materials on the farm. This includes harvesters, farm machinery and tractor and trailers.

(v) A special construction vehicle is a motor vehicle designed specifically for use on construction and demolition sites. This includes bulldozers, diggers, earth levellers, dump trucks. backhoes, front-end loaders, pavers, and mechanical shovels.

(w) A special all-terrain vehicle is a motor vehicle of special design to enable it to negotiate over rough or soft terrain , snow or sand. Examples of special design are high construction, special wheels and tires, tracks, and support on a cushion of air. This includes snow mobiles, All-terrain vehicles (ATV), and dune buggies. It does not include passenger vehicle designated as Sport Utility Vehicles. (SUV)

(x) A watercraft is any device designed for transporting passengers or goods on water. This includes motor or sail boats, ships, and hovercraft.

(y) An aircraft is any device for transporting passengers or goods in the air. This includes hot-air balloons, gliders, helicopters and airplanes.

(z) A military vehicle is any motorized vehicle operating on a public roadway owned by the military and being operated by a member of the military.

Use additional code to identify:
Airbag injury (W22.1)
Type of street or road (Y92.4-)
Use of cellular telephone and other electronic equipment at the time of the transport accident (Y93.C-)

EXCLUDES 1 *agricultural vehicles in stationary use or maintenance (W31.-)*
assault by crashing of motor vehicle (Y03.-)
automobile or motor cycle in stationary use or maintenance- code to type of accident
crashing of motor vehicle, undetermined intent (Y32)
intentional self-harm by crashing of motor vehicle (X82)

EXCLUDES 2 *transport accidents due to cataclysm (X34-X38)*

Pedestrian injured in transport accident (V00-V09)

INCLUDES person changing tire on transport vehicle
person examining engine of vehicle broken down in (on side of) road

EXCLUDES 1 *fall due to non-transport collision with other person (W03)*
pedestrian on foot falling (slipping) on ice and snow (W00.-)
struck or bumped by another person (W51)

4 + V00 Pedestrian conveyance accident
Use additional place of occurrence and activity external cause codes, if known (Y92.-, Y93.-)

EXCLUDES 1 *collision with another person without fall (W51)*
fall due to person on foot colliding with another person on foot (W03)
fall from non-moving wheelchair, nonmotorized scooter and motorized mobility scooter without collision (W05.-)
pedestrian (conveyance) collision with other land transport vehicle (V01-V09)
pedestrian on foot falling (slipping) on ice and snow (W00.-)

The appropriate 7th character is to be added to each code from category V00
A initial encounter
D subsequent encounter
S sequela

5 + V00.0 Pedestrian on foot injured in collision with pedestrian conveyance

7 + V00.01X- Pedestrian on foot injured in collision with roller-skater

7 + V00.02X- Pedestrian on foot injured in collision with skateboarder

7 + V00.09X- Pedestrian on foot injured in collision with other pedestrian conveyance

5 + V00.1 Rolling-type pedestrian conveyance accident

EXCLUDES 1 *accident with babystroller (V00.82-)*
accident with wheelchair (powered) (V00.81-)
accident with motorized mobility scooter (V00.83-)

6 + V00.11 In-line roller-skate accident

7 + V00.111- Fall from in-line roller-skates

7 + V00.112- In-line roller-skater colliding with stationary object

7 + V00.118- Other in-line roller-skate accident

EXCLUDES 1 *roller-skater collision with other land transport vehicle (V01-V09 with 5th character 1)*

6 + V00.12 Non-in- line roller-skate accident

7 + V00.121- Fall from non-in-line roller-skates

7 + V00.122- Non-in-line roller-skater colliding with stationary object

7 + V00.128- Other non-in-line roller-skating accident

EXCLUDES 1 *roller-skater collision with other land transport vehicle (V01-V09 with 5th character 1)*

6 + V00.13 Skateboard accident

7 + V00.131- Fall from skateboard

7 + V00.132- Skateboarder colliding with stationary object

7 + V00.138- Other skateboard accident

EXCLUDES 1 *skateboarder collision with other land transport vehicle (V01-V09 with 5th character 2)*

6 + V00.14 Scooter (nonmotorized) accident

EXCLUDES 1 *motorscooter accident (V20-V29)*

7 + V00.141- Fall from scooter (nonmotorized)

7 + V00.142- Scooter (nonmotorized) colliding with stationary object

7 + V00.148- Other scooter (nonmotorized) accident

EXCLUDES 1 *scooter (nonmotorized) collision with other land transport vehicle (V01-V09 with fifth character 9)*

6 + V00.15 Heelies accident
Rolling shoe
Wheeled shoe
Wheelies accident

7 + V00.151- Fall from heelies

7 + V00.152- Heelies colliding with stationary object

7 + V00.158- Other heelies accident

6 + V00.18 Accident on other rolling-type pedestrian conveyance

7 + V00.181- Fall from other rolling-type pedestrian conveyance

7 + V00.182- Pedestrian on other rolling-type pedestrian conveyance colliding with stationary object

7 + V00.188- Other accident on other rolling-type pedestrian conveyance

5 + V00.2 Gliding-type pedestrian conveyance accident

6 + V00.21 Ice-skates accident

7 + V00.211- Fall from ice-skates

7 + V00.212- Ice-skater colliding with stationary object

7 + V00.218- Other ice-skates accident

EXCLUDES 1 *ice-skater collision with other land transport vehicle (V01-V09 with 5th digit 9)*

6 + V00.22 Sled accident

7 + V00.221- Fall from sled

7 + V00.222- Sledder colliding with stationary object

7 + V00.228- Other sled accident

EXCLUDES 1 *sled collision with other land transport vehicle (V01-V09 with 5th digit 9)*

6 + V00.28 Other gliding-type pedestrian conveyance accident

7 + V00.281- Fall from other gliding-type pedestrian conveyance

7 + V00.282- Pedestrian on other gliding-type pedestrian conveyance colliding with stationary object

7 + V00.288- Other accident on other gliding-type pedestrian conveyance

EXCLUDES 1 *gliding-type pedestrian conveyance collision with other land transport vehicle (V01-V09 with 5th digit 9)*

5 + V00.3 Flat-bottomed pedestrian conveyance accident

6 + V00.31 Snowboard accident

● New ▲ Revised *Manifestation* **4 - 7** Digit Indicators ⊟ Laterality 🅐 Adult (15+ years) 🅜 Maternity (12-55 years) 🅝 Newborn 🅟 Pediatric (0-17 years) ♂ Male ♀ Female
✖ Deleted Unspecified + Additional code

7 + **V00.311-** **Fall from snowboard**

7 + **V00.312-** **Snowboarder colliding with stationary object**

7 + **V00.318-** **Other snowboard accident**

> EXCLUDES 1 *snowboarder collision with other land transport vehicle (V01-V09 with 5th digit 9)*

6 + **V00.32** **Snow-ski accident**

7 + **V00.321-** **Fall from snow-skis**
AHA: (V00.321A) 1Q 2015, 12

7 + **V00.322-** **Snow-skier colliding with stationary object**

7 + **V00.328-** **Other snow-ski accident**

> EXCLUDES 1 *snow-skier collision with other land transport vehicle (V01-V09 with 5th digit 9)*

6 + **V00.38** **Other flat-bottomed pedestrian conveyance accident**

7 + **V00.381-** **Fall from other flat-bottomed pedestrian conveyance**

7 + **V00.382-** **Pedestrian on other flat-bottomed pedestrian conveyance colliding with stationary object**

7 + **V00.388-** **Other accident on other flat-bottomed pedestrian conveyance**

5 + **V00.8** **Accident on other pedestrian conveyance**

6 + **V00.81** **Accident with wheelchair (powered)**

7 + **V00.811-** **Fall from moving wheelchair (powered)**

> EXCLUDES 1 *fall from non-moving wheelchair (W05.0)*

7 + **V00.812-** **Wheelchair (powered) colliding with stationary object**

7 + **V00.818-** **Other accident with wheelchair (powered)**

6 + **V00.82** **Accident with babystroller**

7 + **V00.821-** **Fall from babystroller**

7 + **V00.822-** **Babystroller colliding with stationary object**

7 + **V00.828-** **Other accident with babystroller**

6 + **V00.83** **Accident with motorized mobility scooter**

7 + **V00.831-** **Fall from motorized mobility scooter**

> EXCLUDES 1 *fall from non-moving motorized mobility scooter (W05.2)*

7 + **V00.832-** **Motorized mobility scooter colliding with stationary object**

7 + **V00.838-** **Other accident with motorized mobility scooter**

6 + **V00.89** **Accident on other pedestrian conveyance**

7 + **V00.891-** **Fall from other pedestrian conveyance**

7 + **V00.892-** **Pedestrian on other pedestrian conveyance colliding with stationary object**

7 + **V00.898-** **Other accident on other pedestrian conveyance**

> EXCLUDES 1 *other pedestrian (conveyance) collision with other land transport vehicle (V01-V09 with 5th digit 9)*

4 **V01** **Pedestrian injured in collision with pedal cycle**

> The appropriate 7th character is to be added to each code from category V01
> A   initial encounter
> D   subsequent encounter
> S   sequela

5 **V01.0** **Pedestrian injured in collision with pedal cycle in nontraffic accident**

7 **V01.00X-** **Pedestrian on foot injured in collision with pedal cycle in nontraffic accident**
Pedestrian NOS injured in collision with pedal cycle in nontraffic accident

7 **V01.01X-** **Pedestrian on roller-skates injured in collision with pedal cycle in nontraffic accident**

7 **V01.02X-** **Pedestrian on skateboard injured in collision with pedal cycle in nontraffic accident**

7 **V01.09X-** **Pedestrian with other conveyance injured in collision with pedal cycle in nontraffic accident**
Pedestrian with babystroller injured in collision with pedal cycle in nontraffic accident
Pedestrian on ice-skates injured in collision with pedal cycle in nontraffic accident
Pedestrian on nonmotorized scooter injured in collision with pedal cycle in nontraffic accident
Pedestrian on sled injured in collision with pedal cycle in nontraffic accident
Pedestrian on snowboard injured in collision with pedal cycle in nontraffic accident
Pedestrian on snow-skis injured in collision with pedal cycle in nontraffic accident
Pedestrian in wheelchair (powered) injured in collision with pedal cycle in nontraffic accident
Pedestrian in motorized mobility scooter injured in collision with pedal cycle in nontraffic accident

5 **V01.1** **Pedestrian injured in collision with pedal cycle in traffic accident**

7 **V01.10X-** **Pedestrian on foot injured in collision with pedal cycle in traffic accident**
Pedestrian NOS injured in collision with pedal cycle in traffic accident

7 **V01.11X-** **Pedestrian on roller-skates injured in collision with pedal cycle in traffic accident**

7 **V01.12X-** **Pedestrian on skateboard injured in collision with pedal cycle in traffic accident**

7 **V01.19X-** **Pedestrian with other conveyance injured in collision with pedal cycle in traffic accident**
Pedestrian with babystroller injured in collision with pedal cycle in traffic accident
Pedestrian on ice-skates injured in collision with pedal cycle in traffic accident
Pedestrian on nonmotorized scooter injured in collision with pedal cycle in traffic accident
Pedestrian on sled injured in collision with pedal cycle in traffic accident
Pedestrian on snowboard injured in collision with pedal cycle in traffic accident
Pedestrian on snow-skis injured in collision with pedal cycle in traffic accident
Pedestrian in wheelchair (powered) injured in collision with pedal cycle in traffic accident
Pedestrian in motorized mobility scooter injured in collision with pedal cycle in traffic accident

5 **V01.9** **Pedestrian injured in collision with pedal cycle, unspecified whether traffic or nontraffic accident**

7 **V01.90X-** **Pedestrian on foot injured in collision with pedal cycle, unspecified whether traffic or nontraffic accident**
Pedestrian NOS injured in collision with pedal cycle, unspecified whether traffic or nontraffic accident

7 **V01.91X-** **Pedestrian on roller-skates injured in collision with pedal cycle, unspecified whether traffic or nontraffic accident**

7 **V01.92X-** **Pedestrian on skateboard injured in collision with pedal cycle, unspecified whether traffic or nontraffic accident**

● New   ▲ Revised   *Manifestation*   4-7 Digit Indicators   ⊟ Laterality   Adult (15+ years)   Maternity (12-55 years)   N Newborn   Pediatric (0-17 years)   ♂ Male   ♀ Female
✖ Deleted   Unspecified   + Additional code

☑ V01.99X- **Pedestrian with other conveyance injured in collision with pedal cycle, unspecified whether traffic or nontraffic accident**

Pedestrian with babystroller injured in collision with pedal cycle, unspecified whether traffic or nontraffic accident

Pedestrian on ice-skates injured in collision with pedal cycle unspecified, whether traffic or nontraffic accident

Pedestrian on nonmotorized scooter injured in collision with pedal cycle, unspecified whether traffic or nontraffic accident

Pedestrian on sled injured in collision with pedal cycle unspecified, whether traffic or nontraffic accident

Pedestrian on snowboard injured in collision with pedal cycle, unspecified whether traffic or nontraffic accident

Pedestrian on snow-skis injured in collision with pedal cycle, unspecified whether traffic or nontraffic accident

Pedestrian in wheelchair (powered) injured in collision with pedal cycle, unspecified whether traffic or nontraffic accident

Pedestrian in motorized mobility scooter injured in collision with pedal cycle, unspecified whether traffic or nontraffic accident

④ V02 **Pedestrian injured in collision with two- or three-wheeled motor vehicle**

The appropriate 7th character is to be added to each code from category V02
A   initial encounter
D   subsequent encounter
S   sequela

⑤ V02.0 **Pedestrian injured in collision with two- or three-wheeled motor vehicle in nontraffic accident**

☑ V02.00X- **Pedestrian on foot injured in collision with two- or three-wheeled motor vehicle in nontraffic accident**

Pedestrian NOS injured in collision with two- or three-wheeled motor vehicle in nontraffic accident

☑ V02.01X- **Pedestrian on roller-skates injured in collision with two- or three-wheeled motor vehicle in nontraffic accident**

☑ V02.02X- **Pedestrian on skateboard injured in collision with two- or three-wheeled motor vehicle in nontraffic accident**

☑ V02.09X- **Pedestrian with other conveyance injured in collision with two- or three-wheeled motor vehicle in nontraffic accident**

Pedestrian with babystroller injured in collision with two- or three-wheeled motor vehicle in nontraffic accident

Pedestrian on ice-skates injured in collision with two- or three-wheeled motor vehicle in nontraffic accident

Pedestrian on nonmotorized scooter injured in collision with two- or three-wheeled motor vehicle in nontraffic accident

Pedestrian on sled injured in collision with two- or three-wheeled motor vehicle in nontraffic accident

Pedestrian on snowboard injured in collision with two- or three-wheeled motor vehicle in nontraffic accident

Pedestrian on snow-skis injured in collision with two- or three-wheeled motor vehicle in nontraffic accident

Pedestrian in wheelchair (powered) injured in collision with two- or three-wheeled motor vehicle in nontraffic accident

Pedestrian in motorized mobility scooter injured in collision with two- or three-wheeled motor vehicle in nontraffic accident

⑤ V02.1 **Pedestrian injured in collision with two- or three-wheeled motor vehicle in traffic accident**

☑ V02.10X- **Pedestrian on foot injured in collision with two- or three-wheeled motor vehicle in traffic accident**

Pedestrian NOS injured in collision with two- or three-wheeled motor vehicle in traffic accident

☑ V02.11X- **Pedestrian on roller-skates injured in collision with two- or three-wheeled motor vehicle in traffic accident**

☑ V02.12X- **Pedestrian on skateboard injured in collision with two- or three-wheeled motor vehicle in traffic accident**

☑ V02.19X- **Pedestrian with other conveyance injured in collision with two- or three-wheeled motor vehicle in traffic accident**

Pedestrian with babystroller injured in collision with two- or three-wheeled motor vehicle in traffic accident

Pedestrian on ice-skates injured in collision with two- or three-wheeled motor vehicle in traffic accident

Pedestrian on nonmotorized scooter injured in collision with two- or three-wheeled motor vehicle in traffic accident

Pedestrian on sled injured in collision with two- or three-wheeled motor vehicle in traffic accident

Pedestrian on snowboard injured in collision with two- or three-wheeled motor vehicle in traffic accident

Pedestrian on snow-skis injured in collision with two- or three-wheeled motor vehicle in traffic accident

Pedestrian in wheelchair (powered) injured in collision with two- or three-wheeled motor vehicle in traffic accident

Pedestrian in motorized mobility scooter injured in collision with two- or three-wheeled motor vehicle in traffic accident

⑤ V02.9 **Pedestrian injured in collision with two- or three-wheeled motor vehicle, unspecified whether traffic or nontraffic accident**

☑ V02.90X- **Pedestrian on foot injured in collision with two- or three-wheeled motor vehicle, unspecified whether traffic or nontraffic accident**

Pedestrian NOS injured in collision with two- or three-wheeled motor vehicle, unspecified whether traffic or nontraffic accident

☑ V02.91X- **Pedestrian on roller-skates injured in collision with two- or three-wheeled motor vehicle, unspecified whether traffic or nontraffic accident**

☑ V02.92X- **Pedestrian on skateboard injured in collision with two- or three-wheeled motor vehicle, unspecified whether traffic or nontraffic accident**

☑ V02.99X- **Pedestrian with other conveyance injured in collision with two- or three-wheeled motor vehicle, unspecified whether traffic or nontraffic accident**

Pedestrian with babystroller injured in collision with two- or three-wheeled motor vehicle, unspecified whether traffic or nontraffic accident

Pedestrian on ice-skates injured in collision with two- or three-wheeled motor vehicle, unspecified whether traffic or nontraffic accident

Pedestrian on nonmotorized scooter injured in collision with two- or three-wheeled motor vehicle, unspecified whether traffic or nontraffic accident

Pedestrian on sled injured in collision with two- or three-wheeled motor vehicle, unspecified whether traffic or nontraffic accident

Pedestrian on snowboard injured in collision with two- or three-wheeled motor vehicle, unspecified whether traffic or nontraffic accident

Pedestrian on snow-skis injured in collision with two- or three-wheeled motor vehicle, unspecified whether traffic or nontraffic accident

Pedestrian in wheelchair (powered) injured in collision with two- or three-wheeled motor vehicle, unspecified whether traffic or nontraffic accident

Pedestrian in motorized mobility scooter injured in collision with two- or three-wheeled motor vehicle, unspecified whether traffic or nontraffic accident

● New   ▲ Revised   *Manifestation*   ④-☑ Digit Indicators   ▤ Laterality   Ⓐ Adult (15+ years)   Ⓜ Maternity (12-55 years)   Ⓝ Newborn   Ⓟ Pediatric (0-17 years)   ♂ Male   ♀ Female

✖ Deleted   Unspecified   ✚ Additional code

1112   © 2017 DecisionHealth   2017 ICD-10-CM Expert for Physicians

▣ **V03 Pedestrian injured in collision with car, pick-up truck or van**

The appropriate 7th character is to be added to each code from category V03
A   initial encounter
D   subsequent encounter
S   sequela

▣ **V03.0 Pedestrian injured in collision with car, pick-up truck or van in nontraffic accident**

▦ **V03.00X- Pedestrian on foot injured in collision with car, pick-up truck or van in nontraffic accident**
Pedestrian NOS injured in collision with car, pick-up truck or van in nontraffic accident

▦ **V03.01X- Pedestrian on roller-skates injured in collision with car, pick-up truck or van in nontraffic accident**

▦ **V03.02X- Pedestrian on skateboard injured in collision with car, pick-up truck or van in nontraffic accident**

▦ **V03.09X- Pedestrian with other conveyance injured in collision with car, pick-up truck or van in nontraffic accident**
Pedestrian with babystroller injured in collision with car, pick-up truck or van in nontraffic accident
Pedestrian on ice-skates injured in collision with car, pick-up truck or van in nontraffic accident
Pedestrian on nonmotorized scooter injured in collision with car, pick-up truck or van in nontraffic accident
Pedestrian on sled injured in collision with car, pick-up truck or van in nontraffic accident
Pedestrian on snowboard injured in collision with car, pick-up truck or van in nontraffic accident
Pedestrian on snow-skis injured in collision with car, pick-up truck or van in nontraffic accident
Pedestrian in wheelchair (powered) injured in collision with car, pick-up truck or van in nontraffic accident
Pedestrian in motorized mobility scooter injured in collision with car, pick-up truck or van in nontraffic accident

▣ **V03.1 Pedestrian injured in collision with car, pick-up truck or van in traffic accident**

▦ **V03.10X- Pedestrian on foot injured in collision with car, pick-up truck or van in traffic accident**
Pedestrian NOS injured in collision with car, pick-up truck or van in traffic accident

▦ **V03.11X- Pedestrian on roller-skates injured in collision with car, pick-up truck or van in traffic accident**

▦ **V03.12X- Pedestrian on skateboard injured in collision with car, pick-up truck or van in traffic accident**

▦ **V03.19X- Pedestrian with other conveyance injured in collision with car, pick-up truck or van in traffic accident**
Pedestrian with babystroller injured in collision with car, pick-up truck or van in traffic accident
Pedestrian on ice-skates injured in collision with car, pick-up truck or van in traffic accident
Pedestrian on nonmotorized scooter injured in collision with car, pick-up truck or van in traffic accident
Pedestrian on sled injured in collision with car, pick-up truck or van in traffic accident
Pedestrian on snowboard injured in collision with car, pick-up truck or van in traffic accident
Pedestrian on snow-skis injured in collision with car, pick-up truck or van in traffic accident
Pedestrian in wheelchair (powered) injured in collision with car, pick-up truck or van in traffic accident
Pedestrian in motorized mobility scooter injured in collision with car, pick-up truck or van in traffic accident

▣ **V03.9 Pedestrian injured in collision with car, pick-up truck or van, unspecified whether traffic or nontraffic accident**

▦ **V03.90X- Pedestrian on foot injured in collision with car, pick-up truck or van, unspecified whether traffic or nontraffic accident**
Pedestrian NOS injured in collision with car, pick-up truck or van, unspecified whether traffic or nontraffic accident

▦ **V03.91X- Pedestrian on roller-skates injured in collision with car, pick-up truck or van, unspecified whether traffic or nontraffic accident**

▦ **V03.92X- Pedestrian on skateboard injured in collision with car, pick-up truck or van, unspecified whether traffic or nontraffic accident**

▦ **V03.99X- Pedestrian with other conveyance injured in collision with car, pick-up truck or van, unspecified whether traffic or nontraffic accident**
Pedestrian with babystroller injured in collision with car, pick-up truck or van, unspecified whether traffic or nontraffic accident
Pedestrian on ice-skates injured in collision with car, pick-up truck or van, unspecified whether traffic or nontraffic accident
Pedestrian on nonmotorized scooter injured in collision with car, pick-up truck or van, unspecified whether traffic or nontraffic accident
Pedestrian on sled injured in collision with car, pick-up truck or van in nontraffic accident
Pedestrian on snowboard injured in collision with car, pick-up truck or van, unspecified whether traffic or nontraffic accident
Pedestrian on snow-skis injured in collision with car, pick-up truck or van, unspecified whether traffic or nontraffic accident
Pedestrian in wheelchair (powered) injured in collision with car, pick-up truck or van, unspecified whether traffic or nontraffic accident
Pedestrian in motorized mobility scooter injured in collision with car, pick-up truck or van, unspecified whether traffic or nontraffic accident

▣ **V04 Pedestrian injured in collision with heavy transport vehicle or bus**

EXCLUDES 1 *pedestrian injured in collision with military vehicle (V09.01, V09.21)*

The appropriate 7th character is to be added to each code from category V04
A   initial encounter
D   subsequent encounter
S   sequela

▣ **V04.0 Pedestrian injured in collision with heavy transport vehicle or bus in nontraffic accident**

▦ **V04.00X- Pedestrian on foot injured in collision with heavy transport vehicle or bus in nontraffic accident**
Pedestrian NOS injured in collision with heavy transport vehicle or bus in nontraffic accident

▦ **V04.01X- Pedestrian on roller-skates injured in collision with heavy transport vehicle or bus in nontraffic accident**

▦ **V04.02X- Pedestrian on skateboard injured in collision with heavy transport vehicle or bus in nontraffic accident**

▦ **V04.09X- Pedestrian with other conveyance injured in collision with heavy transport vehicle or bus in nontraffic accident**
Pedestrian with babystroller injured in collision with heavy transport vehicle or bus in nontraffic accident
Pedestrian on ice-skates injured in collision with heavy transport vehicle or bus in nontraffic accident
Pedestrian on nonmotorized scooter injured in collision with heavy transport vehicle or bus in nontraffic accident
Pedestrian on sled injured in collision with heavy transport vehicle or bus in nontraffic accident
Pedestrian on snowboard injured in collision with heavy transport vehicle or bus in nontraffic accident
Pedestrian on snow-skis injured in collision with heavy transport vehicle or bus in nontraffic accident
Pedestrian in wheelchair (powered) injured in collision with heavy transport vehicle or bus in nontraffic accident
Pedestrian in motorized mobility scooter injured in collision with heavy transport vehicle or bus in nontraffic accident

---

● New   ▲ Revised   *Manifestation*   ▣-▦ Digit Indicators   ▤ Laterality   Ⓐ Adult (15+ years)   Ⓜ Maternity (12-55 years)   Ⓝ Newborn   Ⓟ Pediatric (0-17 years)   ♂ Male   ♀ Female
✖ Deleted̶   Unspecified   + Additional code

⑤ **V04.1 Pedestrian injured in collision with heavy transport vehicle or bus in traffic accident**

⑦ **V04.10X- Pedestrian on foot injured in collision with heavy transport vehicle or bus in traffic accident**

Pedestrian NOS injured in collision with heavy transport vehicle or bus in traffic accident

⑦ **V04.11X- Pedestrian on roller-skates injured in collision with heavy transport vehicle or bus in traffic accident**

⑦ **V04.12X- Pedestrian on skateboard injured in collision with heavy transport vehicle or bus in traffic accident**

⑦ **V04.19X- Pedestrian with other conveyance injured in collision with heavy transport vehicle or bus in traffic accident**

Pedestrian with babystroller injured in collision with heavy transport vehicle or bus in traffic accident

Pedestrian on ice-skates injured in collision with heavy transport vehicle or bus in traffic accident

Pedestrian on nonmotorized scooter injured in collision with heavy transport vehicle or bus in traffic accident

Pedestrian on sled injured in collision with heavy transport vehicle or bus in traffic accident

Pedestrian on snowboard injured in collision with heavy transport vehicle or bus in traffic accident

Pedestrian on snow-skis injured in collision with heavy transport vehicle or bus in traffic accident

Pedestrian in wheelchair (powered) injured in collision with heavy transport vehicle or bus in traffic accident

Pedestrian in motorized mobility scooter injured in collision with heavy transport vehicle or bus in traffic accident

⑤ **V04.9 Pedestrian injured in collision with heavy transport vehicle or bus, unspecified whether traffic or nontraffic accident**

⑦ **V04.90X- Pedestrian on foot injured in collision with heavy transport vehicle or bus, unspecified whether traffic or nontraffic accident**

Pedestrian NOS injured in collision with heavy transport vehicle or bus, unspecified whether traffic or nontraffic accident

⑦ **V04.91X- Pedestrian on roller-skates injured in collision with heavy transport vehicle or bus, unspecified whether traffic or nontraffic accident**

⑦ **V04.92X- Pedestrian on skateboard injured in collision with heavy transport vehicle or bus, unspecified whether traffic or nontraffic accident**

⑦ **V04.99X- Pedestrian with other conveyance injured in collision with heavy transport vehicle or bus, unspecified whether traffic or nontraffic accident**

Pedestrian with babystroller injured in collision with heavy transport vehicle or bus, unspecified whether traffic or nontraffic accident

Pedestrian on ice-skates injured in collision with heavy transport vehicle or bus, unspecified whether traffic or nontraffic accident

Pedestrian on nonmotorized scooter injured in collision with heavy transport vehicle or bus, unspecified whether traffic or nontraffic accident

Pedestrian on sled injured in collision with heavy transport vehicle or bus, unspecified whether traffic or nontraffic accident

Pedestrian on snowboard injured in collision with heavy transport vehicle or bus, unspecified whether traffic or nontraffic accident

Pedestrian on snow-skis injured in collision with heavy transport vehicle or bus, unspecified whether traffic or nontraffic accident

Pedestrian in wheelchair (powered) injured in collision with heavy transport vehicle or bus, unspecified whether traffic or nontraffic accident

Pedestrian in motorized mobility scooter injured in collision with heavy transport vehicle or bus, unspecified whether traffic or nontraffic accident

④ **V05 Pedestrian injured in collision with railway train or railway vehicle**

The appropriate 7th character is to be added to each code from category V05

A   initial encounter
D   subsequent encounter
S   sequela

⑤ **V05.0 Pedestrian injured in collision with railway train or railway vehicle in nontraffic accident**

⑦ **V05.00X- Pedestrian on foot injured in collision with railway train or railway vehicle in nontraffic accident**

Pedestrian NOS injured in collision with railway train or railway vehicle in nontraffic accident

⑦ **V05.01X- Pedestrian on roller-skates injured in collision with railway train or railway vehicle in nontraffic accident**

⑦ **V05.02X- Pedestrian on skateboard injured in collision with railway train or railway vehicle in nontraffic accident**

⑦ **V05.09X- Pedestrian with other conveyance injured in collision with railway train or railway vehicle in nontraffic accident**

Pedestrian with babystroller injured in collision with railway train or railway vehicle in nontraffic accident

Pedestrian on ice-skates injured in collision with railway train or railway vehicle in nontraffic accident

Pedestrian on nonmotorized scooter injured in collision with railway train or railway vehicle in nontraffic accident

Pedestrian on sled injured in collision with railway train or railway vehicle in nontraffic accident

Pedestrian on snowboard injured in collision with railway train or railway vehicle in nontraffic accident

Pedestrian on snow-skis injured in collision with railway train or railway vehicle in nontraffic accident

Pedestrian in wheelchair (powered) injured in collision with railway train or railway vehicle in nontraffic accident

Pedestrian in motorized mobility scooter injured in collision with railway train or railway vehicle in nontraffic accident

⑤ **V05.1 Pedestrian injured in collision with railway train or railway vehicle in traffic accident**

⑦ **V05.10X- Pedestrian on foot injured in collision with railway train or railway vehicle in traffic accident**

Pedestrian NOS injured in collision with railway train or railway vehicle in traffic accident

⑦ **V05.11X- Pedestrian on roller-skates injured in collision with railway train or railway vehicle in traffic accident**

⑦ **V05.12X- Pedestrian on skateboard injured in collision with railway train or railway vehicle in traffic accident**

⑦ **V05.19X- Pedestrian with other conveyance injured in collision with railway train or railway vehicle in traffic accident**

Pedestrian with babystroller injured in collision with railway train or railway vehicle in traffic accident

Pedestrian on ice-skates injured in collision with railway train or railway vehicle in traffic accident

Pedestrian on nonmotorized scooter injured in collision with railway train or railway vehicle in traffic accident

Pedestrian on sled injured in collision with railway train or railway vehicle in traffic accident

Pedestrian on snowboard injured in collision with railway train or railway vehicle in traffic accident

Pedestrian on snow-skis injured in collision with railway train or railway vehicle in traffic accident

Pedestrian in wheelchair (powered) injured in collision with railway train or railway vehicle in traffic accident

Pedestrian in motorized mobility scooter injured in collision with railway train or railway vehicle in traffic accident

● New   ▲ Revised   *Manifestation* Unspecified   ④-⑦ Digit Indicators   ⧮ Laterality   ▲ Adult (15+ years)   Ⓜ Maternity (12-55 years)   Ⓝ Newborn   Ⓟ Pediatric (0-17 years)   ♂ Male   ♀ Female
✖ Deleted   ✚ Additional code

S V05.9 Pedestrian injured in collision with railway train or railway vehicle, unspecified whether traffic or nontraffic accident

7 V05.90X- Pedestrian on foot injured in collision with railway train or railway vehicle, unspecified whether traffic or nontraffic accident

Pedestrian NOS injured in collision with railway train or railway vehicle, unspecified whether traffic or nontraffic accident

7 V05.91X- Pedestrian on roller-skates injured in collision with railway train or railway vehicle, unspecified whether traffic or nontraffic accident

7 V05.92X- Pedestrian on skateboard injured in collision with railway train or railway vehicle, unspecified whether traffic or nontraffic accident

7 V05.99X- Pedestrian with other conveyance injured in collision with railway train or railway vehicle, unspecified whether traffic or nontraffic accident

Pedestrian with babystroller injured in collision with railway train or railway vehicle, unspecified whether traffic or nontraffic

Pedestrian on ice-skates injured in collision with railway train or railway vehicle, unspecified whether traffic or nontraffic

Pedestrian on nonmotorized scooter injured in collision with railway train or railway vehicle, unspecified whether traffic or nontraffic

Pedestrian on sled injured in collision with railway train or railway vehicle, unspecified whether traffic or nontraffic

Pedestrian on snowboard injured in collision with railway train or railway vehicle, unspecified whether traffic or nontraffic

Pedestrian on snow-skis injured in collision with railway train or railway vehicle, unspecified whether traffic or nontraffic

Pedestrian in wheelchair (powered) injured in collision with railway train or railway vehicle, unspecified whether traffic or nontraffic

Pedestrian in motorized mobility scooter injured in collision with railway train or railway vehicle, unspecified whether traffic or nontraffic

4 V06 Pedestrian injured in collision with other nonmotor vehicle

| INCLUDES | collision with animal-drawn vehicle, animal being ridden, nonpowered streetcar |
| EXCLUDES 1 | *pedestrian injured in collision with pedestrian conveyance (V00.0-)* |

The appropriate 7th character is to be added to each code from category V06
A   initial encounter
D   subsequent encounter
S   sequela

S V06.0 Pedestrian injured in collision with other nonmotor vehicle in nontraffic accident

7 V06.00X- Pedestrian on foot injured in collision with other nonmotor vehicle in nontraffic accident

Pedestrian NOS injured in collision with other nonmotor vehicle in nontraffic accident

7 V06.01X- Pedestrian on roller-skates injured in collision with other nonmotor vehicle in nontraffic accident

7 V06.02X- Pedestrian on skateboard injured in collision with other nonmotor vehicle in nontraffic accident

7 V06.09X- Pedestrian with other conveyance injured in collision with other nonmotor vehicle in nontraffic accident

Pedestrian with babystroller injured in collision with other nonmotor vehicle in nontraffic accident

Pedestrian on ice-skates injured in collision with other nonmotor vehicle in nontraffic accident

Pedestrian on nonmotorized scooter injured in collision with other nonmotor vehicle in nontraffic accident

Pedestrian on sled injured in collision with other nonmotor vehicle in nontraffic accident

Pedestrian on snowboard injured in collision with other nonmotor vehicle in nontraffic accident

Pedestrian on snow-skis injured in collision with other nonmotor vehicle in nontraffic accident

Pedestrian in wheelchair (powered) injured in collision with other nonmotor vehicle in nontraffic accident

Pedestrian in motorized mobility scooter injured in collision with other nonmotor vehicle in nontraffic accident

S V06.1 Pedestrian injured in collision with other nonmotor vehicle in traffic accident

7 V06.10X- Pedestrian on foot injured in collision with other nonmotor vehicle in traffic accident

Pedestrian NOS injured in collision with other nonmotor vehicle in traffic accident

7 V06.11X- Pedestrian on roller-skates injured in collision with other nonmotor vehicle in traffic accident

7 V06.12X- Pedestrian on skateboard injured in collision with other nonmotor vehicle in traffic accident

7 V06.19X- Pedestrian with other conveyance injured in collision with other nonmotor vehicle in traffic accident

Pedestrian with babystroller injured in collision with other nonmotor vehicle in nontraffic accident

Pedestrian on ice-skates injured in collision with other nonmotor vehicle in traffic accident

Pedestrian on nonmotorized scooter injured in collision with other nonmotor vehicle in traffic accident

Pedestrian on sled injured in collision with other nonmotor vehicle in traffic accident

Pedestrian on snowboard injured in collision with other nonmotor vehicle in traffic accident

Pedestrian on snow-skis injured in collision with other nonmotor vehicle in traffic accident

Pedestrian in wheelchair (powered) injured in collision with other nonmotor vehicle in traffic accident

Pedestrian in motorized mobility scooter injured in collision with other nonmotor vehicle in traffic accident

S V06.9 Pedestrian injured in collision with other nonmotor vehicle, unspecified whether traffic or nontraffic accident

7 V06.90X- Pedestrian on foot injured in collision with other nonmotor vehicle, unspecified whether traffic or nontraffic accident

Pedestrian NOS injured in collision with other nonmotor vehicle, unspecified whether traffic or nontraffic accident

7 V06.91X- Pedestrian on roller-skates injured in collision with other nonmotor vehicle, unspecified whether traffic or nontraffic accident

7 V06.92X- Pedestrian on skateboard injured in collision with other nonmotor vehicle, unspecified whether traffic or nontraffic accident

---

● New   ▲ Revised   *Manifestation*   **4**-**7** Digit Indicators   ▤ Laterality   ▣ Adult (15+ years)   ▣ Maternity (12-55 years)   ▣ Newborn   ▣ Pediatric (0-17 years)   ♂ Male   ♀ Female
✖ Deleted   Unspecified   + Additional code

V06.99X- Pedestrian with other conveyance injured in collision with other nonmotor vehicle, unspecified whether traffic or nontraffic accident

Pedestrian with babystroller injured in collision with other nonmotor vehicle, unspecified whether traffic or nontraffic accident

Pedestrian on ice-skates injured in collision with other nonmotor vehicle, unspecified whether traffic or nontraffic accident

Pedestrian on nonmotorized scooter injured in collision with other nonmotor vehicle, unspecified whether traffic or nontraffic accident

Pedestrian on sled injured in collision with other nonmotor vehicle, unspecified whether traffic or nontraffic accident

Pedestrian on snowboard injured in collision with other nonmotor vehicle, unspecified whether traffic or nontraffic accident

Pedestrian on snow-skis injured in collision with other nonmotor vehicle, unspecified whether traffic or nontraffic accident

Pedestrian in wheelchair (powered) injured in collision with other nonmotor vehicle, unspecified whether traffic or nontraffic accident

Pedestrian in motorized mobility scooter injured in collision with other nonmotor vehicle, unspecified whether traffic or nontraffic accident

V09 Pedestrian injured in other and unspecified transport accidents

The appropriate 7th character is to be added to each code from category V09
A   initial encounter
D   subsequent encounter
S   sequela

V09.0 Pedestrian injured in nontraffic accident involving other and unspecified motor vehicles

V09.00X- Pedestrian injured in nontraffic accident involving unspecified motor vehicles

V09.01X- Pedestrian injured in nontraffic accident involving military vehicle

V09.09X- Pedestrian injured in nontraffic accident involving other motor vehicles

Pedestrian injured in nontraffic accident by special vehicle

V09.1XX- Pedestrian injured in unspecified nontraffic accident

V09.2 Pedestrian injured in traffic accident involving other and unspecified motor vehicles

V09.20X- Pedestrian injured in traffic accident involving unspecified motor vehicles

V09.21X- Pedestrian injured in traffic accident involving military vehicle

V09.29X- Pedestrian injured in traffic accident involving other motor vehicles

V09.3XX- Pedestrian injured in unspecified traffic accident

V09.9XX- Pedestrian injured in unspecified transport accident

Pedal cycle rider injured in transport accident (V10-V19)

INCLUDES any non-motorized vehicle, excluding an animal-drawn vehicle, or a sidecar or trailer attached to the pedal cycle

EXCLUDES 2 *rupture of pedal cycle tire (W37.0)*

V10 Pedal cycle rider injured in collision with pedestrian or animal

EXCLUDES 1 *pedal cycle rider collision with animal-drawn vehicle or animal being ridden (V16.-)*

The appropriate 7th character is to be added to each code from category V10
A   initial encounter
D   subsequent encounter
S   sequela

V10.0XX- Pedal cycle driver injured in collision with pedestrian or animal in nontraffic accident

V10.1XX- Pedal cycle passenger injured in collision with pedestrian or animal in nontraffic accident

V10.2XX- Unspecified pedal cyclist injured in collision with pedestrian or animal in nontraffic accident

V10.3XX- Person boarding or alighting a pedal cycle injured in collision with pedestrian or animal

V10.4XX- Pedal cycle driver injured in collision with pedestrian or animal in traffic accident

V10.5XX- Pedal cycle passenger injured in collision with pedestrian or animal in traffic accident

V10.9XX- Unspecified pedal cyclist injured in collision with pedestrian or animal in traffic accident

V11 Pedal cycle rider injured in collision with other pedal cycle

The appropriate 7th character is to be added to each code from category V11
A   initial encounter
D   subsequent encounter
S   sequela

V11.0XX- Pedal cycle driver injured in collision with other pedal cycle in nontraffic accident

V11.1XX- Pedal cycle passenger injured in collision with other pedal cycle in nontraffic accident

V11.2XX- Unspecified pedal cyclist injured in collision with other pedal cycle in nontraffic accident

V11.3XX- Person boarding or alighting a pedal cycle injured in collision with other pedal cycle

V11.4XX- Pedal cycle driver injured in collision with other pedal cycle in traffic accident

V11.5XX- Pedal cycle passenger injured in collision with other pedal cycle in traffic accident

V11.9XX- Unspecified pedal cyclist injured in collision with other pedal cycle in traffic accident

V12 Pedal cycle rider injured in collision with two- or three-wheeled motor vehicle

The appropriate 7th character is to be added to each code from category V12
A   initial encounter
D   subsequent encounter
S   sequela

V12.0XX- Pedal cycle driver injured in collision with two- or three-wheeled motor vehicle in nontraffic accident

V12.1XX- Pedal cycle passenger injured in collision with two- or three-wheeled motor vehicle in nontraffic accident

V12.2XX- Unspecified pedal cyclist injured in collision with two- or three-wheeled motor vehicle in nontraffic accident

V12.3XX- Person boarding or alighting a pedal cycle injured in collision with two- or three-wheeled motor vehicle

V12.4XX- Pedal cycle driver injured in collision with two- or three-wheeled motor vehicle in traffic accident

V12.5XX- Pedal cycle passenger injured in collision with two- or three-wheeled motor vehicle in traffic accident

V12.9XX- Unspecified pedal cyclist injured in collision with two- or three-wheeled motor vehicle in traffic accident

V13 Pedal cycle rider injured in collision with car, pick-up truck or van

The appropriate 7th character is to be added to each code from category V13
A   initial encounter
D   subsequent encounter
S   sequela

V13.0XX- Pedal cycle driver injured in collision with car, pick-up truck or van in nontraffic accident

V13.1XX- Pedal cycle passenger injured in collision with car, pick-up truck or van in nontraffic accident

V13.2XX- Unspecified pedal cyclist injured in collision with car, pick-up truck or van in nontraffic accident

V13.3XX- Person boarding or alighting a pedal cycle injured in collision with car, pick-up truck or van

V13.4XX- Pedal cycle driver injured in collision with car, pick-up truck or van in traffic accident

V13.5XX- Pedal cycle passenger injured in collision with car, pick-up truck or van in traffic accident

V13.9XX- Unspecified pedal cyclist injured in collision with car, pick-up truck or van in traffic accident

④ V14 Pedal cycle rider injured in collision with heavy transport vehicle or bus

EXCLUDES 1 *pedal cycle rider injured in collision with military vehicle (V19.81)*

The appropriate 7th character is to be added to each code from category V14
A   initial encounter
D   subsequent encounter
S   sequela

☑ **V14.0XX-** Pedal cycle driver injured in collision with heavy transport vehicle or bus in nontraffic accident
☑ **V14.1XX-** Pedal cycle passenger injured in collision with heavy transport vehicle or bus in nontraffic accident
☑ **V14.2XX-** Unspecified pedal cyclist injured in collision with heavy transport vehicle or bus in nontraffic accident
☑ **V14.3XX-** Person boarding or alighting a pedal cycle injured in collision with heavy transport vehicle or bus
☑ **V14.4XX-** Pedal cycle driver injured in collision with heavy transport vehicle or bus in traffic accident
☑ **V14.5XX-** Pedal cycle passenger injured in collision with heavy transport vehicle or bus in traffic accident
☑ **V14.9XX-** Unspecified pedal cyclist injured in collision with heavy transport vehicle or bus in traffic accident

④ V15 Pedal cycle rider injured in collision with railway train or railway vehicle

The appropriate 7th character is to be added to each code from category V15
A   initial encounter
D   subsequent encounter
S   sequela

☑ **V15.0XX-** Pedal cycle driver injured in collision with railway train or railway vehicle in nontraffic accident
☑ **V15.1XX-** Pedal cycle passenger injured in collision with railway train or railway vehicle in nontraffic accident
☑ **V15.2XX-** Unspecified pedal cyclist injured in collision with railway train or railway vehicle in nontraffic accident
☑ **V15.3XX-** Person boarding or alighting a pedal cycle injured in collision with railway train or railway vehicle
☑ **V15.4XX-** Pedal cycle driver injured in collision with railway train or railway vehicle in traffic accident
☑ **V15.5XX-** Pedal cycle passenger injured in collision with railway train or railway vehicle in traffic accident
☑ **V15.9XX-** Unspecified pedal cyclist injured in collision with railway train or railway vehicle in traffic accident

④ V16 Pedal cycle rider injured in collision with other nonmotor vehicle

INCLUDES collision with animal-drawn vehicle, animal being ridden, streetcar

The appropriate 7th character is to be added to each code from category V16
A   initial encounter
D   subsequent encounter
S   sequela

☑ **V16.0XX-** Pedal cycle driver injured in collision with other nonmotor vehicle in nontraffic accident
☑ **V16.1XX-** Pedal cycle passenger injured in collision with other nonmotor vehicle in nontraffic accident
☑ **V16.2XX-** Unspecified pedal cyclist injured in collision with other nonmotor vehicle in nontraffic accident
☑ **V16.3XX-** Person boarding or alighting a pedal cycle injured in collision with other nonmotor vehicle in nontraffic accident
☑ **V16.4XX-** Pedal cycle driver injured in collision with other nonmotor vehicle in traffic accident
☑ **V16.5XX-** Pedal cycle passenger injured in collision with other nonmotor vehicle in traffic accident
☑ **V16.9XX-** Unspecified pedal cyclist injured in collision with other nonmotor vehicle in traffic accident

④ V17 Pedal cycle rider injured in collision with fixed or stationary object

The appropriate 7th character is to be added to each code from category V17
A   initial encounter
D   subsequent encounter
S   sequela

☑ **V17.0XX-** Pedal cycle driver injured in collision with fixed or stationary object in nontraffic accident
☑ **V17.1XX-** Pedal cycle passenger injured in collision with fixed or stationary object in nontraffic accident
☑ **V17.2XX-** Unspecified pedal cyclist injured in collision with fixed or stationary object in nontraffic accident
☑ **V17.3XX-** Person boarding or alighting a pedal cycle injured in collision with fixed or stationary object
☑ **V17.4XX-** Pedal cycle driver injured in collision with fixed or stationary object in traffic accident
☑ **V17.5XX-** Pedal cycle passenger injured in collision with fixed or stationary object in traffic accident
☑ **V17.9XX-** Unspecified pedal cyclist injured in collision with fixed or stationary object in traffic accident

④ V18 Pedal cycle rider injured in noncollision transport accident

INCLUDES fall or thrown from pedal cycle (without antecedent collision)
overturning pedal cycle NOS
overturning pedal cycle without collision

The appropriate 7th character is to be added to each code from category V18
A   initial encounter
D   subsequent encounter
S   sequela

☑ **V18.0XX-** Pedal cycle driver injured in noncollision transport accident in nontraffic accident
☑ **V18.1XX-** Pedal cycle passenger injured in noncollision transport accident in nontraffic accident
☑ **V18.2XX-** Unspecified pedal cyclist injured in noncollision transport accident in nontraffic accident
☑ **V18.3XX-** Person boarding or alighting a pedal cycle injured in noncollision transport accident
☑ **V18.4XX-** Pedal cycle driver injured in noncollision transport accident in traffic accident
☑ **V18.5XX-** Pedal cycle passenger injured in noncollision transport accident in traffic accident
☑ **V18.9XX-** Unspecified pedal cyclist injured in noncollision transport accident in traffic accident

④ V19 Pedal cycle rider injured in other and unspecified transport accidents

The appropriate 7th character is to be added to each code from category V19
A   initial encounter
D   subsequent encounter
S   sequela

⑤ **V19.0 Pedal cycle driver injured in collision with other and unspecified motor vehicles in nontraffic accident**
☑ **V19.00X-** Pedal cycle driver injured in collision with unspecified motor vehicles in nontraffic accident
☑ **V19.09X-** Pedal cycle driver injured in collision with other motor vehicles in nontraffic accident
⑤ **V19.1 Pedal cycle passenger injured in collision with other and unspecified motor vehicles in nontraffic accident**
☑ **V19.10X-** Pedal cycle passenger injured in collision with unspecified motor vehicles in nontraffic accident
☑ **V19.19X-** Pedal cycle passenger injured in collision with other motor vehicles in nontraffic accident
⑤ **V19.2 Unspecified pedal cyclist injured in collision with other and unspecified motor vehicles in nontraffic accident**
☑ **V19.20X-** Unspecified pedal cyclist injured in collision with unspecified motor vehicles in nontraffic accident

Pedal cycle collision NOS, nontraffic
☑ **V19.29X-** Unspecified pedal cyclist injured in collision with other motor vehicles in nontraffic accident

● New ▲ Revised *Manifestation* ④-☑ Digit Indicators ▣ Laterality Ⓐ Adult (15+ years) Ⓜ Maternity (12-55 years) Ⓝ Newborn Ⓟ Pediatric (0-17 years) ♂ Male ♀ Female
✖ Deleted Unspecified ✚ Additional code

2017 ICD-10-CM Expert for Physicians

© 2017 DecisionHealth

1117

☑ V19.3XX- **Pedal cyclist (driver) (passenger) injured in unspecified nontraffic accident**
Pedal cycle accident NOS, nontraffic
Pedal cyclist injured in nontraffic accident NOS

⑤ V19.4 **Pedal cycle driver injured in collision with other and unspecified motor vehicles in traffic accident**

☑ V19.40X- **Pedal cycle driver injured in collision with unspecified motor vehicles in traffic accident**

☑ V19.49X- **Pedal cycle driver injured in collision with other motor vehicles in traffic accident**

⑤ V19.5 **Pedal cycle passenger injured in collision with other and unspecified motor vehicles in traffic accident**

☑ V19.50X- **Pedal cycle passenger injured in collision with unspecified motor vehicles in traffic accident**

☑ V19.59X- **Pedal cycle passenger injured in collision with other motor vehicles in traffic accident**

⑤ V19.6 **Unspecified pedal cyclist injured in collision with other and unspecified motor vehicles in traffic accident**

☑ V19.60X- **Unspecified pedal cyclist injured in collision with unspecified motor vehicles in traffic accident**
Pedal cycle collision NOS (traffic)

☑ V19.69X- **Unspecified pedal cyclist injured in collision with other motor vehicles in traffic accident**

⑤ V19.8 **Pedal cyclist (driver) (passenger) injured in other specified transport accidents**

☑ V19.81X- **Pedal cyclist (driver) (passenger) injured in transport accident with military vehicle**

☑ V19.88X- **Pedal cyclist (driver) (passenger) injured in other specified transport accidents**

☑ V19.9XX- **Pedal cyclist (driver) (passenger) injured in unspecified traffic accident**
Pedal cycle accident NOS

Motorcycle rider injured in transport accident (V20-V29)

INCLUDES	moped
	motorcycle with sidecar
	motorized bicycle
	motor scooter

EXCLUDES 1 *three-wheeled motor vehicle (V30-V39)*

④ V20 **Motorcycle rider injured in collision with pedestrian or animal**

EXCLUDES 1 *motorcycle rider collision with animal-drawn vehicle or animal being ridden (V26.-)*

The appropriate 7th character is to be added to each code from category V20
A initial encounter
D subsequent encounter
S sequela

☑ V20.0XX- **Motorcycle driver injured in collision with pedestrian or animal in nontraffic accident**

☑ V20.1XX- **Motorcycle passenger injured in collision with pedestrian or animal in nontraffic accident**

☑ V20.2XX- **Unspecified motorcycle rider injured in collision with pedestrian or animal in nontraffic accident**

☑ V20.3XX- **Person boarding or alighting a motorcycle injured in collision with pedestrian or animal**

☑ V20.4XX- **Motorcycle driver injured in collision with pedestrian or animal in traffic accident**

☑ V20.5XX- **Motorcycle passenger injured in collision with pedestrian or animal in traffic accident**

☑ V20.9XX- **Unspecified motorcycle rider injured in collision with pedestrian or animal in traffic accident**

④ V21 **Motorcycle rider injured in collision with pedal cycle**

The appropriate 7th character is to be added to each code from category V21
A initial encounter
D subsequent encounter
S sequela

☑ V21.0XX- **Motorcycle driver injured in collision with pedal cycle in nontraffic accident**

☑ V21.1XX- **Motorcycle passenger injured in collision with pedal cycle in nontraffic accident**

☑ V21.2XX- **Unspecified motorcycle rider injured in collision with pedal cycle in nontraffic accident**

☑ V21.3XX- **Person boarding or alighting a motorcycle injured in collision with pedal cycle**

☑ V21.4XX- **Motorcycle driver injured in collision with pedal cycle in traffic accident**

☑ V21.5XX- **Motorcycle passenger injured in collision with pedal cycle in traffic accident**

☑ V21.9XX- **Unspecified motorcycle rider injured in collision with pedal cycle in traffic accident**

④ V22 **Motorcycle rider injured in collision with two- or three-wheeled motor vehicle**

The appropriate 7th character is to be added to each code from category V22
A initial encounter
D subsequent encounter
S sequela

☑ V22.0XX- **Motorcycle driver injured in collision with two- or three-wheeled motor vehicle in nontraffic accident**

☑ V22.1XX- **Motorcycle passenger injured in collision with two- or three-wheeled motor vehicle in nontraffic accident**

☑ V22.2XX- **Unspecified motorcycle rider injured in collision with two- or three-wheeled motor vehicle in nontraffic accident**

☑ V22.3XX- **Person boarding or alighting a motorcycle injured in collision with two- or three-wheeled motor vehicle**

☑ V22.4XX- **Motorcycle driver injured in collision with two- or three-wheeled motor vehicle in traffic accident**

☑ V22.5XX- **Motorcycle passenger injured in collision with two- or three-wheeled motor vehicle in traffic accident**

☑ V22.9XX- **Unspecified motorcycle rider injured in collision with two- or three-wheeled motor vehicle in traffic accident**

④ V23 **Motorcycle rider injured in collision with car, pick-up truck or van**

The appropriate 7th character is to be added to each code from category V23
A initial encounter
D subsequent encounter
S sequela

☑ V23.0XX- **Motorcycle driver injured in collision with car, pick-up truck or van in nontraffic accident**

☑ V23.1XX- **Motorcycle passenger injured in collision with car, pick-up truck or van in nontraffic accident**

☑ V23.2XX- **Unspecified motorcycle rider injured in collision with car, pick-up truck or van in nontraffic accident**

☑ V23.3XX- **Person boarding or alighting a motorcycle injured in collision with car, pick-up truck or van**

☑ V23.4XX- **Motorcycle driver injured in collision with car, pick-up truck or van in traffic accident**

☑ V23.5XX- **Motorcycle passenger injured in collision with car, pick-up truck or van in traffic accident**

☑ V23.9XX- **Unspecified motorcycle rider injured in collision with car, pick-up truck or van in traffic accident**

④ V24 **Motorcycle rider injured in collision with heavy transport vehicle or bus**

EXCLUDES 1 *motorcycle rider injured in collision with military vehicle (V29.81)*

The appropriate 7th character is to be added to each code from category V24
A initial encounter
D subsequent encounter
S sequela

☑ V24.0XX- **Motorcycle driver injured in collision with heavy transport vehicle or bus in nontraffic accident**

☑ V24.1XX- **Motorcycle passenger injured in collision with heavy transport vehicle or bus in nontraffic accident**

☑ V24.2XX- **Unspecified motorcycle rider injured in collision with heavy transport vehicle or bus in nontraffic accident**

☑ V24.3XX- **Person boarding or alighting a motorcycle injured in collision with heavy transport vehicle or bus**

☑ V24.4XX- **Motorcycle driver injured in collision with heavy transport vehicle or bus in traffic accident**

☑ V24.5XX- **Motorcycle passenger injured in collision with heavy transport vehicle or bus in traffic accident**

● New ▲ Revised *Manifestation* ④-☑ Digit Indicators ▣ Laterality Ⓐ Adult (15+ years) Ⓜ Maternity (12-55 years) Ⓝ Newborn (0-17 years) Ⓟ Pediatric ♂ Male ♀ Female
✖ Deleted Unspecified + Additional code

1118 © 2017 DecisionHealth 2017 ICD-10-CM Expert for Physicians

�7 V24.9XX- Unspecified motorcycle rider injured in collision with heavy transport vehicle or bus in traffic accident

�4 **V25 Motorcycle rider injured in collision with railway train or railway vehicle**

The appropriate 7th character is to be added to each code from category V25
A   initial encounter
D   subsequent encounter
S   sequela

�7 V25.0XX- Motorcycle driver injured in collision with railway train or railway vehicle in nontraffic accident
�7 V25.1XX- Motorcycle passenger injured in collision with railway train or railway vehicle in nontraffic accident
�7 V25.2XX- Unspecified motorcycle rider injured in collision with railway train or railway vehicle in nontraffic accident
�7 V25.3XX- Person boarding or alighting a motorcycle injured in collision with railway train or railway vehicle
�7 V25.4XX- Motorcycle driver injured in collision with railway train or railway vehicle in traffic accident
�7 V25.5XX- Motorcycle passenger injured in collision with railway train or railway vehicle in traffic accident
�7 V25.9XX- Unspecified motorcycle rider injured in collision with railway train or railway vehicle in traffic accident

�4 **V26 Motorcycle rider injured in collision with other nonmotor vehicle**

INCLUDES   collision with animal-drawn vehicle, animal being ridden, streetcar

The appropriate 7th character is to be added to each code from category V26
A   initial encounter
D   subsequent encounter
S   sequela

�7 V26.0XX- Motorcycle driver injured in collision with other nonmotor vehicle in nontraffic accident
�7 V26.1XX- Motorcycle passenger injured in collision with other nonmotor vehicle in nontraffic accident
�7 V26.2XX- Unspecified motorcycle rider injured in collision with other nonmotor vehicle in nontraffic accident
�7 V26.3XX- Person boarding or alighting a motorcycle injured in collision with other nonmotor vehicle
�7 V26.4XX- Motorcycle driver injured in collision with other nonmotor vehicle in traffic accident
�7 V26.5XX- Motorcycle passenger injured in collision with other nonmotor vehicle in traffic accident
�7 V26.9XX- Unspecified motorcycle rider injured in collision with other nonmotor vehicle in traffic accident

�4 **V27 Motorcycle rider injured in collision with fixed or stationary object**

The appropriate 7th character is to be added to each code from category V27
A   initial encounter
D   subsequent encounter
S   sequela

�7 V27.0XX- Motorcycle driver injured in collision with fixed or stationary object in nontraffic accident
�7 V27.1XX- Motorcycle passenger injured in collision with fixed or stationary object in nontraffic accident
�7 V27.2XX- Unspecified motorcycle rider injured in collision with fixed or stationary object in nontraffic accident
�7 V27.3XX- Person boarding or alighting a motorcycle injured in collision with fixed or stationary object
�7 V27.4XX- Motorcycle driver injured in collision with fixed or stationary object in traffic accident
�7 V27.5XX- Motorcycle passenger injured in collision with fixed or stationary object in traffic accident
�7 V27.9XX- Unspecified motorcycle rider injured in collision with fixed or stationary object in traffic accident

�4 **V28 Motorcycle rider injured in noncollision transport accident**

INCLUDES   fall or thrown from motorcycle (without antecedent collision)
overturning motorcycle NOS
overturning motorcycle without collision

The appropriate 7th character is to be added to each code from category V28
A   initial encounter
D   subsequent encounter
S   sequela

�7 V28.0XX- Motorcycle driver injured in noncollision transport accident in nontraffic accident
�7 V28.1XX- Motorcycle passenger injured in noncollision transport accident in nontraffic accident
�7 V28.2XX- Unspecified motorcycle rider injured in noncollision transport accident in nontraffic accident
�7 V28.3XX- Person boarding or alighting a motorcycle injured in noncollision transport accident
�7 V28.4XX- Motorcycle driver injured in noncollision transport accident in traffic accident
�7 V28.5XX- Motorcycle passenger injured in noncollision transport accident in traffic accident
�7 V28.9XX- Unspecified motorcycle rider injured in noncollision transport accident in traffic accident

�4 **V29 Motorcycle rider injured in other and unspecified transport accidents**

The appropriate 7th character is to be added to each code from category V29
A   initial encounter
D   subsequent encounter
S   sequela

�5 V29.0 Motorcycle driver injured in collision with other and unspecified motor vehicles in nontraffic accident
  �7 V29.00X- Motorcycle driver injured in collision with unspecified motor vehicles in nontraffic accident
  �7 V29.09X- Motorcycle driver injured in collision with other motor vehicles in nontraffic accident
�5 V29.1 Motorcycle passenger injured in collision with other and unspecified motor vehicles in nontraffic accident
  �7 V29.10X- Motorcycle passenger injured in collision with unspecified motor vehicles in nontraffic accident
  �7 V29.19X- Motorcycle passenger injured in collision with other motor vehicles in nontraffic accident
�5 V29.2 Unspecified motorcycle rider injured in collision with other and unspecified motor vehicles in nontraffic accident
  �7 V29.20X- Unspecified motorcycle rider injured in collision with unspecified motor vehicles in nontraffic accident
    Motorcycle collision NOS, nontraffic
  �7 V29.29X- Unspecified motorcycle rider injured in collision with other motor vehicles in nontraffic accident
�7 V29.3XX- Motorcycle rider (driver) (passenger) injured in unspecified nontraffic accident
    Motorcycle accident NOS, nontraffic
    Motorcycle rider injured in nontraffic accident NOS
�5 V29.4 Motorcycle driver injured in collision with other and unspecified motor vehicles in traffic accident
  �7 V29.40X- Motorcycle driver injured in collision with unspecified motor vehicles in traffic accident
  �7 V29.49X- Motorcycle driver injured in collision with other motor vehicles in traffic accident
�5 V29.5 Motorcycle passenger injured in collision with other and unspecified motor vehicles in traffic accident
  �7 V29.50X- Motorcycle passenger injured in collision with unspecified motor vehicles in traffic accident
  �7 V29.59X- Motorcycle passenger injured in collision with other motor vehicles in traffic accident
�5 V29.6 Unspecified motorcycle rider injured in collision with other and unspecified motor vehicles in traffic accident

● New   ▲ Revised   *Manifestation*   �4-�7 Digit Indicators   ▤ Laterality   ▣ Adult (15+ years)   ▣ Maternity (12-55 years)   ▣ Newborn   ▣ Pediatric (0-17 years)   ♂ Male   ♀ Female
✖ Deleted   Unspecified   + Additional code

2017 ICD-10-CM Expert for Physicians

© 2017 DecisionHealth   1119

☑ V29.60X- Unspecified motorcycle rider injured in collision with unspecified motor vehicles in traffic accident

Motorcycle collision NOS (traffic)

☑ V29.69X- Unspecified motorcycle rider injured in collision with other motor vehicles in traffic accident

⑤ V29.8 Motorcycle rider (driver) (passenger) injured in other specified transport accidents

☑ V29.81X- Motorcycle rider (driver) (passenger) injured in transport accident with military vehicle

☑ V29.88X- Motorcycle rider (driver) (passenger) injured in other specified transport accidents

☑ V29.9XX- Motorcycle rider (driver) (passenger) injured in unspecified traffic accident

Motorcycle accident NOS

Occupant of three-wheeled motor vehicle injured in transport accident (V30-V39)

INCLUDES   motorized tricycle
motorized rickshaw
three-wheeled motor car

EXCLUDES 1   all-terrain vehicles (V86.-)
motorcycle with sidecar (V20-V29)
vehicle designed primarily for off-road use (V86.-)

④ V30 Occupant of three-wheeled motor vehicle injured in collision with pedestrian or animal

EXCLUDES 1   three-wheeled motor vehicle collision with animal-drawn vehicle or animal being ridden (V36.-)

The appropriate 7th character is to be added to each code from category V30
A   initial encounter
D   subsequent encounter
S   sequela

☑ V30.0XX- Driver of three-wheeled motor vehicle injured in collision with pedestrian or animal in nontraffic accident

☑ V30.1XX- Passenger in three-wheeled motor vehicle injured in collision with pedestrian or animal in nontraffic accident

☑ V30.2XX- Person on outside of three-wheeled motor vehicle injured in collision with pedestrian or animal in nontraffic accident

☑ V30.3XX- Unspecified occupant of three-wheeled motor vehicle injured in collision with pedestrian or animal in nontraffic accident

☑ V30.4XX- Person boarding or alighting a three-wheeled motor vehicle injured in collision with pedestrian or animal

☑ V30.5XX- Driver of three-wheeled motor vehicle injured in collision with pedestrian or animal in traffic accident

☑ V30.6XX- Passenger in three-wheeled motor vehicle injured in collision with pedestrian or animal in traffic accident

☑ V30.7XX- Person on outside of three-wheeled motor vehicle injured in collision with pedestrian or animal in traffic accident

☑ V30.9XX- Unspecified occupant of three-wheeled motor vehicle injured in collision with pedestrian or animal in traffic accident

④ V31 Occupant of three-wheeled motor vehicle injured in collision with pedal cycle

The appropriate 7th character is to be added to each code from category V31
A   initial encounter
D   subsequent encounter
S   sequela

☑ V31.0XX- Driver of three-wheeled motor vehicle injured in collision with pedal cycle in nontraffic accident

☑ V31.1XX- Passenger in three-wheeled motor vehicle injured in collision with pedal cycle in nontraffic accident

☑ V31.2XX- Person on outside of three-wheeled motor vehicle injured in collision with pedal cycle in nontraffic accident

☑ V31.3XX- Unspecified occupant of three-wheeled motor vehicle injured in collision with pedal cycle in nontraffic accident

☑ V31.4XX- Person boarding or alighting a three-wheeled motor vehicle injured in collision with pedal cycle

☑ V31.5XX- Driver of three-wheeled motor vehicle injured in collision with pedal cycle in traffic accident

☑ V31.6XX- Passenger in three-wheeled motor vehicle injured in collision with pedal cycle in traffic accident

☑ V31.7XX- Person on outside of three-wheeled motor vehicle injured in collision with pedal cycle in traffic accident

☑ V31.9XX- Unspecified occupant of three-wheeled motor vehicle injured in collision with pedal cycle in traffic accident

④ V32 Occupant of three-wheeled motor vehicle injured in collision with two- or three-wheeled motor vehicle

The appropriate 7th character is to be added to each code from category V32
A   initial encounter
D   subsequent encounter
S   sequela

☑ V32.0XX- Driver of three-wheeled motor vehicle injured in collision with two- or three-wheeled motor vehicle in nontraffic accident

☑ V32.1XX- Passenger in three-wheeled motor vehicle injured in collision with two- or three-wheeled motor vehicle in nontraffic accident

☑ V32.2XX- Person on outside of three-wheeled motor vehicle injured in collision with two- or three-wheeled motor vehicle in nontraffic accident

☑ V32.3XX- Unspecified occupant of three-wheeled motor vehicle injured in collision with two- or three-wheeled motor vehicle in nontraffic accident

☑ V32.4XX- Person boarding or alighting a three-wheeled motor vehicle injured in collision with two- or three-wheeled motor vehicle

☑ V32.5XX- Driver of three-wheeled motor vehicle injured in collision with two- or three-wheeled motor vehicle in traffic accident

☑ V32.6XX- Passenger in three-wheeled motor vehicle injured in collision with two- or three-wheeled motor vehicle in traffic accident

☑ V32.7XX- Person on outside of three-wheeled motor vehicle injured in collision with two- or three-wheeled motor vehicle in traffic accident

☑ V32.9XX- Unspecified occupant of three-wheeled motor vehicle injured in collision with two- or three-wheeled motor vehicle in traffic accident

④ V33 Occupant of three-wheeled motor vehicle injured in collision with car, pick-up truck or van

The appropriate 7th character is to be added to each code from category V33
A   initial encounter
D   subsequent encounter
S   sequela

☑ V33.0XX- Driver of three-wheeled motor vehicle injured in collision with car, pick-up truck or van in nontraffic accident

☑ V33.1XX- Passenger in three-wheeled motor vehicle injured in collision with car, pick-up truck or van in nontraffic accident

☑ V33.2XX- Person on outside of three-wheeled motor vehicle injured in collision with car, pick-up truck or van in nontraffic accident

☑ V33.3XX- Unspecified occupant of three-wheeled motor vehicle injured in collision with car, pick-up truck or van in nontraffic accident

☑ V33.4XX- Person boarding or alighting a three-wheeled motor vehicle injured in collision with car, pick-up truck or van

☑ V33.5XX- Driver of three-wheeled motor vehicle injured in collision with car, pick-up truck or van in traffic accident

☑ V33.6XX- Passenger in three-wheeled motor vehicle injured in collision with car, pick-up truck or van in traffic accident

☑ V33.7XX- Person on outside of three-wheeled motor vehicle injured in collision with car, pick-up truck or van in traffic accident

● New   ▲ Revised   *Manifestation*   ④-☑ Digit Indicators   ▤ Laterality   Ⓐ Adult (15+ years)   Ⓜ Maternity (12-55 years)   Ⓝ Newborn   Ⓟ Pediatric (0-17 years)   ♂ Male   ♀ Female

✖ Deleted   Unspecified   + Additional code

1120   © 2017 DecisionHealth   2017 ICD-10-CM Expert for Physicians

☷ **V33.9XX-** Unspecified occupant of three-wheeled motor vehicle injured in collision with car, pick-up truck or van in traffic accident

◢ **V34** **Occupant of three-wheeled motor vehicle injured in collision with heavy transport vehicle or bus**

EXCLUDES 1 *occupant of three-wheeled motor vehicle injured in collision with military vehicle (V39.81)*

The appropriate 7th character is to be added to each code from category V34
A   initial encounter
D   subsequent encounter
S   sequela

☷ **V34.0XX-** Driver of three-wheeled motor vehicle injured in collision with heavy transport vehicle or bus in nontraffic accident

☷ **V34.1XX-** Passenger in three-wheeled motor vehicle injured in collision with heavy transport vehicle or bus in nontraffic accident

☷ **V34.2XX-** Person on outside of three-wheeled motor vehicle injured in collision with heavy transport vehicle or bus in nontraffic accident

☷ **V34.3XX-** Unspecified occupant of three-wheeled motor vehicle injured in collision with heavy transport vehicle or bus in nontraffic accident

☷ **V34.4XX-** Person boarding or alighting a three-wheeled motor vehicle injured in collision with heavy transport vehicle or bus

☷ **V34.5XX-** Driver of three-wheeled motor vehicle injured in collision with heavy transport vehicle or bus in traffic accident

☷ **V34.6XX-** Passenger in three-wheeled motor vehicle injured in collision with heavy transport vehicle or bus in traffic accident

☷ **V34.7XX-** Person on outside of three-wheeled motor vehicle injured in collision with heavy transport vehicle or bus in traffic accident

☷ **V34.9XX-** Unspecified occupant of three-wheeled motor vehicle injured in collision with heavy transport vehicle or bus in traffic accident

◢ **V35** **Occupant of three-wheeled motor vehicle injured in collision with railway train or railway vehicle**

The appropriate 7th character is to be added to each code from category V35
A   initial encounter
D   subsequent encounter
S   sequela

☷ **V35.0XX-** Driver of three-wheeled motor vehicle injured in collision with railway train or railway vehicle in nontraffic accident

☷ **V35.1XX-** Passenger in three-wheeled motor vehicle injured in collision with railway train or railway vehicle in nontraffic accident

☷ **V35.2XX-** Person on outside of three-wheeled motor vehicle injured in collision with railway train or railway vehicle in nontraffic accident

☷ **V35.3XX-** Unspecified occupant of three-wheeled motor vehicle injured in collision with railway train or railway vehicle in nontraffic accident

☷ **V35.4XX-** Person boarding or alighting a three-wheeled motor vehicle injured in collision with railway train or railway vehicle

☷ **V35.5XX-** Driver of three-wheeled motor vehicle injured in collision with railway train or railway vehicle in traffic accident

☷ **V35.6XX-** Passenger in three-wheeled motor vehicle injured in collision with railway train or railway vehicle in traffic accident

☷ **V35.7XX-** Person on outside of three-wheeled motor vehicle injured in collision with railway train or railway vehicle in traffic accident

☷ **V35.9XX-** Unspecified occupant of three-wheeled motor vehicle injured in collision with railway train or railway vehicle in traffic accident

◢ **V36** **Occupant of three-wheeled motor vehicle injured in collision with other nonmotor vehicle**

INCLUDES collision with animal-drawn vehicle, animal being ridden, streetcar

The appropriate 7th character is to be added to each code from category V36
A   initial encounter
D   subsequent encounter
S   sequela

☷ **V36.0XX-** Driver of three-wheeled motor vehicle injured in collision with other nonmotor vehicle in nontraffic accident

☷ **V36.1XX-** Passenger in three-wheeled motor vehicle injured in collision with other nonmotor vehicle in nontraffic accident

☷ **V36.2XX-** Person on outside of three-wheeled motor vehicle injured in collision with other nonmotor vehicle in nontraffic accident

☷ **V36.3XX-** Unspecified occupant of three-wheeled motor vehicle injured in collision with other nonmotor vehicle in nontraffic accident

☷ **V36.4XX-** Person boarding or alighting a three-wheeled motor vehicle injured in collision with other nonmotor vehicle

☷ **V36.5XX-** Driver of three-wheeled motor vehicle injured in collision with other nonmotor vehicle in traffic accident

☷ **V36.6XX-** Passenger in three-wheeled motor vehicle injured in collision with other nonmotor vehicle in traffic accident

☷ **V36.7XX-** Person on outside of three-wheeled motor vehicle injured in collision with other nonmotor vehicle in traffic accident

☷ **V36.9XX-** Unspecified occupant of three-wheeled motor vehicle injured in collision with other nonmotor vehicle in traffic accident

◢ **V37** **Occupant of three-wheeled motor vehicle injured in collision with fixed or stationary object**

The appropriate 7th character is to be added to each code from category V37
A   initial encounter
D   subsequent encounter
S   sequela

☷ **V37.0XX-** Driver of three-wheeled motor vehicle injured in collision with fixed or stationary object in nontraffic accident

☷ **V37.1XX-** Passenger in three-wheeled motor vehicle injured in collision with fixed or stationary object in nontraffic accident

☷ **V37.2XX-** Person on outside of three-wheeled motor vehicle injured in collision with fixed or stationary object in nontraffic accident

☷ **V37.3XX-** Unspecified occupant of three-wheeled motor vehicle injured in collision with fixed or stationary object in nontraffic accident

☷ **V37.4XX-** Person boarding or alighting a three-wheeled motor vehicle injured in collision with fixed or stationary object

☷ **V37.5XX-** Driver of three-wheeled motor vehicle injured in collision with fixed or stationary object in traffic accident

☷ **V37.6XX-** Passenger in three-wheeled motor vehicle injured in collision with fixed or stationary object in traffic accident

☷ **V37.7XX-** Person on outside of three-wheeled motor vehicle injured in collision with fixed or stationary object in traffic accident

☷ **V37.9XX-** Unspecified occupant of three-wheeled motor vehicle injured in collision with fixed or stationary object in traffic accident

● New   ▲ Revised   *Manifestation*   ◢-☷ Digit Indicators   ▤ Laterality   ▣ Adult (15+ years)   ▥ Maternity (12-55 years)   ▧ Newborn   ▨ Pediatric (0-17 years)   ♂ Male   ♀ Female
✖ Deleted   Unspecified   + Additional code

2017 ICD-10-CM Expert for Physicians

© 2017 DecisionHealth   1121

◢ V38   Occupant of three-wheeled motor vehicle injured in noncollision transport accident

| INCLUDES | fall or thrown from three-wheeled motor vehicle
overturning of three-wheeled motor vehicle NOS
overturning of three-wheeled motor vehicle without collision |

The appropriate 7th character is to be added to each code from category V38
A   initial encounter
D   subsequent encounter
S   sequela

☑ V38.0XX-   Driver of three-wheeled motor vehicle injured in noncollision transport accident in nontraffic accident

☑ V38.1XX-   Passenger in three-wheeled motor vehicle injured in noncollision transport accident in nontraffic accident

☑ V38.2XX-   Person on outside of three-wheeled motor vehicle injured in noncollision transport accident in nontraffic accident

☑ V38.3XX-   Unspecified occupant of three-wheeled motor vehicle injured in noncollision transport accident in nontraffic accident

☑ V38.4XX-   Person boarding or alighting a three-wheeled motor vehicle injured in noncollision transport accident

☑ V38.5XX-   Driver of three-wheeled motor vehicle injured in noncollision transport accident in traffic accident

☑ V38.6XX-   Passenger in three-wheeled motor vehicle injured in noncollision transport accident in traffic accident

☑ V38.7XX-   Person on outside of three-wheeled motor vehicle injured in noncollision transport accident in traffic accident

☑ V38.9XX-   Unspecified occupant of three-wheeled motor vehicle injured in noncollision transport accident in traffic accident

◢ V39   Occupant of three-wheeled motor vehicle injured in other and unspecified transport accidents

The appropriate 7th character is to be added to each code from category V39
A   initial encounter
D   subsequent encounter
S   sequela

⑤ V39.0   Driver of three-wheeled motor vehicle injured in collision with other and unspecified motor vehicles in nontraffic accident

☑ V39.00X-   Driver of three-wheeled motor vehicle injured in collision with unspecified motor vehicles in nontraffic accident

☑ V39.09X-   Driver of three-wheeled motor vehicle injured in collision with other motor vehicles in nontraffic accident

⑤ V39.1   Passenger in three-wheeled motor vehicle injured in collision with other and unspecified motor vehicles in nontraffic accident

☑ V39.10X-   Passenger in three-wheeled motor vehicle injured in collision with unspecified motor vehicles in nontraffic accident

☑ V39.19X-   Passenger in three-wheeled motor vehicle injured in collision with other motor vehicles in nontraffic accident

⑤ V39.2   Unspecified occupant of three-wheeled motor vehicle injured in collision with other and unspecified motor vehicles in nontraffic accident

☑ V39.20X-   Unspecified occupant of three-wheeled motor vehicle injured in collision with unspecified motor vehicles in nontraffic accident

Collision NOS involving three-wheeled motor vehicle, nontraffic

☑ V39.29X-   Unspecified occupant of three-wheeled motor vehicle injured in collision with other motor vehicles in nontraffic accident

☑ V39.3XX-   Occupant (driver) (passenger) of three-wheeled motor vehicle injured in unspecified nontraffic accident

Accident NOS involving three-wheeled motor vehicle, nontraffic
Occupant of three-wheeled motor vehicle injured in nontraffic accident NOS

⑤ V39.4   Driver of three-wheeled motor vehicle injured in collision with other and unspecified motor vehicles in traffic accident

☑ V39.40X-   Driver of three-wheeled motor vehicle injured in collision with unspecified motor vehicles in traffic accident

☑ V39.49X-   Driver of three-wheeled motor vehicle injured in collision with other motor vehicles in traffic accident

⑤ V39.5   Passenger in three-wheeled motor vehicle injured in collision with other and unspecified motor vehicles in traffic accident

☑ V39.50X-   Passenger in three-wheeled motor vehicle injured in collision with unspecified motor vehicles in traffic accident

☑ V39.59X-   Passenger in three-wheeled motor vehicle injured in collision with other motor vehicles in traffic accident

⑤ V39.6   Unspecified occupant of three-wheeled motor vehicle injured in collision with other and unspecified motor vehicles in traffic accident

☑ V39.60X-   Unspecified occupant of three-wheeled motor vehicle injured in collision with unspecified motor vehicles in traffic accident

Collision NOS involving three-wheeled motor vehicle (traffic)

☑ V39.69X-   Unspecified occupant of three-wheeled motor vehicle injured in collision with other motor vehicles in traffic accident

⑤ V39.8   Occupant (driver) (passenger) of three-wheeled motor vehicle injured in other specified transport accidents

☑ V39.81X-   Occupant (driver) (passenger) of three-wheeled motor vehicle injured in transport accident with military vehicle

☑ V39.89X-   Occupant (driver) (passenger) of three-wheeled motor vehicle injured in other specified transport accidents

☑ V39.9XX-   Occupant (driver) (passenger) of three-wheeled motor vehicle injured in unspecified traffic accident

Accident NOS involving three-wheeled motor vehicle

Car occupant injured in transport accident (V40-V49)

| INCLUDES | a four-wheeled motor vehicle designed primarily for carrying passengers
automobile (pulling a trailer or camper) |

| EXCLUDES 1 | *bus (V50-V59)*
minibus (V50-V59)
minivan (V50-V59)
motorcoach (V70-V79)
pick-up truck (V50-V59)
sport utility vehicle (SUV) (V50-V59) |

◢ V40   Car occupant injured in collision with pedestrian or animal

| EXCLUDES 1 | *car collision with animal-drawn vehicle or animal being ridden (V46.-)* |

The appropriate 7th character is to be added to each code from category V40
A   initial encounter
D   subsequent encounter
S   sequela

☑ V40.0XX-   Car driver injured in collision with pedestrian or animal in nontraffic accident

☑ V40.1XX-   Car passenger injured in collision with pedestrian or animal in nontraffic accident

☑ V40.2XX-   Person on outside of car injured in collision with pedestrian or animal in nontraffic accident

☑ V40.3XX-   Unspecified car occupant injured in collision with pedestrian or animal in nontraffic accident

☑ V40.4XX-   Person boarding or alighting a car injured in collision with pedestrian or animal

☑ V40.5XX-   Car driver injured in collision with pedestrian or animal in traffic accident

☑ V40.6XX-   Car passenger injured in collision with pedestrian or animal in traffic accident

☑ V40.7XX-   Person on outside of car injured in collision with pedestrian or animal in traffic accident

7 **V40.9XX-** Unspecified car occupant injured in collision with pedestrian or animal in traffic accident

4 **V41** Car occupant injured in collision with pedal cycle

The appropriate 7th character is to be added to each code from category V41
A   initial encounter
D   subsequent encounter
S   sequela

7 **V41.0XX-** Car driver injured in collision with pedal cycle in nontraffic accident

7 **V41.1XX-** Car passenger injured in collision with pedal cycle in nontraffic accident

7 **V41.2XX-** Person on outside of car injured in collision with pedal cycle in nontraffic accident

7 **V41.3XX-** Unspecified car occupant injured in collision with pedal cycle in nontraffic accident

7 **V41.4XX-** Person boarding or alighting a car injured in collision with pedal cycle

7 **V41.5XX-** Car driver injured in collision with pedal cycle in traffic accident

7 **V41.6XX-** Car passenger injured in collision with pedal cycle in traffic accident

7 **V41.7XX-** Person on outside of car injured in collision with pedal cycle in traffic accident

7 **V41.9XX-** Unspecified car occupant injured in collision with pedal cycle in traffic accident

4 **V42** Car occupant injured in collision with two- or three-wheeled motor vehicle

The appropriate 7th character is to be added to each code from category V42
A   initial encounter
D   subsequent encounter
S   sequela

7 **V42.0XX-** Car driver injured in collision with two- or three-wheeled motor vehicle in nontraffic accident

7 **V42.1XX-** Car passenger injured in collision with two- or three-wheeled motor vehicle in nontraffic accident

7 **V42.2XX-** Person on outside of car injured in collision with two- or three-wheeled motor vehicle in nontraffic accident

7 **V42.3XX-** Unspecified car occupant injured in collision with two- or three-wheeled motor vehicle in nontraffic accident

7 **V42.4XX-** Person boarding or alighting a car injured in collision with two- or three-wheeled motor vehicle

7 **V42.5XX-** Car driver injured in collision with two- or three-wheeled motor vehicle in traffic accident

7 **V42.6XX-** Car passenger injured in collision with two- or three-wheeled motor vehicle in traffic accident

7 **V42.7XX-** Person on outside of car injured in collision with two- or three-wheeled motor vehicle in traffic accident

7 **V42.9XX-** Unspecified car occupant injured in collision with two- or three-wheeled motor vehicle in traffic accident

4 **V43** Car occupant injured in collision with car, pick-up truck or van

The appropriate 7th character is to be added to each code from category V43
A   initial encounter
D   subsequent encounter
S   sequela

5 **V43.0** Car driver injured in collision with car, pick-up truck or van in nontraffic accident

7 **V43.01X-** Car driver injured in collision with sport utility vehicle in nontraffic accident

7 **V43.02X-** Car driver injured in collision with other type car in nontraffic accident

7 **V43.03X-** Car driver injured in collision with pick-up truck in nontraffic accident

7 **V43.04X-** Car driver injured in collision with van in nontraffic accident

5 **V43.1** Car passenger injured in collision with car, pick-up truck or van in nontraffic accident

7 **V43.11X-** Car passenger injured in collision with sport utility vehicle in nontraffic accident

7 **V43.12X-** Car passenger injured in collision with other type car in nontraffic accident

7 **V43.13X-** Car passenger injured in collision with pick-up in nontraffic accident

7 **V43.14X-** Car passenger injured in collision with van in nontraffic accident

5 **V43.2** Person on outside of car injured in collision with car, pick-up truck or van in nontraffic accident

7 **V43.21X-** Person on outside of car injured in collision with sport utility vehicle in nontraffic accident

7 **V43.22X-** Person on outside of car injured in collision with other type car in nontraffic accident

7 **V43.23X-** Person on outside of car injured in collision with pick-up truck in nontraffic accident

7 **V43.24X-** Person on outside of car injured in collision with van in nontraffic accident

5 **V43.3** Unspecified car occupant injured in collision with car, pick-up truck or van in nontraffic accident

7 **V43.31X-** Unspecified car occupant injured in collision with sport utility vehicle in nontraffic accident

7 **V43.32X-** Unspecified car occupant injured in collision with other type car in nontraffic accident

7 **V43.33X-** Unspecified car occupant injured in collision with pick-up truck in nontraffic accident

7 **V43.34X-** Unspecified car occupant injured in collision with van in nontraffic accident

5 **V43.4** Person boarding or alighting a car injured in collision with car, pick-up truck or van

7 **V43.41X-** Person boarding or alighting a car injured in collision with sport utility vehicle

7 **V43.42X-** Person boarding or alighting a car injured in collision with other type car

7 **V43.43X-** Person boarding or alighting a car injured in collision with pick-up truck

7 **V43.44X-** Person boarding or alighting a car injured in collision with van

5 **V43.5** Car driver injured in collision with car, pick-up truck or van in traffic accident

7 **V43.51X-** Car driver injured in collision with sport utility vehicle in traffic accident

7 **V43.52X-** Car driver injured in collision with other type car in traffic accident

7 **V43.53X-** Car driver injured in collision with pick-up truck in traffic accident

7 **V43.54X-** Car driver injured in collision with van in traffic accident

5 **V43.6** Car passenger injured in collision with car, pick-up truck or van in traffic accident

7 **V43.61X-** Car passenger injured in collision with sport utility vehicle in traffic accident
AHA: (V43.61XA) 1Q 2015, 5
AHA: (V43.61XD) 1Q 2015, 5, 7

7 **V43.62X-** Car passenger injured in collision with other type car in traffic accident

7 **V43.63X-** Car passenger injured in collision with pick-up truck in traffic accident

7 **V43.64X-** Car passenger injured in collision with van in traffic accident

5 **V43.7** Person on outside of car injured in collision with car, pick-up truck or van in traffic accident

7 **V43.71X-** Person on outside of car injured in collision with sport utility vehicle in traffic accident

7 **V43.72X-** Person on outside of car injured in collision with other type car in traffic accident

7 **V43.73X-** Person on outside of car injured in collision with pick-up truck in traffic accident

7 **V43.74X-** Person on outside of car injured in collision with van in traffic accident

5 **V43.9** Unspecified car occupant injured in collision with car, pick-up truck or van in traffic accident

7 **V43.91X-** Unspecified car occupant injured in collision with sport utility vehicle in traffic accident

7 **V43.92X-** Unspecified car occupant injured in collision with other type car in traffic accident

7 **V43.93X-** Unspecified car occupant injured in collision with pick-up truck in traffic accident

7 **V43.94X-** Unspecified car occupant injured in collision with van in traffic accident

---

● New ▲ Revised *Manifestation* 4-7 Digit Indicators ▤ Laterality ▣ Adult (15+ years) ▣ Maternity (12-55 years) ▣ Newborn ▣ Pediatric (0-17 years) ♂ Male ♀ Female
✖ Deleted Unspecified ✚ Additional code

V44 Car occupant injured in collision with heavy transport vehicle or bus

> **EXCLUDES 1** *car occupant injured in collision with military vehicle (V49.81)*

The appropriate 7th character is to be added to each code from category V44
A   initial encounter
D   subsequent encounter
S   sequela

V44.0XX- Car driver injured in collision with heavy transport vehicle or bus in nontraffic accident

V44.1XX- Car passenger injured in collision with heavy transport vehicle or bus in nontraffic accident

V44.2XX- Person on outside of car injured in collision with heavy transport vehicle or bus in nontraffic accident

V44.3XX- Unspecified car occupant injured in collision with heavy transport vehicle or bus in nontraffic accident

V44.4XX- Person boarding or alighting a car injured in collision with heavy transport vehicle or bus

V44.5XX- Car driver injured in collision with heavy transport vehicle or bus in traffic accident

V44.6XX- Car passenger injured in collision with heavy transport vehicle or bus in traffic accident

V44.7XX- Person on outside of car injured in collision with heavy transport vehicle or bus in traffic accident

V44.9XX- Unspecified car occupant injured in collision with heavy transport vehicle or bus in traffic accident

V45 Car occupant injured in collision with railway train or railway vehicle

The appropriate 7th character is to be added to each code from category V45
A   initial encounter
D   subsequent encounter
S   sequela

V45.0XX- Car driver injured in collision with railway train or railway vehicle in nontraffic accident

V45.1XX- Car passenger injured in collision with railway train or railway vehicle in nontraffic accident

V45.2XX- Person on outside of car injured in collision with railway train or railway vehicle in nontraffic accident

V45.3XX- Unspecified car occupant injured in collision with railway train or railway vehicle in nontraffic accident

V45.4XX- Person boarding or alighting a car injured in collision with railway train or railway vehicle

V45.5XX- Car driver injured in collision with railway train or railway vehicle in traffic accident

V45.6XX- Car passenger injured in collision with railway train or railway vehicle in traffic accident

V45.7XX- Person on outside of car injured in collision with railway train or railway vehicle in traffic accident

V45.9XX- Unspecified car occupant injured in collision with railway train or railway vehicle in traffic accident

V46 Car occupant injured in collision with other nonmotor vehicle

> **INCLUDES** collision with animal-drawn vehicle, animal being ridden, streetcar

The appropriate 7th character is to be added to each code from category V46
A   initial encounter
D   subsequent encounter
S   sequela

V46.0XX- Car driver injured in collision with other nonmotor vehicle in nontraffic accident

V46.1XX- Car passenger injured in collision with other nonmotor vehicle in nontraffic accident

V46.2XX- Person on outside of car injured in collision with other nonmotor vehicle in nontraffic accident

V46.3XX- Unspecified car occupant injured in collision with other nonmotor vehicle in nontraffic accident

V46.4XX- Person boarding or alighting a car injured in collision with other nonmotor vehicle

V46.5XX- Car driver injured in collision with other nonmotor vehicle in traffic accident

V46.6XX- Car passenger injured in collision with other nonmotor vehicle in traffic accident

V46.7XX- Person on outside of car injured in collision with other nonmotor vehicle in traffic accident

V46.9XX- Unspecified car occupant injured in collision with other nonmotor vehicle in traffic accident

V47 Car occupant injured in collision with fixed or stationary object

The appropriate 7th character is to be added to each code from category V47
A   initial encounter
D   subsequent encounter
S   sequela

▲ V47.0XX- Car driver injured in collision with fixed or stationary object in nontraffic accident

   ✖ V47.01X ~~Driver of sport utility vehicle injured in collision with fixed or stationary object in nontraffic accident~~

   ✖ V47.02X ~~Driver of other type car injured in collision with fixed or stationary object in nontraffic accident~~

▲ V47.1XX- Car passenger injured in collision with fixed or stationary object in nontraffic accident

   ✖ V47.11X ~~Passenger of sport utility vehicle injured in collision with fixed or stationary object in nontraffic accident~~

   ✖ V47.12X ~~Passenger of other type car injured in collision with fixed or stationary object in nontraffic accident~~

▲ V47.2XX- Person on outside of car injured in collision with fixed or stationary object in nontraffic accident

▲ V47.3XX- Unspecified car occupant injured in collision with fixed or stationary object in nontraffic accident

   ✖ V47.31X ~~Unspecified occupant of sport utility vehicle injured in collision with fixed or stationary object in nontraffic accident~~

   ✖ V47.32X ~~Unspecified occupant of other type car injured in collision with fixed or stationary object in nontraffic accident~~

▲ V47.4XX- Person boarding or alighting a car injured in collision with fixed or stationary object

▲ V47.5XX- Car driver injured in collision with fixed or stationary object in traffic accident

   ✖ V47.51X ~~Driver of sport utility vehicle injured in collision with fixed or stationary object in traffic accident~~

   ✖ V47.52X ~~Driver of other type car injured in collision with fixed or stationary object in traffic accident~~

▲ V47.6XX- Car passenger injured in collision with fixed or stationary object in traffic accident

   ✖ V47.61X ~~Passenger of sport utility vehicle injured in collision with fixed or stationary object in traffic accident~~

   ✖ V47.62X ~~Passenger of other type car injured in collision with fixed or stationary object in traffic accident~~

▲ V47.7XX- Person on outside of car injured in collision with fixed or stationary object in traffic accident

▲ V47.9XX- Unspecified car occupant injured in collision with fixed or stationary object in traffic accident

   ✖ V47.91X ~~Unspecified occupant of sport utility vehicle injured in collision with fixed or stationary object in traffic accident~~

   ✖ V47.92X ~~Unspecified occupant of other type car injured in collision with fixed or stationary object in traffic accident~~

V48 Car occupant injured in noncollision transport accident

> **INCLUDES** overturning car NOS
> overturning car without collision

The appropriate 7th character is to be added to each code from category V48
A   initial encounter
D   subsequent encounter
S   sequela

V48.0XX- Car driver injured in noncollision transport accident in nontraffic accident

V48.1XX- Car passenger injured in noncollision transport accident in nontraffic accident

---

● New   ▲ Revised   *Manifestation*   🔢-🔢 Digit Indicators   ▣ Laterality   Ⓐ Adult (15+ years)   Ⓜ Maternity (12-55 years)   Ⓝ Newborn   Ⓟ Pediatric (0-17 years)   ♂ Male   ♀ Female
✖ ~~Deleted~~   Unspecified   + Additional code

▣ V48.2XX-   Person on outside of car injured in noncollision transport accident in nontraffic accident

▣ V48.3XX-   Unspecified car occupant injured in noncollision transport accident in nontraffic accident

▣ V48.4XX-   Person boarding or alighting a car injured in noncollision transport accident

▣ V48.5XX-   Car driver injured in noncollision transport accident in traffic accident

▣ V48.6XX-   Car passenger injured in noncollision transport accident in traffic accident

▣ V48.7XX-   Person on outside of car injured in noncollision transport accident in traffic accident

▣ V48.9XX-   Unspecified car occupant injured in noncollision transport accident in traffic accident

▣ V49   Car occupant injured in other and unspecified transport accidents

The appropriate 7th character is to be added to each code from category V49
A   initial encounter
D   subsequent encounter
S   sequela

▣ V49.0   Driver injured in collision with other and unspecified motor vehicles in nontraffic accident

▣ V49.00X-   Driver injured in collision with unspecified motor vehicles in nontraffic accident

▣ V49.09X-   Driver injured in collision with other motor vehicles in nontraffic accident

▣ V49.1   Passenger injured in collision with other and unspecified motor vehicles in nontraffic accident

▣ V49.10X-   Passenger injured in collision with unspecified motor vehicles in nontraffic accident

▣ V49.19X-   Passenger injured in collision with other motor vehicles in nontraffic accident

▣ V49.2   Unspecified car occupant injured in collision with other and unspecified motor vehicles in nontraffic accident

▣ V49.20X-   Unspecified car occupant injured in collision with unspecified motor vehicles in nontraffic accident
   Car collision NOS, nontraffic

▣ V49.29X-   Unspecified car occupant injured in collision with other motor vehicles in nontraffic accident

▣ V49.3XX-   Car occupant (driver) (passenger) injured in unspecified nontraffic accident
   Car accident NOS, nontraffic
   Car occupant injured in nontraffic accident NOS

▣ V49.4   Driver injured in collision with other and unspecified motor vehicles in traffic accident

▣ V49.40X-   Driver injured in collision with unspecified motor vehicles in traffic accident

▣ V49.49X-   Driver injured in collision with other motor vehicles in traffic accident

▣ V49.5   Passenger injured in collision with other and unspecified motor vehicles in traffic accident

▣ V49.50X-   Passenger injured in collision with unspecified motor vehicles in traffic accident

▣ V49.59X-   Passenger injured in collision with other motor vehicles in traffic accident

▣ V49.6   Unspecified car occupant injured in collision with other and unspecified motor vehicles in traffic accident

▣ V49.60X-   Unspecified car occupant injured in collision with unspecified motor vehicles in traffic accident
   Car collision NOS (traffic)

▣ V49.69X-   Unspecified car occupant injured in collision with other motor vehicles in traffic accident

▣ V49.8   Car occupant (driver) (passenger) injured in other specified transport accidents

▣ V49.81X-   Car occupant (driver) (passenger) injured in transport accident with military vehicle

▣ V49.88X-   Car occupant (driver) (passenger) injured in other specified transport accidents

▣ V49.9XX-   Car occupant (driver) (passenger) injured in unspecified traffic accident
   Car accident NOS
   AHA: (V49.9XXA) 1Q 2015, 11

Occupant of pick-up truck or van injured in transport accident (V50-V59)

INCLUDES   a four or six wheel motor vehicle designed primarily for carrying passengers and property but weighing less than the local limit for classification as a heavy goods vehicle
   minibus
   minivan
   sport utility vehicle (SUV)
   truck
   van

EXCLUDES 1   *heavy transport vehicle (V60-V69)*

▣ V50   Occupant of pick-up truck or van injured in collision with pedestrian or animal

EXCLUDES 1   *pick-up truck or van collision with animal-drawn vehicle or animal being ridden (V56.-)*

The appropriate 7th character is to be added to each code from category V50
A   initial encounter
D   subsequent encounter
S   sequela

▣ V50.0XX-   Driver of pick-up truck or van injured in collision with pedestrian or animal in nontraffic accident

▣ V50.1XX-   Passenger in pick-up truck or van injured in collision with pedestrian or animal in nontraffic accident

▣ V50.2XX-   Person on outside of pick-up truck or van injured in collision with pedestrian or animal in nontraffic accident

▣ V50.3XX-   Unspecified occupant of pick-up truck or van injured in collision with pedestrian or animal in nontraffic accident

▣ V50.4XX-   Person boarding or alighting a pick-up truck or van injured in collision with pedestrian or animal

▣ V50.5XX-   Driver of pick-up truck or van injured in collision with pedestrian or animal in traffic accident

▣ V50.6XX-   Passenger in pick-up truck or van injured in collision with pedestrian or animal in traffic accident

▣ V50.7XX-   Person on outside of pick-up truck or van injured in collision with pedestrian or animal in traffic accident

▣ V50.9XX-   Unspecified occupant of pick-up truck or van injured in collision with pedestrian or animal in traffic accident

▣ V51   Occupant of pick-up truck or van injured in collision with pedal cycle

The appropriate 7th character is to be added to each code from category V51
A   initial encounter
D   subsequent encounter
S   sequela

▣ V51.0XX-   Driver of pick-up truck or van injured in collision with pedal cycle in nontraffic accident

▣ V51.1XX-   Passenger in pick-up truck or van injured in collision with pedal cycle in nontraffic accident

▣ V51.2XX-   Person on outside of pick-up truck or van injured in collision with pedal cycle in nontraffic accident

▣ V51.3XX-   Unspecified occupant of pick-up truck or van injured in collision with pedal cycle in nontraffic accident

▣ V51.4XX-   Person boarding or alighting a pick-up truck or van injured in collision with pedal cycle

▣ V51.5XX-   Driver of pick-up truck or van injured in collision with pedal cycle in traffic accident

▣ V51.6XX-   Passenger in pick-up truck or van injured in collision with pedal cycle in traffic accident

▣ V51.7XX-   Person on outside of pick-up truck or van injured in collision with pedal cycle in traffic accident

▣ V51.9XX-   Unspecified occupant of pick-up truck or van injured in collision with pedal cycle in traffic accident

---

● New   ▲ Revised   *Manifestation*   ▣-▣ Digit Indicators   ⊟ Laterality   Ⓐ Adult (15+ years)   Ⓜ Maternity (12-55 years)   Ⓝ Newborn   Ⓟ Pediatric (0-17 years)   ♂ Male   ♀ Female
✖ Deleted   Unspecified   + Additional code

V52 Occupant of pick-up truck or van injured in collision with two- or three-wheeled motor vehicle

The appropriate 7th character is to be added to each code from category V52
A   initial encounter
D   subsequent encounter
S   sequela

V52.0XX-   Driver of pick-up truck or van injured in collision with two- or three-wheeled motor vehicle in nontraffic accident
V52.1XX-   Passenger in pick-up truck or van injured in collision with two- or three-wheeled motor vehicle in nontraffic accident
V52.2XX-   Person on outside of pick-up truck or van injured in collision with two- or three-wheeled motor vehicle in nontraffic accident
V52.3XX-   Unspecified occupant of pick-up truck or van injured in collision with two- or three-wheeled motor vehicle in nontraffic accident
V52.4XX-   Person boarding or alighting a pick-up truck or van injured in collision with two- or three-wheeled motor vehicle
V52.5XX-   Driver of pick-up truck or van injured in collision with two- or three-wheeled motor vehicle in traffic accident
V52.6XX-   Passenger in pick-up truck or van injured in collision with two- or three-wheeled motor vehicle in traffic accident
V52.7XX-   Person on outside of pick-up truck or van injured in collision with two- or three-wheeled motor vehicle in traffic accident
V52.9XX-   Unspecified occupant of pick-up truck or van injured in collision with two- or three-wheeled motor vehicle in traffic accident

V53 Occupant of pick-up truck or van injured in collision with car, pick-up truck or van

The appropriate 7th character is to be added to each code from category V53
A   initial encounter
D   subsequent encounter
S   sequela

V53.0XX-   Driver of pick-up truck or van injured in collision with car, pick-up truck or van in nontraffic accident
V53.1XX-   Passenger in pick-up truck or van injured in collision with car, pick-up truck or van in nontraffic accident
V53.2XX-   Person on outside of pick-up truck or van injured in collision with car, pick-up truck or van in nontraffic accident
V53.3XX-   Unspecified occupant of pick-up truck or van injured in collision with car, pick-up truck or van in nontraffic accident
V53.4XX-   Person boarding or alighting a pick-up truck or van injured in collision with car, pick-up truck or van
V53.5XX-   Driver of pick-up truck or van injured in collision with car, pick-up truck or van in traffic accident
V53.6XX-   Passenger in pick-up truck or van injured in collision with car, pick-up truck or van in traffic accident
V53.7XX-   Person on outside of pick-up truck or van injured in collision with car, pick-up truck or van in traffic accident
V53.9XX-   Unspecified occupant of pick-up truck or van injured in collision with car, pick-up truck or van in traffic accident

V54 Occupant of pick-up truck or van injured in collision with heavy transport vehicle or bus

EXCLUDES 1   occupant of pick-up truck or van injured in collision with military vehicle (V59.81)

The appropriate 7th character is to be added to each code from category V54
A   initial encounter
D   subsequent encounter
S   sequela

V54.0XX-   Driver of pick-up truck or van injured in collision with heavy transport vehicle or bus in nontraffic accident

V54.1XX-   Passenger in pick-up truck or van injured in collision with heavy transport vehicle or bus in nontraffic accident
V54.2XX-   Person on outside of pick-up truck or van injured in collision with heavy transport vehicle or bus in nontraffic accident
V54.3XX-   Unspecified occupant of pick-up truck or van injured in collision with heavy transport vehicle or bus in nontraffic accident
V54.4XX-   Person boarding or alighting a pick-up truck or van injured in collision with heavy transport vehicle or bus
V54.5XX-   Driver of pick-up truck or van injured in collision with heavy transport vehicle or bus in traffic accident
V54.6XX-   Passenger in pick-up truck or van injured in collision with heavy transport vehicle or bus in traffic accident
V54.7XX-   Person on outside of pick-up truck or van injured in collision with heavy transport vehicle or bus in traffic accident
V54.9XX-   Unspecified occupant of pick-up truck or van injured in collision with heavy transport vehicle or bus in traffic accident

V55 Occupant of pick-up truck or van injured in collision with railway train or railway vehicle

The appropriate 7th character is to be added to each code from category V55
A   initial encounter
D   subsequent encounter
S   sequela

V55.0XX-   Driver of pick-up truck or van injured in collision with railway train or railway vehicle in nontraffic accident
V55.1XX-   Passenger in pick-up truck or van injured in collision with railway train or railway vehicle in nontraffic accident
V55.2XX-   Person on outside of pick-up truck or van injured in collision with railway train or railway vehicle in nontraffic accident
V55.3XX-   Unspecified occupant of pick-up truck or van injured in collision with railway train or railway vehicle in nontraffic accident
V55.4XX-   Person boarding or alighting a pick-up truck or van injured in collision with railway train or railway vehicle
V55.5XX-   Driver of pick-up truck or van injured in collision with railway train or railway vehicle in traffic accident
V55.6XX-   Passenger in pick-up truck or van injured in collision with railway train or railway vehicle in traffic accident
V55.7XX-   Person on outside of pick-up truck or van injured in collision with railway train or railway vehicle in traffic accident
V55.9XX-   Unspecified occupant of pick-up truck or van injured in collision with railway train or railway vehicle in traffic accident

V56 Occupant of pick-up truck or van injured in collision with other nonmotor vehicle

INCLUDES   collision with animal-drawn vehicle, animal being ridden, streetcar

The appropriate 7th character is to be added to each code from category V56
A   initial encounter
D   subsequent encounter
S   sequela

V56.0XX-   Driver of pick-up truck or van injured in collision with other nonmotor vehicle in nontraffic accident
V56.1XX-   Passenger in pick-up truck or van injured in collision with other nonmotor vehicle in nontraffic accident
V56.2XX-   Person on outside of pick-up truck or van injured in collision with other nonmotor vehicle in nontraffic accident
V56.3XX-   Unspecified occupant of pick-up truck or van injured in collision with other nonmotor vehicle in nontraffic accident

---

4 V56.4XX- Person boarding or alighting a pick-up truck or van injured in collision with other nonmotor vehicle

7 V56.5XX- Driver of pick-up truck or van injured in collision with other nonmotor vehicle in traffic accident

7 V56.6XX- Passenger in pick-up truck or van injured in collision with other nonmotor vehicle in traffic accident

7 V56.7XX- Person on outside of pick-up truck or van injured in collision with other nonmotor vehicle in traffic accident

7 V56.9XX- Unspecified occupant of pick-up truck or van injured in collision with other nonmotor vehicle in traffic accident

4 V57 Occupant of pick-up truck or van injured in collision with fixed or stationary object

The appropriate 7th character is to be added to each code from category V57
A   initial encounter
D   subsequent encounter
S   sequela

7 V57.0XX- Driver of pick-up truck or van injured in collision with fixed or stationary object in nontraffic accident

7 V57.1XX- Passenger in pick-up truck or van injured in collision with fixed or stationary object in nontraffic accident

7 V57.2XX- Person on outside of pick-up truck or van injured in collision with fixed or stationary object in nontraffic accident

7 V57.3XX- Unspecified occupant of pick-up truck or van injured in collision with fixed or stationary object in nontraffic accident

7 V57.4XX- Person boarding or alighting a pick-up truck or van injured in collision with fixed or stationary object

7 V57.5XX- Driver of pick-up truck or van injured in collision with fixed or stationary object in traffic accident

7 V57.6XX- Passenger in pick-up truck or van injured in collision with fixed or stationary object in traffic accident

7 V57.7XX- Person on outside of pick-up truck or van injured in collision with fixed or stationary object in traffic accident

7 V57.9XX- Unspecified occupant of pick-up truck or van injured in collision with fixed or stationary object in traffic accident

4 V58 Occupant of pick-up truck or van injured in noncollision transport accident

INCLUDES overturning pick-up truck or van NOS
overturning pick-up truck or van without collision

The appropriate 7th character is to be added to each code from category V58
A   initial encounter
D   subsequent encounter
S   sequela

7 V58.0XX- Driver of pick-up truck or van injured in noncollision transport accident in nontraffic accident

7 V58.1XX- Passenger in pick-up truck or van injured in noncollision transport accident in nontraffic accident

7 V58.2XX- Person on outside of pick-up truck or van injured in noncollision transport accident in nontraffic accident

7 V58.3XX- Unspecified occupant of pick-up truck or van injured in noncollision transport accident in nontraffic accident

7 V58.4XX- Person boarding or alighting a pick-up truck or van injured in noncollision transport accident

7 V58.5XX- Driver of pick-up truck or van injured in noncollision transport accident in traffic accident

7 V58.6XX- Passenger in pick-up truck or van injured in noncollision transport accident in traffic accident

7 V58.7XX- Person on outside of pick-up truck or van injured in noncollision transport accident in traffic accident

7 V58.9XX- Unspecified occupant of pick-up truck or van injured in noncollision transport accident in traffic accident

4 V59 Occupant of pick-up truck or van injured in other and unspecified transport accidents

The appropriate 7th character is to be added to each code from category V59
A   initial encounter
D   subsequent encounter
S   sequela

5 V59.0 Driver of pick-up truck or van injured in collision with other and unspecified motor vehicles in nontraffic accident

7 V59.00X- Driver of pick-up truck or van injured in collision with unspecified motor vehicles in nontraffic accident

7 V59.09X- Driver of pick-up truck or van injured in collision with other motor vehicles in nontraffic accident

5 V59.1 Passenger in pick-up truck or van injured in collision with other and unspecified motor vehicles in nontraffic accident

7 V59.10X- Passenger in pick-up truck or van injured in collision with unspecified motor vehicles in nontraffic accident

7 V59.19X- Passenger in pick-up truck or van injured in collision with other motor vehicles in nontraffic accident

5 V59.2 Unspecified occupant of pick-up truck or van injured in collision with other and unspecified motor vehicles in nontraffic accident

7 V59.20X- Unspecified occupant of pick-up truck or van injured in collision with unspecified motor vehicles in nontraffic accident

Collision NOS involving pick-up truck or van, nontraffic

7 V59.29X- Unspecified occupant of pick-up truck or van injured in collision with other motor vehicles in nontraffic accident

7 V59.3XX- Occupant (driver) (passenger) of pick-up truck or van injured in unspecified nontraffic accident

Accident NOS involving pick-up truck or van, nontraffic
Occupant of pick-up truck or van injured in nontraffic accident NOS

5 V59.4 Driver of pick-up truck or van injured in collision with other and unspecified motor vehicles in traffic accident

7 V59.40X- Driver of pick-up truck or van injured in collision with unspecified motor vehicles in traffic accident

7 V59.49X- Driver of pick-up truck or van injured in collision with other motor vehicles in traffic accident

5 V59.5 Passenger in pick-up truck or van injured in collision with other and unspecified motor vehicles in traffic accident

7 V59.50X- Passenger in pick-up truck or van injured in collision with unspecified motor vehicles in traffic accident

7 V59.59X- Passenger in pick-up truck or van injured in collision with other motor vehicles in traffic accident

5 V59.6 Unspecified occupant of pick-up truck or van injured in collision with other and unspecified motor vehicles in traffic accident

7 V59.60X- Unspecified occupant of pick-up truck or van injured in collision with unspecified motor vehicles in traffic accident

Collision NOS involving pick-up truck or van (traffic)

7 V59.69X- Unspecified occupant of pick-up truck or van injured in collision with other motor vehicles in traffic accident

5 V59.8 Occupant (driver) (passenger) of pick-up truck or van injured in other specified transport accidents

7 V59.81X- Occupant (driver) (passenger) of pick-up truck or van injured in transport accident with military vehicle

7 V59.88X- Occupant (driver) (passenger) of pick-up truck or van injured in other specified transport accidents

7 V59.9XX- Occupant (driver) (passenger) of pick-up truck or van injured in unspecified traffic accident

Accident NOS involving pick-up truck or van

● New   ▲ Revised   *Manifestation*   4-7 Digit Indicators   ▤ Laterality   Ⓐ Adult (15+ years)   Ⓜ Maternity (12-55 years)   Ⓝ Newborn   Ⓟ Pediatric (0-17 years)   ♂ Male   ♀ Female
✖ Deleted   Unspecified   + Additional code

Occupant of heavy transport vehicle injured in transport accident (V60-V69)

INCLUDES	18 wheeler
	armored car
	panel truck
EXCLUDES 1	*bus*
	motorcoach

4 **V60** **Occupant of heavy transport vehicle injured in collision with pedestrian or animal**

> EXCLUDES 1   *heavy transport vehicle collision with animal-drawn vehicle or animal being ridden (V66.-)*

The appropriate 7th character is to be added to each code from category V60
A   initial encounter
D   subsequent encounter
S   sequela

7 **V60.0XX-** Driver of heavy transport vehicle injured in collision with pedestrian or animal in nontraffic accident

7 **V60.1XX-** Passenger in heavy transport vehicle injured in collision with pedestrian or animal in nontraffic accident

7 **V60.2XX-** Person on outside of heavy transport vehicle injured in collision with pedestrian or animal in nontraffic accident

7 **V60.3XX-** Unspecified occupant of heavy transport vehicle injured in collision with pedestrian or animal in nontraffic accident

7 **V60.4XX-** Person boarding or alighting a heavy transport vehicle injured in collision with pedestrian or animal

7 **V60.5XX-** Driver of heavy transport vehicle injured in collision with pedestrian or animal in traffic accident

7 **V60.6XX-** Passenger in heavy transport vehicle injured in collision with pedestrian or animal in traffic accident

7 **V60.7XX-** Person on outside of heavy transport vehicle injured in collision with pedestrian or animal in traffic accident

7 **V60.9XX-** Unspecified occupant of heavy transport vehicle injured in collision with pedestrian or animal in traffic accident

4 **V61** **Occupant of heavy transport vehicle injured in collision with pedal cycle**

The appropriate 7th character is to be added to each code from category V61
A   initial encounter
D   subsequent encounter
S   sequela

7 **V61.0XX-** Driver of heavy transport vehicle injured in collision with pedal cycle in nontraffic accident

7 **V61.1XX-** Passenger in heavy transport vehicle injured in collision with pedal cycle in nontraffic accident

7 **V61.2XX-** Person on outside of heavy transport vehicle injured in collision with pedal cycle in nontraffic accident

7 **V61.3XX-** Unspecified occupant of heavy transport vehicle injured in collision with pedal cycle in nontraffic accident

7 **V61.4XX-** Person boarding or alighting a heavy transport vehicle injured in collision with pedal cycle while boarding or alighting

7 **V61.5XX-** Driver of heavy transport vehicle injured in collision with pedal cycle in traffic accident

7 **V61.6XX-** Passenger in heavy transport vehicle injured in collision with pedal cycle in traffic accident

7 **V61.7XX-** Person on outside of heavy transport vehicle injured in collision with pedal cycle in traffic accident

7 **V61.9XX-** Unspecified occupant of heavy transport vehicle injured in collision with pedal cycle in traffic accident

4 **V62** **Occupant of heavy transport vehicle injured in collision with two- or three-wheeled motor vehicle**

The appropriate 7th character is to be added to each code from category V62
A   initial encounter
D   subsequent encounter
S   sequela

7 **V62.0XX-** Driver of heavy transport vehicle injured in collision with two- or three-wheeled motor vehicle in nontraffic accident

7 **V62.1XX-** Passenger in heavy transport vehicle injured in collision with two- or three-wheeled motor vehicle in nontraffic accident

7 **V62.2XX-** Person on outside of heavy transport vehicle injured in collision with two- or three-wheeled motor vehicle in nontraffic accident

7 **V62.3XX-** Unspecified occupant of heavy transport vehicle injured in collision with two- or three-wheeled motor vehicle in nontraffic accident

7 **V62.4XX-** Person boarding or alighting a heavy transport vehicle injured in collision with two- or three-wheeled motor vehicle

7 **V62.5XX-** Driver of heavy transport vehicle injured in collision with two- or three-wheeled motor vehicle in traffic accident

7 **V62.6XX-** Passenger in heavy transport vehicle injured in collision with two- or three-wheeled motor vehicle in traffic accident

7 **V62.7XX-** Person on outside of heavy transport vehicle injured in collision with two- or three-wheeled motor vehicle in traffic accident

7 **V62.9XX-** Unspecified occupant of heavy transport vehicle injured in collision with two- or three-wheeled motor vehicle in traffic accident

4 **V63** **Occupant of heavy transport vehicle injured in collision with car, pick-up truck or van**

The appropriate 7th character is to be added to each code from category V63
A   initial encounter
D   subsequent encounter
S   sequela

7 **V63.0XX-** Driver of heavy transport vehicle injured in collision with car, pick-up truck or van in nontraffic accident

7 **V63.1XX-** Passenger in heavy transport vehicle injured in collision with car, pick-up truck or van in nontraffic accident

7 **V63.2XX-** Person on outside of heavy transport vehicle injured in collision with car, pick-up truck or van in nontraffic accident

7 **V63.3XX-** Unspecified occupant of heavy transport vehicle injured in collision with car, pick-up truck or van in nontraffic accident

7 **V63.4XX-** Person boarding or alighting a heavy transport vehicle injured in collision with car, pick-up truck or van

7 **V63.5XX-** Driver of heavy transport vehicle injured in collision with car, pick-up truck or van in traffic accident

7 **V63.6XX-** Passenger in heavy transport vehicle injured in collision with car, pick-up truck or van in traffic accident

7 **V63.7XX-** Person on outside of heavy transport vehicle injured in collision with car, pick-up truck or van in traffic accident

7 **V63.9XX-** Unspecified occupant of heavy transport vehicle injured in collision with car, pick-up truck or van in traffic accident

4 **V64** **Occupant of heavy transport vehicle injured in collision with heavy transport vehicle or bus**

> EXCLUDES 1   *occupant of heavy transport vehicle injured in collision with military vehicle (V69.81)*

The appropriate 7th character is to be added to each code from category V64
A   initial encounter
D   subsequent encounter
S   sequela

7 **V64.0XX-** Driver of heavy transport vehicle injured in collision with heavy transport vehicle or bus in nontraffic accident

7 **V64.1XX-** Passenger in heavy transport vehicle injured in collision with heavy transport vehicle or bus in nontraffic accident

7 **V64.2XX-** Person on outside of heavy transport vehicle injured in collision with heavy transport vehicle or bus in nontraffic accident

● New ▲ Revised *Manifestation* 4-7 Digit Indicators ▤ Laterality Ⓐ Adult (15+ years) Ⓜ Maternity (12-55 years) Ⓝ Newborn Ⓟ Pediatric (0-17 years) ♂ Male ♀ Female
✖ Deleted Unspecified + Additional code

1128   © 2017 DecisionHealth   2017 ICD-10-CM Expert for Physicians

☑ V64.3XX- Unspecified occupant of heavy transport vehicle injured in collision with heavy transport vehicle or bus in nontraffic accident

☑ V64.4XX- Person boarding or alighting a heavy transport vehicle injured in collision with heavy transport vehicle or bus while boarding or alighting

☑ V64.5XX- Driver of heavy transport vehicle injured in collision with heavy transport vehicle or bus in traffic accident

☑ V64.6XX- Passenger in heavy transport vehicle injured in collision with heavy transport vehicle or bus in traffic accident

☑ V64.7XX- Person on outside of heavy transport vehicle injured in collision with heavy transport vehicle or bus in traffic accident

☑ V64.9XX- Unspecified occupant of heavy transport vehicle injured in collision with heavy transport vehicle or bus in traffic accident

◢ V65 Occupant of heavy transport vehicle injured in collision with railway train or railway vehicle

The appropriate 7th character is to be added to each code from category V65
A   initial encounter
D   subsequent encounter
S   sequela

☑ V65.0XX- Driver of heavy transport vehicle injured in collision with railway train or railway vehicle in nontraffic accident

☑ V65.1XX- Passenger in heavy transport vehicle injured in collision with railway train or railway vehicle in nontraffic accident

☑ V65.2XX- Person on outside of heavy transport vehicle injured in collision with railway train or railway vehicle in nontraffic accident

☑ V65.3XX- Unspecified occupant of heavy transport vehicle injured in collision with railway train or railway vehicle in nontraffic accident

☑ V65.4XX- Person boarding or alighting a heavy transport vehicle injured in collision with railway train or railway vehicle

☑ V65.5XX- Driver of heavy transport vehicle injured in collision with railway train or railway vehicle in traffic accident

☑ V65.6XX- Passenger in heavy transport vehicle injured in collision with railway train or railway vehicle in traffic accident

☑ V65.7XX- Person on outside of heavy transport vehicle injured in collision with railway train or railway vehicle in traffic accident

☑ V65.9XX- Unspecified occupant of heavy transport vehicle injured in collision with railway train or railway vehicle in traffic accident

◢ V66 Occupant of heavy transport vehicle injured in collision with other nonmotor vehicle

INCLUDES collision with animal-drawn vehicle, animal being ridden, streetcar

The appropriate 7th character is to be added to each code from category V66
A   initial encounter
D   subsequent encounter
S   sequela

☑ V66.0XX- Driver of heavy transport vehicle injured in collision with other nonmotor vehicle in nontraffic accident

☑ V66.1XX- Passenger in heavy transport vehicle injured in collision with other nonmotor vehicle in nontraffic accident

☑ V66.2XX- Person on outside of heavy transport vehicle injured in collision with other nonmotor vehicle in nontraffic accident

☑ V66.3XX- Unspecified occupant of heavy transport vehicle injured in collision with other nonmotor vehicle in nontraffic accident

☑ V66.4XX- Person boarding or alighting a heavy transport vehicle injured in collision with other nonmotor vehicle

☑ V66.5XX- Driver of heavy transport vehicle injured in collision with other nonmotor vehicle in traffic accident

☑ V66.6XX- Passenger in heavy transport vehicle injured in collision with other nonmotor vehicle in traffic accident

☑ V66.7XX- Person on outside of heavy transport vehicle injured in collision with other nonmotor vehicle in traffic accident

☑ V66.9XX- Unspecified occupant of heavy transport vehicle injured in collision with other nonmotor vehicle in traffic accident

◢ V67 Occupant of heavy transport vehicle injured in collision with fixed or stationary object

The appropriate 7th character is to be added to each code from category V67
A   initial encounter
D   subsequent encounter
S   sequela

☑ V67.0XX- Driver of heavy transport vehicle injured in collision with fixed or stationary object in nontraffic accident

☑ V67.1XX- Passenger in heavy transport vehicle injured in collision with fixed or stationary object in nontraffic accident

☑ V67.2XX- Person on outside of heavy transport vehicle injured in collision with fixed or stationary object in nontraffic accident

☑ V67.3XX- Unspecified occupant of heavy transport vehicle injured in collision with fixed or stationary object in nontraffic accident

☑ V67.4XX- Person boarding or alighting a heavy transport vehicle injured in collision with fixed or stationary object

☑ V67.5XX- Driver of heavy transport vehicle injured in collision with fixed or stationary object in traffic accident

☑ V67.6XX- Passenger in heavy transport vehicle injured in collision with fixed or stationary object in traffic accident

☑ V67.7XX- Person on outside of heavy transport vehicle injured in collision with fixed or stationary object in traffic accident

☑ V67.9XX- Unspecified occupant of heavy transport vehicle injured in collision with fixed or stationary object in traffic accident

◢ V68 Occupant of heavy transport vehicle injured in noncollision transport accident

INCLUDES overturning heavy transport vehicle NOS
overturning heavy transport vehicle without collision

The appropriate 7th character is to be added to each code from category V68
A   initial encounter
D   subsequent encounter
S   sequela

☑ V68.0XX- Driver of heavy transport vehicle injured in noncollision transport accident in nontraffic accident

☑ V68.1XX- Passenger in heavy transport vehicle injured in noncollision transport accident in nontraffic accident

☑ V68.2XX- Person on outside of heavy transport vehicle injured in noncollision transport accident in nontraffic accident

☑ V68.3XX- Unspecified occupant of heavy transport vehicle injured in noncollision transport accident in nontraffic accident

☑ V68.4XX- Person boarding or alighting a heavy transport vehicle injured in noncollision transport accident

☑ V68.5XX- Driver of heavy transport vehicle injured in noncollision transport accident in traffic accident

☑ V68.6XX- Passenger in heavy transport vehicle injured in noncollision transport accident in traffic accident

☑ V68.7XX- Person on outside of heavy transport vehicle injured in noncollision transport accident in traffic accident

☑ V68.9XX- Unspecified occupant of heavy transport vehicle injured in noncollision transport accident in traffic accident

● New ▲ Revised *Manifestation* ◢-☑ Digit Indicators ▤ Laterality Ⓐ Adult (15+ years) Ⓜ Maternity (12-55 years) Ⓝ Newborn Ⓟ Pediatric (0-17 years) ♂ Male ♀ Female
✖ Deleted Unspecified + Additional code

2017 ICD-10-CM Expert for Physicians

© 2017 DecisionHealth

1129

V64.3XX- — V68.9XX-

4 V69 **Occupant of heavy transport vehicle injured in other and unspecified transport accidents**

The appropriate 7th character is to be added to each code from category V69
A   initial encounter
D   subsequent encounter
S   sequela

5 V69.0 **Driver of heavy transport vehicle injured in collision with other and unspecified motor vehicles in nontraffic accident**

7 V69.00X- **Driver of heavy transport vehicle injured in collision with unspecified motor vehicles in nontraffic accident**

7 V69.09X- **Driver of heavy transport vehicle injured in collision with other motor vehicles in nontraffic accident**

5 V69.1 **Passenger in heavy transport vehicle injured in collision with other and unspecified motor vehicles in nontraffic accident**

7 V69.10X- **Passenger in heavy transport vehicle injured in collision with unspecified motor vehicles in nontraffic accident**

7 V69.19X- **Passenger in heavy transport vehicle injured in collision with other motor vehicles in nontraffic accident**

5 V69.2 **Unspecified occupant of heavy transport vehicle injured in collision with other and unspecified motor vehicles in nontraffic accident**

7 V69.20X- **Unspecified occupant of heavy transport vehicle injured in collision with unspecified motor vehicles in nontraffic accident**

Collision NOS involving heavy transport vehicle, nontraffic

7 V69.29X- **Unspecified occupant of heavy transport vehicle injured in collision with other motor vehicles in nontraffic accident**

7 V69.3XX- **Occupant (driver) (passenger) of heavy transport vehicle injured in unspecified nontraffic accident**

Accident NOS involving heavy transport vehicle, nontraffic

Occupant of heavy transport vehicle injured in nontraffic accident NOS

5 V69.4 **Driver of heavy transport vehicle injured in collision with other and unspecified motor vehicles in traffic accident**

7 V69.40X- **Driver of heavy transport vehicle injured in collision with unspecified motor vehicles in traffic accident**

7 V69.49X- **Driver of heavy transport vehicle injured in collision with other motor vehicles in traffic accident**

5 V69.5 **Passenger in heavy transport vehicle injured in collision with other and unspecified motor vehicles in traffic accident**

7 V69.50X- **Passenger in heavy transport vehicle injured in collision with unspecified motor vehicles in traffic accident**

7 V69.59X- **Passenger in heavy transport vehicle injured in collision with other motor vehicles in traffic accident**

5 V69.6 **Unspecified occupant of heavy transport vehicle injured in collision with other and unspecified motor vehicles in traffic accident**

7 V69.60X- **Unspecified occupant of heavy transport vehicle injured in collision with unspecified motor vehicles in traffic accident**

Collision NOS involving heavy transport vehicle (traffic)

7 V69.69X- **Unspecified occupant of heavy transport vehicle injured in collision with other motor vehicles in traffic accident**

5 V69.8 **Occupant (driver) (passenger) of heavy transport vehicle injured in other specified transport accidents**

7 V69.81X- **Occupant (driver) (passenger) of heavy transport vehicle injured in transport accidents with military vehicle**

7 V69.88X- **Occupant (driver) (passenger) of heavy transport vehicle injured in other specified transport accidents**

7 V69.9XX- **Occupant (driver) (passenger) of heavy transport vehicle injured in unspecified traffic accident**

Accident NOS involving heavy transport vehicle

Bus occupant injured in transport accident (V70-V79)

INCLUDES motorcoach
EXCLUDES 1 *minibus (V50-V59)*

4 V70 **Bus occupant injured in collision with pedestrian or animal**
    EXCLUDES 1 *bus collision with animal-drawn vehicle or animal being ridden (V76.-)*

The appropriate 7th character is to be added to each code from category V70
A   initial encounter
D   subsequent encounter
S   sequela

7 V70.0XX- **Driver of bus injured in collision with pedestrian or animal in nontraffic accident**

7 V70.1XX- **Passenger on bus injured in collision with pedestrian or animal in nontraffic accident**

7 V70.2XX- **Person on outside of bus injured in collision with pedestrian or animal in nontraffic accident**

7 V70.3XX- **Unspecified occupant of bus injured in collision with pedestrian or animal in nontraffic accident**

7 V70.4XX- **Person boarding or alighting from bus injured in collision with pedestrian or animal**

7 V70.5XX- **Driver of bus injured in collision with pedestrian or animal in traffic accident**

7 V70.6XX- **Passenger on bus injured in collision with pedestrian or animal in traffic accident**

7 V70.7XX- **Person on outside of bus injured in collision with pedestrian or animal in traffic accident**

7 V70.9XX- **Unspecified occupant of bus injured in collision with pedestrian or animal in traffic accident**

4 V71 **Bus occupant injured in collision with pedal cycle**

The appropriate 7th character is to be added to each code from category V71
A   initial encounter
D   subsequent encounter
S   sequela

7 V71.0XX- **Driver of bus injured in collision with pedal cycle in nontraffic accident**

7 V71.1XX- **Passenger on bus injured in collision with pedal cycle in nontraffic accident**

7 V71.2XX- **Person on outside of bus injured in collision with pedal cycle in nontraffic accident**

7 V71.3XX- **Unspecified occupant of bus injured in collision with pedal cycle in nontraffic accident**

7 V71.4XX- **Person boarding or alighting from bus injured in collision with pedal cycle**

7 V71.5XX- **Driver of bus injured in collision with pedal cycle in traffic accident**

7 V71.6XX- **Passenger on bus injured in collision with pedal cycle in traffic accident**

7 V71.7XX- **Person on outside of bus injured in collision with pedal cycle in traffic accident**

7 V71.9XX- **Unspecified occupant of bus injured in collision with pedal cycle in traffic accident**

4 V72 **Bus occupant injured in collision with two- or three-wheeled motor vehicle**

The appropriate 7th character is to be added to each code from category V72
A   initial encounter
D   subsequent encounter
S   sequela

7 V72.0XX- **Driver of bus injured in collision with two- or three-wheeled motor vehicle in nontraffic accident**

7 V72.1XX- **Passenger on bus injured in collision with two- or three-wheeled motor vehicle in nontraffic accident**

7 V72.2XX- **Person on outside of bus injured in collision with two- or three-wheeled motor vehicle in nontraffic accident**

● New ▲ Revised *Manifestation* **4 - 7** Digit Indicators ⊟ Laterality Ⓐ Adult (15+ years) Ⓜ Maternity (12-55 years) Ⓝ Newborn Ⓟ Pediatric (0-17 years) ♂ Male ♀ Female
✖ Deleted Unspecified + Additional code

1130 © 2017 DecisionHealth 2017 ICD-10-CM Expert for Physicians

V69 — V72.2XX-

☑ **V72.3XX-** Unspecified occupant of bus injured in collision with two- or three-wheeled motor vehicle in nontraffic accident

☑ **V72.4XX-** Person boarding or alighting from bus injured in collision with two- or three-wheeled motor vehicle

☑ **V72.5XX-** Driver of bus injured in collision with two- or three-wheeled motor vehicle in traffic accident

☑ **V72.6XX-** Passenger on bus injured in collision with two- or three-wheeled motor vehicle in traffic accident

☑ **V72.7XX-** Person on outside of bus injured in collision with two- or three-wheeled motor vehicle in traffic accident

☑ **V72.9XX-** Unspecified occupant of bus injured in collision with two- or three-wheeled motor vehicle in traffic accident

◁ **V73** **Bus occupant injured in collision with car, pick-up truck or van**

> The appropriate 7th character is to be added to each code from category V73
> A   initial encounter
> D   subsequent encounter
> S   sequela

☑ **V73.0XX-** Driver of bus injured in collision with car, pick-up truck or van in nontraffic accident

☑ **V73.1XX-** Passenger on bus injured in collision with car, pick-up truck or van in nontraffic accident

☑ **V73.2XX-** Person on outside of bus injured in collision with car, pick-up truck or van in nontraffic accident

☑ **V73.3XX-** Unspecified occupant of bus injured in collision with car, pick-up truck or van in nontraffic accident

☑ **V73.4XX-** Person boarding or alighting from bus injured in collision with car, pick-up truck or van

☑ **V73.5XX-** Driver of bus injured in collision with car, pick-up truck or van in traffic accident

☑ **V73.6XX-** Passenger on bus injured in collision with car, pick-up truck or van in traffic accident

☑ **V73.7XX-** Person on outside of bus injured in collision with car, pick-up truck or van in traffic accident

☑ **V73.9XX-** Unspecified occupant of bus injured in collision with car, pick-up truck or van in traffic accident

◁ **V74** **Bus occupant injured in collision with heavy transport vehicle or bus**

> **EXCLUDES 1** *bus occupant injured in collision with military vehicle (V79.81)*

> The appropriate 7th character is to be added to each code from category V74
> A   initial encounter
> D   subsequent encounter
> S   sequela

☑ **V74.0XX-** Driver of bus injured in collision with heavy transport vehicle or bus in nontraffic accident

☑ **V74.1XX-** Passenger on bus injured in collision with heavy transport vehicle or bus in nontraffic accident

☑ **V74.2XX-** Person on outside of bus injured in collision with heavy transport vehicle or bus in nontraffic accident

☑ **V74.3XX-** Unspecified occupant of bus injured in collision with heavy transport vehicle or bus in nontraffic accident

☑ **V74.4XX-** Person boarding or alighting from bus injured in collision with heavy transport vehicle or bus

☑ **V74.5XX-** Driver of bus injured in collision with heavy transport vehicle or bus in traffic accident

☑ **V74.6XX-** Passenger on bus injured in collision with heavy transport vehicle or bus in traffic accident

☑ **V74.7XX-** Person on outside of bus injured in collision with heavy transport vehicle or bus in traffic accident

☑ **V74.9XX-** Unspecified occupant of bus injured in collision with heavy transport vehicle or bus in traffic accident

◁ **V75** **Bus occupant injured in collision with railway train or railway vehicle**

> The appropriate 7th character is to be added to each code from category V75
> A   initial encounter
> D   subsequent encounter
> S   sequela

☑ **V75.0XX-** Driver of bus injured in collision with railway train or railway vehicle in nontraffic accident

☑ **V75.1XX-** Passenger on bus injured in collision with railway train or railway vehicle in nontraffic accident

☑ **V75.2XX-** Person on outside of bus injured in collision with railway train or railway vehicle in nontraffic accident

☑ **V75.3XX-** Unspecified occupant of bus injured in collision with railway train or railway vehicle in nontraffic accident

☑ **V75.4XX-** Person boarding or alighting from bus injured in collision with railway train or railway vehicle

☑ **V75.5XX-** Driver of bus injured in collision with railway train or railway vehicle in traffic accident

☑ **V75.6XX-** Passenger on bus injured in collision with railway train or railway vehicle in traffic accident

☑ **V75.7XX-** Person on outside of bus injured in collision with railway train or railway vehicle in traffic accident

☑ **V75.9XX-** Unspecified occupant of bus injured in collision with railway train or railway vehicle in traffic accident

◁ **V76** **Bus occupant injured in collision with other nonmotor vehicle**

> **INCLUDES** collision with animal-drawn vehicle, animal being ridden, streetcar

> The appropriate 7th character is to be added to each code from category V76
> A   initial encounter
> D   subsequent encounter
> S   sequela

☑ **V76.0XX-** Driver of bus injured in collision with other nonmotor vehicle in nontraffic accident

☑ **V76.1XX-** Passenger on bus injured in collision with other nonmotor vehicle in nontraffic accident

☑ **V76.2XX-** Person on outside of bus injured in collision with other nonmotor vehicle in nontraffic accident

☑ **V76.3XX-** Unspecified occupant of bus injured in collision with other nonmotor vehicle in nontraffic accident

☑ **V76.4XX-** Person boarding or alighting from bus injured in collision with other nonmotor vehicle

☑ **V76.5XX-** Driver of bus injured in collision with other nonmotor vehicle in traffic accident

☑ **V76.6XX-** Passenger on bus injured in collision with other nonmotor vehicle in traffic accident

☑ **V76.7XX-** Person on outside of bus injured in collision with other nonmotor vehicle in traffic accident

☑ **V76.9XX-** Unspecified occupant of bus injured in collision with other nonmotor vehicle in traffic accident

◁ **V77** **Bus occupant injured in collision with fixed or stationary object**

> The appropriate 7th character is to be added to each code from category V77
> A   initial encounter
> D   subsequent encounter
> S   sequela

☑ **V77.0XX-** Driver of bus injured in collision with fixed or stationary object in nontraffic accident

☑ **V77.1XX-** Passenger on bus injured in collision with fixed or stationary object in nontraffic accident

☑ **V77.2XX-** Person on outside of bus injured in collision with fixed or stationary object in nontraffic accident

☑ **V77.3XX-** Unspecified occupant of bus injured in collision with fixed or stationary object in nontraffic accident

☑ **V77.4XX-** Person boarding or alighting from bus injured in collision with fixed or stationary object

☑ **V77.5XX-** Driver of bus injured in collision with fixed or stationary object in traffic accident

☑ **V77.6XX-** Passenger on bus injured in collision with fixed or stationary object in traffic accident

☑ **V77.7XX-** Person on outside of bus injured in collision with fixed or stationary object in traffic accident

☑ **V77.9XX-** Unspecified occupant of bus injured in collision with fixed or stationary object in traffic accident

● New   ▲ Revised   *Manifestation*   ◁-☑ Digit Indicators   ⊟ Laterality   Ⓐ Adult (15+ years)   Ⓜ Maternity (12-55 years)   Ⓝ Newborn   Ⓟ Pediatric (0-17 years)   ♂ Male   ♀ Female
✖ Deleted   Unspecified   + Additional code

2017 ICD-10-CM Expert for Physicians

© 2017 DecisionHealth   1131

4 **V78**   **Bus occupant injured in noncollision transport accident**

> INCLUDES   overturning bus NOS
> overturning bus without collision

> The appropriate 7th character is to be added to each code from category V78
> A   initial encounter
> D   subsequent encounter
> S   sequela

7 **V78.0XX-**   **Driver of bus injured in noncollision transport accident in nontraffic accident**

7 **V78.1XX-**   **Passenger on bus injured in noncollision transport accident in nontraffic accident**

7 **V78.2XX-**   **Person on outside of bus injured in noncollision transport accident in nontraffic accident**

7 **V78.3XX-**   **Unspecified occupant of bus injured in noncollision transport accident in nontraffic accident**

7 **V78.4XX-**   **Person boarding or alighting from bus injured in noncollision transport accident**

7 **V78.5XX-**   **Driver of bus injured in noncollision transport accident in traffic accident**

7 **V78.6XX-**   **Passenger on bus injured in noncollision transport accident in traffic accident**

7 **V78.7XX-**   **Person on outside of bus injured in noncollision transport accident in traffic accident**

7 **V78.9XX-**   **Unspecified occupant of bus injured in noncollision transport accident in traffic accident**

4 **V79**   **Bus occupant injured in other and unspecified transport accidents**

> The appropriate 7th character is to be added to each code from category V79
> A   initial encounter
> D   subsequent encounter
> S   sequela

5 **V79.0**   **Driver of bus injured in collision with other and unspecified motor vehicles in nontraffic accident**

7 **V79.00X-**   **Driver of bus injured in collision with unspecified motor vehicles in nontraffic accident**

7 **V79.09X-**   **Driver of bus injured in collision with other motor vehicles in nontraffic accident**

5 **V79.1**   **Passenger on bus injured in collision with other and unspecified motor vehicles in nontraffic accident**

7 **V79.10X-**   **Passenger on bus injured in collision with unspecified motor vehicles in nontraffic accident**

7 **V79.19X-**   **Passenger on bus injured in collision with other motor vehicles in nontraffic accident**

5 **V79.2**   **Unspecified bus occupant injured in collision with other and unspecified motor vehicles in nontraffic accident**

7 **V79.20X-**   **Unspecified bus occupant injured in collision with unspecified motor vehicles in nontraffic accident**

Bus collision NOS, nontraffic

7 **V79.29X-**   **Unspecified bus occupant injured in collision with other motor vehicles in nontraffic accident**

7 **V79.3XX-**   **Bus occupant (driver) (passenger) injured in unspecified nontraffic accident**

Bus accident NOS, nontraffic
Bus occupant injured in nontraffic accident NOS

5 **V79.4**   **Driver of bus injured in collision with other and unspecified motor vehicles in traffic accident**

7 **V79.40X-**   **Driver of bus injured in collision with unspecified motor vehicles in traffic accident**

7 **V79.49X-**   **Driver of bus injured in collision with other motor vehicles in traffic accident**

5 **V79.5**   **Passenger on bus injured in collision with other and unspecified motor vehicles in traffic accident**

7 **V79.50X-**   **Passenger on bus injured in collision with unspecified motor vehicles in traffic accident**

7 **V79.59X-**   **Passenger on bus injured in collision with other motor vehicles in traffic accident**

5 **V79.6**   **Unspecified bus occupant injured in collision with other and unspecified motor vehicles in traffic accident**

7 **V79.60X-**   **Unspecified bus occupant injured in collision with unspecified motor vehicles in traffic accident**

Bus collision NOS (traffic)

7 **V79.69X-**   **Unspecified bus occupant injured in collision with other motor vehicles in traffic accident**

5 **V79.8**   **Bus occupant (driver) (passenger) injured in other specified transport accidents**

7 **V79.81X-**   **Bus occupant (driver) (passenger) injured in transport accidents with military vehicle**

7 **V79.88X-**   **Bus occupant (driver) (passenger) injured in other specified transport accidents**

7 **V79.9XX-**   **Bus occupant (driver) (passenger) injured in unspecified traffic accident**

Bus accident NOS

Other land transport accidents (V80-V89)

4 **V80**   **Animal-rider or occupant of animal-drawn vehicle injured in transport accident**

> The appropriate 7th character is to be added to each code from category V80
> A   initial encounter
> D   subsequent encounter
> S   sequela

5 **V80.0**   **Animal-rider or occupant of animal drawn vehicle injured by fall from or being thrown from animal or animal-drawn vehicle in noncollision accident**

6 **V80.01**   **Animal-rider injured by fall from or being thrown from animal in noncollision accident**

7 **V80.010-**   **Animal-rider injured by fall from or being thrown from horse in noncollision accident**

7 **V80.018-**   **Animal-rider injured by fall from or being thrown from other animal in noncollision accident**

7 **V80.02X-**   **Occupant of animal-drawn vehicle injured by fall from or being thrown from animal-drawn vehicle in noncollision accident**

Overturning animal-drawn vehicle NOS
Overturning animal-drawn vehicle without collision

5 **V80.1**   **Animal-rider or occupant of animal-drawn vehicle injured in collision with pedestrian or animal**

> EXCLUDES 1   *animal-rider or animal-drawn vehicle collision with animal-drawn vehicle or animal being ridden (V80.7)*

7 **V80.11X-**   **Animal-rider injured in collision with pedestrian or animal**

7 **V80.12X-**   **Occupant of animal-drawn vehicle injured in collision with pedestrian or animal**

5 **V80.2**   **Animal-rider or occupant of animal-drawn vehicle injured in collision with pedal cycle**

7 **V80.21X-**   **Animal-rider injured in collision with pedal cycle**

7 **V80.22X-**   **Occupant of animal-drawn vehicle injured in collision with pedal cycle**

5 **V80.3**   **Animal-rider or occupant of animal-drawn vehicle injured in collision with two- or three-wheeled motor vehicle**

7 **V80.31X-**   **Animal-rider injured in collision with two- or three-wheeled motor vehicle**

7 **V80.32X-**   **Occupant of animal-drawn vehicle injured in collision with two- or three-wheeled motor vehicle**

5 **V80.4**   **Animal-rider or occupant of animal-drawn vehicle injured in collision with car, pick-up truck, van, heavy transport vehicle or bus**

> EXCLUDES 1   *animal-rider injured in collision with military vehicle (V80.910)*
> *occupant of animal-drawn vehicle injured in collision with military vehicle (V80.920)*

7 **V80.41X-**   **Animal-rider injured in collision with car, pick-up truck, van, heavy transport vehicle or bus**

7 **V80.42X-**   **Occupant of animal-drawn vehicle injured in collision with car, pick-up truck, van, heavy transport vehicle or bus**

5 **V80.5**   **Animal-rider or occupant of animal-drawn vehicle injured in collision with other specified motor vehicle**

7 **V80.51X-**   **Animal-rider injured in collision with other specified motor vehicle**

● New   ▲ Revised   *Manifestation*   4 - 7 Digit Indicators   ▤ Laterality   ▲ Adult (15+ years)   Ⓜ Maternity (12-55 years)   Ⓝ Newborn   Ⓟ Pediatric (0-17 years)   ♂ Male   ♀ Female

✖ Deleted   Unspecified   + Additional code

V78 — V80.51X-

1132   © 2017 DecisionHealth   2017 ICD-10-CM Expert for Physicians

External Causes of Morbidity

7 **V80.52X-** Occupant of animal-drawn vehicle injured in collision with other specified motor vehicle

5 **V80.6** Animal-rider or occupant of animal-drawn vehicle injured in collision with railway train or railway vehicle

7 **V80.61X-** Animal-rider injured in collision with railway train or railway vehicle

7 **V80.62X-** Occupant of animal-drawn vehicle injured in collision with railway train or railway vehicle

5 **V80.7** Animal-rider or occupant of animal-drawn vehicle injured in collision with other nonmotor vehicles

6 **V80.71** Animal-rider or occupant of animal-drawn vehicle injured in collision with animal being ridden

7 **V80.710-** Animal-rider injured in collision with other animal being ridden

7 **V80.711-** Occupant of animal-drawn vehicle injured in collision with animal being ridden

6 **V80.72** Animal-rider or occupant of animal-drawn vehicle injured in collision with other animal-drawn vehicle

7 **V80.720-** Animal-rider injured in collision with animal-drawn vehicle

7 **V80.721-** Occupant of animal-drawn vehicle injured in collision with other animal-drawn vehicle

6 **V80.73** Animal-rider or occupant of animal-drawn vehicle injured in collision with streetcar

7 **V80.730-** Animal-rider injured in collision with streetcar

7 **V80.731-** Occupant of animal-drawn vehicle injured in collision with streetcar

6 **V80.79** Animal-rider or occupant of animal-drawn vehicle injured in collision with other nonmotor vehicles

7 **V80.790-** Animal-rider injured in collision with other nonmotor vehicles

7 **V80.791-** Occupant of animal-drawn vehicle injured in collision with other nonmotor vehicles

5 **V80.8** Animal-rider or occupant of animal-drawn vehicle injured in collision with fixed or stationary object

7 **V80.81X-** Animal-rider injured in collision with fixed or stationary object

7 **V80.82X-** Occupant of animal-drawn vehicle injured in collision with fixed or stationary object

5 **V80.9** Animal-rider or occupant of animal-drawn vehicle injured in other and unspecified transport accidents

6 **V80.91** Animal-rider injured in other and unspecified transport accidents

7 **V80.910-** Animal-rider injured in transport accident with military vehicle

7 **V80.918-** Animal-rider injured in other transport accident

7 **V80.919-** Animal-rider injured in unspecified transport accident
Animal rider accident NOS

6 **V80.92** Occupant of animal-drawn vehicle injured in other and unspecified transport accidents

7 **V80.920-** Occupant of animal-drawn vehicle injured in transport accident with military vehicle

7 **V80.928-** Occupant of animal-drawn vehicle injured in other transport accident

7 **V80.929-** Occupant of animal-drawn vehicle injured in unspecified transport accident
Animal-drawn vehicle accident NOS

4 **V81** Occupant of railway train or railway vehicle injured in transport accident

INCLUDES derailment of railway train or railway vehicle
person on outside of train

EXCLUDES 1 *streetcar (V82.-)*

The appropriate 7th character is to be added to each code from category V81
A initial encounter
D subsequent encounter
S sequela

7 **V81.0XX-** Occupant of railway train or railway vehicle injured in collision with motor vehicle in nontraffic accident

EXCLUDES 1 *Occupant of railway train or railway vehicle injured due to collision with military vehicle (V81.83)*

7 **V81.1XX-** Occupant of railway train or railway vehicle injured in collision with motor vehicle in traffic accident

EXCLUDES 1 *Occupant of railway train or railway vehicle injured due to collision with military vehicle (V81.83)*

7 **V81.2XX-** Occupant of railway train or railway vehicle injured in collision with or hit by rolling stock

7 **V81.3XX-** Occupant of railway train or railway vehicle injured in collision with other object
Railway collision NOS

7 **V81.4XX-** Person injured while boarding or alighting from railway train or railway vehicle

7 **V81.5XX-** Occupant of railway train or railway vehicle injured by fall in railway train or railway vehicle

7 **V81.6XX-** Occupant of railway train or railway vehicle injured by fall from railway train or railway vehicle

7 **V81.7XX-** Occupant of railway train or railway vehicle injured in derailment without antecedent collision

5 **V81.8** Occupant of railway train or railway vehicle injured in other specified railway accidents

7 **V81.81X-** Occupant of railway train or railway vehicle injured due to explosion or fire on train

7 **V81.82X-** Occupant of railway train or railway vehicle injured due to object falling onto train
Occupant of railway train or railway vehicle injured due to falling earth onto train
Occupant of railway train or railway vehicle injured due to falling rocks onto train
Occupant of railway train or railway vehicle injured due to falling snow onto train
Occupant of railway train or railway vehicle injured due to falling trees onto train

7 **V81.83X-** Occupant of railway train or railway vehicle injured due to collision with military vehicle

7 **V81.89X-** Occupant of railway train or railway vehicle injured due to other specified railway accident

7 **V81.9XX-** Occupant of railway train or railway vehicle injured in unspecified railway accident
Railway accident NOS

4 **V82** Occupant of powered streetcar injured in transport accident

INCLUDES interurban electric car
person on outside of streetcar
tram (car)
trolley (car)

EXCLUDES 1 *bus (V70-V79)*
motorcoach (V70-V79)
nonpowered streetcar (V76.-)
train (V81.-)

The appropriate 7th character is to be added to each code from category V82
A initial encounter
D subsequent encounter
S sequela

7 **V82.0XX-** Occupant of streetcar injured in collision with motor vehicle in nontraffic accident

7 **V82.1XX-** Occupant of streetcar injured in collision with motor vehicle in traffic accident

7 **V82.2XX-** Occupant of streetcar injured in collision with or hit by rolling stock

7 **V82.3XX-** Occupant of streetcar injured in collision with other object

EXCLUDES 1 *collision with animal-drawn vehicle or animal being ridden (V82.8)*

7 **V82.4XX-** Person injured while boarding or alighting from streetcar

7 **V82.5XX-** Occupant of streetcar injured by fall in streetcar

EXCLUDES 1 *fall in streetcar:*
while boarding or alighting (V82.4)
with antecedent collision (V82.0-V82.3)

7 **V82.6XX-** Occupant of streetcar injured by fall from streetcar

EXCLUDES 1 *fall from streetcar:*
while boarding or alighting (V82.4)
with antecedent collision (V82.0-V82.3)

7 **V82.7XX-** Occupant of streetcar injured in derailment without antecedent collision

EXCLUDES 1 *occupant of streetcar injured in derailment with antecedent collision (V82.0-V82.3)*

● New ▲ Revised *Manifestation* 4-7 Digit Indicators ⊟ Laterality A Adult (15+ years) M Maternity (12-55 years) N Newborn P Pediatric (0-17 years) ♂ Male ♀ Female
✖ Deleted Unspecified + Additional code

2017 ICD-10-CM Expert for Physicians

© 2017 DecisionHealth

1133

4 V82.8XX-   **Occupant of streetcar injured in other specified transport accidents**
    Streetcar collision with military vehicle
    Streetcar collision with train or nonmotor vehicles

7 V82.9XX-   **Occupant of streetcar injured in unspecified traffic accident**
    Streetcar accident NOS

4 V83   **Occupant of special vehicle mainly used on industrial premises injured in transport accident**

> **INCLUDES**   battery-powered airport passenger vehicle
> battery-powered truck (baggage) (mail)
> coal-car in mine
> forklift (truck)
> logging car
> self-propelled industrial truck
> station baggage truck (powered)
> tram, truck, or tub (powered) in mine or quarry

> **EXCLUDES 1**   *special construction vehicles (V85.-)*
> *special industrial vehicle in stationary use or maintenance (W31.-)*

The appropriate 7th character is to be added to each code from category V83
A   initial encounter
D   subsequent encounter
S   sequela

7 V83.0XX-   **Driver of special industrial vehicle injured in traffic accident**

7 V83.1XX-   **Passenger of special industrial vehicle injured in traffic accident**

7 V83.2XX-   **Person on outside of special industrial vehicle injured in traffic accident**

7 V83.3XX-   **Unspecified occupant of special industrial vehicle injured in traffic accident**

7 V83.4XX-   **Person injured while boarding or alighting from special industrial vehicle**

7 V83.5XX-   **Driver of special industrial vehicle injured in nontraffic accident**

7 V83.6XX-   **Passenger of special industrial vehicle injured in nontraffic accident**

7 V83.7XX-   **Person on outside of special industrial vehicle injured in nontraffic accident**

7 V83.9XX-   **Unspecified occupant of special industrial vehicle injured in nontraffic accident**
    Special-industrial-vehicle accident NOS

4 V84   **Occupant of special vehicle mainly used in agriculture injured in transport accident**

> **INCLUDES**   self-propelled farm machinery
> tractor (and trailer)

> **EXCLUDES 1**   *animal-powered farm machinery accident (W30.8-)*
> *contact with combine harvester (W30.0)*
> *special agricultural vehicle in stationary use or maintenance (W30.-)*

The appropriate 7th character is to be added to each code from category V84
A   initial encounter
D   subsequent encounter
S   sequela

7 V84.0XX-   **Driver of special agricultural vehicle injured in traffic accident**

7 V84.1XX-   **Passenger of special agricultural vehicle injured in traffic accident**

7 V84.2XX-   **Person on outside of special agricultural vehicle injured in traffic accident**

7 V84.3XX-   **Unspecified occupant of special agricultural vehicle injured in traffic accident**

7 V84.4XX-   **Person injured while boarding or alighting from special agricultural vehicle**

7 V84.5XX-   **Driver of special agricultural vehicle injured in nontraffic accident**

7 V84.6XX-   **Passenger of special agricultural vehicle injured in nontraffic accident**

7 V84.7XX-   **Person on outside of special agricultural vehicle injured in nontraffic accident**

7 V84.9XX-   **Unspecified occupant of special agricultural vehicle injured in nontraffic accident**
    Special-agricultural vehicle accident NOS

4 V85   **Occupant of special construction vehicle injured in transport accident**

> **INCLUDES**   bulldozer
> digger
> dump truck
> earth-leveller
> mechanical shovel
> road-roller

> **EXCLUDES 1**   *special industrial vehicle (V83.-)*
> *special construction vehicle in stationary use or maintenance (W31.-)*

The appropriate 7th character is to be added to each code from category V85
A   initial encounter
D   subsequent encounter
S   sequela

7 V85.0XX-   **Driver of special construction vehicle injured in traffic accident**

7 V85.1XX-   **Passenger of special construction vehicle injured in traffic accident**

7 V85.2XX-   **Person on outside of special construction vehicle injured in traffic accident**

7 V85.3XX-   **Unspecified occupant of special construction vehicle injured in traffic accident**

7 V85.4XX-   **Person injured while boarding or alighting from special construction vehicle**

7 V85.5XX-   **Driver of special construction vehicle injured in nontraffic accident**

7 V85.6XX-   **Passenger of special construction vehicle injured in nontraffic accident**

7 V85.7XX-   **Person on outside of special construction vehicle injured in nontraffic accident**

7 V85.9XX-   **Unspecified occupant of special construction vehicle injured in nontraffic accident**
    Special-construction-vehicle accident NOS

4 V86   **Occupant of special all-terrain or other off-road motor vehicle, injured in transport accident**

> **EXCLUDES 1**   *special all-terrain vehicle in stationary use or maintenance (W31.-)*
> *sport-utility vehicle (V50-V59)*
> *three-wheeled motor vehicle designed for on-road use (V30-V39)*

The appropriate 7th character is to be added to each code from category V86
A   initial encounter
D   subsequent encounter
S   sequela

5 V86.0   **Driver of special all-terrain or other off-road motor vehicle injured in traffic accident**

7 V86.01X-   **Driver of ambulance or fire engine injured in traffic accident**

7 V86.02X-   **Driver of snowmobile injured in traffic accident**

7 V86.03X-   **Driver of dune buggy injured in traffic accident**

7 V86.04X-   **Driver of military vehicle injured in traffic accident**

7 V86.09X-   **Driver of other special all-terrain or other off-road motor vehicle injured in traffic accident**
    Driver of dirt bike injured in traffic accident
    Driver of go cart injured in traffic accident
    Driver of golf cart injured in traffic accident

5 V86.1   **Passenger of special all-terrain or other off-road motor vehicle injured in traffic accident**

7 V86.11X-   **Passenger of ambulance or fire engine injured in traffic accident**

7 V86.12X-   **Passenger of snowmobile injured in traffic accident**

7 V86.13X-   **Passenger of dune buggy injured in traffic accident**

7 V86.14X-   **Passenger of military vehicle injured in traffic accident**

7 V86.19X-   **Passenger of other special all-terrain or other off-road motor vehicle injured in traffic accident**
    Passenger of dirt bike injured in traffic accident
    Passenger of go cart injured in traffic accident
    Passenger of golf cart injured in traffic accident

5 V86.2   **Person on outside of special all-terrain or other off-road motor vehicle injured in traffic accident**

7 V86.21X-   **Person on outside of ambulance or fire engine injured in traffic accident**

● New   ▲ Revised   *Manifestation*   4-7 Digit Indicators   ⊟ Laterality   A Adult (15+ years)   M Maternity (12-55 years)   N Newborn   P Pediatric (0-17 years)   ♂ Male   ♀ Female
✖ Deleted   Unspecified   + Additional code

1134   © 2017 DecisionHealth   2017 ICD-10-CM Expert for Physicians

7 V86.22X- Person on outside of snowmobile injured in traffic accident

7 V86.23X- Person on outside of dune buggy injured in traffic accident

7 V86.24X- Person on outside of military vehicle injured in traffic accident

7 V86.29X- Person on outside of other special all-terrain or other off-road motor vehicle injured in traffic accident

Person on outside of dirt bike injured in traffic accident

Person on outside of go cart in traffic accident

Person on outside of golf cart injured in traffic accident

5 V86.3 Unspecified occupant of special all-terrain or other off-road motor vehicle injured in traffic accident

7 V86.31X- Unspecified occupant of ambulance or fire engine injured in traffic accident

7 V86.32X- Unspecified occupant of snowmobile injured in traffic accident

7 V86.33X- Unspecified occupant of dune buggy injured in traffic accident

7 V86.34X- Unspecified occupant of military vehicle injured in traffic accident

7 V86.39X- Unspecified occupant of other special all-terrain or other off-road motor vehicle injured in traffic accident

Unspecified occupant of dirt bike injured in traffic accident

Unspecified occupant of go cart injured in traffic accident

Unspecified occupant of golf cart injured in traffic accident

5 V86.4 Person injured while boarding or alighting from special all-terrain or other off-road motor vehicle

7 V86.41X- Person injured while boarding or alighting from ambulance or fire engine

7 V86.42X- Person injured while boarding or alighting from snowmobile

7 V86.43X- Person injured while boarding or alighting from dune buggy

7 V86.44X- Person injured while boarding or alighting from military vehicle

7 V86.49X- Person injured while boarding or alighting from other special all-terrain or other off-road motor vehicle

Person injured while boarding or alighting from dirt bike

Person injured while boarding or alighting from go cart

Person injured while boarding or alighting from golf cart

5 V86.5 Driver of special all-terrain or other off-road motor vehicle injured in nontraffic accident

7 V86.51X- Driver of ambulance or fire engine injured in nontraffic accident

7 V86.52X- Driver of snowmobile injured in nontraffic accident

7 V86.53X- Driver of dune buggy injured in nontraffic accident

7 V86.54X- Driver of military vehicle injured in nontraffic accident

7 V86.59X- Driver of other special all-terrain or other off-road motor vehicle injured in nontraffic accident

Driver of dirt bike injured in nontraffic accident

Driver of go cart injured in nontraffic accident

Driver of golf cart injured in nontraffic accident

5 V86.6 Passenger of special all-terrain or other off-road motor vehicle injured in nontraffic accident

7 V86.61X- Passenger of ambulance or fire engine injured in nontraffic accident

7 V86.62X- Passenger of snowmobile injured in nontraffic accident

7 V86.63X- Passenger of dune buggy injured in nontraffic accident

7 V86.64X- Passenger of military vehicle injured in nontraffic accident

7 V86.69X- Passenger of other special all-terrain or other off-road motor vehicle injured in nontraffic accident

Passenger of dirt bike injured in nontraffic accident

Passenger of go cart injured in nontraffic accident

Passenger of golf cart injured in nontraffic accident

5 V86.7 Person on outside of special all-terrain or other off-road motor vehicle injured in nontraffic accident

7 V86.71X- Person on outside of ambulance or fire engine injured in nontraffic accident

7 V86.72X- Person on outside of snowmobile injured in nontraffic accident

7 V86.73X- Person on outside of dune buggy injured in nontraffic accident

7 V86.74X- Person on outside of military vehicle injured in nontraffic accident

7 V86.79X- Person on outside of other special all-terrain or other off-road motor vehicles injured in nontraffic accident

Person on outside of dirt bike injured in nontraffic accident

Person on outside of go cart injured in nontraffic accident

Person on outside of golf cart injured in nontraffic accident

5 V86.9 Unspecified occupant of special all-terrain or other off-road motor vehicle injured in nontraffic accident

7 V86.91X- Unspecified occupant of ambulance or fire engine injured in nontraffic accident

7 V86.92X- Unspecified occupant of snowmobile injured in nontraffic accident

7 V86.93X- Unspecified occupant of dune buggy injured in nontraffic accident

7 V86.94X- Unspecified occupant of military vehicle injured in nontraffic accident

7 V86.99X- Unspecified occupant of other special all-terrain or other off-road motor vehicle injured in nontraffic accident

All-terrain motor-vehicle accident NOS

Off-road motor-vehicle accident NOS

Other motor-vehicle accident NOS

Unspecified occupant of dirt bike injured in nontraffic accident

Unspecified occupant of go cart injured in nontraffic accident

Unspecified occupant of golf cart injured in nontraffic accident

4 V87 Traffic accident of specified type but victim's mode of transport unknown

EXCLUDES 1 collision involving:
pedal cycle (V10-V19)
pedestrian (V01-V09)

The appropriate 7th character is to be added to each code from category V87
A initial encounter
D subsequent encounter
S sequela

7 V87.0XX- Person injured in collision between car and two- or three-wheeled powered vehicle (traffic)

7 V87.1XX- Person injured in collision between other motor vehicle and two- or three-wheeled motor vehicle (traffic)

7 V87.2XX- Person injured in collision between car and pick-up truck or van (traffic)

7 V87.3XX- Person injured in collision between car and bus (traffic)

7 V87.4XX- Person injured in collision between car and heavy transport vehicle (traffic)

7 V87.5XX- Person injured in collision between heavy transport vehicle and bus (traffic)

7 V87.6XX- Person injured in collision between railway train or railway vehicle and car (traffic)

7 V87.7XX- Person injured in collision between other specified motor vehicles (traffic)

7 V87.8XX- Person injured in other specified noncollision transport accidents involving motor vehicle (traffic)

7 V87.9XX- Person injured in other specified (collision)(noncollision) transport accidents involving nonmotor vehicle (traffic)

● New   ▲ Revised   *Manifestation*   4 - 7 Digit Indicators   ⊟ Laterality   🅰 Adult (15+ years)   🅼 Maternity (12-55 years)   🅽 Newborn   🅿 Pediatric (0-17 years)   ♂ Male   ♀ Female
✖ Deleted   Unspecified   + Additional code

☑ **V88**   **Nontraffic accident of specified type but victim's mode of transport unknown**

> **EXCLUDES 1**   *collision involving:*
> *pedal cycle (V10-V19)*
> *pedestrian (V01-V09)*

> The appropriate 7th character is to be added to each code from category V88
> A   initial encounter
> D   subsequent encounter
> S   sequela

☑ **V88.0XX-**   **Person injured in collision between car and two- or three-wheeled motor vehicle, nontraffic**

☑ **V88.1XX-**   **Person injured in collision between other motor vehicle and two- or three-wheeled motor vehicle, nontraffic**

☑ **V88.2XX-**   **Person injured in collision between car and pick-up truck or van, nontraffic**

☑ **V88.3XX-**   **Person injured in collision between car and bus, nontraffic**

☑ **V88.4XX-**   **Person injured in collision between car and heavy transport vehicle, nontraffic**

☑ **V88.5XX-**   **Person injured in collision between heavy transport vehicle and bus, nontraffic**

☑ **V88.6XX-**   **Person injured in collision between railway train or railway vehicle and car, nontraffic**

☑ **V88.7XX-**   **Person injured in collision between other specified motor vehicle, nontraffic**

☑ **V88.8XX-**   **Person injured in other specified noncollision transport accidents involving motor vehicle, nontraffic**

☑ **V88.9XX-**   **Person injured in other specified (collision)(noncollision) transport accidents involving nonmotor vehicle, nontraffic**

☑ **V89**   **Motor- or nonmotor-vehicle accident, type of vehicle unspecified**

> The appropriate 7th character is to be added to each code from category V89
> A   initial encounter
> D   subsequent encounter
> S   sequela

☑ **V89.0XX-**   **Person injured in unspecified motor-vehicle accident, nontraffic**

Motor-vehicle accident NOS, nontraffic

☑ **V89.1XX-**   **Person injured in unspecified nonmotor-vehicle accident, nontraffic**

Nonmotor-vehicle accident NOS (nontraffic)

☑ **V89.2XX-**   **Person injured in unspecified motor-vehicle accident, traffic**

Motor-vehicle accident [MVA] NOS
Road (traffic) accident [RTA] NOS

☑ **V89.3XX-**   **Person injured in unspecified nonmotor-vehicle accident, traffic**

Nonmotor-vehicle traffic accident NOS

☑ **V89.9XX-**   **Person injured in unspecified vehicle accident**

Collision NOS

Water transport accidents (V90-V94)

☑ **V90**   **Drowning and submersion due to accident to watercraft**

> **EXCLUDES 1**   *civilian water transport accident involving*
> *military watercraft (V94.81-)*
> *fall into water not from watercraft (W16.-)*
> *military watercraft accident in military or war*
> *operations (Y36.0-, Y37.0-)*
> *water-transport-related drowning or submersion*
> *without accident to watercraft (V92.-)*

> The appropriate 7th character is to be added to each code from category V90
> A   initial encounter
> D   subsequent encounter
> S   sequela

☑ **V90.0**   **Drowning and submersion due to watercraft overturning**

☑ **V90.00X-**   **Drowning and submersion due to merchant ship overturning**

☑ **V90.01X-**   **Drowning and submersion due to passenger ship overturning**

Drowning and submersion due to Ferry-boat overturning
Drowning and submersion due to Liner overturning

☑ **V90.02X-**   **Drowning and submersion due to fishing boat overturning**

☑ **V90.03X-**   **Drowning and submersion due to other powered watercraft overturning**

Drowning and submersion due to Hovercraft (on open water) overturning
Drowning and submersion due to Jet ski overturning

☑ **V90.04X-**   **Drowning and submersion due to sailboat overturning**

☑ **V90.05X-**   **Drowning and submersion due to canoe or kayak overturning**

☑ **V90.06X-**   **Drowning and submersion due to (nonpowered) inflatable craft overturning**

☑ **V90.08X-**   **Drowning and submersion due to other unpowered watercraft overturning**

Drowning and submersion due to windsurfer overturning

☑ **V90.09X-**   **Drowning and submersion due to unspecified watercraft overturning**

Drowning and submersion due to boat NOS overturning
Drowning and submersion due to ship NOS overturning
Drowning and submersion due to watercraft NOS overturning

☑ **V90.1**   **Drowning and submersion due to watercraft sinking**

☑ **V90.10X-**   **Drowning and submersion due to merchant ship sinking**

☑ **V90.11X-**   **Drowning and submersion due to passenger ship sinking**

Drowning and submersion due to Ferry-boat sinking
Drowning and submersion due to Liner sinking

☑ **V90.12X-**   **Drowning and submersion due to fishing boat sinking**

☑ **V90.13X-**   **Drowning and submersion due to other powered watercraft sinking**

Drowning and submersion due to Hovercraft (on open water) sinking
Drowning and submersion due to Jet ski sinking

☑ **V90.14X-**   **Drowning and submersion due to sailboat sinking**

☑ **V90.15X-**   **Drowning and submersion due to canoe or kayak sinking**

☑ **V90.16X-**   **Drowning and submersion due to (nonpowered) inflatable craft sinking**

☑ **V90.18X-**   **Drowning and submersion due to other unpowered watercraft sinking**

☑ **V90.19X-**   **Drowning and submersion due to unspecified watercraft sinking**

Drowning and submersion due to boat NOS sinking
Drowning and submersion due to ship NOS sinking
Drowning and submersion due to watercraft NOS sinking

☑ **V90.2**   **Drowning and submersion due to falling or jumping from burning watercraft**

☑ **V90.20X-**   **Drowning and submersion due to falling or jumping from burning merchant ship**

☑ **V90.21X-**   **Drowning and submersion due to falling or jumping from burning passenger ship**

Drowning and submersion due to falling or jumping from burning Ferry-boat
Drowning and submersion due to falling or jumping from burning Liner

☑ **V90.22X-**   **Drowning and submersion due to falling or jumping from burning fishing boat**

☑ **V90.23X-**   **Drowning and submersion due to falling or jumping from other burning powered watercraft**

Drowning and submersion due to falling and jumping from burning Hovercraft (on open water)
Drowning and submersion due to falling and jumping from burning Jet ski

☑ **V90.24X-**   **Drowning and submersion due to falling or jumping from burning sailboat**

☑ **V90.25X-**   **Drowning and submersion due to falling or jumping from burning canoe or kayak**

☑ **V90.26X-** Drowning and submersion due to falling or jumping from burning (nonpowered) inflatable craft

☑ **V90.27X-** Drowning and submersion due to falling or jumping from burning water-skis

☑ **V90.28X-** Drowning and submersion due to falling or jumping from other burning unpowered watercraft

   Drowning and submersion due to falling and jumping from burning surf-board

   Drowning and submersion due to falling and jumping from burning windsurfer

☑ **V90.29X-** Drowning and submersion due to falling or jumping from unspecified burning watercraft

   Drowning and submersion due to falling or jumping from burning boat NOS

   Drowning and submersion due to falling or jumping from burning ship NOS

   Drowning and submersion due to falling or jumping from burning watercraft NOS

⑤ **V90.3** Drowning and submersion due to falling or jumping from crushed watercraft

☑ **V90.30X-** Drowning and submersion due to falling or jumping from crushed merchant ship

☑ **V90.31X-** Drowning and submersion due to falling or jumping from crushed passenger ship

   Drowning and submersion due to falling and jumping from crushed Ferry boat

   Drowning and submersion due to falling and jumping from crushed Liner

☑ **V90.32X-** Drowning and submersion due to falling or jumping from crushed fishing boat

☑ **V90.33X-** Drowning and submersion due to falling or jumping from other crushed powered watercraft

   Drowning and submersion due to falling and jumping from crushed Hovercraft

   Drowning and submersion due to falling and jumping from crushed Jet ski

☑ **V90.34X-** Drowning and submersion due to falling or jumping from crushed sailboat

☑ **V90.35X-** Drowning and submersion due to falling or jumping from crushed canoe or kayak

☑ **V90.36X-** Drowning and submersion due to falling or jumping from crushed (nonpowered) inflatable craft

☑ **V90.37X-** Drowning and submersion due to falling or jumping from crushed water-skis

☑ **V90.38X-** Drowning and submersion due to falling or jumping from other crushed unpowered watercraft

   Drowning and submersion due to falling and jumping from crushed surf-board

   Drowning and submersion due to falling and jumping from crushed windsurfer

☑ **V90.39X-** Drowning and submersion due to falling or jumping from crushed unspecified watercraft

   Drowning and submersion due to falling and jumping from crushed boat NOS

   Drowning and submersion due to falling and jumping from crushed ship NOS

   Drowning and submersion due to falling and jumping from crushed watercraft NOS

⑤ **V90.8** Drowning and submersion due to other accident to watercraft

☑ **V90.80X-** Drowning and submersion due to other accident to merchant ship

☑ **V90.81X-** Drowning and submersion due to other accident to passenger ship

   Drowning and submersion due to other accident to Ferry-boat

   Drowning and submersion due to other accident to Liner

☑ **V90.82X-** Drowning and submersion due to other accident to fishing boat

☑ **V90.83X-** Drowning and submersion due to other accident to other powered watercraft

   Drowning and submersion due to other accident to Hovercraft (on open water)

   Drowning and submersion due to other accident to Jet ski

☑ **V90.84X-** Drowning and submersion due to other accident to sailboat

☑ **V90.85X-** Drowning and submersion due to other accident to canoe or kayak

☑ **V90.86X-** Drowning and submersion due to other accident to (nonpowered) inflatable craft

☑ **V90.87X-** Drowning and submersion due to other accident to water-skis

☑ **V90.88X-** Drowning and submersion due to other accident to other unpowered watercraft

   Drowning and submersion due to other accident to surf-board

   Drowning and submersion due to other accident to windsurfer

☑ **V90.89X-** Drowning and submersion due to other accident to unspecified watercraft

   Drowning and submersion due to other accident to boat NOS

   Drowning and submersion due to other accident to ship NOS

   Drowning and submersion due to other accident to watercraft NOS

④ **V91** Other injury due to accident to watercraft

   | INCLUDES | any injury except drowning and submersion as a result of an accident to watercraft |

   | EXCLUDES 1 | *civilian water transport accident involving military watercraft (V94.81-)* |
   | | *military watercraft accident in military or war operations (Y36, Y37.-)* |

   | EXCLUDES 2 | *drowning and submersion due to accident to watercraft (V90.-)* |

   The appropriate 7th character is to be added to each code from category V91

   A   initial encounter
   D   subsequent encounter
   S   sequela

⑤ **V91.0** Burn due to watercraft on fire

   | EXCLUDES 1 | *burn from localized fire or explosion on board ship without accident to watercraft (V93.-)* |

☑ **V91.00X-** Burn due to merchant ship on fire

☑ **V91.01X-** Burn due to passenger ship on fire

   Burn due to Ferry-boat on fire
   Burn due to Liner on fire

☑ **V91.02X-** Burn due to fishing boat on fire

☑ **V91.03X-** Burn due to other powered watercraft on fire

   Burn due to Hovercraft (on open water) on fire
   Burn due to Jet ski on fire

☑ **V91.04X-** Burn due to sailboat on fire

☑ **V91.05X-** Burn due to canoe or kayak on fire

☑ **V91.06X-** Burn due to (nonpowered) inflatable craft on fire

☑ **V91.07X-** Burn due to water-skis on fire

☑ **V91.08X-** Burn due to other unpowered watercraft on fire

☑ **V91.09X-** Burn due to unspecified watercraft on fire

   Burn due to boat NOS on fire
   Burn due to ship NOS on fire
   Burn due to watercraft NOS on fire

⑤ **V91.1** Crushed between watercraft and other watercraft or other object due to collision

   Crushed by lifeboat after abandoning ship in a collision
   Note: select the specified type of watercraft that the victim was on at the time of the collision

☑ **V91.10X-** Crushed between merchant ship and other watercraft or other object due to collision

☑ **V91.11X-** Crushed between passenger ship and other watercraft or other object due to collision

   Crushed between Ferry-boat and other watercraft or other object due to collision
   Crushed between Liner and other watercraft or other object due to collision

☑ **V91.12X-** Crushed between fishing boat and other watercraft or other object due to collision

☑ **V91.13X-** Crushed between other powered watercraft and other watercraft or other object due to collision

   Crushed between Hovercraft (on open water) and other watercraft or other object due to collision
   Crushed between Jet ski and other watercraft or other object due to collision

---

● New   ▲ Revised   *Manifestation*   ④-☑ Digit Indicators   ⊟ Laterality   Ⓐ Adult (15+ years)   Ⓜ Maternity (12-55 years)   Ⓝ Newborn   Ⓟ Pediatric (0-17 years)   ♂ Male   ♀ Female

✖ Deleted   Unspecified   + Additional code

2017 ICD-10-CM Expert for Physicians

© 2017 DecisionHealth

1137

7 **V91.14X-** **Crushed between sailboat and other watercraft or other object due to collision**

7 **V91.15X-** **Crushed between canoe or kayak and other watercraft or other object due to collision**

7 **V91.16X-** **Crushed between (nonpowered) inflatable craft and other watercraft or other object due to collision**

7 **V91.18X-** **Crushed between other unpowered watercraft and other watercraft or other object due to collision**

Crushed between surfboard and other watercraft or other object due to collision

Crushed between windsurfer and other watercraft or other object due to collision

7 **V91.19X-** **Crushed between unspecified watercraft and other watercraft or other object due to collision**

Crushed between boat NOS and other watercraft or other object due to collision

Crushed between ship NOS and other watercraft or other object due to collision

Crushed between watercraft NOS and other watercraft or other object due to collision

S **V91.2** **Fall due to collision between watercraft and other watercraft or other object**

Fall while remaining on watercraft after collision

Note: select the specified type of watercraft that the victim was on at the time of the collision

EXCLUDES 1   *crushed between watercraft and other watercraft and other object due to collision (V91.1-)*

drowning and submersion due to falling from crushed watercraft (V90.3-)

7 **V91.20X-** **Fall due to collision between merchant ship and other watercraft or other object**

7 **V91.21X-** **Fall due to collision between passenger ship and other watercraft or other object**

Fall due to collision between Ferry-boat and other watercraft or other object

Fall due to collision between Liner and other watercraft or other object

7 **V91.22X-** **Fall due to collision between fishing boat and other watercraft or other object**

7 **V91.23X-** **Fall due to collision between other powered watercraft and other watercraft or other object**

Fall due to collision between Hovercraft (on open water) and other watercraft or other object

Fall due to collision between Jet ski and other watercraft or other object

7 **V91.24X-** **Fall due to collision between sailboat and other watercraft or other object**

7 **V91.25X-** **Fall due to collision between canoe or kayak and other watercraft or other object**

7 **V91.26X-** **Fall due to collision between (nonpowered) inflatable craft and other watercraft or other object**

7 **V91.29X-** **Fall due to collision between unspecified watercraft and other watercraft or other object**

Fall due to collision between boat NOS and other watercraft or other object

Fall due to collision between ship NOS and other watercraft or other object

Fall due to collision between watercraft NOS and other watercraft or other object

S **V91.3** **Hit or struck by falling object due to accident to watercraft**

Hit or struck by falling object (part of damaged watercraft or other object) after falling or jumping from damaged watercraft

EXCLUDES 2   *drowning or submersion due to fall or jumping from damaged watercraft (V90.2-, V90.3-)*

7 **V91.30X-** **Hit or struck by falling object due to accident to merchant ship**

7 **V91.31X-** **Hit or struck by falling object due to accident to passenger ship**

Hit or struck by falling object due to accident to Ferry-boat

Hit or struck by falling object due to accident to Liner

7 **V91.32X-** **Hit or struck by falling object due to accident to fishing boat**

7 **V91.33X-** **Hit or struck by falling object due to accident to other powered watercraft**

Hit or struck by falling object due to accident to Hovercraft (on open water)

Hit or struck by falling object due to accident to Jet ski

7 **V91.34X-** **Hit or struck by falling object due to accident to sailboat**

7 **V91.35X-** **Hit or struck by falling object due to accident to canoe or kayak**

7 **V91.36X-** **Hit or struck by falling object due to accident to (nonpowered) inflatable craft**

7 **V91.37X-** **Hit or struck by falling object due to accident to water-skis**

Hit by water-skis after jumping off of waterskis

7 **V91.38X-** **Hit or struck by falling object due to accident to other unpowered watercraft**

Hit or struck by surf-board after falling off damaged surf-board

Hit or struck by object after falling off damaged windsurfer

7 **V91.39X-** **Hit or struck by falling object due to accident to unspecified watercraft**

Hit or struck by falling object due to accident to boat NOS

Hit or struck by falling object due to accident to ship NOS

Hit or struck by falling object due to accident to watercraft NOS

S **V91.8** **Other injury due to other accident to watercraft**

7 **V91.80X-** **Other injury due to other accident to merchant ship**

7 **V91.81X-** **Other injury due to other accident to passenger ship**

Other injury due to other accident to Ferry-boat

Other injury due to other accident to Liner

7 **V91.82X-** **Other injury due to other accident to fishing boat**

7 **V91.83X-** **Other injury due to other accident to other powered watercraft**

Other injury due to other accident to Hovercraft (on open water)

Other injury due to other accident to Jet ski

7 **V91.84X-** **Other injury due to other accident to sailboat**

7 **V91.85X-** **Other injury due to other accident to canoe or kayak**

7 **V91.86X-** **Other injury due to other accident to (nonpowered) inflatable craft**

7 **V91.87X-** **Other injury due to other accident to water-skis**

7 **V91.88X-** **Other injury due to other accident to other unpowered watercraft**

Other injury due to other accident to surf-board

Other injury due to other accident to windsurfer

7 **V91.89X-** **Other injury due to other accident to unspecified watercraft**

Other injury due to other accident to boat NOS

Other injury due to other accident to ship NOS

Other injury due to other accident to watercraft NOS

4 **V92** **Drowning and submersion due to accident on board watercraft, without accident to watercraft**

EXCLUDES 1   *civilian water transport accident involving military watercraft (V94.81-)*

drowning or submersion due to accident to watercraft (V90-V91)

drowning or submersion of diver who voluntarily jumps from boat not involved in an accident (W16.711, W16.721)

fall into water without watercraft (W16.-)

military watercraft accident in military or war operations (Y36, Y37)

The appropriate 7th character is to be added to each code from category V92

A   initial encounter

D   subsequent encounter

S   sequela

S **V92.0** **Drowning and submersion due to fall off watercraft**

Drowning and submersion due to fall from gangplank of watercraft

Drowning and submersion due to fall overboard watercraft

EXCLUDES 2   *hitting head on object or bottom of body of water due to fall from watercraft (V94.0-)*

• New   ▲ Revised   *Manifestation*   4- 7 Digit Indicators   ⊟ Laterality   Ⓐ Adult (15+ years)   Ⓜ Maternity (12-55 years)   Ⓝ Newborn   Ⓟ Pediatric (0-17 years)   ♂ Male   ♀ Female

✖ Deleted   Unspecified   ✚ Additional code

1138   © 2017 DecisionHealth   2017 ICD-10-CM Expert for Physicians

V92.00X-   **Drowning and submersion due to fall off merchant ship**

V92.01X-   **Drowning and submersion due to fall off passenger ship**

Drowning and submersion due to fall off Ferry-boat

Drowning and submersion due to fall off Liner

V92.02X-   **Drowning and submersion due to fall off fishing boat**

V92.03X-   **Drowning and submersion due to fall off other powered watercraft**

Drowning and submersion due to fall off Hovercraft (on open water)

Drowning and submersion due to fall off Jet ski

V92.04X-   **Drowning and submersion due to fall off sailboat**

V92.05X-   **Drowning and submersion due to fall off canoe or kayak**

V92.06X-   **Drowning and submersion due to fall off (nonpowered) inflatable craft**

V92.07X-   **Drowning and submersion due to fall off water-skis**

> **EXCLUDES 1**   *drowning and submersion due to falling off burning water-skis (V90.27)*
> *drowning and submersion due to falling off crushed water-skis (V90.37)*
> *hit by boat while water-skiing NOS (V94.X)*

V92.08X-   **Drowning and submersion due to fall off other unpowered watercraft**

Drowning and submersion due to fall off surf-board

Drowning and submersion due to fall off windsurfer

> **EXCLUDES 1**   *drowning and submersion due to fall off burning unpowered watercraft (V90.28)*
> *drowning and submersion due to fall off crushed unpowered watercraft (V90.38)*
> *drowning and submersion due to fall off damaged unpowered watercraft (V90.88)*
> *drowning and submersion due to rider of nonpowered watercraft being hit by other watercraft (V94.-)*
> *other injury due to rider of nonpowered watercraft being hit by other watercraft (V94.-)*

V92.09X-   **Drowning and submersion due to fall off unspecified watercraft**

Drowning and submersion due to fall off boat NOS

Drowning and submersion due to fall off ship NOS

Drowning and submersion due to fall off watercraft NOS

S V92.1   **Drowning and submersion due to being thrown overboard by motion of watercraft**

> **EXCLUDES 1**   *drowning and submersion due to fall off surf-board (V92.08)*
> *drowning and submersion due to fall off water-skis (V92.07)*
> *drowning and submersion due to fall off windsurfer (V92.08)*

V92.10X-   **Drowning and submersion due to being thrown overboard by motion of merchant ship**

V92.11X-   **Drowning and submersion due to being thrown overboard by motion of passenger ship**

Drowning and submersion due to being thrown overboard by motion of Ferry-boat

Drowning and submersion due to being thrown overboard by motion of Liner

V92.12X-   **Drowning and submersion due to being thrown overboard by motion of fishing boat**

V92.13X-   **Drowning and submersion due to being thrown overboard by motion of other powered watercraft**

Drowning and submersion due to being thrown overboard by motion of Hovercraft

V92.14X-   **Drowning and submersion due to being thrown overboard by motion of sailboat**

V92.15X-   **Drowning and submersion due to being thrown overboard by motion of canoe or kayak**

V92.16X-   **Drowning and submersion due to being thrown overboard by motion of (nonpowered) inflatable craft**

V92.19X-   **Drowning and submersion due to being thrown overboard by motion of unspecified watercraft**

Drowning and submersion due to being thrown overboard by motion of boat NOS

Drowning and submersion due to being thrown overboard by motion of ship NOS

Drowning and submersion due to being thrown overboard by motion of watercraft NOS

S V92.2   **Drowning and submersion due to being washed overboard from watercraft**

Code first:

any associated cataclysm (X37.0-)

V92.20X-   **Drowning and submersion due to being washed overboard from merchant ship**

V92.21X-   **Drowning and submersion due to being washed overboard from passenger ship**

Drowning and submersion due to being washed overboard from Ferry-boat

Drowning and submersion due to being washed overboard from Liner

V92.22X-   **Drowning and submersion due to being washed overboard from fishing boat**

V92.23X-   **Drowning and submersion due to being washed overboard from other powered watercraft**

Drowning and submersion due to being washed overboard from Hovercraft (on open water)

Drowning and submersion due to being washed overboard from Jet ski

V92.24X-   **Drowning and submersion due to being washed overboard from sailboat**

V92.25X-   **Drowning and submersion due to being washed overboard from canoe or kayak**

V92.26X-   **Drowning and submersion due to being washed overboard from (nonpowered) inflatable craft**

V92.27X-   **Drowning and submersion due to being washed overboard from water-skis**

> **EXCLUDES 1**   *drowning and submersion due to fall off water-skis (V92.07)*

V92.28X-   **Drowning and submersion due to being washed overboard from other unpowered watercraft**

Drowning and submersion due to being washed overboard from surf-board

Drowning and submersion due to being washed overboard from windsurfer

V92.29X-   **Drowning and submersion due to being washed overboard from unspecified watercraft**

Drowning and submersion due to being washed overboard from boat NOS

Drowning and submersion due to being washed overboard from ship NOS

Drowning and submersion due to being washed overboard from watercraft NOS

V93   **Other injury due to accident on board watercraft, without accident to watercraft**

> **EXCLUDES 1**   *civilian water transport accident involving military watercraft (V94.81-)*
> *other injury due to accident to watercraft (V91.-)*
> *military watercraft accident in military or war operations (Y36, Y37.-)*

> **EXCLUDES 2**   *drowning and submersion due to accident on board watercraft, without accident to watercraft (V92.-)*

The appropriate 7th character is to be added to each code from category V93

A   initial encounter

D   subsequent encounter

S   sequela

S V93.0   **Burn due to localized fire on board watercraft**

> **EXCLUDES 1**   *burn due to watercraft on fire (V91.0-)*

V93.00X-   **Burn due to localized fire on board merchant vessel**

V93.01X-   **Burn due to localized fire on board passenger vessel**

Burn due to localized fire on board Ferry-boat

Burn due to localized fire on board Liner

V93.02X-   **Burn due to localized fire on board fishing boat**

● New   ▲ Revised   *Manifestation*   4-7 Digit Indicators   ▣ Laterality   A Adult (15+ years)   M Maternity (12-55 years)   N Newborn   P Pediatric (0-17 years)   ♂ Male   ♀ Female

✖ Deleted   Unspecified   + Additional code

2017 ICD-10-CM Expert for Physicians   © 2017 DecisionHealth   1139

7 V93.03X- **Burn due to localized fire on board other powered watercraft**
Burn due to localized fire on board Hovercraft
Burn due to localized fire on board Jet ski

7 V93.04X- **Burn due to localized fire on board sailboat**

7 V93.09X- **Burn due to localized fire on board unspecified watercraft**
Burn due to localized fire on board boat NOS
Burn due to localized fire on board ship NOS
Burn due to localized fire on board watercraft NOS

5 V93.1 **Other burn on board watercraft**
Burn due to source other than fire on board watercraft
EXCLUDES 1 *burn due to watercraft on fire (V91.0-)*

7 V93.10X- **Other burn on board merchant vessel**

7 V93.11X- **Other burn on board passenger vessel**
Other burn on board Ferry-boat
Other burn on board Liner

7 V93.12X- **Other burn on board fishing boat**

7 V93.13X- **Other burn on board other powered watercraft**
Other burn on board Hovercraft
Other burn on board Jet ski

7 V93.14X- **Other burn on board sailboat**

7 V93.19X- **Other burn on board unspecified watercraft**
Other burn on board boat NOS
Other burn on board ship NOS
Other burn on board watercraft NOS

5 V93.2 **Heat exposure on board watercraft**
EXCLUDES 1 *exposure to man-made heat not aboard watercraft (W92)*
exposure to natural heat while on board watercraft (X30)
exposure to sunlight while on board watercraft (X32)
EXCLUDES 2 *burn due to fire on board watercraft (V93.0-)*

7 V93.20X- **Heat exposure on board merchant ship**

7 V93.21X- **Heat exposure on board passenger ship**
Heat exposure on board Ferry-boat
Heat exposure on board Liner

7 V93.22X- **Heat exposure on board fishing boat**

7 V93.23X- **Heat exposure on board other powered watercraft**
Heat exposure on board hovercraft

7 V93.24X- **Heat exposure on board sailboat**

7 V93.29X- **Heat exposure on board unspecified watercraft**
Heat exposure on board boat NOS
Heat exposure on board ship NOS
Heat exposure on board watercraft NOS

5 V93.3 **Fall on board watercraft**
EXCLUDES 1 *fall due to collision of watercraft (V91.2-)*

7 V93.30X- **Fall on board merchant ship**

7 V93.31X- **Fall on board passenger ship**
Fall on board Ferry-boat
Fall on board Liner

7 V93.32X- **Fall on board fishing boat**

7 V93.33X- **Fall on board other powered watercraft**
Fall on board Hovercraft (on open water)
Fall on board Jet ski

7 V93.34X- **Fall on board sailboat**

7 V93.35X- **Fall on board canoe or kayak**

7 V93.36X- **Fall on board (nonpowered) inflatable craft**

7 V93.38X- **Fall on board other unpowered watercraft**

7 V93.39X- **Fall on board unspecified watercraft**
Fall on board boat NOS
Fall on board ship NOS
Fall on board watercraft NOS

5 V93.4 **Struck by falling object on board watercraft**
Hit by falling object on board watercraft
EXCLUDES 1 *struck by falling object due to accident to watercraft (V91.3)*

7 V93.40X- **Struck by falling object on merchant ship**

7 V93.41X- **Struck by falling object on passenger ship**
Struck by falling object on Ferry-boat
Struck by falling object on Liner

7 V93.42X- **Struck by falling object on fishing boat**

7 V93.43X- **Struck by falling object on other powered watercraft**
Struck by falling object on Hovercraft

7 V93.44X- **Struck by falling object on sailboat**

7 V93.48X- **Struck by falling object on other unpowered watercraft**

7 V93.49X- **Struck by falling object on unspecified watercraft**

5 V93.5 **Explosion on board watercraft**
Boiler explosion on steamship
EXCLUDES 2 *fire on board watercraft (V93.0-)*

7 V93.50X- **Explosion on board merchant ship**

7 V93.51X- **Explosion on board passenger ship**
Explosion on board Ferry-boat
Explosion on board Liner

7 V93.52X- **Explosion on board fishing boat**

7 V93.53X- **Explosion on board other powered watercraft**
Explosion on board Hovercraft
Explosion on board Jet ski

7 V93.54X- **Explosion on board sailboat**

7 V93.59X- **Explosion on board unspecified watercraft**
Explosion on board boat NOS
Explosion on board ship NOS
Explosion on board watercraft NOS

5 V93.6 **Machinery accident on board watercraft**
EXCLUDES 1 *machinery explosion on board watercraft (V93.4-)*
machinery fire on board watercraft (V93.0-)

7 V93.60X- **Machinery accident on board merchant ship**

7 V93.61X- **Machinery accident on board passenger ship**
Machinery accident on board Ferry-boat
Machinery accident on board Liner

7 V93.62X- **Machinery accident on board fishing boat**

7 V93.63X- **Machinery accident on board other powered watercraft**
Machinery accident on board Hovercraft

7 V93.64X- **Machinery accident on board sailboat**

7 V93.69X- **Machinery accident on board unspecified watercraft**
Machinery accident on board boat NOS
Machinery accident on board ship NOS
Machinery accident on board watercraft NOS

5 V93.8 **Other injury due to other accident on board watercraft**
Accidental poisoning by gases or fumes on watercraft

7 V93.80X- **Other injury due to other accident on board merchant ship**

7 V93.81X- **Other injury due to other accident on board passenger ship**
Other injury due to other accident on board Ferry-boat
Other injury due to other accident on board Liner

7 V93.82X- **Other injury due to other accident on board fishing boat**

7 V93.83X- **Other injury due to other accident on board other powered watercraft**
Other injury due to other accident on board Hovercraft
Other injury due to other accident on board Jet ski

7 V93.84X- **Other injury due to other accident on board sailboat**

7 V93.85X- **Other injury due to other accident on board canoe or kayak**

7 V93.86X- **Other injury due to other accident on board (nonpowered) inflatable craft**

7 V93.87X- **Other injury due to other accident on board water-skis**
Hit or struck by object while waterskiing

7 V93.88X- **Other injury due to other accident on board other unpowered watercraft**
Hit or struck by object while surfing
Hit or struck by object while on board windsurfer

7 V93.89X- **Other injury due to other accident on board unspecified watercraft**
Other injury due to other accident on board boat NOS
Other injury due to other accident on board ship NOS
Other injury due to other accident on board watercraft NOS

● New ▲ Revised *Manifestation* 4-7 Digit Indicators ⊟ Laterality Ⓐ Adult (15+ years) Ⓜ Maternity (12-55 years) Ⓝ Newborn Ⓟ Pediatric (0-17 years) ♂ Male ♀ Female
✖ Deleted Unspecified + Additional code

1140   © 2017 DecisionHealth   2017 ICD-10-CM Expert for Physicians

4 **V94** **Other and unspecified water transport accidents**

EXCLUDES 1 *military watercraft accidents in military or war operations (Y36, Y37)*

The appropriate 7th character is to be added to each code from category V94
A   initial encounter
D   subsequent encounter
S   sequela

7 **V94.0XX-** **Hitting object or bottom of body of water due to fall from watercraft**

EXCLUDES 2 *drowning and submersion due to fall from watercraft (V92.0-)*

5 **V94.1** **Bather struck by watercraft**
Swimmer hit by watercraft

7 **V94.11X-** **Bather struck by powered watercraft**

7 **V94.12X-** **Bather struck by nonpowered watercraft**

5 **V94.2** **Rider of nonpowered watercraft struck by other watercraft**

7 **V94.21X-** **Rider of nonpowered watercraft struck by other nonpowered watercraft**
Canoer hit by other nonpowered watercraft
Surfer hit by other nonpowered watercraft
Windsurfer hit by other nonpowered watercraft

7 **V94.22X-** **Rider of nonpowered watercraft struck by powered watercraft**
Canoer hit by motorboat
Surfer hit by motorboat
Windsurfer hit by motorboat

5 **V94.3** **Injury to rider of (inflatable) watercraft being pulled behind other watercraft**

7 **V94.31X-** **Injury to rider of (inflatable) recreational watercraft being pulled behind other watercraft**
Injury to rider of inner-tube pulled behind motor boat

7 **V94.32X-** **Injury to rider of non-recreational watercraft being pulled behind other watercraft**
Injury to occupant of dingy being pulled behind boat or ship
Injury to occupant of life-raft being pulled behind boat or ship

7 **V94.4XX-** **Injury to barefoot water-skier**
Injury to person being pulled behind boat or ship

5 **V94.8** **Other water transport accident**

6 **V94.81** **Water transport accident involving military watercraft**

7 **V94.810-** **Civilian watercraft involved in water transport accident with military watercraft**
Passenger on civilian watercraft injured due to accident with military watercraft

7 **V94.811-** **Civilian in water injured by military watercraft**

7 **V94.818-** **Other water transport accident involving military watercraft**

7 **V94.89X-** **Other water transport accident**

7 **V94.9XX-** **Unspecified water transport accident**
Water transport accident NOS

Air and space transport accidents (V95-V97)

EXCLUDES 1 *military aircraft accidents in military or war operations (Y36, Y37)*

4 **V95** **Accident to powered aircraft causing injury to occupant**

The appropriate 7th character is to be added to each code from category V95
A   initial encounter
D   subsequent encounter
S   sequela

5 **V95.0** **Helicopter accident injuring occupant**

7 **V95.00X-** **Unspecified helicopter accident injuring occupant**

7 **V95.01X-** **Helicopter crash injuring occupant**

7 **V95.02X-** **Forced landing of helicopter injuring occupant**

7 **V95.03X-** **Helicopter collision injuring occupant**
Helicopter collision with any object, fixed, movable or moving

7 **V95.04X-** **Helicopter fire injuring occupant**

7 **V95.05X-** **Helicopter explosion injuring occupant**

7 **V95.09X-** **Other helicopter accident injuring occupant**

5 **V95.1** **Ultralight, microlight or powered-glider accident injuring occupant**

7 **V95.10X-** **Unspecified ultralight, microlight or powered-glider accident injuring occupant**

7 **V95.11X-** **Ultralight, microlight or powered-glider crash injuring occupant**

7 **V95.12X-** **Forced landing of ultralight, microlight or powered-glider injuring occupant**

7 **V95.13X-** **Ultralight, microlight or powered-glider collision injuring occupant**
Ultralight, microlight or powered-glider collision with any object, fixed, movable or moving

7 **V95.14X-** **Ultralight, microlight or powered-glider fire injuring occupant**

7 **V95.15X-** **Ultralight, microlight or powered-glider explosion injuring occupant**

7 **V95.19X-** **Other ultralight, microlight or powered-glider accident injuring occupant**

5 **V95.2** **Other private fixed-wing aircraft accident injuring occupant**

7 **V95.20X-** **Unspecified accident to other private fixed-wing aircraft, injuring occupant**

7 **V95.21X-** **Other private fixed-wing aircraft crash injuring occupant**

7 **V95.22X-** **Forced landing of other private fixed-wing aircraft injuring occupant**

7 **V95.23X-** **Other private fixed-wing aircraft collision injuring occupant**
Other private fixed-wing aircraft collision with any object, fixed, movable or moving

7 **V95.24X-** **Other private fixed-wing aircraft fire injuring occupant**

7 **V95.25X-** **Other private fixed-wing aircraft explosion injuring occupant**

7 **V95.29X-** **Other accident to other private fixed-wing aircraft injuring occupant**

5 **V95.3** **Commercial fixed-wing aircraft accident injuring occupant**

7 **V95.30X-** **Unspecified accident to commercial fixed-wing aircraft injuring occupant**

7 **V95.31X-** **Commercial fixed-wing aircraft crash injuring occupant**

7 **V95.32X-** **Forced landing of commercial fixed-wing aircraft injuring occupant**

7 **V95.33X-** **Commercial fixed-wing aircraft collision injuring occupant**
Commercial fixed-wing aircraft collision with any object, fixed, movable or moving

7 **V95.34X-** **Commercial fixed-wing aircraft fire injuring occupant**

7 **V95.35X-** **Commercial fixed-wing aircraft explosion injuring occupant**

7 **V95.39X-** **Other accident to commercial fixed-wing aircraft injuring occupant**

5 **V95.4** **Spacecraft accident injuring occupant**

7 **V95.40X-** **Unspecified spacecraft accident injuring occupant**

7 **V95.41X-** **Spacecraft crash injuring occupant**

7 **V95.42X-** **Forced landing of spacecraft injuring occupant**

7 **V95.43X-** **Spacecraft collision injuring occupant**
Spacecraft collision with any object, fixed, moveable or moving

7 **V95.44X-** **Spacecraft fire injuring occupant**

7 **V95.45X-** **Spacecraft explosion injuring occupant**

7 **V95.49X-** **Other spacecraft accident injuring occupant**

7 **V95.8XX-** **Other powered aircraft accidents injuring occupant**

7 **V95.9XX-** **Unspecified aircraft accident injuring occupant**
Aircraft accident NOS
Air transport accident NOS

4 **V96** **Accident to nonpowered aircraft causing injury to occupant**

The appropriate 7th character is to be added to each code from category V96
A   initial encounter
D   subsequent encounter
S   sequela

5 **V96.0** **Balloon accident injuring occupant**

7 **V96.00X-** **Unspecified balloon accident injuring occupant**

● New   ▲ Revised   *Manifestation*   4-7 Digit Indicators   ⊟ Laterality   Ⓐ Adult (15+ years)   Ⓜ Maternity (12-55 years)   Ⓝ Newborn   Ⓟ Pediatric (0-17 years)   ♂ Male   ♀ Female
✖ Deleted   Unspecified   + Additional code

☑ V96.01X- **Balloon crash injuring occupant**

☑ V96.02X- **Forced landing of balloon injuring occupant**

☑ V96.03X- **Balloon collision injuring occupant**
Balloon collision with any object, fixed, moveable or moving

☑ V96.04X- **Balloon fire injuring occupant**

☑ V96.05X- **Balloon explosion injuring occupant**

☑ V96.09X- **Other balloon accident injuring occupant**

☑ V96.1 **Hang-glider accident injuring occupant**

☑ V96.10X- **Unspecified hang-glider accident injuring occupant**

☑ V96.11X- **Hang-glider crash injuring occupant**

☑ V96.12X- **Forced landing of hang-glider injuring occupant**

☑ V96.13X- **Hang-glider collision injuring occupant**
Hang-glider collision with any object, fixed, moveable or moving

☑ V96.14X- **Hang-glider fire injuring occupant**

☑ V96.15X- **Hang-glider explosion injuring occupant**

☑ V96.19X- **Other hang-glider accident injuring occupant**

☑ V96.2 **Glider (nonpowered) accident injuring occupant**

☑ V96.20X- **Unspecified glider (nonpowered) accident injuring occupant**

☑ V96.21X- **Glider (nonpowered) crash injuring occupant**

☑ V96.22X- **Forced landing of glider (nonpowered) injuring occupant**

☑ V96.23X- **Glider (nonpowered) collision injuring occupant**
Glider (nonpowered) collision with any object, fixed, moveable or moving

☑ V96.24X- **Glider (nonpowered) fire injuring occupant**

☑ V96.25X- **Glider (nonpowered) explosion injuring occupant**

☑ V96.29X- **Other glider (nonpowered) accident injuring occupant**

☑ V96.8XX- **Other nonpowered-aircraft accidents injuring occupant**
Kite carrying a person accident injuring occupant

☑ V96.9XX- **Unspecified nonpowered-aircraft accident injuring occupant**
Nonpowered-aircraft accident NOS

☑ V97 **Other specified air transport accidents**

The appropriate 7th character is to be added to each code from category V97
A   initial encounter
D   subsequent encounter
S   sequela

☑ V97.0XX- **Occupant of aircraft injured in other specified air transport accidents**
Fall in, on or from aircraft in air transport accident
EXCLUDES 1   *accident while boarding or alighting aircraft (V97.1)*

☑ V97.1XX- **Person injured while boarding or alighting from aircraft**

☑ V97.2 **Parachutist accident**

☑ V97.21X- **Parachutist entangled in object**
Parachutist landing in tree

☑ V97.22X- **Parachutist injured on landing**

☑ V97.29X- **Other parachutist accident**

☑ V97.3 **Person on ground injured in air transport accident**

☑ V97.31X- **Hit by object falling from aircraft**
Hit by crashing aircraft
Injured by aircraft hitting house
Injured by aircraft hitting car

☑ V97.32X- **Injured by rotating propeller**

☑ V97.33X- **Sucked into jet engine**

☑ V97.39X- **Other injury to person on ground due to air transport accident**

☑ V97.8 **Other air transport accidents, not elsewhere classified**
EXCLUDES 1   *aircraft accident NOS (V95.9)*
exposure to changes in air pressure during ascent or descent (W94.-)

☑ V97.81 **Air transport accident involving military aircraft**

☑ V97.810- **Civilian aircraft involved in air transport accident with military aircraft**
Passenger in civilian aircraft injured due to accident with military aircraft

☑ V97.811- **Civilian injured by military aircraft**

☑ V97.818- **Other air transport accident involving military aircraft**

☑ V97.89X- **Other air transport accidents, not elsewhere classified**
Injury from machinery on aircraft

Other and unspecified transport accidents (V98-V99)

EXCLUDES 1   *vehicle accident, type of vehicle unspecified (V89.-)*

☑ V98 **Other specified transport accidents**

The appropriate 7th character is to be added to each code from category V98
A   initial encounter
D   subsequent encounter
S   sequela

☑ V98.0XX- **Accident to, on or involving cable-car, not on rails**
Caught or dragged by cable-car, not on rails
Fall or jump from cable-car, not on rails
Object thrown from or in cable-car, not on rails

☑ V98.1XX- **Accident to, on or involving land-yacht**

☑ V98.2XX- **Accident to, on or involving ice yacht**

☑ V98.3XX- **Accident to, on or involving ski lift**
Accident to, on or involving ski chair-lift
Accident to, on or involving ski-lift with gondola

☑ V98.8XX- **Other specified transport accidents**

☑ V99.XXX- **Unspecified transport accident**

The appropriate 7th character is to be added to code V99
A   initial encounter
D   subsequent encounter
S   sequela

Other external causes of accidental injury (W00-X58)

Slipping, tripping, stumbling and falls (W00-W19)

EXCLUDES 1   *assault involving a fall (Y01-Y02)*
fall from animal (V80.-)
fall (in) (from) machinery (in operation) (W28-W31)
fall (in) (from) transport vehicle (V01-V99)
intentional self-harm involving a fall (X80-X81)

EXCLUDES 2   *at risk for fall (history of fall) Z91.81*
fall (in) (from) burning building (X00.-)
fall into fire (X00-X04, X08-X09)

☑ W00 **Fall due to ice and snow**
INCLUDES   pedestrian on foot falling (slipping) on ice and snow
EXCLUDES 1   *fall on (from) ice and snow involving pedestrian conveyance (V00.-)*
fall from stairs and steps not due to ice and snow (W10.-)

The appropriate 7th character is to be added to each code from category W00
A   initial encounter
D   subsequent encounter
S   sequela

☑ W00.0XX- **Fall on same level due to ice and snow**
AHA: (W00.0XXD) 2Q 2016, 5

☑ W00.1XX- **Fall from stairs and steps due to ice and snow**

☑ W00.2XX- **Other fall from one level to another due to ice and snow**

☑ W00.9XX- **Unspecified fall due to ice and snow**

● New   ▲ Revised   *Manifestation*   �४-☑ Digit Indicators   ⊟ Laterality   Adult (15+ years)   Maternity (12-55 years)   Newborn   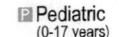 Pediatric (0-17 years)   ♂ Male   ♀ Female

✖ Deleted   + Additional code   Unspecified

1142   © 2017 DecisionHealth

2017 ICD-10-CM Expert for Physicians

V96.01X- — W00.9XX-

④ **W01** **Fall on same level from slipping, tripping and stumbling**

> **INCLUDES** fall on moving sidewalk

> **EXCLUDES 1** *fall due to bumping (striking) against object (W18.0-)*
> *fall in shower or bathtub (W18.2-)*
> *fall on same level NOS (W18.30)*
> *fall on same level from slipping, tripping and stumbling due to ice or snow (W00.0)*
> *fall off or from toilet (W18.1-)*
> *slipping, tripping and stumbling NOS (W18.40)*
> *slipping, tripping and stumbling without falling (W18.4-)*

> The appropriate 7th character is to be added to each code from category W01
> A   initial encounter
> D   subsequent encounter
> S   sequela

⑦ **W01.0XX-** **Fall on same level from slipping, tripping and stumbling without subsequent striking against object**
Falling over animal

⑤ **W01.1** **Fall on same level from slipping, tripping and stumbling with subsequent striking against object**

⑦ **W01.10X-** **Fall on same level from slipping, tripping and stumbling with subsequent striking against unspecified object**

⑥ **W01.11** **Fall on same level from slipping, tripping and stumbling with subsequent striking against sharp object**

⑦ **W01.110-** **Fall on same level from slipping, tripping and stumbling with subsequent striking against sharp glass**

⑦ **W01.111-** **Fall on same level from slipping, tripping and stumbling with subsequent striking against power tool or machine**

⑦ **W01.118-** **Fall on same level from slipping, tripping and stumbling with subsequent striking against other sharp object**

⑦ **W01.119-** **Fall on same level from slipping, tripping and stumbling with subsequent striking against unspecified sharp object**

⑥ **W01.19** **Fall on same level from slipping, tripping and stumbling with subsequent striking against other object**

⑦ **W01.190-** **Fall on same level from slipping, tripping and stumbling with subsequent striking against furniture**

⑦ **W01.198-** **Fall on same level from slipping, tripping and stumbling with subsequent striking against other object**

⑦ **W03.XXX-** **Other fall on same level due to collision with another person**
Fall due to non-transport collision with other person

> **EXCLUDES 1** *collision with another person without fall (W51)*
> *crushed or pushed by a crowd or human stampede (W52)*
> *fall involving pedestrian conveyance (V00-V09)*
> *fall due to ice or snow (W00)*
> *fall on same level NOS (W18.30)*

> The appropriate 7th character is to be added to code W03
> A   initial encounter
> D   subsequent encounter
> S   sequela

> AHA: (WO3.XXXA) 1Q 2015, 9
> AHA: (WO3.XXXA) 4Q 2012, 108
> AHA: (W03.XXXD) 1Q 2015, 10

⑦ **W04.XXX-** **Fall while being carried or supported by other persons**
Accidentally dropped while being carried

> The appropriate 7th character is to be added to code W04
> A   initial encounter
> D   subsequent encounter
> S   sequela

④ **W05** **Fall from non-moving wheelchair, nonmotorized scooter and motorized mobility scooter**

> **EXCLUDES 1** *fall from moving wheelchair (powered) (V00.811)*
> *fall from moving motorized mobility scooter (V00.831)*
> *fall from nonmotorized scooter (V00.141)*

> The appropriate 7th character is to be added to each code from category W05
> A   initial encounter
> D   subsequent encounter
> S   sequela

⑦ **W05.0XX-** **Fall from non-moving wheelchair**
⑦ **W05.1XX-** **Fall from non-moving nonmotorized scooter**
⑦ **W05.2XX-** **Fall from non-moving motorized mobility scooter**

⑦ **W06.XXX-** **Fall from bed**

> The appropriate 7th character is to be added to code W06
> A   initial encounter
> D   subsequent encounter
> S   sequela

⑦ **W07.XXX-** **Fall from chair**

> The appropriate 7th character is to be added to code W07
> A   initial encounter
> D   subsequent encounter
> S   sequela

⑦ **W08.XXX-** **Fall from other furniture**

> The appropriate 7th character is to be added to code W08
> A   initial encounter
> D   subsequent encounter
> S   sequela

④ **W09** **Fall on and from playground equipment**

> **EXCLUDES 1** *fall involving recreational machinery (W31)*

> The appropriate 7th character is to be added to each code from category W09
> A   initial encounter
> D   subsequent encounter
> S   sequela

⑦ **W09.0XX-** **Fall on or from playground slide**
⑦ **W09.1XX-** **Fall from playground swing**
⑦ **W09.2XX-** **Fall on or from jungle gym**
⑦ **W09.8XX-** **Fall on or from other playground equipment**

④ **W10** **Fall on and from stairs and steps**

> **EXCLUDES 1** *Fall from stairs and steps due to ice and snow (W00.1)*

> The appropriate 7th character is to be added to each code from category W10
> A   initial encounter
> D   subsequent encounter
> S   sequela

⑦ **W10.0XX-** **Fall (on)(from) escalator**
⑦ **W10.1XX-** **Fall (on)(from) sidewalk curb**
⑦ **W10.2XX-** **Fall (on)(from) incline**
Fall (on) (from) ramp
⑦ **W10.8XX-** **Fall (on) (from) other stairs and steps**
⑦ **W10.9XX-** **Fall (on) (from) unspecified stairs and steps**

⑦ **W11.XXX-** **Fall on and from ladder**

> The appropriate 7th character is to be added to code W11
> A   initial encounter
> D   subsequent encounter
> S   sequela

⑦ **W12.XXX-** **Fall on and from scaffolding**

> The appropriate 7th character is to be added to code W12
> A   initial encounter
> D   subsequent encounter
> S   sequela

New	▲ Revised							
Deleted	*Manifestation* Unspecified	④-⑦ Digit Indicators + Additional code	▱ Laterality	Ⓐ Adult (15+ years)	Ⓜ Maternity (12-55 years)	Ⓝ Newborn	Ⓟ Pediatric (0-17 years)	♂ Male ♀ Female

2017 ICD-10-CM Expert for Physicians

© 2017 DecisionHealth

1143

W01 — W12.XXX-

☒ **W13**   **Fall from, out of or through building or structure**

The appropriate 7th character is to be added to each code from category W13
A   initial encounter
D   subsequent encounter
S   sequela

☒ **W13.0XX-**   **Fall from, out of or through balcony**
Fall from, out of or through railing

☒ **W13.1XX-**   **Fall from, out of or through bridge**

☒ **W13.2XX-**   **Fall from, out of or through roof**

☒ **W13.3XX-**   **Fall through floor**

☒ **W13.4XX-**   **Fall from, out of or through window**
    EXCLUDES 2   *fall with subsequent striking against sharp glass (W01.110)*

☒ **W13.8XX-**   **Fall from, out of or through other building or structure**
Fall from, out of or through viaduct
Fall from, out of or through wall
Fall from, out of or through flag-pole

☒ **W13.9XX-**   **Fall from, out of or through building, not otherwise specified**
    EXCLUDES 1   *collapse of a building or structure (W20.-)*
fall or jump from burning building or structure (X00.-)

☒ **W14.XXX-**   **Fall from tree**

The appropriate 7th character is to be added to code W14
A   initial encounter
D   subsequent encounter
S   sequela

☒ **W15.XXX-**   **Fall from cliff**

The appropriate 7th character is to be added to code W15
A   initial encounter
D   subsequent encounter
S   sequela

☒ **W16**   **Fall, jump or diving into water**
    EXCLUDES 1   *accidental non-watercraft drowning and submersion not involving fall (W65-W74)*
effects of air pressure from diving (W94.-)
fall into water from watercraft (V90-V94)
hitting an object or against bottom when falling from watercraft (V94.0)
    EXCLUDES 2   *striking or hitting diving board (W21.4)*

The appropriate 7th character is to be added to each code from category W16
A   initial encounter
D   subsequent encounter
S   sequela

☒ **W16.0**   **Fall into swimming pool**
Fall into swimming pool NOS
    EXCLUDES 1   *fall into empty swimming pool (W17.3)*

☒ **W16.01**   **Fall into swimming pool striking water surface**

☒ **W16.011-**   **Fall into swimming pool striking water surface causing drowning and submersion**
    EXCLUDES 1   *drowning and submersion while in swimming pool without fall (W67)*

☒ **W16.012-**   **Fall into swimming pool striking water surface causing other injury**

☒ **W16.02**   **Fall into swimming pool striking bottom**

☒ **W16.021-**   **Fall into swimming pool striking bottom causing drowning and submersion**
    EXCLUDES 1   *drowning and submersion while in swimming pool without fall (W67)*

☒ **W16.022-**   **Fall into swimming pool striking bottom causing other injury**

☒ **W16.03**   **Fall into swimming pool striking wall**

☒ **W16.031-**   **Fall into swimming pool striking wall causing drowning and submersion**
    EXCLUDES 1   *drowning and submersion while in swimming pool without fall (W67)*

☒ **W16.032-**   **Fall into swimming pool striking wall causing other injury**

☒ **W16.1**   **Fall into natural body of water**
Fall into lake
Fall into open sea
Fall into river
Fall into stream

☒ **W16.11**   **Fall into natural body of water striking water surface**

☒ **W16.111-**   **Fall into natural body of water striking water surface causing drowning and submersion**
    EXCLUDES 1   *drowning and submersion while in natural body of water without fall (W69)*

☒ **W16.112-**   **Fall into natural body of water striking water surface causing other injury**

☒ **W16.12**   **Fall into natural body of water striking bottom**

☒ **W16.121-**   **Fall into natural body of water striking bottom causing drowning and submersion**
    EXCLUDES 1   *drowning and submersion while in natural body of water without fall (W69)*

☒ **W16.122-**   **Fall into natural body of water striking bottom causing other injury**

☒ **W16.13**   **Fall into natural body of water striking side**

☒ **W16.131-**   **Fall into natural body of water striking side causing drowning and submersion**
    EXCLUDES 1   *drowning and submersion while in natural body of water without fall (W69)*

☒ **W16.132-**   **Fall into natural body of water striking side causing other injury**

☒ **W16.2**   **Fall in (into) filled bathtub or bucket of water**

☒ **W16.21**   **Fall in (into) filled bathtub**
    EXCLUDES 1   *fall into empty bathtub (W18.2)*

☒ **W16.211-**   **Fall in (into) filled bathtub causing drowning and submersion**
    EXCLUDES 1   *drowning and submersion while in filled bathtub without fall (W65)*

☒ **W16.212-**   **Fall in (into) filled bathtub causing other injury**

☒ **W16.22**   **Fall in (into) bucket of water**

☒ **W16.221-**   **Fall in (into) bucket of water causing drowning and submersion**

☒ **W16.222-**   **Fall in (into) bucket of water causing other injury**

☒ **W16.3**   **Fall into other water**
Fall into fountain
Fall into reservoir

☒ **W16.31**   **Fall into other water striking water surface**

☒ **W16.311-**   **Fall into other water striking water surface causing drowning and submersion**
    EXCLUDES 1   *drowning and submersion while in other water without fall (W73)*

☒ **W16.312-**   **Fall into other water striking water surface causing other injury**

☒ **W16.32**   **Fall into other water striking bottom**

☒ **W16.321-**   **Fall into other water striking bottom causing drowning and submersion**
    EXCLUDES 1   *drowning and submersion while in other water without fall (W73)*

☒ **W16.322-**   **Fall into other water striking bottom causing other injury**

☒ **W16.33**   **Fall into other water striking wall**

☒ **W16.331-**   **Fall into other water striking wall causing drowning and submersion**
    EXCLUDES 1   *drowning and submersion while in other water without fall (W73)*

☒ **W16.332-**   **Fall into other water striking wall causing other injury**

☒ **W16.4**   **Fall into unspecified water**

☒ **W16.41X-**   **Fall into unspecified water causing drowning and submersion**

☒ **W16.42X-**   **Fall into unspecified water causing other injury**

☒ **W16.5**   **Jumping or diving into swimming pool**

☒ **W16.51**   **Jumping or diving into swimming pool striking water surface**

● New   ▲ Revised   *Manifestation*   �४-☒ Digit Indicators   ▤ Laterality   ▲ Adult (15+ years)   Ⓜ Maternity (12-55 years)   Ⓝ Newborn   Ⓟ Pediatric (0-17 years)   ♂ Male   ♀ Femal

✖ ~~Deleted~~   Unspecified   ✚ Additional code

7 **W16.511-** Jumping or diving into swimming pool striking water surface causing drowning and submersion

> EXCLUDES 1 *drowning and submersion while in swimming pool without jumping or diving (W67)*

7 **W16.512-** Jumping or diving into swimming pool striking water surface causing other injury

6 **W16.52** Jumping or diving into swimming pool striking bottom

7 **W16.521-** Jumping or diving into swimming pool striking bottom causing drowning and submersion

> EXCLUDES 1 *drowning and submersion while in swimming pool without jumping or diving (W67)*

7 **W16.522-** Jumping or diving into swimming pool striking bottom causing other injury

6 **W16.53** Jumping or diving into swimming pool striking wall

7 **W16.531-** Jumping or diving into swimming pool striking wall causing drowning and submersion

> EXCLUDES 1 *drowning and submersion while in swimming pool without jumping or diving (W67)*

7 **W16.532-** Jumping or diving into swimming pool striking wall causing other injury

5 **W16.6** Jumping or diving into natural body of water
Jumping or diving into lake
Jumping or diving into open sea
Jumping or diving into river
Jumping or diving into stream

6 **W16.61** Jumping or diving into natural body of water striking water surface

7 **W16.611-** Jumping or diving into natural body of water striking water surface causing drowning and submersion

> EXCLUDES 1 *drowning and submersion while in natural body of water without jumping or diving (W69)*

7 **W16.612-** Jumping or diving into natural body of water striking water surface causing other injury

6 **W16.62** Jumping or diving into natural body of water striking bottom

7 **W16.621-** Jumping or diving into natural body of water striking bottom causing drowning and submersion

> EXCLUDES 1 *drowning and submersion while in natural body of water without jumping or diving (W69)*

7 **W16.622-** Jumping or diving into natural body of water striking bottom causing other injury

5 **W16.7** Jumping or diving from boat

> EXCLUDES 1 *Fall from boat into water -see watercraft accident (V90-V94)*

6 **W16.71** Jumping or diving from boat striking water surface

7 **W16.711-** Jumping or diving from boat striking water surface causing drowning and submersion

7 **W16.712-** Jumping or diving from boat striking water surface causing other injury

6 **W16.72** Jumping or diving from boat striking bottom

7 **W16.721-** Jumping or diving from boat striking bottom causing drowning and submersion

7 **W16.722-** Jumping or diving from boat striking bottom causing other injury

5 **W16.8** Jumping or diving into other water
Jumping or diving into fountain
Jumping or diving into reservoir

6 **W16.81** Jumping or diving into other water striking water surface

7 **W16.811-** Jumping or diving into other water striking water surface causing drowning and submersion

> EXCLUDES 1 *drowning and submersion while in other water without jumping or diving (W73)*

7 **W16.812-** Jumping or diving into other water striking water surface causing other injury

6 **W16.82** Jumping or diving into other water striking bottom

7 **W16.821-** Jumping or diving into other water striking bottom causing drowning and submersion

> EXCLUDES 1 *drowning and submersion while in other water without jumping or diving (W73)*

7 **W16.822-** Jumping or diving into other water striking bottom causing other injury

6 **W16.83** Jumping or diving into other water striking wall

7 **W16.831-** Jumping or diving into other water striking wall causing drowning and submersion

> EXCLUDES 1 *drowning and submersion while in other water without jumping or diving (W73)*

7 **W16.832-** Jumping or diving into other water striking wall causing other injury

5 **W16.9** Jumping or diving into unspecified water

7 **W16.91X-** Jumping or diving into unspecified water causing drowning and submersion

7 **W16.92X-** Jumping or diving into unspecified water causing other injury

4 **W17** **Other fall from one level to another**

> The appropriate 7th character is to be added to each code from category W17
> A   initial encounter
> D   subsequent encounter
> S   sequela

7 **W17.0XX-** Fall into well

7 **W17.1XX-** Fall into storm drain or manhole

7 **W17.2XX-** Fall into hole
Fall into pit

7 **W17.3XX-** Fall into empty swimming pool

> EXCLUDES 1 *fall into filled swimming pool (W16.0-)*

7 **W17.4XX-** Fall from dock

5 **W17.8** Other fall from one level to another

7 **W17.81X-** Fall down embankment (hill)

7 **W17.82X-** Fall from (out of) grocery cart
Fall due to grocery cart tipping over

7 **W17.89X-** Other fall from one level to another
Fall from cherry picker
Fall from lifting device
Fall from mobile elevated work platform [MEWP]
Fall from sky lift
AHA: (W17.89XD) 2Q 2015, 6

4 **W18** **Other slipping, tripping and stumbling and falls**

> The appropriate 7th character is to be added to each code from category W18
> A   initial encounter
> D   subsequent encounter
> S   sequela

5 **W18.0** Fall due to bumping against object
Striking against object with subsequent fall

> EXCLUDES 1 *fall on same level due to slipping, tripping, or stumbling with subsequent striking against object (W01.1-)*

7 **W18.00X-** Striking against unspecified object with subsequent fall

7 **W18.01X-** Striking against sports equipment with subsequent fall

7 **W18.02X-** Striking against glass with subsequent fall

7 **W18.09X-** Striking against other object with subsequent fall

5 **W18.1** Fall from or off toilet

7 **W18.11X-** Fall from or off toilet without subsequent striking against object
Fall from (off) toilet NOS

7 **W18.12X-** Fall from or off toilet with subsequent striking against object

7 **W18.2XX-** Fall in (into) shower or empty bathtub

> EXCLUDES 1 *fall in full bathtub causing drowning or submersion (W16.21-)*

5 **W18.3** Other and unspecified fall on same level

7 **W18.30X-** Fall on same level, unspecified

● New   ▲ Revised   *Manifestation*   4 - 7 Digit Indicators   ▤ Laterality   ▨ Adult (15+ years)   ▨ Maternity (12-55 years)   ▨ Newborn   ▣ Pediatric (0-17 years)   ♂ Male   ♀ Female
Deleted   Unspecified   + Additional code

2017 ICD-10-CM Expert for Physicians   © 2017 DecisionHealth   1145

☑ **W18.31X-**   **Fall on same level due to stepping on an object**
Fall on same level due to stepping on an animal
> **EXCLUDES 1**   *slipping, tripping and stumbling without fall due to stepping on animal (W18.41)*

☑ **W18.39X-**   **Other fall on same level**

Ⓢ **W18.4**   **Slipping, tripping and stumbling without falling**
> **EXCLUDES 1**   *collision with another person without fall (W51)*

☑ **W18.40X-**   **Slipping, tripping and stumbling without falling, unspecified**

☑ **W18.41X-**   **Slipping, tripping and stumbling without falling due to stepping on object**
Slipping, tripping and stumbling without falling due to stepping on animal
> **EXCLUDES 1**   *slipping, tripping and stumbling with fall due to stepping on animal (W18.31)*

☑ **W18.42X-**   **Slipping, tripping and stumbling without falling due to stepping into hole or opening**

☑ **W18.43X-**   **Slipping, tripping and stumbling without falling due to stepping from one level to another**

☑ **W18.49X-**   **Other slipping, tripping and stumbling without falling**

☑ **W19.XXX-**   **Unspecified fall**
Accidental fall NOS

The appropriate 7th character is to be added to code W19
A   initial encounter
D   subsequent encounter
S   sequela

AHA: (W19.XXXD) 4Q 2012, 95

Exposure to inanimate mechanical forces (W20-W49)

> **EXCLUDES 1**   *assault (X92-Y09)*
> *contact or collision with animals or persons (W50-W64)*
> *exposure to inanimate mechanical forces involving military or war operations (Y36.-, Y37.-)*
> *intentional self-harm (X71-X83)*

④ **W20**   **Struck by thrown, projected or falling object**
Code first any associated:
    cataclysm (X34-X39)
    lightning strike (T75.00)
> **EXCLUDES 1**   *falling object in machinery accident (W24, W28-W31)*
> *falling object in transport accident (V01-V99)*
> *object set in motion by explosion (W35-W40)*
> *object set in motion by firearm (W32-W34)*
> *struck by thrown sports equipment (W21.-)*

The appropriate 7th character is to be added to each code from category W20
A   initial encounter
D   subsequent encounter
S   sequela

☑ **W20.0XX-**   **Struck by falling object in cave-in**
> **EXCLUDES 2**   *asphyxiation due to cave-in (T71.21)*

☑ **W20.1XX-**   **Struck by object due to collapse of building**
> **EXCLUDES 1**   *struck by object due to collapse of burning building (X00.2, X02.2)*

☑ **W20.8XX-**   **Other cause of strike by thrown, projected or falling object**
> **EXCLUDES 1**   *struck by thrown sports equipment (W21.-)*

④ **W21**   **Striking against or struck by sports equipment**
> **EXCLUDES 1**   *assault with sports equipment (Y08.0-)*
> *striking against or struck by sports equipment with subsequent fall (W18.01)*

The appropriate 7th character is to be added to each code from category W21
A   initial encounter
D   subsequent encounter
S   sequela

Ⓢ **W21.0**   **Struck by hit or thrown ball**
☑ **W21.00X-**   **Struck by hit or thrown ball, unspecified type**
☑ **W21.01X-**   **Struck by football**

☑ **W21.02X-**   **Struck by soccer ball**
☑ **W21.03X-**   **Struck by baseball**
☑ **W21.04X-**   **Struck by golf ball**
☑ **W21.05X-**   **Struck by basketball**
☑ **W21.06X-**   **Struck by volleyball**
☑ **W21.07X-**   **Struck by softball**
☑ **W21.09X-**   **Struck by other hit or thrown ball**

Ⓢ **W21.1**   **Struck by bat, racquet or club**
☑ **W21.11X-**   **Struck by baseball bat**
☑ **W21.12X-**   **Struck by tennis racquet**
☑ **W21.13X-**   **Struck by golf club**
☑ **W21.19X-**   **Struck by other bat, racquet or club**

Ⓢ **W21.2**   **Struck by hockey stick or puck**
Ⓖ **W21.21**   **Struck by hockey stick**
   ☑ **W21.210-**   **Struck by ice hockey stick**
   ☑ **W21.211-**   **Struck by field hockey stick**
Ⓖ **W21.22**   **Struck by hockey puck**
   ☑ **W21.220-**   **Struck by ice hockey puck**
   ☑ **W21.221-**   **Struck by field hockey puck**

Ⓢ **W21.3**   **Struck by sports foot wear**
☑ **W21.31X-**   **Struck by shoe cleats**
Stepped on by shoe cleats
☑ **W21.32X-**   **Struck by skate blades**
Skated over by skate blades
☑ **W21.39X-**   **Struck by other sports foot wear**

☑✚ **W21.4XX-**   **Striking against diving board**
Use additional code for subsequent falling into water, if applicable (W16.-)

Ⓢ **W21.8**   **Striking against or struck by other sports equipment**
☑ **W21.81X-**   **Striking against or struck by football helmet**
☑ **W21.89X-**   **Striking against or struck by other sports equipment**

☑ **W21.9XX-**   **Striking against or struck by unspecified sports equipment**

④ **W22**   **Striking against or struck by other objects**
> **EXCLUDES 1**   *striking against or struck by object with subsequent fall (W18.09)*

The appropriate 7th character is to be added to each code from category W22
A   initial encounter
D   subsequent encounter
S   sequela

Ⓢ **W22.0**   **Striking against stationary object**
> **EXCLUDES 1**   *striking against stationary sports equipment (W21.8)*

☑ **W22.01X-**   **Walked into wall**
☑ **W22.02X-**   **Walked into lamppost**
☑ **W22.03X-**   **Walked into furniture**
Ⓖ **W22.04**   **Striking against wall of swimming pool**
   ☑ **W22.041-**   **Striking against wall of swimming pool causing drowning and submersion**
> **EXCLUDES 1**   *drowning and submersion while swimming without striking against wall (W67)*
   ☑ **W22.042-**   **Striking against wall of swimming pool causing other injury**
☑ **W22.09X-**   **Striking against other stationary object**

Ⓢ **W22.1**   **Striking against or struck by automobile airbag**
☑ **W22.10X-**   **Striking against or struck by unspecified automobile airbag**
☑ **W22.11X-**   **Striking against or struck by driver side automobile airbag**
☑ **W22.12X-**   **Striking against or struck by front passenger side automobile airbag**
☑ **W22.19X-**   **Striking against or struck by other automobile airbag**

☑ **W22.8XX-**   **Striking against or struck by other objects**
Striking against or struck by object NOS
> **EXCLUDES 1**   *struck by thrown, projected or falling object (W20.-)*

● New   ▲ Revised   *Manifestation*   ④-☑ Digit Indicators   ▤ Laterality   Ⓐ Adult (15+ years)   Ⓜ Maternity (12-55 years)   Ⓝ Newborn   Ⓟ Pediatric (0-17 years)   ♂ Male   ♀ Female
✖ Deleted   Unspecified   ✚ Additional code

1146   © 2017 DecisionHealth   2017 ICD-10-CM Expert for Physician

W23   **Caught, crushed, jammed or pinched in or between objects**

> **EXCLUDES 1**   *injury caused by cutting or piercing instruments (W25-W27)*
> *injury caused by firearms malfunction (W32.1, W33.1-, W34.1-)*
> *injury caused by lifting and transmission devices (W24.-)*
> *injury caused by machinery (W28-W31)*
> *injury caused by nonpowered hand tools (W27.-)*
> *injury caused by transport vehicle being used as a means of transportation (V01-V99)*
> *injury caused by struck by thrown, projected or falling object (W20.-)*

The appropriate 7th character is to be added to each code from category W23
A   initial encounter
D   subsequent encounter
S   sequela

W23.0XX-   **Caught, crushed, jammed, or pinched between moving objects**

W23.1XX-   **Caught, crushed, jammed, or pinched between stationary objects**

W24   **Contact with lifting and transmission devices, not elsewhere classified**

> **EXCLUDES 1**   *transport accidents (V01-V99)*

The appropriate 7th character is to be added to each code from category W24
A   initial encounter
D   subsequent encounter
S   sequela

W24.0XX-   **Contact with lifting devices, not elsewhere classified**
Contact with chain hoist
Contact with drive belt
Contact with pulley (block)

W24.1XX-   **Contact with transmission devices, not elsewhere classified**
Contact with transmission belt or cable

▲ W25.XXX-   **Contact with sharp glass**
Code first any associated:
injury due to flying glass from explosion or firearm discharge (W32-W40)
transport accident (V00-V99)

> **EXCLUDES 1**   *fall on same level due to slipping, tripping and stumbling with subsequent striking against sharp glass (W01.10)*
> *striking against sharp glass with subsequent fall (W18.02)*
>
> **EXCLUDES 2**   *glass embedded in skin (W45)*

The appropriate 7th character is to be added to code W25
A   initial encounter
D   subsequent encounter
S   sequela

▲ W26   **Contact with other sharp objects**

> **EXCLUDES 2**   *sharp object (s) embedded in skin (W45)*

The appropriate 7th character is to be added to each code from category W26
A   initial encounter
D   subsequent encounter
S   sequela

W26.0XX-   **Contact with knife**

> **EXCLUDES 1**   *contact with electric knife (W29.1)*

W26.1XX-   **Contact with sword or dagger**

● W26.2XX-   **Contact with edge of stiff paper**
Paper cut

● W26.8XX-   **Contact with other sharp object(s), not elsewhere classified**
Contact with tin can lid

● W26.9XX-   **Contact with unspecified sharp object(s)**

W27   **Contact with nonpowered hand tool**

The appropriate 7th character is to be added to each code from category W27
A   initial encounter
D   subsequent encounter
S   sequela

W27.0XX-   **Contact with workbench tool**
Contact with auger
Contact with axe
Contact with chisel
Contact with handsaw
Contact with screwdriver

W27.1XX-   **Contact with garden tool**
Contact with hoe
Contact with nonpowered lawn mower
Contact with pitchfork
Contact with rake

W27.2XX-   **Contact with scissors**

W27.3XX-   **Contact with needle (sewing)**

> **EXCLUDES 1**   *contact with hypodermic needle (W46.-)*

W27.4XX-   **Contact with kitchen utensil**
Contact with fork
Contact with ice-pick
Contact with can-opener NOS

W27.5XX-   **Contact with paper-cutter**

W27.8XX-   **Contact with other nonpowered hand tool**
Contact with nonpowered sewing machine
Contact with shovel

W28.XXX-   **Contact with powered lawn mower**
Powered lawn mower (commercial) (residential)

> **EXCLUDES 1**   *contact with nonpowered lawn mower (W27.1)*
>
> **EXCLUDES 2**   *exposure to electric current (W86.-)*

The appropriate 7th character is to be added to code W28
A   initial encounter
D   subsequent encounter
S   sequela

W29   **Contact with other powered hand tools and household machinery**

> **EXCLUDES 1**   *contact with commercial machinery (W31.82)*
> *contact with hot household appliance (X15)*
> *contact with nonpowered hand tool (W27.-)*
> *exposure to electric current (W86)*

The appropriate 7th character is to be added to each code from category W29
A   initial encounter
D   subsequent encounter
S   sequela

W29.0XX-   **Contact with powered kitchen appliance**
Contact with blender
Contact with can-opener
Contact with garbage disposal
Contact with mixer

W29.1XX-   **Contact with electric knife**

W29.2XX-   **Contact with other powered household machinery**
Contact with electric fan
Contact with powered dryer (clothes) (powered) (spin)
Contact with washing-machine
Contact with sewing machine

W29.3XX-   **Contact with powered garden and outdoor hand tools and machinery**
Contact with chainsaw
Contact with edger
Contact with garden cultivator (tiller)
Contact with hedge trimmer
Contact with other powered garden tool

> **EXCLUDES 1**   *contact with powered lawn mower (W28)*

W29.4XX-   **Contact with nail gun**

W29.8XX-   **Contact with other powered powered hand tools and household machinery**
Contact with do-it-yourself tool NOS

4 W30 Contact with agricultural machinery
> INCLUDES animal-powered farm machine
>
> EXCLUDES 1 *agricultural transport vehicle accident*
> *(V01-V99)*
> *explosion of grain store (W40.8)*
> *exposure to electric current (W86.-)*

The appropriate 7th character is to be added to each code from category W30
A   initial encounter
D   subsequent encounter
S   sequela

7 W30.0XX-   Contact with combine harvester
Contact with reaper
Contact with thresher

7 W30.1XX-   Contact with power take-off devices (PTO)

7 W30.2XX-   Contact with hay derrick

7 W30.3XX-   Contact with grain storage elevator
> EXCLUDES 1 *explosion of grain store (W40.8)*

5 W30.8   Contact with other specified agricultural machinery

7 W30.81X-   Contact with agricultural transport vehicle in stationary use
Contact with agricultural transport vehicle under repair, not on public roadway
> EXCLUDES 1 *agricultural transport vehicle accident (V01-V99)*

7 W30.89X-   Contact with other specified agricultural machinery

7 W30.9XX-   Contact with unspecified agricultural machinery
Contact with farm machinery NOS

4 W31 Contact with other and unspecified machinery
> EXCLUDES 1 *contact with agricultural machinery (W30.-)*
> *contact with machinery in transport under own power or being towed by a vehicle (V01-V99)*
> *exposure to electric current (W86)*

The appropriate 7th character is to be added to each code from category W31
A   initial encounter
D   subsequent encounter
S   sequela

7 W31.0XX-   Contact with mining and earth-drilling machinery
Contact with bore or drill (land) (seabed)
Contact with shaft hoist
Contact with shaft lift
Contact with undercutter

7 W31.1XX-   Contact with metalworking machines
Contact with abrasive wheel
Contact with forging machine
Contact with lathe
Contact with mechanical shears
Contact with metal drilling machine
Contact with milling machine
Contact with power press
Contact with rolling-mill
Contact with metal sawing machine

7 W31.2XX-   Contact with powered woodworking and forming machines
Contact with band saw
Contact with bench saw
Contact with circular saw
Contact with molding machine
Contact with overhead plane
Contact with powered saw
Contact with radial saw
Contact with sander
> EXCLUDES 1 *nonpowered woodworking tools (W27.0)*

7 W31.3XX-   Contact with prime movers
Contact with gas turbine
Contact with internal combustion engine
Contact with steam engine
Contact with water driven turbine

5 W31.8   Contact with other specified machinery

7 W31.81X-   Contact with recreational machinery
Contact with roller coaster

7 W31.82X-   Contact with other commercial machinery
Contact with commercial electric fan
Contact with commercial kitchen appliances
Contact with commercial powered dryer (clothes) (powered) (spin)
Contact with commercial washing-machine
Contact with commercial sewing machine
> EXCLUDES 1 *contact with household machinery (W29.-)*
> *contact with powered lawn mower (W28)*

7 W31.83X-   Contact with special construction vehicle in stationary use
Contact with special construction vehicle under repair, not on public roadway
> EXCLUDES 1 *special construction vehicle accident (V01-V99)*

7 W31.89X-   Contact with other specified machinery

7 W31.9XX-   Contact with unspecified machinery
Contact with machinery NOS

4 W32 Accidental handgun discharge and malfunction
> INCLUDES accidental discharge and malfunction of gun for single hand use
> accidental discharge and malfunction of pistol
> accidental discharge and malfunction of revolver
> Handgun discharge and malfunction NOS
>
> EXCLUDES 1 *accidental airgun discharge and malfunction (W34.010, W34.110)*
> *accidental BB gun discharge and malfunction (W34.010, W34.110)*
> *accidental pellet gun discharge and malfunction (W34.010, W34.110)*
> *accidental shotgun discharge and malfunction (W33.01, W33.11)*
> *assault by handgun discharge (X93)*
> *handgun discharge involving legal intervention (Y35.0-)*
> *handgun discharge involving military or war operations (Y36.4-)*
> *intentional self-harm by handgun discharge (X72)*
> *Very pistol discharge and malfunction (W34.09, W34.19)*

The appropriate 7th character is to be added to each code from category W32
A   initial encounter
D   subsequent encounter
S   sequela

7 W32.0XX-   Accidental handgun discharge

7 W32.1XX-   Accidental handgun malfunction
Injury due to explosion of handgun (parts)
Injury due to malfunction of mechanism or component of handgun
Injury due to recoil of handgun
Powder burn from handgun

4 W33 Accidental rifle, shotgun and larger firearm discharge and malfunction
> INCLUDES rifle, shotgun and larger firearm discharge and malfunction NOS
>
> EXCLUDES 1 *accidental airgun discharge and malfunction (W34.010, W34.110)*
> *accidental BB gun discharge and malfunction (W34.010, W34.110)*
> *accidental handgun discharge and malfunction (W32.-)*
> *accidental pellet gun discharge and malfunction (W34.010, W34.110)*
> *assault by rifle, shotgun and larger firearm discharge (X94)*
> *firearm discharge involving legal intervention (Y35.0-)*
> *firearm discharge involving military or war operations (Y36.4-)*
> *intentional self-harm by rifle, shotgun and larger firearm discharge (X73)*

The appropriate 7th character is to be added to each code from category W33
A   initial encounter
D   subsequent encounter
S   sequela

● New   ▲ Revised   *Manifestation*   4-7 Digit Indicators   ▤ Laterality   ▲ Adult (15+ years)   Ⓜ Maternity (12-55 years)   Ⓝ Newborn   Ⓟ Pediatric (0-17 years)   ♂ Male   ♀ Female
✖ Deleted   Unspecified   ✛ Additional code

1148   © 2017 DecisionHealth   2017 ICD-10-CM Expert for Physicians

⑤ **W33.0   Accidental rifle, shotgun and larger firearm discharge**
  ⑦ **W33.00X-   Accidental discharge of unspecified larger firearm**
      Discharge of unspecified larger firearm NOS
  ⑦ **W33.01X-   Accidental discharge of shotgun**
      Discharge of shotgun NOS
  ⑦ **W33.02X-   Accidental discharge of hunting rifle**
      Discharge of hunting rifle NOS
  ⑦ **W33.03X-   Accidental discharge of machine gun**
      Discharge of machine gun NOS
  ⑦ **W33.09X-   Accidental discharge of other larger firearm**
      Discharge of other larger firearm NOS
⑤ **W33.1   Accidental rifle, shotgun and larger firearm malfunction**
    Injury due to explosion of rifle, shotgun and larger firearm (parts)
    Injury due to malfunction of mechanism or component of rifle, shotgun and larger firearm
    Injury due to piercing, cutting, crushing or pinching due to (by) slide trigger mechanism, scope or other gun part
    Injury due to recoil of rifle, shotgun and larger firearm
    Powder burn from rifle, shotgun and larger firearm
  ⑦ **W33.10X-   Accidental malfunction of unspecified larger firearm**
      Malfunction of unspecified larger firearm NOS
  ⑦ **W33.11X-   Accidental malfunction of shotgun**
      Malfunction of shotgun NOS
  ⑦ **W33.12X-   Accidental malfunction of hunting rifle**
      Malfunction of hunting rifle NOS
  ⑦ **W33.13X-   Accidental malfunction of machine gun**
      Malfunction of machine gun NOS
  ⑦ **W33.19X-   Accidental malfunction of other larger firearm**
      Malfunction of other larger firearm NOS
④ **W34   Accidental discharge and malfunction from other and unspecified firearms and guns**

  The appropriate 7th character is to be added to each code from category W34
  A   initial encounter
  D   subsequent encounter
  S   sequela

  ⑤ **W34.0   Accidental discharge from other and unspecified firearms and guns**
    ⑦ **W34.00X-   Accidental discharge from unspecified firearms or gun**
        Discharge from firearm NOS
        Gunshot wound NOS
        Shot NOS
        AHA: (W34.00XS) 1Q 2015, 17
    ⑥ **W34.01   Accidental discharge of gas, air or spring-operated guns**
      ⑦ **W34.010-   Accidental discharge of airgun**
          Accidental discharge of BB gun
          Accidental discharge of pellet gun
      ⑦ **W34.011-   Accidental discharge of paintball gun**
          Accidental injury due to paintball discharge
      ⑦ **W34.018-   Accidental discharge of other gas, air or spring-operated gun**
    ⑦ **W34.09X-   Accidental discharge from other specified firearms**
        Accidental discharge from Very pistol [flare]
  ⑤ **W34.1   Accidental malfunction from other and unspecified firearms and guns**
    ⑦ **W34.10X-   Accidental malfunction from unspecified firearms or gun**
        Firearm malfunction NOS
    ⑥ **W34.11   Accidental malfunction of gas, air or spring-operated guns**
      ⑦ **W34.110-   Accidental malfunction of airgun**
          Accidental malfunction of BB gun
          Accidental malfunction of pellet gun
      ⑦ **W34.111-   Accidental malfunction of paintball gun**
          Accidental injury due to paintball gun malfunction
      ⑦ **W34.118-   Accidental malfunction of other gas, air or spring-operated gun**
    ⑦ **W34.19X-   Accidental malfunction from other specified firearms**
        Accidental malfunction from Very pistol [flare]

⑦ **W35.XXX-   Explosion and rupture of boiler**
    EXCLUDES 1   *explosion and rupture of boiler on watercraft (V93.4)*
    The appropriate 7th character is to be added to code W35
    A   initial encounter
    D   subsequent encounter
    S   sequela
④ **W36   Explosion and rupture of gas cylinder**
    The appropriate 7th character is to be added to each code from category W36
    A   initial encounter
    D   subsequent encounter
    S   sequela
  ⑦ **W36.1XX-   Explosion and rupture of aerosol can**
  ⑦ **W36.2XX-   Explosion and rupture of air tank**
  ⑦ **W36.3XX-   Explosion and rupture of pressurized-gas tank**
  ⑦ **W36.8XX-   Explosion and rupture of other gas cylinder**
  ⑦ **W36.9XX-   Explosion and rupture of unspecified gas cylinder**
④ **W37   Explosion and rupture of pressurized tire, pipe or hose**
    The appropriate 7th character is to be added to each code from category W37
    A   initial encounter
    D   subsequent encounter
    S   sequela
  ⑦ **W37.0XX-   Explosion of bicycle tire**
  ⑦ **W37.8XX-   Explosion and rupture of other pressurized tire, pipe or hose**
⑦ **W38.XXX-   Explosion and rupture of other specified pressurized devices**
    The appropriate 7th character is to be added to code W38
    A   initial encounter
    D   subsequent encounter
    S   sequela
⑦ **W39.XXX-   Discharge of firework**
    The appropriate 7th character is to be added to code W39
    A   initial encounter
    D   subsequent encounter
    S   sequela
④ **W40   Explosion of other materials**
    EXCLUDES 1   *assault by explosive material (X96)*
        explosion involving legal intervention (Y35.1-)
        explosion involving military or war operations (Y36.0-, Y36.2-)
        intentional self-harm by explosive material (X75)
    The appropriate 7th character is to be added to each code from category W40
    A   initial encounter
    D   subsequent encounter
    S   sequela
  ⑦ **W40.0XX-   Explosion of blasting material**
      Explosion of blasting cap
      Explosion of detonator
      Explosion of dynamite
      Explosion of explosive (any) used in blasting operations
  ⑦ **W40.1XX-   Explosion of explosive gases**
      Explosion of acetylene
      Explosion of butane
      Explosion of coal gas
      Explosion in mine NOS
      Explosion of explosive gas
      Explosion of fire damp
      Explosion of gasoline fumes
      Explosion of methane
      Explosion of propane
  ⑦ **W40.8XX-   Explosion of other specified explosive materials**
      Explosion in dump NOS
      Explosion in factory NOS
      Explosion in grain store
      Explosion in munitions
      EXCLUDES 1   *explosion involving legal intervention (Y35.1-)*
          explosion involving military or war operations (Y36.0-, Y36.2-)

● New   ▲ Revised   *Manifestation*   ④-⑦ Digit Indicators   ▤ Laterality   Ⓐ Adult (15+ years)   Ⓜ Maternity (12-55 years)   Ⓝ Newborn   Ⓟ Pediatric (0-17 years)   ♂ Male   ♀ Female
✖ Deleted   Unspecified   ✚ Additional code

External Causes of Morbidity

☷ **W40.9XX-**   **Explosion of unspecified explosive materials**
         Explosion NOS

◢ **W42**   **Exposure to noise**

> The appropriate 7th character is to be added to each code from category W42
> A   initial encounter
> D   subsequent encounter
> S   sequela

☷ **W42.0XX-**   **Exposure to supersonic waves**
☷ **W42.9XX-**   **Exposure to other noise**
         Exposure to sound waves NOS

▲ ◢ **W45**   **Foreign body or object entering through skin**

> INCLUDES   foreign body or object embedded in skin
>   nail embedded in skin
> EXCLUDES 2   *contact with hand tools (nonpowered) (powered) (W27-W29)*
>   *contact with other sharp object (s) (W26.-)*
>   *contact with sharp glass (W25.-)*
>   *struck by objects (W20-W22)*

> The appropriate 7th character is to be added to each code from category W45
> A   initial encounter
> D   subsequent encounter
> S   sequela

☷ **W45.0XX-**   **Nail entering through skin**
✖ ~~**W45.1XX-**~~   ~~**Paper entering through skin**~~
✖ ~~**W45.2XX-**~~   ~~**Lid of can entering through skin**~~
☷ **W45.8XX-**   **Other foreign body or object entering through skin**
         Splinter in skin NOS

◢ **W46**   **Contact with hypodermic needle**

> The appropriate 7th character is to be added to each code from category W46
> A   initial encounter
> D   subsequent encounter
> S   sequela

☷ **W46.0XX-**   **Contact with hypodermic needle**
         Hypodermic needle stick NOS
☷ **W46.1XX-**   **Contact with contaminated hypodermic needle**

◢ **W49**   **Exposure to other inanimate mechanical forces**

> INCLUDES   exposure to abnormal gravitational [G] forces
>   exposure to inanimate mechanical forces NEC
> EXCLUDES 1   *exposure to inanimate mechanical forces involving military or war operations (Y36.-, Y37.-)*

> The appropriate 7th character is to be added to each code from category W49
> A   initial encounter
> D   subsequent encounter
> S   sequela

⑤ **W49.0**   **Item causing external constriction**
   ☷ **W49.01X-**   **Hair causing external constriction**
   ☷ **W49.02X-**   **String or thread causing external constriction**
   ☷ **W49.03X-**   **Rubber band causing external constriction**
   ☷ **W49.04X-**   **Ring or other jewelry causing external constriction**
   ☷ **W49.09X-**   **Other specified item causing external constriction**
☷ **W49.9XX-**   **Exposure to other inanimate mechanical forces**

Exposure to animate mechanical forces (W50-W64)

EXCLUDES 1   *Toxic effect of contact with venomous animals and plants (T63.-)*

◢ **W50**   **Accidental hit, strike, kick, twist, bite or scratch by another person**

> INCLUDES   hit, strike, kick, twist, bite, or scratch by another person NOS
> EXCLUDES 1   *assault by bodily force (Y04)*
>   *struck by objects (W20-W22)*

> The appropriate 7th character is to be added to each code from category W50
> A   initial encounter
> D   subsequent encounter
> S   sequela

☷ **W50.0XX-**   **Accidental hit or strike by another person**
         Hit or strike by another person NOS
☷ **W50.1XX-**   **Accidental kick by another person**
         Kick by another person NOS
☷ **W50.2XX-**   **Accidental twist by another person**
         Twist by another person NOS
         AHA: (W50.2XXA) 1Q 2015, 8
         AHA: (W50.2XXD) 1Q 2015, 8
☷ **W50.3XX-**   **Accidental bite by another person**
         Human bite
         Bite by another person NOS
☷ **W50.4XX-**   **Accidental scratch by another person**
         Scratch by another person NOS

☷ **W51.XXX-**   **Accidental striking against or bumped into by another person**

> EXCLUDES 1   *assault by striking against or bumping into by another person (Y04.2)*
>   *fall due to collision with another person (W03)*

> The appropriate 7th character is to be added to code W51
> A   initial encounter
> D   subsequent encounter
> S   sequela

☷ **W52.XXX-**   **Crushed, pushed or stepped on by crowd or human stampede**
         Crushed, pushed or stepped on by crowd or human stampede with or without fall

> The appropriate 7th character is to be added to code W52
> A   initial encounter
> D   subsequent encounter
> S   sequela

◢ **W53**   **Contact with rodent**

> INCLUDES   contact with saliva, feces or urine of rodent

> The appropriate 7th character is to be added to each code from category W53
> A   initial encounter
> D   subsequent encounter
> S   sequela

⑤ **W53.0**   **Contact with mouse**
   ☷ **W53.01X-**   **Bitten by mouse**
   ☷ **W53.09X-**   **Other contact with mouse**
⑤ **W53.1**   **Contact with rat**
   ☷ **W53.11X-**   **Bitten by rat**
   ☷ **W53.19X-**   **Other contact with rat**
⑤ **W53.2**   **Contact with squirrel**
   ☷ **W53.21X-**   **Bitten by squirrel**
   ☷ **W53.29X-**   **Other contact with squirrel**
⑤ **W53.8**   **Contact with other rodent**
   ☷ **W53.81X-**   **Bitten by other rodent**
   ☷ **W53.89X-**   **Other contact with other rodent**

◢ **W54**   **Contact with dog**

> INCLUDES   contact with saliva, feces or urine of dog

> The appropriate 7th character is to be added to each code from category W54
> A   initial encounter
> D   subsequent encounter
> S   sequela

☷ **W54.0XX-**   **Bitten by dog**
☷ **W54.1XX-**   **Struck by dog**
         Knocked over by dog
☷ **W54.8XX-**   **Other contact with dog**

● New   ▲ Revised   *Manifestation*   ◢-☷ Digit Indicators   ⊟ Laterality   Ⓐ Adult (15+ years)   Ⓜ Maternity (12-55 years)   Ⓝ Newborn   Ⓟ Pediatric (0-17 years)   ♂ Male   ♀ Female
✖ Deleted   Unspecified   + Additional code

1150   © 2017 DecisionHealth   2017 ICD-10-CM Expert for Physicians

④ **W55** **Contact with other mammals**

| INCLUDES | contact with saliva, feces or urine of mammal |

| EXCLUDES 1 | *animal being ridden- see transport accidents*
bitten or struck by dog (W54)
bitten or struck by rodent (W53.-)
contact with marine mammals (W56.-) |

The appropriate 7th character is to be added to each code from category W55
A   initial encounter
D   subsequent encounter
S   sequela

⑤ **W55.0** **Contact with cat**
🔟 **W55.01X-** **Bitten by cat**
🔟 **W55.03X-** **Scratched by cat**
🔟 **W55.09X-** **Other contact with cat**

⑤ **W55.1** **Contact with horse**
🔟 **W55.11X-** **Bitten by horse**
🔟 **W55.12X-** **Struck by horse**
🔟 **W55.19X-** **Other contact with horse**

⑤ **W55.2** **Contact with cow**
Contact with bull
🔟 **W55.21X-** **Bitten by cow**
🔟 **W55.22X-** **Struck by cow**
Gored by bull
🔟 **W55.29X-** **Other contact with cow**

⑤ **W55.3** **Contact with other hoof stock**
Contact with goats
Contact with sheep
🔟 **W55.31X-** **Bitten by other hoof stock**
🔟 **W55.32X-** **Struck by other hoof stock**
Gored by goat
Gored by ram
🔟 **W55.39X-** **Other contact with other hoof stock**

⑤ **W55.4** **Contact with pig**
🔟 **W55.41X-** **Bitten by pig**
🔟 **W55.42X-** **Struck by pig**
🔟 **W55.49X-** **Other contact with pig**

⑤ **W55.5** **Contact with raccoon**
🔟 **W55.51X-** **Bitten by raccoon**
🔟 **W55.52X-** **Struck by raccoon**
🔟 **W55.59X-** **Other contact with raccoon**

⑤ **W55.8** **Contact with other mammals**
🔟 **W55.81X-** **Bitten by other mammals**
🔟 **W55.82X-** **Struck by other mammals**
🔟 **W55.89X-** **Other contact with other mammals**

④ **W56** **Contact with nonvenomous marine animal**

| EXCLUDES 1 | *contact with venomous marine animal (T63.-)* |

The appropriate 7th character is to be added to each code from category W56
A   initial encounter
D   subsequent encounter
S   sequela

⑤ **W56.0** **Contact with dolphin**
🔟 **W56.01X-** **Bitten by dolphin**
🔟 **W56.02X-** **Struck by dolphin**
🔟 **W56.09X-** **Other contact with dolphin**

⑤ **W56.1** **Contact with sea lion**
🔟 **W56.11X-** **Bitten by sea lion**
🔟 **W56.12X-** **Struck by sea lion**
🔟 **W56.19X-** **Other contact with sea lion**

⑤ **W56.2** **Contact with orca**
Contact with killer whale
🔟 **W56.21X-** **Bitten by orca**
🔟 **W56.22X-** **Struck by orca**
🔟 **W56.29X-** **Other contact with orca**

⑤ **W56.3** **Contact with other marine mammals**
🔟 **W56.31X-** **Bitten by other marine mammals**
🔟 **W56.32X-** **Struck by other marine mammals**
🔟 **W56.39X-** **Other contact with other marine mammals**

⑤ **W56.4** **Contact with shark**
🔟 **W56.41X-** **Bitten by shark**
🔟 **W56.42X-** **Struck by shark**
🔟 **W56.49X-** **Other contact with shark**

⑤ **W56.5** **Contact with other fish**
🔟 **W56.51X-** **Bitten by other fish**
🔟 **W56.52X-** **Struck by other fish**
🔟 **W56.59X-** **Other contact with other fish**

⑤ **W56.8** **Contact with other nonvenomous marine animals**
🔟 **W56.81X-** **Bitten by other nonvenomous marine animals**
🔟 **W56.82X-** **Struck by other nonvenomous marine animals**
🔟 **W56.89X-** **Other contact with other nonvenomous marine animals**

🔟 **W57.XXX-** **Bitten or stung by nonvenomous insect and other nonvenomous arthropods**

| EXCLUDES 1 | *contact with venomous insects and arthropods (T63.2-, T63.3-, T63.4-)* |

The appropriate 7th character is to be added to code W57
A   initial encounter
D   subsequent encounter
S   sequela

④ **W58** **Contact with crocodile or alligator**

The appropriate 7th character is to be added to each code from category W58
A   initial encounter
D   subsequent encounter
S   sequela

⑤ **W58.0** **Contact with alligator**
🔟 **W58.01X-** **Bitten by alligator**
🔟 **W58.02X-** **Struck by alligator**
🔟 **W58.03X-** **Crushed by alligator**
🔟 **W58.09X-** **Other contact with alligator**

⑤ **W58.1** **Contact with crocodile**
🔟 **W58.11X-** **Bitten by crocodile**
🔟 **W58.12X-** **Struck by crocodile**
🔟 **W58.13X-** **Crushed by crocodile**
🔟 **W58.19X-** **Other contact with crocodile**

④ **W59** **Contact with other nonvenomous reptiles**

| EXCLUDES 1 | *contact with venomous reptile (T63.0-, T63.1-)* |

The appropriate 7th character is to be added to each code from category W59
A   initial encounter
D   subsequent encounter
S   sequela

⑤ **W59.0** **Contact with nonvenomous lizards**
🔟 **W59.01X-** **Bitten by nonvenomous lizards**
🔟 **W59.02X-** **Struck by nonvenomous lizards**
🔟 **W59.09X-** **Other contact with nonvenomous lizards**
Exposure to nonvenomous lizards

⑤ **W59.1** **Contact with nonvenomous snakes**
🔟 **W59.11X-** **Bitten by nonvenomous snake**
🔟 **W59.12X-** **Struck by nonvenomous snake**
🔟 **W59.13X-** **Crushed by nonvenomous snake**
🔟 **W59.19X-** **Other contact with nonvenomous snake**

⑤ **W59.2** **Contact with turtles**

| EXCLUDES 1 | *contact with tortoises (W59.8-)* |

🔟 **W59.21X-** **Bitten by turtle**
🔟 **W59.22X-** **Struck by turtle**
🔟 **W59.29X-** **Other contact with turtle**
Exposure to turtles

⑤ **W59.8** **Contact with other nonvenomous reptiles**
🔟 **W59.81X-** **Bitten by other nonvenomous reptiles**
🔟 **W59.82X-** **Struck by other nonvenomous reptiles**
🔟 **W59.83X-** **Crushed by other nonvenomous reptiles**
🔟 **W59.89X-** **Other contact with other nonvenomous reptiles**

🔟 **W60.XXX-** **Contact with nonvenomous plant thorns and spines and sharp leaves**

| EXCLUDES 1 | *Contact with venomous plants (T63.7-)* |

The appropriate 7th character is to be added to code W60
A   initial encounter
D   subsequent encounter
S   sequela

● New   ▲ Revised   *Manifestation*   ④-🔟 Digit Indicators   ⊟ Laterality   Ⓐ Adult (15+ years)   Ⓜ Maternity (12-55 years)   Ⓝ Newborn   Ⓟ Pediatric (0-17 years)   ♂ Male   ♀ Female
✖ Deleted   Unspecified   + Additional code
2017 ICD-10-CM Expert for Physicians

© 2017 decisionHealth   1151

⬛ **W61**   **Contact with birds (domestic) (wild)**

> **INCLUDES**   contact with excreta of birds

> The appropriate 7th character is to be added to each code from category W61
> A   initial encounter
> D   subsequent encounter
> S   sequela

   ⬛ **W61.0**   **Contact with parrot**
     ⬛ **W61.01X-**   **Bitten by parrot**
     ⬛ **W61.02X-**   **Struck by parrot**
     ⬛ **W61.09X-**   **Other contact with parrot**
          Exposure to parrots
   ⬛ **W61.1**   **Contact with macaw**
     ⬛ **W61.11X-**   **Bitten by macaw**
     ⬛ **W61.12X-**   **Struck by macaw**
     ⬛ **W61.19X-**   **Other contact with macaw**
          Exposure to macaws
   ⬛ **W61.2**   **Contact with other psittacines**
     ⬛ **W61.21X-**   **Bitten by other psittacines**
     ⬛ **W61.22X-**   **Struck by other psittacines**
     ⬛ **W61.29X-**   **Other contact with other psittacines**
          Exposure to other psittacines
   ⬛ **W61.3**   **Contact with chicken**
     ⬛ **W61.32X-**   **Struck by chicken**
     ⬛ **W61.33X-**   **Pecked by chicken**
     ⬛ **W61.39X-**   **Other contact with chicken**
          Exposure to chickens
   ⬛ **W61.4**   **Contact with turkey**
     ⬛ **W61.42X-**   **Struck by turkey**
     ⬛ **W61.43X-**   **Pecked by turkey**
     ⬛ **W61.49X-**   **Other contact with turkey**
   ⬛ **W61.5**   **Contact with goose**
     ⬛ **W61.51X-**   **Bitten by goose**
     ⬛ **W61.52X-**   **Struck by goose**
     ⬛ **W61.59X-**   **Other contact with goose**
   ⬛ **W61.6**   **Contact with duck**
     ⬛ **W61.61X-**   **Bitten by duck**
     ⬛ **W61.62X-**   **Struck by duck**
     ⬛ **W61.69X-**   **Other contact with duck**
   ⬛ **W61.9**   **Contact with other birds**
     ⬛ **W61.91X-**   **Bitten by other birds**
     ⬛ **W61.92X-**   **Struck by other birds**
     ⬛ **W61.99X-**   **Other contact with other birds**
          Contact with bird NOS

⬛ **W62**   **Contact with nonvenomous amphibians**

> **EXCLUDES 1**   contact with venomous amphibians (T63.81-R63.83)

> The appropriate 7th character is to be added to each code from category W62
> A   initial encounter
> D   subsequent encounter
> S   sequela

   ⬛ **W62.0XX-**   **Contact with nonvenomous frogs**
   ⬛ **W62.1XX-**   **Contact with nonvenomous toads**
   ⬛ **W62.9XX-**   **Contact with other nonvenomous amphibians**

⬛ **W64.XXX-**   **Exposure to other animate mechanical forces**

> **INCLUDES**   exposure to nonvenomous animal NOS

> **EXCLUDES 1**   contact with venomous animal (T63.-)

> The appropriate 7th character is to be added to code W64
> A   initial encounter
> D   subsequent encounter
> S   sequela

Accidental non-transport drowning and submersion (W65-W74)

> **EXCLUDES 1**   accidental drowning and submersion due to fall into water (W16.-)
> accidental drowning and submersion due to water transport accident (V90.-, V92.-)

> **EXCLUDES 2**   accidental drowning and submersion due to cataclysm (X34-X39)

⬛ **W65.XXX-**   **Accidental drowning and submersion while in bath-tub**

> **EXCLUDES 1**   accidental drowning and submersion due to fall in (into) bathtub (W16.211)

> The appropriate 7th character is to be added to code W65
> A   initial encounter
> D   subsequent encounter
> S   sequela

⬛ **W67.XXX-**   **Accidental drowning and submersion while in swimming-pool**

> **EXCLUDES 1**   accidental drowning and submersion due to fall into swimming pool (W16.011, W16.021, W16.031)
> accidental drowning and submersion due to striking into wall of swimming pool (W22.041)

> The appropriate 7th character is to be added to code W67
> A   initial encounter
> D   subsequent encounter
> S   sequela

⬛ **W69.XXX-**   **Accidental drowning and submersion while in natural water**

Accidental drowning and submersion while in lake
Accidental drowning and submersion while in open sea
Accidental drowning and submersion while in river
Accidental drowning and submersion while in stream

> **EXCLUDES 1**   accidental drowning and submersion due to fall into natural body of water (W16.111, W16.121, W16.131)

> The appropriate 7th character is to be added to code W69
> A   initial encounter
> D   subsequent encounter
> S   sequela

⬛ **W73.XXX-**   **Other specified cause of accidental non-transport drowning and submersion**

Accidental drowning and submersion while in quenching tank
Accidental drowning and submersion while in reservoir

> **EXCLUDES 1**   accidental drowning and submersion due to fall into other water (W16.311, W16.321, W16.331)

> The appropriate 7th character is to be added to code W73
> A   initial encounter
> D   subsequent encounter
> S   sequela

⬛ **W74.XXX-**   **Unspecified cause of accidental drowning and submersion**

Drowning NOS

> The appropriate 7th character is to be added to code W74
> A   initial encounter
> D   subsequent encounter
> S   sequela

Exposure to electric current, radiation and extreme ambient air temperature and pressure (W85-W99)

> **EXCLUDES 1**   exposure to:
> failure in dosage of radiation or temperature during surgical and medical care (Y63.2-Y63.5)
> lightning (T75.0-)
> natural cold (X31)
> natural heat (X30)
> natural radiation NOS (X39)
> radiological procedure and radiotherapy (Y84.2)
> sunlight (X32)

⬛ **W85.XXX-**   **Exposure to electric transmission lines**

Broken power line

> The appropriate 7th character is to be added to code W85
> A   initial encounter
> D   subsequent encounter
> S   sequela

● New   ▲ Revised   *Manifestation*   ⬛-⬛ Digit Indicators   ▤ Laterality   Ⓐ Adult (15+ years)   Ⓜ Maternity (12-55 years)   Ⓝ Newborn   Ⓟ Pediatric (0-17 years)   ♂ Male   ♀ Female

✖ Deleted   Unspecified   + Additional code

W61 — W85.XXX-

1152   © 2017 DecisionHealth   2017 ICD-10-CM Expert for Physicians

⊡ W86   Exposure to other specified electric current

The appropriate 7th character is to be added to each code from
category W86
A   initial encounter
D   subsequent encounter
S   sequela

☑ W86.0XX-   Exposure to domestic wiring and appliances
**☑ W86.1XX-   Exposure to industrial wiring, appliances and
electrical machinery**
Exposure to conductors
Exposure to control apparatus
Exposure to electrical equipment and machinery
Exposure to transformers
☑ W86.8XX-   Exposure to other electric current
Exposure to wiring and appliances in or on farm (not
farmhouse)
Exposure to wiring and appliances outdoors
Exposure to wiring and appliances in or on public
building
Exposure to wiring and appliances in or on residential
institutions
Exposure to wiring and appliances in or on schools

⊡ W88   Exposure to ionizing radiation
| EXCLUDES 1 | *exposure to sunlight (X32)* |

The appropriate 7th character is to be added to each code from
category W88
A   initial encounter
D   subsequent encounter
S   sequela

☑ W88.0XX-   Exposure to X-rays
☑ W88.1XX-   Exposure to radioactive isotopes
☑ W88.8XX-   Exposure to other ionizing radiation

▲ ⊡ W89   Exposure to man-made visible and ultraviolet light
| INCLUDES | exposure to welding light (arc) |
| EXCLUDES 1 | *exposure to sunlight (X32)* |

The appropriate 7th character is to be added to each code from
category W89
A   initial encounter
D   subsequent encounter
S   sequela

☑ W89.0XX-   Exposure to welding light (arc)
☑ W89.1XX-   Exposure to tanning bed
**☑ W89.8XX-   Exposure to other man-made visible and ultraviolet
light**
**☑ W89.9XX-   Exposure to unspecified man-made visible and
ultraviolet light**

⊡ W90   Exposure to other nonionizing radiation
| EXCLUDES 1 | *exposure to sunlight (X32)* |

The appropriate 7th character is to be added to each code from
category W90
A   initial encounter
D   subsequent encounter
S   sequela

☑ W90.0XX-   Exposure to radiofrequency
☑ W90.1XX-   Exposure to infrared radiation
☑ W90.2XX-   Exposure to laser radiation
☑ W90.8XX-   Exposure to other nonionizing radiation

☑ W92.XXX-   Exposure to excessive heat of man-made origin

The appropriate 7th character is to be added to code W92
A   initial encounter
D   subsequent encounter
S   sequela

⊡ W93   Exposure to excessive cold of man-made origin

The appropriate 7th character is to be added to each code from
category W93
A   initial encounter
D   subsequent encounter
S   sequela

⑤ W93.0   Contact with or inhalation of dry ice
☑ W93.01X-   Contact with dry ice
☑ W93.02X-   Inhalation of dry ice
⑤ W93.1   Contact with or inhalation of liquid air
☑ W93.11X-   Contact with liquid air
Contact with liquid hydrogen
Contact with liquid nitrogen
☑ W93.12X-   Inhalation of liquid air
Inhalation of liquid hydrogen
Inhalation of liquid nitrogen
**☑ W93.2XX-   Prolonged exposure in deep freeze unit or
refrigerator**
**☑ W93.8XX-   Exposure to other excessive cold of man-made
origin**

**⊡ W94   Exposure to high and low air pressure and changes in
air pressure**

The appropriate 7th character is to be added to each code from
category W94
A   initial encounter
D   subsequent encounter
S   sequela

☑ W94.0XX-   Exposure to prolonged high air pressure
⑤ W94.1   Exposure to prolonged low air pressure
**☑ W94.11X-   Exposure to residence or prolonged visit at high
altitude**
☑ W94.12X-   Exposure to other prolonged low air pressure
⑤ W94.2   Exposure to rapid changes in air pressure during ascent
**☑ W94.21X-   Exposure to reduction in atmospheric pressure
while surfacing from deep-water diving**
**☑ W94.22X-   Exposure to reduction in atmospheric pressure
while surfacing from underground**
**☑ W94.23X-   Exposure to sudden change in air pressure in
aircraft during ascent**
**☑ W94.29X-   Exposure to other rapid changes in air pressure
during ascent**
⑤ W94.3   Exposure to rapid changes in air pressure during descent
**☑ W94.31X-   Exposure to sudden change in air pressure in
aircraft during descent**
**☑ W94.32X-   Exposure to high air pressure from rapid descent
in water**
**☑ W94.39X-   Exposure to other rapid changes in air pressure
during descent**

**☑ W99.XXX-   Exposure to other man-made environmental
factors**

The appropriate 7th character is to be added to code W99
A   initial encounter
D   subsequent encounter
S   sequela

Exposure to smoke, fire and flames (X00-X08)

EXCLUDES 1	*arson (X97)*
EXCLUDES 2	*explosions (W35-W40)*
	lightning (T75.0-)
	transport accident (V01-V99)

⊡ X00   Exposure to uncontrolled fire in building or structure
| INCLUDES | conflagration in building or structure |

Code first:
any associated cataclysm
| EXCLUDES 2 | *Exposure to ignition or melting of nightwear
(X05)* |
| | *Exposure to ignition or melting of other clothing
and apparel (X06.-)* |
| | *Exposure to other specified smoke, fire and
flames (X08.-)* |

The appropriate 7th character is to be added to each code from
category X00
A   initial encounter
D   subsequent encounter
S   sequela

**☑ X00.0XX-   Exposure to flames in uncontrolled fire in building
or structure**
AHA: (X00.0XXD) 2Q 2016, 6
AHA: (X00.0XXS) 2Q 2016, 5; 1Q 2015, 19
**☑ X00.1XX-   Exposure to smoke in uncontrolled fire in building
or structure**

● New   ▲ Revised   *Manifestation*   ⊡-☑ Digit Indicators   ⊟ Laterality   🅐 Adult (15+ years)   🅜 Maternity (12-55 years)   🅝 Newborn   🅟 Pediatric (0-17 years)   ♂ Male   ♀ Female
✖ Deleted   Unspecified   + Additional code

7 X00.2XX- **Injury due to collapse of burning building or structure in uncontrolled fire**
> EXCLUDES 1 *injury due to collapse of building not on fire (W20.1)*

7 X00.3XX- **Fall from burning building or structure in uncontrolled fire**

7 X00.4XX- **Hit by object from burning building or structure in uncontrolled fire**

7 X00.5XX- **Jump from burning building or structure in uncontrolled fire**

7 X00.8XX- **Other exposure to uncontrolled fire in building or structure**

4 X01 **Exposure to uncontrolled fire, not in building or structure**
> INCLUDES exposure to forest fire

The appropriate 7th character is to be added to each code from category X01
A initial encounter
D subsequent encounter
S sequela

7 X01.0XX- **Exposure to flames in uncontrolled fire, not in building or structure**

7 X01.1XX- **Exposure to smoke in uncontrolled fire, not in building or structure**

7 X01.3XX- **Fall due to uncontrolled fire, not in building or structure**

7 X01.4XX- **Hit by object due to uncontrolled fire, not in building or structure**

7 X01.8XX- **Other exposure to uncontrolled fire, not in building or structure**

4 X02 **Exposure to controlled fire in building or structure**
> INCLUDES exposure to fire in fireplace
> exposure to fire in stove

The appropriate 7th character is to be added to each code from category X02
A initial encounter
D subsequent encounter
S sequela

7 X02.0XX- **Exposure to flames in controlled fire in building or structure**

7 X02.1XX- **Exposure to smoke in controlled fire in building or structure**

7 X02.2XX- **Injury due to collapse of burning building or structure in controlled fire**
> EXCLUDES 1 *injury due to collapse of building not on fire (W20.1)*

7 X02.3XX- **Fall from burning building or structure in controlled fire**

7 X02.4XX- **Hit by object from burning building or structure in controlled fire**

7 X02.5XX- **Jump from burning building or structure in controlled fire**

7 X02.8XX- **Other exposure to controlled fire in building or structure**

4 X03 **Exposure to controlled fire, not in building or structure**
> INCLUDES exposure to bon fire
> exposure to camp-fire
> exposure to trash fire

The appropriate 7th character is to be added to each code from category X03
A initial encounter
D subsequent encounter
S sequela

7 X03.0XX- **Exposure to flames in controlled fire, not in building or structure**
AHA: (X03.0XXS) 1Q 2015, 19

7 X03.1XX- **Exposure to smoke in controlled fire, not in building or structure**

7 X03.3XX- **Fall due to controlled fire, not in building or structure**

7 X03.4XX- **Hit by object due to controlled fire, not in building or structure**

7 X03.8XX- **Other exposure to controlled fire, not in building or structure**

7 X04.XXX- **Exposure to ignition of highly flammable material**
Exposure to ignition of gasoline
Exposure to ignition of kerosene
Exposure to ignition of petrol
> EXCLUDES 2 *exposure to ignition or melting of nightwear (X05)*
> *exposure to ignition or melting of other clothing and apparel (X06)*

The appropriate 7th character is to be added to code X04
A initial encounter
D subsequent encounter
S sequela

AHA: (X04.XXA) 2Q 2016, 4

7 X05.XXX- **Exposure to ignition or melting of nightwear**
> EXCLUDES 2 *exposure to uncontrolled fire in building or structure (X00.-)*
> *exposure to uncontrolled fire, not in building or structure (X01.-)*
> *exposure to controlled fire in building or structure (X02.-)*
> *exposure to controlled fire, not in building or structure (X03.-)*
> *exposure to ignition of highly flammable materials (X04.-)*

The appropriate 7th character is to be added to code X05
A initial encounter
D subsequent encounter
S sequela

4 X06 **Exposure to ignition or melting of other clothing and apparel**
> EXCLUDES 2 *exposure to uncontrolled fire in building or structure (X00.-)*
> *exposure to uncontrolled fire, not in building or structure (X01.-)*
> *exposure to controlled fire in building or structure (X02.-)*
> *exposure to controlled fire, not in building or structure (X03.-)*
> *exposure to ignition of highly flammable materials (X04.-)*

The appropriate 7th character is to be added to each code from category X06
A initial encounter
D subsequent encounter
S sequela

7 X06.0XX- **Exposure to ignition of plastic jewelry**
7 X06.1XX- **Exposure to melting of plastic jewelry**
7 X06.2XX- **Exposure to ignition of other clothing and apparel**
7 X06.3XX- **Exposure to melting of other clothing and apparel**

4 X08 **Exposure to other specified smoke, fire and flames**

The appropriate 7th character is to be added to each code from category X08
A initial encounter
D subsequent encounter
S sequela

5 X08.0 **Exposure to bed fire**
Exposure to mattress fire
7 X08.00X- **Exposure to bed fire due to unspecified burning material**
7 X08.01X- **Exposure to bed fire due to burning cigarette**
AHA: (X08.01XS) 1Q 2015, 19
7 X08.09X- **Exposure to bed fire due to other burning material**

5 X08.1 **Exposure to sofa fire**
7 X08.10X- **Exposure to sofa fire due to unspecified burning material**
7 X08.11X- **Exposure to sofa fire due to burning cigarette**
7 X08.19X- **Exposure to sofa fire due to other burning material**

5 X08.2 **Exposure to other furniture fire**
7 X08.20X- **Exposure to other furniture fire due to unspecified burning material**

7 X08.21X-   Exposure to other furniture fire due to burning cigarette

7 X08.29X-   Exposure to other furniture fire due to other burning material

7 X08.8XX-   Exposure to other specified smoke, fire and flames

Contact with heat and hot substances (X10-X19)

EXCLUDES 1   *exposure to excessive natural heat (X30)*
exposure to fire and flames (X00-X09)

4 X10   **Contact with hot drinks, food, fats and cooking oils**

The appropriate 7th character is to be added to each code from category X10
A   initial encounter
D   subsequent encounter
S   sequela

7 X10.0XX-   **Contact with hot drinks**
7 X10.1XX-   **Contact with hot food**
7 X10.2XX-   **Contact with fats and cooking oils**

4 X11   **Contact with hot tap-water**

INCLUDES   contact with boiling tap-water
contact with boiling water NOS

EXCLUDES 1   *contact with water heated on stove (X12)*

The appropriate 7th character is to be added to each code from category X11
A   initial encounter
D   subsequent encounter
S   sequela

7 X11.0XX-   **Contact with hot water in bath or tub**

EXCLUDES 1   *contact with running hot water in bath or tub (X11.1)*

7 X11.1XX-   **Contact with running hot water**
Contact with hot water running out of hose
Contact with hot water running out of tap

7 X11.8XX-   **Contact with other hot tap-water**
Contact with hot water in bucket
Contact with hot tap-water NOS

7 X12.XXX-   **Contact with other hot fluids**
Contact with water heated on stove

EXCLUDES 1   *hot (liquid) metals (X18)*

The appropriate 7th character is to be added to code X12
A   initial encounter
D   subsequent encounter
S   sequela

4 X13   **Contact with steam and other hot vapors**

The appropriate 7th character is to be added to each code from category X13
A   initial encounter
D   subsequent encounter
S   sequela

7 X13.0XX-   **Inhalation of steam and other hot vapors**
7 X13.1XX-   **Other contact with steam and other hot vapors**

4 X14   **Contact with hot air and other hot gases**

The appropriate 7th character is to be added to each code from category X14
A   initial encounter
D   subsequent encounter
S   sequela

7 X14.0XX-   **Inhalation of hot air and gases**
7 X14.1XX-   **Other contact with hot air and other hot gases**

4 X15   **Contact with hot household appliances**

EXCLUDES 1   *contact with heating appliances (X16)*
contact with powered household appliances (W29.-)
exposure to controlled fire in building or structure due to household appliance (X02.8)
exposure to household appliances electrical current (W86.0)

The appropriate 7th character is to be added to each code from category X15
A   initial encounter
D   subsequent encounter
S   sequela

7 X15.0XX-   **Contact with hot stove (kitchen)**
7 X15.1XX-   **Contact with hot toaster**
7 X15.2XX-   **Contact with hotplate**
7 X15.3XX-   **Contact with hot saucepan or skillet**
7 X15.8XX-   **Contact with other hot household appliances**
Contact with cooker
Contact with kettle
Contact with light bulbs

7 X16.XXX-   **Contact with hot heating appliances, radiators and pipes**

EXCLUDES 1   *contact with powered appliances (W29.-)*
exposure to controlled fire in building or structure due to appliance (X02.8)
exposure to industrial appliances electrical current (W86.1)

The appropriate 7th character is to be added to code X16
A   initial encounter
D   subsequent encounter
S   sequela

7 X17.XXX-   **Contact with hot engines, machinery and tools**

EXCLUDES 1   *contact with hot heating appliances, radiators and pipes (X16)*
contact with hot household appliances (X15)

The appropriate 7th character is to be added to code X17
A   initial encounter
D   subsequent encounter
S   sequela

7 X18.XXX-   **Contact with other hot metals**
Contact with liquid metal

The appropriate 7th character is to be added to code X18
A   initial encounter
D   subsequent encounter
S   sequela

7 X19.XXX-   **Contact with other heat and hot substances**

EXCLUDES 1   *objects that are not normally hot, e.g., an object made hot by a house fire (X00-X09)*

The appropriate 7th character is to be added to code X19
A   initial encounter
D   subsequent encounter
S   sequela

Exposure to forces of nature (X30-X39)

7 X30.XXX-   **Exposure to excessive natural heat**
Exposure to excessive heat as the cause of sunstroke
Exposure to heat NOS

EXCLUDES 1   *excessive heat of man-made origin (W92)*
exposure to man-made radiation (W89)
exposure to sunlight (X32)
exposure to tanning bed (W89)

The appropriate 7th character is to be added to code X30
A   initial encounter
D   subsequent encounter
S   sequela

● New   ▲ Revised   *Manifestation*   **4**-**7** Digit Indicators   ⊟ Laterality   **A** Adult (15+ years)   **M** Maternity (12-55 years)   **N** Newborn   **P** Pediatric (0-17 years)   ♂ Male   ♀ Female
✖ Deleted   Unspecified   + Additional code

2017 ICD-10-CM Expert for Physicians   © 2017 DecisionHealth   1155

☑ X31.XXX- Exposure to excessive natural cold
Excessive cold as the cause of chilblains NOS
Excessive cold as the cause of immersion foot or hand
Exposure to cold NOS
Exposure to weather conditions
> **EXCLUDES 1** *cold of man-made origin (W93.-)*
> *contact with or inhalation of dry ice (W93.-)*
> *contact with or inhalation of liquefied gas (W93.-)*

The appropriate 7th character is to be added to code X31
A   initial encounter
D   subsequent encounter
S   sequela

▲☑ X32.XXX- Exposure to sunlight
> **EXCLUDES 1** *man-made radiation (tanning bed) (W89)*

The appropriate 7th character is to be added to code X32
A   initial encounter
D   subsequent encounter
S   sequela

☑ X34.XXX- Earthquake
> **EXCLUDES 2** *tidal wave (tsunami) due to earthquake (X37.41)*

The appropriate 7th character is to be added to code X34
A   initial encounter
D   subsequent encounter
S   sequela

☑ X35.XXX- Volcanic eruption
> **EXCLUDES 2** *tidal wave (tsunami) due to volcanic eruption (X37.41)*

The appropriate 7th character is to be added to code X35
A   initial encounter
D   subsequent encounter
S   sequela

☐ X36 Avalanche, landslide and other earth movements
> **INCLUDES** victim of mudslide of cataclysmic nature
> **EXCLUDES 1** *earthquake (X34)*
> **EXCLUDES 2** *transport accident involving collision with avalanche or landslide not in motion (V01-V99)*

The appropriate 7th character is to be added to each code from category X36
A   initial encounter
D   subsequent encounter
S   sequela

☑ X36.0XX- Collapse of dam or man-made structure causing earth movement
☑ X36.1XX- Avalanche, landslide, or mudslide

☐ X37 Cataclysmic storm

The appropriate 7th character is to be added to each code from category X37
A   initial encounter
D   subsequent encounter
S   sequela

☑ X37.0XX- Hurricane
Storm surge
Typhoon
☑ X37.1XX- Tornado
Cyclone
Twister
☑ X37.2XX- Blizzard (snow)(ice)
☑ X37.3XX- Dust storm
☐ X37.4 Tidalwave
☑ X37.41X- Tidal wave due to earthquake or volcanic eruption
Tidal wave NOS
Tsunami
☑ X37.42X- Tidal wave due to storm
☑ X37.43X- Tidal wave due to landslide

☑ X37.8XX- Other cataclysmic storms
Cloudburst
Torrential rain
> **EXCLUDES 2** *flood (X38)*
☑ X37.9XX- Unspecified cataclysmic storm
Storm NOS
> **EXCLUDES 1** *collapse of dam or man-made structure causing earth movement (X39.0)*

☑ X38.XXX- Flood
Flood arising from remote storm
Flood of cataclysmic nature arising from melting snow
Flood resulting directly from storm
> **EXCLUDES 1** *collapse of dam or man-made structure causing earth movement (X39.0)*
> *tidal wave NOS (X37.41)*
> *tidal wave caused by storm (X37.2)*

The appropriate 7th character is to be added to code X38
A   initial encounter
D   subsequent encounter
S   sequela

☐ X39 Exposure to other forces of nature

The appropriate 7th character is to be added to each code from category X39
A   initial encounter
D   subsequent encounter
S   sequela

▲☐ X39.0 Exposure to natural radiation
> **EXCLUDES 1** *contact with and (suspected) exposure to radon and other naturally occuring radiation (Z77.123)*
> *exposure to man-made radiation (W88-W90)*
> *exposure to sunlight (X32)*
☑ X39.01X- Exposure to radon
☑ X39.08X- Exposure to other natural radiation
☑ X39.8XX- Other exposure to forces of nature

Overexertion and strenuous or repetitive movements (X50)

●☐ X50 Overexertion and strenuous or repetitive movements

The appropriate 7th character is to be added to each code from category X50
A   initial encounter
D   subsequent encounter
S   sequela

●☑ X50.0XX- Overexertion from strenuous movement or load
Lifting heavy objects
Lifting weights
●☑ X50.1XX- Overexertion from prolonged static or awkward postures
Prolonged bending
Prolonged kneeling
Prolonged reaching
Prolonged sitting
Prolonged standing
Prolonged twisting
Static bending
Static kneeling
Static reaching
Static sitting
Static standing
Static twisting
●☑ X50.3XX- Overexertion from repetitive movements
Use of hand as hammer
> **EXCLUDES 2** *Overuse from prolonged static or awkward postures (X50.1)*
●☑ X50.9XX- Other and unspecified overexertion or strenuous movements or postures
Contact pressure
Contact stress

Chapter 20: External Causes of Morbidity

Accidental exposure to other specified factors (X52-X58)

7 X52.XXX- **Prolonged stay in weightless environment**
Weightlessness in spacecraft (simulator)

The appropriate 7th character is to be added to code X52
A   initial encounter
D   subsequent encounter
S   sequela

7 X58.XXX- **Exposure to other specified factors**
Accident NOS
Exposure NOS

The appropriate 7th character is to be added to code X58
A   initial encounter
D   subsequent encounter
S   sequela

Intentional self-harm (X71-X83)

Purposely self-inflicted injury
Suicide (attempted)

4 X71 **Intentional self-harm by drowning and submersion**

The appropriate 7th character is to be added to each code from category X71
A   initial encounter
D   subsequent encounter
S   sequela

7 X71.0XX- **Intentional self-harm by drowning and submersion while in bathtub**
7 X71.1XX- **Intentional self-harm by drowning and submersion while in swimming pool**
7 X71.2XX- **Intentional self-harm by drowning and submersion after jump into swimming pool**
7 X71.3XX- **Intentional self-harm by drowning and submersion in natural water**
7 X71.8XX- **Other intentional self-harm by drowning and submersion**
7 X71.9XX- **Intentional self-harm by drowning and submersion, unspecified**

7 X72.XXX- **Intentional self-harm by handgun discharge**
Intentional self-harm by gun for single hand use
Intentional self-harm by pistol
Intentional self-harm by revolver
    EXCLUDES 1   *Very pistol (X74.8)*

The appropriate 7th character is to be added to code X72
A   initial encounter
D   subsequent encounter
S   sequela

4 X73 **Intentional self-harm by rifle, shotgun and larger firearm discharge**
    EXCLUDES 1   *airgun (X74.01)*

The appropriate 7th character is to be added to each code from category X73
A   initial encounter
D   subsequent encounter
S   sequela

7 X73.0XX- **Intentional self-harm by shotgun discharge**
7 X73.1XX- **Intentional self-harm by hunting rifle discharge**
7 X73.2XX- **Intentional self-harm by machine gun discharge**
7 X73.8XX- **Intentional self-harm by other larger firearm discharge**
7 X73.9XX- **Intentional self-harm by unspecified larger firearm discharge**

4 X74 **Intentional self-harm by other and unspecified firearm and gun discharge**

The appropriate 7th character is to be added to each code from category X74
A   initial encounter
D   subsequent encounter
S   sequela

5 X74.0 **Intentional self-harm by gas, air or spring-operated guns**

7 X74.01X- **Intentional self-harm by airgun**
Intentional self-harm by BB gun discharge
Intentional self-harm by pellet gun discharge
7 X74.02X- **Intentional self-harm by paintball gun**
7 X74.09X- **Intentional self-harm by other gas, air or spring-operated gun**
7 X74.8XX- **Intentional self-harm by other firearm discharge**
Intentional self-harm by Very pistol [flare] discharge
7 X74.9XX- **Intentional self-harm by unspecified firearm discharge**

7 X75.XXX- **Intentional self-harm by explosive material**

The appropriate 7th character is to be added to code X75
A   initial encounter
D   subsequent encounter
S   sequela

7 X76.XXX- **Intentional self-harm by smoke, fire and flames**

The appropriate 7th character is to be added to code X76
A   initial encounter
D   subsequent encounter
S   sequela

4 X77 **Intentional self-harm by steam, hot vapors and hot objects**

The appropriate 7th character is to be added to each code from category X77
A   initial encounter
D   subsequent encounter
S   sequela

7 X77.0XX- **Intentional self-harm by steam or hot vapors**
7 X77.1XX- **Intentional self-harm by hot tap water**
7 X77.2XX- **Intentional self-harm by other hot fluids**
7 X77.3XX- **Intentional self-harm by hot household appliances**
7 X77.8XX- **Intentional self-harm by other hot objects**
7 X77.9XX- **Intentional self-harm by unspecified hot objects**

4 X78 **Intentional self-harm by sharp object**

The appropriate 7th character is to be added to each code from category X78
A   initial encounter
D   subsequent encounter
S   sequela

7 X78.0XX- **Intentional self-harm by sharp glass**
7 X78.1XX- **Intentional self-harm by knife**
7 X78.2XX- **Intentional self-harm by sword or dagger**
7 X78.8XX- **Intentional self-harm by other sharp object**
7 X78.9XX- **Intentional self-harm by unspecified sharp object**

7 X79.XXX- **Intentional self-harm by blunt object**

The appropriate 7th character is to be added to code X79
A   initial encounter
D   subsequent encounter
S   sequela

7 X80.XXX- **Intentional self-harm by jumping from a high place**
Intentional fall from one level to another

The appropriate 7th character is to be added to code X80
A   initial encounter
D   subsequent encounter
S   sequela

4 X81 **Intentional self-harm by jumping or lying in front of moving object**

The appropriate 7th character is to be added to each code from category X81
A   initial encounter
D   subsequent encounter
S   sequela

7 X81.0XX- **Intentional self-harm by jumping or lying in front of motor vehicle**
7 X81.1XX- **Intentional self-harm by jumping or lying in front of (subway) train**
7 X81.8XX- **Intentional self-harm by jumping or lying in front of other moving object**

● New   ▲ Revised   *Manifestation*   4-7 Digit Indicators   ⊟ Laterality   🅰 Adult (15+ years)   Ⓜ Maternity (12-55 years)   Ⓝ Newborn   🅿 Pediatric (0-17 years)   ♂ Male   ♀ Female
✖ Deleted   Unspecified   + Additional code

2017 ICD-10-CM Expert for Physicians   © 2017 DecisionHealth   1157

X52.XXX- — X81.8XX-

4️⃣ **X82** **Intentional self-harm by crashing of motor vehicle**

The appropriate 7th character is to be added to each code from category X82
A   initial encounter
D   subsequent encounter
S   sequela

7️⃣ **X82.0XX-** **Intentional collision of motor vehicle with other motor vehicle**
7️⃣ **X82.1XX-** **Intentional collision of motor vehicle with train**
7️⃣ **X82.2XX-** **Intentional collision of motor vehicle with tree**
7️⃣ **X82.8XX-** **Other intentional self-harm by crashing of motor vehicle**

4️⃣ **X83** **Intentional self-harm by other specified means**
> **EXCLUDES 1** *intentional self-harm by poisoning or contact with toxic substance- See Table of Drugs and Chemicals*

The appropriate 7th character is to be added to each code from category X83
A   initial encounter
D   subsequent encounter
S   sequela

7️⃣ **X83.0XX-** **Intentional self-harm by crashing of aircraft**
7️⃣ **X83.1XX-** **Intentional self-harm by electrocution**
7️⃣ **X83.2XX-** **Intentional self-harm by exposure to extremes of cold**
7️⃣ **X83.8XX-** **Intentional self-harm by other specified means**

Assault (X92-Y09)

> **INCLUDES** homicide
> injuries inflicted by another person with intent to injure or kill, by any means

> **EXCLUDES 1** *injuries due to legal intervention (Y35.-)*
> *injuries due to operations of war (Y36.-)*
> *injuries due to terrorism (Y38.-)*

4️⃣ **X92** **Assault by drowning and submersion**

The appropriate 7th character is to be added to each code from category X92
A   initial encounter
D   subsequent encounter
S   sequela

7️⃣ **X92.0XX-** **Assault by drowning and submersion while in bathtub**
7️⃣ **X92.1XX-** **Assault by drowning and submersion while in swimming pool**
7️⃣ **X92.2XX-** **Assault by drowning and submersion after push into swimming pool**
7️⃣ **X92.3XX-** **Assault by drowning and submersion in natural water**
7️⃣ **X92.8XX-** **Other assault by drowning and submersion**
7️⃣ **X92.9XX-** **Assault by drowning and submersion, unspecified**

7️⃣ **X93.XXX-** **Assault by handgun discharge**
Assault by discharge of gun for single hand use
Assault by discharge of pistol
Assault by discharge of revolver
> **EXCLUDES 1** *Very pistol (X95.8)*

The appropriate 7th character is to be added to code X93
A   initial encounter
D   subsequent encounter
S   sequela

4️⃣ **X94** **Assault by rifle, shotgun and larger firearm discharge**
> **EXCLUDES 1** *airgun (X95.01)*

The appropriate 7th character is to be added to each code from category X94
A   initial encounter
D   subsequent encounter
S   sequela

7️⃣ **X94.0XX-** **Assault by shotgun**
7️⃣ **X94.1XX-** **Assault by hunting rifle**
7️⃣ **X94.2XX-** **Assault by machine gun**
7️⃣ **X94.8XX-** **Assault by other larger firearm discharge**
7️⃣ **X94.9XX-** **Assault by unspecified larger firearm discharge**

4️⃣ **X95** **Assault by other and unspecified firearm and gun discharge**

The appropriate 7th character is to be added to each code from category X95
A   initial encounter
D   subsequent encounter
S   sequela

5️⃣ **X95.0** **Assault by gas, air or spring-operated guns**
7️⃣ **X95.01X-** **Assault by airgun discharge**
Assault by BB gun discharge
Assault by pellet gun discharge
7️⃣ **X95.02X-** **Assault by paintball gun discharge**
7️⃣ **X95.09X-** **Assault by other gas, air or spring-operated gun**
7️⃣ **X95.8XX-** **Assault by other firearm discharge**
Assault by very pistol [flare] discharge
7️⃣ **X95.9XX-** **Assault by unspecified firearm discharge**

4️⃣ **X96** **Assault by explosive material**
> **EXCLUDES 1** *incendiary device (X97)*
> *terrorism involving explosive material (Y38.2-)*

The appropriate 7th character is to be added to each code from category X96
A   initial encounter
D   subsequent encounter
S   sequela

7️⃣ **X96.0XX-** **Assault by antipersonnel bomb**
> **EXCLUDES 1** *antipersonnel bomb use in military or war (Y36.2-)*

7️⃣ **X96.1XX-** **Assault by gasoline bomb**
7️⃣ **X96.2XX-** **Assault by letter bomb**
7️⃣ **X96.3XX-** **Assault by fertilizer bomb**
7️⃣ **X96.4XX-** **Assault by pipe bomb**
7️⃣ **X96.8XX-** **Assault by other specified explosive**
7️⃣ **X96.9XX-** **Assault by unspecified explosive**

7️⃣ **X97.XXX-** **Assault by smoke, fire and flames**
Assault by arson
Assault by cigarettes
Assault by incendiary device

The appropriate 7th character is to be added to code X97
A   initial encounter
D   subsequent encounter
S   sequela

4️⃣ **X98** **Assault by steam, hot vapors and hot objects**

The appropriate 7th character is to be added to each code from category X98
A   initial encounter
D   subsequent encounter
S   sequela

7️⃣ **X98.0XX-** **Assault by steam or hot vapors**
7️⃣ **X98.1XX-** **Assault by hot tap water**
7️⃣ **X98.2XX-** **Assault by hot fluids**
7️⃣ **X98.3XX-** **Assault by hot household appliances**
7️⃣ **X98.8XX-** **Assault by other hot objects**
7️⃣ **X98.9XX-** **Assault by unspecified hot objects**

4️⃣ **X99** **Assault by sharp object**
> **EXCLUDES 1** *assault by strike by sports equipment (Y08.0-)*

The appropriate 7th character is to be added to each code from category X99
A   initial encounter
D   subsequent encounter
S   sequela

7️⃣ **X99.0XX-** **Assault by sharp glass**
7️⃣ **X99.1XX-** **Assault by knife**
7️⃣ **X99.2XX-** **Assault by sword or dagger**
7️⃣ **X99.8XX-** **Assault by other sharp object**
7️⃣ **X99.9XX-** **Assault by unspecified sharp object**
Assault by stabbing NOS

● New ▲ Revised *Manifestation* 4️⃣-7️⃣ Digit Indicators ▭ Laterality 🅰 Adult (15+ years) Ⓜ Maternity (12-55 years) Ⓝ Newborn 🅿 Pediatric (0-17 years) ♂ Male ♀ Female
✖ Deleted Unspecified + Additional code

1158   © 2017 DecisionHealth   2017 ICD-10-CM Expert for Physicians

☑ **Y00.XXX-** **Assault by blunt object**

EXCLUDES 1 *assault by strike by sports equipment (Y08.0-)*

The appropriate 7th character is to be added to code Y00
A   initial encounter
D   subsequent encounter
S   sequela

☑ **Y01.XXX-** **Assault by pushing from high place**

The appropriate 7th character is to be added to code Y01
A   initial encounter
D   subsequent encounter
S   sequela

☐ **Y02** **Assault by pushing or placing victim in front of moving object**

The appropriate 7th character is to be added to each code from category Y02
A   initial encounter
D   subsequent encounter
S   sequela

☑ **Y02.0XX-** **Assault by pushing or placing victim in front of motor vehicle**

☑ **Y02.1XX-** **Assault by pushing or placing victim in front of (subway) train**

☑ **Y02.8XX-** **Assault by pushing or placing victim in front of other moving object**

☐ **Y03** **Assault by crashing of motor vehicle**

The appropriate 7th character is to be added to each code from category Y03
A   initial encounter
D   subsequent encounter
S   sequela

☑ **Y03.0XX-** **Assault by being hit or run over by motor vehicle**

☑ **Y03.8XX-** **Other assault by crashing of motor vehicle**

☐ **Y04** **Assault by bodily force**

EXCLUDES 1 *assault by:*
submersion (X92.-)
use of weapon (X93-X95, X99, Y00)

The appropriate 7th character is to be added to each code from category Y04
A   initial encounter
D   subsequent encounter
S   sequela

☑ **Y04.0XX-** **Assault by unarmed brawl or fight**

☑ **Y04.1XX-** **Assault by human bite**

☑ **Y04.2XX-** **Assault by strike against or bumped into by another person**

☑ **Y04.8XX-** **Assault by other bodily force**
Assault by bodily force NOS

☐ **Y07** **Perpetrator of assault, maltreatment and neglect**
Note: Codes from this category are for use only in cases of confirmed abuse (T74.-)
Selection of the correct perpetrator code is based on the relationship between the perpetrator and the victim

INCLUDES perpetrator of abandonment
perpetrator of emotional neglect
perpetrator of mental cruelty
perpetrator of physical abuse
perpetrator of physical neglect
perpetrator of sexual abuse
perpetrator of torture

☐ **Y07.0** **Spouse or partner, perpetrator of maltreatment and neglect**
Spouse or partner, perpetrator of maltreatment and neglect against spouse or partner

Y07.01 **Husband, perpetrator of maltreatment and neglect**

Y07.02 **Wife, perpetrator of maltreatment and neglect**

Y07.03 **Male partner, perpetrator of maltreatment and neglect**

Y07.04 **Female partner, perpetrator of maltreatment and neglect**

☐ **Y07.1** **Parent (adoptive) (biological), perpetrator of maltreatment and neglect**

Y07.11 **Biological father, perpetrator of maltreatment and neglect**

Y07.12 **Biological mother, perpetrator of maltreatment and neglect**

Y07.13 **Adoptive father, perpetrator of maltreatment and neglect**

Y07.14 **Adoptive mother, perpetrator of maltreatment and neglect**

☐ **Y07.4** **Other family member, perpetrator of maltreatment and neglect**

☐ **Y07.41** **Sibling, perpetrator of maltreatment and neglect**

EXCLUDES 1 *stepsibling, perpetrator of maltreatment and neglect (Y07.435, Y07.436)*

Y07.410 **Brother, perpetrator of maltreatment and neglect**

Y07.411 **Sister, perpetrator of maltreatment and neglect**

☐ **Y07.42** **Foster parent, perpetrator of maltreatment and neglect**

Y07.420 **Foster father, perpetrator of maltreatment and neglect**

Y07.421 **Foster mother, perpetrator of maltreatment and neglect**

☐ **Y07.43** **Stepparent or stepsibling, perpetrator of maltreatment and neglect**

Y07.430 **Stepfather, perpetrator of maltreatment and neglect**

Y07.432 **Male friend of parent (co-residing in household), perpetrator of maltreatment and neglect**

Y07.433 **Stepmother, perpetrator of maltreatment and neglect**

Y07.434 **Female friend of parent (co-residing in household), perpetrator of maltreatment and neglect**

Y07.435 **Stepbrother, perpetrator or maltreatment and neglect**

Y07.436 **Stepsister, perpetrator of maltreatment and neglect**

☐ **Y07.49** **Other family member, perpetrator of maltreatment and neglect**

Y07.490 **Male cousin, perpetrator of maltreatment and neglect**

Y07.491 **Female cousin, perpetrator of maltreatment and neglect**

Y07.499 **Other family member, perpetrator of maltreatment and neglect**

☐ **Y07.5** **Non-family member, perpetrator of maltreatment and neglect**

Y07.50 **Unspecified non-family member, perpetrator of maltreatment and neglect**

☐ **Y07.51** **Daycare provider, perpetrator of maltreatment and neglect**

Y07.510 **At-home childcare provider, perpetrator of maltreatment and neglect**

Y07.511 **Daycare center childcare provider, perpetrator of maltreatment and neglect**

Y07.512 **At-home adultcare provider, perpetrator of maltreatment and neglect**

Y07.513 **Adultcare center provider, perpetrator of maltreatment and neglect**

Y07.519 **Unspecified daycare provider, perpetrator of maltreatment and neglect**

☐ **Y07.52** **Healthcare provider, perpetrator of maltreatment and neglect**

Y07.521 **Mental health provider, perpetrator of maltreatment and neglect**

Y07.528 **Other therapist or healthcare provider, perpetrator of maltreatment and neglect**
Nurse perpetrator of maltreatment and neglect
Occupational therapist perpetrator of maltreatment and neglect
Physical therapist perpetrator of maltreatment and neglect
Speech therapist perpetrator of maltreatment and neglect

Y07.529 **Unspecified healthcare provider, perpetrator of maltreatment and neglect**

● New ▲ Revised *Manifestation* ☐-☑ Digit Indicators ⊟ Laterality Ⓐ Adult (15+ years) Ⓜ Maternity (12-55 years) Ⓝ Newborn Ⓟ Pediatric (0-17 years) ♂ Male ♀ Female
✖ Deleted Unspecified + Additional code

External Causes of Morbidity

Y07.53   Teacher or instructor, perpetrator of maltreatment and neglect
          Coach, perpetrator of maltreatment and neglect
Y07.59   Other non-family member, perpetrator of maltreatment and neglect
Y07.9   Unspecified perpetrator of maltreatment and neglect

Y08   Assault by other specified means

The appropriate 7th character is to be added to each code from category Y08
A   initial encounter
D   subsequent encounter
S   sequela

Y08.0   Assault by strike by sport equipment
Y08.01X-   Assault by strike by hockey stick
Y08.02X-   Assault by strike by baseball bat
Y08.09X-   Assault by strike by other specified type of sport equipment
Y08.8   Assault by other specified means
Y08.81X-   Assault by crashing of aircraft
Y08.89X-   Assault by other specified means

Y09   Assault by unspecified means
Assassination (attempted) NOS
Homicide (attempted) NOS
Manslaughter (attempted) NOS
Murder (attempted) NOS

Event of undetermined intent (Y21-Y33)

Undetermined intent is only for use when there is specific documentation in the record that the intent of the injury cannot be determined. If no such documentation is present, code to accidental (unintentional)

Y21   Drowning and submersion, undetermined intent

The appropriate 7th character is to be added to each code from category Y21
A   initial encounter
D   subsequent encounter
S   sequela

Y21.0XX-   Drowning and submersion while in bathtub, undetermined intent
Y21.1XX-   Drowning and submersion after fall into bathtub, undetermined intent
Y21.2XX-   Drowning and submersion while in swimming pool, undetermined intent
Y21.3XX-   Drowning and submersion after fall into swimming pool, undetermined intent
Y21.4XX-   Drowning and submersion in natural water, undetermined intent
Y21.8XX-   Other drowning and submersion, undetermined intent
Y21.9XX-   Unspecified drowning and submersion, undetermined intent

Y22.XXX-   Handgun discharge, undetermined intent
Discharge of gun for single hand use, undetermined intent
Discharge of pistol, undetermined intent
Discharge of revolver, undetermined intent
            EXCLUDES 2   *very pistol (Y24.8)*

The appropriate 7th character is to be added to code Y22
A   initial encounter
D   subsequent encounter
S   sequela

Y23   Rifle, shotgun and larger firearm discharge, undetermined intent
            EXCLUDES 2   *airgun (Y24.0)*

The appropriate 7th character is to be added to each code from category Y23
A   initial encounter
D   subsequent encounter
S   sequela

Y23.0XX-   Shotgun discharge, undetermined intent
Y23.1XX-   Hunting rifle discharge, undetermined intent
Y23.2XX-   Military firearm discharge, undetermined intent
Y23.3XX-   Machine gun discharge, undetermined intent

Y23.8XX-   Other larger firearm discharge, undetermined intent
Y23.9XX-   Unspecified larger firearm discharge, undetermined intent

Y24   Other and unspecified firearm discharge, undetermined intent

The appropriate 7th character is to be added to each code from category Y24
A   initial encounter
D   subsequent encounter
S   sequela

Y24.0XX-   Airgun discharge, undetermined intent
BB gun discharge, undetermined intent
Pellet gun discharge, undetermined intent
Y24.8XX-   Other firearm discharge, undetermined intent
Paintball gun discharge, undetermined intent
Very pistol [flare] discharge, undetermined intent
Y24.9XX-   Unspecified firearm discharge, undetermined intent

Y25.XXX-   Contact with explosive material, undetermined intent

The appropriate 7th character is to be added to code Y25
A   initial encounter
D   subsequent encounter
S   sequela

Y26.XXX-   Exposure to smoke, fire and flames, undetermined intent

The appropriate 7th character is to be added to code Y26
A   initial encounter
D   subsequent encounter
S   sequela

Y27   Contact with steam, hot vapors and hot objects, undetermined intent

The appropriate 7th character is to be added to each code from category Y27
A   initial encounter
D   subsequent encounter
S   sequela

Y27.0XX-   Contact with steam and hot vapors, undetermined intent
Y27.1XX-   Contact with hot tap water, undetermined intent
Y27.2XX-   Contact with hot fluids, undetermined intent
Y27.3XX-   Contact with hot household appliance, undetermined intent
Y27.8XX-   Contact with other hot objects, undetermined intent
Y27.9XX-   Contact with unspecified hot objects, undetermined intent

Y28   Contact with sharp object, undetermined intent

The appropriate 7th character is to be added to each code from category Y28
A   initial encounter
D   subsequent encounter
S   sequela

Y28.0XX-   Contact with sharp glass, undetermined intent
Y28.1XX-   Contact with knife, undetermined intent
Y28.2XX-   Contact with sword or dagger, undetermined intent
Y28.8XX-   Contact with other sharp object, undetermined intent
Y28.9XX-   Contact with unspecified sharp object, undetermined intent

Y29.XXX-   Contact with blunt object, undetermined intent

The appropriate 7th character is to be added to code Y29
A   initial encounter
D   subsequent encounter
S   sequela

● New   ▲ Revised   *Manifestation*   ◀-▼ Digit Indicators   ▤ Laterality   Ⓐ Adult (15+ years)   Ⓜ Maternity (12-55 years)   Ⓝ Newborn   Ⓟ Pediatric (0-17 years)   ♂ Male   ♀ Female
✖ Deleted   Unspecified   + Additional code

1160   © 2017 DecisionHealth   2017 ICD-10-CM Expert for Physicians

☑ **Y30.XXX-** **Falling, jumping or pushed from a high place, undetermined intent**
Victim falling from one level to another, undetermined intent

The appropriate 7th character is to be added to code Y30
A   initial encounter
D   subsequent encounter
S   sequela

☑ **Y31.XXX-** **Falling, lying or running before or into moving object, undetermined intent**

The appropriate 7th character is to be added to code Y31
A   initial encounter
D   subsequent encounter
S   sequela

☑ **Y32.XXX-** **Crashing of motor vehicle, undetermined intent**

The appropriate 7th character is to be added to code Y32
A   initial encounter
D   subsequent encounter
S   sequela

☑ **Y33.XXX-** **Other specified events, undetermined intent**

The appropriate 7th character is to be added to code Y33
A   initial encounter
D   subsequent encounter
S   sequela

Legal intervention, operations of war, military operations, and terrorism (Y35-Y38)

④ **Y35** **Legal intervention**

| INCLUDES | any injury sustained as a result of an encounter with any law enforcement official, serving in any capacity at the time of the encounter, whether on-duty or off-duty. Includes: injury to law enforcement official, suspect and bystander |

The appropriate 7th character is to be added to each code from category Y35
A   initial encounter
D   subsequent encounter
S   sequela

⑤ **Y35.0** **Legal intervention involving firearm discharge**

⑥ **Y35.00** **Legal intervention involving unspecified firearm discharge**
Legal intervention involving gunshot wound
Legal intervention involving shot NOS

☑ **Y35.001-** **Legal intervention involving unspecified firearm discharge, law enforcement official injured**

☑ **Y35.002-** **Legal intervention involving unspecified firearm discharge, bystander injured**

☑ **Y35.003-** **Legal intervention involving unspecified firearm discharge, suspect injured**

⑥ **Y35.01** **Legal intervention involving injury by machine gun**

☑ **Y35.011-** **Legal intervention involving injury by machine gun, law enforcement official injured**

☑ **Y35.012-** **Legal intervention involving injury by machine gun, bystander injured**

☑ **Y35.013-** **Legal intervention involving injury by machine gun, suspect injured**

⑥ **Y35.02** **Legal intervention involving injury by handgun**

☑ **Y35.021-** **Legal intervention involving injury by handgun, law enforcement official injured**

☑ **Y35.022-** **Legal intervention involving injury by handgun, bystander injured**

☑ **Y35.023-** **Legal intervention involving injury by handgun, suspect injured**

⑥ **Y35.03** **Legal intervention involving injury by rifle pellet**

☑ **Y35.031-** **Legal intervention involving injury by rifle pellet, law enforcement official injured**

☑ **Y35.032-** **Legal intervention involving injury by rifle pellet, bystander injured**

☑ **Y35.033-** **Legal intervention involving injury by rifle pellet, suspect injured**

⑥ **Y35.04** **Legal intervention involving injury by rubber bullet**

☑ **Y35.041-** **Legal intervention involving injury by rubber bullet, law enforcement official injured**

☑ **Y35.042-** **Legal intervention involving injury by rubber bullet, bystander injured**

☑ **Y35.043-** **Legal intervention involving injury by rubber bullet, suspect injured**

⑥ **Y35.09** **Legal intervention involving other firearm discharge**

☑ **Y35.091-** **Legal intervention involving other firearm discharge, law enforcement official injured**

☑ **Y35.092-** **Legal intervention involving other firearm discharge, bystander injured**

☑ **Y35.093-** **Legal intervention involving other firearm discharge, suspect injured**

⑤ **Y35.1** **Legal intervention involving explosives**

⑥ **Y35.10** **Legal intervention involving unspecified explosives**

☑ **Y35.101-** **Legal intervention involving unspecified explosives, law enforcement official injured**

☑ **Y35.102-** **Legal intervention involving unspecified explosives, bystander injured**

☑ **Y35.103-** **Legal intervention involving unspecified explosives, suspect injured**

⑥ **Y35.11** **Legal intervention involving injury by dynamite**

☑ **Y35.111-** **Legal intervention involving injury by dynamite, law enforcement official injured**

☑ **Y35.112-** **Legal intervention involving injury by dynamite, bystander injured**

☑ **Y35.113-** **Legal intervention involving injury by dynamite, suspect injured**

⑥ **Y35.12** **Legal intervention involving injury by explosive shell**

☑ **Y35.121-** **Legal intervention involving injury by explosive shell, law enforcement official injured**

☑ **Y35.122-** **Legal intervention involving injury by explosive shell, bystander injured**

☑ **Y35.123-** **Legal intervention involving injury by explosive shell, suspect injured**

⑥ **Y35.19** **Legal intervention involving other explosives**
Legal intervention involving injury by grenade
Legal intervention involving injury by mortar bomb

☑ **Y35.191-** **Legal intervention involving other explosives, law enforcement official injured**

☑ **Y35.192-** **Legal intervention involving other explosives, bystander injured**

☑ **Y35.193-** **Legal intervention involving other explosives, suspect injured**

⑤ **Y35.2** **Legal intervention involving gas**
Legal intervention involving asphyxiation by gas
Legal intervention involving poisoning by gas

⑥ **Y35.20** **Legal intervention involving unspecified gas**

☑ **Y35.201-** **Legal intervention involving unspecified gas, law enforcement official injured**

☑ **Y35.202-** **Legal intervention involving unspecified gas, bystander injured**

☑ **Y35.203-** **Legal intervention involving unspecified gas, suspect injured**

⑥ **Y35.21** **Legal intervention involving injury by tear gas**

☑ **Y35.211-** **Legal intervention involving injury by tear gas, law enforcement official injured**

☑ **Y35.212-** **Legal intervention involving injury by tear gas, bystander injured**

☑ **Y35.213-** **Legal intervention involving injury by tear gas, suspect injured**

⑥ **Y35.29** **Legal intervention involving other gas**

☑ **Y35.291-** **Legal intervention involving other gas, law enforcement official injured**

☑ **Y35.292-** **Legal intervention involving other gas, bystander injured**

☑ **Y35.293-** **Legal intervention involving other gas, suspect injured**

⑤ **Y35.3** **Legal intervention involving blunt objects**
Legal intervention involving being hit or struck by blunt object

⑥ **Y35.30** **Legal intervention involving unspecified blunt objects**

☑ **Y35.301-** **Legal intervention involving unspecified blunt objects, law enforcement official injured**

● New   ▲ Revised   *Manifestation*   ④-☑ Digit Indicators   ▤ Laterality   Ⓐ Adult (15+ years)   Ⓜ Maternity (12-55 years)   Ⓝ Newborn   Ⓟ Pediatric (0-17 years)   ♂ Male   ♀ Female
✖ Deleted   Unspecified   + Additional code

External Causes of Morbidity

7 Y35.302- Legal intervention involving unspecified blunt objects, bystander injured

7 Y35.303- Legal intervention involving unspecified blunt objects, suspect injured

6 Y35.31 Legal intervention involving baton

7 Y35.311- Legal intervention involving baton, law enforcement official injured

7 Y35.312- Legal intervention involving baton, bystander injured

7 Y35.313- Legal intervention involving baton, suspect injured

6 Y35.39 Legal intervention involving other blunt objects

7 Y35.391- Legal intervention involving other blunt objects, law enforcement official injured

7 Y35.392- Legal intervention involving other blunt objects, bystander injured

7 Y35.393- Legal intervention involving other blunt objects, suspect injured

5 Y35.4 Legal intervention involving sharp objects
Legal intervention involving being cut by sharp objects
Legal intervention involving being stabbed by sharp objects

6 Y35.40 Legal intervention involving unspecified sharp objects

7 Y35.401- Legal intervention involving unspecified sharp objects, law enforcement official injured

7 Y35.402- Legal intervention involving unspecified sharp objects, bystander injured

7 Y35.403- Legal intervention involving unspecified sharp objects, suspect injured

6 Y35.41 Legal intervention involving bayonet

7 Y35.411- Legal intervention involving bayonet, law enforcement official injured

7 Y35.412- Legal intervention involving bayonet, bystander injured

7 Y35.413- Legal intervention involving bayonet, suspect injured

6 Y35.49 Legal intervention involving other sharp objects

7 Y35.491- Legal intervention involving other sharp objects, law enforcement official injured

7 Y35.492- Legal intervention involving other sharp objects, bystander injured

7 Y35.493- Legal intervention involving other sharp objects, suspect injured

5 Y35.8 Legal intervention involving other specified means

6 Y35.81 Legal intervention involving manhandling

7 Y35.811- Legal intervention involving manhandling, law enforcement official injured

7 Y35.812- Legal intervention involving manhandling, bystander injured

7 Y35.813- Legal intervention involving manhandling, suspect injured

6 Y35.89 Legal intervention involving other specified means

7 Y35.891- Legal intervention involving other specified means, law enforcement official injured

7 Y35.892- Legal intervention involving other specified means, bystander injured

7 Y35.893- Legal intervention involving other specified means, suspect injured

5 Y35.9 Legal intervention, means unspecified

7 Y35.91X- Legal intervention, means unspecified, law enforcement official injured

7 Y35.92X- Legal intervention, means unspecified, bystander injured

7 Y35.93X- Legal intervention, means unspecified, suspect injured

4 Y36 **Operations of war**

INCLUDES	injuries to military personnel and civilians caused by war, civil insurrection, and peacekeeping missions
EXCLUDES 1	*injury to military personnel occurring during peacetime military operations (Y37.-)* *military vehicles involved in transport accidents with non-military vehicle during peacetime (V09.01, V09.21, V19.81, V29.81, V39.81, V49.81, V59.81, V69.81, V79.81)*

The appropriate 7th character is to be added to each code from category Y36
A   initial encounter
D   subsequent encounter
S   sequela

AHA: 3Q 2014, 5

5 Y36.0 War operations involving explosion of marine weapons

6 Y36.00 War operations involving explosion of unspecified marine weapon
War operations involving underwater blast NOS

7 Y36.000- War operations involving explosion of unspecified marine weapon, military personnel

7 Y36.001- War operations involving explosion of unspecified marine weapon, civilian

6 Y36.01 War operations involving explosion of depth-charge

7 Y36.010- War operations involving explosion of depth-charge, military personnel

7 Y36.011- War operations involving explosion of depth-charge, civilian

6 Y36.02 War operations involving explosion of marine mine
War operations involving explosion of marine mine, at sea or in harbor

7 Y36.020- War operations involving explosion of marine mine, military personnel

7 Y36.021- War operations involving explosion of marine mine, civilian

6 Y36.03 War operations involving explosion of sea-based artillery shell

7 Y36.030- War operations involving explosion of sea-based artillery shell, military personnel

7 Y36.031- War operations involving explosion of sea-based artillery shell, civilian

6 Y36.04 War operations involving explosion of torpedo

7 Y36.040- War operations involving explosion of torpedo, military personnel

7 Y36.041- War operations involving explosion of torpedo, civilian

6 Y36.05 War operations involving accidental detonation of onboard marine weapons

7 Y36.050- War operations involving accidental detonation of onboard marine weapons, military personnel

7 Y36.051- War operations involving accidental detonation of onboard marine weapons, civilian

6 Y36.09 War operations involving explosion of other marine weapons

7 Y36.090- War operations involving explosion of other marine weapons, military personnel

7 Y36.091- War operations involving explosion of other marine weapons, civilian

5 Y36.1 War operations involving destruction of aircraft

6 Y36.10 War operations involving unspecified destruction of aircraft

7 Y36.100- War operations involving unspecified destruction of aircraft, military personnel

7 Y36.101- War operations involving unspecified destruction of aircraft, civilian

● New   ▲ Revised   *Manifestation*   **4 - 7** Digit Indicators   ⊟ Laterality   🅰 Adult (15+ years)   Ⓜ Maternity (12-55 years)   Ⓝ Newborn   🅿 Pediatric (0-17 years)   ♂ Male   ♀ Female
✖ Deleted   Unspecified   + Additional code

1162   © 2017 DecisionHealth   2017 ICD-10-CM Expert for Physicians

⑥ **Y36.11** **War operations involving destruction of aircraft due to enemy fire or explosives**
War operations involving destruction of aircraft due to air to air missile
War operations involving destruction of aircraft due to explosive placed on aircraft
War operations involving destruction of aircraft due to rocket propelled grenade [RPG]
War operations involving destruction of aircraft due to small arms fire
War operations involving destruction of aircraft due to surface to air missile

⑦ **Y36.110-** **War operations involving destruction of aircraft due to enemy fire or explosives, military personnel**

⑦ **Y36.111-** **War operations involving destruction of aircraft due to enemy fire or explosives, civilian**

⑥ **Y36.12** **War operations involving destruction of aircraft due to collision with other aircraft**

⑦ **Y36.120-** **War operations involving destruction of aircraft due to collision with other aircraft, military personnel**

⑦ **Y36.121-** **War operations involving destruction of aircraft due to collision with other aircraft, civilian**

⑥ **Y36.13** **War operations involving destruction of aircraft due to onboard fire**

⑦ **Y36.130-** **War operations involving destruction of aircraft due to onboard fire, military personnel**

⑦ **Y36.131-** **War operations involving destruction of aircraft due to onboard fire, civilian**

⑥ **Y36.14** **War operations involving destruction of aircraft due to accidental detonation of onboard munitions and explosives**

⑦ **Y36.140-** **War operations involving destruction of aircraft due to accidental detonation of onboard munitions and explosives, military personnel**

⑦ **Y36.141-** **War operations involving destruction of aircraft due to accidental detonation of onboard munitions and explosives, civilian**

⑥ **Y36.19** **War operations involving other destruction of aircraft**

⑦ **Y36.190-** **War operations involving other destruction of aircraft, military personnel**

⑦ **Y36.191-** **War operations involving other destruction of aircraft, civilian**

⑤ **Y36.2** **War operations involving other explosions and fragments**
EXCLUDES 1 *war operations involving explosion of aircraft (Y36.1-)*
war operations involving explosion of marine weapons (Y36.0-)
war operations involving explosion of nuclear weapons (Y36.5-)
war operations involving explosion occurring after cessation of hostilities (Y36.8-)

⑥ **Y36.20** **War operations involving unspecified explosion and fragments**
War operations involving air blast NOS
War operations involving blast NOS
War operations involving blast fragments NOS
War operations involving blast wave NOS
War operations involving blast wind NOS
War operations involving explosion NOS
War operations involving explosion of bomb NOS

⑦ **Y36.200-** **War operations involving unspecified explosion and fragments, military personnel**

⑦ **Y36.201-** **War operations involving unspecified explosion and fragments, civilian**

⑥ **Y36.21** **War operations involving explosion of aerial bomb**

⑦ **Y36.210-** **War operations involving explosion of aerial bomb, military personnel**

⑦ **Y36.211-** **War operations involving explosion of aerial bomb, civilian**

⑥ **Y36.22** **War operations involving explosion of guided missile**

⑦ **Y36.220-** **War operations involving explosion of guided missile, military personnel**

⑦ **Y36.221-** **War operations involving explosion of guided missile, civilian**

⑥ **Y36.23** **War operations involving explosion of improvised explosive device [IED]**
War operations involving explosion of person-borne improvised explosive device [IED]
War operations involving explosion of vehicle-borne improvised explosive device [IED]
War operations involving explosion of roadside improvised explosive device [IED]

⑦ **Y36.230-** **War operations involving explosion of improvised explosive device [IED], military personnel**

⑦ **Y36.231-** **War operations involving explosion of improvised explosive device [IED], civilian**

⑥ **Y36.24** **War operations involving explosion due to accidental detonation and discharge of own munitions or munitions launch device**

⑦ **Y36.240-** **War operations involving explosion due to accidental detonation and discharge of own munitions or munitions launch device, military personnel**

⑦ **Y36.241-** **War operations involving explosion due to accidental detonation and discharge of own munitions or munitions launch device, civilian**

⑥ **Y36.25** **War operations involving fragments from munitions**

⑦ **Y36.250-** **War operations involving fragments from munitions, military personnel**

⑦ **Y36.251-** **War operations involving fragments from munitions, civilian**

⑥ **Y36.26** **War operations involving fragments of improvised explosive device [IED]**
War operations involving fragments of person-borne improvised explosive device [IED]
War operations involving fragments of vehicle-borne improvised explosive device [IED]
War operations involving fragments of roadside improvised explosive device [IED]

⑦ **Y36.260-** **War operations involving fragments of improvised explosive device [IED], military personnel**

⑦ **Y36.261-** **War operations involving fragments of improvised explosive device [IED], civilian**

⑥ **Y36.27** **War operations involving fragments from weapons**

⑦ **Y36.270-** **War operations involving fragments from weapons, military personnel**

⑦ **Y36.271-** **War operations involving fragments from weapons, civilian**

⑥ **Y36.29** **War operations involving other explosions and fragments**
War operations involving explosion of grenade
War operations involving explosions of land mine
War operations involving shrapnel NOS

⑦ **Y36.290-** **War operations involving other explosions and fragments, military personnel**

⑦ **Y36.291-** **War operations involving other explosions and fragments, civilian**

⑤ **Y36.3** **War operations involving fires, conflagrations and hot substances**
War operations involving smoke, fumes, and heat from fires, conflagrations and hot substances
EXCLUDES 1 *war operations involving fires and conflagrations aboard military aircraft (Y36.1-)*
war operations involving fires and conflagrations aboard military watercraft (Y36.0-)
war operations involving fires and conflagrations caused indirectly by conventional weapons (Y36.2-)
war operations involving fires and thermal effects of nuclear weapons (Y36.53-)

⑥ **Y36.30** **War operations involving unspecified fire, conflagration and hot substance**

⑦ **Y36.300-** **War operations involving unspecified fire, conflagration and hot substance, military personnel**

⑦ **Y36.301-** **War operations involving unspecified fire, conflagration and hot substance, civilian**

⑥ **Y36.31** **War operations involving gasoline bomb**
War operations involving incendiary bomb
War operations involving petrol bomb

● New ▲ Revised *Manifestation* ④-⑦ Digit Indicators ⊟ Laterality Ⓐ Adult (15+ years) Ⓜ Maternity (12-55 years) Ⓝ Newborn (0-17 years) Ⓟ Pediatric (0-17 years) ♂ Male ♀ Female
✖ Deleted Unspecified + Additional code

2017 ICD-10-CM Expert for Physicians

© 2017 DecisionHealth   1163

7 Y36.310- War operations involving gasoline bomb, military personnel

7 Y36.311- War operations involving gasoline bomb, civilian

6 Y36.32 War operations involving incendiary bullet

7 Y36.320- War operations involving incendiary bullet, military personnel

7 Y36.321- War operations involving incendiary bullet, civilian

6 Y36.33 War operations involving flamethrower

7 Y36.330- War operations involving flamethrower, military personnel

7 Y36.331- War operations involving flamethrower, civilian

6 Y36.39 War operations involving other fires, conflagrations and hot substances

7 Y36.390- War operations involving other fires, conflagrations and hot substances, military personnel

7 Y36.391- War operations involving other fires, conflagrations and hot substances, civilian

5 Y36.4 War operations involving firearm discharge and other forms of conventional warfare

6 Y36.41 War operations involving rubber bullets

7 Y36.410- War operations involving rubber bullets, military personnel

7 Y36.411- War operations involving rubber bullets, civilian

6 Y36.42 War operations involving firearms pellets

7 Y36.420- War operations involving firearms pellets, military personnel

7 Y36.421- War operations involving firearms pellets, civilian

6 Y36.43 War operations involving other firearms discharge
War operations involving bullets NOS

EXCLUDES 1 *war operations involving munitions fragments (Y36.25-)*
war operations involving incendiary bullets (Y36.32-)

7 Y36.430- War operations involving other firearms discharge, military personnel

7 Y36.431- War operations involving other firearms discharge, civilian

6 Y36.44 War operations involving unarmed hand to hand combat

EXCLUDES 1 *war operations involving combat using blunt or piercing object (Y36.45-)*
war operations involving intentional restriction of air and airway (Y36.46-)
war operations involving unintentional restriction of air and airway (Y36.47-)

7 Y36.440- War operations involving unarmed hand to hand combat, military personnel

7 Y36.441- War operations involving unarmed hand to hand combat, civilian

6 Y36.45 War operations involving combat using blunt or piercing object

7 Y36.450- War operations involving combat using blunt or piercing object, military personnel

7 Y36.451- War operations involving combat using blunt or piercing object, civilian

6 Y36.46 War operations involving intentional restriction of air and airway

7 Y36.460- War operations involving intentional restriction of air and airway, military personnel

7 Y36.461- War operations involving intentional restriction of air and airway, civilian

6 Y36.47 War operations involving unintentional restriction of air and airway

7 Y36.470- War operations involving unintentional restriction of air and airway, military personnel

7 Y36.471- War operations involving unintentional restriction of air and airway, civilian

6 Y36.49 War operations involving other forms of conventional warfare

7 Y36.490- War operations involving other forms of conventional warfare, military personnel

7 Y36.491- War operations involving other forms of conventional warfare, civilian

5 Y36.5 War operations involving nuclear weapons
War operations involving dirty bomb NOS

6 Y36.50 War operations involving unspecified effect of nuclear weapon

7 Y36.500- War operations involving unspecified effect of nuclear weapon, military personnel

7 Y36.501- War operations involving unspecified effect of nuclear weapon, civilian

6 Y36.51 War operations involving direct blast effect of nuclear weapon
War operations involving blast pressure of nuclear weapon

7 Y36.510- War operations involving direct blast effect of nuclear weapon, military personnel

7 Y36.511- War operations involving direct blast effect of nuclear weapon, civilian

6 Y36.52 War operations involving indirect blast effect of nuclear weapon
War operations involving being thrown by blast of nuclear weapon
War operations involving being struck or crushed by blast debris of nuclear weapon

7 Y36.520- War operations involving indirect blast effect of nuclear weapon, military personnel

7 Y36.521- War operations involving indirect blast effect of nuclear weapon, civilian

6 Y36.53 War operations involving thermal radiation effect of nuclear weapon
War operations involving direct heat from nuclear weapon
War operation involving fireball effects from nuclear weapon

7 Y36.530- War operations involving thermal radiation effect of nuclear weapon, military personnel

7 Y36.531- War operations involving thermal radiation effect of nuclear weapon, civilian

6 Y36.54 War operation involving nuclear radiation effects of nuclear weapon
War operation involving acute radiation exposure from nuclear weapon
War operation involving exposure to immediate ionizing radiation from nuclear weapon
War operation involving fallout exposure from nuclear weapon
War operation involving secondary effects of nuclear weapons

7 Y36.540- War operation involving nuclear radiation effects of nuclear weapon, military personnel

7 Y36.541- War operation involving nuclear radiation effects of nuclear weapon, civilian

6 Y36.59 War operation involving other effects of nuclear weapons

7 Y36.590- War operation involving other effects of nuclear weapons, military personnel

7 Y36.591- War operation involving other effects of nuclear weapons, civilian

5 Y36.6 War operations involving biological weapons

6 Y36.6X War operations involving biological weapons

7 Y36.6X0- War operations involving biological weapons, military personnel

7 Y36.6X1- War operations involving biological weapons, civilian

5 Y36.7 War operations involving chemical weapons and other forms of unconventional warfare

EXCLUDES 1 *war operations involving incendiary devices (Y36.3-, Y36.5-)*

6 Y36.7X War operations involving chemical weapons and other forms of unconventional warfare

7 Y36.7X0- War operations involving chemical weapons and other forms of unconventional warfare, military personnel

7 Y36.7X1- War operations involving chemical weapons and other forms of unconventional warfare, civilian

5 Y36.8 War operations occurring after cessation of hostilities
War operations classifiable to categories Y36.0-Y36.8 but occurring after cessation of hostilities

---

● New   ▲ Revised   *Manifestation*   4-7 Digit Indicators   ▤ Laterality   ▲ Adult (15+ years)   Ⓜ Maternity (12-55 years)   Ⓝ Newborn   Ⓟ Pediatric (0-17 years)   ♂ Male   ♀ Female
✖ Deleted   Unspecified   + Additional code

⑥	Y36.81	Explosion of mine placed during war operations but exploding after cessation of hostilities
⑦	Y36.810-	Explosion of mine placed during war operations but exploding after cessation of hostilities, military personnel
⑦	Y36.811-	Explosion of mine placed during war operations but exploding after cessation of hostilities, civilian
⑥	Y36.82	Explosion of bomb placed during war operations but exploding after cessation of hostilities
⑦	Y36.820-	Explosion of bomb placed during war operations but exploding after cessation of hostilities, military personnel
⑦	Y36.821-	Explosion of bomb placed during war operations but exploding after cessation of hostilities, civilian
⑥	Y36.88	Other war operations occurring after cessation of hostilities
⑦	Y36.880-	Other war operations occurring after cessation of hostilities, military personnel
⑦	Y36.881-	Other war operations occurring after cessation of hostilities, civilian
⑥	Y36.89	Unspecified war operations occurring after cessation of hostilities
⑦	Y36.890-	Unspecified war operations occurring after cessation of hostilities, military personnel
⑦	Y36.891-	Unspecified war operations occurring after cessation of hostilities, civilian
⑤	Y36.9	Other and unspecified war operations
⑦	Y36.90X-	War operations, unspecified
⑦	Y36.91X-	War operations involving unspecified weapon of mass destruction [WMD]
⑦	Y36.92X-	War operations involving friendly fire
④	Y37	Military operations

INCLUDES   injuries to military personnel and civilians occurring during peacetime on military property and during routine military exercises and operations

EXCLUDES 1   *military aircraft involved in aircraft accident with civilian aircraft (V97.81-)*
military vehicles involved in transport accident with civilian vehicle (V09.01, V09.21, V19.81, V29.81, V39.81, V49.81, V59.81, V69.81, V79.81)
military watercraft involved in water transport accident with civilian watercraft (V94.81-)
war operations (Y36.-)

The appropriate 7th character is to be added to each code from category Y37
A   initial encounter
D   subsequent encounter
S   sequela

⑤	Y37.0	Military operations involving explosion of marine weapons
⑥	Y37.00	Military operations involving explosion of unspecified marine weapon
		Military operations involving underwater blast NOS
⑦	Y37.000-	Military operations involving explosion of unspecified marine weapon, military personnel
⑦	Y37.001-	Military operations involving explosion of unspecified marine weapon, civilian
⑥	Y37.01	Military operations involving explosion of depth-charge
⑦	Y37.010-	Military operations involving explosion of depth-charge, military personnel
⑦	Y37.011-	Military operations involving explosion of depth-charge, civilian
⑥	Y37.02	Military operations involving explosion of marine mine
		Military operations involving explosion of marine mine, at sea or in harbor
⑦	Y37.020-	Military operations involving explosion of marine mine, military personnel
⑦	Y37.021-	Military operations involving explosion of marine mine, civilian
⑥	Y37.03	Military operations involving explosion of sea-based artillery shell

⑦	Y37.030-	Military operations involving explosion of sea-based artillery shell, military personnel
⑦	Y37.031-	Military operations involving explosion of sea-based artillery shell, civilian
⑥	Y37.04	Military operations involving explosion of torpedo
⑦	Y37.040-	Military operations involving explosion of torpedo, military personnel
⑦	Y37.041-	Military operations involving explosion of torpedo, civilian
⑥	Y37.05	Military operations involving accidental detonation of onboard marine weapons
⑦	Y37.050-	Military operations involving accidental detonation of onboard marine weapons, military personnel
⑦	Y37.051-	Military operations involving accidental detonation of onboard marine weapons, civilian
⑥	Y37.09	Military operations involving explosion of other marine weapons
⑦	Y37.090-	Military operations involving explosion of other marine weapons, military personnel
⑦	Y37.091-	Military operations involving explosion of other marine weapons, civilian
⑤	Y37.1	Military operations involving destruction of aircraft
⑥	Y37.10	Military operations involving unspecified destruction of aircraft
⑦	Y37.100-	Military operations involving unspecified destruction of aircraft, military personnel
⑦	Y37.101-	Military operations involving unspecified destruction of aircraft, civilian
⑥	Y37.11	Military operations involving destruction of aircraft due to enemy fire or explosives
		Military operations involving destruction of aircraft due to air to air missile
		Military operations involving destruction of aircraft due to explosive placed on aircraft
		Military operations involving destruction of aircraft due to rocket propelled grenade [RPG]
		Military operations involving destruction of aircraft due to small arms fire
		Military operations involving destruction of aircraft due to surface to air missile
⑦	Y37.110-	Military operations involving destruction of aircraft due to enemy fire or explosives, military personnel
⑦	Y37.111-	Military operations involving destruction of aircraft due to enemy fire or explosives, civilian
⑥	Y37.12	Military operations involving destruction of aircraft due to collision with other aircraft
⑦	Y37.120-	Military operations involving destruction of aircraft due to collision with other aircraft, military personnel
⑦	Y37.121-	Military operations involving destruction of aircraft due to collision with other aircraft, civilian
⑥	Y37.13	Military operations involving destruction of aircraft due to onboard fire
⑦	Y37.130-	Military operations involving destruction of aircraft due to onboard fire, military personnel
⑦	Y37.131-	Military operations involving destruction of aircraft due to onboard fire, civilian
⑥	Y37.14	Military operations involving destruction of aircraft due to accidental detonation of onboard munitions and explosives
⑦	Y37.140-	Military operations involving destruction of aircraft due to accidental detonation of onboard munitions and explosives, military personnel
⑦	Y37.141-	Military operations involving destruction of aircraft due to accidental detonation of onboard munitions and explosives, civilian
⑥	Y37.19	Military operations involving other destruction of aircraft
⑦	Y37.190-	Military operations involving other destruction of aircraft, military personnel
⑦	Y37.191-	Military operations involving other destruction of aircraft, civilian

---

● New   ▲ Revised   *Manifestation*   ④-⑦ Digit Indicators   ⊟ Laterality   Ⓐ Adult (15+ years)   Ⓜ Maternity (12-55 years)   Ⓝ Newborn   Ⓟ Pediatric (0-17 years)   ♂ Male   ♀ Female
✖ Deleted   Unspecified   ✚ Additional code

External Causes of Morbidity

Y37.2 — **Y37.431-**

⑤ **Y37.2 Military operations involving other explosions and fragments**
> **EXCLUDES 1** *military operations involving explosion of aircraft (Y37.1-)*
> *military operations involving explosion of marine weapons (Y37.0-)*
> *military operations involving explosion of nuclear weapons (Y37.5-)*

⑥ **Y37.20 Military operations involving unspecified explosion and fragments**
Military operations involving air blast NOS
Military operations involving blast NOS
Military operations involving blast fragments NOS
Military operations involving blast wave NOS
Military operations involving blast wind NOS
Military operations involving explosion NOS
Military operations involving explosion of bomb NOS

⑦ **Y37.200- Military operations involving unspecified explosion and fragments, military personnel**

⑦ **Y37.201- Military operations involving unspecified explosion and fragments, civilian**

⑥ **Y37.21 Military operations involving explosion of aerial bomb**

⑦ **Y37.210- Military operations involving explosion of aerial bomb, military personnel**

⑦ **Y37.211- Military operations involving explosion of aerial bomb, civilian**

⑥ **Y37.22 Military operations involving explosion of guided missile**

⑦ **Y37.220- Military operations involving explosion of guided missile, military personnel**

⑦ **Y37.221- Military operations involving explosion of guided missile, civilian**

⑥ **Y37.23 Military operations involving explosion of improvised explosive device [IED]**
Military operations involving explosion of person-borne improvised explosive device [IED]
Military operations involving explosion of vehicle-borne improvised explosive device [IED]
Military operations involving explosion of roadside improvised explosive device [IED]

⑦ **Y37.230- Military operations involving explosion of improvised explosive device [IED], military personnel**

⑦ **Y37.231- Military operations involving explosion of improvised explosive device [IED], civilian**

⑥ **Y37.24 Military operations involving explosion due to accidental detonation and discharge of own munitions or munitions launch device**

⑦ **Y37.240- Military operations involving explosion due to accidental detonation and discharge of own munitions or munitions launch device, military personnel**

⑦ **Y37.241- Military operations involving explosion due to accidental detonation and discharge of own munitions or munitions launch device, civilian**

⑥ **Y37.25 Military operations involving fragments from munitions**

⑦ **Y37.250- Military operations involving fragments from munitions, military personnel**

⑦ **Y37.251- Military operations involving fragments from munitions, civilian**

⑥ **Y37.26 Military operations involving fragments of improvised explosive device [IED]**
Military operations involving fragments of person-borne improvised explosive device [IED]
Military operations involving fragments of vehicle-borne improvised explosive device [IED]
Military operations involving fragments of roadside improvised explosive device [IED]

⑦ **Y37.260- Military operations involving fragments of improvised explosive device [IED], military personnel**

⑦ **Y37.261- Military operations involving fragments of improvised explosive device [IED], civilian**

⑥ **Y37.27 Military operations involving fragments from weapons**

⑦ **Y37.270- Military operations involving fragments from weapons, military personnel**

⑦ **Y37.271- Military operations involving fragments from weapons, civilian**

⑥ **Y37.29 Military operations involving other explosions and fragments**
Military operations involving explosion of grenade
Military operations involving explosions of land mine
Military operations involving shrapnel NOS

⑦ **Y37.290- Military operations involving other explosions and fragments, military personnel**

⑦ **Y37.291- Military operations involving other explosions and fragments, civilian**

⑤ **Y37.3 Military operations involving fires, conflagrations and hot substances**
Military operations involving smoke, fumes, and heat from fires, conflagrations and hot substances
> **EXCLUDES 1** *military operations involving fires and conflagrations aboard military aircraft (Y37.1-)*
> *military operations involving fires and conflagrations aboard military watercraft (Y37.0-)*
> *military operations involving fires and conflagrations caused indirectly by conventional weapons (Y37.2-)*
> *military operations involving fires and thermal effects of nuclear weapons (Y36.53-)*

⑥ **Y37.30 Military operations involving unspecified fire, conflagration and hot substance**

⑦ **Y37.300- Military operations involving unspecified fire, conflagration and hot substance, military personnel**

⑦ **Y37.301- Military operations involving unspecified fire, conflagration and hot substance, civilian**

⑥ **Y37.31 Military operations involving gasoline bomb**
Military operations involving incendiary bomb
Military operations involving petrol bomb

⑦ **Y37.310- Military operations involving gasoline bomb, military personnel**

⑦ **Y37.311- Military operations involving gasoline bomb, civilian**

⑥ **Y37.32 Military operations involving incendiary bullet**

⑦ **Y37.320- Military operations involving incendiary bullet, military personnel**

⑦ **Y37.321- Military operations involving incendiary bullet, civilian**

⑥ **Y37.33 Military operations involving flamethrower**

⑦ **Y37.330- Military operations involving flamethrower, military personnel**

⑦ **Y37.331- Military operations involving flamethrower, civilian**

⑥ **Y37.39 Military operations involving other fires, conflagrations and hot substances**

⑦ **Y37.390- Military operations involving other fires, conflagrations and hot substances, military personnel**

⑦ **Y37.391- Military operations involving other fires, conflagrations and hot substances, civilian**

⑤ **Y37.4 Military operations involving firearm discharge and other forms of conventional warfare**

⑥ **Y37.41 Military operations involving rubber bullets**

⑦ **Y37.410- Military operations involving rubber bullets, military personnel**

⑦ **Y37.411- Military operations involving rubber bullets, civilian**

⑥ **Y37.42 Military operations involving firearms pellets**

⑦ **Y37.420- Military operations involving firearms pellets, military personnel**

⑦ **Y37.421- Military operations involving firearms pellets, civilian**

⑥ **Y37.43 Military operations involving other firearms discharge**
Military operations involving bullets NOS
> **EXCLUDES 1** *military operations involving munitions fragments (Y37.25-)*
> *military operations involving incendiary bullets (Y37.32-)*

⑦ **Y37.430- Military operations involving other firearms discharge, military personnel**

⑦ **Y37.431- Military operations involving other firearms discharge, civilian**

⑥ **Y37.44** **Military operations involving unarmed hand to hand combat**

> **EXCLUDES 1** *military operations involving combat using blunt or piercing object (Y37.45-)*
> *military operations involving intentional restriction of air and airway (Y37.46-)*
> *military operations involving unintentional restriction of air and airway (Y37.47-)*

⑦ **Y37.440-** Military operations involving unarmed hand to hand combat, military personnel

⑦ **Y37.441-** Military operations involving unarmed hand to hand combat, civilian

⑥ **Y37.45** **Military operations involving combat using blunt or piercing object**

⑦ **Y37.450-** Military operations involving combat using blunt or piercing object, military personnel

⑦ **Y37.451-** Military operations involving combat using blunt or piercing object, civilian

⑥ **Y37.46** **Military operations involving intentional restriction of air and airway**

⑦ **Y37.460-** Military operations involving intentional restriction of air and airway, military personnel

⑦ **Y37.461-** Military operations involving intentional restriction of air and airway, civilian

⑥ **Y37.47** **Military operations involving unintentional restriction of air and airway**

⑦ **Y37.470-** Military operations involving unintentional restriction of air and airway, military personnel

⑦ **Y37.471-** Military operations involving unintentional restriction of air and airway, civilian

⑥ **Y37.49** **Military operations involving other forms of conventional warfare**

⑦ **Y37.490-** Military operations involving other forms of conventional warfare, military personnel

⑦ **Y37.491-** Military operations involving other forms of conventional warfare, civilian

⑤ **Y37.5** **Military operations involving nuclear weapons**

> Military operation involving dirty bomb NOS

⑥ **Y37.50** **Military operations involving unspecified effect of nuclear weapon**

⑦ **Y37.500-** Military operations involving unspecified effect of nuclear weapon, military personnel

⑦ **Y37.501-** Military operations involving unspecified effect of nuclear weapon, civilian

⑥ **Y37.51** **Military operations involving direct blast effect of nuclear weapon**

> Military operations involving blast pressure of nuclear weapon

⑦ **Y37.510-** Military operations involving direct blast effect of nuclear weapon, military personnel

⑦ **Y37.511-** Military operations involving direct blast effect of nuclear weapon, civilian

⑥ **Y37.52** **Military operations involving indirect blast effect of nuclear weapon**

> Military operations involving being thrown by blast of nuclear weapon
> Military operations involving being struck or crushed by blast debris of nuclear weapon

⑦ **Y37.520-** Military operations involving indirect blast effect of nuclear weapon, military personnel

⑦ **Y37.521-** Military operations involving indirect blast effect of nuclear weapon, civilian

⑥ **Y37.53** **Military operations involving thermal radiation effect of nuclear weapon**

> Military operations involving direct heat from nuclear weapon
> Military operation involving fireball effects from nuclear weapon

⑦ **Y37.530-** Military operations involving thermal radiation effect of nuclear weapon, military personnel

⑦ **Y37.531-** Military operations involving thermal radiation effect of nuclear weapon, civilian

⑥ **Y37.54** **Military operation involving nuclear radiation effects of nuclear weapon**

> Military operation involving acute radiation exposure from nuclear weapon
> Military operation involving exposure to immediate ionizing radiation from nuclear weapon
> Military operation involving fallout exposure from nuclear weapon
> Military operation involving secondary effects of nuclear weapons

⑦ **Y37.540-** Military operation involving nuclear radiation effects of nuclear weapon, military personnel

⑦ **Y37.541-** Military operation involving nuclear radiation effects of nuclear weapon, civilian

⑥ **Y37.59** **Military operation involving other effects of nuclear weapons**

⑦ **Y37.590-** Military operation involving other effects of nuclear weapons, military personnel

⑦ **Y37.591-** Military operation involving other effects of nuclear weapons, civilian

⑤ **Y37.6** **Military operations involving biological weapons**

⑥ **Y37.6X** **Military operations involving biological weapons**

⑦ **Y37.6X0-** Military operations involving biological weapons, military personnel

⑦ **Y37.6X1-** Military operations involving biological weapons, civilian

⑤ **Y37.7** **Military operations involving chemical weapons and other forms of unconventional warfare**

> **EXCLUDES 1** *military operations involving incendiary devices (Y36.3-, Y36.5-)*

⑥ **Y37.7X** **Military operations involving chemical weapons and other forms of unconventional warfare**

⑦ **Y37.7X0-** Military operations involving chemical weapons and other forms of unconventional warfare, military personnel

⑦ **Y37.7X1-** Military operations involving chemical weapons and other forms of unconventional warfare, civilian

⑤ **Y37.9** **Other and unspecified military operations**

⑦ **Y37.90X-** Military operations, unspecified

⑦ **Y37.91X-** Military operations involving unspecified weapon of mass destruction [WMD]

⑦ **Y37.92X-** Military operations involving friendly fire

④+ **Y38** **Terrorism**

> These codes are for use to identify injuries resulting from the unlawful use of force or violence against persons or property to intimidate or coerce a Government, the civilian population, or any segment thereof, in furtherance of political or social objective
>
> *Use additional code for place of occurrence (Y92.-)*

> The appropriate 7th character is to be added to each code from category Y38
>
> A   initial encounter
> D   subsequent encounter
> S   sequela

⑤+ **Y38.0** **Terrorism involving explosion of marine weapons**

> Terrorism involving depth-charge
> Terrorism involving marine mine
> Terrorism involving mine NOS, at sea or in harbor
> Terrorism involving sea-based artillery shell
> Terrorism involving torpedo
> Terrorism involving underwater blast

⑥+ **Y38.0X** **Terrorism involving explosion of marine weapons**

⑦+ **Y38.0X1-** Terrorism involving explosion of marine weapons, public safety official injured

⑦+ **Y38.0X2-** Terrorism involving explosion of marine weapons, civilian injured

⑦+ **Y38.0X3-** Terrorism involving explosion of marine weapons, terrorist injured

⑤+ **Y38.1** **Terrorism involving destruction of aircraft**

> Terrorism involving aircraft burned
> Terrorism involving aircraft exploded
> Terrorism involving aircraft being shot down
> Terrorism involving aircraft used as a weapon

⑥+ **Y38.1X** **Terrorism involving destruction of aircraft**

⑦+ **Y38.1X1-** Terrorism involving destruction of aircraft, public safety official injured

⑦+ **Y38.1X2-** Terrorism involving destruction of aircraft, civilian injured

---

● New   ▲ Revised   *Manifestation*   ④-⑦ Digit Indicators   ⊟ Laterality   🅰 Adult (15+ years)   🅼 Maternity (12-55 years)   🅽 Newborn   🅿 Pediatric (0-17 years)   ♂ Male   ♀ Female
✖ Deleted   Unspecified   + Additional code

7 + Y38.1X3- Terrorism involving destruction of aircraft, terrorist injured

5 + Y38.2 Terrorism involving other explosions and fragments
Terrorism involving antipersonnel (fragments) bomb
Terrorism involving blast NOS
Terrorism involving explosion NOS
Terrorism involving explosion of breech block
Terrorism involving explosion of cannon block
Terrorism involving explosion (fragments) of artillery shell
Terrorism involving explosion (fragments) of bomb
Terrorism involving explosion (fragments) of grenade
Terrorism involving explosion (fragments) of guided missile
Terrorism involving explosion (fragments) of land mine
Terrorism involving explosion of mortar bomb
Terrorism involving explosion of munitions
Terrorism involving explosion (fragments) of rocket
Terrorism involving explosion (fragments) of shell
Terrorism involving shrapnel
Terrorism involving mine NOS, on land

> **EXCLUDES 1** *terrorism involving explosion of nuclear weapon (Y38.5)*
> *terrorism involving suicide bomber (Y38.81)*

6 + Y38.2X Terrorism involving other explosions and fragments
7 + Y38.2X1- Terrorism involving other explosions and fragments, public safety official injured
7 + Y38.2X2- Terrorism involving other explosions and fragments, civilian injured
7 + Y38.2X3- Terrorism involving other explosions and fragments, terrorist injured

5 + Y38.3 Terrorism involving fires, conflagration and hot substances
Terrorism involving conflagration NOS
Terrorism involving fire NOS
Terrorism involving petrol bomb

> **EXCLUDES 1** *terrorism involving fire or heat of nuclear weapon (Y38.5)*

6 + Y38.3X Terrorism involving fires, conflagration and hot substances
7 + Y38.3X1- Terrorism involving fires, conflagration and hot substances, public safety official injured
7 + Y38.3X2- Terrorism involving fires, conflagration and hot substances, civilian injured
7 + Y38.3X3- Terrorism involving fires, conflagration and hot substances, terrorist injured

5 + Y38.4 Terrorism involving firearms
Terrorism involving carbine bullet
Terrorism involving machine gun bullet
Terrorism involving pellets (shotgun)
Terrorism involving pistol bullet
Terrorism involving rifle bullet
Terrorism involving rubber (rifle) bullet

6 + Y38.4X Terrorism involving firearms
7 + Y38.4X1- Terrorism involving firearms, public safety official injured
7 + Y38.4X2- Terrorism involving firearms, civilian injured
7 + Y38.4X3- Terrorism involving firearms, terrorist injured

5 + Y38.5 Terrorism involving nuclear weapons
Terrorism involving blast effects of nuclear weapon
Terrorism involving exposure to ionizing radiation from nuclear weapon
Terrorism involving fireball effect of nuclear weapon
Terrorism involving heat from nuclear weapon

6 + Y38.5X Terrorism involving nuclear weapons
7 + Y38.5X1- Terrorism involving nuclear weapons, public safety official injured
7 + Y38.5X2- Terrorism involving nuclear weapons, civilian injured
7 + Y38.5X3- Terrorism involving nuclear weapons, terrorist injured

5 + Y38.6 Terrorism involving biological weapons
Terrorism involving anthrax
Terrorism involving cholera
Terrorism involving smallpox

6 + Y38.6X Terrorism involving biological weapons
7 + Y38.6X1- Terrorism involving biological weapons, public safety official injured
7 + Y38.6X2- Terrorism involving biological weapons, civilian injured
7 + Y38.6X3- Terrorism involving biological weapons, terrorist injured

5 + Y38.7 Terrorism involving chemical weapons
Terrorism involving gases, fumes, chemicals
Terrorism involving hydrogen cyanide
Terrorism involving phosgene
Terrorism involving sarin

6 + Y38.7X Terrorism involving chemical weapons
7 + Y38.7X1- Terrorism involving chemical weapons, public safety official injured
7 + Y38.7X2- Terrorism involving chemical weapons, civilian injured
7 + Y38.7X3- Terrorism involving chemical weapons, terrorist injured

5 + Y38.8 Terrorism involving other and unspecified means
7 + Y38.80X- Terrorism involving unspecified means
Terrorism NOS

6 + Y38.81 Terrorism involving suicide bomber
7 + Y38.811- Terrorism involving suicide bomber, public safety official injured
7 + Y38.812- Terrorism involving suicide bomber, civilian injured

6 + Y38.89 Terrorism involving other means
Terrorism involving drowning and submersion
Terrorism involving lasers
Terrorism involving piercing or stabbing instruments
7 + Y38.891- Terrorism involving other means, public safety official injured
7 + Y38.892- Terrorism involving other means, civilian injured
7 + Y38.893- Terrorism involving other means, terrorist injured

5 + Y38.9 Terrorism, secondary effects
Note: This code is for use to identify conditions occurring subsequent to a terrorist attack not those that are due to the initial terrorist attack

6 + Y38.9X Terrorism, secondary effects
7 + Y38.9X1- Terrorism, secondary effects, public safety official injured
7 + Y38.9X2- Terrorism, secondary effects, civilian injured

Complications of medical and surgical care (Y62-Y84)

> **INCLUDES** complications of medical devices
> surgical and medical procedures as the cause of abnormal reaction of the patient, or of later complication, without mention of misadventure at the time of the procedure

Misadventures to patients during surgical and medical care (Y62-Y69)

> **EXCLUDES 1** *surgical and medical procedures as the cause of abnormal reaction of the patient, without mention of misadventure at the time of the procedure (Y83-Y84)*
> **EXCLUDES 2** *breakdown or malfunctioning of medical device (during procedure) (after implantation) (ongoing use) (Y70-Y82)*

4 Y62 Failure of sterile precautions during surgical and medical care
Y62.0 Failure of sterile precautions during surgical operation
Y62.1 Failure of sterile precautions during infusion or transfusion
Y62.2 Failure of sterile precautions during kidney dialysis and other perfusion
Y62.3 Failure of sterile precautions during injection or immunization
Y62.4 Failure of sterile precautions during endoscopic examination
Y62.5 Failure of sterile precautions during heart catheterization
Y62.6 Failure of sterile precautions during aspiration, puncture and other catheterization
Y62.8 Failure of sterile precautions during other surgical and medical care
Y62.9 Failure of sterile precautions during unspecified surgical and medical care

4 Y63 Failure in dosage during surgical and medical care
> **EXCLUDES 2** *accidental overdose of drug or wrong drug given in error (T36-T50)*
Y63.0 Excessive amount of blood or other fluid given during transfusion or infusion

---

● New   ▲ Revised   *Manifestation*   **4 - 7** Digit Indicators   ▣ Laterality   Ⓐ Adult (15+ years)   Ⓜ Maternity (12-55 years)   Ⓝ Newborn   Ⓟ Pediatric (0-17 years)   ♂ Male   ♀ Female
✖ Deleted   Unspecified   + Additional code

External Causes of Morbidity

Y63.1   Incorrect dilution of fluid used during infusion

Y63.2   Overdose of radiation given during therapy

Y63.3   Inadvertent exposure of patient to radiation during medical care

Y63.4   Failure in dosage in electroshock or insulin-shock therapy

Y63.5   Inappropriate temperature in local application and packing

Y63.6   Underdosing and nonadministration of necessary drug, medicament or biological substance

> **GUIDELINES**   Section I.C.19.e.5)(c)
> Noncompliance (Z91.12-, Z91.13-) or complication of care (Y63.6-Y63.9) codes are to be used with an underdosing code to indicate intent, if known.

Y63.8   Failure in dosage during other surgical and medical care

> **GUIDELINES**   Section I.C.19.e.5)(c)
> Noncompliance (Z91.12-, Z91.13-) or complication of care (Y63.6-Y63.9) codes are to be used with an underdosing code to indicate intent, if known.

Y63.9   Failure in dosage during unspecified surgical and medical care

> **GUIDELINES**   Section I.C.19.e.5)(c)
> Noncompliance (Z91.12-, Z91.13-) or complication of care (Y63.6-Y63.9) codes are to be used with an underdosing code to indicate intent, if known.

Y64   Contaminated medical or biological substances

Y64.0   Contaminated medical or biological substance, transfused or infused

Y64.1   Contaminated medical or biological substance, injected or used for immunization

Y64.8   Contaminated medical or biological substance administered by other means

Y64.9   Contaminated medical or biological substance administered by unspecified means
     Administered contaminated medical or biological substance NOS

Y65   Other misadventures during surgical and medical care

Y65.0   Mismatched blood in transfusion

Y65.1   Wrong fluid used in infusion

Y65.2   Failure in suture or ligature during surgical operation

Y65.3   Endotracheal tube wrongly placed during anesthetic procedure

Y65.4   Failure to introduce or to remove other tube or instrument

Y65.5   Performance of wrong procedure (operation)

   Y65.51   Performance of wrong procedure (operation) on correct patient
     Wrong device implanted into correct surgical site
> **EXCLUDES 1**   *performance of correct procedure (operation) on wrong side or body part (Y65.53)*

   Y65.52   Performance of procedure (operation) on patient not scheduled for surgery
     Performance of procedure (operation) intended for another patient
     Performance of procedure (operation) on wrong patient

   Y65.53   Performance of correct procedure (operation) on wrong side or body part
     Performance of correct procedure (operation) on wrong side
     Performance of correct procedure (operation) on wrong site

Y65.8   Other specified misadventures during surgical and medical care

Y66   Nonadministration of surgical and medical care
   Premature cessation of surgical and medical care
> **EXCLUDES 1**   *DNR status (Z66)*
> *palliative care (Z51.5)*

Y69   Unspecified misadventure during surgical and medical care

Medical devices associated with adverse incidents in diagnostic and therapeutic use (Y70-Y82)

> **INCLUDES**   breakdown or malfunction of medical devices (during use) (after implantation) (ongoing use)

> **EXCLUDES 2**   *breakdown or malfunctioning of medical device (after implantation) (during procedure) (ongoing use) (Y70-Y82)*
> *later complications following use of medical devices without breakdown or malfunctioning of device (Y83-Y84)*
> *misadventure to patients during surgical and medical care, classifiable to (Y62-Y69)*
> *surgical and other medical procedures as the cause of abnormal reaction of the patient, or of later complication, without mention of misadventure at the time of the procedure (Y83-Y84)*

Y70   Anesthesiology devices associated with adverse incidents

Y70.0   Diagnostic and monitoring anesthesiology devices associated with adverse incidents

Y70.1   Therapeutic (nonsurgical) and rehabilitative anesthesiology devices associated with adverse incidents

Y70.2   Prosthetic and other implants, materials and accessory anesthesiology devices associated with adverse incidents

Y70.3   Surgical instruments, materials and anesthesiology devices (including sutures) associated with adverse incidents

Y70.8   Miscellaneous anesthesiology devices associated with adverse incidents, not elsewhere classified

Y71   Cardiovascular devices associated with adverse incidents

Y71.0   Diagnostic and monitoring cardiovascular devices associated with adverse incidents

Y71.1   Therapeutic (nonsurgical) and rehabilitative cardiovascular devices associated with adverse incidents

Y71.2   Prosthetic and other implants, materials and accessory cardiovascular devices associated with adverse incidents

Y71.3   Surgical instruments, materials and cardiovascular devices (including sutures) associated with adverse incidents

Y71.8   Miscellaneous cardiovascular devices associated with adverse incidents, not elsewhere classified

Y72   Otorhinolaryngological devices associated with adverse incidents

Y72.0   Diagnostic and monitoring otorhinolaryngological devices associated with adverse incidents

Y72.1   Therapeutic (nonsurgical) and rehabilitative otorhinolaryngological devices associated with adverse incidents

Y72.2   Prosthetic and other implants, materials and accessory otorhinolaryngological devices associated with adverse incidents

Y72.3   Surgical instruments, materials and otorhinolaryngological devices (including sutures) associated with adverse incidents

Y72.8   Miscellaneous otorhinolaryngological devices associated with adverse incidents, not elsewhere classified

Y73   Gastroenterology and urology devices associated with adverse incidents

Y73.0   Diagnostic and monitoring gastroenterology and urology devices associated with adverse incidents

Y73.1   Therapeutic (nonsurgical) and rehabilitative gastroenterology and urology devices associated with adverse incidents

Y73.2   Prosthetic and other implants, materials and accessory gastroenterology and urology devices associated with adverse incidents

Y73.3   Surgical instruments, materials and gastroenterology and urology devices (including sutures) associated with adverse incidents

Y73.8   Miscellaneous gastroenterology and urology devices associated with adverse incidents, not elsewhere classified

Y74   General hospital and personal-use devices associated with adverse incidents

Y74.0   Diagnostic and monitoring general hospital and personal-use devices associated with adverse incidents

● New   ▲ Revised   *Manifestation*   🔢-🔢 Digit Indicators   ⊟ Laterality   🅰 Adult (15+ years)   🅼 Maternity (12-55 years)   🅽 Newborn   🅿 Pediatric (0-17 years)   ♂ Male   ♀ Female
✖ Deleted   Unspecified   ✚ Additional code

2017 ICD-10-CM Expert for Physicians   © 2017 DecisionHealth   1169

Y63.1 — Y74.0

Y74.1 Therapeutic (nonsurgical) and rehabilitative general hospital and personal-use devices associated with adverse incidents

Y74.2 Prosthetic and other implants, materials and accessory general hospital and personal-use devices associated with adverse incidents

Y74.3 Surgical instruments, materials and general hospital and personal-use devices (including sutures) associated with adverse incidents

Y74.8 Miscellaneous general hospital and personal-use devices associated with adverse incidents, not elsewhere classified

◢ **Y75** Neurological devices associated with adverse incidents

Y75.0 Diagnostic and monitoring neurological devices associated with adverse incidents

Y75.1 Therapeutic (nonsurgical) and rehabilitative neurological devices associated with adverse incidents

Y75.2 Prosthetic and other implants, materials and neurological devices associated with adverse incidents

Y75.3 Surgical instruments, materials and neurological devices (including sutures) associated with adverse incidents

Y75.8 Miscellaneous neurological devices associated with adverse incidents, not elsewhere classified

◢ **Y76** Obstetric and gynecological devices associated with adverse incidents

Y76.0 Diagnostic and monitoring obstetric and gynecological devices associated with adverse incidents ♀

Y76.1 Therapeutic (nonsurgical) and rehabilitative obstetric and gynecological devices associated with adverse incidents ♀

Y76.2 Prosthetic and other implants, materials and accessory obstetric and gynecological devices associated with adverse incidents ♀

Y76.3 Surgical instruments, materials and obstetric and gynecological devices (including sutures) associated with adverse incidents ♀

Y76.8 Miscellaneous obstetric and gynecological devices associated with adverse incidents, not elsewhere classified ♀

◢ **Y77** Ophthalmic devices associated with adverse incidents

Y77.0 Diagnostic and monitoring ophthalmic devices associated with adverse incidents

Y77.1 Therapeutic (nonsurgical) and rehabilitative ophthalmic devices associated with adverse incidents

Y77.2 Prosthetic and other implants, materials and accessory ophthalmic devices associated with adverse incidents

Y77.3 Surgical instruments, materials and ophthalmic devices (including sutures) associated with adverse incidents

Y77.8 Miscellaneous ophthalmic devices associated with adverse incidents, not elsewhere classified

◢ **Y78** Radiological devices associated with adverse incidents

Y78.0 Diagnostic and monitoring radiological devices associated with adverse incidents

Y78.1 Therapeutic (nonsurgical) and rehabilitative radiological devices associated with adverse incidents

Y78.2 Prosthetic and other implants, materials and accessory radiological devices associated with adverse incidents

Y78.3 Surgical instruments, materials and radiological devices (including sutures) associated with adverse incidents

Y78.8 Miscellaneous radiological devices associated with adverse incidents, not elsewhere classified

◢ **Y79** Orthopedic devices associated with adverse incidents

Y79.0 Diagnostic and monitoring orthopedic devices associated with adverse incidents

Y79.1 Therapeutic (nonsurgical) and rehabilitative orthopedic devices associated with adverse incidents

Y79.2 Prosthetic and other implants, materials and accessory orthopedic devices associated with adverse incidents

Y79.3 Surgical instruments, materials and orthopedic devices (including sutures) associated with adverse incidents

Y79.8 Miscellaneous orthopedic devices associated with adverse incidents, not elsewhere classified

◢ **Y80** Physical medicine devices associated with adverse incidents

Y80.0 Diagnostic and monitoring physical medicine devices associated with adverse incidents

Y80.1 Therapeutic (nonsurgical) and rehabilitative physical medicine devices associated with adverse incidents

Y80.2 Prosthetic and other implants, materials and accessory physical medicine devices associated with adverse incidents

Y80.3 Surgical instruments, materials and physical medicine devices (including sutures) associated with adverse incidents

Y80.8 Miscellaneous physical medicine devices associated with adverse incidents, not elsewhere classified

◢ **Y81** General- and plastic-surgery devices associated with adverse incidents

Y81.0 Diagnostic and monitoring general- and plastic-surgery devices associated with adverse incidents

Y81.1 Therapeutic (nonsurgical) and rehabilitative general- and plastic-surgery devices associated with adverse incidents

Y81.2 Prosthetic and other implants, materials and accessory general- and plastic-surgery devices associated with adverse incidents

Y81.3 Surgical instruments, materials and general- and plastic-surgery devices (including sutures) associated with adverse incidents

Y81.8 Miscellaneous general- and plastic-surgery devices associated with adverse incidents, not elsewhere classified

◢ **Y82** Other and unspecified medical devices associated with adverse incidents

Y82.8 Other medical devices associated with adverse incidents

Y82.9 Unspecified medical devices associated with adverse incidents

Surgical and other medical procedures as the cause of abnormal reaction of the patient, or of later complication, without mention of misadventure at the time of the procedure (Y83-Y84)

EXCLUDES 1 *misadventures to patients during surgical and medical care, classifiable to (Y62-Y69)*

EXCLUDES 2 *breakdown or malfunctioning of medical device (after implantation) (during procedure) (ongoing use) (Y70-Y82)*

◢ **Y83** Surgical operation and other surgical procedures as the cause of abnormal reaction of the patient, or of later complication, without mention of misadventure at the time of the procedure

Y83.0 Surgical operation with transplant of whole organ as the cause of abnormal reaction of the patient, or of later complication, without mention of misadventure at the time of the procedure

Y83.1 Surgical operation with implant of artificial internal device as the cause of abnormal reaction of the patient, or of later complication, without mention of misadventure at the time of the procedure

Y83.2 Surgical operation with anastomosis, bypass or graft as the cause of abnormal reaction of the patient, or of later complication, without mention of misadventure at the time of the procedure

Y83.3 Surgical operation with formation of external stoma as the cause of abnormal reaction of the patient, or of later complication, without mention of misadventure at the time of the procedure

Y83.4 Other reconstructive surgery as the cause of abnormal reaction of the patient, or of later complication, without mention of misadventure at the time of the procedure

Y83.5 Amputation of limb(s) as the cause of abnormal reaction of the patient, or of later complication, without mention of misadventure at the time of the procedure

Y83.6 Removal of other organ (partial) (total) as the cause of abnormal reaction of the patient, or of later complication, without mention of misadventure at the time of the procedure

Y83.8 Other surgical procedures as the cause of abnormal reaction of the patient, or of later complication, without mention of misadventure at the time of the procedure

Y83.9 Surgical procedure, unspecified as the cause of abnormal reaction of the patient, or of later complication, without mention of misadventure at the time of the procedure

◢ **Y84** Other medical procedures as the cause of abnormal reaction of the patient, or of later complication, without mention of misadventure at the time of the procedure

---

● New ▲ Revised *Manifestation* ◢-◤ Digit Indicators ▭ Laterality ▤ Adult (15+ years) Ⓜ Maternity (12-55 years) Ⓝ Newborn ▣ Pediatric (0-17 years) ♂ Male ♀ Female
✖ Deleted Unspecified + Additional code

1170   © 2017 DecisionHealth   2017 ICD-10-CM Expert for Physicians

Y84.0 Cardiac catheterization as the cause of abnormal reaction of the patient, or of later complication, without mention of misadventure at the time of the procedure

Y84.1 Kidney dialysis as the cause of abnormal reaction of the patient, or of later complication, without mention of misadventure at the time of the procedure

Y84.2 Radiological procedure and radiotherapy as the cause of abnormal reaction of the patient, or of later complication, without mention of misadventure at the time of the procedure

Y84.3 Shock therapy as the cause of abnormal reaction of the patient, or of later complication, without mention of misadventure at the time of the procedure

Y84.4 Aspiration of fluid as the cause of abnormal reaction of the patient, or of later complication, without mention of misadventure at the time of the procedure

Y84.5 Insertion of gastric or duodenal sound as the cause of abnormal reaction of the patient, or of later complication, without mention of misadventure at the time of the procedure

Y84.6 Urinary catheterization as the cause of abnormal reaction of the patient, or of later complication, without mention of misadventure at the time of the procedure

Y84.7 Blood-sampling as the cause of abnormal reaction of the patient, or of later complication, without mention of misadventure at the time of the procedure

Y84.8 Other medical procedures as the cause of abnormal reaction of the patient, or of later complication, without mention of misadventure at the time of the procedure
  AHA: 4Q 2014, 24

Y84.9 Medical procedure, unspecified as the cause of abnormal reaction of the patient, or of later complication, without mention of misadventure at the time of the procedure

Supplementary factors related to causes of morbidity classified elsewhere (Y90-Y99)

Note: These categories may be used to provide supplementary information concerning causes of morbidity. They are not to be used for single-condition coding.

Y90 Evidence of alcohol involvement determined by blood alcohol level
  Code first:
    any associated alcohol related disorders (F10)

Y90.0 Blood alcohol level of less than 20 mg/100 ml

Y90.1 Blood alcohol level of 20-39 mg/100 ml

Y90.2 Blood alcohol level of 40-59 mg/100 ml

Y90.3 Blood alcohol level of 60-79 mg/100 ml

Y90.4 Blood alcohol level of 80-99 mg/100 ml

Y90.5 Blood alcohol level of 100-119 mg/100 ml

Y90.6 Blood alcohol level of 120-199 mg/100 ml

Y90.7 Blood alcohol level of 200-239 mg/100 ml

Y90.8 Blood alcohol level of 240 mg/100 ml or more

Y90.9 Presence of alcohol in blood, level not specified

Y92 Place of occurrence of the external cause
  The following category is for use, when relevant, to identify the place of occurrence of the external cause. Use in conjunction with an activity code.
  Place of occurrence should be recorded only at the initial encounter for treatment

Y92.0 Non-institutional (private) residence as the place of occurrence of the external cause
  EXCLUDES 1 *abandoned or derelict house (Y92.89)*
    home under construction but not yet occupied (Y92.6-)
    institutional place of residence (Y92.1-)

Y92.00 Unspecified non-institutional (private) residence as the place of occurrence of the external cause

Y92.000 Kitchen of unspecified non-institutional (private) residence as the place of occurrence of the external cause

Y92.001 Dining room of unspecified non-institutional (private) residence as the place of occurrence of the external cause

Y92.002 Bathroom of unspecified non-institutional (private) residence single-family (private) house as the place of occurrence of the external cause

Y92.003 Bedroom of unspecified non-institutional (private) residence as the place of occurrence of the external cause

Y92.007 Garden or yard of unspecified non-institutional (private) residence as the place of occurrence of the external cause

Y92.008 Other place in unspecified non-institutional (private) residence as the place of occurrence of the external cause

Y92.009 Unspecified place in unspecified non-institutional (private) residence as the place of occurrence of the external cause
  Home (NOS) as the place of occurrence of the external cause

Y92.01 Single-family non-institutional (private) house as the place of occurrence of the external cause
  Farmhouse as the place of occurrence of the external cause
  EXCLUDES 1 *barn (Y92.71)*
    chicken coop or hen house (Y92.72)
    farm field (Y92.73)
    orchard (Y92.74)
    single family mobile home or trailer (Y92.02-)
    slaughter house (Y92.86)

Y92.010 Kitchen of single-family (private) house as the place of occurrence of the external cause

Y92.011 Dining room of single-family (private) house as the place of occurrence of the external cause

Y92.012 Bathroom of single-family (private) house as the place of occurrence of the external cause

Y92.013 Bedroom of single-family (private) house as the place of occurrence of the external cause

Y92.014 Private driveway to single-family (private) house as the place of occurrence of the external cause

Y92.015 Private garage of single-family (private) house as the place of occurrence of the external cause

Y92.016 Swimming-pool in single-family (private) house or garden as the place of occurrence of the external cause

Y92.017 Garden or yard in single-family (private) house as the place of occurrence of the external cause

Y92.018 Other place in single-family (private) house as the place of occurrence of the external cause

Y92.019 Unspecified place in single-family (private) house as the place of occurrence of the external cause

Y92.02 Mobile home as the place of occurrence of the external cause

Y92.020 Kitchen in mobile home as the place of occurrence of the external cause

Y92.021 Dining room in mobile home as the place of occurrence of the external cause

Y92.022 Bathroom in mobile home as the place of occurrence of the external cause

Y92.023 Bedroom in mobile home as the place of occurrence of the external cause

Y92.024 Driveway of mobile home as the place of occurrence of the external cause

Y92.025 Garage of mobile home as the place of occurrence of the external cause

Y92.026 Swimming-pool of mobile home as the place of occurrence of the external cause

Y92.027 Garden or yard of mobile home as the place of occurrence of the external cause

Y92.028 Other place in mobile home as the place of occurrence of the external cause

Y92.029 Unspecified place in mobile home as the place of occurrence of the external cause

Y92.03 Apartment as the place of occurrence of the external cause
  Condominium as the place of occurrence of the external cause
  Co-op apartment as the place of occurrence of the external cause

Y92.030 Kitchen in apartment as the place of occurrence of the external cause

● New ▲ Revised *Manifestation* ◄-► Digit Indicators ▭ Laterality Ⓐ Adult (15+ years) Ⓜ Maternity (12-55 years) Ⓝ Newborn Ⓟ Pediatric (0-17 years) ♂ Male ♀ Female
✖ Deleted Unspecified ✚ Additional code

2017 ICD-10-CM Expert for Physicians

© 2017 DecisionHealth   1171

Y92.031   Bathroom in apartment as the place of occurrence of the external cause

Y92.032   Bedroom in apartment as the place of occurrence of the external cause

Y92.038   Other place in apartment as the place of occurrence of the external cause

Y92.039   Unspecified place in apartment as the place of occurrence of the external cause

⑥ Y92.04   Boarding-house as the place of occurrence of the external cause

Y92.040   Kitchen in boarding-house as the place of occurrence of the external cause

Y92.041   Bathroom in boarding-house as the place of occurrence of the external cause

Y92.042   Bedroom in boarding-house as the place of occurrence of the external cause

Y92.043   Driveway of boarding-house as the place of occurrence of the external cause

Y92.044   Garage of boarding-house as the place of occurrence of the external cause

Y92.045   Swimming-pool of boarding-house as the place of occurrence of the external cause

Y92.046   Garden or yard of boarding-house as the place of occurrence of the external cause

Y92.048   Other place in boarding-house as the place of occurrence of the external cause

Y92.049   Unspecified place in boarding-house as the place of occurrence of the external cause

⑥ Y92.09   Other non-institutional residence as the place of occurrence of the external cause

Y92.090   Kitchen in other non-institutional residence as the place of occurrence of the external cause

Y92.091   Bathroom in other non-institutional residence as the place of occurrence of the external cause

Y92.092   Bedroom in other non-institutional residence as the place of occurrence of the external cause

Y92.093   Driveway of other non-institutional residence as the place of occurrence of the external cause

Y92.094   Garage of other non-institutional residence as the place of occurrence of the external cause

Y92.095   Swimming-pool of other non-institutional residence as the place of occurrence of the external cause

Y92.096   Garden or yard of other non-institutional residence as the place of occurrence of the external cause

Y92.098   Other place in other non-institutional residence as the place of occurrence of the external cause

Y92.099   Unspecified place in other non-institutional residence as the place of occurrence of the external cause

⑤ Y92.1   Institutional (nonprivate) residence as the place of occurrence of the external cause

Y92.10   Unspecified residential institution as the place of occurrence of the external cause

⑥ Y92.11   Children's home and orphanage as the place of occurrence of the external cause

Y92.110   Kitchen in children's home and orphanage as the place of occurrence of the external cause

Y92.111   Bathroom in children's home and orphanage as the place of occurrence of the external cause

Y92.112   Bedroom in children's home and orphanage as the place of occurrence of the external cause

Y92.113   Driveway of children's home and orphanage as the place of occurrence of the external cause

Y92.114   Garage of children's home and orphanage as the place of occurrence of the external cause

Y92.115   Swimming-pool of children's home and orphanage as the place of occurrence of the external cause

Y92.116   Garden or yard of children's home and orphanage as the place of occurrence of the external cause

Y92.118   Other place in children's home and orphanage as the place of occurrence of the external cause

Y92.119   Unspecified place in children's home and orphanage as the place of occurrence of the external cause

⑥ Y92.12   Nursing home as the place of occurrence of the external cause

Home for the sick as the place of occurrence of the external cause

Hospice as the place of occurrence of the external cause

Y92.120   Kitchen in nursing home as the place of occurrence of the external cause

Y92.121   Bathroom in nursing home as the place of occurrence of the external cause

Y92.122   Bedroom in nursing home as the place of occurrence of the external cause

Y92.123   Driveway of nursing home as the place of occurrence of the external cause

Y92.124   Garage of nursing home as the place of occurrence of the external cause

Y92.125   Swimming-pool of nursing home as the place of occurrence of the external cause

Y92.126   Garden or yard of nursing home as the place of occurrence of the external cause

Y92.128   Other place in nursing home as the place of occurrence of the external cause

Y92.129   Unspecified place in nursing home as the place of occurrence of the external cause

⑥ Y92.13   Military base as the place of occurrence of the external cause

EXCLUDES 1   *military training grounds (Y92.83)*

Y92.130   Kitchen on military base as the place of occurrence of the external cause

Y92.131   Mess hall on military base as the place of occurrence of the external cause

Y92.133   Barracks on military base as the place of occurrence of the external cause

Y92.135   Garage on military base as the place of occurrence of the external cause

Y92.136   Swimming-pool on military base as the place of occurrence of the external cause

Y92.137   Garden or yard on military base as the place of occurrence of the external cause

Y92.138   Other place on military base as the place of occurrence of the external cause

Y92.139   Unspecified place military base as the place of occurrence of the external cause

⑥ Y92.14   Prison as the place of occurrence of the external cause

Y92.140   Kitchen in prison as the place of occurrence of the external cause

Y92.141   Dining room in prison as the place of occurrence of the external cause

Y92.142   Bathroom in prison as the place of occurrence of the external cause

Y92.143   Cell of prison as the place of occurrence of the external cause

Y92.146   Swimming-pool of prison as the place of occurrence of the external cause

Y92.147   Courtyard of prison as the place of occurrence of the external cause

Y92.148   Other place in prison as the place of occurrence of the external cause

Y92.149   Unspecified place in prison as the place of occurrence of the external cause

⑥ Y92.15   Reform school as the place of occurrence of the external cause

Y92.150   Kitchen in reform school as the place of occurrence of the external cause

Y92.151   Dining room in reform school as the place of occurrence of the external cause

Y92.152   Bathroom in reform school as the place of occurrence of the external cause

Y92.153   Bedroom in reform school as the place of occurrence of the external cause

Y92.154   Driveway of reform school as the place of occurrence of the external cause

Y92.155   Garage of reform school as the place of occurrence of the external cause

Y92.156   Swimming-pool of reform school as the place of occurrence of the external cause

Y92.157   Garden or yard of reform school as the place of occurrence of the external cause

Y92.158   Other place in reform school as the place of occurrence of the external cause

● New   ▲ Revised   *Manifestation*   ④-⑦ Digit Indicators   ⊟ Laterality   Ⓐ Adult (15+ years)   Ⓜ Maternity (12-55 years)   Ⓝ Newborn   Ⓟ Pediatric (0-17 years)   ♂ Male   ♀ Female

✖ Deleted   Unspecified   ✚ Additional code

1172   © 2017 DecisionHealth   2017 ICD-10-CM Expert for Physicians

Y92.159 Unspecified place in reform school as the place of occurrence of the external cause

Ⓖ **Y92.16** School dormitory as the place of occurrence of the external cause

> EXCLUDES 1 *reform school as the place of occurrence of the external cause (Y92.15-)*
> *school buildings and grounds as the place of occurrence of the external cause (Y92.2-)*
> *school sports and athletic areas as the place of occurrence of the external cause (Y92.3-)*

Y92.160 Kitchen in school dormitory as the place of occurrence of the external cause

Y92.161 Dining room in school dormitory as the place of occurrence of the external cause

Y92.162 Bathroom in school dormitory as the place of occurrence of the external cause

Y92.163 Bedroom in school dormitory as the place of occurrence of the external cause

Y92.168 Other place in school dormitory as the place of occurrence of the external cause

Y92.169 Unspecified place in school dormitory as the place of occurrence of the external cause

Ⓖ **Y92.19** Other specified residential institution as the place of occurrence of the external cause

Y92.190 Kitchen in other specified residential institution as the place of occurrence of the external cause

Y92.191 Dining room in other specified residential institution as the place of occurrence of the external cause

Y92.192 Bathroom in other specified residential institution as the place of occurrence of the external cause

Y92.193 Bedroom in other specified residential institution as the place of occurrence of the external cause

Y92.194 Driveway of other specified residential institution as the place of occurrence of the external cause

Y92.195 Garage of other specified residential institution as the place of occurrence of the external cause

Y92.196 Pool of other specified residential institution as the place of occurrence of the external cause

Y92.197 Garden or yard of other specified residential institution as the place of occurrence of the external cause

Y92.198 Other place in other specified residential institution as the place of occurrence of the external cause

Y92.199 Unspecified place in other specified residential institution as the place of occurrence of the external cause

Ⓢ **Y92.2** School, other institution and public administrative area as the place of occurrence of the external cause

Building and adjacent grounds used by the general public or by a particular group of the public

> EXCLUDES 1 *building under construction as the place of occurrence of the external cause (Y92.6)*
> *residential institution as the place of occurrence of the external cause (Y92.1)*
> *school dormitory as the place of occurrence of the external cause (Y92.16-)*
> *sports and athletics area of schools as the place of occurrence of the external cause (Y92.3-)*

Ⓖ **Y92.21** School (private) (public) (state) as the place of occurrence of the external cause

Y92.210 Daycare center as the place of occurrence of the external cause

Y92.211 Elementary school as the place of occurrence of the external cause

Kindergarten as the place of occurrence of the external cause

Y92.212 Middle school as the place of occurrence of the external cause

Y92.213 High school as the place of occurrence of the external cause

AHA: 4Q 2012, 108

Y92.214 College as the place of occurrence of the external cause

University as the place of occurrence of the external cause

Y92.215 Trade school as the place of occurrence of the external cause

Y92.218 Other school as the place of occurrence of the external cause

Y92.219 Unspecified school as the place of occurrence of the external cause

Y92.22 Religious institution as the place of occurrence of the external cause

Church as the place of occurrence of the external cause
Mosque as the place of occurrence of the external cause
Synagogue as the place of occurrence of the external cause

Ⓖ **Y92.23** Hospital as the place of occurrence of the external cause

> EXCLUDES 1 *ambulatory (outpatient) health services establishments (Y92.53-)*
> *home for the sick as the place of occurrence of the external cause (Y92.12-)*
> *hospice as the place of occurrence of the external cause (Y92.12-)*
> *nursing home as the place of occurrence of the external cause (Y92.12-)*

Y92.230 Patient room in hospital as the place of occurrence of the external cause

Y92.231 Patient bathroom in hospital as the place of occurrence of the external cause

Y92.232 Corridor of hospital as the place of occurrence of the external cause

Y92.233 Cafeteria of hospital as the place of occurrence of the external cause

Y92.234 Operating room of hospital as the place of occurrence of the external cause

Y92.238 Other place in hospital as the place of occurrence of the external cause

Y92.239 Unspecified place in hospital as the place of occurrence of the external cause

Ⓖ **Y92.24** Public administrative building as the place of occurrence of the external cause

Y92.240 Courthouse as the place of occurrence of the external cause

Y92.241 Library as the place of occurrence of the external cause

Y92.242 Post office as the place of occurrence of the external cause

Y92.243 City hall as the place of occurrence of the external cause

Y92.248 Other public administrative building as the place of occurrence of the external cause

Ⓖ **Y92.25** Cultural building as the place of occurrence of the external cause

Y92.250 Art Gallery as the place of occurrence of the external cause

Y92.251 Museum as the place of occurrence of the external cause

Y92.252 Music hall as the place of occurrence of the external cause

Y92.253 Opera house as the place of occurrence of the external cause

Y92.254 Theater (live) as the place of occurrence of the external cause

Y92.258 Other cultural public building as the place of occurrence of the external cause

Y92.26 Movie house or cinema as the place of occurrence of the external cause

Y92.29 Other specified public building as the place of occurrence of the external cause

Assembly hall as the place of occurrence of the external cause
Clubhouse as the place of occurrence of the external cause

Ⓢ **Y92.3** Sports and athletics area as the place of occurrence of the external cause

Ⓖ **Y92.31** Athletic court as the place of occurrence of the external cause

> EXCLUDES 1 *tennis court in private home or garden (Y92.09)*

● New ▲ Revised *Manifestation* ❹-❼ Digit Indicators ▤ Laterality Ⓐ Adult (15+ years) Ⓜ Maternity (12-55 years) Ⓝ Newborn Ⓟ Pediatric (0-17 years) ♂ Male ♀ Female
✖ Deleted Unspecified + Additional code

2017 ICD-10-CM Expert for Physicians

© 2017 DecisionHealth   1173

Y92.159 — Y92.31

Y92.310   Basketball court as the place of occurrence of the external cause

Y92.311   Squash court as the place of occurrence of the external cause

Y92.312   Tennis court as the place of occurrence of the external cause

Y92.318   Other athletic court as the place of occurrence of the external cause

⑥ Y92.32   Athletic field as the place of occurrence of the external cause

Y92.320   Baseball field as the place of occurrence of the external cause

Y92.321   Football field as the place of occurrence of the external cause

Y92.322   Soccer field as the place of occurrence of the external cause

Y92.328   Other athletic field as the place of occurrence of the external cause
Cricket field as the place of occurrence of the external cause
Hockey field as the place of occurrence of the external cause

⑥ Y92.33   Skating rink as the place of occurrence of the external cause

Y92.330   Ice skating rink (indoor) (outdoor) as the place of occurrence of the external cause

Y92.331   Roller skating rink as the place of occurrence of the external cause

Y92.34   Swimming pool (public) as the place of occurrence of the external cause

> **EXCLUDES 1**   *swimming pool in private home or garden (Y92.016)*

Y92.39   Other specified sports and athletic area as the place of occurrence of the external cause
Golf-course as the place of occurrence of the external cause
Gymnasium as the place of occurrence of the external cause
Riding-school as the place of occurrence of the external cause
Stadium as the place of occurrence of the external cause

▲ ⑤ Y92.4   Street, highway and other paved roadways as the place of occurrence of the external cause

> **EXCLUDES 1**   *private driveway of residence (Y92.014, Y92.024, Y92.043, Y92.093, Y92.113, Y92.123, Y92.154, Y92.194)*

⑥ Y92.41   Street and highway as the place of occurrence of the external cause

Y92.410   **Unspecified street and highway as the place of occurrence of the external cause**
Road NOS as the place of occurrence of the external cause

Y92.411   **Interstate highway as the place of occurrence of the external cause**
Freeway as the place of occurrence of the external cause
Motorway as the place of occurrence of the external cause

Y92.412   **Parkway as the place of occurrence of the external cause**

Y92.413   **State road as the place of occurrence of the external cause**

Y92.414   **Local residential or business street as the place of occurrence of the external cause**

Y92.415   **Exit ramp or entrance ramp of street or highway as the place of occurrence of the external cause**

⑥ Y92.48   Other paved roadways as the place of occurrence of the external cause

Y92.480   **Sidewalk as the place of occurrence of the external cause**

Y92.481   **Parking lot as the place of occurrence of the external cause**

Y92.482   **Bike path as the place of occurrence of the external cause**

Y92.488   **Other paved roadways as the place of occurrence of the external cause**

⑤ Y92.5   Trade and service area as the place of occurrence of the external cause

> **EXCLUDES 1**   *garage in private home (Y92.015)*
> *schools and other public administration buildings (Y92.2-)*

⑥ Y92.51   Private commercial establishments as the place of occurrence of the external cause

Y92.510   **Bank as the place of occurrence of the external cause**

Y92.511   **Restaurant or café as the place of occurrence of the external cause**

Y92.512   **Supermarket, store or market as the place of occurrence of the external cause**

Y92.513   **Shop (commercial) as the place of occurrence of the external cause**

⑥ Y92.52   Service areas as the place of occurrence of the external cause

Y92.520   **Airport as the place of occurrence of the external cause**

Y92.521   **Bus station as the place of occurrence of the external cause**

Y92.522   **Railway station as the place of occurrence of the external cause**

Y92.523   **Highway rest stop as the place of occurrence of the external cause**

Y92.524   **Gas station as the place of occurrence of the external cause**
Petroleum station as the place of occurrence of the external cause
Service station as the place of occurrence of the external cause

⑥ Y92.53   Ambulatory health services establishments as the place of occurrence of the external cause

Y92.530   **Ambulatory surgery center as the place of occurrence of the external cause**
Outpatient surgery center, including that connected with a hospital as the place of occurrence of the external cause
Same day surgery center, including that connected with a hospital as the place of occurrence of the external cause

Y92.531   **Health care provider office as the place of occurrence of the external cause**
Physician office as the place of occurrence of the external cause

Y92.532   **Urgent care center as the place of occurrence of the external cause**

Y92.538   **Other ambulatory health services establishments as the place of occurrence of the external cause**

Y92.59   Other trade areas as the place of occurrence of the external cause
Office building as the place of occurrence of the external cause
Casino as the place of occurrence of the external cause
Garage (commercial) as the place of occurrence of the external cause
Hotel as the place of occurrence of the external cause
Radio or television station as the place of occurrence of the external cause
Shopping mall as the place of occurrence of the external cause
Warehouse as the place of occurrence of the external cause

⑤ Y92.6   Industrial and construction area as the place of occurrence of the external cause

Y92.61   **Building [any] under construction as the place of occurrence of the external cause**

Y92.62   **Dock or shipyard as the place of occurrence of the external cause**
Dockyard as the place of occurrence of the external cause
Dry dock as the place of occurrence of the external cause
Shipyard as the place of occurrence of the external cause

Y92.63   **Factory as the place of occurrence of the external cause**
Factory building as the place of occurrence of the external cause
Factory premises as the place of occurrence of the external cause
Industrial yard as the place of occurrence of the external cause

Y92.64   **Mine or pit as the place of occurrence of the external cause**
Mine as the place of occurrence of the external cause

● New   ▲ Revised   *Manifestation*   ④-⑦ Digit Indicators   ⊟ Laterality   Ⓐ Adult (15+ years)   Ⓜ Maternity (12-55 years)   Ⓝ Newborn   Ⓟ Pediatric (0-17 years)   ♂ Male   ♀ Female

✖ Deleted   Unspecified   ✚ Additional code

1174   © 2017 DecisionHealth   2017 ICD-10-CM Expert for Physicians

Y92.65   Oil rig as the place of occurrence of the external cause
Pit (coal) (gravel) (sand) as the place of occurrence of the external cause

Y92.69   Other specified industrial and construction area as the place of occurrence of the external cause
Gasworks as the place of occurrence of the external cause
Power-station (coal) (nuclear) (oil) as the place of occurrence of the external cause
Tunnel under construction as the place of occurrence of the external cause
Workshop as the place of occurrence of the external cause

⑤ **Y92.7**   Farm as the place of occurrence of the external cause
Ranch as the place of occurrence of the external cause
EXCLUDES 1   *farmhouse and home premises of farm (Y92.01-)*

Y92.71   Barn as the place of occurrence of the external cause

Y92.72   Chicken coop as the place of occurrence of the external cause
Hen house as the place of occurrence of the external cause

Y92.73   Farm field as the place of occurrence of the external cause

Y92.74   Orchard as the place of occurrence of the external cause

Y92.79   Other farm location as the place of occurrence of the external cause

⑤ **Y92.8**   Other places as the place of occurrence of the external cause

⑥ **Y92.81**   Transport vehicle as the place of occurrence of the external cause
EXCLUDES 1   *transport accidents (V00-V99)*

Y92.810   Car as the place of occurrence of the external cause

Y92.811   Bus as the place of occurrence of the external cause

Y92.812   Truck as the place of occurrence of the external cause

Y92.813   Airplane as the place of occurrence of the external cause

Y92.814   Boat as the place of occurrence of the external cause

Y92.815   Train as the place of occurrence of the external cause

Y92.816   Subway car as the place of occurrence of the external cause

Y92.818   Other transport vehicle as the place of occurrence of the external cause

⑥ **Y92.82**   Wilderness area

Y92.820   Desert as the place of occurrence of the external cause

Y92.821   Forest as the place of occurrence of the external cause

Y92.828   Other wilderness area as the place of occurrence of the external cause
Swamp as the place of occurrence of the external cause
Mountain as the place of occurrence of the external cause
Marsh as the place of occurrence of the external cause
Prairie as the place of occurrence of the external cause

⑥ **Y92.83**   Recreation area as the place of occurrence of the external cause

Y92.830   Public park as the place of occurrence of the external cause

Y92.831   Amusement park as the place of occurrence of the external cause

Y92.832   Beach as the place of occurrence of the external cause
Seashore as the place of occurrence of the external cause

Y92.833   Campsite as the place of occurrence of the external cause

Y92.834   Zoological garden (Zoo) as the place of occurrence of the external cause

Y92.838   Other recreation area as the place of occurrence of the external cause

Y92.84   Military training ground as the place of occurrence of the external cause

Y92.85   Railroad track as the place of occurrence of the external cause

Y92.86   Slaughter house as the place of occurrence of the external cause

Y92.89   Other specified places as the place of occurrence of the external cause
Derelict house as the place of occurrence of the external cause

Y92.9   Unspecified place or not applicable

④ **Y93**   **Activity codes**
Note: Category Y93 is provided for use to indicate the activity of the person seeking healthcare for an injury or health condition, such as a heart attack while shoveling snow, which resulted from, or was contributed to, by the activity. These codes are appropriate for use for both acute injuries, such as those from chapter 19, and conditions that are due to the long-term, cumulative effects of an activity, such as those from chapter 13. They are also appropriate for use with external cause codes for cause and intent if identifying the activity provides additional information on the event. These codes should be used in conjunction with codes for external cause status (Y99) and place of occurrence (Y92).
This section contains the following broad activity categories:
Y93.0 Activities involving walking and running
Y93.1 Activities involving water and water craft
Y93.2 Activities involving ice and snow
Y93.3 Activities involving climbing, rappelling, and jumping off
Y93.4 Activities involving dancing and other rhythmic movement
Y93.5 Activities involving other sports and athletics played individually
Y93.6 Activities involving other sports and athletics played as a team or group
Y93.7 Activities involving other specified sports and athletics
Y93.A Activities involving other cardiorespiratory exercise
Y93.B Activities involving other muscle strengthening exercises
Y93.C Activities involving computer technology and electronic devices
Y93.D Activities involving arts and handcrafts
Y93.E Activities involving personal hygiene and interior property and clothing maintenance
Y93.F Activities involving caregiving
Y93.G Activities involving food preparation, cooking and grilling
Y93.H Activities involving exterior property and land maintenance, building and construction
Y93.I Activities involving roller coasters and other types of external motion
Y93.J Activities involving playing musical instrument
Y93.K Activities involving animal care
Y93.8 Activities, other specified
Y93.9 Activity, unspecified

⑤ **Y93.0**   **Activities involving walking and running**
EXCLUDES 1   *activity, walking an animal (Y93.K1)*
activity, walking or running on a treadmill (Y93.A1)

Y93.01   Activity, walking, marching and hiking
Activity, walking, marching and hiking on level or elevated terrain
EXCLUDES 1   *activity, mountain climbing (Y93.31)*

Y93.02   Activity, running

⑤ **Y93.1**   **Activities involving water and water craft**
EXCLUDES 1   *activities involving ice (Y93.2-)*

Y93.11   Activity, swimming

Y93.12   Activity, springboard and platform diving

Y93.13   Activity, water polo

Y93.14   Activity, water aerobics and water exercise

Y93.15   Activity, underwater diving and snorkeling
Activity, SCUBA diving

Y93.16   Activity, rowing, canoeing, kayaking, rafting and tubing
Activity, canoeing, kayaking, rafting and tubing in calm and turbulent water

Y93.17   Activity, water skiing and wake boarding

Y93.18   Activity, surfing, windsurfing and boogie boarding
Activity, water sliding

Y93.19   Activity, other involving water and watercraft
Activity involving water NOS
Activity, parasailing
Activity, water survival training and testing

⑤ **Y93.2** **Activities involving ice and snow**
> EXCLUDES 1 *activity, shoveling ice and snow (Y93.H1)*

Y93.21 **Activity, ice skating**
Activity, figure skating (singles) (pairs)
Activity, ice dancing
> EXCLUDES 1 *activity, ice hockey (Y93.22)*

Y93.22 **Activity, ice hockey**

Y93.23 **Activity, snow (alpine) (downhill) skiing, snow boarding, sledding, tobogganing and snow tubing**
> EXCLUDES 1 *activity, cross country skiing (Y93.24)*

Y93.24 **Activity, cross country skiing**
Activity, nordic skiing

Y93.29 **Activity, other involving ice and snow**
Activity involving ice and snow NOS

⑤ **Y93.3** **Activities involving climbing, rappelling and jumping off**
> EXCLUDES 1 *activity, hiking on level or elevated terrain (Y93.01)*
> *activity, jumping rope (Y93.56)*
> *activity, trampoline jumping (Y93.44)*

Y93.31 **Activity, mountain climbing, rock climbing and wall climbing**

Y93.32 **Activity, rappelling**

Y93.33 **Activity, BASE jumping**
Activity, Building, Antenna, Span, Earth jumping

Y93.34 **Activity, bungee jumping**

Y93.35 **Activity, hang gliding**

Y93.39 **Activity, other involving climbing, rappelling and jumping off**

⑤ **Y93.4** **Activities involving dancing and other rhythmic movement**
> EXCLUDES 1 *activity, martial arts (Y93.75)*

Y93.41 **Activity, dancing**
AHA: 4Q 2012, 108

Y93.42 **Activity, yoga**

Y93.43 **Activity, gymnastics**
Activity, rhythmic gymnastics
> EXCLUDES 1 *activity, trampolining (Y93.44)*

Y93.44 **Activity, trampolining**

Y93.45 **Activity, cheerleading**

Y93.49 **Activity, other involving dancing and other rhythmic movements**

⑤ **Y93.5** **Activities involving other sports and athletics played individually**
> EXCLUDES 1 *activity, dancing (Y93.41)*
> *activity, gymnastic (Y93.43)*
> *activity, trampolining (Y93.44)*
> *activity, yoga (Y93.42)*

Y93.51 **Activity, roller skating (inline) and skateboarding**

Y93.52 **Activity, horseback riding**

Y93.53 **Activity, golf**

Y93.54 **Activity, bowling**

Y93.55 **Activity, bike riding**

Y93.56 **Activity, jumping rope**

Y93.57 **Activity, non-running track and field events**
> EXCLUDES 1 *activity, running (any form) (Y93.02)*

Y93.59 **Activity, other involving other sports and athletics played individually**
> EXCLUDES 1 *activities involving climbing, rappelling, and jumping (Y93.3-)*
> *activities involving ice and snow (Y93.2-)*
> *activities involving walking and running (Y93.0-)*
> *activities involving water and watercraft (Y93.1-)*

⑤ **Y93.6** **Activities involving other sports and athletics played as a team or group**
> EXCLUDES 1 *activity, ice hockey (Y93.22)*
> *activity, water polo (Y93.13)*

Y93.61 **Activity, american tackle football**
Activity, football NOS

Y93.62 **Activity, american flag or touch football**

Y93.63 **Activity, rugby**

Y93.64 **Activity, baseball**
Activity, softball

Y93.65 **Activity, lacrosse and field hockey**
AHA: 1Q 2015, 9

Y93.66 **Activity, soccer**

Y93.67 **Activity, basketball**

Y93.68 **Activity, volleyball (beach) (court)**

Y93.6A **Activity, physical games generally associated with school recess, summer camp and children**
Activity, capture the flag
Activity, dodge ball
Activity, four square
Activity, kickball

Y93.69 **Activity, other involving other sports and athletics played as a team or group**
Activity, cricket

⑤ **Y93.7** **Activities involving other specified sports and athletics**

Y93.71 **Activity, boxing**

Y93.72 **Activity, wrestling**

Y93.73 **Activity, racquet and hand sports**
Activity, handball
Activity, racquetball
Activity, squash
Activity, tennis

Y93.74 **Activity, frisbee**
Activity, ultimate frisbee

Y93.75 **Activity, martial arts**
Activity, combatives

Y93.79 **Activity, other specified sports and athletics**
> EXCLUDES 1 *sports and athletics activities specified in categories Y93.0-Y93.6*

⑤ **Y93.A** **Activities involving other cardiorespiratory exercise**
Activities involving physical training

Y93.A1 **Activity, exercise machines primarily for cardiorespiratory conditioning**
Activity, elliptical and stepper machines
Activity, stationary bike
Activity, treadmill

Y93.A2 **Activity, calisthenics**
Activity, jumping jacks
Activity, warm up and cool down

Y93.A3 **Activity, aerobic and step exercise**

Y93.A4 **Activity, circuit training**

Y93.A5 **Activity, obstacle course**
Activity, challenge course
Activity, confidence course

Y93.A6 **Activity, grass drills**
Activity, guerilla drills

Y93.A9 **Activity, other involving cardiorespiratory exercise**
> EXCLUDES 1 *activities involving cardiorespiratory exercise specified in categories Y93.0-Y93.7*

⑤ **Y93.B** **Activities involving other muscle strengthening exercises**

Y93.B1 **Activity, exercise machines primarily for muscle strengthening**

Y93.B2 **Activity, push-ups, pull-ups, sit-ups**

Y93.B3 **Activity, free weights**
Activity, barbells
Activity, dumbbells

Y93.B4 **Activity, pilates**

Y93.B9 **Activity, other involving muscle strengthening exercises**
> EXCLUDES 1 *activities involving muscle strengthening specified in categories Y93.0-Y93.A*

⑤ **Y93.C** **Activities involving computer technology and electronic devices**
> EXCLUDES 1 *activity, electronic musical keyboard or instruments (Y93.J-)*

Y93.C1 **Activity, computer keyboarding**
Activity, electronic game playing using keyboard or other stationary device

Y93.C2 **Activity, hand held interactive electronic device**
Activity, cellular telephone and communication device
Activity, electronic game playing using interactive device
> EXCLUDES 1 *activity, electronic game playing using keyboard or other stationary device (Y93.C1)*

Y93.C9 **Activity, other involving computer technology and electronic devices**

⑤ **Y93.D** **Activities involving arts and handcrafts**
> EXCLUDES 1 *activities involving playing musical instrument (Y93.J-)*

Y93.D1 **Activity, knitting and crocheting**

Y93.D2 **Activity, sewing**

Y93.D3 **Activity, furniture building and finishing**
Activity, furniture repair

● New   ▲ Revised   *Manifestation*   ④-⑦ Digit Indicators   ▣ Laterality   Ⓐ Adult (15+ years)   Ⓜ Maternity (12-55 years)   Ⓝ Newborn   Ⓟ Pediatric (0-17 years)   ♂ Male   ♀ Female
✖ Deleted   Unspecified   ✚ Additional code

Y93.D9   Activity, other involving arts and handcrafts

⑤ **Y93.E**   **Activities involving personal hygiene and interior property and clothing maintenance**

> **EXCLUDES 1**   *activities involving cooking and grilling (Y93.G-)*
> *activities involving exterior property and land maintenance, building and construction (Y93.H-)*
> *activities involving caregiving (Y93.F-)*
> *activity, dishwashing (Y93.G1)*
> *activity, food preparation (Y93.G1)*
> *activity, gardening (Y93.H2)*

Y93.E1   **Activity, personal bathing and showering**
Y93.E2   **Activity, laundry**
Y93.E3   **Activity, vacuuming**
Y93.E4   **Activity, ironing**
Y93.E5   **Activity, floor mopping and cleaning**
Y93.E6   **Activity, residential relocation**
> Activity, packing up and unpacking involved in moving to a new residence

Y93.E8   **Activity, other personal hygiene**
Y93.E9   **Activity, other interior property and clothing maintenance**

⑤ **Y93.F**   **Activities involving caregiving**
> Activity involving the provider of caregiving

Y93.F1   **Activity, caregiving, bathing**
Y93.F2   **Activity, caregiving, lifting**
Y93.F9   **Activity, other caregiving**

⑤ **Y93.G**   **Activities involving food preparation, cooking and grilling**

Y93.G1   **Activity, food preparation and clean up**
> Activity, dishwashing

Y93.G2   **Activity, grilling and smoking food**
Y93.G3   **Activity, cooking and baking**
> Activity, use of stove, oven and microwave oven

Y93.G9   **Activity, other involving cooking and grilling**

⑤ **Y93.H**   **Activities involving exterior property and land maintenance, building and construction**

Y93.H1   **Activity, digging, shoveling and raking**
> Activity, dirt digging
> Activity, raking leaves
> Activity, snow shoveling

Y93.H2   **Activity, gardening and landscaping**
> Activity, pruning, trimming shrubs, weeding

Y93.H3   **Activity, building and construction**
Y93.H9   **Activity, other involving exterior property and land maintenance, building and construction**

⑤ **Y93.I**   **Activities involving roller coasters and other types of external motion**

Y93.I1   **Activity, roller coaster riding**
Y93.I9   **Activity, other involving external motion**

⑤ **Y93.J**   **Activities involving playing musical instrument**
> Activity involving playing electric musical instrument

Y93.J1   **Activity, piano playing**
> Activity, musical keyboard (electronic) playing

Y93.J2   **Activity, drum and other percussion instrument playing**
Y93.J3   **Activity, string instrument playing**
Y93.J4   **Activity, winds and brass instrument playing**

⑤ **Y93.K**   **Activities involving animal care**

> **EXCLUDES 1**   *activity, horseback riding (Y93.52)*

Y93.K1   **Activity, walking an animal**
Y93.K2   **Activity, milking an animal**
Y93.K3   **Activity, grooming and shearing an animal**
Y93.K9   **Activity, other involving animal care**

⑤ **Y93.8**   **Activities, other specified**

Y93.81   **Activity, refereeing a sports activity**
Y93.82   **Activity, spectator at an event**
Y93.83   **Activity, rough housing and horseplay**
> AHA: 1Q 2015, 8

Y93.84   **Activity, sleeping**
● **Y93.85**   **Activity, choking game**
> Activity, blackout game
> Activity, fainting game
> Activity, pass out game

Y93.89   **Activity, other specified**

Y93.9   **Activity, unspecified**

Y95   **Nosocomial condition**
> AHA: 4Q 2013, 119

④ **Y99**   **External cause status**

> Note: A single code from category Y99 should be used in conjunction with the external cause code(s) assigned to a record to indicate the status of the person at the time the event occurred.

Y99.0   **Civilian activity done for income or pay**
> Civilian activity done for financial or other compensation

> **EXCLUDES 1**   *military activity (Y99.1)*
> *volunteer activity (Y99.2)*

Y99.1   **Military activity**

> **EXCLUDES 1**   *activity of off duty military personnel (Y99.8)*

Y99.2   **Volunteer activity**

> **EXCLUDES 1**   *activity of child or other family member assisting in compensated work of other family member (Y99.8)*

Y99.8   **Other external cause status**
> Activity NEC
> Activity of child or other family member assisting in compensated work of other family member
> Hobby not done for income
> Leisure activity
> Off-duty activity of military personnel
> Recreation or sport not for income or while a student
> Student activity

> **EXCLUDES 1**   *civilian activity done for income or compensation (Y99.0)*
> *military activity (Y99.1)*

> AHA: 4Q 2012, 108

Y99.9   **Unspecified external cause status**

● New   ▲ Revised   *Manifestation*   ④-⑦ Digit Indicators   ⑤ Laterality   Ⓐ Adult (15+ years)   Ⓜ Maternity (12-55 years)   Ⓝ Newborn   Ⓟ Pediatric (0-17 years)   ♂ Male   ♀ Female

✖ Deleted   Unspecified   + Additional code

2017 ICD-10-CM Expert for Physicians

© 2017 DecisionHealth   1177

Y93.D9 — Y99.9

CHAPTER 21: FACTORS INFLUENCING HEALTH STATUS AND CONTACT WITH HEALTH SERVICES (Z00-Z99)

Note: Z codes represent reasons for encounters. A corresponding procedure code must accompany a Z code if a procedure is performed. Categories Z00-Z99 are provided for occasions when circumstances other than a disease, injury or external cause classifiable to categories A00-Y89 are recorded as 'diagnoses' or 'problems'. This can arise in two main ways:

a) When a person who may or may not be sick encounters the health services for some specific purpose, such as to receive limited care or service for a current condition, to donate an organ or tissue, to receive prophylactic vaccination (immunization), or to discuss a problem which is in itself not a disease or injury.

b) When some circumstance or problem is present which influences the person's health status but is not in itself a current illness or injury.

GUIDELINES Section I.C.21.a

Z codes are for use in any healthcare setting. Z codes may be used as either a first-listed (principal diagnosis code in the inpatient setting) or secondary code, depending on the circumstances of the encounter. Certain Z codes may only be used as first-listed or principal diagnosis.

CODING TIP ✓ Aftercare Z codes should not be used for aftercare of injuries. For aftercare of an injury, assign the injury code with the appropriate 7th character, usually "D" if the condition meets the definition of aftercare (patient requires continued care during the healing or recovery phase or long term consequences of the disease/injury).

This chapter contains the following blocks:

Z00-Z13	Persons encountering health services for examinations
Z14-Z15	Genetic carrier and genetic susceptibility to disease
Z16	Resistance to antimicrobial drugs
Z17	Estrogen receptor status
Z18	Retained foreign body fragments
Z19	Hormone sensitivity malignancy status
Z20-Z29	Persons with potential health hazards related to communicable diseases
Z30-Z39	Persons encountering health services in circumstances related to reproduction
Z40-Z53	Encounters for other specific health care
Z55-Z65	Persons with potential health hazards related to socioeconomic and psychosocial circumstances
Z66	Do not resuscitate status
Z67	Blood type
Z68	Body mass index (BMI)
Z69-Z76	Persons encountering health services in other circumstances
Z77-Z99	Persons with potential health hazards related to family and personal history and certain conditions influencing health status

Persons encountering health services for examinations (Z00-Z13)

Note: Nonspecific abnormal findings disclosed at the time of these examinations are classified to categories R70-R94.

EXCLUDES 1 examinations related to pregnancy and reproduction (Z30-Z36, Z39.-)

Z00 Encounter for general examination without complaint, suspected or reported diagnosis

EXCLUDES 1 encounter for examination for administrative purposes (Z02.-)

EXCLUDES 2 encounter for pre-procedural examinations (Z01.81-)
special screening examinations (Z11-Z13)

Z00.0 Encounter for general adult medical examination
Encounter for adult periodic examination (annual) (physical) and any associated laboratory and radiologic examinations

EXCLUDES 1 encounter for examination of sign or symptom- code to sign or symptom
general health check-up of infant or child (Z00.12-)

Z00.00 Encounter for general adult medical examination without abnormal findings
Encounter for adult health check-up NOS
AHA: 1Q 2016, 36-37

+ Z00.01 Encounter for general adult medical examination with abnormal findings
Use additional code to identify abnormal findings
AHA: 1Q 2016, 35, 36

Z00.1 Encounter for newborn, infant and child health examinations

+ Z00.11 Newborn health examination
Health check for child under 29 days old
Use additional code to identify any abnormal findings
EXCLUDES 1 health check for child over 28 days old (Z00.12-)

+ Z00.110 Health examination for newborn under 8 days old
Health check for newborn under 8 days old

+ Z00.111 Health examination for newborn 8 to 28 days old
Health check for newborn 8 to 28 days old
Newborn weight check

Z00.12 Encounter for routine child health examination
Encounter for development testing of infant or child
Health check (routine) for child over 28 days old
EXCLUDES 1 health check for child under 29 days old (Z00.11-)
health supervision of foundling or other healthy infant or child (Z76.1-Z76.2)
newborn health examination (Z00.11-)

+ Z00.121 Encounter for routine child health examination with abnormal findings
Use additional code to identify abnormal findings
AHA: 1Q 2016, 34, 35

Z00.129 Encounter for routine child health examination without abnormal findings
Encounter for routine child health examination NOS
AHA: 1Q 2016, 34-35

Z00.2 Encounter for examination for period of rapid growth in childhood

Z00.3 Encounter for examination for adolescent development state
Encounter for puberty development state

Z00.5 Encounter for examination of potential donor of organ and tissue

Z00.6 Encounter for examination for normal comparison and control in clinical research program
Examination of participant or control in clinical research program

Z00.7 Encounter for examination for period of delayed growth in childhood

Z00.70 Encounter for examination for period of delayed growth in childhood without abnormal findings

+ Z00.71 Encounter for examination for period of delayed growth in childhood with abnormal findings
Use additional code to identify abnormal findings

Z00.8 Encounter for other general examination
Encounter for health examination in population surveys

Z01 Encounter for other special examination without complaint, suspected or reported diagnosis
Note: Codes from category Z01 represent the reason for the encounter. A separate procedure code is required to identify any examinations or procedures performed

INCLUDES routine examination of specific system

EXCLUDES 1 encounter for examination for administrative purposes (Z02.-)
encounter for examination for suspected conditions, proven not to exist (Z03.-)
encounter for laboratory and radiologic examinations as a component of general medical examinations (Z00.0-)
encounter for laboratory, radiologic and imaging examinations for sign (s) and symptom(s) - code to the sign(s) or symptom(s)

EXCLUDES 2 screening examinations (Z11-Z13)

Z01.0 Encounter for examination of eyes and vision
EXCLUDES 1 examination for driving license (Z02.4)

Z01.00 Encounter for examination of eyes and vision without abnormal findings
Encounter for examination of eyes and vision NOS

+ Z01.01 Encounter for examination of eyes and vision with abnormal findings
Use additional code to identify abnormal findings

Z01.1 Encounter for examination of ears and hearing

Z01.10 Encounter for examination of ears and hearing without abnormal findings
Encounter for examination of ears and hearing NOS

● New ▲ Revised *Manifestation* ◀-▶ Digit Indicators ▤ Laterality Ⓐ Adult (15+ years) Ⓜ Maternity (12-55 years) Ⓝ Newborn Ⓟ Pediatric (0-17 years) ♂ Male ♀ Female
~~Deleted~~ Unspecified + Additional code

017 ICD-10-CM Expert for Physicians
© 2017 DecisionHealth
1179

⑥ Z01.11 **Encounter for examination of ears and hearing with abnormal findings**

Z01.110 **Encounter for hearing examination following failed hearing screening**

+ Z01.118 **Encounter for examination of ears and hearing with other abnormal findings**
Use additional code to identify abnormal findings

Z01.12 **Encounter for hearing conservation and treatment**

⑤ Z01.2 **Encounter for dental examination and cleaning**

Z01.20 **Encounter for dental examination and cleaning without abnormal findings**
Encounter for dental examination and cleaning NOS

+ Z01.21 **Encounter for dental examination and cleaning with abnormal findings**
Use additional code to identify abnormal findings

⑤ Z01.3 **Encounter for examination of blood pressure**

Z01.30 **Encounter for examination of blood pressure without abnormal findings**
Encounter for examination of blood pressure NOS

+ Z01.31 **Encounter for examination of blood pressure with abnormal findings**
Use additional code to identify abnormal findings

⑤ Z01.4 **Encounter for gynecological examination**
| **EXCLUDES 2** | *pregnancy examination or test (Z32.0-) routine examination for contraceptive maintenance (Z30.4-)* |

⑥ + Z01.41 **Encounter for routine gynecological examination**
Encounter for general gynecological examination with or without cervical smear
Encounter for gynecological examination (general) (routine) NOS
Encounter for pelvic examination (annual) (periodic)
Use additional code:
for screening for human papillomavirus, if applicable, (Z11.51)
for screening vaginal pap smear, if applicable (Z12.72)
to identify acquired absence of uterus, if applicable (Z90.71-)
| **EXCLUDES 1** | *gynecologic examination status-post hysterectomy for malignant condition (Z08) screening cervical pap smear not a part of a routine gynecological examination (Z12.4)* |

▲ + Z01.411 **Encounter for gynecological examination (general) (routine) with abnormal findings** ♀
Use additional code to identify abnormal findings

▲ + Z01.419 **Encounter for gynecological examination (general) (routine) without abnormal findings** ♀

Z01.42 **Encounter for cervical smear to confirm findings of recent normal smear following initial abnormal smear** ♀

⑤ Z01.8 **Encounter for other specified special examinations**

⑥ Z01.81 **Encounter for preprocedural examinations**
Encounter for preoperative examinations
Encounter for radiological and imaging examinations as part of preprocedural examination

Z01.810 **Encounter for preprocedural cardiovascular examination**

Z01.811 **Encounter for preprocedural respiratory examination**

Z01.812 **Encounter for preprocedural laboratory examination**
Blood and urine tests prior to treatment or procedure

Z01.818 **Encounter for other preprocedural examination**
Encounter for preprocedural examination NOS
Encounter for examinations prior to antineoplastic chemotherapy

Z01.82 **Encounter for allergy testing**
| **EXCLUDES 1** | *encounter for antibody response examination (Z01.84)* |

Z01.83 **Encounter for blood typing**
Encounter for Rh typing

Z01.84 **Encounter for antibody response examination**
Encounter for immunity status testing
| **EXCLUDES 1** | *encounter for allergy testing (Z01.82)* |

Z01.89 **Encounter for other specified special examinations**

④ Z02 **Encounter for administrative examination**

Z02.0 **Encounter for examination for admission to educational institution**
Encounter for examination for admission to preschool (education)
Encounter for examination for re-admission to school following illness or medical treatment

Z02.1 **Encounter for pre-employment examination**

Z02.2 **Encounter for examination for admission to residential institution**
| **EXCLUDES 1** | *examination for admission to prison (Z02.89)* |

Z02.3 **Encounter for examination for recruitment to armed forces**

Z02.4 **Encounter for examination for driving license**

Z02.5 **Encounter for examination for participation in sport**
| **EXCLUDES 1** | *blood-alcohol and blood-drug test (Z02.83)* |

Z02.6 **Encounter for examination for insurance purposes**

⑤ Z02.7 **Encounter for issue of medical certificate**
| **EXCLUDES 1** | *encounter for general medical examination (Z00-Z01, Z02.0-Z02.6, Z02.8-Z02.9,)* |

Z02.71 **Encounter for disability determination**
Encounter for issue of medical certificate of incapacity
Encounter for issue of medical certificate of invalidity

Z02.79 **Encounter for issue of other medical certificate**

⑤ Z02.8 **Encounter for other administrative examinations**

Z02.81 **Encounter for paternity testing**

Z02.82 **Encounter for adoption services**

+ Z02.83 **Encounter for blood-alcohol and blood-drug test**
Use additional code for findings of alcohol or drugs in blood (R78.-)

Z02.89 **Encounter for other administrative examinations**
Encounter for examination for admission to prison
Encounter for examination for admission to summer camp
Encounter for immigration examination
Encounter for naturalization examination
Encounter for premarital examination
| **EXCLUDES 1** | *health supervision of foundling or other healthy infant or child (Z76.1-Z76.2)* |

Z02.9 **Encounter for administrative examinations, unspecified**

④ Z03 **Encounter for medical observation for suspected diseases and conditions ruled out**
This category is to be used when a person without a diagnosis is suspected of having an abnormal condition, without signs or symptoms, which requires study, but after examination and observation, is ruled out. This category is also for use for administrative and legal observation status.
| **EXCLUDES 1** | *contact with and (suspected) exposures hazardous to health (Z77.-) newborn observation for suspected condition, ruled out (P00-P04) person with feared complaint in whom no diagnosis is made (Z71.1) signs or symptoms under study- code to signs or symptoms* |

Z03.6 **Encounter for observation for suspected toxic effect from ingested substance ruled out**
Encounter for observation for suspected adverse effect from drug
Encounter for observation for suspected poisoning

⑤ Z03.7 **Encounter for suspected maternal and fetal conditions ruled out**
Encounter for suspected maternal and fetal conditions not found
| **EXCLUDES 1** | *known or suspected fetal anomalies affecting management of mother, not ruled out (O26.-, O35.-, O36.-, O40.-, O41.-)* |

Z03.71 **Encounter for suspected problem with amniotic** ♀
cavity and membrane ruled out
Encounter for suspected oligohydramnios ruled out
Encounter for suspected polyhydramnios ruled out

Z03.72 **Encounter for suspected placental problem** ♀
ruled out

Z03.73 **Encounter for suspected fetal anomaly ruled out** ♀

● New   ▲ Revised   *Manifestation*   ④-⑦ Digit Indicators   ▤ Laterality   ⒶAdult (15+ years)   ⓂMaternity (12-55 years)   ⓃNewborn   ⓅPediatric (0-17 years)   ♂ Male   ♀ Female
✖ Deleted   Unspecified   + Additional code

Z03.74   **Encounter for suspected problem with fetal growth ruled out** ♀ Ⓜ

Z03.75   **Encounter for suspected cervical shortening ruled out** ♀ Ⓜ

Z03.79   **Encounter for other suspected maternal and fetal conditions ruled out** ♀ Ⓜ

Ⓢ Z03.8   **Encounter for observation for other suspected diseases and conditions ruled out**

Ⓖ Z03.81   **Encounter for observation for suspected exposure to biological agents ruled out**

Z03.810   **Encounter for observation for suspected exposure to anthrax ruled out**

Z03.818   **Encounter for observation for suspected exposure to other biological agents ruled out**

Z03.89   **Encounter for observation for other suspected diseases and conditions ruled out**

▣ Z04   **Encounter for examination and observation for other reasons**

> | INCLUDES | encounter for examination for medicolegal reasons |

This category is to be used when a person without a diagnosis is suspected of having an abnormal condition, without signs or symptoms, which requires study, but after examination and observation, is ruled-out. This category is also for use for administrative and legal observation status.

Z04.1   **Encounter for examination and observation following transport accident**

> | EXCLUDES 1 | *encounter for examination and observation following work accident (Z04.2)* |

Z04.2   **Encounter for examination and observation following work accident**

Z04.3   **Encounter for examination and observation following other accident**

Ⓢ Z04.4   **Encounter for examination and observation following alleged rape**

Encounter for examination and observation of victim following alleged rape

Encounter for examination and observation of victim following alleged sexual abuse

Z04.41   **Encounter for examination and observation following alleged adult rape** Ⓐ

Suspected adult rape, ruled out

Suspected adult sexual abuse, ruled out

Z04.42   **Encounter for examination and observation following alleged child rape** Ⓟ

Suspected child rape, ruled out

Suspected child sexual abuse, ruled out

Z04.6   **Encounter for general psychiatric examination, requested by authority**

Ⓢ Z04.7   **Encounter for examination and observation following alleged physical abuse**

Z04.71   **Encounter for examination and observation following alleged adult physical abuse** Ⓐ

Suspected adult physical abuse, ruled out

> | EXCLUDES 1 | *confirmed case of adult physical abuse (T74.-)* |
> | | *encounter for examination and observation following alleged adult sexual abuse (Z04.41)* |
> | | *suspected case of adult physical abuse, not ruled out (T76.-)* |

Z04.72   **Encounter for examination and observation following alleged child physical abuse** Ⓟ

Suspected child physical abuse, ruled out

> | EXCLUDES 1 | *confirmed case of child physical abuse (T74.-)* |
> | | *encounter for examination and observation following alleged child sexual abuse (Z04.42)* |
> | | *suspected case of child physical abuse, not ruled out (T76.-)* |

Z04.8   **Encounter for examination and observation for other specified reasons**

Encounter for examination and observation for request for expert evidence

Z04.9   **Encounter for examination and observation for unspecified reason**

Encounter for observation NOS

● ▣ Z05   **Encounter for observation and evaluation of newborn for suspected diseases and conditions ruled out**

This category is to be used for newborns, within the neonatal period (the first 28 days of life), who are suspected of having an abnormal condition unrelated to exposure from the mother or the birth process, but without signs or symptoms, and which, after examination and observation, is ruled out.

> | EXCLUDES 2 | *newborn observation for suspected condition, related to exposure from the mother or birth process (P00-P04)* |

● Z05.0   **Observation and evaluation of newborn for suspected cardiac condition ruled out** Ⓝ

● Z05.1   **Observation and evaluation of newborn for suspected infectious condition ruled out** Ⓝ

● Z05.2   **Observation and evaluation of newborn for suspected neurological condition ruled out** Ⓝ

● Z05.3   **Observation and evaluation of newborn for suspected respiratory condition ruled out** Ⓝ

● Ⓢ Z05.4   **Observation and evaluation of newborn for suspected genetic, metabolic or immunologic condition ruled out**

● Z05.41   **Observation and evaluation of newborn for suspected genetic condition ruled out** Ⓝ

● Z05.42   **Observation and evaluation of newborn for suspected metabolic condition ruled out** Ⓝ

● Z05.43   **Observation and evaluation of newborn for suspected immunologic condition ruled out** Ⓝ

● Z05.5   **Observation and evaluation of newborn for suspected gastrointestinal condition ruled out** Ⓝ

● Z05.6   **Observation and evaluation of newborn for suspected genitourinary condition ruled out** Ⓝ

● Ⓢ Z05.7   **Observation and evaluation of newborn for suspected skin, subcutaneous, musculoskeletal and connective tissue condition ruled out**

● Z05.71   **Observation and evaluation of newborn for suspected skin and subcutaneous tissue condition ruled out** Ⓝ

● Z05.72   **Observation and evaluation of newborn for suspected musculoskeletal condition ruled out** Ⓝ

● Z05.73   **Observation and evaluation of newborn for suspected connective tissue condition ruled out** Ⓝ

● Z05.8   **Observation and evaluation of newborn for other specified suspected condition ruled out** Ⓝ

● Z05.9   **Observation and evaluation of newborn for unspecified suspected condition ruled out** Ⓝ

+ Z08   **Encounter for follow-up examination after completed treatment for malignant neoplasm**

Medical surveillance following completed treatment

Use additional code to identify any acquired absence of organs (Z90.-)

Use additional code to identify the personal history of malignant neoplasm (Z85.-)

> | EXCLUDES 1 | *aftercare following medical care (Z43-Z49, Z51)* |

+ Z09   **Encounter for follow-up examination after completed treatment for conditions other than malignant neoplasm**

Medical surveillance following completed treatment

Use additional code to identify any applicable history of disease code (Z86.-, Z87.-)

> | EXCLUDES 1 | *aftercare following medical care (Z43-Z49, Z51)* |
> | | *surveillance of contraception (Z30.4-)* |
> | | *surveillance of prosthetic and other medical devices (Z44-Z46)* |

AHA: 1Q 2015, 8

▣ Z11   **Encounter for screening for infectious and parasitic diseases**

Screening is the testing for disease or disease precursors in asymptomatic individuals so that early detection and treatment can be provided for those who test positive for the disease.

> | EXCLUDES 1 | *encounter for diagnostic examination-code to sign or symptom* |

Z11.0   **Encounter for screening for intestinal infectious diseases**

Z11.1   **Encounter for screening for respiratory tuberculosis**

Z11.2   **Encounter for screening for other bacterial diseases**

Z11.3   **Encounter for screening for infections with a predominantly sexual mode of transmission**

> | EXCLUDES 2 | *encounter for screening for human immunodeficiency virus [HIV] (Z11.4)* |
> | | *encounter for screening for human papillomavirus (Z11.51)* |

| New | ▲ Revised | *Manifestation* | ▣-❼ Digit Indicators | ▣ Laterality | Ⓐ Adult (15+ years) | Ⓜ Maternity (12-55 years) | Ⓝ Newborn | Ⓟ Pediatric (0-17 years) | ♂ Male | ♀ Female |
| Deleted | | Unspecified | + Additional code | | | | | | | |

Z11.4 Encounter for screening for human immunodeficiency virus [HIV]

Z11.5 Encounter for screening for other viral diseases

EXCLUDES 2 *encounter for screening for viral intestinal disease (Z11.0)*

Z11.51 Encounter for screening for human papillomavirus (HPV)

Z11.59 Encounter for screening for other viral diseases

Z11.6 Encounter for screening for other protozoal diseases and helminthiases

EXCLUDES 2 *encounter for screening for protozoal intestinal disease (Z11.0)*

Z11.8 Encounter for screening for other infectious and parasitic diseases

Encounter for screening for chlamydia
Encounter for screening for rickettsial
Encounter for screening for spirochetal
Encounter for screening for mycoses

Z11.9 Encounter for screening for infectious and parasitic diseases, unspecified

Z12 Encounter for screening for malignant neoplasms

Screening is the testing for disease or disease precursors in asymptomatic individuals so that early detection and treatment can be provided for those who test positive for the disease.

Use additional code to identify any family history of malignant neoplasm (Z80.-)

EXCLUDES 1 *encounter for diagnostic examination-code to sign or symptom*

Z12.0 Encounter for screening for malignant neoplasm of stomach

Z12.1 Encounter for screening for malignant neoplasm of intestinal tract

Z12.10 Encounter for screening for malignant neoplasm of intestinal tract, unspecified

Z12.11 Encounter for screening for malignant neoplasm of colon

Encounter for screening colonoscopy NOS

Z12.12 Encounter for screening for malignant neoplasm of rectum

Z12.13 Encounter for screening for malignant neoplasm of small intestine

Z12.2 Encounter for screening for malignant neoplasm of respiratory organs

Z12.3 Encounter for screening for malignant neoplasm of breast

Z12.31 Encounter for screening mammogram for malignant neoplasm of breast

EXCLUDES 1 *inconclusive mammogram (R92.2)*

AHA: 1Q 2015, 24

Z12.39 Encounter for other screening for malignant neoplasm of breast

Z12.4 Encounter for screening for malignant neoplasm of cervix ♀

Encounter for screening pap smear for malignant neoplasm of cervix

EXCLUDES 1 *when screening is part of general gynecological examination (Z01.4-)*

EXCLUDES 2 *encounter for screening for human papillomavirus (Z11.51)*

Z12.5 Encounter for screening for malignant neoplasm of prostate ♂

Z12.6 Encounter for screening for malignant neoplasm of bladder

Z12.7 Encounter for screening for malignant neoplasm of other genitourinary organs

Z12.71 Encounter for screening for malignant neoplasm of testis ♂

Z12.72 Encounter for screening for malignant neoplasm of vagina ♀

Vaginal pap smear status-post hysterectomy for non-malignant condition

Use additional code to identify acquired absence of uterus (Z90.71-)

EXCLUDES 1 *vaginal pap smear status-post hysterectomy for malignant conditions (Z08)*

Z12.73 Encounter for screening for malignant neoplasm of ovary ♀

Z12.79 Encounter for screening for malignant neoplasm of other genitourinary organs

Z12.8 Encounter for screening for malignant neoplasm of other sites

Z12.81 Encounter for screening for malignant neoplasm of oral cavity

Z12.82 Encounter for screening for malignant neoplasm of nervous system

Z12.83 Encounter for screening for malignant neoplasm of skin

Z12.89 Encounter for screening for malignant neoplasm of other sites

Z12.9 Encounter for screening for malignant neoplasm, site unspecified

Z13 Encounter for screening for other diseases and disorders

Screening is the testing for disease or disease precursors in asymptomatic individuals so that early detection and treatment can be provided for those who test positive for the disease.

EXCLUDES 1 *encounter for diagnostic examination-code to sign or symptom*

Z13.0 Encounter for screening for diseases of the blood and blood-forming organs and certain disorders involving the immune mechanism

Z13.1 Encounter for screening for diabetes mellitus

Z13.2 Encounter for screening for nutritional, metabolic and other endocrine disorders

Z13.21 Encounter for screening for nutritional disorder

Z13.22 Encounter for screening for metabolic disorder

Z13.220 Encounter for screening for lipid disorders

Encounter for screening for cholesterol level
Encounter for screening for hypercholesterolemia
Encounter for screening for hyperlipidemia

Z13.228 Encounter for screening for other metabolic disorders

Z13.29 Encounter for screening for other suspected endocrine disorder

EXCLUDES 1 *encounter for screening for diabetes mellitus (Z13.1)*

Z13.4 Encounter for screening for certain developmental disorders in childhood

Encounter for screening for developmental handicaps in early childhood

EXCLUDES 1 *routine development testing of infant or child (Z00.1-)*

Z13.5 Encounter for screening for eye and ear disorders

EXCLUDES 2 *encounter for general hearing examination (Z01.1-)*
encounter for general vision examination (Z01.0-)

Z13.6 Encounter for screening for cardiovascular disorders

Z13.7 Encounter for screening for genetic and chromosomal anomalies

EXCLUDES 1 *genetic testing for procreative management (Z31.4-)*

Z13.71 Encounter for nonprocreative screening for genetic disease carrier status

Z13.79 Encounter for other screening for genetic and chromosomal anomalies

Z13.8 Encounter for screening for other specified diseases and disorders

EXCLUDES 2 *screening for malignant neoplasms (Z12.-)*

Z13.81 Encounter for screening for digestive system disorders

Z13.810 Encounter for screening for upper gastrointestinal disorder

Z13.811 Encounter for screening for lower gastrointestinal disorder

EXCLUDES 1 *encounter for screening for intestinal infectious disease (Z11.0)*

Z13.818 Encounter for screening for other digestive system disorders

Z13.82 Encounter for screening for musculoskeletal disorder

Z13.820 Encounter for screening for osteoporosis

Z13.828 Encounter for screening for other musculoskeletal disorder

Z13.83 Encounter for screening for respiratory disorder NEC

EXCLUDES 1 *encounter for screening for respiratory tuberculosis (Z11.1)*

Z13.84 Encounter for screening for dental disorders

Z13.85 Encounter for screening for nervous system disorders

● New ▲ Revised *Manifestation* ✕ Deleted Unspecified + Additional code / Digit Indicators ▣ Laterality ▣ Adult (15+ years) ▣ Maternity (12-55 years) ▣ Newborn ▣ Pediatric (0-17 years) ♂ Male ♀ Female

1182   © 2017 DecisionHealth   2017 ICD-10-CM Expert for Physicians

Z13.850   Encounter for screening for traumatic brain
injury
Z13.858   Encounter for screening for other nervous
system disorders
Z13.88   **Encounter for screening for disorder due to
exposure to contaminants**
> EXCLUDES 1 *those exposed to contaminants without
suspected disorders (Z57.-, Z77.-)*
Z13.89   **Encounter for screening for other disorder** ☒
Encounter for screening for genitourinary disorders
Z13.9   **Encounter for screening, unspecified**

Genetic carrier and genetic susceptibility to disease (Z14-Z15)

⊞ **Z14   Genetic carrier**
⊞ **Z14.0   Hemophilia A carrier**
Z14.01   **Asymptomatic hemophilia A carrier**
Z14.02   **Symptomatic hemophilia A carrier**
Z14.1   **Cystic fibrosis carrier**
Z14.8   **Genetic carrier of other disease**
⊞ + **Z15   Genetic susceptibility to disease**
> INCLUDES   confirmed abnormal gene
>
> *Use additional code, if applicable, for any associated family
history of the disease (Z80-Z84)*
>
> EXCLUDES 1 *chromosomal anomalies (Q90-Q99)*
>
> GUIDELINES   Section I.C.21.c.3)
> Codes from category Z15 should not be used as principal or
first-listed codes. If the patient has the condition to which
he/she is susceptible, and that condition is the reason for
the encounter, the code for the current condition should be
sequenced first.

⊞ + **Z15.0   Genetic susceptibility to malignant neoplasm**
> Code first:
> , if applicable, any current malignant neoplasm
(C00-C75, C81-C96)
> *Use additional code, if applicable, for any personal history of
malignant neoplasm (Z85.-)*

+ **Z15.01   Genetic susceptibility to malignant neoplasm of
breast**
> CODING TIP ✓   Assign Z15.01 for a patient who
has prophylactic breast removal due to genetic
susceptibility to breast cancer.

+ **Z15.02   Genetic susceptibility to malignant neoplasm of
ovary** ♀
+ **Z15.03   Genetic susceptibility to malignant neoplasm of
prostate** ♂
+ **Z15.04   Genetic susceptibility to malignant neoplasm of
endometrium** ♀
+ **Z15.09   Genetic susceptibility to other malignant neoplasm**
⊞ + **Z15.8   Genetic susceptibility to other disease**
+ **Z15.81   Genetic susceptibility to multiple endocrine
neoplasia [MEN]**
> EXCLUDES 1 *multiple endocrine neoplasia [MEN]
syndromes (E31.2-)*

+ **Z15.89   Genetic susceptibility to other disease**

Resistance to antimicrobial drugs (Z16)

⊞ **Z16   Resistance to antimicrobial drugs**
> Note: The codes in this category are provided for use as additional
codes to identify the resistance and non-responsiveness of a
condition to antimicrobial drugs.
> Code first:
> the infection
> EXCLUDES 1 *Methicillin resistant Staphylococcus aureus
infection (A49.02)*
> *Methicillin resistant Staphylococcus aureus
infection in diseases classified elsewhere
(B95.62)*
> *Methicillin resistant Staphylococcus aureus
pneumonia (J15.212)*
> *Sepsis due to Methicillin resistant Staphylococcus
aureus (A41.02)*

> GUIDELINES   Section I.C.1.c
> Many bacterial infections are resistant to current antibiotics.
It is necessary to identify all infections documented as
antibiotic resistant. Assign a code from category Z16,
Resistance to antimicrobial drugs, following the infection
code only if the infection code does not identify drug
resistance.

⊞ **Z16.1   Resistance to beta lactam antibiotics**
Z16.10   **Resistance to unspecified beta lactam antibiotics**
Z16.11   **Resistance to penicillins**
Resistance to amoxicillin
Resistance to ampicillin
> GUIDELINES   Section I.C.e.1)(a)
> When a patient is diagnosed with an infection that
is due to methicillin resistant Staphylococcus
aureus (MRSA), and that infection has a
combination code that includes the causal
organism (e.g., sepsis, pneumonia) assign the
appropriate combination code for the condition.
>
> Do not assign code B95.62, MRSA infection as the
cause of diseases classified elsewhere, as an
additional code, because the combination code
includes the type of infection and the MRSA
organism. Do not assign a code from subcategory
Z16.11, Resistance to penicillins, as an additional
diagnosis.

Z16.12   **Extended spectrum beta lactamase (ESBL)
resistance**
Z16.19   **Resistance to other specified beta lactam antibiotics**
Resistance to cephalosporins
⊞ **Z16.2   Resistance to other antibiotics**
Z16.20   **Resistance to unspecified antibiotic**
Resistance to antibiotics NOS
Z16.21   **Resistance to vancomycin**
Z16.22   **Resistance to vancomycin related antibiotics**
Z16.23   **Resistance to quinolones and fluoroquinolones**
Z16.24   **Resistance to multiple antibiotics**
Z16.29   **Resistance to other single specified antibiotic**
Resistance to aminoglycosides
Resistance to macrolides
Resistance to sulfonamides
Resistance to tetracyclines
⊞ **Z16.3   Resistance to other antimicrobial drugs**
> EXCLUDES 1 *resistance to antibiotics (Z16.1-, Z16.2-)*

Z16.30   **Resistance to unspecified antimicrobial drugs**
Drug resistance NOS
Z16.31   **Resistance to antiparasitic drug(s)**
Resistance to quinine and related compounds
Z16.32   **Resistance to antifungal drug(s)**
Z16.33   **Resistance to antiviral drug(s)**
⊞ **Z16.34   Resistance to antimycobacterial drug(s)**
Resistance to tuberculostatics
Z16.341   **Resistance to single antimycobacterial drug**
Resistance to antimycobacterial drug NOS
Z16.342   **Resistance to multiple antimycobacterial drugs**
Z16.35   **Resistance to multiple antimicrobial drugs**
> EXCLUDES 1 *Resistance to multiple antibiotics only
(Z16.24)*

Z16.39   **Resistance to other specified antimicrobial drug**

Estrogen receptor status (Z17)

⊞ **Z17   Estrogen receptor status**
> Code first:
> malignant neoplasm of breast (C50.-)
> CODING TIP ✓   When a patient has breast cancer and the
estrogen receptor status is specified, the appropriate code
from category Z17 should be assigned to indicate the ER
positive or negative status. Breast cancers that are ER+
may be treated with selective estrogen receptor modulators
(SERMs). When SERM therapy is also present in an ER+
breast cancer patient, an additional Z code may be assigned
to identify SERM therapy (Z79.810).

Z17.0   **Estrogen receptor positive status [ER+]**
Z17.1   **Estrogen receptor negative status [ER-]**

Retained foreign body fragments (Z18)

⬛ Z18   Retained foreign body fragments

> **INCLUDES**   embedded fragment (status)
> embedded splinter (status)
> retained foreign body status

> **EXCLUDES 1**   *artificial joint prosthesis status (Z96.6-)*
> *foreign body accidentally left during a procedure (T81.5-)*
> *foreign body entering through orifice (T15-T19)*
> *in situ cardiac device (Z95.-)*
> *organ or tissue replaced by means other than transplant (Z96.-, Z97.-)*
> *organ or tissue replaced by transplant (Z94.-)*
> *personal history of retained foreign body fully removed Z87.821*
> *superficial foreign body (non-embedded splinter) - code to superficial foreign body, by site*

⬛ Z18.0   Retained radioactive fragments

  Z18.01   Retained depleted uranium fragments

  Z18.09   Other retained radioactive fragments
    Other retained depleted isotope fragments
    Retained nontherapeutic radioactive fragments

⬛ Z18.1   Retained metal fragments

> **EXCLUDES 1**   *retained radioactive metal fragments (Z18.01-Z18.09)*

  Z18.10   Retained metal fragments, unspecified
    Retained metal fragment NOS

  Z18.11   Retained magnetic metal fragments

  Z18.12   Retained nonmagnetic metal fragments

Z18.2   Retained plastic fragments
  Acrylics fragments
  Diethylhexylphthalates fragments
  Isocyanate fragments

⬛ Z18.3   Retained organic fragments

  Z18.31   Retained animal quills or spines

  Z18.32   Retained tooth

  Z18.33   Retained wood fragments

  Z18.39   Other retained organic fragments

⬛ Z18.8   Other specified retained foreign body

  Z18.81   Retained glass fragments

  Z18.83   Retained stone or crystalline fragments
    Retained concrete or cement fragments

  Z18.89   Other specified retained foreign body fragments

Z18.9   Retained foreign body fragments, unspecified material

Hormone sensitivity malignancy status (Z19)

● ⬛ Z19   Hormone sensitivity malignancy status
> Code first:
> malignant neoplasm - see Table of Neoplasms, by site, malignant

● Z19.1   Hormone sensitive malignancy status

● Z19.2   Hormone resistant malignancy status
  Castrate resistant prostate malignancy status

Persons with potential health hazards related to communicable diseases (Z20-Z29)

⬛ Z20   Contact with and (suspected) exposure to communicable diseases

> **EXCLUDES 1**   *carrier of infectious disease (Z22.-)*
> *diagnosed current infectious or parasitic disease -see Alphabetic Index*

> **EXCLUDES 2**   *personal history of infectious and parasitic diseases (Z86.1-)*

> **GUIDELINES**   **Section I.C.21.c.1)**
> Category Z20 indicates contact with, and suspected exposure to, communicable diseases. These codes are for patients who do not show any sign or symptom of a disease but are suspected to have been exposed to it by close personal contact with an infected individual or are in an area where a disease is epidemic. Category Z77 indicates contact with and suspected exposures hazardous to health.
>
> Contact/exposure codes may be used as a first-listed code to explain an encounter for testing, or, more commonly, as a secondary code to identify a potential risk.

⬛ Z20.0   Contact with and (suspected) exposure to intestinal infectious diseases

  Z20.01   Contact with and (suspected) exposure to intestinal infectious diseases due to Escherichia coli (E. coli)

  Z20.09   Contact with and (suspected) exposure to other intestinal infectious diseases

Z20.1   Contact with and (suspected) exposure to tuberculosis

Z20.2   Contact with and (suspected) exposure to infections with a predominantly sexual mode of transmission

Z20.3   Contact with and (suspected) exposure to rabies

Z20.4   Contact with and (suspected) exposure to rubella

Z20.5   Contact with and (suspected) exposure to viral hepatitis

Z20.6   Contact with and (suspected) exposure to human immunodeficiency virus [HIV]

> **EXCLUDES 1**   *asymptomatic human immunodeficiency virus [HIV]*
> *HIV infection status (Z21)*

Z20.7   Contact with and (suspected) exposure to pediculosis, acariasis and other infestations

⬛ Z20.8   Contact with and (suspected) exposure to other communicable diseases

  ⬛ Z20.81   Contact with and (suspected) exposure to other bacterial communicable diseases

    Z20.810   Contact with and (suspected) exposure to anthrax

    Z20.811   Contact with and (suspected) exposure to meningococcus

    Z20.818   Contact with and (suspected) exposure to other bacterial communicable diseases

  ⬛ Z20.82   Contact with and (suspected) exposure to other viral communicable diseases

    Z20.820   Contact with and (suspected) exposure to varicella

    Z20.828   Contact with and (suspected) exposure to other viral communicable diseases

  Z20.89   Contact with and (suspected) exposure to other communicable diseases

Z20.9   Contact with and (suspected) exposure to unspecified communicable disease

Z21   Asymptomatic human immunodeficiency virus [HIV] infection status
  HIV positive NOS
  Code first:
    Human immunodeficiency virus [HIV] disease complicating pregnancy, childbirth and the puerperium, if applicable (O98.7-)

> **EXCLUDES 1**   *acquired immunodeficiency syndrome (B20)*
> *contact with human immunodeficiency virus [HIV] (Z20.6)*
> *exposure to human immunodeficiency virus [HIV] (Z20.6)*
> *human immunodeficiency virus [HIV] disease (B20)*
> *inconclusive laboratory evidence of human immunodeficiency virus [HIV] (R75)*

> **GUIDELINES**   **Section I.C.1.a.2)(f)**
> Patients previously diagnosed with any HIV illness (B20) should never be assigned to R75 or Z21, Asymptomatic human immunodeficiency virus [HIV] infection status.

> **GUIDELINES**   **Section I.C.1.a.2)(d)**
> Z21, Asymptomatic human immunodeficiency virus [HIV] infection status, is to be applied when the patient without any documentation of symptoms is listed as being "HIV positive," "known HIV," "HIV test positive," or similar terminology. Do not use this code if the term "AIDS" is used or if the patient is treated for any HIV-related illness or is described as having any condition(s) resulting from his/her HIV positive status; use B20 in these cases.

▲ ⬛ Z22   Carrier of infectious disease

> **INCLUDES**   colonization status
> suspected carrier

> **EXCLUDES 2**   *carrier of viral hepatitis (B18.-)*

Z22.0   Carrier of typhoid

Z22.1   Carrier of other intestinal infectious diseases

Z22.2   Carrier of diphtheria

⬛ Z22.3   Carrier of other specified bacterial diseases

  Z22.31   Carrier of bacterial disease due to meningococci

  ⬛ Z22.32   Carrier of bacterial disease due to staphylococci

---

● New   ▲ Revised   *Manifestation*   ⬛-🔢 Digit Indicators   ⊟ Laterality   🅐 Adult (15+ years)   Ⓜ Maternity (12-55 years)   Ⓝ Newborn   🅿 Pediatric (0-17 years)   ♂ Male   ♀ Female
✖ Deleted   Unspecified   + Additional code

GUIDELINES Section I.C.1.e.1)(c)
Assign code Z22.322 for patients documented as having MRSA colonization. Assign code Z22.321 for patient documented as having MSSA colonization. Colonization is not necessarily indicative of a disease process or as the cause of a specific condition the patient may have unless documented as such by the provider.

Z22.321 **Carrier or suspected carrier of Methicillin susceptible Staphylococcus aureus**
MSSA colonization

Z22.322 **Carrier or suspected carrier of Methicillin resistant Staphylococcus aureus**
MRSA colonization

GUIDELINES Section I.C.1.e.1)(d)
If a patient is documented as having both MRSA colonization and infection during a hospital admission, code Z22.322 and a code for the MRSA infection may both be assigned.

⑥ Z22.33 **Carrier of bacterial disease due to streptococci**

▲ Z22.330 **Carrier of Group B streptococcus**
EXCLUDES 1 *Carrier of streptococcus group B (GBS) complicating pregnancy, childbirth and the puerperium (O99.82-)*

Z22.338 **Carrier of other streptococcus**

Z22.39 **Carrier of other specified bacterial diseases**

Z22.4 **Carrier of infections with a predominantly sexual mode of transmission**

Z22.6 **Carrier of human T-lymphotropic virus type-1 [HTLV-1] infection**

Z22.8 **Carrier of other infectious diseases**

Z22.9 **Carrier of infectious disease, unspecified**

Z23 **Encounter for immunization**
Note: procedure codes are required to identify the types of immunizations given
Code first:
any routine childhood examination

GUIDELINES Section I.C.21.c.2)
Code Z23 is for encounters for inoculations and vaccinations. It indicates that a patient is being seen to receive a prophylactic inoculation against a disease. Procedure codes are required to identify the actual administration of the injection and the type(s) of immunizations given. Code Z23 may be used as a secondary code if the inoculation is given as a routine part of preventive health care, such as a well-baby visit.

④ Z28 **Immunization not carried out and underimmunization status**
INCLUDES vaccination not carried out

⑤ Z28.0 **Immunization not carried out because of contraindication**

Z28.01 **Immunization not carried out because of acute illness of patient**

Z28.02 **Immunization not carried out because of chronic illness or condition of patient**

Z28.03 **Immunization not carried out because of immune compromised state of patient**

Z28.04 **Immunization not carried out because of patient allergy to vaccine or component**

Z28.09 **Immunization not carried out because of other contraindication**

Z28.1 **Immunization not carried out because of patient decision for reasons of belief or group pressure**
Immunization not carried out because of religious belief

⑤ Z28.2 **Immunization not carried out because of patient decision for other and unspecified reason**

Z28.20 **Immunization not carried out because of patient decision for unspecified reason**

Z28.21 **Immunization not carried out because of patient refusal**

Z28.29 **Immunization not carried out because of patient decision for other reason**

Z28.3 **Underimmunization status**
Delinquent immunization status
Lapsed immunization schedule status

⑤ Z28.8 **Immunization not carried out for other reason**

Z28.81 **Immunization not carried out due to patient having had the disease**

Z28.82 **Immunization not carried out because of caregiver refusal**
Immunization not carried out because of guardian refusal
Immunization not carried out because of parent refusal
EXCLUDES 1 *immunization not carried out because of caregiver refusal because of religious belief (Z28.1)*

Z28.89 **Immunization not carried out for other reason**

Z28.9 **Immunization not carried out for unspecified reason**

● ④ Z29 **Encounter for other prophylactic measures**
Excludes 1: desensitization to allergens (Z51.6)
prophylactic surgery (Z40.-)

● ⑤ Z29.1 **Encounter for prophylactic immunotherapy**
Encounter for administration of immunoglobulin

● Z29.11 **Encounter for prophylactic immunotherapy for respiratory syncytial virus (RSV)**

● Z29.12 **Encounter for prophylactic antivenin**

● Z29.13 **Encounter for prophylactic Rho(D) immune globulin**

● Z29.14 **Encounter for prophylactic rabies immune globin**

● Z29.3 **Encounter for prophylactic fluoride administration**

● Z29.8 **Encounter for other specified prophylactic measures**

● Z29.9 **Encounter for prophylactic measures, unspecified**

Persons encountering health services in circumstances related to reproduction (Z30-Z39)

④ Z30 **Encounter for contraceptive management**

⑤ Z30.0 **Encounter for general counseling and advice on contraception**

⑥ Z30.01 **Encounter for initial prescription of contraceptives**
EXCLUDES 1 *encounter for surveillance of contraceptives (Z30.4-)*

Z30.011 **Encounter for initial prescription of contraceptive pills** ♀

Z30.012 **Encounter for prescription of emergency contraception** ♀
Encounter for postcoital contraception

Z30.013 **Encounter for initial prescription of injectable contraceptive** ♀

Z30.014 **Encounter for initial prescription of intrauterine contraceptive device** ♀
EXCLUDES 1 *encounter for insertion of intrauterine contraceptive device (Z30.430, Z30.432)*

● Z30.015 **Encounter for initial prescription of vaginal ring hormonal contraceptive** ♀

● Z30.016 **Encounter for initial prescription of transdermal patch hormonal contraceptive device** ♀

● Z30.017 **Encounter for initial prescription of implantable subdermal contraceptive** ♀

▲ Z30.018 **Encounter for initial prescription of other contraceptives** ♀
Encounter for initial prescription of barrier contraception
Encounter for initial prescription of diaphragm

Z30.019 **Encounter for initial prescription of contraceptives, unspecified** ♀

Z30.02 **Counseling and instruction in natural family planning to avoid pregnancy**

Z30.09 **Encounter for other general counseling and advice on contraception**
Encounter for family planning advice NOS

Z30.2 **Encounter for sterilization**

⑤ Z30.4 **Encounter for surveillance of contraceptives**

Z30.40 **Encounter for surveillance of contraceptives, unspecified**

Z30.41 **Encounter for surveillance of contraceptive pills** ♀
Encounter for repeat prescription for contraceptive pill

Z30.42 **Encounter for surveillance of injectable contraceptive** ♀

⑥ Z30.43 **Encounter for surveillance of intrauterine contraceptive device**

Z30.430 **Encounter for insertion of intrauterine contraceptive device** ♀

● New ▲ Revised *Manifestation* ④-⑦ Digit Indicators ▤ Laterality ▣ Adult (15+ years) ▣ Maternity (12-55 years) ▣ Newborn ▣ Pediatric (0-17 years) ♂ Male ♀ Female
✖ Deleted Unspecified + Additional code

Z30.431	**Encounter for routine checking of intrauterine contraceptive device**	♀
Z30.432	**Encounter for removal of intrauterine contraceptive device**	♀
Z30.433	**Encounter for removal and reinsertion of intrauterine contraceptive device**	♀
	Encounter for replacement of intrauterine contraceptive device	
● Z30.44	**Encounter for surveillance of vaginal ring hormonal contraceptive device**	♀
● Z30.45	**Encounter for surveillance of transdermal patch hormonal contraceptive device**	♀
● Z30.46	**Encounter for surveillance of implantable subdermal contraceptive**	♀
	Encounter for checking, reinsertion or removal of implantable subdermal contraceptive	
▲ Z30.49	**Encounter for surveillance of other contraceptives**	♀
	Encounter for surveillance of barrier contraception	
	Encounter for surveillance of diaphragm	
Z30.8	**Encounter for other contraceptive management**	♀
	Encounter for postvasectomy sperm count	
	Encounter for routine examination for contraceptive maintenance	

EXCLUDES 1 *sperm count following sterilization reversal (Z31.42)*
sperm count for fertility testing (Z31.41)

Z30.9	**Encounter for contraceptive management, unspecified**	
▣ **Z31**	**Encounter for procreative management**	

EXCLUDES 1 *complications associated with artificial fertilization (N98.-)*
female infertility (N97.-)
male infertility (N46.-)

Z31.0	**Encounter for reversal of previous sterilization**	
▣ Z31.4	**Encounter for procreative investigation and testing**	

EXCLUDES 1 *postvasectomy sperm count (Z30.8)*

Z31.41	**Encounter for fertility testing**	
	Encounter for fallopian tube patency testing	
	Encounter for sperm count for fertility testing	
Z31.42	**Aftercare following sterilization reversal**	
	Sperm count following sterilization reversal	
▣＋ Z31.43	**Encounter for genetic testing of female for procreative management**	
	Use additional code for recurrent pregnancy loss, if applicable (N96, O26.2-)	

EXCLUDES 1 *nonprocreative genetic testing (Z13.7-)*

＋ Z31.430	**Encounter of female for testing for genetic disease carrier status for procreative management**	♀
＋ Z31.438	**Encounter for other genetic testing of female for procreative management**	♀
▣ Z31.44	**Encounter for genetic testing of male for procreative management**	

EXCLUDES 1 *nonprocreative genetic testing (Z13.7-)*

Z31.440	**Encounter of male for testing for genetic disease carrier status for procreative management**	♂
Z31.441	**Encounter for testing of male partner of patient with recurrent pregnancy loss**	♂
Z31.448	**Encounter for other genetic testing of male for procreative management**	♂
Z31.49	**Encounter for other procreative investigation and testing**	
Z31.5	**Encounter for genetic counseling**	
▣ Z31.6	**Encounter for general counseling and advice on procreation**	
Z31.61	**Procreative counseling and advice using natural family planning**	
Z31.62	**Encounter for fertility preservation counseling**	
	Encounter for fertility preservation counseling prior to cancer therapy	
	Encounter for fertility preservation counseling prior to surgical removal of gonads	
Z31.69	**Encounter for other general counseling and advice on procreation**	
● Z31.7	**Encounter for procreative management and counseling for gestational carrier**	♀Ⓜ

EXCLUDES 1 *pregnant state, gestational carrier (Z33.3)*

▣ Z31.8	**Encounter for other procreative management**	

Z31.81	**Encounter for male factor infertility in female patient**	♀
Z31.82	**Encounter for Rh incompatibility status**	
	AHA: 3Q 2015, 40	
	AHA: 4Q 2014, 17	
＋ Z31.83	**Encounter for assisted reproductive fertility procedure cycle**	♀
	Patient undergoing in vitro fertilization cycle	
	Use additional code to identify the type of infertility	

EXCLUDES 1 *pre-cycle diagnosis and testing - code to reason for encounter*

Z31.84	**Encounter for fertility preservation procedure**	
	Encounter for fertility preservation procedure prior to cancer therapy	
	Encounter for fertility preservation procedure prior to surgical removal of gonads	
Z31.89	**Encounter for other procreative management**	
Z31.9	**Encounter for procreative management, unspecified**	
▣ **Z32**	**Encounter for pregnancy test and childbirth and childcare instruction**	
▣ Z32.0	**Encounter for pregnancy test**	
Z32.00	**Encounter for pregnancy test, result unknown**	♀
	Encounter for pregnancy test NOS	
Z32.01	**Encounter for pregnancy test, result positive**	♀Ⓜ
Z32.02	**Encounter for pregnancy test, result negative**	♀
Z32.2	**Encounter for childbirth instruction**	
Z32.3	**Encounter for childcare instruction**	
	Encounter for prenatal or postpartum childcare instruction	
▣ **Z33**	**Pregnant state**	
▲ Z33.1	**Pregnant state, incidental**	♀Ⓜ
	Pregnant state NOS	

EXCLUDES 1 *complications of pregnancy (O00-O9A)*
pregnant state, gestational carrier (Z33.3)

GUIDELINES **Section I.C.15.a.1)**
Should the provider document that the pregnancy is incidental to the encounter, then code Z33.1 should be used in place of any chapter 15 codes. It is the provider's responsibility to state that the condition being treated is not affecting the pregnancy.

Z33.2	**Encounter for elective termination of pregnancy**	♀Ⓜ

EXCLUDES 1 *early fetal death with retention of dead fetus (O02.1)*
late fetal death (O36.4)
spontaneous abortion (O03)

● Z33.3	**Pregnant state, gestational carrier**	♀Ⓜ

EXCLUDES 1 *encounter for procreative management and counseling for gestational carrier (Z31.7)*

▣ **Z34**	**Encounter for supervision of normal pregnancy**	

EXCLUDES 1 *any complication of pregnancy (O00-O9A)*
encounter for pregnancy test (Z32.0-)
encounter for supervision of high risk pregnancy (O09.-)

▣ Z34.0	**Encounter for supervision of normal first pregnancy**	
Z34.00	**Encounter for supervision of normal first pregnancy, unspecified trimester**	♀Ⓜ
Z34.01	**Encounter for supervision of normal first pregnancy, first trimester**	♀Ⓜ
Z34.02	**Encounter for supervision of normal first pregnancy, second trimester**	♀Ⓜ
Z34.03	**Encounter for supervision of normal first pregnancy, third trimester**	♀Ⓜ
▣ Z34.8	**Encounter for supervision of other normal pregnancy**	
Z34.80	**Encounter for supervision of other normal pregnancy, unspecified trimester**	♀Ⓜ
Z34.81	**Encounter for supervision of other normal pregnancy, first trimester**	♀Ⓜ
Z34.82	**Encounter for supervision of other normal pregnancy, second trimester**	♀Ⓜ
Z34.83	**Encounter for supervision of other normal pregnancy, third trimester**	♀Ⓜ
	AHA: 4Q 2014, 17	
▣ Z34.9	**Encounter for supervision of normal pregnancy, unspecified**	
Z34.90	**Encounter for supervision of normal pregnancy, unspecified, unspecified trimester**	♀Ⓜ
Z34.91	**Encounter for supervision of normal pregnancy, unspecified, first trimester**	♀Ⓜ

● New   ▲ Revised   *Manifestation*   ▣-▯ Digit Indicators   ▭ Laterality   Ⓐ Adult (15+ years)   Ⓜ Maternity (12-55 years)   Ⓝ Newborn   Ⓟ Pediatric (0-17 years)   ♂ Male   ♀ Female
✖ Deleted   Unspecified   ＋ Additional code

1186   © 2017 DecisionHealth   2017 ICD-10-CM Expert for Physicians

Z34.92 Encounter for supervision of normal pregnancy, ♀Ⓜ
unspecified, second trimester

Z34.93 Encounter for supervision of normal pregnancy, ♀ⓂⓂ
unspecified, third trimester

Z36 Encounter for antenatal screening of mother ♀ⓂⓂ

EXCLUDES 1 *abnormal findings on antenatal screening of
mother (O28.-)*
diagnostic examination- code to sign or symptom
*encounter for suspected maternal and fetal
conditions ruled out (Z03.7-)*
*suspected fetal condition affecting management of
pregnancy - code to condition in Chapter 15*
EXCLUDES 2 *genetic counseling and testing (Z31.43-, Z31.5)*
routine prenatal care (Z34)

▲ ④ **Z3A** Weeks of gestation
Note: Codes from category Z3A are for use, only on the maternal
record, to indicate the weeks of gestation of the pregnancy, if
known.
Code first:
complications of pregnancy, childbirth and the puerperium
(O00-O9A)
AHA: 2Q 2013, 33

⑤ **Z3A.0** Weeks of gestation of pregnancy, unspecified or less than
10 weeks

Z3A.00 Weeks of gestation of pregnancy not specified ♀Ⓜ
AHA: 3Q 2014, 18

Z3A.01 Less than 8 weeks gestation of pregnancy ♀Ⓜ

Z3A.08 8 weeks gestation of pregnancy ♀Ⓜ

Z3A.09 9 weeks gestation of pregnancy ♀Ⓜ

⑤ **Z3A.1** Weeks of gestation of pregnancy, weeks 10-19

Z3A.10 10 weeks gestation of pregnancy ♀Ⓜ

Z3A.11 11 weeks gestation of pregnancy ♀Ⓜ

Z3A.12 12 weeks gestation of pregnancy ♀Ⓜ

Z3A.13 13 weeks gestation of pregnancy ♀Ⓜ

Z3A.14 14 weeks gestation of pregnancy ♀Ⓜ

Z3A.15 15 weeks gestation of pregnancy ♀Ⓜ

Z3A.16 16 weeks gestation of pregnancy ♀Ⓜ

Z3A.17 17 weeks gestation of pregnancy ♀Ⓜ

Z3A.18 18 weeks gestation of pregnancy ♀Ⓜ

Z3A.19 19 weeks gestation of pregnancy ♀Ⓜ

⑤ **Z3A.2** Weeks of gestation of pregnancy, weeks 20-29

Z3A.20 20 weeks gestation of pregnancy ♀Ⓜ

Z3A.21 21 weeks gestation of pregnancy ♀Ⓜ

Z3A.22 22 weeks gestation of pregnancy ♀Ⓜ

Z3A.23 23 weeks gestation of pregnancy ♀Ⓜ

Z3A.24 24 weeks gestation of pregnancy ♀Ⓜ

Z3A.25 25 weeks gestation of pregnancy ♀Ⓜ

Z3A.26 26 weeks gestation of pregnancy ♀Ⓜ

Z3A.27 27 weeks gestation of pregnancy ♀Ⓜ

Z3A.28 28 weeks gestation of pregnancy ♀Ⓜ
AHA: 4Q 2014, 17

Z3A.29 29 weeks gestation of pregnancy ♀Ⓜ

⑤ **Z3A.3** Weeks of gestation of pregnancy, weeks 30-39

Z3A.30 30 weeks gestation of pregnancy ♀Ⓜ

Z3A.31 31 weeks gestation of pregnancy ♀Ⓜ

Z3A.32 32 weeks gestation of pregnancy ♀Ⓜ

Z3A.33 33 weeks gestation of pregnancy ♀Ⓜ

Z3A.34 34 weeks gestation of pregnancy ♀Ⓜ

Z3A.35 35 weeks gestation of pregnancy ♀Ⓜ

Z3A.36 36 weeks gestation of pregnancy ♀Ⓜ

Z3A.37 37 weeks gestation of pregnancy ♀Ⓜ
AHA: 4Q 2014, 18

Z3A.38 38 weeks gestation of pregnancy ♀Ⓜ
AHA: 2Q 2016, 34

Z3A.39 39 weeks gestation of pregnancy ♀Ⓜ

⑤ **Z3A.4** Weeks of gestation of pregnancy, weeks 40 or greater

Z3A.40 40 weeks gestation of pregnancy ♀Ⓜ
AHA: 2Q 2014, 9

Z3A.41 41 weeks gestation of pregnancy ♀Ⓜ

Z3A.42 42 weeks gestation of pregnancy ♀Ⓜ
AHA: 4Q 2014, 23

Z3A.49 Greater than 42 weeks gestation of pregnancy ♀Ⓜ
AHA: 4Q 2014, 23

④ **Z37** Outcome of delivery
This category is intended for use as an additional code to identify
the outcome of delivery on the mother's record. It is not for use
on the newborn record.
EXCLUDES 1 *stillbirth (P95)*

Z37.0 Single live birth ♀Ⓜ
AHA: 2Q 2016, 34
AHA: 4Q 2014, 18
AHA: 2Q 2014, 9

Z37.1 Single stillbirth ♀Ⓜ

Z37.2 Twins, both liveborn ♀Ⓜ

Z37.3 Twins, one liveborn and one stillborn ♀Ⓜ

Z37.4 Twins, both stillborn ♀Ⓜ

⑤ **Z37.5** Other multiple births, all liveborn

Z37.50 Multiple births, unspecified, all liveborn ♀Ⓜ

Z37.51 Triplets, all liveborn ♀Ⓜ

Z37.52 Quadruplets, all liveborn ♀Ⓜ

Z37.53 Quintuplets, all liveborn ♀Ⓜ

Z37.54 Sextuplets, all liveborn ♀Ⓜ

Z37.59 Other multiple births, all liveborn ♀Ⓜ

⑤ **Z37.6** Other multiple births, some liveborn

Z37.60 Multiple births, unspecified, some liveborn ♀Ⓜ

Z37.61 Triplets, some liveborn ♀Ⓜ

Z37.62 Quadruplets, some liveborn ♀Ⓜ

Z37.63 Quintuplets, some liveborn ♀Ⓜ

Z37.64 Sextuplets, some liveborn ♀Ⓜ

Z37.69 Other multiple births, some liveborn ♀Ⓜ

Z37.7 Other multiple births, all stillborn ♀Ⓜ

Z37.9 Outcome of delivery, unspecified ♀Ⓜ
Multiple birth NOS
Single birth NOS

④ **Z38** Liveborn infants according to place of birth and type
of delivery
This category is for use as the principal code on the initial record
of a newborn baby. It is to be used for the initial birth record
only. It is not to be used on the mother's record.
AHA: 2Q 2015, 15

⑤ **Z38.0** Single liveborn infant, born in hospital
Single liveborn infant, born in birthing center or other health
care facility

Z38.00 Single liveborn infant, delivered vaginally Ⓝ

Z38.01 Single liveborn infant, delivered by cesarean Ⓝ

Z38.1 Single liveborn infant, born outside hospital Ⓝ

Z38.2 Single liveborn infant, unspecified as to place of birth Ⓝ
Single liveborn infant NOS

⑤ **Z38.3** Twin liveborn infant, born in hospital

Z38.30 Twin liveborn infant, delivered vaginally Ⓝ

Z38.31 Twin liveborn infant, delivered by cesarean Ⓝ

Z38.4 Twin liveborn infant, born outside hospital Ⓝ

Z38.5 Twin liveborn infant, unspecified as to place of birth Ⓝ

⑤ **Z38.6** Other multiple liveborn infant, born in hospital

Z38.61 Triplet liveborn infant, delivered vaginally Ⓝ

Z38.62 Triplet liveborn infant, delivered by cesarean Ⓝ

Z38.63 Quadruplet liveborn infant, delivered vaginally Ⓝ

Z38.64 Quadruplet liveborn infant, delivered by cesarean Ⓝ

Z38.65 Quintuplet liveborn infant, delivered vaginally Ⓝ

Z38.66 Quintuplet liveborn infant, delivered by cesarean Ⓝ

Z38.68 Other multiple liveborn infant, delivered
vaginally Ⓝ

Z38.69 Other multiple liveborn infant, delivered by
cesarean Ⓝ

Z38.7 Other multiple liveborn infant, born outside hospital Ⓝ

Z38.8 Other multiple liveborn infant, unspecified as to place
of birth Ⓝ

④ **Z39** Encounter for maternal postpartum care and
examination

Z39.0 Encounter for care and examination of mother ♀Ⓜ
immediately after delivery
Care and observation in uncomplicated cases when the
delivery occurs outside a healthcare facility
EXCLUDES 1 *care for postpartum complication- see
Alphabetic index*

● New   ▲ Revised   *Manifestation*   ④-⑦ Digit Indicators   ▤ Laterality   ▣ Adult   Ⓜ Maternity   Ⓝ Newborn   ▣ Pediatric   ♂ Male   ♀ Female
✖ Deleted   Unspecified   + Additional code   (15+ years)   (12-55 years)   (0-17 years)

Z39.1   **Encounter for care and examination of lactating mother** ♀ Ⓜ
Encounter for supervision of lactation
EXCLUDES 1 *disorders of lactation (O92.-)*

Z39.2   **Encounter for routine postpartum follow-up** ♀ Ⓜ

Encounters for other specific health care (Z40-Z53)

Categories Z40-Z53 are intended for use to indicate a reason for care. They may be used for patients who have already been treated for a disease or injury, but who are receiving aftercare or prophylactic care, or care to consolidate the treatment, or to deal with a residual state
EXCLUDES 2 *follow-up examination for medical surveillance after treatment (Z08-Z09)*

Ⓐ **Z40**   **Encounter for prophylactic surgery**
EXCLUDES 1 *organ donations (Z52.-)*
therapeutic organ removal-code to condition

Ⓢ **+ Z40.0** **Encounter for prophylactic surgery for risk factors related to malignant neoplasms**
Admission for prophylactic organ removal
Use additional code to identify risk factor

+ Z40.00   **Encounter for prophylactic removal of unspecified organ**

+ Z40.01   **Encounter for prophylactic removal of breast**

+ Z40.02   **Encounter for prophylactic removal of ovary** ♀

+ Z40.09   **Encounter for prophylactic removal of other organ**

Z40.8   **Encounter for other prophylactic surgery**

Z40.9   **Encounter for prophylactic surgery, unspecified**

Ⓐ **Z41**   **Encounter for procedures for purposes other than remedying health state**

Z41.1   **Encounter for cosmetic surgery**
Encounter for cosmetic breast implant
Encounter for cosmetic procedure
EXCLUDES 1 *encounter for plastic and reconstructive surgery following medical procedure or healed injury (Z42.-)*
encounter for post-mastectomy breast implantation (Z42.1)

Z41.2   **Encounter for routine and ritual male circumcision** ♂

Z41.3   **Encounter for ear piercing**

Z41.8   **Encounter for other procedures for purposes other than remedying health state**

Z41.9   **Encounter for procedure for purposes other than remedying health state, unspecified**

Ⓐ **Z42**   **Encounter for plastic and reconstructive surgery following medical procedure or healed injury**
EXCLUDES 1 *encounter for cosmetic plastic surgery (Z41.1)*
encounter for plastic surgery for treatment of current injury - code to relevent injury

Z42.1   **Encounter for breast reconstruction following mastectomy** Ⓐ
EXCLUDES 1 *deformity and disproportion of reconstructed breast (N65.1-)*

Z42.8   **Encounter for other plastic and reconstructive surgery following medical procedure or healed injury**

Ⓐ **Z43**   **Encounter for attention to artificial openings**
INCLUDES closure of artificial openings
passage of sounds or bougies through artificial openings
reforming artificial openings
removal of catheter from artificial openings
toilet or cleansing of artificial openings
EXCLUDES 1 *artificial opening status only, without need for care (Z93.-)*
complications of external stoma (J95.0-, K94.-, N99.5-)
EXCLUDES 2 *fitting and adjustment of prosthetic and other devices (Z44-Z46)*

CODING TIP ✓ When assigning a code from Z43 for an encounter for attention to artificial openings, such as a tracheostomy or cystostomy, the plan of care should include interventions for the treatment of the artificial opening.

CODING TIP ✓ Assign codes from category Z43 when reason for encounter is to provide active care/intervention to the artificial opening. Do not use codes in the Z43 category with status ostomy codes (Z93) or when there is a complication with the ostomy.

Z43.0   **Encounter for attention to tracheostomy**
Z43.1   **Encounter for attention to gastrostomy**
Z43.2   **Encounter for attention to ileostomy**
Z43.3   **Encounter for attention to colostomy**
Z43.4   **Encounter for attention to other artificial openings of digestive tract**
Z43.5   **Encounter for attention to cystostomy**
Z43.6   **Encounter for attention to other artificial openings of urinary tract**
Encounter for attention to nephrostomy
Encounter for attention to ureterostomy
Encounter for attention to urethrostomy
Z43.7   **Encounter for attention to artificial vagina**
Z43.8   **Encounter for attention to other artificial openings**
Z43.9   **Encounter for attention to unspecified artificial opening**

Ⓐ **Z44**   **Encounter for fitting and adjustment of external prosthetic device**
INCLUDES removal or replacement of external prosthetic device
EXCLUDES 1 *malfunction or other complications of device - see Alphabetical Index*
presence of prosthetic device (Z97.-)

Ⓢ **Z44.0** **Encounter for fitting and adjustment of artificial arm**

Ⓖ **Z44.00**   **Encounter for fitting and adjustment of unspecified artificial arm**

Ⓔ **Z44.001**   **Encounter for fitting and adjustment of unspecified right artificial arm**

Ⓔ **Z44.002**   **Encounter for fitting and adjustment of unspecified left artificial arm**

Ⓔ **Z44.009**   **Encounter for fitting and adjustment of unspecified artificial arm, unspecified arm**

Ⓖ **Z44.01**   **Encounter for fitting and adjustment of complete artificial arm**

Ⓔ **Z44.011**   **Encounter for fitting and adjustment of complete right artificial arm**

Ⓔ **Z44.012**   **Encounter for fitting and adjustment of complete left artificial arm**

Ⓔ **Z44.019**   **Encounter for fitting and adjustment of complete artificial arm, unspecified arm**

Ⓖ **Z44.02**   **Encounter for fitting and adjustment of partial artificial arm**

Ⓔ **Z44.021**   **Encounter for fitting and adjustment of partial artificial right arm**

Ⓔ **Z44.022**   **Encounter for fitting and adjustment of partial artificial left arm**

Ⓔ **Z44.029**   **Encounter for fitting and adjustment of partial artificial arm, unspecified arm**

Ⓢ **Z44.1** **Encounter for fitting and adjustment of artificial leg**

Ⓖ **Z44.10**   **Encounter for fitting and adjustment of unspecified artificial leg**

Ⓔ **Z44.101**   **Encounter for fitting and adjustment of unspecified right artificial leg**

Ⓔ **Z44.102**   **Encounter for fitting and adjustment of unspecified left artificial leg**

Ⓔ **Z44.109**   **Encounter for fitting and adjustment of unspecified artificial leg, unspecified leg**

Ⓖ **Z44.11**   **Encounter for fitting and adjustment of complete artificial leg**

Ⓔ **Z44.111**   **Encounter for fitting and adjustment of complete right artificial leg**

Ⓔ **Z44.112**   **Encounter for fitting and adjustment of complete left artificial leg**

Ⓔ **Z44.119**   **Encounter for fitting and adjustment of complete artificial leg, unspecified leg**

Ⓖ **Z44.12**   **Encounter for fitting and adjustment of partial artificial leg**

Ⓔ **Z44.121**   **Encounter for fitting and adjustment of partial artificial right leg**

Ⓔ **Z44.122**   **Encounter for fitting and adjustment of partial artificial left leg**

Ⓔ **Z44.129**   **Encounter for fitting and adjustment of partial artificial leg, unspecified leg**

Ⓢ **Z44.2** **Encounter for fitting and adjustment of artificial eye**
EXCLUDES 1 *mechanical complication of ocular prosthesis (T85.3)*

Ⓔ **Z44.20**   **Encounter for fitting and adjustment of artificial eye, unspecified**

● New   ▲ Revised   *Manifestation*   Ⓐ-❼ Digit Indicators   ⊟ Laterality   Ⓐ Adult (15+ years)   Ⓜ Maternity (12-55 years)   Ⓝ Newborn   Ⓟ Pediatric (0-17 years)   ♂ Male   ♀ Female
✖ ~~Deleted~~   Unspecified   + Additional code

Z44.21   Encounter for fitting and adjustment of artificial right eye

Z44.22   Encounter for fitting and adjustment of artificial left eye

Z44.3   **Encounter for fitting and adjustment of external breast prosthesis**

> **EXCLUDES 1**   *complications of breast implant (T85.4-)*
> *encounter for adjustment or removal of breast implant (Z45.81-)*
> *encounter for initial breast implant insertion for cosmetic breast augmentation (Z41.1)*
> *encounter for breast reconstruction following mastectomy (Z42.1)*

Z44.30   **Encounter for fitting and adjustment of external breast prosthesis, unspecified breast** ♀

Z44.31   **Encounter for fitting and adjustment of external right breast prosthesis** ♀

Z44.32   **Encounter for fitting and adjustment of external left breast prosthesis** ♀

Z44.8   **Encounter for fitting and adjustment of other external prosthetic devices**

Z44.9   **Encounter for fitting and adjustment of unspecified external prosthetic device**

Z45   **Encounter for adjustment and management of implanted device**

> **INCLUDES**   removal or replacement of implanted device

> **EXCLUDES 1**   *malfunction or other complications of device - see Alphabetical Index*
> *presence of prosthetic and other devices (Z95-Z97)*

> **EXCLUDES 2**   *encounter for fitting and adjustment of non-implanted device (Z46.-)*

Z45.0   **Encounter for adjustment and management of cardiac device**

▲ **Z45.01**   **Encounter for adjustment and management of cardiac pacemaker**

Encounter for adjustment and management of cardiac resynchronization therapy pacemaker (CRT-P)

> **EXCLUDES 1**   *encounter for adjustment and management of automatic implantable cardiac defibrillator with synchronous cardiac pacemaker (Z45.02)*

Z45.010   **Encounter for checking and testing of cardiac pacemaker pulse generator [battery]**
Encounter for replacing cardiac pacemaker pulse generator [battery]

Z45.018   **Encounter for adjustment and management of other part of cardiac pacemaker**

▲ **Z45.02**   **Encounter for adjustment and management of automatic implantable cardiac defibrillator**
Encounter for adjustment and management of automatic implantable cardiac defibrillator with synchronous cardiac pacemaker
Encounter for adjustment and management of cardiac resynchronization therapy defibrillator (CRT-D)

Z45.09   **Encounter for adjustment and management of other cardiac device**

Z45.1   **Encounter for adjustment and management of infusion pump**

Z45.2   **Encounter for adjustment and management of vascular access device**
Encounter for adjustment and management of vascular catheters

> **EXCLUDES 1**   *encounter for adjustment and management of renal dialysis catheter (Z49.01)*

> **CODING TIP ✓**   This code is used for routine care of vascular access devices, including peripheral, PICC and central lines. Do not use this code if the line is complicated. See T80 for complications.

Z45.3   **Encounter for adjustment and management of implanted devices of the special senses**

Z45.31   **Encounter for adjustment and management of implanted visual substitution device**

Z45.32   **Encounter for adjustment and management of implanted hearing device**

> **EXCLUDES 1**   *Encounter for fitting and adjustment of hearing aide (Z46.1)*

Z45.320   **Encounter for adjustment and management of bone conduction device**

Z45.321   **Encounter for adjustment and management of cochlear device**

Z45.328   **Encounter for adjustment and management of other implanted hearing device**

Z45.4   **Encounter for adjustment and management of implanted nervous system device**

Z45.41   **Encounter for adjustment and management of cerebrospinal fluid drainage device**
Encounter for adjustment and management of cerebral ventricular (communicating) shunt

Z45.42   **Encounter for adjustment and management of neuropacemaker (brain) (peripheral nerve) (spinal cord)**

Z45.49   **Encounter for adjustment and management of other implanted nervous system device**
AHA: 3Q 2014, 20

Z45.8   **Encounter for adjustment and management of other implanted devices**

Z45.81   **Encounter for adjustment or removal of breast implant**
Encounter for elective implant exchange (different material) (different size)
Encounter removal of tissue expander without synchronous insertion of permanent implant

> **EXCLUDES 1**   *complications of breast implant (T85.4-)*
> *encounter for initial breast implant insertion for cosmetic breast augmentation (Z41.1)*
> *encounter for breast reconstruction following mastectomy (Z42.1)*

Z45.811   **Encounter for adjustment or removal of right breast implant** ♀

Z45.812   **Encounter for adjustment or removal of left breast implant** ♀

Z45.819   **Encounter for adjustment or removal of unspecified breast implant** ♀

Z45.82   **Encounter for adjustment or removal of myringotomy device (stent) (tube)**

Z45.89   **Encounter for adjustment and management of other implanted devices**
AHA: 4Q 2014, 27, 28

Z45.9   **Encounter for adjustment and management of unspecified implanted device**

Z46   **Encounter for fitting and adjustment of other devices**

> **INCLUDES**   removal or replacement of other device

> **EXCLUDES 1**   *malfunction or other complications of device - see Alphabetical Index*

> **EXCLUDES 2**   *encounter for fitting and management of implanted devices (Z45.-)*
> *issue of repeat prescription only (Z76.0)*
> *presence of prosthetic and other devices (Z95-Z97)*

Z46.0   **Encounter for fitting and adjustment of spectacles and contact lenses**

Z46.1   **Encounter for fitting and adjustment of hearing aid**

> **EXCLUDES 1**   *encounter for adjustment and management of implanted hearing device (Z45.32-)*

Z46.2   **Encounter for fitting and adjustment of other devices related to nervous system and special senses**

> **EXCLUDES 2**   *encounter for adjustment and management of implanted nervous system device (Z45.4-)*
> *encounter for adjustment and management of implanted visual substitution device (Z45.31)*

Z46.3   **Encounter for fitting and adjustment of dental prosthetic device**
Encounter for fitting and adjustment of dentures

Z46.4   **Encounter for fitting and adjustment of orthodontic device**

Z46.5   **Encounter for fitting and adjustment of other gastrointestinal appliance and device**

> **EXCLUDES 1**   *encounter for attention to artificial openings of digestive tract (Z43.1-Z43.4)*

Z46.51   **Encounter for fitting and adjustment of gastric lap band**

Z46.59   **Encounter for fitting and adjustment of other gastrointestinal appliance and device**

Z46.6   **Encounter for fitting and adjustment of urinary device**

> **EXCLUDES 2**   *attention to artificial openings of urinary tract (Z43.5, Z43.6)*

● New   ▲ Revised   *Manifestation*   **4**-**7** Digit Indicators   ▣ Laterality   Ⓐ Adult (15+ years)   Ⓜ Maternity (12-55 years)   Ⓝ Newborn   Ⓟ Pediatric (0-17 years)   ♂ Male   ♀ Female

✖ Deleted   Unspecified   + Additional code

CODING TIP ✓ Code Z46.6 includes removal and intermittent catheterization as well as indwelling catheter care.

⑤ Z46.8 **Encounter for fitting and adjustment of other specified devices**

Z46.81 **Encounter for fitting and adjustment of insulin pump**
Encounter for insulin pump instruction and training
Encounter for insulin pump titration

Z46.82 **Encounter for fitting and adjustment of non-vascular catheter**

Z46.89 **Encounter for fitting and adjustment of other specified devices**
Encounter for fitting and adjustment of wheelchair

Z46.9 **Encounter for fitting and adjustment of unspecified device**

④ Z47 **Orthopedic aftercare**
EXCLUDES 1 *aftercare for healing fracture-code to fracture with 7th character D*

+ Z47.1 **Aftercare following joint replacement surgery**
Use additional code to identify the joint (Z96.6-)

Z47.2 **Encounter for removal of internal fixation device**
EXCLUDES 1 *encounter for adjustment of internal fixation device for fracture treatment- code to fracture with appropriate 7th character*
encounter for removal of external fixation device- code to fracture with 7th character D
infection or inflammatory reaction to internal fixation device (T84.6-)
mechanical complication of internal fixation device (T84.1-)

⑤ Z47.3 **Aftercare following explantation of joint prosthesis**
Aftercare following explantation of joint prosthesis, staged procedure
Encounter for joint prosthesis insertion following prior explantation of joint prosthesis
AHA: 1Q 2015, 17

Z47.31 **Aftercare following explantation of shoulder joint prosthesis**
EXCLUDES 1 *acquired absence of shoulder joint following prior explantation of shoulder joint prosthesis (Z89.23-)*
shoulder joint prosthesis explantation status (Z89.23-)

Z47.32 **Aftercare following explantation of hip joint prosthesis**
EXCLUDES 1 *acquired absence of hip joint following prior explantation of hip joint prosthesis (Z89.62-)*
hip joint prosthesis explantation status (Z89.62-)
AHA: 1Q 2015, 17

Z47.33 **Aftercare following explantation of knee joint prosthesis**
EXCLUDES 1 *acquired absence of knee joint following prior explantation of knee prosthesis ()*
knee joint prosthesis explantation status (Z89.52-)

⑤ Z47.8 **Encounter for other orthopedic aftercare**

+ Z47.81 **Encounter for orthopedic aftercare following surgical amputation**
Use additional code to identify the limb amputated (Z89.-)
CODING TIP ✓ This code is only used for planned amputations. Do not assign Z47.81 for care following a traumatic amputation or when a surgical amputation is complicated by infection, dehiscence, or other complication.

Z47.82 **Encounter for orthopedic aftercare following scoliosis surgery**

Z47.89 **Encounter for other orthopedic aftercare**
AHA: 1Q 2015, 8

④ Z48 **Encounter for other postprocedural aftercare**
EXCLUDES 1 *encounter for follow-up examination after completed treatment (Z08-Z09)*
EXCLUDES 2 *encounter for attention to artificial openings (Z43.-)*
encounter for fitting and adjustment of prosthetic and other devices (Z44-Z46)

⑤ Z48.0 **Encounter for attention to dressings, sutures and drains**
EXCLUDES 1 *encounter for planned postprocedural wound closure (Z48.1)*

Z48.00 **Encounter for change or removal of nonsurgical wound dressing**
Encounter for change or removal of wound dressing NOS

Z48.01 **Encounter for change or removal of surgical wound dressing**
AHA: 4Q 2015, 38

Z48.02 **Encounter for removal of sutures**
Encounter for removal of staples
AHA: 1Q 2015, 6

Z48.03 **Encounter for change or removal of drains**

Z48.1 **Encounter for planned postprocedural wound closure**
EXCLUDES 1 *encounter for attention to dressings and sutures (Z48.0-)*

⑤ Z48.2 **Encounter for aftercare following organ transplant**

Z48.21 **Encounter for aftercare following heart transplant**
Z48.22 **Encounter for aftercare following kidney transplant**
Z48.23 **Encounter for aftercare following liver transplant**
Z48.24 **Encounter for aftercare following lung transplant**

⑥ Z48.28 **Encounter for aftercare following multiple organ transplant**

Z48.280 **Encounter for aftercare following heart-lung transplant**
Z48.288 **Encounter for aftercare following multiple organ transplant**

⑥ Z48.29 **Encounter for aftercare following other organ transplant**

Z48.290 **Encounter for aftercare following bone marrow transplant**
Z48.298 **Encounter for aftercare following other organ transplant**

+ Z48.3 **Aftercare following surgery for neoplasm**
Use additional code to identify the neoplasm
CODING TIP ✓ When coding Z48.3, an additional code should be assigned to identify the neoplasm. If it is unclear if the neoplasm has been eradicated or if there are plans to continue treatment for the neoplastic disease, assign the appropriate code from Chapter 2 to indicate the neoplasm. If documentation indicates that the neoplasm has been eradicated clearly, assign the appropriate Z85 code to report personal history of neoplasm.

⑤ Z48.8 **Encounter for other specified postprocedural aftercare**

⑥ Z48.81 **Encounter for surgical aftercare following surgery on specified body systems**
These codes identify the body system requiring aftercare. They are for use in conjunction with other aftercare codes to fully explain the aftercare encounter. The condition treated should also be coded if still present.
EXCLUDES 1 *aftercare for injury- code the injury with 7th character D*
aftercare following surgery for neoplasm (Z48.3)
EXCLUDES 2 *aftercare following organ transplant (Z48.2-)*
orthopedic aftercare (Z47.-)

Z48.810 **Encounter for surgical aftercare following surgery on the sense organs**
Z48.811 **Encounter for surgical aftercare following surgery on the nervous system**
EXCLUDES 2 *encounter for surgical aftercare following surgery on the sense organs (Z48.810)*
Z48.812 **Encounter for surgical aftercare following surgery on the circulatory system**
AHA: 4Q 2012, 96-97
Z48.813 **Encounter for surgical aftercare following surgery on the respiratory system**
Z48.814 **Encounter for surgical aftercare following surgery on the teeth or oral cavity**
Z48.815 **Encounter for surgical aftercare following surgery on the digestive system**
AHA: 4Q 2015, 38

Z48.816   Encounter for surgical aftercare following surgery on the genitourinary system

    EXCLUDES 1   *encounter for aftercare following sterilization reversal (Z31.42)*

Z48.817   Encounter for surgical aftercare following surgery on the skin and subcutaneous tissue

    AHA: 1Q 2015, 6

Z48.89   Encounter for other specified surgical aftercare

▲ ⁴ Z49   Encounter for care involving renal dialysis

    Code also:

      associated end stage renal disease (N18.6)

⑤ Z49.0   Preparatory care for renal dialysis

    Encounter for dialysis instruction and training

Z49.01   Encounter for fitting and adjustment of extracorporeal dialysis catheter

    Removal or replacement of renal dialysis catheter

    Toilet or cleansing of renal dialysis catheter

Z49.02   Encounter for fitting and adjustment of peritoneal dialysis catheter

⑤ Z49.3   Encounter for adequacy testing for dialysis

Z49.31   Encounter for adequacy testing for hemodialysis

Z49.32   Encounter for adequacy testing for peritoneal dialysis

    Encounter for peritoneal equilibration test

▲ ⁴ Z51   Encounter for other aftercare and medical care

    Code also:

      condition requiring care

    EXCLUDES 1   *follow-up examination after treatment (Z08-Z09)*

    GUIDELINES   Section I.C.2.e.2)

If a patient admission/encounter is solely for the administration of chemotherapy, immunotherapy or radiation therapy, assign code Z51.0, Encounter for antineoplastic radiation therapy, or Z51.11, Encounter for antineoplastic chemotherapy, or Z51.12, Encounter for antineoplastic immunotherapy as the first-listed or principal diagnosis.

If a patient receives more than one of these therapies during the same admission more than one of these codes may be assigned, in any sequence. The malignancy for which the therapy is being administered should be assigned as a secondary diagnosis.

    CODING TIP ✓   Only the provider administering the radiation, chemotherapy or immunotherapy may assign a code from category Z51 to report encounter for radiation, chemotherapy, or immunotherapy.

Z51.0   Encounter for antineoplastic radiation therapy

    GUIDELINES   Section I.C.2.e.3)

When a patient is admitted for the purpose of radiotherapy, immunotherapy or chemotherapy and develops complications such as uncontrolled nausea and vomiting or dehydration, the principal or first-listed diagnosis is Z51.0 or Z51.11 or Z51.12, followed by any codes for the complications.

⑤ Z51.1   Encounter for antineoplastic chemotherapy and immunotherapy

    EXCLUDES 2   *encounter for chemotherapy and immunotherapy for nonneoplastic condition - code to condition*

Z51.11   Encounter for antineoplastic chemotherapy

    AHA: 3Q 2015, 19

Z51.12   Encounter for antineoplastic immunotherapy

Z51.5   Encounter for palliative care

● Z51.6   Encounter for desensitization to allergens

⑤ Z51.8   Encounter for other specified aftercare

    EXCLUDES 1   *holiday relief care (Z75.5)*

    AHA: 4Q 2012, 96, 97

Z51.81   Encounter for therapeutic drug level monitoring

    Code also:

      any long-term (current) drug therapy (Z79.-)

    EXCLUDES 1   *encounter for blood-drug test for administrative or medicolegal reasons (Z02.83)*

Z51.89   Encounter for other specified aftercare

⁴ Z52   Donors of organs and tissues

    INCLUDES   autologous and other living donors

    EXCLUDES 1   *cadaveric donor - omit code examination of potential donor (Z00.5)*

    AHA: 4Q 2012, 99-100

⑤ Z52.0   Blood donor

⑥ Z52.00   Unspecified blood donor

Z52.000   Unspecified donor, whole blood

Z52.001   Unspecified donor, stem cells

Z52.008   Unspecified donor, other blood

⑥ Z52.01   Autologous blood donor

Z52.010   Autologous donor, whole blood

Z52.011   Autologous donor, stem cells

Z52.018   Autologous donor, other blood

⑥ Z52.09   Other blood donor

    Volunteer donor

Z52.090   Other blood donor, whole blood

Z52.091   Other blood donor, stem cells

Z52.098   Other blood donor, other blood

⑤ Z52.1   Skin donor

Z52.10   Skin donor, unspecified

Z52.11   Skin donor, autologous

Z52.19   Skin donor, other

⑤ Z52.2   Bone donor

Z52.20   Bone donor, unspecified

Z52.21   Bone donor, autologous

Z52.29   Bone donor, other

Z52.3   Bone marrow donor

Z52.4   Kidney donor

Z52.5   Cornea donor

Z52.6   Liver donor

    AHA: 4Q 2012, 99-100

⑤ Z52.8   Donor of other specified organs or tissues

⑥ Z52.81   Egg (Oocyte) donor

Z52.810   Egg (Oocyte) donor under age 35, anonymous recipient   ♀ Ⓜ

    Egg donor under age 35 NOS

Z52.811   Egg (Oocyte) donor under age 35, designated recipient   ♀ Ⓜ

Z52.812   Egg (Oocyte) donor age 35 and over, anonymous recipient   ♀ Ⓜ

    Egg donor age 35 and over NOS

Z52.813   Egg (Oocyte) donor age 35 and over, designated recipient   ♀ Ⓜ

Z52.819   Egg (Oocyte) donor, unspecified   ♀ Ⓜ

Z52.89   Donor of other specified organs or tissues

Z52.9   Donor of unspecified organ or tissue

    Donor NOS

⁴ Z53   Persons encountering health services for specific procedures and treatment, not carried out

⑤ Z53.0   Procedure and treatment not carried out because of contraindication

Z53.01   Procedure and treatment not carried out due to patient smoking

Z53.09   Procedure and treatment not carried out because of other contraindication

Z53.1   Procedure and treatment not carried out because of patient's decision for reasons of belief and group pressure

⑤ Z53.2   Procedure and treatment not carried out because of patient's decision for other and unspecified reasons

Z53.20   Procedure and treatment not carried out because of patient's decision for unspecified reasons

Z53.21   Procedure and treatment not carried out due to patient leaving prior to being seen by health care provider

Z53.29   Procedure and treatment not carried out because of patient's decision for other reasons

●⑤ Z53.3   Procedure converted to open procedure

● Z53.31   Laparoscopic surgical procedure converted to open procedure

● Z53.32   Thoracoscopic surgical procedure converted to open procedure

● Z53.33   Arthroscopic surgical procedure converted to open procedure

● Z53.39   Other specified procedure converted to open procedure

Z53.8   Procedure and treatment not carried out for other reasons

Z53.9   Procedure and treatment not carried out, unspecified reason

● New   ▲ Revised   *Manifestation*   ④-⑦ Digit Indicators   ▤ Laterality   Ⓐ Adult (15+ years)   Ⓜ Maternity (12-55 years)   Ⓝ Newborn   Ⓟ Pediatric (0-17 years)   ♂ Male   ♀ Female

✖ Deleted   Unspecified   + Additional code

2017 ICD-10-CM Expert for Physicians   © 2017 DecisionHealth   1191

Persons with potential health hazards related to socioeconomic and psychosocial circumstances (Z55-Z65)

④ Z55   Problems related to education and literacy

> **EXCLUDES 1**   *disorders of psychological development (F80-F89)*

Z55.0   Illiteracy and low-level literacy

Z55.1   Schooling unavailable and unattainable

Z55.2   Failed school examinations

Z55.3   Underachievement in school

Z55.4   Educational maladjustment and discord with teachers and classmates

Z55.8   Other problems related to education and literacy
Problems related to inadequate teaching

Z55.9   Problems related to education and literacy, unspecified
Academic problems NOS

④ Z56   Problems related to employment and unemployment

> **EXCLUDES 2**   *occupational exposure to risk factors (Z57.-)*
> *problems related to housing and economic circumstances (Z59.-)*

Z56.0   Unemployment, unspecified

Z56.1   Change of job   Ⓐ

Z56.2   Threat of job loss

Z56.3   Stressful work schedule

Z56.4   Discord with boss and workmates

Z56.5   Uncongenial work environment
Difficult conditions at work

Z56.6   Other physical and mental strain related to work

⑤ Z56.8   Other problems related to employment

    Z56.81   Sexual harassment on the job

    Z56.82   Military deployment status   Ⓐ
Individual (civilian or military) currently deployed in theater or in support of military war, peacekeeping and humanitarian operations

    Z56.89   Other problems related to employment

Z56.9   Unspecified problems related to employment
Occupational problems NOS

④ Z57   Occupational exposure to risk factors

Z57.0   Occupational exposure to noise

Z57.1   Occupational exposure to radiation

Z57.2   Occupational exposure to dust

⑤ Z57.3   Occupational exposure to other air contaminants

    Z57.31   Occupational exposure to environmental tobacco smoke

> **EXCLUDES 2**   *exposure to environmental tobacco smoke (Z77.22)*

    Z57.39   Occupational exposure to other air contaminants

Z57.4   Occupational exposure to toxic agents in agriculture
Occupational exposure to solids, liquids, gases or vapors in agriculture

Z57.5   Occupational exposure to toxic agents in other industries
Occupational exposure to solids, liquids, gases or vapors in other industries

Z57.6   Occupational exposure to extreme temperature

Z57.7   Occupational exposure to vibration

Z57.8   Occupational exposure to other risk factors

Z57.9   Occupational exposure to unspecified risk factor

④ Z59   Problems related to housing and economic circumstances

> **EXCLUDES 2**   *problems related to upbringing (Z62.-)*

Z59.0   Homelessness

Z59.1   Inadequate housing
Lack of heating
Restriction of space
Technical defects in home preventing adequate care
Unsatisfactory surroundings

> **EXCLUDES 1**   *problems related to the natural and physical environment (Z77.1-)*

Z59.2   Discord with neighbors, lodgers and landlord

Z59.3   Problems related to living in residential institution
Boarding-school resident

> **EXCLUDES 1**   *institutional upbringing (Z62.2)*

Z59.4   Lack of adequate food and safe drinking water
Inadequate drinking water supply

> **EXCLUDES 1**   *effects of hunger (T73.0)*
> *inappropriate diet or eating habits (Z72.4)*
> *malnutrition (E40-E46)*

Z59.5   Extreme poverty

Z59.6   Low income

Z59.7   Insufficient social insurance and welfare support

Z59.8   Other problems related to housing and economic circumstances
Foreclosure on loan
Isolated dwelling
Problems with creditors

Z59.9   Problem related to housing and economic circumstances, unspecified

④ Z60   Problems related to social environment

Z60.0   Problems of adjustment to life-cycle transitions
Empty nest syndrome
Phase of life problem
Problem with adjustment to retirement [pension]

Z60.2   Problems related to living alone

Z60.3   Acculturation difficulty
Problem with migration
Problem with social transplantation

Z60.4   Social exclusion and rejection
Exclusion and rejection on the basis of personal characteristics, such as unusual physical appearance, illness or behavior.

> **EXCLUDES 1**   *target of adverse discrimination such as for racial or religious reasons (Z60.5)*

Z60.5   Target of (perceived) adverse discrimination and persecution

> **EXCLUDES 1**   *social exclusion and rejection (Z60.4)*

Z60.8   Other problems related to social environment

Z60.9   Problem related to social environment, unspecified

④ Z62   Problems related to upbringing

> **INCLUDES**   current and past negative life events in childhood
> current and past problems of a child related to upbringing

> **EXCLUDES 2**   *maltreatment syndrome (T74.-)*
> *problems related to housing and economic circumstances (Z59.-)*

Z62.0   Inadequate parental supervision and control

Z62.1   Parental overprotection

⑤ Z62.2   Upbringing away from parents

> **EXCLUDES 1**   *problems with boarding school (Z59.3)*

    Z62.21   Child in welfare custody   Ⓟ
Child in care of non-parental family member
Child in foster care

> **EXCLUDES 2**   *problem for parent due to child in welfare custody (Z63.5)*

    Z62.22   Institutional upbringing
Child living in orphanage or group home

    Z62.29   Other upbringing away from parents

Z62.3   Hostility towards and scapegoating of child   Ⓟ

Z62.6   Inappropriate (excessive) parental pressure

⑤ Z62.8   Other specified problems related to upbringing

    ⑥ Z62.81   Personal history of abuse in childhood

        Z62.810   Personal history of physical and sexual abuse in childhood

> **EXCLUDES 1**   *current child physical abuse (T74.12, T76.12)*
> *current child sexual abuse (T74.22, T76.22)*

        Z62.811   Personal history of psychological abuse in childhood

> **EXCLUDES 1**   *current child psychological abuse (T74.32, T76.32)*

        Z62.812   Personal history of neglect in childhood

> **EXCLUDES 1**   *current child neglect (T74.02, T76.02)*

        Z62.819   Personal history of unspecified abuse in childhood

> **EXCLUDES 1**   *current child abuse NOS (T74.92, T76.92)*

    ⑥ Z62.82   Parent-child conflict

        Z62.820   Parent-biological child conflict
Parent-child problem NOS

● New   ▲ Revised   *Manifestation*   ④-⑦ Digit Indicators   ▣ Laterality   Ⓐ Adult (15+ years)   Ⓜ Maternity (12-55 years)   Ⓝ Newborn   Ⓟ Pediatric (0-17 years)   ♂ Male   ♀ Female

✖ Deleted   Unspecified   + Additional code

1192   © 2017 DecisionHealth   2017 ICD-10-CM Expert for Physicians

Z62.821   Parent-adopted child conflict
Z62.822   Parent-foster child conflict
⑥ Z62.89   Other specified problems related to upbringing
Z62.890   Parent-child estrangement NEC
Z62.891   Sibling rivalry
Z62.898   Other specified problems related to upbringing
Z62.9   Problem related to upbringing, unspecified

④ Z63   Other problems related to primary support group, including family circumstances
EXCLUDES 2   *maltreatment syndrome (T74.-, T76)*
parent-child problems (Z62.-)
problems related to negative life events in childhood (Z62.-)
problems related to upbringing (Z62.-)

Z63.0   Problems in relationship with spouse or partner
EXCLUDES 1   *counseling for spousal or partner abuse problems (Z69.1)*
counseling related to sexual attitude, behavior, and orientation (Z70.-)

Z63.1   Problems in relationship with in-laws
⑤ Z63.3   Absence of family member
EXCLUDES 1   *absence of family member due to disappearance and death (Z63.4)*
absence of family member due to separation and divorce (Z63.5)

Z63.31   Absence of family member due to military deployment
Individual or family affected by other family member being on military deployment
EXCLUDES 1   *family disruption due to return of family member from military deployment (Z63.71)*

Z63.32   Other absence of family member
Z63.4   Disappearance and death of family member
Assumed death of family member
Bereavement
AHA: 1Q 2014, 25

Z63.5   Disruption of family by separation and divorce
Marital estrangement
Z63.6   Dependent relative needing care at home
⑤ Z63.7   Other stressful life events affecting family and household
Z63.71   Stress on family due to return of family member from military deployment
Individual or family affected by family member having returned from military deployment (current or past conflict)

Z63.72   Alcoholism and drug addiction in family
Z63.79   Other stressful life events affecting family and household
Anxiety (normal) about sick person in family
Health problems within family
Ill or disturbed family member
Isolated family

Z63.8   Other specified problems related to primary support group
Family discord NOS
Family estrangement NOS
High expressed emotional level within family
Inadequate family support NOS
Inadequate or distorted communication within family

Z63.9   Problem related to primary support group, unspecified
Relationship disorder NOS

④ Z64   Problems related to certain psychosocial circumstances
Z64.0   Problems related to unwanted pregnancy   ♀Ⓜ
Z64.1   Problems related to multiparity   ♀
Z64.4   Discord with counselors
Discord with probation officer
Discord with social worker

④ Z65   Problems related to other psychosocial circumstances
Z65.0   Conviction in civil and criminal proceedings without imprisonment
Z65.1   Imprisonment and other incarceration
Z65.2   Problems related to release from prison
Z65.3   Problems related to other legal circumstances
Arrest
Child custody or support proceedings
Litigation
Prosecution
Z65.4   Victim of crime and terrorism
Victim of torture

Z65.5   Exposure to disaster, war and other hostilities   Ⓐ
EXCLUDES 1   *target of perceived discrimination or persecution (Z60.5)*
Z65.8   Other specified problems related to psychosocial circumstances
Z65.9   Problem related to unspecified psychosocial circumstances

Do not resuscitate status (Z66)

Z66   Do not resuscitate
DNR status

Blood type (Z67)

④ Z67   Blood type
⑤ Z67.1   Type A blood
Z67.10   Type A blood, Rh positive
Z67.11   Type A blood, Rh negative
⑤ Z67.2   Type B blood
Z67.20   Type B blood, Rh positive
Z67.21   Type B blood, Rh negative
⑤ Z67.3   Type AB blood
Z67.30   Type AB blood, Rh positive
Z67.31   Type AB blood, Rh negative
⑤ Z67.4   Type O blood
Z67.40   Type O blood, Rh positive
Z67.41   Type O blood, Rh negative
⑤ Z67.9   Unspecified blood type
Z67.90   Unspecified blood type, Rh positive
Z67.91   Unspecified blood type, Rh negative
AHA: 3Q 2015, 40

Body mass index [BMI] (Z68)

④ Z68   Body mass index [BMI]
Kilograms per meters squared
Note: BMI adult codes are for use for persons 21 years of age or older
BMI pediatric codes are for use for persons 2-20 years of age. These percentiles are based on the growth charts published by the Centers for Disease Control and Prevention (CDC)

CODING TIP ✓   BMI adult codes are for use in persons 21 years of age or older. Pediatric BMI codes (Z69.5-) are for use in persons aged 2-20 years of age. Percentiles are based on growth charts published by the CDC. BMI code assignment may be based on documentation from clinicians other than the physician.

CODING TIP ✓   When coding weight loss, obesity, overweight or morbid obesity, it is recommended to calculate and code the associated BMI. BMI may be calculated and coded based upon documentation from clinicians other than physician.

Z68.1   Body mass index (BMI) 19 or less, adult   Ⓐ
⑤ Z68.2   Body mass index (BMI) 20-29, adult
Z68.20   Body mass index (BMI) 20.0-20.9, adult   Ⓐ
Z68.21   Body mass index (BMI) 21.0-21.9, adult   Ⓐ
Z68.22   Body mass index (BMI) 22.0-22.9, adult   Ⓐ
Z68.23   Body mass index (BMI) 23.0-23.9, adult   Ⓐ
Z68.24   Body mass index (BMI) 24.0-24.9, adult   Ⓐ
Z68.25   Body mass index (BMI) 25.0-25.9, adult   Ⓐ
Z68.26   Body mass index (BMI) 26.0-26.9, adult   Ⓐ
Z68.27   Body mass index (BMI) 27.0-27.9, adult   Ⓐ
Z68.28   Body mass index (BMI) 28.0-28.9, adult   Ⓐ
Z68.29   Body mass index (BMI) 29.0-29.9, adult   Ⓐ
⑤ Z68.3   Body mass index (BMI) 30-39, adult
Z68.30   Body mass index (BMI) 30.0-30.9, adult   Ⓐ
Z68.31   Body mass index (BMI) 31.0-31.9, adult   Ⓐ
Z68.32   Body mass index (BMI) 32.0-32.9, adult   Ⓐ
Z68.33   Body mass index (BMI) 33.0-33.9, adult   Ⓐ
Z68.34   Body mass index (BMI) 34.0-34.9, adult   Ⓐ
Z68.35   Body mass index (BMI) 35.0-35.9, adult   Ⓐ
Z68.36   Body mass index (BMI) 36.0-36.9, adult   Ⓐ
Z68.37   Body mass index (BMI) 37.0-37.9, adult   Ⓐ
Z68.38   Body mass index (BMI) 38.0-38.9, adult   Ⓐ

Factors Influencing Health Status and Contact With Health Services

| | |

Z68.39 Body mass index (BMI) 39.0-39.9, adult ⓐ

Ⓢ **Z68.4** Body mass index (BMI) 40 or greater, adult
- **Z68.41** Body mass index (BMI) 40.0-44.9, adult ⓐ
- **Z68.42** Body mass index (BMI) 45.0-49.9, adult ⓐ
- **Z68.43** Body mass index (BMI) 50-59.9 , adult ⓐ
- **Z68.44** Body mass index (BMI) 60.0-69.9, adult ⓐ
- **Z68.45** Body mass index (BMI) 70 or greater, adult ⓐ

Ⓢ **Z68.5** Body mass index (BMI) pediatric
- **Z68.51** Body mass index (BMI) pediatric, less than 5th percentile for age ⓟ
- **Z68.52** Body mass index (BMI) pediatric, 5th percentile to less than 85th percentile for age ⓟ
- **Z68.53** Body mass index (BMI) pediatric, 85th percentile to less than 95th percentile for age ⓟ
- **Z68.54** Body mass index (BMI) pediatric, greater than or equal to 95th percentile for age ⓟ

Persons encountering health services in other circumstances (Z69-Z76)

④ **Z69** Encounter for mental health services for victim and perpetrator of abuse
> INCLUDES counseling for victims and perpetrators of abuse

Ⓢ **Z69.0** Encounter for mental health services for child abuse problems

⑥ **Z69.01** Encounter for mental health services for parental child abuse
- **Z69.010** Encounter for mental health services for victim of parental child abuse ⓟ
- **Z69.011** Encounter for mental health services for perpetrator of parental child abuse
> EXCLUDES 1 encounter for mental health services for non-parental child abuse (Z69.02-)

⑥ **Z69.02** Encounter for mental health services for non-parental child abuse
- **Z69.020** Encounter for mental health services for victim of non-parental child abuse ⓟ
- **Z69.021** Encounter for mental health services for perpetrator of non-parental child abuse

Ⓢ **Z69.1** Encounter for mental health services for spousal or partner abuse problems
- **Z69.11** Encounter for mental health services for victim of spousal or partner abuse
- **Z69.12** Encounter for mental health services for perpetrator of spousal or partner abuse

Ⓢ **Z69.8** Encounter for mental health services for victim or perpetrator of other abuse
- **Z69.81** Encounter for mental health services for victim of other abuse
  Encounter for rape victim counseling
- **Z69.82** Encounter for mental health services for perpetrator of other abuse

④ **Z70** Counseling related to sexual attitude, behavior and orientation
> INCLUDES encounter for mental health services for sexual attitude, behavior and orientation
> EXCLUDES 2 contraceptive or procreative counseling (Z30-Z31)

Z70.0 Counseling related to sexual attitude
Z70.1 Counseling related to patient's sexual behavior and orientation
  Patient concerned regarding impotence
  Patient concerned regarding non-responsiveness
  Patient concerned regarding promiscuity
  Patient concerned regarding sexual orientation
Z70.2 Counseling related to sexual behavior and orientation of third party
  Advice sought regarding sexual behavior and orientation of child
  Advice sought regarding sexual behavior and orientation of partner
  Advice sought regarding sexual behavior and orientation of spouse
Z70.3 Counseling related to combined concerns regarding sexual attitude, behavior and orientation
Z70.8 Other sex counseling
  Encounter for sex education
Z70.9 Sex counseling, unspecified

④ **Z71** Persons encountering health services for other counseling and medical advice, not elsewhere classified
> EXCLUDES 2 contraceptive or procreation counseling (Z30-Z31)
> sex counseling (Z70.-)

Z71.0 Person encountering health services to consult on behalf of another person
  Person encountering health services to seek advice or treatment for non-attending third party
> EXCLUDES 2 anxiety (normal) about sick person in family (Z63.7)
> expectant (adoptive) parent(s) pre-birth pediatrician visit (Z76.81)

Z71.1 Person with feared health complaint in whom no diagnosis is made
  Person encountering health services with feared condition which was not demonstrated
  Person encountering health services in which problem was normal state
  'Worried well'
> EXCLUDES 1 medical observation for suspected diseases and conditions proven not to exist (Z03.-)

Z71.2 Person consulting for explanation of examination or test findings
➕ **Z71.3** Dietary counseling and surveillance
  Use additional code for any associated underlying medical condition
  Use additional code to identify body mass index (BMI), if known (Z68.-)

Ⓢ➕ **Z71.4** Alcohol abuse counseling and surveillance
  Use additional code for alcohol abuse or dependence (F10.-)
➕ **Z71.41** Alcohol abuse counseling and surveillance of alcoholic
➕ **Z71.42** Counseling for family member of alcoholic
  Counseling for significant other, partner, or friend of alcoholic

Ⓢ➕ **Z71.5** Drug abuse counseling and surveillance
  Use additional code for drug abuse or dependence (F11-F16, F18-F19)
➕ **Z71.51** Drug abuse counseling and surveillance of drug abuser
➕ **Z71.52** Counseling for family member of drug abuser
  Counseling for significant other, partner, or friend of drug abuser

➕ **Z71.6** Tobacco abuse counseling
  Use additional code for nicotine dependence (F17.-)
Z71.7 Human immunodeficiency virus [HIV] counseling
Ⓢ **Z71.8** Other specified counseling
> EXCLUDES 2 counseling for contraception (Z30.0-)
> counseling for genetics (Z31.5)
> counseling for procreative management (Z31.6-)
- **Z71.81** Spiritual or religious counseling
- **Z71.89** Other specified counseling
Z71.9 Counseling, unspecified
  Encounter for medical advice NOS

④ **Z72** Problems related to lifestyle
> EXCLUDES 2 problems related to life-management difficulty (Z73.-)
> problems related to socioeconomic and psychosocial circumstances (Z55-Z65)

Z72.0 Tobacco use
  Tobacco use NOS
> EXCLUDES 1 history of tobacco dependence (Z87.891)
> nicotine dependence (F17.2-)
> tobacco dependence (F17.2-)
> tobacco use during pregnancy (O99.33-)

Z72.3 Lack of physical exercise
Z72.4 Inappropriate diet and eating habits
> EXCLUDES 1 behavioral eating disorders of infancy or childhood (F98.2.-F98.3)
> eating disorders (F50.-)
> lack of adequate food (F59.4)
> malnutrition and other nutritional deficiencies (E40-E64)

Ⓢ **Z72.5** High risk sexual behavior
  Promiscuity
> EXCLUDES 1 paraphilias (F65)
- **Z72.51** High risk heterosexual behavior
- **Z72.52** High risk homosexual behavior

● New ▲ Revised *Manifestation* ④-⑦ Digit Indicators ▭ Laterality ⓐ Adult (15+ years) Ⓜ Maternity (12-55 years) Ⓝ Newborn ⓟ Pediatric (0-17 years) ♂ Male ♀ Female
✖ Deleted Unspecified ➕ Additional code

1194   © 2017 DecisionHealth   2017 ICD-10-CM Expert for Physicians

Z72.53   **High risk bisexual behavior**

Z72.6   **Gambling and betting**

> **EXCLUDES 1**   *compulsive or pathological gambling (F63.0)*

🅢 **Z72.8**   **Other problems related to lifestyle**

    🅖 **Z72.81**   **Antisocial behavior**

> **EXCLUDES 1**   *conduct disorders (F91.-)*

      Z72.810   **Child and adolescent antisocial behavior** 🄿

         Antisocial behavior (child) (adolescent) without manifest psychiatric disorder

         Delinquency NOS

         Group delinquency

         Offenses in the context of gang membership

         Stealing in company with others

         Truancy from school

      Z72.811   **Adult antisocial behavior** 🄰

         Adult antisocial behavior without manifest psychiatric disorder

    🅖 **Z72.82**   **Problems related to sleep**

      Z72.820   **Sleep deprivation**

         Lack of adequate sleep

> **EXCLUDES 1**   *insomnia (G47.0-)*

      Z72.821   **Inadequate sleep hygiene**

         Bad sleep habits

         Irregular sleep habits

         Unhealthy sleep wake schedule

> **EXCLUDES 1**   *insomnia (F51.0-, G47.0-)*

      Z72.89   **Other problems related to lifestyle**

         Self-damaging behavior

Z72.9   **Problem related to lifestyle, unspecified**

🄳 **Z73**   **Problems related to life management difficulty**

> **EXCLUDES 2**   *problems related to socioeconomic and psychosocial circumstances (Z55-Z65)*

Z73.0   **Burn-out**

Z73.1   **Type A behavior pattern**

Z73.2   **Lack of relaxation and leisure**

Z73.3   **Stress, not elsewhere classified**

    Physical and mental strain NOS

> **EXCLUDES 1**   *stress related to employment or unemployment (Z56.-)*

Z73.4   **Inadequate social skills, not elsewhere classified**

Z73.5   **Social role conflict, not elsewhere classified**

Z73.6   **Limitation of activities due to disability**

> **EXCLUDES 1**   *care-provider dependency (Z74.-)*

🅢 **Z73.8**   **Other problems related to life management difficulty**

    🅖 **Z73.81**   **Behavioral insomnia of childhood**

      Z73.810   **Behavioral insomnia of childhood, sleep-onset association type** 🄿

      Z73.811   **Behavioral insomnia of childhood, limit setting type** 🄿

      Z73.812   **Behavioral insomnia of childhood, combined type** 🄿

      Z73.819   **Behavioral insomnia of childhood, unspecified type** 🄿

    Z73.82   **Dual sensory impairment**

    Z73.89   **Other problems related to life management difficulty**

Z73.9   **Problem related to life management difficulty, unspecified**

🄳 **Z74**   **Problems related to care provider dependency**

> **EXCLUDES 2**   *dependence on enabling machines or devices NEC (Z99.-)*

🅢 **Z74.0**   **Reduced mobility**

    Z74.01   **Bed confinement status**

      Bedridden

    Z74.09   **Other reduced mobility**

      Chairridden

      Reduced mobility NOS

> **EXCLUDES 2**   *wheelchair dependence (Z99.3)*

Z74.1   **Need for assistance with personal care**

Z74.2   **Need for assistance at home and no other household member able to render care**

Z74.3   **Need for continuous supervision**

Z74.8   **Other problems related to care provider dependency**

Z74.9   **Problem related to care provider dependency, unspecified**

🄳 **Z75**   **Problems related to medical facilities and other health care**

Z75.0   **Medical services not available in home**

> **EXCLUDES 1**   *no other household member able to render care (Z74.2)*

Z75.1   **Person awaiting admission to adequate facility elsewhere**

Z75.2   **Other waiting period for investigation and treatment**

Z75.3   **Unavailability and inaccessibility of health-care facilities**

> **EXCLUDES 1**   *bed unavailable (Z75.1)*

Z75.4   **Unavailability and inaccessibility of other helping agencies**

Z75.5   **Holiday relief care**

Z75.8   **Other problems related to medical facilities and other health care**

Z75.9   **Unspecified problem related to medical facilities and other health care**

🄳 **Z76**   **Persons encountering health services in other circumstances**

Z76.0   **Encounter for issue of repeat prescription**

    Encounter for issue of repeat prescription for appliance

    Encounter for issue of repeat prescription for medicaments

    Encounter for issue of repeat prescription for spectacles

> **EXCLUDES 2**   *issue of medical certificate (Z02.7)*
> *repeat prescription for contraceptive (Z30.4-)*

Z76.1   **Encounter for health supervision and care of foundling**

Z76.2   **Encounter for health supervision and care of other healthy infant and child** 🄿

    Encounter for medical or nursing care or supervision of healthy infant under circumstances such as adverse socioeconomic conditions at home

    Encounter for medical or nursing care or supervision of healthy infant under circumstances such as awaiting foster or adoptive placement

    Encounter for medical or nursing care or supervision of healthy infant under circumstances such as maternal illness

    Encounter for medical or nursing care or supervision of healthy infant under circumstances such as number of children at home preventing or interfering with normal care

Z76.3   **Healthy person accompanying sick person**

Z76.4   **Other boarder to healthcare facility**

> **EXCLUDES 1**   *homelessness (Z59.0)*

Z76.5   **Malingerer [conscious simulation]**

    Person feigning illness (with obvious motivation)

> **EXCLUDES 1**   *factitious disorder (F68.1-)*
> *peregrinating patient (F68.1-)*

🅢 **Z76.8**   **Persons encountering health services in other specified circumstances**

    Z76.81   **Expectant parent(s) prebirth pediatrician visit**

      Pre-adoption pediatrician visit for adoptive parent(s)

    Z76.82   **Awaiting organ transplant status**

      Patient waiting for organ availability

    Z76.89   **Persons encountering health services in other specified circumstances**

      Persons encountering health services NOS

      AHA: 2Q 2014, 10

Persons with potential health hazards related to family and personal history and certain conditions influencing health status (Z77-Z99)

Code also:

any follow-up examination (Z08-Z09)

▲ 🄳 **Z77**   **Other contact with and (suspected) exposures hazardous to health**

> **INCLUDES**   contact with and (suspected) exposures to potential hazards to health

> **EXCLUDES 2**   *contact with and (suspected) exposure to communicable diseases (Z20.-)*
> *exposure to (parental) (environmental) tobacco smoke in the perinatal period (P96.81)*
> *newborn affected by noxious substances transmitted via placenta or breast milk (P04.-)*
> *occupational exposure to risk factors (Z57.-)*
> *retained foreign body (Z18.-)*
> *retained foreign body fully removed (Z87.821)*
> *toxic effects of substances chiefly nonmedicinal as to source (T51-T65)*

● New   ▲ Revised   *Manifestation*   Unspecified   ✖ Deleted   🄳-🄻 Digit Indicators   + Additional code   ▤ Laterality   🄰 Adult (15+ years)   🄼 Maternity (12-55 years)   🄽 Newborn (0-17 years)   🄿 Pediatric   ♂ Male   ♀ Female

2017 ICD-10-CM Expert for Physicians   © 2017 DecisionHealth   1195

GUIDELINES   Section I.C.21.c.1)

Category Z20 indicates contact with, and suspected exposure to, communicable diseases. These codes are for patients who do not show any sign or symptom of a disease but are suspected to have been exposed to it by close personal contact with an infected individual or are in an area where a disease is epidemic. Category Z77 indicates contact with and suspected exposures hazardous to health.

Contact/exposure codes may be used as a first-listed code to explain an encounter for testing, or, more commonly, as a secondary code to identify a potential risk.

⑤ Z77.0   Contact with and (suspected) exposure to hazardous, chiefly nonmedicinal, chemicals

⑥ Z77.01   Contact with and (suspected) exposure to hazardous metals

Z77.010   Contact with and (suspected) exposure to arsenic

Z77.011   Contact with and (suspected) exposure to lead

Z77.012   Contact with and (suspected) exposure to uranium

> **EXCLUDES 1**   *retained depleted uranium fragments (Z18.01)*

Z77.018   Contact with and (suspected) exposure to other hazardous metals
Contact with and (suspected) exposure to chromium compounds
Contact with and (suspected) exposure to nickel dust

⑥ Z77.02   Contact with and (suspected) exposure to hazardous aromatic compounds

Z77.020   Contact with and (suspected) exposure to aromatic amines

Z77.021   Contact with and (suspected) exposure to benzene

Z77.028   Contact with and (suspected) exposure to other hazardous aromatic compounds
Aromatic dyes NOS
Polycyclic aromatic hydrocarbons

⑥ Z77.09   Contact with and (suspected) exposure to other hazardous, chiefly nonmedicinal, chemicals

Z77.090   Contact with and (suspected) exposure to asbestos

Z77.098   Contact with and (suspected) exposure to other hazardous, chiefly nonmedicinal, chemicals
Dyes NOS

⑤ Z77.1   Contact with and (suspected) exposure to environmental pollution and hazards in the physical environment

⑥ Z77.11   Contact with and (suspected) exposure to environmental pollution

Z77.110   Contact with and (suspected) exposure to air pollution

Z77.111   Contact with and (suspected) exposure to water pollution

Z77.112   Contact with and (suspected) exposure to soil pollution

Z77.118   Contact with and (suspected) exposure to other environmental pollution

⑥ Z77.12   Contact with and (suspected) exposure to hazards in the physical environment

Z77.120   Contact with and (suspected) exposure to mold (toxic)

Z77.121   Contact with and (suspected) exposure to harmful algae and algae toxins
Contact with and (suspected) exposure to (harmful) algae bloom NOS
Contact with and (suspected) exposure to blue-green algae bloom
Contact with and (suspected) exposure to brown tide
Contact with and (suspected) exposure to cyanobacteria bloom
Contact with and (suspected) exposure to Florida red tide
Contact with and (suspected) exposure to pfiesteria piscicida
Contact with and (suspected) exposure to red tide

Z77.122   Contact with and (suspected) exposure to noise

Z77.123   Contact with and (suspected) exposure to radon and other naturally occuring radiation

> **EXCLUDES 2**   *radiation exposure as the cause of a confirmed condition (W88-W90, X39.0-)*
> *radiation sickness NOS (T66)*

Z77.128   Contact with and (suspected) exposure to other hazards in the physical environment

⑤ Z77.2   Contact with and (suspected) exposure to other hazardous substances

Z77.21   Contact with and (suspected) exposure to potentially hazardous body fluids

Z77.22   Contact with and (suspected) exposure to environmental tobacco smoke (acute) (chronic)
Exposure to second hand tobacco smoke (acute) (chronic)
Passive smoking (acute) (chronic)

> **EXCLUDES 1**   *nicotine dependence (F17.-)*
> *tobacco use (Z72.0)*

> **EXCLUDES 2**   *occupational exposure to environmental tobacco smoke (Z57.31)*

Z77.29   Contact with and (suspected) exposure to other hazardous substances
AHA: 2Q 2016, 34

Z77.9   Other contact with and (suspected) exposures hazardous to health

④ Z78   Other specified health status

> **EXCLUDES 2**   *asymptomatic human immunodeficiency virus [HIV] infection status (Z21)*
> *postprocedural status (Z93-Z99)*
> *sex reassignment status (Z87.890)*

Z78.0   Asymptomatic menopausal state   ♀ Ⓐ
Menopausal state NOS
Postmenopausal status NOS

> **EXCLUDES 2**   *symptomatic menopausal state (N95.1)*

Z78.1   Physical restraint status

> **EXCLUDES 1**   *physical restraint due to a procedure - omit code*

Z78.9   Other specified health status

▲ ④ Z79   Long term (current) drug therapy

> **INCLUDES**   long term (current) drug use for prophylactic purposes

Code also:
any therapeutic drug level monitoring (Z51.81)

> **EXCLUDES 2**   *drug abuse and dependence (F11-F19)*
> *drug use complicating pregnancy, childbirth, and the puerperium (O99.32-)*
> *long term (current) use of oral antidiabetic drugs (Z79.84)*
> *long term (current) use of oral hypoglycemic drugs (Z79.84)*

GUIDELINES   Section I.C.21.c.3)

Codes from this category [Z79] indicate a patient's continuous use of a prescribed drug (including such things as aspirin therapy) for the long-term treatment of a condition or for prophylactic use. It is not for use for patients who have addictions to drugs. This subcategory is not for use of medications for detoxification or maintenance programs to prevent withdrawal symptoms in patients with drug dependence (e.g., methadone maintenance for opiate dependence). Assign the appropriate code for the drug dependence instead.

Assign a code from Z79 if the patient is receiving a medication for an extended period as a prophylactic measure (such as for the prevention of deep vein thrombosis) or as treatment of a chronic condition (such as arthritis) or a disease requiring a lengthy course of treatment (such as cancer). Do not assign a code from category Z79 for medication being administered for a brief period of time to treat an acute illness or injury (such as a course of antibiotics to treat acute bronchitis).

CODING TIP ✓   Codes classifiable to category Z79 should not be assigned as primary diagnoses. When the management of any of these medications is integral to the plan of care, consider the confirmed diagnosis for which the patient is under treatment with the medication. This diagnosis should be coded, with a code from Z79 as an additional diagnosis.

● New   ▲ Revised   *Manifestation*   ④-⑦ Digit Indicators   ▤ Laterality   Ⓐ Adult (15+ years)   Ⓜ Maternity (12-55 years)   Ⓝ Newborn   Ⓟ Pediatric (0-17 years)   ♂ Male   ♀ Female
✖ Deleted   Unspecified   + Additional code

1196   © 2017 DecisionHealth   2017 ICD-10-CM Expert for Physicians

Ⓢ **Z79.0** **Long term (current) use of anticoagulants and antithrombotics/antiplatelets**
> EXCLUDES 2   *long term (current) use of aspirin (Z79.82)*

Z79.01   **Long term (current) use of anticoagulants**

Z79.02   **Long term (current) use of antithrombotics/antiplatelets**

Z79.1   **Long term (current) use of non-steroidal anti-inflammatories (NSAID)**
> EXCLUDES 2   *long term (current) use of aspirin (Z79.82)*

Z79.2   **Long term (current) use of antibiotics**

Z79.3   **Long term (current) use of hormonal contraceptives**
Long term (current) use of birth control pill or patch

Z79.4   **Long term (current) use of insulin**
> GUIDELINES   Section I.C.4.a.3)
> If the documentation in a medical record does not indicate the type of diabetes but does indicate that the patient uses insulin, code E11, Type 2 diabetes mellitus, should be assigned. Code Z79.4 should also be assigned to indicate that the patient uses insulin. Code Z79.4 should not be assigned if insulin is given temporarily to bring a type 2 patient's blood sugar under control during an encounter.

> GUIDELINES   Section I.C.15.i
> Code Z79.4 should not be assigned with codes from subcategory O24.4 [pregnancy-induced, gestational diabetes]

Ⓢ **Z79.5**   **Long term (current) use of steroids**

Z79.51   **Long term (current) use of inhaled steroids**

Z79.52   **Long term (current) use of systemic steroids**

Ⓢ **Z79.8**   **Other long term (current) drug therapy**

Ⓖ + **Z79.81**   **Long term (current) use of agents affecting estrogen receptors and estrogen levels**
Code first, if applicable:
malignant neoplasm of breast (C50.-)
malignant neoplasm of prostate (C61)
Use additional code, if applicable, to identify:
estrogen receptor positive status (Z17.0)
family history of breast cancer (Z80.3)
genetic susceptibility to malignant neoplasm (cancer) (Z15.0-)
personal history of breast cancer (Z85.3)
personal history of prostate cancer (Z85.46)
postmenopausal status (Z78.0)
> EXCLUDES 1   *hormone replacement therapy (postmenopausal) (Z79.890)*

+ **Z79.810**   **Long term (current) use of selective estrogen receptor modulators (SERMs)**
Long term (current) use of raloxifene (Evista)
Long term (current) use of tamoxifen (Nolvadex)
Long term (current) use of toremifene (Fareston)

+ **Z79.811**   **Long term (current) use of aromatase inhibitors**
Long term (current) use of anastrozole (Arimidex)
Long term (current) use of exemestane (Aromasin)
Long term (current) use of letrozole (Femara)

+ **Z79.818**   **Long term (current) use of other agents affecting estrogen receptors and estrogen levels**
Long term (current) use of estrogen receptor downregulators
Long term (current) use of fulvestrant (Faslodex)
Long term (current) use of gonadotropin-releasing hormone (GnRH) agonist
Long term (current) use of goserelin acetate (Zoladex)
Long term (current) use of leuprolide acetate (leuprorelin) (Lupron)
Long term (current) use of megestrol acetate (Megace)

Z79.82   **Long term (current) use of aspirin**

Z79.83   **Long term (current) use of bisphosphonates**

● **Z79.84**   **Long term (current) use of oral hypoglycemic drugs**
Long term (current) use of oral antidiabetic drugs
> EXCLUDES 2   *long term (current) use of insulin (Z79.4)*

Ⓖ **Z79.89**   **Other long term (current) drug therapy**

Z79.890   **Hormone replacement therapy (postmenopausal)** ♀

▲ **Z79.891**   **Long term (current) use of opiate analgesic**
Long term (current) use of methadone for pain management
> EXCLUDES 1   *methadone use NOS (F11.9-)*
> *use of methadone for treatment of heroin addiction (F11.2-)*

Z79.899   **Other long term (current) drug therapy**
AHA: 4Q 2015, 34
AHA: 3Q 2015, 21-22

④ **Z80**   **Family history of primary malignant neoplasm**
> GUIDELINES   Section I.C.21.c.4)
> There are two types of history Z codes, personal and family. Personal history codes explain a patient's past medical condition that no longer exists and is not receiving any treatment, but that has the potential for recurrence, and therefore may require continued monitoring.
>
> Family history codes are for use when a patient has a family member(s) who has had a particular disease that causes the patient to be at higher risk of also contracting the disease. Personal history codes may be used in conjunction with follow-up codes and family history codes may be used in conjunction with screening codes to explain the need for a test or procedure. History codes are also acceptable on any medical record regardless of the reason for visit. A history of an illness, even if no longer present, is important information that may alter the type of treatment ordered.

Z80.0   **Family history of malignant neoplasm of digestive organs**
Conditions classifiable to C15-C26

Z80.1   **Family history of malignant neoplasm of trachea, bronchus and lung**
Conditions classifiable to C33-C34

Z80.2   **Family history of malignant neoplasm of other respiratory and intrathoracic organs**
Conditions classifiable to C30-C32, C37-C39

Z80.3   **Family history of malignant neoplasm of breast**
Conditions classifiable to C50.-

Ⓢ **Z80.4**   **Family history of malignant neoplasm of genital organs**
Conditions classifiable to C51-C63

Z80.41   **Family history of malignant neoplasm of ovary** ♀

Z80.42   **Family history of malignant neoplasm of prostate** ♂

Z80.43   **Family history of malignant neoplasm of testis** ♂

Z80.49   **Family history of malignant neoplasm of other genital organs**

Ⓢ **Z80.5**   **Family history of malignant neoplasm of urinary tract**
Conditions classifiable to C64-C68

Z80.51   **Family history of malignant neoplasm of kidney**

Z80.52   **Family history of malignant neoplasm of bladder**

Z80.59   **Family history of malignant neoplasm of other urinary tract organ**

Z80.6   **Family history of leukemia**
Conditions classifiable to C91-C95

Z80.7   **Family history of other malignant neoplasms of lymphoid, hematopoietic and related tissues**
Conditions classifiable to C81-C90, C96.-

Z80.8   **Family history of malignant neoplasm of other organs or systems**
Conditions classifiable to C00-C14, C40-C49, C69-C79

Z80.9   **Family history of malignant neoplasm, unspecified**
Conditions classifiable to C80.1

④ **Z81**   **Family history of mental and behavioral disorders**
> GUIDELINES   Section I.C.21.c.4)
> There are two types of history Z codes, personal and family. Personal history codes explain a patient's past medical condition that no longer exists and is not receiving any treatment, but that has the potential for recurrence, and therefore may require continued monitoring.
>
> Family history codes are for use when a patient has a family member(s) who has had a particular disease that causes the patient to be at higher risk of also contracting the disease. Personal history codes may be used in conjunction with follow-up codes and family history codes may be used in conjunction with screening codes to explain the need for a test or procedure. History codes are also acceptable on any medical record regardless of the reason for visit. A history of an illness, even if no longer present, is important information that may alter the type of treatment ordered.

● New   ▲ Revised   *Manifestation*   ④-⑦ Digit Indicators   ▣ Laterality   Ⓐ Adult (15+ years)   Ⓜ Maternity (12-55 years)   Ⓝ Newborn (0-17 years)   Ⓟ Pediatric   ♂ Male   ♀ Female
✖ Deleted   Unspecified   + Additional code

2017 ICD-10-CM Expert for Physicians   © 2017 DecisionHealth   1197

Z81.0   **Family history of intellectual disabilities**
Conditions classifiable to F70-F79

Z81.1   **Family history of alcohol abuse and dependence**
Conditions classifiable to F10.-

Z81.2   **Family history of tobacco abuse and dependence**
Conditions classifiable to F17.-

Z81.3   **Family history of other psychoactive substance abuse and dependence**
Conditions classifiable to F11-F16, F18-F19

Z81.4   **Family history of other substance abuse and dependence**
Conditions classifiable to F55

Z81.8   **Family history of other mental and behavioral disorders**
Conditions classifiable elsewhere in F01-F99

⬛ **Z82**   **Family history of certain disabilities and chronic diseases (leading to disablement)**

GUIDELINES   Section I.C.21.c.4)

There are two types of history Z codes, personal and family. Personal history codes explain a patient's past medical condition that no longer exists and is not receiving any treatment, but that has the potential for recurrence, and therefore may require continued monitoring.

Family history codes are for use when a patient has a family member(s) who has had a particular disease that causes the patient to be at higher risk of also contracting the disease. Personal history codes may be used in conjunction with follow-up codes and family history codes may be used in conjunction with screening codes to explain the need for a test or procedure. History codes are also acceptable on any medical record regardless of the reason for visit. A history of an illness, even if no longer present, is important information that may alter the type of treatment ordered.

Z82.0   **Family history of epilepsy and other diseases of the nervous system**
Conditions classifiable to G00-G99

Z82.1   **Family history of blindness and visual loss**
Conditions classifiable to H54.-

Z82.2   **Family history of deafness and hearing loss**
Conditions classifiable to H90-H91

Z82.3   **Family history of stroke**
Conditions classifiable to I60-I64

⬛ **Z82.4**   **Family history of ischemic heart disease and other diseases of the circulatory system**
Conditions classifiable to I00-I52, I65-I99

Z82.41   **Family history of sudden cardiac death**

Z82.49   **Family history of ischemic heart disease and other diseases of the circulatory system**

Z82.5   **Family history of asthma and other chronic lower respiratory diseases**
Conditions classifiable to J40-J47
EXCLUDES 2   *family history of other diseases of the respiratory system (Z83.6)*

⬛ **Z82.6**   **Family history of arthritis and other diseases of the musculoskeletal system and connective tissue**
Conditions classifiable to M00-M99

Z82.61   **Family history of arthritis**

Z82.62   **Family history of osteoporosis**

Z82.69   **Family history of other diseases of the musculoskeletal system and connective tissue**

⬛ **Z82.7**   **Family history of congenital malformations, deformations and chromosomal abnormalities**
Conditions classifiable to Q00-Q99

Z82.71   **Family history of polycystic kidney**

Z82.79   **Family history of other congenital malformations, deformations and chromosomal abnormalities**

Z82.8   **Family history of other disabilities and chronic diseases leading to disablement, not elsewhere classified**

⬛ **Z83**   **Family history of other specific disorders**
EXCLUDES 2   *contact with and (suspected) exposure to communicable disease in the family (Z20.-)*

GUIDELINES   Section I.C.21.c.4)

There are two types of history Z codes, personal and family. Personal history codes explain a patient's past medical condition that no longer exists and is not receiving any treatment, but that has the potential for recurrence, and therefore may require continued monitoring.

Family history codes are for use when a patient has a family member(s) who has had a particular disease that causes the patient to be at higher risk of also contracting the disease. Personal history codes may be used in conjunction with follow-up codes and family history codes may be used in conjunction with screening codes to explain the need for a test or procedure. History codes are also acceptable on any medical record regardless of the reason for visit. A history of an illness, even if no longer present, is important information that may alter the type of treatment ordered.

Z83.0   **Family history of human immunodeficiency virus [HIV] disease**
Conditions classifiable to B20

Z83.1   **Family history of other infectious and parasitic diseases**
Conditions classifiable to A00-B19, B25-B94, B99

Z83.2   **Family history of diseases of the blood and blood-forming organs and certain disorders involving the immune mechanism**
Conditions classifiable to D50-D89

Z83.3   **Family history of diabetes mellitus**
Conditions classifiable to E08-E13

⬛ **Z83.4**   **Family history of other endocrine, nutritional and metabolic diseases**
Conditions classifiable to E00-E07, E15-E88

Z83.41   **Family history of multiple endocrine neoplasia [MEN] syndrome**

● **Z83.42**   **Family history of familial hypercholesterolemia**

Z83.49   **Family history of other endocrine, nutritional and metabolic diseases**

⬛ **Z83.5**   **Family history of eye and ear disorders**

⬛ **Z83.51**   **Family history of eye disorders**
Conditions classifiable to H00-H53, H55-H59
EXCLUDES 2   *family history of blindness and visual loss (Z82.1)*

Z83.511   **Family history of glaucoma**

Z83.518   **Family history of other specified eye disorder**

Z83.52   **Family history of ear disorders**
Conditions classifiable to H60-H83, H92-H95
EXCLUDES 2   *family history of deafness and hearing loss (Z82.2)*

Z83.6   **Family history of other diseases of the respiratory system**
Conditions classifiable to J00-J39, J60-J99
EXCLUDES 2   *family history of asthma and other chronic lower respiratory diseases (Z82.5)*

⬛ **Z83.7**   **Family history of diseases of the digestive system**
Conditions classifiable to K00-K93

Z83.71   **Family history of colonic polyps**
EXCLUDES 1   *family history of malignant neoplasm of digestive organs (Z80.0)*

Z83.79   **Family history of other diseases of the digestive system**

⬛ **Z84**   **Family history of other conditions**

GUIDELINES   Section I.C.21.c.4)

There are two types of history Z codes, personal and family. Personal history codes explain a patient's past medical condition that no longer exists and is not receiving any treatment, but that has the potential for recurrence, and therefore may require continued monitoring.

Family history codes are for use when a patient has a family member(s) who has had a particular disease that causes the patient to be at higher risk of also contracting the disease. Personal history codes may be used in conjunction with follow-up codes and family history codes may be used in conjunction with screening codes to explain the need for a test or procedure. History codes are also acceptable on any medical record regardless of the reason for visit. A history of an illness, even if no longer present, is important information that may alter the type of treatment ordered.

Z84.0   **Family history of diseases of the skin and subcutaneous tissue**
Conditions classifiable to L00-L99

● New   ▲ Revised   *Manifestation*   ⬛-⬛ Digit Indicators   ⊟ Laterality   Ⓐ Adult (15+ years)   Ⓜ Maternity (12-55 years)   Ⓝ Newborn   Ⓟ Pediatric (0-17 years)   ♂ Male   ♀ Female

✖ Deleted   Unspecified   + Additional code

Z84.1   **Family history of disorders of kidney and ureter**
     Conditions classifiable to N00-N29

Z84.2   **Family history of other diseases of the genitourinary system**
     Conditions classifiable to N30-N99

Z84.3   **Family history of consanguinity**

⑤ Z84.8   **Family history of other specified conditions**

     Z84.81   **Family history of carrier of genetic disease**

     ● Z84.82   **Family history of sudden infant death syndrome**
         Family history of SIDS

     Z84.89   **Family history of other specified conditions**

▲ ④ ✚ Z85   **Personal history of malignant neoplasm**
     Code first:
        any follow-up examination after treatment of malignant neoplasm (Z08)
     Use additional code to identify:
        alcohol use and dependence (F10.-)
        exposure to environmental tobacco smoke (Z77.22)
        history of tobacco dependence (Z87.891)
        occupational exposure to environmental tobacco smoke (Z57.31)
        tobacco dependence (F17.-)
        tobacco use (Z72.0)

     EXCLUDES 2   *personal history of benign neoplasm (Z86.01-)*
         personal history of carcinoma-in-situ (Z86.00-)

     GUIDELINES   Section I.C.21.c.4)
There are two types of history Z codes, personal and family. Personal history codes explain a patient's past medical condition that no longer exists and is not receiving any treatment, but that has the potential for recurrence, and therefore may require continued monitoring.

Family history codes are for use when a patient has a family member(s) who has had a particular disease that causes the patient to be at higher risk of also contracting the disease. Personal history codes may be used in conjunction with follow-up codes and family history codes may be used in conjunction with screening codes to explain the need for a test or procedure. History codes are also acceptable on any medical record regardless of the reason for visit. A history of an illness, even if no longer present, is important information that may alter the type of treatment ordered.

     GUIDELINES   Section I.C.2.m
When a primary malignancy has been excised but further treatment, such as an additional surgery for the malignancy, radiation therapy or chemotherapy is directed to that site, the primary malignancy code should be used until treatment is completed.

When a primary malignancy has been previously excised or eradicated from its site, there is no further treatment (of the malignancy) directed to that site, and there is no evidence of any existing primary malignancy, a code from category Z85 should be used to indicate the former site of the malignancy.

     CODING TIP ✓   The codes in this section are commonly referred to as the 'history of cancer' codes. 'History' in this case means the cancer has been eradicated from its primary site. It does not necessarily mean the patient no longer has cancer. The cancer may have already metastasized to other sites.

⑤ ✚ Z85.0   **Personal history of malignant neoplasm of digestive organs**

   ✚ Z85.00   **Personal history of malignant neoplasm of unspecified digestive organ**

   ✚ Z85.01   **Personal history of malignant neoplasm of esophagus**
       Conditions classifiable to C15

   ⑥ ✚ Z85.02   **Personal history of malignant neoplasm of stomach**

     ✚ Z85.020   **Personal history of malignant carcinoid tumor of stomach**
       Conditions classifiable to C7A.092

     ✚ Z85.028   **Personal history of other malignant neoplasm of stomach**
       Conditions classifiable to C16

   ⑥ ✚ Z85.03   **Personal history of malignant neoplasm of large intestine**

     ✚ Z85.030   **Personal history of malignant carcinoid tumor of large intestine**
       Conditions classifiable to C7A.022-C7A.025, C7A.029

     ✚ Z85.038   **Personal history of other malignant neoplasm of large intestine**
       Conditions classifiable to C18

   ⑥ ✚ Z85.04   **Personal history of malignant neoplasm of rectum, rectosigmoid junction, and anus**

     ✚ Z85.040   **Personal history of malignant carcinoid tumor of rectum**
       Conditions classifiable to C7A.026

     ✚ Z85.048   **Personal history of other malignant neoplasm of rectum, rectosigmoid junction, and anus**
       Conditions classifiable to C19-C21

   ✚ Z85.05   **Personal history of malignant neoplasm of liver**
       Conditions classifiable to C22

   ⑥ ✚ Z85.06   **Personal history of malignant neoplasm of small intestine**

     ✚ Z85.060   **Personal history of malignant carcinoid tumor of small intestine**
       Conditions classifiable to C7A.01-

     ✚ Z85.068   **Personal history of other malignant neoplasm of small intestine**
       Conditions classifiable to C17

   ✚ Z85.07   **Personal history of malignant neoplasm of pancreas**
       Conditions classifiable to C25

   ✚ Z85.09   **Personal history of malignant neoplasm of other digestive organs**

⑤ ✚ Z85.1   **Personal history of malignant neoplasm of trachea, bronchus and lung**

   ⑥ ✚ Z85.11   **Personal history of malignant neoplasm of bronchus and lung**

     ✚ Z85.110   **Personal history of malignant carcinoid tumor of bronchus and lung**
       Conditions classifiable to C7A.090

     ✚ Z85.118   **Personal history of other malignant neoplasm of bronchus and lung**
       Conditions classifiable to C34

   ✚ Z85.12   **Personal history of malignant neoplasm of trachea**
       Conditions classifiable to C33

⑤ ✚ Z85.2   **Personal history of malignant neoplasm of other respiratory and intrathoracic organs**

   ✚ Z85.20   **Personal history of malignant neoplasm of unspecified respiratory organ**

   ✚ Z85.21   **Personal history of malignant neoplasm of larynx**
       Conditions classifiable to C32

   ✚ Z85.22   **Personal history of malignant neoplasm of nasal cavities, middle ear, and accessory sinuses**
       Conditions classifiable to C30-C31

   ⑥ ✚ Z85.23   **Personal history of malignant neoplasm of thymus**

     ✚ Z85.230   **Personal history of malignant carcinoid tumor of thymus**
       Conditions classifiable to C7A.091

     ✚ Z85.238   **Personal history of other malignant neoplasm of thymus**
       Conditions classifiable to C37

   ✚ Z85.29   **Personal history of malignant neoplasm of other respiratory and intrathoracic organs**

   ✚ Z85.3   **Personal history of malignant neoplasm of breast**
       Conditions classifiable to C50.-

⑤ ✚ Z85.4   **Personal history of malignant neoplasm of genital organs**
       Conditions classifiable to C51-C63

   ✚ Z85.40   **Personal history of malignant neoplasm of unspecified female genital organ**   ♀

   ✚ Z85.41   **Personal history of malignant neoplasm of cervix uteri**   ♀

   ✚ Z85.42   **Personal history of malignant neoplasm of other parts of uterus**   ♀

   ✚ Z85.43   **Personal history of malignant neoplasm of ovary**   ♀

   ✚ Z85.44   **Personal history of malignant neoplasm of other female genital organs**   ♀

   ✚ Z85.45   **Personal history of malignant neoplasm of unspecified male genital organ**   ♂

   ✚ Z85.46   **Personal history of malignant neoplasm of prostate**   ♂

   ✚ Z85.47   **Personal history of malignant neoplasm of testis**   ♂

   ✚ Z85.48   **Personal history of malignant neoplasm of epididymis**   ♂

   ✚ Z85.49   **Personal history of malignant neoplasm of other male genital organs**   ♂

⑤ ✚ Z85.5   **Personal history of malignant neoplasm of urinary tract**
       Conditions classifiable to C64-C68

● New   ▲ Revised   *Manifestation*   ④-⑦ Digit Indicators   ⊟ Laterality   Ⓐ Adult (15+ years)   Ⓜ Maternity (12-55 years)   Ⓝ Newborn   Ⓟ Pediatric (0-17 years)   ♂ Male   ♀ Female
✖ Deleted   Unspecified   ✚ Additional code

+ **Z85.50** **Personal history of malignant neoplasm of unspecified urinary tract organ**

+ **Z85.51** **Personal history of malignant neoplasm of bladder**

⑥+ **Z85.52** **Personal history of malignant neoplasm of kidney**

> EXCLUDES 1   *personal history of malignant neoplasm of renal pelvis (Z85.53)*

+ **Z85.520** **Personal history of malignant carcinoid tumor of kidney**
Conditions classifiable to C7A.093

+ **Z85.528** **Personal history of other malignant neoplasm of kidney**
Conditions classifiable to C64

+ **Z85.53** **Personal history of malignant neoplasm of renal pelvis**

+ **Z85.54** **Personal history of malignant neoplasm of ureter**

+ **Z85.59** **Personal history of malignant neoplasm of other urinary tract organ**

+ **Z85.6** **Personal history of leukemia**
Conditions classifiable to C91-C95

> EXCLUDES 1   *leukemia in remission C91.0-C95.9 with 5th character 1*

⑤+ **Z85.7** **Personal history of other malignant neoplasms of lymphoid, hematopoietic and related tissues**

+ **Z85.71** **Personal history of Hodgkin lymphoma**
Conditions classifiable to C81

+ **Z85.72** **Personal history of non-Hodgkin lymphomas**
Conditions classifiable to C82-C85

+ **Z85.79** **Personal history of other malignant neoplasms of lymphoid, hematopoietic and related tissues**
Conditions classifiable to C88-C90, C96

> EXCLUDES 1   *multiple myeloma in remission (C90.01)*
> *plasma cell leukemia in remission (C90.11)*
> *plasmacytoma in remission (C90.21)*

> GUIDELINES   Section I.C.2.n
> The categories for leukemia, and category C90, Multiple myeloma and malignant plasma cell neoplasms, have codes indicating whether or not the leukemia has achieved remission. There are also codes Z85.6, Personal history of leukemia, and Z85.79, Personal history of other malignant neoplasms of lymphoid, hematopoietic and related tissues. If the documentation is unclear, as to whether the leukemia has achieved remission, the provider should be queried.

▲⑤+ **Z85.8** **Personal history of malignant neoplasms of other organs and systems**
Conditions classifiable to C00-C14, C40-C49, C69-C75, C7A.098, C76-C79

⑥+ **Z85.81** **Personal history of malignant neoplasm of lip, oral cavity, and pharynx**

+ **Z85.810** **Personal history of malignant neoplasm of tongue**

+ **Z85.818** **Personal history of malignant neoplasm of other sites of lip, oral cavity, and pharynx**

+ **Z85.819** **Personal history of malignant neoplasm of unspecified site of lip, oral cavity, and pharynx**

⑥+ **Z85.82** **Personal history of malignant neoplasm of skin**

+ **Z85.820** **Personal history of malignant melanoma of skin**
Conditions classifiable to C43

+ **Z85.821** **Personal history of Merkel cell carcinoma**
Conditions classifiable to C4A

+ **Z85.828** **Personal history of other malignant neoplasm of skin**
Conditions classifiable to C44

⑥+ **Z85.83** **Personal history of malignant neoplasm of bone and soft tissue**

+ **Z85.830** **Personal history of malignant neoplasm of bone**

+ **Z85.831** **Personal history of malignant neoplasm of soft tissue**

> EXCLUDES 2   *personal history of malignant neoplasm of skin (Z85.82-)*

⑥+ **Z85.84** **Personal history of malignant neoplasm of eye and nervous tissue**

+ **Z85.840** **Personal history of malignant neoplasm of eye**

+ **Z85.841** **Personal history of malignant neoplasm of brain**

+ **Z85.848** **Personal history of malignant neoplasm of other parts of nervous tissue**

⑥+ **Z85.85** **Personal history of malignant neoplasm of endocrine glands**

+ **Z85.850** **Personal history of malignant neoplasm of thyroid**

+ **Z85.858** **Personal history of malignant neoplasm of other endocrine glands**

+ **Z85.89** **Personal history of malignant neoplasm of other organs and systems**

+ **Z85.9** **Personal history of malignant neoplasm, unspecified**
Conditions classifiable to C7A.00, C80.1

④ **Z86** **Personal history of certain other diseases**
Code first:
any follow-up examination after treatment (Z09)

> GUIDELINES   Section I.C.21.c.4)
> There are two types of history Z codes, personal and family. Personal history codes explain a patient's past medical condition that no longer exists and is not receiving any treatment, but that has the potential for recurrence, and therefore may require continued monitoring.
>
> Family history codes are for use when a patient has a family member(s) who has had a particular disease that causes the patient to be at higher risk of also contracting the disease. Personal history codes may be used in conjunction with follow-up codes and family history codes may be used in conjunction with screening codes to explain the need for a test or procedure. History codes are also acceptable on any medical record regardless of the reason for visit. A history of an illness, even if no longer present, is important information that may alter the type of treatment ordered.

⑤ **Z86.0** **Personal history of in-situ and benign neoplasms and neoplasms of uncertain behavior**

> EXCLUDES 2   *personal history of malignant neoplasms (Z85.-)*

▲⑥ **Z86.00** **Personal history of in-situ neoplasm**
Conditions classifiable to D00-D09

Z86.000 **Personal history of in-situ neoplasm of breast**

▲ **Z86.001** **Personal history of in-situ neoplasm of cervix uteri** ♀
Personal history of cervical intraepithelial neoplasia III [CIN III]

▲ **Z86.008** **Personal history of in-situ neoplasm of other site**
Personal history of vaginal intraepithelial neoplasia III [VAIN III]
Personal history of vulvar intraepithelial neoplasia III [VIN III]

⑥ **Z86.01** **Personal history of benign neoplasm**

Z86.010 **Personal history of colonic polyps**

Z86.011 **Personal history of benign neoplasm of the brain**

Z86.012 **Personal history of benign carcinoid tumor**

Z86.018 **Personal history of other benign neoplasm**

Z86.03 **Personal history of neoplasm of uncertain behavior**

⑤ **Z86.1** **Personal history of infectious and parasitic diseases**
Conditions classifiable to A00-B89, B99

> EXCLUDES 1   *personal history of infectious diseases specific to a body system*
> *sequelae of infectious and parasitic diseases (B90-B94)*

Z86.11 **Personal history of tuberculosis**

Z86.12 **Personal history of poliomyelitis**

Z86.13 **Personal history of malaria**

Z86.14 **Personal history of Methicillin resistant Staphylococcus aureus infection**
Personal history of MRSA infection

Z86.19 **Personal history of other infectious and parasitic diseases**

Z86.2 **Personal history of diseases of the blood and blood-forming organs and certain disorders involving the immune mechanism**
Conditions classifiable to D50-D89

⑤ **Z86.3** **Personal history of endocrine, nutritional and metabolic diseases**
Conditions classifiable to E00-E88

Z86.31 **Personal history of diabetic foot ulcer**

> EXCLUDES 2   *current diabetic foot ulcer (E08.621, E09.621, E10.621, E11.621, E13.621)*

● New   ▲ Revised   *Manifestation*   ④-⑦ Digit Indicators   ▤ Laterality   ▣ Adult (15+ years)   Ⓜ Maternity (12-55 years)   Ⓝ Newborn   ▣ Pediatric (0-17 years)   ♂ Male   ♀ Female
✖ ~~Deleted~~   Unspecified   + Additional code

1200   © 2017 DecisionHealth   2017 ICD-10-CM Expert for Physicians

Z86.32   Personal history of gestational diabetes ♀
          Personal history of conditions classifiable to O24.4-
          EXCLUDES 1   *gestational diabetes mellitus in current pregnancy (O24.4-)*

Z86.39   Personal history of other endocrine, nutritional and metabolic disease

⑤ Z86.5   Personal history of mental and behavioral disorders
          Conditions classifiable to F40-F59

Z86.51   Personal history of combat and operational stress ▲ reaction

Z86.59   Personal history of other mental and behavioral disorders

⑤ Z86.6   Personal history of diseases of the nervous system and sense organs
          Conditions classifiable to G00-G99, H00-H95

Z86.61   Personal history of infections of the central nervous system
          Personal history of encephalitis
          Personal history of meningitis

Z86.69   Personal history of other diseases of the nervous system and sense organs

⑤ Z86.7   Personal history of diseases of the circulatory system
          Conditions classifiable to I00-I99
          EXCLUDES 2   *old myocardial infarction (I25.2)*
                        personal history of anaphylactic shock (Z87.892)
                        postmyocardial infarction syndrome (I24.1)

⑥ Z86.71 Personal history of venous thrombosis and embolism

Z86.711   Personal history of pulmonary embolism

Z86.718   Personal history of other venous thrombosis and embolism

Z86.72   Personal history of thrombophlebitis

Z86.73   Personal history of transient ischemic attack (TIA), and cerebral infarction without residual deficits
          Personal history of prolonged reversible ischemic neurological deficit (PRIND)
          Personal history of stroke NOS without residual deficits
          EXCLUDES 1   *personal history of traumatic brain injury (Z87.820)*
                        sequelae of cerebrovascular disease (I69.-)

          GUIDELINES   Section I.C.9.d.3)
          Codes from category I69, Sequela of cerebrovascular disease, should not be assigned if the patient does not have neurologic deficits. Assign Z86.73, Personal history of transient ischemic attack (TIA) and cerebral infarction
          AHA: 4Q 2012, 92-93

Z86.74   Personal history of sudden cardiac arrest
          Personal history of sudden cardiac death successfully resuscitated

Z86.79   Personal history of other diseases of the circulatory system

④ Z87   Personal history of other diseases and conditions
          Code first:
            any follow-up examination after treatment (Z09)

          GUIDELINES   Section I.C.21.c.4)
          There are two types of history Z codes, personal and family. Personal history codes explain a patient's past medical condition that no longer exists and is not receiving any treatment, but that has the potential for recurrence, and therefore may require continued monitoring.

          Family history codes are for use when a patient has a family member(s) who has had a particular disease that causes the patient to be at higher risk of also contracting the disease. Personal history codes may be used in conjunction with follow-up codes and family history codes may be used in conjunction with screening codes to explain the need for a test or procedure. History codes are also acceptable on any medical record regardless of the reason for visit. A history of an illness, even if no longer present, is important information that may alter the type of treatment ordered.

⑤ Z87.0   Personal history of diseases of the respiratory system
          Conditions classifiable to J00-J99

Z87.01   Personal history of pneumonia (recurrent)

Z87.09   Personal history of other diseases of the respiratory system

⑤ Z87.1   Personal history of diseases of the digestive system
          Conditions classifiable to K00-K93

Z87.11   Personal history of peptic ulcer disease

Z87.19   Personal history of other diseases of the digestive system

Z87.2   Personal history of diseases of the skin and subcutaneous tissue
          Conditions classifiable to L00-L99
          EXCLUDES 2   *personal history of diabetic foot ulcer (Z86.31)*

⑤ Z87.3   Personal history of diseases of the musculoskeletal system and connective tissue
          Conditions classifiable to M00-M99
          EXCLUDES 2   *personal history of (healed) traumatic fracture (Z87.81)*

⑥ Z87.31 Personal history of (healed) nontraumatic fracture

Z87.310   Personal history of (healed) osteoporosis fracture
          Personal history of (healed) fragility fracture
          Personal history of (healed) collapsed vertebra due to osteoporosis

          GUIDELINES   Section I.C.13.d.1)
          Category M81, Osteoporosis without current pathological fracture, is for use for patients with osteoporosis who do not currently have a pathologic fracture due to the osteoporosis, even if they have had a fracture in the past. For patients with a history of osteoporosis fractures, status code Z87.310, Personal history of (healed) osteoporosis fracture, should follow the code from M81.

Z87.311   Personal history of (healed) other pathological fracture
          Personal history of (healed) collapsed vertebra NOS
          EXCLUDES 2   *personal history of osteoporosis fracture (Z87.310)*

Z87.312   Personal history of (healed) stress fracture
          Personal history of (healed) fatigue fracture

Z87.39   Personal history of other diseases of the musculoskeletal system and connective tissue

⑤ Z87.4   Personal history of diseases of genitourinary system
          Conditions classifiable to N00-N99

▲ ⑥ Z87.41 Personal history of dysplasia of the female genital tract
          EXCLUDES 1   *personal history of intraepithelial neoplasia III of female genital tract (Z87.001, Z87.008)*
                        personal history of malignant neoplasm of female genital tract (Z85.40-Z85.44)

Z87.410   Personal history of cervical dysplasia ♀

Z87.411   Personal history of vaginal dysplasia ♀

Z87.412   Personal history of vulvar dysplasia ♀

Z87.42   Personal history of other diseases of the female genital tract ♀

⑥ Z87.43 Personal history of diseases of male genital organs

Z87.430   Personal history of prostatic dysplasia
          EXCLUDES 1   *personal history of malignant neoplasm of prostate (Z85.46)*

Z87.438   Personal history of other diseases of male genital organs

⑥ Z87.44 Personal history of diseases of urinary system
          EXCLUDES 1   *personal history of malignant neoplasm of cervix uteri (Z85.41)*

Z87.440   Personal history of urinary (tract) infections

Z87.441   Personal history of nephrotic syndrome

Z87.442   Personal history of urinary calculi
          Personal history of kidney stones

Z87.448   Personal history of other diseases of urinary system

⑤ Z87.5   Personal history of complications of pregnancy, childbirth and the puerperium
          Conditions classifiable to O00-O9A
          EXCLUDES 2   *recurrent pregnancy loss (N96)*

Z87.51   Personal history of pre-term labor ♀ Ⓜ
          EXCLUDES 1   *current pregnancy with history of pre-term labor (O09.21-)*

Z87.59   Personal history of other complications of pregnancy, childbirth and the puerperium ♀
          Personal history of trophoblastic disease

● New   ▲ Revised   *Manifestation*   ④-⑦ Digit Indicators   ▣ Laterality   Ⓐ Adult (15+ years)   Ⓜ Maternity (12-55 years)   Ⓝ Newborn   Ⓟ Pediatric (0-17 years)   ♂ Male   ♀ Female
✖ Deleted   Unspecified   + Additional code

2017 ICD-10-CM Expert for Physicians

© 2017 DecisionHealth

1201

⑤ Z87.7 **Personal history of (corrected) congenital malformations**
Conditions classifiable to Q00-Q89 that have been repaired or corrected

> **EXCLUDES 1** *congenital malformations that have been partially corrected or repair but which still require medical treatment - code to condition*
>
> **EXCLUDES 2** *other postprocedural states (Z98.-)*
> *personal history of medical treatment (Z92.-)*
> *presence of cardiac and vascular implants and grafts (Z95.-)*
> *presence of other devices (Z97.-)*
> *presence of other functional implants (Z96.-)*
> *transplanted organ and tissue status (Z94.-)*

⑥ Z87.71 **Personal history of (corrected) congenital malformations of genitourinary system**

    Z87.710 **Personal history of (corrected) hypospadias** ♂

    Z87.718 **Personal history of other specified (corrected) congenital malformations of genitourinary system**

⑥ Z87.72 **Personal history of (corrected) congenital malformations of nervous system and sense organs**

    Z87.720 **Personal history of (corrected) congenital malformations of eye**

    Z87.721 **Personal history of (corrected) congenital malformations of ear**

    Z87.728 **Personal history of other specified (corrected) congenital malformations of nervous system and sense organs**

⑥ Z87.73 **Personal history of (corrected) congenital malformations of digestive system**

    Z87.730 **Personal history of (corrected) cleft lip and palate**

    Z87.738 **Personal history of other specified (corrected) congenital malformations of digestive system**

Z87.74 **Personal history of (corrected) congenital malformations of heart and circulatory system**

Z87.75 **Personal history of (corrected) congenital malformations of respiratory system**

Z87.76 **Personal history of (corrected) congenital malformations of integument, limbs and musculoskeletal system**

⑥ Z87.79 **Personal history of other (corrected) congenital malformations**

    Z87.790 **Personal history of (corrected) congenital malformations of face and neck**

    Z87.798 **Personal history of other (corrected) congenital malformations**

⑤ Z87.8 **Personal history of other specified conditions**

> **EXCLUDES 2** *personal history of self harm (Z91.5)*

    Z87.81 **Personal history of (healed) traumatic fracture**

> **EXCLUDES 2** *personal history of (healed) nontraumatic fracture (Z87.31-)*

⑥ Z87.82 **Personal history of other (healed) physical injury and trauma**
Conditions classifiable to S00-T88, except traumatic fractures

    Z87.820 **Personal history of traumatic brain injury**

> **EXCLUDES 1** *personal history of transient ischemic attack (TIA) , and cerebral infarction without residual deficits (Z86.73)*

    Z87.821 **Personal history of retained foreign body fully removed**

    Z87.828 **Personal history of other (healed) physical injury and trauma**

⑥ Z87.89 **Personal history of other specified conditions**

    Z87.890 **Personal history of sex reassignment**

    Z87.891 **Personal history of nicotine dependence**

> **EXCLUDES 1** *current nicotine dependence (F17.2-)*

    Z87.892 **Personal history of anaphylaxis**
Code also allergy status such as:
allergy status to drugs, medicaments and biological substances (Z88.-)
allergy status, other than to drugs and biological substances (Z91.0-)

    Z87.898 **Personal history of other specified conditions**

AHA: 1Q 2013, 21

④ Z88 **Allergy status to drugs, medicaments and biological substances**

> **EXCLUDES 2** *Allergy status, other than to drugs and biological substances (Z91.0-)*

Z88.0 **Allergy status to penicillin**

Z88.1 **Allergy status to other antibiotic agents status**

Z88.2 **Allergy status to sulfonamides status**
AHA: 3Q 2015, 23

Z88.3 **Allergy status to other anti-infective agents status**

Z88.4 **Allergy status to anesthetic agent status**

Z88.5 **Allergy status to narcotic agent status**

Z88.6 **Allergy status to analgesic agent status**

Z88.7 **Allergy status to serum and vaccine status**

Z88.8 **Allergy status to other drugs, medicaments and biological substances status**

Z88.9 **Allergy status to unspecified drugs, medicaments and biological substances status**

④ Z89 **Acquired absence of limb**

> **INCLUDES** amputation status
> postprocedural loss of limb
> post-traumatic loss of limb
>
> **EXCLUDES 1** *acquired deformities of limbs (M20-M21)*
> *congenital absence of limbs (Q71-Q73)*

⑤ Z89.0 **Acquired absence of thumb and other finger(s)**

⑥ Z89.01 **Acquired absence of thumb**

    ☰ Z89.011 **Acquired absence of right thumb**

    ☰ Z89.012 **Acquired absence of left thumb**

    ☰ Z89.019 **Acquired absence of unspecified thumb**

⑥ Z89.02 **Acquired absence of other finger(s)**

> **EXCLUDES 2** *acquired absence of thumb (Z89.01-)*

    ☰ Z89.021 **Acquired absence of right finger(s)**

    ☰ Z89.022 **Acquired absence of left finger(s)**

    ☰ Z89.029 **Acquired absence of unspecified finger(s)**

⑤ Z89.1 **Acquired absence of hand and wrist**

⑥ Z89.11 **Acquired absence of hand**

    ☰ Z89.111 **Acquired absence of right hand**

    ☰ Z89.112 **Acquired absence of left hand**

    ☰ Z89.119 **Acquired absence of unspecified hand**

⑥ Z89.12 **Acquired absence of wrist**
Disarticulation at wrist

    ☰ Z89.121 **Acquired absence of right wrist**

    ☰ Z89.122 **Acquired absence of left wrist**

    ☰ Z89.129 **Acquired absence of unspecified wrist**

⑤ Z89.2 **Acquired absence of upper limb above wrist**

⑥ Z89.20 **Acquired absence of upper limb, unspecified level**

    ☰ Z89.201 **Acquired absence of right upper limb, unspecified level**

    ☰ Z89.202 **Acquired absence of left upper limb, unspecified level**

    ☰ Z89.209 **Acquired absence of unspecified upper limb, unspecified level**
Acquired absence of arm NOS

⑥ Z89.21 **Acquired absence of upper limb below elbow**

    ☰ Z89.211 **Acquired absence of right upper limb below elbow**

    ☰ Z89.212 **Acquired absence of left upper limb below elbow**

    ☰ Z89.219 **Acquired absence of unspecified upper limb below elbow**

⑥ Z89.22 **Acquired absence of upper limb above elbow**
Disarticulation at elbow

    ☰ Z89.221 **Acquired absence of right upper limb above elbow**

    ☰ Z89.222 **Acquired absence of left upper limb above elbow**

    ☰ Z89.229 **Acquired absence of unspecified upper limb above elbow**

⑥ Z89.23 **Acquired absence of shoulder**
Acquired absence of shoulder joint following explantation of shoulder joint prosthesis, with or without presence of antibiotic-impregnated cement spacer

    ☰ Z89.231 **Acquired absence of right shoulder**

    ☰ Z89.232 **Acquired absence of left shoulder**

● New   ▲ Revised   *Manifestation*   ④-❼ Digit Indicators   ☰ Laterality   Ⓐ Adult (15+ years)   Ⓜ Maternity (12-55 years)   Ⓝ Newborn   Ⓟ Pediatric (0-17 years)   ♂ Male   ♀ Female

✖ Deleted   Unspecified   + Additional code

1202   © 2017 DecisionHealth   2017 ICD-10-CM Expert for Physicians

Z89.239   Acquired absence of unspecified shoulder

☐ Z89.4   Acquired absence of toe(s), foot, and ankle

   ☐ Z89.41   Acquired absence of great toe

     ☐ Z89.411   Acquired absence of right great toe

     ☐ Z89.412   Acquired absence of left great toe

     ☐ Z89.419   Acquired absence of unspecified great toe

   ☐ Z89.42   Acquired absence of other toe(s)

     EXCLUDES 2   *acquired absence of great toe (Z89.41-)*

     ☐ Z89.421   Acquired absence of other right toe(s)

     ☐ Z89.422   Acquired absence of other left toe(s)

     ☐ Z89.429   Acquired absence of other toe(s), unspecified side

   ☐ Z89.43   Acquired absence of foot

     ☐ Z89.431   Acquired absence of right foot

     ☐ Z89.432   Acquired absence of left foot

     ☐ Z89.439   Acquired absence of unspecified foot

   ☐ Z89.44   Acquired absence of ankle

     Disarticulation of ankle

     ☐ Z89.441   Acquired absence of right ankle

     ☐ Z89.442   Acquired absence of left ankle

     ☐ Z89.449   Acquired absence of unspecified ankle

☐ Z89.5   Acquired absence of leg below knee

   ☐ Z89.51   Acquired absence of leg below knee

     ☐ Z89.511   Acquired absence of right leg below knee

     ☐ Z89.512   Acquired absence of left leg below knee

     ☐ Z89.519   Acquired absence of unspecified leg below knee

   ☐ Z89.52   Acquired absence of knee

     Acquired absence of knee joint following explantation of knee joint prosthesis, with or without presence of antibiotic-impregnated cement spacer

     ☐ Z89.521   Acquired absence of right knee

     ☐ Z89.522   Acquired absence of left knee

     ☐ Z89.529   Acquired absence of unspecified knee

☐ Z89.6   Acquired absence of leg above knee

   ☐ Z89.61   Acquired absence of leg above knee

     Acquired absence of leg NOS

     Disarticulation at knee

     ☐ Z89.611   Acquired absence of right leg above knee

     ☐ Z89.612   Acquired absence of left leg above knee

     ☐ Z89.619   Acquired absence of unspecified leg above knee

   ☐ Z89.62   Acquired absence of hip

     Acquired absence of hip joint following explantation of hip joint prosthesis, with or without presence of antibiotic-impregnated cement spacer

     Disarticulation at hip

     ☐ Z89.621   Acquired absence of right hip joint

     ☐ Z89.622   Acquired absence of left hip joint

     ☐ Z89.629   Acquired absence of unspecified hip joint

Z89.9   Acquired absence of limb, unspecified

☐ **Z90**   **Acquired absence of organs, not elsewhere classified**

   INCLUDES   postprocedural or post-traumatic loss of body part NEC

   EXCLUDES 1   *congenital absence - see Alphabetical Index*

   EXCLUDES 2   *postprocedural absence of endocrine glands (E89.-)*

☐ Z90.0   Acquired absence of part of head and neck

   Z90.01   Acquired absence of eye

   Z90.02   Acquired absence of larynx

   Z90.09   Acquired absence of other part of head and neck

     Acquired absence of nose

     EXCLUDES 2   *teeth (K08.1)*

☐ Z90.1   Acquired absence of breast and nipple

   ☐ Z90.10   Acquired absence of unspecified breast and nipple

   ☐ Z90.11   Acquired absence of right breast and nipple

   ☐ Z90.12   Acquired absence of left breast and nipple

   ☐ Z90.13   Acquired absence of bilateral breasts and nipples

Z90.2   Acquired absence of lung [part of]

Z90.3   Acquired absence of stomach [part of]

☐ Z90.4   Acquired absence of other specified parts of digestive tract

▲ ☐ + Z90.41   Acquired absence of pancreas

   Code also:

     exocrine pancreatic insufficiency (K86.81)

   Use additional code to identify any associated:

     insulin use (Z79.4)

     diabetes mellitus, postpancreatectomy (E13.-)

   GUIDELINES   Section I.C.4.a.6)(b)(i)

   For postpancreatectomy diabetes mellitus (lack of insulin due to the surgical removal of all or part of the pancreas), assign code E89.1, Postprocedural hypoinsulinemia. Assign a code from category E13 and a code from subcategory Z90.41-, Acquired absence of pancreas, as additional codes.

   + Z90.410   Acquired total absence of pancreas

     Acquired absence of pancreas NOS

   + Z90.411   Acquired partial absence of pancreas

   Z90.49   Acquired absence of other specified parts of digestive tract

Z90.5   Acquired absence of kidney

Z90.6   Acquired absence of other parts of urinary tract

   Acquired absence of bladder

☐ Z90.7   Acquired absence of genital organ(s)

   EXCLUDES 1   *personal history of sex reassignment (Z87.890)*

   EXCLUDES 2   *female genital mutilation status (N90.81-)*

   ☐ Z90.71   Acquired absence of cervix and uterus

     Z90.710   Acquired absence of both cervix and uterus   ♀

       Acquired absence of uterus NOS

       Status post total hysterectomy

     Z90.711   Acquired absence of uterus with remaining cervical stump   ♀

       Status post partial hysterectomy with remaining cervical stump

     Z90.712   Acquired absence of cervix with remaining uterus   ♀

   ☐ Z90.72   Acquired absence of ovaries

     Z90.721   Acquired absence of ovaries, unilateral   ♀

     Z90.722   Acquired absence of ovaries, bilateral   ♀

   Z90.79   Acquired absence of other genital organ(s)

☐ Z90.8   Acquired absence of other organs

   Z90.81   Acquired absence of spleen

   Z90.89   Acquired absence of other organs

☐ **Z91**   **Personal risk factors, not elsewhere classified**

   EXCLUDES 2   *contact with and (suspected) exposures hazardous to health (Z77.-)*

     exposure to pollution and other problems related to physical environment (Z77.1-)

     personal history of physical injury and trauma (Z87.81, Z87.82-)

     occupational exposure to risk factors (Z57.-)

☐ Z91.0   Allergy status, other than to drugs and biological substances

   EXCLUDES 2   *Allergy status to drugs, medicaments, and biological substances (Z88.-)*

   ☐ Z91.01   Food allergy status

     EXCLUDES 2   *food additives allergy status (Z91.02)*

     Z91.010   **Allergy to peanuts**

     Z91.011   **Allergy to milk products**

       EXCLUDES 1   *lactose intolerance (E73.-)*

     Z91.012   **Allergy to eggs**

     Z91.013   **Allergy to seafood**

       Allergy to shellfish

       Allergy to octopus or squid ink

     Z91.018   **Allergy to other foods**

       Allergy to nuts other than peanuts

   Z91.02   **Food additives allergy status**

   ☐ Z91.03   Insect allergy status

     Z91.030   **Bee allergy status**

     Z91.038   **Other insect allergy status**

   ☐ Z91.04   Nonmedicinal substance allergy status

     Z91.040   **Latex allergy status**

       Latex sensitivity status

     Z91.041   **Radiographic dye allergy status**

       Allergy status to contrast media used for diagnostic X-ray procedure

---

New	▲ Revised	*Manifestation*	☐-☐ Digit Indicators	☐ Laterality	☒ Adult (15+ years)	☒ Maternity (12-55 years)	☒ Newborn	☒ Pediatric (0-17 years)	♂ Male	♀ Female
◄ Deleted	Unspecified		+ Additional code							

Z91.048   Other nonmedicinal substance allergy status

Z91.09   Other allergy status, other than to drugs and biological substances

⑤ **Z91.1**   Patient's noncompliance with medical treatment and regimen

Z91.11   Patient's noncompliance with dietary regimen

⑥ **Z91.12**   Patient's intentional underdosing of medication regimen

Code first:

underdosing of medication (T36-T50) with fifth or sixth character 6

EXCLUDES 1   *adverse effect of prescribed drug taken as directed- code to adverse effect poisoning (overdose) -code to poisoning*

GUIDELINES   Section I.C.19.e.5)(c)

Noncompliance (Z91.12-, Z91.13-) or complication of care (Y63.6-Y63.9) codes are to be used with an underdosing code to indicate intent, if known.

CODING TIP ✓   A code from Z91.12- or Z91.13- should be assigned when underdosing has been identified and coded in the plan of care/medical record.

Z91.120   Patient's intentional underdosing of medication regimen due to financial hardship

Z91.128   Patient's intentional underdosing of medication regimen for other reason

⑥ **Z91.13**   Patient's unintentional underdosing of medication regimen

Code first:

underdosing of medication (T36-T50) with fifth or sixth character 6

EXCLUDES 1   *adverse effect of prescribed drug taken as directed- code to adverse effect poisoning (overdose) -code to poisoning*

GUIDELINES   Section I.C.19.e.5)(c)

Noncompliance (Z91.12-, Z91.13-) or complication of care (Y63.6-Y63.9) codes are to be used with an underdosing code to indicate intent, if known.

CODING TIP ✓   A code from Z91.12- or Z91.13- should be assigned when underdosing has been identified and coded in the plan of care/medical record.

Z91.130   Patient's unintentional underdosing of medication regimen due to age-related debility

Z91.138   Patient's unintentional underdosing of medication regimen for other reason

Z91.14   Patient's other noncompliance with medication regimen

Patient's underdosing of medication NOS

Z91.15   Patient's noncompliance with renal dialysis

Z91.19   Patient's noncompliance with other medical treatment and regimen

⑤ **Z91.4**   Personal history of psychological trauma, not elsewhere classified

GUIDELINES   Section I.C.21.c.4)

There are two types of history Z codes, personal and family. Personal history codes explain a patient's past medical condition that no longer exists and is not receiving any treatment, but that has the potential for recurrence, and therefore may require continued monitoring.

Family history codes are for use when a patient has a family member(s) who has had a particular disease that causes the patient to be at higher risk of also contracting the disease. Personal history codes may be used in conjunction with follow-up codes and family history codes may be used in conjunction with screening codes to explain the need for a test or procedure. History codes are also acceptable on any medical record regardless of the reason for visit. A history of an illness, even if no longer present, is important information that may alter the type of treatment ordered.

⑥ **Z91.41**   Personal history of adult abuse

EXCLUDES 2   *personal history of abuse in childhood (Z62.81-)*

Z91.410   Personal history of adult physical and sexual abuse   Ⓐ

EXCLUDES 1   *current adult physical abuse (T74.11, T76.11) current adult sexual abuse (T74.21, T76.11)*

Z91.411   Personal history of adult psychological abuse   Ⓐ

Z91.412   Personal history of adult neglect   Ⓐ

EXCLUDES 1   *current adult neglect (T74.01, T76.01)*

Z91.419   Personal history of unspecified adult abuse   Ⓐ

Z91.49   Other personal history of psychological trauma, not elsewhere classified

Z91.5   Personal history of self-harm

Personal history of parasuicide

Personal history of self-poisoning

Personal history of suicide attempt

GUIDELINES   Section I.C.2

There are two types of history Z codes, personal and family. Personal history codes explain a patient's past medical condition that no longer exists and is not receiving any treatment, but that has the potential for recurrence, and therefore may require continued monitoring.

Family history codes are for use when a patient has a family member(s) who has had a particular disease that causes the patient to be at higher risk of also contracting the disease. Personal history codes may be used in conjunction with follow-up codes and family history codes may be used in conjunction with screening codes to explain the need for a test or procedure. History codes are also acceptable on any medical record regardless of the reason for visit. A history of an illness, even if no longer present, is important information that may alter the type of treatment ordered.

⑤ **Z91.8**   Other specified personal risk factors, not elsewhere classified

GUIDELINES   Section I.C.2

There are two types of history Z codes, personal and family. Personal history codes explain a patient's past medical condition that no longer exists and is not receiving any treatment, but that has the potential for recurrence, and therefore may require continued monitoring.

Family history codes are for use when a patient has a family member(s) who has had a particular disease that causes the patient to be at higher risk of also contracting the disease. Personal history codes may be used in conjunction with follow-up codes and family history codes may be used in conjunction with screening codes to explain the need for a test or procedure. History codes are also acceptable on any medical record regardless of the reason for visit. A history of an illness, even if no longer present, is important information that may alter the type of treatment ordered.

Z91.81   History of falling

At risk for falling

GUIDELINES   Section I.C.18.d

Code R29.6, Repeated falls, is for use for encounters when a patient has recently fallen and the reason for the fall is being investigated. Code Z91.81, History of falling, is for use when a patient has fallen in the past and is at risk for future falls. When appropriate, both codes R29.6 and Z91.81 may be assigned together.

● New   ▲ Revised   *Manifestation*   **4 - 7** Digit Indicators   ⊟ Laterality   Ⓐ Adult (15+ years)   Ⓜ Maternity (12-55 years)   Ⓝ Newborn   Ⓟ Pediatric (0-17 years)   ♂ Male   ♀ Female

✖ Deleted   Unspecified   + Additional code

CODING TIP ✓ Use this code when a patient has fallen in the past and is at risk for future falls. In some cases, it may be appropriate to assign R29.6, Repeated falls, on the same claim with Z91.81 if the patient is experiencing current, repeated falls and the intent of the episode is to investigate and treat the falls. Z91.81 may not be first listed on hospital claims.

Z91.82   Personal history of military deployment
Individual (civilian or military) with past history of military war, peacekeeping and humanitarian deployment (current or past conflict)
Returned from military deployment

Z91.83   Wandering in diseases classified elsewhere
Code first underlying disorder such as:
Alzheimer's disease (G30.-)
autism or pervasive developmental disorder (F84.-)
intellectual disabilities (F70-F79)
unspecified dementia with behavioral disturbance (F03.9-)

Z91.89   Other specified personal risk factors, not elsewhere classified

🄳 Z92   Personal history of medical treatment
EXCLUDES 2   *postprocedural states (Z98.-)*

Z92.0   Personal history of contraception
EXCLUDES 1   *counseling or management of current contraceptive practices (Z30.-)*
long term (current) use of contraception (Z79.3)
presence of (intrauterine) contraceptive device (Z97.5)

🄢 Z92.2   Personal history of drug therapy
EXCLUDES 2   *long term (current) drug therapy (Z79.-)*

Z92.21   Personal history of antineoplastic chemotherapy
Z92.22   Personal history of monoclonal drug therapy
Z92.23   Personal history of estrogen therapy
🄶 Z92.24   Personal history of steroid therapy
Z92.240   Personal history of inhaled steroid therapy
Z92.241   Personal history of systemic steroid therapy
Personal history of steroid therapy NOS
Z92.25   Personal history of immunosupression therapy
EXCLUDES 2   *personal history of steroid therapy (Z92.24)*

Z92.29   Personal history of other drug therapy
Z92.3   Personal history of irradiation
Personal history of exposure to therapeutic radiation
EXCLUDES 1   *exposure to radiation in the physical environment (Z77.12)*
occupational exposure to radiation (Z57.1)

🄢 Z92.8   Personal history of other medical treatment
Z92.81   Personal history of extracorporeal membrane oxygenation (ECMO)
Z92.82   Status post administration of tPA (rtPA) in a different facility within the last 24 hours prior to admission to current facility
Code first condition requiring tPA administration, such as:
acute cerebral infarction (I63.-)
acute myocardial infarction (I21.-, I22.-)
AHA: 4Q 2013, 124

Z92.83   Personal history of failed moderate sedation
Personal history of failed conscious sedation
EXCLUDES 2   *failed moderate sedation during procedure (T88.52)*

● **Z92.84   Personal history of unintended awareness under general anesthesia**
EXCLUDES 2   *unintended awareness under general anesthesia during procedure (T88.53)*

Z92.89   Personal history of other medical treatment
🄳 Z93   Artificial opening status
EXCLUDES 1   *artificial openings requiring attention or management (Z43.-)*
complications of external stoma (J95.0-, K94.-, N99.5-)

CODING TIP ✓ Assign codes from category Z93 to indicate artificial openings which are present but do not require intervention or management by the agency. Do not use codes in the Z93 category with attention to artificial opening codes (Z43) codes for the same ostomy or when the ostomy is complicated.

Z93.0   Tracheostomy status
AHA: 4Q 2013, 129
Z93.1   Gastrostomy status
Z93.2   Ileostomy status
Z93.3   Colostomy status
Z93.4   Other artificial openings of gastrointestinal tract status
🄢 Z93.5   Cystostomy status
Z93.50   Unspecified cystostomy status
Z93.51   Cutaneous-vesicostomy status
Z93.52   Appendico-vesicostomy status
Z93.59   Other cystostomy status
Z93.6   Other artificial openings of urinary tract status
Nephrostomy status
Ureterostomy status
Urethrostomy status
Z93.8   Other artificial opening status
Z93.9   Artificial opening status, unspecified

🄳 Z94   Transplanted organ and tissue status
INCLUDES   organ or tissue replaced by heterogenous or homogenous transplant
EXCLUDES 1   *complications of transplanted organ or tissue - see Alphabetical Index*
EXCLUDES 2   *presence of vascular grafts (Z95.-)*

Z94.0   Kidney transplant status
GUIDELINES   Section I.C.14.a.2)
Patients who have undergone kidney transplant may still have some form of chronic kidney disease (CKD) because the kidney transplant may not fully restore kidney function. Therefore, the presence of CKD alone does not constitute a transplant complication. Assign the appropriate N18 code for the patient's stage of CKD and code Z94.0, Kidney transplant status. If a transplant complication such as failure or rejection or other transplant complication is documented, see section I.C.19.g for information on coding complications of a kidney transplant. If the documentation is unclear as to whether the patient has a complication of the transplant, query the provider.

Z94.1   Heart transplant status
EXCLUDES 1   *artificial heart status (Z95.812)*
heart-valve replacement status (Z95.2-Z95.4)

Z94.2   Lung transplant status
Z94.3   Heart and lungs transplant status
Z94.4   Liver transplant status
Z94.5   Skin transplant status
Autogenous skin transplant status
Z94.6   Bone transplant status
Z94.7   Corneal transplant status
🄢 Z94.8   Other transplanted organ and tissue status
Z94.81   Bone marrow transplant status
Z94.82   Intestine transplant status
Z94.83   Pancreas transplant status
Z94.84   Stem cells transplant status
Z94.89   Other transplanted organ and tissue status
Z94.9   Transplanted organ and tissue status, unspecified

🄳 Z95   Presence of cardiac and vascular implants and grafts
EXCLUDES 1   *complications of cardiac and vascular devices, implants and grafts (T82.-)*

▲ **Z95.0   Presence of cardiac pacemaker**
Presence of cardiac resynchronization therapy (CRT-P) pacemaker
EXCLUDES 1   *adjustment or management of cardiac device (Z45.0-)*
adjustment or management of cardiac pacemaker (Z45.0)
presence of automatic (implantable) cardiac defibrillator with synchronous cardiac pacemaker (Z95.810)

▲ **Z95.1   Presence of aortocoronary bypass graft**
Presence of coronary artery bypass graft

● New   ▲ Revised   *Manifestation*   🄳-🄻 Digit Indicators   ⬡ Laterality   Ⓐ Adult (15+ years)   Ⓜ Maternity (12-55 years)   Ⓝ Newborn   Ⓟ Pediatric (0-17 years)   ♂ Male   ♀ Female
✖ Deleted   Unspecified   + Additional code

Z95.2 **Presence of prosthetic heart valve**
Presence of heart valve NOS

Z95.3 **Presence of xenogenic heart valve**

Z95.4 **Presence of other heart-valve replacement**

Z95.5 **Presence of coronary angioplasty implant and graft**
> EXCLUDES 1 *coronary angioplasty status without implant and graft (Z98.61)*

⑤ Z95.8 **Presence of other cardiac and vascular implants and grafts**

⑥ Z95.81 **Presence of other cardiac implants and grafts**

▲ Z95.810 **Presence of automatic (implantable) cardiac defibrillator**
Presence of automatic (implantable) cardiac defibrillator with synchronous cardiac pacemaker
Presence of cardiac resynchronization therapy defibrillator (CRT-D)
Presence of cardioverter-defibrillator (ICD)

Z95.811 **Presence of heart assist device**

Z95.812 **Presence of fully implantable artificial heart**

Z95.818 **Presence of other cardiac implants and grafts**

⑥ Z95.82 **Presence of other vascular implants and grafts**

Z95.820 **Peripheral vascular angioplasty status with implants and grafts**
> EXCLUDES 1 *peripheral vascular angioplasty without implant and graft (Z98.62)*

Z95.828 **Presence of other vascular implants and grafts**
Presence of intravascular prosthesis NEC

Z95.9 **Presence of cardiac and vascular implant and graft, unspecified**

④ Z96 **Presence of other functional implants**
> EXCLUDES 2 *complications of internal prosthetic devices, implants and grafts (T82-T85)*
> *fitting and adjustment of prosthetic and other devices (Z44-Z46)*

Z96.0 **Presence of urogenital implants**

Z96.1 **Presence of intraocular lens**
Presence of pseudophakia

⑤ Z96.2 **Presence of otological and audiological implants**

Z96.20 **Presence of otological and audiological implant, unspecified**

Z96.21 **Cochlear implant status**

Z96.22 **Myringotomy tube(s) status**

Z96.29 **Presence of other otological and audiological implants**
Presence of bone-conduction hearing device
Presence of eustachian tube stent
Stapes replacement

Z96.3 **Presence of artificial larynx**

⑤ Z96.4 **Presence of endocrine implants**

Z96.41 **Presence of insulin pump (external) (internal)**

Z96.49 **Presence of other endocrine implants**

Z96.5 **Presence of tooth-root and mandibular implants**

⑤ Z96.6 **Presence of orthopedic joint implants**

Z96.60 **Presence of unspecified orthopedic joint implant**

⑥ Z96.61 **Presence of artificial shoulder joint**

⊟ Z96.611 **Presence of right artificial shoulder joint**

⊟ Z96.612 **Presence of left artificial shoulder joint**

⊟ Z96.619 **Presence of unspecified artificial shoulder joint**

⑥ Z96.62 **Presence of artificial elbow joint**

⊟ Z96.621 **Presence of right artificial elbow joint**

⊟ Z96.622 **Presence of left artificial elbow joint**

⊟ Z96.629 **Presence of unspecified artificial elbow joint**

⑥ Z96.63 **Presence of artificial wrist joint**

⊟ Z96.631 **Presence of right artificial wrist joint**

⊟ Z96.632 **Presence of left artificial wrist joint**

⊟ Z96.639 **Presence of unspecified artificial wrist joint**

⑥ Z96.64 **Presence of artificial hip joint**
Hip-joint replacement (partial) (total)

⊟ Z96.641 **Presence of right artificial hip joint**

⊟ Z96.642 **Presence of left artificial hip joint**
AHA: 1Q 2015, 16

⊟ Z96.643 **Presence of artificial hip joint, bilateral**

⊟ Z96.649 **Presence of unspecified artificial hip joint**

⑥ Z96.65 **Presence of artificial knee joint**

⊟ Z96.651 **Presence of right artificial knee joint**

⊟ Z96.652 **Presence of left artificial knee joint**

⊟ Z96.653 **Presence of artificial knee joint, bilateral**

⊟ Z96.659 **Presence of unspecified artificial knee joint**

⑥ Z96.66 **Presence of artificial ankle joint**

⊟ Z96.661 **Presence of right artificial ankle joint**

⊟ Z96.662 **Presence of left artificial ankle joint**

⊟ Z96.669 **Presence of unspecified artificial ankle joint**

⑥ Z96.69 **Presence of other orthopedic joint implants**

⊟ Z96.691 **Finger-joint replacement of right hand**

⊟ Z96.692 **Finger-joint replacement of left hand**

⊟ Z96.693 **Finger-joint replacement, bilateral**

⊟ Z96.698 **Presence of other orthopedic joint implants**

Z96.7 **Presence of other bone and tendon implants**
Presence of skull plate

⑤ Z96.8 **Presence of other specified functional implants**

Z96.81 **Presence of artificial skin**

Z96.89 **Presence of other specified functional implants**

Z96.9 **Presence of functional implant, unspecified**

④ Z97 **Presence of other devices**
> EXCLUDES 1 *complications of internal prosthetic devices, implants and grafts (T82-T85)*
> *fitting and adjustment of prosthetic and other devices (Z44-Z46)*
> EXCLUDES 2 *presence of cerebrospinal fluid drainage device (Z98.2)*

Z97.0 **Presence of artificial eye**

⑤ Z97.1 **Presence of artificial limb (complete) (partial)**

⊟ Z97.10 **Presence of artificial limb (complete) (partial), unspecified**

⊟ Z97.11 **Presence of artificial right arm (complete) (partial)**

⊟ Z97.12 **Presence of artificial left arm (complete) (partial)**

⊟ Z97.13 **Presence of artificial right leg (complete) (partial)**

⊟ Z97.14 **Presence of artificial left leg (complete) (partial)**

⊟ Z97.15 **Presence of artificial arms, bilateral (complete) (partial)**

⊟ Z97.16 **Presence of artificial legs, bilateral (complete) (partial)**

Z97.2 **Presence of dental prosthetic device (complete) (partial)**
Presence of dentures (complete) (partial)

Z97.3 **Presence of spectacles and contact lenses**

Z97.4 **Presence of external hearing-aid**

▲ Z97.5 **Presence of (intrauterine) contraceptive device**   ♀ Ⓜ
> EXCLUDES 1 *checking, reinsertion or removal of implantable subdermal contraceptive (Z30.46)*
> *checking, reinsertion or removal of intrauterine contraceptive device (Z30.43-)*

Z97.8 **Presence of other specified devices**

④ Z98 **Other postprocedural states**
> EXCLUDES 2 *aftercare (Z43-Z49, Z51)*
> *follow-up medical care (Z08-Z09)*
> *postprocedural complication - see Alphabetical Index*

Z98.0 **Intestinal bypass and anastomosis status**
> EXCLUDES 2 *bariatric surgery status (Z98.84)*
> *gastric bypass status (Z98.84)*
> *obesity surgery status (Z98.84)*

Z98.1 **Arthrodesis status**

Z98.2 **Presence of cerebrospinal fluid drainage device**
Presence of CSF shunt

Z98.3 **Post therapeutic collapse of lung status**
Code first:
underlying disease

⑤+ Z98.4 **Cataract extraction status**
Use additional code to identify intraocular lens implant status (Z96.1)
> EXCLUDES 1 *aphakia (H27.0)*

⊟+ Z98.41 **Cataract extraction status, right eye**

⊟+ Z98.42 **Cataract extraction status, left eye**

⊟+ Z98.49 **Cataract extraction status, unspecified eye**

⑤ Z98.5 **Sterilization status**
> EXCLUDES 1 *female infertility (N97.-)*
> *male infertility (N46.-)*

Z98.51 **Tubal ligation status**   ♀

Z98.52 **Vasectomy status**   ♂ Ⓐ

⑤ Z98.6 **Angioplasty status**

● New   ▲ Revised   *Manifestation*   ④-⑦ Digit Indicators   ⊟ Laterality   Ⓐ Adult (15+ years)   Ⓜ Maternity (12-55 years)   Ⓝ Newborn   Ⓟ Pediatric (0-17 years)   ♂ Male   ♀ Female
✖ Deleted   Unspecified   + Additional code

1206   © 2017 DecisionHealth   2017 ICD-10-CM Expert for Physicians

Z98.61 Coronary angioplasty status
> EXCLUDES 1 *coronary angioplasty status with implant and graft (Z95.5)*

Z98.62 Peripheral vascular angioplasty status
> EXCLUDES 1 *peripheral vascular angioplasty status with implant and graft (Z95.820)*

Z98.8 Other specified postprocedural states

Z98.81 Dental procedure status

Z98.810 Dental sealant status

Z98.811 Dental restoration status
Dental crown status
Dental fillings status

Z98.818 Other dental procedure status

Z98.82 Breast implant status
> EXCLUDES 1 *breast implant removal status (Z98.86)*

Z98.83 Filtering (vitreous) bleb after glaucoma surgery status
> EXCLUDES 1 *Inflammation (infection) of postprocedural bleb (H59.4-)*

Z98.84 Bariatric surgery status
Gastric banding status
Gastric bypass status for obesity
Obesity surgery status
> EXCLUDES 1 *bariatric surgery status complicating pregnancy, childbirth, or the puerperium (O99.84)*
> EXCLUDES 2 *intestinal bypass and anastomosis status (Z98.0)*

Z98.85 Transplanted organ removal status
Transplanted organ previously removed due to complication, failure, rejection or infection
> EXCLUDES 1 *encounter for removal of transplanted organ -code to complication of transplanted organ (T86.-)*

> GUIDELINES **Section I.C.21.c.3)**
Assign code Z98.85, Transplanted organ removal status, to indicate that a transplanted organ has been previously removed. This code should not be assigned for the encounter in which the transplanted organ is removed. The complication necessitating removal of the transplant organ should be assigned for that encounter.

Z98.86 Personal history of breast implant removal

Z98.87 Personal history of in utero procedure

Z98.870 Personal history of in utero procedure during pregnancy ♀
> EXCLUDES 2 *complications from in utero procedure for current pregnancy (O35.7) supervision of current pregnancy with history of in utero procedure during previous pregnancy (O09.82-)*

Z98.871 Personal history of in utero procedure while a fetus

▲ **Z98.89 Other specified postprocedural states**

● **Z98.890 Other specified postprocedural states**
Personal history of surgery, not elsewhere classified

● **Z98.891 History of uterine scar from previous surgery** ♀
> EXCLUDES 1 *Maternal care due to uterine scar from previous surgery (O34.2-)*

Z99 Dependence on enabling machines and devices, not elsewhere classified
> EXCLUDES 1 *cardiac pacemaker status (Z95.0)*

Z99.0 Dependence on aspirator

Z99.1 Dependence on respirator
Dependence on ventilator

Z99.11 Dependence on respirator [ventilator] status
AHA: 1Q 2015, 21

Z99.12 Encounter for respirator [ventilator] dependence during power failure
> EXCLUDES 1 *mechanical complication of respirator [ventilator] (J95.850)*

▲ **Z99.2 Dependence on renal dialysis**
Hemodialysis status
Peritoneal dialysis status
Presence of arteriovenous shunt for dialysis
Renal dialysis status NOS
> EXCLUDES 1 *encounter for fitting and adjustment of dialysis catheter (Z49.0-)*
> EXCLUDES 2 *noncompliance with renal dialysis (Z91.15)*
AHA: 1Q 2016, 12-13

Z99.3 Dependence on wheelchair
Wheelchair confinement status
Code first cause of dependence, such as:
  muscular dystrophy (G71.0)
  obesity (E66.-)

Z99.8 Dependence on other enabling machines and devices

Z99.81 Dependence on supplemental oxygen
Dependence on long-term oxygen
AHA: 4Q 2013, 129

Z99.89 Dependence on other enabling machines and devices
Dependence on machine or device NOS

New ▲ Revised *Manifestation* 4-7 Digit Indicators Laterality Adult (15+ years) Maternity (12-55 years) Newborn Pediatric (0-17 years) Male Female Deleted Unspecified + Additional code

2017 ICD-10-CM Expert for Physicians   © 2017 DecisionHealth   1207

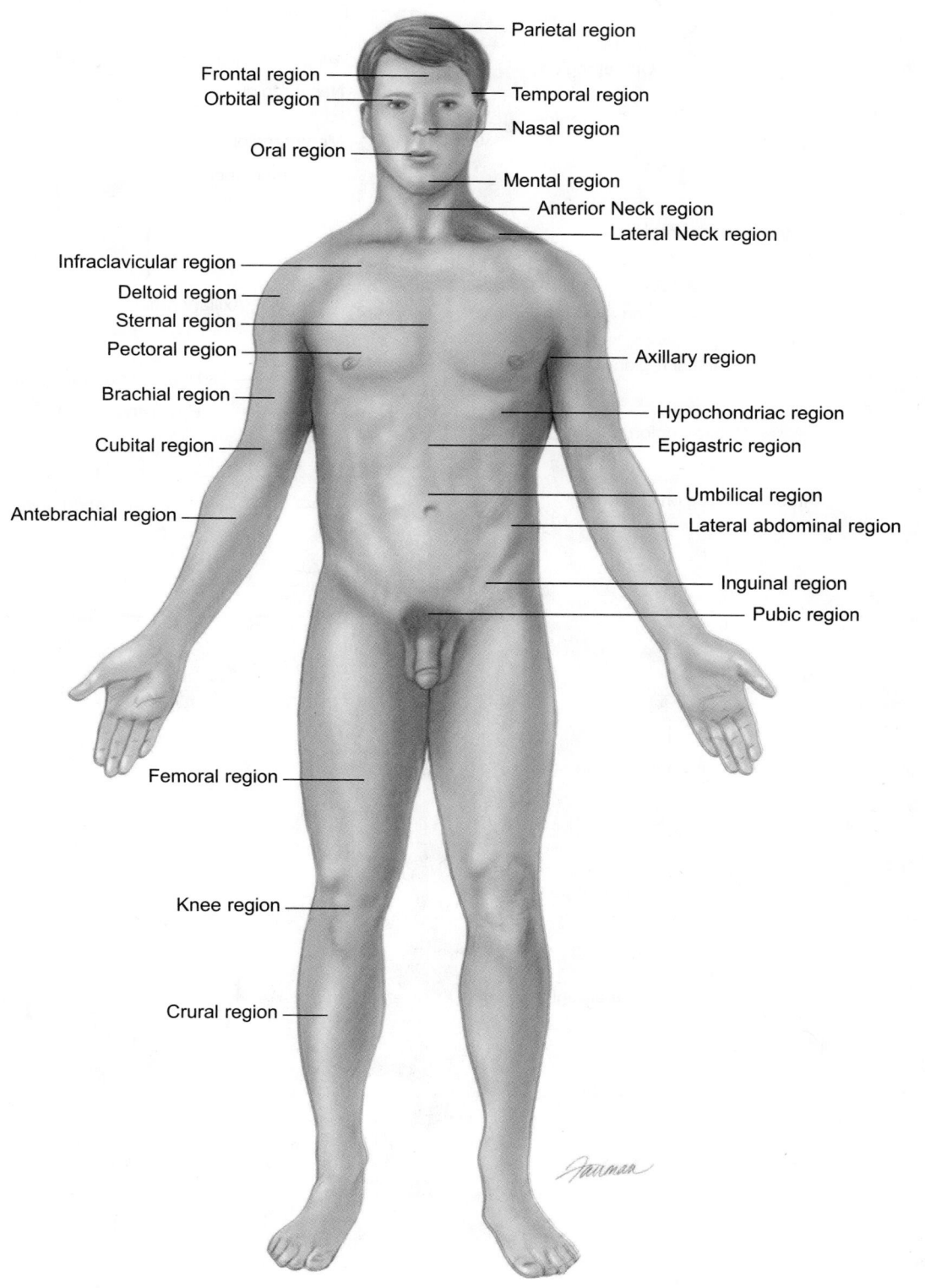

Male Figure
(Anterior View)

Parietal region

Frontal region

Orbital region

Temporal region

Nasal region

Oral region

Mental region

Anterior Neck region

Lateral Neck region

Infraclavicular region

Deltoid region

Sternal region

Pectoral region

Axillary region

Brachial region

Hypochondriac region

Cubital region

Epigastric region

Umbilical region

Antebrachial region

Lateral abdominal region

Inguinal region

Pubic region

Femoral region

Knee region

Crural region

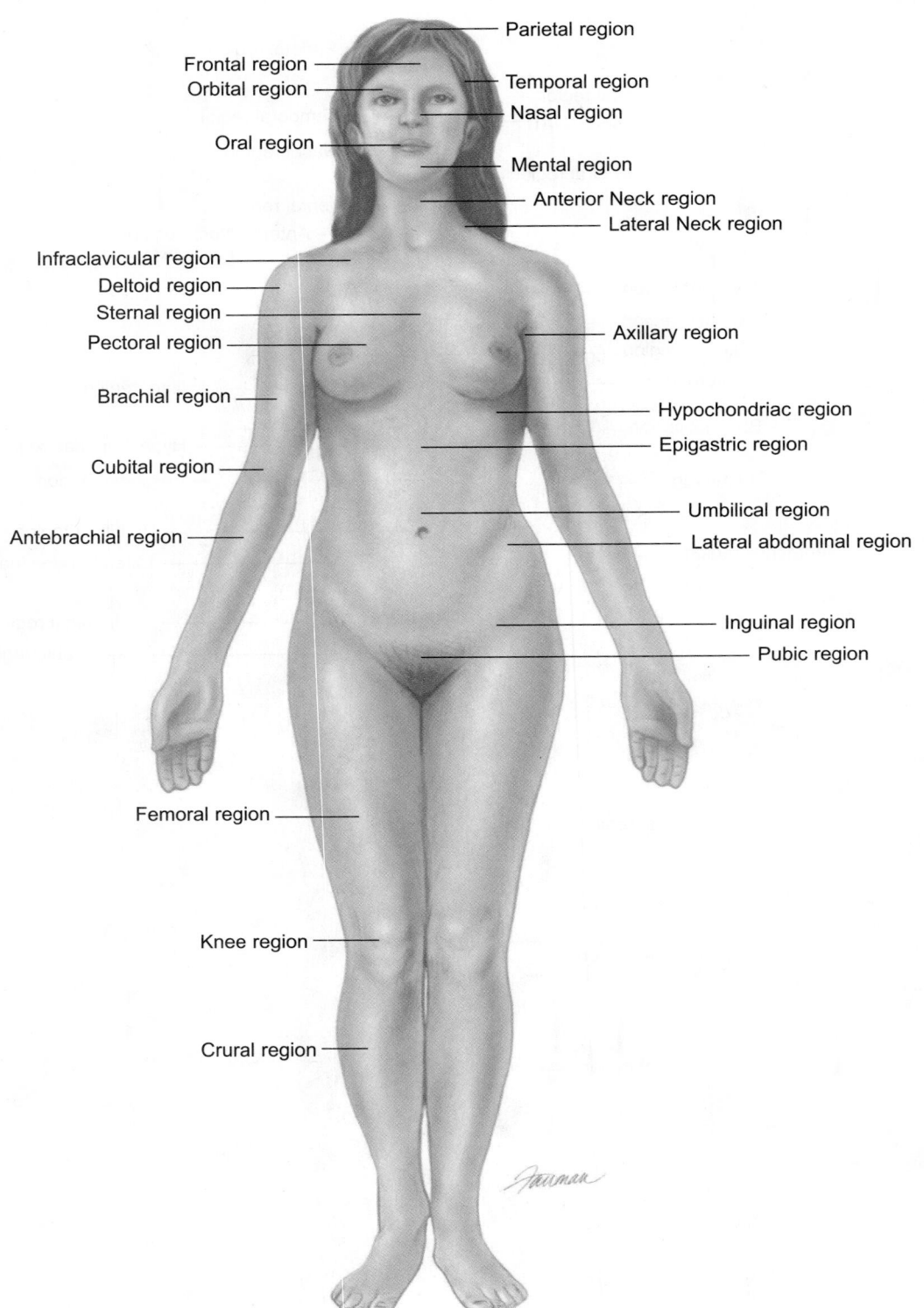

Female Figure
(Anterior View)

Parietal region

Frontal region

Temporal region

Orbital region

Nasal region

Oral region

Mental region

Anterior Neck region

Lateral Neck region

Infraclavicular region

Deltoid region

Sternal region

Pectoral region

Axillary region

Brachial region

Hypochondriac region

Epigastric region

Cubital region

Umbilical region

Antebrachial region

Lateral abdominal region

Inguinal region

Pubic region

Femoral region

Knee region

Crural region

Female Breast

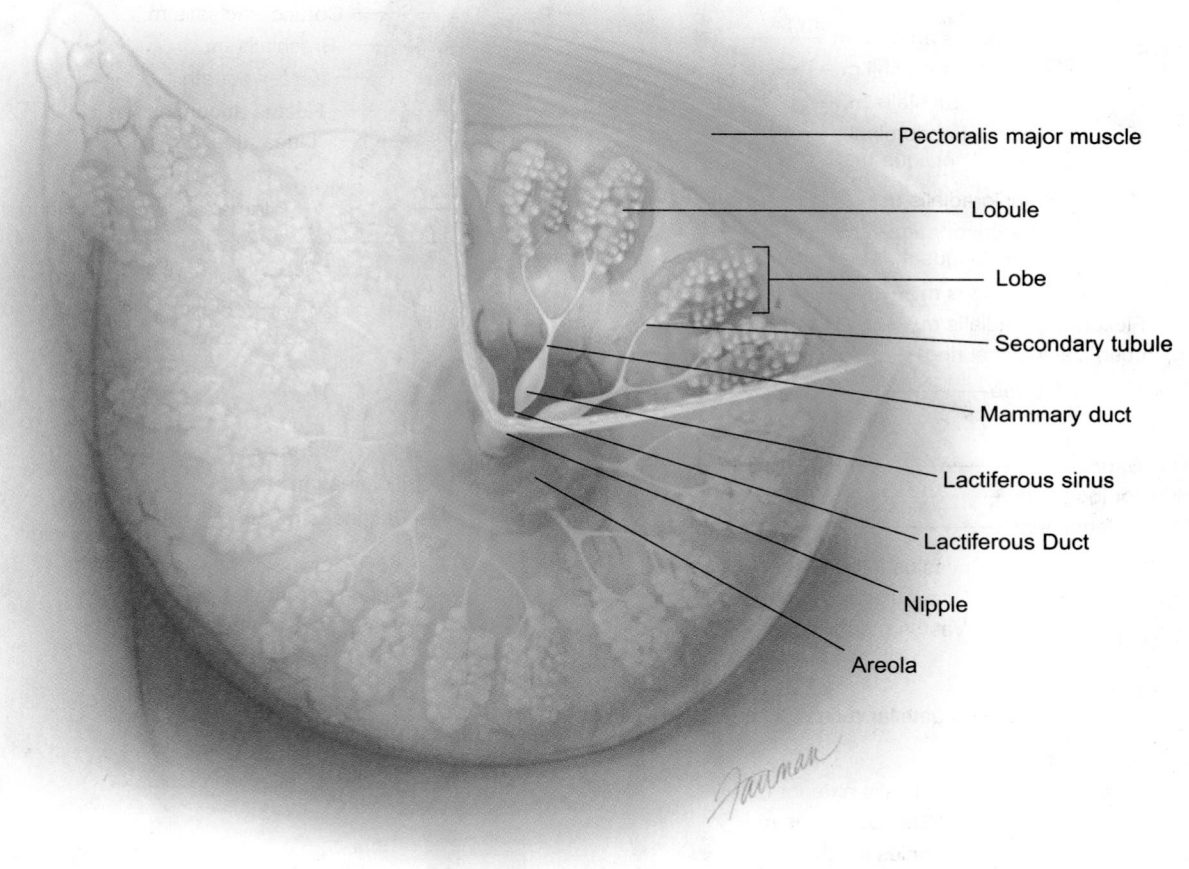

Pectoralis major muscle

Lobule

Lobe

Secondary tubule

Mammary duct

Lactiferous sinus

Lactiferous Duct

Nipple

Areola

Muscular System
(Anterior View)

Temporalis m.
Orbicularis oculi m.
Masseter m.
Buccinator m.
Sternocleidomastoid m.
Trapezius m.

Frontalis m.
Zygomaticus minor m.
Zygomaticus major m.
Orbicularis oris m.
Depressor anguli oris m.
Levator scapulae m.

Deltoid m.
Pectoralis major m.
Serratus anterior m.
Biceps brachii m.
Brachialis m.
External abdominal oblique m.
Brachioradialis m.
Extensor carpi radialis longus m.
Palmaris longus m.
Flexor carpi radialis m.
Superficial inguinal ring
Tensor fasciae latae m.
Sartorius m.
Adductor longus m.
Rectus femoris m.
Vastus lateralis m.
Iliotibial tract
Vastus medialis m.
Gracilis m.
Lateral patellar retinaculum
Tibialis anterior m.
Gastrocnemius m.
Peronius longus m.
Peronius brevis m.
Soleus m.
Extensor digitorum longus m.
Extensor hallucis longus m.
Extensor hallucis brevis m.

Pectoralis minor m.
Internal intercostal mm.
Coracobrachialis m.
Brachialis m.
Rectus sheath
Rectus abdominus m.
Linea alba
Internal abdominal oblique m.
Transversus abdominus m.
Palmaris longus m.
Flexor pollicis longus m.
Flexor digitorum superficialis m.
Abductor pollicis brevis m.
Flexor pollicis brevis m.
Abductor digiti minimi m.
Iliopsoas m.
Pectineus m.
Adductor brevis m.
Adductor magnus m.
Vastus lateralis m.
Vastus medialis m.
Patella
Patellar ligament
Medial patellar retinaculum
Tibia
Flexor digitorum longus m.
Abductor hallucis m.

Scanne

Muscular System
(Posterior View)

Galea aponeurotica

Temporalis m.

Occipitotemporalis m.

Sternocleidomastoid m.

Occipitalis m.

Splenius capitis m.

Splenius cervicis m.

Trapezius m.

Deltoid m.

Infraspinatus m.

Teres minor m.

Teres major m.

Triceps m.

Latissimus dorsi m.

Brachioradialis m.

Extensor carpi
radialis longus m.

Flexor carpi ulnaris m.

Extensor digitorum m.

Extensor carpi
radialis brevis m.

Extensor carpi ulnaris m.

Abductor pollicis longus m.

Extensor pollicis
brevis m.

Extensor pollicis
longus t.

Gluteus medius m.

Gluteus maximus m.

Adductor
magnus m.

Biceps femoris m.

Iliotibial tract

Semitendinosis m.

Semimembranosis m.

Gastrocnemius m.

Soleus m.

Peroneus longus m.

Calcaneal t. (Achilles)

Levator scapulae m.

Supraspinatus m.

Rhomboid minor m.

Rhomboid major m.

Spinalis thoracis m.

Iliocostalis thoracis m.

Longissimus thoracis m.

Serratus posterior inferior m.

External abdominal oblique m.

Anconius m.

Supinator m.

Gluteus minimus m.

Piriformis m.

Superior gemellus m.

Obturator internus m.

Inferior gemellus m.

Quadratus femoris m.

Adductor magnus m.

Gracilis m.

Biceps femoris m.

Semimembranosus m.

Gastrocnemius m. (cut)

Plantaris m. (cut)

Popliteus m.

Soleus m. (cut)

Tibialis posterior m.

Flexor digitorum longus m.

Flexor hallucis longus m.

Peroneus longus m.

Peroneus brevis m.

Anatomy Illustrations

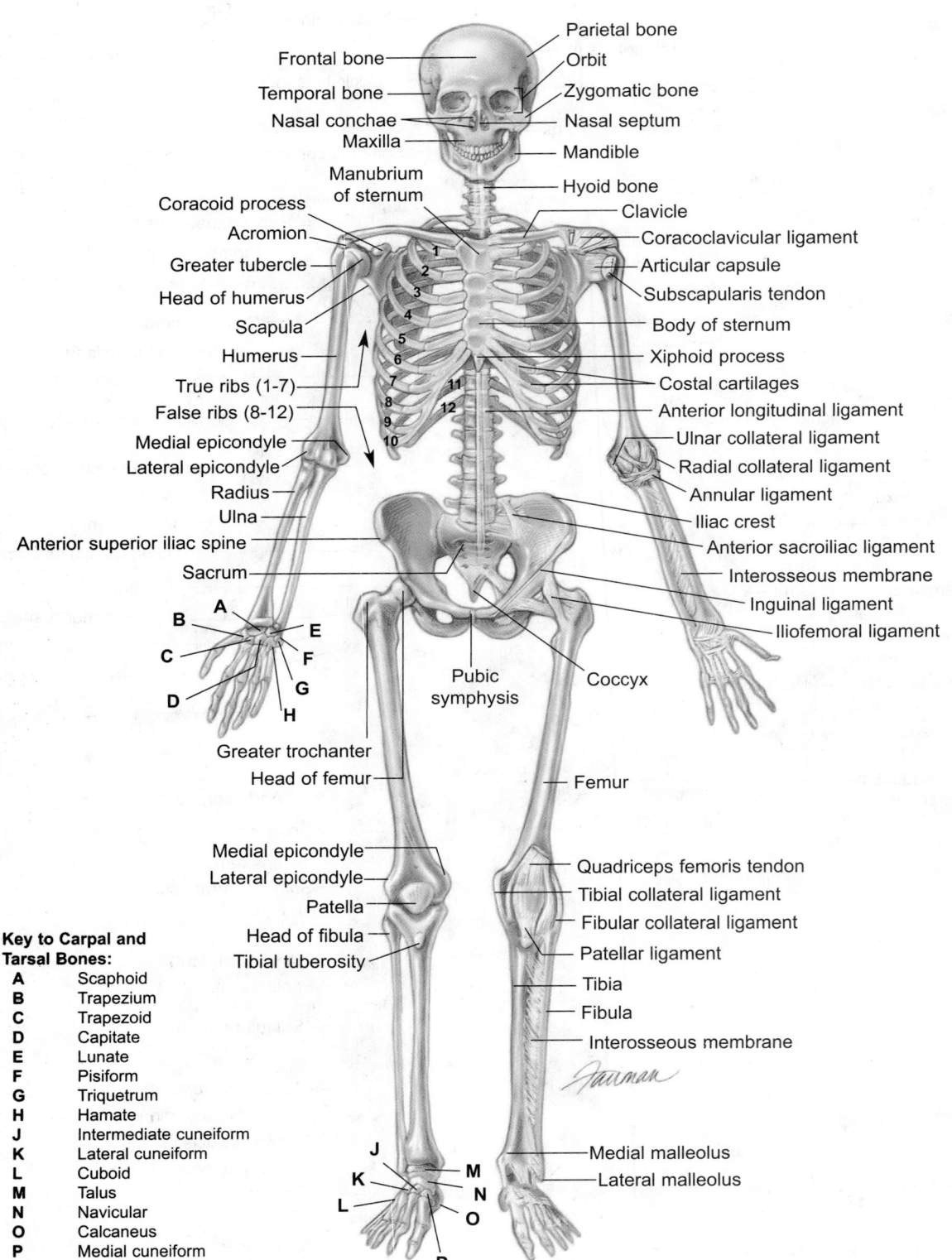

Skeletal System
(Anterior View)

Parietal bone

Frontal bone

Orbit

Temporal bone

Zygomatic bone

Nasal conchae

Nasal septum

Maxilla

Mandible

Manubrium of sternum

Hyoid bone

Coracoid process

Clavicle

Acromion

Coracoclavicular ligament

Greater tubercle

Articular capsule

Head of humerus

Subscapularis tendon

Scapula

Body of sternum

Humerus

Xiphoid process

True ribs (1-7)

Costal cartilages

False ribs (8-12)

Anterior longitudinal ligament

Medial epicondyle

Ulnar collateral ligament

Lateral epicondyle

Radial collateral ligament

Radius

Annular ligament

Ulna

Iliac crest

Anterior superior iliac spine

Anterior sacroiliac ligament

Sacrum

Interosseous membrane

Inguinal ligament

Iliofemoral ligament

Pubic symphysis

Coccyx

Greater trochanter

Head of femur

Femur

Medial epicondyle

Quadriceps femoris tendon

Lateral epicondyle

Tibial collateral ligament

Patella

Fibular collateral ligament

Head of fibula

Patellar ligament

Tibial tuberosity

Tibia

Fibula

Interosseous membrane

Medial malleolus

Lateral malleolus

Key to Carpal and Tarsal Bones:

A	Scaphoid
B	Trapezium
C	Trapezoid
D	Capitate
E	Lunate
F	Pisiform
G	Triquetrum
H	Hamate
J	Intermediate cuneiform
K	Lateral cuneiform
L	Cuboid
M	Talus
N	Navicular
O	Calcaneus
P	Medial cuneiform

Skeletal System
(Posterior View)

Parietal bone
Occipital bone
Temporal bone
Atlas (C1)
Axis (C2)

Mastoid process
Mandible

Clavicle

Supraspinous fossa
Acromion
Infraspinatus tendon
Teres minor tendon
Scapula

1
2
3
4
5
6
7
8
9
10
11
12

Scapular notch
Spine of scapula
Greater tubercle
Head of humerus
Infraspinous fossa
Humerus

Ulnar collateral ligament
Radial collateral ligament
Annular ligament
Radius
Ulna
Ilium
Posterior sacroiliac ligament
Iliofemoral ligament
Ischiofemoral ligament
Sacrotuberous ligament

Medial epicondyle
Lateral epicondyle
Head of radius
Olecranon of ulna
Posterior superior iliac spine
Sacrum
Greater sciatic notch
Head of femur
Greater trochanter

E
A
F
B
C
G
D

Metacarpals

Phalanges

Tibial colateral ligament
Medial meniscus
Anterior cruciate ligament
Fibular collateral ligament
Lateral meniscus
Posterior cruciate ligament

Medial epicondyle
Lateral epicondyle
Lateral condyles
Head of fibula
Medial condyles
Tibia
Fibula

Interosseous membrane

Key to Carpal Bones:

A	Lunate
B	Triquetrum
C	Hamate
D	Capitate
E	Scaphoid
F	Trapezium
G	Trapezoid

Medial malleolus
Lateral malleolus
Metatarsals
Talus
Calcaneus

Posterior tibiofibular ligament
Posterior talofibular ligament
Calcaneal (Achilles) tendon

Skeletal System
(Vertebral Column – Left Lateral View)

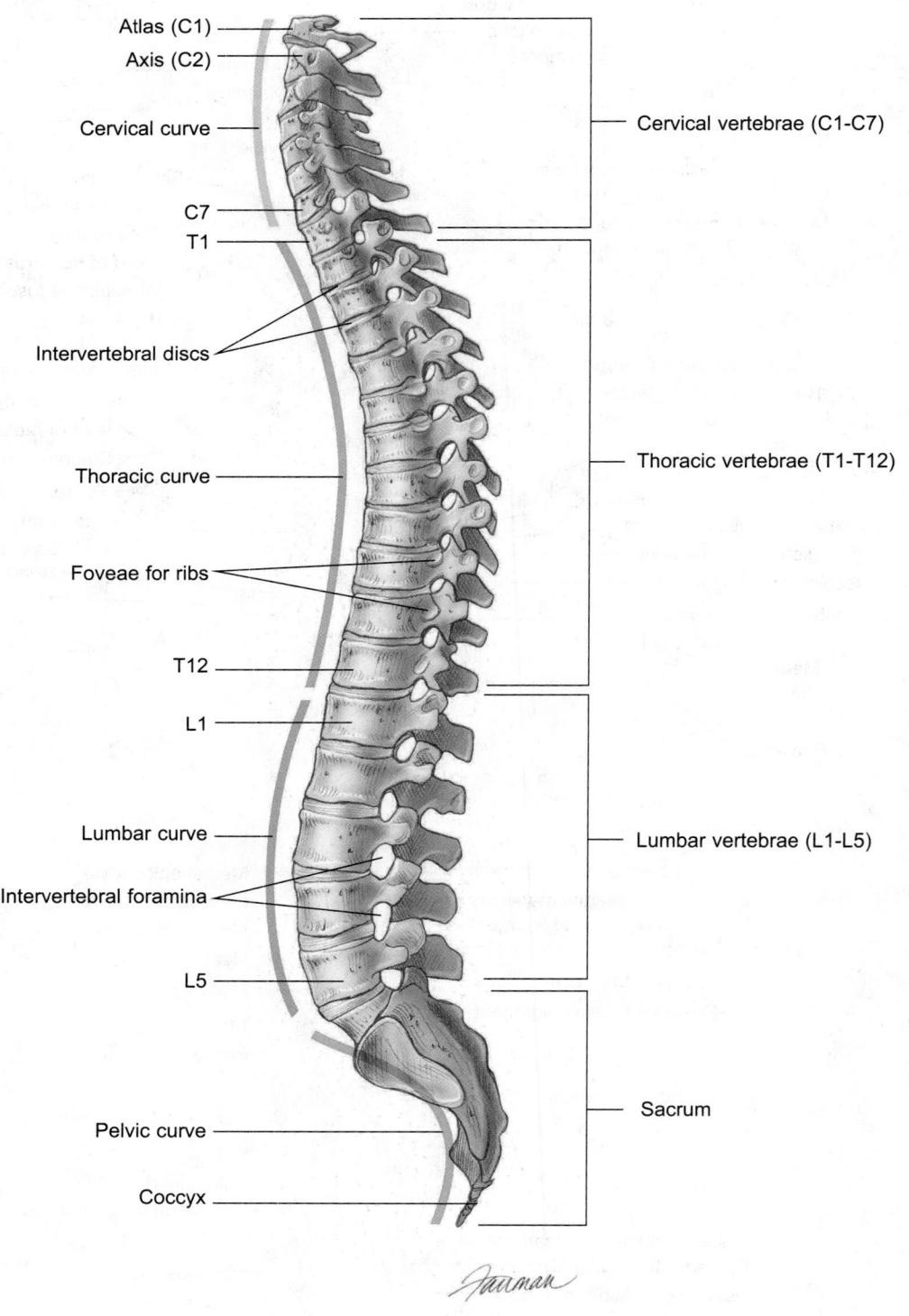

Atlas (C1)

Axis (C2)

Cervical curve

Cervical vertebrae (C1-C7)

C7

T1

Intervertebral discs

Thoracic curve

Thoracic vertebrae (T1-T12)

Foveae for ribs

T12

L1

Lumbar curve

Lumbar vertebrae (L1-L5)

Intervertebral foramina

L5

Sacrum

Pelvic curve

Coccyx

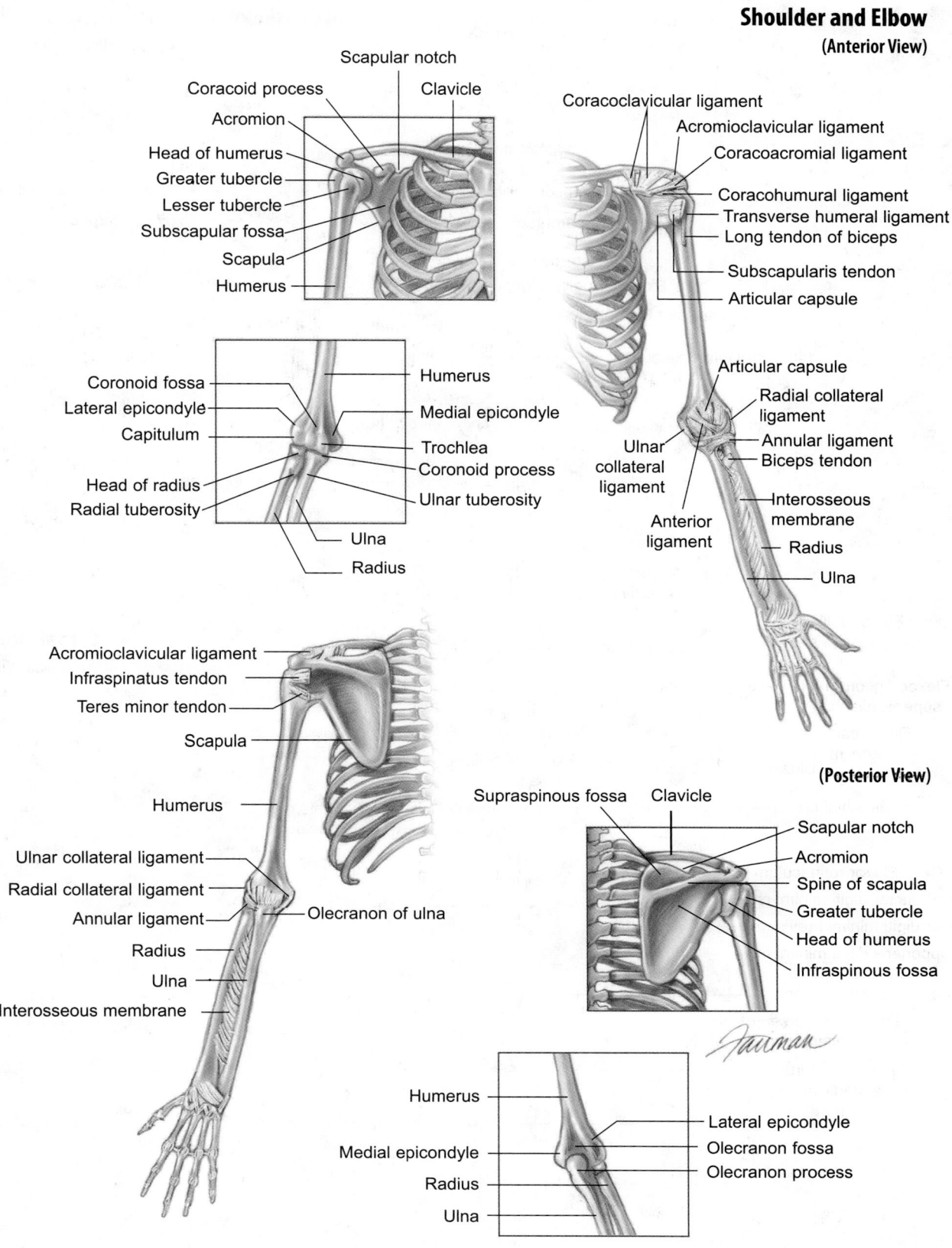

Shoulder and Elbow
(Anterior View)

Scapular notch
Coracoid process
Clavicle
Acromion
Head of humerus
Greater tubercle
Lesser tubercle
Subscapular fossa
Scapula
Humerus

Coracoclavicular ligament
Acromioclavicular ligament
Coracoacromial ligament
Coracohumural ligament
Transverse humeral ligament
Long tendon of biceps
Subscapularis tendon
Articular capsule

Coronoid fossa
Lateral epicondyle
Capitulum
Head of radius
Radial tuberosity
Humerus
Medial epicondyle
Trochlea
Coronoid process
Ulnar tuberosity
Ulna
Radius

Articular capsule
Radial collateral ligament
Annular ligament
Biceps tendon
Ulnar collateral ligament
Interosseous membrane
Anterior ligament
Radius
Ulna

Acromioclavicular ligament
Infraspinatus tendon
Teres minor tendon
Scapula
Humerus
Ulnar collateral ligament
Radial collateral ligament
Annular ligament
Olecranon of ulna
Radius
Ulna
Interosseous membrane

(Posterior View)

Supraspinous fossa
Clavicle
Scapular notch
Acromion
Spine of scapula
Greater tubercle
Head of humerus
Infraspinous fossa

Humerus
Medial epicondyle
Radius
Ulna
Lateral epicondyle
Olecranon fossa
Olecranon process

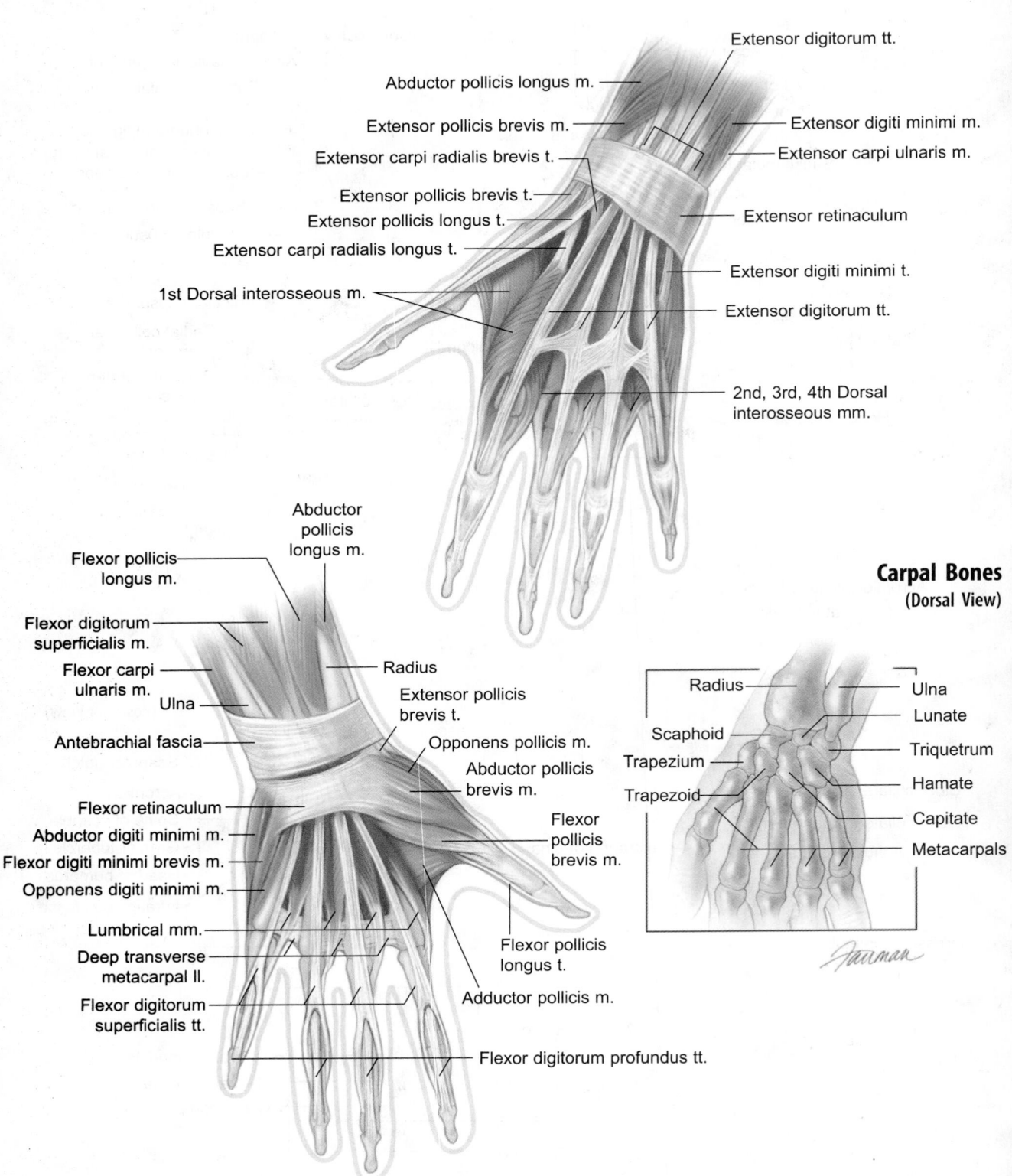

Musculoskeletal System – Hand and Wrist
(Dorsal and Palmar Views)

Extensor digitorum tt.

Abductor pollicis longus m.

Extensor pollicis brevis m.

Extensor carpi radialis brevis t.

Extensor pollicis brevis t.

Extensor pollicis longus t.

Extensor carpi radialis longus t.

1st Dorsal interosseous m.

Extensor digiti minimi m.

Extensor carpi ulnaris m.

Extensor retinaculum

Extensor digiti minimi t.

Extensor digitorum tt.

2nd, 3rd, 4th Dorsal interosseous mm.

Abductor pollicis longus m.

Flexor pollicis longus m.

Flexor digitorum superficialis m.

Flexor carpi ulnaris m.

Ulna

Antebrachial fascia

Flexor retinaculum

Abductor digiti minimi m.

Flexor digiti minimi brevis m.

Opponens digiti minimi m.

Lumbrical mm.

Deep transverse metacarpal ll.

Flexor digitorum superficialis tt.

Radius

Extensor pollicis brevis t.

Opponens pollicis m.

Abductor pollicis brevis m.

Flexor pollicis brevis m.

Flexor pollicis longus t.

Adductor pollicis m.

Flexor digitorum profundus tt.

Carpal Bones
(Dorsal View)

Radius

Scaphoid

Trapezium

Trapezoid

Ulna

Lunate

Triquetrum

Hamate

Capitate

Metacarpals

Fairman

Musculoskeletal System – Hip and Knee
(Anterior and Posterior Views)

Posterior sacroiliac ligament

Ilium

Sacrotuberous ligament

Iliofemoral ligament

Ischiofemoral ligament

Femur

Ischium

Posterior superior iliac spine

Sacrum

Greater sciatic notch

Sacral promontory

Sacrum

Iliac crest

Anterior superior iliac spine

Ilium

Anterior inferior iliac spine

Greater trochanter

Head of femur

Lesser trochanter

Spine of ischium

Obturator foramen

Pubis

Anterior longitudinal ligament

Iliolumbar ligament

Anterior scaroiliac ligament

Coccyx

Sacrotuberous ligament

Sacrospinous ligament

Iliofemoral ligament

Pubofemoral ligament

Inguinal ligament

Obturator membrane

Pubic symphysis

Femur

Medial epicondyle

Lateral epicondyle

Patella

Lateral condyles

Head of fibula

Tibial tuberosity

Medial condyles

Quadriceps femoris tendon

Medial patellar retinaculum

Fibular collateral ligament

Tibial collateral ligament

Lateral patellar retinaculum

Patellar ligament

Tibia

Fibula

Interosseous membrane

Tibial collateral ligament

Medial meniscus

Anterior cruciate ligament

Fibular collateral ligament

Lateral meniscus

Posterior cruciate ligament

Femur

Tibia

Fibula

Musculoskeletal System – Foot and Ankle

Tibialis anterior m.

Extensor digitorum longus m.

Tibia

Fibula

Superior extensor retinaculum

Medial malleolus

Lateral malleolus

Inferior extensor retinaculum

Extensor digitorum brevis m.

Extensor hallicus brevis m.

Peronius tertius m.

Extensor hallicus longus t.

Tuberosity of 5th metatarsal

Extensor digitorum longus tt.

Abductor hallucis m.

Extensor digitorum brevis m.

Dorsal interosseus mm.

Opponens digiti minimi m.

Middle phalanges

Distal phalanges

Proximal phalanges

Metatarsals

Medial cuneiform

Intermediate cuneiform

Lateral cuneiform

Navicular

Cuboid

Talus

Calcaneus

Vascular System

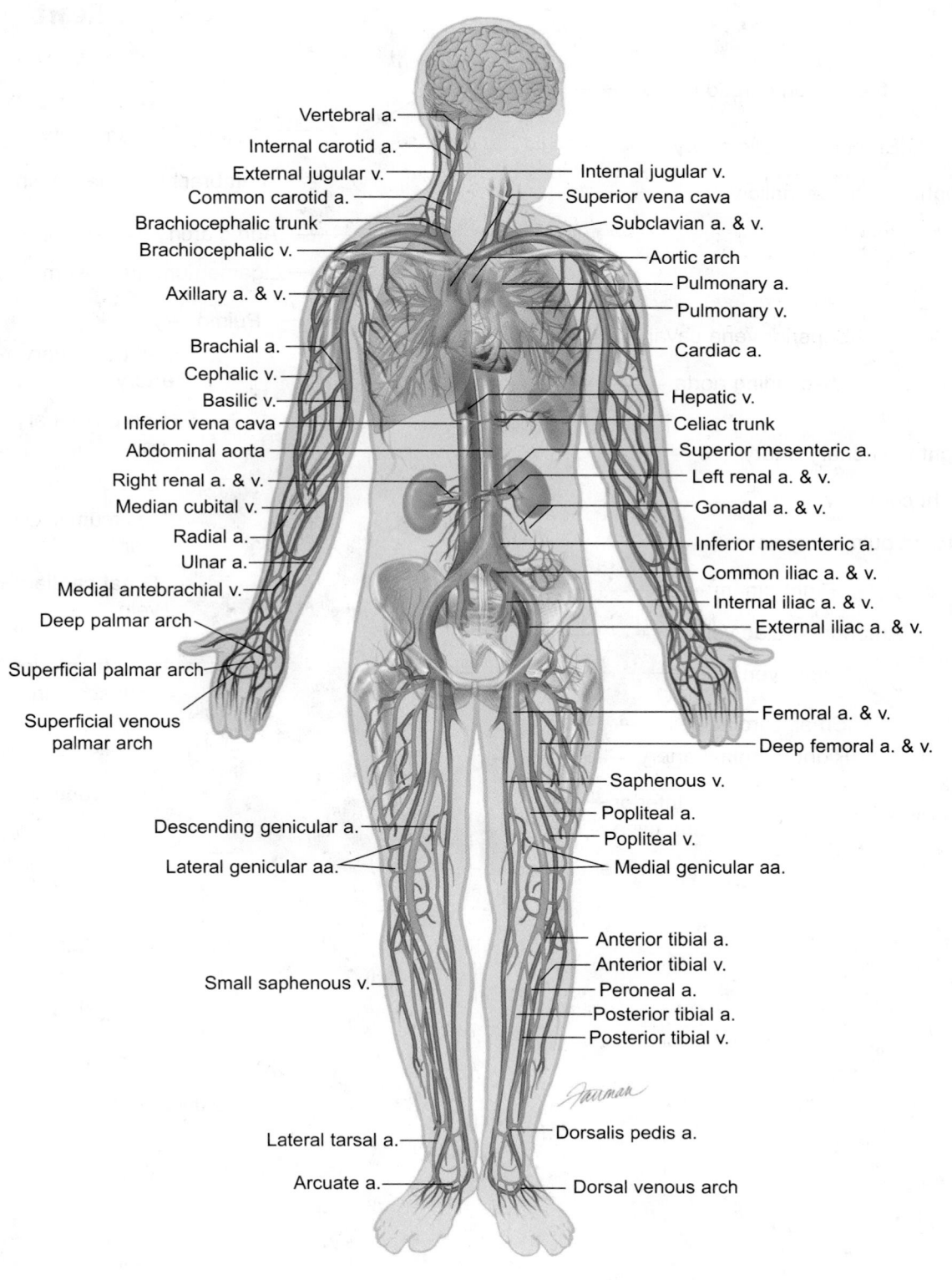

Vertebral a.
Internal carotid a.
External jugular v.
Common carotid a.
Brachiocephalic trunk
Brachiocephalic v.
Axillary a. & v.
Brachial a.
Cephalic v.
Basilic v.
Inferior vena cava
Abdominal aorta
Right renal a. & v.
Median cubital v.
Radial a.
Ulnar a.
Medial antebrachial v.
Deep palmar arch
Superficial palmar arch
Superficial venous palmar arch
Descending genicular a.
Lateral genicular aa.
Small saphenous v.
Lateral tarsal a.
Arcuate a.

Internal jugular v.
Superior vena cava
Subclavian a. & v.
Aortic arch
Pulmonary a.
Pulmonary v.
Cardiac a.
Hepatic v.
Celiac trunk
Superior mesenteric a.
Left renal a. & v.
Gonadal a. & v.
Inferior mesenteric a.
Common iliac a. & v.
Internal iliac a. & v.
External iliac a. & v.
Femoral a. & v.
Deep femoral a. & v.
Saphenous v.
Popliteal a.
Popliteal v.
Medial genicular aa.
Anterior tibial a.
Anterior tibial v.
Peroneal a.
Posterior tibial a.
Posterior tibial v.
Dorsalis pedis a.
Dorsal venous arch

Heart
(External View)

Left common carotid artery

Brachiocephalic artery

Right brachiocephalic vein

Left subclavian artery

Left brachiocephalic vein

Aortic arch

Ligamentum arteriosum

Superior vena cava

Ascending aorta

Pulmonary trunk

Left pulmonary artery

Left pulmonary vein

Right pulmonary artery

Right coronary artery

Right pulmonary vein

Right atrium

Anterior cardiac vein

Right ventricle

Small cardiac vein

Right marginal artery

Inferior vena cava

Descending aorta

Left auricle

Circumflex artery

Great cardiac vein

Left anterior descending artery

Left ventricle

Apex

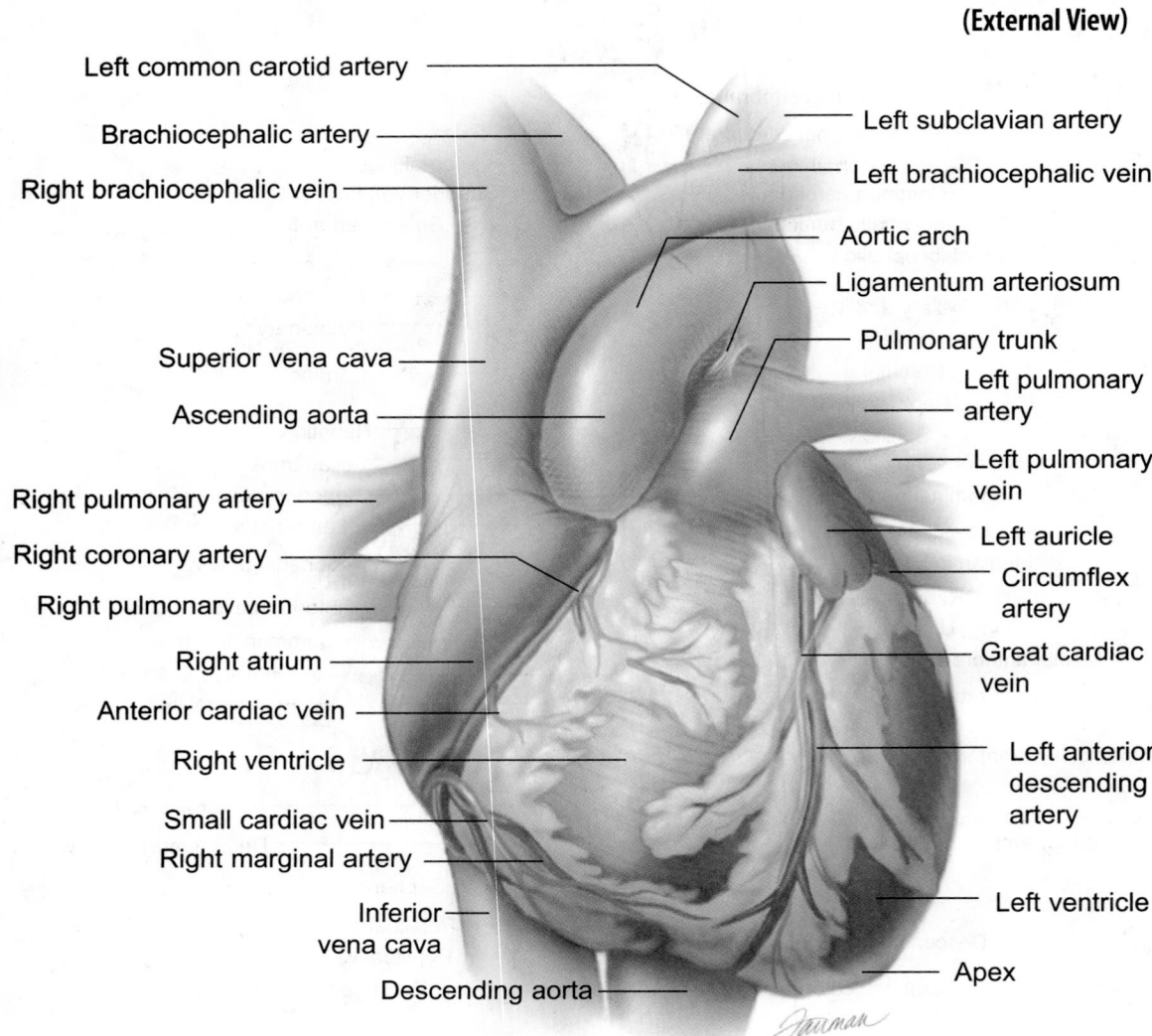

Heart
(Internal View)

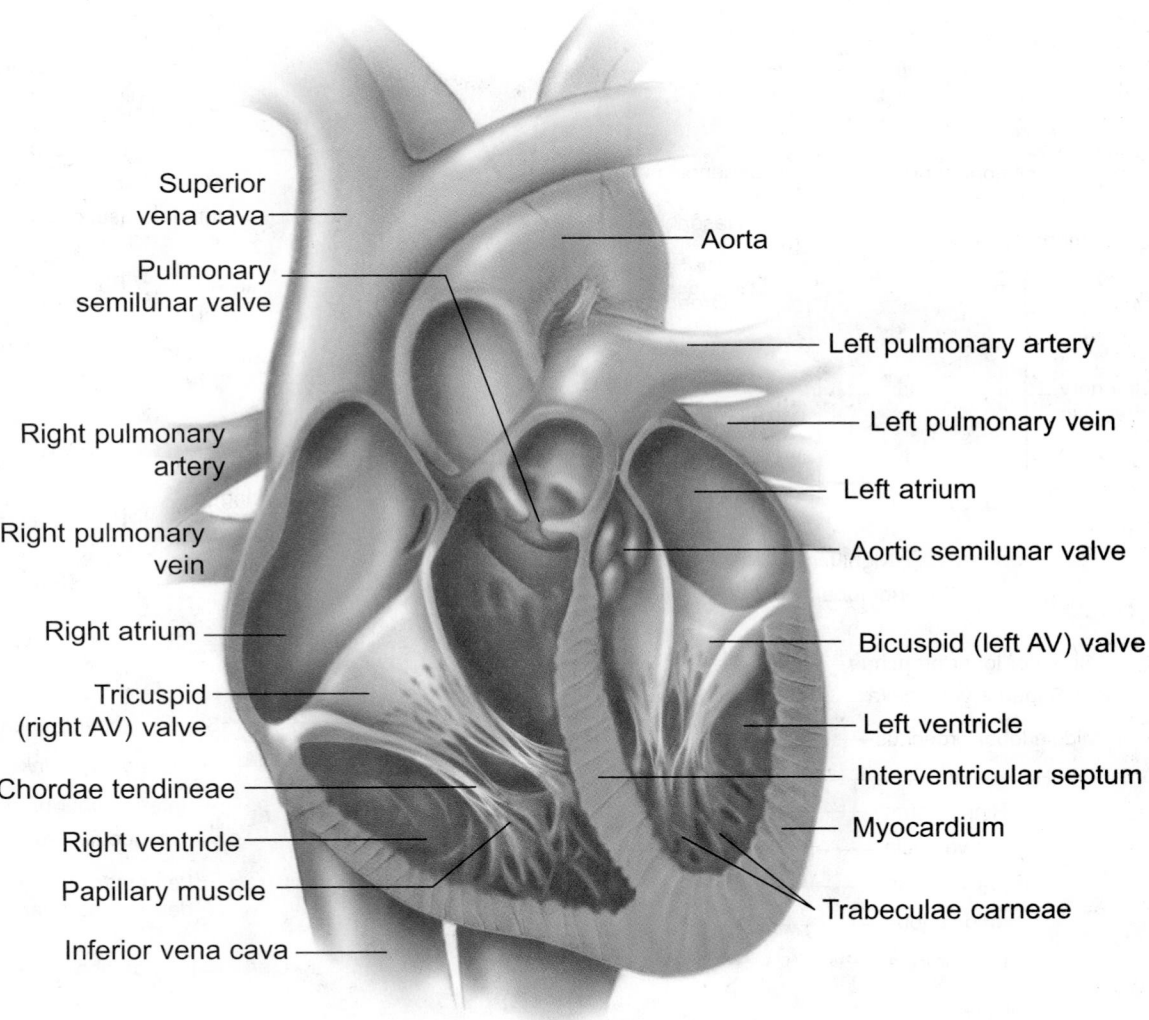

Superior vena cava

Pulmonary semilunar valve

Right pulmonary artery

Right pulmonary vein

Right atrium

Tricuspid (right AV) valve

Chordae tendineae

Right ventricle

Papillary muscle

Inferior vena cava

Aorta

Left pulmonary artery

Left pulmonary vein

Left atrium

Aortic semilunar valve

Bicuspid (left AV) valve

Left ventricle

Interventricular septum

Myocardium

Trabeculae carneae

Respiratory System

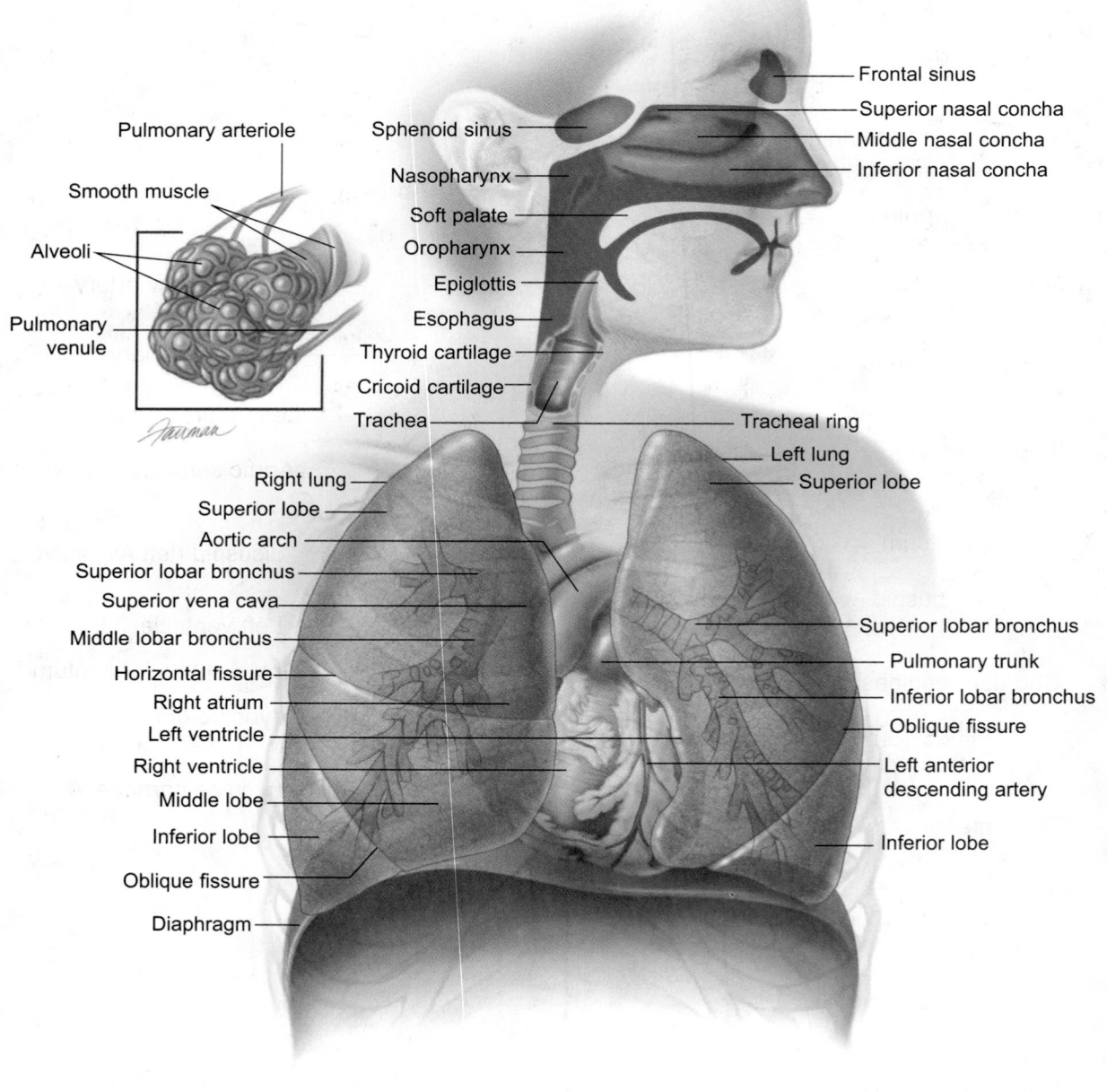

Pulmonary arteriole

Smooth muscle

Alveoli

Pulmonary venule

Sphenoid sinus

Nasopharynx

Soft palate

Oropharynx

Epiglottis

Esophagus

Thyroid cartilage

Cricoid cartilage

Trachea

Frontal sinus

Superior nasal concha

Middle nasal concha

Inferior nasal concha

Tracheal ring

Left lung

Superior lobe

Right lung

Superior lobe

Aortic arch

Superior lobar bronchus

Superior vena cava

Middle lobar bronchus

Horizontal fissure

Right atrium

Left ventricle

Right ventricle

Middle lobe

Inferior lobe

Oblique fissure

Diaphragm

Superior lobar bronchus

Pulmonary trunk

Inferior lobar bronchus

Oblique fissure

Left anterior descending artery

Inferior lobe

Digestive System

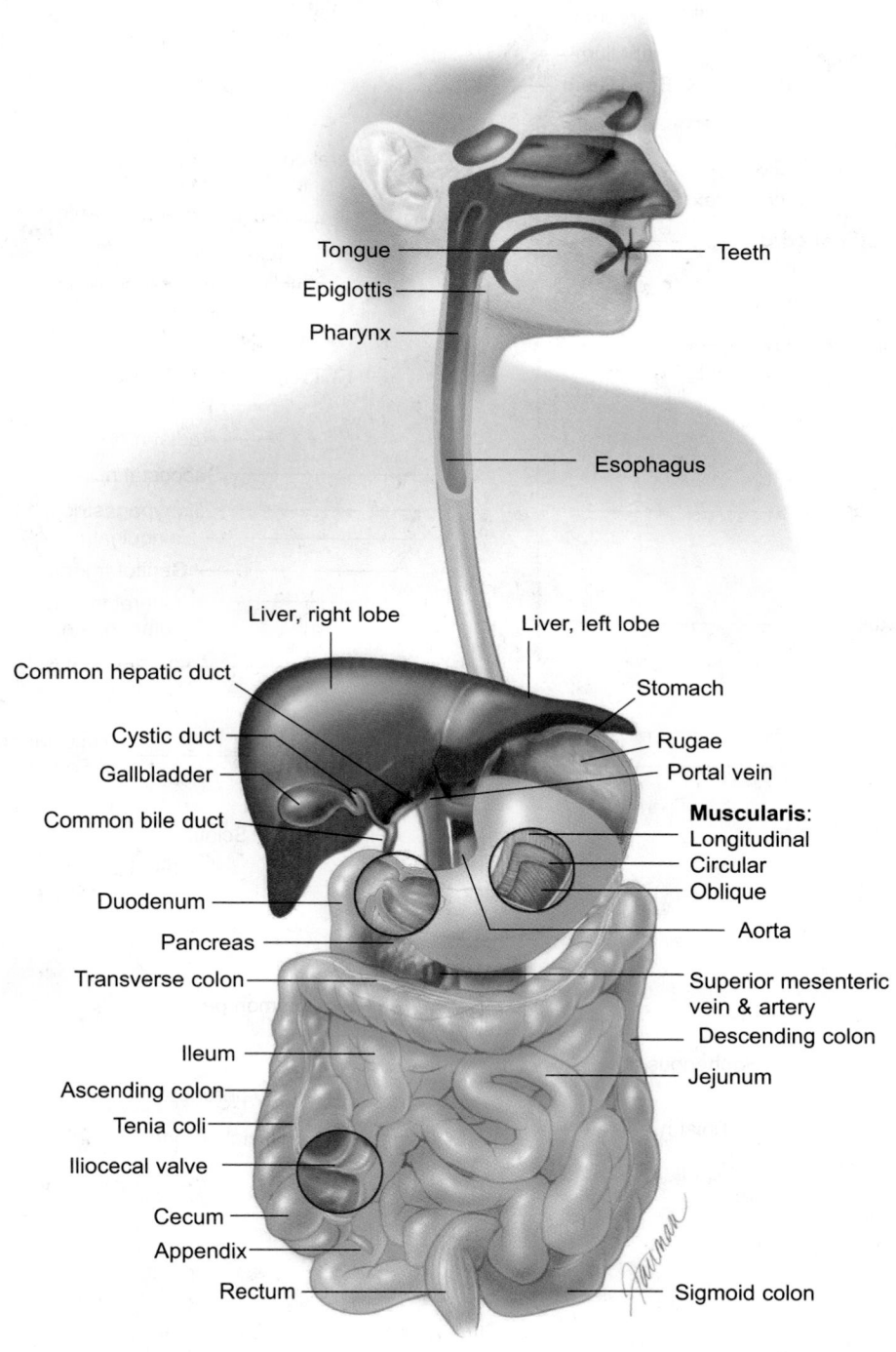

Tongue — Teeth

Epiglottis

Pharynx

Esophagus

Liver, right lobe — Liver, left lobe

Common hepatic duct — Stomach

Cystic duct — Rugae

Gallbladder — Portal vein

Common bile duct — **Muscularis:**
Longitudinal
Circular
Oblique

Duodenum

Pancreas — Aorta

Transverse colon — Superior mesenteric vein & artery

Ileum — Descending colon

Ascending colon — Jejunum

Tenia coli

Iliocecal valve

Cecum

Appendix

Rectum — Sigmoid colon

Nervous System

Brain
(Inferior View)

Cerebrum

Anterior communicating a.

Anterior cerebral a.

Internal carotid a.

Middle cerebral a.

Posterior communicating a.

Posterior cerebral a.

Superior cerebellar a.

Pontine aa.

Basilar a.

Pons

Vertebral a.

Anterior inferior cerebellar a.

Anterior spinal a.

Cerebellum

Posterior inferior cerebellar a.

Spinal cord

Olfactory bulb

Olfactory tract (I)

Optic chiasm

Optic n. (II)

Pituitary gland

Oculomotor n. (III)

Trochlear n. (IV)

Trigeminal n. (V)

Abducens n. (VI)

Facial n. (VII)

Vestibulo-cochlear n.(VIII)

Glosso-pharyngeal n. (IX)

Vagus n. (X)

Hypoglossal n. (XII)

Accessory n. (XI)

Cervical n. I

Medulla oblongata

Cervical n. II

Trigeminal Nerve (V) branches:
A   Ophthalmic branch
B   Maxillary branch
C   Mandibular branch

The Right Eye
(Transverse Section)

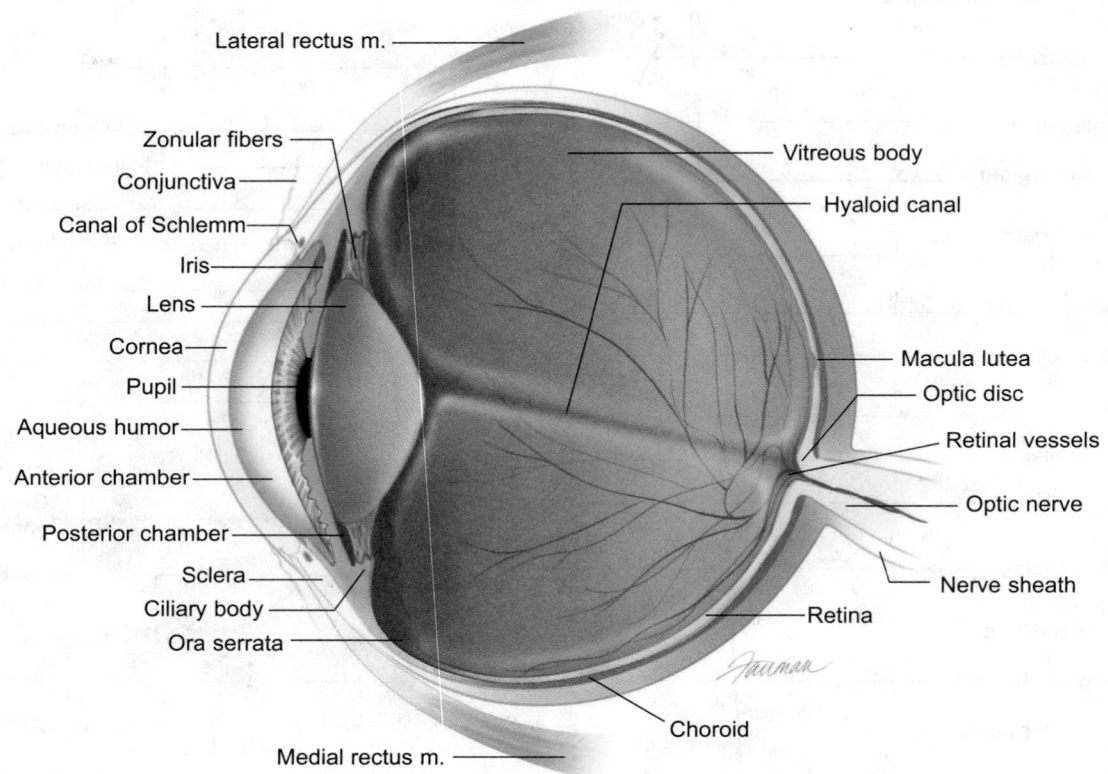

Lateral rectus m.

Zonular fibers

Conjunctiva

Canal of Schlemm

Iris

Lens

Cornea

Pupil

Aqueous humor

Anterior chamber

Posterior chamber

Sclera

Ciliary body

Ora serrata

Medial rectus m.

Vitreous body

Hyaloid canal

Macula lutea

Optic disc

Retinal vessels

Optic nerve

Nerve sheath

Retina

Choroid

The Right Ear

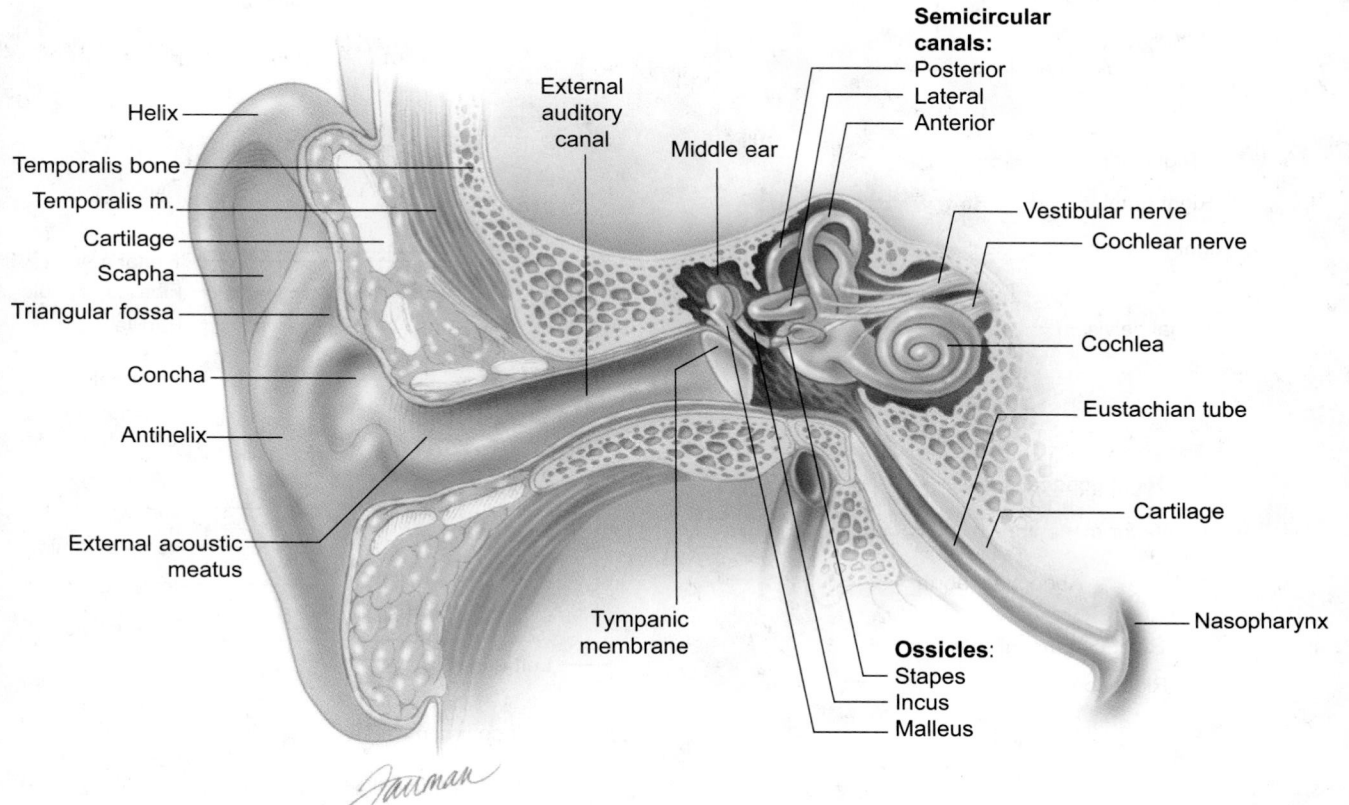

Helix

Temporalis bone

Temporalis m.

Cartilage

Scapha

Triangular fossa

Concha

Antihelix

External acoustic
meatus

External
auditory
canal

Middle ear

Tympanic
membrane

**Semicircular
canals:**
Posterior
Lateral
Anterior

Vestibular nerve

Cochlear nerve

Cochlea

Eustachian tube

Cartilage

Nasopharynx

Ossicles:
Stapes
Incus
Malleus

Urinary System

Celiac trunk

Supererior mesenteric a.

Adrenal gland

Inferior vena cava

Adrenal gland

Right kidney

Right renal v.

Right renal aa.

Renal pelvis

Left kidney

Renal a.

Fibrous capsule

Papilla

Minor calyx

Branches of renal artery

Major calyx

Cortex

Renal pyramid

Renal column

Renal pelvis

Right gonadal a.& v.

Inferior mesenteric a.

Abdominal aorta

Right common iliac v.

Right common iliac a.

Left ureter

Left common iliac a.

Left common iliac v.

Urinary bladder

Opening of ureter

Trigone

Urethra

Male Genital System

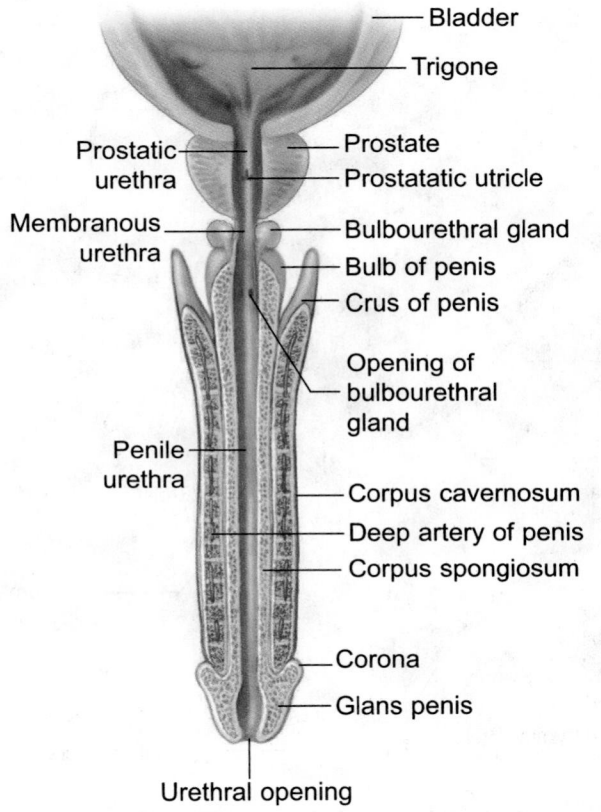

Bladder
Trigone
Prostatic urethra
Prostate
Prostatatic utricle
Membranous urethra
Bulbourethral gland
Bulb of penis
Crus of penis
Opening of bulbourethral gland
Penile urethra
Corpus cavernosum
Deep artery of penis
Corpus spongiosum
Corona
Glans penis
Urethral opening

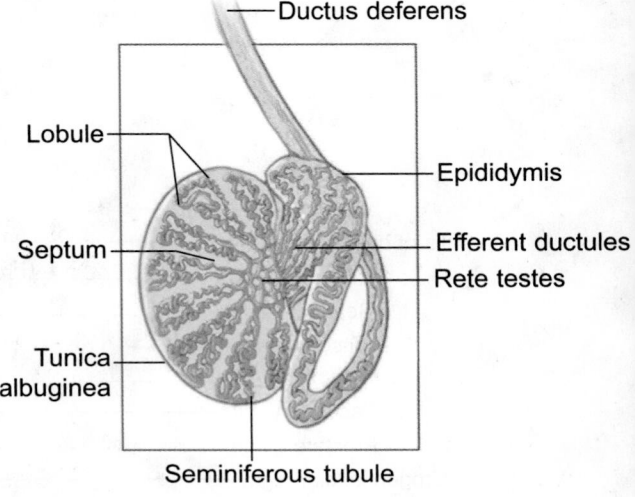

Ductus deferens
Lobule
Epididymis
Septum
Efferent ductules
Rete testes
Tunica albuginea
Seminiferous tubule

Male Genital System

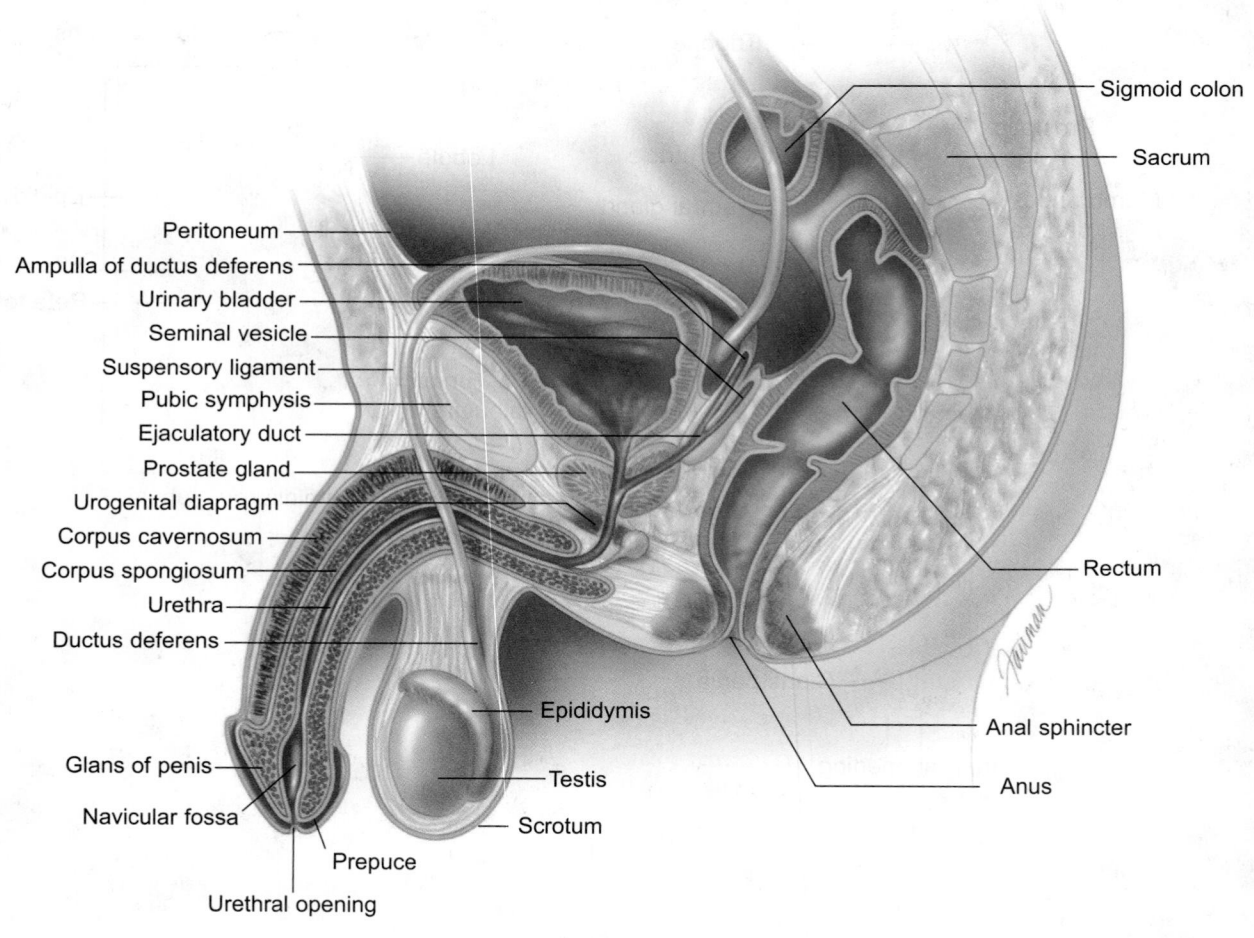

Peritoneum

Ampulla of ductus deferens

Urinary bladder

Seminal vesicle

Suspensory ligament

Pubic symphysis

Ejaculatory duct

Prostate gland

Urogenital diapragm

Corpus cavernosum

Corpus spongiosum

Urethra

Ductus deferens

Glans of penis

Navicular fossa

Urethral opening

Prepuce

Epididymis

Testis

Scrotum

Sigmoid colon

Sacrum

Rectum

Anal sphincter

Anus

Female Genital System

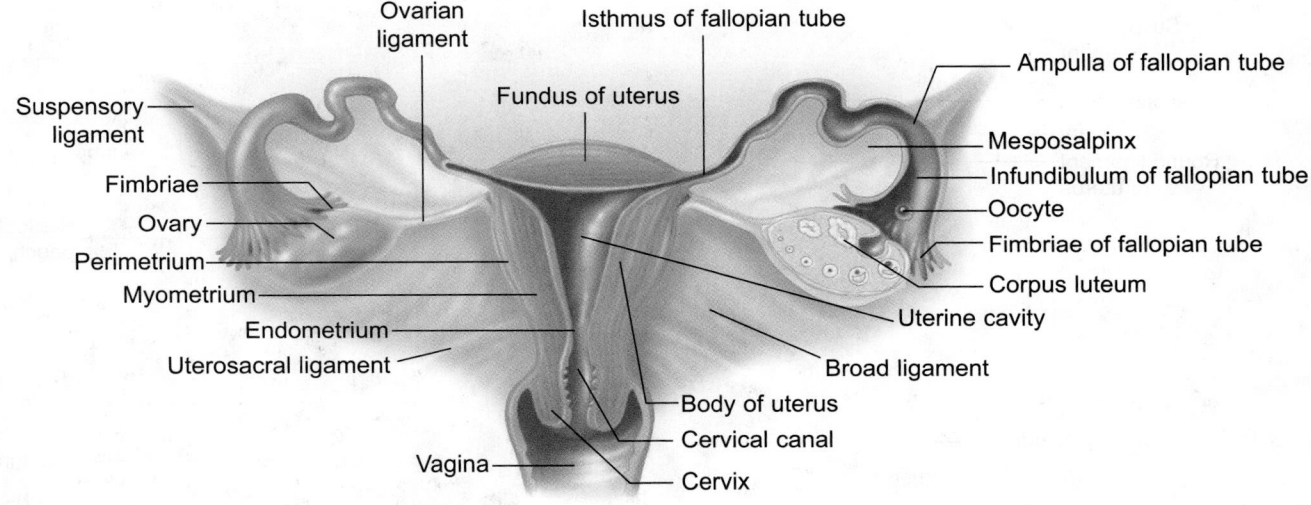

Ovarian ligament

Isthmus of fallopian tube

Fundus of uterus

Ampulla of fallopian tube

Suspensory ligament

Mesposalpinx

Fimbriae

Infundibulum of fallopian tube

Ovary

Oocyte

Perimetrium

Fimbriae of fallopian tube

Myometrium

Corpus luteum

Endometrium

Uterine cavity

Uterosacral ligament

Broad ligament

Body of uterus

Cervical canal

Vagina

Cervix

Female Genital System

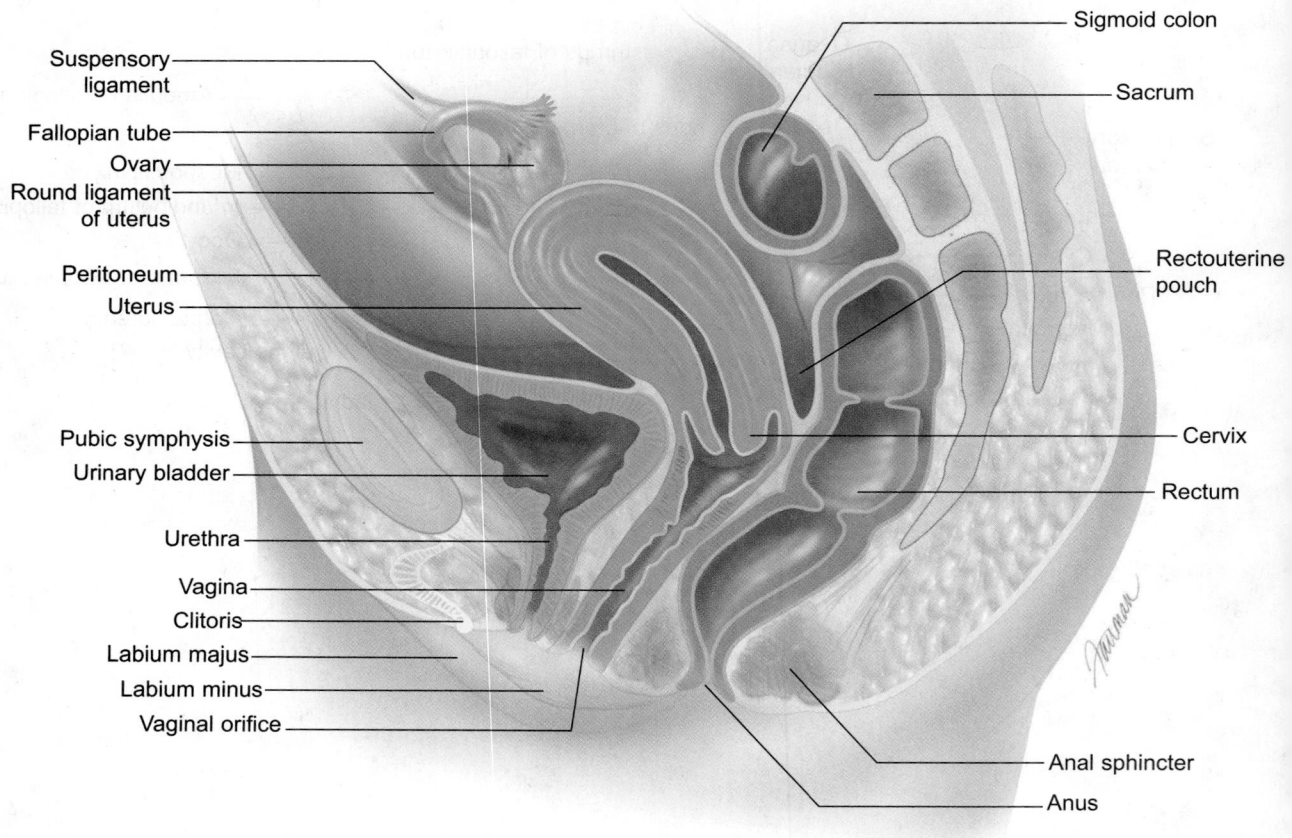

Suspensory ligament

Fallopian tube

Ovary

Round ligament of uterus

Peritoneum

Uterus

Pubic symphysis

Urinary bladder

Urethra

Vagina

Clitoris

Labium majus

Labium minus

Vaginal orifice

Sigmoid colon

Sacrum

Rectouterine pouch

Cervix

Rectum

Anal sphincter

Anus

Female Reproductive System – Pregnancy
(Lateral View)

Diaphragm

Liver

Transverse colon

Stomach

Pancreas

Placenta

Uterus

Amniotic fluid

Umbilical cord

Small intestine

Sacrum

Sigmoid colon

Coccyx

Rectum

Cervix

Vagina

Bladder

Pubic symphysis

Urethra

Cerebral Vasculature

Right anterior cerebral artery

Left anterior cerebral artery

Anterior communicating artery

Circle of Willis

Left middle cerebral artery

Right middle cerebral artery

Posterior communicating artery

Basilar artery

Posterior cerebral artery

Right external carotid artery

Left external carotid artery

Right internal carotid artery

Left internal carotid artery

Vertebral arteries

Common carotid arteries